Williams Obstetrics

22ND EDITION

NOTICE

Medicine is an ever-changing science. As new research and clinical experience broaden our knowledge, changes in treatment and drug therapy are required. The authors and the publisher of this work have checked with sources believed to be reliable in their efforts to provide information that is complete and generally in accord with the standards accepted at the time of publication. However, in view of the possibility of human error changes in medical sciences, neither the editors nor the publisher nor any other party who has been involved in the preparation or publication of this work warrants that the information contained herein is in every respect accurate or complete, and they disclaim all responsibility for any errors or omissions or for the results obtained from use of the information contained in this work. Readers are encouraged to confirm the information contained herein with other sources. For example and in particular, readers are advised to check the product information sheet included in the package of each drug they plan to administer to be certain that the information contained in this work is accurate and that changes have not been made in the recommended dose or in the contraindications for administration. This recommendation is of particular importance in connection with new or infrequently used drugs.

Williams Obstetrics

22ND EDITION

F. Gary Cunningham, MD

Professor and Chairman, Department of Obstetrics & Gynecology
Beatrice & Miguel Elias Distinguished Chair in
Obstetrics & Gynecology
The University of Texas Southwestern Medical Center at Dallas
Chief of Obstetrics & Gynecology
Parkland Memorial Hospital
Dallas, Texas

Kenneth J. Leveno, MD

Jack A. Pritchard Distinguished Professor of Obstetrics & Gynecology
Vice-Chair for Maternal-Fetal Medicine
The University of Texas Southwestern Medical Center at Dallas
Chief of Obstetrics
Parkland Memorial Hospital
Dallas, Texas

Steven L. Bloom, MD

Associate Professor, Department of Obstetrics & Gynecology
The University of Texas Southwestern Medical Center at Dallas
Associate Director of Obstetrics
Parkland Memorial Hospital
Dallas, Texas

John C. Hauth, MD

Professor and Chairman, Department of
Obstetrics & Gynecology
J. Marion Sims Chair in Obstetrics & Gynecology
University of Alabama at Birmingham
Birmingham, Alabama

Larry Gilstrap III, MD

Professor and Chairman,
Department of Obstetrics & Gynecology, and
Reproductive Sciences
Emma Sue Hightower Professor of Obstetrics & Gynecology
The University of Texas-Houston Medical School
Houston, Texas

Katharine D. Wenstrom, MD

Professor, Department of Obstetrics & Gynecology
Director, Division of Maternal-Fetal Medicine
University of Alabama at Birmingham
Birmingham, Alabama

McGraw-Hill
Medical Publishing Division

New York   Chicago   San Francisco   Lisbon   London   Madrid   Mexico City
Milan   New Delhi   San Juan   Seoul   Singapore   Sydney   Toronto

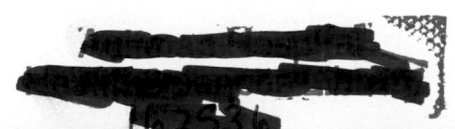

Williams Obstetrics, Twenty-Second Edition

1234567890   DOW/DOW   098765

ISBN: 0-07-141315-4

This book was set in New Times Roman by TechBooks.
The editors were Andrea Seils, and Karen G. Edmonson, and Karen Davis.
The production supervisor was Richard Ruzycka.
The cover designer was Janice Bielawa.
The indexer was Coughlin Editorial Services.
RR Donnelley & Sons was printer and binder.

This book is printed on acid-free paper.

Library of Congress Cataloging-in-Publication Data

Williams obstetrics / [edited by] F. Gary Cunningham . . . [et al.].—22nd ed.
    p. ; cm.
  Includes bibliographical references and index.
  ISBN 0-07-141315-4 (alk. paper)
  1. Obstetrics. I. Title: Obstetrics. II. Cunningham, F. Gary. III. Williams, J. Whitridge (John Whitridge), 1866–1931.
  [DNLM: 1. Obstetrics. WQ 100 W7283 2005]
RG524.W7 2005
618.2—dc22
                                        2004061105

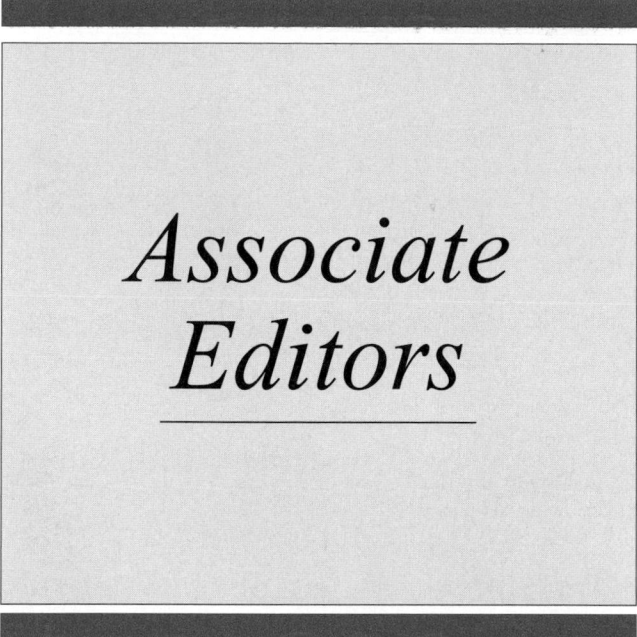

Associate Editors

Dwight Rouse, MD, MSPH
Professor of Obstetrics & Gynecology
Director Obstetrical Complication Clinics
Division of Maternal-Fetal Medicine
University of Alabama at Birmingham
Birmingham, Alabama

Bill Rainey, PhD
Professor of Obstetrics & Gynecology
The University of Texas Southwestern Medical
Center at Dallas
Dallas, Texas

Cathy Spong, MD
Chief, Pregnancy and Perinatology Branch
Maternal-Fetal Medicine Units Network Program Officer
National Institutes of Health
Bethesda, Maryland

George D. Wendel, Jr., MD
Alvin "Bud" Brekken Professor of Obstetrics & Gynecology
Vice-Chair for Education
Professor of Obstetrics & Gynecology
Division of Maternal-Fetal Medicine
The University of Texas Southwestern Medical Center at Dallas
Dallas, Texas

This 22nd edition of Williams Obstetrics is dedicated to those who work tirelessly to provide and improve health care for women and their unborn children. We especially applaud our faculty, residents, nurses, nurse practitioners, and nurse midwives, as well as the frequently unlauded but vital supporting team members who give selflessly to provide the best possible care for indigent women with the least possible resources. We are fortunate to have many such individuals working at the institutions with which we are proudly associated. We also recognize the efforts of many health-care administrators as well as elected and appointed officials who strive to provide these less fortunate women with good obstetrical care and with contraceptive options. At the same time, it is our fervent hope that those who actively impede this progress will eventually come to understand the societal benefits that accrue from fulfilling these lofty goals.

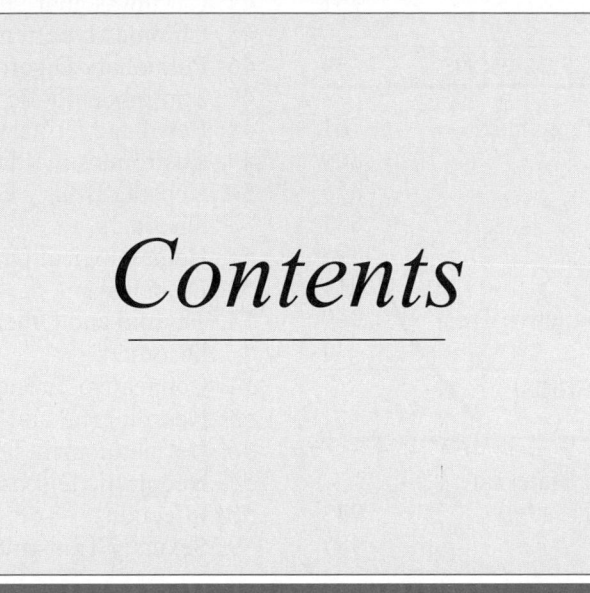

Contents

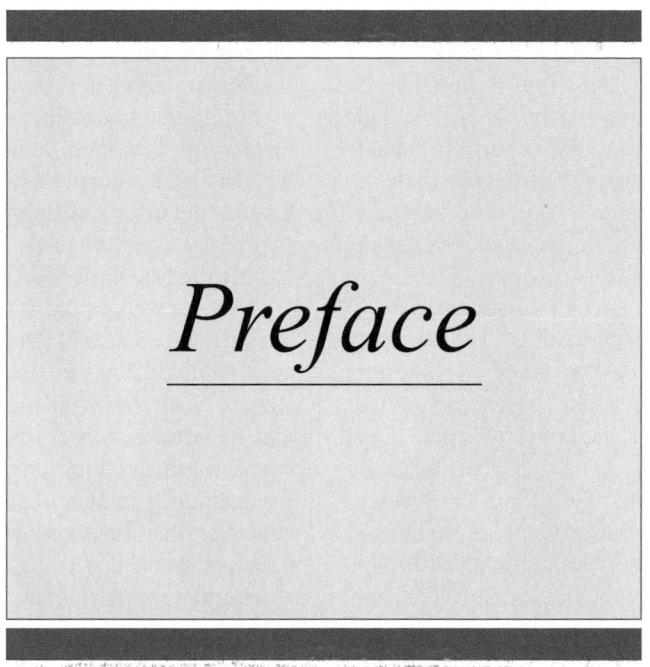

Preface

In previous editions of *Williams Obstetrics*, we have emphasized that obstetrics, originally born as a technical specialty, began to accrue scientific-based underpinnings during the last half of the 20th century. And over the past three decades, evidence-based medicine became embraced and is now firmly inculcated into clinical obstetrics. Accordingly, we again acknowledge the many fruitful efforts of the National Institute of Child Health and Human Development (NICHD) to encourage and support basic science and clinical research in obstetrical specialties. In updating this text, we relied heavily on investigations performed by members of the Maternal-Fetal Medicine Units Network. We also applaud the efforts of the American Gynecological and Obstetrical Society, the Society for Maternal-Fetal Medicine, the Society for Gynecological Investigation, and the American Board of Obstetrics and Gynecology to support the scientific and fiscal health of young clinical investigators.

Evidence-based medicine can be a two-edged sword. How does the busy practitioner keep up with many innovations that seemingly appear daily into our clinical literature? Who is the arbiter of their incorporation into clinical obstetrics? Should observations that satisfy the mathematical definition of statistical significance, but that have limited clinical significance, be employed nationwide as the "standard of care"? To us, the obvious answer is "no." And so we applaud our professional organizations such as the American College of Obstetricians and Gynecologists for their pragmatism and wisdom in recommendation of protocols for clinical management that inevitably do become the "standard." For our part, in this book

we have attempted to perform a balanced review of the literature to present readers with pros and cons of different management methods so that they may select options that are best suited to their available resources. We have also tried to avoid dogmatism which unfortunately dominated the practice of obstetrics for several decades of the 20th century. At the same time, we are proud to be associated with academic teaching services that are disciplined examples of evidence-based obstetrics. Although none of these services is perfect in any sense of the definition, we draw heavily on our combined clinical observations when recommending management options. We do however emphasize that these recommendations do not necessarily represent a sole method of management.

We have added new editors to further balance the breadth of obstetrics with a depth to ensure our self-imposed mandate of citing scientific underpinning of evidence-based clinical medicine. One imperative was a suitable replacement(s) for Dr. Norman Gant who needed more time as Executive Director of the American Board of Obstetrics and Gynecology. Joining us from the University of Texas Southwestern Medical Center is Dr. Steve Bloom who is director of Labor & Delivery at Parkland Hospital and who is responsible for overseeing the welfare of the more than 15,000 women who are delivered there annually. Dr. Bill Rainey is a nationally recognized scientist in reproductive and developmental biology who has made many valuable contributions to our knowledge of fetal physiology and labor initiation. Dr. George Wendel is director of the largest residency program in the country and he has also accrued an enviable reputation in the fields of obstetrical and perinatal infections, especially sexually transmitted diseases. Joining us from the University of Alabama at Birmingham, Dr. Dwight Rouse is an accomplished perinatal epidemiologist who provides depth to our myriad analyses of evidence-based outcomes. We are also fortunate to be joined by Dr. Cathy Spong from the National Institute of Child Health and Human Development who brings substantive dimension drawn from her extensive experiences accrued with the Maternal Fetal Medicine Units Network.

As in the past, we have relied heavily on the expertise of many of our colleagues and hopefully we cite all of them for their scholarly contributions. Drs. Judith Head and Khurram Rehman added insight into basic science principles of fetal and placental development, perinatal physiology, and the initiation of parturition. Dr. Marlene Corton provided new illustrations for pelvic anatomy and physiology. Dr. Beverly Rogers helped with a scholarly update of the placenta and its pathology. Considerable advice for obstetrical anesthesia was given by our colleagues Drs. Don Wallace, Shiv Sharma, and Elaine Sidawi. Dr. John Schorge lent substantive insight into gestational trophoblastic disease and Drs. David Hemsell and Chuck Rolle helped to review ectopic pregnancy. Dr. Jodi Dashe was inexhaustible in her efforts to continually update citations concerning all matters genetic. And she along with Drs. Diane Twickler and Rigoberto Santos lent their considerable knowledge and experiences with ultrasonography and Doppler technology as well as with many beautiful photographs. Dr. Jim Alexander provided useful suggestions concerning the conduct of normal and abnormal labor as well as analgesia for labor. Review of information concerning contraception and sterilization was provided by Drs. Gretchen Stuart, Barry Schwarz, and Stephen Heartwell. Help with the topics of obstetrical critical care as well as imaging techniques and cerebral blood flow measurement in eclamptic women came from Dr. Gerda Zeeman who is now at the University of Groeningen in The Netherlands. Dr. Nicole Yost provided insight into gastrointestinal disorders as well as preterm birth. Dr. Brian Casey shared his considerable clinical and research expertise with diabetes and thyroid disorders complicating pregnancy. Dr. Jeanne Sheffield was immensely helpful with constant updating of recommendations from the Centers for Disease Control and Prevention for treatment of sexually transmitted diseases and other infections.

It would be impossible to put together a 5000-page typed manuscript without a dedicated team to bring these efforts together. We are deeply indebted to Ms. Connie Utterback for her untiring efforts as Production Coordinator. With the help of Ms. Minnie Tregaskis, Ms. Cynthia Allen, Ms. Marsha Congleton, Ms. Kym Morris, Ms. Dina Trujillano, Ms. Ellen Watkins, as well as the late Ms. Jeanette Cogburn, who we miss greatly, the Dallas group kept the lights burning late into many nights. They were aided by Ms. Belinda Rials and Ms. Rhonda Scott in Birmingham, and Ms. Gerri Lopez in Houston. Expert artistic help was provided by Mr. Scott Bodell who had lent his talents on previous editions. Finally, we were fortunate and privileged to have the expert help of Dr. Barbara Hoffman who served as copy and rewrite editor, English and grammar tutor, and eagle-eyed proofreader who helped to keep us honest with hundreds of randomized controlled trials.

These past few years have been most challenging for those of us dedicated to academic obstetrics; medical student, resident, and fellow training; and contributions to clinical and basic research. Imposition of pounds and mounds of forms and paperwork for Medicare, Medicaid, HIPAA, RRC, billing compliance, and managed care, along with major cuts in funding for health care in general, and indigent health care specifically, have required new dimensions of time taken away from clinical duties. We thus are indebted to all of those who took up the slack to allow us more time to devote to this edition. We especially cite the efforts of Drs. Barry Schwarz, Karen Bradshaw, Morris Bryant, and Robert Coleman as well as Ms. Judy Wagers and Ms. Janice Walton.

This is the second edition of *Williams Obstetrics* for which we have been privileged to work closely with the excellent team at McGraw-Hill. Led by Ms. Andrea Seils, we thoroughly enjoyed our interactions with Ms. Karen Davis and Mr. John Williams who have been immensely helpful.

Finally, we thank our families and friends for allowing us to impinge on their time to perform "book duties." We appreciate their patience and encouragement.

Williams Obstetrics

22ND EDITION

I

Overview

1

Obstetrics in Broad Perspective

In the 10th edition of *Williams Obstetrics,* Eastman described the word *obstetrics* as being derived from the Latin *obstetrix,* meaning *midwife.* The word also is connected with the verb *obstare*—to *stand by or in front of.* The rationale for this derivation is that the midwife stood by or in front of the parturient. It is intriguing to consider that the derivation of *obstetrics* may have its origins in the evolution of the human species. To do so, we examine the thought-provoking observations of Rosenberg and Trevathan (2002). Their hypothesis dwells on two characteristics that set humans apart from other mammals, that is, that humans are the only mammals that walk on two legs, and that for body size, we have the largest brains. Also, unlike the females of other mammalian species, including other primates, women routinely seek assistance when they give birth.

Rosenberg and Trevathan (2002) propose that women's need for birthing assistance may be the result of this evolved bipedalism and large brain. The challenge of birth for many primates, and especially for humans, is that the size of the newborn's head is very close to the size of the passage through which it must travel. The series of rotations described in Chapter 17 that the human fetus must undergo during childbirth are thought to be related to the evolution of upright locomotion as well as the larger brain. Because of pelvic changes necessary to accommodate bipedalism, the human fetus must negotiate a birth canal that is not constant in cross-section. The pelvic inlet, where the fetus begins its transit, is widest from side to side. Midway through the pelvis, however, the orientation shifts 90 degrees and the widest dimension of the pelvis is from anterior to posterior. This change in pelvic dimensions means that the fetus must negotiate a series of turns as it passes through the birth canal so that its largest dimensions—the head and shoulders—are always aligned with the widest dimension of the birth canal. As a consequence of this rotation, human fetuses predominantly assume the occiput anterior position at delivery. In contrast, occiput posterior delivery is characteristic for nonhuman primates with smaller brains and correspondingly smaller head size. For example, in monkeys, the neonate is born looking up into its mother's face, which makes it possible for the mother to reach down and guide the newborn out of the birth canal. She can also wipe mucus from the baby's face to assist its breathing.

Thus, Rosenberg and Trevathan (2002) propose that human parturients require assistance because they cannot mechanically manage delivery of the occiput anterior vertex without help. They suggest that the triple challenge of a big-brained neonate, a maternal pelvis designed for walking upright, and a rotational delivery in which the infant emerges facing backward were natural selection pressures that favored humans seeking assistance—hence, *obstetrics.*

In the broader sense, obstetrics is concerned with reproduction of the society of humans. The specialty aims to promote health and well-being as the branch of medicine that is concerned with pregnancy, labor, and the puerperium in both normal and abnormal circumstances. The importance of obstetrics is attested to by the observation that maternal and neonatal outcomes are universally used as an index of the quality of health and life in human society. With this in mind, we provide a synopsis of the current state of maternal and newborn health in the United States. Following this is a perspective on some of the forces affecting obstetrics in these early years of the 21st century.

VITAL STATISTICS

The vital statistics of the United States are collected and published through a decentralized, cooperative system (Tolson and colleagues, 1991). Responsibility for the registration of births, deaths, fetal deaths, marriages, divorces, annulments, and induced terminations of pregnancy is vested in the individual states and certain separate governmental entities. The system comprises 57 registration areas: each state, the District of Columbia, New York City, American Samoa, Guam, the Northern Mariana Islands, Puerto Rico, and the Virgin Islands.

The first standard certificates for the registration of live births and deaths were developed in 1900. An act of Congress in 1902 established the Bureau of the Census to develop a system for the annual collection of vital statistics. The overall objective was to develop and maintain a system for registration that is uniform in such matters as forms, procedures, and statistical methodology. The Bureau retained the authority for producing national vital statistics until 1946, when the function was transferred to the United States Public Health Service. It is presently assigned to the Division of Vital Statistics of the National Center for Health Statistics (NCHS). The standard certificate of live birth was substantially revised in 1989 to include much more information on medical and lifestyle risk factors and also obstetrical care practices. Currently, more than 99 percent of births in the United States are registered.

The NCHS is part of the Centers for Disease Control and Prevention (CDC). Its function is to collaborate with colleagues in state vital statistics offices to revise the certificates of live birth and fetal death. This process generally is carried out every 10 to 15 years. Revisions were initiated in some states in 2003, and full implementation in all states will begin in phases over several years. The 2003 revision focuses on fundamental changes in the way the data are collected to accomplish greater accuracy. Changes also include a format conducive to electronic processing, to collect more explicit parental demographic data, and to improve selection of information regarding antepartum and intrapartum complications. Some examples of new data to be collected include that related to uterine rupture, blood transfusion, and pregnancy resulting from infertility treatment.

DEFINITIONS. The uniform use of standard definitions is encouraged by the World Health Organization as well as the American Academy of Pediatrics and the American College of Obstetricians and Gynecologists (2002). Such uniformity allows comparison of data not only between states or regions of the country, but also between countries. It is recommended that United States statistics include all fetuses and neonates born weighing at least 500 g, whether alive or dead. It must be clarified, however, that the states are not uniform in their definition of fetal death. For example, 28 states stipulate that fetal deaths beginning at 20 weeks' gestation should be recorded, eight states report all products of conception as fetal deaths, and still others use birthweights of 350 g, 400 g, or 500 g or greater to identify fetal deaths.

Definitions recommended by the NCHS and the CDC are as follows:

- **Perinatal period.** The period after birth of an infant weighing 500 g or more and ending at 28 completed days after birth. When perinatal rates are based on gestational age, rather than birthweight, it is recommended that the perinatal period be defined as commencing at 20 weeks.
- **Birth.** The complete expulsion or extraction from the mother of a fetus, irrespective of whether the umbilical cord has been cut or the placenta is attached. Fetuses weighing less than 500 g are usually not considered as births, but rather are termed abortuses for purposes of vital statistics.
- **Birthweight.** The weight of a neonate determined immediately after delivery or as soon thereafter as feasible. It should be expressed to the nearest gram.
- **Birth rate.** The number of live births per 1000 population.
- **Fertility rate.** The number of live births per 1000 females aged 15 through 44 years.
- **Live birth.** The term used to record a birth whenever the newborn at or sometime after birth breathes spontaneously, or shows any other sign of life such as a heartbeat or definite spontaneous movement of voluntary muscles. Heartbeats are to be distinguished from transient cardiac contractions, and respirations are to be distinguished from fleeting respiratory efforts or gasps.
- **Stillbirth or fetal death.** The absence of signs of life at or after birth.
- **Neonatal death.** *Early* neonatal death refers to death of a liveborn neonate during the first 7 days after birth. *Late* neonatal death refers to death after 7 days but before 29 days.
- **Stillbirth rate or fetal death rate.** The number of stillborn neonates per 1000 neonates born, including live births and stillbirths.
- **Neonatal mortality rate.** The number of neonatal deaths per 1000 live births.
- **Perinatal mortality rate.** The number of stillbirths plus neonatal deaths per 1000 total births.

- **Infant death.** All deaths of liveborn infants from birth through 12 months of age.
- **Infant mortality rate.** The number of infant deaths per 1000 live births.
- **Low-birthweight.** A newborn whose weight is less than 2500 g.
- **Very-low-birthweight.** A newborn whose weight is less than 1500 g.
- **Extremely-low-birthweight.** A newborn whose weight is less than 1000 g.
- **Term neonate.** A neonate born anytime after 37 completed weeks of gestation and up until 42 completed weeks of gestation (260 to 294 days).
- **Preterm neonate.** A neonate born before 37 completed weeks (the 259th day).
- **Postterm neonate.** A neonate born anytime after completion of the 42nd week, beginning with day 295.
- **Abortus.** A fetus or embryo removed or expelled from the uterus during the first half of gestation—20 weeks or less—and weighing less than 500 g.
- **Induced termination of pregnancy.** The purposeful interruption of an intrauterine pregnancy with the intention other than to produce a liveborn neonate, and which does not result in a live birth. This definition excludes retention of products of conception following fetal death.
- **Direct maternal death.** The death of the mother resulting from obstetrical complications of pregnancy, labor, or the puerperium, and from interventions, omissions, incorrect treatment, or a chain of events resulting from any of these factors. An example is maternal death from exsanguination after uterine rupture.
- **Indirect maternal death.** A maternal death not directly due to an obstetrical cause, but resulting from previously existing disease, or a disease that developed during pregnancy, labor, or the puerperium, but which was aggravated by maternal physiological adaptation to pregnancy. An example is maternal death from complications of mitral valve stenosis.
- **Nonmaternal death.** Death of the mother resulting from accidental or incidental causes not related to pregnancy. An example is death from an automobile accident or concurrent malignancy.
- **Maternal mortality ratio.** The number of maternal deaths that result from the reproductive process per 100,000 live births. Used more commonly, but less accurately, are the terms *maternal mortality rate* or *maternal death rate.* The term *ratio* is more accurate because it includes in the numerator the number of deaths regardless of pregnancy outcome—for example, live births, stillbirths, ectopic pregnancies—while the denominator includes the number of live births.

In 1987, the CDC collaborated with the Maternal Mortality Special Interest Group of the American College of

Obstetricians and Gynecologists, the Association of Vital Records and Health Statistics, and state and local health departments to initiate the National Pregnancy Mortality Surveillance System. Two new terms were introduced:

- **Pregnancy-associated death.** The death of any woman, from any cause, while pregnant or within 1 calendar year of termination of pregnancy, regardless of the duration and the site of pregnancy.
- **Pregnancy-related death.** A pregnancy-associated death resulting from (1) complications of the pregnancy itself, (2) the chain of events initiated by the pregnancy that led to death, or (3) aggravation of an unrelated condition by the physiological or pharmacological effects of the pregnancy that subsequently caused death.

PREGNANCY IN THE UNITED STATES

Data from diverse sources have been used to provide the following snapshot of pregnancy during the early years of the 21st century in the United States.

In 2002, the fertility rate of women aged 15 to 44 years was 64.8 live births per 1000 women (Sutton and colleagues, 2004). The fertility rate has been trending downward for Caucasian, African-American, and Hispanic women since 1990, when the rate was 70.9 per 1000. The rates of reproduction since 1990 were below replacement births, indicating a population decline (Hamilton, 2004). This decline, however, has been compensated by considerable net migration into the United States. For example, there were more than 1 million migrants each year from 2000 to 2002.

There were 4,021,726 live births in 2002, which when offset by 2,447,864 deaths, resulted in a net population increase of 1.6 million people (Kochanek and colleagues, 2004; Martin and colleagues, 2003). The 2002 birth rate for the United States fell to the lowest rate ever recorded at 13.9 per 1000 population. Hispanic women accounted for more than 1 in 5 births. American women average 3.2 pregnancies over their lifetimes, and 1.8 of these are considered wanted pregnancies (Ventura and colleagues, 1999). After exclusion of fetal losses and induced terminations, American women on average deliver 2.0 live births in a lifetime. Using 1996 as an example, there were 6.24 million pregnancies in the United States; 62 percent ended with live births, 22 percent ended by induced terminations, and 16 percent were spontaneous abortions (Fig. 1–1).

Prenatal care is a major component of the U.S. health care scene. In 2001, delivery was the second leading cause of hospitalization behind heart disease (Hall and DeFrances, 2003). The average length of hospital stay for all deliveries was 2.5 days. Prenatal care was the fourth leading reason for office visits to physicians and accounted for nearly 20 million visits in 2001 (Cherry and co-authors, 2003). Nondelivery hospitalizations have decreased substantially since the late 1980s

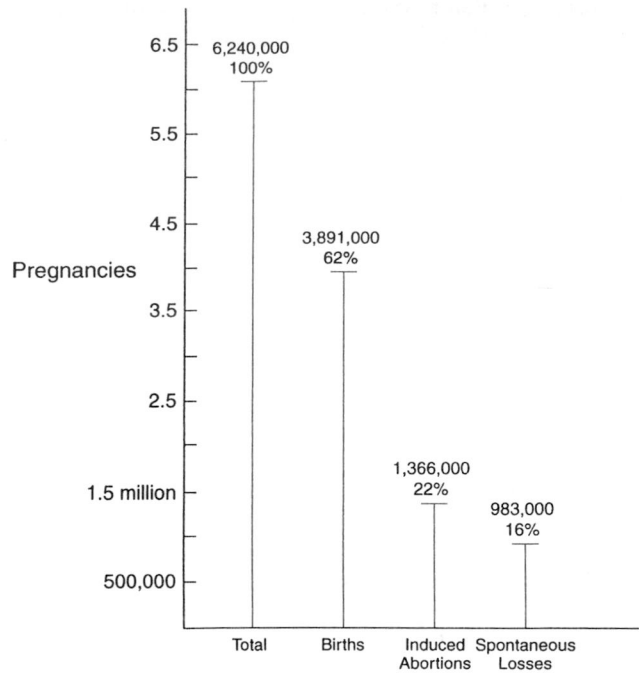

FIGURE 1–1. Results of 6,240,000 pregnancies in the United States, 1996. (Data from Ventura and colleagues, 1999.)

due to efforts to minimize expenditures. The leading indication for hospitalization unrelated to delivery was preterm labor. Nicholson and co-workers (2000) estimated that the total national cost of hospitalization for preterm labor that did not eventuate in delivery was $360 million in 1996 dollars. This sum increased to $820 million when women with preterm labor who actually delivered early were added.

HEALTHY PEOPLE 2010

In 1991, the U.S. Department of Health and Human Services issued a report titled *Healthy People 2000*. In this report, 17 goals were proposed to improve the health of mothers and infants by the year 2000. Unfortunately, progress was made in only eight of these areas. Notable gains were made in the areas of infant death, fetal death, cesarean delivery (particularly repeat cesareans), breast feeding, prenatal care, hospitalization for pregnancy complications, tobacco abstinence during pregnancy, and screening for fetal abnormalities and genetic disorders. Although no progress was made toward four other goals, there also was no regression in these areas, which included maternal deaths, fetal alcohol syndrome, and low-birthweight neonates. For the remaining five objectives, unfortunately, movement was away from the target.

New objectives for maternal and infant health have been promulgated for the current decade as *Healthy People 2010*. Some of these goals are shown in Table 1–1. One other goal is a new indicator of maternal health: maternal morbidity during labor and delivery (Danel and colleagues, 2003).

TABLE 1–1 Some Goals for Mothers and Infants for the United States in 2010

Outcome	Baseline 1997	Goal 2010
Fetal deaths before 20 weeks (per 1000)	6.8	4.1
Neonatal deaths before 29 days (per 1000)	4.8	2.9
Maternal deaths (per 100,000)	8.4	3.3

From *Healthy People 2010*, Centers for Disease Control and Prevention and the Health Resources and Services Administration (2000).

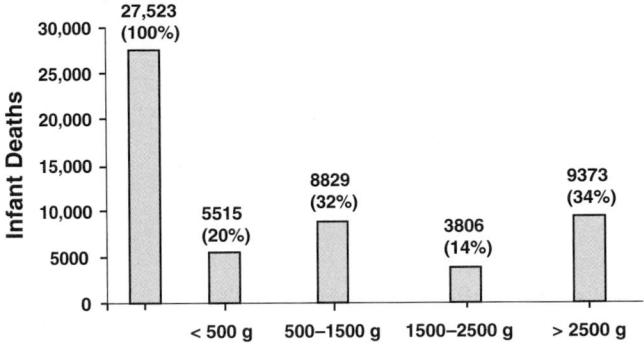

FIGURE 1–3. Infant deaths from birth through 12 months according to birthweight—United States, 2001. (Data from Matthews and co-workers, 2003.)

INFANT DEATHS. There were 27,523 infant deaths in 2001, and as shown in Figure 1–2, two thirds of these were neonatal deaths within the first 28 days of life. When analyzed by birthweight, two thirds of infant deaths were in low-birthweight neonates (Fig. 1–3). Of particular interest are those births less than 500 g, for which neonatal intensive care can now be offered. In 2001, there were 6450 liveborn infants weighing less than 500 g; 86 percent of these infants died during the first 28 days of life. Of the 1044 who survived the first 28 days of life, 934—11 percent of all births less than 500 g—survived infancy.

There were 27,977 infant deaths in 2002 for a rate of 7.0 per 1000 live births compared with 6.8 in 2001 (Kochanek and Smith, 2004). This slight increase in infant mortality between 2001 and 2002 is the first numerical increase since the period that included 1957 through 1978. The increase was concentrated in the neonatal period, particularly the first week of life. The percentage of neonates born preterm and low birthweight rose in 2002, continuing a long-term upward trend. St. John and associates (2000) have estimated the total cost of initial care in the United States for all newborns as $10.2 billion annually. Almost 60 percent of this expenditure is attributed to preterm births before 37 weeks, and 12 percent is spent on neonates born between 24 and 26 weeks.

MATERNAL DEATHS. The health of pregnant women also is an important indicator of national health care. In 2002, a total of 336 maternal deaths were identified by vital statistics (Kochanek and Smith, 2004). Importantly and unfortunately, it is estimated that more than half of maternal deaths are not recorded as such (Koonin and colleagues, 1997). One major accomplishment of obstetrical care was that the risk of death from pregnancy complications decreased almost 99 percent during the 20th century. The ratio of approximately 850 maternal deaths per 100,000 live births in 1900 decreased to 7.5 in 1982 (Chang and colleagues, 2003). Since 1982, however, maternal mortality in the United States has not decreased further.

As shown in Figure 1–4, maternal mortality is related to age and race. Shown in Table 1–2 are the causes of pregnancy-related maternal deaths. Hemorrhage and infection are prominent causes of death in ectopic pregnancies and abortions, whereas hypertension, embolism, hemorrhage, and infection are the leading causes of maternal death in women delivered after midpregnancy. There continues to be significant disparity with increased maternal deaths in minority and indigent populations (Anachebe and Sutton, 2003).

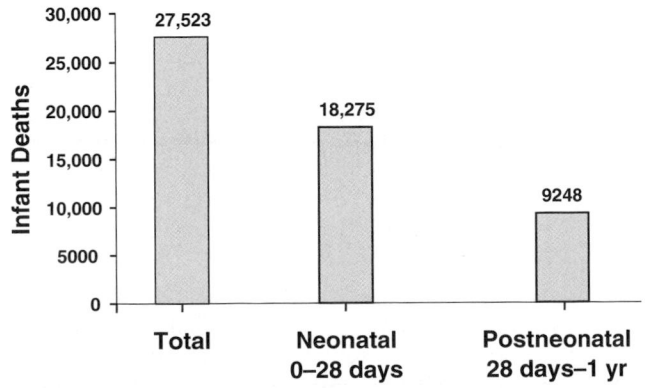

FIGURE 1–2. Infant deaths from birth through 12 months—United States, 2001. (Data from Matthews and colleagues, 2003.)

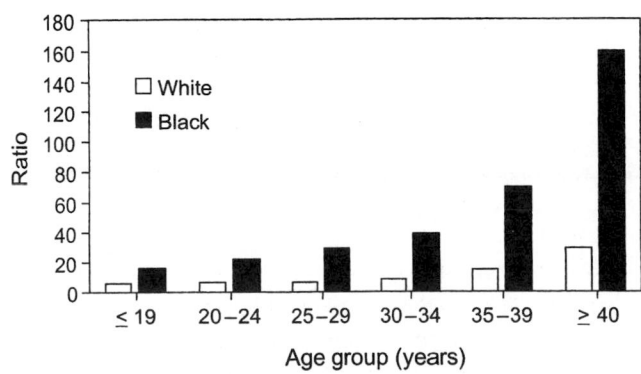

FIGURE 1–4. Pregnancy-related maternal mortality ratios by age and race—United States, 1991–1999. Deaths per 100,000 live births. (From Chang and colleagues, 2003, with permission.)

TABLE 1–2 Causes of 4200 Pregnancy-Related Deaths in the United States, 1991–1999

Cause	Percent
Embolism	19.6
Hemorrhage	17.2
Hypertensive disorders	15.7
Infection	12.6
Cardiomyopathy	8.3
Cerebrovascular accident	5.0
Anesthesia	1.6
Other[a]	19.2
Unknown	0.7

[a] The majority of the other medical conditions were cardiovascular, pulmonary, and neurological problems.
From Chang and colleagues (2003).

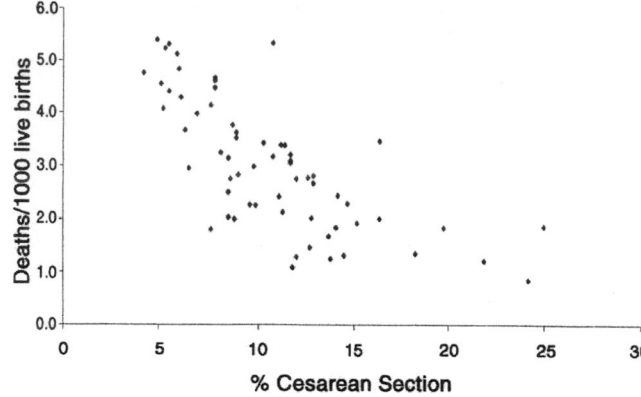

FIGURE 1–5. Scatter plot of cesarean delivery rate versus perinatal death rate in three Dublin hospitals, 1979–2000. (From Matthews and co-authors, 2003, with permission.)

PERSPECTIVES ON OBSTETRICS

There are a number of areas in obstetrics in which societal factors—whether within society at large or within the profession of obstetrics—are influencing reproduction in the United States. Many of these are stimulated or influenced by economics, politics, and religion. There is very much *right* with obstetrics. Three examples were cited by Dr. John Gibbons (2003) in his presidential address to the American College of Obstetricians and Gynecologists: advances in basic science, clinical practice, and social dynamics of women's health care. At the same time, he also cited three serious problems, among them recruitment of medical students, changes in residency training, and the new face of private and academic practice. Frigoletto and Greene (2002) have also provided a thoughtful review of those changes, and we now include some of these that currently have an impact on obstetrics as a specialty.

RISING CESAREAN DELIVERY RATE. In 2002, the cesarean delivery rate climbed to the highest level ever reported in the United States—26.1 percent (Martin and colleagues, 2003). The escalation in the total cesarean delivery rate was fueled by both a rise in the primary cesarean delivery rate and a steep decline in the rate of vaginal birth after cesarean (VBAC) delivery. The forces involved in these changes in cesarean delivery rates are multifactorial and complex. For example, as discussed in Chapter 17, the major indication for primary cesarean delivery is dystocia, and there is evidence that this diagnosis has increased. This increase, at least in part, is due to greater maternal size, lower parity, and more advanced age. The sharp decline in VBAC deliveries is likely related to the uterine rupture risk associated with VBAC and attendant legal pressures (see Chap. 26). In defense of cesarean delivery, Matthews and co-authors (2003) have reported a consistent association between increasing cesarean delivery rates and falling perinatal death rates (Fig. 1–5).

Other forces undoubtedly involved in the record rate of cesarean deliveries include routine cesarean delivery for breech presentation (see Chap. 24) and increased induction of labor (see Chap. 22). An emerging factor is patient choice—or cesarean delivery on request. An emerging impetus for such requests is the desire to prevent pelvic floor injury, thus reducing the incidence of incontinence of stool, flatus, and urine, as well as pelvic organ prolapse (Minkoff and Chervenak, 2003).

WOMEN IN OBSTETRICS. The gender of the obstetrical workforce in the United States has undergone a rapid transformation in the past 20 years (Benedetti and colleagues, 2004). The proportion of women practitioners has increased from 12 percent in 1980 to 32 percent in 2000 and is expected to increase to 50 percent by 2014 (American College of Obstetricians and Gynecologists, 1999). Currently, more than 70 percent of obstetrical residents are women (Association of American Medical Colleges, 2003). Good things undoubtedly will accrue from these changes. Frigoletto and Greene (2002) have identified some of these benefits, which include (1) meeting the preferences of many patients for female obstetricians, (2) heightened sensitivity to the need to balance the demands of work and raising a family, and (3) safer patient care by decreasing often inhumanely long work hours. As described so aptly by Dr. Vivian Dickerson (2004) in her presidential address to the American College of Obstetricians and Gynecologists: "... who we are transcends gender."

That said, there are also concerns about these changes (Chan and Willett, 2004). For example, female obstetricians-gynecologists are less likely to continue to practice obstetrics because of concerns about balance between work and family life. One potential consequence of this phenomenon is that the increasing proportion of women in the obstetrical workforce will ultimately lead to a decline in the availability of obstetricians as early as 2010 (Pearse and colleagues, 2001a).

MEDICAL STUDENTS AND OBSTETRICAL RESIDENCIES. The declining number of medical school graduates for residency training in obstetrics and gynecology is

TABLE 1–3 Business Versus Professional Values

Business Values	Professional Values
Profit	Service
Competition	Advocacy
Responsible to stockholders	Responsible to those served: altruism
Services driven by the market	Services driven by a body of knowledge
Standards set by external forces	Standards set and maintained internally
Consumerism	Humanism
Short-term goals	Long-term goals
Giving society what it thinks it wants	Meeting societal needs

From Swick (2001).

TABLE 1–4 Liability Insurance Premiums for Obstetricians-Gynecologists, 1970–2001

Year	Mean Liability Insurance Premium
1970	$2,237
1980	$9,000
1985	$23,300
1990	$37,808
1995	$29,186
2001	$35,200

From Lockwood (2002).

of concern. This decline has been attributed to multiple reasons identified in the survey by Pearse and co-workers (2001b). The most commonly cited reason was lifestyle and family issues (45 percent), followed closely by malpractice issues (41 percent), and low reimbursement (35 percent).

According to Zuger (2004) the entire profession of medicine has been similarly affected. Dissatisfaction with the practice of medicine increased from 15 percent in 1973 to as high as 40 percent by 1995. And in a follow-up survey in 2001, 58 percent of physicians described "declining enthusiasm" and 87 percent felt that the overall morale of physicians had declined since the first survey in 1981 (Kaiser Family Foundation, 2003). Cited as the major reason for physician dissatisfaction was the deleterious effect on the quality of medical practice by managed care. The malpractice crisis—more accurately, the *liability crisis*—also was frequently cited. In their recent survey, Bettes and co-workers (2004) cited pressures from liability insurance costs as having a more negative impact on satisfaction than managed care. According to Zuger (2004), even those physicians who were not financially burdened cited defensive medicine to thwart potential litigation as being "widely deplored as a growing blight on medical practice."

We conclude, as did Gibbons (2003), that our specialty has not done an adequate job of emphasizing the positive and satisfying aspects to our students. We need to remind them that obstetricians practice in groups that provide reasonable call schedules. The mandate for 80-hour workweeks for residents intersects with the increasing emphasis on lifestyle and patient safety issues (Gaba and Howard, 2002).

PROFESSIONALISM AND MARKET FORCES. Swick (2001), delivering the President's Program at the 2000 Annual Meeting of the American College of Obstetricians and Gynecologists, observed that "Medicine today is under siege from market forces in the new corporate age and that its professional values, indeed, its very identity as a profession, are under threat." Shown in Table 1–3 is the juxtaposition of business versus professional values. Swick concluded that the profession of medicine, viz., obstetrics, must exercise professionalism by advocating the interests of our patients. We are in complete accord.

MEDICAL LIABILITY. Lockwood (2002) has reviewed the professional liability crisis in American obstetrics. The average obstetrician is sued 2.5 times during his or her career and about 75 percent of obstetricians have been sued at least once. Almost 50 percent of obstetrical claims were for neurologically impaired infants or stillbirths. About half of the claims are dropped by the plaintiff attorney or found to be without merit. There has been a steady escalation, however, in the value of awards, with the median award now nearly 1 million dollars. As shown in Table 1–4, professional liability insurance premiums have continued to escalate after a brief respite in the mid-1990s. According to Lockwood (2002), the cost of malpractice coverage passed on to patients added $350 to annual health care premiums for the average American family!

The furor raised by the most outrageous payouts has caused a grassroots tort reform that has been successful in limiting noneconomical damages in some states. Despite this, the American Medical Association recently identified 18 states in which availability of affordable liability insurance was a grave concern (Mello and colleagues, 2003). Contrary to what is alleged by the relatively small number of plaintiff attorneys who personally profit from huge settlements, the crisis has resulted in sparse or no medical care in some areas. Could it be possible that this has caused more morbidity, mortality, and pain and suffering than bad medical outcomes, with or without errors in judgment? Some physicians may take solace in knowing that a 1999 study identified increasing rates of unhappiness among lawyers over the past decade, and that many were planning to leave their profession (Schlitz and associates, 1999). Hopefully this will include the most avaricious plaintiff attorneys!

TECHNOLOGY. Since 1983, when the first infant was conceived from in vitro fertilization (IVF) in the United States, the use of IVF and related procedures—assisted reproductive technology—has increased substantially (Schieve and colleagues, 2002). This technology has resulted in record numbers of multiple births, especially higher-order multiples involving three or more fetuses, with all of the attendant complications. Starting about 1998, the rate of higher-order multiple births began to decline slightly (Martin and colleagues, 2003). This decline likely can be attributed to national guidelines published in 1997 recommending transfer of fewer embryos (Jain and colleagues, 2004). Another effect of technology is the rapid evolution in the maternal–fetal relationship due to advances in imaging, prenatal diagnostics, genetic screening, and fetal surgery (van Dis, 2003).

BIRTHS TO IMMIGRANTS. Persons born outside the United States comprised an estimated 11 percent of the population in 2000, and approximately 20 percent of all U.S. births in 2000 were to women in this population (Sappenfield and colleagues, 2002). Hispanic women, particularly immigrants from Mexico, accounted for most of the births to persons born outside the United States. Women born outside the United States had better birth outcomes than their state-born racial or ethnic counterparts. The reasons for the improved outcomes are unclear. One theory is that women who immigrate are healthier than those who do not. Surgeon General Richard Carmona has called for an end to health care delivery inequalities for Hispanics and African-Americans (*Dallas Morning News,* August 17, 2002).

UNINSURED PEOPLE. The number of people in the United States without health insurance and the consequent strain on the entire health care system constitute a major public policy issue (McLellan, 2003). It is estimated that nearly one third of the nonelderly population, or about 7 million people, lacked health insurance for some part of 2001 and 2002. Hispanics and African-Americans were most likely to be uninsured. Approximately 80 percent of the uninsured were in working families. Factors implicated in this public health crisis include the economic revolution in medicine, whereby the pressure for profitability is closing the doors on the uninsured and concentrating them in public facilities (Ferrer, 2001). This phenomenon already has had a significant impact on pregnant women. For example, 40 percent of the births in Dallas County, Texas, occur at Parkland Hospital, which is the only public facility for the uninsured. Unfortunately, current attitudes about taxes have decimated the budgets of many of these public hospitals.

ABORTION. Even before President George W. Bush had a chance to sign the Partial Birth Abortion Act of 2003, opponents had filed court challenges to block its implementation. Indeed, as of June 2004, at least one court has ruled this act to be unconstitutional. The editorial board of *The Lancet* (2003) has suggested that the Partial Birth Abortion Act will only serve to further divide the United States over the issue of abortion. It is important to recognize that abortion can have a significant effect on infant mortality. Liu and colleagues

(2002) analyzed the impact of prenatal diagnosis and resultant pregnancy terminations in Canada between 1991 and 1998. A large decrease in infant deaths due to congenital anomalies was associated with a decline in the overall infant mortality in Canada.

BIRTH CONTROL. In its legislative agenda, the Bush administration has taken aim at the recent innovation in birth control consisting of over-the-counter availability of the *morning-after pill.* Barr Pharmaceuticals applied to the Food and Drug Administration for nonprescription sales of *Plan B,* which is described in Chapter 32 (see p. 745). During a joint session, the Nonprescription Drug Advisory Committee and the Committee for Reproductive Health Drugs approved the application for over-the-counter sales by a vote of 23 to 4. Presumably concerned about "teenager abuse," and presumably with political pressure from within the Bush administration, the application was denied. Appropriate umbrage has been expressed by Dickerson (2004), Drazen and colleagues (2004), Lockwood and Greene (2004), and Steinbrook (2004).

Governmental interference with women's reproductive rights is not new, of course. In 1998, Congress considered the Title X Parental Notification Act, which would mandate parental notification for minors seeking contraception at federally funded clinics. In the study by Reddy and colleagues (2002), this would have dissuaded almost half of girls younger than 17 years of age from seeking testing or treatment for human immunodeficiency virus (HIV) infection or other sexually transmitted disease. As usual, poor women would suffer disparately.

THE FUTURE. Early into the 21st century, our specialty finds itself faced not only with the many complicated social issues just discussed, but also with many of the same fundamental clinical questions that puzzled our predecessors. What initiates labor at term? What initiates labor prematurely? What causes preeclampsia, and can it be prevented?

As discussed throughout this 22nd edition of *Williams Obstetrics,* much has been accomplished to begin to answer these and other important questions. That said, however, a massive amount of work remains. In our view, the future of obstetrics relies on our continued ability to attract talented individuals to the specialty. And although there are several reasons to question whether one should dedicate one's life to obstetrics, we agree with the description chosen by Dr. John Gibbons (2003). In his previously cited presidential address to the American College of Obstetricians and Gynecologists, he described obstetrics as "vital," "fascinating," and "satisfying." We would add that it is also "incredibly fun." Thus, our hope for the future is that we will continue to attract individuals who will dedicate themselves to this special field and join in the quest to help women safely through pregnancy, thus guaranteeing the best possible beginning for the children of the next generation.

REFERENCES

American Academy of Pediatrics and the American College of Obstetricians and Gynecologists: Guidelines for Perinatal Care, 5th ed. Washington, DC, AAP and ACOG, 2002

American College of Obstetricians and Gynecologists: Ways to increase the role of women in the college. ACOG Clin 3:1, 1999

Anachebe JF, Sutton MY: Racial disparities in reproductive health outcomes. Am J Obstet Gynecol 188:S37, 2003

Association of American Medical Colleges: Women in U.S. Academic medicine statistics 2001–2002. Available at: http://www.aamc.org./members/wim/statistics/stats02/start.htm. Accessed February 25, 2003

Benedetti TJ, Baldwin LM, Andrilla CH, et al: The productivity of Washington State's obstetrician-gynecologist workforce: Does gender make a difference? Obstet Gynecol 103:499, 2004

Bettes BA, Strunk AL, Coleman VH, Schulkin J: Professional liability and other career pressures: Impact on obstetrican—gynecologists' career satisfaction. Obstet Gynecol 103:967, 2004

Centers for Disease Control and Prevention and Health Resources and Service Administration: Maternal, infant, and child health. In: Healthy People 2010, conference ed. Atlanta, Ga, CDC, 2000

Chan BJ, Willett J: Factors influencing participation in obstetrics by obstetrician-gynecologists. Obstet Gynecol 103:493, 2004

Chang J, Elam-Evans LD, Berg CJ, et al: Pregnancy-related mortality surveillance—United States, 1991–1999. MMWR 52(SS-2):4, 2003

Cherry DK, Burk CW, Woodwell DA: National Ambulatory Medical Care Survey: 2001 Summary: Advance data from vital and health statistics, Vol 51, No. 337. Hyattsville, Md, National Center for Health Statistics, 2003

Danel I, Berg C, Johnson CH, Atrash H: Magnitude of maternal morbidity during labor and delivery: United States, 1993–1997. Am J Public Health 93:631, 2003

Dickerson VM: The tolling of the bell: women's health, women's rights. Obstet Gynecol 104:653, 2004

Drazen JM, Greene MF, Wood AJJ: The FDA, politics, and plan B. N Engl J Med 350:1561, 2004

Editorial Board of Lancet: USA continues war over abortion. Lancet 362:1509, 2003

Ferrer RL: Within the system of no-system. JAMA 286:2513, 2001

Frigoletto FD, Greene MF: Is there a sea change ahead for obstetrics and gynecology? Obstet Gynecol 100:1342, 2002

Gaba DM, Howard SK: Fatigue among clinicians and the safety of patients. N Engl J Med 346:1249, 2002

Gibbons JM Jr: Springtime for obstetrics and gynecology: Will the specialty continue to blossom? Obstet Gynecol 102:443, 2003

Hall NJ, DeFrances CJ: 2001 National Hospital Discharge Survey: Advance data from vital and health statistics, Vol 51, No. 332. Hyattsville, Md, National Center for Health Statistics, 2003

Hamilton BE: Reproduction rates for 1990–2002 and intrinsic rates for 1990–2001: United States. National Vital Statistics Reports, Vol 52, No.17. Hyattsville, Md, National Center for Health Statistics, 2004

Jain T, Missmer SA, Harnstein MD: Trends in embryo-transfer practice and in outcomes of the rise of assisted reproductive technology in the United States. N Engl J Med 350:1639, 2004

Kaiser Family Foundation: National survey of physicians part III: Doctors' opinions about their profession. March 2002. Available at: http://www.kff.org/kaiserpolls/20020426c-index.cfm. Accessed December 8, 2003

Kochanek KD, Smith BL: Deaths: Preliminary data of 2002. National Vital Statistics Reports, Vol 52, No. 13. Hyattsville, Md, National Center for Health Statistics, 2004

Koonin LM, MacKay AP, Berg CJ, et al: Pregnancy-related mortality surveillance—United States, 1987–1990. MMWR 46:127, 1997

Liu S, Joseph KS, Kramer MS, et al: Relationship of prenatal diagnosis and pregnancy termination to overall infant mortality in Canada. JAMA 287:1561, 2002

Lockwood CJ: Confronting the professional liability crisis (part 1). Contemp Ob/Gyn, April 2002, p 13

Lockwood CJ, Greene MF: Playing politics with women's health: The FDA and Plan B. Contemp Ob/Gyn, July 2004, p 11

Martin JA, Hamilton BE, Sutton PD, et al: Births: Final data for 2002. National Vital Statistics Reports, Vol 52, No. 10. Hyattsville, Md, National Center for Health Statistics, 2003

Matthews TG, Crowley P, Chong A, et al: Rising caesarean section rates: A cause for concern? Br J Obstet Gynaecol 110:346, 2003

McLellon F: Uninsured people in USA put a strain on health system. Lancet 361:938, 2003

Mello MM, Studder DM, Brennan TA: The new medical malpractice crisis. N Engl J Med 348:2281, 2003

Minkoff H, Cheruenak FA: Elective pricing cesarean delivery. N Engl J Med 348:946, 2003

Nicholson WK, Frick KD, Powe NR: Economic burden of hospitalizations for preterm labor in the United States. Obstet Gynecol 96:95, 2000

Pearse WH, Haffner WH, Primack A: Effect of gender on the obstetric-gynecologic work force. Obstet Gynecol 97:794, 2001a

Pearse WH, Haffner WH, Primack A: Why are ob/gyn residencies losing their allure? Contemp Ob/Gyn, October 2001b, p 146

Reddy DM, Fleming R, Swain C: Effect of mandatory parental notification on adolescent girls' use of sexual health care services. JAMA 288:710, 2002

Rosenberg KR, Trevathan WR: The evaluation of human birth. Sci Am 13:80, 2003

Rosenberg K, Trevathan W: Birth, obstetrics and human evolution. BJOG 109:1199, 2002

Sappenfield B, Ferre C, Slyasu MMBS: State-specific trend in US live births to women born outside the 50 states and the District of Columbia—United States, 1990 and 2000. MMWR 51:1091, 2002

Schieve LA, Jeng G, Wilcox LS, et al: Use of assisted reproductive technology—United States, 1996 and 1998. MMWR 51:97, 2002

Schiltz P: On being a happy, healthy, and ethical member of an unhappy, unhealthy, and unethical profession. Vanderbilt Law Rev 52:871, 1999

St. John EB, Nelson KG, Cliver SP, et al: Cost of neonatal care according to gestational age at birth and survival status. Am J Obstet Gynecol 182:170, 2000

Steinbrook R: Waiting for plan B—The FDA and nonprescription use of emergency contraception. N Engl J Med 350:2327, 2004

Sutton PD, Mathews TJ: Trends in characteristics in births by state: United States, 1990, 1995, and 2000–2002. National Vital Statistics Reports, Vol 52, No.1. Hyattsville, Md, National Center for Health Statistics, 2004

Swick HM: Professionalism: A key to weathering the storm. Obstet Gynecol 98:156, 2001

Tolson GC, Barnes JM, Gay GA, et al: The 1989 revision of the US Standard Certificates and Reports. Monthly Vital Statistics Report 40:1, 1991

U.S. Department of Health and Human Services: Healthy People 2000. DHHS Publication No. HRSA-M-CH-91-2. Washington, DC, DHHS, 1991

van Dis J: The maternal–fetal relationship. JAMA 289:1696, 2003

Ventura SJ, Mosher WD, Curtin SC, et al: Highlights of trends in pregnancies and pregnancy rates by outcome: Estimates for the United States, 1976–96. National Vital Statistics Report, Vol 47, No. 29. Hyattsville, Md, National Center for Health Statistics, 1999

Zuger A: Dissatisfaction with medical practice. N Engl J Med 350:69, 2004

Anatomy and Physiology

2

Maternal Anatomy

The organs of reproduction of women are classified as either external or internal. There may be marked variation in anatomical structures in a given woman, and this is especially true for major blood vessels and nerves.

EXTERNAL GENERATIVE ORGANS

The *pudenda*—commonly designated the *vulva*—includes all structures visible externally from the pubis to the perineum, that is, the mons pubis, labia majora and minora, clitoris, hymen, vestibule, urethral opening, and various glandular and vascular structures (Fig. 2–1). The embryology of the external genitalia is discussed in Chapter 4 (see Fig. 4–17, p. 113).

MONS PUBIS. The mons pubis, or mons veneris, is the fat-filled cushion that lies over the symphysis pubis. After puberty, the skin of the mons pubis is covered by curly hair that forms the escutcheon. In women, it is distributed in a triangular area, the base of which is formed by the upper margin of the symphysis. In men, the escutcheon is not so well circumscribed.

LABIA MAJORA. These structures vary somewhat in appearance, principally according to the amount of fat that is contained within the tissues. Embryologically, the labia majora are homologous with the male scrotum. The round ligaments terminate at the upper borders. After repeated childbearing, the labia majora are less prominent. They are 7 to 8 cm in length, 2 to 3 cm in width, and 1 to 1.5 cm in thickness, and are somewhat tapered at the lower extremities. In children and nulliparous women (see Fig. 2–1), the labia majora usually lie in close apposition, whereas in multiparous women, they may gape widely. They are continuous directly with the mons pubis above and merge into the perineum posteriorly at a site where they are joined medially to form the *posterior commissure*.

Before puberty, the outer surface of the labia is similar to that of the adjacent skin, but after puberty the labia are

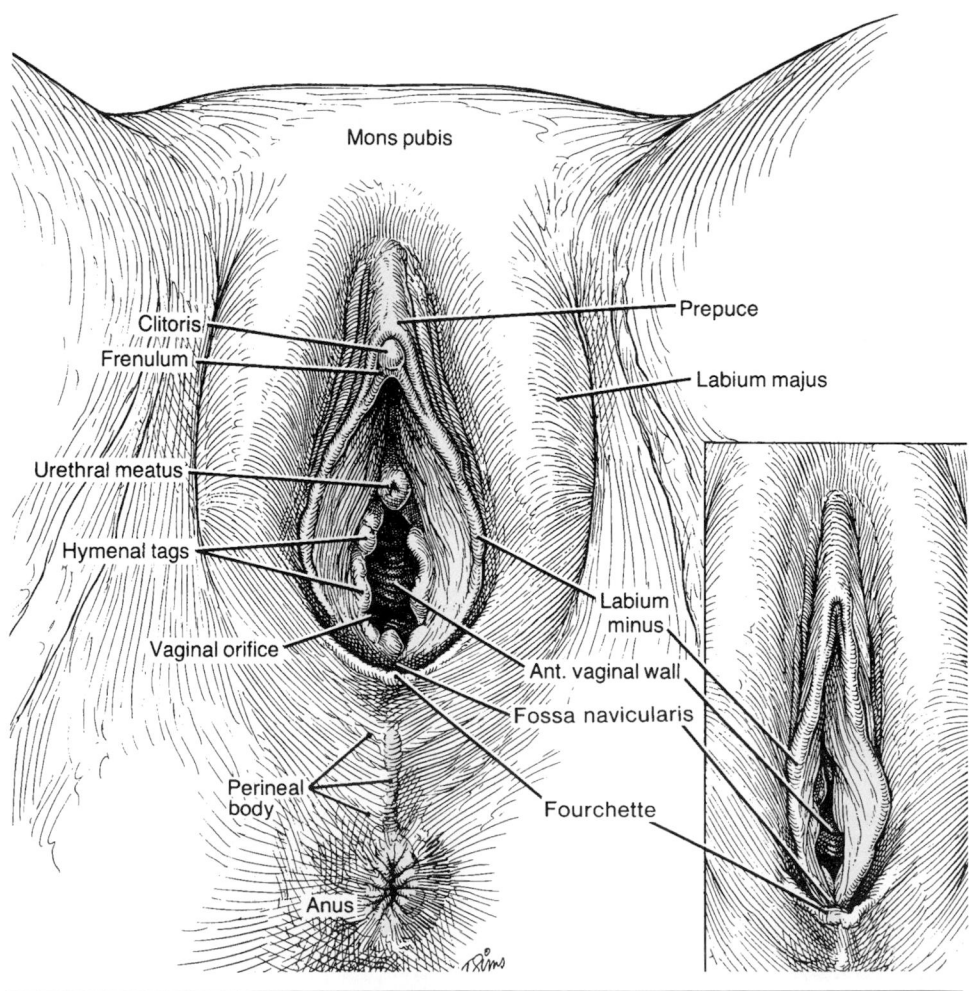

FIGURE 2–1. External female reproductive organs. The lower anterior vaginal wall is visible through the labia minora. In nulliparous women, the vaginal orifice is not so readily visible *(inset)* because of the close apposition of the labia minora.

covered with hair. In nulliparous women, the inner surface is moist and resembles a mucous membrane, whereas in multiparous women, the inner surface becomes more skinlike. The labia majora are richly supplied with sebaceous glands. Beneath the skin, there is a layer of dense connective tissue that is rich in elastic fibers and adipose tissue but is nearly void of muscular elements. Unlike the squamous epithelium of the vagina and cervix, there are epithelial appendages in parts of the vulvar skin. A mass of fat beneath the skin provides the bulk of the volume of the labium, and this tissue is supplied with a rich plexus of veins.

LABIA MINORA. The labia minora vary greatly in size and shape. In nulliparous women, they usually are not visible behind the nonseparated labia majora. In multiparas, it is common for the labia minora to project beyond the labia majora.

Each labium minus is a thin fold of tissue that is moist and reddish, similar in appearance to a mucous membrane. The labia minora are covered by stratified squamous epithelium. Although there are no hair follicles in the labia minora, there are many sebaceous follicles and, occasionally, a few sweat glands. The interior of the labial folds is composed of connective tissue with many vessels and some smooth muscular fibers. They are supplied with a variety of nerve endings and are extremely sensitive. The tissues of the labia minora converge superiorly, where each is divided into two lamellae; the lower pair fuse to form the *frenulum of the clitoris*, and the upper pair merge to form the *prepuce*. Inferiorly, the labia minora extend to approach the midline as low ridges of tissue that fuse to form the *fourchette.*

CLITORIS. The clitoris is the principal female erogenous organ. It is the homologue of the penis and is located near the superior extremity of the vulva. This erectile organ projects downward between the branched extremities of the labia minora. The clitoris is composed of a glans, a corpus, and two crura. The glans is made up of spindle-shaped cells, and in the body there are two corpora cavernosa, in the walls of which are smooth muscle fibers. The long, narrow crura arise from the inferior surface of the ischiopubic rami and fuse just below the middle of the pubic arch to form the corpus.

The clitoris rarely exceeds 2 cm in length. Its free end is pointed downward and inward toward the vaginal opening. The glans is usually less than 0.5 cm in diameter and is covered by stratified squamous epithelium that is richly supplied with nerve endings. The vessels of the erectile clitoris are connected with the vestibular bulbs.

There is a delicate network of free nerve endings in the labia majora, labia minora, and clitoris (Krantz, 1958). Tactile discs are found in abundance in these areas. Genital corpuscles, which are mediators of erotic sensation, vary considerably in number. These structures are abundant in the labia minora and in the skin that overlies the glans clitoris.

VESTIBULE. The vestibule is an almond-shaped area that is enclosed by the labia minora laterally and extends from the clitoris to the fourchette. The vestibule is the functionally mature female structure of the urogenital sinus of the embryo. In the mature state, the vestibule usually is perforated by six openings: the urethra, the vagina, the two ducts of the Bartholin glands, and, at times, the two ducts of the paraurethral glands, also called the *Skene ducts and glands* (Fig. 2–2). The posterior portion of the vestibule between the fourchette and the vaginal opening is called the *fossa navicularis,* and it is usually observed only in nulliparous women.

The pair of *Bartholin glands* (see Fig. 2–2) are about 0.5 to 1 cm in diameter, and each is situated beneath the vestibule on either side of the vaginal opening. They are the *major vestibular glands,* and the ducts are 1.5 to 2 cm long and open on the sides of the vestibule just outside the lateral margin of the vaginal orifice. At times of sexual arousal, they secrete mucoid material. These glands may harbor *Neisseria gonorrhoeae* or other bacteria, which in turn may cause infection and a Bartholin gland abscess.

Urethral Opening. The lower two thirds of the urethra lies immediately above the anterior vaginal wall. The urethral opening or meatus is in the midline of the vestibule, 1 to 1.5 cm below the pubic arch, and a short distance above the vaginal opening. Ordinarily, the *paraurethral ducts,* also known as the *Skene ducts,* open onto the vestibule on either side of the urethra (see Fig. 2–2). The ducts occasionally open on the posterior wall of the urethra just inside the meatus.

Vestibular Bulbs. Embryologically, the vestibular bulbs correspond to the anlage of the corpus spongiosum of the penis. These are almond-shaped aggregations of veins, 3 to 4 cm long, 1 to 2 cm wide, and 0.5 to 1 cm thick, that lie beneath the mucous membrane on either side of the vestibule. They are in close apposition to the ischiopubic rami and are partially covered by the ischiocavernosus and constrictor vaginae muscles. The vestibular bulbs terminate interiorly at about the middle of the vaginal opening and extend upward toward the clitoris. During childbirth, they may be injured and may even rupture to form a vulvar hematoma.

Vaginal Opening and Hymen. In most virginal women, the vaginal opening most often is hidden by the overlapping labia minora. There are marked differences in shape and consistency of the hymen, which is composed mainly of elastic and collagenous connective tissue. Both the outer and inner surfaces are covered by stratified squamous epithelium. The hymen has no glandular or muscular elements, and it is not richly supplied with nerve fibers.

In the newborn, the hymen is very vascular and redundant. In pregnant women, its epithelium is thick, and the tissue is rich in glycogen. After menopause, the epithelium is thin, and focal cornification may develop. In adult women, the hymen is a membrane of various thickness that surrounds the

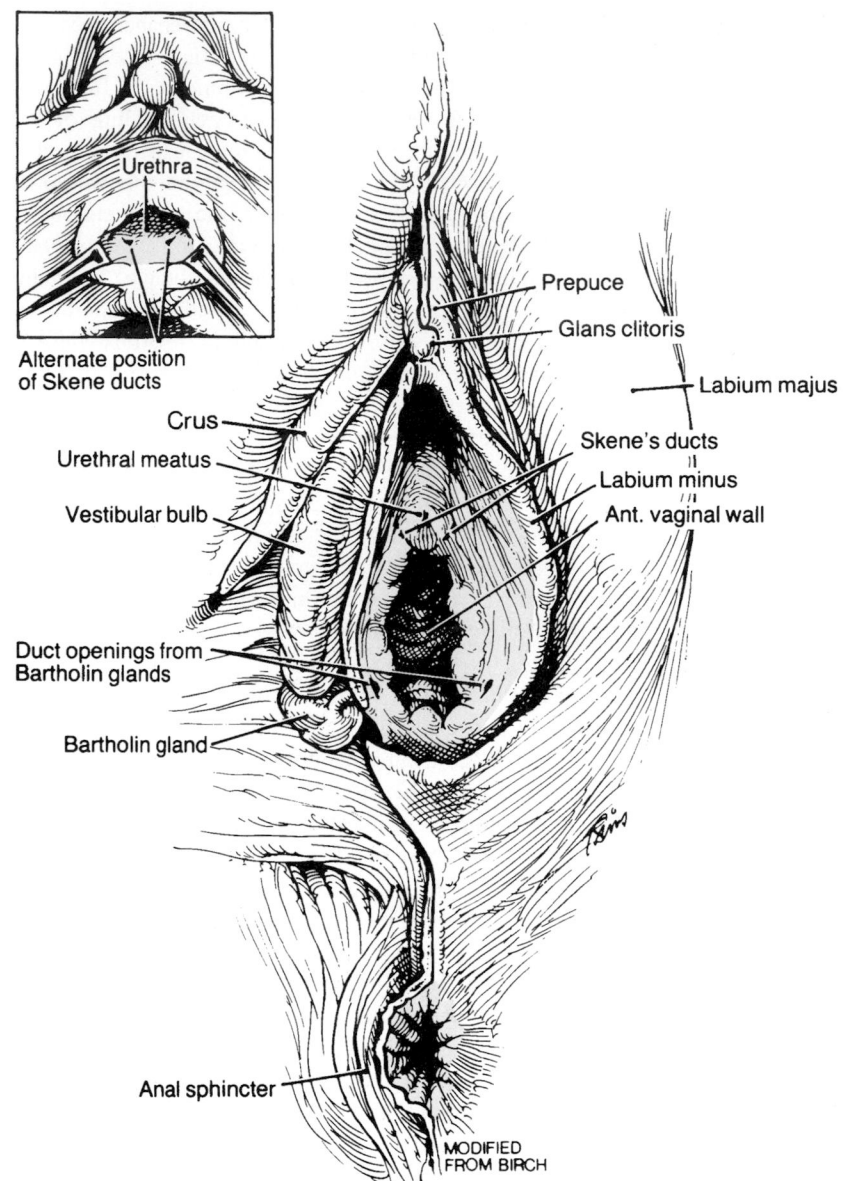

Urethra

Alternate position
of Skene ducts

Crus

Urethral meatus

Vestibular bulb

Duct openings from
Bartholin glands

Bartholin gland

Anal sphincter

Prepuce

Glans clitoris

Labium majus

Skene's ducts

Labium minus

Ant. vaginal wall

MODIFIED
FROM BIRCH

FIGURE 2–2. The external genitalia with the skin and subcutaneous tissue removed from the right side.

vaginal opening more or less completely. Its aperture varies in diameter from pinpoint size to one that admits the tip of one or even two fingers.

The appearance of the hymen cannot be used to determine whether a woman has begun sexual activity. A fimbriated type of hymen in virginal women may be indistinguishable from one that has been penetrated during intercourse. As a rule, however, it is torn at several sites during first coitus, usually in the posterior portion. Identical tears may occur by other penetration, for example, tampons used during menstruation. The edges of the torn tissue soon cicatrize, and the hymen becomes divided permanently into two or more portions that are separated by narrow sulci. Occasionally with hymenal rupture, there may be profuse bleeding.

Changes produced in the hymen by childbirth are usually readily recognizable. Over time, the hymen consists of several

cicatrized nodules of various sizes. *Imperforate hymen* is a rare lesion in which the vaginal orifice is occluded completely, causing retention of menstrual blood (see Chap. 40, p. 950).

VAGINA. This musculomembranous structure extends from the vulva to the uterus and is interposed anteriorly and posteriorly between the urinary bladder and the rectum (Fig. 2–3). The upper portion of the vagina arises from the müllerian ducts, and the lower portion is formed from the urogenital sinus. Anteriorly, the vagina is separated from the bladder and urethra by connective tissue, often referred to as the *vesicovaginal septum.* Posteriorly, between the lower portion of the vagina and the rectum, there are similar tissues that together form the *rectovaginal septum.* The upper fourth of the vagina is separated from the rectum by the *rectouterine pouch,* also called the *cul-de-sac of Douglas.*

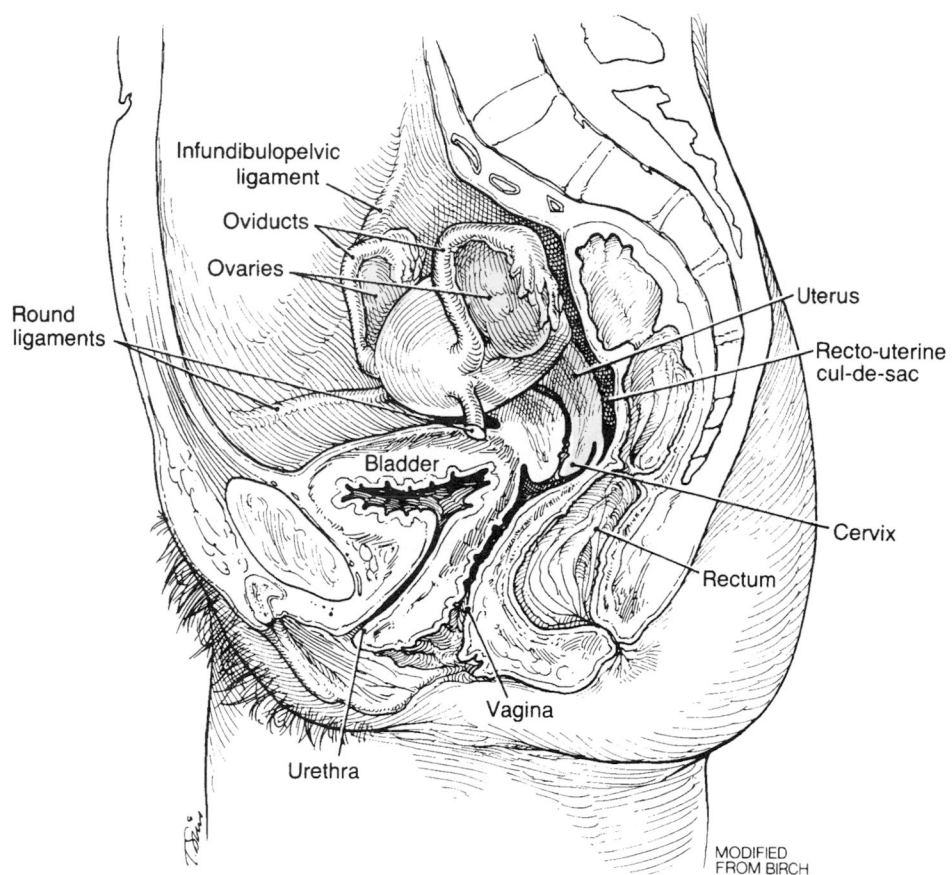

Infundibulopelvic ligament

Oviducts

Ovaries

Round ligaments

Uterus

Recto-uterine cul-de-sac

Bladder

Cervix

Rectum

Vagina

Urethra

MODIFIED FROM BIRCH

FIGURE 2–3. Sagittal section of the pelvis of an adult woman showing relations of pelvic viscera.

Normally, the anterior and posterior vaginal walls lie in contact, with only a slight space intervening between the lateral margins. Vaginal length varies considerably, but commonly, the anterior and posterior vaginal walls are, respectively, 6 to 8 cm and 7 to 10 cm in length. The upper end of the vaginal vault is subdivided into the anterior, posterior, and two lateral fornices by the uterine cervix. These are of considerable clinical importance because the internal pelvic organs usually can be palpated through their thin walls. Moreover, the posterior fornix provides surgical access to the peritoneal cavity.

Prominent midline longitudinal ridges project into the vaginal lumen from the anterior and posterior walls. In nulliparous women, numerous transverse ridges, or *rugae,* extend outward from and almost at right angles to the longitudinal ridges. In postmenopausal multiparous women, the vaginal walls often are smooth.

The vaginal mucosa is composed of noncornified stratified squamous epithelium. Beneath the epithelium is a thin fibromuscular coat, usually consisting of an inner circular layer and an outer longitudinal layer of smooth muscle. A thin layer of connective tissue beneath the mucosa and the muscularis is rich in blood vessels. It is controversial whether this connective tissue—often referred to as *perivaginal endopelvic fascia*—is a definite fascial plane in the strict anatomical sense.

There are no vaginal glands. After giving birth, fragments of stratified epithelium occasionally are embedded in the vaginal connective tissue. They may form *vaginal inclusion cysts,* which are not true glands. In the absence of glands, the vagina is kept moist by a small amount of secretion from the cervix. During pregnancy, there is copious, acidic vaginal secretion, which normally consists of a curdlike product of exfoliated epithelium and bacteria. *Lactobacillus* species are also recovered in higher concentrations than in nonpregnant women (Larsen and Galask, 1980; McGregor and French, 2000).

The vagina has an abundant vascular supply. The upper third is supplied by the cervicovaginal branches of the uterine arteries, the middle third by the inferior vesical arteries, and the lower third by the middle rectal and internal pudendal arteries. The vaginal artery may branch directly from the internal iliac artery. An extensive venous plexus immediately surrounds the vagina and follows the course of the arteries. Lymphatics from the lower third of the vagina, along with those of the vulva, drain primarily into the inguinal lymph nodes. Those from the middle third drain into the internal iliac nodes, and those from the upper third drain into the iliac nodes.

PERINEUM. The many structures that make up the perineum are illustrated in Figure 2–4. Most of the support of

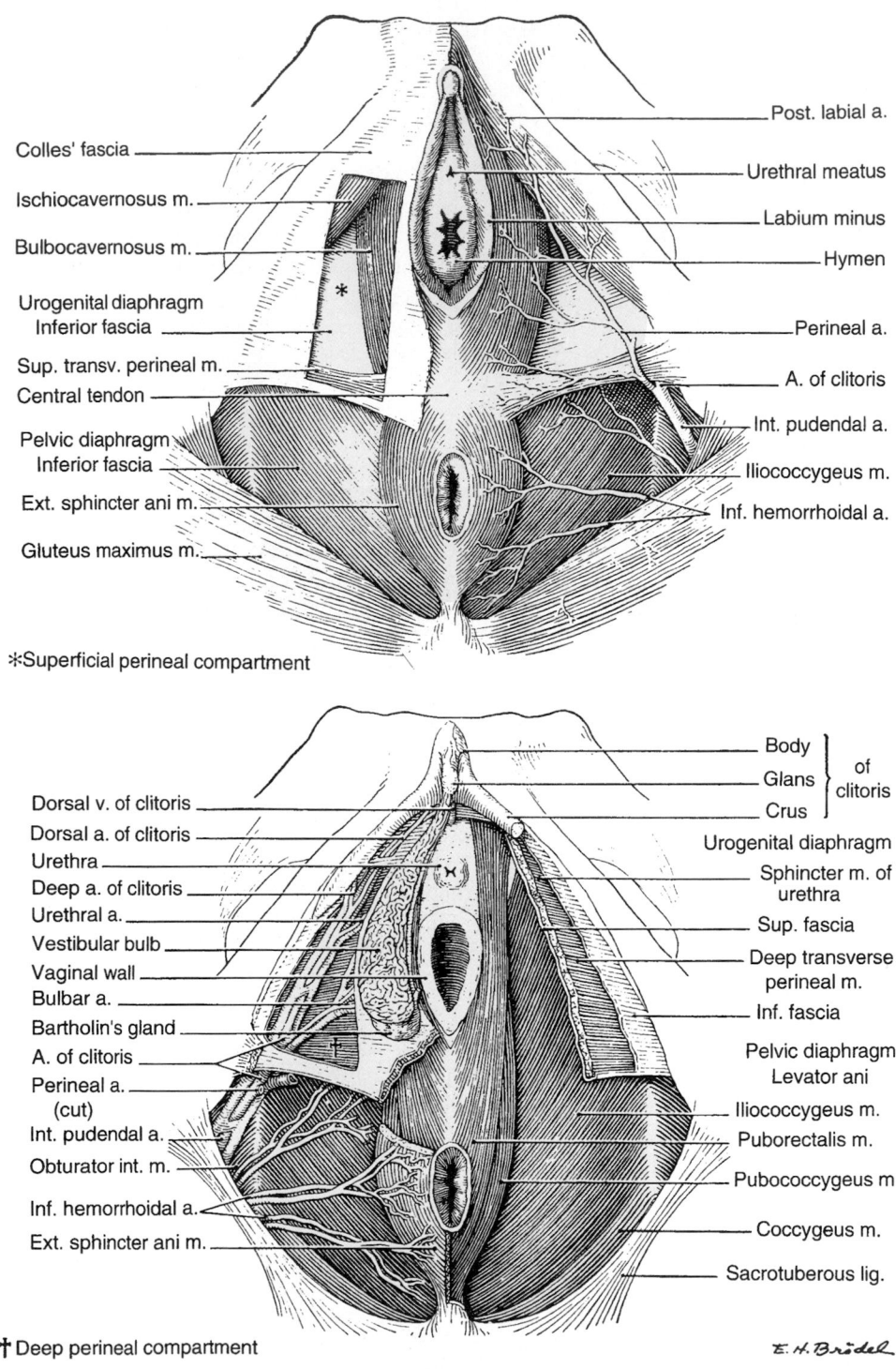

Colles' fascia

Ischiocavernosus m.

Bulbocavernosus m.

Urogenital diaphragm
Inferior fascia

Sup. transv. perineal m.
Central tendon

Pelvic diaphragm
Inferior fascia

Ext. sphincter ani m.

Gluteus maximus m.

Post. labial a.

Urethral meatus

Labium minus

Hymen

Perineal a.

A. of clitoris

Int. pudendal a.

Iliococcygeus m.

Inf. hemorrhoidal a.

✳Superficial perineal compartment

Dorsal v. of clitoris
Dorsal a. of clitoris
Urethra
Deep a. of clitoris
Urethral a.
Vestibular bulb
Vaginal wall
Bulbar a.
Bartholin's gland
A. of clitoris
Perineal a.
(cut)
Int. pudendal a.
Obturator int. m.
Inf. hemorrhoidal a.
Ext. sphincter ani m.

Body ⎫
Glans ⎬ of clitoris
Crus ⎭
Urogenital diaphragm
Sphincter m. of urethra
Sup. fascia
Deep transverse perineal m.
Inf. fascia
Pelvic diaphragm
Levator ani
Iliococcygeus m.
Puborectalis m.
Pubococcygeus m
Coccygeus m.
Sacrotuberous lig.

† Deep perineal compartment

E. H. Bridel

FIGURE 2–4. The perineum. The more superficial components are illustrated above and the deeper structures below. (a. = artery; Ext. = external; Int. = internal; lig. = ligament; m. = muscle; Post. = posterior; Sup. = superior; transv. = transverse; v = vein.)

the perineum is provided by the pelvic and urogenital diaphragms. The *pelvic diaphragm* consists of the levator ani muscles plus the coccygeus muscles posteriorly. The levator ani muscles form a broad muscular sling that originates from the posterior surface of the superior pubic rami, from

the inner surface of the ischial spine, and between these two sites, from the obturator fascia. Some of these muscle fibers are inserted around the vagina and rectum to form efficient functional sphincters. In a recent study utilizing magnetic resonance imaging, Tunn (2003) and Hoyte (2004) and their

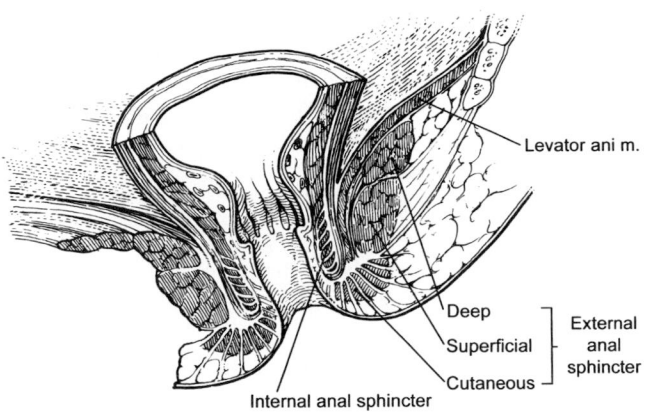

FIGURE 2–5. Anatomy of the anorectum, drawn to show relations of the internal anal sphincter, the external anal sphincter, and the levator ani muscles.

colleagues used magnetic-resonance imaging and reported significant variation in the levator ani muscle, endopelvic fascia, and urethral support in nulliparous women. The *urogenital diaphragm* is external to the pelvic diaphragm and includes the triangular area between the ischial tuberosities and the symphysis. The urogenital diaphragm is made up of the deep transverse perineal muscles, the constrictor of the urethra, and the internal and external fascial coverings.

The external anal sphincter is shown in Figure 2–4, where its proximity to the posterior vaginal fourchette is apparent. The relationship of the internal and external sphincter is shown in Figure 2–5. Damage to either sphincter increases the likelihood of rectal incontinence following vaginal delivery (Delancey and co-workers, 1997). Repair of the disrupted sphincter is shown in Figure 17–36 (see p. 438).

The major blood supply to the perineum is via the internal pudendal artery and its branches. These include the inferior rectal artery and posterior labial artery. The innervation of the perineum is primarily via the pudendal nerve and its branches. The pudendal nerve originates from the S2, S3, and S4 level of the spinal cord.

Perineal Body. The median raphe of the levator ani, between the anus and the vagina, is reinforced by the central tendon of the perineum. The bulbocavernosus, superficial transverse perineal, and external anal sphincter muscles also converge on the central tendon. Thus, these structures contribute to the perineal body, which provides much of the support for the perineum.

INTERNAL GENERATIVE ORGANS

UTERUS. The nonpregnant uterus is situated in the pelvic cavity between the bladder anteriorly and the rectum posteriorly. Almost the entire posterior wall of the uterus is covered by serosa, or peritoneum, the lower portion of which forms the anterior boundary of the *recto-uterine cul-de-sac,* or pouch of Douglas. Only the upper portion of the anterior wall of the uterus is so covered (Fig. 2–6). The lower portion is united to the posterior wall of the bladder by a well-defined loose layer of connective tissue (see Fig. 2–3).

Size and Shape. The uterus resembles a flattened pear in shape (see Fig. 2–6). It consists of two major but unequal parts: an upper triangular portion, the *body,* or corpus; and a lower, cylindrical, or fusiform portion, the *cervix,* which projects into the vagina. The *isthmus* is that portion of the uterus between the internal cervical os and the endometrial cavity. It is of special obstetrical significance because it forms the lower uterine segment during pregnancy. The oviducts,

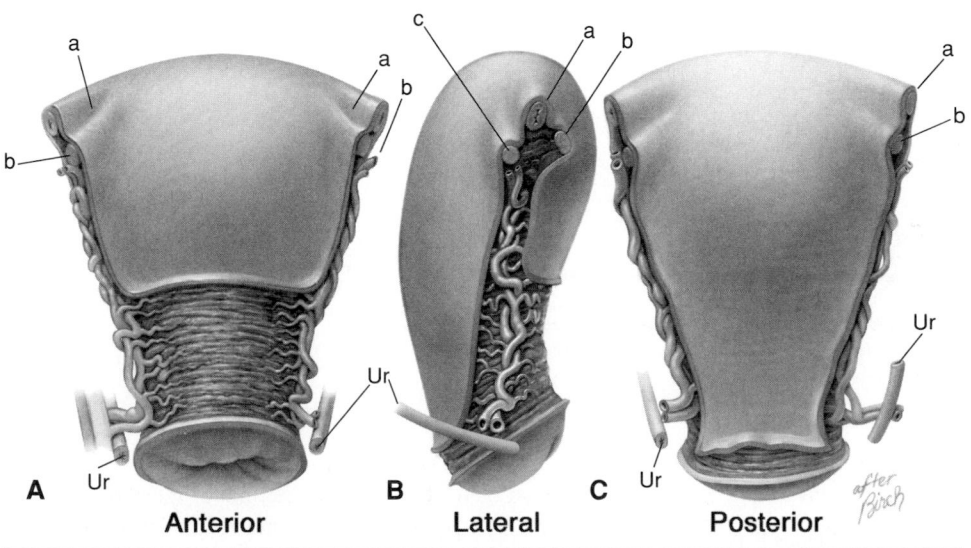

FIGURE 2–6. Anterior **(A)**, right lateral **(B)**, and posterior **(C)** views of the uterus of an adult woman. (a = oviduct; b = round ligament; c = ovarian ligament; Ur = ureter.)

or fallopian tubes, emerge from the *cornua* of the uterus at the junction of the superior and lateral margins. The convex upper segment between the points of insertion of the fallopian tubes is called the *fundus*. The round ligaments insert below the tubes on the anterior side. They are covered by a fold of peritoneum that extends to the pelvic sidewall. These folds are called the *broad ligaments*, however, they do not constitute the anatomical definition of a ligament.

The prepubertal uterus varies in length from 2.5 to 3.5 cm (Orsini and colleagues, 1984). The uterus of adult nulliparous women is from 6 to 8 cm in length as compared with 9 to 10 cm in multiparous women. Uteri of nonparous women average 50 to 70 g, and those of parous women average 80 g or more (Langlois, 1970). In the premenarchal girl, the body of the uterus is only half as long as the cervix. In nulliparous women, the two are about equal in length. In multiparous women, the cervix is only a little more than a third of the total length of the organ. After menopause, uterine size decreases as a consequence of atrophy of both myometrium and endometrium.

The bulk of the body of the uterus, but not the cervix, is composed of muscle. The inner surfaces of the anterior and posterior walls lie almost in contact, and the cavity between these walls forms a mere slit. The cervical canal is fusiform and is open at each end by small apertures, the *internal os* and the *external os*.

Congenital Anomalies. Abnormal müllerian fusion may give rise to a number of uterine anomalies that are discussed in Chapter 40 (see p. 950).

Pregnancy-Induced Uterine Changes. Pregnancy stimulates remarkable uterine growth due to hypertrophy of muscle fibers. The weight of the uterus increases from 70 g to about 1100 g at term. Its total volume averages about 5 L. The uterine fundus, a previously flattened convexity between tubal insertions, now becomes dome shaped (Fig. 2–7). The round ligaments now appear to insert at the junction of the middle and upper thirds of the organ. The fallopian tubes elongate, but the ovaries grossly appear unchanged.

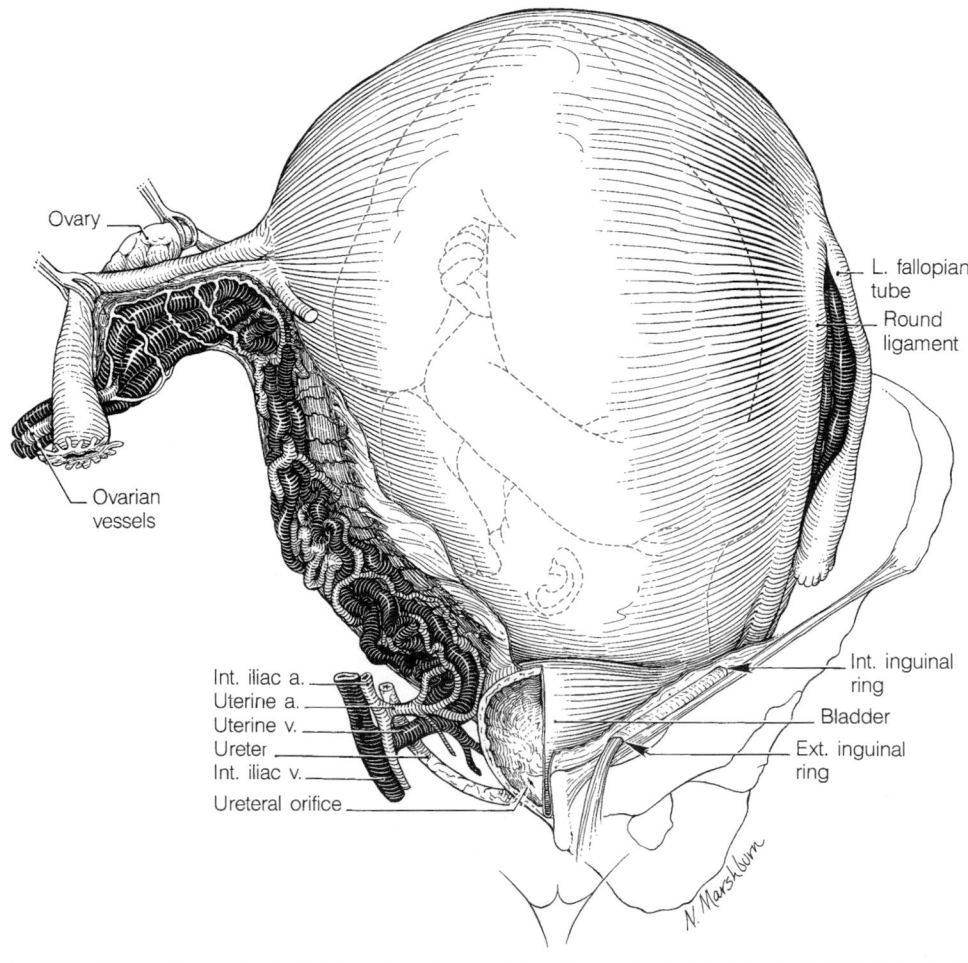

FIGURE 2–7. Uterus of near-term pregnancy. The fundus is now dome shaped, and the tubes and round ligaments appear to insert in the upper middle portion of the uterine body. Note the markedly hypertrophied vascular supply. (a. = artery; Ext. = external; Int. = internal; L. = left; v. = vein.)

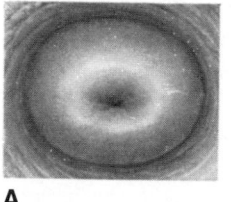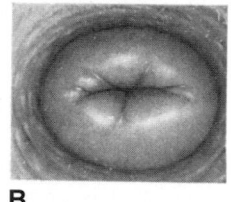

A   **B**

FIGURE 2–8. A. Cervical external os of a nonparous woman. **B.** Cervical external os of a parous woman.

Cervix. Anteriorly, the upper boundary of the cervix is the internal os, which corresponds to the level at which the peritoneum is reflected upon the bladder. The supravaginal segment is covered by peritoneum on its posterior surface. This segment is attached to the cardinal ligaments anteriorly, and it is separated from the overlying bladder by loose connective tissue. The other segment is the lower vaginal portion of the cervix, also called the *portio vaginalis.*

Before childbirth, the external cervical os is a small, regular, oval opening. After childbirth, the orifice is converted into a transverse slit that is divided such that there are the so-called anterior and posterior lips of the cervix. If torn deeply during delivery, it might heal in such a manner that it appears to be irregular, nodular, or stellate (Fig. 2–8). These changes are sufficiently characteristic to permit an examiner to ascertain with some certainty whether a given woman has borne children by vaginal delivery.

The mucosa of the cervical canal is composed of a single layer of very high ciliated columnar epithelium that rests on a thin basement membrane. Numerous cervical glands extend from the surface of the endocervical mucosa directly into the subjacent connective tissue. These glands furnish the thick, tenacious cervical secretions. If the ducts of the cervical glands are occluded, retention cysts, known as *nabothian cysts,* are formed.

Body of the Uterus. The wall of the body of the uterus is composed of serosal, muscular, and mucosal layers. The serosal layer is formed by the peritoneum that covers the uterus. It is firmly adherent except at sites just above the bladder and at the lateral margins, where the peritoneum is deflected to form the broad ligaments.

ENDOMETRIUM. This mucosal layer lines the uterine cavity in nonpregnant women. It is a thin, pink, velvet-like membrane that on close examination is found to be perforated by a large number of minute ostia of the uterine glands. The endometrium normally varies greatly in thickness, and measures from 0.5 mm to as much as 5 mm. It is composed of surface epithelium, glands, and interglandular mesenchymal tissue in which there are numerous blood vessels.

The epithelium of the endometrial surface is made up of a single layer of closely packed, high columnar, ciliated cells. The tubular *uterine glands* are invaginations of the epithelium. The glands extend through the entire thickness of the endometrium to the myometrium, which is occasionally penetrated for a short distance. Histologically, the inner glands resemble the epithelium of the surface and are lined by a single layer of columnar, partially ciliated epithelium that rests on a thin basement membrane. The glands secrete a thin, alkaline fluid. The connective tissue of the endometrium, between the surface epithelium and the myometrium, is a mesenchymal stroma. Histologically, the stroma varies remarkably throughout the ovarian cycle.

After menopause, the endometrium is atrophic and the epithelium flattens. The glands gradually disappear, and the interglandular tissue becomes more fibrous.

The vascular architecture of the uterus and the endometrium is of signal importance in pregnancy. The uterine and ovarian arteries branch and penetrate the uterine wall obliquely inward and reach its middle third. They then ramify in a plane that is parallel to the surface and are therefore named the *arcuate arteries* (DuBose and colleagues, 1985). Radial branches extend from the arcuate arteries at right angles and enter the endometrium to become *coiled or spiral arteries.* Also from the radial arteries, *basal arteries* branch at a sharp angle (Fig. 2–9). The coiled arteries supply most of the midportion and all of the superficial third of the endometrium. The walls of these vessels are responsive (sensitive) to the action of a number of hormones, especially by vasoconstriction, and thus probably serve an important role in the mechanism(s) of menstruation. The straight basal endometrial arteries extend only into the basal layer of the endometrium and are not responsive to hormonal action.

MYOMETRIUM. The myometrium makes up the major portion of the uterus. It is composed of bundles of smooth muscle united by connective tissue in which there are many elastic fibers. According to Schwalm and Dubrauszky (1966), the number of muscle fibers of the uterus progressively diminishes caudally such that, in the cervix, muscle comprises only

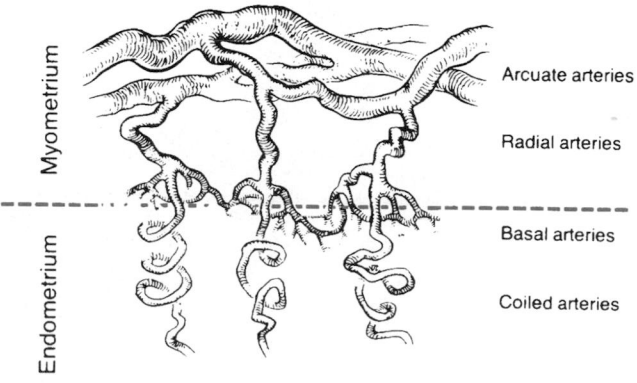

FIGURE 2–9. Stereographic representation of myometrial and endometrial arteries in the macaque. Above, parts of myometrial arcuate arteries from which myometrial radial arteries course toward the endometrium. Below, the larger endometrial coiled arteries and the smaller endometrial basal arteries. (From Okkels and Engle, 1938.)

10 percent of the tissue mass. In the inner wall of the body of the uterus, there is relatively more muscle than in the outer layers; and in the anterior and posterior walls, there is more muscle than in the lateral walls. During pregnancy, the upper myometrium undergoes marked hypertrophy, but there is no significant change in cervical muscle content.

LIGAMENTS. The *broad ligaments* are made up of two winglike structures that extend from the lateral margins of the uterus to the pelvic walls. They divide the pelvic cavity into anterior and posterior compartments. Each broad ligament consists of a fold of peritoneum. The inner two thirds of the superior margin form the *mesosalpinx,* to which the fallopian tubes are attached. The outer third of the superior margin, which extends from the fimbriated end of the oviduct to the pelvic wall, forms the *infundibulopelvic ligament* or *suspensory ligament of the ovary,* through which the ovarian vessels traverse.

At the lateral margin of each broad ligament, the peritoneum is reflected onto the side of the pelvis. The thick base of the broad ligament is continuous with the connective tissue of the pelvic floor. The densest portion is usually referred to as the *cardinal ligament*—also called the *transverse cervical ligament* or the *Mackenrodt ligament*—and is composed of connective tissue that medially is united firmly to the supravaginal portion of the cervix.

A vertical section through the uterine end of the broad ligament is triangular, and the uterine vessels and ureter are found within its broad base (Fig. 2–10). In its lower part, it is widely attached to the connective tissues that are adjacent to

the cervix, that is, the *parametrium.* The upper part is made up of three folds that nearly cover the oviduct, the utero-ovarian ligament, and the round ligament.

The *round ligaments* extend from the lateral portion of the uterus, arising somewhat below and anterior to the origin of the oviducts. Each round ligament is located in a fold of peritoneum that is continuous with the broad ligament and extends outward and downward to the inguinal canal, through which it passes to terminate in the upper portion of the labium majus. In nonpregnant women, the round ligament varies from 3 to 5 mm in diameter, and is composed of smooth muscle cells. The round ligament corresponds embryologically to the gubernaculum testis of men. During pregnancy, the round ligaments undergo considerable hypertrophy and increase appreciably in both length and diameter.

Each *uterosacral ligament* extends from an attachment posterolaterally to the supravaginal portion of the cervix to encircle the rectum and inserts into the fascia over the sacrum. Umek and colleagues (2004) used MR-imaging to describe anatomical variations of these ligaments. The ligaments are composed of connective tissue and some smooth muscle and are covered by peritoneum. They form the lateral boundaries of the pouch of Douglas.

BLOOD VESSELS. The vascular supply of the uterus is derived principally from the uterine and ovarian arteries. The uterine artery, a main branch of the internal iliac artery—referred to in the past as the hypogastric artery—enters the base of the broad ligament and makes its way medially to the side of the

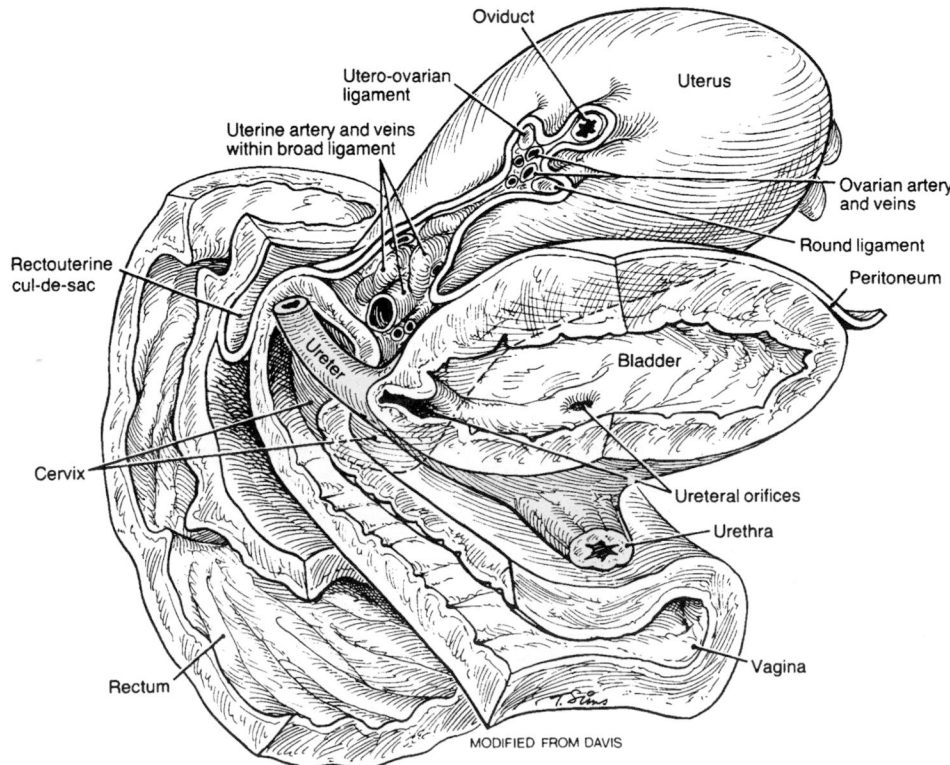

Oviduct
Utero-ovarian ligament
Uterine artery and veins within broad ligament
Uterus
Rectouterine cul-de-sac
Ovarian artery and veins
Round ligament
Peritoneum
Ureter
Bladder
Cervix
Ureteral orifices
Urethra
Rectum
Vagina

MODIFIED FROM DAVIS

FIGURE 2–10. Vertical section through the uterine end of the right broad ligament.

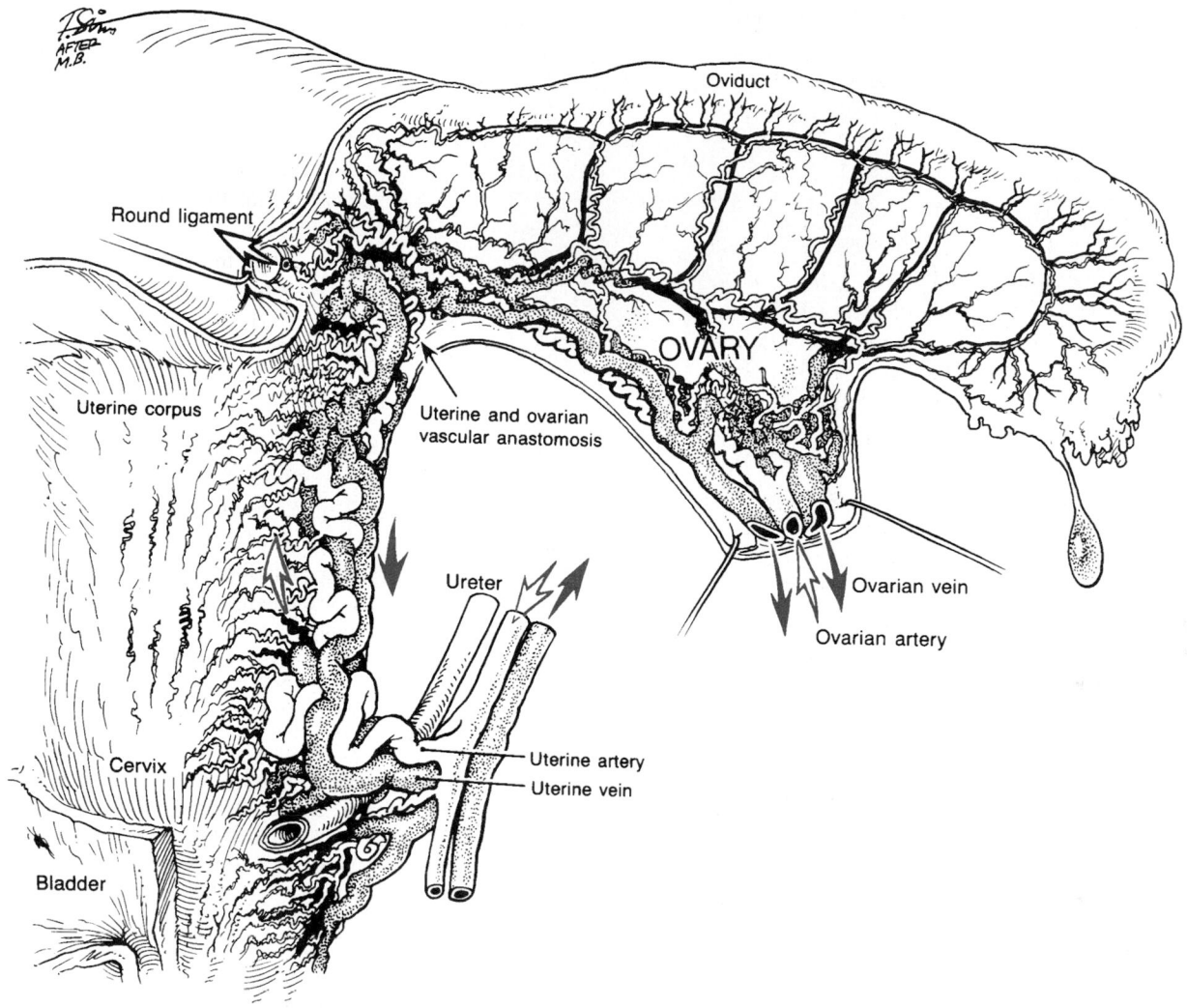

FIGURE 2–11. Blood supply to the left ovary, left oviduct, and left side of the uterus. The ovarian and uterine vessels anastomose freely. Note the uterine artery and vein crossing over the ureter that lies immediately adjacent to the cervix.

uterus. Immediately adjacent to the supravaginal portion of the cervix, the uterine artery divides. The smaller cervicovaginal artery supplies blood to the lower cervix and upper vagina. The main branch turns abruptly upward and extends as a highly convoluted vessel that traverses along the margin of the uterus. A branch of considerable size extends to the upper portion of the cervix, and numerous other branches penetrate the body of the uterus. Just before the main branch of the uterine artery reaches the oviduct, it divides into three terminal branches. The ovarian branch of the uterine artery anastomoses with the terminal branch of the ovarian artery; the tubal branch makes its way through the mesosalpinx and supplies part of the oviduct; and the fundal branch is distributed to the uppermost uterus.

About 2 cm lateral to the cervix, the uterine artery crosses over the ureter (Figs. 2–6 and 2–11). The proximity of the uterine artery and vein to the ureter at this point is of great

surgical significance. Because of their close proximity, the ureter may be injured or ligated during a hysterectomy when the vessels are clamped and ligated.

A major portion of the blood supply to the pelvis is via the branches of the internal iliac artery, as shown in the arteriogram in Figure 2–12. In addition to the uterine artery, other branches of the anterior and posterior divisions of the internal iliac artery include those listed in Table 2–1.

The *ovarian artery* is a direct branch of the aorta. It enters the broad ligament through the infundibulopelvic ligament. At the ovarian hilum, it divides into a number of smaller branches that enter the ovary. Its main stem, however, traverses the entire length of the broad ligament very near the mesosalpinx and makes its way to the upper lateral portion of the uterus. Here it anastomoses with the ovarian branch of the uterine artery. There are numerous additional communications among the arteries on both sides of the uterus.

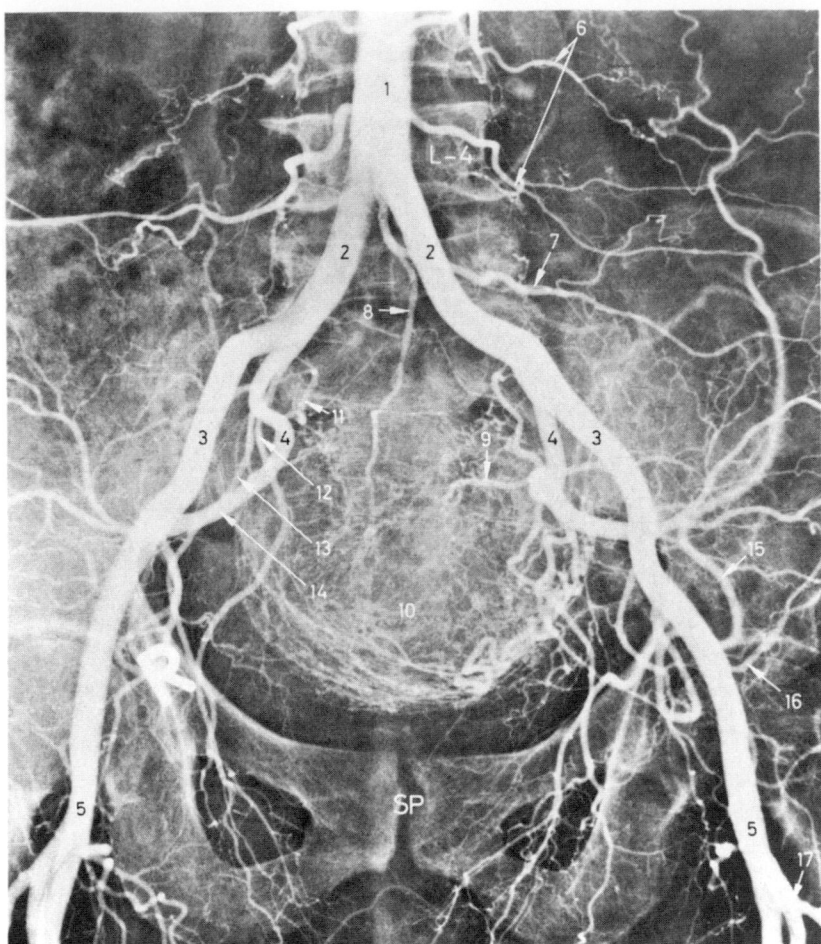

FIGURE 2–12. Iliac arteriogram. It can be seen that the bifurcation of the aorta (1) into the two common iliac arteries (2) occurs at the lower border of the body of the L4 vertebra. The common iliac vessels branch into external (3) and internal (4) iliac arteries. The internal iliac artery (4) on each side serves a number of branches to the pelvis, perineum, and gluteal region, whereas the external iliac artery (3), after giving off the inferior epigastric (15) and deep circumflex iliac (16) arteries, becomes the femoral artery below the inguinal ligament. (Also shown: 5 = femoral artery; 6 = lumbar arteries; 7 = iliolumbar artery; 8 = median sacral artery; 9 = uterine artery; 10 = uterus; 11 = lateral sacral artery; 12 = obturator artery; 13 = internal pudendal artery; 14 = superior gluteal artery; 17 = deep femoral artery; L4 = fourth lumbar vertebra; SP = symphysis pubis.) (From Wicke, 1982.)

When the uterus is in a contracted state, its numerous venous lumens are collapsed, however, in injected specimens the greater part of the uterine wall appears to be occupied by dilated venous sinuses. On either side, the arcuate veins unite to form the *uterine vein,* which empties into the internal iliac vein and thence into the common iliac vein. Some of the blood from the upper uterus, the ovary, and the upper part of the broad ligament is collected by several veins. Within the broad ligament, these veins form the large *pampiniform plexus* that terminates in the ovarian vein. The right ovarian vein empties into the vena cava, whereas the left ovarian vein empties into the left renal vein. During pregnancy, there is marked hypertrophy of the blood supply to the uterus, as shown in Figure 2–7.

LYMPHATICS. The endometrium is abundantly supplied with true lymphatic vessels that are confined largely to the basal layer. The lymphatics of the underlying myometrium are increased in number toward the serosal surface and form an abundant lymphatic plexus just beneath it. Lymphatics from the cervix terminate mainly in the hypogastric nodes, which are situated near the bifurcation of the common iliac vessels. The lymphatics from the body of the uterus are distributed to two groups of nodes. One set of vessels drains into the internal iliac nodes. The other set, after joining certain lymphatics from the ovarian region, terminates in the periaortic lymph nodes.

INNERVATION. The nerve supply to the pelvic area is derived principally from the sympathetic nervous system, but also partly from the cerebrospinal and parasympathetic systems. The parasympathetic system is represented on either side by the pelvic nerve, which is made up of a few fibers that are

TABLE 2–1 Branches of the Internal Iliac Artery

Anterior Division	Posterior Division
Uterine	Superior gluteal
Umbilical	Lateral sacral
Uterine vesical	Iliolumbar
Obturator	
Internal pudendal	
Inferior gluteal	
Middle vesical	
Middle rectal	
Vaginal	

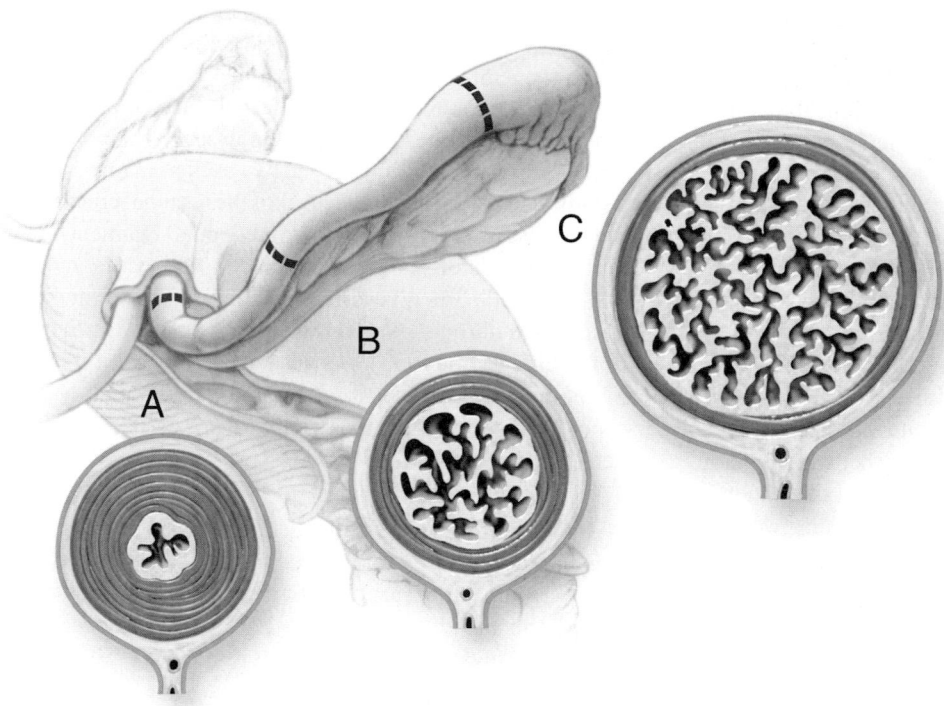

FIGURE 2–13. The oviduct of an adult woman with cross-sectioned illustrations of the gross structure of the epithelium in several portions: **(A)** isthmus, **(B)** ampulla, and **(C)** infundibulum.

derived from the second, third, and fourth sacral nerves. It loses its identity in the *cervical ganglion of Frankenhäuser.* The sympathetic system enters the pelvis by way of the internal iliac plexus that arises from the aortic plexus just below the promontory of the sacrum. After descending on either side, it also enters the uterovaginal plexus of Frankenhäuser, which is made up of ganglia of various sizes, but particularly of a large ganglionic plate that is situated on either side of the cervix and just above the posterior fornix in front of the rectum.

Branches from these plexuses supply the uterus, bladder, and upper vagina. In the 11th and 12th thoracic nerve roots, there are sensory fibers from the uterus that transmit the painful stimuli of contractions to the central nervous system. The sensory nerves from the cervix and upper part of the birth canal pass through the pelvic nerves to the second, third, and fourth sacral nerves, whereas those from the lower portion of the birth canal pass primarily through the pudendal nerve. Knowledge of the innervation of dermatomes and its clinical application to providing epidural or spinal analgesia for labor and vaginal or cesarean delivery is illustrated in Figures 19–1 and 19–3 (see pp. 477 and 480).

OVIDUCTS. More commonly called the *fallopian tubes,* the oviducts vary in length from 8 to 14 cm. They are covered by peritoneum, and their lumen is lined by mucous membrane. Each tube is divided into an *interstitial portion, isthmus, ampulla,* and *infundibulum.* The interstitial portion is embodied within the muscular wall of the uterus. The isthmus, or the narrow portion of the tube that adjoins the uterus, passes gradually into the wider, lateral portion, or *ampulla.* The *infundibulum,* or fimbriated extremity, is the funnel-shaped opening of the distal end of the fallopian tube (Fig. 2–13). The oviduct varies considerably in thickness; the narrowest portion of the isthmus measures from 2 to 3 mm in diameter, and the widest portion of the ampulla measures from 5 to 8 mm. The fimbriated end of the infundibulum opens into the abdominal cavity. One projection, the *fimbria ovarica,* which is considerably longer than the other fimbriae, forms a shallow gutter that approaches or reaches the ovary.

The musculature of the fallopian tube is arranged in an inner circular and an outer longitudinal layer. In the distal portion, the two layers are less distinct and, near the fimbriated extremity, are replaced by an interlacing network of muscular fibers. The tubal musculature undergoes rhythmic contractions constantly, the rate of which varies with the hormonal changes of the ovarian cycle. The greatest frequency and intensity of contractions is reached during transport of ova.

The oviducts are lined by a single layer of columnar cells, some of them ciliated and others secretory. The ciliated cells are most abundant at the fimbriated extremity, elsewhere, they are found in discrete patches. There are differences in the proportions of these two types of cells in different phases of the ovarian cycle. Because there is no submucosa, the epithelium is in close contact with the underlying muscle. In the tubal mucosa, there are cyclical histological changes similar to those of the endometrium, but much less striking. The mucosa is arranged in longitudinal folds that are more complex toward the fimbriated end. On cross sections through the uterine portion, four simple folds are found that form a figure that resembles a Maltese cross. The isthmus has a more complex pattern. In the ampulla, the lumen is occupied almost completely by the arborescent mucosa, which consists of very complicated folds (see Fig. 2–13). The current produced by the tubal cilia is such that the direction of flow is toward the uterine cavity. Tubal peristalsis is believed to be an extraordinarily important factor in transport of the ovum.

The tubes are supplied richly with elastic tissue, blood vessels, and lymphatics. Sympathetic innervation of the tubes is extensive, in contrast to their parasympathetic innervation.

Diverticula may extend occasionally from the lumen of the tube for a variable distance into the muscular wall and reach almost to the serosa. These diverticula may play a role in the development of ectopic pregnancy (see Chap. 10, p. 256).

Embryological Development of the Uterus and Oviducts.
The uterus and tubes arise from the müllerian ducts, which first appear near the upper pole of the urogenital ridge in the fifth week of embryonic development (Fig. 2–14). This ridge is composed of the mesonephros, gonad, and associated ducts. The first indication of the development of the müllerian duct is a thickening of the coelomic epithelium at about the level of the fourth thoracic segment. This thickening becomes the

fimbriated extremity of the fallopian tube, which invaginates and grows caudally to form a slender tube at the lateral edge of the urogenital ridge. In the sixth week of embryonic life, the growing tips of the two müllerian ducts approach each other in the midline; they reach the urogenital sinus 1 week later. At that time, a fusion of the two müllerian ducts to form a single canal is begun at the level of the inguinal crest, that is, the gubernaculum (primordium of the round ligament). Thus, the upper ends of the müllerian ducts produce the oviducts and the fused parts give rise to the uterus. The vaginal canal is not patent throughout its entire length until the sixth month of fetal life (Koff, 1933). Because of the clinical importance of anomalies that arise from abnormal fusion and dysgenesis of these structures, their embryogenesis is discussed in detail in Chapter 40 (see Fig. 40–1, p. 951).

OVARIES. Compared with each other, as well as between women, the ovaries vary considerably in size. During childbearing years, they are from 2.5 to 5 cm in length, 1.5 to 3 cm in breadth, and 0.6 to 1.5 cm in thickness. After menopause, ovarian size diminishes remarkably. The position of the ovaries also varies, but they usually are situated in the upper part of the pelvic cavity and rest in a slight depression on the lateral wall of the pelvis between the divergent external and internal iliac vessels—the *ovarian fossa of Waldeyer.* The ovary is attached to the broad ligament by the *mesovarium.* The *utero-ovarian ligament* extends from the lateral and posterior portion of the uterus, just beneath the tubal insertion, to the uterine pole of the ovary. Usually, it is several

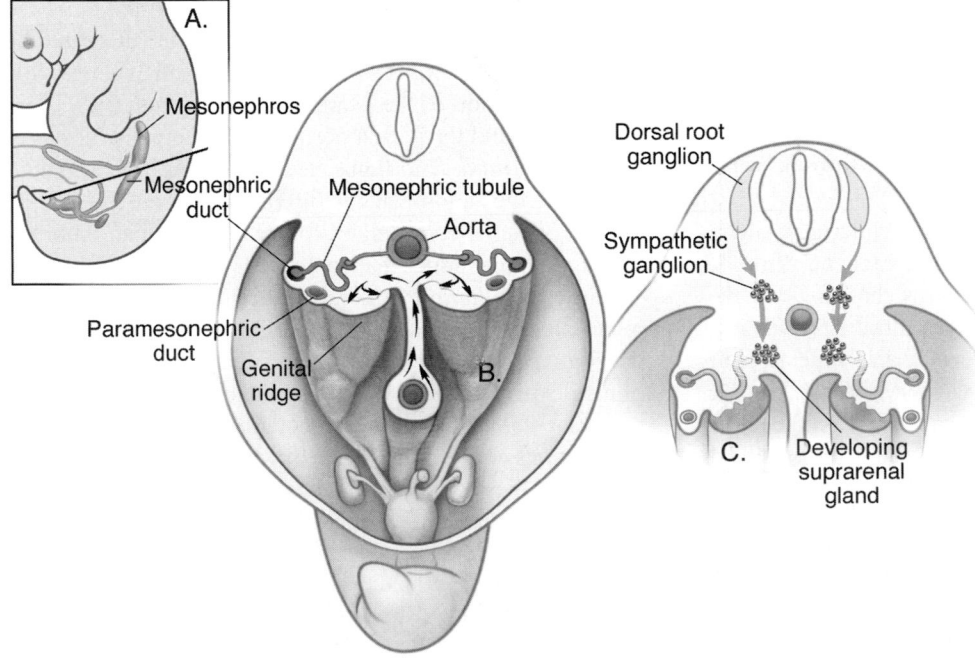

FIGURE 2–14. A. Cross section of an embryo at 4 to 6 weeks. **B.** Large ameboid primordial germ cells migrate *(arrows)* from the yolk sac to the area of germinal epithelium, within the genital ridge. **C.** Migration of sympathetic cells from the spinal ganglia to a region above the developing kidney. (After Moore and colleagues, 2000.)

centimeters long and 3 to 4 mm in diameter. It is covered by peritoneum and is made up of muscle and connective tissue fibers. The *infundibulopelvic* or *suspensory ligament of the ovary* extends from the upper or tubal pole to the pelvic wall; through it course the ovarian vessels and nerves.

In young women, the exterior surface of the ovary is smooth, with a dull white surface through which glisten several small, clear follicles. As the woman ages, the ovaries become more corrugated, and in elderly women, the exterior surfaces may be convoluted markedly.

The ovary consists of two portions, the cortex and medulla. The cortex is the outer layer, which varies in thickness with age and becomes thinner with advancing years. It is in this layer that the ova and graafian follicles are located. The cortex is composed of spindle-shaped connective tissue cells and fibers, among which are scattered primordial and graafian follicles in various stages of development. As the woman ages, the follicles become less numerous. The outermost portion of the cortex, which is dull and whitish, is designated the *tunica albuginea.* On its surface, there is a single layer of cuboidal epithelium, the *germinal epithelium of Waldeyer.*

The medulla is the central portion, which is composed of loose connective tissue that is continuous with that of the mesovarium. There are a large number of arteries and veins in the medulla and a small number of smooth muscle fibers that are continuous with those in the suspensory ligament.

The ovaries are supplied with both sympathetic and parasympathetic nerves. The sympathetic nerves are derived primarily from the ovarian plexus that accompanies the ovarian vessels. Others are derived from the plexus that surrounds the ovarian branch of the uterine artery. The ovary is richly supplied with nonmyelinated nerve fibers, which for the most part accompany the blood vessels. These are merely vascular nerves, whereas others form wreaths around normal and atretic follicles, and these give off many minute branches that have been traced up to, but not through, the membrana granulosa.

Embryology. The earliest sign of a gonad is one that appears on the ventral surface of the embryonic kidney at a site between the eighth thoracic and fourth lumbar segments at about 4 weeks. The coelomic epithelium is thickened, and clumps of cells are seen to bud off into the underlying mesenchyme. This circumscribed area of the coelomic epithelium is called the *germinal epithelium.* By the fourth to sixth week, however, there are many large ameboid cells in this region that have migrated into the body of the embryo from the yolk sac (see Fig. 2–14). These *primordial germ cells* are distinguishable by their large size and certain morphological and cytochemical features.

When the primordial germ cells reach the genital area, some enter the germinal epithelium and others mingle with the groups of cells that proliferate from it or lie in the mesenchyme. By the end of the fifth week, rapid division of all these types of cells results in development of a prominent *genital ridge.* The ridge projects into the body cavity medially to a fold in which there are the mesonephric (wolffian) and the müllerian ducts (Fig. 2–15). By the seventh week, it is separated from the mesonephros except at the narrow central zone, the future hilum, where the blood vessels enter. At this time, the sexes can be distinguished, because the testes can be recognized by well-defined radiating strands of cells (sex cords). These cords are separated from the germinal epithelium by mesenchyme that is to become the tunica albuginea. The sex cords, which consist of large germ cells and smaller epithelioid cells derived from the germinal epithelium, develop into the seminiferous tubules and tubuli rete. The latter establishes connection with the mesonephric tubules that develop into the epididymis. The mesonephric ducts become the vas deferens.

In the female embryo, the germinal epithelium continues to proliferate for a much longer time. The groups of cells thus formed lie at first in the region of the hilum. As connective tissue develops between them, these appear as sex cords. These cords give rise to the medullary cords and persist for variable times (Forbes, 1942). By the third month, medulla and cortex are defined (see Fig. 2–15). The bulk of the organ is made up of cortex, a mass of crowded germ and epithelioid cells that show some signs of grouping, but there are no distinct cords as in the testis. Strands of cells extend from the germinal epithelium into the cortical mass, and mitoses are numerous. The rapid succession of mitoses soon reduces the size of the germ cells to the extent that these no longer are differentiated clearly from the neighboring cells. These germ cells are now called *oogonia.*

By the fourth month, some germ cells in the medullary region begin to enlarge. These are called *primary oocytes* at the beginning of the phase of growth that continues until maturity is reached. During this period of cell growth, many oocytes undergo degeneration, both before and after birth. A single layer of flattened follicular cells that were derived originally from the germinal epithelium soon surrounds the primary oocytes. These structures are now called *primordial follicles* and are seen first in the medulla and later in the cortex. Some follicles begin to grow even before birth, and some are believed to persist in the cortex almost unchanged until menopause.

By 8 months, the ovary has become a long, narrow, lobulated structure that is attached to the body wall along the line of the hilum by the *mesovarium,* in which lies the *epoöphoron.* The germinal epithelium has been separated for the most part from the cortex by a band of connective tissue—*tunica albuginea*—which is absent in many small areas where strands of cells, usually referred to as *cords of Pflüger,* are in contact with the germinal epithelium. Among these cords are cells believed by many investigators to be oogonia that have come to resemble the other epithelial cells as a result of repeated mitoses. In the underlying cortex, there are two distinct zones. Superficially, there are nests of germ cells in synapsis, interspersed with Pflüger cords and strands of connective

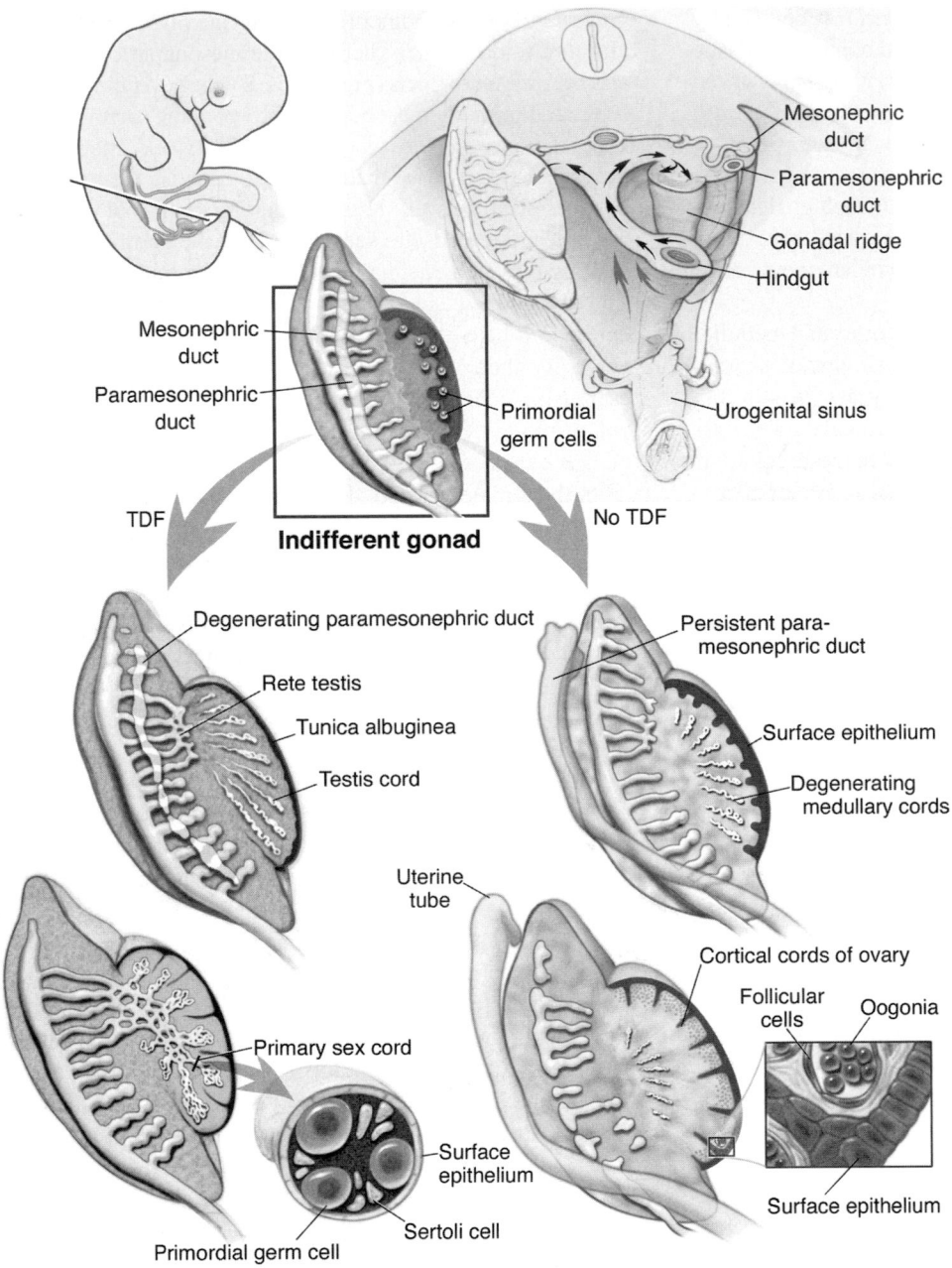

FIGURE 2–15. Continuation of sexual differentiation of the embryo. See text for explanation. (After Moore and colleagues, 2000.)

tissue. In the deeper zone, there are many groups of germ cells in synapsis, as well as primary oocytes, prospective follicular cells, and a few primordial follicles.

At term, the various types of ovarian cells in the human female fetus may still be found.

Histology. From the first stages of its development until after the menopause, the ovary undergoes constant change. The number of oocytes at the onset of puberty has been estimated variously at 200,000 to 400,000. Because only one ovum

ordinarily is cast off during each ovarian cycle, it is evident that a few hundred ova suffice for purposes of reproduction.

The glandular elements of ovaries of adult women include interstitial, thecal, and luteal cells. The interstitial glandular elements are formed from cells of the theca interna of degenerating or atretic follicles; the thecal glandular cells are formed from the theca interna of ripening follicles; and the true luteal cells are derived from the granulosa cells of ovulated follicles and from the undifferentiated stroma that surround them.

The huge store of primordial follicles at birth is exhausted gradually after sexual maturation and through the reproductive span. Block (1952) found that there is a gradual decline from a mean of 439,000 oocytes in girls younger than 15 years to a mean of 34,000 in women older than 36 years. In young girls, the greater portion of the ovary is composed of the cortex, which is filled with large numbers of closely packed primordial follicles. In young women, the cortex is relatively thinner but still contains a large number of primordial follicles. Each primordial follicle is made up of an oocyte and its surrounding single layer of epithelial cells, which are small and flattened, spindle-shaped, and somewhat sharply differentiated from the still smaller and spindly cells of the surrounding stroma.

The oocyte is a large, spherical cell in which there is clear cytoplasm and a relatively large nucleus located near the center of the ovum. In the nucleus, there are one large and several smaller nucleoli, and numerous masses of chromatin. In adult women, the diameter of the smallest oocytes averages 33 μm, and that of the nuclei, 20 μm.

EMBRYOLOGICAL REMNANTS. There are a number of vestigial wolffian structures that are identified after embryogenesis of the female reproductive system. Some of these occasionally cause clinical concerns. The *parovarium* can be found in the scant loose connective tissue within the broad ligament in the vicinity of the mesosalpinx. It comprises a number of narrow vertical tubules that are lined by ciliated epithelium. These tubules connect at the upper ends with a longitudinal duct that extends just below the oviduct to the lateral margin of the uterus, where it ends blindly near the internal os. This canal is the remnant of the wolffian (mesonephric) duct in women and is called the *Gartner duct.* The parovarium, also a remnant of the wolffian duct, is homologous embryologically with the caput epididymis in men. The cranial portion of the parovarium is the *epoöphoron,* or *organ of Rosenmüller;* the caudal portion, or *paroöphoron,* is a group of vestigial mesonephric tubules that lie in or around the broad ligament. It is homologous embryologically with the paradidymis of men. The paroöphoron in adult women usually disappears.

SURGICAL ANATOMY. Shown in Figure 2–16 are illustrations of female pelvic surgical anatomy. The figure depicts a nonpregnant uterus, and details of a peripartum hysterectomy are discussed in Chapter 25 (see p. 599).

THE BONY PELVIS

In both women and men, the pelvis forms the bony ring through which body weight is transmitted to the lower extremities, but in women it has a special form that adapts it to childbearing (Fig. 2–17). The pelvis is composed of four bones: the sacrum, coccyx, and two innominate bones. Each innominate bone is formed by the fusion of the ilium, ischium, and pubis. The innominate bones are joined to the sacrum at the sacroiliac synchondroses and to one another at the symphysis pubis.

PELVIC ANATOMY. The false pelvis lies above the linea terminalis and the true pelvis below this anatomical boundary (see Fig. 2–17). The false pelvis is bounded posteriorly by the lumbar vertebra and laterally by the iliac fossa. In front, the boundary is formed by the lower portion of the anterior abdominal wall.

The true pelvis is the portion important in childbearing. It is bounded above by the promontory and alae of the sacrum, the linea terminalis, and the upper margins of the pubic bones, and below by the pelvic outlet. The cavity of the true pelvis can be described as an obliquely truncated, bent cylinder with its greatest height posteriorly. Its anterior wall at the symphysis pubis measures about 5 cm, and its posterior wall, about 10 cm (Figs. 2–18 and 2–19).

The walls of the true pelvis are partly bony and partly ligamentous. The posterior boundary is the anterior surface of the sacrum, and the lateral limits are formed by the inner surface of the ischial bones and the sacrosciatic notches and ligaments. In front, the true pelvis is bounded by the pubic bones, the ascending superior rami of the ischial bones, and the obturator foramen.

The sidewalls of the true pelvis of an adult woman converge somewhat. Extending from the middle of the posterior margin of each ischium are the ischial spines. These are of great obstetrical importance because the distance between them usually represents the shortest diameter of the pelvic cavity. They also serve as valuable landmarks in assessing the level to which the presenting part of the fetus has descended into the true pelvis. The sacrum forms the posterior wall of the pelvic cavity. Its upper anterior margin corresponds to the promontory that may be felt during bimanual pelvic examination in women with a small pelvis. It can provide a landmark for clinical pelvimetry. Normally the sacrum has a marked vertical and a less pronounced horizontal concavity, which in abnormal pelves may undergo important variations. A straight line drawn from the promontory to the tip of the sacrum usually measures 10 cm, whereas the distance along the concavity averages 12 cm.

The descending inferior rami of the pubic bones unite at an angle of 90 to 100 degrees to form a rounded arch under which the fetal head must pass.

PELVIC JOINTS

Symphysis Pubis. Anteriorly, the pelvic bones are joined together by the symphysis pubis. This structure consists of fibrocartilage and the superior and inferior pubic ligaments; the latter are frequently designated the *arcuate ligament of the pubis* (Fig. 2–20).

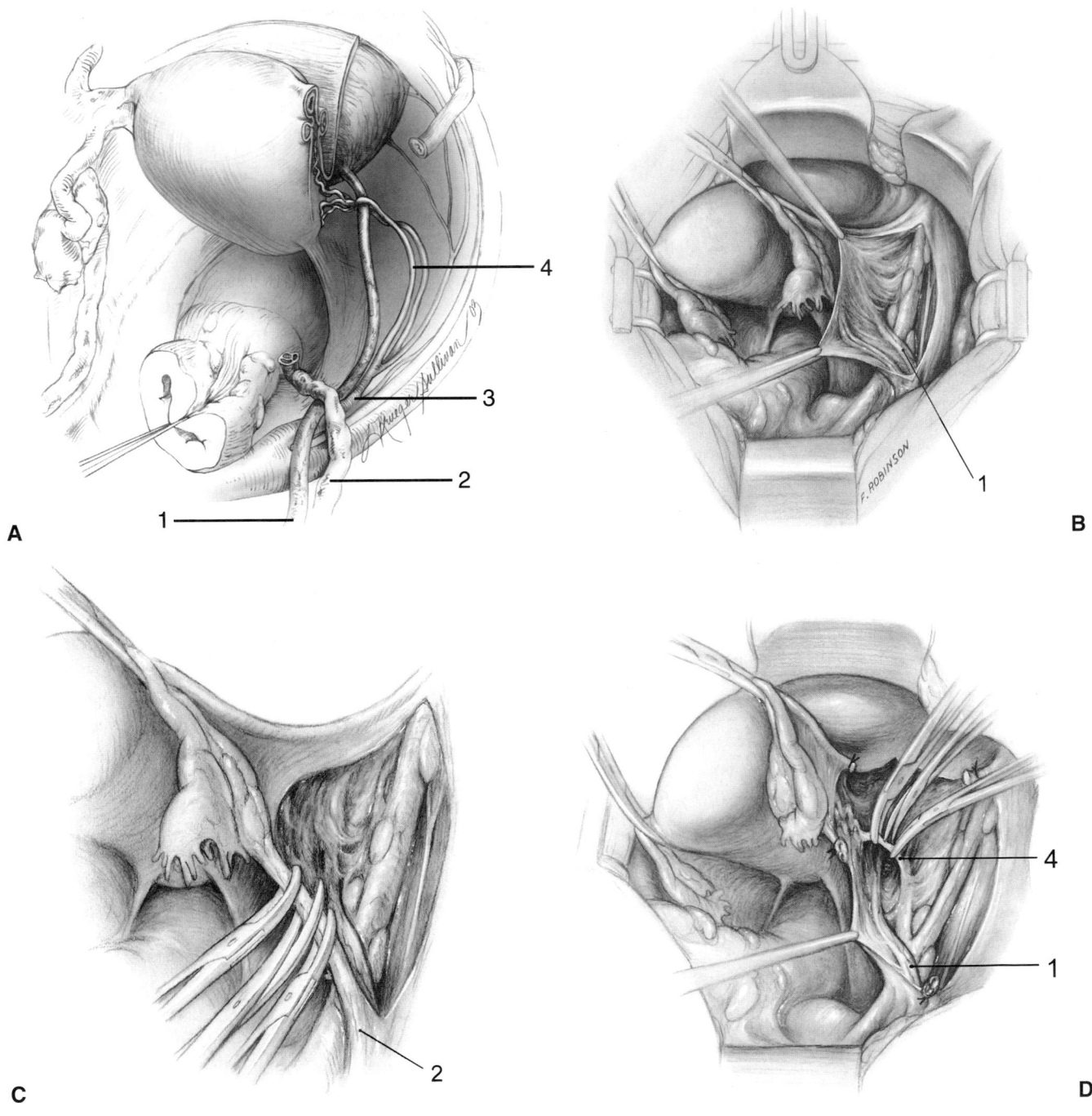

FIGURE 2–16. Pelvic retroperitoneal anatomy. **A.** Dissected right retroperitoneal space illustrating the course of the pelvic ureter. The right uterine adnexa have been transected adjacent to the uterus, the ovarian vessels have been severed just distal to the pelvic brim, and the peritoneum has been removed from the right pelvic sidewall and the right portion of the bladder. The ureter (1) enters the pelvis by crossing over the bifurcation of the common iliac artery just medial to the ovarian vessels (2). It then descends medial to the branches of the internal iliac artery (3). The ureter then courses through the cardinal ligament and passes under the uterine artery (4, "water under the bridge") approximately 1 to 2 cm lateral to the cervix at the level of the internal cervical os. The origin of the uterine artery from the internal iliac artery (3) is shown. The ureter then courses medially toward the base of the bladder. The distal part of the ureter is associated with the upper portion of the anterior vaginal wall. **B.** The retroperitoneal space has been entered and the peritoneum is retracted medially to show the ureter (1) crossing over the external and internal iliac artery bifurcation. Note that the ureter remains attached to the peritoneum of the pelvic sidewall and the medial leaf of the broad ligament. **C.** The ovarian vessels (2) are clamped and transected after visualization of the ureter. **D.** The uterine artery (4) is being clamped and transected. Note the ureter (1) crossing under this vessel lateral to the cervix. (Figs. B, C, and D from Nelson, 1977, with permission.)

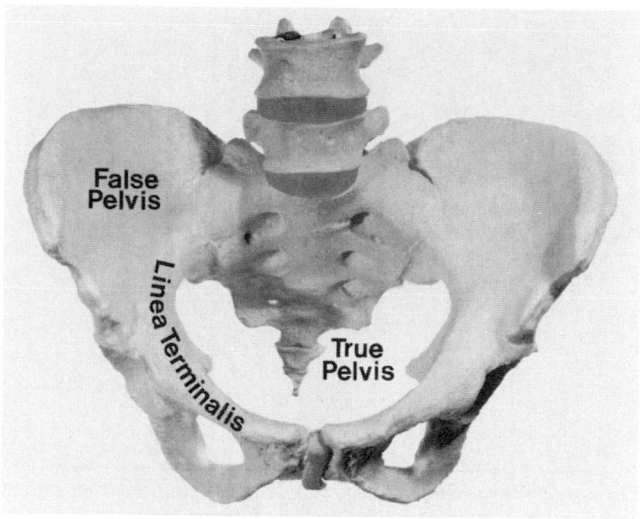

FIGURE 2–17. Normal female pelvis with the false and true pelves identified.

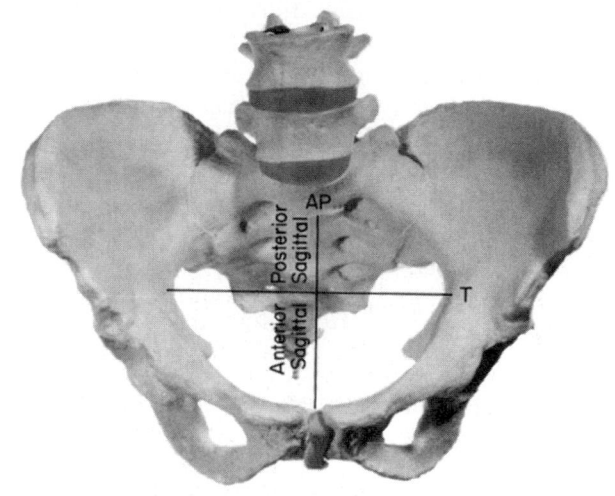

FIGURE 2–19. Adult female pelvis. Anteroposterior (AP) and transverse (T) diameters of the pelvic inlet are illustrated, as well as the posterior sagittal diameter of the inlet.

Sacroiliac Joints. Posteriorly, the pelvic bones are joined by the articulations between the sacrum and the iliac portion of the innominate bones to form the sacroiliac joints. These joints also have a certain degree of mobility.

Relaxation of the Pelvic Joints. During pregnancy, relaxation of these joints likely results from hormonal changes. Abramson and co-workers (1934) observed that relaxation of the symphysis pubis commenced in women in the first half of pregnancy and increased during the last 3 months. They also observed that this laxity began to regress immediately after parturition and that regression was completed within 3 to 5 months. The symphysis pubis also increases

in width during pregnancy—more so in multiparas than in primigravidas—and returns to normal soon after delivery.

There are important changes in sacroiliac joint mobility. Borell and Fernstrom (1957) demonstrated that the rather marked mobility of the pelvis at term was caused by an upward gliding movement of the sacroiliac joint. The displacement, which is greatest in the dorsal lithotomy position, may increase the diameter of the outlet by 1.5 to 2.0 cm. **This is the main justification for placing a woman in this position for a vaginal delivery.** The increase in the diameter of the pelvic outlet, however, occurs only if the sacrum is allowed to rotate posteriorly, that is, only if the sacrum is not forced anteriorly by the weight of the maternal pelvis against the

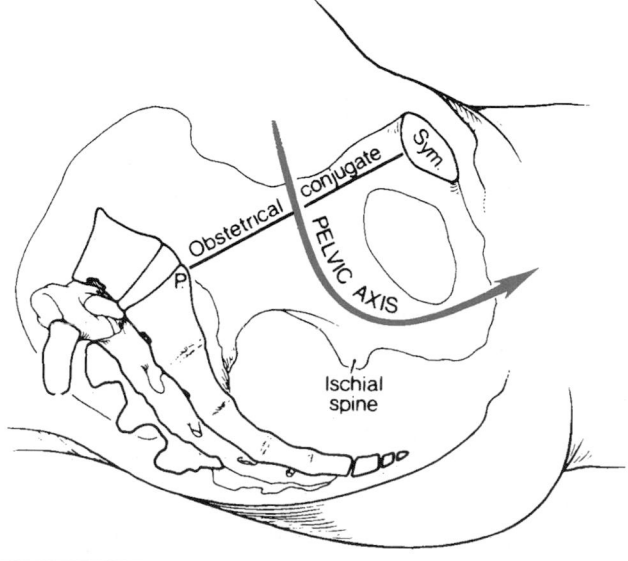

FIGURE 2–18. The cavity of the true pelvis is comparable to an obliquely truncated, bent cylinder with its greatest height posteriorly. Note the curvature of the pelvic axis.

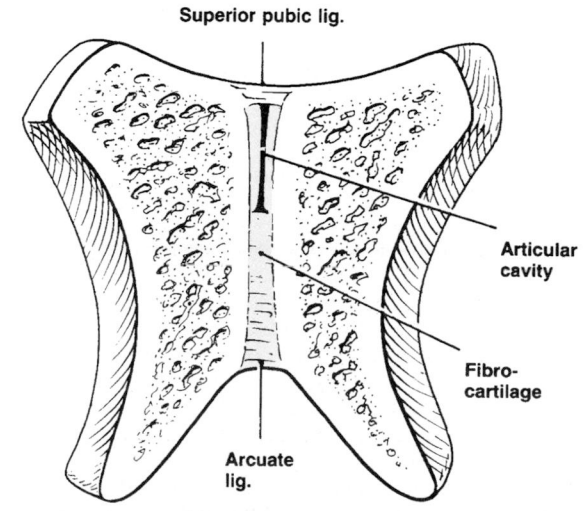

FIGURE 2–20. Frontal section through the symphysis pubis. (lig. = ligament.) (Redrawn from Spalteholz, 1933.)

delivery table or bed (Russell, 1969, 1982). Sacroiliac joint mobility is also the likely reason that the McRoberts maneuver often is successful in releasing an obstructed shoulder in a case of shoulder dystocia (see Chap. 20, p. 513). These changes have also been attributed to the success of the modified squatting position to hasten second-stage labor (Gardosi and co-workers, 1989). The squatting position may increase the interspinous diameter and the diameter of the pelvic outlet (Russell, 1969, 1982). These latter observations are unconfirmed, but this position is assumed for birth in many primitive societies.

PLANES AND DIAMETERS OF THE PELVIS. The pelvis is described as having four imaginary planes:

1. The plane of the pelvic inlet—the superior strait.
2. The plane of the pelvic outlet—the inferior strait.
3. The plane of the midpelvis—the least pelvic dimensions.
4. The plane of greatest pelvic dimension—of no obstetrical significance.

Pelvic Inlet. The pelvic inlet (superior strait) is bounded posteriorly by the promontory and alae of the sacrum, laterally by the linea terminalis, and anteriorly by the horizontal pubic rami and the symphysis pubis (Figs. 2–21 and 2–22; see also Figs. 2–18 and 2–19). The inlet of the female pelvis typically is more nearly round than ovoid. Caldwell and co-workers (1934) identified radiographically a nearly round or *gynecoid* pelvic inlet in approximately 50 percent of white women.

Four diameters of the pelvic inlet are usually described: anteroposterior, transverse, and two obliques. The obstetrically

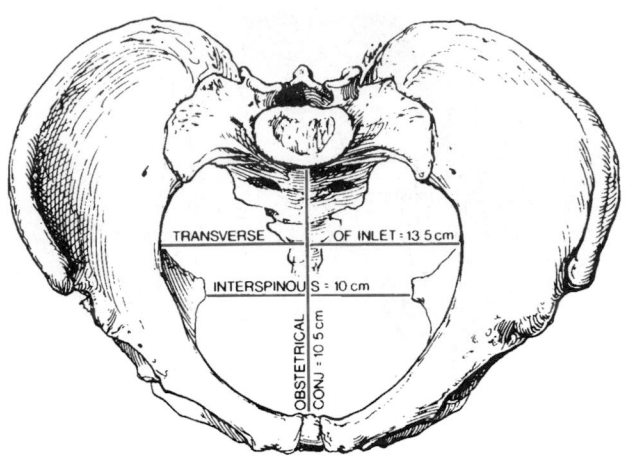

FIGURE 2–22. Adult female pelvis demonstrating anteroposterior and transverse diameters of the pelvic inlet and transverse (interspinous) diameter of the midpelvis. The obstetrical conjugate is normally greater than 10 cm.

important anteroposterior diameter is the shortest distance between the promontory of the sacrum and the symphysis pubis, and is designated the *obstetrical conjugate* (see Figs. 2–18, 2–19, and 2–21). Normally, this measures 10 cm or more.

The transverse diameter is constructed at right angles to the obstetrical conjugate and represents the greatest distance between the linea terminalis on either side. It usually intersects the obstetrical conjugate at a point about 4 cm in front of the promontory (Fig. 2–19). The segment of the obstetrical conjugate from the intersection of these two lines to the promontory is designated the *posterior sagittal diameter* of the inlet.

Each of the two oblique diameters extends from one of the sacroiliac synchondroses to the iliopectineal eminence on the opposite side. They average less than 13 cm.

The anteroposterior diameter of the pelvic inlet that has been identified as the *true conjugate* does not represent the shortest distance between the promontory of the sacrum and the symphysis pubis (see Fig. 2–21). The shortest distance is the obstetrical conjugate, which is the shortest anteroposterior diameter through which the head must pass in descending through the pelvic inlet (see Figs. 2–18, 2–19, and 2–21). The obstetrical conjugate cannot be measured directly with the examining fingers. For clinical purposes, the obstetrical conjugate is estimated indirectly by subtracting 1.5 to 2 cm from the diagonal conjugate. The latter is determined by measuring the distance from the lower margin of the symphysis to the promontory of the sacrum (see Fig. 2–21).

Midpelvis. The midpelvis is measured at the level of the ischial spines—the midplane, or plane of least pelvic dimensions. It is of particular importance following engagement of the fetal head in obstructed labor. The interspinous diameter, 10 cm or somewhat more, is usually the smallest diameter of

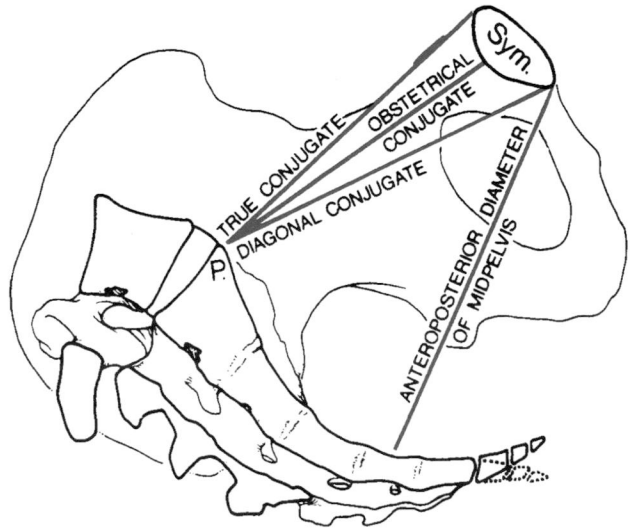

FIGURE 2–21. Three anteroposterior diameters of the pelvic inlet are illustrated: the true conjugate, the more important obstetrical conjugate, and the clinically measurable diagonal conjugate. The anteroposterior diameter of the midpelvis is also shown. (P = sacral promontory; Sym = symphysis pubis.)

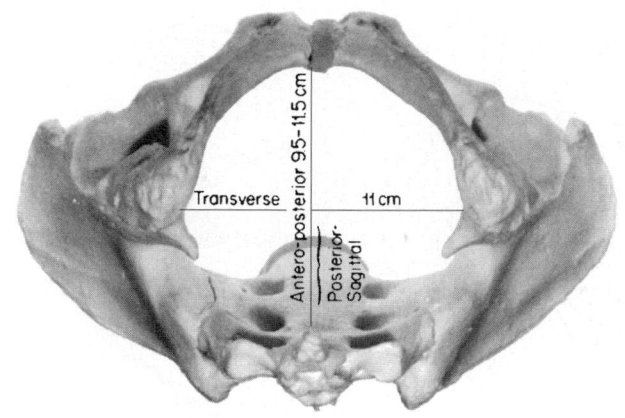

FIGURE 2–23. Pelvic outlet with diameters marked. Note that the anteroposterior diameter may be divided into anterior and posterior sagittal diameters.

the pelvis. The anteroposterior diameter through the level of the ischial spines normally measures at least 11.5 cm. Its posterior component (posterior sagittal diameter), between the sacrum and the line created by the interspinous diameter, is usually at least 4.5 cm (Fig. 2–22).

Pelvic Outlet. The pelvic outlet consists of two approximately triangular areas that are not in the same plane. They have a common base, which is a line drawn between the two ischial tuberosities (Fig. 2–23). The apex of the posterior

triangle is at the tip of the sacrum, and the lateral boundaries are the sacrosciatic ligaments and the ischial tuberosities. The anterior triangle is formed by the area under the pubic arch. Three diameters of the pelvic outlet usually are described: the anteroposterior, transverse, and posterior sagittal.

PELVIC SHAPES. In the past, x-ray pelvimetry was used frequently in women with suspected cephalopelvic disproportion or fetal malpresentation. Caldwell and Moloy (1933, 1934) developed a classification of the pelvis that is still used. The classification is based on the shape of the pelvis, and its familiarity helps the clinician understand better the mechanisms of labor.

The *Caldwell–Moloy classification* is based on measurement of the greatest transverse diameter of the inlet and its division into anterior and posterior segments. The shapes of these are used to classify the pelvis as gynecoid, anthropoid, android, or platypelloid (Fig. 2–24). The character of the posterior segment determines the type of pelvis, and the character of the anterior segment determines the tendency. These are both determined because many pelves are not pure but are mixed types; for example, a gynecoid pelvis with an android tendency means that the posterior pelvis is gynecoid and the anterior pelvis is android in shape.

From viewing the four basic types in Figure 2–24, the configuration of the gynecoid pelvis would intuitively seem suited for delivery of most fetuses. Indeed, Caldwell and co-workers (1939) reported that the gynecoid pelvis was found

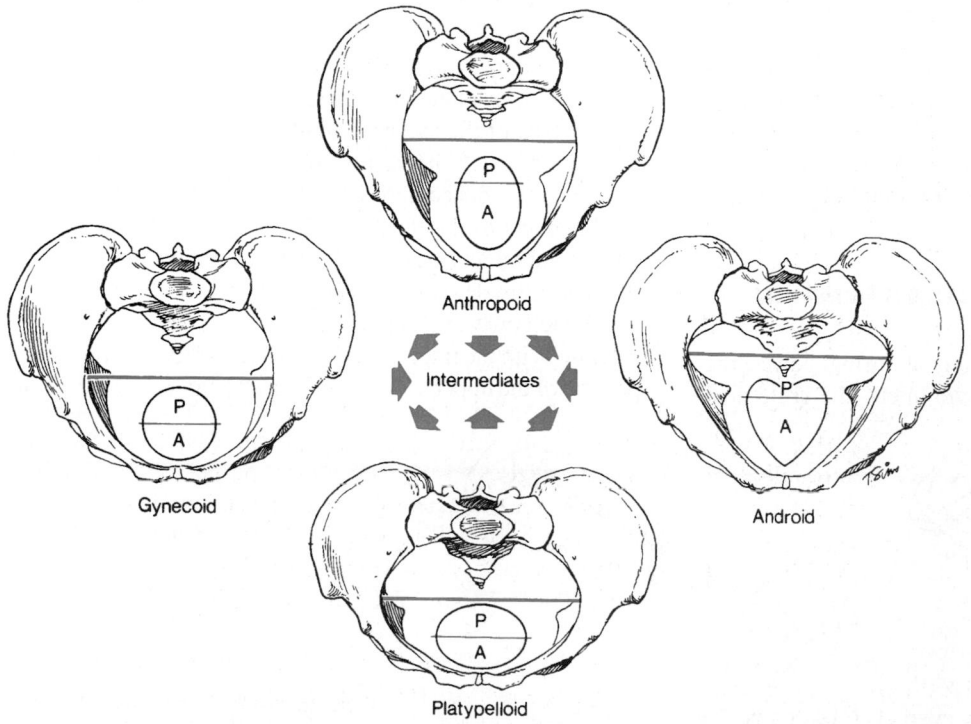

FIGURE 2–24. The four parent pelvic types of the Caldwell–Moloy classification. A line passing through the widest transverse diameter divides the inlets into posterior (P) and anterior (A) segments.

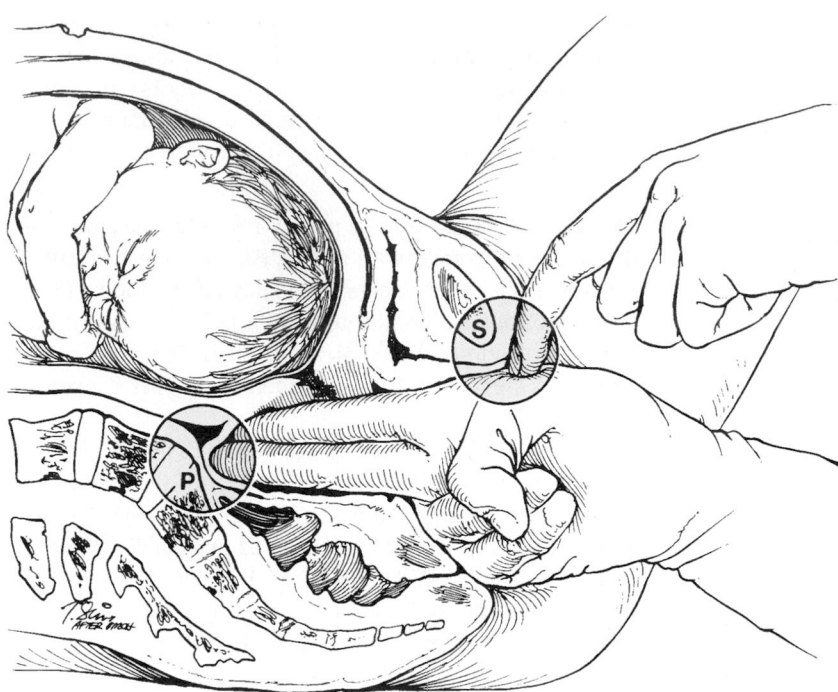

FIGURE 2–25. Vaginal examination to determine the diagonal conjugate. (P = sacral promontory; S = symphysis pubis.)

in almost 50 percent of women. In contrast, in the android pelvis, the posterior sagittal diameter at the inlet is much shorter than the anterior sagittal diameter, limiting the use of the posterior space by the fetal head. Moreover, the anterior portion is narrow and triangular. The extreme android pelvis presages a poor prognosis for vaginal delivery. In the anthropoid pelvis, the anteroposterior diameter of the inlet is greater than the transverse. This results in an oval anteroposteriorly, with the anterior segment somewhat narrow and pointed. Variations of anthropoid-type pelves are found in about one third of women. The *platypelloid pelvis* has a flattened gynecoid shape with short anteroposterior and wide transverse diameters. Pure varieties are found in fewer than 3 percent of women.

PELVIC SIZE AND ITS CLINICAL ESTIMATION

Pelvic Inlet Measurements. In many abnormal pelves, the anteroposterior diameter of the pelvic inlet—the obstetrical conjugate—is considerably shortened. The diagonal conjugate is clinically estimated by measuring the distance from the sacral promontory to the lower margin of the symphysis pubis (Figs. 2–25 and 2–26). Two fingers of the dominant hand are introduced into the vagina. The mobility of the coccyx is first evaluated. The anterior surface of the sacrum is next palpated from below upward and its vertical and lateral curvatures noted. In normal pelves, only the last three sacral vertebrae can be felt without indenting the perineum. Conversely, in markedly contracted pelves, the entire anterior surface of the sacrum usually is readily palpable. Next, in order to reach the sacral promontory, the examiner's elbow must be flexed and the perineum forcibly indented by the knuckles of the third and fourth fingers. The index and the second fingers are carried up and over the anterior surface of the sacrum. By deeply inserting the wrist, the promontory may be felt by the tip of the second finger as a projecting bony margin. With the finger closely applied to the most prominent portion of the upper sacrum, the vaginal hand is elevated until

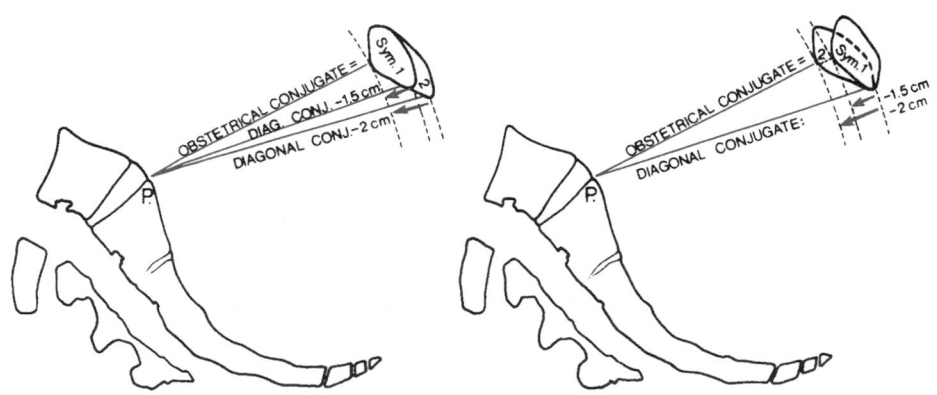

FIGURE 2–26. Variations in length of the diagonal conjugate dependent on height and inclination of the symphysis pubis. (P. = sacral promontory; Sym. = symphysis pubis.)

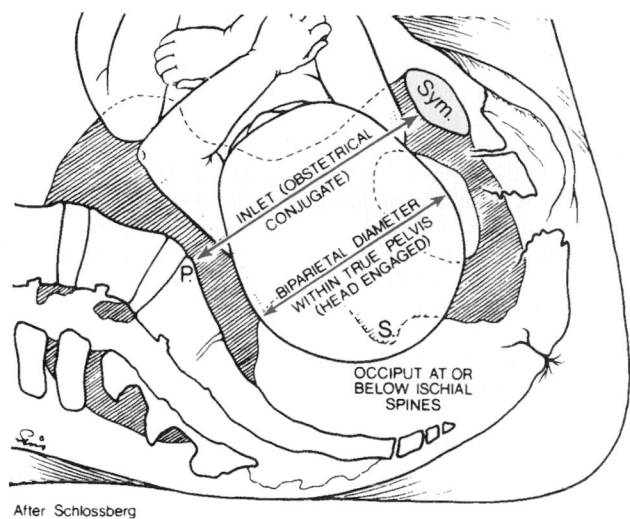

After Schlossberg

FIGURE 2–27. When the lowermost portion of the fetal head is at or below the ischial spines, it is usually engaged. Exceptions occur when there is considerable molding, caput formation, or both. (P = sacral promontory; S = ischial spine; Sym = symphysis pubis.)

it contacts the pubic arch. The immediately adjacent point on the index finger is marked, as shown in Figure 2–25. The distance between the mark and the tip of the second finger is the diagonal conjugate. The obstetrical conjugate is computed by subtracting 1.5 to 2.0 cm, depending on the height and inclination of the symphysis pubis, as illustrated in Figure 2–26. If the diagonal conjugate is greater than 11.5 cm, it is justifiable to assume that the pelvic inlet is of adequate size for vaginal delivery of a normal-sized fetus.

Transverse contraction of the inlet can be measured only by imaging pelvimetry. Pelvic contraction is possible even if the anteroposterior diameter is adequate.

Engagement. Descent of the biparietal plane of the fetal head to a level below that of the pelvic inlet is termed *engagement* (Fig. 2–27). When the biparietal—the largest—diameter of the normally flexed fetal head has passed through the inlet, the head is engaged. Although engagement usually is regarded as a phenomenon of labor, in nulliparas it may occur during the last few weeks of pregnancy. When it does so, it is confirmatory evidence that the pelvic inlet is adequate for that fetal head. **With engagement, the fetal head serves as an internal pelvimeter to demonstrate that the pelvic inlet is ample for that fetus.**

Engagement is ascertained by vaginal examination or by abdominal palpation. With vaginal examination, the station of the lowermost part of the fetal head in relation to the level of the ischial spines is determined. If the lowest part of the occiput is at or below the level of the spines, the head usually, but not always, is engaged. The distance from the plane of the pelvic inlet to the level of the ischial spines is approximately 5 cm in most pelves. Although the distance from the biparietal plane of the unmolded fetal head to the vertex is usually only 3 to 4 cm, accurate determination of engagement may be difficult if there is considerable elongation of the fetal head from molding or formation of a *caput succedaneum.*

Abdominal examination is a less satisfactory method to determine engagement. If the biparietal plane of a term-sized infant has descended through the inlet, the examining fingers cannot reach the lowermost part of the head. Thus, when pushed downward over the lower abdomen, the examining fingers will slide over that portion of the head proximal to the biparietal plane (nape of the neck) and diverge. Conversely, if the head is not engaged, the examining fingers can easily palpate the lower part of the head and will converge.

Fixation of the fetal head occurs when descent proceeds to a depth that prevents its free movement when pushed right and then left by both hands placed over the lower abdomen. Fixation is not necessarily synonymous with engagement. Although a head that is freely movable on abdominal examination cannot be engaged, fixation of the head is sometimes seen when the biparietal plane is still 1 cm or more above the pelvic inlet, especially if the head is molded appreciably.

Pelvic Outlet Measurements. An important dimension of the pelvic outlet that is accessible for clinical measurement is the diameter between the ischial tuberosities, variously called the *biischial diameter, intertuberous diameter,* and *transverse diameter of the outlet.* A measurement of more than 8 cm is considered normal. The measurement of the transverse diameter of the outlet can be estimated by placing a closed fist against the perineum between the ischial tuberosities. Usually the closed fist is wider than 8 cm. The shape of the subpubic arch also can be evaluated at the same time by palpating the pubic rami from the subpubic region toward the ischial tuberosities.

Midpelvis Estimation. Clinical estimation of midpelvic capacity by any direct form of measurement is not possible. If the ischial spines are quite prominent, the sidewalls are felt to converge, and the concavity of the sacrum is very shallow, then suspicion of a contraction is aroused.

REFERENCES

Abramson D, Roberts SM, Wilson PD: Relaxation of the pelvic joints in pregnancy. Surg Obstet Gynecol 58:595, 1934

Block E: Quantitative morphological investigation of the follicular system in women. Acta Anat 14:108, 1952

Borell U, Fernstrom I: Movements at the sacroiliac joints and their importance to changes in pelvic dimensions during parturition. Acta Obstet Gynecol Scand 36:42, 1957

Caldwell WE, Moloy HC: Anatomical variations in the female pelvis and their effect in labor with a suggested classification. Am J Obstet Gynecol 26:479, 1933

Caldwell WE, Moloy HC, D'Esopo DA: Further studies on the pelvic architecture. Am J Obstet Gynecol 28:482, 1934

Caldwell WE, Moloy HC, Swenson PC: The use of the roentgen ray in obstetrics, 1. Roentgen pelvimetry and cephalometry; technique of pelviroentgenography. Am J Roentgenol 41:305, 1939

Delancey JOL, Toglia MR, Perucchini D: Internal and external anal sphincter anatomy as it relates to midline obstetric lacerations. Obstet Gynecol 90:924, 1997

DuBose TJ, Hill LW, Hennigan HW Jr, et al: Sonography of arcuate uterine blood vessels. J Ultrasound Med 4:229, 1985

Forbes TR: On the fate of the medullary cords of the human ovary. Contrib Embryol 30:9, 1942

Gardosi J, Hutson N, Lynch CB: Randomised, controlled trial of squatting in the second stage of labour. Lancet 2:74, 1989

Hoyte L, Jakab M, Warfield SK, et al: Levator ani thickness variation in symptomatic and asymptomatic women using magnetic resonance-based 3-dimensional color mapping. Am J Obstet Gynecol 191:856, 2004

Koff AK: Development of the vagina in the human fetus. Contrib Embryol 24:59, 1933

Krantz KE: Innervation of the human vulva and vagina. Obstet Gynecol 13:382, 1958

Langlois PL: The size of the normal uterus. J Reprod Med 4:220, 1970

Larsen B, Galask RP: Vaginal microbial flora: Practical and theoretic relevance. Obstet Gynecol 55:100S, 1980

McGregor JA, French JI: Bacterial vaginosis in pregnancy. Obstet Gynecol Surv 55:S1, 2000

Moore KL, Persaud TVN, Shiota K: Color Atlas of Clinical Embryology, 2nd ed. Philadelphia, Saunders, 2000

Nelson JH: Atlas of Radical Pelvic Surgery, 2nd ed. New York, Appleton, 1977, p 133

Okkels H, Engle ET: Studies on the finer structure of the uterine blood vessels of the macacus monkey. Acta Pathol Microbiol Scand 15:150, 1938

Orsini LF, Salardi S, Pilu G, et al: Pelvic organs in premenarcheal girls: Real-time ultrasonography. Radiology 153:113, 1984

Russell JGB: Moulding of the pelvic outlet. J Obstet Gynaecol Br Commonw 76:817, 1969

Russell JGB: The rationale of primitive delivery positions. Br J Obstet Gynaecol 89:712, 1982

Schwalm H, Dubrauszky V: The structure of the musculature of the human uterus—muscles and connective tissue. Am J Obstet Gynecol 94:391, 1966

Spalteholz: Hand Atlas of Human Anatomy, Vol 1. Philadelphia, Lippincott, 1933

Tunn R, Delancey JO, Howard D, et al: Anatomic variations in the levator ani muscle, endopelvic fascia, and urethra in nulliparas evaluated by magnetic resonance imaging. Am J Obstet Gynecol 188:116, 2003

Umek WH, Morgan DM, Ashton-Miller JA, DeLancey JOL: Quantitative analysis of uterosacral ligament origin and insertion points by magnetic resonance imaging. Obstet Gynecol 103:447, 2004

Wicke L: Atlas of Radiologic Anatomy, 3rd ed. Baltimore, Urban and Schwarzenberg, 1982

3

Implantation, Embryogenesis, and Placental Development

All obstetricians should be aware of the basic reproductive biological processes that are required for women to successfully achieve ovulation, fertilization, and implantation. A number of abnormalities can affect each of these processes and lead to infertility or pregnancy loss. In most women, spontaneous, cyclical ovulation at 25- to 35-day intervals continues throughout almost 40 years between the time of menarche and menopause. For women who never use contraception, there are approximately 400 opportunities for pregnancy, which may occur with sexual intercourse on any of 1200 days (the day of ovulation and the 2 preceding days). This narrow window available for fertilization is controlled by tightly regulated production of ovarian steroids that cause the optimal regeneration of endometrium that begins with the ending of menstruation.

Should fertilization occur, the events that unfold after the initial implantation of the blastocyst onto the surface of the endometrium through to parturition result from a unique interaction between the trophoblasts of the fetus and the endometrium–decidua of the mother. The ability of mother and fetus to coexist as two distinct immunological systems results from endocrine, paracrine, and immunological modification of fetal and maternal tissues in a manner not seen elsewhere. The placenta mediates a unique fetal–maternal communication system, which creates a hormonal environment that helps initially to maintain pregnancy and eventually initiates the events leading to parturition. The following sections address the physiology of the ovarian–endometrial cycle, implantation, the placenta and fetal membranes, and the specialized endocrine arrangements between fetus and mother.

THE OVARIAN–ENDOMETRIAL CYCLE

The endometrium–decidua is the anatomical site of blastocyst apposition, implantation, and placental development. From an evolutionary perspective, the human endometrium is highly developed to accommodate interstitial implantation and a hemochorial type of placentation. Endometrial development of a magnitude similar to that observed in women—that is, with special spiral (or coiling) arteries—is restricted to only a few primates, such as humans, great apes, and Old World monkeys. Trophoblasts of the blastocyst invade these endometrial arteries during implantation and placentation to establish uteroplacental vessels.

These primates are the only mammals that menstruate, which is a process of endometrial tissue shedding with hemorrhage that is dependent on sex steroid hormone–directed changes in blood flow in the spiral arteries. With nonfertile, but ovulatory, ovarian cycles, menstruation effects desquamation of the endometrium. New endometrial growth and development must be initiated with each cycle, so that endometrial maturation corresponds rather precisely with the next pregnancy (implantation) opportunity. There seems to

be a very narrow window of endometrial receptivity to blastocyst implantation in the human that corresponds approximately to menstrual cycle days 20 to 24.

To place repetitive menstruation in perspective, the lifetime cumulative blood loss associated with normal endometrial shedding is 10 to 20 liters or more, an amount of blood that contains at least three times the total body iron content of the average adult woman. The approximately 38-year reproductive lifetime cumulative production of progesterone by corpora lutea and placenta in the woman who has two pregnancies and 450 nonfertile ovarian cycles is about 150,000 mg (150 g), which is similar to the cumulative amount of cortisol secreted by the adrenal cortices during the same 38 years. This incredible investment in endometrial tissue growth provides for regular renewal of the functional portion of this tissue in preparation for the next pregnancy opportunity.

THE OVARIAN CYCLE. The development of predictable, regular, cyclical, and spontaneous ovulatory menstrual cycles is regulated by complex interactions of the hypothalamic–pituitary axis, the ovaries, and the genital tract (Fig. 3–1). The average duration of the cycle in women of reproductive age is approximately 28 days, with a range of 25 to 32 days. The sequence of hormonal events leading to ovulation dictates the menstrual cycle. The cyclical changes in endometrial histology are faithfully reproduced during each ovulatory ovarian cycle.

In 1937, Rock and Bartlett suggested that the histological features of the endometrium were sufficiently characteristic to permit "dating" of the ovarian cycle of the woman from whom the endometrial tissue was obtained. The histological changes that occur in the endometrium during the nonfertile (but ovulatory) menstrual cycle are summarized in Figure 3–2. The follicular (proliferative) phase and the postovulatory (luteal or secretory) phase of the ovarian–endometrial cycle are customarily divided into early and late stages.

Follicular (Preovulatory) Ovarian Phase. In the human ovary, 2 million oocytes are found at birth, and about 400,000 follicles are present at the onset of puberty (Baker, 1963). The remaining follicles are depleted at a rate of approximately 1000 follicles per month until 35 years of age, when this rate accelerates (Faddy and colleagues, 1992). Only 400 follicles are normally ovulated during female reproductive life. Therefore, more than 99.9 percent of follicles undergo the degenerative process known as atresia through a process of cell death termed *apoptosis* (Gougeon, 1996; Hsueh and colleagues, 1994; Kaipia and Hsueh, 1997). Human follicular development consists of several stages, which include the gonadotropin-independent recruitment of primordial follicles from the resting pool and growth of these follicles to the antral stage. This process appears to be under the control of locally produced growth factors. The production of two members of the transforming growth factor-β family, viz., growth differentiation factors 9 and 10, regulates the proliferation and

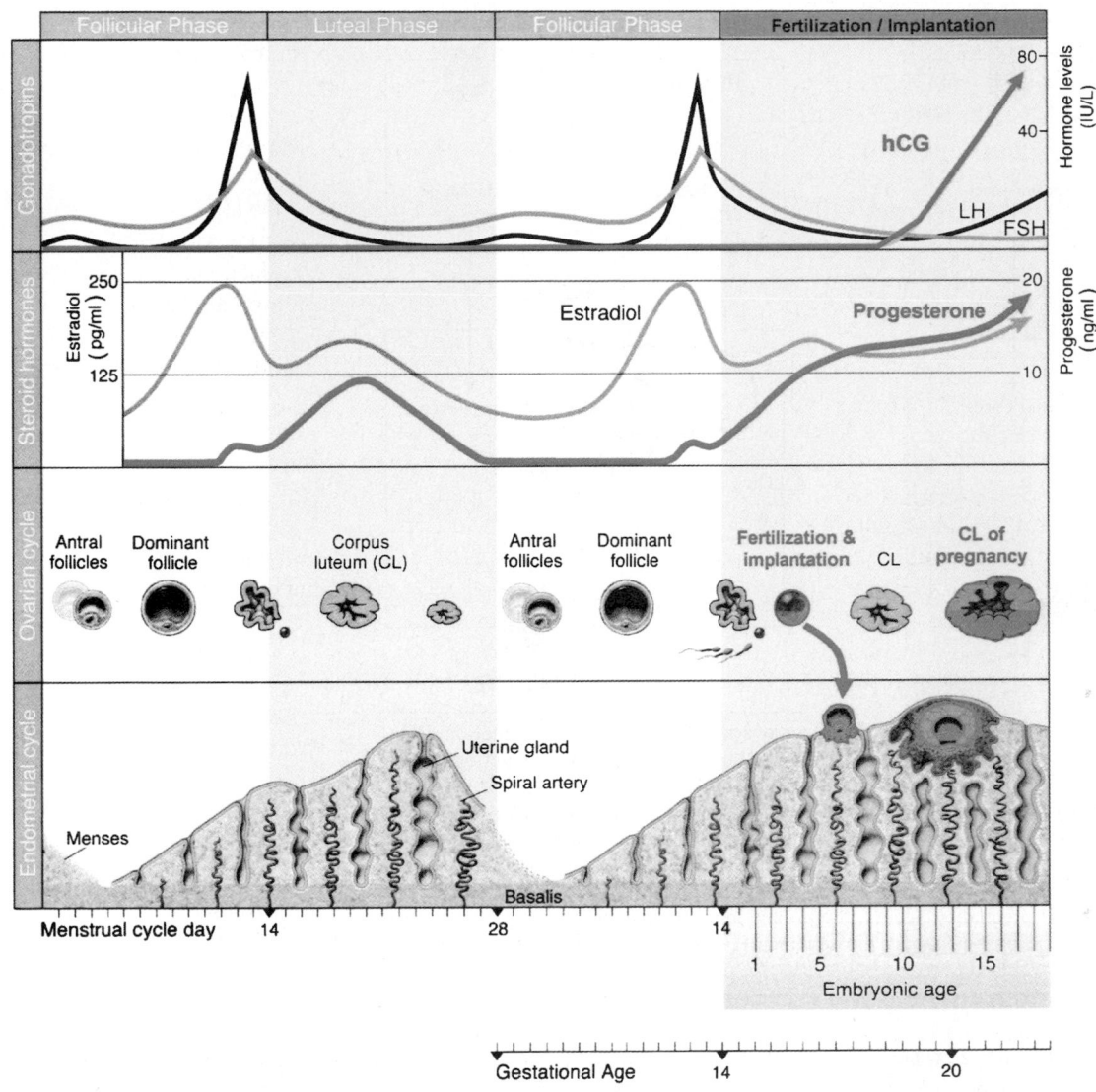

FIGURE 3–1. Gonadotropin control of the ovarian and endometrial cycles. The ovarian–endometrial cycle has been structured as a 28-day cycle. The follicular phase (days 1 to 14) is characterized by rising levels of estrogen, thickening of the endometrium, and selection of the dominant "ovulatory" follicle. During the luteal phase (days 14 to 28), the corpus luteum produces estrogen and progesterone, which prepare the endometrium for implantation. If implantation occurs, the developing blastocysts will begin to produce human chorionic gonadotropin (hCG) and rescue the corpus luteum, thus maintaining progesterone production. (FSH = follicle-stimulating hormone; LH = luteinizing hormone.)

differentiation of the granulosa cells as the primary follicles grow (Aaltonen and colleagues, 1999; Hreinsson and colleagues, 2002). These factors are produced by the oocytes, suggesting that the early steps in follicular development are in part oocyte controlled. As the antral follicles develop, the surrounding stromal cells are recruited in a yet-to-be-defined mechanism to become thecal cells.

Although not required for early stages of follicular development, follicle-stimulating hormone (FSH) is required for further development of large antral follicles (Hillier, 2001). During each ovarian cycle, a group of antral follicles, known as a *cohort,* begins a phase of semisynchronous growth as

a result of their state of maturation at the time of the FSH rise during the late luteal phase of the previous cycle. This FSH rise leading to the development of follicles is called the *selection window* of the ovarian cycle (Macklon and Fauser, 2001). Only the follicles progressing to this stage develop the capacity to produce estrogen.

During the follicular phase, estrogen levels rise in parallel to the growth of the dominant follicle and the increase in its number of granulosa cells (see Fig. 3–1). The granulosa cells are the exclusive site of FSH receptor expression. The increase in circulating FSH during the late luteal phase of the previous cycle stimulates an increase in FSH receptors and,

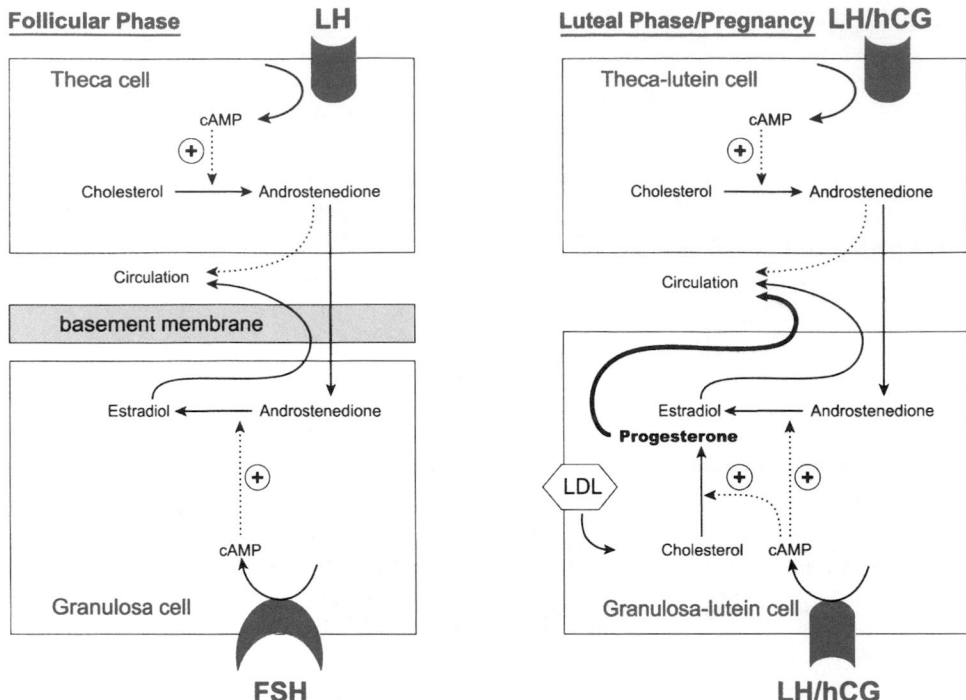

FIGURE 3–2. The two-cell–two-gonadotropin principle of ovarian steroid hormone production. During the follicular phase (*left panel*), luteinizing hormone (LH) controls theca cell production of androstenedione, which diffuses into the adjacent granulosa cells and acts as precursor for estradiol biosynthesis. The capacity for the granulosa cell to convert androstenedione to estradiol is controlled by follicle-stimulating hormone (FSH). After ovulation, the corpus luteum forms and both theca-lutein and granulosa-lutein cells respond to LH. The theca-lutein cells continue to produce androstenedione, while granulosa-lutein cells greatly increase the capacity to produce progesterone as well as to convert androstenedione to estradiol. If pregnancy occurs, the production of human chorionic gonadotropin (hCG) by the placenta rescues the corpus luteum through the LH receptor. (cAMP = cyclic adenosine monophosphate.)

subsequently, the ability to aromatize thecal cell–derived androstenedione into estradiol. The requirement for thecal cells that respond to luteinizing hormone (LH) and granulosa cells that respond to FSH represents the *two-gonadotropin, two-cell hypothesis* for estrogen biosynthesis described by Short (1962) and shown in Figure 3–2. FSH induces the enzyme aromatase and expansion of the antrum of the growing follicles. The follicle within the cohort that is most responsive to FSH is likely to be the first to produce estradiol and initiate expression of LH receptors.

After the appearance of LH receptors, the preovulatory granulosa cells begin to secrete small quantities of progesterone. The preovulatory secretion of progesterone, although somewhat limited, is believed to exert positive feedback on the estrogen-primed pituitary to either cause or help augment release of LH. In addition, during the late follicular phase, LH stimulates thecal cell production of androgens, particularly androstenedione, which are then transferred to the adjacent follicles where they are metabolized to estradiol. During the early follicular phase, the granulosa cells also produce inhibin B, which can feed back on the pituitary to inhibit FSH release (Groome and colleagues, 1996). As the

dominant follicle begins to grow, the production of estradiol and the inhibins increases, resulting in a decline of follicular-phase FSH. This drop in FSH is responsible for the failure of other follicles to reach preovulatory status—*the Graafian follicle stage*—during any one cycle. Thus, 95 percent of plasma estradiol produced at this time is secreted by the dominant follicle, which is destined to ovulate. The contralateral ovary is relatively inactive.

Ovulation. The onset of the gonadotropin surge resulting from increasing secretion of estrogen by preovulatory follicles is a relatively precise predictor of the time of ovulation, occurring some 34 to 36 hours before the release of the ovum from the follicle (see Fig. 3–1). The peak of LH secretion occurs 10 to 12 hours before ovulation and stimulates the resumption of the meiosis process in the ovum with the release of the first polar body. At this time a protrusion of the follicular wall (the stigma) develops, which then ruptures, allowing release of the oocyte–cumulus complex. It has long been suggested that the actual rupture of the follicle is controlled by the plasminogen activator group of proteases (Beers, 1975). Current studies suggest that in response to LH, increased production of progesterone and prostaglandins activates members of both the plasminogen activator and matrix metalloproteinases. Activation of these proteases is likely to play a pivotal role in the weakening of the follicular basement membrane and ovulation (Ny and colleagues, 2002).

Luteal (Postovulatory) Phase of the Ovary. Following ovulation, the corpus luteum develops from the remains of the dominant or *Graafian follicle* in a process referred to as *luteinization.* Rupture of the follicle initiates a series of morphological and chemical changes leading to transformation into the corpus luteum (Browning, 1973). The basement membrane separating the granulosa-lutein and theca-lutein cells breaks down, and by day 2 postovulation, blood vessels and capillaries invade the granulosa cell layer. The rapid neovascularization of the once avascular granulosa may be due to a variety of angiogenic factors. These include vascular endothelial growth factor and others produced in response to LH by the theca-lutein and granulosa-lutein cells (Albrecht and Pepe, 2003; Fraser and Wulff, 2001). During luteinization, these cells undergo hypertrophy and increase their capacity to synthesize hormones (see Figs. 3–1 and 3–2).

That LH is the primary luteotropic factor was well established in studies of hypophysectomized women (Vande Wiele and colleagues, 1970). In these women, the life span of the corpus luteum is dependent on repeated injections of LH or human chorionic gonadotropin (hCG). In addition, LH injections can extend the life span of the corpus luteum in normal women by 2 weeks (Segaloff and colleagues, 1951). In normal cycling women, the corpus luteum is maintained by low-frequency, high-amplitude pulses of LH secreted by gonadotropes in the anterior pituitary (Filicori and colleagues, 1986).

The pattern of hormone secretion by the corpus luteum is different from that of the follicle (see Fig. 3–1). The increased capacity of the granulosa-lutein cells to produce progesterone is the result of increased access to considerably more steroidogenic precursors through blood-borne low-density lipoprotein (LDL)–derived cholesterol (Carr and colleagues, 1981b). It is due as well to changes in the level of steroidogenic acute regulatory protein, which allows rapid use of this cholesterol for progesterone biosynthesis (Devoto and colleagues, 2002). The important role for LDL in progesterone biosynthesis is supported by the observation that women with extremely low levels of LDL cholesterol exhibit low progesterone secretion during the luteal phase (Illingworth and colleagues, 1982). In addition, high-density lipoprotein (HDL) may contribute to progesterone production in granulosa-lutein cells (Ragoobir and colleagues, 2002).

Estrogen levels follow a more complex pattern of secretion. Specifically, just after ovulation, estrogen levels decrease followed by a secondary rise that reaches a peak production of 0.25 mg/day of 17β-estradiol at the midluteal phase. Toward the end of the luteal phase there is a secondary decrease in estradiol production. Ovarian production of progesterone peaks at 25 to 50 mg/day during the midluteal phase. If pregnancy occurs, the corpus luteum continues production of progesterone in response to embryonic hCG, which will bind and activate luteal cell LH receptors (see Fig. 3–2).

The human corpus luteum is a transient endocrine organ that, in the absence of pregnancy, will rapidly regress 9 to 11 days after ovulation. The mechanisms that control luteolysis of the human corpus luteum remain unclear. In part luteolysis results from the combination of decreased levels of circulating LH in the late luteal phase and decreased LH sensitivity of luteal cells (Duncan and colleagues, 1996; Filicori and colleagues, 1986). The role of other luteotropic factors in women is less clear, however, prostaglandin $F_{2\alpha}$ ($PGF_{2\alpha}$) appears to be luteolytic in nonhuman primates as well as in women (Auletta, 1987; Wentz and Jones, 1973). Within the corpus luteum, luteolysis is characterized by a loss of luteal cells due to an increase in apoptotic cell death (Vaskivuo and colleagues, 2002). The endocrine effects, consisting of a dramatic drop in circulating levels of estradiol and progesterone, are critical to allow the follicular development and ovulation of the next ovarian cycle. In addition, the regression of the corpus luteum and drop in circulating steroids signal the endometrium to initiate the molecular events that will lead to menstruation.

ESTROGEN AND PROGESTERONE ACTION. The fluctuating levels of ovarian steroids are the direct cause of the endometrial cycle. Recent advances in the molecular biology of receptors for estrogen and progesterone have greatly improved our understanding of how sex steroids regulate the endometrium. 17β-Estradiol, the most biologically potent naturally occurring estrogen, is secreted by the granulosa cells of the dominant ovarian follicle and luteinized granulosa cells of the corpus luteum (see Figs. 3–1 and 3–2). Estrogen is the essential hormonal signal on which most events in the normal menstrual cycle depend. Estradiol action is complex and appears to involve two classical nuclear hormone receptors, which have been designated estrogen receptor α (ERα) and estrogen receptor β (ERβ) (Katzenellenbogen and colleagues, 2001). These isoforms are the product of separate genes and can exhibit distinct tissue differences in relative expression. Both estradiol-receptor complexes act as transcriptional factors that become associated with the estrogen response element of specific genes. Both share a robust activation by estradiol, but there are differences in the binding of other estrogens, making these receptors targets for selective estrogen receptor modulators.

The interaction with steroid ligands brings about estrogen receptor–specific initiation of gene transcription, which promotes the synthesis of specific messenger RNAs, and thereafter the synthesis of specific proteins. Among the many proteins synthesized in most estrogen-responsive cells are additional estrogen receptors and progesterone receptors. In addition, estradiol has been proposed to act at the cell surface to stimulate nitric oxide production in endothelial cells, leading to the rapid vasoactive properties of estradiol (Shaul, 2002). The ability of estradiol to work in the cell nucleus through classical ligand-regulated nuclear hormone receptors and at the cell surface to cause rapid changes in cell signaling molecules is one explanation for the complex responses seen as a result of estrogen therapies.

It is likely that estradiol and other bioactive estrogens cause replication of the endometrium indirectly (through actions on stromal cells). The expression pattern of ERα and ERβ in the various cellular components of the endometrium has been examined using immunohistochemistry (Lecce and colleagues, 2001). ERβ is expressed in glands, stroma, and vascular cells of the endometrium. ERβ levels are highest during the proliferative phase of the cycle. With the development and widespread use of selective estrogen receptor modulators, the differential expression and roles of the two isoforms of estrogen receptor within the endometrium will need careful study.

The majority of effects of progesterone on the female reproductive tract are mediated through nuclear hormone receptors. Progesterone enters cells by diffusion and in responsive tissues becomes associated with progesterone receptors (Conneely and colleagues, 2002). There are two distinct isoforms of the human progesterone receptor, viz., the progesterone receptor type A (PR-A) and type B (PR-B). Both arise from a single gene, are members of the steroid receptor superfamily of transcription factors, and regulate transcription of target genes. These receptors may have unique actions within cells. When the PR-A and PR-B receptors are co-expressed, it appears that the PR-A can act as an inhibitor of PR-B gene regulation. The repressor effect of PR-A may extend to actions on other steroid receptors, including estrogen receptors. In addition, progesterone may act by receptor-independent nongenomic mechanisms. Membrane receptors for progesterone have been best characterized in human spermatozoa, but their role in other human tissues is not currently clear (Luconi and colleagues, 2002).

The expression patterns of PR-A and PR-B receptors in the human endometrium have been examined using immunohistochemistry (Mote and colleagues, 1999). The endometrial glands and stroma appear to have different expression patterns for PR-A and PR-B, which vary over the menstrual cycle. The glands express both receptors in the proliferative phase, suggesting that both receptors are involved with subnuclear vacuole formation. After ovulation the glands continue to express PR-B through the midluteal phase, suggesting that glandular secretion seen during the luteal phase is PR-B regulated. In contrast, the stroma and predecidual cells express only PR-A throughout the menstrual cycle, suggesting that progesterone-stimulated events within the stroma are mediated by this receptor. Progesterone receptor expression has not been observed in inflammatory cells or in endothelial cells of the endometrial vessels. Dissecting the role of these two receptor isoforms in the regulation of human menstruation may be difficult, however, studies in animal models have given evidence that the PR-A receptor regulates the antiproliferative effects of progesterone seen in the secretory phase. Specifically, ablation of PR-A expression in mice blocks decidualization and implantation. These observations imply that the two progesterone receptor isoforms play distinct roles in the endometrium during the menstrual cycle. In addition, distinct roles for PR-A and PR-B have been proposed for the regulation of the myometrium during the initiation of labor (Mesiano and colleagues, 2002).

THE ENDOMETRIAL CYCLE

Proliferative (Preovulatory) Phase of the Endometrium. Fluctuations in estrogen and progesterone levels produce striking effects on the reproductive tract, particularly the endometrium (Fig. 3–3). Characteristic changes occur in the endometrium during the menstrual cycle, which makes dating of the endometrium possible (Rock and Bartlett, 1937). The growth and functional characteristics of the human endometrium are unique. The epithelial (glandular) cells, the stromal (mesenchymal) cells, and the blood vessels of the endometrium replicate cyclically in reproductive-aged women at a rapid rate. The endometrium is regenerated during each ovarian–endometrial cycle. The superficial endometrium is shed and regenerated almost 400 times during the reproductive lifetime of most women. There is no other example in humans of the cyclical shedding and regrowth of an entire tissue.

Follicular-phase production of estradiol is the most important factor in recovery of the endometrium following menstruation. About two thirds of the functional endometrium is fragmented and shed during menstruation; but reepithelialization is in progress even before menstrual bleeding has ceased. By the fifth day of the endometrial cycle (first day of menses equals day 1), the epithelial surface of the endometrium has been restored and revascularization of the endometrium is in progress. The preovulatory endometrium is characterized by proliferation of vascular endothelial, stromal, and glandular cells (see Fig. 3–3). During the early part of the proliferative phase, the endometrium is thin, usually less than 2 mm in thickness. The glands at this stage are narrow, tubular structures that pursue almost a straight and parallel course from the basal layer toward the surface of the endometrial cavity. Mitotic figures, especially in the glandular epithelium, are identified by the fifth cycle day, and mitotic activity in both epithelium and stroma persists until day 16 to 17 (2 to 3 days after ovulation). Although blood vessels are numerous and prominent, there is no extravascular blood or leukocyte infiltration in the endometrium at this stage.

Clearly, reepithelialization and angiogenesis are important to the cessation of endometrial bleeding at the end of menstruation, and these processes are dependent on tissue regrowth. Estradiol appears to act by inducing growth factor gene expression in stromal cells. Stromal cell proliferation appears to increase through paracrine and autocrine action of estrogen and increased local levels of fibroblast growth

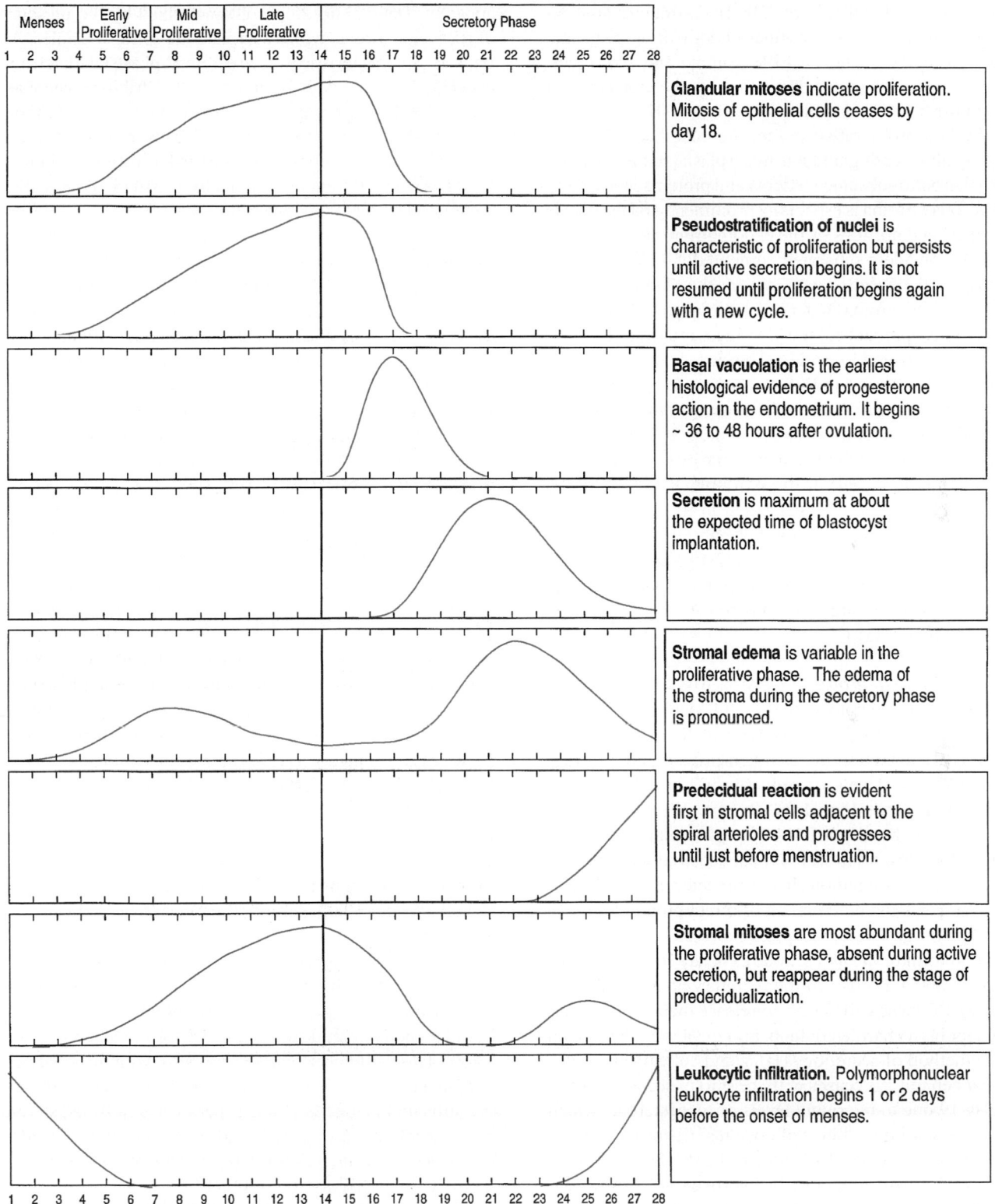

FIGURE 3–3. Dating of the endometrium according to the day of the menstrual cycle during a hypothetical 28-day ovarian cycle. Correlation with the extent of typical morphological findings. (From Noyes and colleagues, 1950.)

factor-9 (Tsai and colleagues, 2002). Estrogens also increase local production of vascular endothelial growth factor (Bausero and colleagues, 1998; Sugino and colleagues, 2002), which causes angiogenesis through the elongation of vessels in the basalis (Gargett and Rogers, 2001).

By the late proliferative phase, the endometrium thickens, the result of both glandular hyperplasia and an increase in stromal ground substance (edema and proteinaceous material). The loose stroma is especially prominent, and the glands in the superficial portions of the endometrium (the functionalis layer) are widely separated compared with those of the deeper zone (the basalis layer), where the glands are more crowded and the stroma is denser. At midcycle, as the time of ovulation is approached, the glandular epithelium has become taller and pseudostratified. The surface epithelial cells acquire numerous microvilli, which increase epithelial surface area, and cilia, which aid in the movement of endometrial secretions in the secretory phase (Ferenczy, 1976).

Day-by-day dating of the endometrium by histological criteria is difficult during the proliferative phase because of the considerable variation among women in the length of this phase of the cycle. In apparently normal, fertile women the follicular phase may be as short as 5 to 7 days or as long as 21 to 30 days. However, the luteal or secretory (postovulatory) phase of the cycle among women is remarkably constant in duration (12 to 14 days).

Secretory (Postovulatory) Phase of the Endometrium.

During the early secretory phase, the dating of the endometrium is based on the histology of the glandular epithelium. After ovulation the estrogen-primed endometrium responds to rising levels of progesterone in a highly predictable manner (see Fig. 3–3). By day 17, glycogen accumulates in the basal portion of the glandular epithelium, creating subnuclear vacuoles and pseudostratification. This is the first sign of ovulation that is reflected in histological changes, and it is likely the result of direct progesterone action through progesterone receptors expressed in the glandular cells (Mote and colleagues, 2000). On day 18, the vacuoles move to the apical portion of the secretory nonciliated cells, and by day 19, these cells begin to release their glycoprotein and mucopolysaccharide contents into the lumen through an apocrine method of secretion (Hafez and colleagues, 1975). Glandular cell mitosis ceases with the start of secretory activity on day 19 due to the rising levels of progesterone, which antagonize the mitotic effects of estrogen. Estradiol action is also decreased because of glandular expression of the type 2 form of 17β-hydroxysteroid dehydrogenase, which converts estradiol to the less active estrogen, estrone (Casey and MacDonald, 1996).

The dating of the cycle in the mid- to late-secretory phase relies on changes seen in the endometrial stroma (see Fig. 3–3). On cycle days 21 to 24, the stroma becomes edematous. On days 22 to 25, stromal cells surrounding the spiral arterioles begin to enlarge, and stromal mitosis becomes apparent. Days 23 to 28 are characterized by the presence of predecidual cells, which surround the spiral arterioles. An important characteristic of the secretory-phase endometrium occurring between days 22 and 25 is the striking change associated with the predecidual transformation of the upper two thirds of the functionalis layer. The glands exhibit extensive coiling and secretions become visible within the lumen. Changes within the endometrium also can mark the so-called window of implantation seen on days 20 to 24. Close examination of the surface epithelial cells during this time has shown a decrease in microvilli and cilia on cell surfaces as well as protrusions of the apical cell surface into the lumen (Nikas, 2003). These protrusions, termed *pinopods,* are an important event in preparation for blastocyst implantation and coincide with changes in the surface glycocalyx that allow acceptance of a blastocyst (Aplin, 2003).

In addition, this secretory phase is highlighted by the continuing growth and development of the spiral arteries. Boyd and Hamilton (1970) emphasized the extraordinary importance of the spiraling or coiled arteries of the human endometrium, pointing out that the British gynecologist William Hunter in 1774 referred to these vessels as the "curling" arteries. The endometrial spiral arteries arise from the arcuate arteries, which are branches of the uterine vessels that lie in the myometrium (see Fig. 2–9; p. 23). The morphological and functional properties of the spiral arteries are unique and essential for establishing the changes in blood flow that permit menstruation or, should fertilization occur, implantation. During the phase of endometrial growth, the spiral arteries lengthen at a rate that is appreciably greater than the rate of increase in endometrial tissue height or thickness (Fig. 3–4). This discordance in growth between the two tissues obliges even greater coiling of the already spiraling vessels. The development of the spiral arteries represents an extraordinary induction of angiogenesis, consisting of widespread sprouting and extension of blood vessels. Perrot-Applanat and associates (1988) described progesterone and estrogen receptors in the smooth muscle cells of the uterine arteries, including the spiral arteries. These investigators further demonstrated that this rapid angiogenesis is regulated in part through estrogen- and progesterone-regulated synthesis of vascular endothelial growth factor (Ancelin and colleagues, 2002). This protein is secreted by cells within the stroma and glandular epithelium and stimulates endothelial cell proliferation and increases vascular permeability. Thus, steroid hormone influences on growth and vasculature are directed to a large degree through the local production of growth factors.

MENSTRUATION. In the catarrhine primates, the midluteal–secretory phase of the endometrial cycle is a critical branch point in the development and differentiation of the endometrium. With rescue of the corpus luteum and continued progesterone secretion, the process of decidualization continues. If, however, the corpus luteum production of progesterone drops as a result of *luteolysis,* the events

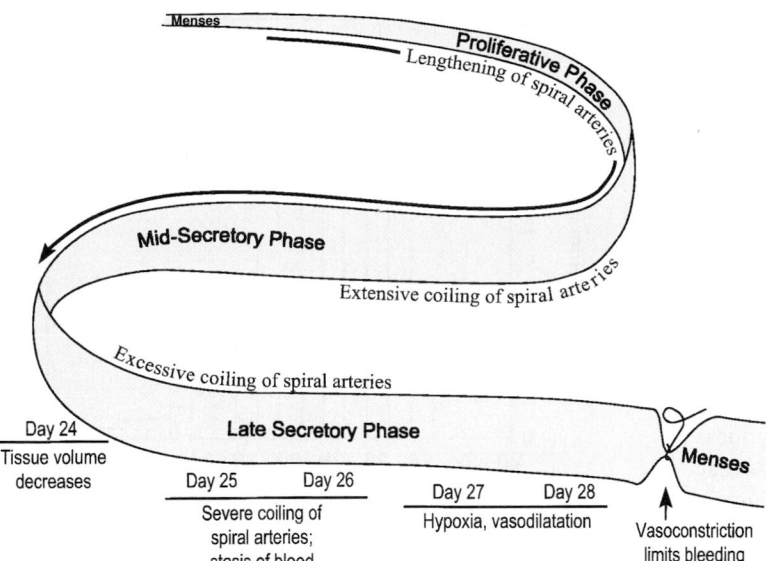

FIGURE 3–4. Modifications in the spiral arteries of the human endometrium during the ovulatory cycle. Changes in blood flow through these vessels facilitate endometrial growth (blue band). Excessive coiling and stasis in blood flow coincides with regression of corpus luteum function, and leads to a decline in endometrial tissue volume. Just prior to the commencement of endometrial bleeding, intense spiral artery vasospasm serves to limit blood loss with menstruation.

leading to menstruation will be initiated. Many of the molecular mechanisms involving endometrial progesterone withdrawal, as well as the subsequent inflammatory response that causes the sloughing of the endometrium, have been defined (Critchley and colleagues, 2001).

A notable histological characteristic of the late premenstrual-phase endometrium is the infiltration of the stroma by polymorphonuclear leukocytes, giving a pseudoinflammatory appearance to the tissue (see Fig. 3–3). The infiltration of neutrophils occurs primarily on the day or two immediately preceding the onset of menstruation. The endometrial stromal and epithelial cells produce interleukin-8 (IL-8), a chemotactic–activating factor for neutrophils (Arici and colleagues, 1993). IL-8 may be one of the agents that serve to recruit neutrophils to the endometrium just prior to the onset of menstruation. Similarly, the endometrium is capable of synthesizing monocyte chemotactic protein-1 (MCP-1), a potent chemoattractant for monocytes (Arici and colleagues, 1995). The rates of synthesis of IL-8 and MCP-1 in endometrial stromal cells appear to be modulated, in part, by circulating sex steroid hormones and local production of transforming growth factor-β (Arici and colleagues, 1996a, 1996b).

The infiltration of leukocytes is considered key to initiation of extracellular matrix breakdown of the functionalis layer. The invading leukocytes secrete enzymes that are members of the matrix metalloproteinase family of proteins. These metalloproteinases add to the proteases already produced by the endometrial stromal cells. The rising level of metalloproteinases tips the balance between proteases and protease inhibitors, effectively initiating degradation of the matrix. This phenomenon has been proposed to initiate the events leading to menstruation (Dong and colleagues, 2002).

A classical study by Markee (1940) described the tissue and vascular changes that occur in endometrium before menstruation. He observed 432 separate cyclical alterations in endometrial tissue explants that he had transplanted to the anterior chamber of the eye of rhesus monkeys. There were marked changes in blood flow to the endometrium during the time of growth regression, which are essential for menstruation. As the regression of the endometrium occurs, the coiling of the spiral arteries becomes sufficiently severe that the resistance to blood flow in these vessels is increased strikingly, causing hypoxia of the endometrium. The resultant stasis is the primary cause of endometrial ischemia and then tissue degeneration. A period of vasoconstriction precedes the onset of menstruation and is the most striking and constant event observed in the menstrual cycle. The intense vasoconstriction of the spiral arteries serves to limit blood loss during menstruation. Blood flow in the spiral arteries appears to be regulated in an endocrine manner by sex steroid hormone–induced modifications of a local (paracrine-mediated) vasoactive peptide system.

Prostaglandins and Menstruation. Prostaglandins are most often synthesized within the same tissue in which they act through autocrine or paracrine mechanisms, or both. Prostaglandins act through a host of separate but specific plasma membrane G-protein–linked receptors that can activate diverse cellular signaling cascades and thus provide an additional level of specificity to the various prostaglandins. Prostaglandins can be degraded rapidly in the tissues of origin, for example, endometrium, in nearby tissues, or in more remote sites such as the lungs in a reaction catalyzed by prostaglandin dehydrogenase (Casey and colleagues, 1980, 1989).

A role for prostaglandins, especially prostaglandin $F_{2\alpha}$ ($PGF_{2\alpha}$), which is a vasoconstrictor, in the initiation of menstruation has been suggested (Abel, 2002). Large amounts of prostaglandins are present in menstrual blood. The administration of $PGF_{2\alpha}$ to women gives rise to symptoms that mimic dysmenorrhea, which is commonly associated with normal menses and likely is caused by myometrial contractions and uterine ischemia. The administration of $PGF_{2\alpha}$ to nonpregnant women also will cause menstruation. This response is believed to be mediated by $PGF_{2\alpha}$-induced vasoconstriction of the endometrial spiral arteries.

Vasoactive Peptides and Menstruation. The actions of a number of peptides may comprise a hormone-responsive paracrine system in the endometrium to regulate spiral artery blood flow. One is the endothelin–enkephalinase system (Casey and MacDonald, 1996). The endothelins—ET-1, ET-2, and ET-3—are small, 21-amino acid peptides. Endothelin-1 (ET-1) is a potent vasoconstrictor that was first identified as a product of vascular endothelial cells (Yanagisawa and colleagues, 1988). The endothelins are degraded by the enzyme enkephalinase. Enkephalinase is localized in endometrial stromal cells, and its specific activity in these cells increases strikingly and in parallel with the increase in blood levels of progesterone after ovulation. The specific activity of enkephalinase in endometrium is highest during the midluteal phase of the ovarian cycle and declines steadily thereafter as the plasma levels of progesterone decrease with regression of the corpus luteum (Casey and colleagues, 1991).

Origin of Menstrual Blood. Menstrual bleeding is of both arterial and venous origin, but arterial bleeding is, quantitatively, appreciably greater than venous. Endometrial bleeding appears to begin by rupture of an arteriole of a coiled artery, with consequent formation of a hematoma. On occasion, however, bleeding takes place by leakage through a spiral artery. When a hematoma forms, the superficial endometrium is distended and then ruptures. Subsequently, fissures develop in the adjacent functionalis layers and blood, as well as fragments of tissue of various sizes, is detached. Although some tissue autolysis occurs, as a rule, fragments of endometrium can be identified in menstrual discharge collected from the vagina. Hemorrhage stops when the arterioles are again constricted. The changes that accompany partial tissue necrosis also serve to seal off the tips of the vessels. Often only the endothelium remains in the superficial portion.

The surface of the endometrium is restored, by growth of the flanges, or collars, that form the everted free ends of the uterine glands (Markee, 1940). These flanges increase in diameter very rapidly, and the continuity of the epithelium is reestablished by the fusion of the edges of these sheets of migrating thin cells.

Interval Between Menses. The modal interval at which menstruation recurs is considered to be 28 days, but there is considerable variation among women in general, as well as in the cycle lengths of a given woman. Marked variation in the intervals between menstrual cycles is not necessarily indicative of infertility. Arey (1939) analyzed the findings of

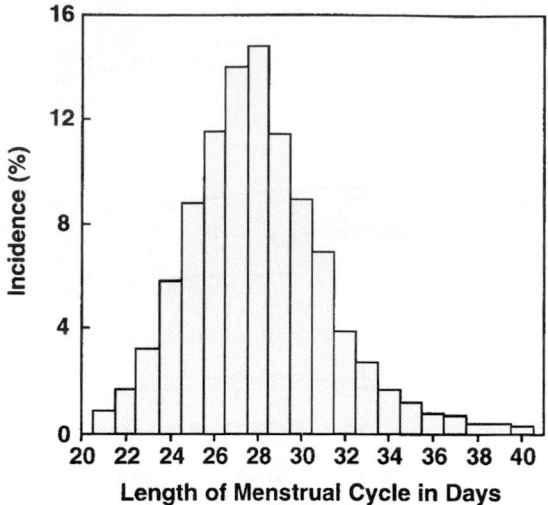

FIGURE 3–5. Duration of menstrual cycle. (Based on distribution data of Arey, 1939, and Haman, 1942.)

12 studies comprising about 20,000 calendar records from 1500 women and concluded that there is no evidence of perfect menstrual cycle regularity. He found that among average adult women, one third of menstrual cycles departed by more than 2 days from the mean of the lengths of all cycles. In Arey's analysis of 5322 cycles in 485 normal women, an average interval of 28.4 days was estimated; his finding for the average cycle length in pubertal girls was longer, 33.9 days. Haman (1942) surveyed 2460 cycles in 150 women who attended a clinic where special attention was directed to recording accurately the length of the menstrual cycles. The distribution curve for menstrual cycle length, computed from averages from both the Haman and Arey studies, is shown in Figure 3–5.

THE DECIDUA OF THE ENDOMETRIUM. The decidua is a specialized, highly modified endometrium of pregnancy and is a function of hemochorial placentation. This form of placentation has in common the process of trophoblast invasion, and therefore considerable research has focused on the interaction between the cells within the decidua and the invading trophoblasts. Decidualization, the transformation of secretory endometrium to decidua, is dependent on the action of estrogen and progesterone and factors secreted by the implanting blastocyst during trophoblast invasion. The special relationship that exists between the decidua and the invading trophoblast seemingly defies the laws of transplantation immunology (Beer and Billingham, 1971). The success of this unique semiallograft not only is of great scientific interest but may involve processes that harbor insights leading to more successful transplantation surgery and perhaps even immunological treatment of neoplasia (Billingham and Head, 1986; Lala and colleagues, 2002).

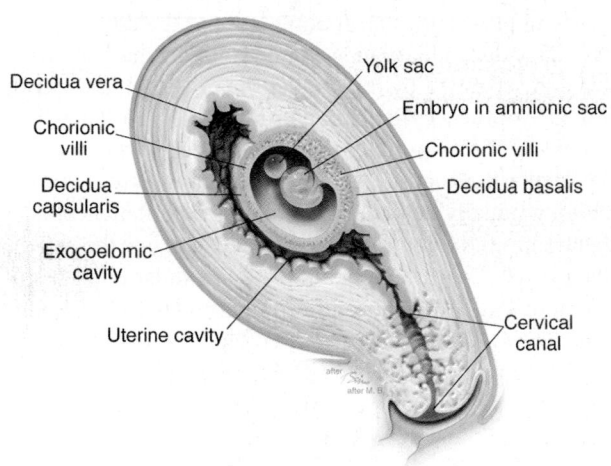

Decidua vera
Chorionic villi
Decidua capsularis
Exocoelomic cavity
Uterine cavity
Yolk sac
Embryo in amnionic sac
Chorionic villi
Decidua basalis
Cervical canal

FIGURE 3–6. Decidualized endometrium covers the early embryo. Three portions of the decidua (basalis, capsularis, and vera or parietalis) also are illustrated.

Decidual Structure. William Hunter, the 18th-century British gynecologist, provided the first scientific description of the *membrana decidua*. According to Damjanov (1985), the term *membrana* denoted its gross anatomical appearance, while *decidua* was added with analogy to deciduous leaves to indicate an ephemeral nature and the fact that it is shed from the rest of the uterus after childbirth. The decidua of pregnancy is composed of three parts based on its anatomical location. The portion of the decidua directly beneath the site of blastocyst implantation is modified by trophoblast invasion and becomes the *decidua basalis*. That portion overlying the enlarging blastocyst, and initially separating it from the rest of the uterine cavity, is the *decidua capsularis* (Fig. 3–6). The decidua capsularis is most prominent during the second month of pregnancy, consisting of decidual cells covered by a single layer of flattened epithelial cells without traces of glands. Internally, this portion of the decidua contacts the avascular, extraembryonic fetal membrane, the *chorion laeve*. The remainder of the uterus is lined by *decidua parietalis*, sometimes called the *decidua vera* at the point in development when decidua capsularis and decidua parietalis are joined.

During the early weeks of pregnancy, there is a space between the decidua capsularis and decidua parietalis because the gestational sac does not fill the entire uterine cavity. By 14 to 16 weeks, the expanding sac has enlarged enough to fill the uterine cavity. With fusion of the decidua capsularis and parietalis, the uterine cavity is functionally obliterated. In early pregnancy, the decidua begins to thicken, eventually attaining a depth of 5 to 10 mm. With magnification, furrows and numerous small openings, representing the mouths of uterine glands, can be detected. Later in pregnancy, as the fetus grows and the amnionic fluid expands, the thickness of the decidua decreases, presumably because of the pressure exerted by the expanding uterine contents.

The decidua parietalis and the decidua basalis, like the secretory endometrium, each are composed of three layers: a surface, or compact zone (zona compacta); a middle portion, or spongy zone (zona spongiosa), with remnants of glands and numerous small blood vessels; and a basal zone (zona basalis). The zona compacta and spongiosa together form the functional zone (zona functionalis). The basal zone remains after delivery and gives rise to new endometrium.

The Decidual Reaction. In human pregnancy, the decidual reaction is completed only with blastocyst implantation. Predecidual changes, however, commence first during the mid-luteal phase in endometrial stromal cells adjacent to the spiral arteries and arterioles, spreading thereafter in waves throughout the mucosa of the uterus and then from the site of implantation. The endometrial stromal cells enlarge to form polygonal or round decidual cells. The nuclei become round and vesicular, and the cytoplasm becomes clear, slightly basophilic, and surrounded by a translucent membrane. Each mature decidual cell becomes surrounded by a pericellular membrane. Thus, the human decidual cells clearly build walls around themselves and possibly around the fetus. The pericellular matrix surrounding the decidual cells may provide for attachment of cytotrophoblasts through cellular adhesion molecules. The pericellular decidual cell membrane also may provide for protection of the decidual cell against selected proteases of the cytotrophoblasts.

Decidual Blood Supply. This supply is changed as a consequence of implantation. The blood supply to the decidua capsularis is lost as the embryo-fetus grows and expands into the uterine cavity. The blood supply to the decidua parietalis through the spiral arteries persists, as in the endometrium during the luteal phase of the cycle. The spiral arteries in the decidua parietalis retain a smooth muscle wall and endothelium and thereby remain responsive to vasoactive agents that act on the smooth muscle or the endothelial cells of these vessels.

The spiral arterial system supplying the decidua basalis directly beneath the implanting blastocyst, and ultimately the intervillous space surrounding the syncytiotrophoblast of the placenta, is altered remarkably. These spiral arterioles and arteries are invaded by the cytotrophoblasts, and during this process the walls of the vessels in the basalis are destroyed, leaving only a shell without smooth muscle or endothelial cells. As a consequence, these vascular conduits of maternal blood—which become the uteroplacental vessels—are not responsive to vasoactive agents. By contrast, the fetal chorionic vessels, which transport blood between the placenta and the fetus, contain smooth muscle and do respond to vasoactive agents.

Decidual Histology. The decidua is composed of a variety of cell types, which varies with the stage of gestation (Loke and King, 1995). The primary cellular components of the decidua are the true decidual cells that differentiated from the endometrial stromal cells and numerous bone marrow–derived cells. The compact layer of the decidua consists of large, closely packed, epithelioid, polygonal, lightly staining cells with round nuclei. Many stromal cells appear stellate, with long protoplasmic processes that anastomose with those of adjacent cells. This is particularly so when the decidua is edematous. Numerous small round cells, which contain very little cytoplasm, are scattered among the decidual cells, especially in early pregnancy. Most of these are a particular type of natural killer lymphocyte and are referred to as *endometrial large granular lymphocytes (LGLs),* in which a special and unusual phenotype has been defined (Vince and Johnson, 2000). These are bone marrow-derived cells that at one time entered endometrium from peripheral blood. But thereafter, these large granular lymphocytes arise primarily by replication in the endometrium in situ at specific times in the menstrual cycle and during the first trimester.

Early in pregnancy, the spongy layer of the decidua consists of large distended glands, often exhibiting marked hyperplasia and separated by minimal stroma. At first, the glands are lined by typical cylindrical uterine epithelium. They have abundant secretory activity that contributes to the nourishment of the blastocyst. As pregnancy progresses, the epithelium gradually becomes cuboidal or even flattened, later degenerating and sloughing to a greater extent into the lumens of the glands. Later in pregnancy the glandular elements of the decidua largely disappear. In comparing the decidua parietalis at 16 weeks with the early proliferative endometrium of a nonpregnant woman, it is clear that there is marked hypertrophy but only slight hyperplasia of the endometrial stroma during decidual transformation.

The decidua basalis contributes to the formation of the basal plate of the placenta, and differs histologically from the decidua parietalis in two important respects (Fig. 3–7). First, the spongy zone of the decidua basalis consists mainly

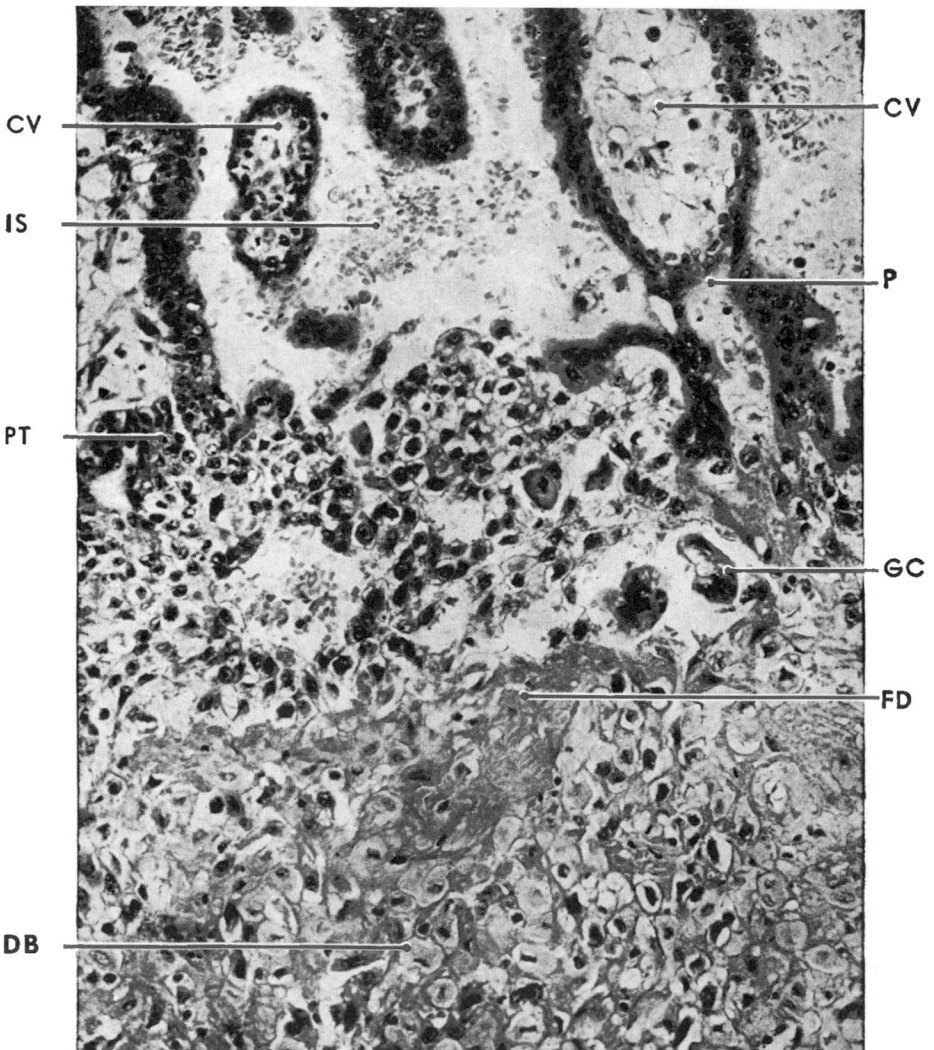

FIGURE 3–7. Section through junction of chorion and decidua basalis at fourth month of gestation. (CV = chorionic villi; DB = decidua basalis; FD = fibrinoid degeneration; GC = giant cell; IS = intervillous space containing maternal blood; P = fastening villus; PT = proliferating trophoblast.)

of arteries and widely dilated veins, but by term, the glands have virtually disappeared. Second, the decidua basalis is invaded by large numbers of interstitial trophoblast cells and trophoblastic giant cells. Although most abundant in the decidua, the giant cells commonly penetrate the upper myometrium. Their number and invasiveness may be so extensive as to be confused with choriocarcinoma by the inexperienced observer.

Where invading trophoblasts meet the decidua, there is a zone of fibrinoid degeneration, the *Nitabuch layer.* Whenever the decidua is defective, as in placenta accreta, the Nitabuch layer is usually absent (see Chap. 35, p. 830). There is also a more superficial, but inconsistent deposition of fibrin—*Rohr stria*—at the bottom of the intervillous space and surrounding the anchoring villi. McCombs and Craig (1964) found that decidual necrosis is a normal phenomenon in the first and probably the second trimester. Thus, necrotic decidua obtained through curettage after spontaneous abortion in the first trimester should not necessarily be interpreted as either a cause or an effect of the pregnancy loss.

Decidual Prolactin Production. Convincing evidence has been presented that the decidua is the source of the prolactin that is present in enormous amounts in amnionic fluid during human pregnancy (Golander and colleagues, 1978; Riddick and colleagues, 1979). Decidual prolactin is not to be confused with placental lactogen (hPL), which is produced only by the syncytiotrophoblast. Rather, decidual prolactin is a product of the same gene that encodes for prolactin that is secreted by the anterior pituitary, and the amino acid sequence of prolactin in both tissues is identical. In decidua, however, an alternative promoter is used within the prolactin gene to initiate transcription (Telgmann and Gellersen, 1998). This alternative prolactin promoter through novel transcription factors is thought to explain the different mechanisms that regulate expression in the decidua versus pituitary (Christian and colleagues, 2002a, 2000b).

The levels of prolactin in amnionic fluid may reach 10,000 ng/mL during the 20th to 24th weeks (Tyson and colleagues, 1972). This is extraordinarily high compared with the 350 ng/mL seen in the fetus or 150 to 200 ng/mL seen in maternal plasma. Prolactin produced in decidua preferentially enters amnionic fluid, and little or none enters maternal blood. This is a classical example of paracrine function between maternal and fetal tissues.

The factors that regulate prolactin production in decidua are not clearly defined. Most of the agents known to inhibit or stimulate anterior pituitary prolactin secretion, including dopamine, dopamine agonists, and thyrotropin-releasing hormone, do not alter the rate of decidual prolactin secretion either in vivo or in vitro. Brosens and colleagues (2000) demonstrated that progestins act synergistically with cyclic adenosine monophosphate on human endometrial stromal cells in culture to increase the expression of prolactin. These findings suggest that the level of progesterone receptor

expression may determine the decidualization process, as marked by prolactin production. It has been reported that arachidonic acid, but not $PGF_{2\alpha}$ or PGE_2, attenuates the rate of decidual prolactin secretion (Handwerger and colleagues, 1981). In addition, a variety of cytokines and growth factors, including ET-1, IL-1, IL-2, and epidermal growth factor, act to decrease decidual prolactin secretion (Chao and colleagues, 1994; Frank and colleagues, 1995).

The exact physiological roles of prolactin produced in decidua are still unknown. Prolactin action is mediated by the relative expression of two unique prolactin receptors as well as the amount of intact (full-length) prolactin protein versus the truncated (16-kDa) form (Jabbour and Critchley, 2001). Receptor expression has been demonstrated in decidua, chorionic cytotrophoblasts, amnionic epithelium, and placental syncytiotrophoblast (Maaskant and colleagues, 1996). Because all (or most) of the prolactin produced in decidua enters amnionic fluid, it has been speculated that there may be a role for this hormone in solute and water transport across the amniochorion, and thus in the maintenance of amnionic fluid volume homeostasis. It also has been shown, however, that prolactin receptors are present in a number of bone marrow–derived immune cells, and that prolactin may act on human T cells in an autocrine or paracrine manner (Pellegrini and colleagues, 1992). Therefore, prolactin produced in decidua may act in regulating immunological functions in this tissue during pregnancy. Prolactin also may play a role in the regulation of angiogenesis that occurs during implantation. In this regard, the intact (full-length) prolactin protein can enhance angiogenesis while the proteolytic fragment (16-kDa) form can inhibit angiogenesis. Thus, the role of prolactin may vary dramatically at different periods of gestation based on the type of receptors expressed and the relative form of prolactin present.

IMPLANTATION AND FORMATION OF THE PLACENTA AND FETAL MEMBRANES

The development of the human placenta is as uniquely intriguing as the embryology of the fetus. During its brief intrauterine existence, the fetus is dependent on the placenta for pulmonary, hepatic, and renal functions. The placenta accomplishes these functions through its unique anatomical association with the mother. The placenta links the mother and fetus by indirect interaction with the maternal blood that spurts out of the uteroplacental vessels. This blood bathes the outer syncytiotrophoblast, allowing exchange of gases and nutrients with fetal capillary blood within the connective tissue at the villous core. Fetal and maternal blood are not mixed in this hemochorial type of placenta. There is also a paracrine system that links the mother and fetus through the anatomical and biochemical juxtaposition of extraembryonic chorion laeve of fetal origin and maternal uterine decidua parietalis tissue. This is an extraordinarily important arrangement for communication between fetus and mother, for maternal immunological acceptance of the conceptus, and possibly for controlling the timing of parturition.

FERTILIZATION AND IMPLANTATION

Ovum Fertilization and Zygote Cleavage. The union of egg and sperm at fertilization represents one of the most important processes in biology. Ovulation frees the secondary oocyte and the adhering cells of the cumulus oophorus from the ovary. Although technically this mass of cells is released into the peritoneal cavity, the oocyte is quickly engulfed by the infundibulum of the fallopian tube. Transport of the oocyte through the fallopian tube toward the uterus is accomplished by directional movement of ciliary action as well as peristalsis. Fertilization occurs in the fallopian tube, and it is generally agreed that fertilization of the ovum must occur a few hours and no more than a day after ovulation. Consequently, spermatozoa must be present in the fallopian tube at the time of oocyte arrival. Almost all pregnancies occur when intercourse occurs during the 2 days preceding or on the day of ovulation. Thus the postovulatory and postfertilization developmental ages are similar. The steps involved to achieve fertilization are highly complex and have been the topic of much research. The molecular mechanisms that allow passage of spermatozoa between the follicular cells, through the zona pellucida, and into the oocyte cytoplasm leading to the formation of the zygote continue to be unraveled and recently have been reviewed (Primakoff and Myles, 2002).

In this chapter, the timing of events in early human development is described as days or weeks postfertilization, viz., postconceptional, rather than using the clinical pregnancy dating convention of weeks from the start of the last menstrual period. As discussed on page 46, the length of the follicular phase of the menstrual cycle is subject to more variability than that of the luteal phase. Thus, 1 week postfertilization corresponds to approximately 3 weeks from the last menstrual period in women with regular 28-day cycles.

After fertilization in the fallopian tube, the mature ovum becomes a zygote—a diploid cell with 46 chromosomes—that then undergoes cleavage into blastomeres (Fig. 3–8). In the two-cell zygote, the blastomeres and the polar body are free in the perivitelline fluid and are surrounded by a thick zona pellucida. The zygote undergoes slow cleavage for 3 days while still within the fallopian tube. As the blastomeres continue to divide, a solid mulberry-like ball of cells, referred to as the *morula,* is produced (Fig. 3–8D). The morula enters the uterine cavity about 3 days after fertilization. The gradual accumulation of fluid between the cells of the morula results in the formation of the early blastocyst.

In a 58-cell blastocyst, the outer cells, called the *trophectoderm,* can be distinguished from the inner cell mass that forms the embryo (Fig. 3–8E). In the earliest stages of the human blastocyst, the wall of the primitive blastodermic vesicle is characterized as consisting of a single layer of ectoderm. As early as 4 to 5 days after fertilization, the 58-cell blastula differentiates into five embryo-producing cells known as the *inner cell mass,* and 53 cells destined to form trophoblasts (Hertig, 1962).

Interestingly, the 107-cell blastocyst is found to be no larger than the earlier cleavage stages, despite the accumulated fluid (Fig. 3–8F). It measured 0.155 mm in diameter, which is similar to the size of the initial postfertilization zygote. At this stage the eight formative, or embryo-producing, cells are surrounded by 99 trophoblastic cells. It is at this stage that the blastocyst is released from the zona pellucida as a result of secretion of specific proteases from the secretory-phase endometrial glands (O'Sullivan and colleagues, 2002).

Release from the zona pellucida allows blastocyst-produced cytokines and hormones to directly influence the receptivity of the endometrium (Lindhard and colleagues, 2002). Evidence has accumulated that IL-1α and IL-1β are secreted by the blastocyst and that these cytokines can directly influence the endometrium. Embryos also have been shown to secrete human chorionic gonadotropin (hCG), which may influence endometrial receptivity (Licht and colleagues, 2001; Lobo and colleagues, 2001). The receptive endometrium is thought to respond by producing leukemia inhibitory factor and colony-stimulating factor-1, which increase trophoblast production of proteases that degrade selected endometrial extracellular matrix proteins and allow trophoblast invasion. Thus, embryo "hatching" is a critical step toward successful pregnancy as it allows association of the trophoblasts with the epithelial cells of the endometrium and the release of trophoblast-produced hormones into the uterine cavity.

Implantation of the Blastocyst. Implantation of the embryo into the wall of the uterus is a common feature of all mammals and in humans occurs six or seven days after fertilization. Successful implantation requires a receptive endometrium that has been appropriately primed with estrogen and progesterone. As shown in Figure 3–1, uterine receptivity toward the blastocyst is limited to days 20 to 24 of the ovarian–endometrial cycle (Bergh and Navot, 1992). The ability of the blastocyst to adhere to the epithelium is mediated by cell surface receptors at the implantation site that interact with receptors on the blastocyst (Carson, 2002; Lessey and Castelbaum, 2002; Lindhard and colleagues, 2002; Paria and colleagues, 2002). The development of the receptive epithelia results from the postovulatory production of estrogen and progesterone by the corpus luteum. If the blastocyst approaches the endometrium after cycle day 24, the potential for adhesion is diminished because of the synthesis of antiadhesive glycoproteins, which prevent receptor interactions (Navot and Bergh, 1991).

At the time of its interaction with the endometrium, the blastocyst is composed of 100 to 250 cells. The blastocyst loosely adheres to the endometrial epithelium, a process called *apposition,* which most commonly occurs on the endometrium of the upper posterior wall of the uterus. Although

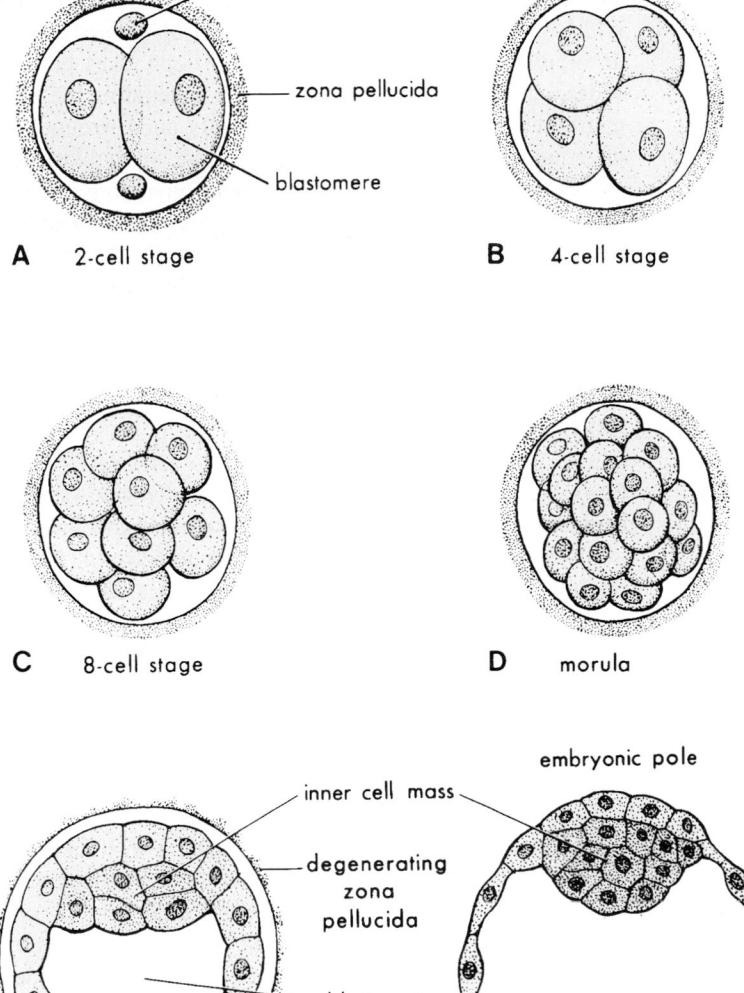

A 2-cell stage

B 4-cell stage

C 8-cell stage

D morula

E early blastocyst

F late blastocyst

FIGURE 3–8. Cleavage of the zygote and formation of the blastocyst. **A** through **D** show various stages of cleavage. The period of the morula begins at the 12- to 16-cell stage and ends when the blastocyst forms, which occurs when there are 50 to 60 blastomeres present. **E** and **F** are sections of blastocysts. The zona pellucida has disappeared by the late blastocyst stage (5 days). The polar bodies shown in **A** are small, nonfunctional cells that soon degenerate. (From Moore, 1988.)

as subsequently discussed, syncytiotrophoblast has not been distinguished prior to human blastocyst implantation, syncytiotrophoblast has been observed in the earliest implanted blastocyst of the macaque monkey (Boyd and Hamilton, 1970). The attachment of the trophectoderm of the blastocyst to the endometrial surface by apposition and adherence appears to be closely regulated by paracrine interactions between these two tissues.

Successful adhesion of the blastocyst to the endometrium also involves modification in the expression of cellular adhesion molecules. The integrins, one of four families of cell adhesion molecules, are cell-surface receptors that mediate the adhesion of cells to extracellular matrix proteins (Lessey and Castelbaum, 2002). Great diversity of cell binding to a host of different extracellular matrix proteins is possible by differential regulation of the integrin system of receptors. An alteration of integrin subunit expression on the endometrial epithelial cells is considered a marker of receptivity for blastocyst attachment.

BIOLOGY OF THE TROPHOBLAST. The formation of the human placenta begins with the trophectoderm, which is the first tissue to differentiate at the morula stage of development, giving rise to a layer of trophoblast cells encircling the blastocyst. From the early blastocyst to term placenta, the trophoblast plays critical roles at the fetal–maternal interface. The trophoblast exhibits the most variable structure, function, and developmental pattern of all placental components.

Its invasiveness provides for attachment of the blastocyst to the decidua; its role in nutrition of the conceptus is reflected in its name; and its function as an endocrine organ in human pregnancy is essential to maternal physiological adaptations and to the maintenance of pregnancy.

Trophoblast Differentiation. By the eighth day postfertilization, after initial implantation of the blastocyst, the trophoblast has differentiated into an outer multinucleated syncytium, the primitive *syncytiotrophoblast,* and an inner layer of primitive mononuclear *cytotrophoblasts.* The cytotrophoblasts are the germinal cells for the syncytium; the latter acts as the primary secretory component within the placenta. Although the ability to undergo DNA synthesis and mitosis, a well-demarcated cell border, and a single nucleus characterize each cytotrophoblast, these characteristics are lacking in the syncytium covering the chorionic villi (Arnholdt and colleagues, 1991). The syncytium has no individual cells, only a continuous syncytial lining. Therefore, the cellular term used is *syncytiotrophoblast,* in which the cytoplasm is amorphous, without cell borders, and the nuclei are multiple and diverse in size and shape. The absence of cell borders facilitates transport across the syncytiotrophoblast, because the control of transport is not dependent on the participation of individual cells.

After implantation is complete, *the trophoblast further differentiates along two main pathways, giving rise to villous and extravillous trophoblast.* Both pathways give rise to populations of trophoblast cells with distinct functions, which come into contact with maternal tissues (Loke and King, 1995). The villous trophoblast, as its name suggests, gives rise to the chorionic villi of the placenta, and primarily functions in the transport of oxygen and nutrients between the fetus and mother. The extravillous trophoblast migrates into the decidua and myometrium and also penetrates maternal vasculature, thus coming into contact with a variety of maternal cell types (Pijnenborg, 1994). The extravillous trophoblast is thus further classified as interstitial trophoblast and endovascular trophoblast. The interstitial trophoblast both invades the maternal decidua, eventually penetrating the myometrium to form placental bed giant cells, and surrounds the maternal spiral arteries. The endovascular trophoblast penetrates the lumen of the spiral arteries (Pijnenborg and colleagues, 1983). Both the formation of chorionic villi and the remarkable process of invasion of maternal tissues by extravillous trophoblast are discussed separately in greater detail in the sections that follow.

EMBRYONIC DEVELOPMENT AFTER IMPLANTATION

Early Trophoblast Invasion. After gentle erosion between epithelial cells of the surface endometrium, the invading trophoblasts burrow deeper into the endometrium, and by the 10th day the blastocyst becomes totally encased within the endometrium. This process of erosion and invasion into the endometrium is carried out actively by the trophoblast cells. *The mechanisms leading to trophoblast invasion into the endometrium are similar to the characteristics of metastasizing malignant cells.* These mechanisms are discussed in more detail on page 58.

One of the earliest implanting blastocysts discovered by Hertig and Rock (1945) is shown in Figure 3–9. It measured only 0.36 by 0.31 mm, and it was believed to have been in the process of penetrating the endometrium, with the thin outer wall of the blastocyst still within the uterine cavity. An implanting blastocyst at a similar stage of development, 9 days after fertilization, is shown in Figure 3–10. It appears to have been flattened in the process of penetrating the uterine epithelium; the enlargement and multiplication of the trophoblasts

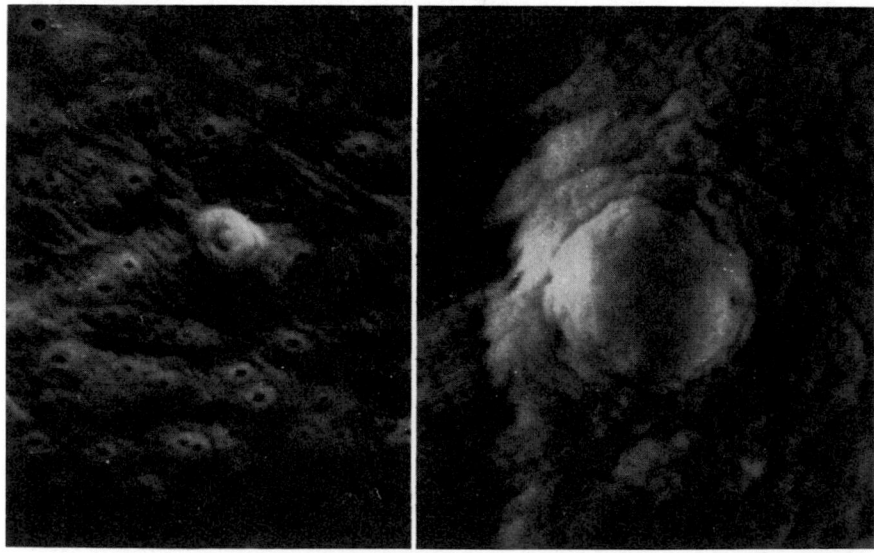

FIGURE 3–9. Low- and high-power photomicrographs of a surface view of an early implanted blastocyst obtained on day 22 of the endometrial cycle, less than 8 days after conception. The site was slightly elevated and measured 0.36 × 0.31 mm. Mouths of uterine glands appear as dark spots surrounded by halos. (From Hertig and Rock, 1945.)

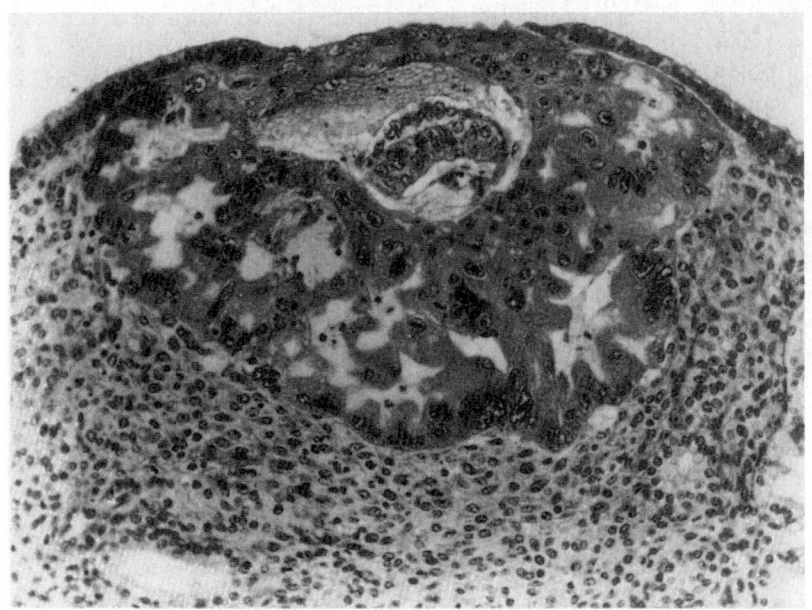

FIGURE 3–10. Section through middle of an implanting embryo at about 9 days. Regeneration of the endometrial epithelium is taking place. Lacunae appear as clear spaces in the large mass of syncytiotrophoblast. The bilaminar embryonic disk is seen. (Carnegie Collection no. 8225.) (From Hertig and Rock, 1944.)

in contact with the endometrium are alone responsible for the increase in size of the implanted blastocyst as compared with that of the free blastocyst.

At 9 days of development (see Figs. 3–9 and 3–10), the wall of the blastocyst that faces toward the uterine lumen is a single layer of flattened cells. The opposite, thicker wall comprises two zones, the trophoblasts and the embryo-forming inner cell mass. As early as 7½ days after fertilization, the inner cell mass, referred to as the embryonic disc, is differentiated into a thick plate of primitive ectoderm and an underlying layer of

endoderm. Some small cells appear between the embryonic disc and the trophoblast, enclosing a space that will become the amnionic cavity.

The embryonic mesenchyme first appears as isolated cells within the cavity of the blastocyst. When the cavity is completely lined with mesoderm, it is termed the *chorionic vesicle,* and its membrane, now called the *chorion,* is composed of trophoblasts and mesenchyme. The amnion and yolk sac, with both epithelial and mesenchymal components, are illustrated in Figures 3–11 and 3–12. The mesenchymal cells within the

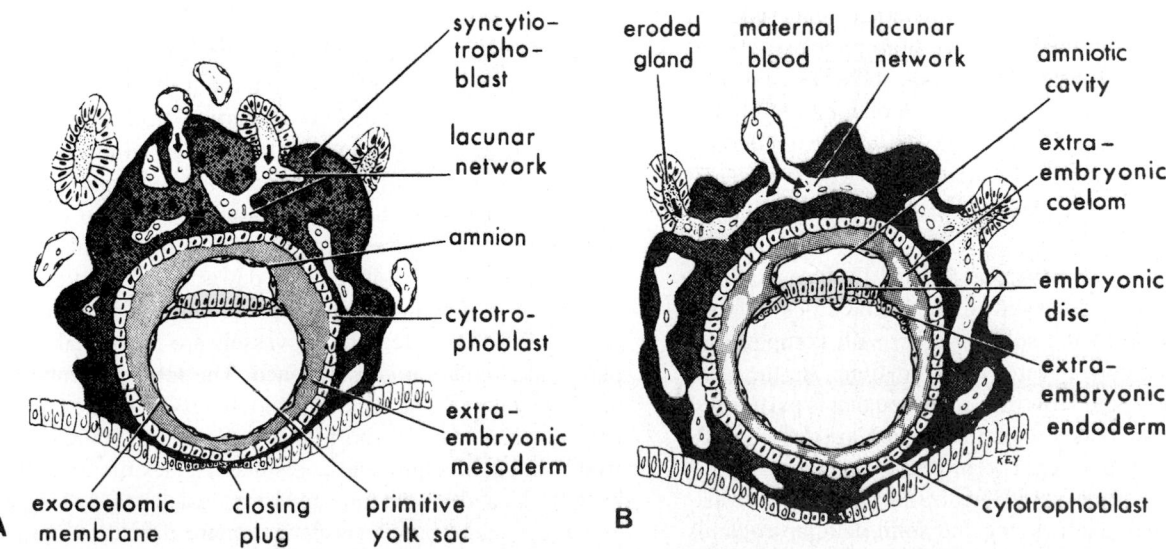

FIGURE 3–11. Drawing of sections through implanted blastocysts. **A.** At 10 days. **B.** At 12 days after fertilization. The stage of development is characterized by the intercommunication of the lacunae filled with maternal blood. Note in **B** that large cavities have appeared in the extraembryonic mesoderm, forming the beginning of the extraembryonic coelom. Also note that extraembryonic endodermal cells have begun to form on the inside of the primitive yolk sac. (From Moore, 1988.)

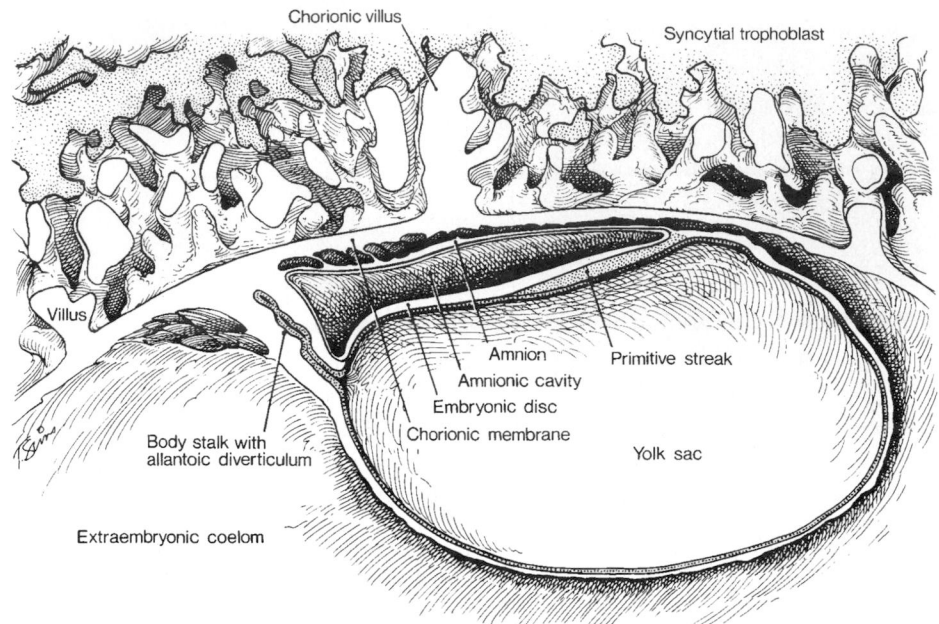

Chorionic villus

Syncytial trophoblast

Villus

Amnion

Amnionic cavity

Primitive streak

Embryonic disc

Chorionic membrane

Yolk sac

Body stalk with allantoic diverticulum

Extraembryonic coelom

FIGURE 3–12. Median view of a drawing of a wax reconstruction of an 18-day-old Mateer-Streeter embryo, showing the amnionic cavity and its relations to chorionic membrane and yolk sac ($\times$ 500). (After Streeter, 1920.)

cavity are the most numerous and eventually will condense to form the body stalk, which serves to join the embryo to the nutrient chorion and later develops into the umbilical cord. The body stalk can be recognized at an early stage, as shown in Figure 3–12, at the caudal end of the embryonic disc.

Lacunae Formation Within the Syncytiotrophoblast. About 12 days after conception, the syncytiotrophoblast of the trophoblast shell is permeated by a system of intercommunicating channels of trophoblastic lacunae, or small cavities. As the embryo enlarges, more maternal tissue (decidua basalis) is invaded by the basal syncytiotrophoblast, including the walls of the superficial decidual capillaries, and these lacunae become filled with maternal blood (see Fig. 3–11). At the same time, the decidual reaction intensifies in the surrounding stroma, which is characterized by enlargement of the decidual stromal cells and glycogen storage.

Development of Primary Villous Stalks. With deeper blastocyst invasion into the decidua, the extravillous cytotrophoblasts give rise to the solid primary villi composed of a cytotrophoblast core covered by syncytium. As the lacunae join, a complicated labyrinth is formed that is partitioned by solid cytotrophoblastic columns, which arise from buds of cytotrophoblast that begin to protrude into the primitive syncytium before 12 days postfertilization. The trophoblast-lined labyrinthine channels and the solid cellular columns form the intervillous space and the primary villous stalks, respectively. The villi initially are located over the entire blastocyst surface, but later disappear except over the most deeply implanted portion, the site destined to form the placenta.

ORGANIZATION OF THE PLACENTA. The term *hemochorial* and the older term *hemochorioendothelial* are used to describe human placentation. The terms are derived as follows: *hemo* refers to maternal blood, which directly bathes the syncytiotrophoblast; *chorio* is for chorion–placenta, which in turn is separated from fetal blood by the *endothelial* wall of the fetal capillaries that traverse the villous core (hence the older term *hemochorioendothelial*). The characteristics of this type of placentation are illustrated in Figures 3–11 and 3–12.

CHORIONIC VILLI. Chorionic villi can first be distinguished in the human placenta on about the 12th day after fertilization. Mesenchymal cords, derived from extraembryonic mesoderm, invade the solid trophoblast columns, forming the secondary villi. After angiogenesis occurs from the mesenchymal cores, the resulting villi are termed *tertiary.* Maternal venous sinuses are tapped early in the implantation process, but until the 14th or 15th day after fertilization, maternal arterial blood does not enter the intervillous space. By about the 17th day, fetal blood vessels are functional, and a placental circulation is established. The fetal–placental circulation is completed when the blood vessels of the embryo are connected with the chorionic blood vessels. Some villi, in which failure of angiogenesis results in a lack of circulation, become distended with fluid and form vesicles. A striking exaggeration of this process is characteristic of the development of hydatidiform mole (see Chap. 11, p. 274).

The trophoblasts of the villus consist of the outer layer of syncytium and an inner layer of cytotrophoblasts, also known as *Langhans cells.* Proliferation of the cytotrophoblasts at the tips of the villi produces the trophoblastic cell columns or

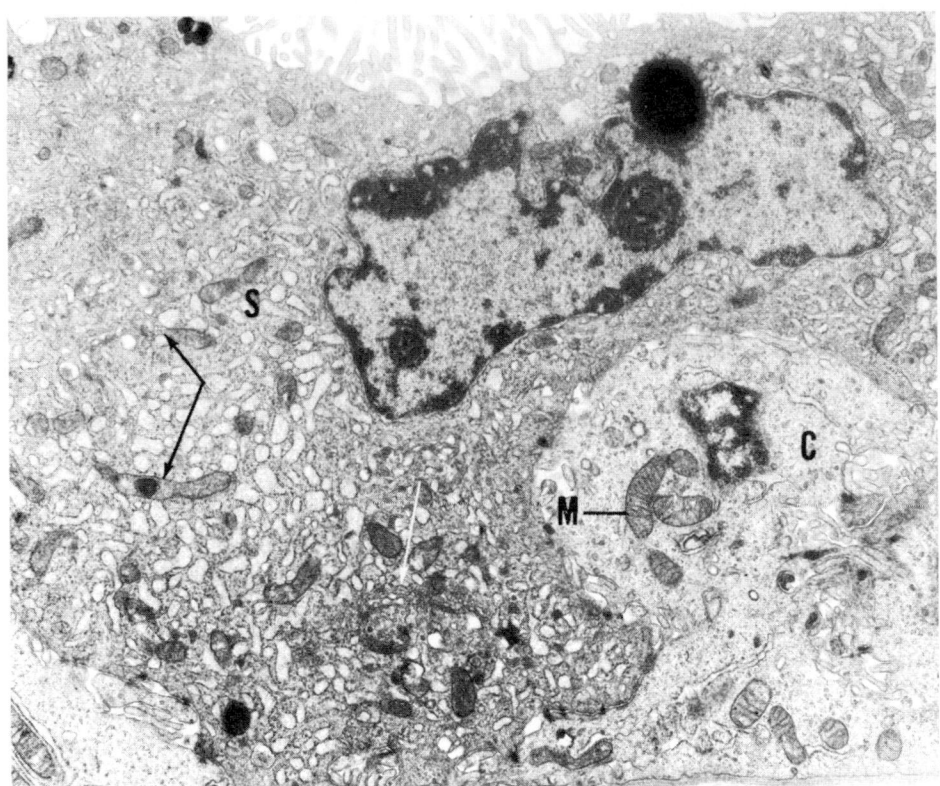

FIGURE 3-13. Electron micrograph of first-trimester human placenta showing well-differentiated syncytiotrophoblast (S) with numerous mitochondria (*black arrows*) and Golgi complexes (*white arrow*). Cytotrophoblast (C) has large mitochondria (M) but few other organelles. At the top, there is a prominent border of microvilli arising from the syncytium.

anchoring villi. These structures are not invaded by fetal mesenchyme but are anchored to the decidua at the basal plate. Thus, the base of the intervillous space, the maternal-facing side, consists of cytotrophoblasts from the cell columns (trabeculae), the covering syncytium of the trophoblast shell, and decidua of the basal plate. The base of the chorionic plate forms the roof of the intervillous space and consists of two layers of trophoblasts externally and fibrous mesoderm internally. The "definitive" chorionic plate is formed by 8 to 10 weeks as the amnionic and primary chorionic plate mesenchyme fuse together. This formation is accomplished by expansion of the amnionic sac, which also surrounds the connective stalk and the allantois and joins these structures to form the umbilical cord (Kaufmann and Scheffen, 1992).

Villus Ultrastructure. The electron microscopic studies of Wislocki and Dempsey (1955) permitted a functional interpretation of the fine structure of the placenta. There are prominent microvilli on the syncytial surface, corresponding to the so-called brush border described by light microscopy (Fig. 3–13). Associated pinocytotic vacuoles and vesicles are related to the absorptive and secretory placental functions. The microvilli act to increase the surface area that will have direct contact with maternal blood. It is the contact between the trophoblastic surface and maternal blood that is the defining characteristic of the hemochorial type of placenta. Depending on the number of trophoblastic epithelial layers, the human

hemochorial placenta can be subdivided into hemodichorial or hemomonochorial (Enders, 1965). The inner layer of the villi—the cytotrophoblasts and the associated basal lamina—is more prominent during the first trimester of gestation (Fig. 3–14). Later in gestation, however, the layer of cytotrophoblasts inside the syncytium is no longer continuous, with only scattered cells present at term, creating a narrower hemomonochorial barrier that facilitates transport of nutrients and oxygen to the fetus.

PLACENTAL DEVELOPMENT

Development of the Chorion and Decidua. In early pregnancy, the villi are distributed over the entire periphery of the chorionic membrane. A blastocyst dislodged from the endometrium at this stage of development appears shaggy (Fig. 3–15). As the blastocyst with its surrounding trophoblasts grows and expands into the decidua, one pole of this mass extends outward toward the endometrial cavity. The opposite, innermost pole enters into the formation of the placenta, that is, the villous trophoblasts and the anchoring cytotrophoblasts. Here the chorionic villi, in contact with the decidua basalis, proliferate to form the chorion frondosum or so-called leafy chorion, the fetal component of the placenta. As the growth of embryonic and extraembryonic tissues continues, the blood supply of the chorion facing the endometrial cavity is restricted, and consequently the villi in contact with

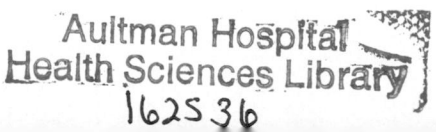

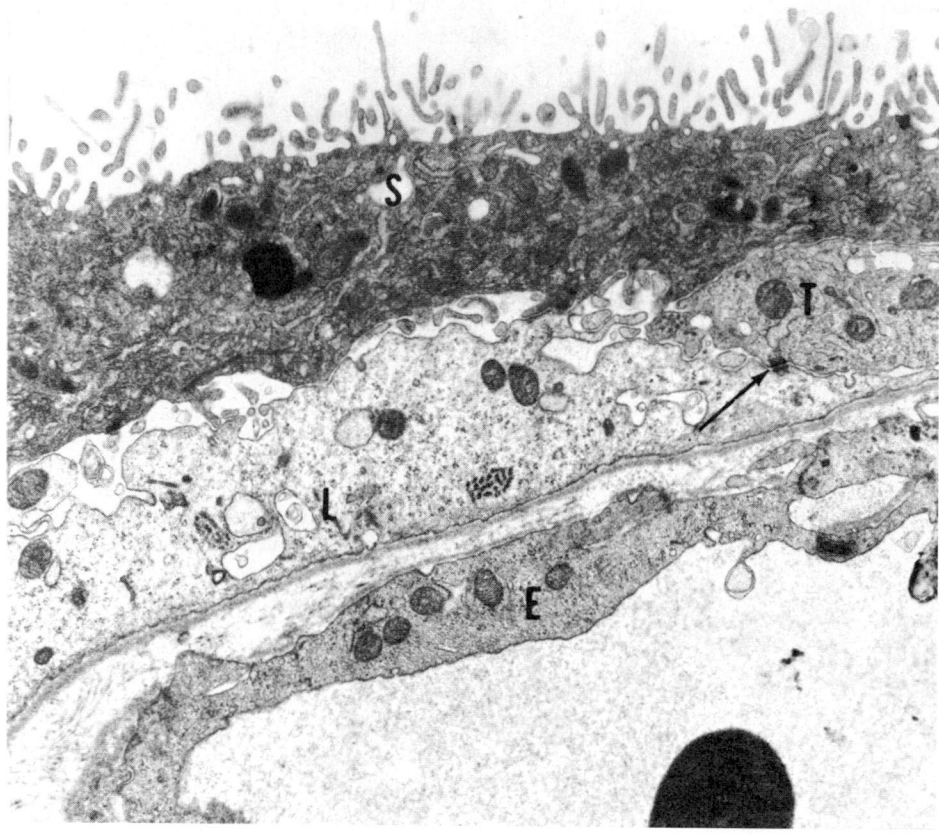

FIGURE 3–14. Term human placenta showing electron-dense syncytium (S), Langhans cells (cytotrophoblasts) (L), transitional cytotrophoblast (T), and capillary endothelium (E). Arrow points to desmosome. (Courtesy of Dr. Ralph M. Wynn.)

the decidua capsularis cease to grow and degenerate. This portion of the chorion becomes the avascular fetal membrane that touches the decidua parietalis, viz., the chorion laeve or so-called smooth chorion. The chorion laeve is generally more nearly translucent than the amnion and rarely exceeds 1 mm thickness. It is composed of cytotrophoblasts and fetal mesodermal (mesenchymal) cells that survive in a relatively low-oxygen atmosphere.

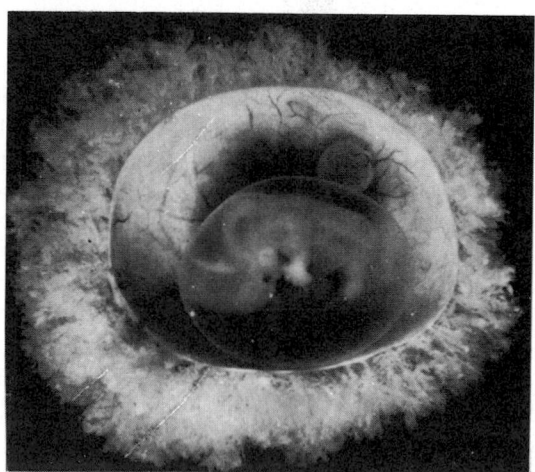

FIGURE 3–15. Human chorionic vesicle at ovulatory age of 40 days. (Carnegie Collection No. 8537.)

Until near the end of the third month, the chorion laeve is separated from the amnion by the exocoelomic cavity. Thereafter, the amnion and chorion are in intimate contact. In the human, the chorion laeve and amnion form an avascular amniochorion, but these two structures are important sites of molecular transfer and metabolic activity. They constitute an important paracrine arm of the fetal–maternal communication system.

With continued expansion of the embryo–fetus, the uterine lumen is obliterated and the chorion laeve becomes contiguous with the entire maternal decidua parietalis that is not occupied by the placenta. As the fetus grows, the decidua capsularis merges with the decidua parietalis. The decidua capsularis, however, is largely lost by pressure and the attendant loss of blood supply. The area of decidua where decidua capsularis and decidua parietalis merge is referred to as the *decidua vera* (see Fig. 3–6).

Trophoblast Invasion of the Endometrium. The extravillous trophoblast cells of the first-trimester placenta are highly invasive. They form columns of cells that extend from the endometrium to the inner third of the myometrium. Development of the hemochorial placenta requires the invasion of the endometrium and the spiral arteries. The invasive ability of these cells results from their ability to secrete numerous proteolytic enzymes capable of digesting the extracellular matrix of the endometrium as well as activating proteinases that are already present in the endometrium. Trophoblasts produce urokinase-type plasminogen activator, which converts plasminogen into the broadly acting serine protease plasmin, which in turn is able to both degrade matrix proteins and activate matrix metalloproteinases. The matrix metalloproteinases are a family of structurally similar enzymes that are secreted as inactive proenzymes. One member of the family, matrix metalloproteinase-9, appears to be critical for human trophoblast invasion, and its production is increased by factors produced by the trophoblasts such as IL-1 and hCG as well as paracrine factors produced by the uterus such as leukemia inhibiting factor and colony-stimulating factor-1 (Bischof and colleagues, 2002; Librach and colleagues, 1991).

The relative ability to invade maternal tissue in the first trimester versus the limited invasiveness seen in the last trimester is controlled by autocrine and paracrine trophoblastic and endometrial factors. Trophoblasts secrete insulin-like growth factor II, which acts in an autocrine manner to promote invasion into the endometrium, whereas decidual cells secrete insulin-like growth factor binding protein type 4, which is able to block this autocrine loop. Thus, the degree of trophoblast invasion is kept under tight control through the regulation of matrix degradation as well as by factors that cause migration of the trophoblasts.

Integrin subunit expression also appears to be important in the control of trophoblast invasion of the endometrium–decidua. Recall that the decidual cell becomes completely encased by a pericellular extracellular matrix membrane. This "wall" around the decidual cell provides the scaffolding for the attachment of the cytotrophoblasts of the anchoring villi described earlier, which are a subset of extravillous trophoblasts. These cells first elaborate selected proteinases that degrade the extracellular matrix of decidua. Thereafter, the expression of a specific group of integrins enables the docking of these cells. The trophoblasts are further secured by the production of fetal fibronectin (Feinberg and colleagues, 1991). This oncofetal fibronectin, or fetal-specific fibronectin (fFN), is a unique glycopeptide of the fibronectin molecule. FFN has been called *trophoblast glue* to suggest a critical role for this protein in the migration and attachment of trophoblasts to maternal decidua. Indeed, the presence of fFN in cervical or vaginal fluid can be used as a prognostic indicator for preterm labor, as discussed in Chapter 36 (see p. 862).

Decidual Spiral Artery Invasion. One of the most remarkable features of human placental development is the extensive modification of the maternal vasculature by trophoblast cells, which are, by definition, of fetal origin. These events occur in the first half of pregnancy and are considered in detail because of their importance in the understanding of uteroplacental blood flow in both normal pregnancy and labor. They are also important in pathological conditions such as preeclampsia and intrauterine growth restriction (see

Chap. 34, p. 763 and Chap. 38, p. 895). These modifications are carried out by two populations of extravillous trophoblast, viz., the interstitial trophoblast surrounding the maternal spiral arteries and the endovascular trophoblast, which penetrates the lumen of the spiral arteries. Early investigators focused on the role of the endovascular trophoblast, however, the function of the interstitial trophoblast has more recently been investigated (Benirschke and Kaufmann, 2000). These cells are now recognized to constitute a major portion of the placental bed, penetrating the decidua and adjacent myometrium (Pijnenborg and colleagues, 1981). They aggregate around the maternal spiral arteries, where their functions may include preparation of the vessels to facilitate invasion by the endovascular trophoblast (Pijnenborg and colleagues, 1983).

The endovascular trophoblast enters the lumen of the maternal spiral arteries, initially forming cellular plugs within the lumen. It then proceeds to destroy the vascular endothelium, and invade and modify the vascular media, where fibrinoid material replaces the smooth muscle and connective tissue of this layer. The spiral arteries later regenerate their endothelium. Hamilton and Boyd (1966) give credit to Friedlander who in 1870 first described the structural changes occurring in the spiral arteries. They noted that the invading endovascular trophoblast can pass several centimeters along the vessel lumen, migrating against arterial flow and pressure. They also found that these vascular changes are not observed in the decidua parietalis, that is, in decidual sites removed from the invading cytotrophoblasts. Of note, the invasion of maternal vascular tissues by trophoblasts involves only the decidual spiral arteries, and not the decidual veins.

Ramsey and Donner (1980) presented a summary of their anatomical studies of the uteroplacental vasculature. The timing of the development of these uteroplacental vessels has been described in waves, or stages, over the course of gestation. The first wave occurs before 12 weeks postfertilization and consists of invasion and modification of the spiral arteries of the decidua, reaching its border with the myometrium. Between 12 to 16 weeks postfertilization, the second wave occurs. This involves invasion of the intramyometrial parts of the spiral arteries, converting narrow-lumen, muscular spiral arteries into dilated, low-resistance uteroplacental vessels. The molecular mechanisms of these crucial events, and their significance in the pathogenesis of preeclampsia and fetal growth restriction, have recently been reviewed by Kaufmann and associates (2003).

Establishment of Maternal Blood Flow. At approximately 1 month after conception, maternal blood enters the intervillous space from the spiral arteries in fountain-like bursts. Thus, maternal blood that is propelled outside of the maternal vessels sweeps over and directly bathes the syncytiotrophoblast. The apical surface of the syncytiotrophoblast consists of a complex microvillous structure that undergoes continual shedding and reformation during pregnancy.

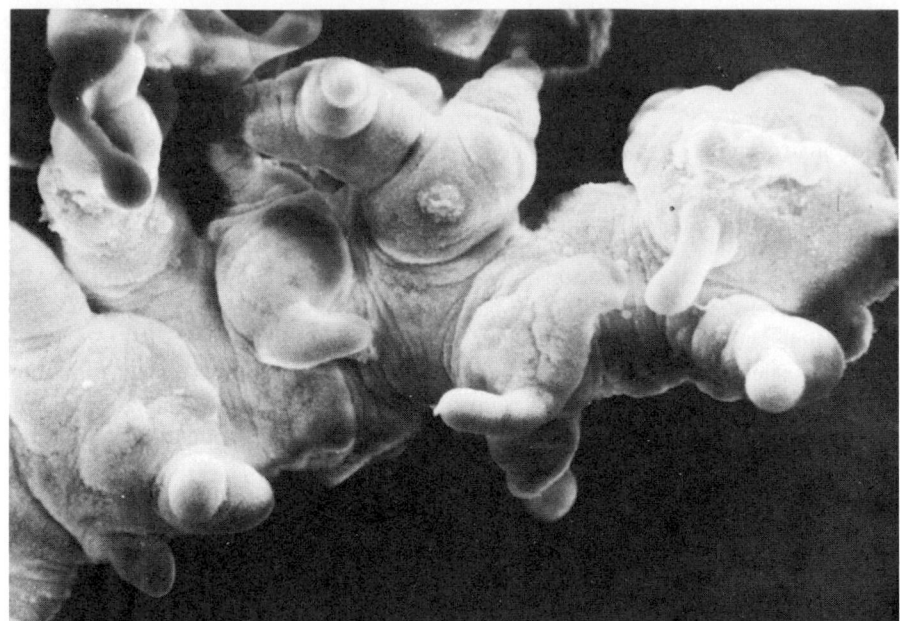

FIGURE 3–16. Scanning electron micrograph of placental villi at 10 to 14 weeks' gestation. Note the larger stem villi and the small syncytial sprouts at various stages of formation. Furrows or creases on the surface also are evident, especially at the bases of larger villi (× 289). (From King and Menton, 1975.)

Villus Branching. Certain villi of the chorion frondosum extend from the chorionic plate to the decidua and serve as *anchoring villi.* Most chorionic villi, however, arborize and end freely in the intervillous space without reaching the decidua (Fig. 3–16). As the placenta develops, the short, thick, early stem villi branch repeatedly, forming progressively finer subdivisions and greater numbers of increasingly small villi (Fig. 3–17). Each of the truncal or main stem villi and their ramifications (rami) constitute a placental *lobule,* or cotyledon. Each lobule is supplied with a single truncal branch of the chorionic artery; and for each lobule, there is a single vein; thus, these lobules constitute the functional units of the placental architecture.

PLACENTAL GROWTH AND MATURATION

PLACENTAL GROWTH. In the first trimester, growth of the placenta is more rapid than that of the fetus, but by approximately 17 weeks postmenstruation (from the last menstrual

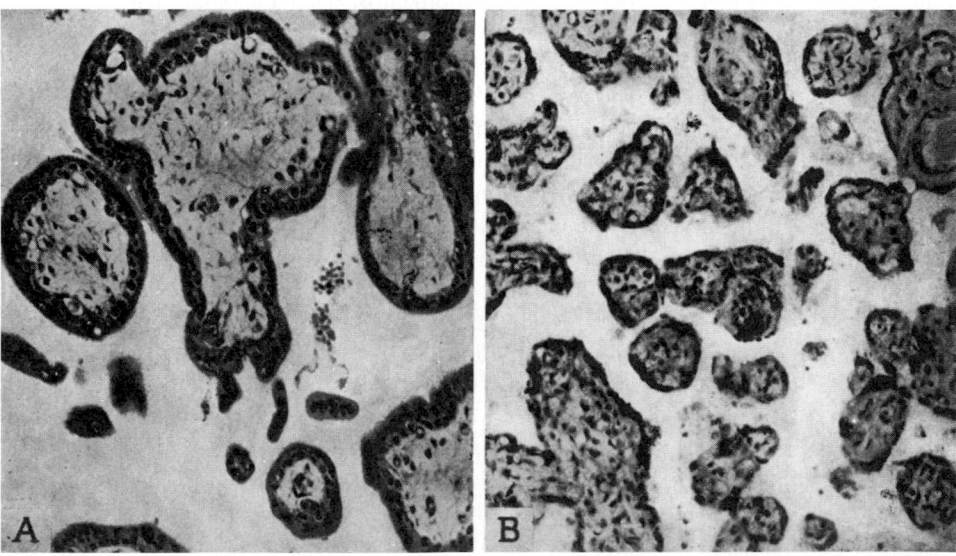

FIGURE 3–17. Comparison of chorionic villi in early and late pregnancy. **A.** About 8 weeks' gestation. Note inner Langhans cells (cytotrophoblasts) and outer syncytial layer. **B.** Term placenta. Syncytial layer is obvious, but Langhans cells (cytotrophoblasts) are difficult to recognize at low magnification in light micrographs.

period), placental and fetal weights are approximately equal. At term, the placental weight may be roughly one sixth that of fetal weight. According to Boyd and Hamilton (1970), the average placenta at term is 185 mm in diameter and 23 mm in thickness, with a volume of 497 mL and a weight of 508 g. These measurements vary widely, and there are multiple variant forms of the human placenta and several types of umbilical cord insertions, which are discussed in Chapter 27.

Viewed from the maternal surface, the number of slightly elevated convex areas, called *lobes,* varies from 10 to 38. These lobes are incompletely separated by grooves of variable depth, overlying the *placental septa,* which arise from folding of the basal plate. These grossly visible lobes have also been referred to as "cotyledons", however, this use should be avoided, because they bear no relation to the functional units supplied by each primary villus, which are termed either *lobules* or *cotyledons.*

The total number of lobes remains the same throughout gestation, and individual lobes continue to grow, although less actively in the final weeks (Crawford, 1959). Placental weights vary considerably, depending on how the placenta is prepared. If the fetal membranes and most of the cord are left attached and the adherent maternal blood clot is not removed, the weight may be greater by nearly 50 percent (Thomson and colleagues, 1969).

PLACENTAL MATURATION. As the villi continue to branch and the terminal ramifications become more numerous and smaller, the volume and prominence of cytotrophoblasts decrease. As the syncytium thins, the fetal vessels become more prominent and lie closer to the surface. The stroma of the villi also exhibits changes as gestation progresses. In placentas of early pregnancy, the branching connective tissue cells are separated by an abundant loose intercellular matrix. Later, the stroma becomes denser and the cells more spindly and more closely packed.

Another change in the stroma involves the infiltration of *Hofbauer cells,* which represent fetal macrophages. These cells are nearly round with vesicular, often eccentric nuclei and very granular or vacuolated cytoplasm. Hofbauer cells are characterized histochemically by intracytoplasmic lipid and by phenotypic markers specific for macrophages. They increase in numbers and maturation state as pregnancy progresses. Although phagocytic, they have an immunosuppressive phenotype (Vince and Johnson, 1996). In addition, they can produce a variety of cytokines and are capable of paracrine regulation of trophoblast functions (Cervar and colleagues, 1999).

Some of the histological changes that accompany placental growth and maturation provide an increased efficiency of transport and exchange to meet increasing fetal metabolic requirements. Among these changes are a decrease in thickness of the syncytium, a significant reduction of cytotrophoblast cells, a decrease in the stroma, an increase in the number of capillaries, and an approximation of these vessels to the syncytial surface. By 4 months, the apparent continuity of the cytotrophoblasts is broken, and at term, the covering of the villi may be focally reduced to a thin layer of syncytium with minimal connective tissue where the fetal capillaries appear to abut the trophoblast. The villi become dominated by thin-walled capillaries.

Other changes in placental architecture, however, can cause a decrease in the efficiency of placental exchange if they include a substantial portion of the exchange area. These changes include thickening of the basal lamina of the trophoblast or capillaries, obliteration of certain fetal vessels, and fibrin deposition on the surface of the villi in the basal and chorionic plates as well as elsewhere in the intervillous space.

FETAL AND MATERNAL BLOOD CIRCULATION IN THE MATURE PLACENTA. Because the placenta functionally represents an intimate approximation of the fetal capillary bed to maternal blood, its gross anatomy primarily concerns vascular relations. The fetal surface of the placenta is covered by the transparent amnion, beneath which the fetal chorionic vessels course. A section through the placenta includes amnion, chorion, chorionic villi and intervillous spaces, decidual (basal) plate, and myometrium (Figs. 3–18, 3–19, and 3–20). The maternal surface of the placenta shown in Figure 3–21 is divided into irregular lobes by furrows produced by septa, which consist of fibrous tissue with sparse vessels confined mainly to their bases. The broad-based septa ordinarily do not reach the chorionic plate, thus providing only incomplete partitions.

Fetal Circulation. Deoxygenated, or "venous-like," fetal blood flows to the placenta through the two umbilical arteries. Where the umbilical cord joins the placenta, the umbilical vessels branch repeatedly beneath the amnion and again within the dividing villi, finally forming capillary networks in the terminal divisions (Fig. 3–22). Blood with significantly higher oxygen content returns from the placenta to the fetus through a single umbilical vein.

The branches of the umbilical vessels that traverse along the fetal surface of the placenta in the chorionic plate are referred to as the *placental surface* or *chorionic vessels.* These vessels are responsive to vasoactive substances, but anatomically, morphologically, histologically, and functionally, they are unique. The chorionic arteries always cross over the chorionic veins. Identification of chorionic artery and vein is most readily recognized by this interesting relationship, but they are difficult to distinguish by histological criteria. In 65 percent of placentas, the chorionic arteries form a fine network supplying the cotyledons—a pattern of disperse-type branching. The remaining 35 percent of arteries radiate to the edge of the placenta without narrowing. Both are end arteries, supplying one cotyledon as each branch turns downward to pierce the chorionic plate.

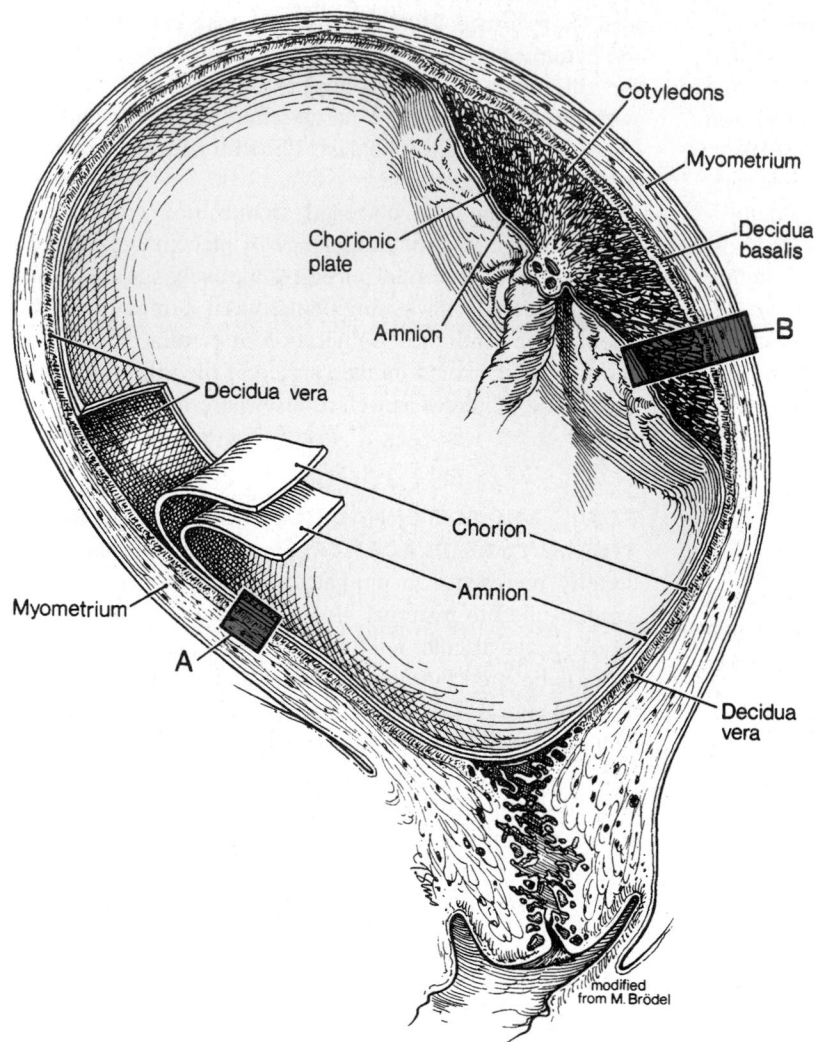

Cotyledons

Myometrium

Chorionic plate

Decidua basalis

Amnion

B

Decidua vera

Chorion

Amnion

Myometrium

A

Decidua vera

modified from M. Brödel

FIGURE 3–18. Uterus of pregnant woman showing normal placenta in situ. **A.** Location of section shown in Figure 3–19. **B.** Location of section shown in Figure 3–20.

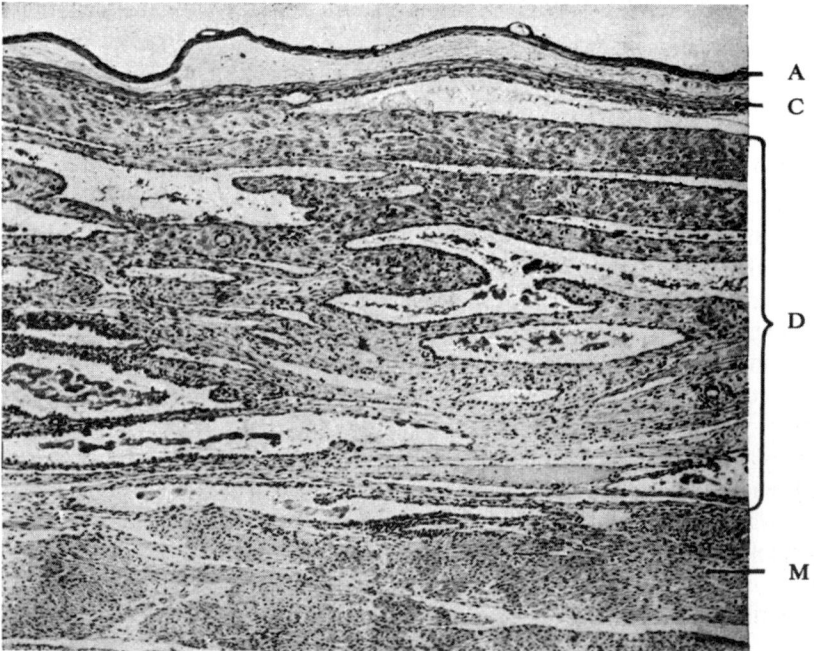

A

C

D

M

FIGURE 3–19. Section of fetal membranes and uterus corresponding to letter **A** in Figure 3–18. (A = amnion; C = chorion laeve; D = decidua parietalis; M = myometrium.)

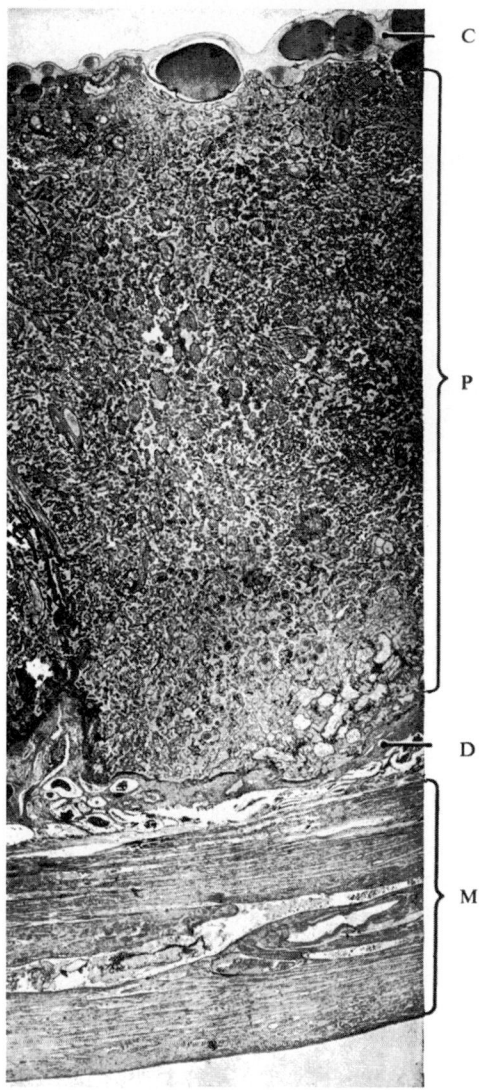

FIGURE 3–20. Section of placenta and uterus corresponding to letter **B** in Figure 3–18. (C = chorionic plate with fetal blood vessels; D = decidua basalis; M = myometrium; P = placental villi.)

The truncal arteries are the perforating branches of the surface arteries that pass through the chorionic plate. Each truncal artery supplies one cotyledon. There is a decrease in smooth muscle of the vessel wall and an increase in the caliber of the vessel as it penetrates through the chorionic plate. The loss in smooth muscle continues as the truncal arteries branch into the rami, and the same is true of the vein walls.

Before 10 weeks, there is no end-diastolic flow pattern within the umbilical artery at the end of the fetal cardiac cycle (Cole and colleagues, 1991a; Fisk and colleagues, 1988; Loquet and colleagues, 1988). At 10 weeks, however, end-diastolic flow appears and is maintained throughout normal pregnancies (Maulik, 1996). Clinically, these are recorded with Doppler ultrasonography as an assessment of fetal well-being (see Chap. 16, p. 401).

Maternal Circulation. Fetal homeostasis is dependent on an efficient maternal–placental circulation. Consequently, investigators have sought to define the factors that regulate the flow of blood into and from the intervillous space. An adequate theory must explain how blood can (1) leave the maternal circulation; (2) flow into an amorphous space lined by syncytiotrophoblast, rather than capillary endothelium; and (3) return through maternal veins without producing arteriovenous-like shunts that would prevent maternal blood from remaining in contact with the villi long enough for adequate exchange. It was not until the studies of Ramsey with Davis (Ramsey and Davis, 1963; Ramsey and Harris, 1966) that a physiological explanation of the placental circulation was available (see Fig. 3–22). These investigators demonstrated, by careful, low-pressure injections of radiocontrast material, that the arterial entrances as well as the venous exits are scattered randomly over the entire base of the placenta.

The physiological maternal–placental circulation is as follows: Maternal blood enters through the basal plate and is driven high up toward the chorionic plate by maternal arterial pressure before lateral dispersion occurs (see Fig. 3–22). After bathing the external microvillous surface of chorionic villi, the maternal blood drains back through venous orifices in the basal plate and enters the uterine veins. Therefore, maternal blood traverses the placenta randomly without preformed channels, propelled by maternal arterial pressure. The previously described processes of trophoblast invasion of the spiral arteries create low-resistance uteroplacental vessels, which can accommodate the massive increase in uterine perfusion over the course of gestation. Generally, the spiral arteries are perpendicular to, but the veins are parallel to, the uterine wall, an arrangement that facilitates closure of the veins during a uterine contraction and prevents squeezing of essential maternal blood from the intervillous space. The number of arterial openings into the intervillous space becomes gradually reduced by cytotrophoblast invasion. According to Brosens and Dixon (1963), there are about 120 spiral arterial entries into the intervillous space at term. These discharge blood in spurts that bathes the adjacent villi (Borell and co-workers, 1958). After the 30th week, a prominent venous plexus, shown in Figure 3–22, separates the decidua basalis from the myometrium, thus participating in providing a plane of cleavage for placental separation.

During uterine contractions, both inflow and outflow are curtailed. Bleker and associates (1975) used serial sonography during normal labor and found that the length, thickness, and surface of the placenta increased during contractions. They attributed these changes to distention of the intervillous spaces by blood as the consequence of relatively greater impairment of venous outflow compared with arterial inflow. During contractions, therefore, a somewhat larger volume of blood is available for exchange even though the rate of flow is decreased. Subsequently, by use of Doppler velocimetry, it was shown that diastolic flow velocity in spiral arteries is

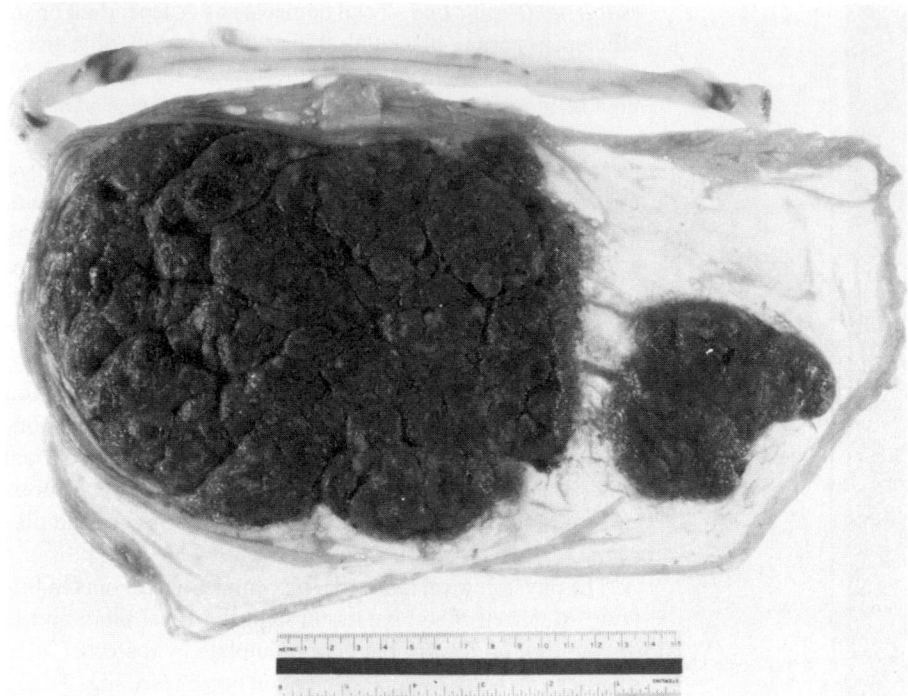

FIGURE 3–21. Maternal surface of a term placenta. Variably discrete, irregularly shaped adjacent lobes are evident plus a large separate (succenturiate) lobe.

diminished during uterine contractions. Therefore, the principal factors regulating blood flow in the intervillous space are arterial blood pressure, intrauterine pressure, the pattern of uterine contractions, and factors that act specifically on the arterial walls.

Breaks in the Placental "Barrier." The placenta does not maintain absolute integrity of the fetal and maternal circulations. This conclusion is evidenced by numerous findings of the passage of cells between mother and fetus in both directions. This situation is best exemplified clinically by erythrocyte D-antigen isoimmunization and the occurrence of *erythroblastosis fetalis,* discussed in Chapter 29 (see p. 663). Typically, a few fetal blood cells are found in maternal blood, but on extremely rare occasions, the fetus exsanguinates into the maternal circulation. Desai and Creger (1963) found that, even under normal conditions, labeled maternal leukocytes and platelets crossed the placenta from mother to fetus. Fetal leukocytes may replicate in the mother, and leukocytes bearing a Y chromosome have been identified in women many years after giving birth to a son (Bianchi and co-workers, 1996; Ciaranfi and colleagues, 1977). These observations have led to the concept of "microchimerism," whereby a variety of fetal cell types may persist in the mother's body for years to decades after a pregnancy. The clinical consequences of fetal cells in the mother are still under debate, however, they may cause maternal autoimmune diseases such as scleroderma, thyroiditis and thyroid failure, and maternal cutaneous eruptions (Aractingi and colleagues, 1998; Lambert and colleagues, 2000; Nelson and colleagues, 1998).

IMMUNOLOGICAL CONSIDERATIONS OF THE FETAL–MATERNAL INTERFACE. Over the past half-century, many attempts to explain the survival of the semiallogenic fetal graft have been proposed. One of the earliest explanations was based on the theory of antigenic immaturity of the embryo-fetus. This explanation was disproved by Billingham (1964), who showed that transplantation (HLA) antigens are demonstrable very early in embryonic life. Another explanation was based on diminished immunological responsiveness of the pregnant woman. There is, however, no evidence for this to be other than an ancillary factor. In a third explanation, the uterus (decidua) is proposed as an immunologically privileged tissue site. This would preclude well-documented advanced ectopic pregnancies, discussed in Chapter 10.

Clearly, the lack of transplantation immunity manifest in the uterus is unique compared with that of other tissues. Therefore, the acceptance and the survival of the conceptus in the maternal uterus must be attributed to an immunological peculiarity of the trophoblasts, not the decidua. The trophoblasts are the only cells of the conceptus in direct contact with maternal tissues or blood, and these tissues are genetically identical with fetal tissues. Several features of trophoblast cells likely contribute to the survival of these cells in an immunologically hostile environment (Thellin and colleagues, 2000). The most important may be the novel aspects of the expression of the HLA system in trophoblasts, coupled with a unique set of uterine lymphocytes.

Immunogenicity of the Trophoblasts. Over 50 years ago, Sir Peter Medawar (1953) suggested that the solution to

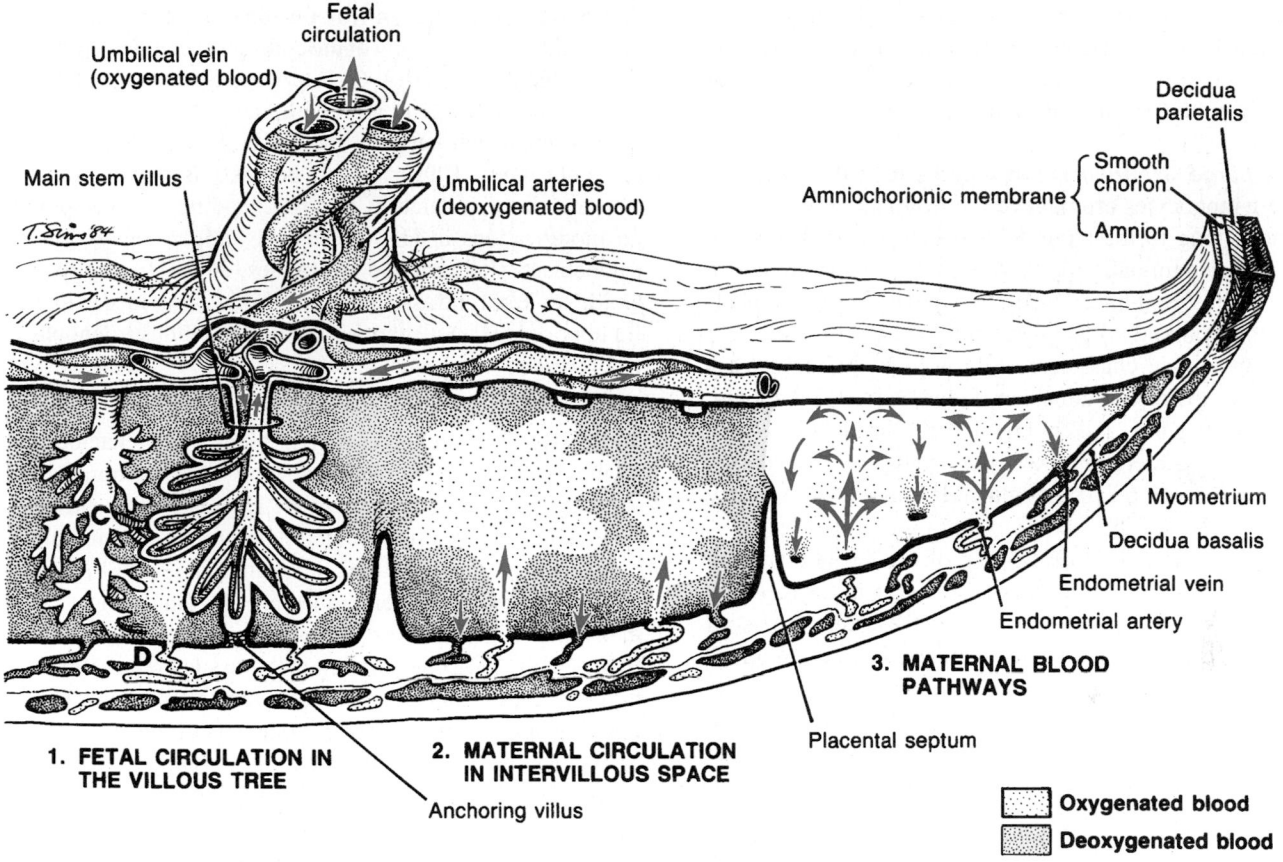

FIGURE 3–22. Schematic drawing of a section through a full-term placenta: **1.** The relation of the villous chorion (C) to the decidua basalis (D) and the fetal–placental circulation. **2.** The maternal blood flows into the intervillous spaces in funnel-shaped spurts, and exchanges occur with the fetal blood as the maternal blood flows around the villi. **3.** The in-flowing arterial blood pushes venous blood into the endometrial veins, which are scattered over the entire surface of the decidua basalis. Note also that the umbilical arteries carry deoxygenated fetal blood to the placenta and that the umbilical vein carries oxygenated blood to the fetus. The cotyledons are separated from each other by placental (decidual) septa. Each cotyledon consists of two or more mainstem villi and their many branches. (Based on Moore, 1988.)

the riddle of the fetal semiallograft might be explained by *immunological neutrality*. The placenta was considered immunologically inert and therefore unable to cause a maternal immune response. Subsequently, many researchers focused on defining the expression of the *major histocompatibility complex (MHC)* antigens on trophoblasts. *Human leukocyte antigens (HLA)* are the human analogue of the major histocompatibility complex. MHC class I and II antigens are absent from villous trophoblasts at all stages of gestation (Weetman, 1999). Thus, these cells do appear to be immunologically inert with regard to fetal–maternal interactions. However, the invasive cytotrophoblasts do express MHC class I molecules and these have been the focus of considerable study.

Trophoblast HLA (MHC) Class I Expression. The HLA genes are the products of multiple genetic loci of the MHC located within the short arm of chromosome 6 (Hunt and Orr,

1992). There are 17 HLA class I genes, including three classical genes, HLA-A, -B, and -C, that encode the major class I (class Ia) transplantation antigens. Three other class I genes, designated HLA-E, -F, and -G, encode class Ib HLA antigens. The remaining DNA sequences appear to be pseudogenes or partial gene fragments.

Moffett-King (2002) reasoned that normal implantation is dependent on controlled trophoblastic invasion of maternal endometrium–decidua and the spiral arteries. Trophoblast invasion must proceed far enough to provide for normal fetal growth and development, and a mechanism for regulating the depth of trophoblast invasion must exist. She suggested that the uterine large granular lymphocytes (LGLs) and the unique expression of three specific HLA class I genes in extravillous cytotrophoblasts act to permit and subsequently to limit the process of trophoblast invasion.

Class I antigens in extravillous cytotrophoblasts are accounted for by the expression of the classical HLA-C and the nonclassical class Ib molecules of HLA-E and HLA-G. To elucidate the importance of HLA-C, HLA-E and HLA-G expression, it is important to understand the nature of the unusual lymphocyte population of the human decidua.

Uterine Large Granular Lymphocytes (LGLs). These distinctive lymphocytes are believed to originate in bone marrow and belong to the natural killer cell lineage. They are by far the predominant population of leukocytes present in midluteal phase endometrium at the expected time of implantation (Johnson and colleagues, 1999). These LGLs have a distinct phenotype characterized by a high surface density of CD56 or neural cell adhesion molecule (Loke and King, 1995; Moffett-King, 2002). The infiltration of LGLs is increased by progesterone as well as stromal cell production of IL-15 and prolactin (Dunn and colleagues, 2002; Gubbay and colleagues, 2002).

Near the end of the luteal phase of nonfertile ovulatory cycles, the nuclei of the uterine LGL begin to disintegrate. With blastocyst implantation, however, these cells persist in large numbers in the decidua during the early weeks of pregnancy. At term, however, there are relatively few LGLs in the decidua. In first-trimester decidua, many LGLs are in close proximity to the extravillous trophoblast. It is speculated that LGLs are involved in the regulation of trophoblast invasion. They secrete large amounts of granulocyte-macrophage–colony-stimulating factor (GM-CSF), suggestive that the LGLs in first-trimester decidua are in an activated state. This has led Jokhi and co-workers (1999) to speculate that GM-CSF may function primarily not to promote trophoblast replication but rather to forestall trophoblast apoptosis. Moreover, expression of angiogenic factors by uterine natural killer cells is suggestive of a potential role for these cells in decidual vascular remodeling (Li and colleagues, 2001). According to this theory, LGLs rather than the T lymphocytes, would bear the primary responsibility for immunosurveillance in decidua.

HLA-G Expression in Human Trophoblasts. HLA-G is expressed only in humans and is distinguished from the HLA class Ia products by a highly restricted tissue distribution. Indeed, HLA-G antigen expression is identified only in extravillous cytotrophoblasts in the decidua basalis and in the chorion laeve (McMaster and colleagues, 1995). HLA-G is not present in villous trophoblasts, either in the syncytium or in the cytotrophoblasts. HLA-G is expressed, however, in cytotrophoblasts that are contiguous with maternal tissues, viz., decidual cells and LGLs. Interestingly the HLA-G gene produces several mRNA transcripts as a result of alternative splicing to yield at least seven isoforms, some soluble and some membrane bound (Carosella and colleagues, 2000). There are few individual DNA variations or polymorphisms in the HLA-G gene sequence, further suggesting an important role for this factor. It has been shown that a soluble major isoform, HLA-G2, is increased during pregnancy (Hunt and colleagues, 2000a, 2000b). Additionally, a recent study of

embryos being used for in vitro fertilization showed that pregnancy did not occur in any of the embryos that did not produce the soluble form of HLA-G (Fuzzi and colleagues, 2002). It may be that HLA-G is immunologically permissive of the antigen mismatch between mother and fetus (LeBouteiller and colleagues, 1999). One hypothesis is that its expression may be stimulated by hypoxia, leading to developmental modifications in HLA-G class I antigen expression on trophoblasts (Kilburn and colleagues, 2000). In that regard, Goldman-Wohl and associates (2000) have provided evidence for abnormal HLA-G expression in extravillous trophoblasts from women with preeclampsia.

AMNION. The amnion at term is a tough and tenacious but pliable membrane. It is the innermost fetal membrane and is contiguous with amnionic fluid. This particular avascular structure occupies a role of incredible importance in human pregnancy. In many obstetrical populations, preterm prematurely ruptured fetal membranes are the single most common antecedent of preterm delivery (see Chap. 6, p. 177, and Chap. 36, p. 864). The amnion is the tissue that provides almost all of the tensile strength of the fetal membranes. Therefore, the development of the components of the amnion that protect against its rupture or tearing is vitally important to successful pregnancy outcome.

Amnion Structure. Bourne (1962) described five separate layers of amnion tissue. The inner surface, which is bathed by amnionic fluid, is an uninterrupted, single layer of cuboidal epithelial cells, believed to be derived from embryonic ectoderm. This epithelium is attached firmly to a distinct basement membrane that is connected to the acellular compact layer, which is composed primarily of interstitial collagens. On the outer side of the compact layer, there is a row of fibroblast-like mesenchymal cells, which are widely dispersed at term. These are probably derived from mesoderm of the embryonic disc. There also are a few fetal macrophages in the amnion. The outermost layer of amnion is the relatively acellular zona spongiosa, which is contiguous with the second fetal membrane, the chorion laeve. The human amnion lacks smooth muscle cells, nerves, lymphatics, and importantly, blood vessels.

Amnion Development. Early in the process of implantation, a space develops between the embryonic cell mass and adjacent trophoblasts (see Fig. 3–11). Small cells that line this inner surface of trophoblasts have been called *amniogenic cells,* the precursors of amnionic epithelium. The human amnion is first identifiable about the seventh or eighth day of embryo development. Initially a minute vesicle (see Fig. 3–11), the amnion develops into a small sac that covers the dorsal surface of the embryo. As the amnion enlarges, it gradually engulfs the growing embryo, which prolapses into its cavity (Benirschke and Kaufmann, 2000).

Distention of the amnionic sac eventually brings it into contact with the interior surface of the chorion laeve. Apposition of the mesoblasts of chorion laeve and amnion near the end of the first trimester then causes an obliteration of the extraembryonic coelom. The amnion and chorion laeve, although slightly adherent, are never intimately connected and usually can be separated easily, even at term.

Amnion Cell Histogenesis. It is now generally accepted that the epithelial cells of the amnion are derived from fetal ectoderm of the embryonic disc. They do not arise by delamination from trophoblasts. This is an important consideration from both embryological and functional perspectives. For example, HLA class I gene expression in amnion is more akin to that in cells of the embryo than that in trophoblasts.

In addition to the epithelial cells that line the amnionic cavity, there is a layer of fibroblast-like (i.e., mesenchymal) cells that are likely derived from embryonic mesoderm. Early in human embryogenesis, the amnionic mesenchymal cells of the amnion lie immediately adjacent to the basal surface of the epithelium. At this time, the amnion surface is a two-cell-layer structure with approximately equal numbers of epithelial and mesenchymal cells. Simultaneously with growth and development, interstitial collagens are deposited between these two layers of cells. This marks the commencement of the formation of the compact layer of the amnion, which also brings about a distinct separation of the two layers of amnion cells.

As the amnionic sac expands to envelop the placenta and then the chorion frondosum at about 10 to 14 weeks, there is a progressive reduction in the compactness of the mesenchymal cells. These cells continue to separate and in the process become rather sparsely distributed. It appears that early in pregnancy the epithelial cells of the amnion replicate at a rate appreciably faster than the mesenchymal cells. At term, the epithelial cells form a continuous uninterrupted epithelium on the fetal surface of the amnion. The mesenchymal cells, however, are widely dispersed, being connected by a fine lattice network of extracellular matrix with the appearance of long slender fibrils.

Amnion Epithelial Cells. The epithelial cells lining the entire amnionic cavity are the cells most commonly studied in investigations of amnion function. The apical surface of the epithelial cells is replete with highly developed microvilli, consistent with a major site of transfer between amnionic fluid and amnion (Fig. 3–23). They also are active metabolically; for example, these epithelial cells are the site of tissue inhibitor of metalloproteinase-1 synthesis, and produce PGE_2 and fetal fibronectin (Rowe and colleagues, 1997). In term pregnancies, the expression of prostaglandin endoperoxide H synthase in amnion has been shown to correlate with elevated fetal fibronectin (Mijovic and co-workers, 2000). As a site of prostaglandin production, the amnionic epithelium participates in the so-called final common pathway of initiation of labor. The epithelial cells may respond to signals derived from the fetus or the mother, and they have been shown to be responsive to a variety of potential endocrine or paracrine modulators. These include oxytocin and vasopressin, which increase PGE_2 production in vitro (Moore and associates, 1988). They may also produce cytokines during the initiation of labor, such as IL-8 (Elliott and colleagues, 2001).

The amnionic epithelium also synthesizes vasoactive peptides, including the vasoconstrictor endothelin as well as the

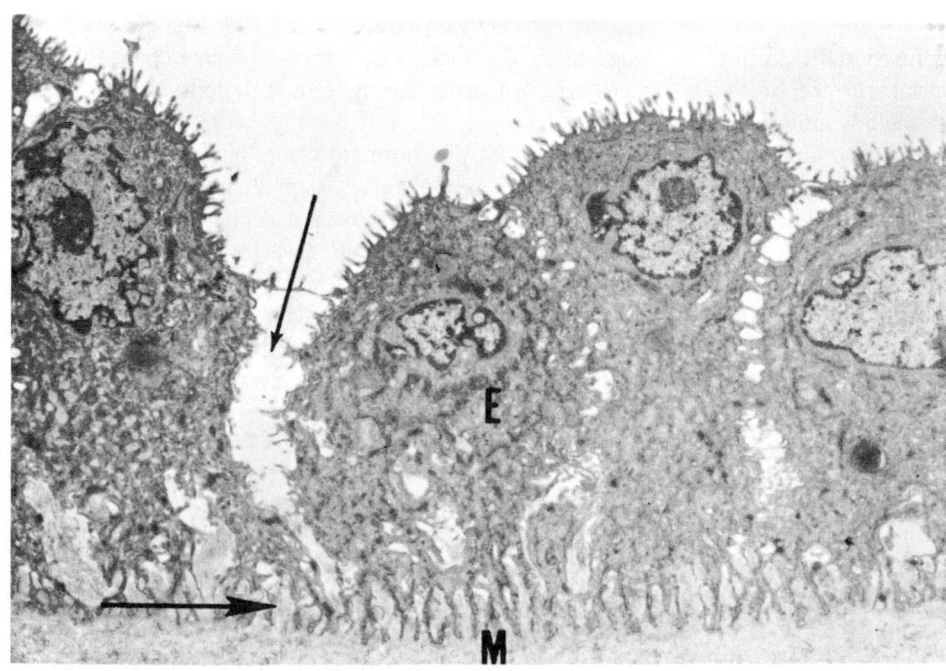

FIGURE 3–23. Electron micrograph of human amnion at term. Epithelium (E) and mesenchyme (M) are shown. Thin arrow indicates intercellular space. Thick arrow points to specializations of basal plasma membranes. (Courtesy of Dr. Ralph M. Wynn.)

vasodilator parathyroid hormone–related protein (Economos and colleagues, 1992; Germain and colleagues, 1992). Amnionic epithelium also produces brain natriuretic peptide and corticotropin-releasing hormone (CRH), which are peptides that are smooth muscle relaxants (Riley and colleagues, 1991; Warren and Silverman, 1995). Thus, the vasoactive peptides produced in amnion may gain access to the adventitial surface of the chorionic vessels. These findings suggest that the placental amnion could be involved in modulating chorionic vessel tone and blood flow. These amnion-derived vasoactive peptides also function in other tissues in diverse physiological processes, including the promotion of cell replication and calcium metabolism. After secretion from the amnion, these bioactive agents can enter amnionic fluid and thereby are available to the fetus by swallowing and fetal thoracic movements.

Amnion Mesenchymal Cells. The mesenchymal cells of the fibroblast layer of amnion are also responsible for major amnion functions. The synthesis of interstitial collagens that make up the compact layer of the amnion, the source of the majority of tensile strength of this membrane, takes place in mesenchymal cells (Casey and MacDonald, 1996). These cells also are highly capable of synthesizing cytokines that include IL-6, IL-8, and monocyte chemoattractant protein-1 (MCP-1). Their synthesis is increased in response to bacterial toxins and IL-1. This functional capacity of amnion mesenchymal cells is an important consideration in the study of amnionic fluid for evidence of labor-associated accumulation of inflammatory mediators (Garcia-Velasco and Arici, 1999). Studies in which isolation of amnion mesenchymal cells from epithelial cells was used demonstrated that the mesenchymal cells may be a far greater source of PGE_2 than epithelial cells (Whittle and colleagues, 2000).

Amnion Anatomy. Reflected amnion is fused to the chorion laeve. Placental amnion covers the fetal surface of the placenta, and thereby is in contact with the adventitial surface of the chorionic vessels. Umbilical amnion covers the umbilical cord. In the conjoined portion of the membranes of diamnionic-dichorionic twin placentas, the fused amnions are separated by fused chorion laeve. Thus, aside from the small area of the membranes immediately over the cervical os, this is the only site at which the reflected chorion laeve is not contiguous with decidua. With diamnionic-monochorionic placentas, there is no intervening tissue between the fused amnions of each twin.

Amnion Tensile Strength. Over 135 years ago, Matthew Duncan examined the nature of the forces involved in fetal membrane rupture. During tests of tensile strength—resistance to tearing and rupture—he found that the decidua and then the chorion laeve gave way long before the amnion ruptured. Indeed, the membranes are quite elastic and can expand to twice normal size during pregnancy (Benirschke and

Kaufmann, 2000). The amnion provides the major strength of the membranes. Moreover, the tensile strength of amnion resides almost exclusively in the compact layer, which is composed of cross-linked interstitial collagens I and III and lesser amounts of collagens V and VI.

Interstitial Collagens. Collagens are the major macromolecules of most connective tissues and the most abundant proteins in the body. Collagen I is the major interstitial collagen in tissues characterized by great tensile strength, such as bone and tendon. In other tissues, collagen III is believed to make a unique contribution to tissue integrity, serving to increase tissue extensibility and tensile strength. For example, the ratio of collagen III to collagen I in the walls of a number of highly extensible tissues—amnionic sac, blood vessels, urinary bladder, bile ducts, intestine, and gravid uterus—is greater than that in nonelastic tissues. Although collagen III provides some of the extensibility of this membrane, elastin microfibrils have been identified (Bryant-Greenwood, 1998). Another unique structural feature of interstitial collagens important to amnion integrity is resistance to proteolytic degradation (Jeffrey, 1991).

Metabolic Functions. The amnion is clearly more than a simple avascular membrane that functions to contain amnionic fluid. It is metabolically active, involved in solute and water transport to maintain amnionic fluid homeostasis, and produces a variety of bioactive compounds, including vasoactive peptides, growth factors, and cytokines. The amnion is responsive both acutely and chronically to mechanical stretch, which alters amnionic gene expression (Nemeth and colleagues, 2000). This in turn potentially triggers both autocrine and paracrine responses, such as increased production of matrix metalloproteinases, IL-8 production, and collagenase activity (Bryant-Greenwood, 1998; Maradny and colleagues, 1996). Such factors may modulate changes in the membrane properties during term or preterm labor.

Amnionic Fluid. The normally clear fluid that collects within the amnionic cavity increases as pregnancy progresses until about 34 weeks, when there is a decrease in volume. An average volume of about 1000 mL is found at term, although this may vary widely from a few milliliters to many liters in abnormal conditions. The origin, composition, circulation, and function of the amnionic fluid are discussed further in Chapters 11 and 31.

UMBILICAL CORD AND RELATED STRUCTURES

Cord Development. The yolk sac and the umbilical vesicle into which it develops are quite prominent early in pregnancy. At first, the embryo is a flattened disc interposed between amnion and yolk sac (see Fig. 3–12). Because the dorsal surface grows faster than the ventral surface, in association with the elongation of the neural tube, the embryo bulges into the

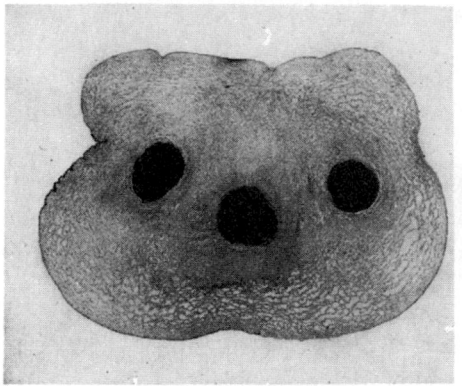
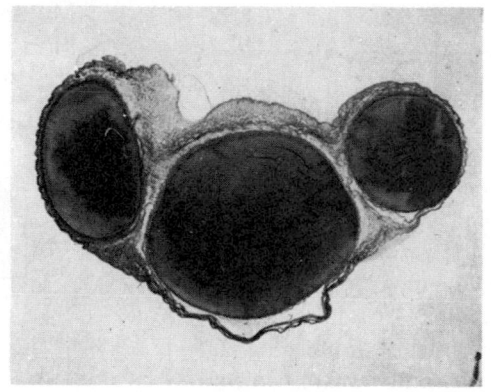

A   **B**

FIGURE 3–24. A. Cross-section of umbilical cord fixed after blood vessels had been emptied. The umbilical vein, carrying oxygenated blood to the fetus, is in the center; on either side are two umbilical arteries carrying deoxygenated blood from the fetus to the placenta. **B.** Cross-section of the same umbilical cord shown in **A**, but through a segment from which the blood vessels had not been emptied. This photograph represents more accurately the conditions in utero. (From Reynolds, 1954.)

amnionic sac and the dorsal part of the yolk sac is incorporated into the body of the embryo to form the gut. The allantois projects into the base of the body stalk from the caudal wall of the yolk sac or, later, from the anterior wall of the hindgut.

As pregnancy advances, the yolk sac becomes smaller and its pedicle relatively longer. By about the middle of the third month, the expanding amnion obliterates the exocoelom, fuses with the chorion laeve, and covers the bulging placental disc and the lateral surface of the body stalk. The latter is then called the *umbilical cord,* or *funis.* Remnants of the exocoelom in the anterior portion of the cord may contain loops of intestine, which continue to develop outside the embryo. Although the loops are later withdrawn into the peritoneal cavity, the apex of the midgut loop retains its connection with the attenuated vitelline duct.

The cord at term normally has two arteries and one vein. The right umbilical vein usually disappears early during fetal development, leaving only the original left vein. Sections of any portion of the cord frequently reveal, near the center, the small duct of the umbilical vesicle, lined by a single layer of flattened or cuboidal epithelial cells. In sections just beyond the umbilicus, but never at the placental end of the cord, another duct representing the allantoic remnant is occasionally found. The intra-abdominal portion of the duct of the umbilical vesicle, which extends from umbilicus to intestine, usually atrophies and disappears, but occasionally it remains patent, forming a Meckel diverticulum. The most common vascular anomaly is the absence of one umbilical artery (see Chap. 27, p. 626).

Cord Structure and Function. The umbilical cord, or funis, extends from the fetal umbilicus to the fetal surface of the placenta or chorionic plate. Its exterior is dull white, moist, and covered by amnion, through which three umbilical

vessels may be seen. Its diameter is 0.8 to 2.0 cm, with an average length of 55 cm and a range of 30 to 100 cm. Generally, cord length less than 30 cm is considered abnormally short (Benirschke and Kaufmann, 2000). Folding and tortuosity of the vessels, which are longer than the cord itself, frequently create nodulations on the surface, or false knots, which are essentially varices. The extracellular matrix is a specialized connective tissue referred to as *Wharton jelly* (Fig. 3–24A). After fixation, the umbilical vessels appear empty, but Figure 3–24B more accurately is representative of the situation in vivo, when the vessels are not emptied of blood. The two arteries are smaller in diameter than the vein. The mesoderm of the cord, which is of allantoic origin, fuses with that of the amnion.

Blood flows from the umbilical vein by two routes—the ductus venosus, which empties directly into the inferior vena cava, and numerous smaller openings into the fetal hepatic circulation—and then into the inferior vena cava by the hepatic vein. The blood takes the path of least resistance through these alternate routes. Resistance in the ductus venosus is controlled by a sphincter situated at the origin of the ductus at the umbilical recess and innervated by a branch of the vagus nerve.

Anatomically, the umbilical cord can be regarded as a component of the fetal membranes. The vessels contained in the cord are characterized by spiraling or twisting. The spiraling may occur in a clockwise (dextral) or anticlockwise (sinistral) direction. The anticlockwise spiral is present in 50 to 90 percent of cases. It is believed that the spiraling serves to prevent clamping, which occurs in all hollow cylinders subjected to torsion. Boyd and Hamilton (1970) note that these twists are not truly spirals, but rather they are cylindrical helices in which a constant curvature is maintained equidistant from the central axis. Benirschke and Kaufmann (2000) reported that 11 is the average number of helices in the cord.

PLACENTAL HORMONES

The production of steroid and protein hormones by human trophoblasts is greater in amount and diversity than that of any single endocrine tissue in all of mammalian physiology. A compendium of the average production rates for various steroid hormones in nonpregnant and in near-term pregnant women is given in Table 3–1. It is apparent that the alterations in steroid hormone production that accompany normal human pregnancy are incredible. The human placenta also synthesizes an enormous amount of protein and peptide hormones: as much as 1 gram of placental lactogen (hPL) every 24 hours, massive quantities of chorionic gonadotropin (hCG), adrenocorticotropin (ACTH), growth hormone variant (hGH-V), parathyroid hormone–related protein (PTH-rP), calcitonin, relaxin, inhibins, activins, and atrial natriuretic peptide, as well as a variety of hypothalamic-like releasing and inhibiting hormones such as thyrotropin-releasing hormone (TRH), gonadotropin-releasing hormone (GnRH), corticotropin-releasing hormone (CRH), somatostatin, and growth hormone–releasing hormone (GHRH).

It is understandable, therefore, that yet another remarkable feature of human pregnancy is the success of the physiological adaptations of pregnant women to the unique endocrine milieu (see Chap. 6). The anatomical parts of the placental arm of the fetal–maternal endocrine communication system are illustrated in Figure 3–25.

HUMAN CHORIONIC GONADOTROPIN (hCG). The so-called pregnancy hormone is a glycoprotein with biological activity very similar to luteinizing hormone (LH), both of which act via the plasma membrane LH–hCG receptor. HCG is produced almost exclusively in the placenta but also is synthesized in fetal kidney, and a number of fetal tissues may

TABLE 3–1 Steroid Production Rates in Nonpregnant and Near-Term Pregnant Woman

	Production Rates (mg/24 hr)	
Steroid[a]	Nonpregnant	Pregnant
17β-Estradiol	0.1–0.6	15–20
Estriol	0.02–0.1	50–150
Progesterone	0.1–40	250–600
Aldosterone	0.05–0.1	0.250–0.600
Deoxycorticosterone	0.05–0.5	1–12
Cortisol	10–30	10–20

[a] Estrogens and progesterone are produced by the placenta. Aldosterone is produced by the maternal adrenal gland in response to the stimulus of angiotensin II. Deoxycorticosterone is produced in extraglandular tissue sites by way of the 21-hydroxylation of plasma progesterone. Cortisol production during pregnancy is not increased, even though the blood levels are elevated because of decreased clearance caused by increased cortisol-binding globulin.

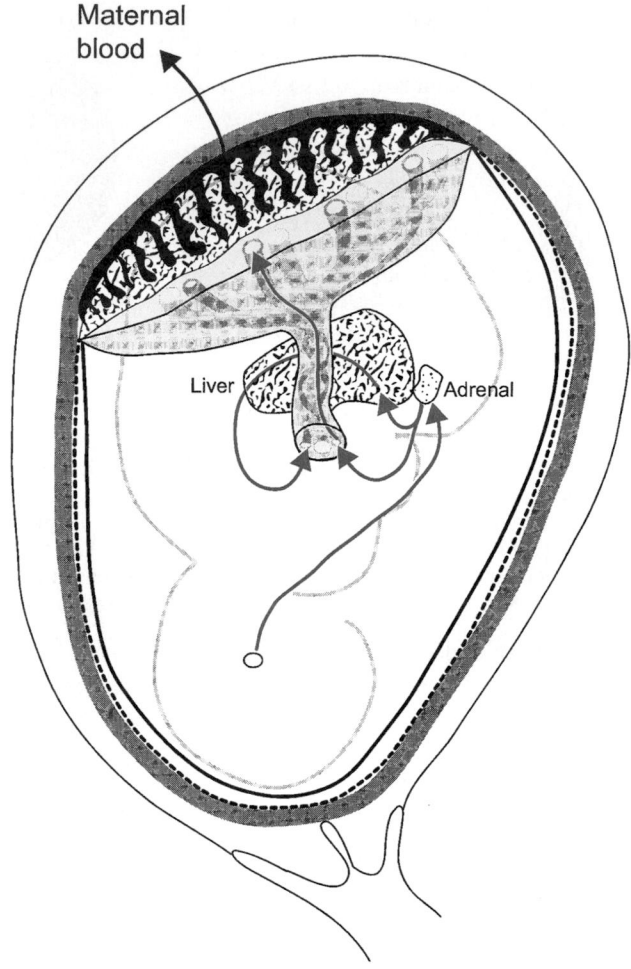

FIGURE 3–25. Anatomical parts of the endocrine component of the placental arm of the fetal–maternal communication system. Adrenocorticotropin hormone from the fetal pituitary gland stimulates fetal adrenal steroidogenesis. Fetal adrenal dehydroepiandrosterone sulfate and 16α-hydroxydehydroepiandrosterone sulfate are transported to the placenta and converted to 17β-estradiol and estriol, respectively. Fetal liver is the major site of production of low-density lipoprotein (LDL) cholesterol, the principal precursor for fetal adrenal steroidogenesis. Cholesterol, derived from LDL in maternal plasma, serves as the precursor for progesterone biosynthesis in the placenta.

produce the β-subunit or intact hCG molecule (McGregor and associates, 1981, 1983).

Various malignant tumors also produce hCG, sometimes in large amounts—especially trophoblastic neoplasms. Chorionic gonadotropin is produced in very small amounts in tissues of men and nonpregnant women, perhaps primarily in the anterior pituitary gland. Nonetheless, the detection of hCG in blood or urine is almost always indicative of pregnancy (see Chap. 8, p. 206).

Chemical Characteristics. Chorionic gonadotropin is a glycoprotein (molecular weight 36,000 to 40,000 d) with the highest carbohydrate (30 percent) content of any human hormone. The carbohydrate component, and especially the terminal sialic acid, protects the molecule from catabolism. The 36-hour plasma half-life of intact hCG is much longer than the 2 hours for LH. The hCG molecule is composed of two dissimilar subunits, designated α (92 amino acids) and β (145 amino acids), which are noncovalently linked. They are held together by electrostatic and hydrophobic forces that can be separated in vitro. Isolated subunits are unable to bind the LH receptor and thus lack biological activity.

This hormone is structurally related to three other glycoprotein hormones—LH, FSH, and TSH. The amino-acid sequence of the α-subunits of all four glycoproteins is identical. The β-subunits, although sharing certain similarities, are characterized by distinctly different amino-acid sequences. Recombination of an α- and a β-subunit of the four glycoprotein hormones gives a molecule with biological activity characteristic of the hormone from which the β-subunit was derived.

Biosynthesis. The synthesis of the α- and the β-chains of hCG is regulated separately. A single gene located on chromosome 6 encodes the α-subunit of all four glycoprotein hormones—hCG, LH, FSH, and TSH. There are seven separate genes on chromosome 19 for the β-hCG–β-LH family. Six of these genes code for β-hCG and one for β-LH, but only three of the β-hCG genes are expressed at significant levels (Miller-Lindholm and colleagues, 1997). Both the α- and β-subunits of hCG are synthesized as larger molecular weight precursors, which are cleaved by microsomal endopeptidases. Once intact hCG is assembled, the molecule is rapidly released from the cell through exocytosis of secretory granules (Morrish and colleagues, 1987).

Cellular Origin of hCG. The origin of hCG appears to vary depending on the time in gestation. At less than 5 weeks, hCG expression is observed in both syncytiotrophoblast and cytotrophoblast cells (Maruo and colleagues, 1992). Later in gestation, when maternal serum levels are at their peak, hCG is produced almost solely in the syncytiotrophoblast (Beck and colleagues, 1986; Kurman and colleagues, 1984). The amounts of hCG mRNA for both α- and β-subunits in syncytiotrophoblast from the first trimester are greater than at term, which may be an important consideration when used as a screening procedure to identify abnormal fetuses (Hoshina and co-workers, 1982).

Molecular Forms of hCG in Plasma and Urine. There are multiple forms of hCG in maternal plasma and urine. Some of these arise as the result of enzymatic degradation, and others are accounted for by modifications during the normal cellular sequence of synthesis and processing of the hCG molecule. The multiple forms of hCG vary enormously in bioactivity and immunoreactivity.

FREE SUBUNITS. The levels of circulating free β-subunit are low to undetectable throughout pregnancy. In part, this is the result of the rate-limiting synthesis of the β-subunit. Free α-subunits that do not combine with the β-subunit are found in the placenta and in maternal plasma. Plasma levels of free α-subunits increase gradually, but steadily, until about 36 weeks, when a plateau is maintained for the remainder of pregnancy. Thus, the secretion of α-hCG roughly corresponds to placental mass, whereas the rate of secretion of the complete hCG molecule is maximal at 8 to 10 weeks' gestation. The plasma concentration of α-hCG, although a minor portion of intact hCG at 10 weeks, can represent 30 to 50 percent during the last trimester (Cole, 1997).

NICKS IN THE hCG MOLECULE. A portion of hCG molecules in serum and urine, as well as purified standard preparations, has been shown to contain so-called nicks, or missing peptide linkages. These nicks occur primarily between β-subunit amino acids 44–45 and 47–48. The extent of nicking in standard preparations from pooled urine is 10 to 20 percent, but in individual samples it varies from 0 to 100 percent (Cole and colleagues, 1991a,b). Their origin is believed to be through enzymatic action on the molecule near the cellular site of β-subunit synthesis. Nicked forms of hCG predominate in cases of gestational trophoblastic neoplasia such as hydatidiform mole or choriocarcinoma (Cole and Butler, 2002). The biological importance of these nicked molecules is unknown but can be an issue of some concern as their detection by commercial immunoassays for hCG is variable (Cole, 1997).

Concentrations of hCG in Serum and Urine. The intact hCG molecule is detectable in plasma of pregnant women about 7 to 9 days after the midcycle surge of LH that precedes ovulation. Thus, it is likely that hCG enters maternal blood at the time of blastocyst implantation. Blood levels increase rapidly, doubling every 2 days, with maximal levels being attained at about 8 to 10 weeks' gestation (Fig. 3–26). Appreciable fluctuations in the levels of plasma hCG are observed on the same day, and evidence has accrued that the trophoblast secretion of protein hormones is episodic (Barnea and Kaplan, 1989; Diaz-Cueto and colleagues, 1994).

Because hCG circulates as multiple highly related isoforms with variable cross-reactivity between commercial assays, there is considerable variation in calculated serum hCG levels among the more than 100 assays. Peak levels reach about 100,000 mIU/mL between the 60th and 80th days after the last menses (see Fig. 3–26). Beginning at about 10 to 12 weeks' gestation, maternal plasma levels of hCG begin to decline, and a nadir is reached by about 20 weeks. Plasma levels are maintained at this lower level for the remainder of pregnancy.

The pattern of appearance of hCG in fetal blood is similar to that in the mother, however, fetal plasma levels are only about 3 percent of those in maternal plasma. The hCG concentration in amnionic fluid early in pregnancy is similar to that in maternal plasma. As pregnancy progresses, the hCG

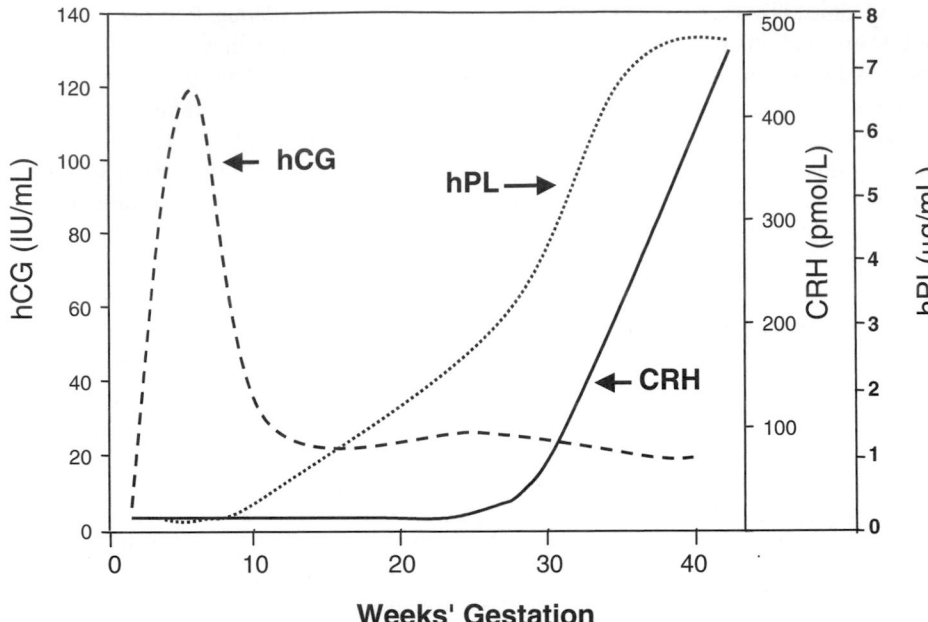

FIGURE 3–26. Distinct profiles for the concentrations of human chorionic gonadotropin (hCG), human placental lactogen (hPL), and corticotropin-releasing hormone (CRH) in serum of women throughout normal pregnancy.

concentration in amnionic fluid declines, so that near term, the levels are only one fifth those in maternal plasma.

Maternal urine hCG also can be monitored and is composed of a variety of degradation products. The primary form of hCG in urine is the terminal degradation product of hCG, the β-core fragment. Its concentrations follow the same general pattern as that in maternal plasma, peaking at about 10 weeks. It is important, however, to recognize that the so-called β-subunit antibody used in most pregnancy tests reacts with both intact hCG, the major form in the plasma, and with fragments of hCG, the major forms found in urine.

Elevated or Depressed hCG Levels in Maternal Plasma or Urine. Significantly higher plasma levels of hCG are sometimes found in women pregnant with multiple fetuses or with a single erythroblastotic fetus resulting from maternal D-antigen isoimmunization. The levels of hCG in plasma and urine may be increased strikingly in women with hydatidiform mole or choriocarcinoma. Relatively higher levels of plasma hCG may be found at midtrimester in women carrying a fetus with Down syndrome, and this finding can be used in biochemical screening tests (see Chap. 13, p. 323). The reason for this is not clear, but it has been speculated that the placentas in these pregnancies are less mature compared with those associated with normal fetuses. Relatively lower levels of hCG in plasma are found with ectopic pregnancies and impending spontaneous abortion.

Regulation of hCG Synthesis. Placental GnRH is likely involved in the regulation of hCG formation. Both GnRH and its receptor are expressed on cytotrophoblasts and syncytiotrophoblast (Wolfahrt and colleagues, 1998). GnRH administration elevates circulating hCG levels, and cultured trophoblast cells respond to GnRH treatment with increased hCG secretion (Iwashita and colleagues, 1993; Siler-Khodr and Khodr, 1981). Pituitary production of GnRH also is regulated by levels of inhibin and activin. In cultured placental cells, activin stimulates and inhibin inhibits the production of GnRH and hCG production, supporting a role for these factors (Petraglia and colleagues, 1989; Steele and colleagues, 1993).

Metabolic Clearance of hCG. The renal clearance of hCG accounts for 30 percent of metabolic clearance and the remainder is cleared by other pathways, likely by metabolism in the liver and kidney (Wehmann and Nisula, 1980). Clearances of β-subunit and α-subunit are about 10-fold and 30-fold, respectively, greater than that of intact hCG. By contrast, renal clearance of these subunits is considerably lower than that of dimeric hCG.

Biological Functions of hCG. Both subunits of hCG are required for normal binding to the LH–hCG receptor in the corpus luteum and the testis. LH–hCG receptors are present in a variety of tissues, and their role there is less defined. The best-known biological function of hCG is the so-called *rescue and maintenance of function of the corpus luteum*—that is, continued progesterone production. Bradbury and colleagues (1950) found that the progesterone-producing life span of the corpus luteum of menstruation could be prolonged perhaps for 2 weeks by hCG administration. This action provides only an incomplete explanation for its physiological role in pregnancy. The maximum plasma hCG concentrations are attained well after hCG-stimulated corpus luteum secretion of progesterone has ceased. Specifically, progesterone luteal synthesis begins to decline at about 6 weeks despite continued and increasing hCG production.

Chorionic gonadotropin stimulates fetal testicular testosterone secretion that is maximum at approximately the same time that maximal levels of hCG are attained. Thus, at a critical time in sexual differentiation of the male fetus, hCG enters fetal plasma from the syncytiotrophoblast, acts as an LH surrogate, and stimulates replication of testicular Leydig cells and testosterone synthesis to *promote male sexual differentiation* (see Chap. 4, p. 113). Before about 110 days, there is no vascularization of the fetal anterior pituitary from the hypothalamus, and thus little LH secretion from the pituitary. HCG acts as LH before this time. Thereafter, as hCG levels fall, pituitary LH maintains a more modest level of fetal testicular stimulation.

There is hCG stimulation of the maternal thyroid gland. In some women with hydatidiform mole or choriocarcinoma, biochemical and clinical evidence of hyperthyroidism sometimes develops (see Chap. 11, p. 277). For a time, this was believed to be due to the formation of *chorionic thyrotropins* by neoplastic trophoblasts. Later, however, it was shown that some forms of hCG bind to the TSH receptors of thyroid cells (Hershman, 1999). Additionally, treatment of normal men with hCG increases thyroid activity. The thyroid-stimulatory activity in plasma of first-trimester pregnant women varies appreciably from sample to sample. Modifications in the oligosaccharides of hCG seem to be important in establishing the capacity of hCG to stimulate thyroid function. Some of the acidic isoforms of hCG stimulate thyroid activity, and some more basic forms also stimulate iodine uptake (Kraiem and colleagues, 1994; Tsuruta and colleagues, 1995; Yoshimura and colleagues, 1994). There is also evidence that the LH–hCG receptor is expressed in the thyroid (Tomer and colleagues, 1992). Thus, the possibility exists that hCG stimulates thyroid activity via the LH–hCG receptor and by the TSH receptor as well.

Other functions include *promotion of relaxin secretion by the corpus luteum* (Duffy and co-workers, 1996). LH–hCG receptors are found in myometrium and in uterine vascular tissue, and it has been hypothesized that hCG may act to *promote uterine vascular vasodilatation and myometrial smooth muscle relaxation* (Kurtzman and colleagues, 2001).

HUMAN PLACENTAL LACTOGEN (hPL). Prolactin-like activity in the human placenta was first described by Ehrhardt in 1936. The protein responsible for this activity was isolated from extracts of human placenta and retroplacental blood (Ito and Higashi, 1961; Josimovich and MacLaren, 1962). Because of the potent lactogenic and growth hormone–like bioactivity, as well as an immunochemical resemblance to human growth hormone, it was first called human placental lactogen or chorionic growth hormone. It also has been referred to as chorionic somatomammotropin. Recently, most authors have used the original name, human placental lactogen (hPL). Grumbach and Kaplan (1964) found, by immunofluorescence studies, that this hormone, like hCG, was concentrated in the syncytiotrophoblast. It is detected in the trophoblast as early as the second or third week after fertilization of the ovum. As with hCG, hPL also is identified in cytotrophoblasts from before 6 weeks (Maruo and associates, 1992).

Chemical Characteristics. Placental lactogen is a single nonglycosylated polypeptide chain with a molecular weight of 22,279 daltons. It is derived from a precursor of 25,000 daltons that contains a 26-amino-acid signal sequence. There are 191 amino-acid residues in placental lactogen, compared with 188 in human growth hormone (hGH). The amino acid sequence in each hormone is strikingly similar, with 96-percent homology. HPL also is structurally similar to human prolactin (hPRL), with an amino-acid sequence similarity of about 67 percent. For these reasons, it has been suggested that the genes for hPL, hPRL, and hGH evolved from a common ancestral gene—probably that of prolactin—by repeated gene duplication (Ogren and Talamantes, 1994).

Gene Structure and Expression. There are five genes in the growth hormone–placental lactogen gene cluster that are linked and located on chromosome 17. Two of these genes, *hPL2* and *hPL3*, both encode hPL, and the amount of mRNA in the term placenta is similar for each. In contrast, the prolactin gene is located on chromosome 6 (Owerbach and colleagues, 1980, 1981). *The production rate of hPL near term, about 1 g/day, is the greatest, by far, of any known hormone in humans.*

Serum Concentration. HPL is demonstrable in the placenta within 5 to 10 days after conception and can be detected in maternal serum as early as 3 weeks after fertilization. Maternal plasma concentration rises steadily until about 34 to 36 weeks and this rise is linked mainly to placental mass. The serum concentration reaches higher levels in late pregnancy (5 to 15 μg/mL) than those of any other known protein hormone (see Fig. 3–26). The half-life of hPL in maternal plasma is between 10 and 30 minutes (Walker and co-workers, 1991).

Very little hPL is detected in fetal blood or in the urine of the mother or newborn. Amnionic fluid levels are somewhat lower than in maternal plasma. Because hPL is secreted primarily into the maternal circulation, with only very small amounts in cord blood, it appears that the role of the hormone in pregnancy, if any, is mediated through actions in maternal rather than in fetal tissues. Nonetheless, there is continuing interest in the possibility that hPL serves select functions in fetal growth.

Regulation of hPL Biosynthesis. The levels of mRNA for hPL in syncytiotrophoblast remain relatively constant throughout pregnancy. This finding is supportive of the idea that the rate of hPL secretion is proportional to placental mass. There are very high plasma levels of hCG in women with trophoblastic neoplasms, but only low levels of hPL in these same women.

Prolonged maternal starvation in the first half of pregnancy leads to an increase in the plasma concentration of hPL. Short-term changes in plasma glucose or insulin, however, have relatively little effect on plasma levels of hPL. In vitro studies using human syncytiotrophoblast suggest that the synthesis of hPL is stimulated by insulin and insulin-like growth factor-1 and inhibited by PGE_2 and $PGF_{2\alpha}$ (Bhaumick and colleagues, 1987; Genbacev and colleagues, 1977).

Metabolic Actions. HPL has putative actions in a number of important metabolic processes. These include:

1. *Maternal lipolysis* and an increase in the levels of circulating free fatty acids, thereby providing a source of energy for maternal metabolism and fetal nutrition.
2. *An anti-insulin or "diabetogenic" action,* leading to an increase in maternal levels of insulin, which favors protein synthesis and provides a readily available source of amino acids for transport to the fetus.
3. *A potent angiogenic hormone*; it also may play an important role in the formation of fetal vasculature (Corbacho and co-workers, 2002).

OTHER PLACENTAL PROTEIN HORMONES

Chorionic Adrenocorticotropin. ACTH, lipotropin, and β-endorphin—all proteolytic products of proopiomelanocortin—are recovered in placental extracts (Genazzani and colleagues, 1975; Odagiri and colleagues, 1979). The physiological role of placental ACTH is unclear. Although maternal plasma levels of ACTH increase during pregnancy, they remain lower than those in men and nonpregnant women, except during labor (Carr and colleagues, 1981a). The placental ACTH is secreted into the mother or fetus during pregnancy, however, maternal ACTH does not cross the placenta to the fetus. Importantly, ACTH produced within the placenta is not under feedback regulation by glucocorticoid, which has been proposed as the rationale for maternal partial resistance to dexamethasone suppression (Nolten and Rueckert, 1981). Corticotropin-releasing hormone (CRH), also produced within the placenta, stimulates the synthesis and release of chorionic ACTH, and placental production of CRH is positively regulated by cortisol, producing a novel positive feedback loop. As discussed later, this system may be important for controlling fetal lung maturation and the timing of parturition.

Relaxin. Expression of relaxin has been demonstrated in human corpus luteum, decidua, and placenta (Bogic and colleagues, 1995). This peptide is synthesized as a single 105 amino-acid preprorelaxin molecule that is cleaved to A and B molecules. Relaxin is structurally similar to insulin and insulin-like growth factor. There are three relaxin genes—H1, H2, and H3—but only H2 and H3 are transcribed in the corpus luteum (Bathgate and associates, 2002; Hudson and colleagues, 1983, 1984). Other tissues, including decidua, placenta, and fetal membranes, express H1 and H2 (Hansell and colleagues, 1991).

The rise in maternal circulating relaxin seen in early pregnancy is attributed to secretion by the corpus luteum, and levels parallel those seen for hCG. The uterine relaxin receptor was recently cloned, which should allow the role of relaxin gene family members to be defined (Hsu and colleagues, 2002). It has been proposed that relaxin along with rising progesterone levels acts on myometrial smooth muscle to promote uterine relaxation and the quiescence observed in early pregnancy (see Chap. 6, p. 163). In addition, the production of relaxin and relaxin-like factors within the placenta and fetal membranes is believed to play an autocrine–paracrine role in regulation of extracellular matrix degradation in the puerperium (Qin and colleagues, 1997a, 1997b).

Parathyroid Hormone-Related Protein (PTH-rP). Circulating levels of PTH-rP are significantly elevated in pregnancy within the maternal but not fetal circulation (Bertelloni and colleagues, 1994; Saxe and colleagues, 1997). Although not clear, many potential functions of this hormone have been proposed. The synthesis of PTH-rP has been demonstrated in several normal adult tissues, especially in reproductive organs, including the myometrium, endometrium, corpus luteum, and lactating mammary tissue. PTH-rP is not produced in the parathyroid glands of normal adults. Placental-derived PTH-rP may have an important autocrine–paracrine role within the fetal–maternal unit as well as on the adjacent myometrium. In the placenta, it may activate receptors on the trophoblast to promote calcium transport for fetal bone growth and ossification.

Growth Hormone Variant (hGH-V). The placenta expresses a growth hormone variant that is not expressed in the pituitary. The gene encoding hGH-V is located in the hGH–hPL gene cluster on chromosome 17. Sometimes referred to as placental growth hormone, hGH-V is a 191-amino-acid protein that differs in 15 amino-acid positions from the sequence for hGH. Placental hGH-V presumably is synthesized in the syncytium, but its pattern of synthesis and secretion during gestation is not precisely known because antibodies against hGH-V cross-react with hGH. It is believed that hGH-V is present in maternal plasma by 21 to 26 weeks, increases in concentration to about 36 weeks, and remains relatively constant thereafter. There is a correlation between the levels of hGH-V in maternal plasma and those of insulin-like growth factor-1, and the secretion of hGH-V by trophoblasts in vitro is inhibited by glucose in a dose-dependent manner (Patel and colleagues, 1995). Overexpression of hGH-V in mice causes severe insulin resistance, and thus it is a likely candidate to mediate insulin resistance of pregnancy (Barbour and associates, 2002).

HYPOTHALAMIC-LIKE RELEASING HORMONES.

For each of the known hypothalamic-releasing or -inhibiting hormones described—GnRH, TRH, CRH, GHRH, and somatostatin—there is an analogous hormone produced in human placenta (Petraglia and colleagues, 1992; Siler-Khodr, 1988). Many investigators have proposed that these substances in placental tissue are indicative of a hierarchy of control in the synthesis of chorionic trophic agents.

Gonadotropin-Releasing Hormone (GnRH). There is a reasonably large amount of immunoreactive GnRH in the placenta (Siler-Khodr, 1988; Siler-Khodr and Khodr, 1978). Interestingly, immunoreactive GnRH was present in cytotrophoblasts but not in the syncytiotrophoblast. Gibbons and co-workers (1975) and Khodr and Siler-Khodr (1980) demonstrated that the human placenta could synthesize both GnRH and TRH in vitro. Placental-derived GnRH functions to regulate trophoblast production of hCG, which is supported by the observation that GnRH levels are higher early in pregnancy. Placental-derived GnRH is also the likely cause of the elevation of maternal levels of circulating GnRH that are seen early in pregnancy (Siler-Khodr and colleagues, 1984).

Corticotropin-Releasing Hormone (CRH). This hormone is a member of a larger family of CRH-related peptides, which includes CRH, urocortin, urocortin II, and urocortin III (Dautzenberg and Hauger, 2002). CRH is produced in nonpregnant women and circulates at the relatively low level of 5 to 10 pmol/L. During pregnancy, levels are significantly elevated and increase to about 100 pmol/L in the early third trimester and to almost 500 pmol/L abruptly during the last 5 to 6 weeks (see Fig. 3–26) (Goland and associates, 1988). Urocortin also is produced by the placenta and secreted into the maternal circulation, but at much lower levels than seen for CRH (Florio and co-workers, 2002). After labor begins, maternal plasma CRH levels increase further by about two- to threefold (Petraglia and colleagues, 1989, 1990).

The biological function of CRH synthesized in the placenta, fetal membranes, and decidua is beginning to be defined. Receptors for CRH are present in many tissues: placenta, adrenal gland, sympathetic ganglia, lymphocytes, gastrointestinal tract, pancreas, gonads, and myometrium. Recent findings suggest that CRH can act through two major families—the type 1 and type 2 CRH receptors (CRH-R1 and CRH-R2). Trophoblast, amnion–chorion, and decidua express both CRH-R1 and CRH-R2 receptors, as well as several variant receptors (Florio and colleagues, 2000). Both CRH and urocortin can increase trophoblast ACTH secretion, supporting an autocrine–paracrine role for these hormones (Petraglia and co-workers, 1999). Large amounts of CRH from trophoblast enter the maternal blood, but there also is a large concentration of a specific CRH-binding protein in maternal plasma, and the bound CRH seems to be biologically inactive.

Other proposed biological roles include the induction of smooth muscle relaxation in vascular and myometrial tissue, and immunosuppression. The physiological reverse, however, induction of myometrial contractions, has been proposed for the rising levels of CRH seen near the end of gestation, leading to the hypothesis that CRH may be involved with the initiation of parturition (Wadhwa and colleagues, 1998). Prostaglandin formation in the placenta, amnion, chorion laeve, and decidua is increased by treatment with CRH (Jones and Challis, 1989), further supporting the potential role of CRH in the timing of parturition.

Glucocorticoids act in the hypothalamus to *inhibit CRH release,* but in the trophoblast, glucocorticoids *stimulate* CRH gene expression. Studies using trophoblast cultures show two- to fivefold increases in CRH mRNA and protein after treatment with glucocorticoids (Jones and colleagues, 1989; Robinson and co-workers, 1988). Thus, a novel positive feedback loop has been considered in the placenta that involves placental CRH stimulation of placental ACTH formation, placental ACTH stimulation of adrenal glucocorticoid formation, and glucocorticoid stimulation of placental CRH expression (Nicholson and King, 2001; Riley and colleagues, 1991).

Growth Hormone–Releasing Hormone (GHRH). Although GHRH has been identified in human placenta, its exact function is not known (Berry and associates, 1992). Another regulator of hGH secretion called *ghrelin* recently was discovered (Horvath and colleagues, 2001). Ghrelin is expressed in the trophoblasts of first-trimester placenta and represents a potential regulator of placental growth hormone production or a paracrine regulator of differentiation (Gualillo and co-workers, 2001).

OTHER PLACENTAL PEPTIDE HORMONES

Leptin. This hormone is normally secreted by adipocytes and initially was believed to be an anti-obesity hormone that decreases food intake and body weight through its receptor in the hypothalamus. It is now known, however, that leptin also regulates bone growth and immune function (Cock and Auwerx, 2003; La Cava and colleagues, 2004). Leptin also is synthesized by both cytotrophoblast cells and syncytiotrophoblast, which explains the increase in circulating levels seen in pregnancy (Henson and Castracane, 2002). Fetal leptin levels are correlated positively with fetal birthweight and are likely to play an important role in fetal development and growth. Maternal serum levels are significantly higher than in nonpregnant women or those seen in the fetal circulation. Currently the relative contribution of leptin from maternal adipose tissue versus placenta is not well defined.

Neuropeptide Y. This small, 36-amino-acid peptide is widely distributed in brain. It also is found in sympathetic neurons innervating the cardiovascular, respiratory, gastrointestinal, and genitourinary systems. Neuropeptide Y has been isolated from placenta and localized in cytotrophoblasts (Petraglia and colleagues, 1989). Receptors for neuropeptide Y have been demonstrated in the placenta, and treatment of placental cells with neuropeptide Y causes the release of CRH (Robidoux and colleagues, 2000).

Inhibin and Activin. Inhibin is a glycoprotein hormone that acts preferentially to inhibit pituitary FSH release. It is produced by human testis and by the granulosa cells of the ovary, including the corpus luteum. Inhibin is a heterodimer with dissimilar α- and β-subunits. The inhibin β-subunit is composed of one of two distinct peptides, βA or βB. The placenta produces inhibin α-, βA-, and βB-subunits with the greatest levels present at term (Petraglia and co-workers, 1991). Placental inhibin production may serve, in conjunction with the large amounts of sex steroid hormones produced in human pregnancy, to inhibit FSH secretion and thereby preclude ovulation during pregnancy. Inhibin may act via GnRH to regulate hCG synthesis and secretion in the placenta (Petraglia and colleagues, 1987).

Activin is closely related to inhibin and is formed by the combination of the two β-subunits. Petraglia and colleagues (1994) found that serum activin A levels decline rapidly after delivery. It is not detectable in fetal blood before labor but is present in umbilical cord blood after labor begins. The receptor for activin is expressed in the placenta and amnion. Chorionic activin and inhibin may serve functions in placental metabolic processes other than GnRH synthesis, but these possibilities continue to be investigated.

PLACENTAL PROGESTERONE PRODUCTION. After 6 to 7 weeks of gestation, very little progesterone is produced in the ovary (Diczfalusy and Troen, 1961). Surgical removal of the corpus luteum or even bilateral oophorectomy during the 7th to 10th week does not cause a decrease in the rate of excretion of urinary pregnanediol, the principal urinary metabolite of progesterone. Before this time, however, removal of the corpus luteum will result in miscarriage unless an exogenous progestin is given (see Chap. 9, p. 234, and Chap. 40, p. 965). After about 8 weeks, the placenta replaces the ovary as the source of progesterone and continues to increase production such that there is a gradual increase in the levels throughout the remainder of pregnancy (Fig. 3–27). By the end of pregnancy, maternal levels of progesterone are 10 to 5000 times those in nonpregnant women, depending on the stage of the ovarian cycle (see Fig. 3–27).

Progesterone Production Rates. Isotope dilution techniques for the measurement of the rates of endogenous hormone production in humans were first applied to the study of progesterone in pregnancy (Pearlman, 1957). The daily production rate of progesterone in late, normal, singleton pregnancies is about 250 mg. The findings of numerous studies using a variety of methodologies have agreed with this value.

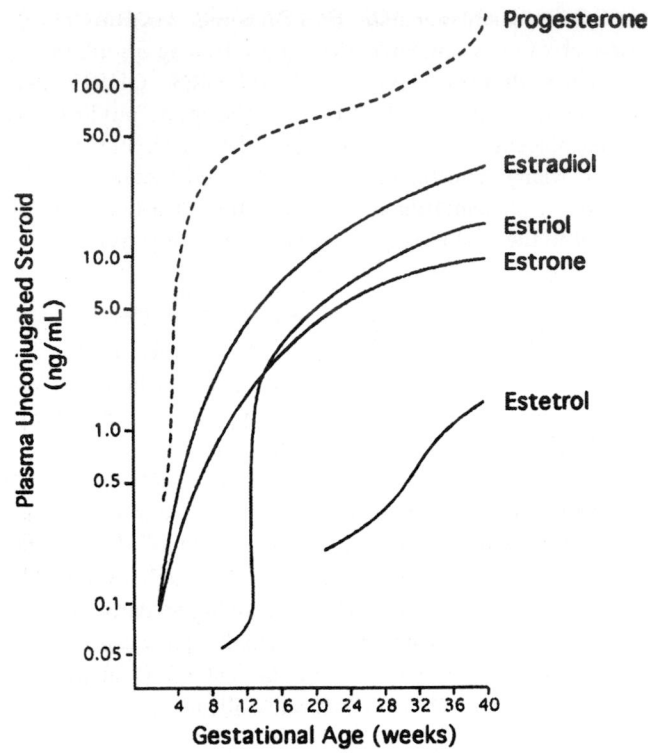

FIGURE 3–27. Plasma levels of progesterone, estradiol, estrone, estetrol, and estriol in women during the course of gestation. (From Mesiano, 2001, with permission.)

In some pregnancies with multiple fetuses, however, the daily progesterone production rate may exceed 600 mg/day.

Source of Cholesterol for Placental Progesterone Biosynthesis. Progesterone is synthesized from cholesterol in a two-step enzymatic reaction. First, cholesterol is converted to pregnenolone within the mitochondria, in a reaction catalyzed by cytochrome P450 cholesterol side-chain cleavage enzyme. Pregnenolone leaves the mitochondria and is converted to progesterone in the endoplasmic reticulum by 3β-hydroxysteroid dehydrogenase. Progesterone is not stored but is released immediately through a process of diffusion.

The placenta produces a prodigious amount of progesterone; nonetheless, there is a limited capacity for the biosynthesis of cholesterol in trophoblast. The incorporation of radiolabeled acetate into cholesterol by placental tissue proceeds at a very slow rate, and the activity of the rate-limiting enzyme in cholesterol biosynthesis, 3-hydroxy-3-methylglutaryl coenzyme A (HMG CoA) reductase, in placental tissue microsomes is low. Thus, the placenta must rely on exogenous cholesterol for progesterone formation. Bloch (1945) and Werbin and co-workers (1957) found that after the intravenous administration of radiolabeled cholesterol to pregnant women, the amount of radioactivity of urinary pregnanediol was similar to that of plasma cholesterol. Hellig and associates (1970) also found that maternal plasma cholesterol was the principal precursor (up to 90 percent) of progesterone biosynthesis in human pregnancy. The trophoblast preferentially uses LDL cholesterol for progesterone biosynthesis (Simpson and Burkhart, 1980; Simpson and colleagues, 1979). This finding was supported by studies in pregnant baboons in which maternal levels of LDL were reduced, leading to a significant drop in placental progesterone production (Henson and associates, 1997). Thus, the formation of placental progesterone occurs through the uptake and use of a maternal circulating precursor. This mechanism is unlike the placental production of estrogens, which relies principally on fetal adrenal precursors.

Progesterone Synthesis and Fetal Well-Being. Although there is a relationship between fetal well-being and placental production of estrogen, this is not the case for placental progesterone. Fetal demise, ligation of the umbilical cord with the fetus and placenta remaining in situ, and anencephaly are all conditions associated with very low maternal plasma levels and urinary excretion of estrogens. In these circumstances, there is not a concomitant decrease in progesterone until some indeterminate time after fetal death. Thus, placental endocrine function, including the formation of protein hormones such as hCG, and progesterone biosynthesis may persist for long periods (weeks) after fetal demise.

Progesterone Metabolism During Pregnancy. The metabolic clearance rate of progesterone in pregnant women is similar to that found in men and nonpregnant women. This is an important consideration in evaluating the role of progesterone in the initiation of parturition (see Chap. 6, p. 168). During pregnancy, there is a disproportionate increase in the plasma concentration of 5α-dihydroprogesterone as a result of synthesis in syncytiotrophoblast from both placenta-produced progesterone and fetal-derived precursor (Dombroski and co-workers, 1997). Thus the ratio of the concentration of this progesterone metabolite to the concentration of progesterone is increased in pregnant women. The mechanisms for this are not defined completely, but may be relevant to the resistance to pressor agents that normally develops in pregnant women (Everett and colleagues, 1978). Progesterone also is converted to the potent mineralocorticoid deoxycorticosterone in pregnant women and in the fetus. The concentration of deoxycorticosterone is increased strikingly in both the maternal and fetal compartments. The extra-adrenal formation of deoxycorticosterone from circulating progesterone accounts for the vast majority of its production in human pregnancy (Casey and MacDonald, 1982a, 1982b).

PLACENTAL ESTROGEN PRODUCTION. The placenta produces huge amounts of estrogens using blood-borne steroidal precursors from the maternal and fetal adrenal glands. Near term, normal human pregnancy is a hyperes-trogenic state of major proportions. The amount of estrogen produced each day by syncytiotrophoblast during the last few weeks of pregnancy is equivalent to that produced in 1 day by the ovaries of no fewer than 1000 ovulatory women. The hyperestrogenic state of human pregnancy is one of continually increasing magnitude as pregnancy progresses, terminating abruptly after delivery.

During the first 2 to 4 weeks of pregnancy, rising levels of hCG maintain production of estradiol in the maternal corpus luteum. The functional activity, viz., production of both progesterone and estrogens, of the maternal ovaries decreases significantly by the seventh week of pregnancy. At this time there is a luteal–placental transition such that, by the seventh week, more than 50 percent of estrogen entering the maternal circulation is produced in the placenta (MacDonald, 1965; Siiteri and MacDonald, 1963, 1966). These studies support the transition of a steroid milieu dependent on the maternal corpus luteum to one dependent on the developing placenta.

Placental Estrogen Biosynthesis. The pathways of estrogen synthesis in the human placenta differ from those in the ovary of nonpregnant women. Estrogen production in the ovary occurs in the follicular and luteal phase through the interaction of theca and granulosa cells. Specifically, androstenedione, synthesized in ovarian theca, is transferred to adjacent granulosa cells for estradiol synthesis. Estradiol production within the corpus luteum of nonpregnant women as well as in early pregnancy continues to require interaction between the luteinized theca and granulosa cells. In human trophoblast, neither cholesterol nor progesterone can serve as precursor for estrogen biosynthesis. A crucial enzyme necessary for sex steroid synthesis, steroid 17α-hydroxylase/17,20-lyase (CYP17), is not expressed in the human placenta. Consequently, the conversion of C_{21}-steroids to C_{19}-steroids, the latter being the immediate and obligatory precursors of estrogens, is not possible.

The C_{19}-steroids, dehydroepiandrosterone (DHEA) and its sulfate (DHEA-S), often are called adrenal androgens, however, these steroids can also act as estrogen precursors (Fig. 3–28). Ryan (1959a) found that there was an exceptionally high capacity of placenta to convert appropriate C_{19}-steroids to estrone and estradiol. The conversion of DHEA-S to estradiol requires placental expression of four key enzymes. First, the placenta expresses high levels of steroid sulfatase (STS), which converts the conjugated DHEA-S to DHEA. DHEA is then acted upon by 3β-hydroxysteroid dehydrogenase type 1 (3βHSD) to produce androstenedione. Cytochrome P_{450} aromatase (CYP19) then converts androstenedione to estrone, which is converted to estradiol by the enzyme 17β-hydroxysteroid dehydrogenase type 1 (17βHSD1). The principal cellular location of STS, 3βHSD, CYP19, and 17βHSD1 is in the syncytiotrophoblast (Bonenfant and colleagues, 2000b; Salido and co-workers, 1990).

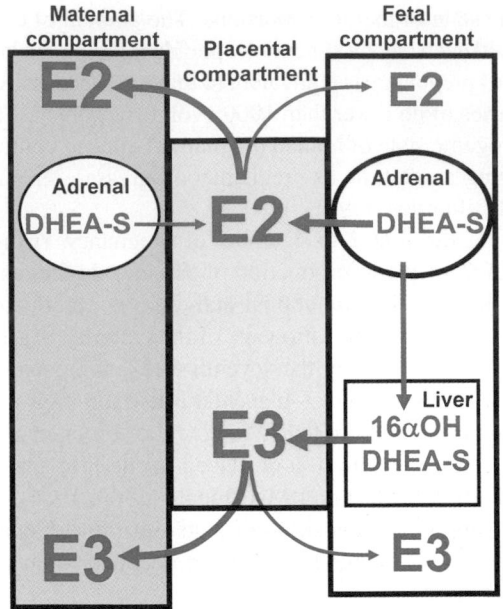

FIGURE 3–28. Schematic presentation of the biosynthesis of estrogens in the human placenta. Dehydroepiandrosterone sulfate (DHEA-S), secreted in prodigious amounts by the fetal adrenal glands, is converted to 16α-hydroxydehydroepiandrosterone sulfate (16αOHDHEA-S) in the fetal liver. These steroids, DHEA-S and 16αOHDHEA-S, are converted in the placenta to estrogens, viz., 17β-estradiol (E2) and estriol (E3). Near term, half of E2 is derived from fetal adrenal DHEA-S and half from maternal DHEA-S. On the other hand, 90 percent of E3 in the placenta arises from fetal 16αOHDHEA-S and only 10 percent from all other sources.

Plasma C₁₉-Steroids as Estrogen Precursors. Frandsen and Stakemann (1961) found that levels of urinary estrogens in women pregnant with an anencephalic fetus were only about one tenth those in urine of pregnant women with a normal fetus. Because of the characteristic absence of the fetal zone of the adrenal cortex in anencephalic fetuses, they reasoned that the glands might provide one or more substances that serve to promote placental estrogen formation. The adrenal glands of anencephalic fetuses are atrophic because of the absence of hypothalamic–pituitary function, which precludes ACTH stimulation.

In subsequent studies, radiolabeled DHEA-S infused into pregnant women was converted to radioactive urinary estrogens in high yield (Baulieu and Dray, 1963; Siiteri and MacDonald, 1963). The large amounts of DHEA-S in plasma and its much longer half-life uniquely qualify it as the principal circulating precursor for placental estradiol synthesis. Gant and co-workers (1971) found that there is a 10- to 20-fold increase in the metabolic clearance rate of plasma DHEA-S in normally pregnant women at term compared with that in men and nonpregnant women. As a consequence, there is a progressive decrease in plasma concentration of DHEA-S as pregnancy progresses (Milewich and co-workers, 1978; Siiteri and MacDonald, 1966). The increase in the metabolic clearance of plasma DHEA-S in pregnant women is

attributable to rapid use as substrate for placental estrogens. Even so, the maternal adrenal glands do not produce sufficient amounts of DHEA-S during pregnancy to account for more than a fraction of total placental estrogen biosynthesis. *The fetal adrenal glands are quantitatively the most important source of placental estrogen precursors in human pregnancy.* A schematic representation of the pathways of estrogen formation in the placenta is presented in Figure 3–28. The estrogen products released from the placenta are dependent on the nature of the substrate available. As discussed below, the nature of the estrogens produced during pregnancy reflects the unique interactions between the fetal adrenal, fetal liver, placenta, and maternal adrenal glands.

FETAL ADRENAL GLANDS. Morphologically, functionally, and physiologically, the human fetal adrenal glands are remarkable organs. Compared with adult organs, the adrenal cortex is the largest organ of the fetus. At term, the fetal adrenal glands weigh the same as those of the adult (Fig. 3–29). More than 85 percent of the fetal gland is composed of a unique fetal zone, which is not found in adults. The daily production of steroids by the fetal adrenal glands near term is estimated to be 100 to 200 mg/day. This compares with steroid secretion in resting adults of 30 to 40 mg/day, demonstrating that the fetal adrenal gland is a truly prodigious steroidogenic tissue.

Contribution to Placental Estrogen Formation. As discussed earlier, women pregnant with an anencephalic fetus excrete little urinary estrogen. This fact, together with the finding of high levels of DHEA-S in cord blood of normal newborns, was suggestive that fetal adrenal cortex is the principal source of placental estrogen precursors. The finding that

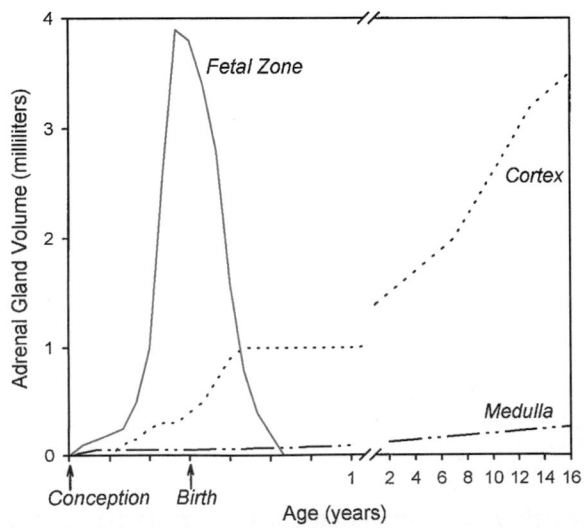

FIGURE 3–29. Size of the adrenal gland and its component parts in utero, during infancy, and during childhood. (Adapted from Bethune, 1974.)

DHEA-S in maternal plasma is converted to estrogen in placenta established this concept. Confirmation was provided by Bolté and co-workers (1964a, 1964b), who demonstrated that radiolabeled DHEA-S perfused through the placenta was converted to estradiol. Near term, about half of the estradiol produced in the placenta arises from maternal and half from fetal plasma DHEA-S (Siiteri and MacDonald, 1966).

Placental Estriol Synthesis. The estrogen products released from the placenta are dependent on the nature of the substrate available. Estradiol is but one placental estrogen secretory product and is the primary estrogen circulating at term. In addition, significant levels of estriol and estetrol are found in the maternal circulation, and they increase, particularly late in gestation. These hydroxylated forms of estrogen are produced in the placenta using substrates formed by the combined efforts of the fetal adrenal gland and liver.

An important component of the fetal–maternal communication system is the fetal liver (Fig. 3–25). The fetal liver expresses high levels of the enzyme 16α-hydroxylase, which acts on adrenal derived steroids. Ryan (1959b) and MacDonald and Siiteri (1965) found that 16α-hydroxylated C_{19}-steroids, particularly 16α-hydroxydehydroepiandrosterone (16-OHDHEA), were converted to estriol by placental tissue (Fig. 3–28). Thus, the disproportionate increase in estriol formation during pregnancy is accounted for by placental synthesis of estriol principally from plasma-borne 16-OHDHEA-S. Near term, the fetus is the source of 90 percent of the placental estriol and estetrol precursor in normal human pregnancy.

Thus, the placenta secretes several estrogens, including estradiol, estrone, estriol, and estetrol. Because of its hemochorial nature, the majority of estrogen produced in the placenta is released into the maternal circulation. Maternal estriol and estetrol are produced by steroid precursors produced almost solely in the fetus, thus, the measure of these steroids can act as an indicator of fetal well-being. However, the low sensitivity and specificity of such tests have diminished their diagnostic value, and they have been supplanted other means of determining fetal well-being (see Chap. 15, p. 373).

Fetal Adrenal Gland Development. The fetal adrenal cortex derives from a common adrenogonadal precursor lineage that also gives rise to the steroid-secreting cells of the gonads. These progenitor cells first appear in the fourth week of gestation within the coelomic epithelium. Soon after, they begin to migrate to the mesonephros, and by 6 to 8 weeks' gestation the cells form the primitive adrenal gland. The factors that control the formation of the primordial adrenal gland are not known. However, it appears that ACTH is not necessary for the early stages of adrenal formation. Specifically, the adrenal gland is formed in the anencephalic fetus as well as in fetuses with mutations in the ACTH receptor.

Fetal Adrenal Morphology. Nearly a century ago, Elliott and Armour (1911) described a histologically unique *fetal zone* in the adrenal cortex. The fetal zone accounts for the bulk of the fetal gland after the first trimester, and it is the source for steroid precursors that are used by the placenta to produce estrogens. The outer zone is called the *neocortex,* or the *definitive zone,* and it is this zone that gives rise to the adult adrenal glomerulosa. Recent studies using immunohistochemistry have been useful in identifying a third region between the neocortex and fetal zone, now called the *transitional zone* (Narasaka and colleagues, 2001). This zone is thought to give rise to the cortisol-producing zona fasciculata seen in the postnatal adrenal gland (Mesiano and co-workers, 1993). The fetal zone of the adrenal gland begins a process of involution commencing immediately after birth. The weight of the adrenal glands decreases strikingly during the first few weeks of life, and the size attained by the fetal glands just before birth is not achieved again until late in adolescence or early adult life.

Fetal Adrenal Gland Growth. The cortex continues to grow throughout gestation and, during the last 5 to 6 weeks of pregnancy, there is a very rapid increase in adrenal size (Fig. 3–29). Relative to body weight, the fetal adrenal glands at term are 25 times larger than those of adults. Because of the enormous size and their very great capacity for steroid synthesis, many investigators have surmised that in addition to ACTH, there must be other growth stimuli for these glands. Indeed, there is a continual decrease in the concentration of immunoreactive ACTH in human fetal plasma as pregnancy progresses and as the fetal adrenal glands are growing at a rapid rate (Winters and associates, 1974). Generally, ACTH acts to promote hypertrophy, but not hyperplasia, of adrenal cells. Despite this, it has been shown that fetal adrenal cells respond to ACTH by secretion of growth factors that appear to stimulate hyperplasia of the fetal zone (Mesiano and colleagues, 1991). ACTH is necessary for the rapid growth of the adrenal gland during the latter part of pregnancy. This is supported by the observation that the adrenal glands in anencephalic fetuses are underdeveloped, indicating that a functional hypothalamic–pituitary system also is needed for normal fetal adrenal function. It also seems likely that the rate of growth of the fetal adrenal glands is influenced by factors secreted by the placenta. This supposition is supported by the continued growth of the fetal adrenal glands throughout gestation, but rapid involution immediately after birth when placenta-derived factors are lost.

Enzymatic Considerations. There is a severe deficiency in the expression of the microsomal enzyme 3α-hydroxysteroid dehydrogenase, Δ^{5-4}-isomerase (3βHSD) in adrenal fetal zone cells (Doody and co-workers, 1990; Rainey and colleagues, 2001). This limits the conversion of pregnenolone to progesterone and of 17α-hydroxypregnenolone to 17α-hydroxyprogesterone, an obligatory step in cortisol biosynthesis. There is, however, very active steroid sulfo-transferase activity in the fetal adrenal glands. As a consequence, the principal secretory products of the fetal adrenal glands are pregnenolone sulfate and DHEA-S. Comparatively, cortisol, which likely arises primarily in the neocortex and transitional zone of the fetal adrenal glands and not in the fetal zone, is a minor secretory product of the fetal adrenal gland until late in gestation.

Fetal Adrenal Steroid Precursor. The precursor for fetal adrenal steroidogenesis is cholesterol. The rate of steroid biosynthesis in the fetal adrenal gland is so great that its steroidogenesis alone is equivalent to one fourth of the total daily LDL cholesterol turnover in adults. The fetal adrenal glands can synthesize cholesterol from two-carbon fragments, that is, acetate. All enzymes involved in cholesterol biosynthesis are elevated compared with that of the adult adrenal gland (Rainey and colleagues, 2001). Thus, the rate of de novo cholesterol synthesis by fetal adrenal tissue is extremely high, however, it is insufficient to account for the steroids produced by these glands. Therefore, cholesterol must be assimilated from the fetal circulation. Plasma cholesterol and its esters are present in the form of very-low-density lipoprotein (VLDL), LDL, and high-density lipoprotein (HDL).

Simpson and colleagues (1979) ascertained that fetal adrenal glands take up lipoproteins as a source of cholesterol for steroidogenesis. HDL was much less effective than LDL, and VLDL was devoid of stimulatory activity. These authors also evaluated the relative contribution of cholesterol synthesized de novo and that of cholesterol derived from LDL uptake. They confirmed that the fetal adrenal glands are highly dependent on circulating LDL as a source of cholesterol for optimum steroidogenesis (Carr and colleagues, 1980, 1982; Carr and Simpson, 1981). A model of cholesterol metabolism in the fetal adrenal glands is shown in Figure 3–30.

The majority of fetal plasma cholesterol arises by de novo synthesis in the fetal liver (Carr and Simpson, 1984). The low level of LDL cholesterol in fetal plasma is not the consequence of impaired fetal LDL synthesis, but instead, it is the result of the rapid use of LDL by the fetal adrenal glands for steroidogenesis (Parker and colleagues, 1980, 1983). In the anencephalic newborn in whom the adrenal glands are atrophic, the levels of LDL cholesterol in umbilical cord plasma are high.

FETAL CONDITIONS THAT AFFECT ESTROGEN PRODUCTION. Several conditions affecting the fetus may alter the availability of substrate for steroid synthesis in placenta. A schematic representation of the pathways of estrogen formation in the placenta is presented in Figure 3–28.

Fetal Demise. It has been known for many decades that death of the human fetus is followed by a striking reduction in the levels of urinary estrogens. Moreover, it was demonstrated that after ligation of the umbilical cord with the fetus and placenta left in situ, there was an abrupt and striking decrease in the production of placental estrogens (Cassmer, 1959). The findings of this classical study were subject to at least two interpretations. The first was that maintenance of the fetal placental circulation is essential to the functional integrity of the placenta. This explanation was unlikely to be correct, however, because the placental production of progesterone was maintained after occlusion of the umbilical cord. A second explanation for the marked decrease in urinary estrogens was that after umbilical cord ligation, an important source of precursors of placental estrogen (but not progesterone) biosynthesis was eliminated—that is, the fetus.

Fetal Anencephaly. In the absence of the fetal zone of the adrenal cortex, as in anencephaly, the rate of formation of

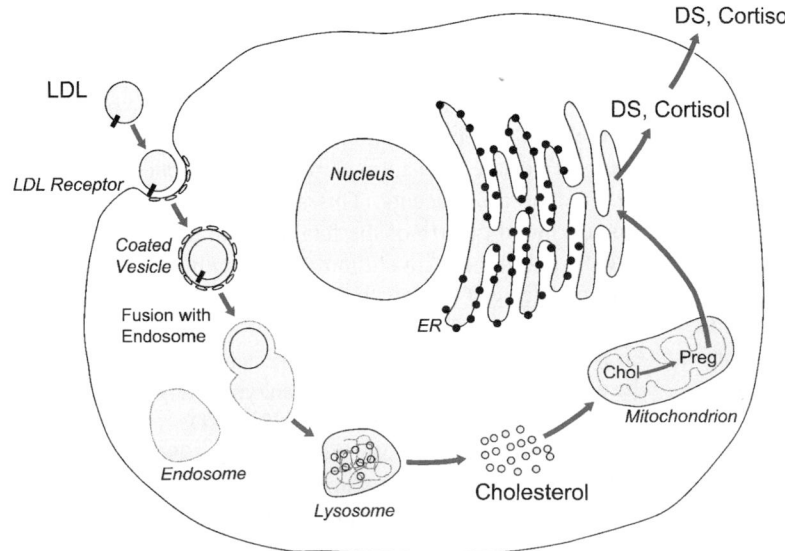

FIGURE 3–30. A model proposed for the regulation of fetal adrenal steroidogenesis, low-density lipoprotein (LDL) use, and cholesterol (chol) metabolism in the human fetal adrenal gland. (DS = dehydroepiandrosterone sulfate; Preg = pregnenolone). DS is produced in the fetal zone and cortisol primarily in the neocortex of the fetal adrenal glands.

placental estrogens (especially estriol) is severely limited because of limited availability of C_{19}-steroid precursors. Verification of the diminished levels of precursors in anencephalic fetuses was provided by the finding of low levels of DHEA-S in cord blood of such newborns (Nichols and colleagues, 1958). Therefore, almost all of the estrogens produced in women pregnant with an anencephalic fetus arise by the placental use of maternal plasma DHEA-S. Furthermore, in such pregnancies the production of estrogens can be increased by the maternal administration of ACTH, which stimulates the rate of DHEA-S secretion by the maternal adrenal. ACTH does not cross the placenta, and thus there is no fetal adrenal stimulation. Finally, placental estrogen production is decreased in women pregnant with an anencephalic fetus when a potent glucocorticoid is given to the mother. This suppresses ACTH secretion and thus decreases the rate of DHEA-S secretion from the maternal adrenal cortex (MacDonald, 1965; MacDonald and Siiteri, 1965). Estriol formation is disproportionately decreased in pregnancies with an anencephalic fetus because the fetal adrenal at term normally provides 90 percent of placental estriol precursor.

Fetal Adrenal Hypoplasia. Congenital adrenal cortical hypoplasia occurs in perhaps 1 in 12,500 births (McCabe, 2001). There appear to be two primary forms of adrenal hypoplasia. The *miniature adult form* is thus named because of the very small cortical zone seen in histological examination. The majority of these cases result from anencephaly or abnormal pituitary function. The *cytomegalic form* is so called because these adrenals, although without the normal fetal adrenal structure, have nodular formation of eosinophilic cells in the fetal zone. Estrogen formation, particularly estriol, in pregnancies with such a fetus is limited and suggests the absence of fetal adrenal C_{19}-precursors for placental estrogen formation. The cytomegalic form results from disruptive mutations in the gene known as the *dosage-sensitive sex reversal–adrenal hypoplasia congenita critical region on the X chromosome, gene 1 (DAX1)* (McCabe, 2001).

Fetal–Placental Sulfatase Deficiency. Placental estrogen formation is generally regulated by the availability of C_{19}-steroid prohormones in fetal and maternal plasma. Specifically, there is no rate-limiting enzymatic reaction in the placental pathway from C_{19}-steroids to estrogen biosynthesis. An exception to this generalization was found by France and Liggins (1969), who were the first to establish that placental sulfatase deficiency is a cause of very low estrogen levels in otherwise normal pregnancies. Sulfatase deficiency precludes the hydrolysis of C_{19}-steroid sulfates, the first enzymatic step in the placental use of these circulating prehormones for estrogen biosynthesis. This deficiency is an X-linked disorder, and all affected fetuses are male. It occurs in an estimated frequency of 1 in 2000 to 5000 births and is associated with delayed onset of labor. It also is associated

with the development of ichthyosis, a scaling skin disorder, in the affected males later in life (Bradshaw and Carr, 1986).

Fetal–Placental Aromatase Deficiency. There are a few well-documented examples of aromatase deficiency (Simpson, 2000). Fetal adrenal DHEA-S, which is produced in large quantities, is converted in the placenta to androstenedione, but in cases of placental aromatase deficiency, androstenedione cannot be converted to estradiol. Rather, androgen metabolites of DHEA produced in the placenta, including androstenedione and some testosterone, are secreted into the maternal or fetal circulation, or both, causing virilization of the mother and the female fetus (Harada and colleagues, 1992; Shozu and associates, 1991). Although pregnancies with aromatase deficiency and a male fetus may be uneventful, these estrogen-deficient males have delayed epiphyseal closure during puberty, and as a consequence, the affected men continue to grow during adulthood, becoming very tall and displaying deficient bone mineralization (Morishima and colleagues, 1995).

Trisomy 21 (Down Syndrome). Second-trimester maternal serum screening for abnormal levels of hCG, alpha-fetoprotein, and other analytes has become universal (see Chap. 13, p. 323). As experience accrued, it was discovered that serum unconjugated estriol levels were low in pregnancies with a Down syndrome fetus (Benn, 2002). The likely reason for this is inadequate formation of C_{19}-steroids in the adrenal glands of these trisomic fetuses. This supposition is supported by reduced DHEA-S levels in both amnionic fluid and maternal serum in Down syndrome pregnancies (Newby and colleagues, 2000).

Deficiency in Fetal LDL Cholesterol Biosynthesis. A successful pregnancy in a woman with beta-lipoprotein deficiency has been described (Parker and co-workers, 1986). The absence of LDL in the maternal serum restricted progesterone formation in both the corpus luteum and placenta. In addition, levels of estriol were lower than normal. Presumably, the diminished estrogen production was the result of decreased fetal LDL formation, which limited fetal adrenal production of estrogen precursor.

Fetal Erythroblastosis. In some cases of severe fetal D-antigen isoimmunization, the levels of estrogens in maternal plasma are elevated above normal for gestational age. This is likely due to an increased placental weight (hypertrophy), which occurs in such pregnancies (see Chap. 29, p. 666).

MATERNAL CONDITIONS THAT AFFECT PLACENTAL ESTROGEN PRODUCTION

Glucocorticoid Treatment. The administration of glucocorticoids in moderate to high doses to pregnant women causes a striking reduction in placental estrogen formation.

Glucocorticoids act to inhibit ACTH secretion by the maternal and fetal pituitary glands, resulting in decreased maternal and fetal adrenal secretion of the placental estrogen precursor, DHEA-S.

Maternal Adrenal Dysfunction. In pregnant women with Addison disease, maternal urinary estrogen levels are decreased (Baulieu and colleagues, 1956). The decrease principally affects estrone and estradiol, because the fetal adrenal contribution to the synthesis of estriol, particularly in the latter part of pregnancy, is quantitatively much more important.

Maternal Ovarian Androgen-Producing Tumors. The extraordinary efficiency of the placenta in the aromatization of C_{19}-steroids may be exemplified by two considerations. First, Edman and associates (1981) found that the placental clearance of maternal plasma androstenedione to estradiol was very similar to estimated placental blood flow. Thus, virtually all of the androstenedione entering the intervillous space is taken up by syncytium and converted to estradiol, and none of this C_{19}-steroid escapes into the fetus. Second, it is relatively rare that a female fetus is virilized in a pregnant woman who is known to have an androgen-secreting ovarian tumor. This finding also indicates that the placenta efficiently converts aromatizable C_{19}-steroids, including testosterone, to estrogens, thus precluding transplacental passage. Indeed, it may be that virilized female fetuses of women with an androgen-producing tumor are cases in which a nonaromatizable C_{19}-steroid androgen is produced by the tumor (e.g., 5α-dihydrotestosterone). Another explanation is that testosterone is produced very early in pregnancy in amounts that exceed the capacity of placental aromatase.

Maternal Renal Disease. Lower levels of estriol in the urine of pregnant women with pyelonephritis may be observed. Presumably this is the consequence of diminished renal clearance, as the maternal serum levels of estrogen are normal in such pregnancies.

Gestational Trophoblastic Disease. In the case of complete hydatidiform mole or choriocarcinoma, there is no fetal adrenal source of C_{19}-steroid precursor for trophoblast estrogen biosynthesis. Consequently, placental estrogen formation is limited to the use of C_{19}-steroids in the maternal plasma, and therefore the estrogen produced is principally estradiol (MacDonald and Siiteri, 1964, 1966). Great variation is observed in the rates of both estradiol and progesterone formation in molar pregnancies. This, however, is not necessarily related to the volume of neoplastic tissue. There is variable disruption of large masses of molar tissue from the uterine wall by blood clots. Consequently, variable amounts of trophoblastic tissue are separated from the maternal blood supply of precursors for estradiol and progesterone formation.

DIRECTIONAL SECRETION OF STEROIDS FROM SYNCYTIOTROPHOBLAST. Estrogens synthesized in the syncytium preferentially enter the maternal circulation. Gurpide and co-workers (1966) reported that more than 90 percent of estradiol and estriol formed in syncytiotrophoblast enters maternal plasma. Gurpide and co-workers (1972) later found that 85 percent or more of placental progesterone enters maternal plasma, and very little maternal plasma progesterone crosses the placenta to the fetus.

The placental estrogens that enter the maternal compartment are estradiol, estrone, and estriol. Estriol synthesized in trophoblasts enters both fetal and maternal plasma, but most (90 percent) enters the mother. There also appears to be preferential transfer of estradiol into the maternal compartment. The major reason for directional movement of newly formed steroid into the maternal circulation is the nature of the hemochorioendothelial form of placentation. In this system, steroids secreted from the syncytiotrophoblast can enter maternal blood directly. Steroids that leave the syncytium toward the fetal compartment, however, do not enter fetal blood directly. First, steroids traveling toward the fetus must traverse the cytotrophoblasts and then enter the connective tissue of the villous core. Steroids in this space can reenter the syncytium. Second, steroids that escape the villous core must then traverse the wall of the fetal capillaries to reach fetal blood. Steroids in the fetal capillaries of the villous core then can reenter the connective tissue of the villous core and then the syncytium. The net result of this hemochorial arrangement is that there is substantially greater entry of steroids into the maternal circulation compared with the amount that enters the fetal blood.

Somewhat surprisingly, there appears to be preferential entry of estrone rather than estradiol into the fetal plasma (Gurpide and colleagues, 1982). One explanation is that the fetal endothelial cells found within the placenta express high levels of 17β-hydroxysteroid dehydrogenase type 2 (17βHSD type 2), the enzyme that converts estradiol to estrone (Bonenfant and co-workers, 2000a; Moghrabi and colleagues, 1997). This enzyme would act as a partial barrier, converting estradiol to estrone as it enters the fetal circulation. In this way, fetal levels of estrone would be composed of the estrone made in the trophoblasts that makes it to the fetal circulation as well as the estradiol that reaches the fetal placental endothelial cells and is converted to estrone. The localization of the 17βHSD type 2 enzyme at the site of fetal–maternal exchange likely serves to protect the fetus from high levels of active estrogens and androgens, principally estradiol and testosterone (Moghrabi and colleagues, 1997).

REFERENCES

Aaltonen J, Laitinen MP, Vuojolainen K, et al: Human growth differentiation factor 9 (GDF-9) and its novel homolog GDF-9B are expressed in oocytes during early folliculogenesis. J Clin Endocrinol Metab 84:2744, 1999

Abel MH: Prostanoids and menstruation. In Baird DT, Michie EA (eds): Mechanisms of Menstrual Bleeding. New York, Raven, 2002, p 139

Albrecht ED, Pepe GJ: Steroid hormone regulation of angiogenesis in the primate endometrium. Front Biosci 8:D416, 2003

Ancelin M, Buteau-Lozano H, Meduri G, et al: A dynamic shift of VEGF isoforms with a transient and selective progesterone-induced expression of VEGF189 regulates angiogenesis and vascular permeability in human uterus. Proc Natl Acad Sci U S A 99:6023, 2002

Aplin JD: MUC-1 glycosylation in endometrium: Possible roles of the apical glycocalyx at implantation. Hum Reprod 2:17, 2003

Aractingi S, Berkane N, Bertheau P, et al: Fetal DNA in skin of polymorphic eruptions of pregnancy. Lancet 352:1898, 1998

Arey LB: The degree of normal menstrual irregularity: An analysis of 20,000 calendar records from 1,500 individuals. Am J Obstet Gynecol 37:12, 1939

Arici A, Head JR, MacDonald PC, et al: Regulation of interleukin-8 gene expression in human endometrial cells in culture. Mol Cell Endocrinol 94:195, 1993

Arici A, MacDonald PC, Casey ML: Modulation of the levels of interleukin-8 messenger ribonucleic acid and interleukin-8 protein synthesis in human endometrial stromal cells by transforming growth factor-beta 1. J Clin Endocrinol Metab 81:3004, 1996a

Arici A, MacDonald PC, Casey ML: Progestin regulation of interleukin-8 mRNA levels and protein synthesis in human endometrial stromal cells. J Steroid Biochem Mol Biol 58:71, 1996b

Arici A, MacDonald PC, Casey ML: Regulation of monocyte chemotactic protein-1 gene expression in human endometrial cells in cultures. Mol Cell Endocrinol 107:189, 1995

Arnholdt H, Meisel F, Fandrey K, et al: Proliferation of villous trophoblast of the human placenta in normal and abnormal pregnancies. Virchows Arch B Cell Pathol Incl Mol Pathol 60:365, 1991

Auletta F: The role of prostaglandin F2a in human luteolysis. Contemp Obstet Gynecol 30:119, 1987

Baker T: A quantitative and cytological study of germ cells in human ovaries. Proc R Soc Lond B Biol Sci 158:417, 1963

Barbour LA, Shao J, Qiao L, et al: Human placental growth hormone causes severe insulin resistance in transgenic mice. Am J Obstet Gynecol 186:512, 2002

Barnea ER, Kaplan M: Spontaneous, gonadotropin-releasing hormone-induced, and progesterone-inhibited pulsatile secretion of human chorionic gonadotropin in the first trimester placenta in vitro. J Clin Endocrinol Metab 69:215, 1989

Bathgate RA, Samuel CS, Burazin TC, et al: Human relaxin gene 3 (H3) and the equivalent mouse relaxin (M3) gene. Novel members of the relaxin peptide family. J Biol Chem 277:1148, 2002

Baulieu EE, Bricaire H, Jayle MF: Lack of secretion of 17-hydroxycorticosteroids in a pregnant woman with Addison's disease. J Clin Endocrinol 16:690, 1956

Baulieu EE, Dray F: Conversion of 3H-dehydroepiandrosterone (3b-hydroxy-D5-androstene-17-one) sulfate to 3H-estrogens in normal pregnant women. J Clin Endocrinol 23:1298, 1963

Bausero P, Cavaillé F, Meduri G, et al: Paracrine action of vascular endothelial growth factor in the human endometrium: Production and target sites, and hormonal regulation. Angiogenesis 2:167, 1998

Beck T, Schweikhart G, Stolz E: Immunohistochemical location of HPL, SP1 and beta-HCG in normal placentas of varying gestational age. Arch Gynecol 239:63, 1986

Beer AE, Billingham RE: Immunobiology of mammalian reproduction. Adv Immunol 14:1, 1971

Beers WH: Follicular plasminogen and plasminogen activator and the effect of plasmin on ovarian follicle wall. Cell 6:379, 1975

Benirschke K, Kaufmann P: Pathology of the Human Placenta, 4th ed. New York, Springer, 2000

Benn PA: Advances in prenatal screening for Down syndrome: I. General principles and second trimester testing. Clin Chim Acta 323:1, 2002

Bergh PA, Navot D: The impact of embryonic development and endometrial maturity on the timing of implantation. Fertil Steril 58:537, 1992

Berry SA, Srivastava CH, Rubin LR, et al: Growth hormone-releasing hormone-like messenger ribonucleic acid and immunoreactive peptide are present in human testis and placenta. J Clin Endocrinol Metab 75:281, 1992

Bertelloni S, Baroncelli GI, Pelletti A, et al: Parathyroid hormone-related protein in healthy pregnant women. Calcif Tissue Int 54:195, 1994

Bethune JE: The Adrenal Cortex, A Scope Monograph. Kalamazoo, Mich, Upjohn, 1974, p 11

Bhaumick B, Dawson EP, Bala RM: The effects of insulin-like growth factor-I and insulin on placental lactogen production by human term placental explants. Biochem Biophys Res Commun 144:674, 1987

Bianchi DW, Zickwolf GK, Weil GJ, et al: Male fetal progenitor cells persist in maternal blood for as long as 27 years postpartum. Proc Natl Acad Sci U S A 93:705, 1996

Billingham RE: Transplantation immunity and the maternal fetal relation. N Engl J Med 270:667, 1964

Billingham RE, Head JR: Recipient treatment to overcome the allograft reaction, with special reference to nature's own solution. Prog Clin Biol Res 224:159, 1986

Bischof P, Meisser A, Campana A: Control of MMP-9 expression at the maternal-fetal interface. J Reprod Immunol 55:3, 2002

Bleker O, Kloostermans G, Mieras D, et al: Intervillous space during uterine contractions in human subjects: An ultrasonic study. Am J Obstet Gynecol 123:697, 1975

Bloch K: The biological conversion of cholesterol to pregnandiol. J Biol Chem 157:661, 1945

Bogic LV, Mandel M, Bryant-Greenwood GD: Relaxin gene expression in human reproductive tissues by in situ hybridization. J Clin Endocrinol Metab 80:130, 1995

Bolté E, Mancuso S, Eriksson G, et al: Studies on the aromatization of neutral steroids in pregnant women, 1. Aromatization of C-19 steroids by placenta perfused in situ. Acta Endocrinol 35:535, 1964a

Bolté E, Mancuso S, Eriksson G, et al: Studies on the aromatization of neutral steroids in pregnant women, 2. Aromatization of dehydroepiandrosterone and of its sulphate administered simultaneously into a uterine artery. Acta Endocrinol 45:560, 1964b

Bonenfant M, Blomquist CR, Provost P, et al: Tissue- and site-specific gene expression of type 2 17beta-hydroxysteroid dehydrogenase: In situ hybridization and specific enzyme activity studies in human placental endothelial cells of the arterial system. J Clin Endocrinol Metab 85:4841, 2000a

Bonenfant M, Provost PR, Drolet R, et al: Localization of type 1 17beta-hydroxysteroid dehydrogenase mRNA and protein in syncytiotrophoblasts and invasive cytotrophoblasts in the human term villi. J Endocrinol 165:217, 2000b

Borell U, Fernstrom I, Westman A: An arteriographic study of the placental circulation. Geburtshilfe Frauenheilkd 18:1, 1958

Bourne GL: The Human Amnion and Chorion. Chicago, Year Book, 1962

Boyd JD, Hamilton WJ: The Human Placenta. Cambridge, England, Heffer, 1970

Bradbury J, Brown W, Guay L: Maintenance of the corpus luteum and physiologic action of progesterone. Recent Prog Horm Res 5:151, 1950

Bradshaw KD, Carr BR: Placental sulfatase deficiency: Maternal and fetal expression of steroid sulfatase deficiency and X-linked ichthyosis. Obstet Gynecol Surv 41:401, 1986

Brosens I, Dixon H: The anatomy of the maternal side of the placenta. Eur J Endocrinol 73:357, 1963

Brosens J, Hayashi N, White J: Progesterone receptor regulates decidual prolactin expression in differentiating human endometrial stromal cells. Eur J Obstet Gynaecol Surv 142:269, 2000

Browning HC: The evolutionary history of the corpus luteum. Biol Reprod 8:128, 1973

Bryant-Greenwood GD: The extracellular matrix of the human fetal membranes: Structure and function. Placenta 19:1, 1998

Carosella ED, Paul P, Moreau P, et al: HLA-G and HLA-E: Fundamental and pathophysiological aspects. Immunol Today 21:532, 2000

Carr BR, Ohashi M, Simpson ER: Low density lipoprotein binding and de novo synthesis of cholesterol in the neocortex and fetal zones of the human fetal adrenal gland. Endocrinology 110:1994, 1982

Carr BR, Parker CR Jr, Madden JD, et al: Maternal plasma adrenocorticotropin and cortisol relationships throughout human pregnancy. Am J Obstet Gynecol 139:416, 1981a

Carr BR, Porter JC, MacDonald PC, et al: Metabolism of low density lipoprotein by human fetal adrenal tissue. Endocrinology 107:1034, 1980

Carr BR, Sadler RK, Rochelle DB, et al: Plasma lipoprotein regulation of progesterone biosynthesis by human corpus luteum tissue in organ culture. J Clin Endocrinol Metab 52:875, 1981b

Carr BR, Simpson ER: Cholesterol synthesis by human fetal hepatocytes: Effect of lipoproteins. Am J Obstet Gynecol 150:551, 1984

Carr BR, Simpson ER: Lipoprotein utilization and cholesterol synthesis by the human fetal adrenal gland. Endocr Rev 2:306, 1981

Carson DD: The glycobiology of implantation. Front Biosci 7:d1535, 2002

Casey ML, Delgadillo M, Cox KA, et al: Inactivation of prostaglandins in human decidua vera (parietalis) tissue: Substrate specificity of prostaglandin dehydrogenase. Am J Obstet Gynecol 160:3, 1989

Casey ML, Hemsell DL, MacDonald PC, et al: NAD+-dependent 15-hydroxyprostaglandin dehydrogenase activity in human endometrium. Prostaglandins 19:115, 1980

Casey ML, MacDonald PC: Extraadrenal formation of a mineralocorticosteroid: Deoxycorticosterone and deoxycorticosterone sulfate biosynthesis and metabolism. Endocr Rev 3:396, 1982a

Casey ML, MacDonald PC: Metabolism of deoxycorticosterone and deoxycorticosterone sulfate in men and women. J Clin Invest 70:312, 1982b

Casey ML, MacDonald PC: The endothelin-parathyroid hormone-related protein vasoactive peptide system in human endometrium: Modulation by transforming growth factor-beta. Hum Reprod 11 Suppl 2:62, 1996

Casey ML, Smith JW, Nagai K, et al: Progesterone-regulated cyclic modulation of membrane metalloendopeptidase (enkephalinase) in human endometrium. J Biol Chem 266:23041, 1991

Cassmer O: Hormone production of the isolated human placenta. Acta Endocrinol (Suppl) 32:45, 1959

Cervar M, Blaschitz A, Dohr G, et al: Paracrine regulation of distinct trophoblast functions in vitro by placental macrophages. Cell Tissue Res 295:297, 1999

Chao HS, Poisner AM, Poisner R, et al: Endothelin-1 modulates renin and prolactin release from human decidua by different mechanisms. Am J Physiol 267:E842, 1994

Christian M, Pohnke Y, Kempf R, et al: Functional association of PR and CCAAT/enhancer-binding protein beta isoforms: Promoter-dependent cooperation between PR-B and liver-enriched inhibitory protein, or liver-enriched activatory protein and PR-A in human endometrial stromal cells. Mol Endocrinol 16:141, 2002a

Christian M, Zhang XH, Schneider-Merck T, et al: Cyclic AMP-induced forkhead transcription factor, FKHR, cooperates with CCAAT/enhancer-binding protein beta in differentiating human endometrial stromal cells. J Biol Chem 277:20825, 2002b

Ciaranfi A, Curchod A, Odartchenko N: [Post-partum survival of fetal lymphocytes in the maternal blood]. Schweiz Med Wochenschr 107:134, 1977

Cock T-A, Auwerx J: Leptin: Cutting the fat off the bone. Lancet 362:1572, 2003

Cole LA: Immunoassay of human chorionic gonadotropin, its free subunits, and metabolites. Clin Chem 43:2233, 1997

Cole LA, Butler S: Detection of hCG in trophoblastic disease. The USA hCG reference service experience. J Reprod Med 47:433, 2002

Cole LA, Kardana A, Andrade-Gordon P, et al: The heterogeneity of human chorionic gonadotropin (hCG). III. The occurrence and biological and immunological activities of nicked hCG. Endocrinology 129:1559, 1991a

Cole LA, Kardana A, Ying FC, et al: The biological and clinical significance of nicks in human chorionic gonadotropin and its free beta-subunit. Yale J Biol Med 64:627, 1991b

Conneely OM, Mulac-Jericevic B, DeMayo F, et al: Reproductive functions of progesterone receptors. Recent Prog Horm Res 57:339, 2002

Corbacho AM, Martinez DLE, Clapp C: Roles of prolactin and related members of the prolactin/growth hormone/placental lactogen family in angiogenesis. J Endocrinol 173:219, 2002

Crawford J: A study of human placental growth with observations on the placenta in erythroblastosis foetalis. Br J Obstet Gynaecol 66:855, 1959

Critchley HO, Kelly RW, Brenner RM, et al: The endocrinology of menstruation—a role for the immune system. Clin Endocrinol (Oxf) 55:701, 2001

Damjanov I: Vesalius and Hunter were right: Decidua is a membrane! Lab Invest 53:597, 1985

Dautzenberg FM, Hauger RL: The CRF peptide family and their receptors: Yet more partners discovered. Trends Pharmacol Sci 23:71, 2002

Desai R, Creger W: Maternofetal passage of leukocytes and platelets in man. Blood 21:665, 1963

Devoto L, Kohen P, Vega M, et al: Control of human luteal steroidogenesis. Mol Cell Endocrinol 186:137, 2002

Diaz-Cueto L, Mendez JP, Barrios-de-Tomasi J, et al: Amplitude regulation of episodic release, in vitro biological to immunological ratio, and median charge of human chorionic gonadotropin in pregnancy. J Clin Endocrinol Metab 78:890, 1994

Diczfalusy E, Troen P: Endocrine functions of the human placenta. Vitam Horm 19:229, 1961

Dombroski RA, Casey ML, MacDonald PC: 5-Alpha-dihydroprogesterone formation in human placenta from 5alpha-pregnan-3beta/alpha-ol-20-ones and 5-pregnan-3beta-yl-20-one sulfate. J Steroid Biochem Mol Biol 63:155, 1997

Dong JC, Dong H, Campana A, et al: Matrix metalloproteinases and their specific tissue inhibitors in menstruation. Reproduction 123:621, 2002

Doody KM, Carr BR, Rainey WE, et al: 3b-hydroxysteroid dehydrogenase/isomerase in the fetal zone and neocortex of the human fetal adrenal gland. Endocrinology 126:2487, 1990

Duffy DM, Hutchison JS, Stewart DR, et al: Stimulation of primate luteal function by recombinant human chorionic gonadotropin and modulation of steroid, but not relaxin, production by an inhibitor of 3 beta-hydroxysteroid dehydrogenase during simulated early pregnancy. J Clin Endocrinol Metab 81:2307, 1996

Duncan WC, McNeilly AS, Fraser HM, et al: Luteinizing hormone receptor in the human corpus luteum: Lack of down-regulation during maternal recognition of pregnancy. Hum Reprod 11:2291, 1996

Dunn CL, Critchley HO, Kelly RW: IL-15 regulation in human endometrial stromal cells. J Clin Endocrinol Metab 87:1898, 2002

Economos K, MacDonald PC, Casey ML: Endothelin-1 gene expression and protein biosynthesis in human endometrium: Potential modulator of endometrial blood flow. J Clin Endocrinol Metab 74:14, 1992

Edman CD, Toofanian A, MacDonald PC, et al: Placental clearance rate of maternal plasma androstenedione through placental estradiol formation: An indirect method of assessing uteroplacental blood flow. Am J Obstet Gynecol 141:1029, 1981

Elliott CL, Allport VC, Loudon JA, et al: Nuclear factor-kappa B is essential for up-regulation of interleukin-8 expression in human amnion and cervical epithelial cells. Mol Hum Reprod 7:787, 2001

Elliott JR, Armour RG: The development of the cortex in the human suprarenal gland and its condition in hemicephaly. J Pathol Bacteriol 15:481, 1911

Enders AC: A comparative study of the fine structure in several hemochorial placentas. Am J Anat 116:29, 1965

Everett RB, Worley RJ, MacDonald PC, et al: Modification of vascular responsiveness to angiotensin II in pregnant women by intravenously infused 5alpha-dihydroprogesterone. Am J Obstet Gynecol 131:352, 1978

Faddy MJ, Gosden RG, Gougeon A, et al: Accelerated disappearance of ovarian follicles in mid-life: Implications for forecasting menopause. Hum Reprod 7:1342, 1992

Feinberg RF, Kliman HJ, Lockwood CJ: Is oncofetal fibronectin a trophoblast glue for human implantation? Am J Pathol 138:537, 1991

Ferenczy A: Studies on the cytodynamics of human endometrial regeneration. I. Scanning electron microscopy. Am J Obstet Gynecol 124:64, 1976

Filicori M, Santoro N, Merriam GR, et al: Characterization of the physiological pattern of episodic gonadotropin secretion throughout the human menstrual cycle. J Clin Endocrinol Metab 62:1136, 1986

Fisk NM, MacLachlan N, Ellis C, et al: Absent end-diastolic flow in first trimester umbilical artery. Lancet 2:1256, 1988

Florio P, Franchini A, Reis FM, et al: Human placenta, chorion, amnion and decidua express different variants of corticotropin-releasing factor receptor messenger RNA. Placenta 21:32, 2000

Florio P, Mezzesimi A, Turchetti V, et al: High levels of human chromogranin A in umbilical cord plasma and amniotic fluid at parturition. J Soc Gynecol Investig 9:32, 2002

France JT, Liggins GC: Placental sulfatase deficiency. J Clin Endocrinol Metab 29:138, 1969

Frandsen VA, Stakemann G: The site of production of oestrogenic hormones in human pregnancy: Hormone excretion in pregnancy with anencephalic foetus. Acta Endocrinol 38:383, 1961

Frank GR, Brar AK, Jikihara H, et al: Interleukin-1 beta and the endometrium: An inhibitor of stromal cell differentiation and possible autoregulator of decidualization in humans. Biol Reprod 52:184, 1995

Fraser HM, Wulff C: Angiogenesis in the primate ovary. Reprod Fertil Dev 13:557, 2001

Fuzzi B, Rizzo R, Criscuoli L, et al: HLA-G expression in early embryos is a fundamental prerequisite for the obtainment of pregnancy. Eur J Immunol 32:311, 2002

Gant NF, Hutchinson HT, Siiteri PK, et al: Study of the metabolic clearance rate of dehydroisoandrosterone sulfate in pregnancy. Am J Obstet Gynecol 111:555, 1971

Garcia-Velasco JA, Arici A: Chemokines and human reproduction. Fertil Steril 71:983, 1999

Gargett CE, Rogers PA: Human endometrial angiogenesis. Reproduction 121:181, 2001

Genazzani AR, Fraioli F, Hurlimann J, et al: Immunoreactive ACTH and cortisol plasma levels during pregnancy. Detection and partial purification of corticotrophin-like placental hormone: The human chorionic corticotrophin (HCC). Clin Endocrinol (Oxf) 4:1, 1975

Genbacev O, Ratkovic M, Kraincanic M, et al: Effect of prostaglandin PGE2alpha on the synthesis of placental proteins and human placental lactogen (HPL). Prostaglandins 13:723, 1977

Germain A, Attaroglu H, MacDonald PC, et al: Parathyroid hormone-related protein mRNA in avascular human amnion. J Clin Endocrinol Metab 75:1173, 1992

Gibbons JM Jr, Mitnick M, Chieffo V: In vitro biosynthesis of TSH- and LH-releasing factors by the human placenta. Am J Obstet Gynecol 121:127, 1975

Goland RS, Wardlaw SL, Blum M, et al: Biologically active corticotropin-releasing hormone in maternal and fetal plasma during pregnancy. Am J Obstet Gynecol 159:884, 1988

Golander A, Hurley T, Barrett J, et al: Prolactin synthesis by human chorion-decidual tissue: A possible source of prolactin in the amniotic fluid. Science 202:311, 1978

Goldman-Wohl DS, Ariel I, Greenfield C, et al: HLA-G expression in extravillous trophoblasts is an intrinsic property of cell differentiation: A lesson learned from ectopic pregnancies. Mol Hum Reprod 6:535, 2000

Gougeon A: Regulation of ovarian follicular development in primates: Facts and hypotheses. Endocr Rev 17:121, 1996

Groome NP, Illingworth PJ, O'Brien M, et al: Measurement of dimeric inhibin B throughout the human menstrual cycle. J Clin Endocrinol Metab 81:1401, 1996

Grumbach MM, Kaplan SL: On placental origin and purification of chorionic growth hormone prolactin and its immunoassay in pregnancy. Trans N Y Acad Sci 27:167, 1964

Gualillo O, Caminos J, Blanco M, et al: Ghrelin, a novel placental-derived hormone. Endocrinology 142:788, 2001

Gubbay O, Critchley HO, Bowen JM, et al: Prolactin induces ERK phosphorylation in epithelial and CD56(+) natural killer cells of the human endometrium. J Clin Endocrinol Metab 87:2329, 2002

Gurpide E, Marks C, de Ziegler D, et al: Asymmetric release of estrone and estradiol derived from labeled precursors in perfused human placentas. Am J Obstet Gynecol 144:551, 1982

Gurpide E, Schwers J, Welch MT, et al: Fetal and maternal metabolism of estradiol during pregnancy. J Clin Endocrinol Metab 26:1355, 1966

Gurpide E, Tseng J, Escarcena L, et al: Fetomaternal production and transfer of progesterone and uridine in sheep. Am J Obstet Gynecol 113:21, 1972

Hafez ES, Ludwig H, Metzger H: Human endometrial fluid kinetics as observed by scanning electron microscopy. Am J Obstet Gynecol 122:929, 1975

Haman JO: The length of the menstrual cycle: A study of 150 normal women. Am J Obstet Gynecol 43:870, 1942

Hamilton W, Boyd J: Trophoblast in human utero-placental arteries. Nature 212:906, 1966

Handwerger S, Barry S, Barrett J, et al: Inhibition of the synthesis and secretion of decidual prolactin by arachidonic acid. Endocrinology 109:2016, 1981

Hansell DJ, Bryant-Greenwood GD, Greenwood FC: Expression of the human relaxin H1 gene in the decidua, trophoblast, and prostate. J Clin Endocrinol Metab 72:899, 1991

Harada N, Ogawa H, Shozu M, et al: Biochemical and molecular genetic analyses on placental aromatase (P-450AROM) deficiency. J Biol Chem 267:4781, 1992

Hellig H, Gattereau D, Lefebvre Y, et al: Steroid production from plasma cholesterol. I. Conversion of plasma cholesterol to placental progesterone in humans. J Clin Endocrinol Metab 30:624, 1970

Henson MC, Castracane VD: Leptin: Roles and regulation in primate pregnancy. Semin Reprod Med 20:113, 2002

Henson MC, Greene SJ, Reggio BC, et al: Effects of reduced maternal lipoprotein-cholesterol availability on placental progesterone biosynthesis in the baboon. Endocrinology 138:1385, 1997

Hershman JM: Human chorionic gonadotropin and the thyroid: Hyperemesis gravidarum and trophoblastic tumors. Thyroid 9:653, 1999

Hertig AT: The placenta: Some new knowledge about an old organ. Obstet Gynecol 20:859, 1962

Hertig AT, Rock J: On the development of the early human ovum, with special reference to the trophoblast of the previllous stage: A description of 7 normal and 5 pathologic ova. Am J Obstet Gynecol 47:149, 1944

Hertig AT, Rock J: Two human ova of the pre-villous stage, having a developmental age of about seven and nine days respectively. Contrib Embryol 31:65, 1945

Hillier SG: Gonadotropic control of ovarian follicular growth and development. Mol Cell Endocrinol 179:39, 2001

Horvath TL, Diano S, Sotonyi P, et al: Minireview: Ghrelin and the regulation of energy balance—a hypothalamic perspective. Endocrinology 142:4163, 2001

Hoshina M, Boothby M, Boime I: Cytological localization of chorionic gonadotropin alpha and placental lactogen mRNAs during development of the human placenta. J Cell Biol 93:190, 1982

Hreinsson JG, Scott JE, Rasmussen C, et al: Growth differentiation factor-9 promotes the growth, development, and survival of human ovarian follicles in organ culture. J Clin Endocrinol Metab 87:316, 2002

Hsu SY, Nakabayashi K, Nishi S, et al: Activation of orphan receptors by the hormone relaxin. Science 295:671, 2002

Hsueh AJ, Billig H, Tsafriri A: Ovarian follicle atresia: A hormonally controlled apoptotic process. Endocr Rev 15:707, 1994

Hudson P, Haley J, John M, et al: Structure of a genomic clone encoding biologically active human relaxin. Nature 301:628, 1983

Hudson P, John M, Crawford R, et al: Relaxin gene expression in human ovaries and the predicted structure of a human preprorelaxin by analysis of cDNA clones. EMBO J 3:2333, 1984

Hunt JS, Jadhav L, Chu W, et al: Soluble HLA-G circulates in maternal blood during pregnancy. Am J Obstet Gynecol 183:682, 2000a

Hunt JS, Orr HT: HLA and maternal-fetal recognition. FASEB J 6:2344, 1992

Hunt JS, Petroff MG, Morales P, et al: HLA-G in reproduction: Studies on the maternal-fetal interface. Hum Immunol 61:1113, 2000b

Illingworth DR, Corbin DK, Kemp ED, et al: Hormone changes during the menstrual cycle in abetalipoproteinemia: Reduced luteal phase progesterone in a patient with homozygous hypobetalipoproteinemia. Proc Natl Acad Sci U S A 79:6685, 1982

Ito Y, Higashi K: Studies on prolactin-like substance in human placenta. Endocrinol Jpn 8:279, 1961

Iwashita M, Kudo Y, Shinozaki Y, et al: Gonadotropin-releasing hormone increases serum human chorionic gonadotropin in pregnant women. Endocr J 40:539, 1993

Jabbour HN, Critchley HOD: Potential roles of decidual prolactin in early pregnancy. Reproduction 121:197, 2001

Jeffrey J: Collagen and collagenase: Pregnancy and parturition. Semin Perinatol 15:118, 1991

Johnson PM, Christmas SE, Vince GS: Immunological aspects of implantation and implantation failure. Hum Reprod 14(suppl 2):26, 1999

Jokhi P, King A, Loke Y: Production of granulocyte/macrophage colony-stimulating factor by human trophoblast cells and by decidual large granular lymphocytes. Hum Reprod 9:1660, 1999

Jones SA, Brooks AN, Challis JR: Steroids modulate corticotropin-releasing hormone production in human fetal membranes and placenta. J Clin Endocrinol Metab 68:825, 1989

Jones SA, Challis JR: Local stimulation of prostaglandin production by corticotropin-releasing hormone in human fetal membranes and placenta. Biochem Biophys Res Commun 159:192, 1989

Josimovich JB, MacLaren JA: Presence in human placenta and term serum of highly lactogenic substance immunologically related in pituitary growth hormone. Endocrinology 71:209, 1962

Kaipia A, Hsueh AJ: Regulation of ovarian follicle atresia. Annu Rev Physiol 59:349, 1997

Katzenellenbogen BS, Sun J, Harrington WR, et al: Structure-function relationships in estrogen receptors and the characterization of novel selective estrogen receptor modulators with unique pharmacological profiles. Ann NY Acad Sci 949:6, 2001

Kaufmann P, Black S, Huppertz B: Endovascular trophoblast invasion: Implications for the pathogenesis of intrauterine growth retardation and preeclampsia. Biol Reprod 69:1, 2003

Kaufmann P, Scheffen I: Placental development. In Polin R, Fox W (eds): Fetal and Neonatal Physiology. Philadelphia, Saunders, 1992, p 47

Khodr GS, Siler-Khodr TM: Placental luteinizing hormone-releasing factor and its synthesis. Science 207:315, 1980

Kilburn B, Wang J, Duniec-Dmuchkowski KZ, et al: Extracellular matrix composition and hypoxia regulate the expression of HLA-G and integrins in a human trophoblast cell line. Biol Reprod 62:739, 2000

King BF, Menton DN: Scanning electron microscopy of human placental villi from early and late in gestation. Am J Obstet Gynecol 122:824, 1975

Kraiem Z, Sadeh O, Blithe DL, et al: Human chorionic gonadotropin stimulates thyroid hormone secretion, iodide uptake, organification, and adenosine 3′,5′-monophosphate formation in cultured human thyrocytes. J Clin Endocrinol Metab 79:595, 1994

Kurman RJ, Young RH, Norris HJ, et al: Immunocytochemical localization of placental lactogen and chorionic gonadotropin in the normal placenta and trophoblastic tumors, with emphasis on intermediate trophoblast and the placental site trophoblastic tumor. Int J Gynecol Pathol 3:101, 1984

Kurtzman JT, Wilson H, Rao CV: A proposed role for hCG in clinical obstetrics. Semin Reprod Med 19:63, 2001

La Cava A, Alviggi C, Matarese G: Unraveling the multiple roles of leptin in inflammation and autoimmunity. J Mol Med 82:4, 2004

Lala PK, Lee BP, Xu G, et al: Human placental trophoblast as an in vitro model for tumor progression. Can J Physiol Pharmacol 80:142, 2002

Lambert NC, Evans PC, Hashizumi TL, et al: Cutting edge: Persistent fetal microchimerism in T lymphocytes is associated with

HLA-DQA1*0501: Implications in autoimmunity. J Immunol 164:5545, 2000

LeBouteiller P, Solier C, Proll J, et al: Placental HLA-G protein expression in vivo: Where and what for? Hum Reprod Update 5:223, 1999

Lecce G, Meduri G, Ancelin M, et al: Presence of estrogen receptor beta in the human endometrium through the cycle: Expression in glandular, stromal, and vascular cells. J Clin Endocrinol Metab 86:1379, 2001

Lessey BA, Castelbaum AJ: Integrins and implantation in the human. Rev Endocr Metab Disord 3:107, 2002

Li XF, Charnock-Jones DS, Zhang E, et al: Angiogenic growth factor messenger ribonucleic acids in uterine natural killer cells. J Clin Endocrinol Metab 86:1823, 2001

Librach CL, Werb Z, Fitzgerald ML, et al: 92-kD type IV collagenase mediates invasion of human cytotrophoblasts. J Cell Biol 113:437, 1991

Licht P, Russu V, Wildt L: On the role of human chorionic gonadotropin (hCG) in the embryo-endometrial microenvironment: Implications for differentiation and implantation. Semin Reprod Med 19:37, 2001

Lindhard A, Bentin-Ley U, Ravn V, et al: Biochemical evaluation of endometrial function at the time of implantation. Fertil Steril 78:221, 2002

Lobo SC, Srisuparp S, Peng X, et al: Uterine receptivity in the baboon: Modulation by chorionic gonadotropin. Semin Reprod Med 19:69, 2001

Loke YM, King A: Human Implantation. Cell Biology and Immunology. Cambridge, Cambridge University Press, 1995

Loquet P, Broughton-Pipkin F, Symonds E, et al: Blood velocity waveforms and placental vascular formation. Lancet 2:1252, 1988

Luconi M, Bonaccorsi L, Bini L, et al: Characterization of membrane nongenomic receptors for progesterone in human spermatozoa. Steroids 67:505, 2002

Maaskant RA, Bogic LV, Gilger S, et al: The human prolactin receptor in the fetal membranes, decidua, and placenta. J Clin Endocrinol Metab 81:396, 1996

MacDonald PC: Placental steroidogenesis. In Wynn RM (ed): Fetal Homeostasis, Vol. I. New York, New York Academy of Sciences, 1965, p 265

MacDonald PC, Siiteri PK: Origin of estrogen in women pregnant with an anencephalic fetus. J Clin Invest 44:465, 1965

MacDonald PC, Siiteri PK: Study of estrogen production in women with hydatidiform mole. J Clin Endocrinol Metab 24:685, 1964

MacDonald PC, Siiteri PK: The in vivo mechanisms of origin of estrogen in subjects with trophoblastic tumors. Steroids 8:589, 1966

Macklon NS, Fauser BC: Follicle-stimulating hormone and advanced follicle development in the human. Arch Med Res 32:595, 2001

Maradny EE, Kanayama N, Halim A, et al: Stretching of fetal membranes increases the concentration of interleukin-8 and collagenase activity. Am J Obstet Gynecol 174:843, 1996

Markee J: Menstruation in intraocular endometrial transplants in the rhesus monkey. Contrib Embryol 28:219, 1940

Maruo T, Ladines-Llave CA, Matsuo H, et al: A novel change in cytologic localization of human chorionic gonadotropin and human placental lactogen in first-trimester placenta in the course of gestation. Am J Obstet Gynecol 167:217, 1992

Maulik D: Doppler ultrasound in obstetrics. Williams Obstetrics, 20 ed. Stamford, Appleton & Lange, 1997, p 1

McCabe ERB: Adrenal hypoplasias and aplasias. In Scriver CR, Beaudet AL, Sly WE, et al (eds): The Metabolic and Molecular Bases of Inherited Disease. New York, McGraw-Hill, 2001, p 4263

McCombs H, Craig M: Decidual necrosis in normal pregnancy. Obstet Gynecol 24:436, 1964

McGregor WG, Kuhn RW, Jaffe RB: Biologically active chorionic gonadotropin: Synthesis by the human fetus. Science 220:306, 1983

McGregor WG, Raymoure WJ, Kuhn RW, et al: Fetal tissue can synthesize a placental hormone. Evidence for chorionic gonadotropin beta-subunit synthesis by human fetal kidney. J Clin Invest 68:306, 1981

McMaster M, Librach C, Zhou Y, et al: Human placental HLA-G expression is restricted to differentiated cytotrophoblasts. J Immunol 154:3771, 1995

Medawar PB: Some immunological and endocrinological problems raised by the evolution of viviparity in vertebrates. Symp Soc Exp Biol 44:1953

Mesiano S: Roles of estrogen and progesterone in human parturition. In Smith R (ed): The Endocrinology of Parturition. Basic Science and Clinical Application. Basel, Karger, 2001, p 86

Mesiano S, Chen EC, Fitter JT, et al: Progesterone withdrawal and estrogen activation in human parturition are coordinated by progesterone receptor A expression in the myometrium. J Clin Endocrinol Metab 87:2924, 2002

Mesiano S, Coulter CL, Jaffe RB: Localization of cytochrome P450 cholesterol side-chain cleavage, cytochrome P450 17-alpha-hydroxylase/17,20-lyase, and 3-beta-hydroxysteroid dehydrogenase isomerase steroidogenic enzymes in human and rhesus monkey fetal adrenal glands: Reappraisal of functional zonation. J Clin Endocrinol Metab 77:1184, 1993

Mesiano S, Mellon SH, Gospodarowicz D, et al: Basic fibroblast growth factor expression is regulated by corticotropin in the human fetal adrenal: A model for adrenal growth regulation. Proc Natl Acad Sci U S A 88:5428, 1991

Mijovic JE, Demianczuk N, Olson DM, et al: Prostaglandin endoperoxide H synthase mRNA expression in the fetal membranes correlates with fetal fibronectin concentration in the cervico-vaginal fluids at term: Evidence of enzyme induction before the onset of labour. Br J Obstet Gynaecol 107:267, 2000

Milewich L, Gomez-Sanchez C, Madden JD, et al: Dehydroisoandrosterone sulfate in peripheral blood of premenopausal, pregnant and postmenopausal women and men. J Steroid Biochem 9:1159, 1978

Miller-Lindholm AK, LaBenz CJ, Ramey J, et al: Human chorionic gonadotropin-beta gene expression in first trimester placenta. Endocrinology 138:5459, 1997

Moffett-King A: Natural killer cells and pregnancy. Nat Rev Immunol 2:656, 2002

Moghrabi N, Head JR, Andersson S: Cell type-specific expression of 17 beta-hydroxysteroid dehydrogenase type 2 in human placenta and fetal liver. J Clin Endocrinol Metab 82:3872, 1997

Moore JJ, Dubyak GR, Moore RM, et al: Oxytocin activates the inositol-phospholipid-protein kinase-C system and stimulates prostaglandin production in human amnion cells. Endocrinology 123:1771, 1988

Moore KL: The Developing Human: Clinically Oriented Embryology, 4th ed. Philadelphia, Saunders, 1988

Morishima A, Grumbach MM, Simpson ER, et al: Aromatase deficiency in male and female siblings caused by a novel mutation and the physiological role of estrogens. J Clin Endocrinol Metab 80:3689, 1995

Morrish DW, Marusyk H, Siy O: Demonstration of specific secretory granules for human chorionic gonadotropin in placenta. J Histochem Cytochem 35:93, 1987

Mote PA, Balleine RL, McGowan EM, et al: Colocalization of progesterone receptors A and B by dual immunofluorescent histochemistry in human endometrium during the menstrual cycle. J Clin Endocrinol Metab 84:2963, 1999

Mote PA, Balleine RL, McGowan EM, et al: Heterogeneity of progesterone receptors A and B expression in human endometrial glands and stroma. Hum Reprod 15(suppl 3):48, 2000

Narasaka T, Suzuki T, Moriya T, et al: Temporal and spatial distribution of corticosteroidogenic enzymes immunoreactivity in developing human adrenal. Mol Cell Endocrinol 174:111, 2001

Navot D, Bergh P: Preparation of the human endometrium for implantation. Ann N Y Acad Sci 622:212, 1991

Nelson JL, Furst DE, Maloney S, et al: Microchimerism and HLA-compatible relationships of pregnancy in scleroderma. Lancet 351:559, 1998

Nemeth E, Tashima LS, Yu Z, et al: Fetal membrane distention: I. Differentially expressed genes regulated by acute distention in amniotic epithelial (WISH) cells. Am J Obstet Gynecol 182:50, 2000

Newby D, Aitken DA, Howatson AG, et al: Placental synthesis of oestriol in Down's syndrome pregnancies. Placenta 21:263, 2000

Nichols J, Lescure OL, Migeon CJ: Levels of 17-hydroxycorticosteroids and 17-ketosteroids in maternal and cord plasma in term anencephaly. J Clin Endocrinol 18:444, 1958

Nicholson RC, King BR: Regulation of CRH gene expression in the placenta. Front Horm Res 27:246, 2001

Nikas G: Cell-surface morphological events relevant to human implantation. Hum Reprod 2:37, 2003

Nolten WE, Rueckert PA: Elevated free cortisol index in pregnancy: Possible regulatory mechanisms. Am J Obstet Gynecol 139:492, 1981

Noyes RW, Hertig AT, Rock J: Dating the endometrial biopsy. Fertil Steril 1:3, 1950

Ny T, Wahlberg P, Brandstrom IJ: Matrix remodeling in the ovary: Regulation and functional role of the plasminogen activator and matrix metalloproteinase systems. Mol Cell Endocrinol 187:29, 2002

O'Sullivan CM, Liu SY, Karpinka JB, et al: Embryonic hatching enzyme strypsin/ISP1 is expressed with ISP2 in endometrial glands during implantation. Mol Reprod Dev 62:328, 2002

Odagiri E, Sherrell BJ, Mount CD, et al: Human placental immunoreactive corticotropin, lipotropin, and beta-endorphin: Evidence for a common precursor. Proc Natl Acad Sci U S A 76:2027, 1979

Ogren L, Talamantes F: The placenta as an endocrine organ: Polypeptides. In Knobil E, Neill JD (eds): The Physiology of Reproduction. New York, Raven, 1994, p 875

Owerbach D, Rutter WJ, Cooke NE, et al: The prolactin gene is located on chromosome 6 in humans. Science 212:815, 1981

Owerbach D, Rutter WJ, Martial JA, et al: Genes for growth hormone, chorionic somatomammotropin, and growth hormones-like gene on chromosome 17 in humans. Science 209:289, 1980

Paria BC, Reese J, Das SK, et al: Deciphering the cross-talk of implantation: Advances and challenges. Science 296:2185, 2002

Parker CR Jr, Carr BR, Simpson ER, et al: Decline in the concentration of low-density lipoprotein-cholesterol in human fetal plasma near term. Metabolism 32:919, 1983

Parker CR Jr, Illingworth DR, Bissonnette J, et al: Endocrinology of pregnancy in abetalipoproteinemia: Studies in a patient with homozygous familial hypobetalipoproteinemia. N Engl J Med 314:557, 1986

Parker CR Jr, Simpson ER, Bilheimer DW, et al: Inverse relation between low-density lipoprotein-cholesterol and dehydroisoandrosterone sulfate in human fetal plasma. Science 208:512, 1980

Patel N, Alsat E, Igout A, et al: Glucose inhibits human placental GH secretion, in vitro. J Clin Endocrinol Metab 80:1743, 1995

Pearlman WH: [16-3H] Progesterone metabolism in advanced pregnancy and in oophorectomized-hysterectomized women. Biochem J 67:1, 1957

Pellegrini I, Lebrun JJ, Ali S, et al: Expression of prolactin and its receptor in human lymphoid cells. Mol Endocrinol 6:1023, 1992

Perrot-Applanat M, Groyer-Picard MT, Garcia E, et al: Immunocytochemical demonstration of estrogen and progesterone receptors in muscle cells of uterine arteries in rabbits and humans. Endocrinology 123:1511, 1988

Petraglia F, Florio P, Benedetto C, et al: Urocortin stimulates placental adrenocorticotropin and prostaglandin release and myometrial contractility in vitro. J Clin Endocrinol Metab 84:1420, 1999

Petraglia F, Gallinelli A, De Vita D, et al: Activin at parturition: Changes of maternal serum levels and evidence for binding sites in placenta and fetal membranes. Obstet Gynecol 84:278, 1994

Petraglia F, Garuti GC, Calza L, et al: Inhibin subunits in human placenta: Localization and messenger ribonucleic acid levels during pregnancy. Am J Obstet Gynecol 165:750, 1991

Petraglia F, Giardino L, Coukos G, et al: Corticotropin-releasing factor and parturition: Plasma and amniotic fluid levels and placental binding sites. Obstet Gynecol 75:784, 1990

Petraglia F, Sawchenko P, Lim AT, et al: Localization, secretion, and action of inhibin in human placenta. Science 237:187, 1987

Petraglia F, Vaughan J, Vale W: Inhibin and activin modulate the release of gonadotropin-releasing hormone, human chorionic gonadotropin, and progesterone from cultured human placental cells. Proc Natl Acad Sci U S A 86:5114, 1989

Petraglia F, Woodruff TK, Botticelli G, et al: Gonadotropin-releasing hormone, inhibin, and activin in human placenta: Evidence for a common cellular localization. J Clin Endocrinol Metab 74:1184, 1992

Pijnenborg R: Trophoblast invasion. Reprod Med Rev 3:53, 1994

Pijnenborg R, Bland JM, Robertson WB, et al: The pattern of interstitial trophoblastic invasion of the myometrium in early human pregnancy. Placenta 2:303, 1981

Pijnenborg R, Bland JM, Robertson WB, et al: Uteroplacental arterial changes related to interstitial trophoblast migration in early human pregnancy. Placenta 4:397, 1983

Primakoff P, Myles DG: Penetration, adhesion, and fusion in mammalian sperm-egg interaction. Science 296:2183, 2002

Qin X, Chua PK, Ohira RH, et al: An autocrine/paracrine role of human decidual relaxin. II. Stromelysin-1 (MMP-3) and tissue inhibitor of matrix metalloproteinase-1 (TIMP-1). Biol Reprod 56:812, 1997a

Qin X, Garibay-Tupas J, Chua PK, et al: An autocrine/paracrine role of human decidual relaxin. I. Interstitial collagenase (matrix metalloproteinase-1) and tissue plasminogen activator. Biol Reprod 56:800, 1997b

Ragoobir J, Abayasekara DR, Bruckdorfer KR, et al: Stimulation of progesterone production in human granulosa-lutein cells by lipoproteins: Evidence for cholesterol-independent actions of high-density lipoproteins. J Endocrinol 173:103, 2002

Rainey WE, Carr BR, Wang ZN, et al: Gene profiling of human fetal and adult adrenals. J Endocrinol 171:209, 2001

Ramsey E, Davis R: A composite drawing of the placenta to show its structure and circulation. Anat Rec 145:366, 1963

Ramsey E, Harris J: Comparison of uteroplacental vasculature and circulation in the rhesus monkey and man. Contrib Embryol 38:59, 1966

Ramsey EM, Donner MW: Placental Vasculature and Circulation. Philadelphia, Saunders, 1980

Reynolds SRM: Hemodynamic characteristics of the fetal circulation. Am J Obstet Gynecol 68:69, 1954

Riddick DH, Luciano AA, Kusmik WF, et al: Evidence for a nonpituitary source of amniotic fluid prolactin. Fertil Steril 31:35, 1979

Riley S, Walton J, Herlick J, et al: The localization and distribution of corticotropin-releasing hormone in the human placenta and fetal membranes throughout gestation. J Clin Endocrinol Metab 72:1001, 1991

Robidoux J, Simoneau L, St Pierre S, et al: Characterization of neuropeptide Y-mediated corticotropin-releasing factor synthesis and release from human placental trophoblasts. Endocrinology 141:2795, 2000

Robinson BG, Emanuel RL, Frim DM, et al: Glucocorticoid stimulates expression of corticotropin-releasing hormone gene in human placenta. Proc Natl Acad Sci U S A 85:5244, 1988

Rock J, Bartlett M: Biopsy studies of human endometrium. JAMA 108:2022, 1937

Rowe T, King L, MacDonald PC, et al: Tissue inhibitor of metalloproteinase-1 and tissue inhibitor of metalloproteinase-2 expression in human amnion mesenchymal and epithelial cells. Am J Obstet Gynecol 176:915, 1997

Ryan KJ: Biological aromatization of steroids. J Biol Chem 234:268, 1959a

Ryan KJ: Metabolism of C-16-oxygenated steroids by human placenta: The formation of estriol. J Biol Chem 234:2006, 1959b

Salido EC, Yen PH, Barajas L, et al: Steroid sulfatase expression in human placenta: Immunocytochemistry and in situ hybridization study. J Clin Endocrinol Metab 70:1564, 1990

Saxe A, Dean S, Gibson G, et al: Parathyroid hormone and parathyroid hormone-related peptide in venous umbilical cord blood of healthy neonates. J Perinat Med 25:288, 1997

Segaloff A, Sternberg W, Gaskill C: Effects of luteotrophic doses of chorionic gonadotropin in women. J Clin Endocrinol Metab 11:936, 1951

Shaul PW: Regulation of endothelial nitric oxide synthase: Location, location, location. Annu Rev Physiol 64:749, 2002

Short R: Steroids in the follicular fluid and the corpus luteum of the mare. A 'two cell type' theory of ovarian steroid synthesis. J Endocrinol 24:59, 1962

Shozu M, Akasofu K, Harada T, et al: A new cause of female pseudohermaphroditism: Placental aromatase deficiency. J Clin Endocrinol Metab 72:560, 1991

Siiteri PK, MacDonald PC: Placental estrogen biosynthesis during human pregnancy. J Clin Endocrinol Metab 26:751, 1966b

Siiteri PK, MacDonald PC: The utilization of circulating dehydroisoandrosterone sulfate for estrogen synthesis during human pregnancy. Steroids 2:713, 1963

Siler-Khodr TM: Chorionic peptides. In McNellis D, Challis JRG, MacDonald PC, et al (eds): The Onset of Labor: Cellular and Integrative Mechanisms. Ithaca, Perinatology Press, 1988, p 213

Siler-Khodr TM, Khodr GS: Content of luteinizing hormone-releasing factor in the human placenta. Am J Obstet Gynecol 130:216, 1978

Siler-Khodr TM, Khodr GS: Dose response analysis of gnRH stimulation of hCG release from human term placenta. Biol Reprod 25:353, 1981

Siler-Khodr TM, Khodr GS, Valenzuela G: Immunoreactive gonadotropin-releasing hormone level in maternal circulation throughout pregnancy. Am J Obstet Gynecol 150:376, 1984

Simpson ER: Genetic mutations resulting in loss of aromatase activity in humans and mice. J Soc Gynecol Investig 7:S18, 2000

Simpson ER, Burkhart MF: Acyl CoA:cholesterol acyl transferase activity in human placental microsomes: Inhibition by progesterone. Arch Biochem Biophys 200:79, 1980

Simpson ER, Carr BR, Parker CR, Jr, et al: The role of serum lipoproteins in steroidogenesis by the human fetal adrenal cortex. J Clin Endocrinol Metab 49:146, 1979

Steele GL, Currie WD, Yuen BH, et al: Acute stimulation of human chorionic gonadotropin secretion by recombinant human activin-A in first trimester human trophoblast. Endocrinology 133:297, 1993

Streeter GL: A human embryo (Mateer) of the presomite period. Contrib Embryol 9:389, 1920

Sugino N, Kashida S, Karube-Harada A, et al: Expression of vascular endothelial growth factor (VEGF) and its receptors in human endometrium throughout the menstrual cycle and in early pregnancy. Reproduction 123:379, 2002

Telgmann R, Gellersen B: Marker genes of decidualization: Activation of the decidual prolactin gene. Hum Reprod Update 4:472, 1998

Thellin O, Coumans B, Zorzi W, et al: Tolerance to the foeto-placental 'graft': Ten ways to support a child for nine months. Curr Opin Immunol 12:731, 2000

Thomson A, Billewicz W, Hytten F: The weight of the placenta in relation to birthweight. Br J Obstet Gynaecol 76:865, 1969

Tomer Y, Huber GK, Davies TF: Human chorionic gonadotropin (hCG) interacts directly with recombinant human TSH receptors. J Clin Endocrinol Metab 74:1477, 1992

Tsai SJ, Wu MH, Chen HM, et al: Fibroblast growth factor-9 is an endometrial stromal growth factor. Endocrinology 143:2715, 2002

Tsuruta E, Tada H, Tamaki H, et al: Pathogenic role of asialo human chorionic gonadotropin in gestational thyrotoxicosis. J Clin Endocrinol Metab 80:350, 1995

Tyson JE, Hwang P, Guyda H, et al: Studies of prolactin secretion in human pregnancy. Am J Obstet Gynecol 113:14, 1972

Vande Wiele RL, Bogumil J, Dyrenfurth I, et al: Mechanisms regulating the menstrual cycle in women. Recent Prog Horm Res 26:63, 1970

Vaskivuo TE, Ottander U, Oduwole O, et al: Role of apoptosis, apoptosis-related factors and 17 beta-hydroxysteroid dehydrogenases in human corpus luteum regression. Mol Cell Endocrinol 194:191, 2002

Vince GS, Johnson PM: Immunobiology of human uteroplacental macrophages—friend and foe? Placenta 17:191, 1996

Vince GS, Johnson PM: Leucocyte populations and cytokine regulation in human uteroplacental tissues. Biochem Soc Trans 28:191, 2000

Wadhwa PD, Porto M, Garite TJ, et al: Maternal corticotropin-releasing hormone levels in the early third trimester predict length of gestation in human pregnancy. Am J Obstet Gynecol 179:1079, 1998

Walker WH, Fitzpatrick SL, Barrera-Saldana HA, et al: The human placental lactogen genes: Structure, function, evolution and transcriptional regulation. Endocr Rev 12:316, 1991

Warren W, Silverman A: Cellular localization of corticotrophin releasing hormone in the human placenta, fetal membranes and decidua. Placenta 16:147, 1995

Weetman AP: The immunology of pregnancy. Thyroid 9:643, 1999

Wehmann RE, Nisula BC: Renal clearance rates of the subunits of human chorionic gonadotropin in man. J Clin Endocrinol Metab 50:674, 1980

Wentz AC, Jones GS: Transient luteolytic effect of prostaglandin F2alpha in the human. Obstet Gynecol 42:172, 1973

Werbin H, Plotz EJ, LeRoy GV, et al: Cholesterol: A precursor of estrone in vivo. J Am Chem Soc 79:1012, 1957

Whittle WL, Gibb W, Challis JR: The characterization of human amnion epithelial and mesenchymal cells: The cellular expression, activity and glucocorticoid regulation of prostaglandin output. Placenta 21:394, 2000

Winters AJ, Oliver C, Colston C, et al: Plasma ACTH levels in the human fetus and neonate as related to age and parturition. J Clin Endocrinol Metab 39:269, 1974

Wislocki GB, Dempsey EW: Electron microscopy of the human placenta. Anat Rec 123:133, 1955

Wolfahrt S, Kleine B, Rossmanith WG: Detection of gonadotrophin releasing hormone and its receptor mRNA in human placental trophoblasts using in-situ reverse transcription-polymerase chain reaction. Mol Hum Reprod 4:999, 1998

Yanagisawa M, Kurihara H, Kimura S, et al: A novel potent vasoconstrictor peptide produced by vascular endothelial cells. Nature 332:411, 1988

Yoshimura M, Pekary AE, Pang XP, et al: Thyrotropic activity of basic isoelectric forms of human chorionic gonadotropin extracted from hydatidiform mole tissues. J Clin Endocrinol Metab 78:862, 1994

4

Fetal Growth and Development

Contemporary obstetrical research focuses on the physiology and pathophysiology of the fetus, its development, and its environment. An important direct result of this research is that the status of the fetus has been elevated to that of a patient who, in large measure, can be given the same meticulous care that obstetricians provide for pregnant women. In the course of these studies it has become apparent that the conceptus is a dynamic force in the pregnancy unit. The contributions of the conceptus to implantation, maternal recognition of pregnancy, immunological acceptance, endocrine function, nutrition, and parturition are enormous, and absolutely essential for successful pregnancy as described in Chapter 3. Normal fetal development is considered in this chapter. Anomalies, injuries, and diseases that affect the fetus and newborn are addressed in detail in Chapter 29. Techniques used to evaluate fetal well-being, or fetal health, are presented in other chapters.

DETERMINATION OF GESTATIONAL AGE

Several different terms are used to define the duration of pregnancy, and thus fetal age, but these are somewhat confusing. They are shown schematically in Figure 4–1. *Gestational age* or *menstrual age* is the time elapsed since the first day of the last menstrual period, a time that actually precedes conception. This starting time, which is usually about 2 weeks before ovulation and fertilization, and nearly 3 weeks before implantation of the blastocyst, has traditionally been used because most women know their last period. The increasing use of infertility therapy has changed this somewhat because ovulation may be known exactly. Embryologists describe embryo-fetal development in *ovulation age,* or the time in days or weeks from ovulation. Another term is *postconceptional age,* nearly identical to ovulation age.

Obstetricians customarily calculate gestational age as menstrual age. About 280 days, or 40 weeks, elapse on average between the first day of the last menstrual period and the

birth of the fetus. This corresponds to $9\frac{1}{3}$ calendar months, or 10 units of 28 days each. The unit of 28 days has been referred to commonly, but imprecisely, as a *lunar month* of pregnancy. Actually, the time from one new moon to the next is $29\frac{1}{2}$ days. A quick estimate of the due date of a pregnancy based on menstrual cycle can be made as follows: add 7 days to the first day of the last menstrual period and subtract 3 months. For example, if the first day of the last menses was July 5th, the due date of this pregnancy is 07-05 + 7 (days) minus 3 (months) = 04-12, or April 12th of the following year. As discussed in Chapter 16 (see p. 392), many women now undergo first- or early second-trimester ultrasound examination to confirm gestational age. In these cases, the sonographic estimate is usually a few days later than that determined by the last period. To rectify this inconsistency—and to reduce the number of pregnancies diagnosed as postterm—some authorities suggest assuming that the average pregnancy is actually 283 days long instead of 280, and thus adding 10 days to the last menses instead of 7 (Olsen and Clausen, 1998).

The period of gestation can also be divided into three units of three calendar months (13 weeks) each, or three *trimesters,* because important obstetrical milestones can be designated conveniently by trimesters. The possibility of spontaneous abortion, for example, is limited principally to the first trimester, whereas the likelihood of infant survival is increased greatly in pregnancies that reach the third trimester.

MORPHOLOGICAL GROWTH

OVUM, ZYGOTE, AND BLASTOCYST. During the first 2 weeks after ovulation, several successive phases of development can be identified: (1) fertilization, (2) formation of free blastocyst, and (3) implantation of the blastocyst. Primitive chorionic villi are formed soon after implantation. With the development of chorionic villi, it is conventional to refer

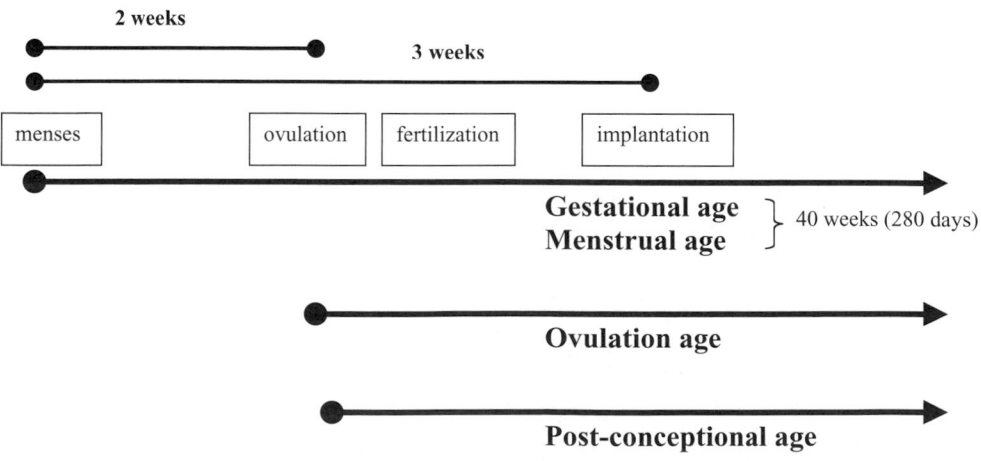

FIGURE 4–1. Terminology used to describe the duration of pregnancy.

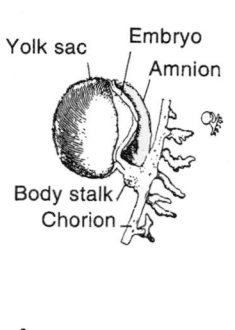

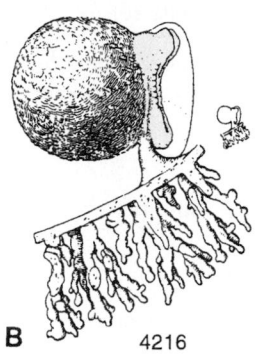

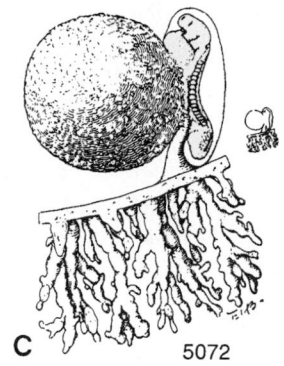

Yolk sac   Embryo
            Amnion

Body stalk
Chorion

A   5960

B   4216

C   5072

FIGURE 4–2. Early human embryos. Only the chorion adjacent to the body stalk is shown. Small outline to the right of each embryo gives its actual size. Ovulation ages: **A.** 19 days (presomite). **B.** 21 days (7 somites). **C.** 22 days (17 somites). (After drawings and models in the Carnegie Institute, drawing identification number noted below each.)

to the products of conception not as a fertilized ovum, or zygote, but as an *embryo.* The early stages of preplacental development and formation of the placenta are described in Chapter 3.

EMBRYO. The embryonic period commences at the beginning of the third week after ovulation and fertilization, which coincides in time with the expected day that the next menstruation would have started. Most pregnancy tests that measure human chorionic gonadotropin (hCG) are positive by this time (see Chap. 8, p. 206), and the embryonic disc is well defined. The body stalk is differentiated; the chorionic sac is approximately 1 cm in diameter (Figs. 4–2 and 4–3). There is a true intervillous space that contains maternal blood and villous cores in which angioblastic chorionic mesoderm can be distinguished.

By the end of the fourth week after ovulation, the chorionic sac is 2 to 3 cm in diameter, and the embryo is about 4 to 5 mm in length (Figs. 4–4, 4–5, and 4–6). Partitioning of the primitive heart begins in the middle of the fourth week. Arm and leg buds are present, and the amnion is beginning to unsheathe the body stalk, which thereafter becomes the umbilical cord.

At the end of the sixth week after fertilization, the embryo is 22 to 24 mm in length, and the head is quite large compared with the trunk. The heart is completely formed. Fingers and

toes are present, and the arms bend at the elbows. The upper lip is complete, and the external ears form definitive elevations on either side of the head.

The end of the embryonic period and the beginning of the fetal period is arbitrarily designated by most embryologists to occur 8 weeks after fertilization, or 10 weeks after the onset of the last menstrual period. At this time, the embryo-fetus is nearly 4 cm long (Fig. 4–7). The major portion of lung development is yet to occur, but few other new major body structures are formed after this time.

FETUS. Development during the fetal period of gestation consists of growth and maturation of structures that were formed during the embryonic period.

12 Gestational Weeks. By the end of the 12th week of pregnancy, when the uterus usually is just palpable above the symphysis pubis, the crown-rump length of the fetus is 6 to 7 cm. Centers of ossification have appeared in most of the fetal bones, and the fingers and toes have become differentiated. Skin and nails have developed and scattered rudiments of hair appear. The external genitalia are beginning to show definitive signs of male or female gender. The fetus begins to make spontaneous movements.

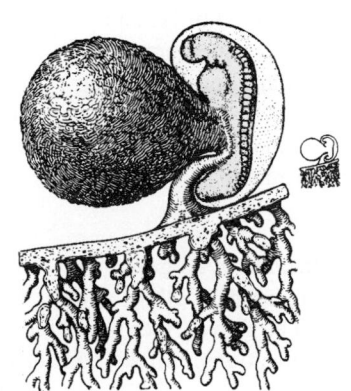

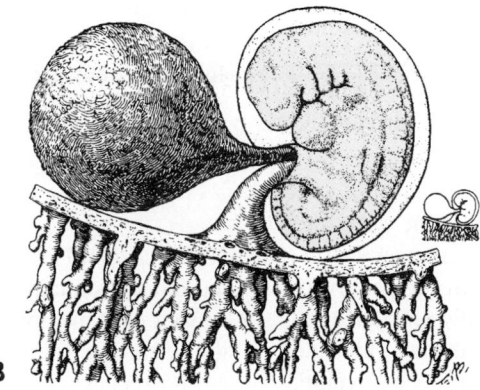

A

B

FIGURE 4–3. Early human embryos. Small outline to the right of each embryo gives its actual size. Ovulation ages: **A.** 22 days. **B.** 23 days. (After drawings and models in the Carnegie Institute.)

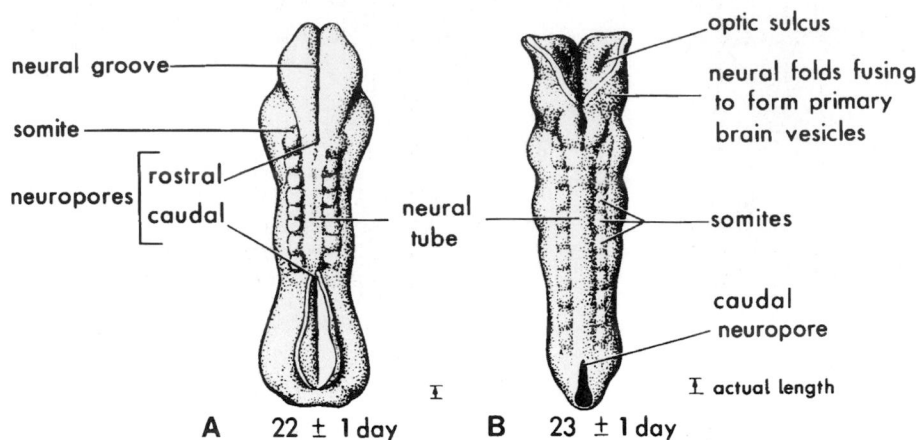

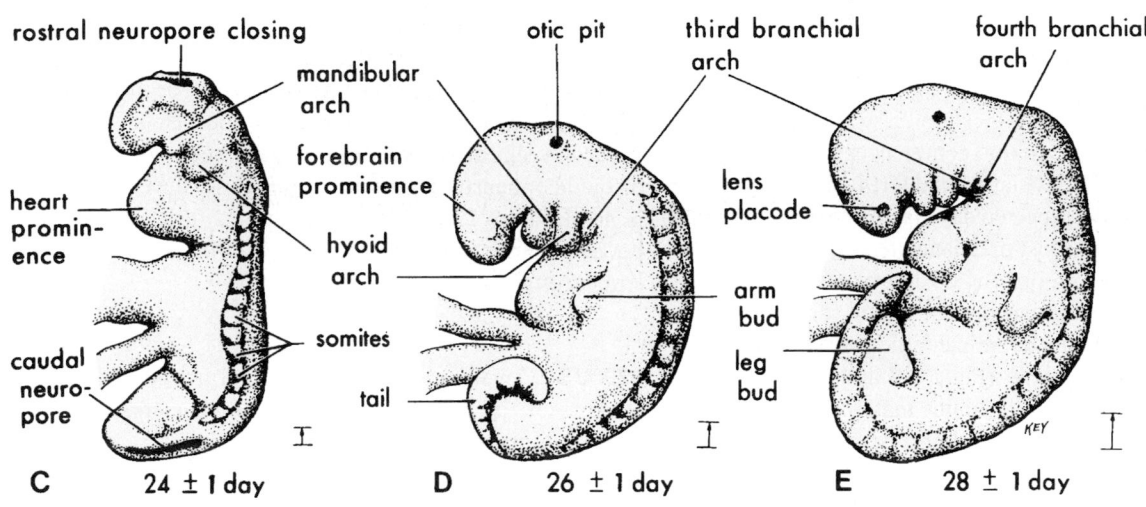

FIGURE 4–4. Three- to four-week-old embryos. **A, B.** Dorsal views of embryos during about 22 to 23 days of development showing 8 and 12 somites, respectively. **C–E.** Lateral views of embryos during 24 to 28 days, showing 16, 27, and 33 somites, respectively. (From Moore, 1988, with permission.)

16 Gestational Weeks. By the end of the 16th week, the crown-rump length of the fetus is 12 cm, and the weight is 110 g. Gender can be correctly determined by experienced observers by inspection of the external genitalia by 14 weeks.

20 Gestational Weeks. The end of the 20th week is the midpoint of pregnancy as estimated from the beginning of the last normal menstrual period. The fetus now weighs somewhat more than 300 g, and the weight begins to increase in a linear manner. The fetal skin has become less transparent, a downy lanugo covers its entire body, and some scalp hair has developed.

24 Gestational Weeks. By the end of the 24th week, the fetus weighs about 630 g. The skin is characteristically wrinkled, and fat deposition begins. The head is still comparatively large, and eyebrows and eyelashes are usually recognizable. The canalicular period of lung development, during which the bronchi and bronchioles enlarge and alveolar ducts develop,

is nearly completed. A fetus born at this time will attempt to breathe, but most will die because the terminal sacs, required for gas exchange, have not yet formed.

28 Gestational Weeks. By the end of the 28th week, a crown-rump length of about 25 cm is attained and the fetus weighs about 1100 g. The thin skin is red and covered with vernix caseosa. The pupillary membrane has just disappeared from the eyes. An infant born at this time moves limbs energetically and cries weakly. The otherwise normal infant of this age has a 90-percent chance of survival without physical or neurological impairment.

32 Gestational Weeks. At the end of 32 gestational weeks, the fetus has attained a crown-rump length of about 28 cm and a weight of about 1800 g. The skin surface is still red and wrinkled. Barring other complications, infants born at this period also usually survive intact.

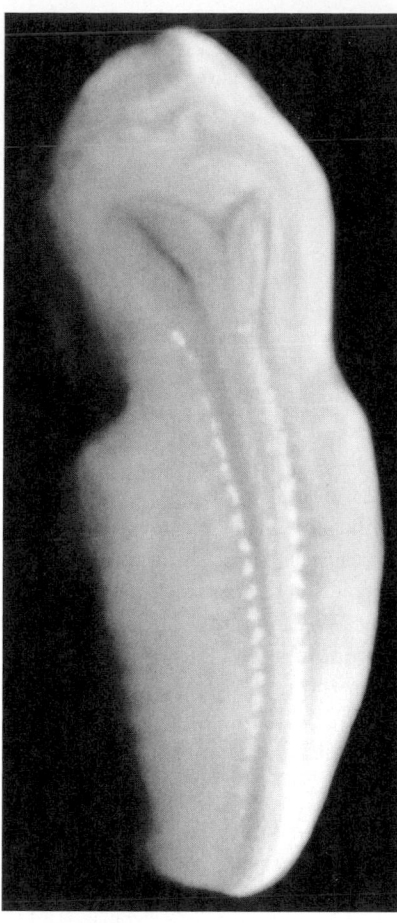

FIGURE 4–5. Photograph of dorsal view of embryo at about 24 to 26 days and corresponding to Figure 4–4B. (From Werth and Tsiaras, 2002, with permission).

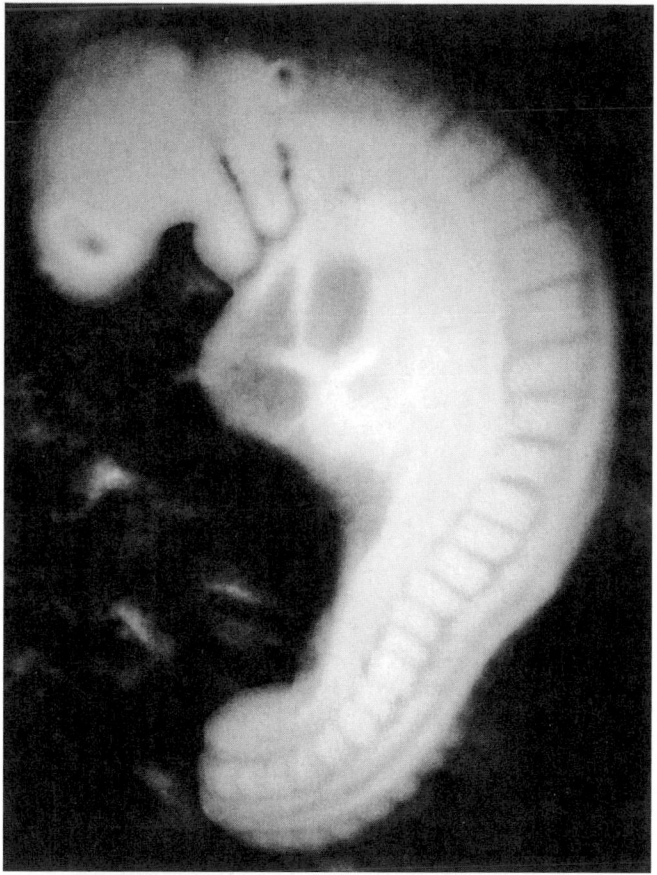

FIGURE 4–6. Photograph of lateral view of embryo at about 28 days and corresponding to Figure 4–4E. (From Werth and Tsiaras, 2002, with permission).

36 Gestational Weeks. At the end of 36 weeks of gestation, the average crown-rump length of the fetus is about 32 cm and the weight is about 2500 g. Because of the deposition of subcutaneous fat, the body has become more rotund, and the previous wrinkled appearance of the face has been lost. Infants born at this time have an excellent chance of survival with proper care.

40 Gestational Weeks. Term is reached at 40 weeks from the onset of the last menstrual period. At this time, the fetus is fully developed. The average crown-rump length of the fetus at term is about 36 cm, and the weight is approximately 3400 g.

Length of Fetus. Because of the variability in the length of the legs and the difficulty of maintaining them in extension, measurements corresponding to the sitting height (crown-to-rump) are more accurate than those corresponding to the standing height. The average sitting height and weight of the fetus at the end of each lunar month were determined by Streeter (1920) from 704 specimens. These values are similar to those shown in Table 4–1. Such values are approximate, but

generally, length is a more accurate criterion of gestational age than weight.

Fetal Head. From an obstetrical viewpoint, the size of the fetal head is important because an essential feature of labor is the adaptation between the fetal head and the maternal bony pelvis. Only a comparatively small part of the head at term is represented by the face. The rest of the head is composed of the firm skull, which is made up of two frontal, two parietal, and two temporal bones, along with the upper portion of the occipital bone and the wings of the sphenoid. These bones are separated by membranous spaces, or *sutures* (Fig. 4–8).

The most important sutures are the frontal, between the two frontal bones; the sagittal, between the two parietal bones; the two coronal, between the frontal and parietal bones; and the two lambdoid, between the posterior margins of the parietal bones and upper margin of the occipital bone. Where several sutures meet, an irregular space forms, which is enclosed by a membrane and designated as a *fontanel* (see Fig. 4–8). The greater, or anterior fontanel, is a lozenge-shaped space that is situated at the junction of the sagittal and the coronal

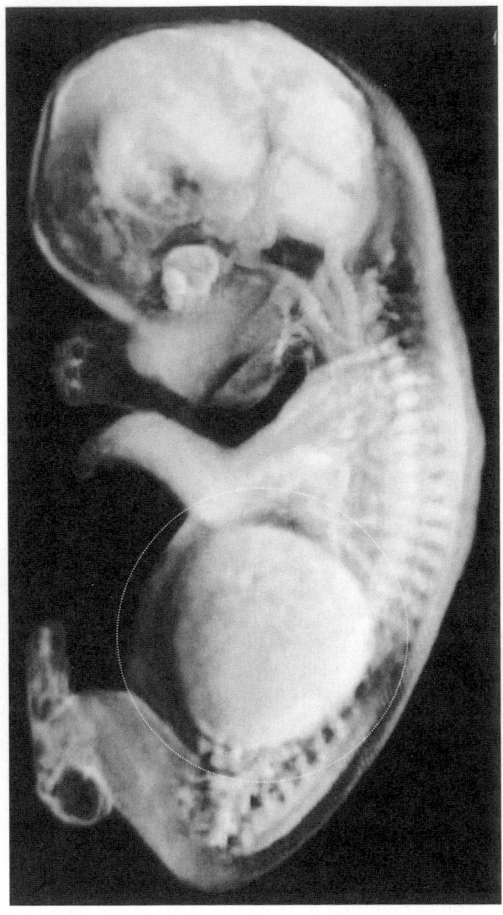

FIGURE 4–7. Lateral view of embryo-fetus at 56 days, which marks the end of the embryonic period and the beginning of the fetal period. The liver is within the dotted-line circle. (From Werth and Tsiaras, 2002, with permission.)

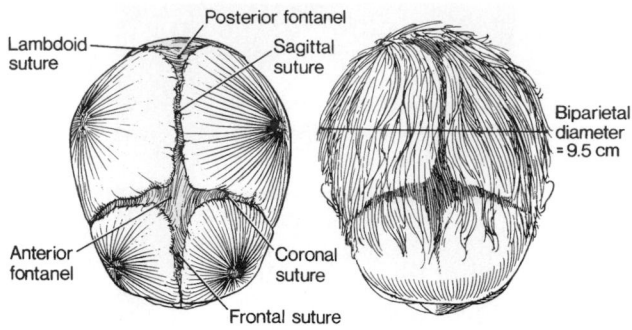

FIGURE 4–8. Fetal head at term showing fontanels, sutures, and the biparietal diameter.

sutures. The lesser, or posterior fontanel, is represented by a small triangular area at the intersection of the sagittal and lambdoid sutures. The localization of these fontanels gives important information concerning the presentation and position of the fetus. The temporal, or casserian fontanels, have no diagnostic significance.

It is customary to measure certain critical diameters and circumferences of the newborn head (Fig. 4–9). The diameters most frequently used, and the average lengths thereof, are:

1. The *occipitofrontal* (11.5 cm), which follows a line extending from a point just above the root of the nose to the most prominent portion of the occipital bone.
2. The *biparietal* (9.5 cm), the greatest transverse diameter of the head, which extends from one parietal boss to the other.

TABLE 4–1 Criteria for Estimating Age During the Fetal Period

Age (wk)		Crown-Rump Length (mm)[a]	Foot Length (mm)[a]	Fetal Weight (g)[b]	Main External Characteristics
Menstrual	Fertilization				
11	9	50	7	8	Eyes closing or closed. Head more rounded. External genitalia still not distinguishable as male or female. Intestines are in umbilical cord.
12	10	61	9	14	Intestines in abdomen. Early fingernail development.
14	12	87	14	45	Sex distinguishable externally. Well-defined neck.
16	14	120	20	110	Head erect. Lower limbs well developed.
18	16	140	27	200	Ears stand out from head.
20	18	160	33	320	Vernix caseosa present. Early toenail development.
22	20	190	39	460	Head and body (lanugo) hair visible.
24	22	210	45	630	Skin wrinkled and red.
26	24	230	50	820	Fingernails present. Lean body.
28	26	250	55	1000	Eyes partially open. Eyelashes present.
30	28	270	59	1300	Eyes open. Good head of hair. Skin slightly wrinkled.
32	30	280	63	1700	Toenails present. Body filling out. Testes descending.
34	32	300	68	2100	Fingernails reach fingertips. Skin pink and smooth.
38	36	340	79	2900	Body usually plump. Lanugo hairs almost absent. Toenails reach toe tips.
40	38	360	83	3400	Prominent chest; breasts protrude. Testes in scrotum or palpable in inguinal canals. Fingernails extend beyond fingertips.

[a]These measurements are average and so may not apply to specific cases; dimensional variations increase with age.
[b]These weights refer to fetuses fixed for about 2 weeks in 10 percent formalin. Fresh specimens weigh about 5 percent less.
From Moore, 1977, with permission.

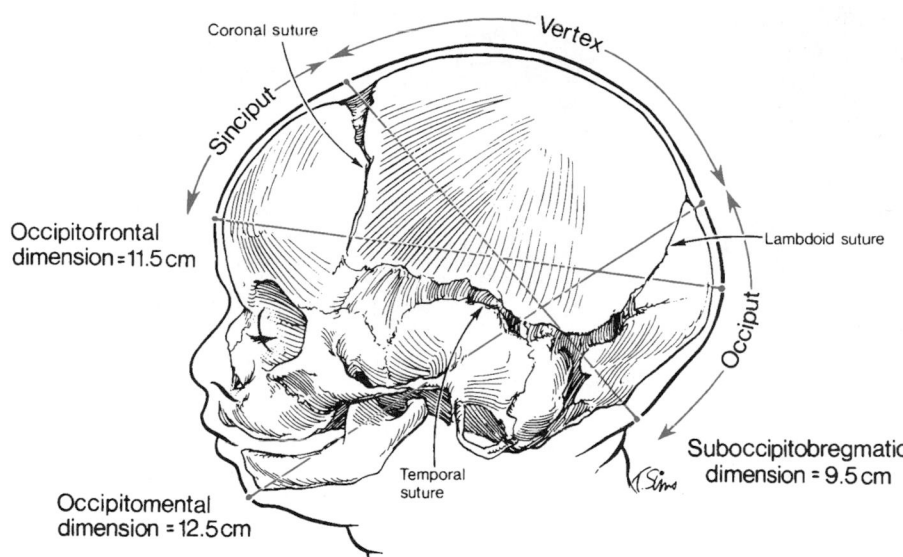

FIGURE 4–9. Diameters of the fetal head at term.

3. The *bitemporal* (8.0 cm), the greatest distance between the two temporal sutures (see Fig. 4–8).
4. The *occipitomental* (12.5 cm), from the chin to the most prominent portion of the occiput.
5. The *suboccipitobregmatic* (9.5 cm), which follows a line drawn from the middle of the large fontanel to the undersurface of the occipital bone just where it joins the neck.

The greatest circumference of the head, which corresponds to the plane of the occipitofrontal diameter, averages 34.5 cm, a size too large to fit through the pelvis without flexion. The smallest circumference, corresponding to the plane of the suboccipitobregmatic diameter, is 32 cm. The bones of the cranium are normally connected only by a thin layer of fibrous tissue that allows considerable shifting or sliding of each bone to accommodate the size and shape of the maternal pelvis. This intrapartum process is termed *molding*. The head position and degree of skull ossification result in a spectrum of cranial plasticity from minimal to great and, in some cases, undoubtedly contribute to fetopelvic disproportion, a leading indication for cesarean delivery (see Chap. 25, p. 591).

Fetal Brain. There is a steady gestational age-related change in the appearance of the fetal brain (Fig. 4–10). It is therefore possible to identify fetal age rather precisely from its external appearance (Dolman, 1977). Myelination of the ventral roots of the cerebrospinal nerves and brainstem begins at approximately 6 months, but the major portion of myelination occurs after birth. The lack of myelin and the incomplete ossification of the fetal skull permit the structure of the brain to be seen with ultrasound throughout gestation.

PLACENTAL ROLE IN FETAL GROWTH

The placenta is the organ of transfer between mother and fetus. At the maternal–fetal interface, there is transfer of oxygen and nutrients from the mother to the fetus. Conversely, there is transfer of carbon dioxide and other metabolic wastes from fetus to mother (see Fig. 3–22, p. 65). There are no direct communications between the fetal blood, which is contained in the fetal capillaries in the intravillous space of the chorionic villi, and the maternal blood, which remains in the intervillous space. The one exception to this dictum is the occasional development of breaks in the chorionic villi, permitting the escape of fetal erythrocytes and leukocytes, in various numbers, into the maternal circulation. This leakage is the mechanism by which some D-negative women become sensitized by the erythrocytes of their D-positive fetus (see Chap. 29, p. 663). Aside from these occasional leaks, however, there is no gross intermingling of the macromolecular constituents of the two circulations. Therefore, bidirectional transfer depends primarily on the processes that permit or facilitate the transport of such substances through the syncytiotrophoblast of the intact chorionic villi.

THE INTERVILLOUS SPACE: MATERNAL BLOOD. The intervillous space is the primary biological compartment of maternal–fetal transfer. Maternal blood in this extravascular compartment directly bathes the trophoblasts. Substances transferred from mother to fetus first enter the intervillous space and are then transported to the syncytiotrophoblast. Substances transported from the fetus to the mother are transferred from the syncytium into the same space. Thus, the chorionic villi and the intervillous space, together, function for the fetus as lung, gastrointestinal tract, and kidney.

The circulation of maternal blood within the intervillous space is described in Chapter 3 (see p. 63). The residual volume of the intervillous space of the term placenta measures about 140 mL. However, before delivery the normal volume of the intervillous space may be twice this value (Aherne and Dunnill, 1966). Uteroplacental blood flow near

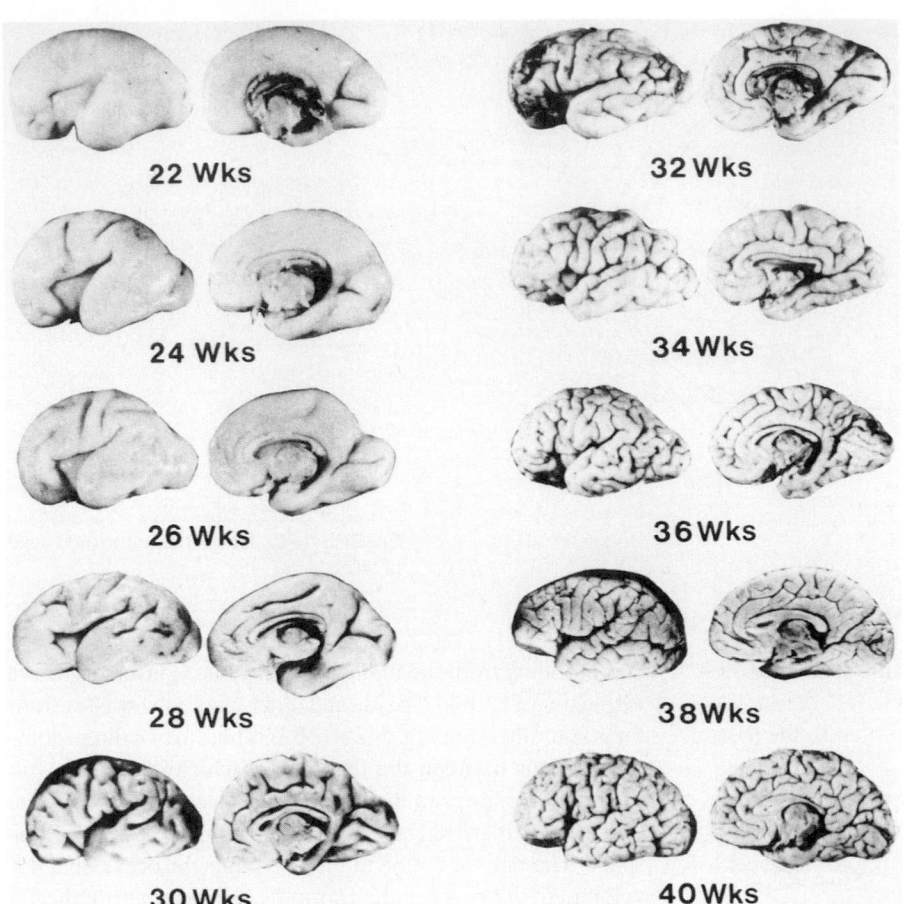

22 Wks

24 Wks

26 Wks

28 Wks

30 Wks

32 Wks

34 Wks

36 Wks

38 Wks

40 Wks

FIGURE 4–10. Characteristic configuration of fetal brains from 22 to 40 weeks of gestation at 2-week intervals. (From Dolman, 1977, with permission.)

term has been estimated to be about 700 to 900 mL/min, with most of the blood apparently going to the intervillous space.

The forceful uterine contractions of active labor cause a reduction in blood flow into the intervillous space, the degree of reduction depending in large measure on the intensity of the contraction. Blood pressure within the intervillous space is significantly less than the uterine arterial pressure, but somewhat greater than uterine venous pressure. Uterine venous pressure, in turn, varies depending on several factors, including maternal position. When supine, for example, pressure in the lower part of the inferior vena cava is elevated, and consequently, pressure in the uterine and ovarian veins, and in turn in the intervillous space, is increased.

PLACENTAL TRANSFER

Chorionic Villus. Substances that pass from maternal blood to fetal blood must traverse (1) syncytiotrophoblast, (2) stroma of the intravillous space, and (3) fetal capillary wall. Although this histological barrier separates the blood in the maternal and fetal circulations, it does not behave in a uniform manner like a simple physical barrier. Throughout pregnancy, syncytiotrophoblast actively or passively permits, facilitates, and adjusts the amount and rate of transfer of a wide range of substances to the fetus. The walls of the villous capillaries

likewise become thinner, and the relative number of fetal vessels increases in relation to the villous connective tissue. It is important to recall that the walls of the fetal placental surface vessels, after branching from the truncal arteries of the chorionic vessels, do not contain smooth muscle cells (see Chap. 3, p. 63). Several attempts have been made to estimate the total surface area of chorionic villi in the human placenta at term. From the planimetric measurements made by Aherne and Dunnill (1966) of the villous surface area of the placenta, it is evident that there is a close correlation with fetal weight. The total surface area at term has been estimated to be approximately 10 m².

Regulation of Placental Transfer. The syncytiotrophoblast is the fetal tissue interface. The maternal-facing surface of this tissue is characterized by a complex microvillus structure. The fetal-facing (basal) cell membrane of the trophoblast is the site of transfer to the intravillous space through which the fetal capillaries traverse. The fetal capillaries are an additional site for transport from the intravillous space into fetal blood, or vice versa.

In determining the effectiveness of the human placenta as an organ of transfer, at least 10 variables are important:

1. The concentration of the substance under consideration in the maternal plasma, and in some instances, the extent

to which it is bound to another compound, such as a carrier protein.

2. The rate of maternal blood flow through the intervillous space.

3. The area available for exchange across the villous trophoblast epithelium.

4. If the substance is transferred by diffusion, the physical properties of the tissue barrier interposed between blood in the intervillous space and in the fetal capillaries.

5. For any substance actively transported, the capacity of the biochemical machinery of the placenta for effecting active transfer, for example, specific receptors on the plasma membrane of the trophoblast.

6. The amount of the substance metabolized by the placenta during transfer.

7. The area for exchange across the fetal capillaries in the placenta.

8. The concentration of the substance in the fetal blood, exclusive of any that is bound.

9. Specific binding or carrier proteins in the fetal or maternal circulation.

10. The rate of fetal blood flow through the villous capillaries.

Mechanisms of Transfer. Most substances with a molecular mass less than 500 d diffuse readily through placental tissue. Molecular weight is clearly important in determining the rate of transfer by diffusion. Simple diffusion, however, is by no means the only mechanism of transfer of low-molecular-weight compounds. The syncytiotrophoblast actively facilitates the transfer of a variety of small compounds, especially those that are in low concentration in maternal plasma but are essential for normal fetal growth and development. Simple diffusion appears to be the mechanism involved in the transfer of oxygen, carbon dioxide, water, and most (but not all) electrolytes. Anesthetic gases also pass through the placenta rapidly by simple diffusion.

Insulin, steroid hormones, and thyroid hormones cross the placenta, but at very slow rates. The hormones synthesized in situ in the trophoblasts enter both the maternal and fetal circulations, but not equally (see Chap. 3). For example, concentrations of chorionic gonadotropin and placental lactogen in fetal plasma are much lower than in maternal plasma. Substances of high molecular weight usually do not traverse the placenta, but there are important exceptions, such as immunoglobulin G—molecular weight 160,000 d—which is transferred by way of a specific trophoblast receptor–mediated mechanism.

Transfer of Oxygen and Carbon Dioxide. In their excellent account of placental transport, Morriss and associates (1994) recall that in 1674, Mayow suggested that the placenta served as the fetal lung. In 1796, Erasmus Darwin, only 22 years after the discovery of oxygen, observed that the color of blood passing through lungs and gills became bright red.

He deduced, from the structure as well as the position of the placenta, that it appeared to be a respiratory organ by which the fetus becomes oxygenated.

The transfer of oxygen across the placenta is blood-flow limited. The placenta supplies about 8 mL O_2/min/kg of fetal weight, and because fetal blood oxygen stores are sufficient for only 1 to 2 minutes, this supply must be continuous (Longo, 1991). Normal values for oxygen, carbon dioxide, and pH in fetal blood are presented in Figure 4–11. Because of the continuous passage of oxygen from maternal blood in the intervillous space to the fetus, its oxygen saturation resembles that in the maternal capillaries. The average oxygen saturation of intervillous blood is estimated to be 65 to 75 percent, with a partial pressure (Po_2) of about 30 to 35 mm

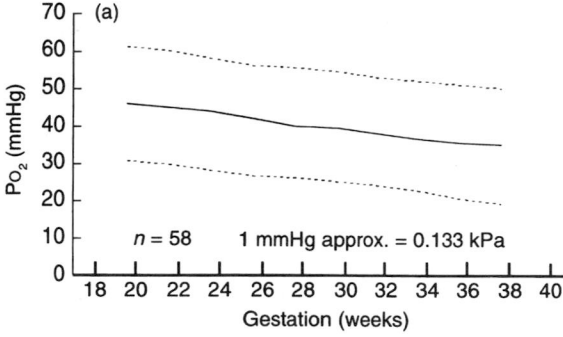

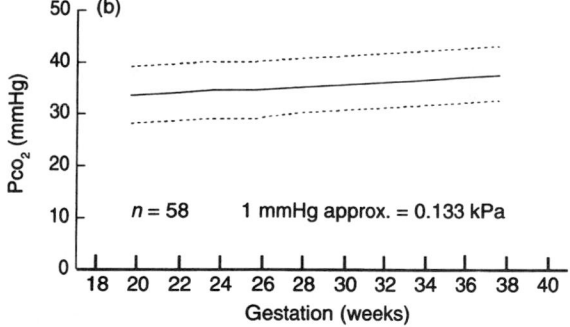

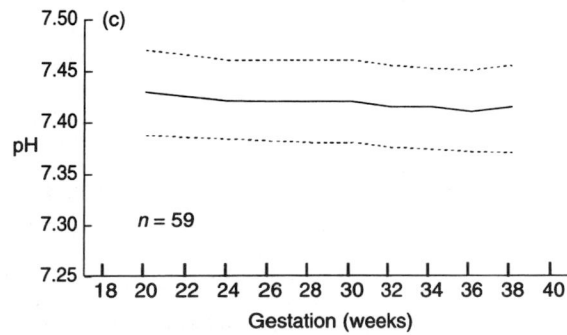

FIGURE 4–11. Umbilical venous oxygen pressure (Po_2) **(a)**, carbon dioxide pressure (Pco_2) **(b)**, and pH **(c)** from cordocentesis on 59 fetuses being evaluated for possible intrauterine infections or hemolysis, and who were found to be healthy at birth and appropriately grown. (From Ramsey, 1996, with permission.)

Hg. The oxygen saturation of umbilical vein blood is similar, but with a somewhat lower oxygen partial pressure.

In general, transfer of fetal carbon dioxide is accomplished by diffusion. The placenta is highly permeable to carbon dioxide, which traverses the chorionic villus more rapidly than oxygen. Near term, the partial pressure of carbon dioxide (P_{CO_2}) in the umbilical arteries is estimated to average about 48 mm Hg, or about 5 mm Hg more than in the maternal intervillous blood. Fetal blood has less affinity for carbon dioxide than does maternal blood, thereby favoring the transfer of carbon dioxide from the fetus to the mother. Also, mild hyperventilation by the pregnant woman results in a fall in P_{CO_2}, favoring a transfer of carbon dioxide from the fetal compartment to maternal blood.

Selective Transfer and Facilitated Diffusion. Although simple diffusion is an important method of placental transfer, the trophoblast and chorionic villus unit demonstrate enormous selectivity in transfer. This results in different concentrations of a variety of metabolites on the two sides of the villus. The concentrations of a number of substances that are not synthesized by the fetus are several times higher in fetal than in maternal blood. Ascorbic acid is a good example of this phenomenon. This relatively low-molecular-weight substance resembles the pentose and hexose sugars and might be expected to traverse the placenta by simple diffusion. The concentration of ascorbic acid, however, is two to four times higher in fetal plasma than in maternal plasma (Morriss and associates, 1994). The unidirectional transfer of iron across the placenta provides another example of transport and sequestration of selected agents. Typically, iron is present in the plasma of the pregnant woman at a lower concentration than in her fetus.

FETAL NUTRITION

During the first 2 months of pregnancy, the embryo consists almost entirely of water. Because of the small amount of yolk in the human ovum, growth of the embryo-fetus from an early stage of development is dependent on nutrients obtained from the mother. During the first few days after implantation, the nutrition of the blastocyst comes from the interstitial fluid of the endometrium and the surrounding maternal tissue. Within the next week, the forerunners of the intervillous space are formed. In the beginning, these are simply lacunae that are filled with maternal blood, but during the third week after fertilization, fetal blood vessels in the chorionic villi appear. During the fourth week, a cardiovascular system has formed, and thereby a true circulation is established both within the embryo and between the embryo and the chorionic villi.

Maternal adaptations to store and transfer nutrients to the fetus are discussed in Chapter 5 and summarized here. The maternal diet is translated into storage forms that are made available to meet the demands for energy, tissue repair, and new growth, including maternal needs for pregnancy. Three major maternal storage depots—the liver, muscle, and adipose tissue—and the storage hormone insulin are intimately involved in the metabolism of the nutrients absorbed from the maternal gut.

Insulin secretion is sustained by increased serum levels of glucose and amino acids. The net effect is storage of glucose as glycogen primarily in liver and muscle, retention of some amino acids as protein, and storage of the excess as fat. Storage of maternal fat peaks in the second trimester, and then declines as fetal demands increase in late pregnancy (Pipe and colleagues, 1979).

During times of fasting, glucose is released from glycogen, but maternal glycogen stores cannot provide an adequate amount of glucose to meet requirements for maternal energy and fetal growth. However, cleavage of triacylglycerols, stored in adipose tissue, provides the mother with energy in the form of free fatty acids. Lipolysis is activated, directly or indirectly, by several hormones, including glucagon, norepinephrine, placental lactogen, glucocorticosteroids, and thyroxine.

GLUCOSE AND FETAL GROWTH. Although the fetus is dependent on the mother for nutrition, the fetus also actively participates in providing for its own nutrition. At midpregnancy, fetal glucose concentration is independent of and may exceed maternal levels (Bozzetti and colleagues, 1988). Glucose is a major nutrient for fetal growth and energy. It is thus logical that mechanisms exist during pregnancy to minimize maternal glucose use so that the limited maternal supply is available to the fetus. It is believed that placental lactogen (hPL), a hormone normally present in abundance in the mother but not the fetus, blocks the peripheral uptake and use of glucose while promoting the mobilization and use of free fatty acids by maternal tissues (see Chap. 3, p. 73).

Glucose Transport. The transfer of D-glucose across cell membranes is accomplished by a carrier-mediated, stereospecific, nonconcentrating process of *facilitated diffusion.* Six separate glucose transport proteins (GLUT) have been discovered. They belong to the 12-transmembrane segment transporter superfamily and are characterized further by tissue-specific distribution (see Chap. 38, p. 895). Transporter proteins for D-glucose—GLUT-1 and GLUT-3—are located in the plasma membrane of the microvilli of human syncytiotrophoblast. GLUT-1 expression is prominent in human placenta, it increases as pregnancy advances, and it is induced by almost all growth factors (Sakata and colleagues, 1995). GLUT-3 is also localized in human syncytiotrophoblast (Hahn and associates, 1995).

Glucose, Insulin, and Fetal Macrosomia. The precise biomolecular events in the pathophysiology of fetal macrosomia are not defined. Nonetheless, it seems clear that fetal hyperinsulinemia is one driving force (Schwartz and colleagues, 1994). As discussed in Chapter 38 (see p. 895), insulin-like growth factor, as well as fibroblast growth factor, also are involved (Giudice and associates, 1995; Hill and colleagues, 1995). Therefore, a hyperinsulinemic state with increased levels of selected growth factors, together with increased expression of GLUT proteins in syncytiotrophoblast, may promote excessive fetal growth.

LACTATE. This substance also is transported across the placenta by facilitated diffusion. By way of co-transport with hydrogen ions, lactate is probably transported as lactic acid.

FREE FATTY ACIDS AND TRIGLYCERIDES. Among mammalian neonates, the human newborn has a large proportion of fat, on average 15 percent of body weight (Kimura, 1991). This finding is indicative that late in pregnancy, a substantial part of the substrate transferred to the human fetus is stored as fat. Neutral fat (triacylglycerols) does not cross the placenta, but glycerol does. It is likely that most fatty acids cross the placenta by simple diffusion. Moreover, fatty acids also are synthesized in the placenta. Lipoprotein lipase is present on the maternal but not on the fetal side of the placenta. This arrangement should favor hydrolysis of triacylglycerols in the maternal intervillous space while preserving these neutral lipids in fetal blood. Fatty acids transferred to the fetus can be converted to triacylglycerols in the fetal liver.

The placental uptake and use of low-density lipoprotein (LDL) was cited in Chapter 3 (see p. 80) as an alternative mechanism for fetal assimilation of essential fatty acids and amino acids. The LDL particles from maternal plasma bind to specific LDL receptors in the coated-pit regions of the microvilli on the maternal-facing side of the syncytiotrophoblast. The large—about 250,000 d—LDL particle is taken up by a process of receptor-mediated endocytosis. The apoprotein and cholesterol esters of LDL are hydrolyzed by lysosomal enzymes in the syncytium to give (1) cholesterol for progesterone synthesis; (2) free amino acids, including essential amino acids; and (3) essential fatty acids, primarily linoleic acid. Indeed, the concentration of arachidonic acid, which is synthesized from linoleic acid in fetal plasma, is greater than that in maternal plasma. Linoleic acid or arachidonic acid, or both, must be assimilated from maternal dietary intake.

AMINO ACIDS. In addition to the hydrolysis of LDL, the placenta concentrates a large number of amino acids (Lemons, 1979). Neutral amino acids from maternal plasma are taken up by trophoblasts by at least three specific processes. Presumably, amino acids are concentrated in the syncytiotrophoblasts and thence transferred to the fetal side by diffusion. Based on data from cordocentesis blood samples, the concentration of amino acids in umbilical cord plasma is greater than in maternal venous or arterial plasma (Morriss and associates, 1994).

PROTEINS. Generally, there is very limited transfer of larger proteins across the placenta. There are important exceptions, for example, immunoglobulin G (IgG) crosses the placenta in large amounts. Another exception is retinol-binding protein. Near term, IgG is present in approximately the same concentrations in cord and maternal sera, but IgA and IgM of maternal origin are effectively excluded from the fetus (Gitlin and colleagues, 1972). Fc receptors are present on trophoblasts, and IgG transport is accomplished by way of these through endocytosis. Increased amounts of IgM are found in the fetus only after the fetal immune system has been provoked into antibody response by infection in the fetus.

IONS AND TRACE METALS. Iodide transport across the placenta is clearly attributable to a carrier-mediated, energy-requiring active process. And indeed, the placenta concentrates iodide. The concentrations of zinc in the fetal plasma also are greater than those in maternal plasma. Conversely, copper levels in fetal plasma are less than those in maternal plasma. This fact is of particular interest because important copper-requiring enzymes are necessary for fetal development.

Placental Sequestration of Heavy Metals. The heavy metal–binding protein, metallothionein-1, is expressed in human syncytiotrophoblast. This protein binds and sequesters a host of heavy metals, including zinc, copper, lead, and cadmium.

The most common source of cadmium in the environment is cigarette smoke. Cadmium levels in maternal blood and placenta are increased with maternal smoking, but there is no increase in cadmium transfer into the fetus. The cadmium concentration in cord blood is less than that in maternal blood, and there is little or no cadmium in fetal liver or kidney. Presumably, the low levels of cadmium in the fetus are attributable to the sequestration of cadmium by metallothionein(s) in trophoblast. This comes about because cadmium acts to increase the transcription of the metallothionein gene(s). Thus, cadmium-induced increases in trophoblast metallothionein levels result in placental cadmium accumulation by sequestration.

Metallothionein also binds and sequesters copper (Cu^{2+}) in placental tissue, thus accounting for the low levels of Cu^{2+} in cord blood (Iyengar and Rapp, 2001). A number of mammalian enzymes require Cu^{2+}, and its deficiency results in inadequate collagen cross-linking and, in turn, diminished tensile strength of tissues. This may be important because the concentration of cadmium in amnionic fluid is similar to that in maternal blood. The incidence of preterm membrane rupture is increased in women who smoke. It is possible that cadmium provokes metallothionein synthesis in amnion, causing sequestration of Cu^{2+} and a pseudocopper deficiency.

Calcium and Phosphorus. These minerals also are actively transported from mother to fetus. A calcium-binding protein is present in placenta. Parathyroid hormone–related protein (PTH-rP), as the name implies, acts as a surrogate PTH in many systems, including the activation of adenylate cyclase and the movement of calcium (Ca^{2+}) (see also Chap. 3, p. 74, and Chap. 6, p. 162). PTH-rP is produced not in normal adult parathyroid glands but rather in the fetal parathyroid and in the placenta and other fetal tissues, especially the fetal kidney. Moreover, PTH is not demonstrable in fetal plasma, but PTH-rP is present. For those reasons, some refer to PTH-rP as the fetal parathormone (Abbas and associates, 1990). There is a Ca^{2+}-sensing receptor in trophoblast, as there is in the parathyroid glands (Juhlin and colleagues, 1990). The expression of PTH-rP in cytotrophoblasts is modulated by the extracellular concentration of Ca^{2+} (Hellman and co-workers, 1992). It seems possible, therefore, that PTH-rP synthesized in decidua, placenta, and other fetal tissues is important in fetal Ca^{2+} transfer and homeostasis.

VITAMINS. The concentration of *vitamin A (retinol)* is greater in fetal than in maternal plasma. Vitamin A in fetal plasma is bound to retinol-binding protein and to prealbumin. Retinol-binding protein is transferred from the maternal compartment across the syncytium. The transport of *vitamin C (ascorbic acid)* across the placenta from mother to fetus is accomplished by an energy-dependent, carrier-mediated process. The levels of the principal *vitamin D (cholecalciferol)* metabolites, including 1,25-dihydroxycholecalciferol, are greater in maternal plasma than are those in fetal plasma. The 1β-hydroxylation of 25-hydroxyvitamin D_3 is known to take place in placenta and in decidua.

FETAL PHYSIOLOGY

AMNIONIC FLUID. In early pregnancy, amnionic fluid is an ultrafiltrate of maternal plasma. By the beginning of the second trimester, it consists largely of extracellular fluid that diffuses through the fetal skin, and thus reflects the composition of fetal plasma (Gilbert and Brace, 1993). After 20 weeks, however, the cornification of fetal skin prevents this diffusion, and amnionic fluid is composed largely of fetal urine. The fetal kidneys start producing urine at 12 weeks, and by 18 weeks they are producing 7 to 14 mL per day. Fetal urine contains more urea, creatinine, and uric acid than fetal plasma. It also contains desquamated fetal cells, vernix, lanugo, and various secretions. Because these are hypotonic, the net effect is decreasing amnionic fluid osmolality with advancing gestation. Pulmonary fluid contributes a small proportion of the amnionic volume, and fluid filtering through the placenta accounts for the rest.

The volume of amnionic fluid at each week of gestation is quite variable. In general, the volume increases by 10 mL per week at 8 weeks and increases up to 60 mL per week at 21 weeks, then declines gradually back to a steady state by 33 weeks (Brace and Wolf, 1989).

Amnionic fluid serves to cushion the fetus, allowing musculoskeletal development and protecting it from trauma. It also maintains temperature and has a minimal nutritive function. Epidermal growth factor (EGF) and EGF-like growth factors, such as transforming growth factor-β, are present in amnionic fluid. Ingestion of amnionic fluid into the gastrointestinal tract and inhalation into the lung may promote growth and differentiation of these tissues. Animal studies have shown that pulmonary hypoplasia can be produced by draining off amnionic fluid, by chronically draining pulmonary fluid through the trachea, and by physically preventing the prenatal chest excursions that mimic breathing (Adzick and associates, 1984; Alcorn and colleagues, 1977). Thus the formation of intrapulmonary fluid and, at least as important, the alternating egress and retention of fluid in the lungs by breathing movements are essential to normal pulmonary development. Clinical implications of oligohydramnios and pulmonary hypoplasia are discussed in Chapter 21 (see p. 530).

FETAL CIRCULATION. The fetal circulation is substantially different from that of the adult and functions smoothly until the moment of birth, when it is required to change dramatically. For example, because fetal blood does not need to enter the pulmonary vasculature to be oxygenated, the major portion of the right ventricular output bypasses the lungs. In addition, the fetal heart chambers work in parallel, not in series, which effectively supplies the brain and heart with more highly oxygenated blood than the rest of the body.

Oxygen and nutrient materials required for fetal growth and maturation are delivered to the fetus from the placenta by the single umbilical vein (Fig. 4–12). The vein then divides into the ductus venosus and the portal sinus. The ductus venosus is the major branch of the umbilical vein and traverses the liver to enter the inferior vena cava directly. Because it does not supply oxygen to the intervening tissues, it carries well-oxygenated blood directly to the heart. In contrast, the portal sinus carries blood to the hepatic veins primarily on the left side of the liver, where oxygen is extracted. The relatively deoxygenated blood from the liver then flows back into the inferior vena cava, which also receives less oxygenated blood returning from the lower body. Blood flowing to the fetal heart from the inferior vena cava, therefore, consists of an admixture of arterial-like blood that passes directly through the ductus venosus and less well-oxygenated blood that returns from most of the veins below the level of the diaphragm. The oxygen content of blood delivered to the heart from the inferior vena cava is thus lower than that leaving the placenta.

In contrast to postnatal life, the ventricles of the fetal heart work in parallel, not in series. Well-oxygenated blood enters the left ventricle, which supplies the heart and brain, and less oxygenated blood enters the right ventricle, which supplies the rest of the body. The two separate circulations are

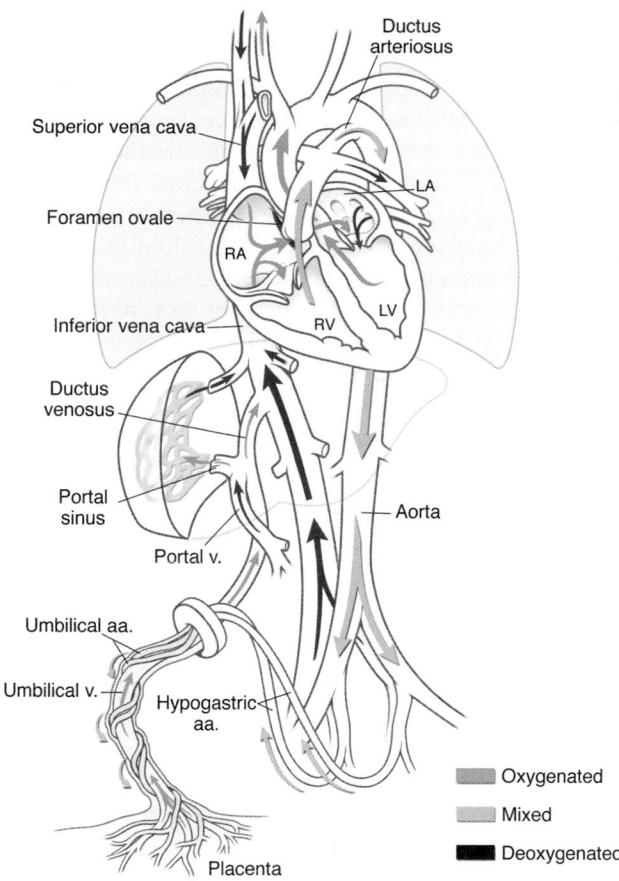

FIGURE 4–12. The intricate nature of the fetal circulation is evident. The degree of oxygenation of blood in various vessels differs appreciably from that in the postnatal state as the consequences of oxygenation being provided by the placenta rather than the lungs and the presence of three major vascular shunts: **1.** Ductus venosus. **2.** Foramen ovale. **3.** Ductus arteriosus.

superior vena cava courses inferiorly and anteriorly as it enters the right atrium, ensuring that less well-oxygenated blood returning from the brain and upper body also will be shunted directly to the right ventricle. Similarly, the ostium of the coronary sinus lies just superior to the tricuspid valve so that less oxygenated blood from the heart also returns to the right ventricle. As a result of this blood flow pattern, blood in the right ventricle is 15 to 20 percent less saturated than blood in the left ventricle.

The major portion, almost 90 percent, of blood exiting the right ventricle is then shunted through the ductus arteriosus to the descending aorta. The high pulmonary vascular resistance and the comparatively lower resistance in the ductus arteriosus and the umbilical–placental vasculature ensure that only about 15 percent of right ventricular output (8 percent of the combined ventricular output) goes to the lungs (Teitel, 1992). Thus, one third of the blood passing through the ductus arteriosus is delivered to the body. The remaining right ventricular output returns to the placenta through the two hypogastric arteries, which distally become the umbilical arteries.

In the placenta, this blood picks up oxygen and other nutrients and is then recirculated back through the umbilical vein. After birth, the umbilical vessels, ductus arteriosus, foramen ovale, and ductus venosus normally constrict or collapse. With the functional closure of the ductus arteriosus and the expansion of the lungs, blood leaving the right ventricle preferentially enters the pulmonary vasculature to become oxygenated before it returns to the left heart. Virtually instantaneously, the ventricles, which had worked in parallel in fetal life, now effectively work in series. The more distal portions of the hypogastric arteries, which course from the level of the bladder along the abdominal wall to the umbilical ring and into the cord as the umbilical arteries, undergo atrophy and obliteration within 3 to 4 days after birth. These become the umbilical ligaments, while the intra-abdominal remnants of the umbilical vein form the ligamentum teres. The ductus venosus constricts by 10 to 96 hours after birth and is anatomically closed by 2 to 3 weeks, resulting in the formation of the ligamentum venosum (Clymann and Heymann, 1981).

FETAL BLOOD

Hemopoiesis. In the very early embryo, hemopoiesis is demonstrable first in the yolk sac. The next major site is the liver, and finally the bone marrow. The contributions made by each site throughout the growth and development of the embryo and fetus are demonstrated graphically in Figure 4–13.

The first erythrocytes released into the fetal circulation are nucleated and macrocytic. The mean cell volume is at least 180 fL in the embryo and normally decreases to 105 to 115 fL at term. The erythrocytes of aneuploid fetuses generally do

maintained by the structure of the right atrium, which effectively directs entering blood to either the left atrium or the right ventricle, depending on its oxygen content. This separation of blood according to its oxygen content is facilitated by the pattern of blood flow in the inferior vena cava. The well-oxygenated blood tends to course along the medial aspect of the inferior vena cava and the less oxygenated blood stays along the lateral vessel wall, facilitating their shunting into opposite sides of the heart. Once this blood enters the atrium, the configuration of the upper interatrial septum, called the *crista dividens,* is such that it preferentially shunts the well-oxygenated blood from the medial side of the inferior vena cava and the ductus venosus through the foramen ovale into the left heart and then to the heart and brain (Dawes, 1962). After these tissues have extracted needed oxygen, the resulting less oxygenated blood returns to the right heart through the superior vena cava.

The less oxygenated blood coursing along the lateral wall of the inferior vena cava enters the right atrium and is deflected through the tricuspid valve to the right ventricle. The

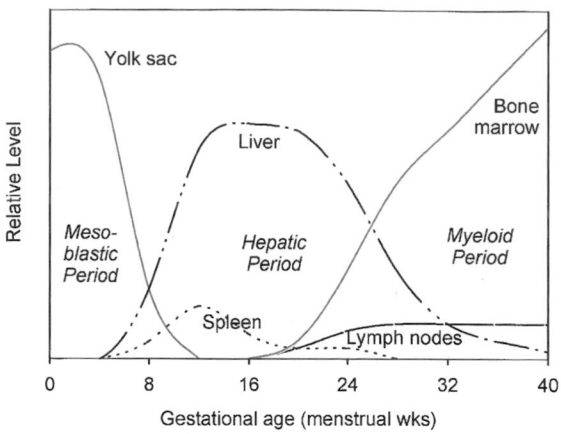

FIGURE 4–13. Sites of hemopoiesis synthesized at various stages of fetal development. (From Brown, 1968, with permission.)

Erythropoiesis. This process is controlled primarily by erythropoietin made by the fetus. Maternal erythropoietin does not cross the placenta. Fetal erythropoietin production is influenced by testosterone, estrogen, prostaglandins, thyroid hormone, and lipoproteins (Stockman and deAlarcon, 1992). Serum levels of erythropoietin increase with fetal maturity, as do the numbers of erythrocytes responsive to it. The exact site of erythropoietin production is disputed, but the fetal liver appears to be an important source until renal production begins. There is a close correlation between the concentration of erythropoietin in amnionic fluid and that in umbilical venous blood obtained by cordocentesis. After birth, erythropoietin normally may not be detectable for up to 3 months.

not undergo this maturation and maintain high mean cell volumes, 130 fL on average (Sipes and associates, 1991). As fetal development progresses, more and more of the circulating erythrocytes are smaller and nonnucleated. As the fetus grows, not only does the volume of blood in the common fetoplacental circulation increase, but hemoglobin concentration rises as well. Hemoglobin content of fetal blood rises to the level of about 12 g/dL at midpregnancy, and at term, it is about 18 g/dL (Walker and Turnbull, 1953). Fetal erythrocytes have a short life span, which progressively lengthens to approximately 90 days at term (Pearson, 1966). As a consequence, red blood cell production is increased. Reticulocytes are initially present at high levels, but decrease to about 4 to 5 percent of the total at term. The fetal erythrocytes differ structurally and metabolically from those of the adult. Fetal erythrocytes are more deformable, which serves to offset their higher viscosity, and contain several enzymes with appreciably different activities (Smith and co-workers, 1981).

Fetal Blood Volume. Precise measurements of human fetoplacental volume are lacking. Usher and associates (1963), however, have measured blood volume of term normal infants very soon after birth and found an average of 78 mL/kg when immediate cord-clamping was conducted. Gruenwald (1967) found the volume of blood of fetal origin contained in the placenta after prompt cord clamping to average 45 mL/kg of fetus. Thus, fetoplacental blood volume at term is approximately 125 mL/kg of fetus.

Fetal Hemoglobin. This respiratory protein is a tetramer composed of two copies each of two different peptide chains. The type of chains determines the type of hemoglobin produced. For example, α and β chains make up normal adult hemoglobin A. During embryonic and fetal life, a variety of α and β chain precursors are produced, resulting in the serial production of several different embryonic hemoglobins. The genes that direct production of the various embryonic versions of these chains are arranged in the order in which they are temporally activated on chromosomes 11 (β-type chains) and 16 (α-type chains). This sequence is shown in Figure 4–14. Each of these genes is turned on and then off during

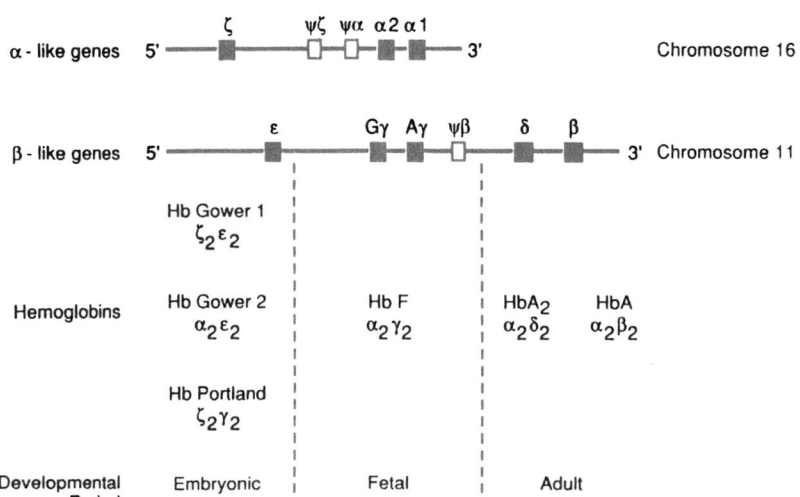

FIGURE 4–14. Schematic drawing of the arrangement of the α and β gene precursors on chromosomes 11 and 16, and the types of hemoglobin made from them. (From Thompson and colleagues, 1991, with permission.)

fetal life, until the α and β genes, which direct the production of hemoglobin A, are permanently activated.

Interestingly, the timing of the production of each of these early hemoglobin versions corresponds to changes in the site of hemoglobin production. As Figure 4–13 illustrates, fetal blood is first produced in the yolk sac, where hemoglobins Gower 1, Gower 2, and Portland are made. Erythropoiesis then moves to the liver, where fetal hemoglobin F is produced. When hemopoiesis finally moves to the bone marrow at around 11 weeks, normal hemoglobin A appears in fetal red blood cells and is present in progressively greater amounts as the fetus matures (Pataryas and Stamatoyannopoulos, 1972).

The final adult version of the α chain is produced exclusively by 6 weeks—after this there are no functional alternative versions. If an α-gene mutation or deletion occurs, there is no alternate α-type chain that could substitute to form functional hemoglobin. In contrast, at least two versions of the β chain—δ and γ—remain in production throughout fetal life and beyond. In the case of a β-gene mutation or deletion, these two other versions of the β chain often continue to be produced, resulting in hemoglobin A_2 or hemoglobin F, which substitute for the abnormal or missing hemoglobin.

The mechanism by which genes are turned off is methylation of the control region, which is discussed in greater detail in Chapter 12 (see p. 305). Thus, the switch from the various embryonic hemoglobins to hemoglobin A likely is associated with methylation of the early globin genes. In some situations, methylation does not occur, and in newborns of diabetic women, there may be persistence of hemoglobin F from hypomethylation of the γ gene (Perrine and associates, 1988). With sickle cell anemia, the γ gene remains unmethylated, and large quantities of fetal hemoglobin continue to be produced (see also Chap. 51, p. 1150).

There is a functional difference between hemoglobins A and F. At any given oxygen tension and at identical pH, fetal erythrocytes that contain mostly hemoglobin F bind more oxygen than do those that contain nearly all hemoglobin A (see Fig. 42–3, p. 992). The major reason for this is that hemoglobin A binds 2,3-diphosphoglycerate (2,3-DPG) more avidly than does hemoglobin F, and this lowers the affinity of hemoglobin A for oxygen (De Verdier and Garby, 1969). The increased oxygen affinity of the fetal erythrocyte results from a lower concentration of 2,3-DPG compared with that of the maternal erythrocyte, in which the 2,3-DPG level is increased during pregnancy.

The amount of hemoglobin F in fetal erythrocytes falls somewhat during the latter weeks of pregnancy. At term, about three fourths of the total hemoglobin normally is hemoglobin F. During the first 6 to 12 months of life, the proportion of hemoglobin F continues to decrease, eventually to reach the low level found in adult erythrocytes. Glucocorticosteroids mediate the switch from fetal to adult hemoglobin, and the effect is irreversible (Zitnik and associates, 1995).

Fetal Coagulation Factors. There are no embryonic forms of the various hemostatic proteins. With the exception of fibrinogen, the fetus starts producing normal, adult-type, procoagulant, fibrinolytic and anticoagulant proteins by about 12 weeks, albeit at appreciably reduced levels. Even with higher levels of these proteins in maternal blood, they do not cross the placenta. The concentrations of several coagulation factors at birth are thus markedly below the levels that develop within a few weeks of life (Corrigan, 1992). Factors that are low in cord blood are II, VII, IX, X, XI, XII, XIII, and fibrinogen. Without prophylactic treatment, the vitamin K–dependent coagulation factors usually decrease even further during the first few days after birth. This decrease is amplified in breast-fed infants and may lead to hemorrhage in the newborn (see Chap. 29, p. 676).

Fetal *fibrinogen,* which appears as early as 5 weeks, has the same amino acid composition as adult fibrinogen but has different properties (Klagsbrun, 1988). It forms a less compressible clot, and the fibrin monomer has a lower degree of aggregation (Heimark and Schwartz, 1988). For reasons unknown, the time for conversion of fibrinogen in plasma to fibrin clot when thrombin is added (thrombin time) is somewhat prolonged compared with that of adults. Fibrinogen levels at birth are somewhat less than those in nonpregnant adults.

Fetal functional *factor XIII (fibrin-stabilizing factor)* levels in plasma are significantly reduced compared with those in normal adults (Henriksson and co-workers, 1974). Severe deficiencies of *factors VIII, IX, XI,* or *XIII* are usually suspected after observing a continuous ooze from the umbilical stump. Nielsen (1969) described low levels of plasminogen and somewhat increased *fibrinolytic activity* in cord plasma compared with maternal plasma. *Platelet* counts in cord blood are in the normal range for nonpregnant adults.

Despite this relative reduction in procoagulant, the fetus seems to be protected from hemorrhage, and fetal bleeding is a rare event. Excessive bleeding does not usually occur even after invasive fetal procedures such as cordocentesis. Ney and colleagues (1989) have shown that amnionic fluid thromboplastins and some factor in Wharton jelly combine to facilitate coagulation at the umbilical cord puncture site.

A variety of thrombophilias, such as protein C, S, or antithrombin III deficiency, or the factor V Leiden mutation may cause thromboses and pregnancy complications in adults (see Chap. 47, p. 1074). If the fetus inherits one of these mutations, thrombosis and infarction can develop. Thorarensen and colleagues (1997) described three neonates with ischemic infarction or hemorrhagic stroke who were heterozygous for factor V Leiden mutation. One had multiple thromboses in the placental vasculature.

Fetal Plasma Proteins. Liver enzymes and other plasma proteins are produced by the fetus, and these levels do not correlate with maternal levels (Weiner and colleagues, 1992).

Concentrations of plasma protein, albumin, lactic dehydrogenase, aspartate aminotransferase, γ-glutamyl transpeptidase, and alanine transferase all increase with gestational age. At birth, the mean total plasma protein and albumin concentrations in fetal blood are similar to maternal levels (Foley and associates, 1978).

ONTOGENY OF THE FETAL IMMUNE RESPONSE.

Infections in utero have provided an opportunity to examine some of the mechanisms of the fetal immune response. Evidence of immunological competence has been reported as early as 13 weeks. Altshuler (1974) described infection of the placenta and fetus by cytomegalovirus with characteristic severe inflammatory cell proliferation as well as viral inclusions. Fetal synthesis of complement late in the first trimester has been demonstrated by Kohler (1973) and confirmed by Stabile and co-workers (1988). All components of complement are produced at an early stage of fetal development. In cord blood at or near term, the average level for most components is about half of the adult value (Adinolfi, 1977).

Fetal Immunocompetence. In the absence of a direct antigenic stimulus, such as infection, the immunoglobulins in the fetus consist almost totally of maternal immunoglobulin G (IgG) transferred across the placenta by receptor-mediated processes in syncytiotrophoblast. Therefore, antibodies in the fetus and the newborn infant are most often reflective of maternal immunological experiences.

Immunoglobulin G. Maternal IgG transport to the fetus begins at about 16 weeks and increases thereafter. The bulk of IgG is acquired during the last 4 weeks of pregnancy (Gitlin, 1971). Accordingly, preterm infants are endowed relatively poorly with maternal antibodies. Newborns begin to produce IgG, but slowly, and adult values are not attained until 3 years of age. In certain situations, the transfer of IgG antibodies from mother to fetus can be harmful rather than protective to the fetus. The classical example is hemolytic disease of the fetus and newborn resulting from D-antigen isoimmunization (see Chap. 29, p. 663).

Immunoglobulin M. In the adult, production of immune globulin M (IgM) in response to an antigenic stimulus is superseded in 1 week or so predominantly by IgG production. In contrast, the IgM response is dominant in the fetus and remains so for weeks to months in the newborn. Because IgM is not transported from mother to fetus, any IgM in the fetus or newborn is that which it produced. Very little IgM is produced by normal, healthy fetuses, and that produced may include antibody to maternal T lymphocytes (Hayward, 1983). Increased levels of IgM are found in newborns with congenital infection such as rubella, cytomegalovirus, or toxoplasmosis. Serum IgM levels in umbilical cord blood and identification of specific antibodies may be useful in the diagnosis of intrauterine infection. Adult levels of IgM are normally attained by 9 months of age.

Immunoglobulin A. Differing from many animals, the human newborn does not acquire much in the way of passive immunity from the absorption of humoral antibodies ingested in colostrum. Nevertheless, immunoglobulin A (IgA) ingested in colostrum provides mucosal protection against enteric infections. This is likely also true for IgA ingested with amnionic fluid before delivery.

Lymphocytes. The immune system begins to mature early in fetal life. B lymphocytes appear in liver by 9 weeks and are present in blood and spleen by 12 weeks. T lymphocytes begin to leave the thymus at about 14 weeks (Hayward, 1983). Despite this, the newborn responds poorly to immunization, and especially poorly to bacterial capsular polysaccharides. This immature response may be due to either deficient response of newborn B cells to polyclonal activators, or lack of T cells that proliferate in response to specific stimuli (Hayward, 1983).

Monocytes. In the newborn, monocytes are able to process and present antigen when tested with maternal antigen-specific T cells.

NERVOUS SYSTEM AND SENSORY ORGANS.

The spinal cord extends along the entire length of the vertebral column in the embryo, but after that it grows more slowly. By 24 weeks, the spinal cord extends to S1, at birth to L3, and in the adult to L1. Myelination of the spinal cord begins in the middle of gestation and continues through the first year of life. Synaptic function is sufficiently developed by the eighth week to demonstrate flexion of the neck and trunk (Temiras and co-workers, 1968). At 10 weeks, local stimuli may evoke squinting, opening of the mouth, incomplete finger closure, and flexion of the toes. Swallowing begins at about 10 weeks, and respiration is evident at 14 to 16 weeks (Miller, 1982). Rudimentary taste buds are present at 7 weeks, and mature receptors are present by 12 weeks (Mistretta and Bradley, 1975). The ability to suck is not present until at least 24 weeks (Lebenthal and Lee, 1983). During the third trimester, integration of nervous and muscular function proceeds rapidly.

The internal, middle, and external components of the ear are well developed by midpregnancy. The fetus apparently hears some sounds in utero as early as 24 to 26 weeks. By 28 weeks, the eye is sensitive to light, but perception of form and color is not complete until long after birth.

GASTROINTESTINAL SYSTEM.

Swallowing begins at 10 to 12 weeks, coincident with the ability of the small intestine to undergo peristalsis and transport glucose actively (Koldovsky and colleagues, 1965; Miller, 1982). Much of the water in swallowed fluid is absorbed, and unabsorbed matter

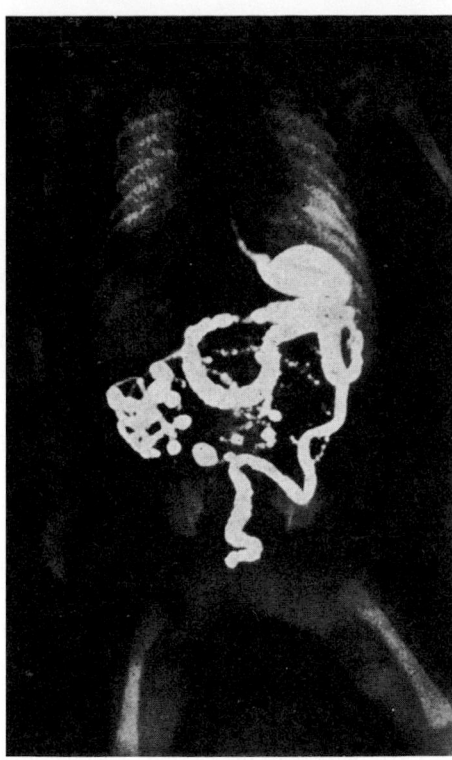

FIGURE 4–15. Radiograph of a 115-g fetus showing radiopaque dye present in the lungs, esophagus, stomach, and entire intestinal tract after injection into the amnionic cavity 26 hours before delivery. This is illustrative not only of intrauterine "respiration" by the fetus but also of active swallowing of amnionic fluid. (From Davis and Potter, 1946, with permission.)

is propelled as far as the lower colon (Fig. 4–15). In late pregnancy, swallowing serves to remove some of the insoluble debris that is normally shed into the amnionic sac and sometimes abnormally excreted into it. It is not clear what stimulates swallowing, but the fetal neural analogue of thirst, gastric emptying, and change in the amnionic fluid composition are potential factors (Boyle, 1992). The fetal taste buds may play a role because saccharin injected into amnionic fluid increases swallowing, whereas injection of a noxious chemical inhibits it (Liley, 1972). Fetal swallowing appears to have little effect on amnionic fluid volume early in pregnancy because the volume swallowed is small compared with the total volume. Late in pregnancy, however, the volume of amnionic fluid appears to be regulated substantially by fetal swallowing, for when swallowing is inhibited, hydramnios is common (see Chap. 21, p. 527). Term fetuses reportedly swallow between 200 and 760 mL per day—an amount comparable to that of the neonate (Pritchard, 1966).

Hydrochloric acid and some digestive enzymes are present in the stomach and small intestine in very small amounts in the early fetus. Intrinsic factor is detectable by 11 weeks, and pepsinogen by 16 weeks. The preterm infant, depending on the gestational age when born, may have transient deficiencies of these enzymes (Lebenthal and Lee, 1983).

Stomach emptying appears to be stimulated primarily by volume. Movement of amnionic fluid through the gastrointestinal system may enhance growth and development of the alimentary canal and condition the fetus for alimentation after birth. Other regulatory factors may be involved, however, because anencephalic fetuses, in whom swallowing is limited, often have normal amnionic fluid volumes and normal-appearing gastrointestinal tracts. The undigested portions of the swallowed debris can be identified in meconium. Gitlin (1974) demonstrated that late in pregnancy, about 0.8 g of soluble protein, approximately half albumin, appears to be ingested by the fetus each day.

Several anomalies can affect normal fetal gastrointestinal function. *Hirschsprung disease,* or *congenital aganglionic megacolon,* prevents the bowel from undergoing parasympathetic-mediated relaxation and thus emptying normally (Watkins, 1992). It may be recognized prenatally by grossly enlarged bowel on sonography. Obstructions such as duodenal atresia, megacystis-microcolon syndrome, or imperforate anus can also prevent the bowel from emptying normally. Meconium ileus, commonly found with fetal cystic fibrosis, is bowel obstruction caused by thick, viscid meconium that blocks the distal ileum.

Meconium. The fetal bowel contents consist of various products of secretion, such as glycerophospholipids from the lung, desquamated fetal cells, lanugo, scalp hair, and vernix. It also contains undigested debris from swallowed amnionic fluid. The dark greenish-black appearance is caused by pigments, especially biliverdin. Meconium passage can result from normal bowel peristalsis in the mature fetus or from vagal stimulation. It can also occur when hypoxia stimulates arginine vasopressin (AVP) release from the fetal pituitary gland. AVP stimulates the smooth muscle of the colon to contract, resulting in intra-amnionic defecation (DeVane and co-workers, 1982; Rosenfeld and Porter, 1985). Small bowel obstruction may lead to vomiting in utero (Shrand, 1972). Fetuses who suffer from congenital chloride diarrhea may have diarrhea in utero, which leads to hydramnios and preterm delivery (Holmberg and associates, 1977).

Liver. Fetal liver enzyme levels increase with gestational age but are present in reduced amounts. The liver has a very limited capacity for converting free bilirubin to bilirubin diglucuronoside (see Chap. 29, p. 672). The more immature the fetus, the more deficient is the system for conjugating bilirubin. Because the life span of fetal erythrocytes is shorter than that of adult erythrocytes, relatively more bilirubin is produced. Most of the bilirubin is transferred to the maternal circulation through the placenta (Bashore and colleagues, 1969). The fetal liver conjugates only a small fraction, which is excreted into the intestine and ultimately oxidized to biliverdin. Unconjugated bilirubin is excreted into the amnionic fluid after 12 weeks and is then transferred across the placenta. Placental transfer, however, is bidirectional. Thus, a pregnant woman with severe hemolytic anemia will have maternal bilirubin that readily passes into the amnionic fluid. On the other hand, conjugated bilirubin is not exchanged to any significant degree between mother and fetus.

Most fetal cholesterol is produced in the fetal liver. Indeed, the large demand for LDL cholesterol by the fetal adrenal glands is met primarily by fetal hepatic synthesis. Glycogen is present in low concentration in the fetal liver during the second trimester, but near term there is a rapid and marked increase to levels two to three times those in the adult liver. After birth, glycogen content falls precipitously.

Pancreas. The discovery of insulin by Banting and Best (1922) came in response to its extraction from the fetal calf pancreas. Insulin-containing granules can be identified in the human fetal pancreas by 9 to 10 weeks, and insulin in fetal plasma is detectable at 12 weeks (Adam and associates, 1969). The fetal pancreas responds to hyperglycemia by increasing plasma insulin (Obenshain and colleagues, 1970). Although the precise role of insulin of fetal origin is not clear, fetal growth must be determined to a considerable extent by the amounts of basic nutrients from the mother with anabolism through the action of fetal insulin. Serum insulin levels are high in newborns of diabetic mothers and in other large-for-gestational-age infants, but insulin levels are low in infants who are small for gestational age (Brinsmead and Liggins, 1979). This relationship is discussed further in Chapter 38 (see p. 895).

Glucagon has been identified in the fetal pancreas at 8 weeks. In the rhesus monkey, hypoglycemia and infused alanine cause an increase in maternal glucagon levels, whereas similar stimuli to the fetus do not. Within 12 hours of birth, however, the infant is capable of responding (Chez and co-workers, 1975). Fetal pancreatic α cells are capable of responding to L-dopa (Epstein and associates, 1977). Therefore, nonresponsiveness to hypoglycemia is likely the consequence of failure of glucagon release rather than inadequate production. This is consistent with findings of the developmental expression of pancreatic genes in the fetus (Mally and associates, 1994).

Most pancreatic enzymes are present by 16 weeks. Trypsin, chymotrypsin, phospholipase A, and lipase are present in the 14-week fetus at low levels, and they increase with gestational age (Werlin, 1992). Amylase has been identified in amnionic fluid at 14 weeks (Davis and associates, 1986). The exocrine function of the fetal pancreas is limited. Physiologically important secretion occurs only after stimulation by a secretogogue such as acetylcholine, which is released locally after vagal stimulation (Werlin, 1992). Cholecystokinin normally is released only after ingestion of protein and thus ordinarily would not be found in the fetus. Its release, however, can be stimulated experimentally. Pritchard (1965) injected radioiodine-labeled albumin into

the amnionic sac, where it was swallowed by the fetus, digested, and absorbed from the fetal intestine.

URINARY SYSTEM. Two primitive urinary systems, the pronephros and the mesonephros, precede the development of the metanephros. The pronephros has involuted by 2 weeks, and the mesonephros is producing urine at 5 weeks and degenerates by 11 to 12 weeks. Failure of these two structures either to form or to regress may result in anomalous development of the definitive urinary system. Between 9 and 12 weeks, the ureteric bud and the nephrogenic blastema interact to produce the metanephros. The kidney and ureter develop from intermediate mesoderm. The bladder and urethra develop from the urogenital sinus. The bladder also develops in part from the allantois.

By week 14, the loop of Henle is functional and reabsorption occurs (Smith and associates, 1992). New nephrons continue to be formed until 36 weeks. In preterm infants, their formation continues after birth. Although the fetal kidneys produce urine, their ability to concentrate and modify the pH is quite limited even in the mature fetus. Fetal urine is hypotonic with respect to fetal plasma and has low concentrations of electrolytes. In the human fetus, the kidneys receive between 2 and 4 percent of the cardiac output compared with 15 to 18 percent in the newborn (Gilbert, 1980).

Renal vascular resistance is high and the filtration fraction is low compared with values in later life (Smith and colleagues, 1992). Fetal renal blood flow and thus urine production are controlled or influenced by the renin-angiotensin system, the sympathetic nervous system, prostaglandins, kallikrein, and atrial natriuretic peptide. The glomerular filtration rate increases with gestational age from less than 0.1 mL/min at 12 weeks to 0.3 mL/min at 20 weeks. In later gestation, the rate remains constant when corrected for fetal weight (Smith and colleagues, 1992). Hemorrhage or hypoxia generally results in a decrease in renal blood flow, glomerular filtration rate, and urine output.

Urine usually is found in the bladder even in small fetuses. The fetal kidneys start producing urine at 12 weeks. By 18 weeks they are producing 7 to 14 mL/day, and at term this increases to 27 mL/hr or 650 mL/day (Wladimiroff and Campbell, 1974). Maternally administered furosemide increases fetal urine formation, whereas uteroplacental insufficiency and other types of fetal stress decrease it. Kurjak and associates (1981) found that fetal glomerular filtration rates and tubular water reabsorption were decreased in 33 percent of growth-restricted infants and in 17 percent of infants of diabetic mothers. All values were normal in anencephalic infants and in those with polyhydramnios.

Obstruction of the urethra, bladder, ureters, or renal pelves can damage renal parenchyma and distort fetal anatomy. With urethral obstruction, the bladder may become sufficiently distended that it ruptures or dystocia results. Kidneys are not essential for survival in utero, but are important in the control of the composition and volume of amnionic fluid. Furthermore, abnormalities that cause chronic anuria are usually accompanied by oligohydramnios and pulmonary hypoplasia. Pathological correlates and prenatal therapy of urinary tract obstruction are discussed in Chapter 13 (see p. 332).

PULMONARY SYSTEM. The timetable of lung maturation and the identification of biochemical indices of functional fetal lung maturity are of considerable interest to the obstetrician. Morphological or functional immaturity of the lung at birth leads to the development of the *respiratory distress syndrome,* and complicates the course and treatment of other neonatal disorders (see Chap. 29, p. 650).

The presence of a sufficient amount of surface-active materials, or *surfactant,* in the amnionic fluid is evidence of fetal lung maturity. As Liggins (1994) emphasized, however, the structural and morphological maturation of fetal lung also is extraordinarily important to proper lung function. It is important, as well, in choosing therapeutic agents used to hasten fetal lung maturation when preterm delivery is likely. Therefore, the two separate but complementary aspects to be considered are anatomical and morphological development of fetal lung as well as its capacity for surfactant formation.

Anatomical Maturation. Like the branching of a tree, lung development proceeds along an established timetable that apparently cannot be hastened by antenatal or neonatal therapy. The limits of viability, therefore, appear to be determined by the usual process of pulmonary growth. There are three essential stages of lung development as described by Moore (1983):

1. During the *pseudoglandular stage,* which entails the growth of the intrasegmental bronchial tree between the 5th and 17th weeks, the lung looks microscopically like a gland.
2. This period is followed by the *canalicular stage,* from 16 to 25 weeks, during which the bronchial cartilage plates extend peripherally. Each terminal bronchiole gives rise to several respiratory bronchioles, and each of these in turn divides into multiple saccular ducts.
3. The final stage is the *terminal sac stage,* during which the alveoli give rise to the primitive pulmonary alveoli, called the terminal sacs. Simultaneously, an extracellular matrix develops from proximal to distal lung segments until term. An extensive capillary network also develops, the lymph system forms, and type II cells begin to produce surfactant. At birth, only about 15 percent of the adult number of alveoli are present, and thus the lung continues to grow, adding more alveoli, from late fetal life up to about 8 years.

Various insults can upset this process, and the timing of the insult determines the outcome. With renal agenesis, for example, no amnionic fluid is present from the beginning of lung growth, and major defects occur in all three stages. The fetus with membrane rupture before 20 weeks and subsequent oligohydramnios usually exhibits nearly normal bronchial branching and cartilage development but has immature alveoli. Membrane rupture occurring after 24 weeks may have little long-term effect on pulmonary structure.

Surfactant. After birth, the terminal sacs must remain expanded despite the pressure imparted by the tissue-to-air interface, and surfactant keeps them from collapsing. There are more than 40 cell types in the lung, but surfactant is formed specifically in the type II pneumonocytes that line the alveoli. These cells are characterized by multivesicular bodies that produce the *lamellar bodies* in which surfactant is assembled. During late fetal life, at a time when the alveolus is characterized by a water-to-tissue interface, the intact lamellar bodies are secreted from the lung and swept into the amnionic fluid during fetal respiratory-like movements, that is, fetal breathing. At birth, with the first breath, an air-to-tissue interface is produced in the lung alveolus. Surfactant uncoils from the lamellar bodies, and it then spreads to line the alveolus to prevent alveolar collapse during expiration. Thus, it is the capacity for fetal lungs to produce surfactant, and not the actual laying down of this material in the lungs in utero, that establishes fetal lung maturity.

SURFACTANT COMPOSITION. Gluck and associates (1967, 1970, 1972) and Hallman and co-workers (1976) found that about 90 percent of surfactant mass (dry weight) is lipid. Proteins account for the other 10 percent. Approximately 80 percent of the glycerophospholipids are phosphatidylcholines (lecithins). The principal active component of surfactant is a specific lecithin—*dipalmitoylphosphatidylcholine (DPPC)*—which accounts for nearly 50 percent. *Phosphatidylglycerol (PG),* the second most surface active component of surfactant, accounts for 8 to 15 percent (Keidel and Gluck, 1975). This component is capable of reducing surface tension in the alveolus, but its precise role is unclear. Infants born with a "mature" lecithin–sphingomyelin (L/S) ratio, but without phosphatidylglycerol, usually do well.

SURFACTANT SYNTHESIS. Biosynthesis takes place in the type II cells. The apoproteins are produced in the endoplasmic reticulum, and the glycerophospholipids are synthesized by cooperative interactions of several cellular organelles. Phospholipid is the primary surface tension–lowering component of surfactant, whereas the surfactant apoproteins serve to facilitate the forming and reforming of a surface film in the alveoli during respiration. The surface properties of the surfactant phospholipids are determined by the composition and degree of saturation of the long-chain fatty acids, the types and amounts of minor lipids and proteins, and the temperature. The regulation of phosphatidylglycerol synthesis is especially important. (Fig. 4–16).

The known surfactant-associated apoproteins are surfactant proteins A, B, and C (Whitsett, 1992). The major one is surfactant A (SP-A), which is a glycoprotein with a molecular

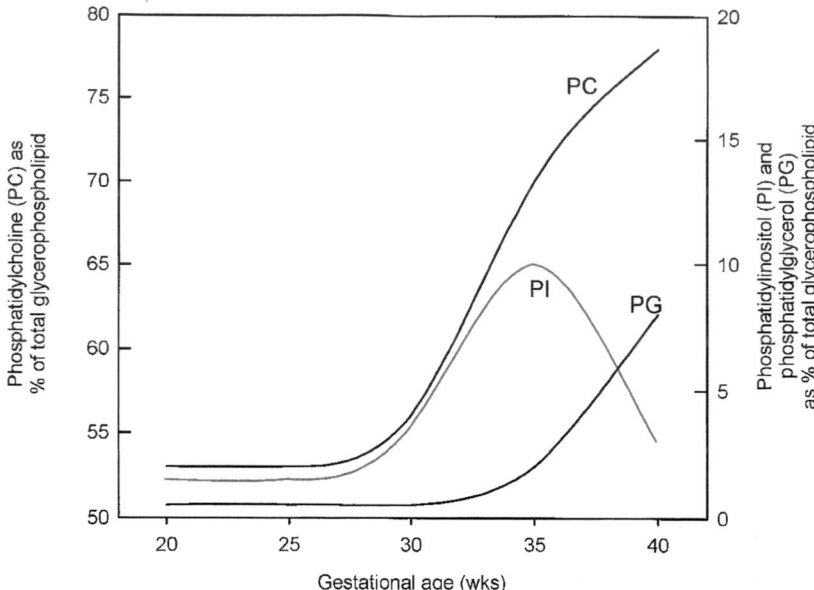

FIGURE 4–16. Relation between the levels of lecithin, or dipalmitoylphosphatidylcholine (PC), phosphatidylinositol (PI), and phosphatidylglycerol (PG) in amnionic fluid as a function of gestational age.

weight of about 28,000 to 35,000 d. It is synthesized in the type II cells, and increased synthesis is related temporally to increased surfactant formation in maturing fetal lungs. The amnionic fluid content of SP-A increases as a function of gestational age and fetal lung maturity. Synthesis of SP-A is increased by treatment of fetal lung tissue with cyclic adenosine monophosphate (AMP) analogues, epidermal growth factors, and triiodothyronine. Increases in surfactant apoprotein synthesis precede the increase in surfactant glycerophospholipid synthesis (Mendelson and associates, 1986).

SP-A gene expression is not detectable at 16 to 20 weeks, but it is demonstrable at 29 weeks (Snyder and colleagues, 1988). More recently, it has been demonstrated that there are two separate SP-A genes on chromosome 10 (SP-A1 and SP-A2). The regulation of synthesis of these two genes is distinctive and different. McCormick and Mendelson (1994) found that the two SP-A genes are differentially regulated. Cyclic AMP is more important in SP-A2 expression (11-fold), whereas dexamethasone caused a decrease in SP-A2 expression.

There are also several smaller apoproteins of about 5000 to 18,000 d. SP-B and SP-C are believed to be important in optimizing the surface-active properties of surfactant. Deletions in the surfactant SP-B gene are not compatible with neonatal survival despite the production of large amounts of surfactant.

CORTICOSTEROIDS AND FETAL LUNG MATURATION. Liggins (1969) observed accelerated lung maturation in lambs that had been treated with glucocorticosteroids prior to preterm birth. Since that time, many investigators have suggested that fetal cortisol is the natural stimulus for lung maturation and augmented surfactant synthesis. Corticosteroids, however, may not be the only stimulus for augmented surfactant for-

mation. For example, respiratory distress syndrome is not always observed in neonates in whom the capacity to secrete cortisol is limited. These situations include those with anencephaly, adrenal hypoplasia, or congenital adrenal hyperplasia. Nevertheless, there is now clinical evidence that glucocorticosteroids administered in large amounts to the woman at certain critical times during gestation effect an increase in the rate of fetal lung maturation. In addition, the advent of neonatal surfactant therapy, either alone or following prenatal corticosteroid treatment, has significantly reduced the incidence of respiratory disease. The use of betamethasone to accelerate fetal lung maturity as well as neonatal surfactant therapy is widely accepted (see Chap. 36, p. 868, and Chap. 29, p. 650).

Respiration. Within a very few minutes after birth, the respiratory system must be able to provide oxygen as well as eliminate carbon dioxide. Respiratory muscles develop early, and movements of the fetal chest wall have been detected by ultrasonic techniques as early as 11 weeks (Boddy and Dawes, 1975). From the beginning of the fourth month, the fetus is capable of respiratory movement sufficiently intense to move amnionic fluid in and out of the respiratory tract.

ENDOCRINE GLANDS

Pituitary Gland. The fetal endocrine system is functional for some time before the central nervous system reaches a state of maturity competent to perform many functions associated with homeostasis (Mulchahey and co-workers, 1987). The fetal endocrine system does not necessarily mimic that of the adult but nonetheless may be one of the first homeostatic systems to develop. The pituitary develops from two different sources. The adenohypophysis develops from the oral ectoderm—Rathke pouch—and the neurohypophysis develops from the neuroectoderm.

ANTERIOR PITUITARY. The adenohypophysis, or anterior pituitary, differentiates into five cell types that secrete six protein hormones: (1) lactotropes, producing prolactin (PRL); (2) somatotropes, producing growth hormone (GH); (3) corticotropes, producing corticotropin (ACTH); (4) thyrotropes, producing thyroid-stimulating hormone (TSH); and (5) gonadotropes, producing luteinizing hormone (LH) and follicle-stimulating hormone (FSH).

ACTH is first detected in the fetal pituitary gland at 7 weeks, and before the end of the 17th week the fetal pituitary gland is able to synthesize and store all pituitary hormones. GH, ACTH, and LH have been identified by 13 weeks. Moreover, the fetal pituitary is responsive to hormones and is capable of secreting these hormones from early in gestation (Grumbach and Kaplan, 1974). Levels of immunoreactive GH are rather high in cord blood, although its role in fetal growth and development is not clear. Anencephalic fetuses, with little pituitary tissue, are not remarkably different in weight from normal fetuses. The fetal pituitary produces and releases β-endorphin in a manner separate from maternal plasma levels (Browning and colleagues, 1983). Furthermore, cord blood levels of β-endorphin and β-lipotropin increase with fetal P_{CO_2}.

NEUROHYPOPHYSIS. The posterior pituitary gland is well developed by 10 to 12 weeks when oxytocin and arginine vasopressin (AVP) are demonstrable. Oxytocin as well as AVP probably function in the fetus to conserve water by actions largely at the level of lung and placenta rather than kidney. Levels of AVP in umbilical cord plasma are increased strikingly compared with the maternal levels (Chard and associates, 1971; Polin and co-workers, 1977). AVP in fetal blood appears to be elevated with fetal stress (DeVane and Porter, 1980; DeVane and co-workers, 1982).

INTERMEDIATE PITUITARY GLAND. There is a well-developed intermediate lobe in the fetal pituitary gland. The cells of this structure begin to disappear before term and are absent from the adult pituitary. The principal secretory products of the intermediate lobe cells are α-melanocyte–stimulating hormone (α-MSH) and β-endorphin. The levels of fetal β-MSH decrease progressively with gestation.

Thyroid Gland. The pituitary–thyroid system is functional by the end of the first trimester. The thyroid gland is able to synthesize hormones by 10 to 12 weeks, and TSH, thyroxine, and thyroid-binding globulin (TBG) have been detected in fetal serum as early as 11 weeks (Ballabio and colleagues, 1989). The placenta actively concentrates iodide on the fetal side, and by 12 weeks and throughout pregnancy, the fetal

thyroid concentrates iodide more avidly than does the maternal thyroid. Thus, maternal administration of either radioiodide or appreciable amounts of ordinary iodide is hazardous after this time. Normal fetal levels of free thyroxine (T_4), free triiodothyronine (T_3), and thyroxin-binding globulin increase steadily throughout gestation (Ballabio and associates, 1989). In comparison to adult levels, by 36 weeks, fetal serum concentrations of TSH are higher, total and free T_3 concentrations are lower, and T_4 is similar. This suggests that the fetal pituitary may not become sensitive to feedback until late in pregnancy (Thorpe-Beeston and co-workers, 1991; Wenstrom and colleagues, 1990).

Fetal thyroid hormone plays a role in the normal development of virtually all fetal tissues, but especially the brain. Its influence is illustrated by congenital hyperthyroidism, which occurs when maternal thyroid-stimulating antibody crosses the placenta to stimulate the fetal thyroid. These fetuses develop tachycardia, hepatosplenomegaly, hematological abnormalities, craniosynostosis, and growth restriction. As children they have perceptual motor difficulties, hyperactivity, and reduced growth (Wenstrom and colleagues, 1990). This relationship is discussed further in Chapter 53 (see p. 1193).

Placental tissue and membranes appear to prevent substantial passage of maternal thyroid hormones to the fetus by rapidly deiodinating maternal T_4 and T_3 to reverse T_3, a relatively inactive thyroid hormone (Vulsma and colleagues, 1989). A number of antithyroid antibodies, however, cross the placenta readily when present in high maternal serum concentrations. Those include the long-acting thyroid stimulators LATS and LATS-protector and thyroid-stimulating immunoglobulin (see Chap. 53, p. 1190). Because maternal thyroid hormones cross the placenta to a very limited degree, congenital hypothyroidism can result in a variety of neonatal problems. These include neurological abnormalities, respiratory difficulties, dysmorphic facies, lethargy and hypotonia, and myxedema of the larynx and epiglottis. These problems typically develop only after birth and can be avoided with prompt thyroid replacement. It was previously believed that normal fetal growth and development that occurred despite fetal hypothyroidism provided evidence that T_4 was not essential for fetal growth. It is now known, however, that growth proceeds normally because small quantities of maternal T_4 prevent antenatal cretinism. Vulsma and colleagues (1989), who studied fetuses with thyroid agenesis, found that fetal T_4 levels were very low and actually represented maternal hormone.

Immediately after birth, there are major changes in thyroid function and metabolism. Atmospheric cooling evokes sudden and marked increase in thyrotropin secretion, which in turn causes a progressive increase in serum T_4 levels that are maximal 24 to 36 hours after birth. There are nearly simultaneous elevations of serum T_3 levels. Failure of these changes to occur, for instance, when the fetus is congenitally hypothyroid, causes multiple problems, including cretinism, a form of mental retardation resulting from postnatal brain injury.

Adrenal Glands. These glands are much larger in relation to total body size in the fetus than in adults. The bulk is made up of the inner or so-called *fetal zone* of the adrenal cortex. The normally hypertrophied fetal zone involutes rapidly after birth. It is scant to absent in rare instances where the fetal pituitary gland is congenitally absent. The function of the fetal adrenal glands and the control of fetal adrenal steroidogenesis of dehydroepiandrosterone sulfate and cortisol are discussed in detail in Chapter 3 (see p. 78).

The fetal adrenal glands also synthesize aldosterone. In one study, aldosterone levels in cord plasma near term exceeded those in maternal plasma, as did renin and renin substrate (Katz and colleagues, 1974). The renal tubules of the newborn, and presumably the fetus, appear relatively insensitive to aldosterone (Kaplan, 1972).

FETAL GENDER

The establishment of the primary gender ratio in humans is impractical, for it would require the recovery and assignment of gender to zygotes that fail to cleave, blastocysts that fail to implant, and early pregnancy losses. Carr (1963) suggested that the primary gender ratio in humans may be unity. However, the secondary ratio—that is, the gender ratio of fetuses that reach viability—usually is quoted as approximately 106 males to 100 females. Studies from industrialized nations more recently suggest that the proportion of male births is dropping. Davis and colleagues (1998) report a significant decline in male births since 1950 in Denmark, Sweden, the Netherlands, the United States, Germany, Norway, and Finland. Allan and co-workers (1997) reviewed the male-to-female ratio for all live births in Canada and found that since 1970, the proportion of males has dropped by 2.2 male births per 1000 live births. In the Atlantic region, the decline was 5.6 male births per 1000.

Theoretically, there should be as many Y-bearing as X-bearing sperm, and thus a primary gender ratio of 1:1 at the time of fertilization. Recent data dispute this, and many factors—among them, differential susceptibility to toxins and other environmental exposures and concomitant medical disorders—have been shown to contribute to gender ratios at conception. Parental age appears to influence the primary gender ratio. For example, Manning and associates (1997) reported that couples with a large age discrepancy more likely have a male offspring. James (1986) theorizes that this may be a result of high stress in urbanized society, which may increase corticotropin secretion, stimulating maternal adrenal androgen secretion that favors male conceptions. If this is not the case, the unbalanced secondary gender ratio can only be explained by the loss of more female than male embryofetuses during the early months of pregnancy.

GENDER ASSIGNMENT AT BIRTH. The first thing that parents in the delivery room want to know is the gender of their infant. If the external genitalia of the newborn are ambiguous, the obstetrician faces a profound dilemma. Griffin and Wilson (1986) state that it is no exaggeration to say that the detection of sexual ambiguity in the newborn constitutes a true medical emergency. An incorrect assignment of gender portends grave psychological and social problems for the infant and family. Furthermore, several endocrinological causes of genital ambiguity are associated with profound blood pressure instability and serious metabolic abnormalities.

It is no longer believed that the proper functional gender assignment for newborns with genital ambiguity can be made in the delivery room. Assignment requires knowledge of the karyotypic sex, gonadal sex, hormonal milieu to which the fetus was exposed, anatomy, and all possibilities for surgical correction. In the past, all infants with a small or likely insufficient phallus were often assigned to the female gender. Based on what is now known of the role of fetal exposure to hormones in establishing gender preference and behavior, it can be seen why such a policy may have caused *gender identity disorder* (Slijper and colleagues, 1998). Thus, it seems best to inform the parents that although their infant appears healthy, the gender will need to be determined by a series of tests. To develop a plan that can assist in determining the cause of ambiguous genitalia, the mechanisms of normal and abnormal sexual differentiation must be considered.

SEXUAL DIFFERENTIATION OF THE EMBRYO-FETUS. Phenotypic gender differentiation is determined by chromosomal makeup acting in conjunction with gonadal development.

Chromosomal Gender. Genetic gender—XX or XY—is established at the time of fertilization. For the first 6 weeks thereafter, however, the development of male and female embryos is morphologically indistinguishable. The differentiation of the primordial gonad into testis or ovary heralds the establishment of gonadal sex (Fig. 4–17).

Gonadal Gender. Primordial germ cells originate in the endoderm of the yolk sac and migrate to the genital ridge to form the indifferent gonad (Simpson, 1997). If a Y chromosome is present, at about 6 weeks after conception the gonad begins developing into a testis. Testes development is directed by a gene located on the short arm of Y, namely *testis-determining factor (TDF),* also called *sex-determining region (SRY).* This gene encodes a transcription factor that acts to modulate the rate of transcription of a number of genes involved in gonadal differentiation. The *SRY* gene is specific to the Y chromosome and is expressed in the human single-cell zygote immediately after ovum fertilization. It is

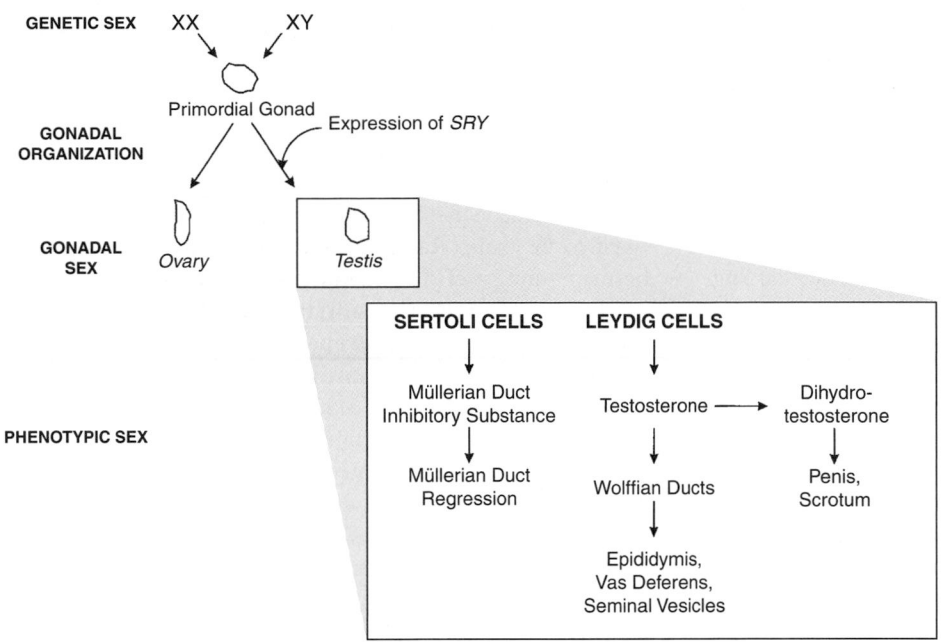

FIGURE 4–17. Gender differentiation. Genetic sex is established at the time of fertilization. At a time thereafter, the primordial gonad differentiates to testis if the *SRY* gene is expressed. The fetal testicular secretions effect male phenotypic gender differentiation.

not expressed in spermatozoa (Fiddler and co-workers, 1995; Gustafson and Donahoe, 1994). In addition, testis development requires a *dose-dependent sex reversal (DDS)* region on the X chromosome, as well as yet unidentified autosomal genes. It is not clear how these genes, or the Y chromosome, direct the biomolecular events involved in gonadal differentiation of the testis.

The contribution of chromosomal gender to gonadal gender is illustrated by several paradoxical conditions. The incidence of 46,XX phenotypic human males is estimated to be about 1 in 20,000 male births (Page and colleagues, 1985). These infants apparently result from translocation of the Y chromosome fragment containing *TDF* to the X chromosome during meiosis of male germ cells (George and Wilson, 1988). Similarly, individuals with XY chromosomes can appear phenotypically female if they carry a mutation in the *TDF (SRY)* gene. There is evidence that genes on Xp are capable of suppressing testicular development, despite the presence of the *SRY* gene. Indeed, this accounts for a form of X-linked recessive gonadal dysgenesis.

The existence of autosomal sex-determining genes is supported by several genetic syndromes in which disruption of an autosomal gene causes, among other things, gonadal dysgenesis. For example, *camptomelic dysplasia,* localized to chromosome 17, is associated with XY phenotypic sex reversal. Similarly, *male pseudohermaphroditism* has been associated with a mutation in the Wilms tumor suppressor gene on chromosome 11.

Phenotypic Gender. After establishment of gonadal gender, phenotypic gender develops very rapidly. It is clear that male phenotypic sexual differentiation is directed by the function of the fetal testis. In the absence of a testis, female differentiation ensues irrespective of the genetic gender. The development of urogenital tracts in both sexes of human embryos is indistinguishable before 8 weeks. Thereafter, development and differentiation of the internal and external genitalia to the male phenotype is dependent on testicular function. The fundamental experiments to determine the role of the testis in male sexual differentiation were conducted by the French anatomist Alfred Jost. Ultimately, he established that the induced phenotype is male and that secretions from the gonads are not necessary for female differentiation. Specifically, the fetal ovary is not required for female sexual differentiation.

Jost and associates (1973) found that if castration of rabbit fetuses was conducted before differentiation of the genital anlagen, all newborns were phenotypic females with female external and internal genitalia. Thus, the müllerian ducts developed into uterus, fallopian tubes, and upper vagina.

If fetal castration was conducted before differentiation of the genital anlagen, and thereafter a testis was implanted on one side in place of the removed gonad, the phenotype of all fetuses was male. Thus, the external genitalia of such fetuses were masculinized. On the side of the testicular implant, the wolffian duct developed into the epididymis, vas deferens, and seminal vesicle. With castration, on the side without the implant, the müllerian duct developed but the wolffian duct did not.

In another experiment, these investigators found that if an androgen pellet was implanted on only the side of the removed gonad, then the external genitalia masculinized. So did the wolffian duct on the side of the androgen pellet. The müllerian duct, however, did not regress. Specifically, the uterine horn and fallopian tube developed despite the androgen implant.

Wilson and Gloyna (1970) and Wilson and Lasnitzki (1971) demonstrated that testosterone action was amplified by conversion to 5α-dihydrotestosterone (5α-DHT). These investigators demonstrated convincingly that in most androgen-responsive tissues, testosterone is converted to 5α-DHT in a reaction catalyzed by the enzyme(s) 5α-reductase. This hormone acts primarily and almost exclusively in the genital tubercle and labioscrotal folds. All of these observations form the basic framework of our understanding of the mechanisms of sexual differentiation of the human embryo-fetus.

Physiological and Biomolecular Basis of Gender Differentiation. Based on these observations, the physiological basis of gender differentiation can be summarized as follows. Genetic gender is established at fertilization. Gonadal gender is determined primarily by factors encoded by genes on the Y chromosome, such as the *SRY* gene. In a manner not yet understood, differentiation of the primitive gonad into a testis is accomplished.

Fetal Testicular Contributions to Male Sexual Differentiation. The fetal testis secretes a proteinaceous substance called *müllerian-inhibiting substance,* a dimeric glycoprotein with a molecular weight of about 140,000 d. It acts locally as a paracrine factor to cause regression of the müllerian duct. Thus, it prevents the development of uterus, fallopian tube, and upper vagina. Fetal testes secrete testosterone, which acts to cause virilization of the external and internal genital anlagen. Müllerian-inhibiting substance is produced by the Sertoli cells of the seminiferous tubules. Importantly, these tubules appear in fetal gonads before differentiation of Leydig cells, which are the cellular site of testosterone synthesis. Thus, müllerian-inhibiting substance is produced by Sertoli cells even before differentiation of the seminiferous tubules, and is secreted as early as 7 weeks. Müllerian duct regression is completed by 9 to 10 weeks, which is before testosterone secretion has commenced. Because it acts locally near its site of formation, if a testis were absent on one side, the müllerian duct on that side would persist and the uterus and fallopian tube would develop on that side.

Fetal Testosterone Secretion. Apparently through stimulation initially by chorionic gonadotropin (hCG), and later by fetal pituitary LH, the fetal testes secrete testosterone. Some investigators are of the view that early embryo-fetal testosterone synthesis is gonadotropin independent. Testosterone acts directly on the wolffian duct to effect the development of the vas deferens, epididymidis, and seminal vesicles. Testosterone also enters fetal blood and acts on the anlagen of the external genitalia. In these tissues, however, testosterone is converted to 5α-DHT, which amplifies the androgen action of testosterone to cause virilization of the external genitalia. Work in marsupials suggests that dihydrotestosterone may be converted to 5α-androstanediol for circulation to the external

genitalia (Leihy and colleagues, 2002; Shaw and associates, 2000).

GENITAL AMBIGUITY OF THE NEWBORN. Ambiguity of the neonatal genitalia is the result of either excessive androgen action in an embryo-fetus that was destined to be female, or inadequate androgen representation for one destined to be male. Rarely, genital ambiguity indicates true hermaphroditism. **If the neonate is a phenotypic male with bilateral cryptorchidism, or if the genitalia are completely ambiguous, congenital adrenal hyperplasia is diagnosed and the neonate treated until appropriate tests confirm it or rule it out.** This is because, of all the causes of genital ambiguity, only congenital adrenal hyperplasia can be life threatening. If not treated immediately, adrenal failure provokes nausea, vomiting, diarrhea, dehydration, and shock (Speroff and co-workers, 1994).

Abnormalities of gender differentiation causing genital ambiguity can be assigned to one of four clinically defined categories that include (1) female pseudohermaphroditism, (2) male pseudohermaphroditism, (3) dysgenetic gonads, including true hermaphroditism, and rarely (4) true hermaphroditism (Low and Hutson, 2003).

Category 1. Female Pseudohermaphroditism. In this condition:

1. Müllerian-inhibiting substance is not produced.
2. Androgen exposure of the embryo-fetus is excessive, but variable, for a fetus genetically predestined to be female.
3. The karyotype is 46,XX.
4. Ovaries are present.

Therefore, by genetic and gonadal gender, all subjects of this category are predestined to be female, and the basic abnormality is androgen excess. Because müllerian-inhibiting substance is not produced, the uterus, fallopian tubes, and upper vagina develop in these subjects.

If affected fetuses were exposed to a small amount of excess androgen reasonably late in fetal development, the only genital abnormality will be slight to modest clitoral hypertrophy, with an otherwise normal female phenotype.

With somewhat greater androgen exposure, clitoral hypertrophy will be more pronounced and posterior labial fusion will develop. With progressively increasing androgen excess occurring somewhat earlier in embryonic development, progressively more severe virilization can be seen. This includes formation of labioscrotal folds; development of a urogenital sinus, in which the vagina empties into the posterior urethra; and even development of a penile urethra with scrotal formation: the empty scrotum syndrome.

The androgenic excess in fetuses with female pseudohermaphroditism most commonly arises as the result of congenital adrenal hyperplasia. These defects in the steroidogenic enzymes that are required in the synthesis of cortisol from cholesterol cause increased secretion of androgenic prehormones by the fetal adrenal cortex. With impaired cortisol synthesis, pituitary ACTH secretion is increased, and excessive ACTH stimulation of the fetal adrenal glands leads to the secretion of large amounts of cortisol precursors, including androgenic prehormones. These prehormones, for example, androstenedione, are converted to testosterone in extra-adrenal fetal tissues. The enzyme deficiency may involve any of several enzymes, but the most common are steroid 21-hydroxylase, 11β-hydroxylase, or 3β-hydroxysteroid dehydrogenase. Deficiency of 3β-hydroxysteroid dehydrogenase prevents synthesis of virtually all steroid hormones. Deficiency of either 17β-hydroxylase or 11β-hydroxylase results in the increased production of deoxycorticosterone, which causes hypertension and hypokalemic acidosis. These forms of congenital adrenal hyperplasia thus constitute medical emergencies.

Another cause of androgen excess in the female embryo-fetus is the transfer of androgen from the maternal compartment. Excess maternal androgen secretion may arise from the ovaries with hyperreactio luteinalis or theca-lutein cysts or tumors such as luteomas, arrhenoblastomas (Sertoli-Leydig cell tumors), or hilar cell tumors. In most of these conditions, however, the female fetus does not become virilized. This is because during most of pregnancy, the fetus is protected from excess maternal androgen by the extraordinary capacity of the syncytiotrophoblast to convert most C_{19}-steroids, including testosterone, to estradiol-17β. The only exception to this generalization is fetal aromatase deficiency, which produces both maternal and fetal virilization (see Chap. 3, p. 81). Drugs ingested in pregnancy also can cause female fetal androgen excess. Most commonly, the drugs implicated are synthetic progestins or anabolic steroids (see Chap. 14, p. 352).

Importantly, all subjects with female pseudohermaphroditism, except those with aromatase deficiency, can be normal, fertile women if the proper diagnosis is made and appropriate and timely treatment is initiated.

Category 2. Male Pseudohermaphroditism. These subjects are characterized by:

1. Production of müllerian-inhibiting substance.
2. Incomplete but variable androgenic representation for a fetus predestined to be male.
3. A 46,XY karyotype.
4. The presence of testes or no gonads.

Incomplete masculinization of the fetus destined to be male is caused by inadequate production of testosterone by the fetal testis. It also may arise from diminished responsiveness of the genital anlagen to normal quantities of androgen, which includes failure of the in situ formation of 5α-DHT in androgen-responsive tissue. Because testes were present, at least at some time in embryonic life, müllerian-inhibiting substance is produced during embryonic life. Thus, the uterus, fallopian tubes, and upper vagina do not develop.

Deficient fetal testicular testosterone production may occur if there is an enzymatic defect of steroidogenesis that involves any one of four enzymes in the biosynthetic pathway for testosterone synthesis. Impaired fetal testicular steroidogenesis can also be caused by an abnormality in the LH-hCG receptor and by Leydig cell hypoplasia.

With embryonic testicular regression, the testes regress during embryonic or fetal life, and there is no testosterone production thereafter (Edman and associates, 1977). These subjects have a spectrum of phenotypes that varies from a normal female with absent uterus, fallopian tubes, and upper vagina, to a normal male phenotype with anorchia.

Androgen resistance, or deficiencies in androgen responsiveness, are caused by an abnormal (or absent) androgen receptor protein, or else by failure of conversion of testosterone to 5α-DHT in such tissues because of deficient enzyme activity (Wilson and MacDonald, 1978).

ANDROGEN INSENSITIVITY SYNDROME. Formerly called *testicular feminization,* this is the most extreme form of the androgen resistance syndrome. These individuals have no tissue responsiveness to androgen. Affected subjects have a female phenotype with a short, blind-ending vagina, no uterus or fallopian tubes, and no wolffian duct structures. At the expected time of puberty, testosterone levels in affected women increase to values similar to normal men. Nonetheless, virilization does not occur, and even pubic and axillary hair do not develop because of end-organ resistance. Presumably, because of androgen resistance at the level of the brain and pituitary, LH levels also are elevated. In response to high concentrations of LH, there is increased testicular secretion of estradiol-17β compared with that in normal men (MacDonald and colleagues, 1979). Increased estrogen secretion and absence of androgen responsiveness act in concert to cause feminization (breast development).

Individuals with *incomplete androgen insensitivity* are slightly responsive to androgen. Although they usually have modest clitoral hypertrophy at birth, at the expected time of puberty, pubic and axillary hair develop but virilization does not occur. These women also develop feminine breasts, presumably through the same endocrine mechanisms as in women with the complete form of the disorder (Madden and co-workers, 1975).

Another group has been referred to as *familial male pseudohermaphroditism, type I* (Walsh and colleagues, 1974). It also is commonly referred to as *Reifenstein syndrome,* but constitutes a spectrum of incomplete genital virilization that can vary from a phenotype similar to that of women with incomplete androgen insensitivity to that of a male phenotype with only a bifid scrotum, infertility, and gynecomastia. In these subjects, androgen resistance is demonstrated by demonstrating diminished 5α-DHT–binding capacity in genital skin.

The gene encoding the androgen receptor protein is located on the X chromosome. More than 100 different mutations of this gene have been demonstrated. This accounts for the wide variability in androgen responsiveness among persons in whom the androgen receptor protein is absent or abnormal, and for the many different mutations associated with one disorder (McPhaul and associates, 1991; Patterson and co-workers, 1994).

An alternate form of androgen resistance is caused by 5α-reductase deficiency in androgen-responsive tissues. Because androgen action in the external genitalia anlagen is mediated by 5α-DHT, persons with this enzyme deficiency have external genitalia that are female but with modest clitoral hypertrophy. But because androgen action in the wolffian duct is mediated directly by testosterone, there are well-developed epididymides, seminal vesicles, and vas deferens, and the male ejaculatory ducts empty into the vagina (Walsh and associates, 1974).

A composite photograph of the external genitalia of subjects with each of four types of androgen resistance is shown in Figure 4–18.

Category 3: Dysgenetic Gonads. This category includes abnormalities of sexual differentiation that have in common several features:

1. Müllerian-inhibiting substance is not produced.
2. Fetal androgen exposure is variable.
3. The karyotype varies among subjects and is commonly abnormal.
4. Neither normal ovaries nor testes are present but rarely, both ovarian and testicular tissues are found.

The uterus, fallopian tubes, and upper vagina are present in all of the subjects in this category.

In the majority, the gonads are dysgenetic. With the most common form of gonadal dysgenesis, *Turner syndrome (46X),* the phenotype is female, but secondary gender characteristics do not develop at the time of expected puberty, and genital infantilism persists. In some persons with dysgenetic gonads, the genitalia are ambiguous, a finding indicating that an abnormal gonad produced androgen, albeit in

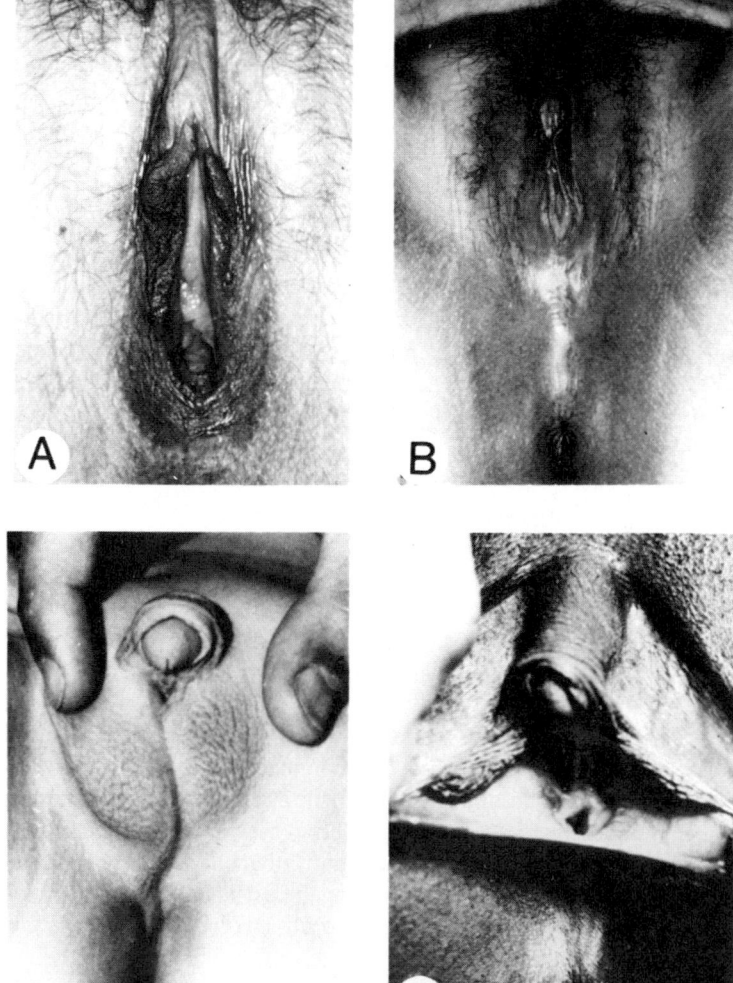

FIGURE 4–18. External genitalia of representative subjects with male pseudohermaphroditism due to androgen resistance. **A.** Testicular feminization from androgen-receptor defect. **B.** Incomplete testicular feminization from androgen-receptor defect. **C.** Familial male pseudohermaphroditism, type I—Reifenstein syndrome, androgen-receptor defect. **D.** 5α-Reductase deficiency from type 2 gene mutation. (From Wilson and MacDonald, 1978, with permission.)

small amounts, during embryonic-fetal life. Generally, there is mixed gonadal dysgenesis in these subjects, and an example is a dysgenetic gonad on one side and an abnormal testis or dysontogenetic tumor on the other side.

Category 4: True Hermaphroditism. In most subjects with true hermaphroditism, the guidelines for category 3 are met. In addition, true hermaphrodites have both ovarian and testicular tissues, and in particular, germ cells (ova and sperm) of both sexes are found in the abnormal gonads.

Preliminary Diagnosis of the Cause of Genital Ambiguity. A preliminary diagnosis of the etiology and pathogenesis of genital ambiguity can be made at the time of birth of an affected child. By physical and ultrasonic examination of the newborn, the experienced examiner can ascertain important findings. These include whether gonads are palpable, and if so, where they are; phallus length and diameter; position of the urethral meatus; degree of labioscrotal fold fusion; and whether there is a vagina, vaginal pouch, or urogenital sinus (Speroff and associates, 1994). If the uterus is present, the diagnosis must be female pseudohermaphroditism, testicular or gonadal dysgenesis, or true hermaphroditism. A family history of congenital adrenal hyperplasia is helpful. If the uterus is not present, the diagnosis is male pseudohermaphroditism. Androgen resistance and enzymatic defects in testicular testosterone biosynthesis are often familial.

REFERENCES

Abbas SK, Pickard DW, Illingworth D, et al: Measurement of PTH-rP protein in extracts of fetal parathyroid glands and placental membranes. J Endocrinol 124:319, 1990

Adam PAJ, Teramo K, Raiha N, et al: Human fetal insulin metabolism early in gestation: Response to acute elevation of the fetal glucose concentration and placental transfer of human insulin-I-131. Diabetes 18:409, 1969

Adinolfi M: Human complement: Onset and site of synthesis during fetal life. Am J Dis Child 131:1015, 1977

Adzick NS, Harrison MR, Glick PL, et al: Experimental pulmonary hypoplasia and oligohydramnios: Relative contributions of lung fluid and fetal breathing movements. J Pediatr Surg 19:658, 1984

Aherne W, Dunnill MS: Morphometry of the human placenta. Br Med Bull 22:1, 1966

Alcorn D, Adamson TM, Lambert TF, et al: Morphological effects of chronic tracheal ligation and drainage in the fetal lamb lung. J Anat 3:649, 1977

Allan BB, Brant R, Seidel JE, et al: Declining sex ratios in Canada. Can Med Assoc J 156:37, 1997

Altshuler G: Immunologic competence of the immature human fetus. Obstet Gynecol 43:811, 1974

Ballabio M, Nicolini U, Jowett T, et al: Maturation of thyroid function in normal human foetuses. Clin Endocrinol 31:565, 1989

Banting FG, Best CH: Pancreatic extracts. J Lab Clin Med 1:464, 1922

Bashore RA, Smith F, Schenker S: Placental transfer and disposition of bilirubin in the pregnant monkey. Am J Obstet Gynecol 103:950, 1969

Boddy K, Dawes GS: Fetal breathing. Br Med Bull 31:3, 1975

Boyle JT: Motility of the upper gastrointestinal tract in the fetus and neonate. In Polin RA, Fox WW (eds): Fetal and Neonatal Physiology. Philadelphia, Saunders, 1992, p 1028

Bozzetti P, Ferrari MM, Marconi AM, et al: The relationship of maternal and fetal glucose concentrations in the human from midgestation until term. Metabolism 37:358, 1988

Brace RA, Wolf EJ: Normal amniotic fluid volume changes throughout pregnancy. Am Obstet Gynecol 161:382, 1989

Brinsmead MW, Liggins GC: Somadomedin-like activity, prolactin, growth hormone and insulin in human cord blood. Aust NZ J Obstet Gynecol 19:129, 1979

Brown AK: Bilirubin metabolism in the developing liver. In Assali NS (ed): Biology of Gestation, Vol II. The Fetus and Neonate. New York, Academic Press, 1968, p 361

Browning AJF, Butt WR, Lynch SS, et al: Maternal plasma concentrations of β-lipotropin, β-endorphin and α-lipotrophin throughout pregnancy. Br J Obstet Gynaecol 90:1147, 1983

Carr D: Chromosome studies in abortuses and stillborn infants. Lancet 2:603, 1963

Chard T, Hudson CN, Edwards CRW, et al: Release of oxytocin and vasopressin by the human foetus during labour. Nature 234:352, 1971

Chez RA, Mintz DH, Reynolds WA, et al: Maternal-fetal plasma glucose relationships in late monkey pregnancy. Am J Obstet Gynecol 121:938, 1975

Clymann RI, Heymann MA: Pharmacology of the ductus arteriosus. Pediatr Clin North Am 28:77, 1981

Corrigan JJ Jr: Normal hemostasis in the fetus and newborn: Coagulation. In Polin RA, Fox WW (eds): Fetal and Neonatal Physiology. Philadelphia, Saunders, 1992, p 1368

Davis DL, Gottlieb MB, Stampnitzky JR: Reduced ratio of male to female births in several industrial countries: A sentinel health indicator? JAMA 279:1018, 1998

Davis ME, Potter EL: Intrauterine respiration of the human fetus. JAMA 131:1194, 1946

Davis MM, Hodes ME, Munsick RA, et al: Pancreatic amylase expression in human pancreatic development. Hybridoma 5:137, 1986

Dawes GS: The umbilical circulation. Am J Obstet Gynecol 84:1634, 1962

DeVane GW, Naden RP, Porter JC, et al: Mechanism of arginine vasopressin release in the sheep fetus. Pediatr Res 16:504, 1982

DeVane GW, Porter JC: An apparent stress-induced release of arginine vasopressin by human neonates. J Clin Endocrinol Metab 51:1412, 1980

De Verdier CH, Garby L: Low binding of 2,3-diphosphoglycerate to hemoglobin F. Scand J Clin Lab Invest 23:149, 1969

Dolman CL: Characteristic configuration of fetal brains from 22 to 40 weeks gestation at two week intervals. Arch Pathol Lab Med 101:193, 1977

Edman CD, Winters AJ, Porter JC, et al: Embryonic testicular regression. A clinical spectrum of XY agonadal individual. Obstet Gynecol 49:208, 1977

Epstein M, Chez RA, Oakes GK, et al: Fetal pancreatic glucagon responses in glucose-intolerant nonhuman primate pregnancy. Am J Obstet Gynecol 127:268, 1977

Fiddler M, Abdel-Rahman B, Rappolee DA, et al: Expression of SRY transcripts in preimplantation human embryos. Am J Med Genet 55:80, 1995

Fisher DA: The unique endocrine milieu of the fetus. J Clin Invest 78:603, 1986

Foley ME, Isherwood DM, McNicol GP: Viscosity, hematocrit, fibrinogen and plasma proteins in maternal and cord blood. Br J Obstet Gynaecol 85:500, 1978

George FW, Wilson JD: Sex determination and differentiation. In Knobil E, Neill J (eds): The Physiology of Reproduction. New York, Raven, 1988, p 3

Gilbert RD: Control of fetal cardiac output during changes in blood volume. Am J Physiol 238:H80, 1980

Gilbert WM, Brace RA: Amniotic fluid volume and normal flows to and from the amniotic cavity. Semin Perinatol 17:150, 1993

Gitlin D: Development and metabolism of the immune globulins. In Kaga BM, Stiehm ER (eds): Immunologic Incompetence. Chicago, Year Book, 1971

Gitlin D: Protein transport across the placenta and protein turnover between amnionic fluid, maternal and fetal circulation. In Moghissi KS, Hafez ESE (eds): The Placenta. Springfield, Ill, Thomas, 1974

Gitlin D, Kumate J, Morales C, et al: The turnover of amniotic fluid protein in the human conceptus. Am J Obstet Gynecol 113:632, 1972

Giudice LC, de-Zegher F, Gargosky SE, et al: Insulin-like growth factors and their binding proteins in the term and preterm human fetus and neonate with normal and extremes of intrauterine growth. J Clin Endocrinol Metab 80:1548, 1995

Gluck L, Kulovich MV, Eidelman AI, et al: Biochemical development of surface activity in mammalian lung, 4. Pulmonary lecithin synthesis in the human fetus and newborn and etiology of the respiratory distress syndrome. Pediatr Res 6:81, 1972

Gluck L, Landowne RA, Kulovich MV: Biochemical development of surface activity in mammalian lung, 3. Structural changes in lung lecithin during development of the rabbit fetus and newborn. Pediatr Res 4:352, 1970

Gluck L, Motoyama EK, Smits HL, et al: The biochemical development of surface activity in mammalian lung, 1. The surface-active phospholipids; the separation and distribution of surface-active lecithin in the lung of the developing rabbit fetus. Pediatr Res 1:237, 1967

Griffin JE, Wilson JD: Disorders of sexual differentiation. In Walsh PC, Gittes RF, Perlmutter AD, Stamey RA (eds): Campbell's Urology. Philadelphia, Saunders, 1986, p 1819

Gruenwald P: Growth of the human foetus. In McLaren A (ed): Advances in Reproductive Physiology. New York, Academic Press, 1967

Grumbach MM, Kaplan SL: Fetal pituitary hormones and the maturation of central nervous system regulation of anterior pituitary function. In Gluck L (ed): Modern Perinatal Medicine. Chicago, Year Book, 1974

Gustafson ML, Donahoe PK: Male sex determination: Current concepts of male sexual differentiation. Annu Rev Med 45:505, 1994

Hahn T, Hartmann M, Blaschitz A, et al: Localisation of the high affinity facilitative glucose transporter protein GLUT 1 in the placenta of human, marmoset monkey (Callithrix jacchus) and rat at different developmental stages. Cell Tissue Res 280:49, 1995

Hallman M, Kulovich MV, Kirkpatrick E, et al: Phosphatidylinositol and phosphatidylglycerol in amniotic fluid: Indices of lung maturity. Am J Obstet Gynecol 125:613, 1976

Hayward AR: The human fetus and newborn: Development of the immune response. Birth Defects 19:289, 1983

Heimark R, Schwartz S: Cellular organization of blood vessels in development and disease. In Ryan U (ed): Endothelial Cells, Vol II. Boca Raton, Fla, CRC Press, 1988, p 103

Hellman P, Ridefelt P, Juhlin C, et al: Parathyroid-like regulation of parathyroid hormone related protein release and cytoplasmic calcium in cytotrophoblast cells of human placenta. Arch Biochem Biophys 293:174, 1992

Henriksson P, Hedner V, Nilsson IM, et al: Fibrin-stabilization factor XIII in the fetus and the newborn infant. Pediatr Res 8:789, 1974

Hill DJ, Tevaarwerk GJ, Caddell C, et al: Fibroblast growth factor 2 is elevated in term maternal and cord serum and amniotic fluid in pregnancies complicated by diabetes: Relationship to fetal and placental size. J Clin Endocrinol Metab 80:2626, 1995

Holmberg C, Perheentupa J, Launiala K, et al: Congenital chloride diarrhea. Arch Dis Child 52:255, 1977

Iyengar CV, Rapp A: Human placenta as a 'dual' biomarker for monitoring fetal and maternal environment with special reference to potentially toxic trace elements. Part 3: Toxic trace elements in placenta and placenta as a biomarker for these elements. Sci Total Environ 280:221, 2001

James WH: Hormonal control of sex ratio. J Theor Biol 118:427, 1986

Jost A, Vigier B, Prepin J: Studies on sex differentiation in mammals. Recent Prog Horm Res 29:1, 1973

Juhlin C, Lundgren S, Johansson H, et al: 500-Kilodalton calcium sensor regulating cytoplasmic Ca2+ in cytotrophoblast cells of human placenta. J Biol Chem 265:8275, 1990

Kaplan S: Disorders of the endocrine system. In Assali NS (ed): Pathophysiology of Gestation, Vol III. Fetal and Neonatal Disorders. New York, Academic Press, 1972

Katz FH, Beck P, Makowski EL: The renin-aldosterone system in mother and fetus at term. Am J Obstet Gynecol 118:51, 1974

Keidel W, Gluck L: Lipid biochemistry and biochemical development of the lung. In Scarpelli E (ed): Pulmonary Physiology of the Fetus, Newborn, and Child. Philadelphia, Lea and Febiger, 1975, p 96

Kimura RE: Lipid metabolism in the fetal-placental unit. In Cowett RM (ed): Principles of Perinatal-Neonatal Metabolism. New York, Springer-Verlag, 1991, p 291

Klagsbrun M: Angiogenesis factors. In Ryan U (ed): Endothelial Cells, Vol II. Boca Raton, Fla, CRC Press, 1988, p 37

Kohler PF: Maturation of the human complement system. J Clin Invest 52:671, 1973

Koldovsky O, Heringova A, Jirsova U, et al: Transport of glucose against a concentration gradient in everted sacs of jejunum and ileum of human fetuses. Gastroenterology 48:185, 1965

Kurjak A, Kirkinen P, Latin V, et al: Ultrasonic assessment of fetal kidney function in normal and complicated pregnancies. Am J Obstet Gynecol 141:266, 1981

Lebenthal E, Lee PC: Interactions of determinants of the ontogeny of the gastrointestinal tract: A unified concept. Pediatr Res 1:19, 1983

Leihy MW, Shaw G, Renfree MD, et al: Administration of 5-alpha-androstane-3 alpha, 17-beta diol to female tammar wallaby pouch young causes development of a mature prostate and male urethra. Endocrinology 143:243, 2002

Lemons JA: Fetal placental nitrogen metabolism. Semin Perinatol 3:177, 1979

Liggins GC: Fetal lung maturation. Aust NZ J Obstet Gynaecol 34:247, 1994

Liggins GC: Premature delivery of fetal lambs infused with glucocorticoids. J Endocrinol 45:515, 1969

Liley AW: Disorders of amniotic fluid. In Assali NS (ed): Pathophysiology of Gestation. New York, Academic Press, 1972

Longo LD: Respiration in the fetal–placental unit. In Cowett RM (ed): Principles of Perinatal-Neonatal Metabolism. New York, Springer-Verlag, 1991, p 304

Low Y, Hutson JM: Rules for clinical diagnosis in babies with ambiguous genitalia. J Paediatr Child Health 39:406, 2003

MacDonald PC, Madden JD, Brenner PF, et al: Origin of estrogen in normal men and in women with testicular feminization. J Clin Endocrinol Metab 49:905, 1979

Madden JD, Walsh PC, MacDonald PC, et al: Clinical and endocrinological characterization of a patient with syndrome of incomplete testicular feminization. J Clin Endocrinol 41:751, 1975

Mally MI, Otonkoski T, Lopez AD, et al: Developmental gene expression in the human fetal pancreas. Pediatr Res 36:537, 1994

Manning JT, Anderton RH, Shutt M: Parental age gap skews child sex ratio. Nature 389:344, 1997

McCormick SM, Mendelson CR: Human SP-A1 and SP-A2 genes are differentially regulated during development and by cAMP and glucocorticoids. Am J Physiol 266:367, 1994

McPhaul MJ, Marcelli M, Tilley WD, et al: Androgen resistance caused by mutations in the androgen receptor gene. FASEB J 5:2910, 1991

Mendelson CR, Chen C, Boggaram V, et al: Regulation of the synthesis of the major surfactant apoprotein in fetal rabbit lung tissue. J Biol Chem 261:9938, 1986

Miller AJ: Deglutition. Physiol Rev 62:129, 1982

Mistretta CM, Bradley RM: Taste and swallowing in utero. Br Med Bull 31:80, 1975

Moore KL: Before We Are Born. Basic Embryology and Birth Defects, 2nd ed. Philadelphia, Saunders, 1983

Moore KL: The Developing Human, 2nd ed. Philadelphia, Saunders, 1977

Moore KL: The Developing Human: Clinically Oriented Embryology, 4th ed. Philadelphia, Saunders, 1988

Morriss FH Jr, Boyd RDH, Manhendren D: Placental transport. In Knobil E, Neill J (eds): The Physiology of Reproduction, Vol II. New York, Raven, 1994, p 813

Mulchahey JJ, DiBlasio AM, Martin MC, et al: Hormone production and peptide regulation of the human fetal pituitary gland. Endocr Rev 8:406, 1987

Ney JA, Fee SC, Dooley SL, et al: Factors influencing hemostasis after umbilical vein puncture in vitro. Am J Obstet Gynecol 160:424, 1989

Nielsen NC: Coagulation and fibrinolysin in normal women immediately postpartum and in newborn infants. Acta Obstet Gynecol Scand 48:371, 1969

Obenshain SS, Adam PAJ, King KC, et al: Human fetal insulin response to sustained maternal hyperglycemia. N Engl J Med 283:566, 1970

Olsen O, Clausen JA: Determination of the expected day of delivery—ultrasound has not been shown to be more accurate than the calendar method. Ugeskr Laeger 160:2088, 1998

Page DC, de la Chapelle A, Weissenbach J: Chromosome Y-specific DNA in related human XX males. Nature 315:224, 1985

Pataryas HA, Stamatoyannopoulos G: Hemoglobins in human fetuses: Evidence for adult hemoglobin production after the 11th gestational week. Blood 39:688, 1972

Patterson MN, McPhaul MJ, Hughes IA: Androgen insensitivity syndrome. Bailleres Clin Endocrinol Metab 8:379, 1994

Pearson HA: Recent advances in hematology. J Pediatr 69:466, 1966

Perrine SP, Greene MF, Cohen RA, et al: A physiological delay in human fetal hemoglobin switching is associated with specific globin DNA hypomethylation. FEBS Lett 228:139, 1988

Pipe NGJ, Smith T, Halliday D, et al: Changes in fat, fat-free mass and body water in human normal pregnancy. Br J Obstet Gynaecol 86:929, 1979

Polin RA, Husain MK, James LS, et al: High vasopressin concentrations in human umbilical cord blood—lack of correlation with stress. J Perinat Med 5:114, 1977

Pritchard JA: Deglutition by normal and anencephalic fetuses. Obstet Gynecol 25:289, 1965

Pritchard JA: Fetal swallowing and amniotic fluid volume. Obstet Gynecol 28:606, 1966

Ramsey, MM: Normal Values in Pregnancy. London, Saunders, 1996

Rosenfeld CR, Porter JC: Arginine vasopressin in the developing fetus. In Albrecht ED, Pepe GJ (eds): Research in Perinatal Medicine, Vol 4. Perinatal Endocrinology. Ithaca, NY, Perinatology Press, 1985, p 91

Sakata M, Kurachi H, Imai T, et al: Increase in human placental glucose transporter-1 during pregnancy. Eur J Endocrinol 132:206, 1995

Schwartz R, Gruppuso PA, Petzold K, et al: Hyperinsulinemia and macrosomia in the fetus of the diabetic mother. Diabetes Care 17:640, 1994

Shaw G, Renfree M, Leihy MW, et al: Prostate formation in a marsupial is mediated by the testicular androgen 5-alpha-androstane-3-alpha, 17-beta-diol. Proc Natl Acad Sci USA 97:12256, 2000

Shrand II: Vomiting in utero with intestinal atresia. Pediatrics 49:767, 1972

Simpson JL: Diseases of the gonads, genital tract, and genitalia. In Rimoin DL, Connor JM, Pyeritz RE (eds): Emery and Rimoin's Principles and Practice of Medical Genetics, Vol I, 3rd ed. New York, Churchill Livingstone, 1997, p 1477

Sipes SL, Weiner CP, Wenstrom KD, et al: The association between fetal karyotype and mean corpuscular volume. Am J Obstet Gynecol 165:1371, 1991

Slijper FM, Drop SL, Molenaar JC, et al: Long-term psychological evaluation of intersex children. Arch Sex Behav 27:125, 1998

Smith CM II, Tukey DP, Krivit W, et al: Fetal red cells (FC) differ in elasticity, viscosity, and adhesion from adult red cells (AC). Pediatr Res 15:588, 1981

Smith FG, Nakamura KT, Segar JL, et al: In Polin RA, Fox WW (eds): Fetal and Neonatal Physiology, Vol 2, Chap. 114. Philadelphia, Saunders, 1992, p 1187

Snyder JM, Kwun JE, O'Brien JA, et al: The concentration of the 35 kDa surfactant apoprotein in amniotic fluid from normal and diabetic pregnancies. Pediatr Res 24:728, 1988

Speroff L, Glass RH, Kase NG: Clinical Gynecologic Endocrinology and Infertility, 5th ed. Baltimore, Williams and Wilkins, 1994

Stabile I, Nicolaides KH, Bach A, et al: Complement factors in fetal and maternal blood and amniotic fluid during the second trimester of normal pregnancy. Br J Obstet Gynaecol 95:281, 1988

Stockman JA III, deAlarcon PA: Hematopoiesis and granulopoiesis. In Polin RA, Fox WW (eds): Fetal and Neonatal Physiology. Philadelphia, Saunders, 1992, p 1327

Streeter GL: Weight, sitting height, head size, foot length, and menstrual age of the human embryo. Contrib Embryol 11:143, 1920

Teitel DF: Physiologic development of the cardiovascular system in the fetus. In Polin RA, Fox WW (eds): Fetal and Neonatal Physiology, Vol I. Philadelphia, Saunders, 1992, p 609

Temiras PS, Vernadakis A, Sherwood NM: Development and plasticity of the nervous system. In Assali NS (ed): Biology of Gestation, Vol VII. The Fetus and Neonate. New York, Academic Press, 1968

Thompson MW, McInnes RR, Willard HF: The hemoglobinopathies: Models of molecular disease. In Thompson MW, McInnes RR, Huntington FW (eds): Thompson and Thompson Genetics in Medicine, 5th ed. Philadelphia, Saunders, 1991, p 247

Thorarensen O, Ryan S, Hunter J, et al: Factor V Leiden mutation: An unrecognized cause of hemiplegic cerebral palsy, neonatal stroke, and placental thrombosis. Ann Neurol 42:372, 1997

Thorpe-Beeston JG, Nicolaides KH, Felton CV, et al: Maturation of the secretion of thyroid hormone and thyroid-stimulating hormone in the fetus. N Engl J Med 324:532, 1991

Usher R, Shephard M, Lind J: The blood volume of the newborn infant and placental transfusion. Acta Paediatr 52:497, 1963

Vulsma T, Gons MH, De Vijlder JJM: Maternal-fetal transfer of thyroxine in congenital hypothyroidism due to a total organification defect or thyroid agenesis. N Engl J Med 321:13, 1989

Walker J, Turnbull EPN: Haemoglobin and red cells in the human foetus and their relation to the oxygen content of the blood in the vessels of the umbilical cord. Lancet 2:312, 1953

Walsh PC, Madden JD, Harrod MJ, et al: Familial incomplete male pseudohermaphroditism, type 2: Decreased dihydrotestosterone formation in pseudovaginal perineoscrotal hypospadias. N Engl J Med 291:944, 1974

Watkins JB: Physiology of the gastrointestinal tract in the fetus and neonate. In Polin RA, Fox WW (eds): Fetal and Neonatal Physiology. Philadelphia, Saunders, 1992, p 1015

Weiner CP, Sipes SL, Wenstrom K: The effect of fetal age upon normal fetal laboratory values and venous pressure. Obstet Gynecol 79:713, 1992

Wenstrom KD, Weiner CP, Williamson RA, et al: Prenatal diagnosis of fetal hyperthyroidism using funipuncture. Obstet Gynecol 76:513, 1990

Werlin SL: Exocrine pancreas. In Polin RA, Fox WW (eds): Fetal and Neonatal Physiology. Philadelphia, Saunders, 1992, p 1047

Werth B, Tsiaras A: From Conception to Birth: A Life Unfolds. New York, Doubleday, 2002

Whitsett JA: Composition of pulmonary surfactant lipids and proteins. In Polin RA, Fox WW (eds): Fetal and Neonatal Physiology. Philadelphia, Saunders, 1992, p 941

Wilson JD, Gloyna RE: The intranuclear metabolism of testosterone in the accessory organs of reproduction. Recent Prog Horm Res 26:309, 1970

Wilson JD, Lasnitzki I: Dihydrotestosterone formation in fetal tissues of the rabbit and rat. Endocrinology 89:659, 1971

Wilson JD, MacDonald PC: Male pseudohermaphroditism due to androgen resistance: Testicular feminization and related syndromes. In Stanbury JB, Wyngaarden JD, Frederickson DS (eds): The Metabolic Basis of Inherited Disease. New York, McGraw-Hill, 1978

Wladimiroff JW, Campbell S: Fetal urine-production rates in normal and complicated pregnancy. Lancet 1:151, 1974

Zitnik G, Peterson K, Stamatoyannopoulos G, et al: Effects of butyrate and glucocorticoids on gamma- to beta-globin gene switching in somatic cell hybrids. Mol Cell Biol 15:790, 1995

5

Maternal Physiology

The anatomical, physiological, and biochemical adaptations to pregnancy are profound. Many of these remarkable changes begin soon after fertilization and continue throughout gestation, and most occur in response to physiological stimuli provided by the fetus. Equally astounding is that the woman who was pregnant is returned almost completely to her prepregnancy state after delivery and lactation. The understanding of these adaptations to pregnancy remains a major goal of obstetrics, and without such knowledge, it is almost impossible to understand the disease processes that can threaten women during pregnancy and the puerperium.

Many of these physiological adaptations could be perceived as abnormal in the nonpregnant woman. For example, cardiovascular changes during pregnancy normally include substantive increases in blood volume and cardiac output, which may mimic thyrotoxicosis. On the other hand, these same adaptations may lead to ventricular failure if there is underlying heart disease. Thus, physiological adaptations of normal pregnancy can be misinterpreted as pathological and can also unmask or worsen preexisting disease.

During normal pregnancy, virtually every organ system undergoes anatomical and functional changes that can alter appreciably the criteria for diagnosis and treatment of diseases. The impact of these marked physiological changes on underlying disease, and vice versa, is considered in detail in Section VIII.

REPRODUCTIVE TRACT

UTERUS. In the nonpregnant woman, the uterus is an almost-solid structure weighing about 70 g and with a cavity of 10 mL or less. During pregnancy, the uterus is transformed into a relatively thin-walled muscular organ of sufficient capacity to accommodate the fetus, placenta, and amnionic fluid. The total volume of the contents at term averages about 5 L but may be 20 L or more, so that by the end of pregnancy the uterus has achieved a capacity that is 500 to 1000 times greater than in the nonpregnant state. The corresponding increase in uterine weight is such that, by term, the organ weighs approximately 1100 g.

During pregnancy, uterine enlargement involves stretching and marked hypertrophy of muscle cells, whereas the production of new myocytes is limited. Accompanying the increase in the size of muscle cells is an accumulation of fibrous tissue, particularly in the external muscle layer, together with a considerable increase in elastic tissue. The network that is formed adds materially to the strength of the uterine wall. Although the walls of the corpus become considerably thicker during the first few months of pregnancy, they actually thin gradually as gestation advances, such that by term they are only about 1.5 cm or even less in thickness. In these later months, the uterus is changed into a muscular sac with thin, soft, readily indentable walls, demonstrable by the ease with which the fetus usually can be palpated.

Early in gestation, uterine hypertrophy probably is stimulated chiefly by the action of estrogen and perhaps that of progesterone. It is apparent that hypertrophy of early pregnancy does not occur entirely in response to mechanical distention by the products of conception, because similar uterine changes are observed with ectopic pregnancy (see Chap. 10, p. 258). But after about 12 weeks, the increase in uterine size is related predominantly in some manner to pressure exerted by the expanding products of conception.

Uterine enlargement is most marked in the fundus. In the early months of pregnancy, the fallopian tubes and ovarian and round ligaments attach only slightly below the apex of the fundus, whereas in the later months, they are located slightly above the middle of the uterus (see Fig. 2–10, p. 24). The position of the placenta also influences the extent of uterine hypertrophy, because the portion of the uterus surrounding the placental site enlarges more rapidly than does the rest.

Arrangement of the Muscle Cells. The uterine musculature during pregnancy is arranged in three strata:

1. An outer hoodlike layer, which arches over the fundus and extends into the various ligaments.
2. A middle layer, composed of a dense network of muscle fibers perforated in all directions by blood vessels.
3. An internal layer, consisting of sphincter-like fibers around the orifices of the fallopian tubes and the internal os of the cervix.

The main portion of the uterine wall is formed by the middle layer, which consists of an interlacing network of muscle fibers between which extend the blood vessels. Each cell in this layer has a double curve, so that the interlacing of any two gives approximately the form of a figure eight. As a result of this arrangement, when the cells contract after delivery, they constrict the penetrating blood vessels and thus act as ligatures.

Uterine Size, Shape, and Position. For the first few weeks, the uterus maintains its original pear shape, but as pregnancy advances, the corpus and fundus assume a more globular form, becoming almost spherical by 12 weeks. Subsequently, the organ increases more rapidly in length than in width and assumes an ovoid shape. By the end of 12 weeks, the uterus has become too large to remain totally within the pelvis. As the uterus continues to enlarge, it contacts the anterior abdominal wall, displaces the intestines laterally and superiorly, and continues to rise, ultimately reaching almost to the liver. With ascent of the uterus from the pelvis, it usually undergoes rotation to the right, and this *dextrorotation* likely is caused by the rectosigmoid on the left side of the pelvis. As the uterus rises, tension is exerted on the broad and round ligaments.

With the pregnant woman standing, the longitudinal axis of the uterus corresponds to an extension of the axis of the pelvic inlet. The abdominal wall supports the uterus and, unless it is quite relaxed, maintains this relation between the long axis of the uterus and the axis of the pelvic inlet. When the pregnant woman is supine, the uterus falls back to rest on the vertebral column and the adjacent great vessels, especially the inferior vena cava and aorta.

Contractility. From the first trimester onward, the uterus undergoes irregular contractions that are normally painless. In the second trimester, these contractions may be detected by bimanual examination. Because attention was first called to this phenomenon in 1872 by J. Braxton Hicks, the contractions have been known by his name. Such contractions appear unpredictably and sporadically, are usually nonrhythmic, and their intensity varies between approximately 5 and 25 mm Hg (Alvarez and Caldeyro-Barcia, 1950). Until the last month of gestation, *Braxton Hicks contractions* are infrequent, but they increase during the last week or two. At this time, the contractions may occur as often as every 10 to 20 minutes and also may assume some degree of rhythmicity. Late in pregnancy, these contractions may cause some discomfort and account for so-called *false labor* (see Chap. 17, p. 424).

Uteroplacental Blood Flow. The delivery of most substances essential for growth and metabolism of the fetus and placenta, as well as removal of most metabolic wastes, is dependent on adequate perfusion of the placental intervillous space (see Chap. 3, p. 61). Placental perfusion is dependent on total uterine blood flow, which is principally from the uterine and ovarian arteries. Uteroplacental blood flow increases progressively during pregnancy, ranging from approximately 450 to 650 mL/min near term (Edman and associates, 1981; Kauppila and co-workers, 1980).

The results of studies conducted in rats by Page and co-workers (2002) suggest that the uterine veins also undergo significant adaptations during pregnancy. Specifically, remodeling of the uterine veins by numerous factors that include reduced elastin content and adrenergic nerve density results in increased venous caliber and distensibility. Logically, such changes are necessary to accommodate massively increased uteroplacental blood flow.

Assali and co-workers (1968), using electromagnetic flow probes placed directly on a uterine artery, studied the effects of labor on uteroplacental blood flow in sheep and dogs at term. They found that uterine contractions, either spontaneous or induced, caused a decrease in uterine blood flow that was approximately proportional to the intensity of the contraction. They also showed that a tetanic contraction caused a precipitous fall in uterine blood flow. Harbert and associates (1969) made a similar observation in gravid monkeys. Uterine contractions appear to affect fetal circulation much less, and Brar and colleagues (1988) reported no adverse effects on umbilical artery flow.

CONTROL OF UTEROPLACENTAL BLOOD FLOW. The progressive increase in maternal–placental blood flow during gestation occurs principally by means of vasodilation, whereas fetal-

placental blood flow is increased by a continuing growth of placental vessels. Palmer and colleagues (1992) showed that uterine artery diameter doubled by 20 weeks and concomitant mean Doppler velocimetry was increased eightfold. It appears likely that vasodilation at this stage of pregnancy is at least in part the consequence of estrogen stimulation. Naden and Rosenfeld (1985) found that 17β-estradiol administration to nonpregnant sheep induced cardiovascular changes similar to those observed in pregnant animals. Using measurements of the uterine artery resistance index, Jauniaux and associates (1994) found that both estradiol and progesterone contributed to the downstream fall in vascular resistance in women with advancing gestational age (see Chap. 16, p. 403).

Other mediators, in addition to estradiol and progesterone, modify vascular resistance during pregnancy, including within the uteroplacental circulation. For example, significant decreases in placental perfusion have been demonstrated in sheep following *catecholamine* infusions (Rosenfeld and co-workers, 1976; Rosenfeld and West, 1977). This response is likely the consequence of greater sensitivity of the uteroplacental vascular bed to epinephrine and norepinephrine when compared with that of the systemic vasculature. In contrast, normal pregnancy is characterized by vascular refractoriness to the pressor effects of *angiotensin II* (see p. 135). This insensitivity serves to increase uteroplacental blood flow (Gant and co-workers, 1973; Rosenfeld and Gant, 1981). *Nitric oxide,* previously termed *endothelium-derived relaxing factor,* is a potent vasodilator released by endothelial cells. It may also have important implications for modifying vascular resistance and, thus, uteroplacental perfusion during pregnancy (Hull and associates, 1994; Seligman and co-workers, 1994). As discussed in Chapter 34 (see p. 769), abnormal synthesis of nitric oxide has been linked to the development of preeclampsia (Savvidou and co-workers, 2003).

CERVIX. As early as 1 month after conception, the cervix begins to undergo pronounced softening and cyanosis. These changes result from increased vascularity and edema of the entire cervix, together with hypertrophy and hyperplasia of the cervical glands. Although the cervix contains a small amount of smooth muscle, its major component is connective tissue. Rearrangement of this collagen-rich connective tissue is necessary to permit functions as diverse as maintenance of a pregnancy to term, dilatation to facilitate delivery, and repair following parturition so that a successful pregnancy can be repeated. The complex dynamic changes that occur in the anatomy and physiology of the cervix as gestation advances were reviewed by Ludmir and Sehdev (2000) and are detailed further in Chapter 6.

As shown in Figure 5–1, the glands of the cervix undergo such marked proliferation that by the end of pregnancy they occupy approximately half of the entire cervical mass, rather than a small fraction as in the nonpregnant state. These normal pregnancy-induced changes represent an extension, or

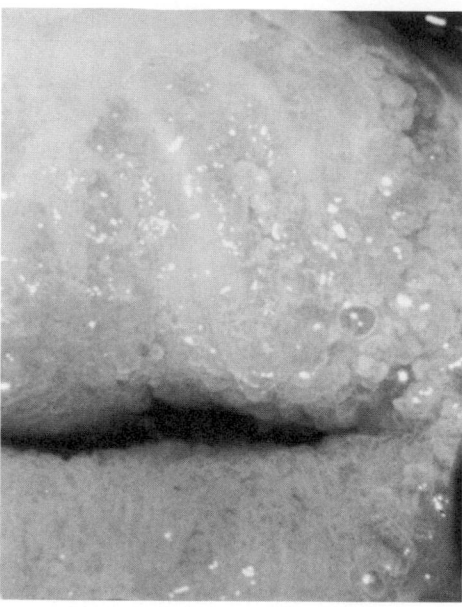

FIGURE 5–1. Cervical eversion of pregnancy as viewed through a colposcope. The eversion represents columnar epithelium on the portio of the cervix. (Courtesy of Dr. Phil DiSaia.)

eversion, of the proliferating columnar endocervical glands. This tissue tends to be red and velvety and bleeds even with minor trauma, such as with taking Pap smears.

The endocervical mucosal cells produce copious amounts of a tenacious mucus that obstruct the cervical canal soon after conception. As discussed on page 131, this mucus is rich in immunoglobulins and cytokines (Kutteh and Franklin, 2001). At the onset of labor, if not before, this *mucus plug* is expelled, resulting in a *bloody show.* Moreover, the consistency of the cervical mucus changes during pregnancy. In the great majority of pregnant women, cervical mucus, spread and dried on a glass slide, is characterized by crystallization, or *beading,* as a result of progesterone. In some women, arborization of the crystals, or *ferning,* is observed as a result of amnionic fluid leakage (see Figs. 8–3 and 8–4, p. 205).

During pregnancy, basal cells near the squamocolumnar junction are likely to be prominent in size, shape, and staining qualities. These changes are considered to be estrogen induced. Because of these basal cell changes, the frequency of less-than-optimal Pap smears is increased in the pregnant woman (Kost and associates, 1993).

OVARIES. Ovulation ceases during pregnancy and the maturation of new follicles is suspended. Ordinarily, only a single corpus luteum of pregnancy can be found in the ovaries of pregnant women. This most likely functions maximally during the first 6 to 7 weeks of pregnancy (4 to 5 weeks postovulation), and thereafter contributes relatively little to progesterone production. These observations have been confirmed by surgical removal of the corpus luteum before 7 weeks (5 weeks postovulation), which results in a rapid

fall in maternal serum progesterone and then spontaneous abortion (Csapo and co-workers, 1973). After this time, however, corpus luteum removal ordinarily does not cause abortion.

A *decidual reaction* on and beneath the surface of the ovaries, similar to that found in the endometrial stroma, is common in pregnancy and may be observed at cesarean delivery. These elevated patches of tissue bleed easily and may, on first glance, resemble freshly torn adhesions. Similar decidual reactions are seen on the posterior uterine serosa and on or within other pelvic or even extrapelvic abdominal organs. Although the ontogeny of such decidual reactions is incompletely understood, Taussig (1906) and others have deduced that these findings likely represent cellular detritus from the endometrium that has passed through the fallopian tubes.

The enormous caliber of the ovarian veins viewed at cesarean delivery is startling. Hodgkinson (1953) found that the diameter of the ovarian vascular pedicle increased during pregnancy from 0.9 cm to approximately 2.6 cm at term.

Relaxin. This protein hormone has structural features that are similar to insulin and insulin-like growth factors I and II. Its major biological action is remodeling of the connective tissue of the reproductive tract, thus allowing accommodation of pregnancy and successful parturition (Weiss and colleagues, 1993). Relaxin is secreted by the corpus luteum, decidua, and placenta in a pattern similar to that of chorionic gonadotropin (hCG). It is also secreted by the heart, and increased levels have been found in association with heart failure (Fisher and co-workers, 2002).

The role of relaxin during human pregnancy is not completely defined, however, it is known to have effects on the biochemical structure of the cervix (Bell and colleagues, 1993). The hormone also affects myometrial contractility, which may be implicated in preterm birth. Increases in peripheral joint laxity during human pregnancy do not correlate with serum relaxin levels (Marnach and co-workers, 2003; Schauberger and colleagues, 1996).

Pregnancy Luteoma. In 1963, Sternberg described a solid ovarian tumor that developed during pregnancy and was composed of large acidophilic luteinized cells. These represented an exaggerated luteinization reaction of the normal ovary. These so-called *luteomas of pregnancy* are variable in size, ranging from microscopic to over 20 cm in diameter (Fig. 5–2). Typical ultrasonographic characteristics include a solid, complex-appearing unilateral or bilateral mass with cystic features that correspond to areas of hemorrhage. It is usually not possible to differentiate luteomas from other solid ovarian neoplasms, such as luteinized thecoma, granulosa cell tumor, or Leydig cell tumor, based on the ultrasound characteristics alone (Choi and associates, 2000). Although luteomas regress after delivery, they may recur in subsequent pregnancies (Shortle and associates, 1987).

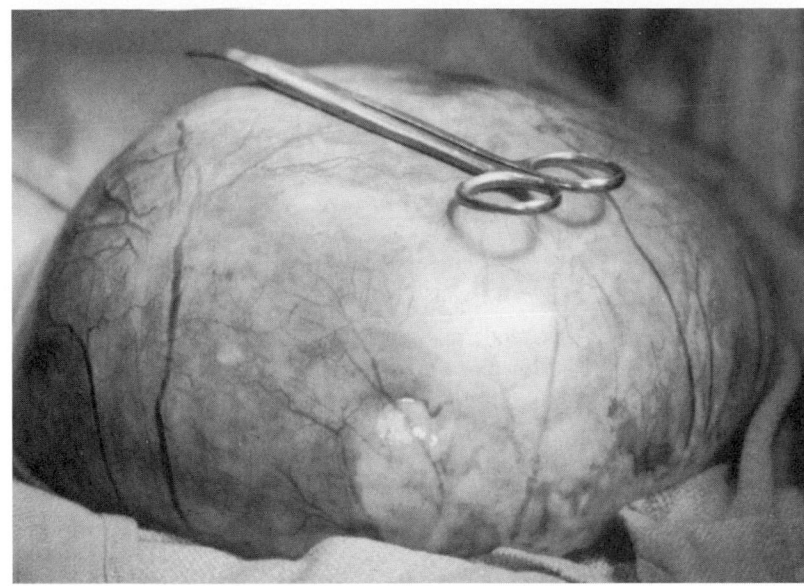

FIGURE 5–2. Large luteoma of pregnancy removed at laparotomy postpartum.

Pregnancy luteomas may result in maternal virilization, but usually the female fetus is not affected. This is presumably because of the protective role of the placenta and its high capacity to convert androgens and androgen-like steroids to estrogens (Edman and co-workers, 1979). Occasionally, however, a female fetus can become virilized (Cohen and associates, 1982).

Theca-Lutein Cysts. These benign ovarian lesions result from exaggerated physiological follicle stimulation, which is termed *hyperreactio luteinalis.* The reaction is associated with markedly elevated serum levels of hCG. Although the cellular pattern of hyperreactio luteinalis is similar to that of a luteoma, these usually bilateral cystic ovaries are moderately to massively enlarged. These are found frequently with gestational trophoblastic disease (see Chap. 11, p. 276). They are more likely in pregnancies associated with a large placenta, for example, diabetes, D-isoimmunization, and multiple fetuses (Tanaka and colleagues, 2001). Theca-lutein cysts have been reported in chronic renal failure as a result of reduced hCG clearance, and in hyperthyroidism as a result of the structural homology between hCG and thyroid-stimulating hormone (Coccia and colleagues, 2003; Gherman and co-workers, 2003). They also are encountered in women with otherwise normal pregnancies but increased hCG concentrations (Bidus and associates, 2002). Their diagnosis and management is discussed in Chapter 40 (see p. 965).

Although usually asymptomatic, hemorrhage into the cysts may cause abdominal pain. In addition, maternal virilization may be seen in up to 25 percent of women (Foulk and associates, 1997). Changes include temporal balding, hirsutism, and clitoromegaly associated with massively elevated levels of androstenedione and testosterone (Bradshaw and co-workers, 1986). The diagnosis typically is based on ultrasonographic findings of bilateral enlarged ovaries containing multiple cysts in the appropriate clinical settings. The condition is self-limited and eventually undergoes spontaneous resolution after delivery. In some women, increased ovarian responsiveness to gonadotropin can be confirmed by several weeks postpartum (Bradshaw and colleagues, 1986).

FALLOPIAN TUBES. The musculature of the fallopian tubes undergoes little hypertrophy during pregnancy. The epithelium of the tubal mucosa, however, becomes somewhat flattened. Decidual cells may develop in the stroma of the endosalpinx, but a continuous decidual membrane is not formed.

VAGINA AND PERINEUM. During pregnancy, increased vascularity and hyperemia develop in the skin and muscles of the perineum and vulva, with softening of the underlying abundant connective tissue. Increased vascularity prominently affects the vagina and results in the violet color characteristic of the *Chadwick sign.* The vaginal walls undergo striking changes, presumably in preparation for the distention that occurs during labor. These changes include a considerable increase in the thickness of the mucosa, loosening of the connective tissue, and hypertrophy of smooth muscle cells. The papillae of the vaginal mucosa also undergo considerable hypertrophy, creating a fine, hobnailed appearance.

The considerably increased volume of cervical secretions within the vagina during pregnancy consists of a somewhat thick, white discharge. The pH is acidic, varying from 3.5 to 6, the result of increased production of lactic acid from glycogen in the vaginal epithelium by the action of *Lactobacillus acidophilus.*

Histopathology. Early in pregnancy the vaginal epithelial cells are similar to those found during the luteal phase. As pregnancy advances, two patterns of response may be seen:

1. Small intermediate cells, called *navicular cells* by Papanicolaou, are found in abundance in small, dense clusters. These ovoid cells contain a vesicular, somewhat elongated nucleus.
2. Vesicular nuclei without cytoplasm, or so-called *naked nuclei,* are evident along with an abundance of *Lactobacillus.*

SKIN

ABDOMINAL WALL. In the later months of pregnancy, reddish, slightly depressed streaks commonly develop in the skin of the abdomen and sometimes in the skin over the breasts and thighs. These are called *striae gravidarum* or *"stretch marks."* In multiparous women, in addition to the reddish striae of the present pregnancy, glistening, silvery lines that represent the cicatrices of previous striae frequently are seen.

Occasionally, the muscles of the abdominal walls do not withstand the tension to which they are subjected, and the rectus muscles separate in the midline, creating a *diastasis recti* of varying extent. If severe, a considerable portion of the anterior uterine wall is covered by only a layer of skin, attenuated fascia, and peritoneum.

PIGMENTATION. In many women, the midline of the abdominal skin—*linea alba*—becomes markedly pigmented, assuming a brownish-black color to form the *linea nigra.* Occasionally, irregular brownish patches of varying size appear on the face and neck, giving rise to *chloasma* or *melasma gravidarum,* which is the so-called mask of pregnancy. Pigmentation of the areolae and genital skin may also be accentuated. These pigmentary changes usually disappear, or at least regress considerably, after delivery (see Chap. 56, p. 1250). Oral contraceptives may cause similar pigmentation. Very little is known of the nature of these pigmentary changes, although melanocyte-stimulating hormone, a polypeptide similar to corticotropin, has been shown to be elevated remarkably from the end of the second month of pregnancy until term. Estrogen and progesterone also are reported to have melanocyte-stimulating effects. These conditions are considered in greater detail in Chapter 56.

VASCULAR CHANGES. Angiomas, called *vascular spiders,* develop in about two thirds of white women and approximately 10 percent of black women. These are minute, red elevations on the skin, particularly common on the face, neck, upper chest, and arms, with radicles branching out from a central lesion. The condition is often designated as nevus, angioma, or telangiectasis. *Palmar erythema* is encountered in pregnancy in about two thirds of white women and one third of black women. The two conditions are of no clinical significance and disappear in most women shortly after pregnancy. They are most likely the consequence of the hyperestrogenemia.

BREASTS

In the early weeks of pregnancy, women often experience breast tenderness and tingling. After the second month, the breasts increase in size, and delicate veins become visible just beneath the skin. The nipples become considerably larger, more deeply pigmented, and more erectile. After the first few months, a thick, yellowish fluid—*colostrum*—can often be expressed from the nipples by gentle massage. During the same months, the areolae become broader and more deeply pigmented. Scattered through the areolae are a number of small elevations, the *glands of Montgomery,* which are hypertrophic sebaceous glands. If the increase in size of the breasts is very extensive, striations similar to those observed in the abdomen may develop. Rarely, breast enlargement may become so pathologically extensive—referred to as *gigantomastia*—that it becomes life threatening and often requires surgical intervention (Vidaeff and associates, 2003). Interestingly, prepregnancy breast size and volume of milk production do not correlate (Hytten, 1995). Histological and functional changes of the breasts induced by pregnancy and lactation are further discussed in Chapter 30 (see p. 699).

METABOLIC CHANGES

In response to the increased demands of the rapidly growing fetus and placenta, the pregnant woman undergoes metabolic changes that are numerous and intense. Certainly no other physiological event in postnatal life induces such profound metabolic alterations. For example, the additional total pregnancy energy demands have been estimated to be as high as 80,000 kcal or about 300 kcal/day (Hytten and Chamberlain, 1991).

WEIGHT GAIN. Most of the increase in weight during pregnancy is attributable to the uterus and its contents, the breasts, and increases in blood volume and extravascular extracellular fluid. A smaller fraction of the increased weight is the result of metabolic alterations that result in an increase in cellular water and deposition of new fat and protein, so-called *maternal reserves.* Hytten (1991) reported that the average weight gain during pregnancy is approximately 12.5 kg or 27.5 lb (Table 5–1). Maternal aspects of weight gain are considered in greater detail in Chapter 8 (see p. 213).

WATER METABOLISM. Increased water retention is a normal physiological alteration of pregnancy. This retention

TABLE 5–1 Analysis of Weight Gain Based on Physiological Events During Pregnancy

Tissues and Fluids	Cumulative Increase in Weight (g) Up To:			
	10 Weeks	20 Weeks	30 Weeks	40 Weeks
Fetus	5	300	1,500	3,400
Placenta	20	170	430	650
Amnionic fluid	30	350	750	800
Uterus	140	320	600	970
Breasts	45	180	360	405
Blood	100	600	1,300	1,450
Extravascular fluid	0	30	80	1,480
Maternal stores (fat)	310	2,050	3,480	3,345
Total	650	40,00	8,500	12,500

Modified from Hytten, 1991, with permission.

is mediated, at least in part, by a fall in plasma osmolality of approximately 10 mOsm/kg induced by a resetting of osmotic thresholds for thirst and vasopressin secretion (Heenan and colleagues, 2003; Lindheimer and Davison, 1995). As shown in Figure 5–3, this phenomenon is functioning by early pregnancy.

At term, the water content of the fetus, placenta, and amnionic fluid amounts to about 3.5 L. Another 3.0 L accumulates as a result of increases in the maternal blood volume and in the size of the uterus and the breasts. Thus, the minimum amount of extra water that the average women accrues during normal pregnancy is about 6.5 L. Clearly demonstrable pitting edema of the ankles and legs is seen in most pregnant women, especially at the end of the day. This accumulation of fluid, which may amount to a liter or so, is caused by

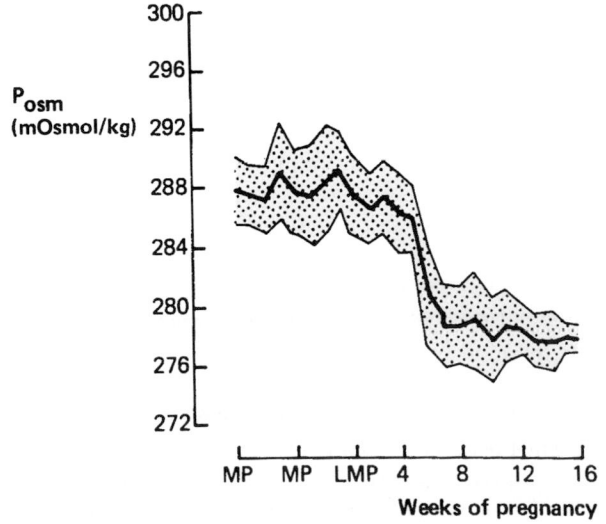

FIGURE 5–3. Mean values (± SD) for plasma osmolality measured at weekly intervals in nine women from preconception to 16 weeks. (LMP = last menstrual period; MP = menstrual period.) (From Davison and colleagues, 1981, with permission.)

an increase in venous pressure below the level of the uterus as a consequence of partial occlusion of the vena cava. A decrease in interstitial colloid osmotic pressure induced by normal pregnancy also favors edema late in pregnancy (Øian and co-workers, 1985).

Longitudinal studies of body composition have shown a progressive increase in total body water and fat mass during pregnancy. It has been known for decades that both initial maternal weight and the weight gained during pregnancy are highly associated with birthweight. It is unclear, however, what role maternal fat or water have in fetal growth. Studies in well-nourished term women suggest that maternal body water, rather than fat, contributes more significantly to infant birthweight (Lederman and co-workers, 1999; Mardones-Santander and associates, 1998).

PROTEIN METABOLISM. The products of conception, the uterus, and maternal blood are relatively rich in protein rather than fat or carbohydrate. At term, the fetus and placenta together weigh about 4 kg and contain approximately 500 g of protein, or about half of the total pregnancy increase (Hytten and Leitch, 1971). The remaining 500 g is added to the uterus as contractile protein, to the breasts primarily in the glands, and to the maternal blood as hemoglobin and plasma proteins.

Mojtahedi and associates (2002) measured nitrogen balance in 12 healthy women before pregnancy and again at 12, 23, and 34 weeks. They found that it increased with gestation, suggesting a more efficient use of dietary protein. In addition, urinary excretion of 3-methylhistidine did not change significantly toward term, indicating that breakdown of maternal muscle is not required to meet the demands of growing maternal and fetal tissues. Supporting the concept that pregnancy is associated with nitrogen conservation, Kalhan and colleagues (2003) found that the turnover rate of the nonessential amino acid serine decreases with advancing gestational age. The daily requirements for dietary protein intake during pregnancy are discussed in Chapter 8 (see p. 215).

CARBOHYDRATE METABOLISM. Normal pregnancy is characterized by mild fasting hypoglycemia, postprandial hyperglycemia, and hyperinsulinemia (Fig. 5–4). The fasting plasma glucose concentration falls somewhat, possibly as a result of the increased plasma levels of insulin observed in pregnancy. This cannot be explained by a decrease in the metabolism of insulin because its half-life during pregnancy is not changed (Lind and associates, 1977).

The increased basal level of plasma insulin in normal pregnancy is associated with several unique responses to glucose ingestion. For example, after an oral glucose meal, gravid women demonstrate both prolonged hyperglycemia and hyperinsulinemia, with a greater suppression of glucagon (Phelps and associates, 1981). This response is consistent with a pregnancy-induced state of peripheral resistance to insulin, the purpose of which is likely to ensure a sustained postprandial supply of glucose to the fetus. Indeed, it has been

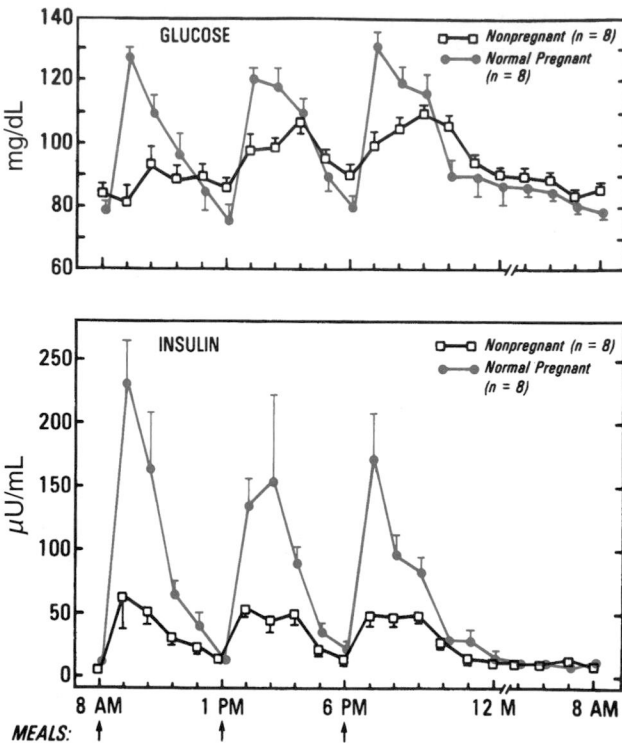

FIGURE 5–4. Diurnal changes in plasma glucose and insulin in normal late pregnancy. (From Phelps and colleagues, 1981, with permission.)

estimated that insulin action in late normal pregnancy is 50 to 70 percent lower than that of healthy, nonpregnant women (Butte, 2000).

The mechanism(s) responsible for insulin resistance is not completely understood. Progesterone and estrogen may act, directly or indirectly, to mediate this resistance. Plasma levels of placental lactogen increase with gestation, and this protein hormone is characterized by growth hormone–like action that may result in increased lipolysis with liberation of free fatty acids (Freinkel, 1980). The increased concentration of circulating free fatty acids also may facilitate increased tissue resistance to insulin.

The pregnant woman changes rapidly from a postprandial state characterized by elevated and sustained glucose levels to a fasting state characterized by decreased plasma glucose and amino acids such as alanine. During fasting, the plasma concentrations of free fatty acids, triglycerides, and cholesterol are higher. Freinkel and colleagues (1985) have referred to this pregnancy-induced switch in fuels from glucose to lipids as *accelerated starvation*. Certainly, when fasting is prolonged in the pregnant woman, these alterations are exaggerated and ketonemia rapidly appears.

FAT METABOLISM. The concentrations of lipids, lipoproteins, and apolipoproteins in plasma increase appreciably during pregnancy. The storage of fat occurs primarily during midpregnancy (Hytten and Thomson, 1968; Pipe and co-workers, 1979). This fat is deposited mostly in central rather than peripheral sites. Later in pregnancy, as fetal nutritional demands increase remarkably, maternal fat storage decreases. Hytten and Thomson (1968) cited some evidence that progesterone may act to reset a lipostat in the hypothalamus, and at the end of pregnancy the lipostat returns to its previous nonpregnant level and the added fat is lost. Such a mechanism for energy storage, theoretically at least, might protect the mother and fetus during time of prolonged starvation or hard physical exertion.

Low-density lipoprotein cholesterol (LDL-C) levels peak at approximately week 36, likely the consequence of the hepatic effects of estradiol and progesterone (Desoye and associates, 1987). High-density lipoprotein cholesterol (HDL-C) peaks at week 25, decreases until week 32, and remains constant for the remainder of pregnancy. The initial increase is believed to be caused by estrogen. Brizzi and colleagues (1999) have suggested that changes in the low-density lipoprotein (LDL) pattern during normal pregnancy might be used to identify those women who later in life may be predisposed to atherogenesis.

During the third trimester, average total serum cholesterol, LDL-C, and HDL-C levels are approximately 245 ± 10 mg/dL, 148 ± 5 mg/dL, and 59 ± 3 mg/dL, respectively (Paradisi and associates, 2002). After delivery, the concentrations of these lipids, as well as lipoproteins and apolipoproteins, decrease at different rates. Lactation speeds the rate of decrease of many of these compounds (Darmady and Postle, 1982).

Leptin. This peptide hormone, primarily secreted by adipose tissue, plays a key role in the regulation of body fat and energy expenditure. During pregnancy, maternal serum leptin levels progressively increase, peaking during the second trimester to plateau at term in concentrations three to four times higher than those in nonpregnant women. This increase is only in part due to the weight gain normally associated with pregnancy, because leptin also is produced by the placenta. Indeed, placental weight is significantly related to leptin levels measured in the umbilical cord blood (Pighetti and co-workers, 2003). Recent investigations have analyzed the relationships between serum leptin levels and preeclampsia as well as fetal growth restriction (Chan, 2003; Lepercq, 2003; Pighetti, 2003; Salomon, 2003, and their many associates). This topic is discussed further in Chapter 38 (see p. 895).

ELECTROLYTE AND MINERAL METABOLISM. During normal pregnancy, nearly 1000 mEq of *sodium* and 300 mEq of *potassium* are retained (Lindheimer and colleagues, 1987). Although the glomerular filtration of sodium and potassium is increased, the excretion of these electrolytes is unchanged during pregnancy as a result of enhanced tubular resorption (Brown and colleagues, 1986, 1988). Although pregnancy is associated with increased total accumulations of sodium and potassium, the serum concentrations of these electrolytes are decreased slightly as a result of the expanded plasma volume, however, they remain very near the range of normal for nonpregnant women (Kametas and colleagues, 2003b).

Total serum *calcium* levels decline during pregnancy, the reduction reflecting lowered plasma albumin concentration and, in turn, the consequent decrease in the amount bound to protein. The levels of serum ionized calcium, however, remain unchanged (Power and associates, 1999). The developing fetus imposes a significant demand on maternal calcium homeostasis. During the third trimester, for example, approximately 200 mg of calcium are deposited in the fetal skeleton per day (Pitkin, 1985). Dietary intake of sufficient calcium (see Table 8–7, p. 215), therefore, is necessary to prevent excess depletion from the mother. This has been reported to be especially important in pregnant adolescents, whose own skeletons are still developing (Repke, 1994).

Serum *magnesium* levels also decline during pregnancy. Bardicef and colleagues (1995) concluded that pregnancy is actually a state of extracellular magnesium depletion. Compared with nonpregnant women, they found that both total and ionized magnesium were significantly lower during normal pregnancy. On the other hand, serum *phosphate* levels are within the nonpregnant range (Kametas and colleagues, 2003b). The renal threshold for inorganic phosphate excretion is elevated in pregnancy due to increased calcitonin (Weiss and colleagues, 1998).

With respect to most other minerals, pregnancy induces little change in their metabolism other than their retention in amounts equivalent to those used for growth of fetal and, to a lesser extent, maternal tissues (see Chap. 4, p. 101, and Chap. 8, p. 216). An important exception, however, is the considerably increased requirement for *iron,* which is discussed later.

HEMATOLOGICAL CHANGES

BLOOD VOLUME. The maternal blood volume increases markedly during pregnancy. In studies of normal women, the blood volumes at or very near term averaged about 40 to 45 percent above their nonpregnant levels (Pritchard, 1965; Whittaker and associates, 1996). The degree of expansion varies considerably. In some women only a modest increase occurs, whereas in others the blood volume nearly doubles. A fetus is not essential for the development of hypervolemia during pregnancy, for increases in blood volume have been demonstrated in some women with hydatidiform mole (Pritchard, 1965).

Pregnancy-induced hypervolemia has several important functions:

1. To meet the demands of the enlarged uterus with its greatly hypertrophied vascular system.

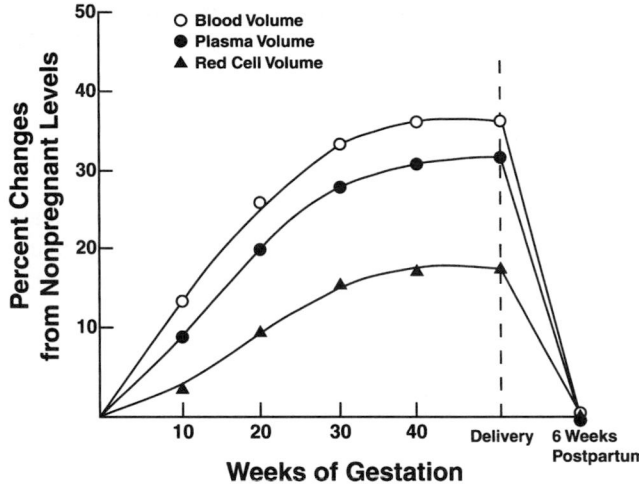

FIGURE 5–5. Changes in total blood volume and its components (plasma and red cell volumes) during pregnancy and postpartum. (From Peck and Arias, 1979, with permission.)

2. To protect the mother, and in turn the fetus, against the deleterious effects of impaired venous return in the supine and erect positions.
3. To safeguard the mother against the adverse effects of blood loss associated with parturition.

Maternal blood volume begins to increase during the first trimester. In fact, by 12 menstrual weeks, the plasma volume expands by approximately 15 percent as compared with that of prepregnancy (Bernstein and co-workers, 2001). As shown in Figure 5–5, maternal blood volume expands most rapidly during the second trimester, and then rises at a much slower rate during the third trimester to plateau during the last several weeks of pregnancy.

Blood volume expansion results from an increase in both plasma and erythrocytes. Although more plasma than erythrocytes is usually added to the maternal circulation, the increase in the volume of erythrocytes is considerable, averaging about 450 mL (Pritchard and Adams, 1960). Moderate erythroid hyperplasia is present in the bone marrow, and the reticulocyte count is elevated slightly during normal pregnancy. As discussed in Chapter 51 (see p. 1144), this change is almost certainly related to the increase in maternal plasma erythropoietin levels, which peak early during the third trimester and correspond to maximal erythrocyte production (Clapp and colleagues, 2003; Harstad and co-workers, 1992).

Hemoglobin Concentration and Hematocrit. In spite of augmented erythropoiesis, hemoglobin concentration and the hematocrit decrease slightly during normal pregnancy. As a result, whole blood viscosity decreases (Huisman and colleagues, 1987). Hemoglobin concentration at term averages 12.5 g/dL and in 6 percent of women it is below 11.0 g/dL (see Fig. 51–1 and Table 51–1). Thus, in most women, a hemoglobin concentration below 11.0 g/dL, especially late in pregnancy, should be considered abnormal and usually due to iron deficiency rather than to hypervolemia of pregnancy.

IRON METABOLISM

Iron Stores. The total iron content of normal adult women ranges from 2.0 to 2.5 g or about half the amount found normally in men. Moreover, the iron stores of normal young women are only about 300 mg (Pritchard and Mason, 1964).

Iron Requirements. The iron requirements of normal pregnancy total approximately 1000 mg. About 300 mg are actively transferred to the fetus and placenta, and about 200 mg are lost through various normal routes of excretion, primarily the gastrointestinal tract. These are obligatory losses and occur even when the mother is iron deficient. The average increase in the total volume of circulating erythrocytes—about 450 mL during pregnancy when iron is available—uses another 500 mg of iron, because 1 mL of normal erythrocytes contains 1.1 mg of iron. Practically all of the iron for these purposes is used during the latter half of pregnancy. Therefore, the iron requirement becomes quite large during the second half of pregnancy, averaging 6 to 7 mg/day (Pritchard and Scott, 1970). Because this amount is not available from body stores in most women, the desired increase in maternal erythrocyte volume and hemoglobin mass will not develop unless exogenous iron is made available in adequate amounts. In the absence of supplemental iron, the hemoglobin concentration and hematocrit fall appreciably as the maternal blood volume increases. Hemoglobin production in the fetus, however, is not impaired, because the placenta obtains iron from the mother even when the mother has severe iron deficiency anemia.

The amount of iron absorbed from diet, together with that mobilized from stores, is usually insufficient to meet the maternal demands imposed by pregnancy. If the nonanemic pregnant woman is not given supplemental iron, serum iron and ferritin concentrations decline during the second half of pregnancy (Fig. 5–6). The somewhat unexpected early pregnancy increases in serum iron and ferritin (see Fig. 5–6) are thought to be due to minimal iron demands during the first trimester as well as to a positive iron balance because of amenorrhea.

Blood Loss. Generally, not all the iron added to the maternal circulation in the form of hemoglobin is lost from the mother. During normal vaginal delivery and through the next few days, only about half of the erythrocytes added to the maternal circulation are lost from the majority of women. These losses are by way of bleeding from the placental implantation site, the episiotomy or lacerations, and in the lochia. On the average, an amount of maternal erythrocytes corresponding to about 500 to 600 mL of predelivery blood is lost during and after vaginal delivery of a single fetus (Pritchard, 1965; Ueland, 1976). The average blood loss associated with cesarean delivery or with the vaginal delivery of twins is about 1000 mL.

IMMUNOLOGICAL AND LEUKOCYTE FUNCTIONS.
As discussed in Chapter 3 (see p. 64), pregnancy has been assumed to be associated with suppression of a variety of humoral and cell-mediated immunological functions in order to accommodate the "foreign" semiallogeneic fetal graft (Thellin and Heinen, 2003). One important mechanism appears to involve the suppression of T-helper (Th) 1 and T-cytotoxic (Tc) 1 cells, which decreases secretion of interleukin (IL)-2, interferon-γ, and tumor necrosis factor-β. In addition, interferon-α, which is present in almost

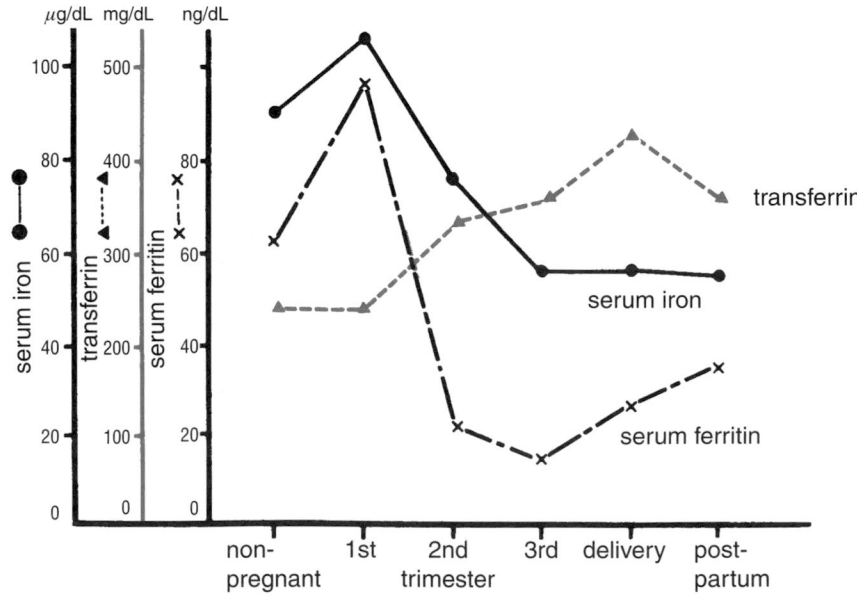

FIGURE 5–6. Indices of iron turnover during pregnancy in women without overt anemia but who were not given iron supplementation. (From Kaneshige, 1981, with permission.)

all fetal tissues and fluids, is most often absent in normally pregnant women (Chard and co-workers, 1986). Moreover, some polymorphonuclear leukocyte chemotaxis and adherence functions are depressed beginning in the second trimester and continuing throughout pregnancy (Krause and associates, 1987). Although this phenomenon is incompletely understood, it may be related, in part, to the recent finding that relaxin impairs neutrophil activation (Masini and co-workers, 2004). It is possible that these depressed leukocyte functions of pregnant women account in part for the improvement observed in some women with autoimmune diseases and the possibly increased susceptibility to certain infections.

Not all aspects of immunological function, however, are depressed. For example, there is upregulation of Th2 cells to increase secretion of IL-4, IL-6, and IL-13 (Michimata and colleagues, 2003). In cervical mucus, peak levels of immunoglobulins A and G (IgA and IgG) are significantly higher during pregnancy compared with normally menstruating women. Similarly, the amount of interleukin-1β found in cervical mucus during pregnancy is approximately 10-fold greater than in the nonpregnant state. Because oral contraceptives have been shown to induce similar changes, Kutteh and Franklin (2001) hypothesized that these immunological changes may be a result of increased estrogen and progesterone. Although such enhanced local reproductive tract immunity may be important for protecting the fetus, the actual clinical significance of these observations is as yet unclear.

The leukocyte count varies considerably during normal pregnancy. Usually it ranges from 5000 to 12,000/μL. During labor and the early puerperium it may become markedly elevated, attaining levels of 25,000/μL or even more, however, it averages 14,000 to 16,000/μL (Taylor and co-workers, 1981). The cause for the marked increase is not known, but the same response occurs during and after strenuous exercise. It probably represents the reappearance of leukocytes previously shunted out of the active circulation.

In addition to normal variations in the leukocyte count, the distribution of cell types is altered significantly during pregnancy. Specifically, during the third trimester, the percentages of granulocytes and CD8 T lymphocytes are significantly increased along with a concomitant reduction in the percentages of CD4 T lymphocytes and monocytes. Moreover, circulating leukocytes undergo significant phenotypic changes including, for example, the upregulation of certain adhesion molecules (Luppi and associates, 2002).

Beginning quite early in pregnancy, the activity of *leukocyte alkaline phosphatase* is increased. Such elevated activity is not peculiar to pregnancy but occurs in a wide variety of conditions, including most inflammatory states. The concentration of *C-reactive protein,* an acute-phase serum reactant, rises rapidly to 1000-fold in response to tissue trauma or inflammation. Watts and colleagues (1991) measured C-reactive protein sequentially during 81 normal pregnancies to establish normative values. Median C-reactive protein values during pregnancy were higher than values for nonpregnant

women, and these values were elevated further in labor. In women not in labor, 95 percent of values were 1.5 mg/dL or less, and gestational age did not affect serum levels. Another marker of inflammation, the *erythrocyte sedimentation rate (ESR),* is increased in normal pregnancy because of elevated plasma globulins and fibrinogen (Hytten and Leitch, 1971). Thus, this test cannot be used to reliably diagnose inflammation during pregnancy. *Complement factors C3 and C4* also are significantly elevated during the second and third trimesters of pregnancy (Gallery and colleagues, 1981).

COAGULATION. In normal pregnancy, the coagulation cascade is in an activated state (Baker and Cunningham, 1999). Evidence of activation includes increased concentrations of all clotting factors, except factors XI and XIII, with increased levels of high-molecular-weight fibrinogen complexes. Considering the substantive physiological increase in plasma volume in normal pregnancy, such increased concentrations represent a markedly augmented production of these procoagulants. For example, plasma fibrinogen (factor I) in normal nonpregnant women averages about 300 mg/dL and ranges from about 200 to 400 mg/dL. During normal pregnancy, fibrinogen concentration increases about 50 percent to average about 450 mg/dL late in pregnancy, with a range from 300 to 600 mg/dL. The percentage of high-molecular-weight fibrinogen is unchanged (Manten and colleagues, 2004). This contributes greatly to the striking increase in the *erythrocyte sedimentation rate.*

High-molecular-weight soluble fibrin–fibrinogen complexes circulate in normal pregnancy, and D-dimer serum concentrations increase with gestational age (Lee and associates, 1996; Nolan and colleagues, 1993). The clotting times of whole blood, however, do not differ significantly in normal pregnant women. Some of the pregnancy-induced changes in the levels of coagulation factors can be duplicated by the administration of estrogen plus progestin contraceptive tablets to nonpregnant women.

Normal pregnancy also involves changes in platelets (Baker and Cunningham, 1999). In a study of almost 7000 healthy women at term, Boehlen and associates (2000) found that the average platelet count was decreased slightly during pregnancy to 213,000/μL compared with 250,000/μL in nonpregnant control women. They defined thrombocytopenia as below the 2.5th percentile, which was 116,000/mL. During normal pregnancy, platelet width and volume increase. Decreased platelet concentrations are partially due to the effects of hemodilution, but they also likely represent increased platelet consumption, leading to a greater proportion of younger, and therefore, larger platelets (Tygart and co-workers, 1986). Further supporting this concept, Hayashi and associates (2002) found that, beginning in midpregnancy, production of thromboxane A$_2$, which induces platelet aggregation, progressively increases.

The end product of the coagulation cascade is fibrin formation, and the main function of the fibrinolytic system is to remove excess fibrin. The inactive precursor plasminogen is activated by plasminogen activators, which are serine proteases that convert plasminogen into plasmin. Their activity is balanced by specific plasma-activator inhibitors present in plasma and platelets. Plasmin activity causes fibrinolysis and produces fibrin degradation products such as D-dimers. Studies of the fibrinolytic system in pregnancy have produced conflicting results, although the majority of evidence suggests that fibrinolytic activity is actually reduced in normal pregnancy, likely related to increased concentrations of plasminogen-activator inhibitors (Baker and Cunningham, 1999; Koh and co-authors, 1993).

Regulatory Proteins. There are a number of natural inhibitors of coagulation, including protein C, protein S, and antithrombin. Inherited or acquired deficiencies of these and other natural regulatory proteins, collectively referred to as thrombophilias, account for more than half of all thromboembolic episodes during pregnancy (Lockwood, 2002). These are discussed in detail in Chapter 47 (see p. 1074).

Activated protein C, along with the co-factors *protein S* and factor V, functions as an anticoagulant by neutralizing the procoagulants factor Va and factor VIIIa (see Fig. 47–1, p. 1075). As normal pregnancy advances, protein C levels remain unchanged. At the same time, resistance to activated protein C increases progressively and is related to a concomitant decrease in free protein S and increase in factor VIII. Specifically, between the first and third trimesters, the levels of activated protein C decrease from about 2.4 to 1.9 U/mL, and free protein S decreases from 0.4 to 0.16 U/mL (Walker and colleagues, 1997). Oral contraceptives also decrease free protein S levels, leading to speculation that the decrease is hormonally mediated. The discovery that the *factor V Leiden mutation* causes resistance to activated protein C has introduced new variables into thrombophilias. In affected women, measurement of this resistance during pregnancy is difficult and DNA testing is recommended.

Levels of *antithrombin* remain relatively constant throughout gestation and the early puerperium (Delorme and associates, 1992).

CARDIOVASCULAR SYSTEM

During pregnancy and the puerperium, the heart and circulation undergo remarkable physiological adaptations. The most important changes in cardiac function occur in the first 8 weeks of pregnancy (McLaughlin and Roberts, 1999). Cardiac output is increased as early as the fifth week of pregnancy, and this initial increase is a function of reduced systemic vascular resistance and an increase in heart rate. Between weeks 10 and 20, notable increases in plasma volume occur such that preload is increased. Ventricular performance during pregnancy is influenced by both the decrease in systemic vascular resistance and changes in pulsatile arterial

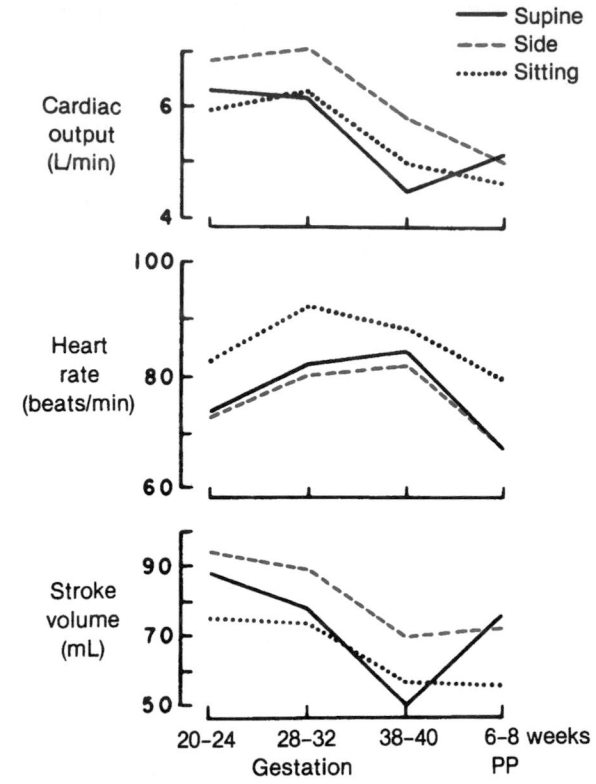

FIGURE 5–7. Effect of maternal posture on hemodynamics. PP = postpartum. (From Ueland and Metcalfe, 1975, with permission.)

flow. Vascular capacity increases, in part, because of an increase in vascular compliance. As discussed in the following section, multiple factors contribute to these changes in overall hemodynamic function, allowing the cardiovascular system to adjust to the physiological demands of the fetus while maintaining maternal cardiovascular integrity. These changes during the last half of pregnancy are graphically summarized in Figure 5–7, which also shows the important effects of maternal posture on hemodynamic events during pregnancy.

HEART. The resting pulse rate increases about 10 beats/min during pregnancy (Stein and co-workers, 1999). As the diaphragm becomes progressively elevated, the heart is displaced to the left and upward, while at the same time it is rotated somewhat on its long axis. As a result, the apex of the heart is moved somewhat laterally from its position in the normal nonpregnant state, and an increase in the size of the cardiac silhouette is found in radiographs (Fig. 5–8). The extent of these changes is influenced by the size and position of the uterus, tone of the abdominal muscles, and configurations of the abdomen and thorax. Furthermore, pregnant women normally have some degree of benign pericardial effusion, which may increase the cardiac silhouette (Enein and colleagues, 1987). Variability of these factors makes it difficult to identify precisely moderate degrees of cardiomegaly by simple radiographic studies. Normal pregnancy induces no

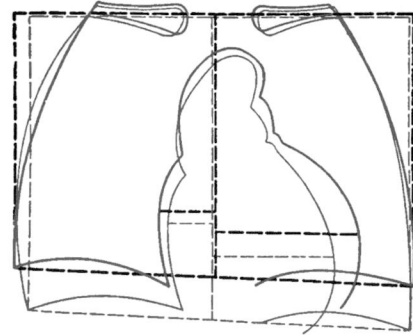

FIGURE 5–8. Change in cardiac outline that occurs in pregnancy. The colored lines represent the relations between the heart and thorax in the nonpregnant woman, and the black lines represent the conditions existing in pregnancy. These findings are based on radiographic findings in 33 women. (From Klafen and Palugyay, 1927, with permission.)

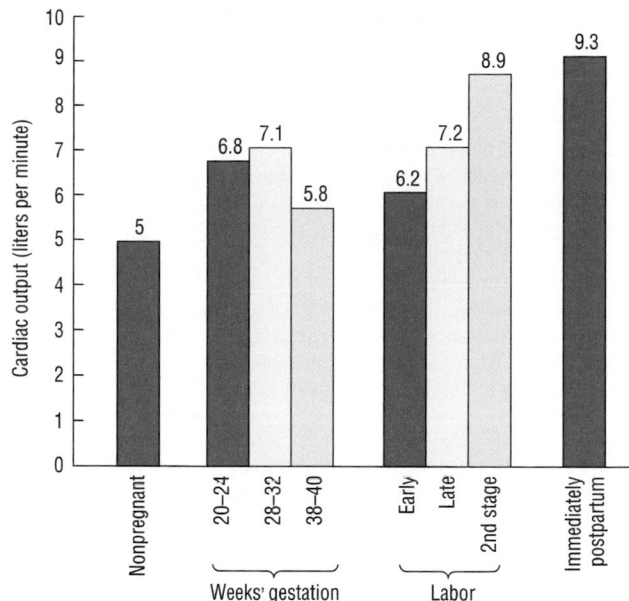

FIGURE 5–9. Cardiac output during three stages of gestation, labor, and immediately postpartum compared with values of nonpregnant women. All values were determined with women in the lateral recumbent position. (Adapted from Ueland and Metcalfe, 1975, with permission.)

characteristic electrocardiographic changes other than slight left-axis deviation as a result of the altered heart position.

Some cardiac sounds may be altered during pregnancy. Cutforth and MacDonald (1966) obtained phonocardiograms at varying stages of pregnancy in 50 normal women. They documented an exaggerated splitting of the first heart sound with increased loudness of both components; no definite changes in the aortic and pulmonary elements of the second sound; and a loud, easily heard third sound. They heard a systolic murmur in 90 percent of pregnant women that was intensified during inspiration in some or expiration in others, and disappeared very shortly after delivery; a soft diastolic murmur transiently in 20 percent; and continuous murmurs arising from the breast vasculature in 10 percent.

Left ventricular size is increased as a result of eccentric enlargement that increases radius-to-wall thickness, and thus end-diastolic dimension (Duvekot and colleagues, 1993). Markedly attenuated afterload manifested by diminished vascular resistance and mean arterial pressure allows the appreciable increase in cardiac output. Because changes in stroke volume are directly proportional to end-diastolic volume, the implication is that the inotropic state of the myocardium changes little during normal pregnancy (Katz and co-workers, 1978). Moreover, Sadaniantz and associates (1996) reported that these changes are not cumulative with subsequent pregnancies. In multifetal pregnancies, compared with singletons, maternal cardiac output is greater by approximately 20 percent because of a greater stroke volume (15 percent) and heart rate (3.5 percent). In addition, left atrial diameter and left ventricular end-diastolic diameter are greater, reflecting the increase in preload (Kametas and co-authors, 2003a). The increased heart rate and inotropic contractility imply that cardiovascular reserve is reduced.

The sustained cardiac changes during pregnancy are similar to acute changes reported for moderate to strenuous exercise. Veille and colleagues (2001) examined the effects of exercise on a stationary bicycle during pregnancy on left-

ventricular diastolic filling. As predicted, exercise-induced tachycardia resulted in decreased ventricular filling time. Interestingly, exercise also was found to be associated with decreased left-ventricular compliance. Although the exact mechanism causing reduced compliance is not known, it may relate to left ventricular wall thickening in response to increased plasma volume.

Cardiac Output. During normal pregnancy, arterial blood pressure and vascular resistance decrease while blood volume, maternal weight, and basal metabolic rate increase. Each of these events would be expected to affect cardiac output. It is now evident that cardiac output *at rest,* when measured in the lateral recumbent position, increases significantly beginning in early pregnancy (Duvekot and colleagues, 1993; Mabie and co-workers, 1994). It continues to increase and remains elevated during the remainder of pregnancy (Fig. 5–9). Typically, cardiac output in late pregnancy is appreciably higher when the woman is in the lateral recumbent position than when she is supine, because in the supine position the large uterus often impedes cardiac venous return. Bamber and Dresner (2003), for example, found cardiac output at term to increase 1200 mL/min—almost 20 percent—when the pregnant woman was moved from her back onto her left side. When she assumes the standing position after sitting, cardiac output falls to the same degree as in the nonpregnant woman (Easterling and associates, 1988).

During the first stage of labor, cardiac output increases moderately, and during the second stage, with vigorous expulsive efforts, it is appreciably greater (see Fig. 5–9). Most

TABLE 5–2 Central Hemodynamic Changes in 10 Normal Nulliparous Women Between 35 and 38 Weeks and Again 11 to 13 Weeks Postpartum

	Pregnant[a]	Postpartum	Change
Mean arterial pressure (mm Hg)	90 ± 6	86 ± 8	No change
Pulmonary capillary wedge pressure (mm Hg)	8 ± 2	6 ± 2	No change
Central venous pressure (mm Hg)	4 ± 3	4 ± 3	No change
Heart rate (beats/min)	83 ± 10	71 ± 10	+ 17%
Cardiac output (L/min)	6.2 ± 1.0	4.3 ± 0.9	+ 43%
Systemic vascular resistance (dyne/sec/cm^{-5})	1210 ± 266	1530 ± 520	– 21%
Pulmonary vascular resistance (dyne/sec/cm^{-5})	78 ± 22	119 ± 47	– 34%
Serum colloid osmotic pressure (mm Hg)	18.0 ± 1.5	20.8 ± 1.0	– 14%
COP–PCWP gradient (mm Hg)	10.5 ± 2.7	14.5 ± 2.5	– 28%
Left ventricular stroke work index (g/m/m^2)	48 ± 6	41 ± 8	No change

COP = colloid osmotic pressure; PCWP = pulmonary capillary wedge pressure.
[a] Measured in lateral recumbent position.
Adapted from Clark and colleagues, 1989, with permission.

of the pregnancy-induced increase is lost very soon after delivery.

Hemodynamic Function in Late Pregnancy. To further elucidate the net changes of normal pregnancy-induced cardiovascular changes, Clark and colleagues (1989) conducted invasive studies to measure hemodynamic function late in pregnancy (Table 5–2). Right heart catheterization was performed in 10 healthy nulliparous women at 35 to 38 weeks, and again at 11 to 13 weeks postpartum. Late pregnancy was associated with the expected increases in heart rate, stroke volume, and cardiac output. Systemic vascular and pulmonary vascular resistance both decreased significantly, as did colloid osmotic pressure. Pulmonary capillary wedge pressure and central venous pressure did not change appreciably between late pregnancy and the puerperium. Thus, as shown in Figure 5–10, although cardiac output is increased,

left ventricular function as measured by stroke work index remains similar to the nonpregnant normal range. Put another way, normal pregnancy is not a continuous "high-output" state.

CIRCULATION AND BLOOD PRESSURE. The posture of the pregnant woman affects arterial blood pressure. Blood pressure in the brachial artery differs when sitting or lying in the lateral recumbent supine position (Bamber and Dresner, 2003). Usually, arterial blood pressure decreases to a nadir at about midpregnancy and rises thereafter. Diastolic pressure decreases more than systolic (Fig. 5–11).

The antecubital *venous pressure* remains unchanged during pregnancy, but in the supine position the femoral venous pressure rises steadily, from 8 cm H_2O early in pregnancy to 24 cm H_2O at term. Employing radiolabeled tracers, Wright

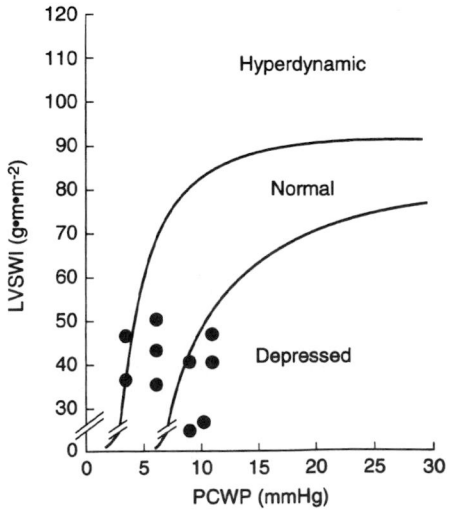

FIGURE 5–10. Relationship between left ventricular stroke work index (LVSWI) (cardiac output) and pulmonary capillary wedge pressure (PCWP) in 10 normal pregnant women in the third trimester. (From Hauth and Cunningham, 1999, with permission.)

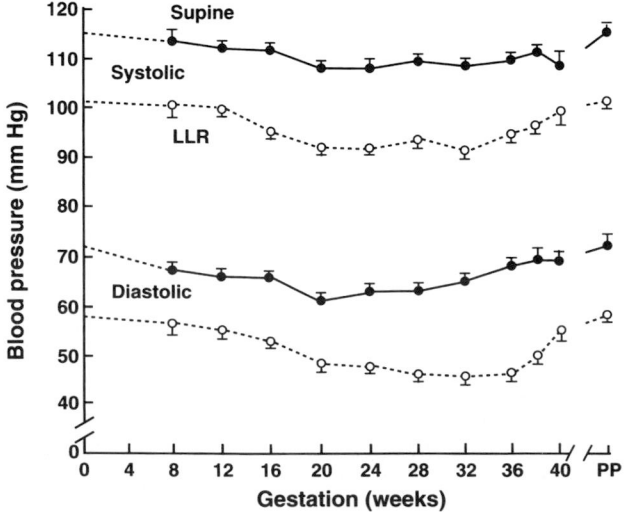

FIGURE 5–11. Sequential changes (± SEM) in blood pressure throughout pregnancy in 69 women in supine (*solid line*) and left lateral recumbent (LLR) positions (*dashed line*). (Adapted from Wilson and colleagues, 1980, with permission.)

and co-workers (1950) demonstrated that blood flow in the legs is retarded during pregnancy except when the lateral recumbent position is assumed. This tendency toward stagnation of blood in the lower extremities during the latter part of pregnancy is attributable to the occlusion of the pelvic veins and inferior vena cava by the enlarged uterus. The elevated venous pressure returns to normal when the pregnant woman lies on her side and immediately after delivery (McLennan, 1943). From a clinical viewpoint, the retarded blood flow and increased lower extremity venous pressure are of great importance. These alterations contribute to the dependent edema frequently experienced by women as they approach term, and to the development of varicose veins in the legs and vulva, as well as hemorrhoids. They also predispose to deep-vein thrombosis, as discussed in Chapter 47 (see p. 1079).

Supine Hypotension. In late pregnancy with the woman in the supine position, the large pregnant uterus rather consistently compresses the venous system that returns blood from the lower half of the body. The results are that cardiac filling may be reduced and cardiac output decreased. In about 10 percent of women, this causes significant arterial hypotension, sometimes referred to as the *supine hypotensive syndrome* (Kinsella and Lohmann, 1994). Moreover, in the supine position, the large pregnant uterus also may compress the aorta sufficiently to lower arterial blood pressure below the level of compression (Bieniarz and associates, 1968). Thus, when the pregnant woman is supine, uterine arterial pressure is significantly lower than that in the brachial artery. In the presence of systemic hypotension, as occurs with spinal analgesia, the decrease in uterine arterial pressure is even more marked than in arteries above the level of aortic compression (see Chap. 19, p. 480).

Renin, Angiotensin II, and Plasma Volume. The renin-angiotensin-aldosterone axis is intimately involved in renal control of blood pressure via salt and water balance. All components of this system are increased in normal pregnancy (Gallery and Lindheimer, 1999). Renin is produced by both the maternal kidney and the uteroplacental unit, and increased renin substrate (angiotensinogen) is produced by both maternal and fetal liver. This increase in angiotensinogen results, in part, from high levels of estrogen production during normal pregnancy. August and colleagues (1995) provided data from first-trimester pregnancies and showed that stimulation of the renin-angiotensin system is important in early blood pressure maintenance.

Gant and associates (1973) conducted a prospective study of vascular reactivity to angiotensin II throughout pregnancy. Normal nulliparas who remained normotensive were refractory to the pressor effects of infused angiotensin II. Conversely, those destined to become hypertensive lost this refractoriness. Later, Gant and co-workers (1974) and Cunningham and associates (1975) found that the increased refractoriness to angiotensin II characteristic of normal preg-

nancy is likely the consequence of individual vessel refractoriness to angiotensin II. That is, in the woman destined to develop preeclampsia, or in the woman already acutely ill with preeclampsia, the increased sensitivity to angiotensin II is the result of an alteration in vessel wall refractoriness rather than the consequence of changes in blood volume or circulating renin-angiotensin levels.

Cardiac Natriuretic Peptides. These include *atrial natriuretic peptide (ANP)* and *B-type natriuretic peptides (BNP)*, which are produced and secreted by cardiomyocytes. In response to stretch of the atrial wall, these peptides are secreted and regulate blood volume by producing significant natriuresis and diuresis. They also promote vasculature smooth muscle relaxation (Clerico and Emdin, 2004). Recently, BNP has been evaluated as a marker for depressed left ventricular systolic function (Heidenreich and associates, 2004).

When the effects of dietary sodium intake and posture are taken into account, plasma levels of ANP during normal gestation are maintained in the nonpregnant range despite the increased plasma volume (Lowe and co-workers, 1992). This physiological adaptation may be important in allowing the expansion of the extracellular fluid volume and the increase in plasma aldosterone concentrations characteristic of normal pregnancy. Moreover, Thomsen and colleagues (1994) investigated 10 healthy primigravid twin pregnancies and reported that all ANP levels were even lower in twin than in singleton pregnancies. These observations may serve to explain in part the relatively increased plasma volume characteristic of women with twins compared with those with singleton fetuses.

C-type natriuretic peptide (CNP) is predominantly secreted by noncardiac tissues. Walther and Stepan (2004) have provided a detailed review of its role during pregnancy. Among its diverse biological functions, the peptide appears to be a major regulator of bone growth in the fetus.

Prostaglandins. Increased production of prostaglandins in normal pregnancy may well play a central role in control of vascular tone, blood pressure, and sodium balance (Gallery and Lindheimer, 1999). Prostaglandin E_2 synthesis in the renal medulla is increased markedly in late pregnancy and is presumed to be natriuretic. Prostacyclin (PGI_2), the principal prostaglandin of endothelium, also is increased in late pregnancy and functions in regulation of blood pressure as well as coagulation. PGI_2 also has been implicated to be a factor in the angiotensin resistance characteristic of normal pregnancy (Friedman, 1988). The ratio of PGI_2 to thromboxane in maternal urine and blood has been considered an important feature in the pathogenesis of preeclampsia (see Chap. 34, p. 769).

Progesterone. The prostaglandin-mediated vascular responsiveness to angiotensin II may be progesterone related. Normally, pregnant women lose their acquired vascular refractoriness to angiotensin II within 15 to 30 minutes after the placenta is delivered. Interestingly, large amounts of intramuscular progesterone, given during late labor, delay this loss. Conversely, intravenously administered progesterone does not restore angiotensin II refractoriness to women with gestational hypertension, however, the infusion of a major progesterone metabolite—5α-dihydroprogesterone—does.

Endothelin. Endothelin-1 is produced in endothelial cells and vascular smooth muscle and is a potent vasoconstrictor that regulates local vasomotor tone (Levin, 1995). Its production is stimulated by angiotensin II, arginine vasopressin, and thrombin. Endothelins, in turn, stimulate secretion of ANP, aldosterone, and catecholamines. As discussed in Chapter 6 (see p. 175), endothelin receptors are present in pregnant and nonpregnant myometrium, and endothelins also have been identified in the amnion, amnionic fluid, decidua, and placental tissue (Kubota and colleagues, 1992; Sagawa and associates, 1994). They likely play an important role in maintaining vascular tone during pregnancy (Ajne and associates, 2003).

Blood Flow in Skin. Increased cutaneous blood flow in pregnancy serves to dissipate excess heat generated by increased metabolism (see Chap. 56, p. 1250).

RESPIRATORY TRACT

The diaphragm rises about 4 cm during pregnancy (see Fig. 5–8). The subcostal angle widens appreciably as the transverse diameter of the thoracic cage increases about 2 cm. The thoracic circumference increases about 6 cm, but not

sufficiently to prevent a reduction in the residual volume of air in the lungs created by the elevated diaphragm. Diaphragmatic excursion is actually greater during pregnancy than when nonpregnant.

PULMONARY FUNCTION. The respiratory rate is little changed during pregnancy, but the *tidal volume, minute ventilatory volume,* and *minute oxygen uptake* increase significantly as pregnancy advances. The *maximum breathing capacity* and *forced* or *timed vital capacity* are not altered appreciably. The *functional residual capacity* and the *residual volume* of air are decreased as a consequence of the elevated diaphragm (Fig. 5–12). *Lung compliance* is unaffected by pregnancy. *Airway conductance* is increased and *total pulmonary resistance* is reduced, possibly as a result of progesterone action. The critical *closing volume,* or the lung volume at which airways in the dependent parts of the lung begin to close during expiration, has been considered to be higher in pregnancy by some investigators, but not by others (DeSwiet, 1991). The increased oxygen requirements and perhaps the increased critical closing volume imposed by pregnancy tend to make respiratory diseases more serious during gestation (see Chap. 46, p. 1056).

At any stage of normal pregnancy, the amount of oxygen delivered into the lungs by the increase in tidal volume clearly exceeds the oxygen need imposed by pregnancy. Moreover, the amount of hemoglobin in the circulation, and in turn the total oxygen-carrying capacity, increases appreciably during normal pregnancy, as does cardiac output. As a consequence, the *maternal arteriovenous oxygen* difference is decreased.

Hankins and colleagues (1999) used pulmonary and radial artery catheters to measure oxygen transport in 10 normal

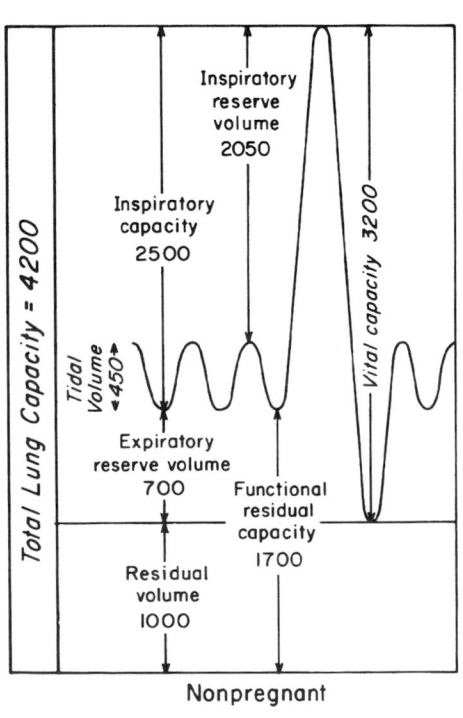
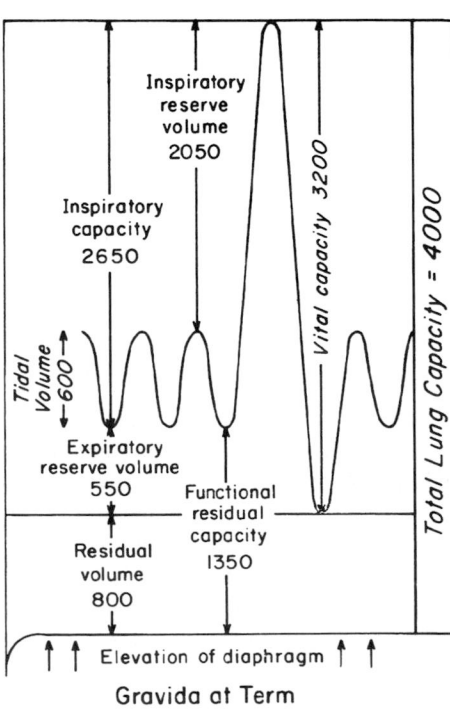

FIGURE 5–12. Respiratory changes during pregnancy. (Reproduced from Bonica, 1967, with permission.)

women between 36 and 38 weeks and again 12 weeks postpartum. The oxygen content of arterial blood was significantly lower in the third trimester than in the postpartum period—12 versus 16 mL/dL, respectively. Although cardiac output was significantly increased consistent with normal pregnancy, its effects on oxygen delivery were negated by a substantially lower hemoglobin content. Thus, the relative or so-called physiological anemia of pregnancy accounted for the lower arterial oxygen content.

McAuliffe and associates (2002) compared pulmonary function in 140 healthy women with singleton pregnancies, 68 women with twins, and 22 women who were not pregnant. No significant differences in respiratory function were observed between the women with twin versus singleton gestations. Compared with nonpregnant women, however, functional reserve capacity and expiratory reserve volume during the third trimester were lower by about 20 and 30 percent, respectively. Moreover, minute ventilation was increased by approximately 30 percent, and this was demonstrable as early as the first trimester.

ACID–BASE EQUILIBRIUM. An increased awareness of a desire to breathe is common even early in pregnancy (Milne and colleagues, 1978). This may be interpreted as dyspnea, which in turn suggests pulmonary or cardiac abnormalities when none exist. The mechanism of physiological dyspnea is thought to be increased tidal volume that lowers the blood P_{CO_2} slightly, which paradoxically causes dyspnea. The increased respiratory effort, and in turn the reduction in P_{CO_2}, during pregnancy is most likely induced in large part by progesterone and to a lesser degree by estrogen. The site of

progestin action appears to be central through a direct stimulatory effect on the respiratory center.

To compensate for the resulting respiratory alkalosis, plasma bicarbonate levels decrease from 26 to about 22 mmol/L. As a result, blood pH is increased only minimally. This increase shifts the oxygen dissociation curve to the left and increases the affinity of maternal hemoglobin for oxygen—the *Bohr effect*—thereby decreasing the oxygen-releasing capacity of maternal blood. Thus, the hyperventilation that results in a reduced maternal P_{CO_2} facilitates transport of carbon dioxide from the fetus to the mother but *appears to impair* release of oxygen from maternal blood to the fetus. The increase in blood pH, however, although minimal, stimulates an increase in 2,3-diphosphoglycerate in maternal erythrocytes (Tsai and de Leeuw, 1982). This counteracts the Bohr effect by shifting the oxygen dissociation curve back to the right, facilitating oxygen release to the fetus.

URINARY SYSTEM

KIDNEY. A remarkable number of changes are observed in the urinary system as a result of pregnancy (Table 5–3). *Kidney size* increases slightly during pregnancy. Bailey and Rolleston (1971), for example, found that the kidney was 1.5 cm longer during the early puerperium than when measured 6 months later using radiographs. The *glomerular filtration rate* and *renal plasma flow* increase early in pregnancy, the former as much as 50 percent by the beginning of the second trimester, and the latter even greater (Lindheimer and co-workers, 2001). Experiments in animals suggest that both

TABLE 5–3 Renal Changes in Normal Pregnancy

Alteration		Clinical Relevance
Increased renal size	Renal length approximately 1 cm greater on radiographs	Postpartum decreases in size should not be mistaken for parenchymal loss
Dilatation of pelves, calyces, and ureters	Resembles hydronephrosis on ultrasound or IVP (more marked on right)	Not to be mistaken for obstructive uropathy; retained urine leads to collection errors; upper urinary tract infections are more virulent; may be responsible for "distention syndrome"; elective pyelography should be deferred to at least 12 weeks postpartum
Increased renal hemodynamics	Glomerular filtration rate and renal plasma flow increase ~ 50%	Serum creatinine and urea nitrogen values decrease during normal gestation; > 0.8 mg/dL (> 72 μmol/L) creatinine already suspect; protein, amino acid, and glucose excretion all increase
Changes in acid–base metabolism	Renal bicarbonate threshold decreases; progesterone stimulates respiratory center	Serum bicarbonate and P_{CO_2} are 4–5 mEq/L and 10 mm Hg lower, respectively, in normal gestation; a P_{CO_2} of 40 mm Hg already represents CO_2 retention
Renal water handling	Osmoregulation altered: osmotic thresholds for AVP release and thirst decrease; hormonal disposal rates increase	Serum osmolality decreases 10 mOsm/L (serum Na ~ 5 mEq/L) during normal gestation; increased metabolism of AVP may cause transient diabetes insipidus in pregnancy

AVP = vasopressin; IVP = intravenous pyelography.
From Lindheimer and colleagues, 2000, with permission.

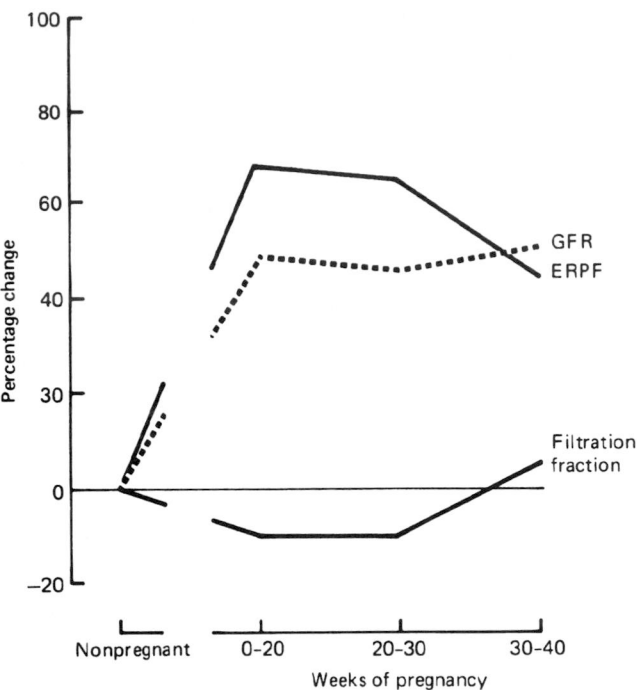

FIGURE 5–13. Relative changes in measures of glomerular filtration rate (GFR), effective renal plasma flow (ERPF), and filtration fraction during normal pregnancy. (From Davison and Dunlop, 1980, with permission.)

relaxin and neuronal nitric oxide synthase may be important for mediating the increased glomerular filtration and plasma flow during pregnancy (Abram and colleagues, 2001; Novak and associates, 2001). As shown in Figure 5–13, elevated glomerular filtration persists until term, even though renal plasma flow decreases during late pregnancy.

Kallikrein, a tissue protease synthesized in cells of the distal renal tubule, is increased in several conditions associated with increased glomerular perfusion in nonpregnant individuals. Platts and colleagues (2000) studied urinary kallikrein excretion rates during human pregnancy and found increased excretion at 18 and 34 weeks, which returned to nonpregnant levels at term. The significance of these fluctuations remains unknown.

As with blood pressure, maternal posture may have a considerable influence on several aspects of renal function. Late in pregnancy, for instance, urinary flow and sodium excretion average less than half the excretion rate in the supine position compared with that in the lateral recumbent position. The impact of posture on glomerular filtration and renal plasma flow is much more variable.

Loss of Nutrients. One unusual feature of the pregnancy-induced changes in renal excretion is the remarkably increased amounts of various nutrients in the urine. Amino acids and water-soluble vitamins are lost in the urine of pregnant women in much greater amounts than in nonpregnant women (Hytten, 1973; Powers and associates, 2004).

Tests of Renal Function. The physiological changes in renal hemodynamics induced during normal pregnancy have several implications for the interpretation of tests of renal function. *Serum creatinine* and *urea nitrogen* levels decrease from a mean of 0.7 and 1.2 mg/dL to 0.5 and 0.9 mg/dL, respectively, *whereas values of 0.9 and 1.4 mg/dL suggest underlying renal disease and should prompt further evaluation* (Lindheimer and associates, 2000). *Creatinine clearance* in pregnancy should be 30 percent higher than the 100 to 115 mL/min normally measured in nonpregnant women (Lindheimer and associates, 2000).

Creatinine clearance is a useful test to estimate renal function in pregnancy provided that complete urine collection is made during an accurately timed period. Incomplete urine concentration tests may give misleading results (Davison and colleagues, 1981). During the day, pregnant women tend to accumulate water in the form of dependent edema, and at night, while recumbent, they mobilize this fluid and excrete it via the kidneys. This reversal of the usual nonpregnant diurnal pattern of urinary flow causes nocturia, and the urine is more dilute than in the nonpregnant state. Failure of a pregnant woman to excrete concentrated urine after withholding fluids for approximately 18 hours does not signify renal damage. In fact, the kidney in these circumstances functions perfectly normally by excreting mobilized extracellular fluid of relatively low osmolality.

Urinalysis. *Glucosuria* during pregnancy is not necessarily abnormal. The appreciable increase in glomerular filtration, together with impaired tubular reabsorptive capacity for filtered glucose, accounts in most cases for glucosuria (Davison and Hytten, 1974). Chesley (1963) calculated that for these reasons alone, about one sixth of all pregnant women should spill glucose in the urine. Even though glucosuria is common during pregnancy, the possibility of diabetes mellitus should not be ignored when it is identified.

Proteinuria normally is not evident during pregnancy except occasionally in slight amounts during or soon after vigorous labor. Higby and associates (1994) measured protein excretion in 270 normal women throughout pregnancy. Their mean 24-hour excretion was 115 mg, and the upper 95-percent confidence limit was 260 mg/day without significant differences by trimester (Fig. 5–14). These authors also showed that albumin excretion is minimal and ranges from 5 to 30 mg/day. Nomograms for urinary microalbumin and creatinine ratios during uncomplicated pregnancies have been developed by Waugh and co-workers (2003).

Hematuria, if not the result of contamination during collection, most often suggests a diagnosis of urinary tract disease (see Chap. 48, p. 1093). Difficult labor and delivery, of course, can cause hematuria because of trauma to the lower urinary tract.

URETERS. After the uterus rises completely out of the pelvis, it rests upon the ureters, laterally displacing and

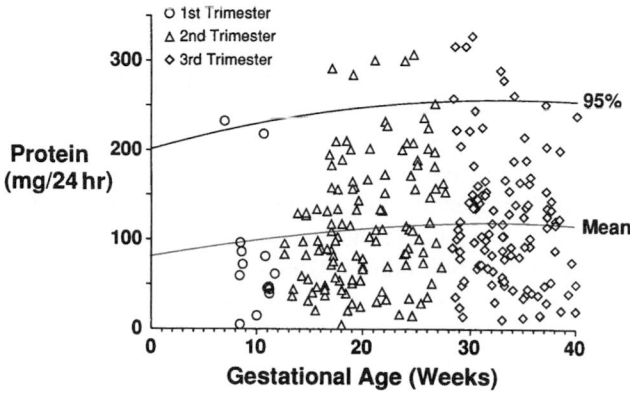

FIGURE 5–14. Scatter plot of all patients showing 24-hour urinary total protein excretion by gestational age. Mean and 95-percent confidence limits are outlined. (From Higby and colleagues, 1994, with permission.)

compressing them at the pelvic brim. Increased intraureteral tonus above this level compared with that of the pelvic portion of the ureter has been identified (Rubi and Sala, 1968). Schulman and Herlinger (1975) found ureteral dilatation to be greater on the right side in 86 percent of pregnant women studied (Fig. 5–15). The unequal degrees of dilatation may

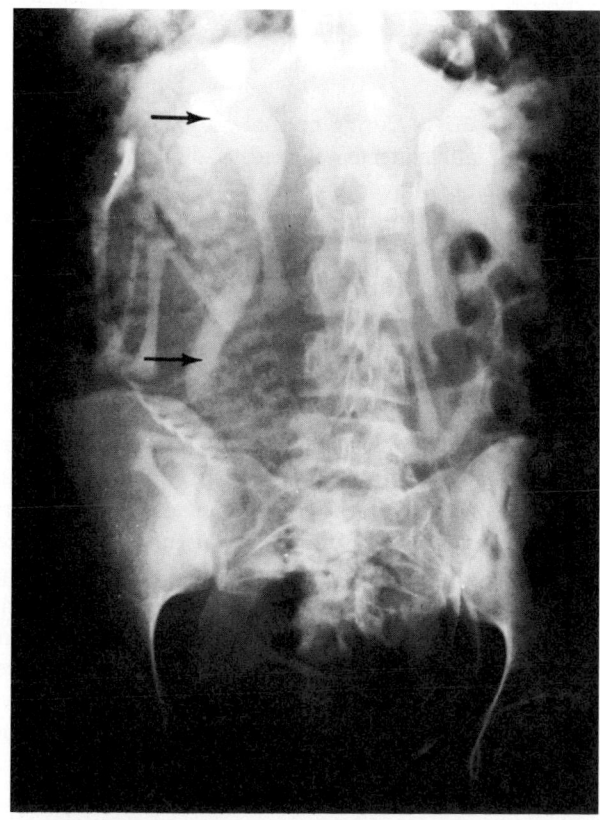

FIGURE 5–15. Normal intravenous pyelogram at 36 weeks. Pregnancy-induced hydronephrosis (*upper arrow*) and hydroureter (*lower arrow*) are more marked on the right. Elongation, dilatation, and peristalsis of the ureter create the appearance of ureteral discontinuity.

result from a cushioning provided the left ureter by the sigmoid colon and perhaps from greater compression of the right ureter as the consequence of dextrorotation of the uterus. The right ovarian vein complex, which is remarkably dilated during pregnancy, lies obliquely over the right ureter and may contribute significantly to right ureteral dilatation.

Another possible mechanism causing hydroureter and hydronephrosis is from an effect of progesterone. Major support for this concept was provided by Van Wagenen and Jenkins (1939), who described further ureteral dilatation after removal of the monkey fetus but with the placenta left in situ. The relatively abrupt onset of dilatation in women at midpregnancy, however, is more consistent with ureteral compression from an enlarging uterus rather than a hormonal effect.

Elongation accompanies distention of the ureter, which is frequently thrown into curves of varying size, the smaller of which may be sharply angulated. These so-called kinks are poorly named, because the term connotes obstruction. They are usually single or double curves, which when viewed in the radiograph taken in the same plane as the curve, appear as more or less acute angulations of the ureter (see Fig. 5–15). Another exposure at right angles nearly always identifies them to be more gentle curves rather than kinks.

BLADDER. There are few significant anatomical changes in the bladder before 12 weeks. From that time onward, however, the increased size of the uterus, together with the hyperemia that affects all pelvic organs, and the hyperplasia of the muscle and connective tissues, elevates the bladder trigone and causes thickening of its posterior, or intraureteric, margin. Continuation of this process to the end of pregnancy produces marked deepening and widening of the trigone. The bladder mucosa undergoes no change other than an increase in the size and tortuosity of its blood vessels.

Using urethrocystometry, Iosif and colleagues (1980) found that bladder pressure in primigravidas increased from 8 cm H_2O early in pregnancy to 20 cm H_2O at term. To compensate for reduced bladder capacity, absolute and functional urethral lengths increased by 6.7 and 4.8 mm, respectively. Finally, to preserve continence, maximal intraurethral pressure increased from 70 to 93 cm H_2O. Still, the majority of women experience urinary incontinence during pregnancy. Indeed, loss of urine is always considered in the differential diagnosis with a question of ruptured membranes.

Nel and co-workers (2001) found that during pregnancy, approximately one fifth of women reported symptoms of stress urinary incontinence for the first time, and Wijma and associates (2001) reported that a similar proportion of nulliparous women actually demonstrate objective evidence of urine leakage. Thorpe and colleagues (1999) found that when pregnant women were asked to compare urinary tract function week by week, they reported a steady deterioration in perceived bladder function.

Toward the end of pregnancy, particularly in nulliparas in whom the presenting part often engages before labor, the entire base of the bladder is pushed forward and upward, converting the normal convex surface into a concavity. As a result, difficulties in diagnostic and therapeutic procedures are greatly increased. In addition, the pressure of the presenting part impairs the drainage of blood and lymph from the base of the bladder, often rendering the area edematous, easily traumatized, and probably more susceptible to infection.

GASTROINTESTINAL TRACT

As pregnancy progresses, the stomach and intestines are displaced by the enlarging uterus. As the result of the positional changes in these viscera, the physical findings in certain diseases are altered. The appendix, for instance, is usually displaced upward and somewhat laterally as the uterus enlarges, and at times it may reach the right flank.

Gastric emptying time, studied using acetaminophen absorption techniques, appears to be unchanged during each trimester and when compared with nonpregnant women (Macfie and colleagues, 1991; Wong and associates, 2002). During labor, however, and especially after administration of analgesic agents, gastric emptying time may be prolonged appreciably. As a result, a major danger of general anesthesia for delivery is regurgitation and aspiration of either food-laden or highly acidic gastric contents (see Chap. 19, p. 490).

Pyrosis (heartburn) is common during pregnancy and is most likely caused by reflux of acidic secretions into the lower esophagus (see Chap. 49, p. 1114). Although the altered position of the stomach probably contributes to its frequent occurrence, lower esophageal sphincter tone also is decreased. In addition, intraesophageal pressures are lower and intragastric pressures higher in pregnant women. At the same time, esophageal peristalsis has lower wave speed and lower amplitude (Ulmsten and Sundström, 1978).

The gums may become hyperemic and softened during pregnancy and may bleed when mildly traumatized, as with a toothbrush. A focal, highly vascular swelling of the gums, the so-called *epulis* of pregnancy, develops occasionally but typically regresses spontaneously after delivery. Most evidence indicates that pregnancy does not incite tooth decay.

Hemorrhoids are fairly common during pregnancy. They are caused in large measure by constipation and elevated pressure in veins below the level of the enlarged uterus.

LIVER. Although the liver in some animals increases in size remarkably during pregnancy, there is no increase during human pregnancy (Combes and Adams, 1971). Histological evaluation of liver biopsies, including examination with the electron microscope, has shown no distinct changes in liver morphology in normal pregnant women (Ingerslev and Teilum, 1946). Despite this, the diameter of the portal vein and its blood flow both increase substantively (Clapp and colleagues, 2000).

Some of the laboratory tests used to evaluate hepatic function yield appreciably different results during normal pregnancy. Moreover, some of the changes are similar to those in nonpregnant patients with liver disease. Total *alkaline phosphatase* activity in serum almost doubles during normal pregnancy, but much of the increase is attributable to heat-stable placental alkaline phosphatase isozymes. Serum aspartate transaminase, alanine transaminase, γ-glutamyl transferase, and bilirubin levels are slightly lower during pregnancy compared with nonpregnant normal values (Girling and colleagues, 1997).

The concentration of serum albumin decreases during pregnancy. Late in pregnancy, for example, albumin concentrations may normally be near 3.0 g/dL compared with approximately 4.3 g/dL in nonpregnant women (Mendenhall, 1970). Total albumin is increased, however, because of a greater volume of distribution. The reduction in albumin concentration, combined with a normal slight increase in serum globulin levels, results in a decrease in the albumin-to-globulin ratio similar to that seen in certain hepatic diseases (see Chapter 50).

Leucine aminopeptidase activity is markedly elevated in serum from pregnant women. The increase results from the appearance of a pregnancy-specific enzyme(s) with distinct substrate specificities (Song and Kappas, 1968). Pregnancy-induced aminopeptidase has oxytocinase and vasopressinase activity.

GALLBLADDER. During normal pregnancy, the contractility of the gallbladder is reduced, leading to an increased residual volume (Braverman and co-workers, 1980). It has been suggested that progesterone impairs gallbladder contraction by inhibiting cholecystokinin-mediated smooth muscle stimulation, the primary regulator of gallbladder contraction. Impaired gallbladder contraction leads to stasis, and this, associated with the increased cholesterol saturation of pregnancy, at least partially explains the increased prevalence of cholesterol stones in multiparous women.

The effects of pregnancy on maternal bile acid serum concentrations have been incompletely characterized despite the long-acknowledged propensity for pregnancy to cause intrahepatic cholestasis and pruritus gravidarum from retained bile salts. Intrahepatic cholestasis has been linked to high circulating levels of estrogen, which inhibit intraductal transport of bile acids (Simon and colleagues, 1996). In addition, increased progesterone and genetic factors have been implicated in the pathogenesis (Lammert and associates, 2000). Cholestasis of pregnancy is described in greater detail in Chapter 50 (see p. 1126).

ENDOCRINE SYSTEM

Some of the most important endocrine changes of pregnancy are discussed elsewhere, especially in Chapter 3.

PITUITARY GLAND. During normal pregnancy the pituitary gland enlarges by approximately 135 percent (Gonzalez and colleagues, 1988). Although it has been suggested that the increase may be sufficient to compress the optic chiasma and reduce visual fields, changes in vision during normal pregnancy are minimal. Scheithauer and colleagues (1990) have provided evidence that the incidence of pituitary prolactinomas is not increased during pregnancy. When these tumors are large before pregnancy—a macroadenoma is 10 mm or greater—then enlargement during pregnancy is more likely (see Chap. 53, p. 1203).

The maternal pituitary gland is not essential for maintenance of pregnancy. Many women have undergone hypophysectomy, completed pregnancy successfully, and undergone spontaneous labor while receiving glucocorticoids along with thyroid hormone and vasopressin.

Growth Hormone. During the first trimester, growth hormone is secreted predominantly from the maternal pituitary gland, and concentrations in serum and amnionic fluid are within nonpregnant values of 0.5 to 7.5 ng/mL (Kletzky and associates, 1985). As early as 8 weeks, growth hormone secreted from the placenta becomes detectable (Lønberg and co-workers, 2003). By about 17 weeks, the placenta is the principal source of growth hormone secretion (Obuobie and co-workers, 2001). Maternal serum values increase slowly from approximately 3.5 ng/mL at 10 weeks to plateau after 28 weeks at approximately 14 ng/mL. Growth hormone in amnionic fluid peaks at 14 to 15 weeks and slowly declines thereafter to reach baseline values after 36 weeks.

Although growth hormone is abundant in the fetal circulation, at least in the second half of gestation, it has not been considered to be a major hormonal regulator of fetal growth (Lønberg and co-workers, 2003). For example, anencephalic fetuses cannot produce significant amounts of pituitary growth hormone, yet they usually have near normal weight and length (Wollmann, 2000). More recently, however, Chellakooty and co-investigators (2004) were the first to demonstrate that the rate of fetal growth, after adjusting for confounding variables, significantly correlated with the increase in placental growth hormone in the latter half of pregnancy. Interestingly, they also found that the gestational age when peak concentrations of placental growth hormone were reached was associated with the onset of labor. After delivery, growth hormone is elevated for some time but at levels lower than during late pregnancy (Spellacy and Buhi, 1969).

Prolactin. Maternal plasma levels of prolactin increase markedly during the course of normal pregnancy. Serum concentration levels are usually 10-fold greater at term—about 150 ng/mL—compared with normal nonpregnant women. Paradoxically, after delivery, the plasma prolactin concentration decreases even in women who are breast feeding. During early lactation, pulsatile bursts of prolactin secretion occur apparently in response to suckling. The physiological cause of the marked increase in prolactin prior to parturition is not entirely certain. It is known, however, that estrogen stimulation increases the number of anterior pituitary lactotrophs and may stimulate the release of prolactin from these cells (Andersen, 1982). Thyroid-releasing hormone also acts to cause an increased prolactin level in pregnant compared with nonpregnant women, but the response decreases as pregnancy advances (Andersen, 1982; Miyamoto, 1984). Serotonin also is believed to increase prolactin, and prolactin-inhibiting factor (dopamine) inhibits its secretion.

The principal function of maternal serum prolactin is to ensure lactation. Early in pregnancy, prolactin acts to initiate DNA synthesis and mitosis of glandular epithelial cells and the presecretory alveolar cells of the breast. Prolactin also increases the number of estrogen and prolactin receptors in these same cells. Finally, prolactin promotes mammary alveolar cell RNA synthesis, galactopoiesis, and production of casein and lactalbumin, lactose, and lipids (Andersen, 1982). Kauppila and co-workers (1987) found that a woman with an isolated prolactin deficiency failed to lactate after two pregnancies, establishing the absolute necessity of prolactin for lactation but not for successful pregnancy outcome.

Prolactin is present in amnionic fluid in high concentrations. Levels of up to 10,000 ng/mL are found at 20 to 26 weeks, thereafter, levels decrease and reach a nadir after 34 weeks. Several investigators have presented convincing evidence that the uterine decidua is the site of prolactin synthesis in amnionic fluid (see Chap. 3, p. 51). Although the exact function of amnionic fluid prolactin is not known, it has been suggested that amnionic fluid prolactin impairs the transfer of water from the fetus into the maternal compartment, thus preventing fetal dehydration during late pregnancy when amnionic fluid is normally hypotonic.

THYROID GLAND. During pregnancy, important changes in thyroidal economy occur that are due to three modifications in the regulation of thyroid hormones. First, pregnancy induces a marked increase in circulating levels of the major thyroxine transport protein, thyroxine-binding globulin, in response to high estrogen levels. Second, several thyroidal stimulatory factors of placental origin are produced in excess. Third, pregnancy is accompanied by a decreased availability of iodide for the maternal thyroid. This finding occurs because of increased renal clearance and excretion that results in a relative iodine-deficiency state.

Also during pregnancy, the thyroid undergoes moderate enlargement caused by glandular hyperplasia and increased vascularity. Glinoer and colleagues (1990) found that mean thyroid volume increased from 12.1 mL in the first trimester to 15.0 mL at delivery. Moreover, total volume was found to be inversely proportional to serum thyrotropin concentrations. These enlargements are not pathological and normal pregnancy does not typically cause significant thyromegaly, thus, any goiter should be investigated.

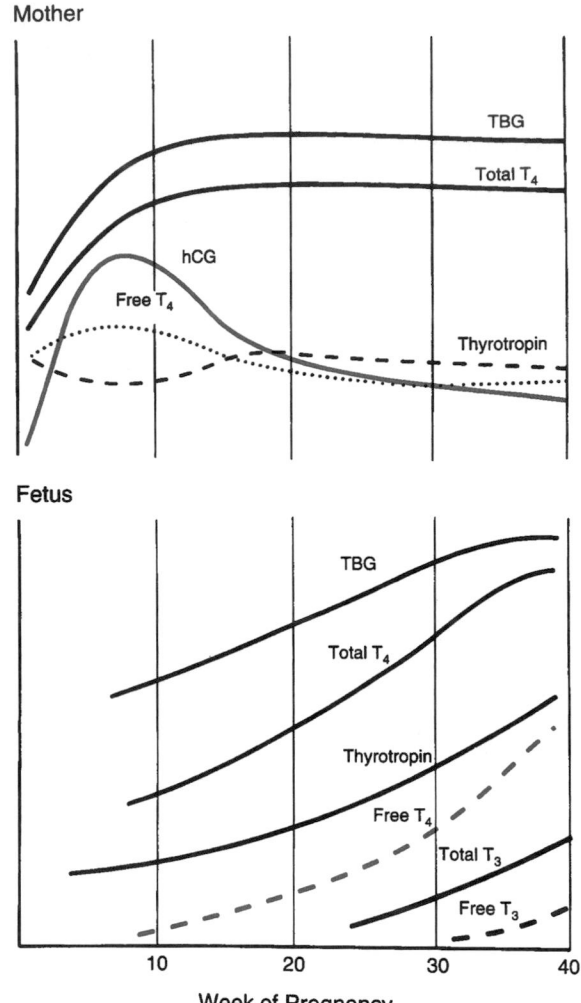

FIGURE 5–16. Relative changes in maternal thyroid function during pregnancy. Maternal changes include a marked and early increase in hepatic production of thyroxine-binding globulin (TBG) and placental production of chorionic gonadotropin (hCG). Increased thyroxine-binding globulin increases serum thyroxine (T$_4$) concentrations, and chorionic gonadotropin has thyrotropin-like activity and stimulates maternal T$_4$ secretion. The transient hCG-induced increase in serum T$_4$ inhibits maternal secretion of thyrotropin. Except for minimally increased free T$_4$ levels when hCG peaks, these levels are essentially unchanged. (T$_3$ = triiodothyronine.) (From Burrow and colleagues, 1994, with permission.)

Changes in thyroid physiology function during pregnancy are detailed in Figure 5–16. Beginning early in the first trimester, thyroxine-binding globulin increases, reaches its zenith at about 20 weeks, and stabilizes at approximately double baseline values for the remainder of pregnancy. Total serum thyroxine (T$_4$) increases sharply beginning between 6 and 9 weeks, and reaches a plateau at 18 weeks. Free serum T$_4$ levels rise slightly and peak along with hCG levels, then they return to normal. The rise in total triiodothyronine (T$_3$) is more pronounced up to 18 weeks, and thereafter, it plateaus. *Thyroid-releasing hormone (TRH)* levels are not increased during normal pregnancy, but this neurotransmitter does cross the placenta and may stimulate the fetal pituitary to secrete thyrotropin (Thorpe-Beeston and associates, 1991).

Interestingly, the secretion of T$_4$ and T$_3$ is not similar for all pregnant women (Glinoer and associates, 1990). Approximately one third of women experience relative hypothyroxinemia, preferential T$_3$ secretion, and higher, albeit normal, serum thyrotropin levels. Thus, there may be considerable variability in thyroidal adjustments during normal pregnancy.

The modifications in serum thyroid-stimulating hormone and hCG as a function of gestational age also are illustrated in Figure 5–16. As discussed in Chapter 3 (see p. 70), the α-subunits of the two glycoproteins are identical whereas the β-subunits, although similar, differ in their amino acid sequence. As a result of this structural similarity, hCG has intrinsic thyrotropic activity, and thus, high serum levels cause thyroid stimulation. Indeed, thyrotropin levels decrease in more than 80 percent of pregnant women, even though levels are in the normal range for nonpregnant women (see Fig. 53–1, p. 1190).

These many complex alterations in thyroid regulation during pregnancy do not appear to alter maternal thyroid status as measured by metabolic studies. Although basal metabolic rate increases progressively during normal pregnancy by as much as 25 percent, most of this increase in oxygen consumption can be attributed to fetal metabolic activity. If fetal body surface area is considered along with that of the mother, the predicted and observed basal metabolic rates are quite similar to nonpregnant women. Fetal thyroid physiology is discussed in Chapter 4 (see p. 111) and thyroid disorders in Chapter 53 (see p. 1190).

PARATHYROID GLANDS. The regulation of calcium concentration is closely interrelated to magnesium, phosphate, parathyroid hormone, vitamin D, and calcitonin physiology. Any alteration of one of these factors is likely to change the others. In a longitudinal investigation of 20 women, More and associates (2003) found that all markers of bone turnover increased during normal pregnancy and failed to reach baseline level by 12 months postpartum. They concluded that the calcium needed for fetal growth and lactation may be drawn at least in part from the maternal skeleton.

Parathyroid Hormone and Calcium. Acute or chronic decreases in plasma calcium or acute decreases in magnesium stimulate the release of parathyroid hormone, whereas increases in calcium and magnesium suppress parathyroid hormone levels. The action of this hormone on bone resorption, intestinal absorption, and kidney reabsorption is to increase extracellular fluid calcium and decrease phosphate.

Parathyroid hormone plasma concentrations decrease during the first trimester and then increase progressively throughout the remainder of pregnancy (Pitkin and associates, 1979). Increased levels likely result from the lower calcium concentration in the pregnant woman. As discussed earlier, this is the result of increased plasma volume, increased glomerular filtration rate, and maternal–fetal transfer of calcium. Ionized calcium is decreased only slightly, and Reitz and co-workers (1977) suggest that during pregnancy a new "set point" is established for ionized calcium and parathyroid hormone. Estrogens also appear to block the action of parathyroid hormone on bone resorption, resulting in another mechanism to increase parathyroid hormone during pregnancy. The net result of these actions is a *physiological hyperparathyroidism* of pregnancy, likely to supply the fetus with adequate calcium.

The potential roles of parathyroid hormone–related peptide production in the fetus, placenta, and maternal tissues are discussed in Chapter 3, p. 74, and Chapter 6, p. 166.

Calcitonin and Calcium. The calcitonin-secreting C cells are derived embryologically from the neural crest and are located predominantly in the perifollicular areas of the thyroid gland. Calcium and magnesium increase the biosynthesis and secretion of calcitonin. Various gastric hormones—gastrin, pentagastrin, glucagon, and pancreoxymin—and food ingestion also increase calcitonin plasma levels.

The known actions of calcitonin generally are considered to oppose those of parathyroid hormone and vitamin D to protect skeletal calcification during times of calcium stress. Pregnancy and lactation cause profound calcium stress, and during these times, calcitonin levels are appreciably higher than in nonpregnant women (Weiss and co-workers, 1998; Whitehead and associates, 1981).

Vitamin D and Calcium. Vitamin D, a hormone that is synthesized in the skin or ingested, is converted by the liver into 25-hydroxyvitamin D_3. This form then is converted in the kidney, decidua, and placenta to 1,25-dihydroxyvitamin D_3, serum levels of which are increased during normal pregnancy (Weisman and co-workers, 1979; Whitehead and associates, 1981). Most likely this form is the biologically active compound, and it stimulates resorption of calcium from bone and absorption from the intestines. Although its control is unclear, the conversion of 25-hydroxyvitamin D_3 to 1,25-dihydroxyvitamin D_3 is facilitated by parathyroid hormone and by low calcium and phosphate plasma levels and opposed by calcitonin.

ADRENAL GLANDS. In normal pregnancy, the maternal adrenal glands undergo little, if any, morphological change.

Cortisol. The serum concentration of circulating cortisol is increased, but much of it is bound by cortisol-binding globulin, or *transcortin*. The rate of adrenal cortisol secretion is not increased, and probably it is decreased compared with that of the nonpregnant state. The metabolic clearance rate of cortisol, however, is lower during pregnancy because its half-life is nearly doubled over that for nonpregnant women (Migeon and associates, 1957). Administration of estrogen, including most oral contraceptives, causes changes in serum cortisol levels and transcortin similar to those of pregnancy.

In early pregnancy, the levels of circulating corticotropin (ACTH) are reduced strikingly. As pregnancy progresses, the levels of ACTH and free cortisol rise. This apparent paradox is not understood completely. Nolten and Rueckert (1981) have presented evidence that the higher free cortisol levels observed in pregnancy are the result of a "resetting" of the maternal feedback mechanism to higher levels. They further propose that this might result from *tissue refractoriness* to cortisol. Keller-Wood and Wood (2001) later suggested that these may result from an antagonistic action of progesterone on mineralocorticoids. Thus, in response to elevated progesterone levels during pregnancy, an elevated free cortisol is needed to maintain homeostasis. Indeed, experiments in pregnant ewes demonstrate that elevated maternal cortisol and aldosterone secretion are necessary to maintain the normal increase in plasma volume during late pregnancy (Jensen and associates, 2002).

Aldosterone. As early as 15 weeks, the maternal adrenal glands secrete considerably increased amounts of aldosterone. By the third trimester, about 1 mg/day is secreted. If sodium intake is restricted, aldosterone secretion is elevated even further (Watanabe and co-workers, 1963). At the same time, levels of renin and angiotensin II substrate normally are increased, especially during the latter half of pregnancy. This scenario gives rise to increased plasma levels of angiotensin II, which by acting on the zona glomerulosa of the maternal adrenal glands, accounts for the markedly elevated aldosterone secretion. It has been suggested that the increased aldosterone secretion during normal pregnancy affords protection against the natriuretic effect of progesterone and atrial natriuretic peptide discussed earlier.

Deoxycorticosterone. Maternal plasma levels of this potent mineralocorticosteroid progressively increase during pregnancy. Indeed, plasma levels of deoxycorticosterone rise to near 1500 pg/mL by term, a more than 15-fold increase (Parker and associates, 1980). This marked elevation is not derived from adrenal secretion, but instead represents increased kidney production resulting from estrogen stimulation. The levels of deoxycorticosterone and its sulfate in fetal blood are appreciably higher than those in maternal blood, which suggests transfer of fetal deoxycorticosterone into the maternal compartment.

Dehydroepiandrosterone Sulfate. As discussed in Chapter 3 (see p. 78), the levels of *dehydroepiandrosterone sulfate* circulating in maternal blood and excreted in the urine are decreased during normal pregnancy. This finding is a consequence of increased metabolic clearance through extensive 16α-hydroxylation in the maternal liver and conversion to estrogen by the placenta.

Androstenedione and Testosterone. Maternal plasma levels of these androgens are increased during pregnancy. This finding is not totally explained by alterations in their metabolic clearance. Maternal plasma androstenedione and testosterone are converted to estradiol in the placenta, which increases their clearance rates. Conversely, the increased sex hormone–binding globulin in plasma of pregnant women retards testosterone clearance. Thus, the plasma production rate of maternal testosterone and androstenedione during human pregnancy are increased. The source of this increased C_{19}-steroid production is unknown, but it likely originates in the ovary. Interestingly, little or no testosterone in maternal plasma enters the fetal circulation as testosterone. Even when massive testosterone levels are found in the circulation of pregnant women, as with androgen-secreting tumors, the testosterone levels in umbilical cord venous plasma are likely to be undetectable. This finding is the result of the near complete conversion of testosterone to 17β-estradiol by the trophoblast (Edman and associates, 1979).

OTHER SYSTEMS

MUSCULOSKELETAL SYSTEM. Progressive lordosis is a characteristic feature of normal pregnancy. Compensating for the anterior position of the enlarging uterus, the lordosis shifts the center of gravity back over the lower extremities. The sacroiliac, sacrococcygeal, and pubic joints have increased mobility during pregnancy. As discussed on page 124, Marnach and co-workers (2003) found that although joint laxity increased during pregnancy, it did not correlate with maternal estradiol, progesterone, or relaxin levels. Joint mobility may contribute to the alteration of maternal posture, and in turn cause discomfort in the lower back. This is especially bothersome late in pregnancy, during which time aching, numbness, and weakness also occasionally are experienced in the upper extremities. This may occur as a result of the marked lordosis with anterior neck flexion and slumping of the shoulder girdle, which in turn produce traction on the ulnar and median nerves (Crisp and DeFrancesco, 1964).

The bones and ligaments of the pelvis undergo remarkable adaptation during pregnancy. In 1934, Abramson and colleagues described the normal relaxation of the pelvic joints, and particularly the symphysis pubis, that occurs during pregnancy (Fig. 5–17). They reported that most relaxation takes place in the first half of pregnancy. Retrogression begins immediately following delivery, and it is usually complete within 3 to 5 months.

EYES. Intraocular pressure decreases during pregnancy, attributed in part to increased vitreous outflow (Sunness, 1988). Corneal sensitivity also is decreased, with the great-

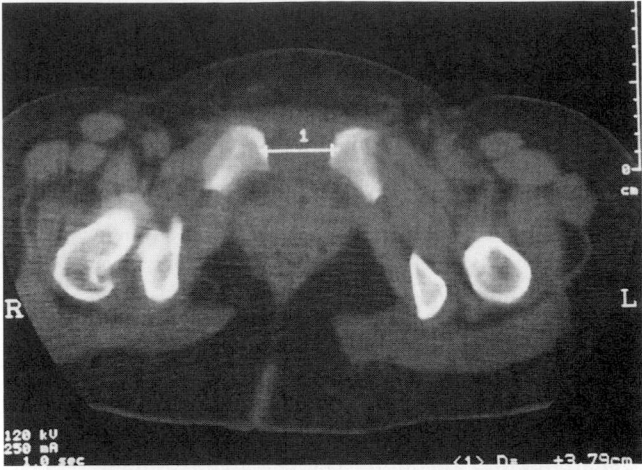
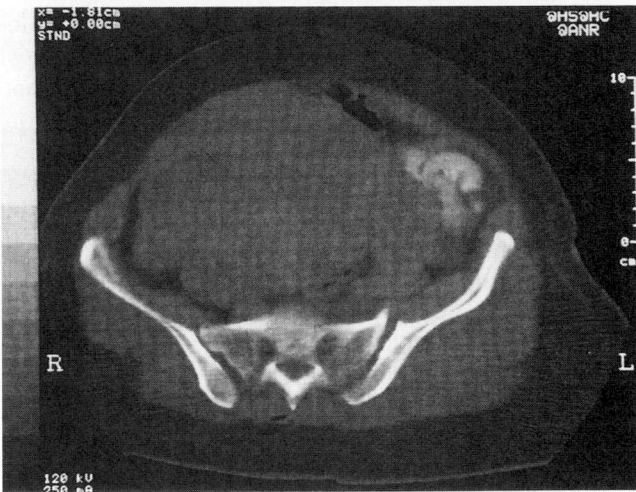

FIGURE 5–17. Computed tomography images demonstrating symphyseal diastasis and widening of the left anterior sacroiliac joint. (From Dunbar and Ries, 2002, with permission.)

est changes late in gestation. Most pregnant women demonstrate a measurable but slight increase in corneal thickness that is thought to be due to edema. Consequently, pregnant women may have difficulty with previously comfortable contact lenses. Brownish-red opacities on the posterior surface of the cornea—*Krukenberg spindles*—have also been observed with a higher than expected frequency during pregnancy. Hormonal effects are postulated as the cause of this increased pigmentation. Other than transient loss of accommodation reported with both pregnancy and lactation, visual function is unaffected by pregnancy. These changes, as well as pathological eye aberrations, were reviewed by Dinn and colleagues (2003).

CENTRAL NERVOUS SYSTEM. Women often report problems with attention, concentration, and memory throughout pregnancy and the early postpartum period. Systematic studies of memory in pregnancy, however, are limited and often anecdotal. Keenan and colleagues (1998) longitudinally investigated memory in pregnant women as well as a matched control group. They found pregnancy-related memory decline, which was limited to the third trimester. This decline was not attributable to depression, anxiety, sleep deprivation, or other physical changes associated with pregnancy. It was transient and quickly resolved following delivery.

Zeeman and co-workers (2003) used magnetic resonance imaging to measure cerebral blood flow across pregnancy in 10 healthy women. They found that mean blood flow bilaterally in the middle and posterior cerebral arteries decreased progressively from 147 and 56 mL/min when nonpregnant to 118 and 44 mL/min late in the third trimester, respectively. The mechanism and clinical significance of this decrease, and whether it relates to the diminished memory observed during pregnancy, is unknown.

Beginning as early as about 12 weeks, and extending through the first 2 months postpartum, women have difficulty going to sleep, frequent awakenings, fewer hours of night sleep, and reduced sleep efficiency (Lee and colleagues, 2000; Swain and colleagues, 1997). Trakada and co-workers (2003) found that during normal pregnancy, the frequency and duration of sleep apnea episodes were decreased significantly compared with those postpartum. In the supine position, however, average Pao_2 levels were lower. The greatest disruption of sleep is encountered postpartum and may contribute to *postpartum blues,* or even frank depression (see Chap. 55, p. 1243).

REFERENCES

Abram SR, Alexander BT, Bennett WA, et al: Role of neuronal nitric oxide synthase in mediating renal hemodynamic changes during pregnancy. Am J Physiol Regul Integr Comp Physiol 281:R1390, 2001

Abramson D, Roberts SM, Wilson PD: Relaxation of the pelvic joints in pregnancy. SGO 58:59S, 1934

Ajne G, Nisell H, Wolff K, et al: The role of endogenous endothelin in the regulation of uteroplacental and renal blood flow during pregnancy in conscious rats. Placenta 24:813, 2003

Alvarez H, Caldeyro-Barcia R: Contractility of the human uterus recorded by new methods. Surg Gynecol Obstet 91:1, 1950

Andersen JR: Prolactin in amniotic fluid and maternal serum during uncomplicated human pregnancy. Dan Med Bull 29:266, 1982

Assali NS, Dilts PV, Pentl AA, et al: Physiology of the placenta. In Assali NS (ed): Biology of Gestation, Vol I. The Maternal Organism. New York, Academic Press, 1968

August P, Mueller FB, Sealey JE, et al: Role of renin–angiotensin system in blood pressure regulation in pregnancy. Lancet 345:896, 1995

Bailey RR, Rolleston GL: Kidney length and ureteric dilatation in the puerperium. J Obstet Gynaecol Br Commonw 78:55, 1971

Baker PN, Cunningham FG: Platelet and coagulation abnormalities. In Lindhemier ML, Roberts JM, Cunningham FG (eds): Chesley's Hypertensive Diseases in Pregnancy, 2nd ed. Stamford, CT, Appleton and Lange, 1999, p 349

Bamber JH, Dresner M: Aortocaval compression in pregnancy: The effect of changing the degree and direction of lateral tilt on maternal cardiac output. Anesth Analg 97:256, 2003

Bardicef M, Bardicef O, Sorokin Y, et al: Extracellular and intracellular magnesium depletion in pregnancy and gestational diabetes. Am J Obstet Gynecol 172:1009, 1995

Bell RJ, Permezel M, MacLennan A, et al: A randomized, double-blind, placebo controlled trial of the safety of vaginal recombinant human relaxin for cervical ripening. Obstet Gynecol 82:328, 1993

Bernstein IM, Ziegler W, Badger GJ: Plasma volume expansion in early pregnancy. Obstet Gynecol 97:669, 2001

Bidus MA, Ries A, Magann EF, et al: Markedly elevated beta-hCG levels in a normal singleton gestation with hyperreactio luteinalis. Obstet Gynecol 99:958, 2002

Bieniarz J, Branda LA, Maqueda E, et al: Aortocaval compression by the uterus in late pregnancy, 3. Unreliability of the sphygmomanometric method in estimating uterine artery pressure. Am J Obstet Gynecol 102:1106, 1968

Boehlen F, Hohlfeld P, Extermann P, et al: Platelet count at term pregnancy: A reappraisal of the threshold. Obstet Gynecol 95:29, 2000

Bonica JJ: Principles and Practice of Obstetric Analgesia and Anesthesia. Philadelphia, FA Davis, 1967

Bradshaw KD, Santos-Ramos R, Rawlins SC, et al: Endocrine studies in a pregnancy complicated by ovarian theca lutein cysts and hyperreactio luteinalis. Obstet Gynecol 67:66S, 1986

Brar HS, Platt LD, DeVore GR, et al: Qualitative assessment of maternal uterine and fetal umbilical artery blood flow and resistance in laboring patients by Doppler velocimetry. Am J Obstet Gynecol 158:952, 1988

Braverman DZ, Johnson ML, Kern F Jr: Effects of pregnancy and contraceptive steroids on gallbladder function. N Engl J Med 302:362, 1980

Brizzi P, Tonolo G, Esposito F, et al: Lipoprotein metabolism during normal pregnancy. Am J Obstet Gynecol 181:430, 1999

Brown MA, Gallery EDM, Ross MR, et al: Sodium excretion in normal and hypertensive pregnancy: A prospective study. Am J Obstet Gynecol 159:297, 1988

Brown MA, Sinosich MJ, Saunders DM, et al: Potassium regulation and progesterone-aldosterone interrelationships in human pregnancy: A prospective study. Am J Obstet Gynecol 155:349, 1986

Burrow GN, Fisher DA, Larsen PR: Maternal and fetal thyroid function. N Engl J Med 331:1072, 1994

Butte NF: Carbohydrate and lipid metabolism in pregnancy: Normal compared with gestational diabetes mellitus. Am J Clin Nutr 7:1256S, 2000

Chan TF, Su JH, Chung YF, et al: Amniotic fluid and maternal serum leptin levels in pregnant women who subsequently develop preeclampsia. Eur J Obstet Gynecol Reprod Biol 108:50, 2003

Chard T, Craig PH, Menabawey M, et al: Alpha interferon in human pregnancy. Br J Obstet Gynaecol 93:1145, 1986

Chellakooty M, Vangsgaard K, Larsen T, et al: A longitudinal study of intrauterine growth and the placental growth hormone (GH)–insulin-like growth factor I axis in maternal circulation. J Clin Endocrinol Metab 89:384, 2004

Chesley LC: Renal function during pregnancy. In Carey HM (ed): Modern Trends in Human Reproductive Physiology. London, Butterworth, 1963

Choi JR, Levine D, Finberg H: Luteoma of pregnancy: Sonographic findings in two cases. J Ultrasound Med 19:877, 2000

Clapp JF III, Little KD, Widness JA: Effect of maternal exercise and fetoplacental growth rate on serum erythropoietin concentrations. Am J Obstet Gynecol 188:1021, 2003

Clapp JF III, Stepanchak W, Tomaselli J, et al: Portal vein blood flow—effects of pregnancy, gravity, and exercise. Am J Obstet Gynecol 183:167, 2000

Clark SL, Cotton DB, Lee W, et al: Central hemodynamic assessment of normal term pregnancy. Am J Obstet Gynecol 161:1439, 1989

Clerico A, Emdin M: Diagnostic accuracy and prognostic relevance of the measurement of cardiac natriuretic peptides: A review. Clin Chem 50:33, 2004

Coccia ME, Pasquini L, Comparetto C, et al: Hyperreactio luteinalis in a woman with high-risk factors: A case report. J Reprod Med 48:127, 2003

Cohen DA, Daughaday WH, Weldon VV: Fetal and maternal virilization associated with pregnancy: A case report and review of the literature. Am J Dis Child 136:353, 1982

Combes B, Adams RH: Disorders of the liver in pregnancy. In Assali NS (ed): Pathophysiology of Gestation, Vol I. New York, Academic Press, 1971

Crisp WE, DeFrancesco S: The hand syndrome of pregnancy. Obstet Gynecol 23:433, 1964

Csapo AI, Pulkkinen MO, Wiest WG: Effects of luteectomy and progesterone replacement therapy in early pregnant patients. Am J Obstet Gynecol 115:759, 1973

Cunningham FG, Cox K, Gant NF: Further observations on the nature of pressor responsivity to angiotensin II in human pregnancy. Obstet Gynecol 46:581, 1975

Cutforth R, MacDonald CB: Heart sounds and murmurs in pregnancy. Am Heart J 71:741, 1966

Darmady JM, Postle AD: Lipid metabolism in pregnancy. Br J Obstet Gynaecol 89:211, 1982

Davison JM, Dunlop W: Renal hemodynamics and tubular function in normal human pregnancy. Kidney Int 18:152, 1980

Davison JM, Hytten FE: Glomerular filtration during and after pregnancy. J Obstet Gynaecol Br Commonw 81:588, 1974

Davison JM, Vallotton MB, Lindheimer MD: Plasma osmolality and urinary concentration and dilution during and after pregnancy: Evidence that lateral recumbency inhibits maximal urinary concentrating ability. Br J Obstet Gynaecol 88:472, 1981

Delorme MA, Burrows RF, Ofosu FA, et al: Thrombin regulation in mother and fetus during pregnancy. Semin Thromb Hemost 18:81, 1992

Desoye G, Schweditsch MO, Pfeiffer KP, et al: Correlation of hormones with lipid and lipoprotein levels during normal pregnancy and postpartum. J Clin Endocrinol Metab 64:704, 1987

DeSwiet M: The respiratory system. In Hytten FE, Chamberlain G (eds): Clinical Physiology in Obstetrics, 2nd ed. Oxford, Blackwell, 1991, p 83

Dinn RB, Harris A, Marcus PS: Ocular changes in pregnancy. Obstet Gynecol Surv 58:137, 2003

Dunbar RP, Ries AM: Puerperal diastasis of the pubic symphysis. A case report. J Reprod Med 47:581, 2002

Duvekot JJ, Cheriex EC, Pieters FA, et al: Early pregnancy changes in hemodynamics and volume homeostasis are consecutive adjustments triggered by a primary fall in systemic vascular tone. Am J Obstet Gynecol 169:1382, 1993

Easterling TR, Schmucker BC, Benedetti TJ: The hemodynamic effects of orthostatic stress during pregnancy. Obstet Gynecol 72:550, 1988

Edman CD, Devereux WP, Parker CR, et al: Placental clearance of maternal androgens: A protective mechanism against fetal virilization. Abstract 112 presented at the 26th annual meeting of the Society for Gynecologic Investigation, San Diego, 1979. Gynecol Invest 67:68, 1979

Edman CD, Toofanian A, MacDonald PC, et al: Placental clearance rate of maternal plasma androstenedione through placental estradiol formation: An indirect method of assessing uteroplacental blood flow. Am J Obstet Gynecol 141:1029, 1981

Enein M, Zina AA, Kassem M, et al: Echocardiography of the pericardium in pregnancy. Obstet Gynecol 69:851, 1987

Fisher C, MacLean M, Morecroft I, et al: Is the pregnancy hormone relaxin also a vasodilator peptide secreted by the heart? Circulation 106:292, 2002

Foulk RA, Martin MC, Jerkins GL, et al: Hyperreactio luteinalis differentiated from severe ovarian hyperstimulation syndrome in a spontaneously conceived pregnancy. Am J Obstet Gynecol 176:1300, 1997

Freinkel N: Banting lecture 1980: Of pregnancy and progeny. Diabetes 29:1023, 1980

Freinkel N, Dooley SL, Metzger BE: Care of the pregnant woman with insulin-dependent diabetes mellitus. N Engl J Med 313:96, 1985

Friedman SA: Preeclampsia: A review of the role of prostaglandins. Obstet Gynecol 71:122, 1988

Gallery EDM, Lindheimer MD: Alterations in volume homeostasis. In Lindhemier ML, Roberts JM, Cunningham FG (eds): Chesley's Hypertensive Diseases in Pregnancy, 2nd ed. Stamford, CT, Appleton and Lange, 1999, p 327

Gallery ED, Raftos J, Gyory AZ, et al: A prospective study of serum complement (C3 and C4) levels in normal human pregnancy: Effect of the development of pregnancy-associated hypertension. Aust N Z J Med 11:243, 1981

Gant NF, Chand S, Whalley PJ, et al: The nature of pressor responsiveness to angiotensin II in human pregnancy. Obstet Gynecol 43:854, 1974

Gant NF, Daley GL, Chand S, et al: A study of angiotensin II pressor response throughout primigravid pregnancy. J Clin Invest 52:2682, 1973

Gherman RB, Mestman JH, Satis AJ, et al: Intractable hyperemesis gravidarum, transient hyperthyroidism and intrauterine growth restriction associated with hyperreactio luteinalis. A case report. J Reprod Med 48:553, 2003

Girling JC, Dow E, Smith JH: Liver function tests in preeclampsia: Importance of comparison with a reference range derived for normal pregnancy. Br J Obstet Gynaecol 104:246, 1997

Glinoer D, de Nayer P, Bourdoux P, et al: Regulation of maternal thyroid during pregnancy. J Clin Endocrinol Metab 71:276, 1990

Gonzalez JG, Elizondo G, Saldivar D, et al: Pituitary gland growth during normal pregnancy: An in vivo study using magnetic resonance imaging. Am J Med 85:217, 1988

Hankins GDV, Clark SL, Uckan E, et al: Maternal oxygen transport variables during the third trimester of normal pregnancy. Am J Obstet Gynecol 180:406, 1999

Harbert GM Jr, Cornell GW, Littlefield JB, et al: Maternal hemodynamics associated with uterine contraction in gravid monkeys. Am J Obstet Gynecol 104:24, 1969

Harstad TW, Mason RA, Cox SM: Serum erythropoietin quantitation in pregnancy using an enzyme-linked immunoassay. Am J Perinatol 9:233, 1992

Hauth JC, Cunningham FG: Preeclampsia-Eclampsia. In Lindhemier MD, Roberts JM, Cunningham FG: Chesley's Hypertensive Disorders in Pregnancy, 2nd ed. Stamford, CT, Appleton & Lange, 1999, p 174

Hayashi M, Inoue T, Hoshimoto K, et al: The levels of five markers of hemostasis and endothelial status at different stages of normotensive pregnancy. Acta Obstet Gynecol Scand 81:208, 2002

Heenan AP, Wolfe LA, Davies GAL, et al: Effects of human pregnancy on fluid regulation responses to short-term exercise. J Appl Physiol 95:2321, 2003

Heidenreich PA, Gubens MA, Fonarow GC, et al: Cost-effectiveness of screening with B-type natriuretic peptide to identify patients with reduced left ventricular ejection fraction. J Am Coll Cardiol 43:1019, 2004

Higby K, Suiter CR, Phelps JY, et al: Normal values of urinary albumin and total protein excretion during pregnancy. Am J Obstet Gynecol 171:984, 1994

Hodgkinson CP: Physiology of the ovarian veins in pregnancy. Obstet Gynecol 1:26, 1953

Huisman A, Aarnoudse JG, Heuvelmans JHA, et al: Whole blood viscosity during normal pregnancy. Br J Obstet Gynaecol 94:1143, 1987

Hull AD, White CR, Pearce WJ: Endothelium-derived relaxing factor and cyclic GMP-dependent vasorelaxation in human chorionic plate arteries. Placenta 15:365, 1994

Hytten FE: Lactation. In: The Clinical Physiology of the Puerperium. London, Farrand Press, 1995, p 59

Hytten FE: The renal excretion of nutrients in pregnancy. Postgrad Med J 49:625, 1973

Hytten FE: Weight gain in pregnancy. In Hytten FE, Chamberlain G (eds): Clinical Physiology in Obstetrics, 2nd ed. Oxford, Blackwell, 1991, p 173

Hytten FE, Chamberlain G: Clinical Physiology in Obstetrics. Oxford, Blackwell, 1991, p 152

Hytten FE, Leitch I: The Physiology of Human Pregnancy, 2nd ed. Philadelphia, Davis, 1971

Hytten FE, Thomson AM: Maternal physiological adjustments. In Assali NS (ed): Biology of Gestation, Vol I. The Maternal Organism. New York, Academic Press, 1968

Ingerslev M, Teilum G: Biopsy studies on the liver in pregnancy, 2. Liver biopsy on normal pregnant women. Acta Obstet Gynecol Scand 25:352, 1946

Iosif S, Ingemarsson I, Ulmsten U: Urodynamic studies in normal pregnancy and in puerperium. Am J Obstet Gynecol 137:696, 1980

Jauniaux E, Johnson MR, Jurkovic D, et al: The role of relaxin in the development of the uteroplacental circulation in early pregnancy. Obstet Gynecol 84:338, 1994

Jensen E, Wood C, Keller-Wood M: The normal increase in adrenal secretion during pregnancy contributes to maternal volume expansion and fetal homeostasis. J Soc Gynecol Investig 9:362, 2002

Kalhan SC, Gruca LL, Parimi PS, et al: Serine metabolism in human pregnancy. Am J Physiol Endocrinol Metab 284:E733, 2003

Kametas NA, McAuliffe F, Krampl E, et al: Maternal cardiac function in twin pregnancy. Obstet Gynecol 102:806, 2003a

Kametas N, McAuliffe F, Krampl E, et al: Maternal electrolyte and liver function changes during pregnancy at high altitude. Clin Chim Acta 328:21, 2003b

Kaneshige E: Serum ferritin as an assessment of iron stores and other hematologic parameters during pregnancy. Obstet Gynecol 57:238, 1981

Katz R, Karliner JS, Resnik R: Effects of a natural volume overload state (pregnancy) on left ventricular performance in normal human subjects. Circulation 58:434, 1978

Kauppila A, Chatelain P, Kirkinen P, et al: Isolated prolactin deficiency in a woman with puerperal alactogenesis. J Clin Endocrinol Metab 64:309, 1987

Kauppila A, Koskinen M, Puolakka J, et al: Decreased intervillous and unchanged myometrial blood flow in supine recumbency. Obstet Gynecol 55:203, 1980

Keenan PA, Yaldoo DT, Stress ME, et al: Explicit memory in pregnant women. Am J Obstet Gynecol 179:731, 1998

Keller-Wood M, Wood CE: Pregnancy alters cortisol feedback inhibition of stimulated ACTH: Studies in adrenalectomized ewes. Am J Physiol Regul Integr Comp Physiol 280:R1790, 2001

Kinsella SM, Lohmann G: Supine hypotensive syndrome. Obstet Gynecol 83:774, 1994

Klafen A, Palugyay J: Vergleichende Untersuchungen über Lage und Ausdehrung von Herz und Lunge in der Schwangerschaft und im Wochenbett. Arch Gynaekol 131:347, 1927

Kletzky OA, Rossman F, Bertolli SI, et al: Dynamics of human chorionic gonadotropin, prolactin, and growth hormone in serum and amniotic fluid throughout normal human pregnancy. Am J Obstet Gynecol 151:878, 1985

Koh SC, Anandakumar C, Montan S, et al: Plasminogen activators, plasminogen activator inhibitors and markers of intravascular coagulation in preeclampsia. Gynecol Obstet Invest 35:214, 1993

Kost ER, Snyder RR, Schwartz LE, et al: The "less than optimal" cytology: Importance in obstetric patients and in a routine gynecologic population. Obstet Gynecol 81:127, 1993

Krause PJ, Ingardia CJ, Pontius LT, et al: Host defense during pregnancy: Neutrophil chemotaxis and adherence. Am J Obstet Gynecol 157:274, 1987

Kubota T, Kamada S, Hirata Y, et al: Synthesis and release of endothelin-1 by human decidual cells. J Clin Endocrinol Metab 75:1230, 1992

Kutteh WH, Franklin RD: Quantification of immunoglobulins and cytokines in human cervical mucus during each trimester of pregnancy. Am J Obstet Gynecol 184:865, 2001

Lammert F, Marschall HU, Glantz A, et al: Intrahepatic cholestasis of pregnancy: Molecular pathogenesis, diagnosis and management. J Hepatol 33:1012, 2000

Lederman SA, Paxton A, Heymsfield SB, et al: Maternal body fat and water during pregnancy: Do they raise infant birth weight? Am J Obstet Gynecol 180:235, 1999

Lee DH, Henderson PA, Blajchman MA: Prevalence of Factor V Leiden in a Canadian blood donor population. Can Med Assoc J 155:285, 1996

Lee KA, Zaffke ME, McEnany G: Parity and sleep patterns during and after pregnancy. Obstet Gynecol 95:14, 2000

Lepercq J, Guerre-Millo M, Andre J, et al: Leptin: A potential marker of placental insufficiency. Gynecol Obstet Invest 55:151, 2003

Levin ER: Endothelins. N Engl J Med 333:356, 1995

Lind T, Bell S, Gilmore E, et al: Insulin disappearance rate in pregnant and non-pregnant women, and in non-pregnant women given GHRIH. Eur J Clin Invest 7:47, 1977

Lindheimer MD, Davison JM: Osmoregulation, the secretion of arginine vasopressin and its metabolism during pregnancy. Eur J Endocrinol 132:133, 1995

Lindheimer MD, Davison JM, Katz AI: The kidney and hypertension in pregnancy: Twenty exciting years. Semin Nephrol 21:173, 2001

Lindheimer MD, Grünfeld J-P, Davison JM: Renal disorders. In Barran WM, Lindheimer MD (eds): Medical Disorders During Pregnancy, 3rd ed. St. Louis, Mosby, 2000, p 39

Lindheimer MD, Richardson DA, Ehrlich EN, et al: Potassium homeostasis in pregnancy. J Reprod Med 32:517, 1987

Lockwood CJ: Inherited thrombophilias in pregnant patients: Detection and treatment paradigm. Obstet Gynecol 99:333, 2002

Lønberg U, Damm P, Andersson A-M, et al: Increase in maternal placental growth hormone during pregnancy and disappearance during parturition in normal and growth hormone-deficient pregnancies. Am J Obstet Gynecol 188:247, 2003

Lowe SA, Macdonald GJ, Brown MA: Acute and chronic regulation of atrial natriuretic peptide in human pregnancy: A longitudinal study. J Hypertens 10:821, 1992

Ludmir J, Sehdev HM: Anatomy and physiology of the uterine cervix. Clin Obstet Gynecol 43:433, 2000

Luppi P, Haluszczak C, Trucco M, et al: Normal pregnancy is associated with peripheral leukocyte activation. Am J Reprod Immunol 47:72, 2002

Mabie WC, DiSessa TG, Crocker LG, et al: A longitudinal study of cardiac output in normal human pregnancy. Am J Obstet Gynecol 170:849, 1994

Macfie AG, Magides AD, Richmond MN, et al: Gastric emptying in pregnancy. Br J Anaesth 67:54, 1991

Manten GTR, Franx A, Sikkema JM, et al: Fibrinogen and high molecular weight fibrinogen during and after normal pregnancy. Thrombosis Res 114:19, 2004

Mardones-Santander F, Salazar G, Rosso P, et al: Maternal body composition near term and birth weight. Obstet Gynecol 91:873, 1998

Marnach ML, Ramin KD, Ramsey PS, et al: Characterization of the relationship between joint laxity and maternal hormones in pregnancy. Obstet Gynecol 101:331, 2003

Masini E, Nistri S, Vannacci A, et al: Relaxin inhibits the activation of human neutrophils: Involvement of the nitric oxide pathway. Endocrinology 145:1106, 2004

McAuliffe F, Kametas N, Costello J, et al: Respiratory function in singleton and twin pregnancy. Br J Obstet Gynaecol 109:765, 2002

McLaughlin MK, Roberts JM: Hemodynamic changes. In Lindhemier ML, Roberts JM, Cunningham FG (eds): Chesley's Hypertensive Diseases in Pregnancy, 2nd ed. Stamford, CT, Appleton and Lange, 1999, p 69

McLennan CE: Antecubital and femoral venous pressure in normal and toxemic pregnancy. Am J Obstet Gynecol 45:568, 1943

Mendenhall HW: Serum protein concentrations in pregnancy. 1. Concentrations in maternal serum. Am J Obstet Gynecol 106:388, 1970

Michimata T, Sakai M, Miyazaki S, et al: Decrease of T-helper 2 and T-cytotoxic 2 cells at implantation sites occurs in unexplained recurrent spontaneous abortion with normal chromosomal content. Hum Reprod 18:1523, 2003

Migeon CJ, Bertrand J, Wall PE: Physiological disposition of 4-C[14] cortisol during late pregnancy. J Clin Invest 36:1350, 1957

Milne JA, Howie AD, Pack AI: Dyspnoea during normal pregnancy. Br J Obstet Gynaecol 85:260, 1978

Miyamoto J: Prolactin and thyrotropin responses to thyrotropin-releasing hormone during the peripartal period. Obstet Gynecol 63:639, 1984

Mojtahedi M, de Groot LC, Boekholt HA, et al: Nitrogen balance of healthy Dutch women before and during pregnancy. Am J Clin Nutr 75:1078, 2002

More C, Bhattoa HP, Bettembuk P, et al: The effects of pregnancy and lactation on hormonal status and biochemical markers of bone turnover. Eur J Obstet Gynecol Reprod Biol 106:209, 2003

Naden RP, Rosenfeld CR: Systemic and uterine responsiveness to angiotensin II and norepinephrine in estrogen-treated nonpregnant sheep. Am J Obstet Gynecol 153:417, 1985

Nel JT, Diedericks A, Joubert G, et al: A prospective clinical and urodynamic study of bladder function during and after pregnancy. Int Urogynecol J Pelvic Floor Dysfunct 12:21, 2001

Nolan TE, Smith RP, DeVoe LD: Maternal plasma D-dimer levels in normal and complicated pregnancies. Obstet Gynecol 81:235, 1993

Nolten WE, Rueckert PA: Elevated free cortisol index in pregnancy: Possible regulatory mechanisms. Am J Obstet Gynecol 139:492, 1981

Novak J, Danielson LA, Kerchner LJ, et al: Relaxin is essential for renal vasodilation during pregnancy in conscious rats. J Clin Invest 107:1469, 2001

Obuobie K, Mullik V, Jones C, et al: McCune-Albright syndrome: Growth hormone dynamics in pregnancy. J Clin Endocrinol Metab 86:2456, 2001

Øian P, Maltau JM, Noddeland H, et al: Oedema-preventing mechanisms in subcutaneous tissue of normal pregnant women. Br J Obstet Gynaecol 92:1113, 1985

Page KL, Celia G, Leddy G, et al: Structural remodeling of rat uterine veins in pregnancy. Am J Obstet Gynecol 187:1647, 2002

Palmer SK, Zamudio S, Coffin C, et al: Quantitative estimation of human uterine artery blood flow and pelvic blood flow redistribution in pregnancy. Obstet Gynecol 80:1000, 1992

Paradisi G, Biaggi A, Ferrazzani S, et al: Abnormal carbohydrate metabolism during pregnancy: Association with endothelial dysfunction. Diabetes Care 25:560, 2002

Parker CR Jr, Everett RB, Whalley PJ, et al: Hormone production during pregnancy in the primigravid patients. II. Plasma levels of deoxycorticosterone throughout pregnancy of normal women and women who developed pregnancy-induced hypertension. Am J Obstet Gynecol 138:626, 1980

Peck TM, Arias F: Hematologic changes associated with pregnancy. Clin Obstet Gynecol 22:785, 1979

Phelps RL, Metzger BE, Freinkel N: Carbohydrate metabolism in pregnancy, 17. Diurnal profiles of plasma glucose, insulin, free fatty acids, triglycerides, cholesterol, and individual amino acids in late normal pregnancy. Am J Obstet Gynecol 140:730, 1981

Pighetti M, Tommaselli GA, D'Elia A, et al: Maternal serum and umbilical cord blood leptin concentrations with fetal growth restriction. Obstet Gynecol 102:535, 2003

Pipe NGJ, Smith T, Halliday D, et al: Changes in fat, fat-free mass and body water in human normal pregnancy. Br J Obstet Gynaecol 86:929, 1979

Pitkin RM: Calcium metabolism in pregnancy and the perinatal periods: A review. Am J Obstet Gynecol 151:99, 1985

Pitkin RM, Reynolds WA, Williams GA, et al: Calcium metabolism in normal pregnancy: A longitudinal study. Am J Obstet Gynecol 133:781, 1979

Platts JK, Meadows P, Jones R, et al: The relation between tissue kallikrein excretion rate, aldosterone and glomerular filtration rate in human pregnancy. Br J Obstet Gynaecol 107:278, 2000

Power ML, Heaney RP, Kalkwarf HJ, et al: The role of calcium in health and disease. Am J Obstet Gynecol 181:1560, 1999

Powers RW, Majors AK, Kerchner LJ, et al: Renal handling of homocysteine during normal pregnancy and preeclampsia. J Soc Gynecol Investig 11:45, 2004

Pritchard JA: Changes in the blood volume during pregnancy and delivery. Anesthesiology 26:393, 1965

Pritchard JA, Adams RH: Erythrocyte production and destruction during pregnancy. Am J Obstet Gynecol 79:750, 1960

Pritchard JA, Mason RA: Iron stores of normal adults and their replenishment with oral iron therapy. JAMA 190:897, 1964

Pritchard JA, Scott DE: Iron demands during pregnancy. In: Iron Deficiency-Pathogenesis: Clinical Aspects and Therapy. London, Academic Press, 1970, p 173

Reitz RE, Daane TA, Woods JR, et al: Calcium, magnesium, phosphorus, and parathyroid hormone interrelationships in pregnancy and newborn infants. Obstet Gynecol 50:701, 1977

Repke JT: Calcium homeostasis in pregnancy. Clin Obstet Gynecol 37:59, 1994

Rosenfeld CR, Barton MD, Meschia G: Effects of epinephrine on distribution of blood flow in the pregnant ewe. Am J Obstet Gynecol 124:156, 1976

Rosenfeld CR, Gant NF Jr: The chronically instrumented ewe: A model for studying vascular reactivity to angiotensin II in pregnancy. J Clin Invest 67:486, 1981

Rosenfeld CR, West J: Circulatory response to systemic infusion of norepinephrine in the pregnant ewe. Am J Obstet Gynecol 127:376, 1977

Rubi RA, Sala NL: Ureteral function in pregnant women, 3. Effect of different positions and of fetal delivery upon ureteral tonus. Am J Obstet Gynecol 101:230, 1968

Sadaniantz A, Saint Laurent L, Parisi AF: Long-term effects of multiple pregnancies on cardiac dimensions and systolic and diastolic function. Am J Obstet Gynecol 174:1061, 1996

Sagawa N, Hasegawa M, Itoh H, et al: Current topic: The role of amniotic endothelin in human pregnancy. Placenta 15:565, 1994

Salomon LJ, Benattar C, Audibert F, et al: Severe preeclampsia is associated with high inhibin A levels and normal leptin levels at 7 to 13 weeks into pregnancy. Am J Obstet Gynecol 189:1517, 2003

Savvidou MD, Hingorani AD, Tsikas D, et al: Endothelial dysfunction and raised plasma concentrations of asymmetric dimethylarginine in pregnant women who subsequently develop pre-eclampsia. Lancet 361:1511, 2003

Schauberger CW, Rooney BL, Goldsmith L, et al: Peripheral joint laxity increases in pregnancy but does not correlate with serum relaxin levels. Am J Obstet Gynecol 174:667, 1996

Scheithauer BW, Sano T, Kovacs KT, et al: The pituitary gland in pregnancy: A clinicopathologic and immunohistochemical study of 69 cases. Mayo Clin Proc 65:461, 1990

Schulman A, Herlinger H: Urinary tract dilatation in pregnancy. Br J Radiol 48:638, 1975

Seligman SP, Buyon JP, Clancy RM, et al: The role of nitric oxide in the pathogenesis of preeclampsia. Am J Obstet Gynecol 171:944, 1994

Shortle BE, Warren MP, Tsin D: Recurrent androgenicity in pregnancy: A case report and literature review. Obstet Gynecol 70:462, 1987

Simon FR, Fortune J, Iwahashi M, et al: Ethinyl estradiol cholestasis involves alterations in expression of liver sinusoidal transporters. Am J Physiol 271:G1043, 1996

Song CS, Kappas A: The influence of estrogens, progestins and pregnancy on the liver. Vitam Horm 26:147, 1968

Spellacy WN, Buhi WC: Pituitary growth hormone and placental lactogen levels measured in normal term pregnancy and at the early and late postpartum periods. Am J Obstet Gynecol 105:888, 1969

Stein PK, Hagley MT, Cole PL, et al: Changes in 24-hour heart rate variability during normal pregnancy. Am J Obstet Gynecol 180:978, 1999

Sternberg WH: Non-functioning ovarian neoplasms. In Grady HG, Smith DE (eds): International Academy of Pathology monograph no. 3. The Ovary. Baltimore, Williams and Wilkins, 1963

Sunness JS: The pregnant woman's eye. Surv Ophthalmol 32:219, 1988

Swain AM, O'Hara MW, Starr KR, et al: A prospective study of sleep, mood, and cognitive function in postpartum and nonpostpartum women. Obstet Gynecol 90:381, 1997

Tanaka Y, Yanagihara T, Ueta M, et al: Naturally conceived twin pregnancy with hyperreactio luteinalis, causing hyperandrogenism and maternal virilization. Acta Obstet Gynecol Scand 80:277, 2001

Taussig FJ: Ectopic decidua formation. Surg Gynecol Obstet 2:292, 1906

Taylor DJ, Phillips P, Lind T: Puerperal haematological indices. Br J Obstet Gynaecol 88:601, 1981

Thellin O, Heinen E: Pregnancy and the immune system: Between tolerance and rejection. Toxicology 185:179, 2003

Thomsen JK, Fogh-Anderson N, Jaszczak P: Atrial natriuretic peptide, blood volume, aldosterone, and sodium excretion during twin pregnancy. Acta Obstet Gynecol Scand 73:14, 1994

Thorpe JM Jr, Norton PA, Wall LL, et al: Urinary incontinence in pregnancy and the puerperium: A prospective study. Am J Obstet Gynecol 181:266, 1999

Thorpe-Beeston JG, Nicolaides KH, Snijders RJM, et al: Fetal thyroid-stimulating hormone response to maternal administration of thyrotropin-releasing hormone. Am J Obstet Gynecol 164:1244, 1991

Trakada G, Tsapanos V, Spiropoulos K: Normal pregnancy and oxygenation during sleep. Eur J Obstet Gynecol Reprod Biol 109:128, 2003

Tsai CH, de Leeuw NKM: Changes in 2,3-diphosphoglycerate during pregnancy and puerperium in normal women and in β-thalassemia heterozygous women. Am J Obstet Gynecol 142:520, 1982

Tygart SG, McRoyan DK, Spinnato JA, et al: Longitudinal study of platelet indices during normal pregnancy. Am J Obstet Gynecol 154:883, 1986

Ueland K: Maternal cardiovascular dynamics, 7. Intrapartum blood volume changes. Am J Obstet Gynecol 126:671, 1976

Ueland K, Metcalfe J: Circulatory changes in pregnancy. Clin Obstet Gynecol 18:41, 1975

Ulmsten U, Sundström G: Esophageal manometry in pregnant and nonpregnant women. Am J Obstet Gynecol 132:260, 1978

Van Wagenen G, Jenkins RH: An experimental examination of factors causing ureteral dilatation of pregnancy. J Urol 42:1010, 1939

Veille JC, Kitzman DW, Millsaps PD, et al: Left ventricular diastolic filling response to stationary bicycle exercise during pregnancy and the postpartum period. Am J Obstet Gynecol 185:822, 2001

Vidaeff AC, Ross PJ, Livingston CK, et al: Gigantomastia complicating mirror syndrome in pregnancy. Obstet Gynecol 101:1139, 2003

Walker MC, Garner PR, Keely EJ, et al: Changes in activated protein C resistance during normal pregnancy. Am J Obstet Gynecol 177:162, 1997

Walther T, Stepan H: C-type natriuretic peptide in reproduction, pregnancy and fetal development. J Endocrinol 180:17, 2004

Watanabe M, Meeker CI, Gray MJ, et al: Secretion rate of aldosterone in normal pregnancy. J Clin Invest 42:1619, 1963

Watts DH, Krohn MA, Wener MH, et al: C-reactive protein in normal pregnancy. Obstet Gynecol 77:176, 1991

Waugh J, Bell SC, Kilby MD, et al: Urinary microalbumin/creatinine ratios: Reference range in uncomplicated pregnancy. Clin Sci 104:103, 2003

Weisman Y, Harell A, Edelstein S, et al: 1α,25-Dihydroxyvitamin D$_3$ and 24,25-dihydroxyvitamin D$_3$ in vitro synthesis by human decidua and placenta. Nature 281:317, 1979

Weiss G, Goldsmith LT, Sachdev R, et al: Elevated first-trimester serum relaxin concentrations in pregnant women following ovarian stimulation predict prematurity risk and preterm delivery. Obstet Gynecol 82:821, 1993

Weiss M, Eisenstein Z, Ramot Y, et al: Renal reabsorption of inorganic phosphorus in pregnancy in relation to the calciotropic hormones. Br J Obstet Gynaecol 105:195, 1998

Whitehead M, Lane G, Young O, et al: Interrelations of calcium-regulating hormones during normal pregnancy. BMJ 283:10, 1981

Whittaker PG, MacPhail S, Lind T: Serial hematologic changes and pregnancy outcome. Obstet Gynecol 88:33, 1996

Wijma J, Weis Potters AE, de Wolf BT, et al: Anatomical and functional changes in the lower urinary tract during pregnancy. Br J Obstet Gynaecol 108:726, 2001

Wilson M, Morganti AA, Zervoudakis I, et al: Blood pressure, the renin-aldosterone system and sex steroids throughout normal pregnancy. Am J Med 68:97, 1980

Wollmann HA: Growth hormone and growth factors during perinatal life. Horm Res 53:50, 2000

Wong CA, Loffredi M, Ganchiff JN, et al: Gastric emptying of water in term pregnancy. Anesthesiology 96:1395, 2002

Wright HP, Osborn SB, Edmonds DG: Changes in rate of flow of venous blood in the leg during pregnancy, measured with radioactive sodium. Surg Gynecol Obstet 90:481, 1950

Zeeman GG, Hatab M, Twickler DM: Maternal cerebral blood flow changes in pregnancies. Am J Obstet Gynecol 189:968, 2003

Parturition

The last few hours of human pregnancy are characterized by uterine contractions that effect dilatation of the cervix and force the fetus through the birth canal. The myometrial contractions of labor are painful, which is why the term *labor pains* is used to describe this process. Before these forceful, painful contractions begin, however, the uterus must be prepared for labor. During the first 36 to 38 weeks of gestation, the myometrium is unresponsive. After this prolonged period of quiescence, a transitional phase is required during which myometrial unresponsiveness is suspended and the cervix is softened and effaced.

The physiological processes that regulate parturition and the onset of labor continue to be defined. It is clear, however, that the onset of labor represents the culmination of a series of biochemical changes in the uterus that result from endocrine and paracrine signals coming from both the mother and the fetus. The relative role of their contributions varies between species, and it is these differences that complicate the determination of the exact underlying factors regulating human parturition. When parturition is abnormal, the result can be preterm labor, dystocia, or postterm pregnancy. Although dystocia and postterm pregnancy can be treated by cesarean delivery, preterm labor remains the major contributor to neonatal mortality and morbidity in developed countries. What follows is a concise view of the process of parturition and the events that regulate its progression to delivery. Because of the impact of preterm delivery on society, the potential physiological causes of preterm birth also are discussed (see also Chap. 36, p. 859).

PHASES OF PARTURITION

Parturition, the bringing forth of young, encompasses all physiological processes involved in birthing: the prelude to (phase 0), the preparation for (phase 1), the process of (phase 2), and recovery from (phase 3) childbirth. From the disparate nature of these physiological processes, it is evident that multiple transformations in uterine function must be accommodated in a timely manner. As shown in Figure 6–1, parturition can be arbitrarily divided into four uterine phases, which correspond to the major physiological transitions of the myometrium and cervix during pregnancy (Casey and MacDonald, 1993, 1997; Challis and associates, 2000). The *phases of parturition* should not be confused with the clinical stages of labor (first, second, and third stages), which comprise phase 2 of parturition.

PHASE 0 OF PARTURITION: UTERINE QUIESCENCE. Beginning even before implantation, a remarkably effective period of myometrial quiescence is imposed. This phase is characterized by uterine smooth muscle tranquility with maintenance of cervical structural integrity. During this phase, which normally characterizes 95 percent of pregnancy, the inherent propensity of the myometrium to contract is held in abeyance. Thus, the uterine myometrial smooth muscle is rendered unresponsive to natural stimuli, and relative contractile paralysis is imposed against a host of mechanical and chemical challenges that otherwise would promote emptying of the uterine contents. The myometrial unresponsiveness of phase 0 continues until near the end of pregnancy, when the myometrium must be awakened from this prolonged parturitional diapause in preparation for labor.

During phase 0 of parturition, as the myometrium is maintained in a quiescent state, the cervix must remain firm and unyielding. The maintenance of cervical anatomical and structural integrity is essential for successful parturition. Preterm cervical dilatation, structural incompetence, or both, may forecast an unfavorable pregnancy outcome that ends most often in preterm delivery (see Chap. 36, p. 860). Indeed, shortening of the cervix between 24 and 28 weeks was associated with an increased risk of preterm delivery (Iams and colleagues, 1996).

Some myometrial contractions occur during the quiescent phase, but they do not normally cause cervical dilatation. These contractions are characterized by unpredictable occurrence, very low intensity, and brief duration. Any discomfort that they produce usually is confined to the lower abdomen and groin. Near the end of pregnancy, as the uterus undergoes preparation for labor, contractions of this type are more common, especially in multiparous women. They are sometimes referred to as *Braxton-Hicks contractions* or *false labor* (see Chap. 17, p. 424).

PHASE 1 OF PARTURITION: PREPARATION FOR LABOR. To prepare the uterus for labor, the myometrial tranquility of phase 0 of parturition must be suspended

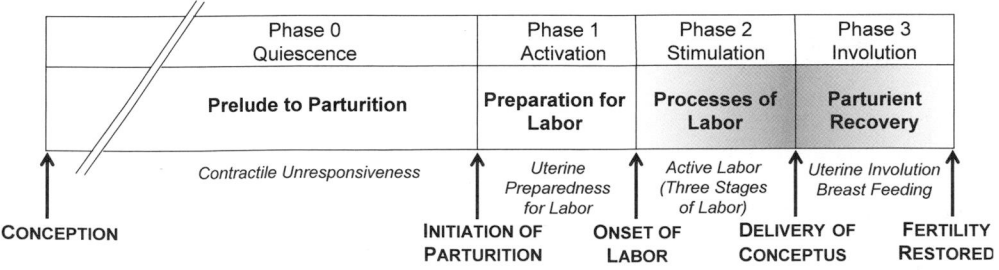

FIGURE 6–1. The phases of parturition and the onset of labor.

through what has been called *uterine awakening* or *activation*. This process is termed *phase 1 of parturition* and represents a progression of changes in the uterus during the last 6 to 8 weeks of pregnancy. It is important to consider that shifting the events associated with phase 1 can cause either preterm or delayed labor. Thus, understanding the modifications in the myometrium and cervix during phase 1 provides a better understanding of events leading to normal labor as well as preterm labor.

Cervical Changes. Although parts of the same organ, the body or fundus of the uterus and the cervix must respond quite differently during pregnancy and parturition. Specifically, it is essential that during most of pregnancy the myometrium be able to stretch but remain quiescent. And, at the same time, the cervix must remain unyielding and reasonably rigid. Then, coincidentally with the initiation of parturition, the cervix must soften, yield, and become more readily dilatable. The fundus must be transformed from the relatively relaxed, unresponsive organ characteristic of most of pregnancy to one that will produce effective contractions that drive the fetus through the yielding (dilatable) cervix and on through the birth canal. Failure of a coordinated interaction between the functions of fundus and cervix is indicative of an unfavorable pregnancy outcome. But despite the apparent reversal of roles between cervix and fundus from before to during labor, it is likely that common agents regulate both.

The cervical modifications during phase 1 of parturition principally involve changes in the connective tissue. These are accompanied by the invasion by inflammatory cells to the extent that the process has been likened to a state of inflammation. Two complementary changes occur to its connective tissues as the cervix softens. The first change relates to the state of the bundles of collagen fibers that act during most of gestation to provide rigid support. Late in gestation there is an increase in collagen breakdown and a rearrangement of the collagen fiber bundles. This process causes a decrease in the number and size of collagen bundles within the cervix. During this same period, there are changes in the relative amounts of the various glycosaminoglycans, particularly hyaluronic acid, a compound associated with the capacity of the cervix to retain water. The second change relates to the striking increase in the amount of hyaluronic acid in the cervix, with a concomitant increase in water. In addition, there is a decrease in dermatan sulfate, which is needed for collagen fiber cross-linking (Cabrol and associates, 1985). Other cervical changes associated with softening include an increased production of cytokines that causes infiltration of leukocytes, which also degrade collagen. The result of these changes is cervical thinning, softening, and relaxation, which allow the cervix to initiate dilatation.

The exact mechanisms that lead to cervical ripening are still being defined, but several candidates have already been used clinically. Prostaglandins E_2 (PGE$_2$) and $F_{2\alpha}$ (PGF$_{2\alpha}$) applied directly to the cervix will induce these same maturational softening changes. Specifically, they cause modification of collagen and alterations in the relative concentration of the glycosaminoglycans. This property is useful clinically, and prostaglandin preparations placed intravaginally adjacent to the cervix effect cervical softening or "ripening" to facilitate the induction of labor (see Chap. 22, p. 537). In some species, but not humans, these events are induced by falling levels of progesterone. However, even in humans, progesterone antagonists will cause cervical softening. As discussed later, humans may have developed unique mechanisms to cause a localized decrease in progesterone action in the cervix and myometrium. Despite the enormous importance of cervical softening to the success of parturition, relatively little is known of the precise sequence (or regulation) of the biochemical processes involved.

Myometrial Changes. The uterine smooth muscle must undergo a series of changes during phase 1 to prepare it for labor. Most relate to its state of contractility. These changes are manifest by a transition from a contractile state characterized predominantly by occasional painless contractions to one in which more frequent contractions develop. This shift probably results from alterations in the expression of key proteins that control myometrial contractility. These have been termed the *contraction-associated proteins (CAPs)*. During phase 1 there is a striking increase in myometrial oxytocin receptors. There are increased numbers and surface areas of myometrial cell gap junction proteins such as connexin-43. Together these changes result in increased uterine irritability and responsiveness to uterotonins.

Another critical change that occurs in phase 1 is the formation of the lower uterine segment. With the development of a well-formed lower segment, the fetal head oftentimes descends to or even through the pelvic inlet—a distinctive event referred to as *lightening*. The abdomen commonly undergoes a change in shape, an event sometimes described by the mother as "the baby dropped." It is also likely that the myometrium in the lower uterine segment is unique from the adjacent myometrium in the upper uterine segment, resulting in distinct roles for each during labor.

PHASE 2 OF PARTURITION: THE PROCESS OF LABOR. Phase 2 is synonymous with active labor, that is, the uterine contractions that bring about progressive cervical dilatation and delivery. Clinically, phase 2 of parturition is customarily divided into the three stages of labor. These stages compose the labor graph commonly used and shown in Figure 6–2. The clinical stages of labor may be summarized as follows:

1. The first stage of labor begins when widely spaced uterine contractions of sufficient frequency, intensity, and duration are attained to bring about effacement of the cervix. This stage of labor ends when the cervix is fully dilated (about 10 cm) to allow passage of the fetal head. The first

Stages of Labor

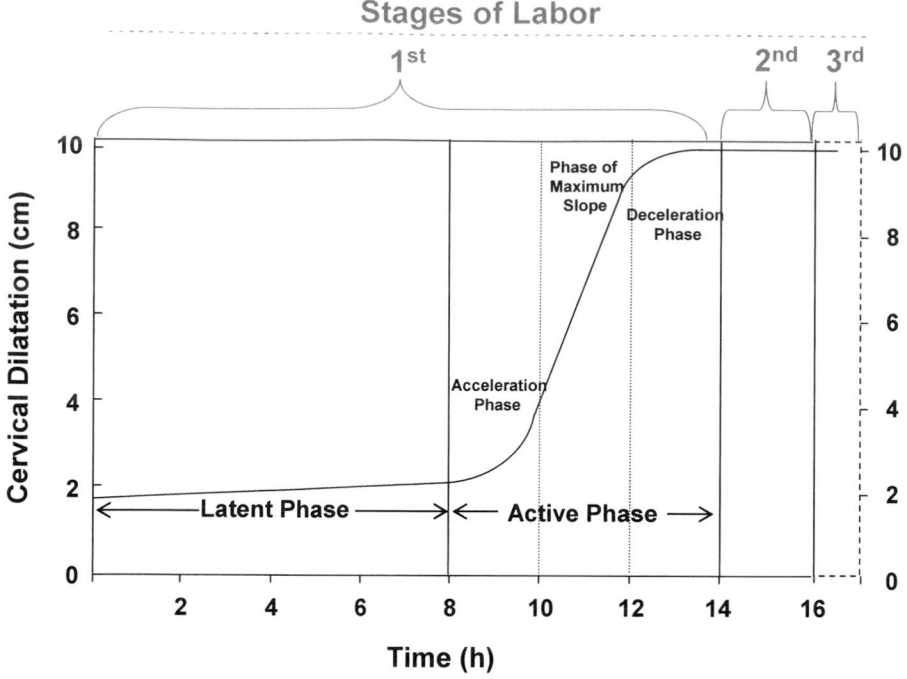

FIGURE 6-2. Composite of the average dilatation curve for nulliparous labor based on analysis of the data derived from the patterns traced from a large, nearly consecutive, series of gravidas. The first stage is divided into a relatively flat latent phase and a rapidly progressive active phase. In the active phase, there are three identifiable component parts: an acceleration phase, a linear phase of maximum slope, and a deceleration phase. (Redrawn from Friedman, 1978.)

stage of labor, therefore, is the stage of cervical effacement and dilatation.

2. The second stage of labor begins when dilatation of the cervix is complete, and ends with delivery of the fetus. Thus, the second stage of labor is the stage of expulsion of the fetus.

3. The third stage of labor begins immediately after delivery of the fetus and ends with the delivery of the placenta and fetal membranes. Thus, the third stage of labor is the stage of separation and expulsion of the placenta.

First Stage of Labor: Clinical Onset of Labor. In some women, the forceful uterine contractions that effect cervical dilatation, fetal descent, and delivery begin suddenly and seemingly without warning. In other women, a rather dependable sign of the initiation of labor is the spontaneous discharge of a small amount of blood-tinged mucus from the vagina. This event represents the extrusion of the mucus plug that had filled the cervical canal during pregnancy, and is referred to as "show" or "bloody show." There is very little blood with the mucus plug, and substantial bleeding is suggestive of an abnormal cause. Passage of the mucus plug indicates that labor is already in progress or likely will ensue during the next several hours to days.

UTERINE CONTRACTIONS CHARACTERISTIC OF LABOR. Unique among physiological muscular contractions, those of uterine smooth muscle during labor are painful. The cause of the pain is not known definitely, but several possibilities have been suggested:

1. Hypoxia of the contracted myometrium (as in angina pectoris).

2. Compression of nerve ganglia in the cervix and lower uterus by the interlocking muscle bundles.

3. Stretching of the cervix during dilatation.

4. Stretching of the peritoneum overlying the fundus.

Compression of nerve ganglia in the cervix and lower uterine segment by the contracting myometrium is an especially attractive hypothesis. Paracervical infiltration with a local anesthetic usually produces appreciable relief of pain during subsequent contractions (see Chap. 19, p. 479). Uterine contractions are involuntary and, for the most part, independent of extrauterine control. Neural blockage from epidural analgesia does not diminish their frequency or intensity. Moreover, the myometrial contractions in paraplegic women are normal, though painless, as in women after bilateral lumbar sympathectomy.

Mechanical stretching of the cervix enhances uterine activity in several species, including humans. This phenomenon has been referred to as the *Ferguson reflex* (Ferguson, 1941). The exact mechanism by which mechanical dilatation of the cervix causes increased myometrial contractility is not clear. Release of oxytocin was suggested as the cause, but this is not proven. Manipulation of the cervix and "stripping" the fetal membranes is associated with an increase in the levels of prostaglandin $F_{2\alpha}$ metabolite (PGFM) in blood which could also increase contractions.

The interval between contractions diminishes gradually from about 10 minutes at the onset of the first stage of labor to as little as 1 minute or less in the second stage. Periods of relaxation between contractions, however, are essential to the welfare of the fetus. Unremitting contractions compromise uteroplacental blood flow sufficiently to cause fetal

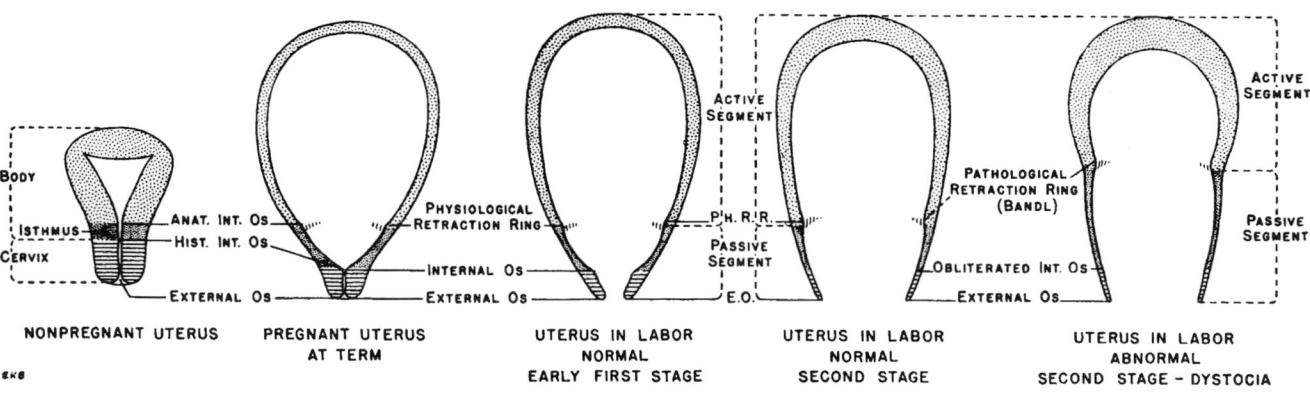

FIGURE 6–3. Sequence of development of the segments and rings in the uterus in pregnant women at term and in labor. Note comparison between the uterus of a nonpregnant woman, the uterus at term, and the uterus during labor. The passive lower segment of the uterine body is derived from the isthmus; the physiological retraction ring develops at the junction of the upper and lower uterine segments. The pathological retraction ring develops from the physiological ring. (Anat. Int. Os = anatomical internal os; E.O. = external os; Hist. Int. Os = histological internal os; Ph.R.R. = physiological retraction ring.)

hypoxemia. In the active phase of labor, the duration of each contraction ranges from 30 to 90 seconds, averaging about 1 minute. There is appreciable variability in the intensity of contractions during normal labor, as emphasized by Schulman and Romney (1970). They recorded the amnionic fluid pressures generated by contractions during spontaneous labor and found the average to be about 40 mm Hg, with variations from 20 to 60 mm Hg (see Chap. 18, p. 466).

FORMATION OF DISTINCT LOWER AND UPPER UTERINE SEGMENTS. During active labor, the divisions of the uterus that were initiated in phase 1 of parturition become increasingly evident. The actively contracting upper segment becomes thicker as labor advances. The lower or passive segment of the uterus and the cervix are relatively inactive compared with the upper segment. It subsequently develops into a much more thinly walled passage for the fetus. The lower segment is analogous to a greatly expanded and thinned-out isthmus in nonpregnant women and thus is not solely a phenomenon of labor. The lower segment develops gradually as pregnancy progresses and then thins remarkably during labor (Figs. 6–3 and 6–4).

By abdominal palpation, even before rupture of the membranes, the two segments can be differentiated during a contraction. The upper uterine segment is quite firm or hard during contractions. The consistency of the lower uterine segment is much less firm, and it is distended and normally much more passive. If the entire wall of uterine musculature, including the lower uterine segment and cervix, were to contract simultaneously and with equal intensity, the net expulsive force would be decreased markedly. Herein lies the importance of the division of the uterus into an actively contracting upper segment and a more passive lower segment that differ not only anatomically but also physiologically.

The upper segment contracts, retracts, and expels the fetus. In response to the force of these contractions, the softened lower uterine segment and cervix dilate and thereby form a greatly expanded, thinned-out muscular and fibromuscular tube through which the fetus can be extruded. The myometrium of the upper uterine segment does not relax to its original length after contractions. Instead, it becomes relatively fixed at a shorter length.

The upper active segment of the uterus contracts down on its diminishing contents, but myometrial tension remains constant. The net effect is to take up slack, thus maintaining the advantage gained in the expulsion of the fetus, and keeping the uterine musculature in firm contact with the intrauterine contents. As the consequence of retraction, each successive contraction commences where its predecessor left off. Thus, the upper part of the uterine cavity becomes slightly smaller with each successive contraction. Because of the successive shortening of the muscular fibers with contractions, the upper active uterine segment becomes progressively thickened throughout the first and second stages of labor (see Fig. 6–3). This process continues and results in an upper uterine segment that is tremendously thickened immediately after delivery. The phenomenon of upper segment retraction is contingent upon a decrease in the volume of its contents. For the contents to be diminished, particularly early in labor when the entire uterus is virtually a closed sac with only a minute opening at the cervical os, the musculature of the lower segment must stretch. This permits increasingly more of the uterine contents to occupy the lower segment, and the upper segment retracts only to the extent that the lower segment distends and the cervix dilates.

Relaxation of the lower uterine segment is not complete, but rather the opposite of retraction. The fibers of the lower segment become stretched with each contraction of the upper segment and after which are not returned to the previous length but remain fixed at the longer length. Importantly, the tension remains essentially the same as before. The

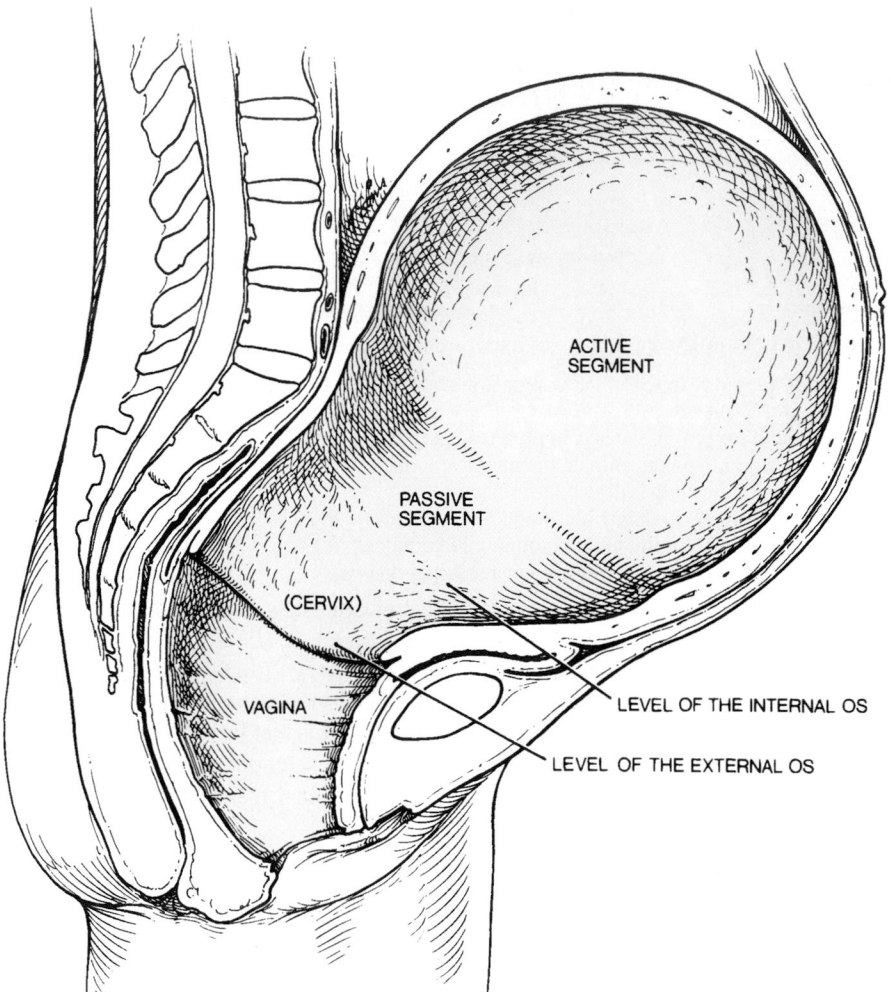

ACTIVE
SEGMENT

PASSIVE
SEGMENT

(CERVIX)

VAGINA

LEVEL OF THE INTERNAL OS

LEVEL OF THE EXTERNAL OS

FIGURE 6–4. The uterus at the time of vaginal delivery. The active upper segment of the uterus retracts about the fetus as the fetus descends through the birth canal. In the passive lower segment, there is considerably less myometrial tone.

musculature still manifests tone, still resists stretch, and still contracts somewhat on stimulation. The successive lengthening of the fibers in the lower segment, as labor progresses, is accompanied by thinning, normally to only a few millimeters in the thinnest part. As a result of the lower segment thinning and concomitant upper segment thickening, a boundary between the two is marked by a ridge on the inner uterine surface—the *physiological retraction ring*. When the thinning of the lower uterine segment is extreme, as in obstructed labor, the ring is very prominent, forming a *pathological retraction ring*. This is an abnormal condition, also known as *Bandl ring*, which is illustrated in Figure 6–3 and discussed further in Chapter 20 (see p. 519). The existence of a gradient of diminishing physiological activity from fundus to cervix was established from measurements of differences in behavior of the upper and lower parts of the uterus during normal labor.

CHANGES IN UTERINE SHAPE DURING LABOR. Each contraction produces an elongation of the uterine ovoid with a concomitant decrease in horizontal diameter. By virtue of this change

in shape, there are important effects on the process of labor. First, the decrease in horizontal diameter produces a straightening of the fetal vertebral column. This presses the upper pole of the fetus firmly against the fundus, whereas the lower pole is thrust farther downward and into the pelvis. The lengthening of the fetal ovoid thus produced has been estimated as between 5 and 10 cm. The pressure exerted in this fashion is known as the *fetal axis pressure*. Second, with lengthening of the uterus, the longitudinal fibers are drawn taut, and because the lower segment and cervix are the only parts of the uterus that are flexible, these are pulled upward over the lower pole of the fetus. This effect on the musculature of the lower segment and on the cervix is an important factor in cervical dilatation.

ANCILLARY FORCES IN LABOR. After the cervix is dilated fully, the most important force in the expulsion of the fetus is that produced by maternal intra-abdominal pressure. Created by contraction of the abdominal muscles simultaneously with forced respiratory efforts with the glottis closed, this is referred to as "pushing." The nature of the force produced is similar to that involved in defecation, but the intensity usually is much greater. The importance of intra-abdominal pressure in fetal expulsion is most clearly attested to by the labors of women who are paraplegic. Such women suffer no pain, although the uterus may contract vigorously. Cervical dilatation, in large measure the result of uterine contractions acting on a softened cervix, proceeds normally. Expulsion of the infant, however, is accomplished more readily when the woman is instructed to bear down during a uterine contraction.

Although increased intra-abdominal pressure is required for the spontaneous completion of labor, it is futile until the cervix is fully dilated. Specifically, it is a necessary auxiliary to contractions in second-stage labor, but pushing accomplishes little in the first stage.

Cervical Changes Induced During the First Stage of Labor. There are three principal structural components of the cervix: collagen, smooth muscle, and the extracellular matrix. Constituents important in modifications at parturition are those in the extracellular matrix, including the glycosaminoglycans, dermatan sulfate, and hyaluronic acid. The smooth muscle content of the cervix is much less than that of the fundus and varies anatomically from 25 to only 6 percent. Before the onset of labor, during the phase of uterine awakening and preparedness, the cervix is softened, which facilitates dilatation once forceful myometrial contractions of labor begin. The effective force of first-stage labor is the uterine contraction, which in turn exerts hydrostatic pressure through the fetal membranes against the cervix and lower uterine segment. In the absence of intact membranes, the

presenting part is forced directly against the cervix and lower uterine segment. As the result of the action of these forces, two fundamental changes—effacement and dilatation—take place in the already softened cervix. For the average-sized fetal head to pass through the cervix, its canal must dilate to a diameter of about 10 cm. At this time, the cervix is said to be completely (or fully) dilated. There may be no fetal descent during cervical effacement, but most commonly the presenting fetal part descends somewhat as the cervix dilates. During second-stage labor, descent of the presenting part typically occurs rather slowly but steadily in nulliparas. In multiparas, however, particularly those of high parity, descent may be rapid.

The "obliteration" or "taking up" of the cervix is the shortening of the cervical canal from a length of about 2 cm to a mere circular orifice with almost paper-thin edges. This process is referred to as *cervical effacement* and takes place from above downward. The muscular fibers at about the level of the internal cervical os are pulled upward, or "taken up," into the lower uterine segment, as the condition of the external os remains temporarily unchanged. As illustrated in Figures 6–5 to 6–8, the edges of the internal os are drawn upward several centimeters to become a part of the lower uterine segment.

Effacement may be compared with a funneling process in which the whole length of a narrow cylinder is converted into a very obtuse, flaring funnel with a small circular orifice for an outlet. As the result of increased myometrial activity during uterine preparedness for labor, appreciable effacement of the softened cervix sometimes is accomplished before active

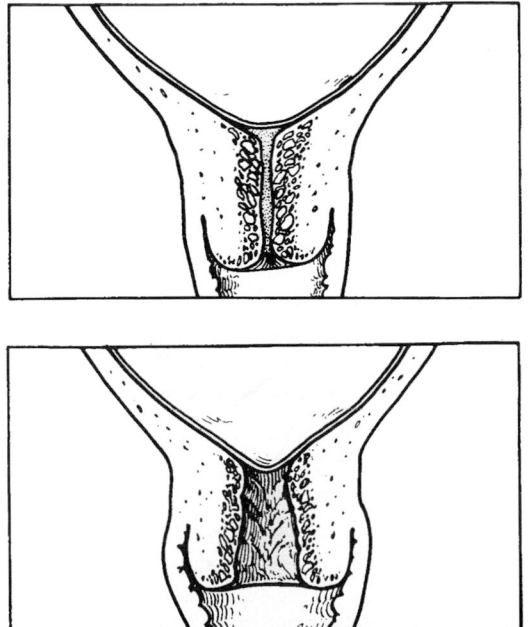

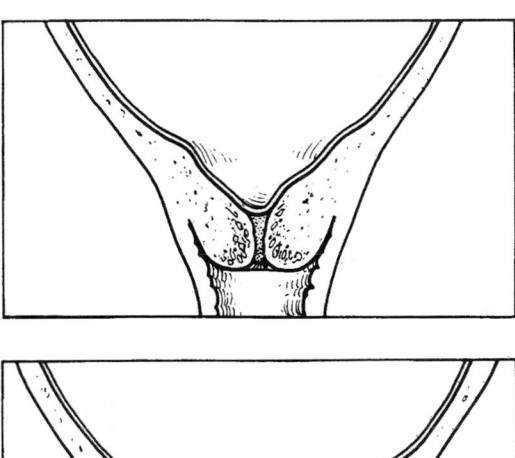

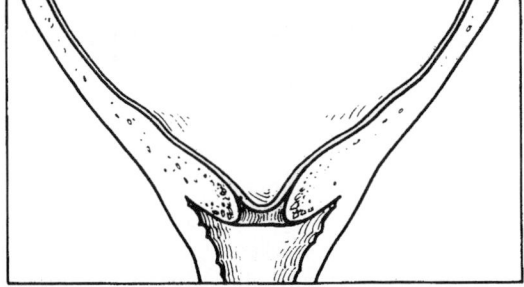

FIGURE 6–5. Cervix near the end of pregnancy but before labor. Top, primigravida; bottom, multipara. Note that the internal os and external cervical os are more dilated in the multipara.

FIGURE 6–6. Beginning effacement of the cervix. Note dilatation of the internal os and funnel-shaped cervical canal. Top, primigravida; bottom, multipara.

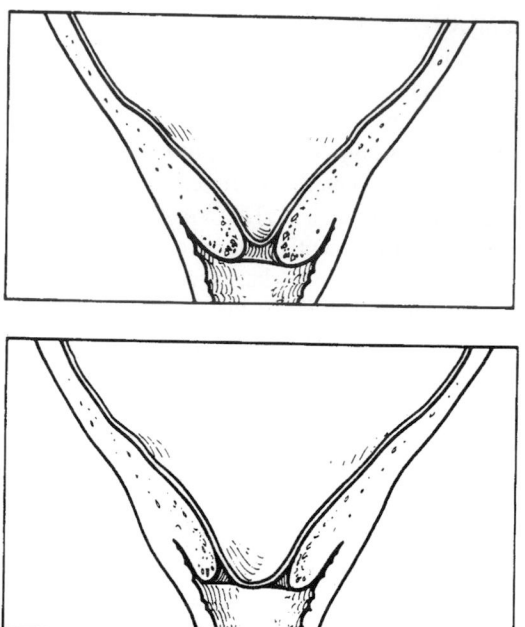

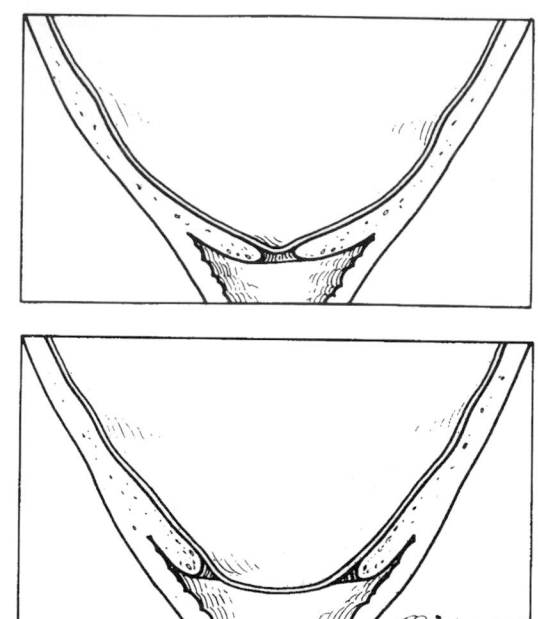

FIGURE 6–7. Further effacement of the cervix. Top, primigravida; bottom, multipara.

FIGURE 6–8. Cervical canal obliterated—that is, the cervix is completely effaced. Top, primigravida; bottom, multipara.

labor begins. Effacement causes expulsion of the mucus plug as the cervical canal is shortened.

Compared with the body of the uterus, the lower uterine segment and the cervix are regions of lesser resistance. Therefore, during a contraction a centrifugal pull is exerted on the cervix leading to distention, a process referred to as *cervical dilatation* (Figs. 6–9 to 6–11). As the uterine contractions cause pressure on the membranes, the hydrostatic action of the amnionic sac in turn dilates the cervical canal like a wedge. In the absence of intact membranes, the pressure of the presenting part against the cervix and lower uterine segment is similarly effective. Early rupture of the membranes does not retard cervical dilatation so long as the presenting part of the fetus is positioned to exert pressure against the cervix and lower uterine segment. The process of cervical effacement and dilatation causes the formation of the forebag of the amnionic fluid, which is later described in detail.

As depicted in Figure 6–2, two phases of cervical dilatation are the latent phase and the active phase. The active phase has been subdivided further as the acceleration phase, the phase of maximum slope, and the deceleration phase (Friedman, 1978). The duration of the latent phase is more variable and sensitive to changes by extraneous factors, such as sedation, which prolongs the latent phase, and myometrial stimulation, which shortens it. The duration of the latent phase has little bearing on the subsequent course of labor, whereas the characteristics of the accelerated phase are usually predictive of the outcome of a particular labor. The completion of cervical dilatation during the active phase of labor is accomplished by cervical retraction about the presenting part of the fetus. After cervical dilatation, the second stage of labor

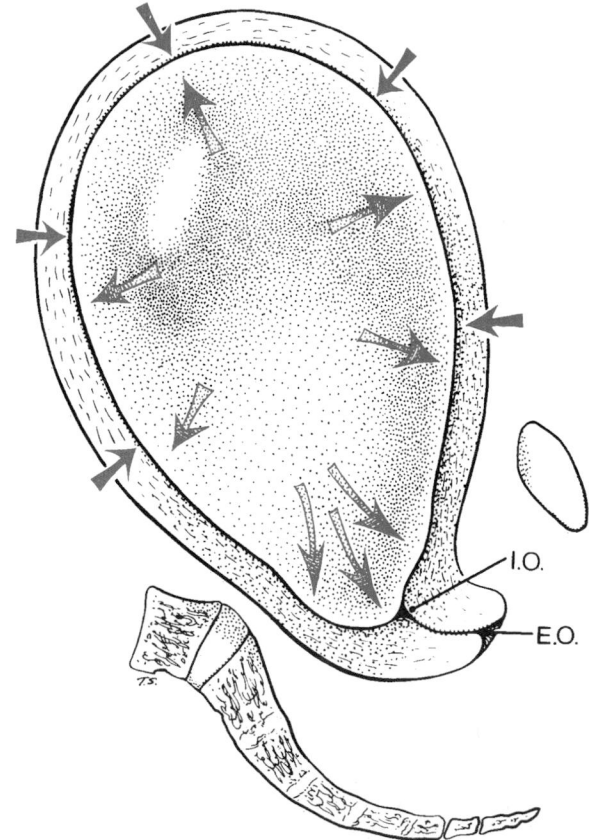

FIGURE 6–9. Hydrostatic action of membranes in effecting cervical effacement and dilatation. In the absence of intact membranes, the presenting part, applied to the cervix and the forming lower uterine segment, acts similarly. In this and Figures 6–10 and 6–11, note changing relations of the external os (E.O.) and internal os (I.O.).

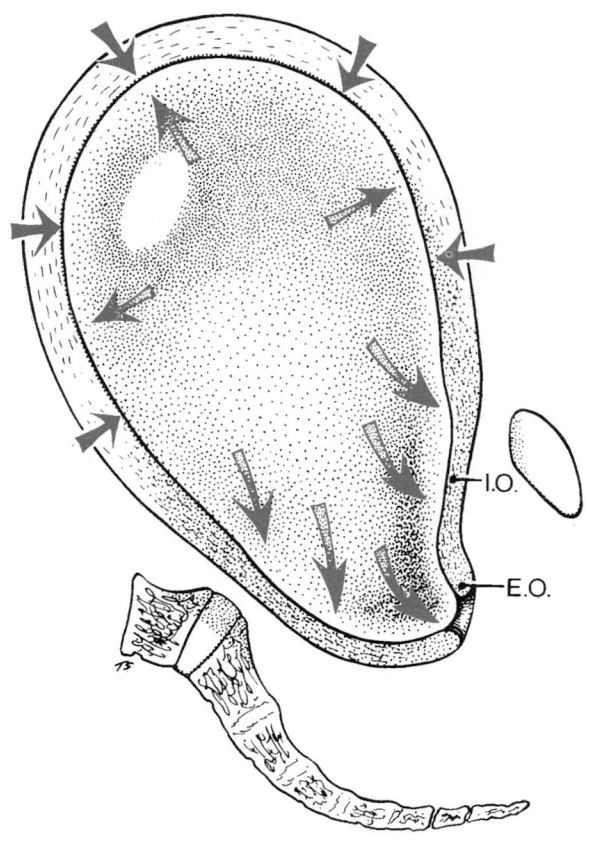

FIGURE 6–10. Hydrostatic action of membranes at completion of effacement. (E.O. = external os; I.O. = internal os.)

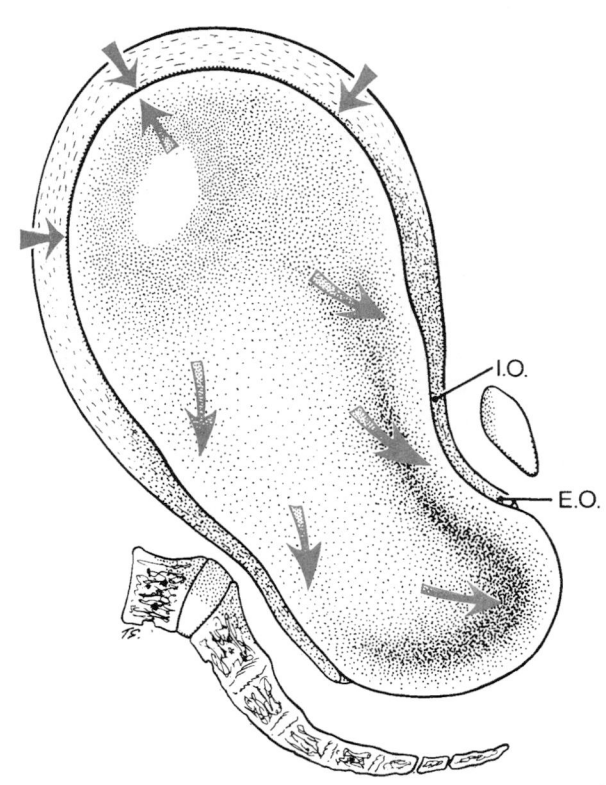

FIGURE 6–11. Hydrostatic action of membranes at full cervical dilatation. (E.O. = external os; I.O. = internal os.)

commences; thereafter, only progressive descent of the presenting fetal part is available to assess the progress of labor.

The Second Stage of Labor: Fetal Descent. In many nulliparas, engagement of the fetal head is accomplished before labor begins, and further descent does not occur until late in labor. In others in whom engagement of the fetal head is initially not so complete, further descent occurs during the first stage of labor. In the descent pattern of normal labor, a typical hyperbolic curve is formed when the station of the fetal head is plotted as a function of the duration of labor. Active descent usually takes place after dilatation has progressed for some time (Figs. 6–2 and 6–12). In nulliparas, increased rates of descent are observed ordinarily during the phase of maximum slope of cervical dilatation. At this time, the speed of descent increases to a maximum, and this is maintained until the presenting part reaches the perineal floor (Friedman, 1978).

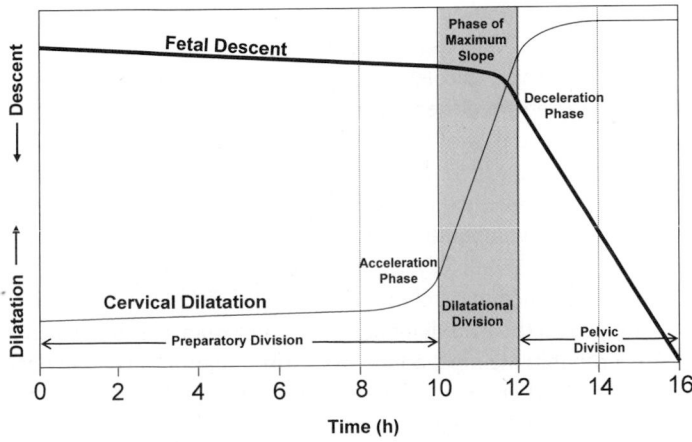

FIGURE 6–12. Labor course divided functionally on the basis of expected evolution of the dilatation and descent curves into (1) a preparatory division, including latent and acceleration phases; (2) a dilatational division, occupying the phase of maximum slope of dilatation; and (3) a pelvic division, encompassing both deceleration phase and second stage while concurrent with the phase of maximum slope of fetal descent. (Redrawn from Friedman, 1978.)

CHANGES IN THE PELVIC FLOOR DURING LABOR. The birth canal is supported and is functionally closed by several layers of tissues that together form the pelvic floor. The most important structures are the levator ani muscle and the fascia covering its upper and lower surfaces, which for practical purposes may be considered as the pelvic floor. This group of muscles closes the lower end of the pelvic cavity as a diaphragm, and thereby a concave upper and a convex lower surface are presented (see Chapter 2, p. 20). The levator ani consists of a pubococcygeus and iliococcygeus portion (Kearney and colleagues, 2004).

The posterior and lateral portions of the pelvic floor, which are not filled out by the levator ani, are occupied bilaterally by the piriformis and coccygeus muscles. The levator ani varies in thickness from 3 to 5 mm, though its margins encircling the rectum and vagina are somewhat thicker. During pregnancy, the levator ani usually undergoes hypertrophy, forming a thick band that extends backward from the pubis and encircles the vagina about 2 cm above the plane of the hymen. On contraction, the levator ani draws both the rectum and the vagina forward and upward in the direction of the symphysis pubis and thereby acts to close the vagina. The more superficial muscles of the perineum are too delicate to serve more than an accessory function.

In the first stage of labor, the membranes, when intact, and the fetal presenting part serve a role in dilating the upper portion of the vagina. The most marked change consists of the stretching of the fibers of the levator ani muscles and the thinning of the central portion of the perineum, which becomes transformed from a wedge-shaped mass of tissue 5 cm in thickness to a thin, almost transparent membranous structure less than 1 cm thick. When the perineum is distended maximally, the anus becomes markedly dilated and presents an opening that varies from 2 to 3 cm in diameter and through which the anterior wall of the rectum bulges. The extraordinary number and size of the blood vessels that supply the vagina and pelvic floor effect a great increase in the amount of blood loss when these tissues are torn.

Third Stage of Labor: Delivery of Placenta and Membranes. The third stage of labor begins immediately after delivery of the fetus and involves the separation and expulsion of the placenta and membranes. As the infant is born, the uterus spontaneously contracts around its diminishing contents. Normally, by the time the infant is completely delivered, the uterine cavity is nearly obliterated and the organ consists of an almost solid mass of muscle, several centimeters thick, above the thinner lower segment. The uterine fundus now lies just below the level of the umbilicus.

This sudden diminution in uterine size is inevitably accompanied by a decrease in the area of the placental implantation site (Fig. 6–13). For the placenta to accommodate itself to this reduced area, it increases in thickness, but because of limited placental elasticity, it is forced to buckle. The resulting tension causes the weakest layer of the decidua—the decidua

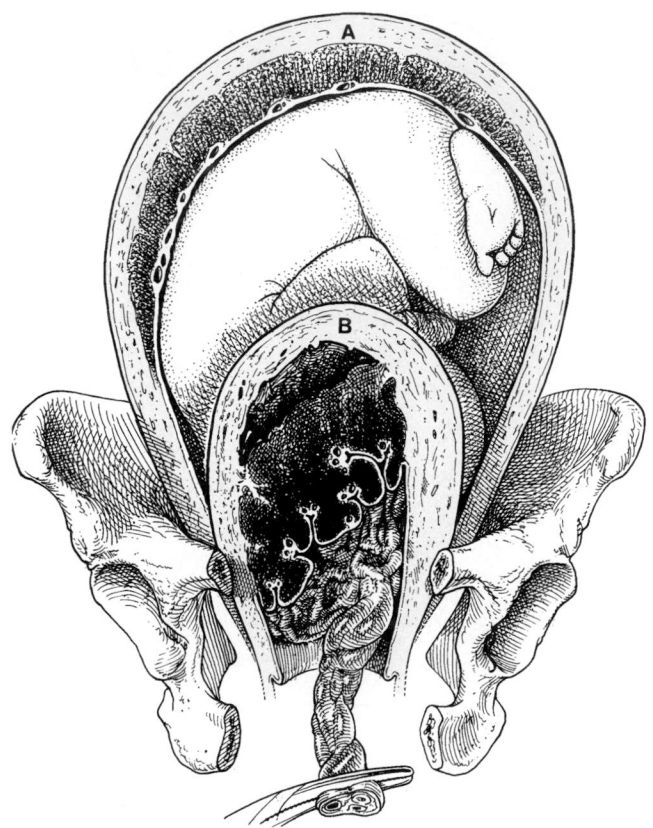

FIGURE 6–13. Diminution in size of the placental site after birth of the infant. **A.** Spatial relations before birth. **B.** Placental spatial relations after birth.

spongiosa—to give way, and cleavage takes place at that site. Therefore, separation of the placenta results primarily from a disproportion created between the unchanged size of the placenta and the reduced size of the underlying implantation site. During cesarean delivery, this phenomenon may be directly observed when the placenta is implanted posteriorly.

Cleavage of the placenta is facilitated greatly by the nature of the loose structure of the spongy decidua, which may be likened to the row of perforations between postage stamps. As separation proceeds, a hematoma forms between the separating placenta and the remaining decidua. The hematoma is usually the result, rather than the cause, of the separation, because in some cases bleeding is negligible. The hematoma may, however, accelerate the process of cleavage. Because the separation of the placenta is through the spongy layer of the decidua, part of the decidua is cast off with the placenta, whereas the rest remains attached to the myometrium. The amount of decidual tissue retained at the placental site varies.

Placental separation ordinarily occurs within a very few minutes after delivery. Brandt (1933) and others, based on results obtained in combined clinical and radiographic studies, supported the idea that because the periphery of the placenta is probably the most adherent portion, separation usually begins elsewhere. Occasionally some degree of separation begins even before the third stage of labor, probably accounting

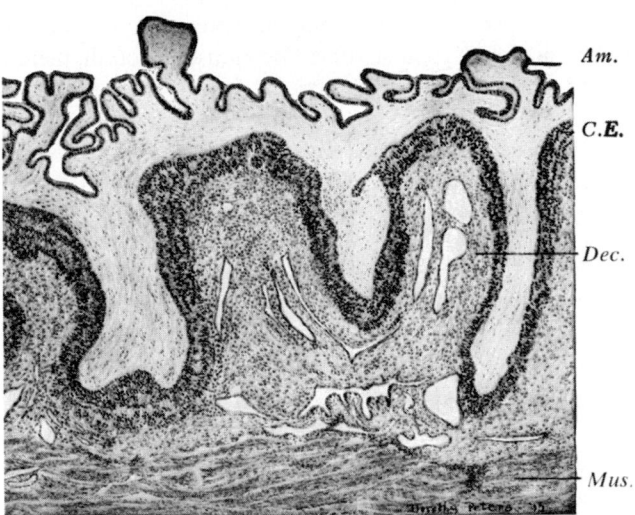

FIGURE 6–14. Folding of membranes as uterine cavity decreases in size. (Am. = amnion; C.E. = cytotrophoblast epithelium of chorion laeve; Dec. = decidua parietalis; Mus. = myometrium.)

for certain cases of fetal heart rate decelerations that occur just before expulsion of the infant.

SEPARATION OF AMNIOCHORION. The great decrease in the surface area of the uterine cavity simultaneously causes the fetal membranes (amniochorion) and the parietal decidua to be thrown into innumerable folds that increase the thickness of this layer from less than 1 mm to 3 to 4 mm. The lining of the uterus early in the third stage indicates that much of the parietal layer of decidua parietalis is included between the folds of the festooned amnion and chorion laeve (Fig. 6–14). The membranes usually remain in situ until the separation of the placenta is nearly completed. These are then peeled off the uterine wall, partly by the further contraction of the myometrium and partly by traction that is exerted by the separated placenta, which lies in the thin lower uterine segment or in the upper portion of the vagina. The body of the uterus at that time normally forms an almost solid mass of muscle, the anterior and posterior walls of which, each measuring 4 to 5 cm in thickness, lie in close apposition such that the uterine cavity is almost obliterated.

PLACENTAL EXTRUSION. After the placenta has separated from its implantation site, the pressure exerted upon it by the uterine walls causes it to slide downward into the lower uterine segment or the upper vagina. In some cases the placenta may be expelled by an increase in abdominal pressure, but women in the recumbent position frequently cannot expel the placenta spontaneously. An artificial means of completing the third stage is therefore generally required. The usual method employed is alternately to compress and elevate the fundus, while exerting minimal traction on the umbilical cord.

When the central, or usual, type of placental separation occurs, the retroplacental hematoma is believed to push the placenta toward the uterine cavity, first the central portion and then the rest. The placenta, thus inverted and weighted with the hematoma, then descends. Because the surrounding membranes are still attached to the decidua, the placenta can descend only by dragging the membranes along as they peel off its periphery. Consequently, the sac formed by the membranes is inverted, with the glistening amnion over the placental surface presenting at the vulva. The retroplacental hematoma either follows the placenta or is found within the inverted sac. In this process, known as the *Schultze mechanism* of placental expulsion, blood from the placental site pours into the inverted sac, not escaping externally until after extrusion of the placenta. In the other method of placental extrusion, known as the *Duncan mechanism,* separation of the placenta occurs first at the periphery, with the result that blood collects between the membranes and the uterine wall and escapes from the vagina. In this circumstance, the placenta descends to the vagina sideways, and the maternal surface is the first to appear at the vulva.

PHASE 3 OF PARTURITION: THE PUERPERIUM. Immediately after delivery, and for about an hour or so thereafter, the myometrium must be held in a state of rigid and persistent contraction and retraction, which effects compression of the large uterine vessels and thrombosis of their lumens. In this coordinated fashion, severe postpartum hemorrhage is prevented. During the early puerperium, a maternal-type behavior pattern develops and maternal–infant bonding begins. The onset of lactogenesis and milk let-down in maternal mammary glands also is, in an evolutionary sense, crucial to the bringing forth of young. Finally, involution of the uterus, which restores this organ to the nonpregnant state, and the reinstitution of ovulation must be accomplished in preparation for the next pregnancy. Four to six weeks usually are required for complete uterine involution; however, this process is dependent on the duration of breast feeding. Infertility usually persists as long as breast feeding is continued because of lactation-induced (prolactin-mediated) anovulation and amenorrhea (see Chap. 32, p. 746).

PHYSIOLOGICAL AND BIOCHEMICAL PROCESSES REGULATING PARTURITION

The physiological processes in human pregnancy that result in the initiation of parturition and the onset of labor remain poorly defined. Presently, there are two general theorems on the mechanisms regulating the initiation of labor. Viewed simplistically, these are the *retreat from pregnancy maintenance* and the *uterotonin induction of parturition* hypotheses. Several combinations of selected tenets of these two postulates are incorporated into the theorems of most investigators.

Some researchers also speculate that the mature human fetus is the source of the initial signal for the commencement of the parturitional process. Other investigators suggest that one or more uterotonins, produced in increased amounts or an elevation in the population of its myometrial receptors, is the proximate cause of the initiation of human parturition. Indeed, an obligatory role for one or more uterotonins is included in most parturition theories, either as a primary or a secondary phenomenon in the final events of childbirth. Both of these suppositions rely on careful regulation of the activity of the myometrial smooth muscle cell contraction. Therefore, a detailed understanding of this critical tissue and its regulation aids in understanding normal and pathological progression of the various phases of parturition.

ANATOMICAL AND PHYSIOLOGICAL CONSIDERATIONS OF THE MYOMETRIUM.

There are unique characteristics of smooth muscle, including myometrium, compared with those of skeletal muscle. Huszar and Walsh (1989) point out that these differences create an advantage for the myometrium in the efficiency of uterine contractions and delivery of the fetus. First, the degree of shortening of smooth muscle cells with contractions may be one order of magnitude greater than that attained in striated muscle cells. Second, forces can be exerted in smooth muscle cells in any direction, whereas the contraction force generated by skeletal muscle is always aligned with the axis of the muscle fibers. Third, smooth muscle is not organized in the same manner as skeletal muscle, viz., in myometrium the thick and thin filaments are found in long, random bundles throughout

the cells. This arrangement facilitates greater shortening and force-generating capacity of smooth muscle. Fourth, there is the advantage that multidirectional force generation in the uterus—fundus versus lower uterine segment—permits versatility in expulsive force directionality that can be brought to bear irrespective of the lie or presentation of the fetus.

REGULATION OF MYOMETRIAL CONTRACTION AND RELAXATION.

The control of myometrial contraction is at the heart of understanding both the maintenance of pregnancy and the onset of labor. The regulation of myometrial cell contraction versus relaxation can be divided temporally into acute and chronic mechanisms. Acutely, the interaction of myosin and actin is essential to muscle contraction. Myosin (Mr about 500,000) is comprised of multiple light and heavy chains and is arranged in thick myofilaments. The interaction of myosin and actin, which causes activation of adenosine triphosphatase, adenosine triphosphate hydrolysis, and force generation, is effected by enzymatic phosphorylation of the 20-kd light chain of myosin (Stull and colleagues, 1988, 1998). This phosphorylation reaction is catalyzed by the enzyme *myosin light chain kinase,* which is activated by calcium (Fig. 6–15). Calcium binds to calmodulin, a calcium-binding regulatory protein, which in turn binds to and activates myosin light chain kinase. In this manner, agents that act on myometrial smooth muscle cells to cause an increase in the intracellular cytosolic concentration of calcium

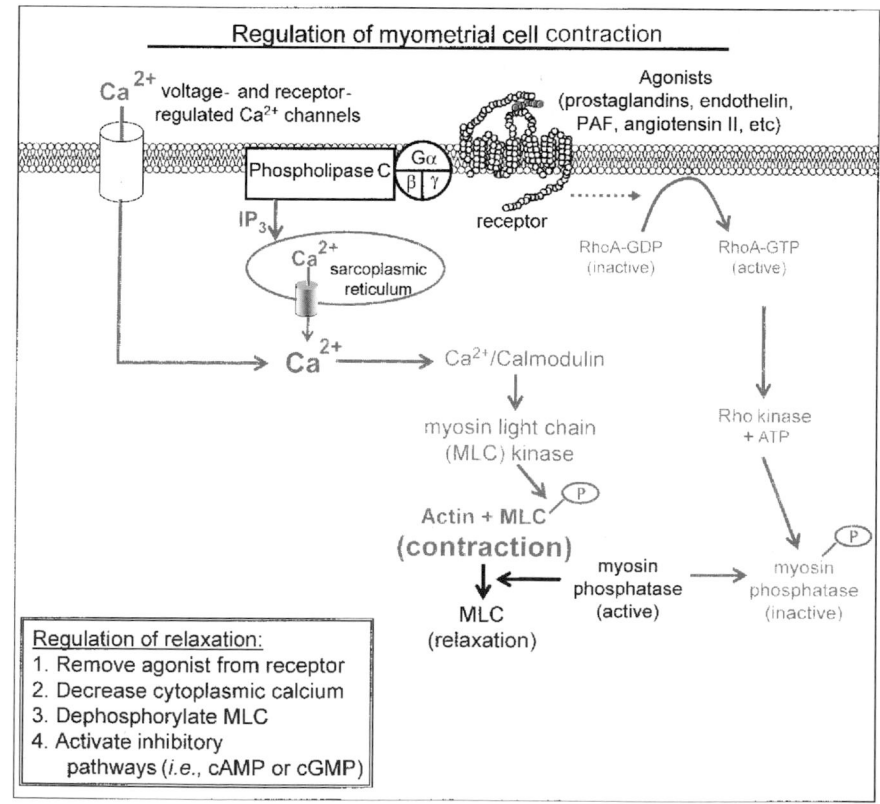

FIGURE 6–15. Regulation of myometrial smooth muscle cell contraction and relaxation. There are numerous agonists that bind cell surface receptors and activate phospholipase C and its production of inositol 1,4,5-trisphosphate (IP$_3$). IP$_3$ will bind receptors on the sarcoplasmic reticulum and cause release of calcium (Ca^{2+}) into the cytoplasm. Ca^{2+} can also be increased through voltage- or receptor-activated channels. Ca^{2+} will activate calmodulin, leading to increased activity of myosin light chain kinase (MLC kinase) and phosphorylation of myosin light chain (MLC). Phosphorylated MLC interacts with actin, activating adenosine triphosphatase and, through the hydrolysis of adenosine triphosphate (ATP), generates the force needed for contraction. Contraction can be sustained by activation of the guanosine triphosphate (GTP)–binding protein, RhoA, and Rho kinase, which will phosphorylate and inhibit myosin phosphatase. Relaxation results from reversal by removal of the ligand from its receptor. Relaxation also can occur through the activity of hormones that inactivate MLC kinase, as has been seen for agents that activate the cyclic adenosine monophosphate (cAMP) or cyclic guanosine monophosphate signaling pathway. (PAF = platelet-activating factor.) (Based on Webb, 2003.)

$([Ca^{2+}]_i)$ promote contraction. The increase in $[Ca^{2+}]_i$ is often transient, but contractions can be prolonged through the inhibition of myosin phosphatase activity by Rho kinase, which is activated in a receptor-dependent fashion (Woodcock and associates, 2004). Conditions that cause a decrease in $[Ca^{2+}]_i$ favor relaxation. Ordinarily, agents that cause an increase in the intracellular concentration of cyclic adenosine monophosphate (cAMP) or cyclic guanosine monophosphate (cGMP) promote uterine relaxation. It is believed that cAMP and cGMP act to cause a decrease in $[Ca^{2+}]_i$, although the exact mechanism(s) is not defined.

Myometrial cell contractions also can be greatly influenced by the chronic action of hormones on the contractile status of the cell. This influence can occur through the effects that mediate the transcription of key genes that repress or enhance the contractility of the cell. Considerable data indicate that uterine activity is influenced through the regulation of the so-called *contraction-associated proteins* (*CAPs*). These proteins include channels associated with smooth muscle excitation and contraction, gap junction components, and uterotonic stimulatory or inhibitory receptors.

Myometrial Gap Junctions. Like other muscle cells, the cellular signals that control myometrial contraction and relaxation can be effectively transferred between cells through intercellular junctional channels. Communication is established between myometrial cells by gap junctions that facilitate the passage of electrical or ionic coupling currents as well as metabolite coupling. The transmembrane channels that make up the gap junctions consist of two protein "hemi-channels," termed *connexons*. Each connexon is hexameric assemblage of a type of protein called a connexin. These pairs of connexons establish a conduit for the exchange of small molecules (Mr less than 1000) and ions between cells.

The physiological importance of optimal numbers (area) of functional permeable gap junctions between myometrial cells is believed to be the establishment of electrical synchrony in the myometrium, which effects coordination of contractions and thereby greater force during labor. As discussed below, the regulated expression of gap junction proteins is one way to regulate uterine quiescence.

Cell Surface Receptors As Regulators of Myometrium. Myometrial cells have developed a unique system of regulatory pathways that rely not only on estrogen and progesterone receptors but also on a variety of cell surface receptors that can directly regulate the contractile state of the cell. The three major classes of cell surface receptors are the G-protein–linked, ion channel–linked, and enzyme-linked. Multiple examples of each class of receptors have been identified in human myometrium, and examples of each class appear to be modified during the phases of parturition. Most of these heptahelical receptors are associated with the

activation of adenylyl cyclase. Other heptahelical receptors in myometrium, however, are more commonly associated with G-protein–mediated activation of phospholipase C, which will lead to increased $[Ca^{2+}]_i$ and myometrial cell contraction. Many G-protein–coupled receptors that participate in regulation of myometrial activity have been characterized. These were reviewed recently by Lopez (2003).

Ligands for the heptahelical receptors include neuropeptides, hormones, and autacoids. Many of these are available to the myometrium during pregnancy in high concentration by several routes: from maternal blood (endocrine), contiguous tissues or adjacent cells (paracrine), or direct synthesis in the myometrial smooth muscle cells (autocrine) (Fig. 6–16). It is important to note that the myometrial response to a hormone can change during the course of pregnancy. Thus, it is conceivable that hormone action on the myometrium is regulated at several levels, including the expression of the heptahelical receptor, its associated G-proteins, or the effector proteins in the plasma membrane. Specifically, the imposition of quiescence (activation of adenylyl cyclase) or the facilitation of contractions (activation of phospholipase C and increased $[Ca^{2+}]_i$) may in some cases be regulated by the same hormone.

A FAIL-SAFE SYSTEM THAT MAINTAINS UTERINE QUIESCENCE. The myometrial smooth muscle is, inherently, a contractile tissue. Isolated strips of myometrium from uteri of nonpregnant women placed in an isotonic water bath contract in a rhythmical fashion without added stimuli, even in the presence of prostaglandin synthase inhibitors (Crankshaw and Dyal, 1994). Therefore, it is difficult to comprehend how the uterus can be expanded to accommodate a 3500-g fetus, 1 liter of amnionic fluid, and 800 g of placenta and membranes without erupting into powerful contractions. The myometrial quiescence of phase 0 of parturition is so remarkable and successful that it probably is induced by multiple independent and cooperative biomolecular processes. Individually, some of these processes may be redundant; that is, pregnancy may continue in the absence of one or more processes that normally contribute to the fail-safe system of pregnancy maintenance.

The physiological investments that must be made to sustain the uterine quiescence of phase 0 are enormous. It is likely that all manner of biomolecular systems—neural, endocrine, paracrine, and autocrine—are called on to implement and coordinate a state of relative uterine unresponsiveness. *Moreover, a complementary fail-safe system that protects the uterus against agents that could perturb the tranquil state of phase 0 also must be in place.*

Phase 0 of human parturition and its quiescent state are likely the result of many factors, including:

1. Actions of estrogen and progesterone via intracellular receptors.

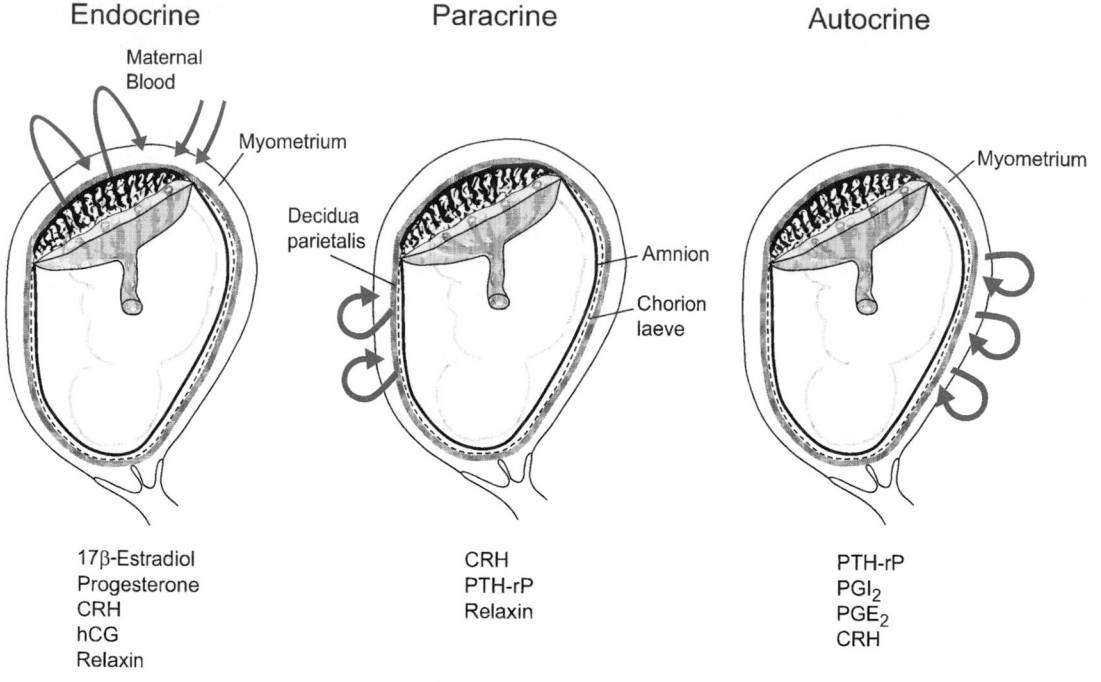

FIGURE 6–16. Theoretical fail-safe system involving endocrine, paracrine, and autocrine mechanisms for the maintenance of phase 0 of parturition, uterine quiescence. (CRH = corticotropin-releasing hormone; hCG = human chorionic gonadotropin; PGE_2 = prostaglandin E_2; PGI_2 = prostaglandin I_2; PTH-rP = parathyroid hormone–related peptide.)

2. Myometrial cell plasma membrane receptor-mediated increases in cAMP.
3. The generation of cGMP.
4. Other systems, including modifications in myometrial cell ion channels.

Because phase 0 is the result of several independent pathways, it is likely that defects—either naturally occurring or pharmacologically induced—in one component of this system might not necessarily preclude the successful maintenance of pregnancy to term (Fig. 6–17).

Progesterone and Estrogen Contributions to Phase 0 of Parturition. In many species the role of the sex steroids is clear—progesterone inhibits and estrogen promotes the events leading to parturition. In humans, however, it seems most likely that both estrogen and progesterone are

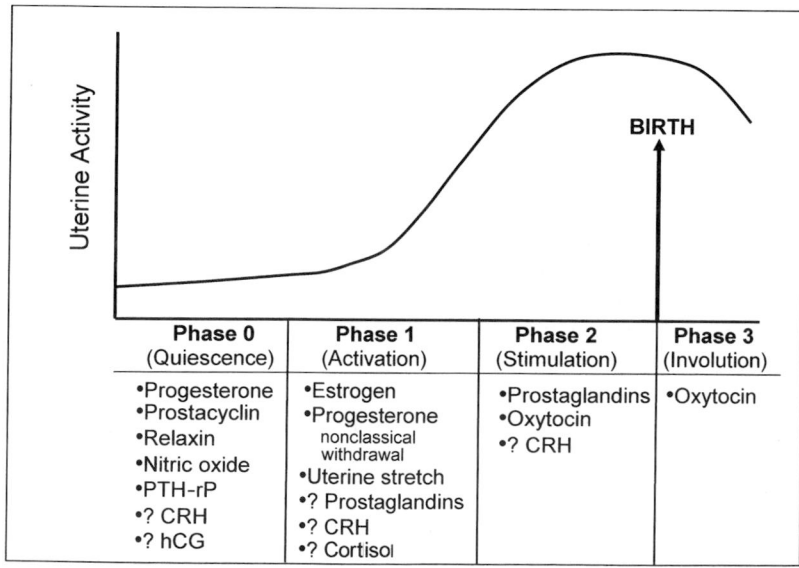

FIGURE 6–17. The key factors thought to regulate the phases of parturition. (CRH = corticotropin-releasing hormone; hCG = human chorionic gonadotrophin; PTH-rP = parathyroid hormone–related peptide.) (Based on Challis and co-workers, 2002.)

components of a broader-based fail-safe biomolecular system that implements and maintains phase 0 of human parturition and thus the maintenance of pregnancy. In many species the removal of progesterone, or *progesterone withdrawal,* directly precedes the progression of phase 0 into phase 1 of parturition. In addition, providing progesterone to some species will delay parturition and decrease myometrial activity (Challis and Lye, 1994). In these species the progestational effects of progesterone have been well studied, leading to a better understanding of why the myometrium of phase 0 is relatively noncontractile.

The plasma levels of estrogen and progesterone in normal human pregnancy are enormous. Both are in great excess of the affinity constants for estrogen and progesterone receptors. For this reason, it is difficult to comprehend how relatively subtle changes in the ratio of the concentrations of these two steroids could modulate physiological processes during human pregnancy. The teleological evidence, however, for a role of the progesterone-to-estrogen ratio in the maintenance of pregnancy and parturition is overwhelming. The rationale for the supraphysiological concentrations of both estrogens and progesterone in human pregnancy is still poorly defined.

It has been presumed for decades that progesterone action is essential for the successful maintenance of pregnancy. Regrettably, however, neither the biomolecular evidence for this nor the role of other agents in promoting uterine quiescence is clearly defined. Because of its action in other mammalian species, however, it is presumed that progesterone acts to establish and maintain the uterine phase 0 of parturition.

The exact role of estrogen in regulating the human uterine contractile state has always proven difficult to elucidate. Defining estrogen action is complicated by the presence of cell surface and nuclear receptors that can respond to estrogen. It would appear, however, that estrogen can act to promote progesterone responsiveness and in doing so promote uterine quiescence. In many responsive tissues, the estrogen receptor, acting via the estrogen response element of the progesterone receptor gene, induces progesterone receptors synthesis.

Steroid Hormone Regulation of Myometrial Cell-to-Cell Communication. Considerable data indicate that progesterone increases uterine quiescence by direct or indirect effects that cause decreased expression of the contraction-associated proteins. Key proteins in the CAP grouping would include channels associated with smooth muscle excitation–contraction, gap junction components, and uterotonic stimulatory receptors. Progesterone has been shown to inhibit expression of the gap junctional protein connexin 43 in several rodent models of labor. Administration of progesterone prevents or delays labor and prevents the normal induction of connexin 43 expression seen at term during uterine activation prior to labor. Inhibition of progesterone activity at midgestation using the progesterone receptor antagonist RU 486 leads

to a premature induction of connexin 43 protein production in the uterus and thus stimulates labor.

Estrogen treatment promotes myometrial gap junction formation in some animals by increasing connexin 43 synthesis. The simultaneous administration of anti-estrogens prevents this (Burghardt and colleagues, 1984). Progesterone treatment also negates the stimulatory effect of estrogen on the development of gap junctions in some animals. Conversely, progesterone antagonists lead to the premature development of gap junctions and preterm labor and delivery (Chwalisz and colleagues, 1991). In myometrial tissue obtained from pregnant women before labor, when the number of gap junctions is small, a spontaneous increase in the number of gap junctions occurs when the tissue is placed in vitro (Hayashi and collaborators, 1985). This suggests that the excised tissue is relieved from a pregnancy endocrine milieu that prevented gap junction development in vivo. The mechanisms leading to increased gap junctions at the time of labor, however, are still unclear. Chow and Lye (1994) found that the level of connexin 43 mRNA in human myometrial tissues increased before labor, between 37 and 40 weeks, and increased further after labor began. Gap junctions also increased in myometrium from laboring women. Interestingly the expression of connexin 43 protein did not increase during gestation or at labor, leaving in question the intracellular regulator of actual gap junction assembly at the time of labor. These processes appear to be regulated in part by estrogen and progesterone.

Heptahelical Receptors That Promote Myometrial Relaxation. The possibility also must be considered that the contractile unresponsiveness imposed on the uterus during most of human pregnancy is ensured by multiple processes that act independently and cooperatively to establish uterine quiescence. A number of heptahelical receptors that nominally are associated with $G_{\alpha s}$-mediated activation of adenylyl cyclase and increased levels of cAMP are present in myometrium. These receptors together with appropriate ligands may act (in concert with sex steroid hormones) as part of a fail-safe system to maintain uterine quiescence, phase 0 of parturition (Price and associates, 2000; Sanborn and colleagues, 1998).

BETA-ADRENORECEPTORS. In studies of the role of cAMP signaling in causing myometrium relaxation, the β-adrenergic receptors have served as prototypes. Most commonly, the β-adrenergic receptors mediate $G_{\alpha s}$-stimulated increases in adenylyl cyclase, increased levels of cAMP, and myometrial cell relaxation. The rate-limiting factor in the β-receptor system is likely the number of β-receptors expressed and the level of adenylyl cyclase expression. The number of G-proteins in most systems far exceeds the number of receptors and effector molecules. The exact role of catecholamines in maintaining uterine quiescence in vivo remains ill defined.

LUTEINIZING HORMONE (LH) AND CHORIONIC GONADOTROPIN (hCG). The heptahelical receptor for LH–hCG has been demonstrated in a number of extragonadal tissues, including myometrial smooth muscle and blood vessels (Lei and co-workers, 1992; Ziecik and colleagues, 1992). Initially, their identification seemed quite aberrant considering the more commonly recognized tissue localization in the ovary and testis. The levels of the LH–hCG receptor in myometrium during pregnancy are greater before than during labor (Zuo and colleagues, 1994). Chorionic gonadotropin acts to activate adenylyl cyclase by way of a plasma membrane receptor–$G_{\alpha s}$-linked system. This causes a decrease in contraction frequency and force and a decrease in tissue-specific myometrial cell gap junctions (Ambrus and Rao, 1994; Eta and co-workers, 1994). Thus, the high circulating levels of hCG during pregnancy may be one mechanism causing uterine quiescence.

RELAXIN. This peptide hormone is a member of the insulin-like growth factor family of proteins, consisting of an A and B chain (Bogic and associates, 1995; Weiss, 1995). There are two separate human relaxin genes, designated H1 and H2. Relaxin in plasma of pregnant women is believed to originate exclusively by secretion from the corpus luteum. Plasma levels of relaxin are greatest and peak at about 1 ng/mL between 8 and 12 weeks, and thereafter decline to lower levels that persist until term. The plasma membrane receptor for relaxin mediates the activation of adenylyl cyclase and promotes myometrial relaxation, but also effects cervical softening. Consequently, it has not been possible to envision a clear-cut role for this hormone in human parturition.

CORTICOTROPIN-RELEASING HORMONE (CRH). This heptahelical receptor is present in myometrium during pregnancy. There are multiple isoforms of the receptor in myometrium, and their affinity and coupling are modified late in pregnancy (Grammatopoulos and associates, 1994, 1995; Hillhouse and colleagues, 1993). CRH is synthesized in the placenta, amnion, decidua, and myometrium. As discussed below, plasma levels of CRH increase during the final 6 to 8 weeks of normal pregnancy in dramatic fashion. Because of this, several investigators have suggested that CRH is involved in the initiation of human parturition (Wadhwa and colleagues, 1998). CRH receptors can signal through either cAMP or calcium, thus CRH may cause relaxation or contraction of myometrial cells depending on the receptor isoform present. It is for that reason that CRH could potentially play the role of a uterorelaxant during phase 0 and a uterotonin in phases 1 and 2 of parturition.

PARATHYROID HORMONE–RELATED PROTEIN (PTH-rP). The receptor for PTH–PTH-rP is a plasma membrane heptahelical receptor. Most often this receptor initiates $G_{\alpha s}$-mediated activation of adenylyl cyclase. PTH-rP is expressed in myometrium, decidua, amnion, and trophoblast. Treatment of human myometrial cells with estrogen and transforming growth factor-β causes an increase in the levels of PTH-rP

mRNA (Casey and associates, 1992; Paspalliaris and associates, 1995). PTH-rP expression in smooth muscle, including myometrium, is increased by muscle stretch (Daifotis and associates, 1992; Yamamoto and colleagues, 1992). Whereas the function of PTH-rP in uterine physiology is not established, it may serve to maximize uterine blood flow during myometrial contractions by its vasorelaxant action (Thiede and colleagues, 1991a, 1991b). PTH-rP also may act on myometrial smooth muscle to facilitate the maintenance of uterine tranquility.

PROSTAGLANDINS. The prostanoids interact with a family of eight different heptahelical receptors, several of which are expressed in the myometrium (Myatt and Lye, 2004). Although prostaglandins most commonly have been considered as uterotonins (see p. 173), prostanoids can sometimes act as smooth muscle relaxants. Because the individual prostanoid can have such diverse effects, it is important to review the major synthetic pathways involved in prostaglandin biosynthesis (Fig. 6–18). Prostaglandins are produced using plasma membrane–derived arachidonic acid, which usually

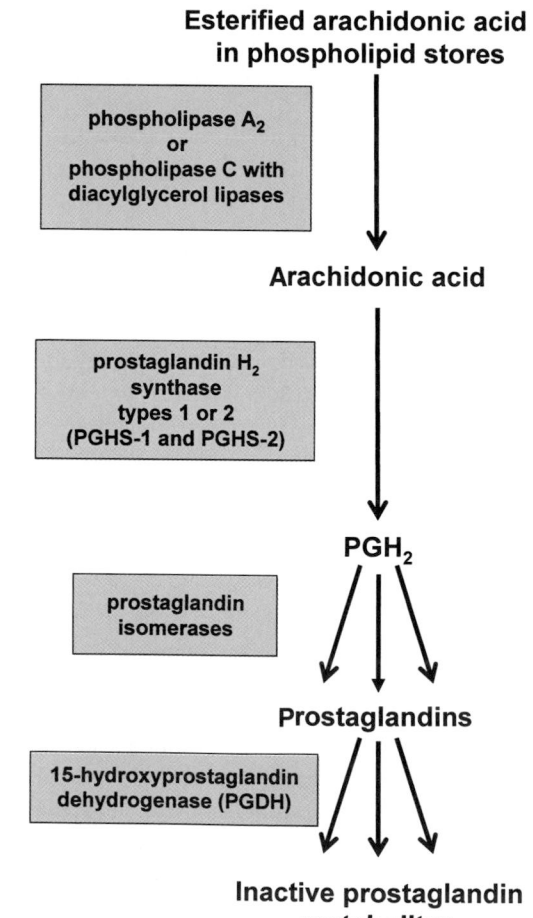

FIGURE 6–18. Overview of the prostaglandin biosynthetic pathway. (PGH_2 = prostaglandin H_2.)

is released by the action of the phospholipases A_2 or C on membrane phospholipids. Arachidonic acid can then act as substrate for both type 1 and type 2 prostaglandin H synthase (PGHS-1 and -2), also called cyclooxygenase-1 and -2. In general PGHS-1 is constitutively expressed, whereas PGHS-2 expression is highly regulated. These two isoforms share 65-percent sequence similarity, and both will convert arachidonic acid to the unstable endoperoxide prostaglandin G_2 and then to prostaglandin H_2. These enzymes are the target of many nonsteroidal anti-inflammatory drugs (NSAIDs), and the ability of these or new specific NSAIDs to act as tocolytics to safely prevent preterm labor is an active area of research (Loudon and co-workers, 2003; Olson, 2003). As substrate for several prostaglandin isomerases, prostaglandin H_2 is converted to active prostaglandins, including PGE_2, $PGF_{2\alpha}$ and PGI_2. The expression of the prostaglandin isomerases is tissue-specific, thus controlling the relative production of the various prostaglandins. However, within a tissue the activity of these enzymes does not appear to be rate limiting. Another important control point for prostaglandin activity is metabolism, which most often occurs through the action of 15-hydroxyprostaglandin dehydrogenase (PGDH). The expression of this enzyme can be regulated in the uterus, which is important because of its ability to rapidly inactivate prostaglandins to their respective 15-keto metabolites.

The effect of prostaglandins on tissue targets is complicated by the fact that there are a number of G-protein–coupled prostaglandin receptors (Coleman and associates, 1994). The prostaglandin family of receptors is classified according to the specificity of binding of a given receptor to a particular prostaglandin. The receptors (and their naturally occurring, preferred ligands) are TP (thromboxane A_2), DP (PGD_2), IP (prostacyclin or PGI_2), FP ($PGF_{2\alpha}$), and EP_1 to EP_4 (PGE_2). The signaling pathways activated by these receptors differ in that DP and IP receptors increase intracellular cAMP, whereas FP receptors increase intracellular calcium. In addition, the EP receptor family has several isoforms, including EP_2 and EP_4, which activate cAMP production, and EP_1 and EP_3, which increase intracellular calcium levels. With this in mind, both PGE_2 and PGI_2 could act to maintain uterine quiescence by increasing cAMP signaling.

Indeed, PGE_2, PGD_2, and PGI_2 have been shown to cause relaxation of vascular smooth muscle and vasodilatation in many circumstances. Thus, either the generation of specific prostaglandins or the relative expression of the various prostaglandin receptors may determine the responses of human myometrium to prostaglandins. For example, Breuiller and co-workers (1991) found that prostanoids stimulate adenylyl cyclase activity in myometrium obtained at 32 to 35 weeks, but not in tissue obtained at 39 to 40 weeks. More recent studies have shown alterations in the expression of the EP receptor isoforms in myometrium in laboring women and baboons (Lyall and associates, 2002; Smith and colleagues, 1998, 2001). In addition to changes with gestation, several studies show that there may be regional

changes in the upper and lower uterine segments. Thus, it is entirely possible that prostanoids contribute to myometrial relaxation at one stage of pregnancy and to regional myometrial contractions—in the fundus—after the initiation of parturition (Myatt and Lye, 2004).

ATRIAL AND BRAIN NATRIURETIC PEPTIDES AND CYCLIC GUANOSINE MONOPHOSPHATE (cGMP). The activation of guanylyl cyclase gives rise to increased intracellular levels of cGMP, which also promotes smooth muscle relaxation (Word and colleagues, 1993). The intracellular levels of cGMP can be stimulated by either of the two forms of atrial natriuretic peptide (ANP) and brain natriuretic peptide (BNP) receptors that are both present in the myometrium during human pregnancy (Itoh and co-workers, 1994). These receptors structurally include the enzymatic activity of guanylyl cyclase and mediate an increase in the cellular levels of cGMP. Specifically, the ANP–BNP receptor molecule is a guanylyl cyclase. BNP is secreted by amnion in large amounts, and ANP is expressed in placenta (Itoh and associates, 1993; Lim and Gude, 1995).

The soluble form of guanylyl cyclase is activated by nitric oxide, which, because of its very hydrophobic nature, readily penetrates the plasma membrane to enter cells. Nitric oxide reacts with iron in the active site of the soluble guanylyl cyclase enzyme, stimulating it to produce cGMP, and acts to cause myometrial relaxation (Izumi and colleagues, 1993). Nitric oxide is synthesized in decidua, myometrial blood vessels, and nerves (Yallampalli and colleagues, 1994a, 1994b). Whether nitric oxide gains access to the myometrium and how the synthesis and action of nitric oxide is regulated as it pertains to a potential contribution to uterine quiescence is not understood.

Accelerated Uterotonin Degradation and Phase 0 of Parturition. In addition to pregnancy-induced compounds that stimulate myometrial cell refractoriness, there are striking increases in the activities of enzymes that degrade or inactivate endogenously produced uterotonins. Some of these uterotonins (and their degredative enzymes) include prostaglandins (e.g., PGDH), endothelins (e.g., enkephalinase), oxytocin (e.g., oxytocinase), histamine (e.g., diamine oxidase), catecholamines (e.g., catechol *O*-methyltransferase), angiotensin-II (e.g., angiotensinases), and platelet-activating factor (PAF) (e.g., PAF-acetylhydrolase). The activities of several of these enzymes are increased by progesterone action and many decrease late in gestation (Bates and co-workers, 1979; Casey and associates, 1980, Germain and colleagues, 1994; Yasuda and Johnston, 1992).

FAIL-SAFE SYSTEMS FOR UTERINE ACTIVATION. The morphological and functional changes in the myometrium and cervix that prepare the uterus for labor are considered phase 1 of parturition. This process is characterized by the development of uterotonin sensitivity, improved intercellular communicability via gap junctions, and alterations in the capacity of myometrial cells to regulate the concentration of cytoplasmic Ca^{2+}. The processes leading to enhanced uterine responsiveness also have been termed *activation* by Challis and associates (2000). There are likely multiple systems responsible for the uterine activation seen during phase 1 (see Fig. 6–17). As the functional contractile capacity of the myometrium is realized and the cervix is ripened, phase 1 merges into phase 2, active labor. Alterations in the timing of these processes are likely to cause preterm and delayed labor, making an understanding of these prelabor events key.

Classical Progesterone Withdrawal Does Not Cause Human Parturition. In many species the drop in maternal plasma progesterone levels, *progesterone withdrawal*, allows activation of the uterus in preparation for labor. This decrease in progesterone levels is associated with an increase in estrogen levels in several species, and this shift in the steroid milieu is thought to have dramatic effects on both the cervix and the myometrium. In primates, however, plasma progesterone levels do not decrease before labor (Challis and Lye, 1994). Plasma levels decline only after delivery of the placenta. Nonetheless, the morphological and functional modifications that prepare the uterus for labor occur in a timely manner in human pregnancy just as in those species in which progesterone withdrawal is a clearly demonstrable endocrine antecedent of parturition.

In species that exhibit progesterone withdrawal, progression of parturition to labor can be blocked by administering progesterone to the mother. In pregnant women, however, there are conflicting reports as to whether or not progesterone administration can delay the timely onset of parturition or prevent preterm labor. The majority of studies suggest that progesterone cannot prevent preterm labor and does not appear to extend labor in the control group (Goldstein and associates, 1989). In contrast, there have been some optimistic reports on the ability of the progesterone metabolite, 17-hydroxyprogesterone, to minimally decrease the incidence of preterm labor in high-risk populations (Johnson and associates, 1979; Keirse, 1990; Meis and co-workers, 2003; Yemini and colleagues, 1985). The fact that 17-hydroxyprogesterone is much less potent than progesterone at binding and activating the progesterone receptor suggests that additional research needs to be done to explain the action of this steroid and how it could prevent the onset of preterm labor.

Progesterone Receptor Antagonists and Human Parturition. When the steroidal antiprogestin RU 486, or mifepristone, is administered to women during the latter phase of the ovarian cycle, it induces menstruation prematurely. It is also quite effective in the induction of abortion during early stages of pregnancy (Avrech and co-workers, 1991). This compound is a classical steroid antagonist, acting at the level of the progesterone receptor. Although less effective in inducing abortion or labor in women later in pregnancy, RU 486 remains effective in ripening the cervix and increasing myometrium sensitivity to uterotonins (Chwalisz and Garfield, 1994; Chwalisz, 1994). Further support for the ability of progesterone withdrawal to effect labor in primates can be found in studies that decreased circulating progesterone by inhibiting the enzyme 3β-hydroxysteroid dehydrogenase, which induced labor (Haluska and associates, 1997; Selinger and co-workers, 1987). One interpretation for these data is that in humans the inhibition of progesterone action is important for activation phase of parturition, but there is a "hidden" or unique form of functional progesterone withdrawal that ends uterine quiescence.

Functional Progesterone Withdrawal in Human Parturition. As an alternative to classical progesterone withdrawal, many researchers have focused on determining if humans have evolved unique mechanisms to inhibit progesterone action. This theory of functional progesterone withdrawal or progesterone antagonism could be mediated in the uterus through several mechanisms, including:

1. Changes in the relative expression of the progesterone receptor or of its two isoforms (PR-A and PR-B).
2. Posttranslational modifications of the progesterone receptor causing decreased activity.
3. Alterations in progesterone receptor activity through changes in the expression of co-activators or co-repressors that directly influence receptor function.
4. Local inactivation of progesterone by steroid-metabolizing enzymes or the synthesis of a natural antagonist.

Indeed, there is experimental evidence that lends support to each of these possible explanations for a functional progesterone withdrawal that could occur in the presence of high circulating progesterone levels. The most obvious possibility would be a late gestational decrease in activity of the progesterone receptor expression that would cause a functional withdrawal. There are now several lines of evidence that suggest that the activity of the progesterone receptor is decreased late in gestation. As was discussed in Chapter 3, there are two isoforms of the progesterone receptor (PR-A and PR-B). The PR-B isoform is more transcriptionally active than the PR-A isoform, which has actually been shown to inhibit PR-B activity. In a series of studies, it has been shown that there is a shift in relative ratio of PR-A to PR-B within the myometrium late in gestation that may be the cause of a functional progesterone withdrawal (Haluska, 2002; Madsen, 2004; Mesiano, 2002; Pieber, 2001, and all of their colleagues). Analysis of the placental membranes for PR-A and PR-B suggests that the ratio is similarly modified in decidua and chorion, but that there is a drop in overall progesterone receptor expression in the amnion (Haluska and co-workers, 2002). The activity of progesterone receptors for gene transcription also is impacted through the levels of several co-activators and co-repressors. It would appear that there is a decrease in co-activators and an increase in co-repressors for the progesterone receptor in late gestation, which would further enhance a functional withdrawal (Allport and co-workers, 2001; Condon and colleagues, 2003).

There is also evidence using rodent models that functional progesterone withdrawal within the cervix results from local inactivation of progesterone. Indeed, if mice are produced without the expression of 5α-reductase, the cervix does not ripen and parturition does not occur (Mahendroo and colleagues, 1999). Finally, there is also some support for antiprogestin-like activities of glucocorticoids on progesterone receptor activity (Karalis and co-workers, 1996). Because glucocorticoids play an important role in the initiation of parturition in several species, examining their potential role as an antiprogestin in humans warrants further study. Taken together, these observations support the concept that humans do undergo a progesterone withdrawal, which results from a decrease in receptor activity.

Oxytocin Receptors. There is still controversy as to whether oxytocin plays a role in the early phases of uterine activation or solely in the expulsive phase of labor. Most studies to evaluate the regulation of myometrial oxytocin receptor synthesis have been performed in the rat and mouse. Disruption of the oxytocin gene in the mouse does not affect parturition, suggesting that at least in this species multiple systems are in place to ensure that parturition occurs. There is little doubt, however, that there is an increase in oxytocin receptors in the myometrium during phase 1 of parturition.

Progesterone and estradiol appear to be the primary regulators of oxytocin receptor expression. Estradiol treatment either in vivo or in myometrial explants causes an increase in myometrial oxytocin receptors. This action is prevented by simultaneous treatment with progesterone (Fuchs and colleagues, 1983). Progesterone also may act within the myometrial cell to increase oxytocin receptor degradation and at the cell surface to inhibit oxytocin activation of its receptor (Bogacki and associates, 2002; Soloff and colleagues, 1983). These data indicate that one of the mechanisms whereby progesterone maintains uterine quiescence is through the inhibition of myometrial oxytocin response.

The increase in oxytocin receptors appears to be mainly regulated either directly or indirectly by estradiol. Estradiol treatment of several species leads to an increase in uterine oxytocin receptors (Blanks and co-workers, 2003; Challis and Lye, 1994). In vitro studies using myometrial cells have shown that estradiol can increase the expression of oxytocin receptors (Adachi and Oku, 1995). The level of oxytocin receptor mRNA in myometrium obtained at caesarean delivery at term is greater than that found in preterm myometrium (Wathes and co-workers, 1999). Thus, the increase in oxytocin receptor number in myometrium at term may be attributable to increased oxytocin gene transcription. An estrogen response element, however, is not present in the oxytocin receptor gene, suggesting that the stimulatory effects of estrogen may occur indirectly. Oxytocin receptors also are present in human endometrium and in decidua at term, and these stimulate prostaglandin production (Fuchs and associates, 1981). Oxytocin receptors also are present, albeit at lower levels, in amnion and chorion–decidual tissues (Benedetto and associates, 1990; Wathes and co-workers, 1999).

FETAL CONTRIBUTIONS TO INITIATION OF PARTURITION. It is intellectually intriguing to envision that the fetus, after appropriate growth and maturation of vital organs, provides the initial signal that sets the parturitional process in motion. Teleologically, this seems to be the most logical manner by which parturition could begin in a timely fashion. A signal from the human fetus could be transmitted in one of several ways, but however accomplished, the end result must include the suspension of uterine quiescence. This system of fetal signals has been most studied in fetal sheep, where the parturitional process is believed to proceed via the fetal brain, pituitary gland, adrenal glands, and fetal blood to the placenta. The human fetus also may provide a signal through a blood-borne agent that acts on the placenta. It is unlikely, however, that the initial signal for phase 1 of parturition is a uterotonin such as oxytocin, prostaglandins, or endothelin-1. Rather, it is more likely that the uterus first must be prepared for labor before a uterotonin can be optimally effective (Casey and MacDonald, 1994).

Role of Uterine Stretch in Parturition. There is now considerable evidence that fetal growth is an important component in the activation of the uterus seen in phase 1 of parturition. During the course of gestation, and in association with fetal growth, there is a significant increase in myometrial tensile stress and amnionic fluid pressure (Fisk and co-workers, 1992). Much of the work demonstrating a role for stretch in the activation of the uterus prior to labor comes from studies in rat models of parturition. In this model, stretch was required for the normal induction of specific contraction-associated proteins (CAPs). Stretch also increased expression of the gap junction protein, connexin 43, as well as oxytocin receptors. Other studies have led to the hypothesis that stretch plays an integrated role with fetal–maternal endocrine cascades in uterine activation prior to labor (Lyall and co-workers, 2002; Ou and colleagues, 1997, 1998).

Support for a role of stretch in human parturition comes from the observation that twin pregnancies are at a much greater risk of preterm labor than singletons (Gardner and co-workers, 1995). In addition, preterm labor is also significantly more common in pregnancies complicated by hydramnios, where uterine stretch would occur (Many and colleagues, 1996). Although the mechanisms causing preterm birth in twin pregnancies and in hydramnios are still debated, a role for uterine stretch must be considered.

The cell signaling systems used by stretch to regulate the myometrial cell continue to be defined. This process, termed *mechanotransduction*, may include activation of cell surface receptors or ion channels, signaling through extracellular matrix, or through the release of autocrine molecules that act directly on the myometrial cells. It appears likely that the elevated expression of CAP genes allows the myometrium to be more responsive to the uterotonins that appear late in gestation at the time of labor.

Fetal Endocrine Cascades Leading to Parturition. The ability of the fetus to provide endocrine signals that set into motion the parturitional process has been demonstrated in several species. More than 30 years ago, Liggins and associates (1967, 1973) demonstrated that the fetus provides the signal for the timely onset of parturition in sheep, and this signal was shown to come from the fetal hypothalamic–pituitary–adrenal axis. It is now well established that parturition in the sheep results from the initiation of an endocrine cascade involving a hypothalamic–pituitary–adrenal–placental axis (Whittle and co-workers, 2001).

Defining the exact mechanisms regulating human parturition has proven more difficult, and all evidence suggests that it is not regulated in the exact manner seen in the sheep. There is considerable evidence, however, that there is a placental–pituitary–adrenal axis that may play a key, albeit different, role in the timing of human parturition. Indeed, activation of the human fetal hypothalamic–pituitary–adrenal axis is considered a critical component of normal parturition. Moreover, premature activation of this axis is considered a cause of many cases of preterm labor (Challis and co-workers, 2000, 2001). As in the sheep, the steroid products of the human fetal adrenal gland are believed to have effects on the placenta and membranes that eventually promote the myometrium to transform from a quiescent to contractile state. If true, then this cascade is an important component of the activation phase of parturition. Current evidence suggests that human parturition is regulated in part through an endocrine cascade that includes the hypothalamic–pituitary–adrenal–placental axis that is quite unique from that seen in the sheep model. A key component in the human may be the unique ability of the placenta to produce large amounts of corticotropin-releasing hormone (CRH).

Actions of CRH on the Fetal Adrenal Gland. As discussed in Chapter 3 (see p. 78), the human fetal adrenal glands are morphologically, functionally, and physiologically remarkable organs. At term, the fetal adrenal glands weigh the same as those in the adult and are similar in size to the adjacent fetal kidney. The daily production of steroids by the fetal adrenal glands near term is estimated to be 100 to 200 mg/day, which is higher than the 30 to 40 mg/day seen in adult adrenals at rest. Within the fetal adrenal gland, steroidogenic function and zonation are different from the adult. For example, significant amounts of cortisol are not produced in the fetal adrenal gland until the last trimester. As a result, fetal cortisol levels increase during the last weeks of gestation (Murphy,

1982). During this same period, levels of dehydroepiandrosterone sulfate (DHEA-S) production also are increasing significantly, leading to increases in maternal estrogens, particularly estriol. The increase in adrenal activity occurs in contrast to fetal adrenocorticotropic hormone (ACTH) levels which do not increase until the stress of actual labor.

This substantial growth and increased steroid synthesis during latter gestation is at a time when fetal plasma ACTH levels appear to decline (Winters and co-workers, 1974). Thus, many investigators have surmised that there must be growth and steroidogenesis stimuli for these glands in addition to ACTH. Two observations have made it extremely likely that factors secreted by the placenta play a key role in the regulation of steroidogenesis during late gestation. First, the fact that ACTH levels do not increase significantly during the last part of gestation makes it likely that growth and differentiation of the fetal adrenal glands are influenced by factors secreted by the placenta. Second, the fetal zone of the adrenal gland undergoes rapid involution immediately after birth when placenta-derived factors are no longer available. Many believe that CRH of placental origin is one of the critical components that facilitates fetal adrenal hypertrophy and increased steroidogenesis late in gestation. Indeed, in vitro studies have shown that CRH is able to stimulate fetal adrenal DHEA-S and cortisol biosynthesis (Parker and associates, 1999; Smith and co-workers, 1998). The ability of CRH to regulate the adrenal glands and of the adrenals to regulate placental production of CRH has led to the idea of a feed-forward endocrine cascade that occurs late in gestation (Fig. 6–19).

Placental CRH Production. In addition to maternal and fetal hypothalamic CRH, an identical CRH hormone is synthesized by the placenta in relatively large amounts (Grino and associates, 1987; Saijonmaa and colleagues, 1988). Unlike hypothalamic CRH, which is under glucocorticoid negative feedback, cortisol has been shown to stimulate placental CRH production both in vitro and in vivo, in humans and other primates (Jones and associates, 1989; Karalis and Majzoub, 1995; Marinoni and associates, 1998). The ability of cortisol to stimulate placental CRH makes it possible to create a feed-forward endocrine cascade that does not end until separation of the fetus from the placenta at delivery. It is this cascade that has been proposed to drive the rise in CRH as well as fetal adrenal steroidogenesis in late gestation.

Maternal plasma CRH levels are low in the first trimester, rising from midgestation to term. In the last 12 weeks of gestation, CRH plasma levels rise exponentially, peaking during labor and then falling precipitously after delivery (Frim and associates, 1988; Goland and co-workers, 1986; Sasaki and colleagues, 1987). Amnionic fluid levels of CRH similarly increase in late gestation. Umbilical cord blood levels of CRH are lower than those in maternal circulation but are still quite substantial and well within the range of concentrations that we and others have found (see below) to stimulate

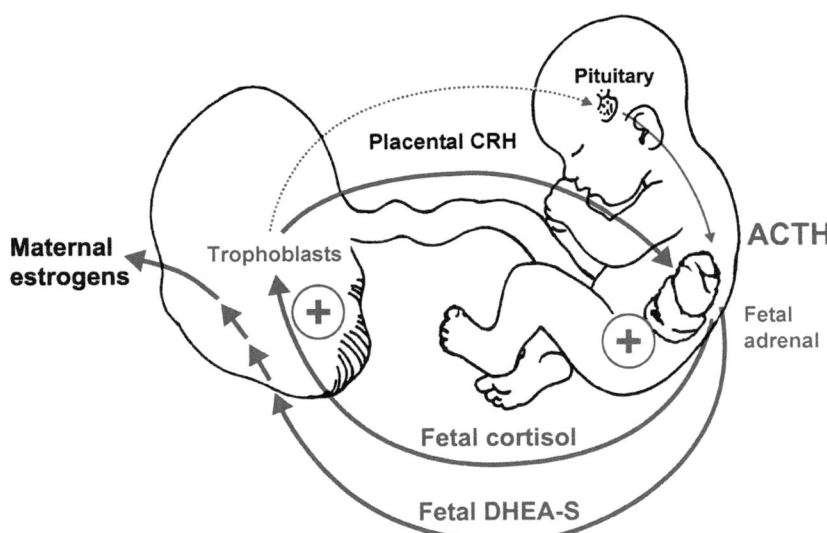

FIGURE 6–19. The placental–fetal adrenal endocrine cascade. In late gestation, placental corticotropin-releasing hormone (CRH) stimulates fetal adrenal production of dehydroepiandrosterone sulfate (DHEA-S) and cortisol. The cortisol stimulates the production of placental CRH, which leads to a feed-forward cascade that enhances adrenal steroid hormone production. (ACTH = adrenocorticotropic hormone.)

fetal adrenal steroidogenesis (Goland and co-workers, 1986, 1993; Perkins and associates, 1995).

CRH is the only trophic hormone–releasing factor to have a specific serum binding protein. During most of pregnancy, it appears that CRH-binding protein (CRH-BP) binds the majority of circulating CRH in the maternal compartment. Binding likely serves to inactivate the ACTH-stimulating activity of placental CRH (Lowry, 1993). During later pregnancy, however, CRH-BP levels in both maternal plasma and amnionic fluid decline when CRH levels are increasing strikingly, giving rise to markedly increased levels of bioavailable CRH (Perkins and co-workers, 1995; Petraglia and associates, 1997).

In pregnancies in which the fetus can be considered to be stressed as a result of various complications, the concentrations of CRH in fetal plasma, amnionic fluid, and maternal plasma are increased over those seen in normal gestation (Berkowitz, 1996; Goland, 1993; McGrath, 2002; Perkins, 1995, and all of their co-workers). The placenta is likely the source for stress-associated increases in CRH because the placental content of CRH has been found to be fourfold higher in placentas from women with preeclampsia than in those from normal pregnancies (Perkins and co-workers, 1995). Moreover, the biological impact of increased CRH levels is likely to be amplified in such instances as a result of subnormal levels of CRH-BP (Petraglia and co-workers, 1996). Such increases in placental CRH production during normal gestation and the excessive secretion of placental CRH in complicated pregnancies may play a role in the normal gestational increases in fetal adrenal cortisol synthesis (Murphy, 1982). It also may result in the supranormal levels of umbilical cord blood cortisol noted to occur in stressed neonates (Falkenberg and colleagues, 1999; Goland and co-workers, 1994).

Potential Roles of CRH in Timing of Parturition. Placental CRH has been proposed to play several roles in the regulation of parturition. First, placental CRH may enhance fetal cortisol production, which would provide positive feedback on the placenta to produce more CRH. The resulting high level of CRH may modulate myometrial contractility. Second, cortisol has been proposed to affect the myometrium indirectly by stimulating the membranes to increase prostaglandin synthesis. Third, CRH has been shown to stimulate fetal adrenal C_{19}-steroid synthesis, leading to increased substrate for placental aromatization. The resulting elevation in estrogens would shift the estrogen-to-progesterone ratio and promote the expression of a series of contractile proteins in the myometrium, leading to a loss of myometrial quiescence.

Some investigators have proposed that the rising level of CRH at the end of gestation reflects a *fetal–placental clock* (McLean and colleagues, 1995). In this regard, the human placenta and fetus, through endocrine events, influence the timing of parturition at the end of normal gestation. The origin for the signals to initiate the onset of parturition in humans remains controversial, in contrast to animal models such as the sheep. The role of cortisol and the feed-forward cascade of placental CRH, however, is an intriguing explanation for the timing of human parturition.

Fetal Anomalies and Delayed Parturition. There is fragmentary evidence that pregnancies with hypoestrogenism are sometimes associated with prolonged gestation. Examples of this include fetal anencephaly, adrenal hypoplasia, and placental sulfatase deficiency. However, the broad range of gestational length in these disorders has left in question the exact role of estrogen in the initiation of human parturition.

Other fetal abnormalities that prevent or severely reduce the entry of fetal urine into amnionic fluid (renal agenesis) or lung secretions (pulmonary hypoplasia) do not prolong human pregnancy. Thus, a fetal signal through the paracrine arm of the fetal–maternal communication system does not appear to be mandated for initiation of parturition.

Anomalies of the brain of the fetal calf, fetal lamb, and sometimes the human fetus delay the normal timing of parturition. With congenital absence of the pituitary gland in the bovine fetus, gestation is prolonged by several weeks. Adrenal hypoplasia in the bovine fetus also is associated with delayed parturition. Rea (1898) observed an association between fetal anencephaly and prolonged human gestation. Malpas (1933) extended these observations and described a human pregnancy with an anencephalic fetus that went to 374 days (53 weeks). He concluded that the association between fetal anencephaly and prolonged human gestation was attributable to anomalous brain–pituitary–adrenal function in the anencephalic fetus. The adrenal glands of the anencephalic fetus are very small, and at term may be only 5 to 10 percent as large as those of a normal fetus. This decrease in size is caused by failure of development of the fetal zone that normally accounts for most of fetal adrenal mass and C_{19}-steroid biosynthesis (see Chap. 3, p. 78). Also, in pregnancies in which the fetal adrenal glands are hypoplastic, the onset of labor may be delayed (Anderson and Turnbull, 1973). These findings were suggestive that in humans, as in sheep, the fetal adrenal glands are important for the timely onset of parturition.

FAIL-SAFE SYSTEMS TO ENSURE SUCCESS OF PHASE 2 OF PARTURITION. Phase 2 of parturition is synonymous with the uterine contractions that bring about progressive cervical dilatation and delivery. Several researchers have investigated the possibility that an increase in the formation of uterotonins is the most likely cause of the initiation of labor. This widely accepted concept represents the *uterotonins theory of the initiation of labor.* Once phase 0 is suspended and uterine phase 1 processes are implemented, a number of uterotonins may be important to the success of phase 2, viz., active labor (see Fig. 6–17). Just as multiple processes likely contribute to the maintenance of the myometrial unresponsiveness of phase 0 of parturition, other processes may contribute jointly to a system to ensure the success of labor. There are many candidate uterotonins for the induction of labor that include oxytocin, prostaglandins, serotonin, histamine, PAF, angiotensin II, and many others. As opposed to the receptor-mediated $G_{\alpha s}$-adenylyl cyclase–linked systems of myometrium that may promote cAMP accumulation, other heptahelical receptors have been identified in myometrium that more commonly activate $G_{\alpha i}$- or $G_{\alpha q}$-mediated processes that eventuate in increased myometrial cell $[Ca^{2+}]_i$. The preceding factors all have been shown to stimulate smooth muscle contraction through such G-protein coupling.

Oxytocin and Phase 2 of Parturition. Late in pregnancy, during phase 1 of parturition, there is a 50-fold or more increase in the number of myometrial oxytocin receptors (Fuchs and associates, 1982; Kimura and co-workers, 1996). This increase coincides with the increase in uterine contractile

responsiveness to oxytocin (Soloff and co-workers, 1979). Also, prolonged gestation is associated with a delay in this increase in these receptors (Fuchs and collaborators, 1984).

Oxytocin, which means *quick birth,* was the first uterotonin to be implicated in the initiation of parturition. In 1906, Sir Henry Dale discovered uterotonic bioactivity in extracts of the posterior pituitary gland. By 1909, the uterotonic property of these extracts was confirmed, and by 1911, they were in use in clinical obstetrics. In 1950, Pierce and du Vigneaud determined the structure of oxytocin, the uterotonic agent of the posterior pituitary. Oxytocin is a nanopeptide synthesized in the magnocellular neurons of the supraoptic and paraventricular neurons. The oxytocin prohormone is transported, with the carrier protein *neurophysin,* along the axons to the neural lobe of the posterior pituitary gland in membrane-bound vesicles for storage and later release. Oxytocin prohormone is converted enzymatically to oxytocin during transport (Gainer and colleagues, 1988; Leake, 1990). Oxytocin does not appear to cause the initiation of parturition, but it may be one of several participants in ensuring the effectiveness of active labor. Oxytocin acts by way of a heptahelical receptor, which likely activates phospholipase (Ku and colleagues, 1995). Oxytocin also is a very important hormone of phase 3 of parturition.

ROLE OF OXYTOCIN IN PHASES 2 AND 3 OF PARTURITION. There is a long history of safe and successful labor induction by oxytocin administration to near-term pregnant women. It was straightforward, therefore, to hypothesize that oxytocin was involved physiologically in the initiation of parturition. Several lines of evidence provided sufficient reasons for suspecting that oxytocin might be involved in the initiation of parturition: the effectiveness of oxytocin in inducing labor at term, the great potency of this uterotonin, and its natural occurrence in humans. More recent discoveries provide additional support for this theory:

1. There is a striking increase in the number of oxytocin receptors in myometrial and decidual tissues near the end of gestation.
2. Oxytocin acts on decidual tissue to promote prostaglandin release.
3. Oxytocin is synthesized directly in decidual and extraembryonic fetal tissues and in the placenta (Chibbar and associates, 1993; Zingg and colleagues, 1995).

Although there is little evidence in favor of a role for oxytocin in phase 1 of parturition, there is a large body of evidence in support of an important role for oxytocin during second-stage labor and the puerperium (phase 3 of parturition). There are increased maternal oxytocin levels (1) during second-stage labor (the end of phase 2 of parturition), (2) in the early postpartum period, and (3) during breast feeding (phase 3 of parturition) (Nissen and co-workers, 1995). This timing of increased oxytocin release is indicative of a role for oxytocin at the end of labor and during the puerperium.

Immediately after delivery of the fetus, placenta, and membranes (completion of uterine phase 2), firm and persistent contraction and retraction of the uterus are essential to prevent postpartum hemorrhage. Oxytocin likely causes persistent contractions. Certainly, maternal plasma oxytocin levels are increased at this time, and the increase in myometrial oxytocin receptors before the onset of labor favors this process.

Oxytocin infusion in women promotes increased levels of mRNAs in myometrium of genes that encode proteins essential for uterine involution. These include interstitial collagenase, monocyte chemoattractant protein-1, interleukin-8 (IL-8), and urokinase plasminogen activator receptor. Therefore, oxytocin action at the end of labor and during phase 3 of parturition may be involved in uterine involution.

Prostaglandins and Phase 2 of Parturition. Many investigators have accepted and fostered the view that prostaglandins, particularly $PGF_{2\alpha}$ and PGE_2, are involved in phase 2 of parturition, the process of labor. Many lines of evidence are supportive of this theory, including:

1. The levels of prostaglandins (or their metabolites) in amnionic fluid, maternal plasma, and maternal urine are increased during labor (Keirse, 1979).
2. The treatment of pregnant women with prostaglandins, by any of several routes of administration, causes abortion or labor at all stages of gestation (Novy and Liggins, 1980).
3. Administration of prostaglandin H synthase type 2 (PGHS-2) inhibitors to pregnant women will delay the time of onset of spontaneous labor and sometimes arrest preterm labor (Loudon and co-workers, 2003).
4. Prostaglandin treatment of myometrial smooth muscle tissues in vitro sometimes causes contraction, dependent on the prostanoid tested and the physiological status of the tissue treated.

Although a critical role for prostaglandins in phase 2 of parturition is clear, their role in phase 1 (activation phase) of noncomplicated pregnancies is less well defined (MacDonald and Casey, 1993). However, like oxytocin, prostaglandins produced directly in or adjacent to myometrial tissue are likely to play a major role in the effectiveness of myometrial contractions of active labor once labor is initiated.

UTERINE EVENTS REGULATING PROSTAGLANDIN PRODUCTION. The production of prostaglandins at the time of labor within the myometrium could be seen as a most efficient mechanism of activating contractions. However, the fetal membranes and placenta also are able to produce prostaglandins. Indeed, prostaglandins, primarily PGE_2 (but also $PGF_{2\alpha}$), are detected in amnionic fluid at all stages of gestation. As the fetus grows, the levels of prostaglandins in amnionic fluid increase gradually. The major increases in amnionic fluid, however, occur after labor begins (MacDonald and Casey, 1993) and are now believed to be the result of an inflammatory response that signals the events leading to active labor.

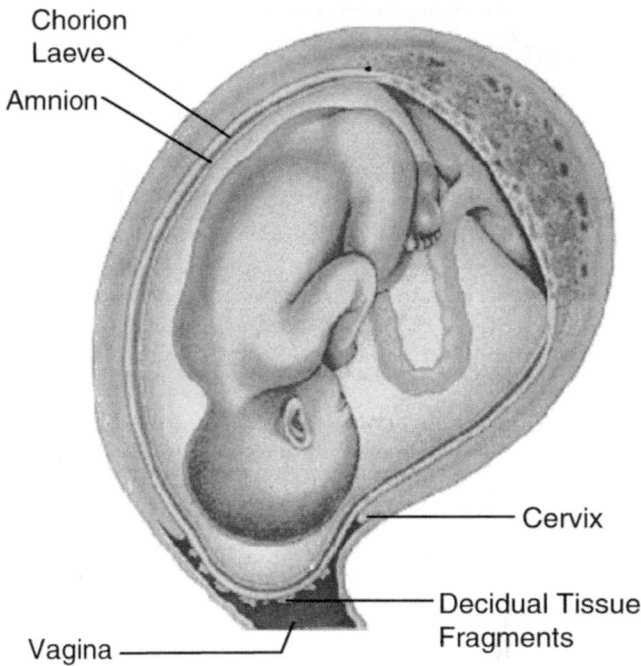

FIGURE 6–20. Sagittal view of the exposed forebag and attached decidual fragments after cervical dilatation during labor. (From MacDonald and Casey, 1996. Illustration by Michael Reingold.)

To understand the source of prostaglandins in amnionic fluid at parturition, the anatomical changes involving the fetal membranes during cervical dilatation must be envisioned. The lowermost pole of the fetal membranes is structurally modified in the formation of the forebag of the amnionic sac. Before labor, the fetal membranes are contiguous with and attached to the uterine decidua vera, which in the lower uterine segment of the uterus is thin and poorly developed. As the lower pole of the amnionic sac is pulled away from the wall of the uterus, fragments of decidua parietalis are torn away but remain attached rather firmly to the outer surface of the chorion laeve (Fig. 6–20).

This normal phenomenon of early labor is complementary to successful cervical dilatation. Membranes that slide readily over the lower uterine segment and partly through the cervix are much more efficacious dilators. As the cervix is opened, the forebag presents through the cervix in the upper vagina, like the tip of a fluid-filled balloon under pressure being pushed through the enlarging diameter of a hollow cylinder. The surface area of the exposed forebag increases as cervical dilatation progresses during phase 2 of parturition. The innermost tissue of the forebag is the avascular amnion, which is bathed by the amnionic fluid on its epithelial surface. The outer surface of the amnion is adherent to the avascular chorion laeve. The traumatized, devascularized decidual tissue fragments that are torn away from the uterus form an irregular lining on the outer surface of the forebag, which presents in the vagina (see Fig. 6–20). Thereafter, the forebag tissues are bathed continuously by the vaginal fluid,

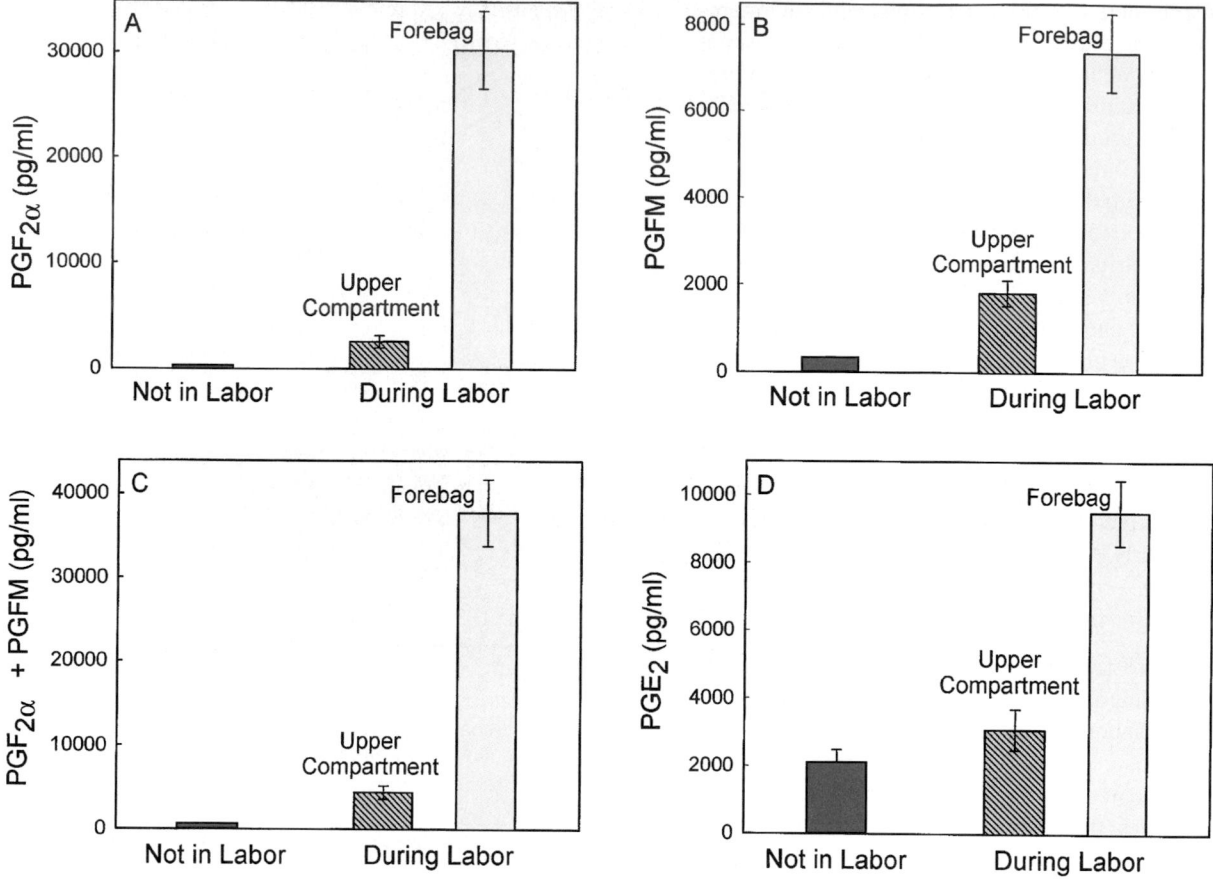

FIGURE 6–21. Mean values of prostaglandin $F_{2\alpha}$ ($PGF_{2\alpha}$; panel A), prostaglandin FM (PGFM; panel B), $PGF_{2\alpha}$ + PGFM (panel C), and prostaglandin E_2 (PGE_2; panel D) in amnionic fluid at term before labor and in the upper and forebag compartments during labor. Values are in labor at all stages of cervical dilatation. (From MacDonald and Casey, 1993, with permission.)

which in all women (pregnant and nonpregnant) contains a large number and variety of microorganisms, bacterial toxins in large amounts, and prostaglandins and cytokines (Cox and associates, 1993b).

Because of (1) trauma to decidual tissues in the formation of the forebag, (2) devascularization of the decidual fragments that are pulled away from the uterus, and (3) the action of the constituents of the vaginal fluids on these tissues, an inflammatory response in the decidual fragments of the forebag develops and is readily demonstrable. During labor, the levels of cytokines in the forebag are much greater than those found in the upper compartment of the amnionic sac (MacDonald and associates, 1991). The cytokines produced in the forebag are thought to greatly enhance the levels of prostaglandins produced by the amnion. This scenario leads to substantially higher levels of prostaglandins in the forebag compartment (Fig. 6–21). The prostaglandins synthesized in forebag tissues also are released into the vagina (Fig. 6–22).

Recent findings of Kemp and co-workers (2002) and Kelly (2002) support the possibility that inflammatory mediators facilitate cervical dilatation and alterations to the lower

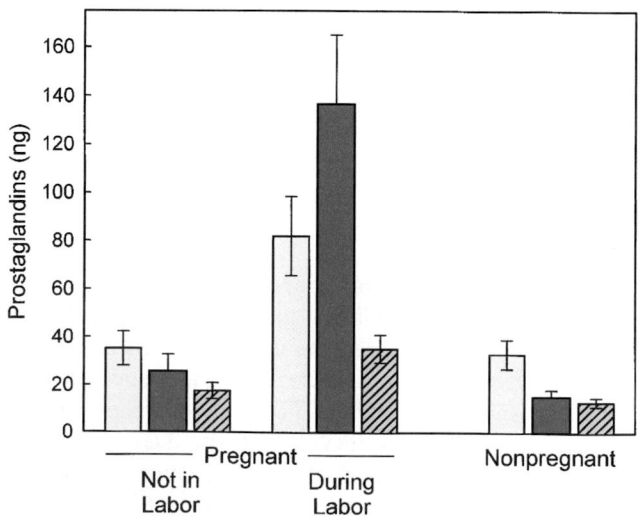

FIGURE 6–22. Prostaglandins recovered from vaginal fluid (by lavage) before and during labor. Prostaglandin E_2 (open bar); prostaglandin $F_{2\alpha}$ (solid bar); prostaglandin FM (hatched bar). (From Cox and associates, 1993b, with permission.)

uterine segment. These cytokines and chemokines lead to further extracellular matrix degradation, increase levels of hyaluronic acid, and cause an influx of leukocytes into the area. Together the increases in cytokines and prostaglandins cause further degradation of the extracellular matrix, thus weakening the fetal membranes. It can be envisioned that they also add to the relatively rapid changes in the cervix that are characteristic of the parturitional process.

Platelet-Activating Factor (PAF). The PAF receptor also is a member of the heptahelical family of transmembrane receptors and acts to increase myometrial cell calcium and promote uterine contractions. The levels of PAF in amnionic fluid are increased during labor, and PAF treatment of myometrial tissue promotes contraction (Billah and Johnston, 1983; Nishihara and associates, 1984; Zhu and colleagues, 1992). It is likely that PAF, like prostaglandins, cytokines, and endothelin-1, is produced in leukocytes as a result of the inflammatory process that develops when cervical dilatation brings about exposure of the traumatized forebag tissues to the vaginal fluids.

The transport of PAF from amnionic fluid to myometrium is uncertain but unlikely. PAF is inactivated enzymatically by PAF-acetylhydrolase. This enzyme is present and possesses high specific activity in macrophages which are present in large numbers in decidua (Prescott and associates, 1990). Thus, the myometrium may be protected from PAF action by PAF-acetylhydrolase in a manner similar to that for uterotonins: oxytocin by oxytocinase, endothelin-1 by enkephalinase, and prostaglandins by prostaglandin dehydrogenase.

Endothelin-1. The endothelins are very powerful inducers of myometrial smooth muscle contraction, and endothelin receptors are demonstrable in myometrial tissue (Word and colleagues, 1990). The endothelin A receptor, preferentially expressed in smooth muscle cells, including the myometrium, acts to effect an increase in intracellular calcium, apparently by linkage to both $G_{\alpha q}$- and $G_{\alpha i}$-subunits of the G-proteins. Endothelin-1 is produced in myometrium, but the exact cellular site of synthesis is not clearly established, and the potential contribution of myometrial endothelin-1 to phase 2 of parturition is not defined.

Endothelin-1 also is synthesized in amnion. Like other uterotonins synthesized in amnion, it is unlikely that endothelin-1 can be transported from reflected amnion (or amnionic fluid), to the myometrium without degradation (Eis and colleagues, 1992). One obstacle to endothelin-1 transport across the fetal membranes is the enzyme enkephalinase (membrane metalloendopeptidase), which is present in chorion laeve and highly active (Germain and associates, 1994). Enkephalinase catalyzes the degradation of endothelin-1 as well as several other small, bioactive peptides—for example, the enkephalins, substance P, and atrial and brain natriuretic peptides. However, in situations such as premature rupture of the fetal membranes, endothelin-1 could then play a role in uterine contraction.

Angiotensin II. There are two heptahelical G-protein–linked angiotensin II receptors (AT1 and AT2) expressed in the uterus. In nonpregnant women, the AT2 receptor is predominant, but in myometrium of pregnant women, it is the AT1 receptor that is preferentially expressed (Cox and associates, 1993a). This fact likely explains why nonpregnant myometrial tissue does not contract in response to angiotensin II treatment (Cox and co-workers, 1996). Most commonly, angiotensin II binding to the plasma membrane receptor on smooth muscle cells evokes contraction. During pregnancy, vascular smooth muscle, which expresses the AT2 receptor, is refractory to the pressor effects of angiotensin II (see Chap. 5, p. 135). In myometrium near term, however, angiotensin II may be another component of the uterotonin system of phase 2 of parturition, acting to promote increased myometrial cell calcium.

CRH, hCG, and PTH-rP. There may be a late pregnancy modification in the receptor for CRH, hCG, or PTH-rP or in their G-protein coupling in myometrium that favors a switch from cAMP formation to increased myometrial cell calcium. Oxytocin acts to attenuate CRH-stimulated accumulation of cAMP in myometrial tissue, and CRH augments the contraction-inducing potency of a given dose of oxytocin in human myometrial strips (Quartero and colleagues, 1991, 1992). CRH also acts to increase myometrial contractile force in response to $PGF_{2\alpha}$ (Benedetto and associates, 1994).

Contribution of Intrauterine Tissues to Parturition. The potential role of amnion, chorion laeve, and decidua vera has been studied to define their participation in promoting initiation of parturition. In uncomplicated pregnancy, an alternative role for these tissues appears to be more likely. The membranes and decidua comprise an important tissue shell around the fetus that serves as a physical, immunological, and metabolic shield that protects against the untimely initiation of parturition. However, late in gestation the fetal membranes have been reported to change and may indeed act to prepare for labor.

AMNION. The amnion provides virtually all of the tensile strength of the membranes, that is, resistance to tearing and rupture (see Chap. 3, p. 66). The avascular amnion is highly resistant to penetration by leukocytes, microorganisms, and neoplastic cells from the maternal compartment. It also constitutes a selective filter to prevent fetal particulate-bound lung and skin secretions from reaching the maternal compartment. In this manner, maternal tissues are protected from constituents in the amnionic fluid that could adversely affect decidual or myometrial function or even maternal well-being, such as seen in amnionic fluid embolism (see Chap. 35, p. 845).

Several bioactive peptides and prostaglandins, which could cause myometrial relaxation or contraction, are synthesized in amnion. It is the late gestation production of prostaglandins that has been most studied. There appears to be an overall increase in amnion prostaglandin biosynthetic capability late in gestation. Amnion does increase its activity for phospholipase A_2 and PGHS-2 late in gestation (Johnson and colleagues, 2002; Smieja and co-workers, 1993). This increase in ability to produce prostaglandins has made it the topic of many hypotheses as a regulator of the events leading to parturition. It is likely that the major source for prostaglandins in the amnionic fluid is the amnion, and a role for amnion-derived factors in uterine quiescence and activation has been proposed. However, it is the transport of prostaglandins and active peptides from amnion through the chorion to access maternal tissues that has been at issue.

CHORION LAEVE. The chorion is similar to the amnion in that it serves primarily as a protective tissue, in this case providing immunological acceptance. In addition, the chorion laeve is enriched with enzymes that inactivate uterotonins such as prostaglandin dehydrogenase (PGDH), oxytocinase, and enkephalinase (Cheung and co-workers, 1990; Germain and associates, 1994). As seen in Figure 6–18, PGDH through its metabolism of active prostaglandins will prevent passage of amnion-derived prostaglandins across the fetal membranes. Thus, during most of gestation the prostaglandins produced by the amnion could be released into the amnionic fluid or metabolized by the adjacent chorion. In cases with rupture of the fetal membranes, this barrier would be lost and prostaglandins could readily have an impact on the adjacent decidua and myometrium. Recent evidence suggests that the level of PGDH found in chorion can be regulated. It is through PGDH regulation that prostaglandins produced in the amnion may play a regulatory role in maternal tissues of uncomplicated pregnancies (Patel and colleagues, 1999; Van Meir and associates, 1996; Wu and co-workers, 2000). It is currently believed that progesterone maintains chorion PGDH expression, whereas cortisol decreases its expression. With this in mind, PGDH would decrease late in gestation as fetal cortisol production increases and as part of progesterone withdrawal. The exact role of fetal membrane-derived peptides or prostaglandins in the initiation of parturition (phase 1) is still under debate; however, these compounds are likely to be important for the process of labor itself (phase 2) and could continue to play a role in involution (phase 3).

DECIDUA PARIETALIS. A metabolic contribution of decidua parietalis to the initiation of parturition has been an appealing possibility for a number of reasons, both anatomical and functional. The generation of uterotonins in decidua that act in a paracrine manner on contiguous myometrium is an interesting option. There are also several lines of evidence that decidual activation is an accompaniment of human parturition (Casey and MacDonald, 1988a, 1988b, 1990; MacDonald and colleagues, 1991). The central question, however, is whether decidual activation precedes or follows the onset of labor. The process of decidual activation appears to be localized to the exposed decidual fragments lining the forebag. Trauma, hypoxia, and exposure of forebag decidua to endotoxin lipopolysaccharide, microorganisms, and interleukin-1β (IL-1β) in the vaginal fluids provoke an inflammatory reaction, which is an inevitable and consistent sequela of labor.

During this inflammatory reaction, a whole series of cytokines is produced that can either increase the production of uterotonins (principally prostaglandins) or act directly on myometrium to cause contraction. These include tumor necrosis factor-α (TNF-α) and interleukins 1, 6, 8, and 12. In addition, these molecules can act as chemokines that recruit neutrophils and eosinophils to the uterus and further increase uterine activity and labor (Keelan and co-workers, 2003).

Regulation of Phase 2 of Parturition: Summary. It is likely that multiple (possibly redundant) processes contribute to the success of phase 2 (active labor) once phase 0 is suspended and phase 1 of parturition is implemented. A variety of myometrial heptahelical receptors may promote uterine quiescence, but there is another group that should inhibit cAMP formation or activate phospholipase C or A_2, or both. The source of regulatory ligands for these receptors varies from endocrine hormones such as oxytocin to locally produced prostaglandins. It is likely that functional progesterone withdrawal modifies the myometrium, perhaps in a regional manner—fundus versus lower uterine segment—such that the heptahelical receptor–G-protein–effector phenotype can contribute to a regional relaxation or contraction in a manner that effectively promotes delivery.

PHYSIOLOGY AND BIOCHEMISTRY OF PRETERM LABOR

As discussed in Chapter 36, preterm birth is one of the major health hazards of humans, being the greatest cause—after congenital anomalies—of neonatal morbidity and mortality. Although there are many conditions that lead to preterm delivery, one can place most of the causes into three major categories:

1. Complications of pregnancy that severely jeopardize fetal and sometimes maternal health often mandate preterm delivery. These medically indicated or iatrogenic causes represent about 25 percent of preterm births.
2. Preterm premature rupture of the fetal membranes (PPROM), which is followed by preterm delivery, causes approximately 25 percent of preterm births.
3. Spontaneous preterm labor in pregnancies with intact fetal membranes represents the largest cause of preterm delivery, accounting for about half of preterm births.

MANDATED PRETERM DELIVERY. All too often, pregnancy complications require a clinical decision to effect preterm delivery rather than continue pregnancy in a deteriorating intrauterine environment. A host of pregnancy disorders may mandate such a choice (Iams, 2003). Most commonly, these complications of pregnancy threaten fetal health so that a continued intrauterine existence will likely result in fetal death. Many examples may be cited, but the most common are maternal hypertension, severe diabetes mellitus, failure of fetal growth, multiple pregnancies, and abruptio placenta. The causes of iatrogenic preterm delivery are further discussed in Chapter 36.

PRETERM PREMATURE RUPTURE OF THE MEMBRANES (PPROM). This nomenclature is used to denote spontaneous rupture of the fetal membranes that occurs before 37 completed weeks and *before the onset of labor.* It is likely that *PPROM* has a variety of causes, but many believe intrauterine infection to be one of the major predisposing events (Gomez and colleagues, 1997; Mercer, 2003).

Recent studies suggest that the pathogenesis of PPROM relates to increased apoptosis of the cellular components of the fetal membranes as well as an elevation in specific proteases in the membranes and amnionic fluid. Much of the tensile strength of the fetal membranes is provided by the extracellular matrix within the amnion. Interstitial amnionic collagens, primarily types I and III, are produced in mesenchymal cells and are the structural component most important for its strength (Casey and MacDonald, 1996). For that reason, the degradation of collagens has been a focus of research.

The matrix metalloproteinase (MMP) family of proteinases is involved with normal tissue remodeling and particularly the degradation of collagens. The MMP-2, MMP-3, and MMP-9 members of this family are found in higher concentrations in amnionic fluid from pregnancies with PPROM (Fortunato and co-workers, 1999a, 2001; Park and colleagues, 2003; Romero and associates, 2002). The activity of the MMPs is in part regulated by tissue inhibitors of matrix metalloproteinases (TIMPs). Interestingly, several of the TIMP family members are found in lower concentrations in amnionic fluid from women with PPROM. The elevation of these proteases at a time when protease inhibitor expression drops further supports the idea that their expression alters the tensile strength of the amnion and increases the incidence of PPROM. Studies using isolated amniochorion explants have demonstrated that the expression of MMPs can be increased by treatment with IL-1, TNF-α, and IL-6 (Fortunato and colleagues, 1999a, 1999b, 2002). Thus, MMP induction may be part of an inflammatory process.

In addition to an increase in collagen breakdown, the amnion from PPROM exhibits a higher degree of cell death than is seen in the term amnion (Arechavaleta-Velasco and colleagues, 2002; Fortunato and Menon, 2003; Fortunato and co-workers, 2001). Markers of apoptosis (programmed cell death) are increased in membranes with PPROM compared with those in normal term membranes. In vitro studies have shown that apoptosis is likely regulated by bacterial endotoxin, IL-1β, and TNF-α. Taken together, these observations suggest that many cases of PPROM result from an activation of collagen breakdown and cell death leading to a weakening of the amnion.

Studies have been undertaken to ascertain the incidence of infection-induced PPROM. The number of positive cultures of amnionic fluid in PPROM supports a role for infection in a significant proportion of cases. A survey of 18 independent studies between 1979 and 2000 that consisted of 1462 women with PPROM indicates that a third had bacteria isolated from amnionic fluid (Goncalves and co-workers, 2002). Because of this, studies have been performed to address prophylactic antimicrobial treatment to prevent PPROM. As discussed in Chapter 36 (see p. 862), although the results of these studies are conflicting, there is evidence that early treatment of some asymptomatic lower genital tract infections, as well as active periodontal inflammation, will reduce the incidence of PPROM and preterm birth. Thus, the evidence is compelling that infection causes a significant proportion of cases of PPROM. The inflammatory response that leads to the weakening of the fetal membranes is now being defined in detail. Current research is being focused on certain mediators of this process that accumulate in amnionic fluid and may provide early markers for women at risk for PPROM.

SPONTANEOUS PRETERM LABOR. Pregnancies with intact fetal membranes and spontaneous preterm labor—for clinical as well as research purposes—must be distinguished from those in which there has been preterm premature membrane rupture. Even so, pregnancies complicated by spontaneous preterm labor do not constitute a homogeneous group characterized singularly by the early initiation of parturition. Among the more common associated findings are multifetal pregnancy, intrauterine infection, bleeding, placental infarction, premature cervical dilatation, cervical incompetence, uterine fundal abnormalities, and fetal anomalies. Severe maternal illness as a result of nonobstetrical infections, autoimmune diseases, and gestational hypertension increase the incidence of preterm labor. These disorders cause about half of spontaneous preterm deliveries, and their relative contribution varies between populations.

Although there are unique aspects to each of the causes of preterm labor, recent studies have suggested that they share certain common denominators. Thus, the fetal or maternal conditions provide important clues to the cause of the premature onset of parturition. It seems important to reemphasize that the actual process of preterm labor should be considered a final step—one that results from premature uterine activation that was initiated weeks before the onset of labor. Indeed, many of the forms of spontaneous preterm labor that result from premature initiation of phase 1 of parturition may be viewed in this light (see Fig. 6–17). Specifically, many of the alterations discussed earlier with regard to normal parturition also occur with preterm labor, including cervical ripening and myometrial activation. Identification of common factors has begun to explain the physiological processes of human parturition at term and preterm. Three major causes of spontaneous preterm labor include uterine distention, maternal–fetal stress, and infection.

Uterine Distention. There is no doubt that multifetal pregnancy as well as hydramnios lead to an increased risk of preterm birth (see Chap. 39, p. 924). As discussed on page 169, uterine stretch can play an important role in the normal process of myometrial activation in preparation for labor. In multifetal gestation or hydramnios, it is likely that early uterine distention acts to initiate expression of contraction-associated proteins (CAPs) in the myometrium. The CAP genes influenced by stretch include those coding for gap junction proteins, such as connexin 43, for oxytocin receptors, and for prostaglandin synthase (Korita and colleagues, 2002; Lyall and co-workers, 2002; Sooranna and associates, 2004). The result of excessive uterine stretch is the premature loss of myometrial quiescence.

In addition to direct action of uterine stretch on the myometrium, these pregnancies also exhibit an early activation of the placental–fetal endocrine cascade shown in Figure 6–19. This cascade results in an early rise in maternal CRH and estrogen levels, which can further enhance the expression of myometrial CAP genes (Warren and co-workers, 1990; Wolfe and colleagues, 1988).

Finally, the influence of uterine stretch also should be considered with regard to the cervix. Cervical length is an important risk factor in multifetal pregnancies (Goldenberg and co-workers, 1996). The premature increase in stretch and endocrine activity that is seen in multifetal gestations may initiate the sequence of events causing a shift in the timing of uterine activation seen in Figure 6–17, including premature cervical ripening.

Maternal–Fetal Stress. The complexities of measuring stress and other moderating psychosocial factors that lead to stress contribute to the difficulty of defining its exact role in preterm birth (Lobel, 1994). There is, however, a large body of evidence that shows a correlation between maternal stress and preterm birth (Hobel and Culhane, 2003; Ruiz and colleagues, 2003). Prospective studies involving women of different ethnicity, socioeconomic, and behavioral risk factors have shown a correlation between stress, low birthweight, and preterm birth (Hedegaard and associates, 1993; Wadhwa and co-workers, 1993, 2001; Zambrana and colleagues, 1999). During recent years, studies showing a correlation between maternal psychological stress and the placental–adrenal endocrine axis have provided a potential mechanism for stress-induced preterm birth (Lockwood, 1999; Wadhwa and associates, 2001).

As discussed earlier, the last trimester is marked by rising maternal serum levels of placental-derived CRH. This hormone works with ACTH to increase adult and fetal adrenal steroid hormone production, including the initiation of fetal cortisol biosynthesis. Rising levels of maternal and fetal cortisol further increase placental CRH secretion, which develops a feed-forward endocrine cascade that does not end until delivery (see Fig. 6–19). In addition, the rising levels of CRH further stimulate fetal adrenal DHEA-S biosynthesis, which acts as substrate to increase maternal circulating estrogens, particularly estriol. It has been hypothesized that a premature rise in cortisol and estrogens causes an early loss of uterine quiescence.

Supporting this hypothesis are numerous studies indicating that spontaneous preterm labor is associated with an early rise in maternal circulating CRH (Holzman, 2001; McGrath, 2002; Moawad, 2002, and all their co-workers). It appears that levels of CRH in term and preterm women are similar; *however,* women destined for preterm labor exhibit a rise in CRH that occurs 2 to 6 weeks earlier (McLean and co-workers, 1995). The rise in CRH has been noted as early as 18 weeks' gestation, leading some to suggest that this assay might provide a useful marker for preterm delivery.

As discussed in Chapter 3 (see p. 75), placental CRH also enters the fetal circulation, albeit at lower levels than those seen in the maternal circulation. In vitro studies have shown that CRH can directly stimulate fetal adrenal production of DHEA-S and cortisol (Parker and colleagues, 1999; Smith and co-workers, 1998). If preterm delivery is associated with premature activation of the fetal adrenal–placental endocrine cascade, it would be hypothesized that maternal estrogen levels would be prematurely elevated. And this is seen for CRH. Moreover, several studies have shown an early rise of serum estriol concentrations in women with subsequent preterm labor (Heine and co-workers, 2000; McGregor and co-workers, 1995). Physiologically, this premature rise in estrogens may alter myometrial quiescence. Taken together, these observations suggest that preterm birth is associated, in many cases, with a maternal–fetal biological stress response. The nature and variety of the stressors that activate this cascade likely are broad. For example, several studies have noted that CRH or estriol levels are prematurely activated in preterm birth due to infection and multifetal pregnancies (Gravett and colleagues, 2000; Warren and co-workers, 1990). Thus, activation of this axis may be considered a common feature for the activation of phase I of parturition. Further study will be needed to define the exact biochemical role of CRH, estrogens, and cortisol in preterm birth, as well as the exact nature of the stressors that lead to the activation of this endocrine cascade.

Infection and Preterm Labor. It has been known for more than 50 years that the administration to animals of bacteria or bacterial endotoxin (e.g., lipopolysaccharide) causes abortion or preterm delivery, which is accompanied by decidual hemorrhage and necrosis (Zahl and Bjerknes, 1943). It was not until many years later, however, that the biomolecular particulars of the inflammatory response were defined in detail (Dudley, 1997; Goldenberg and colleagues, 2000; Romero and co-workers, 2003). Determining the details associated with intrauterine infection during pregnancy has helped provide an attractive explanation as to how infection might cause preterm labor.

There is great interest in the role of infection as a primary cause of preterm labor in pregnancies with intact membranes. It has been estimated that as much as 40 percent of preterm labor may be caused by intrauterine infection. This concept has been promoted because of widespread suspicion that subclinical infection is a common accompaniment and cause of preterm labor. The term *subclinical* has been used to describe the condition in which intrautcrine infection is accompanied by little or no clinical evidence of infection, and at times, microorganisms cannot be recovered from the amnionic fluid (Goncalves and co-workers, 2002; Iams and colleagues, 1987).

The incidence of positive cultures of amnionic fluid during preterm labor varies from 10 to 40 percent, the average being about 13 percent (Goncalves and co-workers, 2002). Importantly, these women were more likely to develop chorioamnionitis and PPROM than women with negative cultures. They are also more likely to have neonates with complications (Hitti and co-workers, 2001). The earlier the onset of preterm labor, the greater is the likelihood of documented amnionic fluid infection (Goldenberg and associates, 2000; Watts and colleagues, 1992). At the same time, however, the incidence of culture-positive amnionic fluids collected by amniocentesis during spontaneous term labor is similar or even greater than it is during preterm labor (Gomez and colleagues, 1994; Romero and co-workers, 1993). It has been suggested that at term, amnionic fluid is infiltrated by bacteria as a consequence of the processes of labor, whereas in preterm pregnancies bacteria represent an important cause of labor. Although plausible, this explanation questions the contribution of fetal infection as a major contributor to preterm birth.

Certainly, there are considerable data to associate chorioamnionitis with preterm labor (Chellam and Rushton, 1985; Goldenberg and associates, 2002; Mueller-Heubach and colleagues, 1990; Üstün and colleagues, 2001). In such infections, the microbes may invade maternal tissue only, and not amnionic fluid. Despite this, endotoxins can stimulate amnionic cells to secrete cytokines that enter amnionic fluid. This scenario may serve to explain the apparently contradictory observations concerning an association between amnionic fluid cytokines and preterm labor, in which microbes were not detectable in the amnionic fluid.

It seems logical that infection-mediated preterm deliveries should be preventable by antimicrobial treatment. However, there continues to be debate on the effectiveness of antimicrobial prophylaxis to prevent spontaneous preterm birth, and as discussed in Chapter 36 (see p. 862), it is recommended in only a few situations to prevent spontaneous preterm delivery (Andrews and associates, 2003; Kenyon and co-workers, 2001, 2003; King and Flenady, 2002).

SOURCES FOR INTRAUTERINE INFECTION. The patency of the female reproductive tract, although essential for achievement of pregnancy and delivery, is theoretically problematic during phase 0 of parturition. It has been suggested that bacteria can gain access to the intrauterine tissues through (1) transplacental transfer of maternal systemic infection, (2) retrograde flow of infection from the peritoneal cavity via the fallopian tubes, or (3) ascending infection with bacteria from the vagina and cervix. The lower pole of the fetal membrane–decidual junction embraces the orifice of the cervical canal, which anatomically is patent to the vagina. This anatomical arrangement provides a passageway for microorganisms to enter intrauterine tissues. For this reason, the ascending route of infection is considered the most common. A thoughtful description of the potential degrees of intrauterine infection has been provided by Goncalves and co-workers (2002). They categorize intrauterine infection into four stages of microbial invasion that include bacterial vaginosis (stage I), decidual infection (stage II), amnionic infection (stage III), and finally fetal systemic infection (stage IV). As expected, progression of these stages is thought to increase the effects on preterm birth as well as neonatal morbidity.

Based on these insights into the process of infection, it is straightforward to construct a theory for the pathogenesis of infection-induced preterm labor (Fig. 6–23). Microorganisms originating in the vagina or cervix, after ascending, colonize the decidua and possibly the fetal membranes, where they then may enter the amnionic sac. Lipopolysaccharide or other toxins elaborated by these bacteria induce cytokine production in cells within the decidua, membranes, or fetus itself. Both lipopolysaccharide and a variety of cytokines that increase due to its presence provoke prostaglandin release from fetal membranes, the decidua, or both. The rise in cytokines and prostaglandins will then influence both cervical ripening and loss of myometrial quiescence with resultant myometrial stimulation (Challis, 2002; Keelan, 2003; Loudon, 2003; Olson, 2003; and all their associates).

MICROBES ASSOCIATED WITH PRETERM BIRTH. Some microorganisms, for example, *Gardnerella vaginalis, Fusobacterium, Mycoplasma hominis,* and *Ureaplasma urealyticum,* are detected more commonly than others in amnionic fluid of women with preterm labor (Gerber, 2003; Hillier, 1988; Romero, 1989; Yoon, 1998, and all their co-workers). This finding was interpreted by some as presumptive evidence that specific microorganisms are more commonly involved as pathogens in the induction of preterm labor. Another interpretation, however, is that given direct access to the membranes after cervical dilatation, selected microorganisms, such

Mechanisms causing infection-induced preterm labor

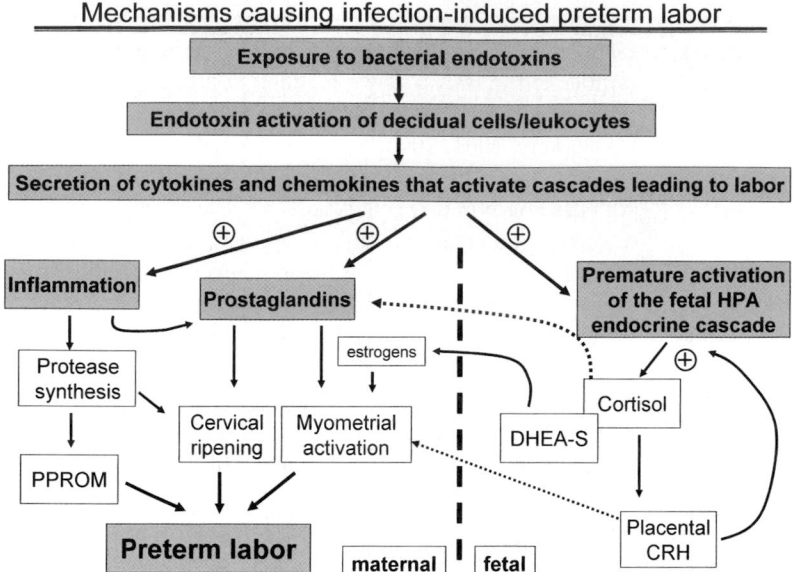

FIGURE 6–23. Potential pathways for infection-induced preterm birth. Exposure to bacterial endotoxins causes an early initiation of the normal processes associated with parturition, including cervical ripening, loss of uterine quiescence, and increased production of uterotonins. (CRH = corticotropin-releasing hormone; DHEA-S = dehydroepiandrosterone sulfate; HPA = hypothalamic–pituitary–adrenal; PPROM = preterm premature rupture of membranes.)

as fusobacteria that are more capable of burrowing through these exposed tissues, will do so. Fusobacteria are found in the vaginal fluid of only 9 percent of women but in 28 percent of positive amnionic fluid cultures from preterm labor pregnancies with intact membranes (Chaim and Mazor, 1992). Further studies are needed to better define the intrauterine site of infection that most influences the timing of delivery as well as why some pregnant women appear more susceptible to microbes associated with bacterial vaginosis.

INTRAUTERINE INFLAMMATORY RESPONSE TO INFECTION. The initial inflammatory response elicited by bacterial toxins is mediated, in large measure, by specific receptors on mononuclear phagocytes, decidual cells, and trophoblasts. These *toll-like receptors* represent a family of receptors that has evolved to recognize pathogen-associated molecules (Janssens and Beyaert, 2003). Toll-like receptors are present in the placenta on trophoblast cells as well as fixed and invading leukocytes (Chuang and Ulevitch, 2000; Holmlund and co-workers, 2002). Under the influence of ligands such as bacterial lipopolysaccharide, these receptors increase the local release of chemokines, cytokines, and prostaglandins as part of an inflammatory response. For example, IL-1β is produced rapidly after lipopolysaccharide stimulation (Dinarello, 2002). IL-1 in turn acts to promote a series of responses that include increased synthesis of other cytokines, viz., TNF-α, IL-6, and IL-8; the proliferation, activation, and migration of leukocytes; modifications in extracellular matrix proteins; and mitogenic and cytotoxic effects, including fever and the acute phase response (El-Bastawissi and colleagues, 2000). IL-1 also acts to promote prostaglandin formation in many tissues, including myometrium, decidua, and amnion (Casey and co-workers, 1990). Thus, there appears to be a cascade

of events once an inflammatory response is initiated that can result in preterm labor.

ORIGIN OF CYTOKINES IN INTRAUTERINE INFECTION. Cytokines within the normal term uterus are likely important for normal and preterm labor. The transfer of cytokines such as IL-1 from decidua across the membranes into amnionic fluid appears to be severely limited. Thus, it is likely that cytokines produced in maternal decidua and myometrium will have effects on that side, whereas cytokines produced in the membranes or in cells within the amnionic fluid will not be transferred to the maternal tissues. In most cases of inflammation resulting from infection, resident and invading leukocytes produce the bulk of cytokines. Indeed, leukocytes—mainly neutrophils, macrophages, and T lymphocytes—infiltrate the cervix, lower uterine segment, and fundus at the time of labor. Other studies have shown that leukocytes invade membranes and cervix with preterm labor. Thus, invading leukocytes may be the major source of cytokines at the time of labor.

Immunohistochemistry studies of cytokine expression have shown that, in the term laboring uterus, both invading leukocytes and certain parenchymal cells produce cytokines. These leukocytes appear to be the primary source of myometrial cytokines, including IL-1, IL-6, IL-8, and TNF-α (Young and co-workers, 2002), although in the decidua both stromal cells and invading leukocytes are likely to contribute because they have been shown to produce IL-1, IL-6, TNF-α, and IL-8. In the cervix, glandular and surface epithelial cells appear to produce IL-6, IL-8, and TNF-α. In fact, IL-8 is considered a critical cytokine in cervical ripening, and it is produced in both epithelial and stromal cells of the cervix.

The presence of cytokines in amnionic fluid and their association with preterm labor has been well documented; however, their exact cellular origin—with or without culturable microorganisms—has not been well defined. Although the rate of IL-1 secretion from forebag decidual tissue is great, Kent and colleagues (1994) found that there is negligible in vivo transfer of radiolabeled IL-1 across the membranes. Amnionic fluid IL-1 probably does not arise from amnion tissue, fetal urine, or fetal lung secretions, but most likely is secreted by mononuclear phagocytes or neutrophils activated and recruited into the amnionic fluid. Therefore, IL-1 in amnionic fluid likely is generated in situ from newly recruited cells. This scenario is supported by immunohistochemical studies that show invading leukocytes are the primary cells expressing IL-1, IL-8, TNF-α, and IL-6 in membranes at the time of labor (Young and co-workers, 2002). Thus, the amount of amnionic fluid IL-1 would be determined by the number of leukocytes recruited, their activational status, or the effect of amnionic fluid constituents on their rate of IL-1 secretion.

Leukocyte infiltration may be regulated by fetal membrane synthesis of specific chemokines. In term labor, there are increased amnionic fluid concentrations of the potent chemoattractant and monocyte-macrophage activator, *monocyte chemotactic protein-1 (MCP-1)*. As is true for prostaglandins and other cytokines, the levels of MCP-1 are much higher in the forebag compared with the upper compartment (Esplin and co-workers, 2003). Levels in preterm labor were significantly higher than those found in normal term amnionic fluid (Jacobsson and colleagues, 2003). It has been proposed that MCP-1 may be the factor that initiates fetal leukocyte infiltration of the placenta and membranes. In addition, the production of MCP-1 may act as a marker for intra-amnionic infection and inflammation.

SUMMARY OF INFECTION AND PRETERM LABOR. It is likely that intrauterine infection causes a significant number of cases currently categorized as idiopathic spontaneous preterm labor. The variety of sites for intrauterine infection—maternal, fetal, or both—and the similarities between the inflammatory responses of preterm and term labor make it difficult to determine the proportion of pregnancies that end prematurely due to infection.

Mechanistically, infection-induced preterm labor should be discussed as a process causing the early initiation of phase 1 of parturition (see Figs. 6–1 and 6–17). This process, illustrated in Figure 6–23, involves the initial exposure to bacterial endotoxins leading to production of cytokines. In the cervix, these cytokines are the cause of infiltration of leukocytes and ripening. Activation of proteases in the cervix promotes cervical dilatation and can, in some cases, weaken the fetal membranes and cause PPROM. Transfer of bacteria or cytokines into the fetal circulation is likely to cause premature activation of CRH and the placental–adrenal endocrine cascade, causing a loss of myometrial quiescence. With continued leukocyte infiltration, proinflammatory cytokines further increase prostaglandins within maternal decidua and myometrium, which then act as uterotonins to cause preterm labor.

REFERENCES

Adachi S, Oku M: The regulation of oxytocin receptor expression in human myometrial monolayer culture. J Smooth Muscle Res. 31:175, 1995

Allport VC, Pieber D, Slater DM, et al: Human labour is associated with nuclear factor-kappaB activity which mediates cyclo-oxygenase-2 expression and is involved with the 'functional progesterone withdrawal'. Mol Hum Reprod 7:581, 2001

Ambrus G, Rao Ch V: Novel regulation of pregnant human myometrial smooth muscle cell gap junctions by human chorionic gonadotropin. Endocrinology 135:2772, 1994

Anderson ABM, Turnbull AC: Comparative aspects of factors involved in the onset of labor in ovine and human pregnancy. In Klopper A, Gardner J (eds): Endocrine Factors in Labour. London, Cambridge University Press, 1973, p 141

Andrews WW, Sibai BM, Thom EA, et al: Randomized clinical trial of metronidazole plus erythromycin to prevent spontaneous preterm delivery in fetal fibronectin-positive women. Obstet Gynecol 101:847, 2003

Arechavaleta-Velasco F, Mayon-Gonzalez J, Gonzalez-Jimenez M, et al: Association of type II apoptosis and 92-kDa type IV collagenase expression in human amniochorion in prematurely ruptured membranes with tumor necrosis factor receptor-1 expression. J Soc Gynecol Investig 9:60, 2002

Avrech OM, Golan A, Weinraub Z, et al: Mifepristone (RU486) alone or in combination with a prostaglandin analogue for termination of early pregnancy: a review. Fertil Steril 56:385, 1991

Bates GW, Edman CD, Porter JC, et al: Catechol-O-methyl-transferase activity in erythrocytes of women taking oral contraceptive steroids. Am J Obstet Gynecol 133:691, 1979

Benedetto MT, DeCicco F, Rossiello F, et al: Oxytocin receptor in human fetal membranes at term and during delivery. J Steroid Biochem 35:205, 1990

Benedetto C, Petraglia F, Marozio L, et al: Corticotropin-releasing hormone increases prostaglandin-$F_{2\alpha}$ activity on human myometrium in vitro. Am J Obstet Gynecol 171:126, 1994

Berkowitz GS, Lapinski RH, Lockwood CJ, et al: Corticotropin-releasing factor and its binding protein: Maternal serum levels in term and preterm deliveries. Am J Obstet Gynecol 174:1477, 1996

Billah MM, Johnston JM: Identification of phospholipid platelet-activating factor (1-0-alkyl-2-acetyl-sn-glycero-3-phosphocholine) in human amnionic fluid and urine. Biochem Biophys Res Commun 113:51, 1983

Blanks AM, Vatish M, Allen MJ, et al: Paracrine oxytocin and estradiol demonstrate a spatial increase in human intrauterine tissues with labor. J Clin Endocrinol Metab 88:3392, 2003

Bogacki M, Silvia WJ, Rekawiecki R, et al: Direct inhibitory effect of progesterone on oxytocin-induced secretion of prostaglandin F (2alpha) from bovine endometrial tissue. Biol Reprod 67:184, 2002

Bogic LV, Mandel M, Bryant-Greenwood GD: Relaxin gene expression in human reproductive tissues by in situ hybridization. J Clin Endocrinol Metab 80:130, 1995

Brandt ML: Mechanism and management of the third stage of labor. Am J Obstet Gynecol 25:662, 1933

Breuiller M, Doualla-Bell F, Litine MH, et al: Disappearance of human myometrial adenylate cyclase activation by prostaglandins at the end of pregnancy. Comparison with beta-adrenergic response. Adv Prostaglandin Thromboxane Leukot Res 21b:811, 1991

Burghardt RC, Mitchell PA, Kurten RC: Gap junction modulation in rat uterus, II. Effects of antiestrogens on myometrial and serosal cells. Biol Reprod 30:249, 1984

Cabrol D, Dallot E, Cedard L, et al: Pregnancy-related changes in the distribution of glycosaminoglycans in the cervix and corpus of the human uterus. Eur J Obstet Gynecol Reprod Biol 20:289, 1985

Casey ML, MacDonald PC: The endocrinology of human parturition. Ann N Y Acad Sci 828:273, 1997

Casey ML, MacDonald PC: Transforming growth factor-beta inhibits progesterone-induced enkephalinase expression in human endometrial stromal cells. J Clin Endocrinol Metab 81:4022, 1996

Casey ML, MacDonald PC: Human parturition. In Bruner JP (ed): Infertility and Reproductive Medicine Clinics of North America. Philadelphia, Saunders, 1994, p 765

Casey ML, MacDonald PC: Human parturition: Distinction between the initiation of parturition and the onset of labor. In Ducsay CA (ed): Seminars in Reproductive Endocrinology. New York, Thieme, 1993, p 272

Casey ML, MacDonald PC: Biomolecular mechanisms in human parturition: Activation of uterine decidua. In d'Arcangues C, Fraser IS, Newton JR, Odlind V (eds): Contraception and Mechanisms of Endometrial Bleeding. Cambridge, England, Cambridge University Press, 1990, p 501

Casey ML, MacDonald PC: Biomolecular processes in the initiation of parturition: Decidual activation. Clin Obstet Gynecol 31:533, 1988a

Casey ML, MacDonald PC: The role of a fetal–maternal paracrine system in the maintenance of pregnancy and the initiation of parturition. In Jones CT (ed): Fetal and Neonatal Development. Ithaca, Perinatology, 1988b, p 521

Casey ML, Mibe M, Erk A, et al: Transforming growth factor-beta 1 stimulation of parathyroid hormone–related protein expression in human uterine cells in culture: mRNA levels and protein secretion. J Clin Endocrinol Metab 74:950, 1992

Casey ML, Cox SM, Word RA, et al: Cytokines and infection-induced preterm labour. Reprod Fertil Devl 2:499, 1990

Casey ML, Hemsell DL, MacDonald PC, et al: NAD$^+$-dependent 15-hydroxyprostaglandin dehydrogenase activity in human endometrium. Prostaglandins 19:115, 1980

Chaim W, Mazor M: Intraamniotic infection with fusobacteria. Arch Gynecol Obstet 251:1, 1992

Challis JR, Sloboda DM, Alfaidy N, et al: Prostaglandins and mechanisms of preterm birth. Reproduction 124:1, 2002

Challis JR, Smith SK: Fetal endocrine signals and preterm labor. Biol Neonate 79:163, 2001

Challis JRG, Lye SJ: Parturition. In Knobil E, Neill JD (eds): The Physiology of Reproduction, 2nd ed, Vol II. New York, Raven, 1994, p 985

Challis JRG, Matthews SG, Gibb W, et al: Endocrine and paracrine regulation of birth at term and preterm. Endocr Rev 21:514, 2000

Chellam VG, Rushton DI: Chorioamnionitis and funiculitis in the placentas of 200 births weighing less than 2.5 kg. Br J Obstet Gynaecol 92:808, 1985

Cheung PY, Walton JC, Tai HH, et al: Immunocytochemical distribution and localization of 15-hydroxyprostaglandin dehydrogenase in human fetal membranes, decidua, and placenta. Am J Obstet Gynecol 163:1445, 1990

Chibbar R, Miller FD, Mitchell BF: Synthesis of oxytocin in amnion, chorion, and decidua may influence the timing of human parturition. J Clin Invest 91:185, 1993

Chow L, Lye SJ: Expression of the gap junction protein connexin-43 is increased in the human myometrium toward term and with the onset of labor. Am J Obstet Gynecol 170:788, 1994

Chuang TH, Ulevitch RJ: Cloning and characterization of a subfamily of human toll-like receptors: hTLR7, hTLR8, and hTLR9. Eur Cytokine Netw 11:372, 2000

Chwalisz K: The use of progesterone antagonists for cervical ripening and as an adjunct to labour and delivery. Hum Reprod Suppl 1:131, 1994

Chwalisz K, Fahrenholz F, Hackenberg M, et al: The progesterone antagonist onapristone increases the effectiveness of oxytocin to produce delivery without changing the myometrial oxytocin receptor concentrations. Am J Obstet Gynecol 165:1760, 1991

Chwalisz K, Garfield RE: Antiprogestins in the induction of labor. Ann N Y Acad Sci 734:387, 1994

Coleman RA, Smith WL, Narumiya S: Eighth International Union of Pharmacology. Classification of prostanoid receptors: Properties, distribution, and structure of the receptor and their subtypes. Pharmacol Rev 46:205, 1994

Condon JC, Jeyasuria P, Faust JM, et al: A decline in the levels of progesterone receptor coactivators in the pregnant uterus at term may antagonize progesterone receptor function and contribute to the initiation of parturition. Proc Natl Acad Sci U S A 100:9518, 2003

Cox BE, Ipson MA, Shaul PW, et al: Myometrial angiotensin II receptor subtypes change during ovine pregnancy. J Clin Invest 92:2240, 1993a

Cox BE, Word RA, Rosenfeld CR: Angiotensin II receptor characteristics and subtype expression in uterine arteries and myometrium during pregnancy. J Clin Endocrinol Metab 81:49, 1996

Cox SM, Casey ML, MacDonald PC: Accumulation of interleukin-1 beta and interleukin-6 in amniotic fluid: A sequela of labour at term and preterm. Hum Reprod Update 3:517, 1997

Cox SM, King MR, Casey ML, et al: Interleukin-1 beta, -1 alpha, and -6 and prostaglandins in vaginal/cervical fluids of pregnant women before and during labor. J Clin Endocrinol Metab 77:805, 1993b

Crankshaw DJ, Dyal R: Effects of some occurring prostanoids and some cyclooxygenase inhibitors on the contractility of the human lower uterine segment in vitro. Can J Physiol Pharmacol 72:870, 1994

Daifotis AG, Weir EC, Dreyer BE: Stretch induced parathyroid hormone–related peptide gene expression in the rat uterus. J Biol Chem 267:23455, 1992

Dale HH: On some physiologic actions of ergot. J Physiol (Lond) 34:163, 1906

Dinarello CA: The IL-1 family and inflammatory diseases. Clin Exp Rheumatol 20:S1, 2002

Dudley DJ: Pre-term labor: An intra-uterine inflammatory response syndrome? J Reprod Immunol 36:93, 1997

Eis AW, Mitchell MD, Myatt L: Endothelin transfer and endothelin effects on water transfer in human fetal membranes. Obstet Gynecol 79:411, 1992

El-Bastawissi AY, Williams MA, Riley DE, et al: Amniotic fluid interleukin-6 and preterm delivery: A review. Obstet Gynecol 95:1056, 2000

Esplin MS, Romero R, Chaiworapongsa T, et al: Amniotic fluid levels of immunoreactive monocyte chemotactic protein-1 increase during term parturition. J Matern Fetal Neonatal Med 14:51, 2003

Eta E, Ambrus G, Rao CV: Direct regulation of human myometrial contractions by human chorionic gonadotropin. J Clin Endocrinol Metab 79:1582, 1994

Falkenberg ER, Davis RO, DuBard M, et al: Effects of maternal infections on fetal adrenal steroid production. Endocr Res 25:239, 1999

Ferguson JKW: A study of the motility of the intact uterus at term. Surg Gynecol Obstet 73:359, 1941

Fisk NM, Ronderos-Dumit D, Tannirandorn Y, et al: Normal amniotic pressure throughout gestation. Br J Obstet Gynaecol 99:18, 1992

Fortunato SJ, Menon R: IL-1 beta is a better inducer of apoptosis in human fetal membranes than IL-6. Placenta 24:922, 2003

Fortunato SJ, Menon R, Lombardi SJ: Role of tumor necrosis factor-alpha in the premature rupture of membranes and preterm labor pathways. Am J Obstet Gynecol 187:1159, 2002

Fortunato SJ, Menon R, Lombardi SJ: Support for an infection-induced apoptotic pathway in human fetal membranes. Am J Obstet Gynecol 184:1392, 2001

Fortunato SJ, Menon R, Lombardi SJ: MMP/TIMP imbalance in amniotic fluid during PROM: An indirect support for endogenous pathway to membrane rupture. J Perinat Med 27:362, 1999a

Fortunato SJ, Menon R, Lombardi SJ: Stromelysins in placental membranes and amniotic fluid with premature rupture of membranes. Obstet Gynecol 94:435, 1999b

Friedman EA: Labor: Clinical Evaluation and Management, 2nd ed. New York, Appleton-Century-Crofts, 1978

Frim DM, Emanuel RL, Robinson BG, et al: J Clin Invest 82:287, 1988

Fuchs AR, Fuchs F, Husslein P, et al: Oxytocin receptors and human parturition. A dual role for oxytocin in the initiation of labor. Science 215:1396, 1982

Fuchs AR, Fuchs F, Husslein P, et al: Oxytocin receptors in the human uterus during pregnancy and parturition. Am J Obstet Gynecol 150:734, 1984

Fuchs AR, Husslein P, Fuchs F: Oxytocin and the initiation of human parturition, 2. Stimulation of prostaglandin production in human decidua by oxytocin. Am J Obstet Gynecol 141:694, 1981

Fuchs AR, Periyasamy S, Alexandrova M, et al: Correlation between oxytocin receptor concentration and responsiveness to oxytocin in pregnant rat myometrium: Effect of ovarian steroids. Endocrinology 113:742, 1983

Gainer H, Alstein M, Whitnall MH, et al: The biosynthesis and secretion of oxytocin and vasopressin. In Knobil E, Neill J (eds): The Physiology of Reproduction, Vol II. New York, Raven, 1988, p 2265

Gardner MO, Goldenberg RL, Cliver SP, et al: The origin and outcome of preterm twin pregnancies. Obstet Gynecol 85:553, 1995

Garfield RE, Hayashi RH, Harper MJ: In vitro studies on the control of human myometrial gap junctions. Int J Gynaecol Obstet 25:241, 1987

Gerber S, Vial Y, Hohlfeld P, et al: Detection of Ureaplasma urealyticum in second-trimester amniotic fluid by polymerase chain reaction correlates with subsequent preterm labor and delivery. J Infect Dis 187:518, 2003

Germain A, Smith J, MacDonald PC, et al: Human fetal membrane contribution to the prevention of parturition: Uterotonin degradation. J Clin Endocrinol Metab 78:463, 1994

Goland RS, Jozak S, Conwell I: Placental corticotropin-releasing hormone and the hypercortisolism of pregnancy. Am J Obstet Gynecol 171:1287, 1994

Goland RS, Jozak S, Warren WB, et al: Elevated levels of umbilical cord plasma corticotropin-releasing hormone in growth-retarded fetuses. J Clin Endocrinol Metab 77:1174, 1993

Goland RS, Wardlaw SL, Stark RI, et al: High levels of corticotropin-releasing hormone immunoactivity in maternal and fetal plasma during pregnancy. J Clin Endocrinol Metab 63:1199, 1986

Goldenberg RL, Andrews WW, Hauth JC: Choriodecidual infection and preterm birth. Nutr Rev 60:S19, 2002

Goldenberg RL, Hauth JC, Andrews WW: Intrauterine infection and preterm delivery. N Engl J Med 342:1500, 2000

Goldenberg RL, Iams JD, Miodovnik M, et al: The preterm prediction study: Risk factors in twin gestations. National Institute of Child Health and Human Development Maternal-Fetal Medicine Units Network. Am J Obstet Gynecol 175:1047, 1996

Goldstein P, Berrier J, Rosen S, et al: A meta-analysis of randomized control trials of progestational agents in pregnancy. Br J Obstet Gynaecol 96:265, 1989

Gomez R, Romero R, Edwin SS, et al: Pathogenesis of preterm labor and preterm premature rupture of membranes associated with intraamniotic infection. Infect Dis Clin North Am 11:135, 1997

Gomez R, Romero R, Glasasso M, et al: The value of amniotic fluid interleukin-6, white blood cell count, and gram stain in the diagnosis of microbial invasion of the amniotic cavity in patients at term. Am J Reprod Immunol 32:200, 1994

Goncalves LF, Chaiworapongsa T, Romero R: Intrauterine infection and prematurity. Ment Retard Dev Disabil Res Rev 8:3, 2002

Grammatopoulos D, Milton NGN, Hillhouse EW: The human myometrial CRH receptor: G proteins and second messengers. Mol Cell Endocrinol 99:245, 1994

Grammatopoulos D, Thompson S, Hillhouse EW: The human myometrium expresses multiple isoforms of the corticotropin-releasing hormone receptor. J Clin Endocrinol Metab 80:2388, 1995

Gravett MG, Hitti J, Hess DL, et al: Intrauterine infection and preterm delivery: Evidence for activation of the fetal hypothalamic-pituitary-adrenal axis. Am J Obstet Gynecol 182:1404, 2000

Grino M, Chrousos GP, Margioris AN: The corticotropin releasing hormone gene is expressed in human placenta. Biochem Biophys Res Commun 148:1208, 1987

Haluska GJ, Wells TR, Hirst JJ, et al: Progesterone receptor localization and isoforms in myometrium, decidua, and fetal membranes from rhesus macaques: Evidence for functional progesterone withdrawal at parturition. J Soc Gynecol Invest 9:125, 2002

Haluska GJ, Cook MJ, Novy MJ: Inhibition and augmentation of progesterone production during pregnancy: Effects on parturition in rhesus monkeys. Am J Obstet Gynecol 176:682, 1997

Hedegaard M, Henriksen TB, Sabroe S, et al: Psychological distress in pregnancy and preterm delivery. BMJ 307:234, 1993

Heine RP, McGregor JA, Goodwin TM, et al: Serial salivary estriol to detect an increased risk of preterm birth. Obstet Gynecol 96:490, 2000

Hillhouse EW, Grammatopoulos D, Milton NGN, Quartero HWP: The identification of a human myometrial corticotropin-releasing hormone receptor that increases in affinity during pregnancy. J Clin Endocrinol Metab 76:736, 1993

Hillier SL, Martius J, Krohn M, et al: A case-control study of chorioamnionic infection and histologic chorioamnionitis in prematurity. N Engl J Med 319:972, 1988

Hitti J, Tarczy-Hornoch P, Murphy J, et al: Amniotic fluid infection, cytokines, and adverse outcome among infants at 34 weeks' gestation or less. Obstet Gynecol 98:1080, 2001

Hobel C, Culhane J: Role of psychosocial and nutritional stress on poor pregnancy outcome. J Nutr 133:1709S, 2003

Holmlund U, Cabers G, Dahlfors AR, et al: Expression and regulation of the pattern recognition receptors Toll-like receptor-2 and Toll-like receptor-4 in the human placenta. Immunology 107:145, 2002

Holzman C, Jetton J, Siler-Khodr T, et al: Second trimester corticotropin-releasing hormone levels in relation to preterm delivery and ethnicity. Obstet Gynecol 97:657, 2001

Huszar G, Walsh MP: Biochemistry of the myometrium and cervix. In Wynn RM, Jollie WP (eds): Biology of the Uterus, 2nd ed. New York, Plenum, 1989, p 355

Iams JD: The epidemiology of preterm birth. Clin Perinatol 30:651, 2003

Iams JD, Clapp DH, Contox DA, et al: Does extraamniotic infection cause preterm labor? Gas-liquid chromatography studies of amniotic fluid in amnionitis, preterm labor, and normal controls. Obstet Gynecol 70:365, 1987

Iams JD, Goldenberg RL, Meis PJ, et al: The length of the cervix and the risk of spontaneous premature delivery. N Engl J Med 334:567, 1996

Itoh H, Sagawa N, Hasegawa M, et al: Brain natriuretic peptide is present in the human amniotic fluid and is secreted from amnion cells. J Clin Endocrinol Metab 76:907, 1993

Itoh H, Sagawa N, Hasegawa M, et al: Expression of biologically active receptors for natriuretic peptides in the human uterus during pregnancy. Biochem Biophys Res Commun 203:602, 1994

Izumi H, Yallampalli C, Garfield RE: Gestational changes in L-arginine-induced relaxation of pregnant rat and human myometrial smooth muscle. Am J Obstet Gynecol 169:1327, 1993

Jacobsson B, Holst RM, Wennerholm UR, et al: Monocyte chemotactic protein-1 in cervical and amniotic fluid: Relationship to microbial invasion of the amniotic cavity, intraamniotic inflammation, and preterm delivery. Am J Obstet Gynecol 189:1161, 2003

Janssens S, Beyaert R: Role of Toll-like receptors in pathogen recognition. Clin Microbiol Rev 16:637, 2003

Johnson JW, Lee PA, Zachary AS, et al: High-risk prematurity—progestin treatment and steroid studies. Obstet Gynecol 54:412, 1979

Johnson RF, Mitchell CM, Giles WB, et al: The in vivo control of prostaglandin H synthase-2 messenger ribonucleic acid expression in the human amnion at parturition. J Clin Endocrinol Metab 87:2816, 2002

Jones SA, Brooks AN, Challis JR: Steroids modulate corticotropin-releasing hormone production in human fetal membranes and placenta. J Clin Endocrinol Metab 68:825, 1989

Karalis K, Goodwin G, Majzoub JA: Cortisol blockade of progesterone: A possible molecular mechanism involved in the initiation of human labor. Nat Med 2:556, 1996

Karalis K, Majzoub JA: Regulation of placental corticotropin-releasing hormone by steroids. Possible implications in labor initiation. Ann N Y Acad Sci 771:551, 1995

Kearney R, Sawhney R, DeLancey JO: Levator ani muscle anatomy evaluated by origin insertion pairs. Obstet Gynecol 104:168, 2004

Keelan JA, Blumenstein M, Helliwell RJ, et al: Cytokines, prostaglandins and parturition—a review. Placenta 24:S33, 2003

Keirse MJNC: Eicosanoids in human pregnancy and parturition. In Mitchell M (ed): Eicosanoids in Reproduction. Boca Raton, Fla, CRC Press, 1990, p 199

Keirse MJNC: Prostaglandins in parturition. In Keirse M, Anderson A, Gravenhorst J (eds): Human Parturition. The Hague, Netherlands, Martinus Nijhoff, 1979, p 101

Kelly RW: Inflammatory mediators and cervical ripening. J Reprod Immunol 57:217, 2002

Kemp B, Menon R, Fortunato SJ, et al: Quantitation and localization of inflammatory cytokines interleukin-6 and interleukin-8 in the lower uterine segment during cervical dilatation. J Asst Reprod Genet 19:215, 2002

Kent AS, Sullivan MH, Elder MG: Transfer of cytokines through human fetal membranes. J Reprod Fertil 100:81, 1994

Kenyon S, Boulvain M, Neilson J: Antibiotics for preterm rupture of membranes. Cochrane Data Base Syst Rev 2:CD001058, 2003

Kenyon SL, Taylor DJ, Tarnow-Mordi W: Broad-spectrum antibiotics for spontaneous preterm labour: The ORACLE II randomised trial. ORACLE Collaborative Group. Lancet 357:989, 2001

Kimura T, Takemura M, Nomura S, et al: Expression of oxytocin receptor in human pregnant myometrium. Endocrinology 137:780, 1996

King J, Flenady: Prophylactic antibiotics for inhibiting preterm labour with intact membranes. Cochrane Database Syst Rev 4:CD000246, 2002

Korita D, Sagawa N, Itoh H, et al: Cyclic mechanical stretch augments prostacyclin production in cultured human uterine myometrial cells from pregnant women: Possible involvement of upregulation of prostacyclin synthase expression. J Clin Endocrinol Metab 87:5209, 2002

Ku CY, Qian A, Wen Y, et al: Oxytocin stimulates myometrial guanosine triphosphatase and phospholipase-C activities via coupling to G alpha q/11. Endocrinology 136:1509, 1995

Leake RD: Oxytocin in the initiation of labor. In Carsten ME, Miller JD (eds): Uterine Function. Molecular and Cellular Aspects. New York, Plenum, 1990, p 361

Lei ZM, Reshef E, Rao CV: The expression of human chorionic gonadotropin/luteinizing hormone receptors in human endometrial and myometrial blood vessels. J Clin Endocrinol Metab 75:651, 1992

Liggins GC, Fairclough RJ, Grieves SA, et al: The mechanism of initiation of parturition in the ewe. Recent Prog Horm Res 29:111, 1973

Liggins GC, Kennedy PC, Holm LW: Failure of initiation of parturition after electrocoagulation of the pituitary of the fetal lamb. Am J Obstet Gynecol 98:1080, 1967

Lim AT, Gude NM: Atrial natriuretic factor production by the human placenta. J Clin Endocrinol Metab 80:3091, 1995

Lobel M. Conceptualizations, measurement, and effects of prenatal maternal stress on birth outcomes. J Behav Med 17:225, 1994

Lockwood CJ: Stress-associated preterm delivery: The role of corticotropin-releasing hormone. Am J Obstet Gynecol 180:S264, 1999

Lopez BA: Mechanisms of labour—biochemical aspects. Br J Obstet Gynaecol 110:39, 2003

Loudon JA, Groom KM, Bennett PR: Prostaglandin inhibitors in preterm labour. Best Pract Res Clin Obstet Gynaecol 17:731, 2003

Lowry PJ: Corticotropin-releasing factor and its binding protein in human plasma. Ciba Found Symp 172:108, 1993

Lyall F, Lye S, Teoh T, et al: Expression of Gsalpha, connexin-43, connexin-26, and EP1, 3, and 4 receptors in myometrium of prelabor singleton versus multiple gestations and the effects of mechanical stretch and steroids on Gsalpha. J Soc Gynecol Investi 9:299, 2002

MacDonald PC, Casey ML: Preterm birth. Sci Am 3:42, 1996

MacDonald PC, Casey ML: The accumulation of prostaglandins (PG) in amniotic fluid is an aftereffect of labor and not indicative of a role for PGE2 and PGE2 alpha in the initiation of human parturition. J Clin Endocrinol Metab 76:1332, 1993

MacDonald PC, Koga S, Casey ML: Decidual activation in parturition: Examination of amniotic fluid for mediators of the inflammatory response. Ann N Y Acad Sci 622:315, 1991

Madsen G, Zakar T, Ku CY, et al: Prostaglandins differentially modulate progesterone receptor-A and -B expression in human myometrial cells: Evidence for prostaglandin-induced functional progesterone withdrawal. J Clin Endocrinol Metab 89:1010, 2004

Mahendroo MS, Porter A, Russell DW, et al: The parturition defect in steroid 5alpha-reductase type 1 knockout mice is due to impaired cervical ripening. Mol Endocrinol 13:981, 1999

Malpas P: Postmaturity and malformation of the fetus. J Obstet Gynaecol Br Emp 40:1046, 1933

Many A, Lazebhnik N, Hill LM: The underlying cause of polyhydramnios determines prematurity. Prenat Diagn 16:55, 1996

Marinoni E, Korebrits C, Di Iorio R, et al: Effect of betamethasone in vivo on placental corticotropin-releasing hormone in human pregnancy. Am J Obstet Gynecol 178:770, 1998

McGrath S, Smith R: Prediction of preterm delivery using plasma corticotrophin-releasing hormone and other biochemical variables. Ann Med 34:28, 2002

McGregor JA, Jackson GM, Lachelin GC, et al: Salivary estriol as risk assessment for preterm labor: A prospective trial. Am J Obstet Gynecol 173:1337, 1995

McLean M, Bisits A, Davies J, et al: A placental clock controlling the length of human pregnancy. Nat Med 1:460, 1995

Meis PJ, Klebanoff M, Thom E, et al: Prevention of recurrent preterm delivery by 17 alpha-hydroxyprogesterone caproate. N Engl J Med 348:2379, 2003

Mercer BM: Preterm premature rupture of the membranes. Obstet Gynecol 101:178, 2003

Mesiano S, Chan EC, Fitter JT, et al: Progesterone withdrawal and estrogen activation in human parturition are coordinated by progesterone receptor A expression in the myometrium. J Clin Endocrinol Metab 87:2924, 2002

Moawad AH, Goldenberg RL, Mercer B, et al: The Preterm Prediction Study: The value of serum alkaline phosphatase, alpha-fetoprotein, plasma corticotropin-releasing hormone, and other serum markers for the prediction of spontaneous preterm birth. Am J Obstet Gynecol 186:990, 2002

Mueller-Heubach E, Rubinstein DN, Schwarz SS: Histologic chorioamnionitis and preterm delivery in different patient populations. Obstet Gynecol 75:622, 1990

Murphy BE: Human fetal serum cortisol levels related to gestational age: Evidence of a midgestational fall and a steep late gestational rise independent of sex or mode of delivery. Am J Obstet Gynecol 144:276, 1982

Myatt L, Lye SJ: Expression, localization and function of prostaglandin receptors in myometrium. Prostaglandins Leukot Essent Fatty Acids 70:137, 2004

Nishihara J, Ishibashi T, Mai Y, et al: Mass spectrometric evidence for the presence of platelet-activating factor (1-0-alkyl-2-sn-glycero-3-phosphocholine) in human amniotic fluid during labor. Lipids 19:907, 1984

Nissen E, Lilja G, Widstrom A-M, et al: Elevation of oxytocin levels early post partum in women. Acta Obstet Gynecol Scand 74:530, 1995

Novy MJ, Liggins GC: Role of prostaglandin, prostacyclin, and thromboxanes in the physiologic control of the uterus and in parturition. Semin Perinatol 4:45, 1980

Olson DM, Zaragoza DB, Shallow MC: Myometrial activation and preterm labour: Evidence supporting a role for the prostaglandin F receptor—a review. Placenta 24:S47, 2003

Ou CW, Chen ZQ, Qi S, et al: Increased expression of the rat myometrial oxytocin receptor messenger ribonucleic acid during labor requires both mechanical and hormonal signals. Biol Reprod 59:1055, 1998

Ou CW, Orsino A, Lye SJ: Expression of connexin-43 and connexin-26 in the rat myometrium during pregnancy and labor is differentially regulated by mechanical and hormonal signals. Endocrinology 138:5398, 1997

Park KH, Chaiworapongsa T, Kim YM, et al: Matrix metalloproteinase 3 in parturition, premature rupture of the membranes, and microbial invasion of the amniotic cavity. J Perinat Med 31:12, 2003

Parker CR Jr, Stankovic AM, Goland RS: Corticotropin-releasing hormone stimulates steroidogenesis in cultured human adrenal cells. Mol Cell Endocrinol 155:19, 1999

Paspalliaris V, Patersen DN, Thiede MA: Steroid regulation of parathyroid hormone–related protein expression and action in the rat uterus. J Steroid Biochem Mol Biol 53:259, 1995

Patel FA, Clifton VL, Chwalisz K, et al: Steroid regulation of prostaglandin dehydrogenase activity and expression in human term placenta and chorio-decidua in relation to labor. J Clin Endocrinol Metab 84:291, 1999

Perkins AV, Wolfe CD, Eben F, et al: Corticotrophin-releasing hormone-binding protein in human fetal plasma. J Endocrinol 146:395, 1995

Petraglia F, Florio P, Benedetto C, et al: High levels of corticotropin-releasing factor (CRF) are inversely correlated with low levels of maternal CRF-binding protein in pregnant women with pregnancy-induced hypertension. J Clin Endocrinol Metab 81:852, 1996

Petraglia F, Florio P, Simoncini T, et al: Cord plasma corticotropin-releasing factor-binding protein (CRF-BP) in term and preterm labour. Placenta 18:115, 1997

Pieber D, Allport VC, Hills F, et al: Interactions between progesterone receptor isoforms in myometrial cells in human labour. Mol Hum Reprod 7:875, 2001

Pierce JG, du Vigneaud V: Studies on high potency oxytocic materials from beef posterior pituitary lobes. J Biol Chem 186:77, 1950

Prescott SM, Zimmerman GA, McIntyre TM: Platelet activating factor. J Biol Chem 265:17381, 1990

Price SA, Pochun I, Phaneuf S, Lopez Bernal A: Adenylyl cyclase isoforms in pregnant and nonpregnant human myometrium. J Endocrinol 164:21, 2000

Quartero HWP, Noort WA, Fry CH, et al: Role of prostaglandins and leukotrienes in the synergistic effect of oxytocin and corticotropin-releasing hormone (CRH) on the contraction force in human gestational myometrium. Prostaglandins 42:137, 1991

Quartero HWP, Strivatsa G, Gillham B: Role for cyclic adenosine monophosphate in the synergistic interaction between oxytocin and corticotrophin-releasing factor in isolated human gestational myometrium. Clin Endocrinol 36:141, 1992

Rea C: Prolonged gestation, acrania, monstrosity and apparent placenta praevia in one obstetrical case. JAMA 30:1166, 1898

Romero R, Chaiworapongsa T, Espinoza J, et al: Fetal plasma MMP-9 concentrations are elevated in preterm premature rupture of the membranes. Am J Obstet Gynecol 187:1125, 2002

Romero R, Chaiworapongsa T, Espinoza J: Micronutrients and intrauterine infection, preterm birth and the fetal inflammatory response syndrome. J Nutr 133:1668S, 2003

Romero R, Durum S, Dinarello CA, et al: Interleukin-1 stimulates prostaglandin biosynthesis by human amnion. Prostaglandins 37:13, 1989

Romero R, Nores J, Mazor M, et al: Microbial invasion of the amniotic cavity during term labor. Prevalence and clinical significance. J Reprod Med 38:543, 1993

Ruiz RJ, Fullerton J, Dudley DJ: The interrelationship of maternal stress, endocrine factors and inflammation on gestational length. Obstet Gynecol Surv 58:415, 2003

Saijonmaa O, Laatikainen T, Wahlstrom T: Corticotrophin-releasing factor in human placenta: Localization, concentration and release in vitro. Placenta 9:373, 1988

Sanborn BM, Yue C, Wang W, et al: G-protein signaling pathways in myometrium: Affecting the balance between contraction and relaxation. Rev Reprod 3:196, 1998

Sasaki A, Shinkawa O, Margioris AN, et al: Immunoreactive corticotropin-releasing hormone in human plasma during pregnancy, labor, and delivery. J Clin Endocrinol Metab 64:224, 1987

Schulman H, Romney SL: Variability of uterine contractions in normal human parturition. Obstet Gynecol 36:215, 1970

Selinger M, Mackenzie IZ, Gillmer MD, et al: Progesterone inhibition in mid-trimester termination of pregnancy: Physiological and clinical effects. Br J Obstet Gynaecol 94:1218, 1987

Smieja Z, Zakar T, Walton JC, et al: Prostaglandin endoperoxide synthase kinetics in human amnion before and after labor at term and following preterm labor. Placenta 14:163, 1993

Smith GC, Wu WX, Nathanielsz PW. Effects of gestational age and labor on expression of prostanoid receptor genes in baboon uterus. Biol Reprod 64:1131, 2001

Smith R, Mesiano S, Chan EC, et al: Corticotropin-releasing hormone directly and preferentially stimulates dehydroepiandrosterone sulfate secretion by human fetal adrenal cortical cells. J Clin Endocrinol Metab 83:2916, 1998

Soloff MS, Alexandrova M, Fernström MJ: Oxytocin receptors: Triggers for parturition and lactation? Science 204:1313, 1979

Soloff MS, Fernström MA, Periyasamy S, et al: Regulation of oxytocin receptor concentration in rat uterine explants by estrogen and progesterone. Can J Biochem Cell Biol 61:625, 1983

Sooranna SR, Lee Y, Kim LU, et al: Mechanical stretch activates type 2 cyclooxygenase via activator protein-1 transcription factor in human myometrial cells. Mol Hum Reprod 10:109, 2004

Stull JT, Lin PJ, Krueger JK, et al: Myosin light chain kinase; functional domains and structural motifs. Acta Physiol Scand 164:471, 1998

Stull JT, Taylor DA, MacKenzie LW, et al: Biochemistry and physiology of smooth muscle contractility. In McNellis D, Challis JRG, MacDonald PC, et al (eds): Cellular and Integrative Mechanisms in the Onset of Labor. An NICHD Workshop. Ithaca, NY, Perinatology, 1988, p 17

Thiede MA, Harm SC, Hasson DM, et al: In vivo regulation of PTH-rP messenger ribonucleic acid in the rat uterus by 17 beta-estradiol. Endocrinology 128:2317, 1991a

Thiede MA, Harm SC, McKee RL, et al: Expression of the PTH-rP gene in the avian oviduct. Endocrinology 129:1958, 1991b

Üstün C, Kocak I, Baris S, et al: Subclinical chorioamnionitis as an etiologic factor in preterm deliveries. Int J Obstet Gynecol 72:109, 2001

Van Meir CA, Sangha RK, Walton JC, et al: Immunoreactive 15-hydroxyprostaglandin dehydrogenase (PGDH) is reduced in fetal membranes from patients at preterm delivery in the presence of infection. Placenta 17:291, 1996

Wadhwa PD, Culhane JF, Rauh V, et al: Stress and preterm birth: Neuroendocrine, immune/inflammatory, and vascular mechanisms. Matern Child Health J 5:119, 2001

Wadhwa PD, Porto M, Garite TJ, et al: Maternal corticotropin-releasing hormone levels in the early third trimester predict length of gestation in human pregnancy. Am J Obstet Gynecol 179:1079, 1998

Wadhwa PD, Sandman CA, Porto M, et al: The association between prenatal stress and infant birth weight and gestational age at birth: A prospective investigation. Am J Obstet Gynecol 169:858, 1993

Warren WB, Goland RS, Wardlaw SL, et al: Elevated maternal plasma corticotropin releasing hormone levels in twin gestation. J Perinat Med 18:39, 1990

Wathes DC, Borwick SC, Timmons PM, et al: Oxytocin receptor expression in human term and preterm gestational tissues prior to and following the onset of labour. J Endocrinol 161:143, 1999

Watts DH, Krohn MA, Hillier SL, et al: The association of occult amniotic fluid infection with gestational age and neonatal outcome among women in preterm labor. Obstet Gynecol 79:351, 1992

Webb RC: Smooth muscle contraction and relaxation. Adv Physiol Educ 27:201, 2003

Weiss G: Relaxin used to produce the cervical ripening of labor. Clin Obstet Gynecol 38:293, 1995

Whittle WL, Patel FA, Alfaidy N, et al: Glucocorticoid regulation of human and ovine parturition: The relationship between fetal hypothalamic-pituitary-adrenal axis activation and intrauterine prostaglandin production. Biol Reprod 64:1019, 2001

Winters AJ, Oliver C, Colston C, et al: Plasma ACTH levels in the human fetus and neonate as related to age and parturition. J Clin Endocrinol Metab 39:269, 1974

Wolfe CD, Patel SP, Linton EA, et al: Plasma corticotrophin-releasing factor (CRF) in abnormal pregnancy. Br J Obstet Gynaecol 95:1003, 1988

Woodcock NA, Taylor CW, Thornton S: Effect of an oxytocin receptor antagonist and rho kinase inhibitor on the [Ca++]$_i$ sensitivity of human myometrium. Am J Obstet Gynecol 190:222, 2004

Word RA, Kamm KE, Stull JT, et al: Endothelin increases cytoplasmic calcium and myosin phosphorylation in human myometrium. Am J Obstet Gynecol 162:1103, 1990

Word RA, Stull JT, Casey ML, et al: Contractile elements and myosin light chain phosphorylation in myometrial tissue from nonpregnant and pregnant women. J Clin Invest 92:29, 1993

Wu WX, Ma XH, Smith GC, et al: Prostaglandin dehydrogenase mRNA in baboon intrauterine tissues in late gestation and spontaneous labor. Am J Physiol Regul Integr Comp Physiol 279:R1082, 2000

Yallampalli C, Byam-Smith M, Nelson SO, et al: Steroid hormones modulate the production of nitric oxide and cGMP in the rat uterus. Endocrinology 134:1971, 1994a

Yallampalli C, Izumi H, Byam-Smith M, et al: An L-arginine-nitric oxide-cyclic guanosine monophosphate system exists in the uterus and inhibits contractility during pregnancy. Am J Obstet Gynecol 170:175, 1994b

Yamamoto M, Harm SC, Grasser WA, et al: Parathyroid hormone–related protein in the rat urinary bladder: A smooth muscle relaxant produced locally in response to mechanical stretch. Proc Natl Acad Sci U S A 89:5326, 1992

Yasuda K, Johnston JM: The hormonal regulation of PAFacetylhydrolase in the rat. Endocrinology 130:708, 1992

Yemini M, Borenstein R, Dreazen E, et al: Prevention of premature labor by 17 alpha-hydroxyprogesterone caproate. Am J Obstet Gynecol 151:574, 1985

Yoon BH, Romero R, Park JS, et al: Microbial invasion of the amniotic cavity with Ureaplasma urealyticum is associated with robust host response in fetal, amniotic, and maternal compartments. Am J Obstet Gynecol 179:1254, 1998

Young A, Thomson AJ, Ledingham M, et al: Immunolocalization of proinflammatory cytokines in myometrium, cervix, and fetal membranes during human parturition at term. Biol Reprod 66:445, 2002

Zahl PA, Bjerknes C: Induction of decidua–placental hemorrhage in mice by the endotoxins of certain gram-negative bacteria. Proc Soc Exp Biol Med 54:329, 1943

Zambrana RE, Dunkel-Schetter C, Collins NL, et al: Mediators of ethnic-associated differences in infant birth weight. J Urban Health 76:102, 1999

Zhu YP, Word RA, Johnston JM: The presence of PAF binding sites in human myometrium and its role in uterine contraction. Am J Obstet Gynecol 166:1222, 1992

Ziecik AJ, Derecka-Reszka K, Rzucidlo SJ: Extragonadal gonadotropin receptors, their distribution and function. J Physiol Pharmacol 43:33, 1992

Zingg HH, Rozen F, Chu K, et al: Oxytocin and oxytocin receptor gene expression in the uterus. Recent Prog Horm Res 50:255, 1995

Zuo J, Lei ZM, Rao CV: Human myometrial chorionic gonadotropin/luteinizing hormone receptors in preterm and term deliveries. J Clin Endocrinol Metab 79:907, 1994

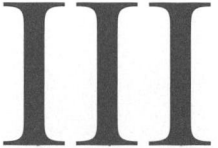

SECTION

Antepartum

7

Preconceptional Counseling

DEFINITION

PRECONCEPTIONAL COUNSELING VISIT

Personal and Family History
Medical History
Social History
Lifestyle and Work Habits
Family History
Immunizations

BENEFITS OF PRECONCEPTIONAL COUNSELING

Unplanned Pregnancy
Chronic Medical Disorders
Genetic Diseases

PRECONCEPTIONAL COUNSELORS

SCREENING TESTS

REFERENCES

In the early part of the 20th century, women with medical problems were often unable to conceive or were advised not to. Discoveries such as insulin and the development of effective antihypertensive medications subsequently made it possible for many of these women to contemplate pregnancy. Obstetrical care of women with medical problems during this time dealt almost exclusively with protecting maternal health, as little was known about pathological influences on fetal development. In the 1960s, research began to focus on the pathophysiology of pregnancy and perinatal outcome. As a result, prenatal care was gradually extended to include fetal concerns, and interest in perinatal research increased dramatically. The etiologies of many maternal and fetal conditions were determined, and research also clarified the genetic origins of many diseases. At the same time, effective contraception was developed, allowing women to postpone pregnancy and limit family size while striving to optimize perinatal outcome. The focus of obstetrical care thus changed once again, from treating maternal and fetal diseases to predicting and preventing them.

In 2000, the Public Health Service released *Healthy People 2010,* a guide for the second nationwide preventive medicine program. The major goals are to increase the quality and years of healthy life and to eliminate health disparities between individuals. More specifically, it strives to improve the health and well-being of women, infants, children, and families.

Preconceptional counseling can play a major role in achieving these goals. As stated in the Department of Health and Human Services report on the program: "Preconceptional screening and counseling offer an opportunity to identify and mitigate maternal risk factors before pregnancy begins." For example, the two leading causes of death in the first year of life—birth defects and disorders caused by preterm birth—can both be significantly reduced or eliminated by the preconceptional initiation of specific preventive strategies. Morbidity caused by a variety of factors, including uncontrolled maternal disease, environmental exposures, and nutritional deficiencies, also can be prevented by preconceptional care. Furthermore, as discussed in Chapter 38 (see p. 904), the intrauterine fetal environment has a tremendous impact on the health and well-being of the adult that fetus will become— the *Barker hypothesis* (Barker, 1994). Thus, optimizing pregnancy conditions and outcomes has long-term health impacts that are only beginning to be apparent. The 1989 Public Health Service Expert Panel on the Content of Prenatal Care rightfully concluded: "The preconceptional visit may be the single most important health care visit when viewed in the context of its effect on pregnancy."

DEFINITION

Preconceptional counseling is preventive medicine for obstetrics. Factors that could potentially affect perinatal outcome are identified, and the woman is advised of her risks.

Whenever possible, a strategy is provided to reduce or eliminate the pathological influences revealed by her family, medical, or obstetrical history, or by specific testing. This chapter reviews data confirming that preconceptional counseling has a measurable positive impact on pregnancy outcome. It also provides a description of the components of a thorough preconceptional assessment. In most cases, specific guidelines for the preconceptional management of a variety of medical, obstetrical, and genetic disorders are provided in chapters pertaining to each topic.

BENEFITS OF PRECONCEPTIONAL COUNSELING

Randomized trials of the efficacy of preconceptional counseling are scarce, partly because withholding such counseling for research purposes would in many cases be considered unethical. In addition, because maternal and perinatal outcomes are dependent on the interaction of a variety of maternal, fetal, and environmental factors, it is often difficult to ascribe pregnancy outcome to a specific intervention (Moos, 2004). Nevertheless, what follows are several prospective and case-control trials that clearly demonstrate that preconceptional counseling improves pregnancy outcome.

UNPLANNED PREGNANCY. To be effective, counseling about potential pregnancy risks and strategies to prevent them must be provided before conception. By the time most women realize they are pregnant—1 to 2 weeks after the first missed period—the fetal spinal cord has already formed and the heart is beating (Moore, 1983). Many prevention strategies, for example, folic acid to prevent neural-tube defects, are ineffective if initiated at this time. The Centers for Disease Control and Prevention (1999) estimate that up to half of all pregnancies are unplanned, and there is evidence that these may be at greatest risk.

Adams and colleagues (1993) conducted a population-based survey of almost 12,500 women in four states and found that women with unintended pregnancies were more likely than those with planned pregnancies to have an indication for preconceptional counseling. Hellerstedt and co-workers (1998) surveyed nearly 7200 pregnant women and found that women with unintended pregnancies were more likely to have high-risk behaviors. Jack and associates (1995) administered a comprehensive risk survey to 136 women at the time of a negative pregnancy test. They found that (1) the majority did not want to be pregnant, (2) half reported a medical or reproductive risk that could adversely affect pregnancy, (3) half reported a genetic risk, and (4) one fourth reported risks for human immunodeficiency virus (HIV) and hepatitis B infection or alcohol or recreational drug use. Unwanted pregnancies are particularly common in the unmarried urban poor (Besculides and Laraque, 2004).

An important measure of the effectiveness of preconceptional counseling is, therefore, its influence in reducing the number of unintended pregnancies. Moos and colleagues (1996) instituted a preconceptional care program for reproductive-aged women who visited a health department clinic and then also studied 1378 women who sought prenatal care. They reported that the 456 women who had preconceptional counseling had a 50-percent greater likelihood of describing their pregnancies as intended compared with that of 309 women with health care but no counseling, and a 65-percent greater likelihood compared with that of women with no health care prior to pregnancy.

CHRONIC MEDICAL DISORDERS

Diabetes Mellitus. Because maternal and fetal pathology associated with hyperglycemia is well known, diabetes is the prototype of a condition for which preconceptional counseling is beneficial. Diabetes-associated risks to both mother and fetus are discussed in detail in Chapter 52 (see p. 1176). Many of these complications can be avoided if conception occurs when glucose control is optimal (Jovanovic and colleagues, 1981). Such control requires either that glucose levels be chronically well regulated—always a goal, but difficult to achieve—or that the woman make necessary changes before attempting conception. Preconceptional counseling can educate her about risks and provide a program designed to reduce them (Bernasko, 2004).

The utility of preconceptional counseling in preventing diabetes-related complications at all stages of pregnancy has been confirmed. Shown in Figure 7–1 are summaries of major studies in which the incidence of anomalies in infants born to diabetic women who received preconceptional counseling was compared with that of women without such counseling. Importantly, all studies showed that counseling is associated with significantly fewer malformations.

Dunne and co-workers (1999) reviewed the impact of preconceptional counseling on other diabetes-related neonatal morbidity. Women who received counseling sought prenatal care earlier, had lower hemoglobin A_{1c} levels, and were less likely to smoke during pregnancy. Their outcomes were compared with those of a cohort of women who did not receive such counseling. Of the women who received counseling, none were delivered before 30 weeks compared with 17 percent in the uncounseled group. In addition, the counseled women had fewer macrosomic infants—25 versus 40 percent; they had no growth-restricted infants compared with 8.5 percent; they had no neonatal deaths compared with 6 percent; and their infants had 50 percent fewer admissions to the intensive care nursery—17 versus 34 percent.

Preconceptional counseling also reduces obstetrical complications and health care costs in diabetic women. In a prospective multicenter observational trial from five Michigan centers, Herman and colleagues (1999) confirmed these benefits. They reported that diabetic women who received preconceptional counseling reported for prenatal care 3 weeks earlier than uncounseled women; they had lower hemoglobin A_{1c} levels; they were significantly less likely to require antepartum hospitalization for diabetes control—8 versus 68 percent; and they had significantly fewer hospitalization days—4.5 versus 15.7. Counseled women also had fewer episodes of hypoglycemia and diabetic ketoacidosis; they had no hypertensive complications; and their postpartum stay was 2 days shorter than that of uncounseled women. These improved outcomes were associated with savings of $34,000 in direct medical costs per patient who received counseling.

Epilepsy. Women with epilepsy are two to three times more likely to have infants with structural anomalies than unaffected women (Chang and McAuley, 1998; Wide and associates, 2004). Some reports indicate that epilepsy itself increases the incidence of congenital anomalies, independent of the effects of antiseizure medication. In a recent study, however, Holmes and colleagues (2001) compared 509 epileptic women who took antiseizure medication during pregnancy to 606 who did not. They found that only infants exposed to anticonvulsant medications had an increased incidence of structural anomalies. Fetuses exposed to one drug had significantly fewer malformations than those exposed to two or more drugs—21 versus 28 percent. By contrast, the incidence of defects in fetuses of epileptic mothers who did not take medication was only 8.5 percent—the same as in fetuses of women without seizure disorders. Preconceptional counseling usually includes recommendations to switch to monotherapy with the least teratogenic medication (Adab and colleagues, 2004; American Academy of Neurology, 1998). The risks of antiseizure medication are described in detail in Chapter 14 (see p. 347).

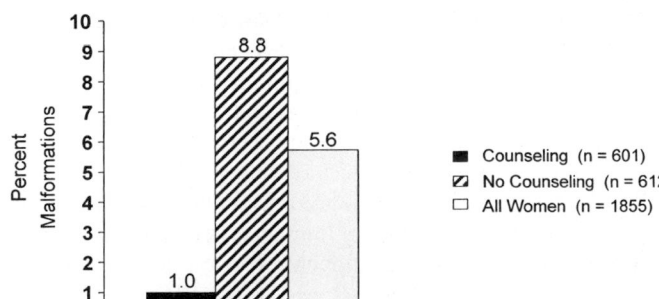

FIGURE 7–1. Major congenital anomalies in diabetic women according to whether they had preconceptional counseling. (Data from Gregory and Tattersall, 1992.)

Epileptic women also are advised to take supplemental folic acid. Biale and Lewenthal (1984) performed a retrospective case-control study to evaluate effects of periconceptional folate supplementation in women taking anticonvulsants. Although 10 of 66 (15 percent) unsupplemented pregnancies resulted in offspring with congenital malformations, none of 33 neonates of supplemented women had anomalies. Depending on the history, a trial period without anticonvulsants also may be recommended.

Other Chronic Diseases. Cox and co-workers (1992) reviewed pregnancy outcomes of 1075 high-risk women who received preconceptional counseling. If they received counseling, 240 women with hypertension, renal disease, thyroid disease, asthma, and heart disease had significantly better outcomes than previous pregnancies. Indeed, 80 percent of those counseled gave birth to a normal infant compared with only 40 percent in the previous uncounseled gestation.

GENETIC DISEASES. Birth defects are currently the leading cause of infant mortality and account for 20 percent of all infant deaths. These defects can be avoided with three types of prevention strategies. The preferred strategy is *primary prevention*—avoidance of causal factors—which is becoming possible for more congenital diseases as their etiologies are discovered. *Secondary prevention*—identifying and terminating affected pregnancies—is an alternative strategy for single-gene disorders and other defects that cannot be prevented. Surgical correction of structural defects is one type of *tertiary prevention,* but it is not possible for most genetic disorders. The benefits of preconceptional counseling usually are measured by comparing the incidence of new cases before and after the initiation of a counseling program. Some examples of congenital conditions that clearly benefit from counseling include neural-tube defects, phenylketonuria, Tay-Sachs disease, and the thalassemias.

Neural-Tube Defects (NTDs). The incidence of these defects is 1 to 2 per 1000 live births, and they are second only to cardiac anomalies as the most frequent structural fetal malformation (see Chap. 12, p. 302). Some NTDs are associated with a specific mutation in the methylene tetrahydrofolate reductase gene (677C $\rightarrow$ T), the adverse effects of which appear to be largely overcome by periconceptional folic acid supplementation (Ou and associates, 1996; van der Put and colleagues, 1995). The Medical Research Council on Vitamin Study Research Group (1991) conducted a randomized double-blind study of preconceptional folic acid therapy at 33 centers in seven European countries. Women with a previous affected child who took supplemental folic acid before conception and throughout the first trimester reduced their NTD recurrence risk by 72 percent. Perhaps more importantly, because 90 to 95 percent of NTDs occur in families with no prior history, Czeizel and Dudas (1992) subsequently

showed that supplementation reduced the a priori risk of a *first* NTD occurrence.

Phenylketonuria (PKU). This disorder is an inborn error of phenylalanine metabolism. It is an example of a disease in which the fetus is not at risk to inherit the disease but may be damaged by the effects of maternal genetic disease. For such conditions, preconceptional counseling regarding strategies to improve the intrauterine environment constitutes primary prevention and may significantly reduce fetal morbidity. Individuals with PKU who eat an unrestricted diet have abnormally high blood phenylalanine levels. This amino acid readily crosses the placenta and can damage developing fetal organs, especially neural and cardiac tissues (see Chap. 12, p. 297). With preconceptional counseling and adherence to a phenylalanine-restricted diet before pregnancy, the incidence of fetal malformations is dramatically reduced (Guttler and colleagues, 1990; Koch and associates, 1990).

The Maternal Phenylketonuria Collaborative Study evaluated the effectiveness of preconceptional care in preventing PKU-related fetal defects (Rouse and co-workers, 1997). Almost 300 women with PKU began a low-phenylalanine diet before pregnancy. Compared with infants whose mothers had poor dietary control, infants of women achieving good control had a lower incidence of microcephaly (6 versus 15 percent), neurological abnormalities (4 versus 14 percent), and cardiac defects (none versus 16 percent). The proportion of women treated preconceptionally increased from 7 to 51 percent from 1984 to 1994 (Platt and colleagues, 2000).

Tay-Sachs Disease. This disease is a severe, autosomal-recessive neurodegenerative disorder that leads to death in childhood. The effectiveness of preconceptional counseling in reducing genetic disease has been most clearly demonstrated in Tay-Sachs disease. In the early 1970s, there were approximately 60 new cases in the United States each year, primarily in individuals of Jewish heritage. An intensive worldwide campaign was initiated to counsel Jewish men and women of reproductive age, to identify carriers through genetic testing, to provide prenatal testing—secondary prevention—for high-risk couples, and even to help heterozygote carriers choose unaffected mates—primary prevention! The outcome of this initiative has been monitored by the National Tay-Sachs Disease and Allied Disorders Association (Kaback and colleagues, 1993). Within 8 years of its inception, nearly 1 million young adults around the world had been tested and counseled, and the incidence of new Tay-Sachs cases has plummeted to only about five new cases per year. Currently, most new cases are in the non-Jewish population.

Thalassemias. These disorders of globin-chain synthesis are the most common single-gene disorders worldwide. Approximately 200 million people carry a gene for one of these hemoglobinopathies (Benz, 2001). Hundreds of mutations have been identified that cause several important thalassemia syndromes, discussed in Chapter 51 (see p. 1154). Some of these could be avoided by both primary and secondary prevention (Fucharoen and associates, 1991; Wong, 1985). In endemic areas such as Mediterranean countries, counseling and other prevention strategies have reduced the incidence of new cases by at least 80 percent (Angastiniotis and Modell, 1998). Experiences with a long-standing counseling program aimed at Montreal high school students at risk were summarized by Mitchell and colleagues (1996). Over a 20-year period, 25,274 students of Mediterranean origin were counseled and tested for β-thalassemia. Within a few years of initiating the preconceptional program, all high-risk couples who requested prenatal diagnosis had already been counseled, and no affected children have been born since that time.

PRECONCEPTIONAL COUNSELORS

Practitioners providing routine health maintenance for reproductive-aged women have the best opportunity to provide preventive counseling. Gynecologists, internists, family practitioners, and pediatricians can do so at the annual examination. The occasion of a negative pregnancy test is a good time for counseling. Jack and associates (1995) administered a comprehensive preconceptional risk survey to 136 women who had a negative pregnancy test in an ambulatory general practice clinic. Almost 95 percent of these women reported at least one problem that could affect a future pregnancy. These included medical or reproductive problems (52 percent), a family history of genetic diseases (50 percent), increased risk of contracting HIV (30 percent), increased risk of contracting hepatitis B and use of illegal substances (25 percent), alcohol use (17 percent), and nutritional risk (54 percent).

Basic preconceptional advice regarding diet, alcohol use, smoking, illicit drug use, vitamin intake, exercise, and other behaviors can be provided by the primary care provider, including the obstetrician-gynecologist. Medical records should be obtained and reviewed. Counselors should be knowledgeable about relevant medical diseases, prior surgery, reproductive disorders, or genetic conditions, and must be able to interpret data and recommendations provided by other specialists. The practitioner who is uncomfortable providing counseling should refer the woman or couple to a counselor with special expertise.

PRECONCEPTIONAL COUNSELING VISIT

PERSONAL AND FAMILY HISTORY. Counseling begins with a thorough review of the medical, obstetrical, social, and family histories. Useful information is more likely to be obtained by asking specific questions about each aspect of the history and about each member of the family than by asking general, open-ended questions. The interview may take 30 minutes to an hour. Some important information can be obtained by questionnaire, ideally at a routine prepregnancy visit. Commercially prepared questionnaires are available that address medical and surgical history; reproductive history, including outcomes of each prior pregnancy; medication use and drug allergies; family history of medical or genetic diseases and reproductive abnormalities; racial or ethnic origin; social risk factors such as alcohol, illicit drugs, smoking, high-risk sexual behavior, and spousal abuse; environmental risk factors such as exposure to pesticides or other chemicals; and home environment and stress inducers. Answers should be reviewed with the patient to ensure appropriate follow-up, including obtaining relevant medical records or consultant notes.

MEDICAL HISTORY. Preconceptional counseling should address all risk factors pertinent to both mother and fetus. General questions to be answered include how pregnancy will affect maternal health, and how a high-risk condition will affect the fetus. Almost any medical, obstetrical, or genetic condition warrants some consideration prior to pregnancy. These conditions should be discussed in terms of general maternal and fetal risks, and suggestions for prepregnancy evaluation should be offered. Finally, advice for improving outcome is provided. More detailed information on specific diseases such as diabetes, hypertension, collagen vascular disorders, and others are found in the relevant chapters.

Genetic Diseases. Women whose ethnic background, race, or personal or family history places them at increased risk to have a fetus with a genetic disease should receive appropriate counseling. This includes the possibility of prenatal diagnosis as discussed in Chapter 13. Women who have a genetic disease usually require additional counseling about their own risks by someone knowledgeable about genetics. This is because genetic conditions are often associated with unique medical problems that may be adversely affected by pregnancy or that can adversely affect pregnancy outcome. They also may benefit from consultation with other specialists, for example, anesthesiologists, cardiologists, or surgeons. A variety of genetic resources can be accessed for detailed information about many inherited disorders.

Reproductive History. This component includes questions regarding infertility; abnormal pregnancy outcomes, including miscarriage, ectopic pregnancy, recurrent pregnancy loss, and preterm delivery; and complications such as preeclampsia or placental abruption. The reproductive history of first-degree relatives also may be helpful. For example, if a patient with recurrent pregnancy loss has other family members with the same history, her risk of carrying a familial translocation or another chromosomal rearrangement is increased. A history suggesting an incompetent cervix or a uterine anomaly should prompt an appropriate evaluation. The need for assisted reproductive technologies should be noted and associated risks discussed (Jackson and associates, 2004). The latter include a significantly increased risk of multiple gestation (see Chap. 39). Counseling regarding intracytoplasmic sperm injection and cryopreservation of embryos also should be provided (Bowen and colleagues, 1998; Hansen and co-workers, 2002). Risk factors for recurrent preterm delivery, preeclampsia, placental abruption, and repeat cesarean delivery are summarized in discussions of these disorders later in this text.

SOCIAL HISTORY

Maternal Age. The mother's age can have an impact on pregnancy at both ends of the reproductive spectrum.

TEENAGE PREGNANCY. According to the American College of Obstetricians and Gynecologists (2003), the pregnancies of women between the ages of 15 and 19 years accounted for about 11 percent of all births in 2001. Teenagers are more likely to be anemic, and they are at increased risk to have growth-restricted infants, preterm labor, and higher infant mortality (Fraser and associates, 1995). The incidence of sexually transmitted diseases—common in adolescents—is even higher during pregnancy (Niccolai and colleagues, 2003). Because most teenage pregnancies are unplanned, teens rarely seek preconceptional counseling.

Teenagers usually are still growing and developing, and thus have greater caloric requirements than older women. The normal or underweight teenager should be advised to increase caloric intake by 400 kcal/day. Alternatively, as discussed in Chapter 43, the obese teenager may not need additional calories. Nonjudgmental questioning may elicit a history of substance abuse. Instructions regarding the identification or prevention of common pregnancy complications should be given.

PREGNANCY AFTER AGE 35. Currently, about 10 percent of pregnancies occur in women in this age group. The older woman is more likely to request preconceptional counseling, either because she has postponed pregnancy and now wishes to optimize her outcome, or because she plans to undergo infertility treatment. In the past, the indelicate term *elderly gravida* was used to arbitrarily define women over 35. Although the term is now passé, certain age-related adverse pregnancy outcomes do begin to increase at this age.

Some studies indicate that after age 35, women are at increased risk for obstetrical complications as well as perinatal morbidity and mortality. There is no doubt that the older woman who has a chronic illness or who is in poor physical condition has increased risks. For the physically fit woman without medical problems, however, the risks are much lower than previously reported.

The influence of socioeconomic and health status on pregnancy outcome in the older woman is illustrated by two studies involving different populations of women. Berkowitz and co-workers (1990) described outcomes of almost 800 privately insured nulliparas, age 35 and older, who were cared for at Mount Sinai Hospital in New York City. These authors reported only slightly increased risks of gestational diabetes, pregnancy-induced hypertension, placenta previa or abruption, and cesarean delivery. The women did not have an increased incidence of preterm delivery, growth-restricted infants, or perinatal death. In contrast, a study from Parkland Hospital, which included nearly 900 socioeconomically disadvantaged women older than 35 years of age, identified a significantly increased incidence of hypertension, diabetes, placenta previa and abruption, preterm delivery, and perinatal mortality (Fig. 7–2). The disparate outcomes in these two groups of women are likely attributable to socioeconomic status, which influences lifestyle and access to health care and thus health status.

Maternal mortality is higher in women age 35 and older, but improved medical care may ameliorate this risk. Buehler and colleagues (1986) reviewed maternal deaths in the United States from 1974 through 1982. From 1974 through 1978, older women had a fivefold increased relative risk of maternal

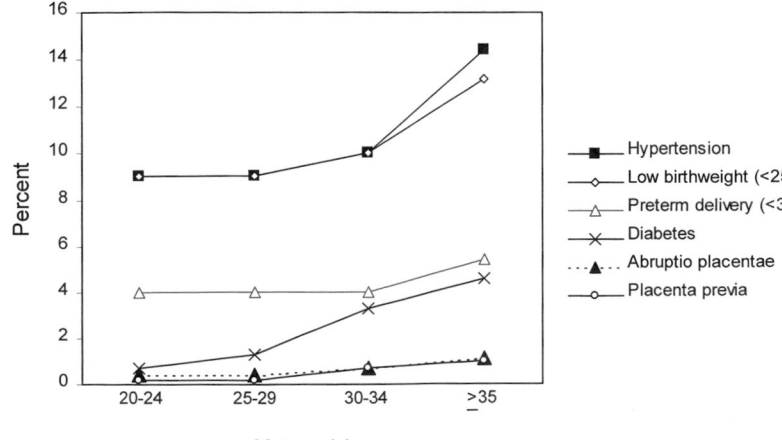

FIGURE 7–2. Incidence of some pregnancy complications in 20,525 women delivered at Parkland Hospital, 1987–1988. (Data from Cunningham and Leveno, 1995.)

death compared with that of younger women. By 1982, however, the mortality rates for older women had decreased by 50 percent. They concluded that this was probably due to improvements in health care.

Maternal age-related fetal risks primarily stem from (1) iatrogenic preterm delivery required for maternal complications such as hypertension and diabetes, (2) spontaneous preterm delivery, (3) fetal growth disorders related to chronic maternal disease or multiple gestation, (4) fetal aneuploidy, and (5) pregnancies resulting from use of assisted reproductive technology.

Most researchers have found that fetal aneuploidy is the only congenital abnormality related to maternal age. A study of 577,000 births in British Columbia by Baird and co-workers (1991) and another of 574,000 live births in Sweden by Pradat (1992) found no association between nonaneuploid structural defects and maternal age. An exception was the study by Hollier and colleagues (2000) of nearly 103,000 pregnancies that included 3885 infants with congenital malformations delivered at Parkland Hospital. They reported that the incidence of nonaneuploid structural abnormalities increased significantly with maternal age. Some contend, however, that ascertainment bias was likely because older mothers commonly underwent targeted ultrasound examination but not amniocentesis, and the study population was enriched with regional referrals for women with malformed fetuses.

Older paternal age is associated with an increased incidence of genetic diseases caused by new autosomal-dominant mutations, but the incidence is still low (see Chap. 12, p. 289). Accordingly, whether targeted ultrasound examinations should be performed solely for advanced maternal or paternal age is controversial.

Although the incidence of dizygotic twinning increases with maternal age, the most important cause of multifetal gestations in older women currently is conception with the use of *assisted reproductive technology* and *ovulation induction.* According to the Centers for Disease Control and Prevention (2002), 0.7 percent of all 3.9 million births in the United States in 1998 were the result of these techniques. More than half of this percentage were multiple infant births, which account for much of the morbidity from preterm delivery and neurological sequelae (Adashi and collaborators, 2003, 2004; Schieve and colleagues, 2002; Strömberg and associates, 2002). Finally, Hansen and co-workers (2002) reported that 8.6 percent of 301 infants conceived using intracytoplasmic sperm injection and 9 percent of 837 infants conceived by in vitro fertilization had major birth defects—compared with 4.2 percent in 4000 control women.

Recreational Drugs and Smoking. Fetal risks associated with alcohol, marijuana, cocaine, amphetamines, and heroin are discussed in Chapter 14 (see p. 363). Alcohol-related mental retardation is currently the only mental retardation syndrome amenable to primary prevention. The first step in preventing this and other types of drug-related fetal damage is the woman's honest assessment of her usage. Questions regarding usage should be asked in a nonjudgmental manner. The alcoholic patient can be identified by asking the well-studied TACE questions, which correlate with DSM-IV criteria for lifetime alcoholism diagnoses (Chang and associates, 1998). TACE is a series of four questions concerning *tolerance* to alcohol, being *annoyed* by comments about their drinking, attempts to *cut down,* and a history of drinking early in the morning—the *eye opener.*

According to the Centers for Disease Control and Prevention (2003), almost one fourth of women who are between the ages of 18 and 44 years smoke cigarettes. Smoking affects fetal growth in a dose-dependent manner. It increases the risk of preterm labor, fetal growth restriction, and low birthweight. It has also been associated with an increased incidence of attention-deficit/hyperactivity disorder and behavioral and learning problems typically identified by school age (American College of Obstetricians and Gynecologists, 1999). Smoking also increases the risk of pregnancy complications related to vascular damage, such as uteroplacental insufficiency and placental abruption (see Chap. 35, p. 811). After counseling, the woman should be provided with a prepregnancy program to reduce or eliminate smoking.

Environmental Exposures. Everyone is exposed to environmental substances, but fortunately only a few agents have an impact on pregnancy outcome. Exposures to infectious organisms and chemicals impart the greatest risk. Examples of high-risk exposures include pregnant nurses exposed to cytomegalovirus or respiratory syncytial virus; day-care workers exposed to parvovirus and rubella; industrial workers exposed to chemicals such as heavy metals or organic solvents; and women living in rural areas exposed to potentially harmful chemicals through pesticide use or contaminated well water.

Methyl mercury is a recently recognized environmental contaminant that is especially important because all pregnant women are potentially at risk. It is now well established that certain kinds of large fish are contaminated (see Chap. 14, p. 355). Mercury is a neurotoxin that readily crosses the placenta and has adverse effects on fetal neurological development. Accordingly, the US Food and Drug Administration (2004) has recommended that pregnant women not eat shark, swordfish, king mackerel, or tilefish and that they consume no more than 12 ounces of other kinds of shellfish or other fish per week. Albacore or "white" tuna has more mercury than other canned tuna. Oken and colleagues (2003) have provided data that since the original FDA advisory, there has been a decline of ingestion by pregnant women of suspect fish species.

LIFESTYLE AND WORK HABITS. A number of personal and work habits as well as lifestyle issues may have an impact on pregnancy outcome.

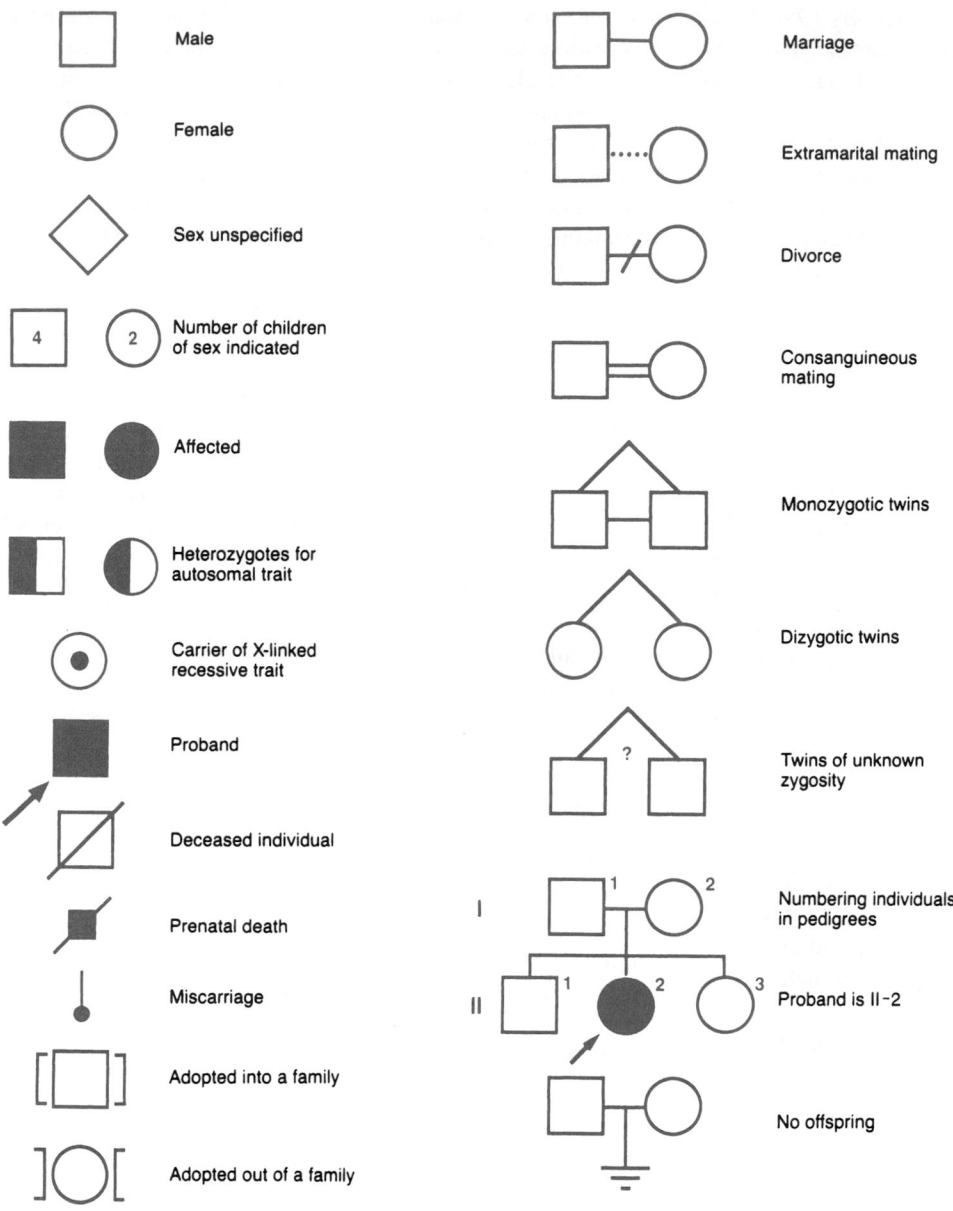

FIGURE 7–3. Symbols used for pedigree construction. (From Thompson and colleagues, 1991, with permission.)

Diet. Pica for ice, laundry starch, clay, dirt, or other nonfood items should be discouraged (see Chap. 8, p. 255). In some cases, it may represent an unusual physiological response to iron deficiency (Federman and colleagues, 1997). Many vegetarian diets are protein deficient but can be corrected by increasing egg and cheese consumption. As discussed in Chapter 43, obesity is associated with a number of maternal complications such as hypertension, preeclampsia, gestational diabetes, labor abnormalities, postterm pregnancy, cesarean delivery, and operative complications (Wolfe, 1998). It is also associated with adverse fetal outcomes, including spina bifida and ventral wall defects, late fetal death, and preterm delivery (Cnattingius and co-workers, 1998).

In addition to nutritional deficiencies, anorexia and bulimia increase the risk of associated maternal problems such as electrolyte disturbances, cardiac arrhythmias, and gastrointestinal pathology (Becker and associates, 1999). In a study of 23 pregnancies in 15 women previously treated for anorexia nervosa or bulimia, Stewart and colleagues (1987) reported that those whose anorexia was not in remission at the time of conception had increased symptoms during pregnancy. They also gained less weight and had smaller infants.

Exercise. There are no data to suggest that exercise is deleterious during pregnancy; thus, conditioned pregnant women usually can continue to exercise throughout gestation

(American College of Obstetricians and Gynecologists, 2002). As pregnancy progresses, balance problems and joint relaxation may predispose to orthopedic injury. The woman should be advised to not exercise to exhaustion, avoid supine positions, avoid activities requiring good balance, augment heat dissipation and fluid replacement, and avoid extreme weather conditions.

Domestic Abuse. Pregnancy can exacerbate interpersonal problems and is a time of increased risk from an abusive partner. As discussed in Chapter 42 (see p. 997), one in six women is abused during pregnancy (Eisenstat and Bancroft, 1999). The interviewer should inquire about risk factors for domestic violence, and should offer intervention as appropriate. Abuse is more likely in women whose partners abuse alcohol or drugs, are recently unemployed, have a poor education or low income, or have a history of arrest (Grisso and colleagues, 1999; Kyriacou and associates, 1999).

FAMILY HISTORY. The most thorough method for obtaining a family history is to construct a pedigree using the symbols shown in Figure 7–3. The health and reproductive status of each "blood relative" should be individually reviewed for medical illnesses, mental retardation, birth defects, infertility, and pregnancy loss. Certain racial, ethnic, or religious backgrounds may indicate increased risk for specific recessive disorders. Although most women can provide some information regarding their history, their understanding may be limited. For example, several studies have shown that pregnant women often fail to report a birth defect in the family or report it incorrectly. Romitti and associates (1997) interviewed 345 women who had a relative with a birth defect and 380 women without such a history. They verified their responses about family history by contacting relatives. Only 30 percent of these 725 women correctly reported familial birth defects. Rasmussen and colleagues (1990) used the Atlanta Birth Defects Registry to identify 4929 women whose child had a verified birth defect. When contacted, only 60 percent accurately reported the defect. It is thus important to verify the type of reported defect or genetic disease by reviewing pertinent medical records or by contacting affected relatives for additional information.

IMMUNIZATIONS. Preconceptional counseling includes assessment of immunity to rubella and hepatitis B. Depending on health status, travel plans, and time of year, other immunizations may be in order (see Table 8–9, p. 222). Vaccines consist of either toxoids (e.g., tetanus); killed bacteria or viruses (e.g., influenza, pneumococcus, hepatitis B, meningococcus, and rabies); or attenuated live viruses (e.g., varicella-zoster, measles, mumps, polio, rubella, chickenpox, yellow fever). Immunization during pregnancy with toxoids or killed bacteria or viruses has not been associated with adverse fetal outcomes (Chutivongse and colleagues, 1995; Czeizel and Rockenbauer, 1999). Alternatively, live-virus vaccines are not recommended during pregnancy and ideally

should be given at least 1 month before attempts to conceive. Women inadvertently given measles, mumps, rubella, or varicella vaccines during pregnancy, however, are not necessarily advised to seek pregnancy termination. Most reports indicate that immunization to any of these agents poses only a theoretical risk to the fetus. Lastly, immunization to smallpox, anthrax, and other bioterrorist diseases should be discussed (see Chap. 8, p. 221).

SCREENING TESTS

Certain laboratory tests may be helpful in assessing the risk of complications during pregnancy. These include basic tests that are usually performed during prenatal care. For example, rubella, varicella, and hepatitis B immune status should be determined so that vaccination can be carried out as part of preconceptional care. A complete blood count with mean red blood cell volume will exclude most serious inherited anemias. Hemoglobin electrophoresis is performed in individuals at increased risk, such as African-Americans for sickle syndromes and women of Mediterranean or Asian origin for thalassemias. Women with Jewish ancestry are candidates for carrier testing for Tay-Sachs and Canavan disease, whereas Caucasians of northern European descent may elect screening for cystic fibrosis. Specific counseling issues pertaining to these genetic diseases are discussed throughout Chapter 12. Partners of women discovered to be carriers of autosomal-recessive diseases should be tested to determine the risk to future offspring. Couples discovered to be at significant increased risk of having an affected child can then contemplate their reproductive options before undertaking a pregnancy.

More specific tests may assist the evaluation of women with certain chronic medical diseases. Examples of some, but certainly not all, chronic diseases that may be assessed by prenatal testing include kidney disease, cardiovascular diseases, and diabetes. In the first example, the outcome of pregnancies complicated by chronic renal disease can be predicted to some extent by the serum creatinine level (Table 7–1). In the

TABLE 7–1 Relationship of Chronic Renal Insufficiency with Pregnancy Outcome (in Percent)

Outcome	Serum Creatinine (mg/dL)		
	Mild <1.5	Moderate 1.5–3.0	Severe ≥3.0
Preterm birth	13	50	100
Perinatal death	5	17	33
Fetal growth restriction	10	20	100
Abortion[a]	11	21	25
Surviving infants	84	62	50

[a] Includes spontaneous miscarriage and induced abortion.
Data from Cunningham (1990), Hou (1985), Imbasciati (1986), Jungers (1986), Katz (1980), Trevisan (2004), and all their coworkers.

TABLE 7–2 **Predictors of Fetal Outcome in 816 Pregnancies Complicated by Maternal Cyanotic Heart Disease**

Predictor	Specifics	Liveborn (%)
Lesion	Single ventricle and/or TCA	31
	Tetralogy of Fallot or pulmonary atresia	33
	Ebstein anomaly, atrial septal defect	86
	Corrected TCA, VSD, and pulmonary stenosis	60
Hemoglobin (g/dL)	≤ 16	71
	17–19	45
	≥ 20	8
Arterial oxygen saturation (%)	≤ 85	12
	85–89	45
	≥ 90	92
Maternal age	≤ 23	35
	24–27	40
	≥ 28	45
Shunt	Yes	51
	No	35

TCA = tricuspid atresia; VSD = ventricular septal defect.
Adapted from Presbitero and colleagues (1994), with permission.

second example, the likelihood that a woman with cyanotic heart disease will have a successful pregnancy outcome can be predicted by a number of factors shown in Table 7–2. The third example is the use of hemoglobin A_{1c} measurement to assess diabetic control during the preceding 6 weeks. This in turn can be used to compute risks for major anomalies (Table 7–3). These figures may be useful in gauging patient compliance and motivation. Although these data are from women with severe diabetes, the incidence of fetal anomalies in women who have gestational diabetes associated with fasting hyperglycemia is increased fourfold compared with nondiabetic control women (Sheffield and associates, 2002). Other specific tests used for the assessment of these and other diseases are discussed more fully in later chapters.

Electromagnetic Energy. There is no evidence in humans or animals that exposure to various electromagnetic fields such as high-voltage power lines, electric blankets, microwave ovens, and cellular phones causes adverse fetal effects (O'Connor, 1999; Robert, 1999). Electrical shock is discussed further in Chapter 41 (see p. 1001).

REFERENCES

Adab N, Tudur SC, Vinten J, et al: Common antiepileptic drugs in pregnancy in women with epilepsy. Cochrane Database Syst Rev CD004848, 2004

Adams MM, Bruce FC, Shulman HB, et al: Pregnancy planning and pre-conception counseling. Obstet Gynecol 82:955, 1993

Adashi EY, Barri PN, Berkowitz R, et al: Infertility therapy-associated multiple pregnancies (births): an ongoing epidemic. Reprod Biomed Online 7:515, 2003

Adashi EY, Ekins MN, Lacousiere Y: On the discharge of Hippocratic obligations: challenges and opportunities. Am J Obstet Gynecol 190:885, 2004

American Academy of Neurology: Practice parameter: Management issues for women with epilepsy (summary statement). Report of the Quality Standards Subcommittee of the American Academy of Neurology. Epilepsia 39:1226, 1998

American College of Obstetricians and Gynecologists: Adolescent Pregnancy Facts. 2003

American College of Obstetricians and Gynecologists: Exercise during pregnancy and the postpartum period. Committee Opinion No. 267, January, 2002.

American College of Obstetricians and Gynecologists: Psychosocial risk factors: Perinatal screening and interaction. Educational Bulletin No. 255, November, 1999

Angastiniotis M, Modell B: Global epidemiology of hemoglobin disorders. Ann NY Acad Sci 850:251, 1998

Baird PA, Saolovnick AD, Yee IM: Maternal age and birth defects: A population study. Lancet 338:527, 1991

Barker DJP: Mothers, Babies and Disease in Later Life. London, BMJ Publishing, 1994

Becker AE, Grinspoon SK, Klibanski A, et al: Eating disorders. N Engl J Med 340:14, 1999

TABLE 7–3 **Relationship of First-Trimester Glycosylated Hemoglobin to Major Congenital Anomalies in 320 Insulin-Dependent Diabetic Women**

Glycohemoglobin (%)	Major Anomalies (%)
4.6–7.6	1.9
7.7–8.6	1.7
8.7–9.9	6.3
10–10.5	9.1
> 10.6	25.0

From Kitzmiller and colleagues (1991).

Benz EJ: Hemoglobinopathies. In Braunwald E, Fauci AS, Kasper DL, et al (eds): Harrison's Principles of Internal Medicine, 15th ed. New York, McGraw-Hill, 2001, p 666

Berkowitz GS, Skovron ML, Lapinski RH, et al: Delayed childbearing and the outcome of pregnancy. N Engl J Med 322:659, 1990

Bernasko J: Contemporary Management of type 1 diabetes mellitus in pregnancy. Obstet Gynecol Surv 59:628, 2004

Besculides M, Laraque F. Unintended pregnancy among the urban poor. J Urban Health 81: 340, 2004

Biale Y, Lewenthal H: Effect of folic acid supplementation on congenital malformations due to anticonvulsive drugs. Eur J Obstet Gynecol Reprod Biol 18:211, 1984

Bobrowski RA, Bottoms SF: Underappreciated risks of the elderly multipara. Am J Obstet Gynecol 172:1764, 1995

Bowen JR, Gibson FL, Leslie GI, et al: Medical and development outcome at 1 year for children conceived by intracytoplasmic sperm injection. Lancet 351:1529, 1998

Buehler JW, Kaunitz AM, Hogue CJR, et al: Maternal mortality in women aged 35 years or older: United States. JAMA 255:53, 1986

Centers for Disease Control and Prevention: Cigarette smoking among adults—United States, 2001. MMWR 52:953, 2003

Centers for Disease Control and Prevention: Insurance coverage of unintended pregnancies resulting in live-born infants. MMWR 48:1, 1999

Centers for Disease Control and Prevention: Use of assisted reproductive technology—United States, 1996 and 1998. MMWR 51:97, 2002.

Chang G, Wilkins-Haug L, Berman S, et al: Alcohol use and pregnancy: Improving identification. Obstet Gynecol 91:892, 1998

Chang S, McAuley JW: Pharmacotherapeutic issues for women of childbearing age with epilepsy. Ann Pharmacol 32:794, 1998

Chutivongse S, Wilde H, Benjavongkulchai M, et al: Postexposure rabies vaccination during pregnancy: Effect on 202 women and their infants. Clin Infect Dis 20:818, 1995

Cnattingius S, Bergstrom R, Lipworth L, et al: Prepregnancy weight and the risk of adverse pregnancy outcomes. N Engl J Med 338:147, 1998

Cox M, Whittle MJ, Byrne A, et al: Prepregnancy counseling: Experience from 1075 cases. Br J Obstet Gynaecol 99:873, 1992

Cunningham FG, Cox SM, Harstad TW, et al: Chronic renal disease and pregnancy outcome. Am J Obstet Gynecol 163:453, 1990

Cunningham FG, Leveno KJ: Childbearing among older women— the message is cautiously optimistic. N Engl J Med 333:1002, 1995

Czeizel AE, Dudas I: Prevention of the first occurrence of neural-tube defects by periconceptional vitamin supplementation. N Engl J Med 327:1832, 1992

Czeizel AE, Rockenbauer M: Tetanus toxoid and congenital abnormalities. Int J Gynaecol Obstet 64:253, 1999

Dunne FP, Brydon P, Smith T, et al: Preconception diabetes care in insulin-dependent diabetes mellitus. QJM 92:175, 1999

Eisenstat SA, Bancroft L: Domestic violence. N Engl J Med 341:886, 1999

Federman DG, Kirsner RS, Federman GS: Pica: Are you hungry for the facts? Conn Med 61:207, 1997

Fraser AM, Brockert JE, Ward RH: Association of young maternal age with adverse reproductive outcomes. N Engl J Med 332:1113, 1995

Fucharoen S, Winichagoon P, Thonglairoam V, et al: Prenatal diagnosis of thalassemia and hemoglobinopathies in Thailand: Experience from 100 pregnancies. Southeast Asian J Trop Med Public Health 22:16, 1991

Gregory R, Tattersall RB: Are diabetic pre-pregnancy clinics worth while? Lancet 340:656, 1992

Grisso JA, Schwarz DF, Hirschinger N, et al: Violent injuries among women in an urban area. N Engl J Med 341:1899, 1999

Guttler F, Lou H, Andresen J, et al: Cognitive development in offspring of untreated and preconceptionally treated maternal phenylketonuria. J Inherited Metab Dis 13:665, 1990

Hansen M, Kurinczuk JJ, Bower C, et al: The risk of major birth defects after intracystoplasmic sperm injection and in vitro fertilization. N Engl J Med 346:725, 2002

Hellerstedt WL, Pirie PL, Lando HA, et al: Differences in preconceptional and prenatal behaviors in women with intended and unintended pregnancies. Am J Public Health 88:663, 1998

Herman WH, Janz NK, Becker MP, et al: Diabetes and pregnancy: Preconception care, pregnancy outcomes, resource utilization and costs. J Reprod Med 44:33, 1999

Hollier LM, Leveno KJ, Kelly MA, et al: Maternal age and malformations in singleton births. Obstet Gynecol 96:701, 2000

Holmes LB, Harvey EA, Coull BA, et al: The teratogenicity of anticonvulsant drugs. N Engl J Med 344:1132, 2001

Hou SH, Grossman SD, Madias NE: Pregnancy in women with renal disease and moderate renal insufficiency. Am J Med 78:185, 1985

Imbasciati E, Pardi G, Capetta P, et al: Pregnancy in women with chronic renal failure. Am J Nephrol 6:193, 1986

Jack BW, Campanile C, McQuade W, et al: The negative pregnancy test. An opportunity for preconception care. Arch Fam Med 4:340, 1995

Jackson RA, Gibson KA, Wu YW, Croughan MS. Perinatal outcomes in singletons following in vitro fertilization: A meta-analysis. Obstet Gynecol. 103:551, 2004

Jovanovic L, Druzin M, Peterson CM: Effect of euglycaemia on the outcome of pregnancy in insulin-dependent diabetic women as compared to normal control subjects. Am J Med 71:921, 1981

Jungers P, Forget D, Henry-Amar M: Chronic renal disease and pregnancy. Adv Nephrol 15:103, 1986

Kaback M, Lim-Steele J, Dabholkar D, et al: Tay Sachs disease: Carrier screening, prenatal diagnosis, and the molecular era. JAMA 270:2307, 1993

Katz AL, Davison JM, Hayslett JP, et al: Pregnancy in women with kidney disease. Kidney Int 18:192, 1980

Kitzmiller JL, Gavin LA, Gin GD, et al: Preconception care of diabetics. JAMA 265:731, 1991

Koch R, Hanley W, Levy H, et al: A preliminary report of the collaborative study of maternal phenylketonuria in the United States and Canada. J Inherit Metab Dis 13:641, 1990

Kyriacou DN, Anglin D, Taliaferro E, et al: Risk factors for injury to women from domestic violence. N Engl J Med 341:1892, 1999

Medical Research Council on Vitamin Study Research Group: Prevention of neural tube defects: Results of the medical research council vitamin study. Lancet 338:131, 1991

Mitchell JJ, Capua A, Clow C, et al: Twenty-year outcome analysis of genetic screening programs for Tay-Sachs and beta-thalassemia disease carriers in high schools. Am J Hum Genet 59:793, 1996

Moore KL: Before We Are Born. Basic Embryology and Birth Defects, 2nd ed. Philadelphia, Saunders, 1983

Moos MK: Preconceptional health promotion: Progress in changing a prevention paradigm. J Perinat Neonatal Nurs 18:2, 2004

Moos MK, Bangdiwala SI, Meibohm AR, et al: The impact of a preconceptional health promotion program on intendedness of pregnancy. Am J Perinatol 13:103, 1996

Niccolai LM, Ethier KA, Kershaw TS, et al: Pregnant adolescents at risk: Sexual behaviors and sexually transmitted disease prevalence. Am J Obstet Gynecol 188:63, 2003

O'Connor ME: Intrauterine effects in animals exposed to radiofrequency and microwave fields. Teratology 59:287, 1999

Oken E, Kleinman KP, Berland WE, et al: Decline in fish consumption among pregnant women after national mercury advisory. Obstet Gynecol 102:346, 2003

Ou CY, Stevenson RE, Brown VK, et al: 5, 10 Methylenetetrahydrofolate reductase genetic polymorphism as a risk factor for neural tube defects. Am J Med Genet 63:610, 1996

Platt LD, Koch R, Hanley WB, et al: The international study of pregnancy outcome in women with maternal phenylketonuria: Report of a 12-year study. Am J Obstet Gynecol 182:326, 2000

Pradat P. Epidemiology of major congenital heart defects in Sweden, 1981–1986. J Epidemiol Community Health 46:211, 1992

Presbitero P, Sommerville J, Stone S, et al: Pregnancy in cyanotic congenital heart disease. Circulation 89:2673, 1994

Public Health Service: Caring for the Future: The Content of Prenatal Care. Washington, DC, Department of Health and Human Services, 1989, p 26

Public Health Service: Healthy People 2010: A Systematic Approach to Health Improvement. Washington, DC, US Department of Health and Human Services, Public Health Service, 2000

Rasmussen SA, Mulinare J, Khoury MJ, et al: Evaluation of birth defect histories obtained through maternal interviews. Am J Hum Genet 46:478, 1990

Robert E: Intrauterine effects of electromagnetic fields (low frequency, mid-frequency RF, and microwave): Review of epidemiologic studies. Teratology 59:292, 1999

Romitti PA, Burns TL, Murray JC: Maternal interview reports of family history of birth defects: Evaluation from a population-based case-control study of orofacial clefts. Am J Med Genet 72:422, 1997

Rouse B, Azen C, Koch R, et al: Maternal phenylketonuria collaborative study (MPKUCS) offspring: Facial anomalies, malformations, and early neurological sequelae. Am J Med Genet 69:89, 1997

Schieve LA, Meikle SF, Ferre C, et al: Low and very low birth weight in infants conceived with use of assisted reproductive technology. N Engl J Med 346:731, 2002

Sheffield JS, Butler-Koster EL, Casey BM, et al: Maternal diabetes mellitus and infant malformations. Obstet Gynecol 100:925, 2002

Smith BL, Martin JA, Ventura SJ: Births and deaths: Preliminary data for July 1997–June 1998. Natl Vital Stat Rep 47:1, 1999

Stewart DE, Raskin J, Garfinkel PE, et al: Anorexia nervosa, bulimia, and pregnancy. Am J Obstet Gynecol 157:1194, 1987

Strömberg B, Dahlquist A, Ericson A, et al: Neurological sequelae in children born after in-vitro fertilisation: A population-based study. Lancet 359:461, 2002

Thompson MW, McInnes RR, Huntington FW (eds): Genetics in Medicine, 5th ed. Philadelphia, Saunders, 1991

Trevisan G, Ramos JG, Martins-Costa S, Barros EJ: Pregnancy in patients with chronic renal insufficiency at Hopital de Clinicas of Porto Alegre, Brazil. Ren Fail 26:29, 2004

US Food and Drug Administration: What you need to know about mercury in fish and shellfish. 2004 EPA and FDA advice for: Women who might become pregnant, women who are pregnant, nursing mother, young children. EPA-823-R-04-005, March 2004. http://cfsan.fda.gov

van der Put NMJ, Steegers-Theunissen RPM, Frosst P, et al: Mutated methylenetetrahydrofolate reductase as a risk factor for spina bifida. Lancet 345:1070, 1995

Wide K, Winbladh B, Kallen B: Major malformations in infants exposed to antiepileptic drugs in utero, with emphasis on carbamazepine and valproic acid: A nation-wide population-based register study. 93:174, 2004

Wolfe H: High prepregnancy body-mass index—a maternal fetal risk factor. N Engl J Med 338:191, 1998

Wong HB: Prevention of thalassaemias in South-East Asia. Ann Acad Med Singapore 14:654, 1985

Yerby MS: Epilepsy and pregnancy. New issues for an old disorder. Neurol Clin 11:777, 1993

8

Prenatal Care

Organized prenatal care in the United States was introduced largely by social reformers and nurses (Merkatz and colleagues, 1990). In 1901, Mrs. William Lowell Putnam of the Boston Infant Social Service Department began a program of nurse visits to women enrolled in the home delivery service of the Boston Lying-in Hospital. This work was so successful that an outpatient prenatal clinic was established in 1911. Former authors of *Williams Obstetrics* were early supporters of prenatal care. In 1915, J. Whitridge Williams reviewed 10,000 consecutive deliveries at Johns Hopkins Hospital and concluded that 40 percent of 705 perinatal deaths could have been prevented by prenatal care. In 1954, Nicholas J. Eastman credited organized prenatal care with having "done more to save mothers' lives in our time than any other single factor" (Speert, 1980). In the 1960s, Jack Pritchard established a network of neighborhood prenatal clinics located in the most underserved communities in Dallas County. In large part because of increased accessibility, approximately 95 percent of medically indigent women now delivering at Parkland Hospital receive prenatal care. Importantly and related, the perinatal mortality rate of women in this system is less than that of the United States overall.

OVERVIEW OF PRENATAL CARE

Almost a century since its introduction, prenatal care has become one of the most frequently used health services in the United States. In 2001, there were approximately 50 million prenatal visits—the median was 12.3 visits per pregnancy—and, as shown in Figure 8–1, many women had 17 or more visits (Martin and associates, 2002b). More than 83 percent

of women began prenatal care during the first trimester, and all but 1.1 percent received some prenatal care. Over the past decade, the largest gains in timely prenatal care have been among minority groups (Fig. 8–2), but disparity continues. Significant obstetrical and medical risk factors or complications identifiable during prenatal care are summarized in Table 8–1. Importantly, many of these complications are *treatable*.

INADEQUATE PRENATAL CARE. A commonly employed system for measuring the adequacy of prenatal care is the Kessner Index (Kessner and colleagues, 1973). As shown in Table 8–2, this index incorporates information from three items recorded on the birth certificate: length of gestation, timing of the first prenatal care visit, and number of visits. Although the index measures the quantity of care better than either the number or timing of prenatal visits alone, it does not measure the quality of care. Similarly, the index does not consider the relative risk of the mother. Despite these limitations, the index remains a useful measure of prenatal care adequacy. Using the Kessner Index, the National Center for Health Statistics concluded that 12 percent of American women delivering in 2000 received inadequate prenatal care (Martin and associates, 2002a).

The Centers for Disease Control and Prevention (2000) analyzed birth certificate data for the years 1989 to 1997 and concluded that half of women with delayed or no prenatal care wanted to begin care earlier. Reasons for inadequate prenatal care varied by social and ethnic group, age, and method of payment. The most common reason cited was that the woman did not know she was pregnant. The second most commonly cited barrier was lack of money or insurance for such care. The third was inability to obtain an appointment.

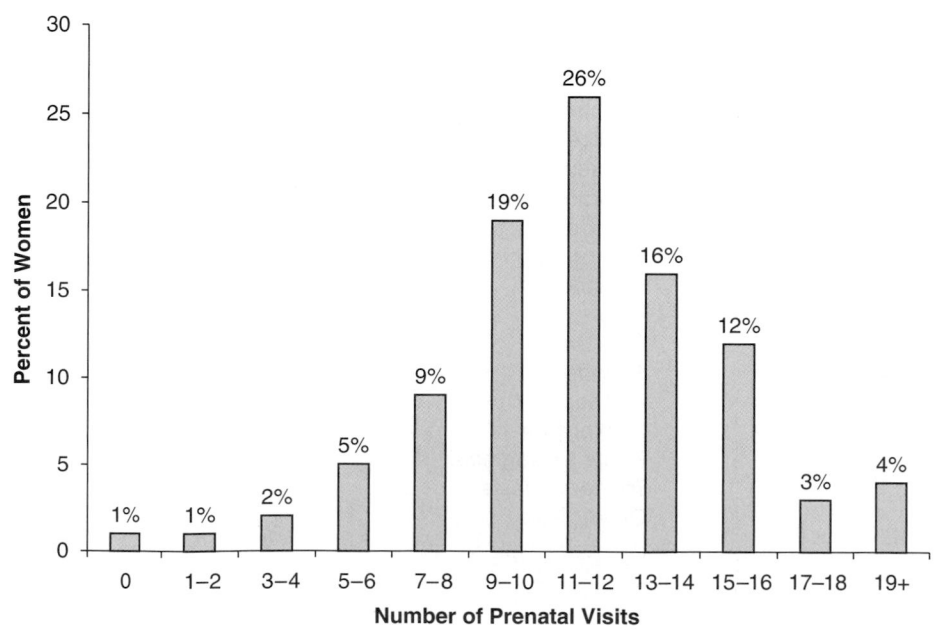

FIGURE 8–1. Frequency distribution of the number of prenatal visits for the United States in 2001. (Adapted from Martin and associates, 2002b.)

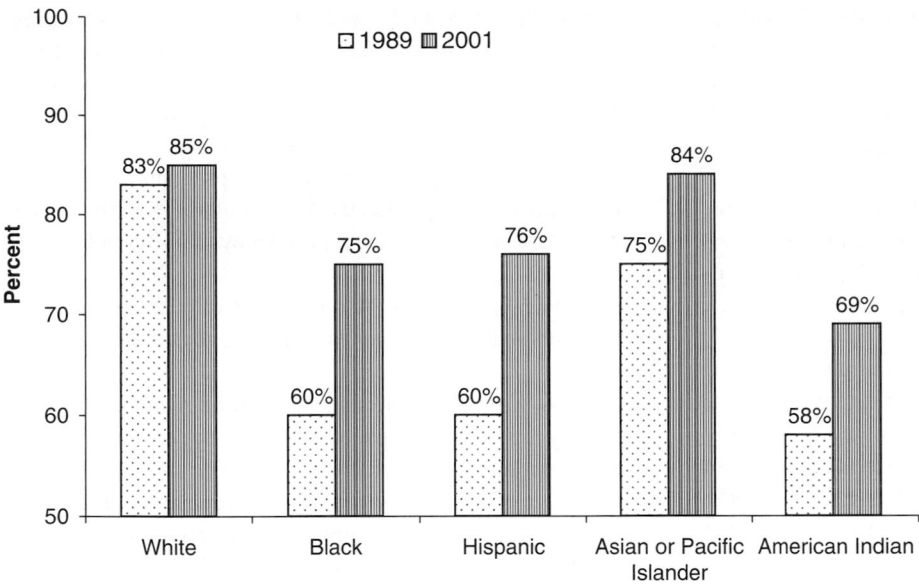

FIGURE 8–2. Percent of women in the United States with prenatal care beginning in the first trimester by ethnicity, 1989 compared with 2001. (Adapted from Martin and associates, 2002b.)

EFFECTIVENESS OF PRENATAL CARE. Over the past several decades, some have concluded that prenatal care offers no benefits, and indeed may be disadvantageous. In an extensive review, Fiscella (1995) found no conclusive evidence that prenatal care improved birth outcomes. Other authors raised concern about the effectiveness of prenatal care because in the 1980s and 1990s, when use of prenatal care increased substantively, the rates of low-birthweight and preterm birth increased in the United States (Kogan and colleagues, 1998).

Conversely, Herbst and associates (2003) found that failure to obtain prenatal care was associated with more than a twofold increased risk of preterm birth. Schramm (1992) compared the costs and benefits of prenatal care in over 12,000 Medicaid patients in Missouri in 1988. He found that for each $1 spent for prenatal care, there were estimated savings of $1.49 in newborn and postpartum costs. Vintzileos and colleagues (2002b) analyzed data for the years 1995 to 1997 from the National Center for Health Statistics to measure the relationship between prenatal care and the risk of fetal

TABLE 8–1 Obstetrical and Medical Risk Factors Detected During Prenatal Care in the United States in 2001

Risk Factor	Births	Percent
Total live births	4,025,933	100
Hypertension due to pregnancy	150,329	3.7
Diabetes	124,242	3.1
Anemia	99,558	2.5
Hydramnios/oligohydramnios	54,694	1.4
Acute or chronic lung disease	48,246	1.2
Genital herpes	33,560	0.8
Chronic hypertension	32,232	0.8
D (Rh) sensitization	26,933	0.7
Cardiac disease	20,698	0.5
Renal disease	12,045	0.3
Incompetent cervix	11,251	0.3
Hemoglobinopathy	3,141	0.1
Total	616,929	15.3

Adapted from Martin and associates, 2002b.

TABLE 8–2 Kessner Index Criteria

Adequate Prenatal Care		
Initial visit in 1st trimester and:		
Weeks at Delivery		**No. of Prenatal Visits**
17	and	2 or more
18–21	and	3 or more
22–25	and	4 or more
26–29	and	5 or more
30–31	and	6 or more
32–33	and	7 or more
34–35	and	8 or more
36–47	and	9 or more
Inadequate Prenatal Care		
Initial visit in 3rd trimester or:		
Weeks at Delivery		**No. of Prenatal Visits**
17–21	and	None
22–29	and	1 or fewer
30–31	and	2 or fewer
32–33	and	3 or fewer
34–47	and	4 or fewer
Intermediate Care		
All other combinations		

Adapted from Kessner and colleagues, 1973, with permission.

death. They found that prenatal care was associated with an overall fetal death rate of 2.7 per 1000 compared with 14.1 per 1000 for women without prenatal care. Stated differently, failure to receive prenatal care increased the adjusted relative risk of stillbirth 3.3-fold. Vintzileos and colleagues (2002a) later reported that prenatal care significantly lowered the rate of neonatal death associated with several high-risk conditions, including placenta previa, fetal growth restriction, and post-term pregnancy. They also found that prenatal care was associated with fewer preterm births (Vintzileos and colleagues, 2003).

It must also be remembered that prenatal care designed during the early 1900s was focused on lowering the extremely high incidence of maternal death. Prenatal care undoubtedly contributed to the dramatic decline in maternal mortality from 690 per 100,000 births in 1920 to 50 per 100,000 by 1955 (Loudon, 1992). As discussed in Chapter 1 (see p. 7), the current maternal mortality rate of about 8 per 100,000 is likely associated with the high utilization of prenatal care. Indeed, in a population-based study from North Carolina, Harper and co-workers (2003) found that the risk of pregnancy-related maternal death was decreased fivefold among recipients of prenatal care.

Logically, the effectiveness of prenatal care cannot be gauged in isolation from other innovations. In the seventh edition of *Williams Obstetrics* (1929), prenatal care was specifically designated as one part of an organized program for pregnant women. Thus, in this context, prenatal care is not an end in itself but an initial step for coordinated intrapartum and postpartum care that often extends even beyond into a woman's later life.

ORGANIZATION OF PRENATAL CARE

The American Academy of Pediatrics and the American College of Obstetricians and Gynecologists (2002) have defined prenatal care as: "A comprehensive antepartum care program that involves a coordinated approach to medical care and psychosocial support that optimally begins before conception and extends throughout the antepartum period." The content of such a comprehensive program includes (1) preconceptional care, (2) prompt diagnosis of pregnancy, (3) initial presentation for pregnancy care, and (4) follow-up prenatal visits.

PRECONCEPTIONAL CARE. Because health during pregnancy depends on health before pregnancy, preconceptional care should logically be an integral part of prenatal care. As discussed in detail in Chapter 7, a comprehensive preconceptional care program has the potential to assist women by reducing risks, promoting healthy lifestyles, and improving readiness for pregnancy.

DIAGNOSIS OF PREGNANCY. The diagnosis of pregnancy usually begins when a woman presents with symptoms, and possibly a positive home urine pregnancy test. Typically, such women receive confirmatory testing for human chorionic gonadotropin (hCG) in urine or blood. There may be presumptive or diagnostic findings of pregnancy on examination. Ultrasound is often used, particularly in those cases in which there is question about pregnancy viability or location.

Signs and Symptoms. A number of clinical findings and symptoms may indicate an early pregnancy.

CESSATION OF MENSES. The abrupt cessation of menstruation in a healthy reproductive-aged woman who previously has experienced spontaneous, cyclical, predictable menses is highly suggestive of pregnancy. There is appreciable variation in the length of the ovarian—and thus menstrual—cycle among women, and even in the same woman. Thus, the absence of menses is not a reliable indication of pregnancy until 10 days or more after the time of expected onset of the menstrual period. When a second menstrual period is missed, the probability of pregnancy is much greater.

Uterine bleeding somewhat suggestive of menstruation occurs occasionally after conception. One or two episodes of bloody discharge, somewhat reminiscent of and sometimes mistaken for menstruation, are not uncommon during the first half of pregnancy. Such episodes are interpreted to be physiological, and likely the consequence of blastocyst implantation.

CHANGES IN CERVICAL MUCUS. If cervical mucus is aspirated, spread on a glass slide, allowed to dry for a few minutes, and examined microscopically, characteristic patterns can be discerned that are dependent on the stage of the ovarian cycle and the presence or absence of pregnancy. From about the 7th to the 18th day of the menstrual cycle, a fernlike pattern of dried cervical mucus is seen (Fig. 8–3). After approximately the 21st day, a different pattern forms that gives a beaded or cellular appearance (Fig. 8–4). This beaded pattern also is usually encountered during pregnancy.

The crystallization of the mucus, which is necessary for the production of the fern pattern, is dependent on an increased concentration of sodium chloride. This concentration, and in turn the presence or absence of the fern pattern, is determined by cervical glandular response to hormonal action. Specifically, cervical mucus is relatively rich in sodium chloride when estrogen, but not progesterone, is being produced. Progesterone secretion—even without a reduction in estrogen secretion—acts promptly to lower sodium chloride concentration to levels at which ferning will not occur. During pregnancy, progesterone usually exerts a similar effect, even though the amount of estrogen produced is enormous. Thus, if copious thin mucus is present and if a fern pattern develops on drying, early pregnancy is unlikely.

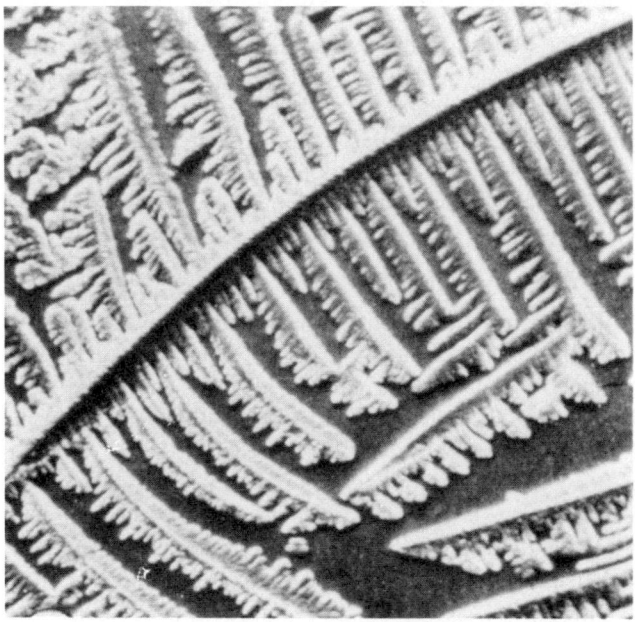

FIGURE 8–3. Scanning electron microscopy of cervical mucus obtained on day 11 of the menstrual cycle. (From Zaneveld and associates, 1975, with permission.)

CHANGES IN THE BREASTS. Generally, the anatomical changes in the breasts that accompany pregnancy are quite characteristic during the first pregnancy (see Chap. 5, p. 126). These are less obvious in multiparas, whose breasts may contain a small amount of milky material or colostrum for months or even years after the birth of their last child, especially if breast feeding was chosen.

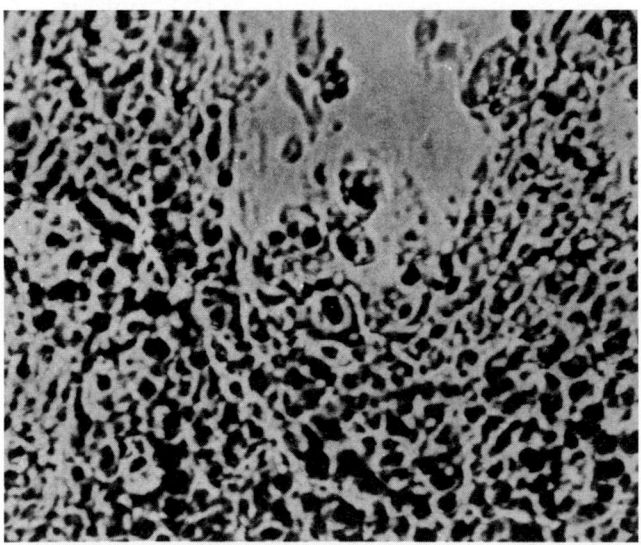

FIGURE 8–4. Photomicrograph of dried cervical mucus obtained from the cervical canal of a woman pregnant at 32 to 33 weeks. The beaded pattern is characteristic of progesterone action on the endocervical gland mucus composition. (Courtesy of Dr. J. C. Ullery.)

DISCOLORATION OF THE VAGINAL MUCOSA. During pregnancy, the vaginal mucosa usually appears dark bluish or purplish-red and congested—the so-called *Chadwick sign* (Chadwick, 1886). This appearance is presumptive evidence of pregnancy, but it is not conclusive.

SKIN CHANGES. Increased pigmentation and changes in appearance of abdominal striae are common to, but not diagnostic of, pregnancy. They may be absent during pregnancy, and they may be seen in women taking estrogen–progestin contraceptives (see Chap. 5, p. 126, and Chap. 56, p. 1250).

CHANGES IN THE UTERUS. During the first few weeks of pregnancy, the increase in uterine size is limited principally to the anteroposterior diameter. By 12 weeks, the body of the uterus is almost globular, and an average uterine diameter of 8 cm is attained. On bimanual examination, the uterus during pregnancy feels doughy or elastic and sometimes becomes exceedingly soft. At about 6 to 8 weeks' menstrual age, on bimanual examination a firm cervix is felt which contrasts the now softer body of the uterus and compressible interposed softened isthmus. This contrast is the *Hegar sign.* The softening at the isthmus may be so marked that the cervix and the body of the uterus seem to be separate organs. In fact, the inexperienced examiner may mistakenly conclude that the cervix is a small uterus, and that the softened body of the fundus is an adnexal mass.

CHANGES IN THE CERVIX. The cervix undergoes increased softening as pregnancy advances. In primigravidas, the consistency of the cervical tissue that surrounds the external os is more similar to that of the lips of the mouth than to that of nasal cartilage characteristic of the nonpregnant cervix. Other conditions, such as estrogen–progestin contraceptives, may cause cervical softening. As pregnancy progresses, the cervical canal may become sufficiently patulous to admit the fingertip.

FETAL HEART ACTION. The fetal heartbeat can be detected by auscultation with a standard nonamplified stethoscope by a mean of 17 weeks, and by 19 weeks in nearly all pregnancies in non-obese women (Jimenez and co-workers, 1979). The fetal heart rate now ranges from 110 to 160 beats/min and is heard as a double sound resembling the tick of a watch under a pillow. Because the fetus moves freely in amnionic fluid, the site on the maternal abdomen where fetal heart sounds can be heard best will vary.

Instruments incorporating Doppler ultrasound are often used to easily detect fetal heart action (see Chap. 18, p. 445). Fetal cardiac action can be detected almost always by 10 weeks with Doppler equipment. Using real-time sonography with a vaginal probe, fetal heart action can be seen following as little as 5 weeks of amenorrhea.

In the later months of pregnancy, the examiner may often hear other sounds, the most common of which are:

1. The funic (umbilical cord) "souffle."
2. The uterine "souffle."
3. Sounds resulting from fetal movement.
4. Maternal pulse.
5. Sounds from maternal intestinal peristalsis.

The *funic souffle* is caused by the rush of blood through the umbilical arteries. It is a sharp, whistling sound that is synchronous with the fetal pulse. It is not heard consistently, even in the same pregnancy. The *uterine souffle* is a soft, blowing sound that is synchronous with the maternal pulse. It is usually heard most distinctly near the lower portion of the uterus. This sound is produced by the passage of blood through the dilated uterine vessels. It also may be heard with any condition in which uterine blood flow is greatly increased, for example, with large uterine myomas or ovarian tumors.

Frequently, the maternal pulse can be heard distinctly by auscultation of the abdomen, and in some women, the pulsation of the aorta is unusually loud. Occasionally the pulse of the mother may become so rapid as to simulate fetal heart sounds.

PERCEPTION OF FETAL MOVEMENTS. At or about 20 weeks, the examiner can begin to detect fetal movements.

Chorionic Gonadotropin. Detection of hCG in maternal blood and urine provides the basis for endocrine tests of pregnancy. This hormone is a glycoprotein with a high carbohydrate content. The molecule is a heterodimer composed of two dissimilar subunits, designated α and β, which are noncovalently linked (see Chap. 3, p. 70). The α-subunit is similar to those of luteinizing hormone (LH), follicle-stimulating hormone (FSH), and thyroid-stimulating hormone (TSH). HCG prevents involution of the corpus luteum, the principal site of progesterone formation during the first 6 weeks.

Trophoblast cells produce hCG in amounts that increase exponentially following implantation. With a sensitive test, the hormone can be detected in maternal plasma or urine by 8 to 9 days after ovulation. The doubling time of plasma hCG concentration is 1.4 to 2.0 days. Levels increase from the day of implantation and reach peak levels at about 60 to 70 days. Thereafter, the concentration declines slowly until a nadir is reached at about 14 to 16 weeks (Fig. 8–5).

MEASUREMENT OF hCG. With the recognition that LH and hCG were both composed of an α- and a β-subunit, but that the β-subunits of each were structurally distinct, antibodies were developed with high specificity for the β-subunit of hCG. This specificity is the basis for detection of hCG in urine or blood. Numerous commercial immunoassays are available for measuring serum and urine levels of hCG, each employing a slightly different combination of antibodies. Although each detects a slightly different mixture of hormone, its free subunits, or its metabolites, all of these immunoassays are appropriate for normal pregnancy testing (Cole, 1998).

One commonly employed technique for detection and quantification of hCG is the *sandwich-type immunoassay.* This test uses a monoclonal antibody against the β-subunit, which is bound to a solid-phase support. The bound antibody is then exposed to hCG in the serum or urine specimen. A second antibody is then added to "sandwich" the bound hCG. In some assays, the second antibody is linked to an enzyme, such as alkaline phosphatase. When substrate for the enzyme is added, a color develops, the intensity of which is proportional to the amount of enzyme and thus to the amount of the second antibody bound. This, in turn, is a function of the amount of hCG in the test sample. The sensitivity for the laboratory detection of hCG in serum is as low as 1.0 mIU/mL using this technique. With extremely sensitive immunoradiometric assays, the detection limit is even lower (Wilcox and associates, 2001).

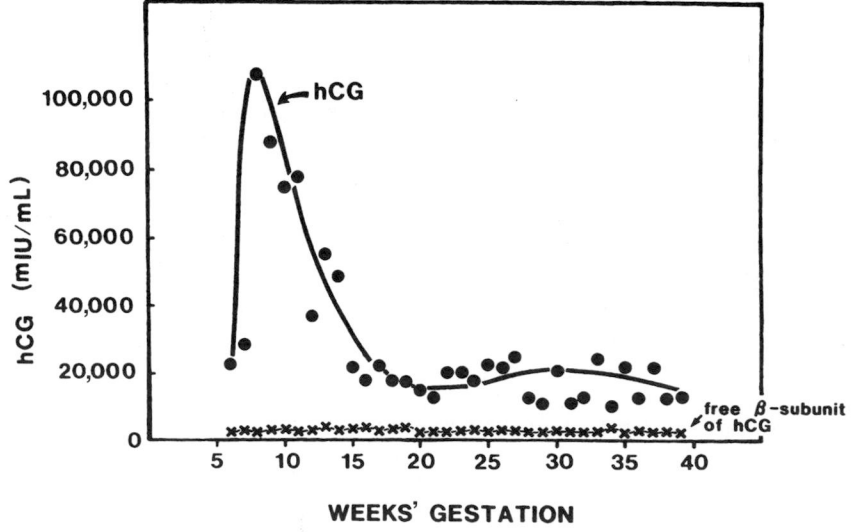

FIGURE 8–5. Mean concentration of chorionic gonadotropin (hCG) in serum of women throughout normal pregnancy. The free β-subunit of hCG is in low concentration throughout pregnancy. (Data from Ashitaka and colleagues, 1980; Selenkow and co-workers, 1971.)

False-positive hCG test results are rare (Braunstein, 2002). However, some women have circulating factors in their serum that may interact with the hCG antibody. The most common are heterophilic antibodies, which are human antibodies directed against animal-derived antigens used in immunoassays. Women who have worked closely with animals are more likely to develop such heterophilic antibodies. The American College of Obstetricians and Gynecologists (2002a) has suggested alternative laboratory techniques if heterophilic antibodies are suspected.

HOME PREGNANCY TESTS. In 1999, approximately 19 million over-the-counter pregnancy test kits were sold in the United States, with sales of about $230 million (Wilcox and associates, 2001). Bastian and colleagues (1998) evaluated published results of 16 home pregnancy test kits, of which only five met their inclusion criteria. If testing was done by volunteers, a mean 91-percent sensitivity was obtained. Importantly, however, actual patients obtained only 75-percent sensitivity.

Cole and colleagues (2004) also questioned the utility of home testing. They found that a detection limit of 12.5 mIU/mL would be required to diagnose 95 percent of pregnancies at the time of missed menses. In their study of the accuracy of 18 different home pregnancy tests, they also found that only one brand had this degree of sensitivity. Two other brands gave false-positive or invalid results. In fact, clearly positive results were given by only 44 percent of the brands at an hCG concentration of 100 mIU/mL. A test capable of detecting this level would be expected to identify only about 15 percent of pregnancies at the time of the missed menses.

Ultrasonic Recognition of Pregnancy. The use of transvaginal sonography has revolutionized imaging of early pregnancy and its growth and development. A gestational sac may be demonstrated by abdominal sonography after only 4 to 5 weeks' menstrual age (Fig. 8–6). By 35 days, all normal sacs should be visible, and after 6 weeks, a heartbeat should be detectable. Up to 12 weeks, the crown-rump length is predictive of gestational age within 4 days. These measurements are discussed in detail in Chapter 16 (see p. 392).

INITIAL PRENATAL EVALUATION. Prenatal care should be initiated as soon as there is a reasonable likelihood of pregnancy. The major goals are:

1. To define the health status of the mother and fetus.
2. To estimate the gestational age of the fetus.
3. To initiate a plan for continuing obstetrical care.

Typical components of the initial visit are summarized in Table 8–3. The initial plan for subsequent care may range from relatively infrequent routine visits to prompt hospitalization because of serious maternal or fetal disease.

Prenatal Record. Use of a standardized record within a perinatal health care system greatly facilitates antepartum and intrapartum management. A prototype is provided by the

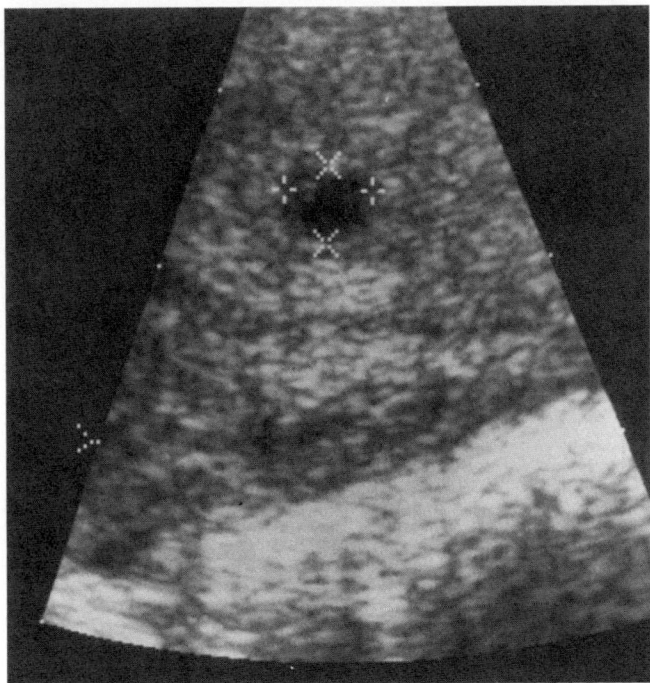

FIGURE 8–6. Abdominal sonogram demonstrating a gestational sac at 4 to 5 weeks' gestational (menstrual) age. (Courtesy of Dr. Diane Twickler.)

American Academy of Pediatrics and the American College of Obstetricians and Gynecologists (2002).

DEFINITIONS. There are several definitions pertinent to establishment of an accurate prenatal record:

• *Nulligravida:* a woman who is not now and never has been pregnant.
• *Gravida:* a woman who is or has been pregnant, irrespective of the pregnancy outcome. With the establishment of the first pregnancy, she becomes a primigravida, and with successive pregnancies, a multigravida.
• *Nullipara:* a woman who has never completed a pregnancy beyond 20 weeks' gestation. She may or may not have been pregnant or may have had a spontaneous or elective abortion(s).
• *Primipara:* a woman who has been delivered only once of a fetus or fetuses born alive or dead with an estimated length of gestation of 20 or more weeks. In the past, a 500-g birthweight threshold was used to define parity. This threshold is no longer as pertinent because of the survival of infants with birthweights less than 500 g.
• *Multipara:* a woman who has completed two or more pregnancies to 20 weeks or more. Parity is determined by the number of pregnancies reaching 20 weeks and not by the number of fetuses delivered. That is, parity is not greater if a single fetus, twins, or quintuplets were delivered, nor lower if the fetus or fetuses were stillborn.

In some locales, the obstetrical history is summarized by a series of digits connected by dashes. These usually refer to

TABLE 8–3 Typical Components of Routine Prenatal Care

	Text Referral	Weeks			
		First Visit	*15–20*	*24–28*	*29–41*
History					
Complete	Chap. 8, p. 209	•			
Updated			•	•	•
Physical examination					
Complete	Chap. 8, p. 210	•			
Blood pressure	Chap. 34, p. 762	•	•	•	•
Maternal weight	Chap. 8, p. 213	•	•	•	•
Pelvic/cervical examination	Chap. 8, p. 210	•			
Fundal height	Chap. 8, p. 212	•	•	•	•
Fetal heart rate and position	Chap. 8, p. 212	•	•	•	•
Laboratory tests					
Hematocrit or hemoglobin	Chap. 51, p. 1144	•		•	
Blood type and Rh factor	Chap. 29, p. 667	•			
Antibody screen	Chap. 29, p. 667	•		A	
Pap smear	Chap. 57, p. 1264	•			
Glucose tolerance test	Chap. 52, p. 1171			•	
Maternal serum AFP screening	Chap. 13, p. 319		B		
Cystic fibrosis screening	Chap. 13, p. 325	B or	B		
Urine protein	Chap. 48, p. 1094	•			
Urine culture	Chap. 48, p. 1095	•			
Rubella titer	Chap. 58, p. 1280	•			
Syphilis test	Chap. 59, p. 1302	•			C
Gonococcal culture	Chap. 59, p. 1305	D			D
Chlamydia culture	Chap. 59, p. 1306	D			D
Hepatitis B surface antigen	Chap. 50, p. 1130	•			
Human immunodeficiency virus (HIV)	Chap. 59, p. 1310	B			
Group B streptococcus culture	Chap. 58, p. 1284				E
Rhogam if D-negative	Chap. 29, p. 671			A	

A Performed at 28 weeks, if indicated.
B Test should be offered.
C High-risk women should be retested at the beginning of the third trimester.
D High-risk women should be screened at the first prenatal visit and again in the third trimester.
E Rectovaginal culture should be obtained between 35 and 37 weeks.

the number of term infants, preterm infants, abortions, and children currently alive. For example, a woman who is para 6–1–2–6 has had six term deliveries, one preterm delivery, and two abortions, and has six children living. Such shorthand is often confusing because no one system is widely adopted.

Normal Pregnancy Duration. The mean duration of pregnancy calculated from the first day of the last normal menstrual period is very close to 280 days, or 40 weeks. In a study of 427,581 singleton pregnancies abstracted in the Swedish Birth Registry, Bergsjø and colleagues (1990) found that the mean duration of pregnancy was 281 days with a standard deviation of 13 days.

It is customary to estimate the expected date of delivery by adding 7 days to the date of the first day of the last normal menstrual period and counting back 3 months (Naegele rule). For example, if the last menstrual period began on September 10, the expected date of delivery would be June 17. It is apparent that pregnancy is erroneously considered to have begun about 2 weeks before ovulation if the duration is so calculated. Nonetheless, clinicians conventionally calculate *gestational age* or *menstrual age* from the first day of the last menstrual period to identify temporal events in pregnancy. Embryologists and other reproductive biologists more often employ *ovulatory age* or *fertilization age,* both of which are typically 2 weeks shorter. Bracken and Belanger (1989) tested the accuracy of various "pregnancy wheels" provided by three pharmaceutical companies and found that such devices were remarkably prone to error. Specifically, incorrect delivery dates were predicted in 40 to 60 percent of estimates, with a 5-day error being typical.

It has become customary to divide pregnancy into three equal *trimesters* of approximately 3 calendar months. Historically, the *first trimester* extended through the completion of 14 weeks, the *second trimester* through 28 weeks, and the third trimester included the 29th through 42nd weeks of pregnancy. Put another way, trimesters can be obtained by division of 42 into three periods of 14 weeks each. There are certain major obstetrical problems that cluster in each of these time periods. For example, the majority of spontaneous abortions take place during the first trimester, whereas most women with hypertensive disorders due to pregnancy are diagnosed during the third trimester.

The clinical use of trimesters to describe the duration of a specific pregnancy is too imprecise. For example, it is inappropriate in cases of uterine hemorrhage to categorize the problem temporally as "third-trimester bleeding." Appropriate management for the mother and her fetus will vary remarkably, depending on whether the bleeding is encountered early or late in the third trimester (see Chap. 35, p. 810). **Precise knowledge of the age of the fetus is imperative for ideal obstetrical management!** Therefore, expert attention must be given to this important measurement. The clinically appropriate unit of measure is *weeks of gestation completed.* Increasingly, clinicians designate gestational age using completed weeks and days, for example, 33 3/7 weeks for 33 completed weeks and 3 days.

History. For the most part, the same essentials go into appropriate history-taking from the pregnant woman as elsewhere in medicine. **Detailed information concerning past obstetrical history is crucial because many prior pregnancy complications tend to recur in subsequent pregnancies.**

The *menstrual history* is extremely important. The woman who spontaneously menstruates regularly every 28 days or so is most likely to ovulate at midcycle. Thus, the gestational age (menstrual age) becomes simply the number of weeks since the onset of the last menstrual period. If her menstrual cycles were significantly longer than 28 to 30 days, ovulation more likely occurred well beyond 14 days. Similarly, if the intervals were much longer and irregular, chronic anovulation is likely to have preceded some of the episodes of vaginal bleeding identified as menses. **Without a history of regular, predictable, cyclic, spontaneous menses that suggest ovulatory cycles, accurate dating of pregnancy by history and physical examination is difficult.**

It is important to ascertain whether or not *steroidal contraceptives* were used before the pregnancy. Because ovulation may not have resumed 2 weeks after the onset of the last withdrawal bleeding, and instead, may have occurred at an appreciably later and highly variable date, using the time of ovulation for predicting the time of conception in this circumstance may be erroneous. Use of ultrasonography in early pregnancy can clarify gestational age in these situations.

Psychosocial Screening. The American College of Obstetricians and Gynecologists (1999b) has concluded that addressing psychosocial issues is an essential step toward improving women's health and birth outcomes. Shown in Table 8–4 is a psychosocial screening tool, recommended for this purpose, that was developed by the Healthy Start Program of the Florida Department of Health.

TABLE 8–4 Psychosocial Prenatal Screening Questions

1. Do you have any problems that prevent you from keeping your health care appointments?
2. How many times have you moved in the past 12 months?
   0   1   2   3   > 3
3. Do you feel unsafe where you live?
4. Do you or any members of your household go to bed hungry?
5. In the past 2 months, have you used any form of tobacco?
6. In the past 2 months, have you used drugs or alcohol (including beer, wine, or mixed drinks)?
7. In the past year, has anyone hit you or tried to hurt you?
8. How do you rate your current stress level—low or high?
9. If you could change the timing of this pregnancy, would you want it earlier, later, not at all, or no change?

From the Florida Department of Health, 1997, with permission.

CIGARETTE SMOKING. Since 1984, the Surgeon General has required four specific, rotating health warnings on all cigarette packages, including: "Smoking by pregnant women may result in fetal injury, premature birth, and low birthweight" (United States Department of Health and Human Services, 2000). Information on maternal smoking during pregnancy has been included on the birth certificate since 1989. According to this information, reported smoking during pregnancy has progressively declined from 20 percent in 1989 to 12 percent in 2001 (Martin and colleagues, 2002b). In 2001, as in previous years, the smoking rate of 19 percent was highest for older teenagers—those aged 18 to 19 years.

Various adverse outcomes have been linked to smoking during pregnancy. Included are spontaneous abortion, low birthweight due to either preterm delivery or fetal growth restriction, infant and fetal deaths, and placental abruption (Ananth, 1996; Centers for Disease Control and Prevention, 2002d; Lin and Santolaya-Forgas, 1998; Martin, 2002b; Ness, 1999, and all their associates). Suggested pathophysiological mechanisms for these adverse pregnancy effects include increased fetal carboxyhemoglobin, reduced uteroplacental blood flow, and fetal hypoxia (Jazayeri and colleagues, 1998; Monheit and co-workers, 1983). To put the smoking problem into a national perspective, in 2001 the incidence of low birthweight among infants born to American women who reported smoking during pregnancy was two-thirds higher than that for nonsmokers—11.9 compared with 7.3 percent. Even among births to women who smoked only 1 to 5 cigarettes daily, 11.3 percent were low birthweight, and this rate was more than 50-percent higher than for nonsmokers (Martin and co-workers, 2002b). Jacqz-Aigrain and associates (2002) found that maternal cigarette consumption correlated directly with levels of cotinine measured in neonatal hair samples.

The most successful efforts for smoking cessation during pregnancy involve interventions that emphasize how to stop smoking. The Food and Drug Administration (FDA) classifies nicotine gum as category C (risk cannot be excluded), and transdermal systems are rated category D (positive evidence of risk). The American College of Obstetricians and Gynecologists (2000) has concluded, however, that it is reasonable to use these nicotine medications during pregnancy if prior non-pharmacological attempts have failed. Optimally, smokers should be treated before conception. Wisborg and co-workers (2000) randomly assigned 250 women who smoked at least 10 cigarettes per day after the first trimester to receive nicotine or placebo patches. Overall, 26 percent stopped smoking, however, no significant differences in smoking cessation, birthweight, or preterm delivery were detected between the nicotine and placebo groups. Of note, no serious adverse effects from the patches were reported, but compliance with the assigned treatments was low.

ALCOHOL AND ILLICIT DRUGS DURING PREGNANCY. Ethanol is a potent teratogen and causes the fetal alcohol syndrome, which is characterized by growth restriction, facial abnormalities, and central nervous system dysfunction (see Chap. 14, p. 346). The Surgeon General recommends that women who are pregnant or considering pregnancy abstain from using any alcoholic beverages.

Alcohol use is substantively underreported on the birth certificate—less than 1 percent of women reported any alcohol use during pregnancy in 2001 (Martin and colleagues, 2002b). According to the Centers for Disease Control and Prevention (2002a), about 13 percent of pregnant women used alcohol in 1999, down from 16 percent in 1995. Unfortunately, rates of binge and frequent drinking during pregnancy have not declined.

Chronic use of large quantities of illicit drugs, including opium derivatives, barbiturates, and amphetamines, is harmful to the fetus. Fetal distress, low birthweight, and drug withdrawal soon after birth are well documented. Often the mother who uses such drugs does not seek prenatal care, and even if she does, she may not admit to the use of such substances. El-Mohandes and associates (2003) have found that when women who use illicit drugs receive prenatal care, the risks for preterm birth and low birthweight are reduced.

The effects of several illicit drugs are considered in detail in Chapter 14 (see p. 363). The American College of Obstetricians and Gynecologists (1999b) has reviewed methods for screening women during pregnancy for use of illicit drugs and for alcohol abuse.

DOMESTIC VIOLENCE SCREENING. The term *domestic violence* usually refers to violence against adolescent and adult females within the context of family or intimate relationships. Such violence has been increasingly recognized as a major public health problem (see also Chap. 42, p. 997). Unfortunately, the majority of abused women continue to be victimized during pregnancy. With the possible exception of preeclampsia, domestic violence is more prevalent than any major medical condition detectable through routine prenatal screening (American Academy of Pediatrics and the American College of Obstetricians and Gynecologists, 2002). In their survey of 4750 women, Janssen and colleagues (2003)

found that 1.2 percent were exposed to physical violence by an intimate partner during pregnancy. This finding was associated with an approximate threefold increased risk of antepartum hemorrhage and fetal growth restriction and an eightfold increased risk of perinatal death.

The American College of Obstetricians and Gynecologists (1999a) has provided methods for screening for domestic violence and recommends their use at the first prenatal visit, then again at least once per trimester, and again at the postpartum follow-up. Webster and Holt (2004) found that a simple, six-question self-report survey is an effective alternative to direct questioning for identifying pregnant women who are experiencing partner violence. Physicians should be familiar with state laws that may require reporting of domestic violence (American Academy of Pediatrics and the American College of Obstetricians and Gynecologists, 2002).

Physical Examination. A thorough, general physical examination should be completed at the initial prenatal encounter. Expected changes in physical examination findings resulting from normal pregnancy are addressed in Chapters 2 and 5.

PELVIC EXAMINATION. The cervix is visualized employing a speculum lubricated with warm water. Bluish-red passive hyperemia of the cervix is characteristic, but not of itself diagnostic, of pregnancy (see p. 205). Dilated, occluded cervical glands bulging beneath the exocervical mucosa, so-called *nabothian cysts,* may be prominent. The cervix is not normally dilated above the level of the internal os. Next, to identify cytological abnormalities, a Pap smear is obtained and specimens for identification of *Neisseria gonorrhoeae* and *Chlamydia trachomatis* are obtained if screening is indicated.

Digital pelvic examination is completed by palpation, with special attention given to the consistency, length, and dilatation of the cervix; to the fetal presentation later in pregnancy; to the bony architecture of the pelvis; and to any anomalies of the vagina and perineum, including cystocele, rectocele, and relaxed or torn perineum. The vulva and contiguous structures are carefully inspected. All cervical, vaginal, and vulvar lesions are evaluated further by appropriate use of colposcopy, biopsy, culture, or dark-field examination. The perianal region should be visualized and digital rectal examination performed.

Laboratory Tests. Recommended routine laboratory tests at the first prenatal encounter are listed in Table 8–3. The Institute of Medicine recommended that a national policy of universal screening be developed for human immunodeficiency virus (HIV) testing, with patient notification, as a routine part of prenatal testing. The American Academy of Pediatrics and the American College of Obstetricians and Gynecologists (2002) support this recommendation. If a woman declines testing, this should be noted in the prenatal record. All pregnant women should also be screened for hepatitis B virus infection. Based on their prospective investigation of

1000 women, Murray and co-workers (2002) concluded that in the absence of hypertension, routine urinalyses beyond the initial prenatal visit were not necessary.

High-Risk Pregnancies. There are many risk factors that can be identified and given appropriate consideration in pregnancy management, and these are shown in Table 8–5. Some conditions may require the involvement of a maternal–fetal medicine subspecialist, geneticist, pediatrician, anesthesiologist, or other medical specialist in the evaluation, counseling, and care of the patient (American Academy of Pediatrics and the American College of Obstetricians and Gynecologists, 2002).

SUBSEQUENT PRENATAL VISITS. Traditionally, the timing of subsequent prenatal visits has been scheduled at intervals of 4 weeks until 28 weeks, and then every 2 weeks until 36 weeks, and weekly thereafter. Women with complicated pregnancies often require return visits at 1- to 2-week intervals. For example, Luke and co-workers (2003) found that a specialized prenatal care program that emphasized nutrition and education and required return visits every 2 weeks resulted in improved outcomes in twin pregnancies. In 1986, the Department of Health and Human Services convened an expert panel to review the content of prenatal care (Rosen and associates, 1991). The panel recommended that the number of prenatal visits be reduced in women at no apparent risk. They suggested that such women would best be served by return visits targeted at specific times; an example is alpha-fetoprotein screening at 16 weeks. Parous women with normal obstetrical histories are seen even less frequently.

The World Health Organization conducted a multicenter randomized trial with almost 25,000 women comparing routine prenatal care with an experimental model designed to minimize visits (Villar and associates, 2001). In the new model, women were seen once in the first trimester and screened for certain risk factors. Those without any anticipated complications—80 percent of the women screened—were seen again at 26, 32, and 38 weeks. Compared with routine prenatal care, which required a median of eight visits, the new model required a median of only five visits. No disadvantages were found in women with fewer visits. These results are consistent with other randomized trials (Clement and co-workers, 1999; McDuffie and colleagues, 1996).

Prenatal Surveillance. At each return visit, steps are taken to determine the well-being of mother and fetus (see Table 8–3). Certain information—for example, assessment of gestational age and accurate measurement of blood pressure (Jones and associates, 2003)—is especially important.

Fetal
- Heart rate(s)
- Size—current and rate of change
- Amount of amnionic fluid
- Presenting part and station (late in pregnancy)
- Activity

TABLE 8–5 Recommended Consultation for Risk Factors Identified in Early Pregnancy[a]

Risk Factor	
Asthma	
Symptomatic on medication	OBG
Severe (multiple hospitalizations)	MFM
Cardiac disease	
Cyanotic, prior myocardial infarction, aortic stenosis, pulmonary hypertension, Marfan syndrome, prosthetic valve, American Heart Association class II or greater	MFM
Other	OBG
Diabetes mellitus	
Class A–C	OBG
Class D or greater	MFM
Drug and alcohol use	MFM
Epilepsy (on medication)	OBG
Family history of genetic problems (Down syndrome, Tay-Sachs disease, phenylketonuria)	MFM
Hemoglobinopathy (SS, SC, S-thalassemia)	MFM
Hypertension	
Chronic, with renal or heart disease	MFM
Chronic, without renal or heart disease	OBG
Prior pulmonary embolus or deep vein thrombosis	OBG
Psychiatric illness	OBG
Pulmonary disease	
Severe obstructive or restrictive	MFM
Moderate	OBG
Renal disease	
Chronic, creatinine $\geq$ 3 mg/dL, $\pm$ hypertension	MFM
Chronic, other	OBG
Requirement for prolonged anticoagulation	MFM
Severe systemic disease	MFM
Obstetrical History and Conditions	
Age $\geq$ 35 years at delivery	OBG
Cesarean delivery, prior classical or vertical incision	OBG
Incompetent cervix	OBG
Prior fetal structural or chromosomal abnormality	MFM
Prior neonatal death	OBG
Prior fetal death	OBG
Prior preterm delivery or preterm ruptured membranes	OBG
Prior low birthweight (< 2500 g)	OBG
Second-trimester pregnancy loss	OBG
Uterine leiomyomata or malformation	OBG
Condylomata (extensive, covering vulva or vaginal opening)	OBG
Initial Laboratory Tests	
Human immunodeficiency virus (HIV)	
Symptomatic or low CD4 count	MFM
Other	OBG
CDE (Rh) or other blood group isoimmunization (excluding ABO, Lewis)	MFM

MFM = Maternal–fetal medicine specialist; OBG = obstetrician–gynecologist.
[a]At the time of consultation, continued patient care should be determined by collaboration with the referring care provider or by transfer of care.
Reproduced from the American Academy of Pediatrics and the American College of Obstetricians and Gynecologists, 2002, with permission.

Maternal

- Blood pressure—current and extent of change
- Weight—current and amount of change
- Symptoms—including headache, altered vision, abdominal pain, nausea and vomiting, bleeding, vaginal fluid leakage, and dysuria
- Height in centimeters of uterine fundus from symphysis
- Vaginal examination late in pregnancy often provides valuable information:
  - Confirmation of the presenting part.
  - Station of the presenting part (see Chap. 17, p. 426).
  - Clinical estimation of pelvic capacity and its general configuration (see Chap. 2, p. 36).
  - Consistency, effacement, and dilatation of the cervix.

Assessment of Gestational Age. One of the most important determinations at prenatal examinations is assessment of fetal age. Precise knowledge of gestational age is important because a number of pregnancy complications may develop for which optimal treatment will depend on fetal age. Fortunately, it is possible to identify this with considerable precision through an appropriately timed, carefully performed clinical examination, coupled with knowledge of the time of onset of the last menstrual period.

FUNDAL HEIGHT. Between 20 and 31 weeks, the height of the uterine fundus, measured in centimeters, correlates closely with gestational age in weeks (Jimenez and co-workers, 1983). Quaranta and associates (1981) and Calvert and colleagues (1982) reported essentially identical observations up to 34 weeks. Obesity, however, may distort this relationship. The fundal height should be measured as the distance over the abdominal wall from the top of the symphysis pubis to the top of the fundus. *The bladder must be emptied before making the measurement.* Worthen and Bustillo (1980), for example, demonstrated that at 17 to 20 weeks, fundal height was 3 cm higher with a full bladder.

FETAL HEART SOUNDS. The fetal heart can first be heard in most women between 16 and 19 weeks when carefully auscultated with a DeLee fetal stethoscope. The ability to hear unamplified fetal heart sounds will depend on factors such as patient size and the examiner's hearing acuity. Herbert and co-workers (1987) reported that the fetal heart was audible by 20 weeks in 80 percent of women. By 21 weeks audible fetal heart sounds were present in 95 percent, and by 22 weeks in all.

ULTRASOUND. When gestational age cannot be clearly identified, sonography is of considerable value. Compared with the last menstrual period, Taipale and Hiilesmaa (2001) found that ultrasonography performed between 8 and 16 weeks was slightly more accurate, by approximately 2 days, for predicting the actual date of delivery. Although controversial, as discussed in Chapter 13 (see p. 326), routine ultrasound is

not currently recommended in low-risk pregnancies by the American Academy of Pediatrics and the American College of Obstetricians and Gynecologists (2002).

Subsequent Laboratory Tests. If the initial results were normal, most tests need not be repeated (see Table 8–3). Maternal serum screening at 16 to 18 weeks (15 to 20 weeks is acceptable) is recommended for detecting open neural-tube defects and some chromosomal anomalies (see Chap. 13, p. 319). Hematocrit (or hemoglobin) determination, along with syphilis serology if it is prevalent in the population, should be repeated at about 28 to 32 weeks (Hollier and co-workers, 2003; Kiss and colleagues, 2004).

Cystic fibrosis carrier screening should be offered to couples with a family history of cystic fibrosis and to Caucasian couples of European or Ashkenazi Jewish descent planning a pregnancy or seeking prenatal care. Ideally, screening is performed before conception or during the first or early second trimester. Information about cystic fibrosis screening also should be provided to patients in other racial and ethnic groups who are at lower risk (see Chap. 13, p. 325).

ANCILLARY PRENATAL TESTS

Gestational Diabetes. All pregnant women should be screened for gestational diabetes mellitus, whether by history, clinical risk factors, or routine laboratory testing. Although laboratory testing between 24 and 28 weeks is the most sensitive approach, there may be pregnant women at low risk who are less likely to benefit from testing (American Academy of Pediatrics and the American College of Obstetricians and Gynecologists, 2002). Gestational diabetes is discussed in Chapter 52 (see p. 1172).

Chlamydial Infection. Women at high risk for *C trachomatis* infection should be screened during the first prenatal visit (American Academy of Pediatrics and the American College of Obstetricians and Gynecologists, 2002). Risk factors include unmarried status, recent change in sexual partner or multiple concurrent partners, age under 25 years, inner-city residence, history or presence of other sexually transmitted diseases, and little or no prenatal care. The United States Preventive Services Task Force (2001) concluded that evidence that screening and treatment of women at risk for chlamydia improves pregnancy outcome is "fair." They concluded that benefits of screening outweigh potential harms. A negative prenatal chlamydia or gonorrhea test should not preclude postpartum screening (Mahon and associates, 2002).

Gonococcal Infection. Risk factors for gonorrhea are similar for those for chlamydia. The American Academy of Pediatrics and the American College of Obstetricians and Gynecologists (2002) recommend that pregnant women with risk factors or symptoms be cultured for *N gonorrhoeae* at an early prenatal visit and again in the third trimester. Treatment is given for gonorrhea as well as possible coexisting chlamydial infection, as outlined in Chapter 59 (see p. 1305).

Fetal Fibronectin. Detection of this protein in vaginal fluid has been used to forecast preterm delivery in women with contractions (see Chap. 36, p. 862). The American College of Obstetricians and Gynecologists (2001b) does not recommend routine screening.

Group B Streptococcal (GBS) Infection. Universal prenatal screening for GBS carriage has been controversial. Based largely on a retrospective study comparing risk-based and culture-based approaches (Schrag and co-workers, 2002), the American College of Obstetricians and Gynecologists (2002c) and the Centers for Disease Control and Prevention (2002c) now recommend that vaginal and rectal GBS cultures be obtained in all women between 35 and 37 weeks. Intrapartum antimicrobial prophylaxis is given for those whose cultures are positive. Women with GBS bacteriuria or a previous infant with invasive disease are given empirical intrapartum prophylaxis. These infections are discussed in detail in Chapter 58 (see p. 1284).

Special Screening for Genetic Diseases. Selected screening can be offered based on maternal age, family history, or the ethnic or racial background of the couple (American College of Obstetricians and Gynecologists, 1995). Examples include testing for Tay-Sachs disease for people of Eastern European Jewish or French Canadian ancestry; β-thalassemia for those of Mediterranean, Southeast Asian, Indian, Pakistani, or African ancestry; α-thalassemia for people of Southeast Asian or African ancestry; and sickle-cell anemia for people of African, Mediterranean, Middle Eastern, Caribbean, Latin American, or Indian descent (see Chap. 7, p. 192).

NUTRITION

Meaningful studies of nutrition in human pregnancy are exceedingly difficult to design. For ethical reasons, experimental dietary deficiency must not be produced deliberately. In those instances in which severe nutritional deficiencies have been induced as a consequence of social, economic, or political disaster, coincidental events often have created many variables, the effects of which are not amenable to quantification. Some past experiences suggest, however, that in otherwise healthy women a state of near starvation is required to establish clear differences in pregnancy outcome.

During the severe European winter of 1944–1945, nutritional deprivation of known intensity prevailed in a well-circumscribed area of the Netherlands occupied by the German military (Stein and associates, 1972). At the lowest point during the *Hunger Winter,* rations reached 450 kcal/day, with generalized rather than selective malnutrition. Smith (1947)

analyzed the outcomes of pregnancies that were in progress during this 6-month famine. Median infant birthweights decreased about 250 g and rose again after food became available. This indicated that birthweight can be influenced significantly by starvation during later pregnancy. The perinatal mortality rate, however, was not altered, nor was the incidence of malformations significantly increased. Interestingly, the frequency of pregnancy "toxemia" was found to decline.

Evidence of impaired brain development has been obtained in some animal fetuses whose mothers had been subjected to intense dietary deprivation. Subsequent intellectual development was studied by Stein and associates (1972) in young Dutch adults whose mothers had been starved during pregnancy. The comprehensive study was made possible because all males at age 19 underwent compulsory examination for military service. It was concluded that severe dietary deprivation during pregnancy caused no detectable effects on subsequent mental performance.

Conversely, there is evidence that maternal weight gain during pregnancy influences birthweight. This was studied by Martin and colleagues (2002b) who used birth certificate data for 2001. As shown in Figure 8–7, nearly two thirds of pregnant women gained 26 lb or more. The median weight gain was 30.5 lb. Maternal weight gain had a positive correlation with birthweight, and women with the greatest risk—14 percent—for delivering an infant weighing less than 2500 g were those with weight gains less than 16 lb. This incidence was 20 percent in African-American women who gained 15 lb or less. Cohen and associates (2001) studied more than 4000 pregnant women and concluded that ethnic differences in pregnancy outcomes were not explained by nutritional variations.

RECOMMENDATIONS FOR WEIGHT GAIN. For the first half of the 20th century, it was recommended that weight gain during pregnancy be limited to less than 20 lb (9.1 kg). It was believed that such restriction would prevent pregnancy hypertensive disorders and fetal macrosomia resulting in operative deliveries. By the 1970s, however, women were encouraged to gain at least 25 lb (11.4 kg) to prevent preterm birth and fetal growth restriction, a recommendation that subsequent research continues to support (Ehrenberg and associates, 2003). In 1990, the Institute of Medicine recommended a weight gain of 25 to 35 lb (11.5 to 16 kg) for women with a normal prepregnancy body mass index (BMI). This index is easily calculated using the chart shown in Figure 43–1 (see p. 1008). Weight gains recommended by the Institute of Medicine (1990) according to prepregnant BMI categories are shown in Table 8–6. The American Academy of Pediatrics and the American College of Obstetricians and Gynecologists (2002) have endorsed these guidelines. Of note, in 2001, almost 1 in 3 women had weight gains outside the Institute of Medicine guidelines (Martin and colleagues, 2002b).

Feig and Naylor (1998) from Canada have challenged recommendations for liberal weight gain in industrial nations.

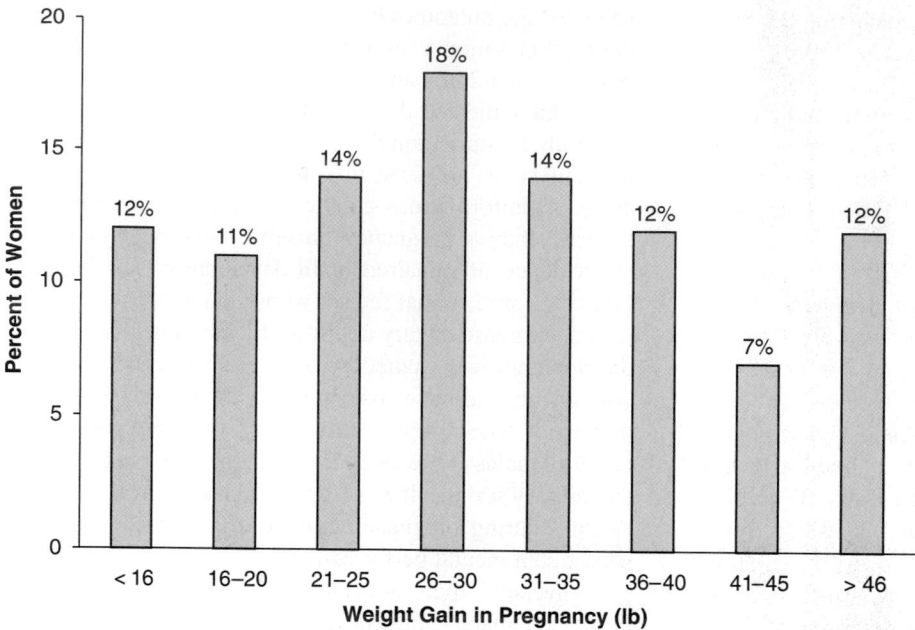

FIGURE 8–7. Maternal weight gain in the United States reported on the birth certificate in 2001. (From Martin and colleagues, 2002b.)

They concluded that these recommendations encourage women to overeat during pregnancy without addressing other causes of low-birthweight infants such as adolescent pregnancy, drug abuse, and heavy smoking. They endorsed the recommendation by the Committee on Medical Aspects of Food Policy (1991) in the United Kingdom that a pregnant woman with a normal BMI should gain 15 to 25 lb during pregnancy.

Disadvantages of excessive maternal weight gain and fetal macrosomia must be considered. Thorsdottir and associates (2002) analyzed pregnancy outcome in relation to weight gain in 615 healthy women with a normal BMI before pregnancy. The frequency of antepartum and intrapartum complications, including fetal macrosomia, was highest among women who gained more than 44 lb (20 kg) during pregnancy. Conversely, these complications were lowest among those whose weight gain was within the range recommended by the Institute of Medicine. Similarly, Rhodes and co-workers (2003) found in their analysis of 1999–2000 United States birth certificate data that excessive weight gain—defined as more than 40 lb—correlated closely with fetal macrosomia.

Weight Retention After Pregnancy. Not all the weight put on during pregnancy is lost during and immediately after parturition (Hytten, 1991). The average-sized normal woman who gains 28 lb (12.5 kg) in pregnancy is about 9 lb (4.4 kg) above her prepregnant weight when discharged postpartum. Schauberger and co-workers (1992) studied prenatal and postpartum weights in 795 women delivered in Wisconsin. Their average weight gain was 28.6 ± 10.6 lb (13.0 ± 4.8 kg). As shown in Figure 8–8, the majority of maternal weight loss was at delivery—about 12 lb (5.5 kg)—and in the ensuing 2 weeks thereafter—about 9 lb (4 kg). An additional 5.5 lb (2.5 kg) was lost between 2 weeks and 6 months postpartum. The average total weight loss resulted in an average retained weight of 3 ± 10.5 lb (1.4 ± 4.8 kg) due to pregnancy. Overall, the more weight gained during pregnancy, the more that was lost postpartum. Parous women retained more of their pregnancy weight, and this is linked to long-term obesity (see Chap. 43, p. 1012). The effect of breast feeding on maternal weight loss was negligible.

Summary of Weight Gain. Perhaps the most remarkable finding about weight gain in pregnancy is that a wide range is compatible with good clinical outcomes. Moreover, departures from "normal" are nonspecific for any outcome in a given individual.

TABLE 8–6 Recommended Ranges of Total Weight Gain for Pregnant Women by Prepregnancy Body Mass Index (BMI) for Singleton Gestation[a]

Weight-for-Height Category		Recommended Total Weight Gain	
Category	BMI	kg	lb
Low	< 19.8	12.5–18	28–40
Normal	19.8–26	11.5–16	25–35
High	26–29	7–11.5	15–25
Obese	> 29	≥ 7	≥ 15

[a]The range for women carrying twins is 35–45 lb (16–20 kg). Young adolescents (< 2 years after menarche) and African-American women should strive for gains at the upper end of the range. Short women (< 62 in. or < 157 cm) should strive for gains at the lower end of the range.
From the Institute of Medicine, 1990, with permission.

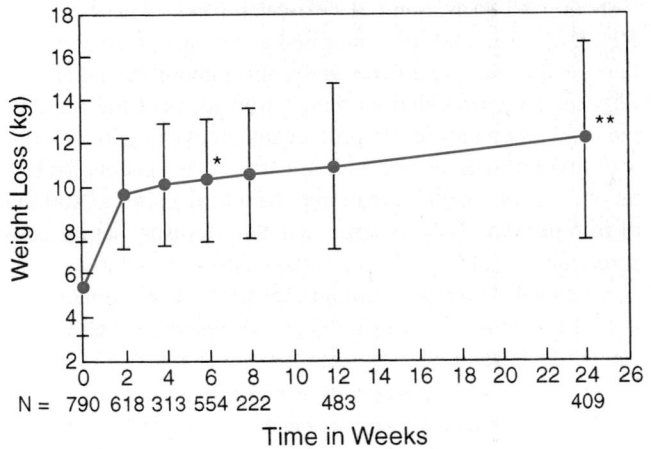

FIGURE 8–8. Cumulative weight loss from last antepartum visit to 6 months postpartum. *Statistically different from 2-week weight loss, **Statistically different from 6-week weight loss. (From Schauberger and co-workers, 1992, with permission.)

RECOMMENDED DIETARY ALLOWANCES. Periodically, the Food and Nutrition Board of the Institute of Medicine recommends dietary allowances for women, including those who are pregnant or lactating. Its latest recommendations (2004) are summarized in Table 8–7. Certain prenatal vitamin–mineral supplements may lead to intakes well in excess of the recommended allowances. Moreover, the use

of excessive supplements—for example, 10 times the recommended daily allowances—which often are self-prescribed, has led to concern about nutrient toxicities during pregnancy. Nutrients that can potentially exert toxic effects include iron, zinc, selenium, and vitamins A, B_6, C, and D. Vitamin and mineral intake more than twice the recommended daily dietary allowance shown in Table 8–7 should be avoided during pregnancy (American Academy of Pediatrics and the American College of Obstetricians and Gynecologists, 2002).

Calories. As shown in Figure 8–9, pregnancy requires an additional 80,000 kcal, which are accumulated primarily in the last 20 weeks. To meet this demand, a caloric increase of 100 to 300 kcal per day is recommended during pregnancy (American Academy of Pediatrics and the American College of Obstetricians and Gynecologists, 2002). Calories are necessary for energy, and whenever caloric intake is inadequate, protein is metabolized rather than being spared for its vital role in fetal growth and development. Total physiological requirements during pregnancy are not necessarily the sum of ordinary nonpregnant requirements plus those specific to pregnancy. For example, the additional energy required during pregnancy may be compensated in whole or in part by reduced physical activity (Hytten, 1991).

Protein. To the basic protein needs of the nonpregnant woman are added the demands for growth and repair of the

TABLE 8–7 Recommended Daily Dietary Allowances for Adolescent and Adult Pregnant and Lactating Women

	Pregnant			Lactating		
	14–18 years	*19–30 years*	*31–50 years*	*14–18 years*	*19–30 years*	*31–50 years*
Fat-soluble vitamins						
Vitamin A	750 μg	770 μg	770 μg	1200 μg	1300 μg	1300 μg
Vitamin D[a]	5 μg	5 μg	5 μg	5 μg	5 μg	5 μg
Vitamin E	15 mg	15 mg	15 mg	19 mg	19 mg	19 mg
Vitamin K[a]	75 μg	90 μg	90 μg	75 μg	90 μg	90 μg
Water-soluble vitamins						
Vitamin C	80 mg	85 mg	85 mg	115 mg	120 mg	120 mg
Thiamine	1.4 mg	1.4 mg	1.4 mg	1.4 mg	1.4 mg	1.4 mg
Riboflavin	1.4 mg	1.4 mg	1.4 mg	1.6 mg	1.6 mg	1.6 mg
Niacin	18 mg	18 mg	18 mg	17 mg	17 mg	17 mg
Vitamin B_6	1.9 mg	1.9 mg	1.9 mg	2 mg	2 mg	2 mg
Folate	600 μg	600 μg	600 μg	500 μg	500 μg	500 μg
Vitamin B_{12}	2.6 μg	2.6 μg	2.6 μg	2.8 μg	2.8 μg	2.8 μg
Minerals						
Calcium[a]	1300 mg	1000 mg	1000 mg	1300 mg	1000 mg	1000 mg
Phosphorus	1250 mg	700 mg	700 mg	1250 mg	700 mg	700 mg
Iron	27 mg	27 mg	27 mg	10 mg	9 mg	9 mg
Zinc	13 mg	11 mg	11 mg	14 mg	12 mg	12 mg
Iodine	220 μg	220 μg	220 μg	290 μg	290 μg	290 μg
Selenium	60 μg	60 μg	60 μg	70 μg	70 μg	70 μg

[a]Recommendations measured as Adequate Intake (AI) instead of Recommended Daily Dietary Allowance (RDA). An AI is set instead of an RDA if insufficient evidence is available to determine an RDA. The AI is based on observed or experimentally determined estimates of average nutrient intake by a group (or groups) of healthy people.
From the Food and Nutrition Board of the Institute of Medicine, National Academy of Sciences, 2004.

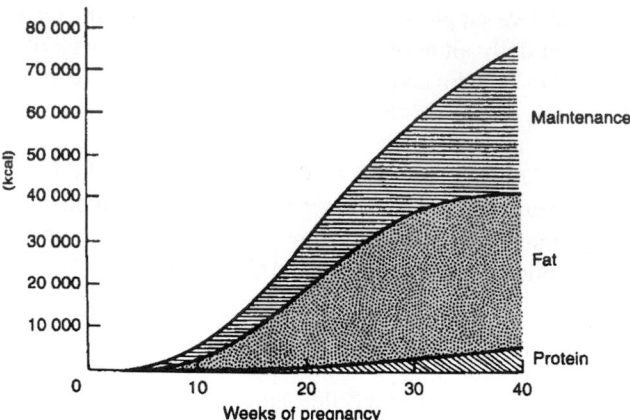

FIGURE 8–9. Cumulative kilocalories of energy required for pregnancy. (From Hytten and Chamberlain, 1991, with permission.)

fetus, placenta, uterus, and breasts, and increased maternal blood volume (see Chap. 5, p. 127). During the second half of pregnancy, about 1000 g of protein are deposited, amounting to 5 to 6 g/day (Hytten and Leitch, 1971). The concentrations of most amino acids in maternal plasma fall markedly, including ornithine, glycine, taurine, and proline (Hytten, 1991). Exceptions during pregnancy are glutamic acid and alanine, which rise in concentration.

Preferably, most protein should be supplied from animal sources, such as meat, milk, eggs, cheese, poultry, and fish, because they furnish amino acids in optimal combinations. Milk and dairy products have long been considered nearly ideal sources of nutrients, especially protein and calcium, for pregnant or lactating women.

Minerals. The intakes recommended by the Food and Nutrition Board of the Institute of Medicine (2004) for a variety of minerals are presented in Table 8–7. With the exception of iron, practically all diets that supply sufficient calories for appropriate weight gain will contain enough minerals to prevent deficiency if iodized food is used.

IRON. The reasons for increased iron requirements during pregnancy are discussed in Chapter 5 (see p. 130). Of the approximately 300 mg of iron transferred to the fetus and placenta and the 500 mg incorporated, if available, into the expanding maternal hemoglobin mass, nearly all is used after midpregnancy. During that time, iron requirements imposed by pregnancy and maternal excretion total about 7 mg per day (Pritchard and Scott, 1970). Very few women have sufficient iron stores to supply this amount, and the diet seldom contains enough iron to meet this demand. For these reasons, the American Academy of Pediatrics and the American College of Obstetricians and Gynecologists (2002) endorse the recommendation by the National Academy of Sciences that at least 27 mg of ferrous iron supplement be given daily to pregnant women. This amount is contained in most prenatal vitamins.

Scott and co-workers (1970) established that as little as 30 mg of elemental iron, supplied as ferrous gluconate, sulfate, or fumarate and taken daily throughout the latter half of pregnancy, provided sufficient iron to meet the requirements of pregnancy and to protect any preexisting iron stores. This amount will also provide for iron requirements for lactation. The pregnant woman may benefit from 60 to 100 mg of iron per day if she is large, has twin fetuses, begins supplementation late in pregnancy, takes iron irregularly, or has a somewhat depressed hemoglobin level. The woman who is overtly anemic from iron deficiency responds well to oral supplementation with iron salts (see Chap. 51, p. 1145).

Because iron requirements are slight during the first 4 months of pregnancy, it is *not necessary* to provide supplemental iron during this time. Withholding iron supplementation during the first trimester of pregnancy avoids the risk of aggravating nausea and vomiting. Ingestion of iron at bedtime or on an empty stomach facilitates absorption and appears to minimize the possibility of an adverse gastrointestinal reaction.

Since 1997, the FDA has required that iron preparations containing 30 mg or more of elemental iron per tablet be packaged as individual doses, such as in blister packages. This regulation is targeted at preventing accidental iron poisoning in children.

CALCIUM. As discussed in Chapter 5 (see p. 129), the pregnant woman retains about 30 g of calcium, most of which is deposited in the fetus late in pregnancy (Pitkin, 1985). This amount of calcium represents only about 2.5 percent of total maternal calcium, most of which is in bone, and which can readily be mobilized for fetal growth. Moreover, Heaney and Skillman (1971) demonstrated increased calcium absorption by the intestine and progressive retention throughout pregnancy. Efforts to prevent preeclampsia using calcium supplementation have not proven efficacious, and it is not recommended for routine use during pregnancy (see Chap. 34, p. 780).

PHOSPHORUS. The ubiquitous distribution of phosphorus ensures an adequate intake during pregnancy. Plasma levels of inorganic phosphorus do not differ appreciably from nonpregnant levels.

ZINC. Severe zinc deficiency may lead to poor appetite, suboptimal growth, and impaired wound healing. Profound zinc deficiency may cause dwarfism and hypogonadism. It may also lead to a specific skin disorder, *acrodermatitis enteropathica,* as the result of a rare, severe congenital zinc deficiency. Although the level of zinc supplementation that is safe for pregnant women has not been clearly established, recommended daily intake during pregnancy is about 12 mg (see Table 8–7).

Goldenberg and colleagues (1995) randomly assigned 580 indigent women to zinc supplementation (25 mg) or placebo beginning at a mean gestational age of 19 weeks. Plasma zinc levels were significantly higher in women who received supplements. Infants born to zinc-supplemented women were slightly larger (mean 125 g) and had a slightly larger head circumference (mean 4 mm). Later, Osendarp and colleagues (2001) randomly assigned 420 women in Bangladesh to receive either zinc supplementation (30 mg daily) or placebo from 12 to 16 weeks' gestation until delivery. Although supplementation did not improve birthweight, low-birthweight infants of mothers who received zinc had reduced risks of acute diarrhea, dysentery, and impetigo. In a follow-up study of these infants at 13 months, zinc supplementation was not found to confer any benefits on developmental outcome (Hamadani and co-workers, 2002).

IODINE. The use of iodized salt and bread products is recommended during pregnancy to offset the increased fetal requirements and maternal renal losses. Despite this, iodine intake has declined substantially in the past 15 years, and it is probably inadequate for some populations (see Chap. 53, p. 1196). Interest in increasing dietary iodine was heightened by reports linking subclinical maternal hypothyroidism to adverse pregnancy outcomes and possible neurodevelopmental defects in children studied at age 7 years (Casey and associates, 2004; Haddow and colleagues, 1999). Severe maternal iodine deficiency predisposes offspring to endemic cretinism, characterized by multiple severe neurological defects (see Chap. 53, p. 1196). In parts of China and Africa where this condition is endemic, iodide supplementation very early in pregnancy prevents cretinism (Cao and colleagues, 1994).

MAGNESIUM. Deficiency of magnesium as the consequence of pregnancy has not been recognized. Undoubtedly, during prolonged illness with no magnesium intake, the plasma level might become critically low, as it would in the absence of pregnancy. We have observed magnesium deficiency during pregnancy complicated by the consequences of previous intestinal bypass surgery. Sibai and co-workers (1989) randomly assigned 400 normotensive primigravid women to 365 mg elemental magnesium supplementation or placebo tablets from 13 to 24 weeks. Supplementation did not improve any measures of pregnancy outcome.

COPPER. Enzymes that contain copper, such as cytochrome oxidase, play key roles in many oxidative processes and hence in the production of most of the energy required for metabolism. Pregnancy has a major effect on maternal copper metabolism, with marked increases in serum ceruloplasmin and plasma copper (Reyes and associates, 2000). Copper deficiency has not been documented in humans during pregnancy. No studies of copper supplementation of pregnant women have been reported, although several prenatal supplements currently marketed provide 2 mg of copper per tablet.

SELENIUM. This mineral is an essential component of the enzyme glutathione peroxidase, which catalyzes the conversion of hydrogen peroxide to water. Selenium is an important defensive component against free radical damage. A severe geochemical deficiency has been identified in a large area of China. Deficiency is manifested by a frequently fatal cardiomyopathy in young children and women of childbearing age. Conversely, selenium toxicity resulting from oversupplementation also has been observed. There is no reported need to supplement selenium in American women.

CHROMIUM. Trace amounts of chromium are believed to serve as a co-factor for insulin by facilitating attachment to peripheral receptors. The extent to which chromium is important in human nutrition remains uncertain, and there are no data suggesting that supplementation is advisable during pregnancy.

MANGANESE. This mineral serves as a co-factor for enzymes such as the glycosyltransferases, which are necessary for the synthesis of polysaccharides and glycoproteins. Manganese deficiency has not been observed in human adults, and supplements are not indicated during pregnancy.

POTASSIUM. The concentration of potassium in maternal plasma decreases by about 0.5 mEq/L by midpregnancy (Brown and colleagues, 1986). Potassium deficiency develops in the same circumstances as when the woman is not pregnant. Prolonged nausea and vomiting may lead to hypokalemia and metabolic alkalosis.

SODIUM. Deficiency during pregnancy is unusual unless diuretics are prescribed or dietary sodium intake is reduced drastically. A normal diet provides an abundance of sodium. Although pregnancy is associated with increased total accumulation of sodium, the serum concentration decreases slightly due to the expanded plasma volume. Sodium excretion remains unchanged, and averages 100 to 110 mEq/day (Brown and colleagues, 1986).

FLUORIDE. The value of supplemental fluoride during pregnancy has been questioned. Maheshwari and co-workers (1983) found that fluoride metabolism is not altered appreciably during the course of pregnancy. Horowitz and Heifetz (1967) investigated the prevalence of caries in temporary and permanent teeth of children with the same postnatal exposure to optimally fluoridated water but different patterns of prenatal exposure. They concluded that there were no additional benefits from maternal ingestion of fluoridated water if the offspring ingested such water from birth.

Fluoride supplementation during pregnancy has not been endorsed by the American Dental Association (Institute of Medicine, 1990). Supplemental fluoride ingested by the lactating woman does not increase the fluoride concentration in her milk (Ekstrand and colleagues, 1981).

Vitamins. The increased requirements for vitamins during pregnancy shown in Table 8–7 usually are supplied by any general diet that provides adequate calories and protein. The exception is folic acid during times of unusual requirements, such as pregnancy complicated by protracted vomiting, hemolytic anemia, or multiple fetuses.

FOLIC ACID. In the United States, approximately 4000 pregnancies are affected by neural-tube defects each year; more than half of these defects could be prevented with daily intake of 400 μg of folic acid throughout the periconceptional period (Centers for Disease Control and Prevention, 1999). Since 1992, the Public Health Service has recommended that all women capable of becoming pregnant consume 400 μg of folic acid daily throughout their childbearing years. The FDA (1996) later established standards fortifying grain products such as cereal, bread, rice, and pasta with folic acid. By putting 140 μg of folic acid into each 100 g of grain products, it was estimated that the folic acid intake of the average American woman of childbearing age would increase 100 μg per day. Because nutritional sources alone are insufficient, however, folic acid supplementation is still recommended (American College of Obstetrician and Gynecologists, 2003b).

Honein and co-workers (2001) compared birth certificate reports of neural-tube defects before and after mandatory fortification. Although other factors may have contributed, they found that the prevalence of neural-tube defects declined almost 20 percent following grain fortification. Ray and associates (2002) reported that the prevalence of neural-tube defects in Ontario, Canada, declined from 1.13 to 0.58 per 1000 births following grain fortification.

There is also evidence that grain fortification is contributing to a rise in the serum folate levels of American women. The Centers for Disease Control and Prevention (2002b) compared serum and red blood cell folate concentrations in childbearing-aged women who participated in National Health and Nutrition Examination Surveys between 1988 and 1994 versus 1999 to 2000. Among the women in the latter group, the median serum folate concentration was increased approximately threefold, and the median red blood cell folate concentration increased approximately twofold. The findings also indicated that a national health objective for 2010—to increase the median red blood cell folate level among women of childbearing age to 220 ng/mL—has been met for many ethnic groups, but not for African-Americans.

A woman with a prior pregnancy complicated by a neural-tube defect can reduce the 3-percent recurrence risk by more than 70 percent if she supplements her daily diet with 4 mg of folic acid for the month before conception and for the first trimester of pregnancy. As emphasized by the American Academy of Pediatrics and the American College of Obstetricians and Gynecologists (2002), this dose should be consumed as a separate supplement, not as multiple multivitamin tablets, to avoid excessive intake of fat-soluble vitamins. Unfortunately, surveys continue to suggest that many women, especially among minorities, remain unaware of the recommendations regarding folic acid supplementation (Perlow, 2001; Rinsky-Eng and Miller, 2002).

The relationship of folic acid deficiency and neural-tube defects as well as other congenital malformations are discussed in detail in Chapters 7 (see p. 192), 12 (see p. 302), and 14 (see p. 345).

VITAMIN A. Dietary intake of vitamin A in the United States appears to be adequate, and routine supplementation during pregnancy is not recommended (American College of Obstetricians and Gynecologists, 1998b). A small number of case reports suggest an association of birth defects with very high doses during pregnancy—10,000 to 50,000 IU daily. These malformations are similar to those produced by the vitamin A derivative isotretinoin (Accutane), which is a potent teratogen in humans (see Chap. 14, p. 350). Beta-carotene, the precursor of vitamin A found in fruits and vegetables, has not been shown to produce vitamin A toxicity.

Radhika and colleagues (2002) examined the effects of vitamin A deficiency in 736 Indian women during the third trimester. Overt deficiency, manifested as night blindness, was observed in approximately 3 percent of the women. Subclinical vitamin A deficiency, defined as a serum retinol concentration below 20 μg/dL without clinical signs, was present in 27 percent. Vitamin A deficiency, whether overt or subclinical, was associated with a significantly increased risk of both maternal anemia and spontaneous preterm birth. The former likely reflected the need for vitamin A to facilitate iron absorption, and the latter possibly reflected increased susceptibility to infection associated with vitamin A deficiency.

VITAMIN B_{12}. The level of vitamin B_{12} in maternal plasma decreases variably in otherwise normal pregnancies (see Chap. 51, p. 1147). This decrease is mostly from a reduction in plasma transcobalamins and is thus prevented only in part by supplementation. Vitamin B_{12} occurs naturally only in foods of animal origin. It is now established that strict vegetarians may give birth to infants whose vitamin B_{12} stores are low. Likewise, because breast milk of a vegetarian mother contains little vitamin B_{12}, the deficiency may become profound in the breast-fed infant (Higginbottom and associates, 1978). Excessive ingestion of vitamin C also can lead to a functional deficiency of vitamin B_{12}.

VITAMIN B_6. Most clinical trials in pregnant women have failed to demonstrate any benefits of vitamin B_6 supplements (Institute of Medicine, 1990). For women at high risk for inadequate nutrition (e.g., substance abuse, adolescents, and those with multifetal gestations), a daily supplement containing 2 mg is recommended.

VITAMIN C. The recommended dietary allowance for vitamin C during pregnancy is 80 to 85 mg/day, or about 20 percent more than when nonpregnant (see Table 8–7). A reasonable diet should readily provide this amount. The maternal plasma level declines during pregnancy, whereas the cord level is higher, a phenomenon observed with most water-soluble vitamins.

PRAGMATIC NUTRITIONAL SURVEILLANCE. Although the science of nutrition continues in its perpetual struggle to identify the ideal amounts of protein, calories, vitamins, and minerals for the pregnant woman and her fetus, those directly responsible for their care may best discharge their duties as follows:

1. In general, advise the pregnant woman to eat what she wants in amounts she desires and salted to taste.
2. Make sure that there is ample food to eat in the case of socioeconomically deprived women.
3. Monitor weight gain, with a goal of about 25 to 35 pounds in women with a normal BMI.
4. Periodically explore food intake by dietary recall to discover the occasional nutritionally absurd diet.
5. Give tablets of simple iron salts that provide at least 27 mg of iron daily. Give folate supplementation before and in the early weeks of pregnancy.
6. Recheck the hematocrit or hemoglobin concentration at 28 to 32 weeks to detect any significant decrease.

COMMON CONCERNS

EXERCISE. In general, it is not necessary for the pregnant woman to limit exercise, provided she does not become excessively fatigued or risk injury. Clapp (1989) reported that 18 conditioned pregnant women actually improved their metabolic efficiency during exercise. Specifically, the amount of oxygen required to complete a treadmill exercise actually decreased during pregnancy. Pivarnik and co-workers (1990) used invasive hemodynamic monitoring and compared cardiovascular responses of seven healthy women to aerobic exercise (cycle or treadmill) during late pregnancy and again 3 months postpartum. Oxygen consumption, heart rate, stroke volume, and cardiac output all increased appropriately in response to exercise. Pivarnik and associates (1994) later showed that pregnant women who exercised regularly had significantly larger blood volumes.

Clapp and associates (2000) randomly assigned 46 women who did not exercise regularly to either no exercise or to weight-bearing exercise beginning at 8 weeks. Exercise consisted of treadmill running, step aerobics, or stair stepper use for 20 minutes three to five times each week. They did this throughout pregnancy at an intensity between 55 and 60 percent of the preconceptional maximum aerobic capacity. Both placental size and birthweight were significantly greater in the exercise group. In contrast, Magann and colleagues (2002) prospectively collected information on exercise behavior in 750 healthy women during their pregnancy. Among working

TABLE 8–8 Absolute and Relative Contraindications to Aerobic Exercise During Pregnancy

Absolute Contraindications
- Hemodynamically significant heart disease
- Restrictive lung disease
- Incompetent cervix or cerclage
- Multifetal gestation at risk for preterm labor
- Persistent second- or third-trimester bleeding
- Placenta previa after 26 weeks of gestation
- Preterm labor during the current pregnancy
- Ruptured membranes
- Preeclampsia or gestational hypertension

Relative Contraindications
- Severe anemia
- Unevaluated maternal cardiac arrhythmia
- Chronic bronchitis
- Poorly controlled type 1 diabetes mellitus
- Extreme morbid obesity
- Extreme underweight (BMI < 12)
- History of extremely sedentary lifestyle
- Fetal growth restriction in current pregnancy
- Poorly controlled hypertension
- Orthopedic limitations
- Poorly controlled seizure disorder
- Poorly controlled hyperthyroidism
- Heavy smoker

BMI = body mass index.
Reproduced from the American College of Obstetricians and Gynecologists, 2002b, with permission.

women, exercise was associated with smaller infants, more dysfunctional labors, and more frequent upper respiratory infections.

The American College of Obstetricians and Gynecologists (2002b) advises a thorough clinical evaluation be conducted before recommending an exercise program. In the absence of contraindications (Table 8–8), pregnant women should be encouraged to engage in regular, moderate-intensity physical activity 30 minutes or more a day. Each activity should be reviewed individually for its potential risk. Activities with a high risk of falling or abdominal trauma should be avoided. Similarly, scuba diving should be avoided because the fetus is at an increased risk for decompression sickness.

With some pregnancy complications, the mother and her fetus may benefit from a sedentary existence. For example, some women with hypertensive disorders caused by pregnancy may benefit from being sedentary (see Chap. 34, p. 781), as may some women pregnant with two or more fetuses (see Chap. 39, p. 936), those suspected of having a growth-restricted fetus (see Chap. 38, p. 903), or those with severe heart disease (see Chap. 44, p. 1021).

EMPLOYMENT. The legal and social movements in the United States to provide equality of opportunity in the workplace have reached women who are or might become pregnant. Annas (1991) reviewed the legal issues involved with employment during pregnancy. Importantly, the United States Supreme Court buttressed the Pregnancy Discrimination Act of 1978 by ruling in 1991 that federal law prohibits employers from excluding women from job categories on the basis that they are or might become pregnant. More than 120 nations around the world currently provide paid maternity leave and health benefits by law, including most industrialized nations except the United States, Australia, and New Zealand (Luke and co-authors, 1999).

The Family and Medical Leave Act (FMLA) was passed in 1993, however, a subsequent report to Congress found that because this leave is without pay, eligible women did not take it for financial reasons. It is estimated that nearly half of childbearing-aged women in the United States are in the labor force. For many, an additional financial strain stems from being pressured to stop working during pregnancy. For example, Frazier and colleagues (2001) found that more than 27 percent of 1635 women were advised to stop working. The most frequent reasons included hypertension, vaginal bleeding, and labor. More than half of the women were instructed to stop working before the seventh month of gestation.

Teitelman and co-workers (1990) evaluated maternal work activity and pregnancy outcome in 4186 women delivered at Yale–New Haven Hospital. Women were classified according to the type of jobs they held. *Standing* jobs, such as those of a cashier, bank teller, or dentist, required standing in the same position for more than 3 hours per day. *Active* jobs, such as physicians, waitresses, and real estate agents, involved continuous or intermittent walking. *Sedentary* jobs, such as librarians, bookkeepers, or bus drivers, required less than 1 hour of standing per day. These authors found that pregnant women who work at jobs that require prolonged standing are at greater risk for preterm delivery, but it did not have any effect on fetal growth.

Mozurkewich and colleagues (2000) reviewed 29 studies with over 160,000 pregnancies. They confirmed a 20- to 60-percent increase in preterm birth, fetal growth restriction, or hypertension associated with physically demanding work. In a prospective study of more than 900 healthy primigravidas, Higgins and associates (2002) found that women who worked were about fivefold more likely to develop preeclampsia. Newman and colleagues (2001) reported the relationship between occupational fatigue and preterm birth in 2929 women with singleton pregnancies studied by the Maternal–Fetal Medicine Units Network. They found that occupational fatigue—estimated by the number of hours standing, intensity of physical and mental demands, and environmental stressors—was associated with an increased risk of preterm membrane rupture. For those women reporting the highest degrees of fatigue, the risk was 7.4 percent.

Common sense dictates that any occupation that subjects the pregnant woman to severe physical strain should be avoided. Ideally, no work or play should be continued to the extent that undue fatigue develops. Adequate periods of rest should be provided during the work period. Women with previous pregnancy complications that are likely to be repetitive, such as low-birthweight infants, probably should minimize physical work. The American Academy of Pediatrics and the American College of Obstetricians and Gynecologists (2002) have concluded that women with uncomplicated pregnancies usually can continue to work until the onset of labor. Furthermore, although a period of 4 to 6 weeks generally is required for return of the physiological condition to normal, they advise that individual circumstances should be considered when recommending resumption of full activity.

TRAVEL. In general, travel by the healthy woman has no harmful effect on pregnancy (Aerospace Medical Association, 2003). Travel in properly pressurized aircraft offers no unusual risk, and in the absence of obstetrical or medical complications, the American College of Obstetricians and Gynecologists (2001a, 2004) has concluded that pregnant women can safely fly up to 36 weeks. It is recommended that pregnant women observe the same precautions for air travel as the general population, including periodic movement of the lower extremities, ambulation at least hourly, and use of seatbelts while seated. Perhaps the greatest risks with travel, especially international travel, are acquiring an infectious disease or developing a complication remote from facilities adequate to manage the complication (Ryan and associates, 2002).

The American College of Obstetricians and Gynecologists (1998a) has formulated guidelines for use of automobile passenger restraints during pregnancy. There is no evidence that safety restraints increase the chance of fetal injury. Indeed, the leading cause of fetal death in a motor accident is the death of the mother (see Chap. 42, p. 997). Therefore, pregnant women should be encouraged to wear properly positioned three-point restraints throughout pregnancy while riding in automobiles. The lap belt portion of the restraining belt should be placed under the woman's abdomen and across her upper thighs. The belt should be as snug as comfortably possible. The shoulder belt also should be snugly applied and positioned between the breasts. Based on limited existing information, the American College of Obstetricians and Gynecologists (1998a) has concluded that it does not appear reasonable to recommend disabling airbags during pregnancy.

BATHING. There are no contraindications to bathing during pregnancy or the puerperium. One caveat is that early pregnancy exposure to a hot tub or Jacuzzi at 100°F or higher has been associated with an increased risk of miscarriage (Li and co-workers, 2003). It also has been linked to neural-tube defects (see Chap. 13, p. 317). During late pregnancy, the heavy uterus usually upsets the balance of the pregnant woman and increases the likelihood of her slipping and falling in the bathtub. For that reason, showers at the end of pregnancy may be preferable.

CLOTHING. It generally has been recommended that the clothing worn during pregnancy be comfortable and nonconstricting. According to fashion experts, however, pregnancy apparel has changed considerably in recent years (Morgan, 2000). One clothing designer stated: "It used to be about covering it up, and now it's about showing it off. Today's maternity chic is body-hugging not body hiding."

The increasing mass of the breasts may make them pendulous and painful, and a well-fitting supporting brassiere may be indicated for comfort. Constricting leg wear should be avoided.

BOWEL HABITS. Constipation is common, presumably because of prolonged transit time and compression of the lower bowel by the uterus or by the presenting part (see Chap. 49, p. 1115). In addition to discomfort caused by passage of hard fecal material, bleeding and painful fissures may develop in the edematous and hyperemic rectal mucosa. There is also greater frequency of *hemorrhoids* and, much less commonly, prolapse of the rectal mucosa.

Women whose bowel habits are normal before pregnancy may prevent constipation during pregnancy. This is done by ingesting sufficient quantities of fluid along with reasonable amounts of daily exercise. This regimen may be supplemented when necessary by a mild laxative, such as prune juice, milk of magnesia, bulk-producing substances, or stool-softening agents.

COITUS. Whenever abortion or preterm labor threatens, coitus should be avoided. Otherwise it has been generally accepted that in healthy pregnant women, sexual intercourse usually is not harmful. Nearly 10,000 women enrolled in a prospective investigation by the Vaginal Infection and Prematurity Study Group were interviewed regarding sexual activity during pregnancy. There was a significantly decreased frequency of sexual intercourse reported with advancing gestation (Read and Klebanoff, 1993). By 36 weeks, 72 percent of these women reported intercourse less than once weekly. Bartellas and colleagues (2000) reported that the decrease was attributed to decreased desire (58 percent) and fear of harm to the pregnancy (48 percent).

Risks from intercourse late in pregnancy have not been clearly delineated. Grudzinskas and co-workers (1979) found no association between gestational age at delivery and the frequency of coitus during the last 4 weeks of pregnancy. Similarly, Sayle and colleagues (2001) found no increased— and actually a decreased—risk of delivery within 2 weeks of intercourse.

On occasion, sexual drive in the face of admonishment against intercourse late in pregnancy has led to sexual practices with disastrous consequences. Aronson and Nelson (1967) described a fatal case of air embolism late in pregnancy as a result of air blown into the vagina during cunnilingus. Other near-fatal cases have been described (Bernhardt and associates, 1988).

DENTITION. Examination of the teeth should be included in the prenatal examination, and good dental hygiene is encouraged. Dental caries are not aggravated by pregnancy. Likewise, pregnancy is not a contraindication to dental treatment.

IMMUNIZATION. Current recommendations for immunizations during pregnancy are summarized in Table 8–9. The American College of Obstetricians and Gynecologists (2003a) stresses that current information on the safety of vaccines given during pregnancy is subject to change and can be verified from the Centers for Disease Control and Prevention website at www.cdc.gov/nip.

Women who are susceptible to rubella during pregnancy should receive MMR (measles-mumps-rubella) vaccination postpartum. There is no contraindication to this vaccination while breast feeding (American College of Obstetricians and Gynecologists, 2002d).

Biological Warfare and Vaccines. The tragic events of September 11, 2001, and the ongoing threat of bioterrorism require familiarity with smallpox and anthrax vaccines during pregnancy. The smallpox vaccine is actually a live attenuated vaccinia virus that is related both to smallpox and to cowpox viruses. Fetal infection from this vaccine, termed *vaccinia,* is a rare complication, but it may result in abortion, stillbirth, or neonatal death. Therefore, in nonemergency circumstances, smallpox vaccination is contraindicated both during pregnancy and in women who desire to become pregnant within 28 days of vaccination (Centers for Disease Control and Prevention, 2003b). If, however, vaccination is inadvertently performed in early pregnancy, this is not grounds for termination (Suarez and Hankins, 2002). If the pregnant woman is at risk because of exposure to smallpox—either as a direct victim of a bioterrorist attack or as a close contact of an individual case—the risks from clinical smallpox substantially outweigh any potential risk from vaccination (Suarez and Hankins, 2002).

Anthrax vaccination has been limited principally to individuals who are occupationally exposed, such as special veterinarians, laboratory workers, and members of the armed forces. The vaccine contains no live virus and thus would not be expected to pose significant risk to the fetus. Wiesen and Littell (2002) studied the reproductive outcomes of 385 women in the United States Army who became pregnant after receiving the anthrax vaccine. They found no adverse effects on fertility or pregnancy outcome.

Smallpox, anthrax, and other infections related to bioterrorism are discussed in Chapter 58 (see p. 1293).

CAFFEINE. In 1980, the FDA advised pregnant women to limit caffeine intake. The Fourth International Caffeine Workshop concluded shortly thereafter that there was no evidence that caffeine caused increased teratogenic or reproductive risks (Dews and colleagues, 1984). In small laboratory animals, caffeine is not a teratogen, but if given in massive doses it potentiates mutagenic effects of radiation and some

TABLE 8–9 Recommendations for Immunization During Pregnancy

Immunobiological Agent	Indications for Immunization During Pregnancy	Dosing Schedule	Comments
Live Attenuated Virus Vaccines			
Measles	Contraindicated—see Immune Globulins below	Single dose, preferably as measles-mumps-rubella (MMR)[a]	Vaccinate susceptible women postpartum. Breast feeding is not a contraindication
Mumps	Contraindicated	Single dose, preferably as MMR	Vaccinate susceptible women postpartum
Rubella	Contraindicated, but congenital rubella syndrome has never been described after vaccination	Single dose, preferably as MMR	Teratogenicity of vaccine is theoretical, not confirmed to date; vaccinate susceptible women postpartum
Poliomyelitis Oral = live attenuated; SC = enhanced-potency inactivated virus[b]	Not routinely recommended for women in the United States, except women at increased risk of exposure	*Primary:* Two doses of enhanced-potency inactivated virus SC at 4–8 wk intervals and a 3rd dose 6–12 mo after 2nd dose *Immediate protection:* One dose oral polio vaccine (in outbreak setting)	Vaccine indicated for susceptible women traveling in endemic area or in other high-risk situations
Yellow fever	Contraindicated except if exposure is unavoidable	Single dose SC	Postponement of travel preferable to vaccination, if possible
Varicella	Contraindicated, but no adverse outcomes reported in pregnancy	Two doses needed, with 2nd dose given 4–8 wk after 1st dose	Teratogenicity of vaccine is theoretical. Vaccination of susceptible women should be considered postpartum
Other			
Influenza	All women, regardless of trimester, who will be pregnant during the influenza season.	One dose IM every year	Inactivated virus vaccine
Rabies	Indications for prophylaxis not altered by pregnancy; each case considered individually	Public health authorities to be consulted for indications, dosage, and route of administration	Killed virus vaccine
Hepatitis B	Preexposure and postexposure for women at risk of infection	Three-dose series IM at 0, 1, and 6 mo	Vaccine produced from purified surface antigen developed by recombinant technology. Used with hepatitis B immune globulin for some exposures. Exposed newborn needs birth dose vaccination and immune globulin ASAP. All infants should receive birth dose of vaccine
Hepatitis A	Preexposure and postexposure if at risk (international travel)	Two-dose schedule 6 mo apart	Inactivated virus
Inactivated Bacterial Vaccines			
Pneumococcus	Indications not altered by pregnancy. Recommended for women with asplenia; metabolic, renal, cardiac, pulmonary diseases; smokers; immunosuppressed	In adults, one dose only; consider repeat dose in 6 yr for high-risk women	Polyvalent polysaccharide vaccine
Meningococcus	Indications not altered by pregnancy; vaccination recommended in unusual outbreaks	One dose; consult public health authorities	Quadrivalent polysaccharide vaccine

Typhoid	Not recommended routinely except for close, continued exposure or travel to endemic areas	Killed vaccine *Primary:* 2 injections, > 4 wk apart *Booster:* 1 dose; schedule not yet determined	Killed or live attenuated oral bacterial vaccine. Oral vaccine preferred
Anthrax	See text discussion	6-dose primary vaccination, then annual booster vaccination	Preparation from cell-free filtrate of *B anthracis*. No dead or live bacteria. Teratogenicity of vaccine theoretical
Toxoids			
Tetanus-diphtheria	Lack of primary series, or no booster within past 10 yr	*Primary:* 2 doses at 1–2-mo interval with 3rd dose 6–12 mo after the 2nd *Booster:* Single dose IM every 10 yr after completion of primary series	Combined tetanus-diphtheria toxoids preferred: adult tetanus–diphtheria formulation. Updating immune status should be part of antepartum care
Specific Immune Globulins			
Hepatitis B	Postexposure prophylaxis	Depends on exposure. See Chap. 50, p. 1130	Usually given with hepatitis B virus vaccine; exposed newborn needs immediate prophylaxis
Rabies	Postexposure prophylaxis	Half dose at injury site, half dose in deltoid	Used in conjunction with rabies killed virus vaccine
Tetanus	Postexposure prophylaxis	1 dose IM	Used in conjunction with tetanus toxoid
Varicella	Should be considered for exposed pregnant women to protect against maternal, not congenital, infection	1 dose IM within 96 hr of exposure	also for newborns or women with varicella within 4 days before or 2 days following delivery
Standard Immune Globulins			
Hepatitis A Hepatitis A virus vaccine should be used with hepatitis A immune globulin	Postexposure prophylaxis	0.02 mL/kg IM for 1 dose of immune globulin	Given ASAP and within 2 wk of exposure; infants born to women who are incubating the virus or are acutely ill at delivery should receive 1 dose of 0.5 mL ASAP after birth
Measles	Postexposure prophylaxis	.25 mL/kg (maximum of 15 mL) for 1 dose	Given within 6 days of exposure

ID = intradermally; IM = intramuscularly; PO = orally; SC = subcutaneously; ASAP = as soon as possible.
[a]Two doses necessary for students entering institutions of higher education, newly hired medical personnel, and travel abroad.
[b]Inactivated polio vaccine recommended for nonimmunized adults at increased risk.
Adapted from the Centers for Disease Control and Prevention, Recommendations of the Advisory Committee on Immunization Practices, 2003a, 2004.

chemicals. When infused intravenously into sheep, caffeine decreases uterine blood flow by 5 to 10 percent (Conover and colleagues, 1983).

The risk of spontaneous abortion related to caffeine consumption is controversial. Klebanoff and co-workers (1999) measured paraxanthine as a biological serum marker of caffeine consumption. They estimated caffeine doses in 487 women with spontaneous abortions and in 2087 controls. Only extremely high serum paraxanthine concentrations were associated with abortion. Such high levels were equivalent to drinking more than 5 cups of coffee per day. Clausson and associates (2002) found no association of moderate caffeine consumption of less than 500 mg daily with low birthweight, fetal growth restriction, or preterm delivery. The American Dietetic Association (2002) recommends that caffeine intake during pregnancy be limited to less than 300 mg daily, or about three, 5-oz cups of percolated coffee.

MEDICATIONS. A number of drugs commonly ingested during pregnancy, and their possible adverse fetal effects, are considered in detail in Chapter 14. Based on interviews with 578 women, Glover and co-workers (2003) found that during pregnancy more than 95 percent took prescription medications and 92 percent self-medicated with over-the-counter preparations. **With rare exceptions, any drug that exerts a systemic effect in the mother will cross the placenta to reach the embryo and fetus.** All physicians should develop the habit of ascertaining the likelihood of pregnancy before prescribing drugs for any woman, because a number of medications in common use are potentially injurious to the embryo and the fetus. Package inserts provided by pharmaceutical companies and approved by the FDA should be consulted before drugs are prescribed for pregnant women.

NAUSEA AND VOMITING. These are common complaints during the first half of pregnancy. Erroneously called *morning sickness,* symptoms usually commence between the first and second missed menstrual period and continue until about 14 to 16 weeks. Although nausea and vomiting tend to be worse in the morning, they may continue throughout the day. Lacroix and co-workers (2000) found that nausea and vomiting were reported by three fourths of pregnant women and lasted an average of 35 days. Half had relief by 14 weeks, and 90 percent by 22 weeks. In 80 percent of the women, nausea lasted all day. It was frequently described to have a character and intensity similar to that experienced by patients undergoing cancer chemotherapy.

The genesis of pregnancy-induced nausea and vomiting is not clear, and it is discussed further in Chapter 49 (see p. 1113). Although high levels of serum hCG have been implicated as causing nausea, this placental hormone is likely a surrogate for increasing estrogen levels which are known to cause such symptoms. Huxley (2000) speculates that nausea and emesis in early gestation have a functional role in promoting and maintaining early placental growth. Specifically,

the reduced caloric intake lowers maternal insulin and insulin growth factor-1 levels and suppresses maternal anabolic synthesis, ensuring that nutrient partitioning favors placental growth.

Seldom is the treatment of nausea and vomiting of pregnancy so successful that the affected expectant mother is afforded complete relief. Fortunately, the unpleasantness and discomfort usually can be minimized. Eating small feedings at more frequent intervals but stopping short of satiation is of value. The smell of certain foods often precipitates or aggravates the symptoms and should be avoided. In some women, vomiting may be so severe that dehydration, electrolyte and acid–base disturbances, and starvation ketosis become serious problems. This condition is termed *hyperemesis gravidarum,* and its management is described in Chapter 49 (see p. 1113).

BACKACHE. Low back pain to some extent is reported in nearly 70 percent of pregnant women (Wang and colleagues, 2004). Minor degrees follow excessive strain or fatigue and excessive bending, lifting, or walking. Orvieto and associates (1994) studied 449 women and reported that back pain increased with duration of gestation. Prior low back pain and obesity were risk factors.

Back pain can be reduced by having women squat rather than bend over when reaching down, providing back support with a pillow when sitting down, and avoiding high-heeled shoes. Severe back pain should not be attributed simply to pregnancy until a thorough orthopedic examination has been conducted. Muscular spasm and tenderness, which often are classified clinically as acute strain or fibrositis, respond well to analgesics, heat, and rest. As discussed in Chapter 53 (see p. 1199), some women with severe back and hip pain may have *pregnancy-associated osteoporosis* (Dunne and colleagues, 1993). Severe pain also has other uncommon causes, such as disc disease, vertebral osteoarthritis, or septic arthritis.

Norén and co-workers (2002) studied the long-term outcomes of 231 women who had some type of back pain during pregnancy. Residual pain 3 years after delivery was reported by approximately 20 percent. Women with combined lumbar back and posterior pelvic pain were at greatest risk for disability, which was attributed to impaired back extensor and hip abductor muscle functions.

VARICOSITIES. These enlarged veins generally result from congenital predisposition and are exaggerated by prolonged standing, pregnancy, and advancing age. Usually varicosities become more prominent as pregnancy advances, as weight increases, and as the length of time spent upright is prolonged. As discussed in Chapter 5 (see p. 134), femoral venous pressure increases appreciably as pregnancy advances. The symptoms produced by varicosities vary from cosmetic blemishes on the lower extremities and mild discomfort at the end of the day to severe discomfort that requires prolonged rest with the feet elevated.

The treatment of varicosities of the lower extremities is generally limited to periodic rest with elevation of the legs, elastic stockings, or both. Surgical correction of the condition during pregnancy generally is not advised, although occasionally the symptoms may be so severe that injection, ligation, or even stripping of the veins is necessary. Vulvar varicosities may be aided by application of a foam rubber pad suspended across the vulva by a belt of the type used with a perineal pad. Rarely, large varicosities may rupture, resulting in profuse hemorrhage.

HEMORRHOIDS. Varicosities of the rectal veins may first appear during pregnancy. More often, pregnancy causes an exacerbation or recurrence of previous hemorrhoids. Their development or aggravation during pregnancy undoubtedly is related to increased pressure in the rectal veins. This is caused by obstruction of venous return by the large uterus as well as by constipation during pregnancy. Pain and swelling usually are relieved by topically applied anesthetics, warm soaks, and stool-softening agents. Thrombosis of a rectal vein can cause considerable pain, but the clot usually can be evacuated by incising the vein wall under topical anesthesia.

HEARTBURN. This symptom is one of the most common complaints of pregnant women and is caused by reflux of gastric contents into the lower esophagus. The increased frequency of regurgitation during pregnancy most likely results from the upward displacement and compression of the stomach by the uterus, combined with relaxation of the lower esophageal sphincter. In most pregnant women, symptoms are mild and are relieved by a regimen of more frequent but smaller meals and avoidance of bending over or lying flat. Antacid preparations may provide considerable relief. Aluminum hydroxide, magnesium trisilicate, or magnesium hydroxide alone or in combination are given. Management for symptoms that do not respond to these simple measures is discussed in Chapter 49 (see p. 1114).

PICA. There has been considerable historical interest in the cravings (pica) of pregnant women for strange foods and, at times, nonfoods such as ice (pagophagia), starch (amylophagia), or clay (geophagia). This desire has been considered by some to be triggered by severe iron deficiency. Although some women crave these items, and although the craving usually is ameliorated after correction of iron deficiency, not all pregnant women with pica are necessarily iron deficient. Indeed, if strange "foods" dominate the diet, iron deficiency will be aggravated or will develop eventually, blurring the distinction between cause and effect.

Patel and colleagues (2004) from the University of Alabama at Birmingham prospectively completed a dietary inventory on more than 3000 women during the second trimester. The prevalence of pica was 4 percent. The most common nonfood items ingested were starch (64 percent), dirt (14 percent), sourdough (9 percent), and ice (5 percent).

The prevalence of anemia was 15 percent in women with pica compared with 6 percent in those without it. Interestingly, the rate of spontaneous preterm birth at less than 35 weeks was twice as high in women with pica.

PTYALISM. Women during pregnancy are occasionally distressed by profuse salivation. The cause of this ptyalism sometimes appears to be stimulation of the salivary glands by the ingestion of starch. This cause should be looked for and eradicated if found. Most cases are unexplained.

FATIGUE. Early in pregnancy, most women complain of fatigue and desire for excessive sleep. The condition usually remits spontaneously by the fourth month of pregnancy and has no special significance. It may be due to the soporific effect of progesterone(s).

HEADACHE. This complaint is common early in pregnancy. A few cases may result from sinusitis or ocular strain caused by refractive errors. In the vast majority, however, no cause can be demonstrated. Treatment is largely symptomatic. By midpregnancy, most headaches decrease in severity or disappear. The clinical and pathological significance of headaches as the consequence of hypertensive disorders later in pregnancy is considered in Chapter 34 (see p. 776). Persistent or severe headaches of other origins, for example, migraine, are discussed in Chapter 55 (see p. 1230).

LEUKORRHEA. Pregnant women commonly develop increased vaginal discharge, which in many instances is not pathological. Increased mucus secretion by cervical glands in response to hyperestrogenemia is undoubtedly a contributing factor. Occasionally, troublesome leukorrhea is the result of an infection caused by trichomonal or yeast vulvovaginal infections.

BACTERIAL VAGINOSIS. Not an infection in the ordinary sense, bacterial vaginosis is a maldistribution of normal vaginal flora. Numbers of lactobacilli are decreased, and overrepresented species tend to be anaerobic bacteria, including *Gardnerella vaginalis, Mobiluncus,* and some *Bacteroides* species. The prevalence of vaginosis during pregnancy varies from 10 to 30 percent, and it is associated with preterm birth. Treatment is reserved for symptomatic women who usually complain of a fishy-smelling discharge. Metronidazole, 500 mg twice daily orally for 7 days, will achieve cure in about 90 percent of cases. Unfortunately, treatment does not reduce preterm birth, and routine screening is not recommended (American College of Obstetricians and Gynecologists, 2001b). These relationships are discussed further in Chapters 36 (see p. 862) and 59 (see p. 1319).

TRICHOMONIASIS. In as many as 20 percent of women, *Trichomonas vaginalis* can be identified during prenatal examination. Symptomatic infection is much less prevalent, and vaginitis is characterized by foamy leukorrhea with pruritus and irritation. Trichomonads are demonstrated readily in fresh vaginal secretions as flagellated, pear-shaped, motile organisms that are somewhat larger than leukocytes.

Metronidazole has proved effective in eradicating *T vaginalis*. The drug may be administered orally or vaginally, and it crosses the placenta and enters the fetal circulation. The possibility of teratogenicity from first-trimester exposure was raised previously. Rosa and colleagues (1987), however, found no increased frequency of birth defects in over 1000 women given metronidazole during early pregnancy (see Chap. 14, p. 360). Even so, many recommend against its use in early pregnancy. Some studies have linked trichomonal infection with preterm birth, however, treatment has not proven to decrease the risk (see Chap. 36, p. 863). Thus, screening and treatment of asymptomatic women is not recommended during pregnancy.

CANDIDIASIS. *Candidia albicans* can be cultured from the vagina in about 25 percent of women approaching term. Asymptomatic colonization requires no treatment, but the organism may sometimes cause an extremely profuse, irritating discharge associated with a pruritic, painfully tender, and edematous vulva. Miconazole, clotrimazole, and nystatin are effective for the treatment of candidiasis during pregnancy (see Chap. 14, p. 359). In some women, infection is likely to recur, thereby requiring repeated treatment during pregnancy. In these cases, symptomatic infection usually subsides after pregnancy.

REFERENCES

Aerospace Medical Association, Medical Guidelines Task Force: Medical guidelines for airline travel, 2nd ed. Aviat Space Environ Med 74:5, 2003

American Academy of Pediatrics and the American College of Obstetricians and Gynecologists: Guidelines for perinatal care, 5th ed. October 2002

American College of Obstetricians and Gynecologists: Immunization during pregnancy. Committee Opinion No. 282, January 2003a

American College of Obstetricians and Gynecologists: Neural tube defects. Practice Bulletin No. 44, July 2003b

American College of Obstetricians and Gynecologists: Avoiding inappropriate clinical decisions based on false-positive human chorionic gonadotropin test results. Committee Opinion No. 278, November 2002a

American College of Obstetricians and Gynecologists: Exercise during pregnancy and the postpartum period. Committee Opinion No. 267, January 2002b

American College of Obstetricians and Gynecologists: Prevention of early-onset group B streptococcal disease in newborns. Committee Opinion No. 279, December 2002c

American College of Obstetricians and Gynecologists: Rubella vaccination. Committee Opinion No. 281, December 2002d

American College of Obstetricians and Gynecologists: Air travel during pregnancy. Committee Opinion No. 264, December 2001a, Reaffirmed 2004

American College of Obstetricians and Gynecologists: Assessment of risk factors for preterm birth. Practice Bulletin No. 31, October 2001b

American College of Obstetricians and Gynecologists: Smoking cessation during pregnancy. Education Bulletin No. 260, September 2000

American College of Obstetricians and Gynecologists: Domestic violence. Educational Bulletin No. 257, December 1999a

American College of Obstetricians and Gynecologists: Psychosocial risk factors: Perinatal screening and intervention. Educational Bulletin No. 255, November 1999b

American College of Obstetricians and Gynecologists: Obstetric aspects of trauma management. Educational Bulletin No. 251, September 1998a

American College of Obstetricians and Gynecologists: Vitamin A supplementation during pregnancy. Committee Opinion No. 196, January 1998b

American College of Obstetricians and Gynecologists: Preconceptional care. Technical Bulletin No. 205, May 1995

American Dietetic Association: Position of the American Dietetic Association: Nutrition and lifestyle for a healthy pregnancy outcome. J Am Diet Assoc 102:1479, 2002

Ananth CV, Savitz DA, Luther ER: Maternal cigarette smoking as a risk factor for placental abruption, placenta previa, and uterine bleeding in pregnancy. Am J Epidemiol 144:881, 1996

Annas GJ: Fetal protection and employment discrimination—the Johnson Controls case. N Engl J Med 325:740, 1991

Aronson ME, Nelson PK: Fatal air embolism in pregnancy resulting from an unusual sex act. Obstet Gynecol 30:127, 1967

Ashitaka Y, Nishimura R, Takemori M, et al: Production and secretion of hCG and hCG subunits by trophoblastic tissue. In Segal S (ed): Chorionic Gonadotropins. New York, Plenum, 1980, p 151

Bartellas E, Crane JMG, Daley M, et al: Sexuality and sexual activity in pregnancy. Br J Obstet Gynaecol 107:964, 2000

Bastian LA, Nanda K, Hasselblad V, et al: Diagnostic efficiency of home pregnancy test kits. A meta-analysis. Arch Fam Med 7:465, 1998

Bergsjø P, Denman DW III, Hoffman HJ, et al: Duration of human singleton pregnancy. A population-based study. Acta Obstet Gynecol Scand 69:197, 1990

Bernhardt TL, Goldmann RW, Thombs PA, et al: Hyperbaric oxygen treatment of cerebral air embolism from orogenital sex during pregnancy. Crit Care Med 16:729, 1988

Bracken MB, Belanger K: Calculation of delivery dates. N Engl J Med 321:1483, 1989

Braunstein GD: False-positive serum human chorionic gonadotropin results: Causes, characteristics, and recognition. Am J Obstet Gynecol 187:217, 2002

Brown MA, Sinosich MJ, Saunders DM, et al: Potassium regulation and progesterone-aldosterone interrelationships in human pregnancy: A prospective study. Am J Obstet Gynecol 155:349, 1986

Calvert JP, Crean EE, Newcombe RG, et al: Antenatal screening by measurement of symphysis–fundus height. BMJ 285:846, 1982

Cao X-Y, Jiang X-M, Dou Z-H, et al: Timing of vulnerability of the brain to iodine deficiency in endemic cretinism. N Engl J Med 331:1739, 1994

Casey BM, Dashe JS, McIntire DD, et al: Pregnancy outcomes in women with subclinical hypothyroidism. Society for Maternal-Fetal Medicine Annual Meeting, New Orleans, La, February 2–7, 2004, Abstract No. 307

Centers for Disease Control and Prevention: Prevention and control of influenza: Recommendations of the advisory committee on immunization practices (ACIP). MMWR 53:10, 2004

Centers for Disease Control and Prevention: Recommendations of the Advisory Committee on Immunization Practices, 2003a. Available at: http://www.cdc.gov/mmwr/preview/mmwrhtml/0002528. Accessed March 4, 2003

Centers for Disease Control and Prevention: Smallpox vaccination and adverse reactions. MMWR 52:RR-4, 2003b

Centers for Disease Control and Prevention: Alcohol use among women of childbearing age—United States, 1991–1999. MMWR 51:273, 2002a

Centers for Disease Control and Prevention: Folate status in women of childbearing age, by race/ethnicity—United States, 1999–2000. MMWR 51:808, 2002b

Centers for Disease Control and Prevention: Prevention of perinatal group B streptococcal disease. MMWR 51:RR-11, 2002c

Centers for Disease Control and Prevention: Women and smoking: A report of the Surgeon General. MMWR 51:RR-12, 2002d

Centers for Disease Control and Prevention: Entry into prenatal care—United States, 1989–1997. MMWR 49:393, 2000

Centers for Disease Control and Prevention: Knowledge and use of folic acid by women of childbearing age—United States 1995–1998. MMWR 48:16, 1999

Chadwick JR: Value of the bluish coloration of the vaginal entrance as a sign of pregnancy. Trans Am Gynecol Soc 11:399, 1886

Clapp JF III: Oxygen consumption during treadmill exercise before, during, and after pregnancy. Am J Obstet Gynecol 161:1458, 1989

Clapp JF III, Kim H, Burciu B, et al: Beginning regular exercise in early pregnancy: Effect on fetoplacental growth. Am J Obstet Gynecol 183:1484, 2000

Clausson B, Granath F, Ekbom A, et al: Effect of caffeine exposure during pregnancy on birth weight and gestational age. Am J Epidemiol 155:429, 2002

Clement S, Candy B, Sikorski J, et al: Does reducing the frequency of routine antenatal visits have long term effects? Follow up of participants in a randomised controlled trial. Br J Obstet Gynaecol 106:367, 1999

Cohen GR, Curet LB, Levine RJ, et al: Ethnicity, nutrition, and birth outcomes in nulliparous women. Am J Obstet Gynecol 185:660, 2001

Cole LA: HCG, its free subunits and its metabolites: Roles in pregnancy and trophoblastic disease. J Reprod Med 43:3, 1998

Cole LA, Khanlian SA, Sutton JM, et al: Accuracy of home pregnancy tests at the time of missed menses. Am J Obstet Gynecol 190:100, 2004

Committee on Medical Aspects of Food Policy: Report of the Panel on Dietary Reference Values: Dietary Reference Values for Food, Energy and Nutrients for the United Kingdom. London, Department of Health, 1991, p 30

Conover WB, Key TC, Resnik R: Maternal cardiovascular response to caffeine infusion in the pregnant ewe. Am J Obstet Gynecol 145:534, 1983

Dews P, Grice HC, Neims A, et al: Report of Fourth International Caffeine Workshop, Athens, 1982. Food Chem Toxicol 22:163, 1984

Dunne F, Walters B, Marshall T, et al: Pregnancy associated osteoporosis. Clin Endocrinol 39:487, 1993

Ehrenberg HM, Dierker L, Milluzzi C, et al: Low maternal weight, failure to thrive in pregnancy, and adverse pregnancy outcomes. Am J Obstet Gynecol 189:1726, 2003

Ekstrand J, Boreus LO, de Chateau P: No evidence of transfer of fluoride from plasma to breast milk. Br Med J (Clin Res Ed) 283:761, 1981

El-Mohandes A, Herman AA, Kl-Khorazaty MN, et al: Prenatal care reduces the impact of illicit drug use on perinatal outcomes. J Perinatol 23:354, 2003

Feig DS, Naylor CD: Eating for two: Are guidelines for weight gain during pregnancy too liberal? Lancet 351:1054, 1998

Fiscella K: Does prenatal care improve birth outcomes? A critical review. Obstet Gynecol 85:468, 1995

Florida Department of Health: Healthy Start Prenatal Risk Screening Instrument. DH No. 3134, September 1997

Food and Drug Administration: Food standards: Amendment of standards of identity for enriched grain products to require addition of folic acid. 61 Federal Register 8781 (1996)

Food and Nutrition Board of the Institute of Medicine: Dietary Reference Intake. National Academy of Sciences, 2004. Available at: http://www.iom.edu/object.file/master/21/372/o.pdf

Frazier LM, Golbeck AL, Lipscomb L: Medically recommended cessation of employment among pregnant women in Georgia. Obstet Gynecol 97:971, 2001

Glover DD, Amonkar M, Rybeck BF, et al: Prescription, over-the-counter, and herbal medicine use in a rural, obstetric population. Am J Obstet Gynecol 188:1039, 2003

Goldenberg RL, Tamura T, Neggers Y, et al: The effect of zinc supplementation on pregnancy outcome. JAMA 274:463, 1995

Grudzinskas JG, Watson C, Chard T: Does sexual intercourse cause fetal distress? Lancet 2:692, 1979

Haddow JE, Palomaki GE, Allan WC, et al: Maternal thyroid deficiency during pregnancy and subsequent neuropsychological development of the child. N Engl J Med 341:549, 1999

Hamadani JD, Fuchs GJ, Osendarp SJ, et al: Zinc supplementation during pregnancy and effects on mental development and behaviour of infants: A follow-up study. Lancet 360:290, 2002

Harper MA, Byington RP, Espeland MA, et al: Pregnancy-related death and health care services. Obstet Gynecol 102:273, 2003

Heaney RP, Skillman TG: Calcium metabolism in normal human pregnancy. J Clin Endocrinol Metab 33:661, 1971

Herbert WNP, Bruninghaus HM, Barefoot AB, et al: Clinical aspects of fetal heart auscultation. Obstet Gynecol 69:574, 1987

Herbst MA, Mercer BM, Beazley D, et al: Relationship of prenatal care and perinatal morbidity in low-birth-weight infants. Am J Obstet Gynecol 189:930, 2003

Higginbottom MC, Sweetman L, Nyhan WL: A syndrome of methylmalonic aciduria, homocystinuria, megaloblastic anemia and neurologic abnormalities in a vitamin B_{12}-deficient breast-fed infant of a strict vegetarian. N Engl J Med 299:317, 1978

Higgins JR, Walshe JJ, Conroy RM, et al: The relation between maternal work, ambulatory blood pressure, and pregnancy hypertension. J Epidemiol Community Health 56:389, 2002

Hollier LM, Hill J, Sheffield JS, et al: State laws regarding prenatal syphilis screening in the United States. Am J Obstet Gynecol 189:1178, 2003

Honein MA, Paulozzi LJ, Mathews TJ, et al: Impact of folic acid fortification of the US food supply on the occurrence of neural tube defects. JAMA 285:2981, 2001

Horowitz HS, Heifetz SB: Effects of prenatal exposure to fluoridation on dental caries. Public Health Rep 82:297, 1967

Huxley RR: Nausea and vomiting in early pregnancy: Its role in placental development. Obstet Gynecol 95:779, 2000

Hytten FE: Weight gain in pregnancy. In Hytten FE, Chamberlain G (eds): Clinical Physiology in Obstetrics, 2nd ed. Oxford, Blackwell, 1991, p 173

Hytten FE, Chamberlain G: Clinical Physiology in Obstetrics, 2nd ed. Oxford, Blackwell, 1991, p 152

Hytten FE, Leitch I: The Physiology of Human Pregnancy, 2nd ed. Oxford, Blackwell, 1971

Institute of Medicine: Nutrition During Pregnancy, 1. Weight Gain; 2. Nutrient Supplements. Washington, DC, National Academy Press, 1990

Jacqz-Aigrain E, Zhang D, Maillard G, et al: Maternal smoking during pregnancy and nicotine and cotinine concentrations in maternal and neonatal hair. Br J Obstet Gynaecol 109:909, 2002

Janssen PA, Holt VL, Sugg NK, et al: Intimate partner violence and adverse pregnancy outcomes: A population-based study. Am J Obstet Gynecol 188:1341, 2003

Jazayeri A, Tsibris JCM, Spellacy WN: Umbilical cord plasma erythropoietin levels in pregnancies complicated by maternal smoking. Am J Obstet Gynecol 178:433, 1998

Jimenez JM, Tyson JE, Reisch JS: Clinical measures of gestational age in normal pregnancies. Obstet Gynecol 61:438, 1983

Jimenez JM, Tyson JE, Santos-Ramos R, et al: Comparison of obstetric and pediatric evaluation of gestational age. Abstract No. 1033, Pediatr Res 13:498, 1979

Jones DW, Appel LJ, Sheps SG, et al: Measuring blood pressure accurately: New and persistent challenges. JAMA 289:1027, 2003

Kessner DM, Singer J, Kalk CE, et al: Infant death: An analysis by maternal risk and health care. In: Contrasts in Health Status, Vol 1. Washington, DC, Institute of Medicine, National Academy of Sciences, 1973, p 59

Kiss H, Widham A, Geusau A, et al: Universal antenatal screening for syphilis: Is it still justified economically? A 10-year retrospective analysis. Eur J Obstet Gynecol Reprod Biol 112:24, 2004

Klebanoff MA, Levine RJ, DerSimonian R, et al: Maternal serum paraxanthine, a caffeine metabolite, and the risk of spontaneous abortion. N Engl J Med 341:1639, 1999

Kogan MD, Martin JA, Alexander GR, et al: The changing pattern of prenatal care utilization in the United States, 1981–1995, using different prenatal care indices. JAMA 279:1623, 1998

Lacroix R, Eason E, Melzack R: Nausea and vomiting during pregnancy: A prospective study of its frequency, intensity, and patterns of change. Am J Obstet Gynecol 182:931, 2000

Li D-K, Janevic T, Odouli R, et al: Hot tub use during pregnancy and the risk of miscarriage. Am J Epidemiol 158:931, 2003

Lin CC, Santolaya-Forgas J: Current concepts of fetal growth restriction: Part I. Causes, classification, and pathophysiology. Obstet Gynecol 92:1044, 1998

Loudon I: Death in Childbirth. New York, Oxford University Press, 1992, p 577

Luke B, Avni M, Min L, et al: Work and pregnancy: The role of fatigue and the "second shift" on antenatal morbidity. Am J Obstet Gynecol 181:1172, 1999

Luke B, Brown MB, Misiunas R, et al: Specialized prenatal care and maternal and infant outcomes in twin pregnancy. Am J Obstet Gynecol 934, 2003

Magann EF, Evans SF, Weitz B, et al: Antepartum, intrapartum, and neonatal significance of exercise on healthy low-risk pregnant working women. Obstet Gynecol 99:466, 2002

Maheshwari UR, King JC, Leybin L, et al: Fluoride balances during early and late pregnancy. J Occup Med 25:587, 1983

Mahon BE, Rosenman MB, Graham MF, et al: Postpartum *Chlamydia trachomatis* and *Neisseria gonorrhoeae* infections. Am J Obstet Gynecol 186:1320, 2002

Martin JA, Hamilton BE, Ventura SJ, et al: Births: Final Data for 2000. Natl Vital Stat Rep 50:1, February 12, 2002a

Martin JA, Hamilton BE, Ventura SJ, et al: Births: Final Data for 2001. Natl Vital Stat Rep 51:2, December 18, 2002b

McDuffie RS Jr, Beck A, Bischoff K, et al: Effect of frequency of prenatal care visits on perinatal outcome among low-risk women. A randomized controlled trial. JAMA 275:847, 1996

Merkatz IR, Thompson JE, Walsh LV: History of prenatal care. In Merkatz IR, Thompson JE (eds): New Perspectives on Prenatal Care. New York, Elsevier, 1990, p 14

Monheit AG, Van Vunakis H, Key TC, et al: Maternal and fetal cardiovascular effects of nicotine infusion in pregnant sheep. Am J Obstet Gynecol 145:290, 1983

Morgan K: Front and center. Dallas Morning News, June 7, 2000

Mozurkewich EL, Luke B, Avni M, et al: Working conditions and adverse pregnancy outcome: A meta-analysis. Obstet Gynecol 95:623, 2000

Murray N, Homer CS, Davis GK, et al: The clinical utility of routine urinalysis in pregnancy: A prospective study. Med J Aust 177:477, 2002

Ness RB, Grisso JA, Hirschinger N, et al: Cocaine and tobacco use and the risk of spontaneous abortion. N Engl J Med 340:333, 1999

Newman RB, Goldenberg RL, Moawad AH, et al: Occupational fatigue and preterm premature rupture of membranes. Am J Obstet Gynecol 184:438, 2001

Norén L, Östgaard S, Johansson G, et al: Lumbar back and posterior pelvic pain during pregnancy: A 3-year follow-up. Eur Spine J 11:267, 2002

Orvieto R, Achiron A, Ben-Rafael Z, et al: Low-back pain of pregnancy. Acta Obstet Gynecol Scand 73:209, 1994

Osendarp SJ, van Raaij JM, Darmstadt GL, et al: Zinc supplementation during pregnancy and effects on growth and morbidity in low birthweight infants: A randomised placebo controlled trial. Lancet 357:1080, 2001

Patel MV, Nuthalapaty FS, Ramsey PS, et al: Pica: A neglected risk factor for preterm birth [abstract]. Obstet Gynecol 103:68S, 2004

Perlow JH: Comparative use and knowledge of preconceptional folic acid among Spanish- and English-speaking patient populations in Phoenix and Yuma, Arizona. Am J Obstet Gynecol 184:1263, 2001

Pitkin RM: Calcium metabolism in pregnancy and the perinatal period: A review. Am J Obstet Gynecol 151:99, 1985

Pivarnik JM, Lee W, Clark SL, et al: Cardiac output responses of primigravid women during exercise determined by the direct Fick technique. Obstet Gynecol 75:954, 1990

Pivarnik JM, Mauer MB, Ayres NA, et al: Effects of chronic exercise on blood volume expansion and hematologic indices during pregnancy. Obstet Gynecol 83:265, 1994

Pritchard JA, Scott DE: Iron demands during pregnancy. In Hallberg L, Harwerth HG, Vannotti A (eds): Iron Deficiency: Pathogenesis, Clinical Aspects, Therapy. New York, Academic Press, 1970

Quaranta P, Currell R, Redman CWG, et al: Prediction of small-for-dates infants by measurement of symphysial-fundal height. Br J Obstet Gynaecol 88:115, 1981

Radhika MS, Bhaskaram P, Balakrishna N, et al: Effects of vitamin A deficiency during pregnancy on maternal and child health. Br J Obstet Gynaecol 109:689, 2002

Ray JG, Meier C, Vermeulen MJ, et al: Association of neural tube defects and folic acid food fortification in Canada. Lancet 360:2047, 2002

Read JS, Klebanoff MA: Sexual intercourse during pregnancy and preterm delivery: Effects of vaginal microorganisms. Am J Obstet Gynecol 168:514, 1993

Reyes H, Báez ME, Gonzáles MC, et al: Selenium, zinc and copper plasma levels in intrahepatic cholestasis of pregnancy, in normal pregnancies and in healthy individuals, in Chile. J Hepatol 32:542, 2000

Rhodes JC, Schoendorf KC, Parker JD: Contribution of excess weight gain during pregnancy and macrosomia to the cesarean delivery rate, 1990–2000. Pediatrics 111:1181, 2003

Rinsky-Eng J, Miller L: Knowledge, use, and education regarding folic acid supplementation: Continuation study of women in Colorado who had a pregnancy affected by a neural tube defect. Teratology 66:S29, 2002

Rosa FW, Baum C, Shaw M: Pregnancy outcomes after first-trimester vaginitis drug therapy. Obstet Gynecol 69:751, 1987

Rosen MG, Merkatz IR, Hill JG: Caring for our future: A report by the expert panel on the content of prenatal care. Obstet Gynecol 77:782, 1991

Ryan ET, Wilson ME, Kain KC: Illness after international travel. N Engl J Med 347:505, 2002

Sayle AE, Savitz DA, Thorp JM Jr, et al: Sexual activity during late pregnancy and risk of preterm delivery. Obstet Gynecol 97:283, 2001

Schauberger CW, Rooney BL, Brimer LM: Factors that influence weight loss in the puerperium. Obstet Gynecol 79:424, 1992

Schrag SJ, Zell ER, Lynfield R, et al: A population-based comparison of strategies to prevent early-onset group B streptococcal disease in neonates. N Engl J Med 347:233, 2002

Schramm WF: Weighing costs and benefits of adequate prenatal care for 12,023 births in Missouri's Medicaid Program, 1988. Public Health Rep 107:647, November–December 1992

Scott DE, Pritchard JA, Saltin AS, et al: Iron deficiency during pregnancy. In Hallberg L, Harwerth HG, Vannottti A (eds): Iron Deficiency: Pathogenesis, Clinical Aspects, Therapy. New York, Academic Press, 1970

Selenkow HA, Varma K, Younger D, et al: Patterns of serum immunoreactive human placental lactogen (IR-HPL) and chorionic gonadotropin (IR-HCG) in diabetic pregnancy. Diabetes 20:696, 1971

Sibai BM, Villar MA, Bray E: Magnesium supplementation during pregnancy: A double-blind randomized controlled clinical trial. Am J Obstet Gynecol 161:115, 1989

Smith CA: Effects of maternal undernutrition upon the newborn infant in Holland (1944–1945). Am J Obstet Gynecol 30:229, 1947

Speert H: Obstetrics and Gynecology in America: A History. Chicago, American College of Obstetricians and Gynecologists, 1980, p 142

Stein Z, Susser M, Saenger G, et al: Nutrition and mental performance. Science 178:708, 1972

Suarez VR, Hankins GD: Smallpox and pregnancy: From eradicated disease to bioterrorist threat. Obstet Gynecol 100:87, 2002

Taipale P, Hiilesmaa V: Predicting delivery date by ultrasound and last menstrual period in early gestation. Obstet Gynecol 97:189, 2001

Teitelman AM, Welch LS, Hellenbrand KG, et al: Effect of maternal work activity on preterm birth and low birth weight. Am J Epidemiol 131:104, 1990

Thorsdottir I, Torfadottir JE, Birgisdottir BE, et al: Weight gain in women of normal weight before pregnancy: Complications in pregnancy or delivery and birth outcome. Obstet Gynecol 99:799, 2002

United States Department of Health and Human Services: Reducing tobacco use: A report of the Surgeon General. Atlanta, Ga, U.S. Department of Health and Human Services, Centers for Disease Control and Prevention, National Center for Chronic Disease Prevention and Health Promotion, Office on Smoking and Health, 2000

United States Preventive Services Task Force: Screening for chlamydial infection: Recommendations and rationale. Am J Prev Med 20:90, 2001

Villar J, Báaqeel H, Piaggio G, et al: WHO antenatal care randomised trial for the evaluation of a new model of routine antenatal care. Lancet 357:1551, 2001

Vintzileos AM, Ananth CV, Smulian JC, et al: The impact of prenatal care on neonatal deaths in the presence and absence of antenatal high-risk conditions. Am J Obstet Gynecol 186:1011, 2002a

Vintzileos AM, Ananth CV, Smulian JC, et al: The impact of prenatal care on preterm births among twin gestations in the United States, 1989–2000. Am J Obstet Gynecol 189:818, 2003

Vintzileos AM, Ananth CV, Smulian JC, et al: Prenatal care and black-white fetal death disparity in the United States: Heterogeneity by high-risk conditions. Obstet Gynecol 99:483, 2002b

Wang SM, Dezinno P, Maranets I, et al: Low back pain during pregnancy: Prevalence, risk factors, and outcomes. Obstet Gynecol 104:65, 2004

Webster J, Holt V: Screening for partner violence: Direct questioning or self-report? Obstet Gynecol 103:299, 2004

Wiesen AR, Littell CT: Relationship between prepregnancy anthrax vaccination and pregnancy and birth outcomes among US Army women. JAMA 287:1556, 2002

Wilcox AJ, Baird DD, Dunson D, et al: Natural limits of pregnancy testing in relation to the expected menstrual period. JAMA 286:1759, 2001

Williams Obstetrics, 7th ed. Stander HJ (ed). New York, Appleton-Century, 1929, p 278

Williams JW: The limitations and possibilities of prenatal care. JAMA 64:95, 1915

Wisborg K, Henriksen TB, Jespersen LB, et al: Nicotine patches for pregnant smokers: A randomized controlled study. Obstet Gynecol 96:967, 2000

Worthen N, Bustillo M: Effect of urinary bladder fullness on fundal height measurements. Am J Obstet Gynecol 138:759, 1980

Zaneveld LJ, Tauber PF, Port C, et al: Scanning electron microscopy of cervical mucus crystallization. Obstet Gynecol 46:419, 1975

9

Abortion

Abortion is the termination of pregnancy, either spontaneously or intentionally, before the fetus develops sufficiently to survive. By convention, abortion is usually defined as pregnancy termination prior to 20 weeks' gestation or less than 500-g birthweight. Definitions vary, however, according to state laws for reporting abortions, fetal deaths, and neonatal deaths.

SPONTANEOUS ABORTION

Abortion occurring without medical or mechanical means to empty the uterus is referred to as *spontaneous*. Another widely used term is *miscarriage*.

PATHOLOGY. Hemorrhage into the decidua basalis, followed by necrosis of tissues adjacent to the bleeding, usually accompanies abortion. If early, the ovum detaches, stimulating uterine contractions that result in its expulsion. When a gestational sac is opened, fluid is commonly found surrounding a small macerated fetus, or alternatively no fetus is visible—the so-called *blighted ovum*.

In later abortions, several outcomes are possible. The retained fetus may undergo *maceration,* in which the skull bones collapse, the abdomen distends with blood-stained fluid, and the internal organs degenerate. The skin softens and peels off in utero or at the slightest touch. Alternatively, when amnionic fluid is absorbed, the fetus may become compressed and desiccated, forming a *fetus compressus.* Occasionally, the fetus may become so dry and compressed that it resembles parchment—a *fetus papyraceous.*

ETIOLOGY. More than 80 percent of abortions occur in the first 12 weeks of pregnancy, and at least half result from chromosomal anomalies. After the first trimester, both the abortion rate and the incidence of chromosomal anomalies decrease (Fig. 9–1).

The risk of spontaneous abortion increases with parity as well as with maternal and paternal age (Warburton and Fraser, 1964; Wilson and associates, 1986). The frequency of clinically recognized abortion increases from 12 percent in women younger than 20 years to 26 percent in those older than 40 years (Fig. 9–2). For the same paternal ages, the frequency increases from 12 to 20 percent. Finally, the incidence of abortion increases if a woman conceives within 3 months following a term birth (Harlap and Shiono, 1980).

The exact mechanisms responsible for abortion are not always apparent, but in the first 3 months of pregnancy, death of the embryo or fetus nearly always precedes spontaneous expulsion of the ovum. For this reason, finding the cause of early abortion involves ascertaining the cause of fetal death. In subsequent months, the fetus frequently does not die before expulsion; therefore, other explanations for its expulsion should be sought.

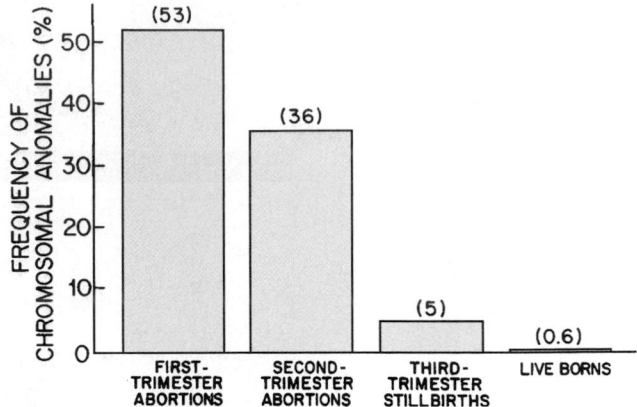

FIGURE 9–1. Frequency of chromosomal anomalies in abortuses and stillbirths for each trimester compared with the frequency of chromosomal anomalies in liveborn infants. The percentage for each group is shown in parentheses. (Data adapted from Fantel, 1980; Warburton, 1980, and their associates.)

FETAL FACTORS

Abnormal Zygotic Development. Early spontaneous abortions commonly display a developmental abnormality of the zygote, embryo, early fetus, or at times the placenta. Of 1000 spontaneous abortions analyzed by Hertig and Sheldon (1943), half demonstrated degenerated or absent embryos, that is, blighted ova (Fig. 9–3). Poland and co-workers (1981) identified morphological disorganization of growth

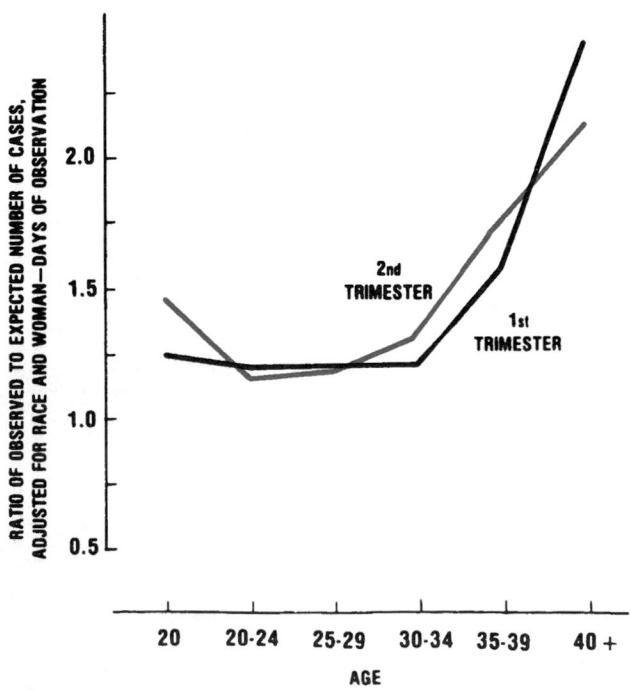

FIGURE 9–2. First- and second-trimester spontaneous abortions by maternal age. (From Harlap and colleagues, 1980, with permission.)

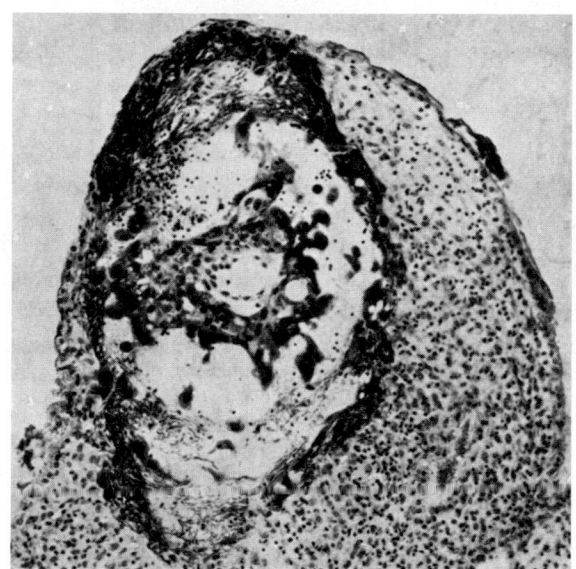

FIGURE 9–3. Abnormal ovum. A cross-section of a defective ovum showing an empty chorionic sac embedded within a polypoid mass of endometrium. (From Hertig and Rock, 1944.)

in 40 percent of abortuses that were expelled spontaneously before 20 weeks.

Aneuploid Abortion. Approximately 50 to 60 percent of embryos and early fetuses that are spontaneously aborted contain chromosomal abnormalities, accounting for most of early pregnancy wastage (Table 9–1). Jacobs and Hassold (1980) reported that approximately 95 percent of chromosomal abnormalities were due to maternal gametogenesis errors and 5 percent to paternal errors.

Autosomal trisomy is the most frequently identified chromosomal anomaly associated with first-trimester abortions

TABLE 9–1 Chromosomal Findings in Abortuses

	Incidence in Percent	
Chromosomal Studies	Kajii et al (1980)	Simpson (1980)
Normal (euploid), 46,XY and 46,XX	46	54
Abnormal (aneuploid)		
Autosomal trisomy	31	22
Monosomy X (45,X)	10	9
Triploidy	7	8
Tetraploidy	2	3
Structural anomaly	3	2
Double trisomy	2	0.7
Triple trisomy	0.4	NL
Others—XXY, monosomy 21	0.8	NL
Autosomal monosomy G	NL	0.1
Mosaic trisomy	NL	1.3
Sex chromosome polysomy	NL	0.2
Abnormality not specified	NL	0.9

NL = not listed.

(see Table 9-1). Although most trisomies result from *isolated nondisjunction,* balanced structural chromosomal rearrangements are present in one partner in 2 to 4 percent of couples with a history of recurrent abortions (American College of Obstetricians and Gynecologists, 2001a). Trisomies for all autosomes except chromosome number 1 have been identified in abortuses, but autosomes 13, 16, 18, 21, and 22 have been found most commonly.

Monosomy X (45,X), the second most frequent chromosomal abnormality, usually results in abortion and much less frequently in liveborn female infants (Turner syndrome). Conversely, autosomal monosomy is rare and incompatible with life.

Triploidy is often associated with hydropic placental (molar) degeneration. Incomplete (partial) hydatidiform moles may contain triploidy or trisomy for only chromosome 16. Although these fetuses frequently abort early, the few carried longer are all grossly malformed. Advanced maternal and paternal age does not increase the incidence of triploidy.

Tetraploid abortuses rarely are liveborn and most often are aborted early in gestation.

Chromosomal structural abnormalities, identified only since the development of banding techniques, infrequently cause abortion. Some of these infants who are liveborn with balanced translocations may appear normal.

Euploid Abortion. Euploid fetuses tend to abort later in gestation than aneuploid ones. Kajii and co-workers (1980) reported that although three fourths of aneuploid abortions occurred before 8 weeks, euploid abortions peaked at about 13 weeks. Stein and associates (1980) presented evidence that the incidence of euploid abortions increased dramatically after maternal age exceeded 35 years.

MATERNAL FACTORS. The causes of euploid abortions are poorly understood, although a variety of medical disorders, environmental conditions, and developmental abnormalities have been implicated.

Infections. Various infections are uncommon causes of abortion in humans (American College of Obstetricians and Gynecologists, 2001a). Although *Brucella abortus* and *Campylobacter fetus* cause chronic abortion in cattle, they are not significant in humans (Sauerwein and associates, 1993). Researchers also found no evidence that either *Listeria monocytogenes* or *Chlamydia trachomatis* produced abortions in humans (Feist and associates, 1999; Osser and Persson, 1996; Paukku and associates, 1999). In the only prospective study of serological conversion, the herpes simplex virus did not increase the incidence of abortion following infection in early pregnancy (Brown and colleagues, 1997).

Serological evidence supporting a role for *Mycoplasma hominis* and *Ureaplasma urealyticum* in abortion was provided by Quinn and co-workers (1983). Conversely, Temmerman and associates (1992) found no link between genital mycoplasma and spontaneous abortion. They did, however, report that spontaneous abortion was independently associated with maternal serological evidence of syphilis and human immunodeficiency virus-1 (HIV-1), and with vaginal colonization with group B streptococci. More recently, van Benthem and associates (2000) reported that women with HIV infection showed no greater risk of spontaneous abortion after being diagnosed with HIV than before. Evidence that *Toxoplasma gondii* causes abortion in humans remains inconclusive. In 2002, Oakeshott and associates reported an association between second- but not first-trimester spontaneous abortion and bacterial vaginosis.

Chronic Debilitating Diseases.

In early pregnancy, fetuses seldom abort secondary to chronic wasting diseases such as tuberculosis or carcinomatosis. Celiac sprue, however, has been reported to cause both male and female infertility and recurrent abortions (Sher and colleagues, 1994).

Endocrine Abnormalities

HYPOTHYROIDISM. Iodine deficiency may be associated with excessive miscarriages (Castañeda and co-workers, 2002). The effects of clinical hypothyroidism on early pregnancy wastage have not been adequately studied (see Chap. 53, p. 1194). Thyroid autoantibodies, however, were associated with an increased incidence of abortion despite the lack of overt hypothyroidism (Dayan and Daniels, 1996; Stagnaro-Green and associates, 1990). Conversely, others have found that women with recurrent abortions have no greater incidence of antithyroid antibodies than normal controls (Esplin and colleagues, 1998; Pratt and associates, 1994). Moreover, Rushworth and colleagues (2000) studied a group of 870 women with recurrent abortion and found that untreated women with antithyroid antibodies were as likely to achieve a live birth as women without antibodies.

DIABETES MELLITUS. The rates of spontaneous abortion and major congenital malformations are both increased in women with insulin-dependent diabetes (Greene, 1999). The risk appears related to the degree of metabolic control in the first trimester. In a prospective study, Mills and associates (1988) reported that excellent glucose control within 21 days of conception resulted in a spontaneous abortion rate similar to that in nondiabetic controls. Poor glucose control, however, resulted in a marked increase in the abortion rate. Craig and co-workers (2002) have reported a higher incidence of insulin resistance in women with recurrent pregnancy loss.

PROGESTERONE DEFICIENCY. Termed *luteal phase defect,* insufficient progesterone secretion by the corpus luteum or placenta has been suggested as a cause of abortion. Deficient progesterone production, however, may be the consequence rather than the cause of early pregnancy failure (Salem and co-workers, 1984). Currently, the diagnostic criteria and

efficacy of therapy for this supposed disorder require validation (American College of Obstetricians and Gynecologists, 2001a). If the corpus luteum is removed surgically, such as for an ovarian tumor, progesterone replacement is indicated in pregnancies less than 8 to 10 weeks (see Chap. 40, p. 966).

Nutrition.

Dietary deficiency of any one nutrient or moderate deficiency of all nutrients do not appear important causes of abortion. Similarly, the nausea and vomiting that develop commonly during early pregnancy and any subsequent weight loss are rarely followed by spontaneous abortion.

Drug Use and Environmental Factors.

A variety of different agents has been reported to be associated with an increased incidence of abortion.

TOBACCO. Smoking has been linked with an increased risk for euploid abortion (Harlap and Shiono, 1980). For women who smoked more than 14 cigarettes a day, the risk was approximately twofold greater than the risk for controls (Kline and associates, 1980). Armstrong and associates (1992) calculated that the abortion risk increased in a linear fashion by a factor of 1.2 for each 10 cigarettes smoked per day, consistent with the factor of 1.4 calculated by Chatenoud and colleagues (1998). Two more recent studies, however, have failed to support this association (Rasch, 2003; Wisborg and colleagues, 2003).

ALCOHOL. Both spontaneous abortion and fetal anomalies may result from frequent alcohol use during the first 8 weeks of pregnancy (Floyd and associates, 1999). Spontaneous abortion rates increased even when alcohol was consumed "in moderation." Kline and co-workers (1980) reported that the abortion rate doubled in women who drank twice a week and tripled in women who consumed alcohol daily compared with the rate for nondrinkers.

Armstrong and colleagues (1992) computed that abortion risk increased by an average of 1.3 for each drink per day. In contrast, Cavallo and associates (1995) and Kesmodel and co-workers (2002) found that a low level of alcohol consumption during pregnancy was not associated with a significant risk for abortion.

CAFFEINE. Armstrong and associates (1992) reported that women who consumed at least 5 cups of coffee per day exhibited a slightly increased risk of abortion, and for those who drank above this daily 5-cup threshold, the risk correlated with the number of cups consumed per day. Similarly, Cnattingius and colleagues (2000) observed a significantly increased abortion risk only in women who consumed at least 500 mg of caffeine a day, or roughly equivalent to 5 cups of coffee. Klebanoff and associates (1999) noted that pregnant women in whom paraxanthine (a caffeine metabolite) levels were extremely elevated experience an almost twofold risk for spontaneous abortion. In their review of 15 studies, Signorello and McLaughlin (2004) deemed the evidence for a causal link between spontaneous abortion and caffeine inconclusive.

RADIATION. In sufficient doses, radiation is a recognized abortifacient. As discussed in Chapter 41 (see p. 977), the human dose to effect abortion is not precisely known.

CONTRACEPTIVES. Oral contraceptives or spermicidal agents used in contraceptive creams and jellies are not associated with an increased incidence of abortion. When intrauterine devices fail to prevent pregnancy, however, the risk of abortion, and specifically septic abortion, increases substantively (see Chap. 32, p. 739).

ENVIRONMENTAL TOXINS. Accurately assessing the relationship between environmental exposures and spontaneous abortion poses challenges. Investigators may encounter difficulties in measuring the intensity and duration of exposure and in establishing when and whether abortion actually occurred. Thus, in most instances, research provides little information to conclusively indict (or absolve) any specific environmental agent. Although this is generally true, work by Barlow and Sullivan (1982) implicated arsenic, lead, formaldehyde, benzene, and ethylene oxide as possible abortifacients. Video display terminals and exposure to the accompanying electromagnetic fields do not adversely affect abortion rates (Schnorr and co-workers, 1991). Similarly, no effects were found with occupational exposure to ultrasound (Taskinen and colleagues, 1990). Rowland and associates (1995) reported an increased risk of spontaneous abortion among dental assistants exposed to 3 or more hours of nitrous oxide per day in offices without gas-scavenging equipment, but not in offices using such equipment. In a meta-analysis of data from the prescavenging era, Boivin (1997) concluded that women occupationally exposed to anesthetic gases exhibited an increased risk of spontaneous abortion.

Immunological Factors. Much attention has focused on the immune system as important in recurrent pregnancy loss. In analyzing compiled studies, Kutteh and Pasquarette (1995) determined that 15 percent of more than 1000 women with recurrent pregnancy loss had recognized autoimmune factors. Two primary pathophysiological models are the *autoimmune theory* (immunity against self) and the *alloimmune theory* (immunity against another person).

AUTOIMMUNE FACTORS. Antiphospholipid antibodies are a family of autoantibodies that bind to negatively charged phospholipids, phospholipid-binding proteins, or a combination of the two (Branch and Khamashta, 2003). They are discussed in more detail in Chapter 54 (see p. 1215). Two of these, lupus anticoagulant and anticardiolipin antibody, have been implicated in spontaneous abortion. Criteria for the diagnosis of the *antiphospholipid syndrome* have been specified by Levine and associates (2002) and are discussed in Chapter 54 (see p. 1217). Recurrent abortion before 12 weeks along with laboratory criteria for anticardiolipin antibodies or lupus anticoagulant satisfy the diagnosis.

Antiphospholipid antibodies can be an immunoglobulin G (IgG), IgA, or IgM isotype. The mechanism of pregnancy loss in women with these antibodies involves placental thrombosis and infarction. In one postulated mechanism, antibodies may inhibit the release of prostacyclin, a potent vasodilator and inhibitor of platelet aggregation. In contrast, platelets produce thromboxane A_2, a vasoconstrictor and platelet aggregator. They have also been shown to inhibit protein C activation, resulting in coagulation and fibrin formation.

Women with both a history of early fetal loss and high levels of these antibodies may suffer a 70-percent abortion recurrence (Dudley and Branch, 1991). In a prospective study of 860 women screened for anticardiolipin antibody in the first trimester, Yasuda and colleagues (1995) reported that only 7 percent tested positive for antibodies. Spontaneous abortion occurred in 25 percent of the antibody-positive group compared with only 10 percent of the negative group. In another study, however, Simpson and associates (1998) found no association between early pregnancy loss and the presence of either anticardiolipin antibody or lupus anticoagulant.

Despite these controversies with early abortion, researchers agree regarding increased second-trimester pregnancy losses and the antiphospholipid syndrome. As further discussed in Chapter 54, p. 1217, this autoimmune condition is characterized by moderate to high levels of antiphospholipid IgG antibodies with variable incidence of thrombosis, thrombocytopenia, and fetal loss (American College of Obstetricians and Gynecologists, 1998; Blumenfeld and Brenner, 1999; Cowchock, 1997; Simpson and associates, 1998).

There are therapies for antiphospholipid syndrome that can increase live birth rates. Two randomized trials support the premise that, compared with treatment with low-dose aspirin alone, treatment with a combination of heparin and low-dose aspirin can improve the chance of live birth in a subsequent pregnancy in women with the syndrome. Kutteh (1996) randomized 50 such women to receive either low-dose aspirin alone or low-dose aspirin with heparin. Women who received both aspirin and heparin had significantly more viable infants—80 versus 44 percent. Rai and colleagues (1997) reported a 77-percent live birth rate with low-dose aspirin and low-dose heparin therapy (5000 units twice a day) versus one of 42 percent with low-dose aspirin alone. In contrast, Farquharson and associates (2002) observed a 72-percent live birth rate using low-dose aspirin alone versus one of 78 percent using low-dose aspirin plus low-dose, low-molecular-weight heparin.

As emphasized by Branch and Khamashta (2003), the discrepant reports are confusing and therapeutic guidelines are blurred. Because of this, we individualize therapy for women who meet the criteria for antiphospholipid syndrome and involve them in the decision-making process. We recommend low-dose aspirin, 81 mg per day, given along with unfractionated heparin, 5000 units subcutaneously twice daily. This therapy, begun when pregnancy is diagnosed, is continued until labor or delivery. Therapies are discussed further in Chapter 54 (see p. 1218).

ALLOIMMUNE FACTORS. Various alloimmune disorders have been posited to cause recurrent abortion, and a variety of therapies to correct these disorders have been put forth. None, however, has withstood rigorous scrutiny, including use of paternal cell immunization, third-party donor leukocytes, trophoblast membranes, and intravenous immunoglobulin (Scott, 2000). Accordingly, we do not endorse the use of immunotherapy for recurrent abortion outside the context of properly conceived, designed, and executed randomized clinical trials.

Inherited Thrombophilia. Several genetic disorders of blood coagulation may increase the risk of thrombosis. Research with the growing number of recognized inherited thrombophilias, such as factor V Leiden mutation, continues to evolve. Many studies of aggregated thrombophilias—including antiphospholipid antibodies—cite excessive recurrent abortions (see Chap. 47, p. 1078). Reports by Carp and associates (2002) and the review by Adelberg and Kuller (2002) cast doubt on the importance of mutant-gene inherited thrombophilias in early spontaneous abortion. Even if these disorders do play an etiological role in abortion, proper treatment trials have not been conducted to determine whether abortion might be prevented.

Conversely, *late abortions,* viz., midpregnancy losses before 20 weeks, are linked to some of these thrombophilias. Although controversial, treatment is thought by many to improve outcomes, as discussed in Chapter 47 (see p. 1074).

Laparotomy. Uncomplicated abdominal or pelvic surgery performed during early pregnancy does not appear to increase the risk of abortion. Certain complications, for example peritonitis, may be the indication for, or the consequence of surgery (see Chap. 41, p. 974). Ovarian tumors generally are removed without interfering with pregnancy. An important exception involves early removal of the corpus luteum cyst or the ovary in which the corpus luteum resides. If performed prior to 10 weeks' gestation, supplemental progesterone is indicated (Chap. 40, p. 966).

Physical Trauma. Clearly, major abdominal trauma can precipitate abortion. Determining the effect of minor trauma on abortion rates, however, poses problems. Minor trauma that fails to interrupt a pregnancy is often forgotten, whereas minor trauma temporally associated with abortion is more likely recalled. In general, trauma contributes minimally to the incidence of abortion.

Uterine Defects

ACQUIRED UTERINE DEFECTS. Even large and multiple uterine leiomyomas usually do not cause abortion. When associated with abortion, their location is more important than their size (see Chap. 40, p. 962). *Asherman syndrome,* characterized by uterine synechiae, usually results from destruction of large areas of endometrium by curettage. If pregnancy follows, the amount of remaining endometrium may be insufficient to support the pregnancy, and abortion may ensue. A hysterosalpingogram that shows characteristic multiple filling defects may indicate Asherman syndrome, but hysteroscopy most accurately and directly identifies this condition (Raziel and colleagues, 1994).

Recommended treatment consists of lysis of the adhesions via hysteroscopy and placement of an intrauterine contraceptive device to prevent recurrence. Some practitioners also recommend continuous high-dose estrogen therapy for 60 to 90 days following adhesiolysis. March and Israel (1981) reported that abortions decreased from 80 to 15 percent with this therapy.

DEVELOPMENTAL UTERINE DEFECTS. Abnormal müllerian duct formation or fusion defects may develop spontaneously or may follow in utero exposure to diethylstilbestrol (see Chap. 40, p. 953). Controversy surrounds the question of whether uterine defects cause abortion, and therefore, whether their correction prevents it (American College of Obstetricians and Gynecologists, 2001a). Thus, corrective procedures of the uterus for the prevention of abortion, if done at all, should be performed as a last resort, with a full understanding that they may lack efficacy.

Incompetent Cervix. Traditionally, the term *incompetent cervix* describes a discrete obstetrical entity. Classically, it is characterized by painless cervical dilatation in the second trimester, with prolapse and ballooning of membranes into the vagina, followed by expulsion of an immature fetus. Unless effectively treated, this sequence may repeat in future pregnancies.

Unfortunately, women with pregnancies that abort in the second trimester often have histories and clinical findings that make it difficult to distinguish true cervical incompetence from other causes of midtrimester pregnancy loss. Almost 1300 women with nonclassical histories of cervical incompetence were studied in a randomized trial that had as its primary outcome delivery before 33 weeks. Cerclage was found to be beneficial, albeit marginally, in that 13 percent of women in the cerclage group delivered prior to 33 weeks versus 17 percent in the noncerclage group (MacNaughton and colleagues, 1993). Thus, for every 25 cerclage procedures, one birth prior to 33 weeks was prevented.

Currently, interest is focused on the use of transvaginal ultrasound to aid in diagnosing cervical incompetence. Multiple studies have demonstrated that certain features of the cervix, primarily cervical length, when measured in the mid-second trimester, may predict preterm delivery. Another feature termed *funneling*—ballooning of the membranes into a dilated internal os, but with a closed external os—also has been assessed (Owen and associates, 2003).

The clinical relevance of these cervical features, however, is uncertain. Three randomized cerclage trials that included women found by transvaginal ultrasound to have either cervical shortening or funneling reported conflicting results. Rust and colleagues (2001) randomized 113 women with a cervical length of less than 25 mm, or with substantial funneling, to undergo either cerclage or expectant management. The incidence of preterm birth was 35 percent in the cerclage group and 36 percent in the control group. Similarly, To and colleagues (2004) reported that following their randomized trial involving cerclage placement in 253 women, the risk of early preterm birth was not significantly reduced. The results of a smaller randomized European trial of 35 women suggested that cerclage might be beneficial (Althuisius and colleagues, 2001).

Unless ongoing studies demonstrate compellingly that cerclage performed for ultrasonographically diagnosed cervical abnormalities prevents preterm delivery, the use of ultrasound to diagnose cervical incompetence is not recommended.

ETIOLOGY. Although the cause of cervical incompetence is obscure, previous trauma to the cervix—especially in the course of dilatation and curettage, conization, cauterization, or amputation—appears to be a factor in some cases. In other instances, abnormal cervical development, including that following exposure to diethylstilbestrol in utero, may play a role (see Chap. 40, p. 957).

TREATMENT. The treatment of classical cervical incompetence is cerclage. The operation is performed to surgically reinforce the weak cervix by some type of purse-string suturing. Bleeding, uterine contractions, or ruptured membranes are usually contraindications to cerclage.

Preoperative Evaluation. Sonography to confirm a living fetus and to exclude major fetal anomalies should precede cerclage. Preoperatively, cervical specimens are tested for gonorrhea and chlamydia. If positive, or if there are other obvious cervical infections, treatment is given. For at least a week before and after surgery, sexual intercourse should be restricted.

Cerclage may be performed prophylactically before cervical dilatation, or emergently after the cervix has dilated. Although prophylactic surgery generally is performed between 12 and 16 weeks, experts disagree as to how late emergency cerclage should be performed. The more advanced the pregnancy, the more likely the risk that surgical intervention will stimulate preterm labor or membrane rupture. We usually do not perform cerclage after about 23 weeks, although others have done so (Caruso and associates, 2000; Terkildsen and colleagues, 2003).

In a 10-year review of 75 emergency cerclage procedures, Chasen and Silverman (1998) reported that 65 percent of infants were delivered at 28 weeks or later, and half delivered after 36 weeks. Only 44 percent of cases with bulging membranes at the time of cerclage reached 28 weeks. Caruso and associates (2000) reported their experience with emergency cerclage from 17 to 27 weeks in 23 women, all with a dilated cervix and protruding membranes. Because only 11 liveborn infants resulted, they concluded that success was unpredictable. Based on their 20-year experience with 116 women undergoing emergency cerclage, Terkildsen and colleagues (2003) reported that nulliparous women and those with bulging membranes were significantly more likely to be delivered before 28 weeks. Paradoxically, cerclage after 22 weeks was associated with a better chance of delivery beyond 28 weeks.

If the clinical indication for cerclage is questionable, these women may be advised to decrease physical activity and abstain from intercourse. Cervical examinations are performed each week or every 2 weeks to assess cervical effacement and dilatation. Unfortunately, rapid effacement and dilatation can develop despite such precautions (Witter, 1984).

Cerclage Procedures. Two types of vaginal operations commonly are used during pregnancy. One is the simple procedure, developed by McDonald (1963) and shown in Figure 9–4. The second, a more complicated operation shown in Figure 9–5, is a modification of the original procedure described by Shirodkar (1955). Compared with historical controls, women with classical histories of cervical incompetence have success rates approaching 85 to 90 percent when either technique is performed prophylactically (Caspi and associates, 1990; Kuhn and Pepperell, 1977). For these reasons, most practitioners reserve the modified Shirodkar procedure for women with a previous failure of the McDonald cerclage or those with structural cervical abnormalities.

During emergency cerclage, moving the prolapsed amnionic sac back into the uterus may facilitate suture placement (Locatelli and associates, 1999). In some cases, filling the bladder with 600 mL of sterile saline through an indwelling Foley catheter will reduce prolapsing membranes. Unfortunately, this maneuver also can carry the cervix cephalad, away from the operating field. Alternatively, placing a Foley catheter with a 30-mL balloon through the cervix and inflating the balloon will deflect the amnionic sac cephalad. The balloon is then deflated gradually as the cerclage stitch is cinched tight.

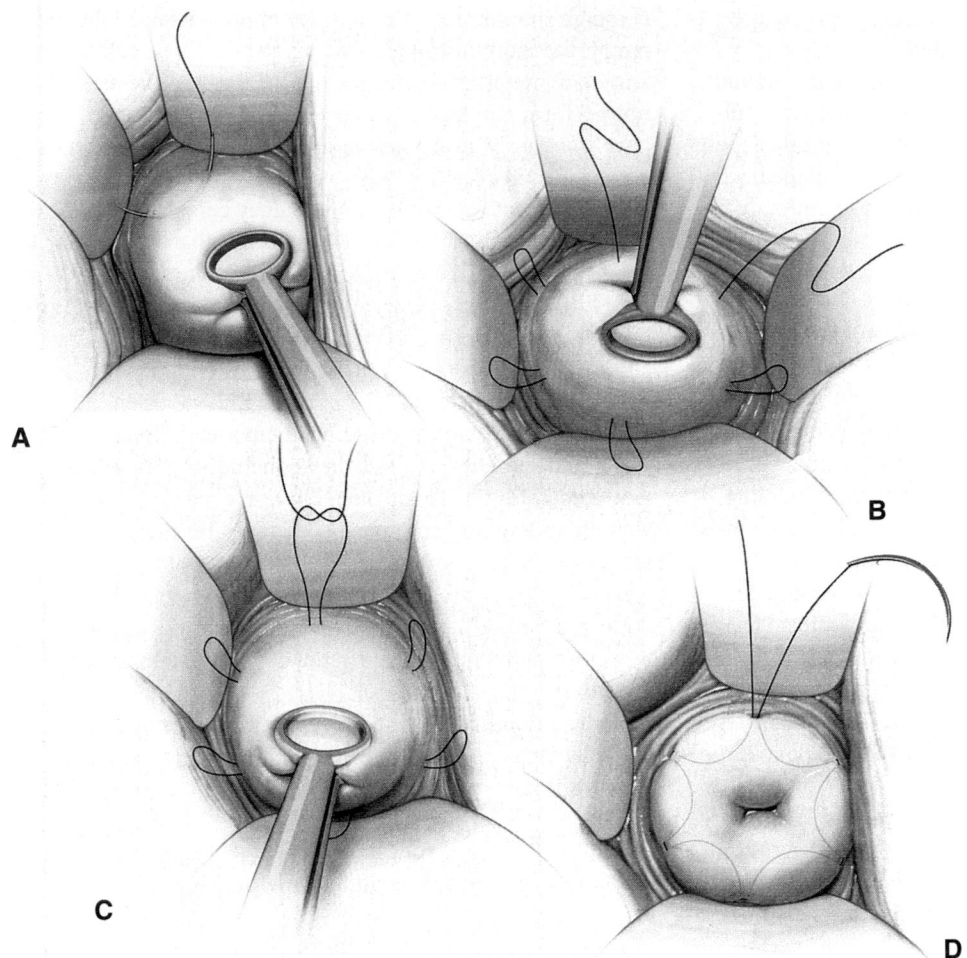

A

B

C

D

FIGURE 9–4. McDonald cerclage procedure for incompetent cervix. **A.** Start of the cerclage procedure with a suture of number 2 monofilament being placed in the body of the cervix very near the level of the internal os. **B.** Continuation of suture placement in the body of the cervix so as to encircle the os. **C.** Completion of encirclement. **D.** The suture is tightened around the cervical canal sufficiently to reduce the diameter of the canal to 5 to 10 mm, and then the suture is tied. The effect of the suture placement on the cervical canal is apparent. Placement somewhat higher may be of value, especially if the first is not in close proximity to the internal os.

Transabdominal cerclage with the suture placed at the uterine isthmus is used in some cases of severe anatomical defects of the cervix or cases of prior transvaginal cerclage failure (Cammarano and colleagues, 1995; Gibb and Salaria, 1995). In a review of 14 retrospective reports, Zaveri and associates (2002) concluded that when a prior transvaginal cerclage failed to prevent preterm delivery, the risk of perinatal death or delivery prior to 24 weeks following transabdominal cerclage (6 percent) was only slightly lower than the risk following repeat transvaginal cerclage (13 percent). Importantly, 3 percent of women who underwent transabdominal cerclage had serious operative complications, whereas there were none in women in the transvaginal group. Although transabdominal cerclage has been performed through the laparoscope, it generally requires laparotomy for initial suture placement and subsequent laparotomy for removal of the suture, for delivery of the fetus, or both.

COMPLICATIONS. Charles and Edward (1981) identified complications, especially infection, to be less frequent when cerclage was performed by 18 weeks. In the large trial of

MacNaughton and colleagues (1993), membrane rupture complicated only 1 of over 600 procedures. Cerclage was associated with higher rates of subsequent hospitalization and tocolysis, as well as a doubling of the incidence of puerperal fever—6 percent versus 3 percent. Thomason and co-workers (1982) found that prophylactic antimicrobials failed to prevent most infection and tocolytics failed to halt most labor. With clinical infection, the suture should be cut, and labor induced or augmented if necessary. Similarly, if signs of imminent abortion or delivery develop, the suture should be released at once. Failure to do so may enable vigorous uterine contractions to tear the uterus or cervix.

Membrane rupture during suture placement or within the first 48 hours following surgery is considered by some practitioners to be an indication to remove the cerclage. Kuhn and Pepperell (1977) reported that membrane rupture in the absence of labor increased the likelihood of serious fetal or maternal infection if the suture was left in situ and delivery delayed. Still, the range of management options spans from observation, to removal of the cerclage and observation, to removal of the cerclage and labor induction (Barth, 1995). Insufficient data limit firm recommendations, and the

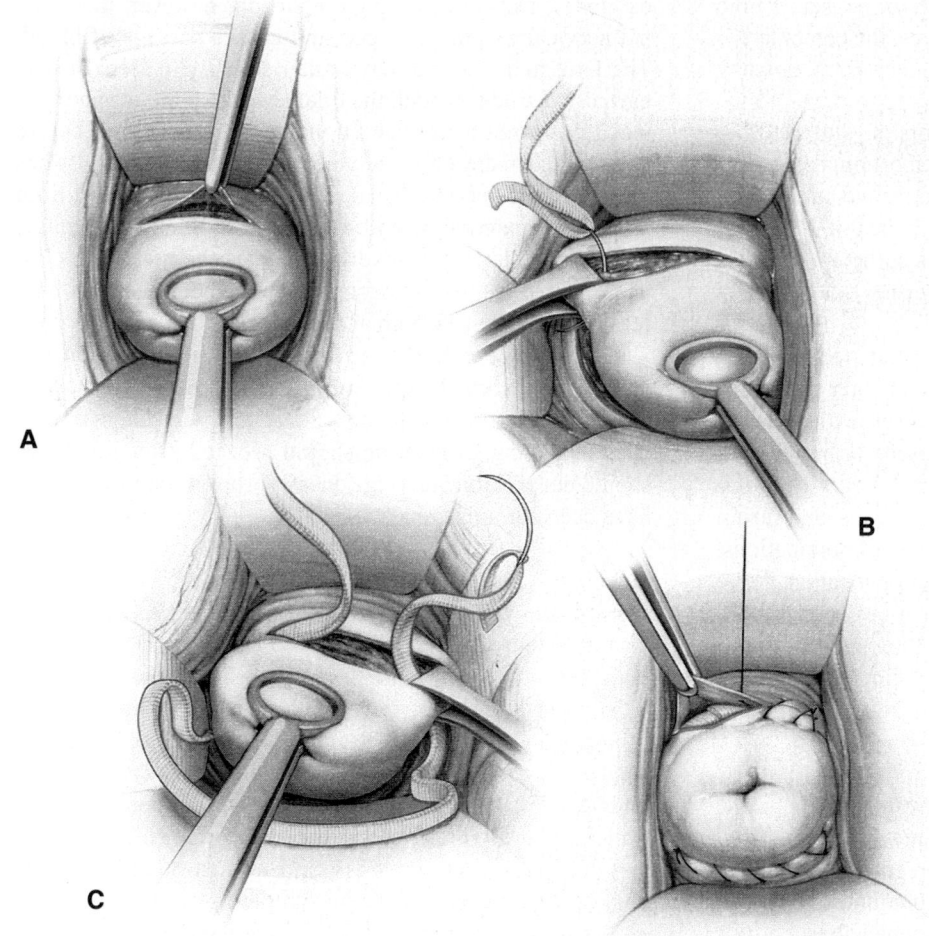

FIGURE 9–5. Modified Shirodkar cerclage for incompetent cervix. **A.** A transverse incision is made in the mucosa overlying the anterior cervix, and the bladder is pushed cephalad. **B.** A 5-mm Mersiline tape on a Mayo needle is passed anteriorly to posteriorly. **C.** The tape is then directed posteriorly to anteriorly on the other side of the cervix. Allis clamps placed so as to bunch the cervical tissue to diminish the distance the needle must travel submucosally facilitate placement of the tape. **D.** The tape is snugly tied anteriorly, after ensuring that all slack has been taken up. The cervical mucosa is then closed with a continuous chromic suture to bury the anterior Mersilene knot.

optimal management of such patients remains controversial (O'Connor and associates, 1999).

Following the modified Shirodkar operation, the suture may be left in place, and delivery affected by cesarean. Conversely, it may be removed, and vaginal delivery permitted.

PATERNAL FACTORS. Little is known about paternal factors in the genesis of spontaneous abortion. Certainly, chromosomal abnormalities in sperm have been associated with abortion (Carrell and colleagues, 2003).

CATEGORIES OF SPONTANEOUS ABORTION. The clinical aspects of spontaneous abortion separate into five subgroups: threatened, inevitable, complete or incomplete, missed, and recurrent abortion.

Threatened Abortion. The clinical diagnosis of threatened abortion is presumed when a bloody vaginal discharge or bleeding appears through a closed cervical os during the first half of pregnancy. Occurring commonly, vaginal spotting or heavier bleeding during early gestation may persist for days or weeks and may affect one out of four or five pregnant women. Overall, approximately half of these pregnancies will abort, although the risk is substantially lower if fetal cardiac activity can be documented (Tongsong and colleagues, 1995). Even without abortion, these fetuses are at increased risk for preterm delivery, low birthweight, and perinatal death (Batzofin, 1984; Funderburk, 1980; Weiss, 2004, and their colleagues). Importantly, the risk of a malformed infant does not appear to be increased.

Some bleeding near the time of expected menses may be physiological. Cervical lesions commonly bleed in early pregnancy, especially after intercourse. Polyps presenting at the external cervical os and decidual reaction in the cervix also tend to bleed in early gestation. Lower abdominal pain and persistent low backache do not accompany bleeding from these benign causes.

Bleeding usually begins first, and cramping abdominal pain follows a few hours to several days later. The pain of abortion may manifest as anterior and clearly rhythmic cramps; as a persistent low backache, associated with a feeling of pelvic pressure; or as a dull, midline, suprapubic discomfort. Whichever form the pain takes, the combination of bleeding and pain predicts a poor prognosis for pregnancy continuation.

Because ectopic pregnancy, ovarian torsion, and the other types of abortion may mimic threatened abortion, the threshold to examine women with vaginal bleeding and pain should be low. If the bleeding is persistent or heavy, a hematocrit should be obtained. If blood loss is sufficient to cause significant anemia or hypovolemia, uterine evacuation is done.

There are no effective therapies for threatened abortion. Bed rest, although often prescribed, does not alter the course of threatened abortion. Acetaminophen-based analgesia may be given to help relieve the pain. As discussed in Chapter 10 (see p. 259), vaginal sonography, serial serum quantitative human chorionic gonadotropin (hCG) levels, and serum progesterone values, used alone or in various combinations, can help ascertain if the fetus is alive and its location. None of these tests, however, especially early in gestation, is 100 percent accurate to confirm fetal death; thus, repeat evaluations over 1 or 2 weeks may be necessary. **Ectopic pregnancy should always be considered in the differential diagnosis of threatened abortion.**

ANTI-D IMMUNOGLOBULIN. We as well as others recommend treatment of D-negative women with anti-D immunoglobulin after abortion because up to 5 percent of D-negative women will become isoimmunized without it (see Chap. 29, p. 663). In D-negative women with threatened abortion, this practice is controversial, because it lacks evidence-based support (American College of Obstetricians and Gynecologists, 1999; Weissman and associates, 2002).

Inevitable Abortion. Gross rupture of the membranes, evidenced by leaking amnionic fluid, in the presence of cervical dilatation signals almost certain abortion. Commonly, either uterine contractions begin promptly, resulting in abortion, or infection develops. Rarely, a gush of fluid from the uterus during the first half of pregnancy is without serious consequence. The fluid may have collected previously between the amnion and chorion. Thus, if a sudden discharge of fluid in early pregnancy occurs before any pain, fever, or bleeding, the woman may be put to bed and observed. If after 48 hours no additional amnionic fluid has escaped, and there is no bleeding, pain, or fever, she may resume her usual activities except for any form of vaginal penetration. If, however, the gush of fluid is accompanied or followed by bleeding, pain, or fever, abortion should be considered inevitable and the uterus emptied.

Complete and Incomplete Abortion. When the placenta, in whole or in part, detaches from the uterus, bleeding ensues. Following complete detachment and expulsion of the conceptus, termed complete abortion, the internal cervical

os closes. During incomplete abortion, however, the internal cervical os remains open and allows passage of blood. The fetus and placenta may remain entirely in utero or may partially extrude through the dilated os. Incomplete abortion may or may not require additional cervical dilatation before curettage. In many cases, retained placental tissue simply lies loosely in the cervical canal, allowing easy extraction from an exposed external os with ring forceps. Suction curettage, as described later, effectively evacuates the uterus. In clinically stable women, expectant management also can be a reasonable option (Blohm and colleagues, 2003).

Hemorrhage from the incomplete abortion of a more advanced pregnancy, though rarely fatal, is occasionally severe. Therefore, in women with more advanced pregnancies or with heavy bleeding, evacuation should proceed promptly. Fever should not prohibit curettage once appropriate antimicrobials have been administered (see p. 247).

Missed Abortion. In this case, the uterus retains dead products of conception behind a closed cervical os for days or even weeks. In the typical instance, early pregnancy appears to be normal, with amenorrhea, nausea and vomiting, breast changes, and growth of the uterus. After fetal death, there may or may not be vaginal bleeding or other symptoms of threatened abortion. For days or weeks, the uterus remains stationary in size, but then gradually becomes smaller. Mammary changes usually regress, and women often lose a few pounds. Many women have no symptoms during this period except persistent amenorrhea. If the missed abortion terminates spontaneously, and most do, the process of expulsion is the same as in any abortion.

After death of the conceptus, management can be individualized, depending on individual circumstances. Expectant, medical, and surgical approaches can all be reasonable options, each with its own merits and disadvantages. Surgery is generally definitive and predictable but is invasive and is not necessary for all women. Expectant and medical management spare some women from curettage, but are associated with unpredictable bleeding and, in some women, the need for unscheduled surgery. These approaches may require more follow-up, may cause significant pain, and may carry time delays, all or one of which some women may not accept.

Nielsen and Hahlin (1995) performed a randomized study comparing expectant management with curettage for missed abortions earlier than 13 weeks. Spontaneous resolution occurred within 3 days in 80 percent of women treated conservatively, although vaginal bleeding averaged 1 day longer. Complications were similar between the groups. Luise and colleagues (2002), in an observational study of almost 1100 women with suspected first-trimester abortion, reported spontaneous resolution in 81 percent. In this study, compared with the report by Nielsen and Hahlin (1995), however, pregnancies were aborted later, and only half of those with a fetal pole or gestational sac aborted within 2 weeks of diagnosis.

Muffley and colleagues (2002) randomized 50 women with pregnancy failure prior to 12 weeks either to dilatation and curettage, or to 800 μg of misoprostol placed in the posterior vaginal fornix and repeated in 24 hours if necessary. Failure of medical therapy, defined as retained gestational sac at 48 hours, occurred in 60 percent of those treated medically. There were no differences between groups in hematocrit level changes or in the time to disappearance of serum hCG levels. One woman in the misoprostol group returned 6 hours after initial dosing with profuse vaginal bleeding.

In another randomized trial, Chung and colleagues (1999) reported that approximately 50 percent of the group given medical treatment subsequently required surgical evacuation. Following abortion completion with medical therapy, vaginal or abdominal ultrasound can be used to document an empty uterine cavity. If significant amounts of material remain within the uterine cavity, curettage should follow.

In some cases after prolonged retention of a dead fetus, serious coagulation defects develop and are more likely if there is fetal death after midpregnancy. Coagulopathies may cause troublesome maternal bleeding from the nose, gums, and sites of slight trauma. The pathogenesis and treatment of these defects are considered in Chapter 35 (see p. 843).

Recurrent Abortion. Defined by various criteria of number and sequence, recurrent abortion in its generally accepted definition refers to three or more consecutive spontaneous abortions. In the majority of cases, repeated spontaneous abortions are likely to be chance phenomena. Accepting an independent risk of spontaneous abortion occurrence to be 15 percent, a second loss could be calculated to occur at a rate of 2.3 percent and a third loss at a rate of 0.34 percent. Confirming this, a study of women physicians reported the occurrences of one, two, and three miscarriages to be 10.4, 2.3, and 0.34 percent, respectively (Alberman, 1988).

The American College of Obstetricians and Gynecologists (2001a) recognizes only two types of tests as having clear value in the investigation of recurrent miscarriage: (1) parental cytogenetic analysis, and (2) lupus anticoagulant and anticardiolipin antibodies assays (see p. 235). Cytogenetics, in addition to providing a potential explanation for the abortions, may identify couples at risk of giving birth to an infant with a deleterious unbalanced chromosomal translocation. Thrombophilia antibody assays rarely identify a treatable condition (see p. 236).

PROGNOSIS. The majority of women who attempt pregnancy after being diagnosed with recurrent abortion will have successful outcomes, with or without treatment. Warburton and Fraser (1964) reported that the likelihood of recurrent abortion was 25 to 30 percent regardless of the number of previous abortions. Poland and associates (1977) noted that if a woman with this diagnosis had previously delivered a liveborn infant, the risk for subsequent recurrent abortion was approximately 30 percent. If, however, a woman had no liveborn infants, and had at least one spontaneous fetal loss, the risk of abortion was 46 percent.

INDUCED ABORTION

Induced abortion is *the medical or surgical termination of pregnancy before the time of fetal viability.* In 2000, a total of 857,475 legal abortions were reported to the Centers for Disease Control and Prevention (2003). These numbers are underestimated because clinics inconsistently report medically induced abortions. Of those reported, about 20 percent involved women aged 19 years or younger, and the majority were younger than 25 years, white, and unmarried. Almost 60 percent of induced abortions were performed during the first 8 weeks, and 88 percent during the first 12 weeks of pregnancy.

HISTORY OF ABORTION. Until the United States Supreme Court decision of 1973, only therapeutic abortions could be performed legally in most states. The most common legal definition of therapeutic abortion until then was termination of pregnancy before the period of fetal viability for the purpose of saving the life of the mother. A few states extended their laws to read "to prevent serious or permanent bodily injury to the mother" or "to preserve the life or health of the woman." Some states allowed abortion if a pregnancy was likely to result in the birth of an infant with grave malformations.

The stringent abortion laws in effect prior to 1973 were of fairly recent origin. Abortion before quickening—the first definite perception of fetal movement, which most often occurs between 16 and 20 weeks' gestation—was either lawful or widely tolerated in both the United States and Great Britain until 1803. In that year, as part of a general restructuring of British criminal law, a statute was enacted that made all induced abortions regardless of gestational age illegal. The Roman Catholic Church's traditional prohibition of abortion did not receive the ultimate sanction of universal law (excommunication) until 1869 (Pilpel and Norwich, 1969).

In this country, it was not until 1821 that Connecticut enacted the first abortion law. Subsequently, abortion became illegal throughout the United States except to save the life of the mother. Because therapeutic abortion to save the life of the woman is rarely necessary or definable, it follows that the great majority of such operations previously performed in this country went beyond legal boundaries. Borgmann and Jones (2000) have extensively reviewed these legal issues.

INDICATIONS. Some indications for therapeutic abortion are discussed with the diseases that commonly lead to the operation. Well-documented indications include persistent heart disease after cardiac decompensation, advanced hypertensive vascular disease, and invasive carcinoma of the cervix. In addition to medical and surgical disorders that may be an indication for termination of pregnancy, there are others. Certainly, in cases of rape or incest, most authorities consider termination to be indicated. Another commonly cited indication is to prevent a viable birth of a fetus with a significant anatomical or mental deformity. The seriousness of fetal deformities is wide ranging and frequently defies social or legal classification.

ELECTIVE (VOLUNTARY) ABORTION. Elective or voluntary abortion is the interruption of pregnancy before viability at the request of the woman but not for reasons of impaired maternal health or fetal disease. Most abortions performed today fall into this category. Approximately one pregnancy is electively aborted for every four live births delivered in the United States (Ventura and colleagues, 2003). The Executive Board of the American College of Obstetricians and Gynecologists (2000) supports the right of women to choose abortion and considers this a medical matter between the woman and her physician.

In 1973, the United States Supreme Court legalized abortion. Several Supreme Court decisions in the history of abortion merit explanation.

Roe v Wade. The legality of elective abortion was established by the Supreme Court in its 1973 decision in *Roe v Wade*. It defined the extent to which states might regulate abortion:

1. For the stage prior to approximately the end of the first trimester, the abortion decision and its effectuation must be left to the medical judgment of the attending physician.
2. For the stage subsequent to approximately the end of the first trimester, the State, in promoting its interest in the health of the mother, may, if it chooses, regulate the abortion procedures in ways that are reasonably related to maternal health.
3. For the stage subsequent to viability, the State, in promoting its interest in the potential of human life, may, if it chooses, regulate, and even proscribe, abortion, except where necessary, in appropriate medical judgment, for the preservation of the life or health of the mother.

Webster v Reproductive Health Services. Since the *Roe v Wade* decision, many different pieces of legislation have been introduced at both the state and national level, and some enacted, to regulate or even dismantle its three provisions. All such attempts were unsuccessful until the United States Supreme Court ruled in the 1989 case *Webster v Reproductive Health Services* that states could place restrictions interfering with the provision of abortion services on such items as

waiting periods, specific informed consent requirements, parental or spousal notification, and hospital requirements. Based on this decision, numerous restrictions now limit choice and access to abortion services. A more recent choice-limiting decision is the federal law banning the poorly defined "partial birth abortion" (see p. 243). At least two federal courts—June 2004 in San Francisco and August 2004 in New York—have ruled the law unconstitutional.

In its statement on abortion policy, the American College of Obstetricians and Gynecologists (2000) affirmed: *The intervention of legislative bodies into medical decision making is inappropriate, ill advised, and dangerous.*

Counseling Before Elective Abortion. Three choices available to a woman considering an abortion include continued pregnancy with its risks and parental responsibilities; continued pregnancy with its risks and its responsibilities of arranged adoption; or the choice of abortion with its risks. Knowledgeable and compassionate counselors should objectively describe and provide information about these choices.

Abortion can be performed either medically or surgically (Table 9–2), and each has distinctive clinical features (Table 9–3). Stubblefield and colleagues (2004) summarized in detail many abortion techniques.

Surgical Techniques for Abortion. A pregnancy may be removed surgically through an appropriately dilated cervix or transabdominally by either hysterotomy or hysterectomy.

DILATATION AND CURETTAGE. Transcervical approaches to surgical abortion require first dilating the cervix and then

TABLE 9–2 Abortion Techniques

Surgical Techniques
Cervical dilatation followed by uterine evacuation
Curettage
Vacuum aspiration (suction curettage)
Dilatation and evacuation (D & E)
Dilatation and extraction (D & X)
Menstrual aspiration
Laparotomy
Hysterotomy
Hysterectomy
Medical Techniques
Intravenous oxytocin
Intra-amnionic hyperosmotic fluid
20% saline
30% urea
Prostaglandins E_2, $F_{2\alpha}$, E_1, and analogues
Intra-amnionic injection
Extraovular injection
Vaginal insertion
Parenteral injection
Oral ingestion
Antiprogesterones—RU 486 (mifepristone) and epostane
Methotrexate—intramuscular and oral
Various combinations of the above

TABLE 9–3 Features of Medical and Surgical Abortion

Medical Abortion	Surgical Abortion
Usually avoids invasive procedure	Invasive procedure
Usually avoids anesthesia	Sedation used if desired
Requires two or more visits	Usually requires one visit
Days to weeks to complete	Complete in a predictable period
Available during early pregnancy	Available during early pregnancy
High success rate (~95%)	High success rate (99%)
Requires follow-up to ensure completion of abortion	Does not require follow-up in all cases
Requires patient participation throughout multistep process	Requires participation in a single-step process

From the American College of Obstetricians and Gynecologists, 2001b, with permission.

evacuating the pregnancy by mechanically scraping out the contents (sharp curettage), by suctioning out the contents (suction curettage), or both. Vacuum aspiration, the most common form of suction curettage, requires a rigid cannula attached to an electric-powered vacuum source. Alternatively, manual vacuum aspiration uses a similar cannula that attaches to a handheld syringe for its vacuum source (Goldberg and associates, 2004). The likelihood of complications increases after the first trimester. These include uterine perforation, cervical laceration, hemorrhage, incomplete removal of the fetus and placenta, and infections. Accordingly, sharp or suction curettage should be performed before 14 to 15 weeks.

Beginning at 16 weeks, fetal size and structure dictate use of the *dilatation and evacuation (D & E)* technique. Wide mechanical cervical dilatation, achieved with metal or hygroscopic dilators, precedes mechanical destruction and evacuation of fetal parts. With complete removal of the fetus, a large-bore vacuum curette is used to remove the placenta and remaining tissue.

A *dilatation and extraction (D & X)* is similar to a dilatation and evacuation except that suction evacuation of the intracranial contents after delivery of the fetal body through the dilated cervix facilitates extraction and minimizes uterine or cervical injury from instruments or fetal bones. In political parlance, this procedure has been termed *partial birth abortion.*

Antimicrobial prophylaxis should be provided to all women undergoing a transcervical surgical abortion. Based on their review of 11 randomized trials, Sawaya and associates (1996) concluded that antimicrobials decreased the risk of infection by approximately 40 percent. No one regimen appears superior. One convenient, inexpensive, and effective regimen is doxycycline, 100 mg orally before the procedure and 200 mg orally after.

In the absence of maternal systemic disease, abortion procedures do not require hospitalization. When abortion is performed outside a hospital setting, capabilities for cardiopulmonary resuscitation and for immediate transfer to a hospital must be available.

Hygroscopic Dilators. Trauma from mechanical dilatation can be minimized by using devices that slowly dilate the cervix. These devices, called *hygroscopic dilators,* draw water from cervical tissues and expand, gradually dilating the cervix. One type of hygroscopic dilators originates from the stems of *Laminaria digitata* or *Laminaria japonica,* a brown seaweed (Fig. 9–6). The stems are cut, peeled, shaped, dried, sterilized, and packaged according to size—small, 3 to 5 mm in diameter; medium, 6 to 8 mm; and large, 8 to 10 mm. The strongly hygroscopic laminaria presumably act by drawing water from proteoglycan complexes, causing the complexes to dissociate, and thereby allowing the cervix to soften and dilate.

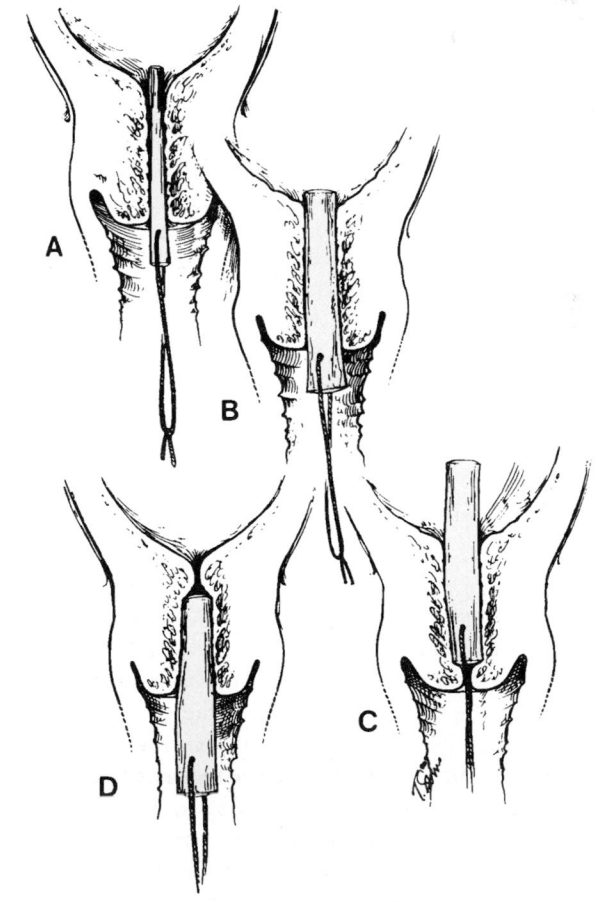

FIGURE 9–6. Insertion of laminaria prior to dilatation and curettage. **A.** Laminaria immediately after being appropriately placed with its upper end just through the internal os. **B.** Several hours later the laminaria is now swollen, and the cervix is dilated and softened. **C.** Laminaria inserted too far through the internal os; the laminaria may rupture the membranes. **D.** Laminaria not inserted far enough to dilate the internal os.

Synthetic hygroscopic dilators, such as Lamicel, a polyvinyl alcohol polymer sponge impregnated with anhydrous magnesium sulfate, also effectively dilate the cervix (Nicolaides and co-workers, 1983).

An interesting dilemma is presented by the woman who has a hygroscopic dilator placed overnight preparatory to elective abortion, but who then changes her mind. Schneider and associates (1991) described this in 7 first-trimester and 14 second-trimester pregnancies. Four patients returned to their original decision and aborted their pregnancies. Of the remaining 17, there were 14 term deliveries, 2 preterm deliveries, and 1 spontaneous abortion 2 weeks later. None of the patients suffered infectious morbidity, including three untreated women with cervical cultures positive for chlamydia. In spite of this generally reassuring report, an attitude of irrevocability with regard to dilator placement and abortion seems prudent.

Technique for Insertion. The cervix is cleansed with povidone-iodine solution and is grasped anteriorly with a tenaculum. A laminaria of the appropriate size is then inserted using a uterine packing forceps so that the tip rests at the level of the internal os (see Fig. 9–6). After 4 to 6 hours, the laminaria will have swollen and will have dilated the cervix sufficiently to allow easier mechanical dilatation and curettage. Cramping frequently accompanies expansion of the laminaria.

Prostaglandins. As an alternative to hygroscopic dilators, various prostaglandin preparations may be placed into the posterior vaginal fornix to facilitate subsequent dilatation. MacIsaac and colleagues (1999) randomized women to 400 μg of misoprostol placed vaginally 4 hours before first-trimester abortion versus laminaria placement. Misoprostol effected equal or greater dilatation, caused less pain on insertion, and produced similar side effects. It is important to emphasize that this 400-μg dose is far in excess of oral or vaginal dosing for labor induction (see Chap. 22, p. 538).

Technique for Dilatation and Curettage. A bimanual examination is performed to determine the size and orientation of the uterus. After speculum insertion, the cervix is swabbed with povidone-iodine or equivalent solution and the anterior cervical lip is grasped with a toothed tenaculum. A local anesthetic, such as 5 mL of 1 or 2 percent lidocaine, is injected bilaterally into the cervix. Alternatively, a paracervical block may be used with dilute vasopressin added to the local anesthetic to decrease blood loss (Keder, 2003).

If required, the cervix is further dilated with Hegar or Pratt dilators until a suction cannula of the appropriate diameter can be inserted. Choosing the most appropriately sized cannula balances competing factors: small cannulas carry the risk of retained intrauterine tissue postoperatively,

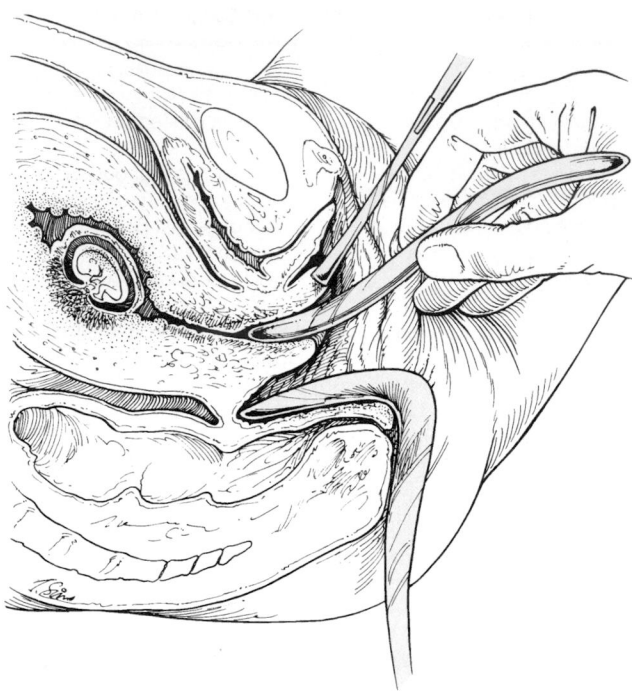

FIGURE 9–7. Dilatation of cervix with a Hegar dilator. Note that the fourth and fifth fingers rest against the perineum and buttocks, lateral to the vagina. This maneuver is a most important safety measure because if the cervix relaxes abruptly, these fingers prevent a sudden and uncontrolled thrust of the dilator, a common cause of uterine perforation.

whereas large cannulas risk cervical injury and more discomfort. The fourth and fifth fingers of the hand introducing the dilator should rest on the perineum and buttocks as the dilator is pushed through the internal os (Fig. 9–7). This technique minimizes forceful dilatation and provides a safeguard against uterine perforation. Uterine sounding measures the depth and inclination of the uterine cavity prior to cannula insertion. The suction cannula is moved toward the fundus, then back toward the os and is turned circumferentially to cover the entire surface of the uterine cavity. When no more tissue is aspirated, a gentle sharp curettage should follow to remove any remaining placental or fetal fragments.

Because uterine perforations rarely occur on the downstroke of instrumentation, and characteristically occur on the insertion of any instrument into the uterus, manipulations should be carried out with the thumb and forefinger only (Fig. 9–8). If beyond 16 weeks' gestation, the fetus is extracted, usually in parts, using Sopher forceps and other destructive instruments. Risks include uterine perforation, cervical laceration, and uterine bleeding due to the larger fetus and placenta and to the thinner uterine walls. Morbidity can be minimized if (1) the cervix is adequately dilated before attempting to remove the products of conception, (2) instruments are introduced into the uterus and manipulated without force, and (3) all tissue is removed.

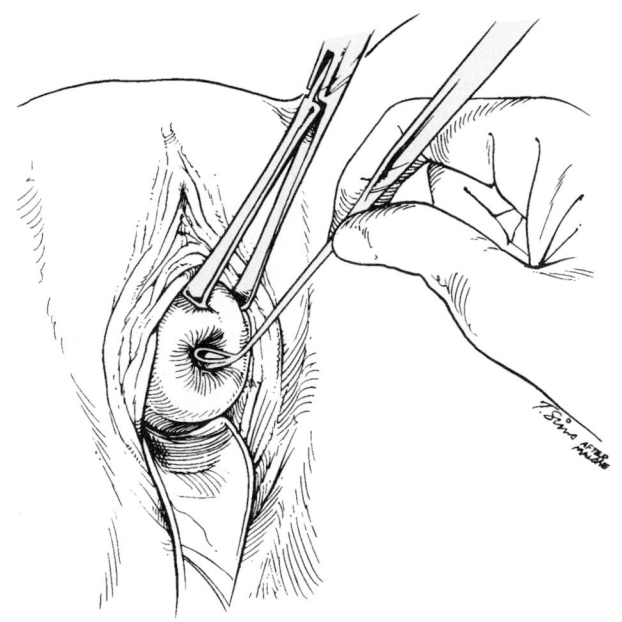

FIGURE 9–8. Introduction of a sharp curet. Note that the instrument is held with the thumb and forefinger; in the upward movement of the curet, only the strength of these two fingers should be used.

Complications. The incidence of uterine perforation associated with elective abortion varies. Two important determinants are the skill of the physician and the position of the uterus, with a much greater likelihood of perforation if the uterus is retroverted. Accidental uterine perforation usually is recognized easily when the instrument passes without resistance deep into the pelvis. Observation may be sufficient if the uterine perforation is small, as when produced by a uterine sound or narrow dilator.

Considerable intra-abdominal damage can be caused by instruments, especially suction and sharp curettes, passed through a uterine defect into the peritoneal cavity (Keegan and Forkowitz, 1982). In this circumstance, laparotomy to examine the abdominal contents is often the safest course of action. Depending on the circumstances, laparoscopy may be substituted. Unrecognized bowel injury can cause severe peritonitis and sepsis (Kambiss and associates, 2000).

Some women may develop cervical incompetence or uterine synechiae following dilatation and curettage. Rarely, abortion performed by curettage on more advanced pregnancies may induce sudden, severe consumptive coagulopathy, which can prove fatal. Those contemplating abortion should understand the potential for these rare but serious complications.

MENSTRUAL ASPIRATION. Aspiration of the endometrial cavity using a flexible 5- or 6-mm Karman cannula and attached syringe within 1 to 3 weeks after a missed menstrual period has been referred to as *menstrual extraction, menstrual induction, instant period, traumatic abortion,* and *mini-abortion.* At this

early stage of gestation, pregnancy can be misdiagnosed, an implanted zygote can be missed by the curette, ectopic pregnancy can be unrecognized, or infrequently, a uterus can be perforated. Even so, Paul and associates (2002) reported a 98-percent success rate in more than 1000 women who underwent this procedure. A positive pregnancy test will eliminate a needless procedure on a nonpregnant woman whose period has been delayed for other reasons.

To identify placenta in the aspirate, MacIsaac and Darney (2000) recommend that the syringe contents be rinsed in a strainer to remove blood, then placed in a clear plastic container with saline and examined with back lighting. Placental tissue macroscopically appears soft, fluffy, and feathery. A magnifying lens, colposcope, or microscope also can improve visualization.

LAPAROTOMY. In a few circumstances, abdominal hysterotomy or hysterectomy for abortion is preferable to either curettage or medical induction. If significant uterine disease is present, hysterectomy may provide ideal treatment. Either hysterotomy with tubal ligation or, on occasion, hysterectomy may be indicated for women who desire pregnancy termination and sterilization. At times, a failed medical induction during the second trimester may necessitate hysterotomy or hysterectomy.

Medical Induction of Abortion. Throughout history, many naturally occurring substances have been tried as abortifacients. Most often, serious systemic illness or even death has resulted rather than abortion. Even today, only a few effective, safe abortifacient drugs are used.

EARLY ABORTION. According to the American College of Obstetricians and Gynecologists (2001b), outpatient medical abortion is an acceptable alternative to surgical abortion in appropriately selected women with pregnancies of less than 49 days' gestation. Beyond this point, the available data, though less robust, support surgical abortion as a preferable method of early abortion. Three medications for early medical abortion have been widely studied and used: the antiprogestin *mifepristone,* the antimetabolite *methotrexate,* and the prostaglandin *misoprostol.* These agents cause abortion by increasing uterine contractility, either by reversing the progesterone-induced inhibition of contractions (mifepristone and methotrexate), or by stimulating the myometrium directly (misoprostol).

Various dosing schemes have proven effective (Table 9–4). Mifepristone or methotrexate is administered initially, and followed after some time interval by misoprostol. Methotrexate and misoprostol are teratogens. Their use thus requires a commitment on the part of both patient and caregiver to complete the abortion, even if surgical evacuation becomes necessary.

Contraindications to medical abortion have evolved from the exclusion criteria of various medical abortion trials. In

TABLE 9–4 Regimens for Medical Termination of Early Pregnancy

Mifepristone plus Misoprostol
Mifepristone, 100–600 mg orally, followed by:
Misoprostol, 400 μg orally or 800 μg vaginally in 6–72 hr

Methotrexate plus Misoprostol
Methotrexate, 50 mg/m² intramuscularly or orally, followed by:
Misoprostol, 800 μg vaginally in 3–7 days; repeated if needed 1 wk after methotrexate initially given

Data from the American College of Obstetricians and Gynecologists, 2001b; Borgatta, 2001; Creinin, 2001, 2004; Pymar, 2001; Schaff, 2000; von Hertzen, 2003; Wiebe, 1999, 2002, and their many colleagues.

addition to specific allergies to the medicines, they have included an in situ intrauterine device, severe anemia, coagulopathy or anticoagulant use, and significant medical conditions, such as active liver disease, cardiovascular disease, and uncontrolled seizure disorders. Additionally, because misoprostol can lower glucocorticoid activity, women with adrenal disease or with disorders requiring glucocorticoid therapy should be excluded (American College of Obstetricians and Gynecologists, 2001b). Women contemplating medical abortion should receive thorough counseling regarding the risks, benefits, and requirements of both medical and surgical approaches.

With the mifepristone regimen, according to the Food and Drug Administration package labeling, the misoprostol is to be provider-administered. Afterward, the woman typically remains in the office for 4 hours, although her activity is not restricted. If the products of conception appear to have been expelled, she is examined to confirm expulsion. If during observation the conceptus does not appear to have been expelled, a pelvic examination is performed before discharge and the woman is rescheduled for an appointment in 1 to 2 weeks. At this later appointment, if both history and physical examination or ultrasound fail to confirm completed abortion, a suction procedure usually is performed.

In regimens employing methotrexate, women typically are seen at least 24 hours after misoprostol administration, and approximately 7 days after methotrexate administration, at which time an ultrasound examination is performed. If the pregnancy persists, another dose of misoprostol is given, and the woman is seen again in 1 week if fetal cardiac activity is present, or in 4 weeks if there is no fetal cardiac activity. If, by the second visit, abortion has not occurred, it usually is completed by suction curettage (American College of Obstetricians and Gynecologists, 2001b).

Bleeding and cramping with medical termination can be significantly worse than symptoms experienced with menses. Adequate pain medication, usually including a narcotic, should be provided. According to the American College of Obstetricians and Gynecologists (2001b), soaking two pads or more per hour for at least 2 hours is a threshold at which

the woman should be instructed to contact her provider to determine whether she needs to be seen.

Early medical abortion is highly effective—90 to 98 percent of women will not require surgical intervention (Kahn and associates, 2000). According to Hausknecht (2003), when mifepristone was given with misoprostol to 80,000 women for medical abortion, only 139 complications were reported to the manufacturer. Unnecessary surgical intervention in women undergoing medical abortion can be avoided if ultrasound results are interpreted appropriately. Specifically, if no gestational sac is present, in the absence of heavy bleeding, intervention in most women is unnecessary. This is true even when, as is common, the uterus contains ultrasonographically evident debris (Cowett and associates, 2004).

SECOND-TRIMESTER ABORTION. Invasive means of second-trimester medical abortion have long been available (see Table 9–2). In the past decade, however, the ability to safely and effectively accomplish noninvasive second-trimester abortion has evolved considerably. Principal among these noninvasive methods are high-dose intravenous oxytocin and vaginal prostaglandin administration, including prostaglandin E_2 suppositories and prostaglandin E_1 (misoprostol) pills. Regardless of method, laminaria placement as shown in Figure 9–6 will shorten the duration (Stubblefield and colleagues, 1975).

Oxytocin. Given as a single agent in high doses, oxytocin will effect second-trimester abortion in 80 to 90 percent of cases. For more than 15 years, the regimen shown in Table 9–5 has been used with a high degree of safety and effectiveness at the University of Alabama. By always mixing the oxytocin in an isotonic solution such as normal saline, and avoiding excessive administration of dilute intravenous solutions, we have not observed hyponatremia or water intoxication.

Prostaglandin E_2. Suppositories of 20-mg prostaglandin E_2 placed in the posterior vaginal fornix are a simple and

TABLE 9–5 Concentrated Oxytocin Protocol for Midtrimester Abortion

50 units oxytocin in 500 mL of normal saline infused over 3 hr; 1-hr diuresis (no oxytocin)
100 units oxytocin in 500 mL of normal saline infused over 3 hr; 1-hr diuresis (no oxytocin)
150 units oxytocin in 500 mL of normal saline infused over 3 hr; 1-hr diuresis (no oxytocin)
200 units oxytocin in 500 mL of normal saline infused over 3 hr; 1-hr diuresis (no oxytocin)
250 units oxytocin in 500 mL of normal saline infused over 3 hr; 1-hr diuresis (no oxytocin)
300 units oxytocin in 500 mL of normal saline infused over 3 hr; 1-hr diuresis (no oxytocin)

Modified from Ramsey and Owen, 2000, with permission.

effective means of effecting second-trimester abortion. This method is not more effective than high-dose oxytocin, and it causes more frequent side effects such as nausea, vomiting, fever, and diarrhea (Owen and associates, 1992). If prostaglandin E_2 is used, an antiemetic such as metoclopramide, an antipyretic such as acetaminophen, and an antidiarrheal such as diphenoxylate/atropine are given either to prevent or to treat symptoms.

Prostaglandin E_1. Misoprostol can be used easily and inexpensively as a single agent for second-trimester pregnancy termination. In their randomized trial, Ramsey and co-workers (2004) administered misoprostol, 600 μg vaginally followed by 400 μg every 4 hours, and reported that this effected abortion significantly faster than concentrated oxytocin given in combination with prostaglandin E_2-median time to abortion 12 versus 17 hours, respectively. Misoprostol achieved abortion within 24 hours in 95 percent of women compared with 85 percent in the other group. Importantly, only 2 percent of women in the misoprostol group required curettage for retained placenta compared with 15 percent in the oxytocin/prostaglandin E_2 group.

The safety of medically induced second-trimester abortion after a previous cesarean delivery was reported by Boulot and associates (1993). At a mean gestational age of almost 24 weeks, 20 of 23 fetuses aborted. At hysterotomy in the three treatment failures, there was one uterine rupture that was successfully repaired. Chapman and colleagues (1996) reported a uterine rupture rate of 3.8 percent in 79 women with a prior cesarean delivery undergoing medical termination at a mean gestational age of 21 weeks.

CONSEQUENCES OF ELECTIVE ABORTION

Maternal Mortality. Legally induced abortion, performed by trained gynecologists, especially when performed during the first 2 months of pregnancy, has a mortality rate of only 0.7 per 100,000 procedures (Bartlett and co-workers, 2004; Gissler and associates, 2004; Grimes, 1994). The relative risk of dying as the consequence of abortion approximately doubles for each 2 weeks after 8 weeks' gestation.

Impact on Future Pregnancies. In a scholarly review of the impact of elective abortion on subsequent pregnancy outcome, Hogue (1986) summarized data from more than 200 publications. Data relating abortion to subsequent pregnancy outcome are observational, and therefore subject to bias and uncontrolled confounding factors. All studies on this topic must be interpreted with these limitations in mind.

Fertility does not appear to be diminished by an elective abortion, except infrequently as a consequence of infection. Vacuum aspiration does not increase the subsequent incidence of second-trimester spontaneous abortion or preterm delivery. Similarly, subsequent ectopic pregnancies are not increased, except possibly in women with preexisting chlamydial infection or in those who develop postabortion infections. Multiple sharp curettage abortion procedures may increase the subsequent risk of placenta previa, whereas vacuum aspiration procedures likely do not (Johnson and co-workers, 2003).

Septic Abortion. Although serious complications of abortion most often occur with criminal abortion, even spontaneous abortion and legal elective abortion continue to be associated with severe and even fatal infections (Barrett and colleagues, 2002). Severe hemorrhage, sepsis, bacterial shock, and acute renal failure have all developed in association with abortion but at a much lower frequency. Uterine infection is the usual outcome, but parametritis, peritonitis, endocarditis, and septicemia may all occur (Vartian and Septimus, 1991).

Among 300 women with septic abortions at Parkland Hospital, one fourth had a positive blood culture result. The organisms were predominantly anaerobic bacteria and coliforms, but others, including *Haemophilus influenzae, Campylobacter jejuni,* and group A streptococcus, also were noted (Denton and Clarke, 1992; Dotters and Katz, 1991; Pinhas-Hamiel and associates, 1991). Treatment of infection includes prompt intravenous administration of broad-spectrum antimicrobials followed by evacuation of the products of conception. If sepsis and shock supervene, then supportive care is essential, as discussed in Chapter 42 (see p. 993). Septic abortion also may lead to disseminated intravascular coagulopathy (see Chap. 35, p. 843).

RESUMPTION OF OVULATION AFTER ABORTION

Ovulation may resume as early as 2 weeks after an abortion. Lähteenmä ki and Luukkainen (1978) detected surges of luteinizing hormone (LH) 16 to 22 days in 15 of 18 women studied. Moreover, plasma progesterone levels, which had plummeted after the abortion, increased soon after the LH surges. These hormonal events agree with histological changes observed in endometrial biopsies (Boyd and Holmstrom, 1972). **Therefore, if pregnancy is to be prevented, effective contraception should be initiated soon after abortion.** If contraception is not desired, Grossman and colleagues (2004) concluded that a visit to assess for complications is not necessary for procedures done before 50 days' gestation.

REFERENCES

Aarts JM, Brons JT, Bruinse HW: Emergency cerclage: A review. Obstet Gynecol Surv 50:459, 1995

Adelberg AM, Kuller JA: Thrombophilias and recurrent miscarriage. Obstet Gynecol Surv 57:703, 2002

Alberman E: The epidemiology of repeated abortion. In Beard RW, Sharp F (eds): Early Pregnancy Loss: Mechanisms and Treatment. London, RCOG, 1988, p 9

Althuisius SM, Dekker GA, Hummel P, et al: Final results of the cervical incompetence prevention randomized cerclage trial (CIPRACT): Therapeutic cerclage with bed rest versus bed rest alone. Am J Obstet Gynecol 185:1106, 2001

American College of Obstetricians and Gynecologists: Management of recurrent early pregnancy loss. Practice Bulletin No. 24, February 2001a

American College of Obstetricians and Gynecologists: Medical management of abortion. Practice Bulletin No. 26, April 2001b

American College of Obstetricians and Gynecologists: Abortion policy. Statement of Policy by the ACOG Executive Board, September 2000

American College of Obstetricians and Gynecologists: Prevention of Rh D alloimmunization. Practice Bulletin No. 4, May 1999

American College of Obstetricians and Gynecologists: Antiphospholipid syndrome. Educational Bulletin No. 244, February 1998

Armstrong BG, McDonald AD, Sloan M: Cigarette, alcohol, and coffee consumption and spontaneous abortion. Am J Public Health 82:85, 1992

Barlow S, Sullivan FM: Reproductive Hazards of Industrial Chemicals: An Evaluation of Animal and Human Data. New York, Academic Press, 1982

Barrett JP, Whiteside JL, Boardman LA: Fatal clostridial sepsis after spontaneous abortion. Obstet Gynecol 99:899, 2002

Barth WH: Operative procedures of the cervix. In Hankins GDV, Clark SL, Cunningham FG, et al (eds): Operative Obstetrics. Norwalk, CT, Appleton & Lange, 1995, p 753

Bartlett LA, Berg CJ, Shulman HB, et al: Risk factors for legal induced abortion-related mortality in the United States. Obstet Gynecol 103:729, 2004

Batzofin JH, Fielding WL, Friedman EA: Effect of vaginal bleeding in early pregnancy on outcome. Obstet Gynecol 63:515, 1984

Blohm F, Fridén B, Platz-Christensen JJ, et al: Expectant management of first-trimester miscarriage in clinical practice. Acta Obstet Gynecol Scand 82:654, 2003

Blumenfeld Z, Brenner B: Thrombophilia-associated pregnancy wastage. Fertil Steril 72:765, 1999

Boivin JF: Risk of spontaneous abortion in women occupationally exposed to anaesthetic gases: A meta-analysis. Occup Environ Med 54:541, 1997

Borgatta L, Burnhill MS, Tyson J, et al: Early medical abortion with methotrexate and misoprostol. Obstet Gynecol 97:11, 2001

Borgmann CE, Jones BS: Legal issues in the provision of medical abortion. Am J Obstet Gynecol 183:S84, 2000

Boulot P, Hoffet M, Bachelard B, et al: Late vaginal induced abortion after a previous cesarean birth: Potential for uterine rupture. Gynecol Obstet Invest 36:87, 1993

Boyd EF Jr, Holmstrom EG: Ovulation following therapeutic abortion. Am J Obstet Gynecol 113:469, 1972

Branch DW, Khamashta MA: Antiphospholipid syndrome: Obstetric diagnosis, management, and controversies. Obstet Gynecol 101:1333, 2003

Brown ZA, Selke S, Zeh J, et al: The acquisition of herpes simplex virus during pregnancy. N Engl J Med 337:509, 1997

Cammarano CL, Herron MA, Parer JT: Validity of indications for transabdominal cervicoisthmic cerclage for cervical incompetence. Am J Obstet Gynecol 172:1871, 1995

Carp H, Dolitzky M, Tur-Kaspa I, et al: Hereditary thrombophilias are not associated with a decreased live birth rate in women with recurrent miscarriage. Fertil Steril 78:58, 2002

Carrell DT, Wilcox AL, Lowy L, et al: Male chromosomal factors of unexplained recurrent pregnancy loss. Obstet Gynecol 101:1229, 2003

Caruso A, Trivellini C, De Carolis S, et al: Emergency cerclage in the presence of protruding membranes: Is pregnancy outcome predictable? Acta Obstet Gynecol Scand 79:265, 2000

Caspi E, Schneider DF, Mor Z, et al: Cervical internal os cerclage: Description of a new technique and comparison with Shirodkar operation. Am J Perinatol 7:347, 1990

Casteñada R, Lechuga D, Ramos RI, et al: Endemic goiter in pregnant women: Utility of the simplified classification of thyroid size by palpation and urinary iodide as screening tests. Br J Obstet Gynaecol 109:1366, 2002

Cavallo F, Russo R, Zotti C, et al: Moderate alcohol consumption and spontaneous abortion. Alcohol 30:195, 1995

Centers for Disease Control and Prevention: Abortion surveillance—United States, 2000. MMWR 52:SS-12, 2003

Chapman S, Crispens MA, Owen J, et al: Complications of midtrimester pregnancy terminations: The effect of prior cesarean delivery. Am J Obstet Gynecol 174:356, 1996

Charles D, Edward WR: Infectious complications of cervical cerclage. Am J Obstet Gynecol 141:1065, 1981

Chasen ST, Silverman NS: Mid-trimester emergent cerclage: A ten year single institution review. J Perinatol 18:338, 1998

Chatenoud L, Parazzini F, Di Cintio E, et al: Paternal and maternal smoking habits before conception and during the first trimester: Relation to spontaneous abortion. Ann Epidemiol 8:520, 1998

Chung TKH, Lee DTSL, Cheung LP, et al: Spontaneous abortion: A randomized, controlled trial comparing surgical evacuation with conservative management using misoprostol. Fertil Steril 71:1054, 1999

Cnattingius S, Signorello LB, Anneren G, et al: Caffeine intake and the risk of first-trimester spontaneous abortion. N Engl J Med 343:1839, 2000

Cowchock S: Autoantibodies and pregnancy loss. N Engl J Med 337:197, 1997

Cowett AA, Cohen LS, Lichtenberg ES, Stika CS: Ultrasound evaluation of the endometrium after medical termination of pregnancy. Obstet Gynecol 103:871, 2004

Craig TB, Ke RW, Kutteh WH: Increase prevalence of insulin resistance in women with a history of recurrent pregnancy loss. Fertil Steril 78:487, 2002

Creinin MD, Fox MC, Teal S, et al: A randomized comparison of misoprostol 6 to 8 hours versus 24 hours after mifepristone for abortion. Obstet Gynecol 103:850, 2004

Creinin MD, Pymar HC, Schwartz JL: Mifepristone 100 mg in abortion regimens. Obstet Gynecol 98:434, 2001

Dayan CM, Daniels GH: Chronic autoimmune thyroiditis. N Engl J Med 335:99, 1996

Denton KJ, Clarke T: Role of Campylobacter jejuni as a placental pathogen. J Clin Pathol 45:171, 1992

Dotters DJ, Katz VL: Streptococcal toxic shock associated with septic abortion. Obstet Gynecol 78:549, 1991

Dudley DJ, Branch W: Antiphospholipid syndrome: A model for autoimmune pregnancy loss. Infert Reprod Med Clin North Am 2:149, 1991

Esplin MS, Branch DW, Silver R, et al: Thyroid autoantibodies are not associated with recurrent pregnancy loss. Am J Obstet Gynecol 179:1583, 1998

Fantel AG, Shepard TH, Vadheim-Roth C, et al: Embryonic and fetal phenotypes: Prevalence and other associated factors in a large study of spontaneous abortion. In Porter IH, Hook EM (eds): Human Embryonic and Fetal Death. New York, Academic Press, 1980, p 71

Farquharson RG, Quenby S, Greaves M: Antiphospholipid syndrome in pregnancy: A randomized, controlled trial of treatment. Obstet Gynecol 100:408, 2002

Feist A, Sydler T, Gebbers JJ, et al: No association of Chlamydia with abortion. J R Soc Med 92:237, 1999

Floyd RL, Decoufle P, Hungerford DW: Alcohol use prior to pregnancy recognition. Am J Prev Med 17:101, 1999

Funderburk SJ, Guthrie D, Meldrum D: Outcome of pregnancies complicated by early vaginal bleeding. Br J Obstet Gynaecol 87:100, 1980

Gibb DM, Salaria DA: Transabdominal cervicoisthmic cerclage in the management of recurrent second trimester miscarriage and preterm delivery. Br J Obstet Gynaecol 102:802, 1995

Gissler M, Berg C, Bouvier-Colle M-H, Buekens P: Pregnancy-associated mortality after birth, spontaneous abortion, or induced abortion in Finland, 1987–2000. Am J Obstet Gynecol 190:422, 2004

Goldberg AB, Dean G, Kang M-S, et al: Manual versus electric vacuum aspiration for early first-trimester abortion: A controlled study of complication rates. Obstet Gynecol 103:101, 2004

Greene MF: Spontaneous abortions and major malformations in women with diabetes mellitus. Semin Reprod Endocrinol 17:127, 1999

Grimes DA: The morbidity and mortality of pregnancy: still risky business. Am J Obstet Gynecol 170:1489, 1994

Grosman D, Ellertson C, Grimes DA, Walker D: Routine follow-up visits after first-trimester induced abortion. Obstet Gynecol 103:738, 2004

Harlap S, Shiono PH: Alcohol, smoking, and incidence of spontaneous abortions in the first and second trimester. Lancet 2:173, 1980

Harlap S, Shiono PH, Ramcharan S: A life table of spontaneous abortions and the effects of age, parity and other variables. In Porter IH, Hook EB (eds): Human Embryonic and Fetal Death. New York, Academic Press, 1980, p 145

Hauskecht R: Mifepristone and misoprostol for early medical abortion: 18 months experience in the United States. Contraception 67:463, 2003

Hertig AT, Rock J: On the development of the early human ovum, with special reference to the trophoblast of the previllous stage: A description of 7 normal and 5 pathologic human ova. Am J Obstet Gynecol 47:149, 1944

Hertig AT, Sheldon WH: Minimal criteria required to prove prima facie case of traumatic abortion or miscarriage: An analysis of 1,000 spontaneous abortions. Ann Surg 117:596, 1943

Hogue CJR: Impact of abortion on subsequent fecundity. Clin Obstet Gynecol 13:95, 1986

Jacobs PA, Hassold TJ: The origin of chromosomal abnormalities in spontaneous abortion. In Porter IH, Hook EB (eds): Human Embryonic and Fetal Death. New York, Academic Press, 1980, p 289

Johnson LG, Mueller BA, Daling JR: The relationship of placenta previa and history of induced abortion. Int J Gynaecol Obstet 81:191, 2003

Kahn JG, Becker BJ, MacIssa L, et al: The efficacy of medical abortion: A meta-analysis. Contraception 61:29, 2000

Kajii T, Ferrier A, Niikawa N, et al: Anatomic and chromosomal anomalies in 639 spontaneous abortions. Hum Genet 55:87, 1980

Kambiss SM, Hibbert ML, Macedonia C, et al: Uterine perforation resulting in bowel infarction: Sharp traumatic bowel and mesenteric injury at the time of pregnancy termination. Milit Med 165:81, 2000

Keder LM: Best practices in surgical abortion. Am J Obstet Gynecol 189:418, 2003

Keegan GT, Forkowitz MJ: A case report: Uretero-uterine fistula as a complication of elective abortion. J Urol 128:137, 1982

Kesmodel U, Wisborg K, Olsen SF, et al: Moderate alcohol intake in pregnancy and the risk of spontaneous abortion. Alcohol Alcohol 37:87, 2002

Klebanoff MA, Levine RJ, DerSimonian R, et al: Maternal serum paraxanthine, a caffeine metabolite, and the risk of spontaneous abortion. N Engl J Med 341:1639, 1999

Kline J, Stein ZA, Shrout P, et al: Drinking during pregnancy and spontaneous abortion. Lancet 2:176, 1980

Kuhn RPJ, Pepperell RJ: Cervical ligation: A review of 242 pregnancies. Aust NZ J Obstet Gynaecol 17:79, 1977

Kutteh WH: Antiphospholipid antibody–associated recurrent pregnancy loss: Treatment with heparin and low-dose aspirin is superior to low-dose aspirin alone. Am J Obstet Gynecol 174:1584, 1996

Kutteh WH, Pasquarette MM: Recurrent pregnancy loss. Adv Obstet Gynecol 2:147, 1995

Lähteenmä ki P, Luukkainen T: Return of ovarian function after abortion. Clin Endocrinol 8:123, 1978

Levine JS, Branch DW, Rauch J: The antiphospholipid syndrome. N Engl J Med 346:752, 2002

Locatelli A, Vergani P, Bellini P, et al: Amnioreduction in emergency cerclage with prolapsed membranes: Comparison of two methods for reducing the membranes. Am J Perinatol 16:73, 1999

Luise C, Jermy K, May C, et al: Outcome of expectant management of spontaneous first trimester miscarriage: Observational study. BMJ 324:873, 2002

MacIsaac L, Darney P: Early surgical abortion: An alternative to and backup for medical abortion. Am J Obstet Gynecol 183:S76, 2000

MacIsaac L, Grossman D, Balistreri E, et al: A randomized controlled trial of laminaria, oral misoprostol, and vaginal misoprostol before abortion. Obstet Gynecol 93:766, 1999

MacNaughton MC, Chalmers IG, Dubowitz V, et al: Final report of the Medical Research Council/Royal College of Obstetricians and Gynaecologists Multicentre Randomized Trial of Cervical Cerclage. Br J Obstet Gynaecol 100:516, 1993

March CM, Israel R: Gestational outcome following hysteroscopic lysis of adhesions. Fertil Steril 36:455, 1981

McDonald IA: Incompetent cervix as a cause of recurrent abortion. J Obstet Gynaecol Br Commonw 70:105, 1963

Mills JL, Simpson JL, Driscoll SG, et al: Incidence of spontaneous abortion among normal women and insulin-dependent diabetic women whose pregnancies were identified within 21 days of conception. N Engl J Med 319:1618, 1988

Muffley PE, Stitely ML, Gherman RB: Early intrauterine pregnancy failure: A randomized trial of medical versus surgical treatment. Am J Obstet Gynecol 187:321, 2002

Nicolaides KH, Welch CC, Koullapis EN, et al: Cervical dilatation by Lamicel—studies on the mechanism of action. Br J Obstet Gynaecol 90:1060, 1983

Nielsen S, Hahlin M: Expectant management of first-trimester spontaneous abortion. Lancet 345:84, 1995

Oakeshott P, Hay P, Hay S, et al: Association between bacterial vaginosis or chlamydial infection and miscarriage before 16 weeks' gestation: Prospective, community based cohort study. BMJ 325:1334, 2002

O'Connor S, Kuller JA, McMahon MJ: Management of cervical cerclage after preterm premature rupture of membranes. Obstet Gynecol Surv 54:391, 1999

Osser S, Persson K: Chlamydial antibodies in women who suffer miscarriage. Br J Obstet Gynaecol 103:137, 1996

Owen J, Hauth JC, Winkler CL, et al: Midtrimester pregnancy termination: A randomized trial of prostaglandin E$_2$ versus concentrated oxytocin. Am J Obstet Gynecol 167:1112, 1992

Owen J, Iams JD, Hauth JC: Vaginal sonography and cervical incompetence. Am J Obstet Gynecol 188:586, 2003

Paukku M, Tulppala M, Puolakkainen M, et al: Lack of association between serum antibodies to Chlamydia trachomatis and a history of recurrent pregnancy loss. Fertil Steril 72:427, 1999

Paul ME, Mitchell CM, Rogers AJ, et al: Early surgical abortion: Efficacy and safety. Am J Obstet Gynecol 187:407, 2002

Pilpel HF, Norwich KP: When should abortion be legal? New York, Public Affairs Committee, No. 429, 1969

Pinhas-Hamiel O, Schiff E, Ben-Baruch G, et al: A life-threatening sexually transmitted Haemophilus influenzae in septic abortion: A case report. Am J Obstet Gynecol 165:66, 1991

Poland BJ, Miller JR, Harris M, et al: Spontaneous abortion: A study of 1961 women and their abortuses. Acta Obstet Gynecol Scand 102:1, 1981

Poland BJ, Miller JR, Jones DC, et al: Reproductive counseling in patients who have had a spontaneous abortion. Am J Obstet Gynecol 127:685, 1977

Pratt D, Novotny M, Kaberlein G, et al: Antithyroid antibodies and the association with non-organ-specific antibodies in recurrent pregnancy loss. Am J Obstet Gynecol 170:956, 1994

Pymar HC, Creinin MD, Schwartz JL: Mifepristone followed on the same day by vaginal misoprostol for early abortion. Contraception 64:87, 2001

Quinn PA, Shewchuck AB, Shuber J, et al: Serologic evidence of Ureaplasma urealyticum infection in women with spontaneous pregnancy loss. Am J Obstet Gynecol 145:245, 1983

Rai R, Cohen H, Dave M, Regan L: Randomised controlled trial of aspirin and aspirin plus heparin in pregnant women with recurrent miscarriage associated with phospholipids antibodies (or antiphospholipid antibodies). BMJ 314:253, 1997

Ramsey PS, Owen J: Midtrimester cervical ripening and labor induction. Clin Obstet Gynecol 43:495, 2000

Ramsey PS, Savage K, Lincoln T, Owen J: Vaginal misoprostol versus concentrated oxytocin and vaginal PGE_2 for second-trimester labor induction. Obstet Gynecol 104:138, 2004

Rasch V: Cigarette, alcohol, and caffeine consumption: Risk factors for spontaneous abortion. Acta Obstet Gynecol Scand 82:182, 2003

Raziel A, Arieli S, Bukovsky I, et al: Investigation of the uterine cavity in recurrent aborters. Fertil Steril 62:1080, 1994

Rowland AS, Baird DD, Shore DL, et al: Nitrous oxide and spontaneous abortion in female dental assistants. Am J Epidemiol 141:531, 1995

Rushworth FH, Backos M, Rai R, et al: Prospective pregnancy outcome in untreated recurrent miscarriages with thyroid autoantibodies. Hum Reprod 15:1637, 2000

Rust OA, Atlas RO, Reed J, et al: Revisiting the short cervix detected by transvaginal ultrasound in the second trimester: Why cerclage may not help. Am J Obstet Gynecol 185:1098, 2001

Salem HT, Ghaneimah SA, Shaaban MM, et al: Prognostic value of biochemical tests in the assessment of fetal outcome in threatened abortion. Br J Obstet Gynaecol 91:382, 1984

Sauerwein RW, Bisseling J, Horrevorts AM: Septic abortion associated with Campylobacter fetus subspecies fetus infection: Case report and review of the literature. Infection 21:33, 1993

Sawaya GF, Grady D, Kerlikowske K, et al: Antibiotics at the time of induced abortion: The case for universal prophylaxis based on a meta-analysis. Obstet Gynecol 87:884, 1996

Schaff EA, Fielding SL, Westhoff C, et al: Vaginal misoprostol administered 1, 2, or 3 days after mifepristone for early medical abortion. A randomized trial. JAMA 284:1948, 2000

Schneider D, Golan A, Langer R, et al: Outcome of continued pregnancies after first and second trimester cervical dilatation by laminaria tents. Obstet Gynecol 78:1121, 1991

Schnorr TM, Grajewski BA, Hornung RW, et al: Video display terminals and the risk of spontaneous abortion. N Engl J Med 324:727, 1991

Scott JR. Immunotherapy for recurrent miscarriage. Cochrane Database of Systematic Reviews. (2):CD000112, 2000

Sher KS, Jayanthi V, Probert CS, et al: Infertility, obstetric and gynaecological problems in coeliac sprue. Dig Dis 12:186, 1994

Shirodkar VN: A new method of operative treatment for habitual abortions in the second trimester of pregnancy. Antiseptic 52:299, 1955

Signorello LB, McLaughlin JK: Maternal caffeine consumption and spontaneous abortion: A review of the epidemiologic evidence. Epidemiology 15:229, 2004

Simpson JL: Genes, chromosomes, and reproductive failure. Fertil Steril 33:107, 1980

Simpson JL, Carson SA, Chesney C, et al: Lack of association between antiphospholipid antibodies and first trimester spontaneous abortion: Prospective study of pregnancies detected within 21 days of conception. Fertil Steril 69:814, 1998

Stagnaro-Green A, Roman SH, Cobin RH, et al: Detection of at-risk pregnancy by means of highly sensitive assays for thyroid autoantibodies. JAMA 264:1422, 1990

Stein Z, Kline J, Susser E, et al: Maternal age and spontaneous abortion. In Porter IH, Hook EB (eds): Human Embryonic and Fetal Death. New York, Academic Press, 1980, p 107

Strauss JH, Wilson M, Caldwell D, et al: Laminaria use in midtrimester abortions induce intra-amniotic prostaglandin F2alpha with urea intravenous oxytocin. Am J Obstet Gynecol 134:260, 1979

Stubblefield PG, Carr-Ellis S, Borgatta L: Methods for induced abortion. Obstet Gynecol 104:174, 2004

Stubblefield PG, Naftolin F, Frigoletto F, Ryan KJ: Laminaria augmentation of intra-amniotic PGF midtrimester pregnancy termination. Prostaglandins 10:413, 1975

Supreme Court of the United States: William Webster v Reproductive Health Services. Opinion No. 88-605, July 3, 1989

Supreme Court of the United States: Jane Roe et al v Henry Wade, District Attorney of Dallas County. Opinion No. 70-18, January 22, 1973

Taskinen H, Kyyrönen P, Hemminki K: Effects of ultrasound, shortwaves, and physical exertion on pregnancy outcome in physiotherapists. J Epidemiol Community Health 44:196, 1990

Temmerman M, Lopita MI, Sanghvi HC, et al: The role of maternal syphilis, gonorrhoea and HIV-1 infections in spontaneous abortion. Int J STD AIDS 3:418, 1992

Terkildsen MFC, Parilla BV, Kumar P, et al: Factors associated with success of emergent second-trimester cerclage. Obstet Gynecol 101:565, 2003

Thomason JL, Sampson MB, Beckman CR, et al: The incompetent cervix: A 1982 update. J Reprod Med 27:187, 1982

To MS, Alfirevic Z, Heath VCF, et al: Cervical cerclage for prevention of preterm delivery in women with short cervix: Randomised controlled trial. Lancet 363:1849, 2004

Tongsong T, Srisomboon J, Wanapirak C, et al: Pregnancy outcome of threatened abortion with demonstrable fetal cardiac activity: A cohort study. J Obstet Gynaecol 21:331, 1995

Vartian CV, Septimus EJ: Tricuspid valve group B streptococcal endocarditis following elective abortion. Rev Infect Dis 13:997, 1991

van Benthem BH, de Vincenzi I, Delmas MC, et al: Pregnancies before and after HIV diagnosis in a european cohort of HIV-infected women. European Study of the Natural History in HIV Infection in Women. AIDS 14:2171, 2000

von Hertzen H, Honkanen H, Piaggio G, et al: WHO multinational study of three misoprostol regimens after mifepristone for early medical abortion. I: Efficacy. Br J Obstet Gynaecol 110:808, 2003

Ventura SJ, Abona JC, Mosher WD, Henshaw S: Revised pregnancy rates, 1990–97, and new rates for 1998–99: United States. Natl Vital Stat Rep 52:1, 2003

Warburton D, Fraser FC: Spontaneous abortion risks in man: Data from reproductive histories collected in a medical genetics unit. Am J Hum Genet 16:1, 1964

Warburton D, Stein Z, Kline J, et al: Chromosome abnormalities in spontaneous abortion: Data from the New York City study. In

Porter IH, Hook EB (eds): Human Embryonic and Fetal Death. New York, Academic Press, 1980, p 261

Weiss JL, Malone, FD, Vidaver J, et al: Threatened abortion: A risk factor for poor pregnancy outcome, a population-based screening study. Am J Obstet Gynecol 190:745, 2004

Weissman AM, Dawson JD, Rijhsinghani A, et al: Non-evidence-based use of Rho(D) immune globulin for threatened abortion by family practice and obstetric faculty physicians. J Reprod Med 47:909, 2002

Wiebe ER: Oral methotrexate compared with injected methotrexate when used with misoprostol for abortion. Am J Obstet Gynecol 181:149, 1999

Wiebe E, Dunn S, Guilbert E, et al: Comparison of abortions induced by methotrexate or mifepristone followed by misoprostol. Obstet Gynecol 99:813, 2002

Wilson RD, Kendrick V, Wittmann BK, et al: Spontaneous abortion and pregnancy outcome after normal first-trimester ultrasound examination. Obstet Gynecol 67:352, 1986

Wisborg K, Kesmodel U, Henriksen TB, et al: A prospective study of maternal smoking and spontaneous abortion. Acta Obstet Gynecol Scand 82:936, 2003

Witter FR: Negative sonographic findings followed by rapid cervical dilatation due to cervical incompetence. Obstet Gynecol 64:136, 1984

Yasuda M, Takakuwa K, Tokunaga A, et al: Prospective studies of the association between anticardiolipin antibody and outcome of pregnancy. Obstet Gynecol 86:555, 1995

Zaveri V, Aghajafari F, Amankwah K, et al: Abdominal versus vaginal cerclage after a failed transvaginal cerclage: A systematic review. Am J Obstet Gynecol 187:868, 2002

10

Ectopic Pregnancy

The blastocyst normally implants in the endometrial lining of the uterine cavity. Implantation anywhere else is an ectopic pregnancy. Almost 2 in 100 pregnancies in the United States are ectopic, and over 95 percent of these involve the oviduct. The risk of death from an extrauterine pregnancy is greater than that for pregnancy that either results in a live birth or is intentionally terminated. Moreover, the chance for a subsequent successful pregnancy is reduced after an ectopic pregnancy. With earlier diagnosis, however, both maternal survival and conservation of reproductive capacity are enhanced.

GENERAL CONSIDERATIONS

RISK FACTORS. There are a number of risk factors for tubal damage and dysfunction (Table 10–1). Prior tubal surgery, either to restore patency or to perform sterilization, confers the highest risk of obstruction (Ankum and colleagues, 1996). After one previous ectopic pregnancy, the chance of another is 7 to 15 percent (Ankum and colleagues, 1996; Coste and associates, 1991). Prior salpingitis—pelvic inflammatory disease—is a common risk factor. Peritubal adhesions subsequent to postabortal or puerperal infection, appendicitis, or endometriosis may cause tubal kinking and narrowing of the lumen and thereby increase the risk of tubal pregnancy (Coste and associates, 1991). Previous cesarean delivery has been linked to a small increase in ectopic pregnancy risk (Hemminki and Meriläinen, 1996).

Hormonal perturbations have been implicated in tubal dysfunction. An increased relative incidence of ectopic

pregnancy has been reported with use of progestin-only oral contraceptives, postovulatory high-dose estrogens to prevent pregnancy (the "morning after pill"), and following ovulation induction (Morris and Van Wagenen, 1973; Ory, 1981; Sivin, 1991).

Assisted Reproduction. Rates of tubal pregnancy are increased following gamete intrafallopian transfer (GIFT) and in vitro fertilization (IVF) to as high as 3 percent (Coste and associates, 1991; Guirgis and Craft, 1991). Moreover, "atypical" implantations—cornual, abdominal, cervical, ovarian, and heterotypic (concomitant uterine and extrauterine pregnancy)—are more common following assisted reproductive procedures.

Failed Contraception. With any form of contraceptive, the *absolute* number of ectopic pregnancies is decreased because pregnancy occurs less often. In some contraceptive failures, however, the relative number of ectopic pregnancies is increased. Examples include some forms of tubal sterilization, intrauterine devices, and progestin-only minipills (Sivin, 1991).

EPIDEMIOLOGY. The rate of ectopic pregnancies per 1000 reported pregnancies increased fourfold in the United States from 1970 to 1992. This increase was greater for nonwhite than for white women, and for both, the incidence increased with age. In 1992, there were 108,800 ectopic pregnancies in the United States—almost 2 percent of all pregnancies. Importantly, ectopic pregnancy accounted for 10 percent of all pregnancy-related deaths (Koonin and colleagues, 1997).

The incidence of ectopic pregnancy for nonwhite women is higher in every age category compared with that for whites, and this disparity increases with age (Fig. 10–1). Overall, in 1989 a nonwhite woman had a 1.4 times increased risk for ectopic pregnancy compared with a white woman. Because of the increasing use of in-office medical therapy for ectopic pregnancy, reliable data on the actual number of ectopic pregnancies in the United States are not available after 1990.

Increasing Ectopic Pregnancy Rates. The reasons for the increased number and rate of ectopic pregnancies in the United States are not entirely clear. Similar increases for the 1970s and 1980s were reported from Eastern Europe, Scandinavia, and Great Britain. Some likely causes include an increase in the following factors:

1. Prevalence of sexually transmitted tubal infection and damage (Brunham and associates, 1992; Maccato and colleagues, 1992).
2. Ascertainment through earlier diagnosis of some ectopic pregnancies otherwise destined to resorb spontaneously (Ong and Wingfield, 1999).

TABLE 10–1 Risk Factors for Ectopic Pregnancy

Risk Factor	Risk[a]
High Risk	
Tubal corrective surgery	21.0
Tubal sterilization	9.3
Previous ectopic pregnancy	8.3
In utero DES exposure	5.6
Intrauterine device	4.2–45
Documented tubal pathology	3.8–21
Moderate Risk	
Infertility	2.5–21
Previous genital infection	2.5–3.7
Multiple partners	2.1
Slight Risk	
Previous pelvic or abdominal surgery	0.93–3.8
Smoking	2.3–2.5
Douching	1.1–3.1
Intercourse before 18 years	1.6

DES = diethylstilbestrol.
[a]Single values are common odds ratio from homogeneous studies; double values are range of values from heterogeneous studies. Modified from Pisarska and Carson, 1999, with permission.

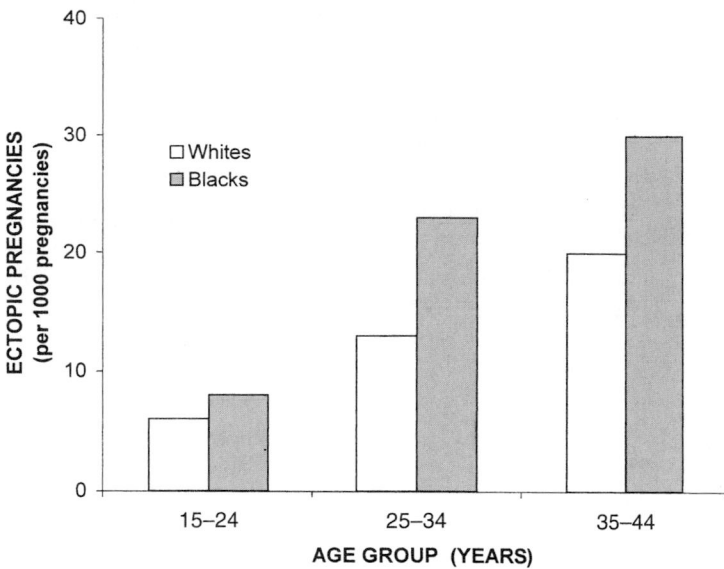

FIGURE 10–1. Ectopic pregnancy rates for white and black women—United States, 1970 through 1990. (Data from Goldner and colleagues, 1993.)

3. Popularity of contraception that predisposes failures to be ectopic.
4. Use of tubal sterilization techniques that increase the likelihood of ectopic pregnancy.
5. Use of assisted reproductive techniques.
6. Use of tubal surgery, including salpingotomy for tubal pregnancy and tuboplasty for infertility.

MORTALITY. Deaths from ectopic pregnancy in the United States decreased from a total of 63 in 1970, to 46 in 1980, and to 30 in 1987. The proportion of all maternal deaths attributed to ectopic pregnancy, however, increased from 8 percent in 1970 to 11 percent in the 3-year period ending 1990

(Koonin and associates, 1997). As shown in Figure 10–2, the death rate from ectopic pregnancy declined markedly from 1970 to 1986 and then plateaued for both white and black women. Over the same time period, the case-fatality rate decreased 10-fold, from 35 per 10,000 ectopic pregnancies in 1970 to 3.8 per 10,000 in 1989. This decrease is likely due to improved diagnosis and management. Anderson and colleagues (2004) report that about one maternal death per year due to ectopic pregnancy occurred in Michigan from 1985 to 1999. Concurrently, black women in the state had an ectopic pregnancy-related mortality ratio 18 times higher than white women. In the United States, ectopic pregnancy is the most common cause of maternal mortality in the first trimester (Centers for Disease Control and Prevention, 1995).

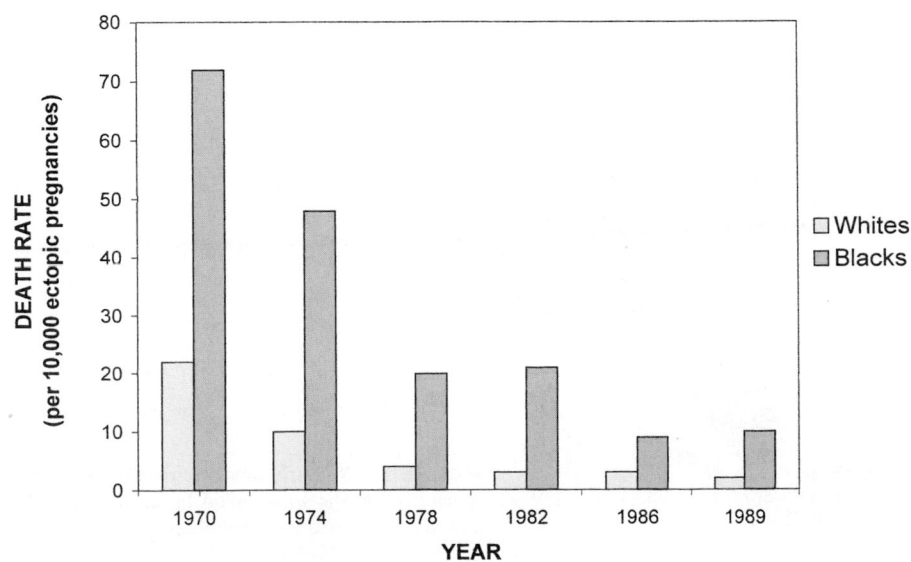

FIGURE 10–2. Death rate from ectopic pregnancy for white and black women—United States, 1970 through 1989. (From Goldner and co-workers, 1993.)

PATHOGENESIS OF ECTOPIC PREGNANCIES

TUBAL PREGNANCY. The fertilized ovum may lodge in any portion of the oviduct, giving rise to ampullary, isthmic, and interstitial tubal pregnancies (see Fig. 2–13, p. 27). In rare instances, the fertilized ovum may implant in the fimbriated extremity. The ampulla is the most frequent site, followed by the isthmus. Interstitial pregnancy accounts for only about 3 percent of all tubal gestations. From these primary types, secondary forms of tubo-abdominal, tubo-ovarian, and broad-ligament pregnancies occasionally develop.

Because the tube lacks a submucosal layer, the fertilized ovum promptly burrows through the epithelium, and the zygote comes to lie within the muscular wall. At the periphery of the zygote is a capsule of rapidly proliferating trophoblast that invades and erodes the subjacent muscularis. At the same time, maternal blood vessels are opened, and blood pours into the spaces lying within the trophoblast or between it and the adjacent tissue. The tubal wall in contact with the zygote offers only slight resistance to invasion by the trophoblast, which soon burrows through it (Fig. 10–3). The embryo or fetus in an ectopic pregnancy is often absent or stunted.

TUBAL ABORTION. The frequency of tubal abortion depends in part on the implantation site. Abortion is common in ampullary tubal pregnancy, whereas rupture is the usual outcome with isthmic pregnancy. The immediate consequence of hemorrhage is further disruption of the connection between the placenta and membranes and the tubal wall. If placental separation is complete, all of the products of conception may be extruded through the fimbriated end into the peritoneal cavity. At this point, hemorrhage may cease and symptoms eventually disappear. Some bleeding usually persists as long as products remain in the oviduct. Blood slowly trickles from the tubal fimbria into the peritoneal cavity and typically pools in the rectouterine cul-de-sac. If the fimbriated extremity is occluded, the fallopian tube may gradually become distended by blood, forming a hematosalpinx.

TUBAL RUPTURE. The invading, expanding products of conception may rupture the oviduct at any of several sites. Before sophisticated methods to measure chorionic gonadotropin were available, many cases of tubal pregnancy ended in rupture during the first trimester. As a rule, whenever there is tubal rupture in the first few weeks, the pregnancy is situated in the isthmic portion of the tube. When the fertilized ovum is implanted well within the interstitial portion, rupture usually occurs later. Rupture is usually spontaneous, but it may be caused by trauma associated with coitus or bimanual examination.

With intraperitoneal rupture, the entire conceptus may be extruded from the tube, or if the rent is small, profuse hemorrhage may occur without extrusion. In either event, the woman commonly shows signs of hypovolemia. If an early conceptus is expelled essentially undamaged into the peritoneal cavity, it may reimplant almost anywhere, establish adequate circulation, survive, and grow. This, however, occurs rarely. Most small conceptuses are resorbed. Occasionally, if larger, they may remain in the cul-de-sac for years as an encapsulated mass, or even become calcified to form a *lithopedion* (Fig. 10–4).

Abdominal Pregnancy. If only the fetus is extruded at the time of rupture, the effect on the pregnancy will vary, depending on the extent of injury sustained by the placenta. The fetus dies if the placenta is damaged appreciably, but if the greater portion of the placenta retains its tubal attachment,

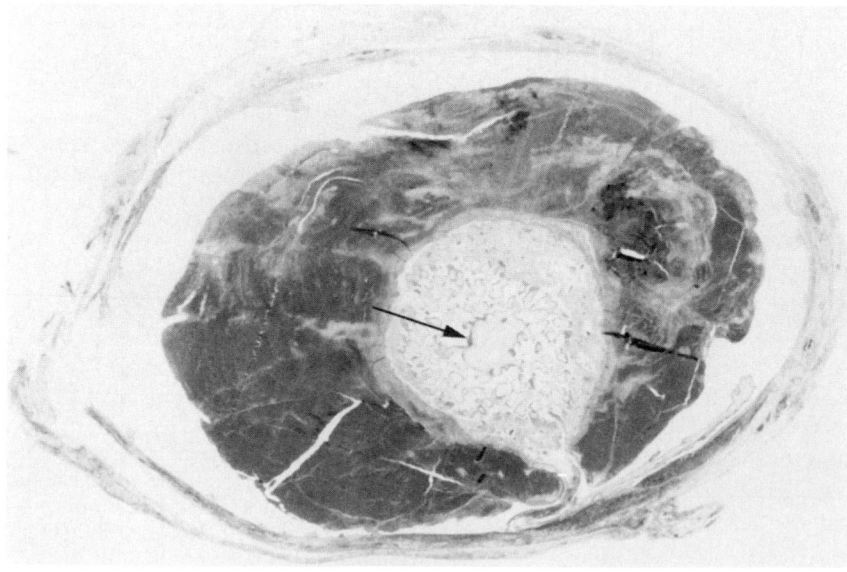

FIGURE 10–3. Early tubal pregnancy. Amnionic sac (*arrow*) is surrounded by chorionic villi, which in turn are encased in blood clot. (Courtesy of Dr. Richard Voet.)

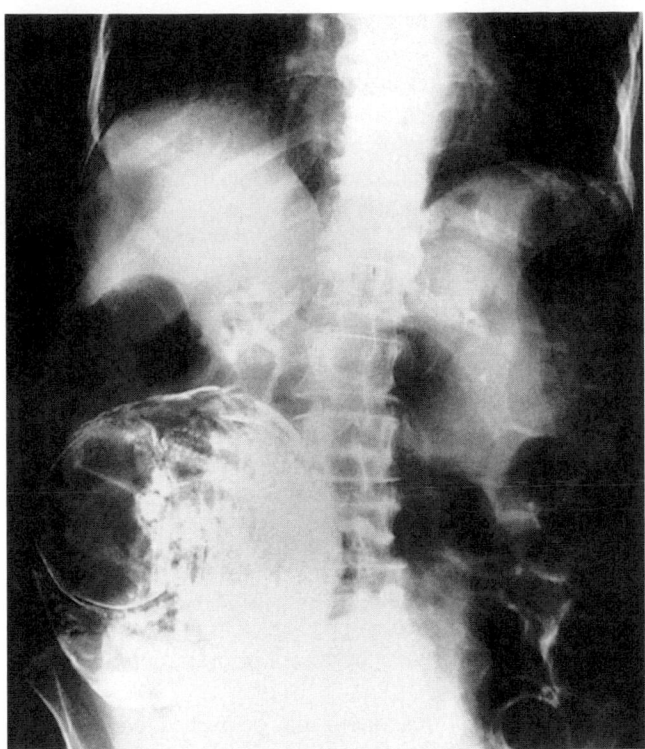

FIGURE 10–4. Abdominal radiograph of a 78-year-old woman demonstrating a lithopedion. (From Berman and Katsiyiannis, 2001, with permission.)

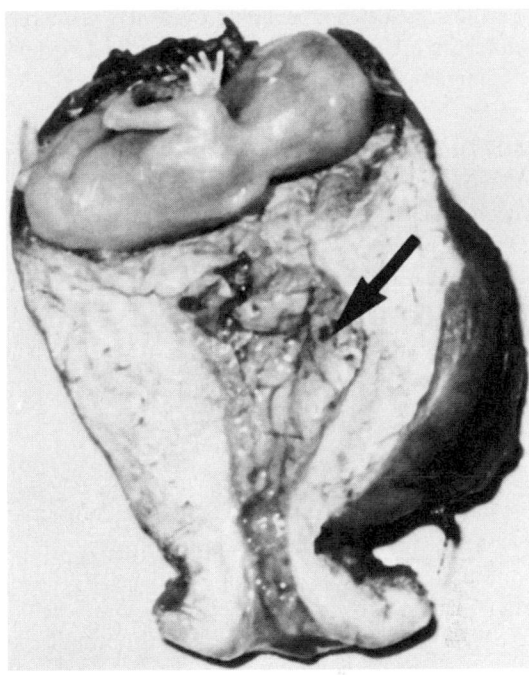

FIGURE 10–5. Right interstitial tubal pregnancy. Fetus weighed 55 g and measured 90 mm crown to rump (14 to 15 weeks' gestational age). Note abundant decidua (*arrow*) filling the uterine cavity. The patient sought medical help because of sudden severe abdominal pain with syncope following intercourse. Hysterectomy and 2000 mL blood transfusion were necessary.

further development is possible. The fetus may then survive for some time, giving rise to an abdominal pregnancy. Typically in such cases, a portion of the placenta remains attached to the tubal wall and the periphery grows beyond the tube and implants on surrounding structures.

Broad-Ligament Pregnancy. When original zygote implantation is toward the mesosalpinx, rupture may occur at the portion of the tube not immediately covered by peritoneum. The gestational contents may be extruded into a space formed between the folds of the broad ligament and then become an intraligamentous or broad-ligament pregnancy.

Interstitial Pregnancy. Implantation within the tubal segment that penetrates the uterine wall results in an interstitial or cornual pregnancy (Fig. 10–5). These account for about 3 percent of all tubal gestations. Although rupture may not occur until up to 16 weeks, all 32 cases reported to the Society of Reproductive Surgeons were diagnosed before 12 weeks (Tulandi and Al-Jaroudi, 2004). Because the implantation site is located between the ovarian and uterine arteries, there is severe hemorrhage. Many fatal ectopic pregnancies are interstitial implantations (Dorfman and associates, 1984). Moon and colleagues (2000) and Tulandi and Al-Jaroudi (2004) described a total of 56 women with an interstitial pregnancy treated with uterus-sparing laparoscopic surgery

or methotrexate. Katz and colleagues (2003) used a combined hysteroscopic and laparoscopic approach to successfully treat two such cases.

MULTIFETAL ECTOPIC PREGNANCY

Heterotypic Ectopic Pregnancy. Tubal pregnancy may be accompanied by a coexisting uterine gestation. Until recently, such heterotypic pregnancies were rare, with an incidence of 1 per 30,000 pregnancies. Currently, because of assisted reproduction, the incidence is likely 1 in 7000 overall, and following ovulation induction it may be as high as 1 in 900 (Glassner and associates, 1990). In vitro fertilization and embryo transfer also increase its incidence (Dimitry and colleagues, 1990; Marcus and associates, 1995).

A heterotypic pregnancy is more likely, and should be considered:

1. After assisted reproductive techniques.
2. With persistent or rising chorionic gonadotropin levels after dilatation and curettage for an induced or spontaneous abortion.
3. When the uterine fundus is larger than menstrual dates.
4. With more than one corpus luteum.
5. With absence of vaginal bleeding in the presence of signs and symptoms of an ectopic pregnancy.

6. When there is ultrasonographic evidence of uterine and extrauterine pregnancy (Kouyoumdjian and Kirkpatrick, 1990; Nugent, 1992).

Multifetal Tubal Pregnancy. Twin tubal pregnancy has been reported with both embryos in the same tube, as well as with one in each tube (Rolle and colleagues, 2004).

TUBO-UTERINE, TUBO-ABDOMINAL, AND TUBO-OVARIAN PREGNANCIES.

These various forms of ectopic pregnancy are very uncommon. A tubo-uterine pregnancy results from the gradual extension into the uterine cavity of products of conception that originally implanted in the interstitial portion of the tube. Tubo-abdominal pregnancy is derived from a tubal pregnancy in which the zygote, originally implanted near the fimbriated end of the tube, gradually extends into the peritoneal cavity. A tubo-ovarian pregnancy occurs when the fetal sac is adherent partly to tubal and partly to ovarian tissue. Such cases arise from zygote development in a tubo-ovarian cyst or in a tube, the fimbriated extremity of which was adherent to the ovary during or soon after fertilization.

CLINICAL FEATURES OF ECTOPIC PREGNANCY

Clinical manifestations of a tubal pregnancy are diverse and depend on whether rupture has occurred. Earlier presentation and more precise diagnostic technology have enabled identification before rupture in most cases. Usually, the woman does not suspect pregnancy, or thinks that she has a normal pregnancy, or that she is having a miscarriage. **In contemporary practice, symptoms and signs of ectopic pregnancy are often subtle or even absent.**

In what used to be considered "classical" cases, normal menstruation is replaced by variably delayed slight vaginal bleeding, or "spotting." With rupture, the woman suddenly is stricken with severe lower abdominal pain, frequently described as sharp, stabbing, or tearing in character. Vasomotor disturbances develop, ranging from vertigo to syncope. There is tenderness on abdominal palpation, and bimanual pelvic examination, especially cervical motion, causes exquisite pain. The posterior vaginal fornix may bulge because of blood in the cul-de-sac, or a tender, boggy mass may be felt to one side of the uterus. Symptoms of diaphragmatic irritation, characterized by pain in the neck or shoulder, especially on inspiration, develop in perhaps 50 percent of women with sizable intraperitoneal hemorrhage.

SYMPTOMS AND SIGNS. Because of earlier diagnosis, the presenting symptoms and physical findings in the woman with an ectopic pregnancy have changed markedly over the past two decades.

Pain. The most frequently experienced symptoms of ectopic pregnancy are pelvic and abdominal pain (95 percent) and amenorrhea with some degree of vaginal spotting or bleeding (60 to 80 percent). With more advanced gestation, Dorfman and associates (1984) reported that gastrointestinal symptoms (80 percent) and dizziness or light-headedness (58 percent) were common. With rupture, pain may be anywhere in the abdomen.

Abnormal Menstruation. Most women experience amenorrhea, however one fourth do not—they mistake the uterine bleeding that frequently occurs with tubal pregnancy for true menstruation. Although profuse vaginal bleeding is suggestive of an incomplete abortion rather than an ectopic gestation, such bleeding occasionally is seen with tubal gestations.

Abdominal and Pelvic Tenderness. Exquisite tenderness on abdominal and vaginal examination, especially on motion of the cervix, is demonstrable in over three fourths of women with ruptured or rupturing tubal pregnancies. Such tenderness, however, may be absent prior to rupture.

Uterine Changes. The uterus may be pushed to one side by an ectopic mass, or if the broad ligament is filled with blood, the uterus may be greatly displaced. In 25 percent of women, the uterus enlarges due to hormonal stimulation of pregnancy (Stabile and Grudzinskas, 1990). The degree to which the endometrium is converted to decidua in the presence of ectopic pregnancy is variable. The finding of uterine decidua without trophoblast suggests ectopic pregnancy but not absolutely, and absence of decidual tissue does not exclude it. Uterine decidual casts are passed by only 5 to 10 percent of women. Their passage may be accompanied by cramps similar to those occurring with a spontaneous abortion.

Blood Pressure and Pulse. Before rupture, vital signs generally are normal. Early responses to moderate hemorrhage range from no change in vital signs to a slight rise in blood pressure, or a vasovagal response with bradycardia and hypotension. Birkhahn and colleagues (2003) noted that in 25 women with ruptured ectopic pregnancy, the majority on presentation had a heart rate of less than 100 beats per minute and a systolic blood pressure greater than 100 mm Hg. Blood pressure will fall and pulse will rise only if bleeding continues and hypovolemia becomes significant. Stabile and Grudzinskas (1990) reviewed several reports totaling almost 2400 women with surgically confirmed ectopic pregnancy. Almost one fourth presented in shock, with a range of from 1 to 50 percent in various series.

Pelvic Mass. On bimanual examination, a pelvic mass, ranging in size from 5 to 15 cm, is palpable in about 20 percent of women. The mass is almost always either posterior or lateral to the uterus, and typically is soft and elastic. With extensive infiltration of blood into the tubal wall, however, the mass may be firm. Pain and tenderness often preclude identification of the mass by palpation. Overzealous and unnecessary bimanual examinations should be avoided so as to avert iatrogenic rupture.

Culdocentesis. This simple technique is used to identify hemoperitoneum. The cervix is pulled toward the symphysis with a tenaculum, and a long 16- or 18-gauge needle is inserted through the posterior fornix into the cul-de-sac. If present, fluid can be aspirated, however, failure to do so is interpreted only as unsatisfactory entry into the cul-de-sac and does not exclude an ectopic pregnancy, either ruptured or unruptured. Fluid containing fragments of old clots, or bloody fluid that does not clot, is compatible with the diagnosis of hemoperitoneum resulting from an ectopic pregnancy. If the blood subsequently clots, it may have been obtained from an adjacent blood vessel rather than from a bleeding ectopic pregnancy.

LABORATORY TESTS

Hemogram. After hemorrhage, depleted blood volume is restored toward normal by hemodilution over the course of a day or longer. Even after substantive hemorrhage, hemoglobin or hematocrit readings may at first show only a slight reduction. Hence, after an acute hemorrhage, a decrease in hemoglobin or hematocrit level over several hours is a more valuable index of blood loss than is the initial reading. In about half of women with ruptured ectopic pregnancies, varying degrees of leukocytosis up to $30,000/\mu L$ may be documented.

Chorionic Gonadotropin Assays. Ectopic pregnancy cannot be diagnosed by a positive pregnancy test alone. The key issue, however, is whether the woman is pregnant. Current serum and urine pregnancy tests that use enzyme-linked immunosorbent assays (ELISAs) are sensitive to levels of chorionic gonadotropin of 10 to 20 mIU/mL, and are positive in over 99 percent of ectopic pregnancies (Kalinski and Guss, 2002; Olshaker, 1996).

Serum Progesterone Levels. A single progesterone measurement can be used to establish that there is a normally developing pregnancy with high reliability. A value exceeding 25 ng/mL excludes ectopic pregnancy with 97.5-percent sensitivity (Lipscomb and co-workers, 1999a; Pisarska and colleagues, 1998). Values below 5 ng/mL occur in only 0.3 percent of normal pregnancies (Mol and colleagues, 1998). Thus, values this low suggest either an intrauterine pregnancy with a dead fetus or an ectopic pregnancy. In many cases, however, progesterone levels range from 5 to 25 ng/mL and are inconclusive (McCord and colleagues, 1996).

ULTRASOUND IMAGING. Ultrasonic imaging is indispensable to confirm the clinical diagnosis of suspected ectopic gestation, its size, and its location.

Abdominal Sonography. Identification of pregnancy products in the fallopian tube is difficult using abdominal sonography. If a gestational sac is clearly identified within the uterine cavity, ectopic pregnancy rarely coexists. Moreover, with sonographic absence of a uterine pregnancy, a positive pregnancy test result, fluid in the cul-de-sac, and an abnormal pelvic mass, ectopic pregnancy is almost certain (Romero and associates, 1988). Unfortunately, ultrasonic findings suggestive of early uterine pregnancy may be apparent in some cases of ectopic pregnancy. A small sac suggestive of a very early pregnancy or a collapsed sac suggesting a dead fetus may actually be a blood clot or decidual cast (Coleman and colleagues, 1985). A uterine pregnancy usually is not recognized using abdominal ultrasound until 5 to 6 menstrual weeks or 28 days after timed ovulation (Batzer and co-workers, 1983). Conversely, demonstration of an adnexal or cul-de-sac mass by sonography is not necessarily helpful. Corpus luteum cysts and matted bowel can have the sonographic appearance of tubal pregnancies. Fetal heart action clearly outside the uterine cavity provides firm evidence of an ectopic pregnancy.

Vaginal Sonography. There has been much improvement in the early diagnosis of ectopic pregnancy using vaginal sonography. Its use results in earlier and more specific diagnoses of uterine pregnancy than abdominal sonography, and it has become the imaging method of choice in early pregnancy. Using a vaginal transducer allows ultrasonic detection of a uterine gestation as early as 1 week after missed menses. When serum chorionic gonadotropin (β-hCG) levels exceed 1000 mIU/mL, a gestational sac is seen half the time (De Cherney and Eichhorn, 1996). Criteria include identification of a 1- to 3-mm or larger gestational sac, eccentrically placed in the uterus, and surrounded by a decidual–chorionic reaction. A fetal pole within the sac is diagnostic, especially when accompanied by fetal heart action.

Vaginal sonography also is used to detect adnexal masses. An ectopic pregnancy may be missed, however, when a tubal mass is small or obscured by bowel (Cacciatore and colleagues, 1990). The reported sensitivity of vaginal sonography for the diagnosis of ectopic pregnancy ranges widely, from only 20 percent to as high as 80 percent (Brown and Doubilet, 1994). Fluid seen in the cul-de-sac increases the likely diagnosis of ectopic pregnancy, and depending on the amount, this likelihood may exceed 50 percent if the fluid is echogenic (Dart and colleagues, 2002).

DIAGNOSIS OF ECTOPIC PREGNANCY

MULTI-MODALITY DIAGNOSIS. During the past three decades, as methods of identifying ectopic pregnancy have evolved and been refined, the majority of ectopic pregnancies—perhaps 80 percent—are diagnosed before

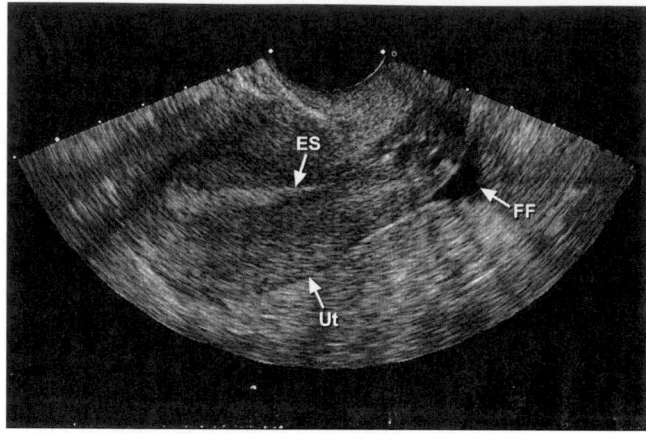

A

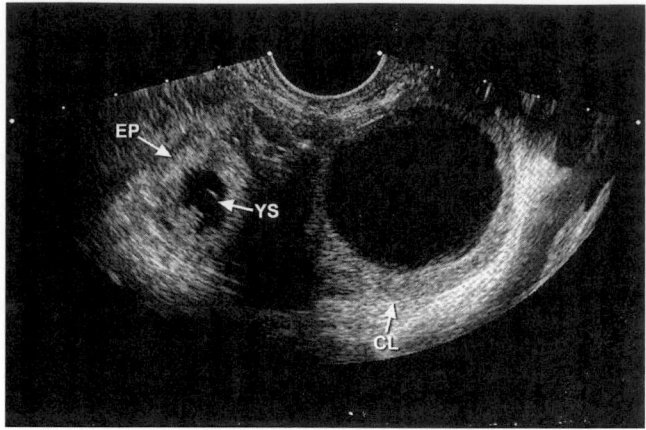

B

FIGURE 10–6. Vaginal sonogram of an ectopic pregnancy. **A.** The uterus (Ut) is seen with a normal endometrial stripe (ES). A small amount of free fluid (FF) is visible in the posterior cul-de-sac. **B.** The tubal ectopic pregnancy (EP) with its yolk sac (YS) is seen along with a corpus luteum (CL) cyst. (Photograph courtesy of Dr. Michelle Robbin.)

rupture. Concurrent with this evolution, the death rate from ectopic pregnancy has decreased appreciably (see Fig. 10–2).

Several algorithms for the diagnosis of ectopic pregnancy have been proposed (Barnhart, 1994, 1999; Kaplan, 1996; McCord, 1996; Stovall, 1989, 1990, 1992, and all their colleagues). All use five key components:

1. Vaginal sonography.
2. Serum β-hCG—both the initial level and the pattern of subsequent rise or decline.
3. Serum progesterone.
4. Uterine curettage.
5. Laparoscopy and, less frequently, laparotomy.

All diagnostic strategies for the unruptured ectopic pregnancy involve trade-offs. For example, strategies that maximize detection of ectopic pregnancy may result in the interruption of one normal pregnancy for every 100 women evaluated. Conversely, those that reduce the potential for interruption of a normal uterine pregnancy will miss more ectopic pregnancies (Gracia and Barnhart, 2001). Those that do not employ curettage result in unnecessary medical or surgical therapy for ectopic pregnancy (Barnhart and colleagues, 2002). **The choice of diagnostic algorithm applies only to hemodynamically stable women; those with presumed rupture should undergo prompt surgical therapy.** In a woman in whom ectopic pregnancy is suspected because of pain, bleeding, and a positive pregnancy test, performance of vaginal sonography is a logical first step. If a live uterine gestation is present, ectopic pregnancy is extremely unlikely. A heterotypic pregnancy is, of course, the rare exception (Hirsch and associates, 1992). Alternatively, if the uterus is empty, an ectopic pregnancy can be diagnosed based on

visualization of an adnexal mass separate from the ovaries (Fig. 10–6).

In the event of a nondiagnostic study, subsequent management can be based on serial serum β-hCG values and repeat vaginal sonography. A number of investigators have described *discriminatory β-hCG levels* (Bateman, 1990; Cacciatore, 1990; Fossum, 1988; Goldstein, 1988; Nyberg, 1987, and all their associates). Above these levels, failure to visualize a uterine pregnancy by transvaginal ultrasound indicates with high reliability that the pregnancy is either ectopic or nonviable. In a study by Barnhart and colleagues (1994), an empty uterus with a serum β-hCG concentration of 1500 mIU/mL or higher was 100-percent accurate in excluding a live uterine pregnancy. Thus, if the initial β-hCG exceeds the discriminatory level, and no live intrauterine pregnancy is identified by vaginal sonography, the differential diagnosis is narrowed to a uterine pregnancy with a dead fetus versus an ectopic pregnancy. Early multifetal gestation, of course, remains a possibility. Uterine curettage will distinguish an ectopic from a nonliving uterine pregnancy. If an embryo, fetus, or placenta is identified, the diagnosis is apparent. When none of these is identified, tubal pregnancy is a probability.

If the initial β-hCG level is below the discriminatory value, early uterine pregnancy is a possibility, and serial assays of β-hCG, in conjunction with repeat vaginal sonography, may prove useful. Kadar and Romero (1987) confirmed earlier work and demonstrated that in women with normal pregnancies, mean doubling time for β-hCG in serum was approximately 48 hours, and the lowest normal value for this increase was 66 percent (Table 10–2). In a series of 287 pregnant women, Barnhart and co-workers more recently (2004) reported a somewhat lower 48-hour minimum rise for a live intrauterine pregnancy of 53 percent, and a 24-hr minimum rise of 24 percent. Kadar and Romero concluded that failure

TABLE 10-2 Lower Normal Limits for Percentage Increase of Serum β-hCG during Early Uterine Pregnancy

Sampling Interval (days)	Increase from Initial Value (%)
1	29
2	66
3	114
4	175
5	255

Modified from Kadar and co-workers (1981) with permission.

to maintain this minimum rate of increased β-hCG production, along with an empty uterus, was suggestive of an ectopic pregnancy. Thus, appropriately selected women in whom ectopic pregnancy is suspected, but whose initial β-hCG is below the discriminatory level, may be followed expectantly. They are seen at 2- to 3-day intervals for further evaluation. If the β-hCG level rises inappropriately, plateaus, or exceeds the discriminatory level without evidence of a uterine pregnancy by vaginal sonography, a live uterine pregnancy can be excluded. Then, distinction between nonliving uterine versus an ectopic pregnancy is made by uterine curettage, or in some cases, by endometrial biopsy. Barnhart and associates (2003) reported that biopsy was less sensitive than curettage.

A single measurement of serum progesterone may clarify the diagnosis when ectopic pregnancy is suspected (McCord and colleagues, 1996; Stovall and associates, 1989, 1992). Its accuracy is crude, and customary thresholds of less than 5 ng/mL and greater than 25 ng/mL neither absolutely refute nor confirm a living uterine pregnancy. Moreover, the capacity to expeditiously measure serum progesterone is not available at all institutions. Another pitfall is that pregnancy using assisted reproductive techniques may be associated with higher than usual serum progesterone levels (Perkins and associates, 2000). This being said, serum levels of at least 25 ng/mL after spontaneous conception provide reassurance that an ectopic pregnancy is *unlikely*. This finding may negate the need for vaginal sonography. Buckley and colleagues (2000), however, reported that serum progesterone was conclusive in only one fourth of women undergoing evaluation for ectopic pregnancy.

SURGICAL DIAGNOSIS

Laparoscopy. Direct visualization of the fallopian tubes and pelvis by diagnostic laparoscopy offers a reliable diagnosis in most cases of suspected ectopic pregnancy, and a ready transition to definitive operative therapy. Compared with laparotomy, laparoscopy is more cost-effective, and there is a shorter postoperative recovery (Gray and colleagues, 1995).

At times, identification of an early unruptured tubal pregnancy may be difficult, even if the tube is fully visualized.

In spite of the low morbidity and quick recovery time, laparoscopy is not without risks or cost. Thus laparoscopy usually is performed when, on the basis of noninvasive test or curettage results, the diagnosis of ectopic pregnancy is fairly certain and medical therapy is not planned.

Laparotomy. Open abdominal surgery is preferred when the woman is hemodynamically unstable, or when laparoscopy is not feasible. Laparotomy should not be delayed while laparoscopy is performed in a woman with obvious abdominal hemorrhage that requires immediate definitive treatment.

TREATMENT AND PROGNOSIS

Over the past two decades, earlier diagnosis and treatment have allowed definitive management of unruptured ectopic pregnancy even before the onset of symptoms. Importantly, early diagnosis, although contributing to a higher incidence, has made many cases of ectopic pregnancy amenable to medical therapy, which is more cost-effective than surgical therapy (Alexander and associates, 1996; Morlock and colleagues, 2000).

ANTI-D IMMUNOGLOBULIN. D-negative women with an ectopic pregnancy who are not sensitized to D-antigen should be given anti-D immunoglobulin.

SURGICAL MANAGEMENT. Higher subsequent pregnancy and lower recurrent ectopic pregnancy rates are observed in women in whom surgery is performed prior to rupture. Laparoscopy is preferred over laparotomy unless the woman is unstable (Tulandi and Saleh, 1999). Even though reproductive outcome is similar, including rates of uterine and recurrent ectopic pregnancies, laparoscopy is more cost-effective and has a shorter recovery time—1.3 versus 3.1 days (Tay and colleagues, 2000).

Tubal surgery for ectopic pregnancy is considered *conservative* when there is tubal salvage. Examples include salpingostomy, salpingotomy, and fimbrial expression of the ectopic pregnancy. *Radical surgery* is defined by salpingectomy. Conservative therapy may increase the subsequent rate of uterine pregnancy at the expense, however, of higher rates of persistently functioning trophoblast (Bangsgaard and colleagues, 2003).

Salpingostomy. This procedure is used to remove a small pregnancy that is usually less than 2 cm in length and located in the distal third of the fallopian tube (Fig. 10–7). A linear incision, 10 to 15 mm in length or less, is made on the antimesenteric border immediately over the ectopic pregnancy. The products usually will extrude from the incision and can be carefully removed or flushed out. Small bleeding sites are controlled with needlepoint electrocautery or laser, and the incision is left unsutured to heal by secondary intention. This procedure is readily performed through a laparoscope.

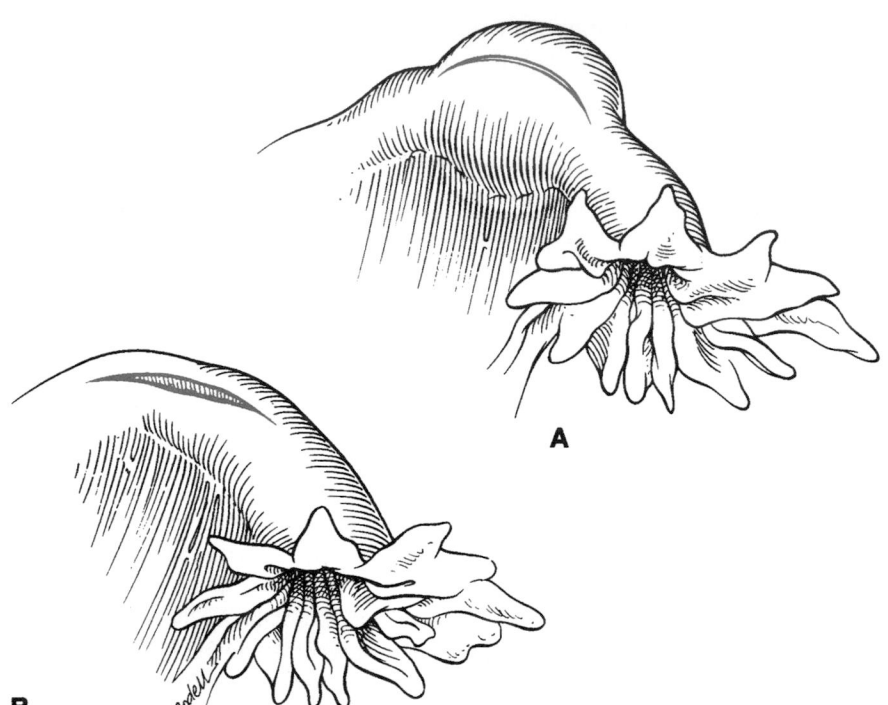

FIGURE 10–7. Linear salpingostomy for ectopic pregnancy. **A.** Linear incision for removal of a small tubal pregnancy in the distal third of the fallopian tube. **B.** Hemostasis is by cautery or laser, and the incision is not sutured. If the incision is closed, the procedure is termed a *salpingotomy.*

Salpingotomy. Seldom performed today, salpingotomy is essentially the same procedure as salpingostomy except that the incision is closed with 7-0 Vicryl or similar suture. According to Tulandi and Saleh (1999), there is no difference in prognosis with or without suturing.

Salpingectomy. Tubal resection can be performed through an operative laparoscope and may be used for both ruptured and unruptured ectopic pregnancies. When removing the oviduct, it is advisable to excise a wedge of the outer third (or less) of the interstitial portion of the tube. This so-called *cornual resection* is done in an effort to minimize the rare recurrence of pregnancy in the tubal stump. Even with cornual resection, however, a subsequent interstitial pregnancy may not be prevented (Kalchman and Meltzer, 1966).

Segmental Resection and Anastomosis. Resection of the ectopic mass and tubal reanastomosis is sometimes used for an unruptured isthmic pregnancy because salpingostomy may cause scarring and subsequent narrowing of the small isthmic lumen (Stangel and associates, 1976).

Persistent Trophoblast. Following salpingostomy, serum β-hCG levels usually fall quickly and are at about 10 percent of preoperative values by day 12 (Hajenius and colleagues, 1995; Vermesh and associates, 1988). Persistent ectopic pregnancy is the result of incomplete removal of trophoblast and complicates 5 to 20 percent of salpingostomies (Graczykowski and Mishell, 1997). If the postoperative day 1 serum β-hCG value is less than 50 percent of the preoperative

value, then persistent ectopic trophoblast rarely is a problem (Spandorfer and co-workers, 1997). According to Seifer (1997), factors that increase the risk of persistent ectopic pregnancy include:

1. Small pregnancies, viz., less than 2 cm.
2. Early therapy, viz., before 42 menstrual days.
3. β-hCG serum levels exceeding 3000 mIU/mL.
4. Implantation medial to the salpingostomy site.

In the face of persistent or increasing β-hCG, additional surgical or medical therapy is necessary.

MEDICAL MANAGEMENT

Systemic Methotrexate. This antineoplastic drug acts as a folic acid antagonist and is highly effective against rapidly proliferating trophoblast (see Chap. 11, p. 282). Tanaka and associates (1982) were first to recommend use of methotrexate for an ectopic interstitial pregnancy. Since then, there have been numerous reports describing successful treatment of all varieties of ectopic pregnancy using a number of methotrexate regimens. In the largest single-center series, Lipscomb and colleagues (1999a) reported a 91-percent success rate in 350 women given methotrexate therapy. Of these, 283 women were given a single dose of methotrexate, 60 women received two doses, six women, three doses, and one woman, four doses.

Active intra-abdominal hemorrhage is a contraindication to chemotherapy. The size of the ectopic mass is also important, and Pisarska and colleagues (1998) recommend that

TABLE 10–3 Methotrexate Therapy for Primary Treatment of Ectopic Pregnancy

Regimen	Follow-up

Single Dose[a]
Methotrexate, 50 mg/m^2 IM
	Measure β-hCG levels days 4 and 7:
	  If difference is $\geq$ 15 percent, repeat weekly until
	    undetectable
	  If difference < 15 percent, repeat methotrexate dose and
	    begin new day 1
	  If fetal cardiac activity present day 7, repeat methotrexate
	    dose, begin new day 1
	  Surgical treatment if β-hCG levels not decreasing or fetal
	    cardiac activity persists after three doses of methotrexate

Variable Dose Methotrexate, 1 mg/kg IM, days 1, 3, 5, 7 Leukovorin, 0.1 mg/kg IM, days 2, 4, 6, 8	Continue alternate-day injections until β-hCG levels decrease 15 percent in 48 hr, or four doses methotrexate given Then, weekly β-hCG until undetectable

β-hCG = β-subunit human chorionic gonadotropin; IM = intramuscularly.
[a] Preferred by editors.
Regimens from Buster and Pisarska (1999), Lipscomb and co-workers (1999b), and Pisarska and colleagues (1998, 1999).

methotrexate not be used if the pregnancy is more than 4 cm. Success is greatest if the gestation is less than 6 weeks, the tubal mass is not more than 3.5 cm in diameter, the fetus is dead, and the β-hCG is less than 15,000 mIU/mL (Lipscomb and colleagues, 1999a; Stovall, 1995). According to the American College of Obstetricians and Gynecologists (1998), contraindications include breast feeding, immunodeficiency, alcoholism, liver or renal disease, blood dyscrasias, active pulmonary disease, and peptic ulcer.

PATIENT SELECTION. Candidates for methotrexate therapy must be hemodynamically stable. They are instructed that:

1. Medical therapy fails in at least 5 to 10 percent of cases, and this rate is higher in pregnancies past 6 weeks' gestation or with a tubal mass greater than 4 cm in diameter.
2. Failure of medical therapy requires retreatment, either medically or with elective surgery. If tubal rupture occurs—a 5- to 10-percent chance—emergency surgery is necessary.
3. If the woman is treated as an outpatient, rapid transportation must be reliably available.

4. Signs and symptoms of tubal rupture such as vaginal bleeding, abdominal and pleuritic pain, weakness, dizziness, or syncope must be reported promptly.
5. Until the ectopic pregnancy is resolved, sexual intercourse is prohibited, alcohol avoided, and folic acid supplements—including prenatal vitamins—should not be taken.

DOSE AND ADMINISTRATION. The two general schemes used for methotrexate administration for ectopic pregnancy are shown in Table 10–3. Although single-dose treatment is easier to administer and monitor than variable-dose methotrexate therapy, it is associated with a higher failure rate, defined as persistent ectopic pregnancy (Table 10–4). In most studies, the methotrexate dose was 50 mg/m^2.

MONITORING TOXICITY. Most regimens are associated with minimal laboratory changes and symptoms, although toxicity may be severe. Kooi and Kock (1992) reviewed 16 studies that reported side effects. All adverse effects were resolved by 3 to 4 days after methotrexate was discontinued. The most common were liver involvement (12 percent), stomatitis (6 percent), and gastroenteritis (1 percent). One woman

TABLE 10–4 Success Rates and Subsequent Pregnancy Following Primary Treatment for Ectopic Pregnancy

Treatment	Studies (no.)	Total Patients	Treatment Success (%)[a]	Tubal Patency (%)[b]	Subsequent Pregnancy (%)	
					Uterine	Ectopic
Conservative laparoscopic surgery	32	1626	93	76	57	13
Variable-dose methotrexate	12	338	93	75	58	7
Single-dose methotrexate	7	393	87	81	61	8

[a] Success defined as resolution of ectopic pregnancy with initial treatment scheme.
[b] Only 12–55% of all women tested for patency.

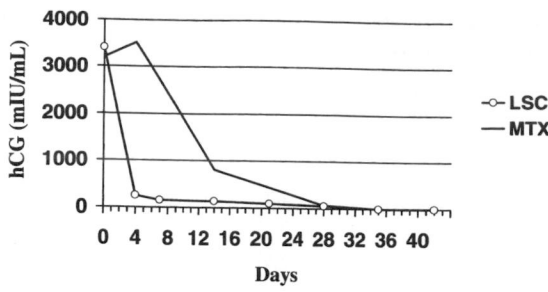

FIGURE 10–8. Comparative pattern of resolution of serum human chorionic gonadotropin (β-hCG) levels after laparoscopic salpingostomy (LSC) and single-dose methotrexate (MTX) treatment of unruptured ectopic pregnancy. (From Saraj and colleagues, 1998, with permission.)

had bone marrow depression. Case reports also describe life-threatening neutropenia and fever, transient drug-induced pneumonitis, and alopecia (Buster and Pisarska, 1999).

MONITORING EFFICACY OF THERAPY. Serum β-hCG levels are the most widely used marker to monitor response to both medical and surgical therapy. Saraj and colleagues (1998) reported serum β-hCG data for women enrolled in their randomized trial. After linear salpingostomy, serum β-hCG levels declined rapidly over days and then more gradually, with a mean resolution time of 20 days. In contrast, after a single intramuscular injection of methotrexate, mean serum β-hCG levels **rose** for the first 4 days, and then gradually declined, with a mean resolution time of 27 days (Fig. 10–8). Lipscomb and colleagues (1998) treated 287 women successfully with methotrexate and found the average time to resolution, defined as serum hCG level less than 15 mIU/mL, was 34 days. The longest time was 109 days.

As shown in Table 10–3, monitoring single-dose therapy calls for serum β-hCG determinations at 4 and 7 days. With variable-dose methotrexate, levels are measured at 48-hour intervals until they fall more than 15 percent. After successful treatment, weekly serum β-hCG determinations are measured until undetectable. Outpatient surveillance is preferred, but if there is any question of safety or compliance, the woman is hospitalized. Failure is judged when the β-hCG level plateaus or rises or tubal rupture occurs. Tubal rupture can occur in the face of declining β-hCG levels.

PERSISTENT ECTOPIC PREGNANCY. Conservative therapy carries with it the risk of initial treatment failure, which requires either additional methotrexate therapy or surgical removal. In three randomized trials, 5 to 14 percent of women treated initially with systemic methotrexate ultimately required surgery, whereas 4 to 20 percent of those treated with laparoscopy eventually received methotrexate for persistent trophoblast (Fernandez, 1998; Hajenius, 1997; Saraj, 1998, and their associates).

An important observation is that 65 to 75 percent of women initially given methotrexate will have increasing pain beginning several days after therapy. This *separation pain* generally is mild and relieved by nonnarcotic analgesics. In a series of 258 women treated with single-dose methotrexate, 53 (20 percent) had pain severe enough to require evaluation in the clinic or emergency room. Ultimately, 10 of these 53 underwent surgical exploration (Lipscomb and colleagues, 1999b). In women with worrisome pain after medical treatment for ectopic pregnancy, careful clinical observation—as an inpatient, if necessary—is warranted. Assessment of serial hematocrits and serum β-hCG levels coupled with vaginal sonography can be used to identify those who require surgical intervention.

Rupture of persistent ectopic pregnancy is the most catastrophic form of primary therapy failure. Its incidence is 5 to 10 percent in women initially treated medically. Lipscomb and associates (1998) described a 14-day mean time to rupture, but one woman had tubal rupture 32 days after single-dose methotrexate therapy.

OTHER TREATMENTS

Direct Injection. Various cytotoxic drugs have been injected directly into the ectopic mass, either by laparoscopy or transvaginally by culdocentesis. However, because of the relative effectiveness of systemic therapy for ectopic pregnancy, its ease of delivery, and widespread experience, direct injection is infrequently employed.

Oral Methotrexate Therapy. Recently Lipscomb and colleagues (2002) evaluated oral methotrexate for the treatment of ectopic pregnancy in two divided doses 2 hours apart for a total dose of 60 mg/m². They reported that the oral medication had a lower success rate and a greater necessity for repeated dosing compared with the single-dose intramuscular regimen.

Expectant Management. Some practitioners choose to observe very early tubal pregnancies that are associated with stable or falling serum β-hCG levels. As many as one third of women with ectopic pregnancies will present with declining β-hCG levels (Shalev and colleagues, 1995). Stovall and Ling (1992) restrict expectant management to women with these criteria:

1. Decreasing serial β-hCG levels.
2. Tubal pregnancies only.
3. No evidence of intra-abdominal bleeding or rupture as assessed by vaginal sonography.
4. Diameter of the ectopic mass not greater than 3.5 cm.

Trio and colleagues (1995) reported spontaneous resolution of ectopic pregnancy in 49 of 67 selected women (73 percent) treated expectantly. Resolution without treatment was more likely if the initial serum β-hCG level was less than 1000 mIU/mL. In another study of 60 women managed expectantly, Shalev and associates (1995) reported spontaneous resolution in 28 (48 percent). **The potentially grave consequences of tubal rupture, coupled with the established safety of medical and surgical therapy, require that expectant therapy be undertaken only in appropriately selected and counseled women.**

ABDOMINAL PREGNANCY

Almost all cases of abdominal pregnancy follow early rupture or abortion of a tubal pregnancy into the peritoneal cavity. The Centers for Disease Control and Prevention estimated that the incidence of abdominal pregnancy is 1 in 10,000 live births (Atrash and co-workers, 1987). At Parkland Hospital, where ectopic pregnancy is common, advanced abdominal pregnancy is rare and encountered in perhaps 1 in 25,000 births. Risk factors for abdominal pregnancy are the same as for ectopic pregnancy in general.

Typically, the growing placenta, after penetrating the oviduct wall, maintains its tubal attachment but gradually encroaches upon and implants in the neighboring serosa. Meanwhile, the fetus continues to grow within the peritoneal cavity. Occasionally, the placenta is found in the general region of

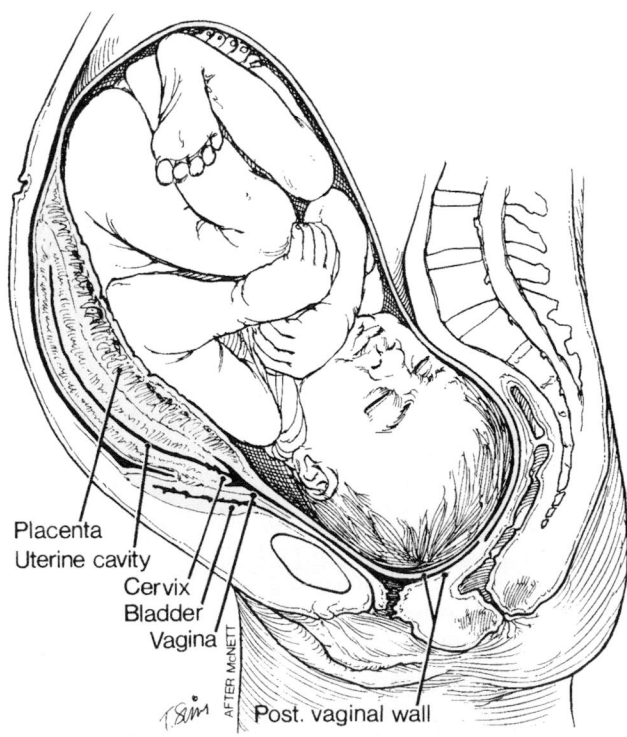

Placenta
Uterine cavity
Cervix
Bladder
Vagina

AFTER McNETT

Post. vaginal wall

FIGURE 10–9. Abdominal pregnancy at term. The placenta is implanted on the posterior wall of the uterus and broad ligament. The enlarged, flattened uterus is located just beneath the anterior abdominal wall. The cervix and vagina are dislodged anteriorly and superiorly by the large fetal head in the cul-de-sac.

the oviduct and over the posterior aspect of the broad ligament and uterus (Fig. 10–9). In other cases, after tubal rupture, the conceptus reimplants elsewhere in the peritoneal cavity.

DIAGNOSIS. Because early rupture or abortion of a tubal pregnancy is the usual antecedent of an abdominal pregnancy, in retrospect, a suggestive history can usually be obtained. These include spotting or irregular bleeding along with abdominal pain that usually was most prominent in one or both lower quadrants (Costa and associates, 1991). Women with an established abdominal pregnancy are likely to be uncomfortable but not sufficiently so to warrant thorough evaluation. Nausea, vomiting, flatulence, constipation, diarrhea, and abdominal pain may each be present in varying degrees. Multiparas may state that the pregnancy does not "feel right." Late in pregnancy, fetal movements may cause pain.

Abnormal fetal positions frequently can be palpated, but the ease of palpating fetal parts is not a reliable sign. Fetal parts sometimes feel exceedingly close to the examining fingers even in normal pregnancies, especially in thin, multiparous women. As depicted in Figure 10–9, the cervix is usually displaced, depending in part on the fetal position, and it may dilate, but appreciable effacement is unusual. The uterus may be outlined over the lower part of the pregnancy mass. Small parts or the fetal head may occasionally be palpated through the vaginal fornices and identified as clearly outside the uterus.

Laboratory Tests. An unexplained transient anemia early in pregnancy may accompany the initial tubal rupture or abortion. An otherwise unexplained increase in the serum alpha-fetoprotein value sometimes is found (Bombard, 1994; Costa, 1991; el Kareh, 1993; Jackson, 1993, and their associates).

Sonography. Ultrasonic findings with an abdominal pregnancy most often do not allow an unequivocal diagnosis to be made. Oligohydramnios is common but nonspecific. In some suspected cases, however, ultrasound findings may be diagnostic; for example, if the fetal head is seen to lie immediately adjacent to the maternal bladder with no interposed uterine tissue (Kurtz and associates, 1982). Even with ideal conditions, however, a sonographic diagnosis of abdominal pregnancy is missed in half of cases (Costa and associates, 1991).

Magnetic Resonance Imaging. This technique can be used to confirm abdominal pregnancy following a suspicious ultrasound examination. It has been described as very accurate and specific by some (Harris and associates, 1988; Wagner and Burchardt, 1995). Even so, in our institutions, abdominal pregnancy has been incorrectly diagnosed as a placenta previa, and an intrauterine pregnancy with degenerating fibroids has been misdiagnosed as an abdominal pregnancy.

Computed Tomography. Costa and associates (1991) maintain that computed tomography is superior to magnetic resonance imaging, but its use is limited because of the concern for fetal radiation. In cases of fetal demise, however, computed tomography may be diagnostic and should be considered (Glew and Sivanesaratnam, 1989).

FETAL OUTCOME. Fetal salvage in an abdominal pregnancy is much the exception rather than the rule, and surviving fetuses may be abnormal. However, in his extensive review of abdominal pregnancies, Stevens (1993) found that survival of infants born after 30 weeks was 63 percent. Moreover, fetal malformations and deformations were only 20 percent. The most common deformations were facial or cranial asymmetry, or both, and various joint abnormalities. The most common malformations were limb deficiency and central nervous system anomalies.

MANAGEMENT. An abdominal pregnancy is life-threatening, and clinical management depends on the gestational age at diagnosis. Some practitioners await fetal viability with in-hospital expectant management if pregnancy is diagnosed after 24 weeks (Cartwright and associates, 1986; Hage and colleagues, 1988). Such management carries a risk for sudden and life-threatening intra-abdominal bleeding. Because of this risk, termination generally is indicated when the diagnosis of abdominal pregnancy is made. In cases where amnionic fluid volume is minimal or absent, and in cases less than 24 weeks, conservative treatment rarely is justified because fetal survival is extremely poor.

The natural history was described in older literature: If the fetus died after reaching a size too large to be resorbed, it would undergo suppuration, mummification, or calcification. If bacteria gained access to the gestational products, particularly when they were adherent to the intestines, this resulted in suppuration. Eventually, the abscess would rupture, and if the woman did not die of peritonitis and septicemia, fetal parts would eventually be extruded through the abdominal wall or more commonly into the intestine or bladder (Emembolu, 1989). In some cases, mummification and lithopedion formation would ensue, and calcified products of conception would be carried for years (see Fig. 10–4). Much more rarely, the fetus would be converted into a yellowish, greasy mass to which the term *adipocere* is applied.

Surgery for abdominal pregnancy may precipitate torrential hemorrhage due to the lack of constriction of hypertrophied blood vessels after placental separation. Condition permitting, management of presumed abdominal pregnancy is best done in a facility with trauma center capabilities. It is essential to have adequate blood immediately available. Preoperatively, two intravenous infusion systems, each capable of delivering large volumes of fluid at a rapid rate, should be functioning. Techniques for monitoring the adequacy of the circulation should be employed, as described in Chapter 35 (see p. 839). If time allows, a mechanical bowel preparation should be done. For optimal exposure, laparotomy generally is performed through a vertical midline incision. In general, the infant should be delivered, and the cord severed close to the placenta.

Management of the Placenta. Partial placental separation can develop spontaneously or, more likely, in the course of the operation while attempting to locate the exact site of placental attachment. Therefore, it is best to avoid unnecessary exploration of surrounding organs. If it is obvious that the placenta can be safely removed, or if there is already hemorrhage from its implantation site, then removal begins immediately. When possible, blood vessels supplying the placenta should be ligated first.

Often, leaving the placenta in place represents the lesser of two evils. This decreases the chance of immediate life-threatening hemorrhage, but at the expense of long-term sequelae. Unfortunately, when left in the abdominal cavity, the placenta commonly causes infection with abscesses, adhesions, intestinal obstruction, and wound dehiscence (Bergstrom and colleagues, 1998; Martin and associates, 1988). Partial urethral obstruction with reversible hydronephrosis has been described (Weiss and Stone, 1994). In another report, Piering and colleagues (1993) described persistent preeclampsia for 99 days until the placenta was removed! In these cases, surgical removal becomes inevitable.

If the placenta is left, its involution may be monitored using ultrasound and serum β-hCG levels (France and Jackson, 1980; Martin and McCaul, 1990). We have used color Doppler ultrasound to follow changes in blood flow to the placenta. In some cases, and usually depending on its size, placental function rapidly declines, and the placenta is resorbed. In one case described by Belfar and associates (1986), placental resorption took over 5 years. Methotrexate use is controversial. It has been recommended to hasten involution but may cause accelerated placental destruction with accumulation of necrotic tissue and infection with abscess formation (Rahman and associates, 1982).

Arterial Catheterization and Embolization. Percutaneous femoral artery catheterization and pelvic angiography, followed by embolization of specific bleeding sites, is discussed in Chapter 35 (see p. 836). This has been lifesaving in some instances of massive pelvic hemorrhage (Kivikoski and associates, 1988; Martin and colleagues, 1990). When the diagnosis is made preoperatively, Kerr and associates (1993) advocate transcatheter embolization of major feeder vessels immediately prior to surgical intervention.

Maternal Prognosis. Maternal mortality is increased substantively compared with normal pregnancy. With appropriate preoperative planning, however, maternal mortality has been reduced from approximately 20 percent to less than 5 percent in the past 20 years (Stevens, 1993).

OVARIAN PREGNANCY

Ectopic pregnancy implanted in the ovary is rare. Traditional risk factors for ovarian ectopic pregnancy are similar to those for tubal pregnancy. Use of an intrauterine contraceptive device seems to be disproportionately associated with ovarian pregnancy (Gray and Ruffolo, 1978; Pisarska and Carson, 1999). Although the ovary can accommodate itself more readily than the fallopian tube to the expanding pregnancy, rupture at an early period is the usual consequence. Nonetheless, there are recorded cases in which ovarian pregnancy went to term, and a few infants survived (Williams and associates, 1982).

DIAGNOSIS. Findings are likely to mimic those of a tubal pregnancy or a bleeding corpus luteum. Serious bleeding is seen in about one third of cases. At surgery, early ovarian pregnancies are likely to be considered corpus luteum cysts or a bleeding corpus luteum. Use of vaginal ultrasound has resulted in the more frequent diagnosis of unruptured ovarian pregnancies (Marcus and Brinsden, 1993; Sidek and colleagues, 1994). Such early diagnosis may allow for a medical approach.

MANAGEMENT. The classical management for ovarian pregnancies has been surgical. Early bleeding for small lesions has been managed by ovarian wedge resection or cystectomy (Schwartz and colleagues, 1993). In the presence of larger lesions, ovariectomy is most often performed. Recently, laparoscopy has been used to resect or to perform laser ablation of ovarian pregnancies (Carter and colleagues, 1993; Goldenberg and associates, 1994). Finally, methotrexate has been used successfully to treat unruptured ovarian pregnancies (Chelmow and associates, 1994; Raziel and Golan, 1993; Shamma and Schwartz, 1992).

CERVICAL PREGNANCY

In the past, cervical pregnancy was a rare form of ectopic gestation. Dees (1966) estimated the incidence to be 1 in 18,000 pregnancies. The incidence is increasing as a result of assisted reproduction, especially after in vitro fertilization and embryo transfer (Ginsburg, 1994; Pattinson, 1994; Peleg, 1994, and their associates). According to Pisarska and Carson (1999), prior dilatation and curettage precedes 70 percent of cases.

In a typical case, the endocervix is eroded by trophoblast, and the pregnancy proceeds to develop in the fibrous cervical wall (Fig. 10–10). The duration of pregnancy depends on the site of implantation. The higher the trophoblast is implanted in the cervical canal, the greater is its capacity to grow and cause hemorrhage.

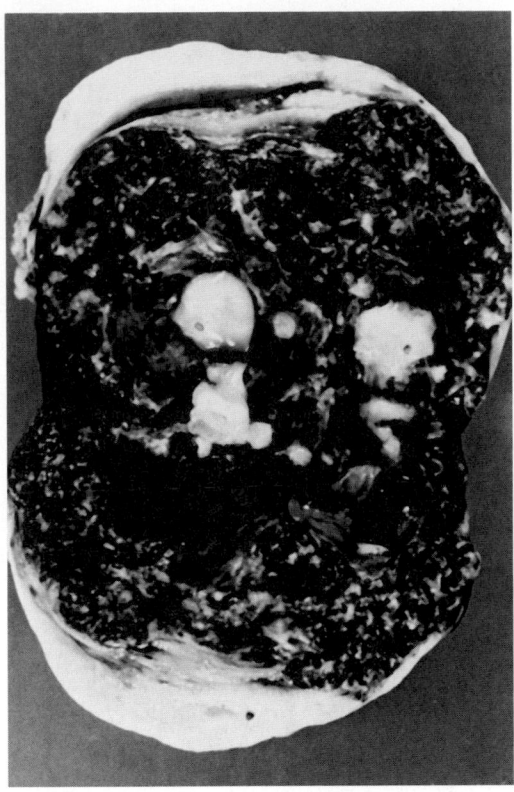

FIGURE 10–10. Cervical pregnancy in situ removed by hysterectomy nearly 3 months after the last normal menstrual period and 1 month after onset of vaginal bleeding. (Courtesy of Drs. D. Rubell and A. Brekken.)

Painless vaginal bleeding is present in 90 percent of cervical pregnancies, and one third of these have massive hemorrhage (Ushakov and colleagues, 1997). Only one fourth have abdominal pain with bleeding. As pregnancy progresses, a distended, thin-walled cervix with a partially dilated external os may be evident. Above the cervical mass, a slightly enlarged uterine fundus may be palpated. Cervical pregnancy rarely extends beyond 20 weeks and usually is surgically terminated because of bleeding. Identification of cervical pregnancy is based on a high degree of clinical suspicion coupled with sonography (Frates and colleagues, 1994; Kligman and associates, 1995). Findings include an empty uterus and a gestation filling the cervical canal (Fig. 10–11). Magnetic resonance imaging can be used to confirm the diagnosis (Bader-Armstrong and associates, 1989; Rafal and co-workers, 1990).

SURGICAL MANAGEMENT. In the past, hysterectomy was often the only choice available because of profuse hemorrhage that accompanied attempts at removal of the cervical pregnancy. With hysterectomy, the risk of urinary tract injury is increased because of the enlarged barrel-shaped cervix. To avoid the morbidity of surgery, and in some cases to preserve fertility, other approaches have been developed.

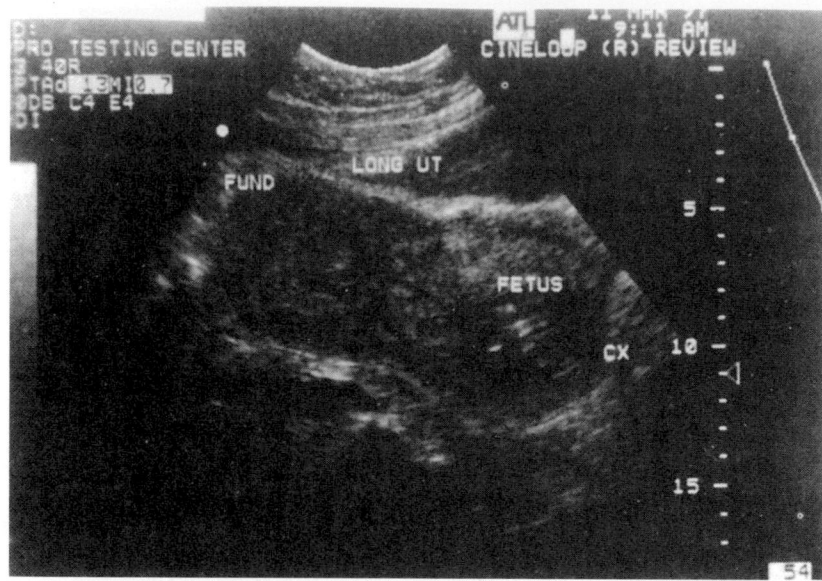

FIGURE 10–11. Sonogram showing longitudinal view of an 11-week cervical pregnancy. (From Eblen and colleagues, 1999, with permission.)

Cerclage. Bernstein and associates (1981) and Bachus and colleagues (1990) successfully managed cervical pregnancy by placing a heavy silk ligature around the cervix, similar to a McDonald cerclage (see Chap. 9, p. 238). More recently, Mashiach and colleagues (2002) described the successful management and resolution of four cervical pregnancies using a Shirodkar cerclage. In one of these cases, a concurrent uterine pregnancy progressed to term and a healthy infant was delivered vaginally.

Curettage and Tamponade. Nolan and associates (1989) and Thomas and co-workers (1991) recommend placement of hemostatic cervical sutures at 3 and 9 o'clock. Suction curettage is then performed, followed immediately by insertion of a Foley catheter into the cervical canal. The 30-mL catheter bulb is inflated, and the vagina is packed tightly with gauze to further tamponade bleeding. A suction catheter tip may be left above the vaginal packing to ensure adequate drainage and to monitor blood loss.

Arterial Embolization. Successful selective preoperative uterine artery embolization using Gelfoam has been described by Lobel and colleagues (1990), Saliken and co-workers (1994), and others. This technique, detailed in Chapter 35 (see p. 836), also has been used successfully to control bleeding after medical therapy (Cosin and associates, 1997; Wong and colleagues, 1999). Kung and colleagues (2004) employed a combination of laparoscopically assisted uterine artery ligation followed by hysteroscopic endocervical resection to successfully treat six cervical pregnancies.

MEDICAL MANAGEMENT. To avoid the risks of uncontrolled hemorrhage, methotrexate and other drug treatments have been used successfully for treatment of cervical pregnancies. In many centers, including ours, chemotherapy is now the first line of therapy in the stable woman. The general guidelines for methotrexate use for ectopic pregnancy are as described earlier (see p. 263). The drug has been injected directly into the gestational sac, with or without potassium chloride to induce fetal death. It has been given systemically in single high-dose therapy with folinic acid rescue, in lower-dose prolonged courses, and as a single low-dose regimen. It also has been given in various combinations, for example, intra-amnionically, after failure of systemic therapy (Kaplan, 1990; Marcovici, 1994; Roussis, 1992; Timor-Tritsch, 1994; Wong, 1999, and their colleagues).

Pregnancies of more than 6 weeks' duration generally require induction of fetal death with potassium chloride or high-dose and prolonged methotrexate therapy. Kung and Chang (1999) reviewed 62 methotrexate-treated cases. The 35 women in whom the fetus was alive had a higher failure rate with single-dose methotrexate. Almost half of these required a surgical procedure compared with 4 percent in the group with a dead fetus.

OTHER SITES OF ECTOPIC PREGNANCY

Primary *splenic pregnancy* was reported by Mankodi and associates (1977). A similar case was reported by Cormio and associates (2003). A few cases of primary *hepatic pregnancy* have been described, including one with a lithopedion (Barbosa Junior Ade A and associates, 1991; Børlum and Blom, 1988; Schlatter and colleagues, 1988). At least four cases of *retroperitoneal pregnancy* have been reported. In the two described by Ferland and associates (1991) and Reid and Steel (2003), pregnancy followed in vitro fertilization and embryo transfer. Varma and co-workers (2003) described the live birth at 35 weeks of an infant whose placenta implanted exclusively on the omentum. Fishman and co-workers (1998) described implantation of a 6-week *diaphragmatic pregnancy* in a women with abdominal and shoulder pain, dyspnea, and a hemothorax. Fylstra and colleagues (2002) recently described an ectopic *cesarean scar pregnancy.* We have also encountered these, and they are in many ways similar to a placenta increta with all of its proclivity to cause torrential hemorrhage (see Chap. 35, p. 830).

REFERENCES

Alexander JM, Rouse DJ, Varner E, et al: Treatment of the small unruptured ectopic pregnancy: A cost analysis of methotrexate versus laparoscopy. Obstet Gynecol 88:123, 1996

American College of Obstetricians and Gynecologists: Medical management of tubal pregnancy. Practice Bulletin No. 3, December, 1998

Anderson FWJ, Hogan JG, Ansbacher R. Sudden death: Ectopic pregnancy mortality. ACOG 103:1218, 2004

Ankum WM, Mol BWJ, Van der Veen F, et al: Risk factors for ectopic pregnancy: A meta-analysis. Fertil Steril 65:1093, 1996

Atrash HK, Friede A, Hogue CJ: Abdominal pregnancy in the United States: Frequency and maternal mortality. Obstet Gynecol 69:333, 1987

Bachus KE, Stone D, Suh B, et al: Conservative management of cervical pregnancy with subsequent fertility. Am J Obstet Gynecol 162:450, 1990

Bader-Armstrong B, Shah Y, Rubens D: Use of ultrasound and magnetic resonance imaging in the diagnosis of cervical pregnancy. J Clin Ultrasound 17:283, 1989

Bangsgaard N, Lund CO, Ottesen B, et al: Improved fertility following conservative surgical treatment of ectopic pregnancy. Br J Obstet Gynaecol 110:765, 2003

Barbosa Junior Ade A, de Freitas LA, Mota MA: Primary pregnancy in the liver: A case report. Pathol Res Pract 187:329, 1991

Barnhart KT, Sammel MD, Rinaudo PF, et al: Symptomatic patients with an early viable intrauterine pregnancy: hCG curves redefined. ACOG 104:50, 2004

Barnhart KT, Gracia CR, Reindl B, et al: Usefulness of Pipelle endometrial biopsy in the diagnosis of women at risk for ectopic pregnancy. Am J Obstet Gynecol 188:906, 2003

Barnhart KT, Katz I, Hummel A, et al: Presumed diagnosis of ectopic pregnancy. Obstet Gynecol 100:505, 2002

Barnhart K, Mennuti MT, Benjamin I, et al: Prompt diagnosis of ectopic pregnancy in an emergency department setting. Obstet Gynecol 84:1010, 1994

Barnhart KT, Simhan H, Kamelle SA: Diagnostic accuracy of ultrasound, above and below the beta-hCG discriminatory zone. Obstet Gynecol 94:583, 1999

Bateman BG, Nunley WC Jr, Kolp LA, et al: Vaginal sonography findings and hCG dynamics of early intrauterine and tubal pregnancies. Obstet Gynecol 75:421, 1990

Batzer FR, Weiner S, Corson SL, et al: Landmarks during the first forty-two days of gestation demonstrated by the beta-subunit of human chorionic gonadotropin and ultrasound. Am J Obstet Gynecol 146:973, 1983

Belfar HL, Kurtz AB, Wapner RJ: Long-term follow-up after removal of an abdominal pregnancy: Ultrasound evaluation of the involuting placenta. J Ultrasound Med 5:521, 1986

Bergstrom R, Mueller G, Yankowitz J: A case illustrating the continued dilemmas in treating abdominal pregnancy and a potential explanation for the high rate of postsurgical febrile morbidity. Gynecol Obstet Invest 46:268, 1998

Berman BJ, Katsiyiannis WT: Images in clinical medicine. A medical mystery. N Engl J Med 345:1176, 2001

Bernstein D, Holzinger M, Ovadia J, et al: Conservative treatment of cervical pregnancy. Obstet Gynecol 58:741, 1981

Birkhahn RH, Gaieta TJ, Van Deusen SK, et al: The ability of traditional vital signs and shock index to identify ruptured ectopic pregnancy. Am J Obstet Gynecol 189:1293, 2003

Bombard AT, Nakagawa S, Runowicz CD, et al: Early detection of abdominal pregnancy by maternal serum AFP screening. Prenat Diagn 14:1155, 1994

Børlum KG, Blom R: Primary hepatic pregnancy. Int J Gynaecol Obstet 27:427, 1988

Brown DL, Doubilet PM: Transvaginal sonography for diagnosing ectopic pregnancy: Positivity criteria and performance characteristics. J Ultrasound Med 13:259, 1994

Brunham RC, Peeling R, Maclean I, et al: Chlamydia trachomatis–associated ectopic pregnancy: Serologic and histologic correlates. J Infect Dis 165:1076, 1992

Buckley RG, King KJ, Disney JD, et al: Serum progesterone testing to predict ectopic pregnancy in symptomatic first-trimester patients. Ann Emerg Med 36:95, 2000

Buster JE, Pisarska MD: Medical management of ectopic pregnancy. Clin Obstet Gynecol 42:23, 1999

Cacciatore B, Stenman UH, Ylöstalo P: Diagnosis of ectopic pregnancy by vaginal ultrasonography in combination with a discriminatory serum hCG level of 1000 IU/L (IRP). Br J Obstet Gynaecol 97:904, 1990

Carter JE, Ekuan J, Kallins GJ: Laparoscopic diagnosis and excision of an intact ovarian pregnancy. A case report. J Reprod Med 38:962, 1993

Cartwright PS, Brown JE, Davis RJ, et al: Advanced abdominal pregnancy associated with fetal pulmonary hypoplasia: Report of a case. Am J Obstet Gynecol 155:396, 1986

Centers for Disease Control and Prevention: Ectopic pregnancy—United States, 1990–1992. MMWR 1:46, 1995

Chelmow D, Gates E, Penzias AS: Laparoscopic diagnosis and methotrexate treatment of an ovarian pregnancy: A case report. Fertil Steril 62:879, 1994

Coleman BG, Baron RL, Arger PH, et al: Ectopic embryo detection using real-time sonography. J Clin Ultrasound 13:545, 1985

Cormio G, Santamato S, Vimercati A, et al: Primary splenic pregnancy: A case report. J Reprod Med 48:479, 2003

Cosin JA, Bean M, Grow D, et al: The use of methotrexate and arterial embolization to avoid surgery in a case of cervical pregnancy. Fertil Steril 67:1169, 1997

Costa SD, Presley J, Bastert G: Advanced abdominal pregnancy. Obstet Gynecol Surv 46:515, 1991

Coste J, Bouyer J, Germain E, et al: Recent declining trend in ectopic pregnancy in France: Evidence of two clinicoepidemiologic entities. Fertil Steril 74:881, 2000

Coste J, Job-Spira N, Fernandez H, et al: Risk factors for ectopic pregnancy: A case-control study in France, with special focus on infectious factors. Am J Epidemiol 133:839, 1991

Dart R, McLean SA, Dart L: Isolated fluid in the cul-de-sac: How well does it predict ectopic pregnancy? Am J Emerg Med 20:1, 2002

De Cherney AH, Eichhorn JH: Severe abdominal pain during early pregnancy in a woman with previous infertility: Case 3-1996. N Engl J Med 334:255, 1996

Dees DH: Cervical pregnancy associated with uterine leiomyomas. South Med J 59:900, 1966

Dimitry ES, Subak-Sharpe R, Mills M, et al: Nine cases of heterotopic pregnancies in 4 years of in vitro fertilization. Fertil Steril 53:107, 1990

Dorfman SF, Grimes DA, Cates W Jr, et al: Ectopic pregnancy mortality, United States, 1979 to 1980: Clinical aspects. Obstet Gynecol 64:386, 1984

Eblen AC, Pridham DD, Tatum CJ Jr: Conservative management of an 11-week cervical pregnancy. A case report. J Reprod Med 44:61, 1999

Egger M, Low N, Smith GD, et al: Screening for chlamydial infections and the risk of ectopic pregnancy in a county in Sweden: Ecological analysis. BMJ 316:1776, 1998

el Kareh A, Beddoe AM, Brown BL: Advanced abdominal pregnancy complicated by bilateral ureteral obstruction. A case report. J Reprod Med 38:900, 1993

Emembolu JO: Celo-intestinal fistulae complicating advanced extra-uterine pregnancy. Int J Gynaecol Obstet 28:177, 1989

Ferland RJ, Chadwick DA, O'Brien JA, et al: An ectopic pregnancy in the upper retroperitoneum following in vitro fertilization and embryo transfer. Obstet Gynecol 78:544, 1991

Fernandez H, Yves Vincent SCA, Pauthier S, et al: Randomized trial of conservative laparoscopic treatment and methotrexate administration in ectopic pregnancy and subsequent fertility. Hum Reprod 13:3239, 1998

Fishman DA, Padilla LA, Joob A, et al: Ectopic pregnancy causing hemothorax managed by thoracoscopy and actinomycin D. Obstet Gynecol 91:837, 1998

Fossum GT, Davajan V, Kletzky OA: Early detection of pregnancy with transvaginal ultrasound. Fertil Steril 49:788, 1988

France JT, Jackson P: Maternal plasma and urinary hormone levels during and after a successful abdominal pregnancy. Br J Obstet Gynaecol 87:356, 1980

Frates MC, Benson CB, Doubilet PM, et al: Cervical ectopic pregnancy: Results of conservative treatment. Radiology 191:773, 1994

Fylstra DL, Pound-Chang T, Miller MG, et al: Ectopic pregnancy within a cesarean delivery scar: A case report. Am J Obstet Gynecol 187:302, 2002

Ginsburg ES, Frates MC, Rein MS, et al: Early diagnosis and treatment of cervical pregnancy in an in vitro fertilization program. Fertil Steril 61:966, 1994

Glassner MJ, Aron E, Eskin BA: Ovulation induction with clomiphene and the rise in heterotopic pregnancies: A report of two cases. J Reprod Med 35:175, 1990

Glew SS, Sivanesaratnam V: Advanced extrauterine pregnancy mimicking intrauterine fetal death: Case reports. Aust NZ J Obstet Gynaecol 29:450, 1989

Goldenberg M, Bider D, Mashiach S, et al: Laparoscopic laser surgery of primary ovarian pregnancy. Hum Reprod 9:1337, 1994

Goldner TE, Lawson HW, Xia Z, et al: Surveillance for ectopic pregnancy—United States, 1970–1989. MMWR 42:73, 1993

Goldstein SR, Snyder JR, Watson C, et al: Vaginal sonography versus serum human chorionic gonadotropin in early detection of pregnancy. Am J Obstet Gynecol 158:608, 1988

Gracia CR, Barnhart KT: Diagnosing ectopic pregnancy: Decision analysis comparing six strategies. Obstet Gynecol 97:464, 2001

Graczykowski JW, Mishell DR Jr: Methotrexate prophylaxis for persistent ectopic pregnancy after conservative treatment by salpingostomy. Obstet Gynecol 89:118, 1997

Gray CL, Ruffolo EH: Ovarian pregnancy associated with intrauterine contraceptive devices. Am J Obstet Gynecol 132:134, 1978

Gray DT, Thorburn J, Lundorff P, et al: A cost-effectiveness study of a randomised trial of laparoscopy versus laparotomy for ectopic pregnancy. Lancet 345:1139, 1995

Guirgis RR, Craft IL: Ectopic pregnancy resulting from gamete intrafallopian transfer and in vitro fertilization. Role of ultrasonography in diagnosis and treatment. J Reprod Med 36:793, 1991

Hage ML, Wall LL, Killam A: Expectant management of abdominal pregnancy. A report of two cases. J Reprod Med 33:407, 1988

Hajenius PJ, Engelsbel S, Mol BW, et al: Randomised trial of systemic methotrexate versus laparoscopic salpingostomy in tubal pregnancy. Lancet 350:774, 1997

Hajenius PJ, Mol BWJ, Ankum WM, et al: Clearance curves of serum human chorionic gonadotropin for the diagnosis of persistent trophoblast. Hum Reprod 10:683, 1995

Harris MB, Angtuaco T, Frazier CN, et al: Diagnosis of a viable abdominal pregnancy by magnetic resonance imaging. Am J Obstet Gynecol 159:150, 1988

Hemminki E, Meriläinen J: Long-term effects of cesarean sections: Ectopic pregnancies and placental problems. Am J Obstet Gynecol 174:1569, 1996

Hirsch E, Cohen L, Hecht BR: Heterotopic pregnancy with discordant ultrasonic appearance of fetal cardiac activity. Obstet Gynecol 79:824, 1992

Jackson S, Hollingworth T, Macpherson M: Elevated serum alpha fetoprotein and normal liquor alpha fetoprotein values in association with an abdominal pregnancy. Aust NZ J Obstet Gynaecol 33:214, 1993

Kadar N, DeVore G, Romero R: The discriminatory hCG "zone." Its use in the sonographic evaluation for ectopic pregnancy. Obstet Gynecol 58:156, 1981

Kadar N, Romero R: Observations on the log human chorionic gonadotropin–time relationship in early pregnancy and its practical implications. Am J Obstet Gynecol 157:73, 1987

Kalchman GG, Meltzer RM: Interstitial pregnancy following homolateral salpingectomy: Report of 2 cases and a review of the literature. Am J Obstet Gynecol 96:1139, 1966

Kalinski MA, Guss DA: Hemorrhagic shock from a ruptured ectopic pregnancy in a patient with a negative urine pregnancy test result. Ann Emerg Med 40:102, 2002

Kaplan BC, Dart RG, Moskos M, et al: Ectopic pregnancy: Prospective study with improved diagnostic accuracy. Ann Emerg Med 28:10, 1996

Kaplan BR, Brandt T, Javaheri G, et al: Nonsurgical treatment of a viable cervical pregnancy with intra-amniotic methotrexate. Fertil Steril 53:941, 1990

Katz DL, Barrett JP, Sanfilippo JS, et al: Combined hysteroscopy and laparoscopy in the treatment of interstitial pregnancy. Am J Obstet Gynecol 188:1113, 2003

Kerr A, Trambert J, Mikhail M, et al: Preoperative transcatheter embolization of abdominal pregnancy: Report of three cases. J Vasc Interv Radiol 4:733, 1993

Kivikoski AI, Martin C, Weyman P, et al: Angiographic arterial embolization to control hemorrhage in abdominal pregnancy: A case report. Obstet Gynecol 71:456, 1988

Kligman I, Adachi TJ, Katz E, et al: Conserving fertility with early management of cervical pregnancy: A case report. J Reprod Med 40:743, 1995

Kooi S, Kock HC: A review of the literature on nonsurgical treatment in tubal pregnancy. Obstet Gynecol Surv 47:739, 1992

Koonin LM, MacKay AP, Berg CJ, et al: Pregnancy-related mortality surveillance—United States, 1987–1990. MMWR 46:17, 1997

Kouyoumdjian A, Kirkpatrick J: Coexistence of an intrauterine pregnancy with both an ectopic pregnancy and salpingitis in the right fallopian tube: A case report. J Reprod Med 35:824, 1990

Kung FT, Chang SY: Efficacy of methotrexate treatment in viable and nonviable cervical pregnancies. Am J Obstet Gynecol 181:1438, 1999

Kung FT, Lin H, Hsu TY, et al: Differential diagnosis of suspected cervical pregnancy and conservative treatment with the combination of laparoscopy-assisted uterine artery ligation and hysteroscopic endocervical resection. Fertility & Sterility 81:1642, 2004

Kurtz AB, Dubbins PA, Wapner RJ, et al: Problem of abnormal fetal position. JAMA 247:3251, 1982

Lipscomb GH, Bran D, McCord ML, et al: Analysis of three hundred fifteen ectopic pregnancies treated with single-dose methotrexate. Am J Obstet Gynecol 178:1354, 1998

Lipscomb GH, McCord ML, Stovall TG, et al: Predictors of success of methotrexate treatment in women with tubal ectopic pregnancies. N Engl J Med 341:1974, 1999a

Lipscomb GH, Meyer NL, Flynn DE, et al: Oral methotrexate for treatment of ectopic pregnancy. Am J Obstet Gynecol 186:1192, 2002

Lipscomb GH, Puckett KJ, Bran D, et al: Management of separation pain after single-dose methotrexate therapy for ectopic pregnancy. Obstet Gynecol 93:590, 1999b

Lobel SM, Meyerovitz MF, Benson CC, et al: Preoperative angiographic uterine artery embolization in the management of cervical pregnancy. Obstet Gynecol 76:938, 1990

Maccato M, Estrada R, Hammill H, et al: Prevalence of active Chlamydia trachomatis infection at the time of exploratory laparotomy for ectopic pregnancy. Obstet Gynecol 79:211, 1992

Mäkinen J: Ectopic pregnancy falls in Finland. Lancet 348:129, 1996

Mankodi RC, Sankari K, Bhatt SM: Primary splenic pregnancy. Br J Obstet Gynaecol 84:634, 1977

Marcovici I, Rosenzweig BA, Brill AI, et al: Cervical pregnancy: Case reports and a current literature review. Obstet Gynecol Surv 49:49, 1994

Marcus SF, Brinsden PR: Analysis of the incidence and risk factors associated with ectopic pregnancy following in vitro fertilization and embryo transfer. Hum Reprod 10:199, 1995

Marcus SF, Brinsden PR: Primary ovarian pregnancy after in vitro fertilization and embryo transfer: Report of seven cases. Fertil Steril 60:167, 1993

Marcus SF, Macnamee M, Brinsden P: Heterotopic pregnancies after in-vitro fertilization and embryo transfer. Hum Reprod 10:1232, 1995

Martin JN Jr, McCaul JF IV: Emergent management of abdominal pregnancy. Clin Obstet Gynecol 33:438, 1990

Martin JN Jr, Ridgway LE III, Connors JJ, et al: Angiographic arterial embolization and computed tomography–directed drainage for the management of hemorrhage and infection with abdominal pregnancy. Obstet Gynecol 76:941, 1990

Martin JN Jr, Sessums JK, Martin RW, et al: Abdominal pregnancy: Current concepts of management. Obstet Gynecol 71:549, 1988

Mashiach S, Admon D, Oelsner G, et al: Cervical Shirodkar cerclage may be the treatment modality of choice for cervical pregnancy. Hum Reprod 17:493, 2002

McCord ML, Muram D, Buster JE, et al: Single serum progesterone as a screen for ectopic pregnancy: Exchanging specificity and sensitivity to obtain optimal test performance. Fertil Steril 66:513, 1996

Mol BWJ, Lijmer JG, Ankum WM, et al: The accuracy of single serum progesterone measurement in the diagnosis of ectopic pregnancy: A meta-analysis. Hum Reprod 13:3220, 1998

Moon HS, Choi YJ, Park YH, et al: New simple endoscopic operations for interstitial pregnancies. Am J Obstet Gynecol 182:114, 2000

Morlock RJ, Lafata JE, Eisenstein D: Cost-effectiveness of single-dose methotrexate compared with laparoscopic treatment of ectopic pregnancy. Obstet Gynecol 95:407, 2000

Morris JM, Van Wagenen G: Interception: The use of postovulatory estrogens to prevent implantation. Am J Obstet Gynecol 115:101, 1973

Nolan TE, Chandler PE, Hess LW, et al: Cervical pregnancy managed without hysterectomy. A case report. J Reprod Med 34:241, 1989

Nugent PJ: Ruptured ectopic pregnancy in a patient with a recent intrauterine abortion. Ann Emerg Med 21:97, 1992

Nyberg DA, Filly RA, Laing FC, et al: Ectopic pregnancy. Diagnosis by sonography correlated with quantitative hCG levels. J Ultrasound Med 6:145, 1987

Olshaker JS: Emergency department pregnancy testing. J Emerg Med 14:59, 1996

Ong S, Wingfield M: Increasing incidence of ectopic pregnancy: Is it iatrogenic? Ir Med J 92:364, 1999

Ory HW: Ectopic pregnancy and intrauterine contraceptive devices: New perspectives. The woman's health study. Obstet Gynecol 57:137, 1981

Pattinson HA, Dunphy BC, Wood S, et al: Cervical pregnancy following in vitro fertilization: Evacuation after uterine artery embolization with subsequent successful intrauterine pregnancy. Aust NZ J Obstet Gynaecol 34:492, 1994

Peleg D, Bar-Hava I, Neuman-Levin M, et al: Early diagnosis and successful nonsurgical treatment of viable combined intrauterine and cervical pregnancy. Fertil Steril 62:405, 1994

Perkins SL, Al-Ramahi M, Claman P: Comparison of serum progesterone as an indicator of pregnancy nonviability in spontaneously pregnant emergency room and infertility clinic patient populations. Fertil Steril 73:499, 2000

Piering WF, Garancis JG, Becker CG, et al: Preeclampsia related to a functioning extrauterine placenta: Report of a case and 25-year follow-up. Am J Kidney Dis 21:310, 1993

Pisarska MD, Carson SA: Incidence and risk factors for ectopic pregnancy. Clin Obstet Gynecol 42:2, 1999

Pisarska MD, Carson SA, Buster JE: Ectopic pregnancy. Lancet 351:1115, 1998

Rafal RB, Kosovsky PA, Markisz JA: Case Report. MR appearance of cervical pregnancy. J Comput Assist Tomogr 14:482, 1990

Rahman MS, Al-Suleiman SA, Rahman J, et al: Advanced abdominal pregnancy—observations in 10 cases. Obstet Gynecol 59:366, 1982

Raziel A, Golan A: Primary ovarian pregnancy successfully treated with methotrexate. Am J Obstet Gynecol 169:1362, 1993

Reid F, Steel M: An exceptionally rare ectopic pregnancy. Br J Obstet Gynaecol 110:222, 2003

Rolle C, Wai C, Hoffman B: Unilateral twin ectopic pregnancy in a patient with multiple sexually transmitted infections. Infect Dis Obstet Gynecol 1:14, 2004

Romero R, Kadar N, Castro D, et al: The value of adnexal sonographic findings in the diagnosis of ectopic pregnancy. Am J Obstet Gynecol 158:52, 1988

Roussis P, Ball RH, Fleischer AC, et al: Cervical pregnancy: A case report. J Reprod Med 37:479, 1992

Saliken JC, Normore WJ, Pattinson HA, et al: Embolization of the uterine arteries before termination of a 15-week cervical pregnancy. Can Assoc Radiol J 45:399, 1994

Saraj AJ, Wilcox JG, Najmabadi S, et al: Resolution of hormonal markers of ectopic gestation: A randomized trial comparing single-dose intramuscular methotrexate with salpingostomy. Obstet Gynecol 92:989, 1998

Schlatter MC, DePree B, Vanderkolk KJ: Hepatic abdominal pregnancy: A case report. J Reprod Med 33:921, 1988

Schwartz LB, Carcangiu ML, DeCherney AH: Primary ovarian pregnancy. A case report. J Reprod Med 38:155, 1993

Seifer DB: Persistent ectopic pregnancy: An argument for heightened vigilance and patient compliance. Fertil Steril 68:402, 1997

Shalev E, Peleg D, Tsabari A, et al: Spontaneous resolution of ectopic tubal pregnancy: Natural history. Fertil Steril 63:15, 1995

Shamma FN, Schwartz LB: Primary ovarian pregnancy successfully treated with methotrexate. Am J Obstet Gynecol 167:1307, 1992

Sidek S, Lai SF, Lim-Tan SK: Primary ovarian pregnancy: Current diagnosis and management. Singapore Med J 35:71, 1994

Sivin I: Alternative estimates of ectopic pregnancy risks during contraception. Am J Obstet Gynecol 165:1900, 1991

Spandorfer SD, Sawin SW, Benjamin I, et al: Postoperative day 1 serum human chorionic gonadotropin level as a predictor of persistent ectopic pregnancy after conservative surgical management. Fertil Steril 68:430, 1997

Stabile I, Grudzinskas JG: Ectopic pregnancy: A review of incidence, etiology and diagnostic aspects. Obstet Gynecol Surv 45:335, 1990

Stangel JJ, Reyniak JV, Stone ML: Conservative surgical management of tubal pregnancy. Obstet Gynecol 48:241, 1976

Stevens CA: Malformations and deformations in abdominal pregnancy. Am J Med Genet 47:1189, 1993

Stovall TG: Medical management should be routinely used as primary therapy for ectopic pregnancy. Clin Obstet Gynecol 38:346, 1995

Stovall TG, Kellerman AL, Ling FW, et al: Emergency department diagnosis of ectopic pregnancy. Ann Emerg Med 19:1098, 1990

Stovall TG, Ling FW: Some new approaches to ectopic pregnancy management. Contemp Obstet Gynecol 37:35, 1992

Stovall TG, Ling FW, Carson SA, et al: Serum progesterone and uterine curettage in differential diagnosis of ectopic pregnancy. Fertil Steril 57:456, 1992

Stovall TG, Ling FW, Cope BJ, et al: Preventing ruptured ectopic pregnancy with a single serum progesterone. Am J Obstet Gynecol 160:1425, 1989

Tanaka T, Hayashi H, Kutsuzawa T, et al: Treatment of interstitial ectopic pregnancy with methotrexate: Report of a successful case. Fertil Steril 37:851, 1982

Tay JI, Moore J, Walker JJ: Ectopic pregnancy. BMJ 320:916, 2000

Thomas RL, Gingold BR, Gallagher MW: Cervical pregnancy. A report of two cases. J Reprod Med 36:459, 1991

Thorburn J: Ectopic pregnancy. The epidemic seems to be over. Lakartidningen 92:4701, 1995

Timor-Tritsch IE, Monteagudo A, Mandeville EO, et al: Successful management of viable cervical pregnancy by local injection of methotrexate guided by transvaginal ultrasonography. Am J Obstet Gynecol 170:737, 1994

Trio D, Strobelt N, Picciolo C, et al: Prognostic factors for successful expectant management of ectopic pregnancy. Fertil Steril 63:469, 1995

Tulandi T, Al-Jaroudi D: Interstitial pregnancy: Results generated from the Society of Reproductive Surgeons. Obstet Gynecol 103:47, 2004

Tulandi T, Saleh A: Surgical management of ectopic pregnancy. Clin Obstet Gynecol 42:31, 1999

Ushakov FB, Elchalal U, Aceman PJ, et al: Cervical pregnancy: Past and future. Obstet Gynecol Surv 52:45, 1997

Varma R, Mascarenhas L, James D. Successful outcome of advanced abdominal pregnancy with exclusive omental insertion. Ultrasound Obst Gyn 12:192, 2003

Vermesh M, Silva PD, Sauer MV, et al: Persistent tubal ectopic gestation: Patterns of circulating beta-human chorionic gonadotropin and progesterone and management options. Fertil Steril 50:584, 1988

Wagner A, Burchardt AJ: MR imaging in advanced abdominal pregnancy. A case report of fetal death. Acta Radiol 36:193, 1995

Weiss RE, Stone NN: Persistent maternal hydronephrosis after intra-abdominal pregnancy. J Urol 152:1196, 1994

Williams PC, Malvar TC, Kraft JR: Term ovarian pregnancy with delivery of a live female infant. Am J Obstet Gynecol 142:589, 1982

Wong YH, Liang EY, Ng TK, et al: A cervical ectopic pregnancy managed by medical treatment and angiographic embolization. Aust NZ J Obstet Gynaecol 39:493, 1999

11

Gestational Trophoblastic Disease

The term *gestational trophoblastic disease* refers to pregnancy-related trophoblastic proliferative abnormalities. In the past, classification of these abnormalities was confusing because it was defined by histological criteria as well as by clinical findings. As experience accrued, it became evident that a histological diagnosis was not necessary to provide effective treatment. Thus, a system has been adopted based principally on clinical findings and serial measurement of serum human chorionic gonadotropin (hCG) levels (Hammond and colleagues, 1973).

In 1983, the World Health Organization Scientific Group on Gestational Trophoblastic Diseases published recommendations for the definition, classification, and staging of trophoblastic disease. This classification was recently updated by the International Federation of Gynecology and Obstetrics (FIGO Oncology Committee, 2002). Gestational trophoblastic disease is divided into two groups, *hydatidiform mole* and *postmolar gestational trophoblastic neoplasia* (Table 11–1). The latter is termed *malignant gestational trophoblastic disease* by the American College of Obstetricians and Gynecologists (2004).

HYDATIDIFORM MOLE (MOLAR PREGNANCY)

Molar pregnancy is characterized histologically by abnormalities of the chorionic villi that consist of trophoblastic proliferation and edema of villous stroma. Moles usually occupy the uterine cavity, however, occasionally they develop in the oviduct and even the ovary (Chauhan and colleagues, 2004; Stanhope and associates, 1983). The absence or presence of a fetus or embryonic elements has been used to describe them as *complete* and *partial moles* (Table 11–2). As emphasized by Benirschke and Kaufmann (2000), in many cases classification may be difficult.

COMPLETE HYDATIDIFORM MOLE. In complete hydatiform mole, the chorionic villi transform into a mass of clear vesicles (Fig. 11–1). The vesicles vary in size from barely visible to a few centimeters and often hang in

TABLE 11–1 Criteria for Diagnosis of Gestational Trophoblastic Disease

Hydatidiform Mole
  Complete
  Partial
Gestational Trophoblastic Neoplasia–Postmolar GTN
1. Plateau of serum hCG level (±10%) for four measurements during a period of 3 weeks or longer—days 1, 7, 14, 21.
2. Rise of serum hCG > 10% during three weekly consecutive measurements or longer, during a period of 2 weeks or more—days 1, 7, 14.
3. The serum hCG level remains detectable for 6 months or more.
4. Histological criteria for choriocarcinoma.

GTN = gestational trophoblastic neoplasia or malignant gestational trophoblastic disease; hCG = human chorionic gonadotropin.
Criteria of the International Federation of Gynecology and Obstetrics (FIGO Oncology Committee, 2002).

clusters from thin pedicles. The histological structure typically shows:

1. Hydropic degeneration and swelling of the villous stroma.
2. Absence of blood vessels in the swollen villi.
3. Proliferation of the trophoblastic epithelium to a varying degree (Fig. 11–2).
4. Absence of fetus and amnion.

Of note, *hydropic* or *molar degeneration,* which may be confused histologically with a true mole, is not considered trophoblastic disease (Berkowitz and associates, 1991).

The chromosomal composition in 85 percent of complete molar pregnancies is 46,XX, with both chromosomes being of paternal origin (Wolf and Lage, 1995). This phenomenon is termed *androgenesis.* Typically, the ovum has been fertilized by a haploid sperm, which then duplicates its own chromosomes after meiosis. The chromosomes of the ovum are either absent or inactivated. Occasionally, the chromosomal pattern in a complete mole may be 46,XY due to dispermic fertilization (Bagshawe and Lawler, 1982; Lawler and colleagues, 1991).

TABLE 11–2 Features of Partial and Complete Hydatidiform Moles

Feature	Partial Mole	Complete Mole
Karyotype	Usually 69,XXX or 69,XXY	46,XX or 46,XY
Pathology		
Embryo-fetus	Often present	Absent
Amnion, fetal red blood cells	Often present	Absent
Villous edema	Variable, focal	Diffuse
Trophoblastic	Variable, focal, slight to moderate	Variable, slight to severe
Clinical presentation		
Diagnosis	Missed abortion	Molar gestation
Uterine size	Small for dates	50% large for dates
Theca-lutein cysts	Rare	25–30%
Medical complications	Rare	Frequent
Gestational trophoblastic neoplasia	<5–10%	20%

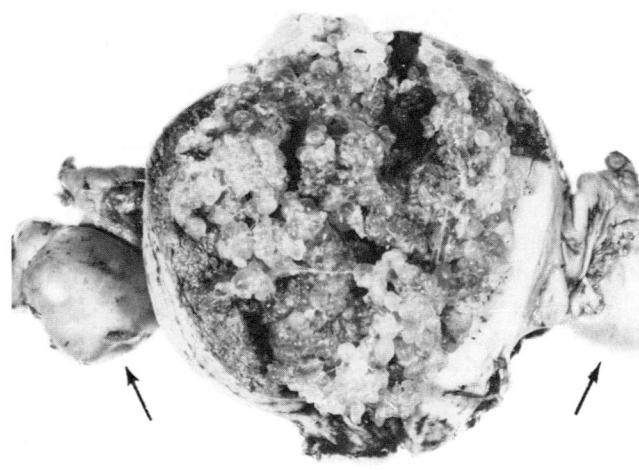

FIGURE 11–1. A complete or classical hydatidiform mole is characterized grossly by an abundance of edematous enlarged chorionic villi but no fetus or fetal membranes. There are theca-lutein cysts in both ovaries (*arrows*).

Lawler and colleagues (1991) described 200 hydatidiform moles—151 were complete and 49 partial moles (Table 11–3). Whereas almost 85 percent of complete moles are diploid, 85 percent of partial moles are triploid. Other variations also have been identified, such as 45,X. Thus, a morphologically complete mole can result from a variety of chromosomal patterns (Wolf and Lage, 1995).

PARTIAL HYDATIDIFORM MOLE. When the hydatidiform changes are focal and less advanced, and some element of fetal tissue is seen, the term *partial hydatidiform mole* is used. There is slowly progressive swelling within the stroma of characteristically avascular chorionic villi, whereas other vascular villi with a functioning fetal–placental circulation are spared (Shapter and McLellan, 2001).

As shown in Table 11–3, the karyotype typically is triploid—69,XXX, 69,XXY, or 69,XYY—these are each composed of one maternal and two paternal haploid sets of chromosomes (Berkowitz and colleagues, 1986, 1991; Wolf and Lage, 1995). Although nontriploid partial moles have been reported, some have questioned whether they exist (Genest and colleagues, 2002). The nonviable fetus of a triploid partial mole typically has multiple malformations (Phillip and co-workers, 2004). Abnormal growth is also common, and in the review by Jauniaux (1999), 82 percent of fetuses had symmetrical growth restriction.

A twin gestation of a complete mole and a normal fetus and placenta is sometimes misdiagnosed as a diploid partial mole (Fig. 11–3). It is important to distinguish between the two, because twin pregnancies consisting of a normal fetus and a complete mole have a substantively increased risk of developing subsequent gestational trophoblastic neoplasia (Bruchim and associates, 2000). Generally, gestational trophoblastic neoplasia follows 20 percent of complete moles, whereas it develops in only 0.5 percent of women after a partial mole (Hancock and Tidy, 2000). In their recent review of 77 such cases, Sebire and colleagues (2002b) reported that 16 percent of women whose pregnancies were terminated, versus 21 percent of those with continued pregnancies, required chemotherapy for gestational trophoblastic neoplasia. In another review, Vejerslev (1991) found that of 113 pregnancies with a hydatidiform mole coexistent with a normal fetus, 45 percent of fetuses progressed to 28 weeks, and fetal survival was 70 percent. Thus, when providing counseling for women with a coexistent mole and a fetus, both cytogenetic and high-resolution ultrasonographic studies are of

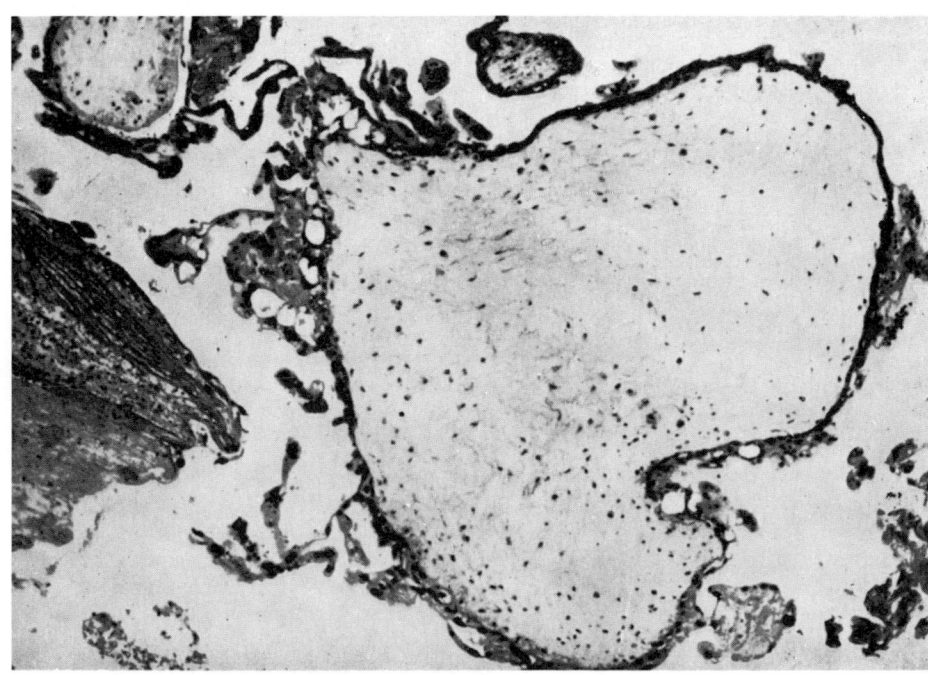

FIGURE 11–2. Photomicrograph of a hydatidiform mole with slight to moderate trophoblastic hyperplasia confined to the syncytium and considered probably benign. (From Smalbraak, 1957.)

TABLE 11–3 Chromosomal Composition of 200 Hydatidiform Moles

Chromosomes	Complete (n = 151) No. (%)	Partial (n = 49) No. (%)
Haploid	1 (0.7)	—
Diploid	128 (85)	1 (2)
Triploid	3 (2)	42 (86)
Tetraploid	—	2 (4)
Unknown	19 (13)	4 (8)

Adapted from Lawler and colleagues (1991), with permission.

paramount importance. The risk of *choriocarcinoma* arising from a partial mole is also low (see Table 11–2). Seckl and associates (2000) described 3000 cases of partial mole and documented only three cases of choriocarcinoma.

HISTOLOGICAL DIAGNOSIS OF HYDATIDIFORM MOLES. Attempts to relate the histological structure of individual complete hydatidiform moles to their subsequent malignant potential have generally been disappointing. For example, Novak and Seah (1954) could not precisely establish such a relationship in 120 cases of uncomplicated hydatidiform mole or in 26 cases of choriocarcinoma that developed after a molar pregnancy.

THECA-LUTEIN CYSTS. In many cases of hydatidiform mole, the ovaries contain multiple theca-lutein cysts. These may vary from microscopic size to 10 cm or more in diameter. Their surfaces are smooth, often yellowish, and lined with lutein cells. The incidence of obvious cysts in association with a mole is reported to be from 25 to 60 percent. They are thought to result from overstimulation of lutein elements by large amounts of hCG secreted by proliferating trophoblastic cells. Montz and colleagues (1988) reported that gestational trophoblastic neoplasia was more likely in women with theca-lutein cysts, especially if bilateral. Cysts, however, are not limited to cases of hydatidiform mole and may be associated with fetal hydrops and placental hypertrophy or with multifetal pregnancy. They may undergo torsion, infarction, and hemorrhage. Because the cysts regress after delivery, oophorectomy should not be performed unless the ovary is extensively infarcted. Large ovarian cysts may be decompressed by aspiration if symptomatic (Berkowitz and Goldstein, 1996).

INCIDENCE AND RISK FACTORS. Hydatidiform mole develops in approximately 1 in 1000 pregnancies in the United States and Europe. Although it has been reported to be more frequent in other countries, especially in parts of Asia, much of this information was obtained from hospital studies (Schorge and associates, 2000). When derived from population studies, the incidence in most of the world is probably similar to that in the United States (Miller and colleagues, 1989; Semer and Macfee, 1995). The role of gravidity, estrogen status, oral contraceptives, and dietary factors in the risk of gestational trophoblastic disease is unclear (Semer and Macfee, 1995).

Age. Sebire and colleagues (2002a) found the incidence of molar pregnancy highest in women aged 15 years or younger, and those aged 45 years or older. In the latter group, the

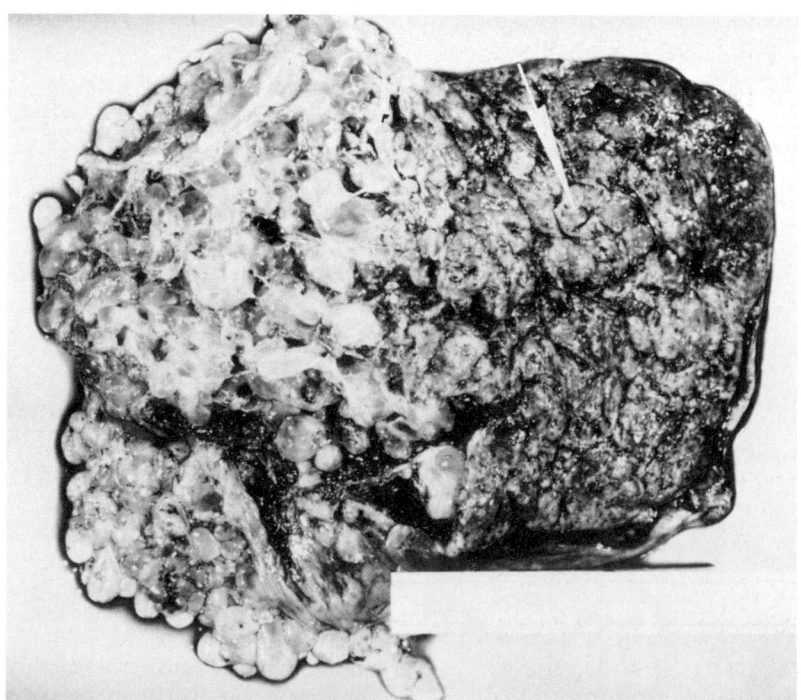

FIGURE 11–3. Molar placenta on the left and normal placenta on the right (*white arrow*). The molar placenta was identified by ultrasonography late in pregnancy when the mother developed preeclampsia. She underwent cesarean delivery of a healthy fetus near term. Most likely, these were twins consisting of a placenta with a fetus from one ovum and a complete mole developing from the other ovum.

relative frequency of the lesion is at least 10 times greater than that at ages 20 to 40 years (Schorge and colleagues, 2000).

Previous Mole. Women with molar pregnancies are at increased risk of developing either a complete or a partial mole in a future pregnancy (Garner and colleagues, 2002). In a review of 12 series totaling almost 5000 deliveries, the frequency of recurrent moles was 1.3 percent (Loret de Mola and Goldfarb, 1995). Garner and colleagues (2002) reported a 1.4 percent frequency of repeat moles in women with a prior complete mole and 2.4 percent in those with a prior partial mole. Repetitive hydatidiform moles in women with different partners would suggest that an oocyte problem leads to molar development (Garner and colleagues, 2002; Tuncer and colleagues, 1999).

CLINICAL COURSE. The clinical presentation of molar pregnancy has changed appreciably during the past 20 years (Coukos and colleagues, 1999; Hancock and Tidy, 2002). The availability of ultrasonography and quantitative measurement of serum hCG levels now allows earlier diagnosis. Symptoms are more likely to be dramatic with a complete mole than with a partial mole.

Bleeding. Uterine bleeding is almost universal, and may vary from spotting to profuse hemorrhage. It may begin just before abortion or, more often, these women may bleed intermittently for weeks and even months. At times there may be considerable hemorrhage concealed within the uterus. Iron-deficiency anemia is common, and a dilutional effect from appreciable pregnancy-induced hypervolemia is present in some women with larger moles.

Uterine Size. The growing uterus often enlarges more rapidly than usual, exceeding in about half of cases that expected from the gestational age. The uterus may be difficult to identify precisely by palpation because of its soft consistency. At times, ovarian theca-lutein cysts are difficult to distinguish from the enlarged uterus.

Fetal Activity. Even though the uterus is enlarged sufficiently to extend well above the symphysis, typically no fetal heart motion is detected. Infrequently, there may be extensive but incomplete molar degeneration in the placenta accompanied by a living fetus.

Gestational Hypertension. Because hypertension caused by pregnancy is rarely seen before 24 weeks, preeclampsia that develops before this gestational age may be from hydatidiform mole or extensive molar degeneration.

Hyperemesis. Significant nausea and vomiting may develop. Of interest, none of the 24 complete moles reported by Coukos and colleagues (1999) were associated with preeclampsia, hyperemesis, or clinical hyperthyroidism.

Thyrotoxicosis. Plasma thyroxine levels in women with molar pregnancy are often elevated, but clinically apparent hyperthyroidism is unusual (see Chap. 53, p. 1194). According to Amir (1984) and Curry (1975) and their colleagues, hyperthyroidism is identified in about 2 percent. In these cases, serum free thyroxine is elevated as the consequence of the thyrotropin-like effect of hCG (Mann and colleagues, 1986).

Embolization. Variable amounts of trophoblastic cells with or without villous stroma escape from the uterus into the venous outflow at the time of molar evacuation (Hankins and colleagues, 1987). The volume may be such as to produce signs and symptoms of acute pulmonary embolism or edema. Embolization with a large amount of trophoblastic tissue is probably uncommon, although fatalities have been described (Delmis and co-workers, 2000). This tissue, though, can subsequently invade the pulmonary parenchyma to establish metastases.

DIAGNOSTIC FEATURES. Spontaneous expulsion is most likely around 16 weeks and is rarely delayed beyond 28 weeks. The greatest diagnostic accuracy is obtained from the characteristic ultrasonographic appearance of hydatidiform mole (Fig. 11–4). Occasionally, other structures may have an appearance similar to that of a mole, including uterine myoma and multifetal pregnancy.

To summarize, the clinical and diagnostic features of a complete hydatidiform mole are:

1. Continuous or intermittent brown or bloody discharge evident by about 12 weeks and usually not profuse.
2. Uterine enlargement out of proportion to the duration of pregnancy in about half of the cases.
3. Absence of fetal parts and fetal heart motion.
4. Characteristic ultrasonographic appearance.
5. Serum hCG level higher than expected for the stage of gestation.
6. Preeclampsia–eclampsia developing before 24 weeks.
7. Hyperemesis gravidarum.

PROGNOSIS. Current mortality from molar pregnancies has been practically reduced to zero by prompt diagnosis and appropriate therapy. Earlier evacuation, however, has not reduced the 20 percent risk for gestational trophoblastic neoplasia (Schorge and co-workers, 2000). The report by Lurain and colleagues (1983) consisted of follow-up of 738 women from 1962 to 1978 after evacuation of a hydatidiform mole. Spontaneous regression was documented in 81 percent, while the remainder developed gestational trophoblastic neoplasia.

TREATMENT. As a result of greater awareness, and certainly of better technology for diagnosis, moles now are terminated more often when they are small. There is time for adequate evaluation of the woman who may be anemic, hypertensive, or hypovolemic. Hydatidiform mole treatment

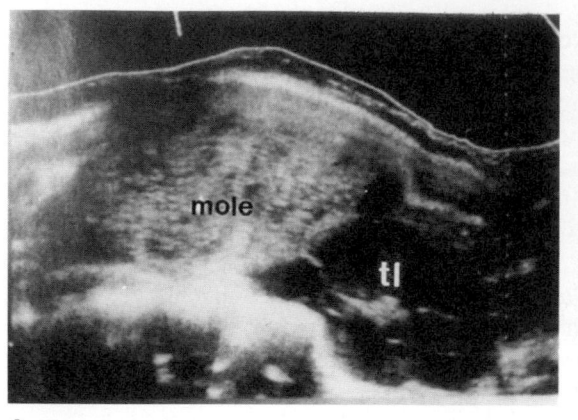
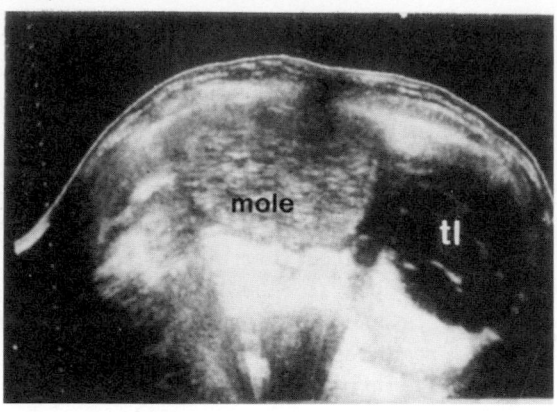

A   **B**

FIGURE 11–4. A. Longitudinal sonogram demonstrating a complete hydatidiform mole that fills a uterus enlarged to well above the umbilicus. A large theca-lutein cyst (tl) is seen above the uterus. **B.** Transverse sonogram of the same woman. (Courtesy of Dr. R. Santos.)

consists of two phases. The first is immediate evacuation of the mole, and the second is subsequent evaluation for persistent trophoblastic proliferation or malignant change. Unless there is other evidence of extrauterine disease, computed tomography or magnetic resonance imaging to evaluate the liver or brain is not performed routinely.

The rare circumstance of twinning with a complete hydatidiform mole plus a fetus and placenta presents an unusual therapeutic dilemma, especially in the absence of karyotypic aberrations or gross fetal anomalies. Neither the risks to the mother nor the likelihood of a healthy offspring have been established if pregnancy is continued (Suzuki and associates, 1980; Vejerslev, 1991).

Prophylactic Chemotherapy. The role of prophylactic chemotherapy for women with a hydatidiform mole is controversial (Bloss and Miller, 1995; Goldstein and Berkowitz, 1995). Such therapy does not improve the long-term prognosis. Moreover, the toxicity from prophylactic chemotherapy may be significant, including death (Bloss and Miller, 1995). Chemoprophylaxis may be considered in women with high-risk complete moles, particularly if serum hCG testing is unavailable or follow-up is impossible (Berkowitz and Goldstein, 1996).

Vacuum Aspiration. Suction evacuation is the treatment of choice for hydatidiform mole, regardless of uterine size (Bloss and Miller, 1995). For large moles, compatible blood should be available and an intravenous system established for its rapid infusion, if needed. Cervical dilating agents may be necessary (see Chap. 9, p. 243). The cervix may be further dilated under anesthesia to a diameter sufficient to allow insertion of a 10- to 12-mm plastic suction curet. After most of the molar tissue has been removed by aspiration, oxytocin is given. After the myometrium has contracted, *thorough but gentle curettage* with a large sharp curet usually is performed. Intraoperative ultrasonographic examination may help document that the uterine cavity has been emptied.

Oxytocin, Prostaglandins, and Hysterotomy. In the United States, labor induction rarely is used for evacuation of hydatidiform moles. In fact, there are many who feel that medical termination and hysterotomy have no role in its management (Miller and co-workers, 1989).

Hysterectomy. If no further pregnancies are desired, then hysterectomy may be preferred to suction curettage. Hysterectomy is a logical procedure in women aged 40 and older, because at least one third develop gestational trophoblastic neoplasia (Tow, 1966; Xia and colleagues, 1980). Although hysterectomy does not eliminate recurrent disease, it appreciably reduces its likelihood.

FOLLOW-UP EVALUATION OF MOLAR PREGNANCY. Close and consistent follow-up for these women is imperative with the following aims:

1. Prevent pregnancy for a minimum of 6 months using hormonal contraception.
2. Monitor serum hCG levels every 2 weeks. Serial measurement of serum hCG is important to detect trophoblastic neoplasia, and even small amounts of trophoblastic tissue can be detected by the assay. These levels should progressively fall to an undetectable level (Fig. 11–5).
3. Chemotherapy is not indicated as long as these serum levels continue to regress. A rise or persistent plateau in the level demands evaluation for gestational trophoblastic neoplasia and usually treatment. An increase signifies trophoblastic proliferation that is most likely malignant unless the woman is again pregnant.
4. Once the hCG level falls to a normal level, test the patient monthly for 6 months; then follow-up is discontinued and pregnancy allowed.

Estrogen–progestin contraceptives or depot-medroxyprogesterone usually are used to prevent a subsequent pregnancy during the period of surveillance. Deicas and associates

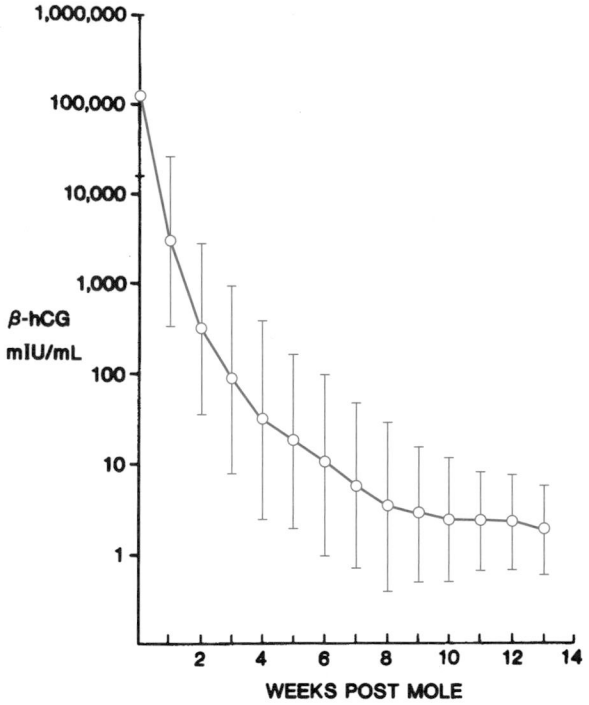

FIGURE 11–5. The mean value and 95-percent confidence limits describing the normal postmolar β-subunit chorionic gonadotropin regression curve. (From Schlaerth and associates, 1981, with permission.)

(1991) studied the effect of contraception on subsequent development of gestational trophoblastic neoplasia in 162 women with hydatidiform mole and 137 with trophoblastic tumor. Oral contraceptives were found to be superior to barrier methods or use of an intrauterine device in decreasing the risk of developing gestational trophoblastic neoplasia. During follow-up, 33 percent of oral contraceptive users developed gestational trophoblastic neoplasia compared with about half who used other methods.

GESTATIONAL TROPHOBLASTIC NEOPLASIA

Also called malignant gestational trophoblastic disease, this term refers to invasive mole, choriocarcinoma, and placental site trophoblastic tumor. Any of these may follow molar pregnancy or normal pregnancy, or develop after abortive outcomes, including ectopic pregnancy. The criteria for diagnosis of postmolar gestational trophoblastic neoplasia are shown in Table 11–1.

ETIOLOGY. Gestational trophoblastic neoplasia almost always develops with or follows some form of pregnancy. Approximately half of cases follow a hydatidiform mole, 25 percent follow an abortion, and 25 percent develop after an apparently normal pregnancy. Of 48 fatal cases from the Brewer Trophoblastic Disease Center, only one third developed in association with a hydatidiform mole (Lurain and co-workers, 1982). The remainder were associated with term or near-term pregnancies, abortions, or ectopic pregnancies. Bailey and colleagues (2003) recently described choriocarcinoma arising from a primary abdominal pregnancy. Rarely, choriocarcinoma may arise from a teratoma.

Malignancy is rarely identified in the placenta of a seemingly normal pregnancy. In a case described by Brewer and Mazur (1981), widespread malignant trophoblastic invasion was evident at 18 weeks, and a primary choriocarcinoma of the placenta was detected. A case in which malignant trophoblastic tissue metastasized to the fetus also has been described (Kruseman and colleagues, 1977). Others have reported intraplacental choriocarcinoma associated with a live fetus (Aonahata and co-workers, 1998; Jacques and associates, 1998).

PATHOLOGY. The diagnosis of gestational trophoblastic neoplasia is made primarily by persistently elevated serum hCG levels. In most cases, there is no tissue to submit for pathological study. Thus, an unusual situation exists in that clinical management is not always dictated by histological findings.

Choriocarcinoma. This extremely malignant form of gestational trophoblastic neoplasia may be considered a carcinoma of the chorionic epithelium. In its growth and metastasis, however, it often behaves like a sarcoma. The characteristic gross picture is that of a rapidly growing mass invading both myometrium and blood vessels that causes hemorrhage and necrosis (Fig. 11–6A). The tumor is dark red or purple and ragged or friable. If it involves the endometrium, then bleeding, sloughing, and infection of the surface usually occur early. Masses of tissue buried in the myometrium may extend outward, appearing on the uterus as dark, irregular nodules that eventually penetrate the peritoneum.

Although cytotrophoblastic and syncytial elements are involved, one or the other may predominate. Microscopically, columns and sheets of these trophoblastic cells penetrate the muscle and blood vessels, sometimes in plexiform arrangement and at other times in complete disorganization, interspersed with clotted blood (Fig. 11–6B). An important diagnostic feature of choriocarcinoma, in contrast to hydatidiform mole or invasive mole, is absence of a villous pattern. Cellular anaplasia exists, but it is not a valuable criterion of malignancy. Factors involved in malignant transformation of the chorion are unknown. In choriocarcinoma, the predisposition of normal trophoblast to invasive growth and erosion of blood vessels is greatly exaggerated.

Metastases often develop early and are generally bloodborne because of the affinity of trophoblastic cells for blood vessels. The most common sites of metastasis are the lungs, in more than 75 percent of cases, and the vagina, in about 50 percent. The vulva, kidneys, liver, ovaries, brain, and bowel also may contain metastases (Fig. 11–7). Ovarian theca-lutein cysts are identified in over one third of cases.

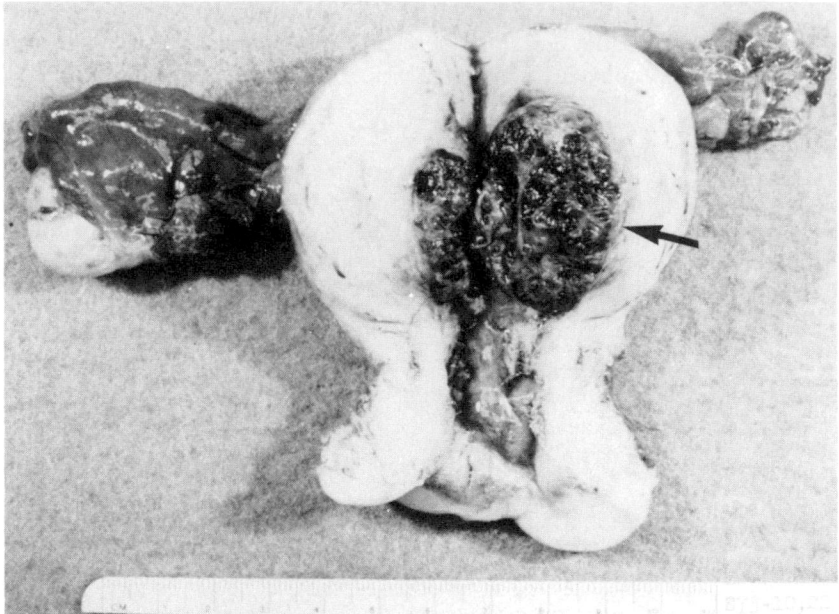

A

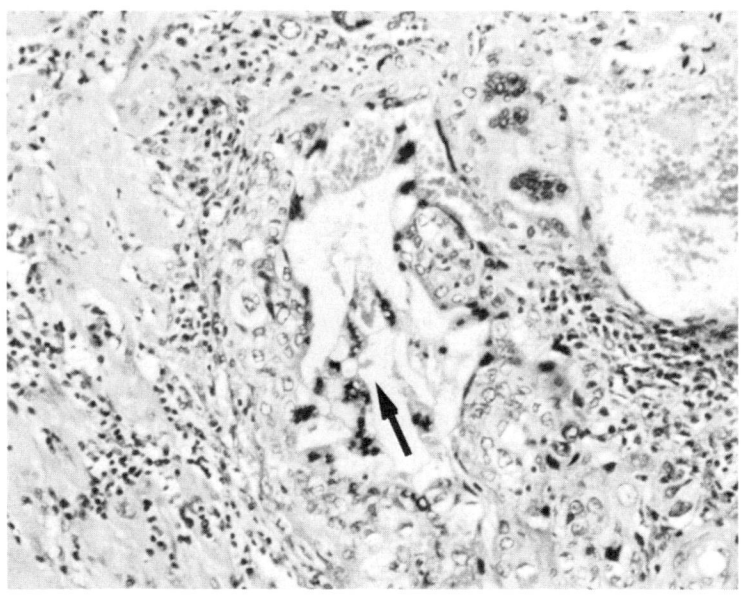

B

FIGURE 11–6. A. Choriocarcinoma (*arrow*) invading the uterus. Persistent trophoblastic disease was demonstrated by curettage subsequent to the expulsion of a hydatidiform mole. When repeated courses of chemotherapy failed to destroy the malignancy, hysterectomy and bilateral salpingo-oophorectomy were performed. The woman was alive without detectable chorionic gonadotropin 10 years later. **B.** Histological characteristics of the same choriocarcinoma. Malignant syncytiotrophoblast and cytotrophoblast without villous stroma invade the myometrium and vascular spaces (*arrow*), accompanied by necrosis and hemorrhage.

Invasive Mole. The distinguishing features of invasive mole are excessive trophoblastic overgrowth and extensive penetration by the trophoblastic cells, including whole villi. These structures penetrate into the depths of the myometrium, sometimes to involve the peritoneum, adjacent parametrium, or vaginal vault. Such moles are locally invasive, but generally lack the pronounced tendency to widespread metastasis typical of choriocarcinoma.

Placental Site Trophoblastic Tumor. Rarely, trophoblastic neoplasia arises from the placental implantation site following a normal term pregnancy, spontaneous or induced abor-

tion, ectopic pregnancy, or molar pregnancy (Feltmate and colleagues, 2001; Moore-Maxwell and Robboy, 2004). The tumor is characterized histologically by predominantly cytotrophoblastic cells, and immunohistochemical staining reveals many prolactin-producing cells and few gonadotropin-producing ones (Miller and associates, 1989). Thus, serum hCG levels may be normal to elevated. Bleeding is the main presenting symptom. Brewer and colleagues (1992) described a placental site trophoblastic tumor associated with erythrocytosis that resolved after hysterectomy. Nigam and co-workers (2004) described a tumor in a postmenopausal woman.

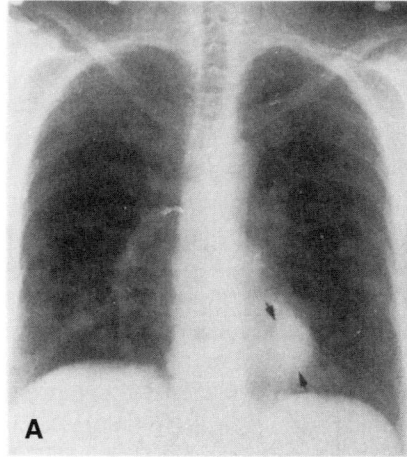

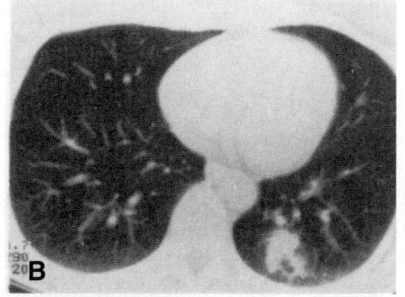

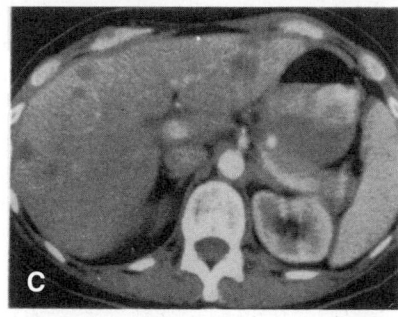

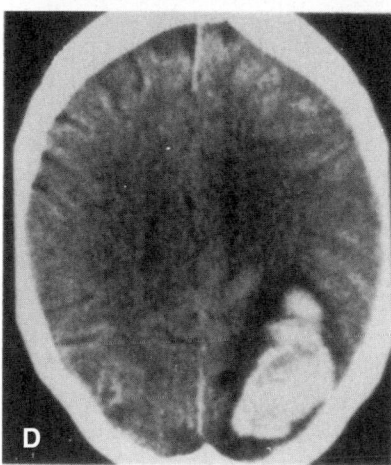

FIGURE 11–7. Metastatic choriocarcinoma. A chest radiograph **(A)** and a computed tomographic (CT) scan **(B)** demonstrate a left lower lobe metastatic lesion having poorly defined, irregular borders ("alveolar type") thought to be secondary to peripheral hemorrhage. **(C)** Abdominal CT scan at the level of the liver shows multiple low-density hepatic metastasis. **(D)** Cranial CT scan of the brain performed without contrast shows a large hemorrhagic metastasis in the left parietal lobe. (From DeBaz and Lewis, 1995, with permission.)

A placental site trophoblastic tumor was detected by Ichikawa and colleagues (2003) at the time of hysterectomy for a large uterine arteriovenous fistula. In another unusual presentation, Wright and colleagues (2002) reported a case of placental site trophoblastic tumor in a woman at 37 weeks' gestation who presented with a pneumothorax caused by a bullous metastatic tumor.

CLINICAL COURSE. The most common finding is irregular bleeding associated with uterine subinvolution. The bleeding may be continuous or intermittent, with sudden and sometimes massive hemorrhage. Uterine perforation caused by invasive trophoblastic growth may cause intraperitoneal hemorrhage (Hancock and Tidy, 2002).

In some cases, the woman presents with a metastatic lesion of the vagina or vulva. Occasionally, it has been impossible to locate choriocarcinoma in the uterus or pelvis because the original lesion has disappeared, leaving only distant metastases. If untreated, choriocarcinoma is invariably fatal.

DIAGNOSIS. Recognition of the possibility of gestational trophoblastic neoplasia is the most important factor in diagnosis. Any case of unusual bleeding after term pregnancy or abortion should be investigated by curettage, and especially with measurements of serum hCG. Solitary or multiple nodules seen in the chest radiograph are suggestive of choriocarcinoma (see Fig. 11–7). Persistent or rising hCG levels in the absence of pregnancy also are indicative of gestational trophoblastic neoplasia.

Anatomical staging before treatment includes pelvic examination, chest radiograph, and computed tomography (CT) scanning of the abdomen and pelvis. CT scanning of the chest and head is recommended only if the chest radiograph is abnormal. Moodley and Moodley (2004) described three women with normal chest radiograph readings but who had lung metastases identified with CT-scanning.

PROGNOSTIC SCORING SYSTEM. The International Federation of Gynecology and Obstetrics recently revised the World Health Organization Prognostic Scoring System (FIGO Oncology Committee, 2002). Scores of 0 to 4 are given according to age; type of antecedent pregnancy and interval from it; serum hCG concentration; size of tumor, site, and number of metastases; and whether previous chemotherapy was given. Low-risk neoplasia generally includes scores of 0 to 6.

Several other prognostic scoring systems and at least one anatomical staging system have been described (Bagshawe, 1976; Kohorn, 2002; Lurain and associates, 1991; Pettersson and colleagues, 1985).

TREATMENT. Single-agent chemotherapy is given for nonmetastatic or low-risk metastatic neoplasia. Methotrexate and other agents effective against malignant tumors, especially actinomycin D, are usually curative. Several regimens have been used with success. Methotrexate has been used with good results when given orally, by intravenous infusions, or by intramuscular injections (Garrett, 2002; Khan, 2003; Soper, 1994, and their colleagues). Single-dose actinomycin D is also highly effective in women with nonmetastatic disease (Lurain and Elfstrand, 1995; Petrilli and associates, 1987). In the ongoing Gynecological Oncology Group Protocol 174, women with low-risk disease are randomized to receive either methotrexate or actinomycin D. Suzuka and colleagues (2001) treated 37 women who had low-risk gestational trophoblastic neoplasia and reported that adjuvant hysterectomy decreased the total dose of chemotherapy needed to achieve primary remission. In some cases, such as with brain metastases, chemotherapy is given along with radiotherapy (Evans and associates, 1995).

High-Risk Trophoblastic Neoplasia. Patients are classified as high risk when the modified WHO prognostic score is 7 or greater. In these women, combination chemotherapy—with its increased toxicity—has produced the highest cure rates. According to Schorge and colleagues (2000) and Lurain (2002), the *EMA-CO regimen* results in response rates of about 90 percent and survival rates of 80 to 100 percent. This regimen is a combination of etoposide, methotrexate, actinomycin, cyclophosphamide, and Oncovin (vincristine). Similar results with EMA-CO were reported recently from the Netherlands by Houwen and associates (2004).

Placental Site Tumors. Hysterectomy is the most efficacious treatment for confirmed placental site trophoblastic tumor (Feltmate and associates, 2001; Miller and colleagues, 1989). It is not necessary to remove the ovaries if they appear normal (Ajithkumar and associates, 2003). Although

chemotherapy is recommended for metastatic disease, it is not as effective as for other gestational trophoblastic neoplasias (Gillespie and colleagues, 2000).

Randall and colleagues (2000) described a woman with a 3-year prolonged remission following recurrent metastatic placental site tumor and chemotherapy. Gillespie and colleagues (2000) treated three women successfully with only hysterectomy for tumor confined to the uterus. Another four were given chemotherapy for metastases, and although two responded, the other two died. Papadopoulos and colleagues (2002) reviewed their 25-year experiences with 34 cases of placental site tumors. Half of these followed a normal pregnancy, 20 percent followed a molar pregnancy, and 15 percent developed after a missed abortion. Of these 34 women, 20 percent died. The two most common factors associated with death were metastatic lung disease and an interval of 4 years or longer between the antecedent pregnancy and diagnosis.

PROGNOSIS. The recent overall cure rate for gestational trophoblastic neoplasia of all severities is about 90 percent. Women with nonmetastatic tumors or low-risk gestational trophoblastic neoplasia are cured virtually 100 percent of the time if single-agent chemotherapy is started as soon as persistent disease is identified (Schorge and colleagues, 2000). Previously cited on page 277 were the remarkable results of Lurain and colleagues (1983) for women treated at the Brewer Trophoblastic Disease Center of Northwestern University. From 1962 to 1978, 738 women with molar pregnancy were managed as generally outlined above. Chemotherapy was given to 142 women (19 percent) for gestational trophoblastic neoplasia. Of this group, 17 percent had an invasive mole and 2 percent had choriocarcinoma. All were living and disease-free 4 to 18 years later.

Women with low-risk metastatic gestational trophoblastic neoplasia who are treated aggressively with single- or multiagent chemotherapy do almost as well as those with nonmetastatic disease (Hammond and colleagues, 1980; Jones, 1987). Women with high-risk metastatic neoplasia have appreciable mortality rates that depend on which factors placed them at high risk (Soper and associates, 1988). Remission rates vary from 45 to 65 percent. Lurain (1987) analyzed 53 deaths from the Brewer Trophoblastic Center and concluded that the three risk factors primarily responsible were: (1) extensive choriocarcinoma at initial diagnosis, (2) lack of appropriately aggressive initial treatment, and (3) failure of currently used chemotherapy to effect neoplasia regression.

PREGNANCY AFTER GESTATIONAL TROPHO-BLASTIC DISEASE. Follow-up surveillance is minimally 6 months for molar pregnancy, 1 year for gestational trophoblastic neoplasia, and up to 2 years for cases with metastases other than to the lung. There is no difficulty with fertility or normal pregnancy outcome following successfully treated gestational trophoblastic disease (Schorge and associates, 2000; Woolas and co-workers, 1998). Women who have been given chemotherapy do not have an increased risk for anomalous fetuses in subsequent pregnancies (Rustin and colleagues, 1984; Song and associates, 1988). The primary concern is that women who had gestational trophoblastic disease are at increased risk for developing it again in a subsequent pregnancy. Berkowitz and colleagues (1987) reported that 1.3 percent of 1048 women treated at the New England Trophoblastic Disease Center developed a second molar pregnancy. Kim and associates (1998) reported that 4.3 percent of 115 Korean women had a second tumor.

REFERENCES

Ajithkumar TV, Abraham EK, Rejnishkumar R, et al: Placental site trophoblastic tumor. Obstet Gynecol Surv 58:484, 2003

American College of Obstetricians and Gynecologists: Bulletin #53. Diagnosis and treatment of gestational trophoblastic disease. Obstet Gynecol 103:1365, 2004

Amir SM, Osathanondh R, Berkowitz RS, et al: Human chorionic gonadotropin and thyroid function in patients with hydatidiform mole. Am J Obstet Gynecol 150:723, 1984

Aonahata M, Masuzawa Y, Tsutsui Y: A case of intraplacental choriocarcinoma associated with placental hemangioma. Pathol Int 48:897, 1998

Bagshawe KD: Risk and prognostic factors in trophoblastic neoplasia. Cancer 38:1373, 1976

Bagshawe KD, Lawler SD: Commentary: Unmasking moles. Br J Obstet Gynaecol 89:255, 1982

Bailey JL, Hinton EA, Ashfaq R, et al: Primary abdominal gestational choriocarcinoma. Obstet Gynecol 102:988, 2003

Benirschke K, Kaufmann P: Pathology of the Human Placenta, 4th ed. New York, Springer-Verlag, 2000

Berkowitz RS, Goldstein DP: Chorionic tumors. N Engl J Med 335:1740, 1996

Berkowitz RS, Goldstein DP, Bernstein MR: Advances in management of partial molar pregnancy. Contemp Obstet Gynecol 36:33, 1991

Berkowitz RS, Goldstein DP, Bernstein MR: Management of partial molar pregnancy. Contemp Obstet Gynecol 27:77, 1986

Berkowitz RS, Goldstein DP, Bernstein MR, et al: Subsequent pregnancy outcome in patients with molar pregnancy and gestational trophoblastic tumors. J Reprod Med 32:680, 1987

Bloss J, Miller D: Gestational trophoblastic disease. In Hankins GDV, Clark SL, Cunningham FG, Gilstrap LC (eds): Operative Obstetrics. Norwalk, CT, Appleton & Lange, 1995, p 695

Brewer CA, Adelson MD, Elder RC: Erythrocytosis associated with a placental-site trophoblastic tumor. Obstet Gynecol 79:846, 1992

Brewer JI, Mazur MT: Gestational choriocarcinoma: Its origin in the placenta during a seemingly normal pregnancy. Am J Surg Pathol 5:267, 1981

Bruchim I, Kidron D, Amiel A, et al: Complete hydatidiform mole and a coexistent viable fetus: Report of two cases and review of the literature. Gynecol Oncol 77:197, 2000

Chauhan S, Diamond MP, Johns DA: A case of molar ectopic pregnancy. Fertil Steril 81:1140, 2004

Coukos G, Makrigiannakis A, Chung J, et al: Complete hydatidiform mole. A disease with a changing profile. J Reprod Med 44:698, 1999

Curry SL, Hammond CB, Tyrey L, et al: Hydatidiform mole: Diagnosis, management, and longtime follow-up of 347 patients. Obstet Gynecol 45:1, 1975

DeBaz BP, Lewis TJ: Imaging of gestational trophoblastic disease. Semin Oncol 22:130, 1995

Deicas RE, Miller DS, Rademaker AW, et al: The role of contraception in the development of postmolar gestational trophoblastic tumor. Obstet Gynecol 78:221, 1991

Delmis J, Pfeifer D, Ivanisecvic M, et al: Sudden death from trophoblastic embolism in pregnancy. Eur J Obstet Gynecol Reprod Biol 92:225, 2000

Evans AC, Soper JT, Clarke-Pearson DL, et al: Gestational trophoblastic disease metastatic to the central nervous system. Gynecol Oncol 59:226, 1995

Feltmate CM, Genest DR, Wise L, et al: Placental site trophoblastic tumor: A 17-year experience at the New England Trophoblastic Disease Center. Gynecol Oncol 82:415, 2001

FIGO Oncology Committee: FIGO staging for gestational trophoblastic neoplasia 2000. Int J Gynecol Obstet 77:285, 2002

Garner EIO, Lipson E, Bernstein MR, et al: Subsequent pregnancy experience in patients with molar pregnancy and gestational trophoblastic tumor. J Reprod Med 47:380, 2002

Garrett AP, Garner EO, Goldstein DP, et al: Methotrexate infusion and folinic acid as primary therapy for nonmetastatic and low-risk metastatic gestational trophoblastic tumors. 15 years of experience. J Reprod Med 47:355, 2002

Genest DR, Ruiz RE, Weremowicz S, et al: Do nontriploid partial hydatidiform moles exist? J Reprod Med 47:363, 2002

Gillespie AM, Liyim D, Goepel JR, et al: Placental site trophoblastic tumour: A rare but potentially curable cancer. Br J Cancer 82:1186, 2000

Goldstein DP, Berkowitz RS: Prophylactic chemotherapy of complete molar pregnancy. Semin Oncol 22:157, 1995

Hammond CB, Borchert I, Tyrey I, et al: Treatment of metastatic trophoblastic disease: Good and poor prognosis. Am J Obstet Gynecol 115:451, 1973

Hammond CB, Weed JC, Currie JL: The role of operation in the current therapy of gestational trophoblastic disease. Am J Obstet Gynecol 136:844, 1980

Hancock BW, Tidy JA: Current management of molar pregnancy. J Reprod Med 47:347, 2002

Hankins GD, Wendel GD, Snyder RR, et al: Trophoblastic embolization during molar evacuation: Central hemodynamic observations. Obstet Gynecol 63:368, 1987

Houwen C, Rietbroek RC, Lok CA, et al: Feasibility of central coordinated EMA/CO for gestational trophoblastic disease in the Netherlands. Br J Obstet Gynaecol 111:143, 2004

Ichikawa Y, Nakauchi T, Sato T, et al: Ultrasound diagnosis of uterine arteriovenous fistula associated with placental site trophoblastic tumor. Ultrasound Obstet Gynecol 21:606, 2003

Jacques SM, Qureshi F, Doss BJ, et al: Intraplacental choriocarcinoma associated with viable pregnancy: Pathologic features and implications for the mother and infant. Pediatr Dev Pathol 1:380, 1998

Jauniaux E: Partial moles: From postnatal to prenatal diagnosis. Placenta 20:379, 1999

Jones WB: Current management of low-risk metastatic gestational trophoblastic disease. J Reprod Med 32:655, 1987

Khan F, Everard J, Ahmed S, et al: Low-risk persistent gestational trophoblastic disease treated with low-dose methotrexate: Efficacy, acute and long-term effects. Br J Cancer 89:2197, 2003

Kim JH, Park DC, Bae SN, et al: Subsequent reproductive experience after treatment for gestational trophoblastic disease. Gynecol Oncol 71:108, 1998

Kohorn EI: Negotiating a staging and risk factor scoring system for gestational trophoblastic neoplasia: A progress report. J Reprod Med 47:445, 2002

Kruseman AC, Lent MV, Blom AH, et al: Choriocarcinoma in mother and child, identified by immunoenzyme histochemistry. Am J Clin Pathol 67:279, 1977

Lawler SD, Fisher RA, Dent J: A prospective genetic study of complete and partial hydatidiform moles. Am J Obstet Gynecol 164:1270, 1991

Loret de Mola JR, Goldfarb JM: Reproductive performance of patients after gestational trophoblastic disease. Semin Oncol 22:193, 1995

Lurain JR: Advances in management of high-risk gestational trophoblastic tumors. J Reprod Med 47:451, 2002

Lurain JR: Causes of treatment failure in gestational trophoblastic disease. J Reprod Med 32:677, 1987

Lurain JR, Brewer JI, Mazur MT, et al: Fatal gestational trophoblastic disease: An analysis of treatment failures. Am J Obstet Gynecol 144:391, 1982

Lurain JR, Brewer JI, Torek EE, et al: Natural history of hydatidiform mole after primary evacuation. Am J Obstet Gynecol 145:591, 1983

Lurain JR, Casanova LA, Miller DS, et al: Prognostic factors in gestational trophoblastic tumors: A proposed new scoring system based on multivariate analysis. Am J Obstet Gynecol 164:611, 1991

Lurain JR, Elfstrand EP: Single-agent methotrexate chemotherapy for the treatment of nonmetastatic gestational trophoblastic tumors. Am J Obstet Gynecol 172:574, 1995

Mann K, Schneider N, Hoermann R: Thyrotropic activity of acidic isoelectric variants of human chorionic gonadotropin and trophoblastic tumors. Endocrinology 118:1558, 1986

Miller DS, Ballon SC, Teng NNH: Gestational trophoblastic diseases. In Brody SA, Ueland K (eds): Endocrine Disorders in Pregnancy. Norwalk, CT, Appleton and Lange, 1989, p 451

Montz FJ, Schlaerth JB, Morrow CP: The natural history of theca lutein cysts. Obstet Gynecol 72:247, 1988

Moodley M, Moodley J: Evaluation of chest X-ray findings to determine metastatic gestational trophoblastic disease according to the proposed new staging system: A case series. J Obstet Gynaecol 24:287, 2004

Moore-Maxwell CA, Robboy SJ: Placental site trophoblastic tumor arising from antecedent molar pregnancy. Gynecol Oncol 92:708, 2004

Nigam S, Singhal N, Kumar Gupta S, et al: Placental site trophoblastic tumor in a postmenopausal female–a case report. Gynecol Oncol 93:550, 2004

Novak E, Seah CS: Choriocarcinoma of the uterus. Am J Obstet Gynecol 67:933, 1954

Papadopoulos AJ, Foskett M, Seckl MJ, et al: Twenty-five years' clinical experience with placental site trophoblastic tumors. J Reprod Med 47:460, 2002

Petrilli ES, Twiggs LB, Blessing JA, et al: Single-dose actinomycin-D treatment for nonmetastatic gestational trophoblastic disease: A prospective phase II trial of the Gynecologic Oncology Group. Cancer 60:2173, 1987

Pettersson F, Kolstad P, Ludwig H: Annual report on the results of treatment in gynecologic cancer. Stockholm, International Federation of Gynecology and Obstetrics, 1985

Philipp T, Grillenberger K, Separovic ER, et al: Effects of triploidy on early human development. Prenat Diagn, 24:276, 2004

Randall TC, Coukos G, Wheeler JE, et al: Prolonged remission of recurrent, metastatic placental site trophoblastic tumor after chemotherapy. Gynecol Oncol 76:115, 2000

Rustin GJ, Booth M, Dent J, et al: Pregnancy after cytotoxic chemotherapy for gestational trophoblastic tumours. BMJ 288: 103, 1984

Schlaerth JB, Morrow CP, Kletzky OA, et al: Prognostic characteristics of serum human chorionic gonadotropin titer regression following molar pregnancy. Obstet Gynecol 58:478, 1981

Schorge JO, Goldstein DP, Bernstein MR, et al: Recent advances in gestational trophoblastic disease. J Reprod Med 45:692, 2000

Sebire NJ, Foskett M, Fisher RA, et al: Risk of partial and complete hydatidiform molar pregnancy in relation to maternal age. Br J Obstet Gynaecol 109:99, 2002a

Sebire NJ, Foskett M, Parainas FJ, et al: Outcome of twin pregnancies with complete hydatidiform mole and healthy co-twin. Lancet 359:2165, 2002b

Seckl MJ, Fisher RA, Salerno G, et al: Choriocarcinoma and partial hydatidiform moles. Lancet 356:36, 2000

Semer DA, Macfee MS: Gestational trophoblastic disease: Epidemiology. Semin Oncol 22:109, 1995

Shapter AP, McLellan R: Gestational trophoblastic disease. Obstet Gynecol Clin North Am 28:805, 2001

Smalbraak J: Trophoblastic Growths. Haarlem, Netherlands, Elsevier, 1957

Song HZ, Wu PC, Wang YE, et al: Pregnancy outcomes after successful chemotherapy for choriocarcinoma and invasive mole: Long-term follow-up. Am J Obstet Gynecol 158:538, 1988

Soper JT, Clarke-Pearson DL, Berchuck A, et al: 5-day methotrexate for women with metastatic gestational trophoblastic disease. Gynecol Oncol 54:76, 1994

Soper JT, Clarke-Pearson D, Hammond CB: Metastatic gestational trophoblastic disease: Prognostic factors in previously untreated patients. Obstet Gynecol 71:338, 1988

Stanhope CR, Stuart GCE, Curtis KL: Primary ovarian hydatidiform mole: Review of the literature and report of a case. Am J Obstet Gynecol 145:886, 1983

Suzuka K, Matsui H, Iitsuka Y, et al: Adjuvant hysterectomy in low-risk gestational trophoblastic disease. Obstet Gynecol 97:431, 2001

Suzuki M, Matsunobu A, Wakita K, et al: Hydatidiform mole with a surviving coexisting fetus. Obstet Gynecol 56:384, 1980

Tow WS: The influence of the primary treatment of hydatidiform mole on its subsequent course. J Obstet Gynaecol Br Commonw 73:544, 1966

Tuncer ZS, Bernstein MR, Wang J, et al: Repetitive hydatidiform mole with different male partners. Gynecol Oncol 75:224, 1999

Vejerslev LO: Clinical management and diagnostic possibilities in hydatidiform mole with coexistent fetus. Obstet Gynecol Surv 46:577, 1991

Wolf NG, Lage JM: Genetic analysis of gestational trophoblastic disease: A review. Semin Oncol 22:113, 1995

Woolas RP, Bower M, Newlands ES, et al: Influence of chemotherapy for gestational trophoblastic disease on subsequent pregnancy outcome. Br J Obstet Gynaecol 105:1032, 1998

World Health Organization Scientific Group on Gestational Trophoblastic Diseases: Gestational Trophoblastic Diseases. Technical Report Series No. 692. Geneva, World Health Organization, 1983

Wright JD, Powell MA, Horowitz NS, et al: Placental site trophoblastic tumor presenting with a pneumothorax during pregnancy. Obstet Gynecol 100:1141, 2002

Xia ZF, Song HZ, Tang MY: Risk of malignancy and prognosis using a provisional scoring system in hydatidiform mole. Chin Med J 93:605, 1980

12

Genetics

Genetics is the study of biological variation. *Medical genetics* is the study of individual variation in the incidence of and susceptibility to medical disorders and birth defects. Disease mechanisms, response to therapy, and genetic testing also are included in this field.

Genetic disease is common. Between 2 and 3 percent of neonates are born with a recognized congenital structural defect, another 3 percent have a defect diagnosed by age 5, and another 8 to 10 percent are discovered to have one or more functional or developmental abnormalities by age 18. In addition, susceptibility to many common diseases often has a genetic basis, and most cancers develop as the result of cumulative mutations. Thus, two thirds of the population will experience a disease with a genetic component in their lifetime. If cancers are included, 91 percent will be affected (Rimoin and colleagues, 1997). The types and estimated frequencies of various categories of genetic conditions by age at diagnosis are listed in Table 12–1. Tests available to diagnose some genetic diseases antenatally and the rationale accompanying their use in pregnancy are described throughout Chapter 13.

The *Human Genome Project*, supported principally by the National Human Genome Research Institute, had the goal of mapping the complete human genome. Sequencing was essentially complete by 2000, and finalized in 2003. Mapping the approximately 40,000 genes that comprise the haploid human genome will no doubt aid studies of normal and abnormal gene function to provide the basis for future diagnosis and therapy. Within our professional lifetimes, it is likely that consideration of each patient's genetic background and specific traits and susceptibilities will become part of routine medical care. Knowledge of genetic principles will thus be essential for all practitioners.

ETIOLOGY OF BIRTH DEFECTS

Birth defects can arise in at least three ways. This is illustrated by Figure 12–1, which shows three similar looking defects that actually arose by three different mechanisms. The first limb defect caused by fusion of the lower extremities is a *malformation*, meaning that the limb was "programmed"

TABLE 12–1 Types and Frequency of Genetic Disease by Age

Type	Frequency by Age 25 (per 1000 live births)	Lifetime Frequency (per 1000 live births)
Chromosomal disorders	1.8	4
Single-gene disorders	3.6	20
Multifactorial disease	46.4	646
Cancer	—	240
Total	52.0	910

Adapted from Baird and colleagues (1988).

to develop abnormally and is thus intrinsically genetically abnormal. In contrast, a *deformation* occurs when a genetically normal structure develops an abnormal shape because of mechanical forces imposed by the uterine environment. An example is an otherwise normal limb that develops contractures because of prolonged oligohydramnios. A *disruption* is a more severe change in form or function that occurs when genetically normal tissue is modified as the result of a specific insult. An example is early amnion rupture causing limb deformities. There are some identical-appearing abnormalities, referred to as *phenocopies*, that have widely varying etiologies, which can make the diagnosis of even relatively simple defects difficult.

Multiple structural defects or developmental abnormalities can occur together in one individual. A cluster of several anomalies or defects can be a *syndrome*, meaning that all the abnormalities have the same cause—for example, trisomy 18. Anomalies also may comprise a *sequence*, meaning that all abnormalities developed sequentially as the result of one initial insult—for example, oligohydramnios leading to pulmonary hypoplasia, limb contractures, and facial deformities. Finally, a group of anomalies may be considered an *association*, meaning that these particular anomalies occur together frequently, but do not seem to be linked etiologically—for example, *CHARGE association*, which is a combination of *c*oloboma, *h*eart defects, *a*tresia choanae, mental *r*etardation, *g*rowth deficiency, and *e*ar anomalies. It is readily apparent that classification of anomalies can be challenging, and reclassification often is required.

CHROMOSOMAL ABNORMALITIES

STANDARD NOMENCLATURE. By convention, karyotypes are reported using nomenclature agreed upon by the genetics community and codified in 1985 by the International System for Human Cytogenetic Nomenclature (ISCN). The total number of chromosomes is listed first and corresponds to the number of centromeres present. This is followed by the sex chromosomes (XX or XY), and then by a description of any variation or abnormality detected. Specific abnormalities are indicated by standard abbreviations, such as *dup (duplicated), der (derivative), t (translocated),* and many more. Each chromosome has a short arm—the "p" or *petit* arm—and a long arm—the "q" arm—named for the next letter in the alphabet. The arms are separated by a centromere. These letters further identify the affected chromosomal components. The standard nomenclature for writing a karyotype is shown in Table 12–2.

Chromosomal abnormalities figure prominently in assessments of the impact of genetic disease, accounting for 50 percent of embryonic deaths, 5 to 7 percent of fetal losses, 6 to 11 percent of stillbirths and neonatal deaths, and 0.9 percent of liveborn children (Hook, 1992; Tolmie, 1995).

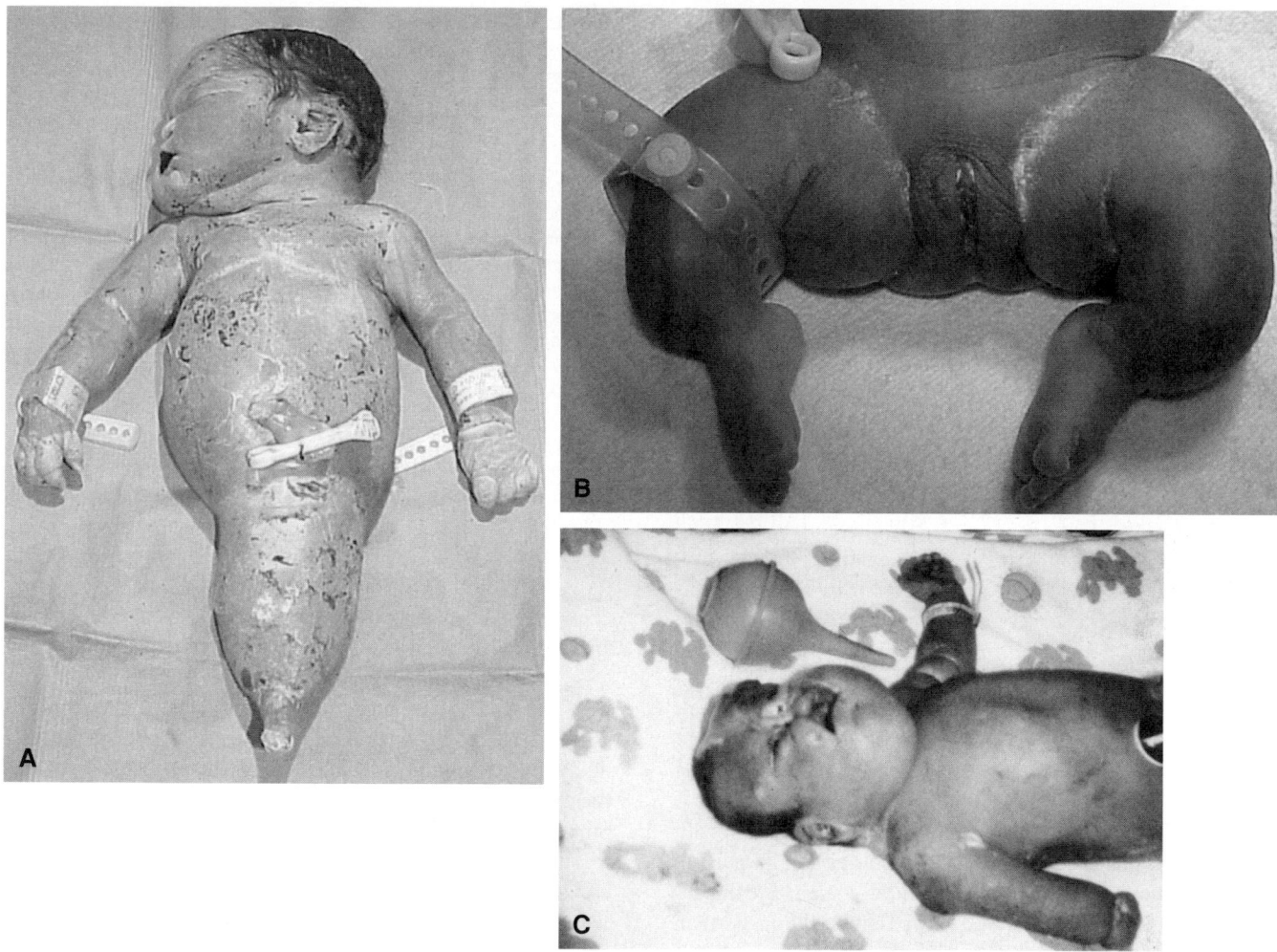

FIGURE 12–1. Examples of three major types of dysmorphogenesis. **A.** Malformation sequence: sircnomelia or fused lower extremities. **B.** Deformation sequence: clubbed feet from prolonged oligo-hydramnios. **C.** Disruption sequence: cephalocele, cleft lip, amputated right arm, and bilateral arm bands from amnionic bands (Photographs courtesy of Dr. Ron Ramus and Dr. Diane Twickler.)

TABLE 12–2 Standard Nomenclature for Chromosome Karyotypes

Karyotypes	Description
46,XY	Normal male chromosome constitution
47,XX,+21	Female with trisomy 21
47,XY,+21/46,XY	Male who is a mosaic of trisomy 21 cells and cells with normal constitution
46,XY,del(4)(p14)	Male with distal deletion of the band designated 14 from the short arm of chromosome 4
46,XX,dup(5p)	Female with duplication of the short arm of chromosome 5
45,XY,−13,−14,t(13q;14q)	Male with a balanced Robertsonian translocation of chromosomes 13 and 14; karyotype shows that one normal 13 and one normal 14 are missing
46,XY,t(11;22)(q23;q22)	Male with a balanced reciprocal translocation between chromosomes 11 and 22; breakpoints are at 11q23 and 22q22
46,XX,inv(3)(p21;q13)	Inversion of chromosome 3 that extends from p21 to q13; because it includes the centromere, this is a pericentric inversion
46,X,r(X)	Female with one normal X chromosome and one ring X chromosome
46,X,I(Xq)	Female with one normal X chromosome and an isochromosome of the long arm of the X chromosome

From Jorde and colleagues (1995), with permission.

TABLE 12-3 Estimates of the Frequency of Chromosomal Abnormalities in a Population of Unselected Newborns

	Incidence per 1000 Births	Per Birth
Sex chromosomes		
Male	1.15	1/870
Female	0.75	1/1333
Autosomal trisomy	1.42	1/700
Structural abnormality		
Unbalanced	0.61	1/1600
Balanced	5.22	1/200
Triploidy	0.02	1/50,000
Total	9.17	1/109

Adapted from Jacobs and colleagues (1992), with permission.

TABLE 12-5 Timing of Loss Due to Common Aneuploidies According to Gestational Age

Chromosomal Defect	Pregnancy Loss (%)		
	Estimated		Observed
	10 Weeks to Birth	16 Weeks to Birth	16 Weeks to Birth
Trisomy 21	47	31	30
Trisomy 18	86	74	86
Trisomy 13	83	71	43
Turner syndrome	76	52	75
47,XXX	~5	~3	0
47,XXY	~5	~3	1
47,XYY	~5	~3	3
Triploidy	>99	>99	100

From Snijders and colleagues (1995), with permission.

ANEUPLOIDY. There are a total of 44 autosomes, arranged in pairs numbered from 1 to 22, and one pair of sex chromosomes. The most obvious or easily recognized chromosomal abnormalities are numerical. In these, the affected individual inherits an extra chromosome—*trisomy;* is missing a chromosome—*monosomy;* or has an abnormal number of haploid chromosomal complements—*polyploidy.* The estimated incidence of aneuploidy and other chromosomal abnormalities in newborns is shown in Table 12–3.

Trisomy. Most trisomies and nonmosaic monosomies result from meiotic nondisjunction. Chromosomes fail to pair up initially, or they pair properly but then fail to separate or separate prematurely (Gardner and Sutherland, 1996; Sherman and colleagues, 1991). The risk of nondisjunction increases with maternal age (Table 12–4). Oocytes are held suspended in midprophase of meiosis I from birth until ovulation—in some cases for 50 years. Aging is thought to break down chiasmata that keep paired chromosomes aligned. When meiosis is completed at the time of ovulation, nondisjunction leads to one resulting gamete receiving two copies of the chromosome in question. This leads to trisomy if fertilized. The other gamete receives no copies and is thus monosomic when fertilized. Although 3 to 4 percent of sperm and 10 to 20 percent of oocytes are aneuploid as the result of meiotic errors, natural selection against these abnormal gametes makes them less likely to result in conception than normal gametes. If fertilization does occur, most aneuploid conceptuses die early.

Although each of the 23 chromosome pairs is equally likely to be involved in a segregation error, only a few trisomies are identified (Kamiguchi and associates, 1993). Some trisomies are associated with such severe abnormalities that they always result in loss before or shortly after implantation. For example, trisomy 1 has never been reported. Trisomy 16 accounts for 16 percent of all first-trimester deaths, but is never seen later. Only autosomal trisomies 13, 18, and 21 result in viable term pregnancies. Even so, the majority of these fetuses are lost before term (Table 12–5). In their review, McIntosh and colleagues (1995) confirmed that one third of Down syndrome fetuses in women aged 35 years and older are lost in the interval between chorionic villus sampling at 10 weeks and amniocentesis at 16 weeks, and half die before term.

TABLE 12-4 Estimated Rates (per 1000 Births) of Cytogenetic Abnormalities by Maternal Age at the Time of Amniocentesis

Maternal Age (years)	47,+21	47,+18	47,+13	47,XXX	47,XXY	Other Clinically Significant	All Abnormalities[a]
33	2.4	0.6	0.4	0.4	0.4	1.1	4.6–5.4
35	4.0	1.0	0.5	0.6	0.6	1.3	7.4–8.0
37	6.7	1.6	0.6	0.8	1.0	1.4	12.1–12.2
40	14.5	3.3	1.0	1.4	1.9	1.7	25.0–23.8
43	31.1	6.6	1.5	2.4	3.8	2.0	51.9–47.5
45	51.8	10.8	2.0	3.4	5.9	2.3	84.3–76.0
47	86.2	16.9	2.7	4.9	9.3	2.6	137–123
49	143.5	26.9	3.6	7.0	14.8	2.9	223–199

[a]The first value of the range given is derived from a regression equation analysis on all abnormalities; the second by adding values for all abnormalitites.
From Hook and co-workers (1983), with permission.

Monosomy. Although nondisjunction leads to an equal number of nullisomic and disomic gametes, there is no clinically recognized association between maternal age and monosomy. The most likely explanation is that monosomy is almost universally incompatible with life, and monosomic conceptuses die prior to implantation (Garber and co-workers, 1996). As a rule, missing chromosomal material is much more devastating to the organism than having extra chromosomal material. One exception is *monosomy X,* or *Turner syndrome,* discussed later. Although it accounts for about 20 percent of first-trimester fetal deaths, a small proportion of cases survive until term.

Polyploidy. Abnormalities of ploidy account for about 20 percent of abortions and are rarely seen in later pregnancies. Two thirds of *triploidy* cases result from fertilization of one egg by two sperm. The remainder are caused by failure of one of the meiotic divisions, resulting in a diploid chromosomal complement in either the egg or, more frequently, the sperm. The origin of the extra set of chromosomes determines the phenotype. If the extra chromosomes are paternal (diandric), the result is usually a partial hydatidiform mole with abnormal fetal structures (see Chap. 11, p. 275). Rarely, a relatively normal-sized fetus develops but the placenta is abnormally large and cystic. These pregnancies frequently are complicated by midtrimester severe preeclampsia. If the extra set of chromosomes is maternal (digynic), a fetus and placenta develop but the fetus is severely growth restricted. Triploid fetuses of either kind are frequently dysmorphic. If a woman had a triploid pregnancy with a fetus that survived past the first trimester, the recurrence risk is 1 to 1.5 percent (Gardner and Sutherland, 1996). This risk justifies offering prenatal diagnosis in subsequent pregnancies (see Chap. 13, p. 315).

Tetraploidy always results in 92,XXXX or 92,XXYY, indicating a postzygotic failure to complete an early cleavage division (Thompson and colleagues, 1991). The recurrence risk for tetraploidy is minimal.

PATERNAL EFFECTS. There is no association between aneuploidy and paternal age, probably because aneuploid sperm cannot fertilize an egg. Advanced paternal age does, however, logarithmically increase the risk of spontaneous new mutations causing autosomal dominant diseases such as neurofibromatosis or achondroplasia (Friedman, 1981). These new mutations also may be a factor in early pregnancy loss. The incidence of new autosomal dominant mutations among newborns whose fathers are 40 years old is at least 0.3 percent. There is some evidence that paternal age also may affect the incidence of isolated structural abnormalities (McIntosh and colleagues, 1995).

Chromosome abnormalities are increased when conception is induced by *intracytoplasmic sperm injection (ICSI).* A study including 2083 such pregnancies evaluated with fetal karyotyping identified 72 chromosomal abnormalities, a rate of 3.5 percent (Van Steirteghem and co-workers, 2002). Of these, 30 were inherited, 15 involved sex chromosome abnormalities, and 28 involved autosomes. In addition, these fetuses are at increased risk to have inherited Y chromosome deletions (In't Velt and colleagues, 1997).

AUTOSOMAL TRISOMIES

Trisomy 21. This trisomy also is called *Down syndrome* after J.L.H. Down, who described it in 1866. A trisomy 21 karyotype, shown in Figure 12–2, is found in 1 in 800 to 1000 newborns. Because it is the most common nonlethal trisomy, this condition is the focus of most genetic

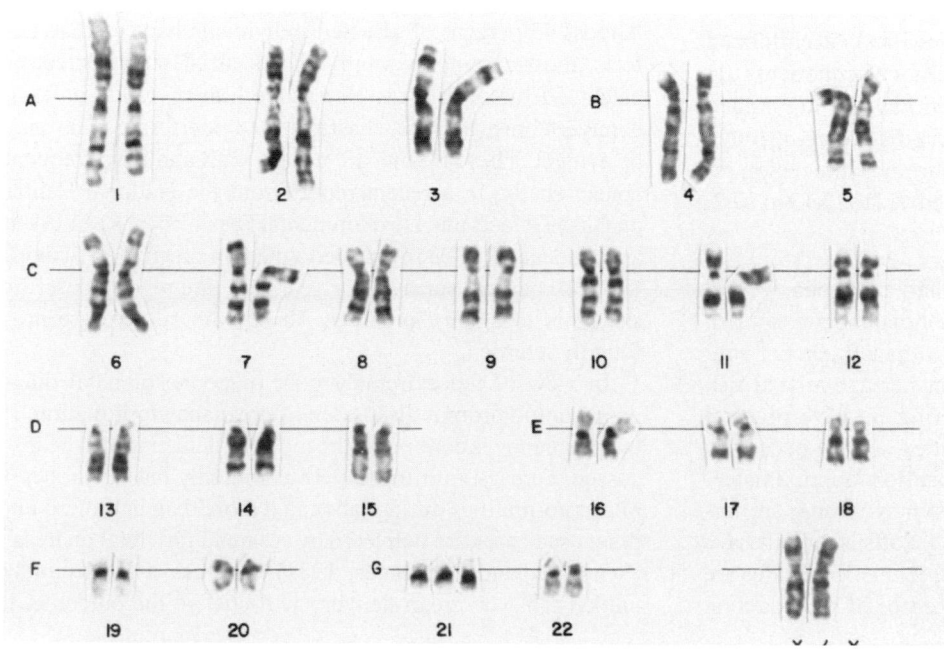

FIGURE 12–2. Abnormal female karyotype with trisomy 21, consistent with Down syndrome; 47,XX+21. (Courtesy of Dr. Nancy R. Schneider.)

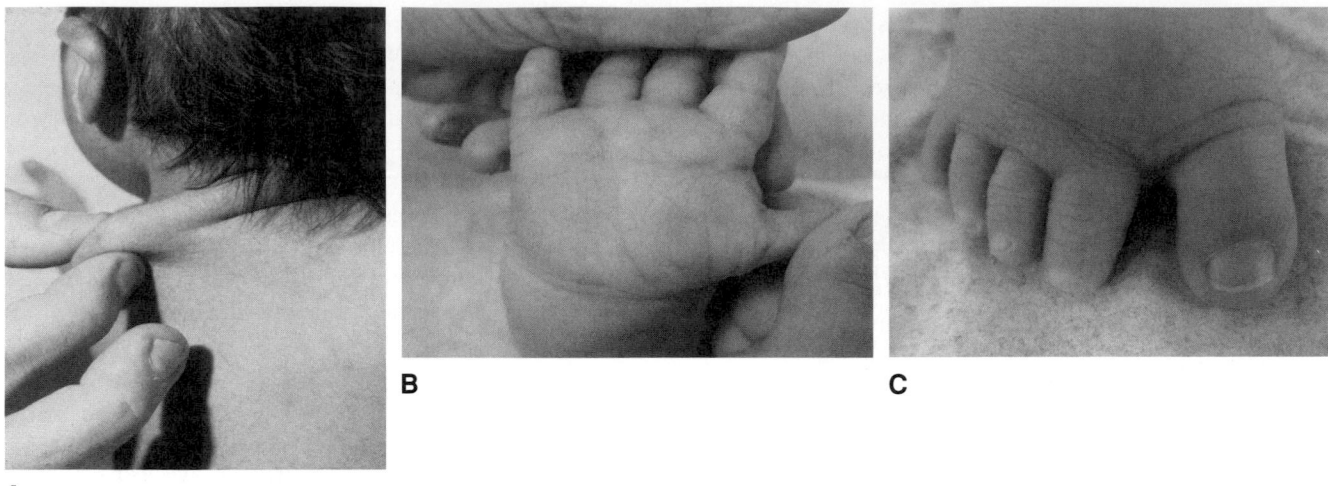

FIGURE 12–3. Trisomy 21 Down syndrome. **A.** Prominent nuchal tissue redundancy. **B.** Transverse palmar crease. **C.** Sandal toe gap. (Photographs courtesy of Dr. Charles Read and Dr. Lewis Waber.)

screening and testing protocols (see Chap. 13, p. 323). Approximately 95 percent of Down syndrome cases result from maternal nondisjunction of chromosome 21—75 percent during meiosis I and 25 percent during meiosis II. The remaining cases result from mosaicism or translocation.

The Down syndrome phenotype includes marked hypotonia, tongue protrusion, a small head with flattened occiput, flat nasal bridge, and epicanthal folds with up-slanting palpebral fissures. There is frequently loose skin at the nape of the neck, short fingers, a single palmar crease, and absence or hypoplasia of the middle phalanx, causing clinodactyly (inward curving) of the fifth finger, and the "sandal toe" gap (Fig. 12–3). Associated major abnormalities include heart defects (particularly endocardial cushion defects) in 30 to 40 percent of cases and gastrointestinal atresias. These children also have a high incidence of neonatal or childhood leukemia and thyroid disease. The intelligence quotient (IQ) ranges from 25 to 50, with a few individuals testing higher, and most affected children have social skills averaging 3 to 4 years ahead of their mental age. The chromosome region responsible for the mental deficit is located at 21q22.13 to 22.2.

RECURRENCE RISK. Once a woman has had a pregnancy complicated by trisomy 21 resulting from nondisjunction, her risk to have another pregnancy with any trisomy is 1 percent until her age-related risk exceeds this; then her age-related risk predominates. This risk justifies offering invasive prenatal diagnosis. Parental chromosomal studies are not necessary unless the trisomy was due to a translocation (approximately 3 percent of cases). Females with Down syndrome are fertile, and approximately one third of their offspring will have Down syndrome (Scharrer and colleagues, 1975). Males are almost always sterile, and only a few cases of reproduction

have been reported (Sheridan and associates, 1989; Zuhlke and co-workers, 1994).

Trisomy 18. Also known as *Edwards syndrome,* trisomy 18 occurs in 1 in 8000 newborns and is three to four times more common in females. The incidence is much higher in the first trimester, but 85 percent of fetuses with this syndrome die between 10 weeks and term. Moreover, trisomy 18 fetuses usually are growth restricted, with a mean birthweight of 2340 g (Snijders and colleagues, 1995).

Striking facial features include prominent occiput, rotated and malformed auricles, short palpebral fissures, and a small mouth. The hands are often held clenched with the second and fifth fingers overlapping the third and fourth (Jones, 1997). Virtually every organ system can be affected by trisomy 18. Almost 95 percent of affected individuals have cardiac defects, most commonly ventricular or atrial septal defect or patent ductus arteriosus. Horseshoe kidney, radial aplasia, hemivertebrae, hernias, diastasis, or imperforate anus may be evident. These infants are usually frail and have frequent apneic spells. In a recent report from the National Center on Birth Defects and Developmental Disabilities, Rasmussen and associates (2003) described a median survival of 14 days. Up to 10 percent survive to 1 year, and rare reports describe survivors to age 10 or older. Those who survive are profoundly retarded.

In view of the extremely poor outcome, prenatal diagnosis should prompt discussion of pregnancy termination. If the pregnancy is continued, the mode of delivery must be discussed. Fetuses with trisomy 18 commonly have fetal heart rate abnormalities during labor, and more than half of all undiagnosed cases are delivered by cesarean for "fetal distress" (Schneider and colleagues, 1981). Because it is extremely unlikely that cesarean delivery will change the outcome, it is reasonable to avoid unnecessary maternal operative morbidity by planning a vaginal delivery regardless of whether the fetus tolerates labor, recognizing that intrapartum fetal demise may occur.

Trisomy 13. Known as *Patau syndrome,* trisomy 13 occurs in approximately 1 in 20,000 births. Common abnormalities include cardiac defects in 80 to 90 percent of cases, and holoprosencephaly in 70 percent. Holoprosencephaly may be accompanied by microcephaly, hypotelorism, and pronounced abnormalities of the orbits, nose, and palate. Affected fetuses also may have abnormal ears, omphalocele, polycystic kidneys, radial aplasia, cutis aplasia, and polydactyly. Rasmussen and colleagues (2003) recently reviewed outcomes of 70 liveborn infants with trisomy 13. They found that the median survival for trisomy 13 liveborn neonates was 7 days. Up to 10 percent survived to 1 year. Counseling regarding prenatal diagnosis and delivery is approached as previously described with trisomy 18.

Other Trisomies. It is rare to see liveborn neonates with other autosomal trisomies, although mosaicism involving a few other autosomal chromosomes has been reported.

SEX CHROMOSOME ABNORMALITIES

XXX and XXY. There have been studies in which children with sex chromosome abnormalities are identified through early screening and then followed prospectively. These studies aid the identification of each specific phenotype. One such study between 1964 and 1974 identified 43 of 40,000 newborns—1 in 930—with sex chromosome aneuploidy (Robinson and colleagues, 1991). They were followed until age 24. Both females with 47,XXX and males with 47,XXY (*Klinefelter syndrome*) had very similar phenotypes. Both tended to be tall. XXX females displayed normal pubertal development and fertility. XXY males, however, did not virilize and required testosterone replacement therapy. They were more likely to be infertile as the result of gonadal dysgenesis and to have gynecomastia and small testicles.

Neither XXX nor XXY is strongly associated with mental retardation, but there is wide variability in intellectual function. The IQ scores ranged from 71 to 122; the mean IQ of XXY males was 95, whereas that of XXX females was 87—both within normal limits, but lower than controls. Most XXX and XXY study subjects had some type of developmental problem or speech disability, neuromotor, or learning disability.

Females with more than three X chromosomes—48,XXXX or 49,XXXXX—are likely to have physical abnormalities that are apparent at birth and to exhibit varying degrees of mental retardation. For both males and females, IQ drops with each additional X chromosome.

47,XYY. These males are phenotypically normal but tall. They generally have normal intelligence, although their IQs may be lower than those of their siblings, and they often have learning disabilities. Early reports indicating that XYY was associated with criminal or violent behavior suffered from ascertainment bias because prisoners or men with serious psychological dysfunction were tested preferentially. In their prospective study, Robinson and colleagues (1997) found only an increased risk of emotional difficulties, including mild depression and increased hyperactivity and aggressiveness in XYY men. Males with more than two Y chromosomes—48,XYYY—or with both additional X and Y chromosomes—48,XXYY or 49,XXXYY—have obvious physical abnormalities and significant mental retardation.

45,X. Called *Turner syndrome,* this is the only monosomy compatible with life. It is the most common aneuploidy in abortuses and accounts for 20 percent of chromosomally abnormal first-trimester abortions. Its prevalence in liveborn neonates is about 1 in 5000 births (Sybert and McCauley, 2004).

There are three distinct phenotypes seen with 45,X. At least 98 percent of conceptuses are so abnormal that they abort in the first trimester. In the majority of the remainder, abnormal ultrasonographic findings such as cystic hygromas (see Fig. 16–8, p. 395) may be detected later, and these findings may be accompanied by hydrops and fetal demise. The third, least common phenotype comprises liveborn individuals, who may have only minor problems. Features of this last group include short stature, broad chest with widely spaced nipples, congenital lymphedema with puffy fingers and toes, low hairline with webbed posterior neck, and minor bone and cartilage abnormalities. Between 30 and 50 percent have a major cardiac malformation, usually aortic coarctation or bicuspid aortic valves. Intelligence is generally in the normal range. 45,X females, however, frequently have visual-spatial organization deficits and difficulty with nonverbal problem solving and with interpretation of subtle social cues (Jones, 1997). Over 90 percent also have ovarian dysgenesis and require life-long hormone replacement beginning just before adolescence.

The tremendous range of phenotypes of Turner syndrome may be explained by a high incidence of mosaicism, with two or more populations of cells identified. About half are 45,X nonmosaic which results from an error in meiosis. The mosaic Turner syndrome stems from an error in mitosis, with one or more populations of cells missing an X chromosome. The live-born infants will have karyotypes like 45,X/46,XX or 45,X/46,XY (Saenger, 1996; Sybert and McCauley, 2004). As many as half of women with Turner syndrome display mosaicism in peripheral blood cells; the remainder may have mosaicism expressed only in tissues that are not routinely tested (Fernandez, 1996; Kim, 1999; Nazarenko, 1999, and their colleagues). If ultimately the majority of cells are 45,X, that individual will have the Turner phenotype, but modified

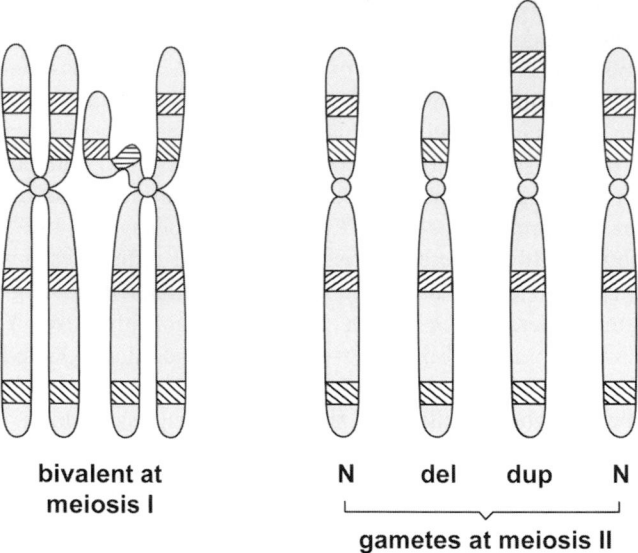

bivalent at meiosis I

N   del   dup   N

gametes at meiosis II

FIGURE 12–4. One mechanism to produce a duplication and a deletion. Similar sequences (crosshatched segments) exist at numerous places along the chromosome. Misalignment of two nonhomologous sequences, followed by illegitimate recombination within these two sequences (X), produces recombinant products that are reciprocally imbalanced: one with a duplication of the chromatin between the two sequences, and the other with a deficiency. (From Gardner and Sutherland, 1996, with permission.)

by the presence of the other cell populations (Koeberl and co-workers, 1995). The missing X chromosome does not appear to be lost randomly—the maternal X is retained in 80 percent of surviving cases (Cockwell and colleagues, 1991; Hassold and associates, 1991).

CHROMOSOMAL DELETIONS. A deletion means that a portion of a chromosome is missing. These errors usually are described by the location of the two break points within the chromosome or, if the deletion is common, by an eponym; for example, *del 5p* also is called *cri du chat syndrome.* Most deletions occur during meiosis and result from malalignment or mismatching during pairing of homologous chromosomes. If the two chromosomes are not aligned properly, the unaligned loop may be deleted (Fig. 12–4). If the mismatch remains and the two chromosomes recombine, the result may be a deletion in one and a duplication in the other. If a deletion is identified in a fetus or child, the parents should be tested to determine whether either carries a balanced translocation that would increase the recurrence risk.

Chromosome Banding. Recognition of a deletion during cytogenetic analysis is facilitated by various staining methods used to create light and dark chromosomal bands. These banding patterns are unique and allow identification of each chromosome and recognition of missing segments. Several genetic conditions have been identified that are caused by

microdeletions—deletions too small to be detected by older methods.

Genes in a deleted chromosomal segment often control several different traits. Thus, *contiguous gene deletion syndromes* usually involve serious but unrelated phenotypic and functional abnormalities. Deletions can occur in any area of any chromosome. Several specific deletions, however, are found more frequently than expected by chance alone, probably because certain regions are predisposed to breakage.

Deletion 4p. Known as *Wolf-Hirschhorn syndrome,* this deletion involves material from the short arm of chromosome number 4. It is characterized by fetal growth restriction, hypotonia, a unique facial appearance, severe mental deficiency, polydactyly, and cutis aplasia. Affected children often have severe seizures and seldom survive childhood. Approximately 85 percent of 4p deletions occur de novo, and in 80 percent the deleted chromosomal material is paternal.

Deletion 5p. Partial deletion of the short arm of chromosome 5 causes *cri du chat syndrome.* Affected infants are growth restricted, hypotonic, and severely retarded. They are sometimes identified by their mewling, high-pitched, catlike cry, attributed to abnormal laryngeal development.

Shprintzen and DiGeorge Phenotypes. These phenotypes both result from the same 22q11.2 microdeletion (Driscoll and colleagues, 1993). Botto and colleagues (2003) recently described a population-based study from the National Center on Birth Defects and Developmental Disabilities. They found the prevalence of 22q11.2 microdeletion to be about 1 in 6000 among whites, blacks, and Asians, and 1 in 3800 among Hispanics. More than 80 percent had heart defects, and one third had major extracardiac anomalies. The deletion accounted for at least 1 in 68 cases of a major heart defect. Shprintzen phenotype also is called *velo-cardio-facial syndrome.* Individuals with this deletion may have cleft palate, velopharyngeal incompetence, prominent nose, a long face with retruded mandible, cardiac defects, learning difficulties, and short stature. By contrast, the DiGeorge phenotype is characterized by thymus hypo- or aplasia, parathyroid hypo- or aplasia, and aortic arch malformations. Typical facies includes short palpebral fissures, micrognathia with a short philtrum, and ear anomalies. Mental development is usually normal.

It has been hypothesized that DiGeorge and Shprintzen phenotypes represent two extremes of a spectrum of abnormalities associated with the identical deletion. It is also possible that each condition represents a separate contiguous gene deletion syndrome of genes located at 22q11.2, but that current cytogenetic methods cannot distinguish differences between the two. Recent data indicate that the 22q11.2 microdeletion also accounts for a large proportion of heart defects in individuals without the extracardiac features of either DiGeorge or Shprintzen syndromes. These include interrupted aortic arch, truncus arteriosus, and Fallot tetralogy.

CHROMOSOMAL TRANSLOCATIONS

Reciprocal Translocations. A reciprocal or double-segment translocation is a rearrangement of chromosomal material in which breaks occur in two different chromosomes, and the fragments are exchanged before the breaks are repaired. The rearranged chromosomes are called *derivative (der) chromosomes.* If no chromosomal material is gained or lost in this process, it is a *balanced translocation.* Although the transposition of chromosomal segments can cause abnormalities due to repositioning of specific genes, in most cases gene function is not affected and the balanced carrier is phenotypically normal. Offspring who inherit either the two normal chromosomes or the two translocated chromosomes also usually have a normal phenotype. Fryns and associates (1992) reported a 6.4 percent total risk (including background) for anomalies with a balanced translocation.

Carriers of a balanced translocation can produce unbalanced gametes that result in abnormal offspring. As shown in Figure 12–5, if one of the translocated chromosomes and one of the normal co-chromosomes are included in the oocyte or sperm, following fertilization, the result is monosomy for part of one chromosome and trisomy for part of another. The observed risk of many specific translocations can be estimated by a genetic counselor, but in general, translocation carriers identified after the birth of an abnormal child have a

5 to 30 percent risk of having unbalanced liveborn offspring. Carriers identified for other reasons, for example, during an infertility workup, only have up to 5 percent risk, probably because their gametes and thus conceptions are so abnormal as to be nonviable.

Robertsonian Translocations. These translocations result when the long arms of two individual acrocentric chromosomes—for example, chromosomes 13 and 14—fuse at the centromere to form one. Translocations may involve any of the acrocentric chromosomes shown in Figure 12–2. These include chromosomes 13, 14, 15, 21, and 22, but almost all involve chromosome 14 (Levitan, 1988). Fusion at the centromeres results in the loss of one centromere and the *satellite regions* which comprise the short arms of each chromosome. These regions contain only genes coding for ribosomal RNA, which also are present in multiple copies on other acrocentric chromosomes. As long as the fused q arms are intact, the translocation carrier is usually phenotypically normal. Because the number of centromeres determines the chromosome count, the typical carrier of a Robertsonian translocation will have only 45 chromosomes.

Robertsonian carriers have reproductive difficulties. If the fused chromosomes are homologous—from the same chromosome pair—the carrier makes only unbalanced gametes. Each egg or sperm contains either both copies of the translocated chromosome, which would result in trisomy if fertilized,

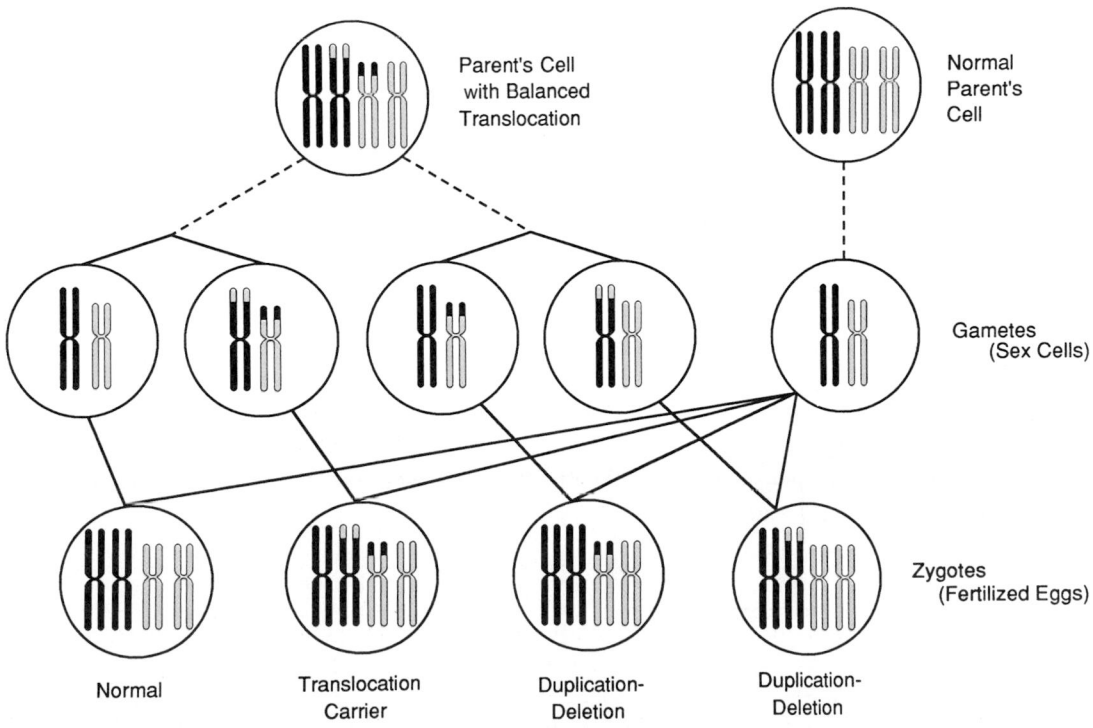

FIGURE 12–5. Gametes produced by a balanced translocation carrier. (From Greenwood Genetics Center, 1995, with permission.)

or no copy, which would result in monosomy. If the fused chromosomes are nonhomologous, four of the six possible gametes (66 percent) would be abnormal. Because some of these abnormal gametes would be nonviable, however, the actual observed incidence of abnormal offspring is only 15 percent if the translocation is carried by the mother, and 2 percent if carried by the father.

Robertsonian translocations are common. Their incidence in newborns is approximately 1 in 1000, which is equal to all other translocations combined. Robertsonian translocations, however, are not a major cause of miscarriage and occur in fewer than 5 percent of couples with recurrent pregnancy loss (Smith and Gaha, 1990). Still, identification of these translocations has tremendous impact on reproductive plans and may have implications for other family members. When a fetus or child is found to have a translocation trisomy, chromosomal studies of both parents should be performed. If neither parent is a carrier and the translocation occurred spontaneously, the recurrence risk is low.

Isochromosomes. These abnormal chromosomes are composed of either two q arms or two p arms of one chromosome fused together. Isochromosomes are thought to arise when the centromere breaks transversely instead of longitudinally during meiosis II or mitosis. They also may result from a meiotic error in a chromosome with a Robertsonian translocation. An isochromosome made of the q arms of an acrocentric chromosome behaves like a homologous Robertsonian translocation,

because no important genetic material is lost. However, such a carrier could produce only abnormal unbalanced gametes. When an isochromosome involves nonacrocentric chromosomes that have p arms containing functional genetic material, the fusion and abnormal centromere break results in two isochromosomes—one composed of both p arms and one composed of both q arms. Because one of these isochromosomes is likely to be lost during cell division, resulting in the deletion of all the genes located on the lost chromosome arm, the carrier is usually phenotypically abnormal and produces abnormal gametes. An example is isochromosome X, which causes the full Turner syndrome phenotype.

CHROMOSOMAL INVERSIONS. Inversions result when two breaks occur in the same chromosome, and the intervening genetic material is inverted before the breaks are repaired. Although no genetic material is lost or duplicated, the rearrangement may alter gene function. *Paracentric inversions* are those in which the inverted material is from only one arm, and the centromere is not within the inverted segment (Fig. 12–6). The carrier makes either normal (balanced) gametes or gametes that are so abnormal as to preclude fertilization. Thus, although infertility may be a problem, the risk of abnormal offspring is extremely low.

Pericentric inversions occur when the breaks are in each arm of the chromosome, so that the inverted chromosome material includes the centromere. Because such inversions cause problems in chromosomal alignment during meiosis, the

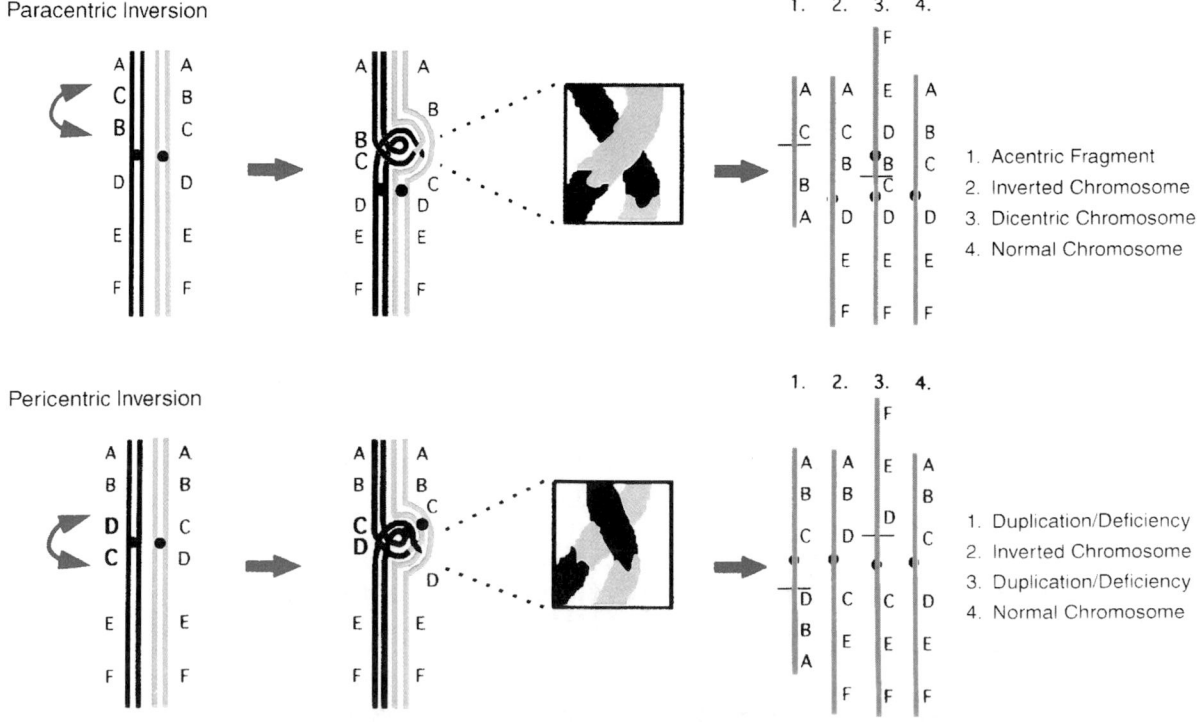

FIGURE 12–6. Meiosis in chromosomes with pericentric and paracentric inversions. (Adapted from Greenwood Genetics Center, 1995, with permission.)

carrier is at high risk to produce abnormal gametes and thus abnormal offspring. The risk can be calculated for each unique inversion, but in general, the observed risk is 5 to 10 percent if ascertainment was prompted after the birth of an abnormal child, and 1 to 3 percent if ascertainment was prompted by some other reason (Gardner and Sutherland, 1996).

RING CHROMOSOMES. When there are deletions from both ends of a chromosome, the ends may unite, forming a ring chromosome. If the deletions are substantial, the carrier is phenotypically abnormal. For example, *ring X chromosome* is associated with the Turner syndrome phenotype.

Telomeres are the physical ends of linear chromosomes. They are specialized nucleoprotein complexes that have important functions, primarily in the protection, replication, and stabilization of the chromosomal ends. If only the telomeres are lost, all important genetic material is retained and the carrier is essentially balanced. The ring, however, prevents normal chromosome alignment during meiosis and thus produces abnormal gametes. It also disrupts cell division, causing abnormal growth of many tissues and leading to small stature, borderline to moderate mental deficiency, and minor dysmorphisms (Gardner and Sutherland, 1996).

A ring chromosome may form de novo or may be inherited from a carrier parent. In all cases of parent-to-child transmission, the mother is the carrier, possibly because a ring chromosome somehow compromises spermatogenesis.

CHROMOSOMAL MOSAICISM. This finding is defined as two or more cytogenetically distinct cell lines in the same individual. In many cases, mosaicism is a cell-culture artifact that must be differentiated from true mosaicism (Claussen and co-workers, 1984). The phenotypic expression of mosaicism depends on many factors, including whether the cytogenetically abnormal cells involve the placenta, the fetus, parts of the fetus, or some combination. Although true mosaicism rarely is encountered in either a fetus or amniocytes, chorionic villus sampling has shown that 2 percent of placentas are mosaic, even though the associated fetus is usually normal (Henderson and associates, 1996). This finding is called *confined placental mosaicism,* and it likely results from nondisjunction during early mitotic divisions in one or more cells destined to become the placenta. It could also result from partial "correction" of a trisomy resulting from a meiotic error, with the extra chromosome lost from all cells destined to become the fetus, but retained in some cells destined to become the placenta. The mechanism causing mosaicism seems to be chromosome specific. Mosaicism involving chromosomes 2, 7, 8, 10, and 12 is usually caused by a mitotic error, whereas that involving chromosomes 9, 16, and 22 tends to result from partial correction of a meiotic error (Robinson and colleagues, 1997).

Confined placental mosaicism may have either positive or negative effects. It may play a role in the survival of some cytogenetically abnormal fetuses. For example, trisomy 13 and 18 fetuses who survive to term may do so only because of early trisomic "correction" in some cells that become trophoblasts. This would favor more normal placental function (Kalousek and co-workers, 1989). Conversely, some cytogenetically normal fetuses may have severe growth restriction because the placenta contains a population of aneuploid cells that impair function (Kalousek and Dill, 1983). It now appears that growth restriction also is influenced by *which* chromosome is lost during the trisomic "correction." If the fetus retains two normal copies of the chromosome in question, but both copies came from the same parent, growth also may be impaired. This event is referred to as *uniparental disomy* and is discussed later.

Gonadal mosaicism is confined to the gonads. It likely arises as the result of a mitotic error in cells destined to become the gonad, resulting in a population of abnormal germ cells. Because spermatogonia and oogonia divide throughout fetal life, and spermatogonia continue to divide throughout adulthood, gonadal mosaicism also could occur as the result of a meiotic error in previously normal dividing germ cells. Gonadal mosaicism may explain de novo autosomal dominant mutations in the offspring of normal parents, causing such diseases as achondroplasia or osteogenesis imperfecta, or X-linked diseases such as Duchenne muscular dystrophy. It also explains the recurrence of such diseases in more than one child in a previously unaffected family. It is because of the potential for gonadal mosaicism that the recurrence risk after the birth of a child with a disease caused by a "new" mutation is approximately 6 percent.

SINGLE-GENE (MENDELIAN) DISORDERS

A mendelian disorder is caused by a mutation or alteration in a single locus or gene, in one or both members of a gene pair. Approximately 0.4 percent of the population has a genetic abnormality caused by a single-gene mutation discovered by age 25, and 2 percent will have a single-gene disorder diagnosed during their lifetime (see Table 12–1). As of 2004, 15,566 monogenic disorders had been identified. Although they are classified according to their mode of inheritance—14,589 autosomal, 868 X-linked, 54 Y-linked, and 61 mitochondrial—it must be emphasized that it is the *phenotype* that is dominant or recessive, not the genes. In some dominant diseases, for example, the normal gene may still be directing the production of normal protein, but the phenotype is determined by protein produced by the abnormal gene. Likewise, the heterozygous carrier of some recessive diseases may produce detectable levels of the abnormal gene product, but he or she does not display features of the disease because the phenotype is directed by the product of the normal co-gene. Some common "single-gene disorders" affecting adults are listed in Table 12–6.

Although transmission patterns of these diseases are consistent with mendelian inheritance, their phenotypes are

TABLE 12–6 Some Relatively Frequent Mendelian Disorders

Autosomal Dominant
Achondroplasia
Acute intermittent porphyria
Adult polycystic kidney disease
Amyotrophic lateral sclerosis
Antithrombin deficiency
BRCA1 and *BRCA2* breast cancer
Ehlers–Danlos syndrome
Factor V Leiden mutation
Familial hypercholesterolemia
Hereditary hemorrhagic telangiectasia
Hereditary spherocytosis
Huntington chorea
Hypertrophic obstructive cardiomyopathy
Long QT syndrome
Marfan syndrome
Multiple endocrine neoplasia type 1 and 2
Myotonic dystrophy
Neurofibromatosis type 1 and 2
Osteogenesis imperfecta tarda
Polyposis of the colon
Retinoblastoma
Tuberous sclerosis
von Willebrand disease

Autosomal Recessive
Albinism
α_1-Antitrypsin deficiency
Congenital adrenal hyperplasia
Cystic fibrosis
Deafness
Friedreich ataxia
Hemochromatosis
Homocystinuria
Phenylketonuria
Sickle cell anemia
Tay–Sachs disease
Thalassemia syndromes
Wilson disease

X Linked
Androgen insensitivity syndrome
Chronic granulomatous disease
Color blindness
Fabry disease
Fragile X syndrome
Glucose-6-phosphate deficiency
Hemophilia A and B
Hypophosphatemic rickets
Muscular dystrophy—Duchenne and Becker
Ocular albinism

strongly influenced by modifying genes and environmental factors. Ironically, although single-gene (mendelian) disorders were the first genetic conditions identified, diseases caused solely by single genes are actually relatively rare.

AUTOSOMAL DOMINANT. If only one member of a gene pair determines the phenotype, that gene is considered to be dominant. Likewise, a gene with a dominant mutation specifies the phenotype in preference to the normal gene.

The carrier of a gene causing an autosomal dominant disease has a 50-percent chance of passing on the affected gene with each conception.

Penetrance. This term describes whether or not the mutant gene is expressed at all. A dominant gene with some kind of recognizable phenotypic expression in all individuals who carry the gene has 100 percent penetrance. If the carrier of the abnormal gene displays *no* features of the associated disease, the gene is not penetrant. Incomplete penetrance, the situation in which some gene carriers express the gene but some do not, is quantitatively expressed by the ratio of gene carriers who have any phenotypic characteristics associated with the altered gene to the total number of gene carriers. A gene that is expressed in some way in 80 percent of individuals who have that gene is 80-percent penetrant. Incomplete or reduced penetrance may explain why some autosomal dominant diseases appear to "skip" generations.

Some mechanisms responsible for reduced penetrance have been identified. For example, in retinoblastoma, reduced penetrance is explained by the fact that an individual carrying the abnormal allele must also acquire a somatic mutation affecting the normal retinoblastoma allele in order to develop the disease. If the normal allele is not mutated, the disease is not penetrant. Another mechanism is delayed onset of disease. For example, because symptoms of Huntington disease may not become apparent until age 40, if the individual carrying the gene died before it had been expressed, the gene would appear to have skipped that generation.

Expressivity. This term refers to the degree to which the phenotypic features are expressed. If all individuals carrying the affected gene do not have identical phenotypes, the gene has *variable expressivity*. Expressivity of a gene can range from complete or severe manifestations to only mild features of the disease. An example of a disease with variable expressivity is neurofibromatosis.

Anticipation. This term describes a phenomenon observed in certain chromosomal diseases such as fragile X syndrome and myotonic dystrophy. Disease symptoms seem to be more severe and to appear at an earlier age in each successive generation. In these cases, the progressively more severe phenotype corresponds to progressively larger gene mutations (discussed later). Other cases of apparent anticipation likely result from ascertainment bias. When an individual with a severe phenotype is identified, the search for other affected family members often reveals milder cases in previous generations.

AUTOSOMAL RECESSIVE. These traits usually are expressed only when both copies of the gene function identically. Thus, autosomal recessive diseases develop only when both gene copies are abnormal. Phenotypic alterations in gene carriers—that is, *heterozygotes*—usually are undetectable clinically but may be recognized at the biochemical or cellular level. For example, many enzyme deficiency diseases are autosomal recessive. The enzyme level in a carrier will be about half of normal, but because enzymes are made in great excess, this reduction usually does not cause disease. It does, however, represent a phenotypic alteration and can be used for screening purposes (see Chap. 13, p. 318). Other recessive conditions do not produce any phenotypic changes in the carrier and can be identified only by molecular methods.

Unless they are screened for a specific disease, such as cystic fibrosis, carriers usually are recognized only after the birth of an affected child or the diagnosis of an affected family member (see Chap. 13, p. 317). A couple whose child has an autosomal recessive disease has a 25-percent recurrence risk with each conception. The likelihood that a normal sibling of an affected child is a carrier of the gene is two out of three; 1/4 of offspring will be homozygous normal, 2/4 will be heterozygote carriers, and 1/4 will be homozygous abnormal—thus, three of four children will be phenotypically normal and two of these three will be carriers.

The carrier child will not have affected children, unless his or her partner is also a carrier (heterozygous) or has the disease (homozygous). Because genes leading to rare autosomal recessive conditions have a low prevalence in the general population, the chance that a partner will be a gene carrier is low unless the couple is related or part of an isolated population (American College of Obstetricians and Gynecologists, 2004).

Inborn Errors of Metabolism. Most of these autosomal recessive diseases result from the absence of a crucial enzyme leading to incomplete metabolism of proteins, sugars, or fats. The metabolic intermediates that build up are toxic to a variety of tissues, resulting in mental retardation or other abnormalities.

PHENYLKETONURIA (PKU). This classical example of an autosomal recessive defect results from diminished or absent phenylalanine hydroxylase activity. Homozygotes are unable to metabolize phenylalanine to tyrosine. If the diet is unrestricted, incomplete protein metabolism leads to abnormally high phenylalanine levels that cause neurological damage and mental retardation. There also is hypopigmented hair, eyes, and skin because phenylalanine competitively inhibits tyrosine hydrolase, which is essential for melanin production. The disease is rare and affects 1 in 10,000 to 15,000 white newborns. There is tremendous geographical and ethnic variation, with incidences ranging from 5 to 190 cases per million.

PKU is notable for two reasons. First, it is one of the few metabolic disorders for which treatment exists. Homozygotes who ingest a phenylalanine-free diet can avoid many of the clinical consequences of the disease. Early diagnosis and limitation of dietary phenylalanine beginning in infancy are essential to prevent neurological damage. Accordingly, all states and many countries now mandate newborn screening

for PKU, and about 100 cases per million births have been identified worldwide. The special diet should be continued indefinitely, as patients who abandon the phenylalanine-free diet may have some decline in IQ.

Women with PKU who plan to conceive and are not already on a phenylalanine-restricted diet should be counseled to adhere to the diet before conception and throughout pregnancy. Phenylalanine readily crosses the placenta, and high maternal serum levels can result in damage to the fetus or pregnancy loss (National Institutes of Health, 2000). Hyperphenylalaninemia causes microcephaly with mental retardation and cardiac defects in the heterozygote fetus who otherwise would not be affected. Importantly, these defects can be prevented with maternal dietary treatment (Williamson and associates, 1981). The Maternal Phenylketonuria Collaborative Study, which enrolled nearly 600 women during 12 years, found that maintenance of serum phenylalanine levels in the 160 to 360 μmol/L (2 to 6 mg/dL) range significantly reduced the risk of fetal abnormalities (Platt and colleagues, 2000).

CONSANGUINITY. Two individuals are considered consanguineous if they have at least one ancestor in common. The term usually refers to an individual mating with a third-degree relative such as a first cousin, a half-uncle or aunt, or a half-niece or nephew, or a more distantly related individual. First-degree relatives share half, second-degree relatives share one fourth, and third-degree relatives (cousins) share one eighth of their genes. Because of the potential for shared deleterious genes, consanguineous unions are at increased risk to produce children with autosomal recessive or multifactorial diseases.

First-cousin marriages, the most frequent consanguineous mating, carry a twofold increased risk of abnormal offspring (4 to 6 percent risk instead of the 2 to 3 percent background risk) if there is no family history of genetic disease. If one of the partners has a sibling with an autosomal recessive disease, the risk of affected offspring is many times higher than if he or she had chosen an unrelated partner. First-cousin marriage is legal in 30 states and is actually preferred in some countries, for example, some parts of the Middle East (Bennett, 1987; Shami and colleagues, 1991). Despite this, there are significant medical, societal, and legal ramifications to first-cousin marriages in the United States. All of these should be addressed by the couple before childbearing with each other.

Incest is defined as a sexual relationship between first-degree relatives such as parent and child or brother and sister and is universally illegal. Progeny of such unions carry the highest risk of abnormal outcome, and up to 40 percent of offspring are abnormal as a result of both recessive and multifactorial disorders (Friere-Maia, 1984; Nadiri, 1979).

CO-DOMINANT GENES. If alleles in a gene pair are different from each other, but both are expressed in the phenotype, they are considered to be co-dominant. An example is the genes responsible for hemoglobinopathies. The individual with one gene directing production of sickle hemoglobin and the other directing production of hemoglobin C produces both S and C hemoglobins. Genes determining human blood type are also co-dominant; both A and B red-cell antigens can be expressed simultaneously in one individual.

X-LINKED AND Y-LINKED GENES. X-linked diseases are usually recessive. The best known X-linked recessive diseases are color blindness, hemophilia A, and Duchenne muscular dystrophy. Women carrying an X-linked recessive gene generally are unaffected, unless unfavorable lyonization—inactivation of one X chromosome in every cell—results in the majority of cells expressing the abnormal gene. When a woman carries a gene causing an X-linked recessive condition, there is a 50 percent chance of passing the gene with each conception. Thus, each son has a 50 percent risk of being affected and each daughter has a 50 percent chance of being a carrier.

Men carrying an X-linked recessive gene usually are affected because they lack a second X chromosome to express the normal dominant gene. When a man has an X-linked disease, none of his sons will be affected because they cannot receive the abnormal X-linked gene from him. As subsequently discussed, for complex reasons, fragile X syndrome does not conform to these rules of X-linked inheritance.

X-linked dominant disorders affect females predominantly because they tend to be lethal in male offspring. Examples include focal dermal hypoplasia, vitamin D–resistant rickets, and incontinentia pigmenti.

The Y chromosome carries genes important for sex determination and a variety of cellular functions such as spermatogenesis and bone development. Deletion of genes on the long arm of the Y chromosome results in severe spermatogenic defects, whereas genes at the tip of the short arm are critical for chromosomal pairing during meiosis and for fertility.

NONMENDELIAN PATTERNS OF INHERITANCE

HEREDITARY UNSTABLE DNA. Mendel's first law states that genes are passed unchanged from parent to progeny. Barring the occurrence of new mutations, that law still applies to many genes or traits. Certain genes, however, are unstable, and their size and consequently their function may be altered as they are transmitted from parent to child.

Fragile X Syndrome. Also called *Martin–Bell syndrome,* fragile X syndrome is the most common form of *familial* mental retardation. By contrast, Down syndrome is the most common *genetic* cause of mental retardation, but it is usually not familial. Fragile X syndrome accounts for 4 to 8 percent of all retardation in males and females in all ethnic and racial groups. The incidence of the full fragile X syndrome is generally cited as 1 in 1000 males and 1 in 2000 females (Rousseau and co-workers, 1995; Turner and colleagues, 1996).

The fragile X mutation is a region of unstable DNA on the X chromosome. The region is best described as a series of CGG (cytosine–guanine–guanine) triplet repeats at Xq27. If the number of repeats and thus the region reaches a critical size, it can be methylated and thus inactivated (Migeon, 1993). When the gene is inactivated, *fragile X mental retardation-1 (FMR-1) protein* is not produced. Although the function of this protein is unknown, it is highly conserved in all species and is most active in brain and testes.

The number of repeats and the degree of methylation determine whether or not an individual is affected (Cutillo, 1994). The absolute number of repeats is less important than whether the number exceeds either of two important thresholds. Individuals carrying 2 to 49 repeats are usually phenotypically normal. Those carrying 50 to 199 repeats have a *premutation,* and although they were previously considered to be normal, three distinct phenotypes have recently been characterized (Hagerman and Hagerman, 2004). These include mild cognitive and behavioral deficits, premature ovarian failure, and a neurodegenerative disorder that affects older adults and has been termed the *fragile X-associated-tremor/ataxia syndrome (FXTAS).* Those with more than 230 repeats have the *full* mutation and, if methylation occurs, are usually affected.

The number of repeats usually remains stable when the gene is transmitted by a male. When transmitted by a female with a premutation, however, the gene can expand during meiosis. The risk of expansion with maternal transmission generally correlates with the number of repeats in the maternal premutation. Thus, if a woman carries a premutation that increases in size as she transmits it to her offspring, it is possible for her child to manifest fragile X syndrome (Cutillo, 1994).

Approximately 80 percent of males and 50 to 70 percent of females carrying the full mutation are mentally handicapped (de Vries and co-workers, 1996; Jones, 1997). Males are moderately to severely affected, with an IQ of 35 to 45, whereas the IQ in females is generally higher (Nelson, 1995). Affected individuals also may have autistic behavior, attention-deficit/hyperactivity disorder, and speech and language problems. The physical phenotype includes a narrow face with large jaw, long prominent ears, and macroorchidism in postpubertal males. Surprisingly, 20 percent of males and 10 percent of females carrying the expanded gene either are unaffected or have a mild phenotype. This phenotypic variability is caused by lyonization (in females) or mosaicism for the size of the expansion, the degree of methylation, or both (Cutillo, 1994).

With the use of restriction endonuclease digestion and Southern blot analysis, as discussed on page 308, the number of CGG repeats and the methylation status of the gene can be accurately determined. Amniocentesis may be preferred for prenatal diagnosis because methylation status may be difficult to determine in chorionic villus cells. It is reasonable to refer individuals with a history of mental retardation, developmental delay of unknown etiology, or autism for genetic evaluation because 2 to 6 percent will be determined to have fragile X (Curry and colleagues, 1997; Wenstrom and associates, 1999). Screening rationale is discussed further in Chapter 13 (see p. 326).

Myotonic Dystrophy. This is the most common form of adult myopathy (Jones, 1997). Affected family members tend to have successively earlier and more severe symptoms with each generation. The affected gene on the long arm of chromosome 9 contains a region of unstable trinucleotide (cytosine–thymine–guanine; CTG) repeats (Buxton and co-workers, 1992). Normal individuals have 3 to 30 repeats, and although they can expand up to 3000, an increase to as few as 40 has been associated with myotonic dystrophy.

There are three distinct myotonic dystrophy phenotypes, depending on the number of repeats. The severity of the phenotype increases as the number of repeats increases from generation to generation, thus accounting for "anticipation." With about 100 repeats there is mild disease, characterized by mild facial muscle weakness and wasting, frontal balding, and cataract formation. With 1300 repeats there is a 90-percent chance of having the full syndrome, which includes proximal muscle weakness, cardiomyopathy, mental retardation, endocrine dysfunction, abnormal facies, and cataract development. Individuals with an intermediate number of repeats, from 200 to 800, have an intermediate phenotype (Gennarelli and colleagues, 1996). The most severe manifestations develop in the congenital form of the disease, which is associated with huge expansions of at least 10 kb. Affected infants are thin and have hypotonia, facial muscle weakness, decreased cry and suck, and respiratory insufficiency, and rarely survive to adulthood. Hydramnios, which results from decreased fetal swallowing, and decreased fetal movement in a patient with facial muscle weakness or frontal balding should arouse suspicion. In contrast to fragile X syndrome, the number of repeats can increase with transmission by either parent and also can decrease when transmitted by a male.

Huntington Disease. This disorder is characterized by progressive chorea, bradykinesia, and rigidity with an insidious deterioration of intellectual function. The mean age at diagnosis is about 40 years. The gene on chromosome 4 contains a region of CAG (cytosine–adenine–guanine) triplet repeats. Normal individuals have 10 to 35 CAG repeats, whereas those with the disease have 36 to 121 repeats. Like myotonic dystrophy, there is a significant correlation between the number of repeats and the age of onset (Andrew and colleagues, 1993). Interestingly, there is also a correlation between *paternal* inheritance and early disease (Clarke, 1990). Thus, the gene appears to be most unstable when transmitted by the father.

Other DNA-Triplet Repeat Diseases. These include Friedreich ataxia, X-linked spinal and bulbar muscular atrophy (Kennedy disease), spinocerebellar ataxia types 1 and 2, dentato-rubro-pallido-luysian atrophy, and Machado–Joseph disease.

IMPRINTING. This term describes the process by which certain genes are inherited in an inactivated or *transcriptionally silent* state (Hall, 1990). This type of gene inactivation is determined by the gender of the transmitting parent and may be reversed in the next generation. Imprinting affects gene expression by *epigenetic control*, that is, it changes the phenotype by altering gene expression and not by permanently altering the genotype. When a gene is inherited in an imprinted state, gene function is necessarily directed entirely by the co-gene inherited from the other parent. Thus, imprinting exerts an effect by controlling the "dosage" of specific genes.

Certain important genes appear to be *monoallelic*. Thus, under normal circumstances only one member of the gene pair is functioning—as opposed to most genes in the genome, which are biallelic. Most of the monoallelic genes identified so far regulate tissue growth. Genes normally expressed only from the paternal allele, such as insulin growth factor 2, tend to be associated with tissue overgrowth and tumor formation, whereas genes normally expressed exclusively from the maternal allele, such as *H19*, result in growth suppression (Tycko, 1994).

The genes inherited from each parent express the parental imprinting in all fetal cells. Then, in the immediate post-zygote period, the inherited methylation pattern in the fetal *germ cells only* is erased, and a new imprinting pattern, corresponding to the gender of the fetus, is imposed. When the fetus reaches adulthood, during reproduction it will pass on the imprinting pattern unique to its own gender.

One example of the effect of imprinting concerns a chromosome deletion at 15q11–13, which causes two very different diseases:

1. *Prader–Willi syndrome* is characterized by obesity and hyperphagia; short stature; small hands, feet, and external genitalia; and mild mental retardation.
2. *Angelman syndrome* includes normal stature and weight, severe mental retardation, absent speech, seizure disorder, ataxia and jerky arm movements, and paroxysms of inappropriate laughter.

Both syndromes are associated with the same deletion, but which of the two different phenotypes occurs depends on whether the missing genetic material was inherited from the mother or the father. If the deleted genetic material was maternal in origin, the result is Angelman syndrome, but if the deleted material was paternally derived, Prader–Willi syndrome results.

There are a number of other examples of imprinting important to obstetricians-gynecologists. *Complete hydatidiform mole,* which has a paternally derived, diploid chromosomal complement, is characterized by the abundant growth of placental tissue, but no fetal structures (see Chap. 11, p. 274). Conversely, *ovarian teratoma,* which has a maternally derived, diploid chromosomal complement, is characterized by the growth of various fetal tissues but no placental structures (Porter and Gilks, 1993). It thus appears that paternal genes are vital for placental development and maternal genes are

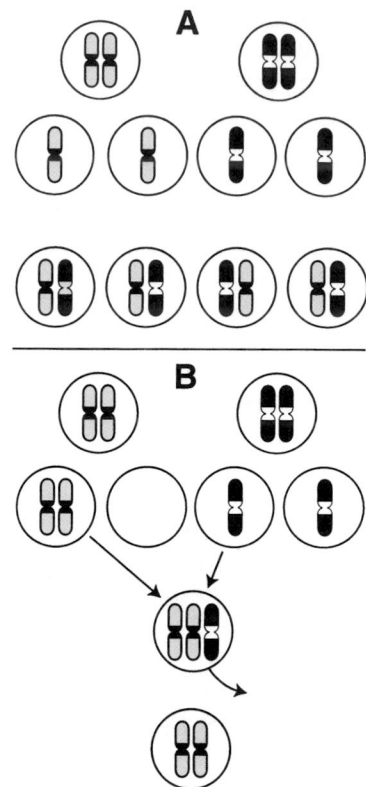

FIGURE 12–7. Diagrammatic representation of how uniparental disomy may arise.

essential for fetal development, but both must be present in every cell for normal fetal growth and development. Imprinting also is operative in some growth disorders and malignancies.

UNIPARENTAL DISOMY. In this situation, both members of one pair of chromosomes are inherited from the same parent (Fig. 12–7). This appears to result from the "correction" of a trisomic zygote by loss of a chromosome. The chromosome transmitted by one parent is lost, and the two chromosomes transmitted by the other parent are retained.

Isodisomy is the unique situation in which an individual receives two identical copies of one chromosome in a pair from one parent. This mechanism explains some cases of cystic fibrosis, in which only one parent was a carrier but the fetus inherited two copies of the same abnormal chromosome from that parent (Spence and co-workers, 1988; Spotila and colleagues, 1992). It also has been implicated in abnormal growth related to placental mosaicism (Robinson and colleagues, 1997).

MITOCHONDRIAL INHERITANCE. Each human cell contains hundreds of mitochondria, each containing its own genome and associated replication systems. In this sense, mitochondria behave autonomously. Interestingly, these organelles are derived exclusively from the mother. Whereas

human oocytes contain approximately 100,000 mitochondria, sperm contain only 100, and these are destined for destruction after fertilization. Each mitochondrion contains multiple copies of a 16.5-kb circular DNA molecule. This DNA encodes 13 peptides that are subunits of proteins required for oxidative phosphorylation, as well as ribosomal and transfer RNAs.

Because mitochondria contain genetic information, mitochondrial inheritance allows the transmission of genes from mother to offspring without the possibility of recombination. If a mitochondrial mutation occurs, it may segregate into a daughter cell during cell division and thus be propagated. Over time, the percentage of mutant mitochondrial DNAs in different cell lines can drift toward either normal or pure mutant (Wallace, 1995). If an oocyte containing largely mutant mitochondrial DNAs is fertilized, the offspring might have a mitochondrial disease. These have a characteristic transmission pattern—individuals of both sexes can be affected, but transmission is only through females. Mitochondrial genetic diseases include *myoclonic epilepsy with ragged red fibers (MERRF), Leber hereditary optic neuropathy, Leigh syndrome,* and *pigmentary retinopathy.*

POLYGENIC AND MULTIFACTORIAL INHERITANCE. *Polygenic traits* are determined by the combined effects of many genes. *Multifactorial traits* are determined by multiple genes and environmental factors. It is now believed that the majority of inherited traits are multifactorial or polygenic. Birth defects caused by such inheritance are recognized by their tendency to recur in families, but not according to a mendelian inheritance pattern. The empirical recurrence risk for first-degree relatives usually is quoted as 2 to 3 percent (Thompson and colleagues, 1991). Multifactorial traits can be classified in several ways, but the most logical is to categorize them as continuously variable traits, threshold traits, or complex disorders of adult life.

Continuously Variable Traits. These traits have a normal distribution in the general population. By convention, abnormality is defined as a trait or measurement greater than two standard deviations above or below the population mean. These are typically measurable or quantitative traits such as height or head size and are believed to result from the individually small effects of many genes combined with environmental factors. Such traits tend to be less extreme in the offspring of affected individuals, because of the statistical principle of regression to the mean.

Threshold Traits. These traits do not appear until a certain threshold of liability is exceeded (Fig. 12–8). Factors creating liability to the malformation are assumed to be continuously distributed, and only individuals at the extreme of this distribution exceed the threshold and have the trait or defect. The phenotypic abnormality is thus an all-or-none phenomenon. Individuals in high-risk families have enough

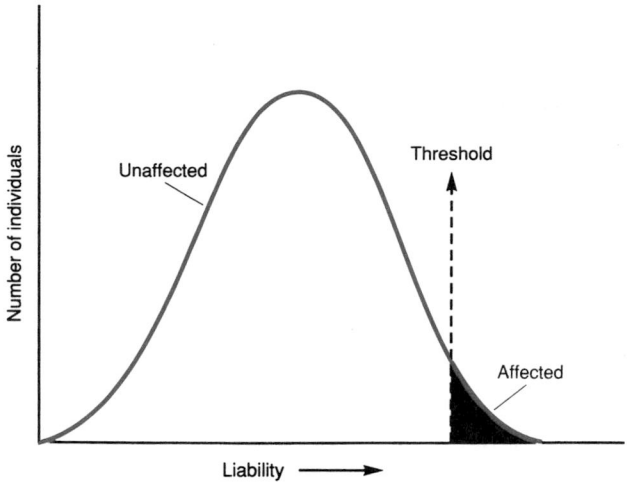

FIGURE 12–8. Example of a threshold trait. Liability to a trait is distributed normally, with a threshold dividing the population into unaffected and affected segments. (From Thompson and colleagues, 1991, with permission.)

abnormal genes or environmental influences that their liability is close to the threshold. Usually for unknown reasons, some factor(s) further increase the liability for certain family members, and the threshold is crossed. Cleft lip and palate and pyloric stenosis are examples of threshold traits.

Certain threshold traits have a predilection for one gender, indicating that males and females have a different liability threshold. An example is pyloric stenosis, which is more common in males. If a female has pyloric stenosis, she or her parents have even more abnormal genes or predisposing factors than is usually necessary to produce pyloric stenosis in males. The recurrence risk for her siblings or for her future children is thus higher than the expected 2 to 3 percent.

Male siblings or offspring would have the highest liability, because they not only will inherit more than the usual number of predisposing genes, but also are the more susceptible sex.

Finally, the recurrence risk of threshold traits is also higher if the defect is severe, again suggesting the presence of more abnormal genes or influences. For example, the recurrence risk after the birth of a child with bilateral cleft lip and palate is 8 percent, compared with only 4 percent associated with unilateral cleft lip without cleft palate (Melnick and associates, 1980).

Complex Disorders of Adult Life. These are traits in which many genes determine the susceptibility to environmental factors, with disease resulting from the most unfavorable combination of both. Examples include common disorders such as heart disease or hypertension. These disorders are usually familial and behave as threshold traits, but with environmental influence as an important cofactor. The genetic mechanisms of many common adult diseases have not yet been elucidated, although in most cases, several associated genes have been identified. In some diseases, the identity of the associated gene provides a clue to pathogenesis, whereas in others the related gene may simply serve as a disease marker. For example, premature cardiovascular disease is associated with the gene for apolipoprotein E, which likely influences the pathology of the disease. In contrast, the association of type 1 diabetes mellitus with HLA-DR3/4 is less clear. Some multifactorial adult-onset diseases and associated genes are listed in Table 12–7.

Examples of Multifactorial or Polygenic Defects. Various isolated structural birth defects and common diseases exhibit multifactorial or polygenic inheritance. All of these traits

TABLE 12–7 Multifactorial Adult-Onset Diseases and Their Associated Mutations

Approach	Disease	Mutation
Working down from the phenotype, using physiological abnormalities	Coronary artery disease	Hypercholesterolemia; combined hyperlipidemia
	Hypertension	Ion transport abnormalities
	Pernicious anemia	Atrophic gastritis
	Peptic ulcer	Hyperpepsinogenemia I
	Lactose intolerance	Lactase deficiency
	Hemochromatosis	Increased iron absorption
	Diabetes mellitus	Glucose intolerance; pancreatic autoimmunity
	Colon cancer	Single adenomatous polyp
Working up from the genotype, using genetic markers	Celiac disease	Associated with HLA-DR3
	Hemochromatosis	Associated with HLA-A3, linked to HLA region (chromosome 6)
	Type 1 diabetes mellitus	Associated with HLA-DR3 and HLA-DR4
	Rheumatoid arthritis	Associated with HLA-DR4
	Ankylosing spondylitis	Associated with HLA-B27
	Alzheimer disease	Linked to amyloid β-protein RFLP (chromosome 21)

From King and associates (1992), with permission.

TABLE 12–8 Characteristics of Multifactorial Traits

* Multiple family members are affected, but there is no specific inheritance pattern
* Risk to first-degree relatives is approximately the population risk squared
* Risk is sharply lower for second-degree relatives and declines rapidly for more distant relatives
* Recurrence risk is higher if more than one family member is affected
* Recurrence risk is higher if defect is severe
* If trait is more frequent in one gender, risk for relatives is higher if person with defect is of less frequently affected gender
* Concordance rate in dizygotic twins is less than one quarter of rate in monozygotic twins
* Recurrence risk is higher if parents are consanguineous

Adapted from Thompson and colleagues (1991).

have certain characteristics that help to distinguish them from disorders with other modes of inheritance, which can be cited in counseling (Table 12–8). When counseling patients regarding risks for a familial multifactorial trait, it is important to consider the degree of relatedness of the affected relative to the *fetus*, not the parents. An affected first-degree relative (the parents or siblings of the fetus) results in a substantial risk increase, but risk declines exponentially with successively more distant relationships. Two examples are neural-tube and cardiac defects.

NEURAL-TUBE DEFECTS. The neural plate extends down the dorsum of the 18-day embryo. It folds and closure is believed to occur in five separate regions, which then fuse (Fig. 12–9). Neural-tube defects likely result from either failure of closure at one or more sites, or failure of two sites to fuse (Golden and Chernoff, 1995).

Isolated or nonsyndromic neural-tube defects are the second most common congenital structural abnormalities after cardiac defects. Worldwide their incidence is 1.4 to 2 per 1000 live births. They also can develop as part of a genetic syndrome or constellation of abnormalities. They are a major cause of stillbirth and neonatal and infant death. With treatment, 80 to 90 percent of infants with isolated spina bifida survive with varying degrees of handicap. Factors that influence eventual neurological function include the size and location of the defect, trauma to exposed neural tissue, timing of surgical closure, degree of associated ventriculomegaly, and occurrence of complications such as infection.

Anencephaly is the most severe defect (Fig. 12–10). It is always lethal and results in stillbirth or early neonatal demise. *Spina bifida* occurs when one or more vertebral arches fail to fuse, so that meninges (*meningocele*) or neural tissue plus meninges (*meningomyelocele*) are exposed (Fig. 12–11). *Rachischisis* describes the lethal situation in which none of the vertebral arches fuse, and the entire spine is open. These lesions, as well as some of their ultrasonographic appearances, are discussed in Chapter 16 (see p. 393).

Neural-tube defects are classical examples of multifactorial inheritance. Their development is influenced by environment, diet, physiological abnormalities such as hyperthermia or hyperglycemia, teratogen exposure, family history, ethnic origin, fetal gender, amnionic fluid nutrients, and various genes. The fact that certain defects are associated with specific risk factors suggests that many genes are likely to be involved in neural-tube development. For example, those associated with type 1 diabetes mellitus are likely to be cranial or cervical-thoracic defects; hyperthermia has been associated with anencephaly; and valproic acid exposure with lumbosacral defects (Becerra and colleagues, 1990; Hunter, 1984; Lindhout and associates, 1992).

Although Hibbard and Smithells (1965) postulated more than 30 years ago that abnormal folate metabolism was responsible for many neural-tube malformations, a specific gene defect only recently has been implicated. A thermolabile variant of the enzyme 5,10-methylene tetrahydrofolate reductase (MTHFR), which plays a key role in folate metabolism, has been associated with neural-tube defects. This enzyme transfers a methyl group from folic acid to convert homocysteine to methionine. One abnormal form of MTHFR carries a mutation at position 677 and has reduced enzymatic activity. Folic acid supplementation likely works by overcoming this relative enzyme deficiency. Because some defects develop in fetuses with normal 677 C → T alleles, and because folic acid supplementation does not prevent all cases, other unknown genes or factors are presumed to be involved. Without folic acid supplementation, the empirical recurrence risk after one affected child is 3 to 4 percent, and after two affected children it is 10 percent. With supplementation, the risk after one affected child decreases by 70 percent to less than 1 percent (Czeizel and Dudas, 1992; MRC Vitamin Study Research Group, 1991).

Importantly, folic acid supplementation may also significantly decrease the incidence of first occurrences of neural-tube defects. Since 1998 the Food and Drug Administration has required fortification of cereal grain products calculated so that the average woman ingests daily an extra 200 μg of folic acid (American College of Obstetricians and Gynecologists, 2003). In the United States, the incidence of neural-tube defects has decreased by one fourth following folic acid fortification (Centers for Disease Control and Prevention, 2004; De Wals and associates, 2003). This relatively small decrease is probably the result of inadequate fortification. Wald (2004) estimates that folic acid supplementation with 5 mg per day would decrease the incidence of neural-tube defects by 85 percent.

CARDIAC DEFECTS. Cardiac anomalies are the most common birth defects worldwide, with an incidence of 8 per 1000 births. They outnumber all other isolated structural defects combined (Burn and Goodship, 1996). The majority of isolated cardiac malformations have traditionally been considered multifactorial, with genetic aspects that were difficult to

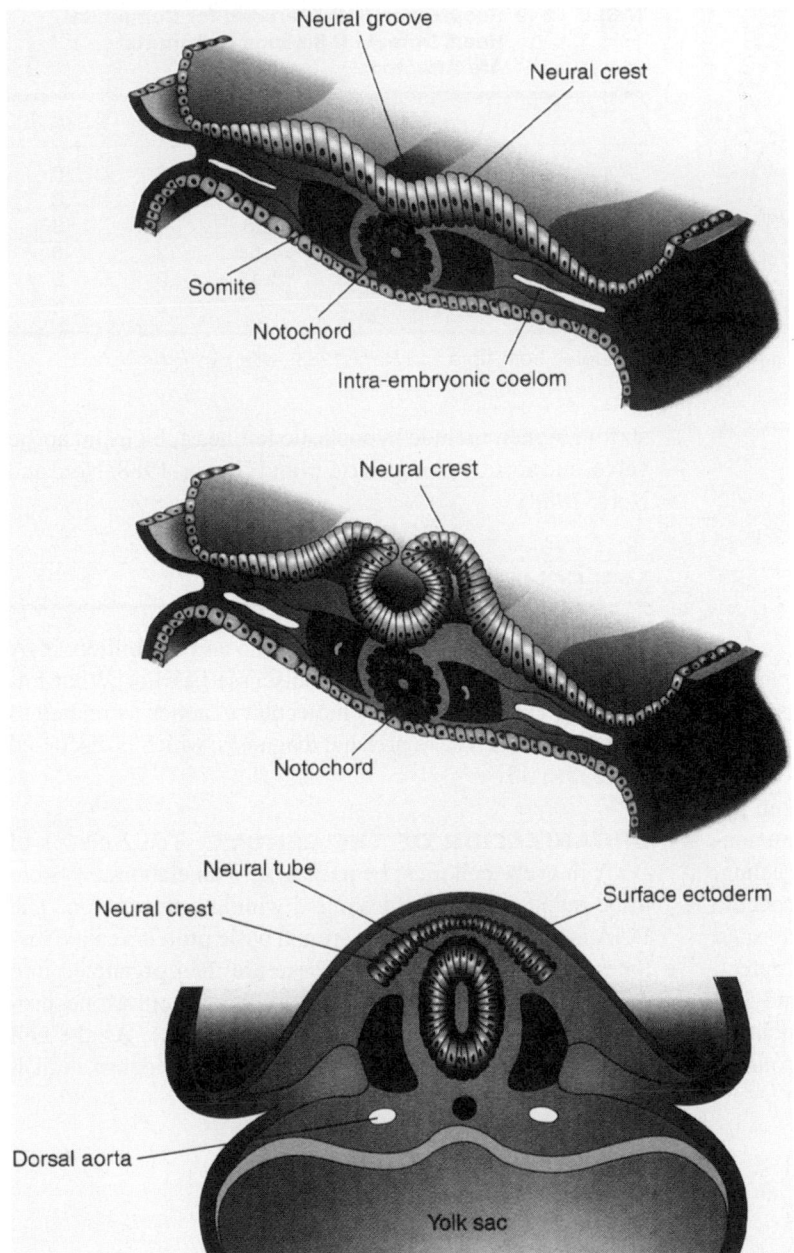

FIGURE 12–9. Schematic representation of neural-tube closure before 28 days of embryonic life. (From Moore and colleagues, 2000, with permission.)

evaluate. In the past, women with severe heart defects often did not reproduce, and many parents whose child had a serious heart defect chose not to have more children. Certain cardiac defects are much more likely to recur than others, and first-degree relatives with heart defects are likely to have the same or similar defect regardless of environmental exposures (see Chap. 13, p. 316).

More than 100 genes believed to be involved in cardiovascular morphogenesis have been identified, including those directing production of various transcription factors, secreted proteins, extracellular proteins, and protein receptors (Chin, 1998). These gene products are likely involved in the development of specific cardiac tissues and structures. For example, clinical and laboratory data indicate that folic acid

and the same MTHFR 677 C $\rightarrow$ T mutation associated with neural-tube defects influence the development of cardiac defects (Wenstrom and co-workers, 2001). As discussed, folic acid provides methyl groups for a number of important cellular processes. One study showed that myocyte DNA in hypoplastic left ventricles was significantly hypomethylated compared with that of normal controls (Wenstrom and co-workers, 2002). Moreover, preconceptional folic acid supplementation appears to reduce their incidence (Czeizel, 1996).

Many other genes likely to be involved in normal and abnormal cardiac development have not yet been identified. Gene deletion syndromes that include cardiac defects provide clues to the function and location of some of these unknown

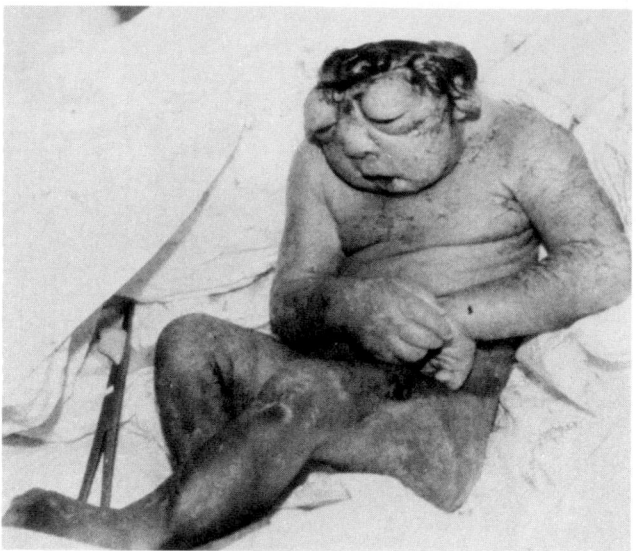

FIGURE 12–10. Anencephalic infant.

genes. For example, an association between the DiGeorge deletion and conotruncal cardiac defects has prompted a search for the causative genes within a small region of chromosome 22q11.2.

Observed recurrence risks, which likely reflect both genetic and environmental influences, for some common congenital heart defects are shown in Table 12–9. For counseling, if the exact nature of the defect is known, the most specific risk should be quoted. Otherwise, couples can be informed of the empirical risk of having a child with a cardiac defect. This is 5 to 6 percent if the mother has the defect, and 2 to 3 percent if the father has the defect (Burn and associates, 1998). Specific defects, which have recurrence risks four- to

TABLE 12–9 Recurrence Risk (Percent) for Congenital Heart Defects if Siblings or Parents Are Affected

	Father	Mother	1 Sibling	2 Siblings
Ventricular septal defects	2	6–10	3	10
Atrial septal defects	1.5	4–4.5	2.5	8
Fallot tetralogy	1.5	2.5	2.5	8
Pulmonary stenosis	2	4–6.5	2	6
Aortic stenosis	3	13–18	2	6
Coarctation	2	4	2	6

Adapted from Nora and Nora (1988), with permission.

sixfold higher, include hypoplastic left heart, bicuspid aortic valve, and aortic coarctation (Lin and Garver, 1988; Nora and Nora, 1988).

MOLECULAR GENETICS

The complexity of the human genome and the billion DNA base pairs that make it up were discussed earlier. What follows is a cursory review of molecular genetics as related to obstetrics as well as to prenatal diagnosis, which is discussed in Chapter 13.

ORGANIZATION OF THE GENOME. The 2 meters of DNA in every cell must be packaged in an elaborate system to be maintained and transmitted without interruption. The DNA is wrapped compactly around basic proteins called histones to form nucleosomes. These are then organized into solenoid structures and looped around a nonhistone protein scaffold to form chromatin (Fig. 12–12). As the cell enters prophase, the chromatin begins to condense until it

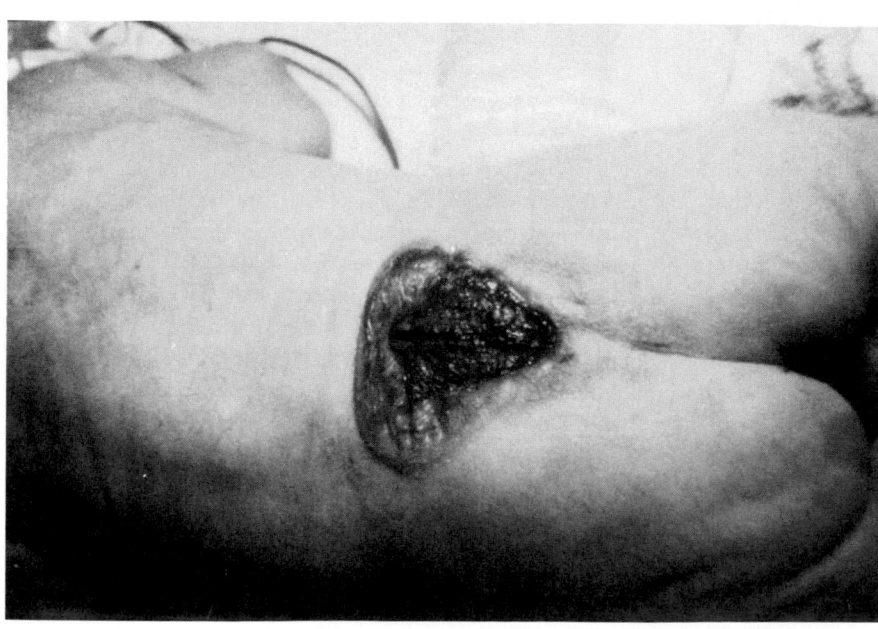

FIGURE 12–11. Large lumbar myeloschisis. (Courtesy of Dr. Victor Klein.)

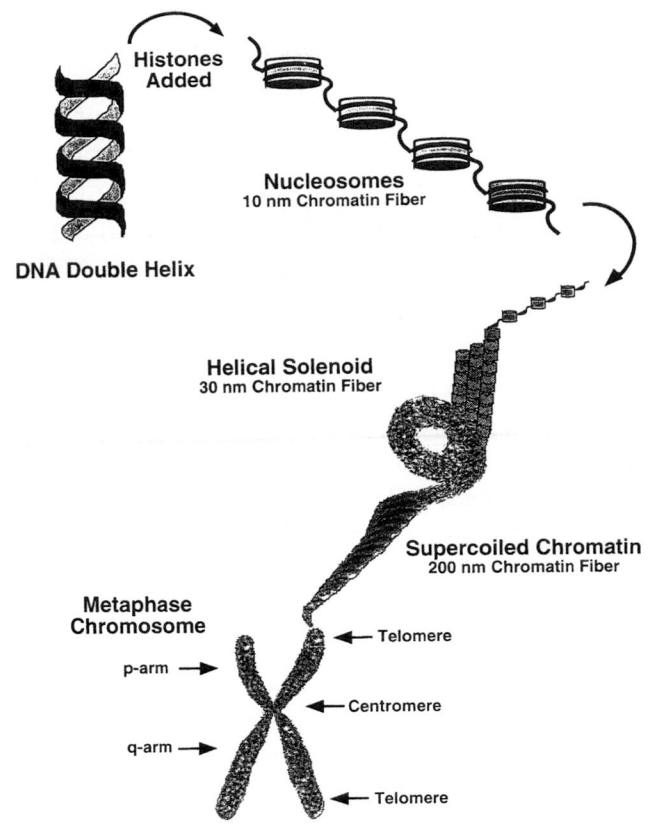

Histones Added

DNA Double Helix

Nucleosomes
10 nm Chromatin Fiber

Helical Solenoid
30 nm Chromatin Fiber

Supercoiled Chromatin
200 nm Chromatin Fiber

Metaphase Chromosome

p-arm →

q-arm →

← Telomere

← Centromere

← Telomere

FIGURE 12–12. Schematic representation of the structural organization of DNA. (Adapted from Elsa and Patel, 1998, with permission.)

assumes the familiar structure of metaphase chromosomes. Each chromosome is composed of densely packed nontranscribed DNA near the centromeres, called *heterochromatin,* and less densely packed transcribed DNA called *euchromatin.*

In humans about 75 percent of the genome is unique, single-copy DNA, and the rest consists of various classes of repetitive DNA. Surprisingly, virtually all of the repetitive DNA and a large portion of the single-copy DNA has no apparent or recognized function. Less than 10 percent of the genome encodes genes! Single-copy DNA is intensely studied because it contains all the genes necessary to make and sustain the organism, and repetitive DNA is of interest because it contains unique markers that identify each individual and can be used to study genetic variation.

CODING DNA: GENES. A gene is a unique series of four types of purine and pyrimidine bases—more generally called *nucleotides*—that specifies the amino acid sequence for a single polypeptide chain of a protein molecule. Within a gene, nucleotide triplets, called *codons,* either code for placement of a specific amino acid within the polypeptide chain or signal the starting or stopping of protein assembly. In the nucleus, codons are *transcribed* from DNA into a single-stranded RNA that corresponds in sequence with one of the strands of the DNA helix. The RNA is processed and transported into the

cytoplasm, where it is *translated* into the amino acid sequence that constitutes a protein. A gene is not one continuous segment of coding DNA, but rather is typically composed of multiple coding sequences called *exons,* interrupted by noncoding regions called *introns* that must be excised prior to translation. Each gene also has a regulatory region called a *promoter,* which is a 5′ untranslated region, and a 3′ untranslated region containing the signal for messenger RNA maturation and function. Posttranslational processing of the protein follows, and the polypeptide chain is folded into a unique three-dimensional structure. Two or more polypeptide chains may combine, or the structure may be chemically modified by the addition of carbohydrate or other moieties.

The vast majority (99.8 percent) of DNA is identical in all humans. There are, however, minor differences that distinguish one person from another. These differences, called *polymorphisms,* generally consist of a single nucleotide substitution present roughly once in every 200 to 500 base pairs. These changes are primarily in noncoding regions of the genome.

Many genes exist in several alternate but normal forms called *alleles.* For example, the Rh and major blood group genes all have several normal alleles. A mutation is an alteration of DNA sequencing within a coding region of a gene that results in an adverse change in protein structure or function. Mutations can be visible chromosomal alterations, such as deletions or insertions, or may involve a substitution in one or more of the purine or pyrimidine bases. Single nucleotide substitutions that result in the wrong amino acid being coded for and selected are called *missense mutations.* Those that create a premature "stop" codon are called *nonsense mutations.* Some mutations cause an error in RNA splicing at the intron–exon splice sites. Diseases caused by a single mutation, such as sickle cell disease, are rare. Because genes coding for the proteins involved in physiological processes are highly redundant, a single mutation located in the coding region of a gene may be clinically silent. Most frequently, pathological phenotypic changes develop only when multiple genes are affected or when specific environmental influences are present.

When newly discovered genes are being analyzed, it can be difficult to distinguish polymorphism in a normal allele from a mutation. For example, more than 6300 variations of the *BRCA1* gene, one of the major genes associated with familial breast and ovarian cancer, have been identified (Hohenstein and Fodde, 2003). It is not currently known whether all of these variations are actually mutations associated with disease, or if some could be polymorphisms or allelic variants (Collins, 1996). The ability to distinguish alleles from mutations is obviously essential to any molecular screening program.

CONTROL OF GENE EXPRESSION: METHYLATION. Genomic DNA methylation is a reversible form of DNA modification that permits control of many aspects of gene expression (Thompson and colleagues, 1991). Its most important function is to control the tissue-specific activation of certain genes. Even though every cell contains the entire genome, genes that are not essential for each specific tissue type are methylated and thus "turned off." The only nucleotide that is methylated is the cytosine of CpG dinucleotide repeats—"p" represents the phosphate backbone of the base pairing. Most CpG dinucleotides are located in gene regulatory regions, where methylation prevents transcription and thus effectively turns off the gene. An example is the globin genes, which are methylated (turned off) in all nonerythroid tissues; thus, only erythrocytes produce hemoglobin (Barsh and Epstein, 1996).

It is likely that both maintenance of methylation and its reversal require the actions of specific enzymes. Methyltransferases capable of adding a methyl group have been identified, but an enzyme capable of removing methyl groups has not (Reik and associates, 2001).

NEW MUTATIONS AND GENE REGULATION. New mutations also are linked to DNA methylation. Although most CpG dinucleotides appear to be located primarily in gene regulatory regions, they are also found within gene coding regions. The function of the CpGs within gene coding regions is not completely understood, but cytosine methylation here does not prevent gene transcription. Once it is methylated, however, the cytosine residue can be deaminated, either spontaneously or as the result of an exogenous mutagen, to become the nucleotide thymine. This thymine may not be recognized as a mutation, and thus not repaired. During DNA replication, this thymine will result in the addition of adenine instead of guanine in the complementary strand. Thus, cytosine methylation can ultimately result in a G to A point mutation (Wajed and Laird, 2001). This specific mutation is extremely common. Methylated CpGs are the single most mutated dinucleotides in the genome, and cause one third of all germline point mutations leading to genetic disease (Mancini and associates, 1997; Ollila and colleagues, 1996; Tornaletti and Pfeifer, 1995). Certain regions of the human genome, termed *hot spots,* have an abundance of CpGs and are especially vulnerable.

CpG dinucleotides have been associated with mutations in a variety of genes. New mutations causing hemophilia A, achondroplasia, mucopolysaccharidosis type II, and some retinoblastomas frequently involve CpG doublets (Mancini and collaborators, 1997; Rathmann and associates, 1996). Other genes with high mutation rates are those causing neurofibromatosis, polycystic kidney disease, and aniridia.

Certain lethal autosomal dominant diseases such as osteogenesis imperfecta or thanatophoric dwarfism *always* result from new mutations. These affected individuals have "reduced reproductive fitness" and are "genetic lethals" who die before they can reproduce.

Other Forms of Gene Regulation. In a small number of genes, the mRNA sequence is modified—termed *mRNA*

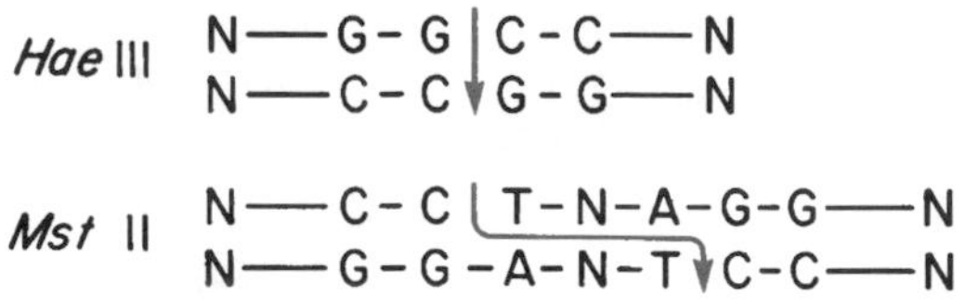

FIGURE 12–13. Restriction endonucleases. *Hae III (H influenzae III)* cleaves a four-base sequence. *Mst II (Microcoleus)* cleaves a seven-base sequence, the center of which is a nonspecific nucleotide, shown here as N.

editing—before it is transcribed, so that it is no longer complementary to its original DNA template (Barsh and Epstein, 1996). The initiation of mRNA translation also can be regulated, controlling the quantity of gene product produced. Finally, rearrangement of DNA can occur and produce a unique functional protein, such as an immunoglobulin (Harriman and colleagues, 1993).

Restriction Fragment Length Polymorphisms (RFLPs). Genomic DNA can be broken into manageable fragments for analysis by bacterial enzymes termed *restriction endonucleases.* Each endonuclease locates and cleaves a specific sequence of base pairs, wherever it occurs along the genome. As shown in Figure 12–13, some enzymes recognize sequences of four nucleotides, some six, and others seven. More than 200 different restriction enzymes have been identified. The number and size of fragments produced by enzyme digestion are determined by the frequency or location of the particular sequences recognized by the enzyme. Each enzyme thus produces its own unique pattern of DNA fragments.

Certain restriction endonuclease sites are the same in all humans. Others, however, are unique to each individual. These unique endonuclease sites, leading to unique DNA fragment lengths, are called *restriction fragment length polymorphisms (RFLPs).* These are not mutations or abnormalities, but are merely individual differences in nucleotide sequences that are present roughly once in every 250 base pairs throughout the genome (Marian, 1995). Each RFLP generally has two alleles and is inherited in mendelian fashion. Because of this, RFLPs can be used for identification purposes, for diagnostic testing, or to confirm or rule out transmission of a specific DNA segment from parent to child.

Repetitive DNA. These segments are characterized by short nucleotide sequences that are repeated many times throughout the genome. These regions are of interest because they include polymorphisms that can be used as markers. They also can be useful for following alleles through a family.

Clustered repetitive DNA makes up 10 to 15 percent of the genome (Elsa and Patel, 1998). These segments are called *simple sequence DNA* or *satellite DNA* because of their physical properties. These segments of DNA include several distinct classes of repeated sequences. One class is characterized by a *variable number of tandem repeats (VNTRs),* consisting of multiple copies of short DNA sequences. *Short tandem repeats (STRs)*, also called *CA dinucleotides* or *GT repeats,* are areas of dinucleotide or trinucleotide repeats scattered throughout the genome. STRs are also highly polymorphic, with 4 to 10 alleles typically identified at each site. VNTRs and STRs are termed more *informative* than RFLPs because their allelic variation makes them more useful for DNA identification.

Interspersed repetitive DNA also occurs randomly and accounts for 15 percent of the genome. These sequences include *short interspersed sequences (SINES)* and *long interspersed sequences (LINES).* All these repetitive sequences can be used to determine the relative locations of markers to each other and to the gene(s) of interest. Thus, they can be used to generate a DNA map.

GENETIC TESTS

Cytogenetic Analysis. Any tissue containing dividing cells or cells that can be stimulated to divide is suitable for cytogenetic analysis. The dividing cells are arrested in metaphase, and the chromosomes are stained to reveal light and dark bands. The unique banding pattern of each chromosome facilitates its identification and detection of any deleted, duplicated, or rearranged segments. The accuracy of cytogenetic analysis increases along with the number of bands produced. Most laboratories now routinely perform high-resolution metaphase banding, which yields 350 to 550 visible bands

per haploid chromosome set. Banding of prophase chromosomes generally yields 850 bands.

Because only dividing cells can be evaluated, the rapidity with which results are obtained correlates with the rapidity of cell growth in culture. Using bone marrow cells, results are usually available in less than 1 day, and adult blood cells yield results in 3 to 4 days. Fetal blood cells often produce results in 1 to 2 days. Amniocytes, which are fetal fibroblasts, sloughed gastrointestinal mucosal cells, and amnion cells, require 7 to 14 days. Skin fibroblasts usually require 3 to 6 weeks, but this is often because the sample is obtained postmortem and stimulation of growth is difficult.

Fluorescence In Situ Hybridization (FISH). This technique provides a rapid method for determining ploidy of select chromosomes or confirming the presence or absence of a specific gene or large DNA sequence (Fig. 12–14). It is not comparable to cytogenetic evaluation because the chromosomes appear squat and the banding patterns are much less distinctive. Chromosome duplications, deletions, and rearrangements often cannot be detected by FISH.

Cells are fixed onto a glass slide, and fluorescently labeled chromosome or gene probes are allowed to hybridize to the fixed chromosomes. Each probe is complementary to a unique area of the chromosome or gene being investigated, thus preventing cross reaction with other chromosomes. If the chromosome or gene of interest is present, hybridization is detected as a bright signal visible by microscopy. The number

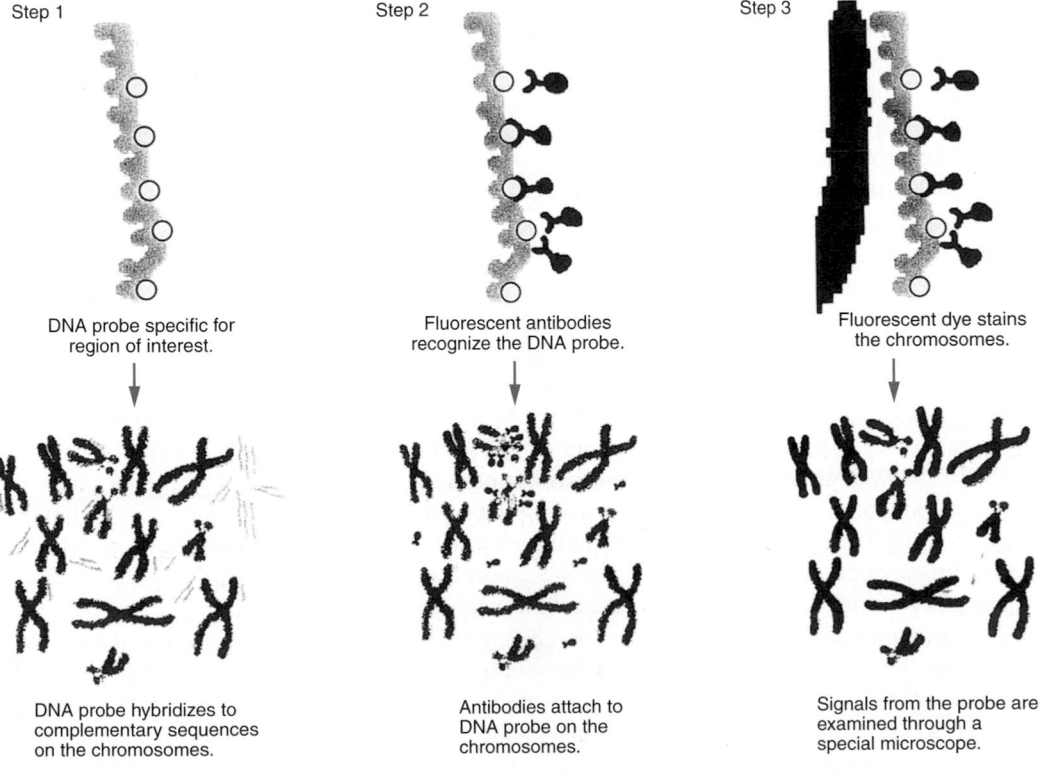

Step 1	Step 2	Step 3
DNA probe specific for region of interest.	Fluorescent antibodies recognize the DNA probe.	Fluorescent dye stains the chromosomes.
DNA probe hybridizes to complementary sequences on the chromosomes.	Antibodies attach to DNA probe on the chromosomes.	Signals from the probe are examined through a special microscope.

FIGURE 12–14. Steps in fluorescence in situ hybridization (FISH). (Adapted from Greenwood Genetics Center, 1995, with permission.)

of signals indicates the number of chromosomes or genes of that type in the cell being analyzed.

The FISH technique usually is used when ploidy status would change clinical management and time constraints prohibit cytogenetic analysis. It also is used to provide fast but preliminary results in order to reduce parental anxiety. The Test and Technology Transfer Committee of the American College of Medical Genetics (2000) recommends that a full karyotype be performed along with all FISH analyses to confirm the ploidy status and to rule out structural chromosomal alterations.

Spectral Karyotype Analysis. This technique is a FISH procedure in which a labeled probe for *every* chromosome is used simultaneously. Chromosomes can be distinguished from each other because each probe emits a unique color. The results are analyzed by computer, making it a rapid and accurate test. It is currently available for research only.

Linkage Analysis. RFLPs, STRs, and other markers can be used to locate a specific gene for research or diagnostic purposes if certain criteria are met (Beaudet and Ballabio, 1994). First, a large family with multiple members affected by the disease in question must be identified. Next, specific markers scattered throughout the genome are selected for study or, if the gene is believed to be located on a specific chromosome, markers on that chromosome are chosen. DNA from each family member is then analyzed to determine whether any of the selected markers are transmitted along with the disease gene. If individuals with the disease have the marker and individuals without the disease do not, the gene causing the disease is said to be linked to the marker, suggesting that they are close to each other on the same chromosome. *Linkage analysis* allows the locations of different genes to be determined, along with their approximate distances from each other.

In cases in which the specific gene has not been identified, linkage analysis can sometimes be used to estimate the likelihood that an individual, for example, a fetus, has inherited the abnormal trait. Linkage analysis, however, is imprecise and depends on family size, availability of family members for testing, and presence of informative markers near the gene.

Complementary DNA (cDNA). When the nucleic acid sequence of a gene or DNA region of interest is known, it can be studied directly using complementary DNA (cDNA), a laboratory-made copy of RNA corresponding to a DNA segment or gene. Many isolated genes or DNA fragments have been collected in cDNA libraries for research and diagnostic use. They are synthesized using reverse transcriptase, an enzyme isolated from tumor viruses, which can synthesize a complementary DNA copy (hence the term *cDNA*) of a nuclear messenger RNA. cDNA is usually single stranded. Importantly, because messenger RNA is the template, it does not contain the introns, which are removed during processing of mRNA. cDNA can be used to locate its corresponding

gene. The cDNA is made using radioactive bases and is then allowed to anneal with the DNA being studied. The radioactive bases allow the DNA probe to be visualized if it bonds successfully, indicating that a matching sequence or identical gene is present.

Fluorescence-Activated Chromosome Sorting (FACS). Large quantities of a specific chromosome can be obtained by FACS. Chromosomes are stained with fluorescent dyes and then passed through a laser beam, which deflects off each chromosome according to its unique intensity. Chromosomes are distinguished from each other by this intensity.

Gel Separation. Once a desired chromosome has been isolated, it can be fragmented with a restriction endonuclease. These fragments can be separated using electrophoresis. Smaller fragments move faster and farther along the gel than larger fragments. The DNA fragments can then be removed from the gel and screened for the gene or DNA sequence of interest.

Polymerase Chain Reaction (PCR). This technique enables the rapid synthesis of large amounts of a specific DNA sequence or gene (Beaudet and Ballabio, 1994). Using PCR, 1 million copies of the original gene or DNA segment can be made in a few hours using minute quantities of DNA. Either the entire gene sequence or the sequences at the beginning and end of the gene, however, must be known. PCR involves three steps that are repeated many times. First, double-stranded DNA is denatured by heating. Then, oligonucleotide primers corresponding to the target sequence on each separated DNA strand are added and anneal to either end of the target sequence. Finally, a mixture of nucleotides and heat-stable DNA polymerase is added to elongate the primer sequence, and new complementary strands of DNA are synthesized. In just a few minutes, the original DNA has been duplicated. The procedure is repeated over and over with exponential amplification of the DNA segment.

Southern Blotting. Named for its inventor, Edward Southern, this technique allows identification of one or several DNA fragments of interest from among the million or so typically obtained by enzyme digestion of the entire human genome. As illustrated in Figure 12–15, it applies the principles of gel separation and cDNA hybridization discussed earlier, but on a much larger scale. The cDNA probe may be a copy of a normal gene, in which case hybridization confirms the presence of the normal gene while lack of hybridization indicates a mutation. Hybridization can occur, however, even with incomplete sequence homology. Therefore, only relatively large mutations or changes such as deletions can be detected by cDNA probes.

The probe could also be a fragment of DNA produced by endonuclease digestion. In this case, individuals with a normal gene would have fragments of a different size from individuals carrying a mutated gene. Basic principles of the

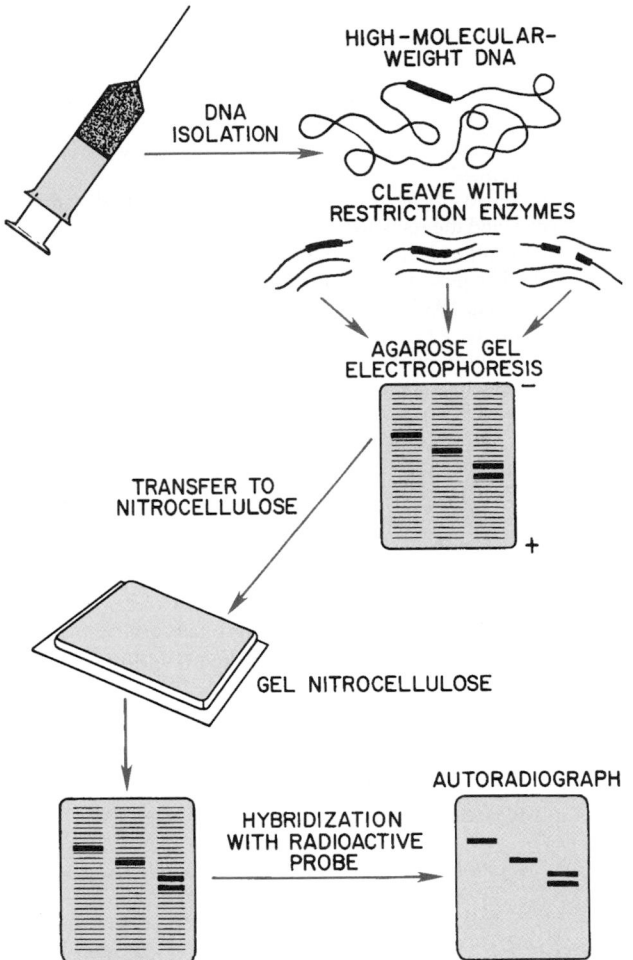

HIGH–MOLECULAR–
WEIGHT DNA

DNA
ISOLATION

CLEAVE WITH
RESTRICTION ENZYMES

AGAROSE GEL
ELECTROPHORESIS

TRANSFER TO
NITROCELLULOSE

GEL NITROCELLULOSE

AUTORADIOGRAPH

HYBRIDIZATION
WITH RADIOACTIVE
PROBE

FIGURE 12–15. Southern blotting analysis. Genomic DNA is isolated from leukocytes or amniocytes and digested with a restriction enzyme. This procedure yields a series of reproducible fragments that are separated by agarose gel electrophoresis. The separated DNA fragments are then transferred ("blotted") to a nitrocellulose membrane that binds DNA. The membrane is treated with a solution containing a radioactive single-stranded nucleic acid probe, which forms a double-stranded nucleic acid complex at membrane sites when homologous DNA is present. These regions are then detected by autoradiography.

Southern blot technique also can be applied to RNA, in which case it is called *Northern blotting,* and to proteins—*Western blotting.*

Allele-Specific Oligonucleotide (ASO) Probes. If a mutation of interest consists of a change in only one or two base pairs, a cDNA probe will not detect it, as discussed earlier. For single-nucleotide mutations, an ASO probe must be used instead. An ASO is a short DNA probe, 15 to 25 bases in length, that is homologous to a specific DNA sequence (Layman, 1992). ASOs can be used instead of cDNA in the Southern blotting technique shown in Figure 12–15. They are useful for testing family members at risk for a small, well-characterized familial mutation.

Multiplex Polymerase Chain Reaction. PCR can be used to amplify any DNA segment, including genes with deletions or mutations, as long as primers spanning the DNA region of interest are available. If various mutations in one gene have been identified in association with a certain disorder, they can all be amplified simultaneously using multiplex PCR.

Oligonucleotide Ligation Assay (OLA). This technique provides great sensitivity in detecting single-base insertions, deletions, or substitutions. Two probes, each corresponding to an adjacent region of the gene in question, are allowed to hybridize to these regions. If the nucleotide sequences of the two probes correspond exactly, they will link together when exposed to DNA ligase, releasing the label attached to one probe. This procedure provides a higher degree of accuracy than can be achieved with single-probe assays (Winn-Deen, 1996).

Ligase Chain Reaction (LCR). This technique is the amplification counterpart of OLA and may be used to screen for many different small or single-gene mutations simultaneously. In a single tube, the specimen is submitted to multiplex PCR and then evaluated with simultaneous OLA analysis for multiple different mutations. LCR is used by many laboratories for cystic fibrosis screening, because it allows simultaneous testing for the entire panel of 25 common mutations (see Chap. 13, p. 325).

Cloning. A clone is a large number of molecules or cells all identical to one ancestral molecule or cell (Lewin, 1997). Cloning refers to the replication of genetic material, although a new definition created by the popular media includes replication of whole animals. Most commonly, cloning involves several laboratory techniques that enable pieces of DNA to be copied in large quantities by vectors within bacteria. These vectors are DNA molecules that replicate autonomously. Restriction enzymes are used to cleave both the DNA sequence of interest and the vector DNA at appropriate sites, and DNA ligase is used to insert the DNA segment into the vector DNA. The inserted DNA is replicated along with the vector DNA, and large quantities of the DNA insert can then be retrieved for study. The first vectors used for cloning were bacterial plasmids, which are circular, double-stranded DNA molecules that replicate separately from bacterial chromosomes.

Plasmids are used for small DNA inserts, usually less than 5 to 10 kb. DNA fragments were later cloned in bacteriophages with inserts up to 20 kb, and in modified plasmids called *cosmids* with inserts up to 50 kb. Burke and colleagues (1987) developed a method to insert 100 to 1000 kb of DNA into a *yeast artificial chromosome (YAC).* These chromosomes have centromeres and telomeres and replicate like normal yeast chromosomes. YAC libraries, with each YAC containing a different fragment of the genome, have been established to greatly simplify gene isolation.

Positional Cloning. This technique is sometimes referred to as *reverse genetics,* because it involves an attempt to clone the gene responsible for a specific disease based on its location, without knowing the nature of the gene product. This attempt is only possible once the gene has been localized to a specific part of a given chromosome, which usually involves narrowing the search to a sequence of over 1 million base pairs (Gelehrter and Collins, 1990). Positional cloning is easier if the affected individual also has a cytogenetic abnormality such as a chromosomal deletion to mark the most likely location. Examples of genes that have been cloned using this technique include those causing cystic fibrosis, Duchenne muscular dystrophy, retinoblastoma, colonic polyposis, neurofibromatosis, and Huntington disease (Beaudet and Ballabio, 1994).

DNA Chips. These chips take advantage of the principles of PCR and nucleic acid hybridization to screen DNA for many genes or mutations simultaneously. Many cDNA probes or ASOs, each representing a different gene mutation, are tagged with differently colored fluorescent dyes and arrayed on a tiny chip. DNA from the tested individual is amplified by PCR and exposed to the probes fixed on the chip. Hybridization to any of the probes is recognized by the color pattern and indicates that the individual carries the mutation represented by that particular cDNA. It is anticipated that this technology will revolutionize genetic screening. For example, although more than 900 mutations causing cystic fibrosis have been identified, patient samples are currently tested only for a panel of 25 of the most common mutations. Using a DNA chip, the patient could be screened for all 900 mutations simultaneously.

Microarrays. DNA chip technology can also be used as a research tool to investigate patterns of gene expression. A microarray platform contains hundreds of oligonucleotides or cDNAs generated from cDNA libraries. Messenger RNA is extracted from the tissue of interest, converted to DNA, labeled with a fluorescent probe, and applied to the microarray. Hybridization to any of the cDNAs is detected and quantified by fluorescence scanning. This technique facilitates analysis and comparison of patterns of gene expression, for example, the genes expressed by the amnion and chorion during preterm versus term labor (Marvin and colleagues, 2002).

REFERENCES

American College of Obstetricians and Gynecologists: Prenatal and preconceptional carrier screening for genetic diseases in individuals of Eastern European Jewish descent. Committee Opinion No. 298, August 2004

American College of Obstetricians and Gynecologists: Neural tube defects. Practice Bulletin No. 44, July 2003

Andrew SE, Goldberg YP, Kremer B: The relationship between trinucleotide repeat length (CAG) and clinical features of Huntington disease. Nat Genet 4:398, 1993

Baird PA, Anderson TW, Newcombe HB, et al: Genetic disorders in children and young adults: A population study. Am J Hum Genet 42:677, 1988

Beaudet AL, Ballabio A: Molecular genetics and medicine. In Isselbacher KJ, Braunwald E, Wilson JD, et al (eds): Harrison's Principles of Internal Medicine, 13th ed. New York, McGraw-Hill, 1994, p 349

Becerra JE, Khoury MJ, Cordero JF, et al: Diabetes mellitus during pregnancy and the risks for specific birth defects: A population-based case-control study. Pediatrics 85:1, 1990

Bennett RL: The genetic risks of incest and consanguinity. Genet Northwest 2:2, 1987

Botto LD, May K, Fernhoff PM, et al: Population-based study of 22q11.2 deletion: Phenotype, incidence, and contribution to major birth defects in the population. Pediatrics 112:101, 2003

Burke DT, Carle CF, Olson MV: Cloning of large segments of exogenous DNA into yeast by means of artificial chromosome vectors. Science 236:806, 1987

Burn J, Brennan P, Little J, et al: Recurrence risks in offspring of adults with major heart defects: Results from first cohort of British collaborative study. Lancet 351:311, 1998

Burn J, Goodship J: Developmental genetics of the heart. Curr Opin Genet Dev 6:322, 1996

Buxton J, Shelbourne P, Davies J: Detection of an unstable fragment of DNA specific to individuals with myotonic dystrophy. Nature 355:547, 1992

Centers for Disease Control and Prevention: Spina bifida and anencephaly before and after folic acid mandate—United States, 1995–1996 and 1999–2000. MMWR 53:362, 2004

Chin AJ: Congenital heart disease. In Jameson JL (ed): Principles of Molecular Medicine. Totowa, NJ, Humana Press, 1998, p 117

Clarke A: Genetic imprinting in clinical genetics. Dev Suppl 1990, p 131

Claussen U, Schafer H, Trampisch HJ: Exclusion of chromosomal mosaicism in prenatal diagnosis. Hum Genet 67:23, 1984

Cockwell A, MacKenzie M, Youings S, et al: A cytogenetic and molecular study of a series of 45 X fetuses and their parents. J Med Genet 28:151, 1991

Collins FS: BRCA1—lots of mutations, lots of dilemmas. N Engl J Med 334:186, 1996

Curry CJ, Stevenson RE, Aughton D, et al: Evaluation of mental retardation: Recommendations of a consensus conference. Am J Med Genet 72:468, 1997

Cutillo DM: Fragile X syndrome. Genet Teratol 2:1, 1994

Czeizel AE: Reduction of urinary tract and cardiovascular defects by periconceptional multivitamin supplementation. Am J Med Genet 62:179, 1996

Czeizel AE, Dudas I: Prevention of the first occurrence of neural-tube defects by periconceptional vitamin supplementation. N Engl J Med 327:1832, 1992

de Vries BB, Weigers AM, Smits APT, et al: Mental status of females with an FMR1 gene full mutation. Am J Hum Genet 58:1025, 1996

De Wals P, Rusen ID, Lee NS, et al: Trend in prevalence of neural tube defects in Quebec. Birth Defects Res Part A 67:919, 2003

Elsa SH, Patel PI: Organization of the human genome, chromosomes, and genes. In Jameson JL (ed): Principles of Molecular Medicine. Totowa, NJ, Humana Press, 1998, p 4

Fernandez R, Mendez J, Pasaro E: Turner syndrome: A study of chromosomal mosaicism. Hum Genet 98:29, 1996

Friedman JM: Genetic disease in the offspring of older fathers. Obstet Gynecol 57:745, 1981

Friere-Maia N: Effects of consanguineous marriages on morbidity and precocious mortality: Genetic counseling. Am J Med Genet 18:401, 1984

Fryns JP, Kleczkowski A, Kubien E, et al: On the excess of mental retardation and/or congenital malformations in apparently balanced reciprocal translocations. A critical review of the Leuven data. Genet Counsel 2:185, 1992

Garber AP, Schreck R, Carlson DE: Fetal loss. In Rimoin DL, Connor JM, Pyeritz RE (eds): Emery and Rimoin's Principles and Practice of Medical Genetics, 3rd ed. New York, Churchill Livingstone, 1996

Gardner RJM, Sutherland GR: Chromosome Abnormalities and Genetic Counseling, 2nd ed. Oxford Monographs on Medical Genetics No. 29. Oxford, Oxford University Press, 1996

Gelehrter TD, Collins FS: Anatomy of the human genome: Gene mapping and linkage. In Gelehrter TD, Collins FS (eds): Principles of Medical Genetics. Baltimore, Williams and Wilkins, 1990, p 193

Gennarelli M, Novelli G, Bassi FA, et al: Prediction of myotonic dystrophy clinical severity based on the number of intragenic [CTG]n trinucleotide repeats. Am J Med Genet 65:342, 1996

Golden JA, Chernoff GF: Multiple sites of anterior neural tube closure in humans: Evidence from anterior neural tube defects (anencephaly). Pediatrics 4:506, 1995

Graham JM Jr: Smith's Recognizable Patterns of Human Deformation, 2nd ed. Philadelphia, Saunders, 1988

Greenwood Genetics Center: Fluorescence in situ hybridization (FISH). In: Counseling Aids for Geneticists, 3rd ed. Greenville, SC, Keys Printing, 1995, p 23

Hagerman PJ, Hagerman RJ: The fragile-X premutation: A maturing perspective. Am J Hum Genet 74:805, 2004

Hall JG: Genomic imprinting: Review and relevance to human diseases. Am J Hum Genet 46:857, 1990

Harriman W, Volk H, Defranoux N, et al: Immunoglobulin class switch recombination. Annu Rev Immunol 11: 361, 1993

Hassold T, Arnovitz K, Jacobs PA, et al: The parental origin of the missing or additional chromosome in 45,X and 47,XXX females. Birth Defects Orig Artic Ser 26:297, 1991

Held KR, Kerber S, Kaminsky E: Mosaicism in 45X Turner syndrome: Does survival in early pregnancy depend on the presence of two sex chromosomes? Hum Genet 88:288, 1992

Henderson KG, Shaw TE, Barrett IJ, et al: Distribution of mosaicism in human placentae. Hum Genet 97:650, 1996

Hibbard ED, Smithells RW: Folic acid metabolism and human embryopathy. Lancet 1:1254, 1965

Hohenstein P, Fodde R: Of mice and (wo)men genotype-phenotype correlations in BRCA1. Hum Mol Genet 15:12, 2003

Hook EB: Prevalence, risks, and recurrence. In Brock DJH, Rodeck CH, Ferguson-Smith MA (eds): Prenatal Diagnosis and Screening. Edinburgh, Churchill Livingstone, 1992, p 351

Hook EB, Cross PK, Schreinemachers DM: Chromosomal abnormality rates at amniocentesis and in live-born infants. JAMA 249:2034, 1983

Hunter AGW: Neural tube defects in Eastern Ontario and Western Quebec: Demography and family data. Am J Med Genet 19:45, 1984

In't Velt P, Halley DJJ, Van Hemel JO, et al: Genetic counseling before intracytoplasmic sperm injection. Lancet 350:490, 1997

Jacobs PA, Browne C, Gregson N, et al: Estimates of the frequency of chromosome abnormalities detectable in unselected newborns using moderate levels of banding. J Med Genet 29:103, 1992

Jones KL: Smith's Recognizable Patterns of Human Malformation, 5th ed. Philadelphia, Saunders, 1997

Jorde LB, Carey JC, White RL: Clinical cytogenetics: The chromosome basis of human disease. In: Medical Genetics. St Louis, Mosby, 1995, p 102

Kalousek DK, Barrett IJ, McGillivray BC: Placental mosaicism and intrauterine survival of trisomies 13 and 18. Am J Hum Genet 44:338, 1989

Kalousek DK, Dill FJ: Chromosomal mosaicism confined to the placenta in human conceptions. Science 221:665, 1983

Kamiguchi Y, Rosenbusch B, Sterzik K, et al: Chromosomal analysis of unfertilized human oocytes prepared by a gradual fixation-air drying method. Hum Genet 90:533, 1993

Kim SS, Jung SC, Kim JH, et al: Chromosome abnormalities in a referred population for suspected chromosomal aberrations: A report of 4117 cases. J Korean Med Sci 14:373, 1999

King RA, Rotter JI, Motulsky AG: The approach to genetic bases of common diseases. In King RA, Rotter JI, Motulsky AG (eds): The Genetic Basis of Common Disease. New York, Oxford University Press, 1992, p 3

Koeberl DD, McGillivray B, Sybert VP: Prenatal diagnosis of 45,X/46,XX mosaicism and 45,X: Implications for postnatal outcome. Am J Hum Genet 57:661, 1995

Layman LC: Basic concepts of molecular biology as applied to pediatric and adolescent gynecology. Obstet Gynecol Clin North Am 19:1, 1992

Levitan M: Textbook of Human Genetics, 3rd ed. New York, Oxford University Press, 1988

Lewin B: DNA biotechnology. In: Genes VI. Oxford, Oxford University Press, 1997, p 623

Lin AE, Garver KL: Genetic counseling for congenital heart defects. J Pediatr 113:1105, 1988

Lindhout D, Omtzigt JGC, Cornel MC: Spectrum of neural tube defects in 34 infants prenatally exposed to antiepileptic drugs. Neurology 42(suppl 5):111, 1992

Mancini D, Singh S, Ainsworth P, et al: Constitutively methylated CpG dinucleotides as mutation hot spots in the retinoblastoma gene (RB1). Am J Hum Genet 61:80, 1997

Marian AJ: Molecular approaches for screening of genetic diseases. Chest 108:255, 1995

Marvin KW, Keelan JA, Eykolt RL, et al: Use of cDNA arrays to generate differential expression profiles for inflammatory genes in human gestational membranes delivered at term and preterm. Mol Hum Reprod 8:399, 2002

McIntosh GC, Olshan AF, Baird PA: Paternal age and the risk of birth defects in offspring. Epidemiology 6:282, 1995

Melnick M, Bixler D, Fogh-Andersen P: Cleft lip +/- cleft palate: An overview of the literature and an analysis of Danish cases born between 1941 and 1968. Am J Med Genet 6:83, 1980

Migeon BR: Role of DNA methylation in X inactivation and the fragile X syndrome. Am J Med Genet 47:685, 1993

Moore KL, Persaud TVN, Shiota K (eds): Color Atlas of Clinical Embryology, 2nd ed. Philadelphia, Saunders, 2000, p 20

MRC Vitamin Study Research Group: Prevention of neural tube defects: Results of the Medical Research Council Vitamin Study. Lancet 338:131, 1991

Nadiri S: Congenital abnormalities in newborns of consanguineous and non-consanguineous parents. Obstet Gynecol 53:195, 1979

National Institutes of Health: Phenylketonuria (PKU): Screening and management. National Institutes of Health Consensus Statement 17:1, October 16–18, 2000

Nazarenko SA, Timoshevsky VA, Sukhanova NN: High frequency of tissue-specific mosaicism in Turner syndrome patients. Clin Genet 56:59, 1999

Nelson DL: The fragile X syndromes. Sem Cell Biol 6:5, 1995

Nora JJ, Nora AH: Updates on counseling the family with a first-degree relative with a congenital heart defect. Am J Med Genet 29:137, 1988

Ollila J, Lappalainen I, Vihinen M: Sequence specificity in CpG mutation hotspots. FEBS Lett 396:119, 1996

Platt LD, Koch R, Hanley WB, et al: The international study of pregnancy outcome in women with maternal phenylketonuria: Report of a 12-year study. Am J Obstet Gynecol 182:326, 2000

Porter S, Gilks CB: Genomic imprinting: A proposed explanation for the different behaviors of testicular and ovarian germ cell tumors. Med Hypotheses 41:37, 1993

Rasmussen SA, Wong L-Y, Yang Q, et al: Population-based analyses of mortality in trisomy 13 and trisomy 18. Pediatrics 111:777, 2003

Rathmann M, Bunge S, Beck M, et al: Mucopolysaccharidosis type II (Hunter syndrome): Mutation "hotspots" in the iduronate-2-sulfatase gene. Am J Hum Genet 59:1202, 1996

Reik W, Dean W, Walter J: Epigenetic reprogramming in mammalian development. Science 293:1089, 2001

Rimoin DL, Connor JM, Pyeritz RE (eds): Emery and Rimoin's Principles and Practice of Medical Genetics, 3rd ed. New York: Churchill Livingstone, 1997, pp 31, 277, 767

Robinson A, Bender BG, Linden MG, et al: Sex chromosome aneuploidy: The Denver prospective study. Birth Defects Orig Artic Ser 26:59, 1991

Robinson WP, Barrett IJ, Bernard L, et al: Meiotic origin of trisomy in confined placental mosaicism is correlated with presence of fetal uniparental disomy, high levels of trisomy in trophoblast, and increased risk of fetal intrauterine growth restriction. Am J Hum Genet 60:917, 1997

Rousseau F, Rouillard P, Morel M-L, et al: Prevalence of carriers of premutation-size alleles of the FMRI gene—and implications for the population genetics of the fragile X syndrome. Am J Hum Genet 57:1006, 1995

Saenger P: Turner's syndrome. N Engl J Med 335:1749, 1996

Scharrer S, Stengel-Rutkowski S, Rodewald-Rudescu A, et al: Reproduction in a female patient with Down's syndrome. Case report of a 46,XY child showing slight phenotypical anomalies born to a 47,XX, +21 mother. Humangenetik 26:207, 1975

Schneider AS, Mennuti MT, Zackai EH: High cesarean section rate in trisomy 18 births: A potential indication for late prenatal diagnosis. Am J Obstet Gynecol 140:367, 1981

Shami SA, Qaisar R, Bittles AH: Consanguinity and adult morbidity in Pakistan. Lancet 338:954, 1991

Sheridan R, Llerena J, Matkins S, et al: Fertility in a male with trisomy 21. J Med Genet 26:294, 1989

Sherman SL, Takaesu N, Freeman SB, et al: Trisomy 21: Association between reduced recombination and nondisjunction. Am J Hum Genet 46:608, 1991

Smith A, Gaha TJ: Data on families of chromosome translocation carriers ascertained because of habitual spontaneous abortion. Aust N Z J Obstet Gynaecol 30:57, 1990

Snijders RJM, Sebire NJ, Nicolaides KH: Maternal age and gestational age-specific risk for chromosomal defects. Fetal Diagn Ther 10:356, 1995

Spence JE, Perciaccante RG, Greig FM, et al: Uniparental disomy as a mechanism for human genetic disease. Am J Hum Genet 42:217, 1988

Spotila LD, Sereda L, Prockop DJ: Partial isodisomy for maternal chromosome 7 and short stature in an individual with a mutation at the COLIA2 locus. Am J Hum Genet 51:1396, 1992

Sybert VP, McCauley E: Turner's syndrome. N Engl J Med 351:1227, 2004

Test and Technology Transfer Committee, American College of Medical Genetics: Technical and clinical assessment of fluorescence in situ hybridization: An ACMG/ASHG position statement. I. Technical considerations. Genet Med 2:356, 2000

Thompson MW, McInnes RR, Huntington FW: Thompson and Thompson—Genetics in Medicine, 5th ed. Philadelphia, Saunders, 1991

Tolmie JL: Chromosome disorders. In Whittle MJ, Connor JM (eds): Prenatal Diagnosis in Obstetric Practice. Oxford, Blackwell Scientific, 1995, p 34

Tornaletti S, Pfeifer GP: Complete and tissue-independent methylation of CpG sites in the p53 gene: Implications for mutations in human cancers. Oncogene 10:1493, 1995

Turner G, Webb T, Wake S, et al: The prevalence of the fragile X syndrome. Am J Med Genet 64:196, 1996

Tycko B: Genomic imprinting: Mechanism and role in human pathology. Am J Pathol 144:431, 1994

Van Steirteghem A, Devroey P, Liebaers I: Intracytoplasmic sperm injection. Mol Cell Endocrinol 186:199, 2002

Wajed SA, Laird PW, De Meester TR: DNA methylation: An alternative pathway to cancer. Ann Surg 234:10, 2001

Wallace DC: 1994 William Allan Award Address. Mitochondrial DNA variation in human evolution, degenerative disease, and aging. Am J Hum Genet 57:201, 1995

Wald NJ: Folic acid and the prevention of neural tube defects. N Engl J Med 350:101, 2004

Wenstrom KD, Descartes M, Franklin J, et al: A five year experience with fragile X screening of high risk gravidas. Am J Obstet Gynecol 181:789, 1999

Wenstrom KD, Faye-Petersen OM, Johanning GL: DNA methylation and tissue cellularity in hypoplastic left ventricles. Am J Obstet Gynecol 187:S68, 2002

Wenstrom KD, Johanning GL, Johnston KE, et al: Association of the C677T methylenetetrahydrofolate reductase mutation and elevated homocysteine levels with congenital cardiac malformations. Am J Obstet Gynecol 184:806, 2001

Williamson ML, Koch R, Azen C, et al: Correlates of intelligence test results in treated phenylketonuric children. Pediatrics 68:161, 1981

Winn-Deen ES: Multi-mutation screening using PCR and ligation—principles and applications. Trends Biotechnol 14:113, 1996

Zuhlke C, Thies U, Braulke I, et al: Down syndrome and male fertility: PCR-derived fingerprinting, serological and andrological investigations. Clin Genet 46:324, 1994

13

Prenatal Diagnosis and Fetal Therapy

The incidence of major abnormalities discovered at birth is 2 to 3 percent. These anomalies cause a significant portion of neonatal deaths, and more than one fourth of all pediatric hospital admissions result from genetic disorders (Lee and colleagues, 2001). Prenatal diagnosis is the science of identifying these structural or functional abnormalities in the developing fetus. With this information, clinicians hope to alter the severity of congenital disease by offering an ever-expanding number of fetal treatments or surveillance as well as optimal delivery for some or consideration of pregnancy termination for others. Diagnostic evaluation typically involves three major categories:

1. Fetuses at high risk for a genetic or congenital disorder.
2. Fetuses at unknown risk for common congenital abnormalities.
3. Fetuses discovered ultrasonographically to have structural or developmental abnormalities.

Current fetal therapy includes optimizing the intrauterine environment and delivery, blood transfusion, administration of medication, amnioreduction, placement of shunts, and surgery. In the near future, hemopoietic stem cell transplantation and other methods for gene therapy likely will be added to this list.

FETUSES AT HIGH RISK FOR GENETIC OR CONGENITAL DISORDERS

FETAL ANEUPLOIDY. At least 8 percent of conceptuses are aneuploid, accounting for 50 percent of first-trimester abortions and 5 to 7 percent of all stillbirths and neonatal deaths (see Chap. 12, p. 288). Chromosomal defects compatible with life but causing significant morbidity are found in 0.65 percent of newborns. Another 0.2 percent have structural chromosomal rearrangements that will eventually affect reproduction (Milunsky, 1992).

Several safe, accurate, and well-established procedures to obtain fetal cells for karyotyping are currently available. The challenge is to determine which women are at high risk for carrying aneuploid fetuses and should be offered one of these tests. Most commonly, "high risk" describes a risk greater than the chance of fetal death associated with the diagnostic procedure being considered. The postamniocentesis pregnancy loss rate is approximately 1 in 200, therefore, amniocentesis for fetal karyotyping would not typically be offered unless the risk of fetal aneuploidy was estimated to be greater than 1 in 200. Women with a risk of carrying an aneuploid fetus high enough to prompt an invasive diagnostic procedure (Table 13–1) include the following:

1. *Women who will be at least 35 years old at the delivery of their singleton pregnancy.* The midtrimester risk, or incidence, of fetal Down syndrome among 35-year-old gravidas is 1 in 250 and rises rapidly with increasing maternal

TABLE 13–1 Women with Risk of Fetal Aneuploidy Significant Enough to Justify Risk of Amniocentesis

Singleton pregnancy at age over 35 years at delivery
Dizygotic twin pregnancy at age over 31 years at delivery
Previous autosomal trisomy birth
Previous 47,XXX or 47,XXY birth
Patient or partner is carrier of chromosome translocation
Patient or partner is carrier of chromosomal inversion
History of triploidy
Some cases with repetitive early pregnancy losses
Patient or partner has aneuploidy
Major fetal structural defect identified by ultrasound

age (Fig. 13–1). The risk of any numerical aneuploidy is 1 in 132 (Table 13–2). The midtrimester incidence is greater than that at term because a large proportion of aneuploid fetuses die spontaneously before reaching term. Consequently, for women aged 35 or older, the risk of fetal Down syndrome at term is 1 in 384 and that of any numeric aneuploidy is 1 in 204.

2. *Women aged at least 31 years at the delivery of their dizygotic twin gestation.* The chance that a pregnancy will be complicated by fetal Down syndrome is greater if there are two fetuses than if there is only one. The risk of trisomy 21 in a twin pregnancy can be calculated by considering the maternal age-related Down syndrome risk,

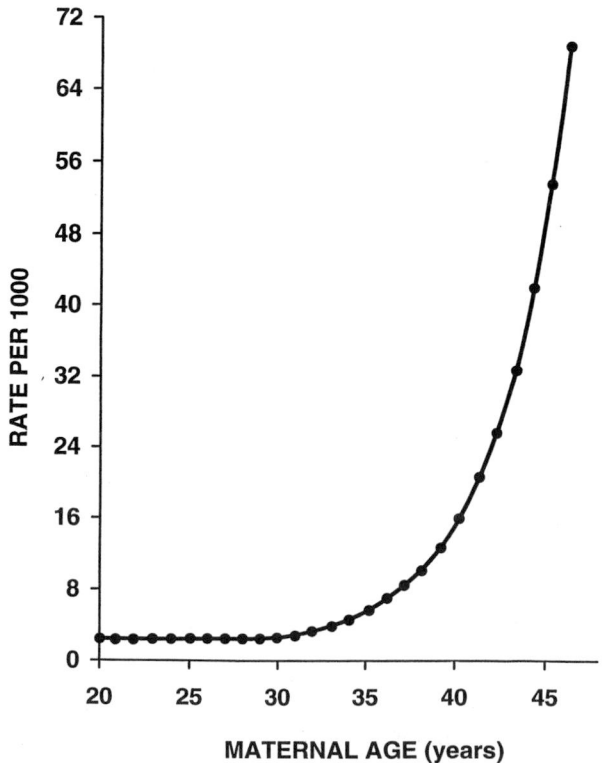

FIGURE 13–1. Maternal age-related incidence of fetal trisomy. (Data from Ferguson-Smith and Yates, 1984.)

TABLE 13–2 Maternal Age-Related Midtrimester Risk of Down Syndrome and All Aneuploidies

Maternal Age	Midtrimester Incidence		Term Liveborn Incidence	
	Down	All Aneuploidies	Down	All Aneuploidies
33	1/417	1/208	1/625	1/345
34	1/333	1/152	1/500	1/278
35	1/250	1/132	1/384	1/204
36	1/192	1/105	1/303	1/167
37	1/149	1/83	1/227	1/130
38	1/115	1/65	1/175	1/103
39	1/89	1/53	1/137	1/81
40	1/69	1/40	1/106	1/63
41	1/53	1/31	1/81	1/50
42	1/41	1/25	1/64	1/39
43	1/31	1/19	1/50	1/30
44	1/25	1/15	1/38	1/24
45	1/19	1/12	1/30	1/19

From Hook and colleagues, 1983, with permission.

the maternal race- and age-related incidence of dizygotic twinning, and the probability that either or both fetuses could be affected. The analysis by Meyers and colleagues (1997) shows that for both white and African-American 31-year-old women, the midtrimester risk of Down syndrome in a dizygotic twin pregnancy is approximately 1 in 190 (Table 13–3). Counseling in this situation should include a discussion of options for pregnancy management if only one fetus is affected, as this may influence the desire for prenatal diagnosis. These options include

TABLE 13–3 Maternal Age-Related Midtrimester Risk of Down Syndrome in One or Both Fetuses of a Dizygotic Twin Pregnancy

Maternal Age	Down Syndrome		All Aneuploidies	
	Midtrimester	Term	Midtrimester	Term
25	1/481	1/679	1/833	1/259
26	1/447	1/636	1/650	1/258
27	1/415	1/599	1/509	1/245
28	1/387	1/566	1/398	1/234
29	1/364	1/535	1/310	1/223
30	1/342	1/508	1/243	1/206
31	1/324	1/483	1/190	1/205
32	1/256	1/409	1/149	1/171
33	1/206	1/319	1/116	1/151
34	1/160	1/257	1/91	1/126
35	1/125	1/199	1/71	1/101
36	1/98	1/153	1/56	1/82
37	1/77	1/118	1/44	1/67
38	1/60	1/92	1/35	1/54
39	1/47	1/72	1/27	1/44
40	1/37	1/56	1/21	1/35
41	1/29	1/44	1/17	1/28
42	1/23	1/33	1/13	1/22

From Meyers and colleagues, 1997, with permission.

aborting the twin pregnancy, selective second-trimester reduction of the affected fetus, continuing the pregnancy with monitoring of only the normal fetus, or continued monitoring of both fetuses.

3. *Women who have previously carried a fetus with an autosomal trisomy.* After having one trisomic fetus, the chance of having another is approximately 1:100 (or 1 percent) until the maternal age-related risk exceeds 1 percent. After that, the age-related risk predominates (Warburton and associates, 1987).

4. *Women who have previously carried a fetus with triple X (47,XXX) or Klinefelter syndrome (47,XXY).* The extra X chromosome in these disorders may be maternal or paternal in origin. As with autosomal trisomies, the recurrence risk is 1:100 until the maternal age-related risk exceeds 1:100, after which the age-related risk predominates (Gardner and Sutherland, 1996). Women whose previous child was 47,XYY are not at high risk for recurrence, because the extra chromosome in this situation is paternal in origin, and paternal errors have minimal chance of recurring. Likewise, 45,X has a very low recurrence risk.

5. *Women or their partners who have a chromosomal translocation.* The risk of having abnormal offspring must be estimated individually, accounting for the chromosomes involved, the gender of the transmitting parent, and the testing method used. For most translocations, the observed risk of an abnormal liveborn neonate is less than the theoretical risk, because a portion of gametes are so abnormal as to either preclude conception or produce only nonviable conceptions. In general, however, translocation carriers identified after the birth of an abnormal neonate have a 5- to 30-percent risk of having another fetus with an unbalanced translocation. In contrast, carriers identified during an infertility evaluation have a much lower risk (0 to 5 percent) because their translocation most likely results in nonviable gametes or embryos (Gardner and Sutherland, 1996).

6. *Women or their partners who are carriers of chromosomal inversions.* The risk for each carrier is individually determined by considering the testing method used, the chromosome involved, and the size of the inversion. In general, the observed risk is approximately 5 to 10 percent if the inversion was detected after the birth of an abnormal neonate and 1 to 3 percent if identified by some other means (Gardner and Sutherland, 1996).

7. *History of triploidy.* Over 99 percent of triploid conceptions are lost in the first or second trimesters. Rarely, a fetus develops. If the triploidy involved a fetus surviving past the first trimester, the recurrence risk is 1 to 1.5 percent, and thus sufficient to prompt prenatal testing (Gardner and Sutherland, 1996).

8. *Repetitive spontaneous first-trimester abortions.* The majority of first-trimester miscarriages result from aneuploidy. A history of one early aneuploid loss does not

increase the maternal age-related risk of a second aneuploid pregnancy. Importantly, the majority of conceptuses from repetitive early abortions are euploid (Morton and associates, 1987; Warburton and colleagues, 1987). In fact, as the number of first-trimester abortions increases, the proportion caused by karyotypic abnormalities decreases (Ogasawara and colleagues, 2000). Accordingly, the value of karyotyping abortuses is unclear. Karyotyping the *parents* may be more helpful, because the few repetitive early abortions associated with a chromosomal abnormality are caused by maternal or paternal inversions or translocations. Identification of such a parental abnormality would allow counseling about the recurrence risk (Warburton and associates, 1987).

9. *Parental aneuploidy.* Women with trisomy 21 or 47,XXX and men with 47,XYY are usually fertile and have a 30-percent risk of having trisomic offspring. In contrast, men with trisomy 21 or 47,XXY are usually sterile.

10. *A fetus with a major structural defect identified by ultrasonography.* This increases the risk of aneuploidy sufficiently to warrant fetal karyotyping, regardless of maternal age or parental karyotypes (Williamson and Pringle, 1987; Wladimiroff and co-workers, 1988).

ISOLATED STRUCTURAL ANOMALIES. Structural malformations that are multifactorial or polygenic in origin have a 2- to 3-percent recurrence risk. Thus, a fetus who is a first-degree relative of an affected individual—usually because it is the sibling of an affected child or the child of an affected parent—has a 2- to 3-percent risk of being similarly affected. Therefore, any parent who is affected or has an affected child should be offered prenatal counseling and diagnostic evaluation. Although the risk conferred by an affected *second-degree* relative of the fetus (i.e., aunt, uncle, grandparent, or half-sibling) is much lower, many of these patients request counseling and testing. In most multifactorial disorders, the risk resulting from affected third-degree relatives (i.e., cousins) is not substantively different from the general population (Thompson and colleagues, 1991). For severe malformations, the evaluation should be completed early in the pregnancy to allow pregnancy termination to be considered. Several kinds of structural defects can be identified by an ultrasonographic examination performed using high-resolution equipment (Table 13–4).

Congenital Heart Defects. These abnormalities are the most common isolated structural defects, with an incidence of 0.7 percent (Burn and colleagues, 1998). Certain specific heart defects or heart defect categories, if present in one fetus, may recur in subsequent pregnancies. Gill and colleagues (2003) studied 6640 pregnancies at risk of recurrent congenital cardiac defect and found that the same defect recurred in 37 percent and a similar defect developed in 44 percent of subsequent fetuses. The abnormalities most like to be associated with recurrence of the same defect were atrioventricular

TABLE 13–4 High-Resolution Ultrasonography for Detection of Fetal Anomalies

Head
 Anencephaly
 Ventriculomegaly–hydrocephaly
 Encephalocele
 Intracranial lesions
Neck
 Cystic hygroma
 Branchial cleft cysts
 Teratomas
Spinal
 Myelomeningocele
 Sacrococcygeal teratomas
Chest
 Diaphragmatic hernia
 Pleural effusion
Gastrointestinal
 Duodenal atresia
 Omphalocele
 Gastroschisis
Urinary Tract
 Bilateral renal agenesis
 Polycystic kidneys
 Multicystic kidneys
Skeletal
 Achondroplasia
 Agenesis or hypoplasia of bones
 Osteogenesis imperfecta
 Camptomelic dysplasia
Cardiac[a]

[a] Frequently requires echocardiography.
Adapted from Vintzileos and colleagues, 1987, with permission.

septal defect, which recurred in 80 percent, and laterality defects, which recurred in 64 percent. Recurrence of a *similar* defect was most likely for left heart defects (47 percent), outflow tract defects (47 percent), and septal defects (60 percent), all of which involve abnormal blood flow patterns.

Prenatal diagnosis typically involves careful evaluation of the heart, usually including echocardiography, at approximately 20 to 22 weeks (see Chap. 16, p. 396). At this gestational age, all cardiac structures can usually be seen, and time remains for a complete evaluation and consideration of pregnancy termination if an anomaly is found. One caveat is that defects associated with abnormal blood flow—generally defects characterized by hypoplasia or atresia—may develop as late as the third trimester (Hornberger and associates, 1996). For this reason, if the initial lesion was in this category (e.g., hypoplastic right or left heart, coarctation of the aorta, or pulmonary or aortic stenosis), then ultrasonographic examinations should be scheduled at 20 to 22 weeks and again in the third trimester.

Neural-Tube Defects. These defects are the second most common congenital malformation in the United States, with an incidence of 1.4 to 2 per 1000 pregnancies (American College of Obstetricians and Gynecologists, 2003). They are

TABLE 13–5 Risk Factors for Neural-Tube Defects

Family history of neural-tube defects
Exposure to certain environmental agents
  Diabetes (hyperglycemia)
  Hyperthermia
  Drugs and medications
Genetic syndrome with known recurrence risk
Some racial or ethnic groups and/or living in high-risk
  geographical regions
Production of anti-folate receptor antibodies

also discussed in Chapter 12 (see p. 302). Women at increased risk of carrying a fetus with a neural-tube defect (NTD) are counseled and offered alpha-fetoprotein testing and targeted ultrasonographic examination as part of the diagnostic evaluation. If the ultrasonographic examination is incomplete or a defect is seen, amniocentesis may be performed to confirm the presence of the defect and to determine the fetal karyotype. Some factors listed in Table 13–5 that are known to increase the risk of NTD include:

1. *Family history of NTDs.* This is the most commonly recognized risk factor, although only 5 percent of all NTDs are familial. The chance of recurrence for a multifactorial NTD is 2 to 3 percent if one first-degree relative is affected and is higher if more than one is affected. The level of risk should be estimated individually for each family, by calculating the number of affected relatives and their degree of relatedness to the fetus (Bonaiti-Pellie and Smith, 1974).

2. *Exposure to certain environmental agents.* A few of these have been implicated in NTD formation. Exposure must occur during the first 28 days of gestation, when the neural tube is developing. *Hyperglycemia,* usually from type 1 diabetes mellitus, increases the risk of NTDs (Becerra and colleagues, 1990). The exact mechanism is unknown, but may involve inhibition of fetal glycolysis, a functional deficiency of arachidonic acid or myoinositol in the developing embryo, or alterations in the yolk sac (Reece and Hobbins, 1986). *Hyperthermia* during neural-tube formation also appears to cause defects. A prolonged increase in maternal core temperature has been reported to increase the relative risk up to sixfold. The duration and intensity of core temperature elevation necessary to produce an effect and the pathophysiology are unknown (Milunsky, 1992). Certain drugs, especially those that disturb folic acid metabolism, are thought to be causative (see Chap. 14, p. 345). *Anticonvulsants,* most notably *valproic acid* and *carbamazepine,* significantly increase malformation risk. *Aminopterin* and *isotretinoin* have been associated with a constellation of abnormalities that can include anencephaly or encephalocele.

3. *History of a genetic syndrome or anatomical anomalies associated with NTDs.* Some inherited syndromes known to contain NTDs include Meckel-Gruber, Roberts–SC phocomelia, Jarco-Levin, and HARDE (hydrocephalus–agyria–retinal dysplasia–encephalocele) syndromes. These are all autosomal recessive with a 25-percent recurrence risk. Trisomies 13 and 18 and triploidy can include NTDs, and all have a 1 percent chance of recurrence (Jones, 1997). Cloacal exstrophy and sacrococcygeal teratoma may be associated with spina bifida. Amnionic bands may cause spina bifida or anencephaly but are believed to occur sporadically and have minimal recurrence risk.

4. *Belonging to a high-risk racial or ethnic group, living in a high-risk geographical region, or both.* The United Kingdom has the highest frequency of NTDs, with a population incidence of almost 1 percent. China, Egypt, and India also have a high frequency. In contrast, the incidence in the United States is 0.2 percent. The frequency of defects in high-risk populations is probably related to both the ethnic (genetic) background of the inhabitants and environmental influences such as diet (see Chap. 12, p. 302). For example, individuals of Celtic origin living in the United States and consuming a vitamin-fortified American diet are at lower risk than those living in the United Kingdom (Main and Mennuti, 1986; Thompson and co-workers, 1991). Moreover, since the fortification of breads and grains was begun in 1998 in this country, there has been a decrease in NTDs (Evans and collaborators, 2004).

5. *Production of anti-folate receptor antibodies.* Rothenberg and colleagues (2004) reported that 9 of 12 women who had a pregnancy complicated by a fetal NTD produced anti-folate receptor antibodies, compared with only 2 of 20 control women. Although cause and effect were not established, these data suggest another mechanism by which periconceptional folic acid supplementation could prevent NTD recurrence.

FAMILIAL GENETIC DISEASE. Couples with a personal or family history of a heritable genetic disorder should be offered genetic counseling and provided with a calculated risk of having an affected fetus. Specific molecular tests for a variety of common genetic diseases are now available (see Chap. 12, p. 307). The risk of a disease for which the responsible gene has not been identified can sometimes be estimated by comparing fetal DNA with that of affected and unaffected family members using *restriction fragment length polymorphism analysis.* The risk of disease for which no laboratory test has been developed may, in some cases, be refined by ultrasonographic examination if the disease is associated with fetal structural abnormalities, or by determination of fetal gender if the disease is X-linked.

A major issue that remains unresolved for many genetic disorders is phenotype prediction. Because of variable penetrance and expressivity, and modification of phenotype by pre- and postnatal environmental influences, identification of a specific disease gene often is not sufficient to allow the phenotype of an affected fetus to be predicted, even when there have been other affected siblings or family members. The phenotype of cystic fibrosis, for example, can vary widely within a family (see Chap. 12, p. 295). Phenotype prediction is especially difficult when there are no living affected family members, or when the disease gene is identified as the result of population screening (see Chap. 12, p. 296).

Ethnic Groups at High Risk. Some otherwise rare recessive genes are found with increased frequency in certain racial or ethnic groups. This increased frequency results from generations who procreate only within their own groups because of religious or ethnic prohibitions or geographical isolation. A phenomenon called the *founder effect* occurs when an otherwise rare gene that is found with increased frequency within a certain population can be traced back to a single family member or small group of ancestors. This effect accounts for the high rate of tyrosinemia in the Lac Saint Jean region of Quebec. Some autosomal recessive diseases are found with increased frequency in ethnic groups living in the United States (Table 13–6).

AFRICAN, MEDITERRANEAN, CARIBBEAN, LATIN AMERICAN, OR MIDDLE EASTERN DESCENT. Several clinically significant hemoglobin gene mutations are more prevalent in patients with ancestry from these areas (see Chap. 51, p. 1150). African-Americans are at increased risk of having sickle cell anemia, which is the most common hemoglobinopathy in the United States. Southeast Asians are at increased risk of carrying hemoglobin E, the second most common abnormal hemoglobin in the world.

MEDITERRANEAN OR ASIAN ORIGIN. These individuals are at increased risk of having α- or β-thalassemia (see Chap. 51, p. 1154).

JEWISH ANCESTRY. These individuals are at increased risk for several diseases, each caused by a different enzyme

deficiency. For example, Tay-Sachs, Canavan, and Gaucher diseases are caused by deficiencies of hexosaminidase A, aspartoacyclase, and glucocerebrosidase, respectively. Carrier rates and screening protocols for these diseases are discussed subsequently.

CAUCASIANS OF NORTHERN EUROPEAN DESCENT. Cystic fibrosis is the most common monogenic disorder in this population. Carrier and fetal screening protocols are discussed on page 325.

SCREENING FOR COMMON CONGENITAL ABNORMALITIES

The vast majority of cases of NTDs, Down syndrome, and many other fetal abnormalities are found in families with no prior history of birth defects. Prenatal evaluation of only women at high risk for these complications would thus fail to identify most affected pregnancies. Couples with no family history of genetic abnormalities can now be offered prenatal screening tests for certain fetal disorders. Screening tests by design do not provide a diagnosis, but rather identify individuals with risk high enough to benefit from a definitive diagnostic test. According to Wald and associates (1997), genetic screening tests should meet criteria generally accepted for other types of screening tests:

1. The disorder is well defined and serious.
2. Treatment or prevention is available but not possible without the screening test.
3. The screening test is cost effective and reliable.
4. The subsequent diagnostic test is reliable.

That said, Caughey and collaborators (2004) interviewed 447 women of all ages with undetermined genetic risk. They reported that half were willing to undergo invasive prenatal diagnostic testing. One third of women aged 35 years or older expressed a willingness to pay partially or completely for such testing. Such requests present a conundrum for prenatal diagnostic centers and each should have a protocol to cover these exigencies.

NEURAL-TUBE DEFECTS (NTDs). At least 95 percent of children with NTDs are born into families with no prior history. Prior to the late 1970s, identification of affected pregnancies was not possible. At that time, Brock and associates (1972, 1973) reported that both amnionic fluid and maternal serum alpha-fetoprotein (AFP) levels were much higher in pregnancies complicated by fetal anencephaly and other NTDs. The first large prospective trial of maternal serum screening was the UK Collaborative Study on Alpha-fetoprotein in Relation to Neural-tube Defects (1977). The utility of maternal serum AFP screening for NTDs was subsequently confirmed by others and adopted in the United States and Europe (Burton and associates, 1983; Haddow and colleagues, 1983; Milunsky and co-workers, 1980).

**TABLE 13–6	Autosomal Recessive Diseases Found with Increased Frequency in Certain Ethnic Groups**

Disease	Heritage of Groups at Increased Risk
Hemoglobinopathies	African, Mediterranean, Caribbean, Latin American, Middle Eastern
Thalassemia	Mediterranean, Asian
Inborn errors of metabolism: Tay-Sachs, Canavan, Gaucher, Niemann-Pick, Fanconi anemia (type C), Bloom syndrome	Ashkenazi Jewish
Cystic fibrosis	Caucasians of northern European descent, Ashkenazi Jewish, Native American (Zuni, Pueblo)
Tyrosinemia, fragile X	French Canadian

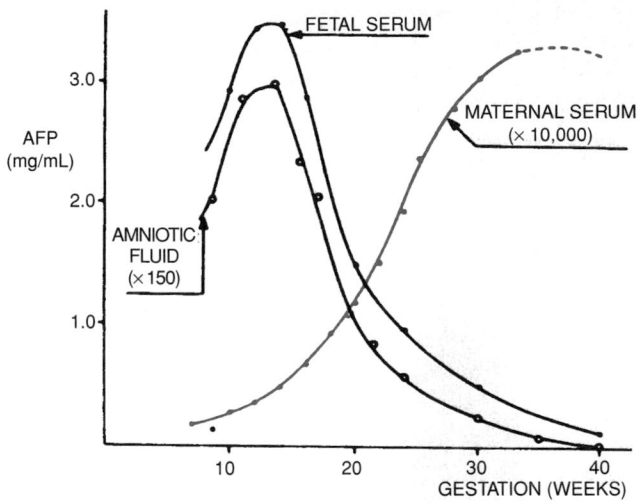

FIGURE 13–2. Maternal and fetal serum and amnionic fluid alpha-fetoprotein (AFP) levels corresponding with gestational age. (From Roberts and colleagues, 1983, with permission.)

Alpha-Fetoprotein (AFP). This glycoprotein is synthesized early in gestation by the fetal yolk sac and later by the fetal gastrointestinal tract and liver (see Chap. 4). It normally circulates in fetal serum and passes into fetal urine and thus into amnionic fluid. Although its function is unknown, AFP is the major serum protein in the embryo-fetus, analogous to albumin. Its concentration increases steadily in both fetal serum

and amnionic fluid until 13 weeks, after which these levels rapidly decrease (Burton, 1988). AFP passes into the maternal circulation by diffusion across the placental membranes and also may be transported via the placental circulation (Brumfield and colleagues, 1990). AFP is found in steadily increasing quantities in maternal serum after 12 weeks (Fig. 13–2). Open fetal body wall defects uncovered by integument permit additional AFP to leak into the amnionic fluid, and maternal serum AFP levels are increased.

Maternal Serum AFP Screening. Maternal screening is offered between 14 and 22 weeks. Maternal serum AFP is measured in nanograms per milliliter and reported as a multiple of the median (MoM) of the unaffected population. Converting the results to MoM normalizes the distribution of AFP levels and permits comparison of results from different laboratories and populations. Factors that influence the maternal serum AFP level include weight, race, and diabetic status, as well as the gestational age and number of fetuses. Using a maternal serum AFP level of 2.0 or 2.5 MoM as the upper limit of normal, most laboratories report a screen-positive rate of 3 to 5 percent, a sensitivity of at least 90 percent, and a positive-predictive value of 2 to 6 percent (Milunsky and associates, 1989).

Evaluation of an elevated maternal serum AFP begins with a basic ultrasonographic examination to determine fetal age and viability and the number of fetuses (Fig. 13–3).

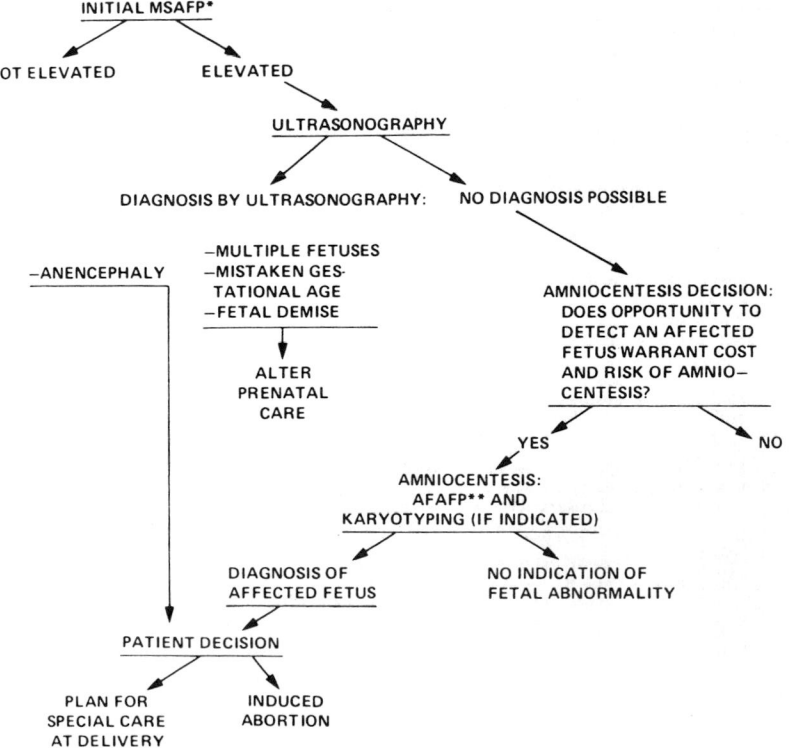

*MSAFP = maternal serum alpha-fetoprotein
**AFAFP = amniotic fluid alpha-fetoprotein

FIGURE 13–3. Algorithm for evaluating an elevated maternal serum alpha-fetoprotein (MSAFP) level. (From Adams and colleagues, 1984, with permission.)

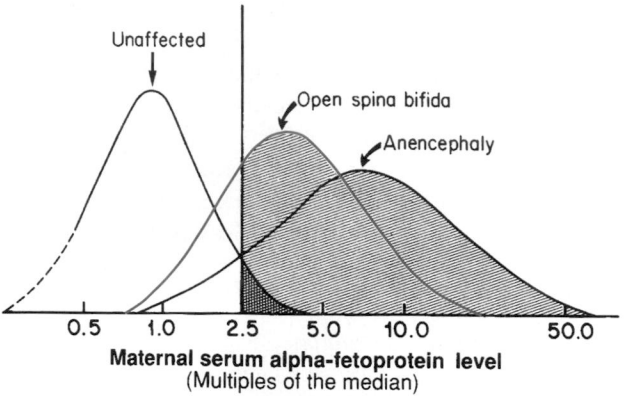

FIGURE 13–4. Maternal serum alpha-fetoprotein levels in single-ton gestations at 16 to 18 weeks. The cutoff value of 2.5 multiples of the median results in both false-positive and false-negative diagnoses. Any cutoff point chosen, however, would result in false-positive (cross-hatched area) and false-negative rates. (Redrawn from American College of Obstetricians and Gynecologists, 1986.)

Underestimating gestational age accounts for a large proportion of abnormal test results. In such cases, the laboratory can usually generate a corrected report when given accurate pregnancy dating criteria. If the initial specimen was obtained prior to 14 weeks, a repeated specimen is necessary. The distributions of maternal serum AFP levels in affected and unaffected pregnancies overlap considerably (Fig. 13–4). If the level falls within the range of the overlap—the *indiscriminate zone* of 2.5 to 3.5 MoM—then repeating the measurement may determine whether the pregnancy is really at risk. Because repeated measurements tend to regress

toward the mean of the population to which they belong, a truly elevated maternal serum AFP level will remain so in the repeated sample, whereas levels from an unaffected pregnancy have a tendency to normalize.

Maternal serum AFP levels greater than 3.5 MoM need not be repeated, because levels this high are outside the AFP distribution of unaffected pregnancies and clearly indicate increased fetal risk. In general, the likelihood that the fetus is affected increases in proportion to the AFP level. In a study of 773 women with elevated serum AFP levels, Reichler and colleagues (1994) reported that there was a progressive increase in the frequency of NTDs, ventral wall defects, and other anomalies as maternal serum AFP levels rose (Fig. 13–5). About 40 percent of pregnancies were abnormal when the AFP level was greater than 7 MoM.

Other Causes of Elevated Maternal Serum AFP Levels. Other causes of elevated levels that can be determined by ultrasonography include fetal death, multiple gestations, structural defects, and placental abnormalities (Table 13–7).

RECOMMENDATIONS FOR SCREENING. The American College of Obstetricians and Gynecologists (2003) recommends that all pregnant women be offered second-trimester maternal serum AFP screening. It should be performed within a protocol that includes quality control, counseling, follow-up, and high-resolution ultrasonography. Because only 1 in 16 to 1 in 33 women with an elevated serum AFP level actually has an affected fetus, women should be counseled regarding the high false-positive rates, the risks of amniocentesis, and the rationale for the screening program.

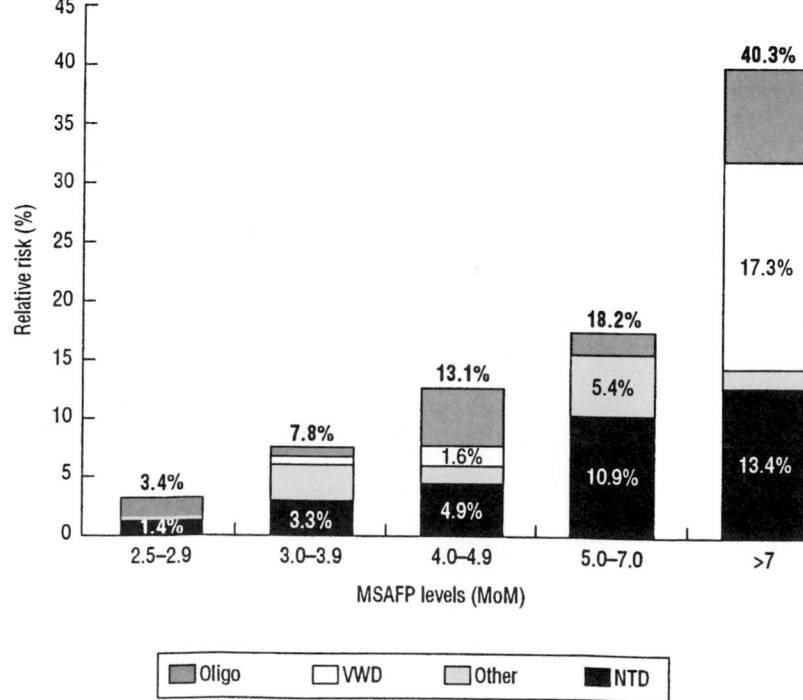

FIGURE 13–5. Distribution of the risk of anomalies and oligohydramnios as a function of elevated maternal serum alpha-fetoprotein levels (MSAFP). (MoM = multiples of median; NTD = neural-tube defect; Oligo = oligohydramnios; Other = subchorionic bleeding, intra-abdominal echogenicity, hydronephrosis, echogenic bowel, dilated kidney, heart defect; VWD = ventral wall defect.) (From Reichler and colleagues, 1994, with permission.)

TABLE 13–7 Conditions Associated with Abnormal Maternal Serum Alpha-Fetoprotein Concentrations

Elevated Levels
Neural-tube defects
Pilonidal cysts
Esophageal or intestinal obstruction
Liver necrosis
Cystic hygroma
Sacrococcygeal teratoma
Abdominal wall defects—omphalocele, gastroschisis
Urinary obstruction
Renal anomalies—polycystic or absent kidneys
Congenital nephrosis
Osteogenesis imperfecta
Congenital skin defects
Cloacal exstrophy
Chorioangioma of placenta
Placental abruption
Placenta accreta
Oligohydramnios
Preeclampsia
Multifetal gestation
Low birthweight
Fetal death
Improper adjustment for low maternal weight
Underestimated gestational age
Maternal hepatoma or teratoma

Low Levels
Chromosomal trisomies
Gestational trophoblastic disease
Fetal death
Improper adjustment for high maternal weight
Overestimated gestational age

Ultrasonographic Examination. After confirming the gestational age and establishing fetal number and viability, the fetus is evaluated by targeted ultrasonography. Anencephaly, other major cranial defects, and most spine defects can be readily identified (Figs. 13–6 and 13–7). In 99 percent of

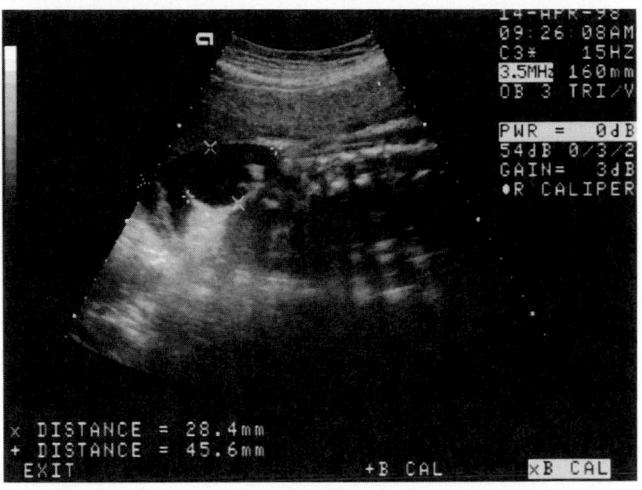

FIGURE 13–7. Lumbosacral view of meningomyelocele. (Courtesy of Dr. Jodi Dashe.)

cases, open spine lesions are associated with one or more of five specific cranial anomalies detected by ultrasonography (Watson and associates, 1991). As detailed in Chapter 16 (see p. 394), these include frontal notching, also called the *lemon sign;* small biparietal diameter; ventriculomegaly; obliteration of the cisterna magna; and elongated cerebellum, the *banana sign* (Fig. 13–8). These cranial anomalies are most clearly visible in the second trimester, and some, such as the lemon sign, may resolve later in pregnancy.

In the early days of AFP screening, an elevated maternal serum AFP level prompted amniocentesis to determine the amnionic fluid AFP level. If the AFP level was elevated, then an assay for acetylcholinesterase was done. These tests were considered diagnostic for fetal NTD. Today, however, nearly 100 percent of NTDs are identified by ultrasonography

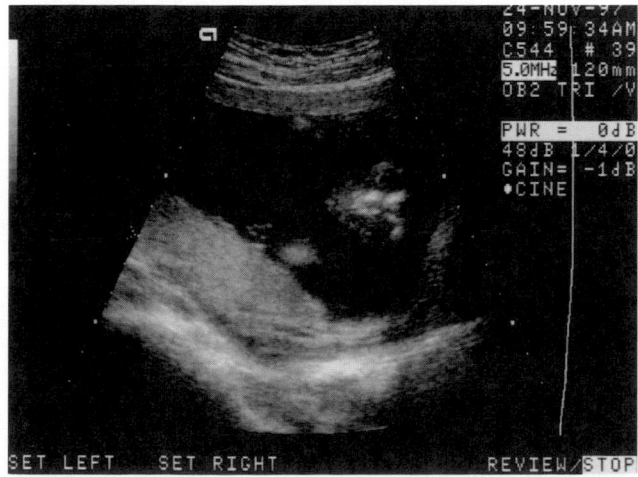

FIGURE 13–6. Anencephalic fetus with the face visualized by sonography. (Courtesy of Dr. Jodi Dashe.)

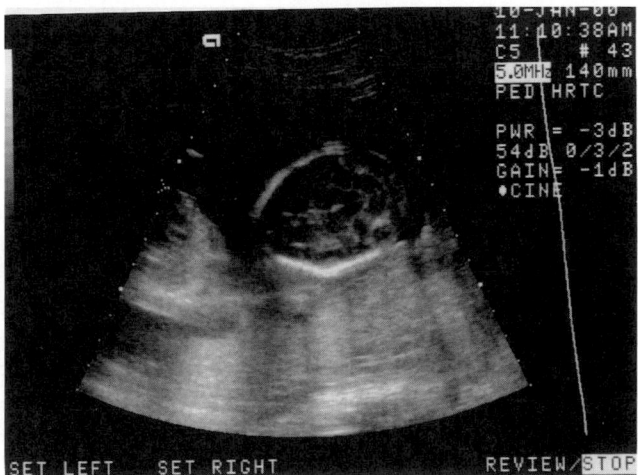

FIGURE 13–8. Cranial ultrasound in a fetus with Arnold–Chiari malformation showing frontal scalloping (lemon sign) on the left and effacement of the cisterna magna (banana sign) on the right. (Courtesy of Dr. Jodi Dashe.)

used alone (Nadel and colleagues, 1990; Sepulveda and associates, 1995). Citing this high detection rate, several authorities conclude that a woman with an elevated maternal serum AFP level and a normal ultrasonographic examination need not undergo amniocentesis for amnionic fluid AFP measurement. Instead, she could be counseled that the risk of an NTD is reduced by 95 percent when no spine defects or cranial findings are seen ultrasonographically (Hogge, 1989; Morrow, 1991; Van den Hof, 1990, and their colleagues).

By contrast, a number of other studies report considerably less than a 100-percent ultrasonographic detection rate for structural fetal anomalies, especially before 22 weeks. For example, only 17 percent of all fetal anomalies were identified in the Routine Antenatal Diagnostic Imaging with Ultrasound (RADIUS) trial (Chap. 16, p. 390). VanDorsten and colleagues (1998) reported only a 48-percent ultrasonographic detection rate for all fetal anomalies diagnosed. Platt and coworkers (1992) reported that 6 of 161 cases of open spina bifida were not recognized in a screening program. Accordingly, many recommend that an amniocentesis for amnionic fluid AFP be offered to all women with elevated maternal serum AFP levels. Women considering amniocentesis should be informed that amnionic fluid AFP measurement will detect only open spine defects, and not the 3 to 5 percent of defects that are covered by skin (Crandall and Matsumoto, 1984).

Amniocentesis. Amnionic fluid AFP levels are measured if an NTD is suspected, if the maternal serum AFP is elevated and the ultrasonographic examination is nondiagnostic, or simply because the maternal serum AFP is elevated, as discussed previously. An elevated amnionic fluid AFP level prompts assay of the same sample for acetylcholinesterase. After ruling out blood contamination, the presence of this enzyme verifies that exposed neural tissue or another open fetal defect is present.

Because NTDs carry a small associated risk of aneuploidy, and aneuploidy would change the prognosis and likely pregnancy management, ultrasonographic identification of a fetal NTD should prompt fetal karyotyping. In a review of more than 17,000 prenatal diagnosis cases, Hume and associates (1996) observed a 2-percent rate of aneuploidy in the 106 fetuses with an isolated NTD. Harmon and colleagues (1995) found that 7 of 43 fetuses with isolated NTDs were aneuploid.

Some clinicians determine the fetal karyotype whenever both maternal serum and amnionic fluid AFP levels are elevated, even if the amnionic fluid acetylcholinesterase assay is negative and an open NTD has thus been ruled out. Gonzalez and associates (1996) reported that in women with elevated serum and amnionic fluid AFP levels and normal ultrasonographic examinations, the incidence of chromosomal abnormalities was elevated fivefold above background risk.

INCIDENTAL FETAL KARYOTYPE. If a woman with a normal targeted ultrasonographic examination has undergone amniocentesis for amnionic fluid AFP just because her maternal serum AFP level was elevated, and the amnionic fluid AFP level is normal, fetal karyotyping is controversial. Thiagarajah and colleagues (1995) studied 658 such women and concluded that there was no justification for routine fetal karyotyping. In contrast, Feuchtbaum and associates (1995) reviewed 8097 pregnancies complicated by elevated maternal serum AFP levels. In the pregnancies in which the elevated maternal serum AFP level was "unexplained" because there was no fetal NTD or ventral wall defect and the amnionic fluid AFP level was normal, the rate of chromosomal anomalies was 1.1 percent, or twice as high as that of the general population.

INCIDENTAL AMNIONIC FLUID AFP MEASUREMENT. When amniocentesis is performed primarily for genetic analysis, amnionic fluid AFP is often routinely measured. This practice may not be cost-effective. Shields and colleagues (1996) reviewed almost 7000 women who underwent second-trimester amniocentesis for fetal karyotyping. They reported that measurement of amnionic fluid AFP did not increase the detection of anomalies. Similarly, Silver and associates (2001) performed a retrospective analysis of 2769 amnionic fluid specimens and reported that incidental amnionic fluid AFP measurement identified only one NTD not detected by ultrasonography. They estimated that routine amnionic fluid AFP measurement cost $219,000 per informative case.

Unexplained Elevated Abnormal Maternal Serum AFP Levels. Even if there are no obvious fetal abnormalities, several large studies have shown that unexplained high maternal serum AFP levels often forecast a poor pregnancy outcome. These outcomes include low birthweight, oligohydramnios, placental abruption, and fetal death (Katz, 1990; Simpson, 1991; Waller, 1991, each with their associates). According to Wenstrom and co-workers (1992), the first maternal serum AFP level is the most predictive, and serial measurements are not helpful. Simpson and colleagues (1991) reported that second-trimester, but not third-trimester, maternal serum AFP elevation levels were associated with preterm ruptured membranes, preterm birth, and low-birthweight infants. Ramus and associates (1996) studied 241 women with unexplained serum AFP elevations and reported that they had a higher incidence of preterm delivery than women who had normal levels—22 versus 11 percent. The incidence of preterm delivery was highest (47 percent) in the 38 women who had both unexplained elevated serum levels and placental sonolucencies on ultrasonographic examination.

Although elevated maternal serum AFP levels in these cases are assumed to result from placental damage or dysfunction, neither the etiology of the elevated maternal serum values nor the most appropriate management for these women is clear. In these cases, no specific program of maternal or fetal surveillance favorably affects pregnancy outcomes (American College of Obstetricians and Gynecologists, 1996; Cunningham and Gilstrap, 1991).

Management of the Fetus with an NTD. Other than termination of pregnancy, options for pregnancies complicated by an NTD have traditionally been limited. Anencephaly, exencephaly, and iniencephaly are lethal, but some women elect to continue these pregnancies. Routine prenatal care is given, but interventions for fetal indications are not recommended as they will not change fetal outcome.

Counseling and decision making in the case of an isolated fetal spine defect are more difficult. Such women may benefit from counseling by a pediatric neurosurgeon, neurologist, or other specialists in pediatric development. The fully informed couple is more likely to make their best decision and to be prepared for the range of possible pregnancy outcomes. With continued pregnancy, antenatal care is designed to detect changes in fetal status that might alter the timing or route of delivery. Generally, the goal is delivery at term, but rapidly increasing ventriculomegaly may prompt delivery before term so that a shunt can be placed. Fetal heart rate testing is problematic because heart rate patterns in anomalous fetuses can be difficult to interpret (Vindla and associates, 1997).

The optimal timing and method of delivery remain controversial. All studies of delivery methods for fetuses with NTDs are retrospective and suffer from various biases. That said, an equal number of reports support cesarean versus vaginal delivery (Bensen and co-workers, 1988; Luthy and colleagues, 1991; Sakala and Andree, 1990). Theoretically, cesarean delivery might reduce the risk of mechanical trauma and infection of the fetal spine and also allow precise timing of delivery so that appropriate consultants can be available. Optimally, the delivery time and method should be determined on a case-by-case basis by the team that ultimately will care for the woman and her neonate. Team members should include maternal–fetal medicine specialists, neonatologists, neurosurgeons, and others. Fetal surgical repair of meningomyelocele is discussed later (see p. 334).

DOWN SYNDROME. Before the mid-1980s, amniocentesis for fetal karyotyping was generally offered only to women aged 35 years and older. After Merkatz and colleagues (1984) reported that pregnancies with fetal Down syndrome were characterized by low maternal serum AFP levels, prenatal NTD screening was expanded to include Down syndrome screening in women aged younger than 35 years. Cuckle (1984) and Haddow (1983) and their associates confirmed this finding, and most NTD screening programs now include Down syndrome screening.

Screening program results show that detection rates are highest when maternal age-related risk is incorporated because it is the most powerful predictor of aneuploidy. Ultimately, the Down syndrome risk for each woman is estimated by multiplying her maternal age-related risk by a likelihood ratio determined by her serum AFP level (New England Regional Genetics Group, 1989). Women with a calculated Down syndrome risk greater than a predetermined threshold are offered amniocentesis for fetal karyotyping. This screening threshold is typically equal to the midtrimester or term Down syndrome risk of a 35-year-old woman.

Multiple-Marker Screening. Fetal aneuploidy alters serum analytes other than AFP. If a fetus has Down syndrome, second-trimester serum levels of chorionic gonadotropin (hCG) are usually higher and those of unconjugated estriol are lower than expected (Bogart and colleagues, 1987; Wald and associates, 1988a, 1988b). The individual predictive values of hCG, estriol, and AFP for detecting Down syndrome are low, but when combined they can frequently distinguish euploid fetuses from those with Down syndrome.

The most common second-trimester screening protocol in current use, variously called the *expanded AFP test, AFP plus, triple screen,* or *multiple-marker screening test,* is based on a composite likelihood ratio determined by levels of all three analytes. The maternal age-related risk is then multiplied by this ratio. The screening threshold chosen may be the midtrimester risk of a 35-year-old woman. More frequently, a threshold is chosen because it results in the optimal combination of a high detection rate with a low screen-positive rate. The risk threshold of about 1:200 is selected most often because, at a 5-percent screen-positive rate, the Down syndrome detection rate is 60 percent in women younger than 35 years. In women older than 35 years, the multiple-marker test detects more than 75 percent of fetuses with Down syndrome and a portion of other aneuploidies as well, although at a detection rate close to 25 percent (Haddow and co-workers, 1994). The multiple-marker test has been validated and has become the preferred second-trimester Down syndrome screening test in most centers (Burton, 1993; Cheng, 1993; Wenstrom, 1993, and their colleagues).

There are several permutations of the multiple-marker test in current use. Some centers offer AFP and hCG testing alone, and others use estriol measurement as a third marker. Some prefer to measure the free β-subunit of hCG (β-hCG) instead of the intact hCG molecule, and others add inhibin as a fourth analyte (Wald and colleagues, 1996; Wenstrom and associates, 1999b). Other multiple-marker screening tests have been used that combine maternal serum analytes, ultrasonographic measurement of the nuchal fold, long bone measurements, and other parameters (Bahado-Singh and colleagues, 2001; Morris and co-workers, 2001). Several investigative protocols are subsequently discussed.

In most series, only 6 percent of all screen-positive samples are associated with an affected fetus. Thus, a positive screening test indicates increased risk but not necessarily fetal Down syndrome. Conversely, a negative screening test indicates *no increased risk,* but does not mean that the fetus is normal. Once gestational age is confirmed by ultrasonography, women with a positive screening test should be offered amniocentesis for karyotyping (American College of Obstetricians and Gynecologists, 1996).

Serum Screening in Women Older than 35 Years. The basis of any multiple-marker algorithm is the maternal age-related risk. Thus, the multiple-marker screening test identifies a higher proportion of fetal Down syndrome cases—at least 80 percent—in women aged 35 years and older than in younger women (Haddow and co-workers, 1994). Although the detection rate increases along with maternal age, so does the screen-positive rate. For example, about 25 percent of women aged 35 years and older will have a test result indicating increased risk. Although some older women will opt for empirical amniocentesis regardless of screening results, others find that serum screening facilitates the decision to undergo invasive testing.

First-Trimester Down Syndrome Screening. Early identification of fetal aneuploidy is desirable for many reasons, including the availability of more options for pregnancy termination. First-trimester screening protocols in current use include maternal serum analyte screening, ultrasonographic evaluation, or a combination of both. Urinary screening has been studied, but the results were disappointing. The most discriminatory first-trimester maternal serum analytes appear to be free β-hCG and pregnancy-associated plasma protein A (PAPP-A) (Haddow and associates, 1998; Wald and colleagues, 1998). Measurement of the nuchal translucency (NT), an echolucent area seen in longitudinal views of the back of the neck, is also highly discriminatory (Snijders and colleagues, 1998). If the NT measurement is expressed as an MoM, it can be combined with serum analytes to calculate a composite risk.

Two large trials of combined first-trimester ultrasonographic and serum screening have documented its efficacy. First Trimester Maternal Serum Biochemistry and Fetal Nuchal Translucency Screening Study, referred to as the "BUN study," reported by Wapner and co-workers (2003) was a multicenter trial that enrolled 8514 women who underwent screening between 74 and 97 days of gestation. Individual risks of fetal Down syndrome and trisomy 18 were calculated based on age, first-trimester levels of free β-hCG and PAPP-A, and NT measurement. Women determined to be screen positive were offered fetal karyotyping. Using a Down syndrome risk cutoff of 1:270, 85 percent of Down syndrome cases were identified at a false-positive rate of 9.4 percent. When the false-positive rate was held at 5 percent, the detection rate was 79 percent. Importantly, 91 percent of trisomy 18 cases were identified at a false-positive rate of 2 percent. Because of the high incidence of spontaneous pregnancy loss in aneuploid pregnancies, performing fetal karyotyping after first-trimester screening likely resulted in the identification of some aneuploid pregnancies that would otherwise have been lost spontaneously. This outcome can be viewed either positively or negatively.

The FASTER (First- and Second-Trimester Evaluation of Risk) trial was reported by Malone and colleagues (2003a, 2003b). This multicenter trial included 33,557 women, and it took a slightly different approach. All women participating in the trial underwent both first-trimester screening—which included free β-hCG, PAPP-A, NT measurement, and maternal age—*and* second-trimester screening with hCG, AFP, estriol, and inhibin, along with maternal age. If either test was positive, fetal karyotyping was offered. The investigators then evaluated the screen-positive and detection rates for first-, second-, and combined first- and second-trimester screening. They found that the best results were obtained when women had combined both first- and second-trimester screening—the Fully Integrated Test—and then underwent definitive testing if its result was positive. The integrated test yielded a Down syndrome detection rate of 90 percent at a screen-positive rate of 5.4 percent. Importantly, the investigators determined that NT measurement was difficult to do accurately and reproducibly (D'Alton and associates, 2003). Further, not only did NT measurement medians vary from center to center and operator to operator, but NT medians obtained by a single operator varied over time. The authors therefore concluded that NT measurement should be performed only by operators with specific training and that measurement medians for individual operators should be monitored carefully and adjusted as necessary.

In addition to drifting NT medians, problems with first-trimester screening include a relatively narrow gestational age window for screening—approximately 10 to 13 weeks—and variability in NT measurement resulting from poor visibility, suboptimal fetal position, or inconsistent measurement technique. Accurate assessment of gestational age is essential. The American College Obstetricians (2004) emphasizes that appropriate training, monitoring systems, and counseling must be provided.

ELECTIVE GENETIC AMNIOCENTESIS IN WOMEN YOUNGER THAN 35 YEARS. Some women younger than 35 years may request amniocentesis for fetal karyotyping despite reassuring maternal serum screening and ultrasonographic findings. Caughey and colleagues (2004) interviewed 447 women of all ages with undetermined genetic risk and reported that half were willing to undergo invasive prenatal diagnostic testing. One third of women aged 35 years or older expressed a willingness to pay partially or completely for such testing. These investigators concluded that guidelines should be expanded to offer testing for a genetic diagnosis, not only for screening. Others believe that each case must be evaluated individually, and each center must develop its own protocol to handle such requests (Pauker and Pauker, 1994).

SCREENING FOR HERITABLE GENETIC DISEASES

The development of molecular tests for various genetic diseases has raised the possibility of population screening. Current debate centers on screening for cystic fibrosis and fragile

X syndrome but will no doubt extend to other conditions as more disease-specific genes are identified.

CYSTIC FIBROSIS (CF). This autosomal recessive disorder is caused by a mutation in the *CFTR* gene that is on the long arm of chromosome 7. The gene encodes a protein called the *cystic fibrosis conductance transmembrane regulator (CFTR)*. As of 2003, over 1300 mutations in this large gene had been described (Cystic Fibrosis Mutation Database, 2004). The CF carrier frequency is about 1 in 29 in Caucasian Americans, 1 in 30 in Native Americans, and 1 in 50 in Hispanics. It ranges from 1 in 90 to 1 in 29 in individuals of Ashkenazi Jewish heritage (National Institutes of Health, 1997). The classical form is marked by abnormal sweat chloride levels, chronic pulmonary disease, pancreatic insufficiency, liver disease, and obstructive azoospermia (Freedman and associates, 2004; Rosenstein and Zeitlin, 1998). Some individuals with CF, however, have mild disease or only a single affected organ—such as chronic pancreatitis (see Chap. 46, p. 1066). This tremendous range of clinical expression likely reflects both the degree to which protein function is changed by the mutation, and variation in exposure and susceptibility to environmental factors. Diagnosing CF prenatally offers little advantage other than to make termination of affected pregnancies possible. Accordingly, CF testing is not included in newborn screening in most states (Wagener and co-workers, 2003).

Carrier Screening. Current technology does not yet allow routine carrier screening for all known mutations. The American College of Obstetricians and Gynecologists and the American College of Medical Genetics (2001) recommend that all couples either planning a pregnancy or seeking prenatal care be counseled about CF screening. Screening should be *offered to* individuals who have an affected first- or second-degree relative or whose reproductive partners have CF, and to couples in whom both partners are Caucasian. Because their CF carrier rate and thus risk of CF is significantly lower, screening should be *made available to* couples of other racial or ethnic backgrounds.

These organizations further recommend that screening include all CF mutations with at least a 0.1 percent incidence in the United States. The ΔF508 mutation, which accounts for 75 percent of cases in Caucasians, and the 5T and W1282X mutations, which account for 50 percent of cases in Ashkenazi Jews, are included. This mutation panel will identify 97 percent of all CF carriers of Ashkenazi Jewish descent, 90 percent of Caucasian carriers of northern European heritage, and 80 percent of Caucasian carriers of European background. It probably will not identify the majority of CF mutations in individuals of other ethnic or racial backgrounds, because the mutations most common in these populations are unknown. Although a negative test does not preclude the possibility of carrying another of the more than 1300 known mutations, it does reduce the risk substantively from the background rate (Table 13–8).

TABLE 13–8 Cystic Fibrosis Carrier Rate by Racial and Ethnic Group, Before and After Screening[a]

Racial or Ethnic Group	Dectection Rate (%)	Estimated Carrier Risk	
		Before Test	After Negative Test
Ashkenazi Jewish	97	1/29	~1 in 930
European Caucasian[b]	80	1/29	~1 in 140
Hispanic American	57	1/46	~1 in 105
African American	69	1/65	~1 in 207
Asian American	NA	1 in 90	NA

NA = not available.
[a]Presented in descending order of level of risk before testing. Assumes recommended panel of mutations tested and that family history is negative for cystic fibrosis.
[b]Represents pooled data. Information for subgroups in this population may differ.
From American College of Obstetricians and Gynecologists and the American College of Medical Genetics, 2001, with permission.

Because CF is a recessive disorder, a fetus must inherit an affected gene from each parent to have the disease. If only one partner undergoes CF screening, the risk of having a child with CF can be calculated assuming that the other partner has the 1 in 29 background risk. Some patients will be reassured by this analysis, especially if the only goal is to determine the risk to the fetus. Testing both partners is more expensive but also more accurate.

Fetal Testing. If both parents are carriers, the fetus can be tested to determine whether it inherited either or both parental mutations. Phenotype prediction is fairly accurate if the mutations are ΔF508 or W1282X. Other mutations are less closely associated with disease symptoms, making phenotype prediction and decisions about the pregnancy difficult. Prognosis is determined primarily by pulmonary status, and there is poor genotype–phenotype correlation between these other mutations and the severity of pulmonary disease.

FRAGILE X SYNDROME. This is the most common cause of *familial* mental retardation, and it is discussed further in Chapter 12 (see p. 298). Although fragile X syndrome is an X chromosome-linked anomaly, inheritance of this syndrome does not conform to the usual rules governing X-linked traits. This is because the fragile X mutation is an unstable region of repeated CGG trinucleotides that can expand when transmitted by a female. When the expansion reaches a critical size—more than 230 repeats—the gene can become methylated and thus turned off. Female carriers of a *premutation*, who have 56 to 229 CGG repeats, are at risk to pass on an expanded gene, and the individual inheriting the expanded gene is at high risk to exhibit fragile X phenotype (Fisch and colleagues, 1995). Premutation carriers are also at risk of developing one of three disorders: carrier females may have mild cognitive or psychological problems; 20 percent of female carriers may have premature ovarian failure; and carrier males older than 50 may develop *fragile-X-associated tremor/ataxia syndrome* (Hagerman and Hagerman, 2004).

Carrier Screening. Based on current knowledge, fragile X syndrome does not meet established criteria for a good screening test. The prevalence of the premutation in the general population is unknown, so it is not clear who should be offered testing. The carrier rate is estimated to be approximately 1 in 700, an incidence that is much lower than that of other genetic diseases for which screening is usually considered (Hagerman and co-workers, 1991). In addition, it is not always possible to predict whether a female carrier will pass on an expanded gene. Studies of Scandinavian kindreds have demonstrated that even large premutations can be passed unchanged through several generations (Holmgren and co-workers, 1988). Finally, phenotype prediction in both male and female fetuses carrying the full mutation is imprecise. Because of favorable lyonization, as many as half of females inheriting the full fragile X mutation will be intellectually normal (de Vries and colleagues, 1996). Mosaicism for either gene size or methylation status results in wide phenotypic variation in both males and females inheriting the gene (see Chap. 12, p. 298).

Testing. It is currently recommended that any individual with unexplained mental retardation be tested for the fragile X mutation, especially if there are clinical findings consistent with the syndrome or a family history (Cutillo, 1994). In this setting, approximately 2 to 6 percent of males and 2 to 4 percent of females will be determined to carry the full mutation (Curry and associates, 1997). Family members of patients with documented fragile X syndrome also should be offered testing. The goal is to identify premutation carriers and allow them to make informed reproductive choices. Based on available data, however, it seems unlikely that it will be cost effective to test relatives of patients with unexplained mental retardation not known to be due to fragile X mutation (Curry and co-workers, 1997; Wenstrom and collaborators, 1999a). Likewise, testing of women without a family history of neurodevelopmental disorders is not recommended by the American College of Obstetricians and Gynecologists (1995).

TAY-SACHS, CANAVAN, AND GAUCHER DISEASES. The carrier rate among individuals of Ashkenazi Jewish heritage is 1 in 30 for Tay-Sachs disease, 1 in 40 for Canavan disease, and 1 in 12 to 1 in 25 for Gaucher disease. Carrier screening for Tay-Sachs and Canavan diseases should be considered for patients of Jewish heritage because these diseases are relatively common, the phenotypes of individuals inheriting the abnormal genes are consistently severe and predictable, and prenatal diagnosis is possible for both. Gaucher disease is more complex because diagnosis requires molecular analysis, but molecular testing cannot determine

which of three phenotypes ranging from mild to severe the fetus will have (Azuri and associates, 1998).

ULTRASONOGRAPHIC SCREENING

INCIDENTAL FINDING OF A MAJOR STRUCTURAL DEFECT. Major structural fetal anomalies or minor dysmorphic features often are discovered during ultrasonographic examinations performed for other indications in pregnancies otherwise at low risk for complications. An isolated malformation may be multifactorial—as in isolated cardiac defects or NTDs—or may be part of a genetic syndrome. If the defect is part of a syndrome, the fetus may have other abnormalities that are undetectable by ultrasonography but that affect the prognosis—for example, mental retardation. Fetal aneuploidy commonly is associated with major anatomical malformations and minor dysmorphic features. The specific aneuploidy risk associated with most major anomalies is high enough to prompt invasive fetal testing (Table 13–9).

The finding of two or more minor structural abnormalities in the same fetus also indicates a risk of aneuploidy sufficient to warrant fetal karyotyping (Williamson and colleagues, 1987; Wladimiroff and associates, 1988). Although some combinations of anomalies may indicate a genetic syndrome not resulting from aneuploidy, fetal karyotyping is still indicated because aneuploidy-associated abnormalities can mimic other syndromes.

ULTRASONOGRAPHIC SCREENING FOR MAJOR STRUCTURAL ANOMALIES. Early second-trimester ultrasonography performed specifically to look for structural fetal abnormalities in women at low risk is controversial. Before this issue can be resolved, the detection and false-negative rates for such screening examinations need to be determined. The largest study to date addressing these issues is the RADIUS trial, reported by Ewigman and colleagues (1993). In this study, the fetuses of almost 16,000 women at low risk for perinatal complications were examined ultrasonographically. Only 17 percent of all major congenital anomalies were detected before 24 weeks, and only 35 percent were detected before delivery (see Chap. 16, p. 390). Others, such as VanDorsten and associates (1998), have reported higher detection rates at tertiary centers (48 percent). Still, it appears that, even under ideal circumstances, the detection rate for major anomalies may not be high enough to warrant screening low-risk women.

ULTRASONOGRAPHIC SCREENING FOR MINOR ABNORMALITIES. By themselves, minor abnormalities or dysmorphisms usually do not affect the fetal prognosis in any substantive way. They can, however, provide important clues that suggest chromosomal abnormalities. To date, dysmorphisms have been studied mostly in women at high

TABLE 13-9 Aneuploidy Risk Associated with Major Structural Fetal Malformations

Defect	Population Incidence	Aneuploidy Risk	Most Common Aneuploidy (Trisomy)
Cystic hygroma	1/120 EU-1/6000 B	60-75%	45X (80%), 21, 18, 13, XXY
Hydrops	1/1500-4000 B	30-80%[a]	13, 21, 18, 45X
Hydrocephalus	3-8/10,000 LB	3-8%	13, 18, triploidy
Hydranencephaly	2/1000 IA	Minimal	
Holoprosencephaly	1/16,000 LB	40-60%	13, 18, 18p-
Cardiac defects	7-9/1000 LB	5-30%	21, 18, 13, 22, 8, 9
Diaphragmatic hernia	1/3500-4000 LB	20-25%	13, 18, 21, 45X
Omphalocele	1/5800 LB	30-40%	13, 18
Gastroschisis	1/10,000-15,000 LB	Minimal	
Duodenal atresia	1/10,000 LB	20-30%	21
Bowel obstruction	1/2500-5000 LB	Minimal	
Bladder outlet obstruction	1-2/1000 B	20-25%	13, 18
Facial cleft	1/700 LB	1%	13, 18, deletions
Limb reduction	4-6/10,000 LB	8%	18
Clubfoot	1.2/1000 LB	20-30%	18, 13, 4p-, 18q-
Single umbilical artery	1%	Minimal	

B = births; EU = early ultrasound; IA = infant autopsy; LB = live births.
[a]30% if diagnosed ≥ 24 weeks; 80% if diagnosed ≤ 17 weeks.
Data from Marchese (1985); Nyberg (1990); Wald (1998); Williamson (1987); Wladimiroff (1988), and all their colleagues.

risk for fetal aneuploidy. Controversy surrounds whether ultrasonographic evaluation for fetal dysmorphisms should be offered as a Down syndrome screening test to women at low risk for aneuploidy instead of or as a supplement to maternal serum screening (Souter and colleagues, 2004). Down syndrome risks resulting from some dysmorphisms detected sonographically in the second trimester are listed in Table 13-10. NT is a first-trimester finding, and a thickened nuchal fold is identified in the second trimester. Other findings include absent nasal bone and a space between the first and second toes—the *sandal gap*.

TABLE 13-10 Down Syndrome Risk Associated with Minor Second-Trimester Fetal Abnormalities and Dysmorphic Features

Ultrasound Marker	Risk (%)	False-Positive (%)
Nuchal fold ≥ 6 mm	38	1.3
Femur length (O/E)	34	5.9
Femur length (BPD/FL)	22	5.9
Humerus length (O/E)	37	5.3
Femur plus humerus (O/E)	36	3.7
Pyelectasis	19	2.4
Hyperechogenic bowel	11	0.7
Ventricular dilatation	6	0
Choroid plexus cyst	0	1.8
Ear length	78	8.0
Fifth midphalanx hypoplasia	75	18.0
Increased iliac length	50	2.0
Short frontal lobe	21	4.8

BPD/FL = biparietal diameter compared with femur length; O/E = observed compared with expected.
Adapted from Wald and colleagues, 1998, with permission.

Nuchal Translucency (NT). This appears to be the best first-trimester discriminator of affected and unaffected pregnancies. It is best seen in the midsagittal plane as a sonolucency at the back of the fetal neck. Although its precise etiology and prognosis are unknown, NT is believed to represent one end of the spectrum of *lymphatic obstruction sequence.* Most data indicate that, even under optimal circumstances, first-trimester NT measurements by themselves typically identify fewer than half of all Down syndrome cases (Brambati and colleagues, 1995; Haddow and Palomaki, 1996). As previously discussed (see p. 324), when NT measurements are expressed as an MoM and incorporated into an algorithm that includes serum analytes and maternal age-related risks, screening efficacy appears to be substantially improved.

Normal measurements are between 0 and 5 mm, with an overlap of 2 to 3 mm between affected and unaffected populations. Accurate measurement requires special training and ongoing monitoring of performance, as discussed earlier. Flexion or extension of the head can change measurements by as much as 0.62 mm, and an unfavorable fetal position or maternal obesity may prevent measurement. Roberts and colleagues (1995) and Haddow and Palomaki (1996) have reported that first-trimester measurement is technically impossible in up to 20 percent of women. In the FASTER trial, NT measurement was not possible in 6 percent of cases (D'Alton and colleagues, 2003).

Nasal Bone. Cicero and colleagues (2001) examined 701 women at 11 to 14 weeks prior to scheduled routine amniocentesis for advanced maternal age or abnormal fetal NT measurements. In this high-risk population, the nasal bone was absent in 73 percent of Down syndrome fetuses but in only 0.5 percent of genetically normal fetuses. In the FASTER trial reported by Malone and colleagues (2003b), which included over 6300 women of average risk who completed first-trimester nasal bone ultrasonography, absence of the nasal bone did not identify any Down syndrome cases.

Modification of Age-Related Risk. Analogous to screening with serum analytes, some investigators believe that certain ultrasonographic markers can be used to modify the maternal age-associated Down syndrome risk (Wald and colleagues, 1998). As an example, Vintzileos and Egan (1995) advocate a second-trimester ultrasonographic screening protocol that includes evaluation for both major structural anomalies and minor dysmorphisms. If no abnormalities are detected, the maternal age-related risk is reduced substantively. For example, a 35-year-old woman with a normal-appearing fetus on a second-trimester ultrasonographic examination would have a Down syndrome risk reduced from 1:274 based on age alone to a risk of 1:4200.

Thus, the primary benefit of ultrasonographic screening appears to be its negative-predictive value. It is problematic that failure to identify a fetal anomaly or dysmorphism, which is used to lower the maternal age-related risk of fetal aneuploidy, also makes this screening test ineffective.

Effect of Maternal Age. As with maternal serum analytes, the aneuploidy risk associated with one ultrasonographic marker can be estimated more accurately by incorporating the age-related risk. Gupta and colleagues (1997) used data from 200,000 ultrasonographic examinations to modify aneuploidy risk in pregnancies with fetal choroid plexus cysts. In women who had multiple-marker screening tests indicating no increased risk, who had otherwise normal-appearing fetuses, and who were younger than 32 years, isolated choroid plexus cysts did not increase the risk of trisomy 18 sufficiently to prompt fetal karyotyping.

DIAGNOSTIC TECHNIQUES

SECOND-TRIMESTER AMNIOCENTESIS. Amniocentesis for genetic diagnosis usually is performed between 14 and 20 weeks. A number of multicenter studies have confirmed its safety and its more than 99-percent diagnostic accuracy for Down syndrome (Canadian Early and Mid-Trimester Amniocentesis Trial Group, 1998; NICHD National Registry for Amniocentesis Study Group, 1976). Typically, ultrasonographic guidance is used to pass a 20- to 22-gauge spinal needle into the amnionic sac while avoiding the placenta, umbilical cord, and fetus. Because the initial 1 or 2 mL of fluid aspirate may be contaminated with maternal cells, it is either discarded or used for amnionic fluid AFP testing. Another approximately 20 mL of fluid is then collected for fetal karyotyping, and the needle is removed. The uterine puncture site is observed for bleeding, and the woman

is shown fetal heart motion and the remaining amnionic fluid at the conclusion of the procedure. The incidence of bloody taps, amnionic fluid leakage, and multiple punctures is inversely related to operator experience (Leschot and co-workers, 1985; Romero and colleagues, 1985).

Complications are infrequent and include transient vaginal spotting or amnionic fluid leakage in 1 to 2 percent and chorioamnionitis in less than 0.1 percent. Needle injuries to the fetus are rare when ultrasonographic guidance is used. Fetal cells obtained during amniocentesis rarely fail to grow in culture, but this is more likely if the fetus is abnormal (Persutte and Lenke, 1995). Fetal loss of 0.5 percent or less has been reported by many investigators, and it does not appear possible to reduce this further (Simpson, 1990; Wilson and colleagues, 1984). Some losses likely result from preexisting abnormalities, such as placental abruption, abnormal placental implantation, uterine anomalies, and infection, and were destined to occur whether or not amniocentesis was performed. For example, Wenstrom and colleagues (1996) analyzed 66 fetal deaths following nearly 12,000 second-trimester amniocenteses, and found that 12 percent were caused by preexisting intrauterine infection. Other postprocedural deaths have no apparent etiology.

EARLY AMNIOCENTESIS. This procedure is performed between 11 and 14 weeks and has been widely studied (Johnson, 1996; Nicolaides, 1994; Shulman, 1994; Sundberg, 1997, and all their associates). The technique is the same as for traditional amniocentesis, although if done before membrane fusion to the uterine wall, puncture of the sac may be difficult. Less fluid can be withdrawn—usually 1 mL for each week of gestation.

For reasons that are not yet clear, early amniocentesis appears to result in significantly higher rates of postprocedural pregnancy loss and other complications than traditional amniocentesis. In the multicenter randomized study by the Canadian Early and Mid-Trimester Amniocentesis Trial Group (1998), the spontaneous abortion rate following early amniocentesis was 2.5 percent compared with that of 0.7 percent after traditional amniocentesis. In an Italian single-center study of 475 early and 3294 midtrimester amniocenteses, Centini and co-workers (2003) reported a miscarriage rate of only 0.4 and 0.3 percent, respectively. In the recently reported randomized trial by the NICHD Early Amniocentesis Trial Group, 3775 women were randomized to either amniocentesis or chorionic villous sampling at 11 to 14 weeks (Philip and colleagues, 2004). The spontaneous loss rate before 20 weeks was 0.9 and 1.5 percent, respectively.

Early amniocentesis has been associated with significantly more positional foot deformities than traditional amniocentesis (Fig. 13–9). A number of large studies cited by Philip and collaborators (2004) report that 0.75 to 1.6 percent of fetuses have talipes equinovarus (clubfoot) after early amniocentesis. This rate is compared with 0.1 percent following traditional amniocentesis and a background rate of 0.1 to 0.3

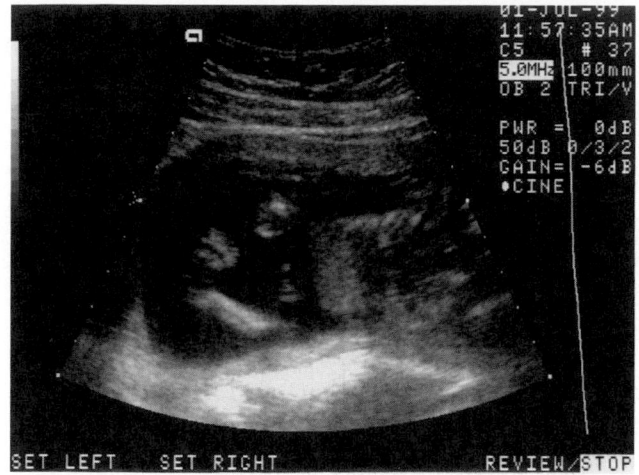

FIGURE 13–9. Clubfoot or talipes equinovarus. (Courtesy of Dr. Jodi Dashe.)

percent. The Canadian study group also found that membrane rupture was more likely after early amniocentesis, and that the incidence of talipes was 15 percent in cases with early postprocedural fluid leakage. Because oligohydramnios was transitory in most cases, at least some of the foot deformities likely resulted from damage to the vascular supply of the developing limb, rather than from oligohydramnios causing positional deformities. Finally, after early amniocentesis,

significantly more cell cultures failed, necessitating an additional amniocentesis in some cases. For all these reasons, many centers no longer perform amniocentesis before 14 weeks.

CHORIONIC VILLUS SAMPLING (CVS). This procedure generally is performed at 10 to 13 weeks. Villi may be obtained transcervically or transabdominally, depending on which route allows easiest access to the placenta (Fig. 13–10). Relative contraindications include vaginal bleeding or spotting, active genital tract infection, extreme uterine ante- or retroflexion, or body habitus precluding easy uterine access or clear ultrasonographic visualization of its contents.

The indications for CVS and amniocentesis are essentially the same, except for a few analyses that specifically require either amnionic fluid or placental tissue. The primary advantage of CVS is that results are available earlier in pregnancy, which lessens parental anxiety when results are normal. It also allows earlier and safer methods of pregnancy termination when they are abnormal.

Complications of CVS are similar to those of amniocentesis. Several randomized and case-control trials have compared the safety of CVS with that of early and midtrimester amniocentesis as well as the safety of transabdominal versus transcervical CVS. Wald and colleagues (1998) summarized eight randomized trials and found that transcervical CVS has a procedure-related fetal death rate 3.7 percent greater than

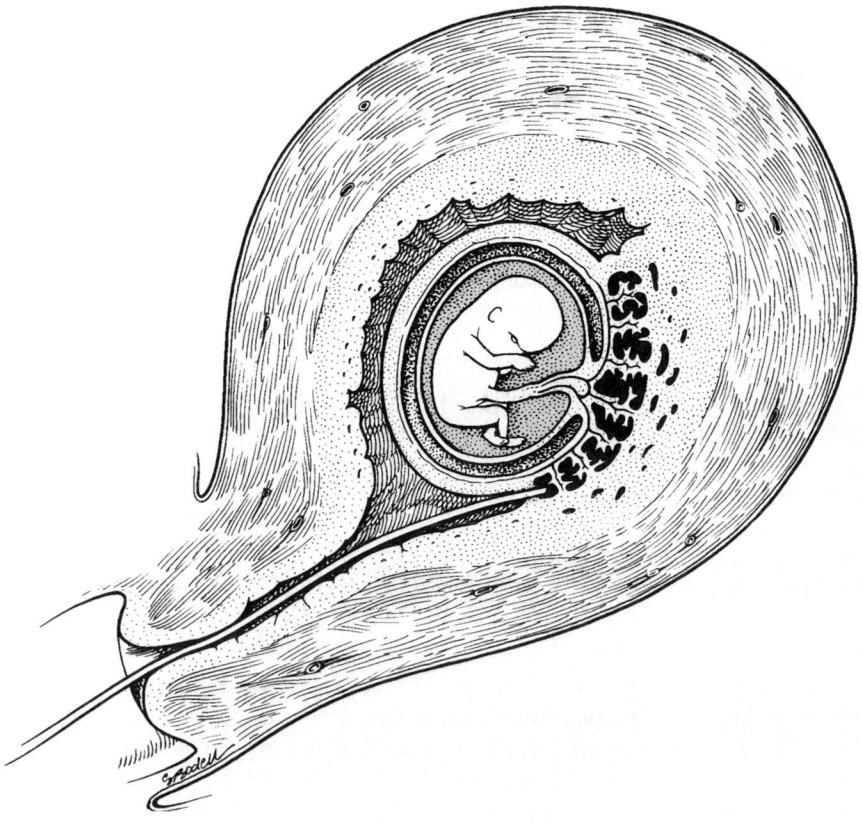

FIGURE 13–10. Transcervical chorionic villus sampling.

that of either transabdominal CVS or traditional amniocentesis. This rate is similar to that for early amniocentesis. In the randomized trial reported by Philip and co-workers (2004), the fetal loss rate associated with transabdominal CVS before 20 weeks was 1.5 percent, compared with that of 0.9 percent for early amniocentesis. In their review of 14 randomized trials, Alfirevic and collaborators (2003) found that midtrimester amniocentesis was safer than either transcervical CVS or early amniocentesis. They recommend transabdominal CVS if early diagnosis is required.

Early reports of an association between CVS and limb-reduction defects, oromandibular defects, and cavernous hemangiomas have been disproved (Burton, 1992; Firth, 1991, 1994; Hsieh, 1995, and their colleagues). When CVS is performed after 9 weeks, Kuliev and colleagues (1996) reported the incidence of limb-reduction defects to be 6 per 10,000—the same as the background incidence. The frequency of oromandibular-limb hypogenesis, however, was increased after CVS when the procedure was performed before 9 weeks (Bianchi and associates, 1993; Kalousek and Dill, 1983).

Laboratory Results. Midtrimester amniocentesis is associated with the lowest incidence of *uninformative results,* which are found in up to 8 percent. This compares with 0.8 to 1.5 percent for transcervical CVS and 0.7 to 1.9 percent for transabdominal CVS (Canadian Collaborative CVS–Amniocentesis Clinical Trial Group, 1989; Philip and co-workers, 2004; Rhoads and colleagues, 1989). Uninformative data usually are the result of an inadequate sample or the detection of *mosaicism,* that is, more than one distinct cell line in a single chorionic villus sample. Such mosaicism rarely represents true fetal mosaicism but usually indicates *confined placental mosaicism,* or *pseudomosaicism* (see Chap. 12, p. 295).

PERCUTANEOUS UMBILICAL CORD BLOOD SAMPLING (PUBS).
Also called *cordocentesis,* this procedure was first described by Daffos and colleagues (1983). Cordocentesis currently is performed primarily for the assessment and treatment of confirmed red cell or platelet alloimmunization and for the analysis of nonimmune hydrops (Fisk and Bower, 1993). If anemia is suspected, Pereira and colleagues (2003) recommended that fetal cerebral artery velocimetry be considered before direct fetal blood sampling. PUBS also can be used to obtain fetal blood cells for genetic analysis when CVS or amniocentesis results are confusing or when rapid diagnosis is necessary. Karyotyping of fetal blood usually can be accomplished within 24 to 48 hours. The sample can also be analyzed as necessary for metabolic and hematological studies, acid–base analysis, viral cultures, polymerase chain reaction and other genetic techniques, and immunological studies.

In this procedure, the operator punctures the umbilical vein, usually at or near its placental origin, with a 22-gauge

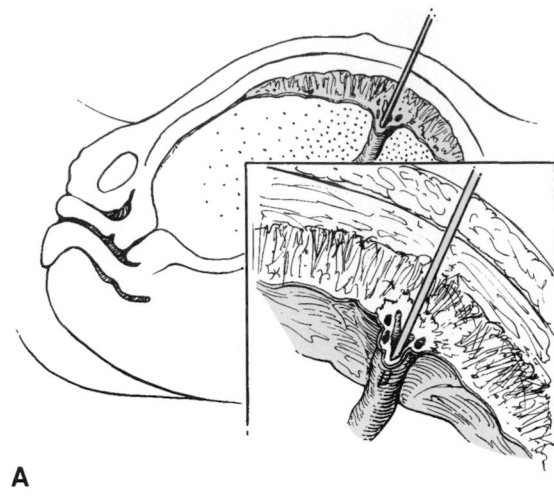

A

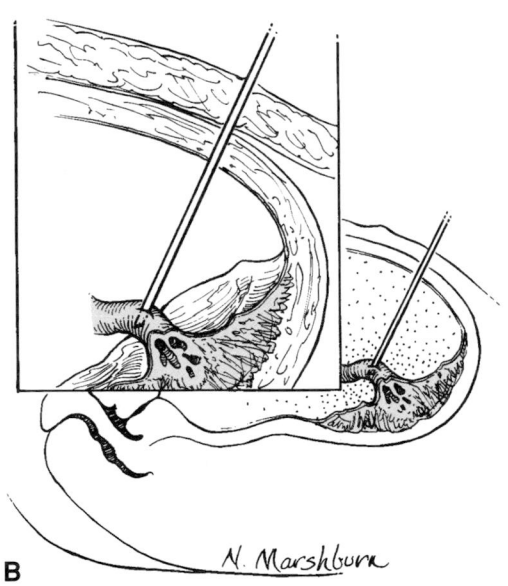

B

FIGURE 13–11. Umbilical cord blood sampling. Access to the umbilical artery or vein varies, depending on both the placental location and the position of cord insertion into the placenta. **A.** With an anterior placenta, the needle may traverse the placenta. **B.** With posterior implantation, the needle usually passes through the amnionic fluid before penetrating an umbilical vessel.

spinal needle under direct ultrasonographic guidance, and blood is withdrawn (Fig. 13–11). A free loop of cord also can be accessed. Arterial puncture should be avoided because it can result in vasospasm and fetal bradycardia.

Complications. The complications of PUBS are similar to those of amniocentesis. Additionally, cord vessel bleeding (50 percent), cord hematoma (17 percent), fetal–maternal hemorrhage (66 percent with an anterior placenta and 17 percent with a posterior placenta), and fetal bradycardia (3 to 12 percent) may result (Ghidini and colleagues, 1993). Most complications are transitory and followed by complete fetal recovery. Some, however, result in fetal death. The overall procedure-related fetal death rate is about 1.4 percent, but varies according to the indication for the procedure and the fetal status at the time of the procedure (Ghidini and colleagues, 1993; Maxwell and associates, 1991).

FETAL TISSUE BIOPSY. There are many genetic conditions for which there is no specific molecular genetic test. Linkage analysis has been used for the diagnosis of familial disorders, but it is possible only if there are living, informative, affected family members (see Chap. 12, p. 308). Prenatal diagnosis of a few conditions sometimes can be accomplished by direct analysis of fetal tissue obtained by ultrasonographically guided biopsy. The technique has been used by Evans and colleagues (1994) for muscle biopsy to diagnose muscular dystrophy or mitochondrial myopathy. Elias and co-workers (1994) used skin biopsy to diagnose epidermolysis bullosa.

PREIMPLANTATION GENETIC DIAGNOSIS. Identification of the genes responsible for certain severe hereditary diseases and in vitro fertilization techniques allow diagnosis of a few such disorders prior to implantation. As a result, only healthy embryos are selected for implantation, and pregnancy termination can be avoided. The technique has been performed to diagnose single-gene disorders such as CF, sickle-cell disease, or thalassemia; determine gender in X-linked diseases; identify aneuploidy associated with advanced maternal age; and detect parentally derived chromosomal rearrangements (Flake, 2003; Grewal and associates, 2004; Jiao and colleagues, 2003; Xu and co-workers, 2004).

Several variations in technique have been reported. Some clinicians favor polar body analysis because the first and second polar bodies normally are expelled, and their removal should not affect fetal development. Because the majority of biopsied polar bodies are in metaphase, the chromosomes in these cells also are suitable for fluorescence in situ hybridization (FISH) analysis (Munne, 2001). A second technique uses the 3-day-old embryo at the 6- to 10-cell stage. It involves *blastomere biopsy* through a hole made in the zona pellucida. Loss of one totipotent cell at this stage supposedly has little or no effect on the developing embryo, although in the report by El-Toukhy and co-workers (2003), there was a lower implantation rate when previously biopsied frozen embryos were thawed and transferred. This technique is still under development and currently is quite complex.

FETAL CELLS IN THE MATERNAL CIRCULATION. Since the 1950s, various types of fetal cells have been identified in the maternal circulation (Douglas and colleagues, 1959). Virtually all pregnant women have at least a small number of fetal cells in their bloodstream (Goldberg, 1997). Isolation of these cells for prenatal analysis might obviate the need for more invasive procedures. Most research in this area focuses on cell sorting techniques, which take advantage of unique cell surface proteins and other characteristics that distinguish fetal from maternal cells. These techniques include *density gradient* or *protein separation, fluorescence-activated cell sorting*, and *magnetic-activated cell sorting*. Nucleated red blood cells are most easily isolated. Fetal cells obtained this way have been evaluated for genetic diseases such as β-thalassemia (Camaschella and associates, 1990) as well as for fetal red cell D-antigen typing (Geifman-Holtzman and colleagues, 1996). Karyotyping using FISH also is possible (Poon and co-workers, 2000; Price and colleagues, 1991). With an aneuploid fetus, Bianchi and colleagues (1997) have reported a sixfold increase in the number of fetal cells in the maternal blood.

Several problems must be resolved before these techniques can be used clinically. Currently, it is difficult to isolate a quantity of fetal cells sufficient for analysis and to isolate a pure sample that does not contain maternal cells. One unique problem is that fetal lymphocytes or stem cells persist in the maternal circulation indefinitely. Thus, it is difficult to determine whether isolated cells come from the current pregnancy or a past one. Indeed, there is evidence that these persistent fetal cells cause certain maternal autoimmune diseases, such as scleroderma and other connective-tissue diseases and thyroiditis (see Chap. 53, p. 1191 and Chap. 54, p. 1210).

FETAL THERAPY

PREGNANCY TERMINATION. It is unfortunate that antenatal therapy is not available for most congenital anomalies. Despite this, the woman and her family may still benefit from prenatal diagnosis because it allows for psychological preparation and for an informed decision about pregnancy termination. In addition to a maternal–fetal medicine or genetics referral, consultation with the appropriate pediatric subspecialist may be helpful. A complete summary of the counseling session should be placed in the medical record. Techniques for singleton pregnancy termination are discussed in Chapter 9 (see p. 242). In some cases, only one fetus of a twin or higher-order multiple gestation is affected, and pregnancy termination in this setting is discussed in Chapter 39 (see p. 941).

TWIN-TO-TWIN TRANSFUSION SYNDROME. This syndrome is a unique problem that complicates about 15 percent of monochorionic twin pregnancies. It occurs as the result of unbalanced vascular anastomoses that connect the two fetal circulations. In the extreme case, one twin is severely growth restricted with no amnionic fluid—the *stuck twin*—while the co-twin is larger, often plethoric, and has hydramnios. The pathophysiology is discussed in greater detail in Chapter 39 (see p. 929). Management options for twin-to-twin transfusion syndrome are limited. They include therapeutic amniocentesis, septostomy, laser occlusion of placental vascular anastomoses, and selective feticide of the donor twin. Unfortunately, with or without therapy, the perinatal death rate is high, and long-term studies indicate severe neurodevelopmental abnormalities in some survivors (Lopriore and colleagues, 2003).

FETAL TRANSFUSION

Isoimmunization. Various techniques for red blood cell transfusion have been used in the treatment of fetal anemia. Ultrasonographically directed transfusion into the umbilical cord vein currently is favored because it has proved effective and safe (Berkowitz, 1986; Nicolaides, 1986; Weiner, 1991, and their colleagues). The fetal–placental volume allows the relatively rapid infusion of a large quantity of blood. Direct ultrasonographic guidance minimizes trauma to the umbilical cord and allows direct fetal monitoring. Prior to the blood infusion, pancuronium and furosemide can be administered directly into the umbilical vein. Pancuronium minimizes trauma by stopping fetal movement and protecting against vagally mediated fetal bradycardia. Furosemide relaxes the capacitance vessels and aids the clearance of excess plasma. The latter is important if there is heart failure with fetal hydrops and hydramnios.

Parvovirus Infection. Some fetuses affected by parvovirus B19 infection, especially those infected before 20 weeks, develop severe transient aplastic anemia with heart failure and hydrops (see Chap. 58, p. 1279). Although an unknown number spontaneously recover, others are severely compromised and die. Some of these moribund fetuses can be rescued with blood transfusion (Peters and Nicolaides, 1990; Sahakian and colleagues, 1991). The hydropic fetus can be evaluated with cordocentesis or cerebral artery Doppler velocimetry and transfusion performed if anemia is confirmed. For confirmation of the diagnosis, parvovirus DNA can be detected in fetal and maternal blood by polymerase chain reaction (Dieck and associates, 1999). Although a single transfusion is all that is required to aid recovery in many cases, fetuses who develop viral myocarditis do not respond to this therapy.

Other Indications. Transfusion may be considered after a severe but not ongoing fetal–maternal hemorrhage. It also has been described in a case of fetal hemoglobin Bart disease (see Chap. 51, p. 1154). Copel and co-workers (1991) have administered platelet transfusion for severe alloimmune thrombocytopenia using the same technique (see Chap. 29, p. 677).

FETAL MEDICAL THERAPY. Sometimes fetal disease can be treated pharmacologically by giving the mother medication that then crosses the placenta. For example, women with Graves disease who have been rendered euthyroid by radioiodine ablation may continue to produce immunoglobulin

G thyroid-stimulating antibodies, which cross the placenta and cause *fetal thyrotoxicosis* (see Chap. 53, p. 1193). Fetal thyroid status can be assessed by cordocentesis and, if hyperthyroidism is confirmed, propylthiouracil administered to the mother crosses the placenta to suppress the fetal thyroid (Wenstrom and associates, 1990).

Another example is the fetus at risk of *congenital adrenal hyperplasia,* an autosomal recessive condition that results in virilization of a female fetus. This outcome can be prevented with maternally administered corticosteroids, which suppress fetal adrenal function (David and Forest, 1984).

A third example is *fetal arrhythmia,* which complicates up to 1 percent of pregnancies (Copel and associates, 2000). Most fetal arrhythmias are tolerated without compromise, or resolve spontaneously (Simpson and colleagues, 1997). The fetus with sustained tachyarrhythmia, however, may experience cardiac decompensation, which can progress to hydrops. Treatment is accomplished by maternal administration of antiarrhythmic agents that cross the placenta in therapeutic doses. Digoxin, verapamil, propranolol, procainamide, quinidine, flecainide, sotalol, and amiodarone have all been used to treat fetal arrhythmias with good results in nonhydropic fetuses (Edwards and colleagues, 1999; Sonesson and associates, 1998). If the fetus is hydropic, some of these drugs may not enter the fetal circulation in sufficient amounts. Strasburger and co-workers (2004), however, found amiodarone effective in most cases. In other cases, medication can be administered directly to the fetus through the umbilical cord or by intramuscular injection in the buttock (Mangione and co-workers, 1999; Parilla and colleagues, 1996).

Congenital Infection. A number of infectious agents can cross the placenta and cause fetal infection with serious consequences. Prompt and effective maternal treatment can improve some or all of the most severe associated fetal morbidity. Treatment of maternal infections that could cause pregnancy complications also constitutes fetal therapy. Diagnosis and treatment of sexually transmitted and other infectious diseases are discussed in Chapters 58 and 59.

FETAL SURGERY. With only a few exceptions, fetal surgery is still in the pioneering stages and is performed in only a few centers. Because it entails substantial fetal and maternal risks, surgery should be considered only when it will improve fetal outcome with certainty, barring unforeseen complications, and when withholding it would be catastrophic. It is important that appropriate selection criteria be established and verified. The procedure must be perfected and tested successfully in experimental animals, preferably primates (Harrison and colleagues, 1980; Moise and associates, 1995). Finally, the efficacy of the technique in humans should be rigorously evaluated prior to its widespread use.

Urinary Shunts. In many cases, the presence of a major urinary tract malformation indicates aneuploidy or another genetic syndrome usually associated with a poor prognosis. Malformations such as cystic dysplasia or renal agenesis cannot be corrected and are associated with oligohydramnios, which prevents development of the fetal lungs (see Chap. 21, p. 530). In contrast, fetuses with certain types of isolated urinary tract obstructive lesions may have the potential for a good prognosis following correction.

Lesions such as posterior urethral valves, urethral atresia, and ureteropelvic junction obstruction often occur with relatively normal kidneys capable of producing normal amounts of urine and thus amnionic fluid. These obstructions, however, can cause renal damage due to prolonged increases in intrarenal pressure and can prevent normal lung development because of oligohydramnios (Adzick and Harrison, 1994). Placement of a double-pigtail catheter— with one end in the fetal bladder and the other in the amnionic cavity—shunts urine into the uterine cavity with restoration of amnionic fluid volume and reduction of intrarenal pressure. In experienced hands, fetal survival after shunt placement is 70 percent (Holzgreve and Evans, 1993). One case in which the catheter was placed transurethrally has been described (Hofmann and co-workers, 2004).

Survivors still may have serious renal pathology because either there is intrinsic renal dysplasia or significant renal damage had already developed by the time obstruction was recognized (Johnson and associates, 1995). Accordingly, the greatest problem with this procedure is selecting appropriate fetuses. Before shunt placement, serial vesicocenteses with urine chemistry analyses can be performed to help determine whether sufficient renal function remains (Johnson and Freedman, 1999). The use of fetal endoscopic cystotomy has been evaluated by Quintero and associates (2000) for complicated cases in which shunting alone is not sufficient.

Thoracic Shunts. Accumulation of thoracic fluid also can cause pulmonary hypoplasia by compressing the developing lung. Some causes include chylothorax, infection, and chest tumors. Survival after thoracic shunt placement for isolated fetal hydrothorax has been reported, but one third of such fetuses will have a poor outcome whether or not a shunt is placed (Hagay and colleagues, 1993).

Intrathoracic masses leading to pulmonary hypoplasia include pulmonary sequestration, congenital cystic adenomatoid malformation, and nonspecific cysts (Harrison and co-workers, 1990). Their diagnosis is considered in Chapter 16 (see p. 396). Fetal goiter or tracheal atresia also may prevent egress of pulmonary fluid. Thoracic shunt placement with variable success has been described for all these entities. Although fluid drainage immediately following the procedure is usually adequate, obstruction or displacement of the shunt can rapidly lead to reaccumulation. Shunt placement in the presence of hydrops is generally not curative, probably because the fetus has already suffered damage, or is moribund at the time of the procedure, or because hydrops itself indi-

cates a more serious abnormality (Adzick and co-workers, 1993; Weiner and colleagues, 1986).

Congenital Diaphragmatic Hernia (CDH). The incidence of this defect in the general population is about 1 in 3700 (Wenstrom and colleagues, 1991). Up to half of these fetuses have genetic syndromes or other associated defects that may be lethal. Approximately 70 percent of those with isolated malformations survive with normal physical and mental function following postnatal surgery and specialized neonatal care (Reickert and colleagues, 1998). Antenatal surgery is presumed to prevent mortality in the 30 percent of fetuses who typically would not survive. Although CDH was one of the first malformations for which ex-utero fetal surgery was performed, the surgical technique has not yet been perfected (Harrison and colleagues, 2003). Importantly, both maternal and fetal surgical outcomes remain suboptimal, whereas the survival rate in neonates treated postnatally continues to improve (Harrison and colleagues, 2003; Wenstrom, 2003). At least three major problems must be overcome:

1. Despite the development of a variety of diagnostic tests, the fetuses with isolated CDH who would not survive despite optimal postnatal care cannot be reliably identified.
2. None of several different antenatal surgical procedures studied has consistently improved neonatal outcome.
3. Virtually all fetuses subjected to antenatal surgery have been delivered preterm, and many before 30 weeks. Such fetuses are thus subjected to the morbidity associated with preterm birth and that associated with surgery itself.

Until these problems can be overcome, antenatal repair of CDH is considered investigational.

Sacrococcygeal Teratoma. This congenital tumor is composed of tissues representing all three germ layers and arises from the totipotent cells in the Hensen node or from ectopic primordial germ cells in the sacral area. These teratomas are vascular, with numerous arteriovenous shunts that can lead to vascular steal syndromes or hemorrhage. Perinatal morbidity and mortality is great due to the associated fetal anemia, heart failure, and hydrops (Altman and colleagues, 1974). Tumors detected early are usually aggressive. Survival is less than 10 percent in fetuses whose tumors are identified before 30 weeks, compared with 75 percent in those whose tumors are discovered later (Malone and co-workers, 1990).

In view of the very poor prognosis for early aggressive lesions, prenatal surgical excision has been attempted, but largely without success (Langer and colleagues, 1989). An alternative approach is to attempt palliative debulking surgery to prevent hydrops, and to defer definitive repair until after birth (Graf and colleagues, 1998).

Congenital Cystic Adenomatoid Malformation and Pulmonary Sequestration. These two pulmonary lesions may be amenable to fetal surgical therapy. Congenital cystic adenomatoid malformations (CCAMs) are pulmonary hamartomas consisting of overgrown terminal bronchioles. Type I has large cysts, type II has multiple small cysts measuring less than 1.2 cm, and type III is full of microcysts, giving the tissue an essentially solid appearance. Type III lesions have the worst prognosis. Pulmonary sequestration occurs when a mass of pulmonary tissue develops completely separated from normal lung and receives its blood supply from the systemic circulation. The intralobar variety is located inside the pleura adjacent to normal lung, whereas the extralobar variety has its own separate pleura, similar to an accessory lobe.

Both of these lesions may enlarge and eventually cause mediastinal shift, pleural effusions, hydramnios, and perinatal death from hydrops or pulmonary hypoplasia. Alternatively, either may regress spontaneously, although this is more likely with sequestration. Hydropic fetuses with either lesion are ideal candidates for fetal surgery because (1) the natural history of these lesions is known, (2) those with a poor prognosis can be readily identified because they are hydropic, and (3) such fetuses do not survive even with aggressive neonatal therapy. Adzick and colleagues (1993) offered fetal surgery to mothers of hydropic fetuses with CCAMs, and reported that the 25 fetuses with large cystic CCAMs and hydrops who were managed expectantly died. In contrast, 13 hydropic fetuses survived after open fetal lobectomy, and 5 of 6 survived with thoracoamnionic shunting.

Neural-Tube Defects. Isolated open spine defects usually result in permanent neurological damage (see Chap. 12, p. 302). The damage likely results from two insults—the "two-hit" hypothesis. The first hit is the defect itself, and the second is neurological damage resulting from chronic exposure of the spine defect to amnionic fluid (Heffez and colleagues, 1990). Several investigators have theorized that antenatal closure or coverage of the spine defect might avert some of the damage. Fetal surgery for this indication is controversial because spina bifida is not a lethal defect, but results in morbidity, including reduced mobility, lack of bowel and bladder control, and need for a ventricular shunt.

The American College of Obstetricians and Gynecologists (2003) cites about 220 fetal surgeries for open spina bifida in the United States from 1997 through 2002. The studies were not randomized, and outcomes were not overly impressive given the risks of surgery. Thus, prenatal surgical closure of a fetal spine defect is currently available only as part of a National Institutes of Health (2003) multicenter research trial entitled *Management of Myelomeningocele Study (MoMS)*. The hypothesis of the study is that fetal surgery results in a decreased incidence of Arnold–Chiari malformation, and thus a reduced need for shunt placement if performed before 25 weeks (Bruner and colleagues, 1999; Tulipan and co-workers, 2003). Unfortunately, fetal surgical repair does not appear to improve lower extremity function (Tubbs and associates, 2003). In addition, there is substantive maternal

morbidity that includes preterm labor and preterm rupture of the membranes, infection, pulmonary edema, and a scar in the contractible portion of the uterus. These complications, along with its uncertain benefit, make it unlikely that fetal surgery for spina bifida will be offered any time soon outside of a research trial.

STEM CELL TRANSPLANTATION

Because immunocompetence in the human fetus does not develop until 18 weeks, it is theorized that the fetus would be tolerant to foreign antigens introduced before that time. For this reason, fetal hemopoietic stem cell transplantation might treat a variety of hematological diseases or serve as a delivery vehicle for gene transfer for the treatment of other genetic conditions. Several animal models have been developed to study fetal bone marrow transplantation. Studies to date have focused on identifying the optimal time interval for transplantation and the best source of hematopoietic stem cells, including fetal liver, umbilical cord blood, and adult bone marrow. Therapeutic fetal bone marrow transplantation has been attempted in the human fetus for such diseases as bare lymphocyte syndrome, severe combined immunodeficiency syndrome, thalassemia, metachromatic leukodystrophy, and D-antigen isoimmunization. Despite limited success, however, research efforts continue (Crombleholme and Bianchi, 1994; Westgren and co-workers, 1996).

GENE TRANSFER

With advances in genetic technologies and progress in the identification of genes responsible for inherited disease, the possibility of gene transfer as definitive therapy for a variety of genetic conditions is being explored. An excellent review by Pergament and Fiddler (1995) provides a detailed summary of fetal gene transfer. Early therapy by gene transfer would be ideal for certain inherited metabolic conditions in which tissue damage begins shortly after or even before birth. In Tay-Sachs disease, for example, central nervous system cells exhibit the characteristic pathology as early as 9 weeks after conception (Grabowski and colleagues, 1984). Early gene therapy also has the potential of requiring only one treatment, which would be definitive and would have a lifetime impact. Finally, healthy children would be assured without having to choose termination of affected pregnancies.

A number of criteria are considered requisite for the development of therapeutic gene transfer. These criteria, which have not yet been met, include that:

1. The normal gene can be inserted into the target cells and remain there long enough to have the desired effect.
2. The level of gene expression in the new gene will be appropriate.

3. The new gene will not harm the cell or the individual (Anderson, 1984). For example, it was recently reported that infants receiving gene therapy for X-linked severe combined immunodeficiency disease developed T-cell leukemia 3 years later (Berns, 2004).

Other unresolved issues include the timing of the procedure, viz., preconceptional, at the time of fertilization, prior to implantation, or during embryogenesis or fetal development; the best DNA vectors to use; the ideal recipient or target cells; and the safest methods. Efficient techniques for in vivo gene targeting have yet to be developed, and the possibility of ex vivo gene transfer raises ethical considerations. Other ethical questions remaining to be resolved include whether or not to target fetal gonadal tissues—which would affect future generations—and how to prevent gene transfer from being used for enhancement of phenotype rather than disease prevention—*eugenics*. Gene transfer is in its earliest experimental stages, and it must be thoroughly investigated in animals and adult humans before it can be extended to fetuses.

REFERENCES

Adams MJ, Windham GC, James LM, et al: Clinical interpretation of maternal serum α-fetoprotein concentrations. Am J Obstet Gynecol 148:241, 1984

Adzick NS, Harrison MR: Fetal surgical therapy. Lancet 343:897, 1994

Adzick NS, Harrison MR, Flake AW, et al: Fetal surgery for cystic adenomatoid malformation of the lung. J Pediatr Surg 28:806, 1993

Alfirevic Z, Sundberg K, Brigham S: Amniocentesis and chorionic villus sampling for prenatal diagnosis. Cochrane Database Syst Rev (3):CD003252, 2003

Altman RP, Randolph JG, Lilly JR: Sacrococcygeal teratoma. American Academy of Pediatrics Surgical Section Survey. J Pediatr Surg 9:389, 1974

American College of Obstetricians and Gynecologists: First-trimester screening for fetal aneuploidy. Committee Opinion No. 296, July 2004

American College of Obstetricians and Gynecologists: Neural tube defects. Practice Bulletin No. 44, July 2003

American College of Obstetricians and Gynecologists: Maternal serum screening. Educational Bulletin No. 228, September 1996

American College of Obstetricians and Gynecologists: Fragile X syndrome. Committee Opinion No. 161, October 1995

American College of Obstetricians and Gynecologists: Prenatal detection of neural tube defects. Technical Bulletin No. 99, 1986

American College of Obstetricians and Gynecologists, American College of Medical Genetics: Preconception and prenatal carrier screening for cystic fibrosis. Clinical and Laboratory Guidelines, October 2001

Anderson WF: Prospects for human gene therapy. Science 226:401, 1984

Azuri J, Elstein D, Lahad A, et al: Asymptomatic Gaucher disease—implications for large-scale screening. Genet Test 2:4, 1998

Bahado-Singh R, Oz UA, Baumgarten A, et al: The comprehensive mid-trimester test (CMT): Highly-sensitive for Down syndrome detection (Abstract 0055). Paper presented at: Society for Maternal–Fetal Medicine; February 5–10, 2001; Reno, Nev

Becerra JE, Khoury MJ, Cordero JF, et al: Diabetes mellitus during pregnancy and the risks for specific birth defects: A population-based case-control study. Pediatrics 85:1, 1990

Bensen JT, Dillard RG, Burton BK: Open spina bifida: Does cesarean section delivery improve prognosis? Obstet Gynecol 71:532, 1988

Berkowitz RL, Chitkara U, Goldberg JD, et al: Intrauterine intravascular transfusions for severe red blood cell isoimmunization: Ultrasound-guided percutaneous approach. Am J Obstet Gynecol 155:574, 1986

Berns A: Good news for gene therapy. N Engl J Med 350:1679, 2004

Bianchi DW, Wilkins-Haug LE, Enders AC, et al: Origin of extraembryonic mesoderm in experimental animals: Relevance to chorionic mosaicism in humans. Am J Med Genet 46:542, 1993

Bianchi DW, Williams JM, Sullivan LM, et al: PCR quantitation of fetal cells in maternal blood in normal and aneuploid pregnancies. Am J Hum Genet 61:822, 1997

Bogart MH, Pandian MR, Jones OW: Abnormal maternal serum chorionic gonadotropin levels in pregnancies with fetal chromosome abnormalities. Prenat Diagn 7:623, 1987

Bonaiti-Pellie C, Smith C: Risks tables for genetic counseling in some common congenital malformations. J Med Genet 11:374, 1974

Brambati B, Cislaghi C, Tului L, et al: First trimester Down's syndrome screening using nuchal translucency: A prospective study in patients undergoing chorionic villus sampling. Ultrasound Obstet Gynecol 5:9, 1995

Brock DJ, Bolton AE, Monaghan JM: Prenatal diagnosis of anencephaly through maternal serum-alpha-fetoprotein measurement. Lancet 2:923, 1973

Brock DJ, Sutcliffe RG: Alpha-fetoprotein in the antenatal diagnosis of anencephaly and spina bifida. Lancet 2:197, 1972

Brumfield CG, Cloud GA, Davis RO, et al: The relationship between maternal serum and amniotic fluid α-fetoprotein in women undergoing early amniocentesis. Am J Obstet Gynecol 163:903, 1990

Bruner JP, Tulipan N, Paschall RL, et al: Fetal surgery for myelomeningocele and the incidence of shunt-dependent hydrocephalus. JAMA 282:1819, 1999

Burn J, Brennan P, Little J, et al: Recurrence risks in offspring of adults with major heart defects: Results from first cohort of British collaborative study. Lancet 351:311, 1998

Burton BK: Elevated maternal serum alpha-fetoprotein (MSAFP): Interpretation and follow-up. Clin Obstet Gynecol 31:293, 1988

Burton BK, Prins GS, Verp MS: A prospective trial of prenatal screening for Down syndrome by means of maternal serum-fetoprotein, human chorionic gonadotropin, and unconjugated estriol. Am J Obstet Gynecol 169:526, 1993

Burton BK, Schulz CJ, Burd LI: Limb anomalies associated with chorionic villus sampling. Obstet Gynecol 79:726, 1992

Burton BK, Sowers SG, Nelson LH: Maternal serum α-fetoprotein screening in North Carolina: Experience with more than twelve thousand pregnancies. Am J Obstet Gynecol 146:439, 1983

Camaschella C, Alfarno A, Gottardi E, et al: Prenatal diagnosis of fetal haemoglobin Lepore-Boston disease on maternal peripheral blood. Blood 75:2101, 1990

Canadian Collaborative CVS–Amniocentesis Clinical Trial Group: Multicentre randomised clinical trial of chorion villus sampling and amniocentesis. Lancet 7:1, 1989

Canadian Early and Mid-Trimester Amniocentesis Trial (CEMAT) Group: Randomised trial to assess safety and fetal outcome of early and midtrimester amniocentesis. Lancet 351:242, 1998

Caughey AB, Washington AE, Gildengorin V, et al: Assessment of demand for prenatal diagnostic test using willingness to pay. Obstet Gynecol 103:539, 2004

Centini G, Rosignoli L, Kenanidis A, et al: A report of early (13 + 0 to 14 + 6 weeks) and midtrimester amniocenteses: 10 years' experience. J Matern Fetal Neonatal Med 14:113, 2003

Cheng EY, Luthy DA, Zebelman AM, et al: A prospective evaluation of a second-trimester screening test for fetal Down syndrome using maternal serum alpha-fetoprotein, hCG, and unconjugated estriol. Obstet Gynecol 81:72, 1993

Cicero S, Curcio P, Papageorghiou A, et al: Absence of nasal bone in fetuses with trisomy 21 at 11–14 weeks of gestation: An observational study. Lancet 358:1665, 2001

Copel JA, Gollin YG, Grannum PA: Alloimmune disorders and pregnancy. Semin Perinatol 15:251, 1991

Copel JA, Liang RI, Demasio K, et al: The clinical significance of the irregular fetal heart rhythm. Am J Obstet Gynecol 182:813, 2000

Crandall BF, Matsumoto M: Routine amniotic fluid α-fetoprotein measurement in 34,000 pregnancies. Am J Obstet Gynecol 149:744, 1984

Crombleholme TM, Bianchi DW: In utero hematopoietic stem cell transplantation and gene therapy. Semin Perinatol 18:376, 1994

Cuckle HS, Wald NJ, Lindenbaum RH: Maternal serum alpha-fetoprotein measurement: A screening test for Down syndrome. Lancet 1:926, 1984

Cunningham FG, Gilstrap LC: Maternal serum alpha-fetoprotein screening. N Engl J Med 325:55, 1991

Curry CJ, Stevenson RE, Aughton D, et al: Evaluation of mental retardation: Recommendations of a consensus conference. Am J Med Genet 72:468, 1997

Cutillo DM: Fragile X syndrome. Genet Teratol 2:1, 1994

Cystic Fibrosis Mutation Database. Available at: www.sickkids.on.ca. Accessed April 2004

D'Alton ME, Malone FD, Lambert-Messerlian G, et al: Maintaining quality assurance for nuchal translucency sonography in a prospective multicenter study: Results from the FASTER Trial [abstract]. Am J Obstet Gynecol 187:S79, 2003

Daffos F, Capella-Pavlovsky M, Forestier F: A new procedure for fetal blood sampling in utero: Preliminary results of fifty-three cases. Am J Obstet Gynecol 146:985, 1983

David M, Forest MG: Prenatal treatment of congenital adrenal hyperplasia resulting from 21-hydroxylase deficiency. J Pediatr 105:799, 1984

de Vries BB, Wiegers AM, Smits AP, et al: Mental status of females with an FMR1 gene full mutation. Am J Hum Genet 58:1025, 1996

Dieck D, Schild RL, Hansmann M, et al: Prenatal diagnosis of congenital parvovirus B19 infection: Value of serological and PCR techniques in maternal and fetal serum. Prenat Diagn 19:1119, 1999

Douglas GW, Thomas L, Carr M, et al: Trophoblasts in the circulating blood during pregnancy. Am J Obstet Gynecol 58:960, 1959

Edwards A, Peek MJ, Curren J: Transplacental flecainide therapy for fetal supraventricular tachycardia in a twin pregnancy. Aust N Z J Obstet Gynaecol 39:110, 1999

El-Toukhy T, Khalaf Y, Al-Darazi K, et al: Effect of blastomere loss on the outcome of frozen embryo replacement cycles. Fertil Steril 79:1106, 2003

Elias S, Emerson DS, Simpson JL, et al: Ultrasound-guided fetal skin sampling for prenatal diagnosis of genodermatoses. Obstet Gynecol 83:337, 1994

Evans MI, Hoffman EP, Cadrin C, et al: Fetal muscle biopsy: Collaborative experience with varied indications. Obstet Gynecol 84:913, 1994

Evans MI, Llurba E, Landsberger EJ, et al: Impact of folic acid fortification in the United States markedly diminished high maternal serum alpha fetoprotein values. Obstet Gynecol 103:474, 2004

Ewigman BG, Crane JP, Frigoletto FD, et al: Effect of prenatal ultrasound screening on perinatal outcome. RADIUS Study Group. N Engl J Med 329:821, 1993

Ferguson-Smith MA, Yates JRW: Maternal age specific rates for chromosome aberrations and factors influencing them: A report of a collaborative European study on 52,965 amniocenteses. Prenat Diagn 4:5, 1984

Feuchtbaum LB, Cunningham G, Waller DK, et al: Fetal karyotyping for chromosome abnormalities after an unexplained elevated maternal serum alpha-fetoprotein screening. Obstet Gynecol 86:248, 1995

Firth HV, Boyd PA, Chamberlain PF, et al: Analysis of limb reduction defects in babies exposed to chorionic villus sampling. Lancet 343:1069, 1994

Firth HV, Boyd PA, Chamberlain P, et al: Severe limb abnormalities after chorion villus sampling at 56–66 days' gestation. Lancet 337:762, 1991

Fisch GS, Snow K, Thibodeau SN, et al: The fragile X premutation in carriers and its effect on mutation size in offspring. Am J Hum Genet 56:1147, 1995

Fisk NM, Bower S: Fetal blood sampling in retreat: A casualty of advances in molecular genetics, cytogenetics, and Doppler imaging. BMJ 307:143, 1993

Flake AW: Stem cell and genetic therapies for the fetus. Semin Pediatr Surg 12:202, 2003

Freedman SD, Blanco PG, Zaman MM, et al: Association of cystic fibrosis with abnormalities in fatty acid metabolism. N Engl J Med 350:605, 2004

Gardner RJM, Sutherland GR: Chromosome Abnormalities and Genetic Counseling, 2nd ed. Oxford Monographs on Medical Genetics No. 29. Oxford, England, Oxford University Press, 1996

Geifman-Holtzman O, Bernstein IM, Berry SM, et al: Fetal RhD genotyping in fetal cells flow sorted from maternal blood. Am J Obstet Gynecol 174:818, 1996

Ghidini A, Sepulveda W, Lockwood CJ, et al: Complications of fetal blood sampling. Am J Obstet Gynecol 168:1339, 1993

Gill HK, Splitt M, Sharland GK, et al: Patterns of recurrence of congenital heart disease: An analysis of 6,640 consecutive pregnancies evaluated by detailed fetal echocardiography. J Am Coll Cardiol 42:923, 2003

Goldberg JD: Fetal cells in maternal circulation: Progress in analysis of a rare event. Am J Hum Genet 61:806, 1997

Gonzalez D, Barret T, Apuzzio J: Utility of routine fetal karyotyping for patients undergoing amniocentesis for elevated maternal serum alpha-fetoprotein. Am J Obstet Gynecol 174:436, 1996

Grabowski GA, Kruse JR, Goldberg JD, et al: First-trimester prenatal diagnosis of Tay–Sachs disease. Am J Hum Genet 36:1369, 1984

Graf JL, Housely HT, Albanese CT, et al: A surprising histological evolution of preterm sacrococcygeal teratoma. J Pediatr Surg 33:177, 1998

Grewal SS, Kahn JP, MacMillan ML, et al: Successful hematopoietic stem cell transplantation for Fanconi anemia from an unaffected HLA-genotype-identical sibling selected using preimplantation genetic diagnosis. Blood 103:1147, 2004

Gupta JK, Khan KS, Thornton JG, et al: Management of fetal choroid plexus cysts. Br J Obstet Gynaecol 104:881, 1997

Haddow JE, Kloza EM, Smith DE, et al: Data from an alpha-fetoprotein pilot screening program in Maine. Obstet Gynecol 62:556, 1983

Haddow JE, Palomaki GE: Down's syndrome screening. Lancet 347:1625, 1996

Haddow JE, Palomaki GE, Knight GJ, et al: Reducing the need for amniocentesis in women 35 years of age or older with serum markers for screening. N Engl J Med 330:1114, 1994

Haddow JE, Palomaki GE, Knight GJ, et al: Screening of maternal serum for fetal Down syndrome in the first trimester. N Engl J Med 338:955, 1998

Hagay Z, Reece EA, Roberts A, et al: Isolated fetal pleural effusion: A prenatal management dilemma. Obstet Gynecol 81:147, 1993

Hagerman PJ, Hagerman RJ: The fragile-X permutation: a maturing perspective. *Am J Hum Genet* 74:805, 2004

Hagerman RJ, Amiri K, Cronister A: Fragile X checklist. Am J Med Genet 38:283, 1991

Harmon JP, Hiett AK, Palmer CG, et al: Prenatal ultrasound detection of isolated neural tube defects: Is cytogenetic evaluation warranted? Obstet Gynecol 86:595, 1995

Harrison MR, Adzick NS, Jennings RW, et al: Antenatal intervention for congenital cystic adenomatoid malformation. Lancet 336:965, 1990

Harrison MR, Jester JA, Ross NA: Correction of congenital diaphragmatic hernia in utero. I. The model: Intrathoracic balloon produces fatal pulmonary hypoplasia. Surgery 88:174, 1980

Harrison MR, Keller RL, Hawgood SM, et al: A randomized trial of fetal endoscopic tracheal occlusion for severe fetal congenital diaphragmatic hernia. N Engl J Med 349:1887, 2003

Heffez DS, Aryanpur J, Hutchins GM, et al: The paralysis associated with myelomeningocele: Clinical and experimental data implicating a preventable spinal cord injury. Neurosurgery 26:987, 1990

Hofmann R, Becker T, Meyer-Wittkopf M, et al: Fetoscopic placement of a transurethral stent for intrauterine obstructive uropathy. J Urol 171:384, 2004

Hogge WA, Thiagarajah S, Ferguson JE, et al: The role of ultrasonography and amniocentesis in the evaluation of pregnancies at risk for neural tube defects. Am J Obstet Gynecol 161:520, 1989

Holmgren G, Blomquist HK, Drugge U, et al: Fragile X families in a northern Swedish county: A genealogical study demonstrating apparent paternal transmission from the 18th century. Am J Med Genet 30:673, 1988

Holzgreve W, Evans MI: Nonvascular needles and shunt placements for fetal therapy. West J Med 159:333, 1993

Hook EB, Cross PK, Schreinemachers DM: Chromosomal abnormality rates at amniocentesis and in live-born infants. JAMA 249:2034, 1983

Hornberger LK, Need L, Benacerraf BR: Development of significant left and right ventricular hypoplasia in the second and third trimester fetus. J Ultrasound Med 15:655, 1996

Hsieh FJ, Shyu MK, Sheu BC, et al: Limb defects after chorionic villus sampling. Obstet Gynecol 85:84, 1995

Hume RF Jr, Drugan A, Reichler A, et al: Aneuploidy among prenatally detected neural tube defects. Am J Med Genet 61:171, 1996

Jacquemont S, Hagerman RJ, Leehey MA, et al: Penetrance of the fragile X-associated tremor/ataxia syndrome in a prematuration carrier population. JAMA 291:460, 2004

Jiao Z, Zhou C, Li J, et al: Birth of healthy children after preimplantation diagnosis of beta-thalassemia by whole-genome amplification. Prenat Diagn 23:646, 2003

Johnson JM, Wilson RD, Winsor RD, et al: The early amniocentesis study: A randomized clinical trial of early amniocentesis versus mid-trimester amniocentesis. Fetal Diagn Ther 11:85, 1996

Johnson MP, Corsi P, Bradfield W, et al: Sequential urinalysis improves evaluation of fetal renal function in obstructive uropathy. Am J Obstet Gynecol 173:59, 1995

Johnson MP, Freedman AL: Fetal uropathy. Curr Opin Obstet Gynecol 11:185, 1999

Jones KL: Smith's Recognizable Patterns of Human Malformation, 5th ed. Philadelphia, Saunders, 1997

Kalousek DK, Dill FJ: Chromosomal mosaicism confined to the placenta in human conceptions. Science 221:665, 1983

Katz VL, Chescheir NC, Cefalo RC: Unexplained elevations of maternal serum alpha-fetoprotein. Obstet Gynecol Surv 45:719, 1990

Kuliev A, Jackson L, Froster U, et al: Chorionic villus sampling safety. Report of World Health Organization/EURO meeting in association with the Seventh International Conference on Early Prenatal Diagnosis of Genetic Diseases, Tel-Aviv, Israel, May 21, 1994. Am J Obstet Gynecol 174:807, 1996

Langer JC, Harrison MR, Schmidt KG, et al: Fetal hydrops and death from sacrococcygeal teratoma: Rationale for fetal surgery. Am J Obstet Gynecol 160:1145, 1989

Lee K, Khoshnood B, Chen L, et al: Infant mortality from congenital malformations in the United States, 1970–1997. Obstet Gynecol 98:620, 2001

Leschot NJ, Verjaal M, Treffers PE: Risks of midtrimester amniocentesis; assessment in 3000 pregnancies. Br J Obstet Gynaecol 92:804, 1985

Lopriore E, Nagel HT, Vandenbussche FP, et al: Long-term neurodevelopmental outcome in twin-to-twin transfusion syndrome. Am J Obstet Gynecol 189:1314, 2003

Luthy DA, Wardinsky T, Shurtleff DB, et al: Cesarean section before the onset of labor and subsequent motor function in infants with meningomyelocele diagnosed antenatally. N Engl J Med 324:662, 1991

Main DM, Mennuti MT: Neural tube defects: Issues in prenatal diagnosis and counseling. Obstet Gynecol 67:1, 1986

Malone FD, Ball RH, Nyberg DA, et al: First-trimester nasal bone evaluation for aneuploidy in an unselected general population: Results from the FASTER Trial [abstract]. Am J Obstet Gynecol 187:S79, 2003a

Malone FD, Wald NJ, Canick JA, et al: First and second trimester evaluation of risk (FASTER) Trial: Principal results of the NICHD multicenter Down syndrome screening study [abstract]. Am J Obstet Gynecol 187:S56, 2003b

Malone PS, Spitz L, Kiely EM, et al: The functional sequelae of sacrococcygeal teratoma. J Pediatr Surg 25:679, 1990

Mangione R, Guyon F, Vergnaud A, et al: Successful treatment of refractory supraventricular tachycardia by repeat intravascular injection of amiodarone in a fetus with hydrops. Eur J Obstet Gynecol Reprod Biol 86:105, 1999

Marchese CA, Carozzi F, Mosso R, et al: Fetal karyotype in malformations detected by ultrasound. Am J Hum Genet 37:A223, 1985

Maxwell DJ, Johnson P, Hurley P, et al: Fetal blood sampling and pregnancy loss in relation to indication. Br J Obstet Gynaecol 98:892, 1991

Merkatz IR, Nitowsky HM, Macri JN, et al: An association between low maternal serum α-fetoprotein and fetal chromosomal abnormalities. Am J Obstet Gynecol 148:886, 1984

Meyers C, Adam R, Dungan J, et al: Aneuploidy in twin gestations: When is maternal age advanced? Obstet Gynecol 89:248, 1997

Milunsky A: Genetic Disorders and the Fetus: Diagnosis, Prevention, and Treatment, 3rd ed. Baltimore, Johns Hopkins University Press, 1992, p 1

Milunsky A, Alpert E, Neff RK, et al: Prenatal diagnosis of neural tube defects. IV. Maternal serum alpha-fetoprotein screening. Obstet Gynecol 55:60, 1980

Milunsky A, Jick SS, Bruell CL, et al: Predictive values, relative risks, and overall benefits of high and low maternal serum α-fetoprotein screening in singleton pregnancies: New epidemiologic data. Am J Obstet Gynecol 161:291, 1989

Moise KJ Jr, Belfort M, Saade G: Iatrogenic gastroschisis in the treatment of diaphragmatic hernia. Am J Obstet Gynecol 172:715, 1995

Morris C, Stringer J, Biggio J, et al: Prenatal screening strategies for Down syndrome. Am J Obstet Gynecol 184:S27, 2001

Morrow RJ, McNay MB, Whittle MJ: Ultrasound detection of neural tube defects in patients with elevated maternal serum alpha-fetoprotein. Obstet Gynecol 78:1055, 1991

Morton NE, Chiu D, Holland C, et al: Chromosome anomalies as predictors of recurrence risk for spontaneous abortion. Am J Med Genet 28:353, 1987

Munne S: Preimplantation genetic diagnosis of structural abnormalities. Mol Cell Endocrinol 183:S55, 2001

Nadel AS, Green JK, Holmes LB, et al: Absence of need for amniocentesis in patients with elevated levels of maternal serum alpha-fetoprotein and normal ultrasonographic examinations. N Engl J Med 323:557, 1990

National Institutes of Health. NICHD study to test surgical technique to repair spinal defect before birth. NIH News Release, April 25, 2003

National Institutes of Health: Genetic testing for cystic fibrosis. NIH Consensus Conference. Washington, DC, 1997

New England Regional Genetics Group Prenatal Collaborative Study of Down Syndrome Screening: Combining maternal serum α-fetoprotein measurements and age to screen for Down syndrome in pregnant women under age 35. Am J Obstet Gynecol 160:575, 1989

NICHD National Registry for Amniocentesis Study Group: Midtrimester amniocentesis for prenatal diagnosis. JAMA 236:1471, 1976

Nicolaides K, Brizot M de L, Patel F, et al: Comparison of chorionic villus sampling and amniocentesis for fetal karyotyping at 10–13 weeks' gestation. Lancet 344:435, 1994

Nicolaides KH, Soothill PW, Rodeck CH, et al: Ultrasound-guided sampling of umbilical cord and placental blood to assess fetal wellbeing. Lancet 1:1065, 1986

Nyberg DA, Resta RG, Luthy DA, et al: Prenatal sonographic findings of Down syndrome: Review of 94 cases. Obstet Gynecol 76:370, 1990

Ogasawara M, Aoki K, Okada S, et al: Embryonic karyotype of abortuses in relation to the number of previous miscarriages. Fertil Steril 73:300, 2000

Parilla BV, Strasburger JF, Socol ML: Fetal supraventricular tachycardia complicated by hydrops fetalis: A role for direct fetal intramuscular therapy. Am J Perinatol 13:483, 1996

Pauker SP, Pauker SG: Prenatal diagnosis—why is 35 a magic number? N Engl J Med 330:1151, 1994

Pereira L, Jenkins TM, Berghella V: Conventional management of maternal red cell alloimmunization compared with management by Doppler assessment of middle cerebral artery peak systolic velocity. Am J Obstet Gynecol 189:1002, 2003

Pergament E, Fiddler M: Prenatal gene therapy: Prospects and issues. Prenat Diagn 15:1303, 1995

Persutte WH, Lenke RR: Failure of amniotic-fluid-cell growth: Is it related to fetal aneuploidy? Lancet 345:96, 1995

Peters MT, Nicolaides KH: Cordocentesis for the diagnosis and treatment of human fetal parvovirus infection. Obstet Gynecol 75:501, 1990

Philip J, Silver RK, Wilson RD, et al: Late first-trimester invasive prenatal diagnosis: Results of an international randomized trial. Am J Obstet Gynecol 103:1164, 2004

Platt LD, Feuchtbaum L, Filly R, et al: The California Maternal Serum α-Fetoprotein Screening Program: The role of ultrasonography in the detection of spina bifida. Am J Obstet Gynecol 166:1328, 1992

Poon LL, Leung TN, Lau TK, et al: Prenatal detection of fetal Down's syndrome from maternal plasma. Lancet 356:1819, 2000

Price JO, Elias S, Wachtel SS, et al: Prenatal diagnosis with fetal cells isolated from maternal blood by multiparameter flow cytometry. Am J Obstet Gynecol 165:1731, 1991

Quintero RA, Morales WJ, Allen MH, et al: Fetal hydrolaparoscopy and endoscopic cystotomy in complicated cases of lower urinary tract obstruction. Am J Obstet Gynecol 183:324, 2000

Ramus R, Martin L, Dowd T, et al: Elevated maternal serum alpha-fetoprotein and placental sonolucencies. Am J Obstet Gynecol 174:423, 1996

Reece EA, Hobbins JC: Diabetic embryopathy: Pathogenesis, prenatal diagnosis and prevention. Obstet Gynecol Surv 41:325, 1986

Reichler A, Hume RF Jr, Drugan A, et al: Risk of anomalies as a function of level of elevated maternal serum α-fetoprotein. Am J Obstet Gynecol 171:1052, 1994

Reickert CA, Hirschl RB, Atkinson JB, et al: Congenital diaphragmatic hernia survival and use of extracorporeal life support at selected level III nurseries with multimodality support. Surgery 123:305, 1998

Rhoads GG, Jackson LG, Schlesselman SE, et al: The safety and efficacy of chorionic villus sampling for early prenatal diagnosis of cytogenetic abnormalities. N Engl J Med 320:609, 1989

Roberts LJ, Bewley S, MacKinson AM, et al: First trimester fetal nuchal translucency: Problems with screening the general population. 1. Br J Obstet Gynaecol 102:381, 1995

Roberts NS, Dunn LK, Weiner S, et al: Midtrimester amniocentesis: Indications, technique, risk and potential for prenatal diagnosis. J Reprod Med 28:167, 1983

Romero R, Jeanty P, Reece EA, et al: Sonographically monitored amniocentesis to decrease intraoperative complications. Obstet Gynecol 65:426, 1985

Rosenstein BJ, Zeitlin PL: Cystic fibrosis. Lancet 351:277, 1998

Rothenberg SP, da Costa MP, Sequeira JM, et al: Autoantibodies against folate receptors in women with a pregnancy complicated by a neural-tube defect. N Engl J Med 350:134, 2004

Sahakian V, Weiner CP, Naides SJ, et al: Intrauterine transfusion treatment of nonimmune hydrops fetalis secondary to human parvovirus B19 infection. Am J Obstet Gynecol 164:1090, 1991

Sakala EP, Andree I: Optimal route of delivery for meningomyelocele. Obstet Gynecol Surv 45:209, 1990

Sepulveda W, Donaldson A, Johnson RD, et al: Are routine alpha-fetoprotein and acetylcholinesterase determinations still necessary at second-trimester amniocentesis? Impact of high-resolution ultrasonography. Obstet Gynecol 85:107, 1995

Shields LE, Uhrich SB, Komarniski CA, et al: Amniotic fluid alpha-fetoprotein determination at the time of genetic amniocentesis: Has it outlived its usefulness? J Ultrasound Med 15:735, 1996

Shulman LP, Elias S, Phillips OP, et al: Amniocentesis performed at 14 weeks' gestation or earlier: Comparison with first-trimester transabdominal chorionic villus sampling. Obstet Gynecol 83:543, 1994

Silver RK, Leeth EA, Check IJ: A reappraisal of amniotic fluid alpha-fetoprotein measurement at the time of genetic amniocentesis and midtrimester ultrasonography. J Ultrasound Med 20:631, 2001

Simpson JL: Incidence and timing of pregnancy losses: Relevance to evaluating safety of early prenatal diagnosis. Am J Med Genet 35:165, 1990

Simpson JL, Elias S, Morgan CD, et al: Does unexplained second trimester (15 to 20 weeks' gestation) maternal serum alpha-fetoprotein elevation presage adverse perinatal outcome? Pitfalls and preliminary studies with late second- and third-trimester maternal serum alpha-fetoprotein. Am J Obstet Gynecol 164:829, 1991

Simpson LL, Marx GR, D'Alton ME: Supraventricular tachycardia in the fetus: Conservative management in the absence of hemodynamic compromise. J Ultrasound Med 16:459, 1997

Snijders RJM, Noble P, Sebire N, et al: UK multicenter project on assessment of risk of trisomy 21 by maternal age and fetal nuchal-translucency thickness at 10–14 weeks of gestation. Lancet 352:343, 1998

Sonesson SE, Fouron JC, Wesslen-Eriksson E, et al: Foetal supraventricular tachycardia treated with sotalol. Acta Paediatr 87:584, 1998

Souter VL, Nyberg DA, Benn PA, et al: Correlation of second-trimester sonographic and biochemical markers. J Ultrasound Med 23:505, 2004

Strasburger JF, Cuneo BF, Michon MM, et al: Amiodarone therapy for drug-refractory fetal tachycardia. Circulation 109:375, 2004

Sundberg K, Bang J, Smidt-Jensen S, et al: Randomised study of risk of fetal loss related to early amniocentesis versus chorionic villus sampling. Lancet 350:697, 1997

Thiagarajah S, Stroud CB, Vavelidis F, et al: Elevated maternal serum α-fetoprotein levels: What is the risk of fetal aneuploidy? Am J Obstet Gynecol 173:388, 1995

Thompson MW, McInnes RR, Huntington WF: Genetics of disorders with multifactorial inheritance. In Thompson MW (ed): Genetics in Medicine, 5th ed. Philadelphia, Saunders, 1991, p 349

Tubbs RS, Chambers MR, Smyth MD, et al: Late gestational intrauterine myelomeningocele repair does not improve lower extremity function. Pediatr Neurosurg 38:128, 2003

Tulipan N, Sutton LN, Bruner JP, et al: The effect of intrauterine myelomeningocele repair on the incidence of shunt-dependent hydrocephalus. Pediatr Neurosurg 38:27, 2003

UK Collaborative Study on Alpha-fetoprotein in Relation to Neural-tube Defects: Maternal serum-alpha-fetoprotein measurement in antenatal screening for anencephaly and spina bifida in early pregnancy. Lancet 11:1323, 1977

Van den Hof MC, Nicolaides KH, Campbell J, et al: Evaluation of the lemon and banana signs in one hundred thirty fetuses with open spina bifida. Am J Obstet Gynecol 162:322, 1990

VanDorsten JP, Hulsey TC, Newman RB, et al: Fetal anomaly detection by second-trimester ultrasonography in a tertiary center. Am J Obstet Gynecol 178:742, 1998

Vindla S, Sahota DS, Coppens M, et al: Computerized analysis of behavior in fetuses with congenital abnormalities. Ultrasound Obstet Gynecol 9:302, 1997

Vintzileos AM, Campbell WA, Nochimson DJ, et al: Antenatal evaluation and management of ultrasonically detected fetal anomalies. Obstet Gynecol 69:640, 1987

Vintzileos AM, Egan JFX: Adjusting the risk for trisomy 21 on the basis of second-trimester ultrasonography. Am J Obstet Gynecol 172:837, 1995

Wagener JS, Sontag MK, Accurso FJ: Newborn screening for cystic fibrosis. Curr Opin Pediatr 15:309, 2003

Wald NJ, Cuckle HS, Densem JW, et al: Maternal serum screening for Down syndrome in early pregnancy. BMJ 297:883, 1988a

Wald NJ, Cuckle HS, Densem JW, et al: Maternal serum unconjugated oestriol as an antenatal screening test for Down's syndrome. Br J Obstet Gynaecol 95:334, 1988b

Wald NJ, Densem JW, George L, et al: Prenatal screening for Down's syndrome using inhibin-A as a serum marker. Prenat Diagn 16:143, 1996

Wald NJ, Kennard A, Hackshaw A, et al: Antenatal screening for Down syndrome. Health Technol Assess 2:1, 1998

Wald NJ, Kennard A, Hackshaw A, et al: Antenatal screening for Down's syndrome. J Med Screen 4:181, 1997

Waller DK, Lustig LS, Cunningham GC, et al: Second-trimester maternal serum alpha-fetoprotein levels and the risk of subsequent fetal death. N Engl J Med 325:6, 1991

Wapner R, Thom E, Simpson JL, et al: First-trimester screening for trisomies 21 and 18. N Engl J Med 349:1405, 2003

Warburton D, Kline J, Stein Z, et al: Does the karyotype of a spontaneous abortion predict the karyotype of a subsequent abortion? Evidence from 273 women with two karyotyped spontaneous abortions. Am J Hum Genet 41:465, 1987

Watson WJ, Chescheir NC, Katz VL, et al: The role of ultrasound in evaluation of patients with elevated maternal serum alpha-fetoprotein: A review. Obstet Gynecol 78:123, 1991

Weiner C, Varner M, Pringle K, et al: Antenatal diagnosis and palliative treatment of nonimmune hydrops fetalis secondary to pulmonary extralobar sequestration. Obstet Gynecol 68:275, 1986

Weiner CP, Williamson RA, Wenstrom KD, et al: Management of fetal hemolytic disease by cordocentesis. II. Outcome of treatment. Am J Obstet Gynecol 165:1302, 1991

Wenstrom KD: Fetal surgery for congenital diaphragmatic hernia. N Engl J Med 349:1887, 2003

Wenstrom KD, Andrews WW, Tamura T, et al: Elevated amniotic fluid interleukin-6 levels at genetic amniocentesis predict subsequent pregnancy loss. Am J Obstet Gynecol 174:830, 1996

Wenstrom KD, Descartes M, Franklin J, et al: A five-year experience with fragile X screening of high-risk gravid women. Am J Obstet Gynecol 181:789, 1999a

Wenstrom KD, Owen J, Chu DC, et al: Prospective evaluation of free β-hCG and dimeric inhibin A for aneuploidy detection. Am J Obstet Gynecol 181:887, 1999b

Wenstrom KD, Sipes SL, Williamson RA, et al: Prediction of pregnancy outcome with single versus serial maternal serum α-fetoprotein tests. Am J Obstet Gynecol 167:1529, 1992

Wenstrom KD, Weiner CP, Hanson JW: A five-year statewide experience with congenital diaphragmatic hernia. Am J Obstet Gynecol 165:838, 1991

Wenstrom KD, Weiner CP, Williamson RA, et al: Prenatal diagnosis of fetal hyperthyroidism using funipuncture. Obstet Gynecol 76:513, 1990

Wenstrom KD, Williamson RA, Grant SS, et al: Evaluation of multiple-marker screening for Down syndrome in a statewide population. Am J Obstet Gynecol 169:793, 1993

Westgren M, Ringden O, Eik-Nes S, et al: Lack of evidence of permanent engraftment after in utero fetal stem cell transplantation in congenital hemoglobinopathies. Transplantation 61:1176, 1996

Williamson RA, Pringle KC: Correcting hydrocephalus and fetal uropathy: How good are the prospects? Contemp Obstet Gynecol 30:77, 1987

Williamson RA, Weiner CP, Patil S, et al: Abnormal pregnancy sonogram: Selective indication for fetal karyotype. Obstet Gynecol 69:15, 1987

Wilson RD, Kendrick V, Wittmann BK, et al: Risk of spontaneous abortion in ultrasonographically normal pregnancies. Lancet 2:290, 1984

Wladimiroff JW, Sachs ES, Reuss A, et al: Prenatal diagnosis of chromosome abnormalities in the presence of fetal structural defects. Am J Med Genet 28:289, 1988

Xu K, Rosenwaks Z, Beaverson K, et al: Preimplantation genetic diagnosis for retinoblastoma: The first reported liveborn. Am J Ophthalmol 137:18, 2004

14

Teratology, Drugs, and Other Medications

A birth defect is defined as a major deviation from normal morphology or function that is congenital in origin. Birth defects are common. Three percent of all newborns born in the United States have a major structural malformation detectable at birth. By 1 year of age, malformations or developmental disorders have been identified in 7 percent. This number increases to 12 to 14 percent by the time children enter school, and to 17 percent before they reach age 18 (Boyle and associates, 1994; Kimmel and colleagues, 1993). Most malformations are not inherited, and less than one third of patients seeking counseling for birth defects have a genetic condition (Hanson, 1996). A smaller proportion—about 10 percent—of congenital abnormalities are caused by teratogens. Only a small number of teratogens have been confirmed (Table 14–1).

TERATOLOGY

A *teratogen* is any agent that acts during embryonic or fetal development to produce a permanent alteration of form or function (Shepard, 1998). Teratology is the study of all environmental contributions to abnormal development. Currently recognized teratogens include chemicals, viruses, environmental agents, physical factors, and drugs. Women commonly ingest medications or drugs while pregnant. In a study of almost 9000 Medicaid prenatal patients in Michigan, Piper and colleagues (1987) reported that each woman received an average of 3.1 prescriptions for drugs other than vitamins. In a more contemporaneous study, Lacroix and colleagues (2000) found that pregnant women each took an average of 13.6 medications. Commonly used drugs include antiemetics, antacids, antihistamines, analgesics, antimicrobials, antihypertensives, tranquilizers, hypnotics, and diuretics. A substantial number of pregnant women also abuse recreational drugs during pregnancy. A study by Vega and colleagues (1993) found that 5.2 percent of 29,494 women presenting for delivery in 202 California hospitals were using one or more illicit drugs, including amphetamines, barbiturates, benzodiazepines, cannabis, cocaine, methadone, opiates, or phencyclidine. Another 6.7 percent were using alcohol, and 8.8 percent smoked cigarettes prior to delivery.

The word *teratogen* is derived from the Greek *teratos,* meaning monster. Because this derivation implies obvious, visible defects, a teratogen is most properly defined as an agent that produces structural abnormalities. Many if not most major structural anomalies are easily recognized at birth, and an association with a specific prenatal exposure is likely to be suspected. Many congenital abnormalities, however, do not become apparent until later. A *hadegen*— after Hades, the god who possessed a helmet conferring invisibility—is an agent that interferes with normal maturation and function of an organ. A *trophogen* is an agent that alters growth. Hadegens and trophogens generally affect processes occurring after organogenesis or even after birth. Chemical or physical exposures that act as hadegens or trophogens are much harder to document. For simplification, most authors use the word *teratogen* to refer to all three types of agents.

EVALUATION OF POTENTIAL TERATOGENS. A birth defect in a newborn exposed prenatally to a certain drug, chemical, or environmental agent naturally arouses concern that the agent was a teratogen. The two approaches used currently to identify teratogenicity after a drug is released for clinical use include follow-up studies and case-control surveillance (Mitchell, 2003). Before such culpability is established, specific criteria, as shown in Table 14–2, must be met:

TABLE 14–1 Drugs or Substances Suspected or Proven to Be Human Teratogens

ACE inhibitors[a]	Kanamycin
Aminopterin	Lithium
Androgens	Methimazole
A-II antagonists[b]	Methotrexate
Busulfan	Misoprostol
Carbamazepine	Penicillamine
Chlorbiphenyls	Phenytoin
Cocaine	Radioactive iodine
Coumarins	Streptomycin
Cyclophosphamide	Tamoxifen
Danazol	Tetracycline
Diethylstilbestrol (DES)	Thalidomide
Ethanol	Tretinoin
Etretinate	Trimethadione
Isotretinoin	Valproic acid

[a]Angiotensin-converting enzyme inhibitors.
[b]Angiotensin II receptor antagonists.
Adapted from Yaffe and Briggs, 2003.

TABLE 14–2 Criteria for Proof of Human Teratogenicity

1. Careful delineation of clinical cases
2. Rare environmental exposure associated with rare defect, with at least three reported cases—easiest if defect is severe
3. Proof that agent acts on embryo or fetus, directly or indirectly
4. Proven exposure to agent at critical time(s) in prenatal development
5. Association must be biologically plausible
6. Consistent findings by two or more epidemiological studies of high quality:
   a. Control of confounding factors
   b. Sufficient numbers
   c. Exclusion of positive and negative bias factors
   d. Prospective studies, if possible
   e. Relative risk of three or more
7. Teratogenicity in experimental, animals, especially primates

Modified from Shepard (2001), Czeizel and Rockenbauer (1997), and Yaffe and Briggs (2003).

The Defect Must Be Completely Characterized. This task preferably is done by a geneticist or dysmorphologist. Many genetic and environmental factors produce similar anomalies. For example, although cleft lip and palate are associated with antenatal hydantoin exposure, there are also more than 200 known genetic causes (Murray, 1995). Identical defects with different etiologies are called *phenocopies* (see Chap. 12, p. 286). Determining the origin of a defect with many known phenocopies can be difficult. In general, it is easiest to prove causation when a rare exposure produces a rare defect, when at least three cases with the same exposure have been identified, and when the defect is relatively severe. For example, it was not difficult to show that isotretinoin is a teratogen because relatively few pregnant women have taken it during pregnancy, and one associated defect—agenesis of the ears—is an otherwise rare and severe abnormality.

The Agent Must Cross the Placenta. It must do so in sufficient quantity to directly influence fetal development or alter maternal or placental metabolism to exert an indirect fetal effect. Placental transfer depends on both maternal metabolism and specific characteristics of the drug, such as protein binding and storage, molecular size, electrical charge, and lipid solubility. Additionally, placental tissue contains an array of enzymes, including cytochrome P_{450}, which may metabolize offending substances. In the first trimester, the placenta also has a relatively thick membrane that slows diffusion (Leppik and Rask, 1988).

Exposure Must Occur During a Critical Developmental Period. Gestation is divided into three periods, and syndromes resulting from teratogen exposure are named accordingly. Exposures within the first 8 weeks result in an *embryopathy*, and after 8 weeks, a *fetopathy*.

1. The *preimplantation period* is the 2 weeks from fertilization to implantation and has traditionally been called the "all or none" period. The zygote undergoes cleavage, and cells divide into an outer and inner cell mass. An insult damaging a large number of cells usually causes death of the embryo. If only a few cells are injured, compensation is usually possible with continued normal development (Clayton-Smith and Donnai, 1996). Animal research studies have shown that some insults, namely those that appreciably diminish the number of cells in the inner cell mass, can produce a dose-dependent diminution in body length or size (Iahnaccone and co-workers, 1987).

2. The *embryonic period,* from the second through the eighth week following conception, encompasses organogenesis and is thus the most crucial with regard to structural malformations. Figure 14–1 illustrates the critical developmental period for each organ system.

3. Maturation and functional development continue after 9 weeks, and during this *fetal period,* certain organs remain vulnerable. For example, the brain remains susceptible throughout pregnancy to environmental influences such as alcohol exposure. Alteration in cardiac blood flow during the fetal period can result in deformations such as hypoplastic left heart or aortic coarctation (Clark, 1984).

There Must Be a Biologically Plausible Association. After consideration of its pharmacology and maternal and fetal metabolism, is it biologically plausible that the suspected

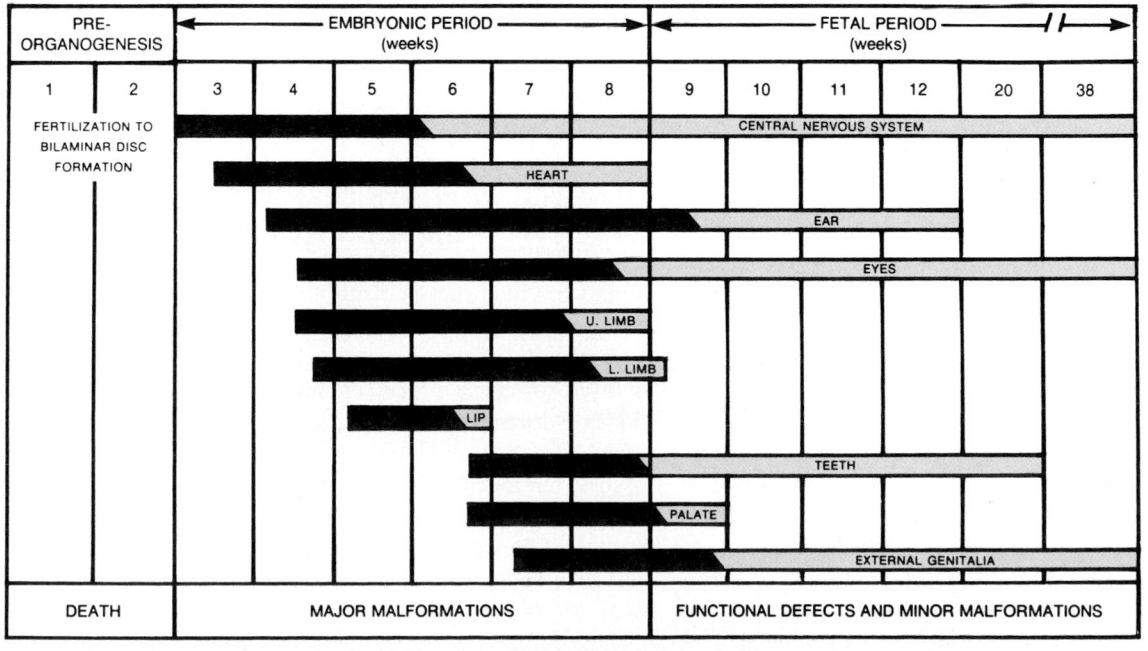

FIGURE 14–1. Timing of organogenesis during the embryonic period. (From Sadler, 1990, with permission.)

agent caused the defect? Because both birth defects and drug or environmental exposures are common, it is always possible that an exposure and a defect are temporally but not causally related. For example, pregnant women frequently express concern about ingesting food or drinks containing aspartame. This compound, however, is metabolized to aspartic acid, which does not cross the placenta; to phenylalanine, which is metabolized; and to methanol, which is produced from aspartame in quantities lower than those released from an equal amount of metabolized fruit juice. Thus, it is not biologically plausible that aspartame is a teratogen.

Epidemiological Findings Must Be Consistent. Recurrent findings of certain abnormalities in association with a possible environmental exposure should prompt suspicion. A current example is first-trimester exposure to some cholesterol-lowering lipophilic statin drugs (Edison and Muenke, 2004). Characteristic abnormalities include fetal wastage, fetal growth restriction, structural abnormalities, and altered neurological function (Hanson, 1996). The initial evaluation of teratogen exposure is usually retrospective, and thus is likely to be hampered by recall bias, inadequate reporting, and incomplete assessment of the exposed population. The investigation is often further confounded by a variety of doses, concomitant drug therapy, and maternal disease(s). Familial and environmental factors can also influence development of birth defects. Thus, an important criterion for proving teratogenicity is that two or more high-quality epidemiological studies report similar findings.

High-quality epidemiological studies are those that are controlled for confounding factors, exclude positive and negative biases, include a sufficient number of cases, and are carried out prospectively. Additionally, a relative risk greater than three is generally necessary to support the hypothesis; a lesser risk should be interpreted with caution (Khouri and colleagues, 1992). An illustration of the advantages of prospective evaluation is the Canadian multicenter study of lithium exposure (Jacobson and colleagues, 1992). Case reports had linked lithium to the rare *Ebstein anomaly.* But when 138 exposed women were carefully evaluated prospectively, there was no increased incidence of birth defects.

Suspected teratogens rarely are evaluated epidemiologically, and as a result, drug safety information frequently is derived from case reports and small series. Nonscientific and biased reporting has contributed to assertions, subsequently proven false, about the safety of many widely used drugs. In many cases these assertions prompted litigation and cessation of manufacture of some very useful drugs. An example is *Bendectin,* a drug that was safe and effective for the treatment of nausea and vomiting in early pregnancy. More than 30 million women used this drug worldwide, and the 3 percent congenital anomaly rate among exposed fetuses was not different from the background rate (McKeigue and associates, 1994). Despite scientific evidence that Bendectin was not teratogenic, it was the subject of numerous lawsuits, and the financial burden of defending these suits forced its withdrawal. Thereafter, hospitalizations for hyperemesis gravidarum increased twofold (Koren and co-workers, 1998).

The Suspected Teratogen Causes a Defect in an Animal. If a drug or environmental exposure causes birth defects in experimental animals, it may be harmful to the human fetus (Brent, 2004a,b). Human teratogenicity is more likely if the agent produces an adverse effect in many different species, especially subhuman primates. That said, drugs under development often are tested in only a few animal species and at the equivalent of toxic human doses, making fetal outcomes difficult to interpret. The problems associated with reliance solely on animal data are illustrated by thalidomide and corticosteroids. Although thalidomide is one of the most potent teratogens ever prescribed, this was not immediately recognized because it produced no defects in mice and rats (Shepard, 1998). Conversely, corticosteroids have been withheld in pregnancy because they cause cleft lip in rodents, even though there is no evidence that they cause human structural malformations (Czeizel and Rockenbauer, 1997).

FOOD AND DRUG ADMINISTRATION CLASSIFICATIONS. To provide therapeutic guidance, a system for rating drug safety in pregnancy was developed by the Food and Drug Administration (FDA). The current FDA system is problematic because many drug ratings have been based on case reports or limited animal data. Moreover, update of these ratings is sometimes slow; for example, oral contraceptives continued to be listed as category X, even after teratogenicity was disproved. Because of these problems, this rating system eventually will be replaced by an evidence-based rating system, currently under development. The most current and accurate information can be obtained from the drug information services offered by many academic centers or through an on-line reproductive toxicity service such as *Reprotox.*

GENETIC AND PHYSIOLOGICAL MECHANISMS OF TERATOGENICITY

Teratogens likely act by disturbing specific pathogenetic processes, leading to cell death, altered tissue growth, or abnormal cellular differentiation. Some teratogens disrupt one or more of these processes, and the effects of combinations of drugs may be additive. Because abnormal physiological processes may be induced in many different cells or tissues, teratogenic exposure commonly results in multiple effects. In addition, different drugs can produce similar phenotypes if they disturb similar pathophysiological processes. The *fetal hydantoin syndrome* illustrates these concepts (see p. 348). Exposure may cause any combination of growth deficiency, borderline mental deficiency, craniofacial abnormalities, hypoplasia of the distal phalanges, and widely spaced nipples. This phenotype also results from prenatal exposure to carbamazepine and is similar to fetal alcohol syndrome (Vorhees and associates, 1988).

Two major mechanisms of teratogenesis are disruption of folic acid metabolism and production of toxic oxidative intermediates.

DISRUPTION OF FOLIC ACID METABOLISM. Several congenital anomalies, including neural-tube defects, cardiac defects, cleft lip and palate, and even Down syndrome, are thought to arise, at least in part, from disturbance of folic acid metabolic pathways. Folic acid is essential for the production of methionine, which is required for methylation reactions and thus production of proteins, lipids, and myelin (Scott and associates, 1994). It is essential for normal meiosis and mitosis. Hydantoin, carbamazepine, valproic acid, and phenobarbital all impair folate absorption or act as antagonists. They can lead to decreased periconceptional folate levels in women with epilepsy and to fetal malformations (Dansky and colleagues, 1987; Hiilesmaa and co-workers, 1983). A recent study by Hernandez-Diaz and colleagues (2000), including 5832 infants with birth defects and 8387 control infants, showed that fetuses who were exposed during embryogenesis to antiseizure medications known to act as folic acid antagonists had a two- to threefold increased risk for oral clefts, cardiac defects, and urinary tract defects. Although periconceptional folate supplementation lowers the malformation rate, women with epilepsy should be given the fewest number of drugs possible during pregnancy as well as folic acid supplementation (Lewis and co-workers, 1998; Zhu and Zhou, 1989).

OXIDATIVE INTERMEDIATES. Hydantoin, carbamazepine, and phenobarbital are metabolized by microsomes to arene oxides or epoxides. These oxidative intermediates normally are detoxified by cytoplasmic *epoxide hydrolase,* but because fetal epoxide hydrolase activity is weak, oxidative intermediates accumulate in fetal tissue (Horning and colleagues, 1974). These free oxide radicals have carcinogenic, mutagenic, and other toxic effects (Buehler and associates, 1990). These effects are dose related and increase with multidrug therapy (Lindhout and co-workers, 1984).

EFFECTS OF MATERNAL DISEASES. The interaction of maternal disease and maternal and fetal genetic composition will determine some drug effects. For example, alcoholic women often have poor nutrition and abuse other drugs. Fetuses exposed to these combined adverse influences are at higher risk of malformation than those exposed to excessive alcohol alone.

FETAL GENETIC COMPOSITION. It is likely that many anomalies now categorized as multifactorial are caused by the interaction of environment and certain altered genes. The most well-known example is the MTHFR 677 C → T mutation, which is associated with neural-tube defects and other malformations, but only when the mother has inadequate folic acid intake. As another example, fetuses exposed to hydantoin are most likely to develop anomalies if they are homozygous for a gene mutation resulting in abnormally low levels of epoxide hydrolase (Buehler and associates, 1990). There is also a reported association between cigarette smoking and isolated cleft palate, but only in individuals with an uncommon polymorphism in the gene for transforming growth factor-1. The risk of clefts in individuals with this allele is increased two- to sevenfold (Hwang and colleagues, 1995; Shaw and co-workers, 1996).

HOMEOBOX GENES. Certain genes are found in all humans and confer equal susceptibility to specific agents. For example, all vertebrates carry groups of highly conserved genes—*homeobox genes*—that share a region of homology. These regulatory genes encode nuclear proteins that act as transcription factors to control the expression of other developmentally important genes (Boncinelli, 1997). They are essential for establishing positional identity of various structures along the body axis from the branchial area to the coccyx. The arrangement of the genes along the chromosome corresponds to the arrangement of the body areas they control and the order in which they are activated. Genes at the 3-prime end control the cranial region and are expressed before those at the 5-prime end, which control the caudal region (Faiella and collaborators, 1994).

During normal embryogenesis, retinoids such as vitamin A activate some of these genes essential for normal growth and tissue differentiation. The potent teratogen, retinoic acid, can activate these genes prematurely, resulting in chaotic gene expression at sensitive stages of development (Soprano and Soprano, 1995). This mechanism has been linked to abnormalities in the hindbrain and limb buds. Valproic acid is believed to preferentially alter the expression of homeobox genes called *Hox genes.* Disregulation of Hox-gene expression by valproic acid may prevent normal closure of the posterior neuropore (Faiella and colleagues, 1994). Interestingly, the affected Hox genes, *Hox d8, d10,* and *d11,* all control posterior structures. This corresponds with clinical observations that most neural-tube defects caused by valproic acid are in the lumbosacral area.

PATERNAL EXPOSURES. There are some paternal exposures to drugs or environmental influences that may increase the risk of adverse fetal outcome (Robaire and Hales, 1993). Several mechanisms have been postulated. One is the induction of a gene mutation or chromosomal abnormality in sperm. Because the process by which germ cells mature into functional spermatogonia takes 64 days, drug exposure at any time during the 2 months prior to conception could result in a mutation. A second possibility is that during intercourse a drug in seminal fluid could directly contact the fetus. Third, paternal germ cell exposure to drugs or environmental agents may alter gene expression (Trasler and Doerksen, 1999).

Some studies support these hypotheses. For example, ethyl alcohol, cyclophosphamide, lead, and certain opiates have been associated with an increased risk of behavioral defects in the offspring of exposed male rodents (Nelson and colleagues, 1996). In humans, paternal environmental exposure to mercury, lead, solvents, pesticides, anesthetic gases, or hydrocarbons has been associated with early pregnancy loss, although the data are of varying quality (Savitz and associates, 1994). Offspring of men employed in the art or textile industries have been reported to be at increased risk for stillbirth, preterm delivery, and growth restriction. Others who may have an increased risk of having anomalous offspring include janitors, woodworkers, firemen, printers, and painters (Olshan and co-workers, 1991; Schnitzer and associates, 1995). There have been no adverse outcomes associated with paternal therapeutic or recreational drug exposure, atomic radiation exposure, or Agent Orange (Centers for Disease Control and Prevention, 1998; Trasler and Doerksen, 1999).

COUNSELING FOR TERATOGEN EXPOSURE

Questions regarding medication and illicit drug use should be part of routine preconceptional and prenatal care (American College of Obstetricians and Gynecologists, 1999). Often women who request genetic counseling for prenatal drug exposure have misconceptions regarding their risk. Koren and colleagues (1989) reported that one fourth of women exposed to nonteratogenic drugs thought they had a 25-percent risk of fetal anomalies—that is, a risk equivalent to thalidomide exposure. Women also may underestimate the background risk of birth defects in the general population. Such misconceptions can be amplified by the referral source, who may exaggerate risk—and even offer pregnancy termination—or by inaccurate reports in the lay press.

Counseling should include possible fetal risks from drug exposure, as well as possible teratogenic risks or genetic implications of the condition for which the drug was prescribed. Importantly, the manner in which information is presented affects the perception of risk. Jasper and colleagues (2001) showed that women given *negative information*—such as a 1 to 3 percent chance of having a malformed newborn—are more likely to perceive an exaggerated risk than women given *positive information*—the 97 to 99 percent chance of having a normal child. Ideally, women should be counseled preconceptionally as discussed throughout Chapter 9. In reality, however, patients often report possible adverse exposures only *after* conception.

With a few notable exceptions, most commonly prescribed drugs and medications can be used with relative safety during pregnancy. For the few drugs believed to be teratogenic, counseling should emphasize *relative risk*. All women have about a 3-percent chance of having a neonate with a birth defect, and although exposure to a confirmed teratogen may increase this risk, it is usually increased by only 1 or 2 percent, or at most

doubled or tripled. The concept of *risk versus benefit* also should be introduced. Some untreated diseases pose a more serious threat to both mother and fetus than any theoretical risks from medication exposure.

KNOWN TERATOGENS

Fortunately, the number of drugs or medications strongly suspected or proven to be human teratogens is small (see Table 14–1). In addition, in nearly every clinical situation potentially requiring therapy with a known teratogen, there are several alternate drugs that can be given with relative safety. New or infrequently used drugs for which there is inadequate safety information should be given in pregnancy only if the benefits clearly outweigh any theoretical risks.

ALCOHOL. Ethyl alcohol is one of the most potent teratogens known. As many as 70 percent of Americans imbibe alcohol socially, and use during pregnancy varies by population. Data from the most recent Behavioral Risk Factor Surveillance System survey indicate an average use of 12.8 percent during pregnancy (Sidhu and Floyd, 2002). Furthermore, although some decline in alcohol use since 1999 has been reported, the amount of binge drinking has not changed. The fetal effects of alcohol abuse have been recognized at least since the 1800s and were first described in a medical journal in 1900 by Sullivan. In 1968, Lemoine and associates reported the wide spectrum of alcohol-related fetal defects, culminating in what is now called *fetal alcohol syndrome* (Table 14–3). According to data from the Birth Defects Monitoring Program, the incidence of fetal alcohol syndrome increased from 1 per 10,000 births in 1979 to more than 6 per 10,000 births in 1993 (Centers for Disease Control and Prevention, 1995). It is one of the most frequent recognizable causes of mental retardation in the United States, a tragedy that could be avoided (Hanson, 1996).

Clinical Characteristics. The affected child may have congenital heart and joint defects, as well as failure to thrive

TABLE 14–3 Features of Fetal Alcohol Syndrome

Behavior disturbances
Brain defects
Cardiac defects
Spinal defects
Craniofacial anomalies
    Absent or hypoplastic philtrum
    Broad upper lip
    Flattened nasal bridge
    Hypoplastic upper lip vermilion
    Micrognathia
    Microphthalmia
    Short nose
    Short palpebral tissues

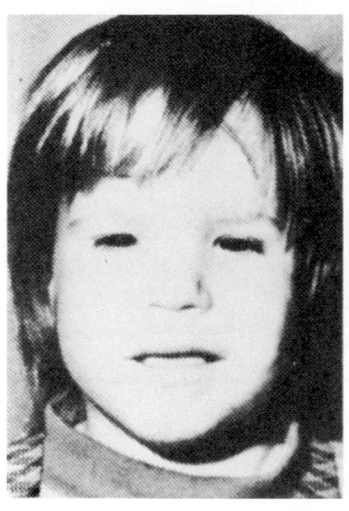 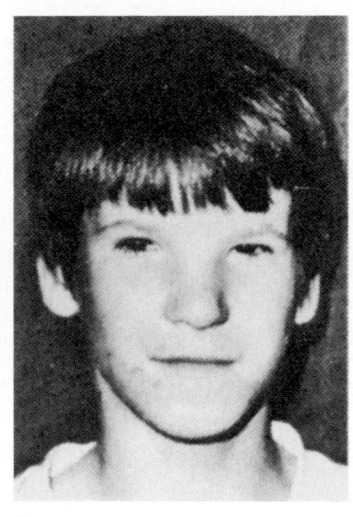 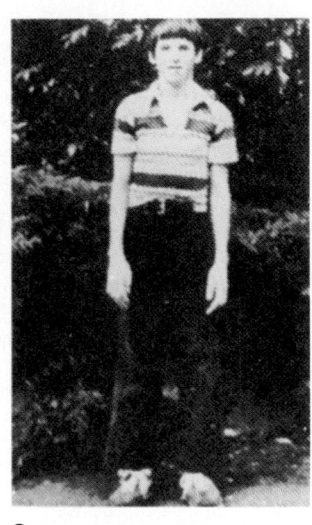

A B C

FIGURE 14–2. Fetal alcohol syndrome. **A.** At 2½ years. **B, C.** At 12 years. Note persistence of short palpebral fissures, epicanthal folds, flat midface, hypoplastic philtrum, and thin upper vermilion border. This individual also has the short, lean prepubertal stature characteristic of young males with fetal alcohol syndrome. (From Streissguth and colleagues, 1985, with permission.)

and persistent irritability in early years. This is followed by developmental delay, growth deficiency, and poor coordination. Other comorbid conditions include mental retardation, attention deficit/hyperactivity disorder, learning disorders, sensory impairment, cerebral palsy, and epilepsy (Burd and colleagues, 2003). The distinctive facial features are shown in Figure 14–2.

Dose Effect. A safe threshold dose for alcohol use during pregnancy has never been established. Current data indicate that women at highest risk to have affected children are those who chronically ingest large quantities and those who engage in binge drinking. This information can be used to reassure women who have inadvertently exposed their fetuses to low levels of alcohol. Although some studies show that fetal injury can result from consuming as little as one to two drinks per day, these studies typically report only the average daily dose and not the dose per occasion, and thus may have obscured the effects of binge drinking. For example, although Jacobson and co-workers (1993) reported that the threshold below which no alcohol-related effects occurred was an average of 0.5 ounce of absolute alcohol per day, they also found that most women with affected children actually drank four to six drinks per occasion. Alcoholic women ingesting eight or more drinks daily throughout pregnancy have a 30- to 50-percent risk of having a child with all the features of fetal alcohol syndrome.

Wass and colleagues (2001) showed that this level of exposure produces anatomical brain abnormalities that may account for some features of the syndrome. They monitored fetal brain growth ultrasonographically in 167 pregnant women and found that 23 percent of the fetuses whose mothers drank an average of 8 ounces of alcohol per day had

a frontal cortex measurement below the 10th percentile for size, compared with only 4 percent of the nonexposed fetuses. Despite these findings, fetal alcohol syndrome cannot be diagnosed prenatally.

Prenatal alcohol exposure also increases the risk of pregnancy complications such as intraventricular hemorrhage and white matter brain damage in preterm neonates (Holzman and colleagues, 1995). Virtually all neonates with the syndrome have significant growth restriction (American College of Obstetricians and Gynecologists, 2000). Maternal age may contribute independently to increased fetal risk. Jacobson and co-workers (1998) have speculated that this susceptibility may be the result of age-related increases in the body fat-to-water ratio and a faster rate of alcohol metabolism in older women.

Fortunately, early cessation of alcohol use may result in amelioration of some of its teratogenic effects. In a prospective study of 60 fetuses exposed to heavy alcohol consumption, Autti-Rämö and colleagues (1992) found no abnormalities in language or mental development in children exposed to heavy drinking only in the first trimester. Those exposed to heavy drinking throughout pregnancy, however, had significantly lower scores in these two areas. Despite this, even low levels of alcohol consumption cannot be recommended during pregnancy. Besides individual variation of "threshold dose," there are confounding effects of maternal age, other drug and environmental exposures, and pregnancy complications.

ANTICONVULSANT MEDICATIONS. Women with epilepsy have an increased risk of fetal malformations. Although some studies suggest increased risk even when

TABLE 14–4 Teratogenic Effects of Common Antiepileptic Drugs

Drug	Teratogenesis	Affected
Phenytoin	Fetal hydantoin syndrome: craniofacial anomalies, fingernail hypoplasia, growth deficiency, developmental delay, cardiac defects, facial clefts	5–11%
Carbamazepine	Fetal hydantoin syndrome; spina bifida	1–2%
Valproate	Neural-tube defects	1–2%
Trimethadione, paramethadione	Craniofacial anomalies, including cleft palate, V-shaped eyebrows, microcephaly, growth deficiency, mental retardation, speech disturbance, cardiac defects	70%
Phenobarbital	Clefts, cardiac anomalies, urinary tract malformations	10–20%
Lamotrigine	Theoretical—lowers fetal folate levels by inhibiting dihydrofolate reductase	?
Topiramate	Theoretical—has produced defects or abnormal pregnancy outcomes in all animals tested, even at low or therapeutic doses	?

the mother is not taking anticonvulsants, others indicate that drug exposure is responsible for most fetal anomalies identified (Holmes and colleagues, 2001; Yerby, 1993). The most frequently reported defects, whether or not the mother takes medication, are orofacial clefts and cardiac malformations. Clefts develop almost 10 times more frequently than in the general population.

Malformations of all types are more prevalent with high serum anticonvulsant concentrations, and polytherapy imposes a higher risk than monotherapy (Dansky and associates, 1980; Omtzigt and colleagues, 1992). A Japanese collaborative study reported that the rate of major fetal malformations was 1.9 percent if women with epilepsy took no anticonvulsants during pregnancy, 5.5 percent if two drugs were taken, 11 percent if three were used, and 23 percent if four were taken (Nakane and colleagues, 1980; Okuma and associates, 1980). Because the need for drug therapy, high serum levels, and multiple medications also reflect severity of maternal disease, it is also possible that at least part of the increased risk is related to the epilepsy itself or some other aspect of the maternal condition.

The most commonly used potentially teratogenic anticonvulsants and their fetal effects are listed in Table 14–4. Several of these medications produce a similar constellation of malformations, typified by the *fetal hydantoin syndrome* shown in Figure 14–3. As discussed earlier, this syndrome results from

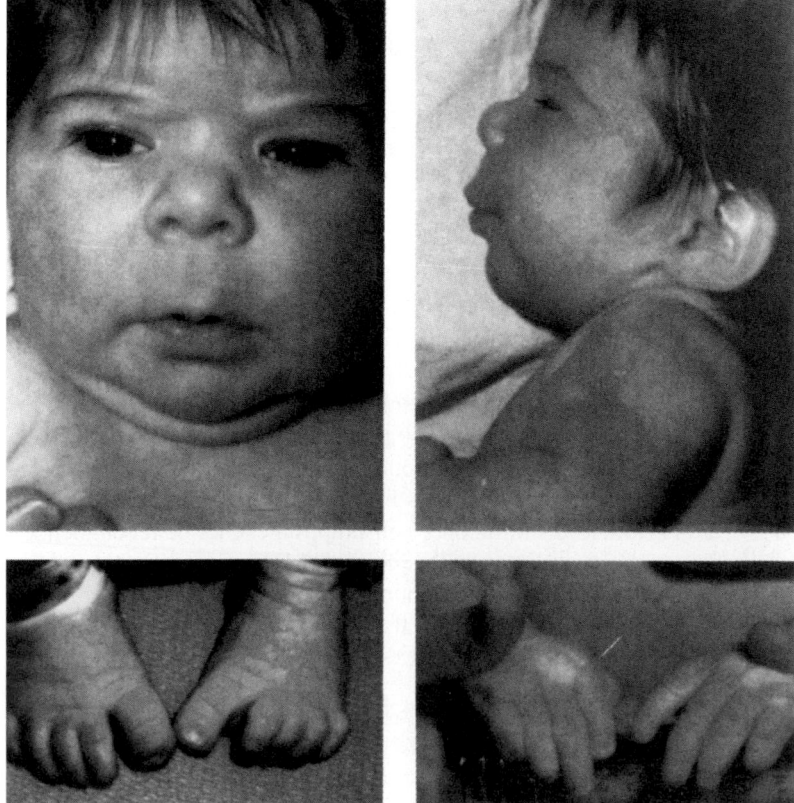

FIGURE 14–3. Fetal hydantoin syndrome. Upper facial features including upturned nose, mild midfacial hypoplasia, and long upper lip with thin vermilion border. Lower distal digital hypoplasia. (From Buehler and colleagues, 1990, with permission.)

the accumulation in fetal tissues of free oxide radicals, which have carcinogenic, mutagenic, and other toxic effects. Data from a Finnish provincial study indicated that monotherapy with carbamazepine did not impair intelligence in offspring who were evaluated when beginning school (Gaily and co-workers, 2004). Other medications, such as *phenobarbital* or *lamotrigine*, act by lowering fetal folate levels and thereby cause defects associated with impaired folic acid metabolism, such as neural-tube defects, oral clefts, cardiac anomalies, and urinary tract malformations (see Chap. 12, p. 302).

WARFARIN COMPOUNDS. These coumarin anticoagulants have a low molecular weight, readily cross the placenta, and can cause significant adverse teratogenic and fetal effects. Hall and co-workers (1980) estimated that one sixth of exposed pregnancies result in an abnormal liveborn neonate, and one sixth result in abortion or stillbirth. Ginsberg and Hirsh (1989) reviewed 186 studies involving 1325 exposed pregnancies and reported that 9 percent of exposed fetuses suffered permanent deformity or disability, and 17 percent of these fetuses died.

Distinct defects with two different etiologies result from exposure during two different developmental periods. If exposed between the sixth and ninth week, the fetus is at increased risk of *warfarin embryopathy*. This is characterized by nasal and midface hypoplasia (Fig. 14–4) and stippled vertebral and femoral epiphyses. Because vitamin K clotting factors are not demonstrable in the embryo at this age, warfarin derivatives are thought to exert their teratogenic effect by inhibiting posttranslational carboxylation of coagulation

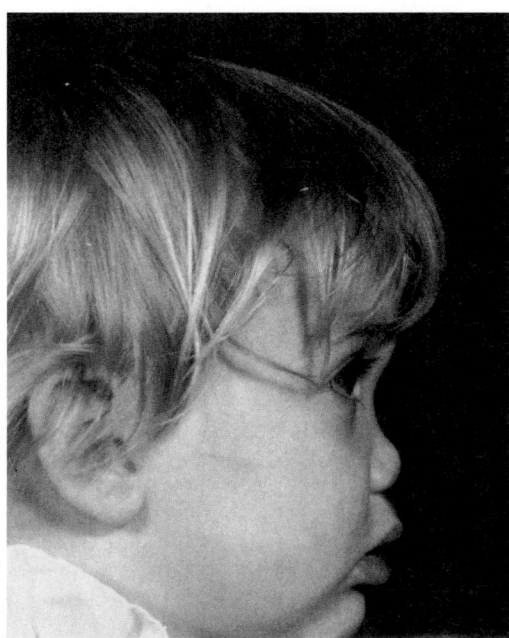

FIGURE 14–4. Warfarin embryopathy or fetal warfarin syndrome: Nasal hypoplasia and depressed nasal bridge. (Courtesy of Dr. Mary Jo Harrod.)

proteins (Hall and associates, 1980). These proteins are called osteocalcins because of their role in embryonic control of calcification, and their deficiency could result in many features of warfarin embryopathy. The syndrome is a phenocopy of *chondrodysplasia punctata*, a group of genetic diseases thought to be caused by inherited defects in osteocalcin (Fig. 14–5). Recent data suggest that the risk of warfarin embryopathy is dose dependent. In a study of 43 women with mechanical heart valves treated with warfarin during 58 pregnancies, Vitale and colleagues (1999) found that warfarin embryopathy and fetal wastage occurred only when a dose exceeding 5 mg was taken throughout the first trimester. In these women, the incidence of embryopathy was 8 percent and the incidence of spontaneous abortion was 72 percent.

During the second and third trimester, the defects associated with fetal exposure to warfarin likely result from hemorrhage leading to disharmonic growth and deformation from scarring in any of several organs (Warkany, 1976). Defects may be regionally extensive and include dorsal midline central nervous system dysplasia, such as agenesis of the corpus callosum, Dandy–Walker malformation, and midline cerebellar atrophy; ventral midline dysplasia such as microphthalmia, optic atrophy, and blindness; and developmental delay and mental retardation (Hall and colleagues, 1980).

ANGIOTENSIN-CONVERTING ENZYME (ACE) IN-HIBITORS. These antihypertensive agents have been associated with many reports of fetal damage. The most frequently associated agent is *enalapril*, although *captopril* and *lisinopril* have been implicated. These drugs disrupt the renin-angiotensin system, which has been shown to be essential for normal renal development. Interruption of angiotensin II type-1 receptor–mediated effects during embryogenesis in experimental animals results in renal papillary and tubular atrophy and a significant impairment in urinary concentrating ability (Guron and Friberg, 2000). ACE inhibitors appear to have similar effects on human fetuses. In addition, they may provoke prolonged fetal hypotension and hypoperfusion, thus initiating a sequence of events leading to renal ischemia, renal tubular dysgenesis, and then anuria (Pryde and colleagues, 1993; Schubiger and associates, 1988). The resulting oligohydramnios prevents normal lung development and causes limb contractures. Reduced perfusion also causes growth restriction, relative limb shortening, and maldevelopment of the calvarium (Barr and Cohen, 1991). Because these changes occur during the fetal period, they are termed *ACE inhibitor fetopathy* (see Chap. 14, p. 343).

There have been reports of cases in which embryonic exposure to an ACE inhibitor has not caused apparent renal abnormalities (Barr, 1994; Lip and colleagues, 1997). One possible explanation for this variable fetal response may be variation in the ACE gene. For example, homozygotes for a 50-base pair deletion in the ACE gene have high serum ACE activity, whereas those homozygous for an insertion of the

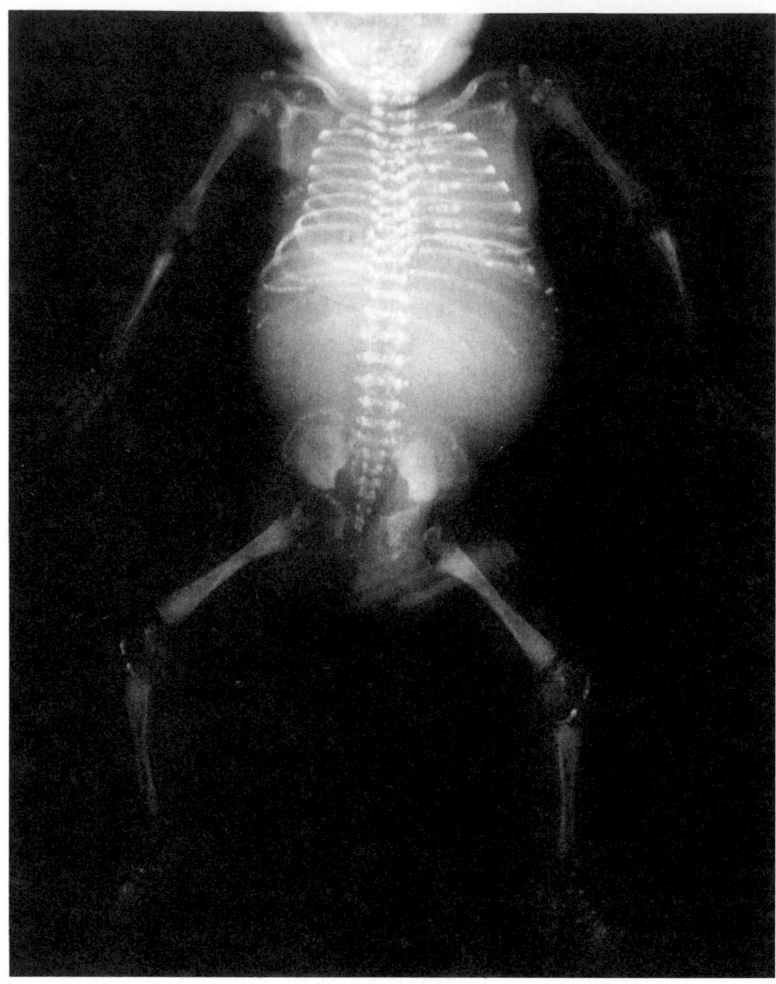

FIGURE 14–5. Fetal radiograph demonstrating the main features of chondrodysplasia punctata: bone stippling of vertebrae; rib ends; iliac, ischial, and pubic bones; epiphyses of the long tubular bones; and patellae. Stippling results from aberrant calcification of cartilage and premature calcification of bone. (From Wessels and Willems, 2002, with permission.)

same fragment have low activity (Lee, 1994; Rigat and associates, 1990). The relationship between ACE exposure and the fetal ACE gene is not yet understood, and ACE exposure during pregnancy should be avoided.

RETINOIDS. Retinoids, especially vitamin A, are essential for normal growth, tissue differentiation, reproduction, and vision (Gudas, 1994). As discussed earlier, retinoids are believed to activate four clusters of homeobox genes during embryogenesis (Soprano and Soprano, 1995).

Vitamin A. There are two forms of vitamin A in nature. *Beta-carotene* is a precursor of provitamin A. It is found in fruits and vegetables and has never been shown to cause birth defects (Oakley and Erickson, 1995). *Retinol* is preformed vitamin A. Many foods contain vitamin A, but animal liver contains the most. It is uncertain whether high doses of vitamin A are teratogenic. Although several reports concerning vitamin A supplementation have associated high doses with congenital anomalies, they have been hampered by small patient numbers, unknown daily dose, and absence of any recognizable pattern of observed defects. Two cohort studies have also

been inconclusive (Conway, 1958; Rothman and co-workers, 1995).

In the largest prospective study, 423 women contacted European Teratology Services to report exposure (Mastroiacovo and associates, 1999). They had ingested from 10,000 to 300,000 IU of vitamin A daily during the first 9 weeks. Only three newborns had birth defects, and there was no relationship between vitamin dose and outcome. Although these data suggest that vitamin A supplements may be safe during pregnancy, vitamin A deficiency is rare in the United States and there is no scientific basis for supplementation. Doses higher than the recommended daily allowance of 5000 IU should be avoided (American College of Obstetricians and Gynecologists, 1995).

ISOTRETINOIN. Some isomers of vitamin A are used chiefly for dermatological disorders because they stimulate epithelial cell differentiation (see Chap. 56, p. 1255). *Isotretinoin,* which is 13-*cis*-retinoic acid, is effective for treatment of cystic acne. It is also considered one of the most potent teratogens in common use. First-trimester exposure is associated with a high rate of fetal loss, and the 26-fold increased malformation

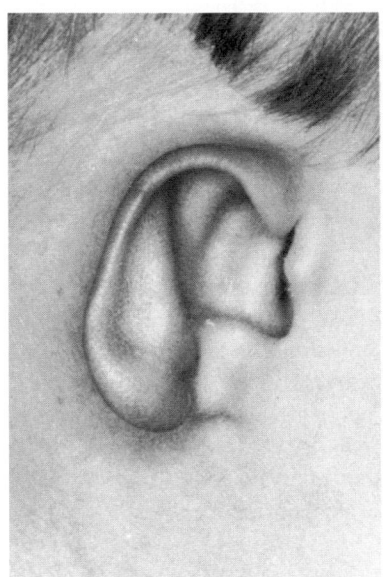 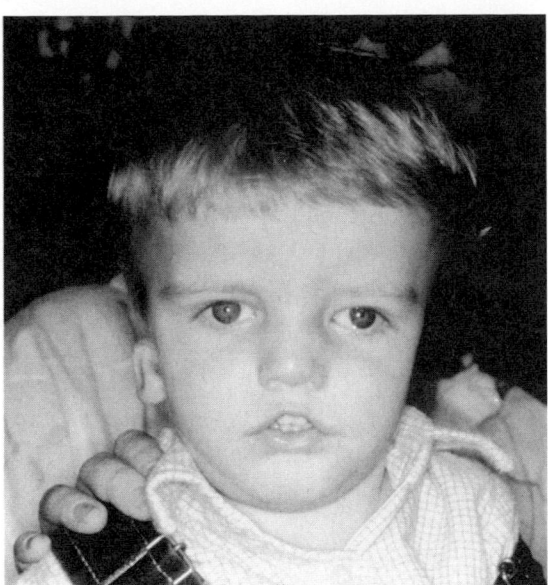

FIGURE 14–6. Isotretinoin embryopathy. *Left:* Bilateral microtia or anotia with stenosis of external ear canal. *Right:* Flat, depressed nasal bridge and ocular hypertelorism. (Photograph courtesy of Dr. Edward Lammer.)

rate in survivors is similar to that for thalidomide (Lammer and co-workers, 1985). Abnormalities have been described only with first-trimester use. Because it is rapidly cleared—the mean serum half-life is 12 hours—anomalies are not increased in women who discontinue therapy before conception (Dai and colleagues, 1989).

Any organ system can be affected by isotretinoin exposure, but malformations typically involve the cranium and face, heart, central nervous system, and thymus. The otherwise extremely rare craniofacial malformation most strongly associated with isotretinoin, microtia or anotia, is bilateral, but often asymmetrical. These defects frequently appear in conjunction with agenesis or stenoses of the external ear canal (Fig. 14–6). Other defects include cleft palate and maldevelopment of the facial bones and cranium. The most frequent cardiac anomalies are conotruncal or outflow tract defects, and hydrocephalus is the most common central nervous system defect. Thymic abnormalities include aplasia, hypoplasia, or malposition.

Dai and colleagues (1992) summarized 433 exposed pregnancies reported to the drug manufacturer. Elective abortion was chosen in half. Of the others exposed before 12 weeks, one third spontaneously aborted and one third resulted in a neonate with at least one major malformation. Importantly, there did not appear to be any safe first-trimester exposure period or dose.

Despite the well-publicized hazards associated with prenatal isotretinoin use, as well as efforts by the manufacturer to highlight these reproductive risks, exposures continue to be reported. A pregnancy test before initiating the drug and a mistake-proof method of birth control such as *Norplant* are now required by many clinics prior to beginning therapy.

Etretinate. This orally administered retinoid is used to treat psoriasis. It is associated with severe anomalies similar to those with isotretinoin. One important difference is that anomalies are observed with etretinate even when conception occurs after discontinuation of therapy. It is lipophilic, has a half-life of 120 days, and has been detected in serum almost 3 years after therapy (DiGiovanna and colleagues, 1984; Thomson and Cordero, 1989). It is unknown how long the teratogenic effects persist, but Lammer (1988) reports that malformations have been described up to 51 weeks after its discontinuation! If possible, women who plan future childbearing should not use this drug. If etretinate is used, Geiger and associates (1994) suggest that women wait at least 2 years after concluding treatment before conceiving.

Tretinoin. This is all-*trans*-retinoic acid, usually prepared as a gel, which is prescribed for treatment of acne vulgaris. It is also available in an oral form, which is used as antineoplastic therapy for acute promyelocytic leukemia at doses 9000 to 14,000 times greater than those used topically. When the gel is used, the skin metabolizes most of the drug with minimal apparent absorption. Jick and colleagues (1993) found no increase in rates of congenital anomalies in 215 neonates born to women who used topical tretinoin during early pregnancy. Four cases have been reported in which first-trimester topical use resulted in fetal defects similar to those associated with isotretinoin (Reprotox, 2003b). In all, however, the doses were unknown and in one case another medication was concurrently used. The oral medication, like other retinoids, is likely to be highly teratogenic although no affected fetuses have been reported to date (Briggs and colleagues, 2002).

HORMONES. The primordial structures that will become the external genitalia are bipotential for the first 9 weeks (see Chap. 4, p. 113). Between 9 and 14 weeks, the testis secretes androgen and the male fetus develops a male perineal phenotype. Because the ovaries do not secrete androgens, the female fetus continues to develop a female phenotype, which is completed by 20 weeks (Speroff and colleagues, 1994). Exposure to exogenous sex hormones before 7 completed weeks generally has no effect on external structures. Between 7 and 12 weeks, however, female genital tissue is responsive to exogenous androgens and exposure can result in full masculinization. The tissue continues to exhibit some response until 20 weeks, with exposure causing partial masculinization or genital ambiguity.

Those areas of the brain with high concentrations of estrogen and androgen receptors are also influenced by hormonal exposure. Hormones program the central nervous system for gender identity, sexual behavior, levels of aggression, and gender-specific play behaviors. The critical period for hormonal influence on behavior is much later than that for the external genitalia, with the degree of behavioral alteration proportional to dose and length of exposure.

Androgens.
An example of the fetal effects from early exposure to androgens is autosomal recessive *congenital adrenal hyperplasia.* Fetal adrenal glands ordinarily begin functioning by 12 weeks, but in this condition, specific enzyme deficiencies prevent the glands from hydroxylating cortisol precursors. Androgenic intermediates accumulate, masculinizing female external genitalia and producing abnormal male genital growth (Chrousos and associates, 1985). Female fetuses exposed early to androgens also develop a more masculine orientation and increased male gender identity (Dittman and co-workers, 1990, 1992; Meyer-Bahlburg and collaborators, 1996; Zucker and associates, 1996). Exposure to exogenous androgens can induce similar fetal effects. In contrast to congenital adrenal hyperplasia, masculinization from exogenous androgens does not progress after birth (Stevenson, 1993b).

TESTOSTERONE AND ANABOLIC STEROIDS. Androgen exposure in reproductive-aged women occurs primarily as the result of anabolic steroid use by athletes to increase lean body mass and muscular strength. The most effective agents are synthetic testosterones, which are taken in doses 10 to 40 times higher than those used therapeutically. In women, these agents cause extreme and irreversible virilization, liver dysfunction, and mood and libido disorders. Exposure of a female fetus results in varying degrees of virilization, including labioscrotal fusion after first-trimester exposure and phallic enlargement with later fetal exposure (Grumbach and Ducharme, 1960; Schardein, 1985). Normal female maturation usually occurs at puberty, although surgery may be necessary to give a more feminine appearance to the virilized genitalia.

ANDROGENIC PROGESTINS. These testosterone derivatives currently are used as contraceptives. In studies of rats and nonhuman primates, antenatal exposure to *medroxyprogesterone acetate,* an intramuscular depot contraceptive, has been associated with virilization of female fetuses and feminization of male fetuses. Fortunately, no association between this agent and any congenital defects in humans has been established. *Norethindrone,* a progesterone-only contraceptive, is estimated to cause female fetus masculinization in 1 percent of exposures (Schardein, 1985).

DANAZOL. This ethinyl testosterone derivative has weak androgenic activity that inhibits the pituitary–ovarian axis. It is prescribed primarily for endometriosis but also is used to treat immune thrombocytopenic purpura, migraine headaches, premenstrual syndrome, and some breast diseases. In a review of its inadvertent use during early pregnancy, Brunskill (1992) reported that 40 percent of 57 exposed female fetuses were virilized. There was a dose-related pattern of clitorimegaly, fused labia, and urogenital sinus malformation, most of which required surgical correction.

Estrogens.
There are many estrogen compounds, and most do not affect fetal development. Oral contraceptives are discussed on page 361.

DIETHYLSTILBESTROL (DES). From 1940 to 1971, between 2 and 10 million pregnant women took DES to "support" high-risk pregnancies (Giusti and co-workers, 1995). The drug later was shown to have no beneficial effects, and its use for this purpose was abandoned. Herbst and colleagues (1971) subsequently reported a series of eight prenatally exposed women who developed vaginal clear-cell adenocarcinoma. Subsequent studies showed that the absolute cancer risk in prenatally exposed women is substantially increased to about 1 per 1000. The Registry for Research on Hormonal Transplacental Carcinogenesis reported that half of 384 cancer patients were exposed before 12 weeks and 70 percent before 17 weeks (Melnick and colleagues, 1987). Malignancy was not dose related, and there was no relationship between location of the tumor and timing of exposure. For these reasons and because its absolute risk is low, some authors categorize DES as an *incomplete carcinogen.*

DES also produces both structural and functional abnormalities (Salle and colleagues, 1996). By 18 weeks, the müllerian-derived cuboidal-columnar epithelium lining the vagina should be replaced by squamous epithelium originating from the urogenital sinus. DES interrupts this transition in up to half of exposed female fetuses, resulting in excess cervical eversion (ectropion) and ectopic vaginal glandular epithelium (adenosis). The Diethylstilbestrol Adenosis Project showed that these lesions have malignant potential, and DES-exposed women have a twofold increase in vaginal and cervical intraepithelial neoplasia (Vessey, 1989).

One fourth of exposed females have structural abnormalities of the cervix or vagina (Robboy and associates, 1984). The embryological mechanism is unknown (Kaufman and co-workers, 1980). The most commonly reported abnormalities include a hypoplastic, T-shaped uterine cavity; cervical collars, hoods, septa, and coxcombs; and "withered" fallopian tubes (Goldberg and Falcone, 1999). As discussed in Chapter 40 (see p. 957), these women are at increased risk for poor pregnancy outcomes related to uterine malformations, decreased endometrial thickness, and reduced uterine perfusion (Kaufman and colleagues, 2000). Exposed men have normal sexual function and fertility, but are at increased risk for epididymal cysts, microphallus, cryptorchidism, and testicular hypoplasia (Stillman, 1982). Recently, Klip and associates (2002) reported that sons of women exposed in utero had an increased risk of hypospadias.

ANTINEOPLASTIC AGENTS

Cyclophosphamide. In the first trimester, this alkylating agent inflicts a chemical insult on developing fetal tissues, resulting in cell death and heritable DNA alterations in surviving cells. Fetal anomalies have been described after exposure during early pregnancy. The most commonly reported are missing and hypoplastic digits on hands and feet. These anomalies are believed to be caused by necrosis of limb buds and DNA damage in surviving cells (Manson and associates, 1982). Other defects include cleft palate, single coronary artery, imperforate anus, and fetal growth restriction with microcephaly (Kirshon and colleagues, 1988). Nurses who administer cyclophosphamide may be at increased risk for fetal loss, but the data are unclear and there are no adequate epidemiological studies (Glantz, 1994). Alkylating agents should be avoided during early pregnancy if possible, but can be given during the second and third trimesters.

Methotrexate and Aminopterin. These drugs alter normal folic acid metabolism, which is essential for cell replication (Sutton and co-workers, 1998). Methotrexate commonly is prescribed as an abortifacient for ectopic pregnancy, and for psoriasis and some connective tissue diseases. Principal features of fetal methotrexate-aminopterin syndrome are growth restriction, failure of calvarial ossification, craniosynostosis, hypoplastic supraorbital ridges, small posteriorly rotated ears, micrognathia, and severe limb abnormalities (Del Campo and associates, 1999). After a review of 20 first-trimester exposures, Feldcamp and Carey (1993) calculated that a dosage of 10 mg/week is necessary to produce abnormalities. This dosage is exceeded during standard therapy for ectopic pregnancy or elective abortion. Ongoing pregnancies after methotrexate treatment, especially if used in conjunction with misoprostol, thus raise concerns about fetal malformations (Creinin and Vittinghoff, 1994).

ANTIMICROBIALS

Tetracyclines. These drugs, including doxycycline and minocycline, may cause yellow-brown discoloration of deciduous teeth or be deposited in fetal long bones (Kutscher and associates, 1966). One acceptable use is treatment of maternal syphilis in penicillin-allergic women for whom desensitization is impractical (see Chap. 59, p. 1304).

Aminoglycosides. Maternal administration can result in toxic fetal blood levels, but this can be avoided by using lower divided doses (Regev and colleagues, 2000). Although both nephrotoxicity and ototoxicity have been reported in preterm newborns and adults treated with *gentamicin* or *streptomycin,* congenital defects resulting from prenatal exposure have not been confirmed.

Sulfonamides. Although these agents readily cross the placenta, fetal blood levels are lower than maternal levels. These drugs can displace bilirubin from protein binding sites, raising theoretical concerns about hyperbilirubinemia in the preterm neonate if used near delivery. There have been no studies documenting an association between sulfonamides and congenital anomalies, even when used in combination with trimethoprim, a folate antagonist (Briggs and colleagues, 2002).

ANTIFUNGALS

Griseofulvin. This oral fungicide is used for treatment of mycotic infections of the skin, nails, and scalp. Animal studies indicate increased anomalies of the central nervous system and skeleton. There have been conflicting reports of a possible association with conjoined twins (Knudsen, 1987; Rosa and associates, 1987a, 1987b).

Fluconazole and Itraconazole. These antifungal agents commonly are used in immunocompromised patients. There have been several reports of congenital malformations associated with fluconazole use during pregnancy. Exposed newborns had skull abnormalities, cleft palate, humeral-radial fusion, and other arm abnormalities, collectively resembling Antley Bixler syndrome (Aleck and Bartley, 1997). The FDA has received reports associating itraconazole with limb defects and other adverse outcomes. Despite this, large cohort studies indicate that neither of these drugs is teratogenic (Bar-Oz and colleagues, 2000; Sorenson and collaborators, 1999).

ANTIVIRALS. *Ribavirin* is given by aerosol inhalation to treat respiratory syncytial virus infections in infants and young children. Pregnant women may be exposed to the drug while working in intensive care nurseries. The drug is highly teratogenic in all animal species studied and consistently produces hydrocephalus and limb abnormalities in rodent models (Johnson, 1990). Although human exposures are rare, the Centers for Disease Control and Prevention and the manufacturers consider it contraindicated for use in pregnancy.

ANTIMALARIALS. *Chloroquine* is valuable as a first-line antimalarial treatment and for chemoprophylaxis. In high doses it is also effective against rheumatoid arthritis and systemic lupus erythematosus. *Quinine* and *quinidine* are reserved for severely ill women with chloroquine-resistant malaria. There has been no increased rate of congenital anomalies in the offspring of mothers given any of these anti-malarial drugs during pregnancy (McGready and co-workers, 2001, 2002). Daily use of chloroquine for lupus and other connective tissue diseases has been shown to cause maternal retinopathy but no adverse fetal effects (Araiza-Casillas and colleagues, 2004; Costedoat-Chalumeau and co-workers, 2003). Second- or third-trimester use of *mefloquine* for asymptomatic malaria treatment has been associated with a fivefold increased risk of stillbirth (Nosten and colleagues, 1999). According to Briggs and colleagues (2002), however, accumulated evidence supports its safety.

TOBACCO. Cigarette smoke contains a number of potential teratogens, including nicotine, cotinine, cyanide, thiocyanate, carbon monoxide, cadmium, lead, and various hydrocarbons. In addition to being fetotoxic, many of these substances have vasoactive effects or reduce oxygen levels.

The most well-documented reproductive outcome related to smoking is a direct dose-response reduction in fetal growth. Newborns of mothers who smoke weigh an average of 200 g less than those of nonsmokers, and heavy smoking results in more severe weight reduction (D'Souza and associates, 1981). Smoking doubles the risk of low birthweight, and increases the risk of a small-for-gestational aged newborn 2.5-fold (Werler, 1997). Women who stop smoking early in pregnancy generally have neonates with normal birthweights (Cliver and co-workers, 1995). Smoking also may cause a slightly increased incidence of subfertility, spontaneous abortion, placenta previa and abruption, and preterm delivery. These effects are discussed in more detail in Chapters 35 (see p. 814), 36 (see p. 859), and 38 (see p. 899).

It is plausible that the vasoactive properties of tobacco smoke could produce congenital defects related to vascular disturbances. Martinez-Frias and colleagues (1999) observed in smokers a twofold risk of Poland sequence, which is caused by an interruption in the vascular supply to one side of the fetal chest and ipsilateral arm. Smoking at least 20 cigarettes a day combined with the use of vasoconstrictive drugs such as amphetamines and decongestants also appears to result in a fourfold risk of gastroschisis and small intestinal atresia (Werler and associates, 2003).

Smoking has been associated with cleft lip and palate in individuals heterozygous or homozygous for an uncommon polymorphism in the transforming growth factor gene (Shaw and colleagues, 1996). When exposed prenatally to cigarette smoke, these individuals have twice the risk of combined cleft lip and palate, and four to seven times the risk for cleft palate alone (Hwang and associates, 1995; Shaw and co-workers, 1996). A study that used the National Vital Statistics System natality data from more than 6 million live births in the United States found an association between maternal smoking and hydrocephaly, microcephaly, omphalocele,

gastroschisis, cleft lip and palate, and hand abnormalities (Honein and colleagues, 2001).

COCAINE. This alkaloid is derived from the leaves of the South American tree *Erythroxylon coca*. It is a highly effective topical anesthetic and local vasoconstrictor. It is also a central nervous system stimulant through sympathomimetic action via dopamine. Cocaine is currently one of the most widely abused drugs in the United States. The National Household Survey on Drug Use, reported by Ebrahim and Gfroerer (2003), found that 6.4 percent of women of childbearing age and 2.8 percent of pregnant women used illicit drugs. Marijuana accounted for 75 percent of drug use, and cocaine for 10 percent. In 1996, the Centers for Disease Control and Prevention determined that 1 in 20 pregnancies was associated with cocaine use.

Most of the adverse outcomes associated with cocaine result from its vasoconstrictive and hypertensive effects. Maternal complications include myocardial infarction, arrhythmias, aortic rupture, stroke, seizure, bowel ischemia, and sudden death. As discussed in Chapter 35 (see p. 814), placental abruption is the most frequently cited cocaine-related pregnancy complication in cocaine abusers, and its incidence is fourfold greater than in nonusers (Chasnoff and colleagues, 1985; Shiono and colleagues, 1995).

The risk of vascular disruption within the embryo, fetus, or placenta is highest *after* the first trimester, and likely accounts for the increased incidence of stillbirth (Hoyme and associates, 1990). A number of cocaine-related congenital anomalies resulting from vascular disruption have been described. These include skull defects, cutis aplasia, porencephaly, subependymal and periventricular cysts, ileal atresia, cardiac anomalies, and visceral infarcts (Cohen and associates, 1994; Little and colleagues, 1989; Stevenson, 1993a). Results from the population-based Atlanta Birth Defects Case-Control Study showed that cocaine use increased the risk of urinary tract defects fourfold (Chavez and colleagues, 1988). Prune-belly anomaly also has been reported (Bingol and co-workers, 1986; Chasnoff and colleagues, 1985, 1988).

Although cocaine has been associated with microcephaly and behavioral abnormalities, there are few prospective studies of its effect on psychomotor development. Singer and colleagues (2002) reported a well-designed, prospective blinded study of 218 cocaine-exposed infants and 197 unexposed controls followed until 2 years. Compared with control infants, the cocaine-exposed infants had significantly more cognitive defects and twice the rate of developmental delay. Cognitive impairments were persistent at age 4 years (Singer and associates, 2004).

Not all studies, however, support the concept of cocaine as a major teratogen. Reports of cocaine-induced limb-reduction defects have been disputed (Hume and co-workers, 1997). One prospective longitudinal cohort study of 272 offspring of crack-cocaine users found no increase in the number or pattern of birth defects (Behnke and co-workers,

2001). Because few reports address dosage or total fetal exposure during pregnancy, it is difficult to estimate the ultimate fetal risk associated with antenatal cocaine use.

THALIDOMIDE. This anxiolytic and sedative drug is likely the most notorious human teratogen. It produces malformations in approximately 20 percent of fetuses exposed during the specific time window from 34 to 50 days menstrual age. Defects primarily are limited to structures derived from the mesodermal layer, such as limbs, ears, cardiovascular system, and bowel musculature. A wide variety of limb-reduction defects have been associated with thalidomide, with upper limbs usually more severely affected. Bone defects range from abnormal shape or size to total absence of a bone or limb segment. Limb-reduction defects may be the result of dysmorphogenesis (as occurs with thalidomide, warfarin, and phenytoin) or of vascular disruption of a normally formed limb (as occurs with misoprostol, chorionic villus sampling, and phenytoin) (Holmes, 2002).

Thalidomide was available from 1956 to 1960 before its teratogenicity, along with several teratological principles, were forcefully demonstrated. Prior to this time, the placenta was believed to be a perfect barrier that was impervious to toxic substances unless given in such high doses as to be lethal to the mother (Dally, 1998). The extreme variability in species susceptibility to drugs and chemicals also had not yet been appreciated. Thus, because thalidomide produced no defects in experimental mice and rats, it was assumed to be safe for humans. The thalidomide experience also demonstrated the close relationship between the timing of exposure and the type of defect (Knapp and co-workers, 1962). For example, upper limb phocomelia developed after exposure occurred during days 27 to 30—coincidental with appearance of the upper limb buds at 27 days. Lower limb phocomelia was associated with exposure during days 30 to 33, gallbladder aplasia with 42 to 43 days, duodenal atresia with 40 to 47 days, and so on for a vast number of malformations.

In the past decade, a number of immunomodulating uses have been found for thalidomide (Franks and associates, 2004). It was approved in 1999 in the United States for the treatment of erythema nodosum leprosum (Ances, 2002). It also has been effective in the treatment of cutaneous lupus erythematosus, chronic graft-versus-host disease, prurigo nodularis, and certain malignancies (Maurer and co-workers, 2004; Pro and associates, 2004). It is recommended that reproductive-aged women taking thalidomide use two highly effective forms of birth control, because thalidomide-affected children continue to be born in countries where the drug is available, despite ample warnings (Castilla and co-investigators, 1996).

METHYL MERCURY. Although not a drug, methyl mercury is a known teratogen. Reports from Minimata, Japan, and from rural Iraq, the sites of two major methyl mercury spills, indicate that the developing nervous system is particularly susceptible to the effects of mercury. Prenatal exposure appears to cause a disturbance in neuronal cell division and migration, resulting in a range of defects from developmental delay and mild neurological abnormalities to microcephaly and severe brain damage (Choi and colleagues, 1978).

Although there have been no recent episodes of large-scale methyl mercury contamination in the United States, pregnant women worldwide are currently at increased risk of exposure. Mercury enters the ecosystem through industrial pollution, which joins surface water and eventually reaches the ocean. Several varieties of older large fish, notably tuna, shark, king mackerel, and tilefish, absorb and retain mercury from the water or ingest it when they eat smaller fish and aquatic organisms. Women who eat these fish ingest mercury as well. Methyl mercury is metabolized to inorganic mercury by intestinal microflora and eliminated by demethylation and fecal excretion. The process is slow, with an elimination half-time of 45 to 70 days (Clarkson, 2002). Women who ingest large quantities of contaminated fish during pregnancy may therefore expose their fetuses to unsafe levels of mercury with the attendant risk of neurological abnormalities. The FDA (2004) currently recommends that pregnant women not eat shark, swordfish, king mackerel, or tilefish. They should also limit ingestion of albacore tuna to 6 ounces per week or to 12 ounces per week of fish and shellfish varieties thought to be low in mercury.

DRUGS COMMONLY USED IN PREGNANCY

Fortunately, as discussed on page 346, only a few drugs taken by pregnant women have adverse fetal effects.

ANALGESICS

Salicylates and Acetaminophen. Almost half of pregnant women use salicylates and acetaminophen. There is some evidence that early spontaneous abortion may be increased with their use (Nielsen and colleagues, 2001). Although two case-control studies have reported an association between first-trimester salicylate use and fetal gastroschisis, most investigators have found no association with any fetal anomalies (CLASP Collaborative Group, 1994; Martinez-Frias and colleagues, 1997).

Because *aspirin* is a potent prostaglandin inhibitor, there is a theoretical concern that fetal exposure could lead to premature closure of the ductus arteriosus. Despite this, and with the massive number of exposures, premature closure has not been reported. DiSessa and colleagues (1994) performed echocardiography from 15 to 40 weeks in 63 fetuses exposed to 60 mg of aspirin given daily to prevent preeclampsia. They consistently found normal ductus flow velocity and cardiac output. *Acetaminophen* also has not been associated with an increased risk of anomalies (Pastore and colleagues, 1999; Thulstrup and associates, 1999).

Other Nonsteroidal Anti-Inflammatory Drugs (NSAIDs). Various NSAIDs have analgesic action, and *ibuprofen, naproxen,* and *ketoprofen* are used most often. *Indomethacin* has been employed as a tocolytic agent (see Chap. 36, p. 871). These drugs are not considered to be teratogenic but they have largely reversible fetal effects when used short term in the third trimester (Parilla, 2004).

In contrast to salicylates, indomethacin can result in constriction of the fetal ductus arteriosus and subsequent pulmonary hypertension in the neonate (Marpeau and associates, 1994; Rasanen and Jouppila, 1995). It also decreases fetal urine output and reduces amnionic fluid volume after prolonged use, presumably by increasing vasopressin levels and responsiveness to it (van der Heijden and colleagues, 1994; Walker and associates, 1994). For these reasons, the drug is used to treat hydramnios (see Chap. 21, p. 530). Most studies have shown that these effects are reversible if the drug is discontinued after 34 weeks (Niebyl, 1991). Case reports have associated indomethacin with other adverse fetal effects such as intraventricular hemorrhage, bronchopulmonary dysplasia, and necrotizing enterocolitis. Some reports indicate that low-birthweight neonates delivered preterm within 48 hours of instituting therapy are at highest risk (Major and associates, 1994; Norton and Vargas, 1993). Studies conducted after neonatal surfactant treatment became available have not confirmed this association (Gardner and colleagues, 1996).

Narcotic Analgesics. Commonly used opioids include meperidine, morphine, codeine, propoxyphene, oxycodone, and hydrocodone. These agents have not been associated with congenital anomalies in humans (Bracken and Holford, 1981; Norton and Vargas, 2003). As with all narcotics, chronic maternal ingestion may be associated with a neonatal withdrawal syndrome (see Chap. 14, p. 364). Butorphanol has been associated with neonatal respiratory depression and withdrawal, and 20 percent of exposed fetuses exhibit a sinusoidal heart rate pattern in utero (Hatjis and Meis, 1986; Welt, 1985).

Migraine Headache Medications. Most medications used to acutely treat migraine headaches cause vasoconstriction. Although ergotamine could theoretically cause anomalies in exposed fetuses, there are conflicting reports about its possible teratogenicity. The case-control study by Czeizel (1989) included 9460 newborns exposed in utero to various medications. This study found an association between first-trimester use and neural-tube defects, but this has not been confirmed by others (Briggs and colleagues, 2002). Third-trimester ergotamine use has been associated with fetal bradycardia, presumably resulting from uterine contractions and decreased uterine blood flow.

Sumatriptan also averts headache by causing vasoconstriction, but in contrast to ergotamine, it does not appear to affect uterine vessels. A study by Kallen and Lygner (2001) of 658 neonates exposed to sumatriptan antenatally found no increased incidence of anomalies. The Sumatriptan and Naratriptin Pregnancy Registries (2002) established by the manufacturer include 316 exposed pregnancies with a 3.8 percent incidence of diverse congenital defects. This rate is similar to the commonly reported background rate.

ANESTHETIC AGENTS

General Anesthesia. All agents used for general anesthesia cross the placenta to some degree. Some local analgesics have the potential for systemic absorption. None of the currently used anesthetic agents is a known teratogen, and exposure during pregnancy is generally brief and at nontoxic levels (Kuczkowski, 2004). A Swedish study that included 720,000 pregnant women who underwent 5405 nonobstetrical operations found no association between anesthesia exposure and adverse fetal outcome (Mazze and Kallen, 1989).

Specific agents that have been evaluated and found to be safe in small studies include *nitrous oxide, halothane, ketamine, methohexital, thiamylal, etomidate, alphaxalone, sodium oxylate,* and *thiopental.* The two most commonly used muscle relaxants, *curare* and *succinylcholine,* likewise have not been associated with teratogenic effects in humans (Friedman, 1988; Heinonen and co-workers, 1977). There have been no epidemiological studies regarding use during pregnancy of *isoflurane, enflurane,* or *methoxyflurane.* Chronic exposure of mouse and rabbit embryos to isoflurane and enflurane at doses resulting in maternal toxicity caused impaired development, but similar effects have not been found in humans (Reprotox, 2000b, 2000c). Older reports suggested that women with an occupational exposure to inhalation agents (e.g., anesthesiologists, surgeons, nurse anesthetists, operating room nurses, dental hygienists) had an increased risk of pregnancy loss or decreased fertility (see Chap. 9, p. 235). Most of these studies had various biases and were conducted before nitrous oxide scavenging equipment was routinely utilized (Boivin, 1997; Friedman, 1988; Rowland and associates, 1992). Exposure is now limited by stringent ventilation and scavenging equipment.

Local Anesthesia. Various local anesthetic agents are used for spinal or epidural analgesia. Fetal malformations have not been associated with exposure to *lidocaine* or the other "-caine" anesthetics (Heinonen and colleagues, 1977). The main concern with these agents is the possibility of associated fetal bradycardia from their affect on diastolic depolarization, or of hyperthermia from maternal malignant hyperthermia. Both could be detrimental to the fetus but would likely not produce structural anomalies (Macaulay and co-workers, 1992; Stavrous and colleagues, 1990).

ANTICOAGULANTS. Deep-vein thrombosis or pulmonary embolus complicates about 1 in 1000 pregnancies (see Chap. 47, p. 1079). As discussed on page 349, warfarin and other *coumarin* derivatives cause embryo-fetal defects and should not be used in pregnancy. Thus, *heparin* is the anticoagulant of choice. It is a group of large (molecular weight 4000 to 30,000), highly polar molecules that do not cross the placenta and thus are not associated with fetal anomalies. Although there are less data regarding the newer low-molecular-weight heparins (molecular weight 4000 to 6000), such as *enoxaparin*, they likewise are not believed to cross the placenta. They have not been associated with fetal malformations, low birthweight, or stillbirth (Fejgin and Lourwood, 1994; Sarensen and colleagues, 2000). Both preparations, however, can cause maternal osteopenia (see Chap. 53, p. 1199).

A number of *thrombolytic agents* have been used during pregnancy. *Urokinase* normally is produced by the ovary and cytotrophoblast, and case reports suggest it can be used safely in pregnancy (Kramer and colleagues 1995; Turrentine and associates, 1995). In two reports of 166 pregnancies, *streptokinase* was not associated with adverse fetal effects (Ludwig, 1973). *Alteplase, tissue plasminogen activator (t-PA)*, is a high-molecular-weight enzyme that likely has no teratogenic risk (Briggs and colleagues, 2002).

ANTIEMETICS. Many agents have been used to treat nausea and vomiting in pregnancy (see Chap. 49, p. 1113). *Bendectin*, a combination of doxylamine and pyridoxine, is the most widely studied, but for reasons discussed on page 344, it is no longer available in the United States. It is, however, available in Canada as *Diclectin*. It also can be reconstituted by combining pyridoxine (vitamin B$_6$) and *doxylamine*, an over-the-counter sleep aid, neither of which is teratogenic (Niebyl, 2000). The piperazines (*meclizine* and *cyclizine*) and the phenothiazines (*chlorpromazine, prochlorperazine, promethazine*, and *metoclopramide*) are also commonly used antiemetics, and none is associated with anomalies (Berkovitch and associates, 2000; Heinonen and colleagues, 1977). *Ondansetron hydrochloride* is highly effective for nausea associated with cancer chemotherapy but it has not been studied during pregnancy. It can be given intravenously or orally and usually is reserved for treatment of hyperemesis refractory to other medications.

ANTIEPILEPTIC DRUGS. Many commonly used anticonvulsants are teratogenic, as discussed on page 347. Ethosuximide and methsuximide are succinimide derivatives used for petit mal seizures. There are no human reproductive studies available and there are no case reports of malformations attributed solely to either of these agents. Information about the safety of newer anticonvulsants, including *felbamate, gabapentin, oxcarbazepine, tiagabin*, and *vigabatrin*, is limited (Briggs and associates, 2002). Based on what is known about the likely mechanisms of teratogenesis of traditional anticonvulsants, some of these newer drugs may prove to be safer for the fetus. For example, none of these new agents has antifolate effects, nor do they result in arene oxide metabolites, and most have minimal or no effect on the cytochrome P$_{450}$ system (Morrell, 1996).

Lamotrigine is from a different drug class but it inhibits dihydrofolate reductase and thus increases the risk for neural-tube defects and other folate-associated anomalies. The interim 2000 report of the Lamotrigine Pregnancy Registry indicated that the drug has a lower teratogenicity risk than other antifolate anticonvulsants (Briggs and co-workers, 2002). A population-based study from Denmark also was reassuring that the drug is likely safe (Sabers and associates, 2004). *Topiramate* is another new anticonvulsant that readily crosses the placenta and causes fetal defects in all animals tested, even at relatively low doses. Human data are lacking, but the drug should be avoided in pregnancy at this time.

ANTIHYPERTENSIVES. Almost 1 percent of pregnant women have some form of cardiovascular disease for which they are given a myriad of drugs and medications. Fortunately, most of these are safe during pregnancy. The majority of these are discussed also in Chapter 45 (see p. 1048).

Undoubtedly *methyldopa* is the agent most widely used during pregnancy for the treatment of chronic hypertension, and its many years of use attest to its safety. *Hydralazine* commonly is used to treat hypertension in women in the latter half of pregnancy without apparent adverse fetal effects. There are no human reproductive studies of *sodium nitroprusside*. It readily crosses the placenta, which could result in the accumulation of cyanide in the fetal liver (Lewis and colleagues, 1977). *Clonidine* is an α-adrenergic antagonist that has been used to treat hypertension in pregnant women without adverse fetal effects (Horvath and co-workers, 1985).

Beta-Adrenergic Antagonists. A number of β-adrenergic blocking agents are used primarily for the treatment of chronic hypertension. These include *propranolol, labetalol, atenolol, metoprolol, nadolol*, and *timolol*. Several are also useful for the chronic treatment of angina pectoris and certain cardiac arrhythmias, and for treatment of hyperthyroidism. Although there is little information regarding their use in early gestation, there appear to be few adverse effects of β-blockers used in the second or third trimesters. There are conflicting reports about a possible association between β-blockers and fetal growth restriction and neonatal hypoglycemia. There are also some reports of transient mild hypotension and symptomatic β-blockade in exposed newborns (Crooks and co-workers, 1998; Reprotox, 2003a; Stevens and Guillet, 1995). Beta-blockers have not been linked to structural fetal anomalies or persistent physiological abnormalities.

Calcium-Channel Blockers. These agents also are used to treat chronic hypertension during pregnancy. Many embryonic processes are calcium dependent and theoretically could also be blocked (Bilozur and Powers, 1982; Lee and Nagel, 1986). *Verapamil* is used to treat hypertension, angina, and supraventricular tachycardias. There has been a report of first-trimester use in association with limb defects in two children, but cause and effect were not established (Magee and associates, 1996). Animal data suggest that second- or third-trimester verapamil use may decrease uterine blood flow (Murad and colleagues, 1985). An association with hypertrophic cardiomyopathy in exposed offspring has been reported (Shen and associates, 1995). Finally, verapamil has been associated with fetal cardiac depression and arrest when used in combination with digoxin for treatment of fetal supraventricular tachycardia (Owen and associates, 1988).

Nifedipine has been associated with pregnancy loss and fetal limb defects, but most reports note no adverse fetal effects (Magee and colleagues, 1996; Sibai and associates, 1992). Other calcium channel antagonists include *diltiazem* and *nicardipine.*

Diuretics. These drugs are prescribed during pregnancy for some women with chronic hypertension and also are given acutely or chronically to treat pulmonary edema. Neither *chlorothiazide* nor *hydrochlorothiazide* has been associated with congenital anomalies (Heinonen and co-workers, 1977; Jick and colleagues, 1981). Thiazide diuretics have been associated with neonatal thrombocytopenia, bleeding, and electrolyte disturbances when given near the time of delivery.

Acetazolamide is a carbonic anhydrase inhibitor used as a diuretic. It also is used to treat glaucoma and epilepsy and to prevent high-altitude sickness. Although the drug has consistently been associated with an unusual type of limb abnormality in rodents, similar defects could not be induced in primates and have not been observed in humans (Heinonen and co-workers, 1977; Hirsch and colleagues, 1983).

Spironolactone is a commonly used potassium-sparing diuretic that has not been widely studied in pregnancy. Acting as an anti-androgen, it causes feminization of male rat fetuses and delayed sexual maturation of female rat fetuses, but these effects have not been observed in humans (Messina and colleagues, 1979).

Ethacrynic acid and *furosemide* are loop diuretics that are not commonly used during pregnancy. Furosemide crosses the placenta and increases fetal urine production. There is some evidence that it stimulates renal synthesis of prostaglandin E_2, which increases the incidence of patent ductus arteriosus in preterm newborns (Green and colleagues, 1983). No adverse fetal effects have been associated with its acute administration. Ethacrynic acid has ototoxic effects in vitro, but there is only one report of associated ototoxicity in vivo (Jones, 1973).

ANTIMICROBIALS. Several bacterial, viral, fungal, and parasitic infections are encountered during pregnancy, and virtually all antimicrobial and chemotherapeutic medications readily cross the placenta.

Antibacterial Agents. As a group, *penicillins* are probably the safest antimicrobials used during pregnancy. They include agents with broad-spectrum activity such as piperacillin and mezlocillin, as well as those combined with the β-lactamase inhibitors, namely, clavulanic acid, sulbactam, and tazobac-

tam. Numerous oral and parenteral *cephalosporins* all cross the placenta, although their half-life is decreased because of increased renal clearance during pregnancy (Gilstrap and colleagues, 1988). No adverse embryo-fetal effects have been reported after many years of use.

Erythromycin is a macrolide often given to penicillin-allergic patients, especially for community-acquired pneumonia (see Chap. 46, p. 1057). Macrolides do not cause fetal anomalies because only small amounts of these drugs reach the fetus. For this reason the erythromycins are not used to treat maternal syphilis (see Chap. 59, p. 1304). *Azithromycin* effectively treats community-acquired pneumonias and chlamydial cervicitis (Peipert, 2003). It also has not been associated with fetal anomalies. *Clindamycin* readily crosses the placenta and may result in significant fetal blood levels (Gilstrap and associates, 1988). There have been few studies of its use during pregnancy, but clinical experience suggests that it is relatively safe. *Vancomycin* is used primarily for bacterial endocarditis prophylaxis in penicillin-allergic patients or for *Clostridium difficile* pseudomembranous colitis. Like the related aminoglycosides, vancomycin is associated with maternal nephrotoxicity and ototoxicity but has not been associated with congenital defects (Hermans and Wilhelm, 1987).

Aztreonam is a monolactam used primarily as an aminoglycoside alternative. It is not associated with either renal or ototoxicity, and although there are no well-controlled human studies, it is not teratogenic in rodents. *Imipenem* is a carbapenem that is effective against aerobic and anaerobic organisms commonly isolated from intra-abdominal and female pelvic infections as well as multiresistant organisms. There are no data regarding its safety during human pregnancy, but it does not appear to be teratogenic in mice, rats, or rabbits.

Chloramphenicol readily crosses the placenta and results in significant fetal blood levels. The incidence of congenital anomalies does not appear to be increased in exposed fetuses (Heinonen and associates, 1977). The *gray baby syndrome,* manifested by cyanosis, vascular collapse, and death, has been reported with large doses of chloramphenicol given to the preterm neonate. It seems unlikely that fetal serum levels obtained from maternal administration would cause this syndrome.

Nitrofurantoin commonly is used for urinary infections during pregnancy. A prospective study of 100 women treated with this drug found no increase in the rate of congenital anomalies (Lenke and colleagues, 1983). Although nitrofurantoin has been associated with hemolytic anemia in women with glucose-6-phosphate dehydrogenase deficiency, we have not observed this in more than 20,000 pregnant women given this drug for asymptomatic bacteriuria.

The quinolones—*ciprofloxacin, norfloxacin, ofloxacin,* and *enoxacin*—are especially useful for treatment of urinary infections. Although there are no well-controlled studies in pregnant women, no teratogenic effects have been demonstrated in animal studies. Fluoroquinolones have an affinity for bone and are reported to be associated with irreversible arthropathy and cartilage erosion in dogs, mice, and rats (Linseman and co-workers, 1995; Lozo and colleagues, 1996). Accordingly, they have not been recommended for use during pregnancy except for the treatment of multiresistant infections. Recently, the American College of Obstetricians and Gynecologists (2001) has recommended ciprofloxacin, 500 mg orally every 12 hours, for maternal prophylaxis after exposure to anthrax (see Chap. 58, p. 1294).

Commonly used tuberculostatic drugs include *rifampicin, isoniazid,* and *ethambutol* (see Chap. 46, p. 1065). *Rifabutin* also is used to treat *Mycobacterium avium complex (MAC)* disease in patients with human immunodeficiency virus (HIV) infection. Snyder and co-workers (1980) reviewed studies of several hundred pregnant women given these drugs and reported no increase in the rate of congenital anomalies.

Antifungal Agents. Vaginal candidiasis is common during pregnancy. Three commonly used agents for its treatment are *clotrimazole, miconazole,* and *nystatin.* There have been no congenital malformations reported in association with their use (Czeizel and co-workers, 2003; Rosa and associates, 1987a). There are no human studies of *butoconazole* use during early pregnancy, however, it is not teratogenic in rodents. *Amphotericin B* is used primarily to treat systemic histoplasmosis, coccidioidomycosis, cryptococcosis, and candidiasis (see Chap. 46, p. 1060). In more than 30 exposed fetuses, there were no congenital anomalies (Dean and associates, 1994).

Antiviral Agents. Experience with use of antiviral medications during pregnancy is growing along with the increasing burden of HIV infections. These agents inhibit host intracellular viral replication through their action on RNA or DNA substrates. A registry chronicling the maternal and fetal effects of these drugs has been established by several drug manufacturers. This registry can be accessed for current information on safety or risks (www.apregistry.com).

Zidovudine, previously called *azidothymidine* or *AZT,* is a thymidine analogue that decreases DNA synthesis by reverse transcriptase inhibition. It is used specifically to treat HIV infections. It has been given to delay the onset of clinical disease in asymptomatic seropositive persons and is used prophylactically following accidental HIV exposure. Transplacental passage of the drug has been documented (Pons and colleagues, 1991). The Antiretroviral Pregnancy Registry Steering Committee (2003) has now acquired information regarding first-trimester exposures, but no increase in anomalies has been seen. The incidence of birth defects was 2.8 percent in zidovudine-exposed newborns compared with that of 3.1 percent in the unexposed control population.

Zalcitabine (ddC), didanosine (ddI), stavudine (d4T), lamivudine (3TC), and *abacavir,* along with zidovudine, are the six currently approved nucleoside (analog reverse)

transcriptase inhibitors (NRTIs). These agents do not appear to cause malformations in animals given nontoxic doses, and there are no reports of defects in exposed human fetuses (Antiretroviral Pregnancy Registry Steering Committee, 2003). These drugs are recommended for use in pregnant women. When combined with protease inhibitors and given along with zidovudine, NRTIs dramatically lower serum viral concentrations, reverse HIV-related complications, and reduce the perinatal transmission rate to 1 percent (Public Health Service Task Force, 2002). This is discussed in detail in Chapter 59 (p. 1313).

The other major class of drugs used to treat HIV infection is the protease inhibitors, including *amprenavir, indinavir, lopinavir, ritonavir, nelfinavir,* and *saquinavir.* There have been no reports of congenital anomalies developing after fetal exposure to these agents. The European Collaborative Study (2000) and the Swiss Mother and Child HIV-1 Cohort Study reported by Mandelbrot and colleagues (2001) found an association between combination therapy and preterm birth. Conversely, a meta-analysis of several studies involving more than 2100 HIV-positive pregnant women did not find such a link (Tuomala and colleagues, 2002).

Enfuviratide inhibits binding or fusion of HIV to host cells. The drug was recently approved for use in combination therapy for adults and children older than 6 years. No teratogenicity was demonstrated in rats or rabbits.

Acyclovir, ganciclovir, and *valacyclovir* are purine nucleoside analogues that inhibit ribonucleotide production. They are effective for treating primary herpes and varicella infections. The Acyclovir Pregnancy Registry (1998) reported the outcome of 1129 pregnancies in which acyclovir was given, including 712 with first-trimester exposure. There was no increase in anomalies and no distinctive pattern of defects. Topical administration of acyclovir results in minimal systemic absorption. There is limited information on ganciclovir, with only 25 first-trimester exposures reported by the Valacyclovir Pregnancy Registry (1998).

Amantadine is used in pregnancy to prevent, modify, or treat influenza infections (see Chap. 46, p. 1059). This drug is embryotoxic and teratogenic in animals at high doses, but data regarding its safety in pregnancy are limited (Centers for Disease Control and Prevention, 2003). Several case reports and case series in which amantadine was given during the first trimester suggest a possible association with cardiac defects, but the information provided is too limited to allow risk assessment (Pandit and colleagues, 1994; Rosa, 1994).

Oseltamivir is a viral neuraminidase inhibitor used to treat influenza. No data on its safety in humans are available. In animals, doses producing blood levels 50 to 100 times higher than those achieved therapeutically caused maternal toxicity and minor fetal skeletal malformations (Reprotox, 2000d).

Interferons are a family of naturally occurring proteins and glycoproteins with antiviral, antineoplastic, and immunomodulating actions. Interferon-α is used during pregnancy for maintenance therapy of chronic myeloid leukemia and essential thrombocytopenia and is effective against some viral infections. Interferons-β 1b and -γ 1b also are used therapeutically. Because interferons-α and -γ 1b inhibit testicular steroidogenesis and may affect ovarian function, they are classified as reproductive hormones (Roberts and colleagues, 1992). Animal studies indicate that interferons have a low potential for teratogenesis. Experience in pregnant women is very limited (Briggs and associates, 2002).

Idoxuridine is a nucleoside analogue that is effective against adenovirus, cytomegalovirus, varicella, and vaccinia viral infections. It has not been investigated in human pregnancy. When tested in rodents, idoxuridine was associated with embryotoxicity and malformations of the eye, palate, head, and limbs (Chaube and Murphey, 1968). *Trifluridine* and *vidarabine,* which were developed originally as antineoplastics, are effective in treating herpesvirus infections, and vidarabine is also effective against poxvirus infections.

Antiparasitic Agents.

Parasitic infections during pregnancy are common, are usually asymptomatic, and in general do not need to be treated until after delivery. *Metronidazole* is a nitroimidazole that is effective for treatment of vaginal trichomoniasis and bacterial vaginosis. Although carcinogenic in rodents and mutagenic in certain bacteria, there was no increase in the rate of congenital anomalies in more than 1700 fetuses exposed to metronidazole during the first trimester (Piper and associates, 1993; Rosa and colleagues, 1987a). In a meta-analysis, Burtin and colleagues (1995) found no increased teratogenic risk. Metronidazole is recommended by the Centers for Disease Control and Prevention (2002) for treatment of trichomoniasis and bacterial vaginosis in pregnancy (see Chap. 59, p. 1319).

Lindane is used topically for the treatment of pediculosis pubis and scabies. It is not teratogenic in a variety of animal species. Approximately 10 percent of the topical adult dose is absorbed systemically, and a portion of this crosses the placenta or accumulates in maternal and fetal tissues (Pompa and associates, 1994; Saxena and colleagues, 1980). Lindane has mild estrogenic qualities, but no fetal effects have been observed. Maternal intoxication from excessive use can lead to maternal restlessness, muscle spasms, and seizures (Meinking and co-workers, 1986). Because of this and its suboptimal effectiveness, some recommend a combination of *pyrethrins* and *piperonyl butoxide* as initial treatment of pediculosis pubis during pregnancy. *Crotamiton* in 10-percent lotion or cream or 6-percent *sulfur in petrolatum* also can be used as first-line treatment for scabies during pregnancy.

Chloroquine, quinine, and mefloquine are first-line antimalarial agents used for treatment and chemoprophylaxis and are discussed on page 353. *Pyrimethamine* is an antiparasitic folic acid antagonist also used to treat malaria. Hengst (1972) reported no increased frequency of malformations in 64 newborns exposed in early pregnancy to pyrimethamine given with sulfadiazine to treat toxoplasmosis. *Spiramycin*

also has been used to treat toxoplasmosis, without evidence of adverse embryo-fetal effects. Unfortunately, these agents neither prevent nor ameliorate all the embryo-fetal effects of toxoplasmosis. Despite antenatal therapy, infected newborns may have chorioretinitis, hydrocephalus, and intracranial calcifications (see Chap. 58, p. 1289).

Mebendazole is effective for treatment of a variety of helminths, including enterobiasis (pinworm), trichuriasis (whipworm), ascariasis (roundworm), and uncinariasis (hookworm), and is used to treat neurocysticercosis. When given at several times the human adult dose, it is teratogenic in animals. In several studies, however, there did not appear to be increased human teratogenic risks (Briggs and co-workers, 2002). *Thiabendazole* is a similar antihelmintic used primarily to treat strongyloidiasis, trichinosis, and cutaneous larval migrans. It also is used as second-line therapy to treat pinworm, whipworm, roundworm, and hookworm infections. There are no adequate human studies, but thiabendazole has not been reported to be teratogenic in animals. *Pyrantel pamoate* is used primarily in the treatment of ascariasis and enterobiasis. It has not been reported as teratogenic in animals, and there are no human studies.

ASTHMA MEDICATIONS. Most medications for treatment of asthma can be used with safety during pregnancy (see Chap. 46, p. 1062). For acute asthma, *epinephrine* and *terbutaline* may be given subcutaneously, as there is little evidence that these agents cause adverse fetal effects. Metaproterenol and albuterol are self-administered by inhalation. There is little information regarding their possible teratogenicity following first-trimester use. Theophylline salts are commonly used bronchodilators and appear to be safe for pregnancy use. *Aminophylline* is the only salt available for parenteral use, but there are numerous oral forms of it that may contain other bronchodilators such as *ephedrine.*

Cromolyn inhibits mast cell histamine release and is given chronically for asthma prophylaxis. A number of studies in pregnant women indicate that first-trimester use does not increase the incidence of congenital anomalies (Briggs and associates, 2002).

Glucocorticoids have long been used for asthma treatment. Inhaled agents, including *beclomethasone* and *triamcinolone,* are now used commonly for maintenance. For flares, oral prednisone may be given as a dose pack, or *methylprednisolone* may be given intravenously. Beclomethasone has not been associated with defects in humans. Two clinical studies that included 101 pregnant women treated with beclomethasone or prednisone or both for severe asthma found no increase in congenital malformation rates (Fitzsimons and colleagues, 1986; Greenberger and Patterson, 1983). Triamcinolone is a more potent teratogen in animals than either hydrocortisone or cortisone, but it has not been associated with adverse human fetal effects (Dombrowski and co-investigators, 1996).

CARDIAC MEDICATIONS. Cardiac glycosides are prescribed for heart failure, atrial fibrillation or flutter, and other supraventricular tachycardias. Although *digoxin* rapidly crosses the placenta, there is no evidence of adverse fetal effects. Antiarrhythmic drugs have been administered both maternally and directly to the fetus in attempts to control fetal tachycardias (Harrigan and associates, 1981; Kerenyi and colleagues, 1980; Weiner and Thompson, 1988). This is discussed in Chapter 13 (see p. 332). *Quinidine* is used to treat supraventricular tachycardias and some ventricular arrhythmias. It readily crosses the placenta and has been given to the mother to treat fetal supraventricular tachycardias (Killeen and Bowers, 1987). The dose used to treat arrhythmias is one tenth the dose used to treat severe malaria and has not been associated with fetal abnormalities.

Several β-blockers may be used to treat supraventricular and ventricular tachycardias, as well as chronic hypertension and hyperthyroidism. As previously discussed, these agents are not believed to be teratogenic. Other drugs used to treat cardiac arrhythmias include *disopyramide, amiodarone, adenosine, bretylium, diltiazem,* local anesthetics (*procainamide, lidocaine,* and *tocainide*), and calcium antagonists (*nifedipine* and *verapamil*). All cross the placenta, and many have been used to treat fetal arrhythmias without adverse effects (Dumesic and colleagues, 1982; Rey and associates, 1985). *Amiodarone* is structurally similar to thyroxine. It readily crosses the placenta at levels that are 10 to 30 percent of maternal serum levels, and because it has been associated with fetal and neonatal hypothyroidism, its use in pregnancy should be avoided (De Catte and co-workers, 1994; Grosso and colleagues, 1998).

HERBAL REMEDIES. It is difficult to estimate the risk or safety of various herbal remedies because they are not regulated as prescription or over-the-counter drugs. Often, the identity and quantity of all ingredients are unknown. Virtually no human or animal studies of their teratogenic potential have been reported, and knowledge of complications has essentially been limited to reports of acute toxicity (Hepner and co-workers, 2002; Sheehan, 1998). Some herbal preparations with physiological and pharmacological effects that could significantly complicate surgery are listed in Table 14–5. Others that have adverse effects when used long term are shown in Table 14–6. Because it is not possible to assess the effects of herbal remedies on the developing fetus, pregnant women should be counseled to avoid these substances.

Several herbal products contain substances with pharmaceutical properties that could theoretically have adverse fetal effects. *Echinacea,* which is believed to have anti-inflammatory properties at high concentrations, causes fragmentation of hamster sperm (Ondrizek and associates, 1999). *Black cohosh,* used to speed labor and treat premenstrual symptoms, contains a chemical that acts similarly to estrogen. *Garlic* and *willow bark* have anticoagulant properties that may intensify the effects of anticoagulant drugs. *Gingko,*

touted as an aid to memory and mental clarity, can interfere with the effects of monoamine oxidase (MAO)–inhibiting drugs and has anticoagulant properties. Real *licorice* contains *glycyrrhizin,* which has hypertensive and potassium-wasting effects. *Valerian* intensifies the effects of prescription sleep aids and anesthetic agents and may cause withdrawal symptoms. *Ginseng,* which is ingested to increase energy, interferes with MAO-inhibiting drugs and promotes hypoglycemia. *Soy* products contain phytoestrogen. *Ephedra,* one of the most dangerous herbal drugs, has both direct and indirect sympathomimetic effects and has been associated with myocardial ischemia and stroke.

Certain herbal remedies are used as abortifacients. For example, *blue* and *black cohosh* appear to directly stimulate uterine musculature. *Pennyroyal* appears to work by irritating the bladder and uterus and causing strong uterine contractions. The drug also can cause liver damage, renal failure, and disseminated intravascular coagulation and has been associated with several maternal deaths (Black, 1985).

HORMONES. Some hormones are teratogenic, as discussed on page 351. *Oral contraceptives* have not been associated with congenital anomalies (Raman-Wilms and colleagues, 1995). A proposed new formulation that includes folic acid may actually reduce the incidence of fetal defects if conception occurs. In 1988, the Food and Drug Administration approved the removal of the package insert rejoinder that warned of birth defects. *Gonadotropin-releasing hormone (GnRH) agonists* have been used to treat infertility and other gynecological conditions. There is little information regarding their use during pregnancy. In a review of five women who were exposed to GnRH agonists during the first trimester, Young and colleagues (1993) reported two abortions and three term pregnancies.

IMMUNOSUPPRESSIVE AGENTS. These agents are given primarily for the treatment of autoimmune disease and for organ transplantation maintenance. Corticosteroids such as prednisone and dexamethasone are discussed on page 360.

Azathioprine is used primarily to prevent reinfection after organ transplantation or to treat inflammatory bowel disease and is not believed to be teratogenic (Briggs and colleagues, 2002). Exposed neonates have an increased risk of growth restriction as well as immune suppression and pancytopenia (Davidson and co-workers, 1985; DeWitte and associates, 1984).

Relatively new immunosuppressants have been isolated from soil fungi. *Cyclosporine* is an immunosuppressant antimicrobial used to prevent rejection of heart, liver, and kidney allografts. The drug causes significant maternal toxicity, especially nephrotoxicity, but it appears to be safe for the fetus (Briggs and co-workers, 2002). Its benefits appear to outweigh any theoretical risks. *Tacrolimus,* also known as *FK506,* is a macrolide antimicrobial that is more potent

TABLE 14–5 Clinically Important Perioperative Effects of Some Herbal Medicines

Herb and Common Name	Pharmacological Action	Perioperative Effects	Preoperative Discontinuation
Echinacea: purple coneflower root	Activation of cell-mediated immunity	Allergic reactions; decreased effectiveness of immunosuppressants; potential for immunosuppression	No data
Ephedra: ma huang	Increased heart rate and blood pressure through direct and indirect sympathomimetic effects	Risk of myocardial ischemia and stroke from tachycardia and hypertension; ventricular arrhythmias with halothane; long-term use depletes endogenous catecholamines and may cause intraoperative hemodynamic instability; life-threatening interaction with monoamine oxidase inhibitors	At least 24 hr before surgery
Feverfew, gingko	Inhibition of platelet aggregation	Potential to increase risk of bleeding	No data
Garlic: ajo	Inhibition of platelet aggregation; increased fibrinolysis	Potential to increase risk of bleeding, especially when combined with drugs that inhibit platelet aggregation	At least 7 days before surgery
Ginger	Inhibition of thromboxane synthase	Potential to increase risk of bleeding	No data
Ginseng: American, Asian, Chinese, or Korean	Lowers blood glucose; inhibition of platelet aggregation	Hypoglycemia; potential to increase risk of bleeding; potential to decrease anticoagulation effect of warfarin	At least 7 days before surgery
Kava: awa, intoxicating pepper, kawa	Sedation, anxiolysis	Potential to increase sedative effect of anesthetics; potential for addiction, tolerance, and withdrawal unstudied	At least 24 hours before surgery
St. John wort: amber, goat weed, hardhay, hypericum, klamatheweed	Inhibition of neurotransmitter reuptake, monoamine oxidase inhibition is unlikely	Induction of cytochrome P_{450} affecting cyclosporine, warfarin, steroids, digoxin, protease inhibitors, and possibly benzodiazepines, calcium-channel blockers, and many other drugs	At least 5 days before surgery
Valerian: all heal, garden heliotrope, vandal root	Sedation	Potential to increase sedative effect of anesthetics; benzodiazepine-like acute withdrawal; potential to increase anesthetic requirements	No data

aPTT = activated partial thromboplastin time; PT = prothrombin time.
Adapted from Ang-Lee and colleagues, 2001, with permission; Hepner and associates, 2002.

TABLE 14–6 Herbal and Dietary Supplement-Induced Diseases with Long-Term Use

Supplement	Alleged Indication	Possible Adverse Effects
DHEA	Aging, fatigue, obesity	Breast and prostate cancer
Echinacea	Common cold	Worsening of autoimmune diseases
Ephedra	Fatigue and obesity	Heart attack, high blood pressure, seizures, stroke
Ginger	Nausea and vomiting	Worsening of bleeding disorders
Glucosamine and chondroitin	Arthritis	Worsening of diabetes
Kava	Anxiety and insomnia	Liver damage
Saw palmetto	Prostate enlargement	Erectile dysfunction
Shark cartilage	Arthritis and cancer	Liver damage
Valerian	Anxiety and insomnia	Liver damage
Vitamin A	High dose: skin aging	Birth defects, osteoporosis, liver damage
Yohimbe	Decreased male sexual desire	High blood pressure, abnormal heart rhythms

DHEA = dehydroepiandrosterone.
From Consumer Reports on Health, 2003, with permission.

than cyclosporine and is used after organ transplantation. It causes abortions and anomalies in some laboring animals, but this has not yet been reported in humans. Documented fetal problems include preterm delivery, growth restriction, hyperkalemia, and nephrotoxicity.

PSYCHOTROPIC DRUGS. Medications used to treat psychiatric illness include sedatives, hypnotics, tranquilizers, antidepressants, and antipsychotics. Some of these are discussed in Chapter 55.

Benzodiazepines. These minor tranquilizers may be required for women who have severe and debilitating anxiety disorders or who are psychotic and violent or agitated. *Diazepam* is the most widely used. It has been associated with an increased risk of cleft palate, limb malformations, and other defects in rodents. Whether or not it has teratogenic effects in human fetuses is controversial, but any effects are likely to be minimal (Briggs and colleagues, 2002; Dolovich and associates, 1998). Other less well-studied agents like *lorazepam* and *midazolam* have not been linked to birth defects. These drugs can cause neonatal depression and somnolence as well as withdrawal symptoms with long-term maternal use or abuse. Also, when used concomitantly with alcohol and other abused substances, there may be adverse fetal effects. In a study of 104,000 pregnant Swedish women, 10 percent of the offspring of women who abused benzodiazepines during pregnancy had birth defects thought to be caused by the additive effects of heavy alcohol use and exposure to other substances (Bergman and colleagues, 1992). *Alprazolam* is a benzodiazepine commonly used for panic disorder. Two studies examining 778 first-trimester exposures found no increase in the incidence of anomalies after antenatal exposure (Schick-Boschetto and Zuber, 1992; St. Clair and Schirmer, 1992). Exposed neonates should be watched for transient withdrawal symptoms.

Lithium salts, especially lithium carbonate, are used for the treatment of manic-depression and other affective illnesses. Reports initially suggested an association between maternal lithium exposure and a cardiac defect called Ebstein anomaly. Subsequent studies found that lithium is not a major teratogen (Cohen and associates, 1994; Jacobson and colleagues, 1992). Lithium can have toxic fetal effects, including diabetes insipidus, hypothyroidism, and hypoglycemia (Pinelli and co-workers, 2002). These can be minimized by monitoring maternal serum levels. It would seem prudent to avoid lithium exposure until at least 6 to 8 weeks' gestation, when organogenesis is completed and cardiac structures have formed (Briggs and colleagues, 2002).

MAO inhibitors are used less frequently today because patients must follow a low tyramine diet and hypertensive crises can develop after dietary indiscretion, as well as after administration of meperidine and some other anesthetic agents. Because such severe adverse reactions are especially undesirable in pregnant women, this class of medication is generally avoided during pregnancy (Mortola, 1989).

Antidepressant Drugs. The most commonly used antidepressants are the *selective serotonin reuptake inhibitors (SSRIs).* The older compounds, *fluoxetine* and *sertraline,* have not been reported to cause birth defects in animals or humans. A summary of almost 800 fluoxetine-exposed pregnancies reported to the manufacturer described rates of early pregnancy loss and congenital abnormalities not different from those in controls. Moreover, there was no specific pattern of defects or a predilection for any particular organ system in the small number of affected offspring (Goldstein and associates, 1993, 1997). In a study evaluating treatment with fluoxetine, there were no differences in rates of malformations or fetal losses (Pastuszak and colleagues, 1993). Because these agents have few side effects compared with other antidepressants, they are a good choice for pregnant women.

Bupropion is not an MAO inhibitor nor is it an SSRI. The interim report by the Bupropion Pregnancy Registry (2000) reported no unusual effects in 90 exposed pregnancies. *Venlafaxine* is another commonly prescribed antidepressant. There are few published data on its fetal effects, but it has not been associated with adverse outcomes (Briggs and colleagues, 2002). *Tricyclic antidepressants* have a long record of use in pregnancy. In the largest study investigating the rate of malformations in more than 1 million fetuses exposed to these antidepressants during pregnancy, no increase in the rate of fetal malformation was found (Rowe, 1973).

Antipsychotic Medications. Many of these agents are *phenothiazines,* which have been used in pregnancy to treat both psychotic disorders and hyperemesis. Most safety information has been derived from their use as antiemetics. Data collected as part of the Collaborative Perinatal Project indicate that *chlorpromazine* and other phenothiazines taken intermittently at low doses for hyperemesis do not increase the risk of fetal malformations (Slone and colleagues, 1977). When taken at high continuous doses for antipsychotic therapy, the safety of these agents is difficult to assess. This is because many affected women take a number of other prescription medications as well as known teratogens such as alcohol, and certain illnesses such as schizophrenia independently increase fetal risk (Elia and colleagues, 1987). Widespread and long-term use of these agents without serious fetal effects suggests that their teratogenic potential is minimal (Briggs and associates, 2002).

RECREATIONAL DRUGS. It has been estimated that from 350,000 to more than 700,000 fetuses may be exposed to illicit substances in utero each year (Chasnoff, 1991; Gomby and Shiono, 1991). *Cocaine* and *alcohol* (see pp. 354 and 346) are potent and commonly used teratogenic substances, but solid data about the risks of other abused substances are lacking (American College of Obstetricians and Gynecologists, 1997). Available information usually is confounded by factors that include poor maternal health, malnutrition, infectious diseases, and polydrug abuse. Several different drugs may be used at the same time, with the combination resulting in a worse outcome than expected with any of the drugs used alone. Furthermore, many illegal substances contain contaminants such as lead, cyanide, cellulose, herbicides, and pesticides. Moreover, substances commonly added as diluents include fine glass beads, powdered sugar, finely ground sawdust, strychnine, arsenic, antihistamines, and even coumadin. Many of these diluents and impurities independently have serious adverse effects on both the mother and her fetus.

Marijuana or *hashish* is used by nearly 15 percent of pregnant women (Abel and Sokol, 1988; Chasnoff and colleagues, 1990). The active ingredient is *delta-9-tetrahydrocannabinol (THC),* which in high doses is teratogenic for animals. However, there is no evidence that marijuana is associated with human anomalies. The birthweight of exposed fetuses has been reported to be lower in some studies but not others (Greenland, 1983; Linn, 1983; Shiono, 1995, and all their colleagues).

Amphetamines are sympathomimetic agents used as central nervous system stimulants, as anorectics, or as treatment for narcolepsy. Various amphetamines are teratogenic at very high doses in mice and rabbits (Reprotox, 2000a). In four cohort studies of 818 women who took amphetamines during early pregnancy, however, the frequencies of major and minor congenital anomalies were no greater than controls (Heinonen and colleagues, 1983; Little and associates, 1988; Milkovich and van den Berg, 1977). *Methamphetamines* are used medically to treat obesity and narcolepsy in adults and hyperkinetic children. These drugs often are used to dilute other illicit drugs. Methamphetamine use has been associated with symmetrical fetal growth restriction but does not appear to increase the frequency of congenital anomalies (Little and colleagues, 1988; Ramin and associates, 1992). Methylamphetamine, known as s*peed, ice, crank,* and *crystal meth,* produces defects in mice, rats, and rabbits, but has not been associated with defects in humans.

In most studies, the frequency of congenital anomalies is not higher among neonates born to mothers addicted to heroin (Little and associates, 1990b). In one cohort study of 830 exposed neonates, the frequency of anomalies was 2.4 percent, similar to the background risk (Ostrea and Chavez, 1979). Other types of morbidity, such as fetal growth restriction, perinatal death, and several perinatal complications, are common in the offspring of narcotic-addicted mothers (Lifschitz and colleagues, 1983; Little and co-workers, 1990b). It is not clear whether these complications are due to fetal heroin exposure or to generally poor maternal health. Postnatal growth of these children appears to be normal in most cases, although the average head circumference is smaller than that of unexposed children, and there may be mild developmental delay or behavioral disturbances (Chasnoff and colleagues, 1986; Lifschitz and co-workers, 1983). Withdrawal symptoms such as tremors, irritability, sneezing, vomiting, fever, diarrhea,

and occasionally seizures are observed in 40 to 80 percent of newborns born to heroin-addicted women (Alroomi and colleagues, 1988). Although these symptoms may be prolonged, they usually persist for fewer than 10 days. Abnormal respiratory function during sleep often persists and may be a factor in the increased incidence of sudden infant death syndrome in exposed newborns (Kandall and associates, 1993).

Methadone, a synthetic opiate narcotic that structurally resembles propoxyphene, is used primarily as maintenance therapy for narcotic addiction. Although large doses are teratogenic in rodents, congenital anomalies were not increased above background in cohort studies and clinical series of neonates born to women on methadone maintenance (Stimmel and Adamsons, 1976). Withdrawal symptoms, however, are frequent and birthweights are often lower than expected (Briggs and colleagues, 2002). Chasnoff and co-workers (1987) compared 52 cocaine-using pregnant women with 73 women who were former heroin addicts maintained on methadone and found a significantly higher rate of preterm labor, rapid labor, abruptio placentae, and meconium staining among cocaine users. Withdrawal from methadone is more severe than from heroin and more protracted—up to 3 weeks—due to the much longer half-life of methadone.

Lysergic acid amides, classically known as *lysergic acid diethylamide (LSD),* are amine alkaloids obtained only through chemical synthesis. There is no evidence that this drug is a human teratogen. Some investigators have found increased frequencies of chromosomal breakage in somatic cells of mothers who used lysergic acid as well as in their prenatally exposed newborns, but such breakage does not appear to correlate with an increased risk for congenital anomalies.

Phencyclidine (PCP), known as *angel dust,* is not associated with congenital anomalies. Neonatal withdrawal, characterized by tremors, jitteriness, and irritability, is observed in more than half of exposed newborns. Golden and colleagues (1987) reported that the incidence of structural malformations was not increased in 94 phencyclidine-exposed infants, but confirmed an increased incidence of newborn behavioral and developmental abnormalities.

"T's and blues" is a street mixture of the narcotic analgesic *pentazocine (Talwin)* and the over-the-counter antihistamine *tripelennamine (Pyribenzamine).* It has not been associated with an increased incidence of congenital anomalies (Little and co-workers, 1990a; von Almen and Miller, 1984).

REFERENCES

Abel EL, Sokol RJ: Marijuana and cocaine use during pregnancy. In Niebyl J (ed): Drug Use in Pregnancy, 2nd ed. Philadelphia, Lea and Febiger, 1988, p 223

Acyclovir Pregnancy Registry: Interim report. Project office. Glaxo Wellcome, Research Triangle Park, NC, July 31, 1998

Aleck KA, Bartley DL: Multiple malformation syndrome following fluconazole use in pregnancy: Report of an additional patient. Am J Med Genet 72:253, 1997

Alroomi LG, Davidson J, Evans TJ, et al: Maternal narcotic abuse and the newborn. Arch Dis Child 63:81, 1988

American College of Obstetricians and Gynecologists: Anthrax. ACOG Guidelines, November 8, 2001.

American College of Obstetricians and Gynecologists: Intrauterine growth restriction. Practice Bulletin No. 12, January 2000

American College of Obstetricians and Gynecologists: Psychosocial risk factors: Perinatal screening and intervention. Educational Bulletin No. 255, November 1999

American College of Obstetricians and Gynecologists: Teratology. Educational Bulletin No. 236, April 1997

American College of Obstetricians and Gynecologists: Vitamin A supplementation during pregnancy. Committee Opinion No. 157, September 1995

Ances BM: New concerns about thalidomide. Obstet Gynecol 99:125, 2002

Ang-Lee MK, Moss J, Yuan CS: Herbal medicines and perioperative care. JAMA 286:208, 2001

Antiretroviral Pregnancy Registry Steering Committee: Antiretroviral Pregnancy Registry International Interim Report for 1 Jan 1989–31 Jan 2003. May 2003

Araiza-Casillas R, Cardenas F, Morales Y, et al: Factors associated with chloroquine-induced retinopathy in rheumatic diseases. Lupus 13:119, 2004

Autti-Rämö I, Korkman M, Hilakivi-Clarke L, et al: Mental development of 2-year-old children exposed to alcohol in utero. J Pediatr 120:740, 1992

Bar-Oz B, Moretti ME, Bishai R, et al: Pregnancy outcome after in utero exposure to itraconazole: A prospective cohort study. Am J Obstet Gynecol 183:617, 2000

Barr M Jr: Teratogen update: Angiotensin-converting enzyme inhibitors. Teratology 50:399, 1994

Barr M, Cohen MM: ACE inhibitor fetopathy and hypocalvaria: The kidney-skull connection. Teratology 44:485, 1991

Behnke M, Eyler FD, Garvan CW, et al: The search for congenital malformations in newborns with fetal cocaine exposure. Pediatrics 107:E74, 2001

Bergman U, Rosa FZ, Baum C, et al: Effects of exposure to benzodiazepine during fetal life. Lancet 340:694, 1992

Berkovitch M, Elbirt D, Addis A, et al: Fetal effects of metoclopramide therapy for nausea and vomiting of pregnancy. N Engl J Med 343:445, 2000

Bilozur M, Powers RD: Two sites for calcium action in compaction of the mouse embryo. Exp Cell Res 142:39, 1982

Bingol N, Fuchs M, Holipas N, et al: Prune belly syndrome associated with maternal cocaine abuse. Am J Hum Genet 39:A51, 1986

Black DR: Pregnancy unaffected by pennyroyal usage. J Am Osteopath Assoc 85:282, 1985

Boivin JF: Risk of spontaneous abortion in women occupationally exposed to anaesthetic gases: A meta-analysis. Occup Environ Med 54:541, 1997

Boncinelli E: Homeobox genes and disease. Curr Opin Genet Dev 7:331, 1997

Boyle CA, Deccoufle PK, Yeargig-Allsopp M: Prevalence and health impact of developmental disabilities in US children. Pediatrics 93:399, 1994

Bracken MB, Holford TR: Exposure to prescribed drugs in pregnancy and association with congenital malformations. Obstet Gynecol 58:336, 1981

Brent RL: Environmental causes of human congenital malformations: the pediatrician's role in dealing with these complex clinical problems caused by a multiplicity of environmental and genetic factors. Pediatrics 113:957, 2004a

Brent RL: Utilization of animal studies to determine the effects and human risks of environmental toxicants (drugs, chemicals, and physical agents). Pediatrics 113:984, 2004b

Briggs GG, Freeman RK, Yaffe SJ: Drugs in Pregnancy and Lactation, 6th ed. Baltimore, Williams and Wilkins, 2002

Brunskill PJ: The effects of fetal exposure to danazol. Br J Obstet Gynaecol 99:212, 1992

Buehler BA, Delimont D, van Waes M, et al: Prenatal prediction of risk of the fetal hydantoin syndrome. N Engl J Med 322:1567, 1990

Bupropion Pregnancy Registry. Interim Report, 1 September 1997 through 31 August 2000. Glaxo Wellcome, December 2000

Burd L, Cotsonas-Hassler TM, Martsolf JT, et al: Recognition and management of fetal alcohol syndrome. Neurotoxicol Teratol 25:681, 2003

Burtin P, Taddio A, Ariburnu O, et al: Safety of metronidazole in pregnancy: A meta-analysis. Am J Obstet Gynecol 172:525, 1995

Castilla EE, Ashton-Prolla O, Barreda-Mejia E, et al: Thalidomide, a current teratogen in South America. Teratology 54:273, 1996

Centers for Disease Control and Prevention: Antiviral agents for influenza: Background information for clinicians. CDC Fact Sheet, December 16, 2003

Centers for Disease Control and Prevention: Sexually-transmitted diseases: Treatment guidelines. MMWR 51:42, 2002

Centers for Disease Control and Prevention: Centers for Disease Control Vietnam Experience Study. Health status of Vietnam veterans III. Reproductive outcomes and child health. JAMA 259:2715, 1998

Centers for Disease Control and Prevention: Population based prevalence of perinatal exposure to cocaine—Georgia, 1994. MMWR 45:887, 1996

Centers for Disease Control and Prevention: Update: Trends in fetal alcohol syndrome United States, 1979–1993. MMWR 44:249, 1995

Chasnoff IJ: Drugs, alcohol, pregnancy, and the neonate: Pay now or pay later. JAMA 266:1567, 1991

Chasnoff IJ, Burns KA, Burns WJ: Cocaine use in pregnancy: Perinatal morbidity and mortality. Neurotoxicol Teratol 9:291, 1987

Chasnoff IJ, Burns KA, Burns WJ, et al: Prenatal drug exposure: Effects on neonatal and infant growth development. Neurotoxicol Teratol 8:357, 1986

Chasnoff IJ, Burns WJ, Schnoll SH, et al: Cocaine use in pregnancy. N Engl J Med 313:666, 1985

Chasnoff IJ, Chisum GM, Kaplan WE: Maternal cocaine use and genitourinary tract malformations. Teratology 37:201, 1988

Chasnoff IJ, Landress HJ, Barrett ME: The prevalence of illicit drug or alcohol use during pregnancy and the discrepancies in mandatory reporting in Pinellas County, Florida. N Engl J Med 322:1202, 1990

Chaube S, Murphy ML: The teratogenic effects of the recent drugs active in cancer chemotherapy. Adv Teratol 3:181, 1968

Chavez GF, Mulinare J, Cordero JF: Maternal cocaine use and the risk for genitourinary tract defects: An epidemiologic approach. Am J Hum Genet 43:A43, 1988

Choi BH, Lapham LW, Amin-Zaki L, et al: Abnormal neuronal migration, deranged cerebellar cortical organization, and diffuse white matter astrocytosis of human fetal brain. A major effect of methyl mercury poisoning in utero. J Neuropathol Neurol 37:719, 1978

Chrousos GP, Evans MI, Loriaux DL, et al: Prenatal therapy in congenital adrenal hyperplasia. Attempted prevention of abnormal external genital masculinization by pharmacologic suppression of the fetal adrenal gland in utero. Ann N Y Acad Sci 458:156, 1985

Clark EB: Neck web and congenital heart defects: A pathogenic association in 45 X-O Turner syndrome? Teratology 29:355, 1984

Clarkson TW: The three modern faces of mercury. Environ Health Perspect 110:11, 2002

CLASP Collaborative Group: CLASP: A randomized trial of low-dose aspirin for the prevention and treatment of preeclampsia among 9364 pregnant women. Lancet 343:619, 1994

Clayton-Smith J, Donnai D: Human malformations. In Rimoin DL, Connor JM, Pyeritz RE (eds): Emery and Rimoin's Principles and Practice of Medical Genetics, 3rd ed. New York, Churchill Livingstone, 1996, p 383

Cliver SP, Goldenberg RL, Lutter R, et al: The effect of cigarette smoking on neonatal anthropometric measurements. Obstet Gynecol 85:625, 1995

Cohen HL, Sloves JH, Laungani S, et al: Neurosonographic findings in full-term infants born to maternal cocaine abusers: Visualization of subependymal and periventricular cysts. J Clin Ultrasound 22:327, 1994a

Cohen LS, Friedman JM, Jefferson JW, et al: A reevaluation of risk of in utero exposure to lithium. JAMA 271:1485, 1994b

Consumer Reports on Health: When good drugs do bad things. Consumer Reports on Health, July 2003, p 8

Conway H: Effect of supplemental vitamin therapy on the limitation of incidence of cleft lip and cleft palate in humans. Plast Reconstr Surg 22:450, 1958

Costedoat-Chalumeau N, Amoura Z, Duhaut P, et al: Safety of hydroxychloroquine in pregnant patients with connective tissue diseases: A study of one hundred thirty-three cases compared with a control group. Arthritis Rheum 48:3207, 2003

Creinin MD, Vittinghoff E: Methotrexate and misoprostol vs misoprostol alone for early abortion: A randomized controlled trial. JAMA 272:1190, 1994

Crooks BN, Deshpande SA, Hall C, et al: Adverse neonatal effects of maternal labetalol treatment. Arch Dis Child Fetal Neonatal Ed 79:150, 1998

Czeizel A: Teratogenicity of ergotamine. J Med Genet 26:69, 1989

Czeizel AE, Kazy Z, Puho E: A population-based case-control teratological study of oral nystatin treatment during pregnancy. Scand J Infect Dis 35:830, 2003

Czeizel AE, Rockenbauer M: Population-based case-control study of teratogenic potential of corticosteroids. Teratology 56:335, 1997

D'Souza SW, Black P, Richards B: Smoking in pregnancy: Associations with skinfold thickness, maternal weight gain, and fetal size at birth. BMJ 282:1661, 1981

Dai WS, Hsu MA, Itri LM: Safety of pregnancy after discontinuation of isotretinoin. Arch Dermatol 125:362, 1989

Dai WS, LaBraico JM, Stern RS: Epidemiology of isotretinoin exposure during pregnancy. J Am Acad Dermatol 26:599, 1992

Dally A: Thalidomide: Was the tragedy preventable? Lancet 351:1197, 1998

Dansky LV, Andermann E, Rosenblatt D, et al: Anticonvulsants, folate levels, and pregnancy outcome: A prospective study. Ann Neurol 21:176, 1987

Dansky LV, Andermann E, Sherwin AL, et al: Maternal epilepsy and congenital malformations: A prospective study with monitoring of plasma anticonvulsant levels during pregnancy. Neurology 3:15, 1980

Davidson JM, Dallagrammatikas H, Parkin JM: Maternal azathioprine therapy and depressed hemopoiesis in the babies of renal allograft patients. Br J Obstet Gynaecol 92:233, 1985

De Catte L, De Wolf D, Smitz J, et al: Fetal hypothyroidism as a complication of amiodarone treatment for persistent fetal supraventricular tachycardia. Prenat Diagn 14:762, 1994

Dean JL, Wolf JE, Ranzini AC, et al: Use of amphotericin B during pregnancy: Case report and review. Clin Infect Dis 18:364, 1994

Del Campo M, Kosaki K, Bennett FC, et al: Developmental delay in fetal aminopterin/methotrexate syndrome. Teratology 60:10, 1999

DeWitte DB, Buick MK, Cyran SE, et al: Neonatal pancytopenia and severe combined immunodeficiency associated with antenatal administration of azathioprine and prednisone. J Pediatr 105:625, 1984

DiGiovanna JJ, Zezh LA, Ruddel ME, et al: Etretinate: Persistent serum levels of a potent teratogen. Clin Res 32:579A, 1984

DiSessa TG, Moretti ML, Khouri A, et al: Cardiac function in fetuses and newborns exposed to low dose aspirin during pregnancy. Am J Obstet Gynecol 171:892, 1994

Dittman RW, Kappes ME, Kappes MH: Sexual behavior in adolescent and adult females with congenital adrenal hyperplasia. Psychoneuroendocrinology 17:153, 1992

Dittman RW, Kappes MH, Kappes ME, et al: Congenital adrenal hyperplasia I: Gender-related behavior and attitudes in female patients and sisters. Psychoneuroendocrinology 15:401, 1990

Dolovich IR, Addis A, Vaillancourt JMR, et al: Benzodiazepine use in pregnancy and major malformations or oral cleft: Meta-analysis of cohort and case-control studies. BMJ 317:839, 1998

Dombrowski MP, Brown CL, Berry SM: Preliminary experience with triamcinolone acetonide during pregnancy. J Matern Fetal Med 5:310, 1996

Dumesic DA, Silverman NH, Tobias S, et al: Transplacental cardioversion of fetal supraventricular tachycardia with procainamide. N Engl J Med 307:1128, 1982

Ebrahim SH, Gfroerer J: Pregnancy-related substance use in the United States during 1996–1998. Obstet Gynecol 101:374, 2003

Edison RJ, Muenke M: Central nervous system and limb abnormalities in case reports of first-trimester statin exposure. N Engl J Med 350:15, 2004

Elia J, Katz IR, Simpson GM: Teratogenicity of psychotherapeutic medications. Psychopharmacol Bull 23:531, 1987

The European Collaborative Study and the Swiss Mother and Child HIV Cohort Study: Combination antiretroviral therapy and duration of pregnancy. AIDS 14:2913, 2000

Faiella A, Zappavigna V, Mavilio F, et al: Inhibition of retinoic acid-induced activation of 3' human HOXB genes by antisense oligonucleotides affects sequential activation of genes located upstream in the four HOX clusters. Proc Natl Acad Sci USA 7:5335, 1994

FDA: Home Page: What you need to know about mercury in fish and shellfish. http://vm.cfsan.fda.gov/~dms/admehg3.html

Fejgin MD, Lourwood DL: Low molecular weight heparins and their use in obstetrics and gynecology. Obstet Gynecol Surv 49:424, 1994

Feldcamp M, Carey JC: Clinical teratology counseling and consultation case report: Low dose methotrexate exposure in the early weeks of pregnancy. Teratology 47:533, 1993

Fitzsimons R, Greenberger PA, Patterson R: Outcome of pregnancy in women requiring corticosteroids for severe asthma. J Allergy Clin Immunol 78:349, 1986

Franks ME, Macpherson GR, Figg WD: Thalidomide. Lancet 363:1802, 2004

Friedman JM: Teratogen update: Anesthetic agents. Teratology 37:69, 1988

Gaily E, Kantola-Sorsa E, Hiilesmaa V, et al: Normal intelligence in children with prenatal exposure to carbamazepine. Neurology 62:28, 2004

Gardner MO, Owen J, Skelly S, et al: Preterm delivery after indomethacin. A risk factor for neonatal complications? J Reprod Med 41:903, 1996

Geiger JM, Baudin M, Saurat JH: Teratogenic risk with etretinate and acitretin treatment. Dermatology 189:109, 1994

Gilstrap LC, Bawdon RE, Burris JS: Antibiotic concentration in maternal blood, cord blood, and placental membranes in chorioamnionitis. Obstet Gynecol 72:124, 1988

Ginsberg JS, Hirsh J: Anticoagulants during pregnancy. Annu Rev Med 40:79, 1989

Giusti RM, Iwamoto K, Hatch EE: Diethylstilbestrol revisited: A review of the long-term health effects. Ann Intern Med 122:778, 1995

Glantz JC: Reproductive toxicology of alkylating agents. Obstet Gynecol Surv 49:709, 1994

Goldberg JM, Falcone T: Effect of diethylstilbestrol on reproductive functions. Fertil Steril 72:1, 1999

Golden NL, Kuhnert BR, Sokol RJ, et al: Neonatal manifestations of maternal phencyclidine exposure. J Perinat Med 15:185, 1987

Goldstein DJ, Corbin LA, Sundell KL: Effects of first-trimester fluoxetine exposure on the newborn. Obstet Gynecol 89:713, 1997

Goldstein DJ, Marvel DE, Lily E: Psychotropic medications during pregnancy: Risk to the fetus. JAMA 270:2177, 1993

Gomby DS, Shiono PH: Estimating the number of substance exposed infants. Future Child 1:17, 1991

Green TP, Thompson TR, Johnson DE, et al: Furosemide promotes patent ductus arteriosus in premature infants with the respiratory-distress syndrome. N Engl J Med 308:743, 1983

Greenberger PA, Patterson R: Beclomethasone dipropionate for severe asthma during pregnancy. Ann Intern Med 98:478, 1983

Greenland S, Richwald GA, Honda GD: The effects of marijuana use during pregnancy, 2. A study in a low-risk home delivery population. Drug Alcohol Depend 11:359, 1983

Grosso S, Berardi R, Cioni M, et al: Transient neonatal hypothyroidism after gestational exposure to amiodarone: A follow-up of two cases. J Endocrinol Invest 21:699, 1998

Grumbach MM, Ducharme JR: The effects of androgens on fetal sexual development. Androgen-induced female pseudohermaphrodism. Fertil Steril 11:157, 1960

Gudas LJ: Retinoids and vertebrate development. J Biol Chem 269:15399, 1994

Guron G, Friberg P: An intact renin-angiotensin system is a prerequisite for normal renal development. J Hypertension 18:123, 2000

Hall JG, Pauli RM, Wilson K: Maternal and fetal sequelae of anticoagulation during pregnancy. Am J Med 68:122, 1980

Hanson JW: Human teratology. In Rimoin DL, Connor JM, Pyeritz RE (eds): Emery and Rimoin's Principles and Practice of Medical Genetics, 3rd ed. New York, Churchill Livingston, 1996, p 697

Harrigan JT, Kangos JJ, Sikka KR, et al: Successful treatment of fetal congestive failure secondary to tachycardia. N Engl J Med 304:1527, 1981

Hatjis CG, Meis PJ: Sinusoidal fetal heart rate pattern associated with butorphanol administration. Obstet Gynecol 67:377, 1986

Heinonen OP, Slone D, Shapiro S: Birth Defects and Drugs in Pregnancy. Littleton, Mass, John Wright Publishing Sciences Group, 1983

Heinonen OP, Slone D, Shapiro S: Birth Defects and Drugs in Pregnancy. Littleton, Mass, Publishing Sciences Group, 1977, p 441

Hengst VP: Investigations of the teratogenicity of Daraprim (pyrimethamine) in humans. Zentralbl Gynakol 94:551, 1972

Hepner DL, Harnett M, Segal S, et al: Herbal medicine use in parturients. Anesth. Anlg 94:690, 2002

Herbst AL, Ulfelder H, Poskanzer DC: Adenocarcinoma of the vagina. Association of maternal stilbestrol therapy. N Engl J Med 284:878, 1971

Hermans PE, Wilhelm MP: Vancomycin. Mayo Clin Proc 62:901, 1987

Hernandez-Diaz S, Werler MM, Walker AM, et al: Folic acid antagonists during pregnancy and the risk of birth defects. N Engl J Med 343:1608, 2000

Hiilesmaa VK, Teramo K, Granstrom ML, et al: Serum folate concentrations in women with epilepsy. BMJ 287:577, 1983

Hirsch KS, Wilson JG, Scott WJ, et al: Acetazolamide teratology and its association with carbonic anhydrase inhibition in the mouse. Teratogenesis Carcinog Mutagen 3:133, 1983

Holmes LB: Teratogen-induced limb defects. Am J Med Genet 112:297, 2002

Holmes LB, Harvey EA, Coull BA, et al: The teratogenicity of anticonvulsant drugs. N Engl J Med 344:1132, 2001

Holzman C, Paneth N, Little R, et al: Perinatal brain injury in premature infants born to mothers using alcohol in pregnancy. Pediatrics 95:66, 1995

Honein MA, Paulozzi LJ, Watkins ML: Maternal smoking and birth defects: Validity of birth certificate data for effect estimation. Public Health Rep 116:327, 2001

Horning MG, Stratton C, Wilson A, et al: Detection of 5-(3,4)-diphenylhydantoin in the newborn human. Anal Lett 4:537, 1974

Horvath JS, Phippard A, Korda A, et al: Clonidine hydrochloride: A safe and effective antihypertensive agent in pregnancy. Obstet Gynecol 66:634, 1985

Hoyme HE, Jones KL, Dixon SD, et al: Prenatal cocaine exposure and fetal vascular disruption. Pediatrics 85:743, 1990

Hume RF Jr, Martin LS, Bottoms SF, et al: Vascular disruption birth defects and history of prenatal cocaine exposure: A case control study. Fetal Diagn Ther 12:292, 1997

Hwang SJ, Beaty TH, Panny SR, et al: Association study of transforming growth factor alpha (TGFα) Tag 1 polymorphism and oral clefts. Am J Epidemiol 14:629, 1995

Iahnaccone PM, Bossert NL, Connelly CS: Disruption of embryonic and fetal development due to preimplantation chemical insults: A critical review. Am J Obstet Gynecol 157:476, 1987

Jacobson JL, Jacobson SW, Sokol RJ, et al: Relation of maternal age and pattern of pregnancy drinking to functionally significant cognitive deficit in infancy. Alcohol Clin Exp Res 22:345, 1998

Jacobson JL, Jacobson SW, Sokol RJ, et al: Teratogenic effects of alcohol on infant development. Alcohol Clin Exp Res 17:174, 1993

Jacobson SJ, Jones K, Johnson K, et al: Prospective multicentre study of pregnancy outcome after lithium exposure during first trimester. Lancet 339:530, 1992

Jasper JD, Goel R, Einarson A, et al: Effects of framing on teratogenic risk perception in pregnant women. Lancet 358:1237, 2001

Jick H, Holmes LB, Hunter JR, et al: First-trimester drug use and congenital disorders. JAMA 246:343, 1981

Jick SS, Terris BZ, Jick H: First trimester topical tretinoin and congenital disorders. Lancet 341:1664, 1993

Johnson EM: The effects of ribavirin on development and reproduction: A critical review of published and unpublished studies in experimental animals. J Am Coll Toxicol 9:551, 1990

Jones HC: Intrauterine ototoxicity: A case report and review of the literature. J Natl Med Assoc 65:201, 1973

Kallen B, Lygner PE: Delivery outcome in women who used drugs for migraine during pregnancy with special reference to sumatriptan. Headache 41:351, 2001

Kandall SR, Gaines J, Habel L, et al: Relationship of maternal substance abuse to subsequent sudden infant death syndrome in offspring. J Pediatr 123:120, 1993

Kaufman RH, Adam E, Binder GL, et al: Upper genital tract changes and pregnancy outcome in offspring exposed in utero to diethylstilbestrol. Am J Obstet Gynecol 137:299, 1980

Kaufman RH, Adam E, Hatch EE, et al: Continued follow-up of pregnancy outcomes in diethylstilbestrol-exposed offspring. Obstet Gynecol 96:483, 2000

Kerenyi TD, Gleicher N, Meller J, et al: Transplacental cardioversion of intrauterine supraventricular tachycardia with digitalis. Lancet 2:393, 1980

Khouri MI, James IM, Flanders WD, et al: Interpretation of recurring weak association obtained from epidemiologic studies of suspected human teratogens. Teratology 46:69, 1992

Killeen AA, Bowers LD: Fetal supraventricular tachycardia treated with high-dose quinidine: Toxicity associated with marked elevation of the metabolite, 3(S)-3-hydroxyquinidine. Obstet Gynecol 70:445, 1987

Kimmel CA, Generoso WM, Thomas RD, et al: A new frontier in understanding the mechanisms of developmental abnormalities. Toxicol Appl Pharmacol 119:159, 1993

Kirshon B, Wasserstrum N, Willis R, et al: Teratogenic effects of first trimester cyclophosphamide therapy. Obstet Gynecol 72:462, 1988

Klip H, Verloop J, van Gool JD, et al: Hypospadias in sons of women exposed to diethylstilbestrol in utero: A cohort study. Lancet 359:1102, 2002

Knapp K, Lenz W, Nowack E: Multiple congenital abnormalities. Lancet 2:725, 1962

Knudsen LB: No association between griseofulvin and conjoined twinning. Lancet 2:1097, 1987

Koren G, Bologa M, Long D, et al: Perception of teratogenic risk by pregnant women exposed to drugs and chemicals during the first trimester. Am J Obstet Gynecol 160:1190, 1989

Koren G, Pastuszak A, Ito S: Drugs in pregnancy. N Engl J Med 338:1128, 1998

Kramer WB, Belfort M, Saade GR, et al: Successful urokinase treatment of massive pulmonary embolism in pregnancy. Obstet Gynecol 86:600, 1995

Kuczkowski KM: Nonobstetric surgery during pregnancy: What are the risks of anesthesia? Obstet Gynecol Surv 59:52, 2004

Kutscher AH, Zegarelli EV, Tovell HM, et al: Discoloration of deciduous teeth induced by administration of tetracycline antepartum. Am J Obstet Gynecol 96:291, 1966

Lacroix I, Damase-Michel C, Lapeyre-Mestre M, et al: Prescription of drugs during pregnancy in France. Lancet 356:1735, 2000

Lammer EJ: Embryopathy in infant conceived one year after termination of maternal etretinate. Lancet 2:1080, 1988

Lammer EJ, Chen DT, Hoar RM, et al: Retinoic acid embryopathy. N Engl J Med 313:837, 1985

Lee EJD: Population genetics of the angiotensin-converting enzyme in Chinese. Br J Clin Pharmacol 37:212, 1994

Lee H, Nagel RG: Toxic and teratologic effects of verapamil on early chick embryos: Evidence for the involvement of calcium in neural tube closure. Teratology 33:203, 1986

Lemoine P: Les enfants de parents alcoholiques. Ovest Med 21:476, 1968

Lenke RR, VanDorsten JP, Schifrin BS: Pyelonephritis in pregnancy: A prospective randomized trial to prevent recurrent disease evaluating suppressive therapy with nitrofurantoin and close surveillance. Am J Obstet Gynecol 146:953, 1983

Leppik IE, Rask CA: Pharmacokinetics of antiepileptic drugs during pregnancy. Semin Neurol 8:240, 1988

Lewis DP, Van Dyke DC, Stumbo PJ, et al: Drug and environmental factors associated with adverse pregnancy outcomes. Part I: Antiepileptic drugs, contraceptives, smoking, and folate. Ann Pharm 32:802, 1998

Lewis PE, Cefalo RC, Naulty JS, et al: Placental transfer and fetal toxicity of sodium nitroprusside. Gynecol Invest 8:46, 1977

Lifschitz MH, Wilson GS, Smith EO, et al: Fetal and postnatal growth of children born to narcotic-dependent women. J Pediatr 102:686, 1983

Lindhout D, Rene JE, Hoppener A, et al: Teratogenicity of antiepileptic drug combinations with special emphasis on epioxidation of carbamazepine. Epilepsia 25:77, 1984

Linn S, Schoenbaum SC, Monson RR, et al: The association of marijuana use with outcome of pregnancy. Am J Public Health 73:1161, 1983

Linseman DA, Hampton LA, Branstetter DG: Quinolone-induced arthropathy in the neonatal mouse. Morphological analysis of articular lesions produced by pipemidic acid and ciprofloxacin. Fundam Appl Toxicol 28:59, 1995

Lip GYH, Churchill D, Beevers M, et al: Angiotensin-coverting-enzyme inhibitors in early pregnancy. Lancet 350:1446, 1997

Little BB, Snell LM, Gilstrap LC, et al: Effects of ts and blues abuse during pregnancy on maternal and infant health status. Am J Perinatol 7:359, 1990a

Little BB, Snell LM, Klein VR, et al: Maternal and fetal effects of heroin addiction during pregnancy. J Reprod Med 35:159, 1990b

Little BB, Snell LM, Klein VR, et al: Cocaine abuse during pregnancy: Maternal and fetal implications. Obstet Gynecol 73:157, 1989

Little BB, Snell LM, Gilstrap LC: Methamphetamine abuse during pregnancy: Outcome and fetal effects. Obstet Gynecol 72:541, 1988

Lozo E, Forster C, Dietz M, et al: Ciprofloxacin and N-methyl-ciprofloxacin induce joint cartilage lesions in immature rats. Teratology 53:32A, 1996

Ludwig H: Results of streptokinase therapy in deep venous thrombosis during pregnancy. Postgrad Med J 49:65, 1973

Macaulay JH, Bond K, Steer PJ: Epidural analgesia in labor and fetal hyperthermia. Obstet Gynecol 80:665, 1992

Magee LA, Schick B, Donnenfeld AE, et al: The safety of calcium channel blockers in human pregnancy: A prospective, multicenter cohort study. Am J Obstet Gynecol 174:823, 1996

Major CA, Lewis DF, Harding JA, et al: Tocolysis with indomethacin increases the incidence of necrotizing enterocolitis in the low-birth-weight neonate. Am J Obstet Gynecol 170:102, 1994

Mandelbrot L, Landreau-Mascaro A, Rekacewicz C, et al: Lamivudine-zidovudine combination for prevention of maternal-infant transmission of HIV-1. JAMA 285:2083, 2001

Manson JM, Papa L, Miller ML, et al: Studies of DNA damage and cell death in embryonic limb buds induced by teratogenic exposure to cyclophosphamide. Teratog Carcinog Mutagen 2:47, 1982

Marpeau L, Bouillie J, Barrat J, et al: Obstetrical advantages and perinatal risks of indomethacin: A report of 818 cases. Fetal Diagn Ther 9:110, 1994

Martinez-Frias ML, Czeizel AE, Rodriguez-Pinilla E, et al: Smoking during pregnancy and Poland sequence: Results of a population-based registry and a case-control registry. Teratology 59:35, 1999

Martinez-Frias ML, Rodriques-Pinilla E, Prieto L: Prenatal exposure to salicylates and gastroschisis: A case-control study. Teratology 56:241, 1997

Mastroiacovo P, Mazzone T, Addis A, et al: High vitamin A intake in early pregnancy and major malformations: A multicenter prospective controlled study. Teratology 59:7, 1999

Maurer T, Poncelet A, Berger T. Thalidomide treatment for prurigo nodularis in human immunodeficiency virus-infected subjects: Efficacy and risk of neuropathy. Arch Dermatol 140:845, 2004

Mazze RI, Kallen B: Reproductive outcome after anesthesia and operation during pregnancy: A registry study of 5405 cases. Am J Obstet Gynecol 161:1178, 1989

McGready R, Cho T, Keo NK, et al: Artemisinin antimalarials in pregnancy: A prospective treatment study of 539 episodes of multidrug-resistant *Plasmodium falciparum*. Clin Infect Dis 33:2009, 2001

McGready R, Thwai KL, Cho T, et al: The effects of quinine and chloroquine antimalaria treatments in the first trimester of pregnancy. Trans R Soc Trop Med Hyg 96:180, 2002

McKeigue PM, Lamm SH, Linn S, et al: Bendectin and birth defects: I. A meta-analysis of the epidemiologic studies. Teratology 50:27, 1994

Meinking TL, Taplin D, Kalter DC, et al: Comparative efficacy of treatments for pediculosis capitis infestations. Arch Dermatol 122:267, 1986

Melnick S, Cole P, Anderson D, et al: Rates and risks of diethylstilbestrol-related clear-cell adenocarcinoma of the vagina and cervix. N Engl J Med 316:514, 1987

Messina M, Biffignandi P, Ghigo E, et al: Possible contraindication of spironolactone during pregnancy. J Endocrinol Invest 2:222, 1979

Meyer-Bahlburg HFL, Gruen RS, New MI, et al: Gender change from female to male in classical congenital adrenal hyperplasia. Horm Behav 3:319, 1996

Milkovich L, van den Berg BJ: Effects of antenatal exposure to anorectic drugs. Am J Obstet Gynecol 129:637, 1977

Mitchell AA: Systematic identification of drugs that cause birth defects—a new opportunity. N Engl J Med 349:26, 2003

Morrell MJ: The new antiepileptic drugs and women: Efficacy, reproductive health, pregnancy, and fetal outcome. Epilepsia 37:S34, 1996

Mortola JF: The use of psychotropic agents in pregnancy and lactation. Psychiatr Clin North Am 12:69, 1989

Murad SH, Tabsh KM, Shilyanski G, et al: Effects of verapamil on uterine blood flow and maternal cardiovascular function in the awake pregnant ewe. Anesth Analg 64:7, 1985

Murray JC: Face facts: Genes, environment, and clefts. Am J Hum Genet 57:3227, 1995

Nakane Y, Okuma T, Takahashi R, et al: Multi-institutional study on the teratogenicity and fetal toxicity of antiepileptic drugs: A report of a collaborative study group in Japan. Epilepsia 21:663, 1980

Nelson BK, Moorman WJ, Schrader SM: Review of experimental male-mediated behavioral and neurochemical disorders. Neurotoxicology 18:611, 1996

Niebyl JR: Management of nausea and vomiting in pregnancy: Traditional therapies. Contemp Ob/Gyn 45:130, 2000

Niebyl JR: Perinatal effects of indomethacin. Biweekly Rev Clin Obstet Gynecol 11:22, 1991

Nielsen GL, Sorensen HT, Larsen H, et al: Risk of adverse birth outcome and miscarriage in pregnant users of non-steroidal anti-inflammatory drugs: Population based observational study and case-control study. BMJ 322:255, 2001

Norton ME, Vargas JE: When a pregnant patient needs analgesics. Contemp Ob/Gyn 48:37, 2003

Nosten F, Vincenti M, Simpson J, et al: The effects of mefloquine treatment in pregnancy. Clin Infect Dis 28:808, 1999

Oakley GP, Erickson JD: Vitamin A and birth defects. N Engl J Med 333:1414, 1995

Okuma T, Takahashi R, Wada T: A collaborative study of the teratogenicity and fetal toxicity of antiepileptic drugs in Japan. In Wada A, Penry JK (eds): Advances in Epileptology: The 10th Epilepsy International Symposium. New York, Raven, 1980, p 511

Olshan AF, Teschke K, Baird PA: Paternal occupation and congenital anomalies. Am J Ind Med 20:447, 1991

Omtzigt JGC, Los RJ, Grobbee DE, et al: The risk of spina bifida aperta after first trimester valproate exposure in a prenatal cohort. Neurology 42(S5):119, 1992

Ondrizek RR, Chan PJ, Patton WC, et al: An alternative medicine study of herbal effects on the penetration of zonafree hamster oocytes and the integrity of sperm deoxyribonucleic acid. Fertil Steril 71:517, 1999

Ostrea EM, Chavez CJ: Perinatal problems (excluding neonatal withdrawal) in maternal drug addiction: A study of 830 cases. J Pediatr 94:292, 1979

Owen J, Clovin EV, Davis RO: Fetal death after successful conversion of fetal supraventricular tachycardia with digoxin and verapamil. Am J Obstet Gynecol 158:1169, 1988

Pandit PB, Chitayat D, Jefferies AL, et al: Tibial hemimelia and tetralogy of Fallot associated with first trimester exposure to amantadine. Reprod Toxicol 8:89, 1994

Parilla BV: Using indomethacin as a tocolytic. Contemp Ob/Gyn 49:90, 2004

Pastore LM, Hertz-Picciotto I, Beaumont JJ: Risk of stillbirth from medications, illnesses and medical procedures. Paediatr Perinat Epidemiol 13:421, 1999

Pastuszak A, Schick-Boschetto B, Ziber C, et al: Pregnancy outcome following first-trimester exposure to fluoxetine. JAMA 269:2246, 1993

Peipert JF: Genital chlamydial infections. N Engl J Med 349:2424, 2003

Pinelli JM, Symington AJ, Cunningham KA, et al: Case report and review of the perinatal implications of maternal lithium use. Am J Obstet Gynecol 187:245, 2002

Piper JM, Baum C, Kennedy DL: Prescription drug use before and during pregnancy in a Medicaid population. Am J Obstet Gynecol 157:148, 1987

Piper JM, Mitchell EF, Ray WA: Prenatal use of metronidazole and birth defects: No association. Obstet Gynecol 82:348, 1993

Pompa G, Fadini L, DiLauro F, et al: Transfer of lindane and pentachlorobenzene from mother to newborn rabbits. Pharmacol Toxicol 74:28, 1994

Pons JC, Taburet AM, Singlas E, et al: Placental passage of azathiothymidine (AZT) during the second trimester of pregnancy: Study by direct fetal blood sampling under ultrasound. Eur J Obstet Gynecol Reprod Biol 40:229, 1991

Pro B, Younes A, Albitar M, et al: Thalidomide for patients with recurrent lymphoma. Cancer 100:1186, 2004

Pryde PG, Sedman AB, Nugent CE, et al: Angiotensin converting enzyme inhibitor fetopathy. J Am Soc Ncphrol 3:1575, 1993

Public Health Service Task Force: Perinatal HIV Guidelines Working Group: Summary of the updated recommendations from the Public Health Service Task Force to reduce perinatal human immunodeficiency virus-1 transmission in the United States. Obstet Gynecol 99:1117, 2002

Raman-Wilms L, Lin-in Tseng A, Wighardt S, et al: Fetal genital effects of first-trimester sex hormone exposure: A meta-analysis. Obstet Gynecol 85:141, 1995

Ramin SM, Little BB, Trimmer KJ, et al: Methamphetamine use during pregnancy. Am J Obstet Gynecol 166:353, 1992

Rasanen J, Jouppila P: Fetal cardiac function and ductus arteriosus during indomethacin and sulindac therapy for threatened preterm labor: A randomized study. Am J Obstet Gynecol 173:20, 1995

Regev RH, Litmanowitz I, Arnon S, et al: Gentamicin serum concentrations in neonates born to gentamicin-treated mothers. Pediat Infect Dis J 19:890, 2000

Reprotox: Reproductive Toxicology Center: Labetalol. 2003a. Available at: http://reprotox.org/data/2175.html

Reprotox: Reproductive Toxicology Center: Tretinoin. 2003b. Available at: http//reprotox.org/data/1428.html

Reprotox: Reproductive Toxicology Center: Amphetamines. 2000a. Available at: http://reprotox.org/data

Reprotox: Reproductive Toxicology Center: Enflurane. 2000b. Available at: http://reprotox.org/data/2680.html

Reprotox: Reproductive Toxicology Center: Isoflurane. 2000c. Available at: http://reprotox.org/data/1252.html

Reprotox: Reproductive Toxicology Center: Oseltamivir. 2000d. Available at: http://reprotox.org/data/4141.html

Rey E, Duperron L, Gautheir R, et al: Transplacental treatment of tachycardia-induced fetal heart failure with verapamil and amiodarone: A case report. Am J Obstet Gynecol 153:311, 1985

Rigat B, Hubert C, Alhenc-Gelas F, et al: An insertion/deletion polymorphism in the angiotensin I-converting enzyme gene accounting for half the variance of serum enzyme levels. J Clin Invest 86:1343, 1990

Robaire B, Hales BF: Paternal exposure to chemicals before conception. BMJ 307:341, 1993

Robboy SJ, Noller KL, O'Brien P, et al: Increased incidence of cervical and vaginal dysplasia in 3,980 diethylstilbestrol-exposed young women. Experience of the National Collaborative Diethylstilbestrol Adenosis Project. JAMA 252:2979, 1984

Roberts RM, Cross JC, Leaman DW: Interferons as hormones of pregnancy. Endocr Rev 13:432, 1992

Rosa F: Amantadine pregnancy experience. Reprod Toxicol 8:531, 1994

Rosa FW, Baum C, Shaw M: Pregnancy outcomes after first trimester vaginitis drug therapy. Obstet Gynecol 69:751, 1987a

Rosa FW, Hernandez C, Carlo WA: Griseofulvin teratology, including two thoracopagus conjoined twins. Lancet 1:171, 1987b

Rothman KJ, Moore LL, Singer MR, et al: Teratogenicity of high vitamin A intake. N Engl J Med 333:1369, 1995

Rowe I: Prescriptions of psychotropic drugs by general practitioners: Antidepressants. Med J Aust 1:642, 1973

Rowland AS, Baird DD, Weinberg CR, et al: Reduced fertility among women employed as dental assistants exposed to high levels of nitrous oxide. N Engl J Med 327:993, 1992

Sabers A, Dam M, A-Rogvi-Hansen B, et al: Epilepsy and pregnancy: Lamotrigine as main drug used. Acta Neurol Scand 109:9, 2004

Sadler TW: Langman's Medical Embryology, 6th ed. Baltimore, Williams and Wilkins, 1990

Salle B, Sergeant P, Awada A, et al: Transvaginal ultrasound studies of vascular and morphological changes in uteri exposed to diethylstilbestrol in utero. Hum Reprod 11:2531, 1996

Sarensen HT, Johnsen SP, Larsen H, et al: Birth outcomes in pregnant women treated with low-molecular-weight heparin. Acta Obstet Gynecol Scand 79:655, 2000

Savitz DA, Sonnenfeld N, Olshan AF: Review of epidemiological studies of paternal occupational exposure and spontaneous abortion. Am J Ind Med 25:361, 1994

Saxena MC, Siddiqui MK, Bhargava AK, et al: Role of chlorinated hydrocarbon pesticides in abortions and premature labour. Toxicology 17:323, 1980

Schardein JL: Congenital abnormalities and hormones during pregnancy: A clinical review. Teratology 22:251, 1985

Schick-Boschetto B, Zuber C: Alprazolam exposure during early human pregnancy. Teratology 45:460, 1992

Schnitzer PG, Olshan AF, Erickson JD: Paternal occupation and risk of birth defects in the offspring. Epidemiology 6:577, 1995

Schubiger G, Flury G, Nussberger J: Enalapril for pregnancy induced hypertension: Acute renal failure in the neonate. Ann Intern Med 108:215, 1988

Scott JM, Weir DG, Molloy A, et al: Folic acid metabolism and mechanisms of neural tube defects. Ciba Foundation Symposium. Manchester, England, John Wiley, 1994, p 181

Shaw GM, Velie EM, Schaffer D: Risk of neural tube defect affected pregnancies among obese women. JAMA 275:1093, 1996

Sheehan DM: Herbal medicines, phytoestrogens and toxicity: Risk: benefit considerations. Proc Soc Exp Biol Med 217:379, 1998

Shen O, Entebi E, Yagel S: Congenital hypertrophic cardiomyopathy associated with in utero verapamil exposure. Prenat Diagn 15:1088, 1995

Shepard TH: Catalog of Teratogenic Agents, 10th ed. Baltimore, Johns Hopkins University Press, 2001

Shiono PH, Klebanoff MA, Nugent RP, et al: The impact of cocaine and marijuana use on low birth weight and preterm birth: A multicenter study. Am J Obstet Gynecol 172:19, 1995

Sibai BM, Barton JR, Sarinoglu C, et al: A randomized prospective comparison of nifedipine and bed rest alone in the management of preeclampsia remote from term. Am J Obstet Gynecol 166:280, 1992

Sidhu JS, Floyd RL: Alcohol use among women of childbearing age—United States, 1991–1999. MMWR 51:273, 2002

Singer LT, Minnes S, Short E, et al: Cognitive outcomes of preschool children with prenatal cocaine exposure. JAMA 292:1021, 2004

Singer LT, Arendt R, Minnes S, et al: Cognitive and motor outcomes of cocaine-exposed infants. JAMA 287:1952, 2002

Slone D, Siskind V, Heinonen OP, et al: Antenatal exposure to the phenothiazines in relation to congenital malformations, perinatal mortality rate, birth weight, and intelligence quotient score. Am J Obstet Gynecol 128:486, 1977

Snyder DE, Layde PM, Johnson MW, et al: Treatment of tuberculosis during pregnancy. Am Rev Respir Dis 122:65, 1980

Soprano DR, Soprano KJ: Retinoids as teratogens. Annu Rev Nutr 15:111, 1995

Sorenson HT, Nelsen GL, Olesen C, et al: Risk of malformations and other outcomes in children exposed to fluconazole in utero. Br J Clin Pharmacol 48:234, 1999

Speroff L, Glass RH, Kase NG: Normal and abnormal sexual development. In: Clinical Gynecologic Endocrinology and Infertility, 5th ed. Baltimore, Williams and Wilkins, 1994, p 321

St. Clair SM, Schirmer RG: First trimester exposure to alprazolam. Obstet Gynecol 80:843, 1992

Stavrous C, Hofmeyer GJ, Boezaart AP: Prolonged fetal bradycardia during epidural analgesia. S Afr Med J 77:66, 1990

Stevens TP, Guillet R: Use of glucagons to treat neonatal low-output congestive heart failure after maternal labetalol therapy. J Pediatr 127:151, 1995

Stevenson RE: Causes of human anomalies: An overview and historical perspective. Human malformations and related anomalies. In Stevenson RE, Hall JG, Goodman RM (eds): Human Malformations and Related Anomalies. New York, Oxford University Press, 1993a, p 3

Stevenson RE: The environmental basis of human anomalies. In Stevenson RE, Hall JG, Goodman RM (eds): Human Malformations and Related Anomalies. New York, Oxford University Press, 1993b, p 137

Stillman RJ: In utero exposure to diethylstilbestrol: Adverse effects on the reproductive tract and reproductive performance in male and female offspring. Am J Obstet Gynecol 142:905, 1982

Stimmel B, Adamsons K: Narcotic dependency in pregnancy. Methadone maintenance compared to use of street drugs. JAMA 235:1121, 1976

Streissguth AP, Clarren SK, Jones KL: Natural history of fetal alcohol syndrome: A 10-year follow-up of eleven patients. Lancet 2:85, 1985

Sullivan WC: The children of the female drunkard. Med Temp Rev 1:72, 1900

Sumatriptan and Naratriptan Pregnancy Registries: Sumatriptan and Naratriptan Pregnancy Registries. International Interim Report: 1 January 1996–30 April 2002. Wilmington, NC, Pharma Research Corporation, July 2002

Sutton C, McIvor RS, Vagt M, et al: Methotrexate-resistant form of dihydroreductase protects transgenic murine embryos from teratogenic effects of methotrexate. Pediatr Dev Pathol 1:503, 1998

Thomson EJ, Cordero JF: The new teratogens: Accutane and other vitamin-A analogs. MCN Am J Matern Child Nurs 14:244, 1989

Thulstrup AM, Sarensen HT, Nielsen GL, et al: Fetal growth and adverse birth outcomes in women receiving prescriptions for acetaminophen during pregnancy. Euro Map Study Group. Am J Perinatol 16:321, 1999

Trasler JM, Doerksen T: Teratogen update: Paternal exposures—reproductive risks. Teratology 60:161, 1999

Tuomala RE, Shapiro DE, Mofenson LM, et al: Antiretroviral therapy during pregnancy and the risk of an adverse outcome. N Engl J Med 346:1863, 2002

Turrentine MA, Braems G, Ramirez MM: Use of thrombolytics for the treatment of thromboembolic disease during pregnancy. Obstet Gynecol Surv 50:534, 1995

Valacyclovir Pregnancy Registry: Interim report. Project office. Glaxo Wellcome, Research Triangle Park, NC, July 31, 1998

van der Heijden BJ, Carlus C, Narcy F, et al: Persistent anuria, neonatal death, and renal microcystic lesions after prenatal exposure to indomethacin. Am J Obstet Gynecol 171:617, 1994

Vega WA, Kolody B, Hwang J, et al: Prevalence and magnitude of perinatal substance exposures in California. N Engl J Med 329:850, 1993

Vessey MP: Epidemiological studies of the effects of diethylstilbestrol. IARC Sci Publ 335, 1989

Vitale N, DeFeo M, De Santo LS, et al: Dose-dependent fetal complications of warfarin in pregnant women with mechanical heart valves. J Am Coll Cardiol 33:1637, 1999

von Almen WF, Miller JM: Ts and blues in pregnancy. J Reprod Med 31:236, 1984

Vorhees CV, Minck Dr, Berry HK: Anticonvulsants and brain development. Prog Brain Res 73:229, 1988

Walker MPR, Moore TR, Brace RA: Indomethacin and arginine vasopressin interaction in the fetal kidney. A mechanism of oliguria. Am J Obstet Gynecol 171:1234, 1994

Warkany J: Warfarin embryopathy. Teratology 14:205, 1976

Wass TS, Persutte WH, Hobbins JC: The impact of prenatal alcohol exposure on frontal cortex development in utero. Am J Obstet Gynecol 185:737, 2001

Weiner CP, Thompson MIB: Direct treatment of fetal supraventricular tachycardia after failed transplacental therapy. Am J Obstet Gynecol 158:570, 1988

Welt SI: Sinusoidal fetal heart rate and butorphanol administration. Am J Obstet Gynecol 152:362, 1985

Werler MM: Teratogen update: Smoking and reproductive outcomes. Teratology 55:382, 1997

Werler MM, Sheehan JE, Mitchell AA: Association of vasoconstrictive exposures with risks of gastroschisis and small intestinal atresia. Epidemiology 14:349, 2003

Wessels MW, Willems PJ: Chondrodysplasia punctata. N Engl J Med 347:110, 2002

Yaffe SJ, Briggs GG: Is this drug going to harm my baby? Contemp Ob/Gyn 48:57, 2003

Yerby MS: Epilepsy and pregnancy. New issues for an old disorder. Neurol Clin 11:777, 1993

Young DC, Snabes MC, Poindexter AN: GnRH agonist exposure during the first trimester of pregnancy. Obstet Gynecol 81:587, 1993

Zhu M, Zhou S: Reduction of the teratogenic effects of phenytoin by folic acid and a mixture of folic acid, vitamins, amino acids: A preliminary trial. Epilepsia 30:246, 1989

Zucker KJ, Bradley SJ, Oliver G, et al. Psychosexual development of women with congenital adrenal hyperplasia. Horm Behav 30:300, 1996

15

Antepartum Assessment

In this chapter, the evolution of techniques employed to forecast fetal well-being is considered. The focus is on testing procedures that depend on fetal physical activities, including movement, breathing, amnionic fluid production, and heart rate. According to the American College of Obstetricians and Gynecologists (1999), the goal of antepartum fetal surveillance is to prevent fetal death. In most cases, a normal test result is highly reassuring, because fetal deaths within 1 week of a normal test are rare. Indeed, negative-predictive values—a true negative test—for most of the tests described are 99.8 percent or higher. In contrast, estimates of the positive-predictive values—a true positive test—for abnormal test results are quite low and range between 10 and 40 percent. Importantly, the widespread use of antepartum fetal surveillance is primarily based on circumstantial evidence because there have been no definitive randomized clinical trials.

FETAL MOVEMENTS

Passive unstimulated fetal activity commences as early as 7 weeks and becomes more sophisticated and coordinated by the end of pregnancy (Vindla and James, 1995). Indeed, beyond 8 menstrual weeks, fetal body movements are never absent for time periods exceeding 13 minutes (DeVries and co-workers, 1985). Between 20 and 30 weeks, general body movements become organized and the fetus starts to show rest-activity cycles (Sorokin and co-workers, 1982). In the third trimester, fetal movement maturation continues until about 36 weeks, when behavioral states are established in 80 percent of normal fetuses. Nijhuis and colleagues (1982) studied fetal heart rate patterns, general body movements, and eye movements and described four fetal behavioral states:

State 1F is a quiescent state (quiet sleep), with a narrow oscillatory bandwidth of the fetal heart rate.

State 2F includes frequent gross body movements, continuous eye movements, and wider oscillation of the fetal heart rate. This state is analogous to rapid eye movement (REM) or active sleep in the neonate.

State 3F includes continuous eye movements in the absence of body movements and no accelerations of the heart rate. The existence of this state is disputed (Pillai and James, 1990a).

State 4F is one of vigorous body movement with continuous eye movements and fetal heart rate accelerations. This state corresponds to the awake state in infants.

Fetuses spend most of their time in states 1F and 2F. For example, at 38 weeks, 75 percent of time is spent in states 1F and 2F (Nijuis and colleagues, 1982).

These behavioral states—particularly 1F and 2F, which correspond to quiet sleep and active sleep—have been used to develop an increasingly sophisticated understanding of fetal behavior. Oosterhof and co-workers (1993) studied fetal

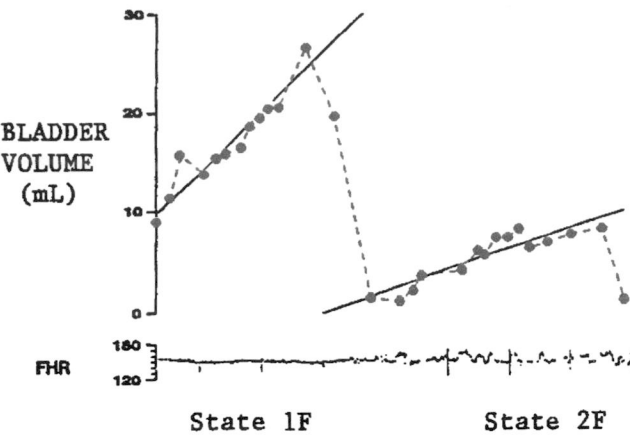

FIGURE 15–1. Fetal bladder volume measurements together with fetal heart rate variation record in relation to 1F or 2F behavior states. State 1F fetal heart rate has a narrow bandwidth consistent with quiet sleep. State 2F heart rate shows wide oscillation of the baseline consistent with active sleep. (Modified from Oosterhof and co-workers, 1993, with permission.)

urine production in normal pregnancies in states 1F or 2F. As shown in Figure 15–1, bladder volumes increased during quiet sleep (state 1F). During state 2F, the fetal heart rate baseline bandwidth increased appreciably, and bladder volume was significantly diminished. The latter occurred due to fetal voiding as well as decreased urine production. These phenomena were interpreted to represent reduced renal blood flow during active sleep. Boito and colleagues (2004) recently reported increasing umbilical vein distention during state 2F, which they interpret to be caused by increased venous pressure from increased flow.

An important determinant of fetal activity appears to be sleep-awake cycles, which are independent of the maternal sleep-awake state. *Sleep cyclicity* has been described as varying from about 20 minutes to as much as 75 minutes. Timor-Tritsch and associates (1978) reported that the mean length of the quiet or inactive state for term fetuses was 23 minutes. Patrick and associates (1982) measured gross fetal body movements with real-time ultrasound for 24-hour periods in 31 normal pregnancies and found the longest period of inactivity to be 75 minutes. Amnionic fluid volume is another important determinant of fetal activity. Sherer and colleagues (1996) assessed the number of fetal movements in 465 pregnancies during biophysical profile testing in relation to amnionic fluid volume estimated using ultrasound. They observed decreased fetal activity with diminished amnionic volumes and suggested that a restricted intrauterine space might physically limit fetal movements.

Sadovsky and colleagues (1979b) studied fetal movements in 120 normal pregnancies and classified the movements into three categories according to both maternal perceptions and independent recordings using piezoelectric sensors. Weak, strong, and rolling movements were described, and their relative contributions to total weekly movements throughout

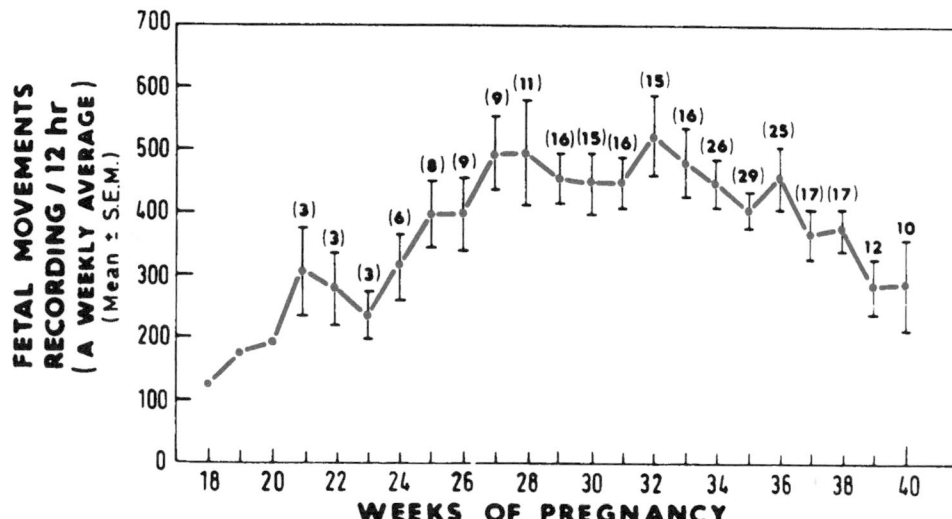

FIGURE 15–2. Weekly average fetal movements calculated from daily fetal movement records during normal pregnancy (means ± SEM). (From Sadovsky and associates, 1979a, with permission.)

the last half of pregnancy were quantified. As pregnancy advances, weak movements decrease and are superseded by more vigorous movements, which increase for several weeks and then subside at term. Presumably, declining amnionic fluid and space account for diminishing activity at term. Figure 15–2 shows fetal movements during the last half of gestation in 127 pregnancies with normal outcomes. The mean number of weekly movements calculated from 12-hour daily recording periods increased from about 200 at 20 weeks to a maximum of 575 movements at 32 weeks. Fetal movements then declined to an average of 282 at 40 weeks. Normal weekly maternal counts of fetal movements ranged between 50 and 950, with large daily variations that included counts as low as 4 to 10 per 12-hour period in normal pregnancies.

CLINICAL APPLICATION. Since 1973, when Sadovsky and Yaffe described seven case reports of pregnancies with decreased fetal activity that preceded fetal death, various methods have been described to quantify fetal movement as a way of prognosticating well-being. Methods include use of a tocodynamometer, visualization with real-time ultrasound, and maternal subjective perceptions. Most investigators have reported excellent correlation between maternally perceived fetal motion and movements documented by instrumentation. For example, Rayburn (1980) found that 80 percent of all movements observed during ultrasonic monitoring were perceived by the mother. In contrast, Johnson and colleagues (1992) reported that beyond 36 weeks, mothers perceived only 16 percent of fetal body movements recorded by a Doppler device. Fetal motions lasting more than 20 seconds were identified more accurately by the mother than shorter episodes.

Although several fetal movement counting protocols have been used, neither the optimal number of movements nor the ideal duration for counting them has been defined. For example, in one method, perception of 10 fetal movements in up to

2 hours is considered normal (Moore and Piaquadio, 1989). In another, women are instructed to count fetal movements for 1 hour a day, and the count is accepted as reassuring if it equals or exceeds a previously established baseline count (Neldam, 1983).

A particularly bothersome clinical situation occurs when women present in the third trimester complaining of subjectively reduced fetal movement. Harrington and colleagues (1998) reported that 7 percent of 6793 women delivered at a London hospital presented with a complaint of decreased fetal movement. Fetal heart rate monitoring tests were employed if ultrasound scans for fetal growth or Doppler velocimetry were abnormal. The pregnancy outcomes for women who complained of decreased fetal movement were not significantly different from those for women without this complaint. Nonetheless, the authors recommended evaluation to reassure the mother.

Grant and co-workers (1989) performed an unparalleled investigation of maternally perceived fetal movements and pregnancy outcome. More than 68,000 pregnancies were randomly assigned between 28 and 32 weeks. Women in the fetal movement arm of the study were instructed by specially employed midwives to record the time needed to feel 10 movements each day. This required an average of 2.7 hours of each day. Women in the control group were informally asked about movements during prenatal visits. Reports of decreased fetal motion were evaluated with tests of fetal well-being. Antepartum death rates for normally formed singletons were similar in the two study groups regardless of prior risk status. Despite the counting policy, most stillborn fetuses were dead by the time the mothers reported for medical attention. Importantly, these investigators did not conclude that maternal perceptions of fetal activity were meaningless. Conversely, they concluded that informal maternal perceptions were as good as formally counted and recorded fetal movement.

FETAL BREATHING

After decades of uncertainty as to whether the fetus normally breathes, Dawes and co-workers (1972) showed small inward and outward flows of tracheal fluid, indicating fetal thoracic movement in sheep. These chest wall movements differed from those following birth in that they were discontinuous. Another interesting feature of fetal respiration was *paradoxical chest wall movement.* As shown in Figure 15–3, during inspiration the chest wall paradoxically collapses and the abdomen protrudes (Johnson and co-authors, 1988). In the newborn or adult, the opposite occurs. One interpretation of the paradoxical respiratory motion might be coughing to clear amnionic fluid debris. Although the physiological basis for the breathing reflex is not completely understood, such exchange of amnionic fluid appears to be essential for normal lung development.

Dawes (1974) identified two types of respiratory movements. The first are *gasps or sighs,* which occurred at a frequency of 1 to 4 per minute. The second, *irregular bursts of breathing,* occurred at rates up to 240 cycles per minute. These latter rapid respiratory movements were associated with REM. Badalian and co-workers (1993) studied the maturation of normal fetal breathing using color flow and spectral Doppler analysis of nasal fluid flow as an index of lung function. They suggested that fetal respiratory rate decreased in conjunction with increased respiratory volume at about 33 to 36 weeks and coincidental with lung maturation.

Many investigators have examined fetal breathing movements using ultrasound to determine whether monitoring chest wall movements might be of benefit to evaluate fetal health. Several variables in addition to hypoxia were found to affect fetal respiratory movements. These included labor—during which it is normal for respiration to cease—hypoglycemia, sound stimuli, cigarette smoking, amniocentesis, impending preterm labor, gestational age, and the fetal heart rate itself.

Because fetal breathing movements are episodic, interpretation of fetal health when respirations are absent may be tenuous. Patrick and associates (1980) performed continuous 24-hour observation periods using real-time ultrasonography in an effort to characterize fetal breathing patterns during the

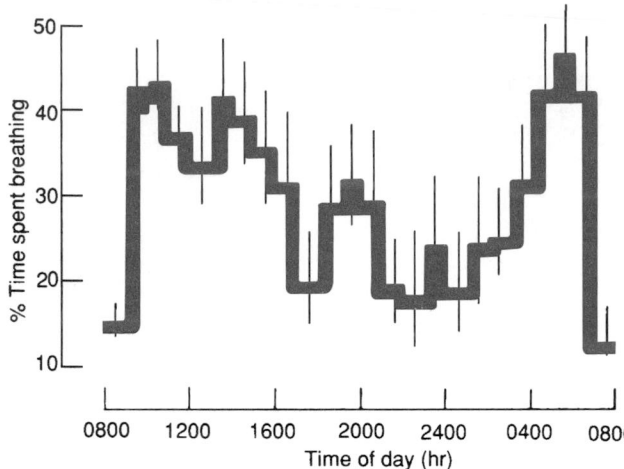

FIGURE 15–4. The percentage of time spent breathing (± SEM) by 11 fetuses at 38 to 39 weeks demonstrated a significant increase in fetal breathing activity after breakfast. Breathing activity diminished over the day and reached its minimum between 1900 and 2400 hours. There was a significant increase in the percentage of time spent breathing between 0400 and 0700 hours, when mothers were asleep. (From Patrick and co-workers, 1980, with permission.)

last 10 weeks of pregnancy. A total of 1224 hours of fetal observation was completed in 51 pregnancies. Figure 15–4 shows the percentage of time spent breathing near term. Clearly, there is diurnal variation, because breathing substantively diminishes during the night. In addition, breathing activity increases somewhat following maternal meals. Total absence of breathing was observed in some of these normal fetuses for up to 122 minutes, indicating that fetal evaluation to diagnose absent respiratory motion may require long periods of observation.

The potential for breathing activity to be an important marker of fetal health is unfulfilled because of the multiplicity of factors that normally affect breathing. Most clinical applications have included assessment of other fetal biophysical indices, such as heart rate. As will be discussed, fetal breathing has become a component of the *biophysical profile.*

CONTRACTION STRESS TESTING

As amnionic fluid pressure increases with uterine contractions, myometrial pressure exceeds collapsing pressure for vessels coursing through uterine muscle, ultimately decreasing blood flow to the intervillous space. Brief periods of impaired oxygen exchange result, and if uteroplacental pathology is present, these elicit late fetal heart rate decelerations (see Chap. 18, p. 452). Contractions also may produce a pattern of variable decelerations as a result of cord compression, suggesting oligohydramnios, which is often a concomitant of placental insufficiency.

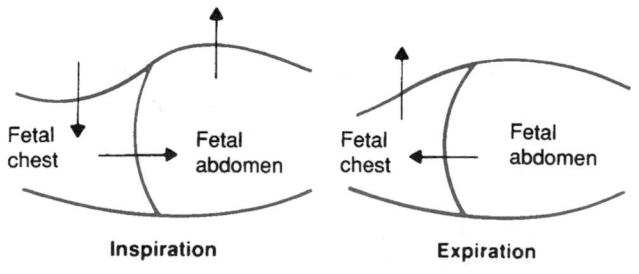

FIGURE 15–3. Paradoxical chest movement with fetal respiration. (From Johnson and co-workers, 1988, with permission.)

Ray and colleagues (1972) used this concept in 66 complicated pregnancies and developed what they termed the *oxytocin challenge test* and later called the *contraction stress test*. Contractions were induced using intravenous oxytocin, and the fetal heart rate response was recorded using standard monitoring. The criterion for a positive (abnormal) test was uniform repetitive fetal heart rate decelerations. These reflected the uterine contraction waveform and had an onset at or beyond the acme of a contraction. Such late decelerations could be the result of uteroplacental insufficiency. The tests were generally repeated on a weekly basis, and the investigators concluded that negative (normal) contraction stress tests forecast fetal health. One disadvantage cited was that the average contraction stress test required 90 minutes to complete.

Fetal heart rate and uterine contractions are recorded simultaneously with an external monitor. If at least three spontaneous contractions of 40 seconds or longer are present in 10 minutes, no uterine stimulation is necessary (American College of Obstetricians and Gynecologists, 1999). Contractions are induced with either oxytocin or nipple stimulation if there are fewer than three in 10 minutes. If oxytocin is preferred, a dilute intravenous infusion is initiated at a rate of 0.5 mU/min and doubled every 20 minutes until a satisfactory contraction pattern is established (Freeman, 1975). The results of the contraction stress test are interpreted according to the criteria shown in Table 15–1.

Nipple stimulation to induce uterine contractions is usually successful for contraction stress testing (Huddleston and associates, 1984). One method recommended by the American College of Obstetricians and Gynecologists (1999) involves the woman rubbing one nipple through her clothing for 2 minutes or until a contraction begins. She is instructed to restart after 5 minutes if the first nipple stimulation did not induce three contractions in 10 minutes. Advantages include reduced cost and shortened testing times. Although Schellpfeffer and associates (1985) reported unpredictable uterine hyperstimulation with fetal distress, others did not find excessive activity to be harmful (Frager and Miyazaki, 1987).

TABLE 15–1 Criteria for Interpretation of the Contraction Stress Test

Negative: no late or significant variable decelerations
Positive: late decelerations following 50% or more of contractions—even if the contraction frequency is fewer than three in 10 min
Equivocal-suspicious: intermittent late decelerations or significant variable decelerations
Equivocal-hyperstimulatory: fetal heart rate decelerations that occur in the presence of contractions more frequent than every 2 min or lasting longer than 90 sec
Unsatisfactory: fewer than three contractions in 10 min or an uninterpretable tracing

From the American College of Obstetricians and Gynecologists, 1999, with permission.

NONSTRESS TESTS

Freeman (1975) and Lee and colleagues (1975) introduced the *nonstress test* to describe fetal heart rate acceleration in response to fetal movement as a sign of fetal health. This test involved the use of Doppler-detected fetal heart rate acceleration coincident with fetal movements perceived by the mother. By the end of the 1970s, the nonstress test had become the primary method of testing fetal health. The nonstress test was much easier to perform, and normal results were used to further discriminate false-positive contraction stress tests. Simplistically, the nonstress test is primarily a test of *fetal condition,* and it differs from the contraction stress test, which is a test of *uteroplacental function.* Currently, nonstress testing is the most widely used primary testing method for assessment of fetal well-being and has also been incorporated into the biophysical profile testing system (see later discussion).

FETAL HEART RATE ACCELERATION. The fetal heart rate normally is increased or decreased by autonomic influences mediated by sympathetic or parasympathetic impulses from brainstem centers. Beat-to-beat variability is also under the control of the autonomic nervous system (Matsuura and colleagues, 1996). Consequently, pathological loss of acceleration may be seen in conjunction with significantly decreased beat-to-beat variability of the fetal heart rate (see Chap. 18, p. 447). Loss of such reactivity, however, is most commonly associated with sleep cycles, discussed earlier, and it also may be caused by central depression from medications or maternal cigarette smoking (Oncken and colleagues, 2002).

The nonstress test is based on the hypothesis that the heart rate of a fetus who is not acidotic as a result of hypoxia or neurological depression will temporarily accelerate in response to fetal movement. Fetal movements during testing are identified by maternal perception and recorded. An example is shown in Figure 15–5. Similarly, Smith and colleagues (1988) observed a decrease in the number of accelerations in preterm fetuses subsequently found to have lower umbilical artery blood Po_2 values.

Gestational age influences acceleration or reactivity of fetal heart rate. Pillai and James (1990b) studied the development of fetal heart rate acceleration patterns during normal pregnancy. The percentage of body movements accompanied by acceleration and the amplitude of these accelerations increased with gestational age (Fig. 15–6). Guinn and colleagues (1998) studied nonstress test results between 25 and 28 weeks in 188 pregnancies that ultimately had normal outcomes. Only 70 percent of these normal fetuses demonstrated the required 15 bpm or more of heart rate acceleration. Lesser degrees of acceleration (i.e., 10 bpm) occurred in 90 percent of the tested pregnancies.

The National Institute of Child Health and Human Development fetal monitoring workshop (1997) has defined acceleration based on gestational age. The acme of acceleration is

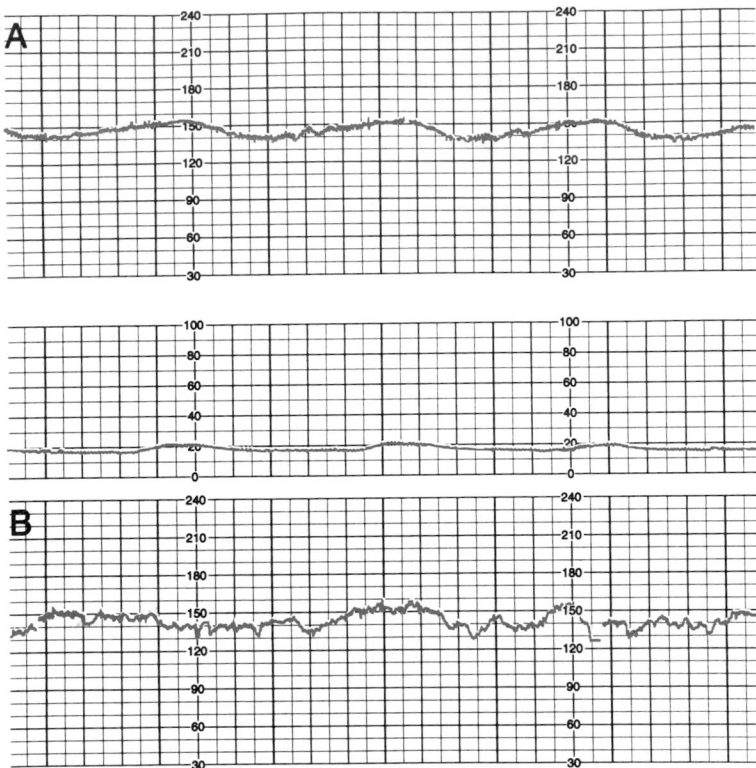

FIGURE 15–5. Antepartum fetal heart rate tracings at 28 weeks' gestation in a woman with diabetic ketoacidosis. Tracing **A**, obtained during maternal and fetal acidemia, shows absence of accelerations, diminished variability, and late decelerations with weak spontaneous contractions. Tracing **B** shows return of normal accelerations and variability of the fetal heart rate following correction of maternal acidemia.

15 bpm or more above the baseline rate, and the acceleration lasts 15 seconds or longer but less than 2 minutes in fetuses at or beyond 32 weeks. Before 32 weeks, accelerations are defined as having an acme 10 bpm or more above baseline for 10 seconds or longer.

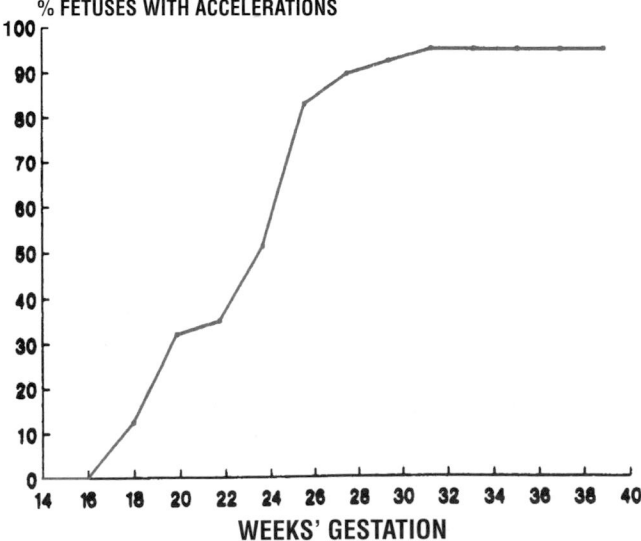

FIGURE 15–6. Percentage of fetuses with at least one acceleration of 15 beats/min sustained for 15 sec with fetal movement. (From Pillai and James, 1990b, with permission.)

NORMAL NONSTRESS TESTS. There have been many different definitions of normal nonstress test results. They vary as to the number, amplitude, and duration of acceleration, as well as the test duration. The definition currently recommended by the American College of Obstetricians and Gynecologists (1999) is two or more accelerations that peak at 15 bpm or more above baseline, each lasting 15 seconds or more, and all occurring within 20 minutes of beginning the test (Fig. 15–7). It was also recommended that accelerations with or without fetal movements be accepted, and that a 40-minute or longer tracing—to account for fetal sleep cycles—should be performed before concluding that there was insufficient fetal *reactivity.* Miller and colleagues (1996b) reviewed fetal outcomes after nonstress tests considered as nonreactive because there was only one acceleration. They concluded that one acceleration was just as reliable in predicting healthy fetal status as were two.

Although a normal number and amplitude of accelerations seems to reflect fetal well-being, "insufficient acceleration" does not invariably predict fetal compromise. Indeed, some investigators have reported false-positive nonstress test rates in excess of 90 percent when acceleration was considered insufficient (Devoe and colleagues, 1986). Because healthy fetuses may not move for periods of up to 75 minutes, Brown and Patrick (1981) considered that a longer duration of nonstress testing might increase the positive-predictive value of an abnormal, or nonreactive test. They concluded that either the test became reactive during a period of time up to

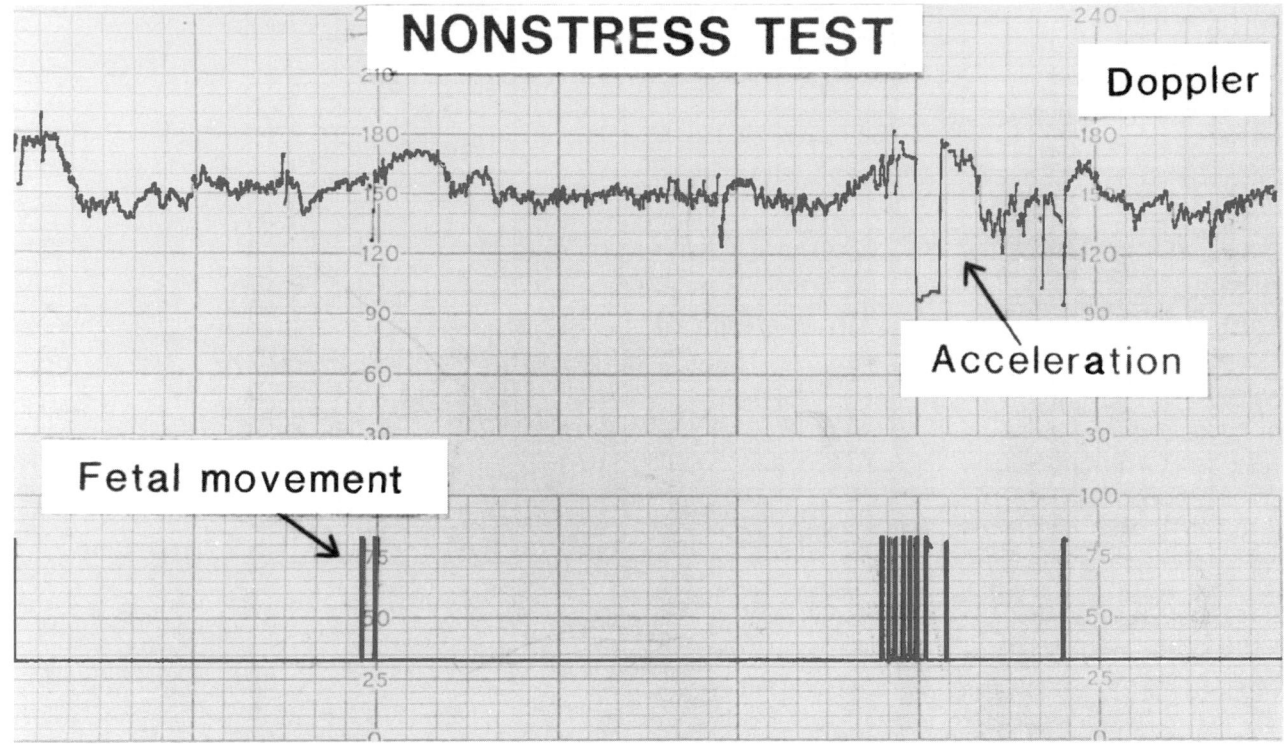

FIGURE 15–7. Reactive nonstress test. Notice increase of fetal heart rate to more than 15 beats/min for longer than 15 sec following fetal movements, indicated by the vertical marks on the lower part of the recording.

80 minutes, or the test remained nonreactive for 120 minutes, indicating that the fetus was very ill.

Not only are there many different definitions of normal nonstress test results, but the reproducibility of interpretations is problematic. For example, Hage (1985) mailed five nonstress tests, blinded to specific patient clinical data, to a national sample of obstetricians for their interpretations. He concluded that although nonstress testing is very popular, the reliability of test interpretation needs improvement. Such problems with subjective interpretation have prompted efforts to computerize analysis of nonstress tests. Pardey and colleagues (2002) developed a computerized system, *Sonicaid Fetal Care,* that they claim is superior to visual subjective interpretation of nonstress tests.

ABNORMAL NONSTRESS TESTS. There are abnormal nonstress test patterns that reliably forecast severe fetal jeopardy. Hammacher and co-workers (1968) described tracings with what they termed a *silent oscillatory pattern.* This pattern consisted of a fetal heart rate baseline that oscillated less than 5 bpm and presumably indicated absent acceleration and beat-to-beat variability. Hammacher considered this pattern ominous.

Visser and associates (1980) described a "terminal cardiotocogram," which included (1) baseline oscillation of less than 5 bpm, (2) absent accelerations, and (3) late

decelerations with spontaneous uterine contractions. These results were very similar to experiences from Parkland Hospital in which absence of accelerations during an 80-minute recording period in 27 fetuses was associated consistently with evidence of uteroplacental pathology (Leveno and associates, 1983). The latter included fetal growth restriction (75 percent), oligohydramnios (80 percent), fetal acidosis (40 percent), meconium (30 percent), and placental infarction (93 percent). Thus, the lack of fetal heart rate acceleration, when not due to maternal sedation, is an ominous finding (Fig. 15–8). Similarly, Devoe and co-workers (1985) concluded that nonstress tests that were nonreactive for 90 minutes were almost invariably (93 percent) associated with significant perinatal pathology.

Interval Between Testing. The interval between tests, originally rather arbitrarily set at 7 days, appears to have been shortened as experience evolved with nonstress testing. According to the American College of Obstetricians and Gynecologists (1999), more frequent testing is advocated by some investigators for women with postterm pregnancy, type 1 diabetes mellitus, fetal growth restriction, or gestational hypertension. In these circumstances, some investigators perform twice-weekly tests, with additional testing performed for maternal or fetal deterioration regardless of time elapsed since the last test. Others perform nonstress tests daily or

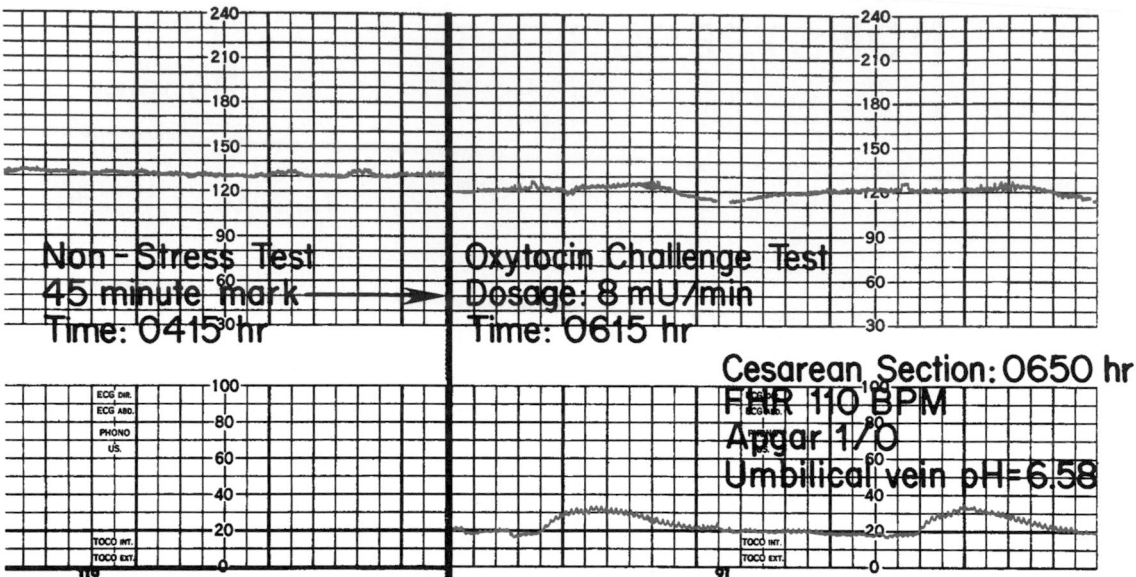

FIGURE 15–8. Nonreactive nonstress test followed by contraction stress test showing mild, late decelerations. Cesarean delivery was performed, and the severely acidemic fetus could not be resuscitated.

even more frequently. For example, Chari and co-workers (1995) recommend daily fetal testing in women with severe preeclampsia remote from term.

Decelerations During Nonstress Testing. Fetal movements commonly produce heart rate decelerations. Timor-Tritsch and co-authors (1978) reported this during nonstress testing in half to two thirds of tracings, depending on the vigor of the fetal motion. Such a high incidence of decelerations inevitably makes interpretation of their significance problematic. Indeed, Meis and co-workers (1986) reported that variable fetal heart rate decelerations during nonstress tests were not a sign of fetal compromise. The American College of Obstetricians and Gynecologists (1999) has concluded that variable decelerations, if nonrepetitive and brief—less than 30 seconds—do not indicate fetal compromise or the need for obstetrical intervention. In contrast, repetitive variable decelerations—at least three in 20 minutes—even if mild, have been associated with an increased risk of cesarean delivery for fetal distress. Decelerations lasting 1 minute or longer have been reported to have an even worse prognosis (Bourgeois and colleagues, 1984; Druzin and colleagues, 1981; Pazos and colleagues, 1982).

Hoskins and associates (1991) attempted to refine interpretation of testing that shows variable decelerations by adding ultrasonic estimation of amnionic fluid volume. The incidence of cesarean delivery for intrapartum fetal distress progressively increased coincidentally with the severity of variable decelerations and diminished amnionic fluid volume. Severe variable decelerations during a nonstress test plus an amnionic fluid index of 5 cm or less resulted in a 75-percent cesarean delivery rate. Fetal distress in labor, however, also frequently developed in those pregnancies with variable decelerations but with normal amounts of amnionic fluid. Similar results were reported by Grubb and Paul (1992).

False-Normal Nonstress Tests. Smith and associates (1987) performed a detailed analysis of the causes of fetal death within 7 days of normal nonstress tests. The most common indication in this study for testing was postterm pregnancy. The mean interval between testing and death was 4 days, with a range of 1 to 7 days. The single most common autopsy finding was meconium aspiration, often associated with some type of umbilical cord abnormality. They concluded that an acute asphyxial insult had provoked fetal gasping. They also concluded that nonstress testing was inadequate to preclude such an acute asphyxial event and that other biophysical characteristics might be beneficial adjuncts. For example, assessment of amnionic fluid volume was considered to be of value. Other ascribed frequent causes of fetal death included intrauterine infection, abnormal cord position, malformations, and placental abruption.

ACOUSTIC STIMULATION TESTS

Loud external sounds have been used to startle the fetus, provoking acceleration of the heart rate—an acoustic stimulation nonstress test. Eller and associates (1995) used a commercially available acoustic stimulator (Corometrics model 146) and measured intrauterine sound levels. Sound intensity between 100 and 105 dB—equivalent to sounds generated by a jet plane at takeoff—was maintained until the stimulator was moved more than 20 cm from the maternal

TABLE 15–2 Components and Their Scores for the Biophysical Profile

Component	Score 2	Score 0
Nonstress test[a]	$\geq$ 2 accelerations of $\geq$ 15 beats/min for $\geq$ 15 sec in 20–40 min	0 or 1 acceleration in 20–40 min
Fetal breathing	$\geq$ 1 episode of rhythmic breathing lasting $\geq$ 30 sec within 30 min	< 30 sec of breathing in 30 min
Fetal movement	$\geq$ 3 discrete body or limb movements within 30 min	< 3 discrete movements
Fetal tone	$\geq$ 1 episode of extension of a fetal extremity with return to flexion, or opening or closing of hand within 30 min	No movements or no extension/flexion
Amnionic fluid volume[b]	Single vertical pocket > 2 cm	Largest single vertical pocket $\leq$ 2 cm

[a] May be omitted if all four ultrasound components are normal.
[b] Further evaluation warranted, regardless of biophysical composite score, if largest vertical amnionic fluid pocket $\leq$ 2 cm.
From the American College of Obstetricians and Gynecologists, 1999, with permission.

abdomen. The acoustic stimulator is positioned on the maternal abdomen and a stimulus of 1 to 2 seconds is applied. This may be repeated up to three times for up to 3 seconds (American College of Obstetricians and Gynecologists, 1999). Perez-Delboy and colleagues (2002) randomized 113 women to nonstress testing with and without vibroacoustic stimulation. Such stimulation shortened the average time for nonstress testing from 24 to 15 minutes.

BIOPHYSICAL PROFILE

Manning and colleagues (1980) proposed the combined use of five fetal biophysical variables as a more accurate means of assessing fetal health than any one used alone. They hypothesized that consideration of five variables could significantly reduce both false-positive and false-negative tests. Required equipment includes a real-time ultrasound device and Doppler ultrasound to record fetal heart rate. Typically, these tests require 30 to 60 minutes of examiner time. Shown in Table 15–2 are the five biophysical components assessed, which include (1) fetal heart rate acceleration, (2) fetal breathing, (3) fetal movements, (4) fetal tone, and (5) amnionic fluid volume. Normal variables were assigned a score of two each and abnormal variables, a score of zero. Thus, the highest score possible for a normal fetus is 10. Kopecky and colleagues

(2000) observed that 10 to 15 mg of morphine sulfate administered to the mother caused a significant decrease in the biophysical score by suppressing fetal breathing and heart rate acceleration.

Manning and colleagues (1987) tested more than 19,000 pregnancies using the biophysical profile interpretation and management shown in Table 15–3. They reported a false-normal test rate, defined as an antepartum death of a structurally normal fetus, of approximately 1 per 1000. More than 97 percent of the pregnancies tested had normal test results. The most common identifiable causes of fetal death after normal biophysical profiles include fetomaternal hemorrhage, umbilical cord accidents, and placental abruption (Dayal and colleagues, 1999). Manning and co-authors (1993) published a remarkable description of 493 fetuses in which biophysical scores were performed immediately before measurement of umbilical venous blood pH values obtained via cordocentesis. Approximately 20 percent of tested fetuses had growth restriction and the remainder had alloimmune hemolytic anemia. As shown in Figure 15–9, a biophysical score of zero was invariably associated with significant fetal acidemia, whereas normal scores of 8 or 10 were associated with normal pH. An equivocal test result—a score of 6—was a poor predictor of abnormal outcome. A decrease from an abnormal result—a score of 2 or 4—to a very abnormal score (zero) was a progressively more accurate predictor of abnormal outcome.

TABLE 15–3 Modified Biophysical Profile Score, Interpretation, and Pregnancy Management

Biophysical Profile Score	Interpretation	Recommended Management
10	Normal, nonasphyxiated	No fetal indication for intervention; repeat test weekly except in diabetic patient and postterm pregnancy (twice weekly)
8 Normal fluid	Normal, nonasphyxiated fetus	No fetal indication for intervention; repeat testing per protocol
8 Oligohydramnios	Chronic fetal asphyxia suspected	Deliver if $\geq$ 37 weeks, otherwise repeat testing
6	Possible fetal asphyxia	If amnionic fluid volume abnormal, deliver If normal fluid at > 36 wk with favorable cervix, deliver If repeat test $\leq$ 6, deliver If repeat test > 6, observe and repeat per protocol
4	Probable fetal asphyxia	Repeat testing same day; if biophysical profile score $\leq$ 6, deliver
0–2	Almost certain fetal asphyxia	Deliver

From Manning and colleagues, 1987, with permission.

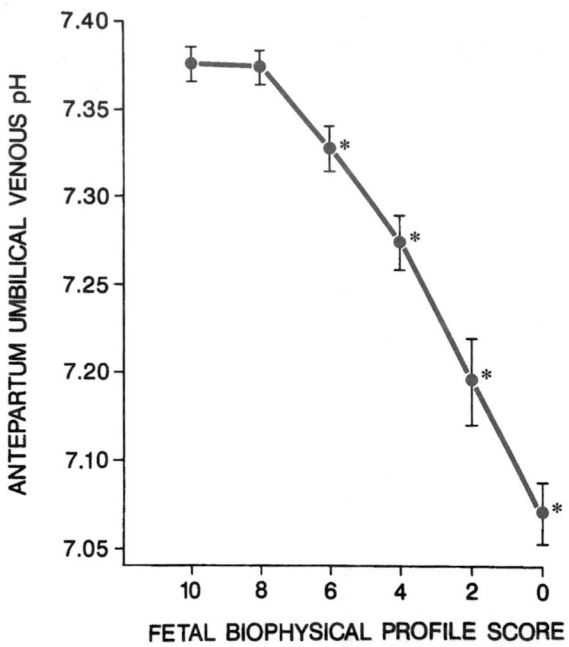

FIGURE 15–9. Mean umbilical vein pH (± 2 SD) in relation to fetal biophysical profile score category. (From Manning and associates, 1993, with permission.)

Salvesen and colleagues (1993) correlated the biophysical profile with umbilical venous blood pH obtained at cordocentesis in 41 pregnancies complicated by diabetes. They also found that abnormal pH was significantly associated with abnormal biophysical profile scores. They concluded, however, that the biophysical profile was of limited value in the prediction of fetal pH, because nine mildly acidemic fetuses had normal antepartum tests. Weiner and colleagues (1996) assessed the meaning of antepartum fetal tests in 135 overtly growth-restricted fetuses and came to a similar conclusion. They found that morbidity and mortality in severe fetal growth restriction were determined primarily by gestational age and birthweight and not by abnormal fetal tests.

MODIFIED BIOPHYSICAL PROFILE. Because the biophysical profile is labor intensive and requires a person trained in ultrasonic visualization of the fetus, Clark and coworkers (1989) used an abbreviated biophysical profile as their first-line antepartum screening test in 2628 singleton pregnancies. Specifically, a vibroacoustic nonstress test was performed twice weekly along with determination of the amnionic fluid index (see Chap. 16, p. 392). An amnionic fluid index of less than 5 cm was considered abnormal. This abbreviated biophysical profile required about 10 minutes to perform, and they concluded that it was a superb method of antepartum surveillance because there were no unexpected fetal deaths.

Nageotte and colleagues (1994) also combined biweekly nonstress tests with the amnionic fluid index and considered 5 cm or less to be abnormal. They performed 17,429 modified

biophysical profiles in 2774 women and concluded that such testing was an excellent method of fetal surveillance. They randomized women with abnormal test results to backup testing with either a complete biophysical profile or a contraction stress test. Contraction stress testing increased intervention for a false-abnormal test. Miller and associates (1996a) reported results with more than 54,000 modified biophysical profiles performed in 15,400 high-risk pregnancies. They described a false-negative rate of 0.8 per 1000 and a false-positive rate of 1.5 percent. Young and co-workers (2003) randomized 683 women to the original biophysical profile or to two modified testing procedures and found no differences in effectiveness between three various methods.

The American College of Obstetricians and Gynecologists (1999) has concluded that the modified biophysical profile test is an acceptable means of antepartum fetal surveillance.

AMNIONIC FLUID VOLUME

Assessment of amnionic fluid has become an integral component in the antepartum assessment of pregnancies at risk for fetal death. This is based on the rationale that decreased uteroplacental perfusion may lead to diminished fetal renal blood flow, decreased urine production, and ultimately, oligohydramnios. As discussed in Chapter 16 (see p. 392), the amnionic fluid index, the deepest vertical pocket, and the 2×2 cm pocket used in the biophysical profile are some ultrasonic techniques used to estimate amnionic fluid volume (Chamberlain, 1984; Manning, 1984; Rutherford, 1987, and their colleagues).

In their review of 42 reports on the amnionic fluid index published between 1987 and 1997, Chauhan and colleagues (1999) concluded that an index of 5.0 cm or less significantly increased the risk of either cesarean delivery for fetal distress or a low 5-minute Apgar score. Similarly, in a retrospective analysis of 6423 pregnancies managed at Parkland Hospital, Casey and colleagues (2000) found that an amnionic fluid index of 5 cm or less was associated with significantly increased perinatal morbidity and mortality. Locatelli and associates (2004) reported excessive low-birthweight infants if there was oligohydramnios so defined.

Not all investigators agree with the concept that an index of 5 cm or less portends more adverse outcomes. Magann and colleagues (1999, 2004) concluded that the index was a poor diagnostic test and that it better predicted normal than abnormal volumes. Driggers and co-workers (2004) and Zhang and collaborators (2004) did not find a correlation with bad outcomes in pregnancies in which the index was below 5 cm. In the only randomized trial reported to date, Conway and colleagues (2000) concluded that nonintervention to permit spontaneous onset of labor was as effective as induction in term pregnancies with amnionic fluid index values of 5 cm or less.

UMBILICAL ARTERY DOPPLER VELOCIMETRY

Doppler ultrasonography is a noninvasive technique to assess blood flow by characterizing downstream impedance (see Chap. 16, p. 400). The umbilical artery systolic–diastolic (S/D) ratio, the most commonly used index, is considered abnormal if it is above the 95th percentile for gestational age or if diastolic flow is either absent or reversed. Absent or reversed end-diastolic flow signifies increased impedance to umbilical artery blood flow (Fig. 15–10 and Fig. 16–20, p. 403). It is reported to result from poorly vascularized placental villi and is seen in the most extreme cases of fetal growth restriction (Todros and co-authors, 1999). Zelop and colleagues (1996) found that perinatal mortality for absent end-diastolic flow was about 10 percent, and for reversed end-diastolic flow, it was approximately 33 percent.

Doppler ultrasonography has been subjected to more extensive assessment with randomized controlled trials than has any previous test of fetal health. Williams and colleagues (2003) randomized 1360 high-risk women to either nonstress testing or Doppler velocimetry. They found a significantly increased incidence of cesarean delivery for fetal distress in the nonstress test group compared with that for those tested with Doppler—8.7 versus 4.6 percent. One interpretation of this finding is that the nonstress test more frequently identified fetuses in jeopardy. The utility of umbilical artery Doppler velocimetry was reviewed by the American College of Obstetricians and Gynecologists (1999, 2000). It was concluded that no benefit has been demonstrated other than in pregnancies with suspected fetal growth restriction. No benefit has been demonstrated for velocimetry for other conditions, such as postterm pregnancy, diabetes mellitus, systemic lupus erythematosus, or antiphospholipid antibody syndrome. Similarly, velocimetry has not proved of value as a screening test for detecting fetal compromise in the general obstetrical population.

It is possible to evaluate blood flow in other vessels in addition to the umbilical vessels (see Chap. 16, p. 401). In the mother, these include velocimetry of the uterine artery (Lees and colleagues, 2001; Vergani and colleagues, 2003). In the fetus, the middle cerebral artery has received particular attention because of observations that the hypoxic fetus achieves *brain sparing* through reduced cerebrovascular impedance and thus increased blood flow. Such brain sparing in growth-restricted fetuses has been documented to undergo reversal in less than 24 hours by Konje and colleagues (2001). They reported that 8 of 17 fetuses with this finding died. Ott and colleagues (1998) randomized 665 women undergoing modified biophysical profiles to either this test alone or combined with middle cerebral to umbilical artery velocity flow ratios. There were no significant differences in pregnancy outcomes between these two study groups. This technique currently is considered investigational by the American College of Obstetricians and Gynecologists (1999).

CURRENT ANTENATAL TESTING RECOMMENDATIONS

According to the American College of Obstetricians and Gynecologists (1999), there is no "best test" to evaluate fetal well-being. Three testing systems—contraction stress test, nonstress test, and biophysical profile—have different end

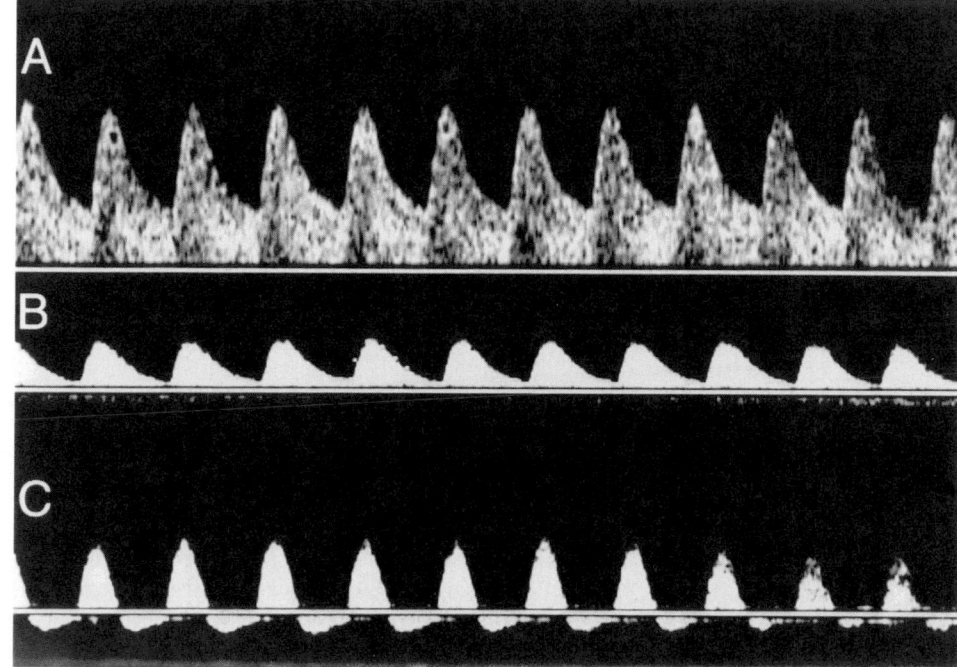

FIGURE 15–10. Three studies of fetal umbilical artery velocimetry. The peaks represent systolic velocity, and the troughs show the diastolic velocity. **A.** Normal velocimetry pattern. **B.** Velocity is zero during diastole (trough reaches the horizontal line). **C.** Arterial velocity is reversed during diastole (trough is below horizontal line). (Courtesy of Dr. Diane Twickler.)

points that are considered, depending on the clinical situation. The American College of Obstetricians and Gynecologists (2002) patient education pamphlet describes these tests of fetal well-being and summarizes as follows: "Monitoring helps you and your doctor during your pregnancy by telling more about the well-being of the baby. If a test result suggests that there may be a problem, this does not always mean that the baby is in trouble. It simply may mean that you need special care or more tests. Discuss any questions you have about monitoring with your doctor."

The most important consideration in deciding when to begin antepartum testing is the prognosis for neonatal survival. The severity of maternal disease is another important consideration. In general, with the majority of high-risk pregnancies, most authorities recommend that testing begin by 32 to 34 weeks. Pregnancies with severe complications might require testing as early as 26 to 28 weeks. The frequency for repeating tests has been arbitrarily set at 7 days, but more frequent testing is often done.

At Parkland Hospital, antepartum fetal heart rate recordings have been limited to about 700 women admitted to the High-Risk Pregnancy Unit each year. Such recordings are often obtained several times throughout the week—for example, Monday, Wednesday, and Friday—in these pregnancies. The primary focus of fetal heart rate assessments is detection of decelerations, and delivery is not withheld simply because accelerations are witnessed. Clinical and ultrasonic estimations of amnionic fluid volume also may be used to assess fetal health. Outpatients do not undergo fetal heart rate testing. If there is concern about fetal movement or amnionic fluid volume, then the woman may be observed in the labor suite with fetal heart rate monitoring. Depending on results, she is either discharged or transferred to the High-Risk Unit, or labor is induced. Despite this limited use of antepartum testing, the fetal death rate in structurally normal infants is quite low in high-risk women. Indeed, most antepartum fetal deaths that we encounter are in low-risk pregnancies, and are attributable to unpreventable causes such as placental abruptions and umbilical cord accidents.

SIGNIFICANCE OF FETAL TESTING. Does antenatal fetal testing really make a difference? Platt and co-workers (1987) reviewed its impact between 1971 and 1985 at Los Angeles County Hospital. During this 15-year period, more than 200,000 pregnancies were managed, and nearly 17,000 of these women underwent antepartum testing of various types. Fetal surveillance increased from less than 1 percent of pregnancies in the early 1970s to 15 percent in the mid-1980s. These authors concluded that such testing was clearly beneficial because the fetal death rate was significantly less in the tested high-risk pregnancies compared with the rate in those not tested.

A contrasting opinion on the benefits of antenatal fetal testing was offered by Thacker and Berkelman (1986). It was their view that efficacy is best evaluated in randomized controlled trials. After reviewing 600 reports, they found only four such trials, all performed with the nonstress test and none with the contraction stress test. The numbers in these four trials were considered too small to detect important benefits. They projected that the costs of such testing exceeded $200 million per year in 1986 and that published studies did not support the use of either test. Enkin and colleagues (2000) reviewed evidence in the Cochrane Library from controlled trials of antepartum fetal surveillance. They concluded that "despite their widespread use, most tests of fetal well-being should be considered of experimental value only rather than validated clinical tools."

Another important and unanswered question is whether antepartum fetal surveillance identifies fetal asphyxia early enough to prevent brain damage. Todd and co-workers (1992) attempted to correlate cognitive development in infants up to the age of 2 years following either abnormal Doppler velocimetry or nonstress tests. Only abnormal nonstress tests were associated with marginally poorer cognitive outcomes. They concluded that by the time fetal compromise is diagnosed with antenatal testing, fetal damage has already been sustained. Low and colleagues (2003) reached a similar conclusion in their study of 36 preterm infants delivered based on antepartum test results. Thornton (2003) randomized 548 preterm pregnancies with abnormal test results to immediate or delayed delivery with a median of 5 days. They found that immediate delivery was associated with neonatal death and delayed delivery with stillbirth.

Manning and co-authors (1998) studied the incidence of cerebral palsy in 26,290 high-risk pregnancies managed with serial biophysical profile testing. They compared these outcomes with those of 58,657 low-risk pregnancies in which antepartum testing was not performed. The rate of cerebral palsy was 1.3 per 1000 in tested pregnancies compared with that of 4.7 per 1000 in untested women. In a prior study, however, Manning and colleagues (1996) had reported that cerebral palsy was significantly associated with low biophysical profile scores, which suggested that identification of the truly compromised fetus may be too late.

Antenatal forecasts of fetal health have clearly been the focus of intense interest for more than two decades. When such testing is reviewed, several themes emerge:

1. Methods of fetal forecasting have evolved continually, a phenomenon that itself suggests dissatisfaction with the precision or efficacy of any given method.
2. The fetal biophysical performance is characterized by wide ranges of normal biological variation, resulting in difficulty determining when such performance should be considered abnormal. *How many movements, respirations, or accelerations? In what time period?* Unable to easily quantify normal fetal biophysical performance, most investigators have resorted to somewhat arbitrary answers to such questions.

3. Despite the invention of increasingly complex testing methods, abnormal results are seldom reliable, prompting many clinicians to use antenatal testing to forecast fetal *wellness* rather than *illness*.

REFERENCES

American College of Obstetricians and Gynecologists: Special tests for monitoring fetal health. Patient Education Pamphlet, January 2002

American College of Obstetricians and Gynecologists: Intrauterine growth restriction. Practice Bulletin No. 12, January 2000

American College of Obstetricians and Gynecologists: Antepartum fetal surveillance. Practice Bulletin No. 9, October 1999

Badalian SS, Chao CR, Fox HE, et al: Fetal breathing-related nasal fluid flow velocity in uncomplicated pregnancies. Am J Obstet Gynecol 169:563, 1993

Boito SM, Ursem MT, Struijk PC, et al: Umbilical venous volume flow and fetal behavioral states in the normally developing fetus. Ultrasound Obstet Gynecol 23:138, 2004

Bourgeois FJ, Thiagarajah S, Harbert GN Jr: The significance of fetal heart rate decelerations during nonstress testing. Am J Obstet Gynecol 150:213, 1984

Brown R, Patrick J: The nonstress test: How long is enough? Am J Obstet Gynecol 141:646, 1981

Casey BM, McIntire DD, Bloom SL, et al: Pregnancy outcomes after antepartum diagnosis of oligohydramnios at or beyond 34 weeks' gestation. Am J Obstet Gynecol 182:909, 2000

Chamberlain PF, Manning FA, Morrison I, et al: Ultrasound evaluation of amniotic fluid volume. II. The relationship of increased amniotic fluid volume to perinatal outcome. Am J Obstet Gynecol 150:250, 1984

Chari RS, Friedman SA, O'Brien JM, et al: Daily antenatal testing in women with severe preeclampsia. Am J Obstet Gynecol 173:1207, 1995

Chauhan SP, Sanderson M, Hendrix NW, et al: Perinatal outcomes and amniotic fluid index in the antepartum and intrapartum periods: A meta-analysis. Am J Obstet Gynecol 181:1473, 1999

Clark SL, Sabey P, Jolley K: Nonstress testing with acoustic stimulation and amnionic fluid volume assessment: 5973 tests without unexpected fetal death. Am J Obstet Gynecol 160:694, 1989

Conway DL, Groth S, Adkins WB, et al: Management of isolated oligohydramnios in the term pregnancy: A randomized clinical trial. Am J Obstet Gynecol 182:S21, 2000

Dawes GS: Breathing before birth in animals and man. An essay in medicine. Physiol Med 290:557, 1974

Dawes GS, Fox HE, Leduc BM, et al: Respiratory movements and rapid eye movement sleep in the foetal lamb. J Physiol 220:119, 1972

Dayal AK, Manning FA, Berck DJ, et al: Fetal death after normal biophysical profile score: An eighteen year experience. Am J Obstet Gynecol 181:1231, 1999

Devoe LD, Castillo RA, Sherline DM: The nonstress test as a diagnostic test: A critical reappraisal. Am J Obstet Gynecol 152:1047, 1986

Devoe LD, McKenzie J, Searle NS, et al: Clinical sequelae of the extended nonstress test. Am J Obstet Gynecol 151:1074, 1985

DeVries JIP, Visser GHA, Prechtl NFR: The emergence of fetal behavior. II. Quantitative aspects. Early Hum Dev 12:99, 1985

Driggers RW, Holcroft CJ, Blakemore KJ, et al: An amniotic fluid index ≤ 5 cm within 7 days of delivery in the third trimester is not associated with decreasing umbilical arterial pH and base excess. J Perinatol 24:72, 2004

Druzin ML, Gratacos J, Keegan KA, et al: Antepartum fetal heart rate testing, 7. The significance of fetal bradycardia. Am J Obstet Gynecol 139:194, 1981

Eller DP, Scardo JA, Dillon AE, et al: Distance from an intrauterine hydrophone as a factor affecting intrauterine sound pressure levels produced by the vibroacoustic stimulation test. Am J Obstet Gynecol 173:523, 1995

Enkin M, Keirse MJNC, Renfrew M, et al: A Guide to Effective Care in Pregnancy and Childbirth, 3rd ed. New York, Oxford University Press, 2000, p 225

Frager NB, Miyazaki FS: Intrauterine monitoring of contractions during breast stimulation. Obstet Gynecol 69:767, 1987

Freeman RK: The use of the oxytocin challenge test for antepartum clinical evaluation of uteroplacental respiratory function. Am J Obstet Gynecol 121:481, 1975

Grant A, Elbourne D, Valentin L, et al: Routine formal fetal movement counting and risk of antepartum late death in normally formed singletons. Lancet 2:345, 1989

Grubb DK, Paul RH: Amnionic fluid index and prolonged antepartum fetal heart rate decelerations. Obstet Gynecol 79:558, 1992

Guinn DA, Kimberlin KF, Wigton TR, et al: Fetal heart rate characteristics at 25 to 28 weeks gestation. Am J Perinatol 15:507, 1998

Hage ML: Interpretation of nonstress tests. Am J Obstet Gynecol 153:490, 1985

Hammacher K, Hüter KA, Bokelmann J, et al: Foetal heart frequency and perinatal condition of the foetus and newborn. Gynaecologia 166:349, 1968

Harrington K, Thompson O, Jorden L, et al: Obstetric outcomes in women who present with a reduction in fetal movements in the third trimester of pregnancy. J Perinat Med 26:77, 1998

Hoskins IA, Frieden FJ, Young BK: Variable decelerations in reactive nonstress tests with decreased amnionic fluid index predict fetal compromise. Am J Obstet Gynecol 165:1094, 1991

Huddleston JF, Sutliff JG, Robinson D: Contraction stress test by intermittent nipple stimulation. Obstet Gynecol 63:669, 1984

Johnson MJ, Paine LL, Mulder HH, et al: Population differences of fetal biophysical and behavioral characteristics. Am J Obstet Gynecol 166:138, 1992

Johnson T, Besigner R, Thomas R: New clues to fetal behavior and well-being. Contemp Ob/Gyn, May 1988

Konje JC, Bell SC, Taylor DT: Abnormal Doppler velocimetry and blood flow volume in the middle cerebral artery in very severe intrauterine growth restriction: Is the occurrence of reversal of compensatory flow too late? Br J Obstet Gynaecol 108:973, 2001

Kopecky EA, Ryan ML, Barrett JFR, et al: Fetal response to maternally administered morphine. Am J Obstet Gynecol 183:424, 2000

Lee CY, DiLoreto PC, O'Lane JM: A study of fetal heart rate acceleration patterns. Obstet Gynecol 45:142, 1975

Lees C, Parra M, Missfelder-Lobos H, et al: Individualized risk assessment for adverse pregnancy outcome by uterine artery Doppler at 23 weeks. Obstet Gynecol 98:369, 2001

Leveno KJ, Williams ML, DePalma RT, et al: Perinatal outcome in the absence of antepartum fetal heart rate acceleration. Obstet Gynecol 61:347, 1983

Locatelli A, Vergani P, Toso L, et al: Perinatal outcome associated with oligohydramnios in uncomplicated term pregnancies. Arch Gynecol Obstet 269:130, 2004

Low JA, Killen H, Derrick EJ: Antepartum fetal complexia in the preterm pregnancy. Am J Obstet Gynecol 188:461, 2003

Magann EF, Chauhan SP, Kinsella MJ, et al: Antenatal testing among 1001 patients at high risk: The role of ultrasonographic estimates of amniotic fluid volume. Am J Obstet Gynecol 180:1330, 1999

Magann EF, Doherty DA, Chauhan SP, et al: How well do the amniotic fluid index and single deepest pocket indices (below the 3rd and 5th and above the 95th and 97th percentiles) predict oligohydramnios and hydramnios? Am J Obstet Gynecol 190:164, 2004

Manning FA, Bondaji N, Harman CR, et al: Fetal assessment based on fetal biophysical profile scoring VIII: The incidence of cerebral palsy in tested and untested perinates. Am J Obstet Gynecol 178:696, 1998

Manning FA, Harman C, Menticoglou S: Fetal biophysical score and cerebral palsy at age 3 years. Am J Obstet Gynecol 174:319, 1996

Manning FA, Harman CR, Morrison I, et al: Fetal assessment based on fetal biophysical profile scoring, IV. An analysis of perinatal morbidity and mortality. Am J Obstet Gynecol 150:245, 1984

Manning FA, Morrison I, Harman CR, et al: Fetal assessment based on fetal biophysical profile scoring: Experience in 19,221 referred high-risk pregnancies, 2. An analysis of false-negative fetal deaths. Am J Obstet Gynecol 157:880, 1987

Manning FA, Platt LD, Sipos L: Antepartum fetal evaluation: Development of a fetal biophysical profile. Am J Obstet Gynecol 136:787, 1980

Manning FA, Snijders R, Harman CR, et al: Fetal biophysical profile score, VI. Correlation with antepartum umbilical venous fetal pH. Am J Obstet Gynecol 169:755, 1993

Matsuura M, Murata Y, Hirano T, et al: The effects of developing autonomous nervous system on FHR variabilities determined by the power spectral analysis. Am J Obstet Gynecol 174:380, 1996

Meis PJ, Ureda JR, Swain M, et al: Variable decelerations during nonstress tests are not a sign of fetal compromise. Am J Obstet Gynecol 154:586, 1986

Miller DA, Rabello YA, Paul RH: The modified biophysical profile: Antepartum testing in the 1990s. Am J Obstet Gynecol 174:812, 1996a

Miller F, Miller D, Paul R, et al: Is one fetal heart rate acceleration during a non-stress test as reliable as two in predicting fetal status? Am J Obstet Gynecol 174:337, 1996b

Moore TR, Piaquadio K: A prospective evaluation of fetal movement screening to reduce the incidence of antepartum fetal death. Am J Obstet Gynecol 160:1075, 1989

Nageotte MP, Towers CV, Asrat T, et al: Perinatal outcome with the modified biophysical profile. Am J Obstet Gynecol 170:1672, 1994

National Institute of Child Health and Human Development Research Planning Workshop. Electronic fetal heart rate monitoring: Research guidelines for interpretation. Am J Obstet Gynecol 177:1385, 1997

Neldam S: Fetal movements as an indicator of fetal well being. Dan Med Bull 30:274, 1983

Nijhuis JG, Prechtl HFR, Martin CB Jr, et al: Are there behavioural states in the human fetus? Early Hum Dev 6:177, 1982

Oncken C, Kranzler H, O'Malley P, et al: The effect of cigarette smoking on fetal heart rate characteristics. Obstet Gynecol 99:751, 2002

Oosterhof H, vd Stege JG, Lander M, et al: Urine production rate is related to behavioural states in the near term human fetus. Br J Obstet Gynaecol 100:920, 1993

Ott WJ, Mora G, Arias F, et al: Comparison of the modified biophysical profile to a "new" biophysical profile incorporating the middle cerebral artery to umbilical artery velocity flow systolic/diastolic ratio. Am J Obstet Gynecol 178:1346, 1998

Pardey J, Moulden M, Redmon CWG: A computer system for numerical analysis of nonstress tests. Am J Obstet Gynecol 186:1095, 2002

Patrick J, Campbell K, Carmichael L, et al: Patterns of gross fetal body movements over 24-hour observation intervals during the last 10 weeks of pregnancy. Am J Obstet Gynecol 142:363, 1982

Patrick J, Campbell K, Carmichael L, et al: Patterns of human fetal breathing during the last 10 weeks of pregnancy. Obstet Gynecol 56:24, 1980

Pazos R, Vuolo K, Aladjem S, et al: Association of spontaneous fetal heart rate decelerations during antepartum nonstress testing and intrauterine growth retardation. Am J Obstet Gynecol 144:574, 1982

Perez-Delboy A, Weiss J, Michels A, et al: A randomized trial of vibroacoustic stimulation for antenatal fetal testing. Am J Obstet Gynecol 187:S146, 2002

Pillai M, James D: Behavioral states in normal mature human fetuses. Arch Dis Child 65:39, 1990a

Pillai M, James D: The development of fetal heart rate patterns during normal pregnancy. Obstet Gynecol 76:812, 1990b

Platt LD, Paul RH, Phelan J, et al: Fifteen years of experience with antepartum fetal testing. Am J Obstet Gynecol 156:1509, 1987

Ray M, Freeman R, Pine S, et al: Clinical experience with the oxytocin challenge test. Am J Obstet Gynecol 114:1, 1972

Rayburn WF: Clinical significance of perceptible fetal motion. Am J Obstet Gynecol 138:210, 1980

Rutherford SE, Phelan JP, Smith CV, et al: The four-quadrant assessment of amniotic fluid volume: An adjunct to antepartum fetal heart rate testing. Obstet Gynecol 70:353, 1987

Sadovsky E, Evron S, Weinstein D: Daily fetal movement recording in normal pregnancy. Riv Obstet Ginecol Practica Med Perinatal 59:395, 1979a

Sadovsky E, Laufer N, Allen JW: The incidence of different types of fetal movement during pregnancy. Br J Obstet Gynaecol 86:10, 1979b

Sadovsky E, Yaffe H: Daily fetal movement recording and fetal prognosis. Obstet Gynecol 41:845, 1973

Salvesen DR, Freeman J, Brudenell JM, et al: Prediction of fetal acidemia in pregnancies complicated by maternal diabetes by biophysical scoring and fetal heart rate monitoring. Br J Obstet Gynaecol 100:227, 1993

Schellpfeffer MA, Hoyle D, Johnson JWC: Antepartum uterine hypercontractility secondary to nipple stimulation. Obstet Gynecol 65:588, 1985

Sherer DM, Spong CY, Ghidini A, et al: In preterm fetuses decreased amniotic fluid volume is associated with decreased fetal movements. Am J Obstet Gynecol 174:344, 1996

Smith CV, Nguyen HN, Kovacs B, et al: Fetal death following antepartum fetal heart rate testing: A review of 65 cases. Obstet Gynecol 70:18, 1987

Smith JH, Anand KJ, Cotes PM, et al: Antenatal fetal heart rate variation in relation to the respiratory and metabolic status of the compromised human fetus. Br J Obstet Gynaecol 95:980, 1988

Sorokin Y, Bottoms SF, Dierker CJ, et al: The clustering of fetal heart rate changes and fetal movements in pregnancies between 20 and 30 weeks gestation. Am J Obstet Gynecol 143:952, 1982

Thacker SB, Berkelman RL: Assessing the diagnostic accuracy and efficacy of selected antepartum fetal surveillance techniques. Obstet Gynecol Surv 41:121, 1986

Thornton JG, The GRIT Study Group: A randomized trial of timed delivery for the compromised preterm fetus: Short term outcomes and Bayesian interpretation. Br J Obstet Gynaecol 110:27, 2003

Timor-Tritsch IE, Dierker LJ, Hertz RH, et al: Studies of antepartum behavioral state in the human fetus at term. Am J Obstet Gynecol 132:524, 1978

Todd AL, Tridinger BJ, Cole MJ, et al: Antenatal tests of fetal welfare and development at age 2 years. Am J Obstet Gynecol 167:66, 1992

Todros T, Sciarrone A, Piccoli E, et al: Umbilical Doppler waveforms and placental villous angiogenesis in pregnancies complicated by fetal growth restriction. Obstet Gynecol 93:499, 1999

Vergani P, Andreotti C, Roncaglia N, et al: Doppler predictors of adverse neonatal outcome in the growth restricted fetus at 34 weeks' gestation or beyond. Am J Obstet Gynecol 189:1007, 2003

Vindla S, James D: Fetal behavior as a test of fetal well-being. Br J Obstet Gynaecol 102:597, 1995

Visser GHA, Redman CWG, Huisjes HJ, et al: Nonstressed antepartum heart rate monitoring: Implications of decelerations after spontaneous contractions. Am J Obstet Gynecol 138:429, 1980

Weiner Z, Divon MY, Katz N, et al: Multi-variant analysis of antepartum fetal test in predicting neonatal outcome of growth retarded fetuses. Am J Obstet Gynecol 174:338, 1996

Williams KP, Farquharson DF, Bebbington M, et al: Screening for fetal well-being in a high-risk pregnant population comparing the nonstress test with umbilical artery Doppler velocimetry: A randomized controlled clinical trial. Am J Obstet Gynecol 188:1366, 2003

Young D, Delaney T, Nogue K, et al: Randomized controlled trial (RCT) of original, modified and selective fetal biophysical profiles [abstract]. Am J Obstet Gynecol 187:S146, 2003

Zelop CM, Richardson DK, Heffner LJ: Outcomes of severely abnormal umbilical artery Doppler velocimetry in structurally normal singleton fetuses. Obstet Gynecol 87:434, 1996

Zhang J, Troendle J, Meikle S, et al: Isolated oligohydramnios is not associated with adverse perinatal outcomes. Br J Obstet Gynaecol 111:220, 2004

16

Ultrasonography and Doppler

The impact of ultrasonography on the practice of obstetrics has been profound. A carefully performed sonographic examination reveals vital information about fetal anatomy, as well as fetal environment, growth, and well-being. Technology has evolved from producing two-dimensional images of the pregnant uterus to using Doppler methods for measurement of maternal and fetal circulation and to creating three-dimensional views of maternal and fetal anatomy.

ULTRASONOGRAPHY IN OBSTETRICS

Since the first obstetrical application of ultrasound imaging by Donald and co-workers (1958), this technique has become indispensable for evaluation of the fetus. According to the National Center for Health Statistics (2002), sonography was used in 67 percent of pregnant women in the United States in 2001.

TECHNOLOGY. The picture displayed on the screen is produced by sound waves reflected back from the imaged structure. Alternating current is applied to a transducer containing piezoelectric crystals, which converts electrical energy to high-frequency sound waves. A water-soluble gel applied to the skin acts as a coupling agent. Sound waves pass through layers of tissue, encounter an interface between tissues of different densities, and are reflected back to the transducer. Converted back into electrical energy, they are displayed on the screen. Dense tissue such as bone produces high-velocity reflected waves, which are displayed as white on the screen. Fluid, however, is anechoic and generates few reflected waves, appearing black on the screen. Images are generated so quickly, more than 40 frames/sec, that the picture on the screen appears to move in real-time.

Higher-frequency transducers yield better image resolution, whereas lower frequencies penetrate tissue more effectively. For example, abdominal scanning is most commonly performed with a 3- to 5-mHz transducer. Obese patients may require a 2-mHz transducer to image the fetus, but the quality of the images (resolution) will be reduced. In early pregnancy, 7- to 10-mHz vaginal transducers may provide excellent resolution because the fetus is close to the transducer.

SAFETY. Ultrasonography should be performed only when there is a valid medical indication, using the lowest possible exposure setting to gain necessary diagnostic information—the ALARA principle or "*as low as reasonably achievable*" (American Institute of Ultrasound in Medicine, 2003). That said, there have been no confirmed damaging biological effects in mammalian tissue demonstrated in the frequency range of medical ultrasound (American Institute of Ultrasound in Medicine, 1991). In the low-intensity range of gray-scale imaging, no fetal harm has been demonstrated in more than 30 years of use (see Chap 9, p. 235).

CLINICAL APPLICATIONS. Obstetrical ultrasound has proven invaluable in a variety of ways, two in particular being more accurate pregnancy dating and detection of fetal anomalies. Several investigators have demonstrated that an estimated gestational age determined sonographically is more accurate than one based on last menstrual period. This alone allows reduction in the number of labor inductions for postterm pregnancy (Waldenstrom and colleagues, 1988). Tunon and colleagues (1996) performed sonography in more than 15,000 unselected women at 18 weeks and decreased the postterm delivery rate from 10 percent to 4 percent. In a randomized study of 218 low-risk women, Bennett and associates (2004) significantly reduced labor induction for postterm pregnancy from 13 to 5 percent.

Accurate dating also may alter the method of pregnancy termination. McGalliard and Gaudoin (2004) reported that there was at least a 1-week discrepancy in 38 percent of 237 women seeking pregnancy termination, and that in many of these cases, a safer method was chosen.

Several investigators have shown that routine sonography can identify at least 35 to 50 percent of major fetal malformations, with a specificity of 90 to 100 percent (Ewigman and colleagues, 1993; Goncalves and colleagues, 1994; Van Dorsten and co-workers, 1998). As technology has improved, attempts to identify fetal anatomy are applied earlier in gestation. Indeed, a complete survey of fetal anatomy can be performed before the end of the first trimester (Michailidis and colleagues, 2002; Whitlow and Economides, 1998). Even so, recently updated practice guidelines of the American Institute of Ultrasound in Medicine (2003) stress that adequate assessment of fetal anatomy is best performed after 18 weeks. Although it may be possible to document normal anatomy before this time, some structures may be difficult to visualize because of fetal size, position, or movement or maternal abdominal scars or obesity. The American College of Obstetricians and Gynecologists (1997) cautions that the sensitivity of ultrasound in detecting fetal anomalies varies in different clinical settings and according to the skill of the sonographer.

FIRST TRIMESTER. Some indications for performing sonography in the first trimester are listed in Table 16–1. Early pregnancy can be evaluated using abdominal or transvaginal sonography, or both. All of the components listed in Table 16–2 should be assessed. As new technical capabilities are developed, greater research emphasis is being placed on first-trimester detection of fetal disorders and even treatment (Bahado-Singh and Cheng, 2004). With transabdominal scanning, the gestational sac is reliably seen in the uterus by 6 weeks, and fetal echoes and cardiac activity by 7 weeks. With transvaginal scanning, these are seen about 1 week earlier.

Early sonography is valuable in diagnosing abnormalities such as anembryonic gestation as well as embryonic demise. With transvaginal examination, cardiac motion usually is observed when the embryo is 5 mm in length. Multifetal

TABLE 16–1 Some Indications for First-Trimester Ultrasound Examination

Confirm intrauterine pregnancy
Evaluate suspected ectopic pregnancy
Define cause of vaginal bleeding
Evaluate pelvic pain
Estimate gestational age
Diagnose or evaluate multiple gestations
Confirm cardiac activity
Assist to chorionic villus sampling, embryo transfer, and
   localization and removal of intrauterine device
Evaluate maternal pelvic masses or uterine abnormalities
Evaluate suspected gestational trophoblastic disease

From the American Institute of Ultrasound in Medicine, 2003, with permission.

gestation can be identified in the first trimester, and this is the optimal time to determine chorionicity. The first trimester also may be the best time to evaluate the uterus, adnexal structures, and cul-de-sac.

Between 11 and 14 weeks, fetal *nuchal translucency* can be accurately measured. This is the maximum thickness of the subcutaneous translucent area between the skin and soft tissue that overlies the fetal spine in the sagittal plane. Measurement of nuchal translucency was described by Nicolaides and colleagues (1992), and has gained widespread use, often in conjunction with maternal serum markers, in the detection of aneuploidy. Wapner and colleagues (2003) recently reported results of their multicenter trial of 8514 pregnancies undergoing first-trimester aneuploidy screening using nuchal translucency along with serum chorionic gonadotropin and pregnancy-associated plasma protein A. They reported detection of 85 percent of cases of Down syndrome with a false-positive rate of 9 percent. Malone and colleagues (2003) reported a multicenter trial in which 33,557 pregnancies underwent first- and second-trimester aneuploidy screening. First-trimester nuchal translucency and serum markers re-

TABLE 16–2 Components of Standard Ultrasound Examination by Trimester

First Trimester	Second and Third Trimester
Gestational sac location	Fetal number
Embryo or yolk sac identification	Presentation
Crown-rump length	Fetal heart motion
Cardiac activity	Placental location
Fetal number, including number of amnions and chorions of multiples when possible	Amnionic fluid volume
	Gestational age assessment
	Fetal weight estimation
Uterus, adnexal, and cul-de-sac evaluation	Evaluation for maternal pelvic masses
	Fetal anatomic survey

Modified from the American Institute of Ultrasound in Medicine, 2003, with permission.

TABLE 16–3 Some Indications for Second- or Third-Trimester Ultrasound Examination

Estimation of gestational age
Evaluation of fetal growth
Vaginal bleeding
Abdominal or pelvic pain
Incompetent cervix
Determination of fetal presentation
Suspected multiple gestation
Adjunct to amniocentesis
Significant uterine size or clinical dates discrepancy
Pelvic mass
Suspected molar pregnancy
Adjunct to cervical cerclage
Suspected ectopic pregnancy
Suspected fetal death
Suspected uterine abnormality
Evaluation of fetal well-being
Suspected hydramnios or oligohydramnios
Suspected abruptio placentae
Adjunct to external cephalic version
Preterm prematurely ruptured membranes or preterm labor
Abnormal biochemical markers
Follow-up observation of identified fetal anomaly
Follow-up evaluation of placental location for suspected
   placenta previa
History of previous congenital anomaly
Serial evaluation of fetal growth in multifetal gestation
Evaluation of fetal condition in late registrants for prenatal care

Adapted from the National Institutes of Health, 1984, by the American Institute of Ultrasound in Medicine, 2003, with permission.

sulted in the detection of 85 percent of Down syndrome cases with a false-positive rate of 7.6 percent. In his review of studies that included over 200,000 pregnancies, Nicolaides (2004) found these to be 87 and 4.2 percent, respectively. When certain criteria are met, the American College of Obstetricians and Gynecologists (2004b) has concluded that first-trimester screening is an acceptable option for trisomy 18 and 21.

SECOND AND THIRD TRIMESTERS. Some of the many indications for second- and third-trimester sonography are listed in Table 16–3. These examinations can be categorized as standard, limited, or specialized. Terms indicate which structures were evaluated and to what extent, and also describe which structures were not evaluated.

Table 16–2 lists the components of a *standard*—also termed *basic*—obstetrical ultrasound examination. A standard examination should be performed or reviewed by an appropriately trained sonologist (American College of Obstetricians and Gynecologists, 1997). It includes a fetal anatomical survey, the components of which are listed in Table 16–4. When multiple gestations are imaged, additional documentation includes the number(s) of chorions and amnions, comparison of fetal sizes, estimation of amnionic fluid volume in each sac, and description of fetal genitalia if visualized. If a complete survey of fetal anatomy cannot

TABLE 16–4 Essential Elements of a Standard Examination of Fetal Anatomy

Head and Neck
   Cerebellum
   Choroid plexus
   Cisterna magna
   Lateral cerebral ventricles
   Midline falx
   Cavum septi pellucidi

Chest
   Four-chamber view of heart
   Evaluation of both outflow tracts if technically feasible

Abdomen
   Stomach—presence, size, and location
   Kidneys
   Bladder
   Umbilical cord insertion into fetal abdomen
   Umbilical cord vessel number

Spine
   Cervical, thoracic, lumbar, and sacral spine

Extremities
   Legs and arms—presence or absence

Gender
   Indicated in low-risk pregnancies only for evaluation of multiple gestations

From the American Institute of Ultrasound in Medicine, 2003, with permission.

be obtained—for example, due to oligohydramnios, fetal position, or maternal obesity—it should be noted.

There are several types of *specialized* examinations. An example includes a detailed anatomical examination, which is performed when an anomaly is suspected on the basis of history, maternal serum screening test abnormalities, or abnormal findings from a standard or limited examination. These examinations are performed and interpreted by a sonologist with special expertise. Other types of examinations include fetal echocardiography, fetal Doppler evaluation, biophysical profile, or additional biometric studies (see Chapter 15, p. 381).

A third type of procedure is the *limited* examination, performed when a specific question requires investigation. Examples include estimation of amnionic fluid volume, placental location, identification of fetal presentation, or determination of fetal viability. In most cases, limited examinations are appropriate only when a prior complete examination is on record (American Institute of Ultrasound in Medicine, 2003).

FETAL MEASUREMENTS. Various formulas and nomograms allow accurate assessment of gestational age and describe normal growth of fetal structures. Modern equipment contains software that provides an estimated gestational age from the crown-rump length measurement in the first trimester. It also estimates both gestational age and fetal weight in the second and third trimester using measurements of the biparietal diameter, head circumference, abdominal circumference, and femur length. Estimates are typically most accurate when multiple parameters are used and when nomograms have been derived from fetuses of the same ethnic or racial background living at similar altitude. Nomograms are available for other fetal structures that may help answer specific questions about organ system abnormalities or syndromes. Examples include length of the fetal ears, kidneys, cerebellum, long bones and feet, and the interocular and binocular distances.

For determining gestational age in the first trimester, the crown-rump length is most accurate. The image should be obtained in a sagittal plane and include neither the yolk sac nor a limb bud. If carefully performed, it has a variation of only 3 to 5 days. Between 14 and 26 weeks, the biparietal diameter (BPD) is usually the most accurate parameter, with a variation of 7 to 10 days. By convention, the BPD is measured from the outer edge of the proximal skull to the inner edge of the distal skull, at the level of the thalami and cavum septi pellucidi. The head circumference (HC) also is measured. If the head shape is flattened (*dolichocephaly*) or rounded (*brachycephaly*), this measurement is more reliable than the BPD. The femur length (FL) correlates well with both BPD and gestational age. The femur is measured with the beam perpendicular to the long axis of the shaft, excluding the epiphysis, and has a variation of 7 to 11 days in the second trimester. The abdominal circumference (AC) is the parameter with the widest variation of 2 to 3 weeks. This is because the AC measurement involves soft tissue rather than bone and is also the parameter most affected by fetal growth. The AC is measured at the skin line in a transverse view of the fetus at the level of the fetal stomach and umbilical vein.

The variability of gestational age estimation increases as pregnancy advances. By the third trimester, all individual measurements become less accurate. Estimates are improved by taking an average of the various parameters—the BPD, HC, AC, and FL. Also, each measurement should be assessed individually; if one measurement is significantly different from the others, it can be excluded from the calculation. The outlier measurement could result from poor visibility, or it could indicate a fetal growth abnormality. If third-trimester ultrasound measurements must be used to determine gestational age, accuracy can be improved by performing serial examinations and documenting normal interval fetal growth.

AMNIONIC FLUID. Determination of the amount of amnionic fluid is an important method of fetal assessment and is discussed in Chapter 15 (see p. 382). When volume is assessed subjectively, oligohydramnios is seen as obvious crowding of the fetus and absence of any significant pockets of fluid. Conversely, hydramnios is an apparent excess of fluid.

Several objective measurement schemes have been used to evaluate amnionic fluid volume. The most widely used is the *amnionic fluid index (AFI),* which is calculated by adding the depth in centimeters of the largest vertical pocket in each of four equal uterine quadrants (Phelan and colleagues, 1987). Reference ranges have been established from 16 weeks onward, and in the majority of normal pregnancies the AFI ranges between 8 and 24 cm (see Table 21–1 and Fig. 21–1, p. 526). Another method is to measure the largest vertical pocket of amnionic fluid. The normal range is 2 to 8 cm; values below 2 cm signify oligohydramnios, whereas those over 8 cm define hydramnios. This latter method is commonly used for twin pregnancies.

NORMAL AND ABNORMAL FETAL ANATOMY

One basic goal of ultrasound evaluation is to categorize fetal components as anatomically normal or abnormal. Poor visualization of a structure allows neither. Deviations from normal anatomy require that a specialized examination be performed. In the discussion that follows, only a few of literally hundreds of fetal anomalies are used as examples of distorted anatomy.

CENTRAL NERVOUS SYSTEM. Anomalies of the fetal brain are among the most common and have the potential to cause serious disability or death. Ultrasonography has proven extremely useful in detecting and characterizing these anomalies. Three transverse (axial) views of the fetal brain are imaged. The transthalamic view shown in Figure 16–1 is used to measure BPD and HC and includes the thalami and cavum septi pellucidi. Moving superiorly yields the transventricular view of the atria of the lateral ventricles, which contain the echogenic choroid plexus (Fig. 16–2). The atrial measurement is normally between 5 and 10 mm from 15 weeks until term. Angling back through the posterior fossa produces the transcerebellar view (Fig. 16–3). Here the cerebellum and cisterna magna are typically measured. Between 15 and 22 weeks, the cerebellar diameter in millimeters is roughly

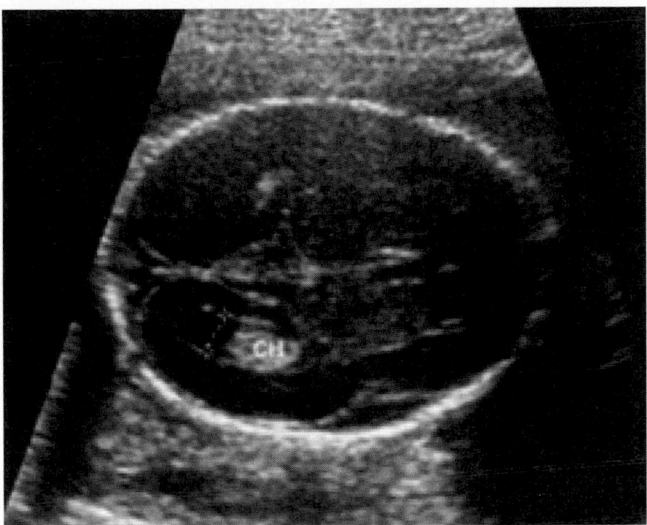

FIGURE 16–2. Transventricular view of the atrium, which is marked by calipers and contains the echogenic choroid plexus (CH). (Courtesy of Dr. Jodi Dashe.)

equivalent to the gestational age in weeks (Goldstein and associates 1987).

Abnormalities detected in any of these three views alert the clinician of a possible fetal brain anomaly. Specialized evaluation may permit accurate diagnosis of relatively subtle anomalies, including neural-tube defects, ventriculomegaly, holoprosencephaly, hydranencephaly, Dandy-Walker malformation, porencephaly, or an intracranial tumor.

Neural-Tube Defects. These malformations are the second most common class of congenital anomalies—cardiac anomalies are the most common. Neural-tube defects occur in about 1.6 per 1000 live births in the United States, and their

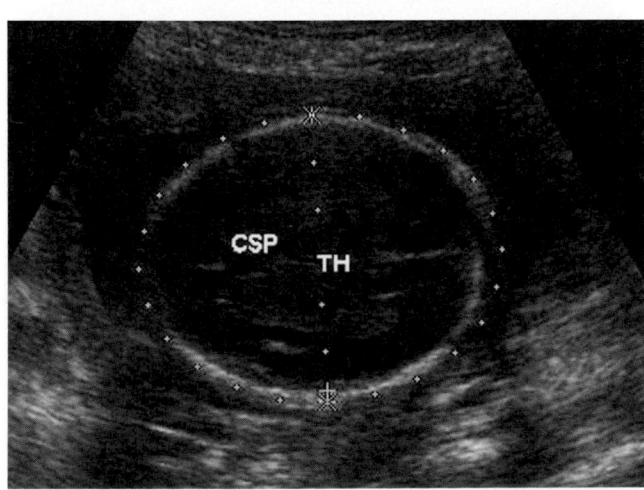

FIGURE 16–1. Transthalamic view showing thalami (TH) and cavum septi pellucidi (CSP). (Courtesy of Dr. Diane Twickler.)

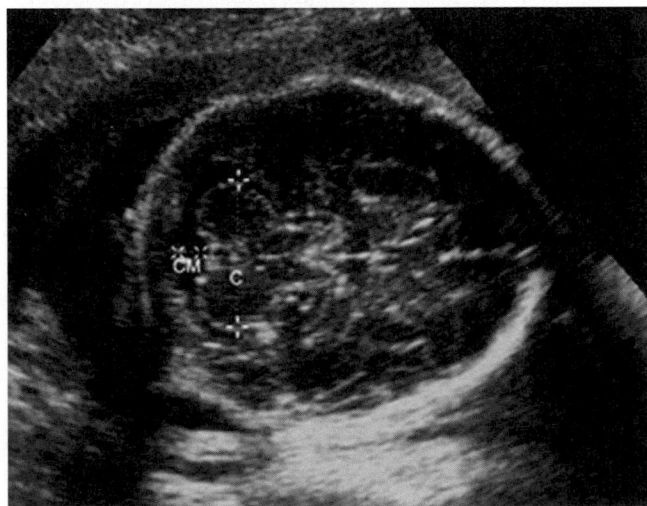

FIGURE 16–3. Transcerebellar view of the posterior fossa, demonstrating measurement of the cerebellum (C) and cisterna magna (CM). (Courtesy of Dr. Jodi Dashe.)

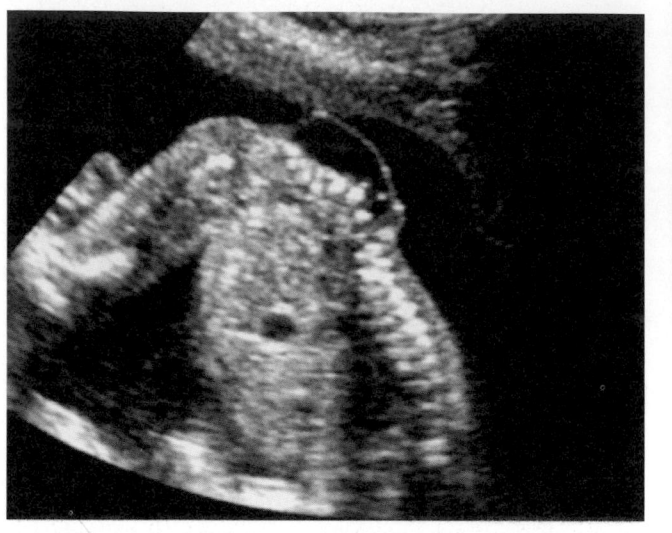

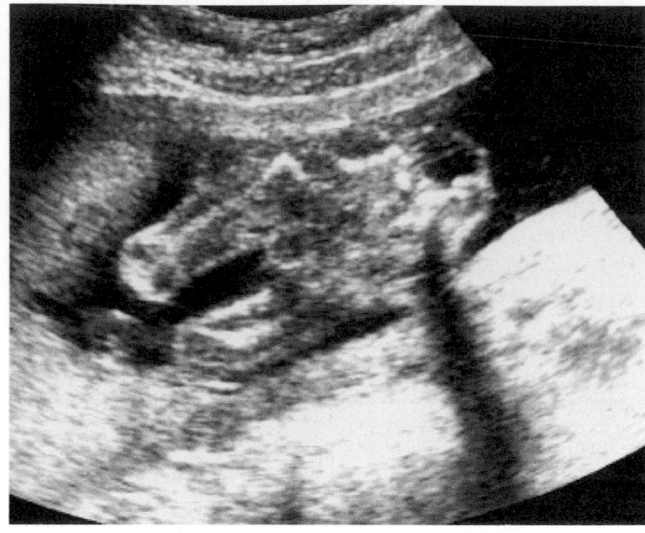

A   B

FIGURE 16–4. Sagittal (*left*) and transverse (*right*) views of the spine in a fetus with a large lumbosacral meningomyelocele. (Courtesy of Dr. Jodi Dashe.)

incidence is as high as 8 per 1000 in the United Kingdom. Defects result from incomplete closure of the neural tube by the sixth week, or the embryonic age of 26 to 28 days. Chapter 13 (see p. 318 and p. 334) discusses diagnosis and management.

Anencephaly is a lethal defect characterized by absence of the brain and cranium above the base of the skull and orbits. It can be diagnosed as early as the first trimester. If visualization is adequate in the second trimester, anencephaly can be diagnosed in virtually all cases (see Fig. 13–6, p. 321). Inability to obtain a view of the biparietal diameter should raise suspicion. Hydramnios from impaired fetal swallowing is common in the third trimester.

Cephalocele is a herniation of meninges and brain tissue through a defect in the cranium, typically an occipital midline defect. Associated hydrocephalus and microcephaly are common, and there is a high incidence of mental impairment. If the fetal head closely abuts the uterine wall, the skull defect may be difficult to image. Cephalocele is an important feature of the autosomal recessive *Meckel-Gruber syndrome*. A cephalocele that is not in the occipital midline may be caused by the *amnionic band sequence*.

Spina bifida is an opening in the vertebrae through which a meningeal sac may protrude. In 90 percent of cases, the sac contains neural elements and the anomaly is termed a *meningomyelocele*. When a meningeal sac alone protrudes through the defect, it is a *meningocele*. Spinal defects usually can be imaged in multiple planes, as shown in Figure 16–4. Transverse images provide the best visualization of the extent of the defect and overlying soft tissue. Movement of the lower extremities does not predict normal function after birth. The *Arnold-Chiari II* malformation associated with spina bifida occurs when downward displacement of the spinal cord pulls a portion of the cerebellum through the foramen magnum

into the upper cervical canal. Classically, fetuses with spina bifida have one or more of the following five cranial signs:

1. Small biparietal diameter.
2. Ventriculomegaly.
3. Frontal bone scalloping or the so-called lemon sign (Fig. 16–5).
4. Elongation and downward displacement of the cerebellum—the so-called banana sign (Fig. 16–6).
5. Effacement or obliteration of the cisterna magna.

When a cranial sign is present but no spinal defect is visualized, amniocentesis for amnionic fluid alpha-fetoprotein and acetylcholinesterase measurement may be diagnostic.

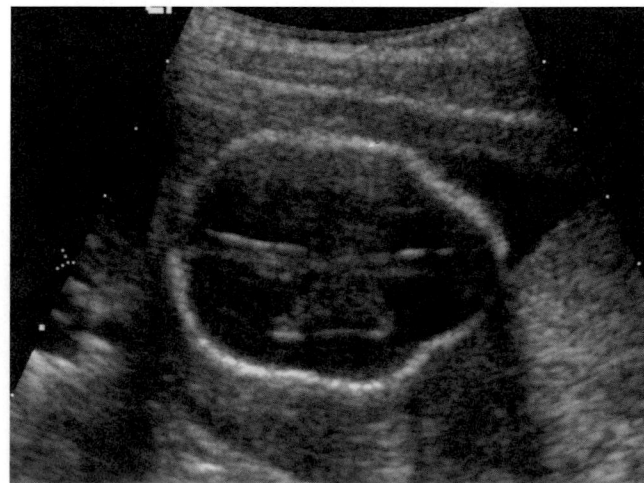

FIGURE 16–5. Frontal scalloping or lemon sign in a fetus with a spinal meningomyelocele. (Photograph courtesy of Dr. Diane Twickler.)

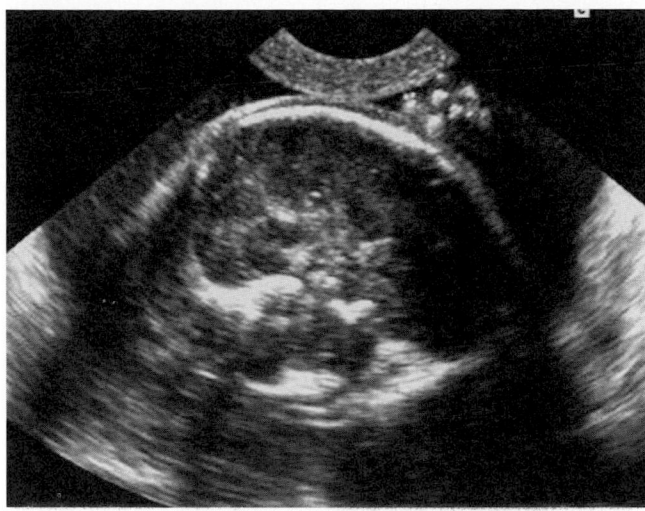

FIGURE 16–6. The banana sign, seen in this fetus with a meningomyelocele, develops when the cerebellum is bowed and inferiorly displaced, causing effacement of the cisterna magna. (Photograph courtesy of Dr. Diane Twickler.)

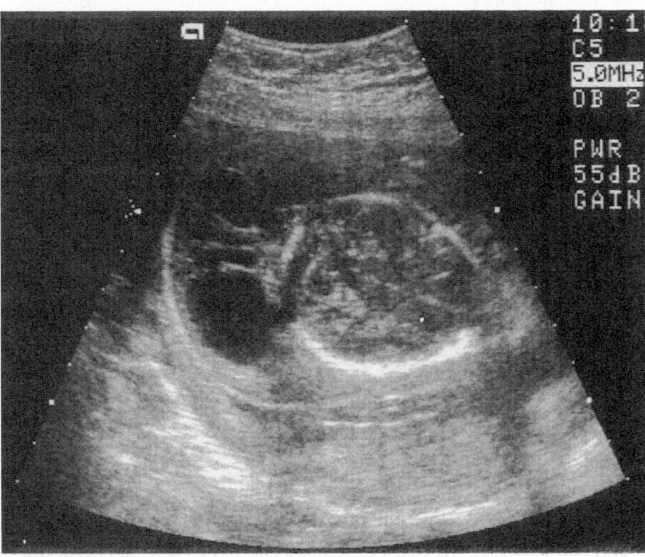

FIGURE 16–8. Large, septated cystic hygromas in a 17-week fetus with Turner syndrome. (Courtesy of Dr. Jodi Dashe.)

Ventriculomegaly. Enlargement of the cerebral ventricles has been viewed as a general marker of abnormal brain development (Callen, 2000; Wyldes and Watkinson, 2004). The lateral ventricle is commonly measured at its *atrium,* which is the confluence of the temporal and occipital horns (see Fig. 16–2). The measurement is relatively constant at 7 mm, with standard deviation of 1 mm, from 15 weeks onward (Heiserman and colleagues, 1991). Mild ventriculomegaly is diagnosed when the atrial width measures 10 to 15 mm, and overt ventriculomegaly when it exceeds 15 mm (Fig. 16–7). A *dangling choroid plexus* characteristically is found in severe cases (Cardoza and associates, 1988a, 1988b; Mahony and colleagues, 1988).

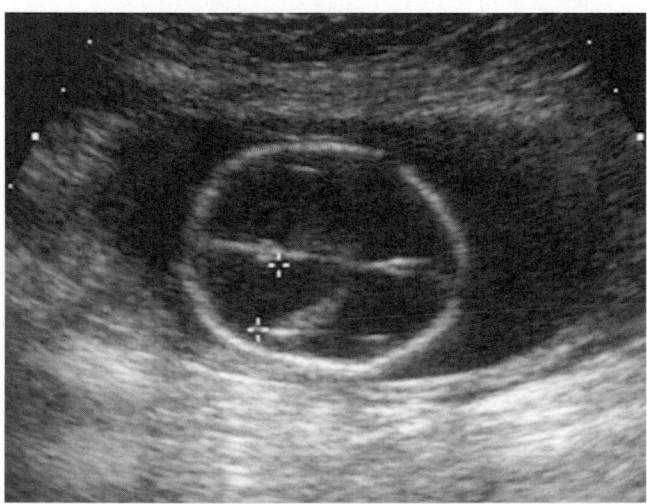

FIGURE 16–7. The atria appear unusually prominent in this fetus with mild ventriculomegaly (caliper measurement 12 mm). (Photograph courtesy of Dr. Diane Twickler.)

Ventriculomegaly may be caused by a wide variety of genetic and environmental insults, and prognosis is determined by both etiology and rate of progression. Generally, the larger the atrium, the greater the likelihood of abnormal outcome. Despite this generalization, Bloom and colleagues (1997) found that 36 percent of infants prenatally diagnosed with isolated and mild ventriculomegaly were developmentally delayed. Initial evaluation of ventricular enlargement includes a thorough examination of fetal anatomy and fetal karyotype and testing for congenital viral infection (Wyldes and Watkinson, 2004).

CYSTIC HYGROMA. This is a congenital malformation of the lymphatic system in which large, often multiseptated, fluid-filled sacs extend from the posterior neck (Fig. 16–8). Cystic hygromas usually develop as part of lymphatic obstruction sequence, in which lymph from the head fails to drain into the jugular vein and collects instead in jugular lymphatic sacs. The enlarged thoracic duct can impinge on the developing heart. In some cases, there are developmental flow-related anomalies such as a hypoplastic left heart or coarctation of the aorta.

In approximately 60 to 70 percent of cases, cystic hygromas are associated with fetal aneuploidy. Turner syndrome (45,X) accounts for 75 percent of these aneuploidies; trisomies 21, 18, and 13 and mosaic aneuploidies account for the remainder (Johnson and colleagues, 1993; Shulman and associates, 1992). They also may be an isolated finding or part of a genetic syndrome, such as *Noonan syndrome.*

Small hygromas may undergo spontaneous resolution, and provided that the fetal karyotype and echocardiography are normal, the prognosis may be good (Shulman and co-workers, 1992; Trauffer and associates, 1994). Conversely,

large, multiseptated lesions rarely resolve, often lead to hydrops fetalis, and have a poor prognosis (Brumfield and colleagues, 1996).

THORAX. The lungs are best visualized after 20 to 25 weeks
and appear as homogeneous structures surrounding the heart.
In the four-chamber view of the chest, they fill approximately
two thirds of the area. A variety of thoracic malformations,
including cystic adenomatoid malformation, extralobar pulmonary sequestration, and bronchogenic cysts, may be visualized sonographically as cystic or solid space-occupying
lesions. Prenatal diagnosis and therapy of these lesions is
discussed in Chapter 13 (see p. 333).

Diaphragmatic Hernia. In 90 percent of cases, these are left-
sided and posterior, and the heart may be pushed to the middle
or right side of the thorax by the stomach or bowel. Associated
findings include absence of the stomach bubble within the abdomen, small abdominal circumference, and bowel peristalsis seen in the fetal chest. Almost half of cases are associated
with other major anomalies or aneuploidy. Thus, a thorough
evaluation of all fetal structures should be performed, along
with amniocentesis. Diagnosis and treatment are discussed
in Chapter 13 (see p. 333).

HEART. As a group, cardiac malformations are the most
common congenital anomalies, with an incidence of about
8 per 1000 live births (see Chap. 12, p. 302). Almost 90
percent of cardiac defects are multifactorial or polygenic,
another 1 to 2 percent are the result of a single-gene disorder or a gene-deletion syndrome, and about 1 to 2 percent
occur after exposure to a teratogen such as isotretinoin, hydantoin, or diabetic hyperglycemia. **As many as 30 to 40 percent of cardiac defects diagnosed prenatally are associated
with chromosomal abnormalities.** Fortunately, up to 50 to
70 percent of aneuploid fetuses have extracardiac anomalies
that are identifiable sonographically. Thus, recognition of a
cardiac malformation should prompt fetal karyotyping. The
most frequently encountered aneuploidies are trisomies 21,
18, and 13, and 45, X (Turner syndrome).

A basic anatomical survey of the heart includes assessment
of a four-chamber view, rate, and rhythm. The four-chamber
view is a transverse plane through the fetal thorax at a level
immediately above the diaphragm (Figs. 16–9 and 16–10).
It allows evaluation of cardiac size, position in the chest and
its axis, atria and ventricles, septum primum, foramen ovale,
interventricular septum, and atrioventricular valves. The two
atria and ventricles should be similar in size, respectively,
and the apex of the heart should form a 45-degree angle with
the left anterior chest wall (see Fig. 16–9). Abnormalities of
cardiac axis should prompt a specialized examination. Smith
and colleagues (1995) found that 75 percent of fetuses with
congenital heart anomalies had a cardiac axis greater than 75
degrees to the left. Ship and co-workers (1995) found that 45

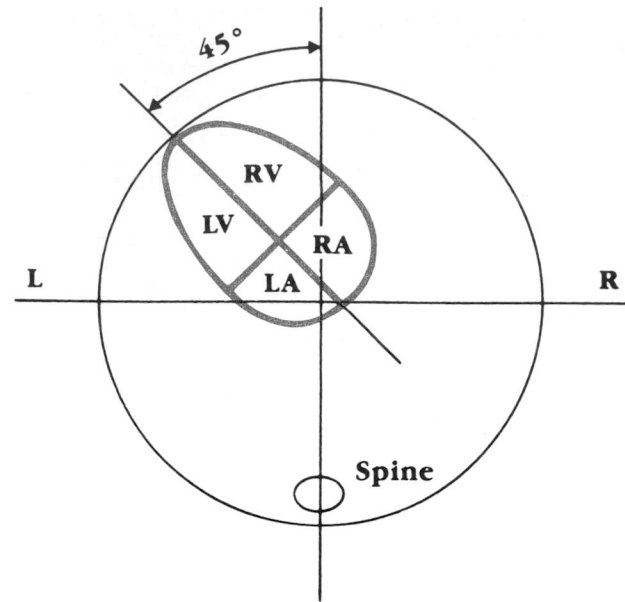

FIGURE 16–9. Measurement of the cardiac axis from the four-
chamber view of the fetal heart. (LA = left atrium; LV = left ventricle; RA = right atrium; RV = right ventricle.) (From Comstock,
1987, with permission.)

percent of those with abnormal hearts had a left axis deviation
exceeding 57 degrees.

A specialized examination with fetal echocardiography is
performed if any of the following are present: abnormal four-
chamber view, arrhythmia, presence of extracardiac anomalies, fetus with a genetic syndrome that includes a cardiac

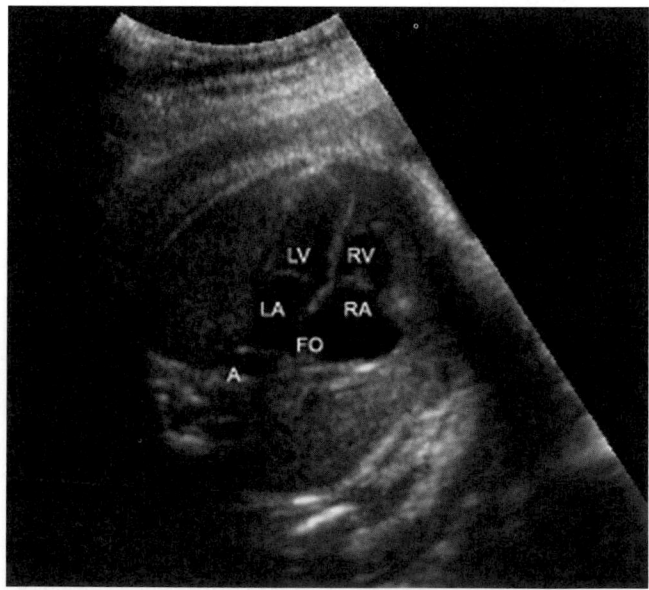

FIGURE 16–10. Four-chamber view of the fetal heart, showing the
location of the left and right atria (LA, RA), left and right ventricles
(LV, RV), foramen ovale (FO), and descending thoracic aorta (A).
(Courtesy of Dr. Jodi Dashe.)

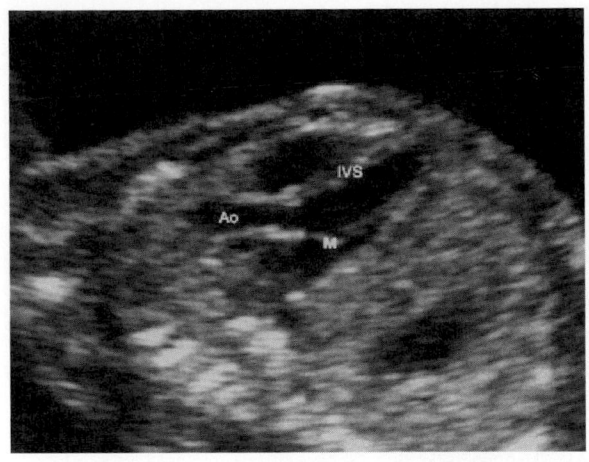
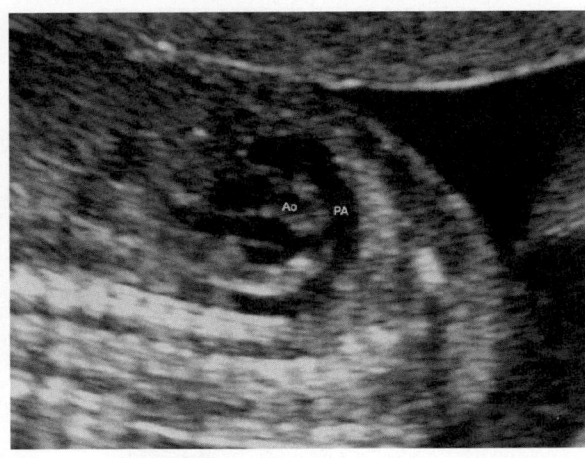

A   **B**

FIGURE 16–11. Views of the left and right ventricular outflow tracts. **A.** The left ventricular outflow tract demonstrates the continuity of the interventricular septum (IVS) and mitral valve (M) with the walls of the aorta (Ao). **B.** The right ventricular outflow tract shows the normal orientation of the aorta (Ao) and pulmonary artery (PA). (Courtesy of Dr. Jodi Dashe.)

defect, parent or sibling with a heart defect, maternal diabetes, teratogen exposure, or nonimmune hydrops. Coco and associates (2004) recommend this also if an isolated echogenic heart focus is visualized.

The American Institute of Ultrasound in Medicine (2003) further recommends that if technically feasible, each standard examination should be attempted to evaluate both left and right ventricular outflow tracts (Fig. 16–11).

Accuracy. Sonographic accuracy depends on the operator, equipment, maternal habitus, fetal gestational age and position, specific cardiac lesion, and whether a standard screening examination or specialized fetal echocardiography is being performed. The prenatal detection rate for cardiac defects ranges from about 15 percent in a low-risk population to 80 percent in a high-risk group (Benacerraf and associates, 1987; Crawford and colleagues, 1988; Ott, 1995). For example, Stoll and colleagues (2002) prospectively studied more than 80,000 pregnancies from Strasbourg, France. They reported that the overall detection of 688 cardiac anomalies in nonaneuploid fetuses was only 20 percent. When there were other malformations, however, the detection rate was 40 percent. It was considerably higher for selected cardiac lesions; for example, 62 percent of cases of hypoplastic left heart and single ventricle were detected.

Overview statistics fail to consider the importance of the type of lesion and the cardiac views imaged. Even under ideal circumstances, small septal defects are consistently missed on screening examinations. When the four-chamber view is the only image taken, anomalies such as Fallot tetralogy and transposition of the great vessels are unlikely to be detected. Incorporation of the outflow tract views shown in Figure 16–11 may improve visualization of the latter anoma-

lies. All women undergoing fetal cardiac evaluation should be counseled regarding its limitations.

GASTROINTESTINAL TRACT. The stomach is visible in 98 percent of fetuses after 14 weeks, and the liver, spleen, gallbladder, and bowel can be identified in many second- and third-trimester fetuses. Nonvisualization of the stomach within the abdomen is associated with a number of abnormalities, such as esophageal atresia, diaphragmatic hernia, abdominal wall defects, and neurological abnormalities that inhibit fetal swallowing. If the stomach is not seen on initial examination, the examination should be repeated. Millener and co-workers (1993), however, found that even with subsequent visualization of the stomach, a third of cases had an abnormal outcome.

The appearance of bowel changes with gestational age. Occasionally it may appear bright, or echogenic, particularly if a higher frequency transducer is used (Vincoff and associates, 1999). Common causes of echogenic bowel include swallowed intra-amnionic blood, malformation, infection, and aneuploidy (Kesrouani and colleagues, 2003). Cystic fibrosis and trisomy 21 also have been associated with echogenic bowel. If this is an isolated finding in a low-risk pregnancy, the risk likely may not be great enough to warrant amniocentesis.

Abdominal Wall Defects. The integrity of the abdominal wall is assessed during the standard examination (Fig. 16–12). Defects are relatively common.

GASTROSCHISIS. This is a full-thickness defect in the abdominal wall. Typically it is located to the right of the umbilical cord insertion, and the bowel herniates into the amnionic cavity (Fig. 16–13). Gastroschisis rarely is associated with

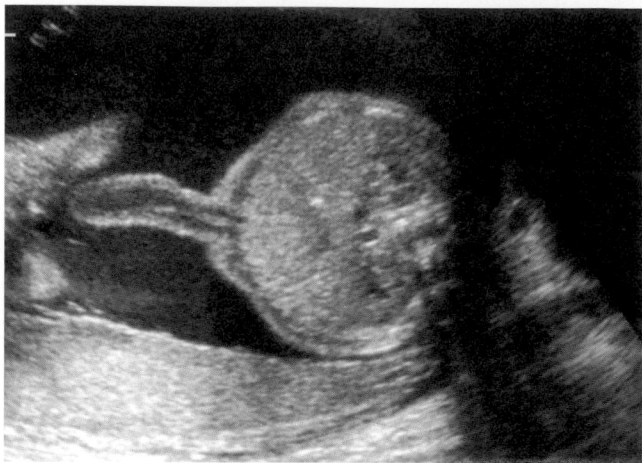

FIGURE 16–12. Transverse sonogram of a second-trimester fetus with an intact anterior abdominal wall and normal cord insertion. (Courtesy of Dr. Jodi Dashe.)

aneuploidy and usually has a survival rate of at least 90 percent (Kitchanan and colleagues, 2000; Nembhard and co-workers, 2001). It is thought to result from an early vascular occlusion that leads to localized abdominal wall ischemia. Associated bowel abnormalities are found in 10 to 30 percent of cases, usually as a result of vascular damage or mechanical trauma (Hoyme and co-workers, 1983). This is the one major anomaly more common in fetuses of younger mothers.

There are two controversies in management of these pregnancies. The first is whether any ultrasound parameter predicts outcome. The second is whether early delivery will prevent bowel damage, ostensibly by limiting bowel exposure to fetal urine. Huang and colleagues (2002) reviewed a series of 57 pregnancies complicated by gastroschisis and concluded that infants delivered at term were able to undergo

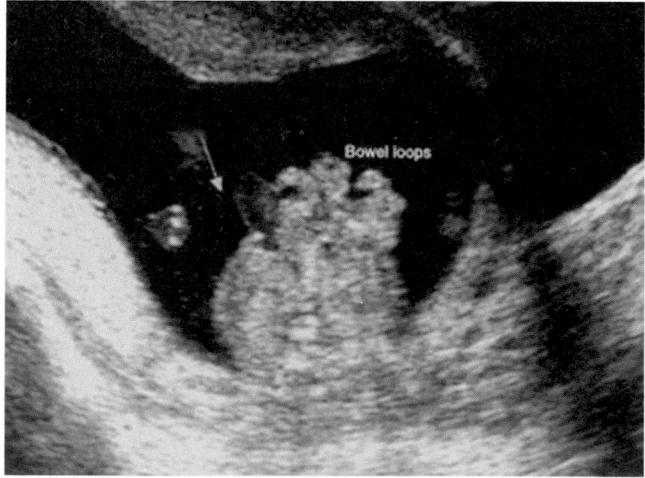

FIGURE 16–13. In this fetus with gastroschisis, extruded bowel loops are floating in the amnionic fluid to the right of the normal umbilical cord insertion site (*arrow*). (Courtesy of Dr. Diane Twickler.)

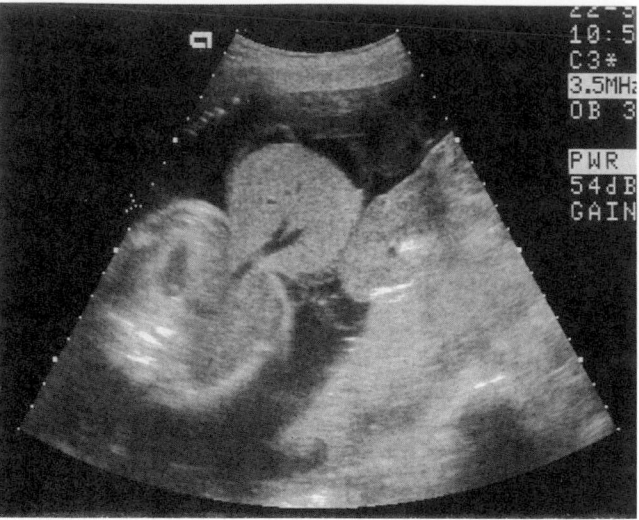

FIGURE 16–14. Transverse view of the abdomen showing an omphalocele as a large abdominal wall defect with exteriorized liver covered by a thin membrane. (Photograph courtesy of Dr. Jodi Dashe.)

earlier defect closure and begin full feedings sooner than those delivered prematurely. Markers of severity that have been evaluated include fetal growth restriction, increased bowel lumen diameter or wall thickness, distention of the stomach, and hydramnios. Japaraj and co-workers (2003) found that only hydramnios was predictive of neonatal bowel complications. Aina-Mumuney and colleagues (2004), however, reported excessive neonatal morbidity if the stomach was dilated prenatally.

OMPHALOCELE. This anomaly occurs when the lateral ectomesodermal folds fail to meet in the midline of the abdomen, leaving the abdominal contents covered only by a two-layered sac of amnion and peritoneum. The umbilical cord inserts into the apex of the sac (Fig. 16–14). In over half of cases, an omphalocele is associated with other major anomalies or aneuploidy. It also may occur as part of a genetic syndrome, such as *Beckwith–Wiedemann* or *pentalogy of Cantrell* (Callen, 2000). The prognosis is determined by the size of the omphalocele and also by the accompanying genetic or structural abnormalities (Heider and colleagues, 2004). For all of these reasons, identification of an omphalocele mandates a complete fetal evaluation, including karyotype.

Gastrointestinal Atresia. Most atresias are characterized by obstruction with proximal bowel dilatation. In general, the more proximal the obstruction, the more likely it is to be associated with hydramnios. *Esophageal atresia* may be suspected when the stomach cannot be visualized and hydramnios is present. In as many as 90 percent of cases, however, there is a *tracheoesophageal fistula* and fluid is able to enter the stomach despite esophageal atresia—thus, prenatal detection is problematic (Pretorius and colleagues, 1987a).

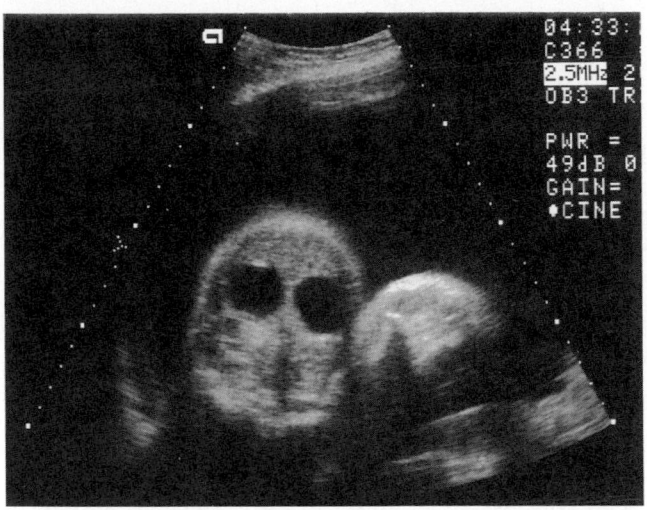

FIGURE 16–15. Double-bubble sign of duodenal atresia is seen on this axial abdominal image of the fetus. (Photograph courtesy of Dr. Jodi Dashe.)

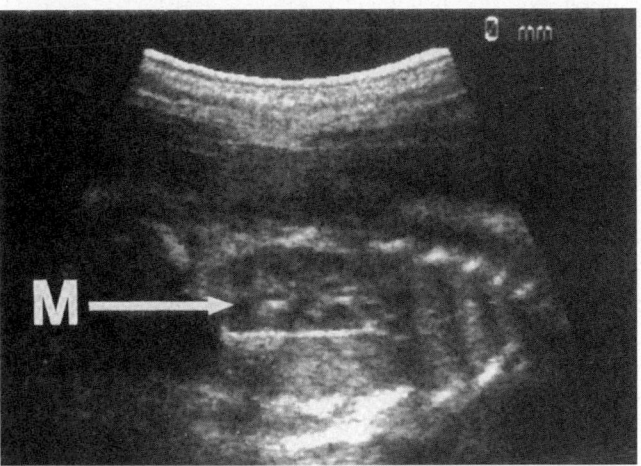

FIGURE 16–16. Longitudinal sonogram of fetal kidney depicting the hypoechoic medullary pyramids (M). (From Lowe and associates, 1990.)

About half of fetuses with esophageal atresia have associated anomalies, including aneuploidy in 20 percent of cases and growth restriction in 40 percent. Cardiac malformations are especially common with this anomaly.

Duodenal atresia occurs in about 1 in 10,000 live births (Robertson and colleagues, 1994). The lesion may be diagnosed prenatally by the demonstration of the so-called *double-bubble sign,* which represents distention of the stomach and the first part of the duodenum (Fig. 16–15). Demonstrating continuity between these two structures will differentiate duodenal atresia from other causes of abdominal cystic structures. About 30 percent of fetuses with duodenal atresia diagnosed antenatally have trisomy 21, and more than half have other anomalies. Obstructions in the lower small bowel usually result in multiple dilated loops, which may have increased peristaltic activity.

Large bowel obstructions and *anal atresia* are less readily diagnosed by ultrasound because hydramnios is not a typical feature and the bowel may not be significantly dilated. The transverse view through the pelvis may reveal the enlarged rectum as a fluid-filled structure between the bladder and the sacrum.

KIDNEYS AND URINARY TRACT. Fetal kidneys are seen as paraspinous masses, frequently as early as 14 weeks, and routinely by 18 weeks (Patten and co-workers, 1990). A longitudinal ultrasonic view is shown in Figure 16–16. Nomograms have been developed that describe kidney dimensions throughout pregnancy (Sagi and associates, 1987). A hypoechoic adrenal gland sits atop each kidney. The placenta and membranes produce amnionic fluid early in pregnancy, but after 16 to 20 weeks, most of the fluid is produced by the kidneys. Fetal urine production increases from 5 mL/hr at 20 weeks to about 50 mL/hr at term

(Rabinowitz and co-workers, 1989). Unexplained oligohydramnios suggests a urinary tract abnormality, whereas normal amnionic fluid volume in the second half of pregnancy suggests urinary tract patency with at least one functioning kidney.

Renal Agenesis. This defect has an incidence of about 1 in 4000 births. No kidneys are seen ultrasonographically at any point during gestation. The adrenal glands typically enlarge and occupy the renal fossae, which Hoffman and colleagues (1992) have aptly termed the *lying down* adrenal sign. Without kidneys, no urine is produced, and the resulting severe oligohydramnios leads to pulmonary hypoplasia, limb contractures, a distinctive compressed face, and death from cord compression or pulmonary hypoplasia. When this combination of abnormalities results from renal agenesis, it is called *Potter syndrome,* after Dr. Edith Potter who described it in 1946. When these abnormalities result from scant amnionic fluid of some other etiology, it is called *oligohydramnios sequence.*

Polycystic Kidney Disease. Of the hereditary polycystic diseases, only autosomal recessive infantile polycystic kidneys may be reliably diagnosed antenatally. As discussed in Chapter 48 (see p. 1102), the autosomal dominant condition usually does not manifest until adulthood, although prenatal diagnosis has been described (Pretorius and associates, 1987b). Infantile polycystic kidney disease is characterized by abnormally large kidneys that fill the fetal abdomen and appear to have a solid, ground-glass texture. The abdominal circumference is enlarged, and there is severe oligohydramnios. The cystic changes can only be identified microscopically.

Multicystic Dysplastic Kidney Disease. These renal changes arise from complete obstruction or atresia at the level of the renal pelvis or proximal ureter prior to 10 weeks (Callen, 2000). The diagnosis usually can be made antenatally by identifying abnormally dense renal parenchyma with multiple peripheral cysts of varying size that do not communicate with each other or with the renal pelvis. This finding should be distinguished from obstructive pyelectasis, in which the fluid-filled areas can be seen to connect. The prognosis for fetuses with multicystic dysplastic kidneys is generally good if findings are unilateral and amnionic fluid volume is normal.

Ureteropelvic Junction Obstruction. This condition is the most common cause of neonatal hydronephrosis and affects males at least twice as often as females. The actual obstruction is generally functional rather than anatomical, and it is bilateral in one third of cases. Unilateral obstruction is associated with an increased risk of anomalies also in the other kidney. Sonographically, only dilatation at the level of the renal pelvis—*pyelectasis*—is visualized. Various measurements taken at all gestational ages are used to predict fetuses who will require postnatal evaluation (Corteville, 1991; Mandell, 1991; Wilson, 1997, and all their colleagues). A commonly used upper limit for the normal pelvis diameter is 4 mm before 20 weeks. If this limit is exceeded, repeat sonography is performed at 34 weeks, and if the pelvis is then greater than 7 mm, neonatal follow-up is warranted. Adra and colleagues (1995) found that two thirds of fetuses with pyelectasis greater than 8 mm had an abnormality at birth. Similarly, Ismaili and associates (2003) reported that a diameter of at least 7 mm in a fetus in the third trimester had a 70-percent positive-predictive value for a renal abnormality in the infant.

Collecting System Duplication. This defect is the most common genitourinary anomaly and affects up to 4 percent of the population. Sonographically, the characteristic obstruction of the upper pole is evident as pyelectasis, often along with a dilated ureter that may be mistaken for a loop of bowel and with an ectopic ureterocele within the bladder. Reflux of the lower pole moiety is common. Prenatal detection permits antimicrobial treatment from birth to minimize urinary infections (Callen, 2000).

Posterior Urethral Valves. This distal obstruction of the urinary tract in male fetuses may have a spectrum of sonographic findings. Characteristically, there is dilatation of the bladder and proximal urethra—with the urethra resembling a keyhole—along with thickening of the bladder wall. Oligohydramnios portends a poor prognosis because of pulmonary hypoplasia. Unfortunately, the outcome is not uniformly good even with a normal amount of fluid. As with other obstructive uropathies, prenatal diagnosis allows some affected fetuses to benefit from early intervention postnatally or even consideration of in utero therapy (see Chap. 13, p. 332).

THREE-DIMENSIONAL ULTRASONOGRAPHY. This technology offers superior views of fetal surface anatomy to be obtained, potentially allowing improved visualization of selected structures such as the face, ear, and extremities. To adequately image a fetal structure in three dimensions, the part must be surrounded by amnionic fluid because crowding by adjacent structures obscures the captured image. Even under ideal circumstances, image processing may take considerably more time than is typically devoted to two-dimensional (2-D) scanning. Further, there are limitations on image resolution, data storage, and manipulation (Michailidis and coworkers, 2001; Pretorius and colleagues, 2001). For these reasons, the American Institute of Ultrasound in Medicine (1999) recommends that 3-D scanning be used as an adjunct to 2-D sonography. There is obvious appeal of a 3-D portrait of the fetal face, however, use of this or any other ultrasound technology when not medically indicated is considered by the Institute and by the American College of Obstetricians and Gynecologists (2004) to be inappropriate and contrary to medical practice.

DOPPLER VELOCIMETRY

The Doppler shift is a phenomenon that occurs when a source of light or sound waves is moving relative to an observer; the observer detects a shift in the wave frequency. Similarly, when sound waves strike a moving target, the frequency of the sound waves reflected back is shifted proportionate to the velocity and direction of the moving target. Because the magnitude and direction of the frequency shift depend on the relative motion of the moving target, the velocity and direction of the target can be determined.

Important to obstetrics, Doppler may be used to determine the volume and rate of blood flow through maternal and fetal vessels. In this situation, the sound source is the ultrasound transducer, the moving target is the column of red blood cells flowing through the circulation, and the reflected sound waves are observed by the ultrasound transducer. Two types—continuous and pulse wave Doppler—are used in medicine.

Continuous wave Doppler equipment has separate crystals: one that transmits a high-frequency sound wave, and another that continuously receives signals. It can record high frequencies using low power output and is easy to use. Unfortunately, it is nonselective, recognizing all signals along its path, and does not allow visualization of the blood vessel(s). In m-mode echocardiography, continuous wave Doppler is used to evaluate motion through time. It defines blood flow through the heart, but because the cardiac structures are not visualized, it requires the correlation of the sequence of waveforms produced with the sequence of structures interrogated by the sound wave.

Pulse wave Doppler has equipment that uses only one crystal, which transmits the signal and then waits until the returning signal is received before transmitting another one.

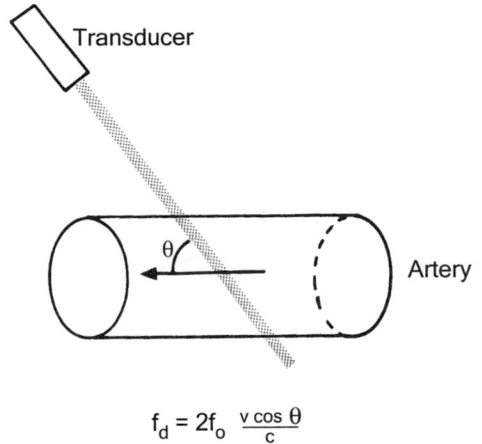

$$f_d = 2f_o \frac{v \cos \theta}{c}$$

FIGURE 16–17. Doppler equation: ultrasound emanating from transducer with initial frequency f_o strikes blood moving at velocity v. Reflected frequency f_d is dependent on angle θ between beam of sound and vessel. (From Copel and associates, 1988.)

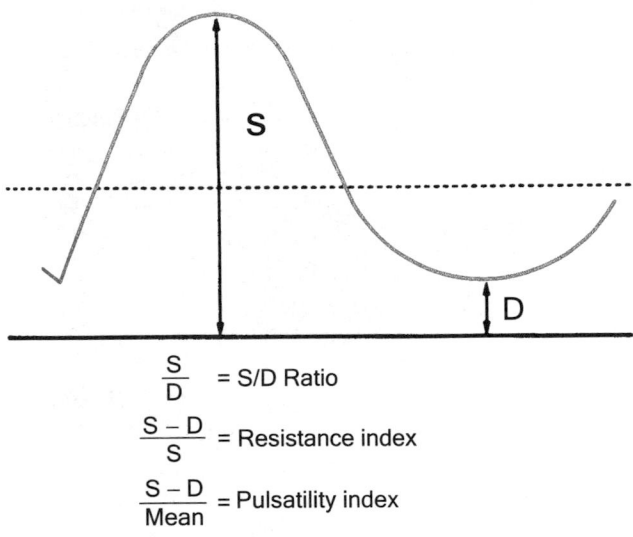

$$\frac{S}{D} = \text{S/D Ratio}$$

$$\frac{S-D}{S} = \text{Resistance index}$$

$$\frac{S-D}{\text{Mean}} = \text{Pulsatility index}$$

FIGURE 16–18. Doppler systolic–diastolic waveform indices of blood flow velocity. The mean is calculated from computer-digitized waveforms. (D = diastole; S = systole.) (From Low, 1991, with permission.)

It is more expensive and requires higher power, but allows precise targeting and visualization of the vessel of interest. Pulse wave Doppler also can be configured to allow color-flow mapping, in which computer software displays blood flowing away from the transducer as blue and blood flowing toward the transducer as red.

Various combinations of continuous wave Doppler, pulse wave Doppler, color-flow Doppler, and real-time ultrasound are commercially available and are loosely referred to as *duplex Doppler.*

CLINICAL APPLICATIONS. The Doppler equation shown in Figure 16–17 contains the variables that affect the Doppler shift. An important source of error when calculating flow or velocity is the angle between sound waves from the transducer and flow within the vessel—termed the *angle of insonation* and abbreviated as theta (θ). Because cosine θ is a component of the equation, measurement error becomes large when the angle of insonation is not close to zero. The practical solution to this problem has been the use of ratios to compare different waveform components—allowing cosine θ to cancel out of the equation. Figure 16–18 is a schematic of the Doppler waveform and describes the three ratios commonly used. The simplest is the *systolic–diastolic ratio (S/D ratio)*, which compares maximum (peak) systolic flow with end-diastolic flow, thereby evaluating downstream impedance to flow.

Virtually every fetal vessel has been insonated in the research setting in an attempt to improve our knowledge of pathophysiology (Detti and colleagues, 2004). Figure 16–19 illustrates several vessels and their corresponding waveforms. The following discussion is limited to selected obstetrical applications.

Umbilical Artery. This vessel normally has forward flow throughout the cardiac cycle, and the amount of flow during diastole increases as gestation advances. Thus the S/D ratio *decreases,* from about 4.0 at 20 weeks to 2.0 at term. The S/D ratio is generally less than 3.0 after 30 weeks (Fleischer and associates, 1986). Umbilical artery Doppler may be a useful adjunct in the management of pregnancies complicated by fetal growth restriction. As presented in Chapter 15 (see p. 383), umbilical artery velocimetry has been subjected to more rigorous assessment than has any previous test of fetal health (Alfirevic and Neilson, 1995). It is, however, not recommended for screening of low-risk pregnancies or for complications other than growth restriction.

Umbilical artery Doppler is considered abnormal if the S/D ratio is above the 95th percentile for gestational age. In extreme cases of growth restriction, end-diastolic flow may become absent or even reversed (Fig. 16–20). These are ominous findings and should prompt a complete fetal evaluation—almost half of cases are due to fetal aneuploidy or a major anomaly (Wenstrom and associates, 1991). In the absence of a reversible maternal complication or a fetal anomaly, reversed end-diastolic flow suggests severe fetal circulatory compromise and usually prompts immediate delivery. Sezik and colleagues (2004) recently reported that fetuses of preeclamptic women who had absent or reversed end-diastolic flow were more likely to have hypoglycemia and polycythemia.

Ductus Arteriosus. Doppler evaluation of the ductus arteriosus has been used primarily to monitor fetuses exposed to indomethacin and other nonsteroidal anti-inflammatory agents. Indomethacin, which is used for tocolysis, causes

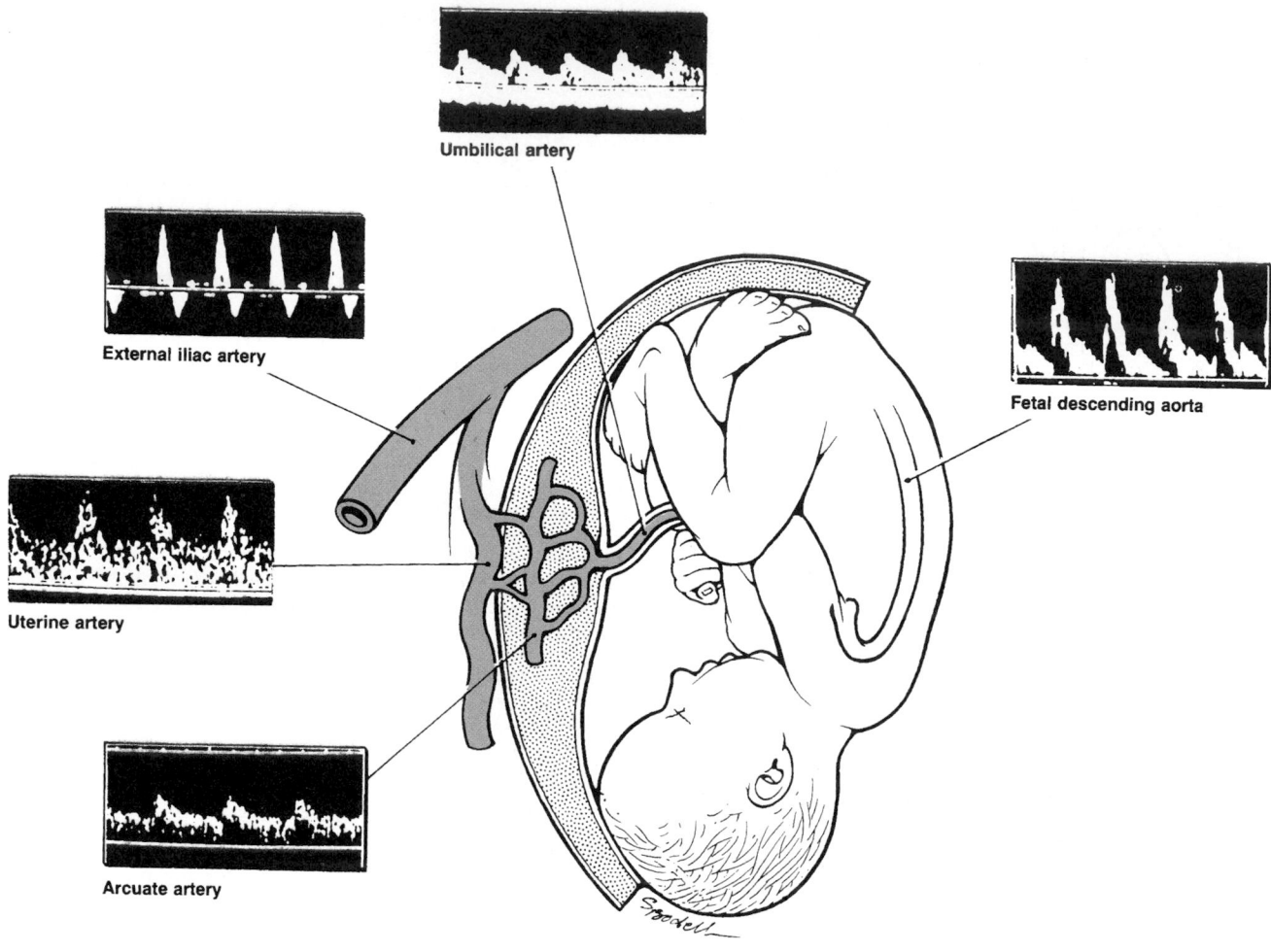

FIGURE 16–19. Doppler waveforms from normal pregnancy. Shown clockwise are normal waveforms from the maternal arcuate, uterine, and external iliac arteries, and from the fetal umbilical artery and descending aorta. Reversed end-diastolic flow velocity is apparent in the external iliac artery, whereas continuous diastolic flow characterizes the uterine and arcuate vessels. Finally, note the greatly diminished end-diastolic flow in the fetal descending aorta. (From Copel and colleagues, 1988.)

constriction of the ductus in sheep and human fetuses (Huhta and colleagues (1987). The resulting increased pulmonary flow may cause reactive hypertrophy of the pulmonary arterioles, and eventually pulmonary hypertension develops (see Chap. 36, p. 871). In a study of 61 indomethacin-treated pregnant women, Vermillion and colleagues (1997) reported that half of exposed fetuses developed ductal constriction. Fortunately, this complication is largely reversible if medication is discontinued before 32 weeks (Moise, 1993).

Middle Cerebral Artery. Peak systolic velocity in the middle cerebral artery is increased with fetal anemia because of increased cardiac output and decreased blood viscosity (Segata and Mari, 2004). Velocity measurements are generally problematic because a high insonating angle introduces considerable error. Middle cerebral artery measurements are an exception, however, because the path of the artery often presents a very low angle of insonation.

Mari and colleagues (1995) performed velocity studies in 135 normal fetuses and 39 with alloimmunization. They reported that all anemic fetuses had peak systolic velocity above the normal mean. This prompted a collaborative study of 376 pregnancies by Mari and colleagues (2000). Using a threshold of 1.50 multiples of the median (MoM), they correctly identified all fetuses with moderate or severe anemia with a false-positive rate of 12 percent. Other investigators have since reported similar results (Abdel-Fattah, 2002; Bahado-Singh, 2000; Cosmi, 2002; Deren and Onderoglu, 2002, and all their associates).

It also has been hypothesized that Doppler evaluation of blood flow through cerebral vessels might be used to detect altered cerebral circulation before there is hypoxemia significant enough to alter the fetal heart rate pattern. The cerebroplacental ratio has been introduced as an indicator of brain sparing in fetuses with growth restriction and as a predictor of adverse perinatal outcome (Bahado-Singh and colleagues,

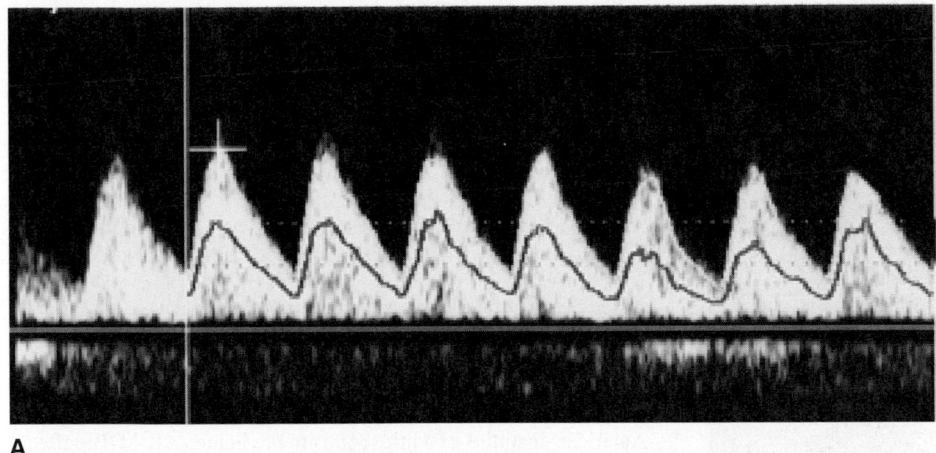

A

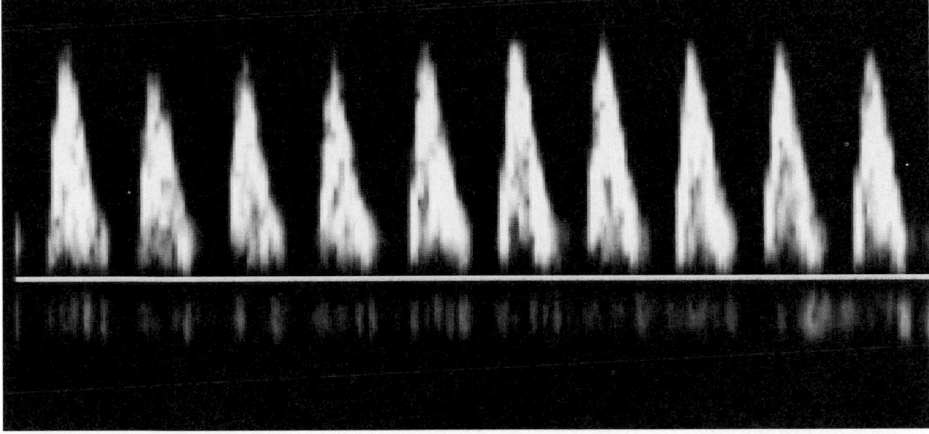

B

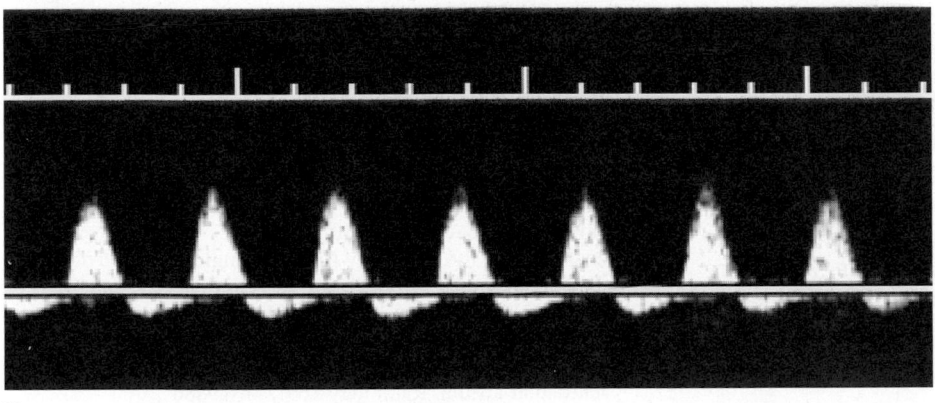

C

FIGURE 16–20. Umbilical artery Doppler waveforms. **A.** Normal diastolic flow. **B.** Absence of end-diastolic flow. **C.** Reversed end-diastolic flow. (Courtesy of Dr. Diane Twickler.)

1999; Gramellini and associates, 1992). Currently, the American College of Obstetricians and Gynecologists (1999) considers antepartum surveillance with cerebral artery Doppler velocimetry to be investigational.

Uterine Artery. Uterine blood flow increases from 50 mL/min early in gestation to 500 to 750 mL/min by term. The uterine artery Doppler waveform is unique and characterized by high diastolic flow velocities similar to those in

systole, and by highly turbulent flow, which displays a spectrum of many different velocities (Fig. 16–21). Increased resistance to flow and development of a diastolic notch have been associated with pregnancy-induced hypertension (Arduini, 1987; Fleischer, 1986; Harrington, 1996; North, 1994, and all their colleagues). In a recent study, Zeeman and co-authors (2003) confirmed that increased impedance of uterine artery velocimetry at 16 to 20 weeks was predictive of superimposed preeclampsia developing in women with

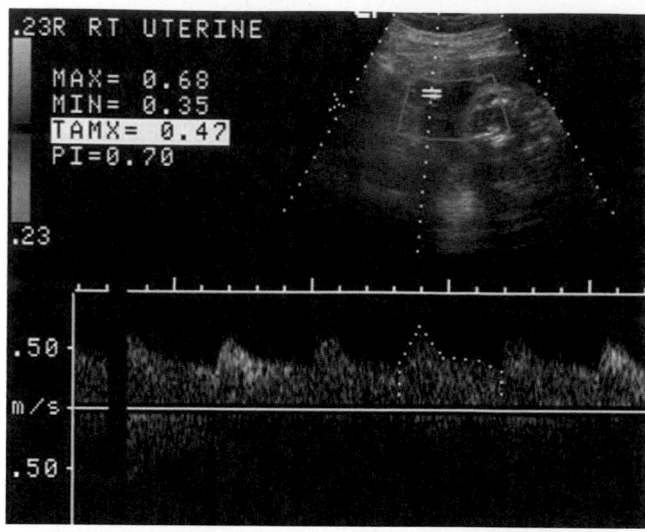

FIGURE 16–21. Normal uterine artery waveform with high-velocity diastolic flow. (Courtesy of Dr. Diane Twickler.)

chronic hypertension. Whether it will be clinically helpful to predict preeclampsia in this manner is yet unclear.

M-MODE ECHOCARDIOGRAPHY

The m-mode is a linear display of the events of the cardiac cycle in real-time. It is used commonly to measure the fetal heart rate, and any deviations from the normal rate and rhythm are readily apparent. If there is an abnormality, an evaluation of cardiac anatomy is performed. M-mode echocardiography may allow precise characterization of an arrhythmia, including separate evaluation of atrial and ventricular waveforms. It can further be used to assess ventricular wall function and functional atrial and ventricular outputs, as well as the timing of these events.

Accurate diagnosis is important because some arrhythmias, for example, supraventricular tachycardia, require medications to prevent or treat heart failure. Others, such as premature atrial contractions, resolve spontaneously without intervention. Antenatal treatment is discussed in Chapter 13 (see p. 332).

REFERENCES

Abdel-Fattah SA, Soothill PW, Carroll SG, et al: Middle cerebral artery Doppler for the prediction of fetal anaemia in cases without hydrops: A practical approach. Br J Radiol 75:726, 2002

Adra AM, Mejides AA, Dennaoui MS, et al: Fetal pyelectasis: Is it always "physiologic"? Am J Obstet Gynecol 173:1263, 1995

Aina-Mumuney AJ, Fischer AC, Blakemore KJ, et al: A dilated fetal stomach predicts a complicated postnatal course in cases of prenatally diagnosed gastroschisis. Am J Obstet Gynecol 190:1326, 2004

Alfirevic Z, Neilson JP: Doppler ultrasonography in high-risk pregnancies: Systematic review with meta-analysis. Am J Obstet Gynecol 172:1379, 1995.

American College of Obstetricians and Gynecologists: Non-medical use of obstetrical ultrasonography. Committee Opinion No. 297, August 2004a

American College of Obstetricians and Gynecologists: First-trimester screening for fetal aneuploidy. Committee Opinion No. 296, July 2004b

American College of Obstetricians and Gynecologists: Antepartum fetal surveillance. Practice Bulletin No. 9, October 1999

American College of Obstetricians and Gynecologists: Routine ultrasound in low-risk pregnancy. Practice Patterns No. 5, August 1997

American Institute of Ultrasound in Medicine: AIUM Practice Guideline for the performance of an antepartum obstetric ultrasound examination. J Ultrasound Med 22:1116, 2003

American Institute of Ultrasound in Medicine: 3-D Technology. Rockville, Md, AIUM, 1999

American Institute of Ultrasound in Medicine: AIUM Bioeffects Committee: Safety Considerations for Diagnostic Ultrasound. Rockville, Md, AIUM, 1991

Arduini D, Rizzo G, Romanini C, et al: Utero-placental blood flow velocity waveforms as predictors of pregnancy-induced hypertension. Eur J Obstet Gynecol Reprod Biol 26:335, 1987

Bahado-Singh RO, Cheng CS: First trimester prenatal diagnosis. Curr Opin Obstet Gynecol 16:177, 2004

Bahado-Singh RO, Kovanci E, Jeffres A, et al: The Doppler cerebroplacental ratio and perinatal outcome in intrauterine growth restriction. Am J Obstet Gynecol 180:750, 1999

Bahado-Singh RO, Oz AU, Hsu C, et al: Middle cerebral artery Doppler velocimetric deceleration angle as a predictor of fetal anemia in Rh-alloimmunized fetuses without hydrops. Am J Obstet Gynecol 183:746, 2000

Benacerraf BR, Pober BR, Sanders SP: Accuracy of fetal echocardiography. Radiology 165:847, 1987

Bennett KA, Crane JM, O'Shea P, et al: First trimester ultrasound screening is effective in reducing postterm labor induction rates: a randomized controlled trial. Am J Obstet Gynecol. 190:1077, 2004

Bloom SL, Bloom DD, DellaNebbia C, et al: The developmental outcome of children with antenatal mild isolated ventriculomegaly. Obstet Gynecol 90:93, 1997

Brumfield CG, Wenstrom KD, Davis RO, et al: Second-trimester cystic hygroma: Prognosis of septated and nonseptated lesions. Obstet Gynecol 88:979, 1996

Callen PW: Ultrasonography in Obstetrics and Gynecology, 4th ed. Philadelphia, Saunders, 2000

Cardoza JD, Filly RA, Podrasky AE: The dangling choroid plexus: A sonographic observation of value in excluding ventriculomegaly. AJR Am J Roentgenol 151:767, 1988a

Cardoza JD, Goldstein RB, Filly RA: Exclusion of fetal ventriculomegaly with a single measurement: The width of the lateral ventricular atrium. Radiology 169:711, 1988b

Coco C, Jeanty P, Jeanty C. An isolated echogenic heart focus is not an indication for amniocentesis in 12,672 unselected patients. J Ultrasound Med 23:489, 2004

Comstock CH: Normal fetal heart axis and position. Obstet Gynecol 70:255, 1987

Copel JA, Grannum PA, Hobbins JC, et al: Doppler ultrasound in obstetrics. Williams Obstetrics, 17th ed (Suppl 16). Norwalk, Conn, Appleton and Lange, 1988

Corteville J, Gray D, Crane J: Congenital hydronephrosis: Correlation of fetal ultrasonographic findings with infant outcome. Am J Obstet Gynecol 165:384, 1991

Cosmi E, Mari G, Delle CL, et al: Noninvasive diagnosis by Doppler ultrasonography of fetal anemia resulting from parvovirus infection. Am J Obstet Gynecol 187:1290, 2002

Crawford DC, Chita SK, Allan LD: Prenatal detection of congenital heart disease: Factors affecting obstetric management and survival. Am J Obstet Gynecol 159:352, 1988

Deren O, Onderoglu L: The value of middle cerebral artery systolic velocity for initial and subsequent management in fetal anemia. Eur J Obstet Gynecol Reprod Biol 101:26, 2002

Detti L, Mari G, Cheng CC, et al: Fetal Doppler velocimetry. Obstet Gynecol Clin North Am 31:201, 2004

Donald I, MacVicar J, Brown TG: Investigation of abdominal masses by pulsed ultrasound. Lancet 7032:1188, 1958

Ewigman BG, Crane P, Frigoletto FD, et al: Effect of prenatal ultrasound screening on perinatal outcome. N Engl J Med 329:821, 1993

Fleischer A, Schulman H, Farmakides G, et al: Uterine artery Doppler velocimetry in pregnant women with hypertension. Am J Obstet Gynecol 154:806, 1986

Goldstein I, Reece EA, Pilu G, et al: Cerebellar measurements with ultrasonography in the evaluation of fetal growth and development. Am J Obstet Gynecol 156:1065, 1987

Goncalves LF, Jeanty P, Piper JM: The accuracy of prenatal ultrasonography in detecting congenital anomalies. Am J Obstet Gynecol 171:1606, 1994

Gramellini D, Folli MC, Raboni S, et al: Cerebral-umbilical Doppler ratio as a predictor of adverse perinatal outcome. Obstet Gynecol 79:416, 1992

Harrington K, Cooper D, Lees C, et al: Doppler ultrasound of the uterine arteries: The importance of bilateral notching in the prediction of pre-eclampsia, placental abruption or delivery of a small-for-gestational-age baby. Ultrasound Obstet Gynecol 7:182, 1996

Heider AL, Strauss RA, Kuller JA. Omphalocele: Clinical outcomes in cases with normal karyotypes. Am J Obstet Gynecol. 190:135, 2004

Heiserman J, Filly RA, Goldstein RB: Effect of measurement errors on sonographic evaluation of ventriculomegaly. J Ultrasound Med 10:121, 1991

Hoffman CK, Filly RA, Callen PW: The "lying down" adrenal sign: A sonographic indicator of renal agenesis or ectopia in fetuses and neonates. J Ultrasound Med 11:533, 1992

Hoyme HE, Jones MC, Jones KL: Gastroschisis: Abdominal wall disruption secondary to early gestational interruption of the omphalomesenteric artery. Semin Perinatol 7:294, 1983

Huang J, Kurkchubasche AG, Carr SR, et al: Benefits of term delivery in infants with antenatally diagnosed gastroschisis. Obstet Gynecol 100:695, 2002

Huhta JC, Moise KJ, Fisher DJ, et al: Detection and quantitation of constriction of the fetal ductus arteriosus by Doppler echocardiography. Circulation 75:406, 1987

Ismaili K, Hall M, Donner C, et al: Results of systematic screening for minor degrees of fetal renal pelvis dilatation in an unselected population. Am J Obstet Gynecol 188:242, 2003

Japaraj RP, Hockey R, Chan FY: Gastroschisis: Can prenatal sonography predict neonatal outcome? Ultrasound Obstet Gynecol 21:329, 2003

Johnson MP, Johnson A, Holzgreve W, et al: First-trimester simple hygroma: Cause and outcome. Am J Obstet Gynecol 168:156, 1993

Kesrouani AK, Guibourdenche J, Muller F, et al: Etiology and outcome of fetal echogenic bowel. Ten years of experience. Fetal Diag and Ther 18:240, 2003

Kitchanan S, Patole SK, Muller R, et al: Neonatal outcome of gastroschisis and exomphalos: A 10-year review. J Paediatr Child Health 36:428, 2000

Low JA: The current status of maternal and fetal blood flow velocimetry. Am J Obstet Gynecol 164:1049, 1991

Lowe TW, Peters MT, Twickler D, et al: Obstetrical sonography

update. Williams Obstetrics, 18th ed (Suppl 6). Norwalk, Conn, Appleton and Lange, 1990

Mahony BS, Nyberg DA, Hirsch JH, et al: Mild idiopathic lateral cerebral ventricular dilatation in utero: Sonographic evaluation. Radiology 169:715, 1988

Malone FD, Wald NJ, Canick JA: First- and second-trimester evaluation of risk (FASTER) trial: Principal results of the NICHD Multicenter Down Syndrome Screening Study [abstract]. Am J Obstet Gynecol 189:S56, 2003

Mandell J, Blyth B, Peters C, et al: Structural genitourinary defects detected in utero. Radiology 178:193, 1991

Mari G, Abuhamad AZ, Uerpairojkit B, et al: Blood flow velocity waveforms of the abdominal arteries in appropriate- and small-for-gestational-age fetuses. Ultrasound Obstet Gynecol 6:15, 1995

Mari G, Deter RL, Carpenter RL, et al: Noninvasive diagnosis by Doppler ultrasonography of fetal anemia due to maternal red-cell alloimmunization. Collaborative Group for Doppler Assessment of the Blood Velocity in Anemic Fetuses. N Engl J Med 342:9, 2000

McGalliard C, Gaudoin M: Routine ultrasound for pregnancy termination requests increases women's choice and reduces inappropriate treatments. Br J Obstet Gynaecol 111:79, 2004

Michailidis GD, Economides DL, Schild RL: The role of three-dimensional ultrasound in obstetrics. Curr Opin Obstet Gynecol 13:207, 2001

Michailidis GD, Papageorgiou P, Economides DL: Assessment of fetal anatomy in the first trimester using two- and three-dimensional ultrasound. Br J Radiol 75:215, 2002

Millener PB, Anderson NG, Chisholm RJ: Prognostic significance of nonvisualization of the fetal stomach by sonography. AJR Am J Roentgenol 160:827, 1993

Moise KJ Jr: Effect of advancing gestational age on the frequency of fetal ductal constriction in association with maternal indomethacin use. Am J Obstet Gynecol 168:1350, 1993

National Center for Health Statistics: National Vital Statistics Reports, Vol 51, No 2, Hyattsville, Md, National Center for Health Statistics, December 18, 2002

Nembhard WN, Waller DK, Sever LE, et al: Patterns of first-year survival among infants with selected congenital anomalies in Texas, 1995–1997. Teratology 64:267, 2001

Nicolaides KH. Nuchal translucency and other first-trimester sonographic markers of chromosomal abnormalities. Am J Obstet Gynecol 191:45, 2004

Nicolaides KH, Azar G, Byrne D, et al: Fetal nuchal translucency: Ultrasound screening for chromosomal defects in the first trimester of pregnancy. BMJ 304:867, 1992

North RA, Ferrier C, Long D, et al: Uterine artery Doppler flow velocity waveforms in the second trimester for the prediction of preeclampsia and fetal growth retardation. Obstet Gynecol 83:378, 1994

Ott WJ: The accuracy of antenatal fetal echocardiography screening in high- and low-risk patients. Am J Obstet Gynecol 172:1741, 1995

Patten RM, Mack LA, Wang KY, et al: The fetal genitourinary tract. Radiol Clin North Am 28:115, 1990

Phelan JP, Ahn MO, Smith CV, et al: Amnionic fluid index measurements during pregnancy. J Reprod Med 32:601, 1987

Potter EL: Bilateral renal agenesis. J Pediatr 29:68, 1946

Pretorius DH, Borok NN, Coffler MS, et al: Three-dimensional ultrasound in obstetrics and gynecology. Radiol Clin North Am 39:499, 2001

Pretorius DH, Drose JA, Dennis MA, et al: Tracheoesophageal fistula in utero: Twenty-two cases. J Ultrasound Med 6:509, 1987a

Pretorius DH, Lee ME, Manco-Johnson ML, et al: Diagnosis of autosomal dominant polycystic kidney disease in utero and in the young infant. J Ultrasound Med 6:249, 1987b

Rabinowitz R, Peters MT, Vyas S, et al: Measurement of fetal urine production in normal pregnancy by real-time ultrasonography. Am J Obstet Gynecol 161:1264, 1989

Robertson FM, Crombleholme TM, Paidas M, et al: Prenatal diagnosis and management of gastrointestinal disorders. Semin Perinatol 18:182, 1994

Sagi J, Vagman I, David MP, et al: Fetal kidney size related to gestational age. Gynecol Obstet Invest 23:1, 1987

Segata M, Mari G: Fetal anemia: New technologies. Curr Opin Obstet Gynecol 16:153, 2004

Sezik M, Tuncay G, Yapar EG: Prediction of adverse neonatal outcomes in preeclampsia by absent or reversed end-diastolic flow velocity in the umbilical artery. Gynecol Obstet Invest 57:109, 2004

Shipp TD, Bromley B, Hornberger LK, et al: Levorotation of the fetal cardiac axis: A clue for the presence of congenital heart disease. Obstet Gynecol 85:97, 1995

Shulman LP, Emerson DS, Felker RE, et al: High frequency of cytogenetic abnormalities in fetuses with cystic hygroma diagnosed in the first trimester. Obstet Gynecol 80:80, 1992

Smith RS, Comstock CH, Kirk JS, et al: Ultrasonographic left cardiac axis deviation: A marker for fetal anomalies. Obstet Gynecol 85:187, 1995

Stoll C, Dott B, Alembik Y, et al: Evaluation and evolution during time of prenatal diagnosis of congenital heart diseases by routine fetal ultrasonographic examination. Ann Genet 45:21, 2002

Trauffer PML, Anderson CE, Johnson A, et al: The natural history of euploid pregnancies with first-trimester cystic hygromas. Am J Obstet Gynecol 170:1279, 1994

Tunon K, Eik-Nes SH, Grottom P: A comparison between ultrasound and a reliable last menstrual period as predictors of the day of delivery in 15,000 examinations. Ultrasound Obstet Gynecol 8:178, 1996

Van Dorsten JP, Hulsey TC, Newman RB, et al: Fetal anomaly detection by second-trimester ultrasonography in a tertiary center. Am J Obstet Gynecol 178:742, 1998

Vermillion ST, Scardo JA, Lashus AG, et al: The effect of indomethacin tocolysis on fetal ductus arteriosus constriction with advancing gestational age. Am J Obstet Gynecol 177:256, 1997

Vincoff NS, Callen PW, Smith-Bindman R, et al: Effect of ultrasound transducer frequency on the appearance of the fetal bowel. J Ultrasound Med 18:799, 1999

Waldenstrom U, Nilsson S, Fall O, et al: Effects of routine one-stage ultrasound screening in pregnancy: A randomized controlled trial. Lancet 2:585, 1988

Wapner R, Thom E, Simpson JL, et al: First-trimester maternal serum biochemistry and fetal nuchal translucency screening (BUN) study group. First-trimester screening for trisomies 21 and 18. N Engl J Med 249:1405, 2003

Wenstrom KD, Weiner CP, Williamson RA: Diverse maternal and fetal pathology associated with absent diastolic flow in the umbilical artery of high-risk fetuses. Obstet Gynecol 77:374, 1991

Whitlow BJ, Economides DL: The optimal gestational age to examine fetal anatomy and measure nuchal translucency in the first trimester. Ultrasound Obstet Gynecol 11:258, 1998

Wilson R, Lynch S, Lessoway V: Fetal pyelectasis: Comparison of postnatal renal pathology with unilateral and bilateral pyelectasis. Prenat Diagn 17:451, 1997

Wyldes M, Watkinson M: Isolated mild fetal ventriculomegaly. Arch Dis Child Fetal Neonatal Ed 89:F9, 2004

Zeeman GG, McIntire DD, Twickler DM: Maternal and fetal artery Doppler findings in women with chronic hypertension who subsequently develop superimposed pre-eclampsia. J Matern Fetal Neonatal Med 14:318, 2003

IV

Labor and Delivery

17

Normal Labor and Delivery

Childbirth is the period from the onset of regular uterine contractions until expulsion of the placenta. The process by which this normally occurs is called *labor*—a term that in the obstetrical context takes on several connotations from the English language. According to the *New Shorter Oxford English Dictionary* (1993), toil, trouble, suffering, bodily exertion, especially when painful, and an outcome of work are all characteristics of *labor* and thus implicated in the process of childbirth. Such connotations all seem appropriate to us and emphasize the need for all attendants to be supportive of the laboring woman's needs, particularly in regard to effective pain relief.

At Parkland Hospital in 2003, only 53 percent of 12,139 women with singleton cephalic presentations at term had a spontaneous labor and delivery. The remainder had ineffective labor requiring augmentation (29 percent) or other medical and obstetrical complications requiring induction of labor. It seems excessive to consider almost 50 percent of parturients as "abnormal" because they did not spontaneously labor and deliver. Hence, the distinction between normal and abnormal is often subjective. This high prevalence of labor abnormalities, however, can be used to underscore the importance of labor events in the successful outcome of pregnancy.

MECHANISMS OF LABOR

At the onset of labor, the position of the fetus with respect to the birth canal is critical to the route of delivery. It is thus of paramount importance to know the fetal position within the uterine cavity at the onset of labor.

LIE, PRESENTATION, ATTITUDE, AND POSITION.
Fetal orientation relative to the maternal pelvis is described in terms of fetal lie, presentation, attitude, and position.

Fetal Lie. The lie is the relation of the long axis of the fetus to that of the mother, and is either *longitudinal* or *transverse*. Occasionally, the fetal and the maternal axes may cross at a 45-degree angle, forming an *oblique* lie, which is unstable

TABLE 17–1 Fetal Presentation in 68,097 Singleton Pregnancies at Parkland Hospital, 1995–1999

Presentation	Percent	Incidence
Cephalic	96.8	
Breech	2.7	1:36
Transverse	0.3	1:335
Compound	0.1	1:1000
Face	0.5	1:2000
Brow	0.01	1:10,000

and always becomes longitudinal or transverse during the course of labor. Longitudinal lies are present in over 99 percent of labors at term. Predisposing factors for transverse lies include multiparity, placenta previa, hydramnios, and uterine anomalies.

Fetal Presentation. The presenting part is that portion of the fetal body that is either foremost within the birth canal or in closest proximity to it. It can be felt through the cervix on vaginal examination. Accordingly, in longitudinal lies, the presenting part is either the fetal head or breech, creating *cephalic* and *breech* presentations, respectively. When the fetus lies with the long axis transversely, the *shoulder* is the presenting part and is felt through the cervix on vaginal examination. Table 17–1 describes the incidences of the various fetal presentations.

CEPHALIC PRESENTATION. Such presentations are classified according to the relationship between the head and body of the fetus (Fig. 17–1). Ordinarily, the head is flexed sharply so that the chin is in contact with the thorax. The occipital fontanel is the presenting part, and this presentation is referred to as a *vertex* or *occiput presentation*. Much less commonly, the fetal neck may be sharply extended so that the occiput and back come in contact and the face is foremost in the birth canal— *face presentation* (see Fig. 20–6, p. 507). The fetal head may assume a position between these extremes, partially flexed

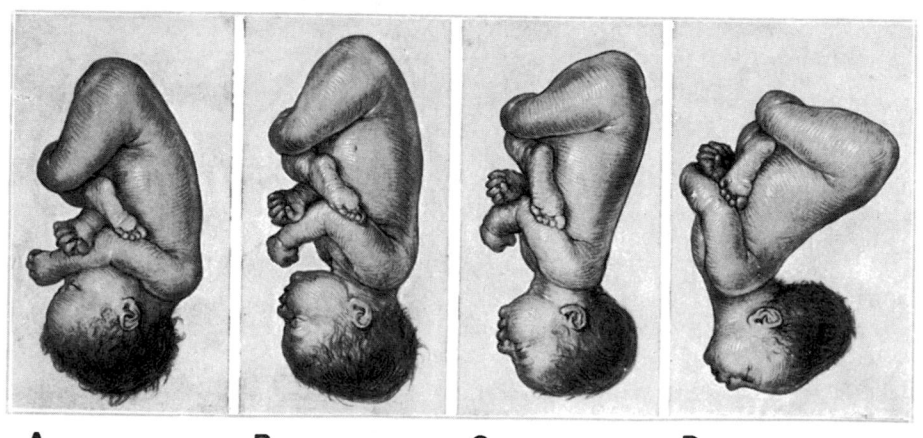

A   **B**   **C**   **D**

FIGURE 17–1. Longitudinal lie. Cephalic presentation. Differences in attitude of the fetal body in **(A)** vertex, **(B)** sinciput, **(C)** brow, and **(D)** face presentations. Note changes in fetal attitude in relation to fetal vertex as the fetal head becomes less flexed.

in some cases, with the anterior (large) fontanel, or bregma, presenting—*sinciput presentation*—or partially extended in other cases to have a *brow presentation* (see Fig. 20–9, p. 508). These latter two presentations are usually transient. As labor progresses, sinciput and brow presentations almost always are converted into vertex or face presentations by neck flexion or extension, respectively. Failure to do so can lead to dystocia, as discussed in Chapter 20.

The term fetus usually presents with the vertex, most logically because the uterus is piriform shaped. Although the fetal head at term is slightly larger than the breech, the entire podalic pole of the fetus—that is, the breech and its flexed extremities—is bulkier and more mobile than the cephalic pole. The cephalic pole is composed of the fetal head only. Until about 32 weeks, the amnionic cavity is large compared with the fetal mass, and there is no crowding of the fetus by the uterine walls. Subsequently, however, the ratio of amnionic fluid volume decreases relative to the increasing fetal mass. As a result, the uterine walls are apposed more closely to the fetal parts.

If presenting by the breech, the fetus often changes polarity to make use of the roomier fundus for its bulkier and more mobile podalic pole. Although the incidence of breech presentation is only a little over 3 percent at term, it is much greater earlier in pregnancy. Scheer and Nubar (1976), using ultrasonography, found the incidence of breech presentation to be 14 percent between 29 and 32 weeks' gestation. Subsequently, the breech converted spontaneously to vertex in increasingly higher percentages as term approached. The high incidence of breech presentation in hydrocephalic fetuses is in accord with this theory, because in this circumstance, the cephalic pole of the fetus is larger than the podalic pole.

BREECH PRESENTATION. When the fetus presents as a breech, the three general configurations are frank, complete, and footling presentations. These all are described in Chapter 24 on management of breech presentations. Breech presentation may result from circumstances that prevent normal version from taking place, for example, a septum that protrudes into the uterine cavity (see Chap. 40, p. 953). A peculiarity of fetal attitude, particularly extension of the vertebral column as seen in frank breeches, also may prevent the fetus from turning. Placentas implanted in the lower uterine segment may distort normal intrauterine anatomy and result in a higher incidence of breech presentation.

Fetal Attitude or Posture. In the later months of pregnancy the fetus assumes a characteristic posture described as attitude or habitus (see Fig. 17–1). As a rule, the fetus forms an ovoid mass that corresponds roughly to the shape of the uterine cavity. The fetus becomes folded or bent upon itself in such a manner that the back becomes markedly convex; the head is sharply flexed so that the chin is almost in contact with the chest; the thighs are flexed over the abdomen; the legs are bent at the knees; and the arches of the feet rest upon the anterior surfaces of the legs. In all cephalic presentations, the arms are usually crossed over the thorax or become parallel to the sides, and the umbilical cord lies in the space between them and the lower extremities. This characteristic posture results from the mode of growth of the fetus and its accommodation to the uterine cavity.

Abnormal exceptions to this attitude occur as the fetal head becomes progressively more extended from the vertex to the face presentation (see Fig. 17–1D). This results in a progressive change in fetal attitude from a convex (flexed) to a concave (extended) contour of the vertebral column.

Fetal Position. Position refers to the relationship of an arbitrarily chosen portion of the fetal presenting part to the right or left side of the maternal birth canal. Accordingly, with each presentation there may be two positions, right or left. The fetal occiput, chin (mentum), and sacrum are the determining points in vertex, face, and breech presentations, respectively (Figs. 17–2 to 17–6). Because the presenting part may be in either the left or right position, there are left and right occipital, left and right mental, and left and right sacral presentations, abbreviated as LO and RO, LM and RM, and LS and RS, respectively.

Varieties of Presentations and Positions. For still more accurate orientation, the relationship of a given portion of the presenting part to the anterior, transverse, or posterior portion of the maternal pelvis is considered. Because the presenting part in right or left positions may be directed anteriorly (A), transversely (T), or posteriorly (P), there are six varieties of each of the three presentations (see Figs. 17–2 to 17–6). Thus, in an occiput presentation, the presentation, position, and variety may be abbreviated in clockwise fashion as:

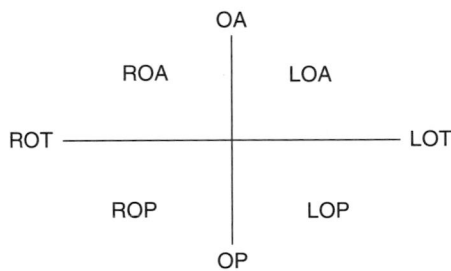

Approximately two thirds of all vertex presentations are in the left occiput position, and one third in the right. In shoulder presentations, the acromion (scapula) is the portion of the fetus arbitrarily chosen for orientation with the maternal pelvis. One example of the terminology sometimes employed for this purpose is illustrated in Figure 17–7. The acromion or back of the fetus may be directed either posteriorly or anteriorly and superiorly or inferiorly (see Chap. 20, p. 509). Because it is impossible to differentiate exactly the several varieties of shoulder presentation by clinical examination, and because such differentiation serves no practical purpose, it is customary to refer to all transverse lies simply as *shoulder presentations.* Another term used is *transverse lie,* with back up or back down.

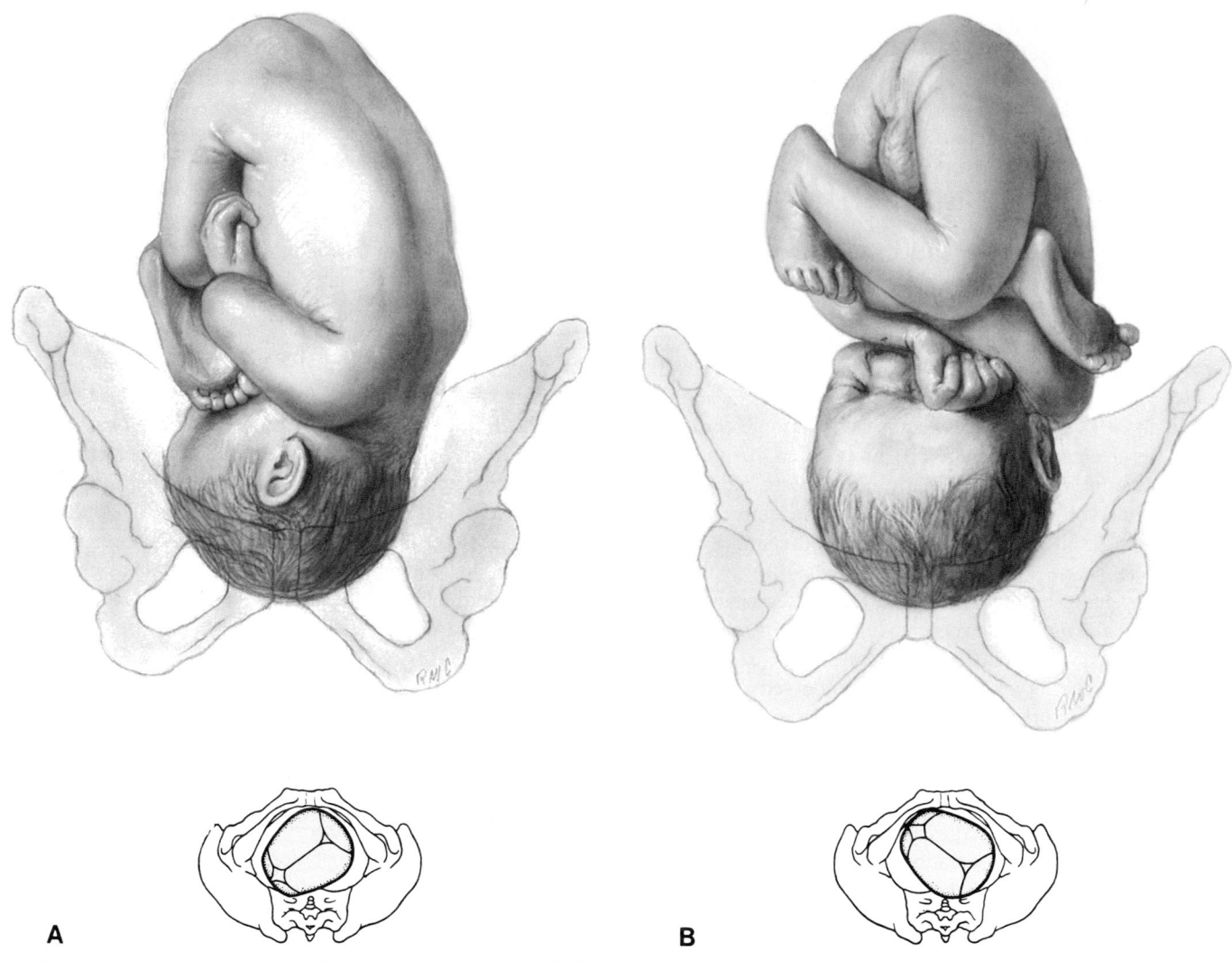

FIGURE 17–2. Longitudinal lie. Vertex presentation. **A.** Left occiput anterior (LOA). **B.** Left occiput posterior (LOP).

DIAGNOSIS OF FETAL PRESENTATION AND POSITION. Several methods can be used to diagnose fetal presentation and position. These include abdominal palpation, vaginal examination, auscultation, and, in certain doubtful cases, imaging studies such as ultrasonography, computed tomography, or magnetic resonance imaging.

Abdominal Palpation—Leopold Maneuvers. Abdominal examination can be conducted systematically employing the four maneuvers described by Leopold and Sporlin in 1894 and shown in Figure 17–8. The mother should be supine and comfortably positioned with her abdomen bared. These maneuvers may be difficult if not impossible to perform and interpret if the patient is obese, if there is excessive amnionic fluid, or if the placenta is anteriorly implanted.

FIRST MANEUVER. This maneuver permits identification of which fetal pole—that is, breech or head—occupies the uterine fundus. The breech gives the sensation of a large, nodular mass, whereas the head feels hard and round and is more mobile and ballottable.

SECOND MANEUVER. After determination of the fetal lie, palms are placed on either side of the maternal abdomen, and gentle but deep pressure is exerted. On one side, a hard, resistant structure is felt—the back—and on the other, numerous small, irregular, mobile parts are felt—the fetal extremities. By noting whether the back is directed anteriorly, transversely, or posteriorly, the orientation of the fetus can be determined.

THIRD MANEUVER. Using the thumb and fingers of one hand, the lower portion of the maternal abdomen is grasped just above the symphysis pubis. If the presenting part is not engaged, a movable mass will be felt, usually the head. The differentiation between head and breech is made as in the first maneuver. If the presenting part is deeply engaged, however, the findings from this maneuver are simply indicative

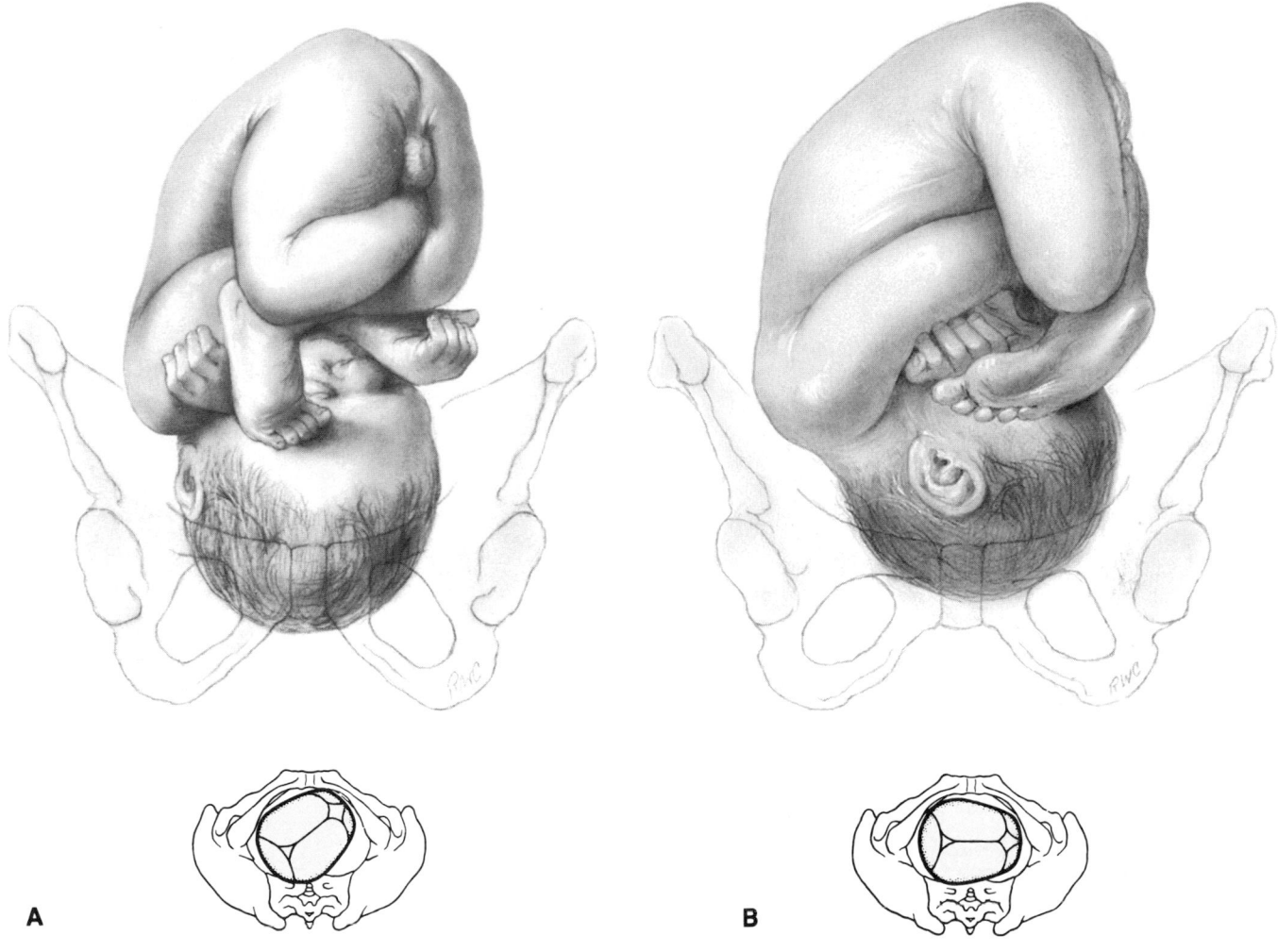

FIGURE 17–3. Longitudinal lie. Vertex presentation. **A.** Right occiput posterior (ROP). **B.** Right occiput transverse (ROT).

that the lower fetal pole is in the pelvis, and details are then defined by the last (fourth) maneuver.

FOURTH MANEUVER. The examiner faces the mother's feet and, with the tips of the first three fingers of each hand, exerts deep pressure in the direction of the axis of the pelvic inlet. In many instances, when the head has descended into the pelvis, the anterior shoulder may be differentiated readily by the third maneuver.

Abdominal palpation can be performed throughout the latter months of pregnancy and during and between the contractions of labor. With experience, it is possible to estimate the size of the fetus. According to Lydon-Rochelle and colleagues (1993), experienced clinicians accurately identify fetal malpresentation using Leopold maneuvers with a high sensitivity (88 percent), specificity (94 percent), positive-predictive value (74 percent), and negative-predictive value (97 percent).

Vaginal Examination. Before labor, the diagnosis of fetal presentation and position by vaginal examination is often inconclusive, because the presenting part must be palpated through a closed cervix and lower uterine segment. With the onset of labor and after cervical dilatation, vertex presentations and their positions are recognized by palpation of the various sutures and fontanels. Face and breech presentations are identified by palpation of the facial features and the fetal sacrum, respectively.

In attempting to determine presentation and position by vaginal examination, it is advisable to pursue a definite routine, comprising four movements:

1. Two fingers of a gloved hand are introduced into the vagina and carried up to the presenting part. The differentiation of vertex, face, and breech is then accomplished readily.
2. If the vertex is presenting, the fingers are directed into the posterior aspect of the vagina. The fingers are then swept forward over the fetal head toward the maternal symphysis (Fig. 17–9). During this movement, the fingers necessarily cross the fetal sagittal suture and its course is delineated.
3. The positions of the two fontanels then are ascertained. The fingers are passed to the most anterior extension of

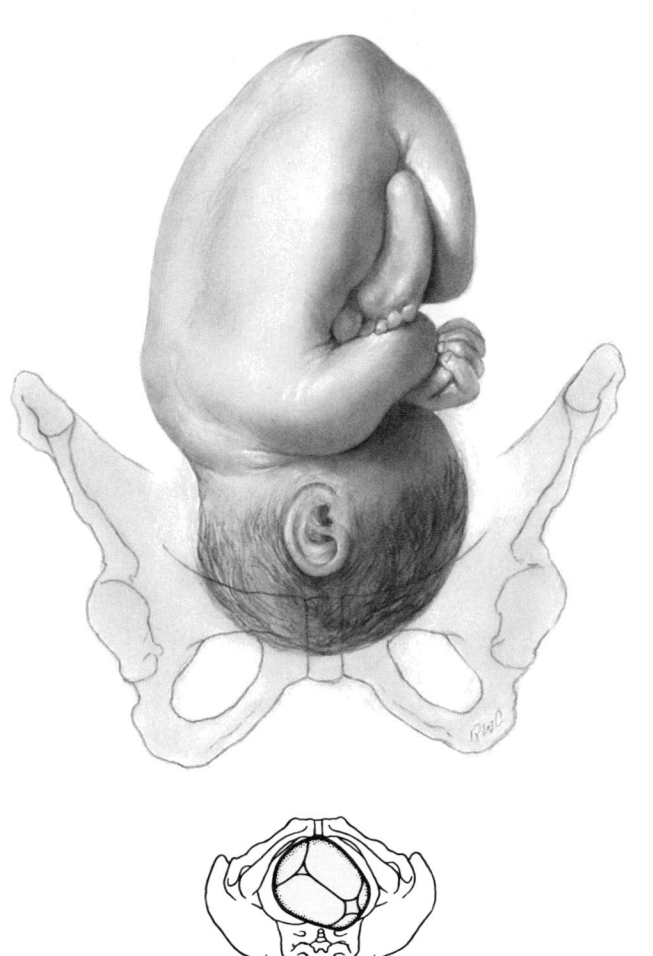

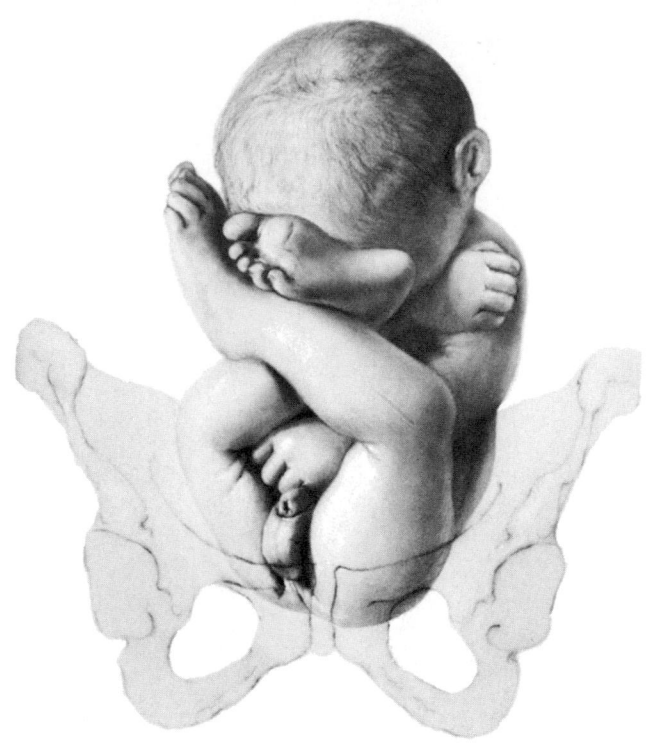

FIGURE 17-6. Longitudinal lie. Breech presentation. Left sacrum posterior (LSP).

FIGURE 17-4. Longitudinal lie. Vertex presentation. Right occiput anterior (ROA).

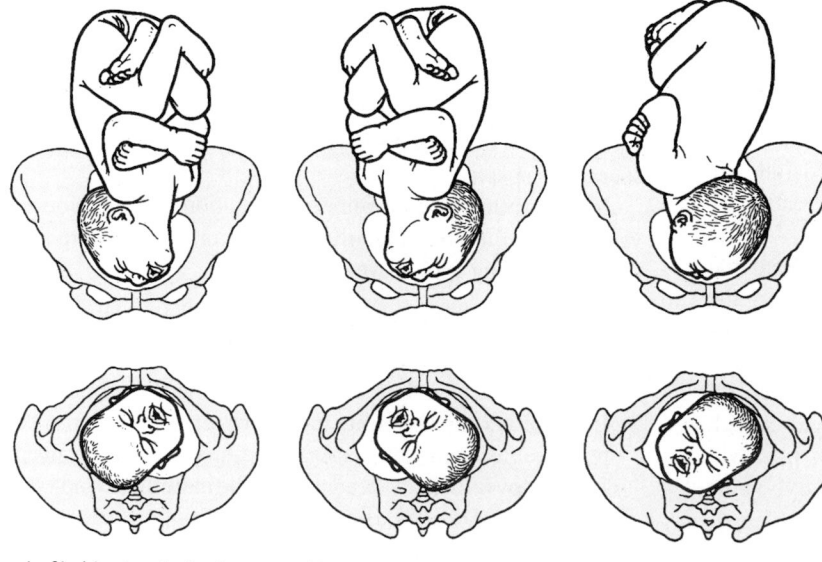

Left Mento-Anterior   Right Mento-Anterior   Right Mento-Posterior

FIGURE 17-5. Longitudinal lie. Face presentation. Left and right anterior and right posterior positions.

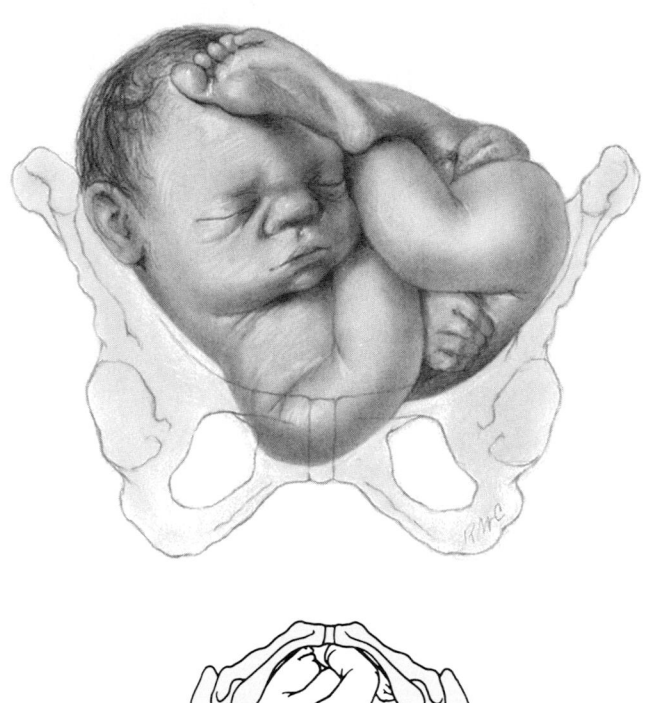

FIGURE 17–7. Transverse lie. Right acromiodorsoposterior (RADP). The shoulder of the fetus is to the mother's right, and the back is posterior.

the sagittal suture, and the fontanel encountered there is examined and identified; then with a sweeping motion, the fingers pass along the suture to the other end of the head until the other fontanel is felt and differentiated (Fig. 17–10).

4. The station, or extent to which the presenting part has descended into the pelvis, can also be established at this time (see p. 426). Using these maneuvers, the various sutures and fontanels are located readily (Fig. 4–8, p. 96).

Auscultation. Although auscultation alone with an aural fetoscope does not provide reliable information concerning fetal presentation and position, auscultatory findings sometimes reinforce results obtained by palpation. The region of the maternal abdomen in which fetal heart sounds are most clearly heard varies according to the presentation and the extent to which the presenting part has descended.

Ultrasonography and Radiography. Ultrasonographic techniques can aid identification of fetal position, especially in obese women or in women with rigid abdominal walls. In some clinical situations, the value of information obtained radiographically far exceeds the minimal risk from a single x-ray exposure (see Chap. 41, p. 977).

LABOR WITH OCCIPUT PRESENTATIONS. In the majority of cases, the vertex enters the pelvis with the sagittal suture lying in the transverse pelvic diameter. The fetus enters the pelvis in the *left occiput transverse (LOT)* position in 40 percent of labors and in the *right occiput transverse (ROT)* position in 20 percent (Caldwell and associates, 1934). In *occiput anterior positions (LOA or ROA),* the head either enters the pelvis with the occiput rotated 45 degrees anteriorly from the transverse position, or subsequently does so. The mechanism of labor in all these presentations is usually similar.

In about 20 percent of labors, the fetus enters the pelvis in an *occiput posterior (OP)* position. The right occiput posterior (ROP) is slightly more common than the left (LOP) (Caldwell and associates, 1934). It appears likely from radiographic evidence that posterior positions are more often associated with a narrow forepelvis. They also are more commonly seen in association with anterior placentation (Gardberg and Tuppurainen, 1994a).

Occiput Anterior Presentation. The positional changes in the presenting part required to navigate the pelvic canal constitute the *mechanisms of labor.* The *cardinal movements of labor* are engagement, descent, flexion, internal rotation, extension, external rotation, and expulsion (Fig. 17–11). During labor, these movements are sequential but also show great temporal overlap. For example, as part of the process of engagement, there is both flexion and descent of the head. It is impossible for the movements to be completed unless the presenting part descends simultaneously. Concomitantly, uterine contractions effect important modifications in fetal attitude, or habitus, especially after the head has descended into the pelvis. These changes consist principally of a straightening of the fetus, with loss of dorsal convexity and closer application of the extremities to the body. As a result, the fetal ovoid is transformed into a cylinder, with the smallest possible cross section typically passing through the birth canal.

ENGAGEMENT. The mechanism by which the biparietal diameter, the greatest transverse diameter of the fetal head in occiput presentations, passes through the pelvic inlet is designated *engagement.* The fetal head may engage during the last few weeks of pregnancy or not until after the commencement of labor. In many multiparous and some nulliparous women, the fetal head is freely movable above the pelvic inlet at the onset of labor. In this circumstance, the head is sometimes referred to as "floating." A normal-sized head usually does not engage with its sagittal suture directed anteroposteriorly. Instead, the fetal head usually enters the pelvic inlet either transversely or obliquely.

ASYNCLITISM. Although the fetal head tends to accommodate to the transverse axis of the pelvic inlet, the sagittal suture, while remaining parallel to that axis, may not lie exactly midway between the symphysis and the sacral promontory. The sagittal suture frequently is deflected either posteriorly toward the promontory or anteriorly toward the symphysis

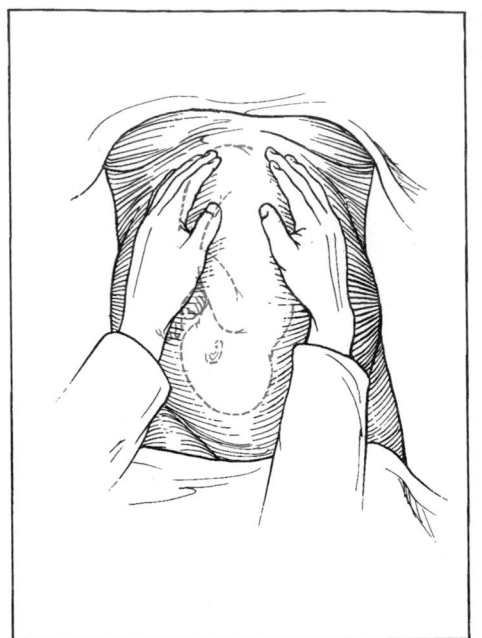

First maneuver

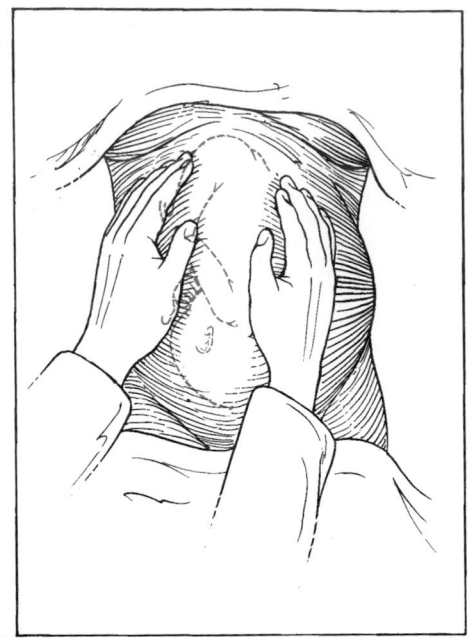

Second maneuver

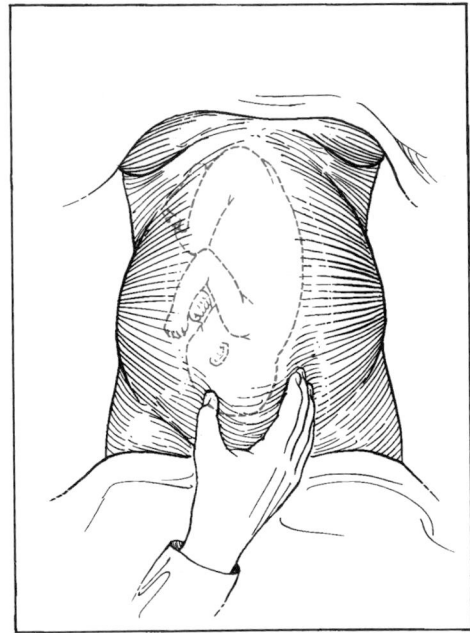

Third maneuver

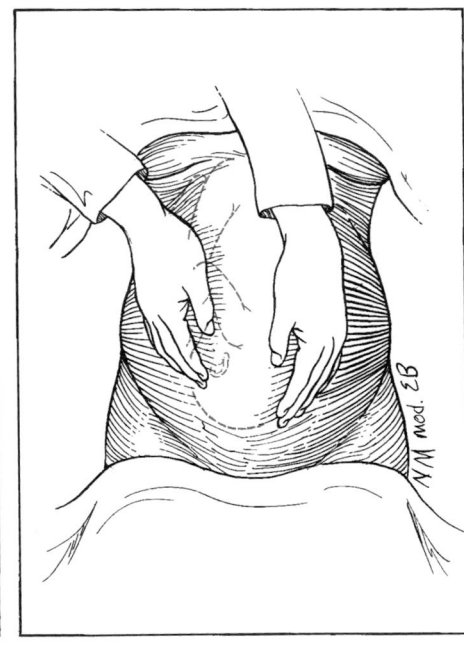

Fourth maneuver

FIGURE 17–8. Longitudinal lie. Left occiput anterior position (LOA) (Leopold maneuvers).

(Fig. 17–12). Such lateral deflection of the head to a more anterior or posterior position in the pelvis is called *asynclitism.* If the sagittal suture approaches the sacral promontory, more of the anterior parietal bone presents itself to the examining fingers, and the condition is called *anterior asynclitism.* If, however, the sagittal suture lies close to the symphysis, more of the posterior parietal bone will present, and the condition is called *posterior asynclitism.* With extreme posterior asynclitism, the posterior ear may be easily palpated.

Moderate degrees of asynclitism are the rule in normal labor, but if severe, the condition may lead to cephalopelvic disproportion even with an otherwise normal-sized pelvis. Successive shifting from posterior to anterior asynclitism aids descent.

DESCENT. This movement is the first requisite for birth of the newborn. In nulliparas, engagement may take place before the onset of labor, and further descent may not follow until the onset of the second stage. In multiparous women, descent usually begins with engagement. Descent is brought about by one or more of four forces: (1) pressure of the amnionic fluid, (2) direct pressure of the fundus upon the breech with

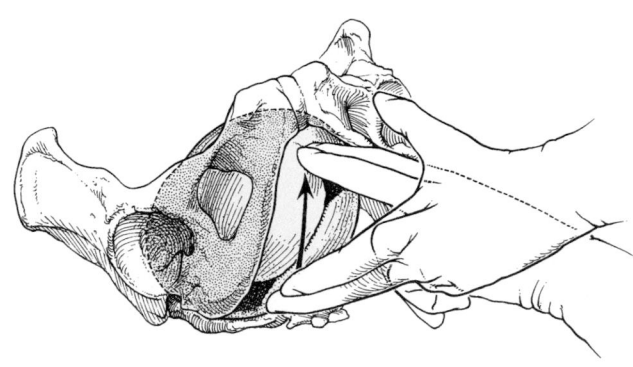

FIGURE 17–9. Locating the sagittal suture by vaginal examination.

contractions, (3) bearing down efforts of maternal abdominal muscles, and (4) extension and straightening of the fetal body.

FLEXION. As soon as the descending head meets resistance, whether from the cervix, walls of the pelvis, or pelvic floor, flexion of the head normally results. In this movement, the chin is brought into more intimate contact with the fetal thorax, and the appreciably shorter suboccipitobregmatic diameter is substituted for the longer occipitofrontal diameter (Figs. 17–13 and 17–14).

INTERNAL ROTATION. This movement consists of a turning of the head in such a manner that the occiput gradually moves toward the symphysis pubis anteriorly from its original position or, less commonly, posteriorly toward the hollow of the sacrum (Figs. 17–15 to 17–17). Internal rotation is essential for the completion of labor, except when the fetus is unusually small.

Calkins (1939) studied more than 5000 women in labor to the time of internal rotation. He concluded that in approximately two thirds, internal rotation is completed by the time the head reaches the pelvic floor; in about one fourth, internal rotation is completed very shortly after the head reaches the pelvic floor; and in about 5 percent, anterior rotation does not take place. When the head fails to turn until reaching the pelvic floor, it typically rotates during the next one or two contractions in multiparas. In nulliparas, rotation usually occurs during the next three to five contractions.

EXTENSION. After internal rotation, the sharply flexed head reaches the vulva and undergoes extension. If the sharply flexed head, on reaching the pelvic floor, did not extend but was driven farther downward, it would impinge on the posterior portion of the perineum and would eventually be forced through the tissues of the perineum. When the head presses upon the pelvic floor, however, two forces come into play. The first, exerted by the uterus, acts more posteriorly, and the second, supplied by the resistant pelvic floor and the symphysis, acts more anteriorly. The resultant vector is in the direction of the vulvar opening, thereby causing head extension. This brings the base of the occiput into direct contact with the inferior margin of the symphysis pubis (see Fig. 17–16).

With progressive distention of the perineum and vaginal opening, an increasingly larger portion of the occiput gradually appears. The head is born as the occiput, bregma, forehead, nose, mouth, and finally the chin pass successively over the anterior margin of the perineum (see Fig. 17–17). Immediately after its delivery, the head drops downward so that the chin lies over the maternal anal region.

EXTERNAL ROTATION. The delivered head next undergoes *restitution.* If the occiput was originally directed toward the left, it rotates toward the left ischial tuberosity; if it was originally directed toward the right, the occiput rotates to the right. Restitution of the head to the oblique position is followed by completion of external rotation to the transverse position, a movement that corresponds to rotation of the fetal body, serving to bring its bisacromial diameter into relation with the anteroposterior diameter of the pelvic outlet. Thus, one shoulder is anterior behind the symphysis and the other is posterior. This movement apparently is brought about by the same pelvic factors that produced internal rotation of the head.

EXPULSION. Almost immediately after external rotation, the anterior shoulder appears under the symphysis pubis, and the perineum soon becomes distended by the posterior shoulder. After delivery of the shoulders, the rest of the body quickly passes.

Occiput Posterior Position. In the great majority of labors in the occiput posterior positions, the mechanism of labor is identical to that observed in the transverse and anterior varieties, except that the occiput has to internally rotate to the symphysis pubis through 135 degrees, instead of 90 and 45 degrees, respectively (see Fig. 17–17).

With effective contractions, adequate flexion of the head, and a fetus of average size, the great majority of posteriorly positioned occiputs rotate promptly as soon as they reach the pelvic floor, and labor is not lengthened appreciably. In perhaps 5 to 10 percent of cases, however, rotation may be incomplete or may not take place at all, especially if the fetus is large (Gardberg and Tuppurainen, 1994b). Poor contractions, faulty flexion of the head, or epidural analgesia,

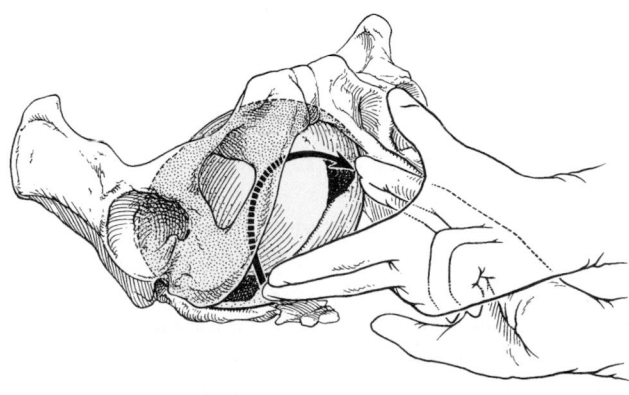

FIGURE 17–10. Differentiating the fontanels by vaginal examination.

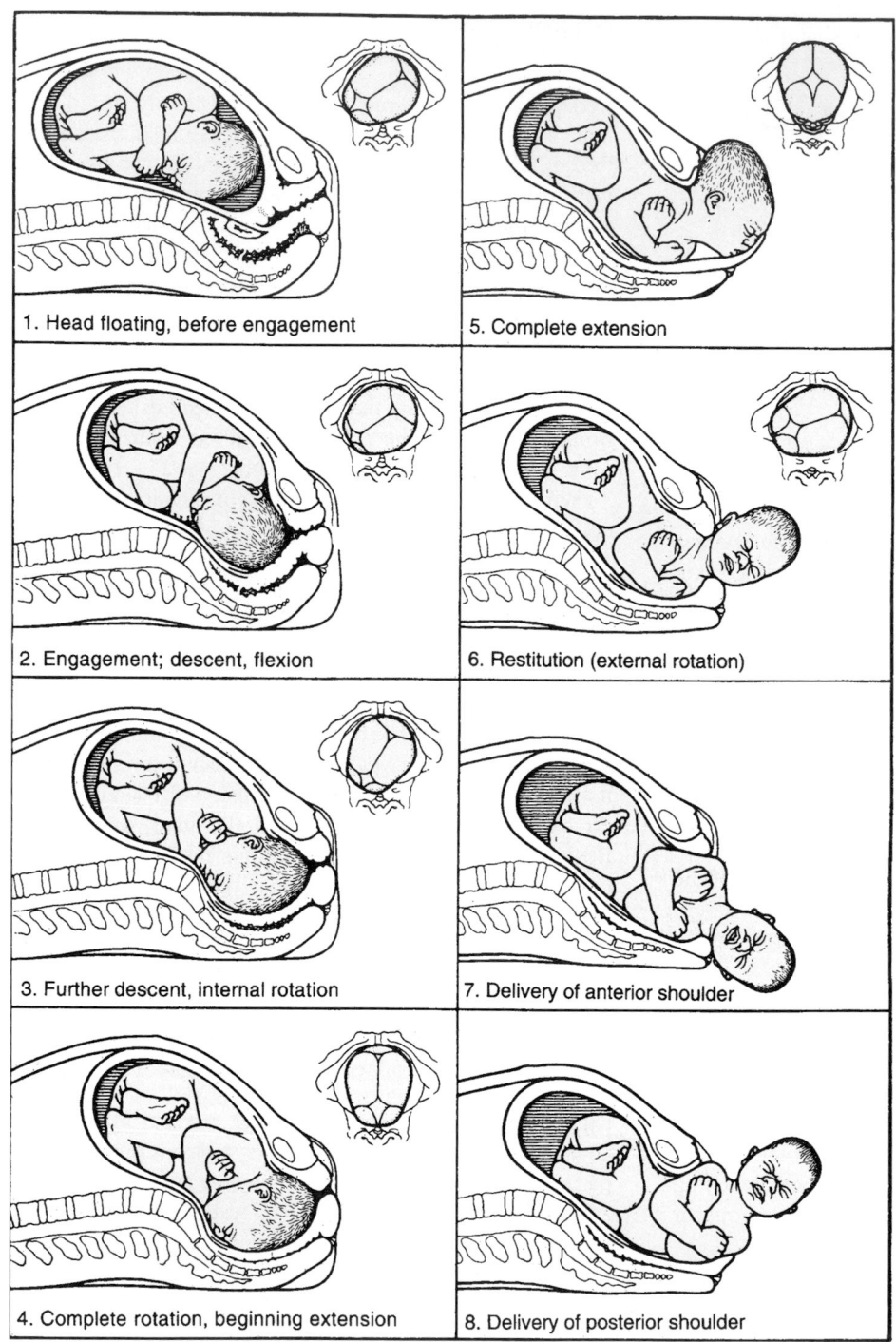

1. Head floating, before engagement

2. Engagement; descent, flexion

3. Further descent, internal rotation

4. Complete rotation, beginning extension

5. Complete extension

6. Restitution (external rotation)

7. Delivery of anterior shoulder

8. Delivery of posterior shoulder

FIGURE 17–11. Cardinal movements in the mechanisms of labor and delivery, left occiput anterior position.

which diminishes abdominal muscular pushing and relaxes the muscles of the pelvic floor, may predispose to incomplete rotation. If rotation is incomplete, transverse arrest results. If no rotation toward the symphysis takes place, the occiput may remain in the direct occiput posterior position, a condition known as *persistent occiput posterior.* Both persistent occiput posterior and transverse arrest represent deviations from the normal mechanisms of labor and are considered further in Chapter 20.

CHANGES IN SHAPE OF THE FETAL HEAD

Caput Succedaneum. In vertex presentations, the fetal head changes shape as the result of labor forces. In prolonged labors before complete cervical dilatation, the portion of the fetal scalp immediately over the cervical os becomes edematous, forming a swelling known as the *caput succedaneum* (Figs. 17–18 and 17–19). It usually attains a thickness of only a few millimeters, but in prolonged labors it may

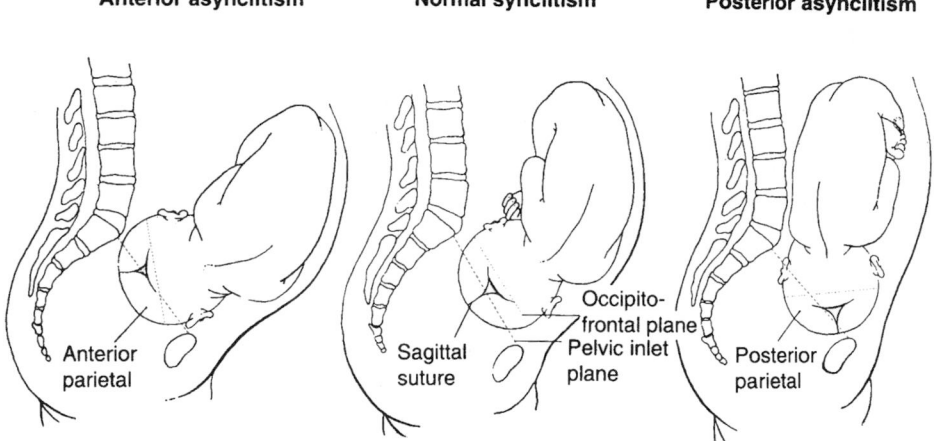

Anterior asynclitism   **Normal synclitism**   **Posterior asynclitism**

Anterior parietal

Sagittal suture

Occipito-frontal plane
Pelvic inlet plane

Posterior parietal

FIGURE 17–12. Synclitism and asynclitism.

be sufficiently extensive to prevent the differentiation of the various sutures and fontanels. More commonly the caput is formed when the head is in the lower portion of the birth canal and frequently only after the resistance of a rigid vaginal outlet is encountered. Because it develops over the most dependent area of the head, one may deduce the original fetal head position by noting the location of the caput succedaneum.

Molding. The change in fetal head shape from external compressive forces is referred to as *molding*. Possibly related to Braxton Hicks contractions, some molding develops before labor. Although taught in previous editions, most studies indicate that there is seldom overlapping of the parietal bones. A "locking" mechanism at the coronal and lambdoidal connections actually prevents such overlapping (Carlan and colleagues, 1991). Molding results in a shortened suboccipi-

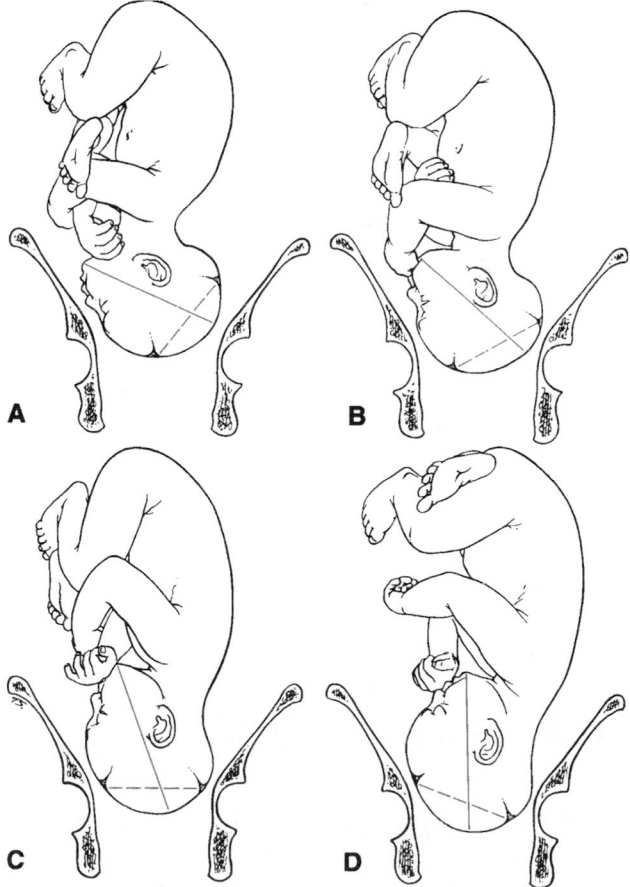

FIGURE 17–14. Four degrees of head flexion. The solid line represents the occipitomental diameter; the broken line connects the center of the anterior fontanel with the posterior fontanel: **(A)** flexion poor, **(B)** flexion moderate, **(C)** flexion advanced, **(D)** flexion complete. Note that with complete flexion, the chin is on the chest, and the suboccipitobregmatic diameter, the shortest anteroposterior diameter of the fetal head, is passing through the pelvic inlet.

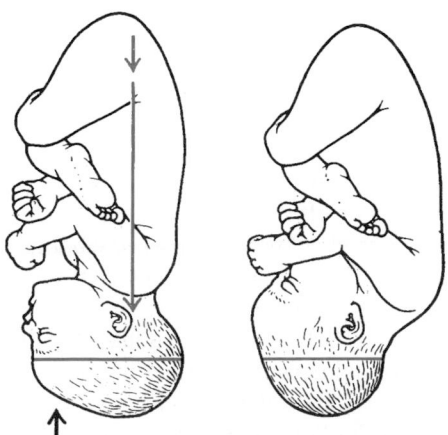

FIGURE 17–13. Lever action produces flexion of the head. Conversion from occipitofrontal to suboccipitobregmatic diameter typically reduces the anteroposterior diameter from nearly 12 to 9.5 cm.

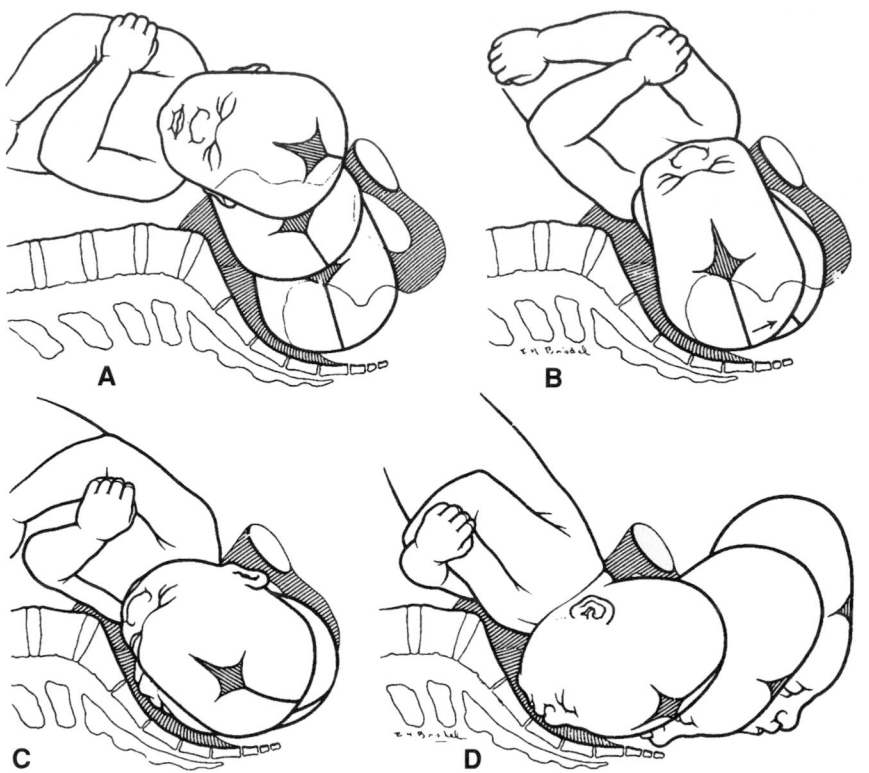

FIGURE 17–15. Mechanism of labor for the left occiput transverse position, lateral view. **A.** Engagement. **B.** Posterior asynclitism at the pelvic brim followed by lateral flexion, resulting in anterior asynclitism **C.** After engagement, further descent **D.** Rotation and extension.

tobregmatic diameter and a lengthened mentovertical diameter. These changes are of greatest importance in women with contracted pelves or asynclitic presentations. In these circumstances, the degree to which the head is capable of molding may make the difference between spontaneous vaginal delivery versus an operative delivery. Some older literature cited severe head molding as a cause for possible cerebral trauma. Because of the multitude of associated factors, for example, prolonged labor with fetal sepsis and acidosis, it is impossible to quantify the effects of molding with any alleged fetal or neonatal neurological sequelae.

CHARACTERISTICS OF NORMAL LABOR

The greatest impediment to understanding normal labor is recognizing its start. The strict definition of labor—*uterine contractions that bring about demonstrable effacement and dilatation of the cervix*—does not easily aid the clinician in determining when labor has actually begun, because this diagnosis is confirmed only retrospectively. Several methods may be used to define its start. One quantifies onset as the clock time when painful contractions become regular. Unfortunately, uterine activity that causes discomfort, but that does not represent true labor, may develop at any time during pregnancy. False labor often stops spontaneously, or it may proceed rapidly into effective contractions.

A second method defines the onset of labor as beginning at the time of admission to the labor unit. At the National Maternity Hospital in Dublin, efforts have been made to codify admission criteria (O'Driscoll and colleagues, 1984). These criteria at term require painful uterine contractions accompanied by any one of the following: (1) ruptured membranes, (2) bloody "show," (3) complete cervical effacement.

In the United States, admission for labor is frequently based on the extent of dilatation accompanied by painful contractions. When a woman presents with intact membranes, cervical dilatation of 3 to 4 cm or greater is presumed to be a

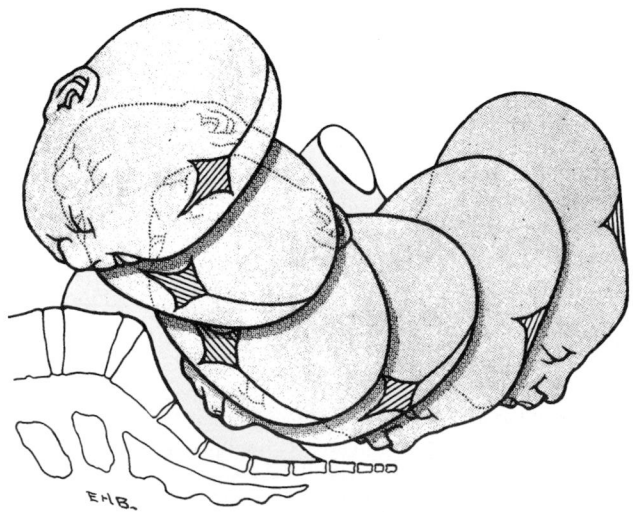

FIGURE 17–16. Mechanism of labor for left occiput anterior position.

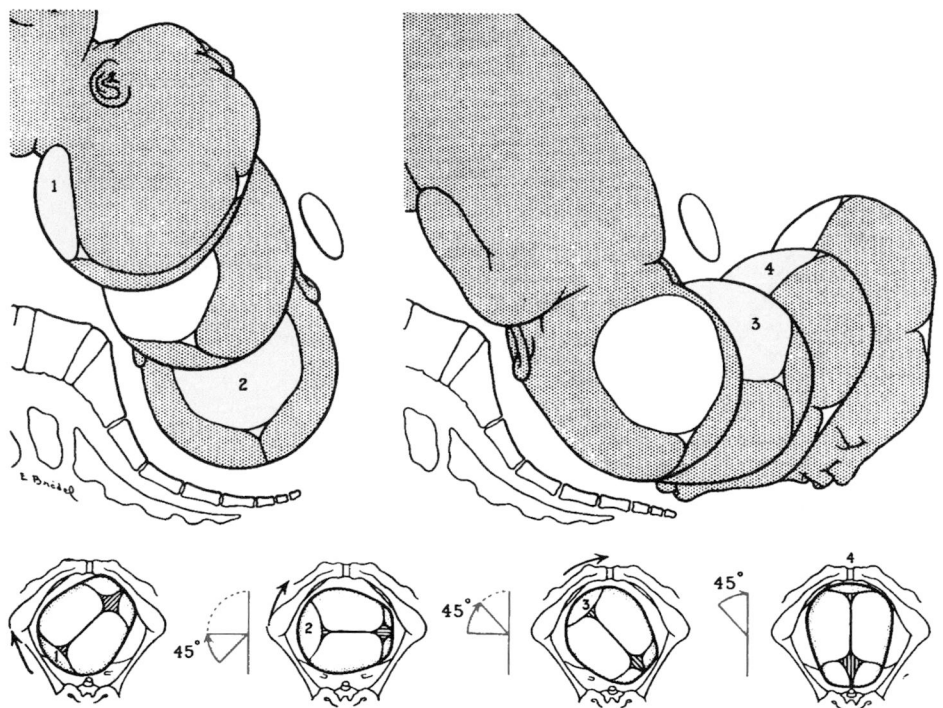

FIGURE 17–17. Mechanism of labor for right occiput posterior position, anterior rotation.

reasonably reliable threshold for the diagnosis of labor. In this case, onset of labor commences with the time of admission. This presumptive method obviates many of the uncertainties in diagnosing labor during earlier stages of cervical dilatation.

FIRST STAGE OF LABOR. Assuming that the diagnosis has been confirmed, then what are the expectations for the progress of normal labor? A scientific approach was begun by Friedman (1954), who described a characteristic sigmoid pattern for labor by graphing cervical dilatation against time. This graphic approach, based on statistical observations, changed labor management.

Friedman developed the concept of three functional divisions of labor to describe the physiological objectives

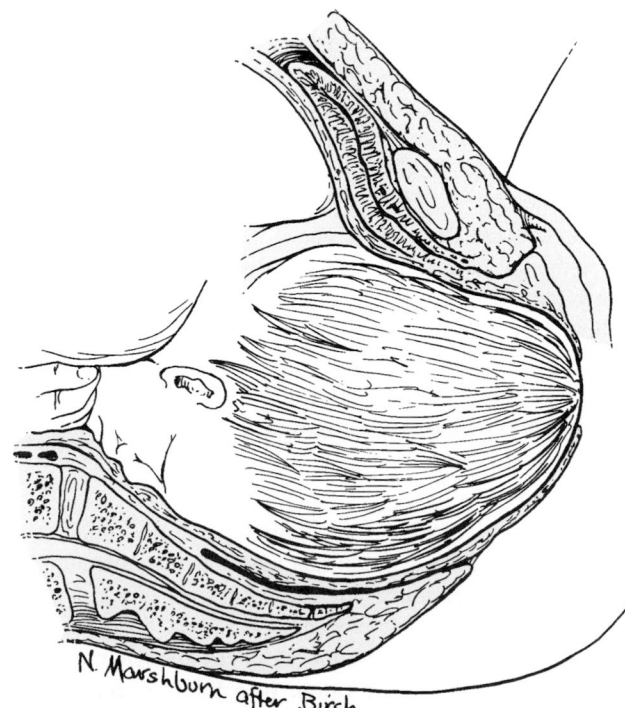

FIGURE 17–18. Formation of caput succedaneum.

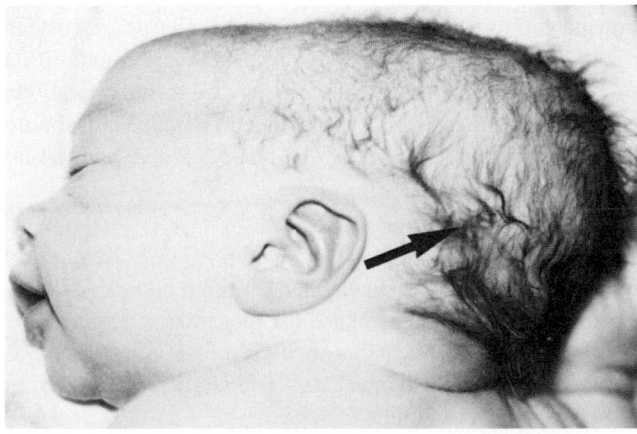

FIGURE 17–19. Considerable molding of the head and caput formation in a recently delivered newborn. The arrow is directed toward the caput succedaneum caused by appreciable scalp edema that overlies the occiput.

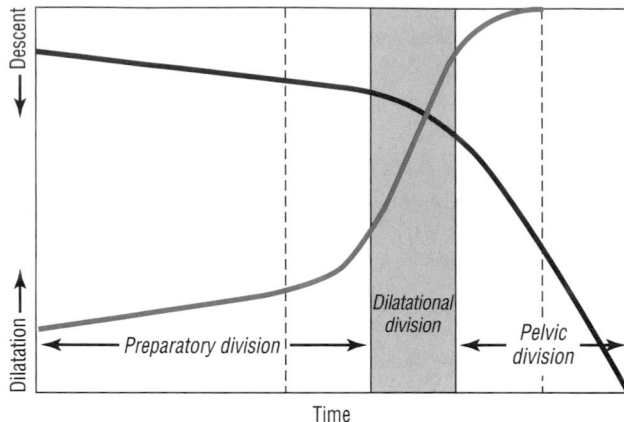

FIGURE 17–20. Labor course divided functionally on the basis of dilatation and descent curves into (1) a preparatory division, including latent and acceleration phases; (2) a dilatational division, occupying the phase of maximum slope of dilatation; and (3) a pelvic division, encompassing both deceleration phase and second stage concurrent with the phase of maximum slope of descent. (Illustration courtesy of Dr. L. Casey; redrawn from Friedman, 1978.)

of each division (Fig. 17–20). Although the cervix dilates little during the *preparatory division,* the connective tissue components of the cervix change considerably. Sedation and conduction analgesia are capable of arresting this division of labor. The *dilatational division,* during which time dilatation proceeds at its most rapid rate, is unaffected by sedation or conduction analgesia. The *pelvic division* commences with the deceleration phase of cervical dilatation. The classical mechanisms of labor that involve the cardinal fetal movements of the cephalic presentation—engagement, flexion, descent, internal rotation, extension, and external rotation—take place principally during the pelvic division. In actual practice, however, the onset of the pelvic division is seldom clearly identifiable.

As shown in Figure 17–20, the pattern of cervical dilatation during the preparatory and dilatational divisions of normal labor is a sigmoid curve. Two phases of cervical dilatation are defined. The *latent phase* corresponds to the preparatory division and the *active phase* to the dilatational division. Friedman subdivided the active phase into the *acceleration phase,* the *phase of maximum slope,* and the *deceleration phase* (Fig. 17–21).

Latent Phase. The onset of latent labor, as defined by Friedman (1972), is the point at which the mother perceives regular contractions. The latent phase for most women ends at between 3 and 5 cm of dilatation. This threshold may be clinically useful, for it defines cervical dilatation limits beyond which active labor can be expected.

Friedman and Sachtleben (1963) defined a *prolonged latent phase* as being greater than 20 hours in the nullipara and 14 hours in the multipara. These are the 95th percentiles. Factors that affect duration of the latent phase include

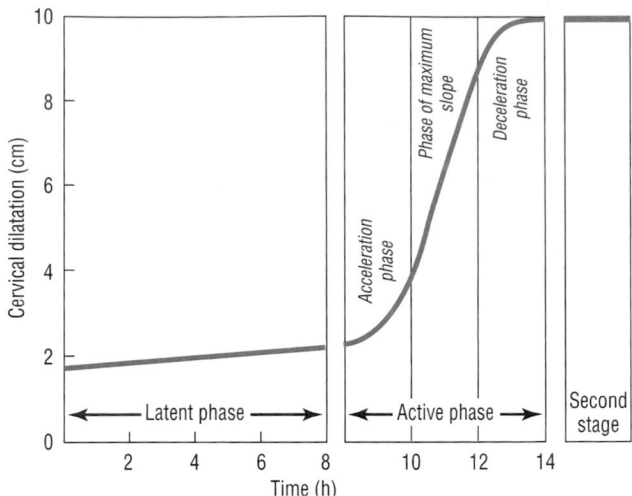

FIGURE 17–21. Composite of the average dilatation curve for nulliparous labor. The first stage is divided into a relatively flat latent phase and a rapidly progressive active phase. In the active phase, there are three identifiable component parts that include an acceleration phase, a linear phase of maximum slope, and a deceleration phase. (Illustration courtesy of Dr. L. Casey; redrawn from Friedman, 1978).

excessive sedation or epidural analgesia; unfavorable cervical condition, that is, thick, uneffaced, or undilated; and false labor. Following strong sedation, 85 percent of women progress to active labor. Another 10 percent cease contracting, and thus had false labor. Finally, 5 percent experience persistence of an abnormal latent phase and require oxytocin stimulation. Amniotomy was discouraged because of the 10 percent incidence of false labor. Sokol and colleagues (1977) reported a 3- to 4-percent incidence of prolonged latent phase, regardless of parity. Friedman (1972) reported that prolongation of the latent phase did not adversely influence fetal or maternal morbidity or mortality, but Chelmow and co-workers (1993) disputed the long-held belief that prolongation of the latent phase is benign.

This concept of a latent phase has great significance in understanding normal human labor because labor is considerably longer when a latent phase is included. To better illustrate this, Figure 17–22 shows eight labor curves from nulliparas in whom labor was diagnosed beginning with their admission, rather than with the onset of regular contractions. When labor is defined similarly, there is remarkable similarity of individual labor curves.

Active Labor. As shown in Figure 17–22, the progress of labor in nulliparous women has particular significance because these curves all reveal a rapid change in the slope of cervical dilatation rates between 3 and 5 cm. **Thus, cervical dilatation of 3 to 5 cm or more, in the presence of uterine contractions, can be taken to reliably represent the threshold for active labor.** Similarly, these curves provide useful guideposts for labor management.

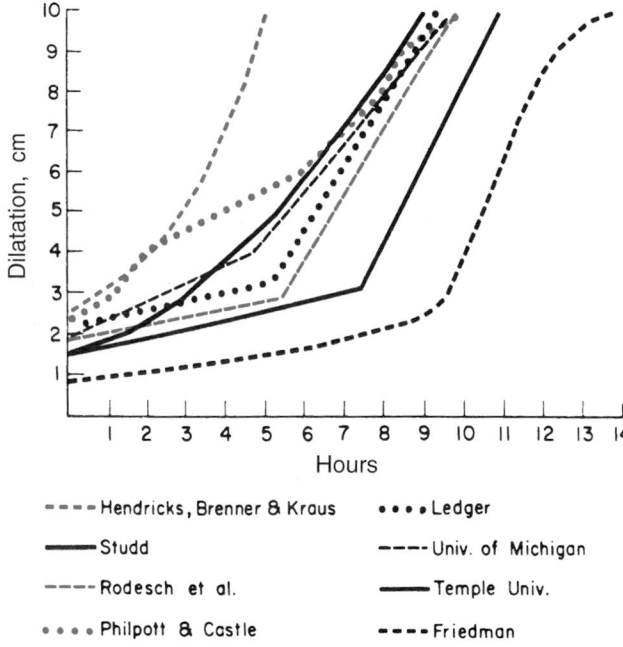

Hours

- - - - Hendricks, Brenner & Kraus   •••• Ledger

———— Studd   - - - - Univ. of Michigan

- - - - Rodesch et al.   ———— Temple Univ.

•••• Philpott & Castle   - - - - Friedman

FIGURE 17–22. Progress of labor in primigravid women from the time of admission. When the starting point on the abscissa begins with admission to the hospital, a latent phase is not observed.

Turning again to Friedman (1955), the mean duration of active-phase labor in nulliparas was 4.9 hours. The standard deviation of 3.4 hours is quite large. Hence, the active phase was reported to have a statistical maximum of 11.7 hours. Indeed, rates of cervical dilatation ranged from a minimum of 1.2 up to 6.8 cm/hr. Friedman (1972) also found that multiparas progress somewhat faster in active-phase labor, with a minimum normal rate of 1.5 cm/hr. His analysis of active-phase labor concomitantly describes rates of fetal descent and cervical dilatation (see Fig. 17–20). Descent begins in the later stage of active dilatation, commencing at about 7 to 8 cm in nulliparas and becoming most rapid after 8 cm.

Active-labor phase abnormalities are quite common. Sokol and co-workers (1977) reported that 25 percent of nulliparous labors were complicated by active-phase abnormalities, whereas 15 percent of multigravidas developed this problem.

Friedman (1972) subdivided active-phase problems into *protraction* and *arrest* disorders. He defined protraction as a *slow rate* of cervical dilatation or descent, which for nulliparas was less than 1.2 cm dilatation per hour or less than 1 cm descent per hour. For multiparas, protraction was defined as less than 1.5 cm dilatation per hour or less than 2 cm descent per hour. He defined arrest as a *complete cessation* of dilatation or descent. *Arrest of dilatation* was defined as 2 hours with no cervical change, and *arrest of descent* as 1 hour without fetal descent.

The prognosis for protraction and arrest disorders differed considerably. Friedman found that about 30 percent of women with protraction disorders had cephalopelvic disproportion,

compared with 45 percent of women in whom an arrest disorder developed. Abnormal labor patterns, diagnostic criteria, and treatment methods according to Cohen and Friedman (1983) are summarized in Table 20–3 (see p. 500).

Factors contributing to both protraction and arrest disorders were excessive sedation, vaginal analgesia, and fetal malposition. In both protraction and arrest disorders, Friedman recommended fetopelvic examination to diagnose cephalopelvic disproportion. Recommended therapy for protraction disorders was expectant management, whereas oxytocin was advised for arrest disorders in the absence of cephalopelvic disproportion.

Remarkably, of the 500 women studied, only 2 percent had cesarean deliveries. Hence, the great majority of active-phase disorders did not result in cesarean delivery. This fact must be kept in mind when considering the significance of various labor abnormalities described by Friedman.

Hendricks and co-workers (1970) challenged Friedman's conclusions about the course of normal human labor. Their principal differences included (1) absence of a latent phase, (2) no deceleration phase, (3) brevity of labor, (4) dilatation at similar rates for nulliparas and multiparas after 4 cm. They disputed the concept of a latent phase because they observed that the cervix dilated and effaced slowly during the 4 weeks preceding labor. According to them, the "latent phase" actually progressed over several weeks. These investigators did observe that labor was relatively rapid; specifically, the average time from admission to complete dilatation was 4.8 hours for nulliparas and 3.2 hours for multiparas.

There have been several reports in which investigators have reassessed Friedman's labor curves. Zhang and colleagues (2002) plotted detailed labor data from 1329 nulliparous women in spontaneous labor at term. The average labor curve differed markedly from the Friedman curve. The cervix dilated more slowly in the active phase, and it took 5.5 hours to progress from 4 cm to 10 cm compared with 2.5 hours in the Friedman curve. Alexander and colleagues (2002), in a study performed at Parkland Hospital, found that epidural analgesia lengthened the active phase of the Friedman labor curve by 1 hour. This increase was the result of a slightly slower but significant rate of cervical dilatation—1.4 cm/hr in women given epidural analgesia compared with 1.6 cm/hr in those without such analgesia. Gurewitsch and colleagues (2002, 2003) studied the labor and descent curves of women with greater and lesser parity. They concluded that poor progress from 4 to 6 cm should not be considered abnormal and that women with high parity should not be expected to progress faster than those with lower parity.

SECOND STAGE OF LABOR. This stage begins when cervical dilatation is complete and ends with fetal delivery. The median duration is about 50 minutes for nulliparas and about 20 minutes for multiparas, but it can be highly variable (Kilpatrick and Laros, 1989). In a woman of higher parity with a previously dilated vagina and perineum, two or three expulsive efforts after full cervical dilatation may suffice to complete delivery. Conversely, in a woman with a contracted pelvis or a large fetus or with impaired expulsive efforts from conduction analgesia or sedation, the second stage may become abnormally long. Abnormalities of the second stage of labor are described in Chapter 20 (see p. 498).

DURATION OF LABOR. Our understanding of the normal duration of human labor may be clouded by the many clinical variables that affect conduct of labor in modern obstetrical units. Kilpatrick and Laros (1989) reported that the mean length of first- and second-stage labor was approximately 9 hours in nulliparous women without regional analgesia, and that the 95th percentile upper limit was 18.5 hours. Corresponding times for multiparous women were a mean of about 6 hours with a 95th percentile maximum of 13.5 hours. These authors defined labor onset as the time when a woman recalled regular, painful contractions every 3 to 5 minutes that led to cervical change.

Spontaneous labor was analyzed in nearly 25,000 women delivered at term at Parkland Hospital in the early 1990s. Almost 80 percent of women were admitted with a cervical dilatation of 5 cm or less. Parity—nulliparous versus multiparous—and cervical dilatation at admission were significant determinants of the length of spontaneous labor. The median time from admission to spontaneous delivery for all parturients was 3.5 hours, and 95 percent of all women delivered within 10.1 hours. These results suggest that normal human labor is relatively short.

SUMMARY OF NORMAL LABOR. Labor is characterized by brevity and considerable biological variation. Active labor can be reliably diagnosed when cervical dilatation is 3 cm or more in the presence of uterine contractions. Once this cervical dilatation threshold is reached, normal progress to delivery can be expected, depending on parity, in the ensuing 4 to 6 hours. Anticipated progress during a 1- to 2-hour second stage is monitored to ensure fetal safety. Finally, most women in spontaneous labor, regardless of parity and if left unaided, will deliver within approximately 10 hours after admission for spontaneous labor. Insufficient uterine activity is a common and correctable cause of abnormal labor progress. **Therefore, when time breaches in normal labor boundaries are the only pregnancy complications, interventions other than cesarean delivery must be considered before resorting to this method of delivery for failure to progress.**

MANAGEMENT OF NORMAL LABOR AND DELIVERY

The ideal management of labor and delivery requires two potentially opposing viewpoints on the part of clinicians. First, birthing should be recognized as a normal physiological

TABLE 17–2 Recommended Nurse-to-Patient Ratios for Labor and Delivery

Nurse-to-Patient Ratio	Clinical Setting
1:2	Patients in labor
1:1	Patients in second-stage labor
1:1	Patients with medical or obstetrical complications
1:2	Oxytocin induction or augmentation of labor
1:1	Initiation of epidural analgesia
1:1	Circulation for cesarean delivery

From the American Academy of Pediatrics and the American College of Obstetricians and Gynecologists (2002), with permission.

process that most women experience without complications. Second, intrapartum complications, often arising quickly and unexpectedly, should be anticipated. Thus, clinicians must simultaneously make every woman and her supporters feel comfortable, yet ensure safety for the mother and newborn should complications suddenly develop. The American Academy of Pediatrics and the American College of Obstetricians and Gynecologists (2002) have collaborated in the development of *Guidelines for Perinatal Care*. These provide detailed information on the appropriate content of intrapartum care, including both personnel and facility requirements. Shown in Table 17–2 are the recommended nurse-to-patient ratios recommended for labor and delivery. Shown in Table 17–3 are the recommended room dimensions for these functions.

ADMISSION PROCEDURES. Pregnant women should be urged to report early in labor rather than to procrastinate until delivery is imminent for fear that they might be experiencing false labor. Early admittance to the labor and delivery unit is important, especially if during antepartum care the woman, her fetus, or both have been identified as being at risk.

Identification of Labor. Although the differential diagnosis between false and true labor is difficult at times, it usually can be made on the basis of the contractions, as follows:

TABLE 17–3 Recommended Minimum Room Dimensions for Labor and Delivery

Function	Net Floor Space (square feet)
Labor	100–160 per bed
LDR	256
Vaginal delivery	350
Cesarean delivery	400

LDR = labor, delivery, and recovery.
From the American Academy of Pediatrics and the American College of Obstetricians and Gynecologists (2002), with permission.

True Labor

- Contractions occur at regular intervals.
- Intervals gradually shorten.
- Intensity gradually increases.
- Discomfort is in the back and abdomen.
- Cervix dilates.
- Discomfort is not stopped by sedation.

False Labor

- Contractions occur at irregular intervals.
- Intervals remain long.
- Intensity remains unchanged.
- Discomfort is chiefly in the lower abdomen.
- Cervix does not dilate.
- Discomfort usually is relieved by sedation.

In those instances when a diagnosis of labor cannot be established with certainty, it is often wise to observe the woman for a longer period of time. The general condition of the mother and fetus should be ascertained accurately by history and physical examination, including blood pressure, temperature, and pulse. The frequency, duration, and intensity of the uterine contractions should be documented, and the time established when they first became uncomfortable. The degree of discomfort that the mother displays is noted. The heart rate, presentation, and size of the fetus should be determined and documented on admission (see Chap. 18, p. 445). Inquiries are made about the status of the fetal membranes and whether there has been any vaginal bleeding. Questions of whether fluid has leaked from the vagina and, if so, how much and when the leakage first commenced also are addressed.

Emergency Medical Treatment and Labor Act (EMTALA). In 1986, Congress enacted EMTALA to ensure public access to emergency services regardless of the ability to pay. All Medicare-participating hospitals with emergency services must provide an appropriate screening examination for any pregnant woman experiencing contractions who comes to the emergency department for evaluation. The most recent iteration of these regulations went into effect on November 10, 2003 (Federal Register, 2003).

The definition of an emergency condition makes specific reference to a pregnant woman who is having contractions. Labor is defined as ". . . the process of childbirth beginning with the latent phase of labor continuing through delivery of the placenta. A woman experiencing contractions is in true labor unless a physician certifies that after a reasonable time of observation the woman is in false labor." A woman in true labor is considered "unstable" for interhospital transfer purposes until the newborn and placenta are delivered. An unstable woman may, however, be transferred at the direction of the patient or when a physician certifies that the benefits of treatment at another facility outweigh the risks of transfer. Physicians and hospitals violating these federal requirements

are subject to civil penalties of up to $50,000 and termination from the Medicare program.

Preadmission and Admission Electronic Fetal Heart Rate Monitoring. As discussed in Chapter 18, electronic fetal heart rate monitoring is routinely used for high-risk pregnancies commencing at admission. Some investigators recommend monitoring women with low-risk pregnancies upon admission as a test of fetal well-being—the so-called *fetal admission test.* If no fetal rate abnormalities are detected, continuous electronic monitoring is replaced by intermittent assessment for the remainder of labor. We are of the view that electronic fetal heart rate monitoring is reasonable in the preadmission evaluation of women who subsequently are discharged. At Parkland Hospital, external electronic monitoring is performed for at least 1 hour before discharging women with false labor.

Home Births. A major emphasis of obstetrical care during the 20th century was the movement to birthing in hospitals rather than in homes. In 2002, 99 percent of 4,021,720 births in the United States took place in hospitals (Martin and colleagues, 2003). A total of 22,980 births were in homes, and the remainder primarily in birthing centers. The results of studies comparing neonatal and perinatal mortality associated with intended home deliveries and with that of hospital deliveries have been conflicting, with most suggesting an increased risk with home delivery. Pang and co-workers (2002) analyzed birth registry information from Washington State during 1989 through 1997 and found that newborns of planned home deliveries were at increased risk of neonatal death. Moreover, prolonged labor and postpartum bleeding were increased in women giving birth at home.

Vital Signs and Review of Pregnancy Record. The maternal blood pressure, temperature, pulse, and respiratory rate are checked for any abnormality, and these are recorded. The pregnancy record is promptly reviewed to identify complications. Any problems identified during the antepartum period and any that were anticipated should be displayed prominently in the pregnancy record.

Vaginal Examination. Most often, *unless there has been bleeding in excess of bloody show,* a vaginal examination is performed. The gloved index and second fingers are then introduced into the vagina (Fig. 17–23). It is important to avoid the anal region and not to withdraw the fingers from the vagina until the examination is completed. The number of vaginal examinations during labor does correlate with infectious morbidity, especially in cases of early membrane rupture.

Detection of Ruptured Membranes. A pregnant woman should be instructed during the antepartum period to be aware of leakage of fluid from the vagina and to report such an event

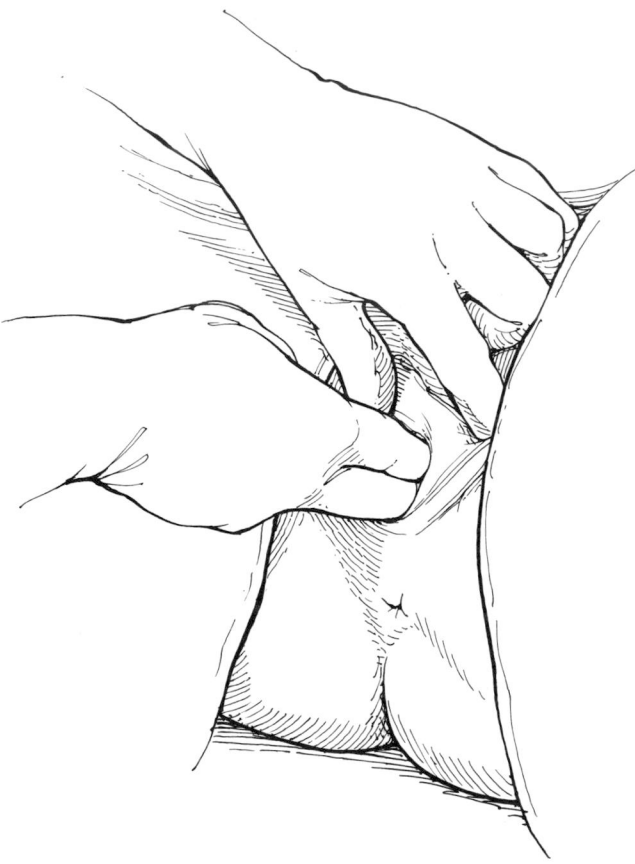

FIGURE 17–23. To perform vaginal examination, the labia have been separated with one hand and the first and second fingers of the other hand are carefully inserted into the introitus.

promptly. Rupture of the membranes is significant for three reasons. First, if the presenting part is not fixed in the pelvis, the possibility of umbilical cord prolapse and cord compression is greatly increased. Second, labor is likely to begin soon if the pregnancy is at or near term. Third, if delivery is delayed for 24 hours or more after membrane rupture, intrauterine infection is more likely.

Using sterile speculum examination, a conclusive diagnosis of rupture of the membranes is made when amnionic fluid is seen pooling in the posterior fornix or clear fluid is passing from the cervical canal (American College of Obstetricians and Gynecologists, 2000). Although several diagnostic tests for the detection of ruptured membranes have been recommended, none is completely reliable. If the diagnosis remains uncertain, another method involves testing the pH of the vaginal fluid. The pH of vaginal secretions normally ranges between 4.5 and 5.5, whereas that of amnionic fluid is usually 7.0 to 7.5. The use of the indicator *nitrazine* for the diagnosis of ruptured membranes is a simple and fairly reliable method. Test papers are impregnated with the dye, and the color of the reaction is interpreted by comparison with a standard color chart. A pH above 6.5 is consistent with ruptured membranes. False-positive test results may occur with coexistent blood,

semen, or bacterial vaginosis and false-negative test results when fluid for analysis is scant (American College of Obstetricians and Gynecologists, 2000).

Other tests have been used as markers for rupture of the membranes. Arborization or ferning of vaginal fluid suggests amnionic rather than cervical fluid. If present, amnionic fluid crystallizes to form a fernlike pattern due to the relative concentrations of sodium chloride, proteins, and carbohydrates in the fluid. Detection of alpha-fetoprotein in the vaginal vault has been used to identify amnionic fluid (Yamada and colleagues, 1998). Unequivocal identification comes from injection of various dyes, including Evans blue, methylene blue, indigo carmine, or fluorescein, into the amnionic sac via abdominal amniocentesis.

Cervical Effacement. The degree of cervical effacement usually is expressed in terms of the length of the cervical canal compared with that of an uneffaced cervix. When the length of the cervix is reduced by one half, it is 50-percent effaced. When the cervix becomes as thin as the adjacent lower uterine segment, it is completely, or 100-percent, effaced.

Cervical Dilatation. This measurement is determined by estimating the average diameter of the cervical opening by sweeping the examining finger from the margin of the cervical opening on one side to that of the opposite side. The diameter traversed is estimated in centimeters. The cervix is said to be dilated fully when the diameter measures 10 cm, because the presenting part of a term-size newborn usually can pass through a cervix this widely dilated.

Position of the Cervix. The relationship of the cervical os to the fetal head is categorized as posterior, midposition, or anterior.

Station. The level of the presenting fetal part in the birth canal is described in relationship to the ischial spines, which are halfway between the pelvic inlet and the pelvic outlet. When the lowermost portion of the presenting fetal part is at the level of the ischial spines, it is designated as being at zero (0) station. In the past, the long axis of the birth canal above the ischial spines was arbitrarily divided into thirds. In 1988, the American College of Obstetricians and Gynecologists began using a classification of station that divides the pelvis above and below the spines into fifths. These divisions represent centimeters above and below the spines. Thus, as the presenting fetal part descends from the inlet toward the ischial spines, the designation is −5, −4, −3, −2, −1, then 0 station. Below the ischial spines, the presenting fetal part passes +1, +2, +3, +4, and +5 stations to delivery. Station +5 cm corresponds to the fetal head being visible at the introitus.

If the leading part of the fetal head is at the 0 station or below, most often the fetal head has engaged; that is, the biparietal plane of the fetal head has passed through the pelvic inlet.

If the head is unusually molded, or if there is an extensive caput formation, or both, engagement might not have taken place even though the head appears to be at 0 station.

Laboratory Studies. When the woman is admitted in labor, most often the hematocrit or hemoglobin concentration should be rechecked. The hematocrit can be measured easily and quickly. At Parkland Hospital, blood is collected in a plain tube from which a heparinized capillary tube is filled immediately. By employing a small microhematocrit centrifuge in the labor and delivery unit, the value can be obtained in 3 minutes. A labeled tube of blood is allowed to clot and is kept available for blood type and screen, if needed, and another tube is used for routine serology. We obtain a urine specimen for protein analysis only in hypertensive women. In some labor units, a voided urine specimen, as free as possible of debris, is examined in all women for protein and glucose. Patients who have had no prenatal care should be considered to be at risk for syphilis, hepatitis B, and human immunodeficiency virus (HIV) (American Academy of Pediatrics and American College of Obstetricians and Gynecologists, 2002). In patients with no prior prenatal care, these laboratory studies, as well as a blood type and antibody screen, should be performed. Some states, for example Texas, now require routine testing for syphilis, hepatitis B, and HIV in all women admitted to labor and delivery units.

MANAGEMENT OF THE FIRST STAGE OF LABOR.

As soon as possible after admittance, the remainder of the general physical examination is completed. The physician can best reach a conclusion about the normalcy of the pregnancy when all examinations, including record and laboratory review, are completed. A rational plan for monitoring labor then can be established based on the needs of the fetus and the mother. If no abnormality is identified or suspected, the mother should be reassured. Because there are marked individual variations in lengths of labor, any precise statement as to its anticipated duration is unwise.

Monitoring Fetal Well-Being During Labor. This subject is discussed in detail in Chapter 18. Briefly, the American Academy of Pediatrics and American College of Obstetricians and Gynecologists (2002) recommend that during the first stage of labor, in the absence of any abnormalities, the fetal heart rate should be checked immediately after a contraction at least every 30 minutes and then every 15 minutes during the second stage. If continuous electronic monitoring is used, the tracing is evaluated at least every 30 minutes during the first stage and at least every 15 minutes during second-stage labor. For women with pregnancies at risk, auscultation is performed at least every 15 minutes during the first stage of labor and every 5 minutes during the second stage. Continuous electronic monitoring may be used with evaluation of the tracing every 15 minutes during the first stage of labor, and every 5 minutes during the second stage.

Uterine Contractions. Although usually assessed by electronic monitoring (see Chap. 18, p. 466), contractions can be both quantitatively and qualitatively evaluated manually. With the palm of the hand resting lightly on the uterus, the examiner determines the time of onset of the contraction. The intensity of the contraction is gauged from the degree of firmness the uterus achieves. At the acme of effective contractions, the finger or thumb cannot readily indent the uterus—a "firm" contraction. Next, the time that the contraction disappears is noted. This sequence is repeated in order to evaluate the frequency, duration, and intensity of uterine contractions.

Maternal Vital Signs. Maternal temperature, pulse, and blood pressure are evaluated at least every 4 hours. If fetal membranes have been ruptured for many hours before the onset of labor, or if there is a borderline temperature elevation, the temperature is checked hourly. Moreover, with prolonged membrane rupture, defined as greater than 18 hours, antimicrobial administration for prevention of group B streptococcal infections is recommended. This is discussed in Chapter 58 (see p. 1285).

Subsequent Vaginal Examinations. During the first stage of labor, the need for subsequent vaginal examinations to identify the status of the cervix and the station and position of the presenting part will vary considerably. When the membranes rupture, an examination should be performed expeditiously if the fetal head was not definitely engaged at the previous vaginal examination. The fetal heart rate should be checked immediately and during the next uterine contraction to help detect occult umbilical cord compression. At Parkland Hospital, periodic pelvic examinations are typically performed at 2- to 3-hour intervals to evaluate the progress of labor (see p. 439).

Oral Intake. Food should be withheld during active labor and delivery. Gastric emptying time is remarkably prolonged once labor is established and analgesics are administered. As a consequence, ingested food and most medications remain in the stomach and are not absorbed, instead, they may be vomited and aspirated (see Chap. 19, p. 490). According to the American Academy of Pediatrics and the American College of Obstetricians and Gynecologists (2002), sips of clear liquids, occasional ice chips, and lip moisturizers are permitted.

Intravenous Fluids. Although it has become customary in many hospitals to establish an intravenous infusion system routinely early in labor, there is seldom any real need for such in the normal pregnant woman at least until analgesia is administered. An intravenous infusion system is advantageous during the immediate puerperium to administer oxytocin prophylactically and at times therapeutically when uterine atony persists. Moreover, with longer labors, the administration of glucose, sodium, and water to the otherwise fasting woman at the rate of 60 to 120 mL/hr prevents dehydration and acidosis.

Garite and colleagues (2000) randomly assigned 195 women in labor to receive either 125 or 250 mL/hr of lactated Ringer or isotonic sodium chloride solution. The mean volume of total intravenous fluid was 2008 mL in the 125 mL/hr group and 2487 mL in the 250 mL/hr group. Labor lasted more than 12 hours in significantly more (26 versus 13 percent) of the women given a 125 mL/hr infusion compared with those given 250 mL/hr.

Maternal Position During Labor. The normal laboring woman need not be confined to bed early in labor. A comfortable chair may be beneficial psychologically and perhaps physiologically. In bed, the laboring woman should be allowed to assume the position she finds most comfortable, which will be lateral recumbency most of the time. She must not be restricted to lying supine. Bloom and colleagues (1998) conducted a randomized trial of walking during labor in more than 1000 women with low-risk pregnancies. They found that walking neither enhanced nor impaired active labor and that it was not harmful.

Analgesia. This topic is discussed in detail in Chapter 19. In general, pain relief should depend on the needs and desires of the woman. The American College of Obstetricians and Gynecologists (2001) has specified optimal goals for anesthesia care in obstetrics.

Amniotomy. If the membranes are intact, there is a great temptation even during normal labor to perform amniotomy. The presumed benefits are more rapid labor, earlier detection of meconium-stained amnionic fluid, and the opportunity to apply an electrode to the fetus or insert a pressure catheter into the uterine cavity. The advantages and disadvantages of amniotomy are discussed in Chapter 22 (see p. 542). Importantly, the fetal head must be well applied to the cervix and not be dislodged from the pelvis during the procedure to avert umbilical cord prolapse.

Urinary Bladder Function. Bladder distention should be avoided, because it can hinder descent of the fetal presenting part and lead to subsequent bladder hypotonia and infection. During each abdominal examination, the suprapubic region should be inspected and palpated to detect distention. If the bladder is readily seen or palpated above the symphysis, the woman should be encouraged to void. At times she can ambulate with assistance to a toilet and successfully void, even though she could not void on a bedpan. If the bladder is distended and she cannot void, catheterization is indicated. Carley and colleagues (2002) found that 51 of 11,332 vaginal deliveries (1 in 200) were complicated by urinary retention. Risk factors included operative vaginal delivery and regional analgesia. Most women resumed normal voiding before discharge from the hospital.

MANAGEMENT OF THE SECOND STAGE OF LA-BOR. With full dilatation of the cervix, which signifies the onset of the second stage of labor, a woman typically begins to bear down, and with descent of the presenting part she develops the urge to defecate. Uterine contractions and the accompanying expulsive forces may last $1\frac{1}{2}$ minutes and recur at an interval no longer than 1 minute. As discussed on page 423, the median duration of the second stage is 50 minutes in nulliparas and 20 minutes in multiparas, but this interval can be highly variable. Monitoring of the fetal heart rate is discussed on page 427, and interpretation of second-stage electronic fetal heart rate patterns is discussed in Chapter 18 (see p. 446).

Maternal Expulsive Efforts. In most cases, bearing down is reflexive and spontaneous during second-stage labor, but occasionally a woman may not employ her expulsive forces to good advantage and coaching is desirable. Her legs should be half-flexed so that she can push with them against the mattress. Instructions should be to take a deep breath as soon as the next uterine contraction begins, and with her breath held, to exert downward pressure exactly as though she were straining at stool. She should not be encouraged to "push" beyond the time of completion of each uterine contraction. Instead, she and her fetus should be allowed to rest and recover.

During this period of active bearing down, the fetal heart rate auscultated immediately after the contraction is likely to be slow, but should recover to normal range before the next expulsive effort. Gardosi and associates (1989) have recommended a squatting or semisquatting position using a specialized pillow. They claim that this shortens second-stage labor by increasing expulsive forces and by increasing the diameter of the pelvic outlet. Eason and colleagues (2000) performed an extensive review of positions and their effect on the incidence of perineal trauma. They found that the supported upright position had no advantages over the recumbent one.

As the head descends through the pelvis, feces frequently are expelled by the woman. With further descent, the perineum begins to bulge and the overlying skin becomes stretched. Now the scalp of the fetus may be visible through the vulvar opening. At this time, the woman and her fetus are prepared for delivery.

The benefits, or lack thereof, for coached pushing during the second stage of labor are discussed in Chapter 20 (see p. 500).

Preparation for Delivery. Delivery can be accomplished with the mother in a variety of positions. The most widely used and often the most satisfactory one is the dorsal lithotomy position. At Parkland Hospital the lithotomy position is not mandated for normal deliveries. In many birthing rooms delivery is accomplished with the woman lying flat on the bed.

For better exposure, leg holders or stirrups are used. In placing the legs in leg holders, care should be taken not to separate the legs too widely or place one leg higher than the other, as this will exert pulling forces on the perineum that might easily result in the extension of a spontaneous tear or an episiotomy into a fourth-degree laceration. The popliteal region should rest comfortably in the proximal portion and the heel in the distal portion of the leg holder. The legs are not strapped into the stirrups, thereby allowing quick flexion of the thighs backward onto the abdomen should shoulder dystocia develop. The legs may cramp during the second stage, in part, because of pressure by the fetal head on nerves in the pelvis. Such cramps may be relieved by changing the position of the leg or by brief massage, but leg cramps should never be ignored.

Preparation for delivery should include vulvar and perineal cleansing. If desired, sterile drapes may be placed in such a way that only the immediate area about the vulva is exposed. In the past, the major reason for care in scrubbing, gowning, and gloving was to protect the laboring woman from the introduction of infectious agents. Although these considerations remain valid, concern today also must be extended to the health care providers, because of the exposure threat to HIV.

SPONTANEOUS DELIVERY

Delivery of the Head. With each contraction, the perineum bulges increasingly, and the vulvovaginal opening becomes more dilated by the fetal head (Fig. 17–24), gradually forming

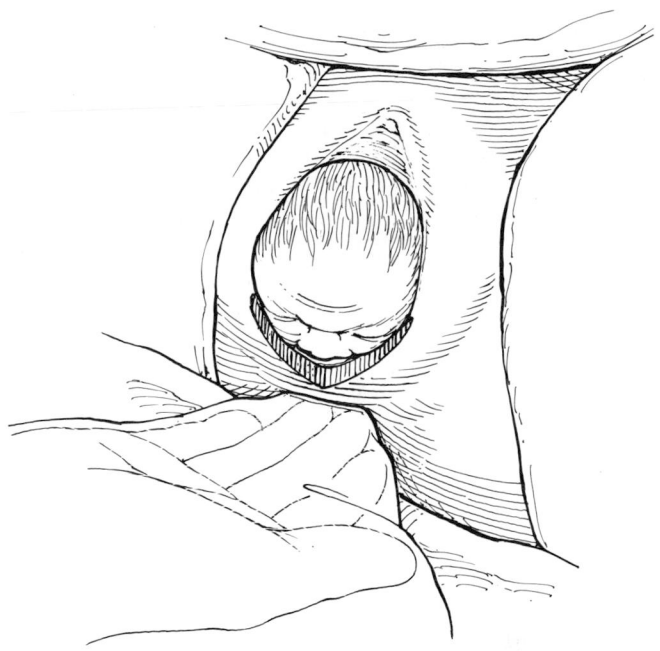

FIGURE 17–25. Delivery of the head. The occiput is being kept close to the symphysis by moderate pressure to the fetal chin at the tip of the maternal coccyx.

an ovoid and finally an almost circular opening (Fig. 17–25). This encirclement of the largest head diameter by the vulvar ring is known as *crowning.*

Unless an episiotomy has been made, as described later in the chapter, the perineum thins and, especially in nulliparous women, may undergo spontaneous laceration. The anus becomes greatly stretched and protuberant, and the anterior wall of the rectum may be easily seen through it. Considerable controversy exists concerning whether an episiotomy should be cut. We advocate individualization and do not routinely cut an episiotomy. It is now clear that an episiotomy will increase the risk of a tear into the external anal sphincter or the rectum, or both. Conversely, anterior tears involving the urethra and labia are much more common in women in whom an episiotomy is not cut. This issue is discussed in detail on page 435.

RITGEN MANEUVER. When the head distends the vulva and perineum enough to open the vaginal introitus to a diameter of 5 cm or more, a towel-draped, gloved hand may be used to exert forward pressure on the chin of the fetus through the perineum just in front of the coccyx. Concurrently, the other hand exerts pressure superiorly against the occiput (Fig. 17–26). Although this maneuver is simpler than that originally described by Ritgen (1855), it is customarily designated the *Ritgen maneuver,* or the *modified Ritgen maneuver.*

This maneuver allows controlled delivery of the head (Fig. 17–27). It also favors extension, so that the head is delivered with its smallest diameters passing through the introitus and

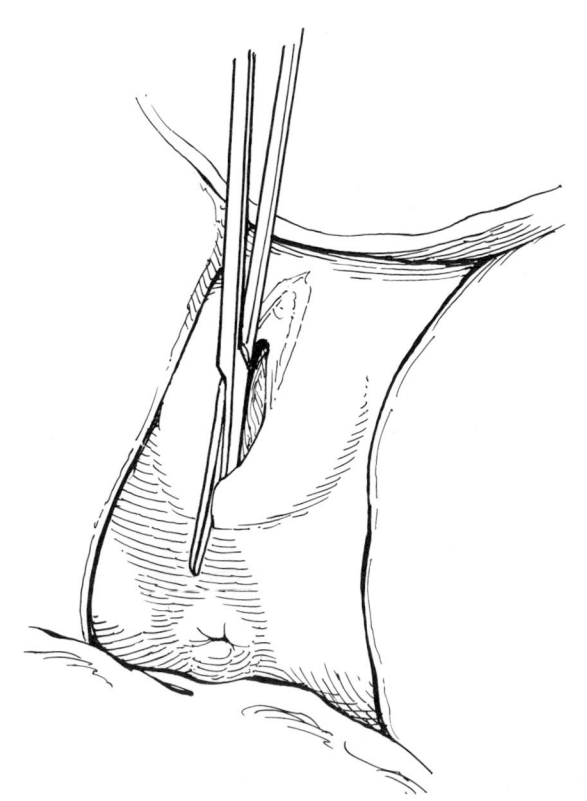

FIGURE 17–24. Vulva partially distended by the fetal head. Midline episiotomy being made.

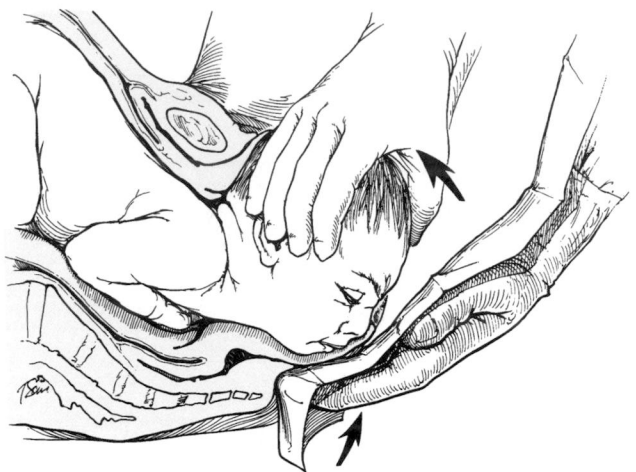

FIGURE 17–26. Near completion of the delivery of the fetal head by the modified Ritgen maneuver. Moderate upward pressure is applied to the fetal chin by the posterior hand covered with a sterile towel while the suboccipital region of the fetal head is held against the symphysis.

over the perineum. Mayerhofer and colleagues (2002) have challenged the use of the Ritgen maneuver on the grounds that this procedure was associated with more third-degree perineal lacerations and more frequent use of episiotomy. They preferred the "hands-poised" method, in which the attendant did not touch the perineum during delivery of the head. This method had similar associated laceration rates and neonatal

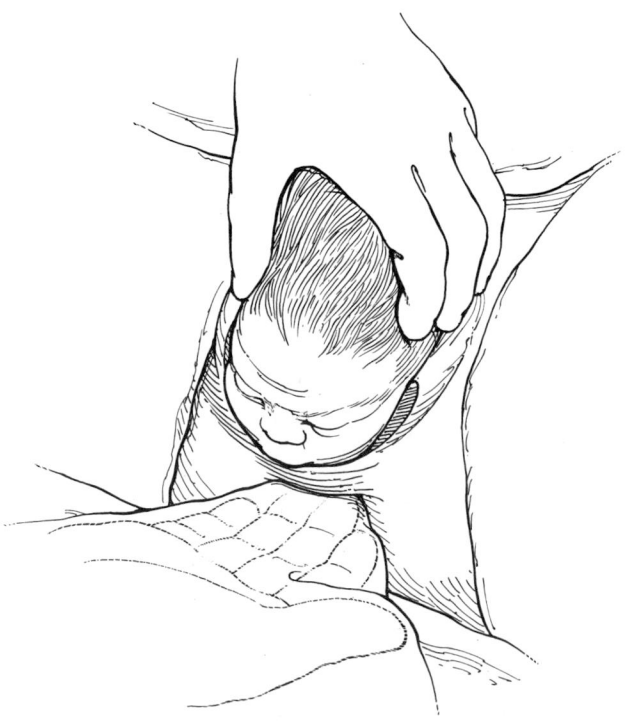

FIGURE 17–27. Delivery of the head; the mouth appears over the perineum.

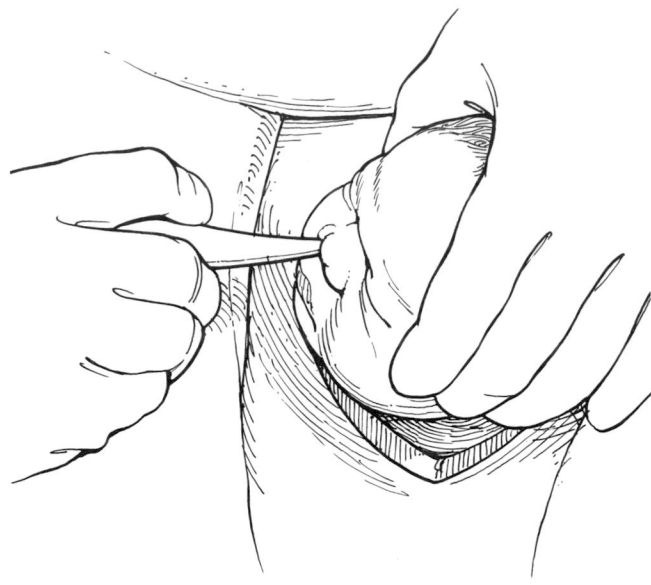

FIGURE 17–28. Aspirating the nose and mouth immediately after delivery of the head.

outcomes as the modified Ritgen maneuver, but with a lower incidence of third-degree tears.

Delivery of the Shoulders. After its delivery, the fetal head falls posteriorly, bringing the face almost into contact with the maternal anus. As described on page 417, the occiput promptly turns toward one of the maternal thighs and the head assumes a transverse position (Fig. 17–28). This movement of restitution (external rotation) indicates that the bisacromial diameter (transverse diameter of the thorax) has rotated into the anteroposterior diameter of the pelvis.

Most often, the shoulders appear at the vulva just after external rotation and are born spontaneously. If delayed, immediate extraction may appear advisable. The sides of the head are grasped with two hands, and gentle downward traction is applied until the anterior shoulder appears under the pubic arch (Fig. 17–29). Some practitioners prefer to deliver the anterior shoulder prior to suctioning the nasopharynx or checking for a nuchal cord to avoid shoulder dystocia. Next, by an upward movement, the posterior shoulder is delivered (see Fig. 17–29).

The rest of the body almost always follows the shoulders without difficulty; but with prolonged delay, its birth may be hastened by moderate traction on the head and moderate pressure on the uterine fundus. Hooking the fingers in the axillae should be avoided because this may injure the nerves of the upper extremity, producing a transient or possibly even a permanent paralysis. Traction, furthermore, should be exerted only in the direction of the long axis of the neonate, for if applied obliquely it causes bending of the neck and excessive stretching of the brachial plexus.

Immediately after delivery of the newborn, there is usually a gush of amnionic fluid, often tinged with blood but not grossly bloody.

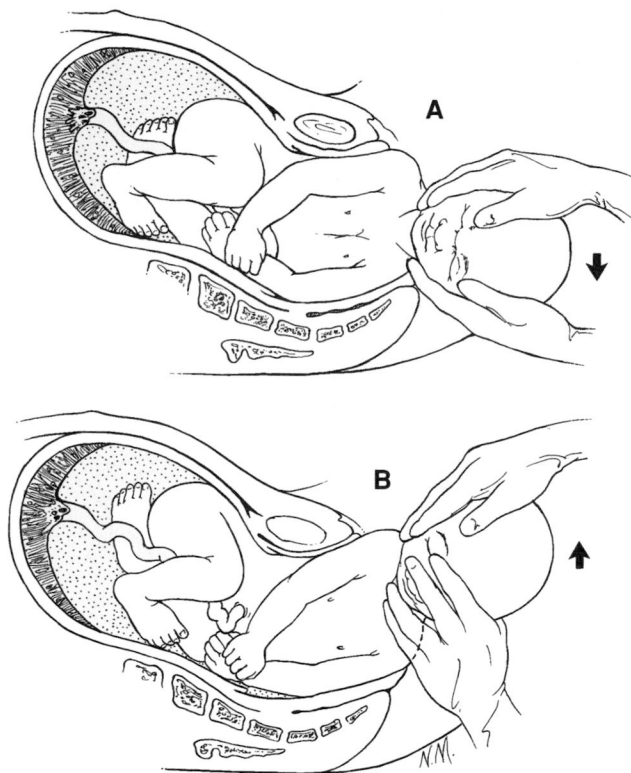

FIGURE 17–29. A. Gentle downward traction to effect descent of the anterior shoulder. **B.** Delivery of the anterior shoulder completed; gentle upward traction to deliver the posterior shoulder.

Clearing the Nasopharynx. To minimize aspiration of amnionic fluid, particulate matter, and blood once the thorax is delivered and the newborn can inspire, the face is quickly wiped and the nares and mouth are aspirated, as demonstrated in Figure 17–28.

Nuchal Cord. Following delivery of the anterior shoulder, a finger should be passed to the fetal neck to determine whether it is encircled by one or more coils of the umbilical cord (Fig. 17–30). Nuchal cords are found in about 25 percent of deliveries and ordinarily do no harm. If a coil of umbilical cord is felt, it should be slipped over the head if loose enough. If applied too tightly, the loop should be cut between two clamps and the neonate promptly delivered.

Clamping the Cord. The umbilical cord is cut between two clamps placed 4 to 5 cm from the fetal abdomen, and later an umbilical cord clamp is applied 2 to 3 cm from the fetal abdomen. A plastic clamp (Double Grip Umbilical Clamp, Hollister) that is safe, efficient, and fairly inexpensive is used at Parkland Hospital.

TIMING OF CORD CLAMPING. If after delivery, the newborn is placed at or below the level of the vaginal introitus for 3 minutes and the fetoplacental circulation is not immediately occluded by clamping the cord, an average of 80 mL of blood

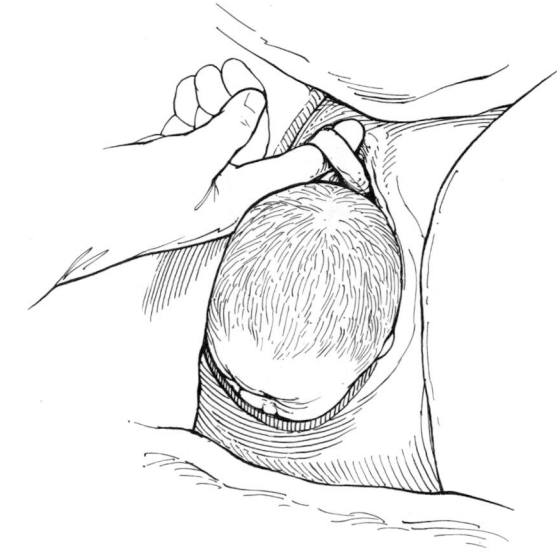

FIGURE 17–30. Cord identified around the neck. It readily slipped over the head.

may be shifted from the placenta to the neonate (Yao and Lind, 1974). This provides about 50 mg of iron, which reduces the frequency of iron deficiency anemia later in infancy.

Accelerated destruction of erythrocytes, as found with maternal alloimmunization, forms additional bilirubin from the added erythrocytes and contributes further to the danger of hyperbilirubinemia (see Chap. 29, p. 667). Although the theoretical risk of circulatory overloading from gross hypervolemia is formidable, especially in preterm and growth-retarded neonates, the addition of placental blood to the otherwise normal newborn's circulation ordinarily docs not cause difficulty.

Our policy is to clamp the cord after first thoroughly clearing the airway, all of which usually requires about 30 seconds. The newborn is not elevated above the introitus at vaginal delivery or much above the maternal abdominal wall at the time of cesarean delivery.

MANAGEMENT OF THE THIRD STAGE OF LABOR. Immediately after delivery of the newborn, the size of the uterine fundus and its consistency are examined. If the uterus remains firm and there is no unusual bleeding, watchful waiting until the placenta separates is the usual practice. Massage is not employed, but the fundus is frequently palpated to make certain that the organ does not become atonic and filled with blood from placental separation.

Signs of Placental Separation. Because attempts to express the placenta prior to its separation are futile and possibly dangerous, the clinician should be alert to the following signs of placental separation:

1. The uterus becomes globular and, as a rule, firmer. This sign is the earliest to appear.

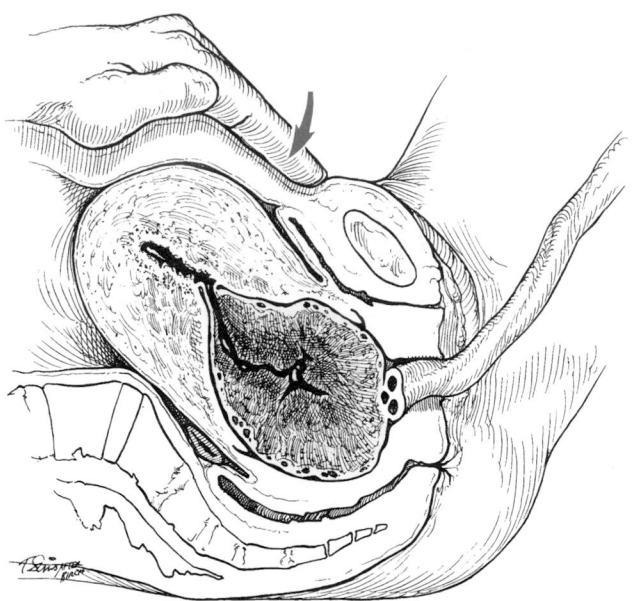

FIGURE 17–31. Expression of placenta. Note that the hand is *not* trying to push the fundus of the uterus through the birth canal! As the placenta leaves the uterus and enters the vagina, the uterus is elevated by the hand on the abdomen (*arrow*) while the cord is held in position. The mother can aid in the delivery of the placenta by bearing down. As the placenta reaches the perineum, the cord is lifted, which in turn, lifts the placenta out of the vagina. Adherent membranes are teased free so as to prevent their being torn off and retained in the birth canal.

2. There is often a sudden gush of blood.
3. The uterus rises in the abdomen because the placenta, having separated, passes down into the lower uterine segment and vagina, where its bulk pushes the uterus upward.
4. The umbilical cord protrudes farther out of the vagina, indicating that the placenta has descended.

These signs sometimes appear within about 1 minute after delivery of the newborn and usually within 5 minutes. When the placenta has separated, it should be determined that the uterus is firmly contracted. The mother may be asked to bear down, and the intra-abdominal pressure may be adequate to expel the placenta. If these efforts fail, or if spontaneous expulsion is not possible because of anesthesia, then after ensuring that the uterus is contracted firmly, pressure is exerted with the hand on the fundus to propel the detached placenta into the vagina, as depicted and described in Figure 17–31. This approach has been termed *physiological management,* as later contrasted with *active management* of the third stage (Thilaganathan and colleagues, 1993).

Delivery of the Placenta. Expression should never be forced before placental separation lest the uterus be turned inside out. **Traction on the umbilical cord must not be used to pull the placenta out of the uterus.** *Inversion* of the uterus is one of the grave complications associated with delivery (see Chap. 35, p. 833). As downward pressure toward the

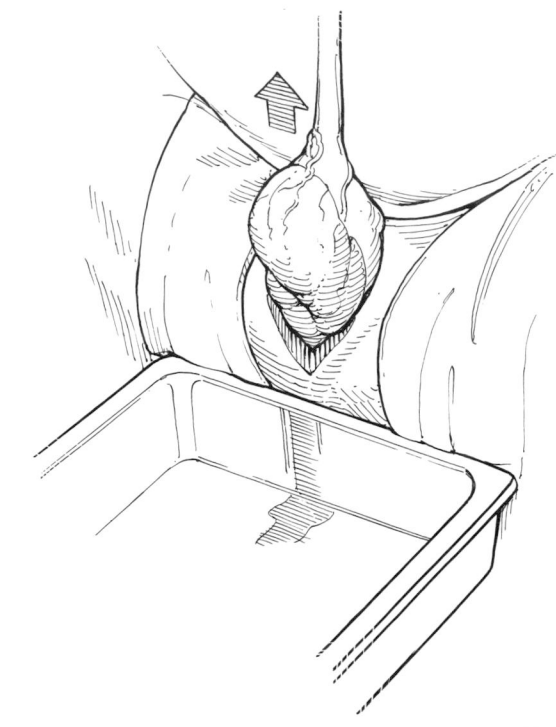

FIGURE 17–32. The placenta is removed from the vagina by lifting the cord.

vagina is applied to the body of the uterus, the umbilical cord is kept slightly taut (see Fig. 17–31). The uterus is then lifted cephalad with the abdominal hand. This maneuver is repeated until the placenta reaches the introitus (Prendiville and associates, 1988b). As the placenta passes through the introitus, pressure on the uterus is stopped. The placenta is then gently lifted away from the introitus (Fig. 17–32). Care is taken to prevent the membranes from being torn off and left behind. If the membranes start to tear, they are grasped with a clamp and removed by gentle teasing (Fig. 17–33). The maternal surface of the placenta should be examined carefully to ensure that no placental fragments are left in the uterus.

MANUAL REMOVAL OF PLACENTA. Occasionally, the placenta will not separate promptly. This is especially common in cases of preterm delivery (Dombrowski and colleagues, 1995). If there is brisk bleeding and the placenta cannot be delivered by the above technique, manual removal of the placenta is indicated, using the safeguards described in Chapter 35. It is unclear as to the length of time that should elapse in the absence of bleeding before the placenta is manually removed. Manual removal of the placenta is practiced sooner and more often than in the past. Some obstetricians practice routine manual removal of any placenta that has not separated spontaneously by the time they have completed delivery of the newborn and care of the cord in women with conduction analgesia. Proof of the benefits of this practice, however, has not been established, and most obstetricians await spontaneous

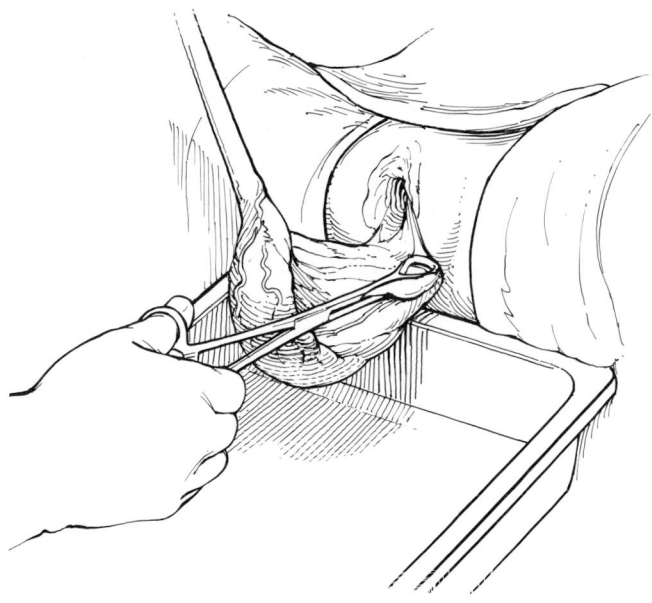

FIGURE 17–33. Membranes that were somewhat adherent to the uterine lining are separated by gentle traction with a ring forceps.

placental separation unless bleeding is excessive. The American College of Obstetricians and Gynecologists (2003b) has concluded that there are no data to either support or refute the use of prophylactic antimicrobials when manual removal of the placenta is performed.

Active Management of the Third Stage. Thilaganathan and associates (1993) compared a regimen of active management with syntometrine (5 units of oxytocin with 0.5 mg of ergometrine) and controlled cord traction with one of physiological management wherein the cord was not clamped and the placenta was delivered by maternal efforts. Among 103 low-risk term deliveries, active management resulted in a reduction in the length of the third stage of labor, but no reduction in blood loss compared with that of physiological management. Mitchell and Elbourne (1993) found that syntometrine administered intramuscularly concurrent with delivery of the anterior shoulder was more effective than oxytocin (5 units intramuscularly) alone in the prevention of postpartum hemorrhage. Duration of the third stage of labor and need for manual removal of the placenta were similar. Side effects of nausea, vomiting, and blood pressure elevations with ergometrine prevented any recommendation for its routine usage.

"Fourth Stage" of Labor. The placenta, membranes, and umbilical cord should be examined for completeness and for anomalies, as described in Chapters 31 and 32. The hour immediately following delivery is critical, and it has been designated by some as the "fourth stage of labor." Even though oxytocics are administered, postpartum hemorrhage as the result of uterine atony is more likely at this time. Consequently,

the uterus and perineum should be frequently evaluated. The American Academy of Pediatrics and the American College of Obstetricians and Gynecologists (2002) recommend that maternal blood pressure and pulse be recorded immediately after delivery and every 15 minutes for the first hour.

Oxytocic Agents. After the uterus has been emptied and the placenta has been delivered, the primary mechanism by which hemostasis is achieved at the placental site is vasoconstriction produced by a well-contracted myometrium. Oxytocin, methylergonovine maleate (Methergine), and prostaglandin analogues are employed in various ways, principally to reduce blood loss by stimulating myometrial contractions.

OXYTOCICS AFTER DELIVERY. Oxytocin, ergonovine, and methylergonovine are all employed widely in the normal third stage of labor, but the timing of their administration differs in various institutions. Oxytocin, and especially ergonovine, given before delivery of the placenta will decrease blood loss (Prendiville and associates, 1988a). There is, however, a significant danger associated with this practice. The use of oxytocin, and especially ergonovine or methylergonovine, before delivery of the placenta may entrap an undiagnosed, undelivered second twin. This may prove injurious, if not fatal, to the entrapped fetus. In most cases following uncomplicated vaginal delivery, the third stage of labor can be conducted with reasonably small blood loss without using these agents before delivery of the placenta.

Several studies have evaluated the use of these agents. Jackson and colleagues (2001) randomly assigned 1486 women to infusions of 20 units of oxytocin diluted in 500 mL normal saline begun before or after delivery of the placenta. There were no benefits to beginning oxytocin before delivery of the placenta. Choy and co-authors (2002) randomly assigned 991 women to receive intravenous oxytocin or intramuscular syntometrine for prevention of third-stage blood loss. They reported oxytocin to be preferable because syntometrine induced hypertension in 3 percent of women. Munn and co-workers (2001) compared two oxytocin dosage regimens for prevention of uterine atony at cesarean delivery. Either 10 units or 80 units of oxytocin in 500 mL of lactated Ringer solution were infused during the 30 minutes following delivery of the newborn. The rate of uterine atony was significantly lower in the high-dose regimen group compared with that of the lower-dose group—19 versus 39 percent, respectively.

If an intravenous infusion is in place, our standard practice has been to add 20 units (2 mL) of oxytocin per liter of infusate. This solution is administered after delivery of the placenta at a rate of 10 mL/min (200 mU/min) for a few minutes until the uterus remains firmly contracted and bleeding is controlled. The infusion rate then is reduced to 1 to 2 mL/min until the mother is ready for transfer from the recovery suite to the postpartum unit. The infusion is usually then discontinued.

OXYTOCIN. The synthetic form of the octapeptide oxytocin is commercially available in the United States as Syntocinon and Pitocin. Each milliliter of injectable oxytocin, which is not effective by mouth, contains 10 USP units. The half-life of intravenously infused oxytocin is approximately 3 minutes.

Before delivery, the spontaneously laboring uterus is typically exquisitely sensitive to oxytocin. With an inappropriate dose of oxytocin, the pregnant uterus may contract so violently as to kill the fetus, rupture itself, or both (see Chap. 22, p. 541). After delivery of the fetus, these dangers no longer exist.

Cardiovascular Effects. Secher and co-workers (1978) consistently observed that, even in healthy women, an intravenous bolus of 10 units of oxytocin caused a transient but marked fall in arterial blood pressure that was followed by an abrupt increase in cardiac output. They concluded that these hemodynamic changes could be dangerous to women already hypovolemic from hemorrhage or who had cardiac disease that limited cardiac output. The same danger is present for women with right-to-left cardiac shunts, because the decrease in systemic resistance would further increase the shunt. **Oxytocin should not be given intravenously as a large bolus,** but rather as a much more dilute solution by continuous intravenous infusion or as an intramuscular injection in a dose of 10 USP units. In cases of postpartum hemorrhage, direct injection into the uterus, either transvaginally or transabdominally, if following a vaginal birth, or directly if at cesarean delivery, has proven effective. The use of nipple stimulation in the third stage of labor also has been shown to increase uterine pressures and to decrease the duration of the third stage of labor and blood loss (Irons and associates, 1994). Indeed, results were similar to those achieved using the combination of oxytocin (5 units) and ergometrine (0.5 mg).

Water Intoxication. The considerable antidiuretic action of oxytocin can cause water intoxication. With high-dose oxytocin, it is possible to produce water intoxication if the oxytocin is administered in a large volume of electrolyte-free aqueous dextrose solution (Whalley and Pritchard, 1963). For example, Schwartz and Jones (1978) described convulsions in both the mother and her newborn following the administration of 6.5 liters of 5-percent dextrose solution and 36 units of oxytocin predelivery. The concentration of sodium in cord plasma was 114 mEq/L.

In general, if oxytocin is to be administered in high doses for a considerable period of time, its concentration should be increased rather than increasing the rate of flow of a more dilute solution (see Chap. 22, p. 540). Consideration also should be given to use of either normal saline or lactated Ringer solution in these circumstances.

ERGONOVINE AND METHYLERGONOVINE. Ergonovine is an alkaloid that is obtained from ergot, a fungus that grows on rye and some other grains, or is synthesized in part from lysergic acid. Methylergonovine is a similar synthetic alkaloid made from lysergic acid. There is no convincing evidence of any appreciable difference in the actions of methylergonovine compared with those of ergonovine, also called ergometrine and ergostetrine. Whether given intravenously, intramuscularly, or orally, these agents are powerful stimulants of myometrial contraction, exerting an effect that may persist for hours. In pregnant women, an intravenous dose of as little as 0.1 mg or an oral dose of only 0.25 mg results in a tetanic uterine contraction that develops almost immediately after intravenous injection of the drug and within a few minutes after intramuscular or oral administration. Moreover, the response is sustained with little tendency toward relaxation. The tetanic effect of both drugs is effective for the prevention and control of postpartum hemorrhage, but it is very dangerous for the fetus and the mother prior to delivery.

The parenteral administration of these alkaloids, especially by the intravenous route, sometimes initiates transient but severe hypertension. Such a reaction is most likely in women who are prone to develop hypertension. Browning (1974) described four instances of serious postdelivery side effects attributable to 0.5 mg of ergonovine administered intramuscularly. Two women promptly became severely hypertensive, the third became hypertensive and convulsed, and the fourth suffered a cardiac arrest. We have seen an instance of such profound vasoconstriction from these compounds when given intravenously that all peripheral pulses were lost, and sodium nitroprusside was required to restore the peripheral circulation. Unfortunately, the mother sustained cerebral hypoxic ischemic injury.

PROSTAGLANDINS. Analogues of prostaglandins are not used routinely for management of third-stage labor. Villar and colleagues (2002) reviewed prophylactic use of misoprostol to prevent postpartum hemorrhage and concluded that oxytocin or oxytocin-ergot preparations are more effective. Other prostaglandins such as 15-methyl prostaglandin $F_{2\alpha}$ are reserved for treatment of hemorrhage, which is discussed in Chapter 35 (see p. 827).

LACERATIONS OF THE BIRTH CANAL. Lacerations of the vagina and perineum are classified as first, second, third, or fourth degree. *First-degree* lacerations involve the fourchette, perineal skin, and vaginal mucous membrane but not the underlying fascia and muscle. *Second-degree* lacerations involve, in addition to skin and mucous membrane, the fascia and muscles of the perineal body but not the anal sphincter (Fig. 17–34). These tears usually extend upward on one or both sides of the vagina, forming an irregular triangular injury. *Third-degree* lacerations extend through the skin, mucous membrane, and perineal body, and involve the anal sphincter. A *fourth-degree* laceration extends through the rectal mucosa to expose the lumen of the rectum. Tears in the region of the urethra that may bleed profusely may also accompany this type of laceration.

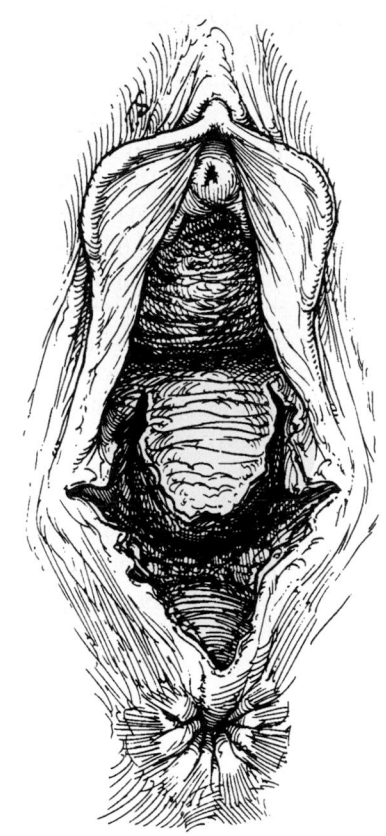

FIGURE 17–34. Deep second-degree laceration of the perineum and vagina.

Because the repair of perineal tears is virtually the same as that of episiotomy incisions, albeit often less satisfactory because of irregular lines of tissue cleavage, the technique of repairing lacerations is discussed in the following section.

EPISIOTOMY AND REPAIR. In a strict sense, episiotomy is incision of the pudenda. Perineotomy is incision of the perineum. In common parlance, however, the term *episiotomy* often is used synonymously with *perineotomy*, a practice that we follow here. The incision may be made in the midline, creating a *median* or *midline episiotomy*, or it may begin in the midline but be directed laterally and downward away from the rectum, termed a *mediolateral episiotomy*.

Purposes of Episiotomy. Although still a common obstetrical procedure, the use of episiotomy has decreased remarkably over the past 25 years. Weber and Meyn (2002) used the National Hospital Discharge Survey to analyze use of episiotomy between 1979 and 1997 in the United States. Approximately 65 percent of women who gave birth vaginally in 1979 had episiotomies compared with 39 percent by 1997. Through the 1970s, it was common practice to cut an episiotomy for almost all women having their first delivery. The reasons for its popularity included substitution of a straight surgical incision, which was easier to repair, for the ragged

laceration that otherwise might result. The long-held beliefs that postoperative pain is less and healing improved with an episiotomy compared with a tear, however, appeared to be incorrect (Larsson and colleagues, 1991).

Another commonly cited but unproven benefit of routine episiotomy was that it prevented pelvic relaxation—that is, cystocele, rectocele, and urinary incontinence. A number of observational studies and randomized trials showed that routine episiotomy is associated with an increased incidence of anal sphincter and rectal tears (Angioli and co-authors, 2000; Argentine Episiotomy Trial Collaborative Group, 1993; Eason and colleagues, 2000; Nager and Helliwell, 2001).

Carroli and Belizan (2000) reviewed the Cochrane Pregnancy and Childbirth Group trials registry. There were six randomized trials of nearly 5000 deliveries in which routine (73-percent rate) versus restricted (28-percent rate) use of episiotomy was evaluated. There were lower rates of posterior perineal trauma, surgical repair, and healing complications in the restricted-use group. Alternatively, the incidence of anterior perineal trauma was lower in the routine-use group. Along with these findings came the realization that episiotomy did not protect the perineal body and contributed to anal sphincter incontinence by increasing the risk of third- and fourth-degree tears. Signorello and associates (2000) reported that fecal and flatus incontinence were increased four- to sixfold in women with an episiotomy compared with findings of a group delivered with an intact perineum. Even when compared with spontaneous lacerations, episiotomy tripled the risk of fecal incontinence and doubled it for flatus incontinence. Episiotomy without extension did not lower this risk. Finally, even with recognition and repair of a third-degree extension, 30 to 40 percent of women have long-term anal incontinence (Gjessing and co-workers, 1998; Poen and colleagues, 1998).

It seems reasonable to conclude that episiotomy should not be performed routinely (Eason and Feldman, 2000). The procedure should be applied selectively for appropriate indications, some of which include fetal indications such as shoulder dystocia and breech delivery; forceps or vacuum extractor deliveries; occiput posterior positions; and in instances where it is obvious that failure to perform an episiotomy will result in perineal rupture. **The final rule is that there is no substitute for surgical judgment and common sense.**

The important variables of episiotomy use include the timing of the incision, the type of incision, and techniques for repair.

Timing of Episiotomy. If performed unnecessarily early, bleeding from the episiotomy may be considerable during the interim between incision and delivery. If it is performed too late, lacerations will not be prevented. It is common practice to perform episiotomy when the head is visible during a contraction to a diameter of 3 to 4 cm (see Fig. 17–24). When used in conjunction with forceps delivery, most practitioners

TABLE 17-4 Midline Versus Mediolateral Episiotomy

Characteristic	Type of Episiotomy	
	Midline	Mediolateral
Surgical repair	Easy	More difficult
Faulty healing	Rare	More common
Postoperative pain	Minimal	Common
Anatomical results	Excellent	Occasionally faulty
Blood loss	Less	More
Dyspareunia	Rare	Occasional
Extensions	Common	Uncommon

perform an episiotomy after application of the blades (see Chap. 23, p. 552).

Midline Versus Mediolateral Episiotomy. The advantages and disadvantages of the two types of episiotomies are summarized in Table 17-4. Except for the important issue of third- and fourth-degree extensions, midline episiotomy is superior. Proper selection of cases can minimize this one disadvantage. In addition to a midline episiotomy, Combs and associates (1990) reported the following factors to be associated with an increased risk of third- and fourth-degree lacerations: nulliparity, second-stage arrest of labor, persistent occiput posterior position, mid or low forceps, use of local anesthetics, and Asian race.

It is reasonable to use a mediolateral episiotomy when a third- or fourth-degree extension is likely, but to employ the midline incision otherwise. Anthony and colleagues (1994), who presented data from the Dutch National Obstetric Database of over 43,000 deliveries, found more than a fourfold decrease in severe perineal lacerations when mediolateral episiotomy was employed compared with midline incision.

Venkatesh and colleagues (1989) reported a 5-percent incidence of third- and fourth-degree perineal tears in 20,500 vaginal deliveries. About 10 percent of these 1040 primary repairs had a postoperative wound disruption, and 67 of the 101 required surgical correction. Goldaber and associates (1993) found that 21 of 390 or 5.4 percent of women with fourth-degree lacerations experienced significant morbidity. There were 7 (1.8 percent) dehiscences, 11 (2.8 percent) infections with dehiscences, and 3 (0.8 percent) infections alone. Although administration of a perioperative 2-g intravenous dose of cefazolin reduced this morbidity, it was not totally eliminated.

Timing of the Episiotomy Repair. The most common practice is to defer episiotomy repair until the placenta has been delivered. This policy permits undivided attention to the signs of placental separation and delivery. A further advantage is that episiotomy repair is not interrupted or disrupted by the obvious necessity of delivering the placenta, especially if manual removal must be performed.

Technique. There are many ways to close an episiotomy incision, but *hemostasis and anatomical restoration without excessive suturing are essential* for success with any method. A technique that commonly is employed is shown in Figure 17-35. The suture material ordinarily used is 3-0 chromic catgut, but Grant (1989) recommends suture composed of derivatives of polyglycolic acid. A decrease in postsurgical pain is cited as the major advantage of the newer materials, despite the occasional later need to remove some of the suture from the site of repair because of pain or dyspareunia. Kettle and co-authors (2002) randomly assigned 1542 women with perineal lacerations or episiotomies to undergo continuous versus interrupted repair with rapidly absorbed polyglactin 910 (Vicryl Rapids, Ethicon) or standard polyglactin 910 sutures. The former typically is absorbed by 42 days and the latter completely absorbed by about 90 days. The continuous method was associated with less perineal pain. The rapidly absorbed material was associated with lower rates of suture removal within 3 months of delivery (3 percent removal versus 13 percent removal for rapidly absorbed versus standard polyglactin). Sanders and co-workers (2002) emphasized that women without regional analgesia can experience high levels of pain during perineal suturing.

FOURTH-DEGREE LACERATION. The technique of repairing a fourth-degree laceration is shown in Figure 17-36. Various techniques have been recommended, but in all instances, it is essential to approximate the torn edges of the rectal mucosa with sutures placed in the muscularis approximately 0.5 cm apart. This muscular layer then is covered with a layer of fascia. Finally, the cut ends of the anal sphincter are isolated, approximated, and sutured together with three or four interrupted stitches. The remainder of the repair is the same as for an episiotomy. The overlapping technique is an alternative method to approximate the external anal sphincter. Despite promising initial results with this technique, more recent data based on a randomized controlled trial do not support that this method yields superior anatomical or functional results over the traditional end-to-end technique (Fitzpatrick and colleagues, 2000; Sultan and co-workers, 1999). Thus, more emphasis should be placed on prevention of anal sphincter lacerations. Postrepair, stool softeners should be prescribed for a week, and enemas should be avoided. Prophylactic antimicrobials should be considered, as described by Goldaber and colleagues (1993). Unfortunately, normal function is not always assured even with correct and complete surgical repair. Some women may experience continuing fecal incontinence caused by injury to the innervation of the pelvic floor musculature (Roberts and co-workers, 1990).

Pain After Episiotomy. Application of ice packs tends to reduce swelling and allay discomfort. Minassian and colleagues (2002) randomly assigned 200 women to receive 5-percent lidocaine ointment versus placebo for relief of postpartum perineal pain. Topical application of lidocaine ointment was not effective in relieving episiotomy or perineal laceration

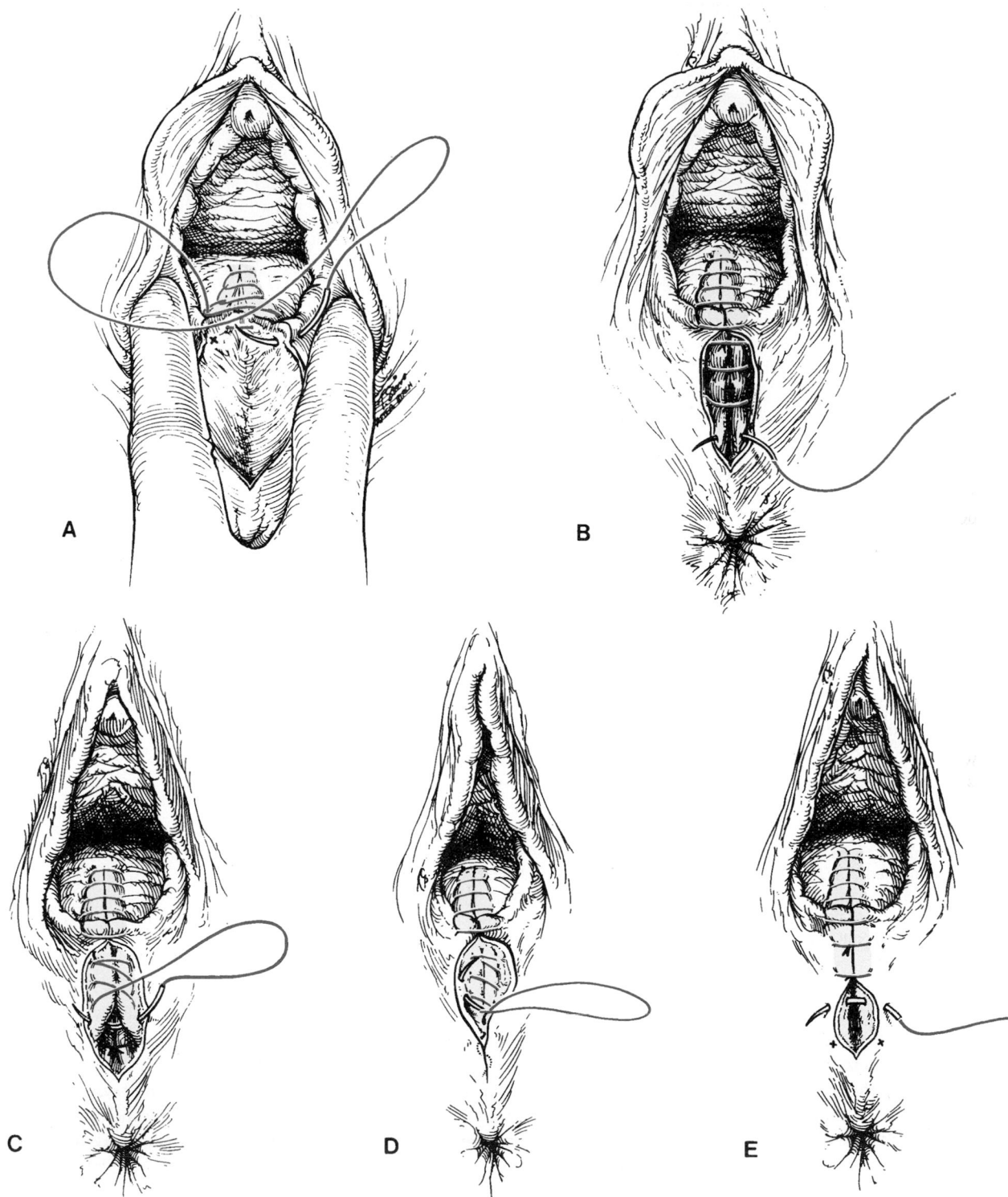

FIGURE 17–35. Repair of midline episiotomy. **A.** Chromic 2-0 or 3-0 suture is used as a continuous suture to close the vaginal mucosa and submucosa. **B.** After closing the vaginal incision and reapproximating the cut margins of the hymenal ring, the suture is tied and cut. Next, three or four interrupted sutures of 2-0 or 3-0 chromic are placed in the fascia and muscle of the incised perineum. **C.** A continuous suture is carried downward to unite the superficial fascia. **D.** Completion of repair. The continuous suture is carried upward as a subcuticular stitch. (An alternative method of closure of skin and subcutaneous fascia is illustrated in E.) **E.** Completion of repair of midline episiotomy. A few interrupted sutures of 3-0 chromic are placed through the skin and subcutaneous fascia and loosely tied. This closure avoids burying two layers of suture in the more superficial layers of the perineum.

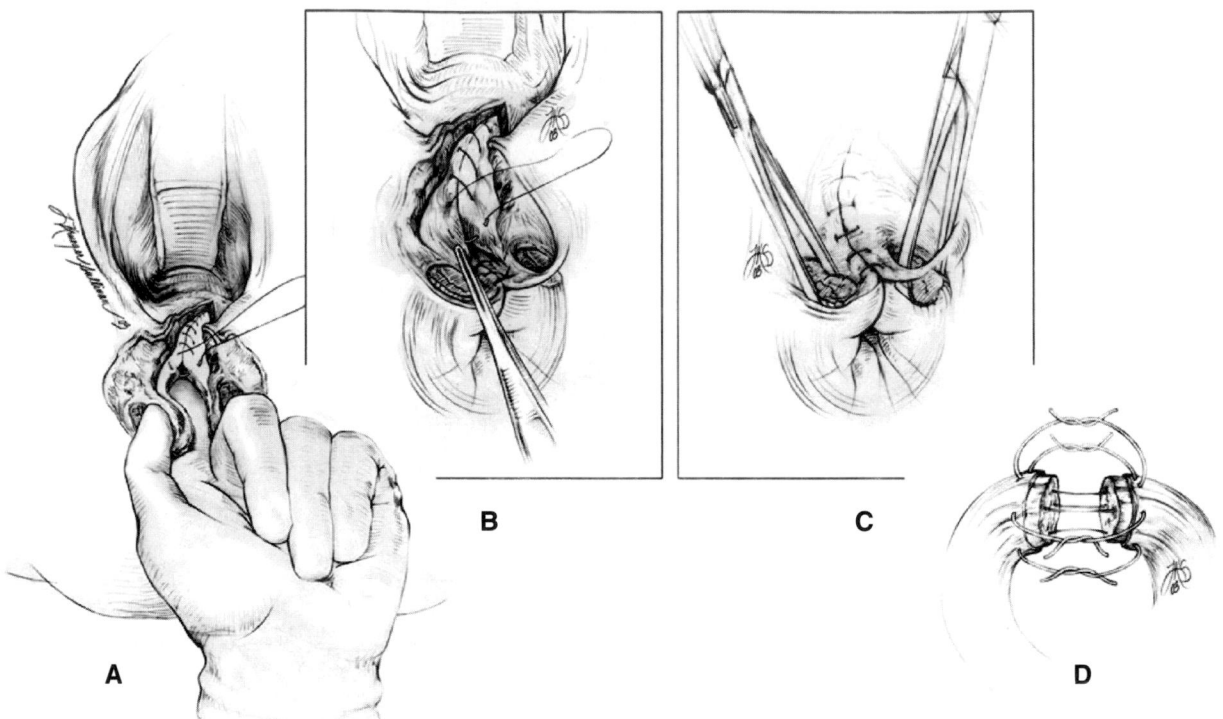

FIGURE 17–36. Layered repair of a fourth-degree perineal laceration. **A.** Approximation of the anorectal mucosa and submucosa in a running or interrupted fashion using fine absorbable suture such as 3-0 or 4-0 chromic or Vicryl. The superior extent of the anterior anal laceration is identified and the sutures are placed through the submucosa of the anorectum approximately 0.5 cm apart down to the anal verge. **B.** A second layer is placed through the rectal muscularis using 3-0 Vicryl suture in a running or interrupted fashion. This "reinforcing layer" should incorporate the torn ends of the internal anal sphincter, which is identified as the thickening of the circular smooth muscle layer at the distal 2 to 3 cm of the anal canal. It can be identified as the glistening white fibrous structure lying between the anal canal submucosa and the fibers of the external anal sphincter (EAS). In many cases, the internal sphincter retracts laterally and must be sought and retrieved for repair. **C.** The disrupted ends of the striated EAS muscle and capsule are then identified and grasped with Allis clamps. The torn ends of the EAS often retract laterally in an asymmetrical fashion as shown. **D.** Traditional end-to-end approximation of the EAS. Four to six simple interrupted 2-0 or 3-0 Vicryl sutures are placed at the 3, 6, 9, and 12 o'clock positions through the EAS muscle and its connective tissue capsule. The sutures through the inferior and posterior portions of the sphincter should be placed first and tied last to facilitate this part of the repair. The remainder of the repair is similar to that described for a midline episiotomy in Figure 17–35.

discomfort. Analgesics such as codeine give considerable relief. **Because pain may be a signal of a large vulvar, paravaginal, or ischiorectal hematoma or perineal cellulitis, it is essential to examine these sites carefully if pain is severe or persistent.** Management of these complications is discussed in Chapter 35.

Signorello and co-workers (2001) surveyed 615 women 6 months postpartum to determine the impact of perineal trauma on sexual functioning. Women whose newborns were delivered over an intact perineum reported the best outcomes in this regard.

LABOR MANAGEMENT PROTOCOLS

O'Driscoll and colleagues (1984) at the National Maternity Hospital in Dublin pioneered the concept that a disciplined,

standardized labor management protocol reduced cesarean deliveries for dystocia. Their overall cesarean delivery rate was 5 percent in the 1970s and 1980s with such management. The approach is now referred to as *active management of labor.* Two of its components—amniotomy and oxytocin—have been widely used, especially in English-speaking countries outside the United States (Thornton and Lilford, 1994). Recently, Impey and Boylan (1999) observed that active management was never intended to reduce the cesarean delivery rate and that the rate had in fact been low (about 5 percent) at the National Maternity Hospital prior to implementation of active management. In their view, active management did serve, however, to prevent the escalating rate of cesarean deliveries in Dublin that developed in the United States and elsewhere. More recently, however, the cesarean delivery rate for nulliparous women who gave birth at the National Maternity Hospital in 1997 has more than doubled to 11.6 percent. This increase was attributed to induction of labor, cesarean delivery for breech presentation, and changing maternal attitudes.

ACTIVE MANAGEMENT OF LABOR. This phrase describes a codified approach to labor diagnosis and management only in nulliparous women. Labor is diagnosed when painful contractions are accompanied by complete cervical effacement, bloody "show," or ruptured membranes. Women with such findings are committed to delivery within 12 hours. Pelvic examination is performed each hour for the next 3 hours, and thereafter at 2-hour intervals. When dilatation has not increased by at least 1 cm/hr, amniotomy is performed. Progress is again assessed at 2 hours and high-dose oxytocin infusion, described in Chapter 22 (see p. 540), is started unless dilatation of at least 1 cm/hr is documented. Women are constantly attended by midwives.

If membranes rupture prior to admission, oxytocin is begun for no progress at the 1-hour mark. No special equipment is used, either to dispense oxytocin or to monitor its effects, and electronic uterine contraction monitoring is not used. Oxytocin is dispensed by gravity regulated by a personal nurse. The solution contains 10 units of oxytocin in 1 L of dextrose and water. The total dose may not exceed 10 units and the infusion rate may not exceed 60 drops/min or 30 to 40 mU/min (15 to 20 drops = 1 mL). In the Irish protocol, scalp blood sampling is used as the definitive test for fetal distress.

López-Zeno and colleagues (1992) prospectively compared active management with the "traditional" approach to labor management practiced at Northwestern Memorial Hospital in Chicago. They randomly assigned 705 nulliparas with uncomplicated pregnancies in spontaneous labor at term. The cesarean delivery rate was statistically different: 10.5 percent with active management and 14.1 percent with the "traditional" approach. Frigoletto and co-workers (1995) also reported a randomized trial of active management in 1934 nulliparous women delivered at Brigham and Women's Hospital in Boston. Although they found that such management somewhat shortened labor, it did not affect the cesarean delivery rate. Similar results were reported by Rogers and colleagues (1997), Sadler and co-authors (2000), and Impey and co-workers (2000). The American College of Obstetricians and Gynecologists (2003a) has concluded that active management of labor may shorten labor, although it has not consistently been shown to reduce rates of cesarean delivery.

World Health Organization Partogram. A *partogram* was designed by the World Health Organization for use in developing countries (Dujardin and co-workers, 1992). Labor is divided into a latent phase, which should last no longer than 8 hours, and an active phase, starting at 3 cm dilatation and during which the rate of dilatation should be no slower than 1 cm/hr. A 4-hour wait is recommended before intervention when the active phase is slow. Labor is graphed, and analysis includes use of alert and action lines.

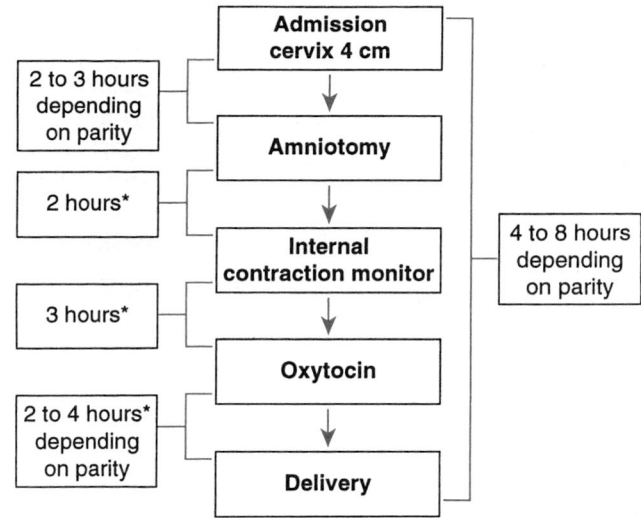

*Depending on progress of cervical dilatation

FIGURE 17–37. Summary of labor management protocol in use at Parkland Hospital. The total admission-to-delivery times are shorter than the potential sum of the intervention intervals because not every woman requires every intervention.

Parkland Hospital Labor Management Protocol. During the 1980s, the obstetrical volume at Parkland Hospital doubled to approximately 15,000 births per year. In response, a second delivery unit designed for women with uncomplicated term pregnancies was developed. This provided a unique opportunity to implement and evaluate a standardized protocol for labor management. Its design was based on the labor management approach that had evolved at our hospital up to that time, which emphasized the implementation of specific, sequential interventions when abnormal labor was suspected. This approach currently is used in both complicated and uncomplicated pregnancies.

Women are admitted when active labor—defined as cervical dilatation of 3 to 4 cm or more in the presence of uterine contractions—is diagnosed or ruptured membranes are confirmed. Management guidelines summarized in Figure 17–37 stipulate that pelvic examinations be performed approximately every 2 hours. Ineffective labor is suspected when the cervix does not dilate within about 2 hours of admission. Amniotomy is then performed and labor progress determined at the next 2-hour evaluation. In women whose labors do not progress, an intrauterine pressure catheter is placed to assess uterine function. Hypotonic contractions and no cervical dilatation after an additional 2 to 3 hours result in stimulation of labor using the high-dose oxytocin regimen described in Chapter 22 (see p. 540). Uterine activity of 200 to 250 Montevideo units is expected for 2 to 4 hours before dystocia is diagnosed.

Dilatation rates of 1 to 2 cm/hr are accepted as evidence of progress after satisfactory uterine activity has been established with oxytocin. As shown in Figure 17–37, this can require up to 8 hours or more before cesarean delivery is performed for dystocia. The cumulative time required to effect this stepwise management approach permits many women to establish effective labor. This management protocol has been evaluated in more than 20,000 women with uncomplicated pregnancies. Cesarean delivery rates in nulliparous and parous women were 8.7 and 1.5 percent, respectively. Importantly, these labor interventions and the relatively infrequent use of cesarean delivery did not jeopardize the fetus-newborn.

REFERENCES

Alexander JM, Sharma SK, McIntire DD, et al: Epidural analgesia lengthens the Friedman active phase of labor. Obstet Gynecol 100:46, 2002

American Academy of Pediatrics and the American College of Obstetricians and Gynecologists: Guidelines for Perinatal Care, 5th ed. Washington, DC, AAP and ACOG, 2002

American College of Obstetricians and Gynecologists: Dystocia and augmentation of labor. Practice Bulletin No. 49, December 2003a

American College of Obstetricians and Gynecologists: Prophylactic antibiotics in labor and delivery. Practice Bulletin No. 47, October 2003b

American College of Obstetricians and Gynecologists: Optimal goals for anesthesia care in obstetrics. Committee Opinion No. 256, May 2001

American College of Obstetricians and Gynecologists: Precis, Obstetrics: An update in obstetrics and gynecology. Washington, DC, ACOG, 2000

Angioli R, Gomez-Marin O, Cantuaria G, et al: Severe perineal lacerations during vaginal delivery: The University of Miami experience. Am J Obstet Gynecol 182:1083, 2000

Anthony S, Buitendijk SE, Zondervan KT, et al: Episiotomies and the occurrence of severe perineal lacerations. Br J Obstet Gynaecol 101:1064, 1994

Argentine Episiotomy Trial Collaborative Group: Routine versus selective episiotomy: A randomized controlled trial. Lancet 342:1515, 1993

Bloom SL, McIntire DD, Kelly MA, et al: Lack of effect of walking on labor and delivery. N Engl J Med 339:76, 1998

Browning DJ: Serious side effects of ergometrine and its use in routine obstetric practice. Med J Aust 1:957, 1974

Caldwell WE, Moloy HC, D'Esopo DA: A roentgenologic study of the mechanism of engagement of the fetal head. Am J Obstet Gynecol 28:824, 1934

Calkins LA: The etiology of occiput presentations. Am J Obstet Gynecol 37:618, 1939

Carlan SJ, Wyble L, Lense J, et al: Fetal head molding: Diagnosis by ultrasound and a review of the literature. J Perinatol 11:105, 1991

Carley ME, Carley JM, Vasdev G, et al: Factors that are associated with clinically overt postpartum urinary retention after vaginal delivery. Am J Obstet Gynecol 187:430, 2002

Carroli G, Belizan J: Episiotomy for vaginal birth. Cochrane Database Syst Rev 2:CD000081, 2000

Chelmow D, Kilpatrick SJ, Laros RK Jr: Maternal and neonatal outcomes after prolonged latent phase. Obstet Gynecol 81:486, 1993

Choy CMY, Lau WC, Tam WH, et al: A randomized controlled trial of intramuscular syntometrine and intravenous oxytocin in the management of the third stage of labor. Br J Obstet Gynaecol 109:173, 2002

Cohen W, Friedman EA (eds): Management of Labor. Baltimore, University Park Press, 1983

Combs CA, Robertson PA, Laros RK: Risk factors for third-degree and fourth-degree perineal lacerations in forceps and vacuum deliveries. Am J Obstet Gynecol 163:100, 1990

Dombrowski MP, Bottoms SF, Saleh AAA, et al: Third stage of labor: Analysis of duration and clinical practice. Am J Obstet Gynecol 172:1279, 1995

Dujardin B, De Schampheleire I, Sene H, et al: Value of the alert and action lines on the partogram. Lancet 339:1336, 1992

Eason E, Feldman P: Much ado about a little cut: Is episiotomy worthwhile? Obstet Gynecol 95:616, 2000

Eason E, Labrecque M, Wells G, et al: Preventing perineal trauma during childbirth: A systematic review. Obstet Gynecol 95:464, 2000

Federal Register, Vol 68, No. 174, p 53222, September 9, 2003

Fitzpatrick M, Behan M, O'Connell PR, et al: A randomized clinical trial comparing primary overlap with approximation repair of third-degree obstetric tears. Am J Obstet Gynecol 183:1220, 2000

Friedman EA: An objective approach to the diagnosis and management of abnormal labor. Bull N Y Acad Med 48:842, 1972

Friedman E: The graphic analysis of labor. Am J Obstet Gynecol 68:1568, 1954

Friedman EA: Labor: Clinical Evaluation and Management, 2nd ed. New York, Appleton-Century-Crofts, 1978

Friedman EA: Primigravid labor: A graphicostatistical analysis. Obstet Gynecol 6:567, 1955

Friedman EA, Kroll BH: Computer analysis of labor progression. V. Effects of fetal presentation and position. J Reprod Med 8:117, 1972

Friedman EA, Sachtleben MR: Amniotomy and the course of labor. Obstet Gynecol 22:755, 1963

Frigoletto FD Jr, Lieberman E, Lang JM, et al: A clinical trial of active management of labor [published correction appears in N Engl J Med 333:1163, 1995]. N Engl J Med 333:745, 1995

Gardberg M, Tuppurainen M: Anterior placental location predisposes for occiput posterior presentation near term. Acta Obstet Gynecol Scand 73:151, 1994a

Gardberg M, Tuppurainen M: Persistent occiput posterior presentation—a clinical problem. Acta Obstet Gynecol Scand 73:45, 1994b

Gardosi J, Hutson N, Lynch CB: Randomised, controlled trial of squatting in the second stage of labour. Lancet 2:74, 1989

Garite TJ, Weeks J, Peters-Phair K, et al: A randomized controlled trial of the effect of increased intravenous hydration on the course of labor in nulliparous women. Am J Obstet Gynecol 183:1544, 2000

Gjessing H, Backe B, Sahlin Y: Third degree obstetric tears; outcome after primary repair. Acta Obstet Gynecol Scand 77:736, 1998

Goldaber KG, Wendel PJ, McIntire DD, et al: Postpartum perineal morbidity after fourth-degree perineal repair. Am J Obstet Gynecol 168:489, 1993

Grant A: The choice of suture materials and techniques for repair of perineal trauma: An overview of the evidence from controlled trials. Br J Obstet Gynaecol 96:1281, 1989

Gurewitsch ED, Diament P, Fong J, et al: The labor curve of the grand multipara: Does progress of labor continue to improve with additional childbearing? Am J Obstet Gynecol 186:1331, 2002

Gurewitsch ED, Johnson E, Allen RH, et al: The descent curve of the grand multiparous woman. Am J Obstet Gynecol 189:1036, 2003

Hendricks CH, Brenner WE: Cardiovascular effects of oxytocic drugs used postpartum. Am J Obstet Gynecol 108:751, 1970

Impey L, Boylan P: Active management of labour revisited. Br J Obstet Gynaecol 106:183, 1999

Impey L, Hobson J, O'Herlihy C: Graphic analysis of actively managed labor: Prospective computation of labor progress in 500 consecutive nulliparous women in spontaneous labor at term. Am J Obstet Gynecol 183:438, 2000

Irons DW, Sriskandabalan P, Bullough CH: A simple alternative to parental oxytocics for the third stage of labor. Int J Gynaecol Obstet 46:15, 1994

Jackson KW, Allbert JR, Schemmer GK, et al: A randomized controlled trial comparing oxytocin administration before and after placental delivery in the prevention of postpartum hemorrhage. Am J Obstet Gynecol 185:873, 2001

Kettle C, Hills RK, Jones P, et al: Continuous versus interrupted perineal repair with standard or rapidly absorbed sutures after spontaneous vaginal birth: A randomized controlled trial. Lancet 359:2217, 2002

Kilpatrick SJ, Laros RK, Jr: Characteristics of normal labor. Obstet Gynecol 74:85, 1989

Larsson P, Platz-Christensen J, Bergman B, et al: Advantage or disadvantage of episiotomy compared with spontaneous perineal laceration. Gynecol Obstet Invest 31:213, 1991

Leopold J: Conduct of normal births through external examination alone. Arch Gynaekol 45:337, 1894

López-Zeno JA, Peaceman AM, Adashek JA, et al: A controlled trial of a program for the active management of labor. N Engl J Med 326:450, 1992

Lydon-Rochelle M, Albers L, Gorwoda J, et al: Accuracy of Leopold maneuvers in screening for malpresentation: A prospective study. Birth 20:132, 1993

Martin JA, Hamilton BE, Sutton PD, et al: Births: Final data for 2002. National Vital Statistics Reports, Vol 52, No. 10. Hyattsville, Md, National Center for Health Statistics, 2003

Mayerhofer K, Bodner-Adler B, Bodner K, et al: Traditional care of the perineum during birth: A prospective, randomized, multicenter study of 1,076 women. J Reprod Med 47:477, 2002

Minassian VA, Jazayeri A, Prien SD, et al: Randomized trial of lidocaine ointment versus placebo for the treatment of postpartum perineal pain. Obstet Gynecol 100:1239, 2002

Mitchell GG, Elbourne DR: The Salford Third Stage Trial. Oxytocin plus ergometrine versus oxytocin alone in the active management of the third stage of labor. Online J Curr Clin Trials 83, 1993

Munn MB, Owen J, Vincent J, et al: Comparison of two oxytocin regimens to prevent uterine atony at cesarean delivery: A randomized controlled trial. Obstet Gynecol 98:386, 2001

Negar CW, Helliwell JP: Episiotomy increases perineal laceration length in primiparous women. Am J Obstet Gynecol 185:444, 2001

New Shorter Oxford English Dictionary. New York, Oxford University Press, 1993

O'Driscoll K, Foley M, MacDonald D: Active management of labor as an alternative to cesarean section for dystocia. Obstet Gynecol 63:485, 1984

Pang YWY, Heffelfinger JD, Huang GJ, et al: Outcomes of planned home births in Washington state: 1989–1996. Obstet Gynecol 100:253, 2002

Poen AC, Felt-Bersma RJ, Strijers RL, et al: Third-degree obstetric perineal tear: Long-term clinical and functional results after primary repair. Br J Surg 85:1433, 1998

Prendiville W, Elbourne D, Chalmers I: The effects of routine oxytocic administration in the management of the third stage of labour:

An overview of the evidence from controlled trials. Br J Obstet Gynaecol 95:3, 1988a

Prendiville WJ, Harding JE, Elbourne DR, et al: The Bristol third stage trial: Active versus physiological management of third stage of labour. Br Med J 297:1295, 1988b

Ritgen G: Concerning his method for protection of the perineum. Monatschrift für Geburtskunde 6:21, 1855. See English translation, Wynn RM: Am J Obstet Gynecol 93:421, 1965

Roberts PL, Coller JA, Schoetz DJ, et al: Manometric assessment of patients with obstetric injuries and fecal incontinence. Dis Colon Rectum 33:16, 1990

Rogers R, Gelson GJ, Miller AC, et al: Active management of labor: Does it make a difference? Am J Obstet Gynecol 177:599, 1997

Sadler LC, Davison T, McCowan LME: A randomized controlled trial and meta-analysis of active management of labour. Br J Obstet Gynaecol 107:909, 2000

Sanders J, Campbell R, Peters TJ: Effectiveness of pain relief during perineal suturing. Br J Obstet Gynaecol 109:1066, 2002

Scheer K, Nubar J: Variation of fetal presentation with gestational age. Am J Obstet Gynecol 125:269, 1976

Schwartz RH, Jones RWA: Transplacental hyponatremia due to oxytocin. Br Med J 1:152, 1978

Secher NJ, Arnso P, Wallin L: Haemodynamic effects of oxytocin (Syntocinon) and methylergometrine (Methergin) on the systemic and pulmonary circulations of pregnant anaesthetized women. Acta Obstet Gynecol Scand 57:97, 1978

Signorello LB, Harlow BL, Chekos AK, et al: Midline episiotomy and anal incontinence: Retrospective cohort study. Br Med J 320:86, 2000

Signorello LB, Harlow BL, Chekos AK, et al: Postpartum sexual functioning and its relationship to perineal trauma: A retrospective cohort study of primiparous women. Am J Obstet Gynecol 184:881, 2001

Sokol RJ, Stojkov J, Chik L, et al: Normal and abnormal labor progress: I. A quantitative assessment and survey of the literature. J Reprod Med 18:47, 1977

Sultan AH, Monga AK, Kumar D, et al: Primary repair of obstetric anal sphincter rupture using the overlap technique. Br J Obstet Gynaecol 106:318, 1999

Thilaganathan B, Cutner A, Latimer J, et al: Management of the third-stage of labour in women at low risk of postpartum haemorrhage. Eur J Obstet Gynecol Reprod Biol 48:19, 1993

Thornton JG, Lilford RJ: Active management of labour: Current knowledge and research issues [published correction appears in Br Med J 309:704, 1994]. Br Med J 309:366, 1994

Venkatesh KS, Ramanujam PS, Larson DM, et al: Anorectal complications of vaginal delivery. Dis Colon Rectum 32:1039, 1989

Villar J, Gülmezoglu AM, Hofmeyr GJ, et al: Systematic review of randomized controlled trials of misoprostol to prevent postpartum hemorrhage. Obstet Gynecol 100:1301, 2002

Weber AM, Meyn L: Episiotomy use in the United States, 1979–1997. Obstet Gynecol 100:1177, 2002

Whalley PJ, Pritchard JA: Oxytocin and water intoxication. JAMA 186:601, 1963

Yamada H, Kishida T, Negishi H, et al: Silent premature rupture of membranes, detected and monitored serially by an AFP kit. J Obstet Gynaecol Res 24:103, 1998

Yao AC, Lind J: Placental transfusion. Am J Dis Child 127:128, 1974

Zhang J, Troendle JF, Yancey MK: Reassessing the labor curve in nulliparous women. Am J Obstet Gynecol 187:824, 2002

18

Intrapartum Assessment

During the late 1960s, continuous electronic fetal monitoring was introduced into obstetrical practice. No longer were intrapartum fetal surveillance and the suspicion of fetal distress based upon periodic auscultation with a fetoscope. Instead, the continuous graph paper portrayal of the fetal heart rate was potentially diagnostic in assessing pathophysiological events affecting the fetus. Indeed, there were great expectations that:

1. Electronic fetal heart rate monitoring provided accurate information.
2. The information was of value in diagnosing fetal distress.
3. It would be possible to intervene to prevent fetal death or morbidity.
4. Continuous electronic fetal heart rate monitoring was superior to intermittent methods.

When first introduced, electronic fetal heart rate monitoring was used primarily in complicated pregnancies, but gradually it came to be used in most pregnancies. By 1978 it was estimated that nearly two thirds of American women were being monitored electronically during labor (Banta and Thacker, 1979). In 2002, approximately 3.4 million American women, comprising 85 percent of all live births, underwent electronic fetal monitoring (Martin and colleagues, 2003). Indeed, fetal monitoring has become the most prevalent obstetrical procedure in the United States.

ELECTRONIC FETAL MONITORING

INTERNAL ELECTRONIC FETAL HEART RATE MONITORING. The fetal heart rate may be measured by attaching a bipolar spiral electrode directly to the fetus (Fig. 18–1). The wire electrode penetrates the fetal scalp,

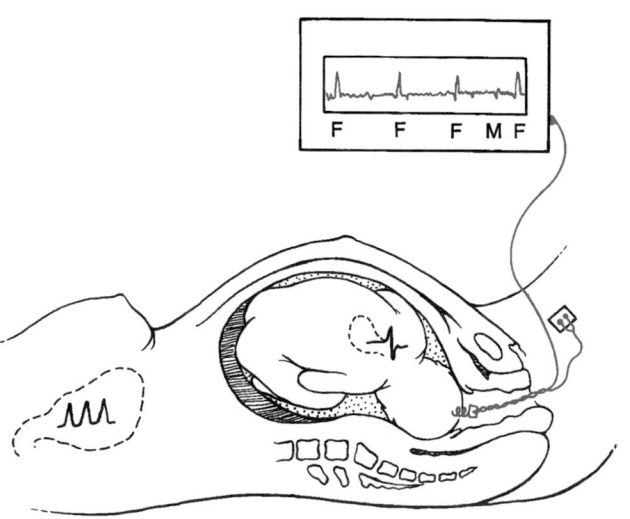

FIGURE 18–1. Schematic representation of a bipolar electrode attached to fetal scalp for detection of fetal QRS complexes (F). Also shown is the maternal heart and corresponding electrical complexes (M) that are detected.

and the second pole is a metal wing on the electrode. Vaginal body fluids create a saline electrical bridge that completes the circuit and permits measurement of the voltage differences between the two poles. The electrical fetal cardiac signal— P wave, QRS complex, and T wave—is amplified and fed into a cardiotachometer for heart rate calculation. The peak R-wave voltage is the portion of the fetal electrocardiogram most reliably detected. The two wires of the bipolar electrode are attached to a reference electrode on the maternal thigh to eliminate electrical interference.

Shown in Figure 18–2 is an example of the method of fetal heart rate processing employed when a scalp electrode is used. Time (t) in milliseconds between fetal R waves is fed into a cardiotachometer, where a new fetal heart rate is set with the arrival of each new R wave. As also shown in Figure 18–2, a premature atrial contraction is computed as a heart rate acceleration because the interval (t_2) is shorter than the preceding one (t_1). The phenomenon of continuous R-to-R wave fetal heart rate computation is known as *beat-to-beat variability*. The physiological event being counted, however, is not a mechanical event corresponding to a heartbeat but rather an electrical event.

Electrical cardiac complexes detected by the electrode include those generated by the mother. Although the maternal electrocardiogram (ECG) signal is approximately five times stronger than the fetal ECG, its amplitude is diminished when it is recorded through the fetal scalp electrode. In a live fetus, this low maternal ECG signal is detected but masked by the fetal ECG. If the fetus is dead, the weaker maternal signal will

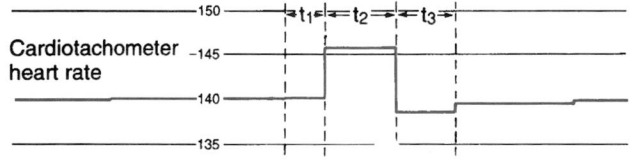

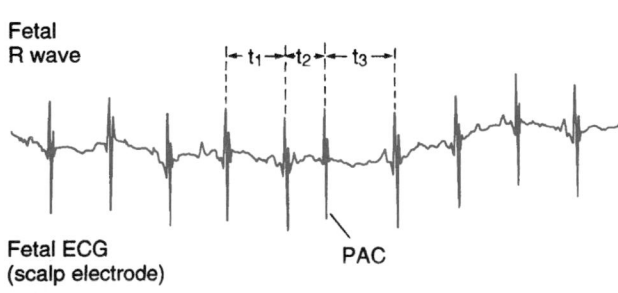

FIGURE 18–2. Schematic representation of fetal electrocardiographic signals used to compute continuing beat-to-beat heart rate with scalp electrodes. Time intervals (t_1, t_2, t_3) in milliseconds between successive fetal R waves are used by cardiotachometer to compute instantaneous fetal heart rate. (PAC = premature atrial contraction.)

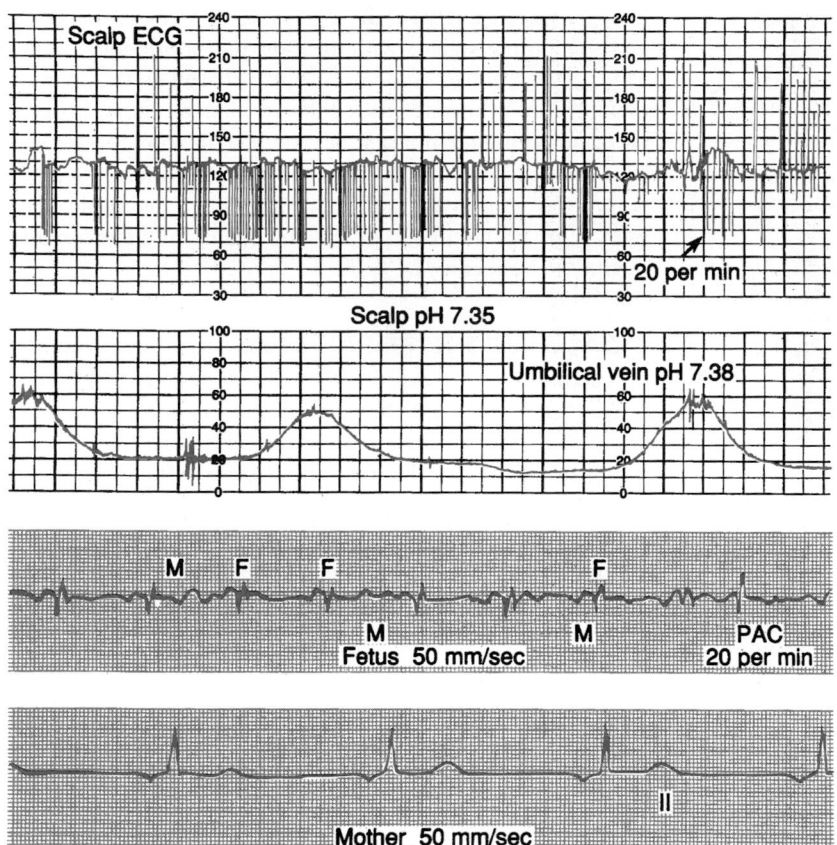

FIGURE 18–3. Standard fetal monitor tracing of heart rate using fetal scalp electrode shown at top. Bottom two tracings represent cardiac electrical complexes detected from fetal scalp and maternal chest wall electrodes. Spiking of the fetal rate in the monitor tracing is due to the premature atrial contractions. (F = fetus; M = mother; PAC = fetal premature atrial contraction.)

be amplified and displayed as the "fetal" heart rate (Freeman and co-authors, 2003). Shown in Figure 18–3 are simultaneous recordings of maternal chest wall ECG signals and fetal scalp electrode ECG signals. This fetus is experiencing premature atrial contractions, which cause the cardiotachometer to rapidly and erratically seek new heart rates, resulting in the "spiking" shown in the standard fetal monitor tracing. Importantly, when the fetus is dead, the maternal R waves are still detected by the scalp electrode as the next best signal and are counted by the cardiotachometer (Fig. 18–4).

EXTERNAL (INDIRECT) ELECTRONIC FETAL HEART RATE MONITORING. The necessity for membrane rupture and uterine invasion may be avoided by use of external detectors to monitor fetal heart action and uterine activity. External monitoring does not provide the precision

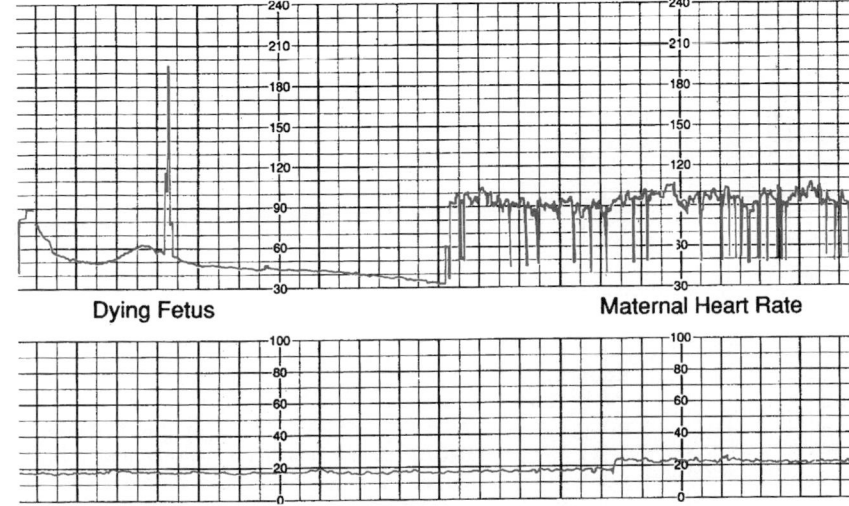

FIGURE 18–4. Placental abruption: The fetal scalp electrode detected the heart rate first of the dying fetus. After fetal death, the maternal electrocardiogram complex is detected and recorded.

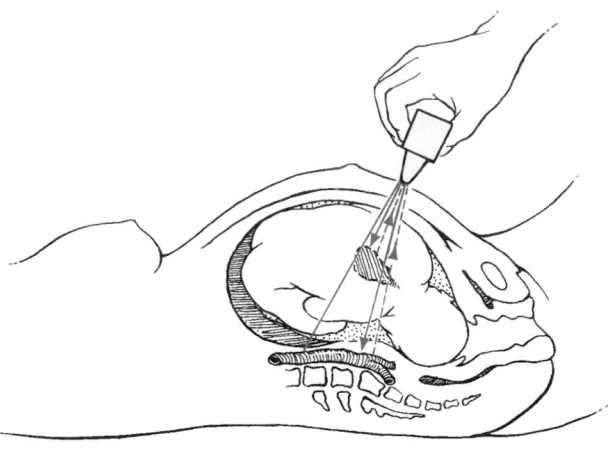

FIGURE 18–5. Ultrasound Doppler principle used externally to measure fetal heart motions. Pulsations of the maternal aorta also may be detected and counted. (Adapted from Klavan and co-authors, 1977, with permission.)

of fetal heart rate measurement or the quantification of uterine pressure afforded by internal monitoring.

The fetal heart rate is detected through the maternal abdominal wall using the *ultrasound Doppler principle* (Fig. 18–5). Ultrasonic waves undergo a shift in frequency as they are reflected from moving fetal heart valves and from pulsatile blood ejected during systole. The unit consists of a transducer that emits ultrasound and a sensor to detect a shift in frequency of the reflected sound. The transducer is placed on the maternal abdomen at a site where fetal heart action is best detected. A coupling gel must be applied because air conducts ultrasound poorly. The device is held in position by a belt. Care should be taken that maternal aortic pulsations are not confused with fetal cardiac motion.

Ultrasound Doppler signals are edited electronically before fetal heart rate data are printed onto the bedside monitor tracing paper. Reflected ultrasound signals from moving fetal heart valves are analyzed through a microprocessor that compares incoming signals with the most recent previous signal. This process, called *autocorrelation*, is based on the premise that the fetal heart rate has regularity whereas "noise" is random and without regularity. Several fetal heart motions must be deemed electronically acceptable by the microprocessor before the fetal heart rate is printed. Such electronic editing has greatly improved the tracing quality of the externally recorded fetal heart rate.

FETAL HEART RATE PATTERNS. It is now generally accepted that interpretation of fetal heart rate patterns can be problematic because of the lack of agreement on definitions and nomenclature (Freeman, 2002). The National Institute of Child Health and Human Development Research Planning Workshop (1997) brought together investigators with expertise in the field to propose standardized, unambiguous definitions for interpretation of fetal heart rate patterns during labor. The definitions proposed as a result of this workshop will be used in this chapter. It is important to recognize that interpretation of electronic fetal heart rate data is based on the visual pattern of the heart rate as portrayed on chart recorder graph paper. Thus, the choice of vertical and horizontal scaling greatly affects the appearance of the fetal heart rate. Scaling factors recommended by the workshop are 30 beats per minute (beats/min or bpm) per vertical cm (range, 30 to 240 beats/min) and 3 cm/min chart recorder paper speed. Fetal heart rate variation is falsely displayed at the slower 1 cm/min paper speed when compared with that of the smoother baseline recorded at 3 cm/min (Fig. 18–6). Thus, pattern recognition can be considerably distorted depending on the scaling factors used.

Baseline Fetal Heart Activity. Baseline fetal heart activity refers to the modal characteristics that prevail apart from periodic accelerations or decelerations associated with

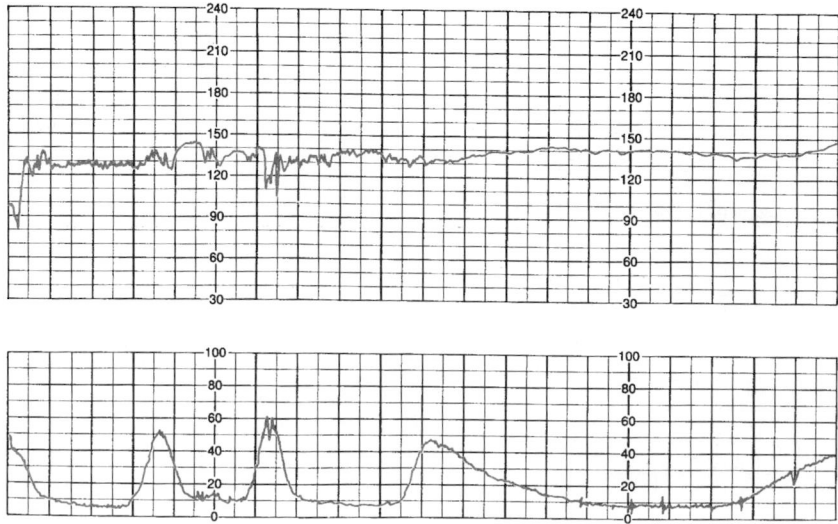

FIGURE 18–6. Fetal heart rate obtained by scalp electrode and recorded at 1 cm/min compared with that of 3 cm/min chart recorder paper speed.

uterine contractions. Descriptive characteristics of baseline fetal heart activity include *rate, beat-to-beat variability, fetal arrhythmia*, and distinct patterns such as *sinusoidal* or *saltatory* fetal heart rates.

RATE. With increasing fetal maturation, the heart rate decreases. This continues postnatally such that the average rate is 90 beats/min by age 8 (Behrman, 1992). Pillai and James (1990) longitudinally studied fetal heart rate characteristics in 43 normal pregnancies. The baseline fetal heart rate decreased an average of 24 beats/min between 16 weeks and term, or approximately 1 beat/min per week. It is postulated that this normal gradual slowing of the fetal heart rate corresponds to maturation of parasympathetic (vagal) heart control (Renou and co-workers, 1969).

The baseline fetal heart rate is the approximate mean rate rounded to increments of 5 beats/min during a 10-minute tracing segment. In any 10-minute window, the minimum interpretable baseline duration must be at least 2 minutes. If the baseline fetal heart rate is less than 110 beats/min, it is termed *bradycardia;* if the baseline rate is greater than 160 beats/min, it is termed *tachycardia*. The average fetal heart rate is considered to be the result of tonic balance between *accelerator* and *decelerator* influences on pacemaker cells. In this concept, the sympathetic system is the accelerator influence, and the parasympathetic system is the decelerator factor mediated via vagal slowing of heart rate (Dawes, 1985). Heart rate also is under the control of arterial chemoreceptors such that both hypoxia and hypercapnia can modulate rate. More severe and prolonged hypoxia, with a rising blood lactate level and severe metabolic acidemia, induces a prolonged fall of heart rate due to direct effects on the myocardium.

BRADYCARDIA. During the third trimester, the normal mean baseline fetal heart rate has generally been accepted to be between 120 and 160 beats/min. The lower normal limit is disputed internationally with some investigators recommending 110 beats/min (Manassiev, 1996). Pragmatically, a rate between 100 and 119 beats/min, in the absence of other changes, usually is not considered to represent fetal compromise. Such low but potentially normal baseline heart rates also have been attributed to head compression from occiput posterior or transverse positions, particularly during second-stage labor (Young and Weinstein, 1976). Such mild bradycardias were observed in 2 percent of monitored pregnancies and averaged about 50 minutes in duration. Freeman and colleagues (2003) have concluded that bradycardia within the range of 80 to 120 beats/min with good variability is reassuring. Interpretation of rates less than 80 beats/min is problematic, and such rates generally are considered nonreassuring.

Some causes of fetal bradycardia include congenital heart block and serious fetal compromise. Figure 18–7 shows bradycardia in a fetus dying from placental abruption. Maternal hypothermia under general anesthesia for repair of a cerebral aneurysm or during maternal cardiopulmonary bypass

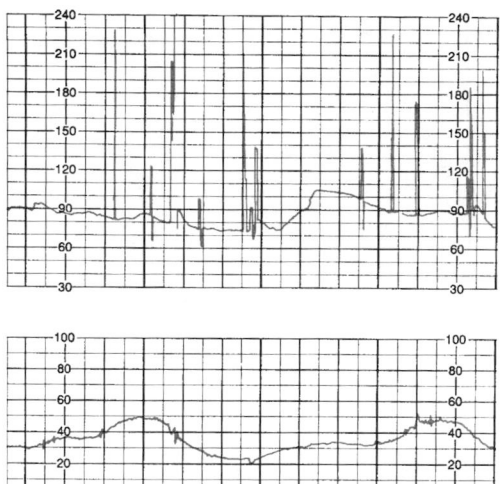

FIGURE 18–7. Fetal bradycardia measured with a scalp electrode in a pregnancy complicated by placental abruption and subsequent fetal death.

for open-heart surgery also can cause fetal bradycardia (see Chap. 44, p. 1023). Sustained fetal bradycardia in the setting of severe pyelonephritis and maternal hypothermia also has been reported (Hankins and co-workers, 1997). These infants apparently are not harmed by several hours of such bradycardia.

TACHYCARDIA. Fetal tachycardia is defined as a baseline heart rate in excess of 160 beats/min. The most common explanation for fetal tachycardia is maternal fever from amnionitis, although fever from any source can increase baseline fetal heart rate. Such infections also have been observed to induce fetal tachycardia before overt maternal fever is diagnosed (Gilstrap and associates, 1987). Fetal tachycardia caused by maternal infection typically is not associated with fetal compromise unless there are associated periodic heart rate changes or fetal sepsis.

Other causes of fetal tachycardia include fetal compromise, cardiac arrhythmias, and maternal administration of parasympathetic (atropine) or sympathomimetic (terbutaline) drugs. The key feature to distinguish fetal compromise in association with tachycardia seems to be concomitant heart rate decelerations. Prompt relief of the compromising event, such as correction of maternal hypotension caused by epidural analgesia, can result in fetal recovery.

WANDERING BASELINE. This baseline rate is unsteady and "wanders" between 120 and 160 beats/min (Freeman and colleagues, 2003). This rare finding is suggestive of a neurologically abnormal fetus and may occur as a preterminal event.

BEAT-TO-BEAT VARIABILITY. Baseline variability is an important index of cardiovascular function and appears to be regulated largely by the autonomic nervous system (Kozuma

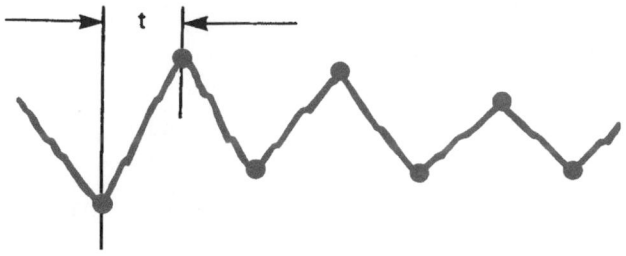

FIGURE 18–8. Schematic representation of short-term beat-to-beat variability measured by a fetal scalp electrode. (t = time interval between successive fetal R waves.) (From Klavan and co-authors, 1977.)

and colleagues, 1997). That is, sympathetic and parasympathetic "push-pull," mediated via the sinoatrial node, produces moment-to-moment or beat-to-beat oscillation of the baseline heart rate. Such irregularity of the heart rate is defined as baseline variability. Variability is further divided into short term and long term.

Short-term variability reflects the instantaneous change in fetal heart rate from one beat—or R wave—to the next. This variability is a measure of the time interval between cardiac systoles (Fig. 18–8). Short-term variability can most reliably be determined to be normally present only when electrocardiac cycles are measured directly with a scalp electrode. *Long-term variability* is used to describe the oscillatory changes that occur during the course of 1 minute and result in the waviness of the baseline (Fig. 18–9). The normal frequency of such waves is three to five cycles per minute (Freeman and co-authors, 2003).

It should be recognized that precise quantitative analysis of both short- and long-term variability presents a number of frustrating problems due to technical and scaling factors. For example, Parer and co-workers (1985) evaluated 22 mathematical formulas designed to quantify heart rate variability and most were unsatisfactory. Consequently, most clinical interpretation is based on visual analysis with subjective judgment of the smoothness or flatness of the baseline. According to Freeman and colleagues (2003), there is no current evidence that the distinction between short- and long-term variability has any clinical relevance. Similarly, the NICHD Workshop (1997) did not recommend differentiating short- and long-term variability because in actual practice they are visually determined as a unit. The workshop panel defined

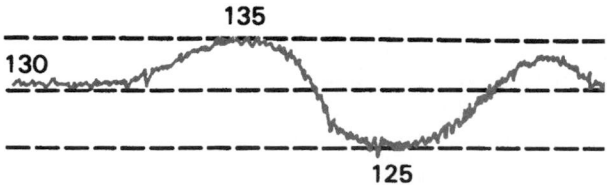

FIGURE 18–9. Schematic representation of long-term beat-to-beat variability of the fetal heart rate ranging between 125 and 135 beats/min. (From Klavan and co-authors, 1977.)

baseline variability as those baseline fluctuations of two cycles per minute or greater. They recommended the criteria shown in Figure 18–10 for quantification of variability. Normal beat-to-beat variability was accepted to be 6 to 25 beats/min.

Several physiological and pathological processes can affect or interfere with beat-to-beat variability. Dawes and co-workers (1981) described increased variability during *fetal breathing*. In healthy infants, short-term variability is attributable to respiratory sinus arrhythmia (Divon and co-workers, 1986). *Fetal body movements* also affect variability (Van Geijn and co-workers, 1980). Pillai and James (1990) reported increased baseline variability with *advancing gestation*. Up to 30 weeks, baseline characteristics were similar during both fetal rest and activity. After 30 weeks, fetal inactivity was associated with diminished baseline variability and conversely, variability was increased during fetal activity. Fetal gender does not affect heart rate variability (Ogueh and Steer, 1998).

It is important to recognize that the baseline fetal heart rate becomes more physiologically fixed (less variable) as the rate increases. Conversely, there is more instability or variability of the baseline at lower heart rates. This phenomenon presumably reflects less cardiovascular physiological wandering as beat-to-beat intervals shorten due to increasing heart rate.

Diminished beat-to-beat variability can be an ominous sign indicating a seriously compromised fetus. Paul and co-workers (1975) reported that loss of variability in combination with decelerations was associated with fetal acidemia. They analyzed variability in the 20 minutes preceding delivery in 194 pregnancies. Decreased variability was defined as 5 or fewer beats/min excursion of the baseline (see Fig. 18–10), whereas acceptable variability exceeded this range. Fetal scalp pH was measured 1119 times in these pregnancies, and mean values were found to be increasingly more acidemic when decreased variability was added to progressively intense heart rate decelerations. For example, mean fetal scalp pH of about 7.10 was found when severe decelerations were combined with 5 beats/min or less variability compared with a pH about 7.20 when greater variability was associated with similarly severe decelerations.

Severe *maternal acidemia* also can cause decreased fetal beat-to-beat variability, as shown in Figure 18–11 in a mother with diabetic ketoacidosis. The precise pathological mechanisms by which fetal hypoxemia results in diminished beat-to-beat variability are not totally understood.

Interestingly, mild degrees of fetal hypoxemia have been reported actually to *increase* variability, at least at the outset of the hypoxic episode (Murotsuki and co-authors, 1997). According to Dawes (1985), it seems probable that the loss of variability is a result of metabolic acidemia that causes depression of the fetal brainstem or the heart itself. Thus, diminished beat-to-beat variability, when a reflection of compromised fetal condition, likely reflects acidemia rather than hypoxia.

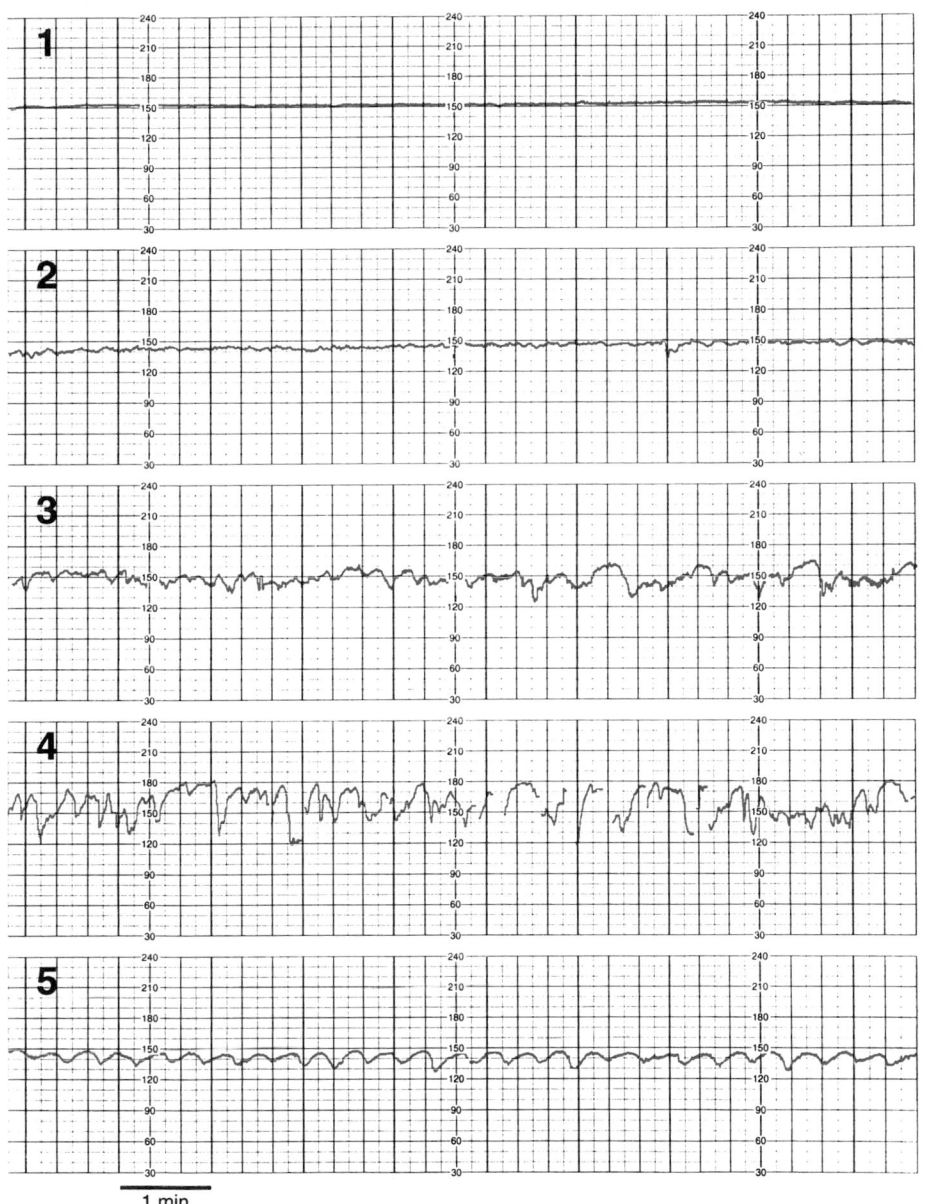

FIGURE 18-10. Grades of baseline fetal heart rate variability (irregular fluctuations in the baseline of 2 cycles per minute or greater) together with a sinusoidal pattern. The sinusoidal pattern differs from variability in that it has a smooth, sinelike pattern of regular fluctuation and is excluded in the definition of fetal heart rate variability. (1) Undetectable, absent variability; (2) minimal ≤ 5 beats/min variability; (3) moderate (normal), 6 to 25 beats/min variability; (4) marked, > 25 beats/min variability; (5) sinusoidal pattern. (From National Institute of Child Health and Human Development Research Planning Workshop, 1997.)

A common cause of diminished beat-to-beat variability is *analgesic drugs* given during labor (see Chap. 19, p. 476). A large variety of central nervous system depressant drugs can cause transient diminished beat-to-beat variability. Included are narcotics, barbiturates, phenothiazines, tranquilizers, and general anesthetics. Diminished variability occurs regularly within 5 to 10 minutes following intravenous meperidine administration, and the effects may last up to 60 minutes or longer depending on the dosage given (Petrie, 1993). Butorphanol given intravenously diminishes fetal heart rate reactivity (Schucker and colleagues, 1996). Hill and colleagues (2003), in a study performed at Parkland Hospital, found that 5 beats/min or less variability occurred in 30 percent of women given continuous intravenous meperidine compared with 7 percent in those given continuous labor epidural analgesia using 0.0625-percent bupivacaine and 2 μg/mL of fentanyl.

Magnesium sulfate, widely used in the United States for tocolysis as well as management of hypertensive women, has been arguably associated with diminished beat-to-beat variability. Hallak and colleagues (1999) randomly assigned 34 normal, nonlaboring women to standard magnesium sulfate infusion versus isotonic saline. Magnesium sulfate was associated with statistically decreased variability only in the third hour of the infusion. However, the average decrease in variability was deemed clinically insignificant because the mean variability was 2.7 beats/min in the third hour of magnesium infusion compared with 2.8 beats/min at baseline. Magnesium sulfate also blunted the frequency of accelerations.

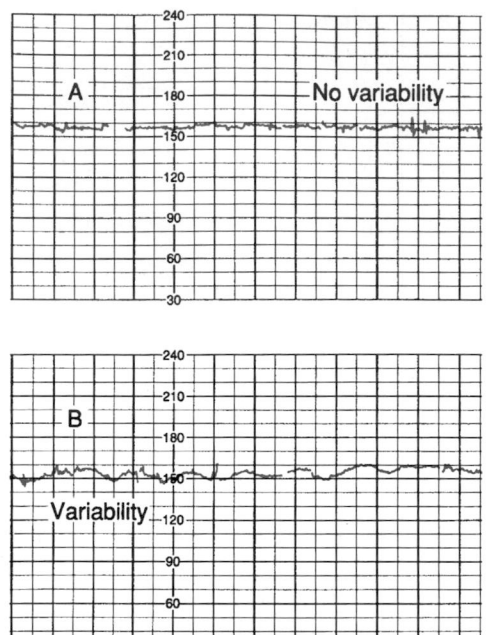

FIGURE 18–11. A. External fetal heart recording showing lack of long-term variability at 31 weeks during maternal diabetic ketoacidosis (pH 7.09). B. Recovery of fetal long-term variability after correction of maternal acidemia.

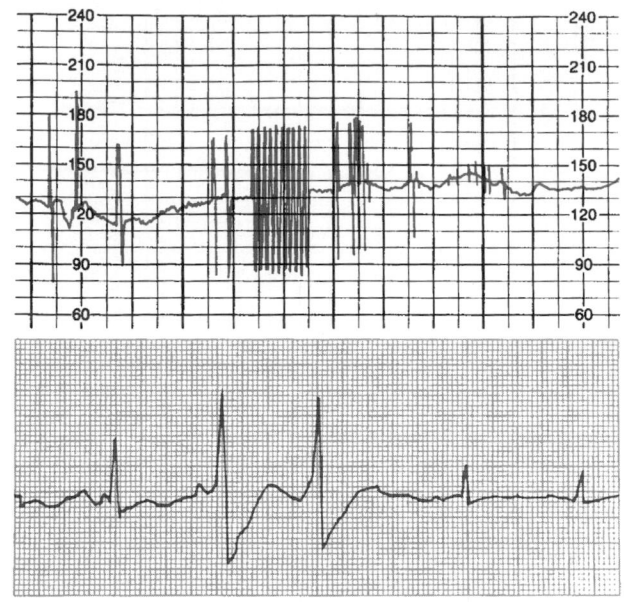

FIGURE 18–12. Internal fetal monitoring at term demonstrated occasional abrupt beat-to-beat fetal heart rate spiking due to erratic extrasystoles shown in the superimposed fetal electrocardiogram. The normal infant was delivered spontaneously and had a normal cardiac rhythm in the nursery.

It is generally believed that reduced baseline heart rate variability is the single most reliable sign of fetal compromise. For example, Smith and co-workers (1988) performed a computerized analysis of beat-to-beat variability in growth-restricted fetuses *before* labor. They observed that diminished variability (4.2 beats/min or less) that was maintained for 1 hour was diagnostic of developing acidemia and imminent fetal death. By contrast, Samueloff and associates (1994) evaluated variability as a predictor of fetal outcome during labor in 2200 consecutive deliveries. They concluded that variability by itself cannot be used as the only indicator of fetal well-being. Conversely, they also concluded that good variability should not be interpreted as necessarily reassuring.

In summary, beat-to-beat variability is affected by a variety of pathological and physiological mechanisms. Variability has considerably different meaning depending on the clinical setting. The development of decreased variability in the absence of decelerations is unlikely to be due to fetal hypoxia (Davidson and co-workers, 1992). A persistently flat fetal heart rate baseline—absent variability—within the normal baseline rate range and without decelerations may reflect a previous insult to the fetus that has resulted in neurological damage (Freeman and colleagues, 2003).

CARDIAC ARRHYTHMIA. When fetal cardiac arrhythmias are first suspected using electronic monitoring, findings can include baseline bradycardia, tachycardia, or most commonly in our experience, *abrupt baseline spiking* (Fig. 18–12). Intermittent baseline bradycardia is frequently due to congenital heart block. As discussed in Chapter 54 (p. 1215), conduction defects, most commonly complete atrioventricular (AV) block, usually are found in association with maternal connective-tissue diseases. Documentation of an arrhythmia can only be accomplished, practically speaking, when scalp electrodes are used. Some fetal monitors can be adapted to output the scalp electrode signals into an electrocardiographic recorder. Because only a single lead is obtained, analysis and interpretation of rhythm and rate disturbances are severely limited.

Southall and co-authors (1980) studied antepartum fetal cardiac rate and rhythm disturbances in 934 normal pregnancies between 30 and 40 weeks. Arrhythmias and episodes of bradycardia less than 100 beats/min, or tachycardia greater than 180 beats/min, were encountered in 3 percent. Most supraventricular arrhythmias are of little significance during labor unless there is coexistent heart failure as evidenced by fetal hydrops. Many supraventricular arrhythmias disappear in the immediate neonatal period, although some are associated with structural cardiac defects. Copel and co-authors (2000) used echocardiography to evaluate 614 fetuses referred for auscultated irregular heart rate without hydrops. Only 10 fetuses (2 percent) were found to have significant arrhythmias, and all but one infant survived.

Boldt and colleagues (2003) followed 292 consecutive fetuses diagnosed with a cardiac arrhythmia through birth and into childhood. Atrial extrasystoles comprised the most common arrhythmia (68 percent), followed by atrial tachycardias (12 percent), atrioventricular block (12 percent), sinus bradycardia (5 percent), and ventricular extrasystoles (2.5 percent). Chromosomal anomalies were found in 1.7 percent of the fetuses. Fetal hydrops developed in 11 percent, and 2 percent had intrauterine deaths. Fetal hydrops was a bad prognostic finding. Overall, 93 percent of the study population was alive at a median follow-up period of 5 years, and 3 percent (7 infants) had neurological handicaps. Almost all (97 percent) of the infants with atrial extrasystoles lived, and none suffered neurological injury. Only 6 percent required postnatal cardiac medications.

Although most fetal arrhythmias are of little consequence during labor when there is no evidence of fetal hydrops, such arrhythmias impair interpretation of intrapartum heart rate tracings. Ultrasonic survey of fetal anatomy as well as echocardiography may be useful. Some clinicians use fetal scalp sampling as an adjunct. Generally, in the absence of fetal hydrops, neonatal outcome is not measurably improved by pregnancy intervention. At Parkland Hospital, intrapartum fetal cardiac arrhythmias, especially in the presence of clear amnionic fluid, are managed conservatively. Freeman and colleagues (2003) have extensively reviewed interpretation of the fetal electrocardiogram during labor.

SINUSOIDAL HEART RATE. A true sinusoidal pattern such as that shown in panel 5 of Figure 18–10 may be observed with serious fetal anemia, whether from D-isoimmunization, ruptured vasa previa, fetomaternal hemorrhage, or twin-to-twin transfusion. Insignificant sinusoidal patterns have been reported following administration of meperidine, morphine, alphaprodine, and butorphanol (Angel, 1984; Egley, 1991; Epstein, 1982, and all their associates). Shown in Figure 18–13 is a sinusoidal pattern seen with maternal meperidine administration. An important characteristic of this pattern when due to narcotics is the sine frequency of 6 cycles per minute. A sinusoidal pattern also has been described with amnionitis, fetal distress, and umbilical cord occlusion (Murphy and

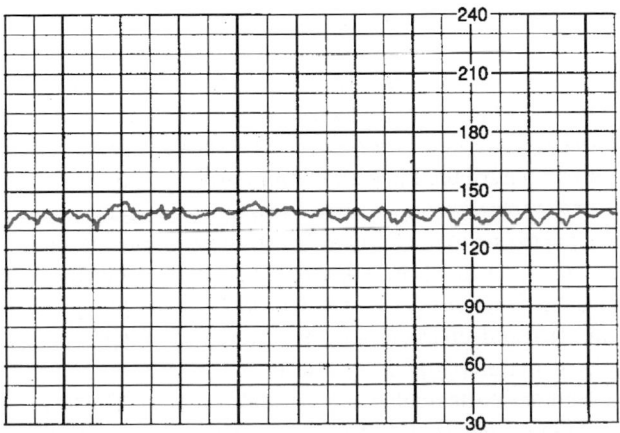

FIGURE 18–13. Sinusoidal fetal heart rate pattern associated with maternal intravenous meperidine administration. Sine waves are occurring at a rate of 6 cycles per minute.

associates, 1991). Young and co-workers (1980a) and Johnson and colleagues (1981) concluded that intrapartum sinusoidal fetal heart patterns were not generally associated with fetal compromise.

Modanlou and Freeman (1982), based on their extensive review, proposed adoption of a strict definition:

1. Stable baseline heart rate of 120 to 160 beats/min with regular oscillations.
2. Amplitude of 5 to 15 beats/min (rarely greater).
3. Long-term variability frequency of 2 to 5 cycles per minute.
4. Fixed or flat short-term variability.
5. Oscillation of the sinusoidal waveform above or below a baseline.
6. Absence of accelerations.

Although these criteria were selected to define a sinusoidal pattern that is most likely ominous, they observed that the pattern associated with alphaprodine is indistinguishable. Other investigators have proposed a classification of sinusoidal heart rate patterns into mild (amplitude 5 to 15 beats/min), intermediate (16 to 24 beats/min), and major (25 or more beats/min) to quantify fetal risk (Murphy and colleagues, 1991; Neesham and co-workers, 1993).

Some investigators have defined intrapartum sine wave–like baseline variation with periods of acceleration as *pseudosinusoidal*. Murphy and co-workers (1991) reported that pseudosinusoidal patterns were seen in 15 percent of monitored labors. Mild pseudosinusoidal patterns were associated with use of meperidine and epidural analgesia. Intermediate pseudosinusoidal patterns were linked to fetal sucking or transient episodes of fetal hypoxia caused by umbilical cord compression. Egley and colleagues (1991) reported that 4 percent of fetuses demonstrated sinusoidal patterns transiently during normal labor. These authors observed patterns for up to 90 minutes in some cases and also in association with oxytocin or alphaprodine usage, or both.

The pathophysiology of sinusoidal patterns is unclear, in part due to various definitions. There seems to be general agreement that *antepartum* sine wave baseline undulation portends severe fetal anemia, however, few D-isoimmunized fetuses develop this pattern (Nicolaides and associates, 1989). The sinusoidal pattern has been reported to develop or disappear after fetal transfusion (Del Valle and associates, 1992; Lowe and co-workers, 1984). Ikeda and colleagues (1999) have proposed, based on studies in fetal lambs, that the sinusoidal fetal heart rate pattern is related to waves of arterial blood pressure, reflecting oscillations in the baroreceptor–chemoreceptor feedback mechanism for control of the circulation.

Periodic Fetal Heart Rate Changes. The periodic fetal heart rate refers to deviations from baseline that are related to uterine contractions. *Acceleration* refers to an increase in fetal heart rate above baseline and *deceleration* to a decrease below baseline rate. The nomenclature most commonly used in the United States is based upon the *timing* of the deceleration in relation to contractions—thus, *early, late,* or *variable* in onset related to the corresponding uterine contraction. The waveform of these decelerations is also significant for pattern recognition. In early and late decelerations, the slope of fetal heart rate change is gradual, resulting in a curvilinear and uniform or symmetrical waveform. With variable decelerations, the slope of fetal heart rate change is abrupt and erratic, giving the waveform a jagged appearance. It has been proposed that decelerations be defined as *recurrent* if they occur with 50 percent or more of contractions in any 20-minute period (NICHD Research Planning Workshop, 1997).

Another system now used less often for description of decelerations is based on the pathophysiological events considered most likely to cause the pattern. In this system, early decelerations are termed *head compression,* late decelerations are termed *uteroplacental insufficiency,* and variable decelerations become *cord compression patterns.* The nomenclature of type I (early), type II (late), and type III (variable) "dips" proposed by Caldeyro-Barcia and co-workers (1973) is not used in the United States.

ACCELERATIONS. An acceleration is a visually apparent abrupt increase—defined as onset of acceleration to a peak in less than 30 seconds—in the fetal heart rate baseline (NICHD Research Planning Workshop, 1997). According to Freeman and co-authors (2003), accelerations most often occur antepartum, in early labor, and in association with variable decelerations. Proposed mechanisms for intrapartum accelerations include fetal movement, stimulation by uterine contractions, umbilical cord occlusion, and fetal stimulation during pelvic examination. Fetal scalp blood sampling and acoustic stimulation also incite fetal heart rate acceleration (Clark and co-workers, 1982). Finally, acceleration can occur during labor without any apparent stimulus. Indeed, accelerations are common in labor and nearly always associated with fetal movement. These accelerations are virtually always reassuring and almost always confirm that the fetus is not acidemic at that time.

Accelerations seem to have the same physiological explanations as beat-to-beat variability in that they represent intact neurohormonal cardiovascular control mechanisms linked to fetal behavioral states. Krebs and co-workers (1982) analyzed electronic heart rate tracings in nearly 2000 fetuses and found sporadic accelerations during labor in 99.8 percent. The presence of fetal heart accelerations during the first or last 30 minutes, or both, was a favorable sign for fetal well-being. The absence of such accelerations during labor, however, is not necessarily an unfavorable sign unless coincidental with other nonreassuring changes. There is about a 50-percent chance of acidemia in the fetus who fails to respond to stimulation in the presence of an otherwise nonreassuring pattern (Clark and colleagues, 1984; Smith and colleagues, 1986).

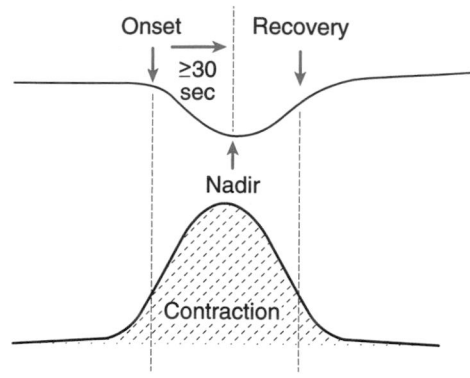

FIGURE 18–14. Features of early fetal heart rate deceleration. Characteristics include gradual decrease in the heart rate with both onset and recovery coincident with the onset and recovery of the contraction. The nadir of the deceleration is 30 seconds or more after the onset of the deceleration.

EARLY DECELERATION. Early deceleration of the fetal heart rate consists of a gradual decrease and return to baseline associated with a contraction (Fig. 18–14). Such early deceleration was first described by Hon (1958). He observed that there was a drop in heart rate with uterine contractions and that this was related to cervical dilatation. He considered these findings to be physiological.

Freeman and co-authors (2003) defined early decelerations as those generally seen in active labor between 4 and 7 cm dilatation. In their definition, the degree of deceleration is generally proportional to the contraction strength and rarely falls below 100 to 110 beats/min or 20 to 30 beats/min below baseline. Such decelerations are uncommon during active labor and are not associated with tachycardia, loss of variability, or other fetal heart rate changes. Importantly, early decelerations are not associated with fetal hypoxia, acidemia, or low Apgar scores.

Head compression probably causes vagal nerve activation as a result of dural stimulation and that mediates the heart rate deceleration (Paul and co-workers, 1964). Ball and Parer (1992) concluded that fetal head compression is a likely cause not only of the deceleration shown in Figure 18–14 but also of those shown in Figure 18–15, which typically occur during second-stage labor. Indeed, they observed that head compression is the likely cause of many variable decelerations classically attributed to cord compression.

LATE DECELERATION. The fetal heart rate response to uterine contractions can be an index of either uterine perfusion or placental function. A late deceleration is a smooth, gradual, symmetrical decrease in fetal heart rate beginning at or after the peak of the contraction and returning to baseline only after the contraction has ended (American College of Obstetricians and Gynecologists, 1995b). In most cases, the onset, nadir, and recovery of the deceleration occur after the beginning, peak, and ending of the contraction, respectively (Fig. 18–16). The magnitude of late decelerations is rarely more than 30 to

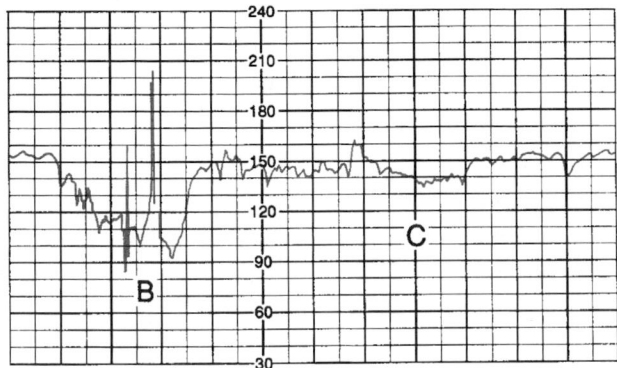

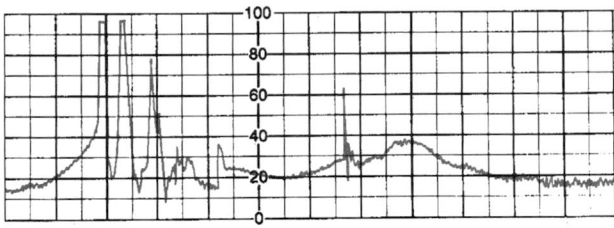

FIGURE 18–15. Two different fetal heart rate patterns during second-stage labor that are likely both due to head compression. Maternal bearing-down efforts correspond to the spikes with uterine contractions. Fetal heart rate deceleration C is consistent with the pattern of head compression shown in Figure 18–12. Deceleration B, however, is "variable" in appearance because of its jagged configuration and may also represent cord occlusion.

40 beats/min below baseline and typically not more than 10 to 20 beats/min. Late decelerations usually are not accompanied by accelerations.

Myers and associates (1973) studied monkeys in which they compromised uteroplacental perfusion by lowering maternal aortic blood pressure. The time interval, or lag period, from the onset of a contraction to the onset of a late deceleration was directly related to basal fetal oxygenation. They

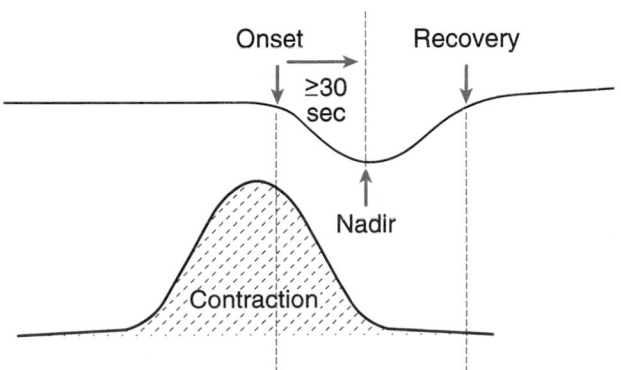

FIGURE 18–16. Features of late fetal heart rate deceleration. Characteristics include gradual decrease in the heart rate with the nadir and recovery occurring after the end of the contraction. The nadir of the deceleration occurs 30 seconds or more after the onset of the deceleration.

demonstrated that the length of the lag phase was predictive of the fetal P_{O_2} but not fetal pH. The lower the fetal P_{O_2} prior to contractions, the shorter the lag phase to onset of late decelerations. This lag period reflected the time necessary for the fetal P_{O_2} to fall below a critical level necessary to stimulate arterial chemoreceptors, which mediated decelerations.

Murata and co-workers (1982) also showed that a late deceleration was the first fetal heart rate consequence of uteroplacental-induced hypoxia. During the course of progressive hypoxia that led to death over 2 to 13 days, the monkey fetuses invariably exhibited late decelerations before the development of acidemia. Variability of the baseline heart rate disappeared as acidemia developed.

A large number of clinical circumstances can result in late decelerations. Generally, any process that causes maternal hypotension, excessive uterine activity, or placental dysfunction can induce late decelerations. The two most common causes are hypotension from epidural analgesia and uterine hyperactivity caused by oxytocin stimulation. Maternal diseases such as hypertension, diabetes, and collagen-vascular disorders can cause chronic placental dysfunction. A rare cause is severe chronic maternal anemia without hypovolemia. Placental abruption can cause acute late decelerations (Fig. 18–17).

VARIABLE DECELERATIONS. The most common deceleration patterns encountered during labor are variable decelerations attributed to umbilical cord occlusion. Melchior and Bernard (1985) identified variable decelerations in 40 percent of over 7000 monitor tracings when labor had progressed to 5 cm dilatation and in 83 percent by the end of the first stage. Variable deceleration of the fetal heart rate is defined as a visually apparent *abrupt* decrease in rate. The onset of deceleration

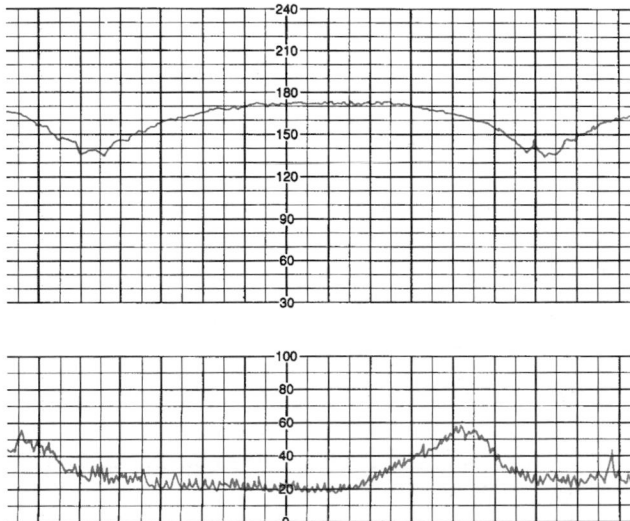

FIGURE 18–17. Late decelerations due to uteroplacental insufficiency resulting from placental abruption. Immediate cesarean delivery was performed. Umbilical artery pH was 7.05 and the P_{O_2} was 11 mm Hg.

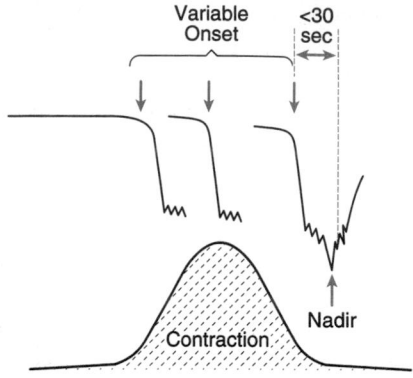

FIGURE 18–18. Features of variable fetal heart rate decelerations. Characteristics include abrupt decrease in the heart rate with onset commonly varying with successive contractions. The decelerations measure ≥ 15 beats/min for 15 seconds or longer with an onset to nadir phase of less than 30 seconds. Total duration is less than 2 minutes.

commonly varies with successive contractions (Fig. 18–18). The duration is less than 2 minutes.

Very early in the development of electronic monitoring, Hon (1959) tested the effects of umbilical cord compression on fetal heart rate (Fig. 18–19). Similar complete occlusion of the umbilical cord in experimental animals produces abrupt, jagged-appearing deceleration of the fetal heart rate (Fig. 18–20). Concomitantly, fetal aortic pressure increases. Itskovitz and co-workers (1983) observed that variable decelerations in fetal lambs occurred only after umbilical blood flow was reduced by at least 50 percent.

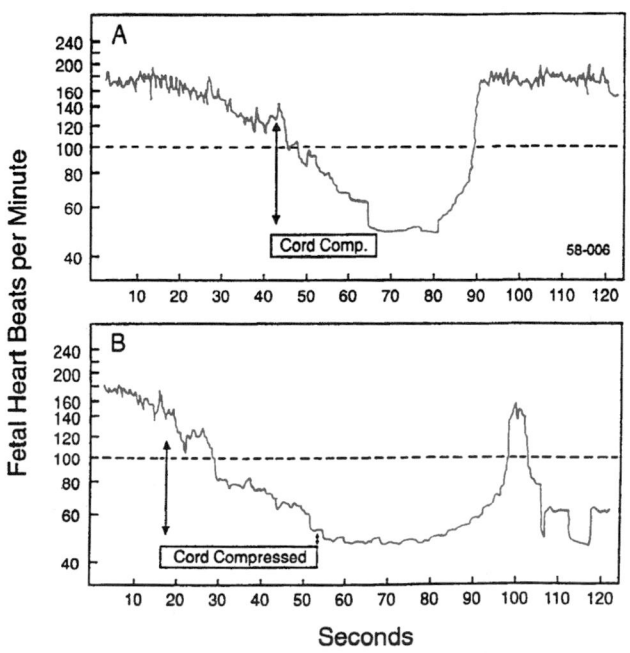

FIGURE 18–19. Fetal heart rate effects of compression of a prolapsed umbilical cord in a 25-week footling breech. Panel **A** shows the effects of 25-second compression compared with those of 40 seconds in panel **B**. (Redrawn from Hon, 1959, with permission.)

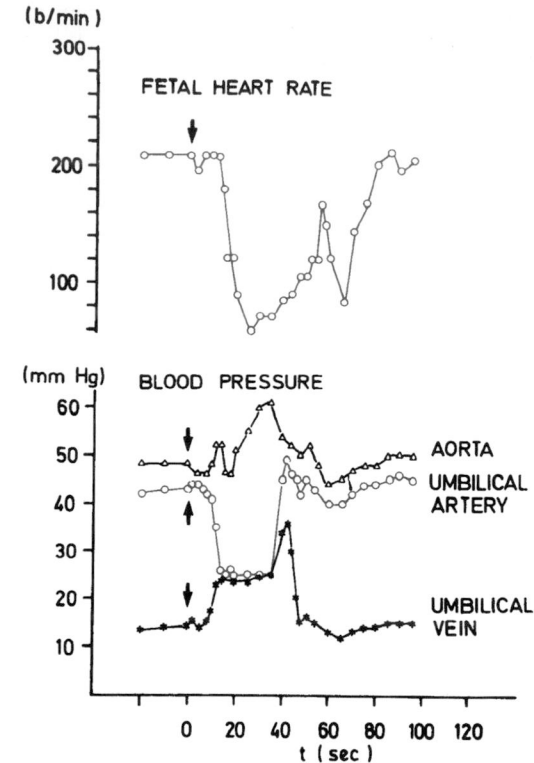

FIGURE 18–20. Total umbilical cord occlusion (*arrow*) in the sheep fetus is accompanied by increase in fetal aortic blood pressure. Blood pressure changes in the umbilical vessels are also shown. (From Kunzel, 1985, with permission.)

Two types of variable decelerations are shown in Figure 18–21. The deceleration denoted by A is very much like that seen with complete umbilical cord occlusion in experimental animals (see Fig. 18–20). Deceleration B, however, has a different configuration because of the "shoulders" of acceleration before and after the deceleration component. Lee and co-workers (1975) proposed that this variation of variable decelerations was caused by differing degrees of partial cord occlusion. In this physiological scheme, occlusion of only the vein reduces fetal blood return, thereby triggering a baroreceptor-mediated acceleration. Subsequent complete occlusion results in fetal systemic hypertension due to obstruction of umbilical artery flow. This stimulates a baroreceptor-mediated deceleration. Presumably, the aftercoming shoulder of acceleration represents the same events occurring in reverse (Fig. 18–22).

Ball and Parer (1992) concluded that variable decelerations are mediated vagally and that the vagal response may be due to chemoreceptor or baroreceptor activity, or both. Partial or complete cord occlusion produces an increase in afterload (baroreceptor) and a decrease in fetal arterial oxygen content (chemoreceptor). These both result in vagal activity leading to deceleration. In fetal monkeys the baroreceptor reflexes appear to be operative during the first 15 to 20 seconds of umbilical cord occlusion followed by decline in P_{O_2} at

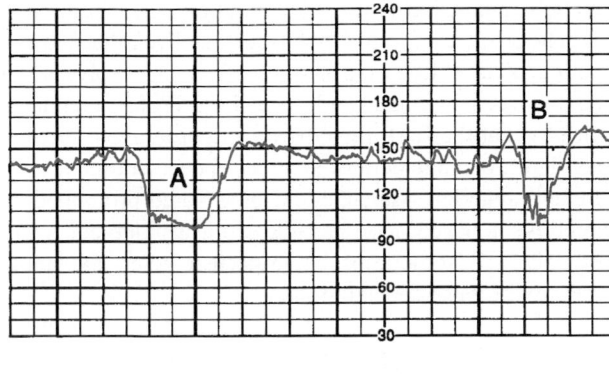

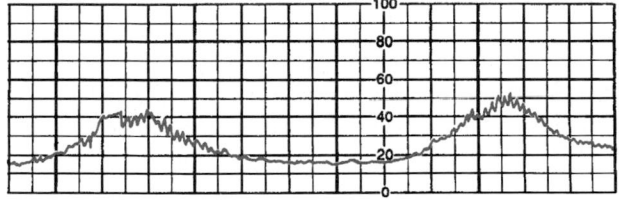

FIGURE 18–21. Varying (variable) fetal heart rate decelerations. Deceleration B exhibits "shoulders" of acceleration compared with deceleration A.

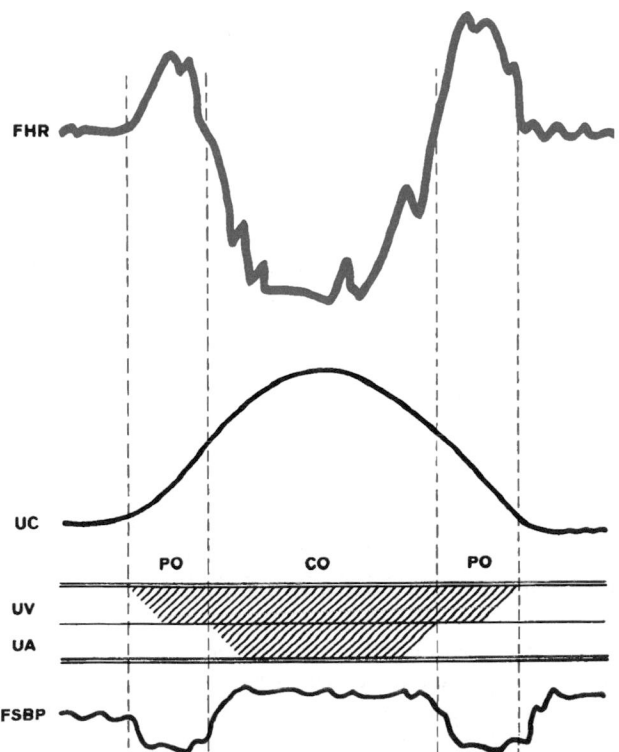

FIGURE 18–22. Schematic representation of the fetal heart rate (FHR) effects of partial occlusion (PO) and complete occlusion (CO) of the umbilical cord. (FSBP = fetal systemic blood pressure; UA = umbilical artery; UC = uterine contraction; UV = umbilical vein.) (From Lee and co-authors, 1975, with permission.)

approximately 30 seconds, which then serves as a chemoreceptor stimulus (Mueller-Heubach and Battelli, 1982).

Thus, variable decelerations represent fetal heart rate reflexes that reflect either blood pressure changes due to interruption of umbilical flow or changes in oxygenation. It is likely that most fetuses have experienced brief but recurrent periods of hypoxia due to umbilical cord compression during gestation. The frequency and inevitability of cord occlusion undoubtedly has provided the fetus with these physiological mechanisms as a means of coping. The great dilemma for the obstetrician in managing variable fetal heart rate decelerations is determining when variable decelerations are pathological. The American College of Obstetricians and Gynecologists (1995b) has defined *significant* variable decelerations as those decreasing to less than 70 beats/min and lasting more than 60 seconds.

Other fetal heart rate patterns have been associated with umbilical cord compression. *Saltatory* baseline heart rate (Fig. 18–23) was first described by Hammacher and co-workers (1968) and linked to umbilical cord complications during labor. Saltatory derives from the Latin and French words meaning "to leap." The pattern consists of rapidly recurring couplets of acceleration and deceleration causing relatively large oscillations of the baseline fetal heart rate. We also observed a relationship between cord occlusion and the saltatory pattern (Leveno and associates, 1984). In the absence of other fetal heart rate findings, these do not signal fetal compromise. *Lambda* is a pattern involving an acceleration followed by a variable deceleration with no acceleration at the

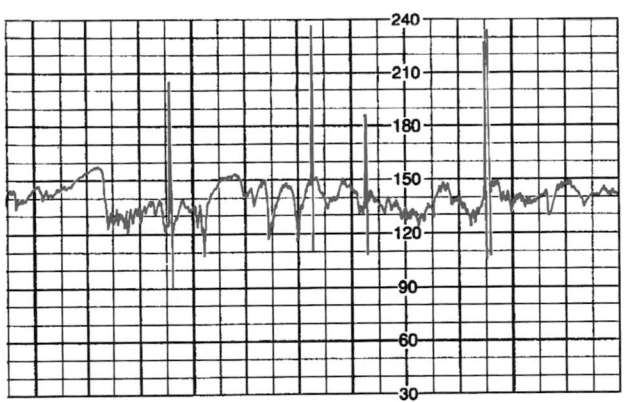

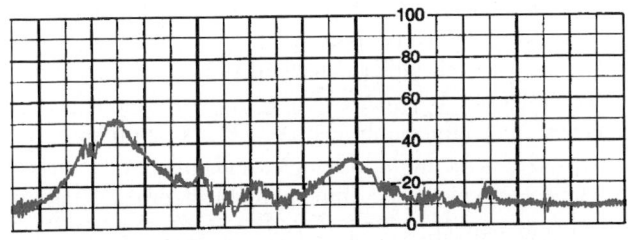

FIGURE 18–23. Saltatory baseline fetal heart rate showing rapidly recurring couplets of acceleration combined with deceleration.

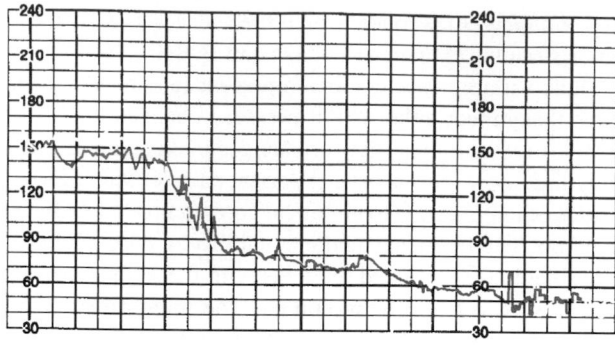

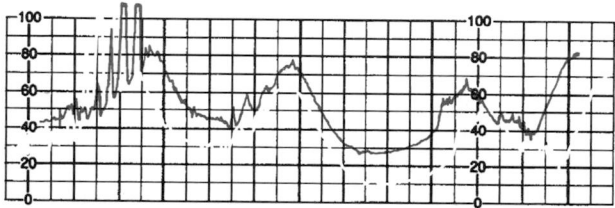

FIGURE 18–24. Prolonged fetal heart rate deceleration due to uterine hyperactivity. Approximately 3 minutes of the tracing are shown, but the fetal heart rate returned to normal after uterine hypertonus resolved. Vaginal delivery later ensued.

end of the deceleration. This pattern typically is seen in early labor and is not ominous (Freeman and colleagues, 2003). This lambda pattern may result from mild cord compression or stretch. *Overshoot* is a variable deceleration followed by acceleration. The clinical significance of this pattern is controversial (Westgate and colleagues, 2001).

PROLONGED DECELERATION. Shown in Figure 18–24, this pattern is defined as an isolated deceleration lasting 2 minutes or longer but less than 10 minutes from onset to return to baseline (NICHD Research Planning Workshop, 1997). Prolonged decelerations are difficult to interpret because they are seen in many different clinical situations. Some of the more common causes include cervical examination, uterine hyperactivity, cord entanglement, and maternal supine hypotension.

Epidural, spinal, or paracervical analgesia may induce prolonged deceleration of the fetal heart rate. For example, Eberle and colleagues (1998) reported that prolonged decelerations occurred in 4 percent of normal parturients given either epidural or intrathecal labor analgesia. Hill and colleagues (2003) observed prolonged deceleration in 1 percent of women given epidural analgesia during labor at Parkland Hospital. Other causes of prolonged deceleration include maternal hypoperfusion or hypoxia from any cause, placental abruption, umbilical cord knots or prolapse, maternal seizures including eclampsia and epilepsy, application of a fetal scalp electrode, impending birth, or even maternal Valsalva maneuver.

The placenta is very effective in resuscitating the fetus if the original insult does not recur immediately. Occasionally,

such self-limited prolonged decelerations are followed by loss of beat-to-beat variability, baseline tachycardia, and even a period of late decelerations, all of which resolve as the fetus recovers. Freeman and co-authors (2003) emphasize rightfully that the fetus may die during prolonged decelerations. Thus, management of prolonged decelerations can be extremely tenuous. Management of isolated prolonged decelerations is based upon bedside clinical judgment, which inevitably will sometimes be imperfect given the unpredictability of these decelerations.

Fetal Heart Rate Patterns During Second-Stage Labor.
Decelerations are virtually ubiquitous. Melchior and Bernard (1985) reported that only 1.4 percent of more than 7000 deliveries did not have fetal heart rate decelerations during second-stage labor. Both cord compression and fetal head compression have been implicated as causes of decelerations and baseline bradycardia during second-stage labor. The high incidence of such patterns minimized their potential significance during the early development and interpretation of electronic monitoring. For example, Boehm (1975) described profound, prolonged fetal heart rate deceleration in the 10 minutes preceding vaginal delivery of 18 healthy infants. Subsequently, Herbert and Boehm (1981) reported another 18 pregnancies with similar prolonged decelerations during second-stage labor, but now associated with one stillbirth and one neonatal death. These experiences attest to the unpredictability of the fetal heart rate during second-stage labor. Spong and colleagues (1998) analyzed the characteristics of second-stage variable fetal heart rate decelerations in 250 deliveries and found that as the total number of decelerations to less than 70 beats/min increased, the 5-minute Apgar score decreased. Put another way, the longer a fetus was exposed to variable decelerations, the lower the Apgar score at 5 minutes.

Picquard and co-workers (1988) analyzed heart rate patterns during second-stage labor in 234 women in an attempt to identify specific patterns to diagnose fetal compromise. Loss of beat-to-beat variability and baseline fetal heart rate less than 90 beats/min were predictive of fetal acidemia. Krebs and co-workers (1981) also found that persistent or progressive baseline bradycardia and baseline tachycardia were associated with low Apgar scores. Gull and colleagues (1996) observed that abrupt fetal heart rate deceleration to less than 100 beats/min, and associated with loss of beat-to-beat variability for 4 minutes or longer, was predictive of fetal acidemia. Thus, abnormal baseline heart rate—either bradycardia or tachycardia, absent beat-to-beat variability, or both—in the presence of second-stage decelerations is associated with increased but not inevitable fetal compromise (Fig. 18–25).

ADMISSION FETAL MONITORING IN LOW-RISK PREGNANCIES. In this application of electronic fetal monitoring, women with low-risk pregnancies are monitored for a short period on admission for labor and continuous monitoring is used only if abnormalities of the fetal heart

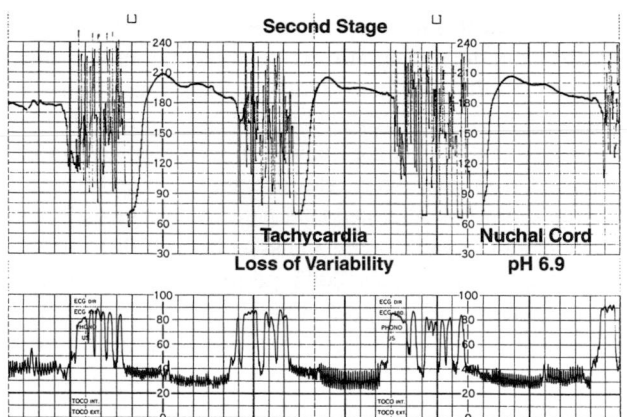

FIGURE 18–25. Cord compression fetal heart rate decelerations in second-stage labor associated with tachycardia and loss of variability. The umbilical cord arterial pH was 6.9.

rate are subsequently identified. Mires and colleagues (2001) randomly assigned 3752 low-risk women in spontaneous labor at the time of admission to either auscultation of the fetal heart rate using Doppler during and immediately after at least one contraction or to 20 minutes of electronic fetal monitoring. Use of admission electronic fetal monitoring did not improve infant outcome. Moreover, its use resulted in increased interventions, including operative delivery. Impey and colleagues (2003) performed a similar study in 8588 low-risk women and also found no improvement in infant outcome. More than half of the women enrolled in these studies, whether they received admission electronic monitoring or auscultation, eventually required continuous monitoring for diagnosed abnormalities in the fetal heart rate.

COMPLICATIONS OF ELECTRONIC FETAL MONITORING. Injury to the fetal scalp or breech by the electrode is rarely a major problem, although application at some other site—such as the eye in case of a face presentation—can prove serious. Rarely, a fetal vessel in the placenta may be ruptured by catheter placement (Trudinger and Pryse-Davies, 1978). Severe cord compression has been described from entanglement with the catheter. Penetration of the placenta, causing hemorrhage and possibly uterine perforation during catheter insertion, has led to serious morbidity, as well as spurious recordings that resulted in inappropriate management.

Both the fetus and the mother may be at increased risk of *infection* as the consequence of internal monitoring. Scalp wounds from the electrode may become infected, and subsequent cranial osteomyelitis has been reported (Eggink and co-investigators, 2004; McGregor and McFarren, 1989). Puerperal infection increased from 12 to 18 percent in externally monitored women compared with those in whom an internal apparatus was used (Faro and associates, 1990). The American Academy of Pediatrics and the American College of Obstetricians and Gynecologists (2002) have recommended that certain maternal infections, including human immunodeficiency virus (HIV), herpes simplex virus, hepatitis B virus, and hepatitis C virus, are relative contraindications to internal fetal heart rate monitoring.

OTHER INTRAPARTUM ASSESSMENT TECHNIQUES

FETAL SCALP BLOOD SAMPLING. According to the American College of Obstetricians and Gynecologists (1995b), measurements of the pH in capillary scalp blood may help to identify the fetus in serious distress. The College also notes that the procedure is now used uncommonly. An illuminated endoscope is inserted through the dilated cervix after ruptured membranes so as to press firmly against the fetal scalp (Fig. 18–26). The skin is wiped clean with a cotton

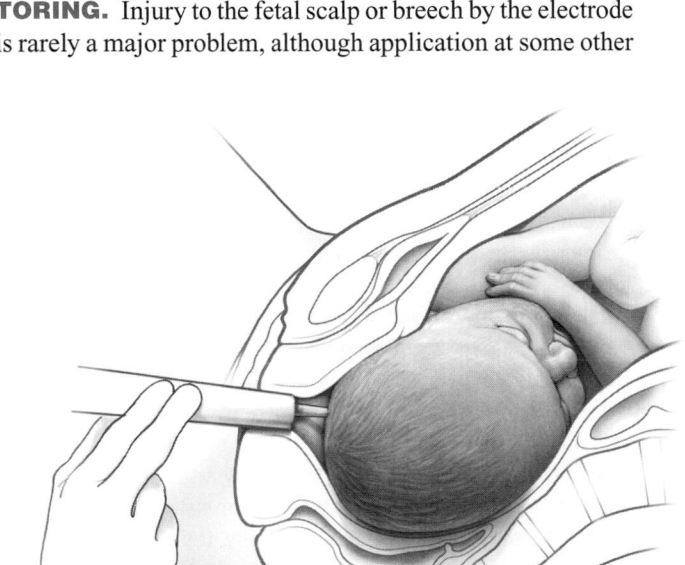

FIGURE 18–26. The technique of fetal scalp sampling using an amnioscope. The end of the endoscope is displaced from the fetal vertex approximately 2 cm to show the disposable blade against the fetal scalp before incision. (Modified from Hamilton and McKeown, 1974, with permission.)

swab and coated with a silicone gel to cause the blood to accumulate as discrete globules. An incision is made through the skin to a depth of 2 mm with a special blade on a long handle. As a drop of blood forms on the surface, it is immediately collected into a heparinized glass capillary tube, and the pH of the blood is measured promptly.

The pH of fetal capillary scalp blood is usually lower than that of umbilical venous blood and approaches that of umbilical arterial blood. Zalar and Quilligan (1979) recommended the following protocol to try to confirm fetal distress: If the pH is greater than 7.25, labor is observed. If the pH is between 7.20 and 7.25, the pH measurement is repeated within 30 minutes. If the pH is less than 7.20, another scalp blood sample is collected immediately and the mother is taken to an operating room and prepared for surgery. Delivery is performed promptly if the low pH is confirmed. Otherwise, labor is allowed to continue and scalp blood samples are repeated periodically. The only benefits reported for scalp pH testing were estimates of fewer cesarean deliveries for fetal distress (Young and co-workers, 1980b). Goodwin and associates (1994), however, in a study of 112,000 deliveries, showed a decrease in the scalp pH sampling rate from approximately 1.8 percent in the mid-1980s to 0.03 percent by 1992 with no increased delivery rate for fetal distress. They concluded that scalp pH sampling was unnecessary. Kruger and colleagues (1999) have advocated use of fetal scalp blood lactate concentration as an adjunct to pH.

SCALP STIMULATION. Clark and associates (1984) have suggested that scalp stimulation is an alternative to scalp blood sampling. This proposal was based on the observation that acceleration of the heart rate in response to pinching of the scalp with an Allis clamp just prior to obtaining blood was invariably associated with a normal pH. Conversely, failure to provoke acceleration was not uniformly predictive of fetal acidemia. Later, Elimian and associates (1997) reported that of 58 cases in which the fetal heart rate accelerated 10 beats/min or more after 15 seconds of gentle digital stroking of the scalp, 100 percent had a scalp pH of 7.20 or greater. Without an acceleration, however, only 30 percent had a scalp pH less than 7.20.

VIBROACOUSTIC STIMULATION. Fetal heart rate acceleration in response to vibroacoustic stimulation has been recommended as a substitute for scalp sampling (Edersheim and colleagues, 1987). The technique involves use of an electronic artificial larynx placed a centimeter or so from, or directly onto, the maternal abdomen (see Chap. 15, p. 380). Response to vibroacoustic stimulation is considered normal if a fetal heart rate acceleration of at least 15 beats/min for at least 15 seconds occurs within 15 seconds after the stimulation and with prolonged fetal movements (Sherer, 1994). Lin and colleagues (2001) prospectively studied vibroacoustic stimulation in 113 women in labor with either moderate to severe variable or late fetal heart rate decelerations. They

concluded that this technique is an effective predictor of fetal acidosis in the setting of variable decelerations. However, the predictability for fetal acidosis in the setting of late decelerations is limited. Other investigators have reported that although vibroacoustic stimulation in second-stage labor is associated with fetal heart rate reactivity, the quality of the response did not predict neonatal outcome or enhance labor management (Anyaegbunam and associates, 1994).

Skupski and colleagues (2002) performed a meta-analysis of reports on intrapartum fetal stimulation tests published between 1966 and 2000. Four types of fetal stimulation were analyzed, including scalp puncture for pH testing, use of an Allis clamp to pinch the fetal scalp, vibroacoustic stimulation, and digital stroking of the scalp. Results were similar for all four methods. These investigators concluded that intrapartum stimulation tests were useful to rule out fetal acidemia. However, they cautioned that these tests are "less than perfect."

FETAL PULSE OXIMETRY. Using technology similar to that of adult pulse oximetry, instrumentation has been developed that may allow assessment of fetal oxyhemoglobin saturation once the membranes are ruptured. A unique pad-like sensor (Fig. 18–27) is inserted through the cervix and positioned against the fetal face, where it is held in place by the uterine wall. As reviewed by Yam and co-authors (2000), this device has been used extensively by many investigators and has been reported to reliably register fetal oxygen saturation in 70 to 95 percent of women throughout 50 to 88 percent of their labors. The lower limit for normal fetal oxygen saturation is generally considered to be 30 percent by most investigators (Gorenberg and colleagues, 2003; Stiller and colleagues, 2002). However, as shown in Figure 18–28, fetal oxygen saturation normally varies greatly when measured in umbilical artery blood (Arikan and colleagues, 2000). Bloom and colleagues (1999) reported that brief, transient fetal oxygen saturations below 30 percent were common during labor because such values were observed in 53 percent of fetuses with normal outcomes. Saturation values below 30 percent, however, when persistent for 2 minutes or longer, were associated with an increased risk of potential fetal compromise.

Garite and colleagues (2000) randomly assigned 1010 women with term pregnancies, and who developed predefined abnormal fetal heart rate patterns, to either conventional fetal monitoring alone or fetal monitoring plus continuous fetal pulse oximetry. Cesarean delivery for fetal distress was performed when pulse oximetry values remained less than 30 percent for the entire interval between two contractions or when the fetal heart rate patterns met predefined guidelines. The use of fetal pulse oximetry significantly reduced the rate of cesarean delivery for nonreassuring fetal status from 10.2 to 4.5 percent. Alternatively, the cesarean delivery rate for dystocia increased significantly from 9 to 19 percent when pulse oximetry was used. There were no neonatal benefits or adverse effects associated with fetal pulse oximetry. In January 2000, the Obstetrics and Gynecology Devices

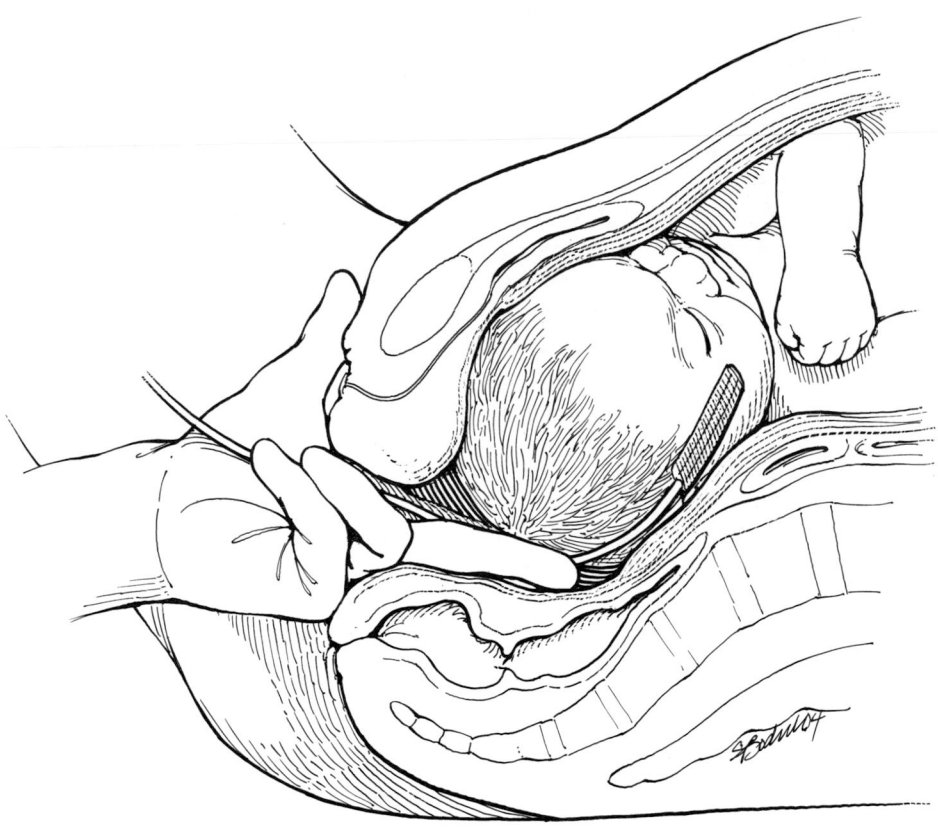

FIGURE 18–27. Schematic diagram of fetal pulse oximeter sensor placement.

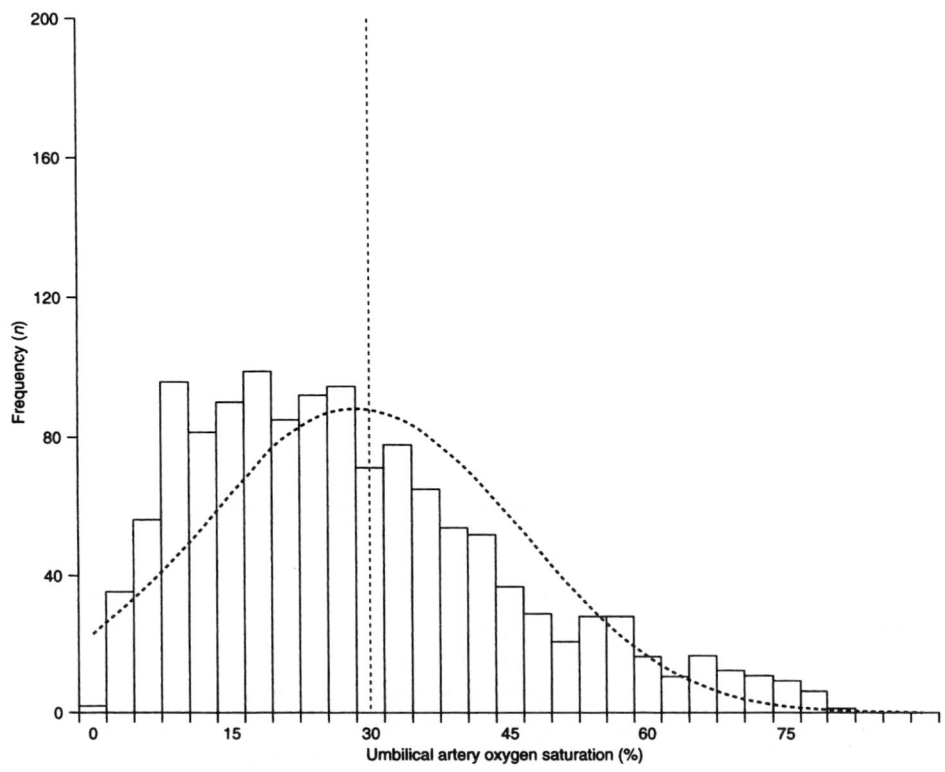

FIGURE 18–28. Frequency distribution of umbilical artery oxygen saturation values in 1281 vigorous newborn infants. Dotted line indicates normal distribution. (From Arikan and colleagues, 2000, with permission.)

Panel of the Medical Devices Advisory Committee of the Food and Drug Administration, based on this randomized study, recommended marketing of the Nellcor N-400 Fetal Oxygen Monitoring System. The American College of Obstetricians and Gynecologists (2001) has recommended that additional randomized trials be conducted to evaluate fetal pulse oximetry before adoption of this devise into clinical practice. The technique currently is being evaluated by the NICHD Maternal–Fetal Medicine Units Network.

FETAL ELECTROCARDIOGRAPHY. Concerns about the validity of continuous electronic fetal monitoring during labor have prompted searches for better methods of monitoring. Because as fetal hypoxia worsens, there are changes in the ST segment and PR interval of the fetal ECG, several investigators have assessed the value of analyzing these parameters as an adjunct to conventional fetal monitoring. The technique requires internal monitoring of the fetal heart rate and special equipment to process the fetal ECG. Westgate and co-workers (1993) studied the benefits of monitoring ST-segment changes in a randomized trial of 2400 pregnancies. Infant outcomes were not improved compared with those with use of conventional fetal monitoring alone, although there was a reduction in the cesarean delivery rate for fetal distress.

In another randomized trial of 4966 Swedish women, Amer-Wåhlin and colleagues (2001) found that the addition of ST analysis to conventional fetal monitoring significantly reduced cesarean delivery rates for fetal distress as well as metabolic acidemia in umbilical artery blood. ST data were collected from all the fetuses in this study. A total of 29 infants had adverse outcomes defined to include death (3), neonatal encephalopathy (7), or metabolic acidemia (19), and 22 of these had abnormal ST waveforms (Norén and colleagues, 2003). A serious confounding factor in interpretation of this study is the long intervals of abnormal fetal heart rate patterns before intervention. For example, the median interval before delivery, and during which time the fetal heart rate pattern was significantly abnormal, was almost 3 hours in the infants with encephalopathy. This may explain why U.S. clinicians shown these very same fetal monitoring tracings more often intervened compared with their European counterparts (Ross and colleagues, 2004). It must be considered that ST abnormalities may occur late in the course of fetal jeopardy, manifest as abnormal heart rate patterns.

INTRAPARTUM DOPPLER VELOCIMETRY. Doppler analysis of the umbilical artery has been studied as another potential adjunct to conventional fetal monitoring. Abnormal Doppler waveforms (see Chap. 16, p. 401), when present, may signify pathological umbilical–placental vessel resistance. Farrell and co-authors (1999) reviewed the literature on the use of intrapartum Doppler velocimetry and concluded that this technique was a poor predictor of adverse perinatal outcomes. They concluded that Doppler velocimetry had little, if any, role in the surveillance of fetal well-being during labor.

"FETAL DISTRESS"

DEFINITION. The term *fetal distress* is too broad and vague to be applied with any precision to clinical situations. Uncertainty about the diagnosis of fetal distress based on interpretation of fetal heart rate patterns has given rise to use of descriptions such as *reassuring* or *nonreassuring*. "Reassuring" suggests a restoration of confidence by a particular pattern, whereas "nonreassuring" suggests inability to remove doubt. These patterns during labor are dynamic, such that they can rapidly change from reassuring to nonreassuring and vice versa. In this situation, obstetricians experience surges of both confidence and doubt. Put another way, most diagnoses of fetal distress using heart rate patterns occur when obstetricians lose confidence or cannot assuage doubts about fetal condition. **These fetal assessments are entirely subjective clinical judgments inevitably subject to imperfection and must be recognized as such.**

Why is diagnosis of fetal distress based on heart rate patterns so tenuous? One explanation is that these patterns are more a reflection of fetal physiology than of pathology. Physiological control of heart rate includes a variety of interconnected mechanisms that depend on blood flow as well as oxygenation. Moreover, the activity of these control mechanisms is influenced by the preexisting state of fetal oxygenation as seen, for example, with chronic placental insufficiency. Importantly, the fetus is tethered by an umbilical cord whereby blood flow is constantly in jeopardy, which demands that the fetus have a strategy for survival. Moreover, normal labor is a process of increasing acidemia (Rogers and colleagues, 1998). Thus, normal labor is a process of repeated fetal hypoxic events resulting inevitably in acidemia. Put another way, and assuming that "asphyxia" can be defined as hypoxia leading to acidemia, normal parturition is an asphyxiating event for the fetus.

DIAGNOSIS. It follows that identification of "fetal distress" based upon fetal heart rate patterns is imprecise and controversial. Experts in interpretation of these patterns so often disagree with each other that one organizer of the NICHD fetal monitoring workshop (1997) lightheartedly compared the experts in attendance with marine iguanas of the Galapagos Islands—"all on the same beach but facing different directions and spitting at one another constantly" (Parer, 1997).

Ayres-de-Campos and colleagues (1999) investigated interobserver agreement on interpretation of fetal heart rate patterns and found that agreement—or conversely, disagreement—was related to whether the pattern was normal, suspicious, or pathological. Specifically, experts agreed on 62 percent of normal patterns, 42 percent of suspicious patterns, and only 25 percent of pathological patterns. Keith and co-workers (1995) asked each of 17 experts to review 50 tracings on two occasions, at least 1 month apart. About 20 percent changed their own interpretations, and approximately 25 percent did not agree with the interpretations of their colleagues. Similarly, Murphy and colleagues (2003) concluded that at least part of the interpretation problem is due to a lack of formalized education in U.S. training programs.

Several research efforts have been aimed at testing the utility of well-defined fetal heart rate classification systems. Berkus and colleagues (1999) retrospectively analyzed fetal heart rate patterns during the last 30 minutes of labor in 1859 term pregnancies. The study was designed to determine if specific patterns, or combinations of patterns, predicted neonatal outcome. Indisputably normal fetal heart rate patterns were recorded within 30 minutes of delivery in only 26 percent of cases. Prolonged bradycardia or tachycardia or fetal heart rate patterns that combined the absence of accelerations with severe variable or late decelerations were associated with an increased incidence of adverse infant outcome. Low and colleagues (1999) analyzed fetal heart rate patterns of term infants born with significant metabolic acidemia, defined as an umbilical artery base deficit greater than 16 mmol/L. Such acidemia was rare, occurring in only 71 of 23,000 births. Patterns with absent baseline variability were the most specific, but identified only 17 percent of the acidemic fetuses.

Dellinger and colleagues (2000) analyzed intrapartum fetal heart rate patterns in 898 pregnancies using a classification system of their design. Fetal heart rate patterns during the hour before delivery were classified as "normal," "stress," or "distress." Fetal "distress" was diagnosed in eight (1 percent) tracings, and 70 percent were classified as "normal." Almost one third were intermediate patterns. Fetal "distress" was classified as patterns with zero variability *plus* late or moderate-to-severe variable decelerations or with baseline rates less than 110 beats/min for 5 minutes or longer. Outcomes such as cesarean delivery, fetal acidemia, and admission to the neonatal intensive care nursery were significantly related to the fetal heart rate pattern. The authors concluded that their classification system accurately predicted normal outcomes for fetuses as well as discriminating true fetal distress. Others have used computers in an effort to improve interpretation of fetal heart rate patterns, with variable results (Agrawal, 2003; Bellver, 2004; Devoe, 2000, and all their co-authors).

In summary, after more than 30 years of experience with interpretation of fetal heart rate patterns, there is finally emerging evidence that some combinations of fetal heart rate characteristics can be meaningfully used to identify normal and severely abnormal fetuses. As shown in Table 18–1, true fetal distress patterns appear to be those in which beat-to-beat variability is zero in conjunction with severe decelerations or persistent baseline rate changes, or both. Fortunately, such fetal distress is rare. One explanation for the persistent failure to scientifically establish the benefits of fetal heart rate monitoring is the rarity of such fetal distress, effectively precluding statistically significant results from clinical trials (Hornbuckle and colleagues, 2000).

TABLE 18–1 NICHD Research Planning Workshop (1997) Fetal Heart Rate Patterns

Pattern	Workshop Interpretations
Normal	Baseline 110–160 beats/min
	Variability 6–25 beats/min
	Accelerations present
	No decelerations
Intermediate	No consensus
Severely abnormal	Recurrent late or variable decelerations with zero variability
	Substantial bradycardia with zero variability

MECONIUM IN THE AMNIONIC FLUID. Obstetrical teaching throughout the past century has included the concept that meconium passage is a potential warning of fetal asphyxia. In 1903, J. Whitridge Williams observed and attributed meconium passage to "relaxation of the sphincter ani muscle induced by faulty aeration of the (fetal) blood." Obstetricians, however, have also long realized that the detection of meconium during labor is problematic in the prediction of fetal distress or asphyxia. In their review, Katz and Bowes (1992) emphasized the prognostic uncertainty of meconium by referring to the topic as a "murky subject." Indeed, although 12 to 22 percent of human labors are complicated by meconium, few such labors are linked to infant mortality. In an investigation from Parkland Hospital, meconium was found to be a "low-risk" obstetrical hazard because the perinatal mortality attributable to meconium was 1 death per 1000 live births (Nathan and co-workers, 1994).

Three theories have been suggested to explain fetal passage of meconium and may, in part, explain the tenuous connection between the detection of meconium and infant mortality. The pathological explanation proposes that fetuses pass meconium in response to hypoxia, and that meconium therefore signals fetal compromise (Walker, 1953). Alternatively, in utero passage of meconium may represent normal gastrointestinal tract maturation under neural control (Mathews and Warshaw, 1979). Third, meconium passage could follow vagal stimulation from common but transient umbilical cord entrapment and resultant increased peristalsis (Hon and colleagues, 1961). Thus, fetal release of meconium also could represent physiological processes.

Ramin and co-authors (1996) studied almost 8000 pregnancies with meconium-stained amnionic fluid delivered at Parkland Hospital. Meconium aspiration syndrome was significantly associated with fetal acidemia at birth. Other significant correlates of aspiration included cesarean delivery, forceps to expedite delivery, intrapartum heart rate abnormalities, depressed Apgar scores, and need for assisted ventilation at delivery. Analysis of the type of fetal acidemia based on umbilical blood gases suggested that the fetal compromise associated with meconium aspiration syndrome was an acute event, because most acidemic fetuses had abnormally increased P_{CO_2} rather than a pure metabolic acidemia.

Interestingly, hypercarbia in fetal lambs has been shown to induce fetal gasping and resultant increased amnionic fluid inhalation (Dawes and co-workers, 1972). Jovanovic and Nguyen (1989) observed that meconium gasped into the fetal lungs caused aspiration syndrome only in asphyxiated animals. Ramin and co-authors (1996) hypothesized that the pathophysiology of meconium aspiration syndrome includes, but is not limited to, fetal hypercarbia, which stimulates fetal respiration leading to aspiration of meconium into the alveoli, and lung parenchymal injury secondary to acidemia-induced alveolar cell damage. In this pathophysiological scenario, meconium in amnionic fluid is a fetal environmental hazard rather than a marker of preexistent compromise. This proposed pathophysiological sequence is not all-inclusive, because it does not account for approximately half of the cases of meconium aspiration syndrome in which the fetus was not acidemic at birth.

Thus, it was concluded that the high incidence of meconium observed in the amnionic fluid during labor often represents fetal passage of gastrointestinal contents in conjunction with normal physiological processes. Although normal, such meconium becomes an environmental hazard when fetal acidemia supervenes. Importantly, such acidemia occurs acutely, and therefore meconium aspiration is unpredictable and likely unpreventable. Moreover, Greenwood and colleagues (2003), in a prospective study of 8394 women with clear amnionic fluid, emphasize that clear fluid is an unreliable sign of fetal well-being.

There is accumulating evidence that many infants with meconium aspiration syndrome have suffered chronic hypoxia before birth (Ghidini and Spong, 2001). For example, Blackwell and colleagues (2001) found that 60 percent of infants diagnosed as having meconium aspiration syndrome had umbilical artery blood pH 7.20 or greater, suggesting that this syndrome was unrelated to the neonatal condition at delivery. Similarly, markers of chronic hypoxia, such as fetal erythropoietin levels and nucleated red blood cells counts in newborn infants, suggest that chronic hypoxia is involved in many cases of meconium aspiration syndrome (Dollberg and colleagues, 2001; Jazayeri and colleagues, 2000).

MANAGEMENT OPTIONS WITH "FETAL DISTRESS." Management for significantly variant fetal heart rate patterns consists of correcting any fetal insult, if possible. Measures suggested by the American College of Obstetricians and Gynecologists (1998) are listed in Table 18–2. Moving the mother to the lateral position, correcting maternal hypotension caused by regional analgesia, and discontinuing oxytocin serve to improve uteroplacental perfusion. Examination is done to rule out prolapsed cord or impending delivery.

Tocolysis. A single intravenous or subcutaneous injection of 0.25 mg of terbutaline sulfate given to relax the uterus has been described as a temporizing maneuver in the manage-

TABLE 18–2 Management Criteria for Nonreassuring Fetal Heart Rate Pattern

The following actions should be documented in the medical record:
1. Repositioning of patient
2. Discontinuation of uterine stimulants and correction of uterine hyperstimulation
3. Vaginal examination
4. Correction of maternal hypotension associated with regional analgesia
5. Notification of anesthesia and nursing staff of need for emergency delivery
6. Monitoring of fetal heart rate—by electronic fetal monitoring or auscultation—in operating room prior to abdominal preparation
7. Request that qualified personnel be in attendance for newborn resuscitation and care[a]
8. Administration of oxygen to mother

[a] Locally acceptable definitions of qualified personnel should be agreed on by authorities at each institution.

ment of nonreassuring fetal heart rate patterns during labor. The rationale for this action is that inhibition of uterine contractions might improve fetal oxygenation, thus achieving in utero resuscitation. Cook and Spinnato (1994) described their experience with terbutaline tocolysis for fetal resuscitation in 368 pregnancies over a 10-year period. Such resuscitation improved fetal scalp blood pH values, although all of these women were delivered by cesarean. These investigators concluded that although the studies were small and rarely randomized, most reported favorable results with terbutaline tocolysis for nonreassuring patterns. Small intravenous doses of nitroglycerin (60 to 180 μg) also have been reported to be beneficial (Mercier and colleagues, 1997).

Amnioinfusion. Gabbe and co-workers (1976) showed in monkeys that removal of amnionic fluid produced variable decelerations and that replenishment of fluid with saline relieved the decelerations. Miyazaki and Taylor (1983) infused saline through the intrauterine pressure catheter in laboring women who had either variable decelerations or prolonged decelerations attributed to cord entrapment. Such therapy improved the heart rate pattern in half of the women studied. Later, Miyazaki and Nevarez (1985) randomly assigned 96 nulliparous women in labor with cord compression patterns and found that those who were treated with amnioinfusion less often required cesarean delivery for fetal distress.

On the basis of many of these early reports, transvaginal amnioinfusion has been extended into three clinical areas:

1. Treatment of variable or prolonged decelerations.
2. Prophylaxis for cases of known oligohydramnios, as with prolonged rupture of membranes.
3. In an attempt to dilute or wash out thick meconium (see Chap. 29, p. 675).

TABLE 18–3 Complications Associated with Amnioinfusion from a Survey of 186 Obstetrical Centers

Complication	Centers Reporting No. (%)
Uterine hypertonus	27 (14)
Abnormal fetal heart rate tracing	17 (9)
Amnionitis	7 (4)
Cord prolapse	5 (2)
Uterine rupture	4 (2)
Maternal cardiac or respiratory compromise	3 (2)
Placental abruption	2 (1)
Maternal death	2 (1)

Adapted from Wenstrom and colleagues (1995), with permission.

Many different amnioinfusion protocols have been reported, but most include a 500 to 800 mL bolus of warmed normal saline followed by a continuous infusion of approximately 3 mL per minute (Owen and co-workers, 1990; Pressman and Blakemore, 1996). In another study, Rinehart and colleagues (2000) randomly gave either 500 mL boluses of normal saline at room temperature alone, or 500 mL boluses plus continuous infusion of 3 mL per minute. Their study included 65 women with variable decelerations, and the investigators found neither method to be superior. Wenstrom and co-authors (1995) surveyed use of amnioinfusion in U.S. teaching hospitals. The procedure was used in 96 percent of the 186 centers surveyed, and it was estimated that 3 to 4 percent of all women delivered at these centers received such infusion. Potential complications of amnioinfusion are summarized in Table 18–3.

PROPHYLACTIC AMNIOINFUSION FOR OLIGOHYDRAMNIOS. Amnioinfusion for oligohydramnios has been used prophylactically in an effort to avoid intrapartum fetal heart rate patterns from umbilical cord occlusion. Nageotte and co-workers (1991) found that such amnioinfusion resulted in significantly decreased frequency and severity of variable decelerations in labor. There was no improvement, however, in the cesarean delivery rate or condition of term infants. In a randomized investigation, Macri and co-workers (1992) studied prophylactic amnioinfusion in 170 term and postterm pregnancies complicated by both thick meconium and oligohydramnios. Amnioinfusion significantly reduced cesarean delivery rates for fetal distress as well as meconium aspiration syndrome. In contrast, Ogundipe and associates (1994) randomly assigned 116 term pregnancies with an amnionic fluid index of less than 5 cm to receive prophylactic amnioinfusion or standard obstetrical care. There were no significant differences in overall cesarean delivery rates, delivery rates for fetal distress, or umbilical gas studies.

AMNIOINFUSION FOR MECONIUM-STAINED AMNIONIC FLUID. Pierce and associates (2000) summarized the results of 13 prospective trials of intrapartum amnioinfusion in 1924 women with moderate to thick meconium-stained fluid. Infants born to women treated by amnioinfusion were significantly less likely to have meconium below the vocal cords and were less likely to develop meconium aspiration syndrome than infants not given amnioinfusion. The cesarean delivery rate was also lower in the amnioinfusion group. Similar results were reported by Rathore and colleagues (2002). In contrast, at the University of Tennessee, amnioinfusion was found not feasible in half of women with moderate or thick meconium who were randomized to this treatment (Usta and colleagues, 1995). These investigators were unable to demonstrate any improvement in neonatal outcomes. Spong and associates (1994) also concluded that, although prophylactic amnioinfusion did dilute meconium, it did not improve perinatal outcome.

FETAL HEART RATE PATTERNS AND BRAIN DAMAGE. Attempts to correlate fetal heart rate patterns with brain damage have been based primarily on studies of infants identified as a result of medicolegal actions. For example, Rosen and Dickinson (1992) analyzed intrapartum fetal heart rate patterns in 55 such cases and found no specific pattern that was correlated with neurological injury. Phelan and Ahn (1994) reported that among 48 fetuses later found to be neurologically impaired, a persistent nonreactive fetal heart rate tracing was already present at the time of admission in 70 percent. They concluded that fetal neurological injury occurred predominately prior to arrival to the hospital. When they looked retrospectively at heart rate patterns in 209 brain-damaged infants, they concluded that there was not a single unique pattern associated with fetal neurological injury (Ahn and co-workers, 1996). Identical results were reported by Williams and Galerneau (2004), who also found that neonatal seizures due to hypoxic ischemic encephalopathy were related to nonspecific abnormal fetal heart rate pattern only when the patterns had been present an average of 72 minutes.

Experimental Evidence. Fetal heart rate patterns necessary for perinatal brain damage have been studied in experimental animals. Myers (1972) described the effects of complete and partial asphyxia in rhesus monkeys in studies of brain damage due to perinatal asphyxia. Complete asphyxia was produced by total occlusion of umbilical blood flow that led to prolonged deceleration (Fig. 18–29). Fetal arterial pH did not reach 7.0 until about 8 minutes after complete cessation of oxygenation and umbilical flow. At least 10 minutes of such prolonged deceleration was required before there was evidence of brain damage in surviving fetuses.

Myers (1972) also produced partial asphyxia in rhesus monkeys by impeding maternal aortic blood flow. This resulted in late decelerations due to uterine and placental hypoperfusion. He observed that several hours of these late decelerations did not damage the fetal brain unless the pH

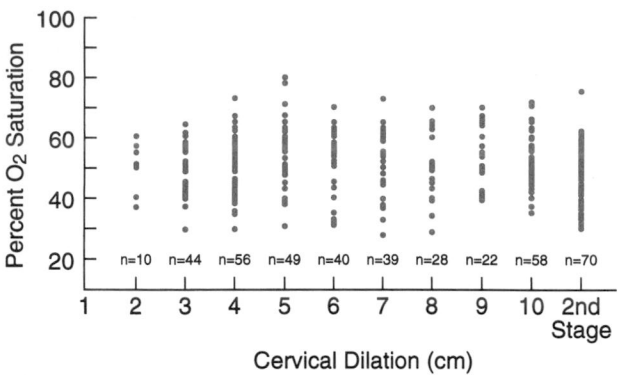

FIGURE 18–29. Prolonged deceleration in a rhesus monkey shown with blood pressure and biochemical changes during total occlusion of umbilical cord blood flow. (Redrawn from Myers, 1972.)

fell below 7.0. Indeed, Adamsons and Myers (1977) reported subsequently that late decelerations were a marker of partial asphyxia long before brain damage occurred.

The most common fetal heart rate pattern during labor, due to umbilical cord occlusion, requires considerable time to significantly affect the fetus in experimental animals. Clapp and colleagues (1988) partially occluded the umbilical cord for 1 minute every 3 minutes in fetal sheep and observed brain damage only after 2 hours. In another experiment in fetal sheep, Westgate and colleagues (2001) totally occluded the umbilical cord for 1 minute every 5 minutes for 4 hours without causing significant acidemia. Total occlusions for 2 minutes every 5 minutes resulted in the rapid onset of progressive fetal metabolic acidemia. The results from experiments such as these suggest that the effects of umbilical cord entrapment depend on the degree of occlusion (partial versus total), the duration of individual occlusions, and the frequency of such occlusions.

Human Evidence. The contribution of intrapartum events to subsequent neurological handicaps has been greatly overestimated (see Chap. 29, p. 654). Nelson and Grether (1998) performed a population-based study of children with disabling spastic cerebral palsy in which the intrapartum records of these children were compared with matched controls. Intrapartum fetal heart rate abnormalities did not distinguish between children with cerebral palsy and normal controls. Badawi and colleagues (1998) performed a case-control population-based study of infants with cerebral palsy in Western Australia. Only 5 percent of the brain-damaged infants had intrapartum factors, which led them to conclude that most cerebral palsy is unrelated to labor events.

Low and co-workers (1989) divided perinatal brain damage found following an asphyxial event into three categories based on microscopic findings:

1. From 18 to 48 hours—neuronal necrosis with pyknosis or lysis of the nucleus in shriveled eosinophilic cells.

2. From 48 to 72 hours—more intense neuronal necrosis with macrophage response.
3. More than 3 days—all the preceding plus astrocytic response with gliosis and in some, early cavitation.

Abnormal brain histopathology was not observed with acute, lethal asphyxia. Moreover, 43 percent of brain damage episodes occurred prior to labor and 25 percent were in the neonatal period. In another investigation, Low and co-workers (1984) estimated that more than 1 hour of fetal hypoxia associated with profound metabolic acidemia—pH less than 7.0—was required before neurological abnormalities could be diagnosed at 6 to 12 months of age. Low and co-workers (1988) identified 37 term infants with profound metabolic acidemia at birth, followed them for 1 year, and found major neurological deficits in 13 percent. Minor deficits were diagnosed in 10 infants, and the remaining 60 percent were normal. These investigators further observed that intrapartum fetal asphyxia with metabolic acidemia at delivery in both the term and preterm fetus was marked by severe complications not only of the central nervous system, but also of the respiratory and renal systems (Low and colleagues, 1994, 1995).

Clearly, for brain damage to occur, the fetus must be exposed to much more than a brief period of hypoxia. Moreover, the hypoxia must cause profound, just barely sublethal metabolic acidemia. Fetal heart rate patterns consistent with these sublethal conditions are fortunately rare. These observations strengthen the position of the American College of Obstetricians and Gynecologists (2003) on the criteria necessary to consider birth asphyxia as a cause of cerebral palsy (Table 18–4). Importantly, spastic quadriplegia and, less commonly, dyskinetic cerebral palsy are the only types of cerebral palsy associated with acute hypoxic intrapartum events. Unilateral brain lesions—hemiplegia or diplegia—are not a result of intrapartum hypoxia.

BENEFITS OF ELECTRONIC FETAL HEART RATE MONITORING. There are several fallacious assumptions behind expectations of improved perinatal outcome with electronic monitoring. One assumption is that fetal distress is a slowly developing phenomenon and that electronic monitoring makes possible early detection of the compromised fetus. This assumption is illogical, viz., how can all fetuses die slowly? Another presumption is that all fetal damage develops in the hospital. Only recently has attention focused on the reality that most damaged fetuses suffered insults before arrival at labor units. The very term *fetal monitor* implies that this inanimate technology in some fashion "monitors." The assumption is made that if a dead or damaged infant is delivered, the tracing strip must provide some clue, because this device was monitoring fetal condition. All of these assumptions led to great expectations and fostered the belief that all dead or damaged neonates were preventable. Parer and King (2000) reviewed reasons why fetal heart rate monitoring did not live up to its expectations. These unwarranted

TABLE 18–4 Criteria to Define an Acute Intrapartum Hypoxic Event as Sufficient to Cause Cerebral Palsy

Essential criteria (must meet all four) :

1. Evidence of metabolic acidosis in fetal umbilical cord arterial blood obtained at delivery (pH < 7 and base deficit ≥ 12 mmol/L
2. Early onset of severe or moderate neonatal encephalopathy in infants born at 34 or more weeks of gestation
3. Cerebral palsy of spastic quadriplegic or dyskinetic type
4. Exclusion of other identifiable etiologies, such as trauma, coagulation disorders, infectious conditions, or genetic disorders

Criteria that collectively suggest intrapartum timing (within close proximity to labor and delivery, e.g., 0–48 hr) but are nonspecific to asphyxial insults:

1. Sentinel (signal) hypoxic event occurring immediately before or during labor
2. Sudden and sustained fetal bradycardia or absence of fetal heart rate variability in presence of persistent, late, or variable decelerations, usually after a hypoxic sentinel event when pattern was previously normal
3. Apgar scores of 0–3 beyond 5 min
4. Onset of multisystem involvement within 72 hr of birth
5. Early imaging study showing evidence of acute nonfocal cerebral abnormality

From the American College of Obstetricians and Gynecologists (2003), with permission.

expectations have greatly fueled litigation in obstetrics. Indeed, Symonds (1994) reported that 70 percent of all liability claims related to fetal brain damage are based on reputed abnormalities seen in the electronic fetal monitor tracing.

By the end of the 1970s, questions about the efficacy, safety, and costs of electronic monitoring were being voiced from the Office of Technology Assessment, the United States Congress, and the Centers for Disease Control and Prevention. Banta and Thacker (2002) have reviewed the last 25 years of controversy on the benefits, or lack thereof, of electronic fetal monitoring. Parer (2003) points out that the controversy continues and that "... to justify our continued use of EFM [electronic fetal monitoring], we need to clean up our house. We must come to some agreement on a national level about interpretation and management."

Parkland Hospital Experience: Selective Versus Universal Monitoring. In July 1982, an investigation began at Parkland Hospital to ascertain whether all women in labor should undergo electronic monitoring (Leveno and co-workers, 1986). In alternating months, universal electronic monitoring was rotated with selective heart rate monitoring, which was the prevailing practice. During the 3-year investigation, 17,410 labors were managed using universal electronic monitoring. No significant differences were found in any perinatal outcomes. There was a significantly small increase in the cesarean delivery rate for fetal distress associated with universal

monitoring. Thus, increased application of electronic monitoring at Parkland Hospital did not improve perinatal results, but it increased the frequency of cesarean delivery for fetal distress.

Summary of Randomized Studies. Thacker and co-authors (1995) identified 12 published randomized clinical trials of electronic fetal monitoring from 1966 to 1994. There were 58,624 total pregnancies included in these studies. These investigators concluded that the benefits once claimed for electronic monitoring are clearly more modest than were believed and appear to be primarily in the prevention of neonatal seizures. Long-term implications of this outcome, however, appear less serious than once believed. Abnormal neurological consequences were not consistently higher among children monitored by auscultation compared with electronic methods. The authors concurred with the position of the American College of Obstetricians and Gynecologists (1995b) on intrapartum fetal surveillance (Table 18–5).

CURRENT RECOMMENDATIONS. The methods most commonly used for intrapartum fetal heart rate monitoring include auscultation with a fetal stethoscope or a Doppler ultrasound device, or continuous electronic monitoring of the heart rate and uterine contractions. No scientific evidence has identified the most effective method, including the frequency or duration of fetal surveillance that ensures optimum results. Summarized in Table 18–5 are the current recommendations of the American College of Obstetricians and Gynecologists (1995b). These recommendations have been reaffirmed by both the American Academy of Pediatrics and the American College of Obstetricians and Gynecologists (2002). Intermittent auscultation or continuous electronic monitoring is considered an acceptable method of intrapartum surveillance in both low- and high-risk pregnancies. The recommended interval between checking the heart rate, however, is longer in the uncomplicated pregnancy. When auscultation is used, it is recommended that it be performed after a contraction and

TABLE 18–5 Guidelines for Intrapartum Fetal Heart Rate Surveillance

Surveillance	Low-Risk Pregnancies	High-Risk Pregnancies
Acceptable methods		
Intermittent auscultation	Yes	Yes
Continuous electronic monitoring (internal or external)	Yes	Yes
Evaluation intervals[a]		
First-stage labor (active)	30 min	15 min[b]
Second-stage labor	15 min	5 min[b]

[a]Following a uterine contraction.
[b]Includes tracing evaluation and charting when continuous electronic monitoring is used.
Adapted from the American College of Obstetricians and Gynecologists (1995b).

for 60 seconds. It also is recommended that a 1-to-1 nurse–patient ratio be used if auscultation is employed.

INTRAPARTUM SURVEILLANCE OF UTERINE ACTIVITY

Analysis of electronically measured uterine activity permits some generalities concerning the relationship of certain contraction patterns to labor outcome. There is considerable normal variation, however, and caution must be exercised before judging true labor or its absence solely from study of a monitor tracing. Uterine muscle efficiency to effect delivery varies greatly. To use an analogy, 100-meter sprinters all have the same muscle groups yet cross the finish line at different times.

INTERNAL UTERINE PRESSURE MONITORING.
Amnionic fluid pressure is measured between and during contractions by a fluid-filled plastic catheter with its distal tip located above the presenting part. The catheter is connected to a strain-gauge pressure sensor adjusted to the same level as the catheter tip in the uterus. The amplified electrical signal produced in the strain gauge by variation in pressure within the fluid system is recorded on a calibrated moving paper strip simultaneously with the fetal heart rate recording. Intrauterine pressure catheters are now available that have the pressure sensor in the catheter tip, which obviates the need for the fluid column.

EXTERNAL MONITORING.
Uterine contractions can be measured by a displacement transducer in which the transducer button, or "plunger," is held against the abdominal wall. As the uterus contracts, the button moves in proportion to the strength of the contraction. This movement is converted into a measurable electrical signal that indicates the *relative* intensity of the contraction—it does not give an accurate measure of intensity. External monitoring can give a good indication of the onset, peak, and end of the contraction.

PATTERNS OF UTERINE ACTIVITY.
Caldeyro-Barcia and Poseiro (1960) from Montevideo, Uruguay, were pioneers who have done much to elucidate the patterns of spontaneous uterine activity throughout pregnancy. Contractile waves of uterine activity were usually measured using intra-amnionic pressure catheters, but early in their studies as many as four simultaneous intramyometrial microballoons also were used to record uterine pressure. They also introduced the concept of *Montevideo units* to define uterine activity (see Chap. 20, p. 498). By this definition, uterine performance is the product of the intensity—increased uterine pressure above baseline tone—of a contraction in millimeters of mercury multiplied by contraction frequency per 10 minutes. For example, three contractions in 10 minutes, each of 50 mm Hg intensity, would equal 150 Montevideo units.

During the first 30 weeks, uterine activity is comparatively quiescent. Contractions are seldom greater than 20 mm Hg, and these have been equated with those first described in 1872 by John Braxton Hicks. Uterine activity increases gradually after 30 weeks, and it is noteworthy that these *Braxton Hicks contractions* also increase in intensity and frequency. Further increases in uterine activity are typical of the last weeks of pregnancy, termed *prelabor.* During this phase, the cervix ripens, presumably as a consequence of increasing uterine contractions (see Chap. 6, p. 153).

According to Caldeyro-Barcia and Poseiro (1960), clinical labor usually commences when uterine activity reaches values between 80 and 120 Montevideo units. This translates into approximately three contractions of 40 mm Hg every 10 minutes. Importantly, there is no clear-cut division between prelabor and labor, but rather a gradual and progressive transition.

During first-stage labor, uterine contractions increase progressively in intensity from about 25 mm Hg at commencement of labor to 50 mm Hg at the end. At the same time, frequency increases from three to five contractions per 10 minutes, and uterine baseline tone from 8 to 12 mm Hg. Uterine activity further increases during second-stage labor, aided by maternal bearing down. Indeed, contractions of 80 to 100 mm Hg are typical and occur as frequently as five to six per 10 minutes. Interestingly, the duration of uterine contractions—60 to 80 seconds—does not increase appreciably from early active labor extending through the second-stage (Pontonnier and colleagues, 1975). Presumably, this constancy of duration serves a fetal respiratory gas-exchange function. That is, functional fetal "breath holding" during a uterine contraction, which results in isolation of the intervillous space where respiratory gas exchange occurs, has a 60- to 80-second limit that remains relatively constant.

Caldeyro-Barcia and Poseiro (1960) also observed empirically that uterine contractions are clinically palpable only after their intensity exceeds 10 mm Hg. Moreover, until the intensity of contractions reaches 40 mm Hg, the uterine wall can readily be depressed by the finger. At greater intensity, the uterine wall then becomes so hard that it resists easy depression. Uterine contractions usually are not associated with pain until their intensity exceeds 15 mm Hg, presumably because this is the minimum pressure required for distending the lower uterine segment and cervix. It follows that Braxton Hicks contractions exceeding 15 mm Hg may be perceived as uncomfortable because distention of the uterus, cervix, and birth canal is generally thought to elicit discomfort.

Hendricks (1968) observed that "the clinician makes great demands upon the uterus." The uterus is expected to remain well relaxed during pregnancy, to contract effectively but intermittently during labor, and then to remain in a state of almost constant contraction for several hours postpartum. Figure 18–30 demonstrates an example of normal uterine activity during labor. As also described by Caldeyro-Barcia

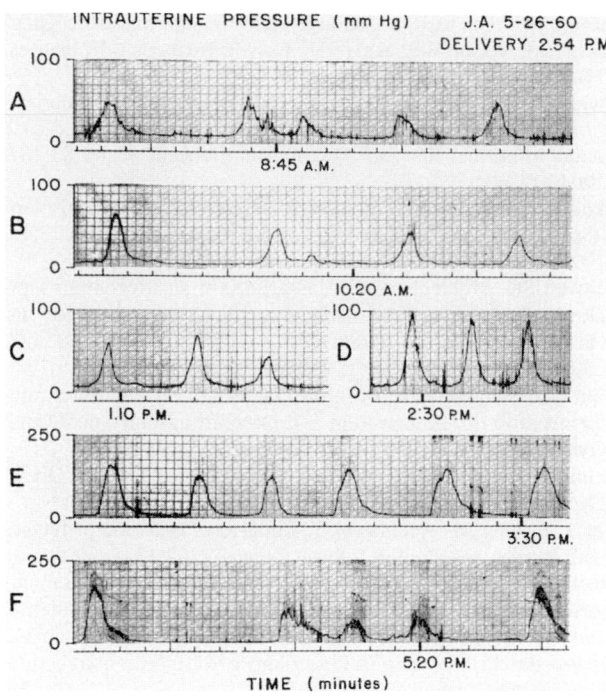

FIGURE 18–30. Intrauterine pressure recorded through a single catheter. **A.** Prelabor. **B.** Early labor. **C.** Active labor. **D.** Late labor. **E.** Spontaneous activity ½ hour postpartum. **F.** Spontaneous activity 2½ hours postpartum. (From Hendricks, 1968.)

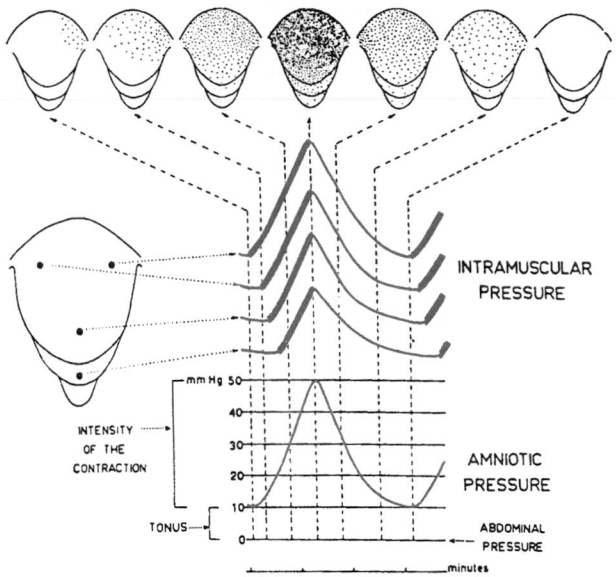

FIGURE 18–31. Schematic representation of the normal contractile wave of labor. Large uterus on the left shows the four points at which intramyometrial pressure was recorded with microballoons. Four corresponding pressure tracings are shown in relation to each other by shading on the small uteri at top. (From Caldeyro-Barcia and Poseiro, 1960.)

and Poseiro (1960), uterine activity progressively and gradually increases from prelabor through late labor. Interestingly, as shown in Figure 18–30, uterine contractions after birth are identical to those resulting in delivery of the infant. Indeed, the pattern of uterine activity is one of gradual subsidence or reverse of that leading up to delivery. It is therefore not surprising that the uterus that performs poorly before delivery is also prone to atony and puerperal hemorrhage.

Origin and Propagation of Contractions. The uterus has not been studied extensively in terms of its nonhormonal physiological mechanisms of function. The normal contractile wave of labor originates near the uterine end of one of the fallopian tubes; thus, these areas act as "pacemakers" (Fig. 18–31). The right pacemaker usually predominates over the left and starts the great majority of contractile waves. Contractions spread from the pacemaker area throughout the uterus at 2 cm/sec, depolarizing the whole organ within 15 seconds. This depolarization wave propagates downward toward the cervix. Intensity is greatest in the fundus, and it diminishes in the lower uterus. This phenomenon is thought to reflect reductions of myometrial thickness from the fundus to the cervix. Presumably, this descending gradient of pressure serves to direct fetal descent toward the cervix as well as to efface the cervix. Importantly, all parts of the uterus are synchronized and reach their peak pressure almost simul-

taneously, giving rise to the curvilinear waveform shown in Figure 18–31.

The pacemaker theory also serves to explain the varying intensity of adjacent coupled contractions shown in panels A and B of Figure 18–30. Such coupling was termed *incoordination* by Caldeyro-Barcia and Poseiro (1960). A contractile wave begins in one cornual-region pacemaker, but does not synchronously depolarize the entire uterus. As a result, another contraction begins in the contralateral pacemaker and produces the second contractile wave of the couplet. These small contractions alternating with larger ones appear to be typical of early labor, and indeed, labor may progress with such uterine activity, albeit at a slower pace. These authors also observed that labor would progress slowly if regular contractions were hypotonic—that is, contractions with intensity less than 25 mm Hg or frequency less than two per 10 minutes. Similar observations were made by Seitchik (1981) in a computer-aided analysis comparing women in active labor with those in arrested labor. Normal labor was characterized by a minimum of three contractions that averaged greater than 25 mm Hg and less than 4-minute intervals between contractions. A lesser amount of uterine activity was associated with arrest of active labor. Prospective diagnosis of hypotonic labor cannot be reliably based simply on a few uterine pressures.

Hauth and co-workers (1986) quantified uterine contraction pressures in 109 women at term who received oxytocin for labor induction or augmentation. Most of these women achieved 200 to 225 Montevideo units, and 40 percent had up to 300 units to effect delivery. The authors suggested that these levels of uterine activity should be sought before consideration of cesarean delivery for presumed dystocia. This recommendation later was endorsed by the American College of Obstetricians and Gynecologists (1995a).

REFERENCES

Adamsons K, Myers RE: Late decelerations and brain tolerance of the fetal monkey to intrapartum asphyxia. Am J Obstet Gynecol 128:893, 1977

Agrawal SK, Doucette F, Gratton R, et al: Intrapartum computerized fetal heart rate parameters and metabolic acidosis at birth. Obstet Gynecol 102:731, 2003

Ahn MO, Korst L, Phelan JP: Intrapartum fetal heart rate patterns in 209 brain damaged infants. Am J Obstet Gynecol 174:492, 1996

American Academy of Pediatrics and the American College of Obstetricians and Gynecologists: Intrapartum and postpartum care of the mother. In Guidelines for Perinatal Care, 5th ed. Washington, DC, AAP and ACOG, 2002

American College of Obstetricians and Gynecologists: Neonatal encephalopathy and cerebral palsy: Defining the pathogenesis and pathophysiology. Washington, DC, ACOG, 2003

American College of Obstetricians and Gynecologists: Fetal pulse oximetry. Committee Opinion No. 258, September 2001

American College of Obstetricians and Gynecologists: Cesarean delivery for nonreassuring fetal status. Criteria Set No. 33, May 1998

American College of Obstetricians and Gynecologists: Dystocia and the augmentation of labor. Technical Bulletin No. 218, December 1995a

American College of Obstetricians and Gynecologists: Fetal heart rate patterns: Monitoring, interpretation, and management. Technical Bulletin No. 207, July 1995b

Amer-Wåhlin I, Hellsten C, Norén H, et al: Cardiotocography only versus cardiotocography plus ST analysis of fetal electrocardiogram for intrapartum fetal monitoring: A Swedish randomized controlled trial. Lancet 358:534, 2001

Angel J, Knuppel R, Lake M: Sinusoidal fetal heart rate patterns associated with intravenous butorphanol administration. Am J Obstet Gynecol 149:465, 1984

Anyaegbunam AM, Ditchik A, Stoessel R, et al: Vibroacoustic stimulation of the fetus entering the second stage of labor. Obstet Gynecol 83:963, 1994

Arikan GM, Scholz HS, Petru F, et al: Cord blood oxygen saturation in vigorous infants at birth: What is normal? Br J Obstet Gynaecol 107:987, 2000

Ayres-de-Campos D, Bernardes J, Costa-Pereira A, et al: Inconsistencies in classification by experts of cardiotocograms and subsequent clinical decision. Br J Obstet Gynaecol 106:1307, 1999

Badawi N, Kurinczuk J, Keogh JM, et al: Intrapartum risk factors for newborn encephalopathy: The Western Australia case-control study. BMJ 317:1554, 1998

Ball RH, Parer JT: The physiologic mechanisms of variable decelerations. Am J Obstet Gynecol 166:1683, 1992

Banta HD, Thacker SB: Assessing the costs and benefits of electronic fetal monitoring. Obstet Gynecol Surv 34:627, 1979

Banta HD, Thacker SB: Electronic fetal monitoring: Lessons from a formative case of health technology assessment. Int J Technol Assess Health Care 18:762, 2002

Behrman RE: The cardiovascular system. In Behrman RE, Kliegman RM, Nelson WE, et al (eds): Nelson Textbook of Pediatrics, 14th ed. Philadelphia, Saunders, 1992, p 1127

Bellver J, Perales A, Maiques V, et al: Can antepartum computerized cardiotocography predict the evolution of intrapartum acid-base status in normal fetuses? Acta Obstet Gynecol Scand 83:267, 2004

Berkus MD, Langer O, Samueloff A, et al: Electronic fetal monitoring: What's reassuring? Acta Obstet Gynecol Scand 78:15, 1999

Blackwell SC, Moldenhauer J, Hassan SS, et al: Meconium aspiration syndrome in term neonates with normal acid-base status at delivery: Is it different? Am J Obstet Gynecol 184:1422, 2001

Bloom SL, Swindle RG, McIntire DD, et al: Fetal pulse oximetry: Duration of desaturation and intrapartum outcome. Obstet Gynecol 93:1036, 1999

Boehm FH: Prolonged end stage fetal heart rate deceleration. Obstet Gynecol 45:579, 1975

Boldt T, Eronen M, Andersson S: Long-term outcome in fetuses with cardiac arrhythmias. Obstet Gynecol 102:1372, 2003

Caldeyro-Barcia R, Mendez-Bauer C, Poseiro JJ, et al: Fetal monitoring in labor. In Walloch HJ, Gold EM, Lis EF (eds): Maternal and Child Health Practices. Springfield, Ill, Thomas, 1973, p 332

Caldeyro-Barcia R, Poseiro JJ: Physiology of the uterine contraction. Clin Obstet Gynecol 3:386, 1960

Clapp JF, Peress NS, Wesley M, et al: Brain damage after intermittent partial cord occlusion in the chronically instrumented fetal lamb. Am J Obstet Gynecol 159:504, 1988

Clark SL, Gimovsky ML, Miller FC: Fetal heart rate response to scalp blood sampling. Am J Obstet Gynecol 14:706, 1982

Clark SL, Gimovsky ML, Miller FC: The scalp stimulation test: A clinical alternative to fetal scalp blood sampling. Am J Obstet Gynecol 148:274, 1984

Cook VD, Spinnato JA: Terbutaline tocolysis prior to cesarean section for fetal distress. J Matern Fetal Med 3:219, 1994

Copel JA, Liang RI, Demasio K, et al: The clinical significance of the irregular fetal heart rhythm. Am J Obstet Gynecol 182:813, 2000

Davidson SR, Rankin JH, Martin CB Jr, et al: Fetal heart rate variability and behavioral state: Analysis by power spectrum. Am J Obstet Gynecol 167:717, 1992

Dawes GS: The control of fetal heart rate and its variability in counts. In Kunzel W (ed): Fetal Heart Rate Monitoring. Berlin, Springer-Verlag, 1985, p 188

Dawes GS, Fox HE, Leduc BM, et al: Respiratory movements and rapid eye movement sleep in the foetal lamb. J Physiol 220:119, 1972

Dawes GS, Visser GHA, Goodman JDS, et al: Numerical analysis of the human fetal heart rate: Modulation by breathing and movement. Am J Obstet Gynecol 140:535, 1981

Del Valle GO, Joffe GM, Izquierdo LA, et al: Acute posttraumatic fetal anemia treated with fetal intravascular transfusion. Am J Obstet Gynecol 166:127, 1992

Dellinger EH, Boehm FH, Crane MM: Electronic fetal heart rate monitoring: Early neonatal outcomes associated with normal rate, fetal stress, and fetal distress. Am J Obstet Gynecol 182:214, 2000

Devoe L, Golde S, Kilman Y, et al: A comparison of visual analyses of intrapartum fetal heart rate tracings according to the new National Institute of Child Health and Human Development guidelines with computer analyses by an automated fetal heart rate monitoring system. Am J Obstet Gynecol 183:361, 2000

Divon MY, Winkler H, Yeh SY, et al: Diminished respiratory sinus arrhythmia in asphyxiated term infants. Am J Obstet Gynecol 155:1263, 1986

Dollberg S, Livny S, Mordecheyev N, et al: Nucleated red blood cells in meconium aspiration syndrome. Obstet Gynecol 97:593, 2001

Eberle RL, Norris MC, Eberle AM, et al: The effect of maternal position on fetal heart rate during epidural or intrathecal labor analgesia. Am J Obstet Gynecol 179:150, 1998

Edersheim TG, Hutson JM, Druzin ML, et al: Fetal heart rate response to vibratory acoustic stimulation predicts fetal pH in labor. Am J Obstet Gynecol 157:1557, 1987

Eggink BH, Richardson CJ, Rowen JL: Gardnerella vaginalis–infected scalp hematoma associated with electronic fetal monitoring. Pediatr Infect Dis J 23:276, 2004

Egley CC, Bowes WA, Wagner D: Sinusoidal fetal heart rate pattern during labor. Am J Perinatol 8:197, 1991

Elimian A, Figueroa R, Tejani N: Intrapartum assessment of fetal well-being: A comparison of scalp stimulation with scalp pH sampling. Obstet Gynecol 89:373, 1997

Epstein H, Waxman A, Gleicher N, et al: Meperidine induced sinusoidal fetal heart rate pattern and reversal with naloxone. Obstet Gynecol 59:225, 1982

Faro S, Martens MG, Hammill HA, et al: Antibiotic prophylaxis: Is there a difference? Am J Obstet Gynecol 162:900, 1990

Farrell T, Chien PFW, Gordon A: Intrapartum umbilical artery Doppler velocimetry as a predictor of adverse perinatal outcome: A systematic review. Br J Obstet Gynaecol 106:783, 1999

Freeman RK: Problems with intrapartum fetal heart rate monitoring interpretation and patient management. Obstet Gynecol 100:813, 2002

Freeman RK, Garite TH, Nageotte MP: Fetal Heart Rate Monitoring, 3rd ed. Philadelphia, Lippincott Williams & Wilkins, 2003

Gabbe SG, Ettinger BB, Freeman RK, et al: Umbilical cord compression associated with amniotomy: Laboratory observations. Am J Obstet Gynecol 126:353, 1976

Garite TJ, Dildy GA, McNamara H, et al: A multicenter controlled trial of fetal pulse oximetry in the intrapartum management of nonreassuring fetal heart rate patterns. Am J Obstet Gynecol 183:1049, 2000

Ghidini A, Spong CY: Severe meconium aspiration syndrome is not caused by aspiration of meconium. Am J Obstet Gynecol 185:931, 2001

Gilstrap LC III, Hauth JC, Hankins GDV, et al: Second stage fetal heart rate abnormalities and type of neonatal acidemia. Obstet Gynecol 70:191, 1987

Goodwin TM, Milner-Masterson L, Paul RH: Elimination of fetal scalp blood sampling on a large clinical service. Obstet Gynecol 83:971, 1994

Gorenberg DM, Pattillo C, Hendi P, et al: Fetal pulse oximetry: Correlation between oxygen desaturation, duration, and frequency and neonatal outcomes. Am J Obstet Gynecol 189:136, 2003

Greenwood C, Lalchandani S, MacQuillan K, et al: Meconium passed in labor: How reassuring is clear amniotic fluid? Obstet Gynecol 102:89, 2003

Gull I, Jaffa AJ, Oren M, et al: Acid accumulation during end-stage bradycardia in term fetuses: How long is too long? Br J Obstet Gynaecol 103:1096, 1996

Hallak M, Martinez-Poyer J, Kruger ML, et al: The effect of magnesium sulfate on fetal heart rate parameters: A randomized, placebo-controlled trial. Am J Obstet Gynecol 181:1122, 1999

Hamilton LA Jr, McKeown MJ: Biochemical and electronic monitoring of the fetus. In Wynn RM (ed): Obstetrics and Gynecology Annual, 1973. New York, Appleton-Century-Crofts, 1974

Hammacher K, Huter K, Bokelmann J, et al: Foetal heart frequency and perinatal conditions of the fetus and newborn. Gynaecologia 166:349, 1968

Hankins GDV, Leicht TL, Van Houk JW: Prolonged fetal bradycardia secondary to maternal hypothermia in response to urosepsis. Am J Perinatol 14:217, 1997

Hauth JC, Hankins GV, Gilstrap LC, et al: Uterine contraction pressures with oxytocin induction/augmentation. Obstet Gynecol 68:305, 1986

Hendricks CH: Uterine contractility changes in the early puerperium. In Anderson GV, Quilligan EJ (eds): Clinical Obstetrics and Gynecology, Thromboembolic Disorders, Physiology of Labor. New York, Harper & Row, 1968, p 125

Herbert CM, Boehm FH: Prolonged end-stage fetal heart deceleration: A reanalysis. Obstet Gynecol 57:589, 1981

Hicks JB: On the contractions of the uterus throughout pregnancy. Trans Obstet Soc Lond 13, 1872

Hill JB, Alexander JM, Sharma SK, et al: A comparison of the effects of epidural and meperidine analgesia during labor on fetal heart rate. Obstet Gynecol 102:333, 2003

Hon EH: The electronic evaluation of the fetal heart rate. Am J Obstet Gynecol 75:1215, 1958

Hon EH: The fetal heart rate patterns preceding death in utero. Am J Obstet Gynecol 78:47, 1959

Hon EH, Bradfield AM, Hess OW: The electronic evaluation of the fetal heart rate. Am J Obstet Gynecol 82:291, 1961

Hornbuckle J, Vail A, Abrams KR, et al: Bayesian interpretation of trials: The example of intrapartum electronic fetal heart rate monitoring. Br J Obstet Gynaecol 107:3, 2000

Ikeda T, Murata Y, Quilligan EJ, et al: Two sinusoidal heart rate patterns in fetal lambs undergoing extracorporeal membrane oxygenation. Am J Obstet Gynecol 180:462, 1999

Impey L, Raymonds M, MacQuillan K, et al: Admission cardiotocography: A randomised controlled trial. Lancet 361:465, 2003

Itskovitz J, LaGamma EF, Rudoloph AM: Heart rate and blood pressure response to umbilical cord compression in fetal lambs with special reference to the mechanisms of variable deceleration. Am J Obstet Gynecol 147:451, 1983

Jazayeri A, Politz L, Tsibris JCM, et al: Fetal erythropoietin levels in pregnancies complicated by meconium passage: Does meconium suggest fetal hypoxia? Am J Obstet Gynecol 183:188, 2000

Johnson TR Jr, Compton AA, Rotmeusch J, et al: Significance of the sinusoidal fetal heart rate pattern. Am J Obstet Gynecol 139:446, 1981

Jovanovic R, Nguyen HT: Experimental meconium aspiration in guinea pigs. Obstet Gynecol 73:652, 1989

Katz VL, Bowes WA: Meconium aspiration syndrome: Reflections on a murky subject. Am J Obstet Gynecol 166:171, 1992

Keith RDF, Beckley S, Garibaldi JM, et al: A multicentre comparative study of 17 experts and an intelligent computer system for managing labour using the cardiotocogram. Br J Obstet Gynaecol 102:688, 1995

Klavan M, Laver AT, Boscola MA: Clinical Concepts of Fetal Heart Rate Monitoring. Waltham, Mass, Hewlett-Packard, 1977

Kozuma S, Watanabe T, Bennet L, et al: The effect of carotid sinus denervation on fetal heart rate variation in normoxia, hypoxia and post-hypoxia in fetal sleep. Br J Obstet Gynaecol 104:460, 1997

Krebs HB, Petres RE, Dunn LJ: Intrapartum fetal heart rate monitoring, 5. Fetal heart rate patterns in the second stage of labor. Am J Obstet Gynecol 140:435, 1981

Krebs HB, Petres RE, Dunn LJ, et al: Intrapartum fetal heart rate monitoring, 6. Prognostic significance of accelerations. Am J Obstet Gynecol 142:297, 1982

Kruger K, Hallberg B, Blennow M, et al: Predictive value of fetal scalp blood lactate concentration and pH as markers of neurologic disability. Am J Obstet Gynecol 181:1072, 1999

Kunzel W: Fetal heart rate alterations in partial and total cord occlusion. In Kunzel W (ed): Fetal Heart Rate Monitoring: Clinical Practice and Pathophysiology. Berlin, Springer-Verlag, 1985, p 114

Lee CV, DiLaretto PC, Lane JM: A study of fetal heart rate acceleration patterns. Obstet Gynecol 45:142, 1975

Leveno KJ, Cunningham FG, Nelson S: Prospective comparison of selective and universal electronic fetal monitoring in 34,995 pregnancies. N Engl J Med 315:615, 1986

Leveno KJ, Quirk JG, Cunningham FG, et al: Prolonged pregnancy: Observations concerning the causes of fetal distress. Am J Obstet Gynecol 150:465, 1984

Lin CC, Vassallo B, Mittendorf R: Is intrapartum vibroacoustic stimulation an effective predictor of fetal acidosis? J Perinat Med 29:506, 2001

Low JA, Galbraith RS, Muir DW, et al: Factors associated with motor and cognitive deficits in children after intrapartum fetal hypoxia. Am J Obstet Gynecol 148:533, 1984

Low JA, Galbraith RS, Muir DW, et al: Motor and cognitive deficits after intrapartum asphyxia in the mature fetus. Am J Obstet Gynecol 158:356, 1988

Low JA, Panagiotopoulos C, Derrick EJ: Newborn complications after intrapartum asphyxia with metabolic acidosis in the preterm fetus. Am J Obstet Gynecol 172:805, 1995

Low JA, Panagiotopoulos C, Derrick EJ: Newborn complications after intrapartum asphyxia with metabolic acidosis in the term fetus. Am J Obstet Gynecol 170:1081, 1994

Low JA, Robertson DR, Simpson LL: Temporal relationships of neuropathologic conditions caused by perinatal asphyxia. Am J Obstet Gynecol 160:608, 1989

Low JA, Victory R, Derrick J: Predictive value of electronic fetal monitoring for intrapartum fetal asphyxia with metabolic acidosis. Obstet Gynecol 93:285, 1999

Lowe TW, Leveno KJ, Quirk JG, et al: Sinusoidal fetal heart rate patterns after intrauterine transfusion. Obstet Gynecol 64:215, 1984

Macri CJ, Schrimmer DB, Leung A, et al: Prophylactic amnioinfusion improves outcome of pregnancy complicated by thick meconium and oligohydramnios. Am J Obstet Gynecol 167:117, 1992

Manassiev N: What is the normal heart rate of a term fetus? Br J Obstet Gynaecol 103:1272, 1996

Martin JA, Hamilton BE, Sutton PD, et al: Births: Final data for 2002. National Vital Statistics Report, Vol 52, No. 1. Hyattsville, Md, National Center for Health Statistics, 2003

Mathews TG, Warshaw JB: Relevance of the gestational age distribution of meconium passage in utero. Pediatrics 64:30, 1979

McGregor JA, McFarren T: Neonatal cranial osteomyelitis: A complication of fetal monitoring. Obstet Gynecol 73:490, 1989

Melchior J, Bernard N: Incidence and pattern of fetal heart rate alterations during labor. In Kunzel W (ed): Fetal Heart Rate Monitoring: Clinical Practice and Pathophysiology. Berlin, Springer-Verlag, 1985, p 73

Mercier FJ, Dounas M, Bouaziz H, et al: Intravenous nitroglycerin to relieve intrapartum fetal distress related to uterine hyperactivity: A prospective observation study. Anesth Analg 84:1117, 1997

Mires G, Williams F, Howie P: Randomised controlled trial of cardiotocography versus Doppler auscultation of fetal heart at admission in labour in low risk obstetric population. BMJ 322:1457, 2001

Miyazaki FS, Nevarez F: Saline amnioinfusion for relief of repetitive variable decelerations: A prospective randomized study. Am J Obstet Gynecol 153:301, 1985

Miyazaki FS, Taylor NA: Saline amnioinfusion for relief of variable or prolonged decelerations. Am J Obstet Gynecol 146:670, 1983

Modanlou H, Freeman RK: Sinusoidal fetal heart rate pattern: Its definition and clinical significance. Am J Obstet Gynecol 142:1033, 1982

Mueller-Heubach E, Battelli AF: Variable heart rate decelerations and transcutaneous PO2 (tc PO2) during umbilical cord occlusion in the fetal monkey. Am J Obstet Gynecol 144:796, 1982

Murata Y, Martin CB, Ikenoue T, et al: Fetal heart rate accelerations and late decelerations during the course of intrauterine death in chronically catheterized rhesus monkeys. Am J Obstet Gynecol 144:218, 1982

Murotsuki J, Bocking AD, Gagnon R: Fetal heart rate patterns in growth-restricted fetal sleep induced by chronic fetal placental embolization. Am J Obstet Gynecol 176:282, 1997

Murphy AA, Halamek LP, Lyell DJ, et al: Training and competency assessment in electronic fetal monitoring: A national survey. Obstet Gynecol 101:1243, 2003

Murphy KW, Russell V, Collins A, et al: The prevalence, aetiology and clinical significance of pseudo-sinusoidal fetal heart rate patterns in labour. Br J Obstet Gynaecol 98:1093, 1991

Myers RE: Two patterns of perinatal brain damage and their conditions of occurrence. Am J Obstet Gynecol 112:246, 1972

Myers RE, Mueller-Heubach E, Adamsons K: Predictability of the state of fetal oxygenation from a quantitative analysis of the components of late deceleration. Am J Obstet Gynecol 115:1083, 1973

Nageotte MP, Bertucci L, Towers CV, et al: Prophylactic amnioinfusion in pregnancies complicated by oligohydramnios: A prospective study. Obstet Gynecol 77:677, 1991

Nathan L, Leveno KJ, Carmody TJ, et al: Meconium: A 1990s perspective on an old obstetric hazard. Obstet Gynecol 83:328, 1994

National Institute of Child Health and Human Development Research Planning Workshop: Electronic fetal heart rate monitoring: Research guidelines for integration. Am J Obstet Gynecol 177:1385, 1997

Neesham DE, Umstad MP, Cincotta RB, et al: Pseudo-sinusoidal fetal heart rate pattern and fetal anemia: Case report and review. Aust N Z J Obstet Gynaecol 33:386, 1993

Nelson KB, Grether JK: Potentially asphyxiating conditions and cerebral palsy in infants of normal birth weight. Am J Obstet Gynecol 179:567, 1998

Nicolaides KH, Sadovsky G, Cetin E: Fetal heart rate patterns in red blood cell isoimmunized pregnancies. Am J Obstet Gynecol 161:351, 1989

Norén H, Amer-Wåhlin I, Hagberg H, et al: Fetal electrocardiography in labor and neonatal outcome: Data from the Swedish randomized controlled trial on intrapartum fetal monitoring. Am J Obstet Gynecol 188:183, 2003

Ogueh O, Steer P: Gender does not affect fetal heart rate variation. Br J Obstet Gynaecol 105:1312, 1998

Ogundipe OA, Spong CY, Ross MG: Prophylactic amnioinfusion for oligohydramnios: A re-evaluation. Obstet Gynecol 84:544, 1994

Owen J, Henson BV, Hauth JC: A prospective randomized study of saline solution amnioinfusion. Am J Obstet Gynecol 162:1146, 1990

Parer JT: Electronic fetal heart rate monitoring: A story of survival. Obstet Gynecol Surv 58:561, 2003

Parer J: NIH sets the terms for fetal heart rate pattern interpretation. OB/Gyn News, September 1, 1997

Parer JT, King T: Fetal heart rate monitoring: Is it salvageable? Am J Obstet Gynecol 182:982, 2000

Parer WJ, Parer JT, Holbrook RH, et al: Validity of mathematical models of quantitating fetal heart rate variability. Am J Obstet Gynecol 153:402, 1985

Paul RH, Snidon AK, Yeh SY: Clinical fetal monitoring, 7. The evaluation and significance of intrapartum baseline FHR variability. Am J Obstet Gynecol 123:206, 1975

Paul WM, Quilligan EJ, MacLachlan T: Cardiovascular phenomena associated with fetal head compression. Am J Obstet Gynecol 90:824, 1964

Petrie RH: Dose/response effects of intravenous meperidine in fetal heart rate variability. J Matern Fetal Med 2:215, 1993

Phelan JP, Ahn MO: Perinatal observations in forty-eight neurologically impaired term infants. Am J Obstet Gynecol 171:424, 1994

Picquard F, Hsiung R, Mattauer M, et al: The validity of fetal heart rate monitoring during the second stage of labor. Obstet Gynecol 72:746, 1988

Pierce J, Gaudier FL, Sanchez-Ramos L: Intrapartum amnioinfusion for meconium-stained fluid: Meta-analysis of prospective clinical trials. Obstet Gynecol 95:1051, 2000

Pillai M, James D: The development of fetal heart rate patterns during normal pregnancy. Obstet Gynecol 76:812, 1990

Pontonnier G, Puech F, Grandjean H, et al: Some physical and biochemical parameters during normal labour. Fetal and maternal study. Biol Neonate 26:159, 1975

Pressman EK, Blakemore KJ: A prospective randomized trial of two solutions for intrapartum amnioinfusion: Effects on fetal electrolytes, osmolality, and acid-base status. Am J Obstet Gynecol 175:945, 1996

Ramin KD, Leveno KJ, Kelly MS, et al: Amnionic fluid meconium: A fetal environmental hazard. Obstet Gynecol 87:181, 1996

Rathore AM, Singh R, Ramji S, et al: Randomised trial of amnioinfusion during labour with meconium stained amniotic fluid. Br J Obstet Gynaecol 109:17, 2002

Renou P, Warwick N, Wood C: Autonomic control of fetal heart rate. Am J Obstet Gynecol 105:949, 1969

Rinehart BK, Terrone DA, Barrow JH, et al: Randomized trial of intermittent or continuous amnioinfusion for variable decelerations. Obstet Gynecol 96:571, 2000

Rogers MS, Mongelli M, Tsang KH, et al: Lipid peroxidation in cord blood at birth: The effect of labour. Br J Obstet Gynaecol 105:739, 1998

Rosen MG, Dickinson JC: The incidence of cerebral palsy. Am J Obstet Gynecol 167:417, 1992

Ross M, Devoe L, Rosen K: Improved intrapartum fetal assessment with addition of ST-segment analysis of fetal heart rate (FHR) tracings: Trial among U.S. clinicians. Am J Obstet Gynecol 189:S183, 2004.

Samueloff A, Langer O, Berkus M, et al: Is fetal heart rate variability a good predictor of fetal outcome? Acta Obstet Gynecol Scand 73:39, 1994

Schucker JL, Sarno AP, Egerman RS, et al: The effect of butorphanol on the fetal heart rate reactivity during labor. Am J Obstet Gynecol 174:491, 1996

Seitchik J: Quantitating uterine contractility in a clinical context. Obstet Gynecol 57:453, 1981

Sherer DM: Blunted fetal response to vibroacoustic stimulation associated with maternal intravenous magnesium sulfate therapy. Am J Perinatol 11:401, 1994

Skupski DW, Rosenberg CR, Eglinton GS: Intrapartum fetal stimulation tests: A meta-analysis. Obstet Gynecol 99:129, 2002

Smith CV, Nguyen HN, Phelan JP, et al: Intrapartum assessment of fetal well-being: A comparison of fetal acoustic stimulation with acid–base determinations. Am J Obstet Gynecol 155:726, 1986

Smith JH, Anand KJ, Cotes PM, et al: Antenatal fetal heart rate variation in relation to the respiratory and metabolic status of the compromised human fetus. Br J Obstet Gynaecol 95:980, 1988

Southall DP, Richards J, Hardwick RA, et al: Prospective study of fetal heart rate and rhythm patterns. Arch Dis Child 55:506, 1980

Spong CY, Ogundipe OA, Ross MG: Prophylactic amnioinfusion for meconium-stained amniotic fluid. Am J Obstet Gynecol 171:931, 1994

Spong CY, Rasul C, Collea JV, et al: Characterization and prognostic significance of variable decelerations in the second stage of labor. Am J Perinatol 15:369, 1998

Stiller R, von Mering R, König V, et al: How well does reflectance pulse oximetry reflect intrapartum fetal acidosis? Am J Obstet Gynecol 186:1351, 2002

Symonds EM: Fetal monitoring: Medical and legal implications for the practitioner. Curr Opin Obstet Gynecol 6:430, 1994

Thacker SB, Stroup DF, Peterson HB: Efficacy and safety of intrapartum electronic fetal monitoring: An update. Obstet Gynecol 86:613, 1995

Trudinger BJ, Pryse-Davies J: Fetal hazards of the intrauterine pressure catheter: Five case reports. Br J Obstet Gynaecol 85:567, 1978

Usta IM, Mercer BM, Aswad NK, et al: The impact of a policy of amnioinfusion for meconium-stained amniotic fluid. Obstet Gynecol 85:237, 1995

Van Geijn HP, Jongsma HN, deHaan J, et al: Heart rate as an indicator of the behavioral state. Am J Obstet Gynecol 136:1061, 1980

Walker J: Foetal anoxia. J Obstet Gynaecol Br Commonw 61:162, 1953

Wenstrom K, Andrews WW, Maher JE: Amnioinfusion survey: Prevalence protocols and complications. Obstet Gynecol 86:572, 1995

Westgate J, Harris M, Curnow JSH, et al: Plymouth randomized trial of cardiotocogram only versus ST waveform plus cardiotocogram for intrapartum monitoring in 2400 cases. Am J Obstet Gynecol 169:1151, 1993

Westgate JA, Bennet L, De Haan HH, et al: Fetal heart rate overshoot during repeated umbilical cord occlusion in sheep. Obstet Gynecol 97:454, 2001

Williams JW: Williams Obstetrics, 1st ed. New York, Appleton, 1903

Williams K, Galerneau F: Comparison of intrapartum fetal heart rate tracings in patients with neonatal seizures vs no seizures, what are the differences? J Perinat Med 32:422, 2004

Yam J, Chua S, Arulkumaran S: Intrapartum fetal pulse oximetry. Part I: Principles and technical issues. Obstet Gynecol Surv 55:163, 2000

Young BK, Katz M, Wilson SJ: Sinusoidal fetal heart rate, 1. Clinical significance. Am J Obstet Gynecol 136:587, 1980a

Young BK, Weinstein HM: Moderate fetal bradycardia. Am J Obstet Gynecol 126:271, 1976

Young DC, Gray JH, Luther ER, et al: Fetal scalp blood pH sampling: Its value in an active obstetric unit. Am J Obstet Gynecol 136:276, 1980b

Zalar RW, Quilligan EJ: The influence of scalp sampling on the cesarean section rate for fetal distress. Am J Obstet Gynecol 135:239, 1979

19

Obstetrical Anesthesia

Pain relief in labor presents unique problems. Labor begins without warning, and obstetrical anesthesia may be required within minutes of a full meal. Vomiting with aspiration of gastric contents is a constant threat that poses serious maternal morbidity and mortality. Moreover, a host of disorders unique to pregnancy, such as preeclampsia, placental abruption, and chorioamnionitis, all superimposed on unique physiological adaptations of pregnancy, are directly affected by the choice of analgesia and anesthesia selected.

Anesthesia complications caused 1.6 percent of pregnancy-related maternal deaths in the United States from 1991 through 1997 (Berg and co-workers, 2003). Data from the Pregnancy Mortality Surveillance Program of the Centers for Disease Control and Prevention indicate that anesthesia-related maternal mortality has declined significantly over the past two decades, from 4.3 per million live births during 1979 to 1981 to less than 2 per million between 1991 and 1999 (Chang and colleagues, 2003; Hawkins and associates, 1997b). The proportion of maternal deaths caused by anesthesia-related complications also has declined from 2.5 percent between 1979 and 1990 to 1.6 percent between 1991 and 1999 (Koonin and associates, 1997).

Several factors likely have contributed to improved safety of obstetrical anesthesia. Eltzschig and associates (2003) and Hawkins and colleagues (1997b) have suggested that the recent trend toward increased use of regional analgesia, rather than general anesthesia, may be the most significant factor. The increased availability of in-house anesthesia coverage almost certainly is another important reason (Hawkins and associates, 1997a). Indeed, inadequate anesthesia services have been identified as a leading and potentially preventable cause of maternal deaths in Japan (Nagaya and associates, 2000).

GENERAL PRINCIPLES

OBSTETRICAL ANESTHESIA SERVICES. The American College of Obstetricians and Gynecologists (2002b) recently reaffirmed its position published jointly with the American Society of Anesthesiologists that a request for pain relief by the woman is sufficient medical indication for its use. The American Academy of Pediatrics and the American College of Obstetricians and Gynecologists (2002) have specified that it is the responsibility of the obstetrician or certified nurse-midwife, in consultation with an anesthesiologist, if appropriate, to develop the most suitable response to accomplish the request for pain relief. Identification of any of the risk factors shown in Table 19–1 should prompt consultation with anesthesia personnel to permit a joint management plan. This plan should include strategies to minimize the need for emergency anesthesia in women for whom such anesthesia would be especially hazardous.

Goals for optimizing obstetrical anesthesia services have been jointly established by the American College of

TABLE 19–1 Maternal Risk Factors That Should Prompt Anesthesia Consultation

Marked obesity
Severe edema or anatomical abnormalities of face, neck, or spine, including trauma or surgery
Abnormal dentition, small mandible, or difficulty opening mouth
Extremely short stature, short neck, or arthritis of the neck
Goiter
Serious maternal medical problems, such as cardiac, pulmonary, or neurological disease
Bleeding disorders
Severe preeclampsia
Previous history of anesthetic complications
Obstetrical complications likely to lead to operative delivery—e.g., placenta previa or higher-order multiple gestation

Adapted from the American Academy of Pediatrics and the American College of Obstetricians and Gynecologists (2002), with permission.

Obstetricians and Gynecologists and the American Society of Anesthesiologists (2001). These goals should be sought by any hospital providing obstetrical care:

1. Availability of a licensed practitioner who is credentialed to administer an appropriate anesthetic whenever necessary and to maintain support of vital functions in an obstetrical emergency.
2. Availability of anesthesia personnel to permit the start of a cesarean delivery within 30 minutes of the decision to perform the procedure.
3. Anesthesia personnel immediately available to perform an emergency cesarean delivery during the active labor of a woman attempting vaginal birth after cesarean (see Chap. 26, p. 610).
4. Appointment of a qualified anesthesiologist to be responsible for all anesthetics administered.
5. Availability of a qualified physician with obstetrical privileges to perform operative vaginal or cesarean delivery during administration of anesthesia.
6. Availability of equipment, facilities, and support personnel equal to that provided in the surgical suite.
7. Immediate availability of personnel, other than the surgical team, to assume responsibility for resuscitation of the depressed newborn (see Chap. 28, p. 634).

To meet these goals, 24-hour in-house anesthesia coverage is usually necessary. Providing such services in smaller facilities is more challenging—a problem underscored by the fact that approximately half of all hospitals providing obstetrical care have fewer than 500 deliveries per year (American College of Obstetricians and Gynecologists, 2001).

Bell and colleagues (2000) calculated the financial burden that may be incurred when trying to provide "24/7" obstetrical anesthesia coverage. Given the average indemnity and Medicaid reimbursement for labor epidural analgesia, they concluded that such coverage could not operate profitably at their tertiary referral institution. Compounding this burden, some third-party payers have denied reimbursement for epidural analgesia in the absence of a specific medical indication. In response, the American College of Obstetricians and Gynecologists and the American Society of Anesthesiologists (2004) issued a joint statement that reimbursement for regional analgesia should not be denied if given *only* for pain relief.

Role of Obstetrician. Every obstetrician should be proficient in local and pudendal analgesia. Regional analgesia may be administered by the properly trained obstetrician in appropriately selected circumstances. In general, however, it is preferable for an anesthesiologist or anesthetist to provide this care so that the obstetrician can focus attention on the concerns for the laboring woman and her fetus. **General anesthesia should be administered only by those with special training.**

PRINCIPLES OF PAIN RELIEF. In a scholarly review, Lowe (2002) emphasized that the experience of labor pain is a highly individual reflection of variable stimuli that are uniquely received and interpreted by each woman individually. These stimuli are modified by emotional, motivational, cognitive, social, and cultural circumstances. The complexity and individuality of the experience suggest that a woman and her caregivers may have a limited ability to anticipate her pain experience prior to labor. Thus, choice among a variety of methods and individualization of pain relief is desirable.

NONPHARMACOLOGICAL METHODS OF PAIN CONTROL. Fear and the unknown potentiate pain. A woman who is free from fear, and who has confidence in the obstetrical staff that cares for her, usually requires smaller amounts of analgesia. Read (1944) emphasized that the intensity of pain during labor is related in large measure to emotional tension. He urged that women be well informed about the physiology of parturition and the various hospital procedures to which they will be subjected during labor and delivery. Lamaze (1970) subsequently described his psychoprophylactic method, which emphasized childbirth as a natural physiological process. Pain often can be lessened by teaching pregnant women relaxed breathing and their labor partners psychological support techniques. These concepts have considerably reduced the use of potent analgesic, sedative, and amnestic drugs during labor and delivery.

When motivated women have been prepared for childbirth, pain and anxiety during labor have been found to be diminished significantly and labors are even shorter (Melzack, 1984; Saisto and associates, 2001). In addition, the presence of a supportive spouse or other family member, of conscientious labor attendants, and of a considerate obstetrician who instills confidence, have all been found to be of considerable benefit. In one study, Kennell and associates (1991) randomly assigned 412 nulliparous women in labor to either continuous emotional support from an experienced companion or to monitoring by an inconspicuous observer who did not interact with the laboring woman. The cesarean delivery rate was significantly lower in the continuous support group compared with that of the hands-off monitored group (8 versus 13 percent), as was the frequency of epidural analgesia for vaginal delivery (8 versus 23 percent).

ANALGESIA AND SEDATION DURING LABOR

When uterine contractions and cervical dilatation cause discomfort, pain relief with a narcotic such as meperidine, plus one of the tranquilizer drugs such as promethazine, is usually appropriate. With a successful program of analgesia and sedation, the mother should rest quietly between contractions. In this circumstance, discomfort usually is felt at the acme of an effective uterine contraction, but the pain is generally not unbearable. Appropriate drug selection and administration of the medications shown in Table 19–2 should safely accomplish these objectives for the great majority of women in labor.

TABLE 19–2 Parenteral Agents for Labor Pain

Agent	Usual Dose	Frequency	Onset	Neonatal Half-Life
Meperidine	25–50 mg (IV)	1–2 hr	5 min	13–22.4 hr
	50–100 mg (IM)	2–4 hr	30–45 min	63 hr for active metabolites
Fentanyl	50–100 μg (IV)	1 hr	1 min	5.3 hr
Nalbuphine	10 mg (IV or IM)	3 hr	2–3 min (IV)	4.1 hr
			15 min (IM)	
Butorphanol	1–2 mg (IV or IM)	4 hr	1–2 min (IV)	Not known
			10–30 min (IM)	Similar to nalbuphine in adults
Morphine	2–5 mg (IV)	4 hr	5 min	7.1 hr
	10 mg (IM)		30–40 min	

IM = intramuscularly; IV = intravenously.
From the American College of Obstetricians and Gynecologists (2002b), with permission.

PARENTERAL AGENTS

Meperidine and Promethazine. Meperidine, 50 to 100 mg, with promethazine, 25 mg, may be administered intramuscularly at intervals of 2 to 4 hours. A more rapid effect is achieved by giving meperidine intravenously in doses of 25 to 50 mg every 1 to 2 hours. Whereas analgesia is maximal about 30 to 45 minutes after an intramuscular injection, it develops almost immediately following intravenous administration. Meperidine readily crosses the placenta, and the half-life is approximately 13 hours or longer in the newborn (American College of Obstetricians and Gynecologists, 2002b). Its depressant effect in the fetus follows closely behind the peak maternal analgesic effect.

In a randomized investigation of epidural analgesia conducted at Parkland Hospital, patient-controlled intravenous analgesia with meperidine was found to be an inexpensive and effective method for labor analgesia (Sharma and colleagues, 1997). Women randomized to self-administered analgesia were given 50-mg meperidine with 25-mg promethazine intravenously as an initial bolus. Thereafter, an infusion pump was set to deliver 15 mg of meperidine every 10 minutes as needed until delivery. The mean and maximum total meperidine doses until delivery were 140 and 500 mg, respectively. One fourth of the women received more than 200 mg of meperidine during their labors. Neonatal sedation, as measured by need for naloxone treatment in the delivery room, was identified in 3 percent of newborns.

Butorphanol (Stadol). This synthetic narcotic, given in 1- to 2-mg doses, compares favorably with 40 to 60 mg of meperidine (Quilligan and colleagues, 1980). The major side effects are somnolence, dizziness, and dysphoria. Neonatal respiratory depression is reported to be less than with meperidine, but care must be taken that the two drugs are not given contiguously because butorphanol antagonizes the narcotic effects of meperidine. Angel and colleagues (1984) and Hatjis and Meis (1986) described a sinusoidal fetal heart rate pattern following butorphanol administration (see Chap. 18, p. 451).

Fentanyl. This short-acting and very potent synthetic opioid may be given in doses of 50 to 100 μg intravenously every hour. Its main disadvantage is a short duration of action, which requires frequent dosing or the use of a patient-controlled intravenous pump. Atkinson and associates (1994) reported that butorphanol provided better initial analgesia than fentanyl and was associated with fewer requests for more medication or for epidural analgesia.

Efficacy and Safety of Parenteral Agents. Bricker and Lavender (2002) have reviewed the effectiveness and safety of parenteral opioids for labor analgesia. Based on their systematic review of 85 investigations, they concluded the following:

1. Meperidine is the most common opioid used worldwide for pain relief in labor.
2. There is no convincing evidence demonstrating that alternative opioids are better.
3. There is no evidence that parenteral opioids influence the length of labor or need for obstetrical intervention.
4. Epidural analgesia provides superior pain relief.

Intravenous and intramuscular sedation are not without risks. Hawkins and colleagues (1997b) reported that 4 of 129 maternal anesthetic-related deaths were from such sedation—one from aspiration, two from inadequate ventilation, and one from overdosage. Moreover, meperidine or other narcotics used during labor may cause newborn respiratory depression.

Narcotic Antagonists. Naloxone is a narcotic antagonist capable of reversing respiratory depression induced by opioid narcotics. It acts by displacing the narcotic from specific receptors in the central nervous system. Withdrawal symptoms may be precipitated in recipients who are physically dependent on narcotics. For this reason, naloxone is contraindicated in a newborn of a narcotic-addicted mother (American Academy of Pediatrics and American College of Obstetricians and Gynecologists, 2002). Naloxone, along with proper ventilation, may be given to reverse respiratory depression in a newborn infant whose mother received narcotics (see Chap. 28, p. 637).

NITROUS OXIDE. A self-administered mixture of 50-percent nitrous oxide (N_2O) and oxygen provides satisfactory analgesia during labor for many women (Rosen, 2002a). Some preparations are premixed in a single cylinder (Entonox), and in others, a blender mixes the two gases from separate tanks (Nitronox). The gases are connected to a breathing circuit through a valve that opens only when the patient inspires. The use of intermittent nitrous oxide for labor pain has been reviewed by Rosen (2002a) and the following technique suggested:

1. Instruct the woman to take slow deep breaths and to begin inhaling 30 seconds before the next anticipated contraction and to cease when the contraction starts to recede.
2. Remove the mask between contractions and encourage her to breathe normally. No one but the patient or knowledgeable personnel should hold the mask.
3. Instruct a caregiver to remain in verbal contact with the patient.
4. Provide the expectation that the pain will likely not be eliminated, but that the gas should provide some relief.
5. Ensure intravenous access, pulse oximetry, and adequate scavenging of exhaled gases.
6. Use with additional caution after previous opioid administration because the combination can more easily render a woman unconscious and unable to protect her airway.

REGIONAL ANALGESIA

Various nerve blocks have been developed over the years to provide pain relief during labor and delivery. They are correctly referred to as *regional analgesics.*

SENSORY INNERVATION OF THE GENITAL TRACT

Uterine Innervation. Pain during the first stage of labor is generated largely from the uterus. Visceral sensory fibers from the uterus, cervix, and upper vagina traverse through the Frankenhäuser ganglion, which lies just lateral to the cervix, into the pelvic plexus, and then to the middle and superior internal iliac plexuses (Fig. 19–1). From there, the fibers travel in the lumbar and lower thoracic sympathetic chains to enter the spinal cord through the white rami communicantes associated with the T10 through T12 and L1 nerves. Early in labor, the pain of uterine contractions is transmitted predominantly through the T11 and T12 nerves.

The motor pathways to the uterus leave the spinal cord at the level of the T7 and T8 vertebrae. Theoretically, any method of sensory block that does not also block the motor pathways to the uterus can be used for analgesia during labor.

Lower Genital Tract Innervation. Pain with vaginal delivery arises from stimuli from the lower genital tract. These are transmitted primarily through the pudendal nerve, the peripheral branches of which provide sensory innervation to the perineum, anus, and the more medial and inferior parts of the vulva and clitoris. The pudendal nerve passes beneath the posterior surface of the sacrospinous ligament just as the ligament attaches to the ischial spine. As discussed in Chapter 2 (see p. 26), the sensory nerve fibers of the pudendal nerve are derived from the ventral branches of the S2 through S4 nerves (see Fig. 19–1).

ANESTHETIC AGENTS. Some of the more commonly used local anesthetics, along with their usual concentrations, doses, and durations of action, are summarized in Table 19–3. Some preparations that contain dilute epinephrine to prolong the action of the anesthetic will also cause symptoms when a test dose is inadvertently given intravenously. The dose of each agent varies widely and is dependent on the particular nerve block and physical status of the woman. The onset, duration, and quality of analgesia can be enhanced by increasing the dose. This can be done safely by only incrementally administering small-volume boluses of the agent and by carefully monitoring for early warning signs of toxicity.

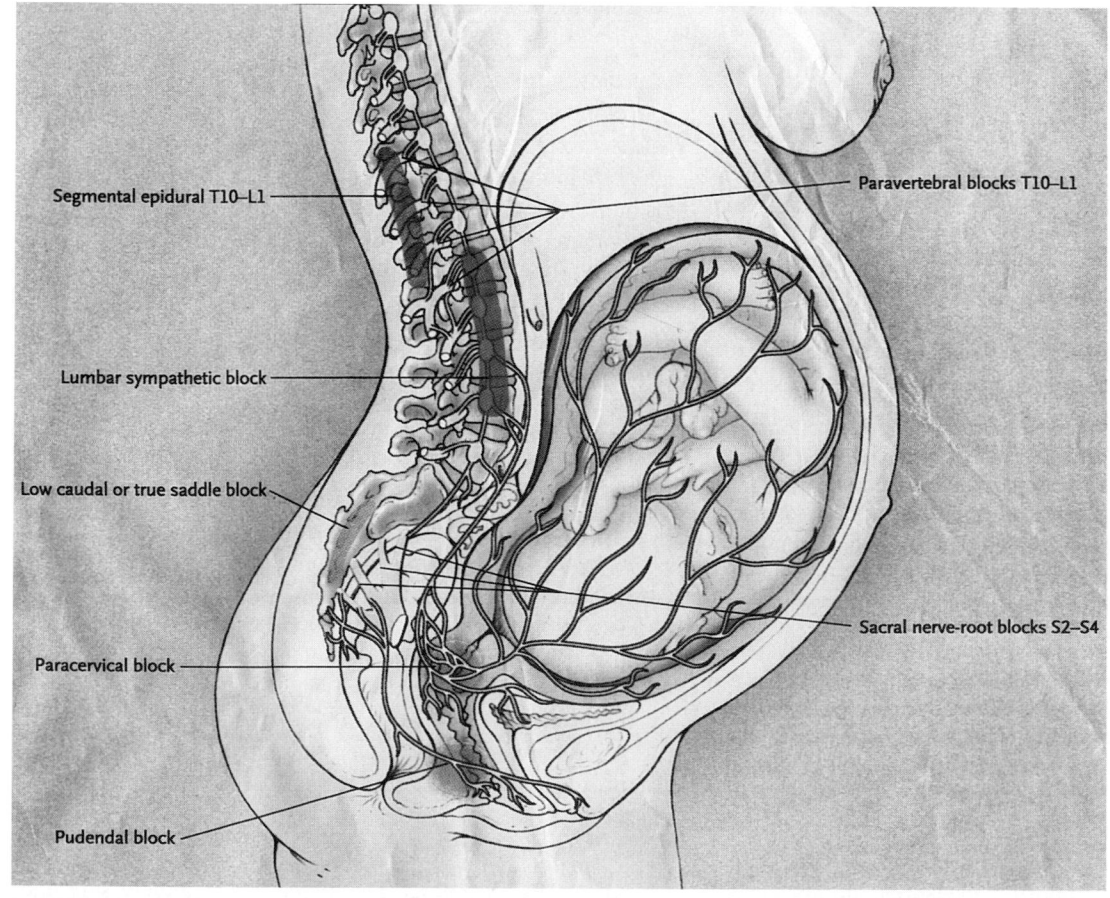

Segmental epidural T10–L1

Lumbar sympathetic block

Low caudal or true saddle block

Paracervical block

Pudendal block

Paravertebral blocks T10–L1

Sacral nerve-root blocks S2–S4

FIGURE 19–1. Pathways of labor pain. (From Eltzschig and associates, 2003, with permission.)

TABLE 19–3 Some Local Anesthetic Agents Used in Obstetrics

Anesthetic Agent	Plain Solutions						
	Usual Concentration (%)	Usual Volume (mL)	Usual Dose (mg)	Onset	Average Duration (min)	Clinical Use	
Amino-esters							
2-Chloroprocaine	1–2	20–30	400–600	Rapid	15–30	Local or pudendal block	
	2–3	15–25	300–750		30–60	Epidural (not subarachnoid) for cesarean delivery	
Tetracaine	0.2	—	4	Slow	75–150	Low spinal block/6% glucose	
	0.5	—	7–10		75–150	Spinal for cesarean delivery/5% glucose	
Amino-amides							
Lidocaine	1	20–30	200–300	Rapid	30–60	Local or pudendal block	
	2	15–30	300–450		60–90	Epidural for cesarean delivery	
	5	1–1.5	50–75		45–60	Spinal for cesarean delivery or puerperal tubal ligation/7.5% glucose	
	5	0.5–1	25–50		30–60	Spinal for vaginal delivery/7.5% glucose	
Bupivacaine	0.5	15–20	50–100	Slow	90–150	Epidural for cesarean delivery	
	0.25	8–10	20–25		60–90	Epidural for labor	
	0.75	1–1.5	7.5–11		60–120	Spinal for cesarean delivery/8.25% glucose	
Ropivacaine	0.5	15–20	75–100	Slow	90–150	Epidural for cesarean delivery	
	0.25	8–10	20–25		60–90	Epidural for labor	

Courtesy of Dr. Shiv Sharma and Dr. Donald Wallace.

Administration of these agents must be followed by appropriate monitoring for adverse reactions, and equipment and personnel to manage these reactions must be immediately available.

Most often, serious toxicity follows inadvertent intravenous injection, but it also may be induced by administration of excessive amounts. Because many of these agents are manufactured in more than one concentration and ampule size, a thorough knowledge of this information is essential for safety. Systemic toxicity from local anesthetics typically manifests in the central nervous and cardiovascular systems.

Central Nervous System Toxicity. Early symptoms are those of stimulation but, as serum levels increase, depression follows. Symptoms may include light-headedness, dizziness, tinnitus, metallic taste, and numbness of the tongue and mouth. Patients may show bizarre behavior, slurred speech, muscle fasciculation and excitation, and ultimately, generalized convulsions, followed by loss of consciousness. The convulsions should be controlled, an airway established, and oxygen delivered. Succinylcholine abolishes the peripheral manifestations of the convulsions and allows tracheal intubation. Thiopental or diazepam act centrally to inhibit convulsions. Magnesium sulfate, administered according to the regimen for eclampsia, also controls convulsions (see Chap. 34, p. 788). Abnormal fetal heart rate patterns, such as late decelerations or persistent bradycardia, may develop from maternal hypoxia and lactic acidosis induced by convulsions. With arrest of the convulsions, administration of oxygen, and application of other supportive measures, the fetus usually recovers more quickly in utero than following immediate

cesarean delivery. Moreover, maternal well-being is usually better served by waiting until the intensity of the hypoxia and the metabolic acidosis have diminished.

Cardiovascular Toxicity. These manifestations generally develop later than those from cerebral toxicity. They do not always follow central nervous system involvement, because they are induced by higher drug levels. The notable exception is bupivacaine, which is associated with the development of neurotoxicity and cardiotoxicity at virtually identical serum drug levels (Mulroy, 2002). Because of this risk of systemic toxicity, use of 0.75-percent solution of bupivacaine for epidural injection was proscribed by the Food and Drug Administration in 1984. Similar to neurotoxicity, cardiovascular toxicity is characterized first by stimulation and then by depression. Accordingly, there is hypertension and tachycardia, which soon is followed by hypotension and cardiac arrhythmias. The latter contribute appreciably to impaired uteroplacental perfusion and fetal distress.

Hypotension is managed initially by turning the woman onto either side to avoid aortocaval compression. A crystalloid solution is infused rapidly along with intravenously administered ephedrine. Emergency cesarean delivery should be considered if maternal vital signs have not been restored within 5 minutes of cardiac arrest (see Chap. 42, p. 1002). As with convulsions, however, the fetus is likely to recover more quickly in utero once maternal cardiac output is reestablished.

PUDENDAL BLOCK. This block is a relatively safe and simple method of providing analgesia for spontaneous

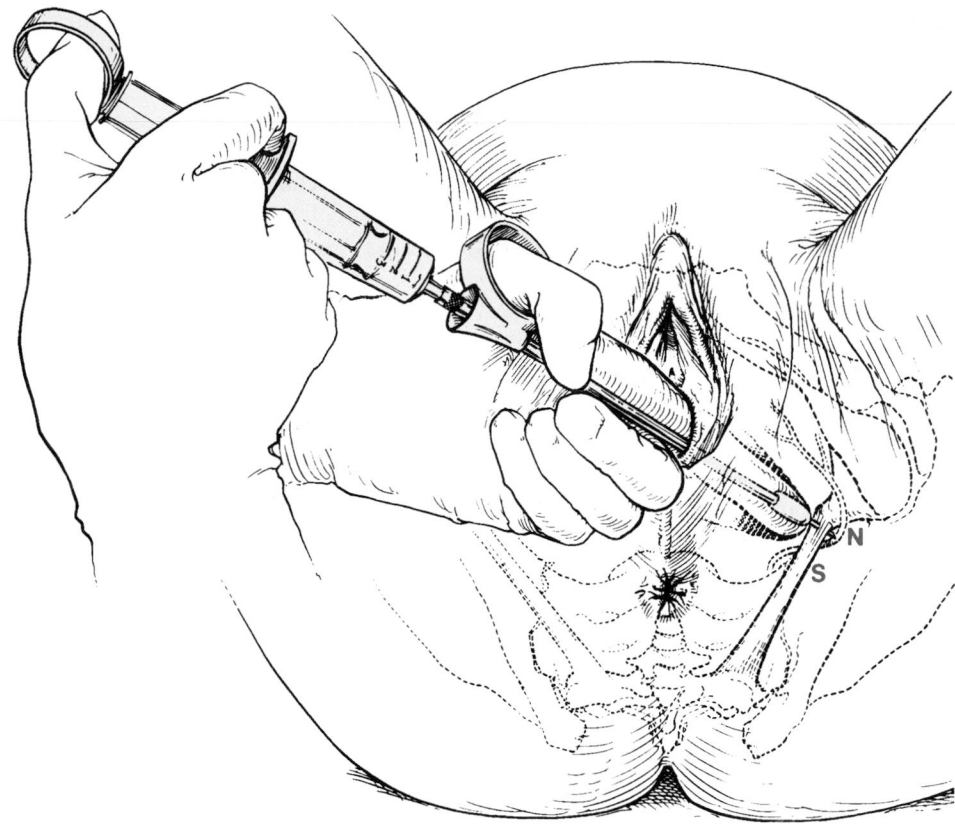

FIGURE 19–2. Local infiltration of the pudendal nerve. Transvaginal technique showing the needle extended beyond the needle guard and passing through the sacrospinous ligament (S) to reach the pudendal nerve (N).

delivery. As shown in Figure 19–2, a tubular introducer that allows 1.0 to 1.5 cm of a 15-cm 22-gauge needle to protrude beyond its tip is used to guide the needle into position over the pudendal nerve. The end of the introducer is placed against the vaginal mucosa just beneath the tip of the ischial spine. The needle is pushed beyond the tip of the director into the mucosa and a mucosal wheal is made with 1 mL of 1-percent lidocaine solution or an equivalent dose of another local anesthetic (see Table 19–3). To guard against intravascular infusion, aspiration is attempted before this and all subsequent injections. The needle is then advanced until it touches the sacrospinous ligament, which is infiltrated with 3 mL of lidocaine. The needle is advanced farther through the ligament, and as it pierces the loose areolar tissue behind the ligament, the resistance of the plunger decreases. Another 3 mL of the anesthetic solution is injected into this region. Next, the needle is withdrawn into the introducer, which is moved to just above the ischial spine. The needle is inserted through the mucosa and the rest of 10 mL of solution is deposited. The procedure is then repeated on the other side.

Within 3 to 4 minutes of the time of injection, the successful pudendal block will allow pinching of the lower vagina and posterior vulva bilaterally without pain. It is often of benefit before pudendal block to infiltrate the fourchette, perineum, and adjacent vagina with 5 to 10 mL of 1-percent lidocaine solution directly at the site where the episiotomy is to be made. Then, if delivery occurs before pudendal block

becomes effective, an episiotomy can be made without pain. By the time of the repair, the pudendal block usually has become effective.

Pudendal block usually does not provide adequate analgesia when delivery requires extensive obstetrical manipulation. Moreover, such analgesia is usually inadequate for women in whom complete visualization of the cervix and upper vagina, or manual exploration of the uterine cavity, are indicated.

Complications. As previously described (see p. 478), intravascular injection of a local anesthetic agent may cause serious systemic toxicity. Hematoma formation from perforation of a blood vessel also may develop. This complication is most likely when there is a coagulopathy (Lee and colleagues, 2004). One example is defective coagulation seen with placental abruption (see Chap. 35, p. 843). Rarely, severe infection may originate at the injection site. The infection may spread posterior to the hip joint, into the gluteal musculature, or into the retropsoas space (Svancarek and associates, 1977).

PARACERVICAL BLOCK. This block usually provides satisfactory pain relief during the first stage of labor. Because the pudendal nerves are not blocked, however, additional analgesia is required for delivery. Usually lidocaine or chloroprocaine, 5 to 10 mL of a 1-percent solution, is injected into the cervix laterally at 3 and 9 o'clock. Bupivacaine is contraindicated because of an increased risk of cardiotoxicity (American Academy of Pediatrics and American College of Obstetricians and Gynecologists, 2002; Rosen, 2002b). Because these anesthetics are relatively short acting, paracervical block may have to be repeated during labor.

Complications. Fetal bradycardia is a worrisome complication that occurs in approximately 15 percent of paracervical blocks (Rosen, 2002b). Bradycardia usually develops within 10 minutes and may last up to 30 minutes. Several investigators stress that bradycardia is not a sign of fetal asphyxia, because it usually is transient and the newborns are in most instances vigorous at birth. There are reports, however, in which fetal scalp blood pH and Apgar scores were sometimes low, and a few fetuses have died. The effect may be the consequence of transplacental transfer of the anesthetic agent or its metabolites and in turn, a depressant effect on the fetal heart. Based on studies in pregnant ewes, Greiss (1976) and Fishburne (1979) and their associates believe that fetal bradycardia results from decreased placental perfusion as the consequence of drug-induced uterine artery vasoconstriction and myometrial hypertonus. Doppler studies have shown an increase in the pulsatility index of the uterine arteries following paracervical block (see Chap. 16, p. 403). These observations further support the hypothesis of drug-induced vasospasm (Manninen and co-workers, 2000). For these reasons, paracervical block should not be used in situations of potential fetal compromise.

SPINAL (SUBARACHNOID) BLOCK. Introduction of a local anesthetic into the subarachnoid space to effect analgesia has long been used for delivery. Advantages include a short procedure time, rapid onset of the block, and high success rate. Because of the smaller subarachnoid space during pregnancy, likely the consequence of engorgement of the internal vertebral venous plexus, the same amount of anesthetic agent in the same volume of solution produces a much higher blockade in parturients than in nonpregnant women.

Vaginal Delivery. Low spinal block is a popular form of analgesia for forceps or vacuum delivery. The level of analgesia should extend to the T10 dermatome, which corresponds to the level of the umbilicus (Fig. 19–3). Blockade to this level provides excellent relief from the pain of uterine contractions (see Fig. 19–1).

Several local anesthetic agents have been used for spinal analgesia. Lidocaine given in a hyperbaric solution produces excellent analgesia and has the advantage of a rapid onset and relatively short duration. Bupivacaine in a dose of 10 to 12 mg in an 8.5-percent dextrose solution provides satisfactory anesthesia to the lower vagina and the perineum for more

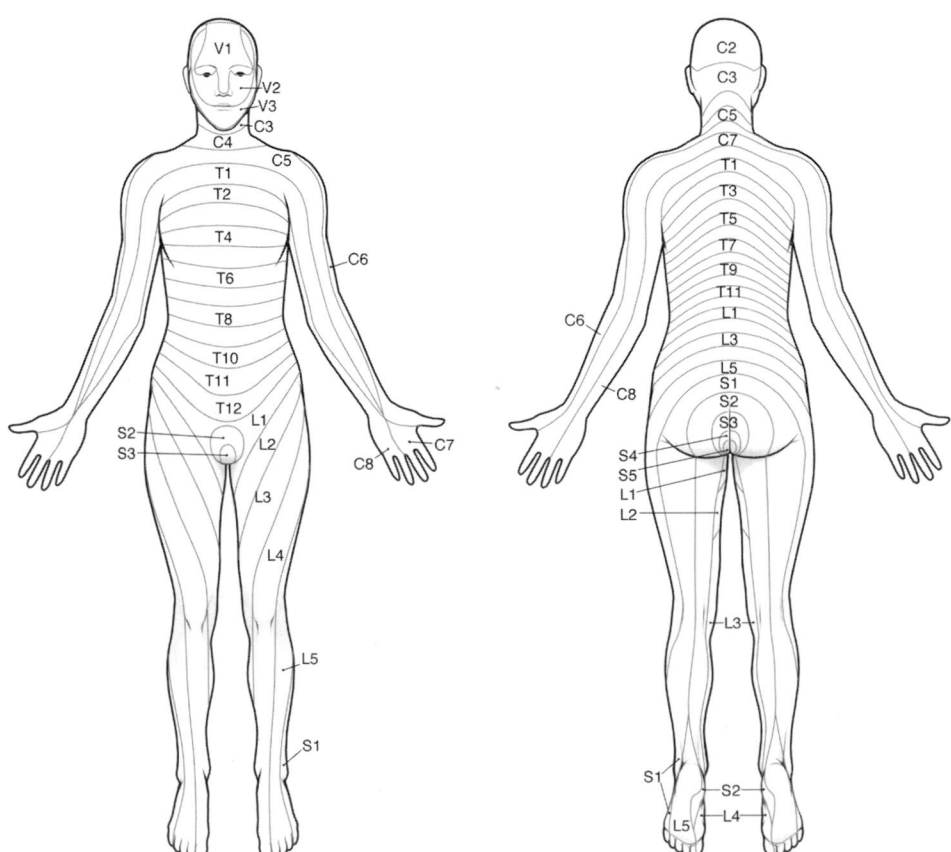

FIGURE 19–3. Dermatome distribution. (Redrawn from Keegan and Garrett, 1948, with permission.)

than 1 hour. Neither is administered until the cervix is fully dilated and all other criteria for safe forceps delivery have been fulfilled (see Chap. 23, p. 550). Preanalgesic intravenous hydration with 1 L of crystalloid solution will prevent or minimize hypotension in many cases.

Cesarean Delivery. A level of sensory blockade extending to the T4 dermatome is desired for cesarean delivery (see Fig. 19–3). Depending on maternal size, 10 to 12 mg of hyperbaric bupivacaine or 50 to 75 mg of hyperbaric lidocaine are administered. The addition of 20 to 25 μg of fentanyl increases the rapidity of the onset of the block and reduces shivering. The addition of 0.2 mg of morphine improves pain control during delivery and postoperatively.

Complications. Shown in Table 19–4 are some of the more common complications associated with regional analgesia. The estimated incidences were derived from 19 studies published between 1987 and 2000, as well as data from the Maternal–Fetal Medicine Units Network, which included more than 50,000 women undergoing cesarean delivery (Bloom and colleagues, 2004). Not listed is that obese women have significantly impaired ventilation (von Ungern-Sternberg and associates, 2004). Clearly, close clinical monitoring is imperative.

HYPOTENSION. This common complication may develop soon after injection of the local anesthetic agent and is the consequence of vasodilatation from sympathetic blockade compounded by obstructed venous return from uterine compression of the vena cava and adjacent large veins. **In the supine position, even in the absence of maternal hypotension measured in the brachial artery, placental blood flow may still be significantly reduced.** Treatment of spinal block hypotension includes uterine displacement, intravenous hydration, and intravenous bolus injections of ephedrine or phenylephrine. The predominant action of ephedrine is to

raise blood pressure by increasing cardiac output rather than vasoconstriction. Phenylephrine is a pure α-agonist which, at least until recently, we have generally avoided because of concerns about potential adverse effects on uterine blood flow. A meta-analysis of seven randomized trials by Lee and colleagues (2002b), however, suggests that the safety profiles of ephedrine and phenylephrine are comparable.

In a randomized trial at Parkland Hospital, Morgan and colleagues (2000) found that infusion of 1000 mL of Ringer lactate during the 20 minutes before spinal injection and 5-mg boluses of ephedrine as needed to maintain normal blood pressure resulted in a mean umbilical artery blood pH of 7.26. In contrast, prophylactic infusions containing diluted ephedrine were associated with significant fetal acidemia—the mean pH was about 7.12. Following a systematic review of 14 reports of elective cesarean deliveries, Lee and colleagues (2002a) question whether routine prophylactic ephedrine is needed. Ngan Kee and associates (2004) have used prophylactic phenylephrine infusion with good results.

HIGH SPINAL BLOCKADE. Most often, complete spinal blockade is the consequence of administration of an excessive dose of local anesthetic agent. This is certainly not always the case, because accidental total spinal block has even occurred following an epidural test dose (Palkar and associates, 1992). In complete spinal block, hypotension and apnea promptly develop and must be immediately treated to prevent cardiac arrest. In the undelivered woman, (1) the uterus is immediately displaced laterally to minimize aortocaval compression; (2) effective ventilation is established, preferably with tracheal intubation; and (3) intravenous fluids and ephedrine are given to correct hypotension.

SPINAL (POSTDURAL PUNCTURE) HEADACHE. Leakage of cerebrospinal fluid from the site of puncture of the meninges is thought to be the major factor in the genesis of spinal headache. Presumably, when the woman sits or stands, the

TABLE 19–4 Complications of Regional Analgesia Techniques

Complication	Incidence (%) from ACOG[a]			Incidence (%) from MFMU[b]		
	Spinal (n = N/A)	Epidural (n = N/A)	Combined[c] (n = N/A)	Spinal (n = 27,319)	Epidural (n = 18,697)	Combined[c] (n = 5,666)
Hypotension[d]	25–67	28–31	—	—	—	—
Postdural puncture headache	1.5–3	2	1–2.8	0.4	0.3	0.4
Pruritus	41–85	1.3–26	41–85	—	—	—
Failed regional block (need for GETA)	—	—	—	1.7	4.0	1.5
High spinal block	—	—	—	0.05	0.08	0.07
Chemical meningitis or epidural abscess or hematoma	—	—	—	0	0	0

GETA = general endotracheal anesthesia; N/A = data not available.
[a]American College of Obstetricians and Gynecologists; incidence based on 19 reports published between 1987–2000.
[b]Maternal–Fetal Medicine Units Network of the National Institute of Child Health and Human Development.
[c]Refers to combined spinal–epidural analgesia technique.
[d]Women were given intravenous prehydration before analgesia was injected.
Data from the American College of Obstetricians and Gynecologists (2002b) and Bloom and colleagues (2004).

diminished volume of cerebrospinal fluid allows traction on pain-sensitive central nervous system structures. This complication can be reduced by using a small-gauge spinal needle and avoiding multiple punctures. In a prospective, randomized study of five different spinal needles, Vallejo and colleagues (2000) concluded that Sprotte and Whitacre needles had the lowest risks of postdural puncture headaches.

There is no good evidence that placing the woman absolutely flat on her back for several hours is effective in preventing headache. Vigorous hydration may be of value, but also without compelling evidence to support its use. The administration of *caffeine,* a cerebral vasoconstrictor, has been shown in randomized studies to afford temporary relief (Sechzer and Abel, 1978; Camann and colleagues, 1990). With severe headache, an *epidural blood patch* is effective. A few milliliters of autologous blood are obtained aseptically by venipuncture without anticoagulant. This is injected into the epidural space at the site of the dural puncture. Relief is immediate and complications uncommon. If the headache does not have the pathognomonic postural characteristics or persists despite treatment with a blood patch, other diagnoses should be considered and appropriate testing performed. For example, Chisholm and Campbell (2001) described a case of superior sagittal sinus thrombosis that manifested as a postural headache. Chan and Paech (2004) have described persistent cerebrospinal fluid leak in three women.

CONVULSIONS. In rare instances, postdural puncture cephalgia is associated with blindness and convulsions. Shearer and colleagues (1995) described eight such cases associated with 19,000 regional analgesic procedures. It is presumed that these too are caused by cerebrospinal fluid hypotension.

BLADDER DYSFUNCTION. With spinal analgesia, bladder sensation is likely to be obtunded and bladder emptying impaired for the first few hours after delivery. As a consequence, bladder distention is a frequent postpartum complication, especially if appreciable volumes of intravenous fluid are given.

OXYTOCICS AND HYPERTENSION. Paradoxically, hypertension from ergonovine or methylergonovine injected following delivery is more common in women who have received a spinal or epidural block.

ARACHNOIDITIS AND MENINGITIS. Local anesthetics are no longer preserved in alcohol, formalin, or other toxic solutes, and disposable equipment is used by most. These practices, coupled with aseptic technique, have made meningitis and arachnoiditis rarities (see Table 19–4). Still, these complications are occasionally documented (Harding and colleagues, 1994; Newton and associates, 1994).

Contraindications to Spinal Analgesia. Shown in Table 19–5 are the absolute contraindications to regional analgesia according to the American College of Obstetricians and

TABLE 19–5 Absolute Contraindications to Regional Analgesia

Refractory maternal hypotension
Maternal coagulopathy
Treatment with once-daily dose of low-molecular-weight heparin within 12 hr
Untreated bacteremia
Skin infection over site of needle placement
Increased intracranial pressure caused by mass lesion

From the American College of Obstetricians and Gynecologists (2002b), with permission.

Gynecologists (2002b). Obstetrical complications that are associated with maternal hypovolemia and hypotension—such as severe hemorrhage—are contraindications to the use of spinal block. The cardiovascular effects of spinal block in the presence of acute blood loss, but in the absence of the hemodynamic effects of pregnancy, have been investigated by Kennedy and co-workers (1968). In 15 nonpregnant volunteers, spinal analgesia to the T5 sensory level was induced twice, the second time after a phlebotomy of 10 mL/kg. In the case of block without hemorrhage, the mean arterial blood pressure fell 10 percent while cardiac output rose slightly. In the case of hemorrhage without block, the mean blood pressure fell to the same degree and again the cardiac output rose slightly. With subarachnoid block administered after the modest hemorrhage, however, the mean arterial pressure fell nearly 30 percent and cardiac output fell 15 percent.

In addition to refractory maternal hypotension, disorders of coagulation and defective hemostasis also preclude the use of spinal analgesia. Similarly, subarachnoid puncture is contraindicated when the skin or underlying tissue at the site of needle entry is infected. Neurological disorders are considered by many to be a contraindication, if for no other reason than that exacerbation of the neurological disease might be attributed without cause to the anesthetic agent. Other maternal conditions, such as significant aortic stenosis or pulmonary hypertension, are also relative contraindications to the use of spinal analgesia (see Chap. 44, pp. 1026 and 1029).

Preeclampsia. As with significant hemorrhage, severe preeclampsia is another complication in which markedly decreased blood pressure can be predicted when subarachnoid analgesia is used. Gambling and Writer (1999) have reviewed the use of spinal analgesia in women with severe preeclampsia. Although they acknowledge it to be quite controversial, they concluded that with severe preeclampsia, epidural analgesia is preferable to a subarachnoid block and especially preferable to a general anesthetic. The latter has inherent risks of difficult intubation due to airway edema and cerebrovascular accidents due to increased blood pressure. As subsequently discussed, hypotension is also a risk with epidural analgesia. Wallace and colleagues (1995) randomly assigned 80 women with severe preeclampsia undergoing cesarean

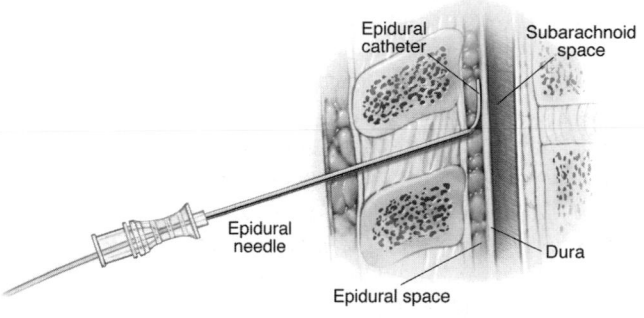

FIGURE 19–4. Introduction of a catheter into the epidural space through a Tuohy needle. (Redrawn from Sharma and Leveno, 2003, with permission.)

delivery to receive general anesthesia or either epidural or spinal–epidural analgesia. There were no differences in maternal or neonatal outcomes, but 30 percent of those given epidural analgesia and 22 percent of those given spinal–epidural blockage developed hypotension, with an average reduction in mean arterial pressure between 15 and 25 percent.

EPIDURAL ANALGESIA. Relief from the pain of labor and childbirth, including cesarean delivery, can be accomplished by injection of a local anesthetic agent into the epidural or peridural space (Fig. 19–4). This potential space contains areolar tissue, fat, lymphatics, and the internal venous plexus. These latter vessels become engorged during pregnancy such that the volume of the epidural space is appreciably reduced. Entry for obstetrical analgesia is usually through a lumbar intervertebral space, and less often through the sacral hiatus and sacral canal for caudal epidural analgesia. Although one injection may be used, these usually are repeated through an indwelling catheter, or they are given by continuous infusion using a volumetric pump.

Continuous Lumbar Epidural Block. Complete analgesia for the pain of labor and vaginal delivery necessitates a block from the T10 to the S5 dermatomes (Figs. 19–1 and 19–3). For cesarean delivery, a block extending from the T4 to the S1 dermatomes is desired. The spread of the anesthetic depends upon the location of the catheter tip; the dose, concentration, and volume of anesthetic agent used, as shown in Table 19–3; and whether the mother is head-down, horizontal, or head-up (Setayesh and colleagues, 2001). Individual variations in the epidural space anatomy also will affect the block, and in some cases, synechiae may preclude a completely satisfactory block. It also should be recognized that the catheter tip might move from its original location during the course of labor.

Technique. One example of the sequential steps and techniques for performance of epidural analgesia is detailed in Table 19–6. Before any injection of the local anesthetic agent,

---

TABLE 19–6 Technique for Labor Epidural Analgesia

1. Informed consent is obtained, and the obstetrician consulted.
2. Monitoring includes the following:
   * Blood pressure every 1–2 min for 15 min after giving a bolus of local anesthetic.
   * Continuous maternal heart rate monitoring during analgesia induction.
   * Continuous fetal heart rate monitoring.
   * Continual verbal communication.
3. Hydration with 500 to 1000 mL of lactated Ringer solution.
4. The woman assumes a lateral decubitus or sitting position.
5. The epidural space is identified with a loss-of-resistance technique.
6. The epidural catheter is threaded 3–5 cm into the epidural space.
7. A test dose of 3 mL of 1.5% lidocaine with 1:200,000 epinephrine or 3 mL of 0.25% bupivacaine with 1:200,000 epinephrine is injected after careful aspiration and after a uterine contraction—this minimizes the chance of confusing tachycardia that results from labor pain with tachycardia from intravenous injection of the test dose.
8. If the test dose is negative, one or two 5-mL doses of 0.25% bupivacaine are injected to achieve a cephalad sensory T10 level.
9. After 15–20 min, the block is assessed using loss of sensation to cold or pinprick. If no block is evident, the catheter is replaced. If the block is asymmetrical, the epidural catheter is withdrawn 0.5–1.0 cm and an additional 3–5 mL of 0.25% bupivacaine is injected. If the block remains inadequate, the catheter is replaced.
10. The woman is positioned in the lateral or semilateral position to avoid aortocaval compression.
11. Subsequently, maternal blood pressure is recorded every 5–15 min. The fetal heart rate is monitored continuously.
12. The level of analgesia and intensity of motor block are assessed at least hourly.

From Glosten (1999), with permission.

---

a test dose is given and the woman is observed for features of toxicity from intravascular injection and for signs of spinal blockade from subarachnoid injection. Only then is a full dose given. Analgesia is maintained by intermittent boluses of similar volume, or small volumes of the drug are delivered continuously by infusion pump. The addition of small doses of a short-acting narcotic, either fentanyl or sufentanil, has been shown to improve analgesic efficacy for labor or cesarean delivery (Chestnut and colleagues, 1988). The rationale for opiate use during labor is to avoid motor block by allowing reduction in the dose of local anesthetic. **Appropriate resuscitation equipment and drugs must be available during administration of epidural analgesia.**

Complications. For most women, epidural analgesia provides unparalleled relief from the pain of labor and delivery. That said, as shown in Table 19–4, there are certain problems inherent in its use and as with spinal blockade, it is imperative that close monitoring, including the level of analgesia, be performed by trained personnel.

TOTAL SPINAL BLOCKADE. Dural puncture with inadvertent subarachnoid injection may cause total spinal block. Personnel and facilities must be immediately available to manage this complication, as described under complications of spinal analgesia (see p. 481).

INEFFECTIVE ANALGESIA. Establishment of effective pain relief with maximum safety takes time. Using currently popular continuous epidural infusion regimens such as 0.125-percent bupivacaine with 2-μg/mL fentanyl, 90 percent of women rate their pain relief as good to excellent, and 95 percent express a desire for the same type of analgesia during a future delivery (Sharma and colleagues, 1997). Alternatively, a few women find epidural analgesia to be inadequate. In a study of 1963 parturients who received epidural analgesia, Hess and associates (2001) found that approximately 12 percent complained of three or more episodes of pain or pressure. Risk factors for such breakthrough pain included nulliparity, heavier fetal weights, and epidural catheter placement at an earlier cervical dilatation. If the epidural analgesia is allowed to dissipate before another injection of anesthetic drug, subsequent pain relief may be delayed, incomplete, or both. In the Maternal–Fetal Medicine Units Network study cited earlier, 4 percent of women initially given epidural analgesia required a general anesthetic for cesarean delivery (Bloom and colleagues, 2004).

At times, perineal analgesia for delivery is difficult to obtain, especially with the lumbar epidural technique. When this condition is encountered, a low spinal or pudendal block or systemic analgesia is added.

HYPOTENSION. By blocking sympathetic tracts, epidurally injected analgesic agents may cause hypotension and decreased cardiac output. In normal pregnant women, hypotension induced by epidural analgesia usually can be prevented by rapid infusion of 500 to 1000 mL of crystalloid solution, or treated successfully as described for spinal analgesia. Danilenko-Dixon and associates (1996) showed that maintaining a lateral position minimized hypotension compared with the supine position. Despite these precautions, hypotension is the most common side effect and is severe enough to require treatment in one third of women (Sharma and colleagues, 1997).

CENTRAL NERVOUS STIMULATION. Convulsions are an uncommon but serious complication, the immediate management of which was described previously.

MATERNAL PYREXIA. Fusi and associates (1989) observed that the mean temperature in laboring women given epidural analgesia was significantly higher than in those given meperidine. Subsequently, a number of randomized and retrospective cohort studies have confirmed an increase in intrapartum fever.

Unfortunately, most investigations are limited by inability to control for other important risk factors, such as length of labor, duration of ruptured membranes, and number of vaginal examinations (Yancey and co-workers, 2001a). With this in mind, the frequency of intrapartum fever was found to be 10 to 15 percent by Lieberman and O'Donoghue (2002).

The precise etiology of maternal hyperthermia with epidural use is unclear. There are two general theories: (1) that fever results from *maternal–fetal infection* or (2) that it is caused by *dysregulation of body temperature*. Infection seems a reasonable explanation, and Dashe and co-workers (1999) studied placental histopathology in these women. After labor with epidural analgesia, they identified intrapartum fever only with placental inflammation. This suggests that fever is due to infection rather than to the analgesia itself. Conversely, other proposed mechanisms include alteration in the hypothalamic thermoregulatory set point, impairment of peripheral thermoreceptor input to the central nervous system with selective blockage of warm stimuli, or imbalance between heat production and heat loss (Yancey and co-workers, 2001a). With the current incomplete understanding of the underlying cause, the clinical significance of the association between epidural use and fever is an undoubtedly higher rate of intrapartum antimicrobial use and perhaps a higher rate of operative delivery.

BACK PAIN. Although an association between epidural analgesia and back pain has been reported by some clinicians, others have not found such a relationship (Breen, 1994; Howell, 2001; MacArthur, 1997, and all their colleagues). In a prospective cohort study, Butler and Fuller (1998) reported that postpartum back pain was common after epidural analgesia, however, persistent or chronic back pain was uncommon. Based on their systematic review of the literature, Lieberman and O'Donoghue (2002) concluded that available data do not support an association between the use of epidural analgesia and development of new, long-term backache.

Effect on Labor. Most studies, including the combined five randomized trials from Parkland Hospital shown in Table 19–7, report that epidural analgesia prolongs labor and increases the need for oxytocin stimulation. Alexander and associates (2002) examined the effects of epidural analgesia on the Friedman (1955) active labor curve, which is described in Chapter 17 (see p. 422). The study included 459 nulliparas randomly assigned to patient-controlled epidural analgesia or patient-controlled intravenous meperidine. Compared with Friedman's original criteria, epidural analgesia prolonged the active phase of labor by 1 hour. As shown in Table 19–7, epidural analgesia also has been found to increase the need for instrumental delivery due to prolonged second-stage labor, however, there were no adverse neonatal effects (Chestnut, 1999; Thorp and Breedlove, 1996). More contemporaneous is the concern for perineal trauma associated with instrumental

TABLE 19–7 **Selected Labor Events in 2703 Nulliparous Women Randomized to Epidural Analgesia or Intravenous Meperidine Analgesia**

Event[a]	Epidural Analgesia (n = 1339)	Intravenous Meperidine (n = 1364)	P Value
Labor Outcomes			
First-stage duration (hr)[b]	8.1 ± 5	7.5 ± 5	.011
Second-stage duration (min)	60 ± 56	47 ± 57	< .001
Oxytocin after analgesia (%)	641 (48)	546 (40)	< .001
Type of Delivery			
Spontaneous vaginal	1027 (77)	1122 (82)	< .001
Forceps	172 (13)	101 (7)	< .001
Cesarean	140 (10.5)	141 (10.3)	.92

[a]Data are presented as n (%) or mean ± SD.
[b]First stage = initiation of analgesia until complete cervical dilatation.
Adapted from Sharma and colleagues (2004), with permission.

delivery. This relationship is discussed in detail in Chapters 17 (see p. 435) and 23 (see p. 556).

FETAL HEART RATE. Hill and colleagues (2003) examined the effects of initiation of epidural analgesia using 0.25-percent bupivacaine on fetal heart rate patterns. Compared with intravenous meperidine, no deleterious effects were identified. In fact, reduced beat-to-beat variability and fewer accelerations were more common in fetuses whose mothers received meperidine (see Chap. 18, p. 449). Based on their systematic review of eight studies, Reynolds and co-workers (2002) found that epidural analgesia was associated with improved neonatal acid–base status compared with that with meperidine.

CESAREAN DELIVERY. A more contentious issue is whether epidural analgesia increases the risk for cesarean delivery. From their review, Sharma and Leveno (2000) found that

several retrospective studies and a few randomized trials concluded that labor epidural analgesia is associated with increased cesarean deliveries. Conversely, others have concluded that the available evidence is insufficient to establish such an association (Eltzschig and associates, 2003; Lieberman and O'Donoghue, 2002; Sharma and colleagues, 2004).

Several studies conducted at Parkland Hospital were designed to answer some of these questions. In the 8-year period from 1995 to 2002, a total of 2703 nulliparous women with term pregnancies in spontaneous labor were studied. There were five trials of various labor epidural analgesia techniques using dilute solutions of local anesthetic as well as methods for administration of meperidine intravenously (Fig. 19–5). Epidural analgesia did not significantly increase cesarean deliveries in any individual trial or in their aggregate. These results are consistent with the belief of many investigators

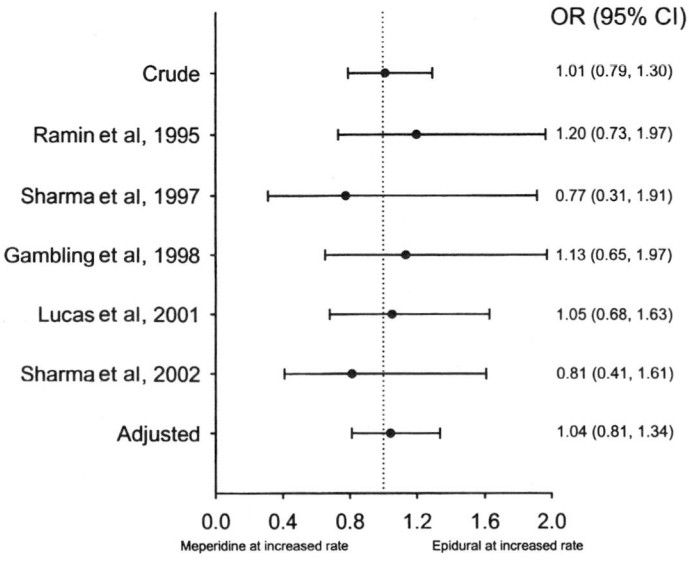

FIGURE 19–5. Results of five studies comparing the incidence of cesarean delivery in women given either epidural analgesia or intravenous meperidine. The individual odds ratios (ORs) with 95-percent confidence intervals (CIs) for each randomized study, as well as overall crude and adjusted ORs with 95-percent CIs, are shown. An OR of less than 1.0 favored epidural over meperidine analgesia. (From Sharma and associates, 2004, with permission.)

that the epidural administration of dilute solutions of local anesthetic is less likely to increase cesarean delivery rates than concentrated solutions (Chestnut, 1997; Thompson and colleagues, 1998).

Yancey and co-workers (1999) described the effects of introduction of an on-demand labor epidural analgesia service at Tripler Army Hospital in Hawaii. In late 1993, a policy change within the Department of Defense required the availability of on-demand labor epidural analgesia in military medical centers. As a result, the incidence of epidural analgesia during labor increased from 1 percent before the policy to 60 percent 2 years after the policy had been implemented. The primary cesarean rate was 13.4 percent before and 13.2 percent after this dramatic change in epidural usage. In a follow-up study, Yancey and co-workers (2001b) reported that fetal malpresentations at the time of vaginal delivery were not more common after epidural usage became prevalent. The only significant difference they found was an increased duration of second-stage labor by approximately 25 minutes (Zhang and co-workers, 2001).

Based on their randomized studies and review of the literature, Sharma and Leveno (2003) and Sharma and colleagues (2004) concluded that epidural analgesia is not associated with an excessive rate of cesarean births. Other investigators have drawn the same conclusion. Leighton and Halpern (2002) performed a meta-analysis of 14 randomized studies involving 2161 women who received epidural analgesia and 2136 who received opioids for labor pain. They found no increase in the cesarean rate attributable to epidural analgesia. The American College of Obstetricians and Gynecologists (2002a) has recently reaffirmed the following statement published jointly with the American Society of Anesthesiologists: "There is no other circumstance where it is considered acceptable for a person to experience severe pain, amenable to safe intervention, while under a physician's care." This statement implies that all women should have access to effective pain relief during labor. We are of the view that the fear of increasing the risk of cesarean delivery should not preclude women from choosing epidural analgesia during labor.

TIMING OF EPIDURAL PLACEMENT. Several retrospective studies have found an association between early epidural placement and a higher rate of cesarean delivery (Lieberman, 1996; Rogers, 1999; Seyb, 1999, and all their co-workers). Conversely, randomized trials comparing early versus late epidural placement in nulliparous women have found no difference in the rates of cesarean birth, forceps delivery, or fetal malposition (Chestnut and associates, 1994a, 1994b; Luxman and colleagues, 1998). The inconsistent findings between retrospective and randomized studies may be caused by confounding variables inherently associated with retrospective study designs (Sharma and Leveno, 2003). Based on their review, Eltzschig and colleagues (2003) recently concluded that there is currently insufficient evidence to justify waiting until a certain degree of cervical dilatation or fetal station is reached

before instituting epidural analgesia. Finally, the American College of Obstetricians and Gynecologists (2002b) has concluded that "women in labor should not be required to reach 4 to 5 cm of cervical dilatation before receiving epidural analgesia."

Safety. The relative safety of epidural analgesia is attested to by the extraordinary experiences reported by Crawford (1985) from the Birmingham Maternity Hospital in England. From 1968 through 1985, over 26,000 women were given epidural analgesia for labor, and there were no maternal deaths. The nine potentially life-threatening complications followed either inadvertent intravenous or intrathecal injection of lidocaine, bupivacaine, or both. Similarly, according to the Confidential Enquiries into Maternal Deaths in the United Kingdom between 1997 and 1999, only one anesthesia-related death was associated with epidural use (Thomas and Cooper, 2002). More recently, no anesthesia-related maternal deaths were recorded among nearly 19,000 women who received epidural analgesia in the Network Study cited earlier (Bloom and colleagues, 2004). Finally, in their Cochrane Library review, Ng and associates (2004) cited a very low incidence of complications.

Contraindications. As with spinal analgesia, contraindications to epidural analgesia include actual or anticipated serious maternal hemorrhage, infection at or near the sites for puncture, and suspicion of neurological disease (see Table 19–5). Rolbin and colleagues (1988) advise against epidural analgesia if the platelet count is below 100,000/μL. Conversely, Rasmus and associates (1989) found no cases in which bleeding was caused by regional analgesia in thrombocytopenic women. They recommended consideration of this method if the patient might be difficult to intubate or ventilate. The American College of Obstetricians and Gynecologists (2002b) has concluded that women with platelet counts of 50,000 to 100,000/μL may be considered potential candidates for regional analgesia.

ANTICOAGULATION. Women receiving anticoagulation therapy who are given regional analgesia are at increased risk for spinal cord hematoma and compression (see Chap. 47, p. 1083). The American College of Obstetricians and Gynecologists (2002b) has recommended the following for women taking anticoagulants:

1. Women receiving unfractionated heparin therapy should be able to receive regional analgesia if they have a normal activated partial thromboplastin time (aPTT).
2. Women receiving prophylactic doses of unfractionated heparin or low-dose aspirin are not at increased risk and can be offered regional analgesia.
3. For women receiving once-daily low-dose low-molecular-weight heparin, regional analgesia should not be placed until 12 hours after the last injection.

4. Low-molecular-weight heparin should be withheld for at least 2 hours after the removal of an epidural catheter.
5. The safety of regional analgesia in women receiving twice-daily low-molecular-weight heparin has not been studied sufficiently, and it is not known whether delaying regional analgesia for 24 hours after the last injection is adequate.

Severe Preeclampsia–Eclampsia. As previously discussed, ideal labor analgesia for women with severe preeclampsia is controversial. Obstetrical concerns include hypotension induced by sympathetic blockade, dangers from pressor agents given to correct hypotension, and potential for pulmonary edema following infusion of large volumes of crystalloid. Conversely, general anesthesia with tracheal intubation may result in severe, sudden hypertension further complicated by pulmonary or cerebral edema or intracranial hemorrhage.

Over the past two to three decades, most obstetrical anesthesiologists have come to favor epidural blockade for labor and delivery in women with severe preeclampsia (Cheek and Samuels, 1991; Gambling and Writer, 1999; Gutsche, 1986). There seems to be no argument that epidural analgesia for women with severe preeclampsia–eclampsia can be safely used when specially trained anesthesiologists and obstetricians are responsible for the woman and her fetus (American College of Obstetricians and Gynecologists, 2002b; Cunningham and Leveno, 1995; Hogg and colleagues, 1999). In a study from Parkland Hospital, Lucas and colleagues (2001) randomly assigned 738 women with hypertension to epidural analgesia or patient-controlled intravenous analgesia during labor. A standardized protocol for prehydration, incremental epidural administration, and ephedrine use was employed. They concluded that labor epidural analgesia was to be considered in women with hypertensive disorders, but that it was not to be considered as *therapy.* In a similar study from the University of Alabama at Birmingham, Head and colleagues (2002) randomly assigned 116 women with severe preeclampsia to receive either intrapartum epidural or patient-controlled intravenous opioid analgesia. Epidural analgesia provided superior pain relief without a significant increase in maternal or neonatal complications.

INTRAVENOUS FLUID PRELOAD. Women with severe preeclampsia have remarkably diminished intravascular volume compared with normal pregnancy (Zeeman and colleagues, 2002). Conversely, total body water is increased because of the capillary leak caused by endothelial cell activation (see Chap. 34, p. 769). This imbalance is manifested as pathological peripheral edema, proteinuria, ascites, and total lung water. For all of these reasons, aggressive volume replacement increases the risk for pulmonary edema, especially in the first 72 hours postpartum (Clark and colleagues, 1985; Cotton and associates, 1986). In one study, Hogg and associates (1999) reported that 3.5 percent of women with severe preeclampsia developed pulmonary edema when preloaded without a

protocol limitation to volume. Importantly, this risk can be reduced or obviated with judicious prehydration—usually with 500 to 1000 mL of crystalloid solution. Specifically, in the study by Lucas and colleagues (2001) cited earlier, there were no instances of pulmonary edema among the 738 women in whom crystalloid preload was limited to 500 mL. Moreover, vasodilation produced by epidural blockade is less abrupt if the analgesia level is achieved slowly with dilute solutions of local anesthetic agents. This allows maintenance of blood pressure while simultaneously avoiding infusion of large volumes of crystalloid.

With vigorous intravenous crystalloid therapy, there is also concern about development of cerebral edema (see Chap. 34, p. 778). Moreover, Heller and co-workers (1983) demonstrated that the majority of cases of *pharyngolaryngeal edema* were related to aggressive volume therapy.

Epidural Opiate Analgesia. Injection of opiates into the epidural space to relieve pain from labor has become popular. Their mechanism of action derives from interaction with specific receptors in the dorsal horn and dorsal roots. Apparently both cerebral and spinal opioid receptors are stimulated by these narcotics (Ackerman and colleagues, 1992).

Opiates alone usually will not provide adequate analgesia, and they most often are given with a local anesthetic agent such as bupivacaine. The major advantages of using such a combination are the rapid onset of pain relief, a decrease in shivering, and less dense motor blockade. Meister and colleagues (2000), in a randomized study of 50 laboring women, compared epidural analgesia with 0.125-percent ropivacaine and fentanyl to 0.125-percent bupivacaine and fentanyl. Both groups had similar labor analgesia, but the ropivacaine group had significantly less motor block.

Side effects are common and include pruritus and urinary retention. Immediate or delayed respiratory depression is worrisome (Ackerman and colleagues, 1992). Naloxone, given intravenously, will abolish these symptoms without affecting the analgesic action. Horta and colleagues (2000) reported a reduction in the incidence of pruritus with droperidol given epidurally in doses of up to 5 mg.

COMBINED SPINAL–EPIDURAL TECHNIQUES. The combination of spinal and epidural techniques has increased in popularity and may provide rapid and effective analgesia for labor as well as for cesarean delivery. As shown in Figure 19–6, an introducer needle is first placed in the epidural space. A small-gauge spinal needle is then introduced through the epidural needle into the subarachnoid space—this is called the *needle-through-needle technique.* A single bolus of an opioid, sometimes in combination with a local anesthetic, is injected into the subarachnoid space, the spinal needle is withdrawn, and an epidural catheter is then placed. The use of a subarachnoid opioid bolus results in the rapid onset of profound pain relief with virtually no motor blockade. The epidural catheter permits repeated dosing of analgesia.

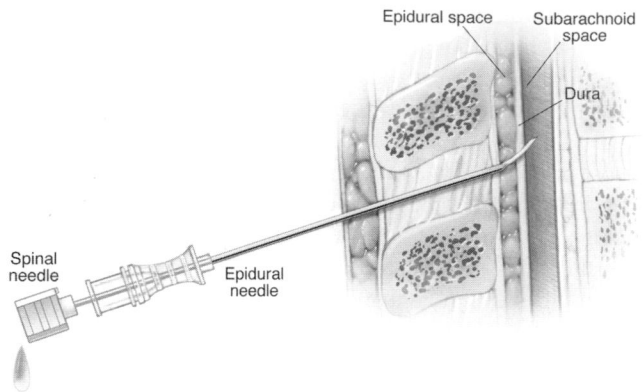

FIGURE 19–6. Combined spinal–epidural block, needle-through-needle technique. An extra-long spinal needle is introduced through a regular Tuohy needle into the subarachnoid space. (Redrawn from Sharma and Leveno, 2003, with permission.)

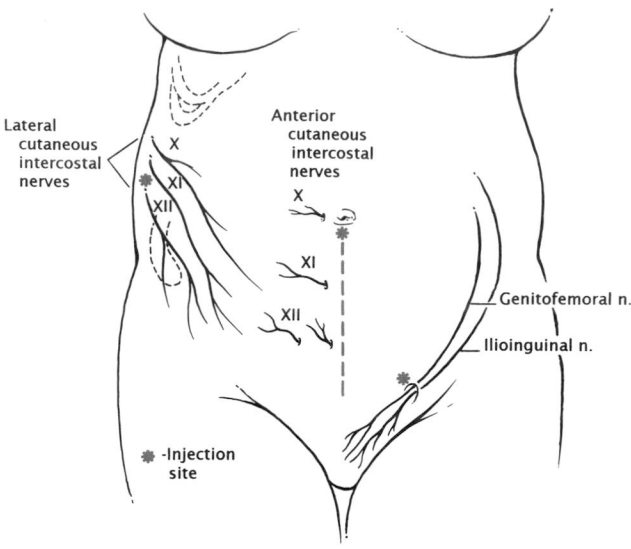

FIGURE 19–7. Local anesthetic block for cesarean delivery. The first injection site is halfway between the costal margin and iliac crest in midaxillary line to block the 10th, 11th, and 12th intercostal nerves. The second site is along the line of proposed skin incision. The third injection at the external inguinal blocks the genitofemoral and ilioinguinal nerves.

In a randomized trial of 110 laboring women, Van de Velde and associates (1999) compared epidural with combined spinal–epidural analgesia and reported that the combined method produced excellent immediate pain relief. Side effects were similar between the two groups. The largest study of the combined technique for laboring women was conducted at Parkland Hospital by Gambling and co-workers (1998). These investigators randomized 1223 women with an uncomplicated term pregnancy to receive either continuous spinal–epidural analgesia or boluses of intravenous meperidine. Rather unexpectedly, emergency cesarean delivery was performed for profound fetal bradycardia in 9 of 616 women (1.4 percent) who had combined spinal–epidural analgesia compared with none of 607 in the meperidine groups ($P <$ .005). Fetal bradycardia typically occurred within 30 minutes of the 10-μg dose of sufentanil, injected intrathecally. None of these women responded to conservative measures such as changing maternal position, oxygen administration, or intravenous ephedrine. Interestingly, none of these cases were associated with maternal hypotension, and none of the infants suffered ill effects. Subsequently, we and others have observed that the risk of fetal bradycardia is minimized with fentanyl, or with a 2.5-μg dose of sufentanil (Mardirosoff and Dumont, 1999).

LOCAL INFILTRATION FOR CESAREAN DELIVERY. Local block is occasionally useful to augment an inadequate or "patchy" regional block that was given in an emergency. On more rare occasions, local infiltration may be used to perform an emergency cesarean to save the life of the fetus in the absence of any anesthesia support.

Technique. In one technique, the skin is infiltrated in the line of the proposed incision, and the subcutaneous, muscle, and posterior rectus sheath layers are injected as the abdomen is opened. A dilute solution of lidocaine—30 mL of 2-percent

with 1:200,000 epinephrine diluted with 60 mL of normal saline—is prepared, and a total of 100 to 120 mL is infiltrated. Injection of large volumes into the fatty layers, which are relatively devoid of nerve supply, is avoided to limit the total dose of local anesthetic needed. To minimize pain, nausea, and hypotension that may accompany intraperitoneal manipulations, each step is accomplished without haste.

A second technique involves a field block of the major branches supplying the abdominal wall, to include the 10th, 11th, and 12th intercostal nerves and the ilioinguinal and genitofemoral nerves (Busby, 1963). As shown in Figure 19–7, the former group of nerves is located at a point midway between the costal margin and iliac crest in the midaxillary line. The latter group is found at the level of the external inguinal ring. Only one skin puncture is made at each of the four sites (right and left sides). At the intercostal block site, the needle is directed horizontally and injection is carried down to the transversalis fascia, avoiding injection of the subcutaneous fat. Approximately 5 to 8 mL of 0.5-percent lidocaine is injected. The procedure is repeated at a 45-degree angle cephalad and caudad at this site. The other side is then injected. At the ilioinguinal and genitofemoral sites, the injection is started at a site 2 to 3 cm from the pubic tubercle at a 45-degree angle. Finally, the skin overlying the planned incision is injected.

GENERAL ANESTHESIA

The increased safety of regional analgesia has increased the relative risk of general anesthesia. The case-fatality rate of general anesthesia for cesarean delivery is estimated to be approximately 32 per million live births compared with 1.9 per million for regional anesthesia (Hawkins and associates, 1997b). Failed intubation occurs in approximately 1 of every 250 general anesthetics administered to pregnant women, a 10-fold higher rate than the nonpregnant population (Barnardo and Jenkins, 2000). The American College of Obstetricians and Gynecologists (2002b) has concluded that this relative increased morbidity and mortality suggest that regional analgesia is the preferred method of pain control and should be used unless contraindicated (see Table 19–5). Indeed, in the Network study that has been cited, 95 percent of more than 50,000 cesarean deliveries were attempted with regional analgesia (Bloom and colleagues, 2004). Trained personnel and specialized equipment—including fiberoptic intubation—are mandatory for the safe use of general anesthesia.

PATIENT PREPARATION. Prior to anesthesia induction, several steps should be taken to help minimize the risk of complications for the mother and fetus. These include the use of antacids, lateral uterine displacement, and preoxygenation.

Antacids. The practice of administering antacids shortly before induction of anesthesia has probably done more to decrease mortality from general anesthesia than any other single practice. Gibbs and Banner (1984) reported that 30 mL of sodium citrate with citric acid (Bicitra), given about 45 minutes before surgery, neutralized gastric contents in nearly 90 percent of women undergoing cesarean delivery. For many years we have recommended administration of 30 mL of Bicitra within a few minutes of the anticipated time of anesthesia induction, either by general or major regional block. If more than 1 hour has passed between when the first dose was given and when anesthesia is induced, then a second dose is given.

Uterine Displacement. As discussed in Chapter 5 (see p. 135), the uterus may compress the inferior vena cava and aorta when the mother is in the supine position. With lateral uterine displacement, the duration of general anesthesia has less effect on neonatal condition than when the woman remains supine (Crawford and colleagues, 1972).

Preoxygenation. Because functional reserve capacity is reduced, pregnant women become hypoxemic more rapidly during periods of apnea than do nonpregnant patients. In order to minimize hypoxia between the time of muscle relaxant injection and intubation, it is important first to replace nitrogen in the lungs with oxygen. This is accomplished by administering 100-percent oxygen via face mask for 2 to 3 minutes prior to anesthesia induction. In an emergency, four vital capacity breaths of 100-percent oxygen via a tight breathing circuit will provide similar benefit (Norris and Dewan, 1985).

INDUCTION OF ANESTHESIA

Thiopental. This thiobarbiturate given intravenously is widely used and offers the advantages of ease and extreme rapidity of induction as well as prompt recovery with minimal risk of vomiting. Thiopental and similar compounds are poor analgesic agents, and the administration of sufficient drug given alone to maintain anesthesia may cause appreciable newborn depression. Thus, thiopental is not used as the sole anesthetic agent, but rather is administered in a dose that induces sleep.

Ketamine. This agent also may be used to render the patient unconscious. Given intravenously in low doses of 0.2 to 0.3 mg/kg, ketamine may be used to produce analgesia and sedation just prior to vaginal delivery. Doses of 1 mg/kg induce general anesthesia. Ketamine may prove useful in women with acute hemorrhage because, unlike thiopental, it is not associated with hypotension. Conversely, it usually causes a rise in blood pressure, and thus it generally should be avoided in women who are already hypertensive. Unpleasant delirium and hallucinations are commonly induced by this agent.

INTUBATION. Immediately after the patient is rendered unconscious, a muscle relaxant is given to facilitate intubation. *Succinylcholine,* a rapid-onset and short-acting agent, commonly is used. Cricoid pressure—the *Sellick maneuver*—is used to occlude the esophagus from induction until intubation is completed by a trained assistant. Before the operation begins, proper placement of the endotracheal tube must be confirmed. Such confirmation includes auscultation of bilateral breath sounds and end-tidal carbon dioxide analysis.

Failed Intubation. Although uncommon, failed intubation is a major cause of anesthesia-related maternal mortality (Wallace and Sidawi, 1997). In their review of 67 maternal deaths associated with general anesthesia, Hawkins and colleagues (1997b) reported that 22 percent were secondary to induction or intubation problems. A history of previous difficulties with intubation as well as a careful assessment of anatomical features of the neck, maxillofacial, pharyngeal, and laryngeal structures may help predict a difficult intubation. Even in cases where the initial assessment of the airway was uneventful, edema may develop intrapartum and present considerable difficulties (Farcon and associates, 1994). Morbid obesity is also a major risk factor for failed or difficult intubation. Of paramount importance is appropriate preoperative preparation to include the immediate availability of specialized equipment, including a variety of different shaped laryngoscopes, laryngeal mask airways, a fiber-optic bronchoscope, a transtracheal ventilation set, as well as liberal use of awake oral intubation techniques (Ezri and associates, 2001; Stamer and co-workers, 2000).

MANAGEMENT. An important principle is to start the operative procedure only after it has been ascertained that tracheal intubation has been successful and that adequate ventilation can be accomplished. Even with an abnormal fetal heart rate pattern, initiation of cesarean delivery will only serve to complicate matters if there is difficult or failed intubation. Frequently, the woman must be allowed to awaken and a different technique used, such as an awake intubation or regional analgesia.

Following failed intubation, the woman is ventilated by mask and cricoid pressure is applied to reduce the chance of aspiration (Cooper and colleagues, 1994). Surgery may proceed with mask ventilation or the woman may be allowed to awaken. In those cases where the woman has been paralyzed, and where ventilation cannot be reestablished by insertion of an oral airway, laryngeal mask airway, or use of a fiberoptic laryngoscope to intubate the trachea, a life-threatening emergency exists. To restore ventilation, percutaneous or even open cricothyrotomy is performed, and jet ventilation begun (Reisner and colleagues, 1999).

GAS ANESTHETICS. Once the endotracheal tube is secured, a 50:50 mixture of nitrous oxide and oxygen is administered to provide analgesia. Usually, a volatile halogenated agent is added to provide amnesia and additional analgesia. The mechanisms of actions of inhaled anesthetics have been reviewed recently by Campagna and colleagues (2003).

Volatile Anesthetics. The most commonly used volatile anesthetic in the United States is *isoflurane*. Both it and *halothane* are potent, nonexplosive agents that produce remarkable uterine relaxation when given in high, inhaled concentrations. Their use in high concentrations is restricted to those uncommon situations in which uterine relaxation is a requisite rather than a hazard. They are used for internal podalic version of the second twin (see Chap. 39, p. 940), breech decomposition (see Chap. 24, p. 579), and replacement of the acutely inverted uterus (see Chap. 35, p. 833). As soon as the maneuver has been completed, anesthetic administration should be stopped and immediate efforts begun to promote myometrial contraction to minimize hemorrhage. Because of cardiodepressant and hypotensive effects, these agents may intensify the adverse effects of maternal hypovolemia. Halothane and isoflurane occasionally have been associated with hepatitis and massive hepatic necrosis (Gunaratnam and associates, 1995).

Anesthesia Gas Exposure and Pregnancy Outcome. Without exception, all anesthetic agents that depress the maternal central nervous system cross the placenta and depress the fetal central nervous system. As a result, personnel responsible for the care of the newborn immediately following delivery with a general anesthetic should be prepared to provide respiratory support (see Chap. 28, p. 634). Ideally, induction-to-delivery time should be minimized when general anesthesia is used (American College of Obstetricians and Gynecologists, 2002b). In one study, Datta and colleagues (1981) concluded that fetal exposure of more than 8 minutes was associated with increased neonatal depression. Kavak and co-workers (2001) randomly assigned 84 women scheduled for elective cesarean delivery to either spinal analgesia or general anesthesia. There were no significant differences in short-term measures of neonatal outcome, including Apgar scores, umbilical artery blood gas determinations, or length of stay. The risks of anesthetic gas exposure associated with nonobstetrical surgery are discussed in Chapter 41 (see p. 974) and the risks of occupational exposure in Chapter 14 (see p. 356).

EXTUBATION. The tracheal tube may be safely removed only if the woman is conscious to a degree that enables her to follow commands and is capable of maintaining oxygen saturation with spontaneous respiration. Typically, the stomach is emptied via a nasogastric tube prior to extubation.

ASPIRATION. Massive gastric acidic inhalation causing pulmonary insufficiency from aspiration pneumonitis was first described by the obstetrician Mendelson, and the syndrome bears his name (Marik, 2001). Such pneumonitis has in the past been the most common cause of anesthetic deaths in obstetrics and therefore deserves special attention. In a survey of maternal deaths between 1979 and 1990, the Centers for Disease Control and Prevention identified that inhalation of gastric contents was associated with 23 percent of the 129 anesthesia-related deaths (Hawkins and colleagues, 1997b). Procedures mentioned previously that are important to effective prophylaxis include use of antacids, skillful intubation accompanied by cricoid pressure, emptying of the stomach with a nasogastric tube, and use of regional analgesia when possible.

Fasting. According to the American Society of Anesthesiologists Task Force on Obstetrical Anesthesia (1999), there are insufficient data regarding fasting times for clear liquids and the risk of pulmonary aspiration during labor. Clear liquids such as water, clear tea, black coffee, carbonated beverages, and fruit juices without pulp may be allowed in uncomplicated laboring women. Obvious solid foods should be avoided. The Task Force also recommended that "a fasting period of 8 hours or more is preferable for uncomplicated parturients undergoing elective cesarean delivery." Despite these precautions, it should be assumed that any woman in labor has both gastric particulate matter as well as acidic contents.

Pathophysiology. In 1952, Teabeaut demonstrated experimentally that if the pH of aspirated fluid was below 2.5, severe chemical pneumonitis developed. It was later demonstrated that the pH of gastric juice of nearly half of women tested intrapartum was below 2.5 (Taylor and Pryse-Davies, 1966). The right mainstem bronchus usually offers the simplest pathway for aspirated material to reach the lung parenchyma, and therefore the right lower lobe is most often involved. In severe cases, there is bilateral widespread involvement.

The woman who aspirates may develop evidence of respiratory distress immediately or as long as several hours after aspiration, depending in part on the material aspirated and the severity of the process. Aspiration of a large amount of solid material causes obvious signs of airway obstruction. Smaller particles without acidic liquid may lead to patchy atelectasis and later to bronchopneumonia.

When highly acidic liquid is inspired, decreased oxygen saturation along with tachypnea, bronchospasm, rhonchi, rales, atelectasis, cyanosis, tachycardia, and hypotension are likely to develop. At the sites of injury, pulmonary capillary leakage results in protein-rich fluid containing numerous erythrocytes exuding from capillaries into the lung interstitium and alveoli to cause decreased pulmonary compliance, shunting of blood, and severe hypoxemia. Radiographic changes may not appear immediately and they may be quite variable, although the right lobe most often is affected. Therefore, chest radiographs alone should not be used to exclude aspiration.

Treatment. The methods recommended for treatment of aspiration have changed appreciably in recent years, indicating that previous therapy was not very successful. Suspicion of aspiration of gastric contents demands very close monitoring for evidence of any pulmonary damage. Respiratory rate and oxygen saturation as measured by pulse oximetry are the most sensitive and earliest indicators of injury.

As much of the inhaled fluid as possible should be immediately wiped out of the mouth and removed from the pharynx and trachea by suction. Saline lavage may further disseminate the acid throughout the lung and is not recommended. If large particulate matter is inspired, bronchoscopy may be indicated to relieve airway obstruction. There is no convincing clinical or experimental evidence that corticosteroid therapy or prophylactic antimicrobial administration is beneficial (Marik, 2001). If clinical evidence of infection develops, however, then vigorous treatment is given. When acute respiratory distress syndrome develops, mechanical ventilation with positive end-expiratory pressure may prove lifesaving (see Chap. 42, p. 991).

REFERENCES

Ackerman WE III, Juneja M, Spinnato JA: Epidural opioids' OB advantages. Contemp Obstet Gynecol 37:68, 1992

Alexander JM, Sharma SK, McIntire DD, et al: Epidural analgesia lengthens the Friedman active phase of labor. Obstet Gynecol 100:46, 2002

American Academy of Pediatrics and American College of Obstetricians and Gynecologists: Guidelines for Perinatal Care, 4th ed. Washington, DC, 2002, p 138–142

American College of Obstetricians and Gynecologists: Analgesia and cesarean delivery rates. Committee Opinion No. 269, February 2002a

American College of Obstetricians and Gynecologists: Obstetric analgesia and anesthesia. Practice Bulletin 36, July 2002b

American College of Obstetricians and Gynecologists: Optimal goals for anesthesia care in obstetrics. Committee Opinion No. 256, May 2001

American College of Obstetricians and Gynecologists: Pain relief during labor. Committee Opinion No. 295, July 2004

American Society of Anesthesiologists Task Force on Obstetrical Anesthesia: Practice guidelines for obstetrical anesthesia. Anesthesiology 90:600, 1999

Angel JL, Knuppel RA, Lake M: Sinusoidal fetal heart rate pattern associated with intravenous butorphanol administration: A case report. Am J Obstet Gynecol 149:465, 1984

Atkinson BD, Truitt LJ, Rayburn WF, et al: Double-blind comparison of intravenous butorphanol (Stadol) and fentanyl (Sublimaze) for analgesia during labor. Am J Obstet Gynecol 171:993, 1994

Barnardo PD, Jenkins JG: Failed tracheal intubation in obstetrics: A 6-year review in the UK region. Anaesthesia 55:690, 2000

Bell ED, Penning DH, Cousineau EF, et al: How much labor is in a labor epidural? Manpower cost and reimbursement for an obstetric analgesia service in a teaching institution. Anesthesiology 92:851, 2000

Berg CJ, Chang J, Callaghan WM, et al: Pregnancy-related mortality in the United States, 1991–1997. Obstet Gynecol 101:289, 2003

Bloom SL, for the NICHD Maternal-Fetal Medicine Units Network: The MFMU cesarean registry: Complications of anesthesia for cesarean delivery. Paper presented at the Society for Maternal-Fetal Medicine Annual Meeting (abstract 41); February 6, 2004; New Orleans, La

Breen TW, Ransil BJ, Groves PA, et al: Factors associated with back pain after childbirth. Anesthesiology 81:29, 1994

Bricker L, Lavender T: Parenteral opioids for labor pain relief: A systematic review. Am J Obstet Gynecol 186:S94, 2002

Busby T: Local anesthesia for cesarean section. Am J Obstet Gynecol 87:399, 1963

Butler R, Fuller J: Back pain following epidural anaesthesia in labour. Can J Anaesth 45:724, 1998

Camann WR, Murray RS, Mushlin PS, et al: Effects of oral caffeine on post-dural puncture headache: A double-blinded, placebo-controlled trial. Anesth Analg 70:181, 1990

Campagna JA, Miller KW, Forman SA: Mechanisms of actions of inhaled anesthetics. N Engl J Med 348:2110, 2003

Chan BO, Paech MJ: Persistent cerebrospinal fluid leak: A complication of the combined spinal-epidural technique. Anesth Analg 98:828, 2004

Chang J, Elam-Evans LD, Berg CJ, et al: Pregnancy-related mortality surveillance—United States, 1991–1999, MMWR 52:1, 2003

Cheek TG, Samuels P: Pregnancy induced hypertension. In Datta S (ed): Anesthesia and Management of High-Risk Pregnancy. St Louis, Mosby-Year Book, 1991

Chestnut DH: Effect on the progress of labor and method of delivery. In Chestnut DH (ed): Obstetric Anesthesia: Principles and Practice, 2nd ed. St Louis: Mosby-Year Book, 1999, p 408

Chestnut DH: Epidural analgesia and the incidence of cesarean section: Time for another close look. Anesthesiology 87:472, 1997

Chestnut DH, McGrath JM, Vincent RD Jr, et al: Does early administration of epidural analgesia affect obstetric outcome in nulliparous women who are in spontaneous labor? Anesthesiology 80:1201, 1994a

Chestnut DH, Owen CL, Bates JN, et al: Continuous infusion epidural analgesia during labor: A randomized, double-blind comparison of 0.625% bupivacaine/0.0002% fentanyl versus 0.125% bupivacaine. Anesthesiology 68:754, 1988

Chestnut DH, Vincent RD Jr, McGrather JM, et al: Does early administration of epidural analgesia affect obstetric outcome in nulliparous women who are receiving intravenous oxytocin? Anesthesiology 80:1193, 1994b

Chisholm ME, Campbell DC: Postpartum postural headache due to superior sagittal sinus thrombosis mistaken for spontaneous intracranial hypotension. Can J Anaesth 48:302, 2001

Clark SL, Divon MY, Phelan JP: Preeclampsia/eclampsia: Hemodynamic and neurologic correlations. Obstet Gynecol 66:337, 1985

Cooper SD, Benumof JL, Ozaki GT: Evaluation of the Bullard laryngoscope using the new intubating stylet: Comparison with conventional laryngoscopy. Anesth Analg 79:965, 1994

Cotton DB, Longmire S, Jones MM, et al: Cardiovascular alterations in severe pregnancy-induced hypertension: Effects of intravenous nitroglycerin coupled with blood volume expansion. Am J Obstet Gynecol 154:1053, 1986

Crawford JS: Some maternal complications of epidural analgesia for labour. Anaesthesia 40:1219, 1985

Crawford JS, Burton M, Davies P: Time and lateral tilt at caesarean section. Br J Anaesth 44:477, 1972

Cunningham FG, Leveno KJ: Obstetrical concerns for anesthetic management of severe preeclampsia. Williams Obstetrics, 19th ed (Suppl 10). Norwalk, Conn, Appleton and Lange, December 1994/January 1995

Danilenko-Dixon DR, Tefft L, Haydon B, et al: The effect of maternal position on cardiac output with epidural analgesia in labor [abstract]. Am J Obstet Gynecol 174:332, 1996

Dashe JS, Rogers BB, McIntire DD, et al: Epidural analgesia and intrapartum fever: Placental findings. Obstet Gynecol 93:341, 1999

Datta S, Ostheimer GW, Weiss JB, et al: Neonatal effect of prolonged anesthetic induction for cesarean section. Obstet Gynecol 58:331, 1981

Eltzschig HK, Lieberman ES, Camann WR: Regional anesthesia and analgesia for labor and delivery. N Engl J Med 348:319, 2003

Ezri T, Szmuk P, Evron S, et al: Difficult airway in obstetric anesthesia: A review. Obstet Gynecol Surv 56:631, 2001

Farcon EL, Kim MH, Marx GF: Changing Mallampati score during labour. Can J Anaesth 41:50, 1994

Fishburne JI Jr, Greiss FC Jr, Hopkinson R, et al: Responses of the gravid uterine vasculature to arterial levels of local anesthetic agents. Am J Obstet Gynecol 133:753, 1979

Friedman EA: Primigravid labor: A graphicostatistical analysis. Obstet Gynecol 6:567, 1955

Fusi L, Steer PJ, Maresh MJA, et al: Maternal pyrexia associated with the use of epidural analgesia in labour. Lancet 1:1250, 1989

Gambling DR, Sharma SK, Ramin SM, et al: A randomized study of combined spinal–epidural analgesia versus intravenous meperidine during labor: Impact on cesarean delivery rate. Anesthesiology 89:1336, 1998

Gambling DR, Writer D: Hypertensive disorders. In Chestnut DH (ed): Obstetric Anesthesia: Principles and Practice, 2nd ed. St Louis, Mosby-Year Book, 1999, p 875

Gibbs CP, Banner TC: Effectiveness of Bicitra® as a preoperative antacid. Anesthesiology 61:97, 1984

Glosten B: Local anesthetic techniques. In Chestnut DH (ed): Obstetric Anesthesia: Principles and Practice, 2nd ed. St Louis, Mosby-Year Book, 1999, p 363

Greiss FC Jr, Still JG, Anderson SG: Effects of local anesthetic agents on the uterine vasculatures and myometrium. Am J Obstet Gynecol 124:889, 1976

Gunaratnam NT, Benson J, Gandolfi AJ, et al: Suspected isoflurane hepatitis in an obese patient with a history of halothane hepatitis. Anesthesiology 83:1361, 1995

Gutsche BB: The experts opine: The role of epidural anesthesia in preeclampsia. Surv Anesthesiol 30:304, 1986

Harding SA, Collis RE, Morgan BM: Meningitis after combined spinal–extradural anaesthesia in obstetrics. Br J Anaesth 73:545, 1994

Hatjis CG, Meis PJ: Sinusoidal fetal heart rate pattern associated with butorphanol administration. Obstet Gynecol 67:377, 1986

Hawkins JL, Gibbs CP, Orleans M, et al: Obstetric anesthesia work force survey, 1981 versus 1992. Anesthesiology 87:135, 1997a

Hawkins JL, Koonin LM, Palmer SK, et al: Anesthesia-related deaths during obstetric delivery in the United States, 1979–1990. Anesthesiology 86:277, 1997b

Head BB, Owen J, Vincent RD, et al: A randomized trial of intrapartum analgesia in women with severe preeclampsia. Obstet Gynecol 99:452, 2002

Heller PJ, Scheider EP, Marx GF: Pharyngolaryngeal edema as a presenting symptom in preeclampsia. Obstet Gynecol 62:523, 1983

Hess PE, Pratt SD, Lucas TP, et al: Predictors of breakthrough pain during labor epidural analgesia. Anesth Analg 93:414, 2001

Hill JB, Alexander JM, Sharma SK, et al: A comparison of the effects of epidural and meperidine analgesia during labor on fetal heart rate. Obstet Gynecol 102:333, 2003.

Hogg B, Hauth JC, Caritis SN, et al: Safety of labor epidural anesthesia for women with severe hypertensive disease. Am J Obstet Gynecol 181:1096, 1999

Horta ML, Ramos L, Goncalves ZR: The inhibition of epidural morphine-induced pruritus by epidural droperidol. Anesth Analg 90:638, 2000

Howell CJ, Kidd C, Roberts W, et al: A randomized controlled trial of epidural compared with non-epidural analgesia in labour. Br J Obstet Gynaecol 108:27, 2001

Kavak ZN, Basgül A, Ceyhan N: Short-term outcome of newborn infants: Spinal versus general anesthesia for elective cesarean section: A prospective randomized study. Eur J Obstet Gynecol Reprod Biol 100:50, 2001

Keegan JJ, Garrett FD: The segmental distribution of the cutaneous nerves in the limbs of man. Anat Rec 102:411, 1948

Kennedy WF Jr, Bonica JJ, Akamatsu TJ, et al: Cardiovascular and respiratory effects of subarachnoid block in the presence of acute blood loss. Anesthesiology 29:29, 1968

Kennell J, Klaus M, McGrath S, et al: Continuous emotional support during labor in a US hospital: A randomized controlled trial. JAMA 265:2197, 1991

Koonin LM, MacKay AP, Berg CJ, et al: Pregnancy-related mortality surveillance—United States, 1987–1990. MMWR 46:17, 1997

Lamaze F: Painless Childbirth: Psychoprophylactic Method. Chicago, Henry Regnery, 1970

Lee LA, Posner KL, Domino KB, et al: Injuries associated with regional anesthesia in the 1980s and 1990s: A closed claims analysis. Anesthesiology 101:143, 2004

Lee A, Ngan Kee WD, Gin T: Prophylactic ephedrine prevents hypotension during spinal anesthesia for cesarean delivery but does not improve neonatal outcome: A quantitative systematic review. Can J Anaesth 49:588, 2002a

Lee A, Ngan Kee WD, Gin T: A quantitative, systematic review of randomized controlled trials of ephedrine versus phenylephrine for the management of hypotension during spinal anesthesia for cesarean delivery. Anesth Analg 94:920, 2002b

Leighton BL, Halpern SH: The effects of epidural analgesia on labor, maternal, and neonatal outcomes: A systematic review. Am J Obstet Gynecol 186:569, 2002

Lieberman E, Lang JM, Cohen A, et al: Association of epidural analgesia with cesarean delivery in nulliparas. Obstet Gynecol 88:993, 1996

Lieberman E, O'Donoghue C: Unintended effects of epidural analgesia during labor: A systematic review. Am J Obstet Gynecol 186:531, 2002

Lowe NK: The nature of labor pain. Am J Obstet Gynecol 106:S16, 2002

Lucas MJ, Sharma SK, McIntire DD, et al: A randomized trial of labor analgesia in women with pregnancy-induced hypertension. Am J Obstet Gynecol 185:970, 2001

Luxman D, Wholman I, Groutz A, et al: The effect of early epidural block administration on the progression and outcome of labor. Int J Obstet Anesth 7:161, 1998

MacArthur AJ, MacArthur C, Weeks SK: Is epidural anesthesia in labor associated with chronic low back pain? A prospective cohort study. Anesth Analg 85:1066, 1997

Manninen T, Aantaa R, Salonen M, et al: A comparison of the hemodynamic effects of paracervical block and epidural anesthesia for labor analgesia. Acta Anaesthesiol Scand 44:441, 2000

Mardirosoff C, Dumont L: Two doses of intrathecal sufentanil (2.5 and 5 μg) combined with bupivacaine and epinephrine for labor analgesia. Anesth Analg 89:1263, 1999

Marik PE: Aspiration pneumonitis and aspiration pneumonia. N Engl J Med 344:665, 2001

Meister GC, D'Angelo R, Owen M, et al: A comparison of epidural analgesia with 0.125% ropivacaine with fentanyl versus 0.125% bupivacaine with fentanyl during labor. Anesth Analg 90:632, 2000

Melzack R: The myth of painless childbirth. Pain 19:321, 1984

Morgan D, Philip J, Sharma S, et al: A neonatal outcome with ephedrine infusions with or without preloading during spinal anesthesia for cesarean section. Society of Anesthesiologists and Perinatologists, Montreal, Quebec, Canada. Anesthesiology (supplement):A5, 2000

Mulroy MF: Systemic toxicity and cardiotoxicity from local anesthetics: Incidence and preventive measures. Reg Anesth Pain Med 27:556, 2002

Ng K, Parsons J, Cyna AM, et al: Spinal versus epidural anaesthesia for caesarean section. Cochrane Database Syst Rev CD003765, 2004

Ngan Kee WD, Khaw KS, Ng FF, et al: Prophylactic phenylephrine infusion for preventing hypotension during spinal anesthesia for cesarean delivery. Anesth Analg 98:815, 2004

Nagaya K, Fetters MD, Ishikawa M, et al: Causes of maternal mortality in Japan. JAMA 283:2661, 2000

Newton JA Jr, Lesnik IK, Kennedy CA: *Streptococcus salivarius* meningitis following spinal anesthesia. Clin Infect Dis 18:840, 1994

Norris MC, Dewan DM: Preoxygenation for cesarean section: A comparison of two techniques. Anesthesiology 62:827, 1985

Palkar NV, Boudreaux RC, Mankad AV: Accidental total spinal block: A complication of an epidural test dose. Can J Anaesth 39:1058, 1992

Quilligan EJ, Keegan KA, Donahue MJ: Double-blind comparison of intravenously injected butorphanol and meperidine in parturients. Int J Gynaecol Obstet 18:363, 1980

Ramin SM, Gambling DR, Lucas MJ, et al: Randomized trial of epidural versus intravenous analgesia during labor. Obstet Gynecol 86:783, 1995

Rasmus KT, Rottman RL, Kotelko DM, et al: Unrecognized thrombocytopenia and regional anesthesia in parturients: A retrospective review. Obstet Gynecol 73:943, 1989

Read GD: Childbirth Without Fear. New York, Harper, 1944, p 192

Reisner LS, Benumof JL, Cooper SD: The difficult airway: Risk, prophylaxis, and management. In Chestnut DH (ed): Obstetric Anesthesia: Principles and Practice, 2nd ed. St Louis, Mosby-Year Book, 1999, p 611

Reynolds F, Sharma SK, Seed PT: Analgesia in labour and fetal acid-base balance: A meta-analysis comparing epidural with systemic opioid analgesia. Br J Obstet Gynaecol 109:1344, 2002

Rogers R, Gilson G, Kammerer-Doak D: Epidural analgesia and active management of labor: Effects on length of labor and mode of delivery. Obstet Gynecol 93:995, 1999

Rolbin SH, Abbott D, Musclow E, et al: Epidural anesthesia in pregnant patients with low platelet counts. Obstet Gynecol 71:918, 1988

Rosen MA: Nitrous oxide for relief of labor pain: A systematic review. Am J Obstet Gynecol 186:S110, 2002a

Rosen MA: Paracervical block for labor analgesia: A brief historic review. Am J Obstet Gynecol 186:S127, 2002b

Saisto T, Salmela-Aro K, Nurmi JE, et al: A randomized controlled trial of intervention in fear of childbirth. Obstet Gynecol 98:820, 2001

Sechzer PH, Abel L: Post-spinal anesthesia headache treated with caffeine. Evaluation with demand method. Part I. Curr Therap Res 24:307, 1978

Setayesh AR, Kholdebarin AR, Moghadam MS, et al: The Trendelenburg position increases the spread and accelerates the onset of epidural anesthesia for cesarean section. Can J Anaesth 48:890, 2001

Seyb ST, Berka RJ, Socol ML, et al: Risk of cesarean delivery with elective induction of labor at term in nulliparous women. Obstet Gynecol 94:600, 1999

Sharma SK, Alexander JM, Messick G, et al: A randomized trial of epidural analgesia versus intravenous meperidine analgesia during labor in nulliparous women. Anesthesiology 96:546, 2002

Sharma SK, Leveno KJ: Regional analgesia and progress of labor. Clin Obstet Gynecol 46:633, 2003

Sharma SK, Leveno KJ: Update: Epidural analgesia during labor does not increase cesarean births. Current Anesthesiology Reports 2:18, 2000

Sharma SK, McIntire DD, Wiley J, et al: Labor analgesia and cesarean delivery. An individual patient meta-analysis of nulliparous women. Anesthesiology 100:142, 2004

Sharma SK, Sidawi JE, Ramin SM, et al: Cesarean delivery: A randomized trial of epidural versus patient-controlled meperidine analgesia during labor. Anesthesiology 87:487, 1997

Shearer VE, Jhaveri HS, Cunningham FG: Puerperal seizures after post-dural puncture headache. Obstet Gynecol 85:255, 1995

Stamer UM, Messerschmidt A, Wulf H, et al: Equipment for the difficult airway in obstetric units in Germany. J Clin Anesthesiol 12:151, 2000

Svancarek W, Chirino O, Schaefer G Jr, et al: Retropsoas and subgluteal abscesses following paracervical and pudendal anesthesia. JAMA 237:892, 1977

Taylor G, Pryse-Davies J: The prophylactic use of antacids in the prevention of the acid pulmonary aspiration syndrome (Mendelson's syndrome). Lancet 1:288, 1966

Teabeaut JR II: Aspiration of gastric contents: An experimental study. Am J Pathol 28:51, 1952

Thomas TA, Cooper GM: Maternal deaths from anaesthesia. An extract from *Why Mothers Die 1997–1999,* The Confidential Enquiries into Maternal Deaths in the United Kingdom. Br J Anaesth 89:499, 2002

Thompson TT, Thorp JM, Mayer D, et al: Does epidural analgesia cause dystocia? J Clin Anesth 10:58, 1998

Thorp JA, Breedlove G: Epidural analgesia in labor: An evaluation of risks and benefits. Birth 23:63, 1996

Vallejo MC, Mandell GL, Sabo DP, et al: Postdural puncture headache: A randomized comparison of five spinal needles in obstetric patients. Anesth Analg 91:916, 2000

Van de Velde M, Mignolet K, Vandermeersch E, et al: Prospective, randomized comparison of epidural and combined spinal analgesia during labor. Acta Anaesthesiol Belg 50:129, 1999

von Ungern-Sternberg BS, Regli A, Bucher E, et al: Impact of spinal anaesthesia and obesity on maternal respiratory function during elective Caesarean section. Anaesthesia 59:743, 2004

Wallace DH, Leveno KJ, Cunningham FG, et al: Randomized comparison of general and regional anesthesia for cesarean delivery in pregnancies complicated by severe preeclampsia. Obstet Gynecol 86:193, 1995

Wallace DH, Sidawi JE: Complications of obstetrical anesthesia. Williams Obstetrics, 20th ed (Suppl 3). Norwalk, Conn, Appleton & Lange, June/July, 1997

Yancey MK, Pierce B, Schweitzer D, et al: Observations on labor epidural analgesia and operative delivery rates. Am J Obstet Gynecol 180:353, 1999

Yancey MK, Zhang J, Schwarz J, et al: Labor epidural analgesia and intrapartum maternal hyperthermia. Obstet Gynecol 98:763, 2001a

Yancey MK, Zhang J, Schweitzer DL, et al: Epidural analgesia and fetal head malposition at vaginal delivery. Obstet Gynecol 97:608, 2001b

Zeeman GG, Cunningham FG: Blood volume expansion in women with antepartum eclampsia. J Soc Gynecol Investig 9:112A, 2002

Zhang J, Yancey MK, Klebanoff MA, et al: Does epidural analgesia prolong labor and increase risk of cesarean delivery? A natural experiment. Am J Obstet Gynecol 185:128, 2001

20

Dystocia

ABNORMAL LABOR

In 2002, the cesarean delivery rate was 26.1 percent—the highest level ever reported for the United States (Martin and co-workers, 2003). According to the American College of Obstetricians and Gynecologists (2003), about 60 percent of cesarean deliveries in the United States are attributable to the diagnosis of dystocia, and thus, its diagnosis has assumed major importance in contemporary obstetrical practice. Dystocia literally means *difficult labor* and is characterized by abnormally slow progress of labor. Generally, abnormal labor is common whenever there is disproportion between the presenting part of the fetus and the birth canal.

Roy (2003) has proposed that the high frequency of dystocia diagnosed contemporaneously results from environmental changes that are developing more rapidly than Darwinian natural selection. Humans are poorly adapted to the affluence of our modern diet, and the result is dystocia. There is some evidence to support this hypothesis. For example, Joseph and colleagues (2003) analyzed changes in maternal characteristics related to the recent increase in primary cesarean deliveries in Nova Scotia. They concluded that the recent increase could be attributed to changes in maternal age, parity, prepregnancy weight, and weight gain during pregnancy. Others also have observed that maternal weight is associated with dystocia (Nuthalapaty and co-workers, 2004; Wilkes and co-workers, 2003).

DYSTOCIA

Dystocia is the consequence of four distinct abnormalities that may exist singly or in combination:

1. Abnormalities of the expulsive forces, either uterine forces insufficiently strong or inappropriately coordinated to efface and dilate the cervix—uterine dysfunction—or inadequate voluntary muscle effort during the second stage of labor.
2. Abnormalities of presentation, position, or development of the fetus.
3. Abnormalities of the maternal bony pelvis—that is, pelvic contraction.
4. Abnormalities of soft tissues of the reproductive tract that form an obstacle to fetal descent (see Chap. 40).

More simply, these abnormalities can be mechanistically simplified into three categories:

1. Abnormalities of the *powers*—uterine contractility and maternal expulsive effort.
2. Abnormalities involving the *passenger*—the fetus.
3. Abnormalities of the *passage*—the pelvis.

Common clinical findings in women with these labor abnormalities are summarized in Table 20–1.

OVERDIAGNOSIS OF DYSTOCIA. Combinations of the abnormalities shown in Table 20–1 often interact to

TABLE 20–1 Common Clinical Findings in Women with Ineffective Labor

Inadequate cervical dilatation or fetal descent
    Protracted labor—slow progress
    Arrested labor—no progress
    Inadequate expulsive effort—ineffective "pushing"
Fetopelvic disproportion
    Excessive fetal size
    Inadequate pelvic capacity
    Malpresentation or position of fetus
Ruptured membranes without labor

produce dysfunctional labor. Today, expressions such as *cephalopelvic disproportion* and *failure to progress* often are used to describe ineffective labors.

The expression *cephalopelvic disproportion* came into use prior to the 20th century to describe obstructed labor resulting from disparity between the dimensions of the fetal head and maternal pelvis such as to preclude vaginal delivery. This term, however, originated at a time when the main indication for cesarean delivery was overt pelvic contracture due to rickets (Olah and Neilson, 1994). Such true disproportion is now rare, and most disproportions are the result of malposition of the fetal head within the pelvis (asynclitism) or of ineffective uterine contractions. True cephalopelvic disproportion is a tenuous diagnosis because two thirds or more of women diagnosed as having this disorder and delivered by cesarean subsequently deliver even larger newborns vaginally (see Chap. 26, p. 612).

Failure to progress in either spontaneous or stimulated labor has become an increasingly popular description of ineffectual labor. This term is used to include lack of progressive cervical dilatation or lack of fetal descent.

As previously stated, dystocia is the most common current indication for primary cesarean delivery. Gifford and colleagues (2000) reported that lack of progress in labor was the reason for 68 percent of unplanned cesarean deliveries for cephalic-presenting fetuses. Notzon and associates (1994) found that 12 percent of American women without prior cesarean delivery were diagnosed as having dystocia requiring abdominal delivery in 1990, and the rate had increased from 7 percent in 1980. A similar change also was reported in the United Kingdom (Leitch and Walker, 1998). Because many women with a primary cesarean delivery for dystocia undergo repeat cesarean delivery in subsequent pregnancies, an estimated 50 to 60 percent of all cesarean deliveries in the United States may be attributable to this diagnosis.

It is generally agreed that dystocia leading to cesarean delivery is overdiagnosed in the United States and elsewhere. Factors leading to increased use of cesarean delivery for dystocia, however, are controversial. Those implicated have included incorrect diagnosis of dystocia, epidural analgesia, fear of litigation, and even clinician convenience (Lieberman and co-workers, 1996; Savage and Francome, 1994; Thorp and colleagues, 1993a).

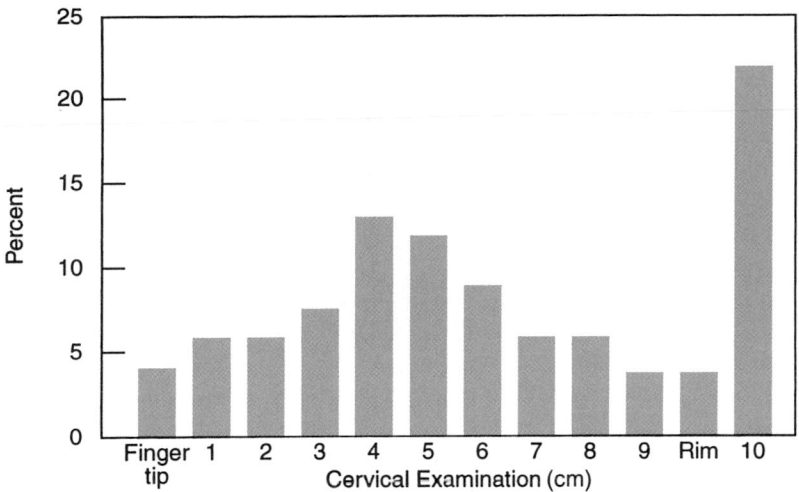

FIGURE 20–1. Distribution of cervical dilatation at the time of cesarean delivery for dystocia. (From Gifford and colleagues, 2000, with permission.)

Variability in the criteria for diagnosis is a major determinant of this increase. For example, Gifford and colleagues (2000) found that almost 25 percent of the cesarean deliveries performed annually in the United States for lack of progress were in women with cervical dilatation of only 0 to 3 cm (Fig. 20–1). According to Stephenson (2000), this practice is contrary to recommendations of the American College of Obstetricians and Gynecologists (1995a) that the cervix be dilated to 4 cm or more before a diagnosis is made. Thus, the diagnosis often is made before the active phase of labor and therefore, before an adequate trial of labor. Another factor implicated is insufficient oxytocin stimulation of labor in women with slow labor (Rouse and colleagues, 1999). King (1993) found that cesarean deliveries for dystocia in private patients in the United Kingdom were related to office hours and surgery schedules, whereas the timing of procedures for fetal distress were evenly distributed throughout the day.

MECHANISMS OF DYSTOCIA. The discussion concerning dystocia by Williams (1903) in the first edition of this text is still true today. Figure 20–2 is from the first edition, and demonstrates the mechanical process of labor and the potential obstacles. The cervix and lower uterus are shown at the end of pregnancy and at the end of labor. At the end of pregnancy, the fetal head, to traverse the birth canal, must encounter a relatively thicker lower uterine segment and undilated cervix. The uterine fundus muscle is less developed and presumably less powerful. Uterine contractions, cervical resistance, and the forward pressure exerted by the leading fetal head are the factors influencing the progress of the first stage of labor (see Chap. 17, p. 421).

After complete cervical dilatation (see Fig. 20–2), however, the mechanical relationship between the fetal head size and position and the pelvic capacity, namely fetopelvic proportion, becomes clearer as the fetus descends. The uterine musculature is much thicker and thus more powerful. Accordingly, abnormalities in fetopelvic proportions become more apparent once the second stage is reached.

Uterine muscle malfunction can result from uterine overdistention or obstructed labor, or both. Thus, ineffective labor is generally accepted as a possible warning sign of fetopelvic disproportion. Simply dividing labor abnormalities into pure *uterine dysfunction* and *fetopelvic disproportion* is incorrect because these two abnormalities are so closely interlinked. Indeed, according to the American College of Obstetricians and Gynecologists (1995a), the bony pelvis is not

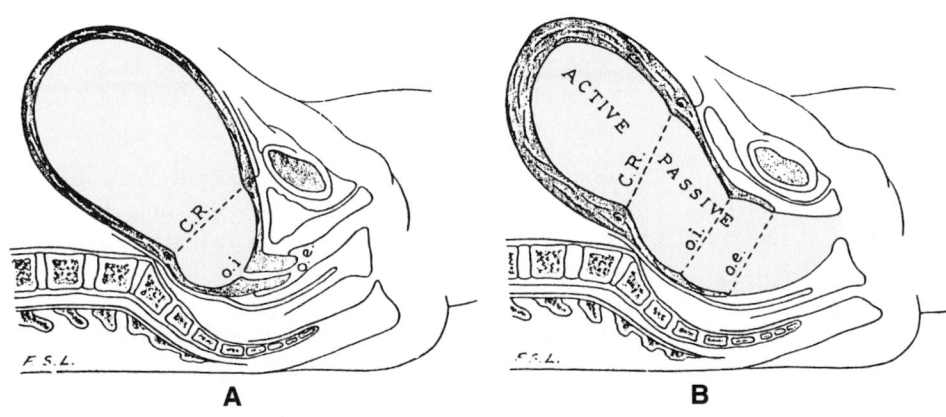

FIGURE 20–2. Diagrams of the birth canal **(A)** at the end of pregnancy and **(B)** during the second stage of labor, showing formation of the birth canal. (C.R. = contraction ring; o.i. = internal cervical os; o.e. = external cervical os.) (From Williams, 1903.)

the factor, with rare exceptions, that limits vaginal delivery. In the absence of objective means of precisely distinguishing these two causes of labor failure, clinicians must rely on a *trial of labor* to determine if labor can be successful in effecting vaginal delivery. Defining the adequacy of a trial of labor is a priority, in our opinion, in moderating the primary cesarean delivery rate for dystocia in the United States.

ABNORMALITIES OF THE EXPULSIVE FORCES

Cervical dilatation and propulsion and expulsion of the fetus is brought about by contractions of the uterus, reinforced during the second stage by voluntary or involuntary muscular action of the abdominal wall—"pushing." Either of these factors may lack intensity and result in delayed or interrupted labor. The diagnosis of uterine dysfunction in the latent phase is difficult and sometimes can be made only in retrospect (see Chap. 17, p. 422). One of the most common errors is to treat women for uterine dysfunction who are not yet in active labor.

There have been three significant advances in the treatment of uterine dysfunction:

1. Realization that undue prolongation of labor may contribute to perinatal morbidity and mortality.
2. Use of dilute intravenous infusion of oxytocin in the treatment of certain types of uterine dysfunction.
3. More frequent use of cesarean delivery rather than difficult midforceps delivery when oxytocin fails or its use is inappropriate.

TYPES OF UTERINE DYSFUNCTION. Reynolds and co-workers (1948) emphasized that uterine contractions of normal labor are characterized by a gradient of myometrial activity, being greatest and lasting longest at the fundus (fundal dominance) and diminishing toward the cervix. Caldeyro-Barcia and colleagues (1950) from Montevideo, Uruguay, inserted small balloons into the myometrium at various levels (see Chap. 18, p. 466). They reported that in addition to a gradient of activity, there was a time differential in the onset of the contractions in the fundus, midzone, and lower uterine segments. Larks (1960) described the stimulus as starting in one cornu and then several milliseconds later in the other, the excitation waves then joining and sweeping over the fundus and down the uterus.

The Montevideo group also ascertained that the lower limit of contraction pressure required to dilate the cervix is 15 mm Hg. This figure is in agreement with the findings of Hendricks and co-workers (1959), who reported that normal spontaneous contractions often exert pressures of about 60 mm Hg. From these observations, it is possible to define two types of uterine dysfunction. In the more common *hypotonic uterine dysfunction,* there is no basal hypertonus and uterine contractions have a normal gradient pattern (synchronous), but the slight rise in pressure during a contraction is insufficient to dilate the cervix. In the other, *hypertonic uterine dysfunction* or *incoordinate uterine dysfunction,* either basal tone is elevated appreciably or the pressure gradient is distorted. Gradient distortion may result from contraction of the midsegment of the uterus with more force than the fundus or from complete asynchronism of the impulses originating in each cornu, or a combination of these two.

Active-Phase Disorders. Labor abnormalities are clinically divided into either slower-than-normal progress—protraction disorder—or complete cessation of progress—arrest disorder. A woman must be in the active phase of labor with cervical dilatation to at least 3 to 4 cm to be diagnosed with either of these. Handa and Laros (1993) diagnosed active-phase arrest, defined as no dilatation for 2 hours or more, in 5 percent of term nulliparas. This incidence has not changed since the 1950s (Friedman, 1978). Inadequate uterine contractions, defined as less than 180 Montevideo units (Fig. 20–3), were diagnosed in 80 percent of women with active-phase arrest.

Protraction disorders are less well described, probably because the time interval necessary before diagnosing slow progress is undefined. The World Health Organization (1994) has proposed a labor management *partograph* in which protraction is defined as less than 1 cm/hr cervical dilatation for a minimum of 4 hours.

The criteria recommended by the American College of Obstetricians and Gynecologists (1995a) for diagnosis of protraction and arrest disorders are shown in Table 20–2. These criteria were adapted from those of Cohen and Friedman (1983), shown in Table 20–3.

Hauth and co-workers (1986, 1991) reported that when labor is effectively induced or augmented with oxytocin, 90 percent of women achieve 200 to 225 Montevideo units, and 40 percent achieve at least 300 Montevideo units. These results suggest that there are certain minimums of uterine activity that should be achieved before performing cesarean delivery for dystocia. Accordingly, the American College of Obstetricians and Gynecologists (1989) has suggested that, before the diagnosis of arrest during first-stage labor is made, both of these criteria should be met:

1. The latent phase has been completed, with the cervix dilated 4 cm or more.
2. A uterine contraction pattern of 200 Montevideo units or more in a 10-minute period has been present for 2 hours without cervical change.

Rouse and colleagues (1999) have recently challenged the "2-hour rule" on the grounds that a longer time, that is, at least 4 hours, is necessary before concluding that the active phase of labor has failed. We agree.

Second-Stage Disorders. As previously noted in Chapter 17 (see p. 416 and Fig. 17–20), fetal descent largely follows complete dilatation. Moreover, the second stage

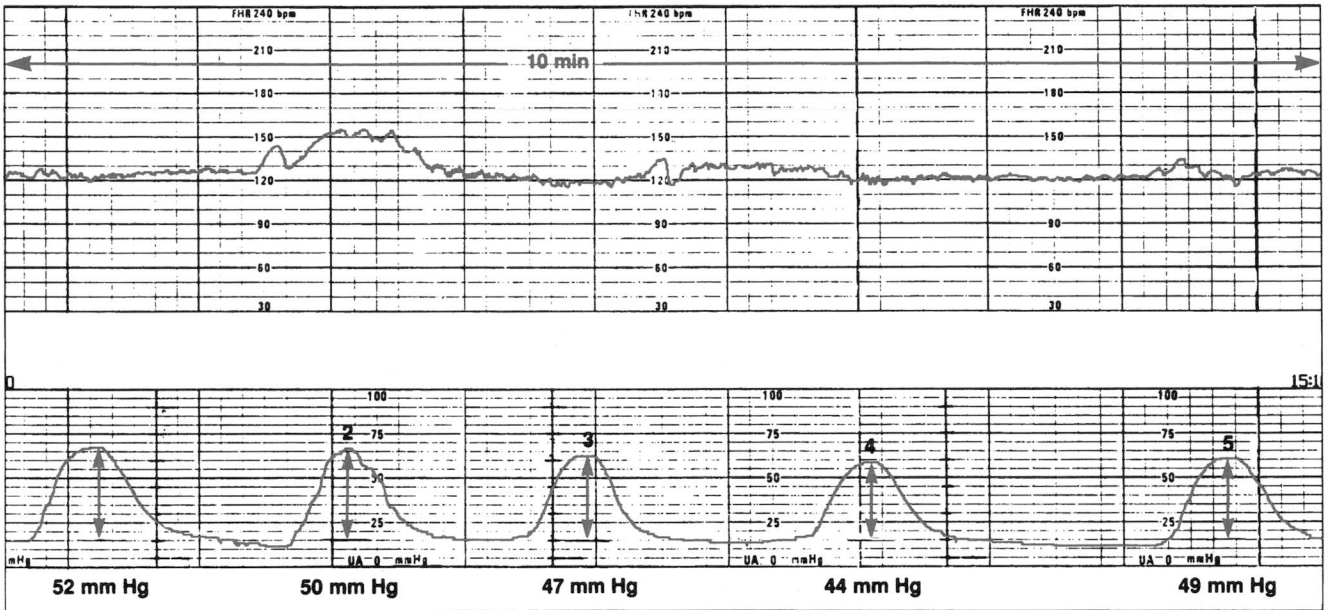

| 52 mm Hg | 50 mm Hg | 47 mm Hg | 44 mm Hg | 49 mm Hg |

FIGURE 20–3. Montevideo units are calculated by subtracting the baseline uterine pressure from the peak contraction pressure for each contraction in a 10-minute window and adding the pressures generated by each contraction. In the example shown, there were five contractions, producing pressure changes of 52, 50, 47, 44, and 49 mm Hg, respectively. The sum of these five contractions is 242 Montevideo units.

incorporates many of the cardinal movements necessary for the fetus to negotiate the birth canal. Accordingly, disproportion of the fetus and pelvis frequently becomes apparent during the second stage.

Until recently, there have been unquestioned second-stage rules that limited its duration. The second stage in nulliparas was limited to 2 hours and extended to 3 hours when regional analgesia was used. For multiparas, 1 hour was the limit, extended to 2 hours with regional analgesia. At Parkland Hospital during 1999, only 6 percent of second-stage labors in nulliparas at term exceeded 2 hours. The second-stage rule of 2 hours was established in American obstetrics by the beginning of the 20th century. It stemmed from concerns about maternal and fetal health, likely regarding infection, and led to difficult forceps operations.

Cohen (1977) investigated the fetal effects of second-stage labor length at Beth Israel Hospital. He included 4403

TABLE 20–2 Criteria for Diagnosis of Abnormal Labor Due to Arrest or Protraction Disorders

Labor Pattern	Nullipara	Multipara
Protraction disorder		
Dilatation	< 1.2 cm/hr	< 1.5 cm/hr
Descent	< 1.0 cm/hr	< 2.0 cm/hr
Arrest disorder		
No dilatation	> 2 hr	> 2 hr
No descent	> 1 hr	> 1 hr

term nulliparas in whom electronic fetal heart rate monitoring was performed. Neonatal mortality was not increased in women whose second-stage labor exceeded 2 hours. Epidural analgesia was used commonly, and this likely accounted for the large number of pregnancies with a prolonged second stage. These data influenced decisions to permit an additional hour for the second stage when regional analgesia was used.

Menticoglou and colleagues (1995b) challenged the prevailing dictums on the duration of the second stage based on their experiences in Winnipeg. These dictums came under scrutiny at their hospitals because of grave neonatal injuries associated with forceps rotations to shorten second-stage labor (Menticoglou and colleagues, 1995a). As a result, they allowed longer second stages in the hope that fewer vaginal operative deliveries would be necessary. Between 1988 and 1992, the second stage of labor exceeded 2 hours in one fourth of 6041 nulliparas at term. Labor epidural analgesia was used in 55 percent. The length of the second stage, even in those lasting up to 6 hours or more, was not related to neonatal outcome. These good results were attributed to careful use of electronic monitoring and scalp pH measurements. They concluded that there is no compelling reason to intervene with a possibly difficult forceps or vacuum extraction because a certain number of hours has elapsed. They offered, however, an important caveat. After 3 hours in the second stage, delivery by cesarean or other operative method increases progressively such that by 5 hours the prospects for spontaneous delivery in the subsequent hour are only 10 to 15 percent.

TABLE 20–3 Abnormal Labor Patterns, Diagnostic Criteria, and Methods of Treatment

Labor Pattern	Diagnostic Criteria		Preferred Treatment	Exceptional Treatment
	Nulliparas	Multiparas		
Prolongation Disorder (Prolonged latent phase)	> 20 hr	> 14 hr	Bed rest	Oxytocin or cesarean delivery for urgent problems
Protraction Disorders				
1. Protracted active-phase dilatation	< 1.2 cm/hr	< 1.5 cm/hr	Expectant and support	Cesarean delivery for CPD
2. Protracted descent	< 1.0 cm/hr	< 2 cm/hr		
Arrest Disorders				
1. Prolonged deceleration phase	> 3 hr	> 1 hr	Oxytocin without CPD	Rest if exhausted
2. Secondary arrest of dilatation				
3. Arrest of descent	> 2 hr	> 2 hr	Cesarean delivery with CPD	Cesarean delivery
4. Failure of descent	> 1 hr, with no descent in deceleration phase or second stage	> 1 hr		

CPD = cephalopelvic disproportion.
Modified from Cohen and Friedman (1983).

Myles and Santolaya (2003) analyzed both the maternal and neonatal consequences of prolonged second stage of labor in 7818 women who gave birth in Chicago between 1996 and 1999. Excluding nonvertex and multiple gestations, 87 percent of the women reached the second stage of labor. Neonatal mortality and morbidity was not related to the length of the second stage. Shown in Table 20–4 are maternal outcomes in relation to the duration of the second stage of labor.

With achievement of full cervical dilatation, the great majority of women cannot resist the urge to "bear down" or "push" each time the uterus contracts. Typically, a laboring woman contracts her abdominal musculature repetitively with vigor to generate increased intra-abdominal pressure throughout the contractions. The combined force created by contractions of the uterus and abdominal musculature propels the fetus downward.

At times, the magnitude of the force created by contractions of abdominal musculature is compromised sufficiently to prevent spontaneous vaginal delivery. Heavy sedation or regional analgesia—lumbar epidural or spinal—is likely to reduce the reflex urge to push, and at the same time may impair the ability to contract the abdominal muscles sufficiently. In other instances, the inherent urge to push is overridden by the intense pain created by bearing down.

Two approaches to maternal pushing during the second stage of labor with epidural analgesia have yielded contradictory results. One approach advocates pushing forcefully once the cervix has completely dilated, regardless of the urge to push. The second favors the delay of pushing until a woman regains the sensory urge to bear down. Fraser and colleagues (2000) found that delayed pushing reduced difficult operative deliveries, whereas Manyonda and colleagues (1990) found the opposite effect. Hansen and colleagues (2002) randomly assigned 252 women with epidural analgesia to one of the two approaches. There were no adverse maternal or neonatal outcomes linked to delayed pushing despite significantly prolonging second-stage labor. Plunkett and colleagues (2003), in a similar study, confirmed these findings.

TABLE 20–4 Clinical Outcomes (in Percent) in Relation to Duration of Second-Stage Labor

Clinical Outcome	Duration of Second Stage		
	< 2 hr (n = 6259)	2–4 hr (n = 384)	> 4 hr (n = 148)
Cesarean delivery	1.2	9.2	34.5
Instrumental delivery	3.4	16.0	35.1
Perineal trauma	3.6	13.4	26.7
Postpartum hemorrhage	2.3	5.0	9.1
Chorioamnionitis	2.3	8.9	14.2

Adapted from Myles and Santolaya (2003).

FETAL STATION AT ONSET OF ACTIVE LABOR. Descent of the fetal biparietal diameter to the level of the maternal pelvic ischial spines (0 station) is defined as engagement (Fig. 2–27, p. 37). Friedman and Sachtleben (1965) reported that there was a significant association between higher station at the onset of labor and subsequent dystocia. They described both protraction and arrested labor disorders in women with fetal head stations above +1 cm and noted that the higher the station at the onset of labor in nulliparas, the more prolonged the labor (Friedman and Sachtleben, 1976). Handa and Laros (1993) found that fetal station at the time of arrested labor was also a risk factor for dystocia. Roshanfekr and associates (1999) analyzed fetal station in 803 nulliparas women with term pregnancies in whom active labor had been diagnosed. About 30 percent of these women presented to the hospital with the fetal head at or below 0 station, and their cesarean delivery rate was 5 percent compared with that of 14 percent for those with higher fetal stations. The prognosis for dystocia, however, was not related to incrementally higher fetal head stations above the pelvic midplane (0 station). Importantly, 86 percent of nulliparous women without fetal head engagement at diagnosis of active labor delivered vaginally. Thus, lack of engagement at the onset of labor, although a statistical risk factor for dystocia, should not be assumed to necessarily predict fetopelvic disproportion. This caveat is especially true for parous women because the head typically descends later in labor.

REPORTED CAUSES OF UTERINE DYSFUNCTION.
Various labor factors have been implicated as causes of uterine dysfunction.

Epidural Analgesia. It is important to emphasize that epidural analgesia can slow labor (Sharma and Leveno, 2000). As shown in Table 20–5, epidural analgesia has been associated with lengthening of both first- and second-stage labor as well as slowing of the rate of fetal descent.

Chorioamnionitis. Because of the association of prolonged labor with maternal intrapartum infection, some clinicians have suggested that infection itself plays a role in the development of abnormal uterine activity. Satin and co-workers (1992) studied the effects of chorioamnionitis on labor stimulation with oxytocin in 266 pregnancies. Chorioamnionitis diagnosed late in labor was found to be a marker of cesarean delivery for dystocia, whereas this was not observed in women diagnosed as having chorioamnionitis early in labor. Specifically, 40 percent of women developing chorioamnionitis after requiring oxytocin for dysfunctional labor later required cesarean delivery for dystocia. It is likely that uterine infection in this clinical setting is a consequence of dysfunctional, prolonged labor rather than a cause of dystocia.

TABLE 20–5 **Effect of Epidural Analgesia on the Progress of Labor in 199 Nulliparous Women Delivered Spontaneously at Parkland Hospital**

Labor	Epidural Analgesia	Meperidine Analgesia	P Value
Cervical dilatation at analgesia, mean	4.1 cm	4.2 cm	NS
Active phase, mean	7.9 hr	6.3 hr	.005
Second stage, mean	60 min	48 min	.03
Fetal descent	4.2 cm/hr	7.9 cm/hr	.003

NS = not stated.
From Alexander and associates (1998).

Maternal Position During Labor. Advocacy for recumbency or ambulation during labor has swung back and forth over time. Proponents of walking during labor report it to shorten labor, decrease rates of oxytocin augmentation, decrease the need for analgesia, and lower the frequency of operative vaginal delivery (Flynn and co-authors, 1978; Read and colleagues, 1981).

According to Miller (1983), the uterus contracts more frequently but with less intensity with the mother in the supine position compared with that of lying on her side. Conversely, contraction frequency and intensity have been reported to increase with sitting or standing. Lupe and Gross (1986) concluded, however, that there is no conclusive evidence that upright maternal posture or ambulation improves labor. They reported that women preferred to lie on their side or sit in bed. Few chose to walk, fewer to squat, and none wanted the knee-chest position. They tended to assume fetal positions in later labor. Most women enthusiastic about ambulation returned to bed when active labor began (Carlson and associates, 1986; Williams and co-workers, 1980).

Bloom and colleagues (1998) conducted a randomized trial to study the effects of walking during first-stage labor. In 1067 women with uncomplicated term pregnancies delivered at Parkland Hospital, these investigators reported that ambulation neither improved nor delayed labor in nulliparous or parous women. Walking during labor did not reduce the need for analgesia, nor was it harmful to the fetus-neonate. Because these results provided no evidence for or against walking during labor, we now give women without complications the option of electing either recumbency or supervised ambulation during labor. The American College of Obstetricians and Gynecologists (2003) has concluded that ambulation in labor is not harmful, and mobility may result in greater comfort.

Birthing Position in Second-Stage Labor. Considerable interest has been shown in alternative second-stage labor birth positions and their effect on labor. Johnson and co-workers (1991) reported that several randomized controlled trials with and without the use of specific birthing aids—for example, birthing chairs—have produced conflicting results and are confounded by observer bias. One reported advantage from avoiding the traditional lithotomy position is an increase in the dimensions of the pelvic outlet. Specifically, Russell (1969) described a 20- to 30-percent increase in the area of the pelvic outlet with squatting compared with that of the supine position. Gupta and co-workers (1991) compared the usual delivery position in the western world—recumbent with the head and shoulders elevated 30 degrees—with the squatting position and found no significant change in the dimensions of either the pelvic inlet or outlet. Crowley and associates (1991) randomly assigned 634 women to deliver in an obstetrical birthing chair and 596 women to deliver in bed. There were no advantages with use of the chair, but hemorrhage was increased in this group. De Jong and co-workers

(1997), in a randomized trial of 517 women, found no increase in hemorrhage with the sitting position. Obstetrical outcomes were not improved by enforcing the upright position for second-stage labor. The main benefits reported were less maternal pain and enhanced maternal satisfaction with the birthing experience. Babayer and coauthors (1998) cautioned that prolonged sitting or squatting during the second stage may cause peroneal neuropathy.

Immersion in Water. This approach has been advocated as a means of relaxation that may contribute to more efficient labor (Odent, 1983). Schorn and colleagues (1993) randomly assigned 96 women at term to immersion in a hot tub with air jets or to prevailing labor management at their hospital. The women were permitted to stay in the tub as long as they desired, and most stayed 30 to 45 minutes. Water immersion did not alter the rate of cervical dilation, length of labor, route of delivery, or analgesia use. Robertson and associates (1998) reported that immersion was not associated with chorioamnionitis or endometritis. Kwee and co-workers (2000) studied the effects of immersion in 20 women and reported that maternal blood pressure decreased, whereas fetal heart rate was unaffected.

RUPTURED MEMBRANES WITHOUT LABOR. Membrane rupture without spontaneous uterine contractions occurs in about 8 percent of term pregnancies. Until recently, management generally included stimulation of contractions when labor did not begin after 6 to 12 hours. This intervention evolved about 40 years ago because of maternal and fetal complications due to amnionitis (Calkins, 1952). Such routine intervention was the accepted practice until challenged by Kappy and co-workers (1979), who reported excessive cesarean delivery in term pregnancies with ruptured membranes managed with labor stimulation compared with that of those managed by expectant observation.

Hannah and co-workers (1996) and Peleg and associates (1999) performed an international randomized investigation of 5042 pregnancies with ruptured membranes at term. They measured the effects of induction versus expectant management and also compared induction with intravenous oxytocin to prostaglandin E_2 gel. There were approximately 1200 pregnancies in each of the four study arms. They concluded that labor induction with intravenous oxytocin was the preferred management. This determination was based on significantly fewer intrapartum and postpartum infections in women whose labor was induced. There were no significant differences in cesarean delivery rates. Subsequent analysis by Hannah and colleagues (2000) indicated increased adverse outcomes when expectant management at home was compared with in-hospital observation. Similar conclusions were reached by Mozurkewich and Wolf (1997) after meta-analysis of reported trials of management of ruptured membrane at term. At Parkland Hospital, labor is induced when ruptured membranes are diagnosed at term.

PRECIPITOUS LABOR AND DELIVERY. Not only can labor be too slow, but it also can be abnormally rapid. Precipitous—that is, extremely rapid—labor and delivery may result from an abnormally low resistance of the soft parts of the birth canal, from abnormally strong uterine and abdominal contractions, or *rarely* from the absence of painful sensations and thus a lack of awareness of vigorous labor.

Definition. According to Hughes (1972), precipitous labor terminates in expulsion of the fetus in less than 3 hours. Using this definition, 79,933 live births (2 percent) were complicated by precipitous labor in the United States during 1998 (Ventura and co-workers, 2000). There is little published information, however, on its maternal and fetal effects. Mahon and colleagues (1994) described 99 pregnancies delivered within 3 hours of labor onset. Short labors, defined as a rate of cervical dilatation of 5 cm/hr or faster for nulliparas and 10 cm/hr for multiparas, were associated with abruption (20 percent), meconium, postpartum hemorrhage, cocaine abuse, and low Apgar scores. Most (93 percent) of the women were multiparas and typically had uterine contractions at intervals less than 2 minutes.

Maternal Effects. Precipitous labor and delivery seldom are accompanied by serious maternal complications if the cervix is effaced appreciably and compliant, the vagina has been stretched previously, and the perineum is relaxed. Conversely, vigorous uterine contractions combined with a long, firm cervix and a noncompliant birth canal may lead to uterine rupture or extensive lacerations of the cervix, vagina, vulva, or perineum. It is in these latter circumstances that the rare condition of *amnionic fluid embolism* most likely develops (see Chap. 35, p. 845). **The uterus that contracts with unusual vigor before delivery is likely to be hypotonic after delivery, with hemorrhage from the placental implantation site as the consequence.** Postpartum hemorrhage from uterine atony is discussed in Chapter 35 (see p. 826).

Effects on Fetus and Neonate. Perinatal mortality and morbidity from precipitous labor may be increased considerably for several reasons. The tumultuous uterine contractions, often with negligible intervals of relaxation, prevent appropriate uterine blood flow and fetal oxygenation. Additionally, resistance of the birth canal may cause intracranial trauma, although this is rare. Acker and colleagues (1988) reported that Erb or Duchenne brachial palsy was associated with such labors in one third of cases. Finally, during an unattended birth, the newborn may fall to the floor and be injured or may need resuscitation that is not immediately available.

Treatment. Unusually forceful spontaneous uterine contractions are not likely to be modified to a significant degree by analgesia. The use of tocolytic agents such as magnesium sulfate is unproven in these circumstances. Use of general anesthesia with agents that impair uterine contractibility, such as halothane and isoflurane, is often excessively heroic. Certainly, any oxytocin agents being administered should be stopped immediately.

FETOPELVIC DISPROPORTION

Fetopelvic disproportion arises from diminished pelvic capacity, excessive fetal size, or more usually, a combination of both.

PELVIC CAPACITY. Any contraction of the pelvic diameters that diminishes the capacity of the pelvis can create dystocia during labor. There may be contractions of the pelvic inlet, the midpelvis, the pelvic outlet, or a generally contracted pelvis caused by combinations of these.

Contracted Pelvic Inlet. The pelvic inlet usually is considered to be contracted if its shortest anteroposterior diameter is less than 10 cm or if the greatest transverse diameter is less than 12 cm. The anteroposterior diameter of the pelvic inlet is commonly approximated by manually measuring the diagonal conjugate, which is about 1.5 cm greater (see Chap. 2, p. 36). Therefore, inlet contraction usually is defined as a diagonal conjugate of less than 11.5 cm.

Using clinical and, at times, imaging pelvimetry, it is important to identify the shortest anteroposterior diameter through which the fetal head must pass. Occasionally, the body of the first sacral vertebra is displaced forward so that the shortest distance may actually be between this abnormal sacral promontory and the symphysis pubis.

Prior to labor, the fetal biparietal diameter has been shown to *average* from 9.5 to as much as 9.8 cm. Therefore, it might prove difficult or even impossible for some fetuses to pass through an inlet that has an anteroposterior diameter of less than 10 cm. Mengert (1948) and Kaltreider (1952), employing x-ray pelvimetry, demonstrated that the incidence of difficult deliveries is increased to a similar degree when either the anteroposterior diameter of the inlet is less than 10 cm or the transverse diameter is less than 12 cm. As expected, when both diameters are contracted, dystocia is much greater than when only one is contracted.

A small woman is likely to have a small pelvis, but she is also likely to have a small neonate. Thoms (1937) studied 362 nulliparas and found the mean birthweight of their offspring was significantly lower (280 g) in women with small pelves than in those with medium or large pelves. In veterinary obstetrics, it frequently has been observed that in most species maternal size rather than paternal size is the important determinant of fetal size.

Normally, cervical dilatation is facilitated by hydrostatic action of the unruptured membranes or, after their rupture, by direct application of the presenting part against the cervix. In contracted pelves, however, when the head is arrested in the pelvic inlet, the entire force exerted by the uterus acts directly on the portion of membranes that overlie the dilating cervix. Consequently, early spontaneous rupture of the membranes is more likely.

After membrane rupture, the absence of pressure by the head against the cervix and lower uterine segment predisposes to less effective contractions. Hence, further dilatation may proceed very slowly or not at all. Cibils and Hendricks (1965) reported that the mechanical adaptation of the fetal passenger to the bony passage plays an important part in determining the efficiency of contractions. The better the adaptation, the more efficient are the contractions. Thus, cervical response to labor provides a prognostic view of the labor outcome in women with inlet contraction.

A contracted inlet plays an important part in the production of abnormal presentations. In normal nulliparas, the presenting part at term commonly descends into the pelvic cavity before the onset of labor. When the inlet is contracted considerably, however, descent usually does not take place until after the onset of labor, if at all. Cephalic presentations still predominate, but because the head floats freely over the pelvic inlet or rests more laterally in one of the iliac fossae, very slight influences may cause the fetus to assume other presentations. **In women with contracted pelves, face and shoulder presentations are encountered three times more frequently, and cord prolapse occurs four to six times more frequently.** Critchlow and colleagues (1994) have quantified the magnitude of risk for cord prolapse in women with cephalopelvic disproportion.

Contracted Midpelvis. This finding is more common than inlet contraction. It frequently causes transverse arrest of the fetal head, which potentially can lead to a difficult midforceps operation or to cesarean delivery.

The obstetrical plane of the midpelvis extends from the inferior margin of the symphysis pubis through the ischial spines and touches the sacrum near the junction of the fourth and fifth vertebrae (see Chap. 2, p. 34). A transverse line theoretically connecting the ischial spines divides the midpelvis into anterior and posterior portions. The former is bounded anteriorly by the lower border of the symphysis pubis and laterally by the ischiopubic rami. The posterior portion is bounded dorsally by the sacrum and laterally by the sacrospinous ligaments, forming the lower limits of the sacrosciatic notch.

Average midpelvis measurements are as follows: *transverse,* or interspinous, 10.5 cm; *anteroposterior,* from the lower border of the symphysis pubis to the junction of S4–S5, 11.5 cm; and *posterior sagittal,* from the midpoint of the interspinous line to the same point on the sacrum, 5 cm. The definition of midpelvic contractions has not been established with the same precision possible for inlet contractions. Even so, the midpelvis is likely contracted when the sum of the interischial spinous and posterior sagittal diameters of the midpelvis—normal, 10.5 plus 5 cm, or 15.5 cm—falls to

13.5 cm or below. This concept was emphasized by Chen and Huang (1982) in evaluating possible midpelvic contraction. There is reason to suspect midpelvic contraction whenever the interischial spinous diameter is less than 10 cm. When it measures less than 8 cm, the midpelvis is contracted.

Although there is no precise manual method of measuring midpelvic dimensions, a suggestion of contraction sometimes can be inferred if the spines are prominent, the pelvic side-walls converge, or the sacrosciatic notch is narrow. Moreover, Eller and Mengert (1947) pointed out that the relationship between the intertuberous and interspinous diameters of the ischium is sufficiently constant that narrowing of the inter-spinous diameter can be anticipated when the intertuberous diameter is narrow. A normal intertuberous diameter, however, does not always exclude a narrow interspinous diameter.

Contracted Pelvic Outlet. This finding usually is defined as an interischial tuberous diameter of 8 cm or less. The pelvic outlet may be roughly likened to two triangles, with the inter-ischial tuberous diameter constituting the base of both. The sides of the anterior triangle are the pubic rami, and its apex is the inferior posterior surface of the symphysis pubis. The posterior triangle has no bony sides but is limited at its apex by the tip of the last sacral vertebra (not the tip of the coccyx). Diminution of the intertuberous diameter with consequent narrowing of the anterior triangle must inevitably force the fetal head posteriorly. Floberg and associates (1987) reported that outlet contractions were found in almost 1 percent of more than 1400 unselected nulliparas with term pregnancies. A contracted outlet may cause dystocia not so much by itself as through the often-associated midpelvic contraction. *Outlet contraction without concomitant midplane contraction is rare.*

Even when the disproportion between the fetal head and the pelvic outlet is not sufficiently great to give rise to severe dystocia, it may play an important part in the production of perineal tears. With increasing narrowing of the pubic arch, the occiput cannot emerge directly beneath the symphysis pubis but is forced increasingly farther down upon the ischiopubic rami. The perineum, consequently, becomes increasingly distended and thus exposed to greater danger of laceration.

Pelvic Fractures and Rare Contractures. Speer and Peltier (1972) reviewed experiences with pelvic fractures and pregnancy. Trauma from automobile collisions was the most common cause of pelvic fractures. With bilateral fractures of the pubic rami, compromise of the birth canal capacity by callus formation or malunion was common. A history of pelvic fracture warrants careful review of previous radiographs and possibly computed tomographic pelvimetry later in pregnancy. Descriptions and illustrations of rare pelvic contractions are provided in the 10th through 17th editions of *Williams Obstetrics.*

Estimation of Pelvic Capacity. The techniques for clinical evaluation using digital examination of the bony pelvis during labor are described in detail in Chapter 2 (p. 36). Briefly, the examiner attempts to judge the anteroposterior diameter of the inlet (the diagonal conjugate), the interspinous diameter of the midpelvis, and the intertuberous distances of the pelvic outlet. A narrow pelvic arch, less than 90 degrees, can signify a narrow pelvis. An unengaged fetal head can indicate either excessive fetal head size or reduced pelvic inlet capacity.

X-RAY PELVIMETRY. The prognosis for successful vaginal delivery in any given pregnancy cannot be established on the basis of x-ray pelvimetry alone, because the pelvic capacity is but one of several factors that determine the outcome (Mengert, 1948). Thus, x-ray pelvimetry is considered to be of limited value in the management of labor with cephalic presentations (American College of Obstetricians and Gynecologists, 1995b).

COMPUTED TOMOGRAPHIC (CT) SCANNING. Advantages of CT pelvimetry, such as that shown in Figure 20–4, compared with those of conventional x-ray pelvimetry include reduced radiation exposure, greater accuracy, and easier performance. With either method, costs are comparable and x-ray exposure is minuscule (see Chap. 41, p. 977). With conventional x-ray pelvimetry, the mean gonadal exposure is estimated to be 885 mrad by the Committee on Radiological Hazards to Patients (Osborn, 1963). Depending on the machine and technique employed, fetal doses with computed tomography may range from 250 to 1500 mrad (Moore and Shearer, 1989).

MAGNETIC RESONANCE IMAGING (MRI). The advantages of MRI pelvimetry include lack of ionizing radiation, accurate measurements, complete fetal imaging, and the potential for evaluating soft tissue dystocia (McCarthy, 1986; Stark and co-workers, 1985). Currently its use is limited because of expense, time involved for adequate imaging studies, and equipment availability.

Sporri and co-workers (1997) used MRI postpartum to measure capacity at each level of the pelvis and ultrasonography intrapartum to measure fetal head dimensions. In this study, "cephalic pelvic disproportion" was defined as arrested labor for more than 4 hours in the presence of normal uterine contractions. "Failure to progress" was diagnosed when there was no labor progress and uterine activity was hypotonic. A fetal head volume exceeding measured pelvic capacity was a frequent finding in women with cephalopelvic disproportion, but not those with failure to progress. Clearly, use of MRI to measure pelvic capacity is investigational.

FETAL DIMENSIONS IN FETOPELVIC DISPROPORTION.

In earlier editions of *Williams Obstetrics,* excessive fetal size as a cause of dystocia in a normally formed pelvis was considered to be 5000 g in the 1st edition (1903) and 4500 g in the 7th and 13th editions (1956, 1966). Despite

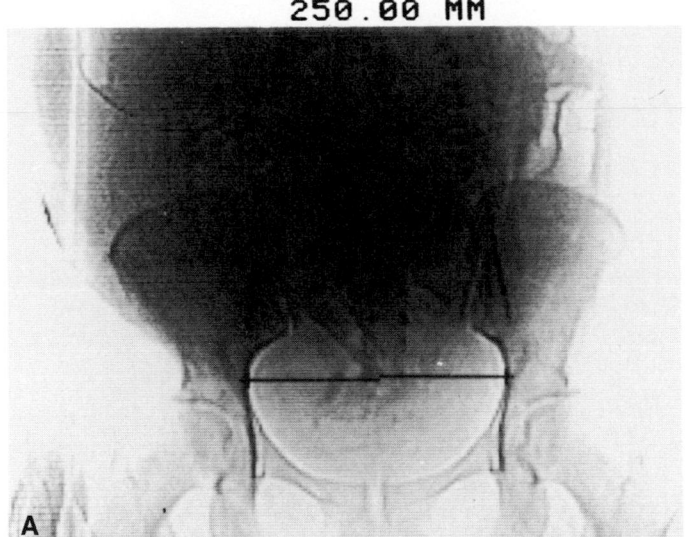

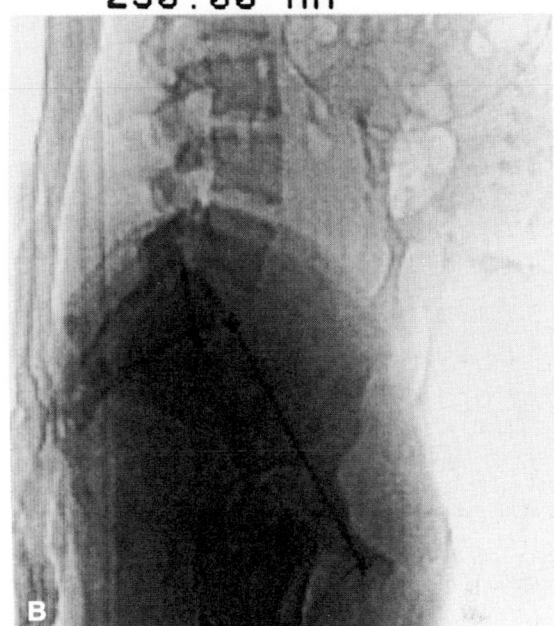

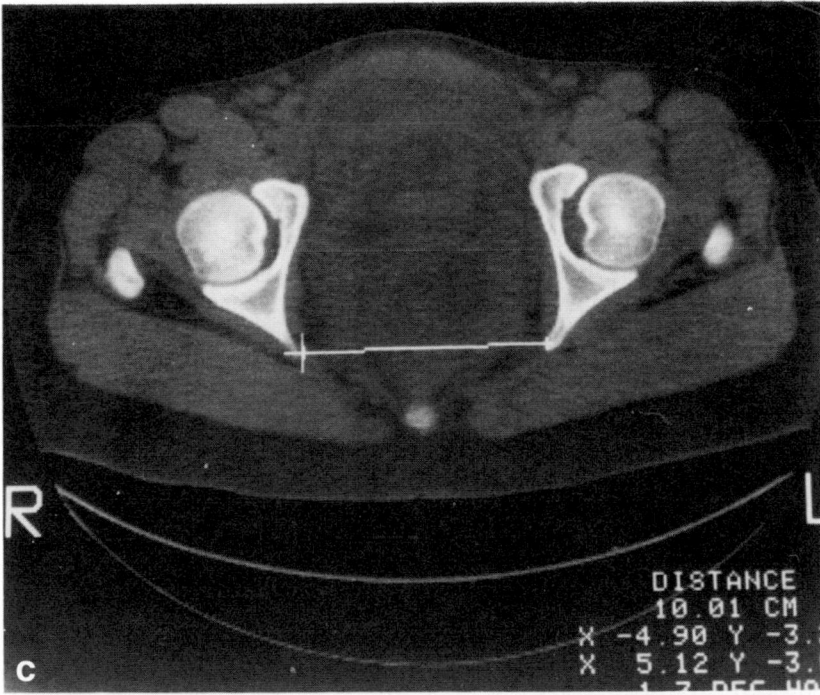

FIGURE 20–4. A. Anteroposterior view of a digital radiograph. Illustrated is the measurement of the transverse diameter of the pelvic inlet using an electronic cursor. The fetal body is clearly outlined. **B.** Lateral view of a digital radiograph. Illustrated are measurements of the anteroposterior diameters of the inlet and midpelvis measurements using the electronic cursor. **C.** An axial computed tomographic section through the midpelvis. The level of the fovea of the femoral heads was ascertained from the anteroposterior digital radiograph because it corresponds to the level of the ischial spines. The interspinous diameter is measured using the electronic cursor. The total fetal radiation dose using the three exposures shown in parts **A** to **C** is approximately 250 mrad.

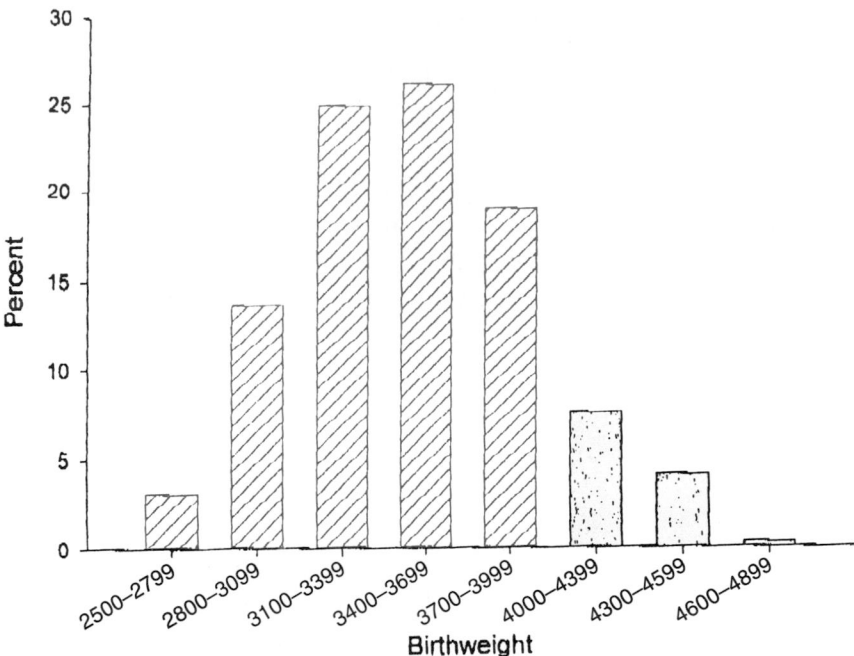

FIGURE 20–5. Birthweight distribution of 362 newborns delivered by cesarean at Parkland Hospital (1989–1999) after a failed attempt to effect vaginal delivery with forceps. Only 12 percent (n = 44) of the newborns weighed ≥ 4000 g (shaded bars).

these variations, the common theme was that fetal size alone is seldom a suitable explanation for failed labor. Now, even with the evolution of remarkable technology, selection of a fetal size threshold to predict fetopelvic disproportion is still elusive. This is because most cases of disproportion occur in fetuses whose weight is well within the range of the general obstetrical population. As shown in Figure 20–5, two thirds of neonates who required cesarean delivery at Parkland Hospital after an attempt at forceps delivery had failed, weighed less than 3700 g (8 lb 2 oz). Thus, fetopelvic disproportion usually is not associated simply with excessive fetal size. Other factors, such as malpositions of the fetal head—for example, occiput position, face and brow presentations—obstruct passage of the fetus through the birth canal.

Estimation of Fetal Head Size. Efforts to clinically and radiographically predict fetopelvic disproportion based on fetal head size have proved disappointing. Müller (1880) and Hillis (1930) both described a clinical maneuver to predict disproportion. In an occiput presentation, the fetal brow and the suboccipital region are grasped through the abdominal wall with the fingers and firm pressure is directed downward in the axis of the inlet. Fundal pressure by an assistant usually is helpful. The effect of the forces on the descent of the head can be evaluated by concomitant vaginal examination. If no disproportion exists, the head readily enters the pelvis, and vaginal delivery can be predicted. Inability to push the head into the pelvis, however, does not necessarily indicate that vaginal delivery is impossible. A clear demonstration of a flexed fetal head that overrides the symphysis pubis, however, is presumptive evidence of disproportion. Thorp and colleagues (1993b) performed a prospective evaluation of

the *Mueller-Hillis maneuver* and concluded that there was no relation between dystocia and failure of descent of the head.

Measurements of fetal head diameters using plain radiographic techniques are not used because of parallax distortions. The biparietal diameter and head circumference can be measured ultrasonographically, and there have been attempts to use this information in the management of dystocia. Thurnau and colleagues (1991) used the fetal-pelvic index to identify labor complications. Unfortunately, the sensitivity of such measurements to predict cephalopelvic disproportion is poor (Ferguson and associates, 1998). We are of the view that there is no currently satisfactory method for accurate prediction of fetopelvic disproportion based on fetal head size.

Face Presentation. With a face presentation, the head is hyperextended so that the occiput is in contact with the fetal back and the chin (mentum) is presenting. The fetal face may present with the chin (mentum) anteriorly or posteriorly, relative to the maternal symphysis pubis. In term-size fetuses, labor progression usually is impeded with mentum posterior face presentations because the fetal brow (bregma) is pressed against the maternal symphysis pubis. This position precludes flexion of the fetal head necessary to negotiate the birth canal (Fig. 20–6). In contrast, flexion of the head and vaginal delivery are typical with mentum anterior presentations. Many mentum posterior presentations convert spontaneously to anterior even in late labor (Duff, 1981).

Cruikshank and White (1973) reported an incidence of 1 in 600, or 0.17 percent. Among more than 70,000 singleton newborns delivered at Parkland Hospital from 1995 through

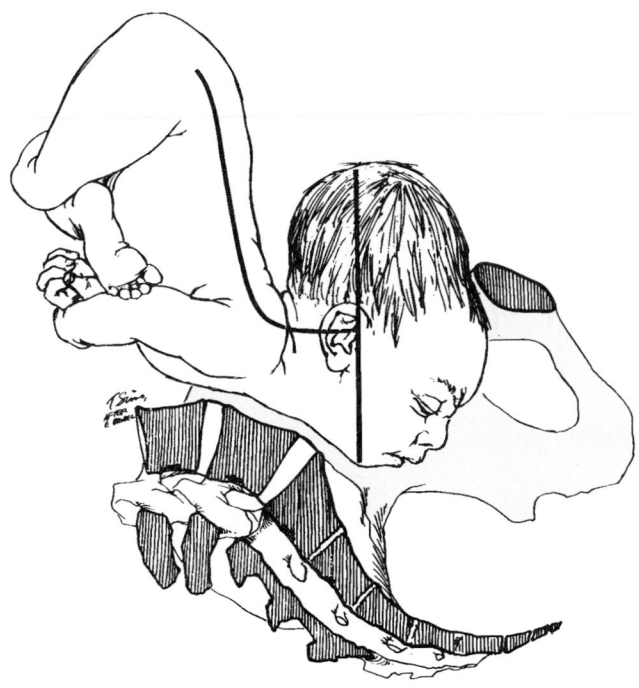

FIGURE 20–6. Face presentation. The occiput is the longer end of the head lever. The chin is directly posterior. Vaginal delivery is impossible unless the chin rotates anteriorly.

1999, 36—or about 1 in 2000—were face presentations at delivery (see Table 17–1, p. 410).

DIAGNOSIS. Face presentation is diagnosed by vaginal examination and palpation of the distinctive facial features of the mouth and nose, the malar bones, and particularly the orbital ridges. As discussed in Chapter 24 (see p. 567), it is possible to mistake a breech for a face presentation, because the anus may be mistaken for the mouth and the ischial tuberosities for the malar prominences. The radiographic demonstration of the hyperextended head with the facial bones at or below the pelvic inlet is characteristic (Fig. 20–7).

ETIOLOGY. Causes of face presentations are numerous, generally stemming from any factor that favors extension or prevents head flexion. In exceptional instances, marked enlargement of the neck or coils of cord about the neck may cause extension. Anencephalic fetuses naturally present by the face. Extended positions develop more frequently when the pelvis is contracted or the fetus is very large. In a series of 141 face presentations studied by Hellman and co-workers (1950), the incidence of inlet contraction was 40 percent. This high incidence of pelvic contraction must be kept in mind when considering management.

In multiparous women, a pendulous abdomen may predispose to face presentation. It permits the back of the fetus to sag forward or laterally, often in the same direction in which the occiput points, thus promoting extension of the cervical

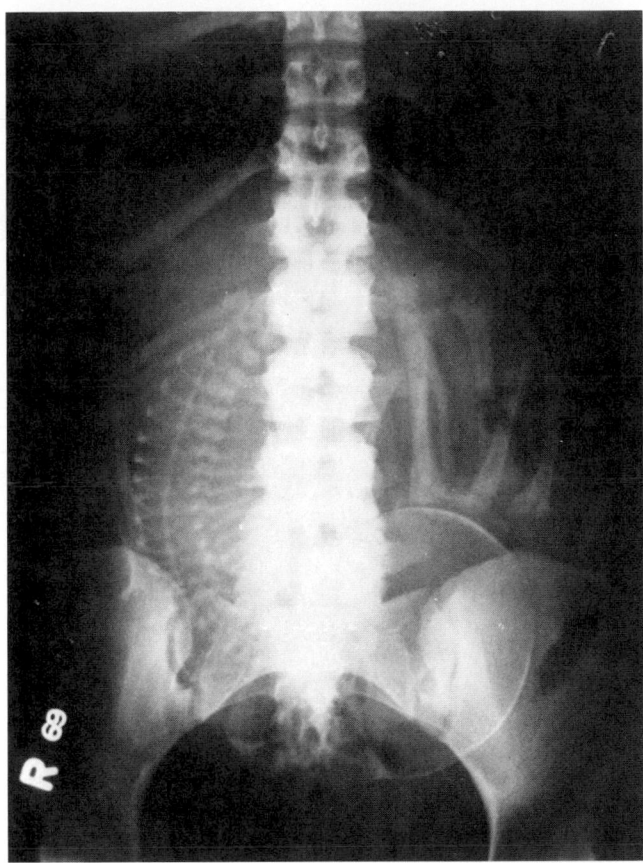

FIGURE 20–7. Radiograph showing face presentation. Note the marked hyperextension of the head and spine of fetus.

and thoracic spine. High parity itself is a predisposing factor (Fuchs and colleagues, 1985).

MECHANISM OF LABOR. Face presentations rarely are observed above the pelvic inlet. The brow generally presents, and it is usually converted into a face presentation after further extension of the head during descent. The mechanism of labor in these cases consists of the cardinal movements of descent, internal rotation, and flexion, and the accessory movements of extension and external rotation (Fig. 20–8). Descent is brought about by the same factors as in cephalic presentations. Extension results from the relation of the fetal body to the deflected head, which is converted into a two-armed lever, the longer arm of which extends from the occipital condyles to the occiput. When resistance is encountered, the occiput must be pushed toward the back of the fetus while the chin descends (see Fig. 20–6).

The objective of internal rotation of the face is to bring the chin under the symphysis pubis. Only in this way can the neck traverse the posterior surface of the symphysis pubis. If the chin rotates directly posteriorly, the relatively short neck cannot span the anterior surface of the sacrum, which measures about 12 cm in length (see Fig. 20–6). Hence, the birth of the head is impossible unless the shoulders enter the pelvis

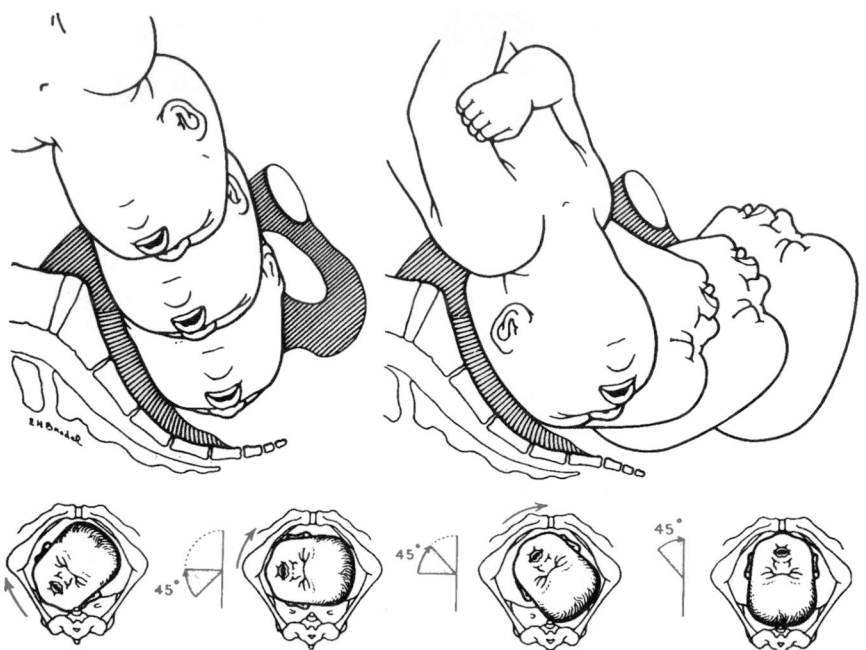

FIGURE 20–8. Mechanism of labor for right mentoposterior position with subsequent rotation of the mentum anteriorly and delivery.

at the same time, an event that is impossible except when the fetus is extremely small or macerated. Internal rotation results from the same factors as in vertex presentations.

After anterior rotation and descent, the chin and mouth appear at the vulva, the undersurface of the chin presses against the symphysis, and the head is delivered by flexion (see Fig. 20–8). The nose, eyes, brow (bregma), and occiput then appear in succession over the anterior margin of the perineum. After birth of the head, the occiput sags backward toward the anus. Next, the chin rotates externally to the side toward which it was originally directed, and the shoulders are born as in cephalic presentations.

Edema may sometimes significantly distort the face. At the same time, the skull undergoes considerable molding, manifested by an increase in length of the occipitomental diameter of the head (see Fig. 20–6).

MANAGEMENT. In the absence of a contracted pelvis, and with effective labor, successful vaginal delivery usually will follow. Fetal heart rate monitoring is probably better done with external devices to avoid damage to the face and eyes. Because face presentations among term-size fetuses are more common when there is some degree of pelvic inlet contraction, cesarean delivery frequently is indicated.

Attempts to convert a face presentation manually into a vertex presentation, manual or forceps rotation of a persistently posterior chin to a mentum anterior position, and internal podalic version and extraction are dangerous and not attempted. Neuman and colleagues (1994) have described intrapartum bimanual conversion of mentoposterior to occipitoanterior presentations in 11 women who refused cesarean delivery.

Brow Presentation. This presentation is the rarest (see Table 17–1, p. 410) and is diagnosed when that portion of the fetal head between the orbital ridge and the anterior fontanel presents at the pelvic inlet. As shown in Figure 20–9, the fetal head thus occupies a position midway between full flexion (occiput) and extension (mentum or face). Except when the fetal head is small or the pelvis is unusually large, engagement of the fetal head and subsequent delivery cannot take place as long as the brow presentation persists.

DIAGNOSIS. The presentation may be recognized by abdominal palpation when both the occiput and chin can be palpated easily, but vaginal examination is usually necessary. The frontal sutures, large anterior fontanel, orbital ridges, eyes, and root of the nose can be felt on vaginal examination. However, neither mouth nor chin is within reach (see Fig. 20–9).

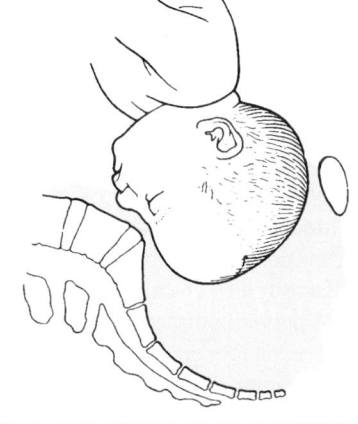

FIGURE 20–9. Brow posterior presentation.

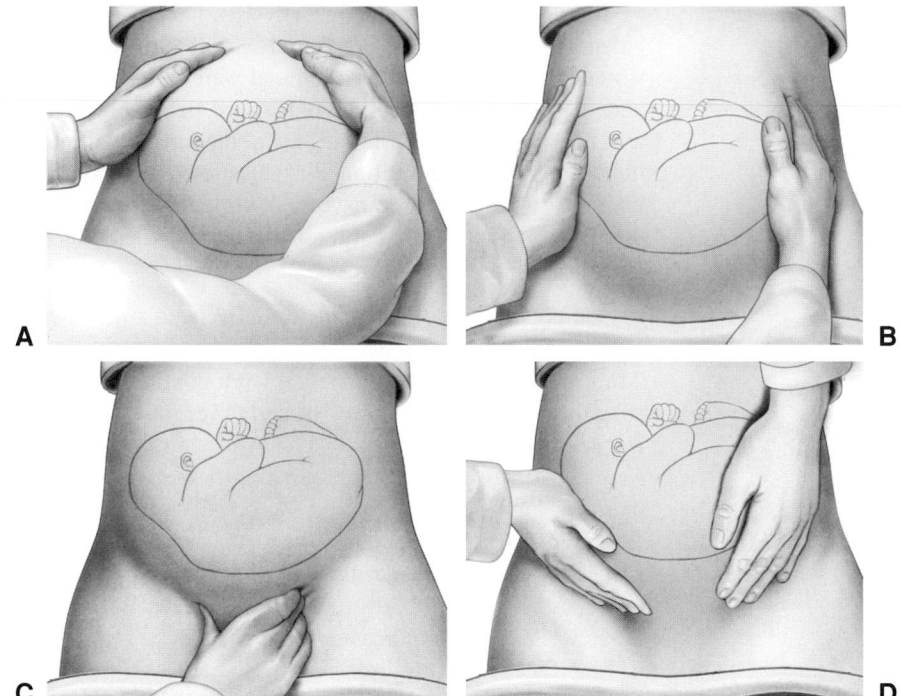

FIGURE 20–10. Palpation in transverse lie, right acromidorsoanterior position. **A.** First maneuver. **B.** Second maneuver. **C.** Third maneuver. **D.** Fourth maneuver.

ETIOLOGY. The causes of persistent brow presentation are the same as those for face presentation. A brow presentation is commonly unstable and often converts to a face or an occiput presentation (Cruikshank and White, 1973).

MECHANISM OF LABOR. With a very small fetus and a large pelvis, labor is generally easy. With a larger fetus, however, it is usually difficult, because engagement is impossible until there is marked molding that shortens the occipitomental diameter or, more commonly, until there is either flexion to an occiput presentation or extension to a face presentation. The considerable molding essential for vaginal delivery of a persistent brow characteristically deforms the head. The caput succedaneum is over the forehead, and it may be so extensive that identification of the brow by palpation is impossible. In these instances, the forehead is prominent and squared, and the occipitomental diameter is diminished.

In transient brow presentations, the prognosis depends on the ultimate presentation. If the brow persists, prognosis is poor for vaginal delivery unless the fetus is small or the birth canal is huge. Principles of management are much the same as those for a face presentation.

Transverse Lie. This position occurs when the long axis of the fetus is approximately perpendicular to that of the mother. When the long axis forms an acute angle, an oblique lie results. The latter is usually only transitory, because either a longitudinal or transverse lie commonly results when labor

supervenes. For this reason, the oblique lie is called an unstable lie in Great Britain.

In transverse lies, the shoulder is usually over the pelvic inlet, with the head lying in one iliac fossa and the breech in the other. In such a *shoulder presentation,* the side of the mother on which the acromion rests determines the designation of the lie as right or left acromial. Moreover, because in either position the back may be directed anteriorly or posteriorly, superiorly or inferiorly, it is customary to distinguish varieties as dorsoanterior and dorsoposterior (Fig. 20–10).

Transverse lie occurred once in 322 singleton deliveries (0.3 percent) at both the Mayo Clinic and the University of Iowa Hospital (Cruikshank and White, 1973; Johnson 1964). At Parkland Hospital, transverse lie was encountered in about 1 in 335 singleton fetuses delivered during a 4-year period (see Table 17–1, p. 410).

DIAGNOSIS. The diagnosis usually is made easily, often by inspection alone. The abdomen is unusually wide, whereas the uterine fundus extends to only slightly above the umbilicus. No fetal pole is detected in the fundus, and the ballottable head is found in one iliac fossa and the breech in the other. The position of the back is readily identifiable. When the back is anterior (see Fig. 20–10), a hard resistance plane extends across the front of the abdomen. When it is posterior, irregular nodulations representing the small parts are felt through the abdominal wall.

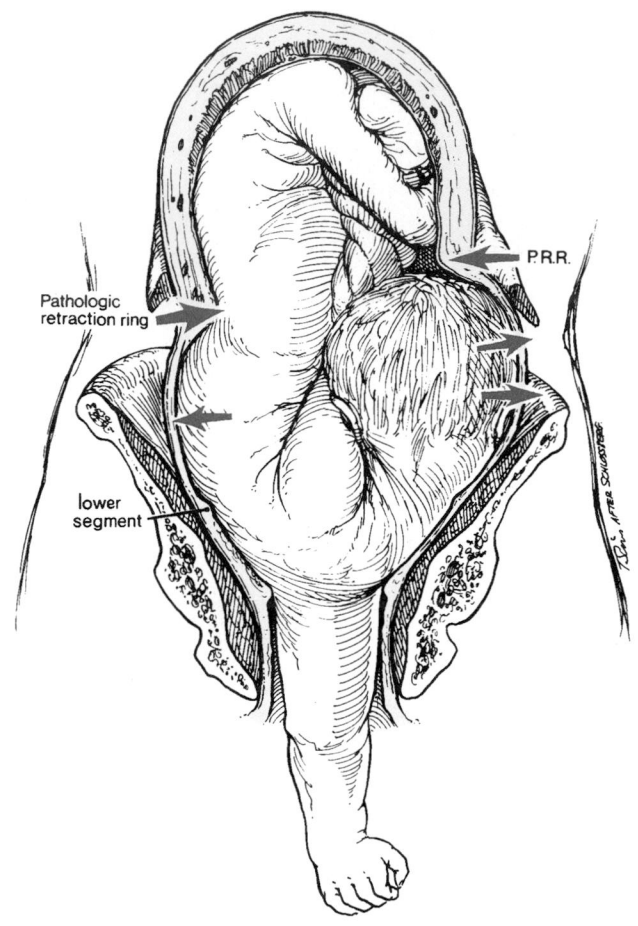

Pathologic
retraction ring

P.R.R.

lower
segment

FIGURE 20–11. Neglected shoulder presentation. A thick muscular band forming a pathological retraction ring has developed just above the thin lower uterine segment. The force generated during a uterine contraction is directed centripetally at and above the level of the pathological retraction ring. This serves to stretch further and possibly to rupture the thin lower segment below the retraction ring. (P.R.R. = pathological retraction ring.)

On vaginal examination, in the early stages of labor, the side of the thorax, if it can be reached, may be recognized by the "gridiron" feel of the ribs. When dilatation is further advanced, the scapula and the clavicle are distinguished on opposite sides of the thorax. The position of the axilla indicates the side of the mother toward which the shoulder is directed. Later in labor, the shoulder will become tightly wedged in the pelvic canal, and a hand and arm frequently prolapse into the vagina and through the vulva (Fig. 20–11).

ETIOLOGY. The common causes of transverse lie are:

1. Abdominal wall relaxation from high parity.
2. Preterm fetus.
3. Placenta previa.
4. Abnormal uterine anatomy.
5. Excessive amnionic fluid.
6. Contracted pelvis.

Women with four or more deliveries have a 10-fold incidence of transverse lie compared with that of nulliparous women. Relaxation of the abdominal wall with a pendulous abdomen allows the uterus to fall forward, deflecting the long axis of the fetus away from the axis of the birth canal into an oblique or transverse position. Placenta previa and pelvic contraction act similarly. A transverse or oblique lie occasionally develops in labor from an initial longitudinal position.

MECHANISM OF LABOR. Spontaneous delivery of a fully developed newborn is impossible with a persistent transverse lie. After rupture of the membranes, if labor continues, the fetal shoulder is forced into the pelvis, and the corresponding arm frequently prolapses (Fig. 20–11). After some descent, the shoulder is arrested by the margins of the pelvic inlet, with the head in one iliac fossa and the breech in the other. As labor continues, the shoulder is impacted firmly in the upper part of the pelvis. The uterus then contracts vigorously in an unsuccessful attempt to overcome the obstacle. With time, a retraction ring rises increasingly higher and becomes more marked. The situation is referred to as a *neglected transverse lie.* If not promptly managed, the uterus eventually ruptures, placing the mother and fetus at grave risk. Even with the best of care, morbidity is increased because of the frequent association with placenta previa, the increased likelihood of cord prolapse, and the necessity for major operative efforts.

If the fetus is small—usually less than 800 g—and the pelvis is large, spontaneous delivery is possible despite persistence of the abnormal lie. The fetus is compressed with the head forced against the abdomen. A portion of the thoracic wall below the shoulder thus becomes the most dependent part, appearing at the vulva. The head and thorax then pass through the pelvic cavity at the same time, and the fetus, which is doubled upon itself, sometimes referred to as *conduplicato corpore*, is expelled.

MANAGEMENT. In general, the onset of active labor in a woman with a transverse lie is an indication for cesarean delivery. Once labor is well established, attempts at conversion to a longitudinal lie by abdominal manipulation will likely not be successful. Before labor or early in labor, with the membranes intact, attempts at external version are worthy of a trial in the absence of other complications that indicate cesarean delivery. Phelan and co-workers (1986) recommend such an attempt only after 39 weeks because of the high (83 percent) spontaneous conversion to a longitudinal lie. If during early labor, the fetal head can be maneuvered by abdominal manipulation into the pelvis, it should be held there during the next several contractions in an attempt to fix the head in the pelvis. If these measures fail, cesarean delivery is performed.

Because neither the feet nor the head of the fetus occupies the lower uterine segment, a low transverse incision into the uterus may lead to difficulty in extraction of a fetus entrapped in the body of the uterus above the level of incision. Therefore,

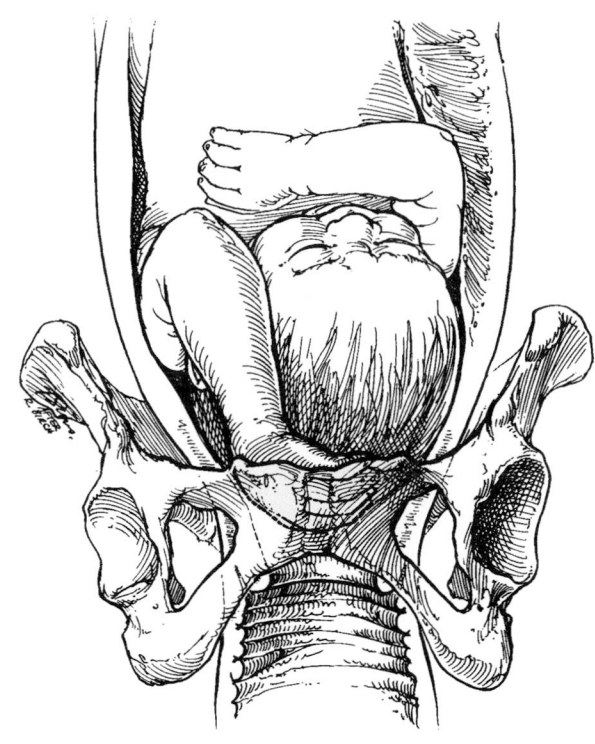

FIGURE 20–12. Compound presentation. The left hand is lying in front of the vertex. With further labor, the hand and arm may retract from the birth canal and the head may then descend normally.

a vertical incision is likely to be indicated (see Chap. 25, p. 598).

Compound Presentation. In a compound presentation, an extremity prolapses alongside the presenting part, with both presenting in the pelvis simultaneously (Fig. 20–12).

INCIDENCE AND ETIOLOGY. Goplerud and Eastman (1953) identified a hand or arm prolapsed alongside the head once in every 700 deliveries. Much less common was prolapse of one or both lower extremities alongside a cephalic presentation or a hand alongside a breech. We identified compound presentations in only 68 of more than 70,000 singleton fetuses delivered from 1995 through 1999, for an incidence of about 1 in 1000 (see Table 17–1, p. 410). Causes of compound presentations are conditions that prevent complete occlusion of the pelvic inlet by the fetal head, including preterm birth (Goplerud and Eastman, 1953).

PROGNOSIS AND MANAGEMENT. Perinatal loss is increased as a result of concomitant preterm delivery, prolapsed cord, and traumatic obstetrical procedures. In most cases, the prolapsed part should be left alone, because most often it will not interfere with labor. Goplerud and Eastman (1953) described 50 cases not associated with a prolapsed cord. In almost half, normal delivery ensued, but there was one fetal death. If the arm is prolapsed alongside the head, the condition should be

observed closely to ascertain whether the arm retracts out of the way with descent of the presenting part. If it fails to retract and if it appears to prevent descent of the head, the prolapsed arm should be pushed gently upward and the head simultaneously downward by fundal pressure. Tebes and co-authors (1999) described a tragic outcome in a newborn delivered spontaneously with the hand alongside the head. The infant developed ischemic necrosis of the presenting forearm, which required amputation.

Persistent Occiput Posterior Position. Most often, occiput posterior positions undergo spontaneous anterior rotation followed by uncomplicated delivery. Although the precise reasons for failure of spontaneous rotation are not known, transverse narrowing of the midpelvis is undoubtedly a contributing factor. Gardberg and associates (1998) used ultrasonography to record the position of the fetal head in 408 term pregnancies at entry into labor (Fig. 20–13). Early in labor, about 15 percent of the fetuses were occiput posterior, and 5 percent were in this position at delivery. Importantly, two thirds of occiput posterior deliveries occurred with fetuses who were occiput anterior at the beginning of labor. Thus, most occiput posterior presentations at delivery are the result of malrotation of occiput anterior position during labor, and most (87 percent) of occiput posterior presentations at the outset of labor spontaneously rotate anteriorly. Induction of labor and epidural analgesia are not factors linked to occiput posterior presentations (Gardberg and associates, 1998).

Labor and delivery need not differ remarkably from that with the occiput anterior. Progress may be determined by assessing cervical dilatation and descent of the head. In most instances, delivery usually can be accomplished without great difficulty once the head reaches the perineum. The possibilities for vaginal delivery are:

1. Spontaneous delivery.
2. Forceps delivery with the occiput directly posterior.
3. Manual rotation to the anterior position followed by spontaneous or forceps delivery.
4. Forceps rotation of the occiput to the anterior position and delivery.

SPONTANEOUS DELIVERY. If the pelvic outlet is roomy and the vaginal outlet and perineum are somewhat relaxed from previous vaginal deliveries, rapid spontaneous delivery often will take place. If the vaginal outlet is resistant to stretch and the perineum is firm, the late first stage or the second stage of labor, or both, may be appreciably prolonged. During each expulsive effort, the head is driven against the perineum to a much greater degree than when anterior. Therefore, forceps delivery often is indicated. A generous episiotomy usually is needed.

FORCEPS DELIVERY AS AN OCCIPUT POSTERIOR. The need for more traction compared with forceps deliveries from the occiput

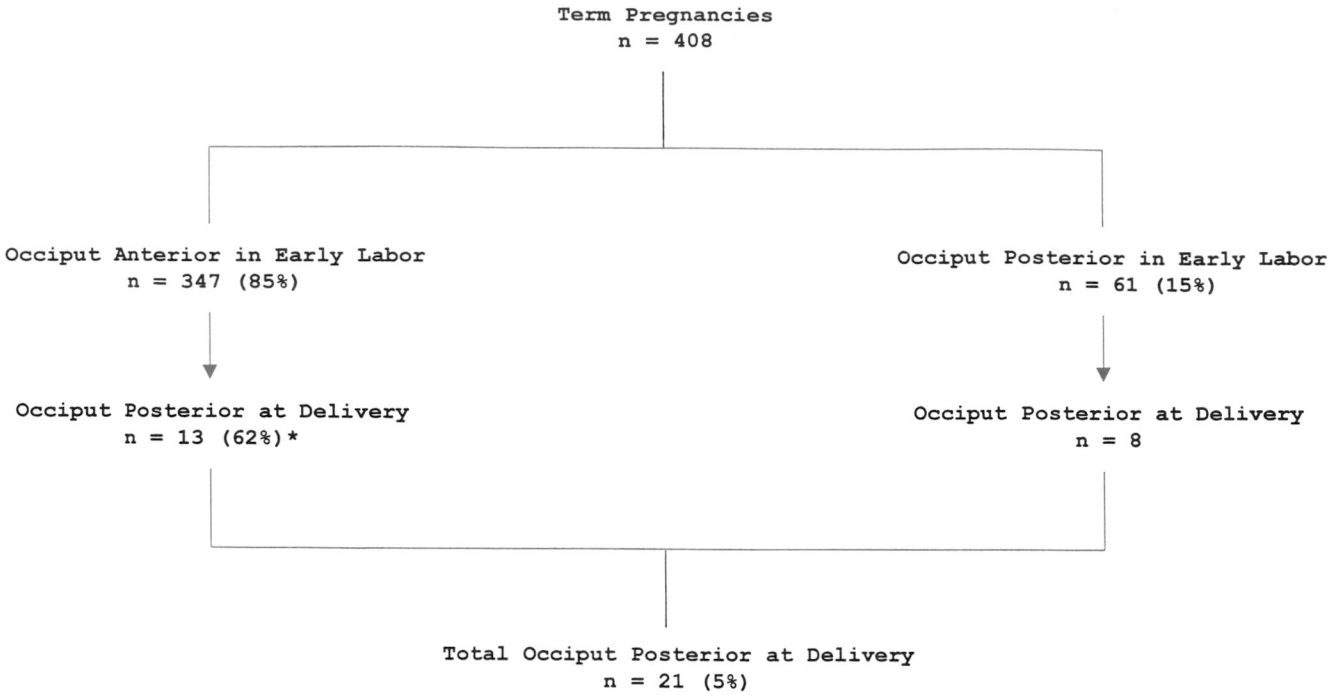

Term Pregnancies
n = 408

Occiput Anterior in Early Labor
n = 347 (85%)

Occiput Posterior in Early Labor
n = 61 (15%)

Occiput Posterior at Delivery
n = 13 (62%)*

Occiput Posterior at Delivery
n = 8

Total Occiput Posterior at Delivery
n = 21 (5%)

* 62% of occiput posterior presentations at delivery were occiput anterior
at the beginning of labor.

FIGURE 20–13. Occiput posterior presentation in early labor compared with presentation at delivery. Ultrasonography was used to determine position of the fetal head in early labor. (From Gardberg and associates, 1998.)

anterior position can be minimized when perineal resistance is lowered by making a larger episiotomy. The use of forceps and a large episiotomy warrant more complete analgesia than may be achieved with pudendal block and local perineal infiltration. The forceps are applied bilaterally along the occipitomental diameter, as described in Chapter 23 (see p. 554).

Infrequently, protrusion of fetal scalp through the introitus is the consequence of marked elongation of the fetal head from molding combined with formation of a large caput succedaneum. The head may not even be engaged—that is, the biparietal diameter may not have passed through the pelvic inlet. In such cases labor is characteristically long and descent of the head is slow. Careful palpation above the symphysis may disclose the fetal head to be above the pelvic inlet. Prompt cesarean delivery is appropriate.

MANUAL ROTATION. The requirements for forceps rotation must be met before performing a manual rotation. When the hand is introduced to locate the posterior ear and thus confirm the posterior position, the occiput often spontaneously rotates toward the anterior position. If not, the head may be grasped with the fingers over one ear and the thumb over the other and rotation of the occiput to the anterior position attempted (see Chap. 23, p. 554).

FORCEPS ROTATION. If the head is engaged, the cervix fully dilated, and the pelvis adequate, forceps rotation may be attempted. These circumstances most likely prevail when expulsive efforts of the mother during the second stage are ineffective. Rotation with forceps is described in Chapter 23 (see p. 555).

Menticoglou and co-workers (1995b) reviewed the obstetrical features of 15 newborns with birth-related high cervical spinal cord injuries in 13 Canadian hospitals between 1982 and 1994. All of these neonates underwent cephalic delivery with forceps rotation of 90 degrees or more from occipitoposterior or occipitotransverse positions. Investigators could not determine whether these serious, albeit rare, fetal injuries resulted from mismanagement or from an intrinsic risk of properly performed forceps rotation. They estimated that this complication developed in less than 1 per 1000 forceps rotations.

OUTCOME. There are notable differences when persistent occiput posterior position is compared with the occiput anterior. Fitzpatrick and colleagues (2001) compared outcomes of 246 women with persistent occiput posterior presentations with those of 13,543 women with occiput anterior positions. Virtually every possible delivery complication was found more frequently in women with persisting occiput posterior presentations. Only 40 percent of these women delivered spontaneously, and cesarean delivery for occiput posterior presentations accounted for 12 percent of all cesarean deliveries performed for dystocia. Similar results were reported by Ponkey and colleagues (2003).

At Parkland Hospital, either manual rotation to the anterior position followed by forceps delivery, or forceps delivery from the occiput posterior position, is used to effect delivery. When neither can be carried out with relative ease, cesarean delivery is performed.

Persistent Occiput Transverse Position. In the absence of a pelvic architecture abnormality, the occiput transverse position is most likely a transitory one because the occiput tends toward the anterior position. Unless hypotonic uterine contractions result, either spontaneously or as the consequence of regional analgesia, spontaneous anterior rotation usually is completed rapidly, thus allowing the choice of spontaneous delivery or delivery with outlet forceps.

DELIVERY. If rotation ceases because of poor expulsive forces and pelvic contractures are absent, vaginal delivery usually can be accomplished readily in a number of ways. The occiput may be manually rotated anteriorly or posteriorly and forceps delivery performed from either the anterior or posterior position. Alternatively, clinicians may apply Kielland forceps to the fetal head in the occiput transverse position (see Chap. 23, p. 555), rotate the occiput to the anterior position, and then deliver the head either with the same forceps or with Simpson or Tucker–McLanc forceps. If failure of spontaneous rotation is caused by hypotonic uterine contractions *without cephalopelvic disproportion,* oxytocin may be infused and closely monitored.

The genesis of the occiput transverse position is not always so simple, or the treatment so benign. With the platypelloid (anteroposteriorly flattened) and the android (heart-shaped) pelves, there may not be adequate room for rotation of the occiput to either the anterior or the posterior position. With the android pelvis, the head may not even be engaged, yet the scalp may be visible through the vaginal introitus as the consequence of considerable molding and caput formation. Consequently, if forceps delivery is attempted, undue force should be avoided.

Shoulder Dystocia. The incidence of shoulder dystocia varies greatly depending on the criteria used for diagnosis. For example, Gross and co-authors (1987) identified that 0.9 percent of almost 11,000 vaginal deliveries were coded for shoulder dystocia at the Toronto General Hospital. True shoulder dystocia, however, diagnosed as such when maneuvers were required to deliver the shoulders in addition to downward traction and episiotomy, was identified in only 24 births (0.2 percent). Significant neonatal trauma was observed only in true shoulder dystocias. Current reports cite an incidence of shoulder dystocia that varies between 0.6 percent and 1.4 percent (American College of Obstetricians and Gynecologists, 2002).

There is some evidence that the incidence of shoulder dystocia increased from 1960 to 1980 (Hopwood, 1982). This is likely due to increasing birthweight. Modanlou and co-workers (1982) showed that neonates experiencing shoulder dystocia had significantly greater shoulder-to-head and chest-to-head disproportions compared with those of equally macrosomic newborns delivered without dystocia. The increased incidence of shoulder dystocia also likely results from increased attention to its appropriate documentation (Nocon and co-workers, 1993).

Use of maneuvers to define shoulder dystocia has been criticized (Beall and associates, 1998; Spong and colleagues, 1995). In deliveries in which shoulder dystocia is anticipated, one or more maneuvers may be used prophylactically, and the diagnosis of shoulder dystocia is therefore not reported. In other cases, one or two maneuvers may be used with rapid resolution of shoulder dystocia and excellent outcome, and the diagnosis may not be recorded. Spong and colleagues (1995) attempted to more objectively define shoulder dystocia by witnessing 250 unselected deliveries and timing the intervals from delivery of the head, to delivery of the shoulders, and to completion of the birth. The incidence defined by the use of obstetrical maneuvers was higher than previously reported (11 percent), and only about half of these were recorded as such by the clinicians. The mean head-to-body delivery time in normal births was 24 seconds compared with 79 seconds in those with shoulder dystocia. They proposed that a head-to-body delivery time exceeding 60 seconds be used to define shoulder dystocia. Gonik and colleagues (2003) have developed computer models to measure the forces necessary to release shoulder dystocia.

MATERNAL CONSEQUENCES. Postpartum hemorrhage, usually from uterine atony, but also from vaginal and cervical lacerations, is the major maternal risk (Benedetti and Gabbe, 1978; Parks and Ziel, 1978).

FETAL CONSEQUENCES. Shoulder dystocia may be associated with significant fetal morbidity and even mortality. Gherman and co-workers (1998) reviewed 285 cases of shoulder dystocia and found 25 percent were associated with fetal injuries. Transient Erb or Duchenne brachial plexus palsies were the most common injury, accounting for two thirds; 38 percent had clavicular fractures; and 17 percent sustained humeral fractures. There was one neonatal death, and four newborns had persistent brachial plexus injuries. In this series, almost half of the cases of shoulder dystocia required a direct fetal manipulation such as the Woods maneuver, in addition to the McRoberts procedure, to effect release of the impacted shoulders. Direct fetal manipulation, however, when compared with use of the McRoberts procedure alone, was not associated with an increased rate of fetal injury.

Brachial Plexus Injury. Injury to the brachial plexus may be localized to the upper or lower part of the plexus (see Chap. 29, p. 683). It usually results from downward traction on the brachial plexus during delivery of the anterior shoulder. Erb palsy results from injury to the spinal nerves C5–6 and sometimes C7. The resultant paralysis of the shoulder and arm muscles causes a hanging upper arm that may be extended at the elbow. Involvement of the lower spinal nerves, C7–T1, always includes injury of the upper nerves and results in a palsy including the hand, which can cause a clawhand deformity. Hardy (1981) studied the prognosis of 36 infants with brachial plexus injuries. Interestingly, shoulder dystocia had been reported in only 10 of these, and two had been delivered abdominally. Nearly 80 percent of these children had complete recovery by 13 months, and none with residual defects had severe sensory or motor deficits in the hand. Jennett and associates (2001, 2002) have presented evidence that brachial plexus injuries may precede delivery itself and may occur even prior to labor. Gherman and colleagues (2003) and Donnelly and co-authors (2002) concluded that these injuries were not predictable before birth.

Clavicular Fracture. Fractured clavicles are relatively common and have been diagnosed in 0.4 percent of newborns delivered vaginally at Parkland Hospital (Roberts and co-workers, 1995). Although at times associated with shoulder dystocia, the clavicle often fractures without any suspect clinical events. Investigators have concluded that isolated fractured clavicles are unavoidable, unpredictable, and of no clinical consequence (Lam and colleagues, 2002).

PREDICTION AND PREVENTION OF SHOULDER DYSTOCIA. There has been considerable evolution in obstetrical thinking about the preventability of shoulder dystocia in the past two decades. Although there are clearly several risk factors associated with shoulder dystocia, identification of individual instances before the fact has proven to be impossible.

Risk Factors. Various maternal, intrapartum, and fetal characteristics have been implicated in the development of shoulder dystocia (Baskett and Allen, 1995; Nesbitt and associates, 1998; Nocon and coauthors, 1993; Robinson and colleagues, 2003). Several maternal risk factors, including obesity, multiparity, and diabetes, all exert their effects because of associated increased birthweight. For example, Keller and co-workers (1991) identified shoulder dystocia in 7 percent of pregnancies complicated by gestational diabetes. Similarly, the association of postterm pregnancy with shoulder dystocia is likely because many fetuses continue to grow after 42 weeks (see Chap. 37, p. 889). Table 20–6 gives the incidence of shoulder dystocia related to birthweight groupings at Parkland Hospital during 1994. Clearly, shoulder dystocia increases with greater birthweight, however, almost half of the newborns with shoulder dystocia weighed less than 4000 g.

TABLE 20–6 Incidence of Shoulder Dystocia According to Birthweight Grouping in Singleton Neonates Delivered Vaginally in 1994 at Parkland Hospital

Birthweight Group	Births	Shoulder Dystocia (%)
≤ 3000 g	2,953	0
3001–3500 g	4,309	14 (0.3)
3501–4000 g	2,839	28 (1.0)
4001–4500 g	704	38 (5.4)
> 4500 g	91	17 (19.0)
All weights	10,896	97 (0.9)

Indeed, Nocon and co-workers (1993) described shoulder dystocia with birth of a 2260-g neonate.

Despite this, some authors advocate identification of macrosomia with ultrasonography and liberal use of cesarean delivery to avoid shoulder dystocia (O'Leary, 1992). Others have disputed the concept that cesarean delivery is indicated for identified large fetuses, even those estimated to weigh in excess of 4500 g. Rouse and Owen (1999) concluded that a prophylactic cesarean delivery policy for macrosomic newborns would require more than 1000 cesarean deliveries and millions of dollars to avert a single permanent brachial plexus injury. The American College of Obstetricians and Gynecologists (2002) has concluded that performing cesarean deliveries for all women suspected of carrying a macrosomic fetus is not appropriate, except possibly for estimated fetal weights over 5000 g in nondiabetic women and over 4500 g in those with diabetes.

Intrapartum complications associated with shoulder dystocia include midforceps delivery and prolonged first- and second-stage labor (Baskett and Allen, 1995; Nocon and co-authors, 1993). Conversely, McFarland and co-workers (1995) found that abnormalities of first- and second-stage labor were not useful clinical predictors of shoulder dystocia. Beall and co-authors (2003) randomly assigned 128 women carrying fetuses estimated to weigh over 3800 g to delivery with or without prophylactic McRoberts maneuvers and found that such use of this maneuver was not beneficial.

Prior Shoulder Dystocia. Ginsberg and Moisidis (2001) identified recurrent shoulder dystocia in 17 percent of women with prior deliveries complicated by shoulder dystocia. In contrast, Baskett and Allen (1995) found the risk to be only 1 to 2 percent for recurrent dystocia. The American College of Obstetricians and Gynecologists (2002) recommends that estimated fetal weight, gestational age, maternal glucose intolerance, and severity of prior neonatal injury should be evaluated and risks and benefits of cesarean delivery discussed with any woman with a history of shoulder dystocia.

Summary. The American College of Obstetricians and Gynecologists (2002) reviewed studies classified according to the evidence-based methods outlined by the United States Preventive Services Task Force. It concluded that the preponderance of current evidence is consistent with the view that:

1. Most cases of shoulder dystocia cannot be accurately predicted or prevented.
2. Elective induction of labor or elective cesarean delivery for all women suspected of carrying a macrosomic fetus is not appropriate.
3. Planned cesarean delivery may be considered for the nondiabetic woman carrying a fetus with an estimated fetal weight exceeding 5000 g or the diabetic woman whose fetus is estimated to weigh more than 4500 g.

MANAGEMENT. Because shoulder dystocia cannot be predicted, the clinician must be well versed in the management principles of this occasionally devastating complication. Reduction in the interval of time from delivery of the head to delivery of the body is of great importance to survival. An initial gentle attempt at traction, assisted by maternal expulsive efforts, is recommended. Some clinicians have advocated

performing a large episiotomy, and adequate analgesia is certainly ideal. After clearing the neonate's mouth and nose, a variety of techniques can be used to free the anterior shoulder from its impacted position beneath the symphysis pubis:

1. Moderate *suprapubic pressure* can be applied by an assistant while downward traction is applied to the fetal head.
2. The *McRoberts maneuver* was described by Gonik and associates (1983) and named for William A. McRoberts, Jr., who popularized its use at the University of Texas at Houston. The maneuver consists of removing the legs from the stirrups and sharply flexing them up onto the abdomen (Fig. 20–14). Gherman and colleagues (2000) analyzed the McRoberts maneuver using x-ray pelvimetry. They found that the procedure caused straightening of the sacrum relative to the lumbar vertebrae, rotation of the symphysis pubis toward the maternal head, and a decrease in the angle of pelvic inclination. Although this does not increase pelvic dimensions, pelvic rotation cephalad tends to free the impacted anterior shoulder. Gonik and co-workers (1989) tested the McRoberts position objectively with laboratory models and found that the maneuver reduced the forces needed to free the fetal shoulder.
3. Woods (1943) reported that, by progressively rotating the posterior shoulder 180 degrees in a corkscrew fashion, the impacted anterior shoulder could be released. This is frequently referred to as the *Woods corkscrew maneuver* (Fig. 20–15).
4. *Delivery of the posterior shoulder* consists of carefully sweeping the posterior arm of the fetus across the chest, followed by delivery of the arm. The shoulder girdle is

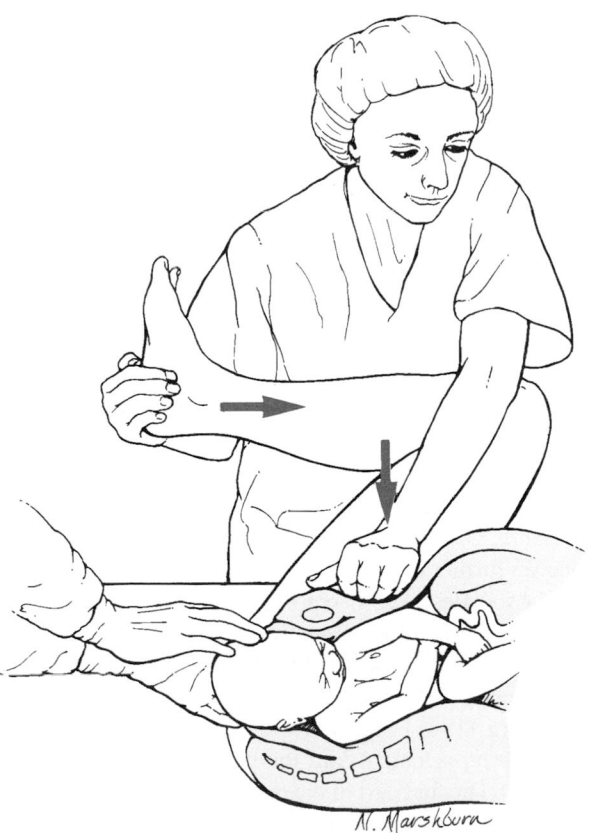

FIGURE 20–14. The McRoberts maneuver. The maneuver consists of removing the legs from the stirrups and sharply flexing the thighs up onto the abdomen, as shown by the horizontal arrow. The assistant is also providing suprapubic pressure simultaneously (*vertical arrow*).

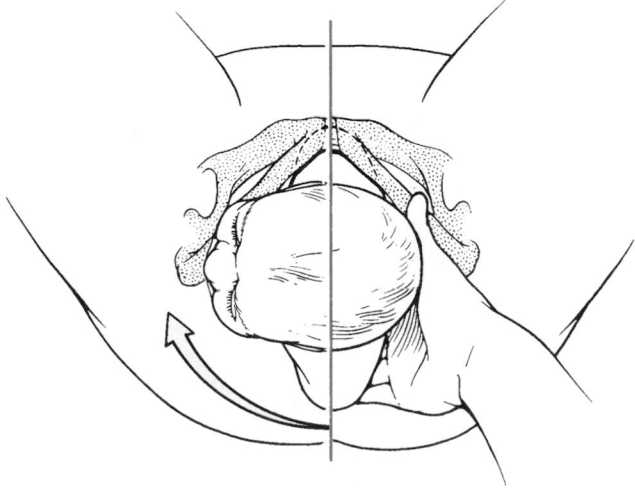

FIGURE 20–15. Woods maneuver. The hand is placed behind the posterior shoulder of the fetus. The shoulder is then rotated progressively 180 degrees in a corkscrew manner so that the impacted anterior is released.

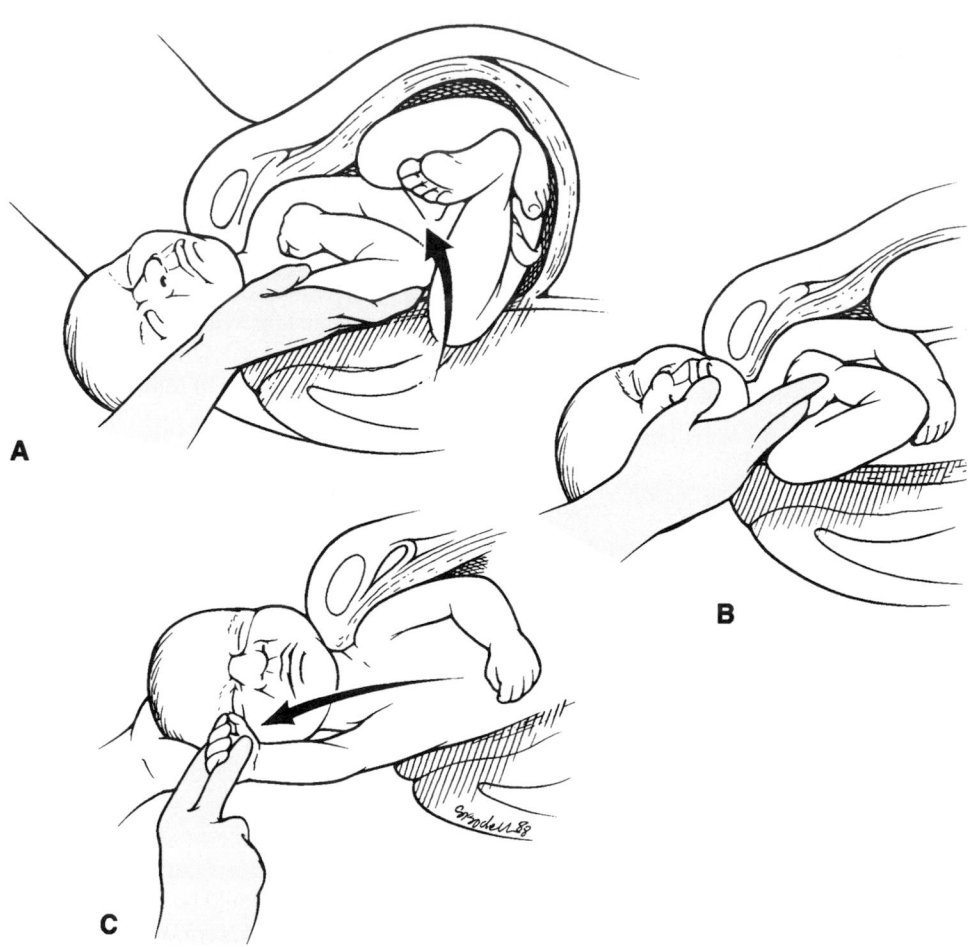

FIGURE 20–16. Shoulder dystocia with impacted anterior shoulder of the fetus. **A.** The operator's hand is introduced into the vagina along the fetal posterior humerus, which is splinted as the arm is swept across the chest, keeping the arm flexed at the elbow. **B.** The fetal hand is grasped and the arm extended along the side of the face. **C.** The posterior arm is delivered from the vagina.

then rotated into one of the oblique diameters of the pelvis with subsequent delivery of the anterior shoulder (Fig. 20–16).

5. Rubin (1964) recommended two maneuvers. First, the fetal shoulders are rocked from side to side by applying force to the maternal abdomen. If this is not successful, the pelvic hand reaches the most easily accessible fetal shoulder, which is then pushed toward the anterior surface of the chest. This maneuver most often results in abduction of both shoulders, which in turn produces a smaller shoulder-to-shoulder diameter and displacement of the anterior shoulder from behind the symphysis pubis (Fig. 20–17).

6. Deliberate *fracture of the clavicle* by pressing the anterior clavicle against the ramus of the pubis can be performed to free the shoulder impaction. In practice, however, it is difficult to deliberately fracture the clavicle of a large neonate. The fracture will heal rapidly and is not nearly as serious as a brachial nerve injury, asphyxia, or death.

7. Hibbard (1982) recommended that pressure be applied to the fetal jaw and neck in the direction of the maternal rectum, with strong fundal pressure applied by an assistant as the anterior shoulder is freed. Strong fundal pressure, however, applied at the wrong time may result in even further impaction of the anterior shoulder. Gross and associates (1987) reported that fundal pressure in the absence of other maneuvers "resulted in a 77 percent complication rate and was strongly associated with (fetal) orthopedic and neurologic damage."

8. Sandberg (1985) reported the *Zavanelli maneuver* for cephalic replacement into the pelvis and then cesarean delivery. The first part of the maneuver consists of returning the head to the occiput anterior or occiput posterior position if the head had rotated from either position. The operator flexes the head and slowly pushes it back into the vagina, following which cesarean delivery is performed. Terbutaline (250 μg subcutaneously) is given to produce uterine relaxation. Sandberg (1999) has subsequently

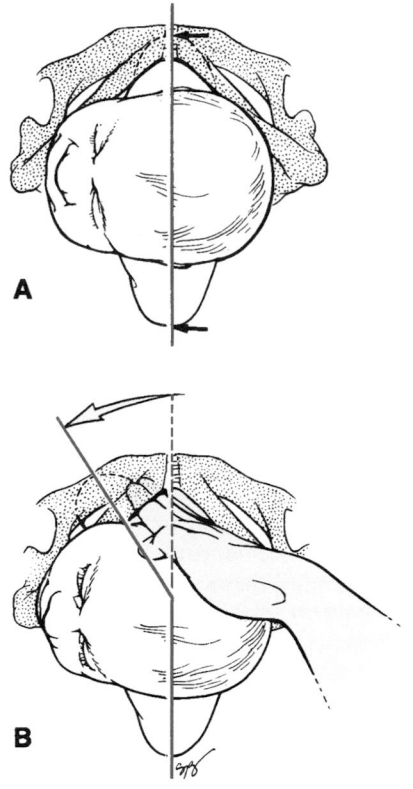

FIGURE 20–17. The second Rubin maneuver. **A.** The shoulder-to-shoulder diameter is shown as the distance between the two small arrows. **B.** The more easily accessible fetal shoulder (the anterior is shown here) is pushed toward the anterior chest wall of the fetus. Most often, this results in abduction of both shoulders, reducing the shoulder-to-shoulder diameter and freeing the impacted anterior shoulder.

reviewed 103 reported cases in which the Zavanelli maneuver was used. This maneuver was successful in 91 percent of cephalic cases and in all cases of breech head entrapments. Fetal injuries were common in the desperate circumstances under which the Zavanelli maneuver was used. There were eight neonatal deaths, six stillbirths, and ten neonates suffered brain damage. Uterine rupture also was reported.

9. *Cleidotomy* consists of cutting the clavicle with scissors or other sharp instruments and is usually used for a dead fetus (Schramm, 1983).

10. *Symphysiotomy* also has been applied successfully, as described by Hartfield (1986). Goodwin and colleagues (1997) reported three cases in which symphysiotomy was performed after the Zavanelli maneuver had failed—all three neonates died and maternal morbidity was significant due to urinary tract injury.

Hernandez and Wendel (1990) suggested use of a *shoulder dystocia drill* to better organize emergency management of an impacted shoulder. The drill is a set of maneuvers performed sequentially as needed to complete vaginal delivery:

1. Call for help—mobilize assistants, an anesthesiologist, and a pediatrician. Initially, a gentle attempt at traction is made. Drain the bladder if it is distended.

2. A generous episiotomy (mediolateral or episioproctotomy) may afford room posteriorly.

3. Suprapubic pressure is used initially by most practitioners because it has the advantage of simplicity. Only one assistant is needed to provide suprapubic pressure while normal downward traction is applied to the fetal head.

4. The McRoberts maneuver requires two assistants. Each assistant grasps a leg and sharply flexes the maternal thigh against the abdomen.

These maneuvers will resolve most cases of shoulder dystocia. If they fail, however, the following steps may be attempted:

5. The Woods screw maneuver.

6. Delivery of the posterior arm is attempted, but if fully extended, this is usually difficult to accomplish.

7. Other techniques generally should be reserved for cases in which all other maneuvers have failed. These include intentional fracture of the anterior clavicle or humerus and the Zavanelli maneuver.

The American College of Obstetricians and Gynecologists (2002) has concluded that there is no evidence that any one maneuver is superior to another in releasing an impacted shoulder or reducing the chance of injury. Performance of the McRoberts maneuver, however, was deemed a reasonable initial approach.

Hydrocephalus as a Cause of Dystocia. Hydrocephalus is an excessive accumulation of cerebrospinal fluid with consequent cranial enlargement. For a number of reasons, discussed in Chapter 13 (see p. 323), it is uncommon with births at term. Associated defects are common, especially neural-tube defects. Normal fetal head circumference at term ranges between 32 and 38 cm. With hydrocephalus, the circumference often exceeds 50 cm and may reach 80 cm. Fluid volume is usually between 500 and 1500 mL, but as much as 5 L may accumulate. Breech presentation is found in at least one third of cases. Whatever the presentation, gross cephalopelvic disproportion is the rule, with dystocia the usual consequence (Figs. 20–18 and 20–19).

Hydrocephalus is somewhat more difficult to diagnose radiographically with a breech presentation, because the outline of a normal fetal head often appears enlarged to a degree suggestive of hydrocephalus. The difficulties inherent in radiological diagnosis are obviated by the use of ultrasonography to measure the diameter of the lateral ventricles and the thickness of the cerebral cortex and to compare the size of the head with that of the thorax and abdomen (Clark and associates, 1985).

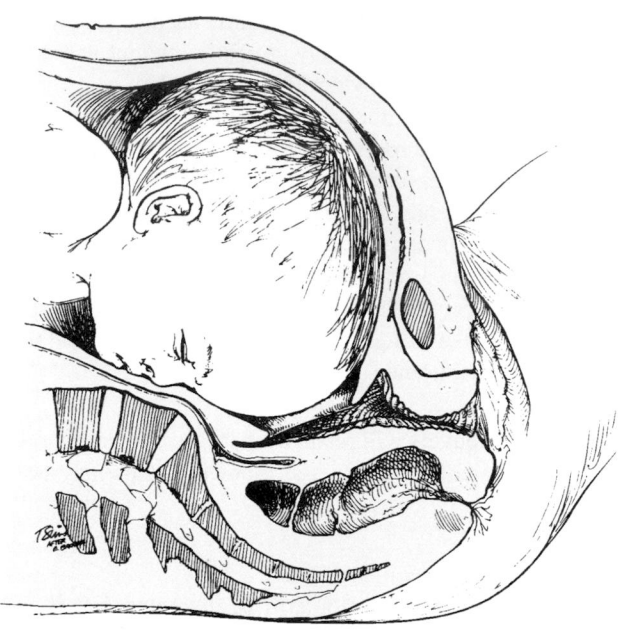

FIGURE 20–18. Severe dystocia from hydrocephalus, cephalic presentation. Note the disparity between the small size of the face and the rest of the cranium.

MANAGEMENT. Most often, the size of the hydrocephalic head must be reduced if the head is to pass through the birth canal. Even with cesarean delivery, it may be desirable to remove cerebrospinal fluid just before incising the uterus to circumvent extensions of a low transverse or vertical incision or to avoid deliberately creating a long vertical uterine incision. Removal of fluid by *cephalocentesis* was a mainstay in the

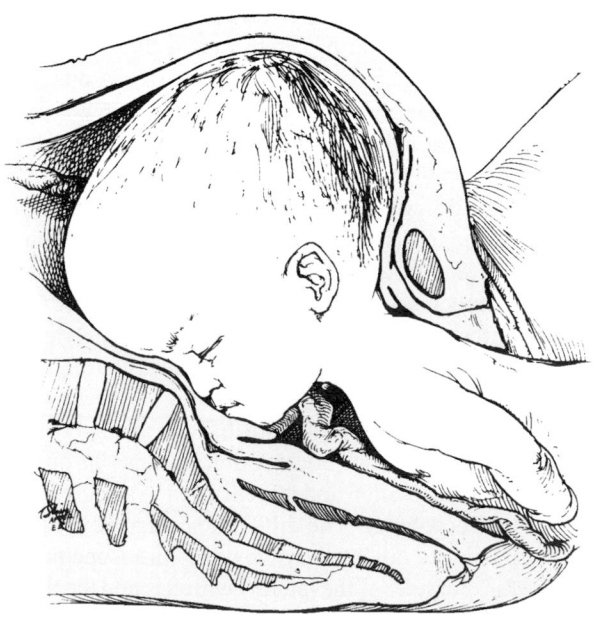

FIGURE 20–19. Severe dystocia from hydrocephalus, breech presentation. Note the distention of the lower uterine segment.

historical management of fetal hydrocephalus with macrocephaly but has come under considerable scrutiny in recent years. Chervenak and colleagues (1985) described results of cephalocentesis in 11 fetuses for whom the procedure was used to permit vaginal or cesarean delivery. Ten of these fetuses died either in utero or within 3 hours of delivery, and seven had intracranial bleeding found at autopsy. Chervenak and McCullough (1986) and Chasen and colleagues (2001) advocate that use of cephalocentesis be limited to fetuses with severe associated abnormalities. They recommended that all others be delivered abdominally. Such management requires precise knowledge of the extent of fetal malformations, which is not always possible.

Technique of Cephalocentesis. The technique varies depending on fetal presentation. With cephalic presentation, as soon as the cervix is dilated 3 to 4 cm, the ventricles may be tapped transvaginally with a needle. An 8-inch, 17-gauge needle is satisfactory for prompt removal of appreciable volumes of cerebrospinal fluid. With a breech presentation, labor can be allowed to progress and the breech and trunk delivered. With the head over the inlet and the face toward the maternal back, the needle is inserted transvaginally just below the anterior vaginal wall and into the aftercoming head through the widened suture line. To protect the birth canal from the needle as it is passed toward the head, the more distal part of the needle, including the point, may be covered with a segment of sterile plastic tubing about 6 inches long cut from an intravenous infusion set. Alternatively, fluid may be withdrawn through a needle inserted via the maternal abdomen into the fetal head. After the bladder is emptied and the skin is cleansed, the needle is inserted in the midline somewhat below the maternal umbilicus and inferior to the top of the fetal skull. The transabdominal approach to remove cerebrospinal fluid also can be used in the event of a cephalic presentation before stimulating labor with oxytocin. The transabdominal approach has also been successfully applied in the breech fetus using ultrasonography to guide the needle (Osathanondh and associates, 1980).

FETAL ABDOMEN AS A CAUSE OF DYSTOCIA. Enlargement of the fetal abdomen sufficient to cause dystocia is usually the result of a *greatly distended bladder* (Fig. 20–20), *ascites,* or *enlargement of the kidneys or liver.* Occasionally, the edematous fetal abdomen may attain such proportions that spontaneous delivery is impossible. Enlargement of the fetal abdomen may escape detection until fruitless attempts at delivery have demonstrated an obstruction. An enlarged abdomen and intra-abdominal accumulation of fluid usually can be diagnosed by ultrasonography. If the diagnosis is made before delivery, the decision must be made whether or not to perform a cesarean delivery (Clark and associates, 1985). In general, fetal prognosis is poor, regardless of the method of delivery.

In nearly 97 percent of such pregnancies, at delivery, the fetus enters the pelvis as a cephalic presentation. In about

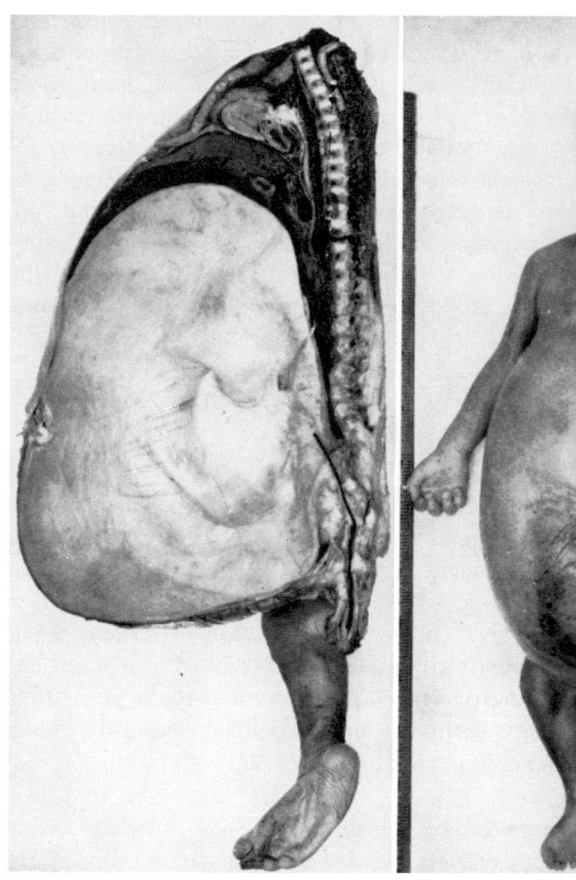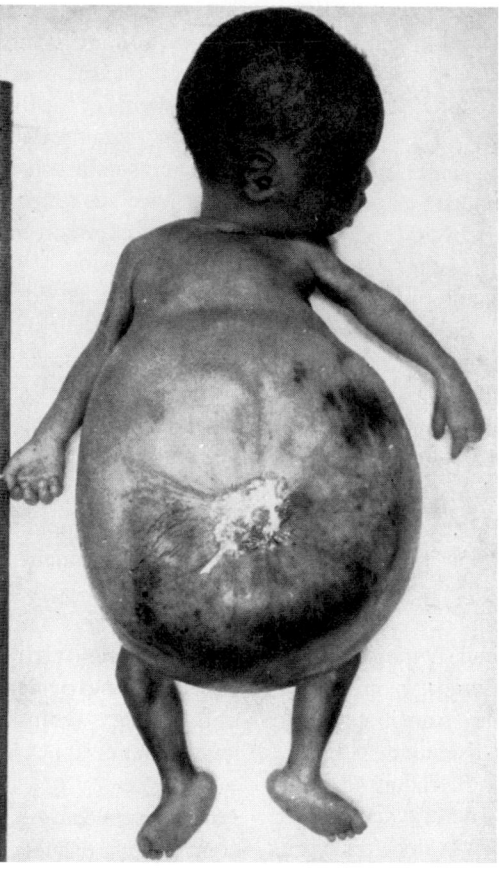

FIGURE 20–20. Fetal abdominal dystocia at 28 weeks caused by an immensely distended bladder. Delivery was made possible by expression of fluid through a bladder perforation at the level of the fetal umbilicus. Section shows the interior of the bladder and compression of organs of abdominal and thoracic cavities. A black thread has been laid in the urethra. (From Savage, 1935.)

3 percent a breech presents, and this is discussed in Chapter 24. In the remaining 0.5 percent, the fetus presents with the long axis either transversely or obliquely, or the head may be extended to present the fetal face or brow.

MATERNAL–FETAL EFFECTS OF DYSTOCIA

Although maternal and fetal effects resulting from dystocia are divided arbitrarily in the following discussion, dystocia may result in serious consequences to either or both simultaneously.

MATERNAL EFFECTS

Intrapartum Infection. Infection may complicate prolonged labor and pose a serious danger to mother and fetus. After membrane rupture, bacteria enter the amnionic fluid, traverse the amnion, and invade decidua and chorionic vessels, thus causing maternal and fetal bacteremia and sepsis. Fetal pneumonia, caused by aspiration of infected amnionic fluid, is another serious consequence. Digital cervical examinations following membrane rupture introduce vaginal bacteria into the uterus (Imseis and co-authors, 1999). These examinations should be limited during labor, especially when dystocia

is suspected. Maternal and fetal infections are discussed in Chapter 31 and Chapters 58 and 59, respectively.

Uterine Rupture. Abnormal thinning of the lower uterine segment creates a serious danger during prolonged labor, particularly in women of high parity and in those with prior cesarean deliveries (see Chap. 35, p. 837). When the disproportion between the fetal head and pelvis is so pronounced that there is no engagement or descent, the lower uterine segment becomes increasingly stretched, and rupture may follow. In such cases, a *pathological retraction ring* may develop (see below) and should prompt immediate abdominal delivery.

Pathological Retraction Ring. Rarely, localized rings or constrictions of the uterus develop in association with prolonged labors. The most common type is the *pathological retraction ring of Bandl,* an exaggeration of the normal retraction ring described in Chapter 6 (see p. 156). It is often the result of obstructed labor, with marked stretching and thinning of the lower uterine segment. The ring may be seen clearly as a uterine indentation and signifies impending rupture of the lower uterine segment (see Fig. 6–3, p. 155). Localized uterine constrictions rarely are seen today because prolonged, obstructed labor is unacceptable. These may still develop occasionally as hourglass constrictions of the uterus following birth of a first twin. The ring can sometimes be relaxed and delivery effected with appropriate general anesthesia, but occasionally prompt cesarean delivery offers a better prognosis for the second twin (see Chap. 39, p. 940).

Fistula Formation. When the presenting part is firmly wedged into the pelvic inlet but does not advance for a considerable time, tissues of the birth canal lying between it and the pelvic wall may be subjected to excessive pressure. Because of impaired circulation, necrosis may result and become evident several days after delivery with the appearance of vesicovaginal, vesicocervical, or rectovaginal fistulas. Most often, pressure necrosis follows a very prolonged second stage of labor. Formerly, when operative delivery was deferred as long as possible, such complications were frequent, but today they are rarely seen except in undeveloped countries.

Pelvic Floor Injury. A long-held belief is that injury to the pelvic floor muscles or to their nerve supply or to the interconnecting fascia is an inevitable consequence of vaginal delivery, particularly if the delivery is difficult. During childbirth the pelvic floor is exposed to direct compression from the fetal head as well as to downward pressure from maternal expulsive efforts. These forces stretch and distend the pelvic floor, resulting in functional and anatomical alterations in the muscles, nerves, and connective tissues. There is accumulating concern that such effects on the pelvic floor during childbirth lead to urinary and anal incontinence and to pelvic organ prolapse (Leitch and Walker, 1998; Sultan and Stanton, 1996). The anal sphincter is torn in 3 to 6 percent of deliveries, and approximately half of these women report subsequent fecal or gas incontinence (Zetterstrom and co-workers, 1999). In continuing studies underway at Parkland Hospital, Casey and colleagues (2004) found that the incidence of symptoms of pelvic floor dysfunction reported within a few months of delivery were increased in women whose newborn was delivered using forceps, in those whose newborn weighed more than 4000 g, and in those who had an episiotomy performed. In a recent poll of English female obstetricians, 30 percent expressed preference for an elective cesarean delivery rather than vaginal delivery and cited avoidance of pelvic floor injury as the explanation for their choice (Wagner, 2000).

Although childbirth undoubtedly plays a significant role in pelvic floor injury, the incidence and types of injuries reported vary widely between studies. Handa and colleagues (2003) found that abnormal pelvic bony architecture was associated with pelvic floor disorders later in life. Currently, there is uncertainty regarding the incidence of childbirth-associated pelvic floor injury, and there is insufficient information as to the relative roles of specific obstetrical antecedents (Samuelsson and associates, 1999).

Postpartum Lower Extremity Nerve Injury. Wong and colleagues (2003) have reviewed neurological injury involving the lower extremities in association with labor and delivery.

Such injuries may manifest as footdrop, which can be secondary to injury at the level of the lumbosacral root, lumbosacral plexus, sciatic nerve, or common peroneal nerve. Components of the lumbosacral plexus cross the pelvic brim and can be compressed by the fetal head or by forceps. Fetal macrosomia and malpresentations such as occiput posterior have been reported to predispose women to footdrop. The most common mechanism of injury, however, is external compression of the peroneal nerves usually caused by inappropriate leg positioning in stirrups especially during a prolonged second stage of labor. Fortunately, symptoms resolve within 6 months of delivery in most women.

FETAL EFFECTS

Caput Succedaneum. If the pelvis is contracted, during labor a large *caput succedaneum* frequently develops on the most dependent part of the fetal head. As shown in Figure 17–19 (see p. 421), this may assume considerable size and lead to serious diagnostic errors. **The caput may reach almost to the pelvic floor while the head is still not engaged. An inexperienced physician may make premature and unwise attempts at forceps delivery.** Typically, even a large caput disappears within a few days after birth.

Fetal Head Molding. Under the pressure of strong uterine contractions, the fetal head changes shape in a process referred to as *molding* (see Fig. 17–19). Factors associated with molding included nulliparity, oxytocin labor stimulation, and delivery with a vacuum extractor. Previously considered an overlapping of the parietal bones, ultrasonographic evidence shows molding to be an unbending or straightening of the parietal bones in combination with an inward movement of the occipital and frontal bone apices (Carlan and colleagues, 1991). These investigators further described a locking mechanism by which the free edges of the cranial bones are forced into one another, preventing further molding and providing protection for the fetal brain. They also observed that severe fetal head molding could develop before labor.

These changes frequently are accomplished without obvious detriment. Alternatively, when the distortion is marked, molding may lead to tentorial tears, laceration of fetal blood vessels, and intracranial hemorrhage. Whitby and colleagues (2004) analyzed nine neonates born with asymptomatic subdural hemorrhages and found that three followed normal vaginal deliveries, suggesting that such hemorrhages are not necessarily evidence of birth trauma. In all nine newborns, hemorrhages resolved spontaneously within 4 weeks. Holland (1922) observed that severe molding could lead to fatal subdural hemorrhage as a result of tears involving the dura mater septa, especially the tentorium cerebelli. Such tears were observed in both normal and complicated deliveries.

Fetal skull bones mold more readily when they are imperfectly ossified. This important feature may explain the differences observed in the course of labor when two apparently similar cases initially present with identical measurements of the pelvis and the fetal head. In one case, the head is softer and more readily molded, and spontaneous delivery results. In the other, the more ossified head retains its original shape, and dystocia develops.

Characteristic pressure marks may form on the scalp, covering the portion of the head that passes over the promontory of the sacrum. From their location, it is frequently possible to ascertain the movements that the head has undergone in passing through the inlet. Rarely, similar marks appear on the portion of the head that has been in contact with the symphysis pubis. Such marks usually disappear within a few days.

Skull fractures occasionally are encountered, usually following forcible attempts at delivery. As discussed in Chapter 29 (see p. 684), the skull also may fracture with spontaneous delivery or even with cesarean delivery (Skajaa and associates, 1987). The fractures are either a shallow groove or a spoon-shaped depression just posterior to the coronal suture. The former is relatively common, but because it involves only the external bone plate, it is not very dangerous. The latter, however, if not surgically corrected, may lead to neonatal death, because it extends through the entire thickness of the skull and may create inner surface projections that exert injurious pressure on the brain. In these cases, it usually is advisable to elevate or remove the depressed portion of the skull.

REFERENCES

Acker DB, Gregory KD, Sachs BP, et al: Risk factors for Erb-Duchenne palsy. Obstet Gynecol 71:389, 1988

Alexander JM, Lucas MJ, Ramin SM, et al: The course of labor with and without epidural analgesia. Am J Obstet Gynecol 178:516, 1998

American College of Obstetricians and Gynecologists: Dystocia and augmentation of labor. Practice Bulletin No. 49, December 2003

American College of Obstetricians and Gynecologists: Shoulder dystocia. Practice Bulletin No. 40, November 2002

American College of Obstetricians and Gynecologists: Dystocia and the augmentation of labor. Technical Bulletin No. 218, December 1995a

American College of Obstetricians and Gynecologists: Guidelines for diagnostic imaging during pregnancy. Committee Opinion No. 158, September 1995b

American College of Obstetricians and Gynecologists: Dystocia. Technical Bulletin No. 137, December 1989

Babayer M, Bodack MP, Creatura C: Common peroneal neuropathy secondary to squatting during childbirth. Obstet Gynecol 91:830, 1998

Baskett TF, Allen AC: Perinatal implications of shoulder dystocia. Obstet Gynecol 86:15, 1995

Beall MH, Spong C, McKay J, et al: Objective definition of shoulder dystocia: A prospective evaluation. Am J Obstet Gynecol 179:934, 1998

Beall MH, Spong CY, Ross MG: A randomized controlled trial of prophylactic maneuvers to reduce head-to-body delivery time in patients at risk for shoulder dystocia. Obstet Gynecol 102:31, 2003

Benedetti TJ, Gabbe SG: Shoulder dystocia. A complication of fetal macrosomia and prolonged second stage of labor with mid-pelvic delivery. Obstet Gynecol 52:526, 1978

Bloom SL, McIntire DD, Kelly MA, et al: Lack of effect of walking on labor and delivery. N Engl J Med 339:76, 1998

Caldeyro-Barcia R, Alvarez H, Reynolds SRM: A better understanding of uterine contractility through simultaneous recording with an internal and a seven channel external method. Surg Obstet Gynecol 91:641, 1950

Calkins LA: Premature spontaneous rupture of the membranes. Am J Obstet Gynecol 64:871, 1952

Carlan SJ, Wyble L, Lense J, et al: Fetal head molding. Diagnosis by ultrasound and a review of the literature. J Perinatol 11:105, 1991

Carlson JM, Diehl JA, Murray MS, et al: Maternal position during parturition in normal labor. Obstet Gynecol 68:443, 1986

Chasen ST, Chervenak FA, McCullough LB: The role of cephalocentesis in modern obstetrics. Am J Obstet Gynecol 185:734, 2001

Chen HY, Huang SC: Evaluation of midpelvic contraction. Int Surg 67:516, 1982

Chervenak FA, Berkowitz RL, Tortona M, et al: The management of fetal hydrocephalus. Am J Obstet Gynecol 151:933, 1985

Chervenak FA, McCullough LB: Ethical analysis of the intrapartum management of pregnancy complicated by fetal hydrocephalus with macrocephaly. Obstet Gynecol 68:720, 1986

Cibils LA, Hendricks CH: Normal labor in vertex presentation. Am J Obstet Gynecol 91:385, 1965

Clark S, DeVore GR, Platt LD: The role of ultrasound in the aggressive management of obstructed labor secondary to fetal malformations. Am J Obstet Gynecol 152:1042, 1985

Cohen W: Influence of the duration of second stage labor on perinatal outcome and puerperal morbidity. Obstet Gynecol 49:266, 1977

Cohen W, Friedman EA (eds): Management of Labor. Baltimore, University Park Press, 1983

Critchlow CW, Leet TL, Benedetti TJ, et al: Risk factors and infant outcomes associated with umbilical cord prolapse: A population-based case control study among births in Washington state. Am J Obstet Gynecol 170:613, 1994

Crowley P, Elbourne D, Ashurst H, et al: Delivery in an obstetric birth chair: A randomized controlled trial. Br J Obstet Gynaecol 98:667, 1991

Cruikshank DP, White CA: Obstetric malpresentations: Twenty years' experience. Am J Obstet Gynecol 116:1097, 1973

De Jong PR, Johanson RB, Baxen P, et al: Randomized trial comparing the upright and supine positions for the second stage of labour. Br J Obstet Gynaecol 104:567, 1997

Donnelly V, Foran A, Murphy J, et al: Neonatal brachial plexus palsy: An unpredictable injury. Am J Obstet Gynecol 187:1209, 2002

Duff P: Diagnosis and management of face presentation. Obstet Gynecol 57:105, 1981

Eller WC, Mengert WF: Recognition of mid-pelvic contraction. Am J Obstet Gynecol 53:252, 1947

Ferguson JE, Newberry YG, DeAngelis GA, et al: The fetal-pelvic index has minimal utility in predicting fetal-pelvic disproportion. Am J Obstet Gynecol 179:1186, 1998

Fitzpatrick M, McQuillan K, O'Herlihy C: Influence of persistent occiput posterior position on delivery outcome. Obstet Gynecol 98:1027, 2001

Floberg J, Belfrage P, Ohlsén H: Influence of pelvic outlet capacity on labor: A prospective pelvimetry study of 1429 unselected primi-paras. Acta Obstet Gynecol Scand 66:121, 1987

Flynn AM, Kelly J, Hollins G, et al: Ambulation in labour. BMJ 2:591, 1978

Fraser WD, Marcoux S, Krauss I, et al: Multicenter, randomized, controlled trial of delayed pushing for nulliparous women in the second stage of labor with continuous epidural analgesia. Am J Obstet Gynecol 182:1165, 2000

Friedman EA: Labor. Clinical Evaluation and Management, 2nd ed. New York, Appleton-Century-Crofts, 1978

Friedman EA, Sachtleben MR: Station of the fetal presenting part II: Effect on the course of labor. Am J Obstet Gynecol 93:530, 1965

Friedman EA, Sachtleben MR: Station of the fetal presenting part IV: Arrest of descent in nulliparas. Obstet Gynecol 47:129, 1976

Fuchs K, Peretz BA, Marcovici R, et al: The grand multipara—is it a problem? Int J Gynaecol Obstet 73:321, 1985

Gardberg M, Laakkonen E, Salevaara M: Intrapartum sonography and persistent occiput posterior position: A study of 408 deliveries. Obstet Gynecol 91:746, 1998

Gherman RB, Ouzounian JG, Goodwin TM: Obstetric maneuvers for shoulder dystocia and associated fetal morbidity. Am J Obstet Gynecol 178:1126, 1998

Gherman RB, Ouzounian JG, Satin AJ, et al: A comparison of shoulder dystocia-associated transient and permanent brachial plexus palsies. Obstet Gynecol 102:544, 2003

Gherman RB, Tramont J, Muffley P, et al: Analysis of McRoberts' maneuver by x-ray pelvimetry. Obstet Gynecol 95:43, 2000

Gifford DS, Morton SC, Fiske M, et al: Lack of progress in labor as a reason for cesarean. Obstet Gynecol 95:589, 2000

Ginsberg NA, Moisidis C: How to predict recurrent shoulder dystocia. Am J Obstet Gynecol 184:1427, 2001

Gonik B, Allen R, Sorab J: Objective evaluation of the shoulder dystocia phenomenon: Effect of maternal pelvic orientation on force reduction. Obstet Gynecol 74:44, 1989

Gonik B, Stringer CA, Held B: An alternate maneuver for management of shoulder dystocia. Am J Obstet Gynecol 145:882, 1983

Gonik B, Zhang N, Grimm MJ: Defining forces that are associated with shoulder dystocia: The use of a mathematic dynamic computer model. Am J Obstet Gynecol 188:1068, 2003

Goodwin TM, Banks E, Millar LK, et al: Catastrophic shoulder dystocia and emergency symphysiotomy. Am J Obstet Gynecol 177:463, 1997

Goplerud J, Eastman NJ: Compound presentation: Survey of 65 cases. Obstet Gynecol 1:59, 1953

Gross SJ, Shime J, Farine D: Shoulder dystocia: Predictors and outcome: A five-year review. Am J Obstet Gynecol 156:334, 1987

Gupta JK, Glanville JN, Johnson N, et al: The effect of squatting on pelvic dimensions. Eur J Obstet Gynecol Reprod Biol 42:19, 1991

Handa VL, Laros RK: Active-phase arrest in labor: Predictors of cesarean delivery in a nulliparous population. Obstet Gynecol 81:758, 1993

Handa VL, Pannu HK, Siddique S, et al: Architectural differences in the bony pelvis of women with and without pelvic floor disorders. Obstet Gynecol 102:1283, 2003

Hannah ME, Hodnett ED, Willan A, et al: Prelabor rupture of the membranes at term: Expectant management at home or in hospital? Obstet Gynecol 96:533, 2000

Hannah M, Ohlsson A, Farine D, et al: International Term PROM Trial: A RCT of induction of labor for prelabor rupture of membranes at term. Am J Obstet Gynecol 174:303, 1996

Hansen SL, Clark SL, Foster JC: Active pushing versus passive fetal descent in the second stage of labor: A randomized controlled trial. Obstet Gynecol 99:29, 2002

Hardy AE: Birth injuries of the brachial plexus: Incidence and prognosis. J Bone Joint Surg [Br] 63:98, 1981

Hartfield VJ: Symphysiotomy for shoulder dystocia. Am J Obstet Gynecol 155:228, 1986

Hauth JC, Hankins GD, Gilstrap LC III: Uterine contraction pressures achieved in parturients with active phase arrest. Obstet Gynecol 78:344, 1991

Hauth JC, Hankins GD, Gilstrap LC III, et al: Uterine contraction pressures with oxytocin induction/augmentation. Obstet Gynecol 68:305, 1986

Hellman LM, Epperson JWW, Connally F: Face and brow presentation: The experience of the Johns Hopkins Hospital, 1896 to 1948. Am J Obstet Gynecol 59:831, 1950

Hendricks CH, Quilligan EJ, Tyler AB, et al: Pressure relationships between intervillous space and amniotic fluid in human term pregnancy. Am J Obstet Gynecol 77:1028, 1959

Hernandez C, Wendel GD: Shoulder dystocia. In Pitkin RM (ed): Clinical Obstetrics and Gynecology, Vol XXXIII. Hagerstown, Pa, Lippincott, 1990, p 526

Hibbard LT: Coping with shoulder dystocia. Contemp Ob/Gyn 20:229, 1982

Hillis DS: Diagnosis of contracted pelvis by the impression method. Surg Gynecol Obstet 51:857, 1930

Holland E: Cranial stress in the foetus during labor. J Obstet Gynaecol Br Emp 29:549, 1922

Hopwood HG: Shoulder dystocia: Fifteen years' experience in a community hospital. Am J Obstet Gynecol 144:162, 1982

Hughes EC: Obstetric-Gynecologic Terminology. Philadelphia, Davis, 1972, p 390

Imseis HM, Trout WC, Gabbe SG: The microbiologic effect of digital cervical examination. Am J Obstet Gynecol 180:578, 1999

Jennett RJ, Tarby TJ: Disuse osteoporosis as evidence of brachial plexus palsy due to intrauterine fetal maladaptation. Am J Obstet Gynecol 185:236, 2001

Jennett RJ, Tarby TJ, Krauss RL: Erb's palsy contrast with Klumpke's and total palsy: Different mechanisms are involved. Am J Obstet Gynecol 186:1216, 2002

Johnson CE: Transverse presentation of the fetus. JAMA 187:642, 1964

Johnson N, Johnson VA, Gupta JK: Maternal positions during labor. Obstet Gynecol Surv 46:428, 1991

Joseph KS, Young DC, Dodds L, et al: Changes in maternal characteristics and obstetric practice and recent increases in primary cesarean delivery. Obstet Gynecol 102:791, 2003

Kaltreider DF: Criteria of midplane contraction. Am J Obstet Gynecol 63:392, 1952

Kappy KA, Cetrulo C, Knuppel RA: Premature rupture of membranes: Conservative approach. Am J Obstet Gynecol 134:655, 1979

Keller JD, Lopez-Zeno JA, Dooley SL, et al: Shoulder dystocia and birth trauma in gestational diabetes: A five year experience. Am J Obstet Gynecol 165:928, 1991

King JF: Obstetric intervention and the economic imperative. Br J Obstet Gynaecol 100:1063, 1993

Kwee A, Graziosi GCM, van Leeuwen JHS, et al: The effect of immersion on haemodynamic and fetal measures in uncomplicated pregnancies of nulliparous women. Br J Obstet Gynaecol 107:663, 2000

Lam MH, Wong GY, Lao TT: Reappraisal of neonatal clavicular fracture: Relationship between infant size and neonatal morbidity. Obstet Gynecol 100:115, 2002

Larks SD: Electrohysterography. Springfield, Ill, Thomas, 1960

Leitch CR, Walker JJ: The rise in caesarean section rate: The same indications but a lower threshold. Br J Obstet Gynaecol 105:621, 1998

Lieberman E, Lang JM, Cohen A, et al: Association of epidural analgesia with cesarean delivery in nulliparas. Obstet Gynecol 88:993, 1996

Lupe PJ, Gross TL: Maternal upright posture and mobility in labor: A review. Obstet Gynecol 67:727, 1986

Mahon TR, Chazotte C, Cohen WR: Short labor: Characteristics and outcome. Obstet Gynecol 84:47, 1994

Manyonda IT, Shaw DE, Drife JO: The effect of delayed pushing in the second stage of labor with continuous lumbar epidural analgesia. Acta Obstet Gynecol Scand 69:291, 1990

Martin JA, Hamilton BE, Sutton PD, et al: Births: Final data for 2002. National Vital Statistics Reports, Vol 52, No. 10. Hyattsville, Md, National Center for Health Statistics, 2003

McCarthy S: Magnetic resonance imaging in obstetrics and gynecology. Magn Reson Imaging 4:59, 1986.

McFarland M, Hod M, Piper JM, et al: Are labor abnormalities more common in shoulder dystocia? Am J Obstet Gynecol 173:1211, 1995

Mengert WF: Estimation of pelvic capacity. JAMA 138:169, 1948

Menticoglou SM, Manning F, Harman C, et al: Perinatal outcomes in relation to second-stage duration. Am J Obstet Gynecol 173:906, 1995a

Menticoglou SM, Perlman M, Manning FA: High cervical spinal cord injury in neonates delivered with forceps: Report of 15 cases. Obstet Gynecol 86:589, 1995b

Miller FC: Uterine motility in spontaneous labor. Clin Obstet Gynecol 26:78, 1983

Modanlou HD, Komatsu G, Dorchester W, et al: Large-for-gestational-age neonates: Anthropometric reasons for shoulder dystocia. Obstet Gynecol 60:417, 1982

Moore MM, Shearer DR: Fetal dose estimates for CT pelvimetry. Radiology 171:265, 1989

Mozurkewich EL, Wolf FM: Premature rupture of membranes at term: A meta-analysis of three management schemes. Obstet Gynecol 89:1035, 1997

Müller: On the frequency and etiology of general pelvic contraction. Arch Gynaek 16:155, 1880

Myles TD, Santolaya J: Maternal and neonatal outcomes in patients with a prolonged second stage of labor. Obstet Gynecol 102:52, 2003

Nesbitt TS, Gilbert WM, Herrchen B: Shoulder dystocia and associated risk factors with macrosomic infants born in California. Am J Obstet Gynecol 179:476, 1998

Neuman M, Beller U, Lavie O, et al: Intrapartum bimanual tocolytic-assisted reversal of face presentation: Preliminary report. Obstet Gynecol 84:146, 1994

Nocon JJ, McKenzie DK, Thomas LJ, et al: Shoulder dystocia: An analysis of risks and obstetric maneuvers. Am J Obstet Gynecol 168:1732, 1993

Notzon FC, Cnattinguis S, Bergsjo P, et al: Cesarean section deliveries in the 1980s: International comparison by indication. Am J Obstet Gynecol 17:495, 1994

Nuthalapaty FS, Rouse DJ, Owen J: The association of maternal weight with cesarean risk, labor duration, and cervical dilation rate during labor induction. Obstet Gynecol 103:452, 2004

O'Leary JA: Shoulder Dystocia and Birth Injury. New York, McGraw-Hill, 1992, p 75

Odent M: Birth under water. Lancet 2:1476, 1983

Olah KSJ, Neilson J: Failure to progress in the management of labour. Br J Obstet Gynaecol 101:1, 1994

Osathanondh R, Birnholz JC, Altman AM, et al: Ultrasonically guided transabdominal encephalocentesis. J Reprod Med 25:125, 1980

Osborn SB: The implications of the Committee on Radiological Hazards to Patients (Adrian Committee), 1. Variations in the radiation dose received by the patient in diagnostic radiology. Br J Radiol 36:230, 1963

Parks DG, Ziel HK: Macrosomia: A proposed indication for primary cesarean section. Obstet Gynecol 52:407, 1978

Peleg D, Hannah ME, Hodnett ED, et al: Predictors of cesarean delivery after prelabor rupture of membranes at term. Obstet Gynecol 93:1031, 1999

Phelan JP, Boucher M, Mueller E, et al: The nonlaboring transverse lie: A management dilemma. J Reprod Med 31:184, 1986

Plunkett BA, Lin A, Wong CA, et al: Management of the second stage of labor in nulliparas with continuous epidural analgesia. Obstet Gynecol 102:109, 2003

Ponkey SE, Cohen AP, Heffner LJ, et al: Persistent fetal occiput posterior position: Obstetric outcomes. Obstet Gynecol 101:915, 2003

Read JA, Miller FC, Paul RH: Randomized trial of ambulation versus oxytocin for labor enhancement: A preliminary report. Am J Obstet Gynecol 139:669, 1981

Reynolds SRM, Heard OO, Bruns P, et al: A multichannel strain-gauge tocodynamometer: An instrument for studying patterns of uterine contractions in pregnant women. Bull Johns Hopkins Hosp 82:446, 1948

Roberts SW, Hernandez C, Maberry MC, et al: Obstetric clavicular fracture: The enigma of normal birth. Obstet Gynecol 86:978, 1995

Robertson PA, Huang LJ, Croughan-Minihane MS, et al: Is there an association between water baths during labor and the development of chorioamnionitis or endometritis? Am J Obstet Gynecol 178:1215, 1998

Robinson H, Tkatch S, Mayes DC, et al: Is maternal obesity a predictor of shoulder dystocia? Obstet Gynecol 101:24, 2003

Roshanfekr D, Blakemore KJ, Lee J, et al: Station at onset of active labor in nulliparous patients and risk of cesarean delivery. Obstet Gynecol 93:329, 1999

Rouse DJ, Owen J: Prophylactic cesarean delivery for fetal macrosomia diagnosed by means of ultrasonography—a Faustian bargain? Am J Obstet Gynecol 181:332, 1999

Rouse DJ, Owen J, Hauth JC: Active-phase labor arrest: Oxytocin augmentation for at least 4 hours. Obstet Gynecol 93:323, 1999

Roy RP: A Darwinian view of obstructed labor. Obstet Gynecol 101:397, 2003

Rubin A: Management of shoulder dystocia. JAMA 189:835, 1964

Russell JG: Moulding of the pelvic outlet. J Obstet Gynaecol Br Commonw 76:817, 1969

Samuelsson EC, Arne Victor FTA, Tibblin G, et al: Signs of genital prolapse in a Swedish population of women 20 to 59 years of age and possible related factors. Am J Obstet Gynecol 180:299, 1999

Sandberg EC: The Zavanelli maneuver: A potentially revolutionary method for the resolution of shoulder dystocia. Am J Obstet Gynecol 152:479, 1985

Sandberg EC: The Zavanelli maneuver: 12 years of recorded experience. Obstet Gynecol 93:312, 1999

Satin AJ, Maberry MC, Leveno KJ, et al: Chorioamnionitis: A harbinger of dystocia. Obstet Gynecol 79:913, 1992

Savage JE: Dystocia due to dilation of the fetal urinary bladder. Am J Obstet Gynecol 29:267, 1935

Savage W, Francome C: British cesarean section rates: Have we reached a plateau? Br J Obstet Gynaecol 101:645, 1994

Schorn MN, McAllister JL, Blanco JD: Water immersion and the effect on labor. J Nurse Midwifery 38:336, 1993

Schramm M: Impacted shoulders—a personal experience. Aust N Z J Obstet Gynaecol 23:28, 1983

Sharma SK, Leveno KJ: Update: Epidural analgesia during labor does not increase cesarean births. Curr Anesth Rep 2:18, 2000

Skajaa K, Hansen ES, Bendix J: Depressed fracture of the skull in a child born by cesarean section. Acta Obstet Gynecol Scand 66:275, 1987

Speer DP, Peltier LF: Pelvic fractures and pregnancy. J Trauma 12:474, 1972

Spong CY, Beall M, Rodrigues D, et al: An objective definition of shoulder dystocia: Prolonged head-to-body delivery intervals and/or the use of ancillary obstetric maneuvers. Obstet Gynecol 86:433, 1995

Sporri S, Hanggi W, Brahetti A, et al: Pelvimetry by magnetic resonance imaging as a diagnostic tool to evaluate dystocia. Obstet Gynecol 89:902, 1997

Stark DD, McCarthy SM, Filly RA, et al: Pelvimetry by magnetic resonance imaging. Am J Radiol 144:947, 1985

Stephenson J: An unkind cut? Health Agencies Update. JAMA 283:2514, 2000

Sultan AH, Stanton SL: Preserving the pelvic floor and perineum during childbirth: Elective cesarean-section? Br J Obstet Gynaecol 103:731, 1996

Tebes CC, Mehta P, Calhoun DA, et al: Congenital ischemic forearm necrosis associated with a compound presentation. J Matern Fetal Med 8:281, 1999

Thoms H: The obstetrical significance of pelvic variations: A study of 450 primiparous women. BMJ 2:210, 1937

Thorp JA, Hu DH, Albin RM, et al: The effect of intrapartum epidural analgesia on nulliparous labor: A randomized, controlled, prospective trial. Am J Obstet Gynecol 169:851, 1993a

Thorp JM Jr, Pahel-Short L, Bowes WA Jr: The Mueller-Hillis maneuver: Can it be used to predict dystocia? Obstet Gynecol 82:519, 1993b

Thurnau GR, Scates DH, Morgan MA: The fetal-pelvic index: A method of identifying fetal-pelvic disproportion in women attempting vaginal birth after previous cesarean delivery. Am J Obstet Gynecol 165:353, 1991

Ventura SJ, Martin JA, Curtin SC, et al: Births: Final data for 1998. National Vital Statistics Reports, Vol 48, No. 3. Hyattsville, Md, National Center for Health Statistics, 2000

Wagner M: Choosing caesarean section. Lancet 356:1677, 2000

Whitby EH, Griffiths PD, Rutter S, et al: Frequency and maternal history of subdural haemorrhages in babies and relation to obstetric factors. Lancet 363:846, 2004

Wilkes PT, Wolf DM, Kronbach DW, et al: Risk factors for cesarean delivery at presentation of nulliparous patients in labor. Obstet Gynecol 102:1352, 2003

Williams JW: Obstetrics: A Textbook for the Use of Students and Practitioners, 1st ed. New York, Appleton, 1903, p 282

Williams RM, Thom MH, Studd JW: A study of the benefits and acceptability of ambulation in spontaneous labor. Br J Obstet Gynaecol 87:122, 1980

Wong CA, Scavone BM, Dugan S, et al: Incidence of postpartum lumbosacral spine and lower extremity nerve injuries. Obstet Gynecol 101:279, 2003

Woods CE: A principle of physics is applicable to shoulder delivery. Am J Obstet Gynecol 45:796, 1943

World Health Organization: Partographic management of labour. Lancet 343:1399, 1994

Zetterstrom J, Lopez A, Auzen B, et al: Anal sphincter tears at vaginal delivery: Risk factors and clinical outcome of primary repair. Obstet Gynecol 94:21, 1999

21

Disorders of Amnionic Fluid Volume

Fetal membranes include the amnion and chorion. Their development, physiology, and histology are detailed in Chapter 3 (see p. 66). Both physiological and pathological events may result in anatomical changes such as meconium staining and chorioamnionitis, which are discussed in Chapter 27 (see p. 624). The most common intrinsic abnormalities that are encountered clinically are too much or too little amnionic fluid—(poly)hydramnios and oligohydramnios, respectively.

NORMAL AMNIONIC FLUID VOLUME

Normally, amnionic fluid volume increases to about 1 L by 36 weeks and decreases thereafter to only 100 to 200 mL or less postterm (Table 21–1). Diminished fluid volume is termed *oligohydramnios*. Somewhat arbitrarily, more than 2 L of amnionic fluid is considered excessive and is termed *hydramnios*. This is sometimes called *polyhydramnios*. In rare instances, the uterus may contain an enormous quantity of fluid, with reports of as much as 15 L. In most instances, chronic hydramnios develops, which is the gradual increase of excessive fluid. In acute hydramnios, the uterus may become markedly distended within a few days.

MEASUREMENT OF AMNIONIC FLUID. Over the past decades, a number of ultrasound methods have been used to measure the amount of amnionic fluid. Phelan and colleagues

TABLE 21–1 Typical Amnionic Fluid Volume

Weeks' Gestation	Fetus (g)	Placenta (g)	Amnionic Fluid (mL)	Percent Fluid
16	100	100	200	50
28	1000	200	1000	45
36	2500	400	900	24
40	3300	500	800	17

From Queenan (1991), with permission.

(1987) described the clinical utility of quantification using the *amnionic fluid index*. This is calculated by adding the vertical depths of the largest pocket in each of four equal uterine quadrants. According to their calculations, significant hydramnios is defined by an index greater than 24 cm. Magann and colleagues (2000) performed a cross-sectional study of longitudinal changes in the amnionic fluid index in normal pregnancies (Fig. 21–1). Porter and associates (1996) and Hill and co-workers (2000) have provided normal values for twin pregnancies (see Chap. 39, p. 936).

The group from the University of Mississippi has performed several investigations to correlate ultrasonic accuracy of predicting abnormal amnionic fluid volume with measurement by dye dilution. Magann and associates (1992) used the dye-dilution technique to measure amnionic fluid in 40 women undergoing amniocentesis in late pregnancy. They found that the amnionic fluid index was reasonably reliable in determining normal or increased amnionic fluid but was

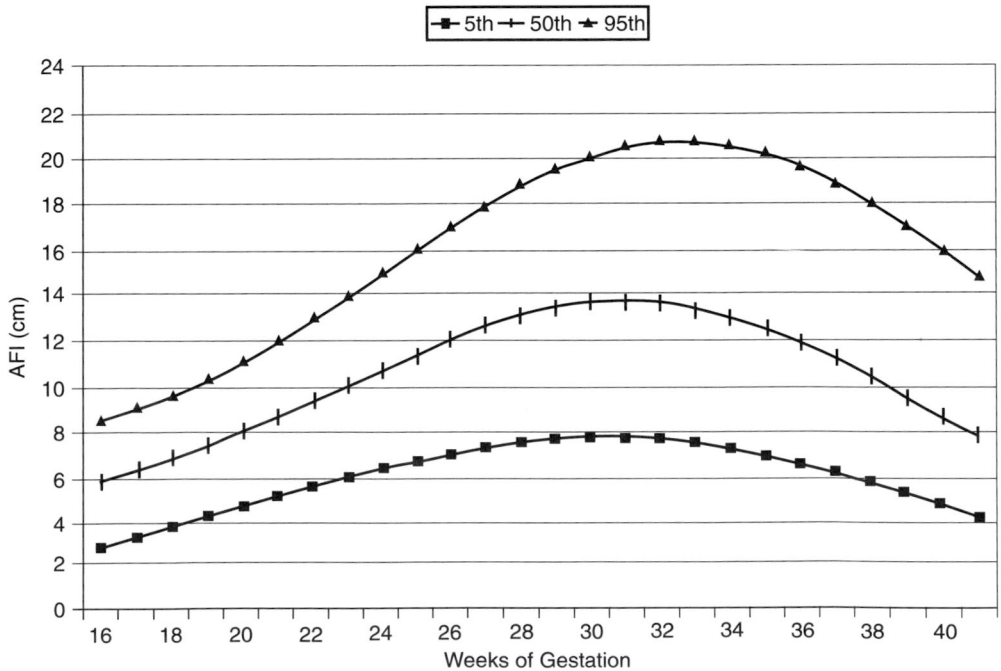

FIGURE 21–1. Normal percentiles for the amnionic fluid index (AFI) from 1400 women. For each gestational week, 50 women were studied. (Data adapted by Schrimmer and Moore, 2002, with permission.)

inaccurate in diagnosing oligohydramnios. In later studies by Chauhan (1997) and Magann (2003a, 2004) and their associates, poor correlation of fluid volume was found with the amnionic fluid index, the two-diameter fluid pocket, and the single deepest pocket methods. Magann and colleagues (2001) evaluated the addition of color Doppler imaging and found that its concurrent use with amnionic fluid index measurements leads to overdiagnosis of oligohydramnios. Peedicayil and colleagues (1994) emphasized that borderline values should be repeated before interventions are undertaken. Morris and colleagues (2003) studied 1584 women at term and found that the amnionic fluid index was superior to the single deepest pocket but had a poor sensitivity for adverse pregnancy outcome. Magann and colleagues (2003b, 2004) also found that amnionic fluid volumes are not predictive of intrapartum or neonatal outcomes.

Several factors may modulate the amnionic fluid index. For example, Yancey and Richards (1994) reported that high altitude (6000 ft) was associated with an increased index. Magann and colleagues (2003c), Deka and Malhotra (2001), Bush and associates (1996), and Kilpatrick and Safford (1993), but not Kerr and associates (1996), showed that maternal hydration increased the index. This effect dissapates by 24 hours (Malhotra and Deka, 2004). Conversely, fluid restriction or dehydration may lower the index. Ross and colleagues (1996) administered 1-deamino-[8-D-arginine] vasopressin (DDAVP) to women with oligohydramnios. This resulted in maternal serum hypoosmolality (285 to 265 mOsm/kg) associated with an increase in the amnionic fluid index from 4 to 8 cm within 8 hours.

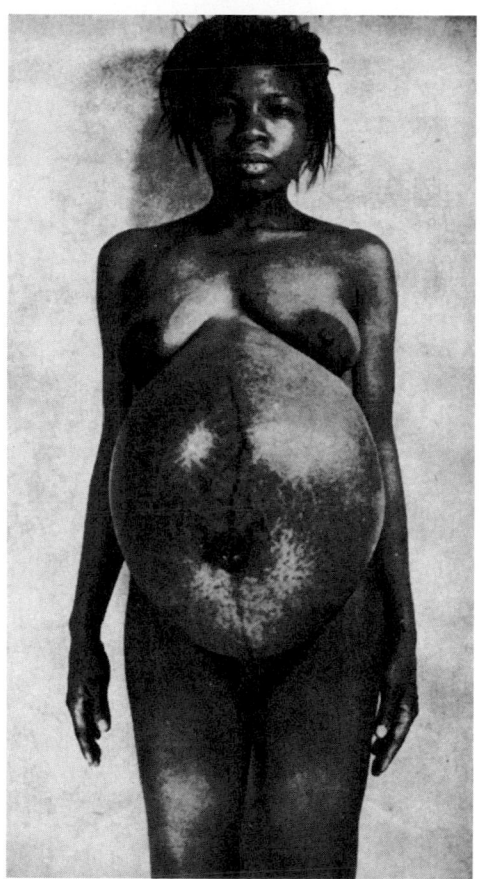

FIGURE 21–2. Advanced degree of hydramnios—5500 mL of amnionic fluid was measured at delivery.

HYDRAMNIOS

INCIDENCE. Hydramnios is identified in about 1 percent of pregnancies. The diagnosis usually is suspected clinically and confirmed by sonographic examination. An extreme example is shown in Figure 21–2. Most investigators define hydramnios as an amnionic fluid index of greater than 24 to 25 cm—corresponding to greater than the 95th or 97.5th percentiles. Using an index of 25 cm or greater, Biggio and colleagues (1999) reported a 1-percent incidence in more than 36,000 women examined at the University of Alabama.

In an earlier study by Hill and associates (1987) from the Mayo Clinic, more than 9000 prenatal patients underwent routine ultrasonic evaluation near the beginning of the third trimester. The incidence of hydramnios was 0.9 percent. Mild hydramnios—defined as pockets measuring 8 to 11 cm in vertical dimension—was present in 80 percent of cases with excessive fluid. Moderate hydramnios—defined as a pocket containing only small parts and measuring 12 to 15 cm deep—was found in 15 percent. Only 5 percent had severe hydramnios, defined by a free-floating fetus found in pockets of fluid of 16 cm or greater. Although two thirds of all cases were idiopathic, the others were associated with fetal anomalies, maternal diabetes, or multifetal gestation. Golan and co-workers (1993) reported remarkably similar findings in nearly 14,000 women.

CAUSES OF HYDRAMNIOS. The degree of hydramnios, as well as its prognosis, is often related to the cause. Many reports are biased because they consist of observations from women referred for targeted ultrasonic evaluation. Others are population based but still may not reflect an accurate incidence unless universal ultrasound screening is performed. In either case, obvious pathological hydramnios frequently is associated with fetal malformations, especially of the central nervous system or gastrointestinal tract. For example, hydramnios accompanies about half of cases of anencephaly and esophageal atresia. In the study by Hill and associates (1987), the cause of mild hydramnios was identified in only 15 percent of cases. Conversely, with moderate or severe hydramnios, the cause was identified in more than 90 percent and fetal anomalies were present in half of these cases. The opposite is not true, however, and in the Spanish Collaborative Study of Congenital Malformations with more than 27,000 anomalous fetuses, only 3.7 percent had hydramnios whereas another 3 percent had oligohydramnios (Martinez-Frias and colleagues, 1999).

TABLE 21–2 Outcomes in Women Identified to Have Hydramnios After 20 Weeks Compared with 36,426 Control Women with a Normal Amnionic Fluid Index

Factor	Amnionic Fluid Index (AFI)			Hydramnios (n = 370)		
	Hydramnios (n = 370)	Normal AFI (n = 36,426)	P	Diabetic (n = 71)	Nondiabetic (n = 299)	P
Perinatal outcomes						
Anomalies	8.4%	0.3%	< .001	0	10.4%	.005
Growth restriction	3.8%	6.7%	.3	0	4.7%	NS
Aneuploidy	1/370	1/3643	.10	0/71	1/299	NS
Mortality	49/1000	14/1000	< .001	0/1000	60/1000	.03
Maternal outcomes						
Cesarean delivery	47%	16.4%	< .001	70%	42%	< .001
Diabetes	19.5%	3.2%	< .001			

NS = not statistically significant.
From Biggio and colleagues (1999).

The population-based study from Birmingham included more than 40,000 women (Biggio and co-workers, 1999). These investigators compared 370 women identified as having hydramnios with more than 36,000 control women having a normal index. As shown in Table 21–2, hydramnios was found to portend a significantly increased risk for adverse outcomes. Most of these were in nondiabetic women with hydramnios.

Damato and colleagues (1993) reported findings from 105 women referred for evaluation of excessive fluid, of whom almost 65 percent had confirmed hydramnios (Table 21–3). There were 47 singletons with one or more abnormalities, viz., gastrointestinal anomalies (15), nonimmune hydrops (12), and central nervous system (12), thoracic (9), skeletal (8), chromosomal (7), and cardiac malformations (4). Among 19 twin pregnancies, 12 involved twin-to-twin transfusion and only two were normal.

Other less common causes of polyhydramnios include fetal pseudohypoaldosteronism, fetal Bartter or hyperprostaglandin E syndrome, nephrogenic diabetes insipidus, placental chorioangioma, sacrococcygeal teratoma, and maternal substance abuse (Narchi and colleagues, 2000; Panting-Kemp and colleagues, 2002).

Using an amnionic fluid index of greater than 24 or 25 cm to define hydramnios, most studies report substantive increases in perinatal mortality. In a report by Carlson and as-

TABLE 21–3 Pregnancy Outcomes in 105 Women Referred for Hydramnios

Largest Pocket (cm)	Abnormal Outcome No. (%)
8.0–9.5	19 (50)
10–11.5	16 (62)
12–13.5	14 (67)
14–15.5	10 (83)
> 16	7 (88)
Total:	66/105 (63)

From Damato and colleagues (1993), with permission.

sociates (1990) of 49 women, there were 14 perinatal deaths, 22 fetal malformations, and six cases of aneuploidy. Brady and colleagues (1992) identified 125 cases of unexplained or idiopathic hydramnios in 5000 population-based pregnancies. Of these, two fetuses had trisomy 18 and two had trisomy 21. Conversely, Panting-Kemp and co-workers (1999) found that idiopathic hydramnios was not associated with increased adverse outcomes except for cesarean delivery.

PATHOGENESIS. Early in pregnancy, the amnionic cavity is filled with fluid very similar in composition to extracellular fluid. During the first half of pregnancy, transfer of water and other small molecules takes place not only across the amnion but also through fetal skin. During the second trimester, the fetus begins to urinate, swallow, and inspire amnionic fluid (Abramovich and colleagues, 1979; Duenhoelter and Pritchard, 1976). These processes have a modulating role in the control of fluid volume. Although the major source of amnionic fluid in hydramnios has most often been assumed to be the amnionic epithelium, no histological changes in amnion or chemical changes in amnionic fluid have been found.

Because the fetus normally swallows amnionic fluid, it has been assumed that this mechanism is one of the ways by which the volume is controlled. The theory gains validity by the nearly constant presence of hydramnios when swallowing is inhibited, as in cases of esophageal atresia. But swallowing is not the only mechanism for preventing hydramnios. Specifically, Pritchard (1966) and Abramovich (1970) found in some instances of gross hydramnios that appreciable volumes of fluid were swallowed.

In cases of anencephaly and spina bifida, increased transudation of fluid from the exposed meninges into the amnionic cavity may result in hydramnios. Another possible explanation in anencephaly, when swallowing is not impaired, is excessive urination caused either by stimulation of cerebrospinal centers deprived of their protective coverings or by lack of antidiuretic effect because of impaired arginine vasopressin secretion. In hydramnios associated with monozygotic twin pregnancy, the hypothesis has been advanced that one fetus usurps the greater part of the circulation common to both twins and develops cardiac hypertrophy, which in turn results in increased urine output (see Chap. 39, p. 929). Naeye and Blanc (1972) identified dilated renal tubules, enlarged bladder, and an increased urinary output in the early neonatal period, suggesting that increased fetal urine production is responsible for hydramnios. Conversely, donor members of twin-to-twin transfusion pairs had dystrophic renal tubules with oligohydramnios.

The hydramnios that commonly develops with maternal diabetes during the third trimester remains unexplained. One explanation is that maternal hyperglycemia causes fetal hyperglycemia, resulting in osmotic diuresis. Bar-Hava and associates (1994) reported that increases in third-trimester amnionic fluid volume in women with gestational diabetes correlated with hyperglycemia the day prior to fluid measurement.

SYMPTOMS. Major maternal symptoms accompanying hydramnios arise from purely mechanical causes and result principally from pressure exerted within the overdistended uterus and upon adjacent organs. When distention is excessive, the mother may suffer from severe dyspnea and, in extreme cases, she may be able to breathe only when upright (see Fig. 21–2). Edema, the consequence of compression of major venous systems by the enlarged uterus, is common, especially in the lower extremities, the vulva, and the abdominal wall. Rarely, oliguria may result from ureteral obstruction by the enlarged uterus (see Chap. 48, p. 1107). Hydramnios associated with fetal hydrops may cause the *mirror syndrome*, whereby the maternal condition mimics the fetus in that she develops edema and mild proteinuria (Carbillon and colleagues, 1997). This was originally described by Ballantyne in 1892, and it is discussed further in Chapter 29 (see p. 674).

With chronic hydramnios, the accumulation of fluid takes place gradually, and the woman may tolerate the excessive abdominal distention with relatively little discomfort. In acute hydramnios, however, distention may lead to disturbances sufficiently serious to be threatening. Acute hydramnios tends to develop earlier in pregnancy than does the chronic form—often as early as 16 to 20 weeks—and it may rapidly expand the hypertonic uterus to enormous size. As a rule, acute hydramnios leads to labor before 28 weeks, or the symptoms become so severe that intervention is mandatory.

DIAGNOSIS. The primary clinical finding with hydramnios is uterine enlargement in association with difficulty in palpating fetal small parts and in hearing fetal heart tones. In severe cases, the uterine wall may be so tense that it is impossible to palpate any fetal parts (see Fig. 21–2). The differentiation between hydramnios, ascites, or a large ovarian cyst usually can be made by ultrasonic evaluation.

PREGNANCY OUTCOME. In general, the more severe the degree of hydramnios, the higher the perinatal mortality rate. Even when sonography and radiography show an apparently normal fetus, the prognosis is still guarded, because fetal malformations and chromosomal abnormalities are common. Furman and co-workers (2000) described substantively increased adverse perinatal outcomes if fetal growth restriction accompanies hydramnios. Perinatal mortality is increased further by preterm delivery, which was more common in women with an anomalous fetus (40 percent). Other conditions adding to bad outcomes are erythroblastosis, maternal diabetes, umbilical cord prolapse, and placental abruption.

The most frequent maternal complications associated with hydramnios are placental abruption, uterine dysfunction, and postpartum hemorrhage. Extensive premature separation of the placenta caused by the decrease in the area of the emptying uterus beneath the placenta sometimes follows escape of massive quantities of amnionic fluid (see Chap. 35, p. 811). Uterine dysfunction and postpartum hemorrhage result from uterine atony consequent to overdistention. Abnormal fetal presentations and operative intervention are also common.

MIDTRIMESTER HYDRAMNIOS. The prognosis of midtrimester hydramnios depends on the severity. Mild hydramnios has a reasonably good outcome. Glantz and co-workers (1994) studied 47 consecutive singleton pregnancies with a single deepest pocket of 6 to 10 cm that was identified at 14 to 27 weeks. Excessive fluid resolved spontaneously in three fourths of these pregnancies, and perinatal outcomes were similar to matched controls without hydramnios. In the group in which hydramnios persisted, 2 of 10 had fetal aneuploidy.

MANAGEMENT. Minor degrees of hydramnios rarely require treatment. Even moderate degrees with some discomfort usually can be managed without intervention until labor ensues or until the membranes rupture spontaneously. If dyspnea or abdominal pain is present, or if ambulation is difficult, hospitalization becomes necessary. Bed rest, diuretics, and water and salt restriction are ineffective. Recently, indomethacin therapy has been used for symptomatic hydramnios.

Amniocentesis. The principal purpose of amniocentesis is to relieve maternal distress, and to that end it is transiently successful. Amnionic fluid also can be tested to predict fetal lung maturity as described in Chapter 29 (see p. 651). Elliott and associates (1994) reported results from 200 therapeutic amniocenteses in 94 women with hydramnios. Common causes included twin-to-twin transfusion (38 percent), idiopathic (26 percent), fetal or chromosomal anomalies (17 percent), and diabetes (12 percent). These authors removed a mean of 1650 mL of fluid at each procedure and gained an average duration to delivery of 7 weeks. Only three procedures were complicated: one woman had ruptured membranes, one developed chorioamnionitis, and another suffered placental abruption after 10 L of fluid was removed. Leung and co-workers (2004) cited a 3.1-percent incidence of complications in 134 rapid aminodrainage procedures.

TECHNIQUE. To remove amnionic fluid, a commercially available plastic catheter that tightly covers an 18-gauge needle is inserted through the locally anesthetized abdominal wall into the amnionic sac, the needle is withdrawn, and an intravenous infusion set is connected to the catheter hub. The opposite end of the tubing is dropped into a graduated cylinder placed at floor level, and the rate of flow of amnionic fluid is controlled with the tubing screw clamp so that about 500 mL/hr is withdrawn. After about 1500 to 2000 mL have been collected, the uterus usually has decreased in size sufficiently that the catheter may be withdrawn from the amnionic sac. At the same time, maternal relief is dramatic and the danger of placental separation from decompression is slight. Using strict aseptic technique, this procedure can be repeated as necessary to make the woman comfortable. Elliott and colleagues (1994) used wall suction and removed 1000 mL over 20 minutes (50 mL/min), however, we prefer more gradual removal.

Amniotomy. The disadvantage inherent in amniotomy during labor is the possibility of cord prolapse and especially of placental abruption. Slow removal of the fluid by amniocentesis helps to obviate these dangers.

Indomethacin Therapy. In their review of several studies, Kramer and colleagues (1994) concluded that indomethacin impairs lung liquid production or enhances absorption, decreases fetal urine production, and increases fluid movement across fetal membranes. Doses employed by most investigators range from 1.5 to 3 mg/kg per day.

Cabrol and associates (1987) used indomethacin therapy for 2 to 11 weeks in eight women with idiopathic hydramnios from 24 to 35 weeks. Hydramnios, defined by at least one 8-cm fluid pocket, improved in all cases. There were no serious adverse effects and the outcomes were good. Mamopoulos and colleagues (1990) treated 15 women— 11 were diabetic—who had hydramnios at 25 to 32 weeks. Amnionic fluid volume decreased in all women after indomethacin was begun. The fluid in the maximum pocket decreased from a mean of 10.7 cm at 27 weeks to 5.9 cm after therapy. The outcome was good in all 15 newborns. Kriplani and colleagues (2001) successfully treated with indomethacin a patient who had polyhydramnios from a placental chorioangioma.

A major concern for the use of indomethacin is the potential for closure of the fetal ductus arteriosus (see Chap. 14, p. 356). Moise and colleagues (1988) reported that 50 percent of 14 fetuses whose mothers received indomethacin had ductal constriction detected by Doppler ultrasound. Persistent constriction was not demonstrated in the studies described earlier in this section, nor has it been described in studies in which indomethacin was given for tocolysis (Kramer and colleagues, 1994).

OLIGOHYDRAMNIOS

In rare instances, the volume of amnionic fluid may fall far below the normal limits and occasionally be reduced to only a few milliliters. In general, oligohydramnios developing early in pregnancy is less common and frequently has a bad prognosis. By contrast, diminished fluid volume may be found often with pregnancies that continue beyond term. Marks and Divon (1992) found oligohydramnios—defined as an amnionic fluid index of 5 cm or less—in 12 percent of 511 pregnancies of 41 weeks or greater. In 121 women studied longitudinally, there was a mean decrease of 25 percent per week in the amnionic fluid index beyond 41 weeks. Gagnon and colleagues (2002) found that chronic severe placental insufficiency caused a reduction in amnionic fluid volume not attributable to reduced fetal urine production. The risk of cord compression, and in turn fetal distress, is increased with diminished fluid in all labors, but especially in postterm pregnancy (Grubb and Paul, 1992; Leveno and colleagues, 1984).

EARLY-ONSET OLIGOHYDRAMNIOS. Several conditions have been associated with diminished amnionic fluid (Table 21–4). Oligohydramnios almost always is evident when there is either obstruction of the fetal urinary tract or renal agenesis. Therefore, anuria almost certainly has an etiological role in such cases. A chronic leak from a defect in the fetal membranes may reduce the volume of fluid appreciably, but most often labor soon ensues. Exposure to angiotensin-converting enzyme inhibitors has been associated with oligohydramnios (see Chap. 14, p. 349). Anywhere from 15 to 25 percent of cases are associated with the fetal anomalies shown in Table 21–5. Pryde and co-workers (2000) were able to visualize fetal structures in only half of women referred for ultrasonic evaluation of midtrimester oligohydramnios. They performed amnioinfusion and were then able to visualize 77 percent of routinely imaged structures. Identification of associated anomalies increased from 12 to 31 percent of fetuses.

TABLE 21–4 Conditions Associated with Oligohydramnios

Fetal	Maternal
Chromosomal abnormalities	Uteroplacental insufficiency
Congenital anomalies	Hypertension
Growth restriction	Preeclampsia
Demise	Diabetes
Postterm pregnancy	**Drugs**
Ruptured membranes	Prostaglandin synthase
Placenta	inhibitors
Abruption	Angiotensin-converting
Twin-to-twin transfusion	enzyme inhibitors
	Idiopathic

From Peipert and Donnenfeld (1991), with permission.

TABLE 21-5 Congenital Anomalies Associated with Oligohydramnios

Amnionic band syndrome
Cardiac—Fallot tetralogy, septal defects
Central nervous system—holoprosencephaly, meningocele, encephalocele, microcephaly
Chromosomal abnormalities: triploidy, trisomy 18, Turner syndrome
Cloacal dysgenesis
Cystic hygroma
Diaphragmatic hernia
Genitourinary—renal agenesis, renal dysplasia, urethral obstruction, bladder exstrophy, Meckel-Gruber syndrome, ureteropelvic junction obstruction, prune-belly syndrome
Hypothyroidism
Skeletal—sirenomelia, sacral agenesis, absent radius, facial clefting
Twin-reversed-arterial-perfusion (TRAP) sequence
Twin-to-twin transfusion
VACTERL (vertebral, anal, cardiac, tracheo-esophageal, renal, limb) association

Adapted from McCurdy and Seeds (1993) and Peipert and Donnenfeld (1991).

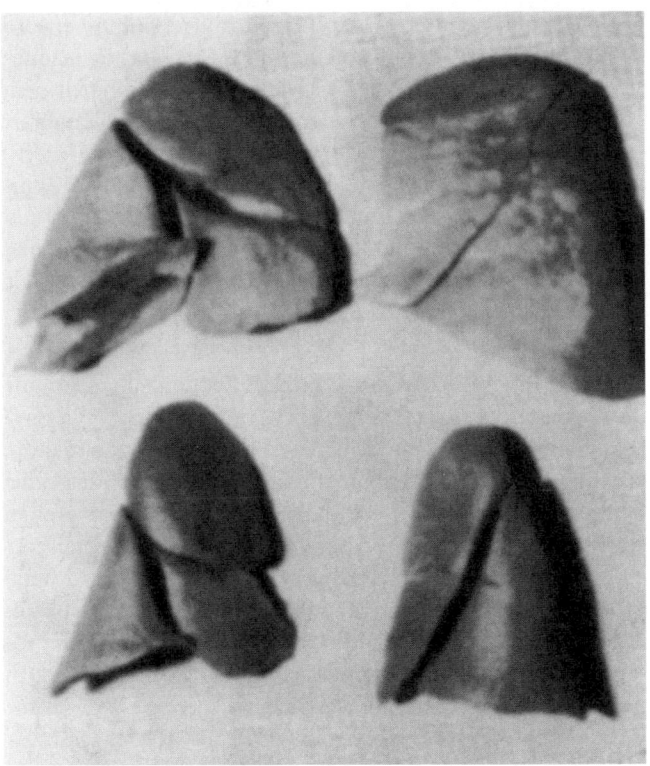

FIGURE 21-3. Normal-sized lungs (top) are shown in comparison with hypoplastic lungs (bottom) of fetuses at the same gestational age. (From Newbould and colleagues, 1994, with permission.)

Prognosis. Fetal outcome is poor with early-onset oligohydramnios. Shenker and colleagues (1991) described 80 pregnancies and only half of these fetuses survived. Mercer and Brown (1986) described 34 midtrimester pregnancies complicated by oligohydramnios diagnosed ultrasonically by the absence of amnionic fluid pockets greater than 1 cm. Nine fetuses (one fourth) had anomalies, and 10 of the 25 who were phenotypically normal either aborted spontaneously or were stillborn because of severe maternal hypertension, restricted fetal growth, or placental abruption. Of the 14 liveborn infants, eight were preterm and seven died. The six infants who were delivered at term did well. Garmel and co-workers (1997) observed that appropriately grown fetuses associated with oligohydramnios prior to 37 weeks had a threefold increase in preterm birth but not of later growth restriction or fetal death.

Newbould and colleagues (1994) described autopsy findings in 89 infants with the oligohydramnios sequence or Potter syndrome. Only 3 percent had a normal renal tract; 34 percent had bilateral renal agenesis; 34 percent, bilateral cystic dysplasia; 9 percent, unilateral agenesis with dysplasia; and 10 percent, minor urinary abnormalities.

Otherwise normal infants may suffer the consequences of early-onset severely diminished amnionic fluid. Adhesions between the amnion may entrap fetal parts and cause serious deformities, including amputation. Moreover, subjected to pressure from all sides, musculoskeletal deformities such as clubfoot are observed frequently.

Pulmonary Hypoplasia. The incidence of pulmonary hypoplasia at birth ranges from 1.1 to 1.4 per 1000 infants (Moessinger and colleagues, 1989). When amnionic fluid is scant, pulmonary hypoplasia, such as that shown in Figure 21-3, is common. Winn and associates (2000) performed a prospective cohort study in 163 cases of oligohydramnios that followed prematurely ruptured membranes at 15 to 28 weeks. Almost 13 percent of fetuses developed pulmonary hypoplasia. This complication was more common as the gestational age at the time of rupture decreased. Kilbride and co-workers (1996) studied 115 women with prematurely ruptured membranes before 29 weeks. There ultimately were seven stillbirths and 40 neonatal deaths for a perinatal mortality of 409 per 1000. The risk of lethal pulmonary hypoplasia was 20 percent. Adverse outcomes were more likely with earlier rupture as well as duration exceeding 14 days.

According to Fox and Badalian (1994) and Lauria and colleagues (1995), there are three possibilities that account for pulmonary hypoplasia. First, thoracic compression may prevent chest wall excursion and lung expansion. Second, lack of fetal breathing movements decreases lung inflow. The third and the most widely accepted model involves a failure to retain intrapulmonary amnionic fluid or an increased outflow with impaired lung growth and development. Albuquerque and colleagues (2002) found a relationship between oligohydramnios and spinal flexion in the human fetus that also may contribute to fetal pulmonary hypoplasia.

The appreciable volume of amnionic fluid demonstrated by Duenhoelter and Pritchard (1976) to be inhaled by the normal fetus suggests a role for the inspired fluid in expansion, and in turn growth, of the lung. Fisk and colleagues (1992), however, concluded that fetal breathing impairment does not cause pulmonary hypoplasia with oligohydramnios. In a unique experiment, McNamara and associates (1995) described findings from two sets of monoamnionic twins with discordant renal anomalies. They provided evidence that normal amnionic fluid volume in the presence of fetal renal obstruction allows normal lung development.

OLIGOHYDRAMNIOS IN LATE PREGNANCY. As shown in Table 21–1 and Figure 21–1, amnionic fluid volume diminishes normally after 35 weeks. Management of oligohydramnios in late pregnancy depends on the clinical situation. An evaluation for fetal anomalies and growth is critical. In a pregnancy complicated by oligohydramnios and fetal growth restriction, close fetal surveillance is important because of associated morbidity, and delivery is recommended for fetal or maternal indications. Although gestational age is considered in this decision, evidence for fetal or maternal compromise usually overrides potential complications from preterm delivery. Oligohydramnios detected before 36 weeks in the presence of normal fetal anatomy and growth may be managed expectantly in conjunction with antepartum fetal testing discussed in Chapter 15.

Oz and colleagues (2002) investigated the etiology of oligohydramnios in postterm pregnancy. They found a reduction in renal artery end-diastolic velocity, suggesting that increased arterial impedance is an important factor. Using an amnionic fluid index of less that 5 cm, Casey and co-workers (2000) found an incidence of oligohydramnios of 2.3 percent in more than 6400 pregnancies undergoing sonography after 34 weeks at Parkland Hospital. They confirmed previous observations that this finding is associated with an increased risk of adverse perinatal outcomes (Table 21–6). Conversely,

using the RADIUS trial database, Zhang and colleagues (2004) reported that oligohydramnios of this degree was not associated with adverse perinatal outcomes. Similarly, Magann and co-workers (1999) did not find that associated oligohydramnios increased risks for intrapartum complications.

Chauhan and associates (1999) performed meta-analysis of 18 studies comprising more than 10,500 pregnancies in which the intrapartum amnionic fluid index was less than 5 cm. Compared with controls whose index was over 5 cm, women with oligohydramnios had a significantly increased, 2.2-fold, risk for cesarean delivery for fetal distress and a 5.2-fold increased risk for a 5-minute Apgar score of less than 7.

Cord compression during labor is common with oligohydramnios. Sarno and co-workers (1989, 1990) reported that an index of 5 cm or less was associated with a fivefold increased cesarean delivery rate. Baron and colleagues (1995) reported a 50-percent increase in variable decelerations during labor and a sevenfold increased cesarean delivery rate in these women. By contrast, Casey and co-workers (2000) showed a 25-percent increase in nonreassuring fetal heart rate patterns when women with oligohydramnios were compared with normal controls. Moreover, the cesarean rate for pregnancies with this finding increased only from 3 to 5 percent (see Table 21–6).

Divon and associates (1995) studied 638 women with a postterm pregnancy in labor and observed that only those whose amnionic fluid index was 5 cm or less had fetal heart rate decelerations and meconium. Interestingly, Chauhan and collaborators (1995) showed that diminished amnionic fluid index increased the cesarean delivery rate only in women whose labor attendants were made aware of the findings!

Amnioinfusion. Results with intrapartum amnioinfusion to prevent fetal morbidity from meconium-stained fluid—often associated with oligohydramnios—are mixed. Pierce and colleagues (2000) performed meta-analysis of 13 studies with 1924 such women randomized to amnioinfusion or no treatment. They found that amnioinfusion resulted in significantly decreased adverse outcomes: meconium beneath the cords (OR 0.18), meconium aspiration syndrome (OR 0.30), neonatal acidemia (OR 0.42), and cesarean delivery rate (0.74). Conversely, Spong and associates (1994) found no benefits when they compared therapeutic with prophylactic amnioinfusion for meconium. Indeed, meconium aspiration syndrome occurred only in the group undergoing therapeutic amnioinfusion. Surprisingly, only 16 percent of the group randomized to expectant therapy ultimately required amnioinfusion for variable fetal heart rate decelerations. These findings are in agreement with reviews of outcomes before and after amnioinfusion protocols were implemented (DeMeeus and colleagues, 1998; Rogers and colleagues, 1996; Usta and colleagues 1995). Taken together these results suggest that routine prophylactic amnioinfusion for meconium is not warranted.

TABLE 21–6 Pregnancy Outcomes (in Percent) in 147 Women with Oligohydramnios at 34 Weeks

Factor	Oligohydramnios[a] (n = 147)	Normal AFI (n = 6276)	P
Labor induction	42	18	< .001
Nonreassuring FHR	48	39	< .03
Cesarean for FHR	5	3	.18
Stillbirth	14/1000	3/1000	< .03
Neonatal ICU	7	2	< .001
Meconium aspiration	1	0.1	< .001
Neonatal death	5	0.3	< .001
Growth restriction	24	9	< .001
Malformation	10	2.5	< .001

AFI = amnionic fluid index; FHR = fetal heart rate pattern; ICU = intensive care unit.
[a]AFI < 5.0 cm.
From Casey and co-workers (2000).

The American College of Obstetricians and Gynecologists (1995), however, states that either prophylactic or therapeutic amnioinfusion for meconium is reasonable. Wenstrom and associates (1995) surveyed academic obstetrical departments and reported that amnioinfusion is widely performed with relatively few complications. The procedure is discussed in greater detail in Chapter 29 (see p. 676), and the technique is described in Chapter 18 (see p. 462).

REFERENCES

Abramovich DR: Fetal factors influencing the volume and composition of liquor amnii. J Obstet Gynaecol Br Commonw 77:865, 1970

Abramovich DR, Garden A, Jandial L, et al: Fetal swallowing and voiding in relation to hydramnios. Obstet Gynecol 54:15, 1979

Albuquerque CA, Smith KR, Saywers TE, et al: Relations between oligohydramnios and spinal flexion in the human fetus. Early Hum Dev 68:119, 2002

American College of Obstetricians and Gynecologists: Fetal heart rate patterns: Monitoring, interpretation, and management. Technical Bulletin No. 207, July 1995

Ballantyne JW: The diseases and deformities of the foetus. Edinburgh, Scotland, Oliver and Boyd, 1892

Bar-Hava I, Scarpelli SA, Barnhard Y, et al: Amniotic fluid volume reflects recent glycemic status in gestational diabetes mellitus. Am J Obstet Gynecol 171:952, 1994

Baron C, Morgan MA, Garite TJ: The impact of amniotic fluid volume assessed intrapartum on perinatal outcome. Am J Obstet Gynecol 173:167, 1995

Biggio JR Jr, Wenstrom KD, Dubard MB, et al: Hydramnios prediction of adverse perinatal outcome. Obstet Gynecol 94:773, 1999

Brady K, Polzin WJ, Kopelman JN, et al: Risk of chromosomal abnormalities in patients with idiopathic polyhydramnios. Obstet Gynecol 79:234, 1992

Bush J, Minkoff H, McCalla S, et al: The effect of intravenous fluid load on amniotic fluid index in patients with oligohydramnios. Am J Obstet Gynecol 174:379, 1996

Cabrol D, Landesman R, Muller J, et al: Treatment of polyhydramnios with prostaglandin synthetase inhibitor (indomethacin). Am J Obstet Gynecol 157:422, 1987

Carbillon L, Oury JF, Guerin JM, et al: Clinical biologic features of Ballantyne syndrome and the role of placental hydrops. Obstet Gynecol Surv 52: 310, 1997

Carlson DE, Platt LD, Medearis AL, et al: Quantifiable polyhydramnios: Diagnosis and management. Obstet Gynecol 75:989, 1990

Casey BM, McIntire DD, Bloom SL, et al: Pregnancy outcomes after antepartum diagnosis of oligohydramnios at or beyond 34 weeks' gestation. Am J Obstet Gynecol 182:909, 2000

Chauhan SP, Magann EF, Morrison JC, et al: Ultrasonographic assessment of amniotic fluid does not reflect actual amniotic fluid volume. Am J Obstet Gynecol 177:291, 1997

Chauhan SP, Sanderson M, Hendrix NW, et al: Perinatal outcome and amniotic fluid index in the antepartum and intrapartum periods: A meta-analysis. Am J Obstet Gynecol 181:1473, 1999

Chauhan SP, Washburne JF, Magann EF, et al: A randomized study to assess the efficacy of the amniotic fluid index as a fetal admission test. Obstet Gynecol 86:9, 1995

Damato N, Filly RA, Goldstein RB, et al: Frequency of fetal anomalies in sonographically detected polyhydramnios. J Ultrasound Med 12:11, 1993

Deka D, Malhotra B: Role of maternal oral hydration in increasing amniotic fluid volume in pregnant women with oligohydramnios. Int J Gynaecol Obstet 73:155, 2001

DeMeeus JB, D'Halluin G, Bascou V, et al: Prophylactic intrapartum amnioinfusion: A controlled retrospective study of 135 cases. Eur J Obstet Gynecol Reprod Biol 72:141, 1997

Divon MY, Marks AD, Henderson CE: Longitudinal measurement of amniotic fluid index in postterm pregnancies and its association with fetal outcome. Am J Obstet Gynecol 172:142, 1995

Duenhoelter JH, Pritchard JA: Fetal respiration: Quantitative measurements of amnionic fluid inspired near term by human and rhesus fetuses. Am J Obstet Gynecol 125:306, 1976

Elliott JP, Sawyer AT, Radin TG, et al: Large-volume therapeutic amniocentesis in the treatment of hydramnios. Obstet Gynecol 84:1025, 1994

Fisk NM, Talbert DG, Nicolini U, et al: Fetal breathing movements in oligohydramnios are not increased by amnioinfusion. Br J Obstet Gynaecol 99:464, 1992

Fox HE, Badalian SS: Ultrasound prediction of fetal pulmonary hypoplasia in pregnancies complicated by oligohydramnios and in cases of congenital diaphragmatic hernia: A review. Am J Perinatol 11:104, 1994

Furman B, Erez O, Senior L, et al: Hydramnios and small for gestational age: Prevalence and clinical significance. Acta Obstet Gynecol Scand 79:31, 2000

Gagnon R, Harding R, Brace RA: Amniotic fluid and fetal urinary responses to severe placental insufficiency in sheep. Am J Obstet Gynecol 186:1076, 2002

Garmel SH, Chelmow D, Sha SJ, et al: Oligohydramnios and the appropriately grown fetus. Am J Perinatol 14:359, 1997

Glantz JC, Abramowicz JS, Sherer DM: Significance of idiopathic midtrimester polyhydramnios. Am J Perinatol 11:305, 1994

Golan A, Wolman I, Saller Y, et al: Hydramnios in singleton pregnancy: Sonographic prevalence and etiology. Gynecol Obstet Invest 35:91, 1993

Grubb DK, Paul RH: Amniotic fluid index and prolonged antepartum fetal heart rate decelerations. Obstet Gynecol 79:588, 1992

Hill LM, Breckle R, Thomas ML, et al: Polyhydramnios: Ultrasonically detected prevalence and neonatal outcome. Obstet Gynecol 69:21, 1987

Hill LM, Krohn M, Lazebnik N, et al: The amniotic fluid index in normal twin pregnancies. Am J Obstet Gynecol 182:950, 2000

Kerr J, Borgida AF, Hardardottir H, et al: Maternal hydration and its effect on the amniotic fluid index. Am J Obstet Gynecol 174:416, 1996

Kilbride HW, Yeast J, Thibeault DW: Defining limits of survival: Lethal pulmonary hypoplasia after midtrimester premature rupture of membranes. Am J Obstet Gynecol 175:675, 1996

Kilpatrick SJ, Safford KL: Maternal hydration increases amniotic fluid index in women with normal amniotic fluid. Obstet Gynecol 81:49, 1993

Kramer WB, Van den Veyver IB, Kirshon B: Treatment of polyhydramnios with indomethacin. Clin Perinatol 21:615, 1994

Kriplani A, Abbi M, Banerjee N, et al: Indomethacin therapy in the treatment of polyhydramnios due to placental chorioangioma. J Obstet Gynaecol Res 27:245, 2001

Lauria MR, Gonik B, Romero R: Pulmonary hypoplasia: Pathogenesis, diagnosis, and antenatal prediction. Obstet Gynecol 86:466, 1995

Leung WC, Jouannic JM, Hyett J, et al: Procedure-related complications of rapid amniodrainage in the treatment of polyhydramnios. Ultrasound Obstet Gynecol. 23:154, 2004

Leveno KJ, Quirk JG Jr, Cunningham FG, et al: Prolonged pregnancy, 1. Observations concerning the causes of fetal distress. Am J Obstet Gynecol 150:465, 1984

Magann EF, Doherty DA, Chauhan SP, et al: How well do the amniotic fluid index and single deepest pocket indices (below the 3rd and 5th and above the 95th and 97th percentiles) predict oligohydramnios and hydramnios? Am J Obstet Gynecol 190:164, 2004

Magann EF, Chauhan SP, Bofill JA, et al: Comparability of the amniotic fluid index and single deepest pocket measurements in clinical practice. Aust N Z J Obstet Gynaeco 43:75, 2003a

Magann EF, Chauhan SP, Martin JN: Is amniotic fluid volume status predictive of fetal acidosis at delivery? N Z J Obstet Gynaecol 43:129, 2003b

Magann EF, Doherty DA, Chauhan SP, et al: Effect of maternal hydration on amniotic fluid volume. Obstet Gynecol 101:1261, 2003c

Magann EF, Chauhan SP, Barrilleaux PS, et al: Ultrasound estimate of amniotic fluid volume: Color Doppler overdiagnosis of oligohydramnios. Obstet Gynecol 98:71, 2001

Magann EF, Kinsella MJ, Chauhan SP, et al: Does an amniotic fluid index of </r = 5 cm necessitate delivery in high-risk pregnancies? A case-control study. Obstet Gynecol 180:1354, 1999

Magann EF, Nolan TE, Hess LW, et al: Measurement of amniotic fluid volume: Accuracy of ultrasonography techniques. Am J Obstet Gynecol 167:1533, 1992

Magann EF, Sanderson M, Martin JN, et al: The amniotic fluid index, single deepest pocket, and two-diameter pocket in normal human pregnancy. Am J Obstet Gynecol 182:1581, 2000

Malhotra B, Deka D: Duration of the increase in amniotic fluid index (AFI) after acute maternal hydration. Arch Gynecol Obstet 269:173, 2004

Mamopoulos M, Assimakopoulos E, Reece EA, et al: Maternal indomethacin therapy in the treatment of polyhydramnios. Am J Obstet Gynecol 162:1225, 1990

Marks AD, Divon MY: Longitudinal study of the amniotic fluid index in postdated pregnancy. Obstet Gynecol 79:229, 1992

Martinez-Frias ML, Bermejo E, Rodriguez-Pinilla E, et al: Maternal and fetal factors related to abnormal amniotic fluid. J Perinatol 19:514, 1999

McCurdy CM, Seeds JW: Oligohydramnios: Problems and treatment. Semin Perinatol 17:183, 1993

McNamara MF, McCurty CM, Reed KL, et al: The relation between pulmonary hypoplasia and amniotic fluid volume: Lessons learned from discordant urinary tract anomalies in monoamniotic twins. Obstet Gynecol 85:867, 1995

Mercer LJ, Brown LB: Fetal outcome with oligohydramnios in the second trimester. Obstet Gynecol 67:840, 1986

Moessinger AC, Santiago A, Paneth NS, et al: Time-trends in necropsy prevalence and birth prevalence of lung hypoplasia. Paediatr Perinat Epidemiol 3:421, 1989

Moise KJ Jr, Huhta JC, Sharif DS, et al: Indomethacin in the treatment of premature labor: Effects on the fetal ductus arteriosus. N Engl J Med 319:327, 1988

Morris JM, Thompson K, Smithey J, et al: The usefulness of ultrasound assessment of amniotic fluid in predicting adverse outcome in prolonged pregnancy: A prospective blinded observational study. Br J Obstet Gynaecol 110:989, 2003

Moses J, Doherty DA, Magann EF, et al: A randomized clinical trial of the intrapartum assessment of amniotic fluid volume: amniotic fluid index versus the single deepest pocket technique. Am J Obstet Gynecol 190:1564, 2004

Naeye RL, Blanc WA: Fetal renal structure and the genesis of amniotic fluid disorders. Am J Pathol 67:95, 1972

Narchi H, Santos M, Kulayat N: Polyhydramnios as a sign of fetal pseudohypoaldosteronism. Int J Gynaecol Obstet 69:53, 2000

Newbould MJ, Lendon M, Barson AJ: Oligohydramnios sequence: The spectrum of renal malformation. Br J Obstet Gynaecol 101:598, 1994

Oz AU, Holub B, Mendilcioglu I, et al: Renal artery Doppler investigation of the etiology of oligohydramnios in postterm pregnancy. Obstet Gynecol 100:715, 2002

Panting-Kemp A, Nguyen T, Castro L: Substance abuse and polyhydramnios. Am J Obstet Gynecol 187:602, 2002

Panting-Kemp A, Nguyen T, Chang E, et al: Idiopathic polyhydramnios and perinatal outcome. Am J Obstet Gynecol 181:1079, 1999

Peedicayil A, Mathai M, Regi AN, et al: Inter- and intra-observer variation in the amniotic fluid index. Obstet Gynecol 84:848, 1994

Peipert JF, Donnenfeld AE: Oligohydramnios: A review. Obstet Gynecol Surv 46:325, 1991

Phelan JP, Smith CV, Broussard P, et al: Amniotic fluid volume assessment with the four-quadrant technique at 36–42 weeks' gestation. J Reprod Med 32:540, 1987

Pierce J, Gaudier FL, Sanchez-Ramos L: Intrapartum amnioinfusion for meconium-stained fluid: Meta-analysis of prospective clinical trials. Obstet Gynecol 95:1051, 2000

Porter TF, Dildy GA, Blanchard JR, et al: Normal values for amniotic fluid index during uncomplicated twin pregnancy. Obstet Gynecol 87:699, 1996

Pritchard JA: Fetal swallowing and amniotic fluid volume. Obstet Gynecol 28:606, 1966

Pryde PG, Hallak M, Lauria MR, et al: Severe oligohydramnios with intact membranes: An indication for diagnostic amnioinfusion. Fetal Diagn Ther 15:46, 2000

Queenan JT: Polyhydramnios and oligohydramnios. Contemp Obstet Gynecol 36:60, 1991

Rogers MS, Lau TK, Wang CC, et al: Amnioinfusion for the prevention of meconium aspiration during labour. Aust N Z J Obstet Gynaecol 36:407, 1996

Ross MG, Cedars L, Nijland MJM, et al: Treatment of oligohydramnios with maternal 1-deamino-[8-D-arginine] vasopressin–induced plasma hypoosmolality. Am J Obstet Gynecol 174:1603, 1996

Sarno AP, Ahn MO, Brar HS, et al: Intrapartum Doppler velocimetry, amniotic fluid volume, and fetal heart rate as predictors of subsequent fetal distress, 1. An initial report. Am J Obstet Gynecol 161:1508, 1989

Sarno AP, Anh MO, Phelan JP: Intrapartum amniotic fluid volume at term: Association of ruptured membranes, oligohydramnios, and increased fetal risk. J Reprod Med 35:719, 1990

Schrimmer DB, Moore TR: Sonographic evaluation of amniotic fluid volume. Clin Obstet Gynecol 45:1026, 2002

Shenker L, Reed KL, Anderson CF, et al: Significance of oligohydramnios complicating pregnancy. Am J Obstet Gynecol 164:1597, 1991

Spong CY, Ogundipe OA, Ross MG: Prophylactic amnioinfusion for meconium stained amniotic fluid. Am J Obstet Gynecol 171:931, 1994.

Usta IM, Mercer BM, Aswad NK, et al: The impact of a policy of amnioinfusion for meconium-stained amniotic fluid. Obstet Gynecol 85:237, 1995

Wenstrom K, Andrews WW, Maher JE: Amnioinfusion survey: Prevalence, protocols, and complications. Obstet Gynecol 86:572, 1995

Winn HN, Chen M, Amon E, et al: Neonatal pulmonary hypoplasia and perinatal mortality in patients with midtrimester rupture of amniotic membranes—a critical analysis. Am J Obstet Gynecol 182:1638, 2000

Yancey MK, Richards DS: Effect of altitude on the amniotic fluid index. J Reprod Med 39:101, 1994

Zhang J, Troendle J, Meikle S, et al: Isolated oligohydramnios is not associated with adverse perinatal outcomes. BJOG 111:220, 2004

22

Induction of Labor

According to the National Center for Health Statistics, the annual incidence of labor induction or augmentation in the United States almost doubled from 20 percent in 1989 to 38 percent in 2002 (Martin and associates, 2003). The incidence is variable between practices. For example, at Parkland Hospital, approximately 35 percent of labors are induced or augmented. And at the University of Alabama at Birmingham Hospital, from 1996 through 1999, 20 percent of women were given oxytocin for induction and 35 percent for augmentation. This chapter includes a description of various techniques to effect cervical ripening as well as schemata for the induction or augmentation of labor.

GENERAL CONCEPTS

ELECTIVE INDUCTION OF LABOR. There can be no doubt that elective induction for convenience of the practitioner or the patient is becoming more prevalent. Despite this, the American College of Obstetricians and Gynecologists (1999a) does not support this practice, except for logistical reasons such as risk of rapid labor, the woman lives a long distance from the hospital, or for psychosocial indications. One reason is that induced labor is associated with an increased cesarean delivery rate, especially in nulliparas (Luthy and colleagues, 2002; Yeast and associates, 1999). A number of investigators have reported that elective induction consistently results in a two- to threefold risk for cesarean delivery (Hoffman and Sciscione, 2003; Maslow and Sweeny, 2000; Smith and colleagues, 2003).

In the Flanders region of Belgium, 30 percent of women delivering in 1996 and 1997 had induction of labor, and two thirds of these were elective (Cammu and colleagues, 2002). The investigators matched 3683 women who had elective inductions with a similar number of women whose labor was spontaneous. Induction resulted in significantly more cesarean deliveries—9.9 versus 6.5 percent—in part due to an increased incidence of dystocia and "fetal distress." This increase appears to be unchanged even when the cervix is more "favorable." Specifically, in a retrospective cohort study, Hamar and associates (2001) found that the rate of cesarean delivery following elective induction was significantly increased in low-risk women with a Bishop score of 7 or greater compared with women with spontaneous labor. Using a decision-tree model, Kaufman and associates (2001) reported that elective induction resulted in more cesarean deliveries at term and increased costs.

For all of these reasons, we agree that routine elective induction at term cannot be justified. Cesarean delivery imposes increased risk for severe, albeit infrequent, adverse maternal outcomes including death (see Chap. 25, p. 592). If elective induction is considered at term, these risks must be discussed with and consented to by each patient. The American College

of Obstetricians and Gynecologists (1999a) defines term as 38 completed weeks.

INDICATED LABOR INDUCTION. Induction is indicated when the benefits to either the mother or the fetus outweigh those of continuing the pregnancy. Indications include emergent conditions such as ruptured membranes with chorioamnionitis or severe preeclampsia. More common indications include membrane rupture without labor, hypertension, nonreassuring fetal status, and postterm gestation.

Induction for *postterm* or *prolonged pregnancy* is discussed in Chapter 37 (see p. 887). Many clinicians consider this diagnosis, especially at 41 weeks, to be within the normal range of term gestation and that induction of such women is considered elective. This belief is due in part to definitions and methods used to support this diagnosis. For example, in a randomized trial, Bennett and associates (2004) reported that *combined* first- and second-trimester ultrasound examination pregnancy dating, compared with a single second-trimester screening examination, reduced the number of women attaining 41 weeks to 6.7 from 16.3 percent. Savitz and colleagues (2002) described a systematic tendency to overstate gestational age from the last menstrual period compared with that from early ultrasound examination—12.1 percent versus 3.4 percent, respectively. This overstatement most likely reflected delayed ovulation. Menticoglou and Hall (2002) present an elegant and compelling analysis to refute routine induction at 41 weeks as a "nonsensus consensus" and as a "rescue from normalcy."

Although induction is widely practiced for suspected *fetal macrosomia,* there is little evidence that it is of benefit. Sanchez-Ramos and colleagues (2002) conducted a meta-analysis of observational studies in which women with suspected fetal macrosomia were managed expectantly or underwent labor induction. Perinatal outcomes were similar, however, the cesarean delivery rate was significantly lower with expectant management compared with that of induction—8.4 versus 16.6 percent.

Women whose labor is induced have an increased incidence of chorioamnionitis and cesarean delivery compared with those in spontaneous labor. In many cases, it seems that the uterus is simply poorly prepared for labor. One example is an "unripe cervix." It is also likely that the increase in cesarean deliveries associated with induction is influenced by the duration of the induction attempt, especially in the circumstance of an unfavorable cervix (Rouse and colleagues, 2000). The duration for either labor induction or augmentation and successful delivery has received too little attention. More precise data are needed to understand the wide range of individual management. For example, Garcia and associates (2001), after adjustment for case mix, reported that cesarean births were significantly lower at academic medical centers (odds ratio 0.66) compared with those at community hospitals. Doyle and colleagues (2002) reported that cesarean deliveries in a community hospital were twice that of a county hospital. There are other factors too. For example, Bland and co-workers (2001) observed a significant decrease in elective induction with a change from individual practitioner billing to revenue sharing.

Cesarean birth is associated with markedly increased common and uncommon maternal infectious morbidities (Goepfert and colleagues, 2001). These morbidities are further increased in women with overt chorioamnionitis. The need for emergent hysterectomy also is increased. Shellhaas and associates (2001), from the Maternal–Fetal Units Network, reported 146 emergent cesarean hysterectomies amongst 136,948 deliveries—about 1 per 1000 vaginal deliveries versus 1 per 200 cesarean deliveries. Importantly, 41 percent of hysterectomies followed primary cesarean delivery. Uterine atony was the indication for one third of all cesarean hysterectomies, and this indication was more prevalent in women with induced or augmented labor, or in those with chorioamnionitis. Kastner and colleagues (2002) reported similar findings.

CONTRAINDICATIONS. Contraindications to labor induction are similar to those that preclude spontaneous labor or delivery. The most common example is a prior uterine disruption such as a classical incision or some type of uterine surgery that involved the myometrium. Most types of placenta previa preclude labor. Labor prohibition due to fetal factors includes appreciable macrosomia, severe hydrocephalus, malpresentations, or nonreassuring fetal status. The few maternal contraindications are related to small maternal size, distorted pelvic anatomy, and conditions such as active genital herpes infection or cervical cancer.

PREINDUCTION CERVICAL RIPENING

The condition of the cervix—or "favorability"—is important to the success of labor induction. One quantifiable method predictive of an outcome of labor induction is that described by Bishop (1964). Elements of the *Bishop score* are presented in Table 22–1. A score of 9 conveys a high likelihood for a successful induction. Most practitioners would consider that

TABLE 22–1 Bishop Scoring System Used for Assessment of Inducibility

	Factor				
Score	Dilatation (cm)	Effacement (%)	Station (−3 to +3)	Cervical Consistency	Cervical Position
0	Closed	0–30	−3	Firm	Posterior
1	1–2	40–50	−2	Medium	Midposition
2	3–4	60–70	−1	Soft	Anterior
3	≥ 5	> 80	+1, +2	—	—

a woman whose cervix is 2 cm dilated, 80 percent effaced, soft, and midposition, and with the fetal occiput at −1 station would have a successful labor induction.

Unfortunately, women too frequently have an indication for induction but with an unfavorable cervix. As favorability or Bishop score decreases, there is an increasingly unsuccessful induction rate. Thus, considerable research has been directed toward various techniques to "ripen" the cervix prior to stimulation of uterine contractions. For research purposes, a Bishop score of 4 or less identifies an unfavorable cervix, and may be an indication for cervical ripening.

PHARMACOLOGICAL TECHNIQUES

Prostaglandin E₂. Local application of prostaglandin E_2 (dinoprostone) is commonly used for cervical ripening (American College of Obstetricians and Gynecologists, 1999a, 1999b). Prostaglandin E_2 gel (Prepidil) is available in a 2.5-mL syringe for an intracervical application of 0.5 mg of dinoprostone. Owen and colleagues (1991) did a meta-analysis of 18 studies that included 1811 women. They found that prostaglandin E_2 improved Bishop scores and induction-to-delivery times when compared with those of untreated controls. Unfortunately, they found no benefit in lowering the cesarean delivery rate. This finding may be the result of other factors. For example, Ramsey and colleagues (2002) reported that dinoprostone gel was more effective when the vaginal pH was greater than 4.5 compared with that of 4.5 or less.

A 10-mg dinoprostone vaginal insert (Cervidil) also is approved for cervical ripening. The insert provides slower release of medication (0.3 mg/hr) than the gel. As with dinoprostone gel, these inserts will shorten the induction-to-delivery interval (Bolnick and associates, 2004; Rayburn and colleagues, 1992). An advantage of the insert is that it can be removed should hyperstimulation occur.

ADMINISTRATION. Prostaglandin preparations should only be administered in or near the delivery suite and where uterine activity and fetal heart rate monitoring can be performed (American College of Obstetricians and Gynecologists, 1995b). When contractions occur, they are usually apparent in the first hour and show peak activity in the first 4 hours (Bernstein, 1991; Miller and colleagues, 1991). Perry and Leaphart (2004) compared intracervical with intravaginal administration of the insert and found the latter to result in quicker delivery—11.7 versus 16.2 hours. When more than two sequential doses were used, Chan and associates (2004) reported that 59 percent of women required emergency cesarean delivery. Finally, according to manufacturer guidelines, oxytocin induction that follows prostaglandin use for cervical ripening should be delayed for 6 to 12 hours following prostaglandin E_2 administration.

SIDE EFFECTS. Uterine tachysystole has been reported to follow vaginally administered prostaglandin E$_2$ in 1 to 5 percent of women (Brindley and Sokol, 1988; Rayburn, 1989). Because hyperstimulation that can cause fetal compromise may occur when prostaglandins are used with preexisting spontaneous labor, such use is not recommended. When hyperstimulation occurs with the 10-mg insert, its removal by pulling on the tail of the surrounding net will usually reverse this effect. Irrigation to remove the gel preparation has not been helpful.

Prostaglandin E$_1$. Misoprostol (Cytotec) is a synthetic prostaglandin E$_1$, available as a 100- or 200-μg tablet for prevention of peptic ulcers. It has been used "off label" for preinduction cervical ripening and may be administered orally or vaginally. The tablets are stable at room temperature. Misoprostol costs less than $1 per 100-$\mu$g tablet compared with $75 for the 0.5-mg dose of dinoprostone gel.

In October 2000, G. D. Searle & Company notified physicians that misoprostol is not approved for labor induction or abortion. Despite this, in December 2000, the American College of Obstetricians and Gynecologists reaffirmed its recommendation for use of the drug because of proven safety and efficacy.

VAGINAL ADMINISTRATION. Several investigators have reported that misoprostol tablets placed into the vagina were either superior to or equivalent in efficacy when compared with intracervical prostaglandin E$_2$ gel (Gemund and associates, 2004; Wing and co-workers, 1995a, 1995b). The Committee on Obstetrics of the American College of Obstetricians and Gynecologists (1999b) reviewed 19 randomized trials in which more than 1900 women were given intravaginal misoprostol in doses ranging from 25 to 200 μg. The Committee on Obstetrics recommended the use of a 25-μg intravaginal dose, which is one fourth of a 100-μg tablet. The drug is evenly distributed among these quartered tablets. Although Williams and colleagues (2002) showed that accurate dosing with 25 μg is possible if the quartered tablets are individually weighed, this seems unnecessary. Also, although it may lower pH, moistening of misoprostol tablets with 3-percent acetic acid solution does not improve efficacy (Sanchez-Ramos and associates, 2002).

Misoprostol use may decrease the need for oxytocin, achieve higher rates of vaginal delivery within 24 hours of induction, and reduce induction-to-delivery intervals (Sanchez-Ramos and colleagues, 1997). Data from the United Kingdom Cochrane Centre support these recommendations, but the investigators cautioned that increased uterine hyperstimulation with adverse fetal heart rate changes was of concern (Hofmeyr and associates, 1999). A 50-μg misoprostol intravaginal dose was associated with significantly increased tachysystole, meconium passage, and meconium aspiration when compared with prostaglandin E$_2$ gel (Wing and co-workers, 1995a, 1995b). A 25-μg dose was found comparable to dinoprostone (van Gemund and associates, 2004). There

is also an increased cesarean delivery rate due to uterine hyperstimulation when compared with that from dinoprostone (Buser and collaborators, 1997). Uterine rupture has been reported with prostaglandin E$_1$ use in women with a prior cesarean delivery (Wing and colleagues, 1998). Plaut and associates (1999) described uterine rupture in 5 of 89 (6 percent) women with a prior cesarean incision who were induced with misoprostol. This finding is compared with only 1 of 423 such women not given misoprostol. Most now agree that prior uterine surgery, including cesarean delivery, precludes the use of misoprostol (American College of Obstetricians and Gynecologists, 2004).

ORAL ADMINISTRATION. Prostaglandin E$_1$ tablets are also effective when given orally. Windrim and associates (1997) reported oral misoprostol to be of similar efficacy for cervical ripening as intravaginal administration. Wing and collaborators (1999) reported that 50 μg of oral misoprostol was less effective than 25 μg administered vaginally for cervical ripening. Subsequently, Wing and colleagues (2003) and Hall and associates (2002) reported that a 100-μg oral dose was as effective as the 25-μg intravaginal dose. In women with premature rupture of membranes at term, Mozurkewich and colleagues (2003) and Pearson and associates (2002) have reported similar success with labor initiation with either oral misoprostol or standard oxytocin regimens. Lo and co-workers (2003), in a similar group of women at term with prematurely ruptured membranes, found that oral misoprostol predictably induced at least 200 Montevideo units within 30 to 60 minutes, and results were comparable to their standard intravenous oxytocin infusion.

MECHANICAL TECHNIQUES

Transcervical Catheter. Sherman and colleagues (1996) summarized the results of 13 trials with balloon-tipped catheters to effect cervical dilatation and concluded that, with or without saline infusion, the method resulted in rapid improvement in Bishop scores and shorter labors. Several comparative trials have been done. Huang and colleagues (2002) randomized 135 women to labor induction with vaginal misoprostol, an intrauterine extra-amnionic Foley catheter with bulb inflation to 30 mL, or both therapies. Outcomes were similar in all three groups, and there was no apparent benefit of combining these two techniques. Bujold and co-workers (2004) retrospectively compared women with a prior cesarean incision undergoing a trial of labor. They reported a lower incidence of success when induction by Foley catheter was compared with that by oxytocin—56 versus 78 percent. Culver and colleagues (2004) compared oxytocin plus an intracervical Foley catheter to 25 μg of misoprostol administered vaginally every 4 hours in women with a Bishop score less than 6. The mean induction-to-delivery time was significantly shorter in the catheter-plus-oxytocin group—16 versus 22 hours.

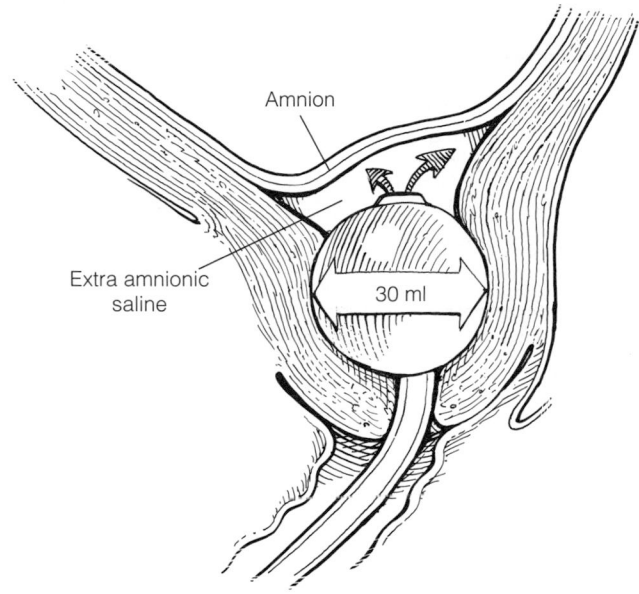

FIGURE 22–1. Extra-amnionic saline infusion (EASI) through 26F Foley catheter placed through the cervix. The 30-mL balloon is inflated with saline and pulled snugly against the internal os and the catheter taped to the thigh.

The addition of *extra-amnionic saline infusion (EASI),* shown in Figure 22–1, has been reported to significantly improve the Bishop score and decrease induction-to-delivery times when compared with that by (1) 50-μg intravaginal misoprostol tablets (Vengalil and colleagues, 1998), (2) 0.5 mg of intracervical prostaglandin E_2 (Goldman and Wigton, 1999; Hemlin and Möller, 1998; Sciscione and associates, 1999), or (3) 50-μg oral misoprostol. Abramovici and co-workers (1999) studied nulliparas with a Bishop score of 5 or less, and reported that 85 percent of those induced by catheter infusion delivered within 24 hours compared with 55 percent of those given misoprostol.

Guinn and colleagues (2000) randomized women to intracervical prostaglandin E_2, laminaria plus intravenous oxytocin, or EASI plus oxytocin. Normal saline was infused through the catheter port at 30 mL/hr. Oxytocin infusion was begun immediately after placement of the catheter. The cesarean delivery rate was similar with all three interventions. The induction-to-delivery mean time of 18 hours with catheter infusion was significantly less than that with laminaria plus oxytocin (21.5 hours) or with prostaglandin E_2 gel (24.8 hours). Mullin and associates (2002) randomized 200 women with no cervical dilatation or effacement to receive 25 μg of misoprostol vaginally every 4 hours compared with EASI plus intravenous oxytocin. The mean induction-to-delivery time was shorter in the catheter-plus-oxytocin group (16.2 versus 22.1 hours). Women given misoprostol had a higher incidence of uterine hyperstimulation.

Hygroscopic Cervical Dilators. Cervical dilatation has been achieved with hygroscopic osmotic cervical dilators

(see Chap. 9, p. 243). These dilators have long been accepted as efficacious when inserted prior to pregnancy termination (Hale and Pion, 1972). More recently, they have also been used for cervical ripening before labor induction in pregnancies with a healthy fetus. Gilson and associates (1996) reported a rapid improvement of cervical favorability in women randomized to hygroscopic dilators prior to oxytocin induction. There was, however, no beneficial effect on the vaginal delivery rate or induction-to-delivery times compared with those of women given oxytocin only. In the randomized study cited earlier, Guinn and co-workers (2000) reported a longer induction-to-delivery time with cervical dilators plus oxytocin compared with that of EASI plus oxytocin. The use of hygroscopic dilators appears to be safe, although anaphylaxis has followed laminaria insertion (Cole and Bruck, 2000; Nguyen and Hoffman, 1995). The attraction of dilators is their low cost and ease of placement and removal.

Membrane Stripping. Induction of labor by membrane "stripping" is a common practice. McColgin and colleagues (1990) reported that stripping was safe and decreased the incidence of postterm gestation. They documented significantly increased serum levels of endogenous prostaglandins with stripping (McColgin and coauthors, 1993). Allott and Palmer (1993) randomized 195 women with normal pregnancies beyond 40 weeks to digital cervical examination either with or without membrane stripping. The women were examined as outpatients. Two thirds of those who underwent stripping entered spontaneous labor within 72 hours compared with one third of the other group. The incidence of ruptured membranes, infection, and bleeding was not increased. Importantly, subsequent induction for postterm pregnancy at 42 weeks was significantly decreased with stripping.

Boulvain and colleagues (1999) reviewed 13 reports that included almost 2000 women who underwent membrane stripping to prevent postterm pregnancy. The risks for maternal and neonatal infection and membrane rupture were similar in intervention versus control groups as were the cesarean delivery rates. Stripping was considered beneficial because women in this group were significantly more likely to deliver within 48 hours, within 1 week, and before 41 weeks, thus, fewer women in the stripping group required labor induction.

SUMMARY OF PREINDUCTION CERVICAL RIPENING. Labor induction frequently is indicated when there is an "unripe" cervix. The preceding preinduction techniques may have some benefit when compared with no attempt at cervical ripening before oxytocin induction. That said, there are few data to support the premise that any of these techniques results in a reduction in cesarean delivery rates or in lower maternal or neonatal morbidity compared with women in whom such techniques are not used.

LABOR INDUCTION AND AUGMENTATION WITH OXYTOCIN

Synthetic oxytocin is one of the most commonly used medications in the United States. It was the first polypeptide hormone synthesized, and the 1955 Nobel Prize in chemistry was awarded for this (DuVigneaud and co-workers, 1953). Regarding labor, it has two uses. *Induction* implies stimulation of contractions before the spontaneous onset of labor, with or without ruptured membranes. *Augmentation* refers to stimulation of spontaneous contractions that are considered inadequate because of failure of progressive cervical dilatation and fetal descent. With oxytocin use, the American College of Obstetricians and Gynecologists (1999a) recommends fetal heart rate and contraction monitoring similar to that for any high-risk pregnancy. Contractions can be monitored either by palpation or by electronic means of recording uterine activity (see Chap. 18, p. 466). Uterine contraction pressures cannot be accurately quantified by palpation (Arrabal and Nagey, 1996).

INTRAVENOUS OXYTOCIN ADMINISTRATION.

The goal of induction or augmentation is to effect uterine activity sufficiently to produce cervical change and fetal descent while avoiding development of a nonreassuring fetal status. Oxytocin should be discontinued if the number of contractions persists with a frequency greater than five in a 10-minute period or seven in a 15-minute period or with a persistent nonreassuring fetal heart rate pattern. Discontinuation of oxytocin nearly always rapidly decreases the frequency of contractions. When oxytocin is stopped, its concentration in plasma rapidly falls because the mean half-life is approximately 5 minutes. Seitchik and co-workers (1984) found that a uterine response occurs within 3 to 5 minutes of beginning an oxytocin infusion and that a plasma steady state is reached in 40 minutes. Response depends on preexisting uterine activity, cervical status, pregnancy duration, and individual biological differences. Caldeyro-Barcia and Poseiro (1960) reported that the uterine response to oxytocin increases from 20 to 30 weeks and increases rapidly at term (see Chap. 18, p. 466).

Oxytocin Dosage. Oxytocin usually is diluted into 1000 mL of a balanced salt solution and administered by infusion pump. A typical oxytocin infusate consists of 10 or 20 units—or 10,000 to 20,000 mU—mixed into 1000 mL of lactated Ringer solution. This mixture results in an oxytocin concentration of 10 or 20 mU/mL, respectively. To avoid bolus administration, the infusion should be inserted into the main intravenous line close to the venipuncture site. The American College of Obstetricians and Gynecologists (1999a) recommends a number of oxytocin regimens for labor stimulation (Table 22–2). Until about 15 years ago, only variations of low-dose protocols were used in the United States. In 1984, O'Driscoll and colleagues described a proto-

TABLE 22–2 Low-Dose and High-Dose Oxytocin Regimen for Stimulation of Labor

Regimen	Starting Dose (mU/min)	Incremental Increase (mU/min)	Dosing Interval (min)
Low-dose	0.5–1	1	30–40
	1–2		15
High-dose	~6	~6	15
	6	6[a], 3, 1	20–40

[a]The incremental increase is reduced to 3 mU/min in presence of hyperstimulation and reduced to 1 mU/min with recurrent hyperstimulation.
From the American College of Obstetricians and Gynecologists (1999a), with permission.

col for the active management of labor that called for oxytocin at a starting dosage of 6 mU/min and advanced in 6-mU/min increments. Following this, various trials during the 1990s compared high-dose (4 to 6 mU/min) versus conventional low-dose (0.5 to 1.5 mU/min) regimens both for labor induction and for augmentation.

At Parkland Hospital, Satin and colleagues (1992) evaluated an oxytocin regimen using an initial and incremental dosage of 6 mU/min compared with one using 1 mU/min. Increases at 20-minute intervals were provided as needed. Among 1112 women undergoing induction, the 6-mU/min regimen resulted in a shorter mean admission-to-delivery time, fewer failed inductions, and no cases of neonatal sepsis. Among 1676 women who had labor augmentation, those who received the 6-mU/min regimen had a shorter duration-to-delivery time, fewer forceps deliveries, fewer cesarean deliveries for dystocia, and decreased intrapartum chorioamnionitis or neonatal sepsis. With this protocol, uterine hyperstimulation is managed by oxytocin discontinuation followed by resumption when indicated and at half the stopping dosage. Thereafter, the dosage is increased at 3 mU/min when appropriate instead of the usual 6-mU/min increase for women without hyperstimulation. No adverse neonatal effects were observed.

Xenakis and colleagues (1995) reported benefits using an incremental oxytocin regimen starting at 4 mU/min. Merrill and Zlatnik (1999) randomized 1307 women for labor induction (816) or augmentation (491) to incremental oxytocin given at either 1.5 or 4.5 mU/min. Women randomized to the 4.5 mU/min dosage had significantly decreased mean durations of induction-to-second-stage labor and induction-to-delivery. Nulliparas randomized to the 4.5 mU/min dosage had a lower cesarean delivery rate for dystocia compared with those at 1.5 mU/min dosage—5.9 versus 11.9 percent.

Thus, benefits favor higher-dose regimens as compared with lower dosages of 0.5 to 1.5 mU/min. In 1990, routine usage of the 6-mU/min oxytocin beginning and incremental dosage was incorporated at Parkland Hospital and continues through today. At the University of Alabama at Birmingham, a 2-mU/min beginning and incremental oxytocin regimen is used. In both cases, these dosages are used for either labor induction or augmentation.

Interval Between Incremental Dosing. Intervals to increase oxytocin dosages vary from 15 to 40 minutes (see Table 22–2). Satin and colleagues (1994) addressed this aspect with a 6-mU/min regimen providing increases at either 20- or 40-minute intervals. Women assigned to the 20-minute interval regimen for labor augmentation had a significant reduction in the rate of cesarean delivery for dystocia compared with that of the 40-minute interval regimen—8 versus 12 percent. In women with labor induction, however, uterine hyperstimulation was significantly more frequent with the 20-minute regimen. Other investigators report incremental increases at even more frequent intervals. Frigoletto and associates (1995) and Xenakis and co-workers (1995) began oxytocin at 4 mU/min with increases as needed every 15 minutes. Merrill and Zlatnik (1999) started with 4.5 mU/min with increases every 30 minutes. López-Zeno and colleagues (1992) began at 6 mU/min with increases every 15 minutes. Thus, there are a number of acceptable oxytocin protocols that appear somewhat dissimilar. But are they? A comparison of protocols from two of our institutions follows.

1. The current Parkland Hospital protocol begins oxytocin at 6 mU/min, with 6-mU/min increases every 40 minutes, but employs flexible dosing based on hyperstimulation.
2. At the University of Alabama at Birmingham, oxytocin for labor induction or augmentation is begun at 2 mU/min and is increased as needed every 15 minutes to 4, 8, 12, 16, 20, 25, and 30 mU/min.

These two regimens, while at first appearing disparate, are similar, viz., if there is no uterine activity, either regimen is delivering 12 mU/min by 45 minutes into the infusion.

Maximal Dosage. The *maximal* effective dose of oxytocin to achieve adequate contractions in all cases is not known. Wen and colleagues (2001) studied 1151 consecutive nulliparas in spontaneous labor or undergoing labor induction and found that the likelihood of progression to a vaginal delivery decreases at and beyond an oxytocin dosage of 36 mU/min. At a dosage of 72 mU/min, however, half of the nulliparas were delivered vaginally. Thus, if contractions are not adequate—less than 200 Montevideo units—and if the fetal status is reassuring and labor has arrested, an oxytocin infusion dose greater than 48 mU/min has no apparent risks.

Risks Versus Benefits. Unless the uterus is scarred, uterine rupture associated with oxytocin infusion is rare, even in parous women (see Chap. 35, p. 837). Flannelly and associates (1993) reported no uterine ruptures with or without oxytocin in 27,829 nulliparas. There were eight instances of overt uterine rupture during labor in 48,718 parous women—only one of these was associated with oxytocin use.

Oxytocin has amino-acid homology similar to arginine vasopressin. Thus, not surprisingly, it has significant antidiuretic action and when infused at 20 mU/min or more, renal free water clearance decreases markedly. If aqueous fluids are infused in appreciable amounts along with oxytocin, *water intoxication* can lead to convulsions, coma, and even death.

Uterine Contraction Pressures. Contraction forces in spontaneously laboring women range from 90 to 390 Montevideo units. The latter are calculated by subtracting the baseline uterine pressure from the peak contraction pressure for each contraction in a 10-minute window and adding the pressures generated by each contraction. Caldeyro-Barcia and associates (1950) and Seitchik and colleagues (1984) found that the mean or median spontaneous uterine contraction pattern resulting in a progression to a vaginal delivery was between 140 and 150 Montevideo units (see Chap. 18, p. 466). However, in the management of active-phase arrest of labor, and with no contraindication to intravenous oxytocin, decisions must be made with knowledge of the safe upper range of uterine activity. Hauth and coworkers (1986) described an effective and safe protocol for oxytocin augmentation for active-phase arrest with which over 90 percent of women achieved an average of at least 200 to 225 Montevideo units. Hauth and associates (1991) later reported that nearly all women in whom arrest of active-phase labor persisted despite oxytocin were able to generate more than 200 Montevideo units. Importantly, despite no labor progression, there were no adverse maternal or newborn effects following cesarean delivery. More data are needed regarding the precise safety and efficacy of contraction patterns in subgroups of women with a prior cesarean delivery, with twins, or with an overdistended uterus.

Duration of Oxytocin Administration. The American College of Obstetricians and Gynecologists (1989, 1995a) has defined arrest in first-stage labor as a completed latent phase along with contractions exceeding 200 Montevideo units for more than 2 hours without cervical change. There are only sparse data to support a more accurate duration to define active-phase arrest. Some investigators have addressed this issue. Arulkumaran and associates (1987) extended the 2-hour limit to better define failed augmentation. Using a 4-hour limit, they reported a cesarean delivery rate of only 1.3 percent in women who continued to have adequate contractions and progressive cervical dilatation of at least 1 cm/hr. In women without progressive cervical dilatation who were allowed another 4 hours of labor, half were delivered vaginally. Rouse and colleagues (1999) prospectively managed 542 women at term with active-phase arrest. Women with other complications were not included. The protocol included an intent to achieve a sustained pattern of at least 200 Montevideo units for a *minimum* of 4 hours. This time frame was extended to 6 hours if activity of 200 Montevideo units or greater could not be sustained. Almost 92 percent of these women were delivered vaginally.

TABLE 22–3 Randomized Clinical Trials of Elective Amniotomy in Early Spontaneous Labor at Term

Study	Number	Mean Dilatation at Amniotomy	Mean Shortening of Labor	Need for Oxytocin	Cesarean Delivery Rate	Abnormal Tracing	Neonatal Effects
				Effects of Amniotomy			
Fraser and co-workers (1993)	925	< 5 cm	125 min	None	None[a]	None	None
Garite and associates (1993)	459	5.5 cm	81 min	Decreased	None[a]	Increased[b]	None
UK Amniotomy Group (1994)	1463	5.1 cm	60 min	None	None	NA	None

NA = not assessed.
[a] No effect on overall rate; cesarean delivery rate for fetal distress significantly increased.
[b] Increased mild and moderate umbilical cord compression patterns.

Rouse and colleagues (2001) extended these observations in 501 spontaneously laboring women at term with active-phase arrest. Using the same protocol, the cesarean delivery rate was only 12 percent. Montevideo units were measured for a total of 1643 hours in these 469 women with arrest of labor in the active phase. Most women with more than 2 hours of labor arrest, but who had sustained uterine activity of 200 Montevideo units or greater, achieved vaginal delivery. These data support the contention that it is safe and effective to allow an active-phase arrest of 4 hours.

Zhang and collaborators (2002) analyzed labor duration from 4 cm to complete dilatation in 1329 nulliparas at term. They found that before dilatation of 7 cm was reached, lack of progress for more than 2 hours was not uncommon in those who delivered vaginally. Alexander and colleagues (2002) reported that epidural analgesia prolonged active labor by 1 hour compared with duration of the active phase as defined by Friedman (1955). Consideration of these changes in the management of labor, especially in nulliparas, may safely reduce the cesarean delivery rate.

AMNIOTOMY. A common indication for amniotomy includes the need for direct monitoring of the fetal heart rate or uterine contractions, or both. To minimize the risk of cord prolapse when membranes are ruptured artificially, care should be taken to avoid dislodging the fetal head. Fundal or suprapubic pressure, or both, may reduce the risk of cord prolapse. Some clinicians prefer to rupture membranes during a contraction. If the vertex is not well applied to the lower uterine segment, a gradual egress of amnionic fluid can be accomplished by several membrane punctures with a 26-gauge needle held with a ring forceps and with direct visualization using a vaginal speculum. The fetal heart rate should be assessed before and immediately after amniotomy.

Elective Amniotomy. Membrane rupture with the intention of accelerating labor is commonly performed. In the investigations presented in Table 22–3, amniotomy at about 5 cm accelerated spontaneous labor by 1 to 2 hours. This procedure was performed without increasing the overall cesarean delivery rate or the use of oxytocin stimulation. Although mild and moderate cord compression patterns were increased follow-

ing amniotomy, cesarean delivery for fetal distress was not increased. Most importantly, there were no adverse perinatal effects.

Amniotomy Induction. Artificial rupture of the membranes can be used to induce labor, but it implies a commitment to delivery. The main disadvantage of amniotomy when used alone for labor induction is the unpredictable and occasionally long interval to the onset of contractions. In a randomized trial, Bakos and Bäckström (1987) found that amniotomy alone or combined with oxytocin was superior to oxytocin alone. Mercer and colleagues (1995) randomized 209 women undergoing oxytocin induction to amniotomy either at 1 to 2 cm dilatation (early amniotomy) or at 5 cm (late amniotomy). Early amniotomy was associated with significantly shorter labor by approximately 4 hours. There was, however, an increased incidence of chorioamnionitis (23 percent) and cord-compression patterns (12 percent) with early amniotomy.

Amniotomy Augmentation. It is common practice to perform amniotomy when labor is abnormally slow. Rouse and coworkers (1994) found that amniotomy with oxytocin augmentation for arrested active-phase labor shortened the time to delivery by 44 minutes compared with that of oxytocin alone. A drawback was that it significantly increased chorioamnionitis. As an adjunct to oxytocin infusion, however, amniotomy did not affect the route of delivery.

ACTIVE MANAGEMENT OF LABOR

This term describes a codified approach to the management of labor, which is discussed in detail in Chapter 17 (see p. 439).

REFERENCES

Abramovici D, Goldwasser S, Mabie BC, et al: A randomized comparison of oral misoprostol versus Foley catheter and oxytocin for induction of labor at term. Am J Obstet Gynecol 181:1108, 1999

Alexander JM, Sharma SK, McIntire D, et al: Epidural analgesia lengthens the Friedman active phase of labor. Obstet Gynecol 100:46, 2002

Allott HA, Palmer CR: Sweeping the membranes: A valid procedure in stimulating the onset of labour? Br J Obstet Gynaecol 100:898, 1993

American College of Obstetricians and Gynecologists: Vaginal birth after cesarean delivery. Practice Bulletin No. 54, July 2004

American College of Obstetricians and Gynecologists: Response to Searle's drug warning on misoprostol. Committee Opinion No. 248, December 2000

American College of Obstetricians and Gynecologists: Induction of labor. Practice Bulletin No. 10, November 1999a

American College of Obstetricians and Gynecologists: Induction of labor with misoprostol. Committee Opinion No. 228, November 1999b

American College of Obstetricians and Gynecologists: Dystocia and the augmentation of labor. Technical Bulletin No. 218, December 1995a

American College of Obstetricians and Gynecologists: Induction of labor. Technical Bulletin No. 217, December 1995b

American College of Obstetricians and Gynecologists: Dystocia. Technical Bulletin No. 137, December 1989

Arrabal PP, Nagey DA: Is manual palpation of uterine contractions accurate? Am J Obstet Gynecol 174:217, 1996

Arulkumaran S, Koh CH, Ingemarsson I, et al: Augmentation of labour—mode of delivery related to cervimetric progress. Aust N Z J Obstet Gynaecol 27:304, 1987

Bakos, O, Bäckström T: Induction of labor: A prospective, randomized study into amniotomy and oxytocin as induction methods in a total unselected population. Acta Obstet Gynecol Scand 66:537, 1987

Bennett KA, Crane JMG, O'Shea P, et al: First trimester ultrasound screening is effective in reducing postterm labor induction rates: A randomized controlled trial. Am J Obstet Gynecol 190:1077, 2004

Bernstein P: Prostaglandin E2 gel for cervical ripening and labour induction: A multi-centre placebo-controlled trial. Can Med Assoc J 145:1249, 1991

Bishop EH: Pelvic scoring for elective induction. Obstet Gynecol 24:266, 1964

Bland ES, Oppenheimer LW, Holmes, et al: The effect of income pooling within a call group on rates of obstetric intervention. Canadian Med Assoc J 164:337, 2001

Bolnick JM, Velazquez MD, Gonzalez JL, et al: Randomized trial between two active labor management protocols in the presence of an unfavorable cervix. Am J Obstet Gynecol 190:124, 2004

Boulvain M, Irion O, Marcoux S, et al: Sweeping of the membranes to prevent post-term pregnancy and to induce labour: A systematic review. Br J Obstet Gynaecol 106:481, 1999

Brindley BA, Sokol RJ: Induction and augmentation of labor. Basis and methods for current practice. Obstet Gynecol Surv 43:730, 1988

Bujold E, Blackwell SC, Gauthier RJ: Cervical ripening with transcervical foley catheter and the risk of uterine rupture. Obstet Gynecol 103:18, 2004

Buser D, Mora G, Arias F: A randomized comparison between misoprostol and dinoprostone for cervical ripening and labor induction in patients with unfavorable cervices. Obstet Gynecol 89:581, 1997

Caldeyro-Barcia R, Alvarez H, Reynolds SRM: A better understanding of uterine contractility through simultaneous recording with an internal and a seven channel external method. Surg Obstet Gynecol 91:641, 1950

Caldeyro-Barcia R, Poseiro JJ: Physiology of the uterine contraction. Clin Obstet Gynecol 3:386, 1960

Cammu H, Marten G, Ruyssinck G, et al: Outcome after elective labor induction in nulliparous women: A matched cohort study. Am J Obstet Gynecol 186:240, 2002

Chan LY, Fu L, Leung TN, et al: Obstetrical outcomes after cervical ripening by multiple doses of vaginal prostaglandin E2. Acta Obstet Gynecol Scand 83:70, 2004

Chyu JK, Strassner HT: Prostaglandin E2 for cervical ripening: A randomized comparison of Cervidil versus Prepidil. Am J Obstet Gynecol 177:606, 1997

Cole DS, Bruck LR: Anaphylaxis after laminaria insertion. Obstet Gynecol 95:1025, 2000

Culver J, Strauss RA, Brody S, et al: A randomized trial comparing vaginal misoprostol versus Foley catheter with concurrent oxytocin for labor induction in nulliparous women. Am J Perinatol 21:139, 2004

Doyle N, Ramin Su, Yeomans E, et al: Cesarean section: Community versus county hospital. Am J Obstet Gynecol 187:S110, 2002

DuVigneaud V, Ressler C, Swan JM, et al: The synthesis of oxytocin. J Am Chem Soc 75:4879, 1953

Flannelly GM, Turner MJ, Rassmussen MJ, et al: Rupture of the uterus in Dublin: An update. J Obstet Gynecol 13:440, 1993

Fraser W, Marcoux S, Moutquin JM, et al: Effect of early amniotomy on the risk of dystocia in nulliparous women. N Engl J Med 328:1145, 1993

Friedman EA: Primigravid labor: A graphicostatistical analysis. Obstet Gynecol 6:567, 1955

Frigoletto FD, Lieberman E, Lang JM, et al: A clinical trial of active management of labor. N Engl J Med 333:745, 1995

Garcia FAR, Miller HB, Huggins GR, et al: Effect of academic affiliation and obstetric volume on clinical outcome and cost of childbirth. Obstet Gynecol 97:567, 2001

Garite TJ, Porto M, Carlson NJ, et al: The influence of elective amniotomy on fetal heart rate patterns and the course of labor in term patients: A randomized study. Am J Obstet Gynecol 168:1827, 1993

Gemund N, Scherjon S, LeCessie S, et al: A randomized trial comparing low dose vaginal misoprostol and dinoprostone for labour induction. Br J Obstet Gynaecol 111:42, 2004

Gilson GJ, Russell DJ, Izquierdo LA, et al: A prospective randomized evaluation of a hygroscopic cervical dilator, Dilapan, in the preinduction ripening of patients undergoing induction of labor. Am J Obstet Gynecol 175:145, 1996

Goepfert A for the NICHD Maternal–Fetal Medicine Units Network: The MFMU cesarean registry: Infectious morbidity following primary cesarean section. Am J Obstet Gynecol 185:S192, 2001

Goldman JB, Wigton TR: A randomized comparison of extraamniotic saline infusion and intracervical dinoprostone gel for cervical ripening. Obstet Gynecol 93:271, 1999

Guinn DA, Goepfert AR, Christine M, et al: Extra-amniotic saline infusion, laminaria, or prostaglandin E2 gel for labor induction with unfavorable cervix: A randomized trial. Obstet Gynecol 96:106, 2000

Hale RW, Pion RJ: Laminaria: An underutilized clinical adjunct. Clin Obstet Gynecol 15:829, 1972

Hall R, Duarte-Gardea M, Harlass F: Oral versus vaginal misoprostol for labor induction. Obstet Gynecol 99:1044, 2002

Hamar B, Mann S, Greenberg P, et al: Low-risk inductions of labor and cesarean delivery for nulliparous and parous women at term. Am J Obstet Gynecol 185:S215, 2001

Hauth JC, Hankins GD, Gilstrap LC III: Uterine contraction pressures achieved in parturients with active phase arrest. Obstet Gynecol 78:344, 1991

Hauth JC, Hankins GD, Gilstrap LC III: Uterine contraction pressures with oxytocin induction/augmentation. Obstet Gynecol 68:305, 1986

Hemlin J, Möller B: Extraamniotic saline infusion is promising in preparing the cervix for induction of labor. Acta Obstet Gynecol Scand 77:45, 1998

Hoffman MK, Sciscione AC: Elective induction with cervical ripening increases the risk of cesarean delivery in multiparous women. Obstet Gynecol 101:7S, 2003

Hofmeyr GJ, Gülmezoglu AM, Alfirevic Z: Misoprostol for induction of labour: A systematic review. Br J Obstet Gynaecol 106:798, 1999

Huang W, Chung J, Rumney P, et al: A prospective, randomized controlled trial comparing misoprostol, Foley catheter, and combination misoprostol-Foley for labor induction. Am J Obstet Gynecol 187:S57, 2002

Kastner ES, Figueroa R, Garry D, et al: Emergency peripartum hysterectomy: Experience at a community teaching hospital. Obstet Gynecol 99:971, 2002

Kaufman K, Bailit J, Grobman W: Elective induction: An analysis of economic and health consequences. Am J Obstet Gynecol 185:S209, 2001

Lo JY, Alexander JM, McIntire DD, et al: Ruptured membranes at term: Randomized, double-blind trial of oral misoprostol for labor induction. Obstet Gynecol 101:685, 2003

López-Zeno JA, Peaceman AM, Adashek JA, et al: A controlled trial of a program for the active management of labor. N Engl J Med 326:450, 1992

Luthy DA, Malmgren JA, Zingheim RW: Increased cesarean section rates associated with elective induction in nulliparous women. Am J Obstet Gynecol 187:S106, 2002

Martin JA, Hamilton BE, Sutton PD, et al: Births: Final data for 2002. National Vital Statistics Reports, Vol 52, No. 10. Hyattsville, Md, National Center for Health Statistics, 2003

Maslow AS, Sweeny AL: Elective induction of labor as a risk factor for cesarean delivery among low-risk women at term. Obstet Gynecol 95:917, 2000

McColgin SW, Bennett WA, Roach H, et al: Parturitional factors associated with membrane stripping. Am J Obstet Gynecol 169:71, 1993

McColgin SW, Hampton HL, McCaul JF, et al: Stripping of membranes at term: Can it safely reduce the incidence of post-term pregnancy? Obstet Gynecol 76:678, 1990

Menticoglou SM, Hall FP: Routine induction of labour at 41 weeks gestation: Nonsensus consensus. Br J Obstet Gynaecol 109:485, 2002

Mercer BM, McNanley T, O'Brien JM, et al: Early versus late amniotomy for labor induction: A randomized trial. Am J Obstet Gynecol 173:1371, 1995

Merrill DC, Zlatnik FJ: Randomized, double-masked comparison of oxytocin dosage in induction and augmentation of labor. Obstet Gynecol 94:455, 1999

Miller AM, Rayburn WF, Smith CV: Patterns of uterine activity after intravaginal prostaglandin E2 during preinduction cervical ripening. Am J Obstet Gynecol 165:1006, 1991

Mozurkewich E, Horrocks J, Daley S, et al: The MisoPROM study: A multicenter randomized comparision of oral misoprostol and oxytocin for premature rupture of membranes at term. Am J Obstet Gynecol 189:1026, 2003

Mullin P, House M, Paul R, et al: A comparison of vaginally administered misoprostol with extra-amnio saline solution infusion for cervical ripening and labor induction. Am J Obstet Gynecol 187:847, 2002

Nguyen MT, Hoffman DR: Anaphylaxis to laminaria. J Allergy Clin Immunol 95:138, 1995

O'Driscoll K, Foley M, MacDonald D: Active management of labor as an alternative to cesarean section for dystocia. Obstet Gynecol 63:485, 1984

Owen J, Winkler CL, Harris BA, et al: A randomized, double-blind trial of prostaglandin E2 gel for cervical ripening and meta-analysis. Am J Obstet Gynecol 165:991, 1991

Pearson M, Hollier L, Shah A, et al: A randomized comparison of oral misoprostol versus intravenous oxytocin for induction of labor with term premature rupture of membranes. Am J Obstet Gynecol 187:S174, 2002

Perry MY, Leaphart WL: Randomized trial of intracervical versus posterior fornix dinoprostone for induction of labor. Obstet Gynecol 103:13, 2004

Plaut MM, Schwartz ML, Lubarsky SL: Uterine rupture associated with the use of misoprostol in the gravid patient with a previous cesarean section. Am J Obstet Gynecol 180:1535, 1999

Ramsey PS, Ogburn PL, Harris DY, et al: Effect of vaginal pH on efficacy of the dinoprostone gel for cervical ripening/labor induction. Am J Obstet Gynecol 187:843, 2002

Rayburn WF: Prostaglandin E2 gel for cervical ripening and induction of labor: A critical analysis. Am J Obstet Gynecol 160:529, 1989

Rayburn WF, Wapner RJ, Barss VA, et al: An intravaginal controlled-release prostaglandin E2 pessary for cervical ripening and initiation of labor at term. Obstet Gynecol 79:374, 1992

Rouse DJ, Owen J, Savage KG, et al: Active phase labor arrest: Revisiting the 2-hour minimum Obstet Gynecol 98:550, 2001

Rouse D, Owen J, Hauth JC: Criteria for failed labor induction: Prospective evaluation of a standardized protocol. Am J Obstet Gynecol 182:S132, 2000

Rouse DJ, Owen J, Hauth JC: Active-phase labor arrest: Oxytocin augmentation for at least 4 hours. Obstet Gynecol 93:323, 1999

Rouse DJ, McCullough C, Wren AL, et al: Active-phase labor arrest: A randomized trial of chorioamnion management. Obstet Gynecol 83:937, 1994

Sanchez-Ramos K, Bernstein S, Kaunitz AM: Expectant management versus labor induction for suspected fetal macrosomia: A systematic review. Obstet Gynecol 100:997, 2002a

Sanchez-Ramos L, Danner CJ, Delke I, et al: The effect of tablet moistening on labor induction with intravaginal misoprostol: A randomized trial. Obstet Gynecol 99:1080, 2002b

Sanchez-Ramos L, Kaunitz AM, Wears RL, et al: Misoprostol for cervical ripening and labor induction: A meta-analysis. Obstet Gynecol 89:633, 1997

Satin AJ, Leveno KJ, Sherman ML, et al: High-dose oxytocin: 20- versus 40-minute dosage interval. Obstet Gynecol 83:234, 1994

Satin AJ, Leveno KJ, Sherman ML, et al: High- versus low-dose oxytocin for labor stimulation. Obstet Gynecol 80:111, 1992

Savitz DA, Terry JW, Dole N, et al: Comparison of pregnancy dating by last menstrual period, ultrasound scanning, and their combination. Am J Obstet Gynecol 187:1660, 2002

Sciscione AC, McCullough H, Manley JS, et al: A prospective, randomized comparison of Foley catheter insertion versus intracervical prostaglandin E2 gel for preinduction cervical ripening. Am J Obstet Gynecol 180:55, 1999

Seitchik J, Amico J, Robinson AG, et al: Oxytocin augmentation of dysfunctional labor, 4. Oxytocin pharmacokinetics. Am J Obstet Gynecol 150:225, 1984

Shellhaas C for the NICHD MFMU Network: The MFMU cesarean registry: Cesarean hysterectomy—its indications, morbidities, and mortality. Am J Obstet Gynecol 185:S123, 2001

Sherman DJ, Frenkel E, Tovbin J, et al: Ripening of the unfavorable cervix with extraamniotic catheter balloon: Clinical experience and review. Obstet Gynecol Surv 51:621, 1996

Smith KM, Hoffman MK, Sciscione A: Elective induction of labor in nulliparous women increases the risk of cesarean delivery. Obstet Gynecol 101:45S, 2003

UK Amniotomy Group: A multicentre randomised trial of amniotomy in spontaneous first labour at term. Br J Obstet Gynaecol 101:307, 1994

van Gemund N, Scherjon S, LeCessie S, et al: A randomised trial comparing low dose vaginal misoprostol and dinoprostone for labour induction. BJOG 111:42, 2004

Vengalil SR, Guinn DA, Olabi NF, et al: A randomized trial of misoprostol and extra-amniotic saline infusion for cervical ripening and labor induction. Obstet Gynecol 91:774, 1998

Wen T, Beceir A, Xenakis E, et al: Is there a maximum effective dose of Pitocin? Am J Obstet Gynecol 185:S212, 2001

Williams MC, Tsibris JC, David G, et al: Dose variation that is associated with approximated one-quarter tablet doses of misoprostol. Am J Obstet Gynecol 187:615, 2002

Windrim R, Bennett K, Mundle W, et al: Oral administration of misoprostol for labor induction: A randomized controlled trial. Obstet Gynecol 89:392, 1997

Wing DA, Ham D, Paul RH: A comparison of orally administered misoprostol with vaginally administered misoprostol for cervical ripening and labor induction. Am J Obstet Gynecol 180:1155, 1999

Wing DA, Jones MM, Rahall A, et al: A comparison of misoprostol and prostaglandin E2 gel for preinduction cervical ripening and labor induction. Am J Obstet Gynecol 172:1804, 1995a

Wing DA, Lovett K, Paul RH: Disruption of prior uterine incision following misoprostol for labor induction in women with previous cesarean delivery. Obstet Gynecol 91:828, 1998

Wing DA, Park MR, Paul RH: A randomized comparison of oral and intravaginal misoprostol for labor induction. Obstet Gynecol 95:905, 2000

Wing DA, Rahall A, Jones MM, et al: Misoprostol: An effective agent for cervical ripening and labor induction. Am J Obstet Gynecol 172:1811, 1995b

Xenakis EMJ, Langer O, Piper JM, et al: Low-dose versus high-dose oxytocin augmentation of labor—a randomized trial. Am J Obstet Gynecol 173:1874, 1995

Yeast JD, Jones A, Poskin M: Induction of labor and the relationship to cesarean delivery: A review of 7001 consecutive inductions. Am J Obstet Gynecol 180:628, 1999

Zhang J, Troendle JF, Yancey MK: Reassessing the labor curve in nulliparous women. Am J Obstet Gynecol 187:824, 2002

23

Forceps Delivery and Vacuum Extraction

The precise incidence of operative vaginal delivery in the United States is unknown, but forceps or vacuum delivery was coded on the birth certificate as the method of delivery for 8 percent of the vaginal births in the United States in 2002 (Martin and colleagues, 2003). Although operative vaginal delivery is still taught in almost all residency programs, there is controversy surrounding this method of delivery (American College of Obstetricians and Gynecologists, 2000; Hankins and colleagues, 1999).

FORCEPS DELIVERY

True forceps were first devised in the late 16th or beginning of the 17th century. The reader is referred to the 19th and earlier editions of *Williams Obstetrics* regarding their history.

DESIGN OF FORCEPS. These instruments basically consist of two crossing branches. Each branch has four components: blade, shank, lock, and handle. Each blade has two curves. The *cephalic curve* conforms to the shape of the fetal head, and the *pelvic curve* corresponds more or less to the axis of the birth canal (Fig. 23–1). Some varieties are *fenestrated* or *pseudofenestrated* to permit a firmer hold on the fetal head.

The blades are connected to the handles by the *shanks,* which are either parallel as in Simpson forceps, or crossing as in Tucker–McLane forceps. The common method of articulation, the *English lock,* consists of a socket located on the shank at the junction with the handle, into which fits a socket similarly located on the opposite shank (Figs. 23–1 and 23–2). A *sliding lock* is used in some forceps, such as Kielland forceps (Fig. 23–3).

CLASSIFICATION OF FORCEPS DELIVERIES. A current classification (American College of Obstetricians and Gynecologists, 2000; American Academy of Pediatrics and American College of Obstetricians and Gynecologists, 2002) for forceps and vacuum operations is summarized in Table

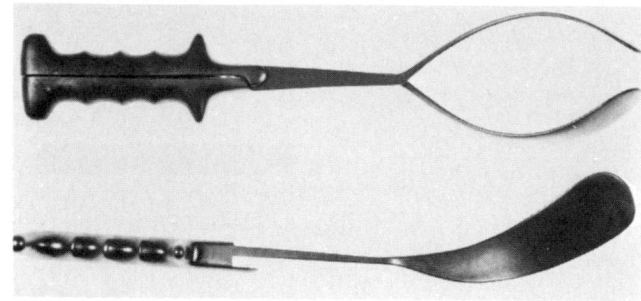

FIGURE 23–2. Tucker–McLane forceps. The blade is solid and the shank is narrow.

23–1. This classification emphasizes the two most important discriminators of risk for both mother and infant: station and rotation. Station is measured in 0 to 5 centimeters, although some clinicians prefer to divide the lower pelvis into thirds—1+, 2+, and 3+, corresponding to +2 cm, +4 cm, and +5 cm, respectively. Deliveries are categorized as outlet, low, and midpelvic procedures. High operations are those in which instruments are applied above 0 station, and thus before engagement. These have no place in contemporary obstetrics.

INCIDENCE OF FORCEPS DELIVERY. In general, there has been a decline in operative vaginal deliveries with a parallel increase in cesarean deliveries over the past two decades (DiMarco and associates, 2000). In a study from the United States National Hospital Discharge Survey, Kozak and Weeks (2002) reported that the cesarean delivery rate—expressed per 100 deliveries—had increased from 16.5 in 1980 to 22.9 in 2000. During this same time period, forceps delivery—expressed per 100 vaginal deliveries—had decreased from 17.7 to 4.0, while the vacuum delivery rate increased from 0.7 to 8.4. Chang and colleagues (2002) studied almost 20,000 deliveries from 1977 to 1999 and reported that the rate of forceps delivery decreased over time while the rate of vacuum delivery increased. These authors also evaluated the impact of gender of the attending physician on

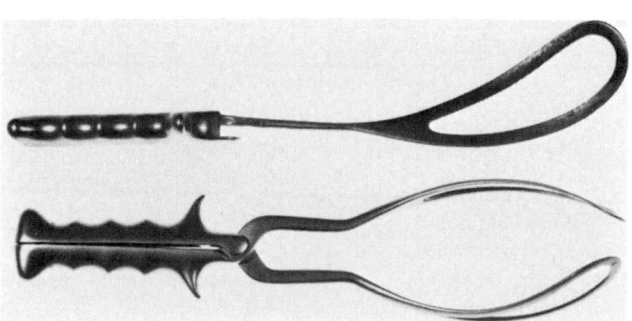

FIGURE 23–1. Simpson forceps. Note the ample pelvic curve in the single blade above and the cephalic curve evident in the articulated blades below. The fenestrated blade and the wide shank in front of the English-style lock characterize the Simpson forceps.

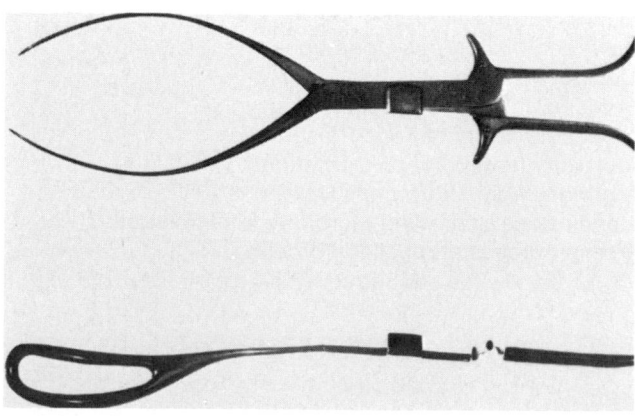

FIGURE 23–3. Kielland forceps. The characteristic features are the sliding lock, minimal pelvic curvature, and light weight.

TABLE 23–1 Classification of Forceps and Vacuum Delivery According to Station and Rotation

Procedure	Criteria
Outlet	1. Scalp is visible at introitus without separating the labia
	2. Fetal skull has reached pelvic floor
	3. Sagittal suture is in anteroposterior diameter or right or left occiput anterior or posterior position
	4. Fetal head is at or on the perineum
	5. Rotation does not exceed 45 degrees
Low	Leading point of fetal skull is at station $\geq$ +2 cm, and not on pelvic floor
	Rotation is 45 degrees or less (left or right occiput anterior to occiput anterior, or left or right occiput posterior to occiput posterior)
	Rotation is greater than 45 degrees
Midpelvic	Station above +2 cm but head is engaged
High	Not included in classification

From the American Academy of Pediatrics and the American College of Obstetricians and Gynecologists (2002).

operative vaginal delivery rates. The authors concluded that gender per se did not have a significant impact on either the forceps or vacuum delivery rate, when controlled for the year in which the procedure was performed.

TRAINING. In a survey of both residency and fellowship training programs by Hankins and colleagues (1999), it was found that residents are still taught operative vaginal delivery with forceps or vacuum, or both. For example, both residents and fellows were expected to be proficient with both instruments for outlet procedures. Importantly, fewer than half of the residency directors expected proficiency with midforceps delivery. Thus, although resident experience obviously varies among programs, it is doubtful that the majority of residents graduating today are adequately trained or skilled in the art of midpelvic delivery with either forceps or vacuum.

EFFECTS OF REGIONAL ANALGESIA ON INSTRUMENTAL DELIVERY.
Epidural analgesia may be associated with failure of spontaneous rotation to an occiput anterior position, as well as slowing of second-stage labor and decreasing maternal expulsive efforts. For example, Kaminski and associates (1987) documented persistent occiput posterior positions in 27 percent of women given epidural analgesia compared with only 8 percent of those not given epidural analgesia. A number of randomized studies have been performed at Parkland Hospital to ascertain the effects of labor analgesia. Five trials that included 2703 nulliparous women were recently analyzed by Sharma and colleagues (2004). Women given epidural analgesia had a twofold increased rate of forceps delivery compared with those given intravenous analgesia—13 versus 7 percent. Similarly, in their

meta-analysis of epidural versus opioid analgesia, Halpern and colleagues (1998) reported that women receiving epidural analgesia were twice as likely to have an instrumental delivery. Both studies are consistent with a comprehensive systematic review performed by Lieberman and O'Donoghue (2002).

FUNCTION OF FORCEPS. Although the most important function of forceps is traction, forceps may be invaluable for rotation, particularly for occiput transverse and posterior positions. In general, Simpson forceps are used to deliver the fetus with a molded head, as is common in nulliparous women. The Tucker–McLane instrument is often used for the fetus with a rounded head, which more characteristically is seen in multiparas. In most situations, however, either instrument is appropriate.

Forces Exerted by the Forceps. The force produced by the forceps on the fetal skull is a complex function of pull and compression by the forceps and friction produced by the maternal tissues. It is impossible to ascertain the amount of force exerted by forceps for an individual patient.

INDICATIONS FOR FORCEPS. Termination of the second stage of labor by forceps delivery or vacuum extraction is indicated in any condition threatening the mother or fetus that is likely to be relieved by delivery (American College of Obstetricians and Gynecologists, 2000). Some maternal indications include heart disease, pulmonary injury or compromise, intrapartum infection, certain neurological conditions, exhaustion, or prolonged second-stage labor. The latter is defined by the American College of Obstetricians and Gynecologists (2002) as more than 3 hours with, and more than 2 hours without, regional analgesia in the nulliparous woman. In the parous woman, a prolonged second stage is defined as more than 2 hours with, and more than 1 hour without, regional analgesia. Shortening of second-stage labor for maternal reasons should generally be accomplished with either outlet or low forceps. Fetal indications for operative vaginal delivery with either forceps or vacuum include prolapse of the umbilical cord, with the other requisites for instrument delivery present; premature separation of the placenta; or a nonreassuring fetal heart rate pattern.

Elective and Outlet Forceps. Forceps generally should not be used electively until the criteria for outlet forceps have been met. The fetal head must be on the perineal floor with the sagittal suture no more than 45 degrees from the anteroposterior diameter. In these circumstances, forceps delivery is a simple and safe operation (Carmona and colleagues, 1995; Hagadorn-Freathy and associates, 1991). Carmona and associates (1995) reported no differences in maternal or infant outcomes with term pregnancies randomized to spontaneous or elective outlet forceps delivery. There is, however,

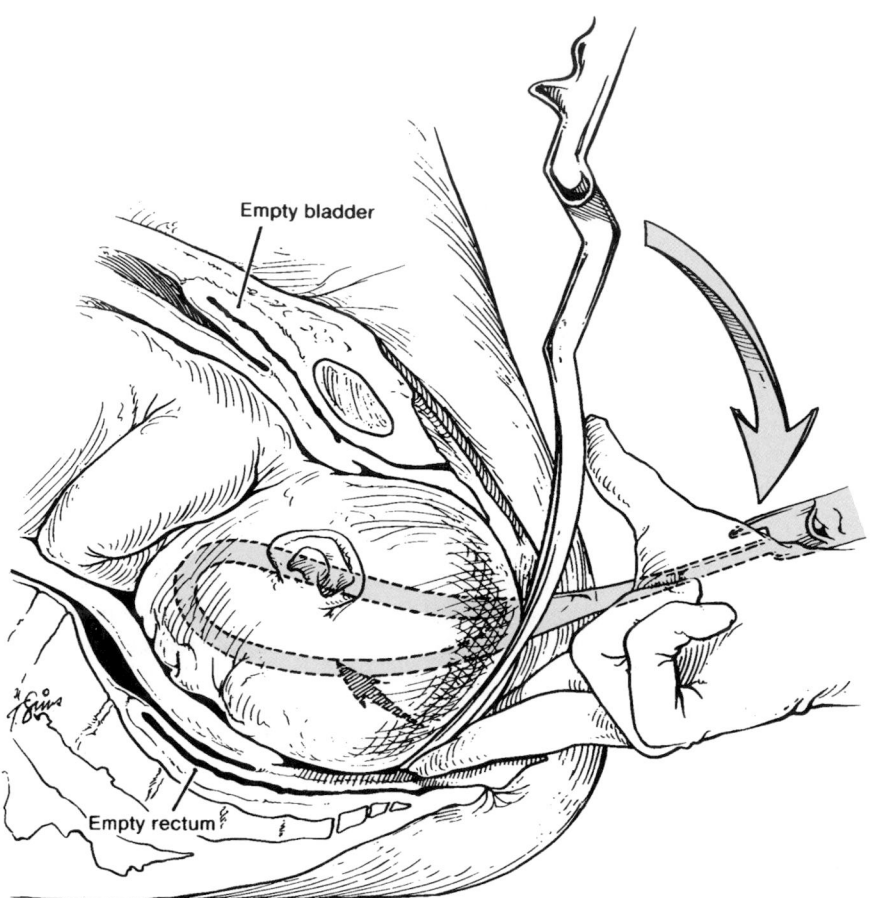

Empty bladder

Empty rectum

FIGURE 23-4. The fetus is presenting as vertex with occiput anterior crowning. The application of the left blade of the Simpson forceps is shown. Next, the right blade is applied and the blades are articulated.

no evidence that use of prophylactic forceps is beneficial in the otherwise normal term labor and delivery.

PROPHYLACTIC OUTLET FORCEPS FOR LOW-BIRTHWEIGHT FETUSES. Fairweather (1981) reported no significant differences in outcomes in neonates who weighed 500 to 1500 g and who were delivered spontaneously or by outlet forceps. Schwartz and colleagues (1983) reported similar findings. Currently, it would appear that there is no obvious advantage to routine outlet forceps delivery of a small fetus.

Prerequisites for Forceps Application. There are at least six prerequisites for successful application of forceps:

1. The head must be engaged. Extensive caput succedaneum formation and molding sometimes make determination of the station of the fetal head difficult. When difficulties of station assignment occur, it is important to realize that a "low-forceps" procedure may actually be a more difficult midforceps operation.
2. The fetus must present as a vertex or by the face with the chin anterior.
3. The position of the fetal head must be precisely known.
4. The cervix must be completely dilated.

5. The membranes must be ruptured.
6. There should be no suspected cephalic–pelvic disproportion.

PREPARATION FOR FORCEPS DELIVERY. Although pudendal block analgesia may prove adequate for outlet forceps operations, either regional analgesia or general anesthesia usually is preferred for low-forceps or midpelvic procedures. The bladder should be emptied.

Forceps Application. Forceps are constructed so that their cephalic curve is closely adapted to the sides of the fetal head (Fig. 23–4). The biparietal diameter of the fetal head corresponds to the greatest distance between the appropriately applied blades. Consequently, the head of the fetus is perfectly grasped only when the long axis of the blades corresponds to the occipitomental diameter. Thus, the major portion of the blade is lying over the face, while the concave margins of the blades are directed toward either the sagittal suture (occiput anterior position) or the face (occiput posterior position). Applied as such, the forceps should not slip, and traction may be applied most advantageously, as illustrated in Figure 23–5. With most forceps, if one blade is applied over the brow and the other over the occiput, the instrument cannot be

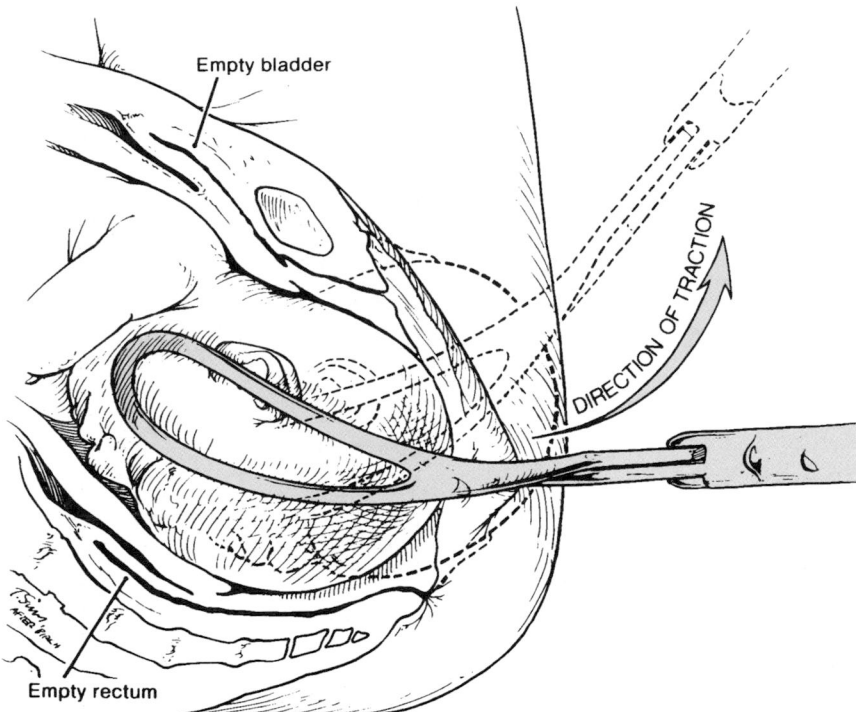

FIGURE 23–5. Occiput anterior. Delivery by outlet forceps (Simpson). The direction of gentle traction for delivery of the head is indicated.

locked, or if locked, the blades slip off when traction is applied (Fig. 23–6). For these reasons, the forceps must be applied directly to the sides of the fetal head along the occipitomental diameter.

Identification of Position. Knowledge of the exact position of the fetal head is essential to a proper cephalic application. With the head low in the pelvis, determination of position is made by examination of the sagittal suture and the fontanels. When the head is at a higher station, an absolute determination can be made by locating the posterior ear.

OUTLET FORCEPS DELIVERY. Delivery by outlet forceps of the occiput anterior fetal head is illustrated in Figures 23–7 through 23–13. In such circumstances, the small (posterior) fontanel is directed toward the symphysis pubis. The

forceps, if applied to the sides of the pelvis, grasp the head ideally. The forceps are applied as follows: Two or more fingers of the right hand are introduced inside the left posterior portion of the vulva and into the vagina beside the fetal head. The handle of the left branch is then grasped between the thumb and two fingers of the left hand and the tip of the blade is gently

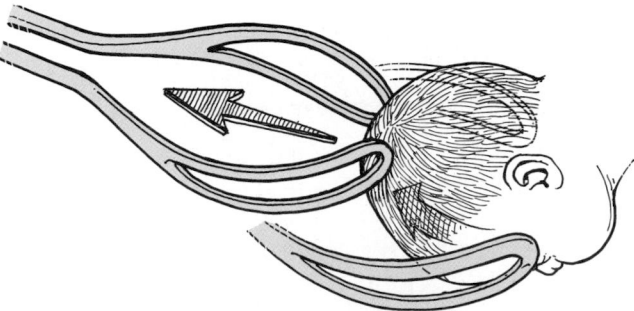

FIGURE 23–6. Incorrect application of forceps, one blade over the occiput and the other over the brow. Forceps cannot be locked and the head is extended with tendency of blades to slip off with traction.

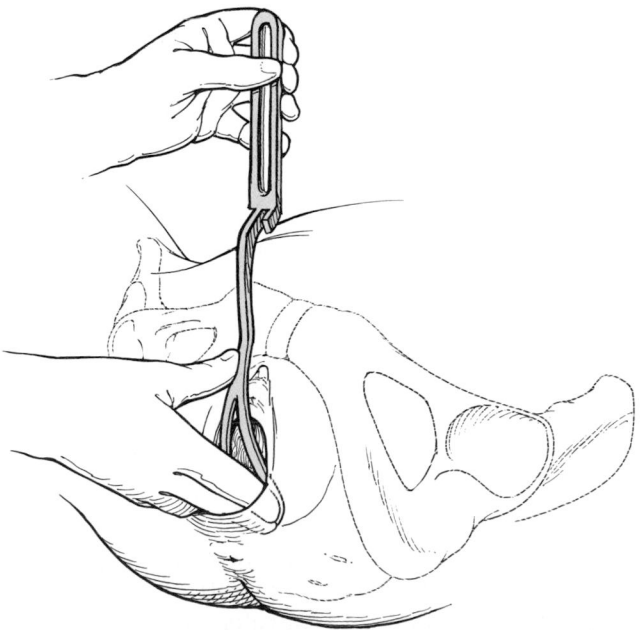

FIGURE 23–7. The left handle of the Simpson forceps is held in the left hand. The blade is introduced into the left side of the pelvis between the fetal head and fingers of the operator's right hand.

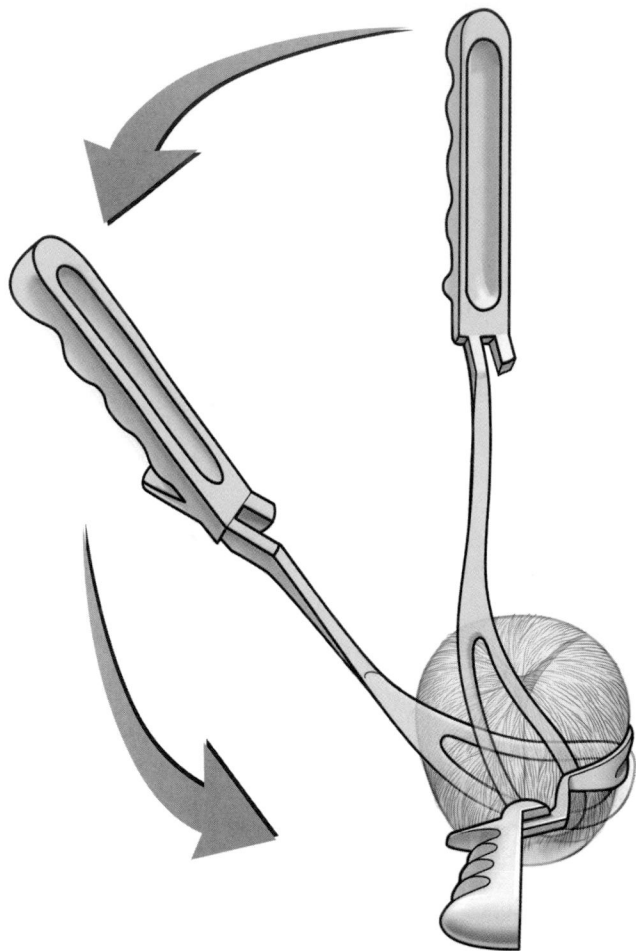

FIGURE 23–8. Continued insertion of left blade. Note the arc of the handles as they rotate to be applied to the mother's left.

passed into the vagina between the fetal head and the palmar surface of the fingers of the right hand (Figs. 23–7 and 23–8). For application of the right blade, two or more fingers of the left hand are introduced into the right, posterior portion of the vagina to serve as a guide for the right blade, which is held in the right hand and introduced into the vagina as described for the left blade. After positioning, the branches are articulated.

Appropriateness of Application. For the occiput anterior position, appropriately applied blades are equidistant from the sagittal suture. In the occiput posterior position, the blades are equidistant from the midline of the face and brow.

Traction. When it is certain that the blades are placed satisfactorily, then gentle, intermittent, horizontal traction is exerted until the perineum begins to bulge. If necessary, rotation to occiput anterior is performed before traction is applied (Figs. 23–9 and 23–10). With traction, as the vulva is distended by the occiput, an episiotomy may be performed if indicated (Fig. 23–11).

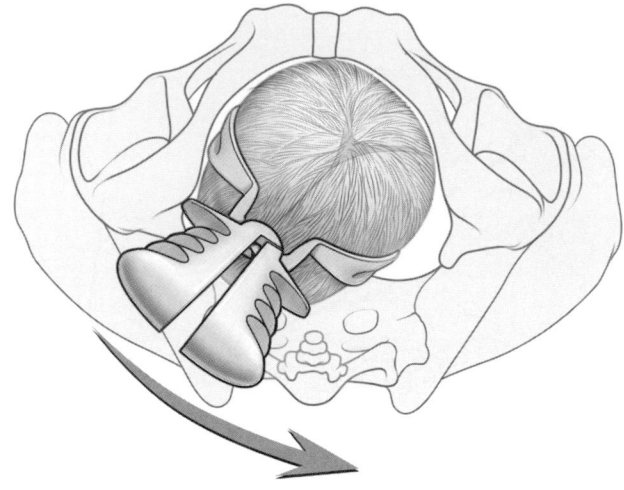

FIGURE 23–9. Forceps have been locked. Vertex is rotated from left occiput anterior to occiput anterior (*arrow*).

More horizontal traction is applied, and the handles are gradually elevated, eventually pointing almost directly upward as the parietal bones emerge (Fig. 23–12). As the handles are raised, the head is extended. During upward traction, the four fingers should grasp the upper surface of the handles and shanks, while the thumb exerts the necessary force on their lower surface. During the birth of the head, spontaneous delivery should be simulated as closely as possible. Traction should therefore be intermittent, and the head should be allowed to recede in intervals, as in spontaneous labor. Except when urgently indicated, as in severe fetal bradycardia, delivery should be sufficiently slow, deliberate, and gentle to prevent undue head compression. It is preferable to apply traction only with each uterine contraction.

After the vulva has been well distended by the head, the delivery may be completed in several ways. Some clinicians keep the forceps in place to control the advance of the head. However, the thickness of the blades adds to the distention of the vulva, thus increasing the likelihood of laceration or

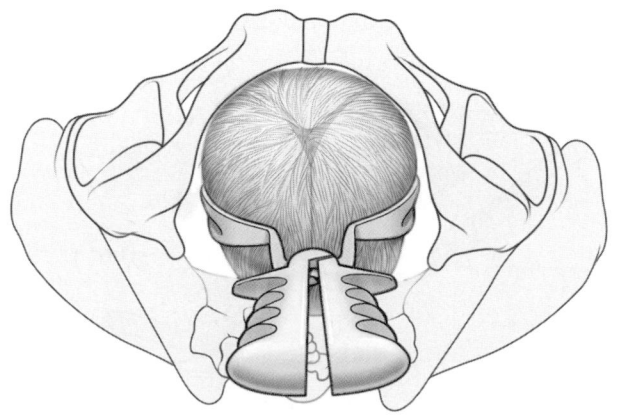

FIGURE 23–10. The vertex is now occiput anterior and the forceps are symmetrically placed and articulated.

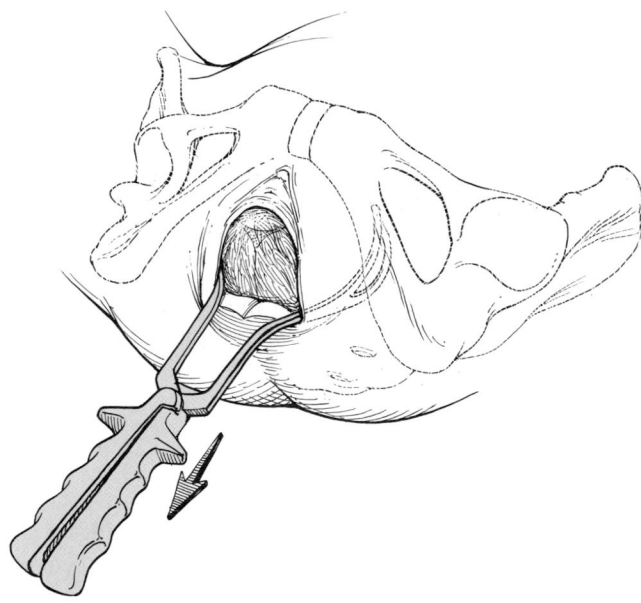

FIGURE 23–11. Horizontal traction.

necessitating a large episiotomy. In such cases, the forceps may be removed and delivery completed by the modified Ritgen maneuver (Fig. 23–13). If the forceps are removed prematurely, the modified Ritgen maneuver may prove to be a tedious and inelegant procedure.

LOW- AND MIDFORCEPS OPERATIONS. When the head lies above the perineum, the sagittal suture usually occupies an oblique or transverse diameter of the pelvis. In such

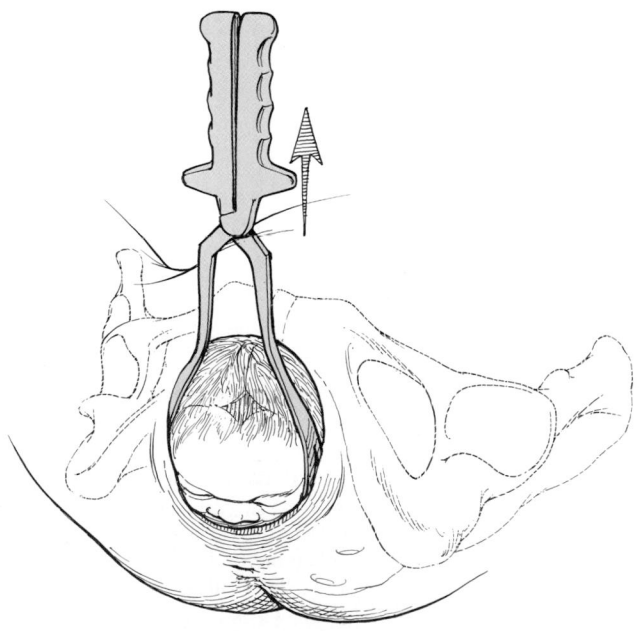

FIGURE 23–12. Upward traction (*arrow*) is applied as the head is delivered. Forceps may be disarticulated after head is delivered.

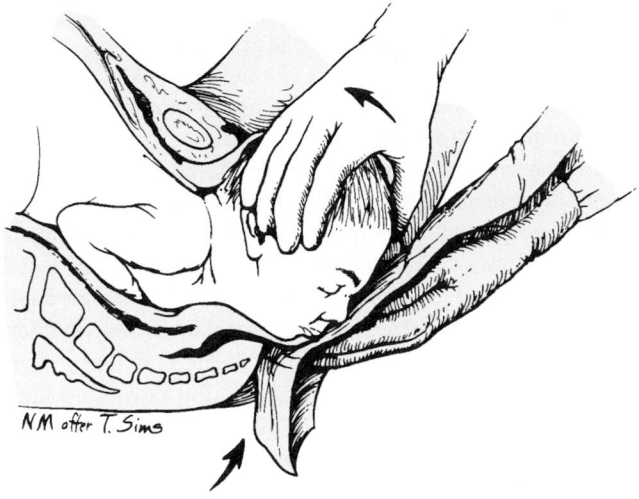

FIGURE 23–13. Forceps have been disarticulated and removed, and modified Ritgen maneuver (*arrow*) is used to complete delivery of the head.

cases, the forceps should always be applied to the sides of the head.

Left Occiput Anterior Position. The right hand, introduced into the left posterior segment of the vagina, should identify the posteriorly located left ear. At the same time, the right hand serves as a guide for introduction of the left branch of the forceps, which is held in the left hand and applied over the left ear. Two fingers of the left hand are then introduced into the right posterior portion of the pelvis.

The right branch of the forceps, held in the right hand, is then introduced along the left hand as a guide. It must then be applied over the anterior ear of the fetus by gently sweeping the blade anteriorly until it lies directly opposite the blade that was introduced first.

Right Occiput Anterior Position. In right positions, the blades are introduced similarly but in opposite directions. After the blades have been applied to the sides of the head, the left handle and shank lie above the right. Consequently, the forceps do not immediately articulate. Locking of the branches is easily effected, however, by rotating the left around the right to bring the lock into proper position.

Occiput Transverse Positions. If the occiput is in a transverse position, the forceps are introduced similarly, with the first blade applied over the posterior ear and the second rotated anteriorly to a position opposite the first. In this case, one blade lies in front of the sacrum and the other behind the symphysis. Simpson or Tucker–McLane forceps (see Figs. 23–1 and 23–2), or one of their modifications, or the specialized Kielland forceps (see Fig. 23–3) may be used.

Rotation from Anterior and Transverse Positions. When the occiput is obliquely anterior, it gradually rotates spontaneously to the symphysis pubis as traction is exerted. When it is directly transverse, however, a rotary motion of the forceps is required. Rotation counterclockwise from the left side toward the midline is required when the occiput is directed toward the left, and in the reverse direction when it is directed toward the right side of the pelvis. Infrequently, when forceps are used in transverse positions in anteroposteriorly flattened (platypelloid) pelves, rotation should not be attempted until the fetal head has reached or approached the pelvic floor. Regardless of the original position of the head, delivery eventually is accomplished by exerting traction downward until the occiput appears at the vulva. After this, the rest of the operation is completed as previously described.

OCCIPUT POSTERIOR POSITIONS. Prompt delivery may at times become necessary when the small (occipital) fontanel is directed toward one of the sacroiliac synchondroses, viz., in right occiput posterior or left occiput posterior positions. When delivery is required in either instance, the head is often imperfectly flexed. In some cases, when the hand is introduced into the vagina to locate the posterior ear, the occiput rotates spontaneously toward the anterior, indicating that manual rotation of the fetal head might easily be accomplished.

Manual Rotation. A hand with the palm upward is inserted into the vagina and the fingers are brought in contact with the side of the fetal head that is to be rotated toward the anterior position, while the thumb is placed over the opposite side of the head. With the occiput in a right posterior position, the left hand is used to rotate the occiput anteriorly in a clockwise direction; the right hand is used for the left occiput posterior position. The head must not be disengaged during rotation.

After the occiput has reached the anterior position, labor may be allowed to continue, or forceps can be used. First one blade is applied to that side of the head that is held by the fingers that are maintaining the occiput in the anterior position. The other blade is immediately applied and delivery accomplished.

Forceps Delivery of Occiput Posterior. If manual rotation cannot be easily accomplished, application of the blades to the head in the posterior position and delivery from the occiput posterior position may be the safest procedure (Fig. 23–14). In many cases, the cause of the persistent occiput posterior position and of the difficulty in accomplishing rotation is an anthropoid pelvis, the architecture of which predisposes to posterior delivery and opposes rotation. When the occiput is directly posterior, horizontal traction should be applied until the base of the nose is under the symphysis. The handles should then be slowly elevated until the occiput gradually emerges over the anterior margin of the perineum. Then, the forceps are directed in a downward motion, and the nose, face, and chin successively emerge from the vulva.

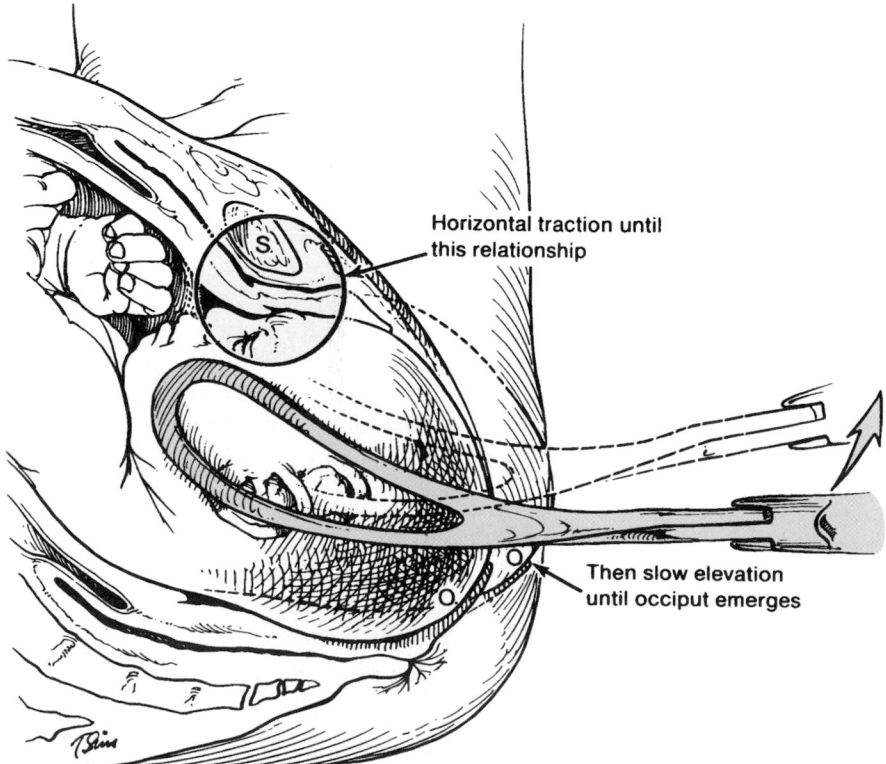

Horizontal traction until this relationship

Then slow elevation until occiput emerges

FIGURE 23–14. Occiput directly posterior. Low forceps (Simpson) delivery as an occiput posterior. (O = occiput, S = symphysis.) The *arrow* illustrates the point at which time the head should be flexed after the bregma passes under the symphysis. It is evident that to prevent serious perineal lacerations, an extensive episiotomy is most often required.

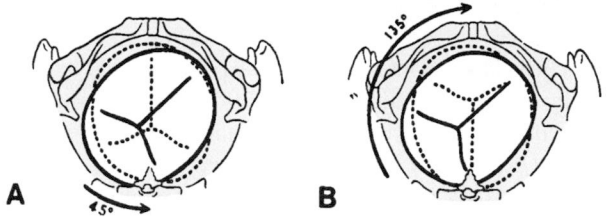

FIGURE 23–15. Rotation of obliquely posterior occiput to sacrum **(A)** and symphysis pubis **(B)**.

Occiput posterior delivery causes greater distention of the vulva, and a large episiotomy may be needed. Pearl and associates (1993) retrospectively reviewed 564 occiput posterior deliveries. These were compared with 1068 controls. The occiput posterior group had a higher incidence of severe perineal lacerations and extensive episiotomy compared with that of the occiput anterior group. Within the occiput posterior group, operative delivery was associated with a higher incidence of severe perineal lacerations (35 versus 16 percent), vaginal lacerations (18 versus 7 percent), and episiotomy (95 versus 74 percent) than was spontaneous delivery. Consequences of these perineal tears are discussed in Chapter 17 (see p. 435). The infants delivered from the occiput posterior position had a higher incidence of Erb (1 percent) and facial nerve (2 percent) palsies than did those delivered from the occiput anterior position.

Forceps Rotations of Occiput Oblique Posterior. Tucker–McLane, Simpson, or Kielland forceps may be used to rotate the fetal head. The oblique occiput may be rotated 45 degrees to the posterior position or 135 degrees to the anterior position (Fig. 23–15). If rotation is performed with Tucker–McLane or Simpson forceps, the head must be flexed, but this is not necessary with Kielland forceps because they have a more straightened pelvic curve. In rotating the occiput anteriorly with Tucker–McLane or Simpson forceps, the pelvic curvature, originally directed upward, at the completion of rotation is inverted and directed posteriorly. Attempted delivery with the instrument in that position is likely to cause vaginal sulcus tears and sidewall lacerations. To avoid such trauma, it is essential to remove and reapply the instrument as described below.

FORCEPS ROTATION OF OCCIPUT TRANSVERSE.
Specialized skill and training are essential when performing this technically difficult operative vaginal procedure. Either standard forceps, such as pseudofenestrated Simpson, or specialized forceps, such as Kielland, are employed. The latter have a sliding lock and almost no pelvic curve (see Fig. 23–3). On each handle is a small knob that indicates the direction of the occiput. The station of the fetal head must be accurately ascertained to be at, or preferably below, the level of the ischial spines, especially in the presence of extreme molding.

Kielland described two methods of applying the anterior blade. In the *wandering* or *gliding* method, the anterior blade is introduced at the side of the pelvis over the brow or face. The blade is then arched around the brow or face to an anterior position, with the handle of the blade held close to the opposite maternal buttock throughout the maneuver. The second blade is introduced posteriorly and the branches are locked. The second method is the *direct* or *classical* application, in which the anterior blade is introduced first with its cephalic curve directed upward, curving under the symphysis. After it has entered sufficiently far into the uterine cavity, it is turned on its axis through 180 degrees to adapt the cephalic curvature to the head. The reader is referred to the second edition of *Operative Obstetrics* (Gilstrap, 2002) for a more detailed description of the technical aspects of Kielland forceps procedures.

FORCEPS DELIVERY OF FACE PRESENTATION.
In the face presentation, with the chin directed toward the symphysis—mentum anterior—forceps occasionally are used to effect vaginal delivery. The blades are applied to the sides of the head along the occipitomental diameter, with the pelvic curve directed toward the neck. Downward traction is exerted until the chin appears under the symphysis. Then, by an upward movement, the face is slowly extracted, with the nose, eyes, brow, and occiput appearing in succession over the anterior margin of the perineum (Fig. 23–16). Forceps should not be applied to the mentum posterior presentation, because vaginal delivery is impossible as such.

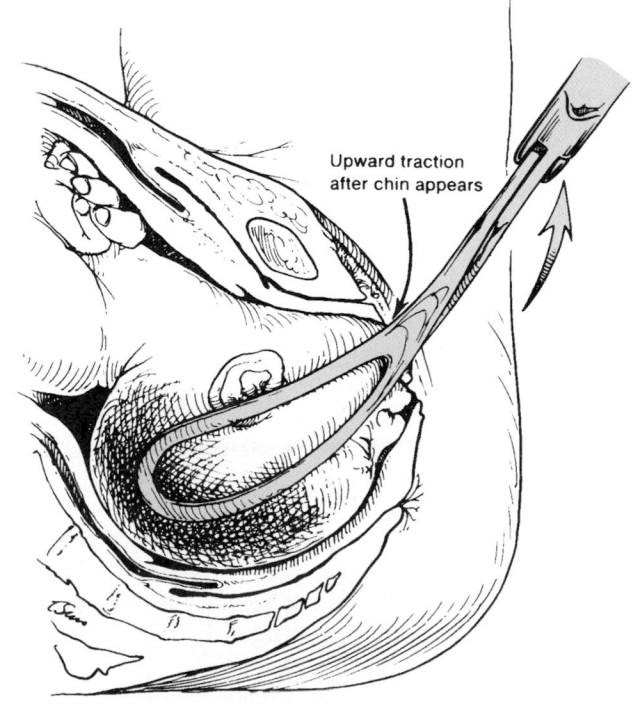

Upward traction after chin appears

FIGURE 23–16. Face presentation, mentum (chin) anterior. Delivery with outlet forceps (Simpson).

MORBIDITY FROM FORCEPS OPERATIONS

Maternal Morbidity. When considering maternal morbidity from operative vaginal delivery, it is important to compare it with the morbidity from cesarean delivery and not to that from spontaneous vaginal delivery. Some generalizations can be made:

1. Elective outlet forceps with rotations not exceeding 45 degrees are associated with little, if any, increase in maternal morbidity (Carmona and colleagues, 1995).
2. Maternal injury increases significantly with rotations of greater than 45 degrees and at higher stations (Hagadorn-Freathy and associates, 1991; Hankins and Rowe, 1996).
3. The need for blood transfusions is increased with operative vaginal delivery, viz., vacuum extraction (6.1 percent) and forceps (4.2 percent), compared with 1.4 percent with uncomplicated cesarean delivery (Sherman and co-workers, 1993).

LACERATIONS AND EPISIOTOMY. The very conditions that lead to the indications for operative vaginal delivery also increase the need for episiotomy. That said, women randomized to delivery with low forceps had no increase in perineal lacerations relative to those delivering spontaneously (Carmona and colleagues, 1995). Conversely, in a retrospective study of over 2 million vaginal deliveries, Handa and colleagues (2001) found a strong association between anal sphincter laceration and operative vaginal delivery. Hagadorn-Freathy and co-workers (1991) reported rates for third- and fourth-degree episiotomy extensions and vaginal lacerations of 13 percent for outlet forceps, 22 percent for low forceps with less than 45 degrees rotation, 44 percent for low forceps with more than 45 degrees rotation, and 37 percent for midforceps deliveries. Similarly, Bofill and colleagues (1996a, 1996b) found a significant association of moderate and severe perineal injuries with indicated operative deliveries, use of forceps versus vacuum extractor, the need for episiotomy, and delivery from other than outlet station.

Robinson and colleagues (1999) studied perineal trauma in 323 women delivered with forceps or vacuum extraction. The incidence of perineal trauma associated with the combination of episiotomy and forceps delivery was not significantly higher than that with forceps delivery alone—46 versus 55 percent, respectively. Vacuum extraction, however, significantly increased such trauma—35 versus 9 percent—with and without episiotomy, respectively. Others report less perineal trauma with the vacuum extractor. Specifically, Low and co-workers (1993) reported vaginal lacerations in 4.3 percent and fourth-degree episiotomy extensions in 1.6 percent of women undergoing vacuum delivery. Loghis and co-workers (1992) reported anal sphincter involvement in 3 percent of vacuum deliveries and vaginal vault extensions in 2.5 percent.

Ecker and colleagues (1997) reported a significant decrease in the episiotomy rate over a 10-year period from 1984 to 1994 for both forceps (96 to 30 percent) and vac-

uum deliveries (89 to 39 percent). During the same time period, there was a decrease in fourth-degree but no change in third-degree lacerations. In a review of over 34,000 vaginal births by Goldberg and colleagues (2002), episiotomy rates decreased significantly from 70 percent in 1983 to 19 percent in 2000. Forceps deliveries, however, were associated with higher episiotomy rates as well as third- and fourth-degree lacerations compared with those of spontaneous delivery.

URINARY AND RECTAL INCONTINENCE. There are a now a number of studies that indicate that even spontaneous vaginal delivery will be followed by urinary and fecal incontinence in some women. In some, incontinence is temporary and improves with time. In others, it persists and may worsen over time. Extensive episiotomies or lacerations, especially of the anal sphincter, are more likely to cause problems with incontinence than spontaneous vaginal delivery alone (Pollack and associates, 2004; Pregazzi and colleagues, 2002). Because forceps deliveries are associated with an increased incidence of episiotomy, episiotomy with second- or third-degree extension, or deep lacerations, it is not surprising that use of forceps has been associated in some reports with a higher rate of incontinence (Eason and colleagues, 2002; Fitzpatrick and colleagues, 2003; Viktrup and Lose, 2001). Thus, the anterior compartment (responsible for bladder function) or the posterior compartment (responsible for anal function) or both may be involved.

Short-term effects of forceps and vacuum deliveries, especially midcavity deliveries, include postpartum urinary retention and bladder dysfunction (Carley and coworkers, 2002). Arya and colleagues (2001) reported that incontinence after forceps delivery was more likely to persist than incontinence associated with vacuum or spontaneous delivery.

Anal sphincter dysfunction, although associated with spontaneous delivery, also is increased with instrumental vaginal delivery, episiotomy extensions, and deep lacerations. Specifically, Eason and colleagues (2000, 2002) evaluated 949 Canadian women 3 months after delivery. Three percent had fecal incontinence, over one fourth had incontinence of flatus, and both were more common in women who had had anal sphincter injuries and forceps delivery. Sultan and colleagues (1993) reported defecatory symptoms in 38 percent of women after forceps delivery, 12 percent following vacuum delivery, and 4 percent delivered spontaneously with either a mediolateral episiotomy or second-degree lacerations. In another study, Sultan and co-workers (1994) reported that half of women who had third-degree tears had anal incontinence or fecal urgency. Endosonographic sphincter defects were seen in 85 percent of those who had a third-degree tear compared with one third of control women without a sphincter tear. In a French study, de Parades and colleagues (2004) identified sonographic sphincter defects in only 13 percent of women with or without an episiotomy or laceration following forceps delivery. Muscle injury is responsible for most anal dysfunction, however, pudendal nerve damage also plays a role (Tetzschner and colleagues, 1998).

Although the short-term effects on anorectal function associated with operative vaginal delivery are of concern, it is unclear what role these have in long-term morbidity. For example, in a 34-year follow-up after forceps delivery, Bollard and colleagues (2003) reported that significant fecal and urinary incontinence was not associated with forceps delivery. In a follow-up of primiparous women 3 to 4 years after delivery, Schraffordt Koops and colleagues (2003) found no difference in fecal incontinence according to the method of vaginal delivery—"normal," forceps, or vacuum. Rieger and associates (1997) documented anal sphincter dysfunction in women following spontaneous delivery. Peschers and colleagues (2003) found that both urinary and anal incontinence symptoms were common after vaginal delivery, occurring in 28 to 42 percent of women, but that vacuum delivery did not increase the risk above that of spontaneous vaginal delivery.

Other factors have been associated with fecal incontinence in older women. Some of these are high parity, menopause, prior hysterectomy, and irritable bowel syndrome (Donnelly and colleagues, 1998; Jackson and associates, 1997). In a 30-year follow-up study, Nygaard and co-workers (1997) documented incontinence of flatus in 31, 43, and 36 percent of women who had experienced a disrupted sphincter, an episiotomy, or cesarean delivery, respectively. Several other investigators have documented sphincter dysfunction in women undergoing cesarean delivery (Fynes and co-workers, 1998; MacArthur and colleagues, 1997).

FEBRILE MORBIDITY. Postpartum metritis is more frequent, and often more severe, in women following cesarean delivery compared with that following operative vaginal delivery (Robertson and colleagues, 1990).

Perinatal Morbidity. Operative vaginal delivery, especially if performed from the midpelvic level, may be associated with increased neonatal morbidity (Table 23–2). Towner and colleagues (1999) studied 583,340 term nulliparous women delivered in California between 1992 and 1994. The third delivered by cesarean, forceps, or vacuum were compared with those delivered spontaneously (Table 23–3). The incidence of intracranial hemorrhage was highest in infants delivered by vacuum, forceps, or cesarean after labor had started. These investigators concluded that abnormal labor was the common risk factor.

White and associates (1996) found a significant association of facial nerve palsy with forceps delivery compared with that following spontaneous or cesarean delivery. Gilbert and co-workers (1999), using the same California data cited above, found that delivery with forceps (3.4-fold) or vacuum (2.7-fold) significantly increased the risk for brachial plexus injury compared with that of spontaneous delivery.

TABLE 23–2 Neonatal Complications with Vacuum and Forceps Delivery

Complications	Method of Delivery	
	Vacuum n = 41 (%)	Forceps n = 40 (%)
Apgar scores		
1 min < 7	4 (10)	4 (10)
5 min < 8	1 (2)	1 (2)
Cephalohematoma		
Mild	6 (15)	3 (10)
Moderate	1 (2)	2 (7)
Caput	14 (34)	7 (14)
Facial mark or injury	1 (2)	7 (18)[a]
Trauma		
Erb palsy (mild)	1 (2)	0
Fractured clavicle	1 (2)	0
Elevated bilirubin	8 (20)	4 (10)
Retinal hemorrhage		
Mild	6/37 (16)	3/36 (8)
Moderate or severe	8/37 (37)	3/36 (8)
Infant stay	3.4 days	3.1 days

[a]Significant difference between rates for vacuum and forceps deliveries.
From Williams and colleagues (1991), with permission.

MORBIDITY FROM MIDFORCEPS DELIVERIES. Numerous studies have described the association of neonatal morbidity and midforceps operations. Several factors must be considered when interpreting these results. First and foremost, most were conducted prior to the redefined classification of forceps in 1988 by the American College of Obstetricians and Gynecologists (2000). Thus, midforceps were not defined clearly and included deliveries from relatively high stations (0 to +1), as well as difficult rotations. Second, spontaneous vaginal deliveries are not appropriate controls for midforceps. Finally, there is no uniformity in the criteria used to define immediate fetal morbidity.

There are a few studies that used the updated 1988 classification. Specifically, Robertson and associates (1990) reported significantly higher neonatal morbidity in the midforceps group compared with that of cesarean delivery.

Hagadorn-Freathy and colleagues (1991) designed a prospective investigation to test the validity of the 1988

TABLE 23–3 Effect of Method of Delivery on Incidence of Neonatal Intracranial Hemorrhage (ICH)

Delivery	ICH
Vacuum and forceps	1 : 280
Forceps	1 : 664
Vacuum	1 : 860
Cesarean with labor	1 : 907
Spontaneous	1 : 1900
Cesarean without labor	1 : 2040

Data from Towner and colleagues (1999).

classification on stratifying fetal risk. They classified 357 forceps deliveries by both the old and new systems and compared outcomes. One example was that facial nerve palsy developed in 1.3 percent of infants delivered by outlet forceps and 3.2 percent of those delivered by midforceps using the 1965 classification. This compared with rates of 0.9 percent for outlet forceps, 1.7 percent for low forceps, and 9.2 percent for midforceps using the 1988 classification. Thus, the 1988 classification can be used to usefully discriminate among the risks associated with outlet, low-, and midpelvic forceps deliveries. Because of increased maternal and neonatal morbidity compared with that of low-forceps operations, midforceps deliveries are seldom performed now.

Long-Term Infant Morbidity. Over decades of their use, forceps have been at the center of an evolving controversy regarding possible long-term infant morbidity. Particularly controversial has been the possible association between forceps delivery and decreased measures of intelligence. Some of the early studies used data from the Collaborative Perinatal Project. In one, Broman and co-workers (1975) controlled for socioeconomic status, race, and gender. They reported that infants delivered by midforceps had slightly higher intelligence scores at 4 years of age compared with those of children delivered spontaneously. Using the same database, Friedman and associates (1977, 1984), analyzed intelligence assessments at no less than 7 years of age. They concluded that children delivered by midforceps had lower mean intelligence quotients (IQs) compared with children delivered by outlet forceps. In yet another report from this same database, Dierker and colleagues (1986) compared long-term outcomes of children delivered by midforceps with those of children delivered by cesarean after dystocia. Clearly, this is the most appropriate control group. The investigators reported that neurodevelopmental disability was not associated with delivery by midforceps.

There are other studies concerning long-term morbidity of midforceps deliveries. In one, Nilsen (1984) evaluated 18-year-old men when they were drafted into the Norwegian Army. The study found that those delivered by Kielland forceps had higher intelligence scores than those delivered spontaneously, by vacuum extraction, or by cesarean. Similar data reported by Seidman and colleagues (1991) from more than 52,000 Israeli Defense Forces draftees are shown in Table 23–4. In a collaborative study of over 3000 school-aged children, Wesley and colleagues (1992) found no significant differences in standardized intelligence scores at age 5 years according to the method of delivery. Assessment included 1746 children delivered spontaneously, 1192 children delivered by either low- or midforceps or vacuum operations, and 114 delivered by midforceps or vacuum extraction.

CONCLUSIONS REGARDING MORBIDITY FROM FORCEPS. It is clear that the greatest risk is incurred with true midforceps operations and when rotations of greater than

TABLE 23–4 Intelligence Test Scores at Age 17 for Subjects Born in Jerusalem Between 1964 and 1970

Type of Delivery	Mean Intelligence Score ($\pm$ SE)	
	Unadjusted	*Adjusted*[a]
Spontaneous (n = 29,136)	105.4 (0.1)	105.7 (0.1)
Forceps (n = 567)	108.2[b] (0.7)	104.6 (0.4)
Vacuum extraction (n = 1207)	109.6[b] (0.5)	105.9 (0.4)
Cesarean delivery (n = 1335)	105.4 (0.4)	103.7[b] (0.1)

SE = Standard error.
[a] Adjusted by multiple regression for confounding effects of sex, birthweight, ethnic origin, birth order, maternal age, and paternal and maternal education and social class.
[b] $p < .0001$ compared with spontaneous delivery.
From Seidman and associates (1991), with permission.

45 degrees are performed. Most studies in which morbid events were reported were from an era when cesarean delivery rates were still around 5 percent. Thus, they undoubtedly included many forceps deliveries that would, in all likelihood, never be attempted today.

The impact of epidural analgesia on the incidence of low- and midforceps deliveries cannot be discounted (Lieberman and O'Donoghue, 2002). The majority of such cases result from inadequate maternal expulsive forces against a relaxed pelvic sling, and thus they are not usually associated with either relative or absolute cephalopelvic disproportion.

Although it is prudent in these cases to allow a longer second stage of labor, in some women and under some circumstances, delivery is indicated sooner. Low-forceps rotations for epidural-associated labor abnormalities are likely to be safer than the same operation performed in women with prolonged labor or midpelvic arrest unassociated with conduction analgesia.

It seems reasonable to conclude that outlet and low-forceps operations with rotation of 45 degrees or less, classified by the scheme proposed by the American College of Obstetricians and Gynecologists (2000), can be performed with safety for both mother and fetus if the basic guidelines set forth in this chapter are carefully observed.

TRIAL OF FORCEPS AND FAILED FORCEPS. If an attempt at operative vaginal delivery is anticipated to be difficult, the attempt should be considered a trial. With an operating room both equipped and staffed for immediate cesarean delivery, the trial may proceed. If a satisfactory application of the forceps cannot be achieved, then the procedure is abandoned and delivery accomplished by use of either vacuum extraction or cesarean. Once application has been achieved, gentle downward pulls are made on the forceps. If there is no descent, the procedure is abandoned. In some situations, vacuum extraction may be successful (Ezenagu and colleagues, 1999). If not deemed safe, or if it also fails to effect vaginal delivery, then cesarean delivery is performed.

In a study of 122 women who had a trial of midcavity forceps or vacuum extraction in a setting with full preparations to proceed to cesarean section, Lowe (1987) found no significant difference in immediate neonatal or maternal morbidity compared with that of 42 women delivered for similar indications by cesarean without such a trial of instrumentation. Conversely, neonatal morbidity was higher in 61 women who had "unexpected" forceps or vacuum failure in which there was no prior preparation for immediate cesarean delivery. Williams and colleagues (1991) reported good outcomes for both mother and infant with use of alternate or sequential forceps and vacuum delivery. They achieved an overall vaginal delivery rate of 97 percent in 99 women, all 35 weeks or greater, who had indications for assisted vaginal delivery. We agree with the American College of Obstetricians and Gynecologists (2000), which cautions that these trials are attempted only if the clinical assessment is highly suggestive of a successful outcome.

VACUUM EXTRACTION

In the United States, the device is referred to as the vacuum extractor, whereas in Europe it is commonly referred to as a *ventouse* (from French, literally, *soft cup*). The theoretical advantages of the vacuum extractor over forceps include the avoidance of insertion of space-occupying steel blades within the vagina and of the requirement for precise positioning over the fetal head; the ability to rotate the fetal head without impinging on maternal soft tissues; and the decreased intracranial pressure during traction. All previously described instruments were unsuccessful until Malmström (1954) applied a new principle, viz., traction on a metal cap designed so that the suction creates an artificial caput, or *chignon,* within the cup that holds firmly and allows adequate traction.

As with forceps choice, the decision to use a metal or a soft cup appears regional. In the United States, the metal cup generally has been replaced by newer soft cup vacuum extractors. As emphasized by Duchon and associates (1998), however, high-pressure vacuum generates large amounts of force regardless of the cup used. The Silastic cup vacuum device is a reusable instrument with a soft, 65-mm-diameter cup. The Mityvac instrument uses a disposable 60-mm-diameter cup (Fig. 23–17), and the CMI Tender Touch uses a 62-mm cup (Fig. 23–18). Bofill and associates (1996b) reported good results with the Mityvac M-cup.

Loghis and colleagues (1992) compared results of 200 women delivered using a metal cup with those of 200 women in whom a pliable cup was used. No differences were found in the rate of birth canal trauma (11 versus 13 percent), major neonatal scalp trauma (6.5 percent versus 5.5 percent), neonatal jaundice (15.5 percent versus 13.5 percent), or Apgar scores. Kuit and co-workers (1993) found the only advantage of the soft cups was a lower incidence of scalp injury. In

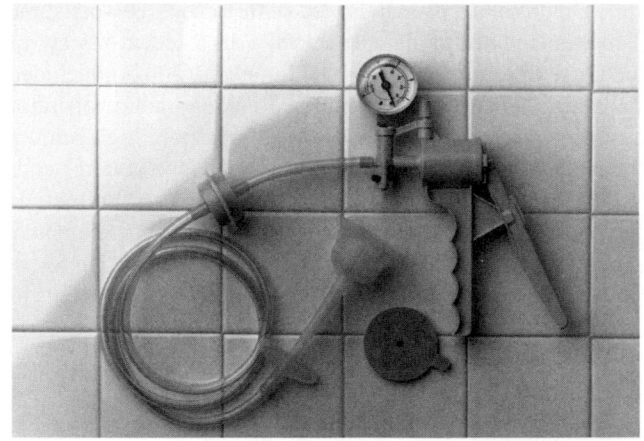

FIGURE 23–17. Mityvac obstetrical vacuum delivery system includes extractor cup and pump. (Photograph reproduced with permission of Prism Enterprises, Inc, Rancho Cucamonga, Calif.)

this study, both rigid and pliable cups had an associated episiotomy extension rate of 14 percent. Vaginal lacerations were 16 percent with rigid cups and 10 percent with pliable cups. Johanson and Menon (2000a) analyzed results from nine randomized trials. They found that soft cups had a higher failure rate (1.65 times) but were associated with less scalp injury (0.45 times) than rigid cups. In a review, Vacca (2002) concluded that randomized trials indicate fewer scalp lacerations with the soft cup, but that the rate of cephalohematomas and subgaleal hemorrhage were similar between soft and rigid cups.

INDICATIONS AND PREREQUISITES. Generally, the indications and prerequisites for the use of the vacuum extractor for delivery are the same as for forceps delivery (American College of Obstetricians and Gynecologists, 2000). The tendency to attempt vacuum deliveries at stations

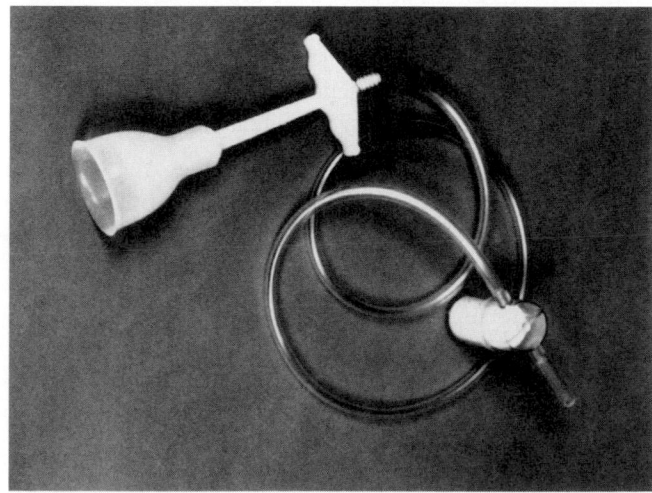

FIGURE 23–18. CMI Tender Touch extractor cup. (Photograph reproduced with permission of Utah Medical Products.)

higher than is usually attempted with forceps is worrisome (Broekhuizen and colleagues, 1987). In a recent review of vacuum extraction, Koscica and Gimovsky (2002) concluded that contraindications to vacuum extraction include operator inexperience, inability to assess fetal position, high station, and suspicion of cephalopelvic disproportion. Relative contraindications for delivery using vacuum extraction include face or other nonvertex presentations, fetal coagulopathy, known macrosomia, and recent scalp blood sampling. Generally, vacuum extraction is reserved for fetuses 34 weeks or older.

TECHNIQUE. Proper cup placement is the most important determinant of success in vacuum extraction. The center of the cup should be over the sagittal suture and about 3 cm in front of the posterior fontanelle toward the face. Anterior placement on the fetal cranium—near the anterior fontanelle rather than over the occiput—will result in cervical spine extension unless the fetus is small. Similarly, asymmetrical placement relative to the sagittal suture may worsen asynclitism. Cup placement for elective use in occiput anterior positions is seldom difficult. In contrast, when the indication for delivery is failure to descend caused by occipital malposition, with or without asynclitism or deflexion, cup placement can be very difficult (Lucas, 1994).

Entrapment of maternal soft tissue predisposes the mother to lacerations and hemorrhage and virtually assures cup "popoff." The full circumference of the cup should be palpated both before and after the vacuum has been created, as well as prior to traction. When using rigid cups, it is recommended that the vacuum be created gradually by increasing the suction by 0.2 kg/cm^2 every 2 minutes until a negative pressure of 0.8 kg/cm^2 is reached. With soft cups, negative pressure can be increased to 0.8 kg/cm^2 over as little as 1 minute (Hankins and associates, 1995; Kuit and colleagues, 1993). Some authors suggest that 0.6 kg/cm^2 is the optimal peak pressure (Lucas, 1994). Listed in Table 23–5 are conversions of various units of pressures used by different instruments.

Traction should be intermittent and coordinated with maternal expulsive efforts. Traction may be initiated by using a two-handed technique, viz., the fingers of one hand are placed against the suction cup, while the other hand grasps

the handle of the instrument. A theoretical advantage of the vacuum cup is that it usually will detach prior to creating tractive forces sufficient to cause fetal injury. Vacuums offer no advantage for avoidance of shoulder dystocia. Manual torque to the cup should be avoided as it may cause cephalohematomas and, with metal cups, "cookie-cutter"–type scalp lacerations. Vacuum extraction should be considered a trial, and without early and clear evidence of descent toward delivery, an alternate delivery approach should be considered. As a general guideline, progressive descent should accompany each traction attempt. Neither data nor consensus are available regarding the number of pulls required to effect delivery, the maximum number of cup detachments that can be tolerated, or optimal total duration of the procedure. A cup pop-off due to technical failure or less than optimal placement should not be equated with a pop-off under ideal conditions of exact cup placement and optimal vacuum maintenance. The former may merit either several additional attempts at placement and delivery or, alternatively, a trial of forceps (Ezenagu and colleagues, 1999; Williams and co-workers, 1991). Conversely, the latter situation is highly suggestive of relative or absolute disproportion or asynclitism. As with forceps procedures, there should be a willingness to abandon attempts at vacuum extraction if satisfactory progress is not made (American College of Obstetricians and Gynecologists, 2000).

COMPLICATIONS. Complications of the vacuum extractor include scalp lacerations and bruising, subgaleal hematomas, cephalohematomas, intracranial hemorrhage, neonatal jaundice, subconjunctival hemorrhage, clavicular fracture, shoulder dystocia, injury of sixth and seventh cranial nerves, Erb palsy, retinal hemorrhage, and fetal death (Broekhuizen and associates, 1987; Galbraith, 1994; Govaert and colleagues, 1992). Significant scalp injuries, hematomas, and resulting hyperbilirubinemia are more common with the metal cup instruments compared with the soft cup devices (American College of Obstetricians and Gynecologists, 2000; Johanson and Menon, 2000a).

In a review by Plauché (1979) of the Malmström vacuum extractor, scalp injury ranged from 0.8 to 33 percent, cephalohematoma from 1 to 26 percent, and subgaleal hemorrhage from 0 to 10 percent. Similar results have been reported by Benjamin and Khan (1993) and Kuit and associates (1993). Conversely, Berkus and associates (1985), found no increase in serious neonatal morbidity, including retinal hemorrhage, for the Silastic vacuum extractor compared with that associated with spontaneous delivery.

The Food and Drug Administration (FDA) issued a Public Health Advisory in 1998 regarding the possible association of vacuum-assisted delivery with serious fetal complications, including death. During a 4-year period, the FDA received reports of nine serious fetal injuries and 12 newborn deaths, which was a significant increase over the preceding 11 years. In a response to this advisory, the American College

TABLE 23–5 Vacuum Pressure Conversions

mm Hg	in Hg	lb/in²	kg/cm²
100	3.9	1.9	0.13
200	7.9	3.9	0.27
300	11.8	5.8	0.41
400	15.7	7.7	0.54
500	19.7	9.7	0.68
600	23.6	11.6	0.82

From Lucas (1994), with permission.

of Obstetricians and Gynecologists (1998) issued a Committee Opinion recommending the continued use of vacuum-assisted delivery devices when appropriate. They estimated that there is approximately one adverse event per 45,455 vacuum extractions per year. Miksovsky and Watson (2001) reviewed obstetrical vacuum extraction.

RECOMMENDATIONS REGARDING VACUUM DELIVERY. Considering the 1998 FDA Public Health Advisory, the following recommendations seem reasonable:

1. The classification of vacuum deliveries should be the same as that utilized for forceps deliveries (including station).
2. The same indications and contraindications utilized for forceps deliveries should be applied to vacuum-assisted deliveries.
3. The vacuum should not be applied to an unengaged vertex, that is, above 0 station.
4. The individual performing or supervising the procedure should be an experienced operator.
5. The operator should be willing to abandon the procedure if it does not proceed easily or if the cup pops off more than three times.

COMPARISON OF VACUUM EXTRACTION WITH FORCEPS

There have been numerous studies comparing vacuum extraction with forceps deliveries. Vacca and associates (1983) conducted a randomized, prospective study comparing metal cup vacuum extraction with forceps delivery. They reported a higher frequency of maternal trauma and blood loss in the forceps group, but an increase in the incidence of neonatal jaundice in the vacuum group. Bofill and colleagues (1996b) randomized 637 women to forceps versus vacuum extraction with the Mityvac M-cup. There were significantly more third- and fourth-degree lacerations (29 versus 12 percent) in the forceps-delivered group. Conversely, the incidence of shoulder dystocia and cephalohematomas was doubled in the vacuum group. Other investigators have found decreased maternal trauma and similar neonatal morbidity in infants delivered by vacuum compared with forceps (Berkus, 1985; Broekhuizen, 1987; Dell, 1985; Williams, 1991, and all their colleagues). Infants delivered with forceps have more marks and bruising from the instrument (Johnson and associates, 2004). Although retinal hemorrhage occasionally is seen with vacuum usage, it has no apparent long-term effects. Johanson and Menon (2000b) analyzed 10 randomized trials and confirmed that vacuum extraction was associated with less maternal but more fetal trauma, for example, cephalohematoma and retinal hemorrhage.

The data are sparse regarding long-term neurological outcome in newborns delivered by vacuum extraction. In the report of an 18-year follow-up by Nilsen (1984), the mean intelligence score of 38 male infants delivered by vacuum was not different from the national average. Seidman and associates (1991) reported in their adjusted analysis a higher mean IQ score at age 17 in those delivered by vacuum or forceps compared with spontaneous delivery (see Table 23–4). Johanson and colleagues (1999) performed a 5-year follow-up of a randomized trial of forceps versus vacuum delivery in over 600 women. Almost half in each group reported urinary incontinence or fecal urgency. These authors also reported that there were no significant differences in child development in the two groups.

REFERENCES

American Academy of Pediatrics and the American College of Obstetricians and Gynecologists. Guidelines for Perinatal Care. 5th ed. Washington, DC, AAP and ACOG, 2002

American College of Obstetricians and Gynecologists: Operative vaginal delivery. Practice Bulletin No. 17, June 2000

American College of Obstetricians and Gynecologists: Delivery by vacuum extraction. Committee on Obstetric Practice, No. 208, 1998

Arya LA, Jackson ND, Myers DL, et al: Risk of new-onset urinary incontinence after forceps and vacuum delivery in primiparous women. Am J Obstet Gynecol 185:1318, 2001

Benjamin B, Khan MRH: Pattern of external birth trauma in southwestern Saudi Arabia. J Trauma 35:737, 1993

Berkus MD, Ramamurthy RS, O'Connor PS, et al: Cohort study of silastic obstetric vacuum cup deliveries, 1. Safety of the instrument. Obstet Gynecol 66:503, 1985

Bofill JA, Rust OA, Devidas M, et al: Prognostic factors for moderate and severe maternal genital tract laceration with operative vaginal delivery. Am J Obstet Gynecol 174:353, 1996a

Bofill JA, Rust OA, Schorr SJ, et al: A randomized prospective trial of the obstetric forceps versus the M-cup. Am J Obstet Gynecol 174:354, 1996b

Bollard RC, Gardiner A, Duthie GS, et al: Anal sphincter injury, fecal and urinary incontinence: A 34-year follow-up after forceps delivery. Dis Colon Rectum 46:1083, 2003

Broekhuizen FF, Washington JM, Johnson F, et al: Vacuum extraction versus forceps delivery: Indications and complications, 1979 to 1984. Obstet Gynecol 69:338, 1987

Broman SH, Nichols PL, Kennedy WA: Preschool IQ: Prenatal and Early Developmental Correlates. Hillside, NJ, Erlbaum, 1975

Carley ME, Carley JM, Vasdev G, et al: Factors that are associated with clinically overt postpartum urinary retention after vaginal delivery. Am J Obstet Gynecol 187:430, 2002

Carmona F, Martinez-Roman S, Manau D, et al: Immediate maternal and neonatal effects of low forceps delivery according to the new criteria of the American College of Obstetricians and Gynecologists compared with spontaneous vaginal delivery in term pregnancies. Am J Obstet Gynecol 173:55, 1995

Chang AL, Noah MS, Laros RK: Obstetric attending physician characteristics and their impact on vacuum and forceps delivery rates: University of California at San Francisco experience from 1977 to 1999. Am J Obstet Gynecol 186:1299, 2002

de Parades V, Etienney I, Thabut D, et al: Anal sphincter injury after forceps delivery: Myth or reality? A prospective ultrasound study of 93 females. Dis Colon Rectum 47:24, 2004

Dell DL, Sightler SE, Plauche WC: Soft cup vacuum extraction: A comparison of outlet delivery. Obstet Gynecol 66:624, 1985

Dierker LJ, Rosen MG, Thompson K, et al: Midforceps deliveries: Long-term outcome of infants. Am J Obstet Gynecol 154:764, 1986

DiMarco CS, Ramsey PS, Williams LH, et al: Temporal trends in operative obstetric delivery: 1992–1999. Obstet Gynecol 95:39S, 2000

Donnelly VS, O'Herlihy C, Campbell DM, et al: Postpartum fecal incontinence is more common in women with irritable bowel syndrome. Dis Colon Rectum 41:586, 1998

Duchon MA, DeMund MA, Brown RH: Laboratory comparison of modern vacuum extractors. Obstet Gynecol 72:155, 1998

Eason E, Labrecque M, Marcoux S, et al: Anal incontinence after childbirth. CMAJ 166:326, 2002

Eason E, Labrecque M, Wells G, et al: Preventing perineal trauma during childbirth: A systematic review. Obstet Gynecol 95:464, 2000

Ecker JL, Tan WM, Bansal RK, et al: Is there a benefit to episiotomy at operative vaginal delivery? Observations over ten years in a stable population. Am J Obstet Gynecol 176:411, 1997

Ezenagu LC, Kakaria R, Bofill JA: Sequential use of instruments at operative vaginal delivery: Is it safe? Am J Obstet Gynecol 180:1446, 1999

Fairweather D: Obstetric management and follow-up of the very low-birth-weight infant. J Reprod Med 26:387, 1981

FDA Public Health Advisory: Need for CAUTION When Using Vacuum Assisted Delivery Devices. May 21, 1998

Fitzpatrick M, Behan M, O'Connell PR, et al: Randomised clinical trial to assess anal sphincter function following forceps or vacuum assisted vaginal delivery. Br J Obstet Gynaecol 110:424, 2003

Friedman EA, Sachtleben MR, Bresky PA: Dysfunctional labor, 12. Long-term effects on the fetus. Am J Obstet Gynecol 127:779, 1977

Friedman EA, Sachtleben-Murray MR, Dahrouge D, et al: Long-term effects of labor and delivery on offspring: A matched-pair analysis. Am J Obstet Gynecol 150:941, 1984

Fynes M, Donnelly VS, O'Connell PR, et al: Cesarean delivery and sphincter injury. Obstet Gynecol 92:496, 1998

Galbraith RS: Incidence of neonatal sixth nerve palsy in relation to mode of delivery. Am J Obstet Gynecol 170:1158, 1994

Gilbert WM, Nesbitt TS, Danielsen B: Associated factors in 1611 cases of brachial plexus injury. Obstet Gynecol 93:536, 1999

Gilstrap LC III: Forceps delivery. In Gilstrap LC III, Cunningham FG, VanDorsten JP (eds): Operative Obstetrics, 2nd ed. New York, McGraw-Hill, 2002

Goldberg J, Holtz D, Hyslop T, et al: Has the use of routine episiotomy decreased? Examination of episiotomy rates from 1983 to 2000. Obstet Gynecol 99:395, 2002

Govaert P, Vanhaesebrouck P, de Praeter C: Traumatic neonatal intracranial bleeding and stroke. Arch Dis Child 67:840, 1992

Hagadorn-Freathy AS, Yeomans ER, Hankins GDV: Validation of the 1988 ACOG forceps classification system. Obstet Gynecol 77:356, 1991

Halpern SH, Leighton BL, Ohisson A, et al: Effect of epidural vs parenteral opioid analgesia on the progress of labor. JAMA 280:2105, 1998

Handa VL, Danielsen BH, Gilbert WM: Obstetric anal sphincter lacerations. Obstet Gynecol 98:225, 2001

Hankins GDV, Clark SL, Cunningham FG, et al: Vacuum delivery. In: Operative Obstetrics. Norwalk, Conn, Appleton & Lange, 1995

Hankins GDV, Rowe TF: Operative vaginal delivery—Year 2000. Am J Obstet Gynecol 175:275, 1996

Hankins GD, Uckan E, Rowe TF, et al: Forceps and vacuum delivery: Expectations of residency and fellowship training program directors. Am J Perinatol 16:23, 1999

Jackson SL, Weber AM, Hull TL, et al: Fecal incontinence in women with urinary incontinence and pelvic organ prolapse. Obstet Gynecol 89:423, 1997

Johanson RB, Heycock E, Carter J, et al: Maternal and child health after assisted vaginal delivery: Five-year follow up of a randomised controlled study comparing forceps and ventouse. Br J Obstet Gynaecol 106:544, 1999

Johanson R, Menon V: Soft versus rigid vacuum extractor cups for assisted vaginal delivery. Cochrane Database Syst Rev 2:CD000446, 2000a

Johanson RB, Menon BK: Vacuum extraction forceps for assisted vaginal delivery. Cochrane Database Syst Rev 2:CD000224, 2000b

Johnson JH, Figueroa R, Garry D, et al: Immediate maternal and neonatal effects of forceps and vacuum assisted deliveries. Obstet Gynecol 103:513, 2004

Kaminski HM, Stafl A, Aiman J: The effect of epidural analgesia on the frequency of instrumental obstetric delivery. Obstet Gynecol 69:770, 1987

Koscica KL, Gimovsky ML: Vacuum extraction. Optimizing outcomes. Reducing legal risk. OBG Management April 2002, p 89

Kozak LJ, Weeks JD: U.S. trends in obstetric procedures, 1990–2000. Birth 29:157, 2002

Kuit JA, Eppinga HG, Wallenburg HCS, et al: A randomized comparison of vacuum extraction delivery with a rigid and a pliable cup. Obstet Gynecol 82:280, 1993

Lieberman E, O'Donoghue C: Unintended effects of epidural analgesia during labor: A systematic review. Am J Obstet Gynecol 186:S31, 2002

Loghis C, Pyrgiotis E, Panayotopoulos N, et al: Comparison between metal cup and silicon rubber cup vacuum extractor. Eur J Obstet Gynecol Reprod Biol 45:173, 1992

Low J, Ng TY, Chew SY: Clinical experience with the silicon cup vacuum extractor. Singapore Med J 34:135, 1993

Lowe B: Fear of failure: A place for the trial of instrumental delivery. Br J Obstet Gynaecol 94:60, 1987

Lucas MJ: The role of vacuum extraction in modern obstetrics (review). Clin Obstet Gynecol 37:794, 1994

MacArthur C, Bick DE, Keighley MR: Faecal incontinence after childbirth. Br J Obstet Gynaecol 104:46, 1997

Malmström T: The vacuum extractor, an obstetrical instrument. Acta Obstet Gynecol Scand Suppl 4:33, 1954

Martin JA, Hamilton BE, Sutton PD, et al: Births: Final data for 2002. National Vital Statistics Report 52:1, 2003

Miksovsky P, Watson WJ: Obstetric vacuum extraction: State of the art in the new millennium. Obstet Gynecol Surv 56:736, 2001

Nilsen ST: Boys born by forceps and vacuum extraction examined at 18 years of age. Acta Obstet Gynecol Scand 63:549, 1984

Nygaard IE, Rao SS, Dawson JD: Anal incontinence after anal sphincter disruption: A 30 year retrospective cohort study. Obstet Gynecol 89:896, 1997

Pearl ML, Roberts JM, Laros RK, et al: Vaginal delivery from the persistent occiput posterior position: Influence on maternal and neonatal morbidity. J Reprod Med 38:955, 1993

Peschers UM, Sultan AH, Jundt K, et al: Urinary and anal incontinence after vacuum delivery. Eur J Obstet Gynecol Reprod Biol 110:39, 2003

Plauché WC: Fetal cranial injuries related to delivery with the Malmström vacuum extractor. Obstet Gynecol 53:750, 1979

Pollack J, Nordenstram J, Brismar S, et al: Anal incontinence after vaginal delivery: A five-year prospective cohort study. Obstet Gynecol 104:1397, 2004

Pregazzi R, Sartore A, Troiano L, et al: Postpartum urinary symptoms: Prevalence and risk factors. Eur J Obstet Gynecol Reprod Biol 103:179, 2002

Rieger N, Schloithe A, Saccone G, et al: The effect of a normal vaginal delivery on anal function. Acta Obstet Gynecol Scand 76:769, 1997

Robertson PA, Laros RK, Zhao RL: Neonatal and maternal outcome in low-pelvic and mid-pelvic operative deliveries. Am J Obstet Gynecol 162:1436, 1990

Robinson JN, Norwitz ER, Cohen AP, et al: Episiotomy, operative vaginal delivery, and significant perinatal trauma in nulliparous women. Am J Obstet Gynecol 181:1180, 1999

Schraffordt Koops SE, Vervest HAM, Oostvogel HJM: Anorectal symptoms after various modes of vaginal delivery. Int Urogynecol J 14:244, 2003

Schwartz DB, Miodovnik M, Lavin JP Jr: Neonatal outcome among low birth weight infants delivered spontaneously or by low forceps. Obstet Gynecol 62:283, 1983

Seidman DS, Laor A, Gale R, et al: Long-term effects of vacuum and forceps deliveries. Lancet 337:1583, 1991

Sharma SK, McIntire DD, Wiley J, et al: Labor analgesia and cesarean delivery: An individual patient meta-analysis of nulliparous women. Anesthesiology 100:142, 2004

Sherman SJ, Greenspoon JS, Nelson JM, et al: Obstetric hemorrhage and blood utilization. J Reprod Med 38:929, 1993

Sultan AH, Kamm MA, Bartram CI, et al: Anal sphincter trauma during instrumental delivery. Int J Gynaecol Obstet 43:263, 1993

Sultan AH, Kamm MA, Hudson CN, et al: Third degree obstetric anal sphincter tears: Risk factors and outcome of primary repair. BMJ 308:887, 1994

Tetzschner T, Sorensen M, Lose G, et al: Anal and urinary incontinence after obstetric and sphincter rupture. Ugeskr Laeger 160:3218, 1998

Towner D, Castro MA, Eby-Wilkens E, et al: Effect of mode of delivery in nulliparous women on neonatal intracranial injury. N Engl J Med 341:1709, 1999

Vacca A: Vacuum-assisted delivery. Best Pract Res Clin Obstet Gynaecol 16:17, 2002

Vacca A, Grant A, Wyatt G, et al: Portsmouth operative delivery trial: A comparison of vacuum extraction and forceps delivery. Br J Obstet Gynaecol 90:1107, 1983

Viktrup L, Lose G: The risk of stress incontinence 5 years after first delivery. Am J Obstet Gynecol 185:82, 2001

Wesley B, Van den Berg B, Reece EA: The effect of operative vaginal delivery on cognitive development. Am J Obstet Gynecol 166:288, 1992

White DA, Pressman EK, Hanna GV, et al: Facial nerve palsy: Frequencies associated with spontaneous, forceps, and cesarean deliveries. Am J Obstet Gynecol 174:353, 1996

Williams MC, Knuppel RA, O'Brien WF, et al: A randomized comparison of assisted vaginal delivery by obstetric forceps and polyethylene vacuum cup. Obstet Gynecol 78:789, 1991

24

Breech Presentation and Delivery

When the buttocks of the fetus enter the pelvis before the head, the presentation is *breech.* The term probably derives from the same word as *britches,* which described a cloth covering the loins and thighs. As shown in Table 24–1, breech presentation is more common remote from term. Most often, however, before the onset of labor the fetus turns spontaneously to a cephalic presentation, so that breech presentation persists in only about 3 to 4 percent of singleton deliveries. Specifically, the annual rate of breech presentation at delivery in nearly 150,000 infants delivered at Parkland Hospital in the 10-year period ending in 2002 was 3.6 percent.

ETIOLOGY

As term approaches, the uterine cavity usually accommodates the fetus in a longitudinal lie with the vertex presenting. Factors other than gestational age that appear to predispose to breech presentation include hydramnios, uterine relaxation associated with great parity, multiple fetuses, oligohydramnios, hydrocephaly, anencephaly, previous breech delivery, uterine anomalies, and pelvic tumors. Fianu and Vaclavinkova (1978) provided sonographic evidence of a much higher prevalence of placental implantation in the cornual-fundal region for breech presentation (73 percent) than for vertex presentations (5 percent). The frequency of breech presentation also is increased with placenta previa, but only a small minority of breech presentations are associated with a previa. No strong correlation has been shown between breech presentation and a contracted pelvis.

COMPLICATIONS

In the persistent breech presentation, an increased frequency of the following complications can be anticipated:

TABLE 24–1 Prevalence of Breech Presentation by Gestational Age

Gestational Age (wks)	Presentation			Breech (%)[a]
	Breech	*Vertex*	Total	
28	218	676	894	24
29	78	296	374	21
30	78	381	459	17
31	29	152	181	13
32	92	637	729	11
33	59	507	566	11
34	6	118	124	5
35	30	392	422	7
36	8	131	139	6
37–40	5	131	136	4

[a]Numbers rounded off.
From Hill (1990), with permission.

1. Perinatal morbidity and mortality from difficult delivery.
2. Low birthweight from preterm delivery, growth restriction, or both.
3. Prolapsed cord.
4. Placenta previa.
5. Fetal, neonatal, and infant anomalies.
6. Uterine anomalies and tumors.

DIAGNOSIS

The varying relations between the lower extremities and buttocks of breech presentations form the categories of frank, complete, and incomplete breech presentations. With a *frank breech* presentation, the lower extremities are flexed at the hips and extended at the knees, and thus the feet lie in close proximity to the head (Fig. 24–1). A *complete breech* presentation differs in that one or both knees are flexed (Fig. 24–2). With *incomplete breech* presentation, one or both hips are not flexed and one or both feet or knees lie below the breech, such that a foot or knee is lowermost in the birth canal (Fig. 24–3). Footling breech is an incomplete breech with one or both feet below the breech.

ABDOMINAL EXAMINATION. Use of the Leopold maneuvers to diagnose presentation is discussed in Chapter 17 (see p. 412) and shown in Figure 17–8. Its accuracy has been reported to be high by some investigators (Lydon-Rochelle and colleagues, 1993) but not others (Thorp and co-workers, 1991). Typically, with the first Leopold maneuver, the hard,

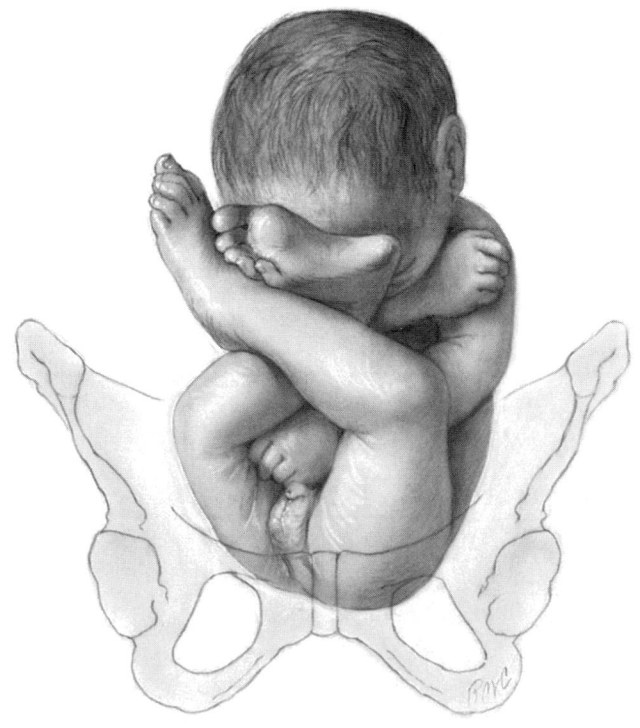

FIGURE 24–1. Frank breech presentation.

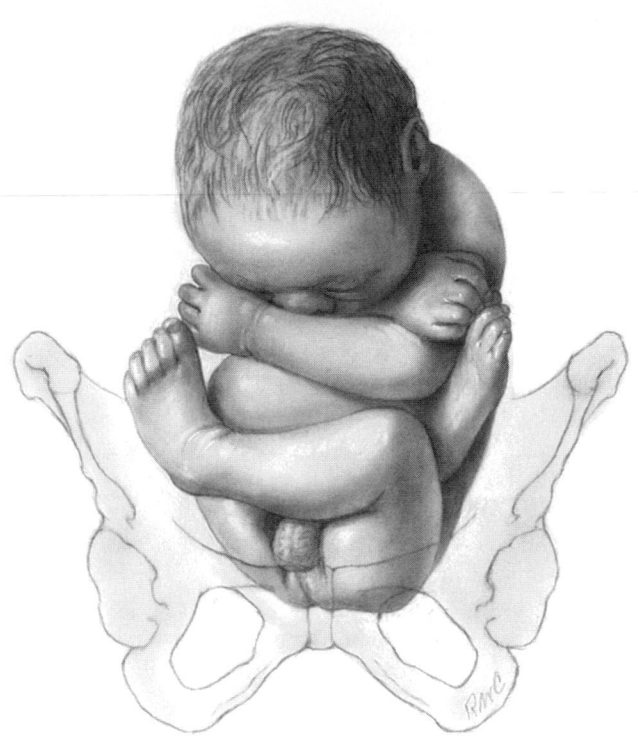

FIGURE 24–2. Complete breech presentation.

round, readily ballotable fetal head is found to occupy the fundus. The second maneuver indicates the back to be on one side of the abdomen and the small parts on the other. On the third maneuver, if engagement has not occurred—the intertrochanteric diameter of the fetal pelvis has not passed through the pelvic inlet—the breech is movable above the pelvic inlet. After engagement, the fourth maneuver shows the firm breech to be beneath the symphysis. Fetal heart sounds usually are heard loudest slightly above the umbilicus, whereas with engagement of the fetal head, the heart sounds are loudest below the umbilicus.

VAGINAL EXAMINATION. With the frank breech presentation, both ischial tuberosities, the sacrum, and the anus usually are palpable, and after further descent, the external genitalia may be distinguished. Especially when labor is prolonged, the buttocks may become markedly swollen, rendering differentiation of face and breech very difficult—the anus may be mistaken for the mouth and the ischial tuberosities for the malar eminences. Careful examination, however, should prevent this error, because the finger encounters muscular resistance with the anus, whereas the firmer, less yielding jaws are felt through the mouth. Furthermore, the finger, upon removal from the anus, sometimes is stained with meconium. The mouth and malar eminences form a triangular shape, whereas the ischial tuberosities and anus are in a straight line. The most accurate information, however, is based on the location of the sacrum and its spinous processes, which establishes the diagnosis of position and variety.

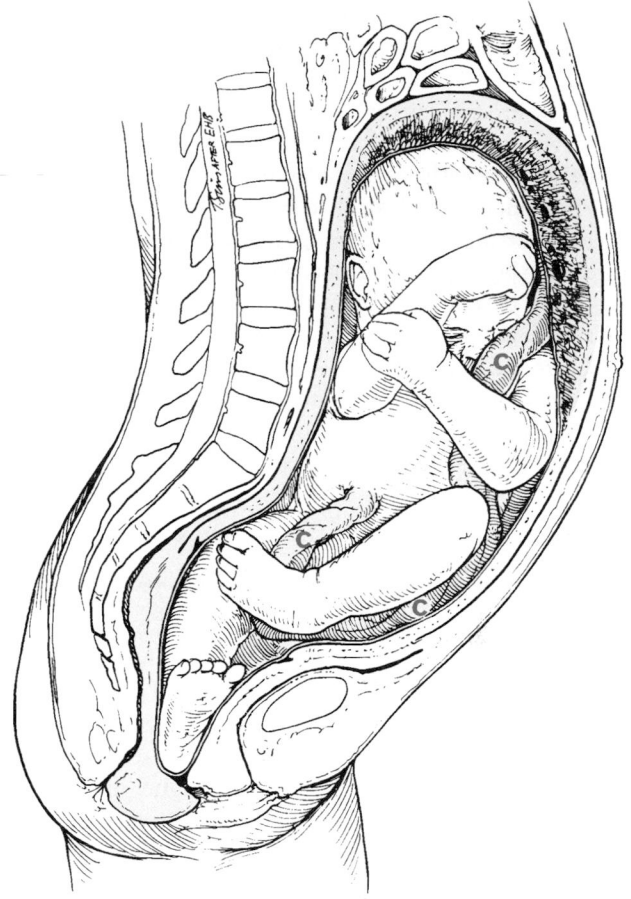

FIGURE 24–3. Double-footling breech presentation in labor with membranes intact. Note possibility of umbilical cord (C) accident at any instant, especially after rupture of membranes.

In complete breech presentations, the feet may be felt alongside the buttocks, and in footling presentations, one or both feet are inferior to the buttocks. In footling presentations, the foot can readily be identified as right or left on the basis of the relation to the great toe. When the breech has descended farther into the pelvic cavity, the genitalia may be felt.

IMAGING TECHNIQUES. Ideally, *ultrasound* should be used to confirm a clinically suspected breech presentation and to identify, if possible, any fetal anomalies. If cesarean delivery is planned, additional imaging is not indicated. If, however, vaginal delivery is considered, the type of breech presentation and the degree of flexion or deflexion of the head is important. Ultrasound also may supply this additional information (Fontenot and associates, 1997; Rojansky and colleagues, 1994). *Computed tomographic (CT) scanning* also can be used and will provide pelvic measurements and configuration at lower doses of radiation than standard radiography (see Chap. 20, p. 504). *Magnetic resonance imaging (MRI)* provides reliable information about pelvic capacity and architecture without ionizing radiation, but it is not always readily available (van Loon and colleagues, 1997).

The role of x-ray pelvimetry in deciding the mode of delivery for breech presentation is controversial (Morrison and co-authors, 1995). Cheng and Hannah (1993) reviewed 15 studies of breech delivery at term in which either x-ray or CT pelvimetry was used as one of the criteria for allowing vaginal delivery. They concluded that although the utility of x-ray pelvimetry was difficult to assess because "permissible" pelvic dimensions varied among studies, in most there was no correlation between pelvic measurements and labor outcome. One study demonstrated that the incidence of complicated labor rose with decreasing pelvic capacity (Ohlsén, 1975). Van Loon and colleagues (1997) reported that although MRI pelvimetry did not significantly lower the overall cesarean rate or improve neonatal outcomes, its use was associated with a lower rate of emergency cesarean delivery.

PROGNOSIS

Both mother and fetus are at greater risk with breech presentation compared with cephalic presentation, but to nowhere near the same degree. In an analysis of 57,819 pregnancies in the Netherlands, Schutte and colleagues (1985) reported that even after correction for gestational age, congenital defects, and birthweight, perinatal mortality was higher in breech infants. They concluded that breech presentation may not be coincidental, but rather is a consequence of poor fetal quality. Nelson and Ellenberg (1986) observed that one third of children with cerebral palsy who were in a breech presentation at birth also had major noncerebral malformations. Finally, Krebs and associates (1999) reported that cerebral palsy in breech-presenting fetuses was not related to the mode of delivery. Thus, obstetrical intervention will not eliminate all mortality and long-term morbidity associated with breech presentation.

MATERNAL MORBIDITY. Because of the greater frequency of operative delivery, including cesarean delivery, there is higher maternal morbidity and slightly higher mortality for pregnancies complicated by persistent breech presentation (Collea and co-authors, 1980). This risk likely is increased even more with emergency surgery instead of elective cesarean delivery (Bingham and Lilford, 1987). Labor length is similar to that with cephalic presentation (Hall and Kohl, 1956).

PERINATAL MORBIDITY AND MORTALITY. The prognosis for the fetus in a breech presentation is considerably worse than when in a vertex presentation. The major contributors to perinatal loss are preterm delivery, congenital anomalies, and birth trauma. Thirty years ago, Brenner and associates (1974) reported that at every stage of gestation and in the neonatal period, neonatal deaths were significantly greater among breeches. Congenital abnormalities

were identified in 6.3 percent of breech deliveries compared with 2.4 percent of nonbreech deliveries. Contemporaneous outcomes, in which careful assessment is made before vaginal delivery is attempted and cesarean delivery rates generally exceed 60 percent, are much improved. Albrechtsen and colleagues (1997) reported that perinatal mortality in 45,579 breech deliveries decreased from 9 percent in the period from 1967 through 1976 to 3 percent in 1987 through 1994. Su and colleagues (2003) reported that avoiding labor augmentation and having an experienced obstetrician present at birth significantly reduces the risk of adverse perinatal outcomes for breech fetuses who undergo vaginal birth.

VAGINAL DELIVERY

Delivery of the breech draws the umbilicus and attached cord into the pelvis, which compresses the cord. Therefore, once the breech has passed beyond the vaginal introitus, the abdomen, thorax, arms, and head must be delivered promptly. This involves delivery of successively less readily compressible parts. With a term fetus, some degree of head molding may be essential for it to negotiate the birth canal successfully. Thus, in certain cases:

1. Delivery may be delayed many minutes while the aftercoming head accommodates to the maternal pelvis, resulting in hypoxia and acidemia, which can become severe; or
2. Delivery may be forced, causing trauma from compression, traction, or both.

With a preterm fetus, the disparity between the size of the head and buttocks is even greater than with a larger fetus. At times, the buttocks and lower extremities of the preterm fetus will pass through the cervix and be delivered, and yet the cervix will not be dilated adequately for the head to escape without trauma (Bodmer and associates, 1986). In this circumstance, *Dührssen incisions* of the cervix, as shown in Figure 24–4, may be lifesaving. Another mechanical problem with breech delivery is entrapment of the fetal arm behind the neck (nuchal arm), which complicates up to 6 percent of vaginal breech deliveries and is associated with increased neonatal mortality (Cheng and Hannah, 1993).

The frequency of cord prolapse is increased when the fetus is small or when the breech is not frank. In the report by Collea and colleagues (1978), the incidence with frank breech presentation was about 0.5 percent, which is similar to 0.4 percent reported for cephalic presentations (Barrett, 1991). In contrast, the incidence of cord prolapse with complete breech presentation was 5 percent, and it was 15 percent with footling breeches. Soernes and Bakke (1986) confirmed earlier observations that umbilical cord length is significantly shorter in breech presentations. Moreover, multiple coils of cord entangling the fetus are more common with breech presentations (Spellacy and associates, 1966). These umbilical

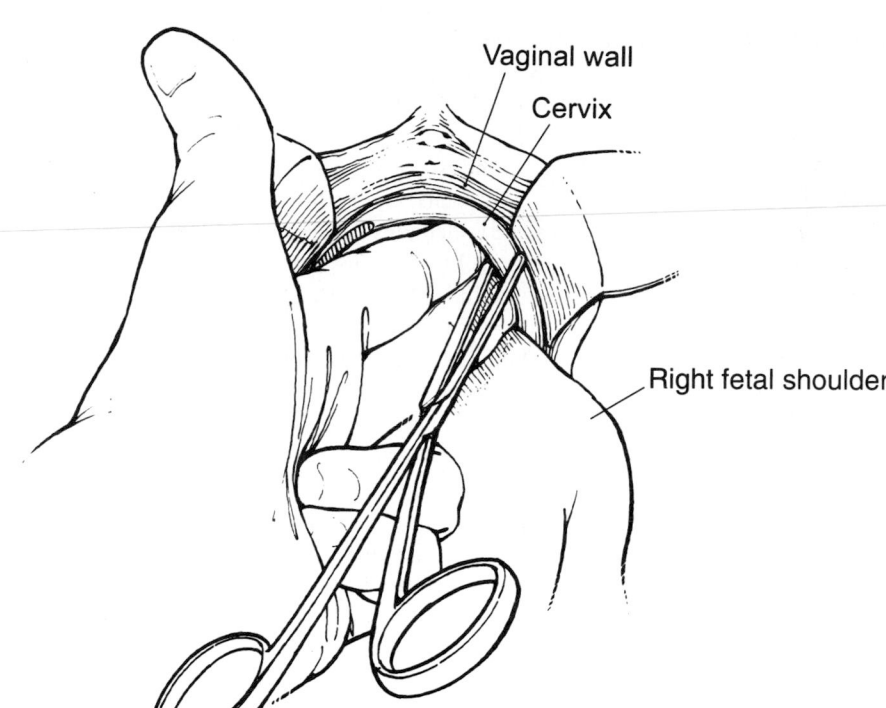

Vaginal wall

Cervix

Right fetal shoulder

FIGURE 24–4. Dührssen incisions at 10 o'clock (already cut) and 2 o'clock (being cut with bandage scissors) to relieve entrapped aftercoming head. Infrequently, an additional incision is required at 6 o'clock. The incisions are so placed as to minimize bleeding from the laterally located cervical branches of the uterine artery. After delivery, the incisions are repaired as described on page 835 (see Fig. 35–27).

cord abnormalities likely play a role both in the development of breech presentation and in the relatively high incidence of a nonreassuring fetal heart rate pattern in labor.

Apgar scores, especially at 1 minute, of vaginally delivered breech infants are generally lower than those of breech infants born by elective cesarean delivery (Flanagan and co-workers, 1987). Compared with cephalic deliveries, umbilical artery blood pH and bicarbonate are lower, and P_{CO_2} is higher (Christian and Brady, 1991). Socol and colleagues (1988), however, concluded that although cesarean delivery improved Apgar scores, it did not improve acid–base status. Flanagan and co-workers (1987) emphasized that ultimate infant outcome for breech birth was not worsened by these significant differences in Apgar scores or acid–base status at birth.

UNFAVORABLE PELVIS. Because there is no time for molding of the aftercoming head, a moderately contracted pelvis that had not previously caused problems in delivery of an average-size cephalic fetus might prove dangerous with a breech. Rovinsky and colleagues (1973) urged not only accurate measurements of the pelvic dimensions but also precise evaluation of the pelvic architecture rather than reliance on pelvic indexes. Gynecoid (round) and anthropoid (elliptical) pelves are favorable configurations, but platypelloid (anteroposteriorly flat) and android (heart-shaped) pelves are not (see Chap. 2, p. 35).

HYPEREXTENSION OF THE FETAL HEAD. In perhaps 5 percent of term breech presentations, the fetal head may be in extreme hyperextension (Fig. 24–5). These presentations have been referred to as the *stargazer fetus*, and in Britain as the *flying foetus*. With such hyperextension, vaginal delivery may result in injury to the cervical spinal cord. In general, marked hyperextension after labor has begun is considered an indication for cesarean delivery (Svenningsen and associates, 1985).

LABOR INDUCTION AND AUGMENTATION. Induction of labor in women with a breech presentation is defended by some clinicians and condemned by others. Brenner and associates (1974) found no significant differences in perinatal mortality and Apgar scores between infants with induced versus spontaneous labor. In oxytocin-augmented labor, however, infant mortality rates were higher and Apgar scores were lower. Fait and colleagues (1998) reported that 12 of 23 women with a breech presentation and an unripe cervix who underwent induction had a successful vaginal delivery with no neonatal complications. At Jackson Memorial Hospital in Miami, oxytocin is used in a manner similar to that for vertex presentations (Diro and associates, 1999). At Parkland Hospital, cesarean delivery is preferred to oxytocin induction or augmentation when there is a viable fetus. Induction may be attempted by amniotomy alone for pregnancies otherwise suitable for a trial of vaginal delivery. At the University of Alabama at Birmingham, oxytocin is employed only if clinical factors are favorable for vaginal delivery, and CT pelvimetry confirms an adequate pelvis.

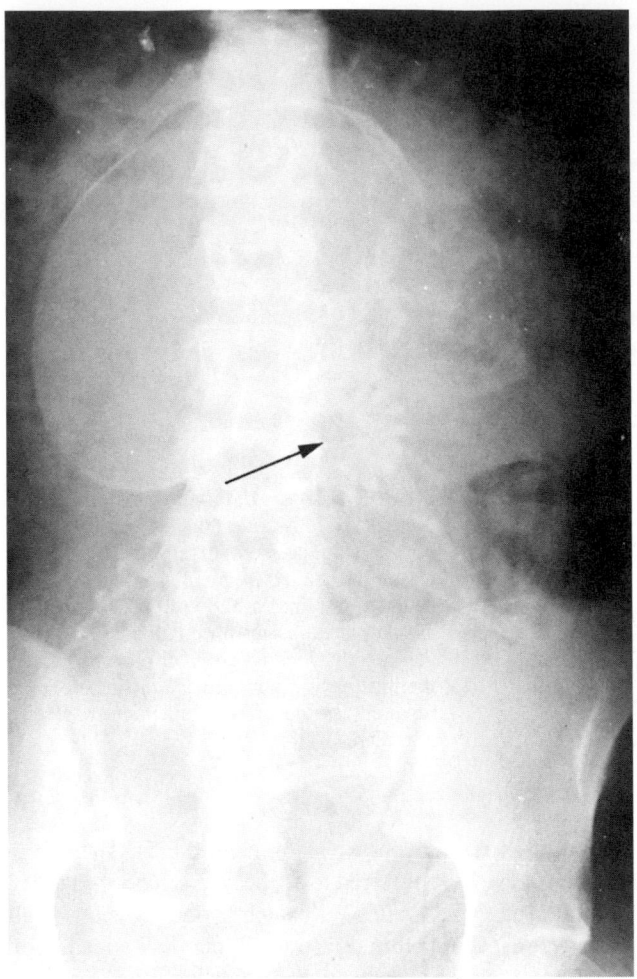

FIGURE 24–5. Radiograph of a fetus presenting as a complete breech and with a markedly hyperextended cervical spine (*arrow*) and head.

FOOTLING BREECH. The possibility of compression of a prolapsed cord or a cord entangled around the extremities as the breech fills the pelvis is a threat to the fetus (see Fig. 24–3).

TERM FETUS. Cheng and Hannah (1993) conducted a systematic search of the world literature regarding term breech delivery and found reports published between 1966 and 1992. A total of 24 studies encompassing 11,721 women were selected because these compared *planned* vaginal with *planned* cesarean delivery for the term, singleton breech fetus. The corrected perinatal mortality rate ranged from 0 to 48 per 1000 births. All but two of the 77 perinatal deaths were in women allowed to deliver vaginally. The main causes of death were head entrapment, cerebral injury and intracranial hemorrhage, cord prolapse, and severe asphyxia. The overall neonatal mortality and morbidity resulting from trauma were increased significantly in the planned vaginal delivery groups, with a typical odds ratio of 3.86. Similarly, Gifford and co-workers (1995b) performed a meta-analysis of out-

comes after term breech delivery. Although acknowledging the many methodological limitations of extant studies, they observed that a trial of labor was associated with an increased risk of perinatal injury or death.

Only two of the 24 reports reviewed by these investigators were randomized trials, and both were from the same institution. Collea and colleagues (1980) reported the results of 208 women with frank breech fetuses at term. Almost half of these women were excluded from further consideration because of possible fetopelvic disproportion based on x-ray pelvimetry. A total of 60 infants eventually were delivered vaginally and all survived, although two sustained brachial plexus injuries. There were no perinatal deaths, but half of the 148 women who had cesarean deliveries experienced significant morbidity compared with only 7 percent of 60 women who were delivered vaginally.

Gimovsky and colleagues (1983) studied 105 nonfrank breech fetuses and reported similar findings. Although these two trials concluded that vaginal breech delivery was relatively safe, only 110 fetuses were actually allowed a trial of labor. As emphasized by Eller and Van Dorsten (1995), this small number does not provide sufficient statistical power to demonstrate differences in uncommon adverse outcomes such as perinatal death and birth injury. Lindqvist and associates (1997), in a nationwide Swedish Registry study from 1991 and 1992, found similar mortality with vaginal compared with cesarean delivery. The opposite conclusion was reached by Rietberg and colleagues (2003) in their study of almost 34,000 term breech births in the Netherlands from 1995 to 1999. After the study by Hannah and colleagues (2000) showed increased neonatal morbidity and mortality, elective cesarean breech delivery in the Netherlands doubled from 31 to 62 percent in 2000 and 2001, respectively (Molkenboer and associates, 2003).

PRETERM FETUS. The aftercoming head of a preterm fetus may be trapped by a cervix that is sufficiently effaced and dilated to allow passage of the thorax but not of the less-compressible head. The consequences of vaginal delivery in this circumstance all too often have been both hypoxia and physical trauma, both of which are especially deleterious to the preterm infant.

There are no randomized studies regarding delivery of the preterm breech fetus. Penn and colleagues (1996) attempted such a study in 26 hospitals in England and discontinued the trial after 17 months because only 13 women could be recruited. Retrospective studies have yielded conflicting results. Bowes and colleagues (1979) and Main and co-workers (1983) found that preterm infants undergoing cesarean delivery had a better prognosis. Others have concluded that vaginal delivery did not significantly increase perinatal mortality (Olshan and co-workers, 1984; Rosen and Chik, 1984; Westgren and co-workers, 1985a). In another study, Wolf and colleagues (1999) compared preterm breech fetuses delivered at two tertiary care facilities in the Netherlands. At one center, vaginal delivery was preferred and the cesarean delivery rate was only 17 percent. At the other center, the cesarean delivery rate was 85 percent. These investigators found no difference in 2-year survival without disability or handicap.

The National Institute of Child Health and Human Development Neonatal Research Network (Malloy and co-workers, 1991) analyzed data from 437 very-low-birthweight breech infants admitted to seven neonatal intensive care centers. After adjusting for several variables, the risk of intraventricular hemorrhage and neonatal death was not significantly affected by the mode of delivery for fetuses weighing less than 1500 g. A similar analysis was reported from the Netherlands by Gravenhorst and co-workers (1993). Perinatal follow-up data were collected on 899 singleton, nonanomalous infants of less than 32 weeks' gestation, with birthweights of less than 1500 g. These investigators could not conclusively resolve whether cesarean delivery was advantageous compared with vaginal delivery of infants.

CURRENT STATUS OF VAGINAL BREECH DELIVERY. In 2002, 87 percent of breech fetuses in the United States were delivered by cesarean (Martin and colleagues, 2002). The number of skilled operators with the ability to safely select and vaginally deliver breech fetuses continues to dwindle. Medicolegal concerns make it difficult to train residents to perform such deliveries, and two groups of investigators who have attempted trials of breech delivery concluded that such studies were likely impossible (Penn and Steer, 1990; Zlatnik, 1993).

As mentioned earlier, Hannah and colleagues (2000) reported results from a multinational randomized trial of planned vaginal versus planned cesarean delivery for women with a term breech presentation. A total of 2083 women were randomized: 1041 to planned cesarean and 1042 to planned vaginal delivery. In the planned vaginal delivery group, 57 percent were actually delivered vaginally. Overall, planned cesarean delivery was associated with a reduction in perinatal mortality from 13 per 1000 to 3 per 1000 and a reduction in "serious" neonatal morbidity from 3.8 to 1.4 percent. Maternal complications were similar between the groups.

On the basis of this international trial, the American College of Obstetricians and Gynecologists (2001) has concluded that, except in cases of "advanced labor" and "imminent delivery," which are not otherwise defined, women with persistent singleton breech presentation at term should undergo a planned cesarean delivery. We have taken issue with this mandate (Hauth and Cunningham, 2002). Our objections center on the College's reliance on the trial of Hannah and colleagues (2000). A number of similar criticisms were discussed in a series of correspondence to the editor of *The Lancet, Obstetrics & Gynecology,* and the *British Medical Journal* (Apuzzio and associates, 2002; Biswas, 2001; Cunha-Filho and Passos, 2001; Leung and Pun, 2001; Premru-Srsen, 2001; Somerset, 2002; Stuart, 2001; Uchide and Murakami, 2001). These issues include that (1) among the 1025 women enrolled

from countries with low perinatal mortality rates, perinatal deaths were infrequent and did not differ significantly between groups—none in 514 women in the planned cesarean compared with 3 of 511 in the planned vaginal delivery group; (2) most components included in the "serious" neonatal morbidity composite do not actually portend long-term disability; (3) fewer than 10 percent of women in the trial underwent pelvimetry using radiography, CT scanning, or MRI; and (4) in over 30 percent of participants, the attitude of the fetal head was determined only by clinical methods.

At least three contemporary single-center studies support a trial of vaginal delivery for selected breech-presenting term fetuses. Irion and associates (1998) reported significantly fewer maternal complications, but no difference in corrected neonatal morbidity or mortality between 385 attempted vaginal breech deliveries—70 percent of whom were delivered vaginally—compared with that of 320 planned cesarean deliveries. Giuliani and associates (2002) reported that in their institution vaginal breech delivery was achieved in half of 699 consecutive, term breech-presenting fetuses, with no short- or long-term differences in outcome for infants delivered vaginally compared with those delivered by cesarean. Alarab and associates (2004) reported no serious adverse neonatal outcomes in 146 term breech infants—one fourth of all their breeches—who were delivered vaginally during 3½ years in their institution.

Based on reports such as these, as well as our collective experiences at Parkland Hospital and the University of Alabama at Birmingham Hospital, women with selected frank breech presentations continue to be offered a trial of vaginal delivery on an individualized basis and with approval of the attending faculty. In these women, fetal weight is estimated to be between 2000 and 3500 g. Under these conditions, between 10 and 20 percent of singleton breeches are delivered vaginally.

Recommendations for Delivery. A diligent search for any other complication, actual or anticipated, that might justify cesarean delivery has become a feature of most philosophies for managing breech delivery. Cesarean delivery is commonly but not exclusively used in the following circumstances:

1. A large fetus.
2. Any degree of contraction or unfavorable shape of the pelvis.
3. A hyperextended head.
4. When delivery is indicated in the absence of spontaneous labor (some clinicians use oxytocin augmentation).
5. Uterine dysfunction (some use oxytocin augmentation).
6. Incomplete or footling breech presentation.
7. An apparently healthy and viable preterm fetus with the mother in either active labor or in whom delivery is indicated.
8. Severe fetal growth restriction.

9. Previous perinatal death or children suffering from birth trauma.
10. A request for sterilization.
11. Lack of an experienced operator.

TECHNIQUES FOR BREECH DELIVERY

LABOR AND SPONTANEOUS DELIVERY. There are fundamental differences between labor and delivery in cephalic and breech presentations. With a cephalic presentation, once the head is delivered, the rest of the body typically follows without difficulty. With a breech, however, successively larger and very much less compressible parts of the fetus are born. Spontaneous complete expulsion of the fetus who presents as a breech, as subsequently described, is seldom accomplished successfully. Therefore, as a rule, vaginal delivery requires skilled participation by the obstetrician for a favorable outcome.

Engagement and descent usually take place with the bitrochanteric diameter in one of the oblique pelvic diameters. The anterior hip usually descends more rapidly than the posterior hip, and when the resistance of the pelvic floor is met, internal rotation of 45 degrees usually follows, bringing the anterior hip toward the pubic arch and allowing the bitrochanteric diameter to occupy the anteroposterior diameter of the pelvic outlet. If the posterior extremity is prolapsed, however, it rotates to the symphysis pubis rather than the anterior hip.

After rotation, descent continues until the perineum is distended by the advancing breech, and the anterior hip appears at the vulva. By lateral flexion of the fetal body, the posterior hip then is forced over the perineum, which retracts over the buttocks, thus allowing the infant to straighten out when the anterior hip is born. The legs and feet follow the breech and may be born spontaneously or with aid.

After the birth of the breech, there is slight external rotation, with the back turning anteriorly as the shoulders are brought into relation with one of the oblique diameters of the pelvis. The shoulders then descend rapidly and undergo internal rotation, with the bisacromial diameter occupying the anteroposterior plane. Immediately following the shoulders, the head, which is normally sharply flexed upon the thorax, enters the pelvis in one of the oblique diameters and then rotates in such a manner as to bring the posterior portion of the neck under the symphysis pubis. The head is then born in flexion.

The breech may engage in the transverse diameter of the pelvis, with the sacrum directed anteriorly or posteriorly. The mechanism of labor in the transverse position differs only in that internal rotation occurs through an arc of 90 rather than 45 degrees. Infrequently, rotation occurs in such a manner that the back of the infant is directed posteriorly instead of anteriorly. Such rotation should be prevented if possible. Although the head may be delivered by allowing the chin and face to pass beneath the symphysis, the slightest traction on the body may cause extension of the head, which increases the diameter of the head that must pass through the pelvis.

METHODS OF VAGINAL DELIVERY. There are three general methods of breech delivery through the vagina:

1. *Spontaneous breech delivery.* The infant is expelled entirely spontaneously without any traction or manipulation other than support of the infant.
2. *Partial breech extraction.* The infant is delivered spontaneously as far as the umbilicus, but the remainder of the body is extracted or delivered with operator traction and assisted maneuvers, with or without maternal expulsive efforts.
3. *Total breech extraction.* The entire body of the infant is extracted by the obstetrician.

The three varieties of breech presentation are illustrated in Figures 24–1, 24–2, and 24–3. Because the technique of breech extraction differs in a complete, incomplete, and frank breech, these are considered subsequently in two separate sections.

MANAGEMENT OF LABOR. During labor, both mother and fetus are at considerably increased risk compared with that of a woman with a cephalic presentation (Kunzel, 1994). A rapid assessment should be made to establish the status of the membranes, labor, and fetal condition. Close surveillance of fetal heart rate and uterine contractions is begun at admission. Immediate recruitment of the necessary nursing, obstetrical, and anesthesia team to accomplish a vaginal or abdominal delivery also should be accomplished. The nursery is notified. A venous catheter is inserted and an infusion begun as soon as the woman arrives in the labor suite. Emergency induction of anesthesia, or hemorrhage from lacerations or from uterine atony, are but two of many reasons that may require immediate intravenous access for the administration of medications, fluids, or blood.

Stage of Labor. Assessment of cervical dilatation and effacement and the station of the presenting part are essential for planning the route of delivery. If labor is too far advanced, there may not be sufficient time to obtain x-ray pelvimetry. This alone, however, should not force the decision for cesarean delivery. Biswas and Johnstone (1993) found that among 267 term breech presentations, satisfactory progress in labor was the best indicator of pelvic adequacy. Nwosu and colleagues (1993) reported similar findings.

Fetal Condition. The presence or absence of gross fetal abnormalities, such as hydrocephaly or anencephaly, can be rapidly ascertained with the use of sonography or radiography. Such efforts will help to ensure that a cesarean delivery is not performed under emergency conditions for an anomalous infant with no chance of survival. If vaginal delivery is planned, the fetal head should not be extended (see Fig. 24–5). As discussed, it is possible to ascertain head flexion and to exclude extension with sonography (Fontenot and colleagues, 1997; Rojansky and co-workers, 1994).

Fetal Monitoring. Guidelines for monitoring the high-risk fetus are applied as discussed in Chapter 17 (p. 427). Thus, the fetal heart rate is recorded at least every 15 minutes. Most clinicians prefer continuous electronic monitoring of fetal heart rate and uterine contractions.

When membranes are ruptured, either spontaneously or artificially, the risk of cord prolapse is appreciably increased. Therefore, a vaginal examination should be performed following rupture to check for cord prolapse. Special attention should be directed to the fetal heart rate for the first 5 to 10 minutes following membrane rupture, to detect occult cord prolapse.

Additional help is required for managing labor and delivery of a breech presentation. For labor, one-on-one nursing is ideal because of the risk of cord prolapse or occlusion, and physicians must be readily available should there be an emergency.

Route of Delivery. Discussions with the woman and planning for the route of delivery may have taken place before admission. If not, they are now accomplished as soon as possible. The choice of abdominal or vaginal delivery is based on the type of breech, flexion of the head, fetal size, quality of uterine contractions, and size of the maternal pelvis (see p. 571). The woman should be informed about all relevant facts and uncertainties before delivery. The obstetrician should consider, and usually abide by, the preferences of the informed parents (Kunzel, 1994).

Timing of Delivery. In general, the capability to proceed with immediate breech extraction when the buttocks or feet appear at the vulva is necessary. This is important because persistent fetal bradycardia is prone to develop from cord compression with further fetal descent through the birth canal. It is essential that the delivery team include:

1. An obstetrician skilled in the art of breech extraction.
2. An associate to assist with the delivery.
3. Anesthesia personnel who can assure adequate analgesia or anesthesia when needed.
4. An individual trained to resuscitate the infant.

Delivery is easier, and in turn, morbidity and mortality are probably lower, when the breech is allowed to deliver spontaneously to the umbilicus. If a nonreassuring fetal heart rate pattern develops before this time, however, a decision must be made whether to perform manual extraction or cesarean delivery. For a favorable outcome with any breech delivery, at the very minimum, the birth canal must be sufficiently large to allow passage of the fetus without trauma. The cervix must be fully dilated, and if not, then a cesarean delivery nearly always is the more appropriate method of delivery when suspected fetal compromise develops.

ASSISTED FRANK BREECH DELIVERY. The frank breech should ideally be allowed to deliver without assistance to at least the level of the umbilicus. Unless there is considerable relaxation of the perineum, an episiotomy should be made. The episiotomy is an important adjunct to any type of breech delivery. As the breech progressively distends the perineum, the posterior hip will deliver, usually from the 6 o'clock position, and often with sufficient pressure to evoke passage of thick meconium at this point (Fig. 24–6). The anterior hip then delivers, followed by external rotation to the sacrum anterior position (Fig. 24–7). The mother should be encouraged to continue to push, as the cord is now drawn well down into the birth canal and likely is being compressed with resultant fetal bradycardia. As the fetus continues to descend, the legs are sequentially delivered by splinting the medial aspect of each femur with the operator's fingers positioned parallel to each femur and by exerting pressure laterally so as to sweep each leg away from the midline.

Following delivery of the legs, the fetal bony pelvis is grasped with both hands, using a cloth towel moistened with warm water. The fingers should rest on the anterior superior iliac crests and the thumbs on the sacrum, minimizing the chance of fetal abdominal soft tissue injury (Fig. 24–8). Maternal expulsive efforts are used in conjunction with continued gentle downward operator rotational traction to effect delivery of the fetus. Gentle downward traction is combined with an initial 90-degree rotation of the fetal pelvis through

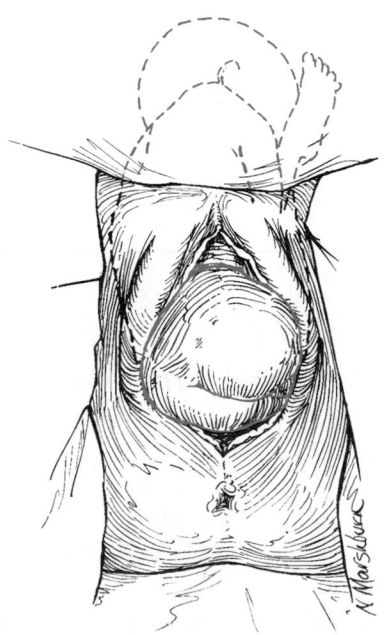

FIGURE 24–6. The posterior hip of the frank breech is delivering over the perineum. A generous midline episiotomy has been cut.

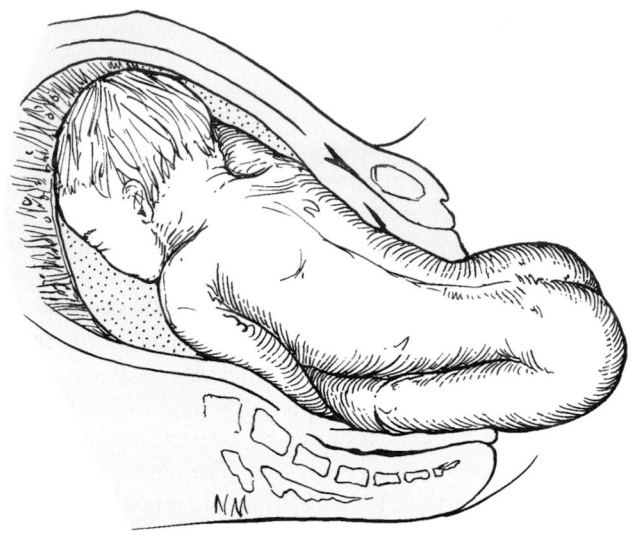

FIGURE 24–7. The anterior hip has now delivered and external rotation has occurred. The fetal thighs remain in flexion, with extension at the knees.

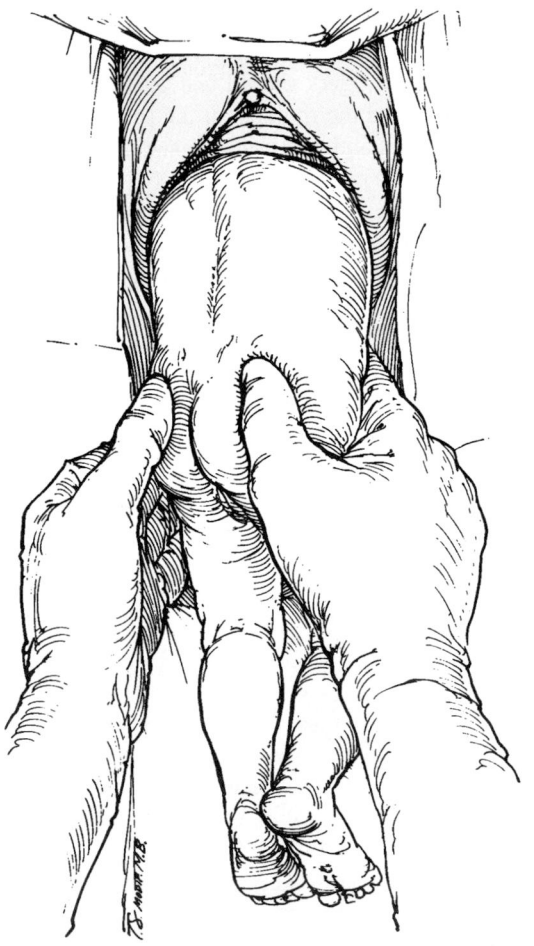

FIGURE 24–8. Delivery of the body. The hands are applied, but not above the pelvic girdle. Gentle downward rotational traction is accomplished until the scapulas are clearly visible.

one arc and then a 180-degree rotation to the other to effect delivery of the scapulas and arms (Figs. 24–9 and 24–10).

The depicted rotational and downward traction maneuvers will decrease the occurrence of persistent nuchal arms, which can complicate all vaginal breech deliveries, prevent further descent, and increase fetal-newborn trauma and morbidity. These maneuvers are frequently most easily effected with the operator at the level of the maternal pelvis and with one knee on the floor. When the scapulas are clearly visible, delivery is then completed as subsequently described for the complete or incomplete breech.

FRANK BREECH EXTRACTION. At times, extraction of a frank breech may be required and can be accomplished by moderate traction exerted by a finger in each groin and facilitated by a generous episiotomy (Fig. 24–11). If moderate traction does not effect delivery of the breech, then vaginal delivery can be accomplished only by breech decomposition. This procedure involves manipulation within the birth canal to convert the frank breech into a footling breech. The procedure is accomplished more readily if the membranes have ruptured recently, and it becomes extremely difficult if considerable time has elapsed since escape of amnionic fluid. In such cases, the uterus may have become tightly contracted over the fetus, and pharmacological relaxation by general anesthesia, intravenous magnesium sulfate, or a

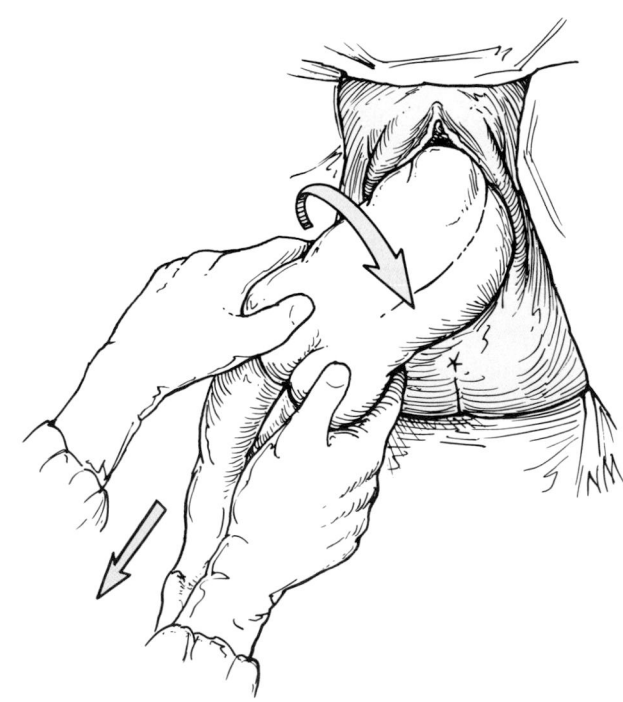

FIGURE 24–9. Clockwise rotation of the fetal pelvis 90 degrees brings the sacrum from anterior to left sacrum transverse. Simultaneously, the application of gentle downward traction effects delivery of the scapula.

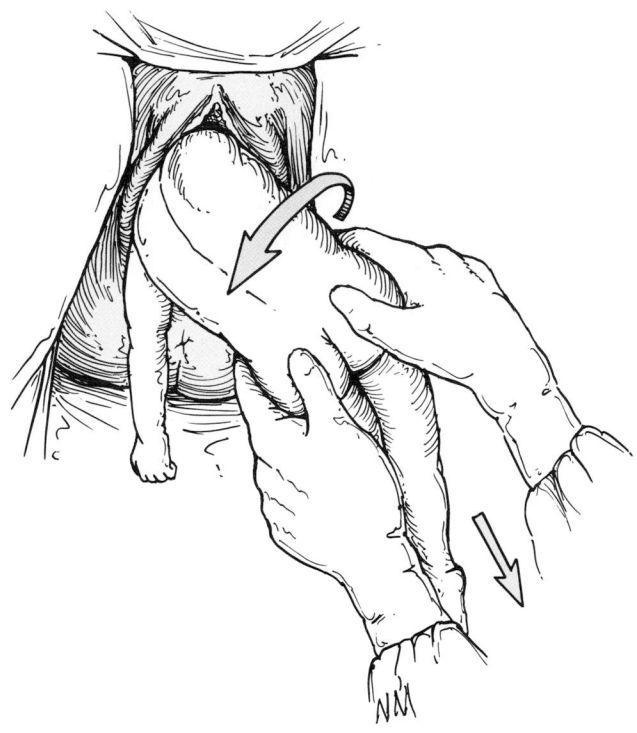

FIGURE 24–10. Counterclockwise rotation from sacrum anterior to right sacrum transverse along with gentle downward traction effects delivery of the right scapula.

beta-mimetic such as terbutaline (250 μg subcutaneously) may be required.

Breech decomposition is accomplished by the maneuver attributed to Pinard (1889). It aids in bringing the fetal feet within reach of the operator. As shown in Figure 24–12, two fingers are carried up along one extremity to the knee to

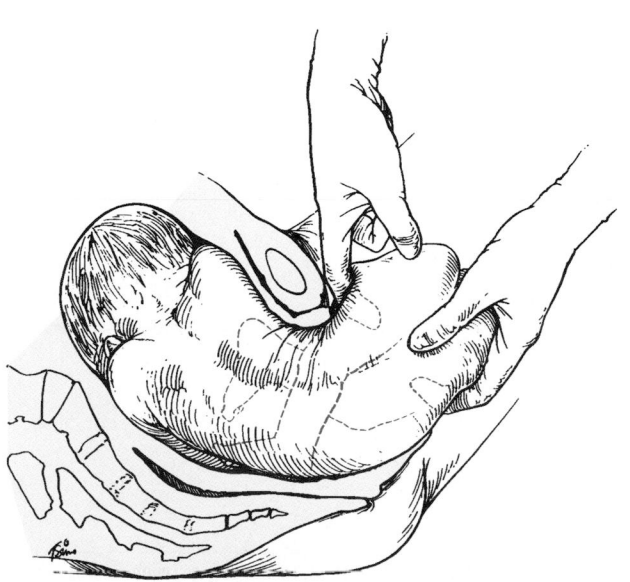

FIGURE 24–11. Extraction of a frank breech using fingers in groins.

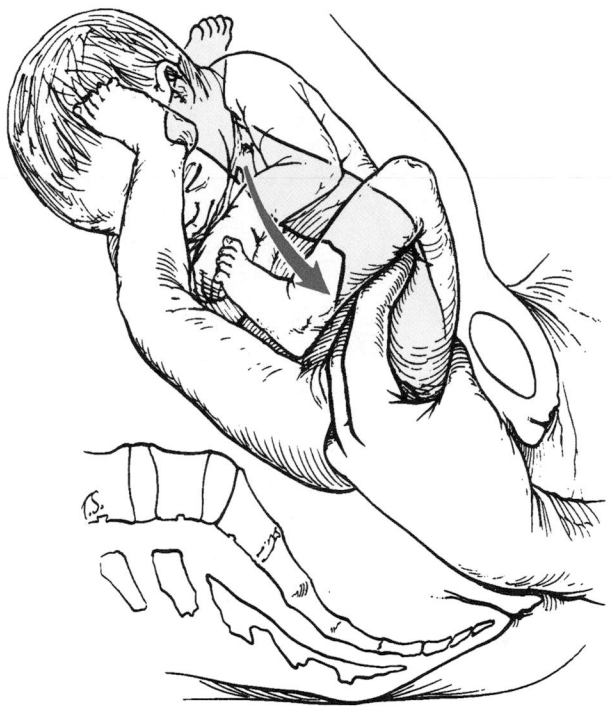

FIGURE 24–12. Frank breech decomposition using the Pinard maneuver. Two fingers are inserted along one extremity to the knee, which is then pushed away from the midline after spontaneous flexion traction is used to deliver a foot into the vagina.

push it away from the midline. Spontaneous flexion usually follows, and the foot of the fetus is felt to impinge on the back of the hand. The fetal foot then may be grasped and brought down.

COMPLETE OR INCOMPLETE BREECH EXTRACTION. During total extraction of a complete or incomplete breech, the hand is introduced through the vagina and both feet of the fetus are grasped. The ankles are held with the second finger lying between them and, with gentle traction, the feet are brought through the vulva. If difficulty is experienced in grasping both feet, first one foot should be drawn into the vagina but not through the introitus, and then the other foot is advanced in a similar fashion (Fig. 24–13). Now both feet are grasped and pulled through the vulva simultaneously.

As the legs begin to emerge through the vulva, downward gentle traction is then continued. As the legs emerge, successively higher portions are grasped, first the calves and then the thighs (Fig. 24–14). When the breech appears at the vulva, gentle traction is applied until the hips are delivered. As the buttocks emerge, the back of the infant usually rotates to the anterior. The thumbs are then placed over the sacrum and the fingers over the hips, and assisted breech delivery is effected, as described previously (see Fig. 24–8). As the scapulas become visible, the back of the infant tends to turn spontaneously toward the side of the mother to which it was originally directed (Fig. 24–15).

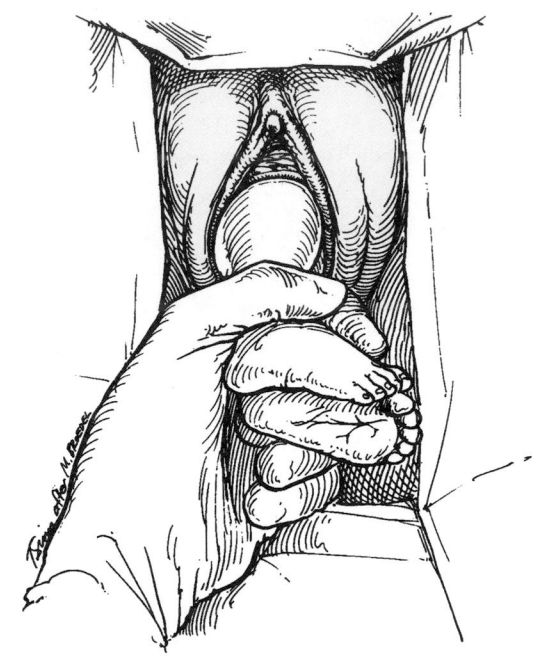

FIGURE 24–13. Complete breech extraction begins with traction on the feet and ankles.

A cardinal rule in successful breech extraction is to **employ steady, gentle, downward rotational traction until the lower halves of the scapulas are delivered outside the vulva, making no attempt at delivery of the shoulders and arms until one axilla becomes visible.** Failure to follow this rule frequently will make an otherwise easy procedure difficult. The appearance of one axilla indicates that the time has arrived for delivery of the shoulders. It makes little difference which shoulder is delivered first, and there are two methods for delivery of the shoulders.

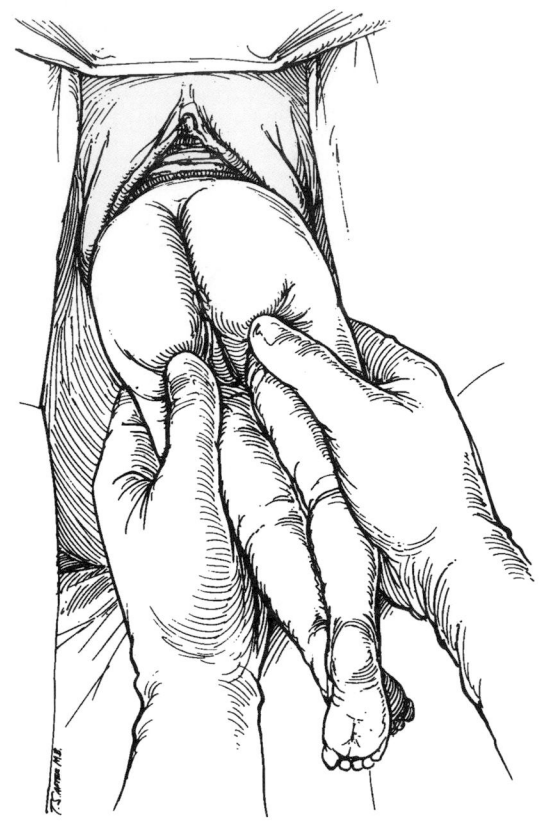

FIGURE 24–14. Complete breech extraction continues with traction on the thighs. A warm, moist towel is most often applied over the fetal parts to reduce slippage from vernix as traction is applied.

In the first method, with the scapulas visible, the trunk is rotated in such a way that the anterior shoulder and arm appear at the vulva and can easily be released and delivered first. In Figure 24–15, the operator is shown rotating the trunk of the

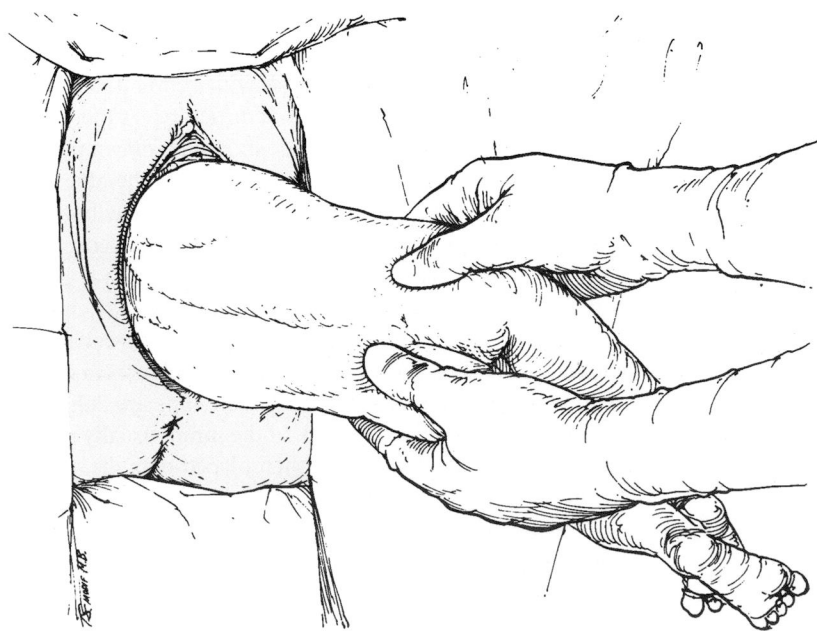

FIGURE 24–15. As breech extraction continues, the scapulas becomes visible and the body rotates, usually to the side of the mother to which it was originally directed.

fetus counterclockwise to deliver the right shoulder and arm. The body of the fetus is then rotated in the reverse direction to deliver the other shoulder and arm.

In the second method, if trunk rotation is unsuccessful, the posterior shoulder must be delivered first. The feet are grasped in one hand and drawn upward over the inner thigh of the mother toward which the ventral surface of the fetus is directed. In this manner, leverage is exerted on the posterior shoulder, which slides out over the perineal margin, usually followed by the arm and hand (Fig. 24–16). Then, by depressing the body of the fetus, the anterior shoulder emerges beneath the pubic arch, and the arm and hand usually follow spontaneously (Fig. 24–17). Thereafter, the back tends to rotate spontaneously in the direction of the symphysis. If upward rotation fails to occur, it is effected by manual rotation of the body. Delivery of the head may then be accomplished.

Unfortunately, the process is not always so simple, and it is sometimes necessary first to free and deliver the arms. These maneuvers are less likely to be required if rotational traction is employed and attempts to deliver the shoulders until an axilla becomes visible are avoided. **Attempts to free the arms immediately after the costal margins emerge should be avoided.**

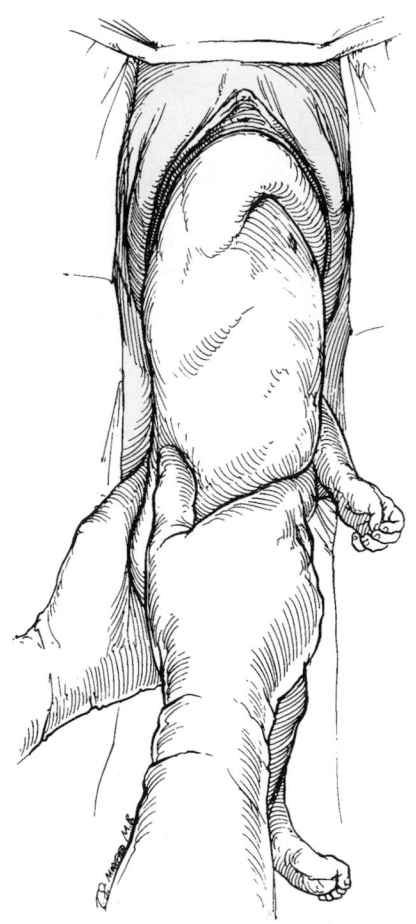

FIGURE 24–17. Breech extraction continues with delivery of the anterior shoulder by downward traction. The anterior arm then may be freed the same way as the posterior arm in Figure 24–16.

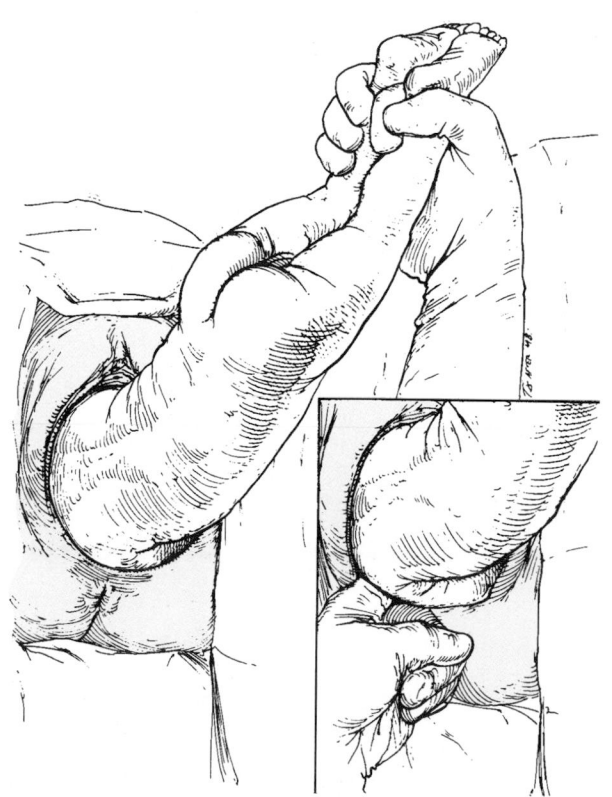

FIGURE 24–16. As breech extraction continues, upward traction is employed, effecting delivery of the posterior shoulder. This is followed by delivery of the posterior arm (*inset*).

There is more space available in the posterior and lateral segments of the normal pelvis than elsewhere. Therefore, in difficult cases, the posterior arm should be freed first. Because the corresponding axilla is already visible, upward traction on the feet is continued, and two fingers of the other hand are passed along the humerus until the elbow is reached (see Fig. 24–16, inset). The fingers are placed parallel to the humerus and used to splint the arm, which is swept downward and delivered through the vulva. To deliver the anterior arm, depression of the body of the infant is sometimes all that is required to allow the anterior arm to slip out spontaneously. In other instances, the anterior arm can be swept down over the thorax using two fingers as a splint. Occasionally, however, the body must be held with the thumbs over the scapulas and rotated to bring the undelivered shoulder near the closest sacrosciatic notch. The legs then are carried upward to bring the ventral surface of the infant to the opposite inner thigh of the mother. Subsequently, the arm can be delivered as described previously. If the arms have become extended over the head, their delivery, although more difficult, usually can be accomplished by the maneuvers just described. In so doing,

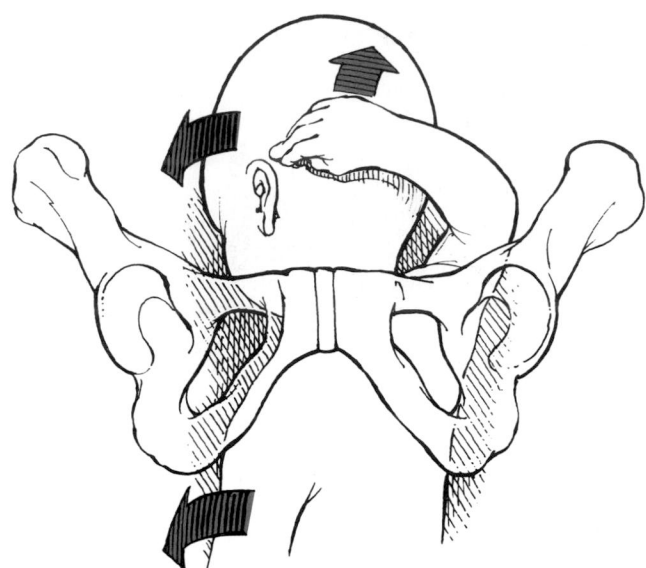

FIGURE 24–18. Reduction of nuchal arm being accomplished by rotating the fetus through half a circle counterclockwise so that the friction exerted by the birth canal will draw the elbow toward the face.

particular care must be taken by the operator to carry the fingers up to the elbow and to use them as a splint to prevent fracture of the humerus.

As discussed earlier, one or both fetal arms occasionally may be found around the back of the neck (nuchal arm) and impacted at the pelvic inlet. In this situation, delivery is more difficult. If the nuchal arm cannot be freed in the manner described, extraction may be facilitated, especially with a single nuchal arm, by rotating the fetus through half a circle in such a direction that the friction exerted by the birth canal will serve to draw the elbow toward the face (Fig. 24–18). Should rotation of the fetus fail to free the nuchal arm(s), it may be

necessary to push the fetus upward in an attempt to release it. If the rotation is still unsuccessful, the nuchal arm often is extracted by hooking a finger(s) over it and forcing the arm over the shoulder, and down the ventral surface for delivery of the arm. In this event, fracture of the humerus or clavicle is very common.

DELIVERY OF THE AFTERCOMING HEAD. The fetal head may be extracted with forceps or by one of the following maneuvers.

Mauriceau Maneuver. The index and middle finger of one hand are applied over the maxilla, to flex the head, while the fetal body rests on the palm of the hand and forearm (Fig. 24–19). The forearm is straddled by the fetal legs. Two fingers of the other hand then are hooked over the fetal neck, and grasping the shoulders, downward traction is applied until the suboccipital region appears under the symphysis. Gentle suprapubic pressure simultaneously applied by an assistant helps keep the head flexed. The body then is elevated toward the maternal abdomen, and the mouth, nose, brow, and eventually the occiput emerge successively over the perineum. **It is emphasized that with this maneuver, the operator uses both hands simultaneously and in tandem to exert continuous downward gentle traction simultaneously on the fetal neck and on the maxilla.** At the same time, appropriate suprapubic pressure applied by an assistant is helpful in delivery of the head (see Fig. 24–19).

Prague Maneuver. Rarely, the back of the fetus fails to rotate to the anterior. When this occurs, rotation of the back to the anterior may be achieved by using stronger traction on the fetal legs or bony pelvis. If the back still remains oriented posteriorly, extraction may be accomplished using the

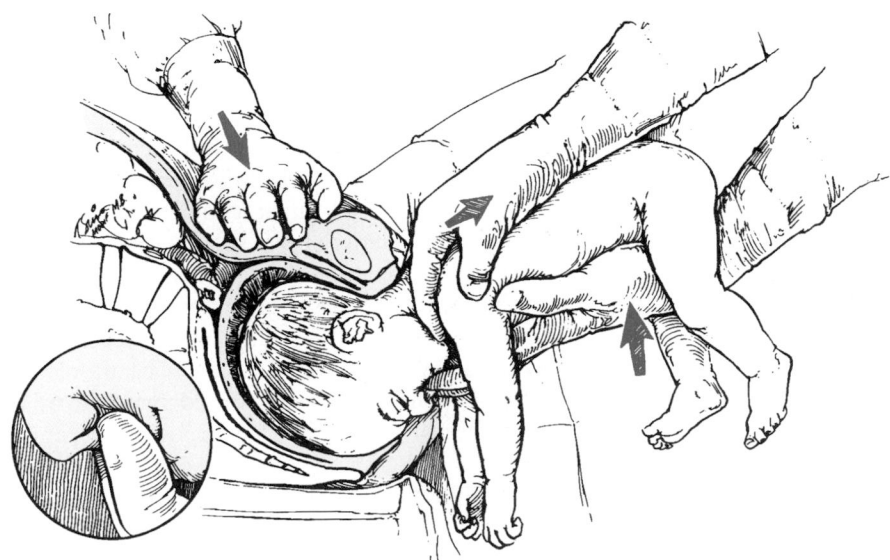

FIGURE 24–19. Delivery of the aftercoming head using the Mauriceau maneuver. Note that as the fetal head is being delivered, flexion of the head is maintained by suprapubic pressure provided by an assistant, and simultaneously by pressure on the maxilla (*inset*) by the operator as traction is applied.

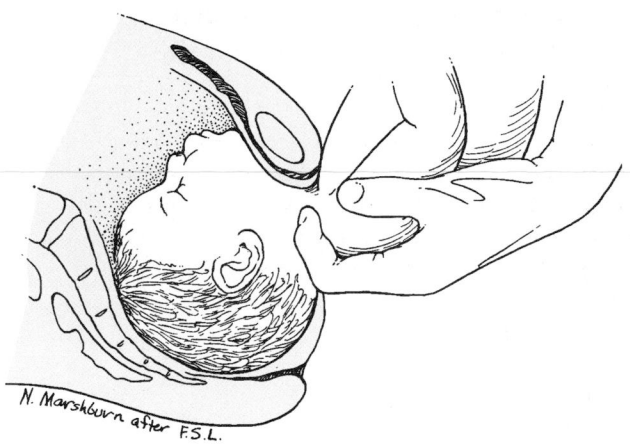

FIGURE 24–20. Delivery of the aftercoming head using the modified Prague maneuver necessitated by failure of the fetal trunk to rotate anteriorly.

Mauriceau maneuver and delivering the fetus back down. If this is impossible, the fetus still may be delivered using the modified Prague maneuver, which, as practiced today, consists of two fingers of one hand grasping the shoulders of the back-down fetus from below while the other hand draws the feet up over the maternal abdomen (Fig. 24–20).

Forceps to Aftercoming Head. Specialized forceps can be used to deliver the aftercoming head. *Piper forceps,* shown in Figure 24–21, or divergent *Laufe forceps* may be applied electively or when the Mauriceau maneuver cannot be accomplished easily. The blades of the forceps should not be applied to the aftercoming head until it has been brought into the pelvis by gentle traction, combined with suprapubic pressure, and is engaged. Suspension of the body of the fetus in a towel effectively holds the fetus and helps keep the arms out of the way.

ENTRAPMENT OF THE AFTERCOMING HEAD. Occasionally, especially with small preterm fetuses, the incompletely dilated cervix will not allow delivery of the aftercoming head. With gentle traction on the fetal body, the cervix, at times, may be manually slipped over the occiput. If this is not successful, then *Dührssen incisions* (see Fig. 24–4) are usually necessary.

Some investigators have recommended intravenous nitroglycerin—typically 100 μg—to provide cervical relaxation for relief of head entrapment (Dufour and colleagues, 1997; Wessen and associates, 1995). There is, however, no compelling evidence of its efficacy for this purpose.

Replacement of the fetus higher into the vagina and uterus, followed by cesarean delivery, can be used successfully to rescue an entrapped breech that cannot be delivered vaginally. Steyn and Pieper (1994) described use of the *Zavanelli maneuver*—cesarean delivery after replacement of the infant back into the uterus—to deliver a healthy 2590-g infant with head entrapment. Sandberg (1999) reviewed 11 breech deliveries in which this maneuver was used.

In some countries, *symphysiotomy* is used to widen the anterior pelvis. In his review, Menticoglou (1990) reported that its use has been associated with good infant outcomes in 80 percent of reported cases. Lack of operator training and the potential to cause serious maternal injury explain its rare use in this country (Goodwin and colleagues, 1997).

ANALGESIA AND ANESTHESIA. Continuous epidural analgesia, as described in Chapter 19, is advocated by some as ideal for women in labor with a breech presentation (Kunzel, 1994; Mokriski, 1994). Confino and colleagues (1985) reviewed the outcomes of 371 nonanomalous singleton breech fetuses delivered vaginally. About 25 percent of these women had been given continuous epidural analgesia, and oxytocin augmentation was necessary to effect delivery in half of them. Although first-stage labor was not longer than in a control group not given epidural analgesia, the second stage was prolonged significantly in women whose fetuses weighed more than 2500 g. It was doubled if the fetus weighed more than 3500 g. Chadha and associates (1992) observed similar effects on labor and an increased incidence of cesarean delivery. These potential disadvantages must be weighed against the advantages of better pain relief and, importantly, increased pelvic relaxation should extensive manipulation be required to effect delivery.

Analgesia for episiotomy and intravaginal manipulations that are needed for breech extraction usually can be accomplished with pudendal block and local infiltration of the perineum. Nitrous oxide plus oxygen inhalation provides further relief from pain. If general anesthesia is required, it can be induced quickly with thiopental plus a muscle relaxant and maintained with nitrous oxide.

Anesthesia for breech decomposition and extraction must provide sufficient relaxation to allow intrauterine manipulations. Although successful decomposition has been accomplished using epidural or spinal analgesia, increased uterine tone may render the operation more difficult. Under such conditions, general anesthesia with a halogenated agent may be required to relax the uterus as well as to provide analgesia.

MORBIDITY AND MORTALITY

MATERNAL INJURIES. Complicated vaginal breech deliveries are associated with increased maternal risks. Manual manipulations within the birth canal increase the risk of infection. Intrauterine maneuvers, especially with a thinned lower uterine segment, or delivery of the aftercoming head through an incompletely dilated cervix may cause rupture of the

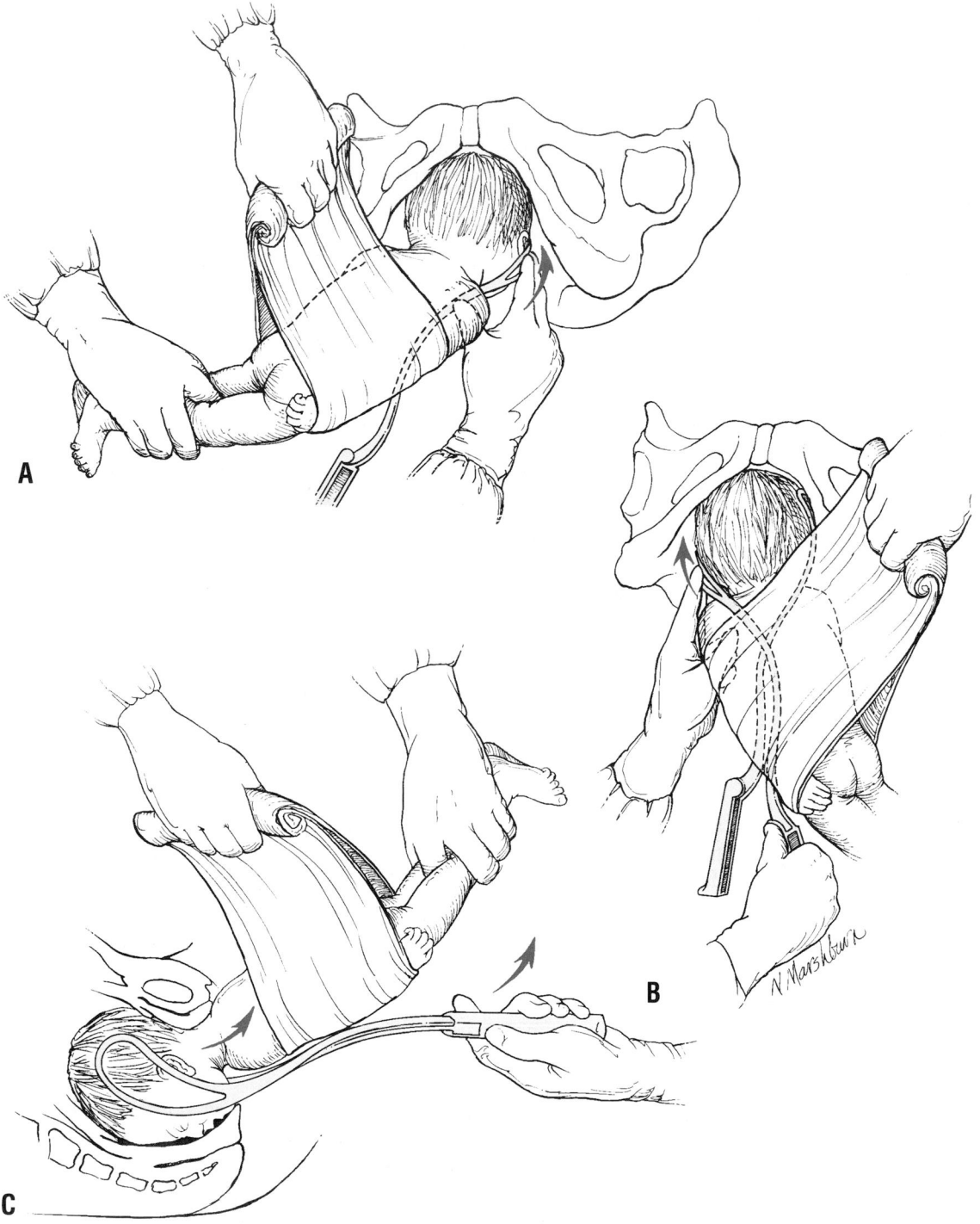

FIGURE 24–21. Piper forceps for delivery of the aftercoming head. Note the direction of movement shown by the arrows. **A.** The fetal body is elevated using a warm towel and the left blade of the forceps is applied to the aftercoming head. **B.** The right blade is applied with the body still elevated. **C.** Forceps delivery of the aftercoming head.

uterus, lacerations of the cervix, or both. Such manipulations also may lead to extensions of the episiotomy and deep perineal tears. Anesthesia sufficient to induce appreciable uterine relaxation may cause uterine atony and, in turn, postpartum hemorrhage.

FETAL INJURIES. Fracture of the humerus and clavicle cannot always be avoided, and fracture of the femur may be sustained during difficult breech extractions (Fig. 24–22). Such fractures are associated with both vaginal and cesarean deliveries (Awwad and colleagues, 1993; Vasa and Kim,

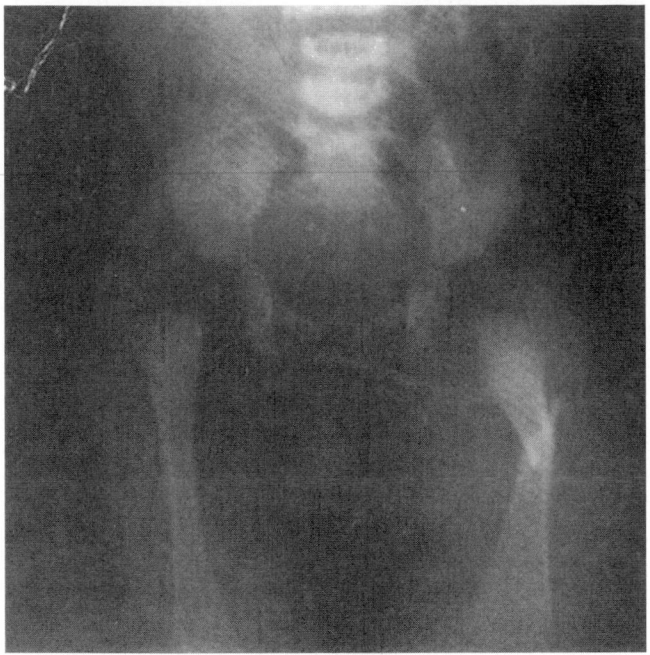

FIGURE 24–22. Midshaft right femoral fracture showing posterior displacement and lateral angulation. Injury occurred with extraction at cesarean delivery. (From Awwad and associates, 1993, with permission.)

1990). Neonatal perineal tears have been reported as a complication of spinal electrode use (Freud and associates, 1993). Hematomas of the sternocleidomastoid muscles occasionally develop after delivery, although they usually disappear spontaneously. More serious problems, however, may follow separation of the epiphyses of the scapula, humerus, or femur. There is no evidence that the incidence of congenital hip dislocations is increased by vaginal delivery of a breech (Clausen and Nielsen, 1988). Bartlett and colleagues (2000) studied early motor development of breech- and control cephalic-presenting infants. They concluded that the mode of delivery did not explain the excess neuromotor impairment detected in breech infants.

Paralysis of the arm may follow pressure on the brachial plexus by the fingers in exerting traction, but more frequently it is caused by overstretching the neck while freeing the arms. Geutjens and colleagues (1996) described 36 newborns with brachial plexus injury following vaginal breech delivery. In 80 percent, there was avulsion of the upper cervical spine roots. This injury cannot be treated by microsurgical nerve grafting and carries a worse prognosis for shoulder function. When the fetus is extracted forcibly through a contracted pelvis, spoon-shaped depressions or actual fractures of the skull may result. Occasionally, even the fetal neck may be broken when great force is employed. Testicular injury, in some cases severe enough to result in anorchia, may occur following vaginal breech delivery (Tiwary, 1989).

VERSION

Version is a procedure in which the fetal presentation is altered by physical manipulation, either substituting one pole of a longitudinal presentation for the other or converting an oblique or transverse lie into a longitudinal presentation. According to whether the head or breech is made the presenting part, the operation is designated *cephalic* or *podalic version,* respectively. In *external version,* the manipulations are performed exclusively through the abdominal wall; in *internal version,* they are accomplished inside the uterine cavity.

EXTERNAL CEPHALIC VERSION. Once very popular, external version has received renewed interest in the past two decades, coincidental with the widespread availability of ultrasound, electronic fetal monitoring, and effective tocolytic agents. In the United States, Van Dorsten and co-workers (1981) rekindled interest in this procedure. And more recently, in conjunction with their recommendation of vaginal delivery for breech, the American College of Obstetricians and Gynecologists (2001) recommended that efforts be made to reduce breech presentation by external cephalic version whenever possible.

The success rate for external cephalic version has ranged from 35 to 85 percent, with an average of about 60 percent (American College of Obstetricians and Gynecologists, 2000). Zhang and co-authors (1993) reviewed 25 selected reports on external cephalic version published between 1980 and 1991. They reported an average success rate of 65 percent. Moreover, they observed that after successful version, almost all fetuses remain cephalic. They estimated that despite version attempts, 37 percent of women identified to have a late pregnancy breech ultimately will require cesarean delivery. Interestingly, several reports suggest that after successful version, the risk of cesarean delivery does not completely revert to the institutional baseline risk for vertex presentations, and that dystocia, malpresentation, and nonreassuring fetal heart patterns may be more common after successful version (Chan and colleagues, 2004; Vézina and associates, 2004).

Application of a policy of external cephalic version has been associated with reductions in the cesarean delivery rate at various institutions. Morrison and co-workers (1986) attempted external cephalic version in 2.3 percent of all pregnancies at the University of Mississippi Medical Center from 1982 to 1984. Compared with the preceding 3 years, they decreased vaginal breech deliveries from 1.8 to 1.1 percent of all pregnancies, and cesarean deliveries for breeches from 2.8 to 1.6 percent. Ben-Arie and colleagues (1995) reported that introduction of an external version protocol at their institution decreased breech presentation at term from 3.9 to 2.4 percent. Decision analysis models suggest that routine use of external cephalic version would reduce not only cesarean births but also costs (Gifford and associates, 1995a; Pollack and Yaffe, 2002).

Indications. In general, when a breech presentation is recognized prior to labor in a woman who has reached 36 weeks' gestation, external cephalic version should be considered. After this point, the likelihood of spontaneous version is low (Hickok and colleagues, 1992; Westgren and co-workers, 1985b). Moreover, if version results in the need for immediate delivery, complications of iatrogenic preterm delivery generally are not severe. An additional consideration in timing the version is that although earlier attempts are more likely to be successful, they also are more likely to be associated with spontaneous reversion to breech (Kornman and associates, 1995; van Veelen and colleagues, 1989).

Version should not be attempted if there is a contraindication to vaginal delivery. Examples include placenta previa or nonreassuring fetal status. A prior uterine incision is a relative contraindication, although in small studies external version was not associated with uterine rupture in women who had previously undergone cesarean delivery (de Meeus and associates, 1998; Flamm and co-workers, 1991; Schachter and colleagues, 1994). At the University of Alabama at Birmingham, decisions about version in women with a prior cesarean incision are individualized with an awareness that repeat cesarean is generally a safe operation. At Parkland Hospital, we do not attempt external version in these women. Obviously, larger studies are needed to better characterize risks versus benefits.

Factors Associated with Successful Version.
Increasing parity is the most consistent factor associated with success of external cephalic version (Zhang and colleagues, 1993). In another study, Hellstrom and co-workers (1990) identified only 3 of 16 variables to be associated with successful external version. The most important factor was parity, followed by fetal presentation, and then the amount of amnionic fluid. Version was more successful in a parous woman who has an unengaged fetus surrounded by a normal amount of amnionic fluid. Boucher and associates (2003) reported a direct relationship between the amnionic fluid index and successful external cephalic version in a prospective observational study of 1361 women who underwent a trial of version. Lau and associates (1997) identified three variables that predicted *failed* version. These were an engaged presenting part, difficulty in palpating the fetal head, and a uterus tense to palpation. In the presence of all three, there were no successes; with two, success was less than 20 percent, however if none was present, the success rate was 94 percent.

Gestational age is also important and earlier attempts increase the chance of success but are associated with an increased rate of spontaneous reversion (Westgren and colleagues, 1985b). Other reported determinants of failed version include diminished amnionic fluid volume, maternal obesity, anterior placenta, cervical dilatation, descent of the breech into the pelvis, and anterior or posterior positioning of the fetal spine (Fortunato and colleagues 1988; Newman and colleagues, 1993).

Transverse Lie.
Women with a transverse lie usually are excluded from analyses of breech version because the overall success rate approaches 90 percent (Newman and colleagues, 1993).

Technique.
External cephalic version should be carried out in an area that has ready access to a facility equipped to perform emergency cesarean deliveries (American College of Obstetricians and Gynecologists, 2000). Real-time ultrasonic examination is performed to confirm nonvertex presentation and adequacy of amnionic fluid volume, to rule out obvious fetal anomalies if not done previously, and to identify placental location. External monitoring is performed to assess fetal heart rate reactivity. D-immune globulin is given if indicated.

A "forward roll" of the fetus usually is attempted first. As shown in Figure 24–23, each hand grasps one of the fetal poles, and the buttocks are elevated from the maternal pelvis and displaced laterally. The buttocks are then gently guided toward the fundus, while the head is directed toward the pelvis. If the forward roll is unsuccessful, then a "backward flip" is attempted. Version attempts are discontinued for excessive discomfort, persistently abnormal fetal heart rate, or after multiple failed attempts. The nonstress test is repeated after version until a normal test result is obtained.

Tocolysis.
Most investigators recommend uterine relaxation with a tocolytic agent, usually terbutaline 250 μg given subcutaneously. Although some have shown a benefit to tocolysis, others have not. Robertson and associates (1987) used ritodrine, Tan and colleagues (1989) used salbutamol, and Yanny and associates (2000) used glyceryl trinitrate—all to no avail. Indeed, in a placebo controlled trial of 99 women, the use of sublingual nitroglycerin was associated with a lower rate of successful version than placebo—48 versus 63 percent—and a higher rate of complications such as hypotension (Bujold and colleagues, 2003). Conversely, in another randomized trial, Fernandez and co-workers (1996) reported that subcutaneous terbutaline significantly increased the success rate of version. It was 27 percent in the control group and 52 percent in the terbutaline group. Marquette and colleagues (1996) reported a benefit of ritodrine infusion, but only in nulliparas. Policies at the University of Alabama at Birmingham and at Parkland Hospital are to administer 250 μg of terbutaline subcutaneously to most women prior to attempted version.

Conduction Analgesia.
Some investigators have reported increased success with version when epidural analgesia is used. In a prospective randomized trial, Schorr and co-workers (1997) found that epidural analgesia given with terbutaline tocolysis was successful in 60 percent of cases, compared with 30 percent in cases in which only terbutaline was given. Mancuso and collaborators (2000) randomized 108 women and reported a success rate of 59 percent with epidural versus one of 33 percent without. Neiger and

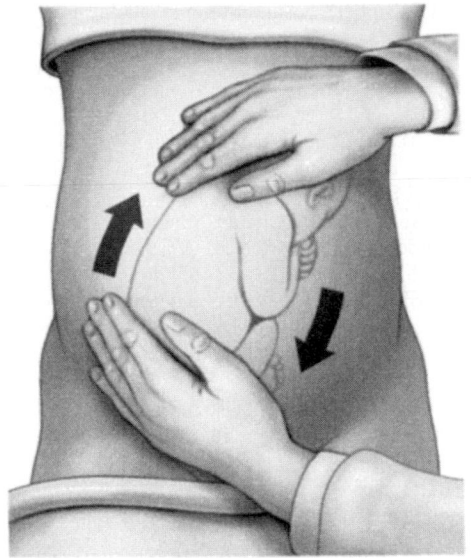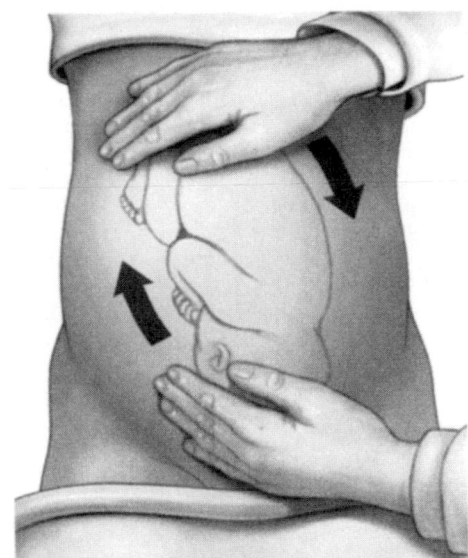

FIGURE 24–23. External cephalic version.

associates (1998) used epidural analgesia after failed versions and reported 56-percent success.

Not all have reported improved success with conduction analgesia. Dugoff and colleagues (1999) randomized 102 women to be given terbutaline, with or without spinal analgesia. The success rates were almost identical, 44 and 42 percent, respectively. Delisle and associates (2001) reported that spinal analgesia did not improve the success rate of external cephalic version in their randomized trial. According to the American College of Obstetricians and Gynecologists (2000), there is not enough consistent evidence to recommend conduction analgesia routinely.

Other Methods. There are some unconventional interventions with reported efficacy that emphasize our lack of understanding regarding the persistence of the breech presentation. Cardini and Weixen (1998) performed a randomized clinical trial to evaluate *moxibustion*—burning the herbal preparation *moxa* to generate heat to stimulate acupuncture point BL67—to promote spontaneous breech version. Women in the intervention group experienced significantly increased fetal movements and more often had a cephalic presentation at delivery. Mehl (1994) prospectively matched 100 women with a breech presentation at 37 to 40 weeks to evaluate *hypnosis* with suggestions for relaxation. Significantly more fetuses of women in the intervention group (81 percent) converted to vertex than in the control group (48 percent). In another study that at least intuitively is comprehensible, Johnson and Elliott (1995) used *acoustic stimulation* to startle breech fetuses to shift their spines laterally for successful manual version attempts.

Complications. Risks of external version include placental abruption, uterine rupture, amnionic fluid embolism, fetomaternal hemorrhage, isoimmunization, preterm labor, fetal

distress, and fetal demise. According to Zhang and colleagues (1993), there have been no reported fetal deaths in the United States resulting directly from external version since 1980. Reported nonfatal complications include fetal heart rate decelerations in almost 40 percent of fetuses and fetomaternal hemorrhage in 4 percent (Phelan and co-workers, 1984; Stine and colleagues, 1985). Scattered case reports have indicated some uncommon complications. Petrikovsky and colleagues (1987) reported a case of fetal brachial plexus injury after successful external version. Stine and co-workers (1985) reported a maternal death due to an amnionic fluid embolism. Rare severe complications notwithstanding, Collaris and Oei (2004) concluded, based on a systematic review of 44 studies, which included 7377 patients from 1990 to 2002, that external cephalic version is a safe procedure for mother and fetus.

INTERNAL PODALIC VERSION. This maneuver is used only for delivery of a second twin. It consists of the insertion of a hand into the uterine cavity to turn the fetus manually. The operator seizes one or both feet and draws them through the fully dilated cervix while using the other hand to transabdominally push the upper portion of the fetal body in the opposite direction. The operation is followed by breech extraction and is discussed in detail in Chapter 39 (see p. 940).

REFERENCES

Alarab M, Regan C, O'Connell MP, et al: Singleton vaginal breech delivery at term: Still a safe option. Obstet Gynecol 103:407, 2004

Albrechtsen S, Rasmussen S, Reigstad H, et al: Evaluation of a protocol for selecting fetuses in breech presentation for vaginal delivery or cesarean section. Am J Obstet Gynecol 177:586, 1997

American College of Obstetricians and Gynecologists: Mode of term singleton breech delivery. Committee Opinion No. 265, December 2001

American College of Obstetricians and Gynecologists: External cephalic version. Practice Bulletin No. 13, February 2000

Apuzzio J, Iffy L, Weiss G: Mode of term singleton breech delivery [letter]. Obstet Gynecol 99:1131, 2002

Awwad JT, Nahhas DE, Karam KS: Femur fracture during cesarean breech delivery. Int J Gynaecol Obstet 43:324, 1993

Barrett JM: Funic reduction for the management of umbilical cord prolapse. Am J Obstet Gynecol 165:654, 1991

Bartlett DJ, Okun NB, Byrne PJ, et al: Early motor development of breech- and cephalic-presenting infants. Obstet Gynecol 95:425, 2000

Ben-Arie A, Kogan S, Schachter M, et al: The impact of external cephalic version on the rate of vaginal and cesarean breech deliveries: A 3-year cumulative experience. Eur J Obstet Gynecol Reprod Biol 63:125, 1995

Bingham P, Lilford RJ: Management of the selected term breech presentation: Assessment of the risks of selected vaginal delivery versus cesarean section for all cases. Obstet Gynecol 69:965, 1987

Biswas A: Term breech trial [correspondence]. Lancet 357:225, 2001

Biswas A, Johnstone MJ: Term breech delivery: Does x-ray pelvimetry help? Aust N Z J Obstet Gynaecol 33:150, 1993

Bodmer B, Benjamin A, McLean FH, et al: Has use of cesarean section reduced the risks of delivery in the preterm breech presentation? Am J Obstet Gynecol 154:244, 1986

Boucher M, Bujold E, Marquette GP, et al: The relationship between amniotic fluid index and successful external cephalic version: A 14-year experience. Am J Obstet Gynecol 189:751, 2003

Bowes WA, Taylor ES, O'Brien M, et al: Breech delivery: Evaluation of method of delivery on perinatal results and maternal morbidity. Am J Obstet Gynecol 135:965, 1979

Brenner WE, Bruce RD, Hendricks CH: The characteristics and perils of breech presentation. Am J Obstet Gynecol 118:700, 1974

Bujold E, Boucher M, Rinfret D, et al: Sublingual nitroglycerin versus placebo as a tocolytic for external cephalic version: A randomized controlled trial in parous women. Am J Obstet Gynecol 189:1070, 2003

Cardini F, Weixin H: Moxibustion for correction of breech presentation: A randomized controlled trial. JAMA 280:1580, 1998

Chadha YC, Mahmood TA, Dick MJ, et al: Breech delivery and epidural analgesia. Br J Obstet Gynaecol 99:96, 1992

Chan LY, Tang JL, Tsoi KF, et al: Intrapartum cesarean delivery after successful external cephalic version: A meta-analysis. Obstet Gynecol 104:155, 2004

Cheng M, Hannah M: Breech delivery at term: A critical review of the literature. Obstet Gynecol 82:605, 1993

Christian SS, Brady K: Cord blood acid–base values in breech-presenting infants born vaginally. Obstet Gynecol 78:778, 1991

Clausen I, Nielsen KT: Breech position, delivery route and congenital hip dislocation. Acta Obstet Gynecol Scand 67:595, 1988

Collaris RJ, Oei SG: External cephalic version: A safe procedure? A systematic review of version-related risks. Acta Obstet Gynecol Scand 83:511, 2004

Collea JV, Chein C, Quilligan EJ: The randomized management of term frank breech presentation: A study of 208 cases. Am J Obstet Gynecol 137:235, 1980

Collea JV, Rabin SC, Weghorst GR, et al: The randomized management of term frank breech presentation: Vaginal delivery vs cesarean section. Am J Obstet Gynecol 131:186, 1978

Confino E, Ismajovich B, Rudick V, et al: Extradural analgesia in the management of singleton breech delivery. Br J Anaesth 57:892, 1985

Cunha-Filho JS, Passos E: Term breech trial [correspondence]. Lancet 357:227, 2001

de Meeus JB, Ellia F, Magnin G: External cephalic version after previous cesarean section: A series of 38 cases. Eur J Obstet Gynecol Reprod Biol 81:65, 1998

Delisle MF, Kamani A, Douglas J, et al: Antepartum external cephalic version under spinal anesthesia: A randomized controlled trial. Am J Obstet Gynecol 185:S115, 2001

Diro M, Puangsricharern A, Royer L, et al: Singleton term breech deliveries in nulliparous and multiparous women: A 5-year experience at the University of Miami-Jackson Memorial Hospital. Am J Obstet Gynecol 181:247, 1999

Dufour PH, Vinatier D, Orazi G, et al: The use of intravenous nitroglycerin for emergency cervico-uterine relaxation. Acta Obstet Gynecol Scand 76:287, 1997

Dugoff L, Stamm CA, Jones OW III, et al: The effect of spinal anesthesia on the success rate of external cephalic version: A randomized trial. Obstet Gynecol 93:345, 1999

Eller DP, Van Dorsten JP: Route of delivery for the breech presentation: A conundrum. Am J Obstet Gynecol 173: 393, 1995

Fait G, Daniel Y, Lessing JB, et al: Can labor with breech presentation be induced? Gynecol Obstet Investig 469:181, 1998

Fernandez CO, Bloom S, Wendel G: A prospective, randomized, blinded comparison of terbutaline versus placebo for singleton, term external cephalic version. Am J Obstet Gynecol 174:326, 1996

Fianu S, Vaclavinkova V: The site of placental attachment as a factor in the aetiology of breech presentation. Acta Obstet Gynecol Scand 57:371, 1978

Flamm BL, Fried MW, Lonky NM, et al: External cephalic version after previous cesarean section. Am J Obstet Gynecol 165:370, 1991

Flanagan TA, Mulchahey KM, Korenbrot CC, et al: Management of term breech presentation. Am J Obstet Gynecol 156:1492, 1987

Fontenot T, Campbell B, Mitchell-Tutt E, et al: Radiographic evaluation of breech presentation: Is it necessary? Ultrasound Obstet 10:338, 1997

Fortunato SJ, Mercer LJ, Guzick DS: External cephalic version with tocolysis: Factors associated with success. Obstet Gynecol 72:59, 1988

Freud E, Orvieto R, Merlob P: Neonatal labioperineal tear from fetal scalp electrode insertion, a case report. J Reprod Med 38:647, 1993

Geutjens G, Gilbert A, Helsen K: Obstetric brachial plexus palsy associated with breech delivery. A different pattern of injury. J Bone Joint Surg [Br] 78:303, 1996

Gifford DS, Keeler E, Kahn KL: Reductions in cost and cesarean rate by routine use of external cephalic version: A decision analysis. Obstet Gynecol 85:930, 1995a

Gifford DS, Morton SC, Fiske M, et al: A meta-analysis of infant outcomes after breech delivery. Obstet Gynecol 85:1047, 1995b

Gimovsky ML, Wallace RL, Schifrin BS, et al: Randomized management of the nonfrank breech presentation at term: A preliminary report. Am J Obstet Gynecol 146:34, 1983

Giuliani A, Scholl WMJ, Basver A, et al: Mode of delivery and outcome of 699 term singleton breech deliveries at a single center. Am J Obstet Gynecol 187:1694, 2002

Goodwin TM, Banks E, Millar LK, et al: Catastrophic shoulder dystocia and emergency symphysiotomy. Am J Obstet Gynecol 177:463, 1997

Gravenhorst JB, Schreuder AM, Veen S, et al: Breech delivery in very preterm and very-low-birthweight infants in the Netherlands. Br J Obstet Gynaecol 100:411, 1993

Hall JE, Kohl SG: Breech presentation: A study of 1456 cases. Am J Obstet Gynecol 72:977, 1956

Hannah ME, Hannah WJ, Hewson SA, et al: Planned caesarean section versus planned vaginal birth for breech presentation at term: A randomised multicentre trial. Lancet 356:1375, 2000

Hauth JC, Cunningham FG: Vaginal breech delivery is still justified. Obstet Gynecol 99:1115, 2002

Hellstrom AC, Nilsson B, Stange L: When does external cephalic version succeed? Acta Obstet Gynecol Scand 69:281, 1990

Hickok DE, Gordon DC, Milberg JA, et al: The frequency of breech presentation by gestational age at birth: A large population-based study. Am J Obstet Gynecol 166:851, 1992

Hill LM: Prevalence of breech presentation by gestational age. Am J Perinatol 7:92, 1990

Irion O, Hirsbrunner Almagbaly PH, Morabia A: Planned vaginal delivery versus elective caesarean section: A study of 705 singleton term breech presentations. Br J Obstet Gynaecol 105:710, 1998

Johnson RL, Elliott JP: Fetal acoustic stimulation, an adjunct to external cephalic version: A blinded, randomized crossover study. Am J Obstet Gynecol 173:1369, 1995

Kornman MT, Kimball KT, Reeves KO: Preterm external cephalic version in an outpatient environment. Am J Obstet Gynecol 172:1734, 1995

Krebs L, Topp M, Langhoff-Roos J: The relation of breech presentation at term to cerebral palsy. Br J Obstet Gynaecol 106:943, 1999

Kunzel W: Recommendations of the FIGO Committee on Perinatal Health on guidelines for the management of breech delivery. Int J Gynaecol Obstet 44:297, 1994

Lau TK, Lo KWK, Wan D, et al: Predictors of successful external cephalic version at term: A prospective study. Br J Obstet Gynaecol 104:798, 1997

Leung WC, Pun TC: Term breech trial [correspondence to the editor]. Lancet 357:225, 2001

Lindqvist A, Norden-Lindeberg S, Hanson U: Perinatal mortality and route of delivery in term breech presentations. Br J Obstet Gynaecol 104:1288, 1997

Lydon-Rochelle M, Albers L, Gorwoda J, et al: Accuracy of Leopold maneuvers in screening for malpresentation: A prospective study. Birth 20:132, 1993

Main DM, Main BK, Maurer MM: Cesarean section versus vaginal delivery for the breech fetus weighing less than 1500 grams. Am J Obstet Gynecol 146:580, 1983

Malloy MH, Onstad L, Wright E: National Institute of Child Health and Human Development Neonatal Research Network: The effect of cesarean delivery on birth outcome in very-low-birthweight infants. Obstet Gynecol 77:498, 1991

Mancuso KM, Yancey MK, Murphy JA, et al: Epidural analgesia for cephalic version: A randomized trial. Obstet Gynecol 95:648, 2000

Marquette GP, Boucher M, Theriault D, et al: Does the use of a tocolytic affect the success rate of external cephalic version? Am J Obstet Gynecol 175:859, 1996

Martin JA, Hamilton BE, Sutton PD, et al: Births: Final data for 2002. National Vital Statistics Reports, Vol 52, No. 10. Hyattsville, Md, National Center for Health Statistics, 2003

Mehl LE: Hypnosis and conversion of the breech to the vertex presentation. Arch Fam Med 3:881, 1994

Menticoglou SM: Symphysiotomy for the trapped aftercoming parts of the breech: A review of the literature and a plea for its use. Aust N Z J Obstet Gynaecol 30:1, 1990

Mokriski B: Abnormal presentation and multiple gestation. In Chestnut DH (ed): Obstetric Anesthesia. St Louis, Mosby, 1994, p 669

Molkenboer JF, Bouchkaert PX, Roumen FJ: Recent trends in breech delivery in the Netherlands. Br J Obstet Gynaecol 110:948, 2003

Morrison JC, Myatt RE, Martin JN, et al: External cephalic version of the breech presentation under tocolysis. Am J Obstet Gynecol 154:900, 1986

Morrison JJ, Sinnatamby R, Hackett GA: Obstetric pelvimetry in the UK: An appraisal of current practice. Br J Obstet Gynaecol 102:748, 1995

Neiger R, Hennessy MD, Patel M: Reattempting failed external cephalic version under epidural anesthesia. Am J Obstet Gynecol 179:1136, 1998

Nelson KB, Ellenberg JH: Antecedents of cerebral palsy: Multivariate analysis of risk. N Engl J Med 315:81, 1986

Newman RB, Peacock BS, Van Dorsten JP: Predicting success of external cephalic version. Am J Obstet Gynecol 169:245, 1993

Nwosu EC, Walkinshaw S, Chia P: Undiagnosed breech. Br J Obstet Gynaecol 100:531, 1993

Ohlsén H: Outcome of term breech delivery in primigravidae. A feto-pelvic breech index. Acta Obstet Gynecol Scand 54:141, 1975

Olshan AF, Shy KK, Luthy DA, et al: Cesarean birth and neonatal mortality in very-low-birthweight infants. Obstet Gynecol 64:267, 1984

Penn ZJ, Steer PJ: Reasons for declining participation in a prospective randomized trial to determine the optimum mode of delivery of the preterm breech. Controlled Clin Trials 11:226, 1990

Penn ZJ, Steer PJ, Grant A: A multicentre randomised controlled trial comparing elective and selective caesarean section for the delivery of the preterm breech infant. Br J Obstet Gynaecol 103:684, 1996

Petrikovsky BM, DeSilva HN, Fumia FD: Erb's palsy and fetal bruising after external cephalic version: Case report. Am J Obstet Gynecol 157:258, 1987

Phelan JP, Stine LE, Mueller ES, et al: Observations of fetal heart rate characteristics related to external cephalic version and tocolysis. Am J Obstet Gynecol 149:658, 1984

Pinard A: On version by external maneuvers. In: Traite de Palper Abdominal. Paris, 1889

Pollack R, Yaffe H: The cesarean birth epidemic: Primary prevention. Am J Obstet Gynecol 187:S82, 2002

Premru-Srsen T: Term breech trial (Correspondence). Lancet 357:225, 2001

Rietberg CC, Elferink-Stinkens PM, Brand R, et al: Term breech presentation in the Netherlands from 1995 to 1999: Mortality and morbidity in relation to the mode of delivery of 33,824 infants. Br J Obstet Gynaecol 110:604, 2003

Robertson AW, Kopelman JN, Read JA, et al: External cephalic version at term: Is a tocolytic necessary? Obstet Gynecol 70:896, 1987

Rojansky N, Tanos V, Lewin A, et al: Sonographic evaluation of fetal head extension and maternal pelvis in cases of breech presentation. Acta Obstet Gynecol Scand 73:607, 1994

Rosen MG, Chik L: The effect of delivery route on outcome of breech presentation. Am J Obstet Gynecol 148:909, 1984

Rovinsky JJ, Miller JA, Kaplan S: Management of breech presentation at term. Am J Obstet Gynecol 115:497, 1973

Sandberg EC: The Zavanelli maneuver: 12 years of recorded experience. Obstet Gynecol 93:312, 1999

Schachter M, Kogan S, Blickstein I: External cephalic version after previous cesarean section. A clinical dilemma. Int J Gynaecol Obstet 45:17, 1994

Schorr SJ, Speights SE, Ross EL, et al: A randomized trial of epidural anesthesia to improve external cephalic version success. Am J Obstet Gynecol 177:1133, 1997

Schutte MF, van Hemel OJS, van de Berg C, et al: Perinatal mortality in breech presentations as compared to vertex presentations in singleton pregnancies: An analysis based upon 57,819 computer-registered pregnancies in the Netherlands. Eur J Obstet Gynecol Reprod Biol 19:391, 1985

Socol ML, Cohen L, Depp R, et al: Apgar scores and umbilical cord arterial pH in the breech neonate. Int J Gynecol Obstet 27:37, 1988

Soernes T, Bakke T: The length of the human umbilical cord in vertex and breech presentations. Am J Obstet Gynecol 154:1086, 1986

Somerset D: Managing term breech deliveries: Term breech trial does not provide unequivocal evidence [letter]. BMJ 324:50, 2002

Spellacy WN, Gravem H, Fisch RO: The umbilical cord complications of true knots, nuchal cords, and cord around the body. Am J Obstet Gynecol 94:1136, 1966

Steyn W, Pieper C: Favorable neonatal outcome after fetal entrapment and partially successful Zavanelli maneuver in a case of breech presentation. Am J Perinatol 11:348, 1994

Stine LE, Phelan JP, Wallace R, et al: Update on external cephalic version performed at term. Obstet Gynecol 65:642, 1985

Stuart IP: Term breech trial [correspondence]. Lancet 357:228, 2001

Su M, McLeod L, Ross S, et al: Factors associated with adverse perinatal outcome in the Term Breech Trial. Am J Obstet Gynecol 189:740, 2003

Svenningsen NW, Westgren M, Ingemarsson I: Modern strategy for the term breech delivery—A study with a 4-year follow-up of the infants. J Perinat Med 13:117, 1985

Tan GW, Jen SW, Tan SL: A prospective randomised controlled trial of external cephalic version comparing two methods of uterine tocolysis with a non-tocolysis group. Singapore Med J 30:155, 1989

Thorp JM Jr, Jenkins T, Watson W: Utility of Leopold maneuvers in screening for malpresentation. Obstet Gynecol 78:394, 1991

Tiwary CM: Testicular injury in breech delivery: Possible implications. Urology 34:210, 1989

Uchide K, Murakami K: Term breech trial [correspondence]. Lancet 357:226, 2001

Van Dorsten JP, Schifrin BS, Wallace RL: Randomized control trial of external cephalic version with tocolysis in late pregnancy. Am J Obstet Gynecol 141:417, 1981

van Loon AJ, Mantingh A, Serlier EK, et al: Randomised controlled trial of magnetic resonance pelvimetry in breech presentation at term. Lancet 350:1799, 1997

van Veelen AJ, Van Cappellen AW, Flu PK, et al: Effect of external cephalic version in late pregnancy on presentation at delivery: A randomized controlled trial. Br J Obstet Gynaecol 96:916, 1989

Vasa R, Kim MR: Fracture of the femur at cesarean section: Case report and review of literature. Am J Perinatol 7:46, 1990

Vézina Y, Bujold E, Varin J, et al: Cesarean delivery after successful external cephalic version of breech presentation at term: A comparative study. Am J Obstet Gynecol 190:763, 2004

Wessen A, Elowsson P, Axemo P, et al: The use of intravenous nitroglycerin for emergency cervico-uterine relaxation. Acta Anaesthesiol Scand 39:847, 1995

Westgren LMR, Songster G, Paul RH: Preterm breech delivery: Another retrospective study. Obstet Gynecol 66:481, 1985a

Westgren M, Edvall H, Nordstrom L, et al: Spontaneous cephalic version of breech presentation in the last trimester. Br J Obstet Gynaecol 92:19, 1985b

Wolf H, Schaap AHP, Bruinse HW, et al: Vaginal delivery compared with caesarean section in early preterm breech delivery: A comparison of long term outcome. Br J Obstet Gynaecol 106:486, 1999

Yanny H, Johanson R, Baldwin KJ, et al: Double-blind randomised controlled trial of glyceryl trinitrate spray for external cephalic version. Br J Obstet Gynaecol 107:562, 2000

Zhang J, Bowes WA, Fortney JA: Efficacy of external cephalic version, including safety, cost-benefit analysis, and impact on the cesarean delivery rate. Obstet Gynecol 82:306, 1993

Zlatnick FJ: The Iowa premature breech trial. Am J Perinatol 10:60, 1993

25

Cesarean Delivery and Peripartum Hysterectomy

Cesarean delivery is defined as the birth of a fetus through incisions in the abdominal wall (laparotomy) and the uterine wall (hysterotomy). This definition does not include removal of the fetus from the abdominal cavity in the case of rupture of the uterus or in the case of an abdominal pregnancy. In some cases, and most often because of emergent complications such as intractable hemorrhage, abdominal hysterectomy is indicated following delivery. When performed at the time of cesarean delivery, the operation is termed *cesarean hysterectomy.* If done within a short time after vaginal delivery, it is termed *postpartum hysterectomy.*

HISTORICAL BACKGROUND

The origin of the term *cesarean* is obscure, and three principal explanations have been suggested.

In the first, according to legend, Julius Caesar was born in this manner, with the result that the procedure became known as the Caesarean operation. Several circumstances weaken this explanation. First, the mother of Julius Caesar lived for many years after his birth in 100 BC, and as late as the 17th century, the operation was almost invariably fatal. Second, the operation, whether performed on the living or the dead, is not mentioned by any medical writer before the Middle Ages. Historical details of the origin of the family name Caesar are found in the monograph by Pickrell (1935).

The second explanation is that the name of the operation is derived from a Roman law, supposedly created in the 8th century BC by Numa Pompilius, ordering that the procedure be performed upon women dying in the last few weeks of pregnancy in the hope of saving the child. This *lex regia*—king's rule or law—later became the *lex caesarea* under the emperors, and the operation itself became known as the caesarean operation. The German term *Kaiserschnitt*—Kaiser cut—reflects this derivation.

The third explanation is that the word *caesarean* was derived sometime in the Middle Age from the Latin verb *caedere, to cut.* This explanation seems most logical, but exactly when it was first applied to the operation is uncertain. Because *section* is derived from the Latin verb *seco,* which also means *cut,* the term *caesarean section* seems tautological—thus *cesarean delivery* is used. In the United States, the *ae* in the first syllable of *caesarean* is replaced with the letter *e.* In the United Kingdom, Australia, and most commonwealth nations, the *ae* is retained.

From the time of Virgil's Aeneas to Shakespeare's Macduff, poets repeatedly have referred to persons "untimely ripped" from their mother's womb. Ancient historians such as Pliny, moreover, say that Scipio Africianus, the conqueror of Hannibal, as well as Martius and Julius Caesar were all born by cesarean. In regard to Julius Caesar, Pliny adds that it was from this circumstance that the surname arose by which the Roman emperors were known. Birth in this extraordinary manner, as described in ancient mythology and legend, was believed to confer supernatural powers and elevated the heroes so born above ordinary mortals.

In evaluating these references to abdominal delivery in antiquity, it is pertinent that no such operation is even mentioned by Hippocrates, Galen, Celsus, Paulus, Soranus, or any other medical writer of those periods. If cesarean delivery actually was employed, it is particularly surprising that Soranus, whose extensive work written in the 2nd century AD covers all aspects of obstetrics, does not refer to it.

Several references to abdominal delivery appear in the Talmud between the 2nd and 6th centuries AD, but whether they had any background in terms of clinical usage is conjectural. There can be no doubt, however, that cesarean delivery in dead women was first practiced soon after the Christian Church gained dominance, as a measure directed at baptism of the child. Confidence in the validity of some of these early reports is rudely shaken, however, when they glibly state that a living, robust child was obtained 8 to 24 *hours* after the death of the mother.

Cesarean deliveries in the living were first recommended, and the current name of the operation used, in the celebrated work of Francois Rousset (1581) entitled *Traité Nouveau de l'Hystérotomotokie ou l'Enfantement Césaerien.* Rousset had never performed or witnessed the operation, and his information was based chiefly on letters from friends. He reported 14 successful cesarean deliveries, a fact in itself difficult to accept. When it is further stated that 6 of the 14 operations were performed on the same woman, the credulity of the most gullible is exhausted!

The apocryphal nature of most early reports on cesarean delivery is stressed because many of them have been accepted without question. Authoritative statements by dependable obstetricians about early use of the operation, however, did not appear in the literature until the mid-17th century. An example is the classical work of the French obstetrician, Francois Mauriceau, first published in 1668. This shows without doubt that the operation was employed on the living in rare and desperate cases, and that it was usually fatal. Details of the history of cesarean deliveries are found in Fasbender's classic text (1906).

The appalling maternal mortality rate of cesarean delivery continued until the beginning of the 20th century. In Great Britain and Ireland, the maternal death rate from the operation in 1865 was 85 percent. In Paris, during the 90 years ending in 1876, not a single mother survived cesarean delivery. Harris (1879) noted that as late as 1879, cesarean deliveries actually were more successful when performed by the patient herself or when the abdomen was ripped open by the horns of a bull! He found nine such cases in the literature with five recoveries, and contrasted them with 12 cesarean deliveries performed in New York City during the same period, with only one recovery.

The turning point in the evolution of cesarean operations came in 1882, when Max Sänger, then a 28-year-old assistant of Credé at Leipzig, introduced suturing of the uterine wall. The long neglect of so simple an expedient had not been from oversight, but stemmed from a deeply rooted belief that sutures in the uterus were superfluous as well as harmful by virtue of serving as the site for severe infection. In meeting these latter objections, Sänger, who had himself used sutures in only one case, documented their value not from the sophisticated medical centers of Europe but from frontier America. There, in outposts from Ohio to Louisiana, 17 cesarean deliveries had been reported in which silver wire sutures had been used, with the survival of eight mothers—an extraordinary record in those days. Thus, hemorrhage was the first and most serious problem to be solved. The review by Eastman (1932) details these findings.

Although the introduction of uterine sutures reduced mortality from the operation from hemorrhage, generalized peritonitis remained the dominant cause of death. Hence, various types of operations were devised to combat this scourge. The earliest was the Porro procedure (1876), which combined subtotal cesarean hysterectomy with marsupialization of the cervical stump. The first extraperitoneal operation was described by Frank in 1907. With various modifications, this technique was introduced by Latzko (1909) and Waters (1940), and it was employed until recent years.

In 1912, Krönig contended that the main advantage of the extraperitoneal technique was that the uterine incision was covered by peritoneum. To accomplish this, he cut through the vesical reflection of the peritoneum from one round ligament to the other and separated it and the bladder from the lower uterine segment. Then, through a vertical median incision, the child was extracted by forceps. The uterine incision was then closed and buried under the vesical peritoneum. With minor modifications, this low-segment technique was introduced into the United States by Beck (1919) and popularized by DeLee (1922) and others. A particularly important modification was recommended by Kerr in 1926, who preferred a transverse rather than a longitudinal uterine incision.

Boley (1991) and Sewell (1993) have provided extensive reviews of the history of cesarean delivery.

CESAREAN DELIVERY

CONTEMPORARY STATUS OF CESAREAN DELIVERY

Frequency. From 1965 through 1988, the cesarean delivery rate in the United States rose progressively from only 4.5 percent of all deliveries to almost 25 percent (U.S. Public Health Service, 1991). Most of this increase took place in the 1970s and early 1980s and occurred throughout the western world (Fig. 25–1). Between 1989 and 1996 the annual rate of cesarean delivery decreased in the United States (Fig. 25–2). This was due in large part to an increased rate of *vaginal*

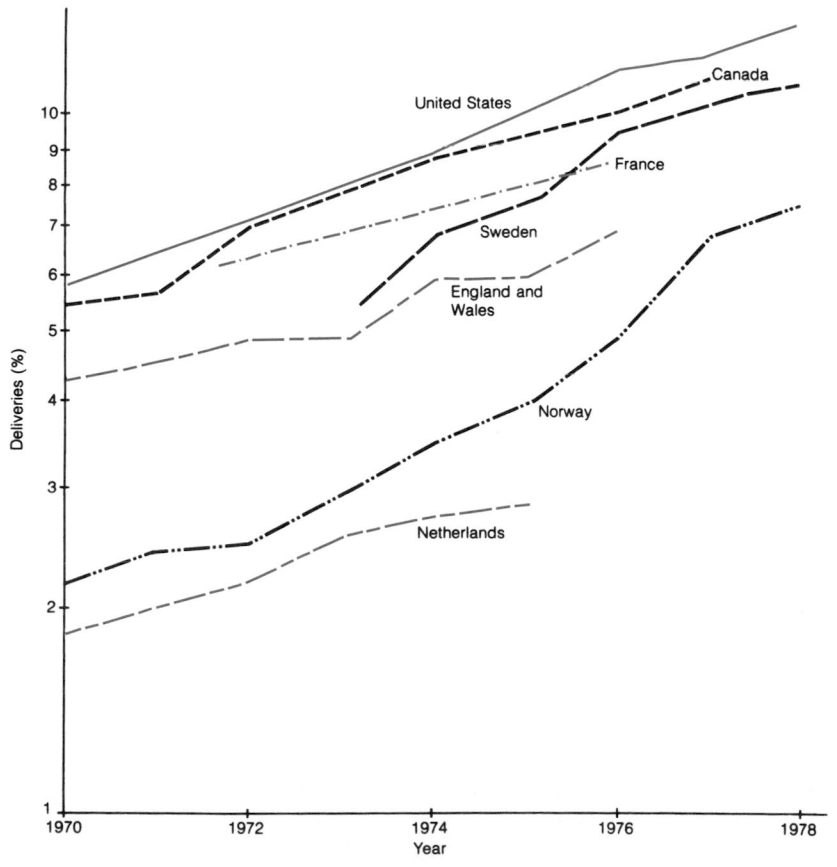

FIGURE 25–1. Percentage of deliveries by cesarean: Selected countries, 1970–1978. (From Smith, 1987, with permission.)

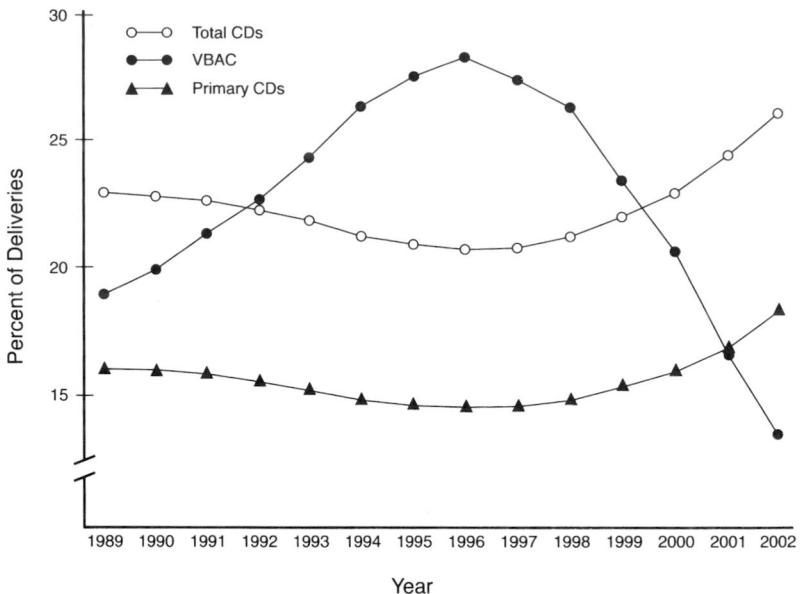

FIGURE 25–2. Total and primary cesarean and vaginal birth after cesarean (VBAC) rates: United States, 1989–2001. The total rate is expressed as the percent of all live births by cesarean delivery (CD). The primary cesarean rate is per 100 live births to women who have not had a previous cesarean. The rate of VBAC delivery is calculated per 100 live births to women with a previous cesarean delivery. (Data from Hamilton and associates, 2003.)

birth after cesarean (VBAC) and to a lesser extent, a small decrease in the primary cesarean rate (see Fig. 25–2). Since 1996, however, the total cesarean rate has increased every year, and in 2002 it was 26.1 percent, the highest rate ever recorded in the United States.

From these figures, it is apparent that the 1991 U.S. Public Health Service goal of an overall cesarean delivery rate of 15 percent by the year 2000 was not achieved. More recently, the American College of Obstetricians and Gynecologists Task Force on Cesarean Delivery Rates (2000) recommended two benchmarks for the United States for the year 2010:

1. A cesarean rate of 15.5 percent for nulliparous women at 37 weeks or more with a singleton cephalic presentation.
2. A vaginal birth rate after a prior cesarean of 37 percent in women at 37 weeks or more with a singleton cephalic presentation who had one prior low-transverse cesarean delivery. The U.S. Department of Health and Human Services (2000) has established similar goals for 2010.

The reasons why the cesarean rate quadrupled between 1965 and 1988 and its continued rise are not completely understood, but some explanations include the following:

1. Women are having fewer children, thus, a greater percentage of births are among *nulliparas*, who are at increased risk for cesarean delivery.
2. The average *maternal age* is rising, and older women, especially nulliparas, are at increased risk of cesarean delivery (Fig. 25–3).
3. The use of *electronic fetal monitoring* is widespread. This technique is associated with an increased cesarean delivery rate compared with intermittent fetal heart rate auscultation (see Chap. 18, p. 444). Although cesarean delivery performed primarily for "fetal distress" comprises only a minority of all such procedures, in many more cases concern for an abnormal, or "nonreassuring," fetal heart rate tracing lowers the threshold for cesarean deliveries performed for abnormal progress of labor.

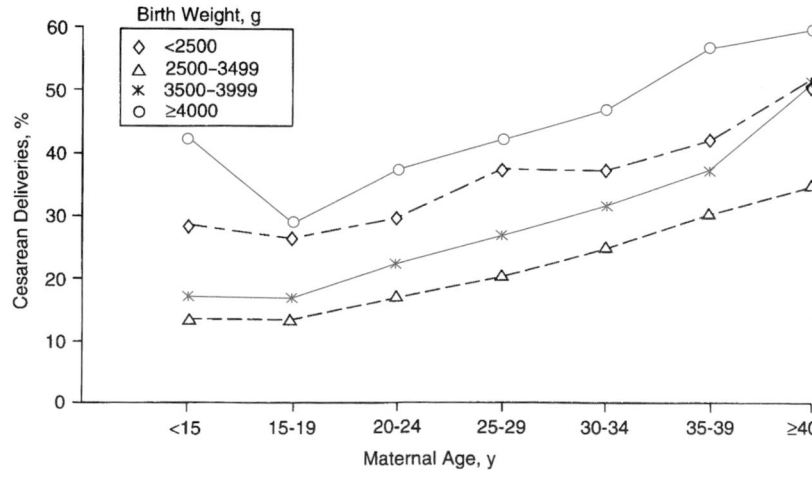

FIGURE 25–3. Primary cesarean delivery rates by maternal age and birthweight among nulliparous women in Washington State, 1987–1990. (From Parrish and co-workers, 1994, with permission.)

4. The vast majority of fetuses presenting as *breech* are now delivered by cesarean (see Chap. 24, p. 571).

5. The incidence of *midpelvic forceps and vacuum deliveries* has decreased (see Chap. 23, p. 548).

6. Rates of *labor induction* continue to rise, and induced labor, especially among nulliparas, increases the risk of cesarean delivery (see Chap. 22, p. 536).

7. The prevalence of *obesity* has risen dramatically, and obesity also increases the risk of cesarean delivery (see Chap. 43, p. 1011).

8. Concern for *malpractice litigation* has contributed significantly to the present cesarean delivery rate. More than a decade ago, it was reported that failure to perform a cesarean delivery and thus avoid adverse neonatal neurological outcome or cerebral palsy was the dominant obstetrical claim in the United States (Physicians Insurance Association of America, 1992). Although more recent data are aggregated differently, they suggest that this picture has changed little. Specifically, in 2001 a brain-damaged infant was the claim responsible for 40 percent of all medicolegal indemnity paid by obstetricians-gynecologists (Physicians Insurance Association of America, 2002). This reality is especially troubling in view of the well-documented lack of association between cesarean delivery and any reduction in childhood neurological problems. According to Foley and colleagues (2002), the incidence of neither neonatal seizures nor cerebral palsy diminished as the rate of cesarean delivery increased (see also Chap. 29, p. 654).

9. Some elective cesarean deliveries are now performed due to concern over pelvic floor injury associated with vaginal birth (Nygaard and Cruikshank, 2003).

Indications. As shown in Table 25–1, repeat cesarean deliveries and those performed for dystocia have been the leading indications in both the United States and other western industrialized countries. Although it is not possible to catalog comprehensively all appropriate indications for cesarean delivery,

TABLE 25–1 **Contribution by Indication to Overall Cesarean Delivery Rate in Four Countries During 1990**

Indications	Cesarean Delivery Rate per 100 Total Deliveries			
	Norway	Scotland	Sweden	United States
Previous cesarean	1.3	3.1	3.1	8.5
Breech	2.1	2.0	1.8	2.6
Dystocia	3.6	4.0	1.7	7.1
Fetal distress	2.0	2.4	1.6	2.3
Other	3.7	2.7	2.4	3.2
Overall cesarean rate	12.8	14.2	10.7	23.6

Modified from Notzon and colleagues (1994), with permission.

over 85 percent are performed because of prior cesarean delivery, dystocia, fetal distress, or breech presentation.

PRIOR CESAREAN DELIVERY. Management of the woman with a prior cesarean delivery is discussed in Chapter 26.

DYSTOCIA. Some form of dystocia is the most frequent indication for cesarean delivery in the United States. An analysis of dystocia as a contributing factor to the cesarean rate is difficult, however, because of the heterogeneity inherent in the condition (see Chap. 20, p. 496). Indeed, there are 16 different ICD-9 (2003) codes applicable to cesarean delivery performed for a labor abnormality! Descriptive terms vary from more precise definitions promulgated by Friedman (1978)—*secondary arrest of dilatation, arrest of descent*—to more ambiguous and commonly used terms such as *cephalopelvic disproportion* and *failure to progress.*

FETAL DISTRESS. Electronic fetal monitoring was employed in 85 percent of labors in the United States in 2002 (Martin and colleagues, 2003). Its use increases the cesarean delivery rate, perhaps by as much as 40 percent (Thacker and associates, 2001). Unfortunately, despite initial optimism, it has become well established that management based on electronic monitoring is no better in reducing the risk of cerebral palsy or perinatal death than that based on intermittent heart rate auscultation. Indeed, the performance of cesarean delivery per se may have no bearing on the neurodevelopmental prognosis of the infant. Scheller and Nelson (1994), in a report from the National Institutes of Health, and Lien and associates (1995) presented data specifically refuting any association between cesarean delivery and either cerebral palsy or seizures.

Pertinent to the diagnosis of fetal distress are the recommendations of the American Academy of Pediatrics and the American College of Obstetricians and Gynecologists (2002) that facilities giving obstetrical care have the capability of initiating a cesarean delivery within 30 minutes of the decision to operate. Misinterpretations of this guideline are common. Specifically, this recommendation addresses facilities and does not govern clinical decision making. There is no nationally recognized standard of care that codifies an acceptable time interval for performance of cesarean delivery. In most instances, operative delivery is not necessary within this 30-minute time frame. Indeed, Bloom and co-workers (2001) from the National Institute of Child Health and Human Development (NICHD) Maternal–Fetal Medicine Units Network reported that 69 percent of 7450 cesareans performed in labor commenced more than 30 minutes after the decision to operate. Moreover, Chauhan and co-workers (1997) and MacKenzie and Cooke (2002) reported that failure to achieve a cesarean delivery decision-to-incision time of less than 30 minutes was not associated with a negative impact on neonatal outcome. On the other hand, when faced with an acute, catastrophic deterioration in fetal condition, cesarean delivery usually is indicated as rapidly as possible and purposeful delays of any time period would be inappropriate.

BREECH PRESENTATION. Management of the breech-presenting fetus is discussed in Chapter 24. Concern for fetal injury, as well as the infrequency with which a breech presentation meets criteria for a trial of labor, make it likely that its contribution to the overall cesarean delivery rate will remain relatively static.

METHODS TO DECREASE CESAREAN DELIVERY RATES.

Several investigators have documented the feasibility of achieving significant reductions in institutional cesarean delivery rates without increased perinatal morbidity or mortality (DeMott, 1990; DeMuylder, 1990; Porreco, 1990; Pridijian, 1991; Sanchez-Ramos, 1990, and all of their co-workers). Programs aimed at reducing the number of cesarean deliveries generally are focused on educating physicians, peer reviewing, encouraging a trial of labor after prior transverse cesarean delivery, and restricting cesarean deliveries for dystocia only to women who meet strictly defined criteria. In a recent randomized study from 34 Latin American hospitals, Althabe and colleagues (2004) reported that a mandatory second opinion was associated with a small but significant reduction in the cesarean delivery rate without an adverse effect on maternal or perinatal morbidity.

MATERNAL MORTALITY AND MORBIDITY.

In the United States, maternal death attributable solely to cesarean delivery is rare. In 1980, Frigoletto and colleagues reported a series of 10,000 consecutive operations with no maternal deaths. In 1988, Sachs and associates observed only seven deaths as a direct result of more than 121,000 cesarean deliveries performed between 1976 and 1984.

Even so, larger data sets attest to the mortality risks. In a population-based case-control study from North Carolina, which encompassed the 7-year period from 1992 to 1998, cesarean delivery was associated with an almost fourfold risk of death, even after controlling for pregnancy complications (Harper and colleagues, 2003). In another study, Hall and Bewley (1999) compiled data from over 2 million births in the United Kingdom from 1994 through 1996. They showed that whereas emergency cesarean delivery was associated with an almost ninefold risk of maternal death relative to that of vaginal delivery, even elective cesarean delivery was associated with an almost threefold risk (Table 25–2). In a recent Network study, Landon and associates (2004) reported a fivefold increased maternal death rate in women with a failed versus successful vaginal delivery who underwent a trial of labor after a prior cesarean delivery.

Maternal morbidity is increased dramatically with cesarean compared with that of vaginal delivery. Principal sources are puerperal infection, hemorrhage, and thromboembolism (Burrows and associates, 2004). Not all morbidity is immediate, and Lydon-Rochelle and colleagues (2000) reported that rehospitalization in the 60 days following cesarean delivery was nearly twice as common as after vaginal delivery—17 versus 10 hospitalizations per 1000 women

TABLE 25–2 Direct Death Rates by Mode of Delivery in the United Kingdom, 1994–1996

Mode of Delivery	Total Births	Total Deaths	Death Rate (per 100,000)	Risk Ratio (95% CI)
Vaginal	1,845,957	38	2.1	1.0
Cesarean				
Elective	153,829	9	5.9	2.84 (1.72–4.70)
Emergency	197,781	36	18.2	8.84 (5.60–13.94)
Total	351,610	45	12.8	6.22 (3.90–9.90)

Adapted from Hall and Bewley (1999), with permission.

delivered. Rajasekar and Hall (1997) reported that the incidence of bladder laceration with cesarean operation was 1.4 per 1000 procedures, and the incidence of ureteral injury was 0.3 per 1000. Although bladder injury was immediately identified, the diagnosis of ureteral injury often was delayed. Uterine infection is relatively common after cesarean delivery. The diagnosis and management of pelvic and wound infections following cesarean delivery are discussed in Chapter 31. As discussed in Chapter 43 (see p. 1011), morbidity associated with cesarean delivery is increased dramatically in obese women.

All of these morbidities, as well as the increased recovery time, result in a twofold increase in costs for cesarean versus vaginal delivery (Henderson and associates, 2001).

PATIENT CHOICE CESAREAN DELIVERY.

As cesarean delivery has become safer and more commonly performed, and women have taken a more active role in their obstetrical care, it has been argued that women should be able to choose to undergo elective cesarean delivery (Harer, 2000). The issue is currently quite contentious. Putative reasons for this choice include avoidance of pelvic floor injury during vaginal birth, reduction in the risk of fetal injury, and convenience (Al-Mufti and colleagues, 1997). Conversely, the motivation of physicians in offering this choice, its medical rationale from both a maternal and fetal-neonatal standpoint, and even the concept of informed free choice have been questioned (Wagner, 2000).

Bewley and Cockburn (2002a, 2000b) found the concept of elective cesarean delivery to lack both ethical and medical merit. Clearly, and usually only with the benefit of hindsight, it can be said that some women and infants who have undergone difficult vaginal birth may have been better served by cesarean delivery instead. In most cases, however, clinically robust means of prospectively identifying otherwise uncomplicated pregnancies in which the woman or her fetus-infant would benefit from elective cesarean delivery are lacking. Minkoff and Chervenak (2003) and Minkhoff and colleagues (2004) concluded that although current evidence does not support routine elective cesarean delivery, it *does* ethically support an obstetrical decision to accede to an *informed* patient's request for such a delivery. At this time, we conclude that it is difficult to justify a *laissez faire* approach to this major operation.

TECHNIQUE FOR CESAREAN DELIVERY. With minor variations, surgical performance of cesarean delivery is comparable worldwide.

Abdominal Incisions. Usually either a midline vertical or a suprapubic transverse incision is used. Only in especial circumstances would a paramedian or midtransverse incision be employed.

Vertical Incision. An infraumbilical midline vertical incision is quickest to make. The incision should be of sufficient length to allow delivery of the infant without difficulty. Therefore, its length should correspond with the estimated fetal size. Sharp dissection is performed to the level of the anterior rectus sheath, which is freed of subcutaneous fat to expose a strip of fascia in the midline about 2 cm wide. Some surgeons prefer to incise the rectus sheath with the scalpel throughout the length of the fascial incision. Others prefer to make a small opening and then incise the fascial layer with scissors. The rectus and the pyramidalis muscles are separated in the midline by sharp and blunt dissection to expose transversalis fascia and peritoneum.

The transversalis fascia and preperitoneal fat are dissected carefully to reach the underlying peritoneum. The peritoneum near the upper end of the incision is opened carefully, either bluntly, or by elevating it with two hemostats placed about 2 cm apart. The tented fold of peritoneum between the clamps is then examined and palpated to be sure that omentum, bowel, or bladder is not adjacent. In women who have had previous intra-abdominal surgery, including cesarean delivery, omentum or bowel may be adherent to the undersurface of the peritoneum. The peritoneum is incised superiorly to the upper pole of the incision and downward to just above the peritoneal reflection over the bladder.

Transverse Incisions. With the modified *Pfannenstiel incision,* the skin and subcutaneous tissue are incised using a lower transverse, slightly curvilinear incision. The incision is made at the level of the pubic hairline and is extended somewhat beyond the lateral borders of the rectus muscles. After the subcutaneous tissue has been separated from the underlying fascia for 1 cm or so on each side, the fascia is incised transversely the full length of the incision. Sequentially, first the superior and then the inferior edge of the fascia is grasped with suitable clamps and elevated by the assistant as the operator separates the fascial sheath from the underlying rectus muscles either bluntly or sharply. Blood vessels coursing between the muscles and fascia are clamped, cut, and ligated, or they are fulgurated with electrocautery. Meticulous hemostasis is imperative. The fascial separation is carried near enough to the umbilicus to permit an adequate midline longitudinal incision of the peritoneum. The rectus muscles are then separated in the midline to expose the underlying peritoneum. The peritoneum is opened as discussed earlier.

The cosmetic advantage of the transverse skin incision is apparent. Whether it is stronger and less likely to undergo dehiscence is debated (Hendrix and co-workers, 2000). There definitely are some disadvantages in its use. Exposure in some women is not as optimal as with a vertical incision, and the latter can more easily be extended to increase exposure—a particular advantage if the woman is obese. With repeat cesarean delivery, reentry through a Pfannenstiel incision usually is more time consuming and difficult because of scarring.

When a transverse incision is desired and more room is needed, the *Maylard incision* provides a safe option (Ayers and Morley, 1987; Giacalone and colleagues, 2002). In this incision, the rectus muscles are divided sharply or with electrocautery. The incision also may be especially useful in women with significant scarring resulting from previous transverse incisions.

Uterine Incisions. Most often the incision is made in the lower uterine segment transversely as described by Kerr in 1926. Occasionally, a low-segment vertical incision as described by Krönig in 1912 may be used. The so-called *classical incision* is a vertical incision into the body of the uterus above the lower uterine segment and reaching the uterine fundus. This incision is seldom used today. For most cesarean deliveries, the transverse incision is the operation of choice. Its advantages are that it (1) is easier to repair, (2) is located at a site least likely to rupture during a subsequent pregnancy, and (3) does not promote adherence of bowel or omentum to the incisional line. If the fetus is not presenting by the vertex, if there are multiple fetuses, or if the fetus is very immature and the woman has had no labor, a lower-segment vertical or even a classical incision may, at times, prove to be advantageous.

TECHNIQUE FOR TRANSVERSE CESAREAN INCISION. Commonly, the uterus is found to be dextrorotated so that the left round ligament is more anterior and closer to the midline than the right. With thick meconium or infected amnionic fluid, some surgeons prefer to lay a moistened laparotomy pack in each lateral peritoneal gutter to absorb fluid and blood that escape from the opened uterus. The rather loose reflection of peritoneum above the upper margin of the bladder and overlying the anterior lower uterine segment—the *bladder flap*—is grasped in the midline with forceps and incised transversely with a scalpel or scissors (Fig. 25–4). Scissors are inserted between the vesicouterine serosa and myometrium of the lower uterine segment and are pushed laterally from the midline, and then withdrawn while partially opening the blades intermittently, to separate a 2-cm-wide strip of serosa, which is then incised. As the lateral margin on each side is approached, the scissors are directed somewhat more cephalad (Fig. 25–5). The lower flap of peritoneum is elevated, and the bladder is gently separated by blunt or sharp dissection from the underlying myometrium (Fig. 25–6). In general, the separation of bladder should not

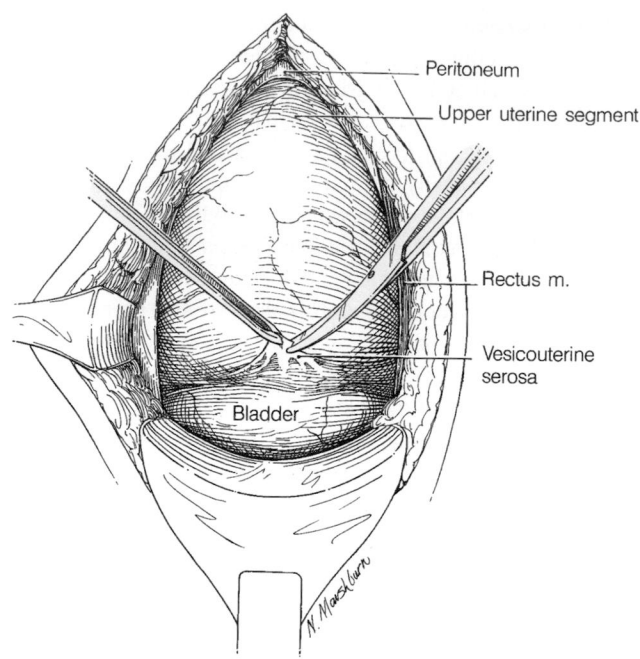

FIGURE 25–4. The loose vesicounterine serosa is grasped with the forceps. The hemostat tip points to the upper margin of the bladder. The retractor is firmly positioned against the symphysis. (m. = muscle.)

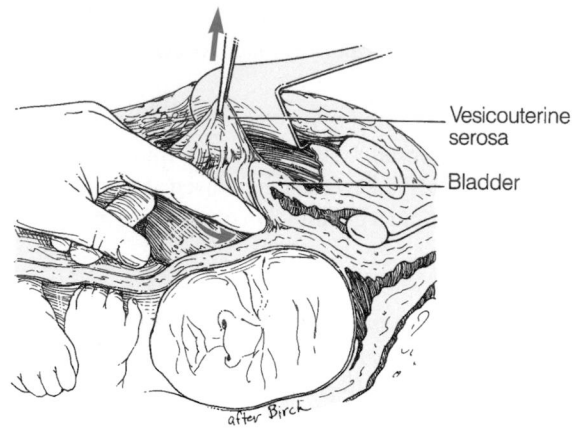

FIGURE 25–6. Cross section showing dissection of the bladder off the uterus to expose the lower uterine segment.

exceed 5 cm in depth and usually should be less. It is possible, especially with an effaced, dilated cervix, to dissect downward so deeply as inadvertently to expose and then enter the underlying vagina rather than the lower uterine segment.

The uterus is entered through the lower uterine segment about 1 cm below the upper margin of the peritoneal reflection. It is important to place the uterine incision relatively higher in women with advanced or complete cervical dilatation to minimize both lateral extension of the incision into the uterine arteries and unintended entry into the vagina. This is done by using the vesicouterine serosal reflection as a guide.

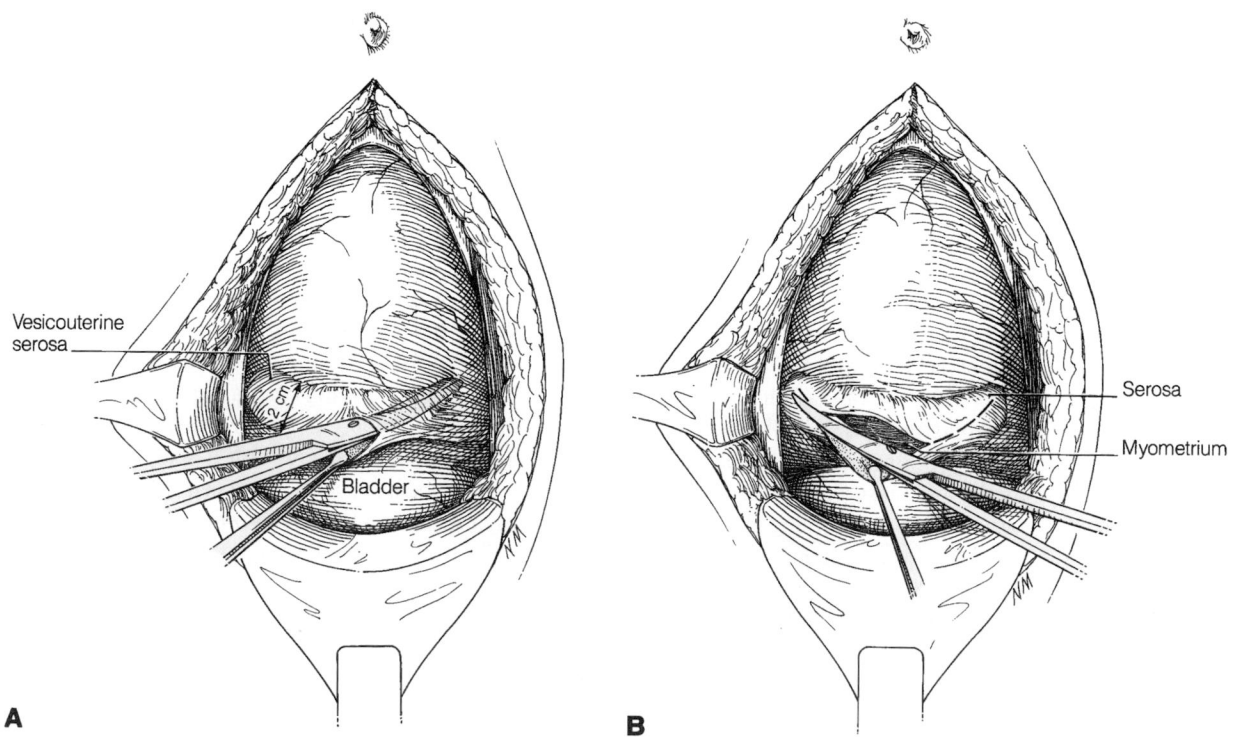

FIGURE 25–5. The loose serosa above the upper margin of the bladder is elevated and incised laterally.

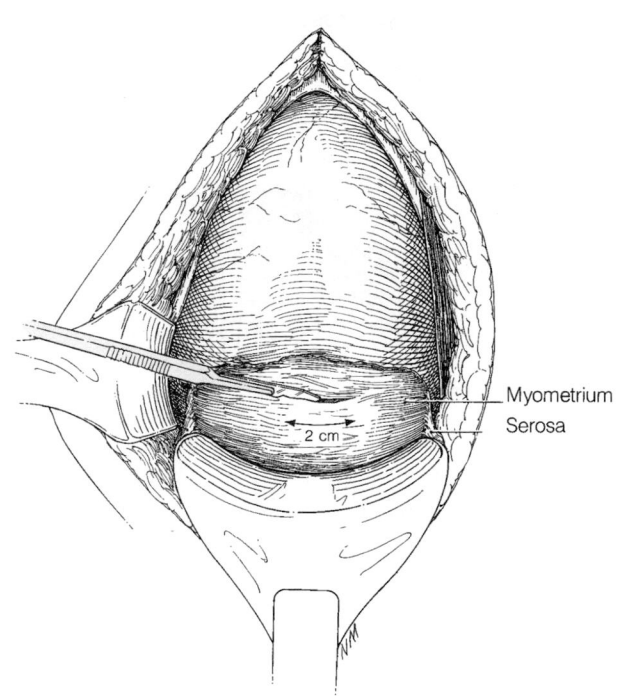

FIGURE 25–7. The myometrium is incised carefully to avoid cutting the fetal head.

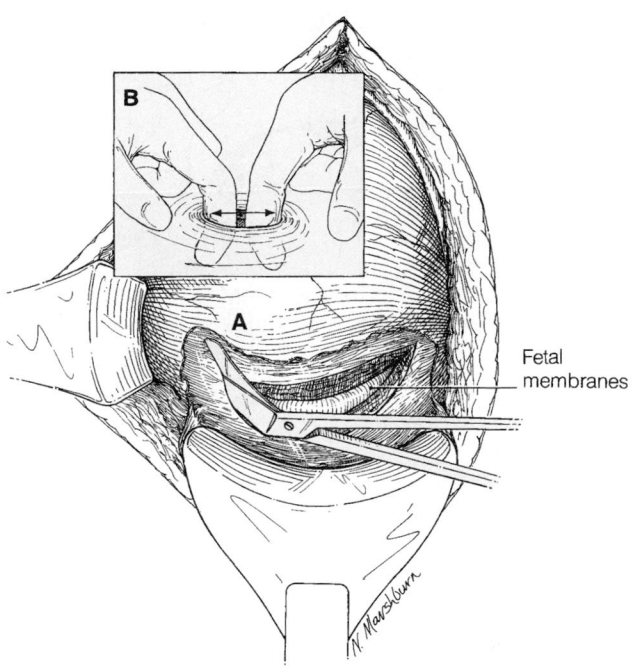

FIGURE 25–8. After entering the uterine cavity, the incision is extended laterally with bandage scissors (**A**) or with the fingers, as shown in **B**.

The uterine incision can be made by a variety of techniques. Each is initiated by using a scalpel to transversely incise the exposed lower uterine segment for 1 to 2 cm in the midline. This must be done carefully to avoid injury to the fetus (Fig. 25–7). Skin laceration was the most common fetal injury seen with 37,110 cesarean deliveries in the Network study reported by Alexander and colleagues (2005). Careful blunt entry using hemostats or fingertip to split the muscle may be helpful. Once the uterus is opened, the incision can be extended by cutting laterally and then slightly upward with bandage scissors. Alternatively, when the lower uterine segment is thin, the incision can be extended by simply spreading the incision, using lateral and upward pressure applied with each index finger (Fig. 25–8). Although Rodriguez and associates (1994) reported that blunt and sharp extensions of the initial uterine incision are equivalent in terms of safety and postoperative complications, Magann and colleagues (2002) reported that sharp dissection increased blood loss and the need for transfusion. **It is very important to make the uterine incision large enough to allow delivery of the head and trunk of the fetus without either tearing into or having to cut into the uterine arteries and veins that course through the lateral margins of the uterus.** If the placenta is encountered in the line of incision, it must be either detached or incised. When the placenta is incised, fetal hemorrhage may be severe; thus, delivery and cord clamping should be performed as soon as possible in such cases.

Delivery of the Infant. In a cephalic presentation, a hand is slipped into the uterine cavity between the symphysis and fetal head, and the head is elevated gently with the fingers and palm through the incision, aided by modest transabdominal fundal pressure (Fig. 25–9). After a long labor with cephalopelvic disproportion, the fetal head may be tightly wedged in the birth canal. Upward pressure exerted by a hand in the vagina by an assistant will help to dislodge the head and allow its delivery above the symphysis. To minimize fetal aspiration of amnionic fluid, exposed nares and mouth are aspirated with a bulb syringe before the thorax is delivered. The shoulders then are delivered using gentle traction plus fundal pressure (Fig. 25–10). The rest of the body readily follows.

After the shoulders are delivered, an intravenous infusion containing about two ampules or 20 units of oxytocin per liter of crystalloid is infused at 10 mL/min until the uterus contracts satisfactorily, after which the rate can be reduced. Bolus doses of 5 to 10 units are avoided because of associated hypotension. Munn and colleagues (2001) studied a much higher initial concentration using a solution of 80 units of oxytocin in 500 mL of crystalloid, which was infused at about 17 mL/min. They reported that this approach significantly reduced the need for additional uterotonic agents.

The cord is clamped, and the infant is given to the team member who will conduct resuscitative efforts as needed. The uterine incision is observed for any vigorously bleeding sites. These should be promptly clamped with Pennington or ring forceps, or similar instruments. The placenta is then delivered unless it has already done so spontaneously. Many surgeons prefer manual removal, but spontaneous delivery with some

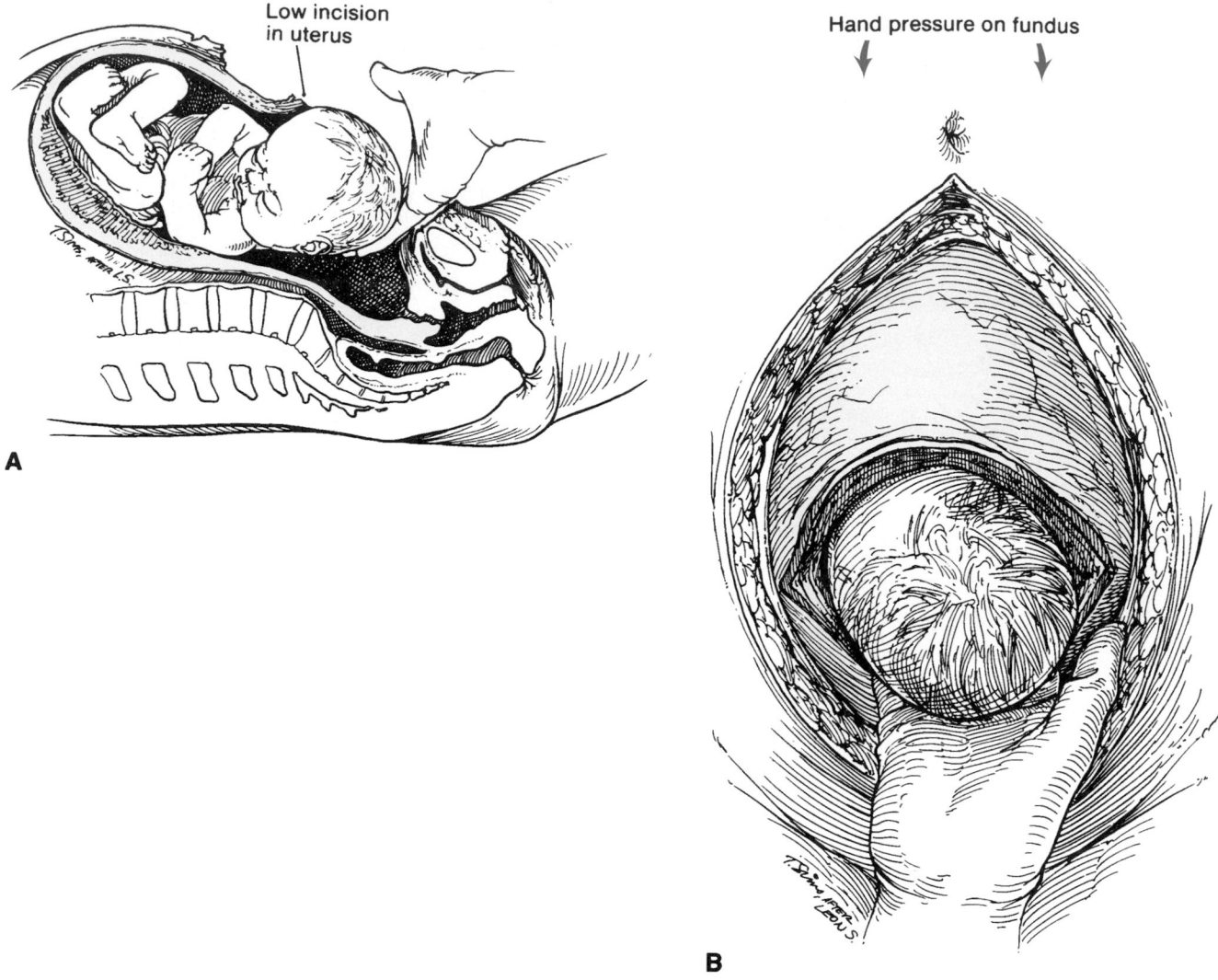

FIGURE 25–9. A. Immediately after incising the uterus and rupturing the fetal membranes, the fingers are insinuated between the symphysis pubis and the fetal head until the posterior surface is reached. The head is lifted carefully anteriorly and, as necessary, superiorly to bring it from beneath the symphysis forward through the uterine and abdominal incisions. **B.** As the fetal head is lifted through the incision, pressure usually is applied to the uterine fundus through the abdominal wall to help expel the fetus.

cord traction (Fig. 25–11) has been shown to reduce the risk of puerperal metritis (Atkinson and colleagues, 1996; Lasley and associates, 1997). Fundal massage, begun as soon as the fetus is delivered, reduces bleeding and hastens placental delivery.

The American Academy of Pediatrics and the American College of Obstetricians and Gynecologists (2002) recommend that "a qualified person who is skilled in neonatal resuscitation should be in the operative delivery room, with all equipment needed for neonatal resuscitation, to care for the neonate." Based on their comparison of 834 cesarean deliveries with 834 low-risk vaginal deliveries, Jacob and Phenninger (1997) reported that, with regional analgesia, there is rarely a need for vigorous infant resuscitation after

elective repeat cesarean delivery or cesarean delivery for dystocia without fetal heart rate abnormalities, and that a pediatrician may not be necessary at such deliveries. At Parkland Hospital, pediatric nurse practitioners attend uncomplicated, scheduled cesarean deliveries.

Repair of the Uterus. After delivery of the placenta, the uterus may be lifted through the incision onto the draped abdominal wall and the fundus covered with a moistened laparotomy pack. Although some clinicians prefer to avoid it, uterine exteriorization often has advantages that outweigh any disadvantages. For example, the relaxed, atonic uterus can be recognized quickly and massage applied. The incision and bleeding points are visualized more easily and repaired,

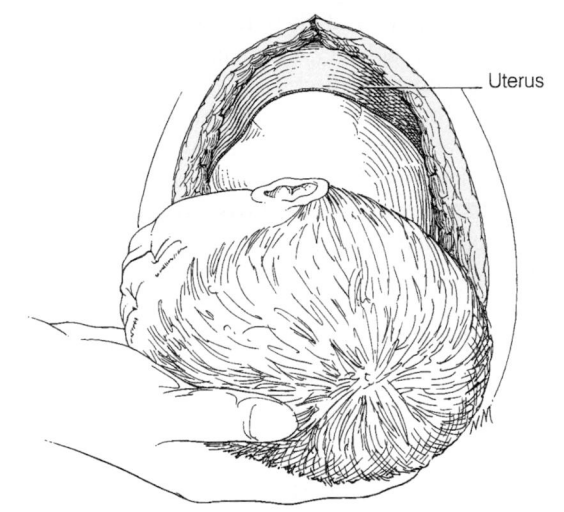

FIGURE 25–10. The shoulders are delivered, and oxytocin infusion is begun.

especially if there have been extensions laterally. Adnexal exposure is superior, and thus tubal sterilization is easier. The principal disadvantage is from discomfort and vomiting caused by traction in cesarean deliveries performed under regional analgesia. Neither febrile morbidity nor blood loss appears to be increased in women undergoing uterine exteriorization prior to repair (Hershey and Quilligan, 1978; Wahab and co-workers, 1999).

Immediately after delivery and inspection of the placenta, the uterine cavity is inspected and either suctioned or wiped out with a gauze pack to remove avulsed membranes, vernix,

clots, and other debris. The upper and lower cut edges and each lateral angle of the uterine incision are examined carefully for bleeding. Individually clamped large vessels are best ligated with a suture ligature. Concern has been expressed by some clinicians that sutures through the decidua may lead to endometriosis in the hysterotomy scar, but this is a rare.

The uterine incision is then closed with one or two layers of continuous 0 or number 1 absorbable suture. Chromic suture is used by most surgeons, but some prefer synthetic nonabsorbable sutures. Hauth and colleagues (1992) randomized 906 women to either one- or two-layer closure using 1-0 chromic gut. A continuous locking one-layer closure required less operative time and fewer additional hemostatic sutures. In a follow-up report of 164 women delivered subsequently, the type of uterine closure did not significantly affect several maternal and fetal complications in the next pregnancy (Chapman and associates, 1997). Similarly, Durnwald and Mercer (2003) reported no uterine ruptures in 182 women who underwent a trial of labor after single-layer closure compared with four ruptures in 340 women (1.2 percent) after double-layer closure. By contrast, Bujold and associates (2002) reported that single-layer closure was associated with a fourfold increased risk of uterine rupture during a subsequent trial of labor. Further study of this issue is needed (see Chap. 26, p. 611).

The initial suture is placed just beyond one angle of the uterine incision. A running-lock suture is then carried out, with each suture penetrating the full thickness of the myometrium (Fig. 25–12). It is important to select carefully the site of each stitch and to avoid withdrawing the needle once it penetrates the myometrium. This minimizes the perforation

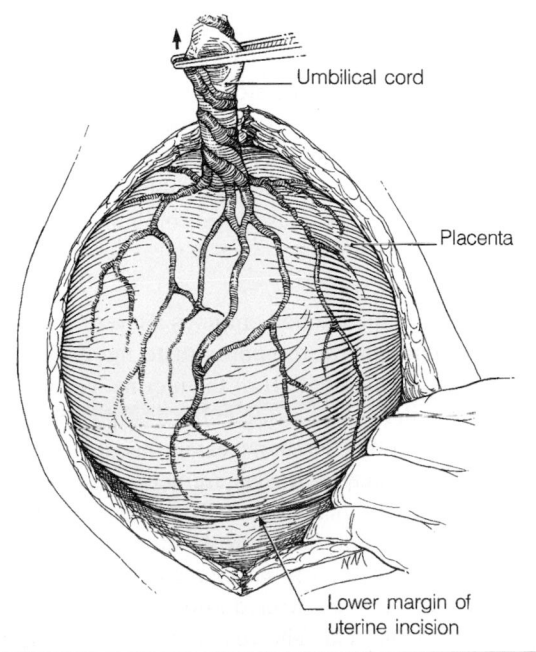

FIGURE 25–11. Placenta bulging through the uterine incision as the uterus contracts.

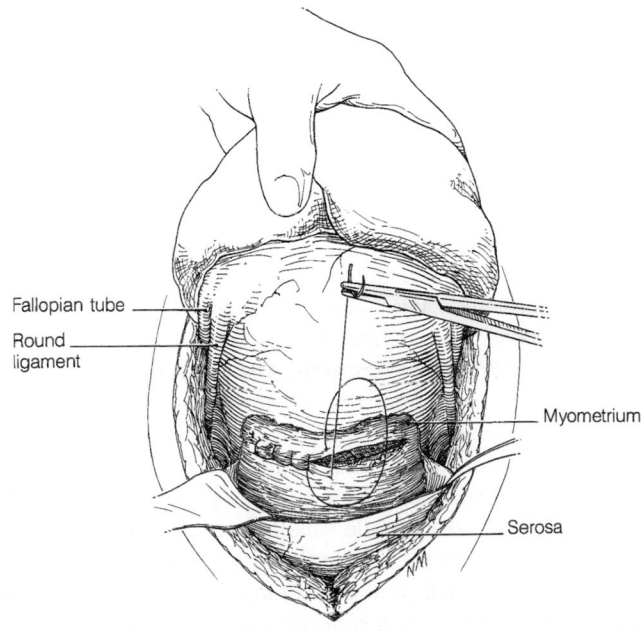

FIGURE 25–12. The cut edges of the uterine incision are approximated with a running-lock suture.

of unligated vessels and subsequent bleeding. The running-lock suture is continued just beyond the opposite incision angle. Especially when the lower segment is thin, satisfactory approximation of the cut edges usually can be obtained with one layer of suture. If approximation is not satisfactory after a single-layer continuous closure, or if bleeding sites persist, then more sutures are required. Either another layer of sutures may be placed so as to achieve approximation and hemostasis, or individual bleeding sites can be secured with figure-of-eight or mattress sutures.

Traditionally, serosal edges overlying the uterus and bladder have been approximated with a continuous 2-0 chromic catgut suture. Multiple randomized trials suggest that omission of this step causes no postoperative complications (Grundsell, 1998; Hull and Varner, 1991; Irion, 1996; Nagele, 1996; Pietrantoni, 1991, and all their associates). Specifically, not approximating the bladder flap is unlikely to increase adhesion formation or long-term morbidity (Roset and colleagues, 2003; Tulandi and Al-Jaroudi, 2003). Data are conflicting as to whether nonclosure of peritoneum decreases postoperative discomfort and need for analgesia (Chanrachakul and colleagues, 2002; Rafique and colleagues, 2002).

If tubal sterilization is to be performed, it is now done as described in Chapter 33 (see p. 752).

Abdominal Closure. All packs are removed, and the paracolic gutters and cul-de-sac are emptied of blood and amnionic fluid using gentle suction. Some surgeons irrigate the gutters and cul-de-sac, especially in the presence of infection or meconium. A small randomized trial by Harrigill and colleagues (2003) supports that this step is not necessary in low-risk women who undergo cesarean delivery in the absence of amnionitis. After the sponge and instrument counts are found to be correct, the abdominal incision is closed in layers. As previously discussed, many surgeons omit the parietal peritoneal closure because it serves little purpose. If there is distended bowel in the incision site, however, we find that peritoneal closure may help to protect the bowel when fascial sutures are placed. As each layer is closed, bleeding sites are located, clamped, and ligated. The rectus muscles are allowed to fall into place, and the subfascial space is meticulously checked for hemostasis. With significant diastasis, the rectus muscles may be approximated with one or two figure-of-eight sutures of 0 or number 1 chromic. The overlying rectus fascia is closed either with interrupted 0 nonabsorbable sutures that are placed lateral to the fascial edges and no more than 1 cm apart, or by continuous, nonlocking suture of a long-lasting absorbable or permanent type.

The subcutaneous tissue usually need not be closed separately if it is less than 2 cm in thickness, and the skin is closed with vertical mattress sutures of 3-0 or 4-0 silk or equivalent suture, with a running 4-0 subcuticular stitch using semipermanent suture, or with skin clips. If the subcutaneous tissue is at least 2 cm thick, it should be closed. In a randomized prospective study of more than 1400 women undergoing cesarean delivery, Bohman and colleagues (1992) reported a significantly decreased frequency of superficial wound disruption when the subcutaneous layer was approximated. Based on their systematic review of six studies, Chelmow and colleagues (2004) concluded that suturing the subcutaneous tissue at cesarean delivery decreases the risk of wound disruption by 34 percent in women with fat thickness greater than 2 cm.

TECHNIQUE FOR CLASSICAL CESAREAN INCISION. Occasionally it is necessary to use a classical incision for delivery. Some indications are:

1. Difficulty in exposing or safely entering the lower uterine segment because the bladder is densely adherent from previous surgery, a myoma occupies the lower uterine segment, or the cervix has been invaded by cancer.
2. Transverse lie of a large fetus, especially if the membranes are ruptured and the shoulder is impacted in the birth canal. A fetus presenting as a back-down transverse lie may be particularly difficult to deliver through a transverse incision.
3. Some cases of placenta previa with anterior implantation, especially in the case where the placenta has grown through a prior uterine incision (placenta percreta).
4. Certain cases in which the fetus is very small, especially if breech, and the lower uterine segment is not thinned out.
5. Massive maternal obesity precluding safe access to the lower uterine segment.

Uterine Incision. A vertical uterine incision is initiated with a scalpel beginning as low as possible, depending on how well the lower segment is thinned out. If adhesions, insufficient exposure, a tumor, or placenta percreta preclude development of a bladder flap, then the incision is made above the level of the bladder. Once uterine entry is made with the scalpel, the incision is extended cephalad with bandage scissors until it is sufficiently long to permit delivery of the fetus. Numerous large vessels that bleed profusely are commonly encountered within the myometrium.

Uterine Repair. One method employs a layer of continuous 0 or 1-0 chromic catgut to approximate the deeper halves of the incision. The outer half of the uterine incision is then closed with similar suture, using either a continuous stitch or figure-of-eight sutures. No unnecessary needle tracts should be made lest myometrial vessels are perforated with subsequent hemorrhage or hematomas. To achieve good approximation and to prevent the suture from tearing through the myometrium, it is helpful to have an assistant compress the uterus on each side of the wound toward the midline as each suture is placed and tied. The edges of the uterine serosa, if not already so, are approximated with continuous 2-0 chromic catgut. The operation is completed as described earlier.

POSTMORTEM CESAREAN DELIVERY. At times, cesarean delivery is performed on a woman who has just died, or who is expected to do so momentarily. The issue of cesarean delivery to aid in cardiopulmonary resuscitation of the mother is further discussed in Chapter 42 (see p. 1002).

PERIPARTUM HYSTERECTOMY

Hysterectomy performed at or following delivery may be lifesaving if there is severe obstetrical hemorrhage. It can be carried out in conjunction with cesarean delivery or following vaginal delivery. One measure of its incidence is from the Maternal–Fetal Medicine Units Network centers. In that study of almost 29,000 cesarean deliveries, Shellhaas and colleagues (2001) reported that hysterectomy was performed in 1 in every 200 cesarean deliveries. Overall, hysterectomy was performed in 1 in every 950 deliveries. During the 9-year period ending with 2002, during which there were almost 129,500 deliveries at Parkland Hospital, peripartum hysterectomy was performed once in every 500 deliveries. The incidence was 1 in 135 for 26,700 cesarean deliveries and about 1 in 1850 for vaginal deliveries. These numbers are similar to those of Kastner and co-workers (2002), who reported an overall rate of peripartum hysterectomy of 1.4 per 1000 deliveries. Similarly, Forna and associates (2004) cited a rate of 0.8 per 1000 deliveries at Grady Hospital.

INDICATIONS. The majority of procedures are performed to arrest hemorrhage from intractable uterine atony, lower-segment bleeding associated with the uterine incision or placental implantation, or a laceration of major uterine vessels. Placenta accreta, often in association with repeat cesarean delivery, and uterine atony are the most common indications today for cesarean or postpartum hysterectomy (Kastner and associates, 2002; Shellhaas and colleagues, 2001). These conditions are discussed in Chapter 35 (see p. 809). Large myomas may preclude satisfactory hysterotomy closure and thus necessitate hysterectomy. Elective indications for peripartum hysterectomy include large or symptomatic myomas and severe cervical dysplasia or carcinoma in situ.

Major complications of peripartum hysterectomy are increased blood loss and the possibility of urinary tract damage. An important factor affecting the complication rate is whether the operation is performed as an elective procedure or as an emergency. As shown in Table 25–3, morbidity associated with emergency hysterectomy is substantively increased. Seago and associates (1999) reported that the rate of intraoperative and postoperative complications among 100 women who underwent planned cesarean hysterectomy was not increased when compared with that of a control group of 37 women who underwent cesarean delivery followed by hysterectomy performed within 6 months.

Although pelvic vessels are appreciably hypertrophied, hysterectomy usually is facilitated by the ease of development of tissue planes in pregnant women. Blood loss is usually appreciable because hysterectomy performed for hemorrhage almost always is torrential. Indeed, as shown in Table 25–3, 90 percent of women undergoing emergency peripartum hysterectomy required transfusions.

TABLE 25–3 Comparison of Morbidity with Elective Versus Emergency Peripartum Hysterectomy

Complications	Complications (%) with Peripartum Hysterectomy	
	Elective[a] (n = 189)	Emergency[b] (n = 231)
Blood transfusions	18	90
Bladder injury	1.5	5
Ureteral injury	0	1.3
Surgical infection	22	30
Death	0	1.3

[a]Data from Plauche (1995).
[b]Data from Kastner (2002), Zelop (1993), Zorlu (1998), and all their colleagues.

TECHNIQUE FOR PERIPARTUM HYSTERECTOMY. Supracervical or total hysterectomy is performed using standard operative techniques. Initially, placement of a self-retaining retractor such as a Balfour is not necessary. Satisfactory exposure is best obtained with cephalad traction on the uterus by an assistant, along with hand-held retractors such as a Richardson or Deaver. The bladder flap is deflected downward to the level of the cervix if possible. After cesarean delivery and placental removal, if the hysterotomy is bleeding appreciably, either it can be sutured, or Pennington or sponge-forceps can be applied for hemostasis. If bleeding is minimal, neither maneuver is necessary.

The round ligaments close to the uterus are divided between Heaney or Kocher clamps and doubly ligated. Either 0 or number 1 sutures can be used. The incision in the vesicouterine serosa that was made to mobilize the bladder is extended laterally and upward through the anterior leaf of the broad ligament to reach the incised round ligaments (Fig. 25–13). The posterior leaf of the broad ligament adjacent to the uterus is perforated just beneath the fallopian tubes, utero-ovarian ligaments, and ovarian vessels (Fig. 25–14A). These vessels then are doubly clamped close to the uterus and divided, and the lateral pedicle is doubly ligated (Fig. 25–14B). The posterior leaf of the broad ligament is divided inferiorly toward the uterosacral ligaments (Fig. 25–15). Next, the bladder and attached peritoneal flap are again deflected and dissected from the lower uterine segment and retracted out of the operative field (Fig. 25–16). If the bladder flap is unusually adherent, as it may be after previous cesarean incisions, careful sharp dissection may be necessary.

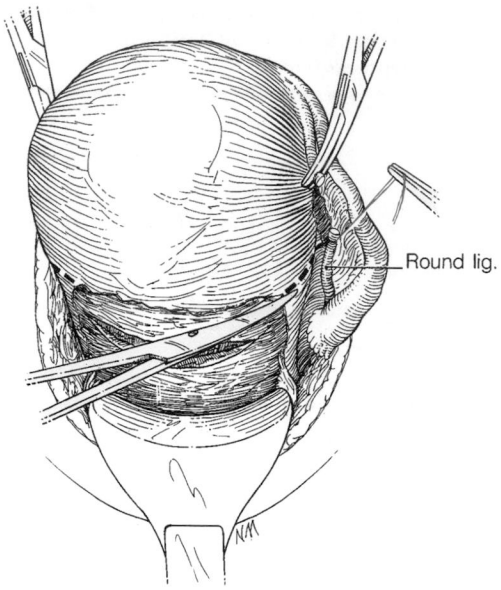

FIGURE 25–13. The incision in the vesicouterine serosa is extended laterally and upward through the anterior leaf of the broad ligament to reach the incised round ligaments.

Special care is necessary from this point on to avoid injury to the ureters, which pass beneath the uterine arteries. To help accomplish this, the assistant places constant traction on the uterus in the direction away from the side on which the uterine vessels are being ligated. The ascending uterine artery and

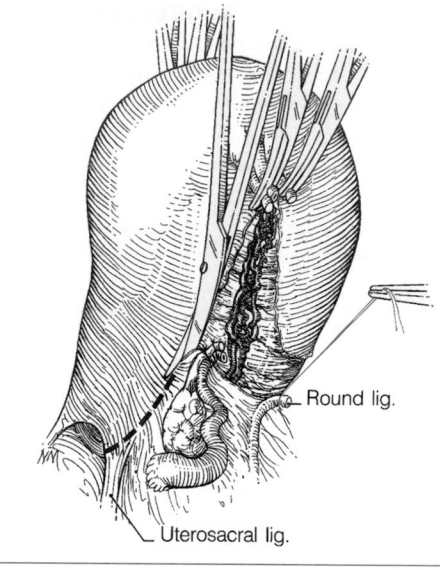

FIGURE 25–15. The posterior leaf of the broad ligament is divided inferiorly toward the uterosacral ligament.

veins on either side are identified near their origin. These pedicles are then doubly clamped immediately adjacent to the uterus, divided, and doubly suture ligated. As shown in Figure 25–17, we prefer to use three heavy clamps, incise the tissue between the most medial and two lateral clamps, and then ligate the two pedicles in the clamps lateral to the uterus.

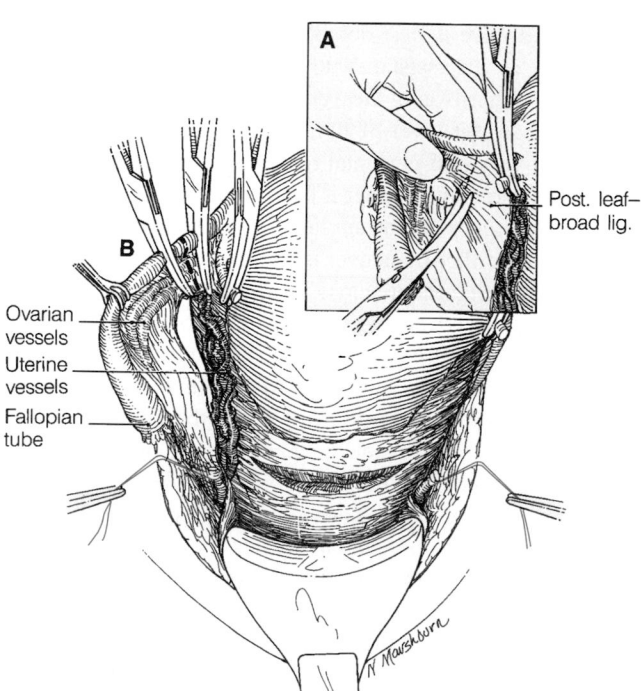

FIGURE 25–14. A. The posterior leaf of the broad ligament adjacent to the uterus is perforated just beneath the fallopian tube, utero-ovarian ligaments, and ovarian vessels. **B.** These then are doubly clamped close to the uterus and divided.

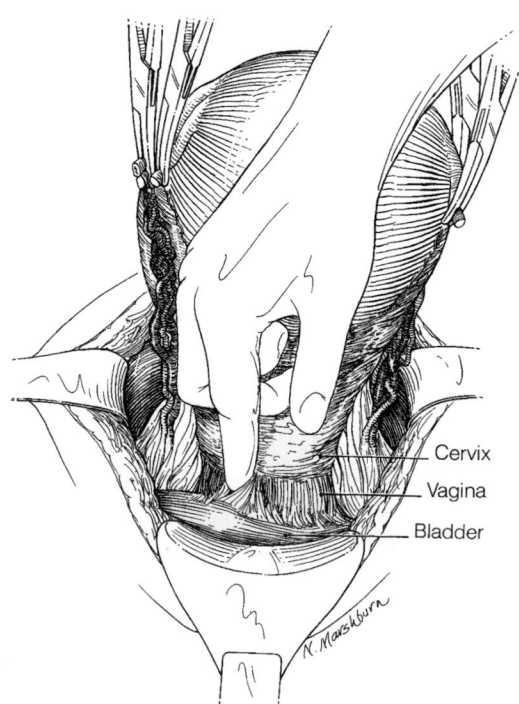

FIGURE 25–16. The bladder is further dissected from the lower uterine segment by blunt dissection with pressure directed toward the lower segment and not the bladder. Sharp dissection may be necessary.

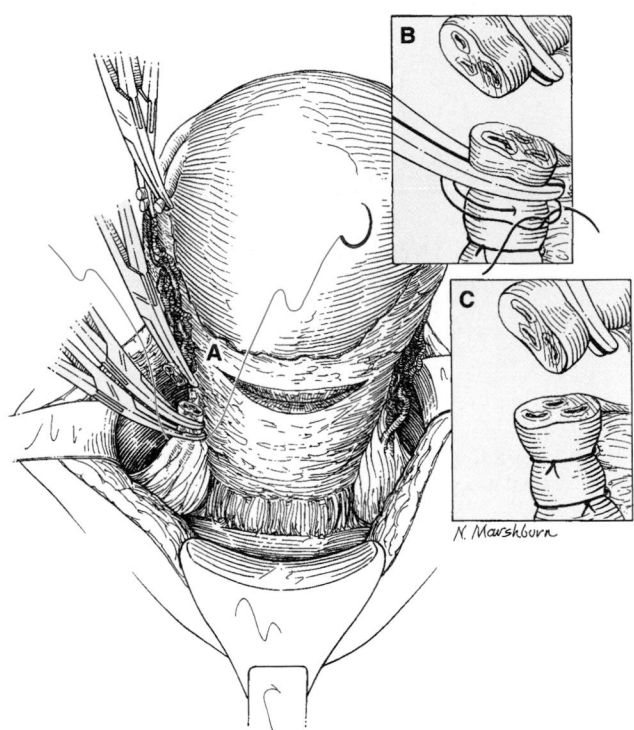

FIGURE 25–17. **A.** The uterine artery and veins on either side are doubly clamped immediately adjacent to the uterus and divided. **B, C.** The vascular pedicle is doubly suture ligated.

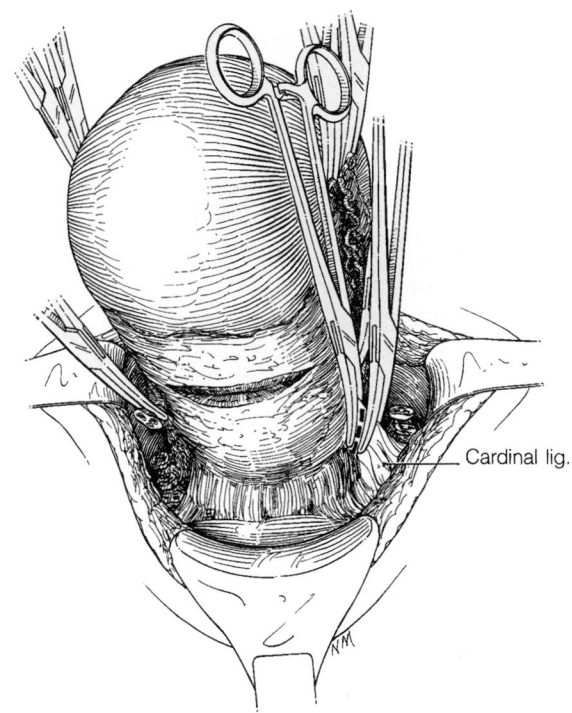

FIGURE 25–18. The cardinal ligaments are clamped, incised, and ligated.

In cases of profuse hemorrhage, it may be more advantageous to rapidly double clamp and divide all of the vascular pedicles between clamps to gain hemostasis and then return to suture ligate all of the pedicles.

Supracervical Hysterectomy. To perform a subtotal hysterectomy, it is necessary only to amputate the body of the uterus at this level. The cervical stump may be closed with continuous or interrupted chromic sutures. Subtotal hysterectomy is often all that is necessary to stop hemorrhage and may be the more prudent operation for selected women (Jones, 1999; Kastner, 2002; Learman, 2003; Munro, 1997, and their associates).

Total Hysterectomy. Even if total hysterectomy is planned, we find it in many cases technically easier to finish the operation after amputating the uterine fundus and placing Ochsner or Kocher clamps on the stump for traction and hemostasis. Self-retaining retractors also are placed at this time. To remove the cervix, it is necessary to mobilize the bladder much more extensively in the midline and laterally. This will help carry the ureters caudad as the bladder is retracted beneath the symphysis and also will prevent laceration or suturing of the bladder during cervical excision and vaginal cuff closure. Before cesarean delivery, the bladder is dissected free for about 2 cm below the lowest margin of the cervix to expose the uppermost part of the vagina. If the cervix is effaced and dilated appreciably, after delivery the cervicovaginal junction

may be identified by a vertical uterine incision made anteriorly in the midline, either through the hysterotomy incision or through an incision made at the level of the ligated uterine vessels. A finger is directed inferiorly through the incision to identify the free margin of the dilated, effaced cervix and the anterior vaginal fornix, and the contaminated glove replaced. Another useful method to identify the cervical margins is to place four metal skin clips or brightly colored sutures at 12, 3, 6, and 9 o'clock positions on the cervical edges prior to hysterectomy.

The cardinal ligaments, uterosacral ligaments, and the many large vessels these ligaments contain are doubly clamped systematically with Heaney-type curved clamps, Ochsner-type straight clamps, or similar instruments (Fig. 25–18). The clamps are placed as close to the cervix as possible, taking care not to include excessive tissue in each clamp. The tissue between the pair of clamps is incised and the distal pedicle suture ligated. These steps are repeated until the level of the lateral vaginal fornix is reached. In this way, the descending branches of the uterine vessels are clamped, cut, and ligated as the cervix is dissected from the cardinal ligaments posteriorly.

Immediately below the level of the cervix, a curved clamp is placed across the lateral vaginal fornix, and the tissue is incised medially to the clamp (Fig. 25–19). The excised lateral vaginal fornix can be simultaneously doubly ligated and sutured to the stump of the cardinal ligament. The entire cervix is then excised from the vagina. The cervix is inspected to

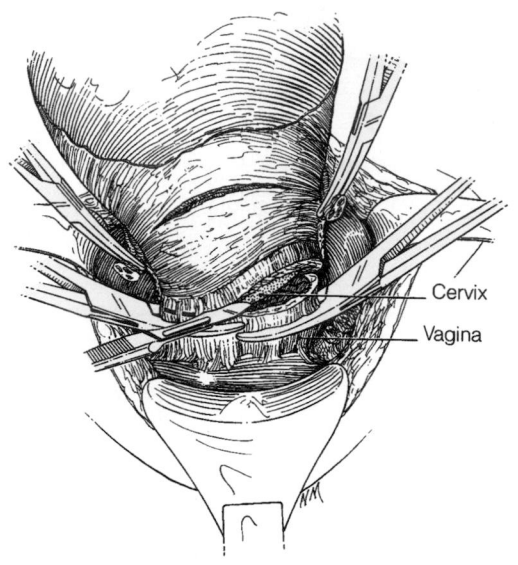

FIGURE 25–19. A curved clamp is placed across the lateral vaginal fornix below the level of the cervix and the tissue incised medially to the point of the clamp.

ensure that it has been completely removed, and the vagina is then repaired. Each of the angles of the lateral vaginal fornix is secured to the cardinal and uterosacral ligaments (Fig. 25–20). Following this step, some surgeons prefer to close the vagina using figure-of-eight chromic catgut sutures. Others achieve hemostasis by using a running-lock stitch of chromic catgut suture placed through the mucosa and adjacent endopelvic fascia around the circumference of the vaginal cuff (Fig. 25–21). The open vagina may promote drainage of fluids that would otherwise accumulate and contribute to hematoma formation and infection.

If a self-retaining retractor has not already been placed, some clinicians choose to insert the instrument at this point. The bowel is then packed out of the field and all sites of incision are examined carefully for bleeding. One technique is to perform a systematic bilateral survey from the fallopian

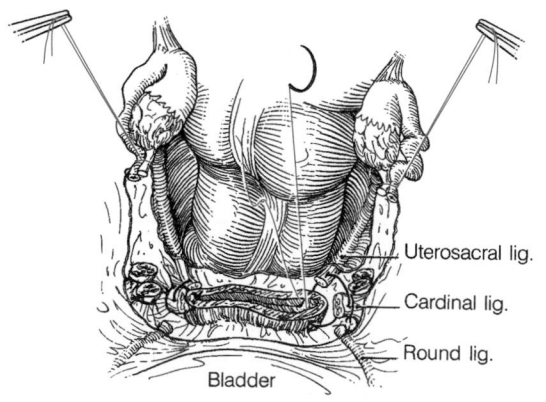

FIGURE 25–20. The lateral angles of the vaginal cuff are secured to the cardinal and uterosacral ligaments.

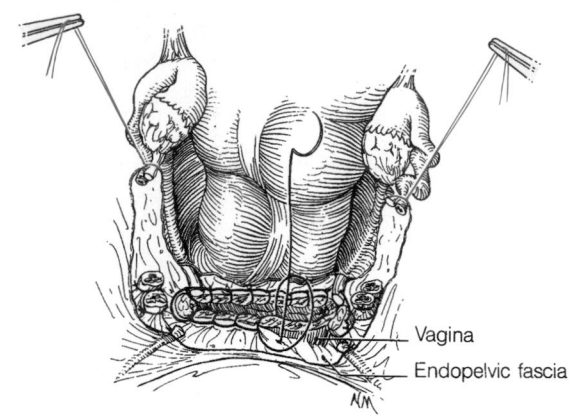

FIGURE 25–21. A running-lock suture is placed through the edge of the vaginal mucosa, circumferentially.

tube and ovarian ligament pedicles to the vaginal vault and bladder flap. Bleeding sites are ligated with care to avoid the ureters.

Some clinicians choose to reperitonealize the pelvis. One method employs a continuous chromic suture starting with the tip of the ligated pedicle of fallopian tube and ovarian ligament, which is inverted retroperitoneally. Sutures are then placed continuously to approximate the leaves of the broad ligament, bury the stump of the round ligament, and to join the cut edge of the vesicouterine peritoneum over the vaginal vault posteriorly to the cut edge of peritoneum above the cul-de-sac. This action is then repeated on the other side. The abdominal wall normally is closed in layers, as previously described.

Oophorectomy. Most studies indicate that in 5 percent of postpartum hysterectomies, one adnexum will have to be removed to stop bleeding (Plauche, 1995). That said, during any hysterectomy, a decision as to the fate of the ovaries must be made. For women who are approaching menopause, the decision is not difficult, but few women who undergo cesarean hysterectomy are of this age.

PERIPARTUM MANAGEMENT

PREOPERATIVE CARE. If cesarean delivery is planned, a sedative, such as secobarbital, 100 mg, may be given at bedtime the night before the operation. In general, no other sedatives, narcotics, or tranquilizers are administered until after the infant is born. Oral intake is stopped at least 8 hours before surgery. The woman scheduled for repeat cesarean delivery typically is admitted the day of surgery and evaluated by the obstetrician and the anesthesiologist. The hematocrit is rechecked, as is the indirect Coombs test. If the latter is positive, then availability of compatible blood must be assured. An antacid, such as Bicitra, 30 mL, is given shortly before placement of conduction analgesia or induction with general anesthesia. This minimizes the risk of lung injury from gastric acid should aspiration occur (see Chap. 19, p. 490). An indwelling bladder catheter is placed. If hair obscures the operative field it should be removed the day of surgery by clipping or shaving. If shaving is performed the night before surgery, the risk of wound infection is increased.

INTRAVENOUS FLUIDS. Requirements for intravenous fluids, including blood during and after cesarean delivery, can vary considerably. The woman of average size with a hematocrit of 30 percent or more and a normally expanded blood and extracellular fluid volume most often will tolerate blood loss up to 2000 mL without difficulty. Unappreciated bleeding through the vagina during the procedure, bleeding concealed in the uterus after its closure, or both, commonly lead to underestimation. Although blood loss averages about 1500 mL with elective cesarean hysterectomy, it is quite variable (Pritchard, 1965). Intravenously administered fluids consist of either lactated Ringer solution or a similar crystalloid solution with 5 percent dextrose. Typically, 1 to 2 L are infused during and immediately after the operation. Throughout the procedure, and subsequently while in the recovery area, the blood pressure and urine flow are monitored closely.

PREVENTION OF POSTOPERATIVE INFECTION. Febrile morbidity is frequent after cesarean delivery. A large number of randomized trials have demonstrated that a single dose of an antimicrobial agent given at the time of cesarean delivery will serve to decrease infection morbidity significantly. This is true of high-risk laboring patients as well as those undergoing elective cesarean delivery (American College of Obstetricians and Gynecologists, 2003). For women in labor or with ruptured membranes, most clinicians recommend a single 2-g dose of a β-lactam drug—either a cephalosporin or an extended-spectrum penicillin—after delivery of the infant. Postoperative pelvic infection is the most frequent cause of febrile morbidity and develops in up to 20 percent of these women despite peripartum prophylactic antimicrobials (Goepfert and associates, 2001). In general, infection rates are higher among government-funded and indigent patients. Treatment of uterine infection and its complications are discussed in Chapter 31.

RECOVERY SUITE. Postoperatively, the amount of bleeding from the vagina must be monitored closely, and the uterine fundus must be identified frequently by palpation to assure that the uterus is remaining firmly contracted. Unfortunately, as conduction analgesia fades or the woman awakens from general anesthesia, palpation of the abdomen is likely to produce considerable discomfort. This can be made more tolerable by giving an effective analgesic intravenously, such as meperidine, 75 to 100 mg, or morphine, 10 to 15 mg. A thick dressing with an abundance of adhesive tape over the abdomen interferes with fundal palpation and massage and

later causes discomfort as the tape is removed. Deep breathing and coughing are encouraged. Once the mother is fully awake, bleeding is minimal, blood pressure is satisfactory, and urine flow is at least 30 mL/hr, she may be sent to her room.

SUBSEQUENT CARE

Analgesia. For the woman of average size, meperidine, 75 to 100 mg, is given intramuscularly as often as every 3 hours as needed for discomfort, or morphine sulfate, 10 to 15 mg, is similarly administered. An antiemetic, such as promethazine, 25 mg, usually is given along with the narcotic. Intravenous meperidine or morphine via a patient-controlled pump is an even more effective alternative to bolus therapy in the immediate postoperative period. The pump typically is programmed to deliver a continuous infusion of drug, which the woman can supplement with intermittent boluses, the frequency of which are determined by the "lock-out" interval (Table 25–4). In a recent trial at Parkland Hospital (Yost and colleagues, 2004), morphine provided superior pain relief to meperidine and was associated with significantly higher rates of breast feeding continuation and infant rooming-in.

Vital Signs. After transfer to her room, the patient is assessed at least hourly for 4 hours and thereafter, at intervals of 4 hours. Blood pressure, pulse, temperature, uterine tone, urine output, and amount of bleeding are evaluated.

Fluid Therapy and Diet. Unless there has been pathological constriction of the extracellular fluid compartment from severe preeclampsia, vomiting, fever, or prolonged labor without adequate fluid intake, or there is sepsis or significant blood loss, the puerperium is characterized by excretion of fluid that was retained during pregnancy. Moreover, with the typical cesarean delivery, significant extracellular fluid sequestration in bowel wall and lumen does not occur, unless it was necessary to pack the bowel away from the operative field or peritonitis develops. Thus, the woman who undergoes cesarean delivery rarely develops fluid sequestration in the so-called third space. Quite the contrary, she normally begins surgery with a physiologically enlarged extravascular volume acquired during pregnancy that she mobilizes and excretes after delivery.

TABLE 25–4 **Typical Settings for Administration of Intravenous Opioids via a Patient-Controlled Analgesia Pump**

Opioid	Bolus Dose (mg)	Lock-Out Interval (min)	Continuous Infusion (mg/hr)
Meperidine	5–15	5–15	5–40
Morphine	0.5–3.0	5–20	1–10

Modified from Lubenow and colleagues (1997), with permission.

Therefore, large volumes of intravenous fluids during and subsequent to surgery are not needed to replace sequestered extracellular fluid. As a generalization, 3 L of fluid should prove adequate during the first 24 hours after surgery. If urine output falls below 30 mL/hr, however, then the woman should be reevaluated promptly. The cause of the oliguria may range from unrecognized blood loss to an antidiuretic effect from infused oxytocin.

Bladder and Bowel Function. The bladder catheter most often can be removed by 12 hours postoperatively or, more conveniently, the morning after surgery. Subsequent ability to empty the bladder before overdistention develops must be monitored as with vaginal delivery.

In uncomplicated cases, solid food may be offered within 8 hours of surgery (Burrows and associates, 1995; Kramer and colleagues, 1996). Although some degree of adynamic ileus follows virtually every abdominal operation, in most cases of cesarean delivery, it is negligible. Symptoms include abdominal distention and gas pains, and an inability to pass flatus or stool. The pathophysiology of postoperative ileus is complex and involves hormonal, neural, and local factors that are incompletely understood (Livingston and Passaro, 1990). If associated with otherwise unexplained fever, an unrecognized bowel injury may be responsible. Treatment for ileus has changed little over the past several decades and involves intravenous fluid and electrolyte supplementation. If severe, nasogastric decompression is necessary. Frequently, a 10-mg bisacodyl rectal suppository provides appreciable relief.

Ambulation. In most instances, by the day after surgery, the woman should get briefly out of bed with assistance at least twice. Ambulation can be timed so that a recently administered analgesic will minimize the discomfort. By the second day she may walk without assistance. Early ambulation lowers the risk of venous thrombosis and pulmonary embolism (see Chap. 47).

Wound Care. The incision is inspected each day, and the skin sutures or clips often can be removed on the fourth day after surgery. However, if there is concern for superficial wound separation, as in the obese patient, the suture or clips should remain in place for 7 to 10 days if they are not causing appreciable skin irritation. By the third postpartum day, bathing by shower is not harmful to the incision. In addition to increasing the risk of wound separation, thick subcutaneous tissue—greater than 3 cm—increases the risk of wound infection (Vermillion and associates, 2000).

Laboratory. The hematocrit is routinely measured the morning after surgery. It is checked sooner when there was unusual blood loss or when there is oliguria or other evidence to suggest hypovolemia. If the hematocrit is decreased significantly from the preoperative level, the measurement is repeated and a search is instituted to identify the cause of the decline. If the hematocrit stabilizes, the mother can ambulate without any difficulty, and if there is little likelihood of further blood loss, iron therapy is preferred to transfusion.

Breast Care. Breast feeding can be initiated the day of surgery. If the mother elects not to breast feed, a binder that supports the breasts without marked compression usually will minimize discomfort (see Chap. 30, p. 699).

Hospital Discharge. Unless there are complications during the puerperium, the mother generally is discharged on the third or fourth postpartum day (see Chap. 30, p. 706). Strong and associates (1993) have presented data suggesting that discharge on day 2 may be appropriate for properly selected and motivated women. The mother's activities during the first week should be restricted to self-care and care of her baby with assistance. Brooten and colleagues (1994) successfully combined early discharge with nurse specialist transitional home care. In many cases, it may be advantageous to perform an initial postpartum evaluation during the first to third week after delivery to search for puerperal complications discussed in Chapters 30 and 32.

REFERENCES

Alexander JM for the NICHD MFMU Network: The MFMU Units Cesarean Registry: Fetal injury associated with cesarean delivery. Presented at the 25th Annual Meeting of the Society for Maternal-Fetal Medicine, Reno/Lake Tahoe NV, 7–12 Feb 2005

Al-Mufti R, McCarthy A, Fisk NM: Survey of obstetricians' personal preference and discretionary practice. Eur J Obstet Gynecol Reprod Biol 73:1, 1997

Althabe F, Belizán JM, Villar J, et al: Mandatory second opinion to reduce rates of unnecessary caesarean sections in Latin America: a cluster randomised controlled trial. Lancet. 12;363:1934, 2004

American Academy of Pediatrics and American College of Obstetricians and Gynecologists: Guidelines for Perinatal Care, 5th ed. Elk Grove, Ill, American Academy of Pediatrics, 2002

American College of Obstetricians and Gynecologists: Prophylactic antibiotics in labor and delivery. Practice Bulletin No. 47, October 2003

American College of Obstetricians and Gynecologists, Task Force on Cesarean Delivery Rates: Evaluation of cesarean delivery. June 2000

Atkinson MW, Owen J, Wren A, et al: The effect of manual removal of the placenta on post-cesarean endometritis. Obstet Gynecol 87:99, 1996

Ayers JWT, Morley GW: Surgical incision for cesarean section. Obstet Gynecol 70:706, 1987

Beck AC: Observations on a series of cases of cesarean section done at the Long Island College Hospital during the past six years. Am J Obstet Gynecol 79:197, 1919

Bewley S, Cockburn J: The unethics of 'request' caesarean section [commentary]. Br J Obstet Gynaecol 109:593, 2002a

Bewley S, Cockburn J: The unfacts of 'request' caesarean section [commentary]. Br J Obstet Gynaecol 109:597, 2002b

Bloom SL for the National Institute of Child Health and Human Development Maternal–Fetal Medicine Units Cesarean Registry: Decision to incision times and infant outcome. Am J Obstet Gynecol 185:S121, 2001

Bohman VR, Gilstrap L, Leveno K, et al: Subcutaneous tissue: To close or not to close at cesarean section. Am J Obstet Gynecol 166:407, 1992

Boley JP: The history of cesarean section. Can Med Assoc J 145:319, 1991

Brooten D, Roncoli M, Finkler S, et al: A randomized trial of early hospital discharge and home follow-up of women having cesarean birth. Obstet Gynecol 84:832, 1994

Bujold E, Bujold C, Hamilton EF, et al: The impact of a single-layer or double-layer closure on uterine rupture. Am J Obstet Gynecol 186:1326, 2002

Burrows LJ, Meyn LA, Weber AM: Maternal morbidity associated with vaginal versus cesarean delivery. Obstet Gynecol. 103:907, 2004

Burrows WR, Gingo AJ Jr, Rose SM, et al: Safety and efficacy of early postoperative solid food consumption after cesarean section. J Reprod Med 40:463, 1995

Chanrachakul B, Hamontri S, Herabutya Y: A randomized comparison of postcesarean pain between closure and nonclosure of peritoneum. Eur J Obstet Gynecol Reprod Biol 101:31, 2002

Chapman SJ, Owen J, Hauth JC: One versus two-layer closure of a low transverse cesarean: The next pregnancy. Obstet Gynecol 89:16, 1997

Chauhan SP, Roach H, Naef RW, et al: Cesarean section for suspected fetal distress: Does the decision-incision time make a difference? J Reprod Med 42:347, 1997

Chelmow D, Rodriguez EJ, Sabatini MM: Suture closure of subcutaneous fat and wound disruption after cesarean delivery: A meta-analysis. Obstet Gynecol. 103:974, 2004

DeLee JB, Cornell EL: Low cervical cesarean section (laparotrachelotomy). JAMA 79:109, 1922

DeMott RK, Sandmire HF: The Green Bay cesarean section study, 1. The physician factor as a determinant of cesarean birth rates. Am J Obstet Gynecol 162:1593, 1990

DeMuylder X, Thiery M: The cesarean delivery rate can be safely reduced in a developing country. Obstet Gynecol 75:60, 1990

Durnwald C, Mercer B: Uterine rupture, perioperative and perinatal morbidity after single-layer and double-layer closure at cesarean delivery. Am J Obstet Gynecol 189:925, 2003

Eastman NJ: The role of frontier America in the development of cesarean section. Am J Obstet Gynecol 24:919, 1932

Fasbender H: Geschichte der Geburtshilfe. Jena, 1906, p 979

Foley M, Alarab M, O'Herlighy C: Neonatal seizures and peripartum deaths: Lack of correlation with cesarean rate [abstract]. Am J Obstet Gynecol 187:S102, 2002

Forna F, Miles AM, Jamieson DJ: Emergency peripartum hysterectomy: A comparison of cesarean and postpartum hysterectomy. Am J Obstet Gynecol 190:1440, 2004

Frank F: Suprasymphysial delivery and its relation to other operations in the presence of contracted pelvis. Arch Gynaekol 81:46, 1907

Friedman EA: Labor, Clinical Evaluation and Management. New York, Appleton, 1978

Frigoletto FD Jr, Ryan KJ, Phillippe M: Maternal mortality rate associated with cesarean section: An appraisal. Am J Obstet Gynecol 136:969, 1980

Giacalone PL, Daures JP, Vignal J, et al: Pfannenstiel versus Maylard incision for cesarean delivery: A randomized controlled trial. Obstet Gynecol 99:745, 2002

Goepfert A for the National Institute of Child Health and Human Development Maternal–Fetal Medicine Units Network: The MFMU Cesarean Registry: Infectious morbidity following primary cesarean section. Am J Obstet Gynecol 185:S192, 2001

Grundsell HS, Rizk DE, Kumar RM: Randomized study of nonclosure of peritoneum in lower segment cesarean section. Acta Obstet Gynecol Scand 77:110, 1998

Hall MH, Bewley S: Maternal mortality and mode of delivery. Lancet 354:776, 1999

Hamilton BE, Martin JA, Sutton PD: Births: Preliminary data for 2002. National Vital Statistics Reports, Vol 51, No. 1. Hyattsville, Md, National Center for Health Statistics, 2003

Harer W: Patient choice caesarean. Am Coll Obstet Gynecol Clin Rev 5:2, 2000

Harper MA, Byington RP, Espeland MA, et al: Pregnancy-related death and health care services. Obstet Gynecol 102:273, 2003

Harrigill KM, Miller HS, Haynes DE: The effect of intraabdominal irrigation at cesarean delivery on maternal morbidity: A randomized trial. Obstet Gynecol 101:80, 2003

Harris RP: Lessons from a study of the cesarean operation in the city and state of New York. Am J Obstet Gynecol 12:82, 1879

Hauth JC, Owen J, Davis RO, et al: Transverse uterine incision closure: One versus two layers. Am J Obstet Gynecol 167:1108, 1992

Henderson J, McCandlish R, Kumiega L, et al: Systematic review of economic aspects of alternative modes of delivery. Br J Obstet Gynaecol 108:149, 2001

Hendrix SL, Schimp V, Martin J, et al: The legendary superior strength of the Pfannenstiel incision: A myth? Am J Obstet Gynecol 182:1446, 2000

Hershey DW, Quilligan EJ: Extraabdominal uterine exteriorization at cesarean section. Obstet Gynecol 52:189, 1978

Hull DB, Varner MW: A randomized study of closure of the peritoneum at cesarean delivery. Obstet Gynecol 77:818, 1991

ICD-9-CM Professional, 6th ed. 2003 ICD-9-CM Vol 1 (October 2002). Salt Lake City, Utah, St. Anthony Publishing, 2003, p 182

Irion O, Luzuy F, Beguin F: Nonclosure of the visceral and parietal peritoneum at caesarean section: A randomised controlled trial. Br J Obstet Gynaecol 103:690, 1996

Jacob J, Phenninger J: Cesarean deliveries: When is a pediatrician necessary? Obstet Gynecol 89:217, 1997

Jones DE, Shackelford DP, Brame RG: Supracervical hysterectomy: Back to the future? Am J Obstet Gynecol 180:513, 1999

Kastner ES, Figueroa R, Garry D, et al: Emergency peripartum hysterectomy: Experience at a community teaching hospital. Obstet Gynecol 99:971, 2002

Kerr JMM: The technic of cesarean section with special reference to the lower uterine segment incision. Am J Obstet Gynecol 12:729, 1926

Kramer R, Van Someren J, Qualls C, et al: Postoperative management of cesarean section patients: The effect of immediate feeding on the incidence of ileus. Obstet Gynecol 88:29, 1996

Krönig B: Transperitonealer cervikaler Kaiserschnitt. In Doderlein A, Krönig B (eds): Operative Gynakologie. 1912, p 879

Landon MB, Hauth JC, Leveno KJ, et al: Maternal and perinatal outcomes associated with a trial of labor after prior cesarean delivery. N Engl J Med 351:25, 2004

Lasley DS, Eblen A, Yancey MK, et al: The effect of placental removal method on the incidence of postcesarean infections. Am J Obstet Gynecol 176:1250, 1997

Latzko W: Ueber den extraperitonealen Kaiserschnitt. Zentralbl Gynaekol 33:275, 1909

Learman LA, Summitt RL, Varner RE, McNeeley SG, et al: A randomized comparison of total or supracervical hysterectomy: Surgical complications and clinical outcomes. Obstet Gynecol 102:453, 2003

Lien JM, Towers CV, Quilligan EJ, et al: Term early-onset neonatal seizures: Obstetric characteristics, etiologic classifications, and perinatal care. Obstet Gynecol 85:163, 1995

Livingston EH, Passaro EP: Postoperative ileus. Dig Dis Sci 35:21, 1990

Lubenow TR, Ivankovich AD, McCarthy RJ: Management of acute postoperative pain. In Barash PG, Cullen BF, Stoelting RK (eds):

Clinical Anesthesia, 3rd ed. Philadelphia, JB Lippincott-Raven, 1997, p 1320

Lydon-Rochelle M, Holt VL, Martin DP, et al: Association between method of delivery and maternal rehospitalization. JAMA 283:2411, 2000

MacKenzie IZ, Cooke I: What is a reasonable time from decision-to-delivery by caesarean section? Evidence from 415 deliveries. Br J Obstet Gynaecol 109:498, 2002

Magann EF, Chauhan SP, Bufkin L, et al: Intra-operative haemorrhage by blunt versus sharp expansion of the uterine incision at caesarean delivery: A randomised clinical trial. Br J Obstet Gynaecol 109:448, 2002

Martin JA, Hamilton BE, Sutton PD, et al: Births: Final data for 2002. National Vital Statistics Reports, Vol 52, No. 10. Hyattsville, Md, National Center for Health Statistics, 2002

Minkoff H, Chervenak FA: Elective primary cesarean delivery. N Engl J Med 348:946, 2003

Minkoff H, Powderly KR, Chervenak F, et al: Ethical dimensions of elective primary cesarean delivery. Obstet Gynecol. 103(2):387, 2004

Munn MB, Owen J, Vincent R, et al: Comparison of two oxytocin regimens to prevent uterine atony at cesarean delivery: A randomized controlled trial. Obstet Gynecol 98:386, 2001

Munro MG: Supracervical hysterectomy: A time for reappraisal. Obstet Gynecol 89:133, 1997

Nagele F, Karas H, Spitzer D, et al: Closure or nonclosure of the visceral peritoneum at cesarean delivery. Am J Obstet Gynecol 174:1366, 1996

Naumann RW, Hauth JC, Owen J, et al: Subcutaneous tissue approximation in relation to wound disruption after cesarean delivery in obese women. Obstet Gynecol 85:412, 1995

Niemann JT: Cardiopulmonary resuscitation. N Engl J Med 327:1085, 1992

Notzon FC, Cnattingius S, Bergsjo P, et al: Cesarean section delivery in the 1980s: International comparison by indication. Am J Obstet Gynecol 170:495, 1994

Nygaard I, Cruikshank DP: Should all women be offered elective cesarean delivery? Obstet Gynecol 102:217, 2003

Parrish K, Holt VL, Easterling TR, et al: Effect of changes in maternal age, parity and birth weight distribution on primary cesarean delivery rates. JAMA 271:443, 1994

Physicians Insurance Association of America: Data Sharing System, Report No. 4. Pennington, NJ, PIAA, 1992

Physicians Insurance Association of America: Risk Management Review, Obstetrics 2002, Rockville, Md. Available at: http://www.thepiaa.org.

Pickrell K: An inquiry into the history of cesarean section. Bull Soc Med Hist (Chicago) 4:414, 1935

Pietrantoni M, Parsons MT, O'Brien WF, et al: Peritoneal closure or non-closure at cesarean. Obstet Gynecol 77:293, 1991

Plauche WC: Obstetric hysterectomy. In Hankins GDV, Clark SL, Cunningham FG, et al (eds): Operative Obstetrics. Norwalk, Conn, Appleton & Lange, 1995, p 333

Pliny the Elder: Natural History, book VII, chap IX. Rackham H, trans. Cambridge, Harvard University Press, 1942

Porreco RP: Meeting the challenge of the rising cesarean birth rate. Obstet Gynecol 75:133, 1990

Porro E: Della Amputazione Utero-ovarica. Milan, 1876

Pridijian G, Hibbard JU, Moawad AH: Cesarean: Changing the trends. Obstet Gynecol 77:195, 1991

Pritchard JA: Changes in the blood volume during pregnancy and delivery. Anesthesiology 26:393, 1965

Rafique Z, Shibli KU, Russell IF, et al: A randomised controlled trial of the closure or non-closure of peritoneum at caesarean section: Effect on post-operative pain. Br J Obstet Gynaecol 109:694, 2002

Rajasekar D, Hall M: Urinary tract injuries during obstetric intervention. Br J Obstet Gynaecol 104:731, 1997

Rodriguez AI, Porter KB, O'Brien WF: Blunt versus sharp expansion of the uterine incision in low-segment transverse cesarean section. Am J Obstet Gynecol 171:1022, 1994

Roset E, Boulvain M, Irion O: Nonclosure of the peritoneum during cesarean section: Long-term follow-up of a randomized controlled trial. Eur J Obstet Gynecol Reprod Biol 108:40, 2003

Rousset F: Traité Nouveau de l'Hystérotomotokie ou l'Enfantement Césarien. Paris, Denys deVal, 1581

Sachs BP, Yeh J, Acker D, et al: Cesarean section-related maternal mortality in Massachusetts, 1954–1985. Obstet Gynecol 71:385, 1988

Sanchez-Ramos L, Kaunitz AM, Peterson HB, et al: Reducing cesarean sections at a teaching hospital. Am J Obstet Gynecol 163:1081, 1990

Sänger M: Der Kaiserschnitt bei Uterusfibromen. Leipzig, 1882

Scheller JM, Nelson KB: Does cesarean delivery prevent cerebral palsy or other neurologic problems of childhood? Obstet Gynecol 83:624, 1994

Seago DP, Roberts WE, Johnson VK, et al: Planned cesarean hysterectomy: A preferred alternative to separate operations. Am J Obstet Gynecol 180:1385, 1999

Sewell JE: Cesarean section—a brief history. Washington, DC, American College of Obstetricians and Gynecologists, 1993

Shellhaas C for the National Institute of Child Health and Human Development Maternal–Fetal Medicine Units Network: The MFMU Cesarean Registry: Cesarean hysterectomy—its indications, morbidities, and mortality. Am J Obstet Gynecol 185:S123, 2001

Smith W: A Profile of Health and Disease in America: Obstetrics, Gynecology, and Infant Mortality. New York, Facts on File Publications, 1987, p 82

Strong TH, Brown WL Jr, Brown WL, et al: Experience with early postcesarean hospital dismissal. Am J Obstet Gynecol 169:116, 1993

Thacker SB, Stroup D, Chang M: Continuous electronic heart rate monitoring for fetal assessment during labor. Cochrane Database of Systematic Reviews 2:CD000063, 2001

Tulandi T, Al-Jaroudi D: Nonclosure of peritoneum: A reappraisal. Am J Obstet Gynecol 189:609, 2003

U.S. Department of Health and Human Services: Healthy People 2010, 2nd ed. With Understanding and Improving Health and Objectives for Improving Health. 2 vols. Washington, DC, U.S. Government Printing Office, November 2000

U.S. Public Health Service: Maternal and Child Health Bureau. Washington, DC, Department of Health and Human Services, 1991. Publication No. HRSA-M-CH 91-2

Vermillion ST, Lamoutte C, Soper DE, et al: Wound infection after cesarean: Effect of subcutaneous tissue thickness. Obstet Gynecol 95:923, 2000

Wagner M: Choosing caesarean section. Lancet 356:1677, 2000

Wahab MA, Karantziz P, Eccersley PS, et al: A randomized, controlled study of uterine exteriorization and repair at cesarean section. Br J Obstet Gynaecol 106:913, 1999

Waters EG: Supravesical extraperitoneal cesarean section: Presentation of a new technique. Am J Obstet Gynecol 39:423, 1940

Yost NP, Bloom SL, Sibley MK, Lo JY, et al: A hospital-sponsored quality improvement study of pain management after cesarean delivery. Am J Obstet Gynecol 190:1341, 2004

Zelop CM, Harlow BL, Frigoletto FD Jr, et al: Emergency peripartum hysterectomy. Am J Obstet Gynecol 168:1443, 1993

Zorlu CG, Turan C, Isik AZ, et al: Emergency hysterectomy in modern obstetric practice. Changing clinical perspective in time. Acta Obstet Gynecol Scand 77:186, 1998

26

Prior Cesarean Delivery

There are few issues in modern obstetrics that have been as controversial as the management of the woman with a prior cesarean delivery. For many decades, a scarred uterus was believed to contraindicate labor out of fear of uterine rupture. In 1916, Cragin made his famous, oft-quoted, and now seemingly excessive pronouncement, "Once a cesarean, always a cesarean." We must remember that when this statement was made, the so-called classical vertical uterine incision was used almost universally. It was not until 1921 that the Kerr transverse incision was recommended. Among Cragin's contemporaries, there were some who did not totally agree with his pronouncement. Writing in the fourth edition of *Williams Obstetrics,* J. Whitridge Williams (1917) termed the statement "an exaggeration." Now, 18 editions and nearly 90 years later, the controversy continues.

The year 1978 was another milestone in the history of prior cesarean delivery. Merrill and Gibbs (1978) reported from the University of Texas at San Antonio that subsequent vaginal delivery was safely attempted in 83 percent of their patients with prior cesarean deliveries. This report served to rekindle interest in vaginal birth after prior cesarean at a time when only 2 percent of American women who had previously undergone cesarean birth were planning vaginal delivery. The report was timely because during this same period, the rates of cesarean delivery in the United States were beginning to increase at an unprecedented rate. Between 1980 and 1988, for example, the rate jumped from 17 to 25 percent—a remarkable 50-percent increase in less than a decade. Meanwhile, evidence had accrued that uterine rupture was infrequent and rarely catastrophic. Thus, in an effort to address this escalation, the American College of Obstetricians and Gynecologists (1988) recommended that, in the absence of a contraindication, a woman with one previous low-transverse cesarean delivery be counseled to attempt

labor in a subsequent pregnancy. Accordingly, the frequency of vaginal birth after cesarean, commonly referred to as *VBAC* and pronounced *vee back,* increased significantly in the United States. As shown in Figure 26–1, by 1996 almost 30 percent of women with a prior cesarean were being delivered vaginally. In 1991, Dr. Roy Pitkin, former editor of *Obstetrics & Gynecology,* wrote that "...without question, the most remarkable change in obstetric practice over the last decade was management of the woman with prior cesarean delivery."

TRIAL OF LABOR VERSUS REPEAT CESAREAN DELIVERY

RISKS AND BENEFITS. Beginning in 1989, as the number of women with prior cesareans attempting vaginal delivery increased, there were a number of reports from around the United States and Canada that suggested that VBAC might be riskier than anticipated (Leveno, 1999). This led Scott (1991) to suggest an "alternative viewpoint on mandatory trial of labor," based on adverse experiences with 12 women in Utah who suffered uterine rupture during a trial of labor. Two women required hysterectomy, there were three perinatal deaths, and two infants suffered significant long-term neurological impairment. Porter and colleagues (1998) subsequently reported that there were 26 uterine ruptures in Salt Lake City between 1990 and 1996 and that 23 percent of the infants were dead or damaged as a result of intrapartum asphyxia. Reports such as these raised serious concern about the safety of this practice and contributed to heightened controversy (Flamm, 1997). These concerns resulted in fewer women with a prior cesarean incision attempting vaginal delivery, which led to a corresponding increase in the overall cesarean delivery rate, again seen in Figure 26–1.

MAGNITUDE OF RISK. Although uterine rupture and its associated complications clearly are increased with a trial of labor, some investigators have argued that these factors should weigh only minimally in the decision to attempt VBAC because the absolute risk of these complications is quite low. For example, Landon and collaborators (2004) from the Maternal–Fetal Medicine Units (MFMU) Network compared the outcomes of nearly 18,000 women who attempted a trial of labor with those of more than 15,000 women who were delivered by elective repeat cesarean. As shown in Table 26–1, although the risk of uterine rupture was higher among the women undergoing a trial of labor, the absolute risk was small. Specifically, the risk of uterine rupture was 7 per 1000. In comparison, however, there were no uterine ruptures in the elective cesarean delivery group. Moreover, the rates of stillbirth and hypoxic ischemic encephalopathy were significantly greater in the trial of labor group.

Smith and associates (2002) measured the risks of intrapartum and neonatal death associated with a trial of labor

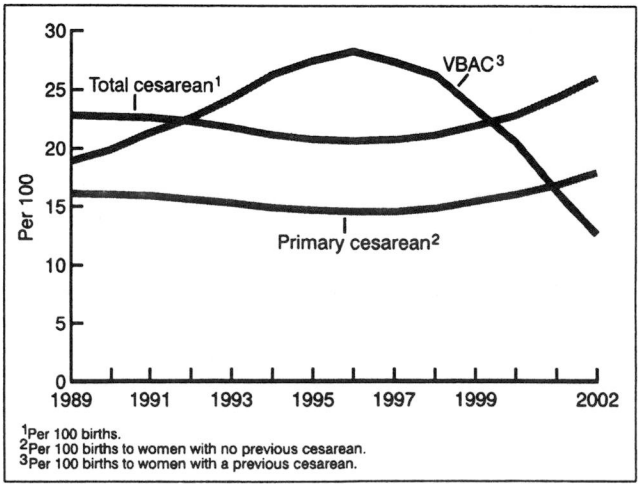

FIGURE 26–1. Total and primary cesarean delivery rate and vaginal birth after previous cesarean (VBAC) rate: United States, 1989–2002. (Reproduced from Hamilton and associates, 2003.)

TABLE 26–1 Complications Associated with a Trial of Labor in Women Delivered at an NICHD Maternal–Fetal Medicine Units Network Center, 1999–2002

Complication	Trial of Labor Group n = 17,898 (%)	Elective Repeat Cesarean Group n = 15,801 (%)	Odds Ratio (95% Confidence Interval)	P value
Uterine rupture	124 (0.7)	0	N/A	< .001
Uterine dehiscence	119 (0.7)	76 (0.5)	1.38 (1.04–1.85)	.03
Hysterectomy	41 (0.2)	47 (0.3)	0.77 (0.51–1.17)	.22
Thromboembolic disease	7 (0.04)	10 (0.1)	0.62 (0.24–1.62)	.32
Transfusion	304 (1.7)	158 (1.0)	1.71 (1.41–2.08)	< .001
Uterine infection	517 (2.9)	285 (1.8)	1.62 (1.40–1.87)	< .001
Maternal death	3	7	0.38 (0.10–1.46)	.21
Antepartum stillbirth[a]				
37–38 weeks	18 (0.1)	8 (0.1)	2.93 (1.27–6.75)	.008
39 weeks or more	16 (0.1)	5 (0.1)	2.70 (0.99–7.38)	.07
Intrapartum stillbirth[a]				
37–38 weeks	1	0	N/A	.43
39 weeks or more	1	0	N/A	1.00
Term HIE[a]	13 (0.08)	0	N/A	.0004
Term neonatal death[a]	13 (0.08)	7 (0.05)	1.82 (0.73–4.57)	.19

HIE = hypoxic ischemic encephalopathy; N/A = not applicable, NICHD = National Institutes of Child Health and Human Development.
[a]Denominator is 15,338 for the trial of labor group and 15,014 for the elective repeat cesarean delivery group.
From Landon and collaborators (2004), with permission.

compared with those of a planned repeat cesarean delivery using a database linking all maternity hospitals in Scotland. Their analysis involved 313,238 term singleton deliveries that were registered between 1992 and 1997 and included 24,529 births from women with a prior cesarean delivery. The risk of delivery-related perinatal death was approximately 1.3 per 1000 among the 15,515 women with a prior cesarean who attempted a vaginal delivery. Although the absolute risk was again small, this rate was *11 times greater* than the risk of perinatal death associated with a planned repeat cesarean.

The results of these and other investigations, including two large systematic reviews by Chauhan and colleagues (2003) and Mozurkewich and Hutton (2000), are congruent. Collectively, they suggest that the absolute risk of uterine rupture attributable to a trial of labor resulting in death or injury to the fetus is about 1 per 1000. The major controversy surrounding the management of women with a prior cesarean thus stems from the question: *Is a 1 per 1000 risk of having an otherwise healthy fetus die or be damaged as a result of a trial of labor acceptable?*

MATERNAL MORBIDITY. Another potential argument in support of VBAC has been that a trial of labor is associated with reduced risks for the mother compared with those of a repeat cesarean delivery. Maternal *mortality* does not appear to differ significantly between women undergoing a trial of labor compared with that of an elective repeat cesarean (Landon and co-workers, 2004; Mozurkewich and Hutton, 2000). Estimates of maternal *morbidity,* however, have produced conflicting results. In the meta-analysis by Mozurkewich and

Hutton (2000), women undergoing a trial of labor were about half as likely to require a blood transfusion or hysterectomy compared with those undergoing an elective repeat cesarean delivery. Conversely, in the MFMU Network study cited earlier, Landon and co-workers (2004) observed that the risks of transfusion and infection were significantly greater for women attempting a trial of labor (see Table 26–1). McMahon and associates (1996), in a population-based study of 6138 women, found that major complications—hysterectomy, uterine rupture, or operative injury—were almost twice as common in women undergoing a trial of labor compared with those of those undergoing an elective second cesarean delivery. Moreover, compared with a successful trial of labor, the risk of these major complications was fivefold greater in women whose attempt at a vaginal delivery failed.

COSTS. Analyses from Northwestern Hospital in Chicago support the safety of VBAC as well as its cost effectiveness in women with one or two prior low-transverse uterine incisions (Grobman and associates, 2000; Socol and Peaceman, 1999). By applying a mathematical model to a hypothetical cohort of 100,000 pregnant women whose only prior delivery was through a low-transverse cesarean incision, a policy of routine repeat cesarean for a second birth was calculated to result in an increased cost of $179 million. Similarly, DiMaio and colleagues (2002) estimated that total hospital costs for mother and newborn were nearly $1100 higher for each elective repeat cesarean compared with that of those who attempted vaginal delivery. Conversely, Clark and colleagues (2000) concluded that "when costs as opposed to charges are considered and the cost of long-term care for neurologically injured infants is taken into account, trial of labor after previous cesarean is unlikely to be associated with a significant cost saving for the health care system."

ELECTIVE REPEAT CESAREAN DELIVERY. As described in Chapter 25 (see p. 592), compared with vaginal delivery, cesarean birth is associated with increased risks, including anesthesia, hemorrhage, damage to the bladder and other organs, pelvic infection, scarring, and other less frequent events. In spite of these potential concerns, an elective repeat cesarean is considered by many women to be preferable to attempting a trial of labor. Frequent reasons for this preference include the convenience of a scheduled delivery and the fear of a prolonged and potentially dangerous labor. Abitbol and associates (1993) studied such preferences by analyzing the results of a program in which women who were candidates for a trial of labor were able to elect their route of delivery following extensive counseling. Information was provided in three separate sessions concerning advantages and disadvantages of VBAC and repeat cesarean delivery. Of the 312 women studied, 125 (40 percent) opted for a repeat cesarean. There were no complications in the elective cesarean group compared with two unanticipated fetal deaths in the VBAC group. All women were interviewed on the day of discharge regarding their delivery experience. Of the women delivered by scheduled cesarean, 93 percent reported that they were satisfied with their choice. This compared with only 53 percent of women who elected a trial of labor and 80 percent of those who had an uncomplicated trial of labor.

Fetal Maturity. If elective repeat cesarean delivery is planned, it is essential that the fetus be mature. The American Academy of Pediatrics and the American College of Obstetricians and Gynecologists (2002) have established guidelines for timing an elective operation. According to these criteria, elective delivery may be considered and fetal maturity assumed if at least one of the criteria outlined in Table 26–2 is met. In all other instances, fetal pulmonary maturity must be documented by amnionic fluid analysis before elective repeat cesarean is undertaken (see Chap. 29, p. 651). Alternatively, the onset of spontaneous labor is awaited.

CANDIDATES FOR A TRIAL OF LABOR

As the foregoing discussion makes clear, a plurality of positions exists regarding the optimal management of the woman with a prior cesarean delivery. Specifically, through 2003, more than 1000 citations were available in the literature— and no randomized trials—addressing subsequent attempts at vaginal delivery. In 1998 and 1999, the American College of Obstetricians and Gynecologists issued updated practice bulletins supporting VBAC but also urging a more cautious approach. In part, their recommendation reads:

> It has become apparent that VBAC is associated with a small but significant risk of uterine rupture with poor outcomes for both mother and infant. . . . These developments, which have led to a more circumspect approach to trial of labor by even the most ardent supporters of VBAC, illustrate the need to reevaluate VBAC recommendations.

Several factors are pertinent to the evaluation of women for a trial of labor to attempt VBAC. The most recent recommendations of the American College of Obstetricians and Gynecologists (2004) for selecting appropriate candidates are listed in Table 26–3. Summarized in the following sections are these and other considerations for the evaluation and management of the woman with a prior cesarean delivery. Such evaluation is particularly challenging given the lack of randomized studies. Indeed, based on their recent review of 100 published studies, Hashima and co-workers (2004) concluded that little high-quality data are available to guide clinical decisions regarding selection of women who are likely to have a successful trial of labor. Following a review of more than 600 articles, Guise and colleagues (2004) reached a similar conclusion.

TABLE 26–2 Establishment of Fetal Maturity Prior to Elective Repeat Cesarean Delivery

Fetal maturity may be assumed if one of the following criteria is met:

1. Fetal heart sounds have been documented for 20 weeks by non-electronic fetoscope or for 30 weeks by Doppler ultrasound
2. It has been 36 weeks since a positive serum or urine chorionic gonadotropin pregnancy test was performed by a reliable laboratory
3. An ultrasound measurement of crown-rump length, obtained at 6–11 weeks, supports current gestational age of 39 weeks or more
4. Clinical history and physical and ultrasound examination performed at 12–20 weeks support current gestational age of 39 weeks or more

From the American Academy of Pediatrics and the American College of Obstetricians and Gynecologists (2002), with permission.

TABLE 26–3 Recommendations of the American College of Obstetricians and Gynecologists Useful for Selection of Candidates for Vaginal Birth After Cesarean Delivery (VBAC)

- No more than 1 prior low-transverse cesarean delivery
- Clinically adequate pelvis
- No other uterine scars or previous rupture
- Physician immediately available throughout active labor who is capable of monitoring labor and performing emergency cesarean delivery
- Availability of anesthesia and personnel for emergency cesarean delivery

From the American College of Obstetricians and Gynecologists (2004), with permission.

TABLE 26–4 Estimated Risks for Uterine Rupture in Women with a Prior Cesarean Delivery

Prior Uterine Incision	Estimated Rupture (%)
Classical	4–9
T-shaped	4–9
Low-vertical	1–7
Low-transverse	0.2–1.5

From the American College of Obstetricians and Gynecologists (1999), with permission.

TYPE OF PRIOR UTERINE INCISION. Women with a transverse scar confined to the lower uterine segment have the lowest risk of symptomatic scar separation during a subsequent pregnancy (Table 26–4). The highest rates of rupture have been reported for incisions extending into the fundus—the classical incision (Fig. 26–2). Importantly, in about one third of women, the classical scar will rupture before the onset of labor. Not infrequently, rupture may take place several weeks before term. In a review of 157 women with a prior classical cesarean, Chauhan and colleagues (2002) reported that one woman had a complete uterine rupture prior to the onset of labor and 15 (9 percent) others suffered a uterine

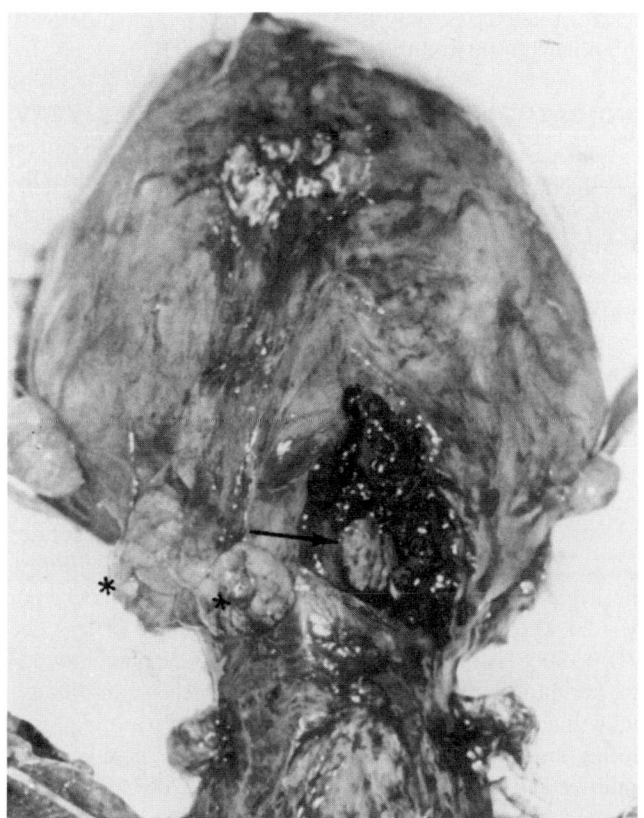

FIGURE 26–2. Ruptured vertical cesarean section scar (*arrow*) identified at time of repeat cesarean delivery early in labor; asterisks indicate some of the sites of densely adherent omentum.

dehiscence (see p. 615). Similarly, we have encountered a term abdominal pregnancy in a woman whose prior classical incision had separated weeks to months before she was delivered by repeat cesarean.

In women with uterine malformations who have undergone cesarean delivery, the risks for uterine rupture in a subsequent pregnancy may be as high as with a classical incision. Specifically, Ravasia and associates (1999) reported the risk of subsequent rupture to be 8 percent in women with unicornuate, bicornuate, didelphic, and septate uterine malformations (see Chap. 40, p. 953).

The risk of uterine rupture in women with a prior vertical incision that did not extend into the fundus is controversial. Martin and co-authors (1997) and Shipp and colleagues (1999) reported that these low-vertical uterine incisions did not have an increased risk for rupture when compared with that of low-transverse incisions. The American College of Obstetricians and Gynecologists (2004) concluded that, although there is limited evidence, women with a prior vertical incision in the lower uterine segment without fundal extension may be candidates for VBAC. This is in contrast to prior classical or T-shaped uterine incisions, which are considered contraindications to VBAC. It seems reasonable to us that, given the very few conditions that call for vertical incisions—for example, preterm delivery with a poorly developed lower uterine segment—these incisions almost invariably extended into the active segment. The unanswered question is: How far upward does the incision have to extend before the risk of rupture is equivalent to a true classical incision? Thus, when preparing an operative report following a vertical uterine incision, it is essential to document its exact extent in a manner that cannot be misunderstood by subsequent surgeons.

Women who have previously sustained a uterine rupture are at increased risk for recurrence. Those with a rupture confined to the lower segment have been reported to have a 6-percent recurrence risk in subsequent labor, whereas those whose prior rupture included the upper uterus have a 32-percent recurrence risk (Reyes-Ceja and associates, 1969; Ritchie, 1971). We are of the view that women with prior uterine ruptures or classical or T-shaped incisions ideally are delivered by cesarean on achievement of fetal pulmonary maturity and prior to the onset of labor, and that such women should be warned of the hazards of unattended labor and signs of possible uterine rupture.

CLOSURE OF PRIOR INCISION. As discussed in Chapter 25 (see p. 597), the low-transverse uterine incision typically is closed in one or two layers. Whether the risk of subsequent uterine rupture is related to the number of layers is controversial. Chapman (1997) and Tucker (1993) and their associates found no relationship between a one- and two-layer closure and risk of subsequent uterine rupture. Although Durnwald and Mercer (2003) also found no increased risk of rupture, uterine dehiscence was more common after single-layer closure. In contrast, Bujold and co-workers (2002) reviewed the operative records of 1980 women who underwent a trial of labor, including 23 (1.2 percent) who experienced uterine rupture. They found that a single-layer closure was associated with nearly a fourfold increased risk of rupture compared with a double-layer closure. The latter consisted of a running-lock suture followed by a running, nonlocking imbricating suture. In response, Vidaeff and Lucas (2003) argued that experimental models of wound healing have not demonstrated any advantages with a double-layer closure. Because of potentially confounding variables inherent in this type of retrospective study, they concluded that the evidence is insufficient to routinely recommend a double-layer closure. There should be further study of the relationship between closure technique and subsequent uterine rupture. This is especially true given the limited available information regarding healing and scarring of cesarean incisions.

Healing of the Cesarean Incision. Williams (1921) believed that the uterus heals by regeneration of the muscular fibers and not by development of scar tissue. Certainly, upon inspection of the unopened uterus at repeat cesarean delivery, there is usually no trace of the former incision, or at most, an almost invisible linear scar. Also, when the uterus is removed and fixed in formalin, there often is no visible scar, or only a shallow vertical furrow in the external and internal surfaces of the anterior uterine wall is seen, with no trace of scar tissue between them.

On the other hand, Schwarz and co-workers (1938) concluded that healing was mainly by fibroblast proliferation. They studied the uterine incision site some days after cesarean incision and observed that as the scar shrinks, connective tissue proliferation becomes less obvious. If the cut surfaces of the uterus are closely apposed, the proliferation of connective tissue is minimal, and the normal relation of smooth muscle to connective tissue gradually is reestablished. Even when the healing is so poor that marked thinning has resulted, the remaining tissue often is entirely muscular.

INTERDELIVERY INTERVAL. It seems logical to assume that the risk of uterine rupture would be increased if the hysterotomy scar did not have sufficient time to heal. Studies of uterine scar healing using magnetic resonance imaging suggest that complete uterine involution and restoration of anatomy may require at least 6 months (Dicle and colleagues, 1997). To explore this issue further, Shipp and associates (2001) retrospectively examined the relationship between interdelivery interval and uterine rupture in 2409 women with one prior cesarean delivery. There were 29 (1.4 percent) cases of uterine rupture. They found that interdelivery intervals of 18 months or less were associated with a threefold increased risk of symptomatic uterine rupture compared with that of those over 18 months.

NUMBER OF PRIOR CESAREAN INCISIONS. The risk of uterine rupture increases with the number of previous cesarean deliveries. Miller and colleagues (1994) stud-

ied 12,707 women undergoing a trial of labor after cesarean delivery. They reported rupture rates of 0.6 percent and 1.8 percent for women with one and two prior cesarean deliveries, respectively. Similarly, in the MFMU Network study by Landon and co-investigators (2004a), uterine rupture was twice as high in women with multiple prior cesareans compared with that of those with only one—1.4 versus 0.7 percent. Caughey and colleagues (1999) compared uterine rupture rates in 3757 women with one prior cesarean delivery with those of 134 women who had two prior cesarean incisions. Although women with a classical incision usually were delivered by elective repeat cesarean, the type of prior uterine incision was not specified. The rate of uterine rupture was increased nearly fivefold in women with two previous cesarean deliveries compared with that of those only with one—3.7 versus 0.8 percent.

Any previous vaginal delivery, either before or following a cesarean birth, significantly improves the prognosis for a subsequent successful VBAC, with either spontaneous or induced labor (Caughey and colleagues, 1998; Grinstead and Grobman, 2004; Hendler and co-workers, 2004). Prior vaginal delivery also lowers the risk of subsequent uterine rupture (Zelop and associates, 2000). Indeed, the most favorable prognostic factor is prior vaginal delivery. The American College of Obstetricians and Gynecologists (2004) has recently taken the position that for women with two prior low-transverse cesarean deliveries, only those with a prior vaginal delivery should be considered for VBAC.

INDICATION FOR PRIOR CESAREAN DELIVERY. The success rate for a trial of labor depends to some extent on the indication for the previous cesarean delivery. Generally, about 60 to 80 percent of trials of labor after prior cesarean birth result in vaginal delivery (American College of Obstetricians and Gynecologists, 2004). In a large series reported by Wing and Paul (1999), 91 percent of women whose first cesarean was for breech presentation had a successful VBAC. When fetal distress was the original indication, the success rate was 84 percent. In those with dystocia as the original indication, Impey and O'Herlihy (1998) reported that even when the strictest criteria are used to diagnose dystocia, a VBAC rate of 68 percent can be achieved.

Hoskins and Gomez (1997) analyzed VBAC success rates in 1917 women in relation to cervical dilation achieved before the original cesarean delivery was performed for dystocia. For women whose cesarean was performed at 5 cm or less, the VBAC success rate was 67 percent. It was 73 percent when the cervix was dilated 6 to 9 cm. The success rate of vaginal delivery fell to 13 percent when dystocia was diagnosed during the second stage. These latter findings seem counterintuitive and, indeed, Bujold and Gauthier (2001) reported a 75-percent VBAC success rate in women who had undergone a prior cesarean for second-stage dystocia.

FETAL MACROSOMIA. It would seem that increasing fetal size would increase the risk of uterine rupture with

VBAC. This, however, remains unproven. Zelop and associates (2001) compared the outcomes of 2749 women undergoing a trial of labor at term. There were 29 (1.1 percent) uterine ruptures. Although not statistically significant, the rate of uterine rupture for women whose infants weighed at least 4000 g was 1.6 percent compared with that of 1.0 percent for those whose infants weighed less. The rate of uterine rupture was even greater (2.4 percent) when the birthweight exceeded 4250 g. Similarly, Elkousy and colleagues (2003) found that for women attempting VBAC who had no previous vaginal deliveries, the relative risk of uterine rupture more than doubled when the birthweight was at least 4000 g.

MATERNAL OBESITY. Carroll and colleagues (2003) found that as maternal weight increased, the rate of VBAC success decreased. In their study, only 4 of 30 women (13 percent) undergoing a trial of labor who weighed more than 300 pounds delivered vaginally. Their observations that puerperal infection was higher in obese women attempting a trial of labor was confirmed by Edwards and associates (2003). Maternal obesity is detailed in Chapter 43.

LABOR AND DELIVERY CONSIDERATIONS

The American Academy of Pediatrics and the American College of Obstetricians and Gynecologists (2002) have formulated the following guidelines for women with a prior cesarean who have chosen a trial of labor:

1. Prompt evaluation of the laboring patient must be performed.
2. Continuous electronic monitoring of fetal heart rate and uterine contractions should be considered (see Chap. 18, p. 444).
3. Personnel familiar with the potential complications of a trial of labor should be vigilant for nonreassuring fetal heart rate patterns and inadequate progress of labor.
4. Attempts should be limited to institutions with physicians immediately available to provide emergency care.

Lavin and co-workers (2002) surveyed all hospitals in Ohio to determine the number that actually had an obstetrician, anesthesia coverage, and a surgical team immediately available—defined as present in the hospital—when a woman was attempting a trial of labor. A complete complement was available in 15, 63, and 100 percent of level I, II, and III institutions, respectively. Because VBAC deliveries were equally distributed among the institutions, the investigators concluded that many women may be attempting VBAC under less than optimal conditions. They recommended that there is a need to examine staffing and referral patterns.

INFORMED CONSENT. No woman should be mandated to undergo a trial of labor. Instead, the risks and benefits of a trial of labor versus a repeat cesarean delivery should be discussed with any woman with a prior uterine incision.

The ultimate decision to attempt a vaginal delivery should be made by the informed patient and her physician. The American Academy of Pediatrics and the American College of Obstetricians and Gynecologists (2002) recommend that the following issues be addressed:

1. Advantages of a successful vaginal delivery, for example, shorter postpartum hospital stay; less painful, more rapid recovery; and others.
2. Contraindications to a trial of labor, for example, prior classical cesarean, placenta previa, and others.
3. Risk of uterine rupture (approximately 1 percent).
4. Increased risk of uterine rupture with more than one prior cesarean delivery, attempts at cervical ripening or labor induction, macrosomia, and oxytocin augmentation.
5. In the event of rupture, there is a 10- to 25-percent risk of significant adverse fetal sequelae.
6. Although catastrophic uterine rupture leading to perinatal death or permanent neonatal injury is rare, occurring less often than 1 per 1000 VBAC attempts, it does occur despite the best available resources.

CERVICAL RIPENING AND LABOR STIMULATION. Any attempt to induce cervical ripening or to induce or augment labor increases the risk of uterine rupture in women undergoing a trial of labor.

Oxytocin. Use of oxytocin to induce or augment labor has been implicated in uterine ruptures in women attempting VBAC. Turner (1997) observed that 13 of the 15 uterine ruptures reported at the Coombe Hospital in Dublin between 1982 and 1991 occurred in women with prior cesareans who had been given an oxytoxic agent, usually for *induction* of labor. In contrast, cautious use of intravenous oxytocin to *augment* labor in women with prior cesarean at this hospital was rarely associated with uterine rupture.

Zelop and associates (1999) analyzed uterine ruptures at Brigham and Women's Hospital after induced or augmented labor in women with one prior cesarean delivery. Rupture occurred in 2.3 percent of those induced compared with 1 and 0.4 percent of those whose labor was augmented or was spontaneous, respectively. They urged caution when using oxytocin for labor stimulation in these women. Goetzl and associates (2001) examined the relationship between the total oxytocin dose and duration of induction and the risk of uterine rupture. Although not significant, oxytocin dose and duration correlated directly with uterine rupture. The investigators concluded, however, that the differences in the dose or patterns of oxytocin use were not substantial enough to develop safer induction protocols.

The American Academy of Pediatrics and the American College of Obstetricians and Gynecologists (2002) have concluded that oxytocin may be used for both labor induction and augmentation with close patient monitoring in women with a prior cesarean delivery undergoing a trial of labor (see Chap. 22, p. 537).

EXPERIENCES AT PARKLAND HOSPITAL. Our experience with uterine ruptures led us to the decision to discontinue the use of oxytocin in women with prior cesarean deliveries. Between 1986 and 1990, a trial of labor was undertaken by 2044 of the 7049 women with prior cesarean deliveries. Of these women, 1482 (73 percent) delivered vaginally. Uterine rupture with part of the fetus extruded outside of the uterus occurred in three women, for a rate of 1.5 per 1000. In another 307 women who received oxytocin during their trial of labor, three uterine ruptures (10 per 1000) occurred. These events prompted a reappraisal of our use of oxytocin and the adoption of a more conservative approach.

Prostaglandins. Several prostaglandin preparations commonly are employed for cervical ripening or labor induction. Recent evidence indicates that their use in women attempting VBAC substantively increases the risk of uterine rupture. For example, Ravasia and colleagues (2000) compared the rupture rates between 172 such women given prostaglandin E_2 gel and 1544 similar women in spontaneous labor. The rate of uterine rupture was significantly greater in the women treated with prostaglandin E_2 gel than in those having spontaneous labor—2.9 percent versus 0.5 percent.

There are only a few reports describing the use of the prostaglandin E_1 analogue misoprostol in women with a prior cesarean delivery. Wing and colleagues (1998) prematurely terminated their randomized study of oxytocin versus misoprostol for labor induction in women with previous cesarean delivery after 2 of the first 17 women randomized to misoprostol experienced a uterine rupture. Sciscione and co-workers (1998) described a case of uterine rupture following misoprostol administration in a woman attempting VBAC. The editors of the *Australian and New Zealand Journal of Obstetrics and Gynaecology* published the report for the stated purpose of warning other investigators of the potential hazards of studying misoprostol in women with a prior cesarean delivery.

Lydon-Rochelle and associates (2001) performed a retrospective, population-based study in Washington State from 1987 through 1996. They included all primiparous women who delivered a live singleton infant by cesarean and who also delivered a second child during the study period. Of the 20,095 women included, 13,115 (65 percent) underwent a trial of labor. As shown in Table 26–5, the risk of uterine rupture was nearly 16-fold greater for women undergoing induction of labor with prostaglandins compared with that of a repeated cesarean delivery without labor. Based in large part on the results of this study, the American College of Obstetricians and Gynecologists (2002, 2004) discourage the use of prostaglandin cervical ripening agents for the induction of labor in these women. They further recommend that if induction of labor in a woman with a prior cesarean delivery is necessary for a clear and compelling clinical indication, the potential increased risk of uterine rupture with prostaglandin use should be discussed with the patient and documented.

As also shown in Table 26–5, Lydon-Rochelle and colleagues (2001) found a threefold risk of uterine rupture associated with spontaneous labor alone compared with the risk associated with elective repeat cesarean delivery. Based on these findings, Greene (2001) editorialized that elective repeat cesarean is the safest route of delivery for the infant.

EPIDURAL ANALGESIA. The use of epidural analgesia for labor in women with a prior cesarean delivery was debated in the past because it was thought that such a technique might mask the pain of uterine rupture. As evidence accrued, however, it was found that less than 10 percent of women with scar separation experience pain and bleeding. Instead, fetal heart rate decelerations are the most likely sign of rupture (Flamm and associates, 1990). Several studies attest to the safety of properly conducted epidural analgesia for labor (Farmer and

TABLE 26–5 Incidence and Relative Risk of Uterine Rupture During a Second Delivery Among Women with a Prior Cesarean Delivery

Mode of Second Delivery	No. of Women	Incidence of Rupture[a] (per 1000)	Relative Risk (95% Confidence Interval)
Repeat cesarean delivery without labor	6,980	1.6	1.0
Spontaneous onset of labor	10,789	5.2	3.3 (1.8–6.0)
Induction of labor without prostaglandins	1,960	7.7	4.9 (2.4–9.7)
Induction of labor with prostaglandins	366	24.5	15.6 (8.1–30.0)

[a] Incidence is expressed as the number of cases of uterine rupture per 1000 women who delivered a singleton infant after a prior cesarean delivery. Women who had repeated cesarean delivery without labor served as the referent group.
Reproduced from Lydon-Rochelle and associates (2001), with permission.

colleagues, 1991; Flamm and associates, 1994). Moreover, vaginal delivery rates are similar among women who receive an epidural for labor compared with those who do not (Flamm and co-workers, 1988; Stovall and colleagues, 1987). The American Academy of Pediatrics and the American College of Obstetricians and Gynecologists (2002) have concluded that epidural analgesia may safely be used during a trial of labor. They further recommend that the anesthesia service be notified whenever a woman with a prior cesarean is admitted in active labor.

UTERINE SCAR EXPLORATION. Although some obstetricians routinely document the integrity of the old scar by palpation following successful vaginal delivery, such uterine exploration is felt by others to be unnecessary. Currently, it is not known what effect documentation of an asymptomatic scar has on subsequent reproduction or route of delivery. There is general agreement, however, that surgical correction of a scar dehiscence is necessary only if significant bleeding is encountered. Asymptomatic separations do not generally require exploratory laparotomy and repair.

EXTERNAL CEPHALIC VERSION. Limited data suggest that external cephalic version for breech presentation may be as successful for women with a prior cesarean as for women without such a history (American Academy of Pediatrics and the American College of Obstetricians and Gynecologists, 2002). Breech presentation and external cephalic version are addressed in Chapter 24 (see p. 581).

UTERINE RUPTURE

CLASSIFICATION. Uterine rupture typically is classified as either *complete* (all layers of the uterine wall separated) or *incomplete* (uterine muscle separated but visceral peritoneum is intact). Incomplete rupture is also commonly referred to as *uterine dehiscence*. As expected, morbidity and mortality are appreciably greater when rupture is complete. Currently, the greatest risk factor for either complete or incomplete uterine rupture is prior cesarean delivery. Indeed, in a review of all cases of uterine rupture in Nova Scotia between 1988 and 1997, Kieser and Baskett (2002) reported that 92 percent occurred in women with a prior cesarean birth. Other causes of uterine rupture are discussed in Chapter 35 (see p. 837).

DIAGNOSIS. Prior to circulatory collapse from hemorrhage, the symptoms and physical findings may appear bizarre unless the possibility of uterine rupture is kept in mind. For example, hemoperitoneum from a ruptured uterus may result in irritation of the diaphragm with pain referred to the chest—leading one to the diagnosis of pulmonary or amnionic fluid embolism instead of uterine rupture. Few women experience cessation of contractions following

uterine rupture, and the use of intrauterine pressure catheters has not been shown to assist reliably in the diagnosis (Rodriguez and associates, 1989). Instead, the most common electronic fetal monitoring finding tends to be sudden, severe heart rate decelerations that may evolve into late decelerations, bradycardia, and undetectable fetal heart action (American Academy of Pediatrics and American College of Obstetricians and Gynecologists, 2002). In the Nova Scotia study cited earlier, 57 percent of the diagnoses were based primarily on fetal heart rate abnormalities (Kieser and Baskett, 2002). Finally, in a recent comparison of fetal heart rate characteristics in 36 cases of uterine rupture versus 100 matched controls, Ridgeway and co-workers (2004) found that bradycardia was the only finding that differentiated uterine rupture from a successful trial of labor.

In a minority of women, the appearance of uterine rupture is identical to that of placental abruption. In most, however, there is remarkably little appreciable pain or tenderness. Also, because most women in labor are treated for discomfort with either narcotics or lumbar epidural analgesia, pain and tenderness may not be readily apparent. The condition usually becomes evident because of signs of fetal distress and occasionally because of maternal hypovolemia from concealed hemorrhage.

In some cases in which the fetal presenting part has entered the pelvis with labor, loss of station may be detected by pelvic examination. If the fetus is partly or totally extruded from the site of uterine rupture, abdominal palpation or vaginal examination may be helpful to identify the presenting part, which will have moved away from the pelvic inlet. A firm contracted uterus may at times be felt alongside the fetus.

PROGNOSIS. With rupture and expulsion of the fetus into the peritoneal cavity, the chances for intact fetal survival are dismal, and reported mortality rates range from 50 to 75 percent. Fetal condition depends on how much placenta is intact, although this likely decreases over minutes. If the fetus is alive at the time of rupture, the only chance of continued survival is afforded by immediate delivery, most often by laparotomy. Otherwise, hypoxia from both placental separation and maternal hypovolemia is inevitable. If rupture is followed by total placental separation, then very few infants will be salvaged.

The maternal prognosis is much better and rupture is seldom fatal. If untreated, however, most women would die from hemorrhage or, less often, later from infection.

Hysterectomy Versus Repair. In cases of scar separation without bleeding following VBAC, exploratory laparotomy is not indicated. With frank rupture during a trial of labor, however, hysterectomy may be required. In two reports by McMahon (1996) and Miller (1997) and their colleagues, 10 to 20 percent of such women required hysterectomy for hemostasis. In selected cases, suture repair with uterine preservation may be performed. Sheth (1968) described outcomes from a series of 66 women in whom repair of a uterine rupture was elected rather than hysterectomy. In 25 instances, the repair was accompanied by tubal sterilization. Thirteen of the 41 mothers who did not have tubal sterilization had a total of 21 subsequent pregnancies, and uterine rupture recurred in four instances. Hysterectomy is described in Chapter 25 (see p. 599), and other techniques to control obstetrical hemorrhage are detailed in Chapter 35 (see p. 809).

REFERENCES

Abitbol MM, Castillo I, Taylor UB, et al: Vaginal birth after cesarean section: The patient's point of view. Am Fam Physician 47:129, 1993

American Academy of Pediatrics and the American College of Obstetricians and Gynecologists: Guidelines for Perinatal Care, 5th ed. Elk Grove, Ill, American Academy of Pediatrics, 2002

American College of Obstetricians and Gynecologists: Induction of labor for vaginal birth after cesarean delivery. Committee Opinion No. 271, April 2002

American College of Obstetricians and Gynecologists: Vaginal birth after previous cesarean delivery. Practice Bulletin No. 54, July 2004

American College of Obstetricians and Gynecologists: Vaginal birth after previous cesarean delivery. Practice Bulletin No. 2, October 1998

American College of Obstetricians and Gynecologists: Guidelines for vaginal delivery after a previous cesarean birth. Committee Opinion No. 64, October 1988

Bujold E, Bujold C, Hamilton EF, et al: The impact of a single-layer or double-layer closure on uterine rupture. Am J Obstet Gynecol 186:1326, 2002

Bujold E, Gauthier RJ: Should we allow a trial of labor after a previous cesarean for dystocia in the second stage of labor? Obstet Gynecol 98:652, 2001

Carroll CS, Magann EF, Chauhan SP, et al: Vaginal birth after cesarean section versus elective repeat cesarean delivery: Weight-based outcomes. Am J Obstet Gynecol 188:1516, 2003

Caughey AB, Shipp TD, Repke JT, et al: Rate of uterine rupture during a trial of labor in women with one or two prior cesarean deliveries. Am J Obstet Gynecol 181:872, 1999

Caughey AB, Shipp TD, Repke JT, et al: Trial of labor after cesarean delivery: The effect of previous vaginal delivery. Am J Obstet Gynecol 179:938, 1998

Chapman SJ, Owen J, Hauth JC: One- versus two-layer closure of a low transverse cesarean: The next pregnancy. Obstet Gynecol 89:16, 1997

Chauhan SP, Magann EF, Wiggs CD, et al: Pregnancy after classic cesarean delivery. Obstet Gynecol 100:946, 2002

Chauhan SP, Martin JN Jr, Henrichs CE, et al: Maternal and perinatal complications with uterine rupture in 142,075 patients who attempted vaginal birth after cesarean delivery: A review of the literature. Am J Obstet Gynecol 189:408, 2003

Clark SL, Scott JR, Porter TF, et al: Is vaginal birth after cesarean less expensive than repeat cesarean delivery? Am J Obstet Gynecol 182:599, 2000

Cragin E: Conservatism in obstetrics. N Y Med J 104:1, 1916

Dicle O, Küçükler C, Pirnar T: Magnetic resonance imaging evaluation of incision healing after cesarean sections. Eur Radiol 7:31, 1997

DiMaio H, Edwards RK, Euliano TY, et al: Vaginal birth after cesarean delivery: An historic cohort cost analysis. Am J Obstet Gynecol 186:890, 2002

Durnwald C, Mercer B: Uterine rupture, perioperative and perinatal morbidity after single-layer and double-layer closure at cesarean delivery. Am J Obstet Gynecol 189:925, 2003

Edwards RK, Harnsberger DS, Johnson IM, et al: Deciding on route of delivery for obese women with a prior cesarean delivery. Am J Obstet Gynecol 189:385, 2003

Elkousy MA, Sammel M, Stevens E, et al: The effect of birth weight on vaginal birth after cesarean delivery success rates. Am J Obstet Gynecol 188:824, 2003

Farmer RM, Kirschbaum T, Potter D, et al: Uterine rupture during trial of labor after previous cesarean section. Am J Obstet Gynecol 165:996, 1991

Flamm BL: Once a cesarean, always a controversy. Obstet Gynecol 90:312, 1997

Flamm BL, Goings JR, Liu Y, et al: Elective repeat cesarean delivery versus trial of labor: A prospective multicenter study. Obstet Gynecol 83:927, 1994

Flamm BL, Lim OW, Jones C, et al: Vaginal birth after cesarean section: Results of a multicenter study. Am J Obstet Gynecol 158:1079, 1988

Flamm BL, Newman LA, Thomas SJ, et al: Vaginal birth after cesarean delivery: Results of a 5-year multicenter collaborative study. Obstet Gynecol 76:750, 1990

Goetzl L, Shipp TD, Cohen A, et al: Oxytocin dose and the risk of uterine rupture in trial of labor after cesarean. Obstet Gynecol 97:381, 2001

Greene MF: Vaginal delivery after cesarean section—is the risk acceptable? N Engl J Med 345:54, 2001

Grinstead J, Grobman WA: Induction of labor after one prior cesarean: Predictors of vaginal delivery. Obstet Gynecol 103:534, 2004

Grobman WA, Peaceman AM, Socol ML: Cost-effectiveness of elective cesarean delivery after one prior low transverse cesarean. Obstet Gynecol 95:745, 2000

Guise J-M, Berlin M, McDonagh M, et al: Safety of vaginal birth after cesarean: A systematic review. Obstet Gynecol 103:420, 2004

Hamilton BE, Martin JA, Sutton PD: Births: Preliminary data for 2002. National Vital Statistics Reports, Vol 51, No. 11. Hyattsville, Md: National Center for Health Statistics, 2003

Hashima JN, Eden KB, Osterweil P, et al: Predicting vaginal birth after cesarean delivery: A review of prognostic factors and screening tools. Am J Obstet Gynecol 190:547, 2004

Hendler I, Gauthier RJ, Bujold E: The effects of prior vaginal delivery compared to prior VBAC on the outcomes of current trial of VBAC [abstract 384]. J Soc Gynecol Investig 11:202A, 2004

Hoskins IA, Gomez JL: Correlation between maximum cervical dilatation at cesarean delivery and subsequent vaginal birth after cesarean delivery. Obstet Gynecol 89:591, 1997

Impey L, O'Herlihy C: First delivery after cesarean delivery for strictly defined cephalopelvic disproportion. Obstet Gynecol 92:799, 1998

Kieser KE, Baskett TF: A 10-year population-based study of uterine rupture. Obstet Gynecol 100:749, 2002

Landon MB, Hauth JC, Leveno KJ, et al: Maternal and perinatal outcomes associated with a trial of labor after prior cesarean delivery. N Engl J Med 351:25, 2004

Lavin JP, DiPasquale L, Crane S, et al: A state-wide assessment of the obstetric, anesthesia, and operative team personnel who are available to manage the labors and deliveries and to treat the complications of women who attempt vaginal birth after cesarean delivery. Am J Obstet Gynecol 187:611, 2002

Leveno KJ: Controversies in OB-Gyn: Should we rethink the criteria for VBAC? Contemp Ob/Gyn, January 1999

Lydon-Rochelle M, Holt VL, Easterling TR, et al: Risk of uterine rupture during labor among women with a prior cesarean delivery. N Engl J Med 345:3, 2001

Martin JN, Perry KG, Roberts WE, et al: The care for trial of labor in the patients with a prior low-segment vertical cesarean incision. Am J Obstet Gynecol 177:144, 1997

McMahon MJ, Luther ER, Bowes WA Jr, et al: Comparison of a trial of labor with an elective second cesarean section. N Engl J Med 335:689, 1996

Merrill BS, Gibbs CE: Planned vaginal delivery following cesarean section. Obstet Gynecol 52:50, 1978

Miller DA, Diaz FG, Paul RH: Vaginal birth after cesarean: A 10-year experience. Obstet Gynecol 84:255, 1994

Miller DA, Goodwin TM, Gherman RB, et al: Intrapartum rupture of the unscarred uterus. Obstet Gynecol 89:671, 1997

Mozurkewich EL, Hutton EK: Elective repeat cesarean delivery versus trial of labor: A meta-analysis of the literature from 1989 to 1999. Am J Obstet Gynecol 183:1187, 2000

Pitkin RM: Once a cesarean? Obstet Gynecol 77:939, 1991

Porter TF, Clark SL, Esplin MS, et al: Timing of delivery and neonatal outcomes in patients with clinically overt uterine rupture during VBAC [abstract 73]. Am J Obstet Gynecol 178:S31, 1998

Ravasia DJ, Brain PH, Pollard JK: Incidence of uterine rupture among women with mullerian duct anomalies who attempt vaginal birth after cesarean delivery. Am J Obstet Gynecol 181:877, 1999

Ravasia DJ, Wood SL, Pollard JK: Uterine rupture during induced trial of labor among women with previous cesarean delivery. Am J Obstet Gynecol 183:1176, 2000

Reyes-Ceja L, Cabrera R, Insfran E, et al: Pregnancy following previous uterine rupture: Study of 19 patients. Obstet Gynecol 34:387, 1969

Ridgeway JJ, Weyrich DL, Benedetti TJ: Fetal heart rate changes associated with uterine rupture. Obstet Gynecol 103:506, 2004

Ritchie EH: Pregnancy after rupture of the pregnant uterus: A report of 36 pregnancies and a study of cases reported since 1932. J Obstet Gynaecol Br Commonw 78:642, 1971

Rodriguez MH, Masaki DI, Phelan JP, et al: Uterine rupture: Are intrauterine pressure catheters useful in the diagnosis? Am J Obstet Gynecol 161:666, 1989

Schwarz O, Paddock R, Bortnick AR: The cesarean scar: An experimental study. Am J Obstet Gynecol 36:962, 1938

Sciscione AC, Nguyen L, Manley JS, et al: Uterine rupture during preinduction cervical ripening with misoprostol in a patient with a previous cesarean delivery. Aust N Z J Obstet Gynecol 38:96, 1998

Scott JR: Mandatory trial of labor after cesarean delivery: An alternative viewpoint. Obstet Gynecol 77:811, 1991

Sheth SS: Results of treatment of rupture of the uterus by suturing. J Obstet Gynaecol Br Commonw 75:55, 1968

Shipp TD, Zelop CM, Repke JT, et al: Interdelivery interval and risk of symptomatic uterine rupture. Obstet Gynecol 97:175, 2001

Shipp TD, Zelop CM, Repke JT, et al: Intrapartum uterine rupture and dehiscence in patients with prior lower uterine segment vertical and transverse incisions. Obstet Gynecol 94:735, 1999

Smith GC, Pell JP, Cameron AD, et al: Risk of perinatal death associated with labor after previous cesarean delivery in uncomplicated term pregnancies. JAMA 287:2684, 2002

Socol ML, Peaceman AM: Vaginal birth after cesarean: An appraisal of fetal risk. Obstet Gynecol 93:674, 1999

Stovall TG, Shaver DC, Soloman SK, et al: Trial of labor in previous cesarean section patients, excluding classical cesarean sections. Obstet Gynecol 70:713, 1987

Tucker JM, Hauth JC, Hodgkins P, et al: Trial of labor after a one- or two-layer closure of a low transverse uterine incision. Am J Obstet Gynecol 168:545, 1993

Turner MJ: Delivery after one previous cesarean section. Am J Obstet Gynecol 176:741, 1997

Vidaeff AC, Lucas MJ: Impact of single- or double-layer closure on uterine rupture [letter]. Am J Obstet Gynecol 188:602, 2003

Williams JW: A critical analysis of 21 years' experience with cesarean section. Bull Johns Hopkins Hosp 32:173, 1921

Williams JW: Obstetrics: A Text-book for the Use of Students and Practitioners, 4th ed. New York, Appleton, 1917

Wing DA, Lovett K, Paul RH: Disruption of prior uterine incision following misoprostol for labor induction in women with previous cesarean delivery. Obstet Gynecol 91:828, 1998

Wing DA, Paul RH: Vaginal birth after cesarean section: Selection and management. Clin Obstet Gynecol 42:836, 1999

Zelop CM, Shipp TD, Repke JT, et al: Effect of previous vaginal delivery on the risk of uterine rupture during a subsequent trial of labor. Am J Obstet Gynecol 183:1184, 2000

Zelop CM, Shipp TD, Repke JT, et al: Outcomes of trial of labor following previous cesarean delivery among women with fetuses weighing > 4000 g. Am J Obstet Gynecol 185:903, 2001

Zelop CM, Shipp TD, Repke JT, et al: Uterine rupture during induced or augmented labor in gravid women with one prior cesarean delivery. Am J Obstet Gynecol 181:882, 1999

27

Abnormalities of the Placenta, Umbilical Cord, and Membranes

With the basic understanding of the process of implantation and placental development presented in Chapter 3 (see p. 51), it is much easier to visualize the development of abnormal placental types. Much of the ever-growing knowledge of primary placental pathology was stimulated by a nucleus of placental pathologists that includes, amongst others, Benirschke, Driscoll, Fox, Naeye, and Salafia. For a detailed account of these disorders, the reader is referred to the Fourth Edition of *Pathology of the Human Placenta* (Benirschke and Kaufmann, 2000).

PLACENTAL ABNORMALITIES

In general, placental and fetal size and weight roughly correlate in a linear fashion. There is also evidence that fetal growth depends on placental weight, which is less with small-for-gestational age infants (Heinonen and colleagues, 2001). According to Mathews and associates (2004), this is not dependent on nutrients (see Chap. 38, p. 895).

ABNORMAL SHAPE OR IMPLANTATION. There are a number of variations of placental shape or implantation, and some have significant clinical impact.

Multiple Placentas with a Single Fetus. The placenta occasionally is separated into lobes. When the division is incomplete and the vessels of fetal origin extend from one lobe to the other before uniting to form the umbilical cord, the condition is termed *placenta bipartita* or *bilobata* (Fig. 27–1). Fox (1978) cited its incidence to be at about 1 in every 350 deliveries. If the two or three distinct lobes are separated entirely, and the vessels remain distinct, the condition is designated *placenta duplex* or *placenta triplex.*

Succenturiate Lobes. This variation describes one or more small accessory lobes that develop in the membranes at a distance from the periphery of the main placenta, to which they usually have vascular connections of fetal origin. It is a smaller version of the bilobed placenta, and although its incidence has been cited by Benirschke and Kaufmann (2000) to be as high as 5 percent, we have encountered these very infrequently. The accessory lobe may sometimes be retained in the uterus after delivery and may cause serious hemorrhage. In some cases, an accompanying vasa previa may cause dangerous fetal hemorrhage at delivery (see p. 627 and also Chap. 35, p. 819).

Membranaceous Placenta. Very rarely, all of the fetal membranes are covered by functioning villi, and the placenta develops as a thin membranous structure occupying the entire periphery of the chorion. This finding is called *placenta membranacea* and also is referred to as *placenta diffusa.* Diagnosis often can be made using sonography. It may occasionally give rise to serious hemorrhage because of associated placenta previa or accreta.

Ring-Shaped Placenta. In fewer than 1 in 6000 deliveries, the placenta is annular in shape, and sometimes a complete ring of placental tissue is present. This development may be a variant of membranaceous placenta. Because of tissue atrophy in a portion of the ring, a horseshoe shape is more common. These abnormalities appear to be associated with a greater likelihood of antepartum and postpartum bleeding and fetal growth restriction.

Fenestrated Placenta. In this rare anomaly, the central portion of a discoidal placenta is missing. In some instances, there is an actual hole in the placenta, but more often the defect involves only villous tissue with the chorionic plate

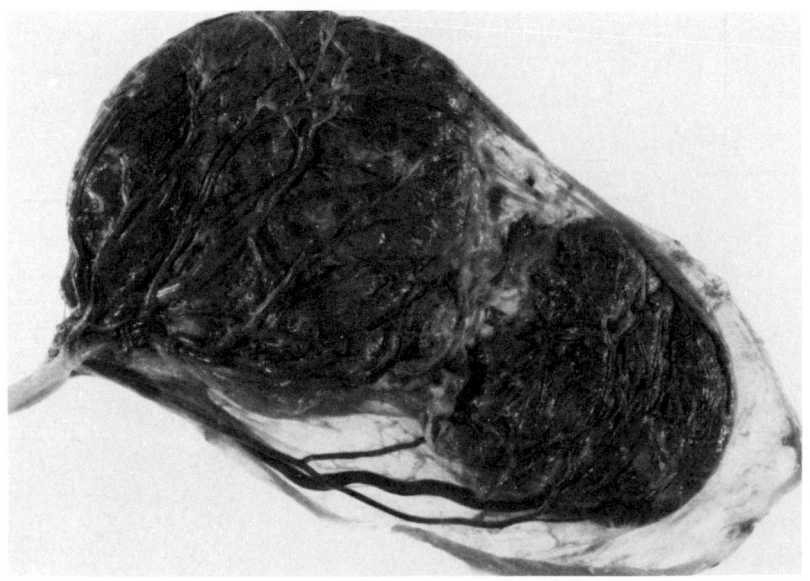

FIGURE 27–1. Bilobed placenta with marginal insertion of the umbilical cord. There also is partial velamentous insertion of the cord with the fetal vessels traversing the membranes to reach the smaller placental lobe on the right.

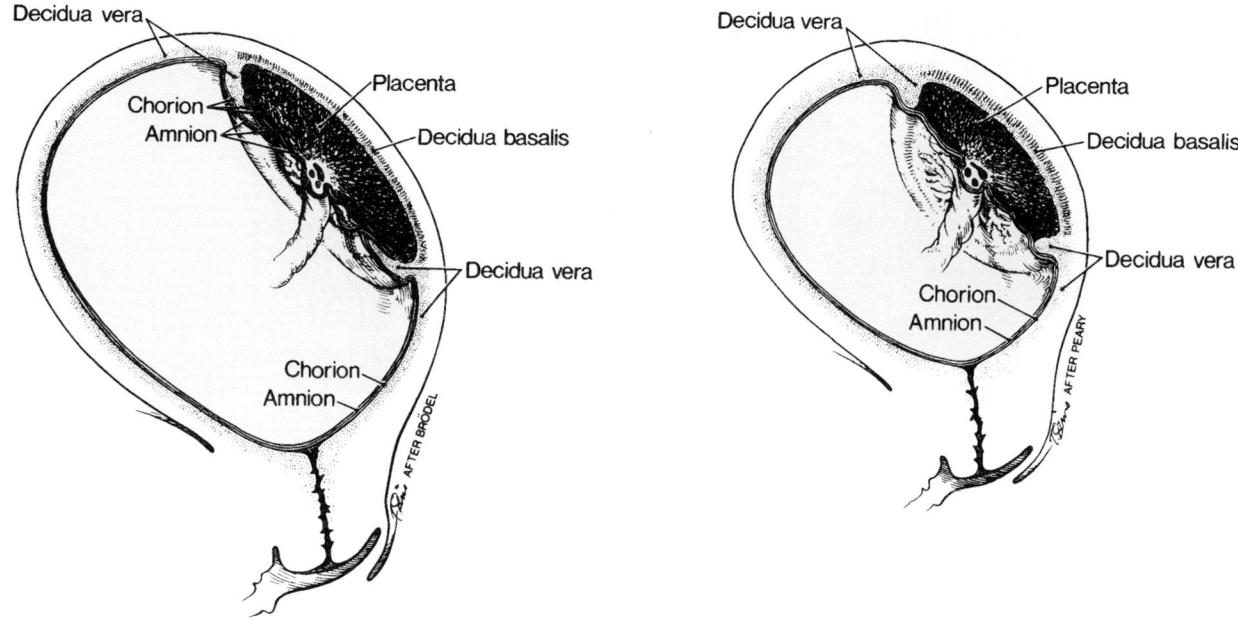

FIGURE 27–2. Circumvallate (*left*) and circummarginate (*right*) varieties of extrachorial placentas.

intact. Clinically, it may be mistakenly considered to indicate that a missing portion of placenta has been retained in the uterus.

Extrachorial Placentation. When the chorionic plate, which is on the fetal side of the placenta, is smaller than the basal plate, which is located on the maternal side, the placental periphery is uncovered and leads to the common designation of *extrachorial placenta* (Fig. 27–2). If the fetal surface of such a placenta presents a central depression surrounded by a thickened, grayish-white ring, it is called a *circumvallate placenta.* The ring is composed of a double fold of amnion and chorion, with degenerated decidua and fibrin in between. Within the ring, the fetal surface presents the usual appearance, except that the large vessels terminate abruptly at the margin of the ring. When the ring does not have the central depression with the fold of membranes, the condition is described as a *circummarginate placenta* (see Fig. 27–2). There is an increased risk with circumvallate placentas of antepartum hemorrhage—both from placental abruption and from fetal hemorrhage—as well as of preterm delivery, perinatal mortality, and fetal malformations (Benirschke, 1974; Lademacher and co-workers, 1981). Adverse clinical outcomes with circummarginate placentas are less well defined.

Placenta Accreta, Increta, and Percreta. These abnormalities are serious variations in which trophoblastic tissues invade the myometrium to varying depths. They are much more likely with placenta previa or with implantation over a prior uterine incision or perforation. Torrential hemorrhage is a frequent complication (see Chap. 25, p. 599, and Chap. 35, p. 830).

DEGENERATIVE PLACENTAL LESIONS. Degenerative lesions may result from trophoblast aging, or impairment of uteroplacental circulation with infarction. Deposition of calcium salts is heaviest on the maternal surface in the basal plate. Further deposition occurs along the septa, and both increase as pregnancy progresses. It is more extensive in smokers whose placentas also have reduced fetal capillary diameters (Larsen and co-workers, 2002). Extensive calcification is found in 10 to 15 percent of all placentas at term (Fig. 27–3). This can be seen with sonography, and Spirt and colleagues (1982) reported that by 33 weeks more than half of placentas have some degree of calcification. It is difficult to correlate the degree of calcium deposition with pregnancy outcome (Benirschke and Kaufmann, 2000).

CIRCULATORY DISTURBANCES. Placental perfusion may be impaired by disruption of uterine vessels, placental vessels, or the intervillous space (Becroft and associates, 2004).

Placental Infarctions. These are the most common placental lesions, and their presence is a continuum from normal changes to extensive and pathological involvement. For example, Salafia and associates (2000) identified infarcts in 10 percent of 500 consecutive placentas from uncomplicated term pregnancies. Almost 90 percent were located at the placental margin and 90 percent were less than 1 cm. These types of limited infarctions result from occlusion of the maternal uteroplacental circulation and usually represent normal aging. Around the edge of nearly every term placenta there is a dense yellowish-white fibrous ring representing a zone of degeneration and necrosis, which is an incidental finding.

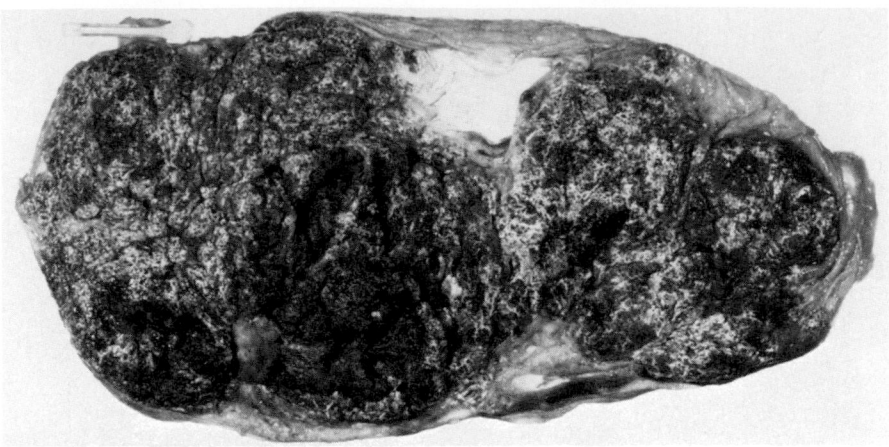

A

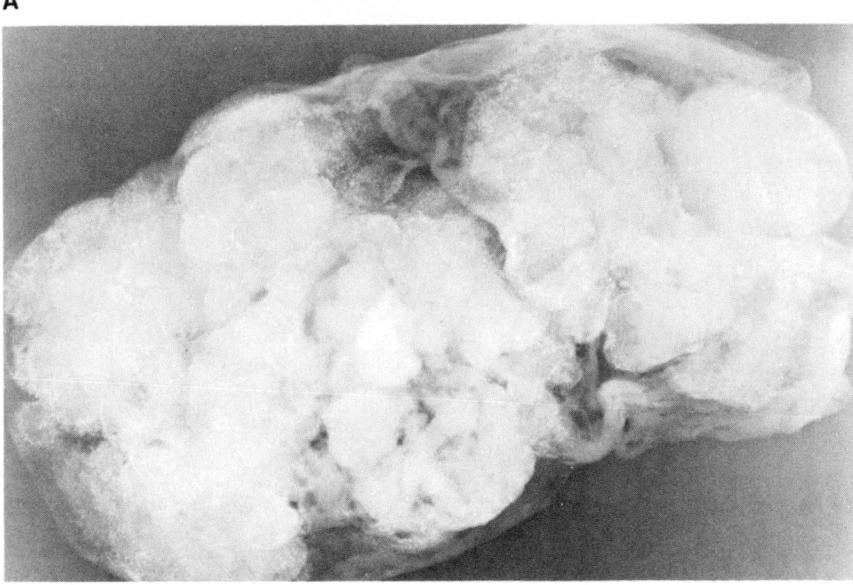

B

FIGURE 27–3. A. Placental calcification is evident as gray plaques on the maternal surface of the placenta. **B.** A radiograph of the same placenta emphasizes the extensive calcification.

Thus, although these infarcts are "normal," if they are numerous, placental insufficiency may develop. When they are thick, centrally located, and randomly distributed, as shown in Figure 27–4, they may be associated with preeclampsia or lupus anticoagulant (Benirschke and Kaufmann, 2000; Many and colleagues, 2001). These conspicuous lesions arise after occlusion of the decidual artery interrupts blood flow to the intervillous space. Necrosis of villous tissue develops from ischemia. Histopathological features include fibrinoid degeneration of the trophoblast, calcification, and ischemic infarction. If decidual artery occlusion is followed by hemorrhage, then *placental abruption* results.

Another type of infarct is found underneath the chorionic plate. These yellowish-white fibrous lesions are usually pyramidal shaped and range from 2 mm to 3 cm across the base. These *subchorionic infarcts* extend downward with their apices in the intervillous space. Similar lesions may be noted about the intercotyledonary septa. Occasionally these lesions meet and form a column of cartilage-like material extending from the maternal surface to the fetal surface. Less frequently, round or oval islands of similar tissue occupy the central portions of the placenta.

Maternal Floor Infarction. This uteroplacental vasculopathy differs from the previously described infarctions in that there are not large areas of villous infarction. Instead, fibrinoid deposition occurs within the decidua basalis and usually is confined to the placental floor. The fibrin, however, can extend into the intervillous space to envelop the villi, which then atrophy. According to Benirschke and Kaufmann (2000), and as shown in Figure 27–5, there frequently is massive net-like fibrin deposition throughout the placenta. It is an uncommon lesion, and Adams-Chapman and colleagues (2002) identified it in 6 per 1000 deliveries. The etiopathogenesis of these lesions is not well defined, although in some cases it is associated with thrombophilia (Katz, 2002; Sebire, 2002, 2003; van der Molen, 2000; Ward, 2000, and all their colleagues). These lesions are considered in further detail in Chapter 47 (see p. 1074).

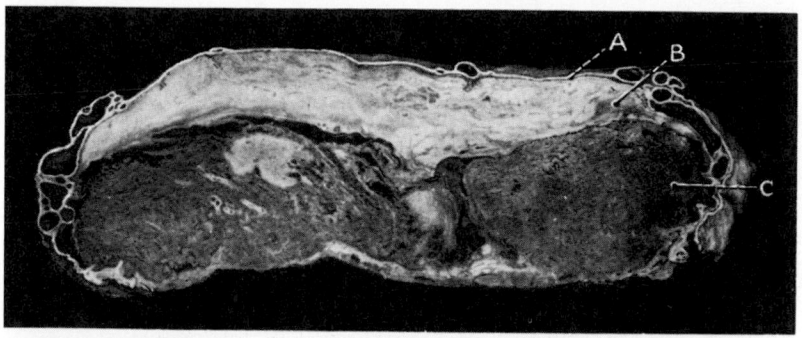

A

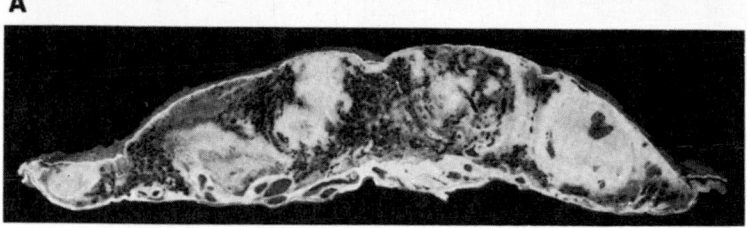

B

FIGURE 27–4. **A.** Placental infarcts. (A = chorioamnionic membrane; B = fibrin deposited locally beneath the chorion; C = normal placental tissue.) In this instance, the infarct was unusually extensive and most likely contributed to fetal death. **B.** Generalized fibrin deposition with little normal tissue remaining.

There is no doubt that maternal floor infarction is associated with fetal growth restriction, abortion, and stillbirths. It is not associated with preeclampsia or placental abruption. There also appears to be an increased incidence of central nervous system injury and neurodevelopmental sequelae in these infants (Adams-Chapman and associates, 2002).

Placental Vessel Thrombosis. When a stem artery from the fetal circulation in the placenta is occluded, it produces a sharply demarcated area of avascularity. Fox (1978) found such single-artery thrombosis in 5 percent of placentas from normal pregnancies and in 10 percent of those from diabetic women. He estimated that thrombosis of a single stem artery will deprive only 5 percent of the villi of their blood supply. Despite this, Benirschke and Kaufmann (2000) found these lesions to be frequently associated with fetal growth restriction and stillbirth.

HYPERTROPHIC LESIONS OF THE CHORIONIC VILLI. Striking enlargement of the chorionic villi is commonly seen in association with severe erythroblastosis and fetal hydrops. It also has been described in maternal diabetes, fetal congestive heart failure, and maternal–fetal syphilis (Sheffield and colleagues, 2002). Many of these conditions are discussed in Chapter 29.

MICROSCOPIC PLACENTAL ABNORMALITIES. Beginning after 32 weeks, clumps of syncytial nuclei are found to project into the intervillous space. These projections are called *syncytial knots* and likely represent apoptosis, although some are artifacts of tangential sectioning of villi (Benirschke and Kaufmann, 2000). The number of *cytotrophoblastic* cells becomes progressively reduced as pregnancy advances. By term, such cells are few and inconspicuous. In some maternal or fetal disorders, numerous cytotrophoblastic cells are found in placentas. Some examples include gestational hypertension, diabetes, and erythroblastosis fetalis.

PLACENTAL INFLAMMATION. Changes that are now recognized as various forms of degeneration and necrosis were formerly described under the term *placentitis.* For example, small placental cysts with grumous contents were formerly thought to be abscesses. Nonetheless, especially in cases of preterm and prolonged membrane rupture, bacteria invade the fetal surface of the placenta. This occurrence is discussed in the section on chorioamnionitis (see p. 625).

TUMORS OF THE PLACENTA

Gestational Trophoblastic Disease. These pregnancy-related trophoblastic proliferative abnormalities are discussed in Chapter 11.

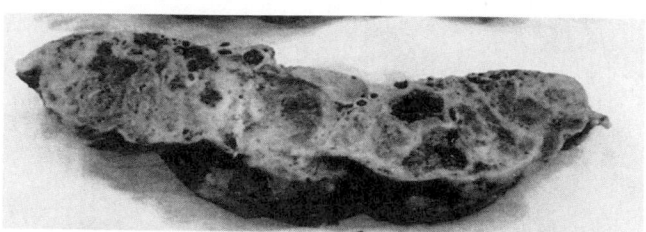

FIGURE 27–5. Section through a 32-week placenta showing maternal floor infarction associated with antiphospholipid antibody syndrome. There is marked thickening of the basal plate, fibrous septa, and massive perivillous fibrin deposition. (From Sebire and colleagues, 2002, with permission.)

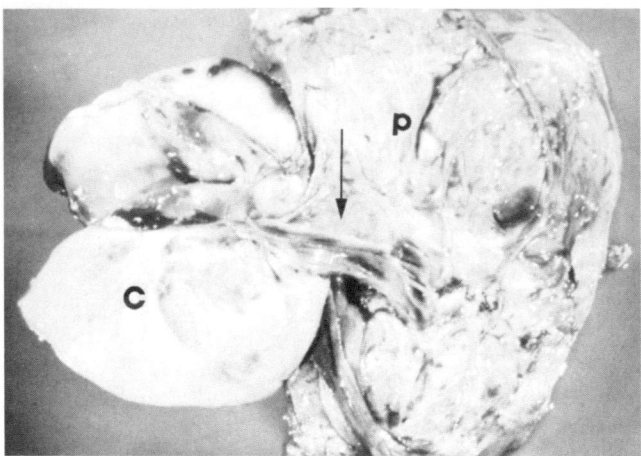

FIGURE 27–6. Placenta (p) and a discrete 450-g chorioangioma (c) connected to the placenta by a vascular stalk (*arrow*). The 34-week fetus was identified by sonography to have marked hydrothorax. Demonstrated in cord blood were severe hypofibrinogenemia, thrombocytopenia, hypoprothrombinemia, and microangiopathic hemolysis. The infant had cardiomegaly, heart failure, pleural effusion, and hepatomegaly. After several cardiac arrests the infant succumbed 3 days after birth.

Chorioangioma (Hemangioma). Various angiomatous tumors ranging widely in size have been described. Because of the resemblance of their components to the blood vessels and stroma of the chorionic villus, the term *chorioangioma,* or *chorangioma,* has been considered the most appropriate designation. These are the only benign tumors of the placenta (Benirschke and Kaufmann, 2000). They most likely are hamartomas of primitive chorionic mesenchyme and have an incidence of about 1 percent. Larger chorioangiomas, such as those shown in Figure 27–6, may be suspected on the basis of certain sonographic findings.

Small growths are usually asymptomatic, but large tumors may be associated with hydramnios or antepartum hemorrhage. Fetal death and malformations are uncommon complications, although there may be a correlation with low birthweight. Stiller and Skafish (1986) described a case with multiple placental chorioangiomas in which a blood group A fetus bled acutely into her O group mother. The mother showed evidence of acute hemolysis without anemia, and the fetus developed a sinusoidal heart rate pattern frequently seen with severe anemia. We have identified an unusual case of severe iron deficiency anemia in the neonate as the consequence of chronic fetal-to-maternal bleeding from multiple small chorioangiomas. Large tumors provide an arteriovenous shunt that can lead to fetal heart failure.

Tumors Metastatic to the Placenta. Malignant tumors rarely metastasize to the placenta. Of those that do, melanoma accounts for nearly one third of reported cases, and leukemias and lymphomas comprise another third (Dildy and associates, 1989; Read and Platzer, 1981). Tumor cells usually are confined within the intervillous space. In a fourth, the

fetus will have metastases. Even so, malignant cells seldom proliferate to cause clinical disease (Altman and associates, 2003; Baergen and colleagues, 1997b).

Embolic Fetal Brain Tissue. Fetal brain tissue occasionally is seen embolized to the placenta or fetal lungs (Baergen and associates, 1997a; Gardiner, 1956). It usually has been described with "traumatic" deliveries. This phenomenon is not without precedent because brain tissue has been found in pulmonary veins following head trauma in older children and adults.

ABNORMALITIES OF THE MEMBRANES

MECONIUM STAINING. The presence of meconium in amnionic fluid is relatively common—it was identified in 12 percent of more than 175,000 liveborn infants by Wiswell and Bent (1993). Benirschke and Kaufmann (2000) described visible meconium-stained placentas in 18 percent of nearly 13,000 consecutive deliveries. The incidence of meconium staining at Parkland Hospital has been remarkably constant, and of almost 250,000 women delivered during the past 20 years, about 20 percent had meconium identified during labor or at delivery. From their review, Ghidini and Spong (2001) cited meconium staining in a median of 14 percent of pregnancies.

Preterm fetuses seldom pass meconium. It is uncommon prior to 38 weeks, after which it increases to 25 to 30 percent after 42 weeks (Table 27–1). Staining of the amnion can be obvious within 1 to 3 hours after meconium passage (Miller and colleagues, 1985). Although more prolonged exposure results in staining of the chorion, umbilical cord, and decidua,

TABLE 27–1 Cumulative Meconium Passage by Gestational Age

Study	Meconium Passage (%)
Eden and associates (1987)	
39 weeks	14
40 weeks	19
42 weeks	26
> 42 weeks	29
Usher and colleagues (1988)	
39–40 weeks	15
41 weeks	27
42 weeks or greater	32
Steer and co-workers (1989)	
< 36 weeks	3
36–39 weeks	13
40–41 weeks	19
42 weeks or greater	23

From Katz and Bowes (1992), with permission.

according to Benirschke and Kaufmann (2000), meconium passage cannot be timed or dated accurately.

In its global sense, meconium passage is associated with increased perinatal morbidity and mortality. Fujikura and Klionsky (1975) identified meconium-stained membranes or fetuses in about 10 percent of 43,000 liveborn infants in the Collaborative Study of Cerebral Palsy. The neonatal mortality rate was 3.3 percent in the group with meconium-stained membranes compared with 1.7 percent in those without such staining. Nathan and co-workers (1994) reviewed perinatal outcomes at Parkland Hospital in more than 8000 women delivered in whom meconium was identified intrapartum. Outcomes were compared with those of more than 34,500 pregnancies with clear amnionic fluid. Perinatal mortality was increased significantly in the meconium group: 1.5 versus 0.3 per 1000. Severe fetal acidemia—cord arterial pH less than 7.0—was significantly more common with meconium-stained fluid: 7 versus 3 per 1000. Moreover, cesarean delivery was doubled in the meconium group: 14 versus 7 percent. These global findings are not applicable to individual cases, but despite this, meconium has assumed great importance in many medicolegal pursuits. Benirschke and Kaufmann (2000) aptly conclude that the legal profession overemphasizes the importance of meconium passage without appreciating its complexity.

Neonatal morbidity and mortality associated with meconium is characterized by the *meconium aspiration syndrome*, which develops in about 10 percent of exposed infants (Ghidini and Spong, 2001). Severe disease requires ventilatory assistance and has a mortality rate of about 10 percent. Although it is commonly held that meconium aspiration syndrome is primarily the result of aspiration of thick, tenacious meconium, Ghidini and Spong (2001) concluded from their review that thin meconium also was associated with respiratory insufficiency.

One serious maternal risk is that meconium associated with amnionic fluid embolism greatly increases maternal mortality from cardiorespiratory failure and consumptive coagulopathy (see Chap. 35, p. 845). Jazayeri and colleagues (2002) also have shown a fourfold risk of puerperal metritis with meconium-stained amnionic fluid.

CHORIOAMNIONITIS. Inflammation of the fetal membranes usually is a manifestation of intrauterine infection. It frequently is associated with prolonged membrane rupture and long labor. Grossly, infection is characterized by clouding of the membranes as shown in Figure 27–7. There also may be a foul odor, depending on bacterial species and concentration. When mono- and polymorphonuclear leukocytes infiltrate the chorion, the resulting microscopical finding is designated *chorioamnionitis*. These cells are maternal in origin. Conversely, if leukocytes are found in amnionic fluid (*amnionitis*), or the umbilical cord (*funisitis*), the cells are fetal in origin (Goldenberg and co-workers, 2000). Before 20 weeks, almost all polymorphonuclear leukocytes are

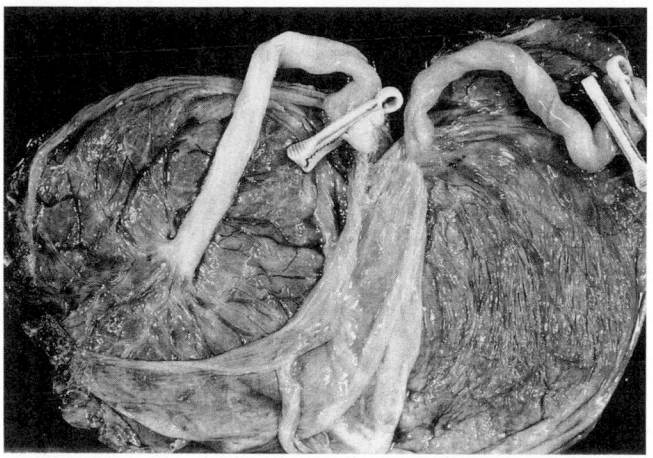

FIGURE 27–7. Chorioamnionitis in a diamnionic dichorionic placenta. Placenta from Twin A on the left was located near the fundus and has a normal luster. Placenta from Twin B has indistinct features caused by clouding of the membranes due to inflammatory exudate. (From Benirschke and Kaufmann, 2000, with permission.)

maternal in origin, but later the inflammatory response is both maternal and fetal (Sampson and colleagues, 1997). Microscopic evidence for inflammation of these structures is much more common in preterm deliveries.

According to some investigators, these findings of inflammation may be nonspecific and are not always associated with other evidence of fetal or maternal infection. For example, Yamada and colleagues (2000) found that meconium-stained fluid is a chemoattractant for leukocytes. Conversely, Benirschke and Kaufmann (2000) believe that microscopic chorioamnionitis is always due to infection.

Management of overt clinical chorioamnionitis is antimicrobial administration and expedient delivery (see Chap. 36, p. 866). Occult chorioamnionitis, caused by a wide variety of microorganisms, frequently is cited as a possible explanation for many otherwise unexplained cases of ruptured membranes, preterm labor, or both. Often, however, it is impossible to verify which occurred first (see Chap. 6, p. 178, and Chap. 36, p. 859).

OTHER ABNORMALITIES. Small *amnionic cysts* lined by typical amnionic epithelium occasionally are formed. The common variety results from fusion of amnionic folds, with subsequent fluid retention.

Amnion nodosum are tiny, light tan, creamy nodules in the amnion made up of vernix caseosa with hair, degenerated squames, and sebum. They result from oligohydramnios and are most commonly found in fetuses with renal agenesis, prolonged preterm ruptured membranes, or in the placenta of the donor fetus with twin-to-twin transfusion syndrome (Benirschke and Kaufmann, 2000).

Amnionic bands are caused when disruption of the amnion leads to formation of bands or strings that entrap the fetus and impair growth and development of the involved structure. Fetal conditions that appear to be the consequence of this phenomenon, including intrauterine amputations, are considered in Chapter 29 (see p. 685).

UMBILICAL CORD ABNORMALITIES

The cord develops in close association with the amnion, as described in Chapter 3 (see p. 68). The cord serves a vital function, but it unfortunately is susceptible to entanglement, compression, and occlusion. Collins and Collins (2000) reported a 1-percent incidence of potentially harmful cord complications.

LENGTH. Cord length at term has appreciable variation, and extremes range from no cord (achordia) to lengths up to 300 cm. Short umbilical cords may be associated with adverse perinatal outcomes such as fetal growth restriction, congenital malformations, intrapartum distress, and a twofold risk of death (Krakowiak and associates, 2004). Excessively long cords are more likely to cause complications such as prolapse. In a study of more than 20,000 placentas, Baergen and colleagues (2001) reported a mean length of 37 cm. They defined excessively long cords to be more than two standard deviations, which was 70 cm or longer. In a retrospective analysis, they compared 926 fetuses with long cords with 200 controls who had normal-length cords. Pregnancies involving a fetus with a long cord were associated with maternal systemic disease and delivery complications. There were more cases of cord entanglement, fetal distress, fetal anomalies, and respiratory distress. Perinatal mortality was increased nearly threefold, albeit with borderline statistical significance.

Determinants of cord length are intriguing. Animal studies and observational studies in human pregnancy support the concept that cord length is influenced positively by both the volume of amnionic fluid and fetal mobility. Heredity is a factor, and 9 percent of women with an excessively long cord in the study by Baergen and colleagues (2001) had such a finding in a subsequent pregnancy. Miller and associates (1981) identified the cord to be shortened appreciably when there had been either chronic fetal constraint from oligohydramnios or decreased fetal movement, such as with Down syndrome or limb dysfunction.

CORD COILING. In most cases, the umbilical vessels course through the cord in a spiraled manner. Several authors have observed a significant increase in various adverse outcomes in fetuses with hypocoiled cords. Some of these are meconium staining, preterm birth, and fetal distress (Strong and colleagues, 1993, 1994). Shen-Schwarz and associates (1996) reported an association between "absent" cord twisting and marginal and velamentous cord insertion. Rana and associates (1995) found a higher incidence of preterm delivery and cocaine abuse in women with hypercoiled cords.

SINGLE UMBILICAL ARTERY. Identification of a *two-vessel cord* is an important observation. **About one fourth of all infants with only one umbilical artery have associated congenital anomalies.** In a review of nearly 350,000 deliveries, Heifetz (1984) found an incidence of a single artery to be 0.63 percent in liveborns, 1.92 percent in neonates with perinatal death, and 3 percent in twins. The incidence is increased considerably in women with diabetes, epilepsy, preeclampsia, antepartum hemorrhage, oligohydramnios, and hydramnios (Leung and Robson, 1989). Two-vessel cords were identified in 1.5 percent of 879 fetuses aborted spontaneously (Byrne and Blanc, 1985). Over half of these had serious malformations, most associated with chromosomal abnormalities.

In many cases, a single umbilical artery is detected by routine ultrasound screening. Hill and co-workers (2001) reported that the number of cord vessels could be quantified ultrasonically in almost 98 percent of cases studied between 17 and 36 weeks. The fetal prognosis depends on whether the two-vessel cord is associated with other abnormalities or whether it is an isolated finding. Coexistent fetal anomalies detected by ultrasound have been reported to be from 10 and 50 percent.

Perinatal prognosis is better when a two-vessel umbilical cord is an *isolated sonographic finding*. In one study, Parilla and colleagues (1995) reported no adverse outcomes in 50 such fetuses. In another report, Budorick and co-workers (2001) found no abnormal karyotypes and only one echocardiographic abnormality in 31 fetuses with a two-vessel cord as an isolated finding. Gossett and associates (2002) reported that 74 such fetuses all had normal echocardiography. Conversely, Catanzarite (1995) described 46 fetuses with this isolated ultrasonographic finding, two of whom had lethal chromosomal abnormalities and a third, a tracheoesophageal fistula.

When a two-vessel cord is a *nonisolated finding,* as many as half of fetuses are aneuploid (Budorick and associates, 2001). There are a number of associated anomalies, and Pavlopoulos and colleagues (1998) reported renal aplasia, limb-reduction defects, and atresia of hollow organs in such fetuses, suggesting a vascular etiology.

Goldkrand and colleagues (1999) performed Doppler velocimetry in 45 fetuses with a two-vessel cord and 124 normal controls. Although velocity indices were all in the normal range, beginning at 26 weeks they were lower in affected fetuses than in those fetuses with normal cords. These investigators later measured blood flow and found that the single artery had volumetric blood flow equal to a normal cord with two arteries (Goldkrand and associates, 2001). They concluded that growth restriction did not occur in anatomically normal fetuses with a single artery. Raio and colleagues (1999) reported an association between a single artery and a reduction of Wharton jelly.

FOUR-VESSEL CORD. Careful inspection may disclose a venous remnant in 5 percent of cases (Fox, 1978). The significance is unknown.

ABNORMALITIES OF CORD INSERTION. The umbilical cord usually is inserted at or near the center of the fetal surface of the placenta.

Furcate Insertion. In this rare anomaly, the umbilical vessels separate from the cord substance before their insertion into the placenta. Because vessels lose cushioning, they are prone to twisting and thrombosis.

Marginal Insertion. Cord insertion at the placental margin is sometimes referred to as a *Battledore placenta.* It is found in about 7 percent of term placentas (Benirschke and Kaufmann, 2000). With the exception of the cord being pulled off during delivery of the placenta, it is of little clinical significance.

Velamentous Insertion. This insertion is of considerable importance. The umbilical vessels separate in the membranes at a distance from the placental margin, which they reach surrounded only by a fold of amnion (Figs. 27–1 and 27–8). Benirschke and Kaufmann (2000) reviewed almost 195,000 deliveries and found an average incidence of 1.1 percent.

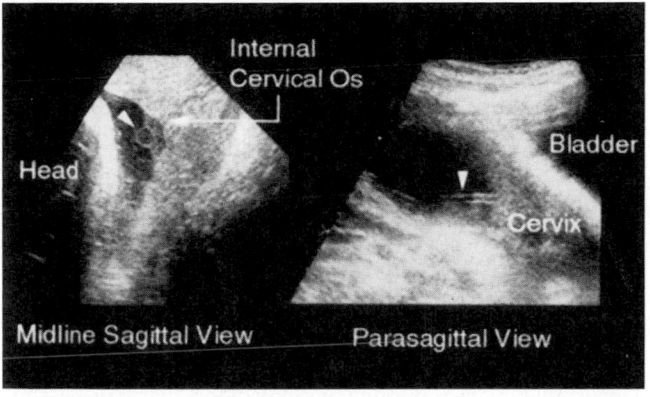

FIGURE 27–9. Grey-scale ultrasonographic scans showing vasa previa. The left figure is a midline sagittal view of the cervix, bladder, and fetal head at 34 weeks' gestation. The aberrant vessel is seen as an echogenic circular structure overlying the internal os. The right figure is a parasagittal view from another woman at 28 weeks. The aberrant vessel (*arrowhead*) is seen as a linear echogenic structure that courses along the amnion adjacent to the cervix. (From Lee and colleagues, 2000, with permission.)

Velamentous insertion occurs much more frequently with twins, and Feldman and associates (2002) identified it in 28 percent of triplets.

Vasa Previa. This finding is associated with velamentous insertion when some of the fetal vessels in the membranes cross the region of the cervical os below the presenting fetal part. Lee and co-workers (2000) attempted to view the internal cervical os with sonography in nearly 94,000 women studied in the second or third trimester. Vasa previa was identified in 18, for an incidence of 1 in about 5200 pregnancies. About half were associated with velamentous insertion and the rest divided between marginal cord insertions and bilobed or succenturiate-lobed placentas (Figs. 27–1 and 27–9). Occasionally, the examiner will be able to palpate or directly visualize a tubular fetal vessel in the membranes overlying the presenting part. Because of a low sensitivity for imaging vasa previa with ultrasound, color Doppler examination is recommended when these are suspected (Harris and Alexander, 2000; Lee and associates, 2000; Nomiyama and colleagues, 1998). In a study of 155 cases by Oyelese and associates (2004), prenatal diagnosis was associated with increased survival—97 versus 44 percent.

With vasa previa, there is considerable potential fetal danger because membrane rupture may be accompanied by tearing of a fetal vessel with exsanguination. In their review, Fung and Lau (1998) found that a low-lying placenta was a risk factor in 80 percent of cases. They also found that antenatal diagnosis was associated with decreased fetal mortality compared with discovery at delivery. Oyelese and colleagues (1999) recommended transvaginal ultrasound with color Doppler for women with risk factors. These included a bilobed, succenturiate, or low-lying placenta; multifetal pregnancy; or pregnancy resulting from in vitro fertilization.

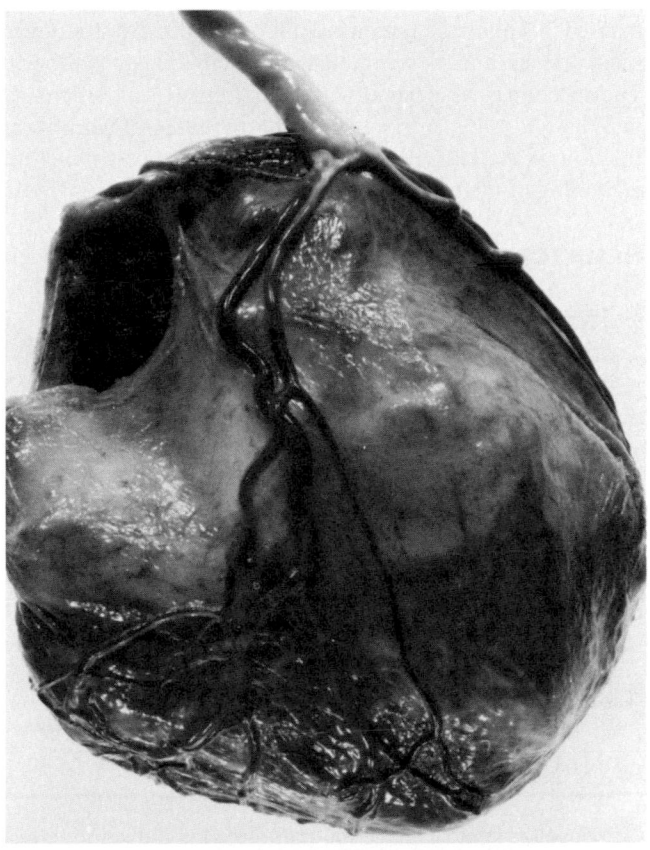

FIGURE 27–8. Velamentous insertion of the cord. The placenta and membranes have been inverted to expose the amnion. Part of the fetal surface of the placenta appears at the bottom of the photograph. Note the large fetal vessels extending from the cord insertion and within the membranes. Finally, note the proximity of the vessels to the site of membrane rupture.

In a prospective study of 45 women with a third-trimester placenta previa, Megier and colleagues (1999) found that 3 of 20 previas located over the internal os also had a vasa previa. In an 8-year survey of more than 90,000 women who had gray-scale ultrasonography, Lee and colleagues (2000) utilized endovaginal and Doppler studies to confirm vasa previa in women whose initial ultrasound showed an "echogenic parallel or circular line near the cervix" (see Fig. 27–9). They were able to detect vasa previa in asymptomatic women as early as the midtrimester.

Whenever there is hemorrhage antepartum or intrapartum, the possibility of vasa previa and a ruptured fetal vessel exists. Unfortunately, the amount of fetal blood that can be shed without killing the fetus is relatively small. Thus, in many cases, fetal death is virtually instantaneous. One approach to detecting fetal blood is to smear the blood on glass slides, stain the smears with Wright stain, and examine for nucleated red cells, which normally are present in cord blood but not maternal blood.

CORD ABNORMALITIES CAPABLE OF IMPEDING BLOOD FLOW.

Several mechanical and vascular abnormalities of the umbilical cord are capable of impairing fetal–placental blood flow.

Knots. *False knots,* which result from kinking of the vessels to accommodate to the length of the cord, should be distinguished from *true knots,* which result from active fetal movements. In nearly 17,000 deliveries in the Collaborative Study on Cerebral Palsy, Spellacy and co-workers (1966) found an incidence of true knots of 1.1 percent. The incidence is especially high in monoamnionic twins. Venous stasis may lead to mural thrombosis and fetal hypoxia, causing death or neurological morbidity. Collins and Collins (2000) estimate a 6 percent incidence of stillbirths when true knots are found.

Loops. The cord frequently becomes coiled around portions of the fetus, usually the neck. This is more likely with longer cords. Several large studies have reported one loop of nuchal cord in 20 to 34 percent of deliveries; two loops in 2.5 to 5 percent; and three loops in 0.2 to 0.5 percent (Kan and Eastman, 1957; Sornes, 1995; Spellacy and associates, 1966). Fortunately, coiling of the cord around the neck is an uncommon cause of antepartum fetal death or neurological damage (Clapp and colleagues, 2003; Nelson and Grether, 1998).

Such entwined cords, however, may cause intrapartum complications. As labor progresses and there is fetal descent, contractions may compress the cord vessels. This causes fetal heart rate decelerations that persist until the contraction ceases (see Chap. 18, p. 453). In labor, 20 percent of fetuses with a nuchal cord have moderate or severe variable heart rate decelerations, and they also are more likely to have a lower umbilical artery pH (Hankins and colleagues, 1987).

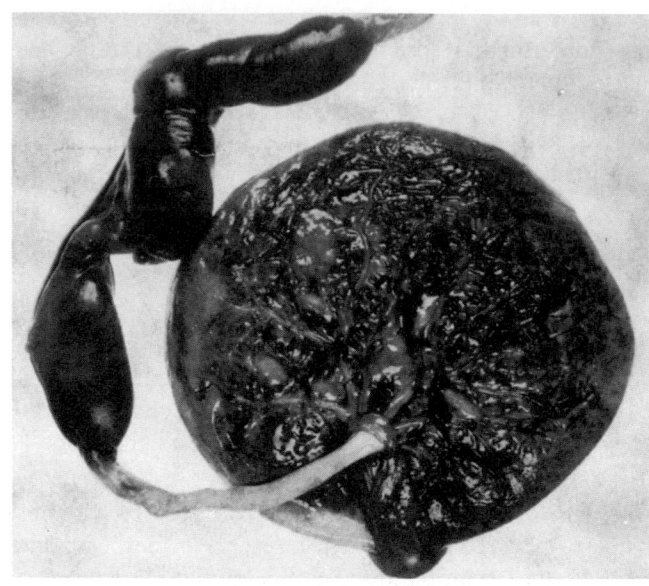

FIGURE 27–10. Hematoma of the umbilical cord.

TORSION AND STRICTURES.

Torsion of the cord is rare. It results from fetal movements during which the cord normally becomes twisted. Occasionally, the torsion is so marked that fetal circulation is compromised. Cord stricture is more serious, and most infants with this finding are stillborn. The stricture is associated with an extreme focal deficiency in Wharton jelly. In monoamnionic twinning, a significant fraction of the high perinatal mortality rate is attributed to entwining of the umbilical cords before labor.

HEMATOMA.

These accumulations of blood are associated with short cords, trauma, and entanglement (Benirschke and Kaufmann, 2000). They may result from the rupture of a varix, usually of the umbilical vein, with effusion of blood into the cord (Fig. 27–10). Hematomas also may be caused by umbilical vessel venipuncture.

CYSTS.

Cord cysts occasionally are found along the course of the cord and are designated true and false, according to their origin. True cysts are quite small and may be derived from remnants of the umbilical vesicle or the allantois. False cysts, which may attain considerable size, result from liquefaction of Wharton jelly. Such cysts that are detected by sonography are difficult to identify precisely.

PATHOLOGICAL EXAMINATION

The development of placental pathology as a discipline has renewed interest in placental examination. In many cases, expert evaluation will help to elucidate the etiopathogenesis of some perinatal outcomes. Although most authorities agree that routine placental examination by a pathologist is not indicated, there still is debate as to which placentas should be submitted. For example, the College of American Pathologists recommends routine examination for a comprehensive and imposing list of maternal, perinatal, and placental conditions (Langston and colleagues, 1997). Conversely, the American College of Obstetricians and Gynecologists (1993) concluded that there are insufficient data to support all of these recommendations. The major concerns are that pathological examination is costly and time consuming and would exhaust resources that could be better spent.

Certainly, all agree that the placenta and cord—including the number of vessels—should be examined grossly following all deliveries. The decision to request pathological examination will depend on clinical and placental findings. The possible correlation(s) of specific placental findings with both short- and long-term neonatal outcomes is unclear at this time.

Although it is our opinion that routine placental examination by a pathologist cannot be justified, there are some obstetrical and perinatal conditions in which placental findings are helpful. For example, when performed in conjunction with fetal autopsy, it may prove useful in determining the cause of stillbirth (see Chap. 29, p. 677). Porter (2000) recommends formal pathological placental examination in the following circumstances: (1) perinatal death, (2) preterm delivery, (3) fetal growth abnormalities, (4) fetal malformations, (5) hydrops, (6) any other fetal disorders, (7) multiple pregnancy, (8) maternal disorders, and (9) gross placental lesions. The protocol used at Parkland Hospital is that the placenta is sent for pathological examination whenever the neonatal resuscitation team is called. The placenta also is examined in all cases of stillborn infants or if there are obvious abnormalities. Thus, the indications are similar to those of Porter (2000). The specimen is accompanied by a completed data sheet with pertinent clinical information.

REFERENCES

Adams-Chapman I, Vaucher YE, Bejar RF, et al: Maternal floor infarction of the placenta: Association with central nervous system injury and adverse neurodevelopmental outcome. J Perinatol 22:236, 2002

Altman JF, Lowe L, Redman B, et al: Placental metastasis of maternal melanoma. J Am Acad Dermatol 49:1150, 2003

American College of Obstetricians and Gynecologists: Committee on Obstetrics: Maternal–Fetal Medicine. Placental Pathology No. 125, July 1993

Baergen RN, Castillo MM, Mario-Singh B, et al: Embolism of fetal brain tissue to the lungs and the placenta. Pediatr Pathol Lab Med 17:159, 1997a

Baergen RN, Johnson D, Moore T, et al: Maternal melanoma metastatic to the placenta. A case report and review of the literature. Arch Pathol Lab Med 121:508, 1997b

Baergen RN, Malicki D, Behling C, et al: Morbidity, mortality, and placental pathology in excessively long umbilical cords: Retrospective study. Pediatr Dev Pathol 4:144, 2001

Becroft DM, Thompson JM, Mitchell EA: Placental infarcts, intervillous fibrin plaques, and intervillous thrombi: Incidences, cooccurrences, and epidemiological associations. Pediatr Dev Pathol 7:26, 2004

Benirschke K: Disease of the placenta. In Gluck L (ed): Modern Perinatal Medicine. Chicago, Year Book, 1974, p 99

Benirschke K, Kaufmann P: Pathology of the Human Placenta, 4th ed. New York, Springer-Verlag, 2000

Budorick NE, Kelly TF, Dunn JA, et al: The single umbilical artery in a high-risk patient population: What should be offered? J Ultrasound Med 20:619, 2001

Byrne J, Blanc WA: Malformations and chromosome anomalies in spontaneously aborted fetuses with single umbilical artery. Am J Obstet Gynecol 151:340, 1985

Catanzarite VA: The clinical significance of a single umbilical artery as an isolated finding on prenatal ultrasound. Obstet Gynecol 86:155, 1995

Clapp JF III, Stepanchak W, Hashimoto K, et al: The natural history of antenatal nuchal cords. Am J Obstet Gynecol 189:488, 2003

Collins JH, Collins CL: The human umbilical cord. In Kingdom J, Jauniaux E, O'Brien S (eds): The Placenta: Basic Science and Clinical Practice. London, RCOG Press, 2000, p 319

Dildy GA III, Moise KJ Jr, Carpenter RJ Jr, et al: Maternal malignancy metastatic to the products of conception: A review. Obstet Gynecol Surv 44:535, 1989

Eden RD, Seifert LS, Winegar A, et al: Perinatal characteristics of uncomplicated postdate pregnancies. Obstet Gynecol 69:296, 1987

Feldman DM, Borgida AF, Trymbulak WP, et al: Clinical implications of velamentous cord insertion in triplet gestations. Am J Obstet Gynecol 186:809, 2002

Fox H: Pathology of the placenta. Monograph, Vol VII. Philadelphia, Saunders, 1978

Fujikura T, Klionsky B: The significance of meconium staining. Am J Obstet Gynecol 121:45, 1975

Fung TY, Lau TK: Poor perinatal outcome associated with vasa previa: Is it preventable? A report of three cases and review of the literature. Ultrasound Obstet Gynecol 12:430, 1998

Gardiner WR: Massive pulmonary embolization of cerebellar cortical tissue. An unusual fetal birth injury. Stanford Med Bull 14:226, 1956

Ghidini A, Spong CY: Severe meconium aspiration syndrome is not caused by aspiration of meconium. Am J Obstet Gynecol 185:931, 2001

Goldenberg RL, Hauth JC, Andrews WW: Intrauterine infection and preterm delivery. N Engl J Med 342:1500, 2000

Goldkrand JW, Lentz SU, Turner AD, et al: Doppler velocimetry in the fetus with a single umbilical artery. J Reprod Med 44:346, 1999

Goldkrand JW, Pettigrew C, Lentz SU, et al: Volumetric umbilical artery blood flow: Comparison of the normal versus the single umbilical artery cord. J Matern Fetal Med 10:116, 2001

Gossett DR, Lantz ME, Chisholm CA: Antenatal diagnosis of single umbilical artery: Is fetal echocardiography warranted? Obstet Gynecol 100:903, 2002

Hankins GD, Snyder RR, Hauth JC, et al: Nuchal cords and neonatal outcome. Obstet Gynecol 70:687, 1987

Harris RD, Alexander RD: Ultrasound of the placenta and umbilical cord. In Callen PW (ed): Ultrasonography in Obstetrics and Gynecology, 4th ed. Philadelphia, Saunders, 2000, p 611

Heifetz SA: Single umbilical artery: A statistical analysis of 237 autopsy cases and a review of the literature. Perspect Pediatr Pathol 8:345, 1984

Heinonen S, Taipale P, Saarikoski S: Weights of placentae from small-for-gestational age infants revisited. Placenta 22:299, 2001

Hill LM, Wibner D, Gonzales P, et al: Validity of transabdominal sonography in the detection of a two-vessel umbilical cord. Obstet Gynecol 98:837, 2001

Jazayeri A, Jazayeri MK, Sahinler M, et al: Is meconium passage a risk factor for maternal infection in term pregnancy? Obstet Gynecol 99:548, 2002

Kan PS, Eastman NJ: Coiling of the umbilical cord around the foetal neck. Br J Obstet Gynaecol 64:227, 1957

Katz VL, Bowes WA Jr: Meconium aspiration syndrome: Reflections on a murky subject. Am J Obstet Gynecol 166:171, 1992

Katz VL, DiTomasso J, Farmer R, et al: Activated protein C resistance associated with maternal floor infarction treated with low-molecular-weight heparin. Am J Perinatol 19:273, 2002

Krakowiak P, Smith EN, de Bruyn G, et al: Risk factors and outcomes associated with a short umbilical cord. Obstet Gynecol 103:119, 2004

Lademacher DS, Vermeulen RCW, Harten JJVD, et al: Circumvallate placenta and congenital malformation. Lancet 1:732, 1981

Langston C, Kaplan C, Macpherson T, et al: Practice guideline for examination of the placenta. Arch Pathol Lab Med 121:449, 1997

Larsen LG, Clausen HV, Jønsson L: Stereologic examination of placentas from mothers who smoke during pregnancy. Am J Obstet Gynecol 186:531, 2002

Lee W, Lee VL, Kirk JS, et al: Vasa previa: Prenatal diagnosis, natural evolution and clinical outcome. Obstet Gynecol 95:572, 2000

Leung AK, Robson WL: Single umbilical artery: A report of 159 cases. Am J Dis Child 143:108, 1989

Many A, Schreiber L, Rosner S, et al: Pathologic features of the placenta in women with severe pregnancy complications and thrombophilia. Obstet Gynecol 98:1041, 2001

Mathews F, Youngman L, Neil A: Maternal circulating nutrient concentrations in pregnancy: Implications for birth and placental weights of term infants. Am J Clin Nutr 79:103, 2004

Megier P, Gorin V, Desroches A: Ultrasonography of placenta previa at the third trimester of pregnancy: Research for signs of placenta accreta/percreta and vasa previa. Prospective color and pulsed Doppler ultrasonography study of 45 cases. J Gynecol Obstet Biol Reprod (Paris) 28:239, 1999

Miller ME, Higginbottom M, Smith DW: Short umbilical cord: Its origin and relevance. Pediatrics 67:618, 1981

Miller PW, Coen RW, Benirschke K: Dating the time interval from meconium passage to birth. Obstet Gynecol 66:459, 1985

Nathan L, Leveno KJ, Carmody TJ III, et al: Meconium: A 1990s perspective on an old obstetric hazard. Obstet Gynecol 83:329, 1994

Nelson KB, Grether JK: Potentially asphyxiating conditions and spastic cerebral palsy in infants of normal birth weight. Am J Obstet Gynecol 179:507, 1998

Nomiyama M, Toyota Y, Kawano H: Antenatal diagnosis of velamentous umbilical cord insertion and vasa previa with color Doppler imaging. Ultrasound Obstet Gynecol 12:426, 1998

Oyelese Y, Catanzarite V, Prefumo F, et al: Vasa previa: the impact of prenatal diagnosis on outcomes. Obstet Gynecol 103:937, 2004

Oyelese KO, Turner M, Lees C, et al: Vasa previa: An avoidable obstetric tragedy. Obstet Gynecol Surv 54:138, 1999

Parilla BV, Tamura RK, MacGregor SN, et al: The clinical significance of a single umbilical artery as an isolated finding on prenatal ultrasound. Obstet Gynecol 85:570, 1995

Pavlopoulos PM, Konstantinidou AE, Agapitos E, et al: Association of single umbilical artery with congenital malformations of vascular etiology. Pediatr Dev Pathol 1:487, 1998

Porter HJ: The role of placental examination as a perinatal investigation. In Kingdom J, Jauniaux E, O'Brien S (eds): The Placenta: Basic Science and Clinical Practice. London, RCOG Press, 2000, p 109

Raio L, Ghezzi F, Di Naro E, et al: Prenatal assessment of Wharton's jelly in umbilical cords with single artery. Ultrasound Obstet Gynecol 14:42, 1999

Rana J, Ebert GA, Kappy KA: Adverse perinatal outcome in patients with an abnormal umbilical coiling index. Obstet Gynecol 85:573, 1995

Read EJ Jr, Platzer PB: Placental metastasis from maternal carcinoma of the lung. Obstet Gynecol 58:387, 1981

Salafia CM, Thorp J, Starzyk KA: Placental pathology in spontaneous prematurity. In Kingdom J, Jauniaux E, O'Brien S (eds): The Placenta: Basic Science and Clinical Practice. London, RCOG Press, 2000, p 174

Sampson JE, Theve RP, Blatman RN, et al: Fetal origin of amniotic fluid polymorphonuclear leukocytes. Am J Obstet Gynecol 176:77, 1997

Sebire NJ, Backos M, El Gaddal S, et al: Placental pathology, antiphospholipid antibodies, and pregnancy outcome in recurrent miscarriage patients. Obstet Gynecol 101:258, 2003

Sebire NJ, Backos M, Goldin RD, et al: Placental massive perivillous fibrin deposition associated with antiphospholipid antibody syndrome. Br J Obstet Gynaecol 109:570, 2002

Sheffield JS, Sánchez PJ, Wendel GD Jr, et al: Placental histopathology of congenital syphilis. Obstet Gynecol 100:126, 2002

Shen-Schwarz S, King E, Benito C, et al: Umbilical cord twist: Relationship with placental gross morphology. Am J Obstet Gynecol 174:361, 1996

Sornes T: Umbilical cord encirclements and fetal growth restriction. Obstet Gynecol 86:725, 1995

Spellacy WN, Gravem H, Fisch RO: The umbilical cord complications of true knots, nuchal coils and cords around the body. Report from the collaborative study of cerebral palsy. Am J Obstet Gynecol 94:1136, 1966

Spirt BA, Cohen WN, Weinstein HM: The incidence of placental calcification in normal pregnancies. Radiology 142:707, 1982

Steer PJ, Eigbe F, Lissauer TJ, et al: Interrelationships among abnormal cardiocograms in labor, meconium staining of the amniotic fluid, arterial cord blood pH and Apgar scores. Obstet Gynecol 74:715, 1989

Stiller AG, Skafish PR: Placental chorioangioma: A rare cause of fetomaternal transfusion with maternal hemolysis and fetal distress. Obstet Gynecol 67:296, 1986

Strong TH Jr, Elliot JP, Radin TG: Noncoiled umbilical blood vessels: A new marker for the fetus at risk. Obstet Gynecol 81:409, 1993

Strong TH, Jarles DL, Vega JS, et al: The umbilical coiling index. Am J Obstet Gynecol 170:29, 1994

Usher RH, Boyd ME, McLean FH, et al: Assessment of fetal risk in postdate pregnancies. Am J Obstet Gynecol 158:259, 1988

van der Molen EF, Arends GE, Nelen WL, et al: A common mutation in the 5,10-methylenetetrahydrofolate reductase gene as a new risk factor for placental vasculopathy. Am J Obstet Gynecol 182:1258, 2000

Ward K: Inherited thrombophilias and placental thrombosis. In Kingdom J, Jauniaux E, O'Brien S (eds): The Placenta: Basic Science and Clinical Practice. London, RCOG Press, 2000, p 139

Wiswell TE, Bent RC: Meconium staining and the meconium aspiration syndrome. Pediatr Clin North Am 40:955, 1993

Yamada T, Minakami H, Matsubara S, et al: Meconium-stained amniotic fluid exhibits chemotactic activity for polymorphonuclear leukocytes in vitro. J Reprod Immunol 46:21, 2000

V

Fetus and Newborn

28

The Newborn Infant

At birth, the infant is subjected to rapid and profound physiological changes. Survival depends on a prompt and orderly conversion to air breathing. For efficient interchange of oxygen and carbon dioxide, the fluid-filled alveoli of the lungs must expand with air, the air must be exchanged by appropriate respiratory motion, and perfusion must be established.

INITIATION OF AIR BREATHING

STIMULI TO BREATHE AIR. The newborn begins to breathe and cry almost immediately after birth, indicating the establishment of active respiration. Factors that appear to influence the first breath of air include:

1. *Physical stimulation,* such as handling the infant during delivery.
2. *Deprivation of oxygen and accumulation of carbon dioxide,* which serve to increase the frequency and magnitude of breathing movements both before and after birth (Dawes, 1974).
3. *Compression of the thorax* during the second stage of labor and vaginal birth, which has been found to force an amount of fluid from the respiratory tract equivalent to about one fourth of the ultimate functional residual capacity (Saunders and Milner, 1978).

Aeration of the newborn lung is not the inflation of a collapsed structure, but instead, the rapid replacement of bronchial and alveolar fluid by air. After delivery, the residual alveolar fluid is cleared through the pulmonary circulation and, to a lesser degree, through the pulmonary lymphatics (Chernick, 1978). Delay in removal of fluid from the alveoli probably contributes to the syndrome of *transient tachypnea of the newborn.* As fluid is replaced by air, the compression of the pulmonary vasculature is reduced considerably and, in turn, resistance to blood flow is lowered. With the fall in pulmonary arterial blood pressure, the ductus arteriosus normally closes.

High negative intrathoracic pressures are required to bring about the initial entry of air into the fluid-filled alveoli. Normally, from the first breath after birth, progressively more residual air accumulates in the lung, and with each successive breath, lower pulmonary opening pressure is required. In the normal mature infant, by about the fifth breath, pressure-volume changes achieved with each respiration are very similar to those of the adult. Thus, the breathing pattern shifts to regular, deeper inhalations from the shallow episodic inspirations characteristic of the fetus and described in Chapter 15 (see p. 376). The presence of surfactant, synthesized by type II pneumocytes, lowers surface tension in the alveoli and thereby prevents the collapse of the lung with each expiration. Lack of sufficient surfactant, common in preterm infants, leads to the prompt development of *respiratory distress syndrome* (see Chap. 29, p. 650).

MANAGEMENT OF DELIVERY

IMMEDIATE CARE. Before and during delivery, careful considerations must be given to several determinants of neonatal well-being that include:

1. Health status of the mother.
2. Prenatal complications, including any suspected fetal malformations.
3. Labor complications.
4. Gestational age.
5. Duration of labor and ruptured membranes.
6. Types, amounts, times, and routes of administration of medications.
7. Type and duration of anesthesia.
8. Any difficulty with delivery.

With delivery of the head, either vaginally or by cesarean, the face should be wiped and the mouth and nares suctioned. A soft rubber syringe or its equivalent is quite suitable. The American Academy of Pediatrics and the American College of Obstetricians and Gynecologists (2002) recommend that at least one person whose primary responsibility is the neonate and who is capable of initiating resuscitation attend every delivery. Either that person or someone else who is immediately available should have the skills required to perform complete resuscitation.

NEWBORN RESUSCITATION. As many as 10 percent of newborn infants require some degree of active resuscitation to stimulate breathing (Kattwinkel, 2000). This is perhaps related to the observation that the risk of death for newborns delivered at home in Washington state between 1989 and 1996 was nearly twice that of those delivered in hospitals (Pang and co-workers, 2002). When deprived of oxygen, either before or after birth, infants demonstrate a well-defined sequence of events leading to apnea. As shown in Figure 28–1, oxygen deprivation results initially in a transient period of rapid breathing. If such deprivation persists, however,

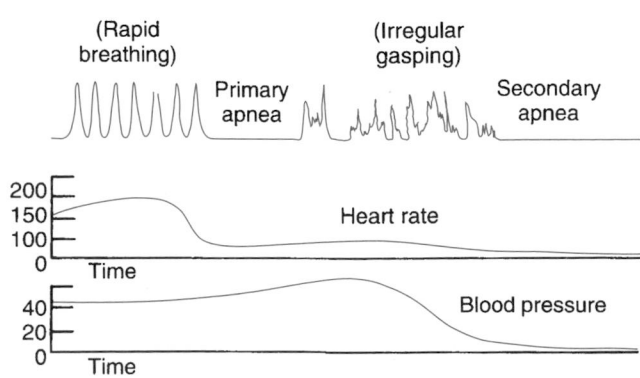

FIGURE 28–1. Physiological changes associated with primary and secondary apnea in the newborn. (Reproduced from Kattwinkel, 2000, with permission.)

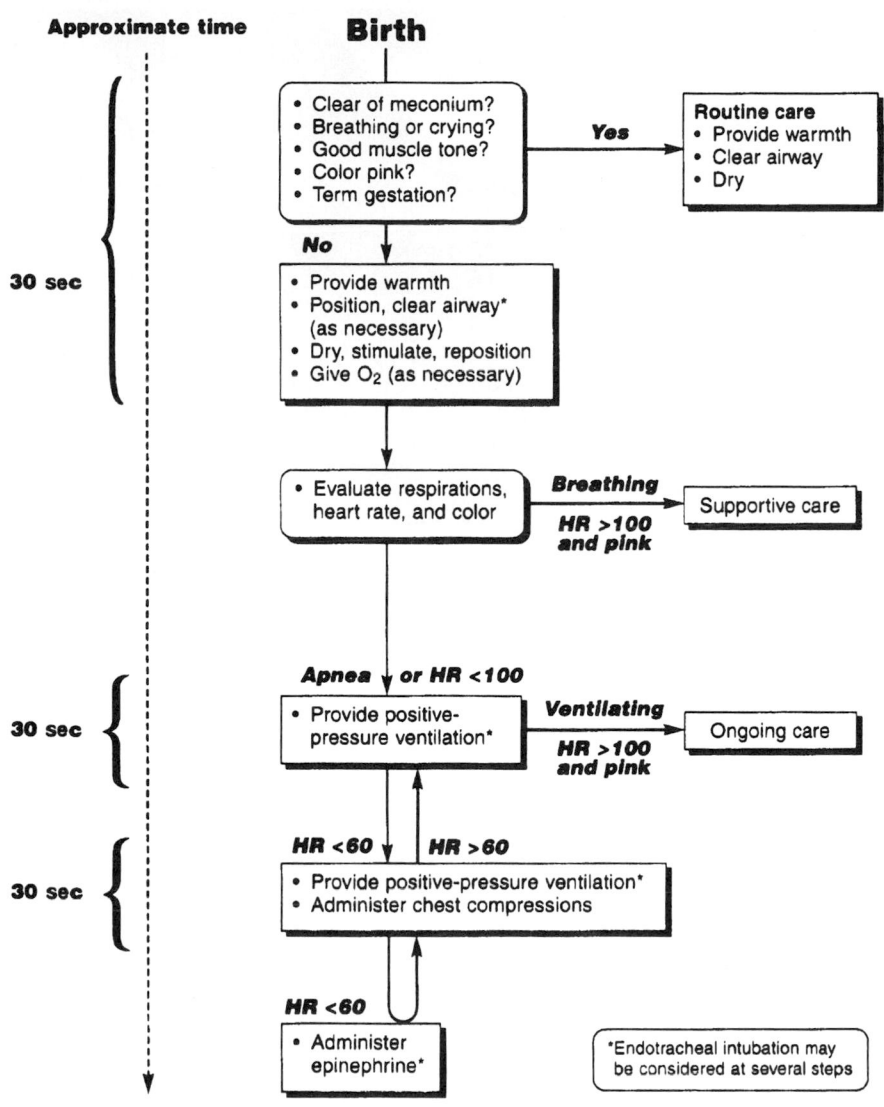

Approximate time

Birth

- Clear of meconium?
- Breathing or crying?
- Good muscle tone?
- Color pink?
- Term gestation?

Yes →

Routine care
- Provide warmth
- Clear airway
- Dry

No

30 sec
- Provide warmth
- Position, clear airway* (as necessary)
- Dry, stimulate, reposition
- Give O$_2$ (as necessary)

- Evaluate respirations, heart rate, and color

Breathing
HR >100 and pink → Supportive care

Apnea or HR <100

30 sec
- Provide positive-pressure ventilation*

Ventilating
HR >100 and pink → Ongoing care

HR <60   HR >60

30 sec
- Provide positive-pressure ventilation*
- Administer chest compressions

HR <60
- Administer epinephrine*

*Endotracheal intubation may be considered at several steps

FIGURE 28–2. Algorithm for resuscitation of the newborn infant. (HR = heart rate.) (Reproduced from Kattwinkel, 2000, with permission.)

breathing stops and the infant enters a stage of apnea known as *primary apnea*. This stage is accompanied by a fall in heart rate and loss of neuromuscular tone. Simple stimulation and exposure to oxygen will usually reverse primary apnea. If oxygen deprivation and asphyxia persist, however, the infant will develop deep gasping respirations, followed by *secondary apnea*. This latter stage is associated with a further decline in heart rate, falling blood pressure, and loss of neuromuscular tone. Infants in secondary apnea will not respond to stimulation and will not spontaneously resume respiratory efforts. Unless ventilation is assisted, death will occur. **Clinically, primary and secondary apnea are indistinguishable; thus, secondary apnea must be assumed and resuscitation of the apneic infant must be started immediately.**

Resuscitation Protocol. The following is a summary of the guidelines for neonatal resuscitation recommended by the American Academy of Pediatrics and the American Heart Association (Kattwinkel, 2000). These guidelines have been endorsed by the American College of Obstetricians and Gynecologists in the *Guidelines for Perinatal Care* (2002). Of note, Wiswell (2003) recently has provided an excellent review summarizing some of the evidence and controversies underlying these guidelines.

BASIC STEPS. As shown in Figure 28–2, the infant is first placed in a warm environment to minimize heat loss. Next, the airway is cleared. If the delivery is complicated by meconium and the infant is not vigorous, endotracheal intubation is recommended as subsequently discussed so that the airway can be suctioned before further resuscitative efforts are performed. The infant is then dried and stimulated after which respiratory effort, heart rate, and color are assessed. In most instances, the infant will take a breath within a few seconds of birth and cry within half a minute. If the infant is breathing, the heart rate is greater than 100 beats/min, and the skin of the central portion of the body and mucus membranes is pink, then routine supportive care is provided.

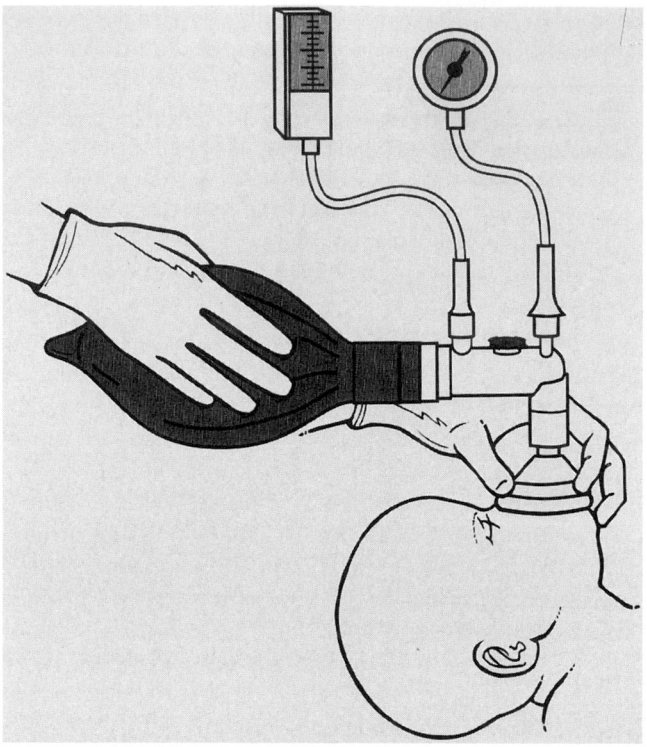

FIGURE 28–3. Correct use of bag-and-mask ventilation. The head should be in a sniffing position with the tip of the nose pointing to the ceiling, and care should be taken to avoid hyperextension of the neck. (Reproduced from Kattwinkel, 2000, with permission.)

VENTILATION. The presence of apnea, gasping respirations, or bradycardia beyond 30 seconds after delivery should prompt administration of *positive-pressure ventilation* (Fig. 28–3). The recommended assisted ventilation rate is 40 to 60 breaths per minute and 30 per minute if chest compressions also are being delivered. Adequate ventilation is indicated by bilateral rise of the chest and auscultation of breath sounds as well as improvement in heart rate and color. If ventilation is inadequate, the infant's head position should be checked (see Fig. 28–3), secretions cleared, and if necessary, inflation pressure increased.

Fetal failure to establish effective respirations may result from a variety of complications, including the following:

1. Fetal hypoxemia or acidosis from any cause.
2. Drugs administered to the mother.
3. Fetal immaturity.
4. Upper airway obstruction.
5. Pneumothorax.
6. Other lung abnormalities, either intrinsic (e.g., hypoplasia) or extrinsic (e.g., diaphragmatic hernia).
7. Aspiration of amnionic fluid contaminated with meconium.
8. Central nervous system developmental abnormality.
9. Septicemia.

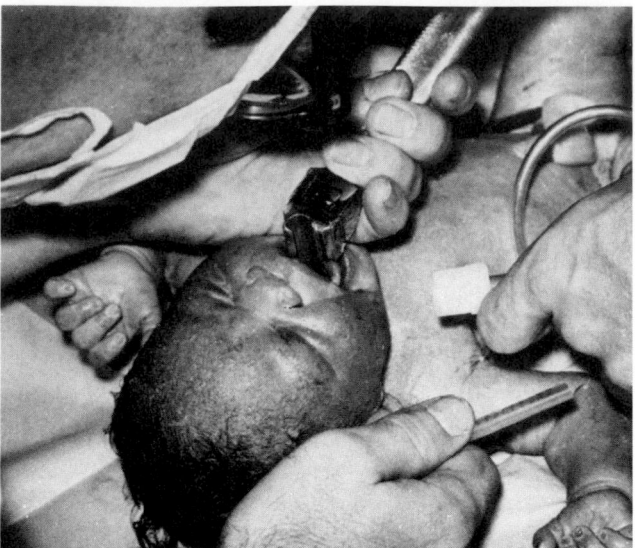

FIGURE 28–4. Use of laryngoscope to insert a tracheal tube under direct vision. Oxygen is being delivered from the curved tube held by an assistant.

ENDOTRACHEAL INTUBATION. If bag-and-mask ventilation is ineffective or prolonged, endotracheal intubation should be performed. Other indications include the need for chest compressions or tracheal administration of medications or special circumstances such as extremely low birthweight or congenital diaphragmatic hernia. A laryngoscope with a straight blade—size 0 for preterm infants, size 1 for term infants—is introduced at the side of the mouth and then directed posteriorly toward the oropharynx (Fig. 28–4). The laryngoscope is next moved gently into the space between the base of the tongue and the epiglottis. Gentle elevation of the tip of the laryngoscope will raise the epiglottis and expose the glottis and the vocal cords. The endotracheal tube is then introduced through the vocal cords. Gentle cricoid pressure may be useful. The suggested tube size and depth of insertion are shown in Table 28–1.

Several steps are taken to ensure that the tube is positioned in the trachea and not the esophagus: observing symmetrical chest wall motion; listening for equal breath sounds, especially in the axillae; and listening for an absence of breath

TABLE 28–1 Suggested Endotracheal Tube Size and Depth of Insertion According to Weight and Gestational Age

Weight (g)	Gestational Age (wk)	Tube Size, Inside diameter (mm)	Depth of Insertion from Upper Lip (cm)
< 1000	< 28	2.5	6–7
1000–2000	28–34	3.0	7–8
2000–3000	34–38	3.5	8–9
> 3000	> 38	3.5–4.0	> 9

From Kattwinkel (2000), with permission.

sounds or a gurgling sound over the stomach. Given that meconium, blood, mucus, and particulate debris in amnionic fluid or in the birth canal may have been inhaled prior to delivery, any foreign material encountered in the tracheal tube should be suctioned immediately.

The resuscitator, using an appropriate ventilation bag attached to the tracheal tube, should deliver puffs of oxygen-rich air into the tube at 1- to 2-second intervals with a force adequate to gently lift the chest wall. Pressures of 25 to 35 cm H_2O typically will expand the alveoli without causing a pneumothorax or pneumomediastinum.

CHEST COMPRESSIONS. If the heart rate remains below 60 beats/min despite adequate ventilation with 100-percent oxygen for 30 seconds, chest compressions are initiated. Compressions are delivered on the lower third of the sternum at a depth sufficient to generate a palpable pulse. A 3:1 ratio of compressions to ventilations is recommended, with 90 compressions and 30 breaths to achieve approximately 120 events each minute. The heart rate is reassessed every 30 seconds, and chest compressions are continued until the spontaneous heart rate is at least 60 beats/min.

MEDICATIONS AND VOLUME EXPANSION. Administration of epinephrine is indicated when the heart rate remains below 60 beats/min after a minimum of 30 seconds of adequate ventilation and chest compressions. Epinephrine is particularly indicated in the presence of asystole. The recommended intravenous or endotracheal dose is 0.1 to 0.3 mL/kg of a 1:10,000 solution. This is repeated every 3 to 5 minutes as indicated.

Volume expansion should be considered when blood loss is suspected, the infant appears to be in shock, or the response to resuscitative measures is inadequate. An isotonic crystalloid solution, such as normal saline or Ringer lactate, is recommended. Symptomatic anemia may require transfusion of red blood cells. The initial dose of either type of volume expander is 10 mL/kg given by slow intravenous push over 5 to 10 minutes.

The routine use of *sodium bicarbonate* during neonatal resuscitation is controversial (Kette and associates, 1991). The hyperosmolarity and CO_2-generating properties of bicarbonate may be detrimental to myocardial and cerebral function. If sodium bicarbonate is used during prolonged arrests

unresponsive to other therapy, it should be administered only after establishment of adequate ventilation and circulation.

Naloxone is a narcotic antagonist indicated for reversal of respiratory depression in a newborn infant whose mother received narcotics within 4 hours of delivery. Adequate ventilation should always be established prior to naloxone administration. The recommended dose of naloxone is 0.1 mg/kg of a 1.0-mg/mL solution. Because the duration of action of narcotics may exceed that of naloxone, continued monitoring of respiratory function is essential, and repeat doses may be necessary to prevent recurrent apnea. Based on their systematic review of nine studies, McGuire and Fowlie (2003) concluded that prophylactic naloxone administration, in the absence of respiratory depression, does not confer any clinical benefits.

Discontinuation of Resuscitation. As expected, infants with cardiopulmonary arrest who do not respond promptly to resuscitation are at great risk for mortality and, if they survive, severe morbidity. For example, Haddad and associates (2000) described 33 infants born without cardiac or respiratory effort that persisted for at least the first 5 minutes of life and in whom resuscitation was attempted. Of the 11 survivors, five had clinical or radiological signs of neurological injury, four were lost to follow-up, and only two had normal neurological development. Given the poor prognosis, the American Academy of Pediatrics and American Heart Association (Kattwinkel, 2000) advise that discontinuation of resuscitative efforts may be appropriate if resuscitation after cardiopulmonary arrest does not result in spontaneous circulation within 15 minutes. Furthermore, resuscitation of newborns after 10 minutes of asystole is very unlikely to result in neurologically intact survival.

METHODS USED TO EVALUATE NEWBORN CONDITION

APGAR SCORE. A useful clinical tool to identify those neonates who require resuscitation as well as to assess the effectiveness of any resuscitative measures is the Apgar scoring system (Apgar, 1953). As shown in Table 28–2, each of the five easily identifiable characteristics—heart rate, respiratory

TABLE 28–2 Apgar Scoring System

Sign	0 Points	1 Point	2 Points
Heart rate	Absent	< 100	> 100
Respiratory effort	Absent	Slow, irregular	Good, crying
Muscle tone	Flaccid	Some flexion of extremities	Active motion
Reflex irritability	No response	Grimace	Vigorous cry
Color	Blue, pale	Body pink, extremities blue	Completely pink

From Apgar (1953).

effort, muscle tone, reflex irritability, and color—is assessed and assigned a value of 0 to 2. The total score, based on the sum of the five components, is determined 1 and 5 minutes after delivery.

The 1-minute Apgar score reflects the need for immediate resuscitation. The 5-minute score, and particularly the change in score between 1 and 5 minutes, is a useful index of the effectiveness of resuscitative efforts. The 5-minute Apgar score also has prognostic significance for neonatal survival, because survival is related closely to the condition of the infant in the delivery room (Apgar and associates, 1958). In an analysis of more than 150,000 infants delivered at Parkland Hospital, Casey and associates (2001b) assessed the contemporaneous significance of the 5-minute score for predicting survival during the first 28 days of life. They found that in term infants the risk of neonatal death was approximately 1 in 5000 for those with Apgar scores of 7 to 10, as compared with approximately 1 in 4 for those with scores of 3 or less. Low 5-minute scores were comparably predictive of neonatal death in preterm infants. They concluded that the Apgar scoring system is as relevant for the prediction of neonatal survival today as it was almost 50 years ago.

There have been attempts to use Apgar scores to define asphyxial injury and to predict subsequent neurological outcome—uses for which the Apgar score was never intended. Such associations are especially difficult to measure given that both asphyxial injury and low Apgar scores are infrequent outcomes. For example, according to U.S. birth certificate records for the year 2002, only 1.4 percent of newborns had a 5-minute score below 7 (Martin and co-workers, 2003). Similarly, in a population-based study of more than 1 million term infants born in Sweden between 1988 and 1997, the incidence of 5-minute Apgar scores of 3 or less was approximately 2 per 1000 (Thorngren-Jerneck and Herbst, 2001).

Despite the methodological challenges, erroneous definitions of asphyxia by many groups were established solely based upon low Apgar scores. The promulgation of such definitions prompted the American College of Obstetricians and Gynecologists and the American Academy of Pediatrics to issue a joint statement in 1986 on the use and misuse of the Apgar score that was reaffirmed in 1996. Important caveats regarding Apgar score interpretation addressed in this statement include the following:

1. Because certain elements of the Apgar score are partially dependent on the physiological maturity of the infant, a healthy preterm infant may receive a low score only because of immaturity (Amon and associates, 1987; Catlin and co-workers, 1986).
2. Given that Apgar scores may be influenced by a variety of factors including, but not limited to, fetal malformations, maternal medications, and infection, to equate the presence of a low Apgar score solely with asphyxia or hypoxia represents a misuse of the score.

TABLE 28–3 Clinical Criteria Necessary to Establish that Acute Neurological Injury in the Newborn Was Related to "Asphyxia" Proximate to Delivery

- Profound metabolic or mixed acidemia (pH < 7.0) determined by an umbilical cord arterial sample, if obtained
- Apgar score of 0–3 for longer than 5 min
- Neonatal neurological manifestations—e.g., seizures, coma, or hypotonia
- Multisystem organ dysfunction—e.g., cardiovascular, gastrointestinal, hematological, pulmonary, or renal system

From the American College of Obstetricians and Gynecologists (1996, 2004), with permission.

3. Correlation of the Apgar score with adverse future neurological outcome increases when the score remains 3 or less at 10, 15, and 20 minutes, but still does not indicate the cause of future disability (Freeman and Nelson, 1988; Nelson and Ellenberg, 1981).
4. The Apgar score alone cannot establish hypoxia as the cause of cerebral palsy (see Chap. 29, p. 655). A neonate who has had an asphyxial insult proximate to delivery that is severe enough to result in acute neurological injury should demonstrate all of the findings listed in Table 28–3.

UMBILICAL CORD BLOOD ACID–BASE STUDIES.

Blood taken from umbilical vessels may be used for acid–base studies to assess the metabolic status of the fetus. Blood collection is performed following delivery by immediately isolating a 10- to 20-cm segment of cord with two clamps near the neonate and two clamps nearer the placenta. The importance of clamping the cord is underscored by the fact that delays of 20 to 30 seconds can alter both the P_{CO_2} and pH (Lievaart and deJong, 1984). The cord is then cut between the two proximal and two distal clamps. *Arterial blood* is drawn from the isolated segment of cord into a 1- to 2-mL commercially prepared plastic syringe containing lyophilized heparin or a similar syringe that has been flushed with a heparin solution containing 1000 U/mL. The needle is capped and the syringe transported, on ice, to the laboratory. Although efforts should be made to transport the blood promptly, neither the pH nor P_{CO_2} change significantly in blood kept at room temperature for up to 60 minutes (Duerbeck and associates, 1992). Chauhan and colleagues (1994) developed mathematical models allowing reasonable prediction of birth acid–base status in properly collected cord blood samples analyzed as late as 60 hours after delivery.

Fetal Acid–Base Physiology. The fetus produces carbonic and organic acids. Carbonic acid (H_2CO_3) is formed by oxidative metabolism of CO_2. The fetus can rapidly clear CO_2 through the placental circulation, and when H_2CO_3 accumulates in fetal blood without an increase in organic acids, the result is *respiratory acidemia*. Organic acids primarily are formed by anaerobic metabolism and include lactic and β-hydroxybutyric acids. These organic acids are cleared slowly from fetal blood, and when they accumulate without an increase in H_2CO_3, the result is *metabolic acidemia*. With the development of metabolic acidemia, bicarbonate (HCO_3^-) decreases because it is used to buffer the organic acid. An increase in H_2CO_3 accompanied by an increase in organic acid (seen as a decrease in HCO_3^-) is known as a *mixed respiratory–metabolic acidemia*.

In the fetus, respiratory and metabolic acidemia, and ultimately tissue acidosis, are most likely part of a progressively worsening continuum. This is different from the adult pathophysiology, in which distinct conditions result in either respiratory (pulmonary disease) or metabolic (diabetes) acidemia. In the fetus, the placenta serves as both the lungs and, to a certain degree, the kidneys. One principal cause of developing acidemia in the fetus is a decrease in uteroplacental perfusion. This results in the retention of CO_2 (respiratory acidemia), and if protracted and severe enough, it ultimately leads to a mixed or metabolic acidemia.

Assuming that maternal pH and blood gases are normal, the actual pH of fetal blood is dependent on the proportion of carbonic and organic acids as well as the amount of bicarbonate, which is the major buffer in blood. This can best be illustrated by the Henderson–Hasselbach equation:

$$pH = pK + \log \frac{[\text{base}]}{[\text{acid}]} \quad \text{or,} \quad pH = pK + \log \frac{HCO_3^-}{H_2CO_3}$$

For clinical purposes, HCO_3^- represents the metabolic component and is reported in mEq/L. The H_2CO_3 concentration represents the respiratory component and is reported as the P_{CO_2} in mmHg. Thus:

$$pH = pK + \log \frac{\text{metabolic } (HCO_3^- \text{ mEq/L})}{\text{respiratory } (P_{CO_2} \text{ mmHg})}$$

Delta base is a calculated number used as a measure of the change in buffering capacity of bicarbonate (HCO_3^-). For example, bicarbonate concentration will be decreased with a metabolic acidemia as it is consumed in order to maintain a normal pH. A *base deficit* occurs when HCO_3^- concentration decreases to below normal levels, and a *base excess* occurs when HCO_3^- values are above normal. Importantly, a mixed respiratory–metabolic acidemia with a large base deficit and a low HCO_3^- (less than 12 mEq/L) is more often associated with a depressed neonate than is a mixed acidemia with a minimal base deficit and a more nearly normal HCO_3^- (American College of Obstetricians and Gynecologists, 1995; Gilstrap and Cunningham, 1994; Ross and Gala, 2002). A nomogram for calculating the delta base has been published by Siggaard-Anderson (1963).

Clinical Diagnosis of Significant Acidemia. Fetal oxygenation and pH generally decline during the course of normal labor (Dildy and co-workers, 1994). Normal umbilical cord blood pH and blood gas values at delivery in term newborns are summarized in Table 28–4. Similar values have been measured in preterm infants (Dickinson and co-workers, 1992; Ramin and associates, 1989; Riley and Johnson, 1993). Using data from over 19,000 deliveries, the lower limits of normal pH in the newborn have been found to range from 7.04 to 7.10 (Boylan and Parisi, 1994). Thus, these values should be considered to define neonatal acidemia. Most fetuses will tolerate intrapartum acidemia with a pH as low as 7.00 without incurring neurological impairment (Freeman and Nelson, 1988; Gilstrap and associates, 1989). Indeed, Goldaber and

TABLE 28–4 Umbilical Cord Blood pH and Blood Gas Values in Normal Term Newborns

	Study			
Values	Yeomans et al (1985)[a] (n = 146)[c]	Ramin et al (1989)[a] (n = 1292)[c]	Riley and Johnson (1993)[b] (n = 3522)[c]	Arikan et al (2000)[a] (n = 1281)
Arterial Blood				
pH	7.28 (0.05)	7.28 (0.07)	7.27 (0.069)	7.25 (7.08)[d]
P_{CO_2} (mm Hg)	49.2 (8.4)	49.9 (14.2)	50.3 (11.1)	50 (75)[e]
HCO_3^- (mEq/L)	22.3 (2.5)	23.1 (2.8)	22.0 (3.6)	—
Base excess (mEq/L)	—	−3.6 (2.8)	−2.7 (2.8)	−4.3 (−11.1)[d]
Venous Blood				
pH	7.35 (0.05)	—	7.34 (0.063)	—
P_{CO_2} (mm Hg)	38.2 (5.6)	—	40.7 (7.9)	—
HCO_3^- (mEq/L)	20.4 (4.1)	—	21.4 (2.5)	—
Base excess (mEq/L)	—	—	−2.4 (2)	—

[a] Infants of selected women with uncomplicated vaginal deliveries.
[b] Infants of unselected women with vaginal deliveries.
[c] Shown as mean ± SD for first three studies.
[d] Shown as median and 2.5 centile.
[e] Shown as median and 97.5 centile.

TABLE 28–5 Umbilical Arterial Blood pH Related to Neonatal Morbidity, Mortality, and Apgar Scores in Term Infants

	Umbilical Artery pH			
	< 7.00 (n = 87)	7.00–7.04 (n = 95)	7.05–7.09 (n = 290)	7.10–7.14 (n = 798)
Complication	No. (%)	No. (%)	No. (%)	No. (%)
Seizure	11 (13)	4 (4.2)	0	2 (0.3)
Neonatal deaths	7 (8)	1 (1.1)	0	3 (0.4)
Intensive care nursery	34 (39)	12 (13)	17 (5.9)	22 (2.8)
Intubated	12 (14)	6 (6.3)	5 (1.7)	5 (0.6)
Apgar scores ≤ 3				
1 min	24 (27.6)	8 (8.4)	12 (4.1)	19 (2.4)
5 min	9 (10.3)	1 (1.1)	1 (0.3)	0

Goldaber and associates (1991), with permission.

associates (1991) found that there were significantly more neonatal deaths and infants with neurological dysfunction if a pH cutoff value of less than 7.00 was used (Table 28–5).

Another important prognostic consideration is the direction of pH change from birth to the immediate neonatal period. Casey and co-workers (2001a) found that the risk of seizures during the first 24 hours of life was reduced fivefold if a cord pH below 7.2 normalized within 2 hours after delivery.

In the fetus, *metabolic acidemia* develops when oxygen deprivation is of sufficient duration and magnitude to require anaerobic metabolism for fetal cellular energy needs. Low and associates (1997) defined fetal acidosis as a base deficit of greater than 12 mmol/L and severe fetal acidosis as a base deficit greater than 16 mmol/L. In the study of over 150,000 newborn infants cited earlier, Casey and associates (2001b) defined metabolic acidemia using umbilical cord blood gas cutoffs that were 2 standard deviations below the mean. Using this criteria, metabolic acidosis was defined as an umbilical artery blood pH less than 7.00 accompanied by a PCO_2 of no more than 76.3 mm Hg, HCO_3^- concentration of no more than 17.7 mmol/L, and base deficit of no more than 10.3 mEq/L. According to the American Academy of Pediatrics and the American College of Obstetricians and Gynecologists (2002), the precise umbilical cord blood pH value that defines *chemically* significant acidemia is not known; however, umbilical artery blood pH values less than 7.00 with a metabolic component and a base deficit of 10 mEq/L or more realistically represent clinically significant metabolic acidosis.

Metabolic acidemia is associated with a high rate of multiorgan dysfunction, and in rare cases such hypoxia-induced metabolic acidemia may be so severe as to cause subsequent neurological impairment. In fact, a fetus without such acidemia cannot by definition have suffered recent hypoxic-induced injury (see Table 28–3). Even severe metabolic acidosis, however, is poorly predictive of subsequent neurological impairment in the term infant. Although metabolic acidosis was associated with an increase in immediate

neonatal complications in a group of infants with depressed 5-minute Apgar scores, Socol and colleagues (1994) found no difference in umbilical artery blood gas measurements among those individuals who developed cerebral palsy and those with subsequent normal neurological outcome. In very-low-birthweight infants—those less than 1000 g—newborn acid–base status may be more closely linked to long-term neurological outcome (Gaudier and co-workers, 1994; Low and associates, 1995). In contrast, Casey and associates (2001b) measured the association between metabolic acidemia, low Apgar scores, and neonatal death in term and preterm infants. Relative to infants with a 5-minute Apgar score of at least 7, the risk of neonatal death was more than 3200-fold greater in term infants with metabolic acidemia and 5-minute scores of 3 or less (Table 28–6).

TABLE 28–6 Relative Risk of Neonatal Death in Preterm and Term Infants with 5-Minute Apgar Scores of 0 to 3 and Various Degrees of Umbilical Artery Blood Acidemia[a]

	Relative Risk (95% CI)[a]	
Characterstic	Preterm Infants	Term Infants
5-min Apgar score of 0–3	59 (40–87)	1460 (835–2555)
Umbilical blood pH		
≤ 7.0	20 (11–34)	180 (97–334)
≤ 6.9	22 (11–46)	708 (381–1320)
≤ 6.8	43 (21–91)	1407 (736–2689)
Metabolic acidemia[b]	38 (17–85)	157 (64–385)
Combined 5-min Apgar score of 0–3 and pH ≤ 7.0	102 (65–160)	3204 (1864–5508)

[a] Infants with 5-minute Apgar scores of 7–10 served as the reference group. CI denotes confidence interval.
[b] Defined by an umbilical artery blood pH of no more than 7.0 with a partial pressure of CO_2 of no more than 76.3 mm Hg, an HCO_3^- concentration of no more than 17.7 mmol/L, and a base deficit of 10.3 or more. These values are 2 SD from the means for all infants.
From Casey and associates (2001b), with permission.

Respiratory acidemia generally develops as a result of an acute interruption in placental gas exchange with subsequent CO_2 retention. Transient umbilical cord compression is the most common antecedent factor in the development of fetal respiratory acidemia. In general, respiratory acidemia does not reflect an insult of potential harm to the fetus. Low and co-workers (1994) found no increase in newborn complications after respiratory acidosis. The degree to which pH is affected by P_{CO_2}, the respiratory component of the acidosis, can be calculated by the following relationship: 10 additional units of P_{CO_2} will lower the pH by 0.08 units (Eisenberg and colleagues, 1987). Thus in a mixed respiratory–metabolic acidemia, the benign respiratory component can be calculated as follows:

> During labor, an acute cord prolapse occurred and the fetus was delivered by cesarean 20 minutes later. The umbilical artery pH at birth was 6.95, with a P_{CO_2} of 89 mm Hg. To calculate the degree to which the cord compression and subsequent impairment of CO_2 exchange affected the pH, the relationship given earlier is applied: 89 mm Hg–49 mm Hg (normal newborn P_{CO_2}) = 40 mm Hg (excess CO_2). To correct pH: $(40 \div 10) \times 0.08 = 0.32$; $6.95 + 0.32 = 7.27$. Therefore, the pH prior to cord prolapse was approximately 7.27, well within normal limits.

Recommendations for Cord Blood Gas Determinations. A cost-effectiveness analysis for universal cord blood gas measurements has not been conducted. In some centers, cord gas analysis is performed in all infants at birth. The American Academy of Pediatrics and American College of Obstetricians and Gynecologists (2002) recommend that cord blood gas and pH analyses be used in select neonates with low Apgar scores to distinguish metabolic acidemia from hypoxia or other causes that might result in a low Apgar score. Although umbilical cord acid–base blood determinations have a low predictability for either immediate or long-term adverse neurological outcome, they are helpful to exclude intrapartum events that may cause acidosis (Gilstrap and Cunningham, 1994).

PREVENTIVE CARE

EYE INFECTION PROPHYLAXIS. A little more than a century ago, it was estimated that as many as 80 percent of children in institutions for the blind had *gonococcal ophthalmia neonatorum* resulting from passage through the birth canal of a mother infected with gonorrhea (Schneider, 1984). In 1884, Credé, a German obstetrician, introduced the practice of instilling into each eye immediately after birth one drop of a 1-percent solution of silver nitrate, which was later washed out with saline. As a result, blindness due to neonatal infection from *Neisseria gonorrhoeae* was largely eliminated. Since that time, a variety of antimicrobials have also proven to be effective, and prophylaxis against gonococcal ophthalmia

neonatorum is now mandatory for all neonates, including those born by cesarean delivery (American Academy of Pediatrics and American College of Obstetricians and Gynecologists, 2002). Current recommendations by the Centers for Disease Control and Prevention (2002a) include a single application of aqueous silver nitrate (1 percent), erythromycin ophthalmic ointment (0.5 percent), or tetracycline ophthalmic ointment (1 percent). For infants born to mothers with untreated gonorrhea, single-dose ceftriaxone, 25 to 50 mg/kg, is given intramuscularly or intravenously, not to exceed 125 mg.

The problem of providing adequate neonatal prophylaxis against *chlamydial conjunctivitis* is much more complex. It is estimated that 12 to 25 percent of infants born vaginally to mothers with an active chlamydial infection will develop conjunctivitis (Teoh and Reynolds, 2003). Although it is reasonable to expect that tetracycline and erythromycin ophthalmic ointments applied at birth should reduce the incidence of chlamydial conjunctivitis, results with these agents and silver nitrate solution have been disappointing. In a study from Kenya, Isenberg and colleagues (1995) showed that 2.5-percent povidone–iodine solution was superior to either 1-percent silver nitrate solution or 0.5-percent erythromycin ointment in preventing chlamydial conjunctivitis. According to the Centers for Disease Control and Prevention (2002a), topical prophylaxis against chlamydial conjunctivitis is inadequate, and any case of conjunctivitis in an infant less than 1 month old should prompt consideration for chlamydial infection.

HEPATITIS B IMMUNIZATION. In 1991, the Centers for Disease Control and Prevention recommended routine immunization of all newborns against hepatitis B prior to hospital discharge. In 1999, routine vaccination of low-risk newborns was suspended because of concerns that the vaccine contained *thimerosal,* a mercury-containing preservative (Clark and co-workers, 2001). A thimerosal-free hepatitis B vaccine became available several months later and the Centers for Disease Control and Prevention (2002a) recommended it for newborn prophylaxis. Use of the vaccine does not appear to increase the number of febrile episodes, sepsis evaluations, or adverse neurological sequelae (Lewis and associates, 2001). If the mother is hepatitis B surface-antigen positive, the neonate should be passively immunized with hepatitis B immune globulin (see Chap. 49, p. 1131).

VITAMIN K. To prevent vitamin K–dependent hemorrhagic disease of the newborn, which is discussed in Chapter 29 (see p. 676), routine intramuscular administration of single-dose vitamin K within 1 hour of birth is recommended by the American Academy of Pediatrics and American College of Obstetricians and Gynecologists (2002).

UNIVERSAL NEWBORN SCREENING. Newborn screening programs began in the early 1960s when Dr. Robert Guthrie developed a test for phenylketonuria (PKU)

Neuromuscular Maturity

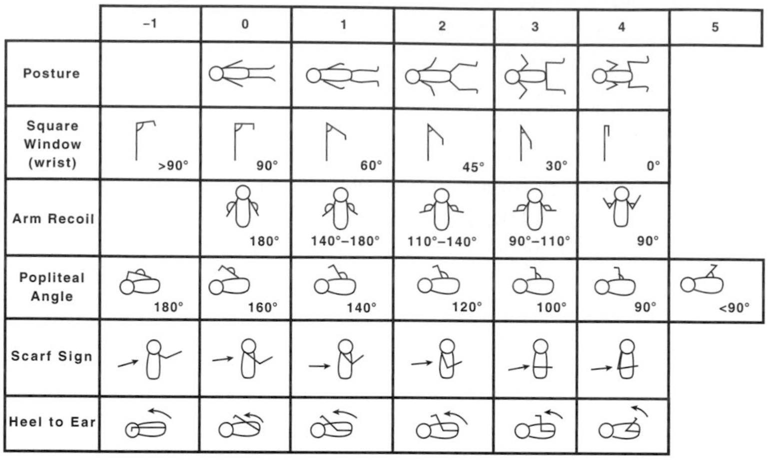

	-1	0	1	2	3	4	5
Posture							
Square Window (wrist)	>90°	90°	60°	45°	30°	0°	
Arm Recoil		180°	140°–180°	110°–140°	90°–110°	90°	
Popliteal Angle	180°	160°	140°	120°	100°	90°	<90°
Scarf Sign							
Heel to Ear							

Physical Maturity

Skin	Sticky triable transparent	gelatinous red, translucent	smooth pink, visible veins	superficial peeling &/or rash, few veins	cracking pale areas rare veins	parchment deep cracking no vessels	leathery cracked wrinkled
Lanugo	none	sparse	abundant	thinning	bald areas	mostly bald	
Plantar Surface	heel–toe 40–50 mm:-1 <40 mm:-2	>50mm no crease	faint red marks	anterior transverse crease only	creases ant. 2/3	creases over entire sole	
Breast	imperceptible	barely perceptible	flat areola no bud	stippled areola 1–2 mm bud	raised areola 3–4 mm bud	full areola 5–10 mm bud	
Eye/Ear	lids fused loosely:-1 tightly:-2	lids open pinna flat stays folded	sl. curved pinna; soft; slow recoil	well–curved pinnal; soft but ready recoil	formed & firm instant recoil	thick cartilage ear stiff	
Genitals male	scrotum flat, smooth	scrotum empyt faint rugae	testes in upper canal rare rugae	testes descending few rugae	testes down good rugae	testes pendulous deep rugae	
Genitals female	clitoris prominent labia flat	prominent clitoris small labia minora	prominent clitoris enlarging minora	majora & minora equally prominent	majora large minora small	majora cover clitoris & minora	

Maturity Rating

score	weeks
-10	20
5	22
0	24
5	26
10	28
15	30
20	32
25	34
30	36
35	38
40	40
45	42
50	44

FIGURE 28–5. Ballard score for estimating gestational age. (Reproduced from Ballard and co-workers, 1991, with permission.)

and a system for collection and transport of blood samples on filter paper (Guthrie and Susi, 1963). Since that time, the term *newborn screening* has referred to biochemical testing for inherited disorders, generally metabolic in origin, that are usually correctable by either drug or dietary interventions (Therrell, 2001). In 2000, all states required mandatory screening for PKU and congenital hypothyroidism and many states required testing for several other disorders, including galactosemia, maple syrup urine disease, homocystinuria, sickle cell disease, and congenital adrenal hyperplasia (American Academy of Pediatrics Newborn Screening Task Force, 2000; March of Dimes, 2002). Using a cost–benefit analysis, Schoen and co-workers (2002) concluded that newborn screening compared favorably with other mass screening programs, including those for breast and prostate cancer. The American College of Obstetricians and Gynecologists (2003) has concluded that newborn screening programs provide an important public health benefit and has advised obstetricians to inform expectant families of the newborn screening process.

ROUTINE NEWBORN CARE

ESTIMATION OF GESTATIONAL AGE. An estimate of the gestational age of the newborn may be made very soon after delivery (Fig. 28–5). The relationship between gestational age and birthweight should be used to identify neonates at risk for complications (McIntire and colleagues, 1999). For example, neonates who are either small- or large-for-gestational age are at increased risk for hypoglycemia and polycythemia, and measurements of blood glucose and hematocrit are indicated (American Academy of Pediatrics and American College of Obstetricians and Gynecologists, 2002).

SKIN CARE. Following delivery, excess vernix, as well as blood and meconium, should be gently wiped off. Any remaining vernix is readily absorbed and disappears entirely within 24 hours. The first bath should be postponed until the temperature of the neonate has stabilized.

UMBILICAL CORD. Loss of water from the Wharton jelly leads to mummification of the umbilical cord shortly after birth. Within 24 hours, the cord stump loses its characteristic bluish-white, moist appearance and soon becomes dry and black. Within several days to weeks, the stump sloughs, leaving a small, granulating wound, which after healing forms the umbilicus. Separation usually takes place within the first 2 weeks, with a range of 3 to 45 days (Novack and colleagues, 1988). The umbilical cord dries more quickly and separates more readily when exposed to air, thus, a dressing is not recommended.

Serious umbilical infections sometimes are encountered. The most likely offending organisms are *Staphylococcus aureus, Escherichia coli,* and group B streptococcus. Because the umbilical stump in such cases may present no outward sign of infection, the diagnosis may be elusive. Strict aseptic precautions should be observed in the immediate care of the cord. In a randomized study of 766 newborns, Janssen and co-workers (2003) showed that triple-dye applied to the cord was superior to soap and water care in preventing colonization and exudate formation.

FEEDING. In many hospitals, infants begin breast feeding in the delivery room. Most term infants thrive best when fed at intervals of every 2 to 4 hours. Preterm or growth-restricted infants require feedings at shorter intervals. In most instances, a 3-hour interval is satisfactory. The proper length of each feeding depends on several factors, such as the quantity of breast milk, the readiness with which it can be obtained from the breast, and the avidity with which the infant nurses. It is generally advisable for the infant to nurse for 5 minutes at each breast for the first 4 days, or until the mother has a supply of milk. After the fourth day, the infant nurses up to 10 minutes on each breast.

A goal established by the U.S. Public Health Service for *Healthy People 2010* is to increase the proportion of mothers who breast feed their infants to 75 percent in the early postpartum period, 50 percent at 6 months, and 25 percent at 12 months (U.S. Department of Health and Human Services, 2000). In 1998, nearly two thirds of mothers chose to breast feed, the highest rate in nearly 30 years, and over 28 percent continued for at least 6 months (American College of Obstetricians and Gynecologists, 2000). Breast feeding is discussed further in Chapter 30 (see p. 699).

Initial Weight Loss. Because most infants actually receive little nutriment for the first 3 or 4 days of life, they progressively lose weight until the flow of maternal milk or other feeding has been established. Preterm infants lose relatively more weight and regain their birthweight more slowly than term infants. Infants who are small-for-gestational age but otherwise healthy regain their initial weight more quickly when fed than preterm infants.

If the normal infant is nourished properly, birthweight usually is regained by the end of the 10th day. Thereafter, the weight typically increases steadily at the rate of about 25 g/day for the first few months. Birthweight doubles by 5 months of age and triples by the end of the first year.

Stools and Urine. For the first 2 or 3 days after birth, the contents of the colon are composed of soft, brownish-green *meconium.* This consists of desquamated epithelial cells from the intestinal tract, mucus, and epidermal cells and lanugo (fetal hair) that have been swallowed along with amnionic fluid. The characteristic color results from bile pigments. During fetal life and for a few hours after birth, the intestinal contents are sterile, but bacteria quickly colonize the bowel.

Meconium stooling is seen in 90 percent of newborns within the first 24 hours, and most of the rest do so within 36 hours. Voiding, although usually occurring shortly after birth, may not occur until the second day. The passage of meconium and urine in the minutes immediately after birth or during the next few hours indicates patency of the gastrointestinal and urinary tracts. Failure of the infant to stool or urinate after these times suggests a congenital defect, such as imperforate anus or a urethral valve. After the third or fourth day, as the consequence of ingesting milk, meconium is replaced by light-yellow homogenous feces with a consistency similar to peanut butter.

ICTERUS NEONATORUM. About one third of all infants, between the second and fifth day of life, develop so-called *physiological jaundice of the newborn.* Serum bilirubin levels at birth are normally 1.8 to 2.8 mg/dL. These levels increase during the next few days but with wide individual variation. Between the third and fourth day, the bilirubin in mature infants commonly exceeds 5 mg/dL, the concentration at which jaundice is usually noticeable. Most of the bilirubin is free, or unconjugated. One cause is immaturity of the hepatic cells, resulting in less conjugation of bilirubin with glucuronic acid leading to reduced excretion in bile (Chap. 29, p. 672). Reabsorption of free bilirubin as the consequence of the enzymatic splitting of bilirubin glucuronide by intestinal conjugase activity in the newborn intestine also appears to contribute significantly to the transient hyperbilirubinemia. In preterm infants, jaundice is more common and usually more severe and prolonged than in term infants, because of even less hepatic enzyme production. Increased erythrocyte destruction from any cause also contributes to hyperbilirubinemia.

CIRCUMCISION. Current scientific evidence suggests that several medical benefits are associated with newborn male circumcision. A review by the American Academy of Pediatrics Task Force on Circumcision (1989) reported that the procedure prevented phimosis, paraphimosis, and balanoposthitis, and it decreased the incidence of penile cancer. The Task Force also cited an increased incidence of cervical cancer among sexual partners of uncircumcised men infected with human papillomavirus. The associations

TABLE 28–7 Contraindications and Relative Contraindications to Routine Newborn Circumcision

Low birthweight (< 2500 g)
Unstable infant
Abnormal body temperature
Abnormal feeding
Bleeding abnormality
Family history of bleeding disorder not ruled out in infant
Hypospadias and outer genitourinary anomalies

From Swaim (2002), with permission.

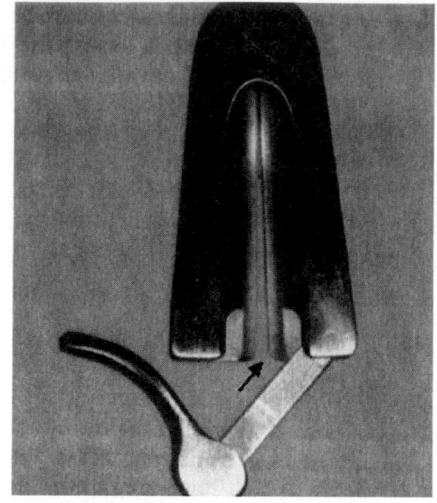

A

between circumcision and reduced risks of penile human papillomavirus infection and cervical cancer in sexual partners have been corroborated by Castellsagué and associates (2002).

The American Academy of Pediatrics (1999), however, has concluded that the existing evidence is insufficient to recommend routine neonatal circumcision, a position that is endorsed by the American College of Obstetricians and Gynecologists (2001). Others have argued that the existing data support a recommendation for routine circumcision (Schoen and associates, 2000). Nevertheless, it is currently recommended that parents should decide what is in the best interest of their own child and should make an informed choice after being given accurate and unbiased information. In 1999, 65 percent of all male infants born in hospitals in the United States were circumcised (Centers of Disease Control and Prevention, 2002b).

Surgical Technique. Newborn circumcision should be performed only on a healthy infant, and some contraindications are listed in Table 28–7. The most commonly used instruments include the Gomco and Mogen clamps and the Plastibell device (Fig. 28–6). Compared with the Gomco procedure, Kaufman and colleagues (2002) reported that the Mogen technique required less time to perform and was associated with less apparent discomfort for the infant. Regardless of the method used, the goal is to remove enough shaft skin and inner preputial epithelium so that the glans is exposed sufficiently to prevent phimosis. In all techniques, (1) the amount of external skin to be removed must be accurately estimated, (2) the preputial orifice must be dilated to visualize the glans and ensure that it is normal, (3) the inner preputial epithelium must be freed from the glans epithelium, and (4) the circumcision device must be left in place long enough to produce hemostasis before amputating the prepuce (Lerman and Liao, 2001). For a detailed description of surgical techniques see *Operative Obstetrics* (Swaim, 2002).

Anesthesia for Circumcision. The American Academy of Pediatrics (1999) recommends that if circumcision is performed, procedural analgesia should be provided. A variety of techniques for pain relief have been described,

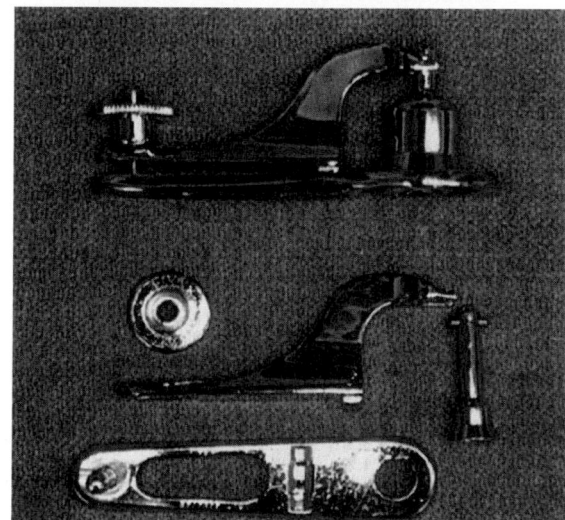

B

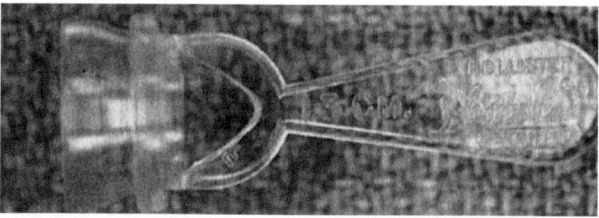

C

FIGURE 28–6. A. Mogen clamp. The arms of the clamp open to 3 mm maximum width (*arrow*). **B.** Gomco clamp, assembled and dissembled. **C.** Plastibell clamp. (Reproduced from Lerman and Liao, 2001, with permission.)

including lidocaine–prilocaine topical cream, local analgesia infiltration, and dorsal penile nerve and ring blocks. Stang and colleagues (1988) reported that dorsal penile nerve block reduced behavioral distress and modified adrenocortical stress response in neonates undergoing circumcision. This observation was confirmed in subsequent clinical studies (Arnett and co-workers, 1990; Fontaine and Toffler, 1991). The results of these studies favor the dorsal penile nerve block and the ring block technique over topical analgesia (Butler-O'Hara, 1998; Hardwick-Smith, 1998; Lander, 1997; Taddio, 1997, and their colleagues). The use of a pacifier dipped in sucrose also appears beneficial (Kaufman and colleagues, 2002).

After appropriate penile cleansing, the *ring block technique* consists of placing a wheal of 1 percent lidocaine at the base of the penis and advancing the needle in a 180-degree arc around the base of the penis first to one side and then the other to achieve a circumferential ring of analgesia. The maximum dose of lidocaine is 1.0 mL. The addition of a buffering agent does not appear to offer a benefit (Newton and co-workers, 1999). **No vasoactive compounds such as epinephrine should ever be added to the local analgesic agent.**

Complications of Circumcision. As with any surgical procedure, there is a risk of bleeding, infection, and hematoma formation. These risks, however, are low (Christakis and colleagues, 2000; Holman and colleagues, 1995). More unusual complications have been reported as isolated cases, including amputation of the distal penile glans during neonatal ritual circumcision (Neulander and colleagues, 1996), infection with human immunodeficiency virus-1 (HIV-1) and other sexually transmitted diseases (Nicoll, 1997), postcircumcision meatal stenosis (Upadhyay and associates, 1998), denudation of the penis (Orozco-Sanchez and Neri-Vela, 1991), penile destruction with electrocautery (Gearhart and Rock, 1989), formation of an epidermal inclusion cyst and urethrocutaneous fistula (Amukele and associates, 2003), and ischemia following the **inappropriate use of lidocaine with epinephrine** (Berens and Pontus, 1990).

ROOMING-IN. A model of maternity care that placed newborns in their mothers' rooms instead of central nurseries, so-called *rooming-in*, first appeared in U.S. hospitals in the early 1940s (Temkin, 2002). In part, rooming-in stems from a trend to make all phases of childbearing as natural as possible and to foster mother–child relationships at an early date. By the end of 24 hours, the mother is generally fully ambulatory. Thereafter, with rooming-in, she can usually provide routine care for herself and her infant. An obvious advantage is her increased ability to assume full care of the infant when she arrives home.

HOSPITAL DISCHARGE. Traditionally, the newborn infant is discharged with its mother, and in most cases, maternal stay has determined that of the infant. In the past decade, the length of stay for the mother following uncomplicated vaginal delivery has declined considerably. Although it is clear that most newborns can be safely discharged within 48 hours, this is not uniformly true. For example, using data from the Canadian Institute for Health Information, Liu and colleagues (2000) examined neonatal readmission rates in over 2.1 million discharges. As the length of hospital stay decreased from 4.2 days in 1990 to 2.7 days in 1997, the readmission rate increased from 27.3 to 38 per 1000 births. Dehydration and jaundice accounted for most of these readmissions. Using Washington state infant discharge data, Malkin and co-workers (2000) found that 28-day mortality was increased fourfold and 1-year mortality increased twofold in infants discharged within 30 hours of birth.

Because of the increased scrutiny regarding short hospital stays, federal legislation—*The Newborns' and Mothers' Health Protection Act of 1996*—was enacted to prohibit insurers from restricting hospital stays for mothers and newborns to less than 2 days for vaginal or 4 days for cesarean deliveries. As a result, the average length of hospital stay for childbirth increased from 2.1 days in 1995 to 2.5 days in 2000. This increase reflected the reduced number of very short hospital stays following childbirth (Hall and Owings, 2002). Mosen and associates (2002) found that implementation of the new legislation was associated with a 6-percent increase in cost; however, neonatal readmission rates within 7 days of discharge decreased by nearly half.

REFERENCES

American Academy of Pediatrics, Newborn Screening Task Force: Newborn screening: A blueprint for the future. Pediatrics 106:389, 2000

American Academy of Pediatrics, Task Force on Circumcision: Circumcision Policy Statement. Pediatrics 103:686, 1999

American Academy of Pediatrics, Task Force on Circumcision: Report of the Task Force on Circumcision. Pediatrics 84:388, 1989

American Academy of Pediatrics, Committee on Fetus and Newborn: Use and abuse of the Apgar score. Pediatrics 78:1148, 1986

American Academy of Pediatrics and the American College of Obstetricians and Gynecologists: Care of the Neonate. In: Guidelines for Perinatal Care, 5th ed. Washington, DC, AAP and ACOG, 2002

American College of Obstetricians and Gynecologists: Inappropriate use of the terms fetal distress and birth asphyxia. Committee Opinion No. 303, October 2004

American College of Obstetricians and Gynecologists: Newborn screening. Committee Opinion No. 287, October 2003

American College of Obstetricians and Gynecologists: Circumcision. Committee Opinion No. 260, October 2001

American College of Obstetricians and Gynecologists: Breastfeeding: Maternal and infant aspects. Educational Bulletin No. 258, July 2000

American College of Obstetricians and Gynecologists: Use and abuse of the Apgar score. Committee Opinion, No. 174, July 1996

American College of Obstetricians and Gynecologists: Umbilical artery blood acid–base analysis. Technical Bulletin No. 216, November 1995

Amon E, Sibai BM, Anderson GD, et al: Obstetric variables predicting survival of the immature newborn ($\leq$ 1000 gm): A five-year experience in a single perinatal center. Am J Obstet Gynecol 156:1380, 1987

Amukele SA, Lee GW, Stock JA, et al: 20-year experience with iatrogenic penile injury. J Urol 170:1691, 2003

Apgar V: A proposal for a new method of evaluation of the newborn infant. Curr Res Anesth Analg 32:260, 1953

Apgar V, Holaday DA, James LS, et al: Evaluation of the newborn infant—second report. JAMA 168:1985, 1958

Arikan GM, Scholz HS, Petru E, et al: Cord blood oxygen saturation in vigorous infants at birth: What is normal? Br J Obstet Gynaecol 107:987, 2000

Arnett RM, Jones JS, Horger EO III: Effectiveness of 1% lidocaine dorsal penile nerve block in infant circumcision. Am J Obstet Gynecol 163:1074, 1990

Ballard JL, Khoury JC, Wedig K, et al: New Ballard score, expanded to include extremely premature infants. J Pediatr 119:417, 1991

Berens R, Pontus SP Jr: A complication associated with dorsal penile nerve block. Reg Anesth 15:309, 1990

Boylan PC, Parisi VM: Fetal acid–base balance. In Creasy RK, Resnik R (eds): Maternal–Fetal Medicine, 3rd ed. Philadelphia, Saunders, 1994

Butler-O'Hara M, LeMoine C, Guillet R: Analgesia for neonatal circumcision: A randomized controlled trial of EMLA cream versus dorsal penile nerve block. Pediatrics 101:691, 1998

Casey BM, Goldaber KG, McIntire DD, et al: Outcomes among term infants when two-hour postnatal pH is compared with pH at delivery. Am J Obstet Gynecol 184:447, 2001a

Casey BM, McIntire DD, Leveno KJ: The continuing value of the Apgar score for the assessment of newborn infants. N Engl J Med 344:467, 2001b

Castellsagué X, Bosch FX, Muñoz N, et al: Male circumcision, penile human papillomavirus infection, and cervical cancer in female partners. N Engl J Med 346:1105, 2002

Catlin EA, Carpenter MW, Brann BS, et al: The Apgar score revisited: Influence of gestational age. J Pediatr 109:865, 1986

Centers for Disease Control and Prevention: National Center for Health Statistics. Trends in circumcisions among newborns. October 2002a. Available at: http://www.cdc.gov/nchs/products/pubs/pubd/hestats/hospbirth.htm

Centers for Disease Control and Prevention: Sexually transmitted diseases treatment guidelines 2002. MMWR 51:63, 2002b

Centers for Disease Control and Prevention: Hepatitis B virus: A comprehensive strategy for eliminating transmission in the United States through universal childhood vaccination: Recommendations of the Immunization Practices Advisory Committee (ACIP). MMWR 40:RR-13, 1991

Chauhan SP, Cowan BD, Meydrech EF, et al: Determination of fetal acidemia at birth from a remote umbilical arterial blood gas analysis. Am J Obstet Gynecol 170:1705, 1994

Chernick V: Fetal breathing movements and the onset of breathing at birth. Clin Perinatol 5:257, 1978

Christakis DA, Harvey E, Zerr DM, et al: A trade-off analysis of routine newborn circumcision. Pediatrics 105:246, 2000

Clark SJ, Cabana MD, Malik T, et al: Hepatitis B vaccination practices in hospital newborn nurseries before and after changes in vaccination recommendations. Arch Pediatr Adolesc Med 155:915, 2001

Credé CSF: Die Verhütung der Augenenzündung der Neugeborenen. Berlin, Hirschwald, 1884

Dawes GS: Breathing before birth in animals or man. N Engl J Med 290:557, 1974

Dickinson JE, Eriksen NL, Meyer BA, et al: The effect of preterm birth on umbilical cord blood gases. Obstet Gynecol 79:575, 1992

Dildy GA, van den Berg PP, Katz M, et al: Intrapartum fetal pulse oximetry: Fetal oxygen saturation trends during labor and relation to delivery outcome. Am J Obstet Gynecol 171:679, 1994

Duerbeck NB, Chaffin DG, Seeds JW: A practical approach to umbilical artery pH and blood gas determinations. Obstet Gynecol 79:959, 1992

Eisenberg MS, Cummins RO, Ho MT: Code blue: Cardiac arrest and resuscitation. Philadelphia, Saunders, 1987, p 146

Fontaine P, Toffler WL: Dorsal penile nerve block for newborn circumcision. Am Fam Physician 43:1327, 1991

Freeman JM, Nelson KB: Intrapartum asphyxia and cerebral palsy. Pediatrics 82:240, 1988

Gaudier FL, Goldenberg RL, Nelson KG, et al: Acid–base status at birth and subsequent neurosensory impairment in surviving 500 to 1000 gm infants. Am J Obstet Gynecol 170:48, 1994

Gearhart JP, Rock JA: Total ablation of the penis after circumcision with electrocautery: A method of management and long-term follow-up. J Urol 142:799, 1989

Gilstrap LC, Cunningham FG: Umbilical cord blood acid–base analysis. In Cunningham FG, MacDonald PC, Gant NF, et al (eds): Williams Obstetrics, 19th ed (suppl 4). Norwalk, Conn, Appleton and Lange, 1994

Gilstrap LC III, Leveno KJ, Burris J, et al: Diagnosis of birth asphyxia on the basis of fetal pH, Apgar score, and newborn cerebral dysfunction. Am J Obstet Gynecol 161:825, 1989

Goldaber KG, Gilstrap LC III, Leveno KJ, et al: Pathologic fetal acidemia. Obstet Gynecol 78:1103, 1991

Guthrie R, Susi A: A simple phenylalanine method for detecting phenylketonuria in large populations of newborn infants. Pediatrics 32:338, 1963

Haddad B, Mercer BM, Livingston JC, et al: Outcome after successful resuscitation of babies born with Apgar scores of 0 at both 1 and 5 minutes. Am J Obstet Gynecol 182:1210, 2000

Hall MJ, Owings MF: 2000 National hospital discharge survey. Advance Data from Vital and Health Statistics; No. 329. Hyattsville, Md: National Center for Health Statistics, 2002

Hardwick-Smith S, Mastrobattista JM, Wallace PA, et al: Ring block for neonatal circumcision. Obstet Gynecol 91:930, 1998

Holman JR, Lewis EL, Ringler RL: Neonatal circumcision techniques. Am Fam Physician 52:511, 1995

Isenberg SJ, Apt L, Wood M: A controlled trial of povidone-iodine as prophylaxis against ophthalmia neonatorum. N Engl J Med 332:562, 1995

Janssen PA, Selwood BL, Dobson SR, et al: To dye or not to dye: A randomized clinical trial of a triple dye/alcohol regime versus dry cord care. Pediatrics 111:15, 2003

Kattwinkel J: Textbook of Neonatal Resuscitation, 4th ed. American Academy of Pediatrics and American Heart Association, 2000

Kaufman GE, Cimo S, Miller LW, et al: An evaluation of the effects of sucrose on neonatal pain with 2 commonly used circumcision methods. Am J Obstet Gynecol 186:564, 2002

Kette F, Weil MH, Gazmuri RJ: Buffer solutions may compromise cardiac resuscitation by reducing coronary perfusion pressure. JAMA 266:2121, 1991

Lander J, Brady-Fryer B, Metcalfe JB, et al: Comparison of ring block, dorsal penile nerve block, and topical anesthesia for neonatal circumcision: A randomized controlled trial. JAMA 278:2157, 1997

Lerman SE, Liao JC: Neonatal circumcision. Pediatr Clin North Am 48:1539, 2001

Lewis E, Shinefield HR, Woodruff BA, et al: Safety of neonatal hepatitis B vaccine administration. Pediatr Infect Dis J 20:1049, 2001

Lievaart M, deJong PA: Acid–base equilibrium in umbilical cord blood and time of cord clamping. Obstet Gynecol 63:44, 1984

Liu S, Wen SW, McMillan D, et al: Increased neonatal readmission rate associated with decreased length of hospital stay at birth in Canada. Can J Public Health 91:46, 2000

Low JA, Lindsay BG, Derrick EJ: Threshold of metabolic acidosis associated with newborn complications. Am J Obstet Gynecol 177:1391, 1997

Low JA, Panagiotopoulos C, Derrick EJ: Newborn complications after intrapartum asphyxia with metabolic acidosis in the preterm fetus. Am J Obstet Gynecol 172:805, 1995

Low JA, Panagiotopoulos C, Derrick EJ: Newborn complications after intrapartum asphyxia with metabolic acidosis in the term fetus. Am J Obstet Gynecol 170:1081, 1994

Malkin JD, Garber S, Broder MS, et al: Infant mortality and early postpartum discharge. Obstet Gynecol 96:183, 2000

March of Dimes: The ob/gyn's role in newborn screening. Contemp Ob/Gyn 67, July 2002

Martin JA, Hamilton BE, Sutton PD, et al: Births: Final data for 2002. National Vital Statistics Reports, Vol 52, No 10. Hyattsville, MD, National Center for Health Statistics, 2003

McGuire W, Fowlie PW: Naloxone for narcotic exposed newborn infants: Systematic review. Arch Dis Child Neonatal Ed 88:308, 2003

McIntire DD, Bloom SL, Casey BM, Leveno KJ: Birth weight in relation to morbidity and mortality among newborn infants. N Engl J Med 340:1234, 1999

Mosen DM, Clark SL, Mundorff MB, et al: The medical and economic impact of the newborns' and mothers' health protection act. Obstet Gynecol 99:116, 2002

Nelson KB, Ellenberg JH: Apgar scores as predictors of chronic neurologic disability. Pediatrics 68:36, 1981

Neulander E, Walfisch S, Kaneti J: Amputation of distal penile glans during neonatal ritual circumcision—a rare complication. Br J Urol 77:924, 1996

Newton CW, Mulnix N, Baer L, et al: Plain and buffered lidocaine for neonatal circumcision. Obstet Gynecol 93:350, 1999

Nicoll A: Routine male neonatal circumcision and risk of infection with HIV-1 and other sexually transmitted diseases. Arch Dis Child 77:194, 1997

Novack AH, Mueller B, Ochs H: Umbilical cord separation in the normal newborn. Am J Dis Child 142:220, 1988

Orozco-Sanchez J, Neri-Vela R: Total denudation of the penis in circumcision. Description of a plastic technique for repair of the penis. Bol Med Hosp Infant Mex 48:565, 1991

Pang JWY, Heffelfinger JD, Huang GJ, et al: Outcomes of planned home births in Washington state: 1989–1996. Obstet Gynecol 100:253, 2002

Ramin SM, Gilstrap LC, Leveno KJ, et al: Umbilical artery acid–base status in the preterm infant. Obstet Gynecol 74:256, 1989

Riley RJ, Johnson JWC: Collecting and analyzing cord blood gases. Clin Obstet Gynecol 36:13, 1993

Ross MG, Gala R: Use of umbilical artery base excess: Algorithm for the timing of hypoxic injury. Am J Obstet Gynecol 187:1, 2002

Saunders RA, Milner AD: Pulmonary pressure/volume relationships during the last phase of delivery and the first postnatal breaths in human subjects. J Pediatr 93:667, 1978

Schneider G: Silver nitrate prophylaxis. Can Med Assoc J 131:193, 1984

Schoen EJ, Baker JC, Colby CJ, et al: Cost-benefit analysis of universal tandem mass spectrometry for newborn screening. Pediatrics 110:781, 2002

Schoen EJ, Wiswell TE, Moses S: New policy on circumcision—cause for concern. Pediatrics 105:620, 2000

Siggaard-Anderson O: Blood acid–base alignment nomogram. Scand J Clin Laborat Invest 15:211, 1963

Socol ML, Garcia PM, Riter S: Depressed Apgar scores, acid–base status, and neurologic outcome. Am J Obstet Gynecol 170:991, 1994

Stang HJ, Gunnar MR, Snellman L, et al: Local anesthesia for neonatal circumcision: Effects on distress and cortisol response. JAMA 259:1507, 1988

Swaim LS: Circumcision. In Gilstrap LC, Cunningham FG, VanDorsten JP (eds): Operative Obstetrics, 2nd ed. New York, McGraw-Hill, 2002, p 657

Taddio A, Stevens B, Craig K, et al: Efficacy and safety of lidocaine-prilocaine cream for pain during circumcision. N Engl J Med 336:1197, 1997

Temkin E: Rooming-in: Redesigning hospitals and motherhood in cold war America. Bull Hist Med 76:271, 2002

Teoh D, Reynolds S: Diagnosis and management of pediatric conjunctivitis. Pediatr Emerg Care 19:48, 2003

Therrell BL Jr: U.S. newborn screening policy dilemmas for the twenty-first century. Mol Genet Metab 74:64, 2001

Thorngren-Jerneck K, Herbst A: Low 5-minute Apgar score: A population-based register study of 1 million term births. Obstet Gynecol 98:65, 2001

U.S. Department of Health and Human Services: Healthy people 2010, Vol II. Washington, DC, USDHHS, Objective 16–19, 2000

Upadhyay V, Hammodat HM, Pease PWB: Post circumcision meatal stenosis: 12 years' experience. N Z Med J 111:57, 1998

Wiswell TE: Neonatal resuscitation. Respir Care 48:288, 2003

Yeomans ER, Hauth JC, Gilstrap LC III, et al: Umbilical cord pH, PCO_2 and bicarbonate following uncomplicated term vaginal deliveries. Am J Obstet Gynecol 151:798, 1985

29

Diseases and Injuries of the Fetus and Newborn

The fetus and newborn infant are susceptible to a large number of diseases. Because many disorders have a different presentation and course in term as compared with preterm infants, these age groups are considered separately in this chapter. Illnesses or disorders that are the direct consequence of maternal disease are considered in other chapters pertinent to specific maternal illnesses. Because most perinatal infections arise as a result of maternal infection or colonization, they are considered in Chapters 58 and 59.

DISEASES OF THE PRETERM FETUS AND NEWBORN

RESPIRATORY DISTRESS SYNDROME. To provide blood gas exchange after birth, the infant's lungs must rapidly fill with air while being cleared of fluid, and the volume of blood that perfuses the lungs must increase remarkably. Some of the fluid is expressed as the chest is compressed during vaginal delivery, and the remainder is absorbed through the pulmonary lymphatics. Sufficient surfactant, synthesized by type II pneumocytes, is essential to stabilize the air-expanded alveoli by lowering surface tension and thereby preventing lung collapse during expiration (see Chap. 4, p. 109). If surfactant is inadequate, respiratory distress develops, and hyaline membranes form in the distal bronchioles and alveoli. Because of this, respiratory distress in the newborn is also termed *hyaline membrane disease.*

Respiratory distress syndrome (RDS) is generally a disease of preterm neonates, although it can occur in term newborns who have sepsis or meconium aspiration. In recent years, RDS has decreased as a cause of neonatal death in the United States as the result of surfactant therapy and administration of antenatal corticosteroids (Jobe, 2004; Martin, 2004). Boys are more likely to develop RDS than girls, and white infants appear to be more frequently and more severely affected than black infants.

Clinical Course. In typical RDS, tachypnea develops, the chest wall retracts, and expiration is accompanied by a grunt and flaring of the nostrils—a combination called *grunting and flaring.* Grunting is common in the newborn whenever there is uneven expansion of the lungs or lower airway obstruction. Shunting of blood through nonventilated lung areas contributes to hypoxemia and to metabolic and respiratory acidosis. Poor peripheral circulation and systemic hypotension may be evident. The chest radiograph shows a diffuse reticulogranular infiltrate with an air-filled tracheobronchial tree (air bronchogram).

Respiratory insufficiency also can be caused by sepsis, pneumonia, meconium aspiration, pneumothorax, persistent fetal circulation, heart failure, and malformations involving thoracic structures, such as diaphragmatic hernia. Recently, Shulenin and colleagues (2004) described surfactant deficiency due to a mutation of the *ABCA3* gene that is involved in surfactant production. Cardiac decompensation in the early newborn period also can have multiple causes, including patent ductus arteriosus and congenital cardiac malformations.

Pathology. Because of inadequate surfactant production, the alveoli are not stable and low pressures cause collapse on end expiration. Nutrition of the lung cells is compromised by hypoxia and systemic hypotension. There may be partial maintenance of the fetal circulation, leading to pulmonary hypertension and a relative right-to-left shunt. Eventually, there is ischemic necrosis of the cells lining the airway. When oxygen therapy is initiated, the pulmonary vascular bed dilates and the shunt (if there is one) reverses. Protein-filled fluid leaks into the alveolar ducts, and the cells lining the alveolar ducts slough. Hyaline membranes composed of fibrin-rich protein and cellular debris line the dilated alveoli and terminal bronchioles, and the epithelium underlying the membrane becomes necrotic.

Treatment. The most important factor influencing survival is admission to a neonatal intensive care unit, which dramatically reduces the number of RDS deaths. Although hypoxemia is indicative of the need for oxygen, excess oxygen can damage the pulmonary epithelium and retina.

Over the years, advances in mechanical ventilation technology have improved neonatal survival. For example, the development of *continuous positive airway pressure (CPAP)* brought about an appreciable reduction in the neonatal mortality rate by preventing the collapse of unstable alveoli and allowing high inspired-oxygen concentrations to be reduced, thereby minimizing toxicity. Disadvantages of CPAP include disturbance of the endothelium and epithelium—caused by overstretching and resulting in barotrauma—and impaired venous return (Verbrugge and Lachmann, 1999). *High-frequency oscillatory ventilation* reduces the risk of barotrauma by using a constant, low-distending pressure and small variations or oscillations to promote alveolar patency. This technique allows optimal lung volume to be maintained and CO_2 to be cleared without damaging alveoli. Although mechanical ventilation has undoubtedly improved survival, it is also an important factor in the genesis of *bronchopulmonary dysplasia* (see p. 651).

Postnatal glucocorticoids have been used for many years to prevent chronic lung disease in these infants. The American Academy of Pediatrics (2002) now recommends against their use because of adverse neuropsychological effects apparent by school age. Yeh and colleagues (2004) recently described significantly impaired motor and cognitive function and school performance in exposed neonates.

SURFACTANT TREATMENT. Administration of exogenous surfactant can prevent hyaline membrane disease. Commercially available preparations contain biological or animal surfactants such as human and bovine (Survanta), calf lung surfactant extract (Infasurf), porcine (Curosurf), or synthetic surfactant (Exosurf). Surfactant therapy has been credited for the largest drop in infant mortality observed in 25 years. It has been used for *prophylaxis* of preterm infants at risk for respiratory distress, as well as for *rescue* of those with established disease.

Jobe (1993) summarized the results of 35 randomized controlled studies of surfactant used for either prophylaxis or rescue therapy and found that it reduced the incidence of pneumothorax and death in the first 28 days of life by 31 to 39 percent. When antenatal corticosteroids and surfactant were given together, there was an even greater reduction in overall death rate and deaths due to respiratory distress syndrome. These findings were confirmed by Kari and associates (1994).

Complications. Persistent hyperoxia injures the lung, especially the alveoli and capillaries. High oxygen concentrations given at high pressures can cause *bronchopulmonary dysplasia,* or *oxygen toxicity lung disease.* This is a chronic condition in which alveolar and bronchiolar epithelial damage leads to hypoxia, hypercarbia, and oxygen dependence, followed by peribronchial and interstitial fibrosis. *Pulmonary hypertension* is another frequent complication. If hyperoxemia is sustained, the infant also is at risk of developing *retinopathy of prematurity,* formerly called *retrolental fibroplasia.* When any of these develop, the likelihood of subsequent neurosensory impairment is substantively increased (Schmidt and colleagues, 2003).

Prevention. With the possible exception of progesterone therapy, no method of prevention or treatment of preterm labor significantly reduces its incidence or improves any index of neonatal outcome (see Chap. 36, p. 869). The National Institutes of Health (1994) concluded that antenatal corticosteroid therapy reduced respiratory distress and intraventricular hemorrhage in preterm infants born between 24 and 32 weeks (see p. 653).

AMNIOCENTESIS FOR FETAL LUNG MATURITY. Delivery for fetal indications is necessary when the risks to the fetus from a hostile intrauterine environment are greater than the risk of respiratory distress, even if the fetus is preterm. If this degree of risk is not present and the criteria for elective delivery at term are not met, amniocentesis is used to confirm fetal lung maturity. The technique is similar to that described for second-trimester amniocentesis in Chapter 13 (see p. 328). Several methods can be used to determine the relative concentration of surfactant-active phospholipids:

1. *Lecithin–sphingomyelin (L/S) ratio.* Lecithin (dipalmitoyl phosphatidylcholine) plus phosphatidylinositol and especially phosphatidylglycerol are important in the formation and stabilization of the surface-active layer that prevents alveolar collapse and respiratory distress (see Chap. 4,

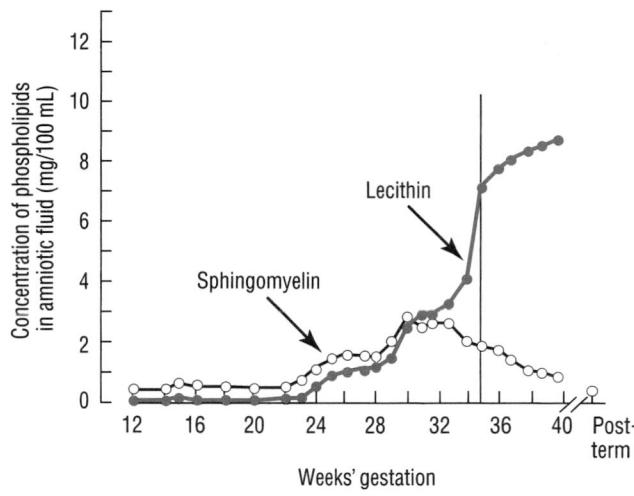

FIGURE 29–1. Changes in mean concentrations of lecithin and sphingomyelin in amnionic fluid during gestation in normal pregnancy. (From Gluck and Kulovich, 1973, with permission.)

p. 109). Before 34 weeks, lecithin and sphingomyelin are present in amnionic fluid in similar concentrations. At about 34 weeks, the concentration of lecithin relative to sphingomyelin begins to rise (Fig. 29–1).

Gluck and co-workers (1971) were the first to report that the risk of neonatal respiratory distress is slight whenever the concentration of lecithin is at least twice that of sphingomyelin (L/S ratio). Conversely, there is increased risk of respiratory distress when this ratio is below 2. Harper and Lorenz (1993) found an immature L/S ratio to be more predictive of the need for ventilatory support than gestational age or birthweight (Table 29–1). Because lecithin and sphingomyelin are found in blood and meconium, contamination with these substances may confound the results. Blood has an L/S ratio of 1.3 to 1.5, and meconium usually lowers the L/S ratio (Buhi and Spellacy, 1975).

2. *Phosphatidylglycerol.* With some pregnancy complications, respiratory distress may develop despite an L/S ratio greater than 2. With diabetes, for example, some clinicians use a number greater than 2 to define maturity or require the presence of phosphatidylglycerol (Ojomo and

TABLE 29–1 Respiratory Support Requirements Compared with Lecithin–Sphingomyelin (L/S) Ratios

L/S Ratio	Mechanical Ventilation (%)	Any Support (%)
<1.0	24	59
1.0–1.5	22	53
1.6–2.0	9	44
2.1–2.5	3	28

Modified from Harper and Lorenz (1993), with permission.

Coustan, 1990). Phosphatidylglycerol is believed to enhance the surface-active properties of lecithin and sphingomyelin (see Chap. 4, p. 109). Its identification in amnionic fluid provides more assurance, but not necessarily an absolute guarantee, that respiratory distress will not develop. Because phosphatidylglycerol is not detected in blood, meconium, or vaginal secretions, these contaminants do not confuse its interpretation.

3. *TDx-FLM.* This automated assay measures the surfactant-to-albumin ratio in uncentrifuged amnionic fluid and gives results in approximately 30 minutes. In a study of 374 consecutive amnionic fluid specimens, Steinfeld and associates (1992) reported that a TDx value of 50 or greater predicted fetal lung maturity in 100 percent of cases. Subsequent investigations by Hagen and associates (1993) and Herbert and co-workers (1993) found the TDx-FLM to be equal or superior to the L/S ratio, foam stability index, or phosphatidylglycerol assessment in predicting both positive and negative tests. Eriksen and associates (1996) reported that, in diabetic women, the TDx-FLM test has a sensitivity, specificity, and negative-predictive value for evaluating fetal lung maturity comparable to the L/S ratio. Many hospitals use the TDx-FLM as their first-line test of pulmonary maturity, followed by the L/S ratio in indeterminant samples.

4. *Other tests.* The *foam stability* or *shake test,* introduced by Clements and associates (1972), depends on the ability of surfactant in amnionic fluid, when mixed appropriately with ethanol, to generate stable foam at the air–liquid interface. Problems with the test include errors caused by slight contamination and frequent false-negative test results. The *Lumadex-FSI test, fluorescent polarization (microviscometry),* and *amnionic fluid absorbance at 650-nm wavelength* have all been used with variable success. The *lamellar body count* is a rapid, simple, and accurate method of assessing fetal lung maturity (Welsch and colleagues, 1996). Measurement of the amnionic fluid concentration of *dipalmitoylphosphatidylcholine (DPPC test)* also has been reported to be highly sensitive and specific for predicting respiratory distress (Alvarez and Ludmir, 1996).

RETINOPATHY OF PREMATURITY. Formerly known as *retrolental fibroplasia,* retinopathy of prematurity had become by 1950 the largest single cause of blindness in this country. After the discovery that the etiology of the disease was hyperoxemia, its frequency decreased remarkably.

The retina vascularizes centrifugally from the optic nerve starting at about the fourth month and continuing until shortly after birth. During the time of vascularization, excessive oxygen induces severe retinal vasoconstriction with endothelial damage and vessel obliteration, especially in the temporal portion. Neovascularization results, and the new vessels penetrate the retina and extend into the vitreous, where they are prone to leak proteinaceous material or burst with subsequent hemorrhage. Adhesions then form, which detach the retina. Precise levels of hyperoxemia that can be sustained without causing retinopathy are not known. That said, retinopathy is unlikely if inhaled air has no more than 40-percent oxygen content. Unfortunately, very immature infants who develop respiratory distress often require high oxygen concentrations to maintain life until respiratory function improves. Importantly, if vascular damage results, it increases threefold the likelihood of later death or neurological disability (Schmidt and co-workers, 2003).

INTRAVENTRICULAR HEMORRHAGE. There are four major categories of neonatal intracranial hemorrhage: *subdural hemorrhage* is usually the result of trauma. *Subarachnoid hemorrhage* and *intracerebellar hemorrhage* usually result from trauma in term infants but in preterm infants are commonly due to hypoxia. *Periventricular–intraventricular hemorrhage* results from either trauma or asphyxia in half of term infants but has no discernible cause in 25 percent of cases (Volpe, 1995). In preterm neonates, the pathogenesis of periventricular hemorrhage is multifactorial and includes hypoxic-ischemic events, anatomical factors, coagulopathy, and many others. The prognosis after hemorrhage depends on the location and extent of the bleeding. For example, subdural and subarachnoid hemorrhage often result in minimal, if any, neurological abnormalities. Bleeding into the parenchyma, however, can cause serious permanent damage.

Periventricular-Intraventricular Hemorrhage. When the fragile capillaries in the germinal matrix rupture, there is bleeding into surrounding tissues, which may extend into the ventricular system and brain parenchyma. Unfortunately, it is a common problem in preterm neonates, especially those born before 32 weeks. These lesions also can develop at later gestational ages and occasionally are seen in term neonates.

Most hemorrhages develop within 72 hours of birth, but they have been observed as late as 24 days (Perlman and Volpe, 1986). Almost half are clinically silent. Most small germinal matrix hemorrhages and those confined to the cerebral ventricles resolve without impairment (Weindling, 1995). Large lesions can result in hydrocephalus or *periventricular leukomalacia,* a correlate of cerebral palsy, discussed later. Because intraventricular hemorrhage usually is recognized within 3 days of delivery, its genesis is often erroneously attributed to birth events. It is important to realize that *prelabor* intraventricular hemorrhage also can occur (Achiron and associates, 1993; Nores and associates, 1996).

PATHOLOGY. The primary pathological process is damage to the germinal matrix capillary network, which predisposes to subsequent extravasation of blood into the surrounding tissue. In preterm infants, this capillary network is especially fragile for several reasons:

1. The subependymal germinal matrix provides poor support for the vessels coursing through it.
2. The venous anatomy in this region causes venous stasis and congestion, which makes the vessel susceptible to bursting with increased intravascular pressure.
3. Vascular autoregulation is impaired before 32 weeks (Volpe and Hill, 1987).

Even if extensive hemorrhage or other complications of preterm birth do not cause death, survivors can have major neurodevelopmental handicaps (Papile and co-workers, 1983). DeVries and colleagues (1985) attribute most long-term sequelae of intraventricular–periventricular hemorrhage to cystic areas called *periventricular leukomalacia*. These areas develop most commonly as a result of ischemia and least commonly in direct response to hemorrhage, and are discussed subsequently.

INCIDENCE AND SEVERITY. The incidence of ventricular hemorrhage depends on gestational age at birth. About half of all neonates born before 34 weeks but only 4 percent of those born at term will have some evidence of hemorrhage (Hayden and associates, 1985). Very-low-birthweight infants have the earliest onset of hemorrhage and the greatest likelihood of involvement of parenchymal tissue, and thus the highest mortality rate (Perlman and Volpe, 1986).

The severity of intraventricular hemorrhage can be assessed by ultrasound and computed tomography. Papile and colleagues (1978) devised the most widely used grading scheme to quantify the extent of the lesion and estimate prognosis:

- *Grade I*—hemorrhage limited to the germinal matrix.
- *Grade II*—intraventricular hemorrhage.
- *Grade III*—hemorrhage with ventricular dilatation.
- *Grade IV*—parenchymal extension of hemorrhage.

Jakobi and colleagues (1992) showed that infants with grade I or II intraventricular hemorrhage had over 90 percent survival rate with a 3.2-percent rate of handicap, the same as control infants of the same age but without hemorrhage. The survival rate for infants with grade III or IV hemorrhage, however, was only 50 percent. Vergani and co-workers (1996) confirmed that very preterm infants are at increased risk of sustaining severe intracranial hemorrhage. The latest figures from the Neonatal Research Network (Lemons and colleagues, 2001), indicate that 30 percent of infants born weighing 501 to 1500 g develop intracranial hemorrhage, with 11 percent of cases being grad III or IV.

CONTRIBUTING FACTORS. Events that predispose to germinal matrix hemorrhage and subsequent periventricular leukomalacia are multifactorial and complex. The preterm fetus has fragile intracranial blood vessels that make it particularly susceptible, and preterm birth is frequently associated with infection, which predisposes to tissue ischemia. Luthy and co-workers (1987) reported a threefold increased risk for grade III or IV hemorrhage when the cord arterial pH was less than 7.2. Respiratory distress syndrome and mechanical ventilation are commonly associated factors. Lesko and colleagues (1986) reported that heparin, often used to maintain vascular catheter patency in intensive care units, was associated with a fourfold increased risk of germinal matrix hemorrhage. In a review of 232 infants who weighed less than 1500 g, Wallin and co-workers (1990) reported that associated postnatal factors include respiratory distress and ventilator therapy.

PREVENTION AND TREATMENT. Administration of corticosteroids at least 24 hours before delivery appears to prevent or reduce the incidence and severity of intraventricular hemorrhage. In a consensus statement developed by a panel of the National Institutes of Health (1994), it was concluded that antenatal corticosteroid therapy reduced mortality, respiratory distress, and intraventricular hemorrhage in preterm infants born between 24 and 32 weeks, and that the benefits were additive with those from surfactant therapy. In addition, the consensus panel concluded that the benefits of antenatal steroid therapy probably extend to preterm premature membrane rupture. After a second Consensus Development Conference held by the National Institutes of Health (2000), it was concluded that repeated courses of antenatal steroids should not be given. Data were considered inadequate to prove any benefit or to document the safety of more than one course (see Chap. 36, p. 868).

The type of corticosteroid administered may be important. Although both betamethasone and dexamethasone cross the placenta in their active form, betamethasone has a longer half-life. This is because it has a larger volume of distribution and is cleared more slowly than dexamethasone (American College of Obstetricians and Gynecologists, 2002). Further, although both medications are associated with a reduced incidence of respiratory distress, only betamethasone has been shown to decrease mortality (Ballard and Ballard, 1995). Consistent with this finding, Cox and associates (1996) found no benefits of dexamethasone with regard to grade III or IV hemorrhage in preterm infants delivered at Parkland Hospital. In another study, Baud and colleagues (1999) found that *betamethasone* decreased the incidence of periventricular leukomalacia, but *dexamethasone* did not. Silver and associates (1996) reported that infants treated with antenatal dexamethasone and born before 30 weeks had fewer grade III and IV hemorrhages after treatment with surfactant, but the comparison group received placebo, not betamethasone.

The efficacy of phenobarbital, vitamin K, vitamin E, or indomethacin in diminishing the frequency and severity of intracranial hemorrhage, when administered either to the neonate or to the mother during labor, remains controversial (Chiswick and colleagues, 1991; Hanigan and colleagues, 1988; Thorp and colleagues, 1995). Data from a variety of sources suggest that magnesium sulfate may prevent the sequelae of periventricular hemorrhage, as discussed on page 658.

It is generally agreed that avoiding significant hypoxia both before and after preterm delivery is of paramount importance (Low and co-workers, 1995). There is presently no convincing evidence, however, that routine cesarean delivery for the preterm fetus presenting cephalic will decrease the incidence of periventricular hemorrhage (Strauss and colleagues, 1985; Tejani and co-workers, 1987; Welch and Bottoms, 1986). For example, Anderson and associates (1992) found no significant difference in the overall *frequency* of hemorrhage in infants whose birthweights were below 1750 g and who were delivered without labor compared with that of those delivered during latent or active labor. Infants delivered of mothers in active labor, however, tended to have more grade III or IV hemorrhages. In contrast, data presented by Ment and associates (1995) suggested a reduction in early intracranial hemorrhage with cesarean delivery.

NECROTIZING ENTEROCOLITIS. This newborn bowel disorder has clinical findings of abdominal distention, ileus, and bloody stools. There is usually radiological evidence of *pneumatosis intestinalis,* which is bowel wall gas formed by invading gas-forming bacteria. Bowel perforation may prompt resection.

The disease is seen primarily in low-birthweight infants but occasionally is encountered in mature neonates. Various causes hypothesized include perinatal hypotension, hypoxia, sepsis, umbilical catheterization, exchange transfusions, and the feeding of cow milk and hypertonic solutions (Kliegman and Fanaroff, 1984). All of these can ultimately lead to occlusive intestinal ischemia. Reperfusion injury also seems to play a role (Czyrko and associates, 1991). Because the disease tends to occur in clusters, some investigators believe that coronaviruses may have an etiological role.

BRAIN DISORDERS. Few events evoke more fear and apprehension in parents and obstetricians than the specter of "brain damage." This term immediately conjures visions of disabling cerebral palsy and hopeless mental retardation. Although most brain disorders or injuries are less horrific, they nevertheless are a major source of psychological and economic damage. The evolution of our understanding of this myriad of brain disorders was presaged by over a century of misconceptions that were accepted by science, medicine, and society.

In 1862, a London orthopedist, William Little, described 47 children with spastic rigidity and concluded that abnormalities of birth could be the cause. Notables such as Sigmund Freud (1897) challenged this view, having observed that abnormal birth processes frequently produced no effects. It was more than 100 years after Little's observations that research was begun in earnest to elucidate the pathophysiology of fetal and neonatal brain damage. The landmark observations of Nelson and Ellenberg (1986a) have subsequently led to the

acceptance—except by plaintiff attorneys—that only a relative few of such cases are caused at the time of birth, and that the majority are not preventable.

The persistence, for so many years, of the presumed birth-injury etiology for cerebral damage was one of the major reasons for the escalating rate of cesarean deliveries in the United States through the 1970s and 1980s. Because cause and effect were not related, this increase in cesarean deliveries did not result in any significant decline in the rate of cerebral palsy.

Brain disorders or damage, including the sequela of cerebral palsy, are a complex and multifactorial process caused by a combination of genetic, physiological, environmental, and obstetrical factors. For years the term *birth asphyxia,* indicating a neurological injury during birth, was applied to many infants inappropriately, however, objective definitions have subsequently evolved. To clarify the potential role of intrapartum events in causing permanent neurological injury, the American College of Obstetricians and Gynecologists (1998, 2004) developed a precise definition of birth asphyxia that includes all of these three:

1. Profound metabolic or mixed acidemia (pH of less than 7.0) determined on an umbilical cord arterial blood sample.
2. Persistent Apgar score of 0 to 3 for longer than 5 minutes.
3. Evidence of neonatal neurological sequelae such as seizures, coma, or hypotonia; or dysfunction of one or more of the following systems: cardiovascular, gastrointestinal, hematological, pulmonary, or renal.

When these three factors are associated with brain injury, they suggest that perinatal *hypoxic ischemic encephalopathy* developed. More importantly, their absence associated with brain injury helped to forge the crucial link between antepartum events that cause the majority of cases of cerebral palsy.

Neonatal Encephalopathy. The American College of Obstetricians and Gynecologists and the American Academy of Pediatrics (2003) recently convened a task force to review scientific data concerning *neonatal encephalopathy* and cerebral palsy. It defined neonatal encephalopathy as some combination of abnormal consciousness, tone, reflexes, feeding, respiration, or seizures in the term or near-term infant. The Task Force concluded that there were many different causes, which may or may not result in permanent sequelae—cerebral palsy being but one. Moreover, cerebral palsy can be attributed to an intrapartum event only if the affected child develops *hypoxic ischemic encephalopathy.* Further, of the several forms of cerebral palsy, only the spastic quadriplegic type can result from an acute interruption of blood supply prior to delivery. Hemiparetic or hemiplegic cerebral palsy, spastic diplegia, and ataxia are unlikely to result from an intrapartum event. Purely dyskinetic or ataxic cerebral palsy, especially when accompanied by a learning disorder, usually has a genetic origin (Nelson and Grether, 1998).

Although there is no doubt that some cases of cerebral palsy arise from intrapartum hypoxic–ischemic events, accumulated data indicate that 70 percent of all cases of neonatal encephalopathy result from an event that occurred *prior* to the onset of labor. To address this, the Task Force developed four essential criteria that, if all are present, define an acute intrapartum event sufficient to cause cerebral palsy:

1. Evidence of metabolic acidosis in fetal umbilical arterial blood obtained at delivery: pH of less than 7.0 and base deficit of at least 12 mmol/L.
2. Early onset of severe or moderate neonatal encephalopathy in infants born at 34 or more weeks.
3. Cerebral palsy of spastic quadriplegic or dyskinetic type.
4. Exclusion of other possible etiologies such as trauma, coagulation disorders, infections, or genetic disorders.

The Task Force also developed five criteria that, if occurring together, suggest that the supposed insult occurred within 0 to 48 hours of delivery:

1. A sentinel hypoxic event occurring immediately before or during labor.
2. Sudden and sustained fetal bradycardia or the absence of fetal heart rate variability in the presence of persistent, late, or variable decelerations, usually after a hypoxic sentinel event when the fetal heart rate pattern was previously normal.
3. Apgar scores of 0 to 2 beyond 5 minutes.
4. Onset of multisystem dysfunction within 72 hours of birth.
5. Early imaging study showing evidence of acute, nonfocal cerebral abnormality.

Gibbs and colleagues (2004) recently reviewed these criteria and offered 12 suggestions for implementation into practice in an obstetrical–neonatal unit.

Cerebral Palsy. This term refers to a group of conditions that are characterized by chronic movement or posture abnormalities, are cerebral in origin, arise early in life, and are nonprogressive (Nelson, 2003). Epilepsy and mental retardation frequently accompany cerebral palsy but usually are not associated with perinatal asphyxia in the absence of cerebral palsy.

Cerebral palsy is commonly classified by the type of neurological dysfunction (spastic, dyskinetic, or ataxic) as well as the number and distribution of limbs involved (quadriplegia, diplegia, hemiplegia, or monoplegia). The major types and frequencies of cerebral palsy are:

1. *Spastic quadriplegia,* which has a strong association with mental retardation and seizure disorders (20 percent).
2. *Diplegia,* which is common in preterm or low-birthweight infants (30 percent).
3. *Hemiplegia* (30 percent).
4. *Choreoathetoid types* (15 percent).

5. *Mixed varieties* (Freeman and Nelson, 1988; Rosen and Dickinson, 1992).

Significant mental retardation, defined as an intelligence quotient (IQ) of less than 50, is associated with 25 percent of cerebral palsy cases.

INCIDENCE AND EPIDEMIOLOGICAL CORRELATES. The incidence of cerebral palsy in developed countries is approximately 2 per 1000 live births (Clark and Hankins, 2003). Importantly, this rate either has remained essentially unchanged or has increased since the 1950s (Freeman and Nelson, 1988; Torfs and colleagues, 1990). In some countries, the incidence has risen because advances in the care of very preterm infants have improved their survival, but with significant handicap (Stanley and Blair, 1991). From their review of 11 studies published from 1985 through 1990, Rosen and Dickinson (1992) reported that the average cumulative rate for cerebral palsy at ages 5 to 7 years was 2.7 per 1000 live births. For infants less than 2500 g, this rate was 15 per 1000; for survivors who weighed 500 to 1500 g at birth, the rate was 13 to 90 per 1000.

Nelson and Ellenberg (1984, 1985, 1986a, 1986b) have made important contributions to our understanding of cerebral palsy. Their studies included data from the Collaborative Perinatal Project, which followed offspring of almost 54,000 pregnancies until age 7. They found that the important antecedents and most commonly associated risk factors for cerebral palsy were (1) evidence of genetic abnormalities, such as maternal mental retardation, fetal microcephaly, and fetal congenital malformations; (2) birthweight less than 2000 g; (3) gestational age at birth less than 32 weeks; and (4) infection. Obstetrical complications were not strongly predictive of cerebral palsy, and indeed, only about 20 percent of affected children had markers of perinatal asphyxia. By contrast, over half had associated congenital malformations, low birthweight, microcephaly, or another explanation for the brain disorder. They concluded that the causes of most cases of cerebral palsy were unknown, and that no foreseeable single intervention would likely prevent a large proportion of cases.

Torfs and associates (1990) reported similar findings in 0.3 percent of over 19,000 children from the California Child Health and Development Studies database who were diagnosed with cerebral palsy. Of these 55 children, 25 percent had neural-tube defects or obvious postnatal causes such as infection or injury. The 22 percent with cerebral palsy who had "perinatal asphyxia," defined erroneously as a time-to-cry interval longer than 5 minutes, also had birth defects, gestational risk factors, or both. The strongest predictors of cerebral palsy included a congenital anomaly, low birthweight, low placental weight, or abnormal fetal position such as face presentation, breech, or transverse lie. The latter is often associated with neurological abnormality. These factors were similar to those identified in the Collaborative Perinatal Project (Table 29–2). Interestingly, low-, mid-, or even high-forceps

TABLE 29–2 Prenatal and Perinatal Risk Factors in Children with Cerebral Palsy

Risk Factors	Risk Ratio	95% CI
Long menstrual cycle (> 36 days)[a]	9.0	2.2–37.1
Hydramnios[a]	6.9	1.0–49.3
Premature placental separation[a]	7.6	2.7–21.1
Intervals between pregnancies < 3 mo or > 3 yr	3.7	1.0–4.4
Birthweight < 2000 g[a]	4.2	1.8–10.2
Breech, face, or transverse lie[a]	3.8	1.6–9.1
Severe birth defect[a]	5.6	8.1–30.0
Nonsevere birth defect	6.1	3.1–11.8
Time to cry more than 5 min[a]	9.0	4.3–18.8
Low placental weight[a]	3.6	1.5–8.4

CI = confidence interval.
[a] Also associated with cerebral palsy in the Collaborative Perinatal Project (Nelson and Ellenberg, 1985, 1986a, 1986b). Adapted from Torfs and associates (1990), with permission.

or cesarean delivery did not correlate with cerebral palsy. Similarly, the Maternal Fetal Medicine Units (MFMU) Network studied nearly 800 infants with birthweights less than 1000 g and showed that only low birthweight and early gestational age correlated with neonatal neurological morbidity (Goepfert and associates, 1996).

Intrapartum Events. The Task Force on Neonatal Encephalopathy determined that only 1.6 cases of cerebral palsy per 10,000 deliveries are attributable solely to intrapartum hypoxia. This finding is supported by many studies. For example, Stanley and Blair (1991) performed a case-control study of all cases of cerebral palsy in Western Australia from 1975 to 1980. They reported that in 92 percent of cases, intrapartum injury as the cause of cerebral palsy was unlikely; in 3.3 percent, it was possible; and in only 4.9 percent was it likely. Phelan and associates (1996) by review of fetal monitor tracings evaluated 209 cases of neonatal neurological impairment and classified 75 percent as nonpreventable.

Consistent with this, data from a variety of sources indicate that continuous electronic fetal monitoring in labor neither predicts nor reduces the risk of cerebral palsy when compared with intermittent auscultation (Clark and Hankins, 2003; Grant and associates, 1989; MacDonald and associates, 1985; Thacker and colleagues, 1995). It was concluded by the American College of Obstetricians and Gynecologists (1995) that "a substantial body of evidence disproves the hypothesis that electronic fetal monitoring would reduce long-term neurological impairment and cerebral palsy in newborns so monitored."

Importantly, there does not appear to be any specific fetal heart rate pattern that predicts cerebral palsy, and a number of studies have found no relationship between the clinician's response to abnormal fetal heart rate patterns and neurological outcome (Melone and associates, 1991; Nelson and co-workers, 1996; Niswander and colleagues, 1984). In fact, an abnormal heart rate pattern in fetuses who ultimately develop cerebral palsy may reflect preexisting neurological abnormality and not ongoing, remedial injury (Phelan and Ahn, 1994). This, in part, accounts for the unchanged incidence of cerebral palsy in the United States, despite a fivefold increase in the cesarean delivery rate since 1965.

Apgar Scores. A variety of data show that Apgar scores alone are generally poor predictors of neurological impairment. Nelson and Ellenberg (1984) studied the interaction between obstetrical complications and a low Apgar score and reported that, in the absence of complications, low Apgar scores alone were not associated with a high level of risk. However, in infants who had 5-minute Apgar scores of 3 or less along with a complicated birth, the incidence of cerebral palsy was increased appreciably. Dijxhoorn and colleagues (1986) reported similar findings. The American College of Obstetricians and Gynecologists (1996) concluded that low Apgar scores at 1 and 5 minutes identify infants who need resuscitation, but that low Apgar scores alone are not evidence for hypoxia sufficient to result in neurological damage (see Chap. 28, p. 637).

Umbilical Cord Blood Gas Studies. As summarized in Chapter 28 (see p. 638), an important part of the definition of neonatal asphyxia is metabolic acidosis. In its absence, significant intrapartum hypoxia or asphyxia generally is excluded. However, when used alone, umbilical cord acid–base determinations have proven no more helpful than the 1- and 5-minute Apgar scores in predicting long-term neurological sequelae. Dijxhoorn and associates (1986) studied 805 term newborns delivered vaginally. They reported that the largest number of neurologically abnormal infants had low Apgar scores but a normal cord arterial pH, indicating that intrapartum hypoxia was not the major cause of neurological morbidity. Other investigators have reported that neither pH measurements nor acidemia alone correlate with long-term neurological outcome in term infants (American College of Obstetricians and Gynecologists, 1992; Fee and associates, 1990).

Data from several studies indicate that a pH of less than 7.0 is the cutoff for clinically significant acidemia (Gilstrap and associates, 1989; Goldaber and associates, 1991). In a later study of more than 150,000 liveborn infants, Casey and co-workers (2001) used umbilical artery pH to assess predictability of neonatal death within 28 days. As the pH fell to 7.0 or less, the likelihood of neonatal death escalated, increasing 1400-fold with a cord pH of 6.8 or lower in term newborns. When the cord pH was 7.0 or less and the 5-minute Apgar score was 0 to 3, the relative risk of neonatal death was 3204!

Nucleated Red Blood Cells. These immature red cells enter the circulation in response to hypoxia or hemorrhage. Their quantification has been proposed as a measure of hypoxia. And, because increased production of nucleated red cells takes place over time, it has been suggested that these counts can be used to measure the duration of hypoxia (Korst and associates, 1996; Naeye and Localio, 1995). Others have not been able to reproduce these findings. Salafia and colleagues (1996) studied 465 preterm newborns and found no correlation between nucleated red cells and hypoxia. Instead, they found these cells to be hematological markers associated with maternal, placental, and newborn infection. Hankins and co-workers (2002) studied 46 fetuses with acute peripartum asphyxia sufficient to result in neonatal encephalopathy. They found that nucleated red cells were elevated in only 41 percent. As summarized by the Task Force on Neonatal Encephalopathy and Cerebral Palsy, the significance of both nucleated erythrocytes and lymphocytes as a marker for hypoxic injury is currently imprecise and unclear.

PERIVENTRICULAR LEUKOMALACIA. This pathological description refers to cystic areas deep in brain white matter that develop after hemorrhagic and ischemic infarction. Tissue ischemia leads to regional necrosis, and because brain tissue does not regenerate, these irreversibly damaged areas appear as echolucent cysts on neuroimaging studies. They generally require at least 2 weeks to develop and have been reported to develop up to 104 days after the initial insult (Goetz and colleagues, 1995). Accordingly, the presence of these cystic areas at birth may help to determine the timing of the hemorrhagic event (Hayakawa and co-workers, 1999).

A variety of clinical and pathological data link severe intraventricular hemorrhage—grade III or IV—and resulting periventricular leukomalacia to cerebral palsy. Grade I or II hemorrhages usually resolve without extensive tissue injury. Luthy and colleagues (1987) reported a 16-fold increased risk of cerebral palsy for low-birthweight infants who had grade III or IV hemorrhage compared with that in infants who had either none or grade I or II hemorrhage. Allan and co-workers (1997) found that the highest rates of cerebral palsy in 505 infants with birthweights between 600 and 1250 g were associated with periventricular leukomalacia (37 percent) and ventriculomegaly (30 percent). DeVries and colleagues (1993) followed 504 infants born at 34 weeks or less. At least two thirds had localized cystic periventricular leukomalacia, and 100 percent of those with extensive cystic areas developed cerebral palsy. Conversely, only 11 percent of those with transient cysts developed cerebral palsy. Hsu and colleagues (1996) showed that the size of the cyst(s) correlates directly with the risk for cerebral palsy. Fujimoto and colleagues (1994) demonstrated that symmetrical cystic lesions convey the highest risk.

Periventricular leukomalacia is more strongly linked to infection and inflammation than to intraventricular hemorrhage. Zupan and colleagues (1996) studied 753 infants born between 24 and 32 weeks, 9 percent of whom developed periventricular leukomalacia. Those born before 28 weeks, or who had inflammatory events during the last days to weeks before delivery, or both, were at highest risk. Perlman and

co-workers (1996) found that periventricular leukomalacia was strongly associated with prolonged membrane rupture, chorioamnionitis, and neonatal hypotension. Spinillo and colleagues (1995, 1998) found a strong association between leukomalacia and a variety of factors, including first-trimester hemorrhage, smoking, urinary infection in labor, preterm labor, low birthweight, neonatal acidosis, meconium staining, and ritodrine therapy for more than 72 hours.

Periventricular Leukomalacia in the Preterm Fetus. Consideration of brain development explains why very preterm infants are most susceptible to intraventricular hemorrhage and periventricular leukomalacia. Before 32 weeks, the vascular anatomy of the brain is composed of two systems, one that penetrates into the cortex—the *ventriculopedal system*—and another that reaches down to the ventricles, but then curves to flow outward—the *ventriculofugal system* (Weindling, 1995). There are no vascular anastomoses connecting these two systems. As a result, the area between these systems, through which the pyramidal tracts pass near the lateral cerebral ventricles, is a watershed area vulnerable to ischemia. Vascular insufficiency before 32 weeks leading to ischemia would affect this watershed area first, and resulting damage of the pyramidal tracts would cause spastic diplegia. After 32 weeks, vascular flow shifts toward the cortex. Thus, hypoxic injury after this time primarily damages the cortical region.

PERINATAL INFECTION. Fetal infection may be the key element in the pathway between preterm birth, intracranial hemorrhage, periventricular leukomalacia, and cerebral palsy (Dammann and Leviton, 1997; Yoon and colleagues, 1997a, 2000, 2001). In the pathway proposed in Figure 29–2, antenatal reproductive tract infection evokes the production of cytokines such as tumor necrosis factor and interleukins-1, -6, and -8. These in turn stimulate prostaglandin production and preterm labor (see Chap. 36, p. 859). Preterm intracranial blood vessels are susceptible to rupture and damage, and the cytokines that stimulate preterm labor also have direct toxic effects on oligodendrocytes and myelin. Vessel rupture, tissue hypoxia, and cytokine-mediated damage result in massive cell death. Glutamate is released, stimulating membrane receptors to allow excess calcium to enter the neurons. High intracellular calcium levels are toxic to white matter, and glutamate may be directly toxic to oligodendroglia (Levene, 1992; Oka and associates, 1993).

Many studies have shown that infection and cytokines can damage the immature brain. Yoon and colleagues (1997a) have shown that inoculation of rabbit embryos with *E coli* causes histological damage in white matter. In another study, these investigators showed that tumor necrosis factor and interleukin-6 were more frequently found in the brains of infants who died with periventricular leukomalacia (Yoon and co-workers, 1997b). Cytokines are strongly linked to white matter lesions even when organisms cannot be demonstrated. In a study of 123 preterm infants, Yoon and colleagues (2000)

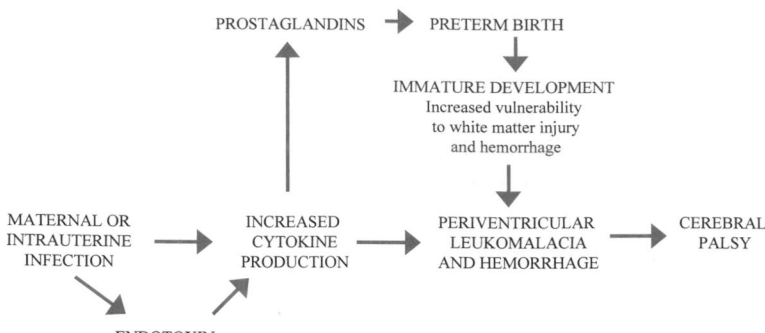

FIGURE 29–2. Schematic representation of the hypothesized pathway between maternal or intrauterine infection, preterm birth, and cerebral palsy. (Courtesy of Dr. Robert Goldenberg.)

demonstrated that only 45 percent of amnionic fluid samples from infants who ultimately developed cerebral palsy contained microorganisms. These same fluids had abnormally elevated levels of interleukin-6 and interleukin-8 in 85 percent of cases.

Infection is important, even when separated from preterm birth. Verma and colleagues (1997) compared 285 infants born after preterm labor and 279 infants born after preterm prematurely ruptured membranes with 149 infants who were delivered preterm for other reasons. The incidence and severity of intraventricular hemorrhage and periventricular leukomalacia were highest in those infants with spontaneous labor or membrane rupture, and were increased even more with chorioamnionitis. Grether and Nelson (1997) performed a population-based case-control study of cerebral palsy in affected children whose birthweight was over 2500 g and who had no congenital brain malformations or genetic abnormalities. They found a ninefold increased risk of cerebral palsy after either intrapartum maternal fever or chorioamnionitis, and a 19-fold risk if there was neonatal infection.

Wu and co-workers (2003) recently described a nested case-control study of over 231,500 singleton infants born at 36 weeks or more. They reported a fourfold increased risk of cerebral palsy if clinical chorioamnionitis was identified. Other independent risk factors were growth restriction (fourfold), black ethnicity (3.6-fold), maternal age over 25 years (2.6-fold), and nulliparity (1.8-fold).

PREVENTION. In preterm infants, corticosteroid therapy may reduce the incidence of intraventricular hemorrhage (see p. 653). In addition, prophylaxis or aggressive treatment of infection may protect against neurological injury. Magnesium sulfate is currently being investigated as another neuroprotective agent. In adults, it has been shown to stabilize intracranial vascular tone, minimize fluctuations in cerebral blood flow, reduce reperfusion injury, and block calcium-mediated intracellular damage (Marret and associates, 1995). Magnesium reduces synthesis of cytokines and bacterial endotoxins and thus also may minimize the inflammatory effects of infection (Grether and Nelson, 1997).

Epidemiological evidence suggests that maternal magnesium sulfate therapy has a fetal neuroprotective effect (Schendel and co-workers, 1996). Some have concluded that this effect may be limited to fetuses delivered early for preeclampsia (Grether and colleagues, 2000). In contrast, however, a recent Australian randomized trial of magnesium sulfate given to 1047 women delivering spontaneously before 30 weeks showed that magnesium exposure improved some perinatal outcomes (Crowther and colleagues, 2003). Although the incidence of both neonatal death and cerebral palsy were improved, the study was not sufficiently powered to make these differences statistically significant. As emphasized by Tyson and Gilstrap (2003), although the 17-percent reduction in death and cerebral palsy reported in this study is encouraging, magnesium for these purposes is still investigational. An ongoing trial conducted by the MFMU Network is the *BEAM (Beneficial Effects of Antenatal Magnesium Sulfate) study* (http://www.nichd.nih.gov/about/womenhealth/premature_birth.cfm).

NEURORADIOLOGICAL IMAGING. Computed tomographic (CT) and magnetic resonance imaging (MRI) scans have been used in older children to define the timing of cerebral injury. Wiklund and colleagues (1991a, 1991b) studied children between 5 and 16 years of age with hemiplegic cerebral palsy, 28 of whom were born preterm and 83 born at term. Only 25 percent of these children had CT findings that were considered normal. In those who had been delivered at term, periventricular atrophy was present in 37 percent and maldevelopment in 17 percent, thus suggesting a *prenatal* injury in over half of cases. In contrast, as many as 70 percent of those delivered preterm had findings that confirmed an insult in early *postnatal* life. Cortical and subcortical injury suggestive of a perinatal injury was found in 19 percent.

Nelson and Lynch (2004) recommend MRI to best identify and characterize neonatal strokes. Truwit and colleagues (1992) performed MRI scans in 40 patients with cerebral palsy. The predominant finding in 80 percent of those born preterm was evidence of periventricular white matter damage. This indicated hypoxic ischemic injury, although its exact chronology was difficult to determine. In contrast, 50 percent of those born at term had findings consistent with antenatal brain damage, including polymicrogyria consistent with midpregnancy injury, and isolated periventricular leukomalacia. In 25 percent of these cases, MRI findings, coupled with

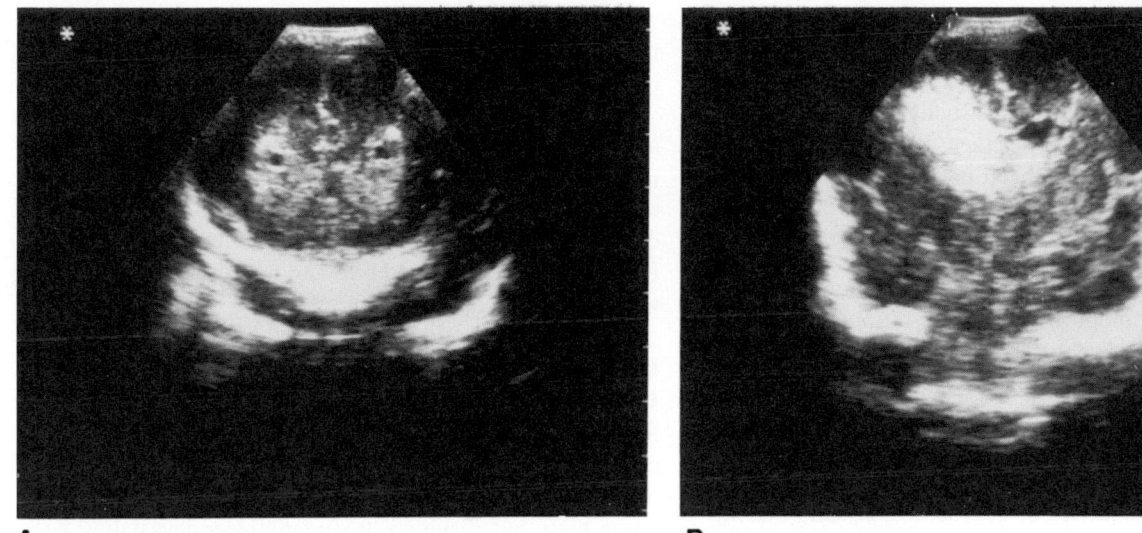

FIGURE 29–3. Preterm infant delivered at 27 weeks because of placental abruption. **A.** Ultrasound scan of the head performed on the first postnatal day shows small bilateral cysts in the periventricular white matter and bilateral germinal-matrix hemorrhages. These findings indicate a much older lesion than one caused by perinatal asphyxia. **B.** Repeat ultrasound of the same infant on day 3 of life showed bilateral intraventricular hemorrhage and a large intraparenchymal echodensity on the right. (Courtesy of Dr. Jeffrey Perlman.)

clinical events, were suggestive of hypoxic ischemic injury at birth.

Cranial ultrasound also provides useful information. The development of periventricular leukomalacia is shown in Figure 29–3. In this case, because cysts take days to weeks to develop, an ultrasound examination performed on day 1 was critical in diagnosing *antenatal* brain injury. Intraventricular hemorrhage was found to be a secondary insult that developed in the nursery. Sometimes head ultrasound reveals findings different but complementary to those of CT scanning. A grade III intraventricular hemorrhage diagnosed at birth by CT scan is shown in Figure 29–4A. A cranial ultrasound examination

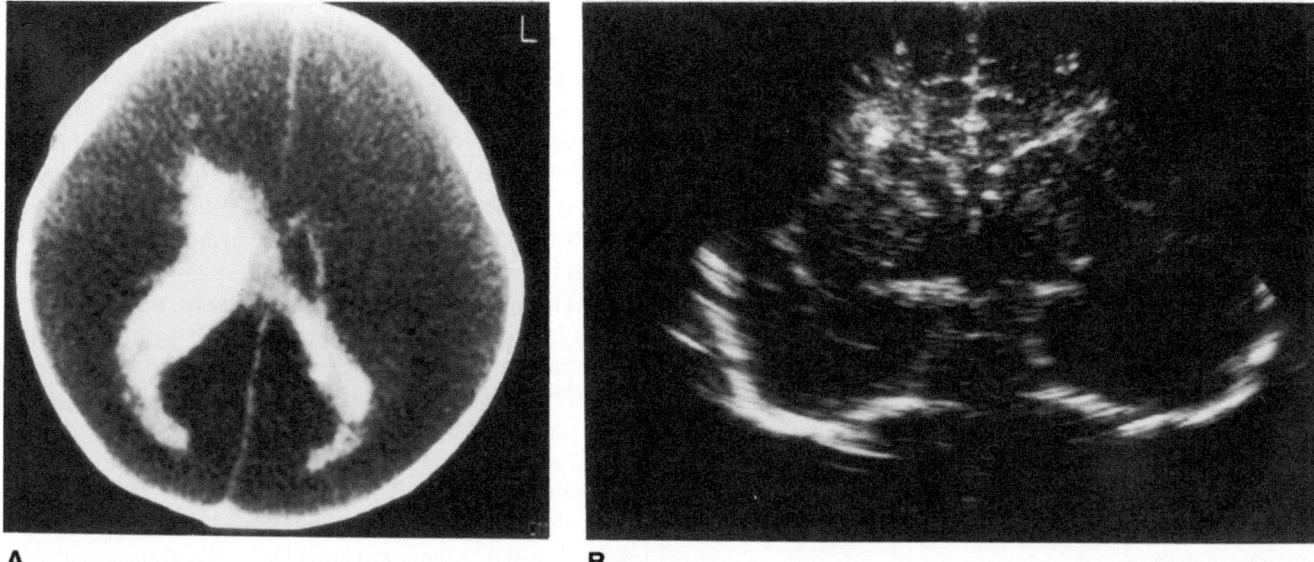

FIGURE 29–4. This term infant was born depressed. **A.** Computed tomographic (CT) scan demonstrates a grade III intraventricular hemorrhage. **B.** Ultrasound scan confirmed intraventricular hemorrhage and in addition, bilateral cystic periventricular leukomalacia was seen, which was not observed on the CT scan. These findings documented a severe antenatal brain insult of 4 to 5 weeks' duration. (From Perlman and Cunningham, 1993.)

done the same day, however, also identified periventricular leukomalacia, thus documenting injury well before birth (Fig. 29–4B).

Neonatal MRI also has been instructive (Battin and associates, 1998; Fedrizzi and colleagues, 1996; Okumura and colleagues, 1997). It also has been used to help determine the most likely time of brain insult in children with cerebral palsy (Jaw and co-workers, 1998).

NEONATAL ENCEPHALOPATHY IN TERM INFANTS. Mature infants also can suffer neurological insults, resulting in permanent compromise. As discussed on page 654, neonatal encephalopathy is a defined syndrome of disturbed neurological function consisting of difficulty in initiating and maintaining respiration, depressed tone and reflexes, subnormal level of consciousness, and frequently seizures. It generally is believed to be the consequence of a hypoxic-ischemic insult, although the timing of the insult is not always known. *Mild encephalopathy* is generally defined as hyperalertness, irritability, jitteriness, and hypertonia and hypotonia; *moderate encephalopathy* includes lethargy, severe hypertonia, and occasional seizures; and *severe encephalopathy* is defined by coma, multiple seizures, and recurrent apnea.

Severe encephalopathy is a more important predictor of cerebral palsy and future cognitive defects than either mild or moderate types (Robertson and Finer, 1985). Poor postnatal brain growth is an early sign of neurological compromise. In one study, Cordes and colleagues (1994) performed serial head circumference measurements of 54 term infants with hypoxic-ischemic encephalopathy. They found that a decrease in the expected head circumference of more than 3.1 percent in the first 4 months of life predicted microcephaly. Permanent impairment was predictable with 90 percent specificity.

MENTAL RETARDATION. Severe mental retardation has a prevalence of 3 per 1000 children. Etiological factors are shown in Table 29–3. Some genetic causes are discussed in Chapter

TABLE 29–3 Some Etiological Factors for Severe Mental Retardation

Factor	Percent
Prenatal	73
Chromosomal	36
Mutant genes	7
Multiple congenital anomalies	20
Acquired infections, diabetes, growth restriction	10
Perinatal	10
Asphyxia or hypoxia	5
Unidentified causes	5
Postnatal	11
Unknown	6

Modified from Rosen and Hobel (1986), with permission.

12. Isolated mental retardation, without epilepsy or cerebral palsy, is associated with perinatal hypoxia in very few cases (Nelson and Ellenberg, 1984, 1985, 1986a, 1986b).

SEIZURE DISORDERS. Although these may accompany cerebral palsy, isolated seizure disorders or epilepsy usually are not caused by perinatal hypoxia. Nelson and Ellenberg (1986b) determined that the major predictors of seizure disorders were fetal malformations—cerebral and noncerebral, family history of seizures, and neonatal seizures.

INFANT OUTCOME IN EXTREME PREMATURE BIRTH. All of the concerns previously described are amplified in infants born at 22 to 25 weeks. Currently, depending on many factors, this gestational age range is considered the limit of viability. Not only is the mortality rate in this age group high, but survivors frequently have devastating neurological, ophthalmological, gastrointestinal, or pulmonary injury. The largest study to date of such infants was conducted by the National Institutes of Health–sponsored Human Development Neonatal Research Network (Lemons and colleagues, 2001). Investigators from 14 tertiary care centers collected data from 1995 and 1996 on 4438 infants who weighed 501 to 1500 grams at birth. The study was limited to liveborn infants and therefore, likely underestimated mortality at the lowest gestational ages. Infants were followed only to hospital discharge. Of the entire cohort, 71 percent were exposed to antenatal steroids and 62 percent to antenatal antimicrobials. After delivery, half were treated with surfactant therapy and one fourth were given corticosteroids for lung disease.

This study provides the most accurate, current data on the outcome of extremely preterm infants. Not surprisingly, the chance of survival until discharge was directly proportional to both gestational age at birth and birthweight (Figs. 29–5 and 29–6). For example, only 25 percent of infants born at 21 to 23 weeks survived, whereas more than 90 percent of those born at 28 weeks or later survived. Also, the incidence of long-term morbidity, including chronic lung disease, grade III or IV intracranial hemorrhage, and necrotizing enterocolitis, was inversely proportional to birthweight and age (Table 29–4). The incidence of chronic morbidity decreased from 63 percent in survivors who weighed 501 to 750 grams at birth, to less than 10 percent in those weighing 1250 to 1500 grams. Hoekstra and co-workers (2004) studied long-term outcomes in 675 survivors born between 23 and 26 weeks. They identified intraventricular hemorrhage and chronic lung disease as being important markers for poor outcomes.

Information on the long-term outcome of similar very-low-birthweight infants was provided by Wood and associates (2000). These investigators followed 283 of 308 survivors born at 25 or fewer completed weeks. Formal assessment at a median of 30 months showed that half had neurological disability. In half of these cases—or 25 percent of the total group—the disability was severe.

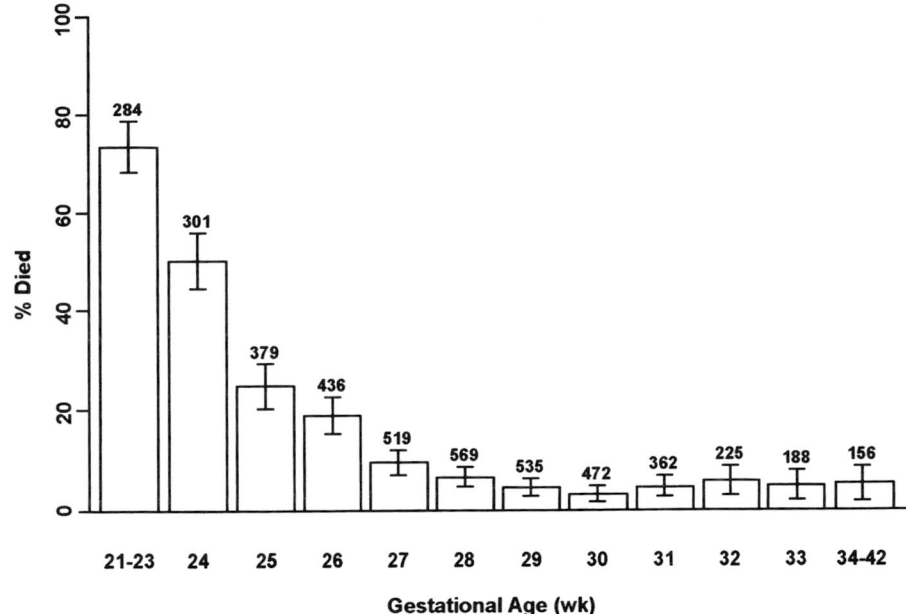

FIGURE 29–5. Mortality before discharge by gestational age among infants born in Neonatal Research Network Centers during 1995 and 1996. Data are expressed as a percentage of infants who died, and 95-percent confidence intervals are shown between bars for each group. (From Lemons and colleagues, 2001, with permission.)

ANEMIA. After 35 weeks, the mean cord hemoglobin concentration is about 17 g/dL and values below 14 g/dL are abnormal. During the first several hours of life, the hemoglobin value may rise by as much as 20 percent due to delayed cord clamping, resulting in an appreciable volume of blood being expressed from the placenta through the cord into the infant. Alternatively, if the placenta is cut or torn, a fetal vessel is perforated or lacerated, or the infant is held well above the level of the placenta for some time before cord clamping, the hemoglobin concentration may fall after delivery.

Fetal-to-Maternal Hemorrhage. Fetal red cells in the maternal circulation can be identified by use of the acid elution principle first described by Kleihauer, Brown, and Betke,

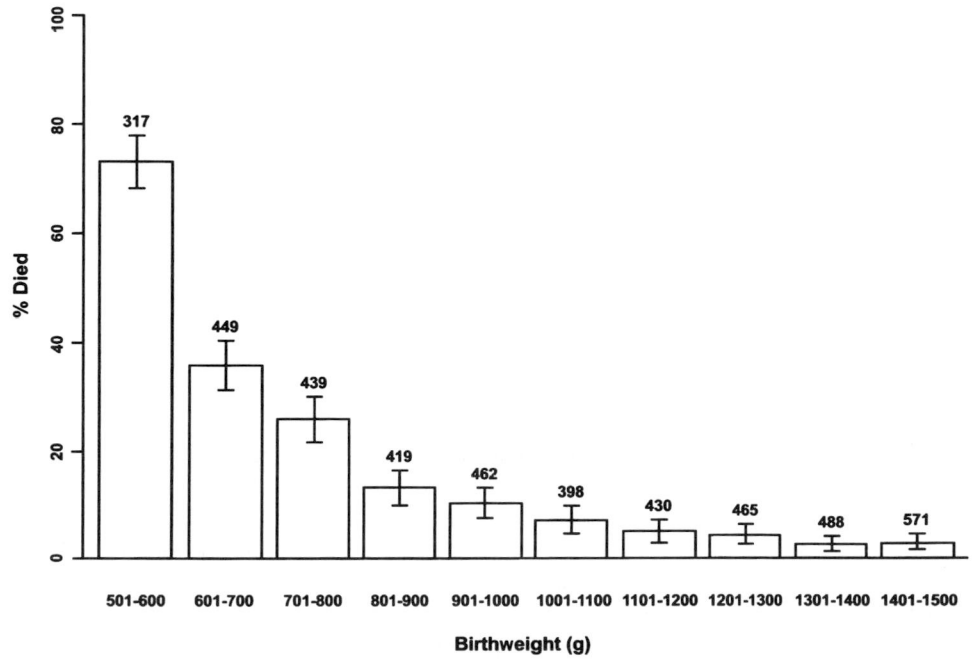

FIGURE 29–6. Mortality before discharge by birthweight among infants born in Neonatal Research Network Centers during 1995 and 1996. Data are expressed as a percentage of infants who died, and 95-percent confidence intervals are shown between bars for each 100-g interval. (From Lemons and co-workers, 2001, with permission.)

TABLE 29–4 Birthweight-Specific Survival and Selected Neonatal Morbidity Among Survivors Born in the NICHD Neonatal Research Network During 1995 and 1996

Factor	Birthweight Categories[a]				
	501–750 g (n = 1002)	751–1000 g (n = 1084)	1001–1250 g (n = 1053)	1251–1500 g (n = 1299)	501–1500 g (n = 4438)
Survivors	540 (54)	935 (86)	992 (94)	1257 (97)	3724 (84)
Survived without morbidity	199 (37)	540 (58)	766 (77)	1132 (90)	2637 (71)
Survived with morbidity	341 (63)	395 (42)	226 (23)	125 (10)	1087 (29)
CLD[b]	189 (35)	245 (26)	121 (12)	71 (6)	626 (17)
Severe ICH[c]	33 (6)	47 (5)	46 (5)	22 (2)	148 (4)
NEC[d]	22 (4)	30 (3)	32 (3)	23 (2)	107 (3)
CLD/severe ICH	56 (10)	39 (4)	19 (2)	6 (0.5)	120 (3)
CLD/NEC	25 (4.6)	26 (2.8)	6 (0.6)	3 (0.2)	60 (1.6)
NEC/severe ICH	9 (1.7)	5 (0.5)	2 (0.2)	0 (0.0)	16 (0.4)
CLD/severe ICH/NEC	7 (1.3)	3 (0.3)	0 (0.0)	0 (0.0)	10 (0.3)

NICHD = National Institute of Child Health and Human Development.
[a]Data expressed as number of infants with percentages in parentheses.
[b]CLD = chronic lung disease at 36 weeks' postmenstrual age.
[c]ICH = intracranial hemorrhage (grades III and IV).
[d]NEC = necrotizing enterocolitis (Bell classification stage ≥ 2).
From Lemons and co-workers (2001), with permission.

or any of several modifications. Fetal erythrocytes contain hemoglobin F, which is more resistant to acid elution than hemoglobin A. After exposure to acid, only fetal hemoglobin remains. Fetal red cells can then be identified by uptake of a special stain and quantified on a peripheral smear (Fig. 29–7).

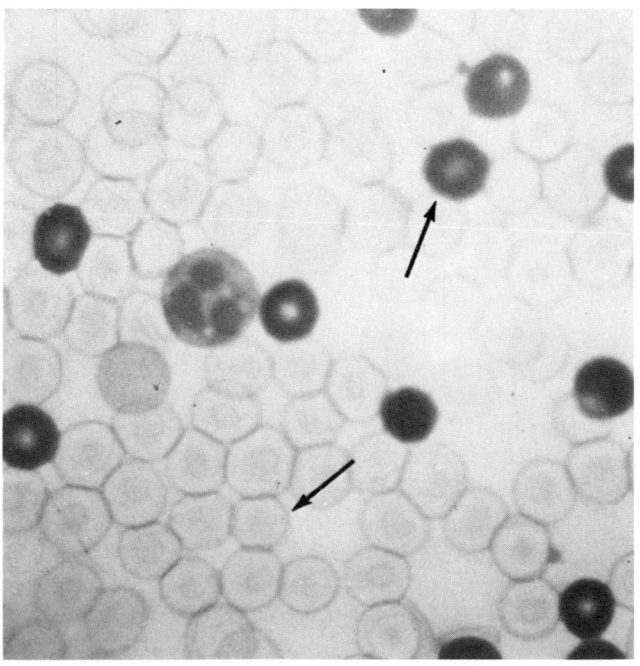

FIGURE 29–7. Massive fetal-to-maternal hemorrhage. After acid-elution treatment, fetal red cells rich in hemoglobin F stain darkly (*upper arrow*), whereas maternal red cells with only very small amounts of hemoglobin F stain lightly (*lower arrow*).

This test is very accurate unless the maternal red cells carry excess fetal hemoglobin as the result of a hemoglobinopathy.

During all pregnancies, very small volumes of blood cells escape from the fetal intravascular compartment across the placental barrier into the maternal intervillous space. This observation is important for several reasons. It is the cause of maternal red cell isoimmunization, as discussed on page 663. Routine fetal-to-maternal cell transfer may someday serve as the basis for a screening test for fetal aneuploidy using maternal peripheral blood (see Chap. 13, p. 331). There is also evidence that persistence of fetal cells in certain maternal tissues, and the immune response they incite, may be the instigating factor in certain autoimmune diseases such as thyroid failure and scleroderma (see Chap. 54, p. 1210).

Choavaratana and colleagues (1997) performed serial Kleihauer–Betke tests in 2000 pregnant women and found that, although the *incidence* of fetal–maternal hemorrhage in each trimester was high, the *volume transfused* from fetus to mother was very small (Table 29–5). Large hemorrhages are uncommon, and Bowman (1985) reported that only 21 of 9000 women had fetal hemorrhage at delivery exceeding 30 mL. Other events that may cause sufficient hemorrhage to incite isoimmunization are shown in Table 29–6.

D-positive fetal red blood cells in D-negative maternal blood can be detected by the rosette test. Maternal red cells are mixed with anti-D antibodies, which coat any fetal (D-positive) cells present in the sample. Indicator red cells bearing the D-antigen are then added, and rosettes form around the fetal cells as the indicator cells attach to them by the antibodies. Rosettes indicate that fetal D-positive cells are present.

TABLE 29–5 Incidence and Volume of Fetal–Maternal Hemorrhage During Pregnancy

Stage of Pregnancy	Hemorrhage (%)	Volume (mL)
First trimester	54	0.07
Second trimester	63	0.08
Third trimester	71	0.13
Delivery	76	0.19

From Choavaratana and colleagues (1997), with permission.

If the fetus becomes severely anemic, a sinusoidal heart rate pattern may develop (see Chap. 18, p 451). Although this pattern is not pathognomonic of fetal anemia, it should prompt immediate evaluation. In general, anemia occurring gradually or chronically, as in isoimmunization, is better tolerated by the fetus than anemia that develops acutely. Chronic anemia may not produce fetal heart rate abnormalities until the fetus is moribund. In contrast, significant acute hemorrhage is poorly tolerated by the fetus and often causes profound neurological fetal impairment.

Acute maternal-fetal hemorrhage results in fetal hypotension, diminished perfusion of vital organs, ischemia, and cerebral infarction. As a result, after an acute hemorrhage, subsequent obstetrical management usually will not change the outcome. De Alemida and Bowman (1994) described 27 cases of fetal–maternal hemorrhage exceeding 80 mL. Despite appropriate management, almost half of these infants died or developed spastic diplegia. In one study, severe fetal-to-maternal hemorrhage caused 5 percent of fetal deaths (Samadi and colleagues, 1996). Although the etiology of such hemorrhage is often undetermined, placental abruption usually is seldom the cause. That said, trauma such as vehicular accidents can cause placental tearing or "fracture," with significant fetal hemorrhage (see Chap. 42, p. 999). The fetal effects of acute hemorrhage also are illustrated by monochorionic twinning. After the death of one monochorionic twin, acute hemorrhage from the living twin into the

TABLE 29–6 Pregnancy Events Causing Fetal–Maternal Hemorrhage

Event	Incidence (%)
Early pregnancy loss	3–5
Elective abortion	6–20
Ectopic pregnancy	5–8
Amniocentesis	4–11
Chorionic villous sampling	8–15
Cordocentesis	30–50
Antepartum trauma	Variable
Placental abruption	Low
Fetal demise	Variable
Manual placental extraction	Variable
External version	Variable

low-resistance circulation of the dead twin can cause such rapid and severe damage that even immediate cesarean delivery does not improve outcome (see Chap. 39, p. 930).

Once fetal–maternal hemorrhage is recognized, the volume of fetal blood lost can be quantified. The volume may influence obstetrical management and is essential to determining the appropriate dose of D-immunoglobulin when the woman is D-negative.

Using basic physiological principles, the amount of fetal hemorrhage may be calculated from the results of a Kleihauer–Betke (KB) stain using the formula:

$$\text{Fetal blood volume} = \frac{\text{MBV} \times \text{maternal Hct} \times \% \text{ fetal cells in KB}}{\text{newborn Hct}}$$

where MBV = maternal blood volume (about 5000 mL in normal-sized normotensive women at term) and Hct = hematocrit. Thus for 1.7-percent positive KB-stained cells in a woman of average size with a hematocrit of 35 percent giving birth to a term infant weighing 3000 g and whose hematocrit is 0.5:

$$\text{Fetal blood volume} = \frac{5000 \times 0.35 \times 0.017}{0.5} = 60 \, \text{mL}$$

The fetal–placental blood volume at term is 125 mL/kg, which is 375 mL for this 3000-g fetus. Thus, this fetus has lost 30 mL of red cells over time into the maternal circulation. This is equivalent to 60 mL of whole blood, because the hematocrit is 50 percent.

ISOIMMUNIZATION. In 1892, Ballantyne established clinicopathological criteria for the diagnosis of hydrops fetalis. In 1932, Diamond, Blackfan, and Baty reported that the fetal anemia in this syndrome was characterized by numerous circulating erythroblasts. Subsequently, the Rhesus factor was discovered by Landsteiner and Weiner in 1940, and Levine and associates confirmed in 1941 that erythroblastosis was due to maternal isoimmunization against paternally inherited fetal factors. The subsequent development of effective maternal prophylaxis was attributed to Finn and associates (1961) in England, and Freda and co-workers (1963) in the United States.

Over 400 red cell antigens have been identified to date. Although some of them are immunologically and genetically important, many are so rare as to be of little clinical significance. Blood banks do not routinely test for any red cell antigen other than the Rhesus and ABO antigens. Any individual who lacks a specific red cell antigen may produce an antibody when exposed to that antigen. Such antibodies can prove harmful to the individual in the case of a blood transfusion or to a fetus during pregnancy. Accordingly, blood banks routinely screen for antibodies.

The vast majority of humans carry at least one red cell antigen inherited from their father but lacking in their mother.

Although the mother could be sensitized if enough fetal erythrocytes reached her circulation to elicit an immune response, isoimmunization is actually rare for the following reasons: (1) low prevalence of red cell antigens; (2) insufficient transplacental passage of fetal antigens or maternal antibodies; (3) maternal–fetal ABO incompatibility, leading to rapid clearance of fetal cells before they elicit an immune response; (4) variable antigenicity; and (5) variable maternal immune response to the antigen, with some antigens provoking only minimal response. Considering all these factors, it is not surprising that there is only an overall 2-percent chance of D-isoimmunization by 6 months postpartum, and that isoimmunization does not always lead to erythroblastosis fetalis.

The incidence of sensitization to red cell antigens at each stage of pregnancy has been studied most extensively in D-negative women. A D-negative woman delivered of a D-positive, ABO-compatible infant has a likelihood of isoimmunization of 16 percent; 2 percent will be immunized by the time of delivery, 7 percent will have anti-D antibody by 6 months postpartum, and the remaining 7 percent will be "sensibilized" (Bowman, 1985). In sensibilized women, anti-D antibodies are produced at such a low level that they are not detected during or after the index pregnancy but instead are identified early in a subsequent pregnancy.

ABO Blood Group System. Although incompatibility for the major blood group antigens A and B is the most common cause of hemolytic disease in the newborn, the resulting anemia is usually very mild. About 20 percent of all infants have an ABO maternal blood group incompatibility, but only 5 percent are clinically affected. ABO incompatibility is different from CDE incompatibility for several reasons:

1. ABO disease frequently is seen in firstborn infants because most group O women have anti-A and anti-B isoagglutinins antedating pregnancy. These antibodies are attributed to exposure to bacteria displaying similar antigens.
2. Most species of anti-A and anti-B antibodies are immunoglobulin M (IgM), which cannot cross the placenta and therefore cannot gain access to fetal erythrocytes. In addition, fetal red cells have fewer A and B antigenic sites than adult cells and are thus less immunogenic. There is no need to monitor antenatal hemolysis with amniocentesis, and no justification for early delivery.
3. The disease is invariably milder than D-isoimmunization and rarely results in significant anemia. Affected infants typically have neonatal anemia and jaundice, which can be treated with phototherapy, and not erythroblastosis fetalis.
4. As a result, ABO isoimmunization is a disease of pediatric rather than obstetrical concern.

ABO isoimmunization can affect future pregnancies but, unlike CDE disease, rarely becomes progressively more severe. Katz and co-workers (1982) identified a recurrence rate

of 87 percent, of whom 62 percent required treatment, most often limited to phototherapy.

Although there is no need for antenatal monitoring, careful neonatal observation is essential because hyperbilirubinemia may require treatment. Treatment usually consists of phototherapy or simple or exchange transfusion with O-negative blood. The usual criteria for diagnosis of neonatal hemolysis due to ABO incompatibility are as follows: (1) the mother is blood group O, with anti-A and anti-B antibodies in her serum, whereas the fetus is group A, B, or AB; (2) jaundice develops within the first 24 hours; (3) there are varying degrees of anemia, reticulocytosis, and erythroblastosis; (4) the Coombs test is positive, although rapid clearance of antibody and antibody-coated cells can result in a negative test; and (5) there has been careful exclusion of other causes of hemolysis.

CDE (Rhesus) Blood Group System. This system includes five red cell proteins or antigens: c, C, D, e, and E. No "d" antigen has been identified, and Rh- or D-negativity is defined as the absence of the D-antigen. There are, however, D-antigen variants that cause hemolytic disease (Bush and associates, 2003; Cannon and colleagues, 2003). The CDE antigens are of considerable clinical importance because most D-negative individuals become immunized after a single exposure. The CDE genes are located on the short arm of chromosome 1 and are inherited as a group, independent of other blood group genes. Like many genes, their incidence varies according to racial origin. Native Americans, Inuits, and Chinese and other Asiatic peoples are almost all D-positive (99 percent). Approximately 92 to 93 percent of African Americans are D-positive, but only 87 percent of Caucasians carry the D-antigen. Of all racial and ethnic groups studied thus far, the Basques show the highest incidence of D-negativity (34 percent).

The C-, c-, E-, and e-antigens have lower immunogenicity than the D-antigen, but they can cause erythroblastosis fetalis. All pregnant women should be tested routinely for the presence or absence of D-antigen on their erythrocytes and for irregular antibodies in their serum. Barss and colleagues (1988) have argued convincingly that this need be done only once during each pregnancy in D-positive women.

Other Blood Group Incompatibilities. Because the routine administration of anti-D immunoglobulin prevents most cases of anti–D-isoimmunization, proportionately more cases of significant antenatal hemolytic disease are now caused by more rare red cell antigens. Such sensitization is suggested by a positive indirect Coombs test performed to screen for abnormal antibodies in maternal serum (Table 29–7).

Several large studies indicate that anti–red cell antibodies are found in 1 percent of pregnancies (Bowell and colleagues, 1986a; Howard and colleagues, 1998). Most of these antibodies (40 to 60 percent) are directed against the CDE genes, with anti-D being most common, followed by anti-E, anti-c, and

TABLE 29–7 Some Red Cell Antigens and Their Propensity to Cause Hemolytic Disease

Blood Group System	Antigen	Severity of Hemolytic Disease	Proposed Management
CDE (Rh)	D	Mild to severe with hydrops fetalis	Amnionic fluid studies
	C	Mild to moderate	Amnionic fluid studies
	c	Mild to severe	Amnionic fluid studies
	E	Mild to severe	Amnionic fluid studies
	e	Mild to moderate	Amnionic fluid studies
I		Not a proven cause of hemolytic disease	
Lewis		Not a proven cause of hemolytic disease	
Kell	K	Mild to severe with hydrops fetalis	Amnionic fluid studies
	k	Mild to severe	Amnionic fluid studies
Duffy	Fy^a	Mild to severe with hydrops fetalis	Amnionic fluid studies
	Fy^b	Not a cause of hemolytic disease	
Kidd	Jk^a	Mild to severe	Amnionic fluid studies
	Jk^b	Mild to severe	Amnionic fluid studies
MNSs	M	Mild to severe	Amnionic fluid studies
	N	Mild	Expectant
	S	Mild to severe	Amnionic fluid studies
	s	Mild to severe	Amnionic fluid studies
	U	Mild to severe	Amnionic fluid studies
Lutheran	Lu^a	Mild	Expectant
	Lu^b	Mild	Expectant
Diego	Di^a	Mild to severe	Amnionic fluid studies
	Di^b	Mild to severe	Amnionic fluid studies
Xg	Xg^a	Mild	Expectant
P	$PP_{1Pk(TJa)}$	Mild to severe	Amnionic fluid studies
Public antigens	Yt^a	Moderate to severe	Amnionic fluid studies
	Yt^b	Mild	Expectant
	Lan	Mild	Expectant
	En^a	Moderate	Amnionic fluid studies
	Ge	Mild	Expectant
	Jr^a	Mild	Expectant
	Co^ar, Berrens, Evans	Severe	Amnionic fluid studies
Private antigens	Co^{a-b}, Batty, Berrens, Evans, Becker, Gonzales, Hunt, Jobbins, Rm, Ven, Wright^b	Mild	Expectant
	Biles, Heibel, Radin, Zd	Moderate	Amnionic fluid studies
	Good, Wright^a	Severe	Amnionic fluid studies

Modified with permission from the American College of Obstetricians and Gynecologists (1990).

anti-C. Anti-Kell antibodies are also frequent. Fortunately, one fourth of these antibodies are from the Lewis system, which does not cause hemolysis because Lewis antigens do not develop on erythrocytes until a few weeks after birth.

KELL ANTIGEN. About 90 percent of Caucasians are Kell negative. Kell type is not routinely determined, and 90 percent of cases of anti-Kell sensitization result from transfusion with Kell-positive blood. As with CDE antigens, Kell sensitization also can occur as the result of maternal–fetal incompatibility (Mayne and associates, 1990). Maternal Kell sensitization is different from D-sensitization because anti-Kell antibodies also attach to fetal erythrocyte precursor cells directly in the bone marrow, thus preventing a hemopoietic response to anemia. This process can cause a more rapid and severe anemia than with anti–D-sensitization (Weiner and Widness, 1996). Because fewer erythrocytes are produced, there is less hemolysis and less amnionic fluid bilirubin. As a result, severe anemia may not be predicted by either the maternal anti-Kell titer or the level of amnionic fluid bilirubin. Caine and Mueller-Heubach (1986) described 13 Kell-sensitized pregnancies with a Kell-positive fetus. Five of these resulted in hydrops or perinatal death, despite favorable amnionic fluid studies 1 week before delivery. Bowman and colleagues (1992a) reviewed 20 Kell-sensitized pregnancies, in which exchange transfusions were required in four and four fetuses died.

Because of this disparate severity of Kell sensitization, some investigators recommend evaluation when the maternal anti-Kell titer is 1:8 or greater, as discussed subsequently. In addition, Weiner and Widness (1996) suggest that the initial evaluation be accomplished by cordocentesis instead of amniocentesis, because fetal anemia from Kell sensitization is usually more severe than indicated by the amnionic fluid bilirubin level.

OTHER ANTIGENS. Kidd (Jk^a), Duffy (Fy^a), c-, E-, and to a lesser extent C-antigens can all cause erythroblastosis as severe as that associated with sensitization to D-antigen (see Table 29–7). Two Duffy antigens have been identified, Fy^a and Fy^b, and some African Americans lack both. Fy^a is the most immunogenic. The Kidd system also has two antigens, Jk^a and Jk^b, with the population distribution as follows: Jk (a+b−), 26 percent; Jk (a−b+), 24 percent; and Jk (a+b+), 50 percent (Alper, 1977). Most cases of isoimmunization to these antigens occur after blood transfusions.

After sensitization to D-antigen, sensitization to the C-antigen is the next most common cause of clinically significant isoimmunization. Although anti–C-isoimmunization most commonly results from previous pregnancies, those fetuses whose mothers have been transfused are more likely to have moderate to severe hemolysis (Bowell and associates, 1986b; Wenk and colleagues, 1986). A third of fetuses with either anti-C or anti-Ce alloimmunization described by Bowman and colleagues (1992b) had hemolysis but none had severe disease. In contrast, Hackney and co-workers (2004) reported that 12 of 46 anti-c isoimmunized fetuses had serious hemolysis, and 8 of these 12 required fetal transfusions.

If an IgG red cell antibody is detected and there is any doubt as to its significance, the clinician should err on the side of caution and the pregnancy should be evaluated. As shown in Table 29–7, many rare or *private antigens* have been associated with severe isoimmunization (Rouse and Weiner, 1990).

Immune Hydrops. The abnormal collection of fluid in more than one area of the fetal body, such as ascites and pleural effusion, is termed *hydrops.* Its causes usually are categorized as immune—such as isoimmunization—and nonimmune. In immune hydrops, excessive and prolonged hemolysis causes anemia, which stimulates marked erythroid hyperplasia of the bone marrow as well as extramedullary hematopoiesis in the spleen and liver with eventual hepatic dysfunction (Nicolini and associates, 1991). There may be cardiac enlargement and pulmonary hemorrhage. Fluid collects in the fetal thorax, abdominal cavity, or skin. The placenta is markedly edematous, enlarged, and boggy, with large, prominent cotyledons and edematous villi. Hydrothorax may be so severe as to restrict lung development, which causes pulmonary compromise after birth. Ascites, hepatomegaly, and splenomegaly may lead to severe dystocia. Hydropic changes are easily seen by sonography (Fig. 29–8).

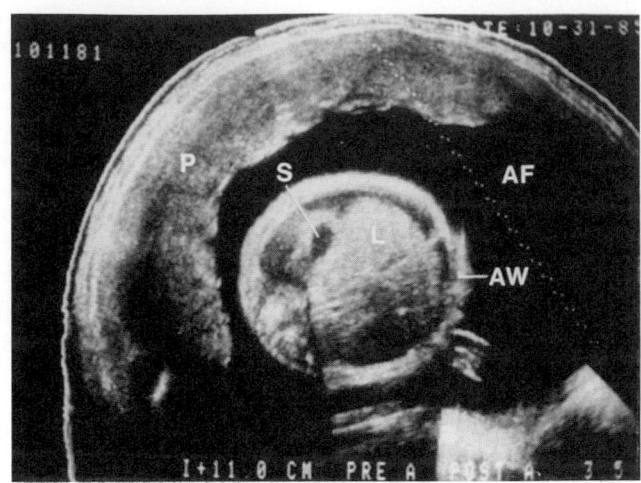

FIGURE 29–8. Transverse sonogram of a hydropic fetus. Illustrated are the edematous fetal abdominal wall (AW) and the fetal liver (L) and stomach (S). Increased amnionic fluid (AF) is apparent, and there is also a large placenta (P). (Courtesy of Dr. R. Santos.)

The precise pathophysiology of hydrops remains unknown. Theories about the inciting pathological event include heart failure from profound anemia and hypoxia, portal hypertension due to hepatic parenchymal disruption caused by extramedullary hemopoiesis, and decreased colloid oncotic pressure resulting from liver dysfunction and hypoproteinemia. The data from several studies indicate that in most cases, the degree and duration of anemia is the major factor causing and influencing the severity of ascites. Secondary factors include hypoproteinemia caused by liver dysfunction and capillary endothelial leakage resulting from tissue hypoxia. Both of these factors lead to protein loss and decreased colloid oncotic pressure, and make the hydrops worse. For example, Nicolaides and colleagues (1985) performed percutaneous umbilical artery blood sampling in 17 severely D-isoimmunized fetuses at 18 to 25 weeks. All fetuses with hydrops had hemoglobin values of less than 3.8 g/dL and plasma protein concentrations less than 2 standard deviations below the normal mean for fetuses of the same age, as well as substantive protein concentrations in ascitic fluid. Conversely, none of the fetuses with hemoglobin values exceeding 4 g/dL were hydropic, even though 6 of 10 also had hypoproteinemia of the same magnitude as the hydropic fetuses. Similarly, Weiner and co-workers (1989) evaluated umbilical venous pressure during 20 antenatal transfusions in isoimmunized pregnancies. They observed that the significantly elevated pressures found in fetuses with immune hydrops normalized within 24 hours of transfusion. Because portal hypertension cannot resolve so rapidly, this suggests that the elevated pressure was actually due to hypoxic myocardial dysfunction, which was reversed by the blood transfusion.

Fetuses with hydrops may die in utero from profound anemia and circulatory failure (Fig. 29–9). One sign of severe anemia and impending death is the sinusoidal fetal heart rate pattern (see Fig. 18–13, p. 451). In addition, hydropic

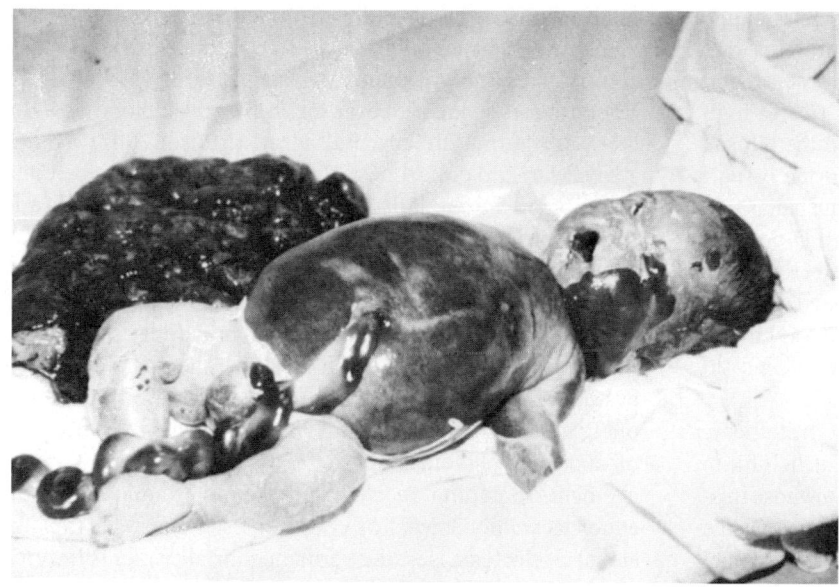

FIGURE 29–9. Severe erythroblastosis fetalis. Hydropic, macerated stillborn infant and characteristically large placenta.

changes in the placenta, leading to placentomegaly, can cause preeclampsia. Because the preeclamptic mother develops severe edema mimicking that of the fetus, this development is referred to as the *mirror syndrome* (see p. 674). The liveborn hydropic infant appears pale, edematous, and limp at birth, and usually requires resuscitation. The spleen and liver are enlarged, and there may be widespread ecchymosis or scattered petechiae. Dyspnea and circulatory collapse are common.

Hyperbilirubinemia. Less severely affected infants may appear well at birth, only to become jaundiced within a few hours. Marked hyperbilirubinemia, if untreated, can cause *kernicterus,* a form of central nervous system damage that specifically affects the basal ganglia and can lead to cerebral palsy. Anemia, in part resulting from impaired erythropoiesis, may persist for many weeks to months in the infant who demonstrates hemolytic disease at birth. In the absence of hypoxia, erythrocyte production normally falls after birth, especially in the preterm infant.

Mortality. Perinatal deaths from hemolytic disease caused by D-isoimmunization have decreased dramatically since adoption of the policy of routine administration of D-immunoglobulin to all D-negative women during or immediately after pregnancy. Survival also has been increased by advances in antenatal and neonatal therapy; the seriously affected fetus can be identified and treated by antenatal transfusions or delivered preterm if necessary (Bowman and colleagues, 1977; Fretts and colleagues, 1992).

Identification of the Isoimmunized Pregnancy. With the exception of ABO incompatibility, which requires only neonatal treatment, the prenatal management of isoimmunization is the same regardless of the inciting antigen. The first step is identifying the woman at risk by performing a blood type and antibody screen at the first prenatal appointment during every pregnancy. Because the antibodies in maternal serum are unbound, they are detected by the *indirect Coombs test.*

In the fetus or neonate, however, the anti–red cell antibodies produced by the mother are absorbed to the D-positive fetal erythrocytes, and thus are identified primarily by the *direct Coombs test.* The absorbed antibodies act as hemolysins, leading to an accelerated rate of red cell destruction. The maternal antibodies detectable in the neonatal circulation at birth gradually disappear over a period of 1 to 4 months. Before these antibodies are cleared, however, they may prevent correct determination of the neonate's blood type; the neonatal red cells may be so thoroughly coated with anti-D antibody that D-antigens are not detectable and the neonate is reported incorrectly to be D-negative.

If the maternal antibody screen reveals the presence of red cell antibodies, they should be identified and their immunoglobulin subtype—either IgG or IgM—determined. Only IgG antibodies are of concern because IgM antibodies cannot cross the placenta or cause fetal hemolysis. If the antibodies are IgG and are known to cause fetal hemolytic anemia (see Table 29–7), the antibody titer should be quantified. A titer above a critical level requires further evaluation. For each antibody, the titer below which the fetus will not die from hemolytic disease is different and is determined individually by each laboratory. For example, the critical titer for anti-D antibodies is usually 1:16; a titer equal to or higher than this indicates the possibility of severe hemolytic disease. Although the critical titers for other antibodies are often assumed to be 1:16 as well, most laboratories have insufficient data to support this assumption. For example, considering two of the more common antibodies, the critical titer for anti-Kell antibody is probably closer to 1:8, whereas the titer for c or E may be 1:32 or higher (see p. 664).

PREDICTING FETAL GENOTYPE. The presence of maternal anti-D antibodies does not necessarily mean that the fetus will be affected or is even D-positive. In a previously sensitized or sensibilized woman, the antibody titer may rise to high levels during a subsequent pregnancy even when the fetus is D-negative, due to the *amnestic response.* Importantly, half of all women with antigen-positive Caucasian husbands can have an antigen-negative baby, because half of all D-positive Caucasian males are heterozygous for D-antigen (Race and Sanger, 1975). In addition, many women sensitized to atypical red cell antigens become immunized after a blood transfusion, and the antigen may not be present on the father's red cells.

For anti-D sensitization, determining whether the father is heterozygous or homozygous for the D-antigen is helpful in determining pregnancy management. The woman whose husband is homozygous for D and thus has a 100 percent chance of having a D-positive infant will be treated differently than the woman whose husband is heterozygous and has only a 50 percent chance of having a positive infant. The most likely paternal genotype—the arrangement of the Rh genes on each paternal chromosome—cannot be determined precisely but can be estimated. The CDE blood group gene locus is located on chromosome 1p34-p36. One gene encodes the C/c and E/e proteins, and a second gene encodes D—recall that there is no "d" gene or gene product. By identifying paternal CDE antigens and considering the most common arrangement of the corresponding genes in men of his race, the father's presumed genotype can be predicted. For example, if the father is CcDe, he could be either homozygous for D (D,D) or heterozygous (D, "d"). If he is white, there is a 94 percent chance that the arrangement of these alleles is CDe/cde; thus, he has a 94 percent chance of being heterozygous for D and a 47 percent (94 ÷ 2) chance of having a D-negative fetus.

If the woman is sensitized by an atypical antigen, the paternal antigen type will determine whether the fetus is at risk. For example, many women producing anti-Kell antibodies are sensitized from a blood transfusion and have a Kell-negative husband. Determining that the father is Kell-negative eliminates the need to monitor the Kell-negative fetus. **Before paternal testing is pursued, it is imperative that any possibility of nonpaternity be disclosed.**

Management of Isoimmunization. Management is individualized after reviewing the obstetrical history. Accurate pregnancy dating is critical, as is determining the gestational age at which fetal anemia developed in the last pregnancy. Anemia tends to occur earlier and be sequentially more severe with every pregnancy. In the first sensitized pregnancy, a positive antibody screen with a titer below the critical level should be followed with repeat titers at timely intervals, usually monthly. Once the critical titer has been met or exceeded, further evaluation is required.

If this is not the first sensitized pregnancy, maternal antibody titers may not be helpful because they may be elevated simply as the result of the *amnestic* response. In these cases,

fetal anemia can be predicted noninvasively using *middle cerebral artery Doppler.* The anemic fetus shunts blood preferentially to the brain to maintain adequate oxygenation. This response can be identified by measuring peak blood flow velocity in the middle cerebral artery (Moise, 2002). In one study, Mari and colleagues (2000) measured middle cerebral artery blood flow serially in 111 fetuses at risk for anemia and in 265 normal fetuses. Doppler was 100-percent sensitive in detection of anemic fetuses, with or without fetal hydrops, and had a false-positive rate of only 12 percent.

If the antibody titer or middle cerebral artery peak blood flow indicate that the fetus is likely to be anemic, then further evaluation is appropriate. Early studies showed that without treatment, isoimmunization has a perinatal mortality rate of about 30 percent (Freda, 1973). With aggressive management, including repeated ultrasound examinations, diagnostic amniocentesis or cordocentesis, and fetal transfusions in selected cases, the perinatal mortality rate is lowered remarkably (Harman and co-workers, 1983; Queenan and colleagues, 1993).

AMNIONIC FLUID EVALUATION. When fetal blood cells undergo hemolysis, breakdown pigments, mostly bilirubin, are present in the supernatant of amnionic fluid. The amount of amnionic fluid bilirubin correlates roughly with the degree of hemolysis and thus indirectly predicts the severity of the fetal anemia. Because the amnionic fluid bilirubin level is low compared with serum levels, the concentration is measured by a continuously recording spectrophotometer and is demonstrable as a change in absorbance at 450 nm, referred to as ΔOD_{450} (Fig. 29–10).

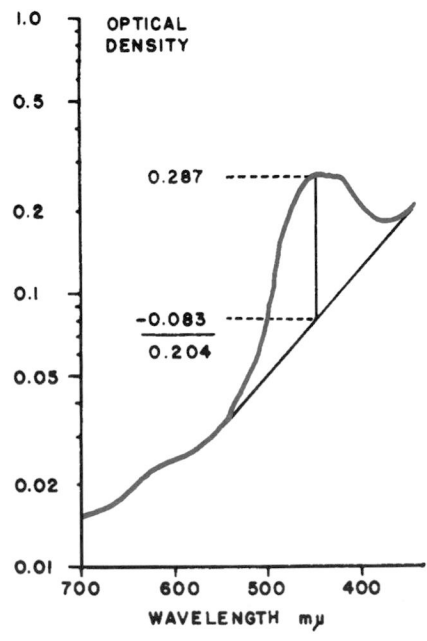

FIGURE 29–10. Spectral absorption curve of amnionic fluid in hemolytic disease.

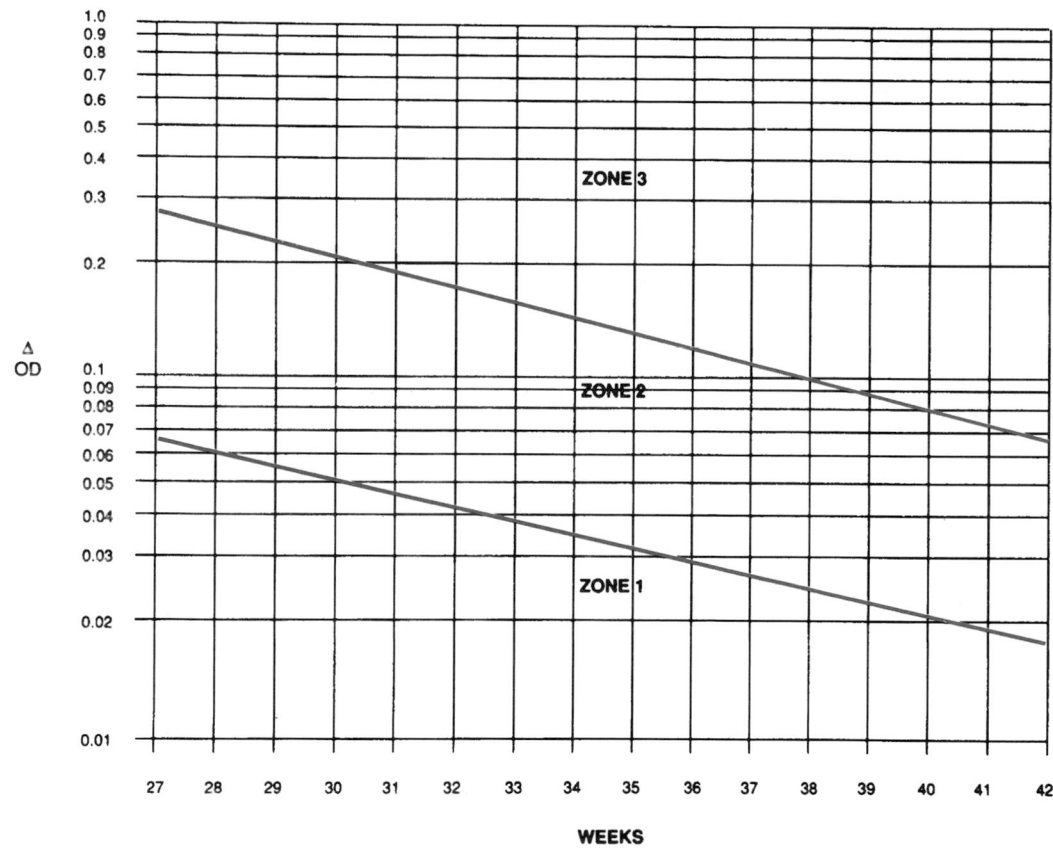

FIGURE 29–11. Liley graph used to depict severity of fetal hemolysis with red cell isoimmunization. (From Liley, 1961, with permission.)

The likelihood that the fetus is anemic is determined by plotting the ΔOD_{450} on a graph, shown in Figure 29–11, that was originated by Liley (1961). He compared ΔOD_{450} measurements with fetal outcome in 101 isoimmunized pregnancies and showed that mild, moderate, or severe fetal anemia could be predicted according to which of three zones the bilirubin level was plotted into. Subsequent studies have correlated these zones with actual fetal hemoglobin concentrations. Optical density values in zone 1 generally indicate a D-negative fetus or one who will have only mild disease. In zone 2, the fetus is at moderate risk. In low zone 2, the expected fetal hemoglobin concentration is between 11.0 and 13.9 g/dL, whereas in upper zone 2, the anticipated hemoglobin level ranges from 8.0 to 10.9 g/dL. Values in zone 3 indicate a severely affected fetus with a hemoglobin level of less than 8.0 g/dL, and without therapy, death is predicted within 7 to 10 days.

A value in zone 3 demands immediate fetal red blood cell transfusion or delivery. Conversely, a value in zone 1 can be followed by a repeated sampling in 2 to 3 weeks and the trend of the two values used to estimate the severity of the hemolytic process. A value in zone 2, however, indicates that severe fetal anemia is possible; this finding should be followed by a repeated sampling within 1 to 2 weeks. If the trend of samples forms a line parallel to the lines on the graph or is decreasing within the zone, either the fetus is unaffected or hemolysis is stable. In these cases, amniocentesis can be repeated at 2- to 3-week intervals until either transfusion or delivery is required (American College of Obstetricians and Gynecologists, 1990). Conversely, if the trend of ΔOD_{450} values is rising within zone 2 or has risen into zone 3, immediate transfusion or delivery is indicated.

Expanded Liley Graph. The original Liley graph was applicable only to pregnancies lasting 27 weeks or more, contemporaneous for the limits of viability at that time. As these limits were expanded, it was necessary to extrapolate the Liley curve back to 18 to 20 weeks. However, this curve cannot simply be extrapolated back to 25 weeks because amnionic fluid bilirubin is normally high at that age. Thus, ΔOD_{450} results plotted on an extrapolated Liley curve do not accurately predict either hemolysis or the fetal hemoglobin level (Nicolaides and colleagues, 1986).

For these reasons, a number of modified Liley curves have been developed for pregnancies of 27 weeks or less. For example, Queenan and colleagues (1993) examined 845 amnionic fluid samples from 75 D-immunized and 520 unaffected pregnancies and constructed a Liley-type curve that begins at 14 weeks (Fig. 29–12). In this graph and others, however, the naturally high amnionic fluid bilirubin level at midpregnancy results in a large "indeterminate" zone. In this zone, bilirubin concentrations do not accurately predict fetal

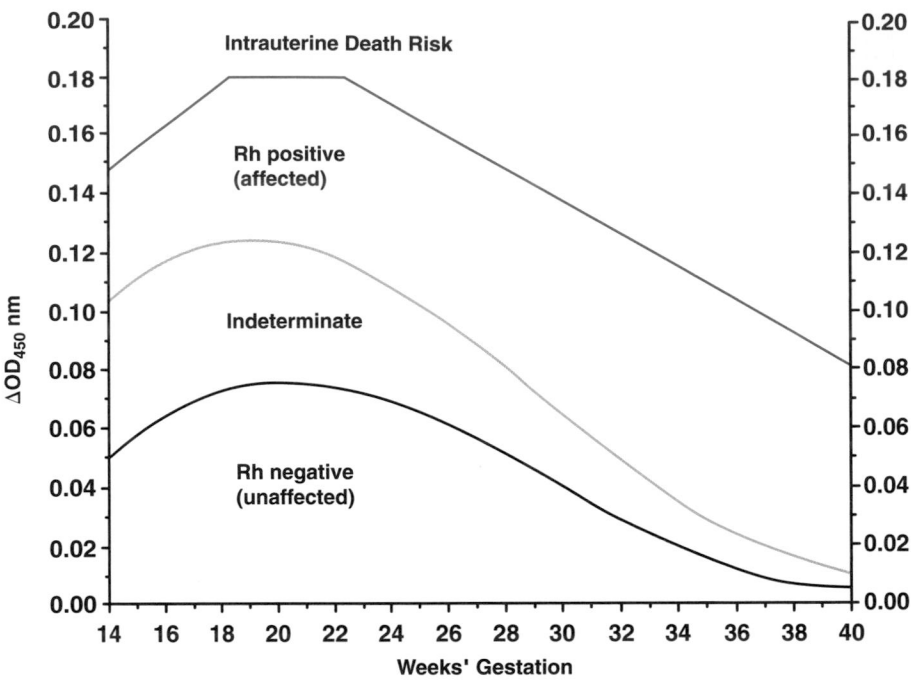

FIGURE 29–12. Proposed amnionic fluid ΔOD_{450} management zones in pregnancies from 14 to 40 weeks. (From Queenan and colleagues, 1993, with permission.)

hemoglobin. For this reason, when evaluation indicates that there is likely to be severe fetal anemia or hydrops before 25 weeks, many clinicians will forego amniocentesis in favor of fetal blood sampling.

FETAL BLOOD SAMPLING. Cordocentesis is performed as described in Chapter 13 (see p. 330). The risk of fetal loss is about 1.4 percent per procedure. Previously, some clinicians used cordocentesis primarily to evaluate all isoimmunized pregnancies. Advantages were that fetal hemoglobin concentration could be accurately determined and fetal blood typing could be accomplished. Currently, however, using molecular genetic techniques, fetal D-antigen type can be determined by testing fetal DNA obtained from amniocytes (Bennett and associates, 1993). This technique is invaluable, especially for pregnancies in which the father is a presumed heterozygote, because in these cases the fetus could be D-negative and one amniocentesis for fetal D typing and ΔOD_{450} measurement might be the only invasive test needed. Greater than 99-percent sensitivity for fetal D-antigen typing is claimed (Van Den Veyver and colleagues, 1996; Yankowitz and co-workers, 1997). Several reference laboratories are now able to analyze amniocytes for the E-, c-, Kell 1, and Kell 2 (Cellano) antigens, as well.

When the ΔOD_{450} measurement or middle cerebral artery Doppler indicates the possibility of fetal anemia, ultrasonography reveals fetal hepatomegaly or hydrops, or fetal testing indicates physiological stress, management is determined by the gestational age. The mature fetus should be delivered, whereas the preterm fetus can be evaluated using diagnostic cordocentesis and transfusion as necessary.

Fetal hemoglobin, hematocrit, reticulocyte count, and indirect Coombs titer also are used to predict the onset of anemia if the fetus is not yet affected (Weiner and associates, 1991a).

Nicolaides and co-workers (1988) recommend that transfusions be commenced when the hemoglobin is at least 2 g/dL below the mean for normal fetuses of corresponding gestational age. Other clinicians perform transfusions when the fetal hematocrit is below 30 percent, which is 2 standard deviations below the mean at all gestational ages (Weiner and co-workers, 1991b). Fetal intraperitoneal and intraumbilical blood transfusions are discussed in Chapter 13 (see p. 332). Various other treatments, such as plasmapheresis, administration of promethazine or D-positive erythrocyte membranes in enteric capsules, or immunosuppression with corticosteroids have been shown to be ineffective.

DELIVERY. Vaginal delivery at or near term is the goal of management. When management includes serial amnionic fluid ΔOD_{450} measurement or fetal transfusions, fetal well-being should be closely monitored (see Chap. 15). With appropriate management, extremely preterm delivery usually can be avoided.

NEONATAL CARE AND OUTCOME. Cord blood is obtained for hemoglobin concentration measurement and direct Coombs testing. If the infant is overtly anemic, it is often best to carry out the initial exchange transfusion promptly, with recently collected type-O, D-negative red cells. For infants who are not overtly anemic, the need for exchange transfusion is determined by the rate of increase in bilirubin concentration, the maturity of the infant, and the presence of other complications. Most fetal transfusion survivors develop normally (Bowman, 1978). Grab and colleagues (1999) reported the long-term outcomes of 35 fetuses who had severe isoimmunization or immune hydrops treated with antenatal intravascular transfusions. One had mild psychomotor disabilities at age 1, and another had delayed speech development. However, at up to 6 years of age, none of the survivors, including those with hydrops, had moderate or severe neurological impairment.

Prevention. Anti–D-immunoglobulin is extracted by cold alcohol fractionation and ultra-filtration of plasma containing high-titer D-antibody. Each dose provides 300 μg of D-antibody as determined by radioimmunoassay. It is given to the D-negative nonsensitized mother to prevent sensitization after any pregnancy-related events that could result in fetal–maternal hemorrhage (see Table 29–6). Up to 2 percent of women with a spontaneous abortion and 5 percent of those undergoing elective termination become isoimmunized without D-immunoglobulin.

ROUTINE ANTEPARTUM ADMINISTRATION. One dose of anti-D immunoglobulin is given prophylactically to all D-negative women at about 28 weeks, and a second dose is given after delivery if the infant is D-positive (American College of Obstetricians and Gynecologists, 1999b). Without such prophylaxis, Bowman and Pollock (1978) showed that 1.8 percent of D-negative women will become isoimmunized by silent fetal–maternal hemorrhage. When such prophylaxis is given, only 0.07 percent of susceptible women are sensitized.

A second dose is required at delivery because the half-life of immunoglobulin is only 24 days and it persists for only 6 weeks. In addition, fetal–maternal hemorrhage is more likely at delivery. Each 300 μg will protect the average-sized mother from fetal hemorrhage of up to 15 mL of D-positive red cells, or 30 mL of fetal whole blood with the usual hematocrit of about 50. The initial dose of 300 μg will produce a weakly positive (1:1 to 1:4) indirect Coombs titer in the mother. As the body mass index increases from over 27 to 40 kg/m^2, serum antibody levels decrease by 30 to 60 percent (Woelfer and co-workers, 2004). Rarely, a small amount of antibody crosses the placenta and results in a weakly positive direct Coombs test in cord and infant blood. This small amount causes negligible hemolysis.

The risk of acquiring a virus such as the human immunodeficiency virus (HIV) as the result of being treated with anti–D-immunoglobulin is extremely low. Individuals who are antibody- or antigen-positive for various hepatitis viruses are excluded from blood donation, donor plasma is tested, and solvent-detergent viral inactivation and nanofiltration eliminate HIV and other viruses (Centers for Disease Control, 1987; Hong and colleagues, 1998; Misbah and Chapel, 1993).

D-negative women who receive blood products are also at risk of becoming sensitized. Although D-negative women should be given only D-negative red cells, platelet transfusions and plasmapheresis can provide sufficient D-antigen to cause sensitization. This can be prevented by an injection of D-immunoglobulin. **When there is doubt about whether to give anti–D-immunoglobulin, it should be given.** Explicitly, anti–D-immunoglobulin, even if not needed, will cause no harm, however, failing to give it when needed can have severe consequences.

LARGE FETAL-TO-MATERNAL HEMORRHAGE. If there is a large fetal–maternal hemorrhage, one dose of D-immunoglobulin may not be sufficient to neutralize the transfused fetal cells. Ness and colleagues (1987) studied 800 D-negative mothers and reported that the incidence of excessive fetal–maternal transfusion exceeding 30 mL of whole blood, the quantity neutralized by one dose of immunoglobulin, was 1 percent. Another 5.6 percent of these pregnancies had fetal–maternal hemorrhage of between 11 and 30 mL. Thus, at least 1 percent, and perhaps more, of susceptible mothers would have been given insufficient immunoglobulin if not tested. Importantly, they determined that if extra D-immunoglobulin is considered only for women with risk factors such as abdominal trauma, placental abruption, placenta previa, intrauterine manipulation, multiple gestation, or manual removal of the placenta, half of women requiring more than the 300-μg dose would be missed. Stedman and co-workers (1986), utilizing the erythrocyte rosette test, reported similar results. Accordingly, the American Association of Blood Banks (Snyder, 1998) recommends that all D-negative women be tested at delivery with the Kleihauer–Betke or rosette test. The dosage of anti–D-immunoglobulin is calculated from the estimated volume of the fetal-to-maternal hemorrhage described on page 663. One 300-μg ampule is given for each 30 mL of fetal blood to be neutralized. To determine if the Rhogam dose was adequate after it is given, the indirect Coombs test is performed. A positive result indicates that there is excess anti–D-immunoglobulin in the maternal serum, thus demonstrating that the dose was sufficient.

D^u-ANTIGEN. Identification of the D^u-antigen may cause confusion or result in designation of the blood type as "weak D-positive." The D^u-antigen is actually a variant of the D-antigen, and women confirmed to be D^u-positive are therefore D-positive and do not need immunoglobulin (American College of Obstetricians and Gynecologists, 1999b). If a D-negative woman delivers a D^u-positive infant, she should be given D-immunoglobulin. As before, if there is any doubt about D-antigen status, then immunoglobin should be given.

MATERNAL-TO-FETAL HEMORRHAGE. It is now recognized that in most pregnancies, small amounts of maternal blood enter the fetal circulation and vice versa. Very rarely, the D-negative fetus is exposed to maternal D-antigen and becomes sensitized as a result. When such a female fetus becomes an adult, she will produce anti-D antibodies indicating sensitization even before or early in her first pregnancy. This mechanism of isoimmunization is called the *grandmother theory* because the fetus in the current pregnancy is jeopardized by antibodies initially provoked by its grandmother's erythrocytes. This scenario accounts for very few cases of D-sensitization. Major blood group (ABO) incompatibility offers appreciable protection against D-sensitization of the fetus. Furthermore, significant maternal-to-fetal hemorrhage is uncommon. D-negative infants born to D-positive mothers are not routinely given D-immunoglobulin prophylaxis.

HYPERBILIRUBINEMIA

Disposal of Bilirubin. Unconjugated or free bilirubin is readily transferred across the placenta from mother to fetus, or vice versa, if the maternal plasma level of unconjugated bilirubin is high. Although bilirubin glucuronide is water soluble and normally is excreted into bile and urine when the plasma level is elevated, unconjugated bilirubin is not excreted this way.

Kernicterus. The great concern over unconjugated hyperbilirubinemia in the newborn, especially if preterm, results from its association with kernicterus. Bilirubin staining of the basal ganglia and hippocampus results in profound degeneration in these regions. Surviving infants show spasticity, muscular incoordination, and varying degrees of mental retardation. There is a positive correlation between unconjugated bilirubin levels above 18 to 20 mg/dL and kernicterus. Despite this, kernicterus may develop at much lower concentrations, especially in very preterm infants.

Factors other than the serum bilirubin concentration that contribute to the development of kernicterus include hypoxia and acidosis. Sepsis contributes to kernicterus. Both hypothermia and hypoglycemia predispose the infant to kernicterus by raising the level of nonesterified fatty acids. These, in turn, compete with bilirubin for binding sites on albumin and inhibit bilirubin conjugation. Although sulfonamides and salicylates also compete for protein-binding sites, and sodium benzoate in injectable diazepam, furosemide, and gentamicin displaces bilirubin from albumin, these drugs are unlikely to lead to kernicterus. Excessive doses of vitamin K analogues may be associated with hyperbilirubinemia. The importance of the serum albumin concentration and the binding sites so provided is obvious.

Physiological Jaundice. By far the most common form of unconjugated nonhemolytic jaundice is so-called physiological jaundice. In the mature infant, the serum bilirubin increases for 3 to 4 days to serum levels of up to 10 mg/dL or so, and then falls rapidly. In preterm infants, the rise is more prolonged and may be more intense.

Treatment. Phototherapy is now widely used to treat hyperbilirubinemia. By some unknown mechanism, light seems to promote hepatic excretion of unconjugated bilirubin. In most instances, phototherapy leads to oxidation of bilirubin, resulting in a lower bilirubin level. Light that penetrates the skin also increases peripheral blood flow, which further enhances photo-oxidation. As much surface area as possible is exposed, the infant is turned every 2 hours, and the temperature is closely monitored to prevent dehydration. The fluorescent bulbs must be the appropriate wavelength, and the eyes should be completely shielded. Serum bilirubin should be monitored for at least 24 hours after discontinuance of phototherapy. Rarely, exchange transfusion is required.

NONIMMUNE HYDROPS FETALIS. Hydrops is defined by the presence of excess fluid in two or more body areas, such as thorax, abdomen, or skin, and is often associated with hydramnios and placental thickening. Because obstetrical ultrasound examination has become routine, hydrops is frequently identified prenatally and in some cases, the etiology is determined. Santolaya and colleagues (1992) identified hydrops in 0.6 percent of 12,572 pregnancies examined with ultrasound, and determined the etiology in 77 percent of cases (Fig. 29–13). Heinonen and colleagues (2000) reported a similar incidence of 1 in 1700, and they were able to determine etiology in 95 percent. In some cases, fetal ascites develops without other features of hydrops and the overall prognosis is better (Favre and co-workers, 2004).

Etiology. A variety of pathogenic mechanisms can lead to hydrops. *Cardiac abnormalities,* either structural defects or arrhythmias, or both, are associated with 20 to 45 percent of cases of nonimmune hydrops (Allan, 1986; Castillo, 1986; Gough, 1986; Santolaya, 1992, and all their co-workers). Fetal heart failure also can result from infection-related myocarditis or hepatitis.

Approximately one third of hydrops cases result from *multiple malformations* or *chromosomal anomalies.* Shulman and colleagues (2000) have reported that the majority of cases of dramatic and extensive subcutaneous edema—so-called *space-suit hydrops*—recognized in the first trimester result from chromosomal abnormalities. Of 30 such fetuses identified at less than 14 weeks of gestation, 87 percent were aneuploid, of which over half involved the sex chromosomes.

About 10 percent of hydrops cases are associated with *twin-to-twin transfusion syndrome* (see Chap. 39, p. 929). In these cases, hydrops can be due to heart failure from volume overload in the recipient twin or myocardial dysfunction from severe anemia in the donor twin. Other causes of severe anemia that can lead to hydrops include parvovirus infection, acute fetal–maternal hemorrhage, or α-thalassemia (American College of Obstetricians and Gynecologists, 1999a). *Inborn errors of metabolism* such as Gaucher disease, GM

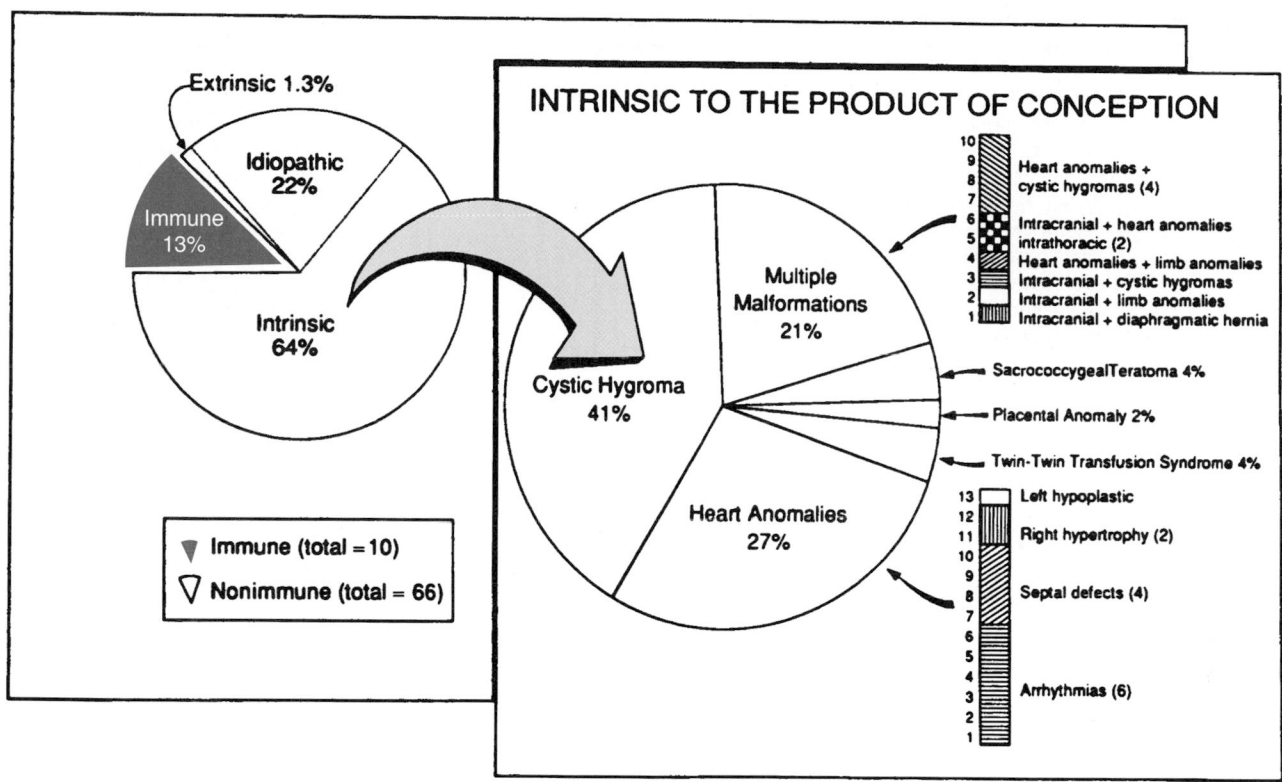

FIGURE 29–13. Classification and cause in 76 cases of fetal hydrops in which the etiology could be diagnosed by ultrasound. (From Santolaya and associates, 1992, with permission.)

1 gangliosidosis, or sialidosis can cause recurrent hydrops (Lefebvre and colleagues, 1999). Rarely, an *anomalous lymph system* can result in lymph accumulating to cause isolated chylothorax or chylous ascites, but these fluid collections do not qualify as hydrops because they involve only one body cavity.

The great variety of causes of hydrops listed by Holzgreve and associates (1984) are presented in Table 29–8. The reported incidence of these causes varies according to the sophistication of the evaluation and the population studied. For example, in San Francisco, which has a large Asian population, 10 percent of hydrops was caused by α-thalassemia (Holzgreve and colleagues, 1984).

Prognosis. Although the outcome for hydrops caused by any of these mechanisms is generally poor, McCoy and colleagues (1995) reviewed 82 cases of nonimmune hydrops attributed to cardiovascular abnormalities (23 percent), aneuploidy (16 percent), thoracic anomalies (13 percent), genetic syndromes (11 percent), anemia and infection (9 percent), twin-to-twin transfusion (6 percent), and idiopathic causes (22 percent). The mortality rate for hydrops evident before 24 weeks was 95 percent. Conversely, fetuses with hydrops who survived to at least 24 weeks, had structurally normal hearts, and were euploid had a survival rate of 20 percent.

Diagnosis. Ultrasound evaluation may provide a diagnosis. Depending on the circumstances, helpful maternal blood tests might include hemoglobin electrophoresis, Kleihauer–Betke test, indirect Coombs test, and serological tests for syphilis, toxoplasmosis, cytomegalovirus, rubella, and parvovirus B19. Cordocentesis is considered for karyotyping, hemoglobin concentration and electrophoresis, evaluation of blood gas and transaminase levels, and serological testing for IgM-specific antibodies to infectious agents. In view of the data from McCoy and associates (1995) described previously, a fetal echocardiogram and karyotype analysis are important in evaluation and predicting prognosis for fetuses who have reached 24 weeks.

Management. In some cases, treatment is possible. Some cardiac arrhythmias can be treated pharmacologically, severe anemia due to fetal–maternal hemorrhage or parvovirus infection can be treated with blood transfusions, and hydrops of one fetus in twin-to-twin transfusion syndrome may resolve with therapeutic amniocentesis (see Chap. 39, p. 929). In most cases, however, hydrops cannot be treated and ultimately proves fatal for the fetus or newborn. In general, when hydrops persists and cardiac abnormalities and aneuploidy have been ruled out, and if the fetus is mature enough that survival is likely, delivery should be accomplished. Very preterm fetuses usually are managed expectantly. Although

TABLE 29–8 Causes of Nonimmune Hydrops Fetalis and Associated Clinical Conditions

Category	Condition	Category	Condition
Cardiovascular	Tachyarrhythmia Congenital heart block Anatomical defects (atrial septal defect, ventricular defect, hypoplastic left heart, pulmonary valve insufficiency, Ebstein subaortic stenosis, dilated heart, atrioventricular canal defect, single ventricle, tetralogy of Fallot, premature closure of foramen ovale, subendocardial fibroelastosis, dextrocardia in combination with pulmonic stenosis)	Urinary	Urethral stenosis or atresia Posterior neck obstruction Spontaneous bladder perforation Prune belly Neurogenic bladder with reflux Ureterocele
Chromosomal	Down syndrome (trisomy 21) Other trisomies Turner syndrome Triploidy	Gastrointestinal	Jejunal atresia Midgut volvulus Malrotation of intestines Duplication of intestinal tract Meconium peritonitis
Malformation syndromes	Thanatophoric dwarfism Arthrogryposis multiplex congenita Asphyxiating thoracic dystrophy Hypophosphatasia Osteogenesis imperfecta Achondroplasia Achondrogenesis Neu–Laxova syndrome Recessive cystic hygroma Saldino–Noonan syndrome Pena–Shokeir type I syndrome	Medications	Antepartum indomethacin (taken to stop preterm labor, causing fetal ductus closure and secondary nonimmune hydrops fetalis)
Hematological	α-Thalassemia Arteriovenous shunts (vascular tumors) Chronic fetomaternal transfusion Kasabach–Merritt syndrome In utero closed-space hemorrhage Caval, portal, or femoral thrombosis	Infections	Cytomegalovirus Toxoplasmosis Syphilis Congenital hepatitis Rubella Parvovirus Leptospirosis Chagas disease
Twin pregnancy	Twin-twin transfusion syndrome Parabiotic (acardiac) twin syndrome		
Respiratory	Diaphragmatic hernia Cystic adenomatous malformation Pulmonary hypoplasia Hamartoma of lung Mediastinal teratoma Congenital chylothorax	Miscellaneous	Amnionic band syndrome Cystic hygroma Congenital lymphedema Polysplenia syndrome Congenital neuroblastoma Tuberous sclerosis Torsion of ovarian cyst Fetal trauma Sacrococcygeal teratoma

Modified from Holzgreve and co-workers (1984), with permission.

hydrops usually persists or worsens with time, it occasionally resolves spontaneously (Mueller-Heubach and Mazer, 1983).

Maternal Complications. A unique complication of hydrops is the maternal *mirror syndrome* (Midgley and Hardrug, 2000). Believed to be caused by vascular changes in the swollen, hydropic placenta, it is called the mirror syndrome because the mother develops preeclampsia with severe edema that is similar to that of the fetus. In these situations, preeclampsia often develops early and only rarely resolves with fetal treatment. Duthie and Walkinshaw (1995) described a woman with parvovirus-associated fetal hydrops and severe preeclampsia whose hypertension resolved at 25 weeks when fetal transfusion reversed the fetal hydrops. In many cases, however, treatment is not possible and delivery is necessary. Preterm labor is common because of hydramnios. Postpartum hemorrhage sometimes occurs as the result of sudden decompression of an overdistended uterus, and retained placenta is common.

FETAL CARDIAC ARRHYTHMIAS. These abnormal heart rhythms are now recognized frequently because of extensive use of real-time ultrasound and Doppler technology. Whereas most arrhythmias are transient and benign, some tachyarrhythmias, if sustained, can result in congestive heart failure, nonimmune hydrops, and fetal death. Sustained bradycardia, although less often associated with hydrops, may signify underlying cardiac pathology that includes structural lesions or autoimmune myocarditis.

Kleinman and associates (1985) summarized their experience with fetal arrhythmias. Premature atrial contractions accounted for two thirds of all cases. Fortunately, this arrhythmia is benign, is related to immaturity, and usually resolves with further development. Rarely, it converts to a sustained supraventricular tachycardia. If the rate is more than 200 beats/min, it may cause cardiac failure, and thus requires treatment as discussed in Chapter 13 (see p. 332).

The prognosis for the fetus with bradycardia is less promising. Bradycardia typically results either from a major structural abnormality or from congenital heart block, including the long QT syndrome (Lin and co-workers, 2004). If a defect is identified by fetal echocardiography, fetal karyotyping should be offered.

Maternal anti–SS-A (anti-Ro) antibody causes half of cases of congenital heart block by binding to tissue in the conduction tracts (Taylor and colleagues, 1986). Intriguing data from Stevens and colleagues (2003) provides evidence that these myocytes may be from maternal engraftment. Such *microchimerism* is considered to be a cause of maternal disease arising from fetal cell engraftment (see Chap. 54, p. 1210). Tissue inflammation provoked by these antibodies leads to permanent damage, and survivors frequently require a pacemaker at birth. Anti–SS-A antibodies can affix to other cardiac tissues as well, and if there is extensive myocarditis, the prognosis is poor. Brucato and co-workers (2003) reviewed 1825 cases of congenital heart block from 38 studies. They reported that in utero diagnosis is associated with a much poorer prognosis and a higher risk of late-onset dilated cardiomyopathy than when the diagnosis is made in childhood. In addition, the recurrence risk of congenital heart block in subsequent pregnancy is high because congenital cases often are associated with anticardiac antibodies. Many of these women have, or subsequently develop, lupus erythematosus or another connective tissue disease. Conversely, of all the women who produce anti–SS-A, only 1 in 20 have fetuses with cardiac disease (see Chap. 54, p. 1215).

Fetal therapy has been attempted for heart block. Robinson and co-workers (2001) used terbutaline to transiently increase the heart rate of seven fetuses with a ventricular rate below 60. Saleeb and colleagues (1999) reviewed the treatment of 50 fetuses with heart block caused by maternal SS-A and SS-B antibodies. They concluded that fluorinated steroids significantly improved outcome and resulted in the resolution of pleural effusions, ascites, or hydrops in 13 of 18 treated cases.

DISEASES OF THE TERM FETUS AND NEONATE

RESPIRATORY DISTRESS SYNDROME. Term infants can have respiratory complications, although these are much less frequent than in those born preterm. Common causes in term infants include sepsis, especially from group B streptococcal disease and intrauterine-acquired pneumonia; persistent pulmonary hypertension of the newborn; meconium aspiration syndrome; and pulmonary hemorrhage.

Advances in neonatal care have improved the survival rate and decreased the morbidity of these conditions. High-frequency oscillatory ventilation improves oxygenation without high ventilatory pressures, and nitric oxide is a specific pulmonary vasodilator that has no effect on systemic vasculature. A meta-analysis of 11 trials of nitric oxide therapy in term or near-term infants with respiratory failure found that nitric oxide significantly improved oxygenation. Its use reduced mortality as well as the need for extracorporeal membrane oxygenation (Finer and Barrington, 2000). Unfortunately, nitric oxide does not appear to have similar beneficial effects for infants born before 34 weeks (Kinsella and co-workers, 1999).

MECONIUM ASPIRATION SYNDROME. This disorder results from peripartum inhalation of meconium-stained amnionic fluid, leading to a chemical pneumonitis with inflammation of pulmonary tissues, mechanical obstruction of the airways, and hypoxia. In severe cases, it progresses to persistent pulmonary hypertension, other morbidity, and death. Even with prompt and appropriate therapy, seriously affected infants frequently die or suffer long-term neurological sequelae.

Risk Factors. In about 20 percent of pregnancies at term, amnionic fluid is contaminated by meconium. In the past, this was considered a sign of "fetal distress" in response to hypoxia. It is now recognized, however, that in the majority of cases, meconium passage indicates a normally maturing gastrointestinal tract, or occurs as the result of vagal stimulation from umbilical cord compression (Nathan and co-workers, 1994). Passage of meconium into a normal amnionic fluid volume results in light meconium staining, and its aspiration before labor is a relatively common occurrence. In healthy, well-oxygenated fetuses, this diluted meconium is readily cleared from the lungs by normal physiological mechanisms. In some infants, however, the inhaled meconium is not cleared, and meconium aspiration syndrome results. It can occur after normal labor, but is more likely when meconium is thick, the pregnancy is postterm, or the fetus is growth-restricted. Putting these together, pregnancies at highest risk are those in which there is diminished amnionic fluid volume, along with cord compression or uteroplacental insufficiency that may cause meconium passage (Davis and co-workers,

1985; Leveno and colleagues, 1984). In these cases, the meconium remains thick and undiluted, and the compromised fetus cannot clear it.

Prevention. Unfortunately, pathological meconium aspiration cannot be predicted by the fetal heart rate tracing (Dooley and colleagues, 1985). However, Carson and colleagues (1976) reported that the incidence of meconium aspiration syndrome could be reduced by *oropharyngeal suctioning* following delivery of the fetal head, but before delivery of the chest. This maneuver is followed by laryngoscopic visualization of the vocal cords and, when meconium is visualized, additional suctioning of the trachea. In this study, meconium aspiration syndrome was reduced but not eliminated, suggesting that delivery factors are not solely responsible. In the almost three decades since this report, this combined obstetrical–pediatric delivery protocol has been the standard of care. Despite this, several investigators reported that strict adherence to this protocol does not reduce the incidence of the syndrome below 2.1 percent (Davis and colleagues, 1985; Wiswell and colleagues, 1990). This observation is explicable for a number of reasons. Murphy and associates (1984) have shown that pulmonary hypertension, the main pathological outcome of meconium aspiration, is characterized by abnormal muscularization of the interacinar arteries. These changes begin well before birth, most likely as the result of a recurring antenatal insult. Consequently, they are unaffected by maneuvers at delivery. Cornish and colleagues (1994) used a baboon model to show that intrapartum meconium aspiration, either alone or combined with peripartum asphyxia, did not produce the kind of pathophysiological effects that could lead to long-term damage or death in the human neonate.

Katz and Bowes (1992) concluded from their review that only chronically asphyxiated fetuses develop meconium aspiration syndrome. They postulated that chronic antepartum asphyxia leads to pulmonary vascular damage, pulmonary hypertension, and persistent fetal circulation. In addition, these infants are unable to clear aspirated meconium. Thus, the 2 percent of infants who do not respond to suctioning at delivery are likely to be those who have sustained such antenatal damage. Similarly, Richey and colleagues (1995) found no correlation between markers of acute asphyxia—umbilical artery pH, lactate, or hypoxanthine—and meconium, but did find that one marker of chronic asphyxia—serum erythropoietin—was significantly elevated in newborns with meconium-stained fluid. This observation was confirmed by Bloom and associates (1996).

Amnioinfusion. Amnioinfusion for meconium may be beneficial only when the meconium is thick and there are recurrent variable decelerations (Spong and colleagues, 1994). On the other hand, it probably poses little or no increased risk (Sadovsky and colleagues, 1989; Wenstrom and coworkers, 1995). Unfortunately, it does not benefit fetuses in whom meconium aspiration syndrome has already developed

before the onset of labor (Byrne and Gau, 1987; Manning and colleagues, 1978). This technique is discussed in Chapter 21 (p. 532) and described in Chapter 18 (p. 462).

Care of the Neonate. According to guidelines of the American Academy of Pediatrics and the American College of Obstetricians and Gynecologists (2002), at delivery the infant's mouth and nares should be carefully suctioned before the shoulders are delivered. A suction bulb is usually adequate. The DeLee trap also can be used, but it should be connected to wall suction and not suctioned by mouth. Although both methods are equally efficacious, even with careful suctioning, 2 to 5 percent of infants with thick meconium develop meconium aspiration syndrome (Locus and colleagues, 1990).

If the infant is depressed, residual meconium in the hypopharynx is removed by suctioning under direct visualization. The trachea is then intubated and meconium suctioned from the lower airway. If the infant is vigorous, there is no evidence that tracheal suctioning is necessary. The stomach can be suctioned of meconium to avoid further meconium aspiration. Although the efficacy of this management in preventing long-term morbidity or mortality is undocumented, it carries little risk when done properly (Yoder, 1994).

HEMORRHAGIC DISEASE OF THE NEWBORN. This disorder is characterized by spontaneous internal or external bleeding, beginning any time after birth. Most hemorrhagic disease results from abnormally low levels of the vitamin K–dependent clotting factors (V, VII, IX, and X), prothrombin, and proteins C and S (Zipursky, 1999). Early bleeding occurs within 48 hours after birth in infants whose mothers took anticonvulsants during pregnancy. In these cases, the depressed factor levels result from their decreased maternal hepatic synthesis, as well as the generally poor transplacental passage of vitamin K. Classical hemorrhagic disease, which becomes apparent from 2 to 5 days after birth, occurs in infants not treated with vitamin K at birth. Late hemorrhage occurs at 2 to 12 weeks in infants who are exclusively breast fed, because breast milk contains very low levels of vitamin K. Other causes include hemophilia, congenital syphilis, sepsis, thrombocytopenia purpura, erythroblastosis, and intracranial hemorrhage.

Prophylaxis. Hemorrhagic disease can be avoided by the intramuscular injection of 1 mg of vitamin K_1 (phytonadione) at delivery. Oral administration is not effective, and maternal administration of vitamin K prior to delivery results in very little transport to the fetus. For treatment of active bleeding, vitamin K is injected intravenously. Reports of an association between the administration of vitamin K to newborns and subsequent development of childhood leukemia have been disproved (Zipursky, 1999).

THROMBOCYTOPENIA. The differential diagnosis of neonatal thrombocytopenia is provided in Table 29–9.

TABLE 29–9 Some Causes of Neonatal Thrombocytopenia

TABLE 29–9 Some Causes of Neonatal Thrombocytopenia

Immune disorders
   Passive—Maternal immune thrombocytopenia, lupus, drugs
   Active—Alloimmune, erythroblastosis fetalis
Infections
Drugs
Congenital
   Thrombocytopenia absent radius (TAR) syndrome
   Fanconi anemia
   Chediak–Higashi disease
   Megakaryocytic hypoplasia
   Leukemia
   Histiocytosis
   Osteopetrosis
Bone marrow disease
Disseminated intravascular coagulation
Inherited
   Wiskott–Aldrich syndrome
   May–Hegglin anomaly

Thrombocytopenia tends to be more severe in preterm fetuses, especially those with respiratory distress and hypoxia or sepsis.

Immune Thrombocytopenia. Rarely, antiplatelet IgG is transferred from the mother, causing thrombocytopenia in the fetus-neonate. In these cases, thrombocytopenia is mild and is found in association with maternal autoimmune disease, especially immune thrombocytopenia. Although corticosteroid therapy usually increases maternal platelet levels, it generally does not affect fetal platelets. Despite this, fetal platelet counts are usually high enough to allow vaginal delivery without an increased risk of intrapartum hemorrhage and without need for fetal platelet sampling (see Chap. 51, p. 1158). Importantly, neonatal platelet levels often fall rapidly after birth, reaching a nadir at 48 to 72 hours of life, making close monitoring in the first days of life essential.

Alloimmune (Isoimmune) Thrombocytopenia. This condition differs from immunological thrombocytopenia in several important ways. It is caused by maternal isoimmunization to fetal platelet antigens in a manner similar to D-antigen isoimmunization (see p. 663). Thus, the maternal platelet count is normal and alloimmunization is not suspected until after the birth of an affected child. Another important difference is that alloimmune fetal thrombocytopenia, even in the first affected infant, is frequently severe, and usually develops before the third trimester. It can thus cause fetal intracranial hemorrhage, even as early as 20 weeks.

Alloimmune thrombocytopenia follows maternal isoimmunization, usually against the platelet antigen HPA-1a—formerly called PL A1—which is found in 98 percent of the population. The susceptible mother lacks this common antigen and becomes immunized when exposed to the fetal platelet antigen. Recall that some degree of fetal–maternal hemorrhage occurs in the majority of pregnancies (see Table 29–5). Based on the incidence of HPA-1a negativity, 1 in 50 pregnancies is at risk. Yet the incidence of alloimmune thrombocytopenia is only 1 in 5000 to 1 in 10,000 live births (Nicolaides and Snijders, 1992; Silver and colleagues, 2000). The paucity of expected cases is explained by the fact that fetal–maternal hemorrhage sufficient to provoke an immune response occurs in only 5 to 10 percent of pregnancies. Other antibodies are also important. Davoren and associates (2004) reported that only 79 percent of these mothers had HPA-1a alloimmunization and 16 percent were due to HPA-5b, HPA-3a, and HPA-1b antibodies.

The diagnosis can be made on clinical grounds if the mother has a normal platelet count and there is no evidence of any immunological disorder, and her infant has thrombocytopenia without evidence of other disease. Fetal alloimmune thrombocytopenia recurs in 70 to 90 percent of subsequent pregnancies, is often severe, and usually develops earlier with each successive pregnancy (Silver and associates, 2000). Fortunately, weekly maternal intravenous infusions of immunoglobulin usually result in fetal platelet levels high enough to allow vaginal delivery (see Chap. 13, p. 332).

Preeclampsia and Eclampsia. Fetal thrombocytopenia is not caused by preeclampsia–eclampsia. Pritchard and colleagues (1987) studied a large number of women with hypertension at Parkland Hospital and identified no cases in which neonatal thrombocytopenia correlated with maternal thrombocytopenia (see Chap. 34, p. 773).

POLYCYTHEMIA AND HYPERVISCOSITY. Neonatal polycythemia and blood hyperviscosity occur as the result of chronic hypoxia in utero, from acute transfusion from the placenta or a twin at delivery, or much more rarely, from maternal–fetal hemorrhage. As the hematocrit rises above 65, blood viscosity markedly increases. Signs and symptoms include plethora, cyanosis, and neurological aberrations. Laboratory findings include hyperbilirubinemia, thrombocytopenia, fragmented erythrocytes, and hypoglycemia. Treatment consists of partial exchange transfusion with plasma to lower the hematocrit.

FETAL DEATH

From the foregoing sections, it is apparent that a number of maternal and fetal conditions can result in fetal demise. With advances in obstetrics, clinical genetics, maternal–fetal and neonatal medicine, and perinatal pathology, a number of stillbirths that previously would have been categorized as "unexplained" can now be attributed to specific causes. In many cases, this information makes management of subsequent pregnancies easier. Ultrasound allows rapid confirmation of fetal death, which frequently prompts labor induction in women with a favorable cervix (see Chap. 22, p. 540).

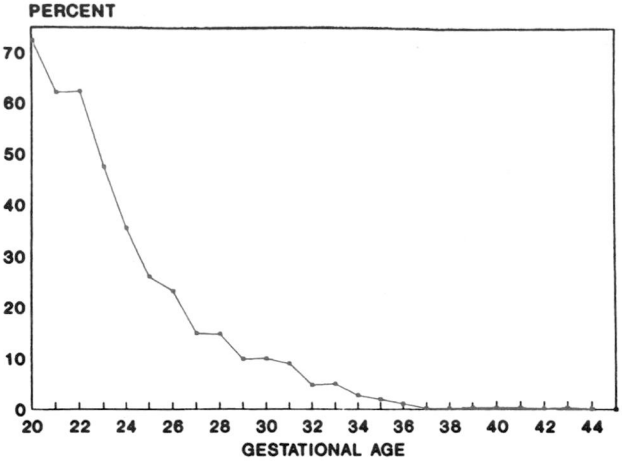

PERCENT

FIGURE 29–14. Relationship between gestational age and incidence of stillbirth. (From Copper and colleagues, 1994, with permission.)

DEFINITION OF FETAL MORTALITY. Stillbirths are much more common with decreasing gestational age. According to Copper and colleagues (1994), almost 80 percent of all stillbirths occur before term, and more than half occur before 28 weeks. Considering this, because statistics on perinatal outcome compiled by the National Center for Health Statistics and others generally include only those dead fetuses and neonates born weighing 500 g or more, the incidence of early stillbirth may actually be even higher than that shown in Figure 29–14.

The stillbirth rate has declined over the past five decades, and the causes of stillbirth also have changed appreciably. Fretts and colleagues (1992) reviewed 709 stillbirths at the Royal Victoria Hospital in Montreal and found that the fetal death rate per 1000 births decreased from 11.5 in the 1960s to 5.1 in the 1980s. The rate due to lethal anomalies declined by almost half between the 1970s and 1980s—from 10.8 to 5.4 per 10,000 births—because deaths of infants with anomalies were "prevented" by early pregnancy terminations. Through the 1980s, commonly recognized causes of fetal death included infection, malformations, fetal growth restriction, and abruptio placentae. Although more than one fourth of all fetal deaths during the 1980s were still unexplained, this number decreased from 38.1 to 13.6 per 10,000 births.

CAUSES OF FETAL DEATH. These can generally be categorized as fetal, placental, or maternal. In the past, because a definable cause could not always be assigned, there was only mild enthusiasm for necropsy. Currently, however, it is recognized that an autopsy performed by a pathologist with expertise in fetal and placental disorders, assisted by a team including maternal–fetal medicine, genetic, and pediatric specialists, often determines the cause of death. Faye-Petersen (1999), Horn (2004), and their colleagues reviewed autopsies performed by such teams, and found that the cause of death was identified in up to 94 percent. Determining the

TABLE 29–10 Categories and Causes of Fetal Death

Fetal (25–40%)
Chromosomal anomalies
Nonchromosomal birth defects
Nonimmune hydrops
Infections—viruses, bacteria, protozoa
Placental (25–35%)
Abruption
Fetal–maternal hemorrhage
Cord accident
Placental insufficiency
Intrapartum asphyxia
Previa
Twin-to-twin transfusion
Chorioamnionitis
Maternal (5–10%)
Antiphospholipid antibodies
Diabetes
Hypertensive disorders
Trauma
Abnormal labor
Sepsis
Acidosis
Hypoxia
Uterine rupture
Postterm pregnancy
Drugs
Unexplained (25–35%)

From Cunningham and Hollier (1997).

cause of death of preterm infants appears to be most difficult (Yudkin and colleagues, 1987). Some causes of fetal death or stillbirth identified by autopsy are shown in Table 29–10.

Fetal Causes. Some type of fetal abnormality accounts for 25 to 40 percent of all stillbirths (Fretts and Usher, 1997; Pauli and Reiser, 1994). These abnormalities include congenital anomalies, infections, malnutrition, nonimmune hydrops, and anti–D-isoimmunization.

The reported incidence of *major congenital malformations* in stillborns is highly variable. It depends on whether necropsy was performed and if so, the experience, interest, and training of the pathologist (Cartlidge and co-workers, 1995). The majority of stillbirths attributed to fetal causes in the Wisconsin Stillbirth Service Program had a major structural malformation identified at autopsy (Pauli and Reiser, 1994). Conversely, in a study of 403 stillbirths reported by Copper and colleagues (1994), malformations were identified prenatally in only 5.6 percent. Faye-Petersen and colleagues (1999) found that one third of fetal deaths were caused by structural anomalies, of which neural-tube defects, hydrops, isolated hydrocephalus, and complex congenital heart disease were the most common. Major structural anomalies, hydrops, and aneuploidy are particularly amenable to antenatal diagnosis.

The incidence of stillbirths caused by fetal infection appears to be remarkably consistent. In five studies totaling 2676 stillbirths, 5.6 percent were attributed to infection (Cartlidge, 1995; Copper, 1994; Fretts, 1992; Lammer, 1989; Pauli and Reiser, 1994, and all of their colleagues). Most were diagnosed as "chorioamnionitis" and others as "fetal or intrauterine sepsis." In indigent and inner-city women, congenital syphilis can be a common cause of fetal death. For example, between 5 and 10 percent of stillbirths at Parkland Hospital are attributable to syphilis (see Chap. 59, p. 1302). Other potentially lethal infections include cytomegalovirus, parvovirus B19, rubella, varicella, and listeriosis.

Placental Causes. Placental abnormalities known to cause fetal death are shown in Table 29–10. Many of these deaths could also be categorized as having maternal or fetal causes. For example, placental abruption is associated with gestational hypertension in about half of cases, and could thus be classified as "maternal." In another example, placental insufficiency could result from aneuploidy or infection and thus be considered "fetal." With these caveats in mind, approximately 15 to 25 percent of fetal deaths are attributed to problems of the placenta, membranes, or cord (Alessandri and colleagues, 1992; Fretts and Usher, 1997).

Placental abruption is the most common single identifiable cause of fetal death (see Chap. 35, p. 812). Fretts and Usher (1997) determined abruption to be the cause of death in 14 percent of stillborns. At Parkland Hospital, about 10 percent of third-trimester stillbirths are the consequence of premature placental separation.

Clinically significant *placental* and *membrane infection* rarely occurs in the absence of significant fetal infection. Exceptions include tuberculosis and malaria. In some cases, microscopic examination of the placenta and membranes may help to identify an infectious cause. Chorioamnionitis is characterized by mononuclear and polymorphonuclear leukocytes infiltrating the chorion. Although some clinicians consider these findings to be nonspecific, Benirschke and Kaufmann (2000) believe that microscopic chorioamnionitis is always due to infection (see Chap. 27, p. 625).

Placental infarcts appear as areas of fibrinoid trophoblastic degeneration, calcification, and ischemic infarction from spiral artery occlusion (see Chap. 27, p. 621). Marginal and subchorionic infarcts are common and usually of no import. Fox (1978) found that one fourth of placentas from uncomplicated term deliveries had infarcts. When there is severe hypertension, two thirds of placentas are so involved. Severe preeclampsia, with or without maternal thrombophilia, frequently results in extensive, centralized infarcts (see Chap. 27, p. 621).

Fetal–maternal hemorrhage sufficient to cause fetal death was reported in 4.7 percent of 319 fetal deaths at Los Angeles County Women's Hospital in which Kleihauer–Betke stains of maternal blood had been performed (Samadi and associates, 1996). Such hemorrhage is common with severe maternal trauma (see Chap. 42, p. 999). Twin-to-twin transfusion is a common cause of fetal death in monochorionic multifetal pregnancy (see Chap. 39, p. 929).

Maternal Causes. Although they appear to make only a small contribution to fetal deaths, maternal factors may be underestimated. This is because pathologies with a strong maternal component, such as placental abruption or isoimmunization, often are attributed to placental or fetal causes. *Hypertensive disorders* and *diabetes* are the two most commonly cited maternal diseases, associated with 5 to 8 percent of stillbirths (Alessandri and colleagues, 1992; Fretts and Usher, 1997).

Lupus anticoagulant and *anticardiolipin antibodies* are associated with decidual vasculopathy, placental infarction, fetal growth restriction, recurrent abortion, and fetal death (see Chap. 54, p. 1215). Although women with these autoantibodies clearly are at increased risk for adverse pregnancy outcomes, very few otherwise unexplained stillbirths can be attributed solely to such antibodies (Haddow and co-workers, 1991; Infante-Rivard and associates, 1991). Some hereditary thrombophilias have been linked with placental abruption, fetal growth restriction, and stillbirths (Procházka and colleagues, 2003; Rey and co-workers, 2003). These disorders are discussed in detail in Chapter 47 (see p. 1074).

EVALUATION OF THE STILLBORN INFANT. Determining the cause of fetal death facilitates the psychological adaptation to a significant loss, helps to assuage the guilt that is part of grieving, makes counseling regarding recurrence more accurate, and may prompt therapy or intervention to prevent a similar outcome in the next pregnancy. Identification of inherited syndromes also provides useful information for other family members.

Clinical Examination. A thorough examination of the fetus, placenta, and membranes should be performed at delivery and recorded in the chart. The details of relevant prenatal events should be provided. Photographs should be taken for the record whenever possible, and a full radiograph of the fetus—a "fetogram"—may be performed. These are especially important in providing anatomical information when the parents decline a full autopsy. The checklist used at Parkland Hospital to format the stillbirth note is outlined in Table 29–11.

Laboratory Evaluation. If autopsy and chromosome studies are performed when indicated, up to 35 percent of stillborn infants are discovered to have major structural anomalies (Faye-Petersen and associates, 1999; Mueller and colleagues, 1983). Another 20 percent have dysmorphic features or skeletal abnormalities (Pauli and Reiser, 1994; Saller and colleagues, 1995). Finally, 8 percent have chromosomal abnormalities. The American College of Obstetricians and Gynecologists (1996) recommends consideration of cytogenetic studies for

TABLE 29–11 Protocol for Examination of Stillborn Infants

Infant Description
  Malformations
  Skin staining
  Degree of maceration
  Color—pale, plethoric
Umbilical Cord
  Prolapse
  Entanglement—neck, arms, legs
  Hematomas or strictures
  Number of vessels
  Length
  Wharton jelly—normal, absent
Amnionic Fluid
  Color—meconium, blood
  Consistency
  Volume
Placenta
  Weight
  Staining—meconium
  Adherent clots
  Structural abnormalities—circumvallate or accessory lobes,
    velamentous insertion
  Edema—hydropic changes
Membranes
  Meconium stained or cloudy
  Thickening

From Cunningham and Hollier (1997).

fetuses with dysmorphic features, inconsistent growth measurements, anomalies, hydrops, or growth restriction. A fetal karyotype also should be performed if either parent is a carrier for a balanced translocation, or if there is a history of recurrent losses or stillbirths in first-degree relatives. Such studies also might be considered in cases in which absolutely no other explanation for the loss is found. If certain types of fetal or placental aneuploidies are detected, such as a chromosome translocation or rearrangement, parental karyotypes also may be indicated.

Appropriate consent must be obtained to take skin and other fetal tissue samples, including fluid obtained by needle postmortem. A total of 3 mL of fetal blood, obtained from the umbilical cord (preferably) or by cardiac puncture is placed into a sterile, heparinized tube for cytogenetic studies. If blood cannot be obtained, a piece of fetal or placental tissue can be substituted, but because it must contain some viable cells that can be stimulated to divide, it cannot be macerated. Skin with attached dermal tissue or fascia from the thigh, inguinal region, or Achilles tendon should measure 1 cm^2 and be washed with sterile saline prior to placement in saline or sterile cytogenetic medium. Placement in formalin or alcohol prevents cytogenetic analysis by killing any remaining viable cells. A full karyotype may not be possible in cases with prolonged intrauterine retention. Fluorescence in situ hybridization, however, might be used to rule out numerical abnormalities or to look for certain common deletions such as

that causing DiGeorge syndrome. Maternal blood should be obtained for Kleihauer–Betke staining, testing for antiphospholipid antibodies and lupus anticoagulant if indicated, and serum glucose to exclude overt diabetes.

Autopsy. Patients should be encouraged to allow a full autopsy, but valuable information also can be obtained from limited studies. A gross external examination, along with photography, radiography, MRI, bacterial cultures, and selective use of chromosomal and histopathology studies often can aid in determining the cause of death (Brookes and coworkers, 1996; Mueller and colleagues, 1983).

A complete autopsy is much more likely to yield valuable information. An analysis of 400 consecutive fetal deaths in Wales found that autopsy altered the presumed cause of death in 13 percent and provided new information in another 26 percent (Cartlidge and Stewart, 1995). Studies from Alabama and New York found that autopsy results changed the recurrence risk estimates and parental counseling in approximately one fourth of cases (Faye-Petersen and colleagues, 1999; Saller and associates, 1995).

In many centers, maternal records and autopsy findings are reviewed on a monthly basis by a stillbirth committee composed of maternal–fetal medicine specialists, neonatologists, clinical geneticists, and perinatal pathologists. If possible, the cause of death is assigned based on available evidence. Most importantly, parents should then be contacted and offered counseling regarding the cause of death, the recurrence risk if any, and strategies to avoid recurrence in future pregnancies.

PSYCHOLOGICAL ASPECTS. Fetal death is psychologically traumatic for the woman and her family. Further stress results from an interval of more than 24 hours between the diagnosis of fetal death and the induction of labor, not seeing her infant for as long as she desires, and having no tokens of remembrance (Radestad and colleagues, 1996). The woman experiencing a stillbirth or even an early miscarriage is at increased risk for postpartum depression and should be closely monitored (see Chap. 55, p. 1243).

PREGNANCY AFTER PREVIOUS STILLBIRTH. Fortunately, there are very few conditions associated with recurrent stillbirth. Other than hereditary disorders, only maternal conditions such as diabetes, chronic hypertension, or hereditary thrombophilia increase risk of recurrence. Several studies have cited rates of recurrent stillbirth that range from 0 to 8 percent, depending on the specific population studied (Freeman, 1985; Samueloff, 1993; Surkan, 2004; Weeks, 1995, and all their colleagues). Losses that occur early in the pregnancy are associated with a higher risk of subsequent adverse outcomes than those that occur late in gestation. Goldenberg and colleagues (1993) studied 95 women who had a pregnancy loss at 13 to 24 weeks and found that almost 40 percent had a preterm delivery in their next pregnancy, 5 percent had a stillbirth, and 6 percent had a neonatal death.

In a national Swedish database study of more than 410,000 deliveries, Surkan and co-workers (2004) found that delivery of a living, growth-restricted term infant was associated with a twofold increased risk of stillbirth in the next pregnancy. For those who had a live growth-restricted preterm infant, the risk was increased to fivefold.

Prenatal Evaluation. Knowledge of the cause of fetal death results in a more precise calculation of individual recurrence risk and in many cases allows a management plan to be made. For example, a cord accident would not be expected to recur. In contrast, aneuploidy generally has a 1-percent recurrence risk, and familial DiGeorge syndrome has a 50-percent recurrence. The latter two could be detected in subsequent pregnancies by chorionic villous sampling or amniocentesis. With proper treatment, infectious causes also would be unlikely to recur.

Maternal medical disorders associated with prior stillbirth are often easily identified. In some cases, intervention either preconceptionally or early in pregnancy improves outcome in subsequent pregnancies (see Chap. 7, p. 193). For example, placental abruption often is associated with chronic hypertension. Although Pritchard and colleagues (1991) demonstrated an abruption recurrence rate of 10 percent, this could possibly be reduced with more stringent blood pressure control or early delivery. Similarly, a significant portion of perinatal mortality is attributable to congenital anomalies occurring in diabetic pregnancies with poor early blood glucose control. Intensive glycemic control in the periconceptional period reduces the incidence of malformations and generally improves outcome (see Chap. 52, p. 1177). Lack of planning can lead to an unexplained pregnancy loss of the type that still accounts for half of stillborns of diabetic mothers (Hanson and Persson, 1993).

There is some evidence that recurrent fetal loss due to antiphospholipid antibodies can be decreased with treatment (see Chap. 54, p. 1218). Testing for antiphospholipid antibodies in women who have an unexplained fetal loss in the second trimester is often helpful, but it is not recommended for the woman with a normally grown, unexplained third-trimester stillborn.

Management. Few studies address management of the woman who has suffered a prior fetal death. At the University of California at Irvine, Freeman and colleagues (1985) evaluated fetal heart rate testing in women with a variety of risk factors, including prior stillbirth. Women with a history of stillbirth were more likely to have a positive contraction stress test than women tested for other indications. The positive tests were mainly in women with hypertension (12 percent) or fetal growth restriction (17 percent). Although there were no recurrent stillbirths, the offspring of women with prior stillborns had an increased incidence of respiratory distress syndrome compared with those of women tested for other reasons. The investigators suggested that early delivery had been performed empirically in women with a previous loss.

A subsequent study by the Irvine group evaluated fetal heart rate testing in women whose only indication was prior stillbirth (Weeks and colleagues, 1995). There was only one recurrent stillbirth and only three fetuses with abnormal testing before 32 weeks among 300 study patients. The investigators found no relationship between the gestational age of the previous stillborn and the incidence or timing of abnormal tests or fetal jeopardy in the subsequent pregnancy. They concluded that antepartum surveillance should begin at 32 weeks or later in the otherwise healthy woman with a history of stillbirth. This is in agreement with recommendations of the American College of Obstetricians and Gynecologists (1999a).

INJURIES OF THE FETUS AND NEWBORN

Considered here are several varieties of birth injuries. Other injuries are described elsewhere in connection with the specific obstetrical complications that lead to or contribute to the injury.

SPONTANEOUS INTRACRANIAL HEMORRHAGE. Fetal or neonatal intracranial hemorrhage can occur at any of several sites (Table 29–12). Isolated intraventricular hemorrhage into the germinal matrix, without associated subarachnoid or subdural bleeding, is the most common type of intracranial hemorrhage. It usually occurs spontaneously as the result of immaturity, and generally does not result from traumatic delivery or obstetrical factors (Hayden and colleagues, 1985). Infants weighing less than 1500 grams are most susceptible. Thorp and colleagues (2001) prospectively studied 12,578 neonates from 23 to 35 weeks and found the incidence of grade III and IV intraventricular hemorrhage was 7.1 percent. The most significant associated factors were early gestational age, antenatal exposure to indomethacin, surfactant use, and need for neonatal transport. The likelihood of severe hemorrhage increased as gestational age at delivery decreased. Antenatal steroid use did not have a significant effect on the development of hemorrhage.

Spontaneous intracranial hemorrhage also has been documented in healthy term neonates (Huang and Robertson, 2004). In a prospective study, Whitby and colleagues (2004) used MRI in such infants and found that 6 percent of those delivered spontaneously, and 28 percent of those delivered by forceps, had a subdural hemorrhage. None of these infants had clinical findings, and hematomas resolved in all by 4 weeks.

The fetal head has considerable plasticity and may undergo appreciable molding during passage through the birth canal. The dimensions of the head actually change during the second stage, with lengthening of the occipitofrontal diameter

TABLE 29–12 **Major Types of Intracranial Hemorrhage in the Newborn**

Type	Gestational Age	Incidence and Severity	Cause(s)
Subdural	Term > preterm	Uncommon Serious	Venous tears Trauma commonly
Primary subarachnoid	Preterm > term	Common Benign	Trauma—term "Hypoxia"—preterm
Intracerebellar	Preterm > term	Uncommon Serious	Multifactorial
Intraventricular	Preterm	Common Serious	Thin-walled vessels of germinal matrix
Miscellaneous	Term > preterm	Uncommon Variable	Multifactorial Trauma, hemorrhagic infarction, coagulopathy, vascular defect, ECMO

ECMO = extracorporeal membrane oxygenation.
Data from Volpe (1995).

of the skull. Rarely, severe molding and marked overlap of the parietal bones can result in tearing of the bridging veins from the cerebral cortex to the sagittal sinus, or rupture of the internal cerebral veins, the vein of Galen at its junctions with the straight sinus, or the tentorium itself. Compression of the skull can stretch the tentorium cerebelli and can tear the vein of Galen or its tributaries. As a result, intracranial hemorrhage may occur even after an apparently uneventful vaginal delivery.

INTRAVENTRICULAR HEMORRHAGE FROM ME-CHANICAL INJURY. Birth trauma is no longer a common cause of intracranial hemorrhage. The elimination of difficult forceps operations and appropriate management of breech delivery have contributed significantly to a reduction in the incidence of all birth injuries, including intracranial hemorrhage. As detailed in Chapter 23 (see p. 558), appropriate use of forceps or vacuum delivery does not lead to increased intracranial hemorrhage or other neonatal injury (American College of Obstetricians and Gynecologists, 2000).

Infants suffering intracranial hemorrhage from mechanical injury, such as subdural hemorrhage from tentorial tears or massive infratentorial hemorrhage, have neurological abnormalities from the time of birth (Volpe, 1995). Severely

affected infants—usually those weighing more than 4000 g—have stupor or coma, nuchal rigidity, and opisthotonus that worsen over minutes to hours. Some infants who are born depressed appear to improve until about 12 hours of age, but then drowsiness, apathy, feeble cry, pallor, failure to nurse, dyspnea, cyanosis, vomiting, and convulsions become evident.

Subarachnoid hemorrhage is usually minor with no symptoms, but seizures with an interictal period may manifest. In some infants, there is catastrophic deterioration. Ultrasound, CT, or MRI of the head are useful for diagnosis and also have contributed appreciably to an understanding of the etiology and frequency of some forms of intracranial hemorrhage (Perlman and Cunningham, 1993).

CEPHALOHEMATOMA. These hematomas are identified in 2.5 percent of all births. They are usually caused by injury to the periosteum of the skull during labor and delivery and rarely develop in the absence of birth trauma (Thacker and colleagues, 1987). In a recent Network study in which 37,100 cesarean delivery outcomes were examined, Alexander and associates (2005) found a 0.3 percent incidence of cephalohematoma. The hemorrhage may develop over one or both parietal bones, and palpable edges can be appreciated as the blood reaches the limits of the periosteum (Fig. 29–15).

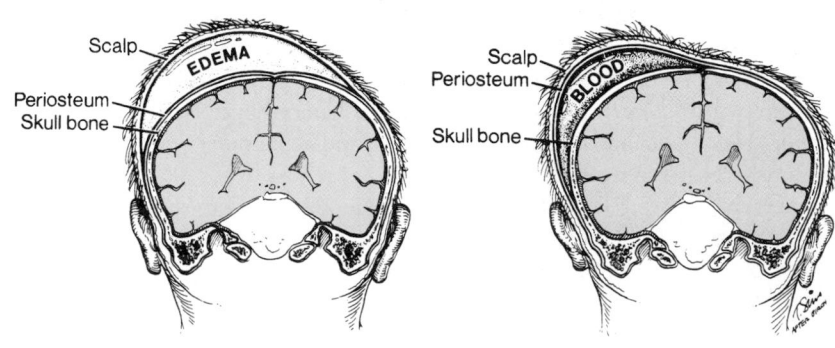

FIGURE 29–15. Difference between a large caput succedaneum (*left*) and cephalohematoma (*right*). In a caput succedaneum, the effusion overlies the periosteum and consists of edema fluid; in a cephalohematoma, it lies under the periosteum and consists of blood.

A cephalohematoma may not be apparent until hours after delivery, when bleeding sufficient to raise the periosteum has occurred. It often grows larger, disappearing only after weeks or even months. In contrast, caput succedaneum, also shown in Figure 29–15, consists of a focal swelling of the scalp from edema that overlies the periosteum. Swelling from caput succedaneum is maximal at birth, rapidly grows smaller, and usually disappears within hours or a few days. Increasing size of the cephalohematoma and other evidence of extensive hemorrhage are indications for additional investigation, including radiographic studies and assessment of coagulation factors.

NERVE INJURIES

Spinal Injury. Overstretching of the spinal cord and associated hemorrhage may follow excessive traction during delivery, and there may be actual fracture or dislocation of the vertebrae. Menticoglou and associates (1995) described 15 neonates with this type of high cervical spinal cord injury and found that all of the injuries were associated with forceps rotations during delivery. Spinal cord injury also can occur during breech delivery.

Brachial Plexus Injury. These injuries are relatively common, complicating between 1 in 500 to 1 in 1000 term births (Boo and colleagues, 1991; Salonen and Uüsitalo, 1990). Three types of brachial plexus damage have been described. Damage to the upper plexus is called *Erb* or *Duchenne paralysis.* It results from damage to C5 and C6 and occasionally C7, leading to paralysis of the deltoid and infraspinatus muscles as well as the flexor muscles of the forearm. The affected arm is held straight and internally rotated, with the elbow extended and the wrist and fingers flexed. The function of the fingers usually is retained. Because lateral head traction is frequently employed to effect delivery of the shoulders in normal vertex presentations, Erb paralysis can occur even when the delivery did not appear to be difficult.

Damage to the lower plexus—C8 and T1—results in *Klumpke's paralysis* in which the hand is flaccid. Total involvement of all brachial plexus nerve roots results in flaccidity of both arm and hand. With this kind of severe damage, there may also be *Horner syndrome* on the affected side—ptosis and pupillary meiosis resulting from interruption of nerve fibers in the cervical sympathetic chain.

The propulsive efforts of normal delivery may cause brachial nerve stretching and damage (Sandmire and DeMott, 2000). In a study of 130 infants with brachial plexus injuries, Ubachs and colleagues (1995) found that cases involving C5 to C6 nerve roots were frequently associated with breech delivery. More extensive damage involving C5 to C7 or C5 to T1 often followed difficult cephalic deliveries. Increasing birthweight and breech delivery are significant risk factors. Unfortunately, and as discussed in detail in Chapter 20 (see p. 513), shoulder dystocia leading to brachial plexus injury cannot be predicted reliably. Thus, it is fortunate indeed that the majority of cases involving nerve stretching or compression resolve with conservative therapy. In cases of complete nerve avulsion, however, normal function does not return.

Facial Paralysis. Pressure on the facial nerve as it emerges from the stylomastoid foramen can cause damage resulting in facial paralysis. The incidence, which has been reported to range from less than 1 to 7.5 per 1000 term births, likely is influenced by the vigor with which the diagnosis is sought (Levine and colleagues, 1984; White and associates, 1996). Facial paralysis may be apparent at delivery or may develop shortly after birth (Fig. 29–16). It can be caused by pressure exerted by the posterior blade when forceps have been

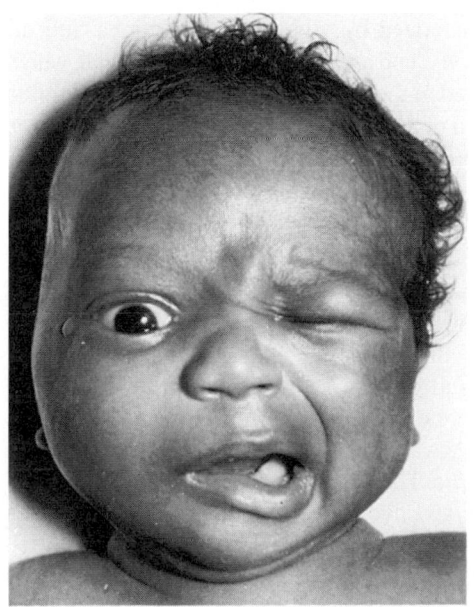

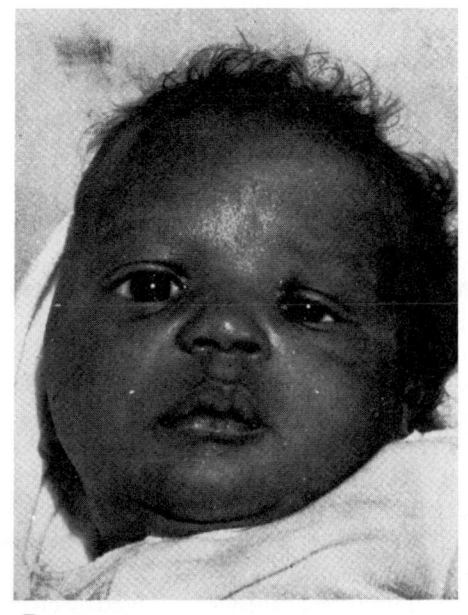

A   **B**

FIGURE 29–16. **A.** Paralysis of the right side of the face 15 minutes after forceps delivery. **B.** Same infant 24 hours later. Recovery was complete in another 24 hours.

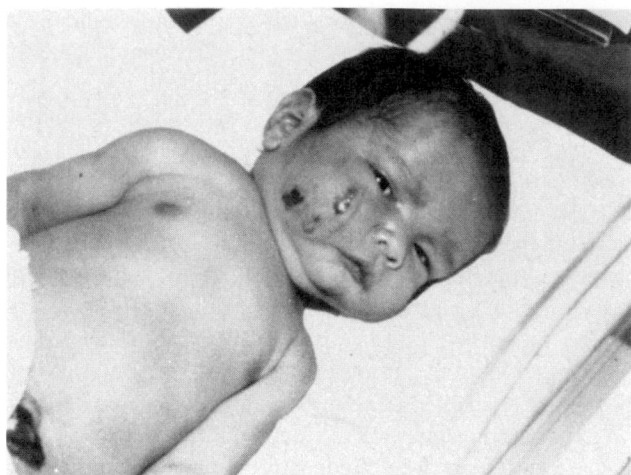

FIGURE 29–17. Healing abrasions and lacerations from a difficult forceps delivery. Palsy of the right facial nerve has nearly cleared.

placed obliquely on the fetal head, in which case the forceps marks indicate the cause of the injury (Fig. 29–17). It also can occur after spontaneous delivery. White and associates (1996) observed that only 18 percent of facial nerve palsies were associated with forceps delivery, and that the majority followed spontaneous vaginal or cesarean delivery. Levine and co-workers (1984) reported that one third of cases followed spontaneous delivery. Spontaneous recovery within a few days is the rule. An increase in injuries to the sixth cranial nerve with resultant lateral rectus ocular muscle paralysis following operative vaginal delivery also has been reported (Galbraith, 1994).

SKELETAL AND MUSCLE INJURIES

Fractures. Clavicular fractures are an unpredictable and unavoidable complication of normal birth. They are surprisingly common, occurring in 3.3 to 18 per 1000 live births (Roberts and associates, 1995; Turpenny and Nimmo, 1993). Chez and colleagues (1994) reported an incidence of 9 per 1000 vaginally delivered newborns and were unable to identify any specific factor that could be changed to avoid such fractures.

Humeral fractures are not common. Difficulty encountered in the delivery of the shoulders in cephalic deliveries and of extended arms in breech deliveries often produce such fractures. Up to 70 percent of cases, however, follow uneventful delivery (Turpenny and Nimmo, 1993). Humeral fractures are often of the greenstick type, although complete fracture with overriding of the bones may occur. Palpation of the clavicles and long bones should be performed on all newborns when a fracture is suspected, and any crepitation or unusual irregularity should prompt radiographic examination.

Femoral fractures are relatively rare and usually associated with breech delivery.

Skull fracture may follow forcible attempts at delivery, especially with forceps, but also can occur during spontaneous

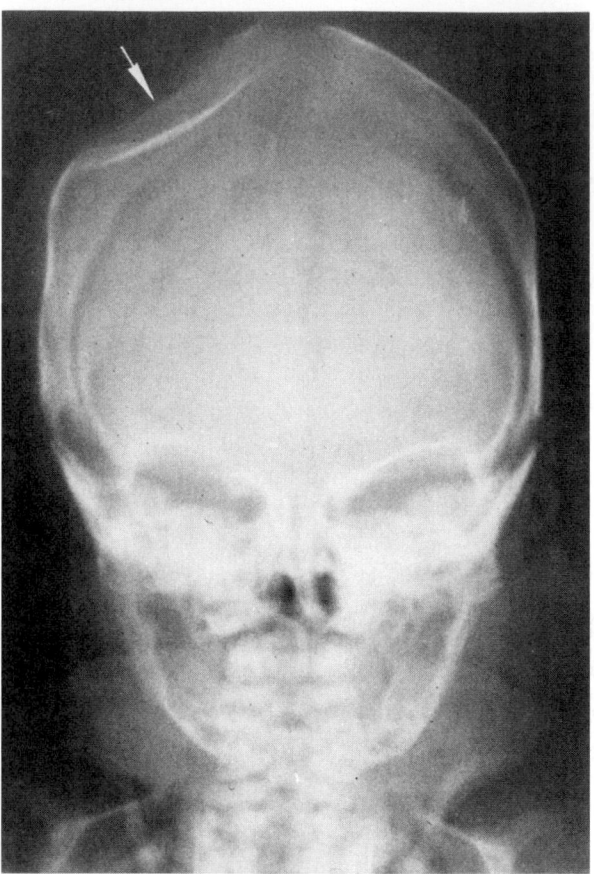

FIGURE 29–18. Depressed skull fracture evident immediately after cesarean delivery. Labor had progressed, and the head was deep in the pelvis. Dislodgment of the head from the birth canal was performed by an assistant using manual pressure upward through the vagina.

or cesarean delivery (Saunders and colleagues, 1979; Skajaa and associates, 1987). In the radiograph shown in Figure 29–18, a focal but marked depressed skull fracture is apparent. Labor was characterized by vigorous contractions, full dilatation of the cervix, and arrest of descent of the head, which was tightly wedged in the pelvis. The fracture likely resulted from compression of the skull against the sacral promontory, from upward pressure from an assistant's hand in the vagina, or as the head was pushed upward out of the birth canal at cesarean delivery. Surgical decompression was successful.

Muscular Injuries. Injury to the sternocleidomastoid muscle may occur, particularly during a breech delivery. There may be a tear of the muscle or the fascial sheath, leading to a hematoma and gradual cicatricial contraction. As the neck lengthens in the process of normal growth, the head is gradually turned toward the side of the injury—a condition known as *torticollis.* This occurs because the damaged muscle is less elastic and does not elongate at the same rate as its normal contralateral counterpart. Roemer (1954) reported that 27 of 44 infants showing this deformity had been delivered by breech or internal podalic version. He postulated that lateral hyperextension sufficient to rupture the sternocleido-mastoid may occur as the aftercoming head passes over the sacral promontory.

CONGENITAL INJURIES

Amnionic Band Syndrome. A free strip of amnion can form a focal ring around an extremity or digit, eventually producing enough constriction to cause damage or even amputation of the encircled structure. The genesis of such bands is debated. Streeter (1930), and others since, maintained that a localized failure of germ plasm or an inherent developmental abnormality of the involved structures is responsible for the abnormalities. Torpin (1968) and others contend that the lesions are the consequence of early rupture of the amnion. Occasionally, the amputated part may be found within the uterus.

Congenital Postural Deformities. Mechanical factors arising from chronically low volumes of amnionic fluid, or restriction of movement imposed by the small size and inappropriate shape of the uterine cavity or the presence of additional fetuses, may deform an otherwise normal fetal structure. Such mechanical deformations include talipes equivarus, or clubfoot; scoliosis; and hip dislocation (Miller and co-workers, 1981). Hypoplastic lungs also can result from oligohydramnios (see Chap. 21, p. 531).

REFERENCES

Achiron R, Pinchas OH, Reichman B, et al: Fetal intracranial haemorrhage: Clinical significance of in-utero ultrasonic diagnosis. Br J Obstet Gynaecol 100:995, 1993

Alessandri LM, Stanley FJ, Garner JB, et al: A case-control study of unexplained antepartum stillbirths. Br J Obstet Gynaecol 99:711, 1992

Alexander JM for the NICHD MFMU Network: The MFMU Units Cesarean Registry: Fetal injury associated with cesarean delivery. Presented at the 25th Annual Meeting of the Society for Maternal-Fetal Medicine, Reno/Lake Tahoe NV, 7–12 Feb 2005

Allan LD, Crawford DC, Sheridan R, et al: Aetiology of non-immune hydrops: The value of echocardiography. Br J Obstet Gynaecol 93:223, 1986

Allan WC, Vohr B, Makuch RW, et al: Antecedents of cerebral palsy in a multicenter trial on indomethacin for intraventricular hemorrhage. Arch Pediatr Adolesc Med 151:580, 1997

Alper CA: Blood groups I. Physiology. In Beck WS (ed): Hematology. Cambridge, Mass, MIT Press, 1977, p 299

Alvarez JG, Ludmir J: Improved DPPC test for the assessment of fetal lung maturity by high-pressure liquid chromatography. Am J Obstet Gynecol 174:473, 1996

American Academy of Pediatrics. Postnatal corticosteroids to treat or prevent chronic lung disease in preterm infants. Pediatrics 109:330, 2002

American Academy of Pediatrics and American College of Obstetricians and Gynecologists: Guidelines for Perinatal Care, 5th ed. Washington, DC, AAP and ACOG Committee on Obstetric Practice, 2002, p 190

American College of Obstetricians and Gynecologists: Inappropriate use of the terms fetal distress and birth asphyxia. Committee Opinion No. 303, October 2004

American College of Obstetricians and Gynecologists: Antenatal corticosteroid therapy for fetal maturation. Committee Opinion No. 273, May 2002

American College of Obstetricians and Gynecologists: Operative vaginal delivery. Practice Bulletin No. 17, June 2000

American College of Obstetricians and Gynecologists: Antepartum fetal surveillance. Practice Bulletin No. 9, October 1999a

American College of Obstetricians and Gynecologists: Prevention of RhD alloimmunization. Clinical Management Guidelines No. 4, May 1999b

American College of Obstetricians and Gynecologists: Inappropriate use of the terms fetal distress and birth asphyxia. Committee Opinion No. 197, February 1998

American College of Obstetricians and Gynecologists: Genetic evaluation of stillbirths and neonatal deaths. Committee Opinion No. 178, November 1996

American College of Obstetricians and Gynecologists: Fetal heart rate patterns: Monitoring, interpretation, and management. Technical Bulletin No. 207, July 1995

American College of Obstetricians and Gynecologists: Fetal and neonatal neurologic injury. Technical Bulletin No. 163, January 1992

American College of Obstetricians and Gynecologists: Management of isoimmunization in pregnancy. Technical Bulletin No. 148, October 1990

American College of Obstetricians and Gynecologists and American Academy of Pediatrics: Neonatal encephalopathy and cerebral palsy. Defining the pathogenesis and pathophysiology. January 2003

Anderson GD, Bada HS, Shaver DC, et al: The effect of cesarean section on intraventricular hemorrhage in the preterm infant. Am J Obstet Gynecol 166:1091, 1992

Ballard PL, Ballard RA: Scientific basis and therapeutic regimens for use of antenatal glucocorticoids. Am J Obstet Gynecol 173:254, 1995

Barss VA, Frigoletto FD, Konugres A: The cost of irregular antibody screening. Am J Obstet Gynecol 159:428, 1988

Battin MR, Maalouf EF, Counsell SJ, et al: Magnetic resonance imaging of the brain in very preterm infants: Visualization of the germinal matrix, early myelination, and cortical folding. Pediatrics 101:957, 1998

Baud O, Foix-L'Helias L, Kaminski M, et al: Antenatal glucocorticoid treatment and cystic periventricular leukomalacia in very premature infants. N Engl J Med 341:1190, 1999

Benirschke K, Kaufmann P (eds): Infectious diseases. In: Pathology of the Human Placenta, 4th ed. New York, Springer-Verlag, 2000, p 468

Bennett PR, Le Van Kim C, Colin Y, et al: Prenatal determination of fetal RhD type by DNA amplification. N Engl J Med 329:607, 1993

Bloom S, Ramin S, Neyman S, et al: Meconium stained amniotic fluid: Is it associated with elevated erythropoietin levels? Am J Obstet Gynecol 174:360, 1996

Boo NY, Lye MS, Kanchanamala M, et al: Brachial plexus injuries in Malaysian neonates: Incidence and associated risk factors. J Trop Pediatr 37:327, 1991

Bowell PJ, Allen DL, Entwistle CC: Blood group antibody screening tests during pregnancy. Br J Obstet Gynaecol 93:1038, 1986a

Bowell PJ, Brown SE, Dike AE, et al: The significance of anti-c alloimmunization. Br J Obstet Gynaecol 93:1044, 1986b

Bowman JM: Controversies in Rh prophylaxis: Who needs Rh immune globulin and when should it be given? Am J Obstet Gynecol 151:289, 1985

Bowman JM: The management of Rh-isoimmunization. Obstet Gynecol 52:1, 1978

Bowman JM, Chown B, Lewis M, et al: Rh isoimmunization, Manitoba, 1963–1975. Can Med Assoc J 116:282, 1977

Bowman JM, Pollock JM: Antenatal Rh prophylaxis: 28 week gestation service program. Can Med Assoc J 118:622, 1978

Bowman JM, Pollock JM, Manning FA, et al: Maternal Kell blood group alloimmunization. Obstet Gynecol 79:239, 1992a

Bowman JM, Pollock JM, Manning FA, et al: Severe anti-C hemolytic disease of the newborn. Am J Obstet Gynecol 166:1239, 1992b

Brookes JAS, Hall-Craggs MA, Sams VR, et al: Noninvasive perinatal necropsy by magnetic resonance imaging. Lancet 348:1139, 1996

Brucato A, Jonzon A, Friedman D, et al: Proposal for a new definition of a congenital complete atrioventricular block. Lupus 12:427, 2003

Buhi WC, Spellacy WN: Effects of blood or meconium on the determination of the amniotic fluid lecithin/sphingomyelin ratio. Am J Obstet Gynecol 121:321, 1975

Bush MC, Gaddipati S, Berkowitz R: Noninvasive management of Rh partial null (D−) to supplement traditional management of Rh isoimmunization. Obstet Gynaecol 102:1145, 2003

Byrne DL, Gau G: In utero meconium aspiration: An unpreventable cause of neonatal death. Br J Obstet Gynecol 94:813, 1987

Caine ME, Mueller-Heubach E: Kell sensitization in pregnancy. Am J Obstet Gynecol 154:85, 1986

Cannon M, Pierce R, Taber EB, et al: Fatal hydrops fetalis caused by anti-D in a mother with partial D. Obstet Gynecol 102:1143, 2003

Carson BS, Losey RW, Bowes WA Jr, et al: Combined obstetric and pediatric approach to prevent meconium aspiration syndrome. Am J Obstet Gynecol 126:712, 1976

Cartlidge PHT, Dawson AT, Stewart JH, et al: Value and quality of perinatal and infant postmortem examination: Cohort analysis of 400 consecutive deaths. BMJ 310:155, 1995

Cartlidge PHT, Stewart JH: Effect of changing the stillbirth definition on evaluation of perinatal mortality rates. Lancet 346:486, 1995

Casey BM, McIntire DD, Leveno KJ: The continuing value of the Apgar score for the assessment of newborn infants. N Engl J Med 344:467, 2001

Castillo RA, Devoe LD, Hadi HA, et al: Nonimmune hydrops fetalis: Clinical experience and factors related to a poor outcome. Am J Obstet Gynecol 155:812, 1986

Centers for Disease Control: Lack of transmission of human immunodeficiency virus through Rho (D) immune globulin (human). MMWR 36:728, 1987

Chez RA, Carlan S, Greenberg SL, et al: Fractured clavicle is an unavoidable event. Am J Obstet Gynecol 174:797, 1994

Chiswick M, Gladman G, Sinha S, et al: Vitamin E supplementation and periventricular hemorrhage in the newborn. Am J Clin Nutr 53:370S, 1991

Choavaratana R, Uer-Areewong S, Makanantakocol S: Fetomaternal transfusion in normal pregnancy and during delivery. J Med Assoc Thai 80:96, 1997

Clark SL, Hankins GD: Temporal and demographic trends in cerebral palsy—fact and fiction. Am J Obstet Gynecol 188:628, 2003

Clements JA, Platzker ACG, Tierney DF, et al: Assessment of the risk of respiratory distress syndrome by a rapid test for surfactant in amniotic fluid. N Engl J Med 286:1077, 1972

Copper RL, Goldenberg RL, DuBard MB, et al: Risk factors for fetal death in white, black, and Hispanic women. Obstet Gynecol 94:490, 1994

Cordes I, Roland EH, Lupton BA, et al: Early prediction of the development of microcephaly after hypoxic ischemic encephalopathy in the full-term newborn. Pediatrics 93:703, 1994

Cornish JD, Dreyer GL, Snyder GE, et al: Failure of acute perinatal asphyxia or meconium aspiration to produce persistent pulmonary hypertension in a neonatal baboon model. Am J Obstet Gynecol 171:43, 1994

Cox SM, Leveno KJ, Cunningham FG, et al: Introduction of corticosteroids for fetal maturation in a large obstetric service: A 2-year before/after comparison. Am J Obstet Gynecol 174:467, 1996

Crowther CA, Hiller JE, Doyle LW, et al: Effect of magnesium sulfate given for neuroprotection before preterm birth. A randomized controlled trial. JAMA 290:2669, 2003

Cunningham FG, Hollier LM: Fetal death. In: Williams Obstetrics, 20th ed (Suppl 4). Norwalk, Conn, Appleton & Lange, August/September 1997

Czyrko C, Steigman C, Turley DL, et al: The role of reperfusion injury in occlusive intestinal ischemia of the neonate: Malonaldehyde-derived fluorescent products and correlation of histology. J Surg Res 51:1, 1991

Dammann O, Leviton A: Maternal intrauterine infection, cytokines, and brain damage in the preterm newborn. Pediatr Res 42:1, 1997

Davis RO, Phillips JB III, Harris BA Jr, et al: Fatal meconium aspiration syndrome occurring despite airway management considered appropriate. Am J Obstet Gynecol 141:731, 1985

Davoren A, Curtis BR, Aster RH, McFarland JG: Human platelet antigen-specific alloantibodies implicated in 1162 cases of neonatal alloimmune thrombocytopenia. Transfusion 44:1220, 2001

de Alemida V, Bowman JM: Massive fetomaternal hemorrhage: Manitoba experience. Obstet Gynecol 83:323, 1994

DeVries LS, Dubowitz V, Lary S, et al: Predictive value of cranial ultrasound in the newborn baby: A reappraisal. Lancet 2:137, 1985

DeVries LS, Eken P, Groenendaal F, et al: Correlation between the degree of periventricular leukomalacia diagnosed using cranial ultrasound and MRI later in infancy in children with cerebral palsy. Neuropediatrics 24:263, 1993

Diamond LK, Blackfan KP, Baty JM: Erythroblastosis fetalis and its association with universal edema of the fetus, icterus gravis neonatorum and anemia of the newborn. J Pediatr 1:269, 1932

Dijxhoorn MJ, Visser GHA, Fidler VJ, et al: Apgar score, meconium and acidemia at birth in relation to neonatal neurological morbidity in term infants. Br J Obstet Gynaecol 86:217, 1986

Dooley SL, Pesavento DJ, Depp R, et al: Meconium below the vocal cords at delivery: Correlation with intrapartum events. Am J Obstet Gynecol 153:767, 1985

Duthie SJ, Walkinshaw SA: Parvovirus associated fetal hydrops: Reversal of pregnancy induced proteinuric hypertension by in utero fetal transfusion. Br J Obstet Gynaecol 102:1011, 1995

Eriksen N, Tey A, Prieto J, et al: Fetal lung maturity in diabetic patients using the TDXFLM assay. Am J Obstet Gynecol 174:348, 1996

Favre R, Dreux S, Dommergues M, et al: Nonimmune fetal ascites: A series of 79 cases. Am J Obstet Gynecol 190:407, 2004

Faye-Petersen OM, Guinn DA, Wenstrom KD: Value of perinatal autopsy. Obstet Gynecol 94:915, 1999

Fedrizzi E, Inverno M, Bruzzone MG, et al: MRI features of cerebral lesions and cognitive functions in preterm spastic diplegic children. Pediatr Neurol 15:207, 1996

Fee SC, Malee K, Deddish R, et al: Severe acidosis and subsequent neurologic status. Am J Obstet Gynecol 162:802, 1990

Finer NN, Barrington KJ: Nitric oxide therapy for the newborn. Semin Perinatol 24:59, 2000

Finn R, Clarke CA, Donohoe W, et al: Experimental studies on the prevention of Rh haemolytic disease. BMJ 1:1486, 1961

Fox H: Pathology of the placenta. Monograph, Vol VI. Philadelphia, Saunders, 1978

Freda V: Hemolytic disease. Clin Obstet Gynecol 16:72, 1973

Freda VJ, Gorman JG, Pollack W: Successful prevention of sensitization to Rh with an experimental anti-Rh gamma2 globulin antibody preparation. Fed Proc 22:374, 1963

Freeman JM, Nelson KB: Intrapartum asphyxia and cerebral palsy. Pediatrics 82:240, 1988

Freeman RK, Dorchester W, Anderson G, et al: The significance of a previous stillbirth. Am J Obstet Gynecol 151:7, 1985

Fretts RC, Boyd ME, Usher RH, et al: The changing pattern of fetal death, 1961–1988. Obstet Gynecol 79:35, 1992

Fretts RC, Usher RH: Causes of fetal death in women of advanced maternal age. Obstet Gynecol 89:40, 1997

Freud S: Infantile Cerebrallahmung. Notnagel's Specielle Pathologie und Therapie 9, Vol XII. Vienna, A. Holder, 1897

Fujimoto S, Yamaguchi N, Togari H, et al: Cerebral palsy of the cystic periventricular leukomalacia in low-birth-weight infants. Acta Paediatr 83:397, 1994

Galbraith RS: Incidence of sixth nerve palsy in relation to mode of delivery. Am J Obstet Gynecol 170:1158, 1994

Gibbs RS, Rosenberg AR, Warren CJ, et al: Suggestions for practice to accompany neonatal encephalopathy and cerebral palsy. Obstet Gynecol 103:778, 2004

Gilstrap LC III, Leveno KJ, Burris J, et al: Diagnosis of asphyxia on the basis of fetal pH, Apgar score, and newborn cerebral dysfunction. Am J Obstet Gynecol 161:825, 1989

Gluck L, Kulovich MV: Lecithin-sphingomyelin ratios in amniotic fluid in normal and abnormal pregnancy. Am J Obstet Gynecol 115:539, 1973

Gluck L, Kulovich MV, Borer RC Jr, et al: Diagnosis of the respiratory distress syndrome by amniocentesis. Am J Obstet Gynecol 109:440, 1971

Goepfert AR, Goldenberg RL, Hauth JC, et al: Obstetrical determinants of neonatal neurological morbidity. Am J Obstet Gynecol 174:470, 1996

Goetz MC, Gretebeck RJ, Oh KS, et al: Incidence, timing, and follow-up of periventricular leukomalacia. Am J Perinatol 12:325, 1995

Goldaber KG, Gilstrap LC 3rd, Leveno KJ, et al: Pathologic fetal acidemia. Obstet Gynecol 78:1103, 1991

Goldenberg RL, Mayberry SK, Cooper RL, et al: Pregnancy outcome following a second-trimester loss. Obstet Gynecol 81:444, 1993

Gough JD, Keeling JW, Castle B, et al: The obstetric management of non-immunological hydrops. Br J Obstet Gynaecol 93:226, 1986

Grab D, Paulus WE, Bommer A, et al: Treatment of fetal erythroblastosis by intravascular transfusions: Outcome at 6 years. Obstet Gynecol 93:165, 1999

Grant A, O'Brien N, Joy MT, et al: Cerebral palsy among children born during the Dublin randomized trial of intrapartum monitoring. Lancet 2:1233, 1989

Grether JK, Hoogstrate J, Walsh-Greene E, et al: Magnesium sulfate for tocolysis and risk of spastic cerebral palsy in premature children born to women without preeclampsia. Am J Obstet Gynecol 183:717, 2000

Grether JK, Nelson KB: Maternal infection and cerebral palsy in infants of normal birth weight. JAMA 278:207, 1997

Hackney DN, Knudtson EJ, Rossi KQ, et al: Management of pregnancies complicated by anti-c isoimmunization. Obstet Gynecol 103:24, 2004

Haddow JE, Rote NS, Dostal-Johnson D, et al: Lack of an association between late fetal death and antiphospholipid antibody measurements in the second trimester. Am J Obstet Gynecol 165:1308, 1991

Hagen E, Link JC, Arias F: A comparison of the accuracy of the TDx-FLM assay, lecithin–sphingomyelin ratio, and phosphatidyl glycerol in the prediction of neonatal respiratory distress syndrome. Obstet Gynecol 82:1004, 1993

Hanigan WC, Kennedy G, Roemisch F, et al: Administration of indomethacin for the prevention of periventricular–intraventricular hemorrhage in high-risk neonates. J Pediatr 112:941, 1988

Hankins GD, Koen S, Gei AF, et al: Neonatal organ system injury in acute birth asphyxia sufficient to result in neonatal encephalopathy. Obstet Gynecol 99:688, 2002

Hanson J, Persson B: Outcome of pregnancies complicated by type 1 insulin-dependent diabetes in Sweden: Acute pregnancy complications, neonatal mortality and morbidity. Am J Perinatol 4:330, 1993

Harman CR, Manning FA, Bowman JM, et al: Severe Rh disease—poor outcome is not inevitable. Am J Obstet Gynecol 145:823, 1983

Harper MA, Lorenz WB Jr: Immature lecithin/sphingomyelin ratios and respiratory course. Am J Obstet Gynecol 168:495, 1993

Hayakawa F, Okumura A, Kato T, et al: Determination of timing of brain injury in preterm infants with periventricular leukomalacia with serial neonatal electroencephalography. Pediatrics 104:1077, 1999

Hayden CK, Shattuck KE, Richardson CJ, et al: Subependymal germinal matrix hemorrhage in full-term neonates. Pediatrics 75:714, 1985

Heinonen S, Ruynamen M, Kirkinen P: Etiology and outcome of second trimester nonimmunological fetal hydrops. Scand J Obstet Gynecol 79:15, 2000

Herbert WNP, Chapman JE, Schnoor MM: Role of the TDx FLM assay in fetal lung maturity. Am J Obstet Gynecol 168:808, 1993

Hoekstra RE, Ferrara TB, Couser RJ, et al: Survival and long-term neurodevelopmental outcome of extremely premature infants born at 23–26 weeks' gestational age at a tertiary center. Pediatrics 113:e1, 2004

Holzgreve W, Curry CJR, Golbus MS, et al: Investigation of non-immune hydrops fetalis. Am J Obstet Gynecol 150:805, 1984

Hong F, Ruiz R, Price H, et al: Safety profile of WinRho anti-D. Semin Hematol 35:9, 1998

Horn LC, Langner A, Stiehl P, et al: Identification of the causes of intrauterine death during 310 consecutive autopsies. Eur J Obstet Gynecol Reprod Biol 113:134, 2004

Howard H, Martlew V, McFadyen I, et al: Consequences for fetus and neonate of maternal red cell allo-immunization. Arch Dis Child Fetal Neonat Ed 78:F62, 1998

Hsu N, Hung KL, Tsai ML, et al: The association of periventricular echodensity of cerebral palsy in preterm infants. Chung-Hua Min Kuo Hsiao Erh Koi Hsueh Hui Tsa Chih 37:433, 1996

Huang AH, Robertson RL: Spontaneous superficial parenchymal and leptomeningeal hemorrhage in term neonates. Am J Neuroradiol 25:469, 2004

Infante-Rivard C, David M, Gautheir R, et al: Lupus anticoagulants, anticardiolipin antibodies, and fetal loss: A case-control study. N Engl J Med 325:1063, 1991

Jakobi P, Weissman A, Zimmer EZ, et al: Survival and long-term morbidity in preterm infants with and without a clinical diagnosis of periventricular, intraventricular hemorrhage. Eur J Obstet Gynecol Reprod Biol 46:73, 1992

Jaw TS, Jong YJ, Sheu RS, et al: Etiology, timing of insult, and neuropathology of cerebral palsy evaluated with magnetic resonance imaging. J Formos Med Assoc 97:239, 1998

Jobe AH: Postnatal corticosteroids for preterm infants—do what we say, not what we do. N Engl J Med 350:1349, 2004

Jobe AH: Pulmonary surfactant therapy. N Engl J Med 328:861, 1993

Kari MA, Hallman M, Eronen M, et al: Prenatal dexamethasone treatment in conjunction with rescue therapy of human surfactant: A randomized placebo-controlled multicentered study. Pediatrics 93:730, 1994

Katz LV, Bowes WA: Meconium aspiration syndrome: Reflections on a murky subject. Am J Obstet Gynecol 166:171, 1992

Katz MA, Kanto WP Jr, Korotkein JH: Recurrence rate of ABO hemolytic disease of the newborn. Obstet Gynecol 59:611, 1982

Kinsella JP, Walsh WF, Bose CL, et al: Inhaled nitric oxide in premature neonates with severe hypoxaemic respiratory failure: A randomised controlled trial. Lancet 354:2126, 1999

Kleinman CS, Copel JA, Weinstein EM, et al: In utero diagnosis and treatment of fetal supraventricular tachycardia. Semin Perinatol 9:113, 1985

Kliegman RM, Fanaroff AA: Necrotizing enterocolitis. N Engl J Med 310:1093, 1984

Korst LM, Ahn MO, Phelan JP: Nucleated red blood cells: An update on the marker for fetal asphyxia. Am J Obstet Gynecol 174:318, 1996

Lammer EJ, Brown LE, Anderka MT, et al: Classification and analysis of fetal deaths in Massachusetts. JAMA 261:1757, 1989

Landsteiner K, Weiner AS: An agglutinable factor in human blood recognized by immune sera for rhesus blood. Proc Soc Exp Biol Med 43:223, 1940

Lefebvre G, Wehbe G, Heron D, et al: Recurrent nonimmune hydrops fetalis: A prepresentation of sciatic acid storage disease. Genet Couns 10:277, 1999

Lemons JA, Bauer CR, Oh W, et al: Very low birth weight outcomes of the National Institute of Child Health and Human Development Neonatal Research Network, January 1995 through December 1996. Pediatrics 107:1, 2001

Lesko SM, Mitchell AA, Epstein MF, et al: Heparin use as a risk factor for intraventricular hemorrhage in low-birth-weight infants. N Engl J Med 314:1156, 1986

Levene M: Role of excitatory amino acid antagonists in the management of birth asphyxia. Biol Neonate 62:248, 1992

Leveno KJ, Quirk JG Jr, Cunningham FG, et al: Prolonged pregnancy. I. Observations concerning the causes of fetal distress. Am J Obstet Gynecol 150:465, 1984

Levine MG, Holroyde J, Woods JR, et al: Birth trauma: Incidence and predisposing factors. Obstet Gynecol 63:792, 1984

Levine P, Katzin KM, Burnham L: Isoimmunization in pregnancy: Its possible bearing on the etiology of erythroblastosis fetalis. JAMA 116:825, 1941

Liley AW: Liquor amnii analysis in management of pregnancy complicated by rhesus sensitization. Am J Obstet Gynecol 82:1359, 1961

Lin MT, Hsieh FJ, Shyu MK, et al: Postnatal outcome of fetal bradycardia without significant cardiac abnormalities. Am Heart J 147:540, 2004

Locus P, Yeomans E, Crosby U: The efficacy of bulb versus DeLee suction at deliveries complicated by meconium stained amniotic fluid. Perinatology 7:87, 1990

Low JA, Panagiotopoulos C, Derrick EJ: Newborn complications after intrapartum asphyxia with metabolic acidosis in the preterm fetus. Am J Obstet Gynecol 172:805, 1995

Luthy DA, Shy KK, Strickland D, et al: Status of infants at birth and risk for adverse neonatal events and long-term sequelae: A study in low birthweight infants. Am J Obstet Gynecol 157:676, 1987

MacDonald D, Grant A, Sheridan-Pereira M, et al: The Dublin randomized controlled trial of intrapartum fetal heart rate monitoring. Am J Obstet Gynecol 152:524, 1985

Manning FA, Schrieber J, Turkel SB: Fatal meconium aspiration "in utero": A case report. Am J Obstet Gynecol 132:111, 1978

Mari G, Deter RL, Carpenter RL, et al: Noninvasive diagnosis by Doppler ultrasonography of fetal anemia due to maternal red-cell alloimmunization. N Engl J Med 342:9, 2000

Marret S, Gressens P, Gadisseux JF, et al: Prevention by magnesium of excitotoxic neuronal death in the developing brain: An animal model for clinical intervention studies. Dev Med Child Neurol 34:473, 1995

Martin RJ: Nitric oxide for preemies—not so fast. N Engl J Med 349:2157, 2004

Mayne KM, Bowell PJ, Pratt GA: The significance of anti-Kell sensitization in pregnancy. Clin Lab Haematol 12:379, 1990

McCoy MC, Katz VL, Could N, et al: Non-immune hydrops after 20 weeks' gestation: Review of 10 years' experience with suggestions for management. Obstet Gynecol 85:578, 1995

Melone PJ, Ernest JM, O'Shea MD Jr, et al: Appropriateness of intrapartum fetal heart rate management and risk of cerebral palsy. Am J Obstet Gynecol 165:272, 1991

Ment LR, Oh W, Ehrenkranz RA, et al: Antenatal steroids, delivery mode and intraventricular hemorrhage in preterm infants. Am J Obstet Gynecol 172:795, 1995

Menticoglou SM, Perlman M, Manning FA: High cervical spinal cord injury in neonates delivered with forceps: Report of 15 cases. Obstet Gynecol 86:589, 1995

Midgley DY, Hardrug K: The mirror syndrome. Eur J Obstet Gynecol Reprod Biol 8:201, 2000

Miller ME, Graham JM Jr, Higginbotton MC, et al: Compression-related defects from early amnion rupture: Evidence for mechanical teratogenesis. J Pediatr 98:292, 1981

Misbah SA, Chapel HM: Adverse effects of intravenous immunoglobulin. Drug Saf 9:254, 1993

Moise KJ Jr: Management of rhesus alloimmunization in pregnancy. Review. Obstet Gynecol 100:600, 2002

Mueller RF, Sybert VP, Johnson J, et al: Evaluation of a protocol for postmortem examination of stillbirths. N Engl J Med 309:586, 1983

Mueller-Heubach E, Mazer J: Sonographically documented disappearance of fetal ascites. Obstet Gynecol 61:253, 1983

Murphy JD, Vawter GF, Reid LM: Pulmonary vascular disease in fatal meconium aspiration. J Pediatr 194:758, 1984

Naeye RL, Localio AR: Determining the time before birth when ischemia and hypoxemia initiated cerebral palsy. Obstet Gynecol 86:713, 1995

Nathan L, Leveno KJ, Carmody TJ, et al: Meconium: A 1990s perspective on an old obstetric hazard. Obstet Gynecol 83:329, 1994

National Institutes of Health: Antenatal corticosteroids revisited: Repeat courses. NIH Consensus Statement Online 17(2):1, August 17–18, 2000

National Institutes of Health: Consensus Development Conference on the effects of corticosteroids for fetal maturation on perinatal outcomes. Consensus Development Conference statement. Bethesda, Md, NIH, 1994

Nelson KB: Can we prevent cerebral palsy? N Engl J Med 349:1765, 2003

Nelson KB, Lynch JK: Stroke in newborn infants. Lancet Neurol 3:150, 2004

Nelson KB, Dambrosia JM, Ting TY, et al: Uncertain value of electronic fetal monitoring in predicting cerebral palsy. N Engl J Med 334:613, 1996

Nelson KB, Ellenberg JH: Antecedents of cerebral palsy: Multivariate analysis of risk. N Engl J Med 315:81, 1986a

Nelson KB, Ellenberg JH: Antecedents of cerebral palsy: Univariate analysis of risks. Am J Dis Child 139:1031, 1985

Nelson KB, Ellenberg JH: Antecedents of seizure disorders in early childhood. Am J Dis Child 140:1053, 1986b

Nelson KB, Ellenberg JH: Obstetric complications as risk factors for cerebral palsy or seizure disorders. JAMA 251:1843, 1984

Nelson KB, Grether JK: Potentially asphyxiating conditions and spastic cerebral palsy in infants of normal birth weight. Am J Obstet Gynecol 179:507, 1998

Ness PM, Baldwin ML, Niebyl JR: Clinical high-risk designation does not predict excess fetal–maternal hemorrhage. Am J Obstet Gynecol 156:154, 1987

Nicolaides KH, Clewell WH, Mibashan RS, et al: Fetal haemoglobin measurement in the assessment of red cell isoimmunization. Lancet 1:1073, 1988

Nicolaides KH, Rodeck CH, Mibashan RS, et al: Have Liley charts outlived their usefulness? Am J Obstet Gynecol 155:90, 1986

Nicolaides KH, Snijders RJM: Cordocentesis. In Evans MI (ed): Reproductive Risks and Prenatal Diagnosis. Norwalk, Conn, Appleton & Lange, 1992, p 201

Nicolaides KH, Warenski JC, Rodeck CH: The relationship of fetal plasma protein concentration and hemoglobin level to the development of hydrops in rhesus isoimmunization. Am J Obstet Gynecol 152:341, 1985

Nicolini U, Nicolaides P, Tannirandorn Y, et al: Fetal liver dysfunction in Rh alloimmunization. Br J Obstet Gynaecol 98:287, 1991

Niswander K, Henson G, Elbourne D, et al: Adverse outcome of pregnancy and the quality of obstetric care. Lancet 2:827, 1984

Nores J, Roberts A, Carr S: Prenatal diagnosis and management of fetuses with intracranial hemorrhage. Am J Obstet Gynecol 174:424, 1996

Ojomo EO, Coustan DR: Absence of evidence of pulmonary maturity at amniocentesis in term infants of diabetic mothers. Am J Obstet Gynecol 163:954, 1990

Oka A, Belliveau MJ, Rosenberg PA, et al: Vulnerability of oligodendroglia to glutamate: Pharmacology, mechanisms, and prevention. J Neurosc 13:1441, 1993

Okumura A, Kato T, Juno K, et al: MRI findings in patients with spastic cerebral palsy. II: Correlation with type of cerebral palsy. Dev Med Child Neurol 39:369, 1997

Papile LA, Burstein J, Burstein R, et al: Incidence and evolution of subependymal and intraventricular hemorrhage: A study of infants with birth weights less than 1500 gm. J Pediatr 92:529, 1978

Papile LA, Munsick-Bruno G, Schaefer A: Relationship of cerebral intraventricular hemorrhage and early childhood neurologic handicaps. J Pediatr 103:273, 1983

Pauli RM, Reiser CA: Wisconsin Stillbirth Service Program: II. Analysis of diagnoses and diagnostic categories in the first 1,000 referrals. Am J Med Genet 50:135, 1994

Perlman JM, Cunningham FG: Fetal and neonatal hypoxic ischemic cerebral injury. In: Williams Obstetrics, 18th ed (Suppl 21). Norwalk, Conn, Appleton & Lange, December/January 1993

Perlman JM, Risser R, Broyles RS: Bilateral cystic periventricular leukomalacia in the premature infant: Associated risk factors. Pediatrics 97:822, 1996

Perlman JM, Volpe JJ: Intraventricular hemorrhage in extremely small premature infants. Am J Dis Child 140:1122, 1986

Phelan JP, Ahn MO: Perinatal observations in forty-eight neurologically impaired term infants. Am J Obstet Gynecol 171:424, 1994

Phelan JP, Ahn MO, Korst L, et al: Is intrapartum fetal brain injury in the term fetus preventable? Am J Obstet Gynecol 174:318, 1996

Pritchard JA, Cunningham FG, Pritchard SA, et al: How often does maternal preeclampsia–eclampsia incite thrombocytopenia in the fetus? Obstet Gynecol 69:292, 1987

Pritchard JA, Cunningham FG, Pritchard SA, et al: On reducing the frequency of severe abruptio placentae. Am J Obstet Gynecol 165:1345, 1991

Procházka M, Happach C, Maršál K, et al: Factor V Leiden in pregnancies complicated by placental abruption. Br J Obstet Gynaecol 110:462, 2003

Queenan JT, Thomas PT, Tomai TP, et al: Deviation in amniotic fluid optical density at a wavelength of 450 nm in Rh isoimmunized pregnancies from 14 to 40 weeks' gestation: A proposal for clinical management. Am J Obstet Gynecol 168:1370, 1993

Race RR, Sanger R: Blood Groups in Man, 6th ed. Oxford, England, Blackwell, 1975

Radestad I, Steineck G, Nordin C, et al: Psychological complications after stillbirth—influence of memories and immediate management: Population based study. BMJ 312:1505, 1996

Rey E, Kahn SR, David M, et al: Thrombophilic disorders and fetal loss: A meta-analysis. Lancet 361:901, 2003

Reznikoff-Etievant MF, Muller JY, Julien F, et al: An immune response gene liked to MHC in man. Tissue Antigens 22:312, 1983

Richey S, Ramin SM, Bawdon RE, et al: Markers of acute and chronic asphyxia in infants with meconium-stained amniotic fluid. Am J Obstet Gynecol 172:1212, 1995

Roberts SW, Hernandez C, Maberry MC, et al: Obstetric clavicular fracture: The enigma of normal birth. Obstet Gynecol 86:978, 1995

Robertson C, Finer N: Term infants with hypoxic-ischemic encephalopathy: Outcome at 3.5 years. Dev Med Child Neurol 27:473, 1985

Robinson BV, Ettedgui JA, Sherman FS: Use of terbutaline in the treatment of complete heart block in the fetus. Cardiol Young 11:683, 2001

Roemer RJ: Relation of torticollis to breech delivery. Am J Obstet Gynecol 67:1146, 1954

Rosen MG, Dickinson JC: The incidence of cerebral palsy. Am J Obstet Gynecol 167:417, 1992

Rosen MG, Hobel CJ: Prenatal and perinatal factors associated with brain disorders. Obstet Gynecol 68:416, 1986

Rouse D, Weiner C: Ongoing fetomaternal hemorrhage treated by serial fetal intravascular transfusions. Obstet Gynecol 76:974, 1990

Sadovsky Y, Amon E, Bade ME, et al: Prophylactic amnioinfusion during labor complicated by meconium: A preliminary report. Am J Obstet Gynecol 161:613, 1989

Salafia CM, Minior UK, Pezzullo JC, et al: Premature rupture of membranes and premature labor neonatal nucleated crythrocyte number (nRBCs) is related to histologic acute inflammation and not to placental markers of hypoxia. Am J Obstet Gynecol 174:318, 1996

Saleeb S, Copel J, Friedman D, et al: Comparison of treatment with fluorinated glucocorticoids to the natural history of autoantibody–associated congenital heart block: Retrospective review of the research registry for neonatal lupus. Arthritis Rheum 42:2335, 1999

Saller DN Jr, Lesser KB, Harrel U, et al: The clinical utility of the perinatal autopsy. JAMA 273:663, 1995

Salonen IS, Uüsitalo R: Birth injuries: Incidence and predisposing factors. Z Kinderchir 45:133, 1990

Samadi R, Miller D, Settlage R, et al: Massive fetomaternal hemorrhage and fetal death: Is it predictable? Am J Obstet Gynecol 174:391, 1996

Samueloff A, Xenakis EMJ, Berkus MD, et al: Recurrent stillbirth: Significance and characteristics. J Reprod Med 88:883, 1993

Sandmire HF, DeMott RK: Erb's palsy: Concepts of causation. Obstet Gynecol 95:941, 2000

Santolaya J, Alley D, Jaffe R, et al: Antenatal classification of hydrops fetalis. Obstet Gynecol 79:256, 1992

Saunders BS, Lazoritz S, McArtor RD, et al: Depressed skull fracture in the neonate. J Neurosurg 50:512, 1979

Schendel DE, Berg CJ, Yeargin-Allsopp M, et al: Prenatal magnesium sulfate exposure and the risk for cerebral palsy or mental retardation among very low-birth-weight children aged 3 to 5 years. JAMA 276:1805, 1996

Schmidt B, Asztalos EV, Roberts RS, et al: Impact of bronchopulmonary dysplasia, brain injury, and severe retinopathy on the outcome of extremely low-birth-weight infants at 18 months. JAMA 289:1124, 2003

Shulenin S, Nogee LM, Annilo T, et al: ABCA3 gene mutations in newborns with fatal surfactant deficiency. N Engl J Med 350:1296, 2004

Shulman LP, Phillips OP, Emerson DS, et al: Fetal "space-suit" hydrops in the first trimester: Differentiating risk for chromosome abnormalities by delineating characteristics of nuchal translucency. Prenat Diagn 20:30, 2000

Silver RK, Vyskocil C, Solomon SL, et al: Randomized trial of antenatal dexamethasone in surfactant-treated infants delivered before 30 weeks' gestation. Obstet Gynecol 87:683, 1996

Silver RM, Porter TF, Branch DW, et al: Neonatal alloimmune thrombocytopenia: Antenatal management. Am J Obstet Gynecol 182:1233, 2000

Skajaa K, Hansen ES, Bendix J: Depressed fracture of the skull in a child born by cesarean section. Acta Obstet Gynecol Scand 66:275, 1987

Snyder EL: Prevention of hemolytic disease of the newborn due to anti-D. Prenatal/perinatal testing and Rh immune globulin administration. Am Assoc Blood Banks Assoc Bull 98:1 (Level III), 1998

Spinillo A, Capuzzo E, Stronati M, et al: Obstetric risk factors for periventricular leukomalacia among preterm infants. Br J Obstet Gynaecol 105:865, 1998

Spinillo A, Ometto A, Bottino R, et al: Antenatal risk factors for germinal matrix hemorrhage and intraventricular hemorrhage in preterm infants. Eur J Obstet Gynecol Reprod Biol 60:13, 1995

Spong CY, Ogundipe OA, Ross MG: Prophylactic amnioinfusion for meconium stained amniotic fluid. Am J Obstet Gynecol 171:931, 1994

Stanley FJ, Blair E: Why have we failed to reduce the frequency of cerebral palsy? Med J Aust 154:623, 1991

Stedman CM, Baudin JC, White CA, et al: Use of the erythrocyte rosette test to screen for excessive fetomaternal hemorrhage in Rh-negative women. Am J Obstet Gynecol 154:1363, 1986

Steinfeld JD, Samuels P, Bulley MA, et al: The utility of the TDx test in the assessment of fetal lung maturity. Obstet Gynecol 79:460, 1992

Stevens AM, Hermes HM, Rutledge JC, et al: Myocardial-tissue-specific phenotype of maternal microchimerism in neonatal lupus congenital heart block. Lancet 362:1617, 2003

Strauss A, Kirz D, Modanlou HD, et al: Perinatal events and intraventricular/subependymal hemorrhage in the very low-birth-weight infant. Am J Obstet Gynecol 151:1022, 1985

Streeter GL: Focal deficiencies in fetal tissues and their relation to intrauterine amputations. Contrib Embryol 22:1, 1930

Surkan PJ, Stephansson O, Dickman PW, et al: Previous preterm and small-for-gestational-age births and the subsequent risk of stillbirth. N Engl J Med 350:754, 2004

Taylor PV, Scott JS, Gerlis LM, et al: Maternal antibodies against fetal cardiac antigens in congenital complete heart block. N Engl J Med 315:667, 1986

Tejani N, Verma U, Hameed C, et al: Method and route of delivery in the low-birth-weight vertex presentation correlated with early periventricular/intraventricular hemorrhage. Obstet Gynecol 69:1, 1987

Thacker KE, Lim T, Drew JH: Cephalhaematoma: A 10-year review. Aust N Z J Obstet Gynaecol 27:210, 1987

Thacker SB, Stroup DF, Peterson HB: Efficacy and safety of intrapartum electronic fetal monitoring: An update. Obstet Gynecol 86:613, 1995

Thorp JA, Ferette-Smith D, Gaston L, et al: Antenatal vitamin K and phenobarbital for preventing intracranial hemorrhage in the premature newborn: A randomized double-blind placebo-controlled trial. Am J Obstet Gynecol 172:253, 1995

Thorp JA, Jones PG, Clark RH, et al: Perinatal factors associated with severe intracranial hemorrhage. Am J Obstet Gynecol 185:859, 2001

Torfs CP, van den Berg B, Oechsli FW, et al: Prenatal and perinatal factors in the etiology of cerebral palsy. J Pediatr 116:615, 1990

Torpin R: Fetal malformations caused by amnion rupture during gestation. Springfield, Ill, Thomas, 1968

Truwit CL, Barkovich AJ, Koch TK, et al: Cerebral palsy: MR findings in 40 patients. AJNR Am J Neuroradiol 13:67, 1992

Turpenny PD, Nimmo A: Fractured clavicle of the newborn in a population with a high prevalence of grand-multiparity: Analysis of 78 consecutive cases. Br J Obstet Gynaecol 100:338, 1993

Tyson JE, Gilstrap LC: Hope for perinatal prevention of cerebral palsy. JAMA 290:2730, 2003

Ubachs JMH, Slooff ACJ, Peeters LLH: Obstetric antecedents of surgically treated obstetric brachial plexus injuries. Br J Obstet Gynaecol 102:813, 1995

Van Den Veyver IB, Subramanian SB, Hudson KM, et al: Prenatal diagnosis of the RhD fetal blood type on amniotic fluid by polymerase chain reaction. Obstet Gynecol 87:419, 1996

Verbrugge SJ, Lachmann B: Mechanisms of ventilation-induced lung injury: Physiological rationale to prevent it. Monaldi Arch Chest Dis 54:22, 1999

Vergani P, Strobetl N, Locatelli A, et al: Clinical significance of fetal intracranial hemorrhage. Am J Obstet Gynecol 175:536, 1996

Verma U, Tejani N, Klein S, et al: Obstetric antecedents of intraventricular hemorrhage and periventricular leukomalacia in the low-birth-weight neonate. Am J Obstet Gynecol 176:275, 1997

Volpe JJ: Neurology of the Newborn, 3rd ed. Philadelphia, Saunders, 1995, p 373

Volpe JJ, Hill A: Neurologic disorders. In Avery GB (ed): Neonatology, 3rd ed. Philadelphia, JB Lippincott, 1987, p 1073

Wallin LA, Rosenfeld CR, Laptook AR, et al: Neonatal intracranial hemorrhage, 2. Risk factor analysis in an inborn population. Early Hum Dev 23:129, 1990

Weeks JW, Asrat T, Morgan MA, et al: Antepartum surveillance for a history of stillbirth: When to begin? Am J Obstet Gynecol 172:486, 1995

Weindling M: Periventricular haemorrhage and periventricular leukomalacia. Br J Obstet Gynaecol 102:278, 1995

Weiner CP, Pelzer GD, Heilskov J, et al: The effect of intravascular transfusion on umbilical venous pressure in anemic fetuses with and without hydrops. Am J Obstet Gynecol 161:1498, 1989

Weiner CP, Wenstrom KD, Sipes SL, et al: Risk factors for cordocentesis and fetal intravascular transfusion. Am J Obstet Gynecol 165:1020, 1991a

Weiner CP, Widness JA: Decreased fetal erythropoiesis and hemolysis in Kell hemolytic anemia. Am J Obstet Gynecol 174:547, 1996

Weiner CP, Williamson RA, Wenstrom KD, et al: Management of fetal hemolytic disease by cordocentesis: I. Prediction of fetal anemia. Am J Obstet Gynecol 165:546, 1991b

Welch RA, Bottoms SF: Reconsideration of head compression and intraventricular hemorrhage in the vertex very low-birth-weight fetus. Obstet Gynecol 68:29, 1986

Welsch C, Woods J, Yancey M, et al: The efficacy of a rapid lamellar body count assay in predicting fetal lung maturity. Am J Obstet Gynecol 174:335, 1996

Wenk RE, Goldstein P, Felix JK: Alloimmunization by hr′ (c), hemolytic disease of newborns, and perinatal management. Obstet Gynecol 67:623, 1986

Wenstrom KD, Andrews WW, Maher JE: Amnioinfusion survey: Prevalence, protocols, and complications. Obstet Gynecol 86:572, 1995

Whitby EH, Griffiths PD, Rutter S, et al: Frequency and natural history of subdural haemorrhages in babies and relation to obstetrical factors. Lancet 363:846, 2004

White DA, Pressman EK, Hanna GV, et al: Facial nerve palsy—frequencies associated with spontaneous, forceps and cesarean deliveries. Am J Obstet Gynecol 174:353, 1996

Wiklund LM, Uvebrant P, Flodmark O: Computed tomography as an adjunct in etiological analysis of hemiplegic cerebral palsy, 1. Children born preterm. Neuropediatrics 22:50, 1991a

Wiklund LM, Uvebrant P, Flodmark O: Computed tomography as an adjunct in etiological analysis of hemiplegic cerebral palsy, 2. Children born at term. Neuropediatrics 22:121, 1991b

Wiswell TE, Tuggle JM, Turner BS: Meconium aspiration syndrome: Have we made a difference? Pediatrics 85:715, 1990

Woelfer B, Schuchter K, Janisiw M, et al: Postdelivery levels of anti-D IgG prophylaxis in mothers depend on maternal body weight. Transfusion 44:512, 2004

Wood NS, Marlow N, Costeloe K, et al: Neurologic and developmental disability after extremely preterm birth. N Engl J Med 343:378, 2000

Wu YW, Escobar GJ, Grether JK, et al: Chorioamnionitis and cerebral palsy in term and near-term infants. JAMA 290:2677, 2003

Yankowitz J, Li S, Weiner CP: Polymerase chain reaction determination of RhC, Rhc, and RhE blood types: An evaluation of accuracy and clinical utility. Am J Obstet Gynecol 176:1107, 1997

Yeh TF, Lin YJ, Lin HC, et al: Outcomes at school age after postnatal dexamethasone therapy for lung disease of prematurity. N Engl J Med 350:1304, 2004

Yoder BA: Meconium stained amniotic fluid and respiratory complications: Impact of selective tracheal suction. Obstet Gynecol 83:77, 1994

Yoon BH, Kim CJ, Romero R, et al: Experimentally induced intrauterine infection causes fetal brain white matter lesions in rabbits. Am J Obstet Gynecol 177:797, 1997a

Yoon BH, Romero R, Kim CJ, et al: High expression of tumor necrosis factor-alpha and interleukin-6 in periventricular leukomalacia. Am J Obstet Gynecol 177:406, 1997b

Yoon BH, Romero R, Moon JB, et al: Clinical significance of intra-amniotic inflammation in patients with preterm labor and intact membranes. Am J Obstet Gynecol 185:1130, 2001

Yoon BH, Romero R, Park JS, et al: Fetal exposure to an intra-amniotic inflammation and the development of cerebral palsy at the age of three years. Am J Obstet Gynecol 182:675, 2000

Yudkin PL, Wood L, Redman CWG: Risk of unexplained stillbirth at different gestational ages. Lancet 1:1192, 1987

Zipursky A: Prevention of vitamin K deficiency bleeding in newborns [review]. Br J Haematol 104:430, 1999

Zupan V, Gonzalez P, Lacaze-Masmonteil T, et al: Periventricular leukomalacia: Risk factors revisited. Dev Med Child Neurol 38:1061, 1996

VI

The Puerperium

30

The Puerperium

The puerperium is strictly defined as the period of confinement during and just after birth. By popular use, however, the meaning usually includes the six subsequent weeks (Hughes, 1972).

CLINICAL AND PHYSIOLOGICAL ASPECTS OF THE PUERPERIUM

UTERINE CHANGES

Uterine Vessels. Successful pregnancy requires a massive increase in uterine blood flow. To provide for this, arteries and veins within the uterus, and especially those of the placental site, enlarge remarkably, as do transport vessels to and from the uterus. Within the uterus, growth of new vessels also provides for the marked increase in blood flow. After delivery, the caliber of extrauterine vessels decreases to equal, or at least closely approximates, that of the prepregnant state. Within the puerperal uterus, larger blood vessels are obliterated by hyaline changes, gradually resorbed, and replaced by smaller ones. Minor vestiges of the larger vessels, however, may persist for years.

Cervix and Lower Uterine Segment. During labor, the outer cervical margin, which corresponds to the external os, is usually lacerated, especially laterally. The cervical opening contracts slowly, and for a few days immediately after labor readily admits two fingers. By the end of the first week, it has narrowed. As the opening narrows, the cervix thickens, and a canal reforms. At the completion of involution, however, the external os does not completely resume its pregravid appearance. It remains somewhat wider, and typically, bilateral depressions at the site of lacerations remain as permanent changes that characterize the parous cervix. Furthermore, cervical epithelium undergoes considerable remodeling as a result of childbirth. Ahdoot and colleagues (1998) found that approximately 50 percent of women with high-grade dysplasia demonstrated regression after vaginal delivery.

The markedly thinned-out lower uterine segment contracts and retracts, but not as forcefully as the body of the uterus. Over the course of a few weeks, the lower segment is converted from a clearly distinct substructure of the uterus, large enough to accommodate the fetal head, into a barely discernible uterine isthmus located between the uterine corpus above and the internal cervical os below.

Involution of the Uterine Corpus. Immediately after placental expulsion, the fundus of the contracted uterus is slightly below the umbilicus. The uterine body then consists mostly of myometrium covered by serosa and lined by basal decidua. The anterior and posterior walls, in close apposition, each measure 4 to 5 cm in thickness (Buhimschi and colleagues, 2003). Because its vessels are compressed by the contracted myometrium, the puerperal uterus on section

appears ischemic when compared with the reddish-purple hyperemic pregnant organ. Two days after delivery, the uterus begins to shrink, and within 2 weeks it has descended into the cavity of the true pelvis. It regains its previous nonpregnant size about 4 weeks after delivery. Immediately postpartum, the uterus weighs approximately 1000 g. As the consequence of *involution,* 1 week later it weighs about 500 g, decreasing at the end of the second week to about 300 g, and soon thereafter to 100 g or less. The total number of muscle cells does not decrease appreciably, but instead, the individual cells decrease markedly in size. The involution of the connective tissue framework occurs equally rapidly.

Because separation of the placenta and membranes involves the spongy layer, the decidua basalis is not sloughed. The decidua that remains has striking variations in thickness, has an irregular jagged appearance, and is infiltrated with blood, especially at the placental site (Fig. 30–1).

AFTERPAINS. In primiparas, the puerperal uterus tends to remain tonically contracted, whereas in multiparas, the uterus often contracts vigorously at intervals, giving rise to *afterpains.* They are more pronounced as parity increases (Holdcroft and colleagues, 2003). They worsen when the infant suckles, likely because of oxytocin release. Usually, they decrease in intensity and become mild by the third day.

LOCHIA. Early in the puerperium, sloughing of decidual tissue results in a vaginal discharge of variable quantity; this is termed *lochia.* It consists of erythrocytes, shredded decidua, epithelial cells, and bacteria. For the first few days after delivery, there is blood sufficient to color it red—*lochia rubra.* After 3 or 4 days, lochia becomes progressively pale in color—*lochia serosa.* After about the 10th day, because of an admixture of leukocytes and reduced fluid content, lochia assumes a white or yellowish-white color—*lochia alba.*

Lochia persists for up to 4 weeks and may stop and resume up to 8 weeks after delivery (Oppenheimer and colleagues, 1986; Visness and co-workers, 1997). Maternal age, parity, infant weight, and breast feeding do not influence the duration of lochia. Moreover, routine administration of oxytocic agents beyond the immediate postpartum period neither diminishes blood loss nor hastens uterine involution (Newton and Bradford, 1961).

Endometrial Regeneration. Within 2 or 3 days after delivery, the remaining decidua becomes differentiated into two layers. The superficial layer becomes necrotic, and it is sloughed in the lochia. The basal layer adjacent to the myometrium remains intact and is the source of new endometrium. The endometrium arises from proliferation of the endometrial glandular remnants and the stroma of the interglandular connective tissue.

Endometrial regeneration is rapid, except at the placental site. Within a week or so, the free surface becomes covered by epithelium, and the entire endometrium is restored during

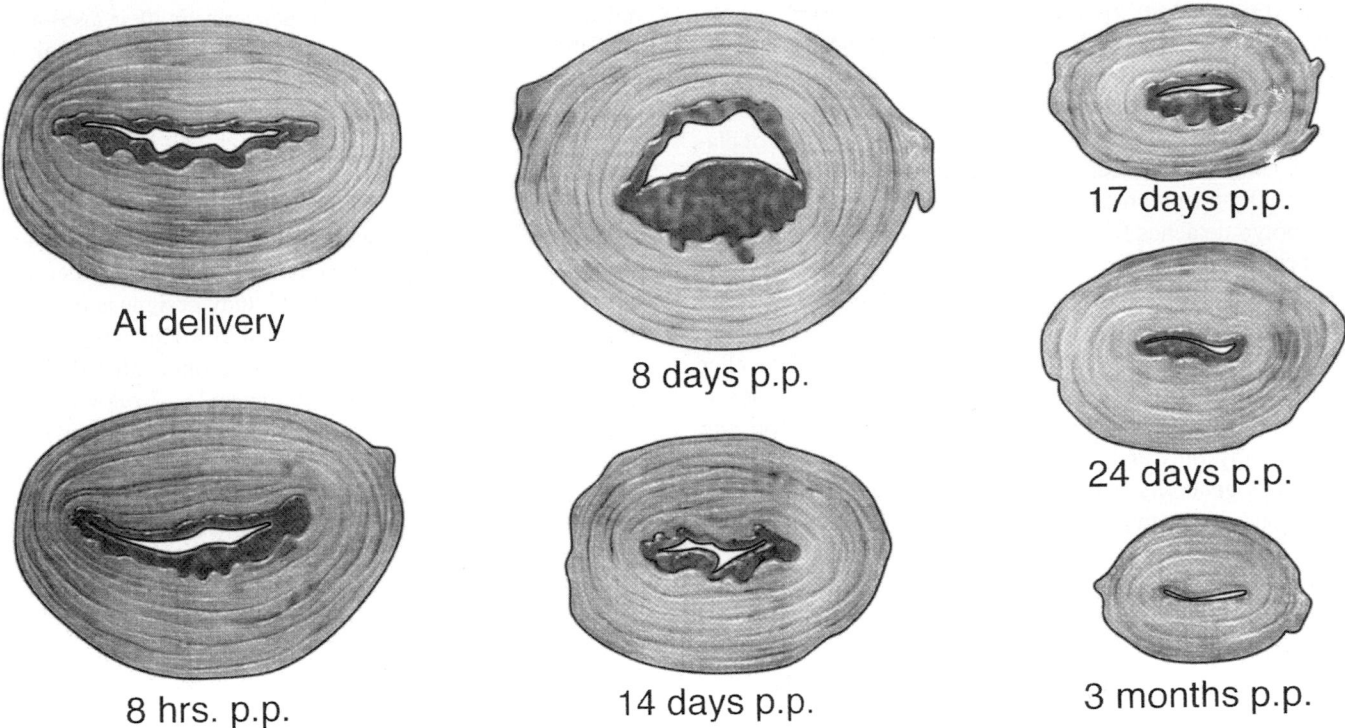

At delivery

8 days p.p.

17 days p.p.

8 hrs. p.p.

14 days p.p.

24 days p.p.

3 months p.p.

FIGURE 30–1. Cross sections of uteri made at the level of the involuting placental site at varying times after delivery. p.p. = postpartum. (Redrawn from Williams, 1931.)

the third week. Sharman (1953) identified fully restored endometrium in all biopsy specimens obtained from the 16th postpartum day onward. Histological endometritis is part of the normal reparative process. Similarly, in almost half of postpartum women, fallopian tubes, between 5 and 15 days, demonstrate microscopical inflammatory changes characteristic of acute salpingitis. These changes, however, do not reflect infection, but rather are part of the normal involutional process (Andrews, 1951).

SUBINVOLUTION. This term describes an arrest or retardation of involution. It is accompanied by prolongation of lochial discharge and irregular or excessive uterine bleeding, which sometimes may be profuse. On bimanual examination, the uterus is larger and softer than would be expected. Some causes of subinvolution are retention of placental fragments and pelvic infection. Because most cases of subinvolution result from local causes, they are usually amenable to early diagnosis and treatment. Ergonovine (Ergotrate) or methylergonovine (Methergine), 0.2 mg every 3 to 4 hours for 24 to 48 hours, is recommended by some clinicians, but its efficacy is questionable. On the other hand, metritis responds to oral antimicrobial therapy. Wager and colleagues (1980) reported that almost a third of cases of late postpartum uterine infection are caused by *Chlamydia trachomatis*; thus, azithromycin or doxycycline therapy may be appropriate.

Andrew and colleagues (1989) described 25 cases of hemorrhage between 7 and 40 days postpartum associated with noninvoluted uteroplacental arteries. These abnormal arteries were filled with thrombi and lacked an endothelial lining. Perivascular trophoblasts were also present in the walls of these vessels, and the authors postulated that subinvolution, at least with regard to the placental vessels, may represent an aberrant interaction between uterine cells and trophoblast.

Placental Site Involution. Complete extrusion of the placental site takes up to 6 weeks (Williams, 1931). This process is of great clinical importance, for when it is defective, late-onset puerperal hemorrhage may ensue. Immediately after delivery, the placental site is about the size of the palm of the hand, but it rapidly decreases thereafter. By the end of the second week, it is 3 to 4 cm in diameter. Within hours of delivery, the placental site normally consists of many thrombosed vessels that ultimately undergo organization (see Fig. 30–1).

Williams (1931) described placental site involution as involving a process of exfoliation, which is in great part brought about by the undermining of the implantation site by growth of endometrial tissue. Thus, involution is not brought about by absorption in situ. Exfoliation consists of both extension and "downgrowth" of endometrium from the margins of the placental site and the development of endometrial tissue from the glands and stroma that are left deep in the decidua basalis after placental separation. Anderson and Davis (1968) concluded that placental site exfoliation is brought about as the consequence of sloughing of infarcted and necrotic superficial tissues followed by a reparative process.

Late Postpartum Hemorrhage. Serious uterine hemorrhage occasionally develops 1 to 2 weeks into the puerperium. This hemorrhage most often is the result of abnormal involution of the placental site. It may also be caused by retention of a portion of the placenta. Usually the retained piece of placenta undergoes necrosis with deposition of fibrin and may eventually form a so-called *placental polyp.* As the eschar of the polyp detaches from the myometrium, hemorrhage may be brisk.

In a study by Lee and associates (1981) of 3822 women delivered during a 1-year period at Henry Ford Hospital, 27 women (0.7 percent) had significant uterine bleeding after the first postpartum day. In 20 of these women, the uterus was judged to be empty by ultrasonographic evaluation, and importantly, only one woman had retained placental tissue.

It has generally been accepted that prompt curettage is necessary for treatment of late postpartum hemorrhage. However, because curettage for late puerperal hemorrhage usually does not remove identifiable placental tissue, it may actually worsen the hemorrhage by traumatizing the implantation site and inciting more bleeding. Thus, initial treatment may be best directed to medical control of the bleeding with intravenous oxytocin, ergonovine, methylergonovine, or prostaglandins (Adrinopoulos and Mendenhall, 1983). In general, curettage is carried out only if appreciable bleeding persists or recurs after medical management.

URINARY TRACT CHANGES. Normal pregnancy is associated with an appreciable increase in extracellular water, and the diuresis that occurs postpartum is a physiological reversal of this process. This regularly occurs between the second and fifth days and corresponds with loss of residual pregnancy hypervolemia. In preeclampsia, both retention of fluid antepartum and diuresis postpartum may be greatly increased (see Chap. 34, p. 774).

The puerperal bladder has an increased capacity and a relative insensitivity to intravesical fluid pressure. Overdistention, incomplete emptying, and excessive residual urine are common. The paralyzing effect of analgesics, especially epidural and spinal blocks, is often contributory. The dilated ureters and renal pelves return to their prepregnant state over the course of 2 to 8 weeks after delivery (see Chap. 5, p. 138). Urinary tract infection is thus a concern because residual urine and bacteriuria in a traumatized bladder, coupled with the dilated renal pelves and ureters, create optimal conditions for development of infection. Kerr-Wilson and colleagues (1984) studied the effect of labor on postpartum bladder function using urodynamic techniques. They concluded that if labor was not prolonged, and **if catheterization was done promptly for bladder distention, bladder hypotonia did not occur.** Yip and colleagues (1997) demonstrated a positive correlation between duration of the first and second stage of labor and postvoid residual bladder volume as assessed by ultrasound on the first postpartum day. Carley and colleagues (2002) reported that overt postpartum urinary retention com-

plicated 1 in every 200 vaginal deliveries in their institution and that most cases resolved before hospital dismissal. In their study, instrument-assisted delivery and regional analgesia were independently correlated with the risk of urinary retention.

Incontinence. Increasing attention has been focused on the potential for the development of urinary incontinence subsequent to pregnancy. Although the literature is difficult to interpret due to the multiplicity of study designs and definitions of incontinence, 3 to 26 percent of women report daily episodes of incontinence in the 3 to 6 months after delivery (Farrell and colleagues, 2001; Wijma and co-workers, 2003; Wilson and associates, 1996). In one study, Viktrup and Lose (1993) followed 305 nulliparous women during pregnancy and postpartum. Seven percent reported the development of stress incontinence after delivery, which correlated with obstetrical factors such as length of second-stage labor, infant head circumference, birthweight, and episiotomy. Impaired muscle function in or around the urethra as a result of vaginal delivery was proposed as the pathophysiology underlying puerperal incontinence. At one-year follow-up, stress incontinence persisted in fewer than half.

Rortveit and colleagues (2003) performed a retrospective cohort study and found that women whose deliveries had all been vaginal had a 70-percent higher risk of incontinence than women whose deliveries had all been by cesarean. They cautioned, however, that for an individual woman, a decision to deliver all her infants by cesarean would decrease her risk of moderate or severe incontinence from 10 percent to only 5 percent, and that there was no evidence that this effect would persist past 50 years of age.

VAGINAL OUTLET RELAXATION AND UTERINE PROLAPSE. Early in the puerperium, the vagina and its outlet form a capacious, smooth-walled passage that gradually diminishes in size but rarely returns to nulliparous dimensions. Rugae reappear by the third week. The hymen is represented by several small tags of tissue, which during cicatrization are converted into the *myrtiform caruncles.*

Extensive lacerations of the perineum during delivery are followed by relaxation of the vaginal outlet. Even when external lacerations are not visible, stretching may lead to marked relaxation. Moreover, changes in pelvic support during parturition predispose to uterine prolapse and to urinary stress incontinence. In general, operative correction is postponed until childbearing is ended, unless serious disability, notably urinary stress incontinence, results in symptoms sufficient to require intervention.

PERITONEUM AND ABDOMINAL WALL. The broad and round ligaments require considerable time to recover from the stretching and loosening that occurred during pregnancy. As a result of the rupture of elastic fibers in the skin and the prolonged distention caused by the pregnant uterus, the abdominal wall remains soft and flaccid. Several weeks are required for these structures to return to normal. Recovery is aided by exercise. Except for silvery striae, the abdominal wall usually resumes its prepregnancy appearance. When muscles remain atonic, however, the abdominal wall also remains lax. There may be a marked separation of the rectus muscles or *diastasis recti*. In this condition, the midline abdominal wall is formed only by peritoneum, attenuated fascia, subcutaneous fat, and skin.

BLOOD AND FLUID CHANGES. Rather marked leukocytosis and thrombocytosis occur during and after labor. The leukocyte count sometimes reaches $30,000/\mu L$, with the increase predominantly from granulocytes. There is also a relative lymphopenia and an absolute eosinopenia. Normally, during the first few postpartum days, hemoglobin concentration and hematocrit fluctuate moderately. If they fall much below the levels present just prior to labor, a considerable amount of blood has been lost (see Chap. 35, p. 839). By 1 week after delivery, the blood volume has returned nearly to its nonpregnant level. Robson and colleagues (1987) showed that cardiac output remains elevated for at least 48 hours postpartum. Most likely this is due to increased stroke volume from venous return, because the heart rate falls at the same time. By 2 weeks, these changes have returned to normal nonpregnant values.

Pregnancy-induced changes in blood coagulation factors persist for variable periods during the puerperium. Elevation of plasma fibrinogen is maintained at least through the first week, and hence, so is the sedimentation rate.

Weight Loss. In addition to the loss of about 5 to 6 kg due to uterine evacuation and normal blood loss, there is usually a further decrease of 2 to 3 kg through diuresis. Chesley and co-workers (1959) demonstrated a decrease in sodium space of about 2 L during the first week postpartum. According to Schauberger and co-investigators (1992), most women approach their self-reported prepregnancy weight 6 months after delivery but still retain an average surplus of 1.4 kg (3 lb). Smith and colleagues (1994) reported on a cohort of women who were followed over a 5-year period. Women who had a single pregnancy and were at least 12 months postpartum had gained an average of 2 to 3 kg more weight and had greater increases in their waist-to-hip ratio (a measure of adiposity) than those who had remained nulliparous. Indigent women are more likely to retain weight gained during pregnancy (Olson and associates, 2003). Deleterious effects of weight gain are discussed in Chapter 43 (see p. 1009).

MAMMARY GLANDS

BREAST ANATOMY. Each mature mammary gland is composed of 15 to 25 lobes. The lobes are arranged radially

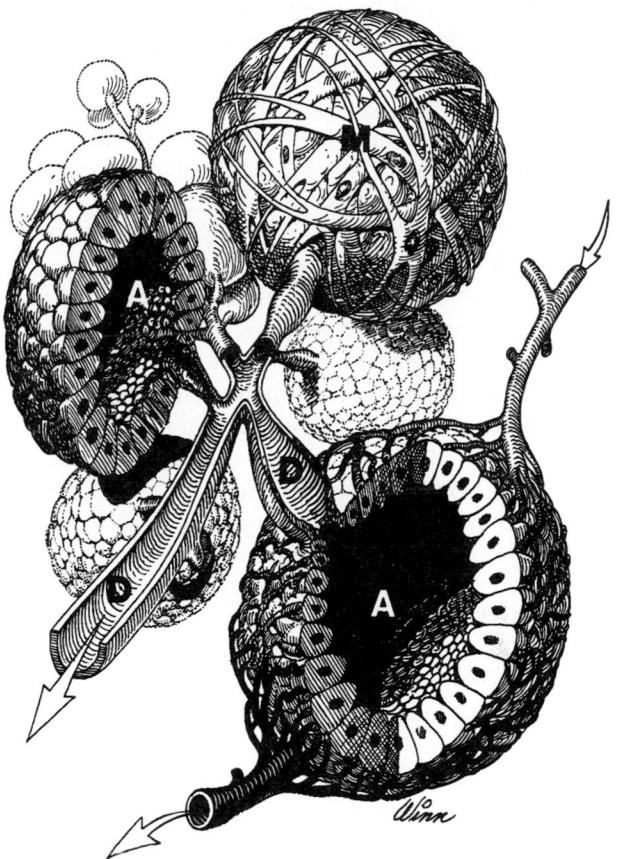

FIGURE 30–2. Graphic demonstration of the alveolar and ductal system. Note the myoepithelial fibers (M) that surround the outside of the uppermost alveolus. The secretions from the glandular elements are extruded into the lumen of the alveoli (A) and ejected by the myoepithelial cells into the ductal system (D), which empties through the nipple. Arterial blood supply to the alveolus is identified by the upper right arrow and venous drainage by the arrow beneath. (Courtesy of Dr. John C. Porter.)

and are separated from one another by varying amounts of fat. Each lobe consists of several lobules, which in turn are made up of large numbers of alveoli (Fig. 30–2). Every alveolus is provided with a small duct that joins others to form a single larger duct for each lobe. These lactiferous ducts open separately on the nipple, where they may be distinguished as minute but distinct orifices. The alveolar secretory epithelium synthesizes the various milk constituents.

BREAST FEEDING. After delivery, the breasts begin to secrete colostrum, which is a deep lemon-yellow-colored liquid. It usually can be expressed from the nipples by the second day.

Colostrum and Milk

COLOSTRUM. Compared with mature milk, colostrum contains more minerals and protein, much of which is globulin, but less sugar and fat. Colostrum secretion persists for about 5 days, with gradual conversion to mature milk during the ensuing 4 weeks. Antibodies are demonstrable in colostrum, and its content of immunoglobulin A (IgA) may offer protection for the newborn against enteric pathogens. Other host resistance factors that are found in colostrum and milk include complement, macrophages, lymphocytes, lactoferrin, lactoperoxidase, and lysozymes.

MILK. Human milk is a suspension of fat and protein in a carbohydrate-mineral solution. Gestational weight gain has little, if any, impact on the subsequent milk quantity or quality (Institute of Medicine, 1990). A nursing mother easily makes 600 mL of milk per day. Milk is isotonic with plasma, with lactose accounting for half of the osmotic pressure. Major proteins, including α-lactalbumin, β-lactoglobulin, and casein, are also present. Essential amino acids are derived from blood, and nonessential amino acids are derived in part from blood or synthesized in the mammary gland. Most milk proteins are unique and not found elsewhere.

Whey is milk serum and has been shown to contain large amounts of interleukin-6 (IL-6) (Saito and co-workers, 1991). Peak levels were found in colostrum, and there was a positive correlation between its concentration and the number of mononuclear cells in human milk. In addition, IL-6 was associated closely with local IgA production by the breast. *Prolactin* appears to be actively secreted into breast milk (Yuen, 1988). *Epidermal growth factor (EGF)* has also been identified in human milk (Koldovsky and associates, 1991; McCleary, 1991). Because EGF is not destroyed by gastric proteolytic enzymes, it may be absorbed orally and promote growth and maturation of intestinal mucosa.

There are major changes in milk composition by 30 to 40 hours postpartum, including a sudden increase of lactose concentration. Some lactose enters the maternal circulation and is excreted by the kidney. This may be misinterpreted as glucosuria unless specific glucose oxidase is used in testing. Fatty acids are synthesized in the alveoli from glucose and are secreted by an apocrine-like process.

All vitamins except K are found in human milk, but in variable amounts, and maternal dietary supplementation increases the secretion of most of these (American Academy of Pediatrics, 1981). Vitamin K administration to the infant soon after delivery is required to prevent hemorrhagic disease of the newborn (see Chap. 29, p. 676).

Endocrinology of Lactation.

The precise humoral and neural mechanisms involved in lactation are complex. Progesterone, estrogen, and placental lactogen, as well as prolactin, cortisol, and insulin, appear to act in concert to stimulate the growth and development of the milk-secreting apparatus of the mammary gland (Porter, 1974). With delivery, there is an abrupt and profound decrease in the levels of progesterone and estrogen, which removes the inhibitory influence of progesterone on the production of α-lactalbumin by the rough endoplasmic reticulum. The increased α-lactalbumin serves to stimulate lactose synthase and ultimately to increase milk lactose. Progesterone withdrawal also allows prolactin to act unopposed in its stimulation of α-lactalbumin production.

The intensity and duration of subsequent lactation are controlled, in large part, by the repetitive stimulus of nursing. Prolactin is essential for lactation; for example, women with extensive pituitary necrosis, or *Sheehan syndrome*, do not lactate (see Chap. 53, p. 1203). Although plasma prolactin falls after delivery to levels lower than during pregnancy, each act of suckling triggers a rise in levels (McNeilly and associates, 1983). Presumably a stimulus from the breast curtails the release of prolactin-inhibiting factor from the hypothalamus, and this, in turn, transiently induces increased prolactin secretion.

The neurohypophysis secretes oxytocin in pulsatile fashion. This stimulates milk expression from a lactating breast by causing contraction of myoepithelial cells in the alveoli and small milk ducts. Milk ejection, or *letting down*, is a reflex initiated especially by suckling, which stimulates the neurohypophysis to liberate oxytocin (McNeilly and associates, 1983). Milk let-down may be provoked even by the cry of the infant and can be inhibited by fright or stress.

In women who become pregnant but who continue to breast feed, milk composition undergoes progressive alterations suggesting gradual loss of metabolic and secretory breast activity (Hartmann and Prosser, 1984).

Immunological Consequences of Breast Feeding.

Antibodies are present in human colostrum and milk but are poorly absorbed, if at all, by infants. For example, no serum antibodies have been detected in infants fed milk containing a high titer of anti-D antibodies. This does not lessen the importance of some of the antibodies in breast milk. The predominant immunoglobulin in milk is secretory IgA. This macromolecule is secreted across mucous membranes and has important antimicrobial functions. For example, human milk contains secretory IgA antibodies against *Escherichia coli,* and breast-fed infants are less prone to enteric infections than bottle-fed infants (Cravioto and associates, 1991). It has been suggested that IgA exerts its action by preventing bacterial adherence to epithelial cell surfaces, thus preventing tissue invasion (Samra and associates, 1991). Moreover, human milk also provides protection against rotavirus infections, which cause up to 50 percent of cases of gastroenteritis among infants in the United States (Newburg and associates, 1998).

Much attention has been directed to an elucidation of the role of maternal breast milk lymphocytes in the immunological processes of the newborn. Milk contains both T and B lymphocytes, but the T lymphocytes appear to differ from those found in blood. Specifically, milk T lymphocytes are almost exclusively composed of cells that exhibit specific membrane antigens, including the LFA-1 high-memory T-cell phenotype. These memory T cells appear to be another mechanism by which the neonate benefits from maternal immunological experience (Bertotto and associates, 1990). Lymphocytes in colostrum undergo blastoid transformation in vitro following exposure to specific antigens. In experimental animals, Beer and Billingham (1976) observed a transmission of viable lymphocytes from mother to infant through breast milk. As mentioned earlier, IL-6 is present in colostrum and appears to stimulate an increase in mononuclear cells in breast milk (Saito and co-workers, 1991).

Nursing. Between 1930 and the late 1960s, there was a dramatic decline in the percentage of American mothers who breast fed (Yaffe, 1994). In 1930, 80 percent of children were breast fed compared with only 20 percent in 1972. The picture has improved since then. Currently in the United States, more than 60 percent of infants are breast fed, and the number is increasing (American College of Obstetricians and Gynecologists, 2000).

Human milk is ideal food for neonates. It provides species- and age-specific nutrients for the infant. In addition to the proper balance of nutrients, immunological factors, and antibacterial properties, human milk contains factors that act as biological signals for promoting cellular growth and differentiation (American College of Obstetricians and Gynecologists, 2000). With limited sun exposure, however, infants who are breast fed exclusively may become vitamin D deficient. Thus supplementation with 200 IU of vitamin D per day for the first two months for such infants is recommended by the American Academy of Pediatrics (Gartner and Greer, 2003).

In 1997, the American Academy of Pediatrics published the policy statement on the infant benefits of nursing shown in Table 30–1. For both mother and infant, the benefits of breast feeding are likely long-term. For example, women who breast feed have a lower risk of breast cancer, and their children have increased adult intelligence independent of a wide range of possible confounding factors (Collaborative Group on Hormonal Factors in Breast Cancer, 2002; Mortensen and

TABLE 30–1 **American Academy of Pediatrics Policy Statement: Research on Established and Potential Protective Effects of Human Milk and Breast Feeding on Infants**

Research in the United States, Canada, Europe, and other developed countries, among predominantly middle-class populations, provides strong evidence that human milk feeding decreases the incidence and/or severity of diarrhea, lower respiratory infection, otitis media, bacteremia, bacterial meningitis, botulism, urinary tract infection, and necrotizing enterocolitis. There are a number of studies that show a possible protective effect of human milk feeding against sudden infant death syndrome, insulin-dependent diabetes mellitus, Crohn disease, ulcerative colitis, lymphoma, allergic diseases, and other chronic digestive diseases. Breast feeding has also been related to possible enhancement of cognitive development.

From the American Academy of Pediatrics (1997), with permission.

associates, 2002). A goal of the United States Public Health Service for year 2010 is to increase the proportion of mothers who breast feed to 75 percent. Educational initiatives can be effective. Kramer and colleagues (2001) demonstrated that the systematic promotion of breast feeding leads to higher rates and longer durations of breast feeding.

In most instances, even though the supply of milk at first appears insufficient, it becomes adequate if suckling is continued. An exception is that 65 percent of women who have undergone augmentation mammoplasty have lactation insufficiency (Hurst, 1996). This problem is more likely if the implant incision was periareolar (Chez and Friedman, 2000). Aerobic exercise performed four or five times per week beginning 6 to 8 weeks postpartum had no adverse effect on amounts or immunological contents of milk (Dewey and co-workers, 1994; Lovelady and associates, 2003). Weight loss of approximately 0.5 kg per week in the first 3 months postpartum does not affect infant growth of exclusively breast feeding, overweight women (Lovelady and co-workers, 2000).

According to Chez and Friedman (2000), a number of Internet resources are available for breast feeding mothers. These include the American Academy of Pediatrics (www.aap.org) and La Leche League International (www.lalecheleague.org).

LACTATION INHIBITION. Approximately 40 percent of American women currently elect not to breast feed, and many experience considerable breast pain and engorgement. Milk leakage, engorgement, and breast pain peak at 3 to 5 days postpartum (Spitz and associates, 1998). As many as 10 percent report severe pain up to 14 days postpartum, and 25 to 50 percent of all women use analgesia for breast pain relief. In 1989, an advisory committee of the Food and Drug Administration, taking the view that there is no need for pharmacological therapy for lactation suppression, recommended that medications should no longer be used for lactation suppression. In part, this decision was because *bromocriptine*, a commonly used drug for lactation inhibition, had been associated with strokes, myocardial infarctions, seizures, and psychiatric disturbances. Evidence to support these associations, however, is tenuous at best (Morgans, 1995). Nevertheless, the manufacturer voluntarily removed lactation suppression as an indication for bromocriptine (Food and Drug Administration, 1994).

The woman who does not desire to breast feed should be reassured that stopping milk production is not a major problem. During the stage of engorgement, the breasts become painful and should be supported with a well-fitting brassiere. Ice packs and oral analgesics for 12 to 24 hours may be required to relieve discomfort. Breast binders are used at Parkland Hospital for these women, and patient-supplied "sports bras" are used at the University of Alabama Hospital.

CONTRACEPTION FOR BREAST FEEDING WOMEN. Three weeks after delivery, ovulation may resume, even in lactating

TABLE 30–2 Recommendations for Hormonal Contraception if Used by Breast Feeding Women

- Progestin-only oral contraceptives prescribed or dispensed at discharge from the hospital to be started 2–3 weeks postpartum—for example, the first Sunday after the newborn is 2 weeks of age.
- Depot medroxyprogesterone acetate initiated at 6 weeks postpartum.[a]
- Hormonal implants inserted at 6 weeks postpartum.
- Combined estrogen–progestin contraceptives, if prescribed, should not be started before 6 weeks postpartum, and only when lactation is well established and the infant's nutritional status well monitored.

[a]There are certain clinical situations in which earlier initiation might be considered.
From the American College of Obstetricians and Gynecologists (2000), with permission.

women. Its resumption depends on individual biological variation as well as the intensity of breast feeding. Progestin-only contraceptives—mini-pills and depot medroxyprogesterone—do not affect the quality or decrease milk volume. They are considered the hormonal contraceptives of choice for breast feeding women by the American College of Obstetricians and Gynecologists (2000). Although estrogen-progestin contraceptives have been shown to reduce the quantity and quality of breast milk, under the proper circumstances they can be used by breast feeding women. These methods are summarized in Table 30–2.

CONTRAINDICATIONS TO BREAST FEEDING. Nursing is contraindicated in women who take street drugs or do not control their alcohol use; have an infant with galactosemia; have human immunodeficiency virus (HIV) infection; have active, untreated tuberculosis; take certain medications; or are undergoing treatment for breast cancer (American College of Obstetricians and Gynecologists, 2000). Breast feeding has been recognized for some time as a mode of HIV transmission (Ziegler and colleagues, 1985). Nduati and colleagues (2000) randomly assigned 401 HIV-seropositive mother–infant pairs in Kenya to formula or breast feeding. At 2 years of age, the rate of viral infection in children who were breast fed was 37 percent—significantly higher than in children who were formula fed, in whom the rate was 21 percent.

Other viral infections do not contraindicate breast feeding. For example, maternal cytomegalovirus infection is not a contraindication, because virus and antibodies are present in breast milk. Likewise, although hepatitis B virus is excreted in milk, breast feeding is not contraindicated if hepatitis B immune globulin is given to infants of seropositive mothers (American College of Obstetricians and Gynecologists, 2000). Maternal hepatitis C infection is also not a contraindication to breast feeding, and the 4-percent risk of infant transmission is the same for breast- and bottle-fed infants (Centers for Disease Control and Prevention, 1998).

Women with active herpes simplex virus may suckle their infants if there are no breast lesions and if particular care is directed to hand washing before nursing.

CARE. The nipples require little attention in the puerperium other than cleanliness and attention to fissures. Because dried milk is likely to accumulate and irritate the nipples, cleaning of the areola with water and mild soap is helpful before and after nursing. When the nipples are irritated, it may be necessary to use a nipple shield for 24 hours or longer. Although inverted or retracted nipples may be troublesome, these can usually be teased out by gently pulling with the finger and thumb. This is best begun during pregnancy to prepare the nipples for subsequent nursing. Proper technique for positioning the mother and infant during nursing has been reviewed by the American College of Obstetricians and Gynecologists (2000). This includes proper techniques for *latch-on* of the infant during suckling.

DRUGS SECRETED IN MILK. Most drugs given to the mother are secreted in breast milk. Many factors influence their excretion, including the concentration of drugs in plasma, degree of protein binding, plasma and milk pH, degree of ionization, lipid solubility, and molecular weight. The amount of drug ingested by the infant typically is small. The ratio of drug concentrations in breast milk to those in maternal plasma is the *milk-to-plasma drug-concentration ratio*. Most drugs have a milk-to-plasma ratio of 1 or less, about 25 percent have a ratio of more than 1, and about 15 percent have a ratio greater than 2 (Ito, 2000).

The American Academy of Pediatrics and the American College of Obstetricians and Gynecologists (2002) agree that cytotoxic drugs may interfere with the cellular metabolism of the infant and potentially cause immune suppression or neutropenia, affect growth, or, at least theoretically, increase the risk of cancer. These include cyclophosphamide; cyclosporine; doxorubicin, which is concentrated in breast milk; and methotrexate. Other drugs that have been associated with significant effects on some nursing infants and therefore should be used with caution are shown in Table 30–3. If a medication presents a concern, then it should be ascertained whether the drug therapy is necessary, whether a safer alternative is available, and whether neonatal exposure can be minimized by having the mother take the medication immediately after breast feeding (American Academy of Pediatrics and the American College of Obstetricians and Gynecologists, 2002).

Radioactive isotopes of copper, gallium, indium, iodine, sodium, and technetium rapidly appear in breast milk. The American Academy of Pediatrics and the American College of Obstetricians and Gynecologists (2002) recommend consultation with a nuclear medicine physician before performing a diagnostic study using these isotopes. The goal is to use a radionuclide with the shortest excretion time in breast milk. The mother should pump her breasts before the study and store enough milk in a freezer for feeding the infant. After

TABLE 30–3 Drugs That Have Been Associated with Significant Effects on Some Nursing Infants

Drug	Reported Effect[a]
Acebutolol	Hypotension, bradycardia, tachypnea
5-Aminosalicylic acid	Diarrhea (one case)
Aspirin (salicylates)	Metabolic acidosis (one case)
Atenolol	Cyanosis, bradycardia
Bromocriptine	Suppresses lactation, may be hazardous to the mother
Clemastine	Drowsiness, irritability, refusal to feed, high-pitched cry, neck stiffness (one case)
Ergotamine	Vomiting, diarrhea, convulsions—doses used in migraine medications
Lithium	A third to half therapeutic blood concentration in infants
Phenindione	Anticoagulant—increased prothrombin and partial thromboplastin time in one infant—not used in United States
Phenobarbital	Sedation; infantile spasms after weaning from milk containing phenobarbital; methemoglobinemia (one case)
Primidone	Sedation, feeding problems
Sulfasalazine	Bloody diarrhea (one case)

[a] Blood concentration in the infant may be of clinical importance.
From the American Academy of Pediatrics and the American College of Obstetricians and Gynecologists, 2002, with permission.

the study, she should pump her breasts to maintain milk production but discard all milk produced during the time that radioactivity is present. This ranges from 15 hours up to 2 weeks, depending on the isotope used.

Breast Fever. For the first 24 hours after commencement of lactation, it is not unusual for the breasts to become distended, firm, and nodular. These findings may be accompanied by a transient elevation of temperature. Puerperal fever from breast engorgement is common. Almeida and Kitay (1986) reported that 13 percent of all postpartum women had fever that ranged from 37.8 to 39°C from this cause. Fever seldom persisted for longer than 4 to 16 hours. The incidence and severity of breast engorgement, and fever associated with it, were lower if treatment was given for lactation suppression. **Other causes of fever, especially those due to infection, must be excluded.** Treatment consists of supporting the breasts with a binder or brassiere, applying an ice bag, and an analgesic. Pumping of the breast or manual expression of milk may be necessary at first, but in a few days the condition is usually alleviated and the infant is able to nurse normally (see p. 699).

Mastitis. Parenchymatous infection of the mammary glands is a rare complication antepartum but is occasionally observed during the puerperium and lactation. It is estimated to occur in anywhere from 2 to 33 percent of breast feeding

women (Barbosa-Cesnik and associates, 2003). Symptoms of suppurative mastitis seldom appear before the end of the first week postpartum and, as a rule, not until the third or fourth week. Infection almost invariably is unilateral, and marked engorgement usually precedes the inflammation. The first sign of inflammation is chills or actual rigor, soon followed by fever and tachycardia. The breast becomes hard and reddened, and the woman complains of severe pain. About 10 percent of women with mastitis develop an abscess. Constitutional symptoms attending a mammary abscess are generally severe, but in some cases the first indication of the true diagnosis often is afforded by the detection of fluctuation. Ultrasonography may be helpful to detect an abscess.

ETIOLOGY. The most commonly isolated organism is *Staphylococcus aureus*. Matheson and colleagues (1988) cultured it from 40 percent of women with mastitis. Other commonly isolated organisms are coagulase-negative staphylococci and viridans streptococci. The immediate source of organisms that cause mastitis is almost always the infant's nose and throat. With nursing, bacteria enter the breast through the nipple at the site of a fissure or abrasion, which may be quite small. In cases of true mastitis, the infecting organism can usually be cultured from milk. Toxic shock syndrome secondary to mastitis caused by *S aureus* has been reported (Demey and associates, 1989; Fujiwara and Endo, 2001).

Suppurative mastitis among nursing mothers has at times reached epidemic levels. Such outbreaks most often coincide with the appearance of a new strain of antibiotic-resistant *Staphylococcus,* an example being methicillin-resistant *S aureus* (MRSA). Typically, the infant becomes infected after contact with nursery personnel who are colonized. Attendants' hands are the major source of contamination of the newborn. The colonization of staphylococci in the infant may be totally asymptomatic or may locally involve the umbilicus or the skin. Occasionally the organisms cause a life-threatening systemic infection.

TREATMENT. Abscess formation is more common with *S aureus* infection (Matheson and associates, 1988). Provided that appropriate therapy is started before suppuration begins, the infection usually resolves within 48 hours. Before initiating antimicrobial therapy, some clinicians recommend that milk be expressed from the affected breast onto a swab and cultured. By so doing, the organism can be identified and its antimicrobial sensitivities ascertained. Results of such cultures also provide information mandatory for a successful program for surveillance of nosocomial infections.

The initial choice of antimicrobial is undoubtedly influenced to a considerable degree by the current experience with staphylococcal infections at the institution. That said, most are community-acquired organisms, and even staphylococcal infections are usually sensitive to penicillin or a cephalosporin (American College of Obstetricians and Gynecologists, 2000). Dicloxacillin, 500 mg orally four times daily, may be started empirically (Hindle, 1994). Erythromycin is given to women who are penicillin sensitive. If the infection is caused by resistant, penicillinase-producing staphylococci, or if resistant organisms are suspected while awaiting the results of culture, an antimicrobial such as vancomycin, which is effective against MRSA, should be given. Even though clinical response may be prompt and striking, treatment should be continued for 10 to 14 days.

Marshall and colleagues (1975) demonstrated the importance of continued breast feeding. They reported that the only three abscesses that developed in 65 women with mastitis were in 15 women who chose to wean their infants. Thomsen and co-workers (1984) observed that vigorous milk expression was sufficient treatment alone in half of women with mastitis. Early therapy and continued lactation was successful in avoiding abscess formation in all 20 women described by Niebyl and co-investigators (1978). If the infected breast is too tender to allow suckling, gently pumping until nursing can be resumed is recommended. Sometimes the infant will not nurse on the inflamed breast. This probably is not related to any changes in the taste of the milk but is secondary to engorgement and edema, which can make the areola harder to grip. Pumping can alleviate this. When nursing bilaterally, it is best to begin suckling on the uninvolved breast. This allows let-down to commence before moving to the tender breast.

Breast Abscess. Clinical suspicion for abscess development is either from failure of defervescence within 48 to 72 hours or development of a palpable mass. Traditional therapy is surgical drainage, which usually requires general anesthesia. The incision should be made corresponding to skin lines for a good cosmetic result (Stehman, 1990). In early cases, a single incision over the most dependent portion of the area of fluctuation is usually sufficient, but multiple abscesses require several incisions, and a finger should be inserted to break up the walls of the locules. The resulting cavity is loosely packed with gauze, which should be replaced at the end of 24 hours by a smaller pack. A less invasive alternative is ultrasonographic-guided needle aspiration using local anesthesia, which has success rates of 80 to 90 percent (Karstrup, 1993; O'Hara, 1996; Schwarz, 2001, and all their associates).

Galactocele. Exceptionally, as the result of the clogging of a duct by inspissated secretion, milk may accumulate in one or more lobes of the breast. The amount is ordinarily limited, but an excess may form a fluctuant mass that may give rise to pressure symptoms. They may resolve spontaneously or require aspiration.

Supernumerary Breasts. One in every few hundred women has one or more accessory breasts (*polymastia*). The supernumerary breasts may be so small as to be mistaken for pigmented moles, or when without a nipple, for a lipoma. They rarely attain considerable size. They are likely to be situated in pairs on either side of the midline of the thoracic or abdominal walls, usually below the main breasts. They are also found in the axillae, and more rarely on other portions of the body, such as the shoulder, flank, groin, or thigh. When arranged symmetrically, two or four are most common, although 10 have been described. Polymastia has no obstetrical significance, although occasionally the enlargement of supernumerary breasts in the axillae may result in considerable discomfort.

Abnormalities of the Nipples. In some women, the lactiferous ducts open directly into a depression at the center of the areola. In marked cases of depressed nipple, nursing is not possible. When the depression is not very deep, the breast may occasionally be made available by use of a breast pump. More frequently, the nipple, although not depressed, is greatly inverted. In such a case, daily attempts should be made during the last few months of pregnancy to draw the nipple out, using traction with fingers.

Nipples that are normal in shape and size may become fissured. In such cases, the fissures almost invariably render nursing painful, sometimes with a deleterious influence on the secretory function. Moreover, such lesions provide a convenient portal of entry for pyogenic bacteria. For these reasons, every effort should be made to heal such fissures, particularly by protecting them from further injury with a nipple shield and topical medication. If such measures are of no avail, the infant should not be permitted to nurse on the affected side. Instead, the breast should be emptied regularly with a suitable pump until the lesions are completely healed.

Abnormalities of Secretion. There are marked individual variations in the amount of milk secreted, many of which are dependent not on the general health and appearance of the woman but on the development of the glandular portions of the breasts. Rarely, there is complete lack of mammary secretion (*agalactia*). Occasionally, the mammary secretion is excessive (*polygalactia*).

CARE OF THE MOTHER DURING THE PUERPERIUM

HOSPITAL CARE. For the first hour after delivery, blood pressure and pulse should be taken every 15 minutes, or more frequently if indicated. The amount of vaginal bleeding is monitored, and the fundus should be palpated to ensure that it is well contracted. If relaxation is detected, the uterus should be massaged through the abdominal wall until it remains contracted. Blood may accumulate within the uterus without external bleeding. This may be detected early by identifying uterine enlargement with serial and frequent fundal palpation during the first few hours. Because the likelihood of significant hemorrhage is greatest immediately postpartum, even in normal cases, a trained attendant should remain with the mother for at least 1 hour after delivery. Identification and management of postpartum hemorrhage is discussed in Chapter 35.

If regional analgesia or general anesthesia is used, the mother should be observed in an appropriately equipped and staffed recovery area.

Early Ambulation. Early ambulation is an accepted puerperal practice. Women are out of bed within a few hours after delivery. The many confirmed advantages of early ambulation include less frequent bladder complications and constipation. As discussed in Chapter 47 (see p. 1074), early ambulation has reduced the frequency of puerperal venous thrombosis and pulmonary embolism (Toglia and Weg, 1996). For at least the first ambulation, an attendant should be present in case the woman should become syncopal.

Care of the Vulva. The patient should be instructed to cleanse the vulva from anterior to posterior (vulva toward anus). An ice bag applied to the perineum may help reduce edema and discomfort during the first several hours after episiotomy repair. Beginning about 24 hours after delivery, moist heat as provided with warm sitz baths can be used to reduce local discomfort. Tub bathing after uncomplicated delivery is allowed.

Bladder Function. Bladder filling after delivery may be quite variable. In most hospitals, intravenous fluids are infused during labor and for an hour after delivery. Oxytocin, in doses that have an antidiuretic effect, is commonly infused after placental delivery. As a consequence of infused fluid and the sudden withdrawal of the antidiuretic effect of oxytocin, rapid bladder filling is common. Moreover, both bladder sensation and capability to empty spontaneously may be diminished by anesthesia, especially conduction analgesia, as well as by episiotomy, lacerations, or hematomas. It is not surprising, therefore, that urinary retention with bladder overdistention is a common complication of the early puerperium. In a prospective observational study, Ching-Chung and colleagues (2002) reported this complication in 4 percent of term women delivered vaginally. On long-term follow-up, only 3 of 114 women had persistent urinary symptoms.

Prevention of bladder overdistention demands observation after delivery to ensure that the bladder does not overfill and that with each voiding it empties adequately. The bladder may be palpated as a cystic mass suprapubically, or the enlarged bladder may be evident abdominally only indirectly, as a consequence of its elevating the uterine fundus above the umbilicus.

If the woman has not voided within 4 hours after delivery, it is likely that she cannot. The woman who has trouble voiding initially is likely to have further trouble. In such women, the likelihood of hematomas of the genital tract must be considered. Whenever the bladder becomes overdistended, an indwelling catheter should be left in place until the factors causing the retention have abated. Even without a demonstrable cause, it usually is best to leave the catheter in place for at least 24 hours, so as to empty the bladder completely. This prevents recurrence as well as allows recovery of normal bladder tone and sensation. When the catheter is removed, it is necessary subsequently to demonstrate ability to void appropriately. If the woman cannot void after 4 hours, she should be catheterized and urine volume measured. If there is more than 200 mL of urine, it is apparent that the bladder is not functioning appropriately. The catheter should be left in place and the bladder drained for another day. If less than 200 mL of urine is obtained, the catheter can be removed and the bladder rechecked subsequently as described. Harris and colleagues (1977) reported that 40 percent of such women develop bacteriuria; and thus, a short course of antimicrobial therapy seems reasonable after the catheter is removed.

Subsequent Discomfort. The discomfort from cesarean delivery, its causes, and its management are considered in Chapter 25 (see p. 589). During the first few days after vaginal delivery, the mother may be uncomfortable for a variety of reasons, including afterpains, episiotomy and lacerations, breast engorgement, and at times, postspinal puncture headache. It is helpful to provide codeine, 60 mg; aspirin, 600 mg; or acetaminophen, 500 mg, preferably in combinations, at intervals as frequent as every 3 hours during the first few days after delivery. Uterine contractions are commonly accentuated during nursing, giving rise at times to troublesome afterpains.

An episiotomy or lacerations may be uncomfortable, as discussed in Chapter 17 (see p. 434). Early application of an ice bag may minimize swelling and discomfort. Most women also appear to obtain a measure of relief from the periodic application of a local anesthetic spray. Severe discomfort usually indicates a problem such as a hematoma within the first day or so and infection after the third or fourth day. For these reasons, severe pain warrants careful examination. The episiotomy incision normally is firmly healed and nearly asymptomatic by the third week.

Depression. It is fairly common for a mother to exhibit some degree of depressed mood a few days after delivery. This situation is termed *postpartum blues,* and it likely is the consequence of a number of factors:

1. The emotional letdown that follows the excitement and fears that most women experience during pregnancy and delivery.
2. The discomforts of the early puerperium.
3. Fatigue from loss of sleep during labor and postpartum.
4. Anxiety over her capabilities for caring for her infant after leaving the hospital.
5. Fears that she has become less attractive.

In the great majority of cases, effective treatment need be nothing more than anticipation, recognition, and reassurance. This mild disorder is self-limited and usually remits after 2 to 3 days, although it sometimes persists for up to 10 days. Should postpartum blues persist or worsen, a careful search should begin for symptoms of major depression, which can occur in almost 20 percent of puerperal women (Josefsson and associates, 2001). If severe, prompt consultation is carried out as discussed in Chapter 55 (see p. 1243). Similarly, suicidal or infanticidal ideation is dealt with emergently. Postpartum depression is likely to recur and warrants pharmacological prophylaxis beginning late in future pregnancies.

Abdominal Wall Relaxation. If the abdomen is unusually flabby or pendulous, an ordinary girdle is often satisfactory. An abdominal binder does not help restore the figure. Exercises to restore abdominal wall tone may be started any time after vaginal delivery and as soon as abdominal soreness diminishes after cesarean delivery.

Diet. There are no dietary restrictions for women who have been delivered vaginally. Two hours after a normal vaginal delivery, if there are no complications likely to necessitate an anesthetic, the woman should be allowed to eat if she desires. The diet of lactating women, compared with that consumed during pregnancy, should be increased in calories and protein, as recommended by the Food and Nutrition Board of the National Research Council (see Chap. 8, p. 215). If the mother does not breast feed, dietary requirements are the same as for a nonpregnant woman.

It is standard practice in our hospitals to continue iron supplementation for at least 3 months after delivery and to check the hematocrit at the first postpartum visit.

Thromboembolic Disease. Perhaps half of thromboembolic events associated with pregnancy develop in the puerperium (see Chap. 47, p. 1074). The frequency of deep venous thrombosis and pulmonary embolism complicating pregnancy and the puerperium has decreased in recent years.

Obstetrical Neuropathies. Pressure on branches of the lumbosacral nerve plexus during labor may be manifest by complaints of intense neuralgia or cramplike pains extending down one or both legs as soon as the head begins to descend into the pelvis. If the nerve is injured, pain continues after delivery and may be accompanied by variable degrees of sensory loss or muscle paralysis supplied by the damaged nerve.

In a recent investigation from Northwestern University, Wong and colleagues (2003) carefully evaluated 6048 consecutively delivered women and found that 56 (approximately 1 percent) had a confirmed new nerve injury. Lateral femoral cutaneous neuropathies were the most common (24), followed by femoral neuropathies (14). A motor deficit was present in a third of injuries. Nulliparity and prolonged

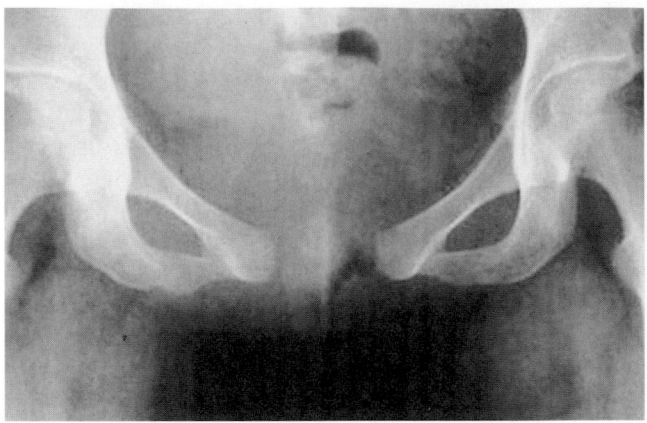

FIGURE 30–3. Radiograph demonstrating a 5-cm diastasis of the symphysis pubis immediately after vaginal delivery. The woman was treated conservatively with analgesics and ambulation as tolerated. Pain diminished over several weeks, and 6 months later, a repeat radiograph showed a 1-cm symphyseal gap. (From Chang and Markman, 2002, with permission.)

second-stage of labor were independent risk factors for nerve injury. In addition, women with injuries pushed longer in the semi-Fowler position than those without. The median duration of symptoms was 2 months, with a range of 2 weeks to 18 months.

Pelvic Joint Separation. Separation of the symphysis pubis or one of the sacroiliac synchondroses during labor may be followed by pain and marked interference with locomotion (Fig. 30–3). Estimates of their frequency vary widely from 1 in 600 to 1 in 30,000 deliveries (Reis and colleagues, 1932; Taylor and Sonson, 1986). In our experience, it is rare and likely closer to the latter incidence. When symptomatic, the onset of pain is acute at delivery. Treatment is generally conservative, with rest in a lateral decubitus position and an appropriately fitted pelvic binder. Occasionally, surgery may be necessary when symphyseal separation is more than 4 cm (Kharrazi and colleagues, 1997). Recurrence is more than 50 percent in subsequent pregnancy, and Culligan and associates (2002) recommend that cesarean delivery be considered.

Immunizations. The D-negative woman who is not isoimmunized and whose infant is D-positive is given 300 μg of anti-D immune globulin shortly after delivery (see Chap. 29, p. 671). Women who are not already immune to rubella or rubeola measles are excellent candidates for combined measles-mumps-rubella vaccination before discharge (see Chap. 8, p. 221). Unless contraindicated, a diphtheria-tetanus toxoid booster injection is also given to postpartum women prior to discharge at Parkland Hospital.

Time of Discharge. Following vaginal delivery, if there are *no complications*, hospitalization is seldom warranted for more than 48 hours. Before discharge, the woman should receive instructions concerning the anticipated normal physiological changes of the puerperium, including lochia patterns, weight loss from diuresis, and when to expect milk letdown. She also should receive instructions concerning what to do if she becomes febrile, has excessive vaginal bleeding, or develops leg pain, swelling, or tenderness. Any shortness of breath or chest pain warrants immediate concern.

EARLY DISCHARGE. As discussed in Chapter 1 (see p. 6), the issue of third-party payers dictating inappropriately short lengths of hospital stays following labor and delivery is now regulated by Federal law. In 2003, the norms are hospital stays of up to 48 hours following uncomplicated vaginal delivery and up to 96 hours following uncomplicated cesarean delivery (American Academy of Pediatrics and the American College of Obstetricians and Gynecologists, 2002). In 1980, the average stay for a woman following vaginal delivery was 3.2 days. This had decreased to 1.7 days by 1995 but had increased to 2.1 days by 1997 (Neergaard, 1999). Despite this, in 1997, 25 percent of new mothers (951,000) had a hospital stay of 1 day or less. This seems acceptable if this was indeed their choice.

Contraception. During the hospital stay, a concerted effort should be made to provide family planning education. Steroidal contraception and its effects on lactation are discussed on page 701. Other forms of contraception are discussed in Chapter 32 and sterilization procedures in Chapter 33.

If the woman does not nurse her child, menses usually return within 6 to 8 weeks. At times, however, it is difficult clinically to assign a specific date to the first menstrual period after delivery. A minority of women bleed small to moderate amounts intermittently, starting soon after delivery. Using histological dating of the endometrium, Sharman (1966) identified ovulation as early as 42 days after delivery. In another study, Perez and associates (1972) did so as early as 36 days. **The necessity for instituting contraceptive techniques for sexually active women is obvious.**

Ovulation is much less frequent in women who breast feed compared with those who do not. In fact, menses may not appear if the infant is nursed, but great variations are observed. In lactating women, the first period may occur as early as the second or as late as the 18th month after delivery. Campbell and Gray (1993) analyzed daily urine specimens to determine ovulation in 92 women. The results of this detailed description of the return of ovarian activity in breast feeding and non–breast feeding women are shown in Figure 30–4. Clearly, there is delayed resumption of ovulation with breast feeding, although as already emphasized, early ovulation is not precluded by persistent lactation. Other findings included the following:

1. Resumption of ovulation was frequently marked by return of normal menstrual bleeding.

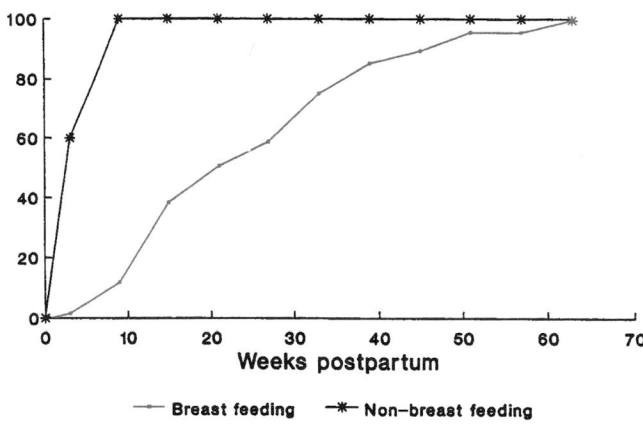

FIGURE 30–4. Cumulative proportion of breast feeding and non–breast feeding women who ovulated during the first 60 weeks following delivery. (From Campbell and Gray, 1993, with permission.)

2. Breast feeding episodes lasting 15 minutes seven times each day delayed resumption of ovulation.
3. Ovulation can occur without bleeding.
4. Bleeding can be anovulatory.
5. The risk of pregnancy in breast feeding women was approximately 4 percent per year.

HOME CARE

Coitus. There is no definite time after delivery when coitus should be resumed. Resumption of intercourse *too soon* may prove to be unpleasant, if not frankly painful, due to incomplete healing of the episiotomy or lacerations. Glazener (1997) surveyed resumption of sexual activity in 1075 British women and found that 70 percent had intercourse within 8 weeks of delivery. The median interval between delivery and intercourse was 5 weeks, but the range was 1 to 12 weeks. Difficulties frequently cited for not resuming intercourse included concern about perineal pain, bleeding, and fatigue. In another survey, Barrett and colleagues (2000) reported that almost 90 percent of 484 primiparous women had resumed sexual activity by 6 months. Although 65 percent of these reported problems, only 15 percent discussed these with a professional.

The best rule to follow is one of common sense. After 2 weeks, coitus may be resumed *based on the patient's desire and comfort.* The women should be advised that breast feeding causes a prolonged period of suppressed estrogen production with a resulting vaginal atrophy and dryness. Such a physiological state results in decreased vaginal lubrication during sexual arousal.

Infant Follow-up. Arrangements must be made to ensure that the neonate receives appropriate follow-up care. Any neonate discharged early should be term, normal, and have stable vital signs. All laboratory studies should be normal, including direct Coombs test, bilirubin, hemoglobin and

TABLE 30–4 Puerperal Morbidity in Percent Reported by Women After Hospital Discharge

Morbidity	By 8 Weeks Postpartum	2 to 18 Months Postpartum
Tiredness	59	54
Breast problems	36	20
Anemia	25	7
Backache	24	20
Hemorrhoids	23	15
Headache	22	15
Tearfulness/depression	21	17
Constipation	20	7
Stitches breaking down	16	—
Vaginal discharge	15	8
Others[a]	2–7	1–8
At least one of the above	87	76

[a] Includes abnormal bleeding, urinary incontinence, urinary infection, difficulty voiding, and hypertension.
From Glazener and co-workers (1995), with permission.

hematocrit, and blood glucose. Abnormal maternal serological tests (e.g., syphilis and hepatitis B surface antigen) should be addressed. Initial hepatitis B vaccine should be administered, and all screening tests required by law should be performed. These always include testing for hypothyroidism and phenylketonuria (PKU). If subsequent PKU retesting is required after the neonate has consumed milk, the mother must be so instructed. Finally, the importance of subsequent neonatal and well-baby care should be stressed and an emphasis placed on infant immunizations.

Late Maternal Morbidity. MacArthur and colleagues (1991), while studying the possible sequelae of labor epidural analgesia, uncovered a vast reservoir of previously unreported morbidity of considerable duration in puerperal women. Following this report, Glazener and co-workers (1995) surveyed health problems in 1249 British mothers after discharge and up to 18 months. Of these, only 3 percent required readmission to the hospital within 8 weeks of delivery. Importantly, 87 percent had milder health problems during the first 8 weeks and 76 percent continued to have a variety of problems for up to 18 months (Table 30–4). Although these self-perceived health problems declined with time, indicating return of health, they did so more slowly than generally assumed.

More recently, Lydon-Rochelle and colleagues (2001) and Thompson and colleagues (2002) reported similar findings. Clearly, maternal morbidity following delivery is extensive and heretofore underrecognized. Glazener and co-authors (1995) called for a greater awareness of the needs of puerperal women as they convalesce from birthing. As an example of how these needs can be met, Chiarelli and Cockburn (2002) designed a randomized trial of a multifaceted intervention, which included pelvic floor exercises. They reported that this intervention was effective in reducing the prevalence and severity of postpartum urinary incontinence.

Follow-up Care. By the time of discharge, women who had a normal delivery and puerperium can resume most activities, including bathing, driving, and household functions. Jimenez and Newton (1979) tabulated cross-cultural information on 202 societies from different international geographic regions. Postnatally, most societies did not restrict maternal work activity, and about half expected a return to full duties within 2 weeks. Tulman and Fawcett (1988) reported, however, that only half of women regained their usual level of energy by 6 weeks postpartum. Women who delivered vaginally were twice as likely to have normal energy levels at this time compared with those with a cesarean delivery. Ideally, the care and nurturing of the neonate should be provided by the mother with ample help from the father. For the mother to provide this care, her presence at home with the infant precludes her early return to full-time work or school.

Women discharged after delivery at Parkland Hospital are given an appointment for follow-up examination during the third postpartum week. This has proven quite satisfactory to identify any abnormalities of the later puerperium as well as to initiate contraceptive practices. Lu and Prentice (2002) have shown that women who did not receive prenatal care are three to four times more likely to miss postpartum appointments than other women.

Estrogen plus progestin oral contraceptives started at this time have proven to be effective without increased morbidity. Moreover, the frequencies of uterine perforation, expulsions, and pregnancies when intrauterine devices were inserted during the third week postpartum were no greater than when the devices were inserted 3 months or more postpartum. Family planning techniques, sterilization, and follow-up care are further discussed in Chapters 32 and 33.

REFERENCES

Adrinopoulos GC, Mendenhall HW: Prostaglandin $F_{2\alpha}$ in the management of delayed postpartum hemorrhage. Am J Obstet Gynecol 146:217, 1983

Ahdoot D, Van Nostrand KM, Nguyen NJ, et al: The effect of route of delivery on regression of abnormal cervical cytologic findings in the postpartum period. Am J Obstet Gynecol 178:1116, 1998

Almeida OD Jr, Kitay DZ: Lactation suppression and puerperal fever. Am J Obstet Gynecol 154:940, 1986

American Academy of Pediatrics, American College of Obstetricians and Gynecologists: Guidelines for Perinatal Care, 5th ed. American Academy of Pediatrics, Elk Grove Village, IL; American College of Obstetricians and Gynecologists, Washington, DC, 2002, pp 154, 229

American Academy of Pediatrics, Committee on Nutrition: Nutrition and lactation. Pediatrics 68:435, 1981

American Academy of Pediatrics, Work Group on Breastfeeding. Breastfeeding and the use of human milk. Pediatrics 100:1035, 1997

American College of Obstetricians and Gynecologists: Breast feeding: Maternal and infant aspects. Education Bulletin No. 258, July, 2000

Anderson WR, Davis J: Placental site involution. Am J Obstet Gynecol 102:23, 1968

Andrew AC, Bulmer JN, Wells M, et al: Subinvolution of the utero-placental arteries in the human placental bed. Histopathology 15:395, 1989

Andrews MC: Epithelial changes in the puerperal fallopian tube. Am J Obstet Gynecol 62:28, 1951

Barbosa-Cesnik C, Schwartz K, Foxman B: Lactation mastitis. JAMA 289:1609, 2003

Barrett G, Pendry E, Peacock J, et al: Women's sexual health after childbirth. BJOG 107:186, 2000

Beer AE, Billingham RE: The immunobiology of mammalian reproduction. Englewood Cliffs, NJ, Prentice-Hall, 1976, p 198

Bertotto A, Gerli R, Fabietti G, et al: Human breast milk T lymphocytes display the phenotype and functional characteristics of memory T cells. Eur J Immunol 20:1877, 1990

Buhimschi CS, Buhimschi IA, Manlinow AM, et al: Myometrial thickness during human labor and immediately post partum. Am J obstet Gynecol 188:553, 2003

Campbell OMR, Gray RH: Characteristics and determinants of postpartum ovarian function in women in the United States. Am J Obstet Gynecol 169:55, 1993

Carley ME, Carley JM, Vasdev G, et al: Factors that are associated with clinically overt postpartum urinary retention after vaginal delivery. Am J Obstet Gynecol 187:430, 2002

Centers for Disease Control and Prevention: Recommendations for prevention and control of hepatitis C virus (HCV) infection and HCV-related chronic disease. MMWR 47:1, 1998

Centers for Disease Control and Prevention: Measles prevention: Recommendations of the Immunization Practice Advisory Committee. MMWR (suppl) 38:1, 1989

Chang D, Markman BS: Spontaneous resolution of a pubic-symphysis diastasis. N Engl J Med 346:39, 2002

Chesley LC, Valenti C, Uichano L: Alterations in body fluid compartments and exchangeable sodium in early puerperium. Am J Obstet Gynecol 77:1054, 1959

Chez RA, Friedman AK: Offering effective breastfeeding advice. Contemp Ob/Gyn 45:32, 2000

Chiarelli P, Cockburn J: Promoting urinary continence in women after delivery: Randomised controlled trial. BMJ 324:1241, 2002

Ching-Chung L, Shuenn-Dhy C, Ling-Hong T, et al: Postpartum urinary retention: Assessment of contributing factors and long-term clinical impact. Aust N Z J Obstet Gynaecol 42:365, 2002

Collaborative Group on Hormonal Factors in Breast Cancer: Breast cancer and breastfeeding: Collaborative reanalysis of individual data from 47 epidemiological studies in 30 countries, including 50,302 women with breast cancer and 96,973 women without the disease. Lancet 360:187, 2002

Cravioto A, Tello A, Villafan H, et al: Inhibition of localized adhesion of enteropathogenic *Escherichia coli* to HEp-2 cells by immunoglobulin and oligosaccharide fractions of human colostrum and breast milk. J Infect Dis 163:1247, 1991

Culligan P, Hill S, Heit M: Rupture of the symphysis pubis during vaginal delivery followed by two subsequent uneventful pregnancies. Obstet Gynecol 100:1114, 2002

Demey HE, Hautekeete MI, Buytaert P, Bossaert LL: Mastitis and toxic shock syndrome. A case report. Acta Obstet Gynecol Scand 68:87, 1989

Dewey KG, Lovelady CA, Nommsen-Rivers LA, et al: A randomized study of the effects of aerobic exercise by lactating women on breast-milk volume and composition. N Engl J Med 330:449, 1994

Farrell SA, Allen VM, Baskett TF: Parturition and urinary incontinence in primiparas. Obstet Gynecol 97:350, 2001

Food and Drug Administration: Bromocriptine indication withdrawn. FDA Medical Bulletin, 24:2, 1994

Food and Drug Administration, Fertility and Maternal Health Drugs Advisory Committee: Summary minutes. Prevention of post-partum breast engorgement with sex hormones and bromocriptine. Washington, DC: U.S. Food and Drug Administration, 1989

Fujiwara Y, Endo S: A case of toxic shock syndrome secondary to mastitis caused by methicillin-resistant Staphylococcus aureus. Kansenshogaku Zasshi 75:898, 2001

Gartner LM, Greer FR: Prevention of rickets and vitamin D deficiency: New guidelines for vitamin D intake. Pediatrics 111:908, 2003

Gherman RB, Goodwin TM, Leung B, et al: Incidence, clinical characteristics, and timing of objectively diagnosed venous thromboembolism during pregnancy. Obstet Gynecol 94:730, 1999

Glazener CMA: Sexual function after childbirth: Women's experiences, persistent morbidity and lack of professional recognition. Br J Obstet Gynaecol 104:330, 1997

Glazener CM, Abdalla M, Stroud P, et al: Postnatal maternal morbidity: Extent, causes, prevention and treatment. Br J Obstet Gynaecol 102:282, 1995

Harris RE, Thomas VL, Hui GW: Postpartum surveillance for urinary tract infection: Patients at risk of developing pyelonephritis after catheterization. South Med J 70:1273, 1977

Hartmann PE, Prosser CG: Physiological basis of longitudinal changes in human milk yield and composition. Fed Proc 43:2448, 1984

Hindle WH: Other benign breast problems. Clin Obstet Gynecol 37:916, 1994

Holdcroft A, Snidvongs S, Cason A, et al: Pain and uterine contractions during breast feeding in the immediate post-partum period increase with parity. Pain 104:589, 2003

Hughes EC: Obstetric-Gynecologic Terminology, 1st ed. American College of Obstetricians and Gynecologists. Philadelphia, Davis, 1972

Hurst NM: Lactation after augmentation mammoplasty. Obstet Gynecol 87:30, 1996

Institute of Medicine: Nutrition During Pregnancy. Washington, DC, National Academy of Science, 1990, p 202

Ito S: Drug therapy for breast-feeding women. N Engl J Med 343:118, 2000

Jimenez MH, Newton N: Activity and work during pregnancy and the postpartum period: A cross-cultural study of 202 societies. Am J Obstet Gynecol 135:171, 1979

Josefsson A, Berg G, Nordin C, Sydsjo G: Prevalence of depressive symptoms in late pregnancy and postpartum. Acta Obstet Gynecol Scand 80:251, 2001

Karstrup S, Solvin J, Nolsoe CP, et al: Acute puerperal breast abscesses. US-guided drainage. Radiology 188:807, 1993

Kerr-Wilson RH, Thompson SW, Orr JW, et al: Effect of labor on the postpartum bladder. Obstet Gynecol 64:115, 1984

Kharrazi FD, Rodgers WB, Kennedy JG, Lhowe DW: Parturition-induced pelvic dislocation: A report of four cases. J Orthop Trauma 11:277, 1997

Koldovsky O, Britton J, Grimes J, Schaudies P: Milk-borne epidermal growth factor (EGF) and its processing in developing gastrointestinal tract. Endocr Regul 25:58, 1991

Kramer MS, Chalmers B, Hodnett ED, et al: Promotion of breast-feeding intervention trial (PROBIT): A randomized trial in the Republic of Belarus. JAMA 285:413, 2001

Lee CY, Madrazo B, Drukker BH: Ultrasonic evaluation of the postpartum uterus in the management of postpartum bleeding. Obstet Gynecol 58:227, 1981

Lovelady CA, Hunter CP, Geigerman C: Effect of exercise on immunologic factors in breast milk. Pediatrics 111:E148, 2003

Lovelady CA, Garner KE, Moreno KL, Williams JP: The effect of weight loss in overweight, lactating women on the growth of their infant. N Engl J Med 342:449, 2000

Lu MC, Prentice J: The postpartum visit: Risk factors for nonuse and association with breast-feeding. Am J Obstet Gynecol 187:1329, 2002

Lydon-Rochelle MT, Holt VL, Martin DP: Delivery method and self-reported postpartum general health status among primiparous women. Paediatr Perinat Epidemiol 15:232, 2001

MacArthur C, Lewis M, Knox EG: Health after childbirth. Br J Obstet Gynaecol 98:1193, 1991

Marshall BR, Hepper JK, Zirbel CC: Sporadic puerperal mastitis—an infection that need not interrupt lactation. JAMA 344:1377, 1975

Matheson I, Aursnes I, Horgen M, et al: Bacteriological findings and clinical symptoms in relation to clinical outcome in puerperal mastitis. Acta Obstet Gynecol Scand 67:723, 1988

McCleary MJ: Epidermal growth factor: An important constituent of human milk. J Hum Lact 7:123, 1991

McNeilly AS, Robinson ICA, Houston MJ, Howie PW: Release of oxytocin and prolactin in response to suckling. BMJ (Clin Res Ed) 286:257, 1983

Morgans D: Bromocriptine and postpartum lactation suppression. Br J Obstet Gynaecol 102:851, 1995

Mortensen EL, Michaelsen KF, Sanders SA, Reinisch JM: The association between duration of breastfeeding and adult intelligence. JAMA 287:2365, 2002

Mulic-Lutvica A, Bekuretsion M, Bakos O, et al: Ultrasonic evaluation of the uterus and uterine cavity after normal, vaginal delivery. Ultrasound Obstet Gynecol 18:491, 2001

Nduati R, John G, Mbori-Hgacha D, et al: Effect of breastfeeding and formula feeding on transmission of HIV-1: A randomized clinical trial. JAMA 283:1167, 2000

Neergaard L: Longer stays for new moms. Available at: Abcnews.go.com/sections/living/dailynews/childbirth990609, 1999

Newburg DS, Peterson JA, Ruiz-Palacias GM, et al: Role of human-milk lactadherin in protection against symptomatic rotavirus infection. Lancet 351:1160, 1998

Newton M, Bradford WM: Postpartal blood loss. Obstet Gynecol 17:229, 1961

Niebyl JR, Spence MR, Parmley TH: Sporadic (nonepidemic) puerperal mastitis. J Reprod Med 20:97, 1978

O'Hara RJ, Dexter SPL, Fox JN: Conservative management of infective mastitis and breast abscesses after ultrasonographic assessment. Br J Surg 83:1413, 1996

Olson CM, Strawderman MS, Hinton PS, et al: Gestational weight gain and postpartum behavior associated with weight change from early pregnancy to 1y postpartum. Int J Obes Relat Metab Disord 27:117, 2003

Oppenheimer LW, Sherriff EA, Goodman JDS, et al: The duration of lochia. Br J Obstet Gynaecol 93:754, 1986

Perez A, Vela P, Masnick GS, Potter RG: First ovulation after childbirth: The effect of breastfeeding. Am J Obstet Gynecol 114:1041, 1972

Porter JC: Proceedings: Hormonal regulation of breast development and activity. J Invest Dermatol 63:85, 1974

Reis RA, Baer JL, Arens RA, Stewart E: Traumatic separation of the symphysis pubis during spontaneous labor: With a clinical and x-ray study of the normal symphysis pubis during pregnancy and the puerperium. Surg Gynecol Obstet 55:336, 1932

Robson SC, Dunlop W, Hunter S: Haemodynamic changes during the early puerperium. BMJ (Clin Res Ed) 294:1065, 1987

Rortveit G, Daltveit AK, Hannestad YS, Hunskaar S: Urinary incontinence after vaginal delivery or cesarean section. N Engl J Med 348:10, 2003

Saito S, Maruyama M, Kato Y, et al: Detection of IL-6 in human milk and its involvement in IgA production. J Reprod Immunol 20:267, 1991

Samra HK, Ganguly NK, Mahajan RC: Human milk containing specific secretory IgA inhibits binding of *Giardia lamblia* to nylon and glass surfaces. J Diarrhoeal Dis Res 9:100, 1991

Schauberger CW, Rooney BL, Brimer LM: Factors that influence weight loss in the puerperium. Obstet Gynecol 79:424, 1992

Schwarz RJ, Shrestha R: Needle aspiration of breast abscesses. Am J Surg 182:117, 2001

Sharman A: Ovulation in the post-partum period. Excerpta Medica International Congress Series, No. 133, 1966, p 158

Sharman A: Postpartum regeneration of the human endometrium. J Anat 87:1, 1953

Smith DE, Lewis CE, Caveny JL, et al: Longitudinal changes in adiposity associated with pregnancy. The CARDIA study. Coronary artery risk development in young adults study. JAMA 271:1747, 1994

Spitz AM, Lee NC, Peterson HB: Treatment for lactation suppression: Little progress in one hundred years. Am J Obstet Gynecol 179:1485, 1998

Stehman FB: Infections and inflammations of the breast. In Hindle WH (ed): Breast Disease for Gynecologists. Norwalk, CT, Appleton & Lange, 1990, p 151

Taylor RN, Sonson RD: Separation of the pubic symphysis. An underrecognized peripartum complication. J Reprod Med 31:203, 1986

Thompson JF, Roberts CL, Currie M, et al: Prevalence and persistence of health problems after childbirth: Associations with parity and method of birth. Birth 29:83, 2002

Thomsen AC, Espersen T, Maigaard S: Course and treatment of milk stasis, noninfectious inflammation of the breast, and infectious mastitis in nursing women. Am J Obstet Gynecol 149:492, 1984

Toglia MR, Weg JG: Venous thromboembolism and pregnancy. N Engl J Med 335:108, 1996

Tulman L, Fawcett J: Return of functional ability after childbirth. Nurs Res 37:77, 1988

Viktrup L, Lose G: Epidural anesthesia during labor and stress incontinence after delivery. Obstet Gynecol 82:984, 1993

Visness CM, Kennedy KI, Ramos R: The duration and character of postpartum bleeding among breast-feeding women. Obstet Gynecol 89:159, 1997

Wager GP, Martin DH, Koutsky L, et al: Puerperal infectious morbidity: Relationship to route of delivery and to antepartum *Chlamydia trachomatis* infection. Am J Obstet Gynecol 138:1028, 1980

Wijma J, Potters AE, Wolf BT, et al: Anatomical and functional changes in the lower urinary tract following spontaneous vaginal delivery. Br J Obstet Gynaecol 110:658, 2003

Williams JW: Regeneration of the uterine mucosa after delivery with especial reference to the placental site. Am J Obstet Gynecol 22:664, 1931

Wilson PD, Herbison RM, Herbison GP: Obstetric practice and the prevalence of urinary incontinence three months after delivery. Br J Obstet Gynaecol 103:154, 1996

Wong CA, Scavone BM, Dugan S, et al: Incidence of postpartum lumbosacral spine and lower extremity nerve injuries. Obstet Gynecol 101:279, 2003

Yaffe SJ: Introduction. In Briggs GG, Freeman RK, Yaffe SJ (eds): Drugs in Pregnancy and Lactation, 4th ed. Baltimore, Williams & Wilkins, 1994

Yip SK, Brieger G, Hin LY, Chung T: Urinary retention in the postpartum period. Acta Obstet Gynecol Scand 76:667, 1997

Yuen BH: Prolactin in human milk: The influence of nursing and the duration of postpartum lactation. Am J Obstet Gynecol 158:583, 1988

Ziegler JB, Cooper DA, Johnston RO, Gold J: Postnatal transmission of AIDS-associated retrovirus from mother to infant. Lancet 1:896, 1985

31

Puerperal Infection

Puerperal infection is a general term used to describe any bacterial infection of the genital tract after delivery. The earliest reference to puerperal infection is found in the works of Hippocrates from the 5th century BC. In his discussion of women, *De Muliebrum Morbis,* he described the condition and attributed it to retention of bowel contents. The history of puerperal infection is discussed in greater detail in previous editions of *Williams Obstetrics.*

Along with preeclampsia and obstetrical hemorrhage, puerperal infection formed the lethal triad of causes of maternal deaths for many decades of the 20th century. Fortunately, because of effective antimicrobials, maternal deaths from infection have become uncommon. Berg and associates (2003) reported results from the Pregnancy Mortality Surveillance System, which contained 3201 maternal deaths in the United States from 1991 through 1997. Infection made up 13 percent of pregnancy-related deaths and was the fifth leading cause of death.

PUERPERAL FEVER

Puerperal morbidity is defined as follows: a *temperature of 38.0°C (100.4°F) or higher, which occurs on any 2 of the first 10 days postpartum, exclusive of the first 24 hours, and which is taken orally by a standard technique at least four times daily.* This definition developed from one proposed by the Joint Committee on Maternal Welfare, which was originally convened in 1919 (Mussey and colleagues, 1935).

Differential Diagnosis. A number of factors can cause fever in the puerperium. **Most persistent fevers after childbirth are caused by genital tract infection.** Filker and Monif (1979) reported that only about 20 percent of women febrile within the first 24 hours after giving birth vaginally were subsequently diagnosed with pelvic infection. This was in contrast to 70 percent of those undergoing cesarean delivery. It must be emphasized that a high-spiking fever (39°C or higher) developing within the first 24 hours after giving birth may be associated with virulent pelvic infection caused by either group A or group B streptococcus. Other causes of puerperal fever that should be considered include breast engorgement; respiratory complications such as atelectasis, aspiration pneumonia, and bacterial pneumonia; acute pyelonephritis; and thrombophlebitis. About 15 percent of all women develop postpartum fever from breast engorgement. This rarely exceeds 39°C in the first few postpartum days and usually lasts no longer than 24 hours.

Atelectasis or alveolar collapse is caused by hypoventilation and is best prevented by patients coughing and deep breathing on a fixed schedule following surgery. Fever associated with atelectasis is thought to be due to infection by normal flora that proliferate distal to obstructing mucous plugs. Following aspiration, women most often develop a high-spiking fever, varying degrees of wheezing, and in most instances, obvious signs of hypoxemia (Marik, 2001).

Acute pyelonephritis has a variable clinical picture, and in puerperal women, the first sign of renal infection may be a temperature elevation, followed later by costovertebral angle tenderness, nausea, and vomiting. Minor temperature elevations in puerperal women may also occasionally be caused by superficial or deep venous thrombosis of the legs.

UTERINE INFECTION

Postpartum uterine infection has been called variously *endometritis, endomyometritis,* and *endoparametritis.* Because infection actually involves not only the decidua but also the myometrium and parametrial tissues, the preferred term is *metritis with pelvic cellulitis.*

PREDISPOSING FACTORS. The route of delivery is the single most significant risk factor for the development of uterine infection (Burrows and associates, 2004; Koroukian, 2004).

Vaginal Delivery. Compared with cesarean delivery, metritis following vaginal delivery is relatively uncommon. A 6-month survey during 1987 of nearly 5000 women whose infants were delivered vaginally at Parkland Hospital showed that only 1.3 percent received treatment for metritis. When data from women at high risk—defined by prolonged membrane rupture and labor, multiple cervical examinations, and internal fetal monitoring—were analyzed separately, the incidence of metritis after vaginal delivery was nearly 6 percent. If there is intrapartum chorioamnionitis, the risk of infection increases to 13 percent (Maberry and colleagues, 1991). Other risk factors for metritis following vaginal delivery include any adverse perinatal outcomes, such as stillbirth, low birthweight, preterm delivery, and serious neonatal morbidity (Libombo and colleagues, 1994).

Cesarean Delivery. The incidence of metritis following surgical delivery varies with socioeconomic factors, and over the years this has been altered substantively by almost universal use of perioperative antimicrobials. For all women at high risk for pelvic infection following cesarean delivery, the American College of Obstetricians and Gynecologists (2003) recommends single-dose perioperative antimicrobial prophylaxis. This is discussed in Chapter 25 (see p. 603). **The use of single-dose perioperative antimicrobial prophylaxis has done more to decrease the incidence and severity of postcesarean delivery pelvic infections than any other innovation in the past 25 years.**

Prior to use of antimicrobial prophylaxis, Sweet and Ledger (1973) reported an overall incidence of uterine infection of 13 percent among affluent women who underwent cesarean delivery at the University of Michigan Hospital. In indigent women who underwent cesarean delivery at Wayne

County Hospital, however, they reported the incidence to be 27 percent. Cunningham and associates (1978) found an overall incidence of about 50 percent in women who had cesarean delivery at Parkland Hospital. Important risk factors for infection included long duration of labor and membrane rupture, multiple cervical examinations, and internal fetal monitoring.

Women with all of these factors, whose infants were delivered for cephalopelvic disproportion, and who were not given perioperative prophylaxis had an incidence of serious pelvic infection that was nearly 90 percent (DePalma and colleagues, 1982; Gilstrap and Cunningham, 1979). Women readmitted to the hospital with postpartum metritis or wound infections are more likely to have undergone cesarean delivery (Lydon-Rochelle and colleagues, 2000).

Other Risk Factors. It is generally accepted that pelvic infection is more common in women of lower socioeconomic status compared with middle- or upper-class patients. Goldenberg and associates (1996) have shown significant racial differences in vaginal colonization with potential pathogens during pregnancy, although the precise reasons for these differences are unclear.

The evidence that *anemia* increases the likelihood of infection is not conclusive (Cook and Lynch, 1986). The results obtained from both animal and in vitro experiments are consistent with the view that iron-deficiency anemia does not predispose to infection, and some believe it may actually prevent infection. The role of *nutrition* in the genesis of infection is also unclear, although cell-mediated immunity is impaired in malnourished laboratory animals.

Bacterial colonization of the lower genital tract with certain microorganisms—for example, group B streptococcus, *Chlamydia trachomatis, Mycoplasma hominis,* and *Gardnerella vaginalis*—has been associated with an increased risk of postpartum infection. Watts and associates (1990) and Jacobsson and colleagues (2002) reported an increased risk of puerperal metritis in women with bacterial vaginosis. Andrews and colleagues (1995) reported that colonization of intact membranes with *Ureaplasma urealyticum* significantly increased the risk for infection following cesarean delivery.

Other factors that are associated with an increased risk of infection include cesarean delivery for *multifetal gestation* (Suonio and Huttunen, 1994), *young maternal age and nulliparity* (Magee and associates, 1994), *prolonged labor induction* (Tran and colleagues, 2000), *obesity* (Myles and co-workers, 2002), and *meconium-stained amnionic fluid* (Jazayeri and colleagues, 2002).

BACTERIOLOGY. Most female pelvic infections are caused by bacteria indigenous to the female genital tract. Over the past decade, there have been reports of group A β-hemolytic streptococcus causing toxic shock–like syndrome and life-threatening infection (Nathan and Leveno, 1994; Stefonek and colleagues, 2001). Anteby and associates (1999) reported experiences with 47 women who had group

TABLE 31–1 Bacteria Commonly Responsible for Female Genital Infections

Aerobes
 Group A, B, and D streptococci
 Enterococcus
 Gram-negative bacteria—*Escherichia coli,*
  Klebsiella, and *Proteus* species
 Staphylococcus aureus
 Staphylococcus epidermidis
 Gardnerella vaginalis
Anaerobes
 Peptococcus species
 Peptostreptococcus species
 Bacteroides fragilis group
 Prevotella species
 Clostridium species
 Fusobacterium species
 Mobiluncus species
Other
 Mycoplasma species
 Chlamydia trachomatis
 Neisseria gonorrhoeae

A streptococcal infections and found that a prominent risk factor was prematurely ruptured membranes. In two reviews of group A infections by Crum (2002) and Udagawa (1999) and their colleagues, women in whom infection was manifested before, during, or within 12 hours of delivery had a mortality of almost 90 percent, and associated fetal mortality was more than 50 percent.

Common Pathogens. Bacteria commonly responsible for female genital tract infections are listed in Table 31–1. Usually multiple species of bacteria are isolated. Although they are typically considered to be of relatively low virulence, they may become pathogenic within hematomas and devitalized tissue.

Although the cervix routinely harbors such bacteria, the uterine cavity is usually sterile before rupture of the amnionic sac. As the consequence of labor and delivery and associated manipulations, the amnionic fluid and perhaps the uterus commonly become contaminated with anaerobic and aerobic bacteria (Fig. 31–1). Gilstrap and Cunningham (1979) cultured amnionic fluid obtained at cesarean delivery in women in labor with membranes ruptured more than 6 hours. They identified anaerobic and aerobic organisms in 63 percent of cultured samples, anaerobes alone in 30 percent, and aerobes alone in 7 percent. Predominant anaerobic organisms were *Peptostreptococcus* and *Peptococcus* species in 45 percent, *Bacteroides* species in 9 percent, and *Clostridium* species in 3 percent. Gram-positive aerobic cocci also were common; *Enterococcus* was isolated in 14 percent, and group B streptococcus in 8 percent. *Escherichia coli* comprised 9 percent of isolates. An average of 2.5 organisms was identified from each specimen. Sherman and co-workers (1999) showed that bacterial isolates at cesarean delivery correlated with those taken at 3 days postpartum when metritis had developed.

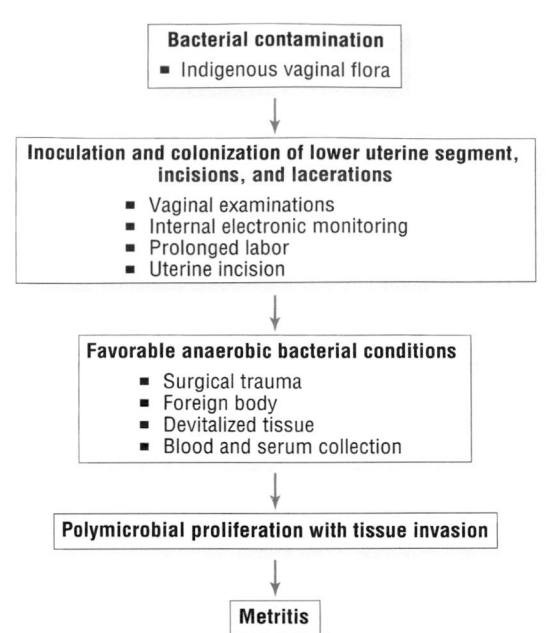

FIGURE 31–1. Pathogenesis of metritis following cesarean delivery. (Data from Gilstrap and Cunningham, 1979.)

The role of other organisms such as chlamydia, mycoplasma, and ureaplasma in the etiology of these infections is unclear. Chlamydial infections have been implicated in late-onset, indolent metritis (Ismail and associates, 1985). In addition, Jacobsson and colleagues (2002) reported that the risk of puerperal infection was tripled in a group of Swedish women with bacterial vaginosis in early pregnancy.

Bacterial Cultures. Routine pretreatment genital tract cultures are of little clinical utility, and they add significantly to hospitalization costs. Similarly, the utility of routine blood cultures is questionable. In two earlier studies, blood cultures were positive in only 13 percent of women at Parkland Hospital and 24 percent at Los Angeles County Hospital who had postcesarean pelvic infections (Cunningham and colleagues, 1978; DiZerega and co-workers, 1979). From Finland, Kankuri and associates (2003) described culture-proven bacteremia in 5 percent of almost 800 women with suspected puerperal sepsis.

PATHOGENESIS. Puerperal infection following vaginal delivery primarily involves the placental implantation site and the decidua and adjacent myometrium. The pathogenesis of uterine infection following cesarean delivery is that of an infected surgical incision (see Fig. 31–1). Bacteria that colonize the cervix and vagina gain access to amnionic fluid during labor, and postpartum they invade devitalized uterine tissue. Parametrial cellulitis next follows with infection of the pelvic retroperitoneal fibroareolar connective tissue. The process is usually limited to the paravaginal tissue and rarely extends deeply into the pelvis.

CLINICAL COURSE. Fever is believed proportional to the extent of infection and sepsis syndrome (see Chap. 42, p. 993). **Fever is the most important criterion for the diagnosis of postpartum metritis.** Temperature commonly exceeds 38 to 39°C. Chills may accompany fever and suggest bacteremia, which is documented in 10 to 20 percent of women with pelvic infection following cesarean delivery. Women usually complain of abdominal pain, and parametrial tenderness is elicited on abdominal and bimanual examination. Although an offensive odor may develop, many women have foul-smelling lochia without evidence for infection. Other infections, notably those due to group A β-hemolytic streptococci, are frequently associated with scanty, odorless lochia. Leukocytosis may range from 15,000 to 30,000 cells/μL. The average increase in the leukocyte count postpartum following cesarean delivery is 22 percent (Hartmann and co-workers, 2000).

TREATMENT

Management. If mild metritis develops after the woman has been sent home following vaginal delivery, treatment with an oral antimicrobial agent is usually sufficient. For moderate to severe infections, however, including those following cesarean delivery, intravenous therapy with a broad-spectrum antimicrobial regimen is indicated. Improvement follows in 48 to 72 hours in nearly 90 percent of women treated with one of several regimens. Persistence of fever after this interval mandates a careful search for causes of refractory pelvic infection. Complications of metritis that cause persistent fever despite appropriate therapy include a parametrial phlegmon or an area of intense cellulitis, a surgical incisional or pelvic abscess, an infected hematoma, and septic pelvic thrombophlebitis. In our experience, persistent fever is seldom due to antimicrobial-resistant bacteria or to drug side effects.

Typically, a patient is discharged after she has been afebrile for at least 24 hours. Further oral antimicrobial therapy is not needed (Dinsmoor and colleagues, 1991; French and Smaill, 2002).

Specific Antimicrobial Treatment. Although therapy is empirical, initial treatment following cesarean delivery is directed against most of the mixed flora that typically cause puerperal infections (see Table 31–1). Such broad-spectrum antimicrobial coverage is often not necessary to treat infection following vaginal delivery, and as many as 90 percent of these infections respond to regimens such as ampicillin plus gentamicin. In contrast, anaerobic coverage must be included for infections following cesarean delivery (Table 31–2).

In 1979, DiZerega and colleagues compared the effectiveness of clindamycin plus gentamicin with penicillin G plus gentamicin for treatment of pelvic infections following cesarean delivery. Women given the *clindamycin-gentamicin* regimen had a 95-percent rate of infection resolution, and this regimen now is considered by most to be the standard by which others are measured (French and Smaill, 2002).

TABLE 31–2 Antimicrobial Regimens for Pelvic Infection Following Cesarean Delivery

Regimen	Comments
Clindamycin 900 mg + gentamicin 1.5 mg/kg, q8h intravenously	"Gold standard," 90–97% efficacy, once-daily gentamicin dosing acceptable
plus ampicillin	Added to regimen with sepsis syndrome or suspected enterococcal infection
Clindamycin + aztreonam	Gentamicin substitute with renal insufficiency
Extended-spectrum penicillins	Piperacillin, ampicillin/sulbactam
Extended-spectrum cephalosporins	Cefotetan, cefoxitin, cefotaxime
Imipenem + cilastatin	Reserved for special indications

Because enterococcal infections may persist despite this standard therapy, many add ampicillin to the clindamycin-gentamicin regimen, either initially or if there is no response by 48 to 72 hours (Walmer and colleagues, 1988). Over the past decade, vancomycin-resistant enterococcal infections have been problematic in nonobstetrical units (Murray, 2000).

Brumfield and colleagues (2000) at the University of Alabama at Birmingham reaffirmed the efficacy of this standard regimen given to 322 women with postcesarean pelvic infections. Many authorities recommend that serum gentamicin levels be periodically monitored. Liu and associates (1999) compared multiple-dosing versus once-daily dosing with gentamicin and found that both provided adequate serum levels. Fortunately, once-daily dosing avoids the need for routine measurement. In a randomized clinical trial, Livingston and colleagues (2003) reported that once-daily dosing with both clindamycin and gentamicin had a similar cure rate as every eight-hour dosing with the two drugs. Because of the potential for nephrotoxicity and ototoxicity with gentamicin in the event of diminished glomerular filtration, some clinicians have recommended a combination of clindamycin and a second-generation cephalosporin to treat such women. Others have recommended a combination of clindamycin and aztreonam, a monobactam compound with activity similar to the aminoglycosides.

The spectra of *β-lactam antimicrobials* include activity against many anaerobic pathogens. Some examples include cephalosporins such as cefoxitin, cefotetan, cefotaxime, as well as extended-spectrum penicillins such as piperacillin, ticarcillin, and mezlocillin. Beta-lactam antimicrobials are inherently safe, and except for allergic reactions, are free of major toxicity. The *β-lactamase inhibitors*, clavulanic acid, sulbactam, and tazobactam, have been combined with ampicillin, amoxicillin, ticarcillin, and piperacillin to extend their spectra.

Metronidazole has superior in vitro activity against most anaerobes. This agent given with ampicillin and an aminoglycoside provides coverage against most organisms encountered in serious pelvic infections.

Imipenem is a carbapenem that has broad-spectrum coverage against the majority of organisms associated with metritis. It is used in combination with *cilastatin*, which inhibits renal metabolism of imipenem. Although this combination is effective in most cases of metritis, it seems reasonable from both a medical and an economical standpoint to reserve it for more serious infections.

PREVENTION OF INFECTION

The use of perioperative antimicrobial prophylaxis has remarkably reduced the rate of postoperative infection after cesarean delivery. For example, prophylactic antimicrobials reduce the rate of puerperal endometritis by 70 to 80 percent (Chelmow and colleagues, 2001; Smaill and Hofmeyr, 2003). The observed benefit applies to both elective and nonelective cesarean delivery and also includes a reduction in abdominal incisional infections. Single agents such as ampicillin and first-generation cephalosporins are ideal prophylactic antimicrobials (American College of Obstetricians and Gynecologists, 2003). Using broad-spectrum agents or a multiple-dose regimen gives no apparent benefit (Hopkins and Smaill, 2003).

A number of locally applied antimicrobials have been studied to assess their efficacy in preventing puerperal infection. Vaginal irrigation with *chlorhexidine* intrapartum did reduce the incidence of postpartum infection (Rouse and colleagues, 1997; Sweeten and associates, 1997). Conversely, *povidone–iodine* irrigation before cesarean delivery had no effect on the incidence of fever, metritis, or abdominal incisional infection (Reid and associates, 2001). In a blinded, placebo-controlled trial, Pitt and colleagues (2001) applied 5 grams of *metronidazole gel* preoperatively as an adjunct to perioperative antimicrobial prophylaxis. They reported reduction in the rate of metritis from 17 to 7 percent with the gel but no effect on febrile morbidity or abdominal incisional infections.

Mercer and associates (1997) for the Maternal–Fetal Medicine Network reported no change in the incidence of pelvic infections in women with preterm prematurely ruptured membranes who were given antimicrobials. These patients received either placebo or intravenous ampicillin plus erythromycin for 48 hours followed by oral amoxicillin plus erythromycin for 5 days. A secondary analysis of the Network study was done by Andrews and associates (2003b) to evaluate the effectiveness of antimicrobial treatment to prevent preterm delivery in fetal fibronectin-positive women. They reported that metronidazole plus erythromycin decreased postpartum metritis in these women from 5.2 percent to 2.1 percent.

Antepartum treatment of asymptomatic women with vaginal infections has not been shown to prevent postpartum metritis. In another Network study, Carey and associates

(2000) reported that antepartum treatment of asymptomatic bacterial vaginosis had no effect on puerperal infection rates. Similarly, Klebanoff and colleagues (2001) found that metritis rates in women treated for second-trimester asymptomatic *Trichomonas vaginalis* infection were no different from those in placebo-treated women.

Limited data hinder the assessment of surgical techniques to decrease puerperal infections. Lifting the uterus out of the abdomen to close the uterine incision did not appreciably affect the infection rate in two small studies (Enkin and Wilkinson, 2002). In another small study, changing of gloves by the surgical team after placental delivery reduced postcesarean wound infections (Ventolini and associates, 2004). No differences in postoperative infection rates were found between single- versus two-layer uterine closure at cesarean delivery (Hauth and colleagues, 1992). Similarly, uterine or abdominal incisional infection rates were not affected by peritoneal closure or nonclosure at cesarean delivery (Tulandi and Al-Jaroudi, 1993; Wilkinson and Enkin, 1999b). Finally, although closure of the subcutaneous tissue in obese women decreased separation, it had no effect on rates of hematoma formation or infection (Chelmow, 2004; Magann, 2002; Naumann, 1995, each with their colleagues).

COMPLICATIONS OF PELVIC INFECTIONS

In more than 90 percent of women, metritis responds to treatment within 48 to 72 hours. In the other women, several complications may arise.

WOUND INFECTIONS. The incidence of abdominal incisional infections following cesarean delivery ranges from 3 to 15 percent, with an average of about 6 percent (Chaim and associates, 2000; Owen and Andrews, 1994). When prophylactic antimicrobials are given, however, the incidence is less than 2 percent (Andrews and colleagues, 2003a). According to Soper and co-workers (1992), wound infection is the most common cause of antimicrobial failure in women treated for metritis. Risk factors for wound infections include obesity, diabetes, corticosteroid therapy, immunosuppression, anemia, and poor hemostasis with hematoma formation.

Abdominal incisional abscesses that develop following cesarean delivery usually cause fever on about the fourth postoperative day. In many cases, these are preceded by uterine infection, and fever persists from the first or second postoperative day or later. Wound erythema and drainage may also be present. Organisms causing these infections are usually the same as those isolated from amnionic fluid at cesarean delivery, but hospital-acquired pathogens may also be the cause (Emmons and colleagues, 1988; Owen and Andrews, 1994). Treatment includes antimicrobials and surgical drainage, with careful inspection to ensure that the abdominal fascia is intact.

Wound Dehiscence. Disruption or dehiscence refers to separation of the fascial layer. McNeeley and colleagues (1998) studied 8590 women undergoing cesarean delivery at Hutzel Hospital in Detroit. They reported fascial dehiscence in about 1 in 300 operations. Most disruptions manifest on about the fifth postoperative day with serosanguineous discharge. Two thirds of 27 fascial dehiscences identified by McNeeley and associates (1998) were associated with concurrent fascial infection and tissue necrosis.

Fascial dehiscence is a serious complication. Treatment includes secondary closure of the incision in the operating room with adequate anesthesia.

Necrotizing Fasciitis. Fortunately, this most serious of wound infections is rare, but it is associated with high mortality. These infections may involve abdominal incisions following cesarean delivery, or may complicate episiotomy or perineal lacerations. As the name implies, there is significant tissue necrosis. Of the risk factors for fasciitis summarized by Owen and Andrews (1994), three of these—*diabetes, obesity*, and *hypertension*—are relatively common in pregnant women. Infections may be caused by a single virulent bacterial species such as group A β-hemolytic streptococcus, but more commonly they are polymicrobial. Synnestvedt and colleagues (2003) have described a woman with streptococcal puerperal sepsis who developed a recurrent genital infection with group A organisms. Occasionally, necrotizing infections are caused by rarely encountered pathogens (Barber and Swygert, 2000; Swartz, 2004).

At the University of Alabama, Goepfert and colleagues (1997) reviewed their experiences from 1987 through 1994. There were nine cases of necrotizing fasciitis in 5048 cesarean deliveries—a rate of 1.8 per 1000 cesarean deliveries. In two women, the infection was fatal. In a report from Brigham and Women's and Massachusetts General Hospitals, Schorge and colleagues (1998) described five women with fasciitis following cesarean delivery. None of these women had predisposing risk factors, and none died.

Zimbelman and co-workers (1999) reported preliminary observations that clindamycin given with a β-lactam antimicrobial may be the most effective regimen. Adjunctive treatment includes promptly debriding wide margins of the fascial incision. With extensive resection, synthetic mesh may be required to close the fascial incision (Gallup and Meguiar, 2004; McNeeley and associates, 1998).

PERITONITIS. Occasionally, this condition is encountered following cesarean delivery complicated by metritis with uterine incisional necrosis and dehiscence. It also is sometimes seen in women with a prior cesarean delivery who then give birth vaginally. Likewise, a parametrial or adnexal abscess may rupture and produce generalized peritonitis.

With puerperal peritonitis, abdominal rigidity may not be prominent because of abdominal wall laxity from pregnancy. Pain may be severe. Frequently, the first symptoms

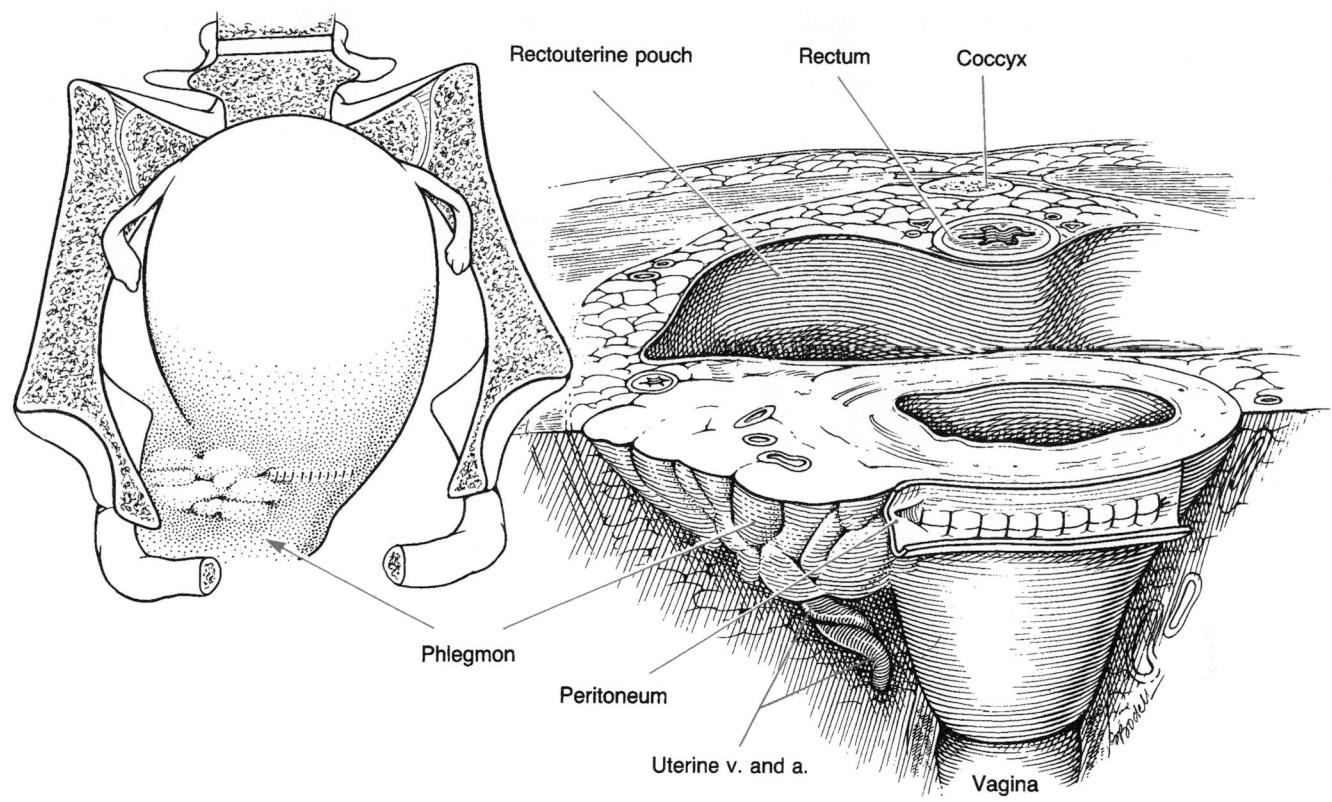

FIGURE 31–2. Parametrial phlegmon. Cellulitis in the right parametrium begins adjacent to the cesarean incision and extends to the pelvic sidewall. On pelvic examination, the phlegmon is palpable as a firm, three-dimensional mass.

of peritonitis are those of *adynamic ileus,* which usually is absent or mild following uncomplicated cesarean delivery. Thus, there may be marked bowel distention. If the infection begins in an intact uterus and extends into the peritoneum, antimicrobial treatment alone usually suffices. Conversely, peritonitis caused by uterine incisional necrosis or by a bowel lesion is treated surgically along with antimicrobial therapy.

ADNEXAL INFECTIONS. An *ovarian abscess* rarely develops from puerperal infection, presumably from bacterial invasion through a rent in the ovarian capsule (Wetchler and Dunn, 1985). The abscess is usually unilateral, and women typically present 1 to 2 weeks after delivery.

PARAMETRIAL PHLEGMON. In some women in whom metritis develops following cesarean delivery, parametrial cellulitis is intensive and forms an area of induration, termed a *phlegmon,* within the leaves of the broad ligament (Fig. 31–2). These infections should be considered when fever persists longer than 72 hours despite intravenous antimicrobial therapy (DePalma and colleagues, 1982). Kindig and colleagues (1998) described such an infection with uterine dehiscence occurring 6 weeks postpartum.

Areas of parametrial cellulitis are more often unilateral, and they frequently may remain limited to the base of the broad ligament. If, however, the inflammatory reaction is more intense, cellulitis extends along natural lines of cleavage. The most common form of extension is laterally, along the base of the broad ligament, with a tendency to extend to the lateral pelvic wall. Posterior extension may involve the rectovaginal septum, producing a firm mass posterior to the cervix.

Severe cellulitis of the uterine incision may cause necrosis and separation. Extrusion of purulent material commonly leads to peritonitis. Because puerperal metritis with cellulitis is typically a retroperitoneal infection, evidence of peritonitis suggests the possibility of uterine incisional necrosis, or less commonly a bowel injury or other lesion.

In most women with a phlegmon, clinical improvement follows continued treatment with a broad-spectrum antimicrobial regimen. These women usually remain febrile for 5 to 7 days, and in some cases even longer. Absorption of the induration may take several days to weeks. Surgery is reserved for women in whom uterine incisional necrosis is suspected. Hysterectomy and surgical debridement are usually difficult, and there is often appreciable blood loss. In rare cases, uterine debridement and resuturing of the incision are feasible (Rivlin and colleagues, 2004). Frequently, the cervix and lower uterine segment are involved with an intensive inflammatory process that extends to the pelvic sidewall to encompass one or both ureters. The adnexa are

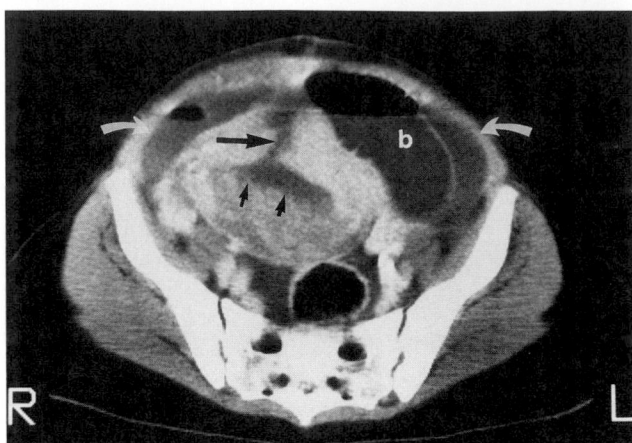

FIGURE 31–3. Pelvic computed tomography scan of dehiscence caused by infection of a vertical cesarean incision. Endometrial fluid (*small black arrows*) communicates with parametrial fluid (*curved white arrows*) through the uterine dehiscence (*black arrow*). A dilated bowel loop (b) is adjacent to the uterus on the left. (Courtesy of Dr. Diane Twickler.)

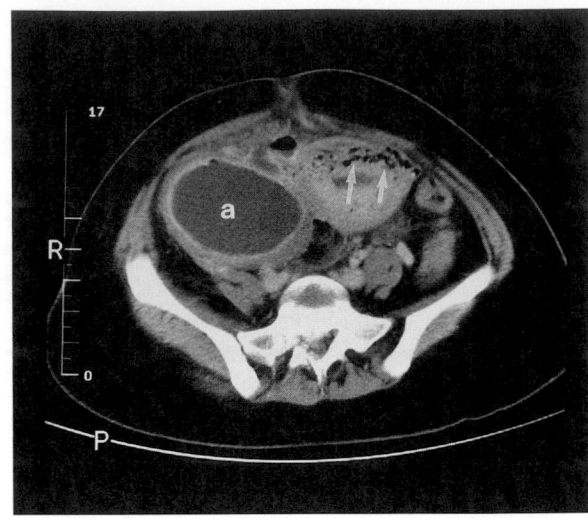

FIGURE 31–4. Pelvic computed tomography scan showing necrosis of the uterus with gas in the myometrium (*arrows*) and a large right-sided parametrial abscess (a). (Courtesy of Dr. Diane Twickler.)

seldom involved, and one or both ovaries usually may be conserved.

Imaging Studies. Brown and colleagues (1991) described the use of computed tomography (CT) in 74 women to assess pelvic infections refractory to standard antimicrobial therapy. They found at least one abnormal radiological finding in 75 percent of these women. Twickler and associates (1997) found that CT with contrast and magnetic resonance imaging (MRI) effectively image ovarian vein thrombosis. Using MRI, Maldjian and associates (1999) studied 50 women with persistent low-grade fever following cesarean delivery. Bladder flap hematomas were found in two thirds, three women had parametrial edema, and two had a pelvic hematoma.

Sometimes evidence of uterine incisional dehiscence can be detected using CT scanning (Figs. 31–3 and 31–4). These radiological findings must be interpreted within the clinical context, because apparent uterine incisional defects can be visualized after cesarean delivery with no other evidence of infection or other complications (Twickler and colleagues, 1991).

PELVIC ABSCESS. Rarely, a parametrial phlegmon suppurates, forming a fluctuant broad ligament mass that may point above the Poupart ligament. These abscesses may dissect anteriorly and be amenable to needle drainage directed by CT imaging (see Fig. 31–4). Occasionally they dissect posteriorly to the rectovaginal septum, where surgical drainage is easily affected by colpotomy incision. *Psoas abscess* may rarely follow delivery. Its management includes antimicrobial therapy, and percutaneous drainage may be required (Shahabi and colleagues, 2002).

Sometimes following cesarean delivery, collections of blood develop under the bladder flap (Maldjian and

associates, 1999). Hematomas may also form in the broad ligament near the uterine incision. These may become infected and require drainage.

SEPTIC PELVIC THROMBOPHLEBITIS. The pathogenesis of suppurative pelvic thrombophlebitis was described by Collins and colleagues (1951) in 70 women cared for from 1937 through 1946 at Charity Hospital in New Orleans. Septic embolization was common in these women and caused a third of maternal deaths during that period. With the advent of antimicrobial therapy, the mortality and need for surgical therapy for these infections diminished.

Pathogenesis. Puerperal infection may extend along venous routes and cause thrombosis (Fig. 31–5). Lymphangitis often coexists. The ovarian veins may then become involved because they drain the upper uterus, which most often includes veins draining the placental site. The experiences of Witlin and Sibai (1995) and Brown and colleagues (1999) suggested that puerperal septic thrombophlebitis is likely to involve one or both ovarian venous plexuses (Fig. 31–6). In a fourth of women, the clot extends into the inferior vena cava, and occasionally extends to the renal vein.

Incidence. During a five-year survey of 45,000 women who gave birth at Parkland Hospital, Brown and associates (1999) found an incidence of septic pelvic thrombophlebitis of 1:9000 with vaginal and 1:800 with cesarean delivery. The overall incidence of 1:3000 deliveries was similar to the 1:2000 reported by Dunnihoo and colleagues (1991).

Clinical Findings. Women with septic pelvic thrombophlebitis usually display some clinical improvement of their pelvic infection following antimicrobial treatment.

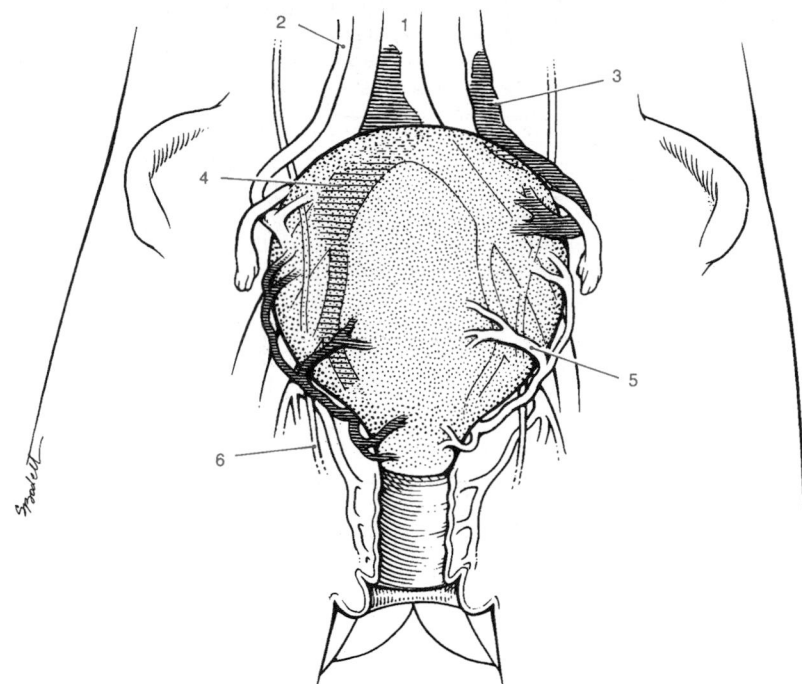

FIGURE 31–5. Routes of extension of septic pelvic thrombophlebitis. Any pelvic vessels and the inferior vena cava may be involved: (1) inferior vena cava; (2) right ovarian vein; (3) left ovarian vein; (4) clot in right common iliac vein which extends from the uterine and internal iliac veins and into the inferior vena cava; (5) left uterine vein; and (6) right ureter.

However, they continue to have fever. They may be asymptomatic except for chills. In some women, the cardinal symptom of ovarian vein thrombophlebitis is pain typically manifested on the second or third postpartum day (Munsick and Gillanders, 1981). In some cases, a tender mass is palpable lateral to the uterine cornu on either side.

Diagnosis is usually by either pelvic CT or MRI (Sheffield and Cunningham, 2001; Twickler and associates, 1997).

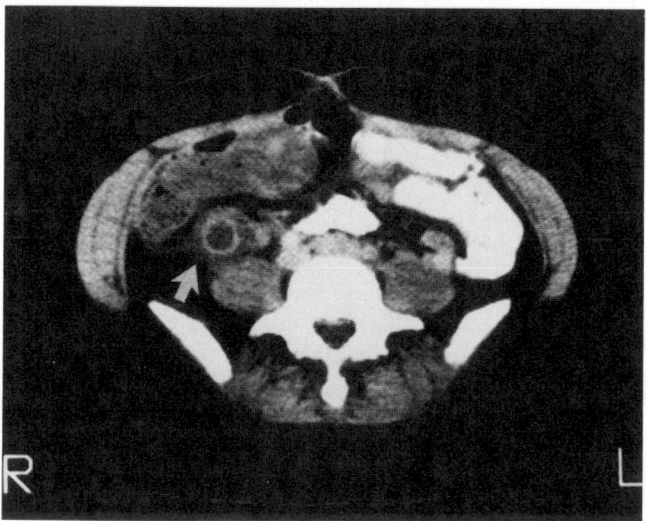

FIGURE 31–6. Pelvic computed tomography scan with intravenous and oral contrast shows enlargement of right ovarian vein, low density of lumen, and vessel-wall enhancement consistent with thrombosis (*arrow*). Associated low-density area surrounding vein represents perivascular edema. (From Brown and colleagues, 1999, with permission.)

Using both imaging techniques, Brown and co-workers (1999) found that 20 percent of 69 women with metritis who had fever despite 5 days of appropriate therapy had was confirmed septic pelvic phlebitis. Before imaging methods were available to confirm venous involvement, the *heparin challenge test* was advocated. Supposedly after intravenous heparin was given, if the temperature decreased, this was taken as diagnostic of pelvic phlebitis and heparin treatment was continued (Josey and Staggers, 1974). This was subsequently disproved by Brown and colleagues (1986), who showed that despite withholding heparin from 6 of 11 women with CT-proven pelvic thrombophlebitis, continued antimicrobial therapy resulted in clinical resolution. Conversely, in the five women given heparin along with antimicrobial drugs, the prolonged febrile course was not appreciably abbreviated. Witlin and Sibai (1995) reported similar observations in 11 women with ovarian vein thrombophlebitis. In a follow-up randomized study of 14 women by Brown and associates (1999), the addition of heparin to antimicrobial therapy for septic pelvic thrombophlebitis did not hasten recovery or improve outcome.

INFECTIONS OF THE PERINEUM, VAGINA, AND CERVIX

Episiotomy infections are not often encountered because the operation is performed much less frequently now than in the past (see Chap. 17, p. 435). For example, Owen and Hauth (1990) described only 10 episiotomy infections among 20,000 deliveries at the University of Alabama at Birmingham. With infection, dehiscence is a concern. Ramin and colleagues (1992) reported that 0.5 percent of episiotomy wounds developed dehiscence at Parkland Hospital, and 80 percent of these were due to infection. No data suggest that dehiscence is related to faulty repair.

Serious infection is more likely in women who sustain a fourth-degree laceration. Goldaber and colleagues (1993) described 390 such women of whom 5.4 percent had morbidity; 2.8 percent had infection and dehiscence, 1.8 percent had only dehiscence, and 0.8 percent had only infection. Although life-threatening septic shock is rare, it may still occur as a result of an infected episiotomy (Soltesz and colleagues, 1999).

PATHOGENESIS AND CLINICAL COURSE. Episiotomy dehiscence is most commonly associated with infection. Other factors include coagulation disorders, smoking, and human papillomavirus infection (Ramin and Gilstrap, 1994). Local pain and dysuria, with or without urinary retention, are common symptoms. Ramin and colleagues (1992), evaluating a series of 34 women with episiotomy dehiscence, reported that the most common findings were pain (65 percent), purulent discharge (65 percent), and fever (44 percent). In extreme cases, the entire vulva may become edematous, ulcerated, and covered with exudate.

Vaginal lacerations may become infected directly or by extension from the perineum. The mucosa becomes red and swollen and may then become necrotic and slough. Parametrial extension may result in lymphangitis.

Cervical lacerations are common, and the cervix normally harbors potentially pathogenic organisms. When infected, deep lacerations often extend directly into the tissue at the base of the broad ligament, and infections may cause lymphangitis, parametritis, and bacteremia.

TREATMENT. Infected episiotomies, like other infected surgical wounds, should be treated by establishing drainage. In most cases, sutures are removed and the infected wound opened. In some women with obvious cellulitis but no purulence, broad-spectrum antimicrobial therapy with close observation is appropriate. Hauth and colleagues (1986) were the first to advocate early repair after evidence of infection subsided. Subsequently, other studies have attested to the efficacy of such practice. Hankins and co-workers (1990) described early repair of episiotomy dehiscence in 31 women. The average duration from dehiscence to episiotomy repair was 6 days. All but two women had a successful repair, and both of them developed a pinpoint rectovaginal fistula treated successfully with a small rectal flap. Ramin and colleagues (1992) reported successful early repair of episiotomy dehiscence associated with infection in 32 of 34 women (94 percent).

Technique for Early Repair. A preoperative protocol for early repair is summarized in Table 31–3. **Prior to attempting early repair of episiotomy dehiscence, the surgical wound must be properly cleaned and free of infection.**

TABLE 31–3 Preoperative Protocol for Early Repair of Episiotomy Dehiscence

Intravenous antimicrobial therapy until afebrile
Remove sutures and open wound entirely
Wound care
    Sedation as indicated
    2% lidocaine jelly applied to wound
    Debridement of all necrotic tissue
    Scrub wound twice daily with a povidone–iodine
    Sitz bath several times daily or hydrotherapy
Mechanical bowel preparation day before surgery—for 4th-degree repairs, NPO the evening before surgery

From Ramin and Gilstrap (1994), with permission.

As shown in Figure 31–7, once the surface of the episiotomy wound is free of infection and exudate and covered by pink granulation tissue, secondary repair can be accomplished. Good tissue mobility must be accomplished, including identification and mobilization of the anal sphincter muscle. Secondary closure of the episiotomy is accomplished in layers as described for primary episiotomy closure (see Chap. 17, p. 436). Postoperative care includes local wound care, low-residue diet, stool softeners that avoid diarrhea, and nothing per vagina or rectum until healed.

NECROTIZING FASCIITIS. A rare but frequently fatal complication of perineal and vaginal wound infections is deep soft tissue infection involving muscle and fascia. These may also complicate vulvar infections in diabetic and immunocompromised women but may develop in otherwise healthy women. The microbiology of these serious perineal infections

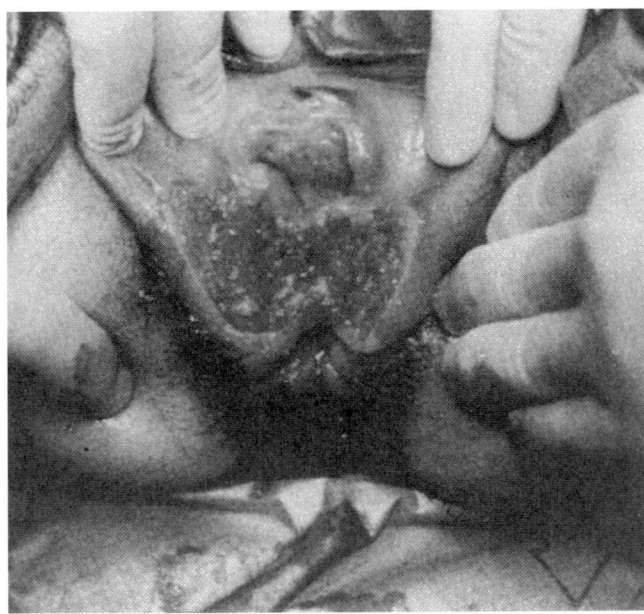

FIGURE 31–7. Dehiscence of fourth-degree episiotomy. Secondary repair is done when the wound surface is free of exudate and covered by pink granulation tissue. (From Ramin and Gilstrap, 1994, with permission.)

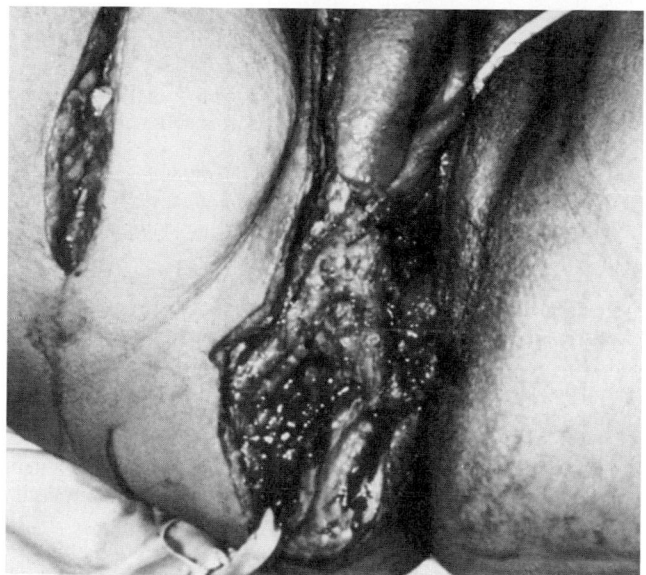

FIGURE 31–8. Necrotizing fasciitis complicating episiotomy infection. Three days postpartum this woman had severe perineal pain and edema of the episiotomy site. Prompt extensive debridement was carried out. Bacteria cultured from the infected episiotomy included *Escherichia coli, Streptococcus viridans,* group D streptococcus, *Corynebacterium* species, *Bacteroides fragilis,* and *Clostridium* species. Blood cultures were positive for *Bacteroides fragilis.*

appears to be similar to those that cause other pelvic infections, as well as necrotizing fasciitis of the abdominal incision described previously. Although uncommon today, Shy and Eschenbach (1979) reported that episiotomy necrotizing fasciitis was responsible for 20 percent of 15 maternal deaths in King County, Washington, in the 1970s.

Necrotizing fasciitis of the episiotomy site may involve any of the several superficial or deep perineal fascial layers, and thus it may extend to the thighs, buttocks, and abdominal wall (Fig. 31–8). Although some virulent infections, for example, from group A β-hemolytic streptococci, may develop early after delivery, these infections usually do not cause symptoms until 3 to 5 days afterward. Clinical findings vary, and it is frequently difficult to differentiate superficial perineal infections from deep fascial ones. A high index of suspicion, with surgical exploration if the diagnosis is uncertain, may be lifesaving. We aggressively pursue early exploration. Certainly, if myofascitis progresses, the woman may become very ill from septicemia, profound hemoconcentration from capillary leakage with circulatory failure commonly occurs, and death may soon follow. Early diagnosis, surgical debridement, antimicrobials, and intensive care are of paramount importance in the successful treatment of necrotizing soft tissue infections (Gallup and Meguiar, 2004; Urschel, 1999).

Aggressive surgical treatment is indicated and includes extensive debridement of all infected tissue, leaving wide margins of healthy tissue. This may include extensive vulvar debridement with unroofing and excision of abdominal,

thigh, or buttock fascia (see Fig. 31–8). **Mortality is virtually universal without surgical treatment, and it approaches 50 percent even if extensive debridement is performed.**

TOXIC SHOCK SYNDROME

This acute febrile illness with severe multisystem derangement has a case-fatality rate of 10 to 15 percent. The illness is usually characterized by fever, headache, mental confusion, diffuse macular erythematous rash, subcutaneous edema, nausea, vomiting, watery diarrhea, and marked hemoconcentration. Renal failure followed by hepatic failure, disseminated intravascular coagulation, and circulatory collapse may follow in rapid sequence. During recovery, the rash-covered areas undergo desquamation. *Staphylococcus aureus* has been recovered from almost all afflicted persons, and a staphylococcal exotoxin, termed *toxic shock syndrome toxin-1,* causes the syndrome by provoking profound endothelial injury.

In many cases, infection is not documented, and colonization of a mucosal surface is the only finding. Nearly 10 percent of pregnant women have vaginal colonization with *S aureus,* and thus it is not surprising that the disease develops in postpartum women (Guerinot and co-workers, 1982). McGregor and colleagues (1988) have described almost identical findings in women with infection complicated by *Clostridium sordellii* colonization.

More recently, as discussed on page 713, there have been reports of *streptococcal toxic shock syndrome* associated with group A β-hemolytic streptococcal infection. Preliminary data implicate serotypes M1 and M3 as particularly virulent (Beres and associates, 2004; Okumura and collaborators, 2004). A delay in diagnosis described by Schummer and Schummer (2002) resulted in a maternal death. Crum and colleagues (2002) reported an antepartum infection at 34 weeks' gestation causing fetal distress and neonatal death.

Principal therapy for toxic shock is supportive, while allowing reversal of capillary endothelial injury (see Chap. 42, p. 994). The toxins are potent, and the mortality rate correspondingly high (Hotchkiss and Karl, 2003). In severe cases, treatment requires massive fluid replacement, mechanical ventilation with positive end-expiratory pressure (Catanzarite and associates, 2001), and renal dialysis. Antimicrobial therapy with antistaphylococcal drugs is given. With evidence for uterine infection, antimicrobial therapy must include agents used for all puerperal infections. Cases of streptococcal toxic shock syndrome often require hysterectomy.

REFERENCES

American College of Obstetricians and Gynecologists: Prophylactic antibiotics in labor and delivery. Practice Bulletin No. 47, October, 2003

Andrews WW, Hauth JC, Cliver SP, et al: Randomized clinical trial of extended spectrum antibiotic prophylaxis with coverage for *Ureaplasma urealyticum* to reduce post-cesarean delivery endometritis. Obstet Gynecol 101:1183, 2003a

Andrews WW, Shah SR, Goldenberg RL, et al: Association of post-cesarean delivery endometritis with colonization of the chorioamnion by *Ureaplasma urealyticum.* Obstet Gynecol 85:509, 1995

Andrews WW, Sibai BM, Thom EA, et al: Randomized clinical trial of metronidazole plus erythromycin to prevent spontaneous preterm delivery in fetal fibronectin-positive women. Obstet Gynecol 101:847, 2003b

Anteby EY, Yagel S, Hanoch J, et al: Puerperal and intrapartum group A streptococcal infection. Infect Dis Obstet Gynecol 7:276, 1999

Barber GR, Swygert JS: Necrotizing fasciitis due to *Photobacterium damsela* in a man lashed by a stingray. N Engl J Med 342:824, 2000

Beres SB, Sylva GL, Sturdevant DE, et al: Genome-wide molecular dissection of serotype M3 group A Streptococcus strains causing two epidemics of invasive infections. Proc Natl Acad Sci USA 101:11833, 2004

Berg CJ, Chang J, Callaghan WM, et al: Pregnancy-related mortality in the United States, 1991–1997. Obstet Gynecol 101:289, 2003

Brown CEL, Dunn DH, Harrell R, et al: Computed tomography for evaluation of puerperal infection. Surg Gynecol Obstet 172:2, 1991

Brown CEL, Lowe TW, Cunningham FG, et al: Puerperal pelvic thrombophlebitis: Impact on diagnosis and treatment using x-ray computed tomography and magnetic resonance imaging. Obstet Gynecol 68:789, 1986

Brown CEL, Stettler RW, Twickler D, et al: Puerperal septic pelvic thrombophlebitis: Incidence and response to heparin therapy. Am J Obstet Gynecol 181:143, 1999

Brumfield CG, Hauth JC, Andrews WW: Puerperal infections following cesarean delivery: Evaluation of a standardized protocol. Am J Obstet Gynecol 182:1147, 2000

Burrows LJ, Meyn LA, Weber AM: Maternal morbidity associated with vaginal versus cesarean delivery. Obstet Gynecol 103:907, 2004

Carey JC, Klebanoff MA, Hauth JC, et al: Metronidazole to prevent preterm delivery in pregnant women with asymptomatic bacterial vaginosis. N Engl J Med 342:534, 2000

Catanzarite V, Willms D, Wong D, et al: Acute respiratory distress syndrome in pregnancy and the puerperium: Causes, courses, and outcomes. Obstet Gynecol 97:760, 2001

Chaim W, Bashiri A, Bar-David J, et al: Prevalence and clinical significance of postpartum endometritis and wound infection. Infect Dis Obstet Gynecol 8:77, 2000

Chelmow D, Ruehli MS, Huang E: Prophylactic use of antibiotics for non-laboring patients undergoing cesarean delivery with intact membranes: A meta-analysis. Am J Obstet Gynecol 184:656, 2001

Chelmow D, Rodriguez EJ, Sabatini MM: Suture closure of subcutaneous fat and wound disruption after cesarean delivery: A meta-analysis. Obstet Gynecol 103:974, 2004

Collins CG, McCallum EA, Nelson EW, et al: Suppurative pelvic thrombophlebitis: 1. Incidence, pathology, etiology; 2. Symptomatology and diagnosis; 3. Surgical techniques: A study of 70 patients treated by ligation of the inferior vena cava and ovarian veins. Surgery 30:298, 1951

Cook JD, Lynch SR: The liabilities of iron deficiency. Blood 68:803, 1986

Crum NF, Chun HM, Gaylord TG, et al: Group A streptococcal toxic shock syndrome developing in the third trimester of pregnancy. Infect Dis Obstet Gynecol 10:209, 2002

Cunningham FG, Hauth JC, Strong JD, et al: Infectious morbidity following cesarean: Comparison of two treatment regimens. Obstet Gynecol 52:656, 1978

DePalma RT, Cunningham FG, Leveno KJ, et al: Continuing investigation of women at high risk for infection following cesarean delivery. Obstet Gynecol 60:53, 1982

Dinsmoor MJ, Newton ER, Gibbs RS: A randomized, double-blind placebo-controlled trial of oral antibiotic therapy following intravenous antibiotic therapy for postpartum endometritis. Obstet Gynecol 77:60, 1991

DiZerega G, Yonekura L, Roy S, et al: A comparison of clindamycin-gentamicin and penicillin gentamicin in the treatment of post-cesarean section endomyometritis. Am J Obstet Gynecol 134:238, 1979

Dunnihoo DR, Gallaspy JW, Wise RB, et al: Postpartum ovarian vein thrombophlebitis: A review. Obstet Gynecol Surv 46:415, 1991

Emmons SL, Krohn M, Jackson M, et al: Development of wound infections among women undergoing cesarean section. Obstet Gynecol 72:559, 1988

Enkin MW, Wilkinson C: Single versus two layer suturing for closing the uterine incision at cesarean section. Cochrane Library, Chichester, Wiley Issue 1, 2002

Filker R, Monif GRG: The significance of temperature during the first 24 hours postpartum. Obstet Gynecol 53:359, 1979

French LM, Smaill FM: Antibiotic regimens for endometritis after delivery. Cochrane Library, Chichester, Wiley Issue 1, 2002

Gallup DG, Meguiar RV: Coping with necrotizing fasciitis. Contemp Ob/Gyn 49:38, 2004

Gilstrap LC III, Cunningham FG: The bacterial pathogenesis of infection following cesarean section. Obstet Gynecol 53:545, 1979

Goepfert AR, Guinn DA, Andrews WW, et al: Necrotizing fasciitis after cesarean section. Obstet Gynecol 89:409, 1997

Goldaber KG, Wendel PJ, McIntire DD, et al: Postpartum perineal morbidity after fourth degree perineal repair. Am J Obstet Gynecol 168:489, 1993

Goldenberg RL, Klebanoff MA, Nugent R, et al: Bacterial colonization of the vagina during pregnancy in four ethnic groups. Am J Obstet Gynecol 174:1618, 1996

Guerinot GT, Gitomer SD, Sanko SR: Postpartum patient with toxic shock syndrome. Obstet Gynecol 59:43S, 1982

Hankins GDV, Hauth JC, Gilstrap LC, et al: Early repair of episiotomy dehiscence. Obstet Gynecol 75:48, 1990

Hartmann KE, Barrett KE, Reid VC, et al: Clinical usefulness of white blood cell count after cesarean delivery. Obstet Gynecol 96:295, 2000

Hauth JC, Gilstrap LC III, Ward SC, et al: Early repair of an external sphincter ani muscle and rectal mucosal dehiscence. Obstet Gynecol 67:806, 1986

Hauth JC, Owen J, Davis RO: Transverse uterine incision closure: One versus two layers. Am J Obstet Gynecol 167:1108, 1992

Hopkins L, Smaill F: Antibiotic prophylaxis regimens and drugs for cesarean section. Cochrane Library, Chichester, Wiley Issue 1, 2003

Hotchkiss RS, Karl IE: The pathophysiology and treatment of sepsis. N Engl J Med 348:138, 2003

Ismail MA, Chandler AE, Beem ME: Chlamydial colonization of the cervix in pregnant adolescents. J Reprod Med 30:549, 1985

Jacobsson B, Pernevi P, Chidekel L, et al: Bacterial vaginosis in early pregnancy may predispose for preterm birth and postpartum endometritis. Acta Obstet Gynecol Scand 81:1006, 2002

Jazayeri A, Jazayeri MK, Sahinler M, et al: Is meconium passage a risk factor for maternal infection in term pregnancies? Obstet Gynecol 99:548, 2002

Josey WE, Staggers SR Jr: Heparin therapy in septic pelvic thrombophlebitis: A study of 46 cases. Am J Obstet Gynecol 120:228, 1974

Kankuri E, Kurki T, Carlson P, et al: Incidence, treatment and outcome of peripartum sepsis. Acta Obstet Gynecol Scand 82:730, 2003

Kindig M, Cardwell M, Lee T: Delayed postpartum uterine dehiscence. Case report. J Reprod Med 43:591, 1998

Klebanoff MA, Carey JC, Hauth JC, et al: Failure of metronidazole to prevent preterm delivery among pregnant women with asymptomatic *Trichomonas vaginalis* infection. N Engl J Med 345:487, 2001

Libombo A, Folgosa E, Bergstrom S: Risk factors in puerperal endometritis-myometritis. An incident case-referent study. Gynecol Obstet Invest 38:198, 1994

Liu C, Abate B, Reyes M, et al: Single daily dosing of gentamicin: Pharmacokinetic comparison of two dosing methodologies for postpartum endometritis. Infect Dis Obstet Gynecol 7:133, 1999

Livingston JC, Llata E, Rinehart E, et al: Gentamicin and clindamycin therapy in postpartum endometritis: The efficacy of daily dosing versus dosing every 8 hours. Am J Obstet Gynecol 188:149, 2003

Lydon-Rochelle M, Holt VL, Martin DP, et al: Association between method of delivery and maternal rehospitalization. JAMA 283:2411, 2000

Koroukian SM: Relative risk of postpartum complications in the Ohio Medicaid population: Vaginal versus cesarean deliver. Med Care Res Rev 61:203, 2004

Maberry MC, Gilstrap LC, Bawdon RE, et al: Anaerobic coverage for intra-amnionic infection: Maternal and perinatal impact. Am J Perinatol 8:338, 1991

Magann EF, Chauhan SP, Rodts-Palenik S, et al: Subcutaneous stitch closure versus subcutaneous drain to prevent wound disruption after cesarean delivery: A randomized clinical trial. Am J Obstet Gynecol 186:1119, 2002

Magee KP, Blanco JD, Graham JM, et al: Endometritis after cesarean: The effect of age. Am J Perinatol 11:24, 1994

Maldjian C, Adam R, Maldjian J, et al: MRI appearance of the pelvis in the post cesarean-section patient. Magn Reson Imaging 17:223, 1999

Marik PE: Aspiration pneumonitis and aspiration pneumonia. N Engl J Med 344:665, 2001

McGregor JA, Soper D, Lovell G: A toxic shock-like syndrome caused by *Clostridia sordelli* affecting postpartum women. Abstract 30 presented at meeting of Infectious Disease Society in Obstetrics and Gynecology, Aspen, CO, August 1988

McNeeley SG Jr, Hendrix SL, Bennett SM, et al: Synthetic graft placement in the treatment of fascial dehiscence with necrosis and infection. Am J Obstet Gynecol 179:1430, 1998

Mercer BM, Miodovnik M, Thurnau GR, et al: Antibiotic therapy for reduction of infant morbidity after preterm premature rupture of the membranes. A randomized control trial. JAMA 278:989, 1997

Munsick RA, Gillanders LA: A review of the syndrome of puerperal ovarian vein thrombophlebitis. Obstet Gynecol Surv 36:57, 1981

Murray BE: Vancomycin-resistant enterococcal infections. N Engl J Med 342:710, 2000

Mussey RD, DeNormandie RL, Adair FL: The American Committee on Maternal Welfare, Inc: Its organization, purposes and activities. Am J Obstet Gynecol 28:754, 1935

Myles TD, Gooch J, Santolaya J: Obesity as an independent risk factor for infectious morbidity in patients who undergo cesarean delivery. Obstet Gynecol 100:959, 2002

Nathan L, Leveno KJ: Group A streptococcal puerperal sepsis: Historical review and 1990s resurgence. Infect Dis Obstet Gynecol 1:252, 1994

Naumann RW, Hauth JC, Owen J, et al: Subcutaneous tissue approximation in relation to wound disruption after cesarean delivery in obese women. Obstet Gynecol 85:412, 1995

Okumura K, Schroff R, Campbell R, et al: Group A streptococcal puerperal sepsis with retroperitoneal involvement developing in a late postpartum woman: Case report. Am Surg. 70:730, 2004

Owen J, Andrews WW: Wound complications after cesarean section. Clin Obstet Gynecol 27:842, 1994

Owen J, Hauth JC: Episiotomy infection and dehiscence. In Gilstrap LC III, Faro S (eds): Infections in Pregnancy. New York, Liss, 1990, p 61

Pitt C, Sanchez-Ramos L, Kaunitz AM: Adjunctive intravaginal metronidazole for the prevention of postcesarean endometritis: A randomized controlled trial. Obstet Gynecol 98:745, 2001

Ramin SM, Gilstrap LC: Episiotomy and early repair of dehiscence. Clin Obstet Gynecol 37:816, 1994

Ramin SM, Ramus R, Little B, et al: Early repair of episiotomy dehiscence associated with infection. Am J Obstet Gynecol 167:1104, 1992

Reid VC, Hartmann KE, McMahon M, et al: Vaginal preparation with povidone iodine and postcesarean infections morbidity: A randomized controlled trial. Obstet Gynecol 97:147, 2001

Rivlin ME, Carroll CS, Morrison JC: Conservative surgery for uterine incisional necrosis complicating cesarean delivery. Obstet Gynecol 103:1105, 2004

Rouse DJ, Hauth JC, Andrews WW, et al: Chlorhexidine vaginal irrigation for the prevention of peripartal infection: A placebo-controlled randomized clinical trial. Am J Obstet Gynecol 176:617, 1997

Schorge JO, Granter SR, Lerner LH, et al: Postpartum and vulvar necrotizing fasciitis: Early clinical diagnosis and histopathologic correlation. J Reprod Med 43:586, 1998

Schummer W, Schummer C: Two cases of delayed diagnosis of postpartal streptococcal toxic shock syndrome. Infect Dis Obstet Gynecol 10:217, 2002

Shahabi S, Klein JP, Rinaudo PF: Primary psoas abscess complicating a normal vaginal delivery. Obstet Gynecol 99:906, 2002

Sheffield JS, Cunningham FG: Detecting and treating septic pelvic thrombophlebitis. Contemp Ob/Gyn 3:15, 2001

Sherman D, Lurie S, Betzer M, et al: Uterine flora at cesarean and its relationship to postpartum endometritis. Obstet Gynecol 94:787, 1999

Shy KK, Eschenbach DA: Fatal perineal cellulitis from an episiotomy site. Obstet Gynecol 52:293, 1979

Smaill F, Hofmeyr GJ: Antibiotic prophylaxis for cesarean section. Cochrane Library, Chichester, Wiley Issue 1, 2003

Soltesz S, Biedler A, Ohlmann P, et al: Puerperal sepsis due to infected episiotomy wound. Zentralbl Gynakol 121:441, 1999

Soper DE, Brockwell WJ, Dalton HP: The importance of wound infection in antibiotic failures in the therapy of postpartum endometritis. Surg Gynecol Obstet 174:265, 1992

Stefonek KR, Maerz LL, Nielsen MP, et al: Group A streptococcal puerperal sepsis preceded by positive surveillance cultures. Obstet Gynecol 98:846, 2001

Suonio S, Huttunen M: Puerperal endometritis after abdominal twin delivery. Acta Obstet Gynecol Scand 73:313, 1994

Swartz MN: Cellulitis. N Engl J Med 350:904, 2004

Sweet RL, Ledger WJ: Puerperal infectious morbidity. A two year review. Am J Obstet Gynecol 117:1093, 1973

Sweeten KM, Eriksen NL, Blanco JD: Chlorhexidine versus sterile water vaginal wash during labor to prevent peripartum infection. Am J Obstet Gynecol 176:426, 1997

Synnestvedt M, Muller F, Gaustad P, et al: Recurrent group A streptococcal genital infection after puerperal sepsis. Scand J Infect Dis 35:509, 2003

Tran TS, Jamulitrat S, Chongsuvivatwong V, et al: Risk factors for postcesarean surgical site infection. Obstet Gynecol 95:367, 2000

Tulandi T, Al-Jaroudi D: Nonclosure of peritoneum: A reappraisal. Am J Obstet Gynecol 189:609, 2003

Twickler DM, Setiawan AT, Evans RS, et al: Imaging of puerperal septic thrombophlebitis: Prospective comparison of MR imaging, CT, and sonography. Am J Roentgenol 169:1039, 1997

Twickler DM, Setiawan AT, Harrell RS, et al: CT appearance of the pelvis after cesarean section. Am J Roentgenol 156:523, 1991

Udagawa H, Oshio Y, Shimizu Y: Serious group A streptococcal infection around delivery. Obstet Gynecol 94:153, 1999

Urschel JD: Necrotizing soft tissue infections. Postgrad Med J 75:645, 1999

Ventolini F, Neiger R, McKenna D: Decreasing infectious morbidity in cesarean delivery by changing gloves. J Reprod Med 49:13, 2004

Walmer D, Walmer KR, Gibbs RS: Enterococci in post-cesarean endometritis. Obstet Gynecol 71:159, 1988

Watts DH, Krohn MA, Hillier SL, et al: Bacterial vaginosis as a risk factor for post-cesarean endometritis. Obstet Gynecol 75:52, 1990

Wetchler SJ, Dunn LJ: Ovarian abscess. Report of a case and a review of the literature. Obstet Gynecol Surv 40:476, 1985

Wilkinson CS, Enkin MW: Manual removal of placenta at caesarean section. Cochrane Library, Chichester, Wiley Issue 1, 1999a

Wilkinson CS, Enkin MW: Peritoneal non-closure at caesarean section. Cochrane Library, Chichester, Wiley Issue 1, 1999b

Witlin AG, Sibai BM: Postpartum ovarian vein thrombosis after vaginal delivery: A report of 11 cases. Obstet Gynecol 85:775, 1995

Zimbelman J, Palmer A, Todd J: Improved outcome of clindamycin compared with beta-lactam antibiotic treatment for invasive *Streptococcus pyogenes* infections. Pediatr Infect Dis J 18:1096, 1999

32

Contraception

The approach to reproductive health in the United States has often been manipulated and constrained by forces from outside the medical community. Social, religious, and political groups have been particularly intrusive and coercive in the area of family planning, although at any given time, the majority of fertile American women would prefer to avoid pregnancy. Such intrusion and coercion is almost certainly counterproductive. At least 10 states and the U.S. Congress have considered legislation requiring parental notification for prescribed contraceptives. Reddy and colleagues (2002) surveyed adolescents and found that 60 percent would stop using all sexual health care services if their parents had to be informed that they were seeking contraception. The adolescents also indicated that they would also delay testing or treatment for human immunodeficiency virus (HIV) infection and other sexually transmitted diseases if parental consent were required. Even in the United States, women are denied access to family planning services. Only in the last few years have some insurance carriers begun to cover the cost of contraceptives. In the United States, access for indigent women to reproductive services is frequently a political decision, and not a medical or even a financial one.

Fortunately, a wide variety of effective methods of regulating fertility is currently available. None is completely without side effects or categorically without danger—for example, latex condoms can initiate anaphylactic reactions. That said, **contraception poses less risk than does pregnancy** (Table 32–1). In fact, for the vast majority of women, it is safer to use contraception than it is to drive an automobile (Hatcher and colleagues, 1998).

NEED FOR CONTRACEPTION

Pregnancy rates for sexually active fertile women who do not use contraception approach 90 percent at 1 year. Because ovulation often precedes menarche, young women who do not want to be pregnant should be advised to use contraception whenever they begin sexual activity. Contraceptive advice for the woman nearing menopause is more difficult to provide because it is not easy to predict when fertility has ended. Results of a study by Metcalf (1979) indicate that *when menstruation remained regular, there was evidence of ovulation in almost every cycle.* Oligomenorrhea or increasing cycle length was associated with a diminished frequency of ovulation, but even the presence of hot flushes, amenorrhea, and elevated gonadotropin levels did not absolutely guarantee that ovulation would not occur.

CONTRACEPTIVE METHODS

Methods of variable effectiveness currently used in the United States include:

1. Oral steroidal contraceptives
2. Injected steroidal contraceptives
3. Intrauterine devices (IUDs)
4. Transdermal and transvaginal steroidal contraceptives
5. Physical, chemical, or barrier techniques
6. Preejaculatory withdrawal
7. Sexual abstinence around the time of ovulation
8. Breast feeding
9. Permanent sterilization

The most recent nationally representative data concerning contraceptive use were collected in 1995 (Fig. 32–1). Estimates of the failure rate *during the first year of use* are given in Table 32–2. Effective education, as well as motivation, can appreciably reduce the cited failure rates (Vessey and co-workers, 1982). **Elective abortion is not a**

TABLE 32–1 Birth-Related or Method-Related Deaths per 100,000 Fertile Women

	Age Group					
	15–19	*20–24*	*25–29*	*30–34*	*35–39*	*40–44*
Pregnancy	4.7	5.4	4.8	6.3	11.7	20.6
Abortion	2.1	2.0	1.6	1.9	2.8	5.3
IUD	0.2	0.3	0.2	0.1	0.3	0.6
Periodic abstinence	1.4	1.3	0.7	1.0	1.0	1.9
Withdrawal	0.9	1.7	0.9	1.3	0.8	1.5
Condom	0.6	1.2	0.6	0.9	0.5	1.0
Diaphragm/cap	0.6	1.1	0.6	0.9	1.6	3.1
Sponge	0.8	1.5	0.8	1.1	2.2	4.1
Spermicides	1.6	1.9	1.4	1.9	1.5	2.7
Oral contraceptives	0.8	1.3	1.1	1.8	1.0	1.9
Implants/injectables	0.2	0.6	0.5	0.8	0.5	0.6
Tubal sterilization	1.3	1.2	1.1	1.1	1.2	1.3
Vasectomy	0.1	0.1	0.1	0.1	0.1	0.2

IUD = intrauterine device.
From Harlap and associates, 1991, with permission.

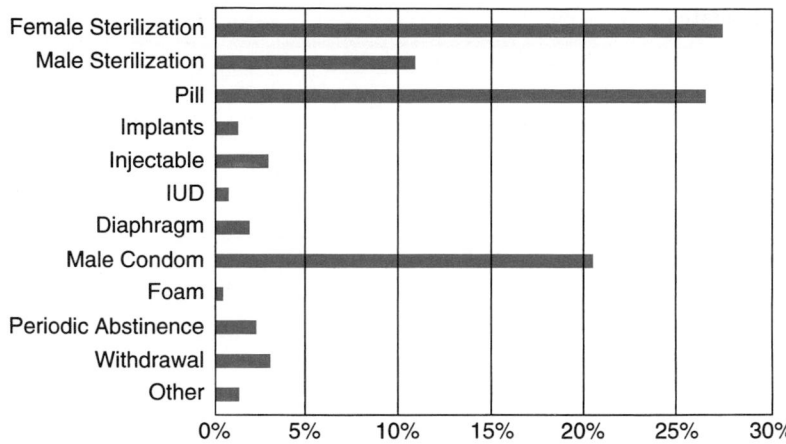

FIGURE 32–1. Contraceptive use in the United States circa 1995 for users aged 15 to 44. Data from Piccinino and Mosher (1998). (IUD = intrauterine device.) (From the Association of Professors of Gynecology and Obstetrics, 1999, with permission.)

TABLE 32–2 Contraceptive Failure Rates During the First Year of Use

Method	Percent of Women with Pregnancy	
	Lowest Expected	*Typical*
None	**85.0**	**85.0**
Combination pill	0.1	7.6
Progestin-only pill ("mini-pill")	0.5	3.0
Intrauterine devices		
Mirena levonorgestrel device	0.1	0.1
ParaGard T 380A	0.6	0.8
Patch	0.05	0.2
Injectable progestin	0.3	3.1
NuvaRing (vaginal ring)	0.7	
Female sterilization	0.05	0.05
Male sterilization	0.1	0.15
Spermicides	6.0	25.7
Periodic abstinence		
Calendar	9.0	20.5
Ovulation method	3.0	
Symptothermal	2.0	
Postovulation	1.0	
Withdrawal	4.0	23.6
Cervical cap		
Parous women	20.0	40.0
Nulliparous women	9.0	20.0
Sponge		
Parous women	20.0	40.0
Nulliparous women	9.0	20.0
Diaphragm plus spermicide	6.0	12.1
Condom		
Male	3.0	13.9
Female	5.0	21.0
Emergency contraception	> 75% reduction	

Modified from Speroff and Darney, 2001, with permission.

contraceptive technique. It serves, at times, as a less than ideal remedy for contraceptive failure or neglect (see Chap. 9, p. 241).

HORMONAL CONTRACEPTIVES

These contraceptives are currently available in a wide variety of oral, injectable, transdermal (patch), and transvaginal (ring) forms. Oral contraceptives are a combination of estrogen and progestin (*the pill*) or progestin only (*mini-pill*). The other forms contain progestins alone or a combination of estrogen and progestin. Unfortunately, no reliable reversible male hormonal contraceptives have been developed (Kamischke and Nieschlag, 2004).

ESTROGEN PLUS PROGESTIN CONTRACEPTIVES. Oral contraceptives are the most frequently used method of hormonal contraception, and an almost bewildering variety are marketed (Table 32–3). Generic formulations have become more popular. In 1990, generic oral contraceptives accounted for only 3.6 percent of prescriptions, and by 2001, this value had increased to 18 percent (Keith and associates, 2001). Oral contraceptives typically consist of a combination of an estrogen and a progestational agent taken daily for 3 weeks and then omitted for 1 week, during which time there is withdrawal uterine bleeding. Longer durations of active hormone administration, designed to minimize the number of menses, have been investigated (Miller and Hughes, 2003). One such extended-cycle product—Seasonale—is now available in the United States.

Mechanisms of Action. The contraceptive actions of combination oral contraceptives are multiple, but the most important effect is to prevent ovulation by suppression of hypothalamic gonadotropin-releasing factors, which in turn prevents pituitary secretion of follicle-stimulating and luteinizing hormones. Progestin prevents ovulation by suppressing luteinizing hormone. Progestins also thicken cervical

TABLE 32–3 Oral Contraceptives Available in the United States

Product Name	Manufacturer	Estrogen Type	Estrogen Dose μg (days)	Progestin Type	Progestin Dose mg (days)[a]
Monophasic Preparations					
20 μg estrogen					
Alesse	Wyeth-Ayerst	EE	20	Levonorgestrel	0.10
Levlite	Berlex	EE	20	Levonorgestrel	0.10
Loestrin 1/20	Parke-Davis	EE	20	Norethindrone acetate	1.00
30–35 μg estrogen					
Desogen	Organon	EE	30	Desogestrel	0.15
Leven	Berlex	EE	30	Levonorgestrel	0.15
Levora	Watson	EE	30	Levonorgestrel	0.15
Lo/Ovral	Wyeth-Ayerst	EE	30	Norgestrel	0.30
Low-Ogestrel	SCS Pharmaceuticals	EE	30	Norgestrel	0.30
Nordette	Wyeth-Ayerst	EE	30	Levonorgestrel	0.15
Ortho-Cept	Ortho-McNeil	EE	30	Desogestrel	0.15
Brevicon	Searle	EE	35	Norethindrone	0.50
Demulen 1/35	Searle	EE	35	Ethynodiol diacetate	1.00
Loestrin 1.5/30	Parke-Davis	EE	30	Norethindrone acetate	1.50
Modicon	Ortho-McNeil	EE	35	Norethindrone	0.50
Necon 0.5/35	Watson	EE	35	Norethindrone	0.50
Necon 1/35	Watson	EE	35	Norethindrone	1.00
Nelova 0.5/35E	Warner Chilcott	EE	35	Norethindrone	0.50
Nelova 1/35E	Warner Chilcott	EE	35	Norethindrone	1.00
Norinyl 1 + 35	Searle	EE	35	Norethindrone	1.00
Ortho-Cyclen	Ortho-McNeil	EE	35	Norgestimate	0.25
Ortho-Novum 1/35	Ortho-McNeil	EE	35	Norethindrone	1.00
Ovcon-35	Bristol-Myers Squibb	EE	35	Norethindrone	0.40
Zovia 1/35E	Watson	EE	35	Ethynodiol diacetate	1.00
50 μg estrogen					
Ovral	Wyeth-Ayerst	EE	50	Norgestrel	0.50
Demulen 1/50	Searle	EE	50	Ethynodiol diacetate	1.00
Necon 1/50	Watson	Mes	50	Norethindrone	1.00
Nelova 1/50M	Warner Chilcott	Mes	50	Norethindrone	1.00
Norinyl 1 + 50	Searle	Mes	50	Norethindrone	1.00
Ortho-Novum 1/50	Ortho-McNeil	Mes	50	Norethindrone	1.00
Ovcon 50	Bristol-Myers Squibb	EE	50	Norethindrone	1.00
Zovia 1/50E	Watson	EE	50	Ethynodiol diacetate	1.00
Multiphasic Preparations					
20 μg estrogen					
Mircette	Organon	EE	20 (21) 0 (2) 10 (5)	Desogestrel	0.15
30–35 μg estrogen					
Ortho Tri-Cyclen	Ortho-McNeil	EE	35 (21)	Norgestimate	0.18 (7) 0.215 (7) 0.25 (7)
Ortho Tri-Cyclen Lo	Ortho-McNeil	EE	25 (21)	Norgestimate	0.18 (7) 0.215 (7) 0.25 (7)
Tri-Levlen	Berlex	EE	30 (6) 40 (5) 30 (10)	Levonorgestrel	0.05 (6) 0.075 (5) 0.125 (10)
Triphasil	Wyeth-Ayerst	EE	30 (6) 40 (5) 30 (10)	Levonorgestrel	0.05 (6) 0.075 (5) 0.125 (10)
Trivora	Watson	EE	30 (6) 40 (5) 30 (10)	Levonorgestrel	0.05 (6) 0.075 (5) 0.125 (10)

TABLE 32–3 Oral Contraceptives Available in the United States (Continued)

Product Name	Manufacturer	Estrogen Type	Estrogen Dose μg (days)	Progestin Type	Progestin Dose mg (days)[a]
Estrostep	Parke-Davis	EE	20 (5) 30 (7) 35 (9)	Norethindrone acetate	1.00
Jenest	Organon	EE	35 (21)	Norethindrone	0.50 (7) 1.00 (14)
Necon 10/11	Watson	EE	35 (21)	Norethindrone	0.50 (10) 1.00 (11)
Nelova 10/11	Warner Chilcott	EE	35 (21)	Norethindrone	0.50 (10) 1.00 (11)
Ortho-Novum 7/7/7	Ortho-McNeil	EE	35 (21)	Norethindrone	0.5 (7) 0.75 (7) 1.00 (7)
Tri-Norinyl	Searle	EE	35 (21)	Norethindrone	0.5 (7) 1.00 (9) 0.50 (5)
Progestin-Only Preparations					
Ovrette	Wyeth-Ayerst	None		Norgestrel	0.075 (c)
Micronor	Ortho-McNeil	None		Norethindrone	0.35 (c)
Nor-QD	Watson	None		Norethindrone	0.35 (c)
Extended-Cycle Preparation[b]					
Seasonale	Barr	EE	30 (84)	Levonorgestrel	0.15 (84)

EE = ethinyl estradiol; Mes = mestranol.
[a]Numbers in parentheses = number of days at a particular dose. (c) = continuous use.
[b]12 weeks of active pills, 1 week of inert pills.
Modified from Wallach and Grimes, 2000, with permission.

mucus, thereby retarding sperm passage. In addition, they render the endometrium unfavorable to implantation. Estrogen prevents ovulation by suppressing the release of follicle-stimulating hormone. A second effect is to stabilize the endometrium, which prevents breakthrough bleeding.

The net effect of estrogen and progestin is extremely effective ovulation suppression, inhibition of sperm migration through cervical mucus, and creation of an unfavorable endometrium for implantation. Thus, estrogen plus progestin containing combined oral contraceptives provide virtually absolute protection against conception *when taken daily for 3 out of every 4 weeks.*

Pharmacology. In the United States, the only *estrogens* available are *ethinyl estradiol* and much less commonly, its 3-methyl ether, *mestranol.* The exact conversion factor for potency of ethinyl estradiol to mestranol is not definitely known but probably is 1.2 to 1.5.

Almost all currently available *progestins* are 19-nortestosterone derivatives, and one is an aldosterone derivative. Although individual progestins are initially chosen because of their progestational potencies, they are often compared and prescribed based on their presumed estrogenic, antiestrogenic, and especially their androgenic effects. However, a scientific basis for such selective prescribing is lacking (Wallach and Grimes, 2000). All progestins reduce

serum free testosterone, and they inhibit 5α-reductase and the conversion of testosterone to its active metabolite, dihydrotestosterone. Thus, all progestins are expected to have salutary effects on androgen-related conditions such as acne (Wallach and Grimes, 2000).

Dosage. Since oral contraceptives have come into use, their estrogen and progestin contents have been reduced remarkably. This is important, because most adverse effects are dose related. The lowest acceptable dose is governed by the ability to prevent unacceptable breakthrough bleeding. Although daily estrogen content varies from 20 to 50 μg of ethinyl estradiol, the vast majority contain 35 μg or less (see Table 32–3). The amount of progestin varies in two ways:

1. Among older, well-evaluated formulations, the progestin dose remains constant during the cycle (*monophasic*).
2. In some newer preparations, the progestin (and in some, the estrogen) dose varies during the cycle (*biphasic and triphasic*).

Ideally, women should begin taking combination oral contraceptives on the first day of a menstrual cycle, in which case a back-up contraceptive method is unnecessary. The more traditional "Sunday start" during the first week of a menstrual cycle necessitates use of a back-up method for 1 week to ensure that conception does not occur.

To obtain maximum effectiveness and promote regular use, most suppliers offer dispensers that provide 21 sequentially and individually wrapped, color-coded tablets containing hormones, followed by seven inert tablets of another color. It is important for maximum contraceptive efficiency and for peace of mind that each woman adopt an effective scheme for ensuring daily (or nightly) self-administration. One technique is to keep a pill supply and toothbrush close to each other and to swallow a pill at tooth brushing time, either in the morning or in the evening. If one dose is missed, contraception is likely not minimized if higher-dose monophasic estrogen and progestin pills are used. It may be desirable to double the next dose to minimize breakthrough bleeding and to stay on schedule. If several doses are missed, or lower-dose pills are used, an effective barrier technique should be used. The pill may be restarted after withdrawal bleeding. Alternatively, a new pack can be started with a barrier method as back-up for a week. If withdrawal bleeding does not occur, the woman should continue to take the pills but seek medical attention to rule out pregnancy.

PHASIC PILLS. These preparations were developed in an effort to reduce the amount of total progestin per cycle without sacrificing contraceptive efficacy or cycle control. The reduction is achieved by beginning with a low dose of progestin and increasing it later in the contraceptive cycle. Theoretically, the lower total dose should result in fewer progestin-attributable metabolic changes and adverse side effects. Similarly, the estrogen dose may be kept constant or increased later in the cycle. In all phasic preparations, estrogen doses are between 20 and 40 μg of ethinyl estradiol (see Table 32–3).

Despite the advantages, both theoretical and actual, there are distinct disadvantages to triphasic formulations. These include confusion due to multicolored pills and breakthrough bleeding or spotting, which likely is increased compared with that of monophasic pills (Hatcher and colleagues, 1990; Woods and associates, 1992).

Drug Interactions. Oral contraceptives interfere with the actions of some drugs (Table 32–4). Conversely, some drugs decrease the contraceptive effectiveness of combination oral contraceptives (Table 32–5). Phenytoin and rifampin are believed to increase breakthrough bleeding and reduce contraceptive effectiveness of pills containing less than 50 μg of ethinyl estradiol (Hatcher and colleagues, 1998). Although package inserts for some broad-spectrum antimicrobials such as ampicillin and tetracycline warn that they may reduce the efficacy of oral contraceptives, this likely is not true. Because vitamin C competes for active sulfate in the intestinal wall and increases the bioavailability of ethinyl estradiol, erratic use of vitamin C can result in breakthrough bleeding (Kubba and Guillebaud, 1993).

TABLE 32–4 Drugs Whose Effectiveness Is Influenced by Combination Oral Contraceptives

Interacting Drug	Documentation	Management
Analgesics		
Acetaminophen	Adequate	Larger doses of analgesic may be required
Aspirin	Probable	Larger doses of analgesic may be required
Meperidine	Suspected	Smaller doses of analgesic may be required
Morphine	Probable	Larger doses of analgesic may be required
Anticoagulants		
Dicumarol, warfarin	Controversial	
Antidepressants		
Imipramine	Suspected	Decrease dose about a third
Tranquilizers		
Diazepam	Suspected	Decrease dose
Alprazolam		
Temazepam	Possible	May need to increase dose
Other benzodiazepines	Suspected	Observe for increased effect
Anti-inflammatories		
Corticosteroids	Adequate	Watch for potentiation of effects and decrease dose accordingly
Bronchodilators		
Aminophyline	Adequate	Reduce starting dose by a third
Theophylline		
Caffeine		
Antihypertensives		
Cyclopenthiazide	Adequate	Increase dose
Guanethidine		
Metoprolol	Suspected	May need to lower dose
Antimicrobials		
Troleandomycin	Suspected liver damage	Avoid
Cyclosporine	Possible	May use smaller dose

Adapted from Wallach and Grimes, 2000, with permission.

TABLE 32–5 Drugs That May Reduce Combined Oral Contraceptive Efficacy

Interacting Drug	Documentation
Antituberculous agent	
Rifampin	Established
Antifungal agent	
Griseofulvin	Strongly suspected
Anticonvulsants and sedatives	
Phenytoin, mephenytoin, phenobarbital, primidone, carbamazepine, ethosuximide	Strongly suspected; clinical trial data lacking
Antimicrobials	
Tetracycline, doxycycline	Two small studies find no association
Penicillins	No association documented
Ciprofloxacin	No effect on efficacy of a 30 μg ethinyl estradiol plus desogestrel oral contraceptive
Ofloxacin	No effect on efficacy of a 30 μg ethinyl estradiol plus levonorgestrel oral contraceptive

Adapted from Wallach and Grimes, 2000, with permission.

Safety. In general, oral contraceptives have proven to be safe for most women (see Table 32–1). The possibility of adverse effects from "the pill" has received so much attention for so long that the major negative health consequence among users may be the anxiety created by unbalanced media coverage! Unfortunately, physicians as well as the public are frequently confused by the many and often conflicting reports.

Beneficial Effects. When used reliably, there is no more effective rapidly reversible form of contraception than the combined estrogen plus progestin pill (see Table 32–2). Some of the associated noncontraceptive benefits include the following:

1. Increased bone density.
2. Reduced menstrual blood loss and anemia.
3. Decreased risk of ectopic pregnancy.
4. Improved dysmenorrhea from endometriosis.
5. Fewer premenstrual complaints.
6. Decreased risk of endometrial and ovarian cancer.
7. Reduction in various benign breast diseases.
8. Inhibition of hirsutism progression.
9. Improvement of acne.
10. Prevention of atherogenesis.
11. Decreased incidence and severity of acute salpingitis.
12. Improvement in rheumatoid arthritis.

Possible Adverse Effects. A number of metabolic changes, often qualitatively similar to those of pregnancy, have been identified in women taking oral contraceptives. For example, total plasma thyroxine and thyroid-binding proteins are elevated. Plasma cortisol concentration increases with a nearly comparable increase in transcortin. Therefore, it is extremely important that these pregnancy-like effects be considered when evaluating laboratory tests in women using oral contraceptives.

LIPOPROTEINS AND LIPIDS. In general, the combination oral contraceptives increase triglycerides and total cholesterol. Estrogen decreases the concentration of low-density lipoprotein cholesterol and increases high-density lipoprotein cholesterol. Some progestins cause the reverse (Stadel, 1981). Despite this, the clinical consequences of these perturbations have almost certainly been overstated (Hoppe, 1990). Oral contraceptives are not atherogenic, and their impact on lipids, irrespective of individual formulation, is inconsequential for the vast majority of women (Wallach and Grimes, 2000).

CARBOHYDRATE METABOLISM. With older, higher-dose oral contraceptive formulations, deterioration in glucose tolerance, mediated principally by the progestin component, was a legitimate clinical concern. With current formulations, such concern is no longer warranted (Speroff and Darney, 2001). In healthy women, large prospective studies with long-term follow-up have demonstrated that oral contraceptives do not increase the risk of diabetes (Hannaford and Kay, 1989; Rimm and associates, 1992). Moreover, oral contraceptives do not increase the risk that women with a history of gestational diabetes will progress to adult-onset diabetes (Kjos and colleagues, 1998).

PROTEIN METABOLISM. Estrogens increase hepatic production of a variety of *globulins.* Increased *angiotensinogen* production appears to be dose related, and its conversion by renin to angiotensin I has been suspected to be associated with so-called "pill-induced hypertension" (see p. 733). Fibrinogen, and likely factors II, VII, IX, X, XII, and XIII, are increased in direct proportion to estrogen dose (Comp, 1996; Kaunitz, 1999b). The relationship of these increased clotting factors to venous and arterial thrombosis is discussed on page 732. The incidence of both forms of thrombosis appears to be estrogen-dose related (Mann, 1982).

LIVER DISEASE. *Cholestasis* and *cholestatic jaundice* are uncommon complications in users of oral contraceptives. If they develop, signs and symptoms clear when the medication is stopped. It appears that oral contraceptives may accelerate the development of gallbladder disease in women who are susceptible, but there is no overall increased long-term risk (Royal College of General Practitioners, 1982; Strom and colleagues, 1986). There is no reason to withhold oral contraceptives from women who have recovered from viral hepatitis.

NEOPLASIA. **A stimulatory effect on some cancers is always a concern with female sex steroids.** However, a number of studies indicate that it is unlikely that hormonal contraception causes cancer (Cancer and Steroid Hormone Study, 1986, 1987a, 1987b; Prentice and Thomas, 1987; Schlesselman and colleagues, 1988). In fact, a protective effect against ovarian and endometrial cancer has been shown in these studies. However, there are conflicting reports concerning the risks of premalignant and malignant changes of the liver, cervix, and breast.

In the past, use of estrogen plus progestin contraceptives has been linked circumstantially with the development of *hepatic focal nodular hyperplasia* and benign hepatic *adenoma*. These associations were observed in women using high-dose estrogen-containing formulations for prolonged periods. Reassuringly, large studies conducted in women taking contemporary low-dose oral contraceptives do not support an association with hepatic adenoma (Hannaford and associates, 1997; Heinemann and colleagues, 1998). Finally, an association between prolonged oral contraceptive use and *hepatocellular carcinoma* in women younger than 50 years of age was reported (Neuberger and associates, 1986). In contrast, conclusions derived from a multicenter World Health Organization study (1989) support the view that there is no increased risk.

There is a correlation between the risk of *cervical dysplasia* and oral contraceptive use, and the risk of invasive cancer increases after 5 years of use (Thomas and Ray, 1996; Vessey and associates, 1983b; Zondervan and co-workers, 1996). It is unclear if these associations have a causal basis. For example, oral contraceptive users are not protected from exposure to human papillomavirus, and they are more frequently screened cytologically for cervical cancer. Thus, they may be more likely to be diagnosed with dysplasia (Butterworth and associates, 1992).

In addition, it is unclear whether oral contraceptives contribute to the development of *breast cancer.* In the largest study, there was no increased risk for breast cancer among oral contraceptive users (Cancer and Steroid Hormone Study, 1986). Moreover, risk did not vary according to preparation or duration of use. The Collaborative Group on Hormonal Factors in Breast Cancer (1996) reanalyzed data from 54 studies that included more than 53,000 women with breast cancer and more than 100,000 without the disease. The study found a small but significantly increased relative risk of breast

cancer in women who were taking combined oral contraceptives or who had stopped within 10 years. The relative risk was 1.24 for current users, 1.16 for those 1 to 4 years after stopping, and 1.07 for those 5 to 9 years after stopping. The risk was not influenced by age at first use, duration of use, family history of breast cancer, first use prior to pregnancy, or the dose or type of hormone used. The lack of correlation with these factors calls into question the causal nature of the association. In this study, tumors associated with oral contraceptive use tended to be to be less aggressive and to be detected at an earlier stage, a finding consistent with the possibility that the increased risk of breast cancer was due to greater surveillance among users. In a recent case-control study (4575 cases and 4682 controls), there was no relationship between either current or past oral contraceptive use and breast cancer (Marchbanks and colleagues, 2002).

NUTRITION. Aberrations in the levels of several *nutrients,* similar to changes induced by normal pregnancy, have been described for women who use oral contraceptives. Lower plasma levels in users compared with those in nonusers have been described by some investigators for ascorbic acid, folic acid, vitamin B_6 (pyridoxine), vitamin B_{12}, niacin, riboflavin, and zinc. An adequate diet, however, is sufficient prophylaxis against any detrimental deficiency (Mooij and co-workers, 1991).

CARDIOVASCULAR EFFECTS. A number of infrequent but significant cardiovascular risks are associated with hormonal contraceptive use.

The risk of *deep vein thrombosis* and *pulmonary embolism* is increased in women who use oral contraceptives (Realini and Goldzieher, 1985; Stadel, 1981). These risks clearly are estrogen-dose related and are decreased with the use of formulations containing 20 to 35 μg of ethinyl estradiol (Westhoff, 1998). Mishell (2000) performed a scholarly evidence-based review of the risks of venous thromboembolism in oral contraceptive users. After analyzing six epidemiologically sound studies, he estimated that the risk is increased three- to fourfold in users but not in former users. Importantly, the baseline risk is low—about 1 per 10,000 woman-years—and thus the incidence with oral contraceptives of 3.0 to 4.0 per 10,000 woman-years is still quite low. Once again, the risk is clearly lower than the incidence of 5.7 per 10,000 woman-years estimated for pregnancy.

The enhanced risk of thromboembolism appears to decrease rapidly once the contraceptive is stopped. Women who develop thromboembolism while taking estrogen-containing contraceptives, however, also appear to be at increased risk during pregnancy and the early puerperium. Those most at risk for venous thrombosis and embolism include women with protein C or S deficiencies (Comp, 1996). Other clinical factors that increase the risk of venous thrombosis and embolism are hypertension, obesity, diabetes, smoking, and a sedentary lifestyle (Hatcher and associates, 1998).

Contraceptive use during the month before a major operative procedure appears to increase the risk of postoperative thromboembolism significantly.

According to the World Health Organization Collaborative Study (1998), *ischemic and hemorrhagic strokes* are uncommon in nonsmoking women younger than 35 years of age. Their incidence is 10 and 24 events per 1 million woman years, respectively. The earlier reports by Lidegaard and colleagues (1993, 1998) that the risk of cerebral thromboembolism was increased in women using low-dose estrogen contraceptives stimulated a number of focused studies. At least five subsequent studies concluded that the use of such compounds by healthy, nonsmoking women is not associated with an increased risk of thrombotic or hemorrhagic strokes (Mishell, 2000; Petitti and co-workers, 1996; Schwartz and associates, 1998; World Health Organization Collaborative Study, 1996). Conversely, women who have hypertension, smoke, or have migraine headaches *and* use oral contraceptives have an increased risk of strokes (Mishell, 2000; Schwartz and colleagues, 1998).

An association between oral contraceptives and *hypertension* was apparent by the late 1960s. Several reports appeared of the occasional woman who, while using an estrogen–progestin oral contraceptive, became overtly hypertensive. Usually blood pressure returned to normal when the medication was stopped. Oral contraceptives, presumably the estrogen component, were shown to increase plasma angiotensinogen (renin substrate) to levels near those found in normal pregnancy. Although the great majority of women using oral contraceptives demonstrate these changes, most do not become hypertensive. Current low-dose oral contraceptive formulations rarely, if ever, cause clinically significant hypertension (Blumenstein, 1980; Chasan-Taber and colleagues, 1996; Kovacs, 1986; Nichols, 1993, and their co-workers). Most certainly, the development of hypertension during pregnancy does not preclude subsequent use of oral contraceptives.

Oral contraceptives containing low-dose estrogen and low-androgenic progestins are not associated with an increased risk of *myocardial infarction* in nonsmokers (Lewis, 1996; Mishell, 2000; Petitti, 1998; Sidney, 1996, 1998; World Health Organization Collaborative Study, 1997, and all their colleagues). In fact, the American College of Obstetricians and Gynecologists (2000b) states there is no contraindication to oral contraceptives in nonsmoking women older than 35 years of age. Finally, the Food and Drug Administration (FDA) revised their labeling of oral contraceptives to remove restrictions for nonsmoking women older than 40 years of age. It is important to recognize that smoking is an independent risk factor for myocardial infarction, and that smoking and oral contraceptives act synergistically to increase this risk, especially beyond 35 years of age (Craft and Hannaford, 1989).

Oral contraceptives have no predictable effect on the frequency or severity of *migraine headaches*. They may, however, add to the already increased risk of stroke faced by women with migraine headaches and neurological symptoms or aura (Chang and associates, 1999). Therefore, most clinicians prefer to avoid combined oral contraceptives in such women, although in certain women, the risks of pregnancy may warrant their use. For other woman with migraine headaches, a progestin-only pill may be more appropriate, because it does not increase the risk of stroke (Speroff and Darney, 2001).

Effects on Reproduction. *Postpill amenorrhea* after combination contraception discontinuation is likely reflective of a preexisting problem (Wallach and Grimes, 2000). At least 90 percent of women who previously ovulated regularly begin to do so within 3 months after discontinuance of oral contraceptives.

There is no evidence that estrogen–progestin preparations are teratogenic. Rothman and Louik (1978) and Savolainen and associates (1981) found no increase in major malformations in infants whose mothers had used oral contraceptives during conception. Similarly, Lammer and Cordero (1986) found no association between major malformations and contraceptive exposure in early pregnancy (see Chap. 14, p. 361).

LACTATION. Data concerning the interaction of combination oral contraceptives and lactation are limited. Very small quantities of the hormones are excreted in breast milk, but no adverse effects on infants have been noted. There is concern that these agents reduce the volume of breast milk, although a recent review confirms the ambiguity of these data (Truitt and colleagues, 2003). Because progestin-only oral contraceptives have little effect on lactation and provide excellent contraception, they are preferred for up to 6 months in women who are breast feeding their infants exclusively (see p. 746). A woman who is breast feeding only intermittently should use effective contraception beginning as soon as 3 weeks postpartum (Kaunitz, 1997).

Other Effects. *Cervical mucorrhea,* likely due to cervical ectopy, is fairly common in response to the estrogen component (Critchlow and colleagues, 1995). The mucus at times may be irritating to the vagina and vulva. *Vaginitis* or *vulvovaginitis,* especially that caused by *Candida,* also may develop.

Hyperpigmentation of the face and forehead (also known as *chloasma*) is more likely in women who demonstrated such a change during pregnancy (see Chap. 56, p. 1250). This is seen much less commonly with the transition to low-dose estrogen formulations. As discussed, low-dose oral contraceptives may improve acne.

Uterine *myomas* do not increase in size with oral contraceptive use (Wise and colleagues, 2004). Although *weight gain* is reported as a side effect by some women, low-dose oral contraceptives do not promote an appreciable weight increase (Gallo and associates, 2004). Low-dose estrogen

TABLE 32–6 **Contraindications and Warnings About the Use of Combination Oral Contraceptives**

CONTRAINDICATIONS: Combination contraceptives should not be used in women with:
Thrombophlebitis or thromboembolic disorders
History of deep vein thrombophlebitis or thrombotic disorders
Cerebrovascular or coronary artery disease
Thrombogenic cardiac valvulopathies
Thrombogenic heart arrhythmias
Diabetes with vascular involvement
Uncontrolled hypertension
Known or suspected breast carcinoma
Carcinoma of the endometrium or other known or suspected estrogen-dependent neoplasia
Undiagnosed abnormal genital bleeding
Cholestatic jaundice of pregnancy or jaundice with pill use
Hepatic adenomas or carcinomas, or active liver disease as long as liver function has not returned to normal
Known or suspected pregnancy

WARNINGS:
Cigarette smoking increases the risk of serious cardiovascular side effects from oral contraceptive use. This risk increases with age and with the extent of smoking (in epidemiological studies, smoking 15 or more cigarettes per day was associated with a significantly increased risk) and is quite marked in women older than 35 years of age. Women who use oral contraceptives should be strongly advised not to smoke.

From Physicians Desk Reference, 2004.

formulations are not associated with *depression,* and indeed, may cause it to improve (Goldzeiher and Zamah, 1995; Vessey and associates, 1985).

Multiple studies have been conducted to evaluate the relationship between the use of oral and injectable contraceptives and the risk of *HIV infection.* Although most of these have methodological limitations, on balance they do not suggest increased risk (Stephenson, 1998). On the other hand, hormonal contraception does not *prevent* the transmission of HIV infection or any other viral infection.

Risk of Death. Mortality associated with oral contraceptives is very low if the woman is younger than 35 years of age, has no systemic illness, and does not smoke (see Table 32–1). Porter and associates (1987) reported only one death attributed to oral contraceptive use in nearly 55,000 woman-years from the Group Health Cooperative of Puget Sound.

Postpartum Use. Women who do not breast feed, especially those who have undergone an abortion, may ovulate before 6 weeks after pregnancy (see Chap. 30, p. 701). There is an advantage, therefore, to starting oral contraceptives before the traditional "6-week postpartum check." On the other hand, increased risks of adverse effects, especially venous thromboembolism, might be anticipated from use of estrogen–progestin contraceptives earlier in the puerperium. The use of 35 μg or smaller estrogen doses has reduced this risk greatly. Thus far, in our now extensive experience in which oral contraceptives have been started during the third week postpartum, there has been no evidence of increased morbidity or mortality.

Contraindications. It could be argued that because pregnancy is usually more dangerous than oral contraception, then no contraindication to oral contraceptives should be considered absolute. Pragmatically, considering the multiplicity of alternative contraceptive methods, if a contraindication listed in Table 32–6 is present, combined oral contraceptive pills should probably not be prescribed or used.

Transdermal Administration. The recently approved patch (Evra) is applied to the buttocks, upper outer arm, lower abdomen, or upper torso but avoiding the breasts (Fig. 32–2). It delivers 150 μg of the progestin norelgestromin and 20 μg of ethinyl estradiol daily. A new patch is applied weekly for 3 weeks, followed by a patch-free week to allow for withdrawal bleeding.

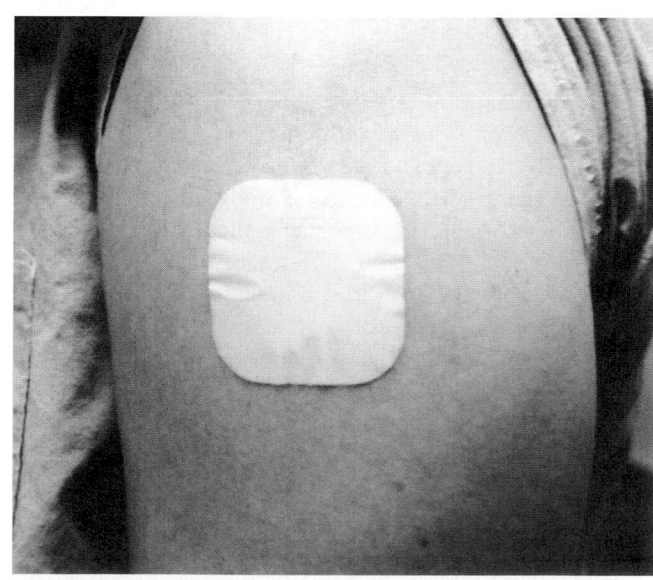

FIGURE 32–2. Evra transdermal contraceptive patch.

Audet and co-workers (2001) found that the patch was slightly more effective than a low-dose oral contraceptive in preventing pregnancy—1.2 versus 2.2 pregnancies per 100 woman-years. Although the patch was well tolerated and safe overall, dysmenorrhea, breast tenderness, and breakthrough bleeding in the first two cycles were more frequent in the women who received the patch. Almost 5 percent of the patches required replacement for either complete (1.8 percent) or partial (2.8 percent) detachment. In about 3 percent of women, the patch caused an application site reaction severe enough to limit usage.

Data suggest that woman who weigh 90 kg or more who use the patch are at increased risk for contraceptive failure. Of 15 failures reported, five women met this threshold, even though they constituted less than 3 percent of the study population (Zieman and associates, 2002). This translates to a relative risk of failure of 16 or more. This may also reflect a phenomenon general to hormone contraceptives as Holt and colleagues (2002) reported that obesity increases the chance of failure.

Therefore, the patch seems to provide an effective alternative hormonal contraceptive method for women who prefer weekly application rather than daily dosing, find the transdermal method of delivery acceptable, and weigh less than 90 kg. Its metabolic and physiological effects should be substantively the same as with low-dose oral contraceptives, although the accumulated experience with the patch is small compared with that of combination oral contraceptives.

Transvaginal Administration. In 2001, the FDA approved for use an intravaginal hormonal contraceptive ring (NuvaRing). This flexible polymer ring has an outer diameter of 54 mm and an inner diameter of 50 mm (Fig. 32–3). The core of this ring contains ethinyl estradiol and the progestin etonogestrel, which are released at rates of 15 μg and 120 μg per day, respectively. Although this release results

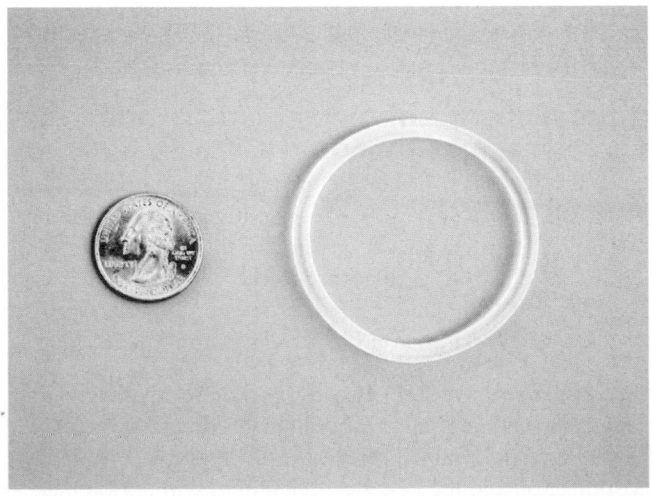

FIGURE 32–3. NuvaRing: estrogen-progestin-releasing vaginal contraceptive ring.

in systemic hormone levels lower than comparable low-dose oral contraceptive formulations, ovulation inhibition is complete (Mulders and Dieben, 2001). The ring is highly effective, and in one study, the failure rate was 0.65 per 100 woman-years (Roumen and colleagues, 2001).

The ring is placed within 5 days of the onset of menses and is removed after 3 weeks of use for 1 week to allow withdrawal bleeding. Breakthrough bleeding is uncommon. Almost 20 percent of women and 35 percent of men reported being able to feel the ring during intercourse. If this is bothersome, the ring may be removed for intercourse but should be replaced within 3 hours. Before dispensing, the rings are refrigerated, and once dispensed, their shelf life is 4 months (Burkman, 2002).

PROGESTATIONAL CONTRACEPTIVES

Oral Progestins. So-called *mini-pills* are oral progestin-only contraceptives that are taken daily. Unlike combined oral contraceptives, they do not reliably inhibit ovulation. Rather, their effectiveness depends more on alterations in cervical mucus and effects on the endometrium. Because the mucus changes do not last longer than 24 hours, mini-pills should be taken at the same time every day to be maximally effective. These contraceptives have not achieved widespread popularity because of a much higher incidence of irregular bleeding and a somewhat higher pregnancy rate than combined contraceptives (see Table 32–2). Improved effectiveness has been reported for married and, in a progressive fashion, older women (Guillebaud, 1985).

BENEFITS. Progestin-only pills have minimal if any effect on carbohydrate metabolism or coagulation, and they do not cause or exacerbate hypertension. They may be ideal for some women who are at increased risk of cardiovascular complications. This includes women with a history of thrombosis, hypertension, or migraine headaches, or who are older than 35 years of age and who smoke. The mini-pill is often an excellent choice for lactating women. In combination with breast feeding, it is virtually 100 percent effective for up to 6 months and does not impair milk production (Betrabet and colleagues, 1987; Shikary and associates, 1987).

DISADVANTAGES. The major drawback of progestin-only pills is contraceptive failure. With these failures, there is a relative increase in the proportion of ectopic pregnancies (Sivin, 1991). Irregular uterine bleeding is another distinct disadvantage and may manifest as amenorrhea, spotting, breakthrough bleeding, or prolonged periods of amenorrhea or menorrhagia. Functional ovarian cysts develop with a greater frequency in women using these agents, although they do not usually necessitate intervention.

A distinct disadvantage is that these contraceptives must be taken at the same or nearly the same time daily (Guillebaud, 1985). **If a progestin-only pill is taken even 4 hours**

TABLE 32–7 Medications That Contraindicate Progestin-Only Oral Contraceptives

Carbamazepine (Tegretol)
Felbamate
Oxcarbazepine
Phenobarbital
Phenytoin (Dilantin)
Primidone (Mysoline)
Rifabutin
Rifampicin (Rifampin)
Topiramate
Vigabatrin
Possibly ethosuximide, griseofulvin, and troglitazone

From Speroff and Darney, 2001, with permission.

late, a **back-up form of contraception must be used for the next 48 hours.** Also, their effectiveness is decreased by the medications shown in Table 32–7. Women taking any of these medications should not use this form of contraception. Finally, unlike combined oral contraceptives, the mini-pill does not improve acne and may even worsen it in some women.

CONTRAINDICATIONS. Progestin-only pills are contraindicated in women with unexplained uterine bleeding, especially in older women.

Injectable Progestin Contraceptives. Depot medroxyprogesterone acetate (Depo-Provera) and norethindrone ethanthate (Norgest) have been used effectively worldwide for many years. Depo-Provera was approved for contraceptive use in the United States in 1992. Norgest is not yet available. The mechanisms of action of both drugs are multiple and similar to those for oral administration. They include ovulation inhibition, increased viscosity of cervical mucus, and stimulation of an endometrium unfavorable for ovum implantation (Mishell, 1996).

Depot medroxyprogesterone is injected deeply into the upper outer quadrant of the buttock without massage to ensure that the drug is released slowly. The usual dose is 150 mg every 90 days. An additional contraceptive method should be used for at least 2 weeks after the initial injection.

BENEFITS AND DISADVANTAGES. Injected progestins have contraceptive effectiveness comparable with or better than combined oral contraceptives, a long duration of action, and minimal to no impairment of lactation (American College of Obstetricians and Gynecologists, 2000a). Iron-deficiency anemia is less likely in long-term users, probably as a result of amenorrhea which develops after 5 years in 80 percent of women (Gardner and Mishell, 1970).

The principal disadvantages of depot progestins include irregular menstrual bleeding and prolonged anovulation after discontinuation, resulting in delayed fertility resumption. Cromer and associates (1994) reported that one fourth of women discontinued its use in the first year because of

irregular bleeding. After the injections are stopped, one fourth of women do not resume regular menses for up to 1 year (Gardner and Mishell, 1970).

The reported risks of breast cancer are conflicting. Skegg and colleagues (1995) pooled the results of the New Zealand and World Health Organization case-control studies. These studies included almost 1800 women with breast cancer and 14,000 controls. Within the first 5 years of use, the contraceptive was associated with a twofold risk of cancer, but overall the risk was not increased. Cervical and hepatic malignancy does not appear to be increased, and the risk of ovarian and endometrial cancers is decreased (Earl and David, 1994; Kaunitz, 1996). The risk of cervical carcinoma in situ may be increased (Thomas and colleagues, 1995).

Although weight gain is often attributed to Depo-Provera, conclusive evidence is lacking (Mainwaring, 1995; Moore, 1995; Taneepanichskul, 1998, and their associates). Breast tenderness is reported by some users, as is depression, although a causal link for the latter has not been demonstrated.

In long-term users of depot medroxyprogesterone, loss of bone mineral density is a potential problem (Scholes and colleagues, 1999). This concern is probably most relevant for teenagers because bone density increases most rapidly from 10 to 30 years of age (Cromer and colleagues, 1996; Sulak and Kaunitz, 1999). Reassuringly, bone loss appears to be reversible after discontinuation of therapy (Cundy and colleagues, 1994).

Progestin Implants (Norplant System). This system provides levonorgestrel in six silastic containers that are implanted subdermally. Its contraceptive effectiveness persists for 60 months, at which point the system should be removed (Hatcher and colleagues, 1998). Despite the effectiveness, safety, and patient satisfaction with this excellent contraceptive, its use waned dramatically in the United States after becoming the target of personal injury lawyers. Based on spurious allegations such as "illness" related to the silicone in the rods, a climate of litigation developed around this system, and currently, it is no longer available. A fund has been established by the manufacturer to ensure medical access for removal.

INJECTABLE MEDROXYPROGESTERONE ACETATE/ESTRADIOL CYPIONATE. This agent, marketed under the trade name Lunelle, contains 25 mg of medroxyprogesterone acetate plus 5 mg of estradiol cypionate (Kaunitz, 1999a). One injection is given monthly. Oettinger and associates (2005) described preliminary good results with subcutaneously implanted estradiol pellets (25 mg) in various numbers and norethindrone-induced withdrawal bleeding.

Mechanism of Action. The drug inhibits ovulation and suppresses endometrial proliferation (Aedo and co-workers, 1985). Estradiol values reach a peak level by 3 to 4 days postinjection and then decline, leading to withdrawal bleeding 20 to 25 days after injection (Garceau and colleagues, 2000).

Effectiveness. Only six method failures in 70,000 woman-years of use have been reported (Hall and co-workers, 1994). This is an effectiveness similar to that seen following female sterilization procedures.

Advantages and Disadvantages. Return to fertility after discontinuation is more rapid compared with depot progestins. Almost 85 percent of women who attempt pregnancy conceive within 12 months of discontinuation (Kaunitz, 1999a). Breakthrough bleeding occurs less often, but amenorrhea is more frequent than with oral contraceptives (Garceau and colleagues, 2000). After 3 months, bleeding irregularities appear to be less common than with depot progesterone injections (Kaunitz, 1999a).

Monthly injections are a drawback for some women. The interval between injections should not exceed 33 days. Other effects are similar to those for depot medroxyprogesterone injections (Cuong and My Huong, 1996; Sang and colleagues, 1995; World Health Organization, 1988, 1993). Because of its estrogen component, Lunelle is likely to decrease lactation, and depot progestin may be a better choice for the woman who is breast feeding. Injectable estrogen–progestin contraception may promote weight gain. In one comparative trial, combination oral contraceptives were associated with no weight gain at one year, compared with 2 to 8 lb with Lunelle (Kaunitz and colleagues, 1999).

Metabolic Effects. Perturbations in the coagulation system with Lunelle are minimal and likely of no clinical consequence. There have been no reports of stroke, thromboembolic events, anaphylaxis, or myocardial infarction (Kaunitz, 1999a). Although slight variations in lipid values have been reported, they have not been clinically important (Nelson, 2000). No studies of bone density have as yet been reported.

Contraindications. These are similar to those for combined oral contraceptives as shown in Table 32–6. Although still FDA-approved, this method has not been available in the United States since late 2002 because of manufacturing problems.

MECHANICAL METHODS OF CONTRACEPTION

INTRAUTERINE DEVICES. At one time in the United States, approximately 7 percent of sexually active women used an intrauterine device (IUD) for contraception. The two devices currently approved for use in this country are shown in Figure 32–4. Unwanted pregnancies during the first year of perfect use are 0.6 percent for the copper-containing ParaGard T 380A and 0.1 percent for the levonorgestrel-containing Mirena. Respective typical failure rates are 0.8 percent and 0.1 percent.

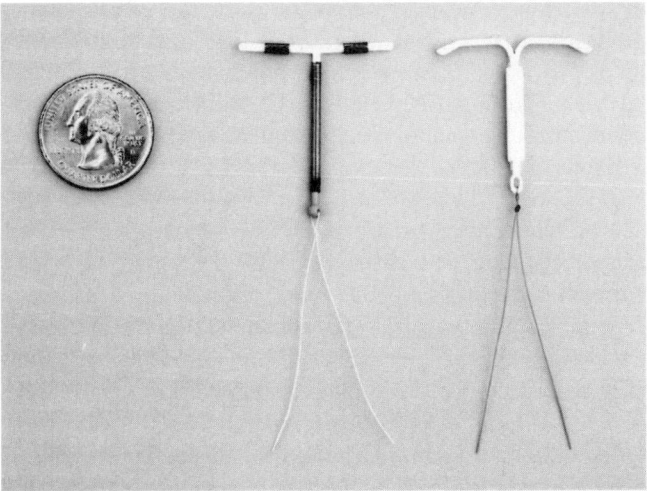

FIGURE 32–4. Intrauterine contraceptive devices available in 2004: Copper-containing ParaGard T 380A (*left*) and levonorgestrel-releasing Mirena (*right*). (Courtesy of Ortho Pharmaceutical, Raritan, NJ, and Berlex Laboratories, Montvale, NJ.)

With new information on safety, the IUD is once again gaining in popularity for several reasons:

1. Both ParaGard and Mirena are "use and forget" effective reversible contraceptive methods that do not have to be replaced for 10 and 5 years, respectively.
2. It is now better established that the major actions of IUDs are contraceptive, not abortifacient.
3. The risk of pelvic infections is markedly reduced with the currently used monofilament string and with techniques to ensure safer insertion.
4. The risk of an associated ectopic pregnancy has been clarified. Specifically, the contraceptive effect decreases the absolute number of ectopic pregnancies by about 50 percent compared with that of women not using contraception (World Health Organization, 1985, 1987). With failure, however, pregnancy is more likely to be ectopic (Furlong, 2002).
5. Legal liability appears to be less because the FDA currently classifies available IUDs as drugs (Mishell and Sulak, 1997). As such, the manufacturers must provide product information to be read by women prior to insertion. Signed consent forms that include a reasonable list of risks and benefits are also required.

Types of Intrauterine Devices. IUDs that are *chemically inert* are composed of a nonabsorbable material, most often polyethylene, and impregnated with barium sulfate for radiopacity. IUDs that are *chemically active* have continuous elution of copper or a progestational agent. At the present time, only chemically active IUDs are available.

LEVONORGESTREL DEVICE (MIRENA). This device releases levonorgestrel into the uterus at a relatively constant rate of 20 μg/day, which reduces the systemic effects of the progestin. It is a T-shaped polyethylene structure that has its stem wrapped with a cylinder of polydimethylsiloxane/levonorgestrel mixture (see Fig. 32–4). A permeable membrane surrounds the mixture to regulate the rate of hormone release.

COPPER DEVICE (PARAGARD T 380A). This device is composed of polyethylene and barium sulfate. The stem is wound with 314 mm^2 of fine copper wire, and the arms each have 33-mm^2 copper bracelets, thus totaling 380 mm^2 of copper. Two strings extend from the base of the stem (see Fig. 32–4). Originally blue, the strings are now off-white.

Mechanisms of Action. These mechanisms have not been defined precisely and are the subject of ongoing controversy. Interference with successful implantation of the fertilized ovum, which at one time was believed to be the main mode of action, is less important than prevention of fertilization (Mishell and Sulak, 1997; Stanford and Mikolajczyk, 2002). The intense local inflammatory response induced in the uterus, especially by copper-containing devices, leads to lysosomal activation and other inflammatory actions that are spermicidal (Alvarez and associates, 1988; Ortiz and Croxatto, 1987). In the unlikely event that fertilization does occur, the same inflammatory actions are directed against the blastocyst. Finally, the endometrium is transformed into a hostile site for implantation.

In long-time users of progestin devices, the endometrium becomes atrophic. There may be a major effect in preventing fertilization by spermicidal action, speeding ovum transport through the fallopian tube, or both (Alvarez and co-workers, 1988; Ortiz and Croxatto, 1987). The progestin may interfere with sperm penetration through thickened cervical mucus, and it inhibits ovulation, but not consistently (Nilsson and colleagues, 1984).

Effectiveness. IUDs have 1-year continuation rates equal to those of oral contraceptives. This almost certainly is due to the effectiveness of IUDs and a once-only approach to contraception. Their effectiveness is similar overall to that of tubal sterilization (American College of Obstetricians and Gynecologists, 2003a). Importantly, the unintended pregnancy rate decreases progressively after the first year of use (Vessey and associates, 1983a). The levonorgestrel-containing Mirena has a typical-user failure rate of 0.1 percent, which is lower than that of the copper-containing ParaGard (Rowe, 1992).

Other Beneficial Effects. The Mirena device reduces menstrual blood loss and can even be used to treat menorrhagia. Moreover, reduced blood loss is often associated with a reduction in dysmenorrhea. Overall, despite the higher upfront costs of IUDs, extended use makes their long-term cost-effectiveness competitive with other forms of contraception.

Women with contraindications to combination oral contraceptives can often use these devices. The device is also reported to reduce the incidence of pelvic infections and to be useful for women with uterine fibroids (Toivonen and associates, 1991; van den Hurk and O'Brien, 1999).

Adverse Effects. Numerous complications have been described with use of various IUDs. For the most part, however, common side effects have not been serious, and serious side effects have not been common. Moreover, with extended use and advancing user age, unintended pregnancy, expulsion, and bleeding complications decrease in frequency.

UTERINE PERFORATION AND ABORTION. The earliest adverse effects are those associated with insertion. They include clinically apparent or silent *uterine perforation,* which occurs while sounding the uterus or during insertion. Another adverse effect is *abortion of an unsuspected pregnancy.* The frequency of these complications depends on operator skill and the precautions taken to detect pregnancy. Perforations occur at a rate of approximately 1 per 1000 insertions (World Health Organization, 1987). Although devices may migrate spontaneously into and through the uterine wall, most perforations occur, or at least begin, at the time of insertion.

UTERINE CRAMPING AND BLEEDING. *Cramping* and some *bleeding* are common soon after insertion. These persist for variable periods. Cramping can be minimized by administering a nonsteroidal anti-inflammatory agent approximately 1 hour prior to insertion. The occasional increase in cramping with menses is controlled in a similar manner.

MENORRHAGIA. *Menstrual blood loss* is commonly doubled with use of the ParaGard device, and this may cause iron-deficiency anemia. Most providers measure hemoglobin concentration or hematocrit annually. Menorrhagia is a troubling side effect, and approximately 10 to 15 percent of women using the copper device have it removed because of this problem (Hatcher and associates, 1998). In contrast, the Mirena device is associated with progressive amenorrhea, which is reported by 30 percent of women after 2 years and by 60 percent after 12 years (Ronnerdag and Odlind, 1999).

INFECTION. A variety of *pelvic infections,* in some cases fatal, have been described with IUDs. These include *septic abortion,* which mandates immediate curettage. *Tubo-ovarian abscesses*—sometimes unilateral—have been described. With suspected infection, the IUD should be removed, and the woman treated with effective antimicrobials. Because of the risk of severe pelvic infections and sterility, IUD use has historically been discouraged for women younger than 25 years of age or those of low parity. According to Vessey and associates (1983a), prolonged impairment of fertility is not observed after removing the device from parous women. Long-term use by nulliparous women, however, has been associated with some degree of subfertility (Doll and co-workers, 2001). Even so, nulliparous women in mutually monogamous relationships may safely use the IUD (Speroff and Darney, 2001). That said, Lee and Rubin (1988) reported that married women and those with only one sexual partner had no higher risk of developing pelvic infection than controls *after* the first 4 months of use.

The major risk of infection is at the time of insertion and does not increase with long-term use. There is a small increased risk of pelvic infection for up to the first 20 days following insertion (Farley and associates, 1992). There currently is no consensus whether antimicrobial administration at the time of insertion reduces the incidence of infection (Sinei, 1990; Walsh, 1998, and their associates). Because of this, the American College of Obstetricians and Gynecologists (2001a) does not recommend prophylaxis with insertion. Long-term use of current IUDs is associated with pelvic infection rates comparable with those associated with oral contraceptives. Any infection after 45 to 60 days should be considered sexually transmitted and appropriately treated.

Actinomyces-like structures identified in Papanicolaou smears and the prolonged use of IUDs have been linked. Fiorino (1996) cited an incidence of 7 percent of *Actinomyces* seen on cytology smears from users of IUDs compared with less than 1 percent in nonusers. The clinical importance of this finding is not clear. In most studies, an increased prevalence of *Actinomyces israelii* or similar organisms was apparent only after several years. Women who developed a pelvic abscess caused by this organism had used the device for a mean of 8 years before symptoms developed.

In the absence of symptoms, the incidental finding of actinomyces by cytology is problematic. Because antimicrobial therapy is not effective with the IUD in place, some clinicians choose to remove the device, although there is no evidence that this prevents infection (Fiorino, 1996). Most clinicians agree, however, that if signs or symptoms of infection develop in women who harbor actinomyces, the device should be removed and antimicrobial therapy instituted.

Pregnancy with a Device In Utero. It is important to identify all pregnant women who might be using an IUD. For up to about 14 weeks, the tail of the device may be visible through the cervix, and if it can be seen, it should be removed. This action reduces subsequent complications such as late abortion, sepsis, and preterm birth. Tatum and co-workers (1976) reported the abortion rate to be 54 percent with the device left in place compared with one of 25 percent if it was promptly removed. Moreover, if the device remained, the frequency of low birthweight, chiefly from preterm delivery, was 20 percent, compared with that of about 5 percent if removed. Vessey and associates (1979) confirmed these observations. If the tail of the device is not visible, attempts to locate and remove the device may result in abortion, although some practitioners have successfully used ultrasonography to assist in the removal of devices without visible strings. After fetal viability has been reached, it is unclear whether it is better to remove an IUD in which the string is visible or leave it in place; both pro and con arguments can be made. Fetal malformations have not been reported to be increased with a device in place.

Second-trimester abortion with an IUD in place is more likely to be septic than one without an IUD (Lewit, 1970; Vessey and associates, 1974). Sepsis may be fulminant and is often fatal. Because of these risks, the woman should be offered the option of pregnancy termination. Women pregnant with a device in utero who demonstrate any evidence of uterine infection are treated with intensive antimicrobial therapy and prompt uterine evacuation. In women who give birth with a device in place, appropriate steps should be taken at delivery to identify it and ensure its removal.

Ectopic Pregnancies. Although the IUD prevents most intrauterine pregnancies, the device provides less protection against extrauterine nidation (Furlong, 2002).

Contraindications. Manufacturers' contraindications to the use of the IUD are listed in Table 32–8. Because the progestin

TABLE 32–8 Contraindications to Use of an Intrauterine Device

General
Pregnancy or suspicion of pregnancy
Abnormalities of the uterus resulting in distortion of the uterine cavity
Acute pelvic inflammatory disease or a history of pelvic inflammatory disease
Postpartum endometritis or infected abortion in the past 3 months
Known or suspected uterine or cervical malignancy, including unresolved, abnormal Pap smear
Genital bleeding of unknown etiology
Untreated acute cervicitis or vaginitis, as well as bacterial vaginosis, until infection is controlled
Patient or her partner has multiple sexual partners
Conditions associated with increased susceptibility to infections with microorganisms. These include, but are not limited to, leukemia, acquired immunodeficiency syndrome (AIDS), and intravenous drug abuse.
Genital actinomycosis
A previously inserted intrauterine device (IUD) that has not been removed

Specific
ParaGard T 380A is contraindicated when one or more of the following conditions exist (because of its copper content):
Wilson disease
Copper allergy
Mirena insertion is contraindicated when one or more of the following conditions exist:
Hypersensitivity to any component of this product
Known or suspected carcinoma of the breast
History of ectopic pregnancy or condition that would predispose to ectopic pregnancy

Modified from Physicians Desk Reference, 2004.

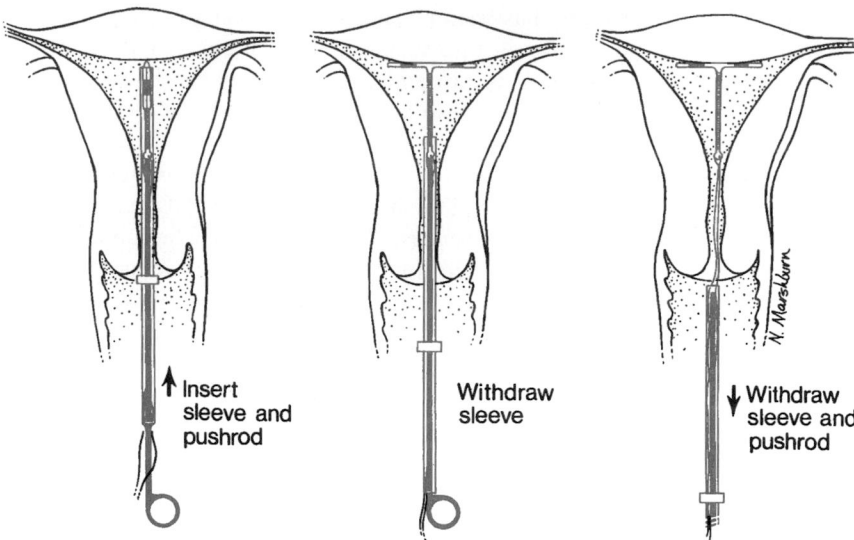

Insert sleeve and pushrod

Withdraw sleeve

Withdraw sleeve and pushrod

FIGURE 32–5. Insertion of ParaGard T 380A using the withdrawal technique.

released by the Mirena device may inhibit tubal mobility, a previous ectopic pregnancy or predisposing risk factors are considered contraindications.

Procedures for Insertion. The FDA requires that before an IUD is inserted, the woman must be given a brochure detailing the side effects and apparent risks associated with its use. Most devices have a special inserter, usually a sterile graduated plastic tube into which the device is drawn just before insertion (Fig. 32–5). Timing of insertion influences the ease of placement as well as the pregnancy and expulsion rates. Insertion near the end of normal menstruation, when the cervix is usually softer and the canal somewhat more dilated, may facilitate insertion and at the same time exclude early pregnancy. Insertion, however, need not be limited to this time. For the woman who is sure she is not pregnant and does not want to be pregnant, insertion may be carried out at any time.

Insertion immediately or very soon after delivery is followed by an unsatisfactorily high expulsion rate. The recommendation has been made, therefore, to withhold insertion for at least 8 weeks to reduce expulsion as well as to minimize the risk of perforation. In our extensive experiences, however, earlier insertion has not led to perforation or expulsion rates significantly higher than for insertion more remote from pregnancy. In the absence of infection, the device may be inserted immediately after early abortion.

A satisfactory technique for insertion of the ParaGard device is as follows:

1. Determine whether there are contraindications, counsel the woman regarding various problems associated with device use, and obtain written consent.
2. Administer a nonsteroidal anti-inflammatory agent with or without codeine to allay cramps.

3. Perform a pelvic examination to identify the position and size of the uterus and adnexa. If abnormalities are found, they should be evaluated, because the IUD may be contraindicated. Mucopurulent discharge and significant vaginitis should be appropriately treated and resolved before insertion.
4. **Make sure that the device is not loaded into its inserter tube more than 5 minutes before insertion.** The malleable arms tend to retain the "memory" of the inserter.
5. Wipe the cervix and the vaginal walls with an antiseptic solution. Then grasp the cervix with a vertically oriented single-tooth tenaculum—one tooth in the canal and one atop the cervix. Use sterile instruments and a sterile device. The cervical canal and uterine cavity are first straightened by applying gentle traction on the tenaculum, and the uterus is sounded to identify the direction and depth of the uterine cavity.
6. Adjust the movable flange on the barrel of the inserter to the sounded depth, from external cervical os to fundus. As shown in Figure 32–5, the inserter, with the IUD contained within its most distal portion, is then gently inserted to the fundus. After rotating the inserter so that the device is positioned high in the transverse plane of the uterus, the inserter is removed while the device is held in the fundus by the plastic rod within the inserter. **Thus, the device is not pushed out of the tube, but rather it is held in place by the rod while the inserter tube is withdrawn.**
7. Cut the marker tail 2 cm from the external os, remove the tenaculum, observe for bleeding from the tenaculum puncture sites, and if there is no bleeding, remove the speculum.
8. Advise the woman to report any apparent adverse effects promptly.

The Mirena device requires some modifications to this technique, which are described in detail in its package insert. Specifically, the arms of the device are released in the uterus *prior* to advancing the device 1.5 to 2 cm to the fundus. This is accomplished by setting the flange to the sounded uterine depth, and using it to gauge, based on its 1.5 to 2 cm distance from the external os, when to release the arms.

Expulsion. Loss of the IUD from the uterus is most common during the first month. The woman should be instructed to palpate the strings protruding from the cervix by either sitting on the edge of a chair or squatting down and then advancing the middle finger into the vagina until the cervix is reached. The woman should be examined again in about a month, usually after menses, for appropriate placement by identifying the tail protruding from the cervix. Barrier contraception may be desirable during this time, especially if a device has been expelled previously.

Lost Device. When the tail of an IUD cannot be visualized, the device may have been expelled, or it may have perforated the uterus. In either event, pregnancy is possible. Conversely, the tail simply may be in the uterine cavity along with a normally positioned device. Often, gentle probing of the uterine cavity with a Randall stone clamp or a rod with a terminal hook retrieves the string. **Never assume that the device has been expelled unless it was seen.**

When the tail is not visible and the device is not felt by gentle probing of the uterine cavity, sonography can be used to ascertain if the device is within the uterine cavity. If these findings are negative or inconclusive, then a radiograph of the abdomen and pelvis is taken with a sound inserted into the uterine cavity. Instillation of radiocontrast for hysterography may be done. Hysteroscopy is yet another alternative. Obviously none of these maneuvers except sonography should be performed during early pregnancy.

An open device of inert material, such as the Lippes Loop, located outside the uterus may or may not do harm. Perforations of large and small bowel and bowel fistulas, with attendant morbidity, have been reported remote from insertion. An extrauterine copper-bearing device induces an intense local inflammatory reaction and adhesions. Chemically inert devices usually are removed easily from the peritoneal cavity by laparoscopy or colpotomy. Copper-bearing devices are more firmly adherent, and laparotomy may be necessary.

A device may penetrate the uterine wall to varying degrees. Part of the device may extend into the peritoneal cavity, or part may remain firmly fixed in the myometrium. A device also may penetrate into the cervix and actually protrude into the vagina.

Replacement. The ParaGard device is approved for 10 years of continuous use and the Mirena device for 5 years.

BARRIER METHODS. For many years, condoms, vaginal spermicidal agents, and vaginal diaphragms have been used for contraception with variable success (see Table 32–2).

Male Condom. These products provide effective contraception, and their failure rate with strongly motivated couples has been as low as 3 or 4 per 100 couple-years of exposure (Vessey and co-workers, 1982). Generally, and during the first year of use especially, the failure rate is much higher (see Table 32–2). Women older than 30 years of age have had fewer unintended pregnancies than those younger than 25 years of age (Trussell and colleagues, 1990).

When used properly, condoms provide considerable but not absolute protection against a broad range of sexually transmitted diseases, including HIV, gonorrhea, syphilis, herpes, chlamydia, and trichomoniasis. They also may prevent and ameliorate premalignant cervical changes, probably by blocking transmission of human papillomavirus (Population Reports, 1982). Because the Centers for Disease Control and Prevention recommend condoms for couples at risk for HIV infection, including those with multiple sex partners, their use has escalated exponentially since the mid-1980s.

The contraceptive effectiveness of the male condom is enhanced appreciably by a reservoir tip and, theoretically, by the addition of spermicidal lubricant to the condom. The contraceptive effectiveness is further improved by the addition of an intravaginal spermicidal agent. Such agents, as well as those used for lubrication, should be water-based, because oil-based products destroy latex condoms and diaphragms (Waldron, 1989).

Speroff and Darney (2001) emphasize the following key steps to ensure maximal condom effectiveness:

1. They must be used with every coital act.
2. Placement should occur before contact of the penis with the vagina.
3. Withdrawal must occur with the penis still erect.
4. The base of the condom must be held during withdrawal.
5. Either an intravaginal spermicide or a condom lubricated with spermicide should be used.

LATEX SENSITIVITY. Some individuals are sensitive to latex. Condoms made from lamb intestines are effective, but they do not provide protection against infection. Fortunately, a nonallergenic condom was developed using synthetic thermoplastic elastomer, similar to that used in surgical gloves (Mason, 1992). Polyurethane condoms are effective against sexually transmitted diseases but have a significantly higher breakage and slippage rate than latex condoms (Frezieres and colleagues, 1998; Waldron, 1991). In a randomized trial of 901 couples, Steiner and colleagues (2003) documented breakage and slippage at 8.4 percent with polyurethane condoms compared with that of 3.2 percent with latex condoms. Respective 6-month typical pregnancy probabilities were 9.0 compared with that of 5.4 percent.

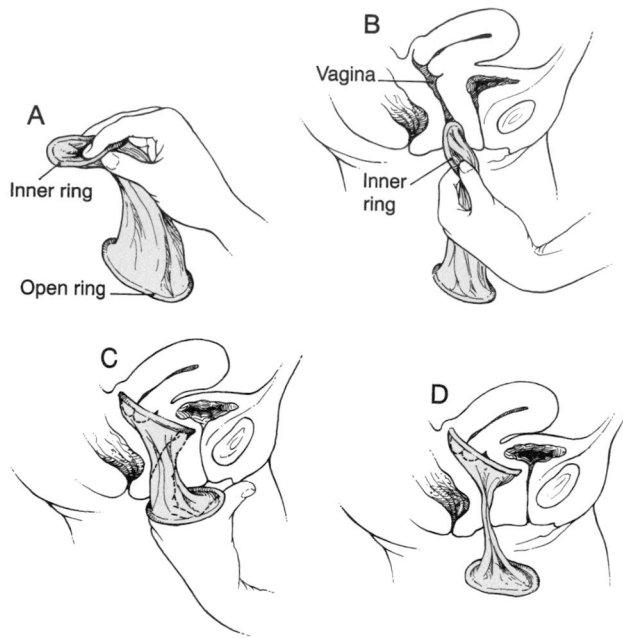

FIGURE 32–6. FC Female Condom insertion and positioning. **A.** Inner ring is squeezed for insertion. **B.** Sheath is inserted similarly to a diaphragm. **C.** Inner ring is pushed up as far as it can go with index finger. **D.** Vaginal pouch is in place. (Courtesy of Wisconsin Pharmacal Company, Jackson, WI.)

Female Condom (Vaginal Pouch). Before approval for marketing, a vaginal pouch must be proven to prevent pregnancy and sexually transmitted diseases. The only female condom available is marketed as the FC Female Condom. It is a polyurethane sheath with one flexible polyurethane ring at each end. The open ring remains outside the vagina, and the closed internal ring is fitted under the symphysis like a diaphragm (Fig. 32–6). In vitro tests have shown the condom to be impermeable to HIV, cytomegalovirus, and hepatitis B virus. It has a 0.6 percent breakage rate. The slippage and displacement rate is about 3 percent compared with that of 3 to 8 percent for male condoms. It has an acceptability rate of about 60 percent for women and 80 percent for men. The pregnancy rate is higher than with the male condom (see Table 32–2).

Spermicides. These contraceptives are marketed variously as creams, jellies, suppositories, films, and foam in aerosol containers. They are used widely in the United States, especially by women who find other methods unacceptable. They are useful especially for women who need temporary protection, for example, during the first week after starting oral contraceptives or while nursing. Most agents can be purchased without a prescription.

Typically, spermicides function by providing a physical barrier to sperm penetration as well as a chemical spermicidal action. The active ingredient is nonoxynol-9 or octoxynol-9. Raymond and colleagues (2004) showed that products with

100 mg of nonoxynol-9 were most effective. **Spermicides must be deposited high in the vagina in contact with the cervix shortly before intercourse.** Their duration of maximal effectiveness is usually no more than 1 hour. Thereafter they must be reinserted before repeat intercourse. Douching should be avoided for at least 6 hours after intercourse.

High pregnancy rates are primarily attributable to inconsistent use rather than to method failure. Even if inserted regularly and correctly, however, foam preparations probably result in 5 to 12 pregnancies per 100 woman-years of use (Trussell and associates, 1990). Spermicides in current use may provide partial protection against some sexually transmitted diseases such as gonorrhea (Feldblum and Fortney, 1988). They are not teratogenic (Briggs and colleagues, 2002).

Diaphragm Plus Spermicide. The diaphragm consists of a circular rubber dome of various diameters supported by a circumferentially placed metal spring. It can be very effective when used in combination with spermicidal jelly or cream. The spermicide is applied to the superior surface both along the rim and centrally. The device is then placed in the vagina so that the cervix, vaginal fornices, and anterior vaginal wall are partitioned effectively from the remainder of the vagina and the penis. At the same time, the centrally placed spermicidal agent is held against the cervix by the diaphragm. When appropriately positioned, the rim is lodged superiorly deep in the posterior vaginal fornix, and inferiorly the rim lies in close proximity to the inner surface of the symphysis immediately below the urethra (Fig. 32–7). If the diaphragm is too small, it does not remain in place. If it is too large, it is uncomfortable when it is forced into position. Cystocele or uterine prolapse is very likely to result in instability and therefore expulsion. Because the variables of size and spring

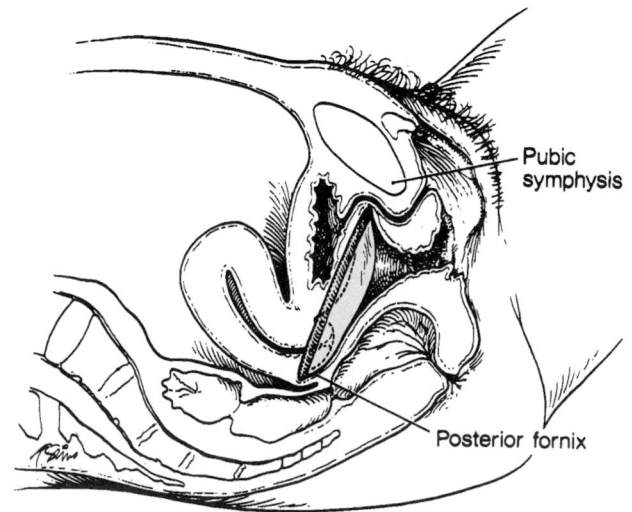

FIGURE 32–7. A diaphragm in place creates a physical barrier between the vagina and cervix and, importantly, provides for intimate contact between the contraceptive jelly or cream and the cervix.

flexibility must be specified, the diaphragm is available only by prescription (Allen, 2004).

The diaphragm and spermicidal agent can be inserted hours before intercourse, but if more than 6 hours elapse, additional spermicide should be placed in the upper vagina for maximum protection and be reapplied before each coital episode. The diaphragm should not be removed for at least 6 hours after intercourse. Because *toxic shock syndrome* has been described following its use, it may be worthwhile to remove the diaphragm at 6 hours, or at least the next morning, to minimize this uncommon event (Alcid and associates, 1982).

The diaphragm requires a high level of motivation for proper use. Vessey and colleagues (1982) reported a pregnancy rate of only 1.9 to 2.4 per 100 woman-years for motivated users. Bounds and associates (1995), in a small study, reported a much higher failure rate of 12.3 per 100 woman-years. The unintended pregnancy rate is lower in women older than 35 years of age than in those younger than 30 years of age. Diaphragm use results in a lower incidence of sexually transmitted diseases compared with that of condom use (Rosenberg and colleagues, 1992). Conversely, diaphragm use is associated with a slight increase in the rate of urinary infections (Hatcher and associates, 1998).

Contraceptive Sponge. After being off the market in the United States for 8 years, the Today contraceptive sponge is again available. It is sold over-the-counter. It consists of a nonoxynol-9–impregnated polyurethane disc that can be inserted for up to 24 hours prior to intercourse. After moistening, it is placed directly against the cervix. While in place, it provides contraception regardless of the frequency of coitus. It should remain in place for 6 hours after intercourse. Although the sponge is perhaps more convenient than the diaphragm or condom, it is less effective (see Table 32–2).

Cervical Cap. The Prentif cavity-rim cervical cap was approved for use by the FDA in 1988. The flexible, cup-like device is made of natural rubber and is fitted around the base of the cervix. It can be self-inserted and allowed to remain in place for up to 48 hours. It should be used with a spermicide applied once at insertion. If properly fitted and used correctly, the cap is comparable in effectiveness to the diaphragm (Bernstein and associates, 1982; Richwald and colleagues, 1989). However, it is relatively costly, and overall, incorrect fitting and/or improper placement make the cap less effective than the diaphragm plus spermicide (see Table 32–2).

PERIODIC (RHYTHMIC) ABSTINENCE. Because the human ovum is probably susceptible to successful fertilization for only about 12 to 24 hours after ovulation, periodic abstinence has intuitive appeal as a means of birth control. Pregnancy rates, however, with various methods of periodic abstinence—rhythm, natural family planning, or fertility awareness—have been estimated from 5 to 40 per 100 woman-years (Population Reports, 1981). In other words, the unwanted pregnancy rate during the first year of use is approximately 20 percent (see Table 32–2).

Calendar Rhythm Method. Ovulation most often occurs about 14 days before the onset of the next menstrual period. Unfortunately, this is not necessarily 14 days *after* the onset of the last menstrual period. Therefore, the *calendar rhythm method* is not reliable. The International Planned Parenthood Federation (1982) concluded that "couples electing to use periodic abstinence should, however, be clearly informed that the method is not considered an effective method of family planning."

Temperature Rhythm Method. The temperature rhythm method relies on *slight* changes—sustained 0.4 degree Fahrenheit increases—in the morning basal body temperature that usually occur just before ovulation. This method is much more likely to be successful if, during each menstrual cycle, intercourse is avoided until well after the ovulatory temperature rise. For this method to be most effective, the woman must abstain from intercourse from the first day of menses through the third day after the increase in temperature. For obvious reasons, this is not a popular method! With excellent compliance, however, the unwanted pregnancy is about 2 percent the first year.

Cervical Mucus Rhythm Method. The so-called *Billings method* depends on awareness of vaginal "dryness" and "wetness." These are the consequence of changes in the amount and quality of cervical mucus at different times in the menstrual cycle. Abstinence is required from the beginning of menses until 4 days after slippery mucus is identified. Although this method has not achieved popularity, when it is used accurately, the first-year failure rate is approximately 3 percent.

Symptothermal Method. This method combines the use of changes in cervical mucus (onset of fertile period), changes in basal body temperature (end of fertile period), and calculations to estimate the time of ovulation. Although this method is more complex to learn and apply, it does not appreciably improve reliability. The use of home kits to detect luteal hormone increases in the urine on the day prior to ovulation may improve the accuracy of periodic abstinence methods (Hatcher and associates, 1998).

Natural Family Planning Methods. For the interested reader, the December 1991 supplement to the *American Journal of Obstetrics and Gynecology* was devoted to the subject of natural family planning. Clearly, proper instruction is critical for natural family planning methods to be successful. Complex charting is involved, and these charts, as well as detailed advice, are available online from the National

Fertility Awareness and Natural Family Planning Service for the United Kingdom (http://www.fertilityuk.org) and The Natural Family Site, BYG Publishing (http://www.bygpub.com/natural).

SPECIAL CONSIDERATIONS IN CONTRACEPTION

A number of unique circumstances present special challenges for assuming contraceptive efficacy while minimizing undesirable effects.

CONTRACEPTION IN ADOLESCENTS. A discussion of the biological antecedents of teenage pregnancy was presented in Chapter 3 (see p. 40). Briefly stated, menarche has decreased from approximately 17 years of age in the mid-1800s to near 12 years of age in 2001. Unfortunately, this means that reproductive function is established sooner than the psychological understanding of the consequences of sexual activity. This far too often results in intermittent spontaneous sexual encounters and a naive perception of the risks of pregnancy and sexually transmitted diseases (Cromer and associates, 1996; Sulak and Haney, 1993).

Contraception is most often sought more than a year after sexual activity has begun (Mosher and McNally, 1991). Concerns over confidentiality and lack of money deter adolescents from seeking and obtaining contraception (American College of Obstetricians and Gynecologists, 2003b). Both barriers are surmountable and in most cases should not impede access to contraception. Indeed, in the majority of states, minors have explicit legal authority to consent to contraceptive services, and in many areas, publicly funded clinics provide free contraception to adolescents (Alan Guttmacher Institute, 2002).

Combination Oral Contraceptives. As a method, these agents are the best choice for adolescents because they provide effective contraception, increase bone density, and can be used to improve acne and regulate irregular menses. The obvious disadvantage is the daily requirement of taking a pill.

Long-Acting Methods. Injectable depot *medroxyprogesterone* is an effective contraceptive that also may be considered a "use and forget" method for 3 months. The disadvantages include the need for injection every 3 months, menstrual irregularities, and loss of bone mass (Sulak and Kaunitz, 1999).

Barrier Methods. Despite their obvious advantage of providing some protection against sexually transmitted diseases, barrier methods are not good choices for adolescents because they require preplanning and motivation for proper use. Such methods, especially vaginal spermicides and male condoms, should be considered primarily as back-up contraceptives and protective methods for sexually transmitted diseases.

CONTRACEPTIVE CHOICES FOR WOMEN OLDER THAN 35 YEARS OF AGE. Although fertility decreases beginning at 35 to 40 years of age, these women are still at risk for unwanted pregnancy and sexually transmitted diseases. Henshaw (1998) reported that half of all pregnancies in women in their 40s are unintended, and that 65 percent of these are terminated.

Combination Oral Contraceptives. These agents, especially the newer low-dose estrogen compounds, when used by nonsmokers without systemic disease, are highly effective, are well tolerated, provide many health benefits, and are associated with minimal risk (Beck, 1995; Speroff and Sulak, 1995). According to the American College of Obstetricians and Gynecologists (2000b), healthy, nonsmoking women may use combination oral contraceptives containing less than 50 μg of estrogen until menopause.

Injectable Depot Medroxyprogesterone. This is a highly effective hormonal contraceptive. It can also be used by some women who cannot for medical reasons take combination oral contraceptives (Speroff and Sulak, 1995).

Intrauterine Devices. IUDs are a logical choice for an older woman who has completed her family and is in a monogamous relationship.

Barrier Techniques and Spermicidal Agents. These methods can be used as either primary or back-up contraception. Their effectiveness improves with advancing age after 40, likely because of diminished fertility.

CONTRACEPTION IN WOMEN WITH MEDICAL CONDITIONS. Pregnancies in women with medical complications often result in dangers that far exceed those seen with most forms of contraception (American College of Obstetricians and Gynecologists, 2000b). The choice of the most effective and safest method of contraception, however, is dependent on the basic pathophysiology of the disease and how pregnancy affects it. Only with such knowledge can the appropriate contraceptive be prescribed or a recommendation for sterilization be made. For these reasons, contraceptive and sterilization recommendations are made throughout this book when individual diseases are discussed.

EMERGENCY CONTRACEPTION. Many women present for contraceptive care following consensual but unprotected sexual intercourse and in some cases aggravated sexual assault. In these situations, a number of methods substantially decrease the likelihood of an unwanted pregnancy when used correctly.

Hormonal Emergency Contraception (morning-after pill or Yuzpe method). The high unintended pregnancy rate in the United States has become the focus of public health attention. To address this problem, there have been some recent rapid changes in the availability of hormonal

TABLE 32–9 **Prescriptive Equivalents of Specifically Designed Products and Common Oral Contraceptives for Use as Emergency Contraception**

Trade Name	Formulation	No. of Pills/Dose[a]
Specifically Designed Products		
Plan B	0.75 mg levonorgestrel	1
Preven	0.05 mg ethinyl estradiol	2
	0.25 mg levonorgestrel	
Common Oral Contraceptives		
Ovrette	0 mg ethinyl estradiol	20
	0.075 mg norgestrel	
Ogestrel	0.05 mg ethinyl estradiol	2
	0.50 mg norgestrel	
Ovral	0.05 mg ethinyl estradiol	2
	0.50 mg norgestrel	
Low-Ogestrel	0.03 mg ethinyl estradiol	4
	0.30 mg norgestrel	
Lo/Ovral	0.03 mg ethinyl estradiol	4
	0.30 mg norgestrel	
Nordette	(light orange pills)	4
	0.03 mg ethinyl estradiol	
	0.15 mg levonorgestrel	
Levlen	(light orange pills)	4
	0.03 mg ethinyl estradiol	
	0.15 mg levonorgestrel	
Levora	0.03 mg ethinyl estradiol	4
	0.15 mg levonorgestrel	
Tri-Levlen	(yellow pills only)	4
	0.03 mg ethinyl estradiol	
	0.125 mg levonorgestrel	
Triphasil	(yellow pills only)	4
	0.03 mg ethinyl estradiol	
	0.125 mg levonorgestrel	
Trivora	(pink pills only)	4
	0.03 mg ethinyl estradiol	
	0.125 mg levonorgestrel	
Alesse	0.02 mg ethinyl estradiol	5
	0.1 mg levonorgestrel	
Levlite	0.02 mg ethinyl estradiol	5
	0.1 mg levonorgestrel	

[a] Treatment consists of two doses taken 12 hours apart. Use of an antiemetic agent before taking the medication lessens the risk of nausea, which is a common side effect.
From American College of Obstetricians and Gynecologists, 2001b, with permission.

emergency contraception. Three hormonal methods are currently available: the Yuzpe method, which consists of commonly available combination oral contraceptives; and two products designed specifically for this purpose, one consisting of an estrogen and progestin combination and the other a progestin-only product.

YUZPE AND ESTROGEN–PROGESTIN COMBINATIONS. In 1997, the FDA approved a number of combined oral contraceptive regimens for use as emergency contraception (Table 32–9), and in 1998, the FDA approved the Preven Emergency Contraceptive Kit. It contains a pregnancy test and four oral contraceptive tablets each containing 50 μg of ethinyl estradiol and 0.25 mg of levonorgestrel. Two tablets are taken within 72 hours of intercourse, followed 12 hours later by the second dose. The regimen is more effective the sooner it is taken after unprotected intercourse. All oral hormone regimens shown in Table 32–9 follow the same dosage schedule.

PROGESTIN-ONLY PREPARATION. Plan B is a progestin-only regimen that consists of two tablets each containing 0.75 mg levonorgestrel. The first dose is taken within 72 hours of unprotected coitus and the second dose 12 hours later (see Table 32–9). This regimen resulted in a crude pregnancy rate of 1.1 compared with that of 3.2 percent in a similar group of women treated with the Yuzpe regimen. The manufacturer of Plan B applied to the FDA to request the product to be sold over the counter. Wai and colleagues (2005) showed that a 24-hour interval between the doses was also effective.

According to the Task Force on Postovulatory Methods of Fertility Regulation (1998), mini-pill progestins are more effective than combination estrogen-progestin pills. The Ovrette method consists of 20 pills taken as one dose within

72 hours of unprotected intercourse followed in 12 hours by a second dose of 20 pills (see Table 32–9). Each dose of 20 pills contains 1.5 mg of norgestrel. This method has proven to be effective and is less likely to cause nausea and vomiting. Jackson and colleagues (2003) reported that *advanced* provision of emergency contraception increased its use without adversely affecting the use of routine contraception.

Access to emergency contraception has not been universal. Trussell and colleagues (2000) found that only 75 percent of attempts to access care through the Emergency Contraception Hotline were successful. Physicians can register to be included as a resource, and patients can obtain referrals on the Hotline at 1-888-NOT-2-LATE (888-668-2528) or the Emergency Contraception Website (http://www.not-2late.com).

In spite of sound published evidence, compelling arguments such as those by Grimes (2002), and a 23 to 4 affirming vote by its two advisory committees, the FDA in 2004 decided to deny over-the-counter status to levonorgestrel emergency contraception. This decision has been widely decried as politically motivated (Drazen and colleagues, 2004; Grimes, 2004).

MECHANISM OF ACTION. The major mechanism is inhibition or delay of ovulation (Food and Drug Administration, 1997). Other mechanisms include alteration of the endometrium, sperm penetration, and tubal motility. **Established pregnancies are not harmed.**

Emergency hormone contraceptive regimens are highly effective and decrease the risk of pregnancy by 75 percent (Trussell and associates, 1996, 1998b). Thus, if 100 women had unprotected intercourse during the second to third week of their menstrual cycle, eight would be expected to conceive. With appropriate use of one of the regimens shown in Table 32–9, only two would actually conceive.

Nausea and vomiting are major problems due to the estrogen in these regimens. Trussell and associates (1998a) reported nausea in 50 percent of women and vomiting in 20 percent. For this reason, we routinely prescribe an oral antiemetic at least 1 hour before each dose. Raymond and colleagues (2000) conducted a randomized trial and found that 1-hour pretreatment with 50-mg meclizine given orally decreased nausea substantially. Ragan and associates (2003) found that 10 mg of oral metoclopramide decreased both nausea and cramping compared with that of placebo. If vomiting occurs within 2 hours of a dose, the dose must be repeated.

Copper-Containing Intrauterine Devices. Fasoli and co-workers (1989) summarized nine studies that included results from 879 women who accepted some type of copper-containing IUD as a sole method of postcoital contraception. The only pregnancy reported aborted spontaneously. Trussell and Stewart (1998) reported that when the IUD was inserted up to 5 days after unprotected intercourse, the failure rate was 1 percent. A secondary advantage is that this method also puts in place an effective 5- to 10-year method of contraception.

Mifepristone (RU 486) and Epostane. These medications are discussed in Chapter 9 (see p. 245). They should be ideal for postcoital contraception, because they either block progesterone production (epostane) or interfere with its action (mifepristone). Implantation prevented by either mechanism results in so-called *menstrual induction.*

Ashok and colleagues (2002) reported that a single 100-mg dose of mifepristone was more effective than the Yuzpe regimen, with crude pregnancy rates of 0.6 versus 3.6 percent, respectively. There were also fewer side effects with mifepristone. Although hormonal regimens must be used within 72 hours of unprotected intercourse, mifepristone is effective up to 17 days after intercourse (Weiss, 1993). Grimes and Cook (1992) propose that that wider availability of mifepristone for postcoital contraception would result in a lowering of the induced abortion rate.

Failure of Emergency Contraception. Any postcoital contraceptive method is associated with failures, which likely can be reduced by employing a barrier technique until the next menses to prevent fertilization after use of the postcoital method. If menstruation is delayed for more than 3 weeks past its expected onset, pregnancy is likely.

LACTATION

Breast feeding is important to infant health and to child-spacing. For mothers who are nursing, ovulation during the first 10 weeks after delivery is unlikely (Pérez, 1981). Nursing, however, is not a reliable method of family planning for women whose infants are on a daytime-only feeding schedule. **Waiting for first menses involves a risk of pregnancy, because ovulation usually antedates menstruation.** Certainly, after the first menses, contraception is essential unless the woman desires pregnancy. Estrogen–progestin contraceptives may reduce both the rate and the duration of milk production. The benefits from prevention of pregnancy by the use of combined oral contraceptives would appear to outweigh the risks in selected patients. According to the American College of Obstetricians and Gynecologists (2000a), progestin-only oral contraceptives are the preferred choice in most cases (see p. 733). IUDs have been recommended for the lactating sexually active woman. The rate of uterine perforation is very slightly increased in lactating women with IUDs, perhaps as a consequence of vigorous myometrial contractions from the release of oxytocin in response to suckling (Heartwell and Schlesselman, 1983).

REFERENCES

Aedo AR, Landgren BM, Johannisson E, et al: Pharmacokinetic and pharmacodynamic investigations with monthly injectable contraceptive preparations. Contraception 31:453, 1985

Alan Guttmacher Institute: State policies in brief. Minors' access to contraceptive services. New York, AGI, 2002. Available at: http://www.agi-usa.org/pubs/spib_MACS.pdf. Accessed December 30, 2002

Alcid DV, Kothari N, Quinn EP, et al: Toxic-shock syndrome associated with diaphragm use for only nine hours. Lancet 1:1363, 1982

Allen RE: Diaphragm fitting. Am Fam Physician 69:97, 2004

Alvarez F, Brache V, Fernandez E, et al: New insights on the mode of action of intrauterine contraceptive devices in women. Fertil Steril 49:768, 1988

American College of Obstetricians and Gynecologists: Benefits and risks of sterilization. Practice Bulletin No. 46, September 2003a

American College of Obstetricians and Gynecologists: Health Care for Adolescents. Washington, DC, ACOG Women's Health Care Physicians, 2003b, pp 39–40

American College of Obstetricians and Gynecologists: Antibiotic prophylaxis for gynecologic procedures. Practice Bulletin No. 23, January 2001a

American College of Obstetricians and Gynecologists: Emergency oral contraception. Practice Bulletin No. 25, March 2001b

American College of Obstetricians and Gynecologists: Breastfeeding: Maternal and infant aspects. Educational Bulletin No. 258, July 2000a

American College of Obstetricians and Gynecologists: The use of hormonal contraception in women with coexisting medical conditions. Practice Bulletin No. 18, July 2000b

Ashok PW, Stalder C, Wagaarachchi PT, et al: A randomized study comparing a low dose of mifepristone and the Yuzpe regimen for emergency contraception. Br J Obstet Gynaecol 109:553, 2002

Association of Professors of Gynecology and Obstetrics: Education Series on Women's Health Issues: Contraception, February, 1999

Audet MC, Moreau M, Koltun WD, et al: Evaluation of contraceptive efficacy and cycle control of a transdermal contraceptive patch vs an oral contraceptive: A randomized controlled trial. JAMA 285:2347, 2001

Beck WW: Use of oral contraceptives in women in their 40s. Clin Obstet Gynecol 15:46, 1995

Bernstein G, Kilzer LH, Coulson AH, et al: Studies of cervical caps. Contraception 26:443, 1982

Betrabet SS, Shikary ZK, Toddywalla VS, et al: ICMR Task Force Study on hormonal contraception. Transfer of norethindrone (NET) and levonorgestrel (LNG) from a single tablet into the infant's circulation through the mother's milk. Contraception 35:517, 1987

Blumenstein BA, Douglas MB, Hall WD: Blood pressure changes and oral contraceptive use: A study of 2,676 black women in the southeastern United States. Am J Epidemiol 112:539, 1980

Bounds W, Guillebaud J, Dominik R, et al: The diaphragm with and without spermicide. A randomized, comparative efficacy trial. J Reprod Med 40:764, 1995

Briggs GG, Freeman RK, Yaffe SJ: Drugs in Pregnancy and Lactation, 6th ed. Baltimore, Williams & Wilkins, 2002

Burkman RT: Rationale for new contraceptive methods. The Female Patient (Suppl), August 2002

Butterworth CE Jr, Hatch KD, Macaluso M, et al: Folate deficiency and cervical dysplasia. JAMA 267:528, 1992

Cancer and Steroid Hormone Study of the Centers for Disease Control and the National Institute of Child Health and Development: Combination oral contraceptive use and the risk of endometrial cancer. JAMA 257:796, 1987a

Cancer and Steroid Hormone Study of the Centers for Disease Control and the National Institute of Child Health and Development: Oral-contraceptive use and the risk of breast cancer. N Engl J Med 315:405, 1986

Cancer and Steroid Hormone Study of the Centers for Disease Control and the National Institute of Child Health and Development:

The reduction in risk of ovarian cancer associated with oral-contraceptive use. N Engl J Med 316:650, 1987b

Chang CL, Donagy M, Poulter N, et al: Migraine and stroke in young women: Case-control study. BMJ 318:13, 1999

Chasan-Taber L, Willett WC, Manson JE, et al: Prospective study of oral contraceptives and hypertension among women in the United States. Circulation 94:483, 1996

Collaborative Group on Hormonal Factors in Breast Cancer: Breast cancer and hormonal contraceptives: Collaborative reanalysis of individual data on 53,297 women with breast cancer and 100,239 women without breast cancer from 54 epidemiological studies. Lancet 347:1713, 1996

Comp PC: Coagulation and thrombosis with OC use: Physiology and clinical relevance. Dialogues Contracept 5:1, 1996

Craft P, Hannaford PC: Risk factors for acute myocardial infarction in women: Evidence from the Royal College of General Practitioners' Oral Contraceptive Study. BMJ 298:165, 1989

Critchlow CW, Wölner-Hanssen P, Eschenback DA, et al: Determinants of cervical ectopia and of cervicitis: Age, oral contraception, specific cervical infection, smoking, and douching. Am J Obstet Gynecol 173:534, 1995

Cromer BA, Blair JM, Mahan JD, et al: A prospective comparison of bone density in adolescent girls receiving depot medroxyprogesterone acetate (Depo-Provera), levonorgestrel (Norplant), or oral contraceptives. J Pediatr 129:671, 1996

Cromer BA, Smith RD, Blair JM, et al: A prospective study of adolescents who choose among levonorgestrel implant (Norplant), medroxyprogesterone acetate (Depo-Provera), or the combined oral contraceptive pill as contraception. Pediatrics 94:687, 1994

Cundy T, Cornish J, Evans MC, et al: Recovery of bone density in women who stop using medroxyprogesterone acetate. BMJ 308:247, 1994

Cuong DT, My Huong NT: Comparative phase III clinical trial of two injectable contraceptive preparations, depot medroxyprogesterone acetate and Cyclofem, in Vietnamese women. Contraception 54:169, 1996

Doll H, Vessey M, Painter R: Return of fertility in nulliparous women after discontinuation of the intrauterine device: Comparison with women discontinuing other methods of contraception. Br J Obstet Gynaecol 108:304, 2001

Drazen JM, Greene MF, Wood AJJ: The FDA, politics, and Plan B. N Engl J Med 350:1561, 2004

Earl DT, David DJ: Depo-Provera: An injectable contraceptive. Am Fam Physician 49:891, 1994

Farley TMM, Rosenberg MJ, Rowe PJ, et al: Intrauterine devices and pelvic inflammatory disease: An international perspective. Lancet 339:785, 1992

Fasoli M, Parazzini F, Cecchetti G, et al: Post-coital contraception: An overview of published studies. Contraception 39:459, 1989

Feldblum PJ, Fortney JA: Condoms, spermicides and the transmission of human immunodeficiency virus: A review of the literature. Am J Public Health 78:52, 1988

Fiorino AS: Intrauterine contraceptive device–associated actinomycotic abscess and Actinomyces detection on cervical smear. Obstet Gynecol 87:142, 1996

Food and Drug Administration: Prescription drug products. Certain combined oral contraceptives for use as postcoital emergency contraception: notice. Federal Register, February 25, 62:8609, 1997

Frezieres RG, Walsh TL, Nelson AL, et al: Breakage and acceptability of a polyurethane condom: A randomized, controlled study. Fam Plann Perspect 30:73, 1998

Furlong LA: Ectopic pregnancy risk when contraception fails. J Reprod Med 47:881, 2002

Gallo MF, Grimes DA, Schulz KF, et al: Combination estrogen-progestin contraceptives and body weight: Systematic review of randomized controlled trials. Obstet Gynecol 103:359, 2004

Garceau RJ, Wajszczuk CP, Kaunitz AM: Bleeding patterns of women using Lunelle monthly contraceptive injections (medroxyprogesterone acetate and estradiol cypionate injectable suspension) compared with those of women using Ortho-Novum 7/7/7 oral contraceptive (norethindrone/ethinyl estradiol triphasic) or other oral contraceptives. Contraception 62:289, 2000

Gardner JM, Mishell DR Jr: Analysis of bleeding patterns and resumption of fertility following discontinuation of a long-acting injectable contraceptive. Fertil Steril 21:286, 1970

Goldzeiher JW, Zamah NM: Oral contraceptive side effects: Where's the beef? Contraception 52:327, 1995

Grimes DA: Emergency contraception: Politics trumps science at the US Food and Drug Administration. Obstet Gynecol 104:220, 2004

Grimes DA: Switching emergency contraception to over-the-counter status. N Engl J Med 347:846, 2002

Grimes DA, Cook RJ: Mifepristone (RU 486)—an abortifacient to prevent abortion? N Engl J Med 327:1088, 1992

Guillebaud J: Contraception: Your Questions Answered. New York, Pitman, 1985

Hall PE, Task Force on Research on Introduction and Transfer of Technologies for Fertility Regulation, Special Programme of Research, Development and Research Training in Human Reproduction, World Health Organization, Geneva, Switzerland: The introduction of Cyclofem into national family planning programmes: Experience from studies in Indonesia, Jamaica, Mexico, Thailand and Tunisia. Contraception 49:489, 1994

Hannaford PC, Kay CR: Oral contraceptives and diabetes mellitus. BMJ 299:1315, 1989

Hannaford PC, Kay CR, Vessey MP, et al: Combined oral contraceptives and liver disease. Contraception 55:145, 1997

Harlap S, Kost K, Forrest JD: Preventing pregnancy, protecting health: A new look at birth control choices in the US. The Alan Guttmacher Institute 1, 1991

Hatcher RA, Stewart F, Trussell J, et al: Contraceptive Technology, 15th ed. New York, Irvington, 1990, p 370

Hatcher RA, Trussell J, Stewart F, et al: Contraceptive Technology, 17th ed. New York, Ardent Media, 1998, pp 230, 322, 384, 409–414, 424–425, 439, 449–450, 467, 520

Heartwell SF, Schlesselman S: Risk of uterine perforation among users of intrauterine devices. Obstet Gynecol 61:31, 1983

Heinemann LA, Weimann A, Gerken G, et al: Modern oral contraceptive use and benign liver tumors: The German Benign Liver Tumor Case-Control Study. Eur J Contracep Reprod Health Care 3:194, 1998

Henshaw SK: Unintended pregnancy in the United States. Fam Plann Perspect 30:24, 1998

Holt VL, Cushing-Haugen KL, Daling JR: Body weight and risk of oral contraceptive failure. Obstet Gynecol 99:820, 2002

Hoppe G: The clinical relevance of oral contraceptive pill-induced plasma lipid changes: Facts and fiction. Am J Obstet Gynecol 163:388, 1990

International Planned Parenthood Federation, International Medical Advisory Panel: Statement on periodic abstinence for family planning. IPPF Med Bull 18:2, 1982

Jackson RA, Schwarz EB, Freedman L, et al: Advance supply of emergency contraception: Effect on use and usual contraction—a randomized trial. Obstet Gynecol 102:8, 2003

Kamischke A, Nieschlag E: Progress towards hormonal male contraception. Trends Pharmacol Sci 25:49, 2004

Kaunitz AM: Considering postpartum contraception and the role of lactation. Dialogues Contracept 5:5, 1997

Kaunitz AM: Depot medroxyprogesterone acetate contraception and the risk of breast and gynecologic cancer. J Reprod Med 45:419, 1996

Kaunitz AM: Medroxyprogesterone acetate/estradiol cypionate: Overview of a new contraceptive. Dialogues Contracept 6:1, 1999a

Kaunitz AM: Oral contraceptive use and venous thromboembolism: Translating epidemiologic data into clinical practice. ACOG Clin Rev 4:1, 1999b

Kaunitz AM, Garceau RJ, Cromie MA, and the Lunelle Study Group: Comparative safety, efficacy, and cycle control of Lunelle monthly contraceptive injection (medroxyprogesterone acetate and estradiol cypionate injectable suspension) and Ortho-Novum 7/7/7 oral contraceptive (norethindrone/ethinyl estradiol triphasic). Contraception 60:179, 1999

Keith LG, Oleszczuk JJ, Ahranjani M: A critical assessment of generic substitution for the obstetrician-gynecologist. Int J Fertil Womens Med 46:286, 2001

Kjos SL, Peters RK, Xiang A, et al: Contraception and the risk of type 2 diabetes mellitus in Latina women with prior gestational diabetes mellitus. JAMA 280:533, 1998

Kovacs L, Bartfai G, Apro G, et al: The effect of the contraceptive pill on blood pressure: A randomized controlled trial of three progestogen-oestrogen combinations in Szeged, Hungary. Contraception 33:69, 1986

Kubba A, Guillebaud J: Combined oral contraceptives: Acceptability and effective use. BMJ 49:140, 1993

Lammer EJ, Cordero JF: Exogenous sex hormone exposure and the risk for major malformations. JAMA 255:3128, 1986

Lee NC, Rubin GL: The intrauterine device and pelvic inflammatory disease revisited: New results from the woman's health study. Obstet Gynecol 72:1, 1988

Lewis MA, Spitzer WO, Heinemann LAJ, et al: Third generation oral contraceptives and risk of myocardial infarction: An international case-control study. BMJ 312:88, 1996

Lewit S: Outcome of pregnancy with an intrauterine device. Contraception 2:47, 1970

Lidegaard Ø: Oral contraception and risk of a cerebral thromboembolic attack: Results of a case-control study. BMJ 306:956, 1993

Lidegaard Ø, Edström B, Kreiner S: Oral contraceptives and venous thromboembolism. Contraception 57:291, 1998

Mainwaring R, Hales HA, Stevenson K, et al: Metabolic parameters, bleeding, and weight changes in U.S. women using progestin only contraceptives. Contraception 51:149, 1995

Mann JI: Progestogens in cardiovascular disease: An introduction to the epidemiologic data. Am J Obstet Gynecol 142:752, 1982

Marchbanks PA, McDonald JA, Wilson HG, et al: Oral contraceptives and the risk of breast cancer. N Engl J Med 346:2025, 2002

Mason V (ed): New contraceptive methods: The good, the bad, and the ugly. Contracept Tech Update 13:101, 1992

Metcalf MG: Incidence of ovulatory cycles in women approaching the menopause. J Biosoc Sci 11:39, 1979

Miller L, Hughes JP: Continuous combination oral contraceptive pills to eliminate withdrawal bleeding: A randomized trial. Obstet Gynecol 101:653, 2003

Mishell DR Jr: Oral contraceptives and cardiovascular events: Summary and application of data. Int J Fertil 45:121, 2000

Mishell DR Jr: Pharmacokinetics of depot medroxyprogesterone acetate contraception. J Reprod Med 41:381, 1996

Mishell DR Jr, Sulak PJ: The IUD: Dispelling the myths and assessing the potential. Dialogues Contracept 5:1, 1997

Mooij PN, Thomas CMG, Doesburg WH, et al: Multivitamin supplementation in oral contraceptive users. Contraception 44:277, 1991

Moore LL, Valuck R, McDougall C, et al: A comparative study of one-year weight gain among users of medroxyprogesterone acetate, levonorgestrel implants, and oral contraceptives. Contraception 52:215, 1995

Mosher WD, McNally JW: Contraceptive use at first premarital intercourse: United States, 1965–1988. Fam Plann Perspect 23:108, 1991

Mulders TM, Dieben T: Use of the novel combined contraceptive vaginal ring NuvaRing for ovulation inhibition. Fertil Steril 75:865, 2001

Nelson AL: Selecting a contraceptive method: Role of MPA/E2C. J Reprod Med 45:879, 2000

Neuberger J, Forman D, Doll R, et al: Oral contraceptives and hepatocellular carcinoma. BMJ 292:1355, 1986

Nichols M, Robinson G, Bounds W, et al: Effect of four combined oral contraceptives on blood pressure in the pill-free interval. Contraception 47:367, 1993

Nilsson CG, Lahteenmaki P, Luukkainen T: Ovarian function in amenorrheic and menstruating users of a levonorgestrel-releasing intrauterine device. Fertil Steril 41:52, 1984

Oettinger M, Barak S, Oettinger-Barak O, et al: Subcutaneous implantation of pure crystalline estradiol pellets for conception control. Gynecol Obstet Invest 59:119, 2005

Ortiz ME, Croxatto HB: The mode of action of IUDs. Contraception 36:37, 1987

Pérez A: Natural family planning: Postpartum period. Int J Fertil 26:219, 1981

Petitti DB, Sidney S, Bernstein A, et al: Stroke in users of low-dose oral contraceptives. N Engl J Med 335:8, 1996

Petitti DB, Sidney S, Quesenberry CP: Oral contraceptive use and myocardial infarction. Contraception 57:143, 1998

Physicians Desk Reference 2004. Montvale, NJ, 2004

Piccinino LJ, Mosher WD: Trends in contraceptive use in the United States: 1982–1995. Fam Plann Perspect 30:4,46 1998

Population Reports: Periodic abstinence: How well do new approaches work? Series L, No. 3, September 1981, p 33

Population Reports: Update on condoms—products, protection, promotion. Series H, No. 6, September–October 1982, p 121

Porter JB, Jick H, Walker AM: Mortality among oral contraceptive users. Obstet Gynecol 70:29, 1987

Prentice RL, Thomas DB: On the epidemiology of oral contraceptives and disease. Adv Cancer Res 49:285, 1987

Ragan RE, Rock RW, Buck HW: Metoclopramide pretreatment attenuates emergency contraceptive-associated nausea. Am J Obstet Gynecol 188:330, 2003

Raymond ER, Chen PL, Luoto J: Contraceptive effectiveness and safety in five nonoxynol-9 spermicides: A randomized trial. Obstet Gynecol 103:430, 2004

Raymond EG, Creinin MD, Barnhart KT, et al: Meclizine for prevention of nausea associated with use of emergency contraceptive pills: A randomized trial. Obstet Gynecol 95:271, 2000

Realini JP, Goldzieher JW: Oral contraceptives and cardiovascular disease: A critique of the epidemiologic studies. Am J Obstet Gynecol 152:729, 1985

Reddy DM, Fleming F, Swain C: Effect of mandatory parental notification on adolescent girls' use of sexual health care services. JAMA 73:1, 2002

Richwald GA, Greenland S, Gerber MM, et al: Effectiveness of the cavity-rim cervical cap: Results of a large clinical study. Obstet Gynecol 74:143, 1989

Rimm EB, Manson JE, Stampfer MJ, et al: Oral contraceptive use and the risk of type 2 (non-insulin-dependent) diabetes mellitus in a large prospective study of women. Diabetologia 35:967, 1992

Ronnerdag M, Odlind V: Health effects of long-term use of the intrauterine levonorgestrel-releasing system. Acta Obstet Gynecol Scand 78:716, 1999

Rosenberg MJ, Davidson AJ, Chen JH, et al: Barrier contraceptives and sexually transmitted diseases in women: A comparison of female-dependent methods and condoms. Am J Public Health 82:669, 1992

Rothman KJ, Louik C: Oral contraceptives and birth defects. N Engl J Med 299:522, 1978

Roumen F, Apter D, Mulders TM, et al: Efficacy, tolerability and acceptability of a novel contraceptive vaginal ring releasing etonogestrel and ethinyl estradiol. Hum Reprod 16:469, 2001

Rowe PJ: Research on Intrauterine Devices. Annual Technical Report 1991. Geneva, Switzerland, Special Programme of Research, Development and Research Training in Human Reproduction, World Health Organization, 1992, p 127

Royal College of General Practitioners' Oral Contraceptive Study: Oral contraceptives and gallbladder disease. Lancet 2:957, 1982

Sang GW, Shao QX, Ge RS, et al: A multi-centered phase III comparative clinical trial of Mesigyna, Cyclofem and Injectable No. 1 given by intramuscular injection to Chinese women. II: The comparison of bleeding patterns. Contraception 51:185, 1995

Savolainen E, Saksela E, Saxen L: Teratogenic hazards of oral contraceptives analyzed in a national malformation register. Am J Obstet Gynecol 140:521, 1981

Schlesselman JJ, Stadel BV, Murray P, et al: Breast cancer in relation to early use of oral contraceptives: No evidence of latent effect. JAMA 259:1828, 1988

Scholes D, Lacroix AZ, Ott SM, et al: Bone mineral density in women using depot medroxyprogesterone acetate for contraception. Obstet Gynecol 93:233, 1999

Schwartz SM, Petitti DB, Siscovick DS, et al: Stroke and use of low-dose oral contraceptives in young women. A pooled analysis of two US studies. Stroke 29:2277, 1998

Shikary ZK, Betrabet SS, Patel ZM, et al: ICMR Task Force Study on hormonal contraception. Transfer of levonorgestrel (LNG) administered through different drug delivery systems from the maternal circulation via breast milk. Contraception 35:477, 1987

Sidney S, Petitti DB, Quesenberry CP Jr, et al: Myocardial infarction in users of low-dose oral contraceptives. Obstet Gynecol 88:939, 1996

Sidney S, Siscovick DS, Petitti DB, et al: Myocardial infarction and use of low-dose oral contraceptives. A pooled analysis of 2 US studies. Circulation 98:1058, 1998

Sinei SKA, Schulz KF, Lamptey PR, et al: Preventing IUD-related pelvic infection: The efficacy of prophylactic doxycycline at insertion. Br J Obstet Gynaecol 97:412, 1990

Sivin I: Alternative estimates of ectopic pregnancy risks during contraception. Am J Obstet Gynecol 165:1900, 1991

Skegg DCG, Noonan EA, Paul C, et al: Depot medroxyprogesterone acetate and breast cancer. JAMA 273:799, 1995

Speroff L, Darney PD: A Clinical Guide for Contraception, 3rd ed. Philadelphia, Lippincott Williams & Wilkins, 2001, pp 66, 99, 240, 284

Speroff L, Sulak PJ: Contraception in the later reproductive years: A valid aspect of preventive health care. Dialogues Contracept 4:1, 1995

Stadel BV: Oral contraceptives and cardiovascular disease. N Engl J Med 305:612, 1981

Stanford JB, Mikolajczyk RT: Mechanisms of action of intrauterine devices: Update and estimation of postfertilization effects. Obstet Gynecol 187:1699, 2002

Steiner MJ, Dominik R, Rountree W, et al: Contraceptive effectiveness of a polyurethane condom and a latex condom: A randomized controlled trial. Obstet Gynecol 101:539, 2003

Stephenson JM: Systematic review of hormonal contraception and risk of HIV transmission: When to resist meta-analysis. AIDS 12:545, 1998

Strom BL, Tamragouri RN, Morse ML, et al: Oral contraceptives and other risk factors for gallbladder diseases. Clin Pharmacol Ther 39:335, 1986

Sulak PJ, Haney AF: Unwanted pregnancies: Understanding contraceptive use and benefits in adolescents and older women. Am J Obstet Gynecol 168:2042, 1993

Sulak PJ, Kaunitz AM: Hormonal contraception and bone mineral density. Dialogues Contracept 6:1, 1999

Taneepanichskul S, Reinprayoon D, Khaosaad P: Comparative study of weight change between long-term DMPA and IUD acceptors. Contraception 58:149, 1998

Task Force on Postovulatory Methods of Fertility Regulation: Randomized controlled trial of levonorgestrel versus the Yuzpe regimen of combined oral contraceptives for emergency contraception. Lancet 352:428, 1998

Tatum HJ, Schmidt FH, Jain AK: Management and outcome of pregnancies associated with Copper-T intrauterine contraceptive device. Am J Obstet Gynecol 126:869, 1976

Thomas DB, Ray RM: World Health Organization Collaborative Study of Neoplasia and Steroid Contraceptives: Oral contraceptives and invasive adenocarcinomas and adenosquamous carcinomas of the uterine cervix. Am J Epidemiol 144:281, 1996

Thomas DB, Ye Z, Ray RM, WHO Collaborative Study of Neoplasia and Steroid Contraceptives: Cervical carcinoma in situ and use of depo-medroxyprogesterone acetate (DMPA). Contraception 51:25, 1995

Toivonen J, Luukkainen T, Allonen H: Protective effect of intrauterine release of levonorgestrel on pelvic infections: Three years' comparative experience of levonorgestrel and copper-releasing intrauterine devices. Obstet Gynecol 77:261, 1991

Truitt ST, Fraser AB, Grimes DA, et al: Hormonal contraception during lactation: Systematic review of randomized controlled trials. Contraception 68:233, 2003

Trussell J, Duran V, Shochet T, et al: Access to emergency contraception. Obstet Gynecol 95:267, 2000

Trussell J, Ellertson C, Stewart F: Emergency contraception. A cost-effective approach to preventing pregnancy. Women Health Primary Care 1:52, 1998a

Trussell J, Ellertson C, Stewart F: The effectiveness of the Yuzpe regimen of emergency contraception. Fam Plann Perspect 28:58, 1996

Trussell J, Hatcher RA, Cates W Jr, et al: Contraceptive failure in the United States: An update. Stud Fam Plann 21:51, 1990

Trussell J, Rodriguez G, Ellertson C: New estimates of the effectiveness of the Yuzpe regimen of emergency contraception. Contraception 57:363, 1998b

Trussell J, Stewart F: An update on emergency contraception. Dialogues Contracept 5:1, 1998

van den Hurk PJ, O'Brien S: Non-contraceptive use of the levonorgestrel-releasing intrauterine system. Obstet Gynaecol 1:13, 1999

Vessey MP, Johnson B, Doll R, et al: Outcome of pregnancy in women using intrauterine devices. Lancet 1:495, 1974

Vessey MP, Lawless M, McPherson K, et al: Fertility after stopping use of intrauterine contraceptive device. BMJ 286:106, 1983a

Vessey MP, Lawless M, Yeates D: Efficacy of different contraceptive methods. Lancet 1:841, 1982

Vessey MP, McPherson K, Lawless M, et al: Neoplasia of the cervix uteri and contraception: A possible adverse effect of the pill. Lancet 2:930, 1983b

Vessey MP, McPherson K, Lawless M, et al: Oral contraception and serious psychiatric illness: Absence of an association. Br J Psychiatry 146:45, 1985

Vessey MP, Meisler L, Flavel R, et al: Outcome of pregnancy in women using different methods of contraception. Br J Obstet Gynaecol 86:548, 1979

Wai Ngai S, Fan S, Li S, et al: A randomized trial to compare 24 h versus 12 h double dose regimen of levonorgestrel for emergency contraception. Hum Reprod 20:307, 2005

Waldron T: Newer, innovative condoms may help increase compliance. Contracept Tech Update 12:171, 1991

Waldron T: Tests show commonly used substances harm latex condoms. Contracept Tech Update 10:20, 1989

Wallach M, Grimes DA (eds): Modern oral contraception. Updates from The Contraception Report. Totowa, New Jersey, Emron, 2000, pp 26, 90, 194–195

Walsh T, Grimes D, Frezieres R, et al: Randomized controlled trial of prophylactic antibiotics before insertion of intrauterine devices. Lancet 351:1005, 1998

Weiss BD: RU 486: The progesterone antagonist. Arch Fam Med 2:63, 1993

Westhoff CL: Oral contraceptives and thrombosis: An overview of study methods and recent results. Am J Obstet Gynecol 179:S38, 1998

Wise LA, Palmer JR, Harlow BL, et al: Reproductive factors, hormonal contraception, and risk of uterine leiomyomata in African-American women: A prospective study. Am J Epidemiol 159:113, 2004

Woods ER, Grace E, Havens KK, et al: Contraceptive compliance with a levonorgestrel triphasic and a norethindrone monophasic oral contraceptive in adolescent patients. Am J Obstet Gynecol 166:901, 1992

World Health Organization Collaborative Study of Cardiovascular Disease and Steroid Hormone Contraception: Acute myocardial infarction and combined oral contraceptives: Results of an international multi-center case-control study. Lancet 349:1202, 1997

World Health Organization Collaborative Study of Cardiovascular Disease and Steroid Hormone Contraception: Cardiovascular disease and use of oral and injectable progestogen-only contraceptives and combined injectable contraceptives. Results of an international, multicenter, case-control study. Contraception 57:315, 1998

World Health Organization Collaborative Study of Cardiovascular Disease and Steroid Hormone Contraception: Ischaemic stroke and combined oral contraceptives: Results of an international, multi-center case-control study. Lancet 348:498, 1996

World Health Organization Special Programme of Research, Development and Research Training in Human Reproduction, Task Force on Intrauterine Devices for Fertility Regulation: A multinational case-control study of ectopic pregnancy. Clin Reprod Fertil 3:131, 1985

World Health Organization Task Force on Long-Acting Systemic Agents for Fertility Regulation, Special Programme of Research, Development and Research Training on Human Reproduction: A multi-centered phase III comparative study of two hormonal contraceptive preparations given once-a-month by intramuscular injection. I: Contraceptive efficacy and side effects. Contraception 37:1, 1988

World Health Organization: Facts about once-a-month injectable contraceptives: Memorandum from a WHO meeting. Bull WHO 71:677, 1993

World Health Organization: Injectable contraceptives: Their role in family planning, monograph. Geneva, WHO, 1990

World Health Organization: Combined oral contraceptives and liver cancer. Int J Cancer 43:254, 1989

World Health Organization: Mechanism of action, safety and efficacy of intrauterine devices. Technical Report No. 753, Geneva, Switzerland, WHO, 1987

Zieman M, Guillebaud J, Weisberg E, et al: Contraceptive efficacy and cycle control with the Ortho Evra/Evra transdermal system: The analysis of pooled data. Fertil Steril 77:S13, 2002

Zondervan KT, Carpenter LM, Painter R, et al: Oral contraceptives and cervical cancer—further findings from the Oxford Family Planning Association Contraceptive Study. Brit J Cancer 73:1291, 1996

33

Sterilization

Surgical sterilization has become the most popular form of contraception. The volume of sterilization procedures cannot be tracked accurately in the United States because most interval tubal sterilizations and vasectomies are performed in ambulatory centers. Westhoff and Davis (2000), however, citing data from the National Survey of Family Growth, estimate that about 700,000 tubal sterilizations are performed annually. Unfortunately, there are still excessive federal rules and regulations that discourage voluntary sterilization among financially underprivileged women. Several important multicenter studies of voluntary sterilization have been performed by investigators of the U.S. Collaborative Review of Sterilization (CREST) and the Centers for Disease Control and Prevention. Many of their observations are subsequently described.

FEMALE STERILIZATION

Female sterilization is the contraceptive method of choice for 28 percent of couples in the United States (American College of Obstetricians and Gynecologists, 2003). It is usually accomplished by occlusion or division of the fallopian tubes. This can be performed at any time, but at least half of tubal sterilization procedures are performed in conjunction with cesarean or vaginal delivery (MacKay and associates, 2001). Nonpuerperal tubal sterilization is usually accomplished via laparoscopy in an outpatient surgical center.

PUERPERAL TUBAL STERILIZATION. The oviducts are accessible at the umbilicus directly beneath the abdominal wall for several days after delivery. Thus, puerperal tubal sterilization is technically simple, and hospitalization need not be prolonged. Some practitioners prefer to perform sterilization immediately following delivery (Bucklin and Smith, 1999), although others wait for 12 to 24 hours. At Parkland and the University of Alabama Hospitals, puerperal tubal ligation is performed in the obstetrical surgical suite the morning after delivery. This minimizes the hospital stay but allows the likelihood of postpartum hemorrhage to diminish. In addition, the status of the newborn can be better ascertained.

The first tubal sterilization reported in the United States, performed 120 years ago, consisted of a silk ligature placed around the tubes about 1 inch from their uterine attachment after a cesarean delivery (Lungren, 1881). It soon was apparent that ligation without tubal resection had an unacceptably high failure rate, and a variety of techniques are now used to disrupt tubal patency.

Irving Procedure. This procedure is the most difficult to perform but the least likely to fail. The cut oviduct is separated from the mesosalpinx sufficiently to free a medial segment of tube (Fig. 33–1A). The freed distal stump of the proximal tubal segment is buried within a tunnel created in the

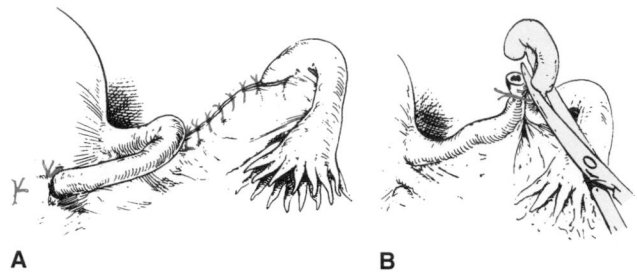

A   **B**

FIGURE 33–1. Techniques for tubal sterilization. **A. Irving procedure**: the medial cut end of the oviduct is buried in the myometrium posteriorly, and the distal cut end is buried in the mesosalpinx. **B. Pomeroy procedure**: a loop of oviduct is ligated, and the knuckle of tube above the ligature is excised.

myometrium posteriorly, and the proximal end of the distal tubal segment is buried within the mesosalpinx.

Pomeroy Procedure. This is the simplest method of dividing the tube (Fig. 33–1B). Plain catgut is used to ligate the knuckle of tube to ensure prompt absorption of the ligature and subsequent separation of the severed tubal ends. Even so, ectopic pregnancy in the distal segment can occur (Berker and colleagues, 2002).

Parkland Procedure. This procedure, shown in Figure 33–2, was developed in the 1960s. It was designed to avoid the initial intimate approximation of the cut ends of the oviduct inherent with the Pomeroy procedure.

SURGICAL TECHNIQUE. A small infraumbilical incision is made. The oviduct is identified by grasping its midportion with a Babcock clamp, and the distal fimbria is identified. This prevents confusing the round ligament with the midportion of the oviduct. **Whenever the oviduct is inadvertently dropped, it is mandatory to repeat this identification procedure.** An avascular site in the mesosalpinx adjacent to the oviduct is then perforated with a small hemostat, and the jaws are opened to separate the oviduct from the adjacent mesosalpinx for about 2.5 cm (see Fig. 33–2). The freed oviduct is ligated proximally and distally with 0-chromic suture, and the intervening segment of about 2 cm is excised and inspected for hemostasis. Both segments are submitted for histological confirmation. During four decades, the failure rate has been less than 1 in 400 procedures.

Other Procedures. The *Madlener technique* and the *Kroener fimbriectomy* for tubal sterilization are rarely used today because of high failure rates (Pati and Cullins, 2000). In most cases, failures are due to recanalization of the proximal portion of the tube.

Failure Rates. Puerperal sterilization fails for two major reasons.

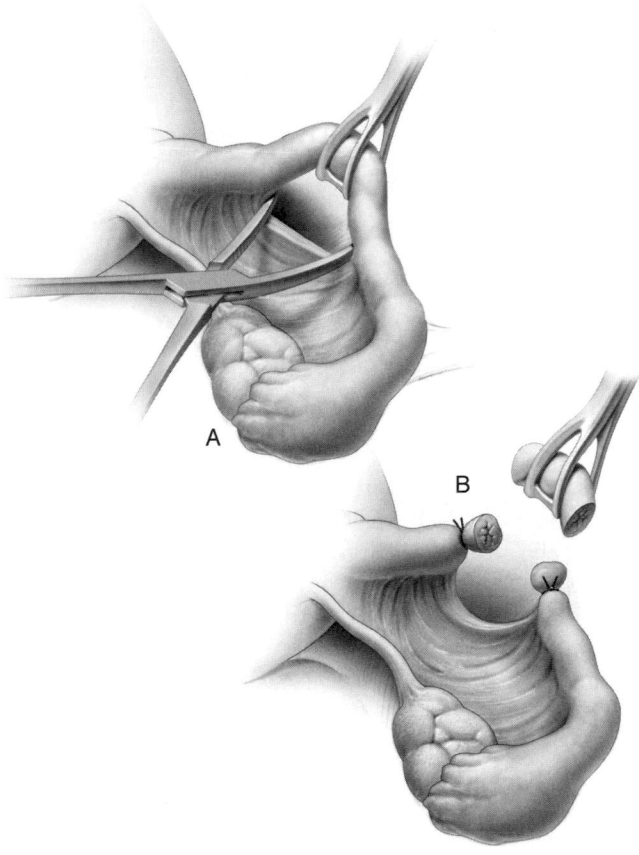

FIGURE 33–2. Parkland tubal ligation: The avascular mesosalpinx is opened by blunt dissection. A 2-cm midsegment of tube is ligated with 0-chromic suture and divided between the sutures.

1. Surgical errors, which include transection of the round ligament instead of the oviduct or partial transection of the oviduct.
2. Formation of a fistulous tract between the severed tubal stumps or spontaneous reanastomosis.

In their first report, investigators from the CREST study described follow-up of 10,863 women who had undergone tubal sterilization from 1978 through 1986. The failure rates for various procedures are summarized in Figure 33–3. It is readily apparent that puerperal sterilization is highly effective, with a short- and long-term failure rate that is better than most interval procedures. Some clinicians have reported an increased failure rate for sterilization at the time of cesarean delivery; however, we have identified no such differences with the technique of tubal sterilization used at Parkland Hospital (see Fig. 33–2).

NONPUERPERAL (INTERVAL) TUBAL STERILIZA-TION.
Techniques for nonpuerperal tubal sterilization, including modifications, basically consist of:

1. Ligation and resection at laparotomy, as described earlier for puerperal sterilization.

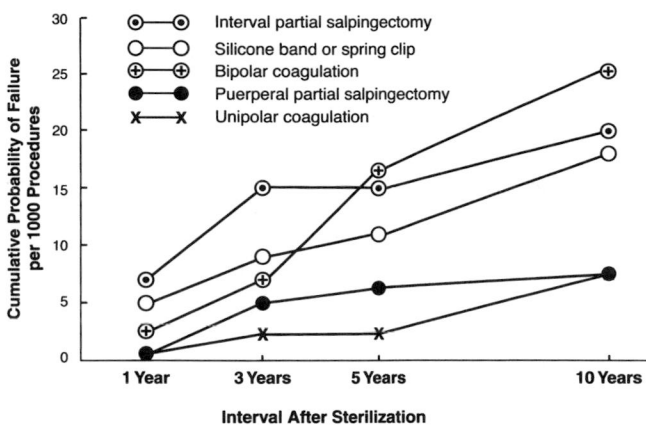

FIGURE 33–3. Data from the U.S. Collaborative Review of Sterilization (CREST) shows the cumulative probability of pregnancy per 1000 procedures for five methods of tubal sterilization. (Data from Peterson and colleagues, 1996.)

2. The application of a variety of permanent rings or clips to the fallopian tubes, usually by laparoscopy.
3. Electrocoagulation of a segment of the tubes, again usually through a laparoscope.

Surgical Approaches. A number of approaches and techniques may be used to perform nonpuerperal tubal sterilization. In developed countries, laparoscopic techniques are most often used. In the United States, laparoscopic tubal ligation is the leading method of female sterilization (American College of Obstetricians and Gynecologists, 2003). The procedure is frequently performed in an ambulatory surgical setting under general anesthesia with tracheal intubation. In almost all cases, the woman can be discharged several hours later. The actual disruption of tubal continuity is accomplished using loops, clips, and electrocauterization with or without transection of the tube. Because electrocauterization destroys a large segment of tube, surgical reversal is usually difficult and often not possible.

"Minilaparotomy" using a 3-cm suprapubic incision is also popular, especially in resource-poor countries (Kulier and colleagues, 2002). The peritoneal cavity can also be entered through the posterior vaginal fornix—*colpotomy* or *culdotomy*—to perform tubal interruption. This approach is not commonly used today.

Major morbidity is rare with either minilaparotomy or laparoscopy. In the study by Kulier and associates (2002), minor morbidity was twice as common in women who had minilaparotomies.

Laparoscopic Methods of Tubal Interruption. A number of techniques or devices can be used to accomplish tubal sterilization via laparoscopy. Details of these have been provided by a number of reviews (Gilstrap and associates, 2002; Pati and Cullins, 2000).

Electrocoagulation is used for destruction of a segment of tube and can be accomplished with either unipolar or bipolar electrical current. Although unipolar electrocoagulation has the lowest long-term failure rate (see Fig. 33–3), it also has the highest serious complication rate. For this reason, bipolar coagulation is favored by most clinicians (American College of Obstetricians and Gynecologists, 2003).

Mechanical methods of tubal occlusion can be accomplished with a silicone rubber band such as the Falope Ring and the Tubal Ring; the spring-loaded Hulka-Clemens Clip (also known as the Wolf Clip); or the silicone-lined titanium Filshie Clip. Sokal and co-workers (2000) compared the Tubal Ring and Filshie Clip in a randomized trial of 2746 women. They reported similar rates of safety and a 1-year pregnancy rate of 1.7 per 1000 women. All these methods have favorable long-term success rates (see Fig. 33–3). When done via laparoscopy, these procedures are technically more difficult, and they have significantly higher failure rates before experience is gained (Peterson and colleagues, 2001).

Operative Complications. Principal hazards are anesthetic complications, inadvertent injury of adjacent structures, the rare occurrence of pulmonary embolism, and sterilization failure with subsequent intrauterine or ectopic pregnancy (see Chap. 10). Because of improved safety with anesthetic and laparoscopic techniques, the case-fatality rates for tubal sterilization have diminished appreciably over the past 2 decades. For example, from 1977 to 1981, Peterson and co-workers (1983) estimated the case-fatality frequency to be 8 per 100,000 procedures. Fifteen years later, Hatcher and colleagues (1998) reported mortality rates of approximately 1.5 per 100,000 for laparoscopic sterilizations. Using the CREST database, Jamieson and co-workers (2000) reported an overall complication rate of 0.9 to 1.6 per 100 laparoscopic interval sterilization procedures. Unintended laparotomy was done in about 1 per 100 procedures.

Failure Rates. The reasons for interval tubal failures are not always apparent, but some are:

1. Surgical errors likely account for 30 to 50 percent of cases.
2. An occlusion method failure may be due to fistula formation, especially with electrocautery procedures. Faulty clips may not be occlusive enough, or the fallopian tube may spontaneously undergo reanastomosis.
3. Equipment failure, such as a defective electrical current for the electrocautery, may be a causative factor.
4. The woman was already pregnant at the time of surgery—a so-called *luteal phase pregnancy.*

As shown in Figure 33–3, some sterilization methods have lower failure rates than others. Even with the same procedure, there are variations in failure rate. For example, when fewer than three tubal sites are coagulated, the five-year cumulative probability of pregnancy is about 12 per 1000 procedures.

This compares with only 3 per 1000 if three or more sites are coagulated (Peterson and associates, 1999).

The lifetime increased cumulative failure rates over time are supportive that failures after 1 year are not likely due to technical errors. Soderstrom (1985) found that most sterilization failures were not preventable. The American College of Obstetricians and Gynecologists (1996) concluded that "pregnancies after sterilization may occur without any technical errors."

Long-Term Complications. In addition to the 15-year cumulative pregnancy rates shown in Figure 33–3, there are other long-term adverse effects.

ECTOPIC PREGNANCY. Approximately half of the pregnancies that follow a failed electrocoagulation procedure were ectopic, compared with only 10 percent following failure of a ring, clip, or tubal resection method (Hatcher and colleagues, 1990; Hendrix and associates, 1999). **Any symptoms of pregnancy in a woman after tubal sterilization must be investigated, and an ectopic pregnancy must be excluded.** Diagnosis and management are discussed in detail in Chapter 10.

POSTTUBAL LIGATION SYNDROME. In 1951, Williams and colleagues described their 22-year experiences with long-term follow-up in women who had undergone tubal ligation. They reported an excessive incidence of menorrhagia and intermenstrual bleeding, a condition that later became known as *posttubal ligation syndrome.* Subsequently, a similar incidence of menstrual dysfunction was reported in women whose husbands had undergone vasectomy (DeStefano and colleagues, 1985; Shy and associates, 1992). Thus, debate over the very existence of a unique syndrome has persisted.

Observations from the CREST study are very informative concerning these issues. Peterson and colleagues (2000) compared long-term outcomes of 9514 women who had undergone tubal sterilization with a cohort of 573 women whose partners had undergone vasectomy. They found that both groups had similar risks for menorrhagia, intermenstrual bleeding, and dysmenorrhea. In fact, they found that women who had undergone sterilization had *decreased* duration and volume of menstrual flow as well as *less* dysmenorrhea. There was, however, an increased incidence of cycle irregularity in the sterilized women. The cause of these findings remains an enigma, although Harlow and co-workers (2002) reported no significant change in serum levels of follicle-stimulating hormone, luteinizing hormone, and estradiol. Timonen and co-workers (2002) reported a transient increase in follicular phase serum estradiol levels that normalized by 12 months.

OTHER EFFECTS. Whether the incidence of *subsequent hysterectomy* is increased in women who have undergone tubal sterilization is controversial (Mall and colleagues, 2002; Pati and Cullins, 2000). In a CREST follow-up study, Hillis and associates (1997) reported that 17 percent of women undergoing tubal sterilization also underwent hysterectomy in the subsequent 14 years. Although the investigators did not compare this incidence with a cohort control, the indications were similar to those for nonsterilized women undergoing hysterectomy.

Westhoff and Davis (2000) concluded that tubal sterilization likely protects against *ovarian cancer*. They found no differences in the incidence of *breast cancer*.

According to Holt and colleagues (2003), the incidence of *functional ovarian cysts* is increased almost twofold following tubal sterilization. Levgur and Duvivier (2000) reported that women who had undergone tubal sterilization were highly unlikely to have subsequent *salpingitis*.

Less objective but important psychological sequelae of sterilization have also been evaluated. In the CREST study, Costello and colleagues (2002) found that tubal ligation did not change *sexual interest or pleasure* in 80 percent of women. In the majority of the 20 percent of women who did report a change, *positive effects* were 10 to 15 times more likely to occur. Invariably, a number of women express *regrets about sterilization*. In the CREST study, Jamieson and co-workers (2002) reported that by 5 years, 7 percent of women who had undergone tubal ligation had regrets. This is not limited to their own sterilization, because 6.1 percent of women whose husbands had undergone vasectomy had similar regrets.

REVERSAL OF TUBAL STERILIZATION. No woman should undergo tubal sterilization believing that subsequent fertility is guaranteed by either surgery or assisted reproductive techniques. These latter procedures are technically difficult, expensive, and not always successful. Success rates vary greatly depending on the age of the woman, the amount of tube remaining, and the technology used. Van Voorhis (2000) reviewed a number of reports and found that pregnancy rates varied from 45 to 90 percent with surgical reversals. For example, pregnancy rates as high as 80 percent have been reported for tubal reanastomosis (Cha and associates, 2001). When neosalpingostomy is done for fimbriectomy reversal, however, successful pregnancies occur in only 30 percent of women (Tourgeman and co-workers, 2001). **Almost 10 percent of women who undergo reversal of tubal sterilization have an ectopic pregnancy.**

Reversal procedures can be done by laparoscopy or laparotomy, and pregnancy rates are similar with either method (Cha and colleagues, 2001). In a cost-effectiveness study from Canada, Hawkins and associates (2002) found laparoscopy to have lower *costs* than laparotomy.

HYSTERECTOMY. For the woman who desires no more children, hysterectomy has many theoretical advantages. In the absence of uterine or other pelvic disease, however, hysterectomy solely for sterilization at the time of cesarean delivery, early in the puerperium, or even remote from pregnancy is difficult to justify.

TRANSCERVICAL STERILIZATION. Sterilization has been performed by using hysteroscopy to visualize the tubal ostia and obliterating them with a variety of compounds or devices.

INTRATUBAL CHEMICAL METHODS. Several compounds are being investigated as useful in tubal sterilization (Ballagh, 2003). Liquid silicone is injected transcervically into the tubes, where it hardens, forming *silicone plugs*. Repeat procedures are necessary in 20 percent of women, however, and continued tubal patency is common. Tubal injections with the adhesive *methylcyanoacrylate* cause inflammation, necrosis, and fibrosis. Insertion of *quinacrine pellets* in more than 100,000 women in other countries has also been used to achieve tubal occlusion. Few well-done studies concerning its efficacy are available, but advantages include minimal complications and low cost. Randic and colleagues (2001) reported cumulative pregnancy rates by 8 years of more than 6 per 100. Because of concerns about carcinogenesis based on a study of 30,000 Vietnamese women, the World Health Organization recommended halting usage of quinacrine (Lippes, 2002). In addition, *erythromycin* placed tubally to incite inflammation has been investigated, but it has an unacceptably high one-year failure rate of 36 percent (Bairagy and Mullick, 2004).

INTRATUBAL DEVICES. Tubes can be occluded by hysteroscopic insertion of some type of mechanical device into the proximal tube. Several of these devices have been evaluated. One of these, Essure, was approved by the Food and Drug Administration in November, 2002. This device is a microinsert that has a stainless steel inner coil enclosed in polyester fibers and an expandable outer coil of Nitinol—a nickel and titanium alloy used in coronary artery stents. The outer coil expands after placement allowing the fiber to also expand, and as tissue grows within the fiber, tubal occlusion results.

Preliminary results with this device and others have been encouraging (Association of Reproductive Health Professionals, 2002). In one study, Cooper and co-workers (2003) used intravenous sedation or paracervical block to insert Essure hysteroscopically. These investigators succeeded in proper insertion in 464 of 507 women (92 percent). None of these women had pregnancies by 9620 woman-months. In a similar study, Kerin and colleagues (2001) reported that 97 percent of women with the device in place after 2 years expressed a satisfaction level of very good to excellent.

Essure use has two major drawbacks: the high cost of the device itself (almost $1000) and the necessity of hysterosalpingography at 3 months to ensure tubal blockage.

MALE STERILIZATION

Nearly a half million men in the United States undergo vasectomy each year (Magnani and colleagues, 1999). Through a small incision in the scrotum, the lumen of the vas deferens

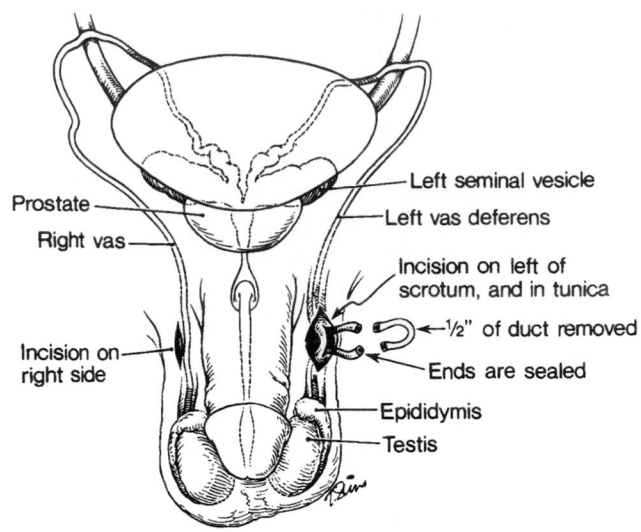

FIGURE 33–4. Anatomy of male reproductive system, showing procedure for vasectomy.

is disrupted to block the passage of sperm from the testes (Fig. 33–4). With local analgesia, the procedure is usually performed within 20 minutes.

In a review, Hendrix and colleagues (1999) found that, compared with vasectomy, female tubal sterilization has a 20-fold increased complication rate, a 10- to 37-fold failure rate, and a 3-fold increased cost. Similarly, in Dallas in 2003, total charges for a vasectomy were $800 compared with almost $6000 for an outpatient laparoscopic tubal ligation.

A disadvantage of vasectomy is that sterility is not immediate. Complete expulsion of sperm stored in the reproductive tract beyond the interrupted vas deferens takes about 3 months or 20 ejaculations (American College of Obstetricians and Gynecologists, 1996). Although most protocols dictate that semen should be analyzed until two consecutive sperm counts are zero, Bradshaw and colleagues (2001) reported that only one azoospermic semen analysis is sufficient evidence of sterility. During the period before azoospermia is documented, another form of contraception must be used.

The failure rate for vasectomy during the first year is 9.4 per 1000 procedures but only 11.4 per 1000 at 2, 3, and 5 years (Jamieson and colleagues, 2004). Failures result from unprotected intercourse too soon after ligation, incomplete occlusion of the vas deferens, or recanalization. A phenomenon termed *transient sperm reappearance* usually is not associated with pregnancy. Haldar and co-workers (2000) described temporary low sperm counts in 20 of 2250 men who had been documented to have azoospermia following vasectomy. Of the 20, the count was less than 10,000/mL, and in the 14 retested one month later, azoospermia was again confirmed. They concluded that spermatozoa present in the distal vas deferens are slowly released, or that microchannels form with sperm granulomas.

RESTORATION OF FERTILITY. Success after vasectomy reversal depends on several factors. Fibrosis increases

with time (Raleigh and colleagues, 2004). A review of several reports suggests that odds for success are about 50 percent, with somewhat higher rates following microsurgical reanastomosis.

LONG-TERM EFFECTS. Other than regrets, long-term consequences are rare (Amundsen and Ramakrishnan, 2004). After vasectomy, antibodies directed at spermatozoa can frequently be identified. Concern was raised about the possibility that the immune response might cause harmful systemic changes. Despite this, studies have not identified an increase in cardiovascular disease, circulating immune complexes, or damage to retinal blood vessels (Giovannucci and colleagues, 1992; Goldacre and co-workers, 1983). Subsequently, Manson and associates (1999) provided data on 1159 physicians from the U.S. Physicians' Health Study. In a 15-year follow-up, there was no difference in the incidence of myocardial infarction or stroke in men with or without vasectomy. On the basis of their review, Schwingl and Guess (2000) also concluded that vasectomy is not followed by accelerated atherogenesis.

There is no convincing evidence of an increased incidence of *testicular cancer* following vasectomy (Giovannucci and colleagues, 1992). Earlier studies found no evidence to associate development of *prostatic carcinoma* after vasectomy (Giovannucci and associates, 1993a, 1993b; Hayes and co-workers, 1993). This changed, however, when Lesko and colleagues (1999) compared follow-up results in 1216 vasectomized men and 1400 controls. They reported an almost twofold risk of prostatic cancer in men younger than 55 years of age, but not in older men. Following this, a population-based Danish cohort study found that prostatic cancer was not increased (Lynge, 2002). These findings indicate, at worst, a weak association that may be explicable by greater scrutiny of men who have undergone vasectomy (Grönberg, 2003).

REFERENCES

American College of Obstetricians and Gynecologists: Benefits and risks of sterilization. Practice Bulletin No. 46, September, 2003

American College of Obstetricians and Gynecologists: Sterilization. ACOG Technical Bulletin No. 222, April, 1996

Amundsen GA, Ramakrishnan K: Vasectomy: A "seminal" analysis. South Med J 97:54, 2004

Association of Reproductive Health Professionals: Clinical proceedings. Clinical update on transcervical sterilization. Washington, DC, 2002

Bairagy NR, Mullick BC: Use of erythromycin for nonsurgical female sterilization in West Bengal, India: A study of 790 cases. Contraception 69:47, 2004

Ballagh SA: Sterilization in the office: The concept now is a reality. Contracept Technol Rep BB #S0315, February 2003

Berker B, Kabukcu C, Dokmeci F: Tubal pregnancy after Pomeroy sterilization. Arch Gynecol Obstet 266:56, 2002

Bradshaw HD, Rosario DJ, James MJ, et al: Review of current practice to establish success after vasectomy. Br J Surg 88:290, 2001

Bucklin BA, Smith CV: Postpartum tubal ligation: Safety, timing and other implications for anesthesia. Anesth Analg 89:1269, 1999

Cha SH, Lee MH, Kim JH, et al: Fertility outcome after tubal anastomosis by laparoscopy and laparotomy. J Am Assoc Gynecol Laparosc 8:348, 2001

Cooper JM, Carignan CS, Cher D, et al: Microinsert nonincisional hysteroscopic sterilization. Obstet Gynecol 102:59, 2003

Costello C, Hillis S, Marchbanks P, et al: The effect of interval tubal sterilization on sexual interest and pleasure. Obstet Gynecol 100:3, 2002

DeStefano F, Perlman JA, Peterson HB, et al: Long term risk of menstrual disturbances after tubal sterilization. Am J Obstet Gynecol 152:835, 1985

Gilstrap LC, Cunningham FG, Van Dorsten P (eds): Obstetric hysterectomy. In Operative Obstetrics, 2nd ed. New York, McGraw-Hill, 2002

Giovannucci E, Ascherio A, Rimm EB, et al: A prospective study of vasectomy and prostate cancer in U.S. men. JAMA 269:876, 1993a

Giovannucci E, Tosteson TD, Speizer FE, et al: A long-term study of mortality in men who have undergone vasectomy. N Engl J Med 326:1392, 1992

Giovannucci E, Tosteson TD, Speizer FE, et al: A retrospective cohort study of vasectomy and prostate cancer in U.S. men. JAMA 269:878, 1993b

Goldacre JM, Holford TR, Vessey MP: Cardiovascular disease and vasectomy. N Engl J Med 308:805, 1983

Grönberg H: Prostate cancer epidemiology. Lancet 361:859, 2003

Haldar N, Cranston D, Turner E, et al: How reliable is a vasectomy? Long-term follow-up of vasectomised men. Lancet 356:43, 2000

Harlow BL, Missmer S, Cramer D, et al: Does tubal sterilization influence the subsequent risk of menorrhagia or dysmenorrhea? Fertil Steril 77:4, 2002

Hatcher RA, Stewart F, Trussell J, et al: Contraceptive Technology, 15th ed. New York, Irvington, 1990, pp 391, 403, 416

Hatcher RA, Trussell J, Stewart F, et al: Contraceptive Technology, 17th ed. New York, Ardent Media, 1998, p 548

Hawkins J, Dube D, Kaplow M, et al: Cost analysis of tubal anastomosis by laparoscopy and by laparotomy. J Am Assoc Gynecol Laparosc 9:120, 2002

Hayes RB, Pottern CM, Greenberg R, et al: Vasectomy and prostate cancer in US blacks and whites. Am J Epidemiol 137:263, 1993

Hendrix NW, Chauhan SP, Morrison JC: Sterilization and its consequences. Obstet Gynecol Surv 54:766, 1999

Hillis SD, Marchbanks PA, Tylor LR, et al: Tubal sterilization and long-term risk of hysterectomy: Findings from the United States Collaborative Review of Sterilization. Obstet Gynecol 89:609, 1997

Holt VL, Cushing-Haugen KL, Daling JR: Oral contraceptives, tubal sterilization, and functional ovarian cyst risk. Obstet Gynecol 102:252, 2003

Jamieson DJ, Costello C, Trussell J, et al: The risk of pregnancy after vasectomy. Obstet Gynecol 103:848, 2004

Jamieson DJ, Hillis SD, Duerr A, et al: Complications of interval laparoscopic tubal sterilization: Findings from the United States Collaborative Review of Sterilization. Obstet Gynecol 96:997, 2000

Jamieson DJ, Kaufman SC, Costello C, et al: A comparison of women's regret after vasectomy versus tubal sterilization. Obstet Gynecol 99:1073, 2002

Kerin JF, Carignan CS, Cher D: The safety and effectiveness of a new hysteroscopic method for permanent birth control: Results of the first Essure pbc clinical study. Aust N Z J Obstet Gynaecol 41:364, 2001

Kulier R, Boulvain M, Walker D, et al: Minilaparotomy and endoscopic techniques for tubal sterilization. Cochrane Database Syst Rev 2002(3):CD001328

Lesko SM, Louik C, Vezina R, et al: Vasectomy and prostate cancer. J Urol 161:1848, 1999

Levgur M, Duvivier R: Pelvic inflammatory disease after tubal sterilization: A review. Obstet Gynecol Surv 55:41, 2000

Lippes J: Quinacrine sterilization: The imperative need for clinical trials. Fertil Steril 77:1106, 2002

Lungren SS: A case of cesarean twice. Am J Obstet Dis Women Child 14:78, 1881

Lynge E: Prostate cancer is not increased in men with vasectomy in Denmark. J Urol 168:488, 2002

MacKay AP, Kieke BA, Koonin LM, et al: Tubal sterilization in the United States, 1994–1996. Fam Plann Perspect 33:161, 2001

Magnani RJ, Haws JM, Morgan GT, et al: Vasectomy in the United States, 1991 and 1995. Am J Public Health 89:92, 1999

Mall A, Shirk G, Van Voorhis BJ: Previous tubal ligation is a risk factor for hysterectomy after rollerball endometrial ablation. Obstet Gynecol 100:659, 2002

Manson JE, Ridker PM, Spelsberg A, et al: Vasectomy and subsequent cardiovascular disease in US physicians. Contraception 59:181, 1999

Pati S, Cullins V: Female sterilization: Evidence. Obstet Gynecol Clin North Am 27:859, 2000

Peterson HB, DeStefano F, Rubin GL, et al: Deaths attributed to tubal sterilization in the United States, 1977 to 1981. Am J Obstet Gynecol 146:131, 1983

Peterson HB, Jeng G, Folger SG, et al: The risk of menstrual abnormalities after tubal sterilization. N Engl J Med 343:1681, 2000

Peterson HB, Xia Z, Hughes JM, et al: The risk of pregnancy after tubal sterilization: Findings from the U.S. Collaborative Review of Sterilization. Am J Obstet Gynecol 174:1161, 1996

Peterson HB, Xia Z, Wilcox LS, et al: Pregnancy after tubal sterilization with bipolar electrocoagulation. U.S. Collaborative Review of Sterilization Working Group. Obstet Gynecol 94:163, 1999

Peterson HB, Xia Z, Wilcox LS, et al: Pregnancy after tubal sterilization with silicone rubber band and spring clip application. Obstet Gynecol 97:205, 2001

Raleigh D, O'Donnell L, Southwick GJ, et al: Stereological analysis of the human testis after vasectomy indicates impairment of spermatogenic efficiency with increasing obstructive interval. Fertil Steril 81:1595, 2004

Randic L, Haller H, Sojat S: Nonsurgical female sterilization: Comparison of intrauterine application of quinacrine alone or in combination with ibuprofen. Fertil Steril 75:830, 2001

Schwingl PJ, Guess HA: Safety and effectiveness of vasectomy. Fertil Steril 73:923, 2000

Shy KK, Stergachis A, Grothaus LG, et al: Tubal sterilization and risk of subsequent hospital admission for menstrual disorders. Am J Obstet Gynecol 166:1698, 1992

Soderstrom RM: Sterilization failures and their causes. Am J Obstet Gynecol 152:395, 1985

Sokal D, Gates D, Amatya R, et al: Two randomized controlled trials comparing the Tubal Ring and Filshie Clip for tubal sterilization. Fertil Steril 74:3, 2000

Timonen S, Tuominin J, Irjala K, et al: Ovarian function and regulation of the hypothalamic-pituitary-ovarian axis after tubal sterilization. J Reprod Med 47:131, 2002

Tourgeman DE, Bhaumik M, Cooke GC, et al: Pregnancy rates following fimbriectomy reversal via neosalpingostomy: A 10-year retrospective analysis. Fertil Steril 76:1041, 2001

Van Voorhis BJ: Comparison of tubal ligation reversal procedures. Clin Obstet Gynecol 43:641, 2000

Westhoff C, Davis A: Tubal sterilization: Focus on the U.S. experience. Fertil Steril 73:913, 2000

Williams EL, Jones HE, Merrill RE: Subsequent course of patients sterilized by tubal ligation. Am J Obstet Gynecol 61:423, 1951

VII

Obstetrical Complications

34

Hypertensive Disorders in Pregnancy

(continued)

Hypertensive disorders complicating pregnancy are common and form one of the deadly triad, along with hemorrhage and infection, that contribute greatly to maternal morbidity and mortality. In 2001, according to the National Center for Health Statistics, gestational hypertension was identified in 150,000 women, or 3.7 percent of pregnancies (Martin and colleagues, 2002). Importantly, Berg and colleagues (2003) reported that almost 16 percent of 3201 pregnancy-related deaths in the United States from 1991 to 1997 were from complications of pregnancy-related hypertension. These investigators also found that black women in this country are 3.1 times as likely to die from preeclampsia as white women.

How pregnancy incites or aggravates hypertension remains unsolved despite decades of intensive research. Indeed, hypertensive disorders remain among the most significant and intriguing unsolved problems in obstetrics. To elucidate these, ongoing research is sponsored by the National Institutes of Child Health and Human Development (NICHD) and its Maternal–Fetal Medicine Units Network. Another important stimulus for research is the International Society for the Study of Hypertension in Pregnancy. The National Heart, Lung, and Blood Institute promotes research and coordination through the National High Blood Pressure Education Program (NHBPEP) and its Working Group for High Blood Pressure in Pregnancy.

TERMINOLOGY AND CLASSIFICATION

The term *gestational hypertension* is used now to describe any form of new-onset pregnancy-related hypertension. It was adopted by the Working Group of the NHBPEP (2000), which proposed a classification system based on clinical simplicity to guide management. The term was chosen to emphasize the cause-and-effect connection between pregnancy and its unique form of hypertension—preeclampsia and eclampsia. It is also meant to be a working term that is purposefully vague, but it should convey that the development of hypertension in a previously normotensive pregnant woman should and must be considered potentially dangerous to both herself and her fetus. In the past several editions of *Williams Obstetrics*, the term *pregnancy-induced hypertension* was used.

It was popularized by Dr. Jack Pritchard to convey the same principles, and it still is used by some interchangeably with gestational hypertension.

The classification of hypertensive disorders complicating pregnancy by the Working Group of the NHBPEP (2000) is shown in Table 34–1. There are five types of hypertensive disease:

1. Gestational hypertension (formerly pregnancy-induced hypertension that included transient hypertension).
2. Preeclampsia.
3. Eclampsia.
4. Preeclampsia superimposed on chronic hypertension.
5. Chronic hypertension.

TABLE 34–1 Diagnosis of Hypertensive Disorders Complicating Pregnancy

Gestational hypertension
BP $\geq$ 140/90 mm Hg for first time during pregnancy
No proteinuria
BP returns to normal < 12 weeks' postpartum
Final diagnosis made only postpartum
May have other signs or symptoms of preeclampsia, for example, epigastric discomfort or thrombocytopenia

Preeclampsia
Minimum criteria
BP $\geq$ 140/90 mm Hg after 20 weeks' gestation
Proteinuria $\geq$ 300 mg/24 hours or $\geq$ 1+ dipstick
Increased certainty of preeclampsia
BP $\geq$ 160/110 mg Hg
Proteinuria 2.0 g/24 hours or $\geq$ 2+ dipstick
Serum creatinine > 1.2 mg/dL unless known to be previously elevated
Platelets < 100,000/mm^3
Microangiopathic hemolysis (increased LDH)
Elevated ALT or AST
Persistent headache or other cerebral or visual disturbance
Persistent epigastric pain

Eclampsia
Seizures that cannot be attributed to other causes in a woman with preeclampsia

Superimposed Preeclampsia (on chronic hypertension)
New-onset proteinuria $\geq$ 300 mg/24 hours in hypertensive women but no proteinuria before 20 weeks' gestation
A sudden increase in proteinuria or blood pressure or platelet count < 100,000/mm^3 in women with hypertension and proteinuria before 20 weeks' gestation

Chronic Hypertension
BP $\geq$ 140/90 mm Hg before pregnancy or diagnosed before 20 weeks' gestation not attributable to gestational trophoblastic disease
or
Hypertension first diagnosed after 20 weeks' gestation and persistent after 12 weeks' postpartum

ALT = alanine aminotransferase; AST = aspartate aminotransferase; BP = blood pressure; LDH = lactate dehydrogenase. Adapted from National High Blood Pressure Education Program Working Group Report on High Blood Pressure in Pregnancy (2000).

An important consideration in this classification is differentiating hypertensive disorders that precede pregnancy from preeclampsia and eclampsia, which are potentially more ominous.

DIAGNOSIS

Hypertension is diagnosed when the resting blood pressure is 140/90 mm Hg or greater; Korotkoff phase V is used to define diastolic pressure. In the past, it had been recommended that an incremental increase of 30 mm Hg systolic or 15 mm Hg diastolic pressure be used as diagnostic criteria, even when absolute values were below 140/90 mm Hg. These criteria are no longer recommended because evidence shows that these women are not likely to suffer increased adverse pregnancy outcomes (Levine and co-workers, 2000; North and colleagues, 1999). That said, women who have a rise of 30 mm Hg systolic or 15 mm Hg diastolic warrant close observation. Edema has been abandoned as a diagnostic criterion because it occurs in too many normal pregnant women to be discriminant.

GESTATIONAL HYPERTENSION. As shown in Table 34–1, the diagnosis of gestational hypertension is made in women whose blood pressure reaches 140/90 mm Hg or greater for the first time during pregnancy but in whom *proteinuria is not identified*. Gestational hypertension is also called *transient hypertension* if preeclampsia does not develop and the blood pressure has returned to normal by 12 weeks' postpartum. In this classification, the final diagnosis that the woman *does not* have gestational hypertension is not made until several weeks after delivery. Thus, gestational hypertension is a diagnosis of exclusion. Importantly, some women with gestational hypertension may later develop other findings of preeclampsia, for example, symptoms such as headaches or epigastric pain, proteinuria, or thrombocytopenia, all of which influence management.

When blood pressure rises appreciably during the latter half of pregnancy, it is dangerous, especially to the fetus, not to act simply because proteinuria has not yet developed. As Chesley (1985) emphasized, 10 percent of eclamptic seizures develop before overt proteinuria is identified. Thus, it is clear that when blood pressure begins to rise, both mother and fetus are at increased risk. Proteinuria is a sign of worsening hypertensive disease, specifically preeclampsia. Overt and persistent proteinuria further increases maternal and fetal risks.

PREECLAMPSIA. This condition is best described as a *pregnancy-specific syndrome* of reduced organ perfusion secondary to vasospasm and endothelial activation. *Proteinuria* is an important sign of preeclampsia, and Chesley (1985) rightfully concluded that the diagnosis is questionable in its absence. Significant proteinuria is defined by 24-hour urinary protein exceeding 300 mg per 24 hours, or persistent

30 mg/dL (1+ dipstick) in random urine samples. The degree of proteinuria may fluctuate widely over any 24-hour period, even in severe cases. Therefore, a single random sample may fail to demonstrate significant proteinuria.

In their extensive study of renal biopsy specimens obtained from hypertensive pregnant women, McCartney and co-workers (1971) invariably found proteinuria when the glomerular lesion considered to be characteristic of preeclampsia was evident. Importantly, both proteinuria and alterations of glomerular histology develop late in the course. It is apparent that preeclampsia becomes evident clinically only near the end of a covert pathophysiological process that may begin as early as implantation.

Thus, the minimum criteria for the diagnosis of preeclampsia are hypertension plus minimal proteinuria. The more severe the hypertension or proteinuria, the more certain is the diagnosis of preeclampsia (see Table 34–1). Similarly, abnormal laboratory findings in tests of renal, hepatic, and hematological function increase the certainty of preeclampsia. In addition, persistent premonitory symptoms of eclampsia, such as headache and epigastric pain, also increase the certainty.

The combination of proteinuria and hypertension during pregnancy markedly increases the risk of perinatal mortality and morbidity (Ferrazzani and associates, 1990). A widely quoted study by Friedman and Neff (1976) of more than 38,000 pregnancies was completed over three decades ago. It showed that diastolic hypertension of 95 mm Hg or greater was associated with a threefold increase in the fetal death rate. Worsening hypertension, especially if accompanied by proteinuria, was more ominous, but proteinuria without hypertension was rather benign. In a recent study, however, Newman and co-workers (2003) reported that worsening proteinuria resulted in increasing preterm delivery, but that neonatal survival was not significantly altered. In contrast, following their analysis of more than 9000 nulliparous women ascertained from the Collaborative Perinatal Project, a large cohort study conducted between 1959 and 1965, Zhang and co-workers (2001) concluded that neither blood pressure severity nor proteinuria were sensitive predictors of adverse outcome.

Epigastric or right upper quadrant pain is thought to result from hepatocellular necrosis, ischemia, and edema that stretches the Glisson capsule. This characteristic pain is frequently accompanied by elevated serum hepatic transaminase levels and usually is a sign to terminate the pregnancy. The pain presages hepatic infarction and hemorrhage or catastrophic rupture of a subcapsular hematoma. Fortunately, hepatic rupture is rare.

Thrombocytopenia is characteristic of worsening preeclampsia, and it probably is caused by platelet activation and aggregation as well as microangiopathic hemolysis induced by severe vasospasm. Evidence of gross hemolysis such as hemoglobinemia, hemoglobinuria, or hyperbilirubinemia is indicative of severe disease.

TABLE 34–2 Indications of Severity of Hypertensive Disorders During Pregnancy

Abnormality	Mild	Severe
Diastolic blood pressure	< 100 mm Hg	110 mm Hg or higher
Proteinuria	Trace to 1+	Persistent 2+ or more
Headache	Absent	Present
Visual disturbances	Absent	Present
Upper abdominal pain	Absent	Present
Oliguria	Absent	Present
Convulsion (eclampsia)	Absent	Present
Serum creatinine	Normal	Elevated
Thrombocytopenia	Absent	Present
Liver enzyme elevation	Minimal	Marked
Fetal growth restriction	Absent	Obvious
Pulmonary edema	Absent	Present

Other factors indicative of severe hypertension include cardiac dysfunction with pulmonary edema as well as obvious fetal growth restriction.

Severity of Preeclampsia. The severity of preeclampsia is assessed by the frequency and intensity of the abnormalities listed in Table 34–2. The more profound these aberrations, the more likely is the need for pregnancy termination. **The differentiation between mild and severe preeclampsia can be misleading because apparently mild disease may progress rapidly to severe disease.**

Although hypertension is a requisite to diagnosing preeclampsia, absolute blood pressure alone is not always a dependable indicator of its severity. For example, young adolescent women may have 3+ proteinuria and convulsions with a blood pressure of 135/85 mm Hg, whereas most women with blood pressures as high as 180/120 mm Hg do not have seizures. A rapid increase in blood pressure followed by convulsions is usually preceded by an unrelenting severe headache or visual disturbances. For this reason, these symptoms are considered ominous.

ECLAMPSIA. The onset of convulsions in a woman with preeclampsia that cannot be attributed to other causes is termed eclampsia. The seizures are generalized and may appear before, during, or after labor. In older studies, in about 10 percent of eclamptic women, especially nulliparas, seizures did not develop until after 48 hours postpartum (Brown and colleagues, 1987; Lubarsky and associates, 1994). As prenatal care improved, many antepartum and intrapartum cases are now prevented, and a more recent study reported that a fourth of eclamptic seizures developed beyond 48 hours postpartum (Chames and co-workers, 2002).

PREECLAMPSIA SUPERIMPOSED ON CHRONIC HYPERTENSION. All *chronic hypertensive disorders*, regardless of their cause, predispose to development of superimposed preeclampsia and eclampsia. These disorders can create difficult problems with diagnosis and management in women who are not seen until after midpregnancy. The diagnosis of chronic underlying hypertension is made when:

1. Hypertension (140/90 mm Hg or greater) is documented antecedent to pregnancy.
2. Hypertension (140/90 mm Hg or greater) is detected before 20 weeks, unless there is gestational trophoblastic disease.
3. Hypertension persists long after delivery (see Table 34–1).

Additional historical factors that help support the diagnosis are multiparity and hypertension complicating a previous pregnancy other than the first. There frequently is also a family history of essential hypertension.

The diagnosis of chronic hypertension may be difficult to make if the woman is not seen until the latter half of pregnancy, because blood pressure decreases during the second and early third trimesters in both normotensive and chronically hypertensive women (see Chap. 45, p. 1045). Thus, a woman with chronic vascular disease, who is seen for the first time at 20 weeks, frequently has blood pressure within the normal accepted range. During the third trimester, however, if blood pressure returns to its former hypertensive level, it presents a diagnostic problem as to whether the hypertension is chronic or induced by pregnancy. In these situations, a search for evidence of end-organ damage from chronic hypertension may help elucidate the underlying cause of hypertension. Examples include left ventricular hypertrophy or retinal changes such as arteriolar narrowing, exudates, or cotton-wool spots.

Some of the many causes of underlying hypertension that are encountered during pregnancy are listed in Table 34–3.

TABLE 34–3 Underlying Causes of Chronic Hypertensive Disorders

Essential familial hypertension (hypertensive vascular disease)
Obesity
Arterial abnormalities
   Renovascular hypertension
   Coarctation of the aorta
Endocrine disorders
   Diabetes mellitus
   Cushing syndrome
   Primary aldosteronism
   Pheochromocytoma
   Thyrotoxicosis
Glomerulonephritis (acute and chronic)
Renoprival hypertension
   Chronic glomerulonephritis
   Chronic renal insufficiency
   Diabetic nephropathy
Connective tissue diseases
   Lupus erythematosus
   Systemic sclerosis
   Periarteritis nodosa
Polycystic kidney disease
Acute renal failure

Essential or familial hypertension is the cause of underlying vascular disease in more than 90 percent of pregnant women. Obesity and diabetes are other common causes. In some women, hypertension develops as a consequence of underlying renal parenchymal disease. Although earlier studies of renal biopsies identified abnormalities, especially in multiparas, Fisher and co-workers (1969) did not confirm a high prevalence of chronic glomerulonephritis.

Depending on its duration, chronic hypertension can lead to ventricular hypertrophy and cardiac decompensation, cerebrovascular accidents, or renal damage. These complications are more likely during pregnancy if there is superimposed preeclampsia, which develops in up to 25 percent of these women (Sibai and colleagues, 1998). The risk of placental abruption is also increased substantively if there is superimposed preeclampsia (see Chap. 35, p. 813). Moreover, the fetuses of women with chronic hypertension are at appreciable risks for growth restriction, preterm delivery, and death.

In some women with chronic hypertension, blood pressure increases to abnormal levels, typically after 24 weeks. If accompanied by proteinuria, then superimposed preeclampsia is diagnosed. Often, superimposed preeclampsia develops earlier in pregnancy than "pure" preeclampsia, and it tends to be more severe and often accompanied by fetal growth restriction. Indicators of severity shown in Table 34–2 are also used to further characterize superimposed preeclampsia.

INCIDENCE AND RISK FACTORS. Gestational hypertension more often affects nulliparous women. Because of the increasing incidence of chronic hypertension with advancing age, older women are at greater risk for superimposed preeclampsia. Thus, women at either end of reproductive age are considered to be more susceptible (see Chap. 7, p. 194).

The incidence of preeclampsia is commonly cited to be about 5 percent, although rather wide variations are reported. The incidence is markedly influenced by parity; it is related to race and ethnicity—and thus to genetic predisposition, and environmental factors likely also play a role. For example, Palmer and associates (1999) reported that living at high altitude in Colorado increased the incidence of preeclampsia. Some investigators have concluded that socioeconomically advantaged women have a lesser incidence of preeclampsia, however, Lawlor and colleagues (2005) did not observe this in an Aberdeen cohort of 3485 women.

The incidence of hypertensive disorders in healthy nulliparous women was carefully studied in a trial of dietary calcium supplementation (Hauth and colleagues, 2000). Of 4302 nulliparous women delivered at or beyond 20 weeks, a fourth developed a pregnancy-related hypertensive disorder. When all nulliparas were considered, preeclampsia was diagnosed in 7.6 percent and severe disease developed in 3.3 percent. By contrast, Vatten and Skjærven (2004) reported an incidence of preeclampsia of 2.6 percent in more than 1.6 million Norwegian nulliparas.

Other risk factors associated with preeclampsia include chronic hypertension as discussed, multifetal gestation, maternal age over 35 years, obesity, and African-American ethnicity (Conde-Agudelo and Belizan, 2000; Sibai and colleagues, 1997; Walker, 2000). The relationship between maternal weight and the risk of preeclampsia is progressive. It increases from 4.3 percent for women with a body mass index less than 19.8 kg/m^2 to 13.3 percent in those with a body mass index greater than 35 kg/m^2. In women with twin gestations compared with those with singletons, the incidence of gestational hypertension (13 versus 6 percent) and the incidence of preeclampsia (13 versus 5 percent) are both significantly increased (Sibai and co-workers, 2000). The incidence is unrelated to zygosity (Maxwell and associates, 2001). Although smoking during pregnancy causes a variety of adverse pregnancy outcomes, ironically, smoking has consistently been associated with a *reduced risk* of hypertension during pregnancy (Bainbridge and associates, 2005; Zhang and colleagues, 1999). Placenta previa has also been reported to reduce the risk of hypertensive disorders in pregnancy (Ananth and colleagues, 1997).

Eclampsia. This condition is somewhat preventable, and its incidence has decreased in the United States because most women now receive adequate prenatal care. For example, in the 15th edition of *Williams Obstetrics* (1976), for the prior 25-year period, the incidence of eclampsia at Parkland Hospital was 1 in 700 deliveries. For the 4-year period from 1983 to 1986, it decreased to 1 in 1150 deliveries, and for the 3-year period ending in 1999, it was approximately 1 in 1750 deliveries (Alexander and associates, 2004). In the National Vital Statistics Report, Ventura and colleagues (2000) estimated that the incidence of eclampsia in the United States in 1998 was about 1 in 3250. In the United Kingdom in 1992, Douglas and Redman (1994) reported that the incidence of eclampsia was 1 in 2000.

ETIOLOGY

Any satisfactory theory concerning the etiology and pathophysiology of preeclampsia must account for the observation that hypertensive disorders due to pregnancy are very much more likely to develop in women who:

1. Are exposed to chorionic villi for the first time.
2. Are exposed to a superabundance of chorionic villi, as with twins or hydatidiform mole.
3. Have preexisting vascular disease.
4. Are genetically predisposed to hypertension developing during pregnancy.

Although chorionic villi are essential, they need not be located within the uterus. A fetus is not a requisite for preeclampsia. Regardless of precipitating etiology, the cascade of events that leads to the preeclampsia syndrome is characterized by a host of abnormalities that result in vascular endothelial damage with vasospasm, transudation of plasma, and ischemic and thrombotic sequelae.

Writings describing eclampsia have been traced as far back as 2200 B.C. (Lindheimer and colleagues, 1999). It is thus not surprising that a number of mechanisms have been proposed to explain its cause. Many of the absurd, and especially the dangerous, thankfully have been discarded. According to Sibai (2003), currently plausible potential causes include the following:

1. Abnormal trophoblastic invasion of uterine vessels.
2. Immunological intolerance between maternal and fetoplacental tissues.
3. Maternal maladaptation to cardiovascular or inflammatory changes of normal pregnancy.
4. Dietary deficiencies.
5. Genetic influences.

ABNORMAL TROPHOBLASTIC INVASION. In normal implantation, the uterine spiral arteries undergo extensive remodeling as they are invaded by endovascular trophoblasts (Fig. 34–1). In preeclampsia, however, there is *incomplete*

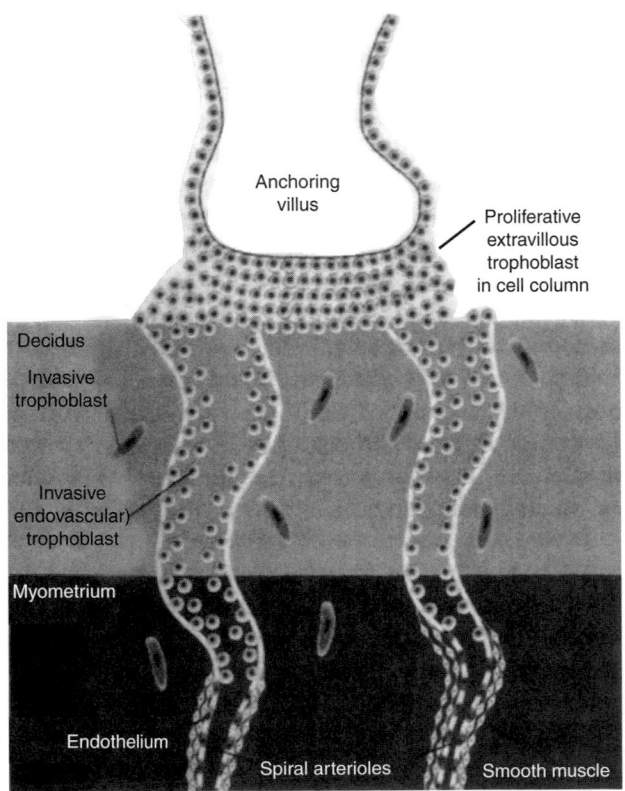

FIGURE 34–1. Normal placental implantation shows proliferation of extravillous trophoblasts, forming a cell column beneath the anchoring villus. The extravillous trophoblasts invade the decidua and extend down the inside of the spiral arteriole. This results in replacement of the endothelium and muscular wall of the vessel and in subsequent enlargement of the blood vessel. (From Rogers and colleagues, 1999, with permission.)

trophoblastic invasion. In this case, decidual vessels, but not myometrial vessels, become lined with endovascular trophoblasts. Meekins and co-workers (1994) described a continuum in the number of spiral arteries with endovascular trophoblasts in placentas of normal women and in those with preeclampsia. Madazli and colleagues (2000) showed that the magnitude of defective trophoblastic invasion of the spiral arteries correlated with the severity of the hypertensive disorder.

Using electron microscopy, De Wolf and co-workers (1980) examined arteries taken from the uteroplacental implantation site. They observed that early preeclamptic changes included endothelial damage, insudation of plasma constituents into vessel walls, proliferation of myointimal cells, and medial necrosis. They found that lipid accumulates first in myointimal cells and then in macrophages. Shown in Figure 34–2, such lipid-laden cells and associated findings have been termed *atherosis* (Hertig, 1945). Typically, the vessels affected by atherosis develop aneurysmal dilatation and are frequently found in association with spiral arterioles that have failed to undergo normal adaptation (Khong, 1991). Obstruction of the spiral arteriolar lumen by atherosis may impair placental blood flow. It is thought that these changes cause placental perfusion to be pathologically diminished, which eventually leads to the preeclampsia syndrome (Lain and Roberts, 2002; Redman and Sargent, 2003).

IMMUNOLOGICAL FACTORS. There is circumstantial evidence to support the theory that preeclampsia is immune mediated. Certainly the microscopic changes at the maternal–placental interface are suggestive of acute graft rejection (Labarrere, 1988). There are also inferential data. For example, the risk of preeclampsia is appreciably enhanced in circumstances where formation of blocking antibodies to placental antigenic sites *might* be impaired. This may arise in situations in which effective immunization by a previous pregnancy is lacking, as in first pregnancies; or in which the number of antigenic sites provided by the placenta is unusually great compared with the amount of antibody, as with multiple fetuses (Beer, 1978). "Immunization" from a prior abortion does not seem to occur. Strickland and associates (1986) analyzed outcomes of over 29,000 pregnancies at Parkland Hospital and reported that hypertensive disorders were decreased only slightly (22 versus 25 percent) in women who previously had miscarried (thus who were previously "immunized") and were now having their first advanced pregnancy. The immunization concept was supported by their observations that preeclampsia developed less often in multiparas who had a prior term pregnancy. Other studies have shown that multiparous women impregnated by a new consort have an increased risk of preeclampsia (Mostello and co-workers, 2002; Trupin and colleagues, 1996).

Dekker and Sibai (1998) have reviewed the possible role of immune maladaptation in the pathophysiology of preeclampsia. Beginning in the early second trimester, women destined

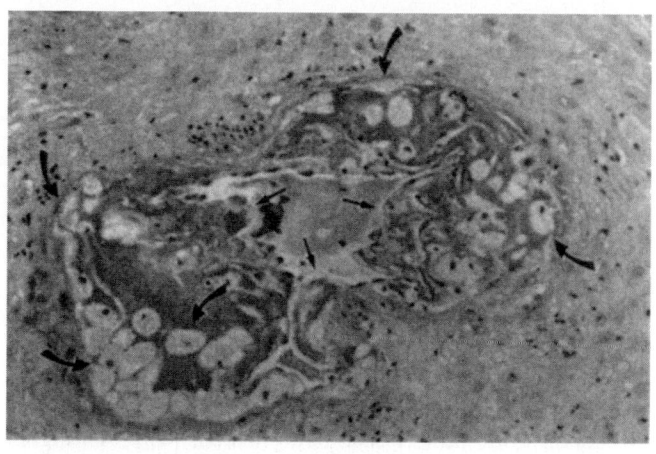

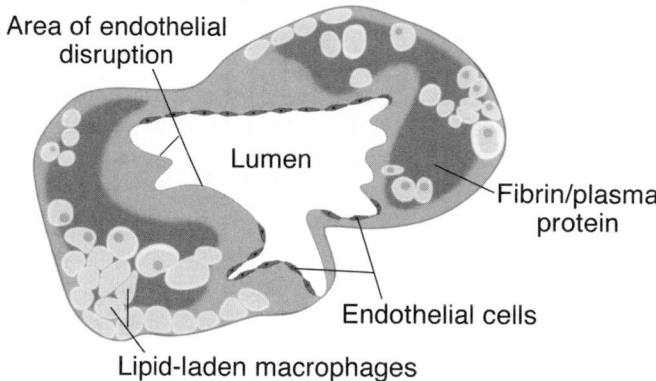

FIGURE 34–2. Atherosis is demonstrated in this blood vessel from the placental bed (left, photomicrograph; right schematic diagram of vessel). Disruption of the endothelium results in a narrowed lumen because of accumulation of plasma proteins and foamy macrophages beneath the endothelium. Some of the foamy macrophages are shown by *curved arrows* in the left photograph and *straight arrows* highlight areas of endothelial disruption. (Modified from Rogers and colleagues, 1999, with permission.)

to develop preeclampsia have a significantly lower proportion of helper T cells (Th$_1$) compared with that of women who remain normotensive (Bardeguez and associates, 1991). This Th$_1$/Th$_2$ imbalance, with Th$_2$ dominance, may be mediated by adenosine, which is found in higher serum levels in preeclamptic compared with normotensive women (Yoneyama and co-workers, 2002). These helper T lymphocytes secrete specific cytokines that promote implantation, and their dysfunction may favor preeclampsia (Hayashi and associates, 2004; Whitecar and colleagues, 2001).

In women with anticardiolipin antibodies, placental abnormalities and preeclampsia develop more commonly (see Chap. 54, p. 1217). This, however, was recently challenged by Branch and associates (2001). According to Katano and colleagues (1996), antibodies associated with β_2-glycoprotein I appear most relevant. Immune complexes and anti-endothelial cell antibodies may also be involved (Taylor and Roberts, 1999).

THE VASCULOPATHY AND THE INFLAMMATORY CHANGES. In many ways, inflammatory changes are a continuation of the placental cause(s) discussed above. In response to placental factors released by ischemic changes, or any other inciting cause, a cascade of events is set in motion (Redman and Sargent, 2003). The decidua also contains an abundance of cells that, when activated, can release noxious agents (Staff and colleagues, 1999). These then serve as mediators to provoke endothelial cell injury.

Redman and colleagues (1999) have proposed that the endothelial cell dysfunction associated with preeclampsia can result from a "generalized perturbation of the normal, generalized maternal intravascular inflammatory adaptation to pregnancy" (Fig. 34–3). In this hypothesis, preeclampsia is considered a disease due to an extreme state of activated

leukocytes in the maternal circulation (Faas and colleagues, 2000; Gervasi and co-workers, 2001). Briefly, cytokines such as tumor necrosis factor-α (TNF-α) and the interleukins may contribute to the oxidative stress associated with preeclampsia. Oxidative stress is characterized by reactive oxygen species and free radicals that lead to formation of

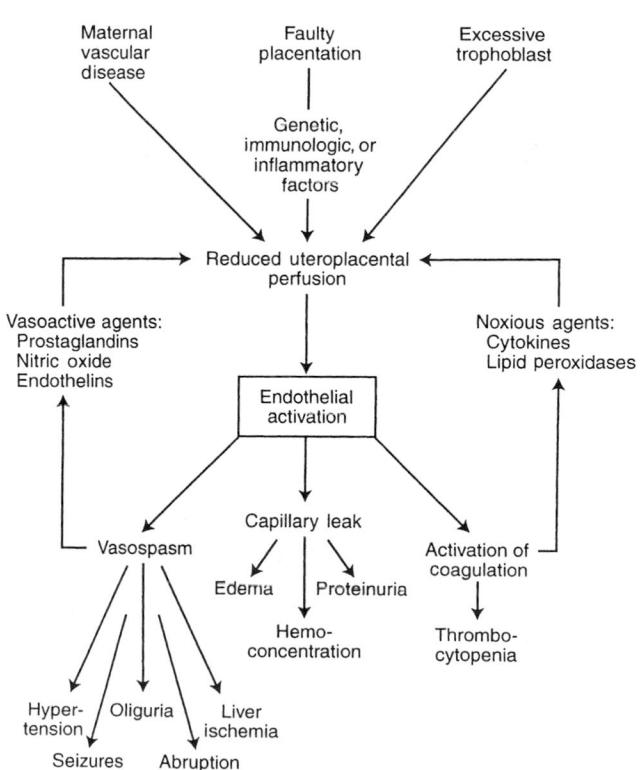

FIGURE 34–3. Pathophysiological considerations in the development of hypertensive disorders due to pregnancy. (Adapted from Friedman and Lindheimer, 1999, with permission.)

self-propagating lipid peroxides (Manten and associates, 2005). These in turn generate highly toxic radicals that injure endothelial cells, modify their nitric oxide production, and interfere with prostaglandin balance.

Not all investigators have confirmed these findings. Diedrich and colleagues (2001) did not detect any lipid hydroperoxides in 38 preeclamptic women, 10 of whom had HELLP syndrome (hemolysis, elevated liver enzymes, low platelets). They did, however, find other evidence of oxidative stress. Other consequences of oxidative stress include production of the lipid-laden macrophage foam cells seen in atherosis (see Fig. 34–2); activation of microvascular coagulation, seen in thrombocytopenia; and increased capillary permeability, seen in edema and proteinuria.

These observations on the effects of oxidative stress in preeclampsia have given rise to increased interest in the potential benefit of antioxidants to prevent preeclampsia (Chappell and colleagues, 1999; Zhang and co-workers, 2002). Antioxidants are a diverse family of compounds that function to prevent overproduction of and damage caused by noxious free radicals. Examples of antioxidants include vitamin E or α-tocopherol, vitamin C (ascorbic acid), and β-carotene. Dietary supplementation with these antioxidants is discussed on page 780.

NUTRITIONAL FACTORS. A number of dietary deficiencies or excesses over the centuries have been blamed as the cause of eclampsia. Dietary taboos that have included meat, protein, purines, fat, dairy products, salt, and other elements have been advocated at times. Observations and theories led to studies of dietary deprivation of various sorts that many times were models of absurdity. In more recent times, sanity and a scientific approach have prevailed. For example, blood pressure in nonpregnant individuals is affected by a number of dietary influences, including minerals and vitamins. Some studies have shown a relationship between dietary deficiencies and the incidence of preeclampsia. This was followed by studies of supplementation with various elements such as zinc, calcium, and magnesium to prevent preeclampsia. Other studies, such as the one by John and co-workers (2002), showed that in the general population a diet high in fruits and vegetables that have antioxidant activity is associated with decreased blood pressure. This is related to the case-control study by Zhang and associates (2002) cited above, in which the incidence of preeclampsia was doubled in women whose daily intake of ascorbic acid was less than 85 mg.

As previously discussed, obesity is a potent risk factor for preeclampsia (see also Chap. 43, p. 1012). Evidence has accrued that obesity in nonpregnant individuals causes endothelial activation and a systemic inflammatory response associated with atherosclerosis (Ross, 1999). In the study of pregnant women by Wolf and colleagues (2001), C-reactive protein, an inflammatory marker, was shown to be increased in obesity, which in turn was associated with preeclampsia.

GENETIC FACTORS. The predisposition to hereditary hypertension undoubtedly is linked to preeclampsia (Ness and colleagues, 2003), and the tendency for preeclampsia–eclampsia is inherited. Chesley and Cooper (1986) studied sisters, daughters, granddaughters, and daughters-in-law of eclamptic women and concluded that preeclampsia–eclampsia is highly heritable. The single-gene model, with a frequency of 0.25, best explained their observations. Other investigators cite possibilities of polygenic inheritance (Trogstad and co-workers, 2004). A Swedish study by Nilsson and co-workers (2004) that included almost 1.2 million births reported a genetic component for gestational hypertension as well as preeclampsia. They reported 60-percent concordance in monozygotic female twin pairs, which was much higher than that found by Treloar and co-workers (2001).

Kilpatrick and associates (1989), but not Hayward and co-workers (1992), reported an association between the histocompatibility antigen HLA-DR4 and proteinuric hypertension. Hoff and associates (1992) concluded that a maternal humoral response directed against fetal anti-HLA-DR immunoglobulin antibody might influence the development of gestational hypertension. A number of single-gene mutations have been studied in women with preeclampsia. For example, Ward (1993) and Zhang (2003) and their associates reported that women heterozygous for the angiotensinogen gene variant T235 had a higher incidence preeclampsia and fetal growth restriction. Morgan and colleagues (1995, 1999) did not confirm this, but they did find that women homozygous for this mutation had abnormal trophoblastic invasion. Some of the inherited thrombophilias predispose some women to preeclampsia (see Table 47–4, p. 1079). Polymorphisms of the genes for TNF, lymphotoxin-α, and interleukin-1β have been studied with varying results (Hefler, 2001; Lachmeijer, 2001; Livingston, 2001b, and all their colleagues).

PATHOGENESIS

VASOSPASM. The concept of vasospasm was advanced by Volhard (1918) based on direct observations of small blood vessels in the nail beds, ocular fundi, and bulbar conjunctivae. It was also surmised from histological changes seen in various affected organs (Hinselmann, 1924; Landesman and co-workers, 1954). Vascular constriction causes resistance and subsequent hypertension. At the same time, endothelial cell damage causes interstitial leakage through which blood constituents, including platelets and fibrinogen, are deposited subendothelially. Wang and colleagues (2002) have also demonstrated disruption of endothelial junctional proteins. Suzuki and co-workers (2003) demonstrated ultrastructural changes in the subendothelial region of resistance arteries in preeclamptic women. With diminished blood flow because of maldistribution, ischemia of the surrounding tissues would lead to necrosis, hemorrhage, and other end-organ disturbances characteristic of the syndrome. Ironically, vasospasm may be worse in women with preeclampsia than in those with the HELLP syndrome (Fischer and colleagues, 2000).

ENDOTHELIAL CELL ACTIVATION.

Over the past two decades, endothelial cell activation has become the centerpiece in the contemporary understanding of the pathogenesis of preeclampsia (see Fig. 34–3). In this scheme, unknown factor(s), likely from the placenta, are secreted into the maternal circulation and provoke activation and dysfunction of the vascular endothelium. The clinical syndrome of preeclampsia is thought to result from these widespread endothelial cell changes (Hayman and associates, 2000; Roberts, 2000; Walker, 2000).

Intact endothelium has anticoagulant properties, and it also blunts the response of vascular smooth muscle to agonists by releasing nitric oxide. Damaged or activated endothelial cells secrete substances that promote coagulation and increase the sensitivity to vasopressors. Further evidence of endothelial activation includes the characteristic changes in glomerular capillary endothelial morphology, increased capillary permeability, and elevated blood concentrations of substances associated with such activation. These latter substances are transferrable, and serum from women with preeclampsia stimulates cultured endothelial cells to produce greater amounts of prostacyclin than serum from normal pregnant women.

Increased Pressor Responses.

Normally, pregnant women develop refractoriness to infused vasopressors (Abdul-Karim and Assali, 1961). Women with early preeclampsia, however, have increased vascular reactivity to infused norepinephrine and angiotensin II (Raab and co-workers, 1956; Talledo and associates, 1968). Moreover, increased sensitivity to angiotensin II clearly precedes the onset of gestational hypertension (Fig. 34–4). Normotensive nulliparas remained

refractory to infused angiotensin II, but those who subsequently became hypertensive lost this refractoriness several weeks before the onset of hypertension. Women with underlying chronic hypertension have almost identical responses (Gant and colleagues, 1977).

PROSTAGLANDINS. A number of prostanoids are central to the pathophysiology of the preeclampsia syndrome. Specifically, the blunted pressor response seen in normal pregnancy is at least partially due to decreased vascular responsiveness mediated by vascular endothelial prostaglandin synthesis. For example, when compared with normal pregnancy, endothelial prostacyclin (PGI_2) production is decreased in preeclampsia. This action appears to be mediated by phospholipase A_2 (Taylor and Roberts, 1999). At the same time, thromboxane A_2 secretion by platelets is increased, and the prostacyclin:thromboxane A_2 ratio decreases. The net result favors increased sensitivity to infused angiotensin II, and ultimately, vasoconstriction. Chavarria and co-workers (2003b) have provided evidence that these changes are apparent as early as 22 weeks in women who later develop preeclampsia.

NITRIC OXIDE. This potent vasodilator is synthesized from L-arginine by endothelial cells. Withdrawal of nitric oxide results in a clinical picture similar to preeclampsia in a pregnant animal model (Conrad and Vernier, 1989; Weiner and associates, 1989). In other animal studies, inhibition of nitric oxide synthesis increases mean arterial pressure, decreases heart rate, and reverses the pregnancy-induced refractoriness to vasopressors. In humans, nitric oxide likely is the compound that maintains the normal low-pressure vasodilated state characteristic of fetoplacental perfusion (Myatt and co-workers, 1992; Weiner and associates, 1992). It also is produced by fetal endothelium and is increased in response to preeclampsia, diabetes, and infection (Parra and associates, 2001; von Mandach and co-workers, 2003).

Preeclampsia is associated with decreased endothelial nitric oxide synthase expression, which increases cell permeability (Wang and colleagues, 2004). There is not decreased nitric oxide release or production prior to the onset of hypertension (Anumba and colleagues, 1999). Its production is increased in severe preeclampsia possibly as a compensatory mechanism for the increased synthesis and release of vasoconstrictors and platelet-aggregating agents (Benedetto and associates, 2000). Thus, increased serum concentrations of nitric oxide in women with preeclampsia are likely the result of hypertension, not the cause (Morris and colleagues, 1996).

ENDOTHELINS. These 21–amino acid peptides are potent vasoconstrictors, and endothelin-1 (ET-1) is the primary isoform produced by human endothelium (Mastrogiannis and co-workers, 1991). Plasma ET-1 is increased in normotensive pregnant women, but women with preeclampsia have even

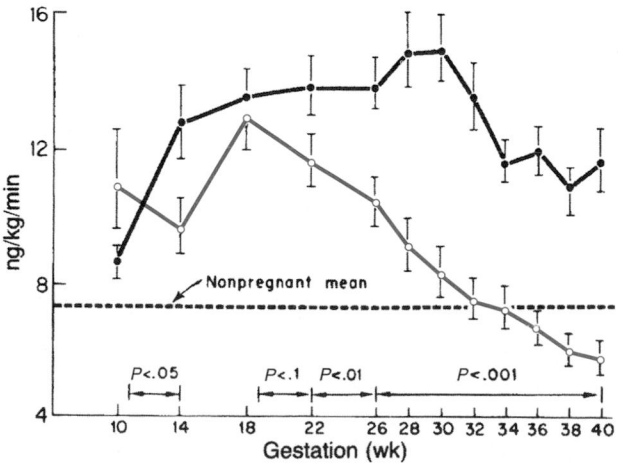

FIGURE 34–4. Comparison of the mean angiotensin II infusion doses required to evoke a pressor response in 120 nulliparous women who remained normotensive (solid circles) and 72 who subsequently developed pregnancy-induced hypertension (open circles). (From Gant and co-workers, 1973, with permission.)

higher levels (Ajne, 2003; Clark, 1992; Nova, 1991, and their associates). According to Taylor and Roberts (1999), the placenta is not the source of increased ET-1 and it likely arises from systemic endothelial activation. Interestingly, treatment of preeclamptic women with magnesium sulfate lowers ET-1 concentrations (Sagsoz and Kucukozkan, 2003).

ANGIOGENIC FACTORS. Several glycosylated glycoproteins are selectively mitogenic for endothelial cells and are thought to be important in mediating the preeclampsia syndrome. Two of these are *vascular endothelial growth factor (VEGF)* and *placental growth factor (PlGF)*. Their secretion increases across normal pregnancy, and they promote angiogenesis and induce nitric oxide and vasodilatory prostaglandins, discussed above. Placental VEGF is important in vasculogenesis and control of microvascular permeability.

Paradoxically, VEGF is increased in serum from women with preeclampsia but its bioavailability is decreased (Baker and associates, 1995; Simmons and co-workers, 2000). In preeclampsia, the gene for *soluble fms-like tyrosine kinase 1 (sFlt1)* is upregulated, and serum levels are increased for up to 48 hours after delivery (Maynard and associates, 2003). Because sFlt1 antagonizes VEGF and PlGF by binding them and decreasing their unbound serum levels, their effects are lost and there is endothelial dysfunction (Luttun and Carmeliet, 2003).

PATHOPHYSIOLOGY

By strict definition, preeclampsia–eclampsia fits the definition of a syndrome: *A group of symptoms or pathological signs which consistently occur together, especially with an (originally) unknown cause* (Oxford English Dictionary, 1993). Although the cause of preeclampsia remains unknown, evidence for it begins to manifest early in pregnancy with covert pathophysiological changes that gain momentum across gestation. Unless delivery supervenes, these changes ultimately result in multiorgan involvement with a clinical spectrum ranging from barely noticeable to one of cataclysmic pathophysiological deterioration that can be life threatening for both mother and fetus. These adverse maternal and fetal effects develop simultaneously. As discussed, these presumably are a consequence of vasospasm, endothelial dysfunction, and ischemia. The myriad of maternal consequences of the preeclampsia syndrome are described in terms of organ systems, but they frequently overlap. It is enigmatic that there are such wide variations of involvement of these systems in individual pregnancies.

CARDIOVASCULAR SYSTEM. Severe disturbances of normal cardiovascular function are common with preeclampsia or eclampsia. These are related to (1) increased cardiac afterload caused by hypertension; (2) cardiac preload, which is substantively affected by pathologically diminished hypervolemia of pregnancy or is iatrogenically increased by intravenous crystalloid or oncotic solutions; and (3) endothelial activation with extravasation into the extracellular space, especially the lung (see Chap. 42, p. 991). In addition, left ventricular mass is increased relative to normal pregnancy (Borghi and colleagues, 2000).

Hemodynamic Changes. The cardiovascular aberrations of hypertensive disorders of pregnancy vary depending on a number of factors. Some of these include severity of hypertension, presence of underlying chronic disease, whether preeclampsia is present, and at what point in the clinical course they are studied. For example, some of these changes precede the onset of hypertension. Bosio and colleagues (1999) used noninvasive Doppler hemodynamic monitoring in a longitudinal study of 400 nulliparous women commencing early in pregnancy. Gestational hypertension developed in 24 women, and 20 others had preeclampsia. Compared with normotensive women, the women who developed preeclampsia had significantly elevated cardiac outputs before hypertension developed. This substantiates earlier observations of Easterling and co-workers (1990), except that the latter group reported increased peripheral resistance during this preclinical phase. With clinical onset of preeclampsia, there was a marked reduction in cardiac output and increased peripheral resistance. By contrast, the women with gestational hypertension maintained their significantly elevated cardiac outputs with development of hypertension.

Much of the data based on invasive hemodynamic studies (Table 34–4) are confounded because of these factors as well as interventions that also may significantly alter these measurements. Thus, variables that define cardiovascular status in women with hypertensive disorders range from high cardiac output with low vascular resistance to low cardiac output with high resistance. Similarly, left ventricular filling pressures, estimated by pulmonary capillary wedge pressure determination, range from low to pathologically high. The studies listed in Table 34–4 are separated into three groups based on clinical management prior to when the initial hemodynamic studies were done:

1. No therapy.
2. Magnesium sulfate and hydralazine without large volumes of intravenous fluid.
3. Magnesium sulfate and hydralazine plus intravenous volume loading.

Ventricular function studies from the investigations in Table 34–4 are plotted in Figure 34–5. Although cardiac function was hyperdynamic in all women, filling pressures varied markedly. Data obtained prior to treatment of preeclampsia identified normal left ventricular filling pressures, high systemic vascular resistances, and hyperdynamic ventricular function. Benedetti (1980) and Hankins (1984) and their associates reported similar findings in women with severe preeclampsia or eclampsia who were being treated with

TABLE 34–4 Severe Preeclampsia and Eclampsia: Associated Hemodynamic Measurements[a]

Therapy	No.	Cardiac Output (L/min)	Pulmonary Capillary Wedge Pressure (mm Hg)	Left Ventricular Stroke Work Index $(g \cdot m^{-2})$	Systemic Vascular Resistance (dyne/sec per cm^{-5})
Before Therapy					
Groenendijk et al (1984)	10	4.66	3.3	44	1943
Visser and Wallenburg (1991)	87	(3.3)[b]	7	NA	3003
Magnesium, Hydralazine, and Fluid Restriction					
Benedetti et al (1980)	10	7.4	6.0	82	1322
Hankins et al (1984)	8	6.7	3.9	66	1357
Magnesium, Hydralazine, and Volume Expansion					
Rafferty and Berkowitz (1980)	3	11.0	7.0	89	780
Phelan and Yurth (1982)	10	9.3	16.0	89	1042

NA = not available.
[a]Values are those reported soon after pulmonary artery catheterization was performed and are the means for each study.
[b]Reported as cardiac index (CI = $L/min/m^{-2}$).

magnesium sulfate and hydralazine, and with intravenous crystalloid restricted to 75 to 100 mL/hour. Cardiac function was normal, and decreased vascular resistance was most likely due to hydralazine treatment.

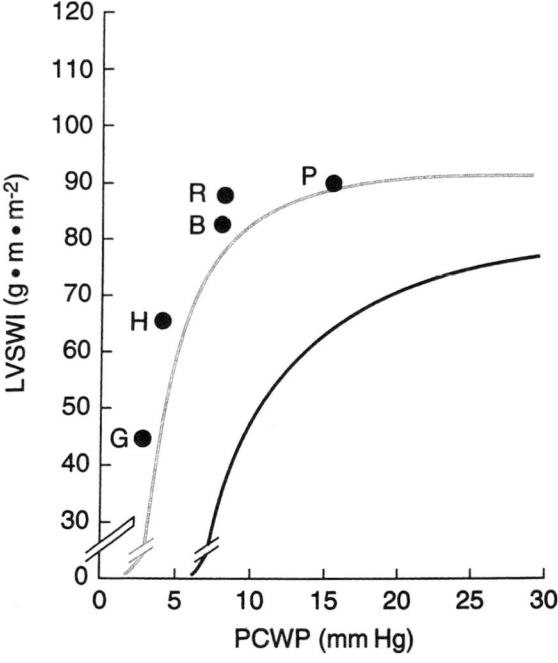

FIGURE 34–5. Ventricular function in severe preeclampsia–eclampsia. Data plotted represent mean values obtained in five of six studies cited in Table 34–4. Left ventricular stroke work index (LVSWI) and pulmonary artery capillary wedge pressure (PCWP) are plotted on a standard ventricular function curve. Points falling within the two solid lines represent normal function, whereas those below represent depressed function. Points above the solid lines represent hyperdynamic ventricular function. Each letter adjacent to the data points is the first initial of the last name of the investigator who reported this value. (From Hauth and Cunningham, 1999, with permission.)

Women similarly treated with magnesium sulfate and hydralazine plus aggressive intravenous therapy or volume expansion had the lowest systemic vascular resistances and highest cardiac outputs. Volume restriction with aggressive hydration results in hyperdynamic ventricular function in most women in both groups, however, there were two responses with respect to left ventricular stroke work index and pulmonary capillary wedge pressure (Fig. 34–6). Women in the fluid restriction group had pulmonary wedge pressures less than 10 mm Hg, and most were less than 5 mm Hg. Thus, hyperdynamic ventricular function was largely a result of low wedge pressures and not a result of augmented myocardial contractility measured as left ventricular stroke work index. By comparison, women given appreciably larger volumes of fluid commonly had filling pressures that exceeded normal, but their ventricular function remained hyperdynamic because of increased cardiac output.

From these studies, it is reasonable to conclude that aggressive fluid administration given to women with severe preeclampsia causes normal left-sided filling pressures to become substantively elevated, while increasing an already normal cardiac output to supranormal levels.

Blood Volume. It has been known for over 75 years that *hemoconcentration* is a hallmark of eclampsia. Zeeman and colleagues (2004b) expanded the previous observations of Pritchard and co-workers (1984) that in eclamptic women the normally expected hypervolemia was severely curtailed or even absent (Fig. 34–7). Women of average size should have a blood volume of nearly 5000 mL during the last several weeks of a normal pregnancy, compared with about 3500 mL when they are not pregnant. With eclampsia, however, much or all of the anticipated excess 1500 mL of blood normally present is absent. Such hemoconcentration is likely the consequence of generalized vasoconstriction and endothelial

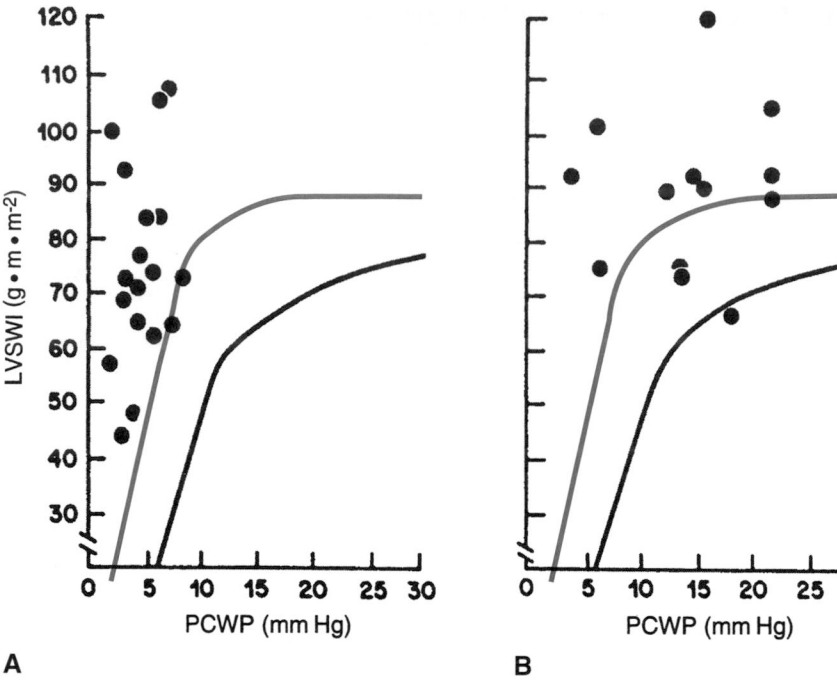

FIGURE 34–6. Ventricular function in women with severe preeclampsia–eclampsia. Left ventricular stroke work index (LVSWI) and pulmonary capillary wedge pressure (PCWP) are plotted. **A.** Restricted intravenous fluids. **B.** Aggressive fluid therapy. (From Hankins and colleagues, 1984, with permission.)

dysfunction with vascular permeability. In women with preeclampsia, and depending on severity, hemoconcentration is usually not as marked, whereas women with gestational hypertension usually have a normal blood volume (Silver and colleagues, 1998; Silver and Seebeck, 1996).

For women with severe hemoconcentration, it was once taught that an acute fall in hematocrit suggested resolution of preeclampsia. However, this usually is the consequence of blood loss, even of normal amounts, at delivery. It may also be partially the result of intense erythrocyte destruction as subsequently described.

In the absence of hemorrhage, the intravascular compartment in eclamptic women is usually not underfilled. Vasospasm and endothelial leakage of plasma has contracted the space to be filled. These changes persist until a variable

amount of time after delivery when the vascular endothelium repairs. Vasodilation then occurs, and as the blood volume increases, the hematocrit usually falls. Thus, women with eclampsia:

1. Are unduly sensitive to vigorous fluid therapy administered in an attempt to expand the contracted blood volume to normal pregnancy levels.
2. Are quite sensitive to even normal blood loss at delivery. (Management in these circumstances is considered in Chapter 35.)

BLOOD AND COAGULATION. Hematological abnormalities develop in some women with preeclampsia. Among these are thrombocytopenia, which at times may become so

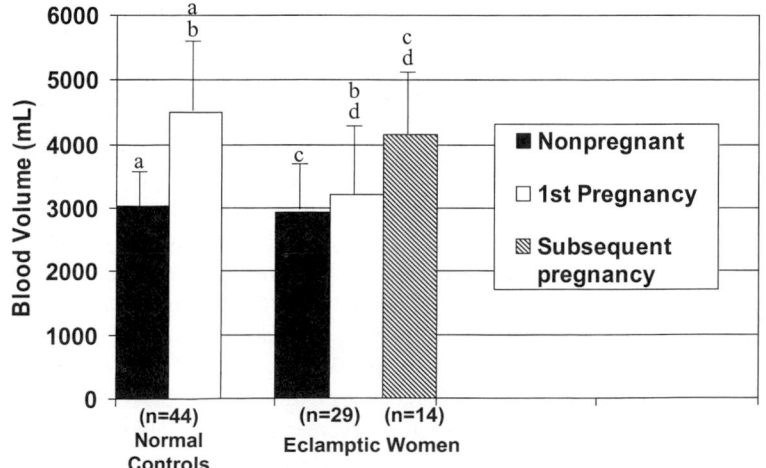

FIGURE 34–7. Bar graph comparing nonpregnant mean blood volumes with those obtained at the time of delivery in a group of women with normal pregnancy, eclampsia in their first pregnancy, and subsequent normal pregnancy in some of the women who had eclampsia. Extensions above bars represent one standard deviation. Comparison between values with identical lowercase letters (namely, a-a, b-b, c-c, d-d) are significant ($P < .001$). (Data from Zeeman and Cunningham, 2002.)

severe as to be life threatening. In addition, the levels of some plasma clotting factors may be decreased, and erythrocytes may display bizarre shapes and undergo rapid hemolysis.

Platelets. Because thrombocytopenia can be induced acutely by preeclampsia–eclampsia, the platelet count is routinely measured in hypertensive pregnant women. The frequency and intensity of maternal thrombocytopenia varies and likely is dependent on the intensity of the disease process, duration of preeclampsia, and the frequency with which platelet counts are performed. Overt thrombocytopenia, defined by a platelet count less than $100,000/\mu L$, indicates severe disease (see Table 34–2). In most cases, delivery is indicated because the platelet count continues to decrease. After delivery, the platelet count increases progressively to reach a normal level within 3 to 5 days.

Thrombocytopenia results from platelet activation, aggregation, and consumption that is accompanied by increased mean platelet volume and decreased life span (Harlow and colleagues, 2002). Levels of platelet-activating factor are increased (Rowland and co-workers, 2000). Platelet production is increased, and *thrombopoietin,* a cytokine that promotes platelet proliferation from megakaryocytes, is increased in preeclampsia with thrombocytopenia (Frolich and associates, 1998). Paradoxically, in most studies, platelet aggregation is decreased compared with the normal increase seen in pregnancy (Baker and Cunningham, 1999). This likely is due to platelet "exhaustion" following in vivo activation. Although the cause(s) is unknown, immunological processes or simply platelet deposition at sites of endothelial damage may be implicated (Pritchard and colleagues, 1976). Platelet-bound and circulating platelet–bindable immunoglobulins are increased, which suggest platelet surface alterations (Samuels and colleagues, 1987).

HELLP SYNDROME. The clinical significance of thrombocytopenia, in addition to any impairment in coagulation, is that it reflects the severity of the pathological process. In general, the lower the platelet count, the higher the maternal and fetal morbidity and mortality (Leduc and co-workers, 1992). In 1954, Pritchard and colleagues called attention to thrombocytopenia accompanied by elevated serum liver transaminase levels in women with eclampsia. Weinstein (1982) later referred to this combination of events as the *HELLP syndrome*—hemolysis (H), elevated liver enzymes (EL), and low platelets (LP)—and this moniker now is used worldwide.

NEONATAL THROMBOCYTOPENIA. Thiagarajah and co-workers (1984) and Weinstein (1985) reported thrombocytopenia in neonates whose mothers had preeclampsia. Conversely, Pritchard and colleagues (1987), in a large clinical study, did *not* observe severe thrombocytopenia in the fetus or infant at or very soon after delivery. In fact, no cases of fetal thrombocytopenia were identified, despite severe maternal thrombocytopenia. **Maternal thrombocytopenia in**

hypertensive women is not a fetal indication for cesarean delivery.

Coagulation. Subtle changes consistent with intravascular coagulation, and less often erythrocyte destruction, commonly are found with preeclampsia and especially eclampsia (Baker and Cunningham, 1999). Since the early description by Pritchard and co-workers (1954) of coagulation abnormalities in women with eclampsia, there is little evidence that these abnormalities are clinically significant (Pritchard and colleagues, 1984). Except for thrombocytopenia, discussed above, laboratory aberrations generally are mild. Unless there is associated placental abruption, plasma fibrinogen levels do not differ remarkably from levels found in normal pregnancy, and fibrin degradation products are elevated only occasionally. Barron and colleagues (1999) found routine laboratory assessment of coagulation, including prothrombin time, activated partial thromboplastin time, and plasma fibrinogen level, to be unnecessary in the management of pregnancy-associated hypertensive disorders. The *thrombin time* is somewhat prolonged in a third of the cases of eclampsia even when elevated levels of fibrin degradation products are not identified. The reason for this elevation is not known, but it has been attributed to hepatic derangements discussed subsequently (Leduc and associates, 1992).

OTHER CLOTTING FACTORS. Clinically concerning deficiency of any of the soluble coagulation factors is very uncommon in preeclampsia–eclampsia unless another event coexists that predisposes to consumptive coagulopathy. Examples include placental abruption or profound hemorrhage due to hepatic infarction.

The *thrombophilias* are clotting factor deficiencies that lead to hypercoagulability. They may be associated with early-onset preeclampsia (see Table 47–4, p. 1079). *Antithrombin* has been reported to be lower in women with preeclampsia compared with normally pregnant women and women with chronic hypertension (Chang and co-workers, 1992). Theories that antithrombin levels might be used to predict development of preeclampsia have not been confirmed (Sen and colleagues, 1994).

Fibronectin, a glycoprotein associated with vascular endothelial cell basement membrane, is elevated in women with preeclampsia (Brubaker and colleagues, 1992). This observation is consistent with the view that preeclampsia causes vascular endothelial injury with subsequent hematological aberrations.

Fragmentation Hemolysis. Severe preeclampsia is frequently accompanied by evidence of hemolysis indicated by elevated serum lactate dehydrogenase levels. Other evidence is from peripheral blood changes that include schizocytosis, spherocytosis, and reticulocytosis (Cunningham and associates, 1985; Pritchard and colleagues, 1954, 1976). These derangements result in part from microangiopathic hemolysis caused by endothelial disruption with platelet adherence and fibrin deposition. Sanchez-Ramos and colleagues (1994) described increased erythrocyte membrane fluidity with HELLP syndrome and postulated that these changes predispose to hemolysis. Erythrocytic membrane changes, increased adhesiveness, and aggregation may also facilitate a hypercoagulable state (Gamzu and co-workers, 2001; Grisaru and associates, 1997).

VOLUME HOMEOSTASIS

Endocrine Changes. Plasma levels of *renin, angiotensin II,* and *aldosterone* are increased during normal pregnancy. With preeclampsia, these values decrease toward the normal nonpregnant range (Weir and colleagues, 1973). With sodium retention, hypertension, or both, renin secretion by the juxtaglomerular apparatus decreases. Renin catalyzes the conversion of angiotensinogen to angiotensin I, which is then transformed into angiotensin II by angiotensin-converting enzyme (ACE). Thus, with preeclampsia, angiotensin II levels decline, resulting in a decrease in aldosterone secretion. Despite this, women with preeclampsia avidly retain infused sodium (Brown and colleagues, 1988b).

Deoxycorticosterone (DOC) is another potent mineralocorticoid that is increased remarkably in third-trimester plasma (see Chap. 5, p. 143). This results from conversion from plasma progesterone rather than increased maternal adrenal secretion. Because of this, DOC is not reduced by sodium retention or hypertension, and it may serve to explain why women with preeclampsia retain sodium.

Vasopressin levels are normal in women with preeclampsia despite decreased plasma osmolality (Dürr and Lindheimer, 1999). During normal pregnancy, serum concentrations of *atrial natriuretic peptide* are maintained in the nonpregnant range despite the increased plasma volume. The peptide is released on atrial wall stretching from blood volume expansion. It is vasoactive and promotes sodium and water excretion, probably by inhibiting aldosterone, renin activity, angiotensin II, and vasopressin. Secretion of atrial natriuretic peptide is increased in women with preeclampsia (Borghi and colleagues, 2000; Gallery and Lindheimer, 1999). Increases in atrial natriuretic peptide following volume expansion result in comparable increases in cardiac output and decreases in peripheral vascular resistance in both normotensive and preeclamptic women (Nisell and associates, 1992). This observation may in part explain observations of a fall in peripheral vascular resistance following volume expansion in preeclamptic women.

Fluid and Electrolyte Changes. The volume of *extracellular fluid,* manifest as edema, in women with severe preeclampsia is usually expanded beyond that of normal pregnant women. The mechanism responsible for pathological fluid retention is thought to be endothelial injury. In addition to generalized edema and proteinuria, these women have reduced plasma oncotic pressure, which creates a filtration

imbalance, further displacing intravascular fluid into the surrounding interstitium.

Electrolyte concentrations do not differ appreciably in women with preeclampsia compared with normal pregnant women unless there has been vigorous diuretic therapy, sodium restriction, or administration of free water with sufficient oxytocin to produce antidiuresis.

Following an eclamptic convulsion, the serum pH and *bicarbonate* concentration are lowered due to lactic acidosis and compensatory respiratory loss of carbon dioxide. The intensity of acidosis relates to the amount of lactic acid produced and its metabolic rate, as well as the rate at which carbon dioxide is exhaled.

KIDNEY. During normal pregnancy, renal blood flow and glomerular filtration rate are increased appreciably (see Chap. 5, p. 137). With development of preeclampsia, a number of reversible anatomical and pathophysiological changes may occur. For example, renal perfusion and glomerular filtration are reduced. Levels that are much less than normal nonpregnant values are the consequence of severe disease. Plasma uric acid concentration is typically elevated, especially in women with severe disease. The elevation exceeds the reduction in glomerular filtration rate and creatinine clearance that accompanies preeclampsia (Chesley and Williams, 1945). Taufield and associates (1987) reported that preeclampsia is associated with diminished urinary excretion of calcium because of increased tubular reabsorption.

Mild to moderately diminished glomerular filtration may result from a reduced plasma volume resulting in plasma creatinine values up to twice those expected for normal pregnancy (from about 0.5 mg/dL to 1.0 mg/dL). In some cases of severe preeclampsia, however, severe intrarenal vasospasm is profound, and plasma creatinine may be elevated several times the nonpregnant normal value—up to 2 to 3 mg/dL (Pritchard and colleagues, 1984). In severe preeclampsia, oliguria develops despite normal ventricular filling pressures (Lee and associates, 1987). In most women, urine sodium concentration is elevated. Urine osmolality, urine:plasma creatinine ratio, and fractional excretion of sodium are also indicative that a prerenal mechanism is involved. Kirshon and co-workers (1988) infused dopamine intravenously into oliguric women with preeclampsia, and this renal vasodilator stimulated increased urine output, fractional sodium excretion, and free water clearance. *Intensive intravenous fluid therapy is not indicated for these women with oliguria.*

Proteinuria. There should be some degree of proteinuria to establish the diagnosis of preeclampsia–eclampsia. Because proteinuria develops late, however, some women may be delivered before it appears. Meyer and colleagues (1994) reported that proteinuria quantification by dipstick was not accurate and recommended 24-hour measurements. Adelberg and co-workers (2001) found that urine protein quantification in 8- and 12-hour samples correlated when there was mild to moderate proteinuria. Use of random urinary protein:creatinine ratio to predict significant proteinuria is controversial. Neithardt and colleagues (2002) and Rodriguez-Thompson and Lieberman (2001) found these determinations to be suitable to predict 24-hour results. Conversely, Durnwald and Mercer (2003) reported that determination of this ratio was not accurate.

Albuminuria is an incorrect term to describe proteinuria of preeclampsia. As with any other glomerulopathy, there is increased permeability to most large-molecular-weight proteins; thus, abnormal albumin excretion is accompanied by other proteins, such as hemoglobin, globulins, and transferrin. Normally, these large protein molecules are not filtered by the glomerulus, and their appearance in urine signifies a glomerulopathic process. Some of the smaller proteins that usually are filtered but reabsorbed are also detected in urine.

Anatomical Changes. Changes identifiable by light and electron microscopy are commonly found in the kidney. Sheehan (1950) observed that the glomeruli were enlarged by about 20 percent. The capillary loops variably are dilated and contracted. The endothelial cells are swollen, and deposited within and beneath them are fibrils that have been mistaken for thickening of the basement membrane.

Most electron microscopy studies of renal biopsies are consistent with glomerular capillary endothelial swelling. These changes, accompanied by subendothelial deposits of protein material, were called *glomerular capillary endotheliosis* by Spargo and associates (1959). The endothelial cells are often so swollen that they block or partially block the capillary lumens. Homogeneous deposits of an electron-dense substance are found between basal lamina and endothelial cells and within the cells themselves. Recently, Strevens and co-workers (2003) questioned whether endotheliosis is pathognomonic of preeclampsia. They identified this lesion on renal biopsies in all 28 women with preeclampsia, in all 8 with gestational hypertension without proteinuria, and in 5 of 12 normotensive controls. The degree of endotheliosis increased with severity of preeclampsia and electron-dense deposits and pronounced endotheliosis were identified only in women with hypertension.

On the basis of immunofluorescent staining, Lichtig and co-workers (1975) identified deposited fibrinogen or its derivatives in 13 of 30 renal biopsy specimens from women with preeclampsia. Kincaid-Smith (1991) found that these deposits disappear progressively in the first week postpartum. Strevens and colleagues (2003) found occasional scarce deposits of immunoglobulin M (IgM), IgA, and C_3 in 32 biopsy specimens.

Renal tubular lesions are common in women with eclampsia, but what has been interpreted as degenerative changes may represent only an accumulation within cells of protein reabsorbed from the glomerular filtrate. The collecting tubules may appear obstructed by casts from derivatives of protein, including, at times, hemoglobin.

Acute renal failure from *acute tubular necrosis* may develop. Such kidney failure is characterized by oliguria or anuria and rapidly developing azotemia (approximately 1 mg/dL increase in serum creatinine per day). Although this is more common in neglected cases, it is invariably induced by hypovolemic shock, usually associated with hemorrhage at delivery, for which adequate blood replacement is not given (see Chap. 48, p. 1106). Drakeley and co-workers (2002) described 72 women with preeclampsia and renal failure, half of whom had HELLP syndrome and a third of whom had placental abruption. Looked at another way, Haddad and colleagues (2000) reported that 5 percent of 183 women with HELLP syndrome developed acute renal failure. Half of these also had a placental abruption, and most had postpartum hemorrhage. Rarely, irreversible *renal cortical necrosis* developed.

LIVER. Hepatic changes in women with fatal eclampsia were described in 1856 by Virchow. The characteristic lesions commonly found were regions of periportal hemorrhage in the liver periphery. In elegant autopsy studies, Sheehan and Lynch (1973) described that infarction accompanied hemorrhage in almost 50 percent of cases. Reports of elevated serum hepatic transaminase levels began with the observations by Pritchard and colleagues (1954), who described these findings in women with eclampsia, hemolysis, and thrombocytopenia. It became appreciated that these changes were also seen in women with severe preeclampsia. As described above, this involvement was later termed *HELLP syndrome* by Weinstein (1985) to call attention to its seriousness.

Anatomical changes with extensive lesions as shown in Figure 34–8 are seldom identified with liver biopsy in nonfatal cases (Barton and colleagues, 1992). Bleeding from these

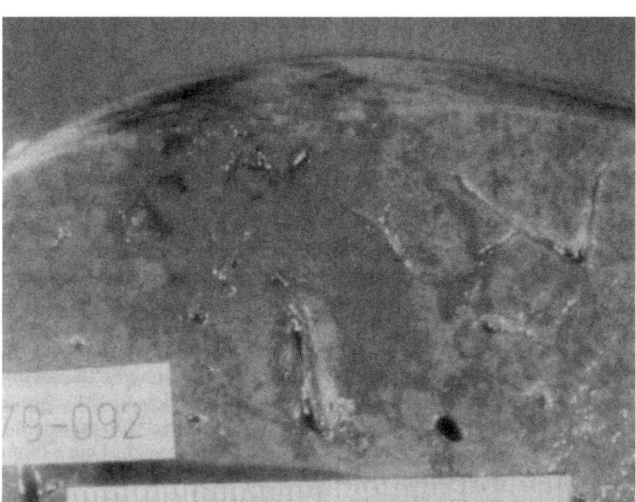

FIGURE 34–8. Gross liver specimen from a woman with preeclampsia who died from severe acidosis and liver failure. Periportal hemorrhagic necrosis was seen microscopically. (From Cunningham, 1993.)

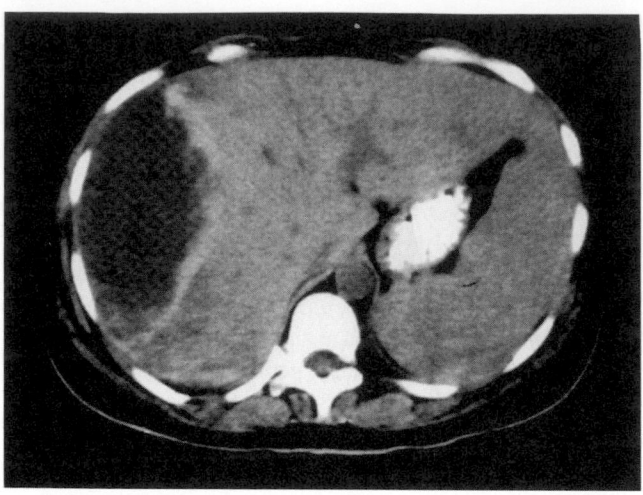

FIGURE 34–9. Computed tomographic scan of liver showing a subcapsular hematoma with a peripheral hyperdense rim corresponding to more recent hemorrhage. (From Wicke and colleagues, 2004, with permission.)

lesions may cause *hepatic rupture*, or they may extend beneath the hepatic capsule and form a *subcapsular hematoma* (Fig. 34–9). These hemorrhages without rupture are probably more common than previously suspected (Manas and colleagues, 1985; Rosen and co-workers, 2003). As subsequently discussed, they are more likely in women with HELLP syndrome.

Most clinicians prefer observation and conservative treatment of hematomas unless hemorrhage is ongoing. That said, in some cases, prompt surgical intervention may be lifesaving. Merchant and associates (2004) reported successful use of recombinant factor VIIa to help control hepatic hemorrhage. Rinehart and co-workers (1999) reviewed 121 cases of spontaneous hepatic rupture associated with preeclampsia, and the mortality rate was 30 percent. One woman cared for at Parkland Hospital survived hepatic rupture after receiving blood and blood products from more than 200 donors along with several laparotomies. Hunter and co-workers (1995) as well as Wicke and colleagues (2004) each described similar women in whom liver transplant was considered lifesaving.

HELLP Syndrome. Because there is no strict definition of the HELLP syndrome, the incidence of the syndrome varies by investigator. In one large study, it was identified in almost 20 percent of women with severe preeclampsia or eclampsia (Sibai and co-workers, 1993b). Earlier reports of severe morbidity and mortality were confirmed by later studies. For example, in a multicenter study, Haddad and colleagues (2000) described 183 women with the syndrome. Adverse outcomes occurred in almost 40 percent of cases, and two women died. Other complications included eclampsia (6 percent), placental abruption (10 percent), acute renal failure (5 percent), pulmonary edema (10 percent), and subcapsular liver hematoma (1.6 percent). Citing autopsy data, Isler and

associates (1999) identified factors contributing to the death of 54 women with HELLP syndrome. These included stroke, coagulopathy, acute respiratory distress syndrome, renal failure, and sepsis.

Some clinicians have advocated corticosteroid therapy for amelioration of HELLP syndrome. Martin and colleagues (2003) reviewed outcomes of almost 500 women cared for at the University of Mississippi. Outcomes of women from 1994 to 2000 (90 percent treated) were considered more favorable than the cohort from 1985 to 1991 (16 percent treated). Unfortunately, there was no untreated control group (Isler and associates, 2001). In a Cochrane Database review, Matchaba and Moodley (2004) concluded that there is insufficient evidence to conclude that adjunctive steroid use is beneficial.

BRAIN. Headaches and visual symptoms are common with severe eclampsia, and associated convulsions define eclampsia. The earliest anatomical descriptions of brain involvement came from autopsy specimens, but imaging and Doppler studies have added new insight into cerebrovascular involvement.

Anatomical Pathology. There are two distinct but related types of cerebral pathology. The first is gross hemorrhage due to ruptured arteries caused by severe hypertension. These can be seen in any woman with gestational hypertension, and preeclampsia is not necessary for their development. These complications are more common in women with underlying chronic hypertension (see Chap. 45, p. 1045). In an older series, Govan (1961) reported that cerebral hemorrhage was the cause of death in 39 of 110 fatal cases of eclampsia.

The second type of cerebral lesion is variably demonstrated with preeclampsia but probably is universal with eclampsia. These are more widespread, focal, and seldom fatal. The principal postmortem lesions are edema, hyperemia, ischemias, thrombosis, and hemorrhage. Sheehan (1950) found hemorrhages, ranging from petechiae to gross bleeding, in 56 percent of the brains of 48 women with eclampsia he examined very soon after death. In addition, he reported that if the brains were examined within an hour after death, they most often displayed normal firmness without obvious edema. This correlates with our clinical and neuroimaging studies in which only 5 percent of 175 eclamptic women had evidence of widespread cerebral edema (Cunningham and Twickler, 2000).

Neuroimaging Studies. With improved computed tomography (CT) and magnetic resonance imaging (MRI) capabilities, Zeeman and colleagues (2004a) reported that nearly all women with eclampsia have abnormal brain findings. Those most commonly seen with CT are hypodense areas in the cortex and correspond to the petechial hemorrhages and infarctions described by Sheehan and Lynch (1973). Several investigators have also described remarkable changes in the area of distribution of the posterior cerebral artery as shown in Figure 34–10 (Brown and colleagues, 1988a; Morriss and

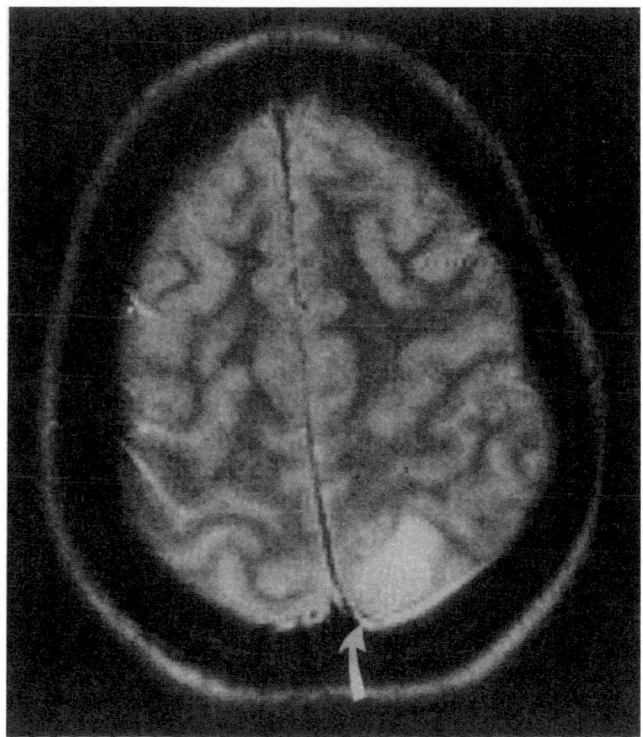

FIGURE 34–10. Magnetic resonance imaging in a 22-year-old woman with eclampsia who had cortical blindness for 96 hours. A high-signal lesion (*arrow*) is apparent in the left occipital lobe. (From Cunningham and associates, 1995, with permission.)

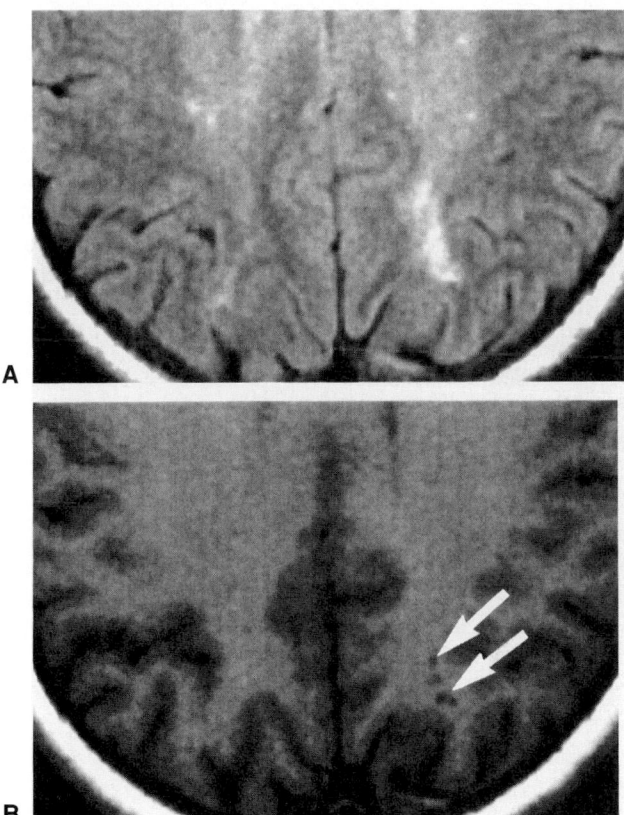

FIGURE 34–11. Follow-up MRIs performed 6 weeks after delivery complicated by eclampsia and in a woman with no residual neurological findings. **A.** There is T2 hyperintensity on FLAIR image in previous areas of vasogenic edema and subcortical infarction. **B.** Corresponding low signal intensity on T1-weighted image (*arrows*) indicates evolution to gliosis or cerebral scarring. (From Zeeman and colleagues, 2004a, with permission.)

associates, 1997). The extent and location of these ischemic and petechial lesions likely influence the severity of the clinical picture. For example, worrisome neurological complications, such as blindness or coma, sometimes occur. It appears that these symptoms represent a continuum of involvement.

Because of clinical resolution in most cases, it was assumed that these findings primarily were areas of edema. This is not the case, however, and recent studies reported that 25 percent of women with eclampsia have areas of cerebral infarction (Loureiro and co-workers, 2003). In another study, Zeeman and colleagues (2004a) evaluated 27 nulliparous women with eclampsia, and all but two had reversible vasogenic edema. In 25 percent, there also were areas of infarction that persisted at follow-up (Fig. 34–11).

Cerebral Blood Flow. Until recently, noninvasive determination of cerebral blood flow was limited to transcranial Doppler ultrasonography. This technology measures blood flow, and *cerebral perfusion pressure* is calculated. Belfort and associates (1999) found that preeclampsia was associated with increased cerebral perfusion pressure counterbalanced by increased cerebrovascular resistance with no net change in cerebral blood flow. In eclampsia, presumably due to loss of autoregulation of cerebral blood flow, there was hyperperfusion similar to that seen in hypertensive encephalopathy unrelated to pregnancy. Women with headaches frequently had

increased cerebral perfusion. The investigators' conclusion that eclampsia is caused by a transient loss of cerebrovascular autoregulation is supported by evidence of widespread low-density areas confirmed by CT and MRI studies (Apollon and co-workers, 2000; Cunningham and Twickler, 2000). Importantly, most studies have not identified appreciable cerebral vasospasm (Morriss, 1997; Rutherford, 2003; Zeeman, 2004b, and all their associates).

MRI techniques have now been developed that allow for accurate measurement of cerebral blood *flow,* and these correlate with invasive procedures. Zeeman and colleagues (2003b) found in normal pregnancy that blood flow decreases beginning early in pregnancy and is 20 percent less than nonpregnant values by late pregnancy. Subsequently, these investigators showed that with preeclampsia, there is hyperperfusion, which at least contributes to vasogenic edema that they identified using MRI.

Blindness. Although visual disturbances are common with severe preeclampsia, blindness is rare with preeclampsia alone. It follows eclamptic convulsions in up to 10 percent of women. Blindness has been reported to develop up to a week or more following delivery (Chambers and Cain, 2004). This condition is also called *amaurosis* (from the Greek *dimming*), and affected women have evidence of extensive occipital lobe vasogenic edema on CT and MRI (see Fig. 34–10). During a 14-year period, 15 such women cared for at Parkland Hospital were described by Cunningham and associates (1995). Blindness lasted from 4 hours to 8 days, but it resolved completely in all cases.

Rarely, permanent visual defects, including blindness, complicate preeclampsia–eclampsia. This can be caused either by cerebral infarction or by retinal artery ischemia and infarction (Lara-Torre and associates, 2002; Moseman and Shelton, 2002).

Retinal detachment may also cause altered vision, although it is usually one-sided and seldom causes total visual loss. Occasionally it coexists with cortical edema and visual defects. Detachment is obvious by examination. Surgical treatment is seldom indicated, the prognosis generally is good, and vision usually returns to normal within a week.

Cerebral Edema. Clinical manifestations suggesting more widespread cerebral edema are worrisome. During a 13-year period, we identified 10 of 175 women with eclampsia at Parkland Hospital who had symptomatic cerebral edema (Cunningham and Twickler, 2000). Symptoms ranged from lethargy, confusion, and blurred vision to obtundation and coma. In some cases, symptoms waxed and waned. Mental status changes generally correlated with the degree of involvement seen with CT and MRI studies. Three women with generalized edema were comatose and had imaging findings of impending transtentorial herniation, and one of these died from herniation.

Clinically, these women are very susceptible to sudden and severe blood pressure elevations, which acutely worsen the widespread vasogenic edema. Thus, careful blood pressure control is essential. Consideration is given for treatment with mannitol or dexamethasone.

Electroencephalography. Sibai and colleagues (1985a) reported that 75 percent of 65 women with eclampsia had nonspecific *electroencephalographic abnormalities* within 48 hours of seizures. Half of the abnormalities persisted longer than 1 week, but most resolved within 3 months.

UTEROPLACENTAL PERFUSION. Compromised uteroplacental perfusion from vasospasm is almost certainly a major culprit in the genesis of increased perinatal morbidity and mortality associated with preeclampsia. Brosens and associates (1972) reported that the mean diameter of myometrial spiral arterioles of 50 normal pregnant women was 500 μm. The same measurement in 36 women with preeclampsia was 200 μm. Attempts to assess human maternal and placental blood flow have been hampered by several obstacles, including inaccessibility of the placenta, the complexity of its venous effluent, and the unsuitability of certain investigative techniques for humans.

Indirect Measurement. The clearance rate of dehydroisoandrosterone sulfate through placental conversion to 17β-estradiol was reported to be an accurate reflection of human placental perfusion (Everett and colleagues, 1980). The placental clearance rate increases with advancing pregnancy, but it decreases before the onset of overt hypertension (Worley and associates, 1975). Subsequently, Fritz and colleagues (1985) reported this method paralleled uteroplacental perfusion in primates.

DOPPLER VELOCIMETRY. Measurement of blood flow velocity through uterine arteries has been used to estimate resistance to uteroplacental blood flow. As described in Chapter 16 (see p. 400), vascular resistance is estimated by comparing arterial systolic and diastolic velocity waveforms. Earlier studies were done to assess this by measuring these ratios from uterine and umbilical arteries in preeclamptic pregnancies. The findings indicated that in some cases, but certainly not all, there was increased resistance (Ducey, 1987; Fleischer, 1986; Hanretty, 1988; Trudinger, 1990, and all their colleagues). Thus, compromised uteroplacental circulation is present in only a few women with preeclampsia. Except for one woman with a previable fetus, all others with abnormal Doppler velocimetry required cesarean delivery for fetal indications. In 50 women with HELLP syndrome, Bush and colleagues (2001) reported that 18 to 36 percent of fetuses had abnormal waveforms.

Matijevic and Johnson (1999) used color pulsed Doppler velocimetry to measure resistance in *uterine spiral arteries*. Impedance was higher in peripheral than in central vessels. This has been termed a "ring-like" distribution. Mean resistance was higher in all women with preeclampsia compared with normotensive controls.

PREDICTION AND PREVENTION

PREDICTION. Measurement in early pregnancy of a variety of biological, biochemical, and biophysical markers implicated in the pathophysiology of preeclampsia has been proposed to predict its development. Investigators have attempted to identify early markers of faulty placentation, reduced placental perfusion, endothelial cell activation and dysfunction, and activation of coagulation. Attempts thus far have resulted in testing strategies with poor sensitivity and with poor positive predictive value for preeclampsia (Conde-Agudelo and colleagues, 2004; Friedman and Lindheimer, 1999; Sibai, 2003; Stamilio and colleagues, 2000). Currently, there are no screening tests for preeclampsia that are reliable, valid, and economical. One goal of the Maternal–Fetal Medicine Units Network is to identify such factors. Selected tests are now discussed.

Roll-Over Test. A hypertensive response induced by having women at 28 to 32 weeks assume the supine position after lying laterally recumbent predicted gestational hypertension (Gant and colleagues, 1974). Women who demonstrated a positive "roll-over" test were also found to be abnormally sensitive to infused angiotensin II (see p. 135). With preeclampsia, rather than gestational hypertension, as the end point, the positive predictive value (true positive) was only 33 percent (Dekker and colleagues, 1990; Friedman and Lindhemier, 1999).

Uric Acid. Elevated serum uric acid levels due to decreased renal urate excretion are frequently found in women with preeclampsia. Jacobson and colleagues (1990) found that plasma uric acid values exceeding 5.9 mg/dL at 24 weeks had a positive predictive value for preeclampsia of 33 percent. Chappell and associates (2002) found it predictive in a small case-control study of high-risk women. In contrast, Weerasekera and Peiris (2003) found that serum uric acid levels did not vary significantly before the detection of hypertension. Because uric acid levels have not even proven useful in differentiating gestational hypertension from preeclampsia, they are not widely used (Lim and co-workers, 1998).

Fibronectin. Endothelial cell activation likely is the cause of elevated serum cellular fibronectin levels in some women with preeclampsia (Brubaker and associates, 1992; Halligan and colleagues, 1994). In a clinical study to predict preeclampsia, Paarlberg and colleagues (1998) found low sensitivity (69 percent) and positive predictive values (12 percent). Chavarria and co-workers (2003a) did four-week sampling beginning at 16 weeks in 378 low-risk nulliparas. The women who subsequently developed preeclampsia had significantly higher levels by 12 weeks but the positive predictive value was only 29 percent, however, the negative predictive value was 98 percent.

Coagulation Activation. Thrombocytopenia and platelet dysfunction are integral features of preeclampsia, as discussed on page 773. Increased destruction causes platelet volumes to increase because of relatively younger, and therefore larger, platelets. Ahmed and associates (1993) found high platelet volumes to be a marker of impending preeclampsia. However, there was substantive overlap with normotensive women. Fibrinolytic activity is normally decreased in pregnancy due to increased plasminogen activator inhibitors (PAI) 1 and 2. In preeclampsia, PAI-1 is increased relative to PAI-2 because of endothelial cell dysfunction (Caron and colleagues, 1991). In the case-control study mentioned above, Chappell and associates (2002) found the PAI-1:PAI-2 ratio to be predictive of preeclampsia in high-risk women.

Oxidative Stress. Increased levels of lipid peroxides, coupled with decreased activity of antioxidants in women with preeclampsia, have raised the possibility that markers of oxidative stress might predict preeclampsia (Walsh, 1994). For example, malondialdehyde is a marker of lipid peroxidation. Other markers are a variety of pro-oxidants or potentiators of pro-oxidants, including iron, transferrin, and ferritin; blood lipids, including triglycerides, free fatty acids, and lipoproteins; and antioxidants, including ascorbic acid and vitamin E (Bainbridge and associates, 2005; Hubel, 1989, 1996; Mikhail, 1994; Powers, 2000, and all their colleagues). Some of these have been studied clinically.

Hyperhomocysteinemia is an independent risk factor for atherosclerosis in women who are not pregnant. According to Rogers and colleagues (1999), this is very similar to implantation site atherosis. Cotter and colleagues (2001, 2003) reported that women with elevated serum homocysteine levels around midpregnancy had a three- to fourfold risk of preeclampsia. Although clinical studies substantiate this association, they have not shown elevated serum homocysteine levels to be a useful predictor (D'Anna, 2004; Hietala, 2001; Zeeman, 2003a, and all their colleagues). Homocysteine levels are influenced by folic acid supplementation (Powers and associates, 2003).

Cytokines. These protein messengers are released by vascular endothelium and leukocytes as well as by macrophages and lymphocytes at the trophoblast–decidua interface. There are over 50 cytokines, and a number of these are elevated in preeclampsia. These include some interleukins and TNF-α. The response to cytokines is the inflammatory process discussed on page 767. A cascade of markers (e.g., C-reactive protein) arise from these reactions, and elevations of their levels have been suggested as possibly predictive of preeclampsia. A number of these have been evaluated in clinical trials but none have yet proved sufficiently predictive (Savvidou and colleagues, 2002; Takacs and associates, 2003).

Placental Peptides. As discussed on page 767, as a result of the inflammatory cascade, a number of peptides are produced by the placenta, and some may prove to be markers for prediction of preeclampsia. Those studied include corticotropin-releasing hormone, chorionic gonadotropin, activin A, and inhibin A (Aquilina, 1999; Ashour, 1997; Cuckle, 1998; Muttukrishna, 1997; Petraglia, 1996, and all their colleagues). The problems with these are similar to those with other markers—namely, they are variably elevated depending on the duration and severity of preeclampsia. Moreover, there usually is substantive overlap with normal pregnant women. For example, Keelan and colleagues (2002) reported that activin A and inhibin A were increased markedly in women who developed preeclampsia. Conversely, other investigators have reported significant overlap of activin A and inhibin A levels in normotensive and preeclamptic pregnancies (Blackburn and associates, 2003; Grobman and Wang, 2000; Zeeman and co-workers, 2002).

As described earlier, the two placentally derived angiogenic factors, VEGF and PlGF, regulate placental development. Both are antagonized by another placental protein, *sFlt1*, whose function is upregulated in women with preeclampsia. Excessively elevated serum levels of sFlt1 have been reported in women with preeclampsia (Levine and associates, 2004b; Maynard and colleagues, 2003).

Thadhani and co-authors (2004) found that first-trimester serum levels of PlGF and sFlt1 could be used to identify women at high risk for preeclampsia. By contrast, Livingston and colleagues (2001a) reported that PlGF levels in early pregnancy were not predictive. Levine and colleagues (2003) and Robinson and Johnson (2003) reported that levels of these two factors correlated with severity and onset of clinical disease. Ecker and colleagues (2003) found that combined first-trimester serum levels of PlGF and sFlt1 were highly predictive of subsequent preeclampsia.

Fetal DNA. Identification of fetal DNA in maternal serum may be predictive of preeclampsia. At the same time that endothelial activation and inflammation occur, fetal cells and cellular material are released into the maternal circulation (Zhong and colleagues, 2001). In a nested, case-control study, Levine and co-workers (2004a) reported that maternal serum levels of cell-free fetal DNA were elevated at two stages. They suggested that screening for fetal DNA in earlier pregnancy may be predictive of subsequent preeclampsia, but that elevations after 28 weeks indicate impending disease.

Uterine Artery Doppler Velocimetry. Measurement of uteroplacental vascular resistance during Doppler ultrasound evaluation of uterine artery impedance in the second trimester has been used as an early screening test for preeclampsia (Bewley and colleagues, 1991; Chappell and Bewley, 1998) (see Chap. 16, p. 400). The rationale for this is based on the presumption that the pathophysiology of preeclampsia includes impaired trophoblastic invasion of the spiral arteries leading to reduction in uteroplacental blood flow. Bower and colleagues (1993) used a two-step screening test beginning at 18 to 22 weeks and its sensitivity for prediction of preeclampsia was 78 percent, but the positive predictive value was only 28 percent. Irion and associates (1998) found uterine artery velocimetry to be an unreliable screening test in low-risk pregnancies. Florio and associates (2003) combined inhibin A and activin A measurements in women with abnormal Doppler findings and reported that the probability of preeclampsia was 86 percent if both hormone markers were elevated and 17 percent if they were both unaltered. Audibert and co-workers (2005) combined second-trimester maternal serum screening for hCG and AFP with uterine artery notching and found sensitivities that ranged from 2 to 40 percent.

PREVENTION. A variety of strategies used to prevent or modify the severity of preeclampsia have been evaluated. In general, none of these have been found to be clinically efficacious (Sibai, 2003).

Dietary Manipulation. One of the earliest research efforts to prevent preeclampsia was salt restriction (De Snoo, 1937). After years of inappropriate salt restriction, followed by years of more inappropriate diuretic therapy, those practices were discarded. Ironically, it was not until relatively recently that the first randomized trial was done by Knuist and colleagues (1998), who showed that a sodium-restricted diet was ineffective in preventing preeclampsia in 361 women.

Early studies performed outside the United States showed that women with low dietary calcium were at significantly increased risk for gestational hypertension (Belizan and Villar, 1980; López-Jaramillo and associates, 1989; Marya and colleagues, 1987). At least 14 randomized trials and a meta-analysis done subsequently showed that prenatal calcium supplementation resulted in a significant reduction in blood pressure and incidence of preeclampsia (Bucher and colleagues, 1996). These were countered, however, by the randomized double-masked NICHD trial. Almost 4600 nulliparous women were given either supplemental calcium or placebo and the incidence of gestational hypertension or preeclampsia was similar in each group (Levine and co-workers, 1997).

Fish oil capsules were given as a supplement in an effort to modify the abnormal prostaglandin balance implicated in the pathophysiology of preeclampsia. The supplement was ineffective in a study of 1474 pregnancies conducted at 19 European hospitals (Olsen and colleagues, 2000).

Low-Dose Aspirin. Early successes of 60-mg aspirin to reduce the incidence of preeclampsia were attributed to selective thromboxane suppression with resultant dominance of endothelial prostacyclin (Hauth and co-workers, 1998; Wallenburg and colleagues, 1986). Subsequent multicenter randomized trials in both low-risk and high-risk women have consistently shown that low-dose aspirin was ineffective in preventing preeclampsia (Caritis, 1998; CLASP Collaborative Group, 1994; Hauth, 1993, 1998; Rotchell, 1998; Sibai, 1993a, and all their colleagues).

Antioxidants. Sera of normal pregnant women contain antioxidant mechanisms that control lipid peroxidation, which has been implicated in endothelial cell dysfunction. Davidge and associates (1992) observed that sera of women with preeclampsia have markedly reduced antioxidant activity. Schiff and colleagues (1996) reported that vitamin E consumption was unrelated to preeclampsia. They found high plasma vitamin E levels in women with preeclampsia and speculated that these were a response to oxidative stress. Chappell and associates (1999) randomly assigned 283 high-risk women at 18 to 22 weeks to treatment with the antioxidants vitamin C or E versus placebo. Therapy significantly reduced endothelial cell activation and led to a significant reduction in preeclampsia compared with that of the control group (17 versus 11 percent). Because of these promising findings, the Maternal–Fetal Medicine Units Network is currently conducting a larger randomized trial.

MANAGEMENT

Basic management objectives for any pregnancy complicated by preeclampsia are:

1. Termination of pregnancy with the least possible trauma to mother and fetus.
2. Birth of an infant who subsequently thrives.
3. Complete restoration of health to the mother.

In certain women with preeclampsia, especially those at or near term, all three objectives are served equally well by induction of labor. **Therefore, the most important information that the obstetrician has for successful management of pregnancy, and especially a pregnancy that becomes complicated by hypertension, is precise knowledge of the age of the fetus.**

EARLY PRENATAL DETECTION. Traditionally, the frequency of prenatal visits is increased during the third trimester to facilitate early detection of preeclampsia. Women with overt hypertension (140/90 mm Hg or greater) are frequently admitted to the hospital for 2 to 3 days to evaluate the severity of new-onset hypertension. Women with persistent severe disease are observed closely, and many are delivered. Conversely, women with mild disease are often managed as outpatients.

Management of women without overt hypertension, but in whom early preeclampsia is suspected during routine prenatal visits, consists primarily of increased surveillance. The protocol used successfully for many years at Parkland Hospital in women with new-onset diastolic blood pressure readings between 81 and 89 mm Hg or sudden abnormal weight gain (more than 2 pounds per week during the third trimester) includes return visits at 3- to 4-day intervals. Such outpatient surveillance is continued unless overt hypertension, proteinuria, visual disturbances, or epigastric discomfort supervene.

ANTEPARTUM HOSPITAL MANAGEMENT. Hospitalization is considered at least initially for women with new-onset hypertension, especially if there is persistent or worsening hypertension or development of proteinuria. A systematic evaluation is instituted to include the following:

1. Detailed examination followed by daily scrutiny for clinical findings such as headache, visual disturbances, epigastric pain, and rapid weight gain.
2. Weight on admittance and every day thereafter.
3. Analysis for proteinuria on admittance and at least every 2 days thereafter.
4. Blood pressure readings in the sitting position with an appropriate-size cuff every 4 hours, except between midnight and morning.
5. Measurements of plasma or serum creatinine, hematocrit, platelets, and serum liver enzymes, the frequency to be determined by the severity of hypertension.
6. Frequent evaluation of fetal size and amnionic fluid volume either clinically or with sonography.

If these observations lead to a diagnosis of severe preeclampsia (see Table 34–2), further management is the same as described subsequently for eclampsia.

Reduced physical activity throughout much of the day is beneficial. Absolute bed rest is not necessary, and sedatives and tranquilizers are not prescribed. Ample, but not excessive, protein and calories should be included in the diet. Sodium and fluid intakes should not be limited or forced. Further management depends on:

1. Severity of preeclampsia, determined by presence or absence of conditions cited.
2. Duration of gestation.
3. Condition of the cervix.

Fortunately, many cases prove to be sufficiently mild and near enough to term that they can be managed conservatively until labor commences spontaneously or until the cervix becomes favorable for labor induction. Complete abatement of all signs and symptoms, however, is uncommon until after delivery. *Almost certainly, the underlying disease persists until after delivery!*

TERMINATION OF PREGNANCY. Delivery is the cure for preeclampsia. Headache, visual disturbances, or epigastric pain are indicative that convulsions may be imminent, and oliguria is another ominous sign. Severe preeclampsia demands anticonvulsant and usually antihypertensive therapy followed by delivery. Treatment is identical to that described subsequently for eclampsia. The prime objectives are to forestall convulsions, to prevent intracranial hemorrhage and serious damage to other vital organs, and to deliver a healthy infant.

When the fetus is known or suspected to be preterm, however, the tendency is to temporize in the hope that a few more weeks in utero will reduce the risk of neonatal death or serious morbidity. As discussed, such a policy certainly is justified in milder cases. Assessments of fetal well-being and placental function have been attempted, especially when there is hesitation to deliver the fetus because of prematurity. Most investigators recommend frequent performance of various tests currently used to assess fetal well-being as described by the American College of Obstetricians and Gynecologists (1999). These include the *nonstress test* or the *biophysical profile*, which are discussed in Chapter 15 (see p. 377 and p. 381). Measurement of the lecithin–sphingomyelin ratio in amnionic fluid may provide evidence of lung maturity. Even when this ratio is less than 2.0, however, respiratory distress may not develop (see Chap. 29, p. 650).

With moderate or severe preeclampsia that does not improve after hospitalization, delivery is usually advisable for the welfare of both mother and fetus. Labor should be induced by intravenous oxytocin. Many clinicians favor preinduction

TABLE 34–5 Summary of Randomized Placebo-Controlled Clinical Trials of Antihypertensive Therapy for Early Mild Hypertension Due to Pregnancy

Study	Study Drug (no.)	Prolongation Pregnancy (days)	Severe Hypertension[a]	Cesarean Delivery (%)	Abruptio Placentae	Mean Birth-weight (g)	Growth Restriction (%)	Neonatal Deaths
Sibai et al (1987a[a])	Labetalol (100)	20.1	5	36	2	2205	19	1
200 inpatients	Placebo (100)	21.3	14[b]	32	0	2260	9[a]	0
Sibai et al (1992[a])	Nifedipine (100)	22.3	9	43	3	2405	8	0
200 outpatients	Placebo (100)	22.5	18[b]	35	2	2510	4	0
Pickles et al (1992)	Labetalol (70)	26.6	6	24	NS	NS	NS	NS
144 outpatients	Placebo (74)	23.1	7	25	NS	NS	NS	NS
Wide-Swensson et al (1995)	Isradipine (54)	23.1	22	26	NS	NS	NS	0
111 outpatients	Placebo (57)	29.8	29	19	NS	NS	NS	0

NS = not stated.
[a]Includes postpartum hypertension.
[b]Significant ($P < .05$) when study drug compared with placebo.

cervical ripening with a prostaglandin or osmotic dilator (see Chap. 22, p. 537). Whenever it appears that labor induction almost certainly will not succeed, or attempts at induction have failed, cesarean delivery is indicated for more severe cases.

For a woman near term, with a soft, partially effaced cervix, even milder degrees of preeclampsia probably carry more risk to the mother and her fetus-infant than does induction of labor by carefully monitored oxytocin infusion. This is not likely to be the case, however, if the preeclampsia is mild but the cervix is firm and closed. The hazards of cesarean delivery may be greater than that of allowing the pregnancy to continue *under close observation* until the cervix is more suitable for induction.

Elective Cesarean Delivery. Once severe preeclampsia is diagnosed, the obstetrical propensity is for prompt delivery. Labor induction to effect vaginal delivery has traditionally been considered to be in the best interest of the mother. Several concerns, including an unfavorable cervix precluding successful induction of labor, a perceived sense of urgency because of the severity of preeclampsia, and the need to coordinate neonatal intensive care, have led some practitioners to advocate cesarean delivery. Alexander and colleagues (1999) reviewed 278 singleton liveborn infants weighing 750 to 1500 g delivered of women with severe preeclampsia at Parkland Hospital. Half of the women had labor induced and the remainder underwent cesarean delivery without labor. Induction was not successful in 35 percent of the women in the induced group, but it was not harmful to their very low-birthweight infants. Similar results were reported by Nassar and colleagues (1998).

ANTIHYPERTENSIVE DRUG THERAPY. The use of antihypertensive drugs in attempts to prolong pregnancy or modify perinatal outcomes in pregnancies complicated by various types and severities of hypertensive disorders has been of considerable interest. Unfortunately, drug treatment for early mild preeclampsia has been disappointing (Table 34–5). Sibai and associates (1987a) performed a well-designed randomized study to evaluate the effectiveness of labetalol and hospitalization compared with hospitalization alone. They evaluated 200 nulliparous women with preeclampsia diagnosed between 26 and 35 weeks. Although women given labetalol had significantly lower mean blood pressures, there were no differences between the groups in terms of mean pregnancy prolongation, gestational age at delivery, or birthweight. The cesarean delivery rates were similar, as were the number of infants admitted to special-care nurseries. **Growth-restricted infants were twice as frequent in women given labetalol compared with those treated by hospitalization alone (19 versus 9 percent).**

At least three other studies have been done to compare either the β-blocking agent, labetalol, or calcium-channel blockers, nifedipine and isradipine, with placebo. As shown in Table 34–5, in none of these studies were any benefits of antihypertensive treatment shown. Von Dadelszen and associates (2000) performed a meta-analysis that included the aforementioned trials for the purpose of determining the relation between fetal growth and antihypertensive therapy. These investigators concluded that treatment-induced decreases in maternal blood pressure may adversely affect fetal growth.

In a somewhat unusual study, Easterling and colleagues (1999) identified 58 women at risk for preeclampsia because they had a high cardiac output at 24 weeks. Cardiac output was measured by Doppler technique and the women were randomly assigned to receive either prophylactic atenolol or placebo. The incidence of preeclampsia was 18 percent in the control group, which was significant compared with 4 percent in the atenolol group.

The use of angiotensin-converting enzyme (ACE) inhibitors during the second and third trimesters should be avoided (see Chap. 14, p. 349). Reported complications include oligohydramnios, fetal growth restriction, bony malformations, limb contractures, persistent patent ductus arteriosus, pulmonary hypoplasia, respiratory distress syndrome, prolonged neonatal hypotension, and neonatal death (Nightingale, 1992). Lip and colleagues (1997) reported that ACE inhibitors taken during early pregnancy do not carry an adverse outlook as long as these drugs are discontinued as soon as possible.

DELAYED DELIVERY WITH SEVERE PREECLAMP-
SIA. Women with severe preeclampsia arc usually delivered without delay. In recent years, a different approach in the treatment of women with severe preeclampsia remote from term has been advocated by several investigators worldwide (Many and colleagues, 1999). This approach advocates conservative or "expectant" management in a selected group of women with the aim of improving infant outcome without compromising the safety of the mother. Aspects of such conservative management always include careful daily, and more frequent, monitoring of the pregnancy in the hospital with or without use of drugs to control hypertension.

Theoretically, antihypertensive therapy has potential usefulness when preeclampsia severe enough to warrant termination of pregnancy develops before neonatal survival is likely. Such management is controversial, and it may be catastrophic. Sibai and colleagues (1985b) attempted to prolong pregnancy because of fetal immaturity in 60 women with severe preeclampsia diagnosed between 18 and 27 weeks. **The total perinatal mortality rate was 87 percent, and although no mothers died, thirteen suffered placental abruption, ten eclampsia, five consumptive coagulopathy, three renal failure, two hypertensive encephalopathy, one intracerebral hemorrhage, and one a ruptured hepatic hematoma.**

Sibai and associates (1994) subsequently performed a randomized controlled trial of expectant versus aggressive management of severe preeclampsia in 95 women at more advanced gestations of 28 to 32 weeks. Women with HELLP

syndrome were specifically excluded from this trial. Aggressive management included glucocorticoid administration for fetal lung maturation followed by delivery in 48 hours. Expectantly managed women were treated with bed rest and either labetalol or nifedipine given orally. Pregnancy was prolonged for a mean of 15.4 days in the expectant management group with an improvement in neonatal outcome. Importantly, 4 percent in each group sustained placental abruption.

In a follow-up nonrandomized study, Abramovici and colleagues (1999) compared infant outcomes for deliveries between 24 and 36 weeks between 133 women with HELLP syndrome and 136 women with severe preeclampsia. Women with HELLP syndrome were subdivided into those with hemolysis plus elevated liver enzymes plus low platelets and those with partial HELLP syndrome, defined as either one or two, but not three, of these laboratory findings. It was concluded that women with partial HELLP syndrome, as well as those with severe preeclampsia, could be managed expectantly. They also concluded that infant outcomes were related to gestational age rather than the hypertensive disorder per se. As shown in Table 34–6, these women were indeed severely hypertensive and had mean diastolic blood pressures of 110 mm Hg. The distinguishing feature between those with HELLP syndrome appears to be the platelet count—the mean value was $52,000/\mu L$ in women with complete HELLP syndrome compared with $113,000/\mu L$ in those with partial HELLP syndrome. Gestational age was about 2 weeks more advanced in women with severe preeclampsia alone compared with those with some degree of HELLP syndrome. Accordingly, neonatal outcomes, in terms of need for mechanical ventilation and neonatal death, were better in women with severe preeclampsia. Fetal growth restriction was not related to the severity of maternal disease and was prevalent in all three groups. Maternal morbidity was not described.

Witlin and associates (2000) later reported that growth restriction adversely affected survival in infants from that institution. Most importantly, the median elapsed time from

TABLE 34–6 Results of Expectant Management of HELLP Syndrome or Severe Preeclampsia Before Term

Outcome	HELLP Syndrome (n = 68)	"Partial" HELLP Syndrome[a] (n = 65)	Severe Preeclampsia (n = 136)
Diastolic BP, mm Hg (mean ± SD)	109 ± 16	110 ± 15	110 ± 15
Platelet count per μL (mean ± SD)	52 ± 21	113 ± 56	199 ± 61
Gestational age in weeks at delivery (mean ± SD)	31 ± 3.2	31 ± 3.3	33 ± 3
Mechanical ventilation of infant (%)	50	40	28
Neonatal death (%)	7	8	4
Fetal growth restriction (%)	28	31	22
Diagnosis-to-delivery (median days)	0	1	2

BP = blood pressure; HELLP = hemolysis, elevated liver enzymes, and low platelet count; SD = standard deviation.
[a]See text for definition.
From Abramovici and colleagues (1999), with permission.

admission to delivery was 0, 1, and 2 days for women with HELLP syndrome, partial HELLP syndrome, or severe preeclampsia, respectively.

Taken in toto, these three studies require comment about repeated claims that expectant management of severe preeclampsia and partial HELLP syndrome is beneficial. First, with expectant management, the interval from admission to delivery is very short, particularly in pregnancies managed subsequent to their report claiming efficacy and safety. Second, it seems possible, even likely, that the gestational age difference between severe preeclampsia and HELLP syndrome is related to the timing of onset of the disease itself. That is, HELLP syndrome may develop earlier in pregnancy than severe preeclampsia. Third, fetal growth restriction is prevalent in women with severe disease and it adversely affects infant survival. Lastly, and most importantly, the authors overlook that the overriding reason to terminate pregnancies with severe preeclampsia is maternal safety. The results shown in Table 34–6 clearly confirm that severe preeclampsia is deleterious for fetal outcome. However, the table provides provide no data suggesting that expectant management is beneficial for the mother.

In a more recent study from Panama, Vigil-De Gracia and colleagues (2003) described the outcomes of 129 women at 24 to 34 weeks with either severe or superimposed preeclampsia in whom efforts were made to delay delivery. Treatment consisted of bed rest, magnesium sulfate for 48 hours, bolus doses of antihypertensive medications to control blood pressures exceeding 160/110 mm Hg, volume expansion, and dexamethasone to promote fetal maturation. Indications for delivery included uncontrollable blood pressure, fetal distress, placental abruption, renal function deterioration, HELLP syndrome, persistent severe symptoms, or attainment of 34 weeks' gestation. The average pregnancy prolongation was 8 days. Although there were no maternal deaths, there were six stillbirths, 11 placental abruptions, and 28 infants diagnosed with growth restriction. Similar results have been described by Visser and Wallenburg (1995). The observations of Chammas and co-workers (2000) provide further data that delay in delivery of the growth-restricted fetus may not be advisable.

Hall and colleagues (2000b) managed 360 women and Haddad and associates (2004), 239 women with severe preeclampsia before 34 weeks. In the first study, the women gained a mean duration of 11 days, but a fourth had major complications: 20 percent had placental abruption, 2 percent had pulmonary edema, and 1.2 percent had eclampsia. In the second study, a median of 5 days was gained with 6 percent having an abruption and 4 percent developing pulmonary edema. Reports such as these serve to emphasize that it is prudent for clinicians to be concerned about maternal as well as fetal safety in women with preterm fetuses. We are reluctant to advise clinicians that it is safe to expectantly manage women with persistent severe hypertension or significant hematological, cerebral, or liver abnormalities due to preeclampsia.

GLUCOCORTICOIDS. In attempts to enhance fetal lung maturation, glucocorticoids have been administered to women with severe hypertension who are remote from term. Treatment does not seem to worsen maternal hypertension, and a decrease in the incidence of respiratory distress and improved fetal survival have been cited (see Chap. 29, p. 650). As discussed on page 776, there are insufficient data to conclude that corticosteroids are beneficial to ameliorate the severity of HELLP syndrome (Matchaba and Moodley, 2004).

There has been only one randomized clinical trial of corticosteroids given to hypertensive women for fetal lung maturation (Amorim and associates, 1999). This trial included 218 women with severe preeclampsia between 26 and 34 weeks who were randomly assigned to be given betamethasone or placebo. Neonatal complications, including respiratory distress, intraventricular hemorrhage, and death, were decreased significantly when betamethasone was given compared with placebo. **But two maternal deaths and 18 stillbirths occurred.** We interpret this report to be an indictment of a strategy in which delivery is delayed in women with severe preeclampsia to allow the administration of glucocorticoids (Bloom and Leveno, 2003).

Thiagarajah and co-authors (1984) were the first to suggest that glucocorticoids might also play a role in treatment of the laboratory abnormalities associated with the HELLP syndrome. O'Brien and associates (2002) and Tompkins and Thiagarajah (1999) later reported that glucocorticoids produced significant but transient improvement in the hematological abnormalities associated with the HELLP syndrome. In the latter study of 52 women between 24 and 34 weeks, platelet counts increased by an average of $23,000/\mu L$. This salutary effect, however, was short-lived, and platelets decreased by an average of $46,000/\mu L$ within 48 hours after completion of treatment. Importantly, few of the women studied had platelet counts less than $100,000/\mu L$ before therapy, and hence, the efficacy of glucocorticoids in women with more severe hematological abnormalities was not extensively tested.

HIGH-RISK PREGNANCY UNIT. An inpatient antepartum unit was established in 1973 by Dr. Peggy Whalley at Parkland Hospital in large part to provide care for women with hypertensive disorders. Initial results from this High-Risk Pregnancy Unit were reported by Hauth (1976) and Gilstrap (1978) and their colleagues. The majority of women hospitalized have a beneficial response characterized by disappearance or improvement of hypertension. **These women are not "cured," because nearly 90 percent have recurrent hypertension before or during labor.** By the end of 2000, almost 8000 nulliparous women with mild to moderate early-onset hypertension during pregnancy had been managed successfully in this unit. Provider costs (*not* charges) for the relatively simple physical facility, modest nursing care, no drugs other than iron and folate supplements, and the very few laboratory tests that are essential are slight compared with the cost of neonatal intensive care for a preterm infant.

HOME HEALTH CARE. Many clinicians believe that further hospitalization is not warranted if hypertension abates within a few days, and this has legitimized third-party payors to refuse hospital reimbursement. Consequently, most women with mild to moderate hypertension, without proteinuria, are managed at home. Such management may continue as long as the disease does not worsen and if fetal jeopardy is not suspected. Sedentary activity throughout the greater part of the day is recommended. These women should be instructed in detail about reporting symptoms. Home blood pressure and urine protein monitoring or frequent evaluations by a visiting nurse may be necessary. Lo and collaborators (2002) cautioned about the use of certain automated home blood pressure monitors that may fail to detect severe hypertension.

Barton and colleagues (1994) used such a home care scheme to manage 592 predominately nulliparous women with mild hypertension. They were 24 to 36 weeks at enrollment. A fourth had proteinuria. Gestation was prolonged for a mean of 4 weeks and 60 percent were delivered after 37 weeks. Importantly, 50 percent developed severe hypertension, and 10 percent had fetal jeopardy. These investigators concluded that in highly motivated women, such management produced results similar to inpatient care. Helewa and associates (1993) reached similar conclusions.

In a study from Parkland Hospital, Horsager and associates (1995) randomly assigned 72 nulliparas with new-onset hypertension from 27 to 37 weeks to continued hospitalization or outpatient care. In all of these women, proteinuria had receded to less than 500 mg per day when randomized. Outpatient management included daily blood pressure monitoring by the patient or her family and weight and spot urine protein were determined three times weekly. A home health nurse visited twice weekly and the women were seen weekly in the clinic. Although perinatal outcomes were similar, development of severe preeclampsia was more common in the home-treated women than in hospitalized women (42 versus 25 percent).

Day-care is another approach that has become common in European countries. It has been evaluated only on a limited basis. Tuffnell and colleagues (1992) randomly assigned 54 women with gestational hypertension after 26 weeks to either day-care or routine management by their individual physicians. Hospitalizations, the development of preeclampsia, and labor inductions were significantly increased in the routine management group. More recently, Turnbull and colleagues (2004) from Australia reported a randomized study of 395 women assigned to either day-care or inpatient management. Almost 95 percent had mild to moderate hypertension; 288 had no proteinuria and 86 had at least 1+ proteinuria at baseline. Perinatal outcomes were good and there were no cases of eclampsia, HELLP syndrome, or neonatal deaths. Routes of delivery and neonatal complications were similar. Surprisingly, costs for either scheme were not significantly different. General satisfaction among the patients favored day-care.

ECLAMPSIA. Preeclampsia complicated by generalized tonic–clonic convulsions is termed eclampsia. Fatal coma without convulsions has also been called eclampsia. However, it is better to limit the diagnosis to women with convulsions and to regard deaths in nonconvulsive cases as due to severe preeclampsia. Once eclampsia has ensued, the risk to both mother and fetus is appreciable. For example, Mattar and Sibai (2000) described the hazards in 399 consecutive women with eclampsia delivered between 1977 and 1998 at their center in Memphis. Major complications included placental abruption (10 percent), neurological deficits (7 percent), aspiration pneumonia (7 percent), pulmonary edema (5 percent), cardiopulmonary arrest (4 percent), acute renal failure (4 percent), and maternal death (1 percent).

Almost without exception, preeclampsia precedes the onset of eclamptic convulsions. Depending on whether convulsions appear before, during, or after labor, eclampsia is designated as antepartum, intrapartum, or postpartum. Eclampsia is most common in the last trimester and becomes increasingly more frequent as term approaches. As discussed on page 764, in more recent years, there has been an increasing shift in the incidence of eclampsia toward the postpartum period. This is presumably related to improved access to prenatal care, earlier detection of preeclampsia, and prophylactic use of magnesium sulfate (Chames and co-workers, 2002). Importantly, other diagnoses including those listed on page 787 should be considered in women with the onset of convulsions more than 48 hours postpartum.

Regardless of the time of onset, the convulsive movements usually begin about the mouth in the form of facial twitchings. After a few seconds, the entire body becomes rigid in a generalized muscular contraction. This phase may persist for 15 to 20 seconds. Suddenly the jaws begin to open and close violently, and soon after, the eyelids as well. The other facial muscles and then all muscles alternately contract and relax in rapid succession. So forceful are the muscular movements that the woman may throw herself out of her bed, and if not protected, her tongue is bitten by the violent action of the jaws (Fig. 34–12). This phase, in which the muscles alternately contract and relax, may last about a minute. Gradually, the muscular movements become smaller and less frequent, and finally the woman lies motionless.

Throughout the seizure the diaphragm has been fixed, with respiration halted. For a few seconds the woman appears to be dying from respiratory arrest, but then she takes a long, deep, stertorous inhalation, and breathing is resumed. Unless treated, the first convulsion is usually the forerunner of others, which may vary in number from one or two in mild cases to even continuous convulsions—status

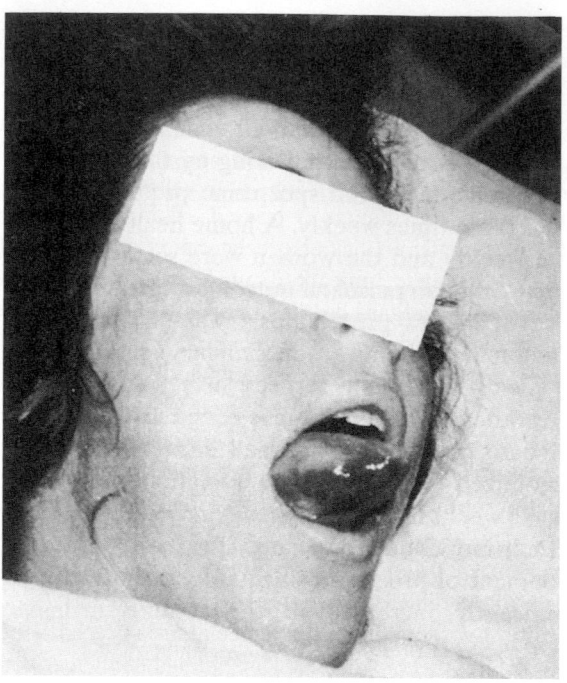

FIGURE 34–12. Hematoma of tongue from laceration during an eclamptic convulsion. Thrombocytopenia may have contributed to the bleeding.

epilepticus—in untreated severe cases. After a seizure, coma then ensues. The woman does not remember the convulsion(s) or, in all probability, events immediately before and afterward. Over time, these memories return.

The duration of coma after a convulsion is variable. When the convulsions are infrequent, the woman usually recovers some degree of consciousness after each attack. As the woman arouses, a semiconscious combative state may ensue. In very severe cases, the coma persists from one convulsion to another, and death may result before she awakens. In rare instances, a single convulsion may be followed by coma from which the woman may never emerge, although, as a rule, death does not occur until after frequent convulsions.

Respirations after an eclamptic convulsion are usually increased in rate and may reach 50 or more per minute, in response presumably to hypercarbia from lactic acidemia, as well as to varying intensities of hypoxia. Cyanosis may be observed in severe cases. High fever is a very grave sign, because it is probably the consequence of a central nervous system hemorrhage.

Proteinuria is almost always present and frequently pronounced. Urine output is likely diminished appreciably, and occasionally anuria develops. Hemoglobinuria is common, but hemoglobinemia is observed only rarely. Often, as shown in Figure 34–13, the edema is pronounced—at times, massive—but it may also be absent.

As with severe preeclampsia, after delivery an increase in urinary output is usually an early sign of improvement. Proteinuria and edema ordinarily disappear within a week (see Fig. 34–13). In most cases, blood pressure returns to normal within a few days to 2 weeks after delivery. The longer hypertension persists postpartum, the more likely that it is the consequence of chronic vascular disease (see Table 34–1).

In antepartum eclampsia, labor may begin spontaneously shortly after convulsions ensue and progress rapidly, sometimes before the attendants are aware that the unconscious or stuporous woman is having effective uterine contractions.

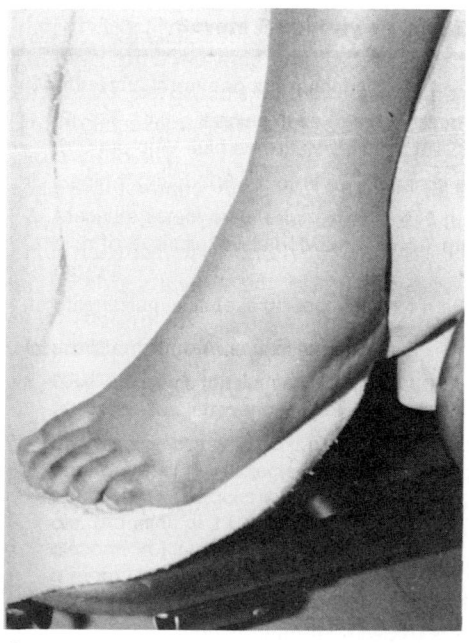

A

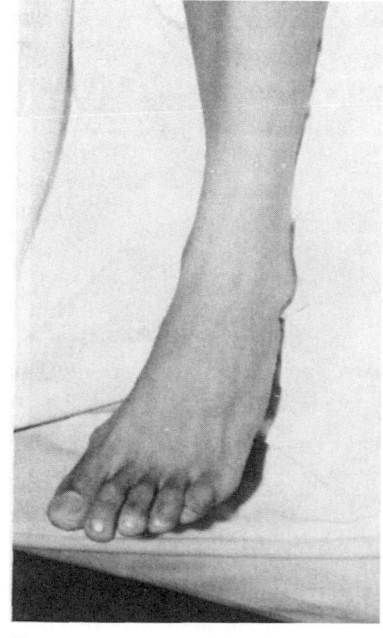

B

FIGURE 34–13. A. Severe edema in a young primigravida with antepartum eclampsia and a markedly reduced blood volume compared with normal pregnancy. **B.** The same woman 3 days after delivery. The remarkable clearance of pedal edema, accompanied by diuresis and a 28-pound weight loss, was spontaneous and unprovoked by any diuretic therapy. (From Cunningham and Pritchard, 1984, with permission.)

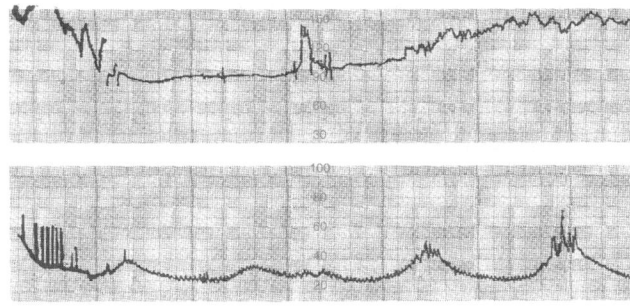

FIGURE 34–14. Fetal bradycardia developing in a woman with an intrapartum eclamptic convulsion. Bradycardia resolved and beat-to-beat variability returned about 5 minutes following the seizure. (From Cantrell and Cunningham, 1994, with permission.)

If the convulsion occurs during labor, contractions may increase in frequency and intensity, and the duration of labor may be shortened. Because of maternal hypoxemia and lactic acidemia caused by convulsions, it is not unusual for fetal bradycardia to follow a seizure (Fig. 34–14). This usually recovers within 3 to 5 minutes; if it persists more than about 10 minutes, another cause, such as placental abruption or imminent delivery, must be considered.

Pulmonary edema may follow eclamptic convulsions. This may be caused by aspiration pneumonitis from inhalation of gastric contents if simultaneous vomiting accompanies convulsions. Alternatively, it may be caused by cardiac failure as the result of a combination of severe hypertension and vigorous intravenous fluid administration.

In some women with eclampsia, sudden death occurs synchronously with a convulsion or follows shortly thereafter, as the result of a massive cerebral hemorrhage (Fig. 34–15). Hemiplegia may result from sublethal hemorrhage. Cerebral hemorrhages are more likely in older women with underlying

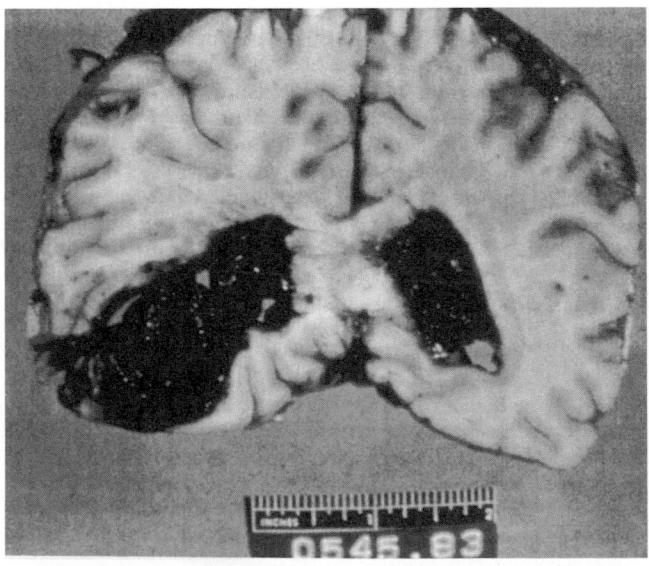

FIGURE 34–15. Hypertensive hemorrhage with eclampsia.

chronic hypertension. Rarely they may be due to a ruptured berry aneurysm or arteriovenous malformation (Witlin and co-workers, 1997a).

In about 10 percent of women, some degree of blindness follows a seizure. Blindness seldom develops spontaneously with preeclampsia. Two causes of blindness or impaired vision are varying degrees of retinal detachment or occipital lobe ischemia and edema. These are discussed in detail on page 777. In both instances, the prognosis for return to normal is good and is usually complete within a week (Cunningham and associates, 1995). About 5 percent of women have substantively altered consciousness, including persistent coma, following a seizure. This is due to extensive cerebral edema, and transtentorial uncal herniation may cause death as discussed on page 778 (Cunningham and Twickler, 2000).

Rarely, eclampsia is followed by psychosis, and the woman becomes violent. This usually lasts for several days to 2 weeks, but the prognosis for return to normal is good, provided there was no preexisting mental illness. Antipsychotic medications in carefully titrated doses have proved effective in the few cases of posteclampsia psychosis treated at Parkland Hospital.

Differential Diagnosis. Generally, eclampsia is more likely to be diagnosed too frequently rather than overlooked, because epilepsy, encephalitis, meningitis, cerebral tumor, cysticercosis, and ruptured cerebral aneurysm during late pregnancy and the puerperium may simulate eclampsia. **Until other such causes are excluded, however, all pregnant women with convulsions should be considered to have eclampsia.**

Prognosis. The prognosis for eclampsia is always serious; it is one of the most dangerous conditions in pregnancy. Fortunately, maternal mortality due to eclampsia has decreased from four decades ago when the rate was between 10 and 15 percent (Eastman and Hellman, 1961). Between 1991 and 1997, approximately 6 percent of maternal deaths in the United States were related to eclampsia; it accounted for at least 207 deaths (Berg and co-workers, 2003). When all hypertensive disorders of pregnancy are considered, the percent of maternal deaths during this same time period was nearly 16 percent (Berg and co-workers, 2003). These facts clearly indicate that eclampsia, as well as severe preeclampsia, should be considered overt threats to maternal life.

Treatment. In 1955, Pritchard initiated a standardized treatment regimen for eclampsia at Parkland Hospital, and this successful approach is still in use today. The results of this regimen employed in 245 women with eclampsia were reported by Pritchard and associates (1984). Most eclampsia regimens used in the United States adhere to a similar philosophy, the tenets of which include:

TABLE 34–7 Intravenous and Intramuscular Magnesium Sulfate Dosage Schedules for Severe Preeclampsia and Eclampsia

Continuous Intravenous Infusion
1. Give 4- to 6-g loading dose of magnesium sulfate diluted in 100 mL of IV fluid administered over 15–20 min.
2. Begin 2 g/hr in 100 mL of IV maintenance infusion.
3. Measure serum magnesium level at 4–6 hr and adjust infusion to maintain levels between 4–7 mEq/L (4.8–8.4 m/dL).
4. Magnesium sulfate is discontinued 24 hr after delivery.

Intermittent Intramuscular Injections
1. Give 4 g of magnesium sulfate (MgSO$_4$ · 7H$_2$O USP) as a 20% solution intravenously at a rate not to exceed 1 g/min.
2. Follow promptly with 10 g of 50% magnesium sulfate solution, one-half (5 g) injected deeply in the upper outer quadrant of both buttocks through a 3-inch-long, 20-gauge needle. (Addition of 1.0 mL of 2% lidocaine minimizes discomfort.) If convulsions persist after 15 min, give up to 2 g more intravenously as a 20% solution at a rate not to exceed 1 g/min. If the woman is large, up to 4 g may be given slowly.
3. Every 4 hr thereafter give 5 g of a 50% solution of magnesium sulfate injected deeply in the upper outer quadrant of alternate buttocks, but only after ensuring that:
   a. the patellar reflex is present
   b. respirations are not depressed
   c. urine output the previous 4 hr exceeded 100 mL
4. Magnesium sulfate is discontinued 24 hr after delivery.

1. Control of convulsions using an intravenously administered loading dose of magnesium sulfate. This is followed either by a continuous infusion of magnesium sulfate or by an intramuscular loading dose and periodic intramuscular injections.

2. Intermittent intravenous or oral administration of an antihypertensive medication to lower blood pressure whenever the diastolic pressure is considered dangerously high. Some clinicians treat at 100 mm Hg, some at 105 mm Hg, and some at 110 mm Hg.
3. Avoidance of diuretics and limitation of intravenous fluid administration unless fluid loss is excessive. Hyperosmotic agents are avoided.
4. Delivery.

MAGNESIUM SULFATE TO CONTROL CONVULSIONS. In more severe cases of preeclampsia, as well as eclampsia, magnesium sulfate administered parenterally is an effective anticonvulsant agent without producing central nervous system depression in either the mother or the infant. It may be given intravenously by continuous infusion or intramuscularly by intermittent injection (Table 34–7). The dosage schedule for severe preeclampsia is the same as for eclampsia. Because labor and delivery is a more likely time for convulsions to develop, women with preeclampsia–eclampsia usually are given magnesium sulfate during labor and for 24 hours postpartum. **Magnesium sulfate is not given to treat hypertension.**

Based on a number of studies cited subsequently, as well as extensive clinical observations, magnesium most likely exerts a specific anticonvulsant action on the cerebral cortex. Typically, the mother stops convulsing after the initial administration of magnesium sulfate and, within an hour or two, regains consciousness sufficiently to be oriented as to place and time.

The magnesium sulfate dosage schedules presented in Table 34–7 usually result in plasma magnesium levels illustrated in Figures 34–16 and 34–17. When magnesium sulfate is

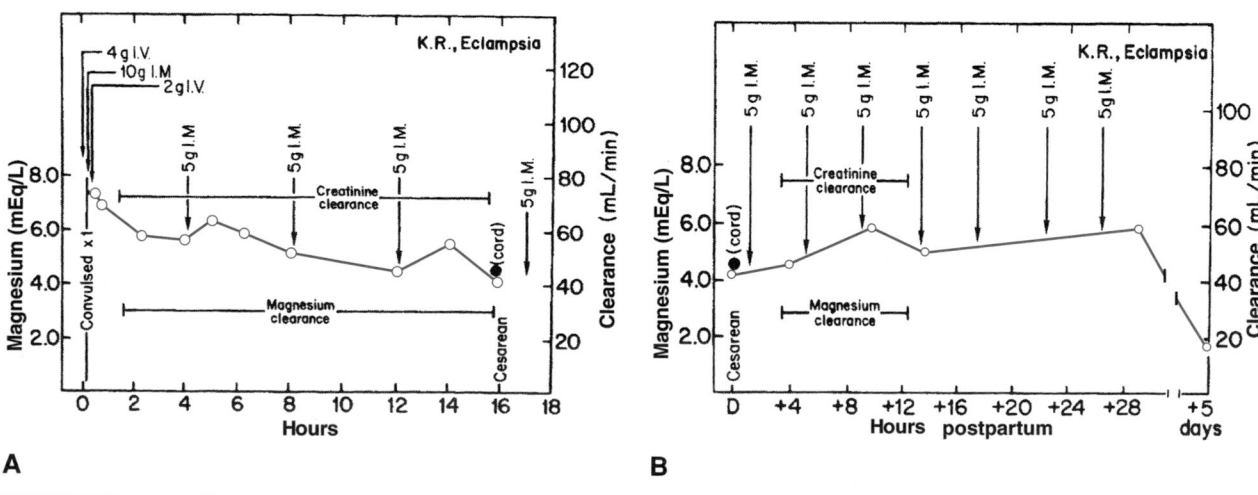

A   **B**

FIGURE 34–16. A. Plasma magnesium levels are plotted for a woman with antepartum eclampsia in whom 4 g of magnesium sulfate intravenously and 10 g intramuscularly were administered at the outset. When she soon convulsed again, 2 g more were injected slowly followed by 5 g intramuscularly every 4 hours, as described in Table 34–7. She did not convulse again. **B.** The same woman as in **A.** Maternal magnesium levels during the first 28 hours postpartum and 4 days after magnesium sulfate was discontinued are plotted. Before and the day after delivery, the renal clearance of magnesium remained relatively constant at about 35 percent of the somewhat depressed creatinine clearance. The mother recovered fully, and the infant thrived. (From Pritchard and associates, 1984, with permission.)

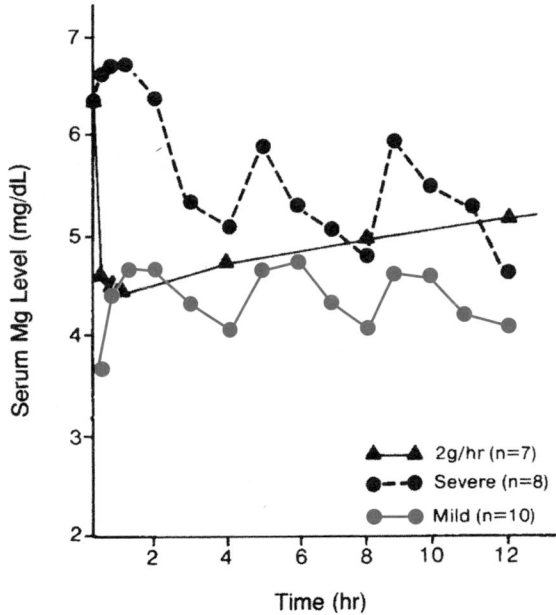

FIGURE 34–17. Comparison of serum magnesium levels following (1) mild preeclampsia—10-g intramuscular loading dose of magnesium sulfate and a 5-g maintenance dose every 4 hours (●–●); (2) severe preeclampsia—4-g intravenous loading dose followed by the same regimen as in (1) (●–●); compared with (3) 4-g intravenous loading dose followed by a continuous infusion of 2 g/hr (▲-▲). (From Sibai and co-workers, 1984, with permission.)

given to arrest and prevent recurrent eclamptic seizures, about 10 to 15 percent of women have a subsequent convulsion. An additional 2-g dose of magnesium sulfate in a 20-percent solution is administered slowly intravenously. In a small woman, an additional 2-g dose may be used once, and twice if needed in a larger woman. In only 5 of 245 women with eclampsia at Parkland Hospital was it necessary to use supplementary medication to control convulsions (Pritchard and associates, 1984). Sodium amobarbital is given slowly intravenously in doses up to 250 mg in women who are excessively agitated in the postconvulsion phase. Thiopental is suitable also. Maintenance magnesium sulfate therapy for eclampsia is continued for 24 hours after delivery. For eclampsia that develops postpartum, magnesium sulfate is administered for 24 hours after the onset of convulsions.

PHARMACOLOGY AND TOXICOLOGY OF MAGNESIUM SULFATE. Magnesium sulfate USP is $MgSO_4 \cdot 7H_2O$ and not $MgSO_4$. Parenterally administered magnesium is cleared almost totally by renal excretion, and magnesium intoxication is avoided by ensuring that urine output is adequate, the patellar or biceps reflex is present, and there is no respiratory depression. Eclamptic convulsions are almost always prevented by plasma magnesium levels maintained at 4 to 7 mEq/L (4.8 to 8.4 mg/dL, or 2.0 to 3.5 mmol/L).

When administered as described in Table 34–7, the drug practically always arrests eclamptic convulsions and prevents their recurrence. The initial intravenous infusion of 4 to 6 g is used to establish a prompt therapeutic level that is maintained by the nearly simultaneous intramuscular injection of 10 g of the compound, followed by 5 g intramuscularly every 4 hours, or by continuous infusion at 2 to 3 g per hour. With these dosage schedules, therapeutically effective plasma levels of 4 to 7 mEq/L are achieved compared with pretreatment plasma levels of less than 2.0 mEq/L.

It should be noted that although laboratories typically report *total* magnesium levels, free or *ionized* magnesium is the active moiety for suppressing neuronal excitability. Taber and colleagues (2002) found that there is a poor correlation between total and ionized magnesium levels. Further studies are necessary to determine whether measurement of ionized, rather than total, magnesium would provide a superior method for surveillance.

Sibai and co-workers (1984) performed a prospective study in which they compared intramuscular and continuous intravenous magnesium sulfate. There was no significant difference between mean magnesium levels observed after intramuscular magnesium sulfate and those observed following a maintenance intravenous infusion of 2 g per hour (see Fig. 34–17). In our experience, a number of women require 3 g/hr to maintain effective plasma levels of magnesium.

Patellar reflexes disappear when the plasma magnesium level reaches 10 mEq/L (about 12 mg/dL) presumably because of a curariform action. This sign serves to warn of impending magnesium toxicity, because a further increase leads to respiratory depression. When plasma levels rise above 10 mEq/L, respiratory depression develops, and at 12 mEq/L or more, respiratory paralysis and arrest follow. Somjen and co-workers (1966) induced in themselves, by intravenous infusion, marked hypermagnesemia, achieving plasma levels up to 15 mEq/L. Predictably, at such high plasma levels, respiratory depression developed that necessitated mechanical ventilation, but depression of the sensorium was not dramatic as long as hypoxia was prevented.

Treatment with calcium gluconate, 1 g intravenously, along with withholding further magnesium sulfate usually reverses mild to moderate respiratory depression. Unfortunately, the effects of intravenously administered calcium may be short-lived. For severe respiratory depression and arrest, prompt tracheal intubation and mechanical ventilation are lifesaving. Direct toxic effects on the myocardium from high levels of magnesium are uncommon. It appears that the cardiac dysfunction associated with magnesium is due to respiratory arrest and hypoxia. With appropriate ventilation, cardiac action is satisfactory even when plasma levels are exceedingly high (McCubbin and colleagues, 1981).

Because magnesium is cleared almost exclusively by renal excretion, plasma magnesium concentration, using the doses described previously, is excessive if glomerular filtration is decreased substantively. The initial standard dose of magnesium sulfate can be safely administered without knowledge of renal function. Renal function is thereafter estimated by measuring plasma creatinine, and whenever it is

1.3 mg/dL or higher, only half of the maintenance intramuscular magnesium sulfate dose outlined in Table 34–7 is given. With this renal impairment dosage, plasma magnesium levels are usually within the desired range of 4 to 7 mEq/L. When magnesium sulfate is being given intravenously by continuous infusion, serum magnesium levels are used to adjust the infusion rate. **With either method, when there is renal insufficiency, plasma magnesium levels must be checked periodically.**

Acute cardiovascular effects of parenteral magnesium ion in women with severe preeclampsia have been studied by Cotton and associates (1986b), who obtained data using pulmonary and radial artery catheterization. After a 4-g intravenous dose given during 15 minutes, mean arterial blood pressure fell slightly, and this was accompanied by a 13-percent increase in cardiac index. Thus, magnesium decreased systemic vascular resistance and mean arterial pressure, and at the same time increased cardiac output, without evidence of myocardial depression. These findings were coincidental with transient nausea and flushing, and the cardiovascular effects persisted for only 15 minutes despite continued infusion of magnesium sulfate at 1.5 g per hour.

Thurnau and colleagues (1987) showed that there was a small but highly significant increase in magnesium concentration in the cerebrospinal fluid after magnesium therapy for preeclampsia. The magnitude of the increase was directly proportional to the corresponding serum concentration. This increase cannot be due to the disease itself, because magnesium levels in the cerebrospinal fluid are unchanged in untreated women with severe preeclampsia when compared with normotensive controls (Fong and associates, 1995).

Lipton and Rosenberg (1994) attribute anticonvulsant effects to blocked neuronal calcium influx through the glutamate channel. Cotton and associates (1992) induced seizure activity in the hippocampus region of rats because it is a region with a low seizure threshold and a high density of N-methyl-D-aspartate (NMDA) receptors. These receptors are linked to various models of epilepsy. Because hippocampal seizures can be blocked by magnesium, it is believed that this implicated the NMDA receptor in eclamptic convulsions (Hallak and colleagues, 1998). Importantly, results such as these suggest that magnesium has a central nervous system effect in blocking seizures.

Uterine Effects. Magnesium ions in relatively high concentration depress myometrial contractility both in vivo and in vitro. With the regimen described earlier and the plasma levels that have resulted, no evidence of myometrial depression has been observed beyond a transient decrease in activity during and immediately after the initial intravenous loading dose. Indeed, Leveno and colleagues (1998) compared labor and delivery outcomes in 480 nulliparous women given phenytoin for preeclampsia with outcomes in 425 similar women given magnesium sulfate. Magnesium sulfate did not significantly alter oxytocin stimulation of labor, admission-

to-delivery intervals, or route of delivery. Similar results have been reported by others (Atkinson and associates, 1995; Szal and co-workers, 1999; Witlin and colleagues, 1997b).

The mechanisms by which magnesium might inhibit uterine contractility are not established but are generally assumed to depend on its effect on intracellular calcium (Watt-Morse and associates, 1995). The regulatory pathway leading to uterine contraction begins with an increase in the intracellular free calcium concentration, which activates myosin light chain kinase (Mizuki and associates, 1993). High concentrations of extracellular magnesium have been reported not only to inhibit calcium entry into myometrial cells but to also lead to high intracellular magnesium levels.

This latter effect has been reported to inhibit calcium entry into the cell—presumably by blocking calcium channels (Mizuki and associates, 1993). These mechanisms for inhibition of uterine contractility appear to be dose dependent, because serum magnesium levels of at least 8 to 10 mEq/L are necessary to inhibit uterine contractions (Watt-Morse and associates, 1995). This likely explains why there is no uterine effect clinically when magnesium sulfate is given for treatment or prophylaxis of eclampsia.

Fetal Effects. Magnesium administered parenterally to the mother promptly crosses the placenta to achieve equilibrium in fetal serum and less so in amnionic fluid (Hallak and colleagues, 1993). Neonatal depression occurs only if there is *severe* hypermagnesemia at delivery. Neonatal compromise after therapy with magnesium sulfate has not been reported (Cunningham and Pritchard, 1984; Green and associates, 1983). Whether magnesium sulfate affects the fetal heart rate pattern, specifically beat-to-beat variability, is controversial (see Chap. 18, p. 449). In a randomized investigation, Hallak and colleagues (1999b) compared an infusion of magnesium sulfate with saline and reported that magnesium was associated with a small but clinically insignificant decrease in heart rate variability.

There has been a suggestion of a possible protective effect of magnesium against cerebral palsy in very-low-birthweight infants (Nelson and Grether, 1995; Schendel and colleagues, 1996). Not all studies, however, have reproduced these findings (Grether and associates, 2000). Such uncertainty underscored the impetus for two large randomized trials designed to assess the fetal effects of magnesium sulfate exposure. In the first trial, conducted at 16 hospitals in Australia and New Zealand, 1062 women with fetuses younger than 30 weeks for whom birth was planned or expected within 24 hours were randomly assigned to receive magnesium sulfate or placebo (Crowther and colleagues, 2003). Nearly all children were evaluated at 2 years of age. Mortality and cerebral palsy were less frequent for infants exposed to magnesium, but the differences were not significant. Substantial gross motor dysfunction, however, was reduced significantly in the magnesium group. Importantly, no serious harmful effects from magnesium were observed. The second trial, with an

Magnesium sulphate versus diazepam

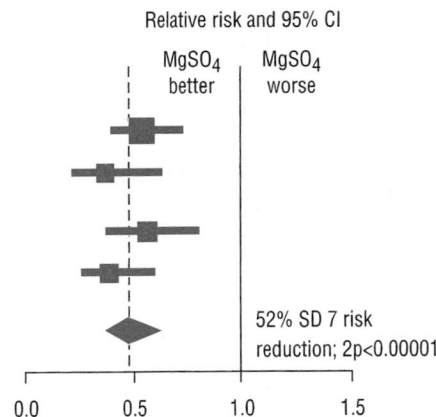

Magnesium sulphate versus phenytoin

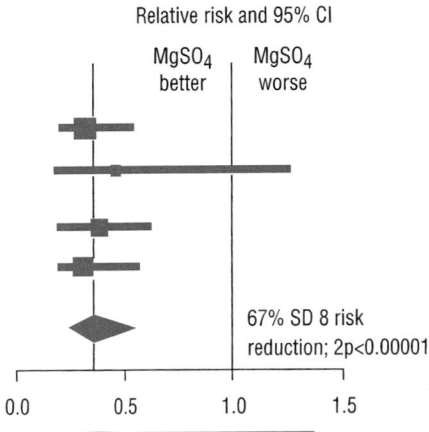

FIGURE 34–18. Effects of magnesium sulfate versus diazepam and phenytoin on recurrent convulsions. (From the Eclampsia Trial Collaborative Group, 1995, with permission.)

even larger sample size, is currently being conducted by the Maternal–Fetal Medicine Units Network.

CLINICAL EFFICACY OF MAGNESIUM SULFATE THERAPY. The multinational Eclampsia Trial Collaborative Group (1995) study was funded in part by the World Health Organization and coordinated by the National Perinatal Epidemiology Unit in Oxford, England. This study involved 1687 women with eclampsia who were randomly allocated to different anticonvulsant regimens. In one study, 453 women were randomly given magnesium sulfate and compared with 452 given diazepam. Another 388 eclamptic women were randomly given magnesium sulfate and compared with 387 women given phenytoin.

As shown in Figure 34–18, women allocated to magnesium sulfate therapy had a 50-percent reduction in recurrent seizures compared with that in those given diazepam. Importantly, as shown in Table 34–8, maternal deaths were reduced in women given magnesium sulfate, and although these differences are clinically impressive, they are not statistically significant. Specifically, there was a 3.8-percent death rate in 453 women randomly allocated to magnesium sulfate compared with a 5.1-percent rate in 452 given diazepam. Maternal and perinatal morbidity were not different between these two groups, and there was no difference in the number of labor inductions or cesarean deliveries.

TABLE 34–8 Maternal Mortality in Eclampsia Trial Collaborative Group

| | | Mortality | |
| | | Maternal | Perinatal |
Regimen	No.	(%)	(Per 1000)
Magnesium sulfate	453	3.8	25
Diazepam	452	5.1	22
Magnesium sulfate	388	2.6	22
Phenytoin	387	5.2	31

From the Eclampsia Trial Collaborative Group (1995).

In a second comparison, also shown in Figure 34–18, women randomly assigned to receive magnesium sulfate compared with phenytoin had a 67-percent reduction in recurrent convulsions. Again shown in Table 34–8, maternal mortality was lower in the magnesium group compared with that in the phenytoin group (2.6 versus 5.2 percent). This clinically impressive decreased maternal mortality of 50 percent again was not significant.

In other comparisons, women allocated to magnesium sulfate therapy were less likely to be artificially ventilated, to develop pneumonia, and to be admitted to intensive care units than those given phenytoin. Neonates of women given magnesium sulfate were significantly less likely to require intubation at delivery and to be admitted to the neonatal intensive care unit compared with infants whose mothers received phenytoin.

The Collaborative Group concluded: "There is now compelling evidence in favour of magnesium sulfate, rather than diazepam or phenytoin, for the treatment of eclampsia." These results are even more impressive when it is emphasized that women in this study who received intravenous magnesium sulfate received only 1 g per hour!

PREVENTION OF ECLAMPSIA. Magnesium sulfate therapy also is superior to phenytoin in *preventing* eclamptic seizures. Lucas and colleagues (1995) reported results of a prospective study from Parkland Hospital in which women with gestational hypertension were randomly allocated to receive magnesium sulfate or phenytoin during labor. The magnesium sulfate therapy consisted of the intramuscular regimen presented in Table 34–7. The phenytoin regimen consisted of a 1000-mg loading dose infused over a 1-hour period, followed by a 500-mg oral dose 10 hours later. Anticonvulsant therapy in both groups was continued for 24 hours postpartum. Ten of the 1089 women randomly assigned to the phenytoin regimen had eclamptic convulsions compared with no convulsions in 1049 women given magnesium sulfate ($P = .004$). Maternal and neonatal outcomes were similar in the two groups. Women given phenytoin who developed eclampsia did so despite "therapeutic" serum levels of 10 to 25 μg/mL.

In an even larger study, more than 10,000 women with preeclampsia in 33 countries were randomly given magnesium sulfate or placebo—the MAGnesium Sulphate for Prevention of Eclampsia, or Magpie trial (Magpie Trial Collaborative Group, 2002). Women allocated to magnesium had a 58-percent lower risk of eclampsia than those given placebo. Stated differently, the overall number of women treated to prevent one case of eclampsia was 91. For women with severe preeclampsia, this number was 63 and for those with milder disease, it was 109. Interestingly, the risk of placental abruption was also significantly lower in the magnesium sulfate group.

Belfort and associates (2003) compared magnesium sulfate and nimodipine, a calcium-channel blocker with specific cerebral vasodilator activity, for the prevention of eclampsia.

In this unblinded randomized trial involving 1650 women with severe preeclampsia, the rate of eclampsia was more than threefold higher for women allocated to the nimodipine group (2.6 versus 0.8 percent).

A number of other studies have helped predict the seizure rate in women with preeclampsia who were not given seizure prophylaxis. Burrows and Burrows (1995) described 467 women not given seizure prophylaxis, and 3.9 percent developed eclampsia. Hall and colleagues (2000a) reported this to be 1.5 percent in 318 preeclamptic women. Coetzee and colleagues (1998) randomly allocated 699 South African women with severe preeclampsia to intravenous magnesium sulfate or to saline placebo. Eclampsia developed in 1 of 30 women given saline, and although the maternal and fetal outcomes were good in both groups, the study was stopped.

Despite proof of its efficacy, there is still debate about whether magnesium sulfate prophylaxis should be given routinely to all hypertensive women in labor (Nelson and Grether, 1995; Robson, 1996). The debate hinges primarily on the belief by some clinicians that a convulsion due to eclampsia does no immediate great harm to most mothers and fetuses. Presumably, those who embrace this view would reserve magnesium sulfate therapy for only those women who develop eclampsia. The unknowns are fetal effects of maternal convulsions. For example, Hallak and associates (1999a) have reported in experimental animals that maternal seizures were associated with fetal brain injury due to maternal hypoxia during the convulsion. Magnesium sulfate prevented this fetal damage.

In the United States, the debate currently centers around which women with preeclampsia should be given prophylaxis. For women with mild preeclampsia, the estimated risk of eclampsia without magnesium prophylaxis is 1 in 100 or less (Lucas and colleagues, 1995). Moreover, in a preliminary study, Livingston and associates (2003) found that magnesium sulfate does not appear to alter the progression of mild preeclampsia to severe preeclampsia.

Because of these findings, we ceased giving intravenous magnesium sulfate as seizure prophylaxis for women with mild gestational hypertension in late 1999. Alexander and co-workers (2003) presented the clinical outcomes in these women for 3-year periods before and after our protocol change. As expected, eclamptic seizures increased in the "after" 3-year period when mildly hypertensive women were not given magnesium. The rate of eclampsia in these women tripled from 2.9 to 9.3 per 1000 mildly hypertensive women. Neonatal outcomes, however, were similar.

The development of eclampsia in these women with mild hypertension and not given magnesium sulfate was not associated with severe maternal morbidity. Despite this, we emphasize two caveats:

1. Severe maternal morbidity due to eclampsia in women with mild hypertension is uncommon and the fact that we did not see such morbidity is likely due to sample size.

Indeed, we are of the view that the very large sample size necessary to definitively address the issue of prophylaxis of maternal morbidity in women with mild hypertension is not feasible. Therefore, this issue will likely never be resolved.

2. The women who developed eclampsia at Parkland Hospital because they did not receive prophylaxis were in a labor-delivery unit with considerable experience in the management of eclampsia. In other settings in which eclampsia is rare, prevention of eclampsia in women with mild hypertension may be preferred as compared with treatment of the convulsing woman.

We currently do not give magnesium sulfate for seizure prophylaxis in women with mild hypertension at Parkland Hospital.

HYDRALAZINE TO CONTROL SEVERE HYPERTENSION. At Parkland Hospital, hydralazine is given intravenously whenever the diastolic blood pressure is 110 mm Hg or higher or the systolic blood pressure is more than 160 mm Hg. Some recommend treatment of diastolic pressures higher than 100 mm Hg and some use 105 mm Hg as a limit (Cunningham and Lindheimer, 1992; Sibai, 1996). Because precise data are lacking, the Working Group of the NHBPEP (2000) suggested the compromise value of persistent systolic pressure exceeding 160 mm Hg or diastolic pressure exceeding 105 mm Hg.

A number of regimens have been used. Hydralazine is administered in 5- to 10-mg doses at 15- to 20-minute intervals until a satisfactory response is achieved. A satisfactory response antepartum or intrapartum is defined as a decrease in diastolic blood pressure to 90 to 100 mm Hg, but not lower lest placental perfusion be compromised. Hydralazine so administered has proven remarkably effective in the prevention of cerebral hemorrhage. At Parkland Hospital, approximately 8 percent of all women with hypertensive disorders are given hydralazine as described, and we estimate that more than 4000 women have been treated. Seldom was another antihypertensive agent needed because of poor response to hydralazine. In many European centers, hydralazine is also favored (Redman and Roberts, 1993).

The tendency to give a larger initial dose of hydralazine when the blood pressure is higher must be avoided. The response to even 5- to 10-mg doses cannot be predicted by the level of hypertension; thus, we always give 5 mg as the initial dose. An example of very severe hypertension in a woman with chronic hypertension complicated by superimposed eclampsia that responded to repeated intravenous injections of hydralazine is shown in Figure 34–19. Hydralazine was injected more frequently than recommended in the protocol, and blood pressure decreased in less than 1 hour from 240–270/130–150 mm Hg to 110/80 mm Hg. Fetal heart rate decelerations characteristic of uteroplacental insufficiency were evident when the pressure fell to 110/80 mm Hg, and persisted until maternal blood pressure increased.

LABETALOL. Intravenous labetalol, an α_1- and nonselective β-blocker, is also used to treat acute hypertension of pregnancy. Mabie and associates (1987) compared intravenous hydralazine with labetalol for blood pressure control in 60 peripartum women. Labetalol lowered blood pressure more rapidly, and associated tachycardia was minimal, but hydralazine lowered mean arterial pressure to safe levels more effectively. We have evaluated labetalol given intravenously for women with severe preeclampsia, and our results are very similar. Our protocol calls for 10 mg intravenously initially. If the blood pressure has not decreased to the desirable level in 10 minutes, then 20 mg is given. The next 10-minute incremental dose is 40 mg followed by another 40 mg, and then 80 mg if a salutary response is not yet achieved.

The Working Group of the NHBPEP (2000) recommends starting with a 20-mg intravenous bolus. If not effective within 10 minutes, this is followed by 40 mg, then 80 mg every 10 minutes but not to exceed a 220-mg total dose per episode treated.

OTHER ANTIHYPERTENSIVE AGENTS. The Working Group of the NHBPEP (2000) recommends *nifedipine* in a 10-mg oral dose to be repeated in 30 minutes if necessary. Scardo and colleagues (1996) gave 10 mg nifedipine orally to 10 women with preeclamptic hypertensive emergencies and reported no hypotension or fetal compromise. Aali and Nejad (2002)

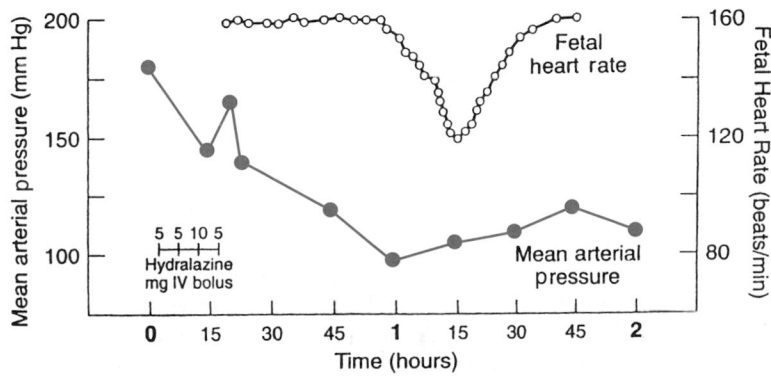

FIGURE 34–19. Effects of acute blood pressure decrease on fetal status. Hydralazine was given at 5-minute intervals instead of 15-minute intervals, and mean arterial pressure decreased from 180 to 90 mm Hg within 1 hour; this change was associated with fetal bradycardia.

found that when nifedipine was compared with hydralazine, fewer doses were required to achieve blood pressure control without increased adverse effects. In contrast, Mabie and colleagues (1988b) administered nifedipine sublingually to 34 women with peripartum hypertension. Its antihypertensive effects were potent and rapid, and two women developed worrisome hypotension. Similar effects in nonpregnant patients have caused cerebrovascular ischemia, myocardial infarction, conduction disturbances, and death. This led Grossman and colleagues (1996) to call for a moratorium on its use in hypertensive emergencies in nonpregnant patients. Vermillion and colleagues (1999) and Scardo and co-workers (1999) compared nifedipine with labetalol in randomized trials and found neither definitively superior to the other.

Belfort and associates (1990) administered the calcium antagonist, *verapamil*, by intravenous infusion at 5 to 10 mg per hour. Mean arterial pressure was lowered by 20 percent. Belfort and co-workers (1996, 2003) reported that *nimodipine* given by continuous infusion as well as orally was effective to lower blood pressure in women with severe preeclampsia. Bolte and colleagues (1998, 2001) reported good results with intravenous *ketanserin*, a selective serotonin$_2$ receptor blocker, in preeclamptic women.

Nitroprusside is not recommended by the Working Group of the NHBPEP (2000) unless there is no response to hydralazine, labetalol, or nifedipine. A continuous infusion is begun with a dose of 0.25 μg/kg/min increased as necessary to 5 μg/kg/min. Fetal cyanide toxicity may occur after 4 hours.

PERSISTENT IMMEDIATE SEVERE POSTPARTUM HYPERTENSION. The potential problem of antihypertensive agents causing serious compromise of placental perfusion and fetal well-being is obviated by delivery. If there is a problem after delivery in controlling severe hypertension and intravenous hydralazine or another agent is being used repeatedly early in the puerperium to control persistent severe hypertension, then other regimens can be used. We have had success with intramuscular hydralazine, usually in 10- to 25-mg doses at 4- to 6-hour intervals. Once repeated blood pressure readings remain near normal, hydralazine is stopped.

If hypertension of appreciable intensity persists or recurs *in these postpartum women*, oral labetalol or a thiazide diuretic are given for as long as necessary. A variety of other antihypertensive agents have been used for this purpose, including other β-blockers and calcium-channel antagonists. The persistence or refractoriness of hypertension is likely due to at least two mechanisms:

1. Underlying chronic hypertension.
2. Mobilization of edema fluid with redistribution into the intravenous compartment.

Labetalol and a diuretic are effective treatment for both mechanisms.

PLASMA EXCHANGE. Over the years, a group at the University of Mississippi Medical Center has described an atypical syndrome in which severe preeclampsia–eclampsia persists despite delivery. Martin and associates (1995) described 18 such women over a 10-year period during which time they delivered nearly 43,000 patients. They advocate single or multiple plasma exchange for these women, and in some cases, 3 L of plasma (representing 12 to 15 donors) were exchanged three times before a response was forthcoming. Other investigators have described cases in which plasma exchange was performed in postpartum women with HELLP syndrome (Förster and colleagues, 2002; Obeidat and associates, 2002). In these cases, however, the distinction between HELLP syndrome and possible thrombotic thrombocytopenic purpura or hemolytic uremic syndrome was not clear (see Chap. 51, p. 1159). In our experience with over 50,000 hypertensive women among nearly 350,000 pregnancies, we have not encountered a syndrome of persistent severe postpartum preeclampsia. In a very few women, persistent hypertension, thrombocytopenia, and renal dysfunction was found to be due to thrombotic microangiopathy (Dashe and colleagues, 1998).

DIURETICS AND HYPEROSMOTIC AGENTS. Potent diuretics further compromise placental perfusion, because their immediate effects include intravascular volume depletion, which most often is already reduced compared with that of normal pregnancy. Therefore, diuretics are not used to lower blood pressure lest they enhance the intensity of the maternal hemoconcentration and its adverse effects on the mother and the fetus (Zondervan and co-authors, 1988). Antepartum use of furosemide or similar drugs typically is limited to the rare instances in which pulmonary edema is identified or strongly suspected.

Once delivery is accomplished, there is a spontaneous diuresis that usually begins within 24 hours in almost all cases of severe preeclampsia and eclampsia. This diuresis results in the disappearance of excessive extravascular fluid over the next 3 to 4 days (see Fig. 34–13).

With infusion of hyperosmotic agents, the potential exists for an appreciable intravascular influx of fluid and, in turn, subsequent escape of intravascular fluid in the form of edema into vital organs, especially the lungs and brain. Moreover, an osmotically active agent that leaks through capillaries into lungs and brain promotes accumulation of edema at these sites. Most importantly, a sustained beneficial effect from their use has not been demonstrated.

FLUID THERAPY. Lactated Ringer solution is administered routinely at the rate of 60 mL to no more than 125 mL per hour unless unusual fluid loss from vomiting, diarrhea, or diaphoresis, or more likely, excessive blood loss at delivery has occurred. Oliguria, common in cases of severe preeclampsia and eclampsia, coupled with the knowledge that maternal blood volume is very likely constricted compared with that of normal pregnancy, makes it tempting to administer intravenous fluids more vigorously. The rationale for controlled, conservative fluid administration is that the typical woman with eclampsia already has excessive extracellular fluid that is inappropriately distributed between the intravascular and extravascular spaces. Infusion of large fluid volumes could and does enhance the maldistribution of extravascular fluid and thereby appreciably increases the risk of pulmonary and cerebral edema (Sciscione and associates, 2003; Sibai and colleagues, 1987b).

PULMONARY EDEMA. Women with severe preeclampsia–eclampsia who develop pulmonary edema most often do so postpartum (Cunningham and colleagues, 1986). Aspiration of gastric contents, the result of convulsions or perhaps from anesthesia, or oversedation, should be excluded, however, the majority of these women have cardiac failure. Some normal pregnancy changes, magnified by preeclampsia–eclampsia, predispose to pulmonary edema. Importantly, plasma oncotic pressure decreases appreciably in normal term pregnancy because of decreases in serum albumin, and oncotic pressure falls even more with preeclampsia (Sciscione and collaborators, 2003; Zinaman and associates, 1985). Moreover, Øian and colleagues (1986) described increased extravascular fluid oncotic pressure in women with preeclampsia, and this favors capillary fluid extravasation. Brown and associates (1989) verified increased capillary permeability in women with preeclampsia. Bhatia and associates (1987) found a correlation between plasma colloid osmotic pressure and fibronectin concentration; this suggested to them that vascular protein loss was the result of increased vascular permeability caused by vessel injury.

The frequent findings of hemoconcentration, as well as the identification of reduced central venous and pulmonary capillary wedge pressures in women with severe preeclampsia, have tempted some investigators to infuse various fluids, starch polymers, or albumin concentrates, or all three, in attempts to expand blood volume and thereby somehow relieve vasospasm and reverse organ deterioration. Thus far, clear-cut evidence of benefits from this approach is lacking, however, serious complications, especially pulmonary edema, have been reported. López-Llera (1982) reported that vigorous volume expansion was associated with a high incidence of pulmonary edema in more than 700 eclamptic women. Benedetti and colleagues (1985) described pulmonary edema in 7 of 10 women with severe preeclampsia who were given colloid therapy. Sibai and colleagues (1987b) cited excessive colloid and crystalloid infusions as causing most of their 37 cases of pulmonary edema associated with severe preeclampsia–eclampsia.

For these reasons, until it is understood how to contain more fluid within the intravascular compartment and, at the same time, less fluid outside the intravascular compartment, we remain convinced that, in the absence of marked fluid loss, fluids can be administered safely only in moderation. To date, no serious adverse effects have been observed from such a policy. Importantly, dialysis for renal failure was not required for any of the more than 400 cases of eclampsia so managed.

INVASIVE HEMODYNAMIC MONITORING. Much of what has been learned within the past decade about cardiovascular and hemodynamic pathophysiological alterations associated with severe preeclampsia–eclampsia has been made possible by invasive hemodynamic monitoring using a flow-directed pulmonary artery catheter. The need for clinical implementation of such technology for women with preeclampsia–eclampsia, however, has not been established. Gilbert and colleagues (2000) described a retrospective review of pulmonary artery catheterization in 17 women with eclampsia. Although they found this procedure subjectively "helpful" in clinical management, all of these women had undergone "multiple interventions," including volume expansion, prior to catheterization.

Use of pulmonary artery catheterization has been reviewed by Clark and Cotton (1988), Hankins and Cunningham (1991), Nolan and colleagues (1992), and Young and Johanson (2001). Two conditions frequently cited as indications for such monitoring are preeclampsia associated with oliguria and preeclampsia associated with pulmonary edema. Perhaps somewhat paradoxically, it is usually vigorous treatment of the oliguria that results in most cases of pulmonary edema.

Because vigorous intravenous hydration and osmotically active agents are avoided at Parkland Hospital in women with severe preeclampsia and eclampsia, hemodynamic monitoring has not been used for the vast majority of these women. Such measures are usually reserved for women with accompanying severe cardiac disease, renal disease, or both, or in cases of refractory hypertension, oliguria, and pulmonary edema. Similar indications are used by Clark and Cotton (1988), Cowles and colleagues (1994), and Easterling and co-workers (1989), as well as recommended by the American College of Obstetricians and Gynecologists (2002). The routine use of such monitoring even if pulmonary edema develops is questionable. Most of these women respond quickly to furosemide given intravenously. Afterload reduction with intermittent doses of intravenous hydralazine to lower blood pressure, as described earlier, may also be necessary, because women with chronic hypertension and severe superimposed preeclampsia are more likely to develop heart failure (Cunningham and colleagues, 1986). As discussed in Chapter 43 (see p. 1011) obese women in these circumstances are even more likely to develop heart failure (Mabie and associates, 1988a).

Invasive monitoring should be considered for those women with multiple clinical factors, such as intrinsic heart disease, advanced renal disease, or both, that might cause pulmonary edema by more than one mechanism. This is particularly relevant if pulmonary edema is inexplicable or refractory to treatment. Still, in most of these cases it is not necessary to perform pulmonary artery catheterization for clinical management.

DELIVERY. To avoid maternal risks from cesarean delivery, steps to effect vaginal delivery are used initially in women with eclampsia. After an eclamptic seizure, labor often ensues spontaneously or can be induced successfully even in women remote from term. An immediate cure does not immediately follow delivery by any route, but serious morbidity is less common during the puerperium in women delivered vaginally.

BLOOD LOSS AT DELIVERY. Hemoconcentration, or lack of normal pregnancy-induced hypervolemia, is an almost predictable feature of severe preeclampsia–eclampsia. **These women, who consequently lack normal pregnancy hypervolemia, are much less tolerant of blood loss than are normotensive pregnant women.** It is of great importance to recognize that an appreciable fall in blood pressure very soon after delivery most often means excessive blood loss and not sudden dissolution of vasospasm. When oliguria follows delivery, the hematocrit should be evaluated frequently to help detect excessive blood loss that, if identified, should be treated appropriately by careful blood transfusion.

ANALGESIA AND ANESTHESIA. In the past, both spinal and epidural analgesia were avoided in women with severe preeclampsia and eclampsia. The primary concern centered on the hypotension induced by sympathetic blockade and, in turn, on dangers from pressor agents or large volumes of intravenous fluid used to correct iatrogenically induced hypotension. For example, rapid infusion of large volumes of crystalloid or colloid, given to counteract maternal hypovolemia caused by a variety of factors, including epidural analgesia, has been implicated as a cause of pulmonary edema (Hogg and co-workers, 1999; Sibai and colleagues, 1987b). There have also been concerns about fetal safety, because sympathetic blockade–induced hypotension can dangerously lower uteroplacental perfusion (Montan and Ingemarsson, 1989). Another concern is that attempts to restore blood pressure pharmacologically with vasopressors may be hazardous

because women with preeclampsia are extremely sensitive to such agents.

As regional analgesia techniques improved during the past decade, epidural analgesia for women with severe preeclampsia was promoted by some proponents to ameliorate vasospasm and lower blood pressure (Gutsche and Cheek, 1993). Moreover, many clinicians who favored epidural blockade believed that general anesthesia was inadvisable because stimulation caused by tracheal intubation may result in sudden hypertension, which may cause pulmonary edema, cerebral edema, or intracranial hemorrhage (Lavies and colleagues, 1989). Other practitioners have also cited that tracheal intubation may be particularly hazardous in women with airway edema due to preeclampsia (Chadwick and Easterling, 1991).

These differing perspectives on the advantages, disadvantages, and safety of the anesthetic method used in the cesarean delivery of women with severe preeclampsia have evolved so that most authorities believe that epidural analgesia is the preferred method (see Chap. 19, p. 487). Wallace and colleagues (1995) evaluated these important issues by conducting a randomized investigation in women with severe preeclampsia cared for at Parkland Hospital. There were 80 women with severe preeclampsia who were to be delivered by cesarean and who were randomized to general anesthesia or epidural or combined spinal–epidural analgesia. Their mean preoperative blood pressure was approximately 170/110 mm Hg, and all had proteinuria. Anesthetic and obstetrical management included antihypertensive drug therapy and limited intravenous fluids and other drug therapy. The infants, whose mean gestational age at delivery was 34.8 weeks, all were born in good condition as assessed by Apgar scores and umbilical arterial blood gas determinations. Maternal hypotension resulting from regional analgesia was managed without excessive intravenous fluid administration. Similarly, maternal blood pressure was managed without severe hypertensive effects in women undergoing general anesthesia (Fig. 34–20). There were no serious maternal or fetal complications

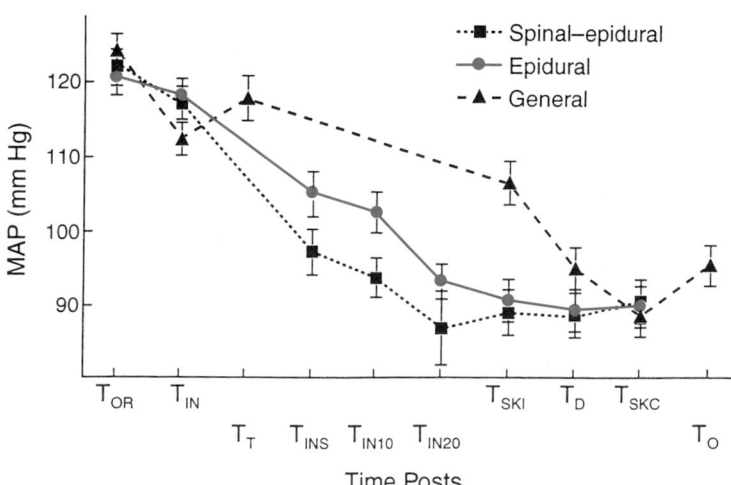

FIGURE 34–20. Blood pressure effects of general anesthesia versus epidural or spinal–epidural analgesia for cesarean delivery in 80 women with severe preeclampsia. [MAP = mean arterial pressure. Time posts (T): OR = operating room, IN = anesthesia induction, T = intubation, SKI = skin incision, D = delivery, SKO = skin closure, O = extubation.] (From Wallace and associates, 1995, with permission.)

TABLE 34–9 Effects of Epidural Analgesia During Labor on Maternal Blood Pressure in Women with Hypertensive Disorders Due to Pregnancy

Outcome	Type of Analgesia		
	Epidural (n = 372)	Meperidine (n = 366)	P-value
Mean maternal BP change	–25 mm Hg	–13 mm Hg	< .001
Ephedrine for hypotension	11%	0	< .001
BP ≥ 160/110 mm Hg develops after analgesia	< 1%	1%	NS

BP = blood pressure; NS = not significant.
From Lucas and colleagues (2001), with permission.

attributable to any of the three anesthetic methods. It was concluded that general as well as regional anesthetic methods are equally acceptable for cesarean delivery in pregnancies complicated by severe preeclampsia if steps are taken to ensure a careful approach to either method. A similar conclusion was reached by Dyer and colleagues (2003) following their randomized study of spinal versus general anesthesia in 70 patients with preeclampsia and a nonreassuring fetal heart rate tracing.

As discussed, the immense popularity and increasing availability of epidural analgesia for labor has led many anesthesiologists as well as obstetricians to develop the viewpoint that epidural analgesia is an important factor in the intrapartum *treatment* of women with preeclampsia (Chadwick and Easterling, 1991; Ramanathan, 1991). To study this issue, Lucas and associates (2001) from Parkland Hospital randomly assigned 738 laboring women at 36 weeks or more who had gestational hypertension of varying severity to epidural analgesia or patient-controlled intravenous meperidine analgesia. Maternal and infant outcomes were similar in the two study groups. As shown in Table 34–9, although epidural analgesia significantly lowered the maternal blood pressure compared with meperidine, this provided no significant benefit in terms of preventing severe hypertension later in labor. It was concluded that epidural analgesia during labor was safe for women with pregnancy-associated hypertensive disorders; it should not be misconstrued to be a therapy for hypertension.

Head and co-workers (2002) from the University of Alabama at Birmingham randomly assigned 116 women with severe preeclampsia to receive either epidural or patient-controlled intravenous meperidine analgesia during labor. Although 9 percent of women who received an epidural required ephedrine for hypotension, pain relief was superior with epidural analgesia and, using a standardized protocol that limited intravenous fluids, there was not a significant increase in other maternal or neonatal complications, including pulmonary edema.

Newsome and colleagues (1986) studied the lowered mean arterial pressure that follows epidural blockade in a group of women with severe preeclampsia. Despite decreased blood pressure, the cardiac index did not fall, and intravenous fluid loading caused elevation of pulmonary capillary wedge pressures as compared with that in women in whom fluids were restricted. It is clear that aggressive volume replacement in these women increases their risk for pulmonary edema, especially in the first 72 hours postpartum (Clark and colleagues, 1985; Cotton and associates, 1986a). When pulmonary edema develops there is also concern for development of cerebral edema. Finally, Heller and co-workers (1983) demonstrated that the majority of cases of pharyngolaryngeal edema seen in women with severe preeclampsia were related to aggressive volume replacement therapy.

LONG-TERM CONSEQUENCES

Women who develop hypertension during pregnancy should be evaluated during the immediate postpartum months and counseled about future pregnancies and also their cardiovascular risk later in life (Working Group of the NHBPEP, 2000). As mentioned earlier, the longer hypertension diagnosed during pregnancy persists postpartum, the greater the likelihood that the cause is underlying chronic hypertension. Indeed, the Working Group has taken the position that hypertension attributable to pregnancy must resolve within 12 weeks of delivery. Persistence of hypertension beyond this time is considered evidence of chronic hypertension (see Chap. 45).

Although hypertension during pregnancy is common, there are few reports concerning the long-term maternal consequences of hypertensive disorders during pregnancy. Most reports are focused on the risk of recurrence of hypertension during a subsequent pregnancy in women affected during a prior pregnancy.

COUNSELING FOR FUTURE PREGNANCIES. Women who have had preeclampsia are more prone to hypertensive complications in future pregnancies (Working Group of the NHBPEP, 2000). Generally, the earlier preeclampsia is diagnosed during the index pregnancy, the greater the likelihood of recurrence. For example, Sibai and colleagues (1986, 1991) found that nulliparous women diagnosed with preeclampsia before 30 weeks have a recurrence risk as high as 40 percent during a subsequent pregnancy.

Sibai and colleagues (1995) found that the recurrence rate for women with one episode of HELLP syndrome was approximately 5 percent. Sullivan and associates (1994) reported a recurrence rate of 27 percent. Our experiences are more in agreement with the lower number. Even if HELLP does not recur, with subsequent preeclampsia there is a high incidence of preterm delivery, fetal growth restriction, placental abruption, and cesarean delivery (Hnat and collaborators, 2002). Multiparous women who develop preeclampsia are at increased risk for recurrence of preeclampsia in subsequent pregnancy compared with nulliparas who develop preeclampsia (Trupin and associates, 1996). Trogstad and associates (2004), using the Medical Birth Registry of

TABLE 34–10 Long-Term Consequences of Eclampsia in 270 Women Followed up to 43 Years After Diagnosis

Outcome	Long-Term Consequences	
	Nulliparas with Eclampsia	*Multiparas with Eclampsia*
Chronic hypertension[a]	Expected incidence	Increased incidence
Death[b]	Expected incidence	Increased 3-fold
Death related to hypertension	29%	80%

[a]Follow-up an average of 33 years after eclampsia diagnosed.
[b]Follow-up an average of 42 years after eclampsia diagnosed.
Adapted from Chesley and colleagues (1976), with permission.

Norway, found that the recurrence risk of preeclampsia for women with a prior singleton versus twin pregnancy complicated by preeclampsia was 14 and 7 percent, respectively.

Women with early-onset severe preeclampsia may have underlying thrombophilias. These disorders, discussed in Chapter 47 (see p. 1074), not only complicate subsequent pregnancies but also have an impact on overall long-term health.

LONG-TERM PROGNOSIS. There is one truly remarkable and unparalleled effort to measure long-term maternal consequences of hypertension due to pregnancy. Chesley and co-workers (1976) identified 270 women with eclampsia delivered at the Margaret Hague Maternity Hospital between 1931 and 1951 and meticulously followed these women through 1974—entailing a follow-up period of up to 43 years in some of the women. As shown in Table 34–10, the long-term cardiovascular prognosis depends on whether eclampsia occurred in nulliparous, compared with multiparous women. Chesley and co-workers (1976) also analyzed the long-term outcome in 54 nulliparous women with eclampsia in their index pregnancy and hypertension again during a subsequent pregnancy compared with that of 100 eclamptic nulliparous who were normotensive during all subsequent pregnancies. Those with recurrent pregnancy hypertension were at increased risk for chronic hypertension, whereas those who remained normotensive during subsequent pregnancies were at decreased risk. Thus, normal blood pressure during subsequent pregnancies serves to define women not at risk for future chronic hypertension. According to the Working Group of the NHBPEP (2000), women experiencing normotensive births have a reduced risk for remote hypertension. Thus, in some respects, repeated pregnancy serves as a screening test for future hypertension. Finally, and importantly, preeclampsia does not cause chronic hypertension (Fisher and colleagues, 1981).

REFERENCES

Aali BS, Nejad SS: Nifedipine or hydralazine as a first-line agent to control hypertension in severe preeclampsia. Acta Obstet Gynecol Scand 81:25, 2002

Abdul-Karim R, Assali NS: Pressor response to angiotonin in pregnant and nonpregnant women. Am J Obstet Gynecol 82:246, 1961

Abramovici D, Friedman SA, Mercer BM, et al: Neonatal outcome in severe preeclampsia at 24 to 36 weeks' gestation: Does the HELLP (hemolysis, elevated liver enzyme, and low platelet count) syndrome matter? Am J Obstet Gynecol 180:221, 1999

Adelberg AM, Miller J, Doerzbacher M, et al: Correlation of quantitative protein measurements in 8-, 12-, and 24-hour urine samples for the diagnosis of preeclampsia. Am J Obstet Gynecol 185:804, 2001

Ahmed Y, van Iddekinge B, Paul C, et al: Retrospective analysis of platelet members and volumes in normal pregnancy and in preeclampsia. Br J Obstet Gynaecol 100:216, 1993

Ajne G, Wolff K, Fyhrquist F, et al: Endothelin converting enzyme (ECE) activity in normal pregnancy and preeclampsia. Hypertens Pregnancy 22:215, 2003

Alexander JM, Bloom SL, McIntire DD, et al: Severe preeclampsia and the very low-birthweight infant: Is induction of labor harmful? Obstet Gynecol 93:485, 1999

Alexander JM, McIntire DD, Leveno KJ, et al: Magnesium sulfate for the prevention of eclampsia in women with mild hypertension. Am J Obstet Gynecol 189:S89, 2003

American College of Obstetricians and Gynecologists: Diagnosis and management of preeclampsia and eclampsia. Practice Bulletin No. 33, January 2002

American College of Obstetricians and Gynecologists: Antepartum fetal surveillance. Practice Bulletin No. 9, October 1999

Amorim MMR, Santos LC, Faúndes A: Corticosteroid therapy for prevention of respiratory distress syndrome in severe preeclampsia. Am J Obstet Gynecol 180:1283, 1999

Ananth CV, Bowes WA, Savitz DA, et al: Relationship between pregnancy-induced hypertension and placenta previa: A population-based study. Am J Obstet Gynecol 177:997, 1997

Anumba DOC, Ford GA, Boys RJ, et al: Stimulated nitric oxide release and nitric oxide sensitivity in forearm arterial vasculature during normotensive and preeclamptic pregnancy. Am J Obstet Gynecol 181:1479, 1999

Apollon KM, Robinson JN, Schwartz RB, et al: Cortical blindness in severe preeclampsia: Computed tomography, magnetic resonance imaging, and single-photon-emission computed tomography findings. Obstet Gynecol 95:1017, 2000

Aquilina J, Barnett A, Thompson O, et al: Second trimester maternal serum inhibin A concentrations as an early marker for preeclampsia. Am J Obstet Gynecol 181:131, 1999

Ashour AMN, Lieberman ES, Wilkins Haug LE, et al: The value of elevated second trimester β-human chorionic gonadotropin in predicting development of preeclampsia. Am J Obstet Gynecol 176:438, 1997

Atkinson MW, Guinn D, Owen J, et al: Does magnesium sulfate affect the length of labor induction in women with pregnancy-associated hypertension. Am J Obstet Gynecol 173:1219, 1995

Audibert F, Benchimol Y, Benattar C, et al: Prediction of preeclampsia or intrauterine growth restriction by second trimester serum screening and uterine Doppler velocimetry. Fetal Diagn Ther 20:48, 2005

Bainbridge SA, Sidle EH, Smith GN: Direct placental effects of cigarette smoke protect women from pre-eclampsia: The specific roles of carbon monoxide and antioxidant systems in the placenta. Med Hypotheses 64:17, 2005

Baker PN, Cunningham FG: Platelet and coagulation abnormalities. In Lindheimer MD, Roberts JM, Cunningham FG (eds): Chesley's Hypertensive Disorders in Pregnancy, 2nd ed. Stamford CT, Appleton & Lange, 1999, p 349

Baker PN, Krasnow J, Roberts JM, et al: Elevated serum levels of vascular endothelial growth factor in patients with preeclampsia. Obstet Gynecol 86:815, 1995

Bardeguez AD, McNerney R, Frieri M, et al: Cellular immunity in preeclampsia: Alterations in T lymphocyte subpopulations during early pregnancy. Obstet Gynecol 77:859, 1991

Barron WM, Heckerling P, Hibbard JU, et al: Reducing unnecessary coagulation testing in hypertensive disorders of pregnancy. Obstet Gynecol 94:364, 1999

Barton JR, Riely CA, Adamec TA, et al: Hepatic histopathologic condition does not correlate with laboratory abnormalities in HELLP syndrome (hemolysis, elevated liver enzymes, and low platelet count). Am J Obstet Gynecol 167:1538, 1992

Barton JR, Stanziano G, Sibai BM: Monitored outpatient management of mild gestational hypertension remote from term. Am J Obstet Gynecol 170:765, 1994

Beer AE: Possible immunologic bases of preeclampsia/eclampsia. Semin Perinatol 2:39, 1978

Belfort MA, Anthony J, Buccimazza A, et al: Hemodynamic changes associated with intravenous infusion of the calcium antagonist verapamil in the treatment of severe gestational proteinuric hypertension. Obstet Gynecol 75:970, 1990

Belfort M, Anthony J, Saade G, et al: A comparison of magnesium sulfate and nimodipine for the prevention of eclampsia. N Engl J Med 348:304, 2003

Belfort MA, Saade GR, Grunewald C, et al: Associates of cerebral perfusion pressure with headache in women with preeclampsia. Br J Obstet Gynaecol 106:814, 1999

Belfort MA, Taskin O, Buhur A, et al: Intravenous nimodipine in the management of severe preeclampsia: Double blind, randomized, controlled clinical trial. Am J Obstet Gynecol 174:451, 1996

Belfort MA, Tooke-Miller C, Allen JC, et al: Changes in flow velocity, resistance indices, and cerebral perfusion pressure in the maternal middle cerebral artery distribution during normal pregnancy. Acta Obstet Gynecol Scand 80:104, 2001

Belizan JM, Villar J: The relationship between calcium intake and edema-, proteinuria-, and hypertension-getosis: An hypothesis. Am J Clin Nutr 33:2202, 1980

Benedetti TJ, Cotton DB, Read JC, et al: Hemodynamic observations in severe preeclampsia with a flow-directed pulmonary artery catheter. Am J Obstet Gynecol 136:465, 1980

Benedetti TJ, Kates R, Williams V: Hemodynamic observations in severe preeclampsia complicated by pulmonary edema. Am J Obstet Gynecol 152:330, 1985

Benedetto C, Marozio L, Neri I, et al: Increased L-citrulline/L-arginine plasma ratio in severe preeclampsia. Obstet Gynecol 96:395, 2000

Berg CJ, Chang J, Callaghan WM, et al: Pregnancy-related mortality in the United States 1991–1997. Obstet Gynecol 101:289, 2003

Bewley S, Cooper D, Campbell S: Doppler investigation of uteroplacental blood flow resistance in the second trimester: A screening study for preeclampsia and intrauterine growth retardation. Br J Obstet Gynaecol 98:871, 1991

Bhatia RK, Bottoms SF, Saleh AA, et al: Mechanisms for reduced colloid osmotic pressure in preeclampsia. Am J Obstet Gynecol 157:106, 1987

Blackburn CA, Keelan JA, Taylor RS, et al: Maternal serum activin A is not elevated before preeclampsia in women who are at high risk. Am J Obstet Gynecol 188:807, 2003

Bloom SL, Leveno KJ: Corticosteroid use in special circumstances: Preterm ruptured membranes, hypertension, fetal growth restriction, multiple fetuses. Clin Obstet Gynecol 46:150, 2003

Bolte AC, Gafar S, van Eyck J, et al: Ketanserin, a better option in the treatment of preeclampsia? Am J Obstet Gynecol 178:S118, 1998

Bolte AC, van Eyck J, Gaffar SF, et al: Ketanserin for the treatment of preeclampsia. J Perinat Med 29:14, 2001

Borghi C, Esposti DD, Immordino V, et al: Relationship of systemic hemodynamics, left ventricular structure and function, and plasma natriuretic peptide concentrations during pregnancy complicated by preeclampsia. Am J Obstet Gynecol 183:140, 2000

Bosio PM, McKenna PJ, Conroy R, et al: Maternal central hemodynamics in hypertensive disorders of pregnancy. Obstet Gynecol 94:978, 1999

Bower S, Bewley S, Campbell S: Improved prediction of preeclampsia by two-stage screening of uterine arteries using the early diastolic notch and color Doppler imaging. Obstet Gynecol 82:78, 1993

Branch DW, Porter TF, Rittenhouse L, et al: Antiphospholipid antibodies in women at risk for preeclampsia. Am J Obstet Gynecol 184:825, 2001

Brosens IA, Robertson WB, Dixon HG: The role of the spiral arteries in the pathogenesis of preeclampsia. Obstet Gynecol Annu 1:177, 1972

Brown CEL, Cunningham FG, Pritchard JA: Convulsions in hypertensive, proteinuric primiparas more than 24 hours after delivery: Eclampsia or some other cause? J Reprod Med 32:499, 1987

Brown CEL, Purdy PD, Cunningham FG: Head computed tomographic scans in women with eclampsia. Am J Obstet Gynecol 159:915, 1988a

Brown MA, Gallery EDM, Ross MR, et al: Sodium excretion in normal and hypertensive pregnancy: A prospective study. Am J Obstet Gynecol 159:297, 1988b

Brown MA, Zammit VC, Lowe SA: Capillary permeability and extracellular fluid volumes in pregnancy-induced hypertension. Clin Sci 77:599, 1989

Brubaker DB, Ross MG, Marinoff D: The function of elevated plasma fibronectin in preeclampsia. Am J Obstet Gynecol 166:526, 1992

Bucher HC, Guyatt GH, Cook RJ, et al: Effect of calcium supplementation on pregnancy-induced hypertension and preeclampsia. JAMA 275:1113, 1996

Burrows RF, Burrows EA: The feasibility of a control population for a randomized control trial of seizure prophylaxis in the hypertensive disorders of pregnancy. Am J Obstet Gynecol 173:929, 1995

Bush KD, O'Brien JM, Barton JR: The utility of umbilical artery Doppler investigation in women with HELLP (hemolysis, elevated liver enzymes, and low platelet count) syndrome. Am J Obstet Gynecol 184:1087, 2001

Cantrell DC, Cunningham FG: Epilepsy complicating pregnancy. Williams Obstetrics, 19th ed (Suppl 8). Norwalk, CT, Appleton & Lange, 1994

Caritis S, Sibai B, Hauth J, et al: Low-dose aspirin to prevent preeclampsia in women at high risk. National Institute of Child

Health and Human Development Network of Maternal–Fetal Medicine Units. N Engl J Med 338:701, 1998

Caron C, Goudemaud J, Marey A, et al: Are haemostatic and fibrinolytic parameters predictors of preeclampsia in pregnancy-associated hypertension? Thromb Haemost 66:410, 1991

Chadwick HS, Easterling T: Anesthetic concerns in the patient with preeclampsia. Semin Perinatol 15:397, 1991

Chambers KA, Cain TW: Postpartum blindness: Two cases. Ann Emerg Med 43:243, 2004

Chames MC, Livingston JC, Ivester TS, et al: Late postpartum eclampsia: A preventable disease? Am J Obstet Gynecol 186:1174, 2002

Chammas MF, Nguyen TM, Li MA, et al: Expectant management of severe preterm preeclampsia: Is intrauterine growth restriction an indication for immediate delivery? Am J Obstet Gynecol 183:853, 2000

Chang CH, Chang FM, Chen CP, et al: Antithrombin III activity in normal and toxemic pregnancies. J Formos Med Assoc 91:680, 1992

Chappell L, Bewley S: Preeclamptic toxaemia: The role of uterine artery Doppler. Br J Obstet Gynaecol 105:379, 1998

Chappell LC, Seed PT, Briley A, et al: A longitudinal study of biochemical variables in women at risk of preeclampsia. Am J Obstet Gynecol 187:127, 2002

Chappell LC, Seed PT, Briley AL, et al: Effect of antioxidants on the occurrence of preeclampsia in women at increased risk: A randomized trial. Lancet 354:810, 1999

Chavarria ME, Lara-González L, González-Gleason A, et al: Maternal plasma cellular fibronectin concentration in normal and preeclamptic pregnancies: A longitudinal study for early prediction of preeclampsia. Am J Obstet Gynecol 189:1212, 2003a

Chavarria ME, Lara-González L, González-Gleason A, et al: Prostacyclin/thromboxane early changes in pregnancies that are complicated by preeclampsia. Am J Obstet Gynecol 188:986, 2003b

Chesley LC: Diagnosis of preeclampsia. Obstet Gynecol 65:423, 1985

Chesley LC, Annitto JE, Cosgrove RA: The remote prognosis of eclamptic women. Sixth periodic report. Am J Obstet Gynecol 124:446, 1976

Chesley LC, Cooper DW: Genetics of hypertension in pregnancy: Possible single gene control of preeclampsia and eclampsia in the descendants of eclamptic women. Br J Obstet Gynaecol 93:898, 1986

Chesley LC, Williams LO: Renal glomerular and tubular function in relation to the hyperuricemia of preeclampsia and eclampsia. Am J Obstet Gynecol 50:367, 1945

Clark BA, Halvorson L, Sachs B, et al: Plasma endothelin levels in preeclampsia: Elevation and correlation with uric acid levels and renal impairment. Am J Obstet Gynecol 166:962, 1992

Clark SL, Cotton DB: Clinical indications for pulmonary artery catheterization in the patient with severe preeclampsia. Am J Obstet Gynecol 158:453, 1988

Clark SL, Divon MY, Phelan JP: Preeclampsia/eclampsia: Hemodynamic and neurologic correlations. Obstet Gynecol 66:337, 1985

CLASP Collaborative Group: A randomized trial of low-dose aspirin for the prevention and treatment of preeclampsia among 9364 pregnant women. Lancet 343:619, 1994

Coetzee EJ, Dommisse J, Anthony J: A randomized controlled trial of intravenous magnesium sulfate versus placebo in the management of women with severe preeclampsia. Br J Obstet Gynaecol 105:300, 1998

Conde-Agudelo A, Belizan JM: Risk factors for pre-eclampsia in a large cohort of Latin American and Caribbean women. Br J Obstet Gynaecol 107:75, 2000

Conde-Agudelo A, Villar J, Lindheimer M: World health organization systematic review of screening tests for preeclampsia. Obstet Gynecol 104:1367, 2004

Conrad KP, Vernier KA: Plasma level, urinary excretion and metabolic production of cGMP during gestation in rats. Am J Physiol 257:R847, 1989

Cotter A, Molloy A, Scott JM, et al: Elevated plasma homocysteine in early pregnancy: A risk factor for the development of nonsevere preeclampsia. Am J Obstet Gynecol 189:391, 2003

Cotter A, Molloy A, Scott JM, et al: Elevated plasma homocysteine in early pregnancy: A risk factor for the development of severe preeclampsia. Am J Obstet Gynecol 185:781, 2001

Cotton DB, Janusz CA, Berman RF: Anticonvulsant effects of magnesium sulfate on hippocampal seizures: Therapeutic implications in preeclampsia–eclampsia. Am J Obstet Gynecol 166:1127, 1992

Cotton DB, Jones MM, Longmire S, et al: Role of intravenous nitroglycerine in the treatment of severe pregnancy-induced hypertension complicated by pulmonary edema. Am J Obstet Gynecol 154:91, 1986a

Cotton DB, Longmire S, Jones MM, et al: Cardiovascular alterations in severe pregnancy-induced hypertension: Effects of intravenous nitroglycerin coupled with blood volume expansion. Am J Obstet Gynecol 154:1053, 1986b

Cowles T, Saleh A, Cotton DB: Hypertensive disorders in pregnancy. In James DK, Steer PJ, Weiner CP, Gonik B (eds): High Risk Pregnancy: Management Options. London, Saunders, 1994, p 253

Crowther CA, Hilles JE, Doyle LW, et al: Effect of magnesium sulfate given for neuroprotection before birth: A randomized controlled trial. JAMA 290:2669, 2003

Cuckle H, Sehmi I, Jones R: Maternal serum inhibin A can predict preeclampsia. Br J Obstet Gynaecol 105:1101, 1998

Cunningham FG: Liver disease complicating pregnancy. Williams Obstetrics, 19th ed (Suppl 1). Norwalk, CT, Appleton & Lange, 1993

Cunningham FG, Pritchard JA: How should hypertension during pregnancy be managed? Experience at Parkland Memorial Hospital. Med Clin North Am 68:505, 1984

Cunningham FG, Lindheimer MD: Hypertension in pregnancy. Current concepts. N Engl J Med 326:927, 1992

Cunningham FG, Twickler D: Cerebral edema complicating eclampsia. Am J Obstet Gynecol 182:94, 2000

Cunningham FG, Fernandez CO, Hernandez C: Blindness associated with preeclampsia and eclampsia. Am J Obstet Gynecol 172:1291, 1995

Cunningham FG, Lowe T, Guss S, et al: Erythrocyte morphology in women with severe preeclampsia and eclampsia. Am J Obstet Gynecol 153:358, 1985

Cunningham FG, Pritchard JA, Hankins GDV, et al: Peripartum heart failure: Idiopathic cardiomyopathy or compounding cardiovascular events? Obstet Gynecol 67:157, 1986

D'Anna R, Baviera G, Corrado F, et al: Plasma homocysteine in early and late pregnancy complicated with preeclampsia and isolated intrauterine growth restriction. Acta Obstet Gynecol Scand 83:155, 2004

Dashe JS, Ramin SM, Cunningham FG: The long-term consequences of thrombotic microangiopathy (thrombotic thrombocytopenic purpura and hemolytic uremic syndrome) in pregnancy. Obstet Gynecol 91:662, 1998

Davidge ST, Hubel CA, Braden RD, et al: Sera antioxidant activity in uncomplicated and preeclamptic pregnancies. Obstet Gynecol 79:897, 1992

De Snoo K: The prevention of eclampsia. Am J Obstet Gynecol 34:911, 1937

De Wolf F, De Wolf-Peeters C, Brosens I, et al: The human placental bed: Electron microscopic study of trophoblastic invasion of spiral arteries. Am J Obstet Gynecol 137:58, 1980

Dekker GA, Makovitz JW, Wallenburg HCS: Prediction of pregnancy-induced hypertensive disorders by angiotensin II sensitivity and supine pressor test. Br J Obstet Gynaecol 97:817, 1990

Dekker GA, Sibai BM: Etiology and pathogenesis of preeclampsia: Current concepts. Am J Obstet Gynecol 179:1359, 1998

Diedrich F, Renner A, Rath W, et al: Lipid hydroperoxides and free radical scavenging enzyme activities in preeclampsia and HELLP (hemolysis, elevated liver enzymes, and low platelet count) syndrome: No evidence for circulating primary products of lipid peroxidation. Am J Obstet Gynecol 185:166, 2001

Douglas KA, Redman CWG: Eclampsia in the United Kingdom. BMJ 309:1395, 1994

Drakeley AJ, Le Roux PA, Anthony J, et al: Acute renal failure complicating severe preeclampsia requiring admission to an obstetric intensive care unit. Am J Obstet Gynecol 186:253, 2002

Ducey J, Schulman H, Farmakides G, et al: A classification of hypertension in pregnancy based on Doppler velocimetry. Am J Obstet Gynecol 157:680, 1987

Durnwald C, Mercer B: A prospective comparison of total protein/creatinine ratio versus 24-hour urine protein in women with suspected preeclampsia. Am J Obstet Gynecol 189:848, 2003

Dürr JA, Lindheimer MD: Control of volume and body tonicity. In Lindheimer MD, Roberts JM, Cunningham FG (eds): Chesley's Hypertensive Disorders in Pregnancy, 2nd ed. Stamford, CT, Appleton & Lange, 1999, p 103

Dyer RA, Els I, Farbas J, et al: Prospective, randomized trial comparing general with spinal anesthesia for cesarean delivery in preeclamptic patients with a nonreassuring fetal heart trace. Anesthesiology 99:561, 2003

Easterling TR, Benedetti TJ, Schmucker BC, et al: Antihypertensive therapy in pregnancy directed by noninvasive hemodynamic monitoring. Am J Perinatol 6:86, 1989

Easterling TR, Benedetti TJ, Schmucker BC, et al: Maternal hemodynamics in normal and preeclamptic pregnancies: A longitudinal study. Obstet Gynecol 76:1061, 1990

Easterling TR, Brateng D, Schmucker B, et al: Prevention of preeclampsia: A randomized trial of atenolol in hyperdynamic patients before onset of hypertension. Obstet Gynecol 93:725, 1999

Eastman NS, Hellman LM: Toxemias of pregnancy. Williams Obstetrics, 12th ed. New York, Appleton-Century-Crofts, Inc., 1961, p 756

Ecker J, Karumanchi A, Roberts J, et al: First-trimester placental growth factor, SFLT-1, and risk for preeclampsia [abstract]. Am J Obstet Gynecol 189:S60, 2003

Eclampsia Trial Collaborative Group: Which anticonvulsant for women with eclampsia? Evidence from the collaborative eclampsia trial. Lancet 345:1455, 1995

Everett RB, Porter JC, MacDonald PC, et al: Relationship of maternal placental blood flow to the placental clearance of maternal plasma dehydroisoandrosterone sulfate through placental estriol formation. Am J Obstet Gynecol 136:435, 1980

Faas MM, Schuiling GA, Linton EA, et al: Activation of peripheral leukocytes in rat pregnancy and experimental preeclampsia. Am J Obstet Gynecol 182:351, 2000

Ferrazzani S, Caruso A, De Carolis S, et al: Proteinuria and outcome of 444 pregnancies complicated by hypertension. Am J Obstet Gynecol 162:366, 1990

Fischer T, Schneider MP, Schobel HP, et al: Vascular reactivity in patients with preeclampsia and HELLP (hemolysis, elevated liver enzymes, and low platelet count) syndrome. Am J Obstet Gynecol 183:1489, 2000

Fisher ER, Pardo V, Paul R, et al: Ultrastructural studies in hypertension, 4. Toxemia of pregnancy. Am J Pathol 55:109, 1969

Fisher KA, Luger A, Spargo BH, et al: Hypertension in pregnancy: Clinical–pathological correlations and remote prognosis. Medicine 60:267, 1981

Fleischer A, Schulman H, Farmakides G, et al: Uterine artery Doppler velocimetry in pregnant women with hypertension. Am J Obstet Gynecol 154:806, 1986

Florio P, Reis FM, Pezzani I, et al: The addition of activin A and inhibin A measurement to uterine artery Doppler velocimetry to improve the early prediction of pre-eclampsia. Ultrasound Obstet Gynecol 21:165, 2003

Fong J, Gurewitsch ED, Vipe L, et al: Baseline serum and cerebrospinal fluid magnesium levels in normal pregnancy and preeclampsia. Obstet Gynecol 85:444, 1995

Förster JG, Peltonen S, Kaaja R, et al: Plasma exchange in severe postpartum HELLP syndrome. Acta Anaesthesiol Scand 46:955, 2002

Friedman SA, Lindheimer MD: Prediction and differential diagnosis. In Lindheimer MD, Roberts JM, Cunningham FG (eds): Chesley's Hypertensive Disorders in Pregnancy, 2nd ed. Stamford, CT, Appleton & Lange, 1999, p 201

Friedman EA, Neff RK: Pregnancy outcome as related to hypertension, edema, and proteinuria. In Lindheimer MD, Katz AI, Zuspan FP (eds): Hypertension in Pregnancy. New York, Wiley, 1976, p 13

Fritz MA, Stanczyk FZ, Novy MJ: Relationship of uteroplacental blood flow to the placental clearance of maternal dehydroepiandrosterone through estradiol formation in the pregnant baboon. J Clin Endocrinol Metab 61:1023, 1985

Frolich MA, Datta S, Corn SB: Thrombopoietin in normal pregnancy and preeclampsia. Am J Obstet Gynecol 179:100, 1998

Gallery EDM, Lindheimer MD: Alterations in volume homeostasis. In Lindheimer MD, Roberts JM, Cunningham FG (eds): Chesley's Hypertensive Disorders in Pregnancy, 2nd ed. Stamford, CT, Appleton & Lange, 1999, p 327

Gamzu R, Rotstein R, Fusman R, et al: Increased erythrocyte adhesiveness and aggregation in peripheral venous blood of women with pregnancy-induced hypertension. Obstet Gynecol 98:307, 2001

Gant NF, Chand S, Worley RJ, et al: A clinical test useful for predicting the development of acute hypertension in pregnancy. Am J Obstet Gynecol 120:1, 1974

Gant NF, Daley GL, Chand S, et al: A study of angiotensin II pressor response throughout primigravid pregnancy. J Clin Invest 52:2682, 1973

Gant NF, Jimenez JM, Whalley PJ, et al: A prospective study of angiotensin II pressor responsiveness in pregnancies complicated by chronic essential hypertension. Am J Obstet Gynecol 127:369, 1977

Gervasi MT, Chaiworapongsa T, Pacora P, et al: Phenotypic and metabolic characteristics of monocytes and granulocytes in preeclampsia. Am J Obstet Gynecol 185:792, 2001

Gilbert WM, Towner DR, Field NT, et al: The safety and utility of pulmonary artery catheterization in severe preeclampsia and eclampsia. Am J Obstet Gynecol 182:1397, 2000

Gilstrap LC, Cunningham FG, Whalley PJ: Management of pregnancy-induced hypertension in the nulliparous patient remote from term. Semin Perinatol 2:73, 1978

Govan ADT: The pathogenesis of eclamptic lesions. Pathol Microbiol 24:561, 1961

Green KW, Key TC, Coen R, et al: The effects of maternally administered magnesium sulfate on the neonate. Am J Obstet Gynecol 146:29, 1983

Grether JK, Hoogstrate J, Walsh-Greene E: Magnesium sulfate for tocolysis and risk of spastic cerebral palsy in premature children born to women without preeclampsia. Am J Obstet Gynecol 183:717, 2000

Grisaru D, Zwang E, Peyser MR, et al: The procoagulant activity of red blood cells from patients with severe preeclampsia. Am J Obstet Gynecol 177:1513, 1997

Grobman WA, Wang EY: Serum levels of activin A and inhibin A and the subsequent development of preeclampsia. Obstet Gynecol 96:390, 2000

Groenendijk R, Trimbros JBM, Wallenburg HCS: Hemodynamic measurements in preeclampsia: Preliminary observations. Am J Obstet Gynecol 150:232, 1984

Grossman E, Messerli FH, Grodzicki T, et al: Should a moratorium be placed on sublingual nifedipine capsules given for hypertensive emergencies and pseudoemergencies? JAMA 276:1328, 1996

Gutsche BB, Cheek TG: Anesthesia considerations in preeclampsia-eclampsia. In Shnider SM, Levinson G (eds): Anesthesia for Obstetrics, 3rd ed. Baltimore, Williams & Wilkins, 1993, p 321

Haddad B, Deis S, Goffinet F, et al: Maternal and perinatal outcomes during expectant management of 239 severe preeclamptic women between 24 and 33 weeks' gestation. Am J Obstet Gynecol 190:1590, 2004

Haddad B, Barton JR, Livingston JC, et al: Risk factors for adverse maternal outcomes among women with HELLP (hemolysis, elevated liver enzymes, and low platelet count) syndrome. Am J Obstet Gynecol 183:444, 2000

Hall DR, Odendaal HJ, Smith M: Is the prophylactic administration of magnesium sulphate in women with pre-eclampsia indicated prior to labour? Br J Obstet Gynaecol 107:903, 2000a

Hall DR, Odendaal HJ, Steyn DW, et al: Expectant management of early onset, severe pre-eclampsia: Maternal outcome. Br J Obstet Gynaecol 107:1252, 2000b

Hallak M, Berry SM, Madincea F, et al: Fetal serum and amniotic fluid magnesium concentrations with maternal treatment. Obstet Gynecol 81:185, 1993

Hallak M, Hotca JW, Evans JB: Magnesium sulfate affects the N-methyl-D-aspartate receptor binding in maternal rat brain. Am J Obstet Gynecol 178:S112, 1998

Hallak M, Kupsky WJ, Hotra JW, et al: Fetal rat brain damage caused by maternal seizure activity: Prevention by magnesium sulfate. Am J Obstet Gynecol 181:828, 1999a

Hallak M, Martinez-Poyer J, Kruger ML, et al: The effect of magnesium sulfate on fetal heart rate parameters: A randomized, placebo-controlled trial. Am J Obstet Gynecol 181:1122, 1999b

Halligan A, Bonnar J, Sheppard B, et al: Haemostatic, fibrinolytic and endothelial variables in normal pregnancies and preeclampsia. Br J Obstet Gynaecol 101:488, 1994

Hankins GDV, Cunningham FG: Severe preeclampsia and eclampsia: Controversies in management. Williams Obstetrics, 18th ed (Suppl 12). Norwalk, CT, Appleton & Lange, 1991

Hankins GDV, Wendel GW Jr, Cunningham FG, et al: Longitudinal evaluation of hemodynamic changes in eclampsia. Am J Obstet Gynecol 150:506, 1984

Hanretty KP, Whittle MJ, Rubin PC: Doppler uteroplacental waveforms in pregnancy-induced hypertension: A re-appraisal. Lancet 1:850, 1988

Harlow FH, Brown MA, Brighton TA, et al: Platelet activation in the hypertensive disorders of pregnancy. Am J Obstet Gynecol 187:688, 2002

Hauth JC, Cunningham FG: Pre-eclampsia–eclampsia. In Lindheimer MD, Roberts JM, Cunningham FG (eds): Chesley's Hypertensive Disorders in Pregnancy, 2nd ed. Stamford, CT, Appleton & Lange, 1999, p 169

Hauth JC, Cunningham FG, Whalley PJ: Management of pregnancy-induced hypertension in the nullipara. Obstet Gynecol 48:253, 1976

Hauth JC, Ewell MG, Levine RJ, et al: Pregnancy outcomes in healthy nulliparas who developed hypertension. Obstet Gynecol 95:24, 2000

Hauth JC, Goldenberg RL, Parker CR Jr, et al: Low-dose aspirin therapy to prevent preeclampsia. Am J Obstet Gynecol 168:1083, 1993

Hauth J, Sibai B, Caritis S, et al: Maternal serum thromboxane B2 concentrations do not predict improved outcomes in high risk pregnancies in a low-dose aspirin trial. Am J Obstet Gynecol 179:1193, 1998

Hayashi M, Hamada Y, Ohkura T: Elevation of granulocyte-macrophage colony-stimulating factor in the placenta and blood in preeclampsia. Am J Obstet Gynecol 190:456, 2004

Hayman R, Warren A, Brockelsby J, et al: Plasma from women with pre-eclampsia induces an in vitro alteration in the endothelium-dependent behaviors of myometrial resistant arteries. Br J Obstet Gynaecol 107:108, 2000

Hayward C, Livingstone J, Holloway S, et al: An exclusion map for preeclampsia: Assuming autosomal recessive inheritance. Am J Hum Genet 50:749, 1992

Head BB, Owen J, Vincent RD Jr, et al: A randomized trial of intrapartum analgesia in women with severe preeclampsia. Obstet Gynecol 99:452, 2002

Hefler LA, Tempfer CB, Gregg AR: Polymorphisms within the interleukin-1β gene cluster and preeclampsia. Obstet Gynecol 97:664, 2001

Helewa M, Heaman M, Robinson M-A, et al: Community-based home-care program for the management of preeclampsia: An alternative. Can Med Assoc J 149:829, 1993

Heller PJ, Scheider EP, Marx GF: Pharyngo-laryngeal edema as a presenting symptom in preeclampsia. Obstet Gynecol 62:523, 1983

Hertig AT: Vascular pathology in the hypertensive albuminuric toxemias of pregnancy. Clinics 4:602, 1945

Hietala R, Turpeinen U, Laatikainen T: Serum homocysteine at 16 weeks and subsequent preeclampsia. Obstet Gynecol 97:527, 2001

Hinselmann H: Die Eklampsie. Bonn, F Cohen, 1924

Hnat MD, Sibai BM, Caritis S, et al: Perinatal outcome in women with recurrent preeclampsia compared with women who develop preeclampsia as nulliparas. Am J Obstet Gynecol 186:422, 2002

Hoff C, Peevy K, Giattina K, et al: Maternal–fetal HLA-DR relationships and pregnancy-induced hypertension. Obstet Gynecol 80:1007, 1992

Hogg B, Hauth JC, Caritis SN, et al: Safety of labor epidural anesthesia for women with severe hypertensive disease. Am J Obstet Gynecol 181:1096, 1999

Horsager R, Adams M, Richey S, et al: Outpatient management of mild pregnancy induced hypertension. Am J Obstet Gynecol 172:383, 1995

Hubel CA, McLaughlin MK, Evans RW, et al: Fasting serum triglycerides, free fatty acids, and malondialdehyde are increased in preeclampsia, are positively correlated, and decrease within 48 hours postpartum. Am J Obstet Gynecol 174:975, 1996

Hubel CA, Roberts JM, Taylor RN, et al: Lipid peroxidation in pregnancy: New perspectives on preeclampsia. Am J Obstet Gynecol 161:1025, 1989

Hunter SK, Martin M, Benda JA, et al: Liver transplant after massive spontaneous hepatic rupture in pregnancy complicated by preeclampsia. Obstet Gynecol 85:819, 1995

Irion O, Masse J, Forest JC, et al: Prediction of preeclampsia, low birthweight for gestation and prematurity by uterine artery blood flow velocity waveforms analysis in low risk nulliparous women. Br J Obstet Gynaecol 105:422, 1998

Isler CM, Barrilleaux PS, Magann EF, et al: A prospective, randomized trial comparing the efficacy of dexamethasone and betamethasone for the treatment of antepartum HELLP (hemolysis, elevated liver enzymes, and low platelet count) syndrome. Am J Obstet Gynecol 184:1332, 2001

Isler CM, Rinehart BK, Terrone DA, et al: Maternal mortality associated with HELLP (hemolysis, elevated liver enzymes, and low platelets) syndrome. Am J Obstet Gynecol 181:924, 1999

Jacobson SL, Imhof R, Manning N, et al: The value of Doppler assessment of the uteroplacental circulation in predicting preeclampsia or intrauterine growth retardation. Am J Obstet Gynecol 162:110, 1990

John JH, Ziebland S, Yudkin P, et al: Effects of fruit and vegetable consumption on plasma antioxidant concentrations and blood pressure: A randomized controlled trial. Lancet 359:1969, 2002

Katano K, Aoki A, Sasa H, et al: Beta 2-glycoprotein I-dependent anticardiolipin antibodies as a predictor of adverse pregnancy outcomes in healthy pregnant women. Hum Reprod 11:509, 1996

Keelan JA, Taylor R, Schellenberg J-C, et al: Serum activin A, inhibin A, and follistatin concentrations in preeclampsia or small for gestational age pregnancies. Obstet Gynecol 99:267, 2002

Khong TY: Acute atherosis in pregnancies complicated by hypertension, small-for-gestational age infants, and diabetes mellitus. Arch Pathol Lab Med 115:722, 1991

Kilpatrick DC, Liston WA, Gibson F, et al: Association between susceptibility to preeclampsia within families and HLA-DR4. Lancet 2:1063, 1989

Kincaid-Smith P: The renal lesion of preeclampsia revisited. Am J Kidney Dis 17:144, 1991

Kirshon B, Lee W, Mauer MB, et al: Effects of low-dose dopamine therapy in the oliguric patient with preeclampsia. Am J Obstet Gynecol 159:604, 1988

Knuist M, Bonsel GJ, Zondervan HA, et al: Low sodium diet and pregnancy-induced hypertension: A multicentre randomized controlled trial. Br J Obstet Gynaecol 105:430, 1998

Labarrere C: Acute atherosis. A histopathological hallmark of immune aggression? Placenta 9:108, 1988

Lachmeijer AMA, Crusius JBA, Pals G, et al: Polymorphisms in the tumor necrosis factor and lymphotoxin-α gene region and preeclampsia. Obstet Gynecol 98:612, 2001

Lain KY, Roberts JM: Contemporary concepts of the pathogenesis and management of preeclampsia. JAMA 287:3183, 2002

Landesman R, Douglas RG, Holze E: The bulbar conjunctival vascular bed in the toxemias of pregnancy. Am J Obstet Gynecol 68:170, 1954

Lara-Torre E, Lee MS, Wolf MA, et al: Bilateral retinal occlusion progressing to long-lasting blindness in severe preeclampsia. Obstet Gynecol 100:940, 2002

Lavies NG, Meiklejohn BH, May AE, et al: Hypertensive and catecholamine response to tracheal intubation in patients with pregnancy-induced hypertension. Br J Anaesth 63:429, 1989

Lawlor DA, Morton SM, Nitsch D, Leon DA: Association between childhood and adulthood socioeconomic position and pregnancy induced hypertension: Results from the Aberdeen children of the 1950s cohort study. J Epidemiol Community Health 59:49, 2005

Leduc L, Wheeler JM, Kirshon B, et al: Coagulation profile in severe preeclampsia. Obstet Gynecol 79:14, 1992

Lee W, Gonik B, Cotton DB: Urinary diagnostic indices in preeclampsia-associated oliguria: Correlation with invasive hemodynamic monitoring. Am J Obstet Gynecol 156:100, 1987

Leveno KJ, Alexander JM, McIntire DD, et al: Does magnesium sulfate given for prevention of eclampsia affect the outcome of labor? Am J Obstet Gynecol 178:707, 1998

Levine RJ, Ewell MG, Hauth JC, et al: Should the definition of preeclampsia include a rise in diastolic blood pressure of $\geq$ 15 mm Hg to a level < 90 mm Hg in association with proteinuria? Am J Obstet Gynecol 183:787, 2000

Levine RJ, Hauth JC, Curet LB, et al: Trial of calcium to prevent preeclampsia. N Engl J Med 337:69, 1997

Levine RJ, Qian C, LeShane ES, et al: Two-stage elevation of cell-free fetal DNA in maternal sera before onset of preeclampsia. Am J Obstet Gynecol 190:707, 2004a

Levine R, Maynard S, Qian C, et al: Acute rise in circulating SFLT-1 may herald preeclampsia [abstract]. Am J Obstet Gynecol 189:S57, 2003

Levine R, Maynard S, Qian C, et al: Circulating angiogenic factors and the risk of preeclampsia. N Engl J Med 350:672, 2004b

Lichtig C, Luger AM, Spargo BH, et al: Renal immunofluorescence and ultrastructural findings in preeclampsia. Clin Res 23:368A, 1975

Lim KH, Friedman SA, Ecker JL, et al: The clinical utility of serum uric acid measurements in hypertensive disease of pregnancy. Am J Obstet Gynecol 178:1067, 1998

Lindheimer MD, Roberts JM, Cunningham FG, et al: Introduction, history, controversies, and definitions. In Lindheimer MD, Roberts JM, Cunningham FG (eds): Chesley's Hypertensive Disorders in Pregnancy, 2nd ed. Stamford, CT, Appleton & Lange, 1999, p 3

Lip GYH, Churchill D, Beevers M, et al: Angiotensin-converting enzyme inhibitors in early pregnancy. Lancet 350:1446, 1997

Lipton SA, Rosenberg PA: Excitatory amino acids as a final common pathway for neurologic disorders. N Engl J Med 330:613, 1994

Livingston JC, Haddad B, Gorski LA, et al: Placenta growth factor is not an early marker for the development of severe preeclampsia. Am J Obstet Gynecol 184:1218, 2001a

Livingston JC, Livingston LW, Ramsey R, et al: Magnesium sulfate in women with mild preeclampsia: A randomized controlled trial. Obstet Gynecol 101:217, 2003

Livingston JC, Park V, Barton JR, et al: Lack of association of severe preeclampsia with maternal and fetal mutant alleles for tumor necrosis factor α and lymphotoxin α genes and plasma tumor necrosis α levels. Am J Obstet Gynecol 184:1273, 2001b

Lo C, Taylor RS, Gamble G, et al: Use of automated home blood pressure monitoring in pregnancy: Is it safe? Am J Obstet Gynecol 187:1321, 2002

López-Jaramillo P, Narváez M, Weigel RM, et al: Calcium supplementation reduces the risk of pregnancy-induced hypertension in an Andes population. Br J Obstet Gynaecol 96:648, 1989

López-Llera M: Complicated eclampsia: Fifteen years' experience in a referral medical center. Am J Obstet Gynecol 142:28, 1982

Lourenço R, Leite CC, Kahhale S, et al: Diffusion imaging may predict reversible brain lesions in eclampsia and severe preeclampsia: Initial experience. Am J Obstet Gynecol 189:1350, 2003

Lubarsky SL, Barto JR, Friedman SA, et al: Late postpartum eclampsia revisited. Obstet Gynecol 83:502, 1994

Lucas MJ, Leveno KJ, Cunningham FG: A comparison of magnesium sulfate with phenytoin for the prevention of eclampsia. N Engl J Med 333:201, 1995

Lucas MJ, Sharma S, McIntire DD, et al: A randomized trial of the effects of epidural analgesia on pregnancy-induced hypertension. Am J Obstet Gynecol 185:970, 2001

Luttun A, Carmeliet P: Soluble VEGF receptor Flt1: The elusive preeclampsia factor discovered? J Clin Invest 111:600, 2003

Mabie WC, Gonzalez AR, Sibai BM, et al: A comparative trial of labetalol and hydralazine in the acute management of severe hypertension complicating pregnancy. Obstet Gynecol 70:328, 1987

Mabie WC, Ratts TE, Ramanathan KB, et al: Circulatory congestion in obese hypertensive women: A subset of pulmonary edema in pregnancy. Obstet Gynecol 72:553, 1988a

Mabie WC, Sibai BM, Anderson GD, et al: Nifedipine in the treatment of severe peripartum hypertension (Abstract #87). Soc Perinat Obstet, February 1988b

Madazli R, Budak E, Calay Z, et al: Correlation between placental bed biopsy findings, vascular cell adhesion molecule and fibronectin levels in preeclampsia. Br J Obstet Gynaecol 107:514, 2000

Magpie Trial Collaborative Group: Do women with pre-eclampsia, and their babies, benefit from magnesium sulphate? The Magpie Trial: A randomized placebo-controlled trial. Lancet 359:1877, 2002

Manas KJ, Welsh JD, Rankin RA, et al: Hepatic hemorrhage without rupture in preeclampsia. N Engl J Med 312:426, 1985

Manten GT, van der Hoek YY, Marko Sikkema J, et al: The role of lipoprotein (a) in pregnancies complicated by pre-eclampsia. Med Hypotheses 64:162, 2005

Many A, Kuperminc MJ, Pausner D, et al: Treatment of severe preeclampsia remote from term: A clinical dilemma. Obstet Gynecol Surv 54:723, 1999

Martin JA, Hamilton BE, Ventura SS, et al: Births: Final data for 2001. National Vital Statistics Report, Vol. 51, No. 2. Hyattsville, Md, National Center for Health Statistics, 2002

Martin JN Jr, Files JC, Blake PG, et al: Postpartum plasma exchange for atypical preeclampsia–eclampsia as HELLP (hemolysis, elevated liver enzymes, and low platelets) syndrome. Am J Obstet Gynecol 172:1107, 1995

Martin JN Jr, Thigpen BD, Rose CH, et al: Maternal benefit of high-dose intravenous corticosteroid therapy for HELLP syndrome. Am J Obstet Gynecol 189:830, 2003

Marya RK, Rathee S, Manrow M: Effect of calcium and vitamin D supplementation on toxaemia of pregnancy. Gynecol Obstet Invest 24:38, 1987

Mastrogiannis DS, O'Brien WF, Krammer J, et al: Potential role of endothelin-1 in normal and hypertensive pregnancies. Am J Obstet Gynecol 165:1711, 1991

Matchaba P, Moodley J: Corticosteroids for HELLP syndrome in pregnancy. Cochrane Database Syst Rev CD002076, 2004

Matthys LA, Coppage KH, Lambers DS, et al: Delayed postpartum preeclampsia: an experience of 151 cases. Am J Obstet Gynecol 190:1464, 2004

Matijevic R, Johnston T: In vivo assessment of failed trophoblastic invasion of the spiral arteries in pre-eclampsia. Br J Obstet Gynaecol 106:78, 1999

Mattar F, Sibai BM: Eclampsia: VIII. Risk factors for maternal morbidity. Am J Obstet Gynecol 182:307, 2000

Maxwell CV, Lieberman E, Norton M, et al: Relatioship of twin zygosity and risk of preeclampsia. Am J Obstet Gynecol 185:819, 2001

Maynard SE, Min J-Y, Merchan J, et al: Excess placental soluble fms-like tyrosine kinase 1 (sFlt1) may contribute to endothelial dysfunction, hypertension, and proteinuria in preeclampsia. J Clin Invest 111:649, 2003

McCartney CP, Schumacher GFB, Spargo BH: Serum proteins in patients with toxemic glomerular lesion. Am J Obstet Gynecol 111:580, 1971

McCubbin JH, Sibai BM, Abdella TN, et al: Cardiopulmonary arrest due to acute maternal hypermagnesemia. Lancet 1:1058, 1981

Meekins JW, Pijnenborg R, Hanssens M, et al: A study of placental bed spiral arteries and trophoblast invasion in normal and severe pre-eclamptic pregnancies. Br J Obstet Gynaecol 101:669, 1994

Merchant SH, Mathew P, Vanderjagt TJ, et al: Recombinant factor VIIa in management of spontaneous subcapsular liver hematoma associated with pregnancy. Obstet Gynecol 103:1055, 2004

Meyer NL, Mercer BM, Friedman SA, et al: Urinary dipstick protein: A poor predictor of absent or severe proteinuria. Am J Obstet Gynecol 170:137, 1994

Mikhail MS, Anyaegbunam A, Garfinkel D, et al: Preeclampsia and antioxidant nutrients: Decreased plasma levels of reduced ascorbic acid, alpha-tocopherol, and beta-carotene in women with preeclampsia. Am J Obstet Gynecol 171:150, 1994

Mizuki J, Tasaka K, Masumoio N, et al: Magnesium sulfate inhibits oxytocin induced calcium mobilization in human puerperal myometrial cells: Possible involvement of intracellular free magnesium concentration. Am J Obstet Gynecol 109:134, 1993

Montan S, Ingemarsson I: Intrapartum fetal heart rate patterns in pregnancies complicated by hypertension. Am J Obstet Gynecol 160:283, 1989

Morgan L, Baker P, Broughton Pipkin F, et al: Preeclampsia and the angiotensinogen gene. Br J Obstet Gynaecol 102:489, 1995

Morgan T, Craven C, Lalouel JM, et al: Angiotensinogen Thr[235] variant is associated with abnormal physiologic change of the uterine spiral arteries in first-trimester decidua. Am J Obstet Gynecol 180:95, 1999

Morris NH, Eaton BM, Dekker G: Nitric oxide, the endothelium, pregnancy and pre-eclampsia. Br J Obstet Gynaecol 103:4, 1996

Morriss MC, Twickler DM, Hatab MR, et al: Cerebral blood flow and cranial magnetic resonance imaging in eclampsia and severe preeclampsia. Obstet Gynecol 89:561, 1997

Moseman CP, Shelton S: Permanent blindness as a complication of pregnancy induced hypertension. Obstet Gynecol 100:943, 2002

Mostello D, Catlin TK, Roman L, et al: Preeclampsia in the parous woman: Who is at risk? Am J Obstet Gynecol 187:425, 2002

Muttukrishna S, Knight PG, Groome NP, et al: Activin-A and inhibin-A as possible endocrine markers for preeclampsia. Lancet 349:1285, 1997

Myatt L, Brewer AS, Langdon G, et al: Attenuation of the vasoconstrictor effects of thromboxane and endothelin by nitric oxide in the human fetal–placental circulation. Am J Obstet Gynecol 166:224, 1992

Nassar AH, Adra AM, Chakhtoura N, et al: Severe preeclampsia remote from term: Labor induction or elective cesarean delivery? Am J Obstet Gynecol 179:1210, 1998

National High Blood Pressure Education Program: Working Group Report on High Blood Pressure in Pregnancy. Am J Obstet Gynecol 183:51, 2000

Neithardt AB, Dooley SL, Borensztajn J: Prediction of 24-hour protein excretion in pregnancy with a single voided urine protein-to-creatinine ratio. Am J Obstet Gynecol 186:883, 2002

Nelson KB, Grether JK: Can magnesium sulfate reduce the risk of cerebral palsy in very low birthweight infants? Pediatrics 95:263, 1995

Ness RB, Markovic N, Bass D, et al: Family history of hypertension, heart disease, and stroke among women who develop hypertension in pregnancy. Obstet Gynecol 102:1366, 2003

Newman MG, Robichaux AG, Stedman CM, et al: Perinatal outcomes in preeclampsia that is complicated by massive proteinuria. Am J Obstet Gynecol 188:264, 2003

Newsome LR, Bramwell RS, Curling PE: Severe preeclampsia: Hemodynamic effects of lumbar epidural anesthesia. Anesth Analg 65:31, 1986

Nightingale FL: Warnings in the use of ACE inhibitors in the second and third trimester of pregnancy. JAMA 267:244, 1992

Nilsson E, Ros HS, Cnattingius S, et al: The importance of genetic and environmental effects for pre-eclampsia and gestational hypertension: A family study. Br J Obstet Gynaecol 111:200, 2004

Nisell H, Carlström K, Cizinsky S, et al: Atrial natriuretic peptide concentrations and hemodynamic effects of acute plasma volume expansion in normal pregnancy and preeclampsia. Obstet Gynecol 79:902, 1992

Nolan TE, Wakefield ML, Devoe LD: Invasive hemodynamic monitoring in obstetrics. A critical review of its indications, benefits, complications, and alternatives. Chest 101:1429, 1992

North RA, Taylor RS, Schellenberg J-C: Evaluation of a definition of preeclampsia. Br J Obstet Gynaecol 106:767, 1999

Nova A, Sibai BM, Barton JR, et al: Maternal plasma level of endothelin is increased in preeclampsia. Am J Obstet Gynecol 165:724, 1991

Obeidat B, MacDougall J, Harding K: Plasma exchange in a woman with thrombotic thrombocytopenic purpura or severe pre-eclampsia. Br J Obstet Gynaecol 109:961, 2002

O'Brien JM, Shumate SA, Satchwell SL, et al: Maternal benefit of corticosteroid therapy in patients with HELLP (hemolysis, elevated liver enzymes, and low platelet count) syndrome: Impact on the rate of regional anesthesia. Am J Obstet Gynecol 186:475, 2002

Øian P, Maltau JM, Noddleland H, et al: Transcapillary fluid balance in preeclampsia. Br J Obstet Gynaecol 93:235, 1986

Olsen SF, Secher NJ, Tabor A, et al: Randomized clinical trials of fish oil supplementation in high risk pregnancies. Br J Obstet Gynaecol 107:382, 2000

Oxford English Dictionary. Oxford, Clarendon Press, 1993

Paarlberg KM, DeJong CLD, Van Geijn HP, et al: Total plasma fibronectin as a marker of pregnancy-induced hypertensive disorders: A longitudinal study. Obstet Gynecol 91:383, 1998

Palmer SK, Moore LG, Young DA, et al: Altered blood pressure and increased preeclampsia at high altitude (3100 meters) in Colorado. Am J Obstet Gynecol 180:1161, 1999

Parra MC, Lees C, Mann GE, et al: Vasoactive mediator release by endothelial cells in intrauterine growth restriction and preeclampsia. Am J Obstet Gynecol 184:497, 2001

Petraglia F, Florio P, Benedetto C, et al: High levels of corticotropin-releasing factor (CRF) are inversely correlated with low levels of maternal CRF-binding protein in pregnant women with pregnancy-induced hypertension. J Clin Endocrinol Metab 81:852, 1996

Phelan JP, Yurth DA: Severe preeclampsia, 1. Peripartum hemodynamic observations. Am J Obstet Gynecol 144:17, 1982

Pickles CJ, Broughton Pipkin F, Symonds EM: A randomised placebo controlled trial of labetalol in the treatment of mild to moderate pregnancy induced hypertension. Br J Obstet Gynaecol 99:964, 1992

Powers RW, Dunbar MS, Gallaher MJ, et al: The 677 C-T methylenetetrahydrofolate reductase mutation does not predict increased maternal homocysteine during pregnancy. Obstet Gynecol 101:762, 2003

Powers RW, Evans RW, Ness RB, et al: Homocysteine is increased in preeclampsia but not in gestational hypertension (Abstract #375). J Soc Gynecol Investig 7(1):(Suppl), 2000

Pritchard JA, Cunningham FG, Mason RA: Coagulation changes in eclampsia: Their frequency and pathogenesis. Am J Obstet Gynecol 124:855, 1976

Pritchard JA, Cunningham FG, Pritchard SA: The Parkland Memorial Hospital protocol for treatment of eclampsia: Evaluation of 245 cases. Am J Obstet Gynecol 148:951, 1984

Pritchard JA, Cunningham FG, Pritchard SA, et al: How often does maternal preeclampsia–eclampsia incite thrombocytopenia in the fetus? Obstet Gynecol 69:292, 1987

Pritchard JA, Weisman R Jr, Ratnoff OD, et al: Intravascular hemolysis, thrombocytopenia and other hematologic abnormalities associated with severe toxemia of pregnancy. N Engl J Med 250:87, 1954

Raab W, Schroeder G, Wagner R, et al: Vascular reactivity and electrolytes in normal and toxemic pregnancy. J Clin Endocrinol 16:1196, 1956

Rafferty TD, Berkowitz RL: Hemodynamics in patients with severe toxemia during labor and delivery. Am J Obstet Gynecol 138:263, 1980

Ramanathan J: Anesthetic considerations in preeclampsia. Clin Perinatol 18:875, 1991

Redman CWG, Roberts JM: Management of pre-eclampsia. Lancet 341:1451, 1993

Redman CWG, Sacks GP, Sargent IL: Preeclampsia: An excessive maternal inflammatory response to pregnancy. Am J Obstet Gynecol 180:499, 1999

Redman CWG, Sargent IL: Pre-eclampsia, the placenta and the maternal systemic inflammatory response—a review. Placenta 17:S21, 2003

Rinehart BK, Terrone DA, Magann EF, et al: Preeclampsia-associated hepatic hemorrhage and rupture: Mode of management related to maternal and perinatal outcome. Obstet Gynecol Surv 54:3, 1999

Roberts JM: Preeclampsia: What we know and what we do not know. Semin Perinatol 24:24, 2000

Robinson C, Johnson D: Placental growth factor: A marker for severity of preeclampsia [abstract]. Am J Obstet Gynecol 189:S85, 2003

Robson SC: Magnesium sulphate: The timing of reckoning. Br J Obstet Gynaecol 103:99, 1996

Rodriguez-Thompson D, Lieberman ES: Use of random urinary protein-to-creatinine ratio for the diagnosis of significant proteinuria during pregnancy. Am J Obstet Gynecol 185:808, 2001

Rogers BB, Bloom SL, Leveno KJ: Atherosis revisited: Current concepts on the pathophysiology of implantation site disorders. Obstet Gynecol Surv 54:189, 1999

Rosen SA, Merchant SH, Vanderjagt TJ, et al: Spontaneous subcapsular liver hematoma associated with pregnancy. Arch Pathol Lab Med 127:1639, 2003

Ross R: Atherosclerosis—an inflammatory disease. N Engl J Med 340:115, 1999

Rotchell YE, Cruickshank JK, Gay MP, et al: Barbados low dose aspirin study in pregnancy (BLASP): A randomized trial for the prevention of pre-eclampsia and its complications. Br J Obstet Gynaecol 105:286, 1998

Rowland BL, Vermillion ST, Roudebush WE: Elevated circulating concentrations of platelet activation factor in preeclampsia. Am J Obstet Gynecol 183:930, 2000

Rutherford JM, Moody A, Crawshaw S, et al: Magnetic resonance spectroscopy in pre-eclampsia: Evidence of cerebral ischaemia. Br J Obstet Gynaecol 110:416, 2003

Sagsoz N, Kucukozkan T: The effect of treatment on endothelin-1 concentration and mean arterial pressure in preeclampsia and eclampsia. Hypertens Pregnancy 22:185, 2003

Samuels P, Main EK, Tomaski A, et al: Abnormalities in platelet antiglobulin tests in preeclamptic mothers and their neonates. Am J Obstet Gynecol 157:109, 1987

Sanchez-Ramos L, Adair CD, Todd JC, et al: Erythrocyte membrane fluidity in patients with preeclampsia and the HELLP syndrome: A preliminary study. J Matern Fetal Invest 4:237, 1994

Savvidou MD, Lees CC, Parra M, et al: Levels of C-reactive protein in pregnant women who subsequently develop pre-eclampsia. Br J Obstet Gynaecol 109:297, 2002

Scardo JA, Vermillion ST, Hogg BB, et al: Hemodynamic effects of oral nifedipine in preeclampsia hypertensive emergencies. Am J Obstet Gynecol 175:336, 1996

Scardo JA, Vermillion ST, Newman RB, et al: A randomized, double-blind, hemodynamic evaluation of nifedipine and labetalol in preeclamptic hypertensive emergencies. Am J Obstet Gynecol 181:862, 1999

Schendel DE, Berg CJ, Yeargin-Allsopp M, et al: Prenatal magnesium sulfate exposure and the risk for cerebral palsy or mental retardation among very low birthweight children aged 3 to 5 years. JAMA 276:1805, 1996

Schiff E, Friedman SA, Stampfer M, et al: Dietary consumption and plasma concentrations of vitamin E in pregnancies complicated by preeclampsia. Am J Obstet Gynecol 175:1024, 1996

Sciscione AC, Ivester T, Largoza M, et al: Acute pulmonary edema in pregnancy. Obstet Gynecol 101:511, 2003

Sen C, Madazh R, Kavuzlu C, et al: The value of antithrombin-III and fibronectin in hypertensive disorders of pregnancy. J Perinat Med 22:29, 1994

Sheehan HL: Pathological lesions in the hypertensive toxaemias of pregnancy. In Hammond J, Browne FJ, Wolstenholme GEW (eds): Toxaemias of Pregnancy, Human and Veterinary. Philadelphia, Blakiston, 1950

Sheehan HL, Lynch JB (eds): Cerebral lesions. In: Pathology of Toxaemia of Pregnancy. Baltimore, Williams & Wilkins, 1973

Sibai BM: Diagnosis and management of gestational hypertension and preeclampsia. Obstet Gynecol 102:181, 2003

Sibai BM: Treatment of hypertension in pregnant women. N Engl J Med 335:257, 1996

Sibai BM, Barton JR, Akl S, et al: A randomized prospective comparison of nifedipine and bed rest alone in the management of preeclampsia remote from term. Am J Obstet Gynecol 167:879, 1992

Sibai BM, Caritis SN, Thom E, et al: Prevention of preeclampsia with low-dose aspirin in healthy, nulliparous pregnant women. N Engl J Med 329:1213, 1993a

Sibai BM, El-Nazer A, Gonzalez-Ruiz A: Severe preeclampsia–eclampsia in young primigravid women: Subsequent pregnancy outcome and remote prognosis. Am J Obstet Gynecol 155:1011, 1986

Sibai BM, Ewell M, Levine RJ, et al: Risk factors associated with preeclampsia in healthy nulliparous women. Am J Obstet Gynecol 177:1003, 1997

Sibai BM, Gonzalez AR, Mabie WC, et al: A comparison of labetalol plus hospitalization versus hospitalization alone in the management of preeclampsia remote from term. Obstet Gynecol 70:323, 1987a

Sibai BM, Graham JM, McCubbin JH: A comparison of intravenous and intramuscular magnesium sulfate regimens in preeclampsia. Am J Obstet Gynecol 150:728, 1984

Sibai BM, Hauth J, Caritis S, et al: Hypertensive disorders in twin versus singleton gestations. Am J Obstet Gynecol 182:938, 2000

Sibai BM, Lindheimer M, Hauth J, et al: Risk factors for preeclampsia, abruptio placentae, and adverse neonatal outcome among women with chronic hypertension. N Engl J Med 339:667, 1998

Sibai BM, Mabie BC, Harvey CJ, et al: Pulmonary edema in severe preeclampsia–eclampsia: Analysis of thirty-seven consecutive cases. Am J Obstet Gynecol 156:1174, 1987b

Sibai BM, Mercer B, Sarinoglu C: Severe preeclampsia in the second trimester: Recurrence risk and long-term prognosis. Am J Obstet Gynecol 165:1408, 1991

Sibai BM, Mercer BM, Schiff E, et al: Aggressive versus expectant management of severe preeclampsia at 28 to 32 weeks' gestation: A randomized controlled trial. Am J Obstet Gynecol 171:818, 1994

Sibai BM, Ramadan MK, Chari RS, et al: Pregnancies complicated by HELLP syndrome (hemolysis, elevated liver enzymes, and low platelets): Subsequent pregnancy outcome and long-term prognosis. Am J Obstet Gynecol 172:125, 1995

Sibai BM, Ramadan MK, Usta I, et al: Maternal morbidity and mortality in 442 pregnancies with hemolysis, elevated liver enzymes, and low platelets (HELLP syndrome). Am J Obstet Gynecol 169:1000, 1993b

Sibai BM, Spinnato JA, Watson DL, et al: Eclampsia, 4. Neurological findings and future outcome. Am J Obstet Gynecol 152:184, 1985a

Sibai BM, Taslimi M, Abdella TN, et al: Maternal and perinatal outcome of conservative management of severe preeclampsia in midtrimester. Am J Obstet Gynecol 152:32, 1985b

Silver H, Seebeck M: Comparison of methods of blood volume measurement in normotensive and preeclamptic pregnancies. Am J Obstet Gynecol 174:452, 1996

Silver HM, Seebeck M, Carlson R: Comparison of total blood volume in normal, preeclamptic, and non-proteinuric gestational hypertensive pregnancy by simultaneous measurement of red blood cell and plasma volumes. Am J Obstet Gynecol 179:87, 1998

Simmons LA, Hennessy A, Gillin AG, et al: Uteroplacental blood flow and placental vascular endothelial growth factor in normotensive and preeclamptic pregnancy. Br J Obstet Gynaecol 107:678, 2000

Somjen G, Hilmy M, Stephen CR: Failure to anesthetize human subjects by intravenous administration of magnesium sulfate. J Pharmacol Exp Ther 154:652, 1966

Spargo B, McCartney CP, Winemiller R: Glomerular capillary endotheliosis in toxemia of pregnancy. Arch Pathol 68:593, 1959

Staff AC, Ranheim T, Khoury J, et al: Increased contents of phospholipids, cholesterol, and lipid peroxides in decidua basalis in women with preeclampsia. Am J Obstet Gynecol 180:587, 1999

Stamilio DM, Sehder HM, Morgan MA, et al: Can antenatal clinical and biochemical markers predict the development of severe preeclampsia? Am J Obstet Gynecol 182:589, 2000

Strevens H, Wide-Swensson D, Hansen A, et al: Glomerular endotheliosis in normal pregnancy and pre-eclampsia. Br J Obstet Gynaecol 110:831, 2003

Strickland DM, Guzick DS, Cox K, et al: The relationship between abortion in the first pregnancy and the development of pregnancy-induced hypertension in the subsequent pregnancy. Am J Obstet Gynecol 154:146, 1986

Sullivan CA, Magann EF, Perry KG Jr, et al: The recurrence risk of the syndrome of hemolysis, elevated liver enzymes, and low platelets (HELLP) in subsequent gestations. Am J Obstet Gynecol 171:940, 1994

Suzuki Y, Yamamoto T, Mabuchi Y, et al: Ultrastructural changes in omental resistance artery in women with preeclampsia. Am J Obstet Gynecol 189:216, 2003

Szal SE, Croughan-Minibane MS, Kilpatrick SJ: Effect of magnesium prophylaxis and preeclampsia on the duration of labor. Am J Obstet Gynecol 180:1475, 1999

Taber EB, Tan L, Chao CR, et al: Pharmacokinetics of ionized versus total magnesium in subjects with preterm labor and preeclampsia. Am J Obstet Gynecol 186:1017, 2002

Takacs P, Green KL, Nikaeo A, et al: Increased vascular endothelial cell production of interleukin-6 in severe preeclampsia. Am J Obstet Gynecol 188:740, 2003

Talledo OE, Chesley LC, Zuspan FP: Renin-angiotensin system in normal and toxemic pregnancies, 3. Differential sensitivity to angiotensin II and norepinephrine in toxemia of pregnancy. Am J Obstet Gynecol 100:218, 1968

Taufield PA, Ales KL, Resnick LM, et al: Hypocalciuria in preeclampsia. N Engl J Med 316:715, 1987

Taylor RN, Roberts JM: Endothelial cell dysfunction. In Lindheimer MD, Roberts JM, Cunningham FG (eds): Chesley's Hypertensive Disorders in Pregnancy, 2nd ed. Stamford, CT, Appleton & Lange, 1999, p 395

Thadhani R, Mutter WP, Wolf M, et al: First trimester placental growth factor and soluble fms-like tyrosine kinase 1 and risk for preeclampsia. J Clin Endocrinol Metab 89:770, 2004

Thiagarajah S, Bourgeois FJ, Harbert GM, et al: Thrombocytopenia in preeclampsia: Associated abnormalities and management principles. Am J Obstet Gynecol 150:1, 1984

Thurnau GR, Kemp DB, Jarvis A: Cerebrospinal fluid levels of magnesium in patients with preeclampsia after treatment with intravenous magnesium sulfate: A preliminary report. Am J Obstet Gynecol 157:1435, 1987

Tompkins MJ, Thiagarajah S: HELLP (hemolysis, elevated liver enzymes, and low platelet count) syndrome: The benefit of corticosteroids. Am J Obstet Gynecol 181:304, 1999

Treloar SA, Cooper DW, Brennecke SP, et al: An Australian twin study of the genetic basis of preeclampsia and eclampsia. Am J Obstet Gynecol 184:374, 2001

Trogstad L, Skrondal A, Stoltenberg C, et al: Recurrence risk of preeclampsia in twin and singleton pregnancies. Am J Med Genet 126A:41, 2004

Trudinger BJ, Cook CM: Doppler umbilical and uterine flow waveforms in severe pregnancy hypertension. Br J Obstet Gynaecol 97:142, 1990

Trupin LS, Simon LP, Eskenazi B: Change in paternity: A risk factor for preeclampsia in multiparas. Epidemiology 7:240, 1996

Tuffnell DJ, Lilford RJ, Buchan PC, et al: Randomized controlled trial of day care for hypertension in pregnancy. Lancet 339:224, 1992

Turnbull DA, Wilkinson C, Gerard K, et al: Clinical, psychosocial, and economic effects of antenatal day care for three medical complications of pregnancy: A randomized controlled trial of 395 women. Lancet 363:1104, 2004

Vatten LJ, Skjærven R: Is pre-eclampsia more than one disease? Br J Obstet Gynaecol 111:298, 2004

Ventura SJ, Martin JA, Curtin SC, et al: Births: Final data for 1998. National Vital Statistics Reports, Vol. 48, No. 3. Hyattsville, Md, National Center for Health Statistics, 2000

Vermillion ST, Scardo JA, Newman RB, et al: A randomized, double-blind trial of oral nifedipine and intravenous labetalol in hypertensive emergencies of pregnancy. Am J Obstet Gynecol 181:858, 1999

Vigil-De Gracia P, Montufar-Rueda C, Ruiz J: Expectant management of severe preeclampsia and preeclampsia superimposed on chronic hypertension between 24 and 34 weeks' gestation. Eur J Obstet Gynecol Reprod Biol 107:24, 2003

Virchow R: Gesammette Abhandlungen zur Wissenschaftlichen Medicin. Frankfurt AM, Meidinger Sohn, 1856, p 778

Visser W, Wallenburg HC: Central hemodynamic observations in untreated preeclamptic patients. Hypertension 17:1072, 1991

Visser W, Wallenburg HC: Temporizing management of severe preeclampsia with and without the HELLP syndrome. Br J Obstet Gynaecol 102:111, 1995

Volhard F: Die doppelseitigen haematogenen Nierenerkrankungen. Berlin, Springer, 1918

von Dadelszen P, Ornstein MP, Bull SB, et al: Fall in mean arterial pressure and fetal growth restriction in pregnancy hypertension: A meta-analysis. Lancet 355:87, 2000

von Mandach U, Lauth D, Huch R: Maternal and fetal nitric oxide production in normal and abnormal pregnancy. J Matern Fetal Neonatal Med 13:22, 2003

Walker JJ: Pre-eclampsia. Lancet 356:1260, 2000

Wallace DH, Leveno KJ, Cunningham FG, et al: Randomized comparison of general and regional anesthesia for cesarean delivery in pregnancies complicated by severe preeclampsia. Obstet Gynecol 86:193, 1995

Wallenburg HC, Dekker GA, Makovitz JW, et al: Low-dose aspirin prevents pregnancy-induced hypertension and preeclampsia in angiotensin-sensitive primigravidae. Lancet 1:1, 1986

Walsh SC: Lipid peroxidation in pregnancy. Hypertens Preg 13:1, 1994

Wang Y, Gu Y, Granger DN, et al: Endothelial junctional protein redistribution and increased monolayer permeability in human umbilical vein endothelial cells isolated during preeclampsia. Am J Obstet Gynecol 186:214, 2002

Wang Y, Gu Y, Zhang Y, et al: Evidence of endothelial dysfunction in preeclampsia. Decreased endothelial nitric oxide synthase expression is associated with increased cell permeability in endothelial cells from preeclampsia. Am J Obstet Gynecol 190:817, 2004

Ward K, Hata A, Jeunemaitre X, et al: A molecular variant of angiotensinogen associated with preeclampsia (comment). Nat Genet 4:59, 1993

Watt-Morse ML, Caritis SN, Kridgen PL: Magnesium sulfate is a poor inhibitor of oxytocin-induced contractility in pregnant sheep. J Matern Fetal Med 4:139, 1995

Weerasekera DS, Peiris H: The significance of serum uric acid, creatinine and urinary microprotein levels in predicting pre-eclampsia. J Obstet Gynaecol 23:17, 2003

Weiner C, Martinez E, Zhu LK, et al: In vitro release of endothelium-derived relaxing factor by acetylcholine is increased during the guinea pig pregnancy. Am J Obstet Gynecol 161:1599, 1989

Weiner CP, Thompson LP, Liu KZ, et al: Endothelium derived relaxing factor and indomethacin-sensitive contracting factor alter arterial contractile responses to thromboxane during pregnancy. Am J Obstet Gynecol 166: 1171, 1992

Weinstein L: Preeclampsia-eclampsia with hemolysis, elevated liver enzymes, and thrombocytopenia. Obstet Gynecol 66:657, 1985

Weinstein L: Syndrome of hemolysis, elevated liver enzymes and low platelet count: A severe consequence of hypertension in pregnancy. Am J Obstet Gynecol 142:159, 1982

Weir RJ, Brown JJ, Fraser R, et al: Plasma renin, renin substrate, angiotensin II, and aldosterone in hypertensive disease of pregnancy. Lancet 1:291, 1973

Whitecar PW, Boggess KA, McMahon MJ, et al: Altered expression of TCR-CD3zeta induced by sera from women with preeclampsia. Am J Obstet Gynecol 185:812, 2001

Wicke C, Pereira PL, Neeser E, et al: Subcapsular liver hematoma in HELLP syndrome: Evaluation of diagnostic and therapeutic options—a unicenter study. Am J Obstet Gynecol 190:106, 2004

Wide-Swensson DH, Ingemarsson I, Lunnell NO, et al: Calcium channel blockade (isradipine) in treatment of hypertension in pregnancy: A randomized placebo-controlled study. Am J Obstet Gynecol 173:872, 1995

Williams Obstetrics, 15th ed. Pritchard JA, MacDonald PC (eds). New York, Appleton-Century-Crofts, 1976, p 413

Witlin AG, Friedman SA, Egerman RS, et al: Cerebrovascular disorders complicating pregnancy beyond eclampsia. Am J Obstet Gynecol 176:1139, 1997a

Witlin AG, Friedman SA, Sibai BA: The effect of magnesium sulfate therapy on the duration of labor in women with mild preeclampsia at term: A randomized, double-blind, placebo-controlled trial. Am J Obstet Gynecol 176:623, 1997b

Witlin AG, Saade GR, Mattar F, et al: Predictors of neonatal outcome in women with severe preeclampsia or eclampsia between 24 and 33 weeks' gestation. Am J Obstet Gynecol 182:607, 2000

Wolf M, Kettyle E, Sandler L, et al: Obesity and preeclampsia: The potential role of inflammation. Obstet Gynecol 98:757, 2001

Worley RJ, Everett RB, MacDonald PC, et al: Placental clearance of dehydroisoandrosterone sulfate and pregnancy outcome in three categories of hospitalized patients with pregnancy-induced hypertension. Gynecol Obstet Invest 6:28, 1975

Yoneyama Y, Suzuki S, Sawa R, et al: Relation between adenosine and T-helper1/T-helper 2 imbalance in women with preeclampsia. Obstet Gynecol 99:641, 2002

Young P, Johanson R: Haemodynamic, invasive and echocardiographic monitoring in the hypertensive parturient. Best Pract Res Clin Obstet Gynaecol 15:605, 2001

Zeeman GG, Cunningham FG: Blood volume expansion in women with antepartum eclampsia. Presented at the Annual Meeting of the Society for Gynecologic Investigation, Los Angeles, CA, March 18, 2002

Zeeman GG, Alexander JM, McIntire DD, et al: Homocysteine plasma concentration levels for the prediction of preeclampsia in women with chronic hypertension. Am J Obstet Gynecol 189:574, 2003a

Zeeman GG, Alexander JM, McIntire DD, et al: Inhibin-A levels and severity of hypertensive disorders due to pregnancy. Obstet Gynecol 100:140, 2002

Zeeman GG, Fleckenstein JL, Twickler DM, et al: Cerebral infarction in eclampsia. Am J Obstet Gynecol 190:714, 2004a

Zeeman GG, Hatab M, Twickler DM: Increased large-vessel cerebral blood flow in severe preeclampsia by magnetic resonance (MR) evaluation. Presented at the 24th Annual Meeting of the Society for Maternal-Fetal Medicine, New Orleans, LA, February 2, 2004b

Zeeman GG, Hatab M, Twickler DM: Maternal cerebral blood flow changes in pregnancy. Am J Obstet Gynecol 189:968, 2003b

Zhang C, Williams MA, King IB, et al: Vitamin C and the risk of preeclampsia—results from dietary questionnaire and plasma assay. Epidemiology 13:382, 2002

Zhang J, Klebanoff MA, Levine RJ, et al: The puzzling association between smoking and hypertension during pregnancy. Am J Obstet Gynecol 181:1407, 1999

Zhang J, Klebanoff MA, Roberts JM: Prediction of adverse outcomes by common definitions of hypertension in pregnancy. Obstet Gynecol 97:261, 2001

Zhang XQ, Varner M, Dizon-Townson D, et al: A molecular variant of angiotensinogen is associated with idiopathic intrauterine growth restriction. Obstet Gynecol 101:237, 2003

Zhong XY, Laivuori H, Livingston JC, et al: Elevation of both maternal and fetal extracellular circulating deoxyribonucleic acid concentrations in the plasma of pregnant women with preeclampsia. Am J Obstet Gynecol 184:414, 2001

Zinaman M, Rubin J, Lindheimer MD: Serial plasma oncotic pressure levels and echoencephalography during and after delivery in severe preeclampsia. Lancet 1:1245, 1985

Zondervan HA, Oosting J, Smorenberg-Schoorl ME, et al: Maternal whole blood viscosity in pregnancy hypertension. Gynecol Obstet Invest 25:83, 1988

35

Obstetrical Hemorrhage

Obstetrics is "bloody business." Even though hospitalization for delivery and the availability of blood for transfusion have dramatically reduced the maternal mortality rate, death from hemorrhage still remains a leading cause of maternal mortality. From 1991 through 1997 in the United States, hemorrhage was a direct cause of more than 18 percent of 3201 pregnancy-related maternal deaths, as ascertained from the Pregnancy Mortality Surveillance System of the Centers for Disease Control and Prevention (Berg and colleagues, 2003). Similarly, in the United Kingdom, hemorrhage was the major factor in more than 150 maternal deaths between 1985 and 1996 (Bonnar, 2000). Moreover, in both countries, hemorrhage is a leading reason for admission of pregnant women to intensive care units (Gilbert, 2003; Hazelgrove, 2001; Zeeman, 2003, and all their associates). In countries with fewer resources, the contribution of hemorrhage to maternal mortality is even more striking (Jegasothy, 2002; Rahman and co-workers, 2002). Indeed, hemorrhage has been identified as the single most important cause of maternal death worldwide, accounting for almost half of all postpartum deaths in developing countries (McCormick and colleagues, 2002).

Undoubtedly, there has been great improvement in mortality from hemorrhage with modernization of American obstetrics. For example, Sachs and associates (1987) reported that maternal deaths from obstetrical hemorrhage in Massachusetts declined tenfold from the mid-1950s to the mid-1980s. Similarly, maternal mortality due to hemorrhage at Grady Memorial Hospital in Atlanta decreased from 13 percent between 1949 and 1971 to 6 percent between 1972 and 2000 (Ho and associates, 2002).

Causes of maternal death from hemorrhage are shown in Table 35–1. Fatal hemorrhage is most likely in circumstances in which blood or components are not available immediately. For example, Singla and associates (2001) reported that women who are Jehovah's Witnesses are at a 44-fold increased risk of maternal death because of hemorrhage. The establishment and maintenance of facilities that allow prompt administration of blood are absolute requirements for acceptable obstetrical care. Hemorrhage may be *antepartum,* such as with placenta previa or placental abruption, or more likely *postpartum,* from uterine atony or genital tract lacerations.

TABLE 35–1 Causes of 763 Pregnancy-related Deaths Due to Hemorrhage

Causes of Hemorrhage	Number (%)
Placental abruption	141 (19)
Laceration/uterine rupture	125 (16)
Uterine atony	115 (15)
Coagulopathies	108 (14)
Placenta previa	50 (7)
Uterine bleeding	47 (6)
Placenta accreta/increta/percreta	44 (6)
Retained placenta	32 (4)

From Chichakli and colleagues (1999), with permission.

Incidence and Predisposing Conditions. Because of inexact terminology, the incidence of obstetrical hemorrhage cannot be determined precisely. Combs and colleagues (1991b) defined hemorrhage by a postpartum hematocrit drop of 10 volumes percent or by need for transfusion. Using these criteria, the incidence was 3.9 percent for women delivered vaginally. In women undergoing cesarean delivery, it was 6 to 8 percent (Combs and associates, 1991a; Naef and co-workers, 1994). In a study at Beth Israel Hospital, Klapholz (1990) reviewed over 30,000 deliveries from 1976 to 1986. The incidence of transfusion decreased over the years; in 1976 it was 4.6 percent, but by 1986 it was 1.9 percent.

Table 35–2 lists the many clinical circumstances in which risk of hemorrhage is appreciably increased. It is apparent that serious hemorrhage may occur at any time throughout pregnancy and the puerperium. The time of bleeding is widely used to classify obstetrical hemorrhage; the term *third-trimester* bleeding, however, is imprecise, and its use is not recommended. One factor not generally considered as "predisposing" to exsanguination is the lack of availability of obstetrical and anesthetic services. According to Bonnar (2000), the majority of deaths from hemorrhage in the United Kingdom cited earlier were associated with substandard care. Nagaya and associates (2000) reviewed 197 maternal deaths in Japan in the 2-year period spanning 1991 and 1992. Hemorrhage caused 40 percent of these deaths, and the investigators concluded that many of these were preventable because they were associated with inadequate obstetrical facilities.

ANTEPARTUM HEMORRHAGE

Slight vaginal bleeding is common during active labor. This "bloody show" is the consequence of effacement and dilatation of the cervix, with tearing of small veins. Uterine bleeding from a site above the cervix before delivery is cause for concern. The bleeding may be the consequence of some separation of a placenta implanted in the immediate vicinity of the cervical canal—*placenta previa.* It may come from separation of a placenta located elsewhere in the uterine cavity—*placental abruption.* Rarely, the bleeding may be the consequence of velamentous insertion of the umbilical cord with rupture and hemorrhage from a fetal blood vessel at the time of rupture of the membranes—*vasa previa.*

The source of uterine bleeding that originates above the level of the cervix is not always identified. In that circumstance, the bleeding typically begins with little or no other symptomatology, and then stops, and at delivery no anatomical cause is identified. Almost always the bleeding must have been the consequence of slight marginal separation of the placenta that did not expand. **The pregnancy in which such bleeding occurs remains at increased risk for a poor outcome even though the bleeding soon stops and placenta previa appears to have been excluded by sonography.** Lipitz and colleagues (1991) studied 65 consecutive

TABLE 35–2 Conditions That Predispose to or Worsen Obstetrical Hemorrhage

Abnormal Placentation	**Uterine Atony**
Placenta previa	Overdistended uterus
Placental abruption	Large fetus
Placenta accreta/increta/percreta	Multiple fetuses
Ectopic pregnancy	Hydramnios
Hydatidiform mole	Distention with clots
Trauma During Labor and Delivery	Anesthesia or analgesia
Episiotomy	Halogenated agents
Complicated vaginal delivery	Conduction analgesia with hypotension
Low- or midforceps delivery	Exhausted myometrium
Cesarean delivery or hysterectomy	Rapid labor
Uterine rupture—risk increased by:	Prolonged labor
Previously scarred uterus	Oxytocin or prostaglandin stimulation
High parity	Chorioamnionitis
Hyperstimulation	Previous uterine atony
Obstructed labor	**Coagulation Defects—Intensify Other Causes**
Intrauterine manipulation	Placental abruption
Midforceps rotation	Prolonged retention of dead fetus
Small Maternal Blood Volume	Amnionic fluid embolism
Small women	Saline-induced abortion
Pregnancy hypervolemia not yet maximal	Sepsis syndrome
Pregnancy hypervolemia constricted	Severe intravascular hemolysis
Severe preeclampsia	Massive transfusions
Eclampsia	Severe preeclampsia and eclampsia
Other Factors	Congenital coagulopathies
Obesity	Anticoagulant treatment
Native American ethnicity	
Previous postpartum hemorrhage	

women who had uterine bleeding between 14 and 26 weeks. Almost a fourth had placental abruption or previa. Total fetal loss including abortions and perinatal deaths was 32 percent. Leung and colleagues (2001) found that unexplained antepartum hemorrhage before 34 weeks was associated with a 62-percent risk of delivery within one week when associated with uterine contractions and a 13-percent risk even in the absence of contractions. In pregnancies with hemorrhage after 26 weeks not explained by placental abruption or previa, Ajayi and associates (1992) reported adverse outcomes in a third. For this reason, delivery should be considered in any woman at term with unexplained vaginal bleeding.

PLACENTAL ABRUPTION

Definition. The separation of the placenta from its site of implantation before delivery has been variously called placental abruption, abruptio placentae, and in Great Britain, accidental hemorrhage. The term *premature separation of the normally implanted placenta* is most descriptive because it differentiates the placenta that separates prematurely but that is implanted some distance beyond the cervical internal os from one that is implanted over the cervical internal os—that is, placenta previa. This is cumbersome, however, and hence the shorter term *abruptio placentae*, or *placental abruption*, has been used. The Latin *abruptio placentae*, which means "rending asunder of the placenta," denotes a sudden accident, a clinical characteristic of most cases of this complication.

Some of the bleeding of placental abruption usually insinuates itself between the membranes and uterus, and then escapes through the cervix, causing *external hemorrhage* (Fig. 35–1). Less often, the blood does not escape externally but is retained between the detached placenta and the uterus, leading to *concealed hemorrhage* (see Figs. 35–1 and 35–2). As shown in Figures 35–1 through 35–3, placental abruption may be *total* or *partial*. Placental abruption with concealed hemorrhage carries with it much greater maternal and fetal hazards, not only because of the possibility of consumptive coagulopathy, but also because the extent of the hemorrhage is not appreciated and the diagnosis typically is made later (Chang and co-workers, 2001).

Frequency and Significance. The frequency with which placental abruption is diagnosed varies because of different criteria. The intensity of the abruption often varies depending on how quickly the woman seeks and receives care following the onset of symptoms. With delay, the likelihood of extensive separation causing death of the fetus is increased remarkably.

The reported frequency for placental abruption averages about 1 in 200 deliveries. According to U.S. birth certificate data for the year 2001, the incidence of placental abruption was 1 in 185 deliveries (Martin and co-workers, 2002). At Parkland Hospital from 1988 through 2003, the incidence of abruption in over 235,000 deliveries has been approximately 1 in 290. Both incidence and severity have decreased over

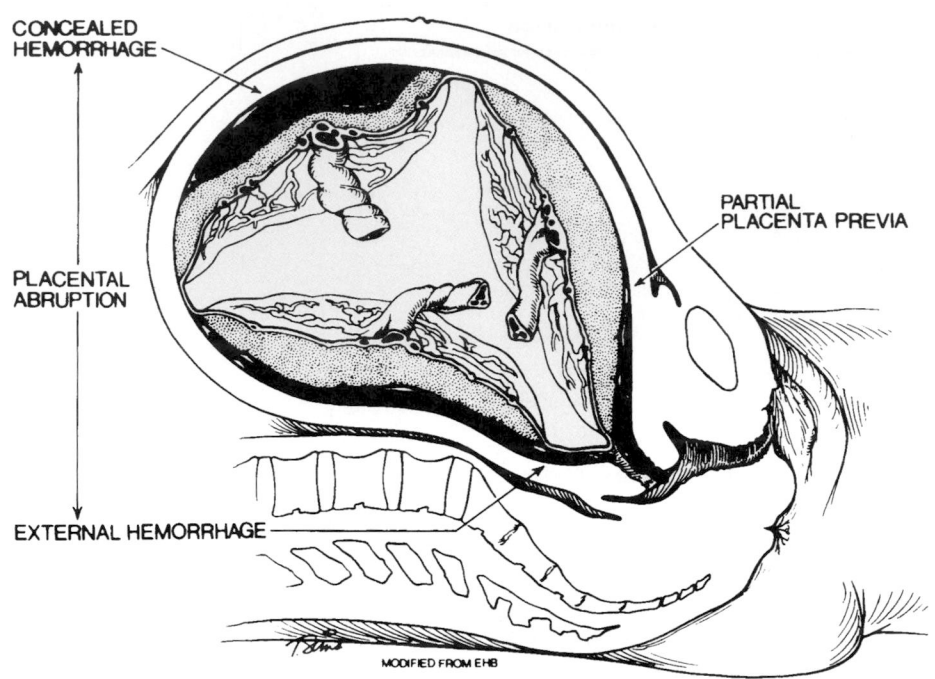

FIGURE 35–1. Hemorrhage from premature placental separation. Upper left: Extensive placental abruption but with the periphery of the placenta and the membranes still adherent, resulting in completely concealed hemorrhage. Lower: Placental abruption with the placenta detached peripherally and with the membranes between the placenta and cervical canal stripped from underlying decidua, allowing external hemorrhage. Right: Partial placenta previa with placental separation and external hemorrhage.

time. Applying the criterion of placental separation so extensive as to kill the fetus, the incidence was 1 in 420 deliveries from 1956 through 1967 (Pritchard and Brekken, 1967). As the number of high-parity women cared for decreased, and community-wide availability of prenatal care as well as emergency transportation improved, the frequency of abruption causing fetal death dropped to about 1 in 830 deliveries from 1974 through 1989 (Pritchard and colleagues, 1991). Between 1996 and 2003, it decreased to about 1 in 1600.

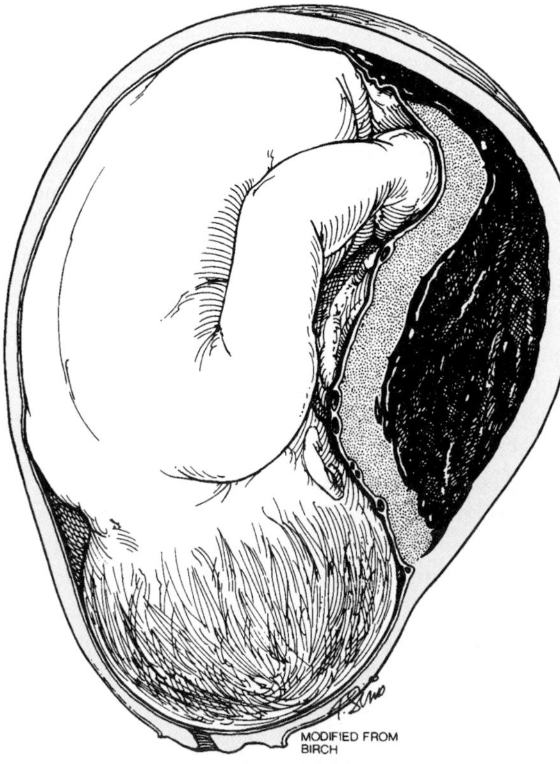

PERINATAL MORBIDITY AND MORTALITY. As stillbirths from other causes have decreased appreciably, those from placental abruption have become especially prominent. For example, of all third-trimester stillbirths at Parkland Hospital between 1992 and 1994, 12 percent were the consequence of placental abruption (Cunningham and Hollier, 1997). This figure has been stable, and from 2000 through 2002, abruption accounted for 10 percent of third-trimester stillbirths among nearly 45,000 deliveries. These frequencies are similar to that described by Fretts and Usher (1997) for the Royal Victoria Hospital in Montreal between 1978 and 1995. Based on their analysis of more than 7 million singleton births delivered in the United States during 1995 and 1996, Ananth and Wilcox (2001) calculated that the perinatal mortality rate associated with placental abruption was 119 per 1000 births compared with 8.2 per 1000 for all others. The high mortality was due in part to the strong association between placental abruption and preterm delivery. Even in those infants delivered at term, however, perinatal mortality was 25-fold higher with placental abruption.

Importantly, if the infant does survive, there may be adverse sequelae. Of the 182 survivors in the study by Abdella and associates (1984), about 15 percent were identified to have significant neurological deficits within the first year of life. Similarly, of the 39 survivors delivered between 26 and 36 weeks followed by Matsuda and co-workers (2003), about

FIGURE 35–2. Total placental abruption with concealed hemorrhage. The fetus is now dead.

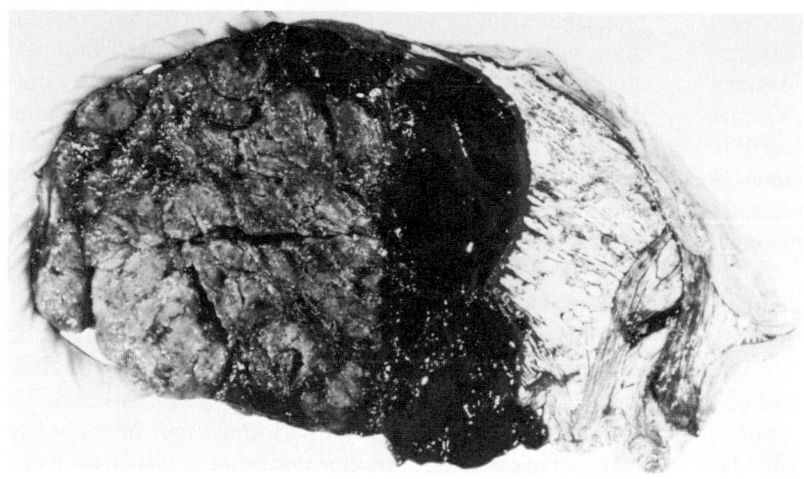

FIGURE 35–3. Partial placental abruption with adherent clot.

20 percent were diagnosed with cerebral palsy compared with 1 percent of gestational age–matched controls.

Etiology. The primary cause of placental abruption is unknown, but there are several associated conditions. Some of these are listed in Table 35–3. As shown in Figure 35–4, the incidence increases with *maternal age*. Although Pritchard and colleagues (1991) have also shown it to be higher in women of *great parity*, Toohey and associates (1995) did not find this in women para 5 or greater. *Race* or ethnicity appears to be important. In the almost 170,000 deliveries studied at Parkland Hospital, abruption was more common in African-American and Caucasian women (1 in 200) than in Asian (1 in 300) or Latin-American women (1 in 450).

By far the most commonly associated condition is some type of *hypertension*. This includes preeclampsia, gestational hypertension, and chronic hypertension. In the earlier Parkland Hospital study of 408 women with placental abruption so severe as to kill the fetus, maternal hypertension was apparent in about 50 percent of the women once the depleted intravascular compartment was adequately refilled (Pritchard and co-workers, 1991). Half of these women had chronic hypertension, and the remainder had gestational hypertension or preeclampsia. Morgan and colleagues (1994) found that hypertensive women were more likely to suffer a more severe abruption. According to Witlin and colleagues (1999), however, the severity of preeclampsia did not correlate with the incidence of abruption in 445 women. From the Maternal–Fetal Medicine Units Network, Sibai and co-workers (1998) reported that 1.5 percent of women with chronic hypertension suffered placental abruption. Ananth and associates (1999a) reported a threefold increased incidence of abruption with chronic hypertension and fourfold with severe preeclampsia. Interestingly, results from the Magpie Trial Collaborative Group (2002) suggests that women with preeclampsia may have a reduced risk of placental abruption when treated with magnesium sulfate (see Chap. 34, p. 792).

TABLE 35–3 Risk Factors for Placental Abruption

Risk Factor	Relative Risk
Increased age and parity	1.3–1.5
Preeclampsia	2.1–4.0
Chronic hypertension	1.8–3.0
Preterm ruptured membranes	2.4–4.9
Multifetal gestation	2.1
Hydramnios	2.0
Cigarette smoking	1.4–1.9
Thrombophilias	3–7
Cocaine use	NA
Prior abruption	10–25
Uterine leiomyoma	NA

NA = not available.
Adapted from Cunningham and Hollier (1997); risk data from Ananth (1999a, 1999b, 2001b); Eskes (2001); Kramer (1997); Kupferminc (1999), and all their associates.

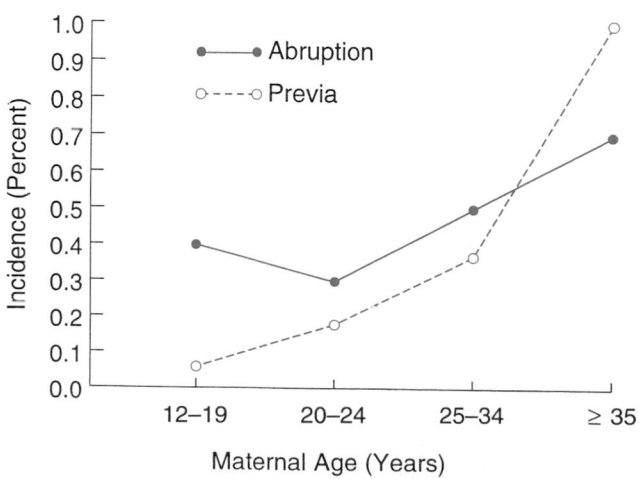

FIGURE 35–4. Incidence of abruptio placentae and placenta previa by maternal age in 169,108 deliveries at Parkland Hospital from 1988 through 1999. (Data courtesy of Dr. Don McIntire.)

There is an increased incidence of abruption with *preterm prematurely ruptured membranes.* Major and colleagues (1995) described an incidence of 5 percent in 756 women with ruptured membranes between 20 and 36 weeks. Kramer and co-workers (1997) found an incidence of 3.1 percent in all patients if membranes were ruptured for longer than 24 hours. In a meta-analysis of 54 studies, Ananth and associates (1996) found a threefold risk of abruption with prematurely ruptured membranes.

In the earliest studies from the Collaborative Perinatal Project, *cigarette smoking* was linked to an increased risk for abruption (Misra and Ananth, 1999; Naeye, 1980). In a meta-analysis of 1.6 million pregnancies, Ananth and colleagues (1999a, 1999b) found a twofold risk for abruption in smokers. This was increased to five- to eightfold if smokers had chronic hypertension, severe preeclampsia, or both. Similar findings have been reported by Odendaal and associates (2001) and Mortensen and colleagues (2001).

Cocaine abuse has been associated with an alarming frequency of placental abruption. In one report of 50 women who abused cocaine during pregnancy, eight stillbirths were caused by placental abruption (Bingol and colleagues, 1987). Addis and associates (2001) systematically reviewed 15 studies of cocaine-using women, all of which showed that placental abruption was more common than in controls.

Over the past decade, a number of inherited or acquired *thrombophilias* have been described that are associated with thromboembolic disorders during pregnancy (see Chap. 47, p. 1074). These clotting disorders also are associated with placental abruption and infarction (Gherman and Goodwin, 2000). For example, Kupferminc and colleagues (1999) found a significantly increased risk of abruption in women with a factor V Leiden or prothrombin gene mutation.

External trauma was implicated in only 3 of 207 cases of placental abruption causing fetal death at Parkland Hospital (see Chap. 42, p. 998). These experiences are similar to those of Kettel (1988) and Stafford (1988) and their co-workers, who stressed that abruption caused by relatively minor trauma may cause fetal jeopardy that is not always associated with immediate evidence of placental separation. In such cases, monitoring for 2 to 6 hours is usually adequate to exclude a subclinical abruption in the absence of uterine contractions, tenderness, or bleeding (American Academy of Pediatrics and American College of Obstetricians and Gynecologists, 2002).

Uterine leiomyomas, especially if located behind the placental implantation site, predispose to abruption (see Chap. 40, p. 963). Rice and associates (1989) reported that 8 of 14 women with retroplacental myomas developed placental abruption; four women had stillborn infants. In contrast, abruption developed in only 2 of 79 women whose myoma was not retroplacental.

Recurrent Abruption. Pritchard and co-workers (1970) identified a recurrence rate of severe abruption in 1 in 8

pregnancies. Importantly, of the 14 recurrent placental abruptions, eight caused fetal death for a second time. Furuhashi and colleagues (2002) analyzed subsequent pregnancy outcomes from 27 women who had a prior placental abruption. Of the six (22 percent) recurrences, four were at a gestational age 1 to 3 weeks earlier than the first abruption. Management of the subsequent pregnancy is made difficult in that placental separation may suddenly occur at any time, even remote from term. In the majority of cases, moreover, fetal well-being is normal beforehand, and thus currently available methods of fetal evaluation are usually not predictive (Toivonen and colleagues, 2002). In an extreme example, Seski and Compton (1976) documented both a normal nonstress test and a normal contraction stress test performed four hours before the onset of placental abruption that promptly killed the fetus.

Pathology. Placental abruption is initiated by hemorrhage into the decidua basalis. The decidua then splits, leaving a thin layer adherent to the myometrium. Consequently, the process in its earliest stages consists of the development of a decidual hematoma that leads to separation, compression, and the ultimate destruction of the placenta adjacent to it (see Chap. 27, p. 621). In its early stage, there may be no clinical symptoms. The condition is discovered only on examination of the freshly delivered organ, which has a circumscribed depression measuring a few centimeters in diameter on its maternal surface, and is covered by dark, clotted blood. Undoubtedly, it takes at least several minutes for these anatomical changes to materialize. Thus, a very recently separated placenta may appear no different from a normal placenta at delivery. According to Benirschke and Kaufmann (2000), and in our experiences, the "age" of the retroplacental clot cannot be determined exactly.

In some instances, a decidual spiral artery ruptures to cause a retroplacental hematoma, which as it expands disrupts more vessels to separate more placenta. The area of separation rapidly becomes more extensive and reaches the margin of the placenta. Because the uterus is still distended by the products of conception, it is unable to contract sufficiently to compress the torn vessels that supply the placental site. The escaping blood may dissect the membranes from the uterine wall and eventually appear externally or may be completely retained within the uterus (see Figs. 35–1 and 35–2).

CONCEALED HEMORRHAGE. Retained or concealed hemorrhage is likely when:

1. There is an effusion of blood behind the placenta but its margins still remain adherent.
2. The placenta is completely separated yet the membranes retain their attachment to the uterine wall.
3. Blood gains access to the amnionic cavity after breaking through the membranes.

4. The fetal head is so closely applied to the lower uterine segment that the blood cannot make its way past it.

Most often, however, the membranes are gradually dissected off the uterine wall, and blood sooner or later escapes.

CHRONIC PLACENTAL ABRUPTION. In some women, hemorrhage with retroplacental hematoma formation is somehow arrested completely without delivery. We have been able to document this phenomenon by labeling maternal red cells with [51]chromium. This technique demonstrated that red blood cells concealed as a 400-mL clot within the uterus at delivery 3 weeks later contained no chromium and therefore were shed before.

FETAL-TO-MATERNAL HEMORRHAGE. Bleeding with placental abruption is almost always maternal. In nontraumatic placental abruption, evidence of fetal-to-maternal hemorrhage was found in 20 percent of 78 cases; in all instances, it was less than 10 mL (Stettler and colleagues, 1992). Significant fetal bleeding is more likely to be seen with traumatic abruption (see Chap. 42, p. 998). **In this circumstance, fetal bleeding results from a tear or fracture in the placenta rather than from the placental separation itself.** Pearlman and associates (1990) found that fetal bleeding averaged 12 mL in a third of women with a traumatic abruption. Stettler and colleagues (1992) reported that there was fetal-to-maternal hemorrhage of 80 to 100 mL in 3 of 8 cases of traumatic placental abruption.

Clinical Diagnosis. It is emphasized that the signs and symptoms of placental abruption can vary considerably. For example, external bleeding can be profuse, yet placental separation may not be so extensive as to compromise the fetus directly. Rarely, there may be no external bleeding but the placenta may be completely sheared off and the fetus dead as the direct consequence. In one very unusual case, a multiparous woman near term presented to the Parkland Hospital obstetrical emergency room because of nosebleed. There was no abdominal or uterine pain or tenderness and no vaginal bleeding, but her fetus was dead. Her blood did not clot, and the plasma fibrinogen level was 25 mg/dL. Labor was induced, and at delivery a total abruption with fresh clots was found.

Hurd and co-workers (1983), in a prospective study of placental abruption, identified the frequency of a variety of pertinent signs and symptoms (Table 35–4). Bleeding and abdominal pain were the most frequent findings. **In 22 percent of cases, idiopathic preterm labor was considered to be the diagnosis until subsequent fetal death or distress developed.** Other findings included back pain, uterine tenderness, frequent uterine contractions, and persistent uterine hypertonus.

Studies consistently demonstrate that ultrasound infrequently confirms the diagnosis of abruption. For example, Sholl (1987) confirmed the clinical diagnosis sonographically

TABLE 35–4 Signs and Symptoms Determined Prospectively in 59 Women with Abruptio Placentae

Sign or Symptom	Frequency (%)
Vaginal bleeding	78
Uterine tenderness or back pain	66
Fetal distress	60
Preterm labor[a]	22
High-frequency contractions	17
Hypertonus	17
Dead fetus	15

[a]All treated with tocolytic agents.
From Hurd and associates (1983), with permission.

in only 25 percent of women. Similarly, Glantz and Purnell (2002) calculated a 24-percent sensitivity in 149 consecutive women who underwent sonography to rule out placental abruption. **Importantly, negative findings with ultrasound examination do not exclude placental abruption.**

Shock. It was once held that the shock sometimes seen with placental abruption was out of proportion to the amount of hemorrhage. Supposedly, thromboplastin from decidua and placenta entered the maternal circulation and incited intravascular coagulation and other features of the amnionic fluid embolism syndrome (see p. 845). This sequence is rare, and the intensity of shock is seldom out of proportion to maternal blood loss. Pritchard and Brekken (1967) studied blood loss in 141 women with placental abruption so severe as to kill the fetus and found that it often amounted to at least half of the pregnant blood volume. Neither hypotension nor anemia is obligatory in cases of concealed hemorrhage, even when the acute hemorrhage has achieved considerable magnitude. Oliguria caused by inadequate renal perfusion but responsive to vigorous treatment of hypovolemia may also be observed in these circumstances.

Differential Diagnosis. With severe placental abruption, the diagnosis generally is obvious. Milder and more common forms of abruption are difficult to recognize with certainty, and the diagnosis is often made by exclusion. Unfortunately, neither laboratory tests nor diagnostic methods are available to detect lesser degrees of placental separation accurately. Therefore, with vaginal bleeding complicating a viable pregnancy, it often becomes necessary to rule out placenta previa and other causes of bleeding by clinical inspection and ultrasound evaluation. It has long been taught, perhaps with some justification, that painful uterine bleeding means placental abruption, whereas painless uterine bleeding is indicative of placenta previa. Unfortunately, the differential diagnosis is not that simple. Labor accompanying placenta previa may cause pain suggestive of placental abruption. On the other hand, abruption may mimic normal labor, or it may cause no pain at all. The latter is more likely with a posteriorly implanted placenta. At times, the cause of the vaginal bleeding remains obscure even after delivery.

Consumptive Coagulopathy. One of the most common causes of clinically significant consumptive coagulopathy in obstetrics is placental abruption. Overt *hypofibrinogenemia* (less than 150 mg/dL of plasma) along with elevated levels of fibrinogen–fibrin degradation products, D-dimers, and variable decreases in other coagulation factors are found in about 30 percent of women with placental abruption severe enough to kill the fetus. Such severe coagulation defects are seen less commonly in those cases in which the fetus survives. Our experience has been that serious coagulopathy, when it develops, is usually evident by the time the woman is symptomatic.

The major mechanism is almost certainly the induction of coagulation intravascularly and, to a lesser degree, retroplacentally. Although an appreciable amount of fibrin is commonly deposited within the uterine cavity in instances of severe placental abruption and hypofibrinogenemia, the amounts are insufficient to account for all of the fibrinogen missing from the circulation (Pritchard and Brekken, 1967). Moreover, Bonnar and co-workers (1969) have observed, and we have confirmed, that the levels of fibrin degradation products are higher in serum from peripheral blood than in serum from blood contained in the uterine cavity. The reverse would be anticipated in the absence of significant intravascular coagulation.

An important consequence of intravascular coagulation is the activation of plasminogen to plasmin, which lyses fibrin microemboli, thereby maintaining patency of the microcirculation. In every instance of placental abruption severe enough to kill the fetus, we have identified clearly pathological levels of fibrinogen–fibrin degradation products in maternal serum. At the outset, severe hypofibrinogenemia may or may not be accompanied by overt thrombocytopenia. After repeated blood transfusions, however, thrombocytopenia is common.

Renal Failure. Acute renal failure may be seen in severe forms of placental abruption. This includes those in which treatment of hypovolemia is delayed or incomplete (see Chap. 48, p. 1106). Of 72 pregnant women with acute renal failure described by Drakeley and colleagues (2002), 32 percent had placental abruption. Fortunately, reversible acute tubular necrosis accounts for 75 percent of cases of renal failure (Turney and colleagues, 1989). According to Lindheimer and associates (2000), acute cortical necrosis in pregnancy is usually caused by abruptio placentae, and Grünfeld and Pertuiset (1987) reported that 7 of 19 women with this lesion had placental abruption.

Seriously impaired renal perfusion is the consequence of massive hemorrhage. Because preeclampsia frequently coexists with placental abruption, renal vasospasm is likely intensified (Hauth and Cunningham, 1999). Even when placental

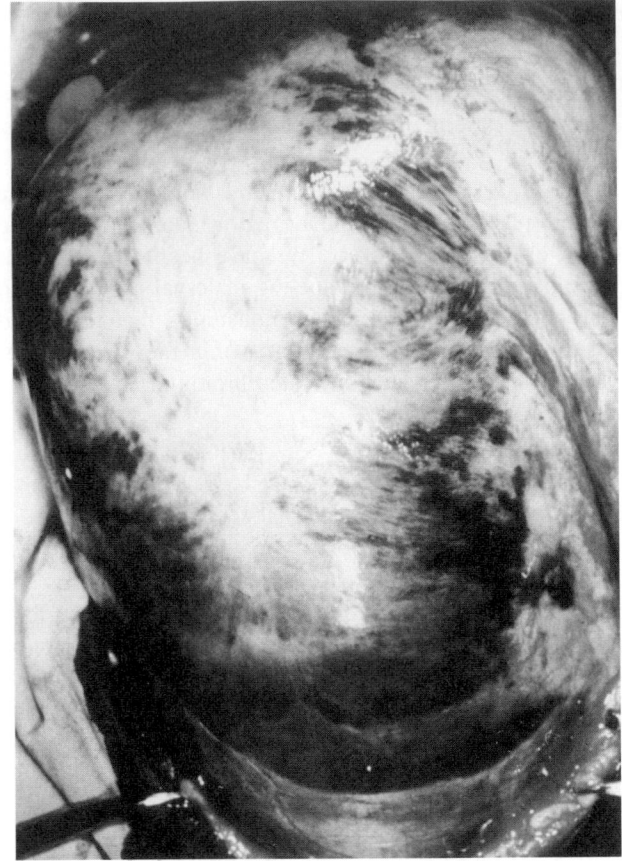

FIGURE 35–5. Couvelaire uterus with total placental abruption before cesarean delivery. Blood had markedly infiltrated much of the myometrium to reach the serosa. After the infant was delivered and the uterus closed, the uterus remained well contracted despite extensive extravasation of blood into the uterine wall.

abruption is complicated by severe intravascular coagulation, prompt and vigorous treatment of hemorrhage with blood and crystalloid solution often prevents clinically significant renal dysfunction. For unknown reasons, even without preeclampsia, *proteinuria* is common, especially with more severe forms of placental abruption. It usually clears soon after delivery.

Couvelaire Uterus. There may be widespread extravasation of blood into the uterine musculature and beneath the uterine serosa (Fig. 35–5). This so-called *uteroplacental apoplexy,* first described by Couvelaire in the early 1900s, is now frequently called *Couvelaire uterus.* Such effusions of blood are also occasionally seen beneath the tubal serosa, in the connective tissue of the broad ligaments, and in the substance of the ovaries, as well as free in the peritoneal cavity. Its precise incidence is unknown because it can be demonstrated conclusively only at laparotomy. These myometrial hemorrhages seldom interfere with uterine contractions sufficiently to produce severe postpartum hemorrhage and are not an indication for hysterectomy.

Management. Treatment for placental abruption varies depending on gestational age and the status of the mother and fetus. With a live and mature fetus, and if vaginal delivery is not imminent, then emergency cesarean delivery is chosen by most clinicians. As discussed in the section Hypovolemic Shock on page 839, with massive external bleeding, intensive resuscitation with blood plus crystalloid and prompt delivery to control the hemorrhage are lifesaving for the mother and, it is hoped, for the fetus. If the diagnosis is uncertain and the fetus is alive but without evidence of fetal compromise, very close observation, with facilities for immediate intervention, can be practiced.

EXPECTANT MANAGEMENT IN PRETERM PREGNANCY. Delaying delivery may prove beneficial when the fetus is immature. Bond and associates (1989) expectantly managed 43 women with placental abruption before 35 weeks, and 31 of them were given tocolytic therapy. The mean time to delivery in all 43 was about 12 days and there were no stillborns. Cesarean delivery was performed in 75 percent of cases.

Women with evidence of very early abruption frequently develop oligohydramnios, either with or without premature membrane rupture. Elliott and associates (1998) described four women with an abruption at a mean gestational age of 20 weeks and who also developed oligohydramnios. They were delivered at an average of 28 weeks.

Lack of ominous decelerations does not guarantee the safety of the intrauterine environment for any period of time. The placenta may further separate at any instant and seriously compromise or kill the fetus unless delivery is performed immediately. Some of the immediate causes of fetal distress from abruptio placentae are shown in Figure 35–6. It is important for the welfare of the distressed fetus that steps be initiated immediately to correct maternal hypovolemia, anemia, and hypoxia so as to restore and maintain the function of any placenta that is still implanted. Little can be done to favorably modify the other causes that contribute to fetal distress except to deliver the fetus.

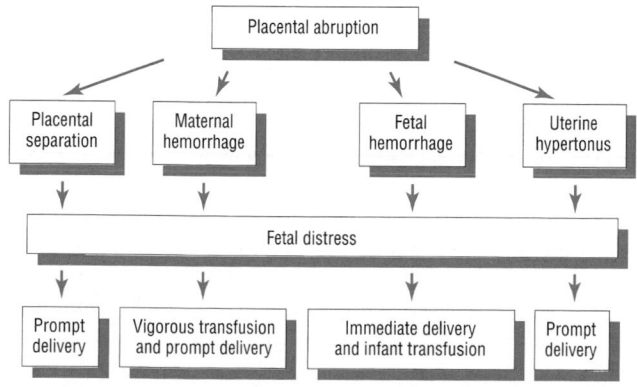

FIGURE 35–6. Various causes of fetal distress from placental abruption and their treatment.

TOCOLYSIS. Some clinicians have advocated tocolysis for the preterm pregnancy complicated by suspected abruption. Hurd and associates (1983) found that abruption went unrecognized for dangerously long periods if tocolysis was initiated. Conversely, Sholl (1987) as well as Combs and co-workers (1992) provided data that tocolysis improved outcome in a highly selected group of preterm pregnancies complicated by partial abruption. Towers and co-workers (1999) administered magnesium sulfate, terbutaline, or both to 95 of 131 women with placental abruption diagnosed before 36 weeks. The perinatal mortality was 5 percent and did not differ from the nontreated group. They concluded that a randomized clinical trial could be safely conducted. Until then, we are of the view that clinically evident placental abruption should be considered a contraindication to tocolytic therapy.

CESAREAN DELIVERY. Rapid delivery of the fetus who is alive but in distress practically always means cesarean delivery. Kayani and colleagues (2003) studied the relationship between the rapidity of delivery and neonatal outcome in 33 singleton pregnancies with a clinically overt placental abruption and fetal bradycardia. Of the 22 neurologically intact survivors, 15 were delivered within 20 minutes of the decision to operate. Of the 11 infants who died or developed cerebral palsy, 8 were delivered beyond 20 minutes of the decision time, suggesting that the speed of response is an important factor in neonatal outcome.

It is important to note that an electrode applied directly to the fetus may rarely provide misleading information, as in the case illustrated in Figure 35–7. At first impression at least, fetal bradycardia of 80 to 90 beats/min, with a degree of beat-to-beat variability, seemed evident. The fetus, however, was dead, and the maternal pulse rate was identical to that recorded through the fetal scalp electrode. Cesarean delivery at this time would likely have proved dangerous for the mother because she was profoundly hypovolemic and had severe consumptive coagulopathy.

VAGINAL DELIVERY. If placental separation is so severe that the fetus is dead, vaginal delivery is preferred unless hemorrhage is so brisk that it cannot be successfully managed even by vigorous blood replacement, or there are other obstetrical complications that prevent vaginal delivery. Serious coagulation defects are likely to prove especially troublesome with cesarean delivery. The abdominal and uterine incisions are prone to bleed excessively when coagulation is impaired. Hemostasis at the placental implantation site depends primarily on myometrial contraction. Therefore, with vaginal delivery, stimulation of the myometrium pharmacologically and by uterine massage causes these vessels to constrict so that serious hemorrhage is avoided even though coagulation defects persist. Moreover, bleeding that does occur is shed through the vagina. In the following example, there was

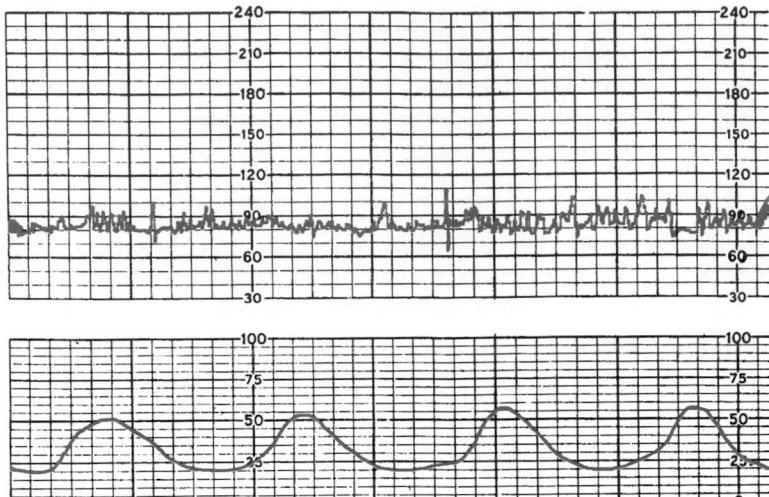

FIGURE 35–7. A recording of uterine pressures and presumed fetal heart rate in a case of placental abruption so severe as to have killed the fetus. The scalp electrode conducted the maternal ECG signal. Note the increased uterine basal tone.

an indication for abdominal delivery despite documented fetal demise:

> Although placental abruption was suspected, because rupture of a prior uterine incision could not be excluded, a repeat cesarean was performed for a 26-week stillborn fetus. The patient had profound hypofibrinogenemia and serious bleeding was encountered from all surgical incisions. Persistent bleeding necessitated hysterectomy followed by internal iliac artery ligation. Lactated Ringer solution was given along with 17 units of blood, 8 units of plasma, and 10 units of platelets to maintain perfusion and treat the coagulopathy.

LABOR. With extensive placental abruption, the uterus is likely to be persistently hypertonic. The baseline intra-amnionic pressure may be 50 mm Hg or higher, with rhythmic increases up to 75 to 100 mm Hg. Because of persistent hypertonus, it may be difficult at times to determine by palpation if the uterus is contracting and relaxing to any degree (Fig. 35–8).

AMNIOTOMY. Rupture of the membranes as early as possible has long been championed in the management of placental abruption. The rationale for amniotomy is that the escape of amnionic fluid might both decrease bleeding from the implantation site and reduce the entry into the maternal circulation of thromboplastin and perhaps activated coagulation factors from the retroplacental clot. There is no evidence, however, that either is accomplished by amniotomy. If the fetus is reasonably mature, rupture of the membranes may hasten delivery. If the fetus is immature, the intact sac may be more efficient in promoting cervical dilatation than is a small fetal part poorly applied to the cervix.

OXYTOCIN. Although baseline hypertonus characterizes myometrial function in most cases of severe placental abruption, if no rhythmic uterine contractions are superimposed, then oxytocin is given in standard doses. Uterine stimulation to effect vaginal delivery provides benefits that override the risks. The use of oxytocin has been challenged on the basis that it

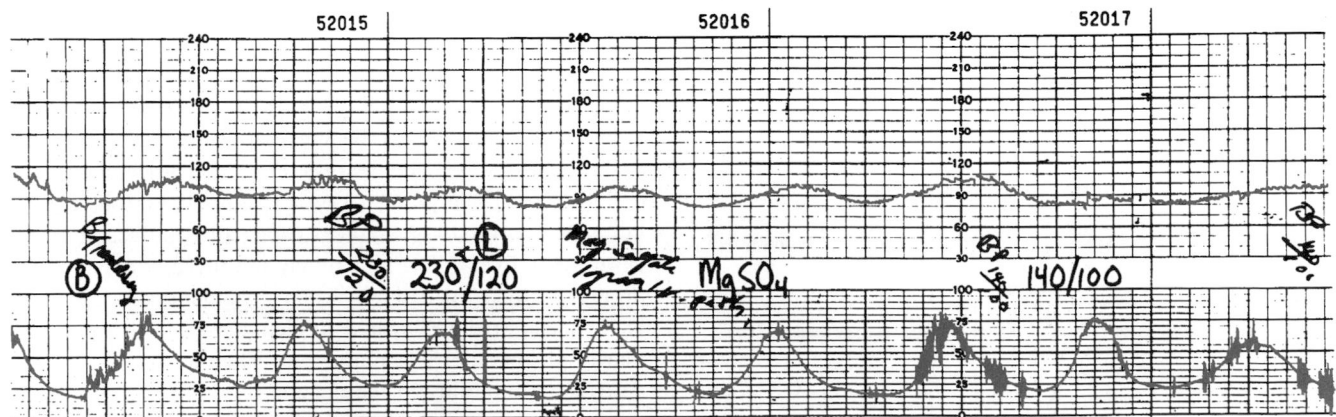

FIGURE 35–8. Placental abruption in a woman with severe preeclampsia. Persistent uterine hypertonus is demonstrated by an elevated baseline pressure of 20 to 25 mm Hg and frequent contractions. The fetal heart rate demonstrates baseline bradycardia with repetitive late decelerations.

might enhance the escape of thromboplastin into the maternal circulation and thereby initiate or enhance consumptive coagulopathy or amnionic fluid embolism syndrome. There is no evidence to support this fear (Clark and colleagues, 1995; Pritchard and Brekken, 1967).

Timing of Delivery After Severe Placental Abruption. When the fetus is dead or previable, there is no evidence that establishing an arbitrary time limit for delivery is necessary. Experiences at both the University of Virginia and Parkland Hospitals indicate that maternal outcome depends on the diligence with which adequate fluid and blood replacement therapy is pursued, rather than on the interval to delivery (Brame and associates, 1968; Pritchard and Brekken, 1967). At the University of Virginia Hospital, women with severe placental abruption who were transfused for 18 hours or more before delivery experienced complications that were neither more numerous nor greater in severity than did the group in which delivery was accomplished sooner. Our observations are similar.

PLACENTA PREVIA

Definition. In placenta previa, the placenta is located over or very near the internal os. Four degrees of this abnormality have been recognized:

1. *Total placenta previa.* The internal cervical os is covered completely by placenta (Fig. 35–9).
2. *Partial placenta previa.* The internal os is partially covered by placenta (see Fig. 35–1; Fig. 35–10).
3. *Marginal placenta previa.* The edge of the placenta is at the margin of the internal os.
4. *Low-lying placenta.* The placenta is implanted in the lower uterine segment such that the placenta edge actually does not reach the internal os but is in close proximity to it.

In another condition, termed *vasa previa,* the fetal vessels course through membranes and present at the cervical os. Vasa previa is an uncommon cause of antepartum hemorrhage and is associated with a high rate of fetal death. It is discussed in detail in Chapter 27 (see p. 627).

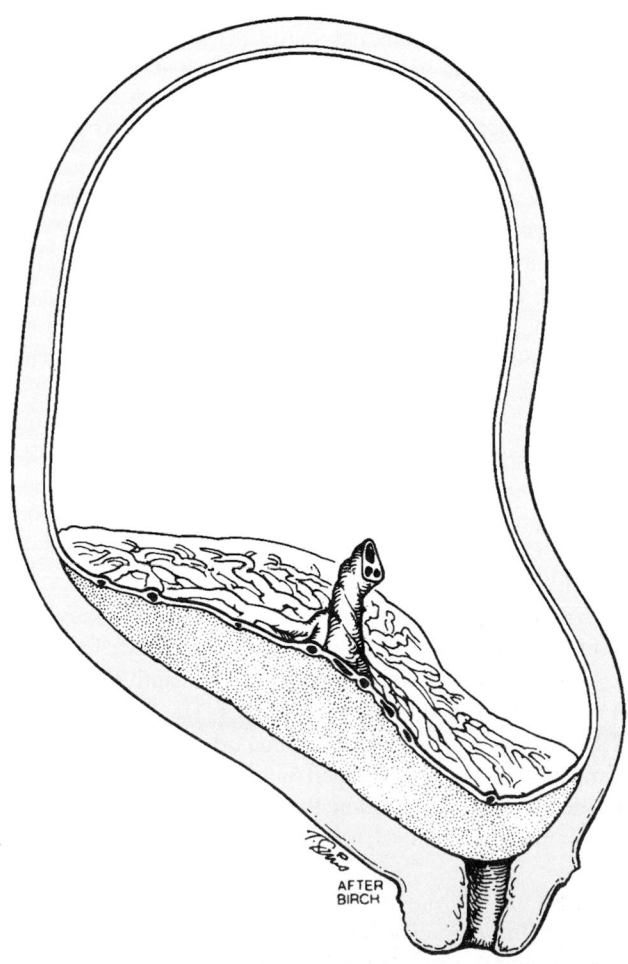

FIGURE 35–9. Total placenta previa. Even with the modest cervical dilatation illustrated, copious hemorrhage would be anticipated.

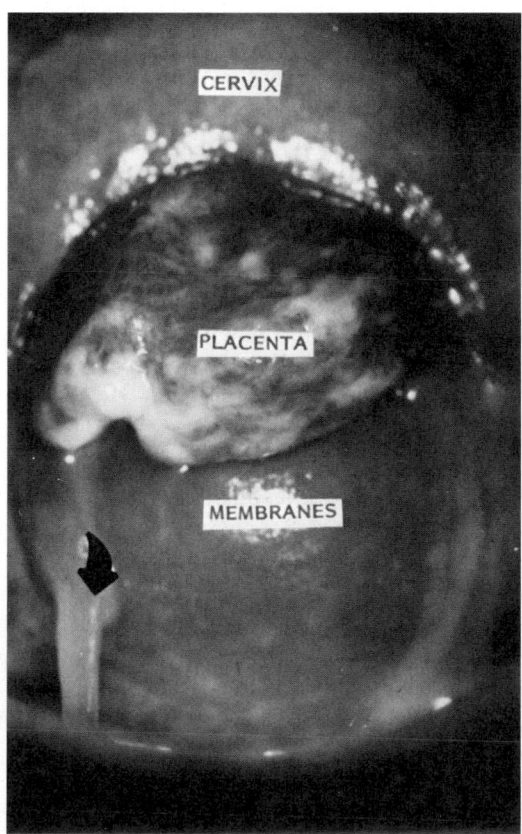

FIGURE 35–10. Partial placenta previa seen through a cervix 3- to 4-cm dilated at 22 weeks' gestation. The arrow points to mucus dripping from the cervix. Uterine cramping was described, but earlier intermittent bleeding had stopped 1 month before. The fetus weighed 410 g when delivered vaginally the next day. Blood loss was not massive. (Photograph courtesy of Dr. Rigoberto Santos.)

The degree of placenta previa depends in large measure on the cervical dilatation at the time of examination. For example, a low-lying placenta at 2-cm dilatation may become a partial placenta previa at 8-cm dilatation because the dilating cervix has uncovered placenta. Conversely, a placenta previa that appears to be total before cervical dilatation may become partial at 4-cm dilatation because the cervix dilates beyond the edge of the placenta (see Fig. 35–10). **Digital palpation to try to ascertain these changing relations between the edge of the placenta and the internal os as the cervix dilates can incite severe hemorrhage!**

With both total and partial placenta previa, a certain degree of spontaneous placental separation is an inevitable consequence of the formation of the lower uterine segment and cervical dilatation. Such separation is associated with hemorrhage from blood vessels so disrupted.

Incidence. According to U.S. birth certificate data for the year 2001, placenta previa complicated 1 in 305 deliveries (Martin and co-workers, 2002). In almost 93,000 deliveries in Nova Scotia, Crane and associates (1999) found the incidence to be 0.33 percent (1 in 300). At Parkland Hospital, the incidence was 0.26 percent (1 in 390) for more than 169,000 deliveries during 12 years. These statistics are remarkably similar considering the lack of precision in definition and identification for reasons already discussed. Moreover, should painless bleeding from focal separation of a placenta implanted in the lower uterine segment but away from a partially dilated cervical os be classified as placenta previa or placental abruption? This question is difficult to answer. Obviously, it is both.

PERINATAL MORBIDITY AND MORTALITY. Preterm delivery is a major cause of perinatal death even with expectant management of placenta previa. Using U.S. linked birth and infant death data sets for 1997, Salihu and associates (2003) found that the neonatal mortality rate was threefold higher in pregnancies complicated by placenta previa primarily because of increased preterm birth. In another large series, Ananth and associates (2003b) reported a comparably increased risk of neonatal death even for those fetuses delivered at term. Some of this risk appears related to fetal growth restriction and limited prenatal care. Although some investigators suggested earlier that congenital malformations are increased with a previa, Crane and co-workers (1999) were the first to confirm this. Their study controlled for maternal age. For reasons that are unclear, fetal anomalies were increased 2.5-fold.

It is also uncertain if there is associated fetal growth restriction with a previa. Brar and colleagues (1988) reported that the incidence was nearly 20 percent. Conversely, Crane and co-workers (1999) found no increased incidence after controlling for gestational age. Ananth and associates (2001a) examined the relationship between placenta previa, fetal growth restriction, and preterm delivery in a large population-based cohort of more than 500,000 singleton births. They found that most of the association between placenta previa and low birthweight is due primarily to preterm birth and, to a lesser extent, growth impairment.

Etiology. Advancing *maternal age* increases the risk of placenta previa. As shown in Figure 35–4, in more than 169,000 deliveries at Parkland Hospital from 1988 through 1999, the incidence of previa increased significantly with each age group. At the extremes, it is 1 in 1500 for women 19 years of age or younger, and it is 1 in 100 for women older than 35 years of age. Frederiksen and colleagues (1999) reported that the incidence of previa increased from 0.3 percent in 1976 to 0.7 percent in 1997. They attributed this to a shift to an older obstetrical population.

Multiparity is associated with previa. In a study of 314 women who were para 5 or greater, Babinszki and collaborators (1999) reported that the 2.2 percent incidence of previa was increased significantly compared with that of women of lower parity. Using U.S. natality figures for 1989 to 1998, Ananth and associates (2003a) found that the rate of placenta previa was 40 percent higher in *multifetal gestations* compared with that of singletons.

Prior cesarean delivery increases the likelihood of placenta previa. Miller and associates (1996) cited a threefold increase of previa in women with prior cesarean delivery in over 150,000 deliveries at Los Angeles County Women's Hospital. The incidence increased with the number of previous cesarean deliveries; it was 1.9 percent with two prior cesarean deliveries and 4.1 percent with three or more. Gesteland and co-workers (2004) and Gilliam and colleagues (2002) also found that the risk of placenta previa increases progressively as parity and number of prior cesarean deliveries increase. Both groups calculated that the likelihood of placenta previa was increased more than eightfold in women with parity greater than four and more than four prior cesareans. Certainly, a prior uterine incision with a previa increases the incidence of *cesarean hysterectomy*. Frederiksen and co-workers (1999) reported a 25-percent hysterectomy rate in women undergoing repeat cesarean for a previa compared with only 6 percent in those undergoing primary cesarean for placenta previa.

Williams and colleagues (1991) found the relative risk of placenta previa to be increased twofold related to *smoking.* These findings were confirmed by Ananth (2003a) and Handler (1994) and all their associates. The Williams group (1991) theorized that carbon monoxide hypoxemia caused compensatory placental hypertrophy. Perhaps related, defective decidual vascularization, the possible result of inflammatory or atrophic changes, is implicated in the development of previa.

Clinical Findings. The most characteristic event in placenta previa is painless hemorrhage, which usually does not appear until near the end of the second trimester or after. Some abortions, however, may result from such an abnormal location of the developing placenta. Frequently, bleeding from placenta previa has its onset without warning, presenting without pain in a woman who has had an uneventful prenatal course. Fortunately, the initial bleeding is rarely so profuse as to prove fatal. Usually it ceases spontaneously, only to recur. In some women, particularly those with a placenta implanted near but not over the cervical os, bleeding does not appear until the onset of labor, when it may vary from slight to profuse hemorrhage and clinically may mimic placental abruption.

The cause of hemorrhage is reemphasized: When the placenta is located over the internal os, the formation of the lower uterine segment and the dilatation of the internal os result inevitably in tearing of placental attachments. The bleeding is augmented by the inherent inability of the myometrial fibers of the lower uterine segment to contract and thereby constrict the torn vessels.

Hemorrhage from the placental implantation site in the lower uterine segment may continue after delivery of the placenta, because the lower uterine segment contracts poorly compared with the uterine body. Bleeding may also result from lacerations in the friable cervix and lower uterine segment, especially following manual removal of a somewhat adherent placenta.

PLACENTA ACCRETA, INCRETA, AND PERCRETA. Placenta previa may be associated with *placenta accreta* or one of its more advanced forms, *placenta increta* or *percreta*. Such abnormally firm attachment of the placenta might be anticipated because of poorly developed decidua in the lower uterine segment. Almost 7 percent of 514 cases of previa reported by Frederiksen and collaborators (1999) had an associated abnormal placental attachment. Biswas and co-workers (1999) performed placental bed biopsies at cesarean delivery in 50 women with previas and 50 control women. Although about 50 percent of specimens from previas showed myometrial spiral arterioles with trophoblastic giant-cell infiltration, only 20 percent from normally implanted placentas had these changes. Placenta accreta is discussed in detail on page 830.

COAGULATION DEFECTS. In our experience, coagulopathy is rare with placenta previa, even when extensive separation from the implantation site has occurred. Wing and colleagues (1996b) studied 87 women with antepartum bleeding from placenta previa and found no evidence of coagulopathy. Presumably thromboplastin that incites intravascular coagulation that commonly characterizes abruptio placentae readily escapes through the cervical canal rather than being forced into the maternal circulation.

Diagnosis. Placenta previa or abruption should always be suspected in women with uterine bleeding during the latter half of pregnancy. The possibility of placenta previa should not be dismissed until appropriate evaluation, including sonography, has clearly proved its absence. The diagnosis of placenta previa can seldom be established firmly by clinical

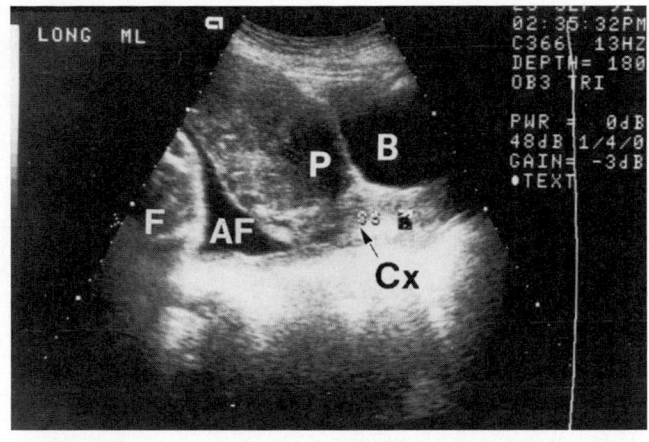

FIGURE 35–11. Partial anterior placenta previa at 36 weeks' gestation. Placenta (P) extends anteriorly and downward toward cervix (Cx). Fetus (F), amnionic fluid (AF), and bladder (B) are seen. (Courtesy of Dr. Rigoberto Santos.)

examination unless a finger is passed through the cervix and the placenta is palpated. **Such examination of the cervix is never permissible unless the woman is in an operating room with all the preparations for immediate cesarean delivery, because even the gentlest examination of this sort can cause torrential hemorrhage.** Furthermore, this type of examination should not be performed unless delivery is planned, for it may cause bleeding that necessitates immediate delivery even though the fetus is immature. This "double set-up" examination is rarely necessary, because placental location can almost always be obtained by sonography.

LOCALIZATION BY SONOGRAPHY. The simplest, most precise, and safest method of placental localization is provided by *transabdominal sonography,* which is used to locate the placenta with considerable accuracy (Figs. 35–11 and 35–12). According to Laing (1996), the average accuracy is about 96 percent, and rates as high as 98 percent have been obtained. **False-positive results are often a result of bladder distention. Therefore, ultrasonic scans in apparently positive cases should be repeated after emptying the bladder.** An uncommon source of error has been identification of abundant placenta implanted in the uterine fundus but failure to appreciate that the placenta was large and extended downward all the way to the internal os of the cervix.

The use of *transvaginal ultrasonography* has substantively improved diagnostic accuracy of placenta previa. Although it may appear dangerous to introduce an ultrasound probe into the vagina of women with placenta previa, the technique has been shown to be safe (Timor-Tritsch and Yunis, 1993). Farine and associates (1988) were able to visualize the internal cervical os in all cases using the transvaginal technique, in contrast to only 70 percent using transabdominal equipment. In later studies comparing abdominal ultrasound with transvaginal imaging, Smith (1997) and Taipale (1998) and their colleagues also found the transvaginal technique to be superior.

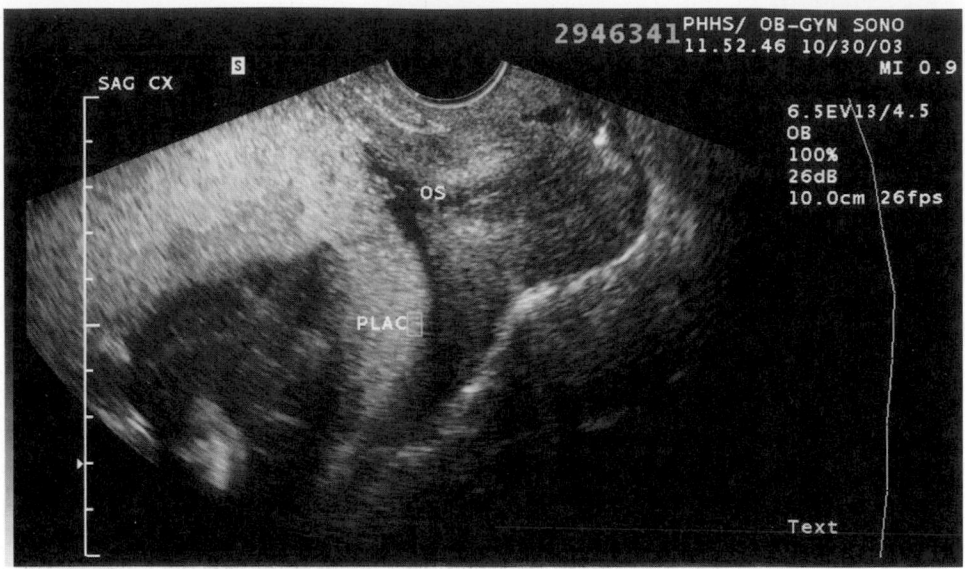

FIGURE 35–12. Total placenta previa at 18 weeks' gestation. Placenta (PLAC) completely overlies the cervical os. (Courtesy of Dr. Rigoberto Santos.)

Hertzberg and associates (1992) demonstrated that *transperineal sonography* allowed visualization of the internal os in all 164 cases examined because transabdominal sonography disclosed a previa or was inconclusive. Placenta previa was correctly excluded in 154 women, and in 10 in whom it was diagnosed sonographically, nine had a previa confirmed at delivery. The positive predictive value was 90 percent and the negative predictive value was 100 percent.

MAGNETIC RESONANCE IMAGING. A number of investigators have used magnetic resonance imaging (MRI) to visualize placental abnormalities, including placenta previa. Although there are many positive attributes of MRI, it is unlikely that this imaging technique will replace ultrasonic scanning for routine evaluation in the near future.

PLACENTAL "MIGRATION." Since the report by King (1973), the apparent peripatetic nature of the placenta has been well established. Sanderson and Milton (1991) found that 12 percent of placentas were "low lying" in 4300 women at 18 to 20 weeks. Of those not covering the internal os, previa did not persist and hemorrhage was not encountered. Conversely, of those covering the os at midpregnancy, about 40 percent persisted as a previa. Thus, placentas that lie close to the internal os, but not over it, during the second trimester, or even early in the third trimester, are unlikely to persist as previas by term.

As shown in Figure 35–13, the likelihood that placenta previa persists after being identified sonographically before 28 weeks is greater in women who have had a prior cesarean delivery (Dashe and colleagues, 2002). In the absence of any other abnormality, sonography need not be frequently repeated simply to follow placental position. Restriction of activity is not necessary unless a previa persists beyond 28 weeks, or becomes clinically apparent before that time.

The mechanism of apparent placental movement is not completely understood. The term *migration* is clearly a misnomer, however, because invasion of chorionic villi into the decidua on either side of the cervical os persists. The apparent movement of the low-lying placenta relative to the internal os probably results from inability to precisely define this relationship in a three-dimensional manner using two-dimensional sonography in early pregnancy. This difficulty is coupled with differential growth of lower and upper myometrial segments as pregnancy progresses. Thus, those

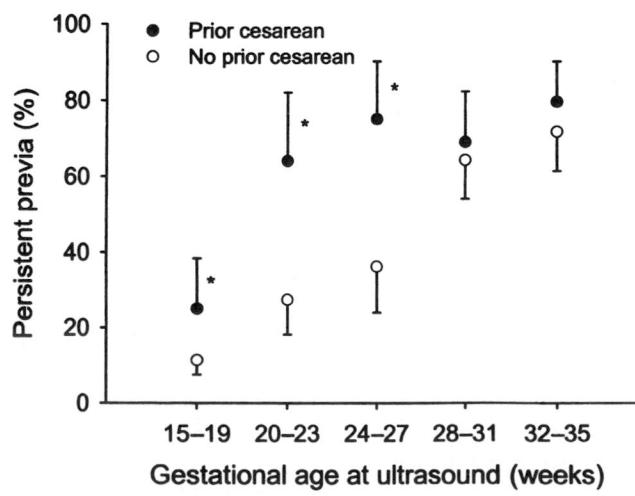

FIGURE 35–13. Percentage of women with persistent placenta previa at delivery according to gestational age at diagnosis and prior cesarean delivery. Error bars represent one direction (half-width) of the 95-percent confidence intervals. (*P < .05 comparing women with prior cesarean delivery with multiparous women with no prior cesarean delivery.) (From Dashe and colleagues, 2002, with permission.)

placentas that "migrate" most likely never had actual circumferential villus invasion that reached the internal cervical os in the first place.

Management. Women with a placenta previa may be considered as follows:

1. Those in whom the fetus is preterm and there is no indication for delivery.
2. Those in whom the fetus is reasonably mature.
3. Those in labor.
4. Those in whom hemorrhage is so severe as to mandate delivery despite fetal immaturity.

Management with a preterm fetus, but with no active uterine bleeding, consists of close observation. For some women, prolonged hospitalization may be ideal, however, the woman is usually discharged after bleeding has ceased and her fetus judged to be healthy. The woman and her family must fully appreciate the problems of placenta previa and be prepared to transport her to the hospital immediately. In properly selected patients, there appears to be no benefit to inpatient versus outpatient management of placenta previa (Mouer, 1994). In another study, Drost and Keil (1994) demonstrated a 50-percent reduction in hospitalization and maternal costs, as well as a 40-percent reduction in cost for mother–infant pairs with outpatient compared with those with inpatient management. Importantly, there were no differences in maternal or fetal morbidity. Wing and colleagues (1996a) reported preliminary results from their randomized clinical trial of inpatient versus home management of 53 women with bleeding from a previa at 24 to 36 weeks. Maternal and perinatal morbidities were similar in each group, but home management saved $15,000 per case. Importantly, 33 (62 percent) of these 53 women had recurrent bleeding, and 28 (52 percent) required expeditious cesarean delivery.

Delivery. Cesarean delivery is necessary in practically all women with placenta previa. Most often, a transverse uterine incision is made. Because fetal bleeding may result from an incision into an anterior placenta, a vertical incision is sometimes recommended. Even when the incision extends through the placenta, however, maternal or fetal outcome is rarely compromised.

An alternative surgical technique that avoids incising the placenta has been described by Ward (2003). Following the uterine incision, a cleavage plane is developed with the forefinger between the uterus and the placenta large enough to deliver the infant. The operator undermines the placenta toward the edge closest to the uterine incision until the membranes are palpable and may be ruptured. Although this approach is intriguing, it has not yet been evaluated in controlled studies.

Because of the poorly contractile nature of the lower uterine segment, there may be uncontrollable hemorrhage following placental removal. This can occur even without

histological confirmation of placenta accreta. Under these circumstances, management appropriate for placenta accreta is indicated (see p. 832). When placenta previa is complicated by degrees of accreta that render control of bleeding from the placental bed difficult by conservative means, other methods of hemostasis are necessary. Oversewing the implantation site with 0 chromic sutures may provide hemostasis. In some women, bilateral uterine or internal iliac artery ligation as described on page 828 may provide hemostasis. Cho and colleagues (1991) have described placing circular interrupted 0 chromic sutures around the lower segment, above and below the transverse incision, which controlled hemorrhage in all eight women in whom this was employed. Druzin (1989) described four cases in which the lower uterine segment was tightly packed with gauze that successfully arrested hemorrhage. The pack was removed transvaginally 12 hours later. Pelvic artery embolization as discussed on page 836 also has gained acceptance (Hansch and colleagues, 1999; Pelage and associates, 1999). If such conservative methods fail, and bleeding is brisk, then hysterectomy is necessary (see Chap. 25, p. 599). **For women whose placenta previa is implanted anteriorly in the site of a prior hysterotomy incision, there is an increased likelihood of associated placenta accreta and need for hysterectomy.**

Prognosis. A marked reduction in maternal mortality from placenta previa has been achieved, a trend that began in 1927 when Bill advocated adequate transfusion and cesarean delivery. Since 1945, when Macafee and Johnson independently suggested expectant therapy for patients remote from term, a similar trend has been evident in perinatal loss. Although half of women are near term when bleeding first develops, preterm delivery still poses a formidable problem for the remainder, because not all women with placenta previa and a preterm fetus can be treated expectantly. Interestingly, Butler and co-workers (2001) found that women with placenta previa who also had maternal serum alpha-fetoprotein levels at least 2.0 multiples of the median (MOM) were at increased risk of bleeding early in the third trimester and of preterm birth.

POSTPARTUM HEMORRHAGE

Hemorrhage following delivery is from excessive bleeding from the placental implantation site, trauma to the genital tract and adjacent structures, or both (Table 35–5). Postpartum hemorrhage is a description of an event rather than a diagnosis, and when encountered, its cause must be determined.

Definition. Traditionally, postpartum hemorrhage has been defined as the loss of 500 mL of blood or more after completion of the third stage of labor. This is unreasonable, because nearly half of all women who are delivered vaginally shed that amount of blood or more when measured

TABLE 35–5 Predisposing Factors and Causes of Immediate Postpartum Hemorrhage

Bleeding from Placental Implantation Site
Hypotonic myometrium—uterine atony
  Some general anesthetics—halogenated hydrocarbons
  Poorly perfused myometrium—hypotension
    Hemorrhage
    Conduction analgesia
  Overdistended uterus—large fetus, twins, hydramnios
  Following prolonged labor
  Following very rapid labor
  Following oxytocin-induced or augmented labor
  High parity
  Uterine atony in previous pregnancy
  Chorioamnionitis
Retained placental tissue
  Avulsed cotyledon, succenturiate lobe
  Abnormally adherent—accreta, increta, percreta

Trauma to the Genital Tract
  Large episiotomy, including extensions
  Lacerations of perineum, vagina, or cervix
  Ruptured uterus

Coagulation Defects
  Intensify all of the above

quantitatively. Blood loss somewhat in excess of 500 mL by accurate measurement is not necessarily unusual for vaginal delivery (Fig. 35–14). Pritchard and associates (1962) found that about 5 percent of women delivering vaginally lost more than 1000 mL of blood. **They also observed that estimated blood loss is commonly only about half the actual loss.** An estimated blood loss in excess of 500 mL in many institutions, therefore, should call attention to mothers who are bleeding excessively and warn the physician that dangerous hemorrhage is imminent.

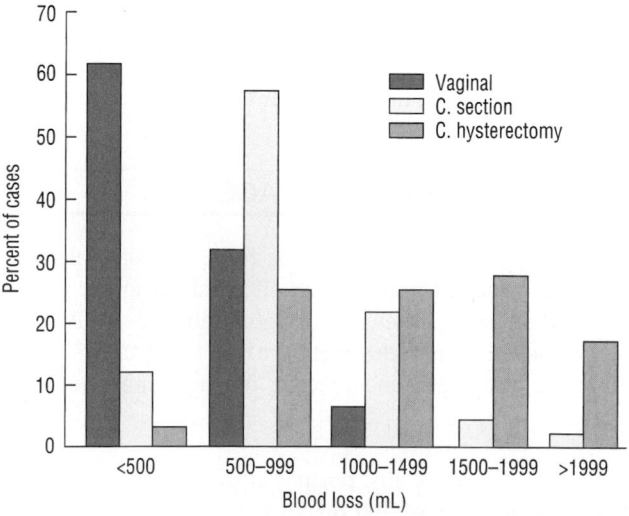

FIGURE 35–14. Blood loss associated with vaginal delivery, repeat cesarean delivery, and repeat cesarean delivery plus hysterectomy. (From Pritchard and associates, 1962, with permission.)

The blood volume of a pregnant woman with normal pregnancy-induced hypervolemia usually increases by 30 to 60 percent, which amounts to 1500 to 2000 mL for an average-sized woman (Pritchard, 1965). Table 35–6 presents an equation that determines this, which we have verified as accurate. A normally pregnant woman tolerates blood loss at delivery that approaches the volume of blood she added during pregnancy without any remarkable decrease in postpartum hematocrit. Thus, if blood loss is less than the amount added by pregnancy, the hematocrit stays the same acutely and eventually increases. **Any time the postpartum hematocrit is lower than one obtained on admission for delivery, blood loss can be estimated as the sum of the calculated pregnancy hypervolemia plus 500 mL for each 3 volumes percent drop in the hematocrit.** In one study, the mean postpartum hematocrit decline ranged from 2.6 to 4.3 volumes percent, and a third of women had no decline or had an actual increase (Combs and colleagues, 1991b). Women undergoing cesarean delivery had a mean drop in hematocrit of 4.2 volume percent, but 20 percent had no decline (Combs and co-workers, 1991a).

Hemorrhage after the first 24 hours is designated *late postpartum hemorrhage* and is discussed in Chapter 30 (see p. 698).

Hemostasis at the Placental Site. Near term, it is estimated that approximately 600 mL/min of blood flows through the intervillous space. With separation of the placenta, there is also separation of the many uterine arteries and veins that carry blood to and from the placenta. Usually, hemostasis in the absence of surgical ligation depends on intrinsic vasospasm and formation of blood clot locally. At the placental implantation site, most important for achieving hemostasis are contraction and retraction of the myometrium to compress the formidable number of relatively large vessels and obliterate their lumens. Adherent pieces of placenta or large blood clots prevent effective contraction and retraction of the myometrium and thereby impair hemostasis at the implantation site. Fatal postpartum hemorrhage can occur from a hypotonic uterus, although the maternal blood coagulation mechanism is quite normal. Conversely, if the myometrium at and adjacent to the denuded implantation site contracts and retracts vigorously, fatal hemorrhage *from the placental implantation site* is unlikely even though the coagulation mechanism is severely impaired.

Clinical Characteristics. Contrary to general opinion, whether postpartum bleeding begins before or after placental delivery, or at both times, there may be no sudden massive hemorrhage but rather steady bleeding that at any given instant appears to be moderate, but persists until serious hypovolemia develops. Especially with hemorrhage after placental delivery, the constant seepage may lead to enormous blood loss.

TABLE 35–6 Calculation of Maternal Total Blood Volume (TBV)

Nonpregnant TBV

$$\frac{[\text{Maternal height (inches)} \times 50] + [\text{Maternal weight (pounds)} \times 25]}{2} = \text{TBV (mL)}$$

Pregnant TBV

Add 50% to nonpregnant TBV but remember normal pregnancy blood volume *increase* varies between 30% and 60% of nonpregnant TBV and increases with gestational age.

Pregnancy TBV increase is less in severe preeclampsia or eclampsia and more with multiple fetuses.

Pregnant TBV in Serious Hemorrhage

Assume acute return to nonpregnant TBV because normal pregnancy hypervolemia has been acutely lost.

From Leveno and colleagues, 2003.

The effects of hemorrhage depend to a considerable degree on the nonpregnant blood volume, magnitude of pregnancy-induced hypervolemia, and degree of anemia at the time of delivery. A treacherous feature of postpartum hemorrhage is the failure of the pulse and blood pressure to undergo more than moderate alterations until large amounts of blood have been lost. The normotensive woman may actually become somewhat hypertensive in response to hemorrhage, at least initially. Moreover, the already hypertensive woman may be interpreted to be normotensive although remarkably hypovolemic. Tragically, the hypovolemia may not be recognized until very late.

The woman with severe preeclampsia or eclampsia does not have normally expanded blood volume. Zeeman and Cunningham (2002) documented a mean increase of only 10 percent in 29 eclamptic women before delivery. Thus, these women are very sensitive to or even intolerant of what may be considered normal blood loss (see Chap. 34, p. 771). **Therefore, when excessive hemorrhage is even suspected in the woman with severe preeclampsia, efforts should be made immediately to identify those clinical and laboratory findings that would prompt vigorous crystalloid and blood replacement.**

In instances in which the fundus has not been adequately monitored after delivery, the blood may not escape vaginally but instead may collect within the uterus. The uterine cavity may thus become distended by 1000 mL or more of blood while an attendant fails to identify the large uterus or, having done so, erroneously massages a roll of abdominal fat. The care of the postpartum uterus, therefore, must not be left to an inexperienced person.

Diagnosis. Except possibly when intrauterine and intravaginal accumulation of blood are not recognized, or in some instances of uterine rupture with intraperitoneal bleeding, the diagnosis of postpartum hemorrhage should be obvious. The differentiation between bleeding from uterine atony and from lacerations is tentatively made on predisposing risk factors and the condition of the uterus (see Table 35–5). If bleeding persists despite a firm, well-contracted uterus, the cause of

the hemorrhage most likely is from lacerations. Bright red blood also suggests lacerations. **To ascertain the role of lacerations as a cause of bleeding, careful inspection of the vagina, cervix, and uterus is essential.**

Sometimes bleeding may be caused by both atony and trauma, especially after major operative delivery. In general, inspection of the cervix and vagina should be performed after every delivery to identify hemorrhage from lacerations. Anesthesia should be adequate to prevent discomfort during such an examination. Examination of the uterine cavity, the cervix, and all of the vagina is essential after internal podalic version and breech extraction. The same is true when unusual bleeding is identified during the second stage of labor.

Sheehan Syndrome. Severe intrapartum or early postpartum hemorrhage is on rare occasions followed by pituitary failure or Sheehan syndrome. The classical case is characterized by failure of lactation, amenorrhea, breast atrophy, loss of pubic and axillary hair, hypothyroidism, and adrenal cortical insufficiency (see Chap. 53, p. 1203). The exact pathogenesis is not well understood, because such endocrine abnormalities do not develop in most women who hemorrhage severely. In some but not all instances of Sheehan syndrome, varying degrees of anterior pituitary necrosis with impaired secretion of one or more trophic hormones account for the endocrine abnormalities. The anterior pituitary of some women who develop hypopituitarism after puerperal hemorrhage does respond to various releasing hormones, which at the least implies impaired hypothalamic function. Moreover, Whitehead (1963) identified specific atrophic changes in hypothalamic nuclei histologically in some cases. Lactation after delivery usually, but not always, excludes extensive pituitary necrosis. In some women, failure to lactate may not be followed until many years later by other symptoms of pituitary insufficiency. In the series reported by Ammini and Mathur (1994), the average duration of onset of symptoms was 5 years.

The incidence of Sheehan syndrome was originally estimated to be 1 per 10,000 deliveries (Sheehan and Murdoch, 1938). It appears to be even less common today (Kovacs,

2003). Bakiri and colleagues (1991) used computed tomography to study 54 women with documented Sheehan syndrome. In all of these, the appearance of the pituitary was abnormal and the sella turcica was either totally or partially empty.

THIRD-STAGE BLEEDING. Some bleeding is inevitable during the third stage as the result of transient partial separation of the placenta. As the placenta separates, blood from the implantation site may escape into the vagina immediately (*Duncan mechanism*), or it may be concealed behind the placenta and membranes (*Schultze mechanism*) until the placenta is delivered.

In the presence of any external hemorrhage during the third stage, the uterus should be massaged if it is not contracted firmly. If the signs of placental separation have appeared, expression of the placenta should be attempted by manual fundal pressure as described in Chapter 17 (see p. 432). Descent of the placenta is indicated by the cord becoming slack. If bleeding continues, manual removal of the placenta is mandatory. **Delivery of the placenta by cord traction, especially when the uterus is atonic, may cause uterine inversion.** Prevention and management of this are discussed in detail on page 833.

Prolonged Third-Stage Bleeding. Occasionally, the placenta does not separate promptly. There is still no definite answer to the question concerning the length of time that should elapse in the absence of bleeding before the placenta is removed manually. Obstetrical tradition has set somewhat arbitrary limits on third-stage duration in attempts to define *abnormally retained placenta* and thus reduce blood loss due to excessively prolonged placental separation. Combs and Laros (1991) studied 12,275 singleton vaginal deliveries and reported the median third-stage duration to be 6 minutes; for 3.3 percent of these women, it was more than 30 minutes. Several measures of hemorrhage, including curettage or transfusion, increased when the third stage was about 30 minutes or longer. Prolonged third-stage labor is discussed in Chapter 17 (see p. 432).

Technique of Manual Removal. Adequate analgesia or anesthesia is mandatory. Aseptic surgical technique should be used. After grasping the fundus through the abdominal wall with one hand, the other hand is introduced into the vagina and passed into the uterus, along the umbilical cord. As soon as the placenta is reached, its margin is located and the ulnar border of the hand insinuated between it and the uterine wall (Fig. 35–15). Then with the back of the hand in contact with the uterus, the placenta is peeled off its uterine attachment by a motion similar to that used in separating the leaves of a book. After its complete separation, the placenta should be grasped with the entire hand, which is then gradually withdrawn. Membranes are removed at the same time by carefully teasing them from the decidua, using ring forceps

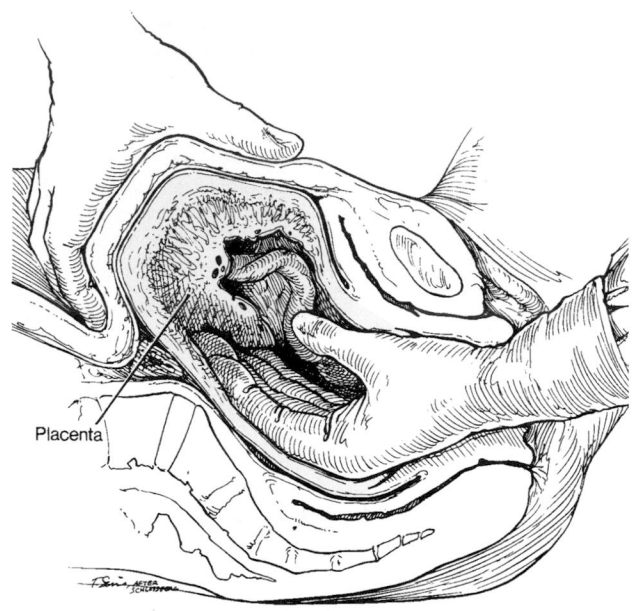

Placenta

FIGURE 35–15. Manual removal of placenta. The fingers are swept from side to side and advanced until the placenta is completely detached.

to grasp them as necessary. Some clinicians prefer to wipe out the uterine cavity with a sponge.

Management after Delivery of Placenta. The fundus should always be palpated following placental delivery to make certain that the uterus is well contracted. If it is not firm, vigorous fundal massage is indicated. Most often, 20 U of oxytocin in 1000 mL of lactated Ringer or normal saline proves effective when administered intravenously at approximately 10 mL/min (200 mU of oxytocin per minute) simultaneously with effective uterine massage. Oxytocin should never be given as an undiluted bolus dose, because serious hypotension or cardiac arrhythmias may occur (see Chap. 17, p. 434).

UTERINE ATONY. Failure of the uterus to contract properly following delivery is a common cause of obstetrical hemorrhage. In many women, uterine atony can at least be suspected well in advance of delivery (see Table 35–5). For example, the overdistended uterus is prone to be hypotonic after delivery. Thus, the woman with a large fetus, multiple fetuses, or hydramnios is prone to hemorrhage from uterine atony. The woman whose labor is characterized by uterine activity that is either remarkably vigorous or barely effective is also likely to bleed excessively from uterine atony after delivery. Similarly, labor either initiated or augmented with oxytocin is more likely to be followed by postdelivery uterine atony and hemorrhage.

The woman of high parity may be at increased risk for uterine atony. Fuchs and colleagues (1985) described the outcomes of nearly 5800 women para 7 or greater. They reported that the 2.7 percent incidence of postpartum hemorrhage in these women was increased fourfold compared with that of the general obstetrical population. Babinszki and colleagues (1999) reported the incidence of postpartum hemorrhage to be 0.3 percent in women of low parity, but it was 1.9 percent in those para 4 or greater. Another risk is if the woman has previously suffered postpartum hemorrhage. Finally, mismanagement of the third stage of labor involves an attempt to hasten delivery of the placenta short of manual removal. **Constant kneading and squeezing of the uterus that already is contracted likely impedes the physiological mechanism of placental detachment, causing incomplete placental separation and increased blood loss.**

Ergot Derivatives. If oxytocin given by rapid infusion as described on page 826 does not prove effective, some clinicians administer intramuscular methylergonovine (0.2 mg). This may stimulate the uterus to contract sufficiently to control hemorrhage. Any superior therapeutic effects of ergot derivatives over oxytocin are speculative, and if these agents are intravenously administered, they may cause dangerous hypertension, especially in women with preeclampsia.

Prostaglandins. The 15-methyl derivative of prostaglandin $F_{2\alpha}$ (carboprost tromethamine) was approved in the mid-1980s by the U.S. Food and Drug Administration (FDA) for treatment of uterine atony. The initial recommended dose is 250 μg (0.25 mg) given intramuscularly, and this is repeated if necessary at 15- to 90-minute intervals up to a maximum of eight doses. Oleen and Mariano (1990) studied use of carboprost for postpartum hemorrhage at 12 cooperating obstetrical units. Arrest of bleeding was considered successful in 208 (88 percent) of 237 women treated. Another 17 women (7 percent) required other oxytocics for control of hemorrhage. The remaining 12 women (5 percent) required surgical intervention.

Carboprost is associated with side effects in about 20 percent of women (Oleen and Mariano, 1990). In descending order of frequency, these include diarrhea, hypertension, vomiting, fever, flushing, and tachycardia. We have encountered serious hypertension in a few women so treated. In addition, Hankins and colleagues (1988) observed that intramuscular carboprost was followed by arterial oxygen desaturation that averaged 10 percent and developed within 15 minutes. They concluded that this was due to pulmonary airway and vascular constriction.

Rectally administered prostaglandin E_2 20-mg suppositories have been used for uterine atony but not studied in clinical trials. A few reports have suggested that misoprostol (Cytotec), a synthetic prostaglandin E_1 analogue, may be effective for the treatment of uterine atony (Abdel-Aleem and associates, 2001; O'Brien and colleagues, 1998). In the larger of these uncontrolled studies, misoprostol (1000 μg) given rectally was effective in 16 of 18 women unresponsive to usual oxytocics. The mean response time was 1.4 minutes.

Misoprostol has also been studied as a potential prophylactic treatment for preventing postpartum hemorrhage. Based on their study of 325 women, Gerstenfeld and Wing (2001) concluded that rectal misoprostol (400 μg) was no more effective than intravenous oxytocin in preventing postpartum hemorrhage. Moreover, Villar and co-workers (2002) found in their systematic review that oxytocin and ergot preparations administered during the third stage of labor were more effective than misoprostol for the prevention of postpartum hemorrhage.

Bleeding Unresponsive to Oxytocics. Continued bleeding after multiple administrations of oxytocics may be from unrecognized genital tract lacerations, including in some cases uterine rupture. Thus, if bleeding persists, no time should be lost in haphazard efforts to control hemorrhage, but the following management should be initiated immediately:

1. Use bimanual uterine compression (Fig. 35–16). The technique consists simply of massage of the posterior aspect of the uterus with the abdominal hand and massage through the vagina of the anterior uterine aspect with the other fist. This procedure controls most hemorrhage.
2. Obtain help!
3. Add a second large-bore intravenous catheter so that crystalloid with oxytocin may be continued at the same time blood is given.
4. Begin blood transfusions. The blood group of every obstetrical patient should be known, if possible, before labor and an indirect Coombs test done to detect erythrocyte antibodies. If the latter is negative, then crossmatching of blood is not necessary (see p. 841). In an extreme emergency, type O D-negative "universal donor" blood is given.

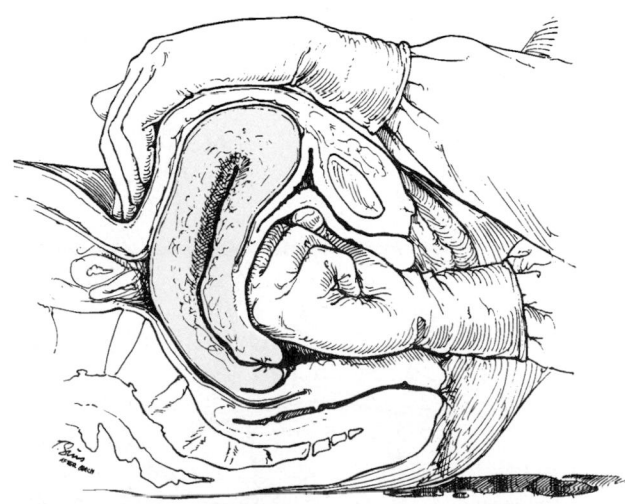

FIGURE 35–16. Bimanual compression of the uterus and massage with the abdominal hand usually effectively controls hemorrhage from uterine atony.

5. Explore the uterine cavity manually for retained placental fragments or lacerations.
6. Thoroughly inspect the cervix and vagina after adequate exposure.
7. Insert a Foley catheter to monitor urine output, which is a good measure of renal perfusion.

Resuscitation is then carried out as described subsequently on page 839. Blood transfusion should be considered in any woman with postpartum hemorrhage in whom abdominal uterine massage and oxytocic agents fail to control the bleeding. With transfusion and simultaneous manual uterine compression and intravenous oxytocin, additional measures are rarely required. Intractable atony may mandate hysterectomy as a lifesaving measure (see Chap. 25, p. 599). Alternatively, uterine artery ligation (Fig. 35–17), internal iliac artery ligation (Figs. 35–18 and 35–19), uterine compression sutures (Fig. 35–20), or angiographic embolization as described on page 836 may prove successful.

INTERNAL ILIAC ARTERY LIGATION. Ligation of the internal iliac arteries at times reduces the hemorrhage appreciably (Allahbadia, 1993; Clark and colleagues, 1985). However, the procedure may be technically difficult and is successful in less than half of the patients in whom it is attempted (American College of Obstetricians and Gynecologists, 1998). With adequate exposure, ligation is accomplished by opening the peritoneum over the common iliac artery and dissecting down to the bifurcation of the external and internal iliac arteries (see Figs. 35–18 and 35–19). The areolar sheath covering the internal iliac artery is incised longitudinally, and a right-angle clamp is carefully passed just beneath the artery. Care must

be taken not to perforate contiguous large veins, especially the internal iliac vein. Suture, usually nonabsorbable, is then inserted into the open clamp, the jaws are locked, the suture is carried around the vessel, and the vessel is securely ligated. Pulsations in the external iliac artery, if present before tying the ligature, should be present afterward as well. If not, pulsations must be identified after arterial hypotension has been successfully treated to ensure that the blood flow through the external iliac vessel has not been compromised by the ligature.

The most important mechanism of action with internal iliac artery ligation is an 85-percent reduction in pulse pressure in those arteries distal to the ligation (Burchell, 1968). This converts an arterial pressure system into one with pressures approaching those in the venous circulation and more amenable to hemostasis via simple clot formation. Bilateral ligation of these arteries does not appear to interfere with subsequent reproduction. Nizard and associates (2003) documented 21 pregnancies in 17 women after bilateral internal iliac artery ligation including three abortions, three miscarriages, two ectopic pregnancies, and 13 normal pregnancies.

UTERINE COMPRESSION SUTURES. In 1997, B-Lynch and colleagues described a surgical technique performed in five women with severe postpartum hemorrhage in which a pair of vertical brace #2 chromic sutures were secured around the uterus, giving the appearance of suspenders, to compress together the anterior and posterior walls (see Fig. 35–20). A simpler modification of the technique has been described by Hayman and associates (2002). We have found this suture to be effective in some cases, however, published experience with these techniques remains limited.

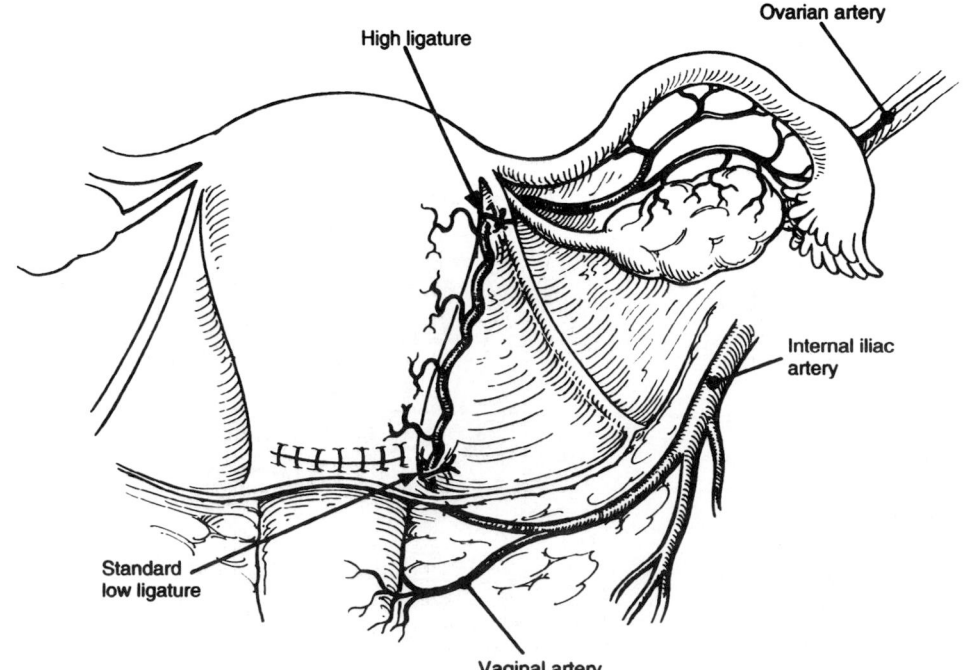

High ligature

Ovarian artery

Internal iliac artery

Standard low ligature

Vaginal artery

FIGURE 35–17. Uterine artery ligation performed superiorly at the approximate junction between the utero-ovarian ligament and the uterus and inferiorly just below the uterine incision. (From Gilstrap, 2002.)

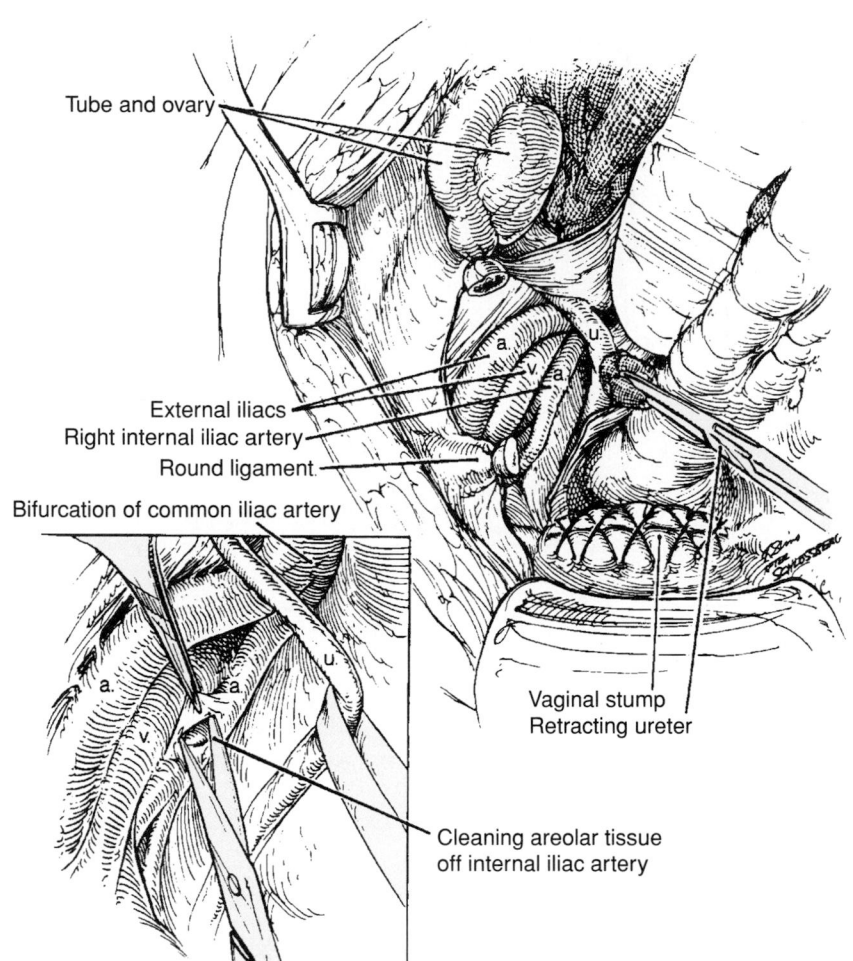

Tube and ovary

External iliacs
Right internal iliac artery
Round ligament
Bifurcation of common iliac artery

Cleaning areolar tissue
off internal iliac artery

Vaginal stump
Retracting ureter

FIGURE 35–18. Ligation of the right internal iliac artery. In the lower left insert, the areolar sheath covering the artery is being opened. (a. = artery; u. = ureter; v. = vein.)

UTERINE PACKING. This technique should be considered in women with refractory postpartum hemorrhage related to uterine atony who wish to preserve fertility. Popular during the first half of the 20th century, uterine packing subsequently fell out of favor because of concerns about concealed bleeding and infection (Hsu and co-workers, 2003). Newer techniques, however, have allayed some of these concerns (Roman and Rebarber, 2003). In one technique, the tip of a no. 24F Foley catheter with a 30-mL balloon is guided into the uterine cavity and filled with 60 to 80 mL of saline. The open tip permits continuous drainage from the uterus. If bleeding subsides, the catheter is typically removed after 12 to 24 hours (Roman and Rebarber, 2003). Alternatively, the uterus or pelvis may be packed directly with gauze (Gilstrap, 2002). After hysterectomy, another technique, the umbrella pack, can be constructed of a sterile x-ray cassette bag, filled with gauze rolls knotted together, providing enough volume to fill the pelvis (Howard and co-workers, 2002). The pack is introduced transabdominally with the stalk exiting the vagina. Mild traction is applied by tying the stalk to a one-liter intravenous fluid bag and hanging the bag over the foot of the bed. An indwelling urinary

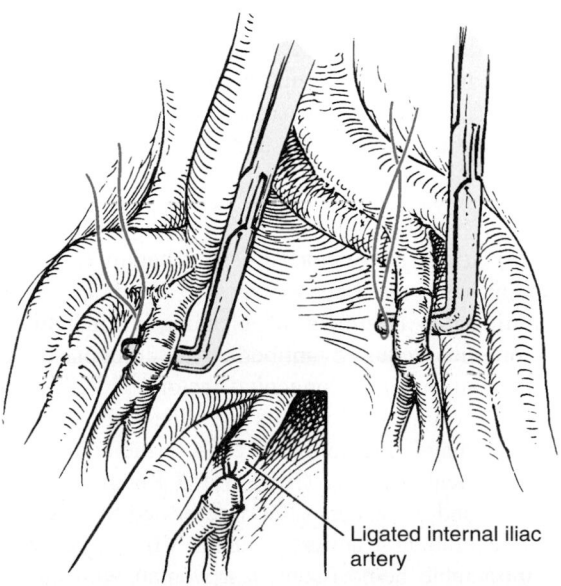

Ligated internal iliac artery

FIGURE 35–19. Ligation of both internal iliac arteries. After the covering sheath has been opened and the artery has been carefully freed from the immediately adjacent veins, a ligature is carried beneath the artery with a right angle clamp and firmly tied.

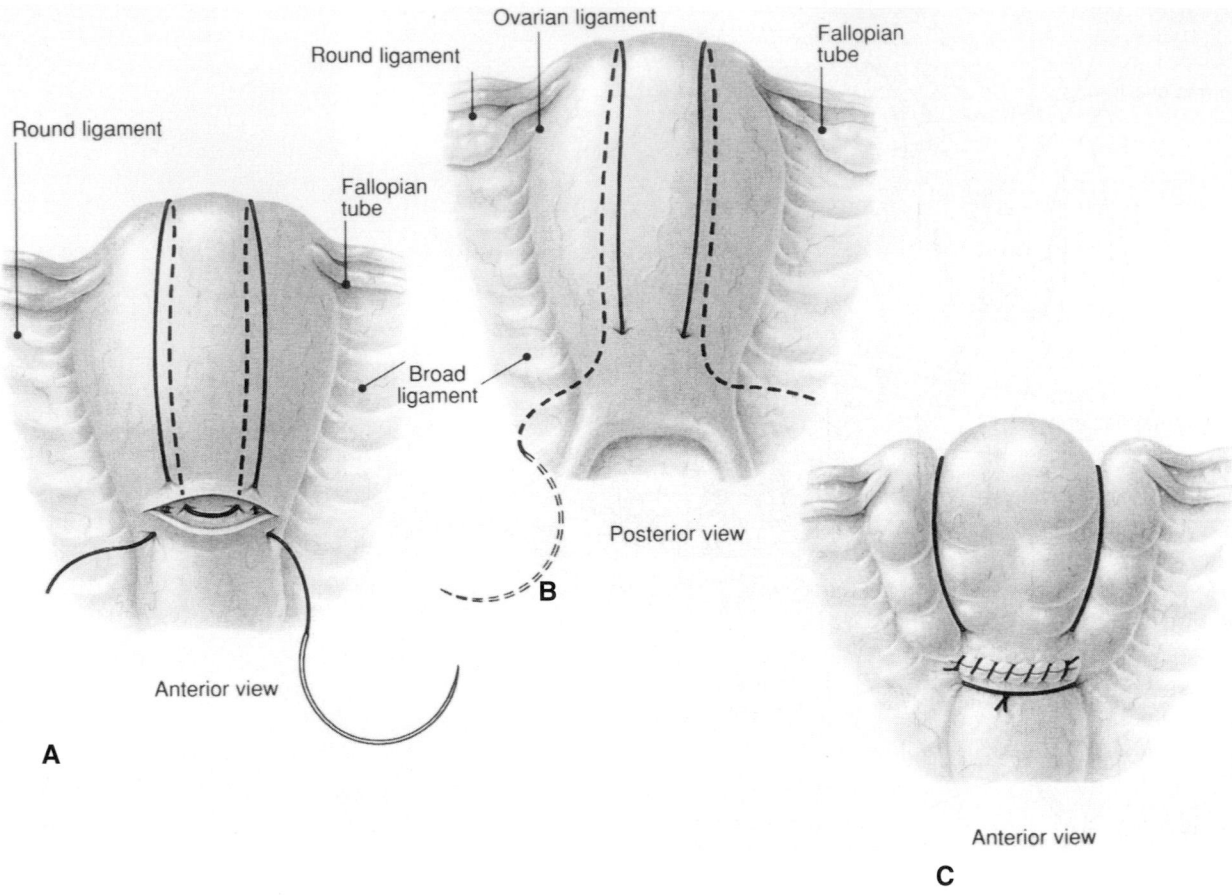

FIGURE 35–20. The B-Lynch uterine compression suture technique. Parts (**A**) and (**B**) demonstrate the anterior and posterior views of the uterus showing application of the suture. Part (**C**) shows the anatomical appearance after completion. (From B-Lynch and colleagues, 1997, with permission.)

catheter is used to monitor urine output and to prevent urinary obstruction. Placement of percutaneous pelvic drains should be considered to monitor ongoing bleeding within the peritoneal cavity (Dildy, 2002). Broad-spectrum antimicrobials should be administered, and the umbrella pack is removed vaginally after 24 hours.

RECOMBINANT ACTIVATED FACTOR VII. This vitamin K–dependent protein has been licensed by the Food and Drug Administration for treatment of bleeding in individuals with hemophilia, acquired antibodies to components of the intrinsic pathway, and congenital factor VII deficiency. Other clinicians have explored its usefulness for the control of hemorrhage due to other causes, including traumatic and surgical bleeding (Branch and Rodgers, 2003). Bouwmeester and associates (2003) described the successful use of recombinant activated factor VII for the treatment of intractable hemorrhage in a woman with uterine atony and vaginal lacerations who did not respond to uterotonic drugs, suturing, ligation of the internal iliac arteries, subtotal hysterectomy, packing of the pelvis, and blood and component transfusions. Although this therapy

looks promising, thrombotic complications have been reported, and additional study clearly is needed (Siegel and associates, 2004).

HEMORRHAGE FROM RETAINED PLACENTAL FRAGMENTS. Immediate postpartum hemorrhage is seldom caused by retained small placental fragments, but a remaining piece of placenta is a common cause of bleeding late in the puerperium. Inspection of the placenta after delivery must be routine. If a portion of placenta is missing, the uterus should be explored and the fragment removed, particularly with continuing postpartum bleeding. Retention of a *succenturiate lobe* is an occasional cause of postpartum hemorrhage (see Chap. 27, p. 620). The late bleeding that may result from a placental polyp is discussed in Chapter 30 (see p. 698).

PLACENTA ACCRETA, INCRETA, AND PERCRETA. In most instances, the placenta separates spontaneously from its implantation site during the first few minutes after delivery of the infant. Very infrequently, detachment is delayed because the placenta is unusually adherent to the implantation

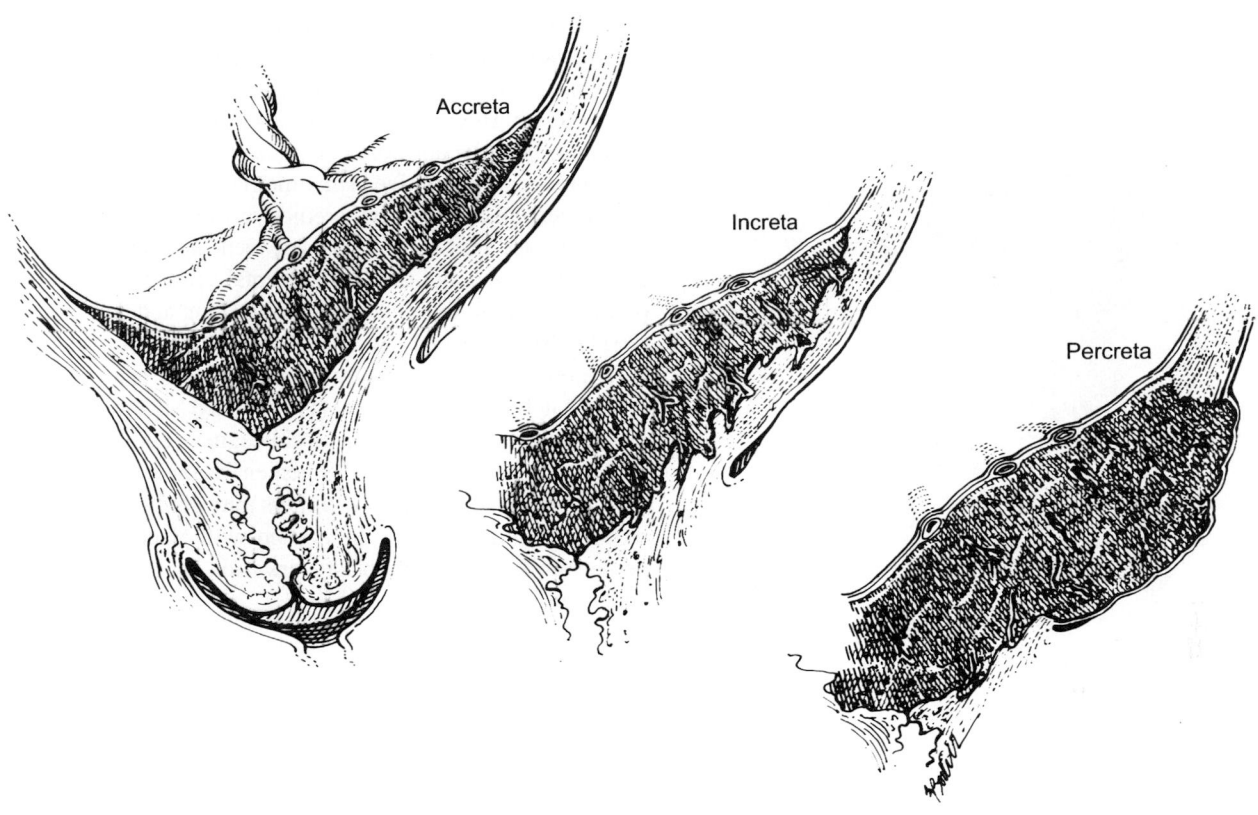

FIGURE 35–21. Placenta accreta, increta, and percreta.

site, with scanty or absent decidua, so that the physiological line of cleavage through the decidual spongy layer is lacking. As a consequence, one or more cotyledons are firmly bound to the defective decidua basalis or even to the myometrium. When the placenta is densely anchored in this fashion, the condition is called placenta accreta.

Definitions. The term *placenta accreta* is used to describe any placental implantation in which there is abnormally firm adherence to the uterine wall. As the consequence of partial or total absence of the decidua basalis and imperfect development of the fibrinoid layer (*Nitabuch layer*), placental villi are attached to the myometrium in *placenta accreta,* actually invade the myometrium in *placenta increta,* or penetrate through the myometrium in *placenta percreta* (Figs. 35–21 and 35–22). The abnormal adherence may involve all of the cotyledons (*total placenta accreta*), a few to several cotyledons (*partial placenta accreta*), or a single cotyledon (*focal placenta accreta*). According to Benirschke and Kaufmann (2000), histological diagnosis of accreta cannot be made from the placenta alone and the entire uterus or curettings with myometrium are necessary.

Significance. An abnormally adherent placenta, although an uncommon condition, assumes considerable significance clinically because of morbidity and, at times, mortality from severe hemorrhage, uterine perforation, and infection.

Indeed, Zelop and colleagues (1993) reported that abnormally adherent placentation caused 65 percent of cases of intractable postpartum hemorrhage requiring emergency peripartum hysterectomy at Brigham and Women's Hospital. The incidence of placenta accreta, increta, and percreta have increased, most likely because of the increased cesarean delivery rate (see Chap. 25, p. 589). The American College of Obstetricians and Gynecologists (2002) estimates that placenta accreta complicates 1 in 2500 deliveries, a 10-fold increase over the past 50 years.

Etiology. Abnormal placental adherence is found when decidual formation is defective. Associated conditions include implantation in the lower uterine segment over a previous surgical scar or after uterine curettage. In a review of 622 cases collected between 1945 and 1969, Fox (1972) noted the following characteristics:

1. Placenta previa was identified in a third of affected pregnancies.
2. A fourth of the women had a prior cesarean delivery.
3. Nearly a fourth had previously undergone curettage.
4. A fourth were gravida 6 or more.

Zaki and associates (1998) found that 10 percent of 112 consecutive cases of placenta previa had associated accreta. Hardardottir and colleagues (1996) observed that almost

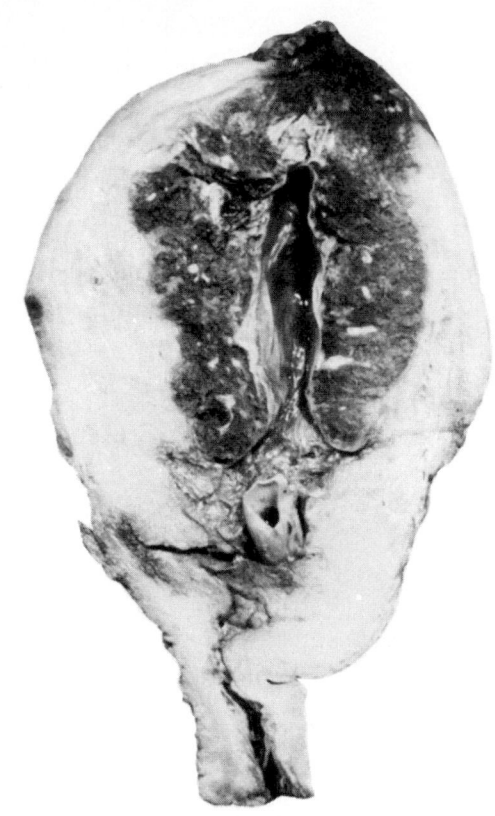

FIGURE 35–22. Placenta percreta. The placenta is fungating through the fundus above the old classical cesarean scar. The variable penetration of the fundus by the placenta is evident. (From Morrison, 1978, with permission.)

50 percent of placentas in women with a prior cesarean delivery had adherent myometrial fibers detected microscopically.

Other risk factors for placenta accreta were analyzed by Hung and co-workers (1999) in their study of over 9300 women screened for Down syndrome at 14 to 22 weeks. Compared with the normal population, they found a 54-fold increased risk for accreta with placenta previa, an 8.3-fold increased risk when maternal serum alpha-fetoprotein levels exceeded 2.5 MoM, a 3.9-fold increased risk when maternal free β-human chorionic gonadotropin (β-hCG) levels were greater than 2.5 MoM, and a 3.2-fold increased risk with maternal age of 35 years of age or older.

Clinical Course and Diagnosis. Early in pregnancy, the maternal serum alpha-fetoprotein level may be increased (see Chap. 13, p. 321). Antepartum hemorrhage is common, but in the great majority of women, bleeding before delivery is the consequence of coexisting placenta previa. Myometrial invasion by placental villi at the site of a previous cesarean scar may lead to uterine rupture before labor (Berchuck and Sokol, 1983; Liang and co-workers, 2003). We have seen this as early as 12 weeks in a woman explored for an ectopic pregnancy. In women whose pregnancies go to term, however, labor will most likely be normal in the absence of an associated placenta previa or an involved uterine scar.

The possibility exists that placenta increta might be diagnosed antepartum. Lam and colleagues (2002) found that ultrasound was only 33-percent sensitive for detecting placenta accreta. However, using ultrasound Doppler color flow mapping, Twickler and colleagues (2000) found that two factors were highly predictive of myometrial invasion (sensitivity of 100 percent and positive predictive value of 78 percent): (1) a distance less than 1 mm between the uterine serosal bladder interface and the retroplacental vessels, and (2) the presence of large intraplacental lakes. Chou and co-workers (2001) also described successful use of three-dimensional color power Doppler imaging for diagnosis of placenta percreta. Maldjian and co-workers (1999) used MRI to diagnose placenta accreta, but Lam and colleagues (2002) reported that its sensitivity was only 38 percent. Baxi and associates (2004) found that elevated D-dimers may predict significant blood loss and morbidity in women with placenta accreta, perhaps reflecting trophoblastic invasion into myometrium and adjacent tissues.

Management. The problems associated with delivery of the placenta and subsequent developments vary appreciably, depending on the site of implantation, depth of myometrial penetration, and number of cotyledons involved. It is likely that focal placenta accreta with implantation in the upper uterine segment develops much more often than is recognized. Either the involved cotyledon is pulled off the myometrium with perhaps somewhat excessive bleeding, or the cotyledon is torn from the placenta and adheres to the implantation site with increased bleeding, immediately or later. According to Benirschke and Kaufmann (2000), this may be one mechanism for formation of so-called placental polyps (see Chap. 30, p. 698).

With more extensive involvement, hemorrhage becomes profuse as delivery of the placenta is attempted. Successful treatment depends on immediate blood replacement therapy as described on page 839 and nearly always prompt hysterectomy. This may be facilitated by fully developing the bladder flap and dissecting it around the percreta if possible prior to delivery. Alternative measures include uterine or internal iliac artery ligation (see p. 828) or angiographic embolization (see p. 836). Karam and colleagues (2003) described use of argon beam coagulation for hemostasis in a woman with placenta percreta with bladder invasion.

With total placenta accreta, there may be very little or no bleeding, at least until manual placental removal is attempted. At times, traction on the umbilical cord inverts the uterus, as described in the next section. Moreover, usual attempts at manual removal do not succeed, because a cleavage plane between the maternal placental surface and the uterine wall cannot be developed. In the past, the most common form of "conservative" management was manual removal of as much placenta as possible and then packing of the uterus. In the review by Fox (1972), 25 percent of women managed conservatively died. Thus, the safest treatment in this circumstance is prompt hysterectomy.

Another possible option for women who are not bleeding significantly is to leave the entire placenta in place. Although this approach has not been studied in depth, Kayem and colleagues (2002) described a case in which they left the placenta in place and also performed uterine artery embolization as prophylaxis against delayed hemorrhage. The placenta was spontaneously resorbed within 6 months, and the patient subsequently had an uncomplicated pregnancy 3 years later. Henrich and co-workers (2002) described a similar case in which the placenta was left in situ, and weekly methotrexate therapy was given postpartum. The placenta spontaneously delivered through the vagina 4 weeks later. Nijman and co-workers (2002) have reviewed other cases in which methotrexate was used to treat retained placenta percreta.

INVERSION OF THE UTERUS. Complete uterine inversion after delivery of the infant is almost always the consequence of strong traction on an umbilical cord attached to a placenta implanted in the fundus (Fig. 35–23). Incomplete uterine inversion may also occur (Fig. 35–24). Contributing to uterine inversion is a tough cord that does not readily break away from the placenta, combined with fundal pressure and a relaxed uterus, including the lower segment and cervix. Placenta accreta may be implicated, although uterine inversion can occur without the placenta being so firmly adherent.

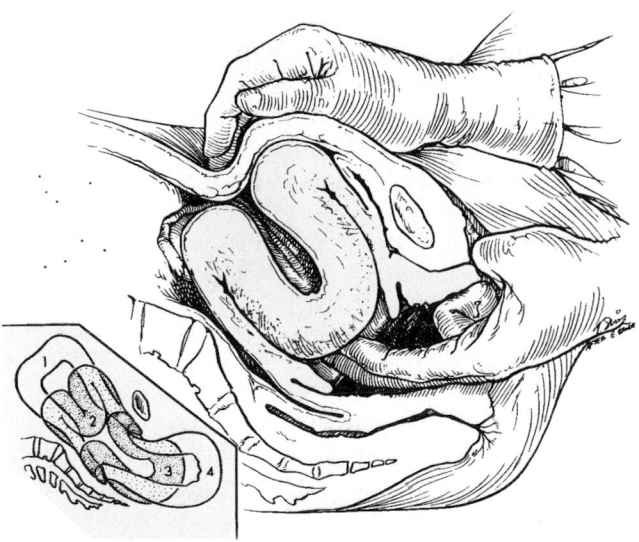

FIGURE 35–24. Incomplete uterine inversion. The diagnosis is made by abdominal palpation of the crater-like depression and vaginal palpation of the fundal wall in the lower segment and cervix. Progressive degrees of inversion are shown in the inset.

Shah-Hosseini and Evrard (1989) reported an incidence of about 1 in 6400 deliveries at the Women and Infants Hospital of Rhode Island. Of the 11 inversions identified, most were in primiparous women. Immediate vaginal replacement of the inverted uterus was successful in nine instances. Platt and Druzin (1981) reported 28 cases in over 60,000 deliveries, for an incidence of about 1 in 2100. On the busy obstetrical service at Parkland Hospital, we encounter several cases annually, and most are in "low-risk" deliveries.

Clinical Course. Uterine inversion is most often associated with immediate life-threatening hemorrhage, and without prompt treatment it may be fatal (Fig. 35–25). In the past it

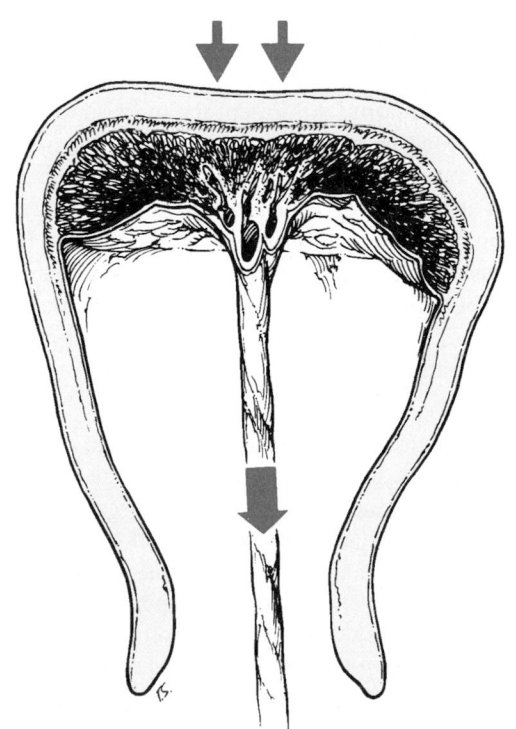

FIGURE 35–23. Most likely site of placental implantation in cases of uterine inversion. With traction on the cord and the placenta still attached, the likelihood of inversion is obvious.

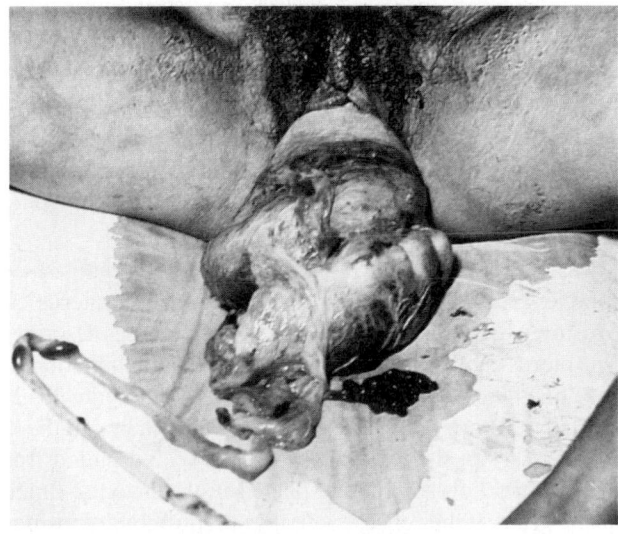

FIGURE 35–25. A fatal case of inverted uterus associated with placenta accreta following delivery at home.

was stated that shock tended to be disproportionate to blood loss. Careful evaluation of the effects from transfusion of large volumes of blood in such cases does not support this concept, but instead makes it very apparent that blood loss in these circumstances was often massive but greatly underestimated (Watson and associates, 1980).

Treatment. Delay in treatment increases the mortality rate appreciably. It is imperative that a number of steps be taken immediately and simultaneously:

1. Assistance, including an anesthesiologist, is summoned immediately.
2. The freshly inverted uterus with placenta already separated from it may often be replaced simply by immediately pushing up on the fundus with the palm of the hand and fingers in the direction of the long axis of the vagina.
3. Preferably two intravenous infusion systems are made operational, and lactated Ringer solution and blood are given to treat hypovolemia.
4. If attached, the placenta is not removed until the infusion systems are operational, fluids are being given, and anesthesia, preferably halothane or enflurane, has been administered. Tocolytic drugs such as terbutaline, ritodrine, or magnesium sulfate have been used successfully for uterine relaxation and repositioning (Catanzarite and associates, 1986; Kovacs and DeVore, 1984; Thiery and Delbeke, 1985). In the meantime, the inverted uterus, if prolapsed beyond the vagina, is replaced within the vagina.
5. After removing the placenta, the palm of the hand is placed on the center of the fundus with the fingers extended to identify the margins of the cervix. Pressure is then applied with the hand so as to push the fundus upward through the cervix.
6. As soon as the uterus is restored to its normal configuration, the agent used to provide relaxation is stopped, and simultaneously oxytocin is started to contract the uterus while the operator maintains the fundus in normal relationship.

Initially, bimanual compression (see Fig. 35–16) aids in control of further hemorrhage until uterine tone is recovered. After the uterus is well contracted, the operator continues to monitor the uterus transvaginally for any evidence of subsequent inversion.

SURGICAL INTERVENTION. Most often, the inverted uterus can be restored to its normal position by the techniques described. If the uterus cannot be reinverted by vaginal manipulation because of a dense constriction ring as shown in Figure 35–26, then laparotomy is imperative. The fundus then may be simultaneously pushed upward from below and pulled from above. A traction suture well placed in the inverted fundus may be of aid. If the constriction ring still prohibits reposition, it is carefully incised posteriorly to expose the fundus. This surgical technique was described by Van Vugt and associates

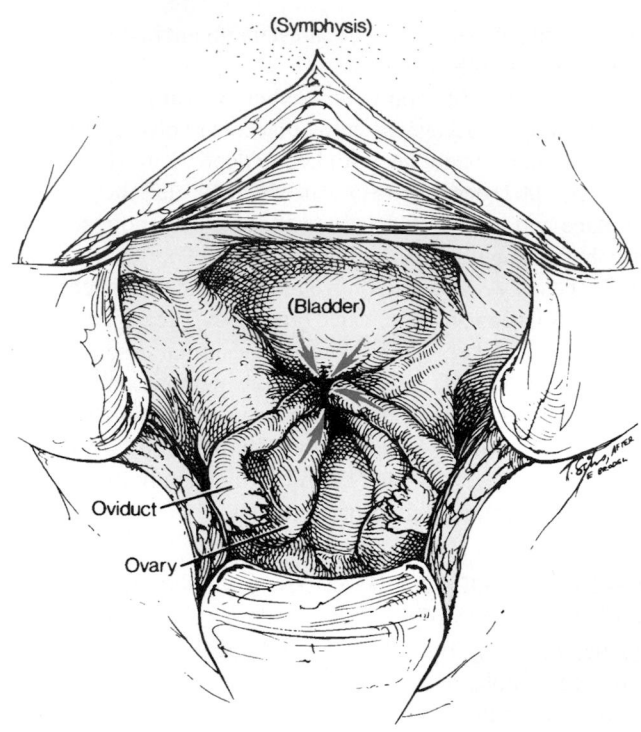

FIGURE 35–26. Completely inverted uterus viewed from above.

(1981). After replacement of the fundus, the anesthetic agent used to relax the myometrium is stopped, oxytocin infusion is begun, and the uterine incision is repaired.

GENITAL TRACT LACERATIONS

Perineal Lacerations. All except the most superficial perineal lacerations are accompanied by varying degrees of injury to the lower portion of the vagina. Such tears may reach sufficient depth to involve the anal sphincter and may extend to varying depths through the walls of the vagina. Bilateral lacerations into the vagina are usually unequal in length and separated by a tongue-shaped portion of vaginal mucosa (see Fig. 17–34). Their repair should form part of every operation for the restoration of a lacerated perineum.

Vaginal Lacerations. Isolated lacerations involving the middle or upper third of the vagina but unassociated with lacerations of the perineum or cervix are observed less commonly. These are usually longitudinal and frequently result from injuries sustained during a forceps or vacuum delivery, but they may even develop with spontaneous delivery. Such lacerations frequently extend deep into the underlying tissues and may give rise to significant hemorrhage, which usually is controlled by appropriate suturing. They may be overlooked unless thorough inspection of the upper vagina is performed. **Bleeding while the uterus is firmly contracted is strong evidence of genital tract laceration, retained placental fragments, or both.**

Lacerations of the anterior vaginal wall in close proximity to the urethra are relatively common. They are often superficial with little to no bleeding, and repair is usually not indicated. If such lacerations are large enough to require extensive repair, difficulty in voiding can be anticipated, and an indwelling catheter is placed.

Injuries to Levator Ani. These are the result of overdistention of the birth canal. Muscle fibers are separated, and diminution in their tonicity may be sufficient to interfere with the function of the pelvic diaphragm. In such cases, pelvic relaxation may develop. If the injuries involve the pubococcygeus muscle, urinary incontinence also may develop (see Chap. 20, p. 520).

Injuries to the Cervix. The cervix is lacerated in over half of all vaginal deliveries (Fahmy and associates, 1991). Most of these are less than 0.5 cm. Deep cervical tears may extend to the upper third of the vagina. In rare instances, however, the cervix may be entirely or partially avulsed from the vagina, with colporrhexis in the anterior, posterior, or lateral fornices. Such injuries sometimes follow difficult forceps rotations or deliveries performed through an incompletely dilated cervix with the forceps blades applied over the cervix. Rarely, cervical tears may extend to involve the lower uterine segment and uterine artery and its major branches, and even through the peritoneum. They may be totally unsuspected, but much more often they become manifest by excessive external hemorrhage or by hematoma formation.

Extensive tears of the vaginal vault should be explored carefully. If there is question of peritoneal perforation, or of retroperitoneal or intraperitoneal hemorrhage, laparotomy should be considered. With damage of this severity, intrauterine exploration for possible rupture is also indicated. Surgical repair is usually required, and effective anesthesia, vigorous blood replacement, and capable assistance are mandatory.

Cervical lacerations up to 2 cm must be regarded as inevitable in childbirth. Such tears heal rapidly and are rarely the source of any difficulty. In healing, they cause a significant change in the round shape of the external os, from circular before labor to appreciably widened after delivery. As the consequence of such tears, there may be eversion of the cervix with exposure of the delicate mucus-producing endocervical glands.

Occasionally, the edematous anterior lip of the cervix may be caught during labor and compressed between the head and the symphysis pubis. If ischemia is severe, the cervical lip may undergo necrosis and separation. More rarely, the entire vaginal portion may be avulsed from the rest of the cervix. Such *annular or circular detachment of the cervix* is uncommon in modern obstetrics.

DIAGNOSIS. A deep cervical tear should always be suspected in women with profuse hemorrhage during and after third-stage labor, particularly if the uterus is firmly contracted. Thorough

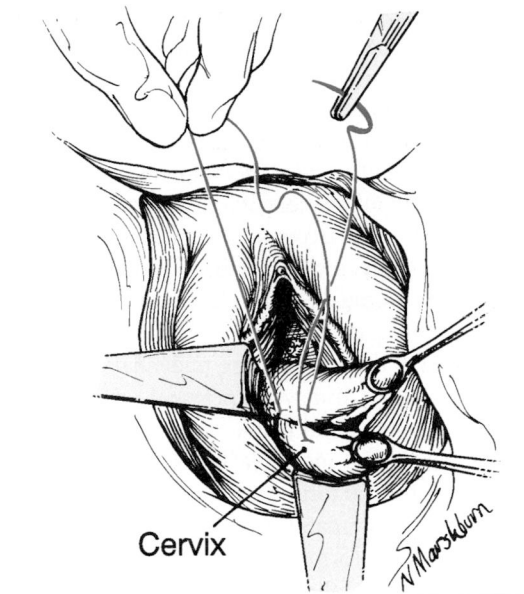

FIGURE 35–27. Cervical laceration exposed for repair.

examination is necessary, and the flabby cervix often makes digital examination alone unsatisfactory. Thus, the extent of the injury can be fully appreciated only after adequate exposure and visual inspection of the cervix. The best exposure is gained by the use of right-angle vaginal retractors by an assistant while the operator grasps the patulous cervix with a ring forceps (Fig. 35–27).

In view of the frequency with which deep tears follow major operative vaginal deliveries, the cervix should be inspected routinely at the conclusion of the third stage after all difficult deliveries, even if there is no bleeding.

TREATMENT. Deep cervical tears require surgical repair. When the laceration is limited to the cervix, or even when it extends somewhat into the vaginal fornix, satisfactory results are obtained by suturing the cervix after bringing it into view at the vulva. Visualization is best accomplished when an *assistant* applies firm downward pressure on the uterus while the operator exerts traction on the lips of the cervix with fenestrated ovum or sponge forceps. Right-angle vaginal wall retractors are often helpful (see Fig. 35–27). Because the hemorrhage usually comes from the upper angle of the wound, the first suture is placed just above the angle. Suturing proceeds outward toward the operator. Associated vaginal lacerations may be tamponaded with gauze packs to retard hemorrhage while cervical lacerations are repaired. Either interrupted or running absorbable sutures are suitable. Overzealous suturing in an attempt to restore the normal cervical appearance may lead to subsequent stenosis during uterine involution. Lichtenberg (2003) described the successful use of angiography for treatment of a high cervical tear after attempted surgical repair failed. This method is discussed on page 836.

PUERPERAL HEMATOMAS. In a review of seven series, the incidence of puerperal hematomas was found to vary from 1 in 300 to 1 in 1000 deliveries (Cunningham, 2002). Nulliparity, episiotomy, and forceps delivery are the most commonly associated risk factors (Propst and Thorp, 1998; Ridgway, 1995). In other cases, hematomas may develop following injury to a blood vessel without laceration of the superficial tissues. These may occur with spontaneous or operative delivery. Occasionally, the hemorrhage is delayed.

Puerperal hematomas may be classified as vulvar, vulvovaginal, paravaginal, or retroperitoneal. Vulvar hematomas most often involve branches of the pudendal artery, including the posterior rectal, transverse perineal, or posterior labial artery, whereas paravaginal hematomas may involve the descending branch of the uterine artery (Zahn and Yeomans, 1990). Infrequently, the torn vessel lies above the pelvic fascia. In that event, the hematoma develops above it. In its early stages, the hematoma forms a rounded swelling that projects into the upper portion of the vaginal canal and may almost occlude its lumen. If the bleeding continues, it dissects retroperitoneally, and thus may form a tumor palpable above the Poupart ligament, or it may dissect upward, eventually reaching the lower margin of the diaphragm. Branches of the uterine artery may be involved with these types of hematomas.

Vulvar Hematomas. These hematomas, such as the one shown in Figure 35–28, and particularly those that develop rapidly, may cause excruciating pain. This often is the first symptom noticed. Moderate-sized hematomas may be absorbed spontaneously. The tissues overlying the hematoma may rupture as a result of necrosis caused by pressure, and profuse hemorrhage may follow. In others, the contents of the hematoma may be discharged in the form of large clots. In the subperitoneal variety, extravasation of blood beneath the peritoneum may be massive and occasionally fatal. Some of these dissect behind the ascending colon up to the hepatic flexure.

DIAGNOSIS. A vulvar hematoma is readily diagnosed by severe perineal pain and usually rapid appearance of a tense, fluctuant, and sensitive tumor of varying size covered by discolored skin. When the mass develops adjacent to the vagina, it may escape detection temporarily. Symptoms of pressure, if not pain or inability to void, should prompt a vaginal examination with discovery of a round, fluctuant tumor encroaching on the lumen. When the hematoma extends upward between the folds of the broad ligament, it may escape detection unless a portion of the tumor can be felt on abdominal palpation or unless hypovolemia develops. These are worrisome because large hematomas have led to death.

TREATMENT. Smaller vulvar hematomas identified after leaving the delivery room may be treated expectantly (Propst and Thorp, 1998). However, if the pain is severe or the hematoma continues to enlarge, the best treatment is prompt incision. This is done at the point of maximal distention along with evacuation of blood and clots and ligation of bleeding points. The cavity may then be obliterated with mattress sutures. Often, no sites of bleeding are identified after the hematoma has been drained. In such cases, the vagina, not the hematoma cavity, is packed for 12 to 24 hours. **With hematomas of the genital tract, blood loss is nearly always considerably more than the clinical estimate.** Hypovolemia and severe anemia should be prevented by adequate blood replacement. In about 50 percent of women with hematomas requiring surgical repair, transfusions are necessary (Zahn and Yeomans, 1990).

Subperitoneal and supravaginal hematomas are more difficult to treat. They can be evacuated by incision of the perineum; but unless there is complete hemostasis, which is difficult to achieve by this route, laparotomy is advisable.

ANGIOGRAPHIC EMBOLIZATION. This technique has become popular for management of intractable puerperal hematomas. It can be used primarily or usually when hemostasis is not obtained by surgical methods. Figure 35–29 shows a case in which embolization was carried out with occlusion of the internal pudendal artery and its vaginal branch as well as the uterine artery. Villella and co-workers (2001) have reviewed other indications for angiographic embolization and also described two women with a vulvovaginal hematoma in which it was used.

Angiographic embolization may also be used in women with intractable postpartum hemorrhage. In the reports by Deux (2001) and Chung (2003) and all their colleagues, the procedure was successful in 55 of 58 such women. Many of them had subsequent successful pregnancies (Goldberg and associates, 2002). Similarly, in their follow-up study of 28 consecutive women who underwent pelvic embolization for postpartum hemorrhage, Ornan and co-workers (2003) reported that all six who attempted pregnancy subsequently

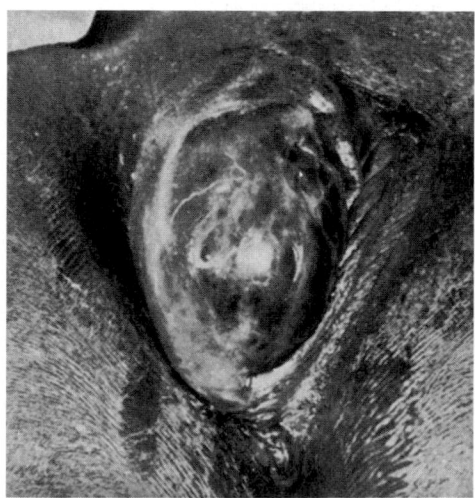

FIGURE 35–28. Vulvar hematoma bulging into the right vaginal wall.

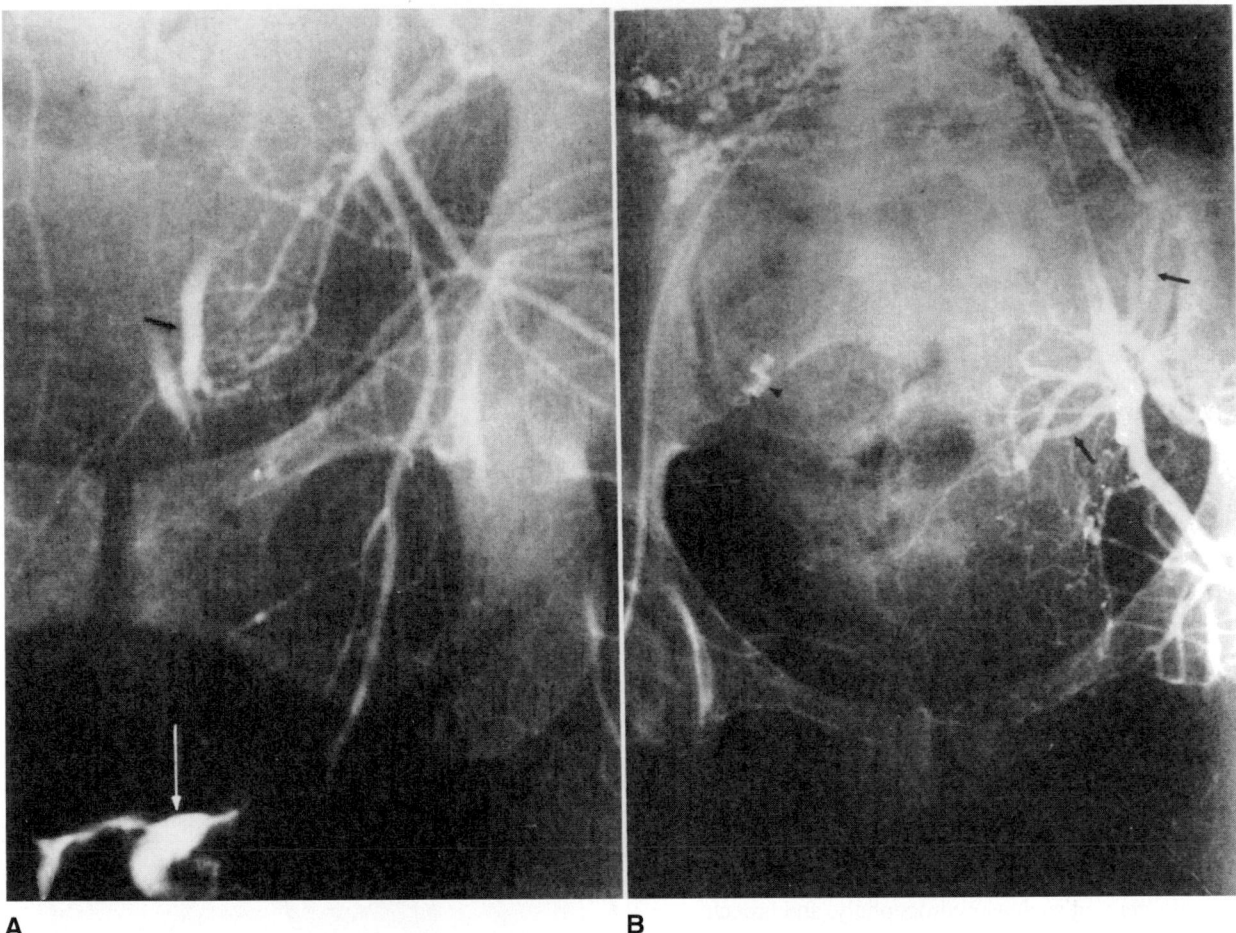

A **B**

FIGURE 35–29. **A.** Selective left internal iliac arteriogram before embolization. Note marked extravasation from vaginal (*black arrow*) and vulvar branches (*white arrow*) of the left internal pudendal artery. **B.** After embolization the branches of the left internal pudendal artery are occluded. Patency of the left uterine artery (*arrows*) and coils in the right internal iliac artery (*arrowhead*) are noted. (From Chin and colleagues, 1989, with permission.)

were successful. No major complications were reported. However, Cottier and co-workers (2002) described a woman who developed ischemic uterine necrosis after arterial embolization for postpartum hemorrhage.

RUPTURE OF THE UTERUS. Uterine rupture may develop as a result of preexisting injury or anomaly, it may be associated with trauma, or it may complicate labor in a previously unscarred uterus. A classification of the etiology of uterine rupture is presented in Table 35–7.

The most common cause of uterine rupture is separation of a previous cesarean hysterotomy scar. This is discussed in detail in Chapter 26 (see p. 608). Other common predisposing factors to uterine rupture are previous traumatizing operations or manipulations such as curettage, perforation, or myomectomy (Fedorkow and colleagues, 1987; Kieser and Baskett, 2002; Pelosi and Pelosi, 1997). Excessive or inappropriate uterine stimulation with oxytocin, a

previously frequent cause, has become uncommon. Mishra and colleagues (1995) described a 43-year-old woman who suffered a ruptured vertical cesarean incision associated with inhaled crack cocaine.

Morbidity and Mortality. Prenatal morbidity and mortality can be substantive with rupture of a prior uterine incision during labor (see Chap. 26, p. 608). Rachagan and colleagues (1991) reported fetal mortality to be almost 70 percent with either spontaneous or traumatic uterine rupture. In 24 women with uterine rupture principally unassociated with prior incisions, Eden and associates (1986) reported one maternal death and a 46-percent perinatal loss. Hysterectomy may be necessary to control hemorrhage.

Traumatic Rupture. Although the uterus is surprisingly resistant to blunt trauma, pregnant women sustaining such trauma to the abdomen should be watched carefully for signs

TABLE 35-7 Classification of Causes of Uterine Rupture

Uterine Injury or Anomaly Sustained Before Current Pregnancy	Uterine Injury or Abnormality During Current Pregnancy

1. Surgery involving the myometrium
  Cesarean delivery or hysterotomy
  Previously repaired uterine rupture
  Myomectomy incision through or to the endometrium
  Deep cornual resection of interstitial oviduct
  Metroplasty
2. Coincidental uterine trauma
  Abortion with instrumentation—curette, sound
  Sharp or blunt trauma—accidents, bullets, knives
  Silent rupture in previous pregnancy
3. Congenital anomaly
  Pregnancy in undeveloped uterine horn
	1. Before delivery
	  Persistent, intense, spontaneous contractions
	  Labor stimulation—oxytocin or prostaglandins
	  Intra-amnionic instillation—saline or prostaglandins
	  Perforation by internal uterine pressure catheter
	  External trauma—sharp or blunt
	  External version
	  Uterine overdistention—hydramnios, multifetal pregnancy
	2. During delivery
	  Internal version
	  Difficult forceps delivery
	  Breech extraction
	  Fetal anomaly distending lower segment
	  Vigorous uterine pressure during delivery
	  Difficult manual removal of placenta
	3. Acquired
	  Placenta increta or percreta
	  Gestational trophoblastic neoplasia
	  Adenomyosis
	  Sacculation of entrapped retroverted uterus

of a ruptured uterus (see Chap. 42, p. 998) as well as a placental abruption (see p. 811). Miller and Paul (1996) found that trauma accounted for a ruptured uterus in only 3 of more than 150 women. In the past, internal podalic version and extraction often caused traumatic rupture during delivery. Other causes of traumatic rupture include difficult forceps delivery, unusual fetal enlargement such as hydrocephaly, and breech extraction (Fig. 35–30).

Spontaneous Rupture. In the study by Miller and Paul (1996), the incidence of spontaneous uterine rupture was only about 1 in 15,000 deliveries. The investigators also found that rupture is more likely in women of high parity (Miller and colleagues, 1997). Oxytocin stimulation of labor has been commonly associated with uterine rupture, especially in women of high parity (Fuchs and co-workers, 1985; Rachagan and associates, 1991). Other uterotonic agents are also implicated. Uterine rupture has resulted from labor induction with prostaglandin E_2 gel or E_1 vaginal tablets (Maymon and associates, 1991; Bennett, 1997). For these reasons, all uterotonic agents should be given with great caution to induce or stimulate labor in women of high parity. Similarly, in women of high parity, a trial of labor with suspected cephalopelvic disproportion, high cephalic presentation, or abnormal presentation such as a brow must be undertaken with caution.

Pathological Anatomy. Excessive stretching of the lower uterine segment with the development of a pathological retraction ring is described in Chapter 20 (see p. 519). Rupture of the previously intact uterus at the time of labor most often involves the thinned-out lower uterine segment. The rent, when it is in the immediate vicinity of the cervix, frequently extends transversely or obliquely. Usually the tear is longitudinal when it occurs in the portion of the uterus adjacent to the broad ligament (see Fig. 35–30). Although developing primarily in the lower uterine segment, it is not unusual for

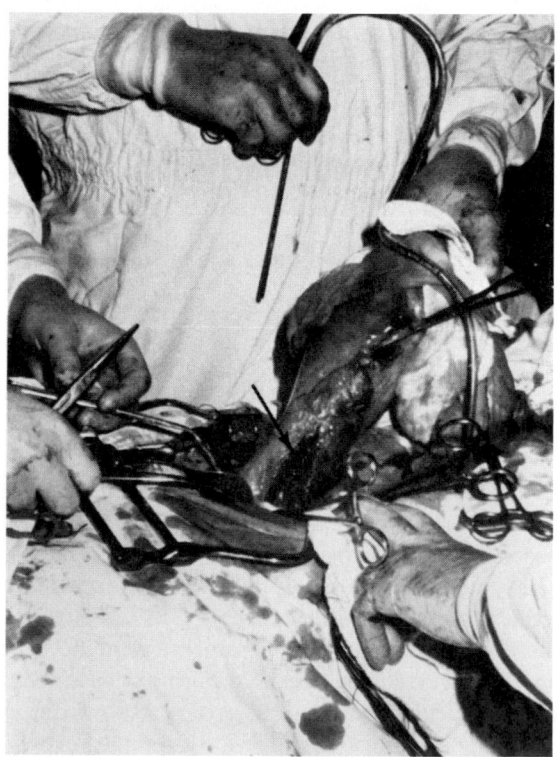

FIGURE 35–30. Ruptured uterus with vaginal breech delivery. At laparotomy, there was extensive bleeding beneath the uterine serosa, bladder, and left broad ligament. The extent of rupture is shown by the *arrow.*

the laceration to extend further upward into the body of the uterus or downward through the cervix into the vagina. At times, the bladder may also be lacerated (Rachagan and colleagues, 1991). After complete rupture, the uterine contents escape into the peritoneal cavity, unless the presenting part is firmly engaged, when only a portion of the fetus may be extruded from the uterus.

In uterine rupture in which the peritoneum remains intact, hemorrhage frequently extends into the broad ligament. In such circumstances, hemorrhage tends to be less severe than with intraperitoneal rupture. Such bleeding, however, may result in a large retroperitoneal hematoma that may involve sufficient blood loss to cause death. Fatal exsanguination may also supervene after rupture of the hematoma relieves the tamponading effect of the intact broad ligament.

Clinical Course and Treatment. Chapter 26 includes a discussion of the various clinical presentations of uterine rupture as well as treatment approaches (see p. 615).

HYPOVOLEMIC SHOCK

Shock from hemorrhage evolves through several stages. Early in the course of massive bleeding, there are decreases in mean arterial pressure, stroke volume, cardiac output, central venous pressure, and pulmonary capillary wedge pressure. Increases in arteriovenous oxygen content difference reflect a relative increase in tissue oxygen extraction, although overall oxygen consumption falls (Bland and colleagues, 1985).

Blood flow to capillary beds in various organs is controlled by arterioles, which are resistance vessels that in turn are partially controlled by the central nervous system. At least 70 percent of total blood volume is contained in venules, which are passive resistance vessels controlled by humoral factors. Catecholamine release during hemorrhage causes a generalized increase in venular tone, resulting in an autotransfusion from this capacitance reservoir (Barber and colleagues, 1999). These changes are accompanied by compensatory increases in heart rate, systemic and pulmonary vascular resistance, and myocardial contractility. In addition, there is redistribution of cardiac output and blood volume by selective, centrally mediated arteriolar constriction. This results in diminished perfusion to the kidneys, splanchnic beds, skin, and uterus, with relative maintenance of blood flow to the heart, brain, adrenal glands, and organs that autoregulate their own flow (Barber and associates, 1999).

As blood volume deficit exceeds 25 percent, compensatory mechanisms usually are inadequate to maintain cardiac output and blood pressure. At this point, additional small losses of blood result in rapid clinical deterioration. Despite an initial increase in *total oxygen extraction* by maternal tissue, maldistribution of blood flow results in *local* tissue hypoxia and metabolic acidosis, producing a vicious cycle of vasoconstriction, organ ischemia, and cellular death.

Hemorrhage also activates lymphocytes and monocytes, which interact with endothelial cells. These events lead to loss of capillary membrane integrity and additional loss of intravascular volume. There is also increased platelet aggregation in hypovolemic shock, resulting in the release of a number of vasoactive mediators that cause small vessel occlusion and further impairment of microcirculatory perfusion.

Often overlooked is the importance of extracellular fluid and electrolyte shifts in both pathophysiology and successful treatment of hypovolemic shock. This involves changes in the cellular transport of various ions, in which sodium and water enter skeletal muscles and cellular potassium is lost to the extracellular fluid (Chiao and colleagues, 1990). Replacement of extracellular fluid is thus an important component of therapy in hypovolemic shock. **Survival is reduced in acute hemorrhagic shock when blood alone, compared with blood and lactated Ringer solution, is administered.**

ESTIMATION OF BLOOD LOSS. Visual inspection is notoriously inaccurate. In some reports, the amount of blood estimated to have been lost by inspection was on average about half the measured loss. Importantly, in obstetrics, part or all of the hemorrhage may be concealed. It is important to realize that in a situation of acute hemorrhage, the immediate hematocrit may not reflect actual blood loss. After the loss of 1000 mL, the hematocrit typically falls only 3 volume percent in the first hour. When resuscitation is given with rapid infusion of intravenous crystalloids, there is rapid equilibration. **During an episode of acute significant hemorrhage, the initial hematocrit is always the highest.** This is true whether it is measured in the delivery room, operating room, or recovery room.

Urine output is one of the most important "vital signs" to follow in the bleeding patient with obstetrical hemorrhage. **In the absence of diuretics, the rate of urine formation, when carefully measured, reflects the adequacy of renal perfusion and, in turn, perfusion of other vital organs, because renal blood flow is especially sensitive to changes in blood volume.** Urine flow of at least 30 mL and preferably 60 mL per hour should be maintained. With potentially serious hemorrhage, an indwelling catheter should be inserted promptly to measure urine flow. Potent diuretics such as furosemide invalidate the relationship between urine flow and renal perfusion. This need not be a problem in the management of the woman who is hemorrhaging, because diuretics should be avoided in a hypovolemic patient. Another effect of furosemide is venodilation, which further reduces cardiac venous return, thereby further compromising cardiac output.

RESUSCITATION AND ACUTE MANAGEMENT. Whenever there is any suggestion of excessive blood loss after delivery, it is essential that steps be taken immediately to identify the presence of uterine atony, retained placental fragments, or genital tract lacerations. It is imperative that at least one or two intravenous infusion systems of large caliber be established promptly to allow rapid administration of crystalloid solutions and blood. An operating room, surgical team, and anesthesiologist should always be immediately available. The management of specific causes of postpartum hemorrhage were discussed earlier in this chapter.

Fluid Replacement. Treatment of serious hemorrhage demands prompt and adequate refilling of the intravascular compartment. Crystalloid solutions typically are used for initial volume resuscitation. Such solutions rapidly equilibrate into the extravascular space and only 20 percent of crystalloid remains in the circulation of critically ill patients after 1 hour (Shoemaker and Kram, 1991). Because of such equilibration, initial fluid infusion should involve about three times as much crystalloid as the estimated blood loss.

There is debate concerning fluid resuscitation of hypovolemic shock with colloid versus crystalloid solutions. In their review, Schierhout and Roberts (1998) found a 4-percent excessive mortality in nonpregnant patients resuscitated with colloid compared with that with crystalloid. The Cochrane Injuries Group Albumin Reviewers (1998) found a 6-percent excess mortality in albumin-treated nonpregnant patients with shock. We concur with Bonnar (2000) that fluid resuscitation should be with crystalloid and blood.

Blood Replacement. Considerable debate also surrounds the hematocrit level or hemoglobin concentration that mandates blood transfusion. According to deliberations of a Consensus Development Conference (1988), cardiac output does not substantively decrease until the hemoglobin concentration falls to about 7 g/dL. Although the committee reported that otherwise healthy anesthetized animals survived isovolemic anemia with hematocrit decreases down to 5 volume percent, they further cited that there was significant functional deterioration well before that point. It is difficult to define a universal hematocrit or hemoglobin value below or

above which transfusion is either mandatory or contraindicated. That said, recommendations of the Consensus Conference should be considered in clinical decision making. According to these guidelines, red blood cells are not infused for moderate anemia in stable women.

For the woman acutely bleeding, we recommend rapid blood infusion if the hematocrit is less than 25 volumes percent. Similarly, Morrison and colleagues (1993) recommend transfusion if the hematocrit is less than 24 volumes percent or if hemoglobin is less than 8 g/dL if there is imminent surgery, acute operative blood loss, acute hypoxia, vascular collapse, or other factors present. Further support for these recommendations was provided by Czer and Shoemaker (1978). In 94 critically ill postoperative patients, mortality rates were lowest when hematocrit values were maintained between 27 and 33 volumes percent.

Hebert and associates (1999) reported results from the Canadian Critical Care Trials Group. A total of 838 critically ill nonpregnant patients were randomized to restrictive red cell transfusions to maintain hemoglobin concentration over 7 g/dL, or to liberal transfusions to maintain the hemoglobin 10 to 12 g/dL. The 30-day mortality rate was similar (19 versus 23 percent in the restrictive versus liberal groups, respectively). In patients who were not as ill (APACHE score 20 or less), however, the 30-day mortality was significantly lower in the restrictive group (9 versus 26 percent). Morrison and colleagues (1991) reported no benefits of red cell transfusions given to women who had suffered postpartum hemorrhage and who were *isovolemic but anemic* with a hematocrit between 18 and 25 volume percent. **Clearly, the level to which a woman is transfused depends not only on the present red cell mass, but also on the likelihood of additional blood loss.**

Whole Blood and Blood Components. Contents and effects of transfusion of various blood components are shown in Table 35–8. **Compatible whole blood is ideal for treatment**

TABLE 35–8 Blood Products Commonly Transfused in Obstetrical Hemorrhage

One Unit	Volume per Unit	Contents per Unit	Effect(s) in Obstetrical Hemorrhage
Whole blood	About 500 mL; Hct~40%	RBCs, plasma, 600–700 mg of fibrinogen, no platelets	Restores TBV and fibrinogen; increases Hct 3–4 volume % per unit
Packed RBCs ("packed cells")	About 250 mL plus additive solutions; Hct~55–80%	RBCs only, no fibrinogen, no platelets	Increases Hct 3–4 volume % per unit
Fresh-frozen plasma	About 250 mL; 30-minute thaw needed before use	Colloid plus about 600–700 mg fibrinogen, no platelets	Restores TBV and fibrinogen
Cryoprecipitate	About 15 mL, frozen	About 200 mg fibrinogen plus other clotting factors, no platelets	About 3000–4000 mg total is needed to restore maternal fibrinogen to > 150 mg/dL
Platelets	About 50 mL, stored at room temperature	One unit has 5.5×10^{10} platelets in 50 mL plasma	6–10 units usually transfused; each increases platelets 5000/μL

Hct = hematocrit; RBCs = red blood cells; TBV = total blood volume.
From Leveno and colleagues, 2003.

of hypovolemia from catastrophic acute hemorrhage. It has a shelf life of 40 days, and 70 percent of the transfused red cells function for at least 24 hours following transfusion. One unit raises the hematocrit by 3 to 4 volume percent. Whole blood replaces many coagulation factors, especially fibrinogen, and its plasma expands hypovolemia from hemorrhage. Importantly, women with severe hemorrhage are resuscitated with fewer blood donor exposures than with packed red cells and components. In a randomized study of 33 nonpregnant patients undergoing liver transplantation, Laine and colleagues (2003) found that whole blood, compared with component therapy, was associated with fewer donor exposures yet provided equally effective therapy for blood loss.

For women who are more stable and do not have massive blood loss, packed red blood cell transfusions are suitable. According to the National Institutes of Health (1993), component therapy provides better treatment because only the specific component needed is given. Accordingly, the infusion of whole banked blood is usually not necessary and is rarely available (Barber and colleagues, 1999; Bonnar, 2000; Laine and collaborators, 2003).

AUTOTRANSFUSION. The safety of intraoperative autologous blood salvage and autotransfusion during cesarean delivery was evaluated in a multicenter historical cohort study by Rebarber and colleagues (1998). When 139 women undergoing cesarean delivery and given autotransfusion were compared with 87 control women, there were no differences in adverse outcomes. Specifically, there was no evidence of respiratory distress or amnionic fluid embolism. The American College of Obstetricians and Gynecologists (2002) now recommends that cell saver technology be considered for women suspected of having a placenta accreta prior to delivery.

DILUTIONAL COAGULOPATHY. When blood loss is massive, replacement with crystalloid solutions and packed red blood cells usually results in a depletion of platelets and soluble clotting factors, leading to a dilutional coagulopathy that clinically is indistinguishable from disseminated intravascular coagulopathy (see p. 843). This impairs hemostasis and further contributes to blood loss. The most frequent coagulation defect found in women with blood loss and multiple transfusions is thrombocytopenia (Counts and colleagues, 1979; Wilson and associates, 1971). Because stored whole blood is deficient in factors V, VIII, XI, and platelets, and all soluble clotting factors are absent from packed red blood cells, severe hemorrhage without factor replacement may also cause hypofibrinogenemia and prolongation of the prothrombin and partial thromboplastin times. In some women, frank consumptive coagulopathy may accompany shock and confuse the distinction between dilutional and consumptive coagulopathy. Fortunately, in most situations encountered in obstetrics, treatment of both types of coagulopathy is the same.

Various algorithms have been proposed to guide the replacement of platelets and clotting factors according to the volume of blood loss, but there is great patient variability. **Component replacement is rarely necessary with acute replacement of 5 to 10 units of packed red blood cells or less.** When blood loss exceeds this amount, consideration should be given to evaluation of platelet count, clotting studies, and plasma fibrinogen concentration. Fortunately, in practice, the level of various clotting factors required for adequate hemostasis is quite minimal.

In the bleeding woman, the platelet count should be maintained above $50,000/\mu L$ with the infusion of platelet concentrates. A fibrinogen level of less than 100 mg/dL or sufficiently prolonged prothrombin or partial thromboplastin times in a woman with surgical bleeding is an indication for fresh-frozen plasma administration in doses of 10 to 15 mL/kg.

TYPE AND SCREEN VERSUS CROSSMATCH. In any woman at significant risk for hemorrhage, typing and screening or crossmatching is essential. The screening procedure involves mixing the maternal serum with standard reagent red cells that contain the antigens with which most of the common clinically significant antibodies react. A crossmatch, on the other hand, involves the use of actual donor erythrocytes rather than standard red cells. Only 0.03 to 0.07 percent of patients who are determined not to have antibodies in a type-and-screen procedure subsequently have antibodies as determined by crossmatch (Boral and colleagues, 1979). Thus, administration of screened blood very rarely results in adverse clinical sequelae. Not performing a crossmatch also decreases blood bank costs. Moreover, blood that is crossmatched is held exclusively for that single potential recipient. With type-and-screening, blood is available for any potential recipient and blood wastage is reduced. For all of these reasons, type and screen is preferred in most obstetrical situations.

PACKED RED BLOOD CELLS. Cells packed from a unit of whole blood have a hematocrit of 60 to 70 volume percent, depending on the method used for preparation and storage. A unit of packed red blood cells contains the same volume of erythrocytes as whole blood and also raises the hematocrit by 3 to 4 volume percent. Packed red blood cell and crystalloid infusion are the mainstays of transfusion therapy for most cases of obstetrical hemorrhage.

PLATELETS. When transfusion is needed, it is preferable to give platelets obtained by apheresis from one donor. In this scheme, the equivalent of platelets from six individual donors is given as a one-unit one-donor transfusion. Such units generally cannot be stored more than 5 days.

If single-donor platelets are not available, random donor platelet packs are used. These are prepared from individual units of whole blood by centrifugation, and then resuspended in 50 to 70 mL of plasma. One unit of random donor platelets contains about 5.5×10^{10} platelets, and six to ten such units are generally transfused. Each unit transfused should raise the platelet count by $5000/\mu L$ (National Institutes of Health, 1993). The donor plasma must be compatible with recipient erythrocytes. Further, because some red blood cells are invariably transfused along with the platelets, only platelets from D-negative donors should be given to D-negative recipients. However, Lin and colleagues (2002) found that transfusion of ABO-nonidentical platelets in nonpregnant patients undergoing cardiovascular surgery was not associated with adverse effects. Platelet transfusion is considered in a bleeding patient with a platelet count below $50,000/\mu L$. In the *nonsurgical patient*, bleeding is rarely encountered if the platelet count exceeds 5000 to $10,000/\mu L$ (Sachs, 1991).

FRESH-FROZEN PLASMA. This component is prepared by separating plasma from whole blood and then freezing it. Approximately 30 minutes are required for the frozen plasma to thaw. It is a source of all stable and labile clotting factors, including fibrinogen. It is often used in the acute treatment of women with consumptive or dilutional coagulopathy. Fresh-frozen plasma is not appropriate for use as a volume expander in the absence of specific clotting factor deficiency. It should be considered in a bleeding woman with a fibrinogen level below 100 mg/dL or with abnormal prothrombin and partial thromboplastin times.

CRYOPRECIPITATE. This component is prepared from fresh-frozen plasma. Cryoprecipitate contains factor VIII: C, factor VIII: von Willebrand factor, fibrinogen factor XIII (about 200 mg), and fibronectin in less than 15 mL of the plasma from which it was derived (American Association of Blood Banks, 1994). Cryoprecipitate is an ideal source of fibrinogen if levels are dangerously low and there is oozing from surgical incisions. There is no advantage to the use of cryoprecipitate for general clotting factor replacement in the bleeding woman instead of fresh-frozen plasma. The exception to this is in states of general factor deficiency where potential volume overload is a problem, and in a few conditions involving deficiency of specific factors.

AUTOLOGOUS TRANSFUSIONS. Under some circumstances, autologous blood storage for transfusion may be considered. In general, however, this has been disappointing. For example, McVay and colleagues (1989) reported observations from 273 pregnant women in whom blood was drawn in the third trimester. Minimal requirements were a hemoglobin concentration 11 g/dL or a hematocrit of 34 volume percent. Unfortunately, almost three fourths of these women donated only one unit, a volume of questionable value.

In many cases, the need for transfusion cannot be predicted. Sherman and colleagues (1992) studied 27 women given two or more transfusions in over 16,000 deliveries. In only 40 percent was an antepartum risk factor identified.

Similar findings were reported by Reyal and associates (2004). Andres and co-workers (1990) and Etchason and associates (1995) concluded that autologous transfusions were not cost effective.

Complications of Blood Transfusion. Each unit of blood or any component is associated with risk of exposure to blood-borne infections. However, during the past several decades, substantial advances have been achieved in blood transfusion safety. Currently, the most serious known risks are administrative error leading to ABO-incompatible blood transfusion, transfusion-related acute lung injury (TRALI), and bacterial and viral transmission (Goodnough, 2003).

HEMOLYTIC TRANSFUSION REACTION. The transfusion of an incompatible blood component may result in acute hemolysis characterized by disseminated intravascular coagulation, acute renal failure, and death. Preventable errors, such as mislabeling of a specimen or transfusing an incorrect patient, are responsible for the majority of these reactions. Although the rate of such errors in the United States is estimated to be 1 in 14,000 units, the rate is likely greater due to underreporting (Goodnough, 2003; Linden and co-workers, 2001).

Signs and symptoms of a transfusion reaction include fever, hypotension, tachycardia, dyspnea, chest or back pain, flushing, severe anxiety, and hemoglobinuria. Immediate supportive measures include stopping the transfusion, treating hypotension and hyperkalemia, administering a diuretic, and alkalinizing the urine. Assays for urine and plasma hemoglobin concentration and an antibody screen help confirm the diagnosis.

TRANSFUSION-RELATED ACUTE LUNG INJURY. TRALI is a life-threatening complication characterized by severe dyspnea, hypoxia, and noncardiogenic pulmonary edema that develops within 6 hours of transfusion (Silliman and associates, 2003). It is estimated to complicate at least 1 in 5000 transfusions. Although the pathogenesis of TRALI is incompletely understood, the mechanisms of injury to the pulmonary capillaries appear to involve lipid products from stored components as well as leukocyte reactions (Kopko and co-workers, 2002; Silliman and associates, 2003). Its management is discussed in Chapter 42, p. 991.

BACTERIAL CONTAMINATION. The transfusion of a contaminated blood component is associated with a 60-percent mortality rate. The most commonly implicated contaminant of red cells is *Yersinia enterocolitica*. In the United States, the risk of bacterial contamination is less than 1 per million units. Currently, the greatest risk of transfusion-transmitted disease is bacterial contamination of platelets, which is estimated to affect as many as 1 in 2000 units (Goodnough, 2003).

VIRAL TRANSMISSION. Fortunately, the most feared infection—*human immunodeficiency virus (HIV)*—is the least common.

With current screening methods using nucleic acid amplification testing, the time period between infection and the first appearance of viral RNA is 11 days for HIV-1 and 8 to 10 days for hepatitis C (Busch and colleagues, 2003). As a result, the risk of HIV infection in screened blood is currently estimated to be 1 in 1.5 to 2 million units transfused; indeed, only four transfusion-transmitted HIV infections have been identified since 1999 (Dodd, 2003). Similarly, the risk of hepatitis C infection is about 1 in 2 million units transfused (Stramer and associates, 2004).

The likelihood of *HIV-2* infection is even less. After implementation of a combined HIV-1/HIV-2 screening of blood donors in 1992, only three units of 74 million tested through 1995 were positive for HIV-2 (Centers for Disease Control and Prevention, 1995). The risk of *hepatitis B* transmission is higher, although it is estimated currently to be less than 1 per 100,000 units transfused (Jackson and colleagues, 2003). The risk of transmitting other infectious diseases with transfusion, such as malaria and cytomegalovirus, is estimated to be less than 1 in 1 million (National Institutes of Health, 1993). More recently, there have been reports of West Nile virus infection acquired via transfusion. Pealer and colleagues (2003) identified 23 confirmed cases between August 2002 and April 2003.

Red-Cell Substitutes. There are three varieties of these substitutes: perfluorochemicals, liposome-encapsulated hemoglobin, and hemoglobin-based oxygen carriers. Their history and development have been reviewed by Cohn (2000) and Wright-Kanuth and Smith (2002). Fluoridated hydrocarbons are biologically inert liquids with relatively high oxygen solubility. The use of such emulsions allows oxygen to be transported and delivered to tissues by simple diffusion. The most commonly used emulsion, Fluosol, must be stored frozen and thawed within 24 hours of use. Clinical benefits of these emulsions are not well established, but they may decrease the need for blood with extensive hemorrhage (Klein, 2000). Liposome-encapsulated hemoglobin has not proved promising. One formulation of a hemoglobin-based oxygen carrier, diaspirin cross-linked hemoglobin (DCLHb), proved to be dangerous (Sloan and colleagues, 1999). Mullon and co-workers (2000) have described successful use of polymerized bovine hemoglobin, HBOC-201, as a blood substitute for nonpregnant women with severe autoimmune hemolytic anemia.

CONSUMPTIVE COAGULOPATHY

In 1901, DeLee reported that "temporary hemophilia" developed in a woman with a placental abruption and another with a long-dead macerated fetus. Observations that extensive placental abruption, as well as other accidents of pregnancy, were frequently associated with hypofibrinogenemia stimulated interest in causes of intense intravascular coagulation. Although these observations were initially almost totally confined to obstetrical cases, subsequently they were made for almost all areas of medicine (Baglin, 1996). These syndromes are commonly termed *consumptive coagulopathy* or *disseminated intravascular coagulation.*

Pregnancy Hypercoagulability. Pregnancy normally induces appreciable increases in the concentrations of coagulation factors I (fibrinogen), VII, VIII, IX, and X (see Chap. 5, p. 131). Other plasma factors and platelets do not change so remarkably. Plasminogen levels are increased considerably, yet plasmin activity antepartum is normally decreased compared with that of the nonpregnant state. Various stimuli act to incite the conversion of plasminogen to plasmin, and one of the most potent is activation of coagulation.

Pathological Activation of Coagulation. In normal circumstances, there is no appreciable continuous physiological intravascular coagulation. During pregnancy, there does appear to be increased activation of platelet, clotting, and fibrinolytic mechanisms. Gerbasi and colleagues (1990) found significant increases in fibrinopeptide A, β-thromboglobulin, platelet factor 4, and fibrinogen–fibrin degradation products. They concluded that this compensated, accelerated intravascular coagulation may serve to maintain the uteroplacental interface.

In pathological states, coagulation may be activated via the extrinsic pathway by thromboplastin from tissue destruction and perhaps via the intrinsic pathway by collagen and other tissue components when there is loss of endothelial integrity (Fig. 35–31). Tissue factor is released and complexes with factor VII. This in turn activates tenase (factor IX) and prothrombinase (factor X) complexes. Common inciting factors in obstetrics include thromboplastin from placental abruption as well as endotoxin and exotoxins. Another mechanism is by direct activation of factor X by proteases, for example, as present in mucin or as produced by neoplasms.

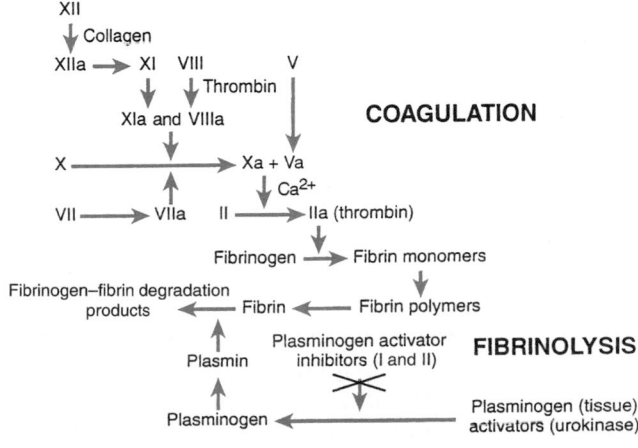

FIGURE 35–31. The coagulation and fibrinolysis cascades. (From Baker and Cunningham, 1999.)

Amnionic fluid contains abundant mucin from fetal squames, and this likely causes rapid defibrination with amnionic fluid embolism.

Consumptive coagulopathy is almost always seen as a complication of an identifiable, underlying pathological process against which treatment must be directed to reverse defibrination. Thus identification and prompt elimination of the source of the coagulopathy is the first priority in dealing with it. With pathological activation of procoagulants that trigger consumptive coagulopathy, there is consumption of platelets and coagulation factors in variable quantities. As a consequence, fibrin may be deposited in small vessels of virtually every organ system. Fortunately, this seldom causes organ failure. Small vessels are protected because coagulation releases fibrin monomers that combine with tissue plasminogen activator and plasminogen, which releases plasmin. In turn, plasmin lyses fibrinogen, fibrin monomer, and fibrin polymers to form a series of fibrinogen–fibrin derivatives. Measured by immunoassay, these are known as fibrin degradation products or split products.

Significance. In addition to bleeding and circulatory obstruction, which may cause ischemia from hypoperfusion, consumptive coagulopathy may be associated with microangiopathic hemolysis. This is caused by mechanical disruption of the erythrocyte membrane within small vessels in which fibrin has been deposited. Varying degrees of hemolysis with anemia, hemoglobinemia, hemoglobinuria, and erythrocyte morphological changes are produced. According to Pritchard and colleagues (1976), this likely causes or contributes to the hemolysis encountered with the so-called *HELLP syndrome,* which is discussed in Chapter 34 (see p. 773).

In obstetrical syndromes involving consumptive coagulopathy, the importance of vigorous restoration and maintenance of the circulation to treat hypovolemia and persistent intravascular coagulation cannot be overemphasized. With adequate perfusion of vital organs, activated coagulation factors and circulating fibrin and fibrin degradation products are promptly removed by the reticuloendothelial system. At the same time, hepatic and endothelial synthesis of procoagulants is promoted.

The likelihood of life-threatening hemorrhage in obstetrical situations complicated by defective coagulation depends not only on the extent of the coagulation defects but—of great importance—on whether the vasculature is intact or disrupted. With gross derangement of blood coagulation, there may be fatal hemorrhage when vascular integrity is disrupted, yet no hemorrhage as long as all blood vessels remain intact.

Clinical and Laboratory Evidence of Defective Hemostasis. Bioassay is an excellent method to clinically detect or suspect significant coagulopathy. **Excessive bleeding at sites of modest trauma characterizes defective hemostasis.** Persistent bleeding from venipuncture sites, nicks from shaving the perineum or abdomen, trauma from insertion of a catheter,

and spontaneous bleeding from the gums or nose are signs of possible coagulation defects. Purpuric areas at pressure sites may indicate incoagulable blood, or more commonly, clinically significant thrombocytopenia. A surgical procedure provides the ultimate bioassay for coagulation. Continuous generalized oozing from the skin, subcutaneous and fascial tissues, and the vascular retroperitoneal space should at least suggest coagulopathy. Such evidence also may be gained by observing continuous oozing from episiotomy incisions or perineal lacerations.

HYPOFIBRINOGENEMIA. In late pregnancy, plasma fibrinogen levels typically are 300 to 600 mg/dL. With consumptive coagulopathy, these high levels may sometimes serve to protect against clinically significant hypofibrinogenemia. To promote clinical coagulation, fibrinogen levels must be about 150 mg/dL. If serious *hypofibrinogenemia* is present, the clot formed from whole blood in a glass tube may initially be soft but not necessarily remarkably reduced in volume. Then, over the next half hour or so, it becomes quite small, so that many of the erythrocytes are extruded and the volume of liquid clearly exceeds that of clot.

FIBRIN AND FIBRINOGEN DERIVATIVES. Fibrin degradation products in serum may be detected by a number of sensitive test systems. Monoclonal antibodies to detect D-dimers are commonly used. With clinically significant consumption coagulopathy, these measurements are always abnormally high.

THROMBOCYTOPENIA. Serious thrombocytopenia is likely if petechiae are abundant, if clotted blood fails to retract over a period of an hour or so, or if platelets are rare in a stained blood smear. Confirmation is provided by platelet count. As discussed in Chapter 34 (see p. 773), there is also *qualitative platelet dysfunction* with severe preeclampsia and eclampsia.

PROTHROMBIN AND PARTIAL THROMBOPLASTIN TIMES. Prolongation of these coagulation tests may be the consequence of appreciable reductions in those coagulants essential for generating thrombin, fibrinogen concentration below a critical level of about 100 mg/dL, or appreciable amounts of circulating fibrinogen–fibrin degradation products. Prolongation of the prothrombin time and partial thromboplastin time need not be the consequence of consumptive coagulopathy.

Heparin. **The infusion of heparin to try to block disseminated intravascular coagulation associated with placental abruption or other situations in which the integrity of the vascular system is compromised is mentioned only to condemn its use.**

Epsilon-Aminocaproic Acid. This agent has been administered in an attempt to control fibrinolysis by inhibiting the conversion of plasminogen to plasmin. Epsilon-aminocaproic acid inhibits the proteolytic action of plasmin on fibrinogen, fibrin monomer, and fibrin polymer (clot). Failure to clear fibrin polymer from the microcirculation could result in organ ischemia and infarction, such as renal cortical necrosis. Its use in most types of obstetrical coagulopathy has not been efficacious and is not recommended.

PLACENTAL ABRUPTION. This is the most common cause of severe consumptive coagulopathy in obstetrics. It is discussed on page 811.

FETAL DEATH AND DELAYED DELIVERY. Although in most women with fetal death, spontaneous labor eventually ensues, most often within 2 weeks, the psychological stress imposed by carrying a dead fetus usually prompts induction of labor at the time of discovery (see Chap. 22). This also obviates the dangers of coagulation defects that may develop.

Coagulation Changes. Prospective studies indicated that gross disruption of the maternal coagulation mechanism rarely developed before less than 1 month after fetal death (Pritchard, 1959, 1973). If the fetus was retained longer, however, about 25 percent of the women developed a coagulopathy. Typically the fibrinogen concentration falls to levels that are normal for the nonpregnant state, and in some cases it falls to potentially dangerous concentrations of 100 mg/dL or less (Pritchard, 1973). The rate of decrease commonly found is demonstrated in Figure 35–32. Simultaneously, fibrin degradation products are elevated in serum. These changes are presumably mediated by thromboplastin from the dead products of conception (Jimenez and Pritchard, 1968; Lerner and associates, 1967). The platelet count tends to decrease in these instances, but severe thrombocytopenia is uncommon even if the fibrinogen level is quite low. Although coagulation defects may correct spontaneously before evacuation, this is unusual and happens quite slowly (Pritchard, 1959).

HEPARIN. Correction of coagulation defects has been accomplished using low doses of heparin (5000 U two to three times daily) under carefully controlled conditions *in women with an intact circulation* (Pacheco and colleagues, 2004). Heparin appropriately administered can block further pathological consumption of fibrinogen and other clotting factors, thereby slowing or temporarily reversing the cycle of consumption and fibrinolysis. Such correction should be undertaken only if the patient is not actively bleeding and with simultaneous steps to effect delivery.

FETAL DEATH IN MULTIFETAL PREGNANCY. It is uncommon that an obvious coagulation derangement develops in multifetal pregnancy complicated by death of at least one fetus and survival of another (Landy and Weingold, 1989). Petersen and Nyholm (1999) followed 22 multifetal pregnancies with one fetal death after the first trimester and did not detect a coagulopathy in any of these cases.

Chescheir and Seeds (1988) reported a woman in whom, following death of one of twin fetuses, there was progressive but transient fall in plasma fibrinogen concentration and rise in fibrin split products. We have encountered only a few such cases at Parkland Hospital, and one is shown in Figure 35–33. Coagulation changes ceased spontaneously, and the surviving fetus, when delivered near term, was healthy. The placenta of the long-dead fetus was filled with fibrin. Most cases are in monochorionic twins with vascular anastomoses (see Chap. 39, p. 928). The survivor twin has an extremely high risk of cerebral palsy and other cerebral impairment (Pharoah and Adi, 2000).

AMNIONIC FLUID EMBOLISM. This is a complex disorder classically characterized by the abrupt onset of hypotension, hypoxia, and consumptive coagulopathy. There is great individual variation in its clinical manifestation, and women are encountered in whom one of these three clinical hallmarks dominates or is entirely absent. The syndrome is uncommon in an absolute sense, however, it is a common cause of maternal death. For example, amnionic fluid embolism was implicated as the cause of death in 275 (9 percent) of the 3201 pregnancy-related maternal deaths ascertained from the Pregnancy Mortality Surveillance System of the Centers for Disease Control and Prevention from 1991 through 1997 (Berg and colleagues, 2003). Using data from 1.1 million deliveries in California, Gilbert and Danielsen (1999) estimated a frequency of about 1 case per 20,000 deliveries.

In obvious cases, the clinical picture frequently is dramatic. Classically, a woman in the late stages of labor or immediately postpartum begins gasping for air, and then rapidly suffers seizure or cardiorespiratory arrest complicated by consumptive coagulopathy, massive hemorrhage, and death.

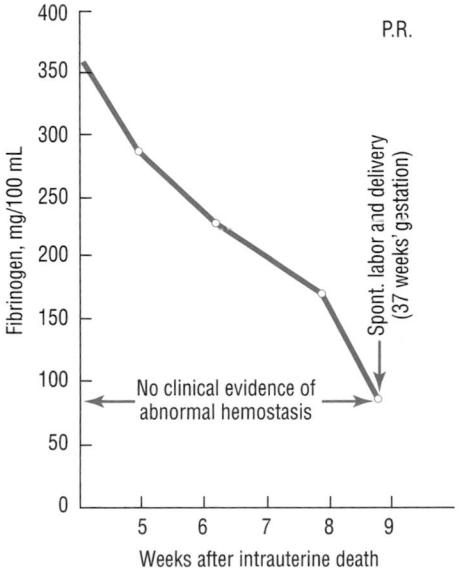

FIGURE 35–32. Slow development of maternal hypofibrinogenemia following fetal death and delayed delivery in Patient P.R. (From Pritchard, 1959, with permission.)

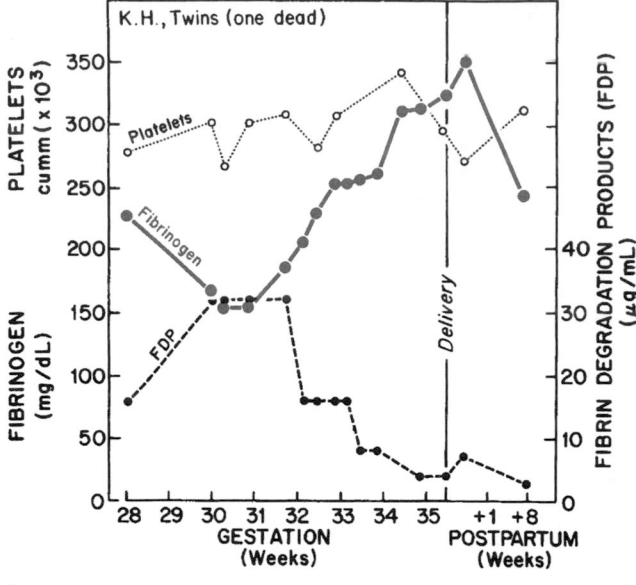

A

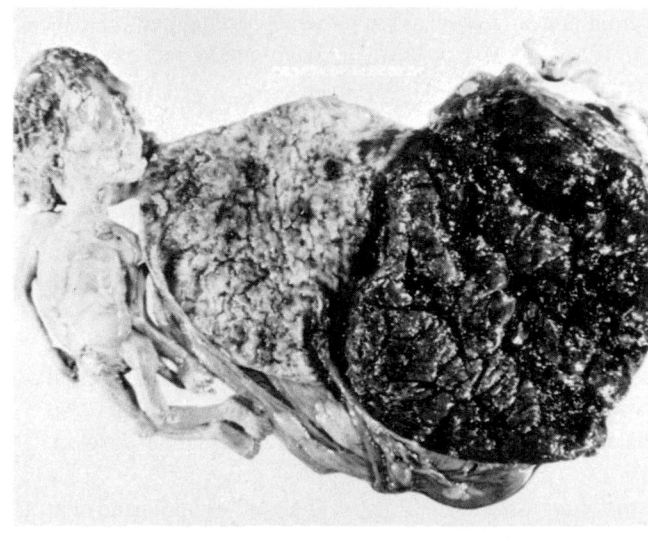

B

FIGURE 35–33. A. Death of one twin was confirmed sonographically at 28 weeks' gestation. Coagulation studies then demonstrated a somewhat low plasma fibrinogen concentration and abnormal amounts of fibrin degradation products. These abnormalities became more intense 2 weeks later. Then, spontaneously, the fibrinogen concentration rose, and the fibrin degradation product levels fell in mirror fashion. The liveborn infant was healthy, and coagulation studies on cord plasma and maternal serum were normal. **B.** The fibrin-filled placenta of the long-dead fetus is apparent. Presumably, the fibrin curtailed the escape of thromboplastin from the dead products into the maternal circulation.

These are unquestionably the most dramatic cases. However, there appears to be variation in the clinical presentation of this condition. For example, we have managed a number of women in whom otherwise uncomplicated vaginal delivery was followed by severe acute consumptive coagulopathy without cardiorespiratory symptoms. Thus, in some women, consumptive coagulopathy appears to be the "forme fruste" of amnionic fluid embolism (Awad and Shorten, 2001; Davies, 1999; Porter and colleagues, 1996). Other features common to amnionic fluid embolism are meconium staining and rapid labor.

Pathogenesis. Amnionic fluid embolism was originally described in 1941 by Steiner and Luschbaugh. Subsequent studies by Adamsons and associates (1971) and Stolte and co-workers (1967) demonstrated that amnionic fluid is innocuous, even when infused in large amounts. Some have suggested that the clinical picture is similar to that seen in human anaphylaxis (Clark and co-workers, 1995).

Amnionic fluid enters the circulation as a result of a breach in the physiological barrier that normally exists between maternal and fetal compartments. Such events appear to be common, if not universal, with both squames of presumed fetal origin and trophoblasts being commonly found in the maternal circulation (Clark and colleagues, 1986; Lee and co-workers, 1986). There may be maternal exposure to various fetal elements during pregnancy termination, following

amniocentesis or trauma, or more commonly during labor or delivery as small lacerations develop in the lower uterine segment or cervix. Alternatively, cesarean delivery affords ample opportunity for mixture of maternal blood and fetal tissue.

In most cases, these events are innocuous. In certain women, however, such exposure initiates a complex series of physiological reactions mimicking those seen in human anaphylaxis and sepsis (Table 35–9). A similar process has been shown for traumatic fat embolism (Peltier, 1984). A complete understanding of the precise pathophysiological cascade

TABLE 35–9 Clinical Findings in 84 Women with Amnionic Fluid Embolism

Clinical Findings	Clark et al (1995) (n = 46)	Weiwen (2000) (n = 38)
Hypotension	43	38
Fetal distress	30/30[a]	NS
Pulmonary edema or ARDS	28/30[a]	11
Cardiopulmonary arrest	40	38
Cyanosis	38	38
Coagulopathy	38	12/16[a]
Dyspnea	22/45[a]	38
Seizure	22	6

[a]Fraction indicates not all patients assessed.
ARDS = acute respiratory distress syndrome; NS = not stated.

remains elusive. In a case-controlled study of nine women with presumed amnionic fluid embolism, Benson and associates (2001) found that some indicators of anaphylaxis—serum tryptase and urinary histamine—were increased in some of the women, yet none had evidence of mast cell degranulation. Of note, complement levels were decreased uniformly, suggesting that complement activation may play an important role. Because such activation also occurs in seriously ill patients with acute respiratory distress syndrome, however, it is not known whether complement activation is a primary or secondary result of amnionic fluid embolism. A number of chemokines and cytokines also likely are important in the pathogenesis. For example, Khong (1998) found intense expression of endothelin-1 in fetal squames recovered from the lungs of two fatal cases.

Pathophysiology. Studies in primates using homologous amnionic fluid injection, as well as a carefully performed study in the goat model, have provided important insights into central hemodynamic aberrations (Adamsons and co-workers, 1971; Hankins and colleagues, 1993; Stolte and colleagues, 1967). The initial phase consists of pulmonary and systemic hypertension. Indeed, in a remarkable case report, Stanten and associates (2003) described the results of a transesophageal echocardiogram performed within 10 minutes of circulatory collapse related to amnionic fluid embolism. The findings, including a massively dilated akinetic right ventricle and a small, vigorously contracting, cavity-obliterated left ventricle, were all consistent with fail-ure to transfer blood from the right to the left heart because of catastrophic pulmonary vasoconstriction. Transient but profound oxygen desaturation is often seen in the initial phase, resulting in neurological injury in most survivors (Harvey and associates, 1996).

Decreased systemic vascular resistance and left ventricular stroke work index occur following this initial phase (Clark and colleagues, 1988). In women who live beyond the initial cardiovascular collapse, a secondary phase of lung injury and coagulopathy often ensues.

The association of uterine hypertonus with cardiovascular collapse appears to be the effect of amnionic fluid embolism rather than the cause (Clark and co-workers, 1995). Indeed, uterine blood flow ceases completely when intrauterine pressures exceed 35 to 40 mm Hg (Towell, 1976). Thus, a hypertonic contraction is the *least* likely time for fetal–maternal exchange to take place. Similarly, there is no causal association between oxytocin use and amnionic fluid embolism, and the frequency of oxytocin use is not increased in these women (American College of Obstetricians and Gynecologists, 1993).

Diagnosis. In the past, the detection of squamous cells or other debris of fetal origin in the central pulmonary circulation was believed to be pathognomonic for amnionic fluid embolism. Indeed, in fatal cases, histopathological findings may be dramatic, especially in those involving meconium-stained amnionic fluid (Fig. 35–34). The detection of such debris, however, may require extensive special staining,

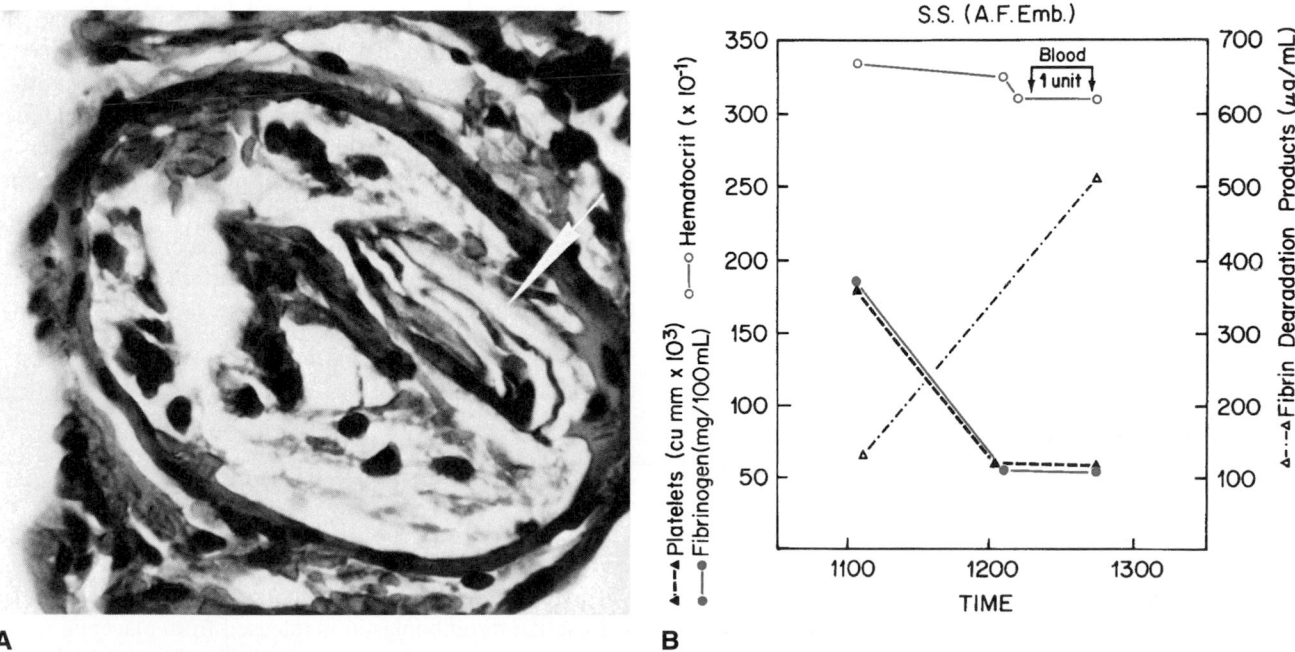

A **B**

FIGURE 35–34. A. Fetal squames (*arrow*) packed into a small pulmonary artery from a fatal case of amnionic fluid embolism. Most of the empty spaces within the vessel were demonstrated by appropriate staining for lipid to have been filled with vernix caseosa. **B.** Levels of fibrinogen, fibrinogen–fibrin degradation products, and platelets during fatal amnionic fluid embolism in patient S.S.

and even then it is often not seen. For example, Hankins and colleagues (2002) injected raw amnionic fluid into eight goats. Using special staining, there was microscopic evidence of pulmonary embolization in only 25 percent. Interestingly, seven other animals who were injected with meconium-stained fluid all had histopathological evidence of embolization. In a study by Clark and associates (1995), fetal elements were detected in 75 percent of autopsies and 50 percent of specimens prepared from concentrated buffy coat aspirates taken antemortem from a pulmonary artery catheter. Further, several studies have demonstrated that squamous cells, trophoblasts, and other debris of fetal origin may commonly be found in the central circulation of women with conditions other than amnionic fluid embolism. Thus, this finding is neither sensitive nor specific, and the diagnosis is generally made by identifying clinically characteristic signs and symptoms. In less typical cases, diagnosis is contingent on careful exclusion of other causes.

Management. Although an initial period of systemic and pulmonary hypertension appears to be involved in amnionic fluid embolism, this phase is transient. Women who survive long enough to receive any treatment other than cardiopulmonary resuscitation should receive therapy directed at oxygenation and support of the failing myocardium. Circulatory support and blood and component replacement are paramount. **There are no data that any type of intervention improves maternal prognosis with amnionic fluid embolism.** In undelivered women suffering cardiac arrest, consideration should be given to emergency perimortem cesarean delivery in an effort to improve newborn outcome. Such decision making is more complex in the woman who is hemodynamically unstable, but who has not suffered cardiac arrest.

Prognosis. The dismal outcomes with amnionic fluid embolism are undoubtedly related to reporting biases. Also, the syndrome likely is underdiagnosed in all but the most severe cases. In the report by Clark and co-workers (1995), there was a 60-percent maternal mortality rate. In the California database of 1.1 million deliveries by Gilbert and Danielson (1999), only 25 percent of reported cases were fatal. Weiwen (2000) has provided preliminary data from 38 cases in the Suzhou region of China; almost 90 percent of these women died. Death can be amazingly rapid, and of the 34 women who died in the series from China, 12 died within 30 minutes.

Profound neurological impairment is common in survivors. **In the cases reported by Clark and colleagues (1995), only 8 percent of women who had a cardiac arrest in conjunction with initial symptoms survived neurologically intact.** Outcome is also poor for fetuses and is related to the cardiac arrest-to-delivery interval. Overall neonatal survival is 70 percent, but almost half suffer residual neurological impairment.

SEPTICEMIA. Infections that lead to bacteremia and septic shock in obstetrics are most commonly due to septic abortion, antepartum pyelonephritis, or puerperal sepsis. Other aspects of septic shock are discussed in Chapter 42 (see p. 993).

Coagulopathy. The lethal properties of bacterial toxins, and especially endotoxins, are undoubtedly mediated largely by disruption of vascular endothelium. It is unclear, however, whether this is the major mechanism that initiates consumptive coagulopathy. For example, in experimental animals, endothelial damage is greatest 24 hours after endotoxin is given, but intravascular coagulation can usually be identified during the first few hours. More likely, endotoxin activates the extrinsic clotting mechanism through cytokine-induced tissue factor expression on the surface of activated monocytes (Levi and colleagues, 1993). The intrinsic route seems unimportant in this role.

Management. The pathophysiology and clinical management of the sepsis syndrome is discussed in detail in Chapter 42 (see p. 993). It has also been reviewed recently by Hotchkiss and Karl (2003). In general, treatment of the inciting cause is followed by reversal of the coagulopathy. In some cases, especially if surgical procedures are performed before sepsis is controlled and the coagulopathy is reversed, treatment with fresh-frozen plasma and platelet packs usually arrests such bleeding. **Heparin therapy is dangerous and should not be given.**

ABORTION. Remarkable blood loss may occur as the consequence of abortion. Hemorrhage during early pregnancy is less likely to be severe unless abortion was induced and the procedure was traumatic. When pregnancy is more advanced, the mechanisms responsible for hemorrhage are most often the same as those described for placental abruption and placenta previa—that is, the disruption of a large number of maternal blood vessels at the site of placental implantation.

Coagulation Defects. Serious disruption of the coagulation mechanism as the consequence of abortion may develop in the following circumstances:

1. Prolonged retention of a dead fetus, as already described.
2. The sepsis syndrome, a notorious cause.
3. Medical induction with a prostaglandin.
4. During instrumental termination of the pregnancy.
5. Intrauterine instillation of hypertonic saline or urea solutions.

The kinds of changes in coagulation that have been identified with abortion induced with *hypertonic solutions* imply at least that thromboplastin is released from placenta, fetus, decidua, or all three by the necrobiotic effect of the hypertonic solutions, which then initiates coagulation within the maternal circulation (Burkman and associates, 1977). Coagulation defects have been observed to develop rarely during induction of abortion with prostaglandin. Saraiya and colleagues (1999) reviewed 62 spontaneous abortion–related deaths reported to the Pregnancy Mortality Surveillance System. Almost 60 percent of deaths were caused by infection, and half of these women had consumptive coagulopathy.

Consumptive coagulopathy has been an uncommon but serious complication among women with *septic abortion*. The incidence of coagulation defects in the past at Parkland Hospital was highest in those with *Clostridium perfringens* sepsis and intense intravascular hemolysis (Pritchard and Whalley, 1971). Management consists of prompt restoration and maintenance of the circulation, and appropriate steps to control the infection, including evacuation of the infected products (see Chap. 9, p. 247).

REFERENCES

Abdel-Aleem H, El-Nashar I, Abdel-Aleem A: Management of severe postpartum hemorrhage with misoprostol. Int J Gynaecol Obstet 72:75, 2001.

Abdella TN, Sibai BM, Hays JM Jr, et al: Perinatal outcome in abruptio placentae. Obstet Gynecol 63:365, 1984

Adamsons K, Mueller-Heubach E, Myers RE: The innocuousness of amniotic fluid infusion in the pregnant rhesus monkey. Am J Obstet Gynecol 109:977, 1971

Addis A, Moretti ME, Ahmed Syed F, et al: Fetal effects of cocaine: An updated meta-analysis. Reprod Toxicol 15:341, 2001

Ajayi RA, Soothill PW, Campbell S, et al: Antenatal testing to predict outcome in pregnancies with unexplained antepartum haemorrhage. Br J Obstet Gynaecol 99:122, 1992

Allahbadia G: Hypogastric artery ligation: A new perspective. J Gynecol Surg 9:35, 1993

American Academy of Pediatrics and American College of Obstetricians and Gynecologists: Guidelines for Perinatal Care, 5th ed., 2002

American Association of Blood Banks: Circular of information for the use of human blood and blood components. American Red Cross 1751, March 1994

American College of Obstetricians and Gynecologists: Placenta accreta. Committee Opinion No. 266, January 2002

American College of Obstetricians and Gynecologists: Postpartum hemorrhage. Educational Bulletin No. 243, January 1998

American College of Obstetricians and Gynecologists: PROLOG Obstetrics, 3rd ed. Washington, DC, American College of Obstetricians and Gynecologists, 1993, p 94

Ammini AC, Mathur SK: Sheehan syndrome: An analysis of possible aetiological factors. Aust NZ J Obstet Gynaecol 34:534, 1994

Ananth CV, Berkowitz GS, Savitz DA, et al: Placental abruption and adverse perinatal outcomes. JAMA 282:1646, 1999a

Ananth CV, Demissie K, Smulian JC, et al: Placenta previa in singleton and twin births in the United States, 1989 through 1998: A comparison of risk factor profiles and associated conditions. Am J Obstet Gynecol 188:275, 2003a

Ananth CV, Demissie K, Smulian JC, et al: Relationship among placenta previa, fetal growth restriction, and preterm delivery: A population-based study. Obstet Gynecol 98:299, 2001a

Ananth CV, Savitz DA, Williams MA: Placental abruption and its association with hypertension and prolonged rupture of membranes: A methodologic review and meta-analysis. Obstet Gynecol 88:309, 1996

Ananth CV, Smulian JC, Demissie K, et al: Placental abruption among singleton and twin births in the United States: Risk factor profiles. Am J Epidemiol 153:771, 2001b

Ananth CV, Smulian JC, Vintzileos AM: Incidence of placental abruption in relation to cigarette smoking and hypertensive disorders during pregnancy: A meta-analysis of observational studies. Obstet Gynecol 93:622, 1999b

Ananth CV, Smulian JC, Vintzileos AM: The effect of placenta previa on neonatal mortality: A population-based study in the United States, 1989 through 1997. Am J Obstet Gynecol 188:1299, 2003b

Ananth CV, Wilcox AJ: Placental abruption and perinatal mortality in the United States. Am J Epidemiol 153:332, 2001

Andres RL, Piacquadio KM, Resnik R: A reappraisal of the need for autologous blood donation in the obstetric patient. Am J Obstet Gynecol 163:1551, 1990

Awad IT, Shorten GD: Amniotic fluid embolism and isolated coagulopathy: Atypical presentation of amniotic fluid embolism. Eur J Anaesthesiol 18:410, 2001

Babinszki A, Kerenyi T, Torok O, et al: Perinatal outcome in grand and great-grand multiparity: Effects of parity on obstetric risk factors. Am J Obstet Gynecol 181:669, 1999

Baglin T: Disseminated intravascular coagulation: Diagnosis and treatment. BMJ 312:683, 1996

Baker PN, Cunningham FG: Platelet and coagulation abnormalities. In Lindheimer ML, Roberts JM, Cunningham FG (eds): Chesley's Hypertensive Disorders in Pregnancy, 2nd ed. Stamford, CT, Appleton & Lange, 1999, p 349

Bakiri F, Bendib S-E, Maoui R, et al: The sella turcica in Sheehan's syndrome: Computerized tomographic study in 54 patients. J Endocrinol Invest 14:193, 1991

Barber A, Shires GT III, Shires GT: Shock. In Schwartz SI, Shires GT, Spencer FC, et al (eds): Principles of Surgery, 7th ed. New York, McGraw-Hill, 1999, p 101

Baxi LV, Liwanpo LI, Fink DJ: D-dimer as a predictor of morbidity in patients with ultrasonographic evidence of placental previa accreta, Abstract 424. J Soc Gynecol Investig 11:215A, 2004

Benirschke K, Kaufmann P (eds): Pathology of the Human Placenta, 4th ed. New York, Springer, 2000, p 554

Bennett BB: Uterine rupture during induction of labor at term with intravaginal misoprostol. Obstet Gynecol 89:832, 1997

Benson MD, Kobayashi H, Silver RK, et al: Immunologic studies in presumed amniotic fluid embolism. Obstet Gynecol 97:510, 2001

Berchuck A, Sokol RJ: Previous cesarean section, placenta increta, and uterine rupture in second-trimester abortion. Am J Obstet Gynecol 145:766, 1983

Berg CJ, Chang J, Callaghan WM, et al: Pregnancy-related mortality in the United States, 1991–1997. Obstet Gynecol 101:289, 2003

Bill AH: The treatment of placenta previa by prophylactic blood transfusion and cesarean section. Am J Obstet Gynecol 14:523, 1927

Bingol N, Fuchs M, Diaz V, et al: Teratogenicity of cocaine in humans. J Pediatr 110:93, 1987

Biswas R, Sawhney H, Dass R, et al: Histopathological study of placental bed biopsy in placenta previa. Acta Obstet Gynecol Scand 78:173, 1999

B-Lynch CB, Coker A, Laval AH, et al: The B-Lynch surgical technique for control of massive postpartum hemorrhage: An alternative to hysterectomy? Five cases reported. Br J Obstet Gynaecol 104:372, 1997

Bland RD, Shoemaker WC, Abraham E, et al: Hemodynamic and oxygen transport patterns in surviving and nonsurviving postoperative patients. Crit Care Med 13:85, 1985

Bond AL, Edersheim TG, Curry L, et al: Expectant management of abruptio placentae before 35 weeks gestation. Am J Perinatol 6:121, 1989

Bonnar J: Massive obstetric haemorrhage. Baillieres Best Pract Res Clin Obstet Gynaecol 14:1, 2000

Bonnar J, McNicol GP, Douglas AS: The behavior of the coagulation and fibrinolytic mechanisms in abruptio placentae. J Obstet Gynaecol Br Commonw 76:799, 1969

Boral LI, Hill SS, Apollon CJ, et al: The type and antibody screen, revisited. Am J Clin Pathol 71:578, 1979

Bouwmeester FW, Jonkhoff AR, Verheijen RHM, et al: Successful treatment of life-threatening postpartum hemorrhage with recombinant activated factor VII. Obstet Gynecol 101:1174, 2003

Brame RG, Harbert GM Jr, McGaughey HS Jr, et al: Maternal risk in abruption. Obstet Gynecol 31:224, 1968

Branch DW, Rodgers GM: Recombinant activated factor VII: A new weapon in the fight against hemorrhage. Obstet Gynecol 101:1155, 2003

Brar HS, Platt LD, DeVore GR, et al: Fetal umbilical velocimetry for the surveillance of pregnancies complicated by placenta previa. J Reprod Med 33:741, 1988

Burchell RC: Physiology of internal iliac artery ligation. J Obstet Gynaecol Br Commonw 75:642, 1968

Burkman RT, Bell WR, Atienza MF, et al: Coagulopathy with midtrimester induced abortion: Association with hyperosmolar urea administration. Am J Obstet Gynecol 127:533, 1977

Busch MP, Kleinman SH, Nemo GJ: Current and emerging infectious risks of blood transfusions. JAMA 289:959, 2003

Butler EL, Dashe JS, Ramus RM: Association between maternal serum alpha-fetoprotein and adverse outcomes in pregnancies with placenta previa. Obstet Gynecol 97:35, 2001

Catanzarite VA, Moffitt KD, Baker ML, et al: New approaches to the management of acute puerperal uterine inversion. Obstet Gynecol 68:7S, 1986

Centers for Disease Control and Prevention: Update: HIV-2 infection among blood and plasma donors—United States, June 1992–June 1995. MMWR 44:603, 1995

Chang YL, Chang SD, Cheng PJ: Perinatal outcome in patients with placental abruption with and without antepartum hemorrhage. Int J Gynaecol Obstet 75:193, 2001

Chescheir NC, Seeds JW: Spontaneous resolution of hypofibrinogenemia associated with death of a twin in utero: A case report. Am J Obstet Gynecol 159:1183, 1988

Chiao JJ, Minei JP, Shires GT III, et al: In vivo myocyte sodium activity and concentration during hemorrhagic shock. Am J Physiol 258:R684, 1990

Chichakli LO, Atrash HK, Mackay AP, et al: Pregnancy-related mortality in the United States due to hemorrhage: 1979–1992. Obstet Gynecol 94:721, 1999

Chin HG, Scott DR, Resnik R, et al: Angiographic embolization of intractable puerperal hematomas. Am J Obstet Gynecol 160:434, 1989

Cho JY, Kim SJ, Cha KY, et al: Interrupted circular suture: Bleeding control during cesarean delivery in placenta previa accreta. Obstet Gynecol 78:876, 1991

Chou MM, Tseng JJ, Ho ES, et al: Three-dimensional color power Doppler imaging in the assessment of uteroplacental neovascularization in placenta previa increta/percreta. Am J Obstet Gynecol 185:1257, 2001

Chung JW, Jeong HJ, Joh JH, et al: Percutaneous transcatheter angiographic embolization in the management of obstetric hemorrhage. J Reprod Med 48:268, 2003

Clark SL, Cotton DB, Gonik B, et al: Central hemodynamic alterations in amniotic fluid embolism. Am J Obstet Gynecol 158:1124, 1988

Clark SL, Hankins GDV, Dudley DA, et al: Amniotic fluid embolism: Analysis of the National Registry. Am J Obstet Gynecol 172:1158, 1995

Clark SL, Pavlova Z, Greenspoon J, et al: Squamous cells in the maternal pulmonary circulation. Am J Obstet Gynecol 154:104, 1986

Clark SL, Phelan JP, Yeh S-Y: Hypogastric artery ligation for obstetric hemorrhage. Obstet Gynecol 66:353, 1985

Cochrane Injuries Group Albumin Reviewers: Human albumin administration in critically ill patients: Systematic review of randomised control trials. BMJ 317:235, 1998

Cohn SM: Blood substitutes in surgery. Surgery 127:599, 2000

Combs CA, Laros RK Jr: Prolonged third stage of labor: Morbidity and risk factors. Obstet Gynecol 77:863, 1991

Combs CA, Murphy EL, Laros RK Jr: Factors associated with hemorrhage in cesarean deliveries. Obstet Gynecol 77:77, 1991a

Combs CA, Murphy EL, Laros RK Jr: Factors associated with postpartum hemorrhage with vaginal birth. Obstet Gynecol 77:69, 1991b

Combs CA, Nyberg DA, Mack LA, et al: Expectant management after sonographic diagnosis of placental abruption. Am J Perinatol 9:170, 1992

Consensus Development Conference: Perioperative red cell transfusion. Bethesda, MD, National Institutes of Health, Vol 7, No. 4, June 27–29, 1988

Cottier JP, Fignon A, Tranquart F, et al: Uterine necrosis after arterial embolization for postpartum hemorrhage. Obstet Gynecol 100:1074, 2002

Counts RB, Haisch C, Simon TL, et al: Hemostasis in massively transfused trauma patients. Ann Surg 190:91, 1979

Crane JMG, Van Den Hof MC, Dodds L, et al: Neonatal outcomes with placenta previa. Obstet Gynecol 93:541, 1999

Cunningham FG: Genital tract lacerations and puerperal hematomas. In Gilstrap LC III, Cunningham FG, Van Dorsten JP (eds): Operative Obstetrics, 2nd ed. New York, McGraw-Hill, 2002, p 223

Cunningham FG, Hollier LM: Fetal death. In: Williams Obstetrics, 20th ed (Suppl 4). Norwalk, CT, Appleton & Lange, August/September 1997

Czer LSC, Shoemaker WC: Optimal hematocrit value in critically ill postoperative patients. Surg Gynecol Obstet 147:363, 1978

Dashe JS, McIntire DD, Ramus RM, et al: Persistence of placenta previa according to gestational age at ultrasound detection. Obstet Gynecol 99:692, 2002

Davies S: Amniotic fluid embolism and isolated disseminated intravascular coagulation. Can J Anaesth 46:456, 1999

DeLee JB: A case of fatal hemorrhagic diathesis, with premature detachment of the placenta. Am J Obstet Gynecol 44:785, 1901

Deux JF, Bazot M, Le Blanche AF, et al: Is selective embolization of uterine arteries a safe alternative to hysterectomy in patients with postpartum hemorrhage? AJR Am J Roentgenol 177:145, 2001

Dildy GA III: Postpartum hemorrhage: New management options. Clin Obstet Gynecol 45:330, 2002

Dodd RY: Emerging infections, transfusion safety, and epidemiology. N Engl J Med 349:1205, 2003

Drakeley AJ, Le Roux PA, Anthony J, et al: Acute renal failure complicating severe preeclampsia requiring admission to an obstetric intensive care unit. Am J Obstet Gynecol 186:253, 2002

Drost S, Keil K: Expectant management of placenta previa: Cost-benefit analysis of outpatient treatment. Am J Obstet Gynecol 170:1254, 1994

Druzin ML: Packing of lower uterine segment for control of postcesarean bleeding in instances of placenta previa. Surg Gynecol Obstet 169:543, 1989

Eden RD, Parker RT, Gall SA: Rupture of the pregnant uterus: A 53-year review. Obstet Gynecol 68:671, 1986

Elliott JP, Gilpin B, Strong TH Jr, et al: Chronic abruption–oligohydramnios sequence. J Reprod Med 43:418, 1998

Eskes TK: Clotting disorders and placental abruption: Homocysteine—a new risk factor. Eur J Obstet Gynecol Reprod Biol 95:206, 2001

Etchason J, Petz L, Keeler E, et al: The cost effectiveness of preoperative autologous blood donations. N Engl J Med 332:719, 1995

Fahmy K, el-Gazar A, Sammour M, et al: Postpartum colposcopy of the cervix: Injury and healing. Int J Gynaecol Obstet 34:133, 1991

Farine D, Fox HE, Jakobson S, et al: Vaginal ultrasound for diagnosis of placenta previa. Am J Obstet Gynecol 159:566, 1988

Fedorkow DM, Nimrod CA, Taylor PJ: Ruptured uterus in pregnancy: A Canadian hospital's experience. Can Med Assoc J 137:27, 1987

Fox H: Placenta accreta, 1945–1969. Obstet Gynecol Surv 27:475, 1972

Frederiksen MC, Glassenberg R, Stika CS: Placenta previa: A 22-year analysis. Am J Obstet Gynecol 180:1432, 1999

Fretts RC, Usher RH: Causes of fetal death in women of advanced maternal age. Obstet Gynecol 89:40, 1997

Fuchs K, Peretz B-A, Marcovici R, et al: The "grand multipara"—is it a problem? A review of 5785 cases. Int J Gynaecol Obstet 23:321, 1985

Furuhashi M, Kurauchi O, Suganuma N: Pregnancy following placental abruption. Arch Gynecol Obstet 267:11, 2002

Gerbasi FR, Bottoms S, Farag A, et al: Increased intravascular coagulation associated with pregnancy. Obstet Gynecol 75:385, 1990

Gerstenfeld TS, Wing DA: Rectal misoprostol versus intravenous oxytocin for the prevention of postpartum hemorrhage after vaginal delivery. Am J Obstet Gynecol 185:878, 2001

Gesteland K, Oshiro B, Henry E, et al: Rates of placenta previa and placental abruption in women delivered only vaginally or only by cesarean section. Abstract No. 403. J Soc Gynecol Investig 11:208A, 2004

Gherman RB, Goodwin TM: Obstetric implications of activated protein C resistance and factor V Leiden mutation. Obstet Gynecol Surv 55:117, 2000

Gilbert TT, Smulian JC, Martin AA, et al: Obstetric admission to the intensive care unit: Outcomes and severity of illness. Obstet Gynecol 102:897, 2003

Gilbert WM, Danielsen B: Amniotic fluid embolism: Decreased mortality in a population-based study. Obstet Gynecol 93:973, 1999

Gilliam M, Rosenberg D, Davis F: The likelihood of placenta previa with greater number of cesarean deliveries and higher parity. Obstet Gynecol 99:976, 2002

Gilstrap LC III: Management of postpartum hemorrhage. In Gilstrap LC III, Cunningham FG, Van Dorsten JP (eds): Operative Obstetrics, 2nd ed. New York, McGraw-Hill, 2002, p 397

Glantz C, Purnell L: Clinical utility of sonography in the diagnosis and treatment of placental abruption. J Ultrasound Med 21:837, 2002

Goldberg J, Pereira L, Berghella V: Pregnancy after uterine artery embolization. Obstet Gynecol 100:869, 2002

Goodnough LT: Risks of blood transfusion. Crit Care Med 31:S678, 2003

Grünfeld JP, Pertuiset N: Acute renal failure in pregnancy: 1987. Am J Kidney Dis 4:359, 1987

Handler AS, Mason ED, Rosenberg DL, et al: The relationship between exposure during pregnancy to cigarette smoking and cocaine use and placenta previa. Am J Obstet Gynecol 170:884, 1994

Hankins GDV, Berryman GK, Scott RT Jr, et al: Maternal arterial desaturation with 15-methyl prostaglandin F2 alpha for uterine atony. Obstet Gynecol 72:367, 1988

Hankins GDV, Snyder RR, Clark SL, et al: Acute hemodynamic and respiratory effects of amniotic fluid embolism in the pregnant goat model. Am J Obstet Gynecol 168:1113, 1993

Hankins GDV, Snyder R, Dinh T, et al: Documentation of amniotic fluid embolism via lung histopathology: Fact or fiction? J Reprod Med 47:1021, 2002

Hansch E, Chitkara U, McAlpine J, et al: Pelvic arterial embolization for control of obstetric hemorrhage: A five-year experience. Am J Obstet Gynecol 180:1454, 1999

Hardardottir H, Borgida AF, Sanders MM, et al: Histologic myometrial fibers adherent to the placenta: Impact of method of placental removal. Am J Obstet Gynecol 174:358, 1996

Harvey C, Hankins G, Clark S: Amniotic fluid embolism and oxygen transport patterns. Am J Obstet Gynecol 174(Part 2):304, 1996

Hauth JC, Cunningham FG: Preeclampsia-eclampsia. In Lindheimer ML, Roberts JM, Cunningham FG (eds): Chesley's Hypertensive Disorders in Pregnancy, 2nd ed. Stamford, CT, Appleton & Lange, 1999, p 179

Hayman RG, Arulkumaran S, Steer PJ: Uterine compression sutures: Surgical management of postpartum hemorrhage. Obstet Gynecol 99:502, 2002

Hazelgrove JF, Price C, Pappachan VJ, et al: Multicenter study of obstetric admissions to 14 intensive care units in southern England. Crit Care Med 29:770, 2001

Hebert PC, Wells G, Blajchman MA, et al: A multicenter, randomized, controlled clinical trial of transfusion requirements in critical care. N Engl J Med 340:409, 1999

Henrich W, Fuchs I, Ehrenstein T, et al: Antenatal diagnosis of placenta percreta with planned in situ retention and methotrexate therapy in a woman infected with HIV. Ultrasound Obstet Gynecol 20:90, 2002

Hertzberg BS, Bowie JD, Carroll BA, et al: Diagnosis of placenta previa during the third trimester: Role of transperineal sonography. AJR Am J Roentgenol 159:83, 1992

Ho EM, Brown J, Graves W, et al: Maternal death at an inner-city hospital, 1949–2000. Am J Obstet Gynecol 187:1213, 2002

Hotchkiss RS, Karl IE: The pathophysiology and treatment of sepsis. N Engl J Med 348:138, 2003

Howard RJ, Straughn JM Jr, Huh WK, et al: Pelvic umbrella pack for refractory obstetric hemorrhage secondary to posterior uterine rupture. Obstet Gynecol 100:1061, 2002

Hsu S, Rodgers B, Lele A, et al: Use of packing in obstetric hemorrhage of uterine origin. J Reprod Med 48:69, 2003

Hung T-II, Shau W-Y, Hsieh C-C, et al: Risk factors for placenta accreta. Obstet Gynecol 93:545, 1999

Hurd WW, Miodovnik M, Hertzberg V, et al: Selective management of abruptio placentae: A prospective study. Obstet Gynecol 61:467, 1983

Jackson BR, Busch MP, Stramer SL, et al: The cost-effectiveness of NAT for HIV, HCV, and HBV in whole-blood donations. Transfusion 43:721, 2003

Jegasothy R: Sudden maternal deaths in Malaysia: A case report. J Obstet Gynaecol Res 28:186, 2002

Jimenez JM, Pritchard JA: Pathogenesis and treatment of coagulation defects resulting from fetal death. Obstet Gynecol 32:449, 1968

Johnson HW: The conservative management of some varieties of placenta previa. Am J Obstet Gynecol 50:248, 1945

Karam AK, Bristow RE, Bienstock J, et al: Argon beam coagulation facilitates management of placenta percreta with bladder invasion. Obstet Gynecol 102:555, 2003

Kayani SI, Walkinshaw SA, Preston C: Pregnancy outcome in severe placental abruption. Br J Obstet Gynaecol 110:679, 2003

Kayem G, Pannier E, Goffinet F, et al: Fertility after conservative treatment of placenta accreta. Fertil Steril 78:637, 2002

Kettel LM, Branch DW, Scott JR: Occult placental abruption after maternal trauma. Obstet Gynecol 71:449, 1988

Khong TY: Expression of endothelin-1 in amniotic fluid embolism and possible pathophysiological mechanism. Br J Obstet Gynaecol 105:802, 1998

Kieser KE, Baskett TF: A 10-year population-based study of uterine rupture. Obstet Gynecol 100:749, 2002

King DL: Placental migration demonstrated by ultrasonography. Radiology 109:167, 1973

Klapholz H: Blood transfusion in contemporary obstetric practice. Obstet Gynecol 75:940, 1990

Klein HG: The prospects for red-cell substitutes. N Engl J Med 342:1666, 2000

Kopko PM, Marshal CS, MacKenzie MR, et al: Transfusion-related acute lung injury: Report of a clinical look-back investigation. JAMA 287:1968, 2002

Kovacs BW, DeVore GR: Management of acute and subacute puerperal uterine inversion with terbutaline sulfate. Am J Obstet Gynecol 150:784, 1984

Kovacs K: Sheehan syndrome. Lancet 361:520, 2003

Kramer MS, Usher RH, Pollack R, et al: Etiologic determinants of abruptio placentae. Obstet Gynecol 89:221, 1997

Kupferminc MJ, Eldor A, Steinman N, et al: Increased frequency of genetic thrombophilia in women with complications of pregnancy. N Engl J Med 340:9, 1999

Laine E, Steadman R, Calhoun L, et al: Comparison of RBCs and FFP with whole blood during liver transplant surgery. Transfusion 43:322, 2003

Laing FC: Ultrasound evaluation of obstetric problems relating to the lower uterine segment and cervix. In Fleischer AC, Manning FA, Jeanty P, et al (eds): Sonography in Obstetrics and Gynecology: Principles and Practice, 5th ed. Stamford, CT, Appleton & Lange, 1996, p 720

Lam G, Kuller J, McMahon M: Use of magnetic resonance imaging and ultrasound in the antenatal diagnosis of placenta accreta. J Soc Gynecol Investig 9:37, 2002

Landy HJ, Weingold AB: Management of a multiple gestation complicated by an antepartum fetal demise. Obstet Gynecol Surv 44:171, 1989

Lee W, Ginsburg KA, Cotton DB, et al: Squamous and trophoblastic cells in the maternal pulmonary circulation identified by invasive hemodynamic monitoring during the peripartum period. Am J Obstet Gynecol 155:999, 1986

Lerner R, Margolin M, Slate WG, et al: Heparin in the treatment of hypofibrinogenemia complicating fetal death in utero. Am J Obstet Gynecol 97:373, 1967

Leung TY, Chan LW, Tam WH, et al: Risk and prediction of preterm delivery in pregnancies complicated by antepartum hemorrhage of unknown origin before 34 weeks. Gynecol Obstet Invest 52:227, 2001

Leveno KJ, Cunningham FG, Gant NF, et al: Williams Manual of Obstetrics, 1st ed. New York, McGraw-Hill, 2003

Levi M, ten Cate H, van der Poll T, et al: Pathogenesis of disseminated intravascular coagulation in sepsis. JAMA 270:975, 1993

Liang H-S, Jeng C-J, Sheen T-C, et al: First-trimester uterine rupture from a placenta percreta. J Reprod Med 48:474, 2003

Lichtenberg ES: Angiography as treatment for a high cervical tear—a case report. J Reprod Med 48:287, 2003

Lin Y, Callum JL, Coovadia AS, et al: Transfusion of ABO-nonidentical platelets is not associated with adverse clinical outcomes in cardiovascular surgery patients. Transfusion 42:166, 2002

Linden JV, Wagner K, Voytovich AE, et al: Transfusion errors in New York State: An analysis of 10 years' experience. Transfusion 40:1207, 2001

Lindheimer MD, Grünfeld JP, Davison JM: Renal disorders. In Barron WM, Lindheimer MD (eds): Medical Disorders During Pregnancy. St Louis, Mosby, 2000, p 39

Lipitz S, Admon D, Menczer J, et al: Midtrimester bleeding: Variables which affect the outcome of pregnancy. Gynecol Obstet Invest 32:24, 1991

Macafee CHG: Placenta praevia: A study of 174 cases. J Obstet Gynaecol Br Emp 52:313, 1945

Magpie Trial Collaborative Group: Do women with pre-eclampsia, and their babies, benefit from magnesium sulphate? The Magpie Trial: A randomised placebo-controlled trial. Lancet 359:1877, 2002

Major CA, deVeciana M, Lewis DF, et al: Preterm premature rupture of membranes and abruptio placentae: Is there an association between these pregnancy complications? Am J Obstet Gynecol 172:672, 1995

Maldjian C, Adam R, Pelosi M, et al: MRI appearance of placenta percreta and placenta accreta. Magn Reson Imaging 17:965, 1999

Martin JA, Hamilton BE, Ventura SJ, et al: Births: Final data for 2001. National Vital Statistics Reports, Vol 51, No. 2. Hyattsville, MD, National Center for Health Statistics, 2002

Matsuda Y, Maeda T, Kouno S: Comparison of neonatal outcome including cerebral palsy between abruption placentae and placenta previa. Eur J Obstet Gynecol Reprod Biol 106:125, 2003

Maymon R, Shulman A, Pomeranz M, et al: Uterine rupture at term pregnancy with the use of intracervical prostaglandin E_2 gel for induction of labor. Am J Obstet Gynecol 165:368, 1991

McCormick ML, Sanghvi HC, McIntosh N: Preventing postpartum hemorrhage in low-resource settings. Int J Gynaecol Obstet 77:267, 2002

McVay PA, Hoag RW, Hoag MS, et al: Safety and use of autologous blood donation during the third trimester of pregnancy. Am J Obstet Gynecol 160:1479, 1989

Miller DA, Diaz FG, Paul RH: Incidence of placenta previa with previous cesarean. Am J Obstet Gynecol 174:345, 1996

Miller DA, Goodwin TM, Gherman RB, et al: Intrapartum rupture of the unscarred uterus. Obstet Gynecol 89:671, 1997

Miller DA, Paul RH: Rupture of the unscarred uterus. Am J Obstet Gynecol 174:345, 1996

Mishra A, Landzberg BR, Parente JT: Uterine rupture in association with alkaloidal ("crack") cocaine abuse. Am J Obstet Gynecol 173:243, 1995

Misra DP, Ananth CV: Risk factor profiles of placental abruption in first and second pregnancies: Heterogeneous etiologies. J Clin Epidemiol 52:453, 1999

Morgan MA, Berkowitz KM, Thomas SJ, et al: Abruptio placentae: Perinatal outcome in normotensive and hypertensive patients. Am J Obstet Gynecol 170:1595, 1994

Morrison JC, Martin RW, Dodson MK, et al: Blood transfusions after postpartum hemorrhage due to uterine atony. J Matern Fetal Invest 1:209, 1991

Morrison JC, Sumrall DD, Chevalier SP, et al: The effect of provider education on blood utilization practices. Am J Obstet Gynecol 169:1240, 1993

Morrison JE: Obstetrics and Gynecology Annual. New York, Appleton-Century-Crofts, 1978, p 113

Mortensen JT, Thulstrup AM, Larsen H, et al: Smoking, sex of the offspring, and risk of placental abruption, placenta previa, and preeclampsia: A population-based cohort study. Acta Obstet Gynecol Scand 80:894, 2001

Mouer JR: Placenta previa: Antepartum conservative management, inpatient versus outpatient. Am J Obstet Gynecol 170:1683, 1994

Mullon J, Giacoppe G, Clagett C, et al: Transfusions of polymerized bovine hemoglobin in a patient with severe autoimmune hemolytic anemia. N Engl J Med 342:1638, 2000

Naef RW III, Chauhan SP, Chevalier SP, et al: Prediction of hemorrhage at cesarean delivery. Obstet Gynecol 83:923, 1994

Naeye RL: Abruptio placentae and placenta previa: Frequency, perinatal mortality, and cigarette smoking. Obstet Gynecol 55:701, 1980

Nagaya K, Fetters MD, Ishikawa M, et al: Causes of maternal mortality in Japan. JAMA 283:2661, 2000

National Institutes of Health: Indications for the use of red blood cells, platelets and fresh frozen plasma. Washington, DC, US Department of Health and Human Services, Pub. No. 89-2974A, August 1993

Nijman RG, Mantingh A, Aarnoudse JG: Persistent retained placenta percreta: Methotrexate treatment and Doppler flow characteristics. Br J Obstet Gynaecol 109:587, 2002

Nizard J, Barrinque L, Frydman R, et al: Fertility and pregnancy outcomes following hypogastric artery ligation for severe postpartum haemorrhage. Hum Reprod 18:844, 2003

O'Brien P, El-Refaey H, Gordon A, et al: Rectally administered misoprostol for the treatment of postpartum hemorrhage unresponsive to oxytocin and ergometrine: A descriptive study. Obstet Gynecol 92:212, 1998

Odendaal HJ, van Schie DL, de Jeu RM: Adverse effects of maternal cigarette smoking on preterm labor and abruption placentae. Int J Gynaecol Obstet 74:287, 2001

Oleen MA, Mariano JP: Controlling refractory atonic postpartum hemorrhage with Hemabate sterile solution. Am J Obstet Gynecol 162:205, 1990

Ornan D, White R, Pollak J, et al: Pelvic embolization for intractable postpartum hemorrhage: Long-term follow-up and implications for fertility. Obstet Gynecol 102:904, 2003

Pacheco LD, Van Hook JW, Gei AF: Disseminated intravascular coagulopathy. In Dildy GA, Belfort MA, Saade GR, et al (eds): Critical Care Obstetrics, 4th ed. Malden, MA, Blackwell Science, 2004, p 404

Pealer LN, Marfin AA, Petersen LR, et al: Transmission of West Nile virus through blood transfusion in the United States in 2002. N Engl J Med 349:1236, 2003

Pearlman MD, Tintinalli JE, Lorenz RP: A prospective controlled study of outcome after trauma during pregnancy. Am J Obstet Gynecol 162:1502, 1990

Pelage J-P, Le Dref O, Jacob D, et al: Selective arterial embolization of the uterine arteries in the management of intractable postpartum hemorrhage. Acta Obstet Gynecol Scand 78:698, 1999

Pelosi MA III, Pelosi MA: Spontaneous uterine rupture at thirtythree weeks subsequent to previous superficial laparoscopic myomectomy. Am J Obstet Gynecol 177:1547, 1997

Peltier LF: Fat embolism: A reappraisal of the problem. Clin Orthop 187:3, 1984

Petersen IR, Nyholm HCJ: Multiple pregnancies with single intrauterine demise. Description of twenty-eight pregnancies. Acta Obstet Gynecol Scand 78:202, 1999

Pharoah POD, Adi Y: Consequences of in-utero death in a twin pregnancy. Lancet 355:1597, 2000

Platt LD, Druzin ML: Acute puerperal inversion of the uterus. Am J Obstet Gynecol 141:187, 1981

Porter TF, Clark SL, Dildy GA, et al: Isolated disseminated intravascular coagulation and amniotic fluid embolism. Am J Obstet Gynecol 174:486, 1996

Pritchard JA: Haematological problems associated with delivery, placental abruption, retained dead fetus, and amniotic fluid embolism. Clin Haematol 2:563, 1973

Pritchard JA: Fetal death in utero. Obstet Gynecol 14:573, 1959

Pritchard JA, Cunningham FG, Pritchard SA, et al: On reducing the frequency of severe abruptio placentae. Am J Obstet Gynecol 165:1345, 1991

Pritchard JA, Cunningham FG, Mason RA: Coagulation changes in eclampsia: Their frequency and pathogenesis. Am J Obstet Gynecol 124:855, 1976

Pritchard JA, Mason R, Corley M, et al: Genesis of severe placental abruption. Am J Obstet Gynecol 108:22, 1970

Pritchard JA, Brekken AL: Clinical and laboratory studies on severe abruptio placentae. Am J Obstet Gynecol 97:681, 1967

Pritchard JA: Changes in the blood volume during pregnancy and delivery. Anesthesiology 26:393, 1965

Pritchard JA, Baldwin RM, Dickey JC, et al: Blood volume changes in pregnancy and the puerperium, 2. Red blood cell loss and changes in apparent blood volume during and following vaginal delivery, cesarean section, and cesarean section plus total hysterectomy. Am J Obstet Gynecol 84:1271, 1962

Pritchard JA, Whalley PJ: Abortion complicated by *Clostridium perfringens* infection. Am J Obstet Gynecol 111:484, 1971

Propst AM, Thorp JM Jr: Traumatic vulvar hematomas: Conservative versus surgical management. South Med J 91:144, 1998

Rachagan SP, Raman S, Balasundram G, et al: Rupture of the pregnant uterus—a 21-year review. Aust NZ J Obstet Gynaecol 31:37, 1991

Rahman MH, Akhter HH, Khan Chowdhury ME, et al: Obstetric deaths in Bangladesh, 1996–1997. Int J Gynaecol Obstet 77:161, 2002

Rebarber A, Lonser R, Jackson S, et al: The safety of intraoperative autologous blood collection and autotransfusion during cesarean section. Am J Obstet Gynecol 179:715, 1998

Reyal F, Sibony O, Oury JF, et al: Criteria for transfusion in severe postpartum hemorrhage: Analysis of practice and risk factors. Eur J Obstet Gynecol Reprod Biol 112:61, 2004

Rice JP, Kay HH, Mahony BS: The clinical significance of uterine leiomyomas in pregnancy. Am J Obstet Gynecol 160:1212, 1989

Ridgway LE: Puerperal emergency: Vaginal and vulvar hematomas. Obstet Gynecol Clin North Am 22:275, 1995

Roman AS, Rebarber A: Seven ways to control postpartum hemorrhage. Contemp Ob/Gyn, March 2003, p 34

Sachs BP, Brown DA, Driscoll SG, et al: Maternal mortality in Massachusetts. Trends and prevention. N Engl J Med 316:667, 1987

Sachs DA: Blood and component therapy in obstetrics. In Clark SL, Cotton DB, Hankins GDV, et al (eds): Critical Care Obstetrics, 2nd ed. Boston, Blackwell, 1991, p 599

Salihu HM, Li Q, Rouse DJ, et al: Placenta previa: Neonatal death after live births in the United States. Am J Obstet Gynecol 188:1305, 2003

Sanderson DA, Milton PJD: The effectiveness of ultrasound screening at 18–20 weeks gestational age for predication of placenta previa. J Obstet Gynaecol 11:320, 1991

Saraiya M, Green CA, Berg CJ, et al: Spontaneous abortion-related deaths among women in the United States—1981–1991. Obstet Gynecol 94:172, 1999

Schierhout G, Roberts I: Fluid resuscitation with colloid or crystalloid solutions in critically ill patients: A systemic review of randomised trials. BMJ 316:961, 1998

Seski JC, Compton AA: Abruptio placentae following a negative oxytocin challenge test. Am J Obstet Gynecol 125:276, 1976

Shah-Hosseini R, Evrard JR: Puerperal uterine inversion. Obstet Gynecol 73:567, 1989

Sheehan HL, Murdoch R: Post-partum necrosis of the anterior pituitary: Pathological and clinical aspects. Br J Obstet Gynaecol 45:456, 1938

Sherman SJ, Greenspoon JS, Nelson JM, et al: Identifying the obstetric patient at high risk of multiple-unit blood transfusions. J Reprod Med 37:649, 1992

Shoemaker WC, Kram HB: Comparison of the effects of crystalloids and colloids on hemodynamic oxygen transport, mortality and morbidity. In Simmons RS, Udeko AJ (eds): Debates in General Surgery. Chicago, Year Book, 1991

Sholl JS: Abruptio placentae: Clinical management in nonacute cases. Am J Obstet Gynecol 156:40, 1987

Sibai BM, Lindheimer M, Hauth J, et al: Risk factors for preeclampsia, abruptio placentae, and adverse neonatal outcomes among women with chronic hypertension. N Engl J Med 339:667, 1998

Siegel LJ, Gerigk L, Tuettenberg J, et al: Cerebral sinus thrombosis in a trauma patient after recombinant activated factor VII infusion. Anesthesiology 100:441, 2004

Silliman CC, Boshkov LK, Mehdizadehkashi Z, et al: Transfusion-related acute lung injury: Epidemiology and a prospective analysis of etiologic factors. Blood 101:454, 2003

Singla AK, Lapinski RH, Berkowitz RL, et al: Are women who are Jehovah's Witnesses at risk of maternal death? Am J Obstet Gynecol 185:893, 2001

Sloan EP, Koenigsberg M, Gens D, et al: Diaspirin cross-linked hemoglobin (DCLHb) in the treatment of severe traumatic hemorrhagic shock: A randomized controlled efficacy trial. JAMA 282:1857, 1999

Smith RS, Lauria MR, Comstock CH, et al: Transvaginal ultrasonography for all placentas that appear to be low-lying or over the internal cervical os. Ultrasound Obstet Gynecol 9:22, 1997

Stafford PA, Biddinger PW, Zumwalt RE: Lethal intrauterine fetal trauma. Am J Obstet Gynecol 159:485, 1988

Stanten RD, Iverson LI, Daugharty TM, et al: Amniotic fluid embolism causing catastrophic pulmonary vasoconstriction: Diagnosis by transesophageal echocardiogram and treatment by cardiopulmonary bypass. Obstet Gynecol 102:496, 2003

Steiner PE, Lushbaugh CC: Maternal pulmonary embolism by amniotic fluid. JAMA 117:1245, 1941

Stettler RW, Lutich A, Pritchard JA, et al: Traumatic placental abruption: A separation from traditional thought. Presented at the American College of Obstetricians and Gynecologists Annual Clinical Meeting, Las Vegas, April 27, 1992

Stolte L, van Kessel H, Seelen J, et al: Failure to produce the syndrome of amniotic fluid embolism by infusion of amniotic fluid and meconium into monkeys. Am J Obstet Gynecol 98:694, 1967

Stramer SL, Glynn SA, Kleinman SH, et al: Detection of HIV-I and HCV infections among antibody-negative blood donors by nucleic acid–amplification testing. N Engl J Med 351:760, 2004

Taipale P, Hiilesmaa V, Ylostalo P: Transvaginal ultrasonography at 18–23 weeks in predicting placenta previa at delivery. Ultrasound Obstet Gynecol 12:422, 1998

Thiery M, Delbeke L: Acute puerperal uterine inversion: Two-step management with a β-mimetic and a prostaglandin. Am J Obstet Gynecol 153:891, 1985

Timor-Tritsch IE, Yunis RA: Confirming the safety of transvaginal sonography in patients suspected of placenta previa. Obstet Gynecol 81:742, 1993

Toivonen S, Heinonen S, Anttila M, et al: Reproductive risk factors, Doppler findings, and outcome of affected births in placental abruption: A population-based analysis. Am J Perinatol 19:451, 2002

Toohey JS, Keegan KA Jr, Morgan MA, et al: The "dangerous multipara": Fact or fiction? Am J Obstet Gynecol 172:683, 1995

Towell ME: Fetal acid–base physiology and intrauterine asphyxia. In Goodwin JW, Godden JO, Chance GW (eds): Perinatal Medicine. Baltimore, Williams & Wilkins, 1976, p 200

Towers CV, Pircon RA, Heppard M: Is tocolysis safe in the management of third-trimester bleeding? Am J Obstet Gynecol 180:1572, 1999

Turney JH, Ellis CM, Parsons FM: Obstetric acute renal failure 1956–1987. Br J Obstet Gynaecol 96:679, 1989

Twickler DM, Lucas MJ, Balis AB, et al: Color flow mapping for myometrial invasion in women with a prior cesarean delivery. J Matern Fetal Med 9:330, 2000

Van Vugt PJH, Baudoin P, Blom VM, et al: Inversio uteri puerperalis. Acta Obstet Gynecol Scand 60:353, 1981

Villar J, Gülmezoglu AM, Hofmeyr GJ, et al: Systematic review of randomized controlled trials of misoprostol to prevent postpartum hemorrhage. Obstet Gynecol 100:1301, 2002

Villella J, Garry D, Levine G, et al: Postpartum angiographic embolization for vulvovaginal hematoma—a report of two cases. J Reprod Med 46:65, 2001

Ward CR: Avoiding an incision through the anterior previa at cesarean delivery. Obstet Gynecol 102:552, 2003

Watson P, Besch N, Bowes WA Jr: Management of acute and subacute puerperal inversion of the uterus. Obstet Gynecol 55:12, 1980

Weiwen Y: Study of the diagnosis and management of amniotic fluid embolism: 38 cases of analysis. Obstet Gynecol 95:385, 2000

Whitehead R: The hypothalamus in post-partum hypopituitarism. J Pathol Bacteriol 86:55, 1963

Williams MA, Mittendorf R, Lieberman E, et al: Cigarette smoking during pregnancy in relation to placenta previa. Am J Obstet Gynecol 165:28, 1991

Wilson RF, Mammem E, Walt AJ: Eight years of experience with massive blood transfusions. Trauma 11:275, 1971

Wing DA, Paul RH, Millar LK: Management of the symptomatic placenta previa: A randomized, controlled trial of inpatient versus outpatient expectant management. Am J Obstet Gynecol 174:305, 1996a

Wing DA, Paul RH, Millar LK: The usefulness of coagulation studies and blood banking in the symptomatic placenta previa. Am J Obstet Gynecol 174:346, 1996b

Witlin AG, Saade GR, Mattar F, et al: Risk factors for abruptio placentae and eclampsia: Analysis of 445 consecutively managed women with severe preeclampsia and eclampsia. Am J Obstet Gynecol 180:1322, 1999

Wright-Kanuth MS, Smith LA: Developments in component therapy: Novel components and new uses for familiar preparations. Clin Lab Sci 15:116, 2002

Zahn CM, Yeomans ER: Postpartum hemorrhage: Placenta accreta, uterine inversion and puerperal hematomas. Clin Obstet Gynecol 33:422, 1990

Zaki ZM, Bahar AM, Ali ME, et al: Risk factors and morbidity in patients with placenta previa accreta compared to placenta previa non-accreta. Acta Obstet Gynecol Scand 77:391, 1998

Zeeman GG, Cunningham FG: Blood volume expansion in women with antepartum eclampsia. J Soc Gynecol Investig 9:112A, 2002

Zeeman GG, Wendel Jr GD, Cunningham FG: A blueprint for obstetric critical care. Am J Obstet Gynecol 188:532, 2003

Zelop CM, Harlow BL, Frigoletto FD Jr, et al: Emergency peripartum hysterectomy. Am J Obstet Gynecol 168:1443, 1993

36

Preterm Birth

Low birthweight defines neonates who are born too small, and *preterm* or *premature birth* are the terms used to define neonates who are born too early. With respect to gestational age, a newborn may be preterm, term, or postterm. With respect to size, a newborn may be normally grown or appropriate for gestational age, small in size or small-for-gestational age, or overgrown and consequently large-for-gestational age. In recent years, the term *small-for-gestational age* has been widely used to categorize newborns whose birthweight is usually below the 10th percentile for gestational age. Other frequently used terms have included *fetal growth restriction* or *intrauterine growth restriction*. The term *large-for-gestational age* has been widely used to categorize newborns whose birthweight is above the 90th percentile for gestational age, and the term *appropriate-for-gestational age* designates newborns whose weight is between the 10th and 90th percentiles. Thus, infants born before term can be small- or large-for-gestational age but still fit the definition of preterm.

In the United States in 2001, almost 28,000 infants died in their first year of life (Table 36–1). Preterm birth, which is defined as delivery before 37 completed weeks, was implicated in approximately two thirds of these deaths. Overall, infant mortality has continued to decline from 1990 to 2000, albeit at a slower rate than in earlier decades (Fig. 36–1). The causes of infant mortality have also declined from 1990 to 2000, except for those associated with preterm birth or low birthweight (Fig. 36–2). Importantly, singleton preterm births in this country have increased only in white non-Hispanic women. Despite this, preterm births in this country remain highest in black women (Fig. 36–3).

CONSIDERATIONS SURROUNDING PRETERM BIRTH

ESTIMATING SURVIVAL. Aside from survival, appreciable physical and intellectual compromise afflicts extremely low-birthweight infants. At what gestational age should obstetrical interventions be practiced?

TABLE 36–1 Infant Mortality in the United States in 2001

	Live Births (%)	Infant Deaths (%)
Total infants	4,026,036 (100)	27,523 (100)
Gestational age at birth		
Less than 32 weeks	77,676 (1.9)	14,060 (51)
32–36 weeks	390,623 (10)	3,538 (13)
37–41 weeks	3,235,790 (80)	8,221 (30)
42 weeks or more	274,065 (7)	809 (2.9)
Unknown	39,882 (1)	894 (3.2)

Adapted from Mathews and colleagues, 2003.

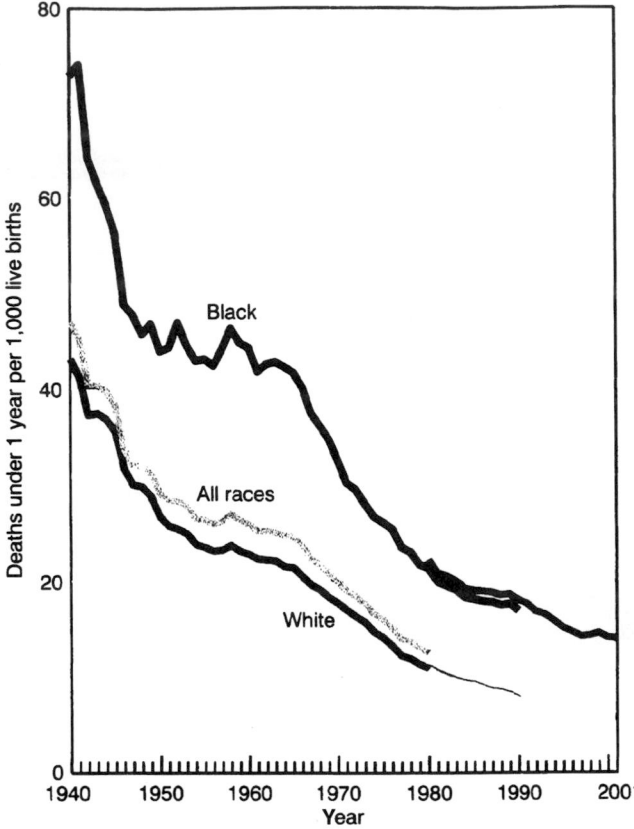

FIGURE 36–1. Infant mortality by race in the United States, 1940–2001, according to the National Vital Statistics Report. (From Arias and colleagues, 2003.)

Improved survival of extremely low-birthweight infants has understandably lowered the "threshold of viability." Stevenson and colleagues (1998) reported outcomes from an inborn cohort of the National Institute of Child Health and

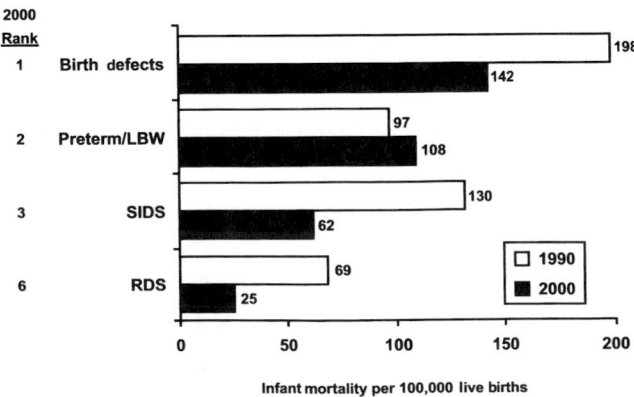

FIGURE 36–2. Selected leading causes of infant mortality and their rank order for the United States, 1990 and 2000. (LBW = low birthweight, SIDS = sudden infant death syndrome, RDS = respiratory disease syndrome.) (From the National Center for Health Statistics, 2000; prepared by the March of Dimes Birth Defects Foundation, 2003.)

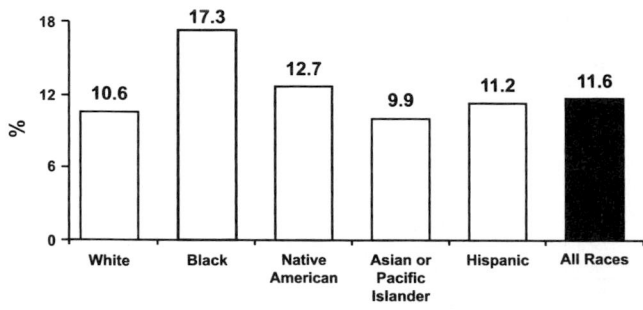

FIGURE 36–3. Preterm births, defined as before 37 weeks, by maternal race/ethnicity for the United States in 2000. (From National Center for Health Statistics, 2002; prepared by the March of Dimes Birth Defects Foundation, 2003.)

Human Development (NICHD) Neonatal Research Network for 1993 and 1994. Death, severe neonatal morbidities, or both were common before 26 weeks, and they were almost universal before 24 weeks. Thus, gestations from 23 to 25 weeks pose the greatest dilemma for providers of obstetrical and newborn care and for their patients.

What is the best management scheme? This question of course cannot be answered, except possibly on an individual basis. Approaches to preterm labor and delivery currently are guided in large part by expectations for survival of the neonate. Perceptions of the potential for survival, however, are often confused by imprecisely known gestational age. For neonates shown in Figure 36–4, the most accurate estimates of gestational age are made from last menses, obstetrical parameters, and ultrasonographical examination (American College of Obstetricians and Gynecologists, 2002). They are considered to be the "best case" outcomes. Perinatal mortality and morbidity decrease markedly from 24 to 26 weeks gestation. Survival increases from approximately 20 percent at 24^0 weeks up to 50 percent at 25^0 weeks, or an increase of almost 4 percent each day.

However, most survival data are based on birthweight, which may vary appreciably between 24 and 26 weeks.

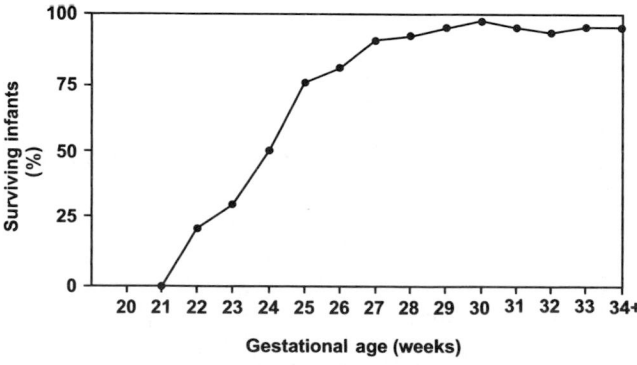

FIGURE 36–4. Neonatal Research Network: Survival of preterm liveborn infants according to gestational age at birth. (Data from Lemons and colleagues, 2001, with permission.)

Neonates born between 24 and 26 weeks can vary in weight from 435 g to 1640 g (Alexander and associates, 1996). The gestational age survival rates for live births during 1995 and 1996 within the NICHD Neonatal Research Network are shown in Figure 36–4. Although survival is possible for newborns weighing 500 to 750 g, many survivors are growth restricted and therefore of more advanced maturity. For example, survival of a 380-g neonate has been reported, but the gestational age was confirmed to be $25^{3/7}$ weeks (Ginsberg and associates, 1990). **Neonatal morbidity and mortality are primarily influenced by gestational age and thus maturity, and less so by birthweight**.

Evans and Levene (2001) described the appreciable selection bias in preterm survival studies. The Neonatal Research Network data reflect an important bias—all neonates were delivered in tertiary university centers and only liveborn infants were included. These rates also exclude deaths after 120 days.

LONG-TERM OUTCOMES. The high rate of significant neonatal morbidity in these very immature neonates and the diminished likelihood of a normal life must be weighed against the *apparent* triumph of survival. A number of investigators have reported long-term outcomes in survivors born at the frontier of viability.

Doyle and colleagues (1994) did a follow-up study of neonates born at 24 to 26 weeks. They reported that only 20 percent were totally free of impairment at 5 years or more. Vohr and co-workers (2000) assessed outcomes at 18 to 22 months in 1151 survivors from the NICHD Neonatal Research Network centers who were born in 1993 and 1994. Their birthweight was 400 to 1000 g. Only 50 percent had a normal neurodevelopmental and sensory assessment, and those with lower birthweights had markedly worse outcomes as predicted by chronic lung disease, grades 3 and 4 intraventricular hemorrhage, and periventricular leukomalacia. Wood and associates (2000) reported similar results in the EPI Cure Study Group of the United Kingdom. They evaluated 283 infants who were born at or before 25 weeks who survived to 30 months of age. Only 1 of 138 infants born during the 22nd week had *no* neurological disability, compared with 11 of 241 (5 percent) of those born during the 23rd week; 45 of 382 (12 percent) of those born during the 24th week; and 98 of 424 (23 percent) of those born during the 25th week. Stoll and colleagues (2004) found that these extremely lowbirthweight newborns compared with similarly matched uninfected neonates had increased associated risks of poor neurodevelopmental and growth outcomes in early childhood.

Hack and Fanaroff (1999) concluded that the limits of viability have been reached and that the continuing toll of major morbidity is of serious concern. In analyzing data collected from three different time periods by the NICHD Neonatal Research Network, Fanaroff and colleagues (2003) found that newborn outcomes at the threshold of viability—24 or 25 weeks or 501 to 750 g—did not improve from 1993 to 1994 compared with 1999 to 2000. This followed a dramatic

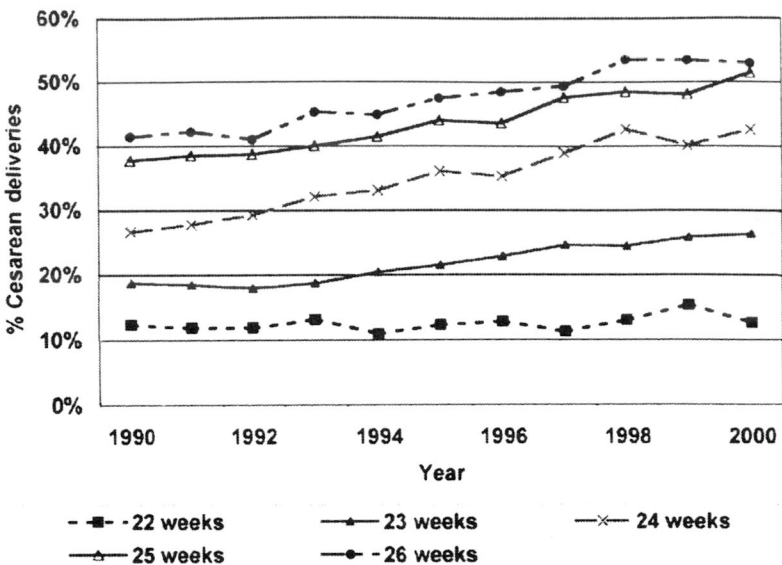

FIGURE 36–5. Cesarean delivery rates for the United States from 1990 to 2000 at 22 to 26 weeks' gestation. Except for 22-week gestations, there is an obvious trend toward increasing cesarean deliveries. (From DeRoche and colleagues, 2002, with permission.)

improvement in both mortality and morbidity between 1987 and 1988 and 1993 to 1994. Similarly, Horbar and colleagues (2002) studied outcomes in 118,448 very-low-birthweight newborns in the Vermont–Oxford Trials Database from 1991 through 1999. There were no additional improvements in mortality or morbidity after 1995, ending a decades-long trend of improving outcomes.

LOWER LIMIT OF SURVIVAL: COUNSELING CONSIDERATIONS. Perinatal care at the threshold of viability, defined as 25 or fewer weeks of gestation, has been reviewed by the American College of Obstetricians and Gynecologists (2002). It concluded that "parents can be counseled that infants delivered before 24 weeks are not likely to survive, and those who do are not likely to survive intact. Disabilities in mental and psychomotor development, neuromotor function, or sensory and communication function are present in approximately one half of survivors." Maternal–fetal transport to a tertiary care center prior to delivery should be considered when possible. Importantly, all members of the health care team should maintain a consistent theme with family members regarding neonatal assessment and prognosis, as well as recommendations and plans for care.

Amon and co-workers (1992) and Bottoms and co-workers (1997) surveyed obstetricians to determine their clinical opinions regarding intrapartum management of the extremely preterm fetus requiring delivery. According to their survey results, cesarean delivery was not performed at less than 24 weeks. Almost 90 percent of respondents were willing to perform cesarean delivery for fetal distress or breech presentation at 26 weeks or 750 g fetal weight. Doron and co-workers (1998) analyzed delivery room decisions by neonatologists to provide or withhold resuscitation between 23 and 26 weeks' gestation. They concluded that resuscitation of these extremely preterm neonates may provide time to gather

additional information about neonatal prognosis and an opportunity for decision making regarding continued care.

The decision not to perform cesarean delivery or use intrapartum monitoring does not necessarily imply that the fetus is "nonviable" or "written off." Kitchen and co-workers (1992) analyzed the outcomes of liveborn neonates weighing 500 to 999 g and found that although 50 percent of newborns survived and only 7 percent were severely disabled, these outcomes were unrelated to the use of cesarean delivery or electronic fetal monitoring.

We believe that these data do not support the aggressive approach to cesarean delivery between 23 and 26 weeks that is described by Redman and Gonik (2002) and that has been documented as the national trend (Fig. 36–5).

UPPER LIMIT FOR ADVERSE OUTCOMES FROM PRETERM DELIVERY. Survival of larger preterm newborns now approaches that for term newborns (see Fig. 36–4; see Table 29–2, p. 656). This raises the question: Is there a birthweight or gestational age threshold after which attempts to delay delivery are unwarranted? DePalma and co-workers (1992) found that the threshold for neonatal mortality at Parkland Hospital was 1600 g, and it was 1900 g for neonatal morbidity. They concluded that aggressive attempts to prevent births for fetuses whose weight estimates exceeded 1900 g offered few apparent benefits. In the United States, 1950 g is the 10th percentile for 34 weeks and the 50th percentile for 32 weeks (see Table 38–1, p. 896). Nationwide, the survival rate for newborns at 34 weeks is within 1 percent of those born at or beyond 37 weeks (American College of Obstetricians and Gynecologists, 1995).

ECONOMIC IMPACT OF PRETERM BIRTH. Resources used to care for low-birthweight newborns is one measure of the financial burden of preterm birth. In the United

States, Lewit and co-workers (1995) found that more than a third of the dollars expended for infant health care during the first year of life is spent on the 7 percent of neonates born who weigh less than 2500 g. Additional expenditures for developmental handicaps during the remainder of childhood should also be considered.

CAUSES OF PRETERM BIRTH

A wide spectrum of causes and demographic factors have been implicated in preterm birth.

MEDICAL AND OBSTETRICAL COMPLICATIONS. The NICHD Maternal–Fetal Medicine Units Network has analyzed the causes of delivery before 37 weeks. The report by Meis and colleagues (1995b, 1998) showed that 28 percent of these preterm singleton births were indicated as being due to several factors; about a half were for preeclampsia; a fourth for fetal distress; and a fourth for fetal growth restriction, placental abruption, or fetal death. The remaining 72 percent were due to spontaneous preterm labor, with or without prematurely ruptured membranes. Kimberlin and colleagues (1999) studied 411 newborns who weighed 1000 g or less and found that outcomes were similar if preterm delivery was indicated or spontaneous.

THREATENED ABORTION. Vaginal bleeding in early pregnancy is associated with increased adverse outcomes. Weiss and associates (2002) reported data on vaginal bleeding at 6 to 13 weeks in nearly 14,000 women. Both light bleeding (described as spotting) and heavy bleeding (similar to menses) were associated with subsequent pregnancy loss prior to 24 weeks, preterm labor, and placental abruption.

LIFESTYLE FACTORS. Cigarette smoking, inadequate maternal weight gain during pregnancy, and illicit drug use play important roles in both the incidence and the outcome of low-birthweight neonates (see Chap. 14). Some of these effects are undoubtedly due to restricted fetal growth, but Hickey and colleagues (1995) linked prenatal weight gain specifically with preterm birth. Other maternal factors implicated include young or advanced maternal age; poverty; short stature; Vitamin C deficiency; and occupational factors such as prolonged walking or standing, strenuous working conditions, and long weekly work hours (Casaneuva, 2005; Gielchinsky, 2002; Kramer, 1995; Luke, 1995; Meis, 1995b; Satin, 1994, and all their colleagues). Santiago and colleagues (2005) found no increased incidence of recurrent preterm birth in women with a history of preterm birth and whose work during their current pregnancies was outside the home or required physical exertion.

Psychological and physical stress have seldom been formally studied but seem intuitively important. Both stress and higher levels of maternal serum cortisol have been associated with spontaneous preterm birth (Copper and colleagues, 1996; Mercer and associates, 2002). Neggers and colleagues (2004) found a significant link between low birthweight and preterm birth in women injured by physical abuse (see Chap. 42, p. 997). McCollum and colleagues (2003), however, reported that maternal depression was not associated with birth prior to 35 weeks.

The association of *cigarette smoking* and fetal growth restriction is unequivocal. The impact of smoking during pregnancy was summarized in a report by the March of Dimes (Berns, 2002). Specifically, 20 percent of low-birthweight neonates, 8 percent of preterm births, and 5 percent of perinatal deaths were caused by smoking. Smoking was associated with a 2- to 5-fold risk of preterm prematurely ruptured membranes, a 1.2- to 2-fold risk of preterm delivery, and a 1.5- to 3.5-fold risk of fetal growth restriction (see Chap. 14, p. 354). Castles and associates (1999) also reviewed five meta-analyses and concluded that smoking increased the incidence of ectopic pregnancy, placental abruption, and placenta previa. Counseling is discussed in Chapter 8 (see p. 209).

GENETIC FACTORS. The recurrent, familial, and racial nature of preterm birth has led to the suggestion that genetics may play a causal role (Hoffman and Ward, 1999). The gene for decidual relaxin is one candidate. Fetal mitochondrial trifunctional protein defects or polymorphism in the interleukin-1 gene complex, β_2-adrenergic receptor, or tumor necrosis factor-α (TNF-α) may also be involved in preterm membrane rupture (Genc, 2002; Landau, 2002; Netta, 2003; Tashima, 2002; Yang, 2002, and all their colleagues). Studies to evaluate gene–environment interactions are also needed. For example, when Bytautiene and colleagues (2003) induced an allergic reaction in pregnant guinea pigs that resulted in preterm delivery, they found that the rate was reduced threefold by pretreatment with an antihistamine and cromolyn sulfate.

CHORIOAMNIONITIS. Infection of the membranes and amnionic fluid caused by a variety of microorganisms has emerged as a possible explanation of some cases of ruptured membranes, preterm labor, or both. Bacteria are recovered by transabdominal amniocentesis from as many as 20 percent of women in preterm labor without overt clinical infection and with intact fetal membranes (Cox and associates, 1996; Watts and co-workers, 1992). Viral products have also been recovered (Reddy and colleagues, 2001). Infection is not limited to amnionic fluid. In studies done at cesarean delivery in 609 women with intact membranes, Hauth and co-workers (1998) confirmed that recovery of organisms from the chorioamnion was significantly increased with spontaneous preterm labor. As shown in Figure 36–6, recovery of pathogens was also inversely correlated with gestational age. The pathogenesis of upper genital tract infection and preterm birth is considered further in Chapter 6 (see p. 178).

The pathway for bacteria to enter amnionic fluid with intact membranes is unclear. Gyr and colleagues (1994) have

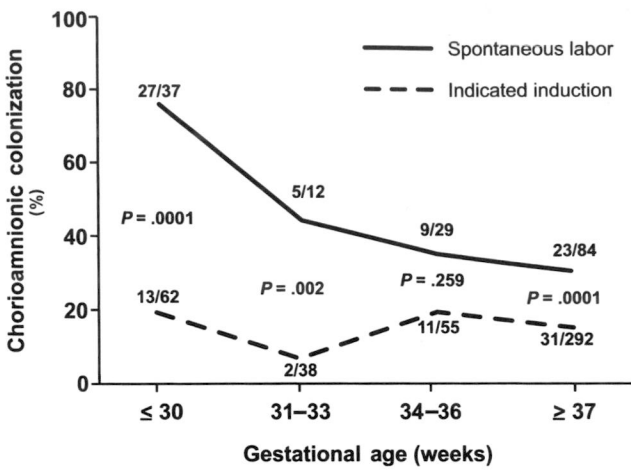

FIGURE 36-6. Chorioamnionic bacterial colonization as a function of gestational age in women with spontaneous labor and in those in whom delivery was indicated for medical or obstetrical complications. The P values represent comparisons between the two groups for each epoch plotted. (From Hauth and colleagues, 1998, with permission.)

shown that *Escherichia coli* can permeate living membranes; thus, they are not an absolute barrier to ascending infection. Another pathway for bacterial initiation of preterm labor may not require bacteria in the amnionic fluid. Cox and co-workers (1993) found that the cytokine network of cell-mediated immunity can be activated within the decidual tissue that lines the presenting fetal membranes. In this scheme, bacterial products such as endotoxin stimulate decidual monocytes to produce cytokines, which in turn stimulate arachidonic acid and then prostaglandin production. Prostaglandins E_2 and $F_{2\alpha}$ act in a paracrine fashion to stimulate adjacent myometrium to contract.

IDENTIFICATION OF WOMEN AT RISK FOR SPONTANEOUS PRETERM LABOR

The first step in prevention of preterm labor is early identification of women at risk. The American College of Obstetricians and Gynecologists (2001) has reviewed selected risk factors to predict spontaneous preterm birth.

RISK-SCORING SYSTEMS. There has been considerable interest in risk-scoring systems to identify women at greatest risk for preterm birth. In their review, Hueston and colleagues (1995) found no benefits of this programmatic approach. Mercer and colleagues (1996) concluded that risk assessment failed to identify most women who deliver preterm neonates. In another study, Klerman and co-workers (2001) randomly assigned 619 Medicaid-eligible black women with a modified risk assessment score for preterm delivery of 10 or higher to receive augmented or customary prenatal care. Mean birthweight and the incidences of preterm delivery and low-birthweight newborns were similar in both groups as well as in the general obstetrical population.

TABLE 36-2 Recurrent Spontaneous Preterm Births According to Prior Outcome in 15,863 Women Delivering Their First and Subsequent Pregnancies at Parkland Hospital

Birth Outcome	Second Birth ≤ 34 Weeks (%)
First birth ≥ 35 weeks	5
First birth ≤ 34 weeks	16
First and second births ≤ 34 weeks	41

Adapted from Bloom and associates, 2001b, with permission.

PRIOR PRETERM BIRTH. Prior preterm delivery strongly correlates with subsequent preterm labor. Shown in Table 36-2 is the incidence of recurrent preterm birth in nearly 16,000 women delivered at Parkland Hospital (Bloom and colleagues, 2001b). The risk of recurrent preterm delivery for women whose first delivery was preterm was increased threefold compared with that of women whose first neonate was born at term. More than a third of women whose first two newborns were preterm subsequently delivered a third preterm newborn. The majority (70 percent) of the recurrent births in this study occurred within 2 weeks of the gestational age of the prior preterm delivery. Importantly, the causes of prior preterm delivery (i.e., preterm labor with intact membranes, preterm membrane rupture, or indicated delivery) also recurred. Although women with prior preterm births were clearly at risk for recurrence, they contributed only 10 percent of the total preterm births. Expressed in another way, 90 percent of the preterm births at Parkland Hospital could not be predicted based on a history of preterm birth.

INCOMPETENT CERVIX. *Cervical incompetence* is a clinical diagnosis characterized by recurrent, painless cervical dilatation and spontaneous midtrimester birth in the absence of spontaneous membrane rupture, bleeding, or infection (American College of Obstetricians and Gynecologists, 2001). It is considered in detail in Chapter 9 (see p. 236).

CERVICAL DILATATION. Asymptomatic cervical dilatation after midpregnancy has gained attention as a risk factor for preterm delivery, although some clinicians consider it to be a normal anatomical variant, particularly in parous women. Recent studies, however, have suggested that parity alone is not sufficient to explain cervical dilatation discovered early in the third trimester. Cook and Ellwood (1996) longitudinally evaluated cervical status with transvaginal ultrasonography between 18 and 30 weeks in both nulliparous and parous women who all subsequently gave birth at term. Cervical length and diameter were identical in both groups throughout these critical weeks. The results of routine cervical examinations performed between 26 and 30 weeks in 185 women

TABLE 36–3 Cervical Dilatation Between 26 and 30 Weeks and Risk of Delivery Before 34 Weeks

| | Preterm Delivery | | | |
| | All Women | Cervical Dilation | | |
Risk Factor/Outcome	(n = 185) no. (%)	< 1 cm (n = 170) no. (%)	2–3 cm (n = 15) no. (%)	Comparison
Prior low birthweight[a]	9 (5)	6 (4)	3 (20)	P < .001
Current pregnancy low birthweight	7 (4)	3 (2)	4 (27)	P < .002

[a]Less than 2200 g (50th percentile for 34 weeks).
From Leveno and associates (1986a), with permission

cared for at Parkland Hospital are shown in Table 36–3. Approximately 25 percent of women whose cervices were dilated 2 or 3 cm delivered prior to 34 weeks. Many of these women had experienced the same complication in earlier pregnancies. Other investigators have verified cervical dilatation as a predictor of increased risk of preterm delivery (Copper and associates, 1995; Papiernik and colleagues, 1986).

Although women with dilatation and effacement in the third trimester are at increased risk for preterm birth, it has not been established that detection improves pregnancy outcome. Buekens and colleagues (1994) randomly assigned 2719 women to undergo routine cervical examinations at each prenatal visit and compared them with 2721 women without examinations. Knowledge of antenatal cervical dilatation did not affect any pregnancy outcome related to preterm birth or the frequency of interventions for preterm labor. The investigators also reported that cervical examinations were not related to preterm membrane rupture. It seems therefore that prenatal cervical examinations are neither beneficial nor harmful.

Ultrasonographic Measurement of Cervical Length. Vaginal-probe ultrasonographic cervical assessment has been evaluated extensively over the past decade. Technique is important, and Yost and colleagues (1999) have cautioned

that special expertise is needed. Iams and co-workers (1996) measured cervical length at approximately 24 weeks and again at 28 weeks in 2915 women not at risk for preterm birth. The mean cervical length at 24 weeks was about 35 mm, and those women with progressively shorter cervices experienced increased rates of preterm birth. In women with a previous birth before 32 weeks, Owen and associates (2001) reported a significant correlation of cervical length at 16 to 24 weeks and subsequent preterm birth before 35 weeks. In a secondary analysis of these data, Yost and colleagues (2004) found that dilatation of 2 to 4 mm identified during second-trimester cervical ultrasonographic scanning independently predicted an increase in births prior to 35 weeks. In their review, Owen and colleagues (2003) concluded that the value of cervical length to predict birth before 35 weeks is apparent only in women at high risk for preterm birth (Table 36–4).

To evaluate the effects of cerclage in women with ultrasonographically measured cervical dilatation, the investigators summarized five retrospective cohort series and two randomized trials (Owen and associates, 2003). Four of the seven reports cited a beneficial effect, and three showed no benefit.

It seems that the use of ultrasonographic cervical measurements can increase the ability to predict spontaneous birth prior to 35 weeks in high-risk women. We agree with Iams

TABLE 36–4 Blinded Observational Studies Comparing Ultrasonographically Determined Cervical Length with the Risk of Preterm Birth

Study	Age at Evaluation (weeks)	n	Population	Age at Endpoint (weeks)	Preterm Birth (%)	Cervical Length Cutoff (mm)	Sensitivity/ Specificity	Positive Predictive Value
Tongsong et al., 1995	28–30	730	Unselected	< 37	12.5	≤ 30	0.31/0.87	0.26
Iams et al., 1996	24	2915	Unselected	< 35	4.3	≤ 25	0.37/0.92	0.18
Taipale et al., 1998	18–22	3694	Unselected	< 35	0.8	≤ 31	0.19/0.91	0.018
Berghella et al., 1997	14–22	96	High-risk	< 35	18	≤ 25	0.59/0.85	0.45
Andrews et al., 2000	15–20	53	High-risk	< 35	30	≤ 22	0.86/1.0	1.0
Owen et al., 2001	16–24	183	High-risk	< 35	26	≤ 25	0.69/0.80	0.55

From Owen and colleagues (2003), with permission.

(2003) that routine cervical ultrasonography currently has no role in the screening of normal-risk pregnant women. The efficacy of cerclage for women with shortened cervical length is inconclusive, and an NICHD multicenter randomized trial concerning this issue is currently underway.

SIGNS AND SYMPTOMS. In addition to painful or painless uterine contractions, symptoms such as pelvic pressure, menstrual-like cramps, watery vaginal discharge, and pain in the low back have been empirically associated with impending preterm birth. Such symptoms are thought by some to be common in normal pregnancy and are therefore often dismissed by patients, clinicians, and nurses. The importance of these signs and symptoms as a harbinger of labor has been emphasized by some but not all investigators (Copper and colleagues, 1990; Iams and associates, 1990; Kragt and Keirse, 1990). Iams and colleagues (1994) found that the signs and symptoms signaling preterm labor, including uterine contraction, appeared only within 24 hours of preterm labor.

AMBULATORY UTERINE MONITORING. Uterine activity monitoring has received considerable interest. An external tocodynamometer is belted around the abdomen and connected to an electronic waist recorder. Uterine activity is transmitted via telephone daily. Women are educated concerning signs and symptoms of preterm labor, and clinicians are kept apprised of their progress.

The 1985 approval of this monitor by the U.S. Food and Drug Administration prompted its widespread clinical use. Subsequently, the American College of Obstetricians and Gynecologists (1995) concluded that the use of this expensive, bulky, and time-consuming system does not reduce the rate of preterm birth. Studies that followed confirmed this conclusion. In the Collaborative Home Uterine Monitoring Study (1995), sham transducers were used in 655 women and outcomes compared with those of 637 women with functioning monitors. The rate of preterm birth was similar in both groups. Iams and colleagues (2002) analyzed data from almost 35,000 hours of daily home monitoring from 306 women. They verified that contraction frequency increased with gestational age but that no pattern efficiently predicted preterm birth.

In a study by Dyson and colleagues (1998), women were randomly assigned to receive weekly contact with a nurse or to use home contraction monitoring. There were no differences in the rates of preterm delivery before 35 weeks or in the incidence of birthweights less than 1500 g or less than 2500 g. Moreover, women who used home monitoring had a significant increase in the number of unscheduled visits and women with twins had increased use of tocolytic therapy.

FETAL FIBRONECTIN. This glycoprotein is produced in 20 different molecular forms by a variety of cell types, including hepatocytes, fibroblasts, and endothelial cells, and by fetal amnion. Present in high concentrations in maternal blood and

in amnionic fluid, it is thought to play a role in intercellular adhesion during implantation and in the maintenance of placental adhesion to the decidua (Leeson and colleagues, 1996). Fetal fibronectin is detected in cervicovaginal secretions in women who have normal pregnancies with intact membranes at term, and it appears to reflect stromal remodeling of the cervix prior to labor.

Lockwood and co-workers (1991) reported that fibronectin detection in cervicovaginal secretions prior to membrane rupture was a possible marker for impending preterm labor. This report stimulated considerable interest in the use of fibronectin assays for the prediction of preterm birth. Fetal fibronectin is measured using an enzyme-linked immunosorbent assay, and values exceeding 50 ng/mL are considered positive. Contamination of the sample by amnionic fluid and maternal blood should be avoided.

A positive value for cervical or vaginal fetal fibronectin assay, even as early as 8 to 22 weeks, has been found to be a powerful predictor of subsequent preterm birth (Goldenberg and co-workers, 2000). In a randomized trial, a negative fibronectin assay in women with threatened preterm labor was associated with fewer admissions and decreased hospital stay (Lowe and associates, 2004).

Subsequent studies of cervicovaginal fibronectin have allowed better assessment of its positive and negative predictive value. Swamy and colleagues (2001) found that in 404 pregnancies, a positive assay result at 22 to 34 weeks had a positive predictive value for delivery within 1 week of 30 percent or within 2 weeks of 41 percent. The negative predictive value was 98 and 96 percent, respectively. The less informative positive predictive value likely results from factors such as cervical manipulation and infection, which can stimulate fetal fibronectin release (Goldenberg and associates, 1996; Jackson and colleagues, 1996; Thorp and Lukes, 1996). These findings may implicate infection in the initiation of preterm labor in some women.

Intervention with Positive Fibronectin Assay. Because the positive predictive value along with evidence that a positive fibronectin assay may suggest infection, Andrews and colleagues (2003) studied the effectiveness of antimicrobial treatment to reduce the incidence of preterm birth. Of 16,317 women screened for fetal fibronectin between 21 and 26 weeks, 6.6 percent had a positive result. In women given antimicrobial treatment or placebo, no differences were observed in rates of spontaneous preterm birth before 37 weeks (14.4 versus 12.4 percent), before 35 weeks (6.9 versus 7.5 percent), or before 32 weeks (4.3 versus 2.2 percent).

BACTERIAL VAGINOSIS. Bacterial vaginosis is not an infection but rather a condition in which the normal, hydrogen peroxide–producing lactobacillus-predominant vaginal flora is replaced with anaerobes, *Gardnerella vaginalis, Mobiluncus* species, and *Mycoplasma hominis* (Hillier and colleagues, 1995; Nugent and co-workers, 1991). Its diagnosis and management are discussed in Chapter 59 (see p. 1319). Using Gram staining, relative concentrations of the bacterial morphotypes characteristic of bacterial vaginosis are determined and graded as the *Nugent score*.

Bacterial vaginosis has been associated with spontaneous abortion, preterm labor, preterm ruptured membranes, chorioamnionitis, and amnionic fluid infection (Hillier, 1995; Kurki, 1992; Leitich, 2003a,b; and all their colleagues). Bacterial vaginosis may precipitate preterm labor by a mechanism similar to that proposed for amnionic fluid infection (Platz-Christensen and co-workers, 1993). In 3600 Danish women, however, when bacterial vaginosis was detected before 24 weeks, it was not related to preterm membrane rupture before 37 weeks or to low birthweight (Thorsen and associates, 1996).

Conflicting reports may relate to the imprecise diagnosis of bacterial vaginosis (Hauth and colleagues, 2003; Simhan and co-workers, 2003). Women with bacterial vaginosis whose vaginal secretions contained *sialidase*, but not *prolidase*, had a significantly increased risk of preterm delivery (Hitti and associates, 2001). Finally, therapy modifies the conditions, and treatment with metronidazole decreased cervical concentrations of interleukin-1β, -6, and -8 (Yudin and colleagues, 2003).

Environmental factors appear to be important in the development of bacterial vaginosis. Exposure to chronic stress, ethnic differences, and frequent or recent douching have all been associated with increased rates of the condition (Culhane and co-workers, 2002; Ness and associates, 2002). Despite this, prospective studies of women who regularly douched reported no relationship with preterm birth (Fiscella and colleagues, 2002; Nuthalapaty and associates, 2003). A gene–environment interaction was identified by Macones and colleagues (2004). Women with bacterial vaginosis who had a susceptible TNF-α genotype had a ninefold increased incidence of preterm birth. Romero and colleagues (2004) have reviewed bacterial vaginosis and the role of genetic epidemiology in the prevention of preterm birth.

From all of these studies there seems no doubt that adverse vaginal flora, such as in bacterial vaginosis, is associated with spontaneous preterm birth. Unfortunately, to date, screening and treatment have not been shown to prevent preterm birth (see p. 869).

LOWER GENITAL TRACT INFECTION. Some investigators have implicated a number of other genital infections as a cause of preterm labor. Meis and co-workers (1995a) evaluated 2929 women at 24 and 28 weeks for *Trichomonas* or *Candida* species. Women who had one or both of these organisms were not at greater risk for preterm birth. Conversely, Cotch and associates (1997) found that the neonates of women with *Trichomonas* had increased risk of having low-birthweight, a 30-percent increased risk of preterm birth, and a twofold risk of perinatal death. Based on this report, Klebanoff and colleagues (2001) evaluated 617 asymptomatic women with tri-

chomoniasis in midtrimester. Preterm birth was significantly *greater* in women randomly assigned to receive metronidazole compared with that of those receiving placebo (19 versus 11 percent).

Chlamydia trachomatis likely does not play a role in increased preterm delivery (see Chap. 59, p. 1306). The MFM Units Network has found no association of preterm birth in women with midtrimester chlamydial infection. Similarly, Goepfert and co-workers (2002) found similar incidences of preterm delivery in women with and without chlamydial or trichomonal infection.In the Vaginal Infections and Prematurity Study, 414 women with chlamydial infection were randomly selected to receive either erythromycin or placebo. Martin and colleagues (1997) found similar incidences of preterm birth. Currently, screening and treatment to prevent preterm birth in women with either *C trachomatis* or *Trichomonas vaginalis* is not recommended.

Finally, other studies implicate nonspecific markers of infection in increasing the risk of preterm birth. In a study of 3160 asymptomatic women, Ramsey and colleagues (2003) found that a midtrimester vaginal Gram-stained smear with an increased polymorphonuclear:epithelial cell ratio was predictive of birth before 35 weeks. Knudtson and associates (2003) reported that nonpregnant women with interpartum chronic endometritis, characterized by plasma cells, were 2.5 times more likely to deliver before 35 weeks in a subsequent pregnancy.

SALIVARY ESTRIOL. Goodwin (1996), Heine (1999), and their co-workers described an association between increased maternal salivary estriol concentration and subsequent preterm birth. We agree with Goodwin (1999) that this test requires further evaluation before it can be recommended for clinical use.

PERIODONTAL DISEASE. Oral bacteria, especially *Fusobacterium nucleatum* and *Capnocytophaga* species, have been associated with upper genital tract infection in pregnant women (Ernest and Wasilauskas, 1985; Wallace, 1986). Offenbacher and associates (1996) found that women with periodontitis had a sevenfold risk of preterm birth compared with that of controls. Hauth and colleagues (2001b) confirmed this in a prospective trial of more than 1300 women assessed at midpregnancy for periodontal inflammation. In each gestational age category, periodontal disease was associated with increased preterm delivery (Table 36–5). Indeed, 24 of the 28 women who delivered before 32 weeks had periodontitis; this is a fourfold increase compared with that of women without disease. Goepfert and colleagues (2004) observed that women who delivered spontaneous before 32 weeks were significantly more likely to have severe periodontal disease than controls.

Boggess and co-workers (2001) found that preterm newborns of mothers with periodontal disease were 23 percent smaller than those of mothers without disease. Devine and

TABLE 36–5 Preterm Birth in 1320 Women with Periodontal Disease

| Preterm Birth | Periodontal Sites of ≥ 3 mm Depth | | |
	0–2 Sites No. (%)	3 Sites No. (%)	Comparison
< 37 weeks	27/589 (4.9)	100/731 (13.7)	P < .0001
< 35 weeks	12/590 (2.0)	46/723 (6.4)	P = .0001
< 34 weeks	9/590 (1.5)	34/723 (4.7)	P = .001
< 32 weeks	4/590 (0.7)	24/723 (3.3)	P = .001

From Hauth and colleagues (2001a), with permission.

TABLE 36–6 Effect of 17α-Hydroxyprogesterone Caproate Versus Placebo to Prevent Recurrent Preterm Birth

| Preterm Delivery | Treatment Group (%) | | Relative Risk (95% CI) | P Value |
	Placebo (n = 153)	17α-OHP (n = 306)		
< 37 weeks	55	36	0.66 (0.54–0.93)	.0001
< 35 weeks	31	21	0.67 (0.48–0.93)	.017
< 32 weeks	20	11	0.58 (0.37–0.91)	.018

Data from Meis and colleagues (2003), with permission.

associates (2001) have suggested that this may be related to decreased maternal antibody titers.

Treatment for Periodontitis. Jeffcoat and colleagues (2003) randomly assigned 366 women with periodontitis at midpregnancy to one of three protocols: simple teeth cleaning and polishing (prophylaxis) plus placebo antimicrobial therapy, deep root scaling and planing (intervention) plus metronidazole, or deep root scaling and planing (intervention) with placebo antimicrobial therapy. The incidence of preterm birth before 35 weeks was 4.9 percent in women who had prophylaxis; 3.3 percent for those who had intervention and metronidazole; and only 0.8 percent in those who had intervention and placebo. There were significantly fewer births before 37 weeks in women who had intervention and placebo (4.1 percent) compared with women who had intervention and metronidazole (12.5 percent).

Two multicenter trials sponsored by the National Institute of Dental and Craniofacial Research are underway to determine whether midpregnancy identification and treatment of women with periodontal disease prevents preterm birth.

ROLE OF PROGESTERONE IN THE MAINTENANCE OF PREGNANCY

Currently, it is accepted that in primate pregnancy, including human pregnancy, progesterone withdrawal does not precede the initiation of parturition. As discussed in Chapter 3 (see p. 76), maternal plasma progesterone levels increase throughout pregnancy. Despite this, the use of progesterone to maintain uterine quiescence and to "block" labor initiation as espoused by Csapo (1956) deserves continued evaluation. Progesterone and estrogen levels vary directly but markedly with gestational age. Taken together, studies have been used to support the concept of an adverse progesterone:estrogen ratio to explain preterm labor (Mazor and colleagues, 1993; Romero and co-workers, 1988). Moreover, progesterone antagonists given at term increase the rate of spontaneous labor (Chwalisz, 1991; Frydman, 1992 and all their colleagues). In animal studies, medroxyprogesterone treatment prevented labor and possessed anti-inflammatory activity in vivo (Elovitz and Wang, 2003, 2004). In that role, activation of both TH_1

and TH_2 cytokine pathways were suppressed in the uterus and cervix. These cytokines are thought to play a role in the maintenance of pregnancy, and later in the initiation of parturition (see Chap. 6, p. 180).

The most commonly used progestin in human clinical trials is 17α-hydroxyprogesterone caproate. Weekly intramuscular administration to women at risk for preterm labor resulted in lower rates of preterm birth and perinatal mortality when compared with that with placebo (Johnson and associates, 1975, 1979; Yemini and co-workers, 1985). Results of the recent report by Meis and collaborators (2003) are shown in Table 36–6. In addition, da Fonseca and colleagues (2003) reported the effectiveness of a 100-mg vaginal suppository of natural progesterone to reduce preterm delivery in high-risk women. Not all investigators have reported improved benefits from progesterone administration (Hauth and colleagues, 1983). The American College of Obstetricians and Gynecologists (2003) has reviewed the use of progesterone to reduce the incidence of preterm birth.

MANAGEMENT OF PRETERM RUPTURED MEMBRANES AND PRETERM LABOR

Women who have been identified as being at risk for preterm birth and women who present with signs and symptoms of preterm labor have become candidates for a number of interventions intended to improve neonatal outcomes. In the absence of maternal or fetal indications warranting intentional delivery, interventions are intended to forestall preterm birth. Although many of these interventions are described in the following sections, they are not necessarily recommended. Some may produce borderline improvement at best, and others are unproven. Many interventions used to delay delivery undergo continuing review by the American College of Obstetricians and Gynecologists (1995, 1998a,b, 2001, 2002).

PRETERM RUPTURED MEMBRANES. Diagnosis of ruptured membranes is detailed in Chapter 17 (see p. 425). Prior to term, the precision of this diagnosis is of great importance. A history of vaginal leakage of fluid, either continuously or as a gush, should prompt a sterile speculum examination to visualize gross vaginal pooling of amnionic fluid, clear fluid from the cervical canal, or both. Confirmation of ruptured membranes is usually accompanied by ultrasonographic examination to assess amnionic fluid volume; to identify the presenting part; and if not previously determined, to estimate gestational age.

Management may be to effect delivery or to await spontaneous labor. It may necessary to decide about administration of either antimicrobials, corticosteroids, or both.

Natural History of Preterm Membrane Rupture. Cox and associates (1988) described pregnancy outcomes of 298 consecutive women who gave birth following spontaneous rupture of membranes between 24 and 34 weeks. Although this complication was identified in only 1.7 percent of pregnancies, it contributed to 20 percent of all perinatal deaths. By the time they presented, 75 percent of the women were already in labor, 5 percent were delivered for other complications, and another 10 percent were delivered within 48 hours. In only 7 percent was delivery delayed 48 hours or more after membrane rupture. This latter subgroup, however, appeared to benefit from delayed delivery, because there were no neonatal deaths. This contrasted with a neonatal death rate of 80 per 1000 in newborns delivered within 48 hours of membrane rupture. Nelson and colleagues (1994) reported similar results.

The time period from preterm rupture of membranes to delivery is inversely proportional to the gestational age when the membranes rupture (Carroll and associates, 1995). As shown in Figure 36–7, very few days were gained when membranes ruptured during the third compared with the second trimester.

Hospitalization. Most clinicians hospitalize women with preterm prematurely ruptured membranes. Concerns about the costs of lengthy hospitalizations are usually moot, because most women enter labor within a week or less after membrane rupture. Carlan and co-workers (1993) randomly assigned 67 pregnant women with ruptured membranes to home or hospital management. No benefits were found for hospitalization, and maternal hospital stays were reduced by 50 percent in those sent home (14 versus 7 days). Importantly, the investigators emphasized that this study was too small to conclude that home management was safe.

Intentional Delivery. Prior to the mid-1970s, labor was usually induced in women with preterm ruptured membranes because of fear of infection. Two randomized trials compared labor induction with expectant management in such pregnancies. Mercer and colleagues (1993) randomly selected 93 women with pregnancies between 32 and 36 weeks to undergo delivery or expectant management. *Fetal lung maturity was documented in all cases.* Intentional delivery reduced the length of maternal hospitalization and also reduced infection rates in both mothers and neonates. Cox and Leveno (1995) similarly apportioned 129 women between 30 and 34 weeks. One fetal death resulted from sepsis in the pregnancies managed expectantly. There were three neonatal deaths among those intentionally delivered; two were due to sepsis and one was due to pulmonary hypoplasia. Thus, neither management approach proved to be superior.

Expectant Management. Despite extensive literature concerning expectant management of preterm ruptured membranes, tocolysis has been used in few studies. In these randomized studies, which assigned women with prematurely ruptured membranes to receive either tocolytic or expectant management, the authors concluded that active interventions did not improve perinatal outcomes (Garite and associates, 1981, 1987; Nelson and co-workers, 1985).

Other considerations with expectant management involve the use of digital cervical examination and cerclage. Alexander and colleagues (2000) compared findings in expectantly managed women between 24 and 32 weeks who had one or two digital cervical examinations with those of women who had no such examinations. Women who were examined digitally had a rupture-to-delivery interval of 3 days compared with 5 days in those who were not examined. This difference did not worsen maternal or neonatal outcomes. McElrath and colleagues (2002) studied 114 women with a cerclage in place who later had ruptured membranes prior to 34 weeks. They were matched with 288 controls who had not received a cerclage. Pregnancy outcomes were equivalent in both groups. As discussed in Chapter 9 (see p. 237), such management is controversial.

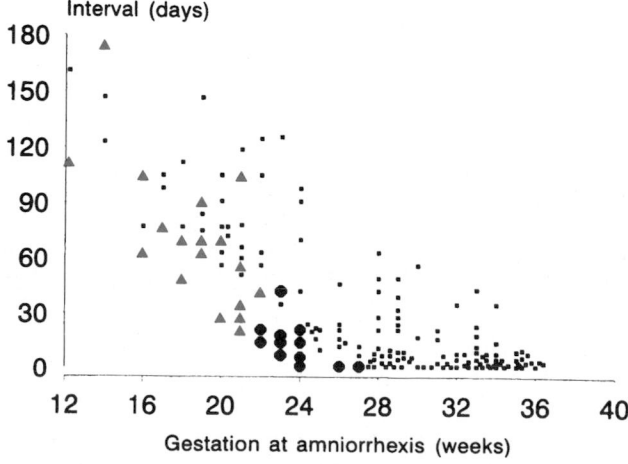

FIGURE 36–7. Relationship of time interval between preterm membrane rupture and delivery in 172 singleton pregnancies. (Squares = survivors; circles = deaths due to prematurity; triangles = deaths due to pulmonary hypoplasia.) (From Carroll and co-workers, 1995, with permission.)

RISKS OF EXPECTANT MANAGEMENT. Maternal and fetal risks vary with the gestational age at membrane rupture and include the consequences of uterine infection and sepsis. When contemplating expectant management before 25 weeks, additional consideration is given to fetal risks of oligo-hydramnios with resultant pulmonary hypoplasia and limb compression deformities (see Chap. 21, p. 531). Morales and Talley (1993) expectantly managed 94 singleton pregnancies with ruptured membranes prior to 25 weeks. They found that 41 percent of infants survived to 1 year of age, however, only 27 percent were neurologically normal. The average time gained was 11 days. Similar results were reported by Farooqi (1998) and Winn (2000) and their associates.

The volume of amnionic fluid remaining after rupture appears to have prognostic importance in pregnancies before 26 weeks. Hadi and associates (1994) described 178 pregnancies with ruptured membranes between 20 and 25 weeks. In 40 percent of women, oligohydramnios developed as defined by the absence of fluid pockets 2 cm or larger. Virtually all women with oligohydramnios delivered before 25 weeks, whereas 85 percent with adequate amnionic fluid volume were delivered in the third trimester. Carroll and colleagues (1995) observed no cases of pulmonary hypoplasia in fetuses born after membrane rupture at 24 weeks or beyond, suggesting that 23 weeks or less is the threshold for the development of lung hypoplasia.

Other risk factors have also been evaluated. Prolonged latency after membrane rupture has not been associated with an increased incidence of fetal neurological damage (McElrath and co-workers, 2003). In neonates born to women with active herpetic lesions who were expectantly managed, the infectious morbidity risk appeared to be outweighed by risks associated with preterm delivery (Major and associates, 2003).

CLINICAL CHORIOAMNIONITIS. If there are no untoward perinatal outcomes from an entangled or prolapsed cord or from placental abruption, most authors, with few exceptions, have found prolonged membrane rupture associated with increased infectious morbidity (Ho and colleagues, 2003). If chorioamnionitis is diagnosed, prompt efforts to effect delivery, preferably vaginally, are initiated. Fever is the only reliable indicator for this diagnosis. A temperature of 38°C (100.4°F) or higher accompanying ruptured membranes implies infection. Maternal leukocytosis alone has not been found to be reliable by most investigators. During expectant management, monitoring for sustained maternal or fetal tachycardia, for uterine tenderness, and for a malodorous vaginal discharge is warranted.

With chorioamnionitis, fetal and neonatal morbidity is substantively increased. Alexander and colleagues (1998) studied 1367 very-low-birthweight neonates delivered at Parkland Hospital. Approximately 7 percent were born to women with overt chorioamnionitis, and their outcomes were compared with those of newborns without clinical infection. Newborns in the infected group had a higher incidence of sepsis, respiratory distress syndrome, early-onset seizures, intraventricular hemorrhage, and periventricular leukomalacia. The investigators concluded that these

very-low-birthweight neonates were vulnerable to neurological injury attributable to chorioamnionitis.

There is other evidence that very small newborns exposed to intrauterine infection are at increased risk. Yoon and colleagues (2000) found that intra-amnionic infection in preterm neonates was related to increased rates of cerebral palsy at 3 years. Petrova and colleagues (2001) studied more than 11 million singleton live births from 1995 to 1997 who were in the database of the National Center for Health Statistics linked birth–infant death cohort. During labor, 1.6 percent of all women had fever, and this was a strong predictor of infection-related death in both term and preterm neonates. Bullard and associates (2002) reported similar results.

ACCELERATED PULMONARY MATURATION. A variety of clinical events—some well defined and others not—were once proposed to accelerate fetal surfactant production (Gluck, 1979). These included chronic renal or cardiovascular disease, hypertensive disorders, heroin addiction, fetal growth restriction, placental infarction, chorioamnionitis, and preterm membrane rupture. Although this view was widely held for many years, subsequent observations do not support this association (Hallak and Bottoms, 1993; Owen and associates, 1990).

ANTIMICROBIAL THERAPY. The proposed microbial pathogenesis for spontaneous preterm labor or ruptured membranes has prompted investigators to give various antimicrobials in an attempt to forestall delivery. Mercer and Arheart (1995) reviewed 13 randomized trials performed to evaluate antimicrobial compared with placebo treatment for women with membranes ruptured before 35 weeks. Meta-analysis indicated that only 3 of 10 outcomes were *possibly* benefited: Fewer women developed chorioamnionitis, fewer newborns developed sepsis, and pregnancy was more often prolonged 7 days in women given antimicrobials. Neonatal survival, however, was unaffected, as was the incidence of necrotizing enterocolitis, respiratory distress, or intracranial hemorrhage.

To further address this issue, the NICHD Maternal–Fetal Medicine Units Network designed a trial to study expectant management combined with a 7-day treatment of either ampicillin, amoxicillin plus erythromycin, or placebo. The women had membrane rupture between 24 and 32 weeks. Neither tocolytics nor corticosteroids were given. Antimicrobial-treated women had significantly fewer newborns with respiratory distress syndrome, necrotizing enterocolitis, and composite adverse outcomes (Mercer and colleagues, 1997). The latency period was significantly longer; 50 percent of women given an antimicrobial regimen remained undelivered after 7 days of treatment compared with only 25 percent of those given a placebo. There was also significant prolongation of pregnancy at 14 and 21 days. Cervicovaginal group B streptococcal colonization did not alter these results.

More recent studies have examined the efficacy of shorter treatment lengths and other antimicrobial combinations.

Three-day treatment compared with 7-day regimens using either ampicillin or ampicillin-sulbactam appeared equally effective in regard to perinatal outcomes (Lewis and associates, 2003; Segel and colleagues, 2003). Similarly, erythromycin compared with placebo offered a range of significant neonatal benefits. The amoxicillin-clavulanate regimen was not recommended, however, because of its association with an increased incidence of necrotizing enterocolitis (Kenyon and colleagues, 2001a).

Prolonged antimicrobial therapy in such pregnancies may have unwanted consequences. Carroll and colleagues (1996) and Mercer and associates (1999) cautioned that such therapy potentially increases the risk for selection of resistant bacteria. Stoll and colleagues (2002) studied 5447 neonates weighing from 400 to 1500 g and born from 1998 to 2000 at centers of the Neonatal Research Network. These were compared with 7606 neonates of similar birthweight born from 1991 to 1993. The overall rate of early-onset sepsis did not change. However, group B streptococcal sepsis decreased in the 1991–1993 group compared with the 1998–2000 group (5.9 to 1.7 per 1000 births), whereas *E coli* sepsis increased (3.2 to 6.8 per 1000 births). Almost 85 percent of coliform isolates from the more recent cohort were ampicillin resistant. Neonates with early-onset sepsis were more likely to die, especially if they were infected with coliforms.

MEMBRANE REPAIR. Use of a gelatin sponge for cervical plugging was described by O'Brien and colleagues (2002) in 15 women with early midtrimester membrane rupture. This technique is still investigational.

Recommended Management of Preterm Membrane Rupture at Parkland Hospital and the University of Alabama at Birmingham. After confirmation of ruptured membranes, the following steps are taken:

1. Cervical dilatation and effacement are estimated visually during a sterile speculum examination.
2. For pregnancies less than 34 weeks, if there are no maternal or fetal indications for delivery, the woman and her fetus are initially observed in the labor unit. Broad-spectrum parenteral antimicrobials are begun to prevent chorioamnionitis. Fetal heart rate and uterine activity are monitored for cord compression, fetal compromise, and early labor.
3. For pregnancies less than 32 weeks, betamethasone (two 12-mg doses intramuscularly 24 hours apart) or dexamethasone (5 mg intramuscularly every 12 hours for four doses) is given.
4. If the fetal status is reassuring, and if labor does not ensue, the woman is usually transferred to an antepartum unit and observed for labor, infection, or fetal jeopardy. We do not use continuous fetal monitoring.
5. For pregnancies 34 weeks or beyond, if labor does not begin spontaneously, then it is induced with intravenous oxytocin unless contraindicated. Cesarean delivery is performed for usual indications, including failed induction of labor.
6. During labor or induction, a parenteral antimicrobial is given for prevention of group B streptococcal infection.

PRETERM LABOR WITH INTACT FETAL MEMBRANES. It is axiomatic that management of preterm labor requires a correct diagnosis.

Diagnosis. Early differentiation between true and false labor is difficult before there is demonstrable cervical effacement and dilatation. Uterine activity alone can be misleading because of *Braxton Hicks contractions* (see Chap. 18, p. 466). These contractions, described as irregular, nonrhythmical, and either painful or painless, can cause considerable confusion in the diagnosis of preterm labor. Not infrequently, women who deliver before term have uterine activity that is attributed to Braxton Hicks contractions, prompting an incorrect diagnosis of false labor. Because uterine contractions alone may be misleading, the American Academy of Pediatrics and the American College of Obstetricians and Gynecologists (1997) proposed the following criteria to document preterm labor:

1. Contractions of four in 20 minutes or eight in 60 minutes plus progressive change in the cervix.
2. Cervical dilatation greater than 1 cm.
3. Cervical effacement of 80 percent or greater.

Management. Women with signs and symptoms of preterm labor with intact membranes are managed much the same as described above for those with preterm ruptured membranes. The cornerstone of treatment is to avoid delivery prior to 34 weeks, if possible. Drugs intended to abate or suppress preterm uterine contractions are subsequently discussed.

AMNIOCENTESIS TO DETECT INFECTION. In centers studying amniocentesis in the management of preterm labor, several tests have been used to diagnose intra-amnionic infection. Romero and colleagues (1993) evaluated the diagnostic value of amnionic fluid containing an elevated leukocyte count, a low glucose level, a high interleukin-6 concentration, or a positive Gram stain result in 120 women with preterm labor and intact fetal membranes. Women with positive amnionic fluid culture results were considered infected. These investigators found that a negative Gram stain reading was the most reliable test to exclude amnionic fluid bacteria; it had a specificity of 99 percent. A high interleukin-6 level was the most sensitive test for detection of amnionic fluids containing bacteria; it had a sensitivity of 82 percent. Other investigators have also found good correlation between amnionic fluid interleukin-6 or leukocyte levels and chorioamnionic infection (Andrews and colleagues, 1995; Yoon and associates, 1996). Despite these associations, it has not been shown that amniocentesis to diagnose infection is associated with improved pregnancy outcomes in women with or without membrane rupture (Feinstein and colleagues, 1986).

GLUCOCORTICOID THERAPY TO ENHANCE FETAL LUNG MATURATION. Corticosteroids accelerated lung maturation in preterm sheep fetuses, and Liggins and Howie (1972) evaluated this treatment in women. Glucocorticoid therapy was effective in lowering the incidence of respiratory distress and neonatal mortality if birth was delayed for at least 24 hours after *initiation* of betamethasone. Its effects persisted for up to 7 days after completion of steroid therapy.

The work by Liggins and Howie (1972) stimulated more than 20 years of fetal lung research. In 1995, a National Institutes of Health Consensus Development Panel recommended corticosteroids for fetal lung maturation in threatened preterm birth. There since has been the nearly universal acceptance and implementation of these recommendations (Leviton and associates, 1999). Evidence supporting the recommendations of this panel is reviewed in Chapter 27 of the 21st edition of *Williams Obstetrics* (2001).

In a later meeting, the Consensus Development Panel concluded that data were insufficient to assess the effectiveness of corticosteroids in pregnancies complicated by hypertension, diabetes, multiple gestation, fetal growth restriction, and fetal hydrops. It concluded, however, that it was reasonable to administer corticosteroids for these complications (Bloom and Leveno, 2003). However, it further determined that data were insufficient to comment on the benefits or risks of repeated treatments. Jobe and Soll (2004) recently suggested that studies to investigate if betamethasone is superior to dexamethasone be performed. Indeed, Spinillo and colleagues (2004) reported that fetal exposure to multiple maternal doses of dexamethasone was associated with a significantly increased risk of leukomalacia and with the overall occurrence of two-year infant neurodevelopmental abnormalities compared with infants exposed to betamethasone.

Subsequent investigators found that corticosteroid treatment was not beneficial for women with preterm prematurely ruptured membranes who were delivered of low- or very-low-birthweight neonates (Chapman and colleagues, 1996; Hershkovitz and colleagues, 2001). Conversely, Thomas and associates (2001) reported that a single course of betamethasone administered to women with preterm ruptured membranes was associated with a significantly reduced incidence of periventricular leukomalacia.

ADVERSE EFFECTS OF CORTICOSTEROIDS. There is controversy surrounding additional effectiveness and safety of weekly glucocorticoid administration. Initially, neither perinatal benefits nor adverse maternal and newborn effects had been associated with multiple- as opposed to single-course therapy (Lee, 2004; Lopez, 2001; Ogunyemi, 2001; Pschirrer, 2001; and all their colleagues). Long-term follow-up studies in the 1970s showed no adverse neurodevelopmental outcomes of exposed children up to 12 years (National Institutes of Health Consensus Development Panel, 1995).

Adverse immediate and long-term effects, however, have now been reported with multiple-course treatment. Investigators have found that early-onset neonatal sepsis, chorioamnionitis, and neonatal death are associated with multiple courses of betamethasone therapy (Lee and associates, 2004; Vermillion and colleagues, 2000).

A randomized NICHD Maternal–Fetal Medicine Units Network trial of single versus weekly courses of betamethasone showed less morbidity in newborns given weekly doses who were delivered before 32 weeks (Wapner and colleagues, 2003). However, this trial was discontinued because repetitive courses adversely impacted both birthweight and the incidence of fetal growth restriction. Esplin and colleagues (2000) compared development of 429 low-birthweight neonates exposed to multiple courses of corticosteroids with that of neonates either exposed to a single course or to no exposure. The investigators found no benefits for repeated doses, however, multiple courses were independently and significantly associated with abnormal psychomotor development. Thorp and co-workers (2001) described a significant reduction in head circumference in newborns exposed to multiple courses of steroids. Bloom and colleagues (2001a) analyzed births at Parkland Hospital and found that dexamethasone-exposed newborns had significantly lower birthweight compared with that of unexposed neonates. Similarly, Mercer and associates (2001) reported a dose-dependent decrease in birthweight and length in neonates exposed to multiple courses. There were 19 growth-restricted fetuses and absent or reversed end-diastolic umbilical artery flow. Maternal betamethasone administration was followed by worsening of these indices in nine fetuses; two died and two had severe acidosis (Simchen and colleagues, 2004). The American College of Obstetricians and Gynecologists (2001) and National Institutes of Health Consensus Panel (2000) subsequently expressed concern about possible adverse fetal and maternal effects of weekly treatment. The former recommended that following the initial therapy, repeated doses after 1 week should be given only when the threat of preterm delivery recurred. The latter recommended that repeated courses of corticosteroids, *including rescue therapy*, should be used only in clinical trials.

Short-term maternal adverse effects include pulmonary edema, infection, and more difficult glucose control in diabetic women. No long-term adverse maternal effects have been reported.

THYROTROPIN-RELEASING HORMONE FOR FETAL LUNG MATURATION. Tri-iodothyronine enhances surfactant synthesis. Knight and colleagues (1994) found that an intravenously administered 400-μg dose of thyrotropin-releasing hormone, given in combination with betamethasone, further augmented lung maturation compared with betamethasone alone. These findings have subsequently been nullified by studies in which women with preterm labor were assigned to receive thyrotropin-releasing hormone plus corticosteroids or to take corticosteroids alone. Investigators found that the incidence of neonatal lung disease was unchanged in women who received thyrotropin-releasing hormone (Ballard and associates, 1998; Crowther and colleagues, 1995). Thus, administration of thyrotropin-releasing hormone is not recommended.

ANTENATAL PHENOBARBITAL AND VITAMIN K. Several investigators have suggested that phenobarbital and vitamin K given to pregnant women may reduce neonatal intracranial hemorrhage. Thorp and colleagues (1995) randomly selected 272 women at risk for preterm birth to receive placebo or phenobarbital and vitamin K. Therapy did not reduce the frequency or severity of intracranial hemorrhage. In a follow-up study, Thorp and colleagues (2003) reported that phenobarbital exposure did not affect intelligence or achievement scores in 291 children tested at 7 years of age. The combination of phenobarbital and vitamin K is not recommended for the prevention of neonatal intraventricular hemorrhage.

Interventions to Delay Preterm Birth

ANTIMICROBIALS. As with preterm ruptured membranes, antimicrobials have been given to arrest preterm labor. Results have been disappointing. A Cochrane meta-analysis by King and Flenady (2000) of 10 randomized trials found no difference in the rates of newborn respiratory distress syndrome or of sepsis between placebo- and antimicrobial-treated groups, but did find an increase in perinatal morbidity in the antimicrobial-treated group. Kenyon and colleagues (2001b) for the ORACLE Collaborative Group, studied 6295 women in spontaneous preterm labor with intact membranes and without evidence of clinical infection. Women were randomly assigned to antimicrobial or placebo therapy. The primary outcomes of neonatal death, chronic lung disease, and major cerebral abnormality were similar in both groups. In his review, Goldenberg (2002) also concluded that antimicrobial treatment of women with preterm labor for the sole purpose of preventing delivery is generally not recommended.

EMERGENCY CERCLAGE. Several researchers support the concept that cervical incompetence and preterm labor are not distinct entities but rather part of a spectrum leading to preterm delivery. Consequently, investigators have evaluated the role of cerclage in the treatment and prevention of preterm birth. Harger (1983) concluded that if cervical incompetence is recognized in threatened preterm labor, emergency cerclage can be attempted, albeit with an appreciable risk of infection and pregnancy loss. Althuisius and associates (2002) randomly assigned 23 women with cervical incompetence prior to 27 weeks to bed rest, with or without emergency McDonald cerclage. Delivery delay was significantly greater in the cerclage group compared with bed rest alone (54 versus 24 days). Terkildsen and associates (2003) studied 116 women who underwent second-trimester emergency cerclage. Nullipar-

ity, membranes extending beyond the external cervical os, and cerclage prior to 22 weeks were associated with a significantly decreased chance of pregnancy continuation to 28 weeks or beyond. Cerclage is discussed further in Chapter 9, p 236.

TREATMENT FOR BACTERIAL VAGINOSIS. Bacterial vaginosis is associated with excess rates of preterm birth (see p. 862). A number of studies have evaluated the effects of various antimicrobials on its eradication. Metronidazole has been evaluated most extensively. Oral metronidazole was found to resolve bacterial vaginosis for at least 10 weeks in 78 percent of treated pregnant women compared with spontaneous resolution in only 37 percent assigned to placebo (Klebanoff and colleagues, 2004a,b).

Clinical studies done to evaluate treatment are conflicting (Leitich and associates, 2003b). Neither the study by McDonald and co-workers (1997) nor the NICHD Maternal–Fetal Medicine Units Network study by Carey and colleagues (2000) found any perinatal benefits from metronidazole treatment. Conversely, in studies of women with prior preterm birth, Hauth and associates (1995, 2001a) found that the incidence of preterm birth was lower in women treated with either metronidazole plus erythromycin or metronidazole plus azithromycin compared with placebo.

Most randomized trials show that intravaginal clindamycin cream used to treat bacterial vaginosis does not prevent preterm birth (Joesoef, 1995; Kekki, 2001; Kurkinen-Raty, 2000; McGregor, 1994, and all their colleagues). Studies in which earlier treatment was initiated are more promising. Ugwumadu and associates (2003) randomly selected 494 women with bacterial vaginosis to receive 300-mg oral clindamycin or placebo twice daily for 5 days. The clindamycin group had fewer pregnancy losses between 13 and 24 weeks and fewer spontaneous preterm births. Ugwumadu and colleagues (2004) reported that prior to 20 weeks oral clindamycin eradicated bacterial vaginosis and intermediate flora in 90 percent of women compared with spontaneous resolution in 31 percent. Lamont and colleagues (2003) also reported that preterm birth was significantly reduced in women treated with clindamycin vaginal cream before 20 weeks (from 10 to 4 percent). Further studies are needed to confirm that treatment for bacterial vaginosis with either oral or vaginal clindamycin is of benefit.

Ralph and colleagues (1999) detected bacterial vaginosis in 190 of 771 women at the time of in vitro fertilization. Women with bacterial vaginosis had a similar rate of conception but an increased risk of first-trimester loss compared with that of uninfected women.

Inhibition of Preterm Labor. Although a number of drugs and other interventions have been used to prevent or inhibit preterm labor, none has been shown to be completely effective. Because of these uncertainties, the American College of Obstetricians and Gynecologists (1998b) has recommended that tocolysis be *considered* when there are regular uterine

contractions plus documented cervical change or appreciable dilatation and effacement.

BED REST. The efficacy of bed rest either in the hospital or at home to prevent preterm labor was reviewed by Goldenberg and colleagues (1994), who found no conclusive evidence that either was helpful. Kovacevich and associates (2000) reported that bed rest for 3 days or more increased thromboembolic complications to 16 per 1000 women compared with only 1 per 1000 with normal ambulation.

HYDRATION AND SEDATION. Helfgott and associates (1994) compared hydration and sedation with bed rest in a randomized trial of 119 women with threatened preterm labor. Women randomly selected to receive 500 mL of crystalloid over 30 minutes and 8 to 12 mg of intramuscular morphine sulfate had outcomes similar to those with bed rest. Although women with preterm contractions treated with 0.25-mg subcutaneous terbutaline may have contractions that cease more quickly and may be discharged significantly earlier compared with women not treated, pregnancy outcomes are similar (Guinn and associates, 1997).

BETA-ADRENERGIC RECEPTOR AGONISTS. A number of compounds react with β-adrenergic receptors to reduce intracellular ionized calcium and prevent activation of myometrial contractile proteins (see Chap. 6, p. 162). In the United States, ritodrine and terbutaline have been used in obstetrics, but only ritodrine had been approved for preterm labor by the U.S. Food and Drug Administration.

Ritodrine. In a multicenter trial, neonates whose mothers were treated with ritodrine for presumed preterm labor had less mortality and respiratory distress, and they achieved a gestational age of 36 weeks or a birthweight of 2500 g more often than did those of untreated mothers (Merkatz and colleagues, 1980). In a randomized trial at Parkland Hospital, Leveno and associates (1986b) allocated 106 women between 24 and 33 weeks to receive either intravenous ritodrine or no tocolysis. Although drug treatment delayed delivery for 24 hours, there were no other benefits. The transient tocolytic effects of ritodrine and its ultimate failure to arrest labor may be due to β-adrenergic receptor desensitization (Hausdorff and co-workers, 1990).

The infusion of β-adrenergic agonists has resulted in frequent and at times, serious and fatal side effects (Table 36–7). Pulmonary edema is of special concern, and its contribution to morbidity is discussed in Chapter 42 (see p. 990). Tocolysis was the third most common cause of acute respiratory distress and death in pregnant women during a 14-year period in Mississippi (Perry and associates, 1996). **The cause of pulmonary edema is multifactorial, and risk factors include tocolytic therapy with β-adrenergic receptor agonists, multifetal gestation, concurrent glucocorticoid therapy, tocolysis for more than 24 hours, and large in-**

TABLE 36–7 Potential Complications of Tocolytic Agents

Beta-adrenergic Agonists
Pulmonary edema
Hyperglycemia
Hypokalemia
Hypotension
Arrhythmias
Myocardial ischemia

Magnesium Sulfate (Toxicity)
Respiratory depression
Weakness diplopia
Muscular paralysis
Cardiac arrest

Indomethacin (Toxicity)
Hepatitis
Renal failure

Nifedipine
Transient hypotension

travenous crystalloid volume infusion. Because β-agonists cause retention of sodium and water, with time (usually 24 to 48 hours), they can lead to volume overload (Hankins and colleagues, 1988). The drugs have been implicated as a cause of increased capillary permeability, disturbance of cardiac rhythm, and myocardial ischemia. Maternal sepsis appreciably increases this risk (see Chap. 42, p. 993).

Schiff and colleagues (1993) challenged the efficacy of oral ritodrine on pharmacokinetic grounds, and its manufacturer discontinued distribution of tablets in 1995. According to the *Federal Register*, ritodrine was withdrawn voluntarily in 2003 by its manufacturer and is not available in the United States.

Terbutaline. This β-agonist is commonly used to forestall preterm labor. Like ritodrine, it can cause pulmonary edema (Angel and associates, 1988). Long-term low-dose terbutaline given by subcutaneous pump in nine pregnancies was described by Lam and colleagues (1988). The Tokos Corporation promptly marketed this approach, and between 1987 and 1993, these pumps were used in nearly 25,000 women with suspected preterm labor (Perry and colleagues, 1995). Adverse reports concerning terbutaline pumps describe a sudden maternal death and a newborn with myocardial necrosis after the mother used the pump for 12 weeks (Fletcher and colleagues, 1991; Hudgens and Conradi, 1993).

Two randomized trials found no benefit for terbutaline pump therapy. In one, Wenstrom and colleagues (1997) randomly assigned 42 women with preterm labor to a terbutaline pump, to a saline pump, or to oral terbutaline. In the other, Guinn and associates (1998) randomly treated 52 women with terbutaline or with saline pump therapy. Terbutaline did not significantly prolong pregnancy, prevent preterm delivery, or improve neonatal outcomes in either of these studies.

Oral terbutaline therapy to prevent preterm delivery has not been effective (How and associates, 1995; Parilla and co-workers, 1993). In a double-blind trial, Lewis and colleagues

(1996) studied 203 women with arrested preterm labor at 24 to 34 weeks. They were randomly assigned to receive 5-mg terbutaline tablets or placebo every 4 hours. Delivery rates at one week were similar in both groups, as was median latency, mean gestational age at delivery, and the incidence of recurrent preterm labor.

OVERVIEW OF BETA-ADRENERGIC DRUGS TO INHIBIT PRETERM LABOR. Analyses of *parenteral* β-agonists to prevent preterm birth have confirmed a delay of delivery for at least 48 hours (Canadian Preterm Labor Investigators Group, 1992). Unfortunately, this delay has not proven to be beneficial. Macones and colleagues (1995) used meta-analysis to assess the efficacy of *oral* β-agonist therapy and found no benefits. Keirse (1995b) suggests that this brief delay may facilitate maternal transport or effect fetal lung maturation with glucocorticoids. Although this is intriguing, no data support this viewpoint.

MAGNESIUM SULFATE. Ionic magnesium in a sufficiently high concentration can alter myometrial contractility. Its role is presumably that of a calcium antagonist. Clinical observations are that magnesium in pharmacological doses may inhibit labor. Steer and Petrie (1977) concluded that intravenously administered magnesium sulfate—a 4-g loading dose followed by a continuous infusion of 2 g/hr—usually arrests labor. In a retrospective study, Elliott (1983) found tocolysis with magnesium sulfate to be 87-percent effective, an extraordinarily high success rate.

There have been only two randomized controlled studies of tocolysis with magnesium sulfate. Cotton and associates (1984) compared magnesium sulfate, ritodrine, and placebo in 54 women in preterm labor. They identified few differences in outcomes. Cox and associates (1990) randomly assigned 156 women to receive magnesium sulfate or normal saline infusions. These women were at appreciable risk, and few reached 33 weeks. Magnesium-treated women and their fetuses had identical outcomes as those given placebo. Because of these findings, this method of tocolysis was abandoned at Parkland Hospital.

Women given magnesium sulfate must be monitored closely for evidence of hypermagnesemia. The pharmacology and toxicology of magnesium are considered in more detail in Chapter 34, p. 789.

Neonatal Effects of Magnesium. Very-low-birthweight neonates (less than 1500 g) whose mothers were treated with magnesium sulfate for preterm labor or preeclampsia had a reduced incidence of cerebral palsy at 3 years (Grether and associates, 2000; Nelson and Grether, 1995). Although it is tempting to link these as cause and effect, in a study from England, where magnesium is not generally used for preeclampsia, Murphy and colleagues (1995) observed that severe preeclampsia or cesarean delivery alone was protective against cerebral palsy. Kimberlin and colleagues (1998) concluded that tocolysis with magnesium was not associated with improved outcomes in 308 newborns with birthweights of less than 1000 g. An ongoing NICHD Maternal–Fetal Medicine Units Network trial was designed to explore any neonatal beneficial effects of antenatal magnesium sulfate therapy (BEAM trial).

Crowther and colleagues (2003) recently reported results from the Australian Collaborative Trial of Magnesium Sulfate. They described outcomes from over 1050 women who gave birth before 30 weeks and who were randomly assigned to receive either intravenous magnesium sulfate or a normal saline placebo. Total neonatal mortality and cerebral palsy at 2 years of age were less frequent in magnesium-exposed infants, albeit with nonsignificant differences. A significant finding was that fewer survivors exposed to magnesium had substantial motor dysfunction at 2 years of age compared with those in the control group (3.4 versus 6.6 percent). The relationships also are considered in Chapter 29 (see p. 658).

PROSTAGLANDIN INHIBITORS. Drugs that inhibit prostaglandins have been of considerable interest because prostaglandins are intimately involved in contractions of normal labor (see Chap. 6, p. 166). Antagonists act by inhibiting prostaglandin synthesis or by blocking their action on target organs. A group of enzymes collectively termed *prostaglandin synthase* is responsible for the conversion of free arachidonic acid to prostaglandins. A number of drugs block this system, including acetylsalicylate and indomethacin.

Indomethacin was first used as a tocolytic for 50 women by Zuckerman and associates (1974). Studies followed that reported the efficacy of indomethacin in halting contractions and delaying preterm birth (Muench and colleagues, 2003; Niebyl and associates, 1980). Morales and co-workers (1989, 1993), however, compared indomethacin with either ritodrine or magnesium sulfate and found no difference in their efficacy to forestall preterm delivery.

Indomethacin is administered orally or rectally. A dose of 50 to 100 mg is followed by a total 24-hour dose not greater than 200 mg. Serum concentrations usually peak 1 to 2 hours after oral administration, whereas levels after rectal administration peak slightly sooner. Most studies have limited indomethacin use to 24 to 48 hours because of concerns about oligohydramnios, which can develop with these doses. If amnionic fluid is monitored, oligohydramnios can be detected early, and it is reversible with discontinuation of indomethacin.

Case-control studies have been performed to assess neonatal effects of indomethacin exposure given for preterm labor. In a study of neonates born before 30 weeks, Norton and colleagues (1993) identified necrotizing enterocolitis in 30 percent of 37 indomethacin-exposed newborns compared with 8 percent of 37 control newborns. Higher incidences of intraventricular hemorrhage and patent ductus arteriosus were also documented in the indomethacin group. The impact of treatment duration and its timing in relation to delivery were not reported. In contrast, several investigators have challenged the association between indomethacin exposure and necrotizing enterocolitis (Muench and co-workers, 2001; Parilla and colleagues, 2000). Finally, Gardner and associates (1996) and Abbasi and co-workers (2003) showed no link between indomethacin use and intraventricular hemorrhage, patent ductus arteriosus, sepsis, necrotizing enterocolitis, or neonatal death.

Schmidt and colleagues (2001) followed 574 newborns who were randomly assigned to receive either indomethacin or placebo to prevent pulmonary hypertension from patent ductus arteriosus. The infants, who weighed 500 to 1000 g, were followed to a corrected age of 18 months. Those given indomethacin had a significantly *reduced* incidence of both patent ductus as well as severe intraventricular hemorrhage. Survival without impairment, however, was similar in both groups. Peck and Lutheran (2003) reported that indomethacin therapy for 7 or more days prior to 33 weeks does not increase the risk of neonatal or childhood medical problems.

CALCIUM CHANNEL BLOCKERS. Myometrial activity is directly related to cytoplasmic free calcium, and a reduction in its concentration inhibits contraction. Calcium channel blockers act to inhibit, by a variety of mechanisms, the entry of calcium through channels in the cell membrane. They were developed to treat hypertension. However, their use in the arrest of preterm labor has been the subject of research since the late 1970s.

Using the Cochrane Database, Keirse (1995a) compared nifedipine and β-agonists and concluded that although nifedipine treatment reduced births of neonates of less than 2500 g, significantly more of these were admitted for intensive care. Other investigators have also concluded that calcium channel blockers, especially nifedipine, are safer and more effective tocolytic agents than beta-mimetics (King and colleagues, 2003; Papatsonis and colleagues, 1997). Oral nifedipine, however, does not significantly prolong pregnancy in women initially treated with intravenous magnesium sulfate for preterm labor (Carr and colleagues, 1999).

Nifedipine-induced decreased vascular resistance can lead to hypotension and decreased uteroplacental perfusion. Parisi and colleagues (1986) described hypercapnia, acidosis, and hypoxemia in fetuses of hypertensive ewes given nicardipine. Similarly, Lirette and associates (1987) observed a fall in uteroplacental blood flow in pregnant rabbits. Childress and Katz (1994) and Papatsonis and colleagues (1997), however, did not find these adverse fetal effects.

The combination of nifedipine with magnesium for tocolysis is potentially dangerous. Ben-Ami and co-workers (1994) and Kurtzman and associates (1993) reported that nifedipine enhances neuromuscular blocking effects of magnesium that can interfere with pulmonary and cardiac function. Smith and colleagues (2000) concluded that nifedipine is effective for severe gestational hypertension or preterm labor but that randomized trials are needed.

ATOSIBAN. This nonapeptide oxytocin analogue is a competitive antagonist of oxytocin-induced contractions. Goodwin and colleagues (1995) described its pharmacokinetics in pregnant women. In randomized clinical trials, however, atosiban failed to improve relevant neonatal outcomes and was linked with significant neonatal morbidity (Moutquin and colleagues, 2000; Romero and associates, 2000). U.S. Food and Drug Administration approval for atosiban use to arrest preterm labor was denied because of concerns regarding efficacy and fetal-newborn safety.

NITRIC OXIDE DONORS. These potent smooth muscle relaxants affect the vasculature, gut, and uterus. In randomized clinical trials, nitroglycerin administered orally, transdermally, or intravenously, was not effective or showed no superiority to other tocolytics. In addition, maternal hypotension was a common side effect (Buhimschi, 2002; Clavin, 1996; El-Sayed, 1999; Lees, 1999, and all their colleagues).

Summary of Tocolytic Use for Preterm Labor. In many women, tocolytics stop contractions temporarily but rarely prevent preterm birth. In a meta-analysis of tocolytic therapy, Gyetvai and colleagues (1999) concluded that although delivery may be delayed long enough for administration of corticosteroids, treatment does not result in any improved perinatal outcomes. Berkman and colleagues (2003) reviewed 60 reports and concluded that tocolytic therapy can prolong gestation, but that beta-mimetics were not better than other drugs and pose potential maternal danger. They also concluded that there were no benefits of maintenance tocolytic therapy.

As a general rule, if tocolytics are given, they should be given concomitantly with corticosteroids. The gestational age range for their use is debated, but because corticosteroids are not generally used after 33 weeks, and because the perinatal outcomes in preterm neonates are generally good after this time, most practitioners do not recommend use of tocolytics at or after 34 weeks (Goldenberg, 2002).

Recommended Management of Preterm Labor. The following considerations should be given to women in preterm labor:

1. Confirmation of preterm labor as detailed on p. 867.
2. For pregnancies less than 34 weeks in women with no maternal or fetal indications for delivery, close observation with monitoring of uterine contractions and fetal heart rate is appropriate, and serial examinations are done to assess cervical changes.
3. For pregnancies less than 34 weeks, glucocorticoids are given for enhancement of fetal lung maturation.
4. For pregnancies less than 34 weeks in women who are not in advanced labor, some practitioners believe it is reasonable to attempt inhibition of contractions to delay delivery while the women are given glucocorticoid therapy

and group B streptococcal prophylaxis. Although tocolytic drugs are not used at Parkland Hospital, they are given at The University of Alabama at Birmingham Hospital.

5. For pregnancies at 34 weeks or beyond, women with preterm labor are monitored for labor progression and fetal well-being.

6. For active labor, an antimicrobial is given for prevention of neonatal group B streptococcal infection.

Intrapartum Management. In general, the more immature the fetus, the greater the risks of labor and delivery.

LABOR. Whether labor is induced or spontaneous, abnormalities of fetal heart rate and uterine contractions should be sought. We prefer continuous electronic monitoring. Fetal tachycardia, especially with ruptured membranes, is suggestive of sepsis. There is some evidence that intrapartum acidemia may intensify some of the neonatal complications usually attributed to preterm delivery. For example, Low and colleagues (1995) observed that intrapartum acidosis—umbilical artery blood pH less than 7.0—had an important role in neonatal complications. Similarly, Kimberlin and colleagues (1996) found that increasing umbilical artery blood acidemia was related to more severe respiratory disease in preterm neonates. Despite this, no effects were found in short-term neurological outcomes that included intracranial hemorrhages.

PREVENTION OF NEONATAL GROUP B STREPTOCOCCAL INFECTIONS. As discussed in Chapter 58 (see p. 1284), group B streptococcal infections are common and dangerous in the preterm neonate. Since 1996, the Centers for Disease Control and Prevention, along with the American College of Obstetricians and Gynecologists, recommend either penicillin G or ampicillin intravenously every 6 hours until delivery for women in preterm labor.

DELIVERY. In the absence of a relaxed vaginal outlet, an episiotomy for delivery may be necessary once the fetal head reaches the perineum. Perinatal outcome data do not support routine forceps delivery to protect the "fragile preterm fetal head." Staff proficient in resuscitative techniques commensurate with the gestational age of the newborn and fully oriented to any specific problems should be present at delivery. Principles of resuscitation described in Chapter 28 are applicable. The importance of the availability of specialized personnel and facilities in the care of preterm newborns is underscored by the improved survival of these neonates when they are delivered in tertiary care centers (American College of Obstetricians and Gynecologists, 2002; Powell and colleagues, 1995).

PREVENTION OF NEONATAL INTRACRANIAL HEMORRHAGE. Preterm newborns frequently have germinal matrix bleeding that can extend to more serious intraventricular hemorrhage (see Chap. 29, p. 652). It was hypothesized that cesarean delivery to obviate trauma from labor and vaginal delivery might prevent these complications. This has not been validated by most subsequent studies. Malloy and colleagues (1991) analyzed 1765 newborns with birthweights less than 1500 g and found that cesarean delivery did not lower the risk of mortality or intracranial hemorrhage. Anderson and colleagues (1988), however, made an interesting observation regarding the role of cesarean delivery in the prevention of neonatal intracranial hemorrhages. These hemorrhages related to whether or not the fetus had been subjected to the active phase of labor, defined as the interval before 5 cm cervical dilatation. They emphasized that avoidance of active-phase labor is impossible in most preterm births because the route of delivery cannot be decided until the active phase labor is firmly established.

REFERENCES

Abbasi S, Gerdes JS, Sehdev HM, et al: Neonatal outcomes after exposure to indomethacin in utero: A retrospective case cohort study. Am J Obstet Gynecol 189:782, 2003

Alexander GR, Himes JH, Kaufman RB, et al: A United States national reference for fetal growth. Obstet Gynecol 87:163, 1996

Alexander JM, Gilstrap LC, Cox SM, et al: Clinical chorioamnionitis and the prognosis for very low birthweight infants. Obstet Gynecol 91:725, 1998

Alexander JM, Merer BM, Miodovnik M, et al: The impact of digital cervical examination on expectantly managed preterm ruptured membranes. Am J Obstet Gynecol 183:1003, 2000

Althuisius SM, Dekker G, Hummel P, et al: Cervical incompetence prevention randomized cerclage trial: Emergency cerclage with bed rest versus bed rest alone. Am J Obstet Gynecol 189:907, 2003

American Academy of Pediatrics and the American College of Obstetricians and Gynecologists: Guidelines for Perinatal Care, 4th ed. 1997, p 100

American College of Obstetricians and Gynecologists: Use of progesterone to reduce preterm birth. Committee Opinion No. 291, November 2003

American College of Obstetricians and Gynecologists: Perinatal care at the threshold of viability. Practice Bulletin No. 38, September 2002

American College of Obstetricians and Gynecologists: Assessment of risk factors for preterm birth. Practice Bulletin No. 31, October 2001

American College of Obstetricians and Gynecologists: Premature rupture of membranes. Practice Bulletin No. 1, June 1998a

American College of Obstetricians and Gynecologists: Procedure: Tocolysis. Criteria Set No. 34, June 1998b

American College of Obstetricians and Gynecologists: Preterm labor. Technical Bulletin No. 206, June 1995

Amon E, Shyken JM, Sibai BM: How small is too small and how early is too early? A survey of American obstetricians specializing in high-risk pregnancies. Am J Perinatol 9:17, 1992

Anderson GD, Bada HS, Sibai BM, et al: The relationship between labor and route of delivery in the preterm infant. Am J Obstet Gynecol 158:1382, 1988

Andrews WW, Copper R, Hauth JC, et al: Mid-trimester cervical ultrasound findings predict recurrent early spontaneous delivery. Obstet Gynecol 95:222, 2000

Andrews WW, Hauth JC, Goldenberg RL, et al: Amniotic fluid interleukin-6: Correlation with upper genital tract microbial colonization and gestational age in women delivered after spontaneous labor versus indicated delivery. Am J Obstet Gynecol 173:606, 1995

Andrews WW, Sibai BM, Thom EA, et al: Randomized clinical trial of metronidazole plus erythromycin to prevent spontaneous preterm delivery in fetal fibronectin-positive women. Obstet Gynecol 101:847, 2003

Angel JL, O'Brien WF, Knuppel RA, et al: Carbohydrate intolerance in patients receiving oral tocolytics. Am J Obstet Gynecol 159:762, 1988

Arias E, Anderson RN, Hsiang-Ching K, et al: Deaths: Final data for 2001. National Vital Statistics Report, Vol 52, No. 3. Hyattsville, MD, National Center for Health Statistics, 2003

Ballard RA, Ballard PL, Cnaan A, et al: Antenatal thyrotropin-releasing hormone to prevent lung disease in preterm infants. N Engl J Med 338:493, 1998

Ben-Ami M, Giladi Y, Shalev E: The combination of magnesium sulphate and nifedipine: A cause of neuromuscular blockade. Br J Obstet Gynaecol 101:262, 1994

Berghella V, Tolosa JE, Kuhlman K, et al: Cervical ultrasonography compared with manual examination as a predictor of preterm delivery. Am J Obstet Gynecol 177:723, 1997

Berkman ND, Thorp JM, Lohr KN, et al: Tocolytic treatment for the management of preterm labor: A review of the evidence. Am J Obstet Gynecol 188:1648, 2003

Berns S: Understanding prematurity. Presentation at the 26th Annual International Neonatal Conference. Miami, FL, 2002

Bloom S, Leveno KJ: Corticosteroid use in special circumstances: Preterm ruptured membranes, hypertension, fetal growth restriction, multiple fetuses. Clin Obstet Gynecol 46:150, 2003

Bloom SL, Sheffield JS, McIntire DD, et al: Antenatal dexamethasone and decreased birth weight. Obstet Gynecol 97:485, 2001a

Bloom SL, Yost NP, McIntire DD, et al: Recurrence of preterm birth in singleton and twin pregnancies. Obstet Gynecol 98:379, 2001b

Boggess K, Murtha A, Lieff S, et al: Maternal periodontal disease is associated with delivery of a small for gestational age infant. Am J Obstet Gynecol 185:S235, 2001

Bottoms SF, Paul RH, Iams JD, et al: Obstetric determinants of neonatal survival: Influence of willingness to perform cesarean delivery on survival of extremely low-birth-weight infants. Am J Obstet Gynecol 176:960, 1997

Buekens P, Alexander S, Boutsen M, et al: Randomised controlled trial of routine cervical examinations in pregnancy. Lancet 344:841, 1994

Buhimschi CS, Buhimschi IA, Malinow AM, et al: Effects of sublingual nitroglycerin on human uterine contractility during the active phase of labor. Am J Obstet Gynecol 187:235, 2002

Bullard I, Vermillion S, Soper D: Clinical intraamniotic infection and the outcome for very low birth weight neonates [abstract]. Am J Obstet Gynecol 187:S73, 2002

Bytautiene E, Romero R, Vedernikov Y, et al: An allergic reaction can induce premature labor and delivery, which can be prevented by treatment with antihistaminics and cromolyn sodium. Am J Obstet Gynecol 189:S71, 2003

Canadian Preterm Labor Investigators Group: Treatment of preterm labor with the beta-adrenergic agonist ritodrine. N Engl J Med 327:308, 1992

Carey JC, Klebanoff MA, Hauth JC, et al: Metronidazole to prevent preterm delivery in pregnant women with asymptomatic bacterial vaginosis. N Engl J Med 342:534, 2000

Carlan SJ, O'Brien WF, Parsons MT, et al: Preterm premature rupture of membranes: A randomized study of home versus hospital management. Obstet Gynecol 81:61, 1993

Carr DB, Clark AL, Kernek K, et al: Maintenance oral nifedipine for preterm labor: A randomized clinical trial. Am J Obstet Gynecol 181:822, 1999

Carroll SG, Blott M, Nicolaides KH: Preterm prelabor amniorrhexis: Outcome of live births. Obstet Gynecol 86:18, 1995

Carroll SG, Papaionnou S, Ntumazah IL, et al: Lower genital tract swabs in the prediction of intrauterine infection in preterm prelabour rupture of the membranes. Br J Obstet Gynaecol 103:54, 1996

Casanueva E, Ripoll C, Meza-Camacho C, et al: Possible interplay between vitamin C deficiency and prolactin in pregnant women with premature rupture of membranes: Facts and hypothesis. Med Hypotheses 64:241, 2005

Castles A, Adams EK, Melvin CL, et al: Effects of smoking during pregnancy: Five meta-analyses. Am J Prev Med 16:208, 1999

Centers for Disease Control and Prevention: Prevention of perinatal group B streptococcal disease: A public health perspective. MMWR 45(RR-7):1, 1996

Chapman S, Hauth JC, Goldenberg RL, et al: Lack of apparent corticosteroid benefits in 1000 g infants born after preterm amnion rupture. Am J Obstet Gynecol 174:316, 1996

Childress CH, Katz VL: Nifedipine and its indications in obstetrics and gynecology. Obstet Gynecol 83:616, 1994

Chwalisz K, Fahrenholz F, Hackenberg M, et al: The progesterone antagonist onapristone increases the effectiveness of oxytocin to produce delivery without changing the myometrial oxytocin receptor concentrations. Am J Obstet Gynecol 165:1760, 1991

Clavin DK, Bayhi DA, Nolan TE, et al: Comparison of intravenous magnesium sulfate and nitroglycerin for preterm labor: Preliminary data. Am J Obstet Gynecol 174:307, 1996

Collaborative Home Uterine Monitoring Study Group: A multicenter randomized controlled trial of home uterine monitoring: Active versus sham device. Am J Obstet Gynecol 173:1170, 1995

Cook CM, Ellwood DA: A longitudinal study of the cervix in pregnancy using transvaginal ultrasound. Br J Obstet Gynaecol 103:16, 1996

Copper RL, Goldenberg RL, Das A, et al: The preterm prediction study: Maternal stress is associated with spontaneous preterm birth at less than thirty-five weeks' gestation. Am J Obstet Gynecol 175:1286, 1996

Copper RL, Goldenberg RL, Davis RO, et al: Warning symptoms, uterine contractions, and cervical examination findings in women at risk of preterm delivery. Am J Obstet Gynecol 162:748, 1990

Copper RL, Goldenberg RL, Dubard MB, et al: Cervical examination and tocodynamometry at 28 weeks' gestation: Prediction of spontaneous preterm birth. Am J Obstet Gynecol 172:666, 1995

Cotch MF, Pastorek JG 2nd, Nugent RP, et al: *Trichomonas vaginalis* associated with low birth weight and preterm delivery. Sex Transm Dis 24:353, 1997

Cotton DB, Strassner HT, Hill LM, et al: Comparison between magnesium sulfate, terbutaline and a placebo for inhibition of preterm labor: A randomized study. J Reprod Med 29:92, 1984

Cox SM, Bohman VR, Sherman ML, et al: Randomized investigation of antimicrobials for the prevention of preterm birth. Am J Obstet Gynecol 174:206, 1996

Cox SM, King MR, Casey ML, et al: Interleukin-1 beta, -1 alpha, and -6 and prostaglandins in vaginal/cervical fluids of pregnant women before and during labor. J Clin Endocrinol Metab 77:805, 1993

Cox SM, Leveno KJ: Intentional delivery versus expectant management with preterm ruptured membranes at 30–34 weeks' gestation. Obstet Gynecol 86:875, 1995

Cox SM, Sherman ML, Leveno KJ: Randomized investigation of magnesium sulfate for prevention of preterm birth. Am J Obstet Gynecol 163:767, 1990

Cox SM, Williams ML, Leveno KJ: The natural history of preterm ruptured membranes: What to expect of expectant management. Obstet Gynecol 71:558, 1988

Crowther CA, Hiller JE, Doyle LW, et al: Effect of magnesium sulfate given for neuroprotection before preterm birth: A randomized controlled trial. JAMA 290:2669, 2003

Crowther CA, Hiller JE, Haslam RR, et al: Australian collaborative trial of antenatal thyrotropin-releasing hormone (ACTOBAT) for prevention of neonatal respiratory disease. Lancet 345:877, 1995

Csapo AI: Progesterone "block." Am J Anat 98:273, 1956

Culhane JF, Rauh V, McCollum KF, et al: Exposure to chronic stress and ethnic differences in rates of bacterial vaginosis among pregnant women. Am J Obstet Gynecol 187:1272, 2002

da Fonseca EB, Bittar RE, Carvalho MHB, et al: Prophylactic administration of progesterone by vaginal suppository to reduce the incidence of spontaneous preterm birth in women at increased risk: A randomized placebo-controlled double-blind study. Am J Obstet Gynecol 188:419, 2003

DePalma RT, Leveno KJ, Kelly MA, et al: Birth weight threshold for postponing preterm birth. Am J Obstet Gynecol 167:1145, 1992

DeRoche ME, Egan JFX, Bolnick AD, et al: Changes in cesarean delivery rates at periviable gestational ages [abstract]. Am J Obstet Gynecol 187:S103, 2002

Devine P, Perez-Delboy A, D'Alton M, et al: Periodontal disease and preterm delivery: A case control study [abstract]. Am J Obstet Gynecol 185:S140, 2001

Doron MW, Veness-Meehan KA, Margolis LH, et al: Delivery room resuscitation decisions for extremely premature infants. Pediatrics 102:574, 1998

Doyle LW, Permezel M, Ford GW, et al: The obstetrician and the extremely immature fetus (24–26 weeks): Outcome to 5 years of age. Aust N Z J Obstet Gynaecol 34:421, 1994

Dyson DC, Danbe KH, Bamber JA, et al: Monitoring women at risk for preterm labor. N Engl J Med 338:15, 1998

Elliott JP: Magnesium sulfate as a tocolytic agent. Am J Obstet Gynecol 147:277, 1983

Elovitz M, Wang Z: Elucidating the mechanisms by which progestational agents prevent preterm birth. Am J Obstet Gynecol 189:S82, 2003

Elovitz M, Wang Z: Medroxyprogesterone acetate, but not progesterone, protects against inflammation-induced parturition and intrauterine fetal demise. Am J Obstet Gynecol 190:693, 2004

El-Sayed Y, Riley ET, Holbrook RH, et al: Randomized comparison of intravenous nitroglycerin and magnesium sulfate for treatment of preterm labor. Obstet Gynecol 93:79, 1999

Ernest JM, Wasilauskas B: Capnocytophaga in the amniotic fluid of a woman in preterm labor with intact membranes. Am J Obstet Gynecol 153:648, 1985

Esplin MS, Fausett MB, Smith S, et al: Multiple courses of antenatal steroids are associated with a delay in long-term psychomotor development in children with birth weights #1500 grams [abstract]. Am J Obstet Gynecol 182:S24, 2000

Evans DJ, Levene MI: Evidence of selection bias in preterm survival studies: A systematic review. Arch Dis Child Fetal Neonatal Ed 84:F79, 2001

Fanaroff AA, Hack M, Walsh MC: The NICHHD Neonatal Research Network: Changes in practice and outcomes. Semin Perinatol 27:281, 2003

Farooqi A, Holmgren PA, Engberg S, et al: Survival and 2-year outcome with expectant management of second trimester rupture of membranes. Obstet Gynecol 92:895, 1998

Feinstein SJ, Vintzileos AM, Lodeiro JG, et al: Amniocentesis with premature rupture of membranes. Obstet Gynecol 68:147, 1986

Fiscella K, Franks P, Kendrick JS, et al: Risk of preterm birth that is associated with vaginal douching. Am J Obstet Gynecol 186:1345, 2002

Fletcher SE, Fyfe DA, Case CL, et al: Myocardial necrosis in a newborn after long-term maternal subcutaneous terbutaline infusion for suppression of preterm labor. Am J Obstet Gynecol 165:1401, 1991

Frydman R, LeLaidier C, Baton C, et al: Labor induction in women at term with mifepristone (RU 486): A double-blind, randomized, placebo-controlled study. Obstet Gynecol 80:972, 1992

Gardner MO, Owen J, Skelly S, et al: Preterm delivery after indomethacin: A risk factor for neonatal complications? J Reprod Med 41:903, 1996

Garite TJ, Freeman RK, Linzey EM, et al: Prospective randomized study of corticosteroids in the management of premature rupture of the membranes and the premature gestation. Am J Obstet Gynecol 141:508, 1981

Garite TJ, Keegan KA, Freeman RK, et al: A randomized trial of ritodrine tocolysis versus expectant management in patients with premature rupture of membranes at 25 to 30 weeks of gestation. Am J Obstet Gynecol 157:388, 1987

Genc MR, Gerber S, Nesin M, et al: Polymorphism in the interleukin-1 gene complex and spontaneous preterm delivery. Am J Obstet Gynecol 187:157, 2002

Gielchinsky Y, Mankuta D, Samueloff A, et al: First pregnancy in women over 45 years of age carries increased obstetrical risk [abstract]. Am J Obstet Gynecol 187:S87, 2002

Ginsberg HG, Goldsmith JP, Stedman CM: Survival of a 380-g infant. N Engl J Med 322:1753, 1990

Gluck L: Fetal lung maturity. Paper presented at the 78th Ross Conference on Pediatric Research, San Diego, May 1979

Goepfert AR, Jeffcoat MK, Andrews, et al: Periodontal disease and upper gential tract inflammation in early spontaneous preterm birth. Obstet Gynecol 104:777, 2004

Goepfert AR, Schwebke J, Andrews W, et al: Perinatal emphasis research center (PERC): Vaginal markers of preterm birth [abstract]. Am J Obstet Gynecol 187:S126, 2002

Goldenberg RL: The management of preterm labor. Obstet Gynecol 100:1020, 2002

Goldenberg RL, Cliver SP, Bronstein J, et al: Bed rest in pregnancy. Obstet Gynecol 84:131, 1994

Goldenberg RL, Klebanoff M, Carey JC, et al: Vaginal fetal fibronectin measurements from 8 to 22 weeks' gestation and subsequent spontaneous preterm birth. Am J Obstet Gynecol 183:469, 2000

Goldenberg RL, Thom E, Moawad AH, et al: The preterm prediction study: Fetal fibronectin, bacterial vaginosis, and peripartum infection. Obstet Gynecol 87:656, 1996

Goodwin TM: A role of estriol in human labor, term and preterm. Am J Obstet Gynecol 180:S208, 1999

Goodwin TM, Jackson GM, McGregor JA, et al: Increased incidence of preterm labor and preterm delivery associated with increased salivary estriol level. Am J Obstet Gynecol 174:326, 1996

Goodwin TM, Millar L, North L, et al: The pharmacokinetics of the oxytocin antagonist atosiban in pregnant women with preterm uterine contractions. Am J Obstet Gynecol 173:913, 1995

Grether JK, Hoogstrate J, Walsh-Greene E, et al: Magnesium sulfate for tocolysis and risk of spastic cerebral palsy in premature children born to women without preeclampsia. Am J Obstet Gynecol 183:717, 2000

Guinn DA, Goepfert AR, Owen J, et al: Management option in women with preterm uterine contractions: A randomized clinical trial. Am J Obstet Gynecol 177:814, 1997

Guinn DA, Goepfert AR, Owen J, et al: Terbutaline pump maintenance therapy for prevention of preterm delivery: A double-blind trial. Am J Obstet Gynecol 179:874, 1998

Gyetvai K, Hannah ME, Hodnett ED, et al: Tocolytics for preterm labor: A systematic review. Obstet Gynecol 94:869, 1999

Gyr TN, Malek A, Mathez-Loic F, et al: Permeation of human chorioamniotic membranes by Escherichia coli in vitro. Am J Obstet Gynecol 170:223, 1994

Hack M, Fanaroff AA: Outcomes of children of extremely low birthweight and gestational age in the 1990s. Early Hum Dev 53:193, 1999

Hack M, Flannery DJ, Schluchter M, et al: Outcomes in young adulthood for very-low-birth-weight infants. N Engl J Med 346:149, 2002

Hadi HA, Hodson CA, Strickland D: Premature rupture of the membranes between 20 and 25 weeks' gestation: Role of amniotic fluid volume in perinatal outcome. Am J Obstet Gynecol 170:1139, 1994

Hallak M, Bottoms SF: Accelerated pulmonary maturation from preterm premature rupture of membranes: A myth. Am J Obstet Gynecol 169:1045, 1993

Hankins GD, Hauth JC, Cissik JH, et al: Effects of ritodrine hydrochloride on arteriovenous blood gas and shunt in healthy pregnant yellow baboons. Am J Obstet Gynecol 158:658, 1988

Harger JM: Cervical cerclage: Patient selection morbidity, and success rates. Clin Perinatol 10: 321, 1983

Hausdorff WP, Caron MG, Lefkowitz RJ: Turning off the signal: Desensitization of beta-adrenergic receptor function. FASEB J 4:2881, 1990

Hauth JC, Andrews WW, Goldenberg RL: Infection-related risk factors predictive of spontaneous preterm labor and birth. Prenat Neonat Med 3:86, 1998

Hauth JC, Cliver S, Hodgkins P, et al: Mid-trimester metronidazole and azithromycin did not prevent preterm birth in women at increased risk: A double-blind trial [abstract]. Am J Obstet Gynecol 185:S86, 2001a

Hauth JC, Gilstrap LC, Brekken AL, et al: The effect of 17 alpha-hydroxyprogesterone caproate on pregnancy outcome in an active-duty military population. Am J Obstet Gynecol 146:187, 1983

Hauth JC, Goldenberg RL, Andrews WW, et al: Reduced incidence of preterm delivery with metronidazole and erythromycin in women with bacterial vaginosis. N Engl J Med 333:1732, 1995

Hauth JC, Jeffcoat M, Cliver SP, et al: Periodontal disease and preterm birth [abstract]. Am J Obstet Gynecol 184:S37, 2001b

Hauth JC, MacPherson C, Carey JC, et al: Early pregnancy threshold vaginal pH and Gram stain scores predictive of subsequent preterm birth in asymptomatic women. Am J Obstet Gynecol 188:831, 2003

Heine RP, McGregor JA, Dullien VK: Accuracy of salivary estriol testing compared to traditional risk factor assessment in predicting preterm birth. Am J Obstet Gynecol 180:S214, 1999

Helfgott AW, Willis DC, Blanco JD: Is hydration and sedation beneficial in the treatment of threatened preterm labor? A preliminary report. J Matern Fetal Med 3:37, 42, 1994

Hershkovitz R, Zmora E, Furman B, et al: Steroid treatment does not alter neonatal morbidity in very-low-birthweight infants [abstract]. Am J Obstet Gynecol 184:S41, 2001

Hickey CA, Cliver SP, McNeal SF, et al: Prenatal weight gain patterns and spontaneous preterm birth among non-obese black and white women. Obstet Gynecol 85:909, 1995

Hillier SL, Nugent RP, Eschenbach DA, et al: Association between bacterial vaginosis and preterm delivery of a low-birthweight infant. N Engl J Med 333:1737, 1995

Hitti J, Cauci S, Noonan C, et al: Vaginal hydrolytic enzyme activity, bacterial vaginosis and risk of early preterm birth among women in preterm labor [abstract]. Am J Obstet Gynecol 185:S193, 2001

Ho M, Ramsey P, Brumfield C, et al: Changes in maternal and neonatal infectious morbidity as latency increases after preterm premature rupture of membranes [abstract]. Obstet Gynecol 101:41S, 2003

Hoffman JD, Ward K: Genetic factors in preterm delivery. Obstet Gynecol Surv 54:203, 1999

Horbar JD, Badger GJ, Carpenter JH, et al: Trends in mortality and morbidity for very low birth weight infants 1991-1999. Pediatrics 110:143, 2002

How HY, Hughes SA, Vogel RL, et al: Oral terbutaline in the outpatient management of preterm labor. Am J Obstet Gynecol 173:1518, 1995

Hudgens DR, Conradi SE: Sudden death associated with terbutaline sulfate administration. Am J Obstet Gynecol 169:120, 1993

Hueston WJ, Knox MA, Eilers G, et al: The effectiveness of preterm-birth prevention educational program for high-risk women: A meta-analysis. Obstet Gynecol 86:705, 1995

Iams JD: Prediction and early detection of preterm labor. Obstet Gynecol 101:402, 2003

Iams JD, Newman RB, Thom EA, et al: Frequency of uterine contractions and the risk of spontaneous preterm birth. N Engl J Med 346:250, 2002

Iams JD, Goldenberg RL, Meis PJ, et al: The length of the cervix and the risk of spontaneous premature delivery. N Engl J Med 334:567, 1996

Iams JD, Johnson FF, Parker M: A prospective evaluation of the signs and symptoms of preterm labor. Obstet Gynecol 84:227, 1994

Iams JD, Stilson R, Johnson FF, et al: Symptoms that precede preterm labor and preterm premature rupture of the membranes. Am J Obstet Gynecol 162:486, 1990

Jackson GM, Edwin SS, Varner MW, et al: Regulation of fetal fibronectin production in human amnion cells. J Soc Gynecol Investig 3:85, 1996

Jeffcoat MK, Hauth JC, Geurs NC, et al: Periodontal disease and preterm birth: Results of a pilot intervention study. J Periodontol 74:1214, 2003

Jobe AH, Soll RF: Choice and dose of corticosteroid for antenatal treatments. Am J Obstet Gynecol 190:878, 2004

Joesoef MR, Hillier SL, Wiknjosastro G, et al: Intravaginal clindamycin treatment for bacterial vaginosis: Effects on preterm delivery and low birth weight. Am J Obstet Gynecol 173:1527, 1995

Johnson JWC, Austin KL, Jones GS, et al: Efficacy of 17α-hydroxyprogesterone caproate in the prevention of premature labor. N Engl J Med 293:675, 1975

Johnson JWC, Lee PA, Zachary AS, et al: High-risk prematurity—progestin treatment and steroid studies. Obstet Gynecol 54:412, 1979

Keirse MJNC: Calcium antagonists vs. betamimetics in preterm labour. In Neilson JP, Crowther C, Hodnett ED, et al (eds): Pregnancy and Childbirth Module. Cochrane Database of Systematic Reviews, Issue 2. Oxford, Update Software, 1995a

Keirse MJNC. New perspectives for the effective treatment of preterm labor. Am J Obstet Gynecol 173:618, 1995b

Kekki M, Kurki T, Pelkonen J, et al: Vaginal clindamycin in preventing preterm birth and peripartal infections in asymptomatic women with bacterial vaginosis: A randomized, controlled trial. Obstet Gynecol 97:643, 2001

Kenyon SL, Taylor DJ, Tarnow-Mordi W, et al: Broad-spectrum antibiotics for preterm, prelabour rupture of fetal membranes: The ORACLE I randomized trial. Lancet 357:979, 2001a

Kenyon SL, Taylor DJ, Tarnow-Mordi, et al: Broad-spectrum antibiotics for spontaneous preterm labour: The ORACLE II randomized trial. Lancet 357:989, 2001b

Kimberlin DF, Hauth JC, Goldenberg RL, et al: Relationship of acid–base status and neonatal morbidity in 1000 g infants. Am J Obstet Gynecol 174:382, 1996

Kimberlin DF, Hauth JC, Goldenberg RL, et al: The effect of maternal magnesium sulfate treatment on neonatal morbidity in 1000 gram infants. Am J Perinatol 15:635, 1998

Kimberlin DF, Hauth JC, Owen J, et al: Indicated versus spontaneous preterm delivery: An evaluation of neonatal morbidity among infants weighing 1000 grams at birth. Am J Obstet Gynecol 180:683, 1999

King J, Flenady V: Antibiotics for preterm labour with intact membranes. Cochrane Database Syst Rev 2:CD000246, 2000

King JF, Flenady V, Papatsonis D, et al: Calcium channel blockers for inhibiting preterm labour: A systematic review of the evidence and a protocol for administration of nifedipine. Aust N Z J Obstet Gynaecol 43:192, 2003

Kitchen WH, Permezel MJ, Doyle LW, et al: Changing obstetric practice and 2-year outcome of the fetus of birthweight under 1000 g. Obstet Gynecol 79:268, 1992

Klebanoff MA, Carey JC, Hauth JC, et al: Failure of metronidazole to prevent preterm delivery among pregnant women with asymptomatic *Trichomonas vaginalis* infection. N Engl J Med 345:487, 2001

Klebanoff MA, Hauth JC, MacPherson CA, et al: Time course of the regression of asymptomatic bacterial vaginosis in pregnancy with and without treatment. Am J Obstet Gynecol 190:363, 2004a

Klebanoff MA, Hillier SL, Nugent RP, et al: Is bacterial vaginosis a stronger risk factor for preterm birth when it is diagnosed earlier in gestation? Am J Obstet Gynecol 2004b (in press)

Klerman LV, Ramey SL, Goldenberg RL, et al: A randomized trial of augmented prenatal care for multiple-risk, Medicaid-eligible African American women. Am J Public Health 91:105, 2001

Knight DB, Liggins GC, Wealthall SR: A randomized, controlled trial of antepartum thyrotropin-releasing hormone and betamethasone in the prevention of respiratory disease in preterm infants. Am J Obstet Gynecol 171:11, 1994

Knudtson E, Senokozlieff M, Ye H: The association of chronic endometritis with preterm birth. Am J Obstet Gynecol 189:S173, 2003

Kovacevich GJ, Gaich SA, Lavin JP, et al: The prevalence of thromboembolic events among women with extended bed rest prescribed as part of the treatment for premature labor or preterm premature rupture of membranes. Am J Obstet Gynecol 182:1089, 2000

Kragt H, Keirse MJ: How accurate is a woman's diagnosis of threatened preterm delivery? Br J Obstet Gynaecol 97:317, 1990

Kramer MS, Coates AL, Michoud MC, et al: Maternal anthropometry and idiopathic preterm labor. Obstet Gynecol 86:744, 1995

Kurki T, Sivonen A, Renkonen OV, et al: Bacterial vaginosis in early pregnancy and pregnancy outcome. Obstet Gynecol 80:173, 1992

Kurkinen-Raty M, Vuopala S, Koskela M, et al: A randomised controlled trial of vaginal clindamycin for early pregnancy bacterial vaginosis. Br J Obstet Gynaecol 107:1427, 2000

Kurtzman JL, Thorp JM Jr, Spielman FJ, et al: Do nifedipine and verapamil potentiate the cardiac toxicity of magnesium sulfate? Am J Perinatol 10:450, 1993

Lam F, Gill P, Smith M, et al: Use of the subcutaneous terbutaline pump for long-term tocolysis. Obstet Gynecol 72:810, 1988

Lamont RF, Duncan SL, Mandal D, et al: Intravaginal clindamycin to reduce preterm birth in women with abnormal genital tract flora. Obstet Gynecol 1001:516, 2003

Landau R, Xie HG, Dishy V, et al: β_2-adrenergic receptor genotype and preterm delivery. Am J Obstet Gynecol 187:1294, 2002

Lee M, Davies J, Guinn D, et al: Single versus weekly courses of antenatal corticosteroids in preterm premature rupture of membranes. Obstet Gynecol 103:274, 2004

Lees CC, Lojacono A, Thompson C, et al: Glyceryl trinitrate and ritodrine in tocolysis: An international multicenter randomized study. Obstet Gynecol 94:403, 1999

Leeson SC, Maresh MJA, Martindale EA, et al: Detection of fetal fibronectin as a predictor of preterm delivery in high risk symptomatic pregnancies. Br J Obstet Gynaecol 103:48, 1996

Leitich H, Bodner-Adler B, Brunbauer M, et al: Bacterial vaginosis as a risk factor for preterm delivery: A meta-analysis. Am J Obstet Gynecol 189:139, 2003a

Leitich H, Brunbauer M, Bodner-Adler B, et al: Antibiotic treatment of bacterial vaginosis in pregnancy: A meta-analysis. Am J Obstet Gynecol 188:752, 2003b

Lemons JA, Bauer CR, Oh W, et al: Very low birth weight outcomes of the National Institute of Child Health and Human Development Neonatal Research Network, January 1995 through December 1996. Pediatrics 107:31, 2001

Leveno KJ, Cox K, Roark ML: Cervical dilatation and prematurity revisited. Obstet Gynecol 68:434, 1986a

Leveno KJ, Klein VR, Guzick DS, et al: Single-centre randomised trial of ritodrine hydrochloride for preterm labour. Lancet 1:1293, 1986b

Leviton LC, Goldenberg RL, Baker CS, et al: Methods to encourage the use of antenatal corticosteroid therapy for fetal maturation: A randomized controlled trial. JAMA 281:46, 1999

Lewis DF, Adair CD, Robichaux AG, et al: Antibiotic therapy in preterm premature rupture of membranes: Are seven days necessary? A preliminary, randomized clinical trial. Am J Obstet Gynecol 188:1413, 2003

Lewis R, Mercer BM, Salama M, et al: Oral terbutaline after parenteral tocolysis: A randomized, double-blind, placebo-controlled trial. Am J Obstet Gynecol 175:834, 1996

Lewit EM, Baker LS, Corman H, et al: The direct cost of low birth weight. Future Child 5:35, 1995

Liggins GC, Howie RN: A controlled trial of antepartum glucocorticoid treatment for prevention of the respiratory distress syndrome in premature infants. Pediatrics 50:515, 1972

Lirette M, Holbrook RH, Katz M: Cardiovascular and uterine blood flow changes during nicardipine HCl tocolysis in the rabbit. Obstet Gynecol 69:79, 1987

Lockwood CJ, Senyei AE, Dische MR, et al: Fetal fibronectin in cervical and vaginal secretions as a predictor of preterm delivery. N Engl J Med 325:669, 1991

Lopez S, Shah J, Verma U, et al: Single- versus multiple-dose antenatal steroids and the effect on blood pressure in low-birth-weight neonates. Am J Obstet Gynecol 184:S47, 2001

Low JA, Panagiotopoulos C, Derrick EJ: Newborn complication after intrapartum asphyxia with metabolic acidosis in the preterm fetus. Am J Obstet Gynecol 172:805, 1995

Lowe MP, Zimmerman B, Hansen W: Prospective randomized controlled trial of fetal fibronectin on preterm labor management in a tertiary care center. Am J Obstet Gynecol 190:358, 2004

Luke B, Mamelle N, Keith L, et al: The association between occupational factors and preterm birth: A United States nurses study. Am J Obstet Gynecol 173:849, 1995

Macones GA, Parry S, Elkousy M, et al: A polymorphism in the promoter region of TNF and bacterial vaginosis: Preliminary evidence of gene-environment interaction in the etiology of spontaneous preterm birth. Am J Obstet Gynecol 190:1504, 2004

Macones GA, Berlin M, Berlin JA: Efficacy of oral beta-agonist maintenance therapy in preterm labor: A meta-analysis. Obstet Gynecol 85:313, 1995

Major CA, Towers CW, Lewis DF, et al: Expectant management of preterm premature rupture of membranes complicated by active recurrent genital herpes. Am J Obstet Gynecol 188:1551, 2003

Malloy MH, Onstad L, Wright E: The effect of cesarean delivery on birth outcome in very low birth weight infants. Obstet Gynecol 77:498, 1991

March of Dimes Birth Defects Foundation: Taking action against prematurity. Contemp Ob/Gyn 143:92, 2003

Martin DH, Eschenbach DA, Cotch MF, et al: Double-blind placebo-controlled treatment trial of Chlamydia trachomatis endocervical infections in pregnant women. Infect Dis Obstet Gynecol 5:10, 1997

Mathews TJ, Menacker F, MacDorman MF: Infant mortality obstetrics from the 2001 period linked birth/infant death data set. National Vital Statistics Reports, Vol 52, No. 2. Hyattsville, MD, National Center for Health Statistics, 2003

Mazor M, Wiznitzer A, Levy J, et al: The relationship between estrogen/progesterone ratio and term human parturitions. Isr J Med Sci 29:97, 1993

McCollum K, Chung E, Culhane J: Maternal depressive symptomatology and preterm birth (< 35 weeks' gestation) among low-income women. Am J Obstet Gynecol 189:S159, 2003

McDonald HM, O'Loughlin JA, Vigneswaran R, et al: Impact of metronidazole therapy on preterm birth in women with bacterial vaginosis flora (Gardnerella vaginalis): A randomised, placebo controlled trial. Br J Obstet Gynaecol 104:1391, 1997

McElrath TF, Allred E, Leviton A: Prolonged latency after preterm premature rupture of membranes: An evaluation of histologic condition and intracranial ultrasonic abnormality in the neonate born at < 28 weeks of gestation. Am J Obstet Gynecol 189:794, 2003

McElrath TF, Norwitz ER, Lieberman ES, et al: Perinatal outcome after preterm premature rupture of membranes with in situ cervical cerclage. Am J Obstet Gynecol 187:1147, 2002

McGregor JA, French JI, Jones W, et al: Bacterial vaginosis is associated with prematurity and vaginal fluid mucinase and sialidase: Results of a controlled trial of topical clindamycin cream. Am J Obstet Gynecol 170:1048, 1994

Meis PJ, Goldenberg RL, Mercer BM, et al: The preterm prediction study: Risk factors for indicated preterm births. Am J Obstet Gynecol 178:562, 1998

Meis PJ, Goldenberg RL, Mercer B, et al: The preterm prediction study: Significance of vaginal infections. Am J Obstet Gynecol 173:1231, 1995a

Meis PJ, Klebanoff M, Thom E, et al: Prevention of recurrent preterm delivery by 17 alpha-hydroxyprogesterone caproate. N Engl J Med 348:2379, 2003

Meis PJ, Michielutte R, Peters TJ, et al: Factors associated with preterm birth in Cardiff, Wales, I. Univariable and multivariable analysis. Am J Obstet Gynecol 173:590, 1995b

Mercer BM, Arheart KL: Antimicrobial therapy in expectant management of preterm premature rupture of the membranes. Lancet 346:1271, 1995

Mercer BM, Ahokas R, Beazley D, et al: Corticol, ACTG, and psychosocial stress in women at high risk for preterm birth [abstract]. Am J Obstet Gynecol 187:S72, 2002

Mercer BM, Carr TL, Beazley DD, et al: Antibiotic use in pregnancy and drug-resistant infant sepsis. Am J Obstet Gynecol 181:816, 1999

Mercer BM, Crocker LG, Boe NM, et al: Induction versus expectant management in premature rupture of the membranes with mature amniotic fluid at 32 to 36 weeks: A randomized trial. Am J Obstet Gynecol 169:775, 1993

Mercer B, Egerman R, Beazley D, et al: Steroids reduce fetal growth: Analysis of a retrospective trial. Am J Obstet Gynecol 186:S7, 2001

Mercer BM, Goldenberg RL, Das A, et al: The preterm prediction study: A clinical risk assessment system. Am J Obstet Gynecol 174:1885, 1996

Mercer BM, Miodovnik M, Thurnau GR, et al: Antibiotic therapy for reduction of infant morbidity after preterm premature rupture of the membranes. JAMA 278:989, 1997

Merkatz IR, Peter JB, Barden TP: Ritodrine hydrochloride: A betamimetic agent for use in preterm labor, II. Evidence of efficacy. Obstet Gynecol 56:7, 1980

Morales WJ, Madhav H: Efficacy and safety of indomethacin compared with magnesium sulfate in the management of preterm labor: A randomized study. Am J Obstet Gynecol 169:97, 1993

Morales WJ, Smith SG, Angel JL, et al: Efficacy and safety of indomethacin versus ritodrine in the management of preterm labor: A randomized study. Obstet Gynecol 74:567, 1989

Morales WJ, Talley T: Premature rupture of membranes < 25 weeks: A management dilemma. Am J Obstet Gynecol 168:503, 1993

Moutquin JM, Sherman D, Cohen H, et al: Double-blind, randomized, controlled trial of atosiban and ritodrine in the treatment of preterm labor: A multicenter effectiveness and safety study. Am J Obstet Gynecol 183:1191, 2000

Muench MV, Baschat AA, Kopelman J, et al: Indomethacin therapy initiated before 24 weeks of gestation for the prevention of preterm birth [abstract]. Obstet Gynecol 101:65S, 2003

Muench V, Harman CR, Baschat AA, et al: Early fetal exposure to long term indomethacin therapy to prevent preterm delivery: Neonatal outcome. Am J Obstet Gynecol 185:S149, 2001

Murphy DJ, Sellers S, MacKenzie IZ, et al: Case-control study of antenatal and intrapartum risk factors for cerebral palsy in very preterm singleton babies. Lancet 346:1449, 1995

National Institutes of Health Consensus Development Conference: Statement on Repeat Courses of Antenatal Corticosteroids. Bethesda, MD. August 17–18, 2000. Available at: http://consensus.nih.gov

National Institutes of Health Consensus Development Panel: Effect of corticosteroids for fetal maturation on perinatal outcomes. JAMA 173:413, 1995

Neggers Y, Goldenberg R, Cliver S, et al: Effects of domestic violence on preterm birth and low birth weight. Acta Obstet Gynecol Scand 83:455, 2004

Nelson KB, Grether JK: Can magnesium sulfate reduce the risk of cerebral palsy in very-low-birthweight infants? Pediatrics 95:263, 1995

Nelson LH, Anderson RL, O'Shea M, et al: Expectant management of preterm premature rupture of the membranes. Am J Obstet Gynecol 171:350, 1994

Nelson LH, Meis PJ, Hatjis CG, et al: Premature rupture of membranes: A prospective, randomized evaluation of steroids, latent phase, and expectant management. Obstet Gynecol 66:55, 1985

Ness RB, Hillier SL, Richter HE: Douching in relation to bacterial vaginosis, lactobacilli, and facultative bacteria in the vagina. Obstet Gynecol 100:765, 2002

Netta D, Fuks A, Godi I: Polymorphism of tumor necrosis factor-α and preterm premature rupture of membranes. Am J Obstet Gynecol 189:S174, 2003

Niebyl JR, Blake DA, White RD, et al: The inhibition of premature labor with indomethacin. Am J Obstet Gynecol 136:1014, 1980

Norton ME, Merrill J, Cooper BA, et al: Neonatal complications after the administration of indomethacin for preterm labor. N Engl J Med 329:1602, 1993

Nugent RP, Krohn MA, Hillier SL: Reliability of diagnosing bacterial vaginosis by a standardized method of gram stain interpretation. J Clin Microbiol 29:297, 1991

Nuthalapaty F, Hauth J, Goldenberg R, et al: Vaginal douching does not increase preterm birth. Obstet Gynecol 101:91S, 2003

O'Brien JM, Barton JR, Milligan DA: An aggressive interventional protocol for early midtrimester premature rupture of the membranes using gelatin sponge for cervical plugging. Am J Obstet Gynecol 187:1143, 2002

Offenbacher S, Katz V, Fertik G, et al: Periodontal infection as a possible risk factor for preterm low birth weight. J Periodontol 67:1103, 1996

Ogunyemi D, Alperson B, Berger J: Effectiveness of antenatal steroids: Is more bad [abstract]? Am J Obstet Gynecol 184:S39, 2001

Owen J, Iams JD, Hauth JC: Vaginal sonography and cervical incompetence. Am J Obstet Gynecol 188:586, 2003

Owen J, Yost N, Berghella V, et al: Mid-trimester endovaginal sonography in women at high risk for spontaneous preterm birth. JAMA 286:1340, 2001

Owen J, Baker SL, Hauth JC, et al: Is indicated or spontaneous preterm delivery more advantageous for the fetus? Am J Obstet Gynecol 163:868, 1990

Papatsonis DN, Van Geijn HP, Ader HJ, et al: Nifedipine and ritodrine in the management of preterm labor: A randomized multicenter trial. Obstet Gynecol 90:230, 1997

Papiernik E, Bouyer J, Collin D, et al: Precocious cervical ripening and preterm labor. Obstet Gynecol 67:238, 1986

Parilla BV, Dooley SL, Minogue JP, et al: The efficacy of oral terbutaline after intravenous tocolysis. Am J Obstet Gynecol 169:965, 1993

Parilla BV, Grobman WA, Holtzman RB, et al: Indomethacin tocolysis and risk of necrotizing enterocolitis. Obstet Gynecol 96:120, 2000

Parisi V, Salina J, Stockman E: Fetal cardiorespiratory responses to maternal administration of nicardipine in the hypertensive ewe. Presented at meeting of the Society of Perinatal Obstetricians, San Antonio, January 30–February 1, 1986

Peck T, Lutheran G: Long-term and short-term childhood health after long-term use of indomethacin in pregnancy. Am J Obstet Gynecol 189:S168, 2003

Perry KG Jr, Morrison JC, Rust OA, et al: Incidence of adverse cardiopulmonary effects with low-dose continuous terbutaline infusion. Am J Obstet Gynecol 173:1273, 1995

Perry KG, Martin RW, Blake PC, et al: Maternal outcome associated with adult respiratory distress syndrome. Am J Obstet Gynecol 174:391, 1996

Petrova A, Demissie K, Rhoads GG, et al: Association of maternal fever during labor with neonatal and infant morbidity and mortality. Obstet Gynecol 98:20, 2001

Platz-Christensen JJ, Mattsby-Baltzer I, Thomsen P, et al: Endotoxin and interleukin-1 alpha in the cervical mucus and vaginal fluid of pregnant women with bacterial vaginosis. Am J Obstet Gynecol 169:1161, 1993

Powell SL, Holt VL, Hickok DE, et al: Recent changes in delivery site of low-birthweight infants in Washington: Impact on birth weight-specific mortality. Am J Obstet Gynecol 173:1585, 1995

Pschirrer ER, Mastrobattista J, Day MC, et al: Single versus multicourse steroids for fetal maturation in women with preterm premature rupture of membranes. Am J Obstet Gynecol 184:S36, 2001

Ralph SG, Rutherford AJ, Wilson JD: Influence of bacterial vaginosis on conception and miscarriage in the first trimester: Cohort study. BMJ 319:220, 1999

Ramsey P, Lyon D, Goepfert A: Midtrimester vaginal polymorphonuclear cell counts compared to PMN to epithelial cell ratios for the prediction of spontaneous preterm birth. Am J Obstet Gynecol 189:S169, 2003

Reddy U, Zlatnik M, Baschat A, et al: Detection of viral deoxyribonucleic acid in amniotic fluid: Predictor of abnormal pregnancy [abstract]. Am J Obstet Gynecol 185:S192, 2001

Redman ME, Gonik B: Cesarean delivery rates at the threshold of viability. Am J Obstet Gynecol 187:873, 2002

Romero R, Chaiworapongsa T, Kuivaniemi H, et al: Bacterial vaginosis, the inflammatory response and the risk of preterm birth: A role for genetic epidemiology in the prevention of preterm birth. Am J Obstet Gynecol 190:1509, 2004

Romero R, Sibai BM, Sanchez-Ramos L, et al: An oxytocin receptor antagonist (atosiban) in the treatment of preterm labor: A randomized, double-blind, placebo-controlled trial with tocolytic rescue. Am J Obstet Gynecol 182:1173, 2000

Romero R, Yoon BH, Mazor M, et al: The diagnostic and prognostic value of amniotic fluid white blood cell count, glucose, interleukin-6 and gram stain in patients with preterm labor and intact membranes. Am J Obstet Gynecol 169:805, 1993

Romero R, Scoccia B, Mazor M, et al: Evidence for a local change in the progesterone/estrogen ratio in human parturition at term. Am J Obstet Gynecol 159:657, 1988

Santiago P, Yost N, Bloom S, et al: Occupational factors and risk for recurrent preterm birth, Presented at the 25th Annual Meeting of the Society for Maternal-Fetal Medicine, Reno, NV, 7–12 February, 2005

Satin AJ, Leveno KJ, Sherman ML, et al: Maternal youth and pregnancy outcomes: Middle school versus high school age groups compared to women beyond the teen years. Am J Obstet Gynecol 171:184, 1994

Schiff E, Sivan E, Terry S, et al: Currently recommended oral regimen for ritodrine tocolysis result in extremely low plasma levels. Am J Obstet Gynecol 169:1059, 1993

Schmidt B, Davis P, Moddemann D, et al: Long-term effects of indomethacin prophylaxis in extremely-low-birth-weight infants. N Engl J Med 344:1966, 2001

Segel SY, Miles AM, Clothier B, et al: Duration of antibiotic therapy after preterm premature rupture of fetal membranes. Am J Obstet Gynecol 189:799, 2003

Simchen MJ, Alkazaleh F, Adamson S, et al: The fetal cardiovascular response to antenatal steroids in severe early-onset intrauterine growth restriction. Am J Obstet Gynecol 190:296, 2004

Simhan HN, Caritis SN, Krohn MA, et al: Elevated vaginal pH and neutrophils are strongly associated with early spontaneous preterm birth. Am J Obstet Gynecol 189:1150, 2003

Smith P, Anthony J, Johanson R: Nifedipine in pregnancy. Br J Obstet Gynaecol 107:299, 2000

Spinillo A, Viazzo F, Colleoni R, et al: Two-year infant neurodevelopmental outcome after single or multiple antenatal courses of corticosteroids to prevent complications of prematurity. Am J Obstet Gynecol 191:217, 2004

St. John EB, Nelson KG, Cliver SP, et al: Cost of neonatal care according to gestational age at birth and survival status. Am J Obstet Gynecol 182:170, 2000

Steer CM, Petrie RH: A comparison of magnesium sulfate and alcohol for the prevention of premature labor. Am J Obstet Gynecol 129:1, 1977

Stevenson DK, Wright LL, Lemons JA, et al: Very low birth weight outcomes of the National Institute of Child Health and Human Development Neonatal Research Network, January 1993 through December 1994. Am J Obstet Gynecol 179:1632, 1998

Stoll BJ, Hansen NI, Adams-Chapman I, et al: Neurodevelopmental and growth impairment among extremely low-birth-weight infants with neonatal infection. JAMA 292:2357, 2004

Stoll BJ, Hansen N, Fanaroff AA, et al: Changes in pathogens causing early-onset sepsis in very-low-birth-weight infants. N Engl J Med 347:240, 2002

Swamy G, Simhan H, Seglin H, et al: The clinical utility of fetal fibronectin [abstract]. Am J Obstet Gynecol 185:S136, 2001

Taipale P, Hiilesmaa V: Sonographic measurement of uterine cervix at 18-22 weeks' gestation and the risk of preterm delivery. Obstet Gynecol 92:902, 1998

Tashima LS, Yamamoto SY, Ysuda M, et al: Decidual relaxins: Gene and protein up-regulation in preterm premature rupture of the membranes by complementary DNA arrays and quantitative immunocytochemistry. Am J Obstet Gynecol 187:785, 2002

Terkildsen MFC, Parilla BV, Kumar P, et al: Factors associated with success of emergent second-trimester cerclage. Obstet Gynecol 101:565, 2003

Thomas N, Chun LY, Nageotte MP, et al: Effects of antenatal betamethasone after preterm premature rupture of membranes between 24 and 32 weeks of gestation [abstract]. Am J Obstet Gynecol 184:S38, 2001

Thorp JA, Clark R, Jones PG, et al: The effect of antenatal steroids on head circumference at birth. Am J Obstet Gynecol 184:S2, 2001

Thorp JA, Ferrette-Smith D, Gaston LA, et al: Combined antenatal vitamin K and phenobarbital therapy for preventing intracranial hemorrhage of newborns less than 34 weeks gestation. Obstet Gynecol 86:1, 1995

Thorp JA, Lukes AG: Predictors of positivity for cervico-fetal fibronectin in patients with symptoms of preterm labor. J Soc Gynecol Investig 3 (Suppl):247, 1996

Thorp JA, O'Connor M, Belden B, et al: Effects of phenobarbital and multiple-dose corticosteroids on developmental outcome at age 7 years. Obstet Gynecol 101:363, 2003

Thorsen P, Molsted K, Jensen IP, et al: Bacterial vaginosis in a population of 3600 pregnant women and relationship to preterm birth. Am J Obstet Gynecol 174:331, 1996

Tongsong T, Kamprapanth P, Srisomboon J, et al: Single transvaginal sonographic measurement of cervical length early in the third trimester as a predictor of preterm delivery. Obstet Gynecol 86:184, 1995

Ugwumadu A, Reid F, Hay P, et al: Natural history of bacterial vaginosis and intermediate flora in pregnancy and effect of oral clindamycin. Obstet Gynecol 104:114, 2004

Ugwumadu A, Manyonda I, Reid F, et al: Effect of early oral clindamycin on late miscarriage and preterm delivery in asymptomatic women with abnormal vaginal flora and bacterial vaginosis: A randomised controlled trial. Lancet 361:983, 2003

Vermillion S, Soper D, Newman R: Neonatal sepsis and death after multiple doses of antenatal betamethasone. Am J Obstet Gynecol 183:810, 2000

Vohr BR, Wright LL, Dusick AM, et al: Neurodevelopmental and functional outcomes of extremely low birth weight infants in the National Institute of Child Health and Human Development Neonatal Research Network, 1993–1994. Pediatrics 105:1216, 2000

Wallace RJ: Capnocytophaga on the fetal surface of the placenta of a patient with ruptured membranes at 39 weeks gestation. Am J Obstet Gynecol 155:228, 1986

Wapner RJ, for the NICHHD MFMU Network: Randomized trial of single vs weekly course of corticosteroids. Am J Obstet Gynecol 189:S56, 2003

Watts DH, Krohn MA, Hillier SL, et al: The association of occult amniotic fluid infection with gestational age and neonatal outcome among women in preterm labor. Obstet Gynecol 79:351, 1992

Weiss JL, Malone FD, Vidaver J, et al: Threatened abortion: A risk factor for poor pregnancy outcome, a population-based screening study. Am J Obstet Gynecol 190:745, 2004

Wenstrom K, Weiner CP, Merrill D, et al: A placebo controlled randomized trial of the terbutaline pump for prevention of preterm delivery. Am J Perinatol 14:87, 1997

Winn HN, Chen M, Amon E, et al: Neonatal pulmonary hypoplasia and perinatal mortality in patients with mid-trimester rupture of amniotic membranes—a critical analysis. Am J Obstet Gynecol 182:1638, 2000

Wood NS, Marlow N, Costeloe K, et al: Neurologic and development disability after extremely preterm birth. N Engl J Med 343:378, 2000

Yang Z, Zhao Y, Bennett MJ, et al: Fetal genotypes and pregnancy outcomes in 35 families with mitochondrial trifunctional protein mutations. Am J Obstet Gynecol 187:715, 2002

Yemini M, Borenstein R, Dreazen E, et al: Prevention of premature labor by 17α-hydroxyprogesterone caproate. Am J Obstet Gynecol 151:574, 1985

Yoon BH, Romero R, Park JS, et al: Fetal exposure to an intra-amniotic inflammation and the development of cerebral palsy at the age of three years. Am J Obstet Gynecol 182:675, 2000

Yoon BH, Yang SH, Jun JK, et al: Maternal blood C-reactive protein, white blood cell count, and temperature in preterm labor: A comparison with amniotic fluid white blood cell count. Obstet Gynecol 87:231, 1996

Yost NP, Owen J, Berghella V, et al: Second-trimester cervical sonography: Features other than cervical length to predict spontaneous preterm birth. Am J Obstet Gynecol 103:457, 2004

Yost NP, Bloom SL, Twickler DM, et al: Pitfalls in ultrasonic cervical length measurement for predicting preterm birth. Obstet Gynecol 93:510, 1999

Yudin MH, Landers DV, Meyn L, et al: Clinical and cervical cytokine response to treatment with oral or vaginal metronidazole for bacterial vaginosis during pregnancy: A randomized trial. Obstet Gynecol 102:527, 2003

Zuckerman H, Reiss U, Rubinstein I: Inhibition of human premature labor by indomethacin. Obstet Gynecol 44:787, 1974

37

Postterm Pregnancy

The terms *postterm, prolonged, postdates,* and *postmature* are often loosely used interchangeably to signify pregnancies that have exceeded a duration considered to be the upper limit of normal. *Postmature* should be used to describe the infant with recognizable clinical features indicating a pathologically prolonged pregnancy. *Postdates* probably should be abandoned, because the real issue in many postterm pregnancies is "post-*what* dates?" Therefore, *postterm* or *prolonged pregnancy* is the preferred expression for an extended pregnancy, and "postmature" is reserved for a specific clinical fetal syndrome. Because few infants from prolonged pregnancies have stigmata of the postmaturity syndrome, use of this term can falsely imply a pathologically prolonged pregnancy.

The standard internationally recommended definition of prolonged pregnancy, endorsed by the American College of Obstetricians and Gynecologists (1997), is 42 completed weeks (294 days) or more from the first day of the last menstrual period. It is important to emphasize the phrase "42 completed weeks." Pregnancies between 41 weeks 1 day and 41 weeks 6 days, although in the 42nd week, do not complete 42 weeks until the seventh day has elapsed. Thus, technically speaking, prolonged pregnancy could begin either on day 294 or on day 295 following the onset of the last menses. Which is it? Day 294 or 295? We cannot resolve this question, and emphasize this dilemma only to ensure that litigators and others understand that some imprecision is inevitable when attempting to define prolonged pregnancy. Amersi and Grimes (1998) have cautioned against use of ordinal numbers such as "42nd week" because of their imprecision. For example, "42nd week" refers to 41 weeks and 1 through 6 days, whereas the cardinal number "42 weeks" refers to precisely 42 completed weeks.

ESTIMATED GESTATIONAL AGE USING MENSTRUAL DATES

The definition of postterm pregnancy as one that persists for 42 weeks or more from the onset of a menstrual period assumes that the last menses was followed by ovulation 2 weeks later. This said, some pregnancies may not actually be postterm, but rather are the result of an error in estimation of gestational age because of faulty recall of the dates of menstruation or delayed ovulation. Thus, there are two categories of pregnancies that reach 42 completed weeks:

1. Those truly 40 weeks past conception.
2. Those of less advanced gestation due to inaccurate estimate of gestational age.

Munster and associates (1992) described a high incidence of large variations in menstrual cycles in normal women. Boyce and associates (1976) studied 317 French women with conceptional basal body temperature profiles and found that 70 percent who completed 42 postmenstrual weeks had less

advanced gestations based on ovulation dates. Blondel and colleagues (2002) analyzed postterm pregnancy rates according to six algorithms for gestational age estimates based on either the last menstrual period, ultrasound at 16 to 18 weeks, or both. This Canadian study included 44,623 women giving birth between 1978 and 1996 at the Royal Victoria Hospital in Montreal. The proportion of births at 42 weeks or longer was 6.4 percent when based on the last menstrual period alone and 1.9 percent when based on ultrasound alone. This raises the possibility that the menstrual dates are frequently inaccurate in predicting postterm pregnancy. The recent study of Bennett and associates (2004) confirmed this. Because a few women ovulate earlier than expected, it is possible that 40 completed postconceptional weeks could be achieved after 41 weeks of amenorrhea.

Therefore, most pregnancies that are reliably 42 completed weeks beyond the last menses probably are not biologically prolonged. Conversely, a few that are not yet 42 weeks might be postterm. These variations in menstrual cycle likely explain, at least partially, why a relatively small proportion of fetuses delivered postterm have evidence of *postmaturity*. Because there is no method to identify pregnancies that are truly prolonged, all pregnancies judged to be 42 completed weeks should be managed as if abnormally prolonged.

INCIDENCE

As shown in Figure 37–1, approximately 7 percent of 4 million infants born in the United States during 2001 were estimated to have been delivered at 42 weeks or more. In comparison, 12 percent of live births were preterm, defined as 36 weeks or less.

Contradictory results have been found concerning the significance of a variety of maternal demographic factors, such as parity, prior postterm birth, socioeconomic class, and age. One interesting feature—the tendency for some mothers to

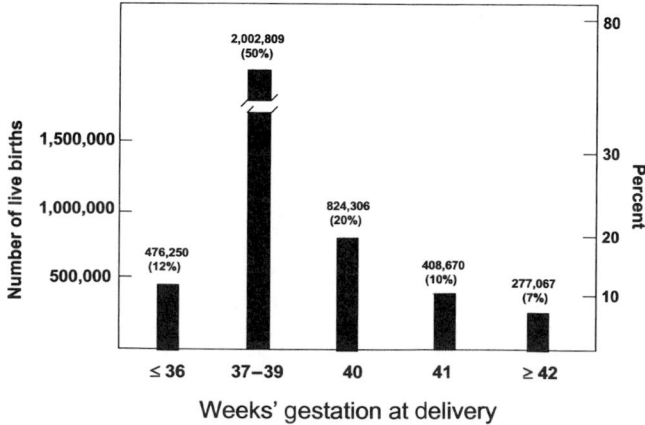

FIGURE 37–1. Gestational age at delivery of 4 million live births in the United States during 2001. (Adapted from Martin and colleagues, 2002.)

have repeated postterm births—suggests that some prolonged pregnancies are biologically determined. In an analysis of 27,677 births to Norwegian women, the incidence of a subsequent postterm birth increased from 10 to 27 percent if the first birth was postterm. This was increased to 39 percent if there had been two previous, successive postterm deliveries (Bakketeig and Bergsjø, 1991). Mogren and colleagues (1999) reported that prolonged pregnancy also recurred across generations in Swedish women. When mother and daughter had had a prolonged pregnancy, the risk for a daughter's subsequent postterm pregnancy was increased two- to threefold. In another Swedish study, Laursen and associates (2004) found that maternal, but not paternal, genes influenced prolonged pregnancy. Fetal–placental factors that have been reported as predisposing to postterm pregnancy include anencephaly, adrenal hypoplasia, and X-linked placental sulfatase deficiency (MacDonald and Siiteri, 1965; Naeye, 1978; Rabe and colleagues, 1983). These cause a lack of the usually high estrogen levels of normal pregnancy (see Chap. 3, p. 77). Finally, reduced cervical nitric oxide release may be a factor (Vaisanen-Tommiska and co-workers, 2004).

PERINATAL MORTALITY

The historical basis for the concept of an upper limit of human pregnancy duration was the observation that perinatal mortality increased after the expected due date was passed. This is best seen when perinatal mortality is analyzed from times before widespread use of interventions for pregnancies exceeding 42 weeks. In two large Swedish studies shown in Figure 37–2, after reaching a nadir at 39 to 40 weeks, perinatal mortality increased as pregnancy exceeded 41 weeks. Lucas and co-workers (1965) compared perinatal outcomes in 6624 postterm pregnancies with those of almost 60,000 singleton pregnancies delivered between 38 and 41 weeks. All components of perinatal mortality—antepartum, intrapartum, and

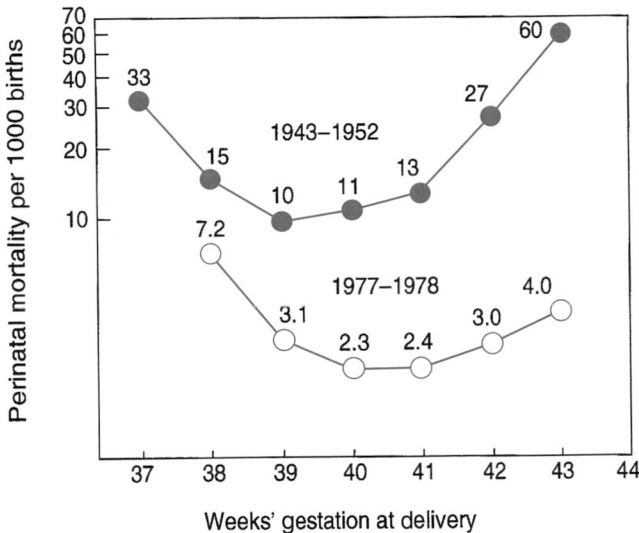

FIGURE 37–2. Perinatal mortality in late pregnancy according to gestational age in Sweden of all births during 1943–1952 compared with those during 1977–1978. The logarithmic scale is used for convenience in depiction. (Adapted from Bakketeig and Bergsjø, 1991, and Lindell, 1956.)

neonatal deaths—were increased at 42 weeks and beyond. The most significant increases occurred intrapartum. The major causes of death included pregnancy hypertension, prolonged labor with cephalopelvic disproportion, "unexplained anoxia," and malformations. Similar outcomes were reported by Olesen and colleagues (2003) in their analysis of 78,022 women with postterm pregnancies delivered before routine labor induction was adopted in Denmark.

Alexander and colleagues (2000a) reviewed 56,317 consecutive singleton pregnancies delivered at 40 or more weeks between 1988 and 1998 at Parkland Hospital. As shown in Table 37–1, labor was induced in 35 percent of pregnancies reaching 42 weeks. The rate of cesarean delivery for dystocia

TABLE 37–1 Pregnancy Outcomes in 56,317 Consecutive Singleton Pregnancies Delivered at or Beyond 40 Weeks from 1988 through 1998 at Parkland Hospital

	Weeks' Gestation			
Outcome	40 (n = 29,136)	41 (n = 16,386)	42 (n = 10,795)	P Value
Maternal outcomes (percent)				
Labor induction	2	7	35	< .001
Cesarean delivery				
Dystocia	7	6	9	< .001
Fetal distress	2	3	4	< .001
Perinatal outcomes (per 1000)				
Neonatal intensive care	4	5	6	< .001
Neonatal seizures	1	1	2	.12
Stillbirth	2	1	2	.84
Neonatal death	0.2	0.2	0.6	.17

Adapted from Alexander and colleagues (2000a).

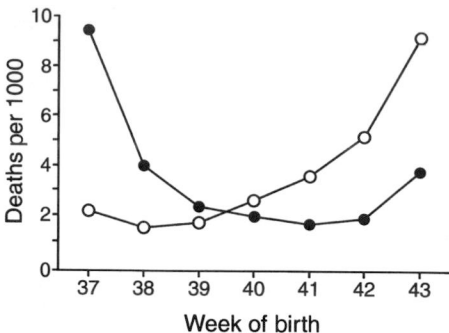

FIGURE 37–3. Perinatal risk index (○) and perinatal mortality rate (●) related to births between 37 and 43 weeks of gestation in Scotland, 1985 through 1996, expressed as deaths per 1000 births. The perinatal risk index is the cumulative probability of perinatal death multiplied by 1000. The perinatal mortality rate is the number of perinatal deaths with delivery in a given gestational week divided by the total number of births in that week multiplied by 1000. (Modified from Smith, 2001, with permission.)

and fetal distress was significantly increased at 42 weeks compared with that of earlier deliveries. More infants were admitted to intensive care in postterm pregnancies. The incidence of neonatal seizures and deaths doubled at 42 weeks. Caughey and Musci (2004) reported similar outcomes in 45,673 pregnancies.

Smith (2001) has challenged analyses such as these because the population at risk for perinatal mortality in a given week consists of all ongoing pregnancies rather than just the births in a given week. Figure 37–3 shows perinatal mortality rates calculated using only births in a given week of gestation from 37 to 43 completed weeks compared with the cumulative probability (perinatal index) of death when all ongoing pregnancies are included in the denominator. Smith found that delivery at 38 weeks was associated with the lowest risk of perinatal death.

PATHOPHYSIOLOGY

Clifford (1954) described a recognizable clinical syndrome that did much to dispel the prevailing obstetrical opinion that prolonged human pregnancy did not exist (Calkins, 1948). Infants, either live or stillborn, demonstrating these clinical characteristics, are now diagnosed to be pathologically *postmature*. Many of the postmature infants described by Clifford died, and many were seriously ill due to birth asphyxia and meconium aspiration. Several survivors were brain damaged. Interestingly, Ballantyne (1902) reported this same postmature infant more than 50 years before Clifford did.

POSTMATURITY SYNDROME. The postmature infant presents a unique and characteristic appearance (Fig. 37–4). Features include wrinkled, patchy, peeling skin; a long, thin body suggesting wasting; and advanced maturity because the infant is open-eyed, unusually alert, and appears old and

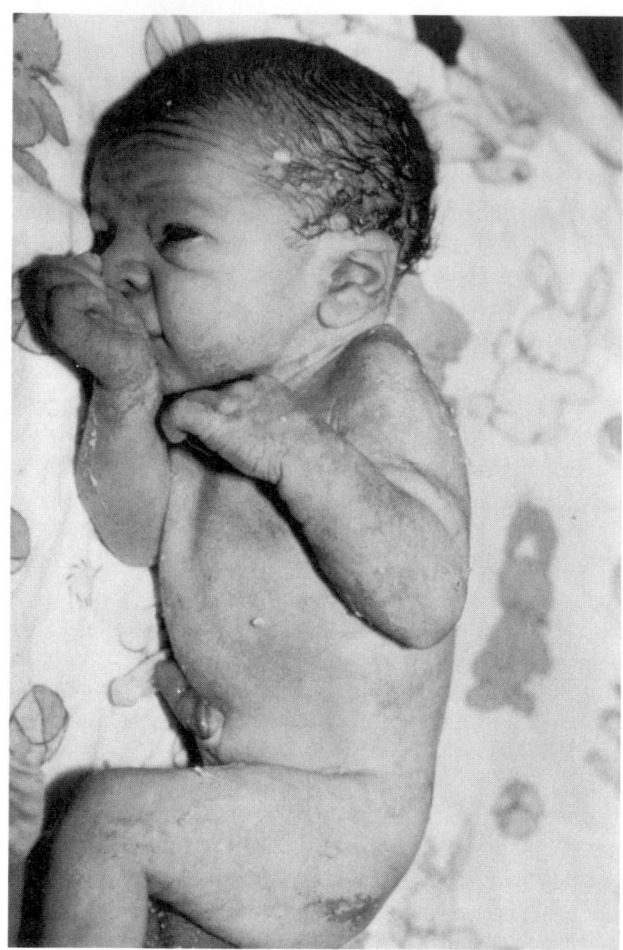

FIGURE 37–4. Postmature infant delivered at 43 weeks of gestation. Thick, viscous meconium coated the desquamating skin. Note the long, thin appearance and wrinkling of the palms of the hands.

worried-looking. Skin wrinkling can be particularly prominent on the palms and soles. The nails are typically quite long. Most such postmature infants are not growth restricted because their birthweight seldom falls below the 10th percentile for gestational age. Severe growth restriction, however, which logically must have preceded completion of 42 weeks, may occur.

The incidence of postmaturity syndrome in infants at 41, 42, or 43 weeks, respectively, has not been conclusively determined. In one of the rare contemporary reports that chronicle postmaturity, Shime and colleagues (1984) found this syndrome in about 10 percent of pregnancies between 41 and 43 weeks. The incidence increased to 33 percent at 44 weeks. Associated oligohydramnios substantially increases the likelihood of postmaturity. Trimmer and colleagues (1990) diagnosed oligohydramnios when the ultrasonic maximum vertical amnionic fluid pocket measured 1 cm or less at 42 weeks and 88 percent of the infants were postmature.

PLACENTAL DYSFUNCTION. Clifford (1954) proposed that the skin changes of postmaturity were due to loss of the protective effects of vernix caseosa. He also attributed

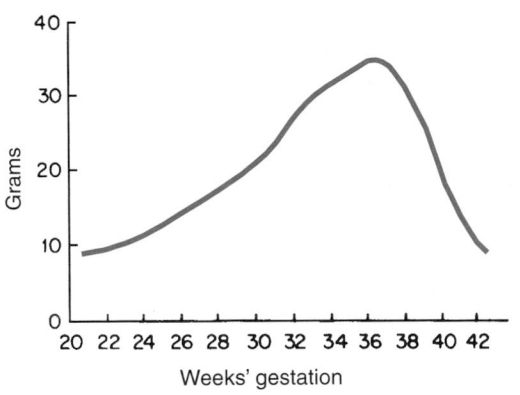

FIGURE 37–5. Mean daily fetal growth during previous week of gestation. (From Jazayeri and co-workers, 1998, with permission.)

the postmaturity syndrome to placental senescence, although he did not find placental degeneration histologically. Still, the concept that postmaturity is due to placental insufficiency has persisted despite an absence of morphological or significant quantitative findings (Larsen and co-workers, 1995; Rushton, 1991). Of interest, Smith and Baker (1999) reported that placental apoptosis—programmed cell death—was significantly increased at 41 to 42 completed weeks compared with that at 36 to 39 weeks. The clinical significance of such apoptosis is unclear at this time.

Jazayeri and co-workers (1998) investigated cord erythropoietin levels in 124 appropriately grown newborns delivered from 37 to 43 weeks. They sought to assess whether fetal oxygenation was compromised due to placental aging in postterm pregnancies. Decreased partial oxygen pressure

is the only known stimulator of erythropoietin. Each woman studied had an uncomplicated labor and delivery. Cord erythropoietin levels were significantly increased in pregnancies reaching 41 weeks or more. Although Apgar scores and umbilical cord blood gases were normal in these infants, the investigators concluded that there was decreased fetal oxygenation in some postterm gestations.

The postterm fetus may continue to gain weight and thus be an unusually large infant at birth. This at least suggests that placental function is not compromised. Indeed, continued fetal growth, although at a slower rate, is characteristic between 38 and 42 weeks (Fig. 37–5). Nahum and colleagues (1995) confirmed that fetal growth continues until at least 42 weeks.

FETAL DISTRESS AND OLIGOHYDRAMNIOS. The principal reasons for increased risks to postterm fetuses were described by Leveno and associates (1984). They reported that both antepartum fetal jeopardy and intrapartum fetal distress were the consequence of cord compression associated with oligohydramnios. In their analysis of 727 postterm pregnancies, intrapartum fetal distress detected with electronic monitoring was not associated with late decelerations characteristic of uteroplacental insufficiency. Instead, one or more prolonged decelerations such as shown in Figure 37–6 preceded three fourths of emergency cesarean deliveries for fetal jeopardy. In all but two cases, there were also variable decelerations (Fig. 37–7). Another common fetal heart rate pattern, although not ominous by itself, was the saltatory baseline shown in Figure 37–8. These findings are consistent with cord occlusion as the proximate cause of fetal distress.

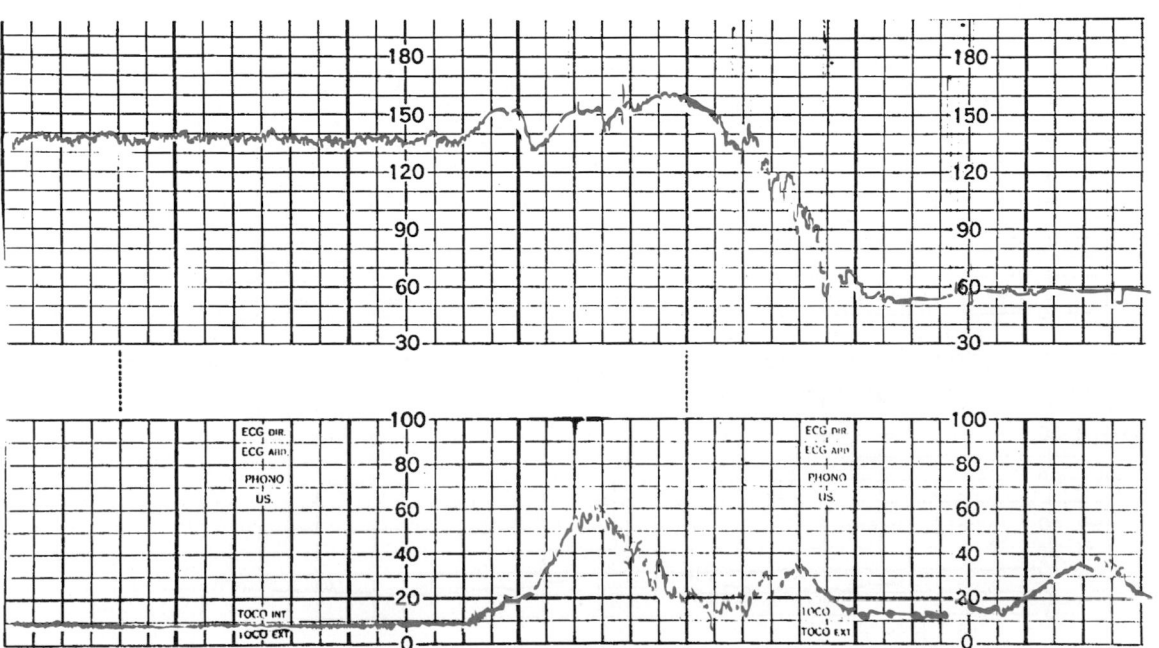

FIGURE 37–6. Prolonged fetal heart rate deceleration prior to emergency cesarean delivery in a postterm pregnancy with oligohydramnios. (From Leveno and co-workers, 1984.)

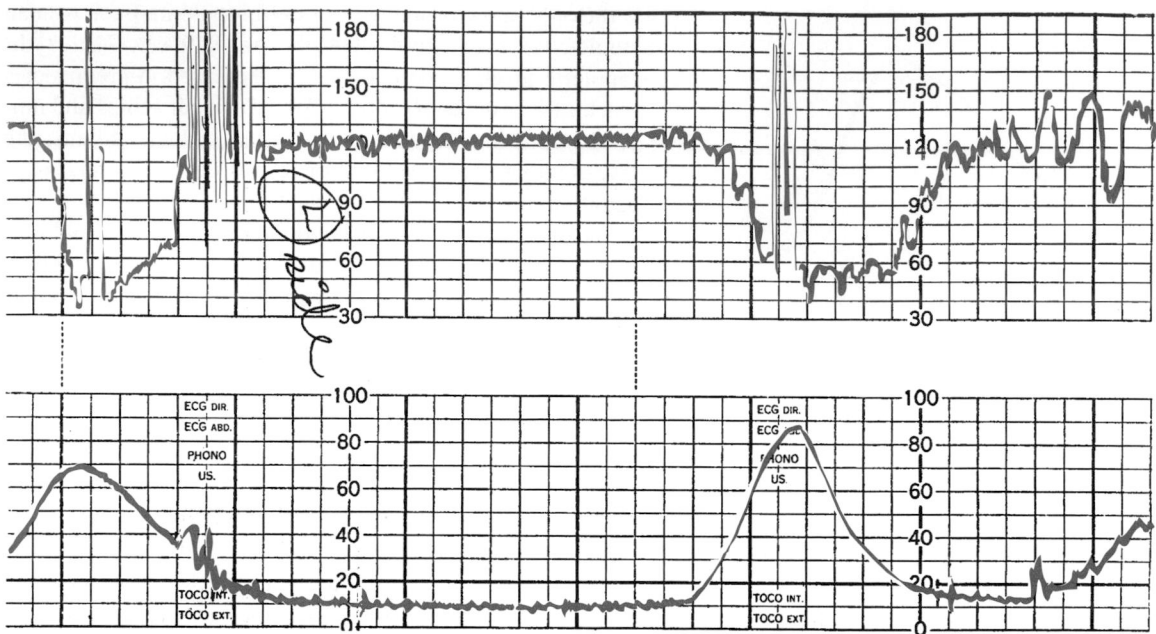

FIGURE 37–7. Severe—less than 70 bpm for 60 seconds or longer—variable decelerations in a postterm pregnancy with oligohydramnios and cesarean delivery for fetal jeopardy. (From Leveno and co-workers, 1984.)

Other correlates found were oligohydramnios and viscous meconium.

Decreased amnionic fluid volume commonly develops as pregnancy advances beyond 42 weeks (Fig. 37–9). It is also likely that meconium release into an already reduced amnionic fluid volume causes thick, viscous meconium

implicated in meconium aspiration syndrome (see Chap. 29, p. 675).

Trimmer and co-workers (1990) measured hourly fetal urine production using sequential ultrasonic bladder volume measurements in 38 pregnancies of 42 weeks or more. Diminished urine production was found to be associated with

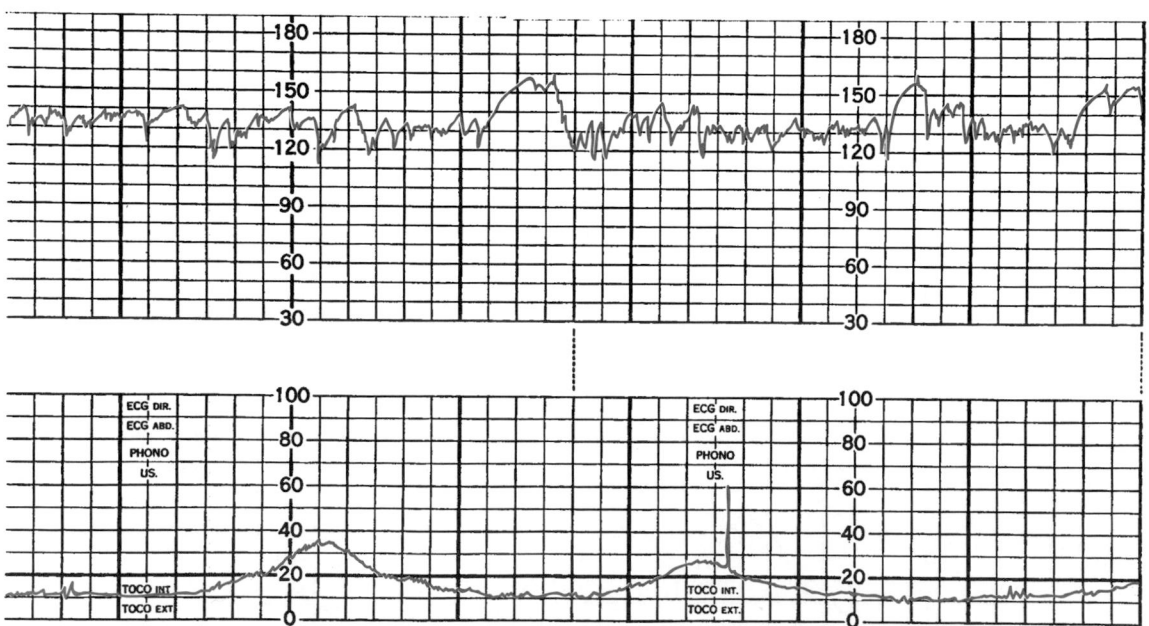

FIGURE 37–8. Saltatory baseline fetal heart rate showing oscillations exceeding 20 bpm and associated with oligohydramnios in a postterm pregnancy. (From Leveno and co-workers, 1984.)

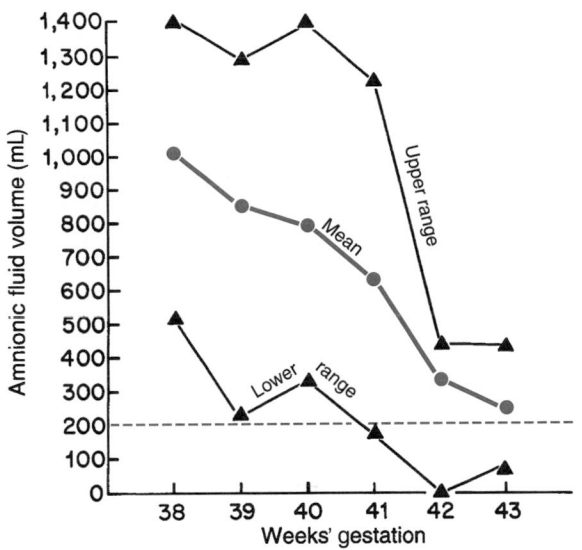

FIGURE 37–9. Volume of amnionic fluid during the last weeks of pregnancy. (Adapted from Elliott and Inman, 1961.)

oligohydramnios. They hypothesized, however, that decreased fetal urine flow was likely the result of preexisting oligohydramnios that limited fetal swallowing. Oz and co-workers (2002), using Doppler waveforms, reported that fetal renal blood flow is reduced in postterm pregnancies with oligohydramnios.

FETAL GROWTH RESTRICTION. Until recently, the clinical significance of fetal growth restriction in the otherwise uncomplicated pregnancy has received little attention. Divon and co-authors (1998) and Clausson and co-workers (1999) analyzed births of almost 700,000 women between 1991 and 1995 using the National Swedish Medical Birth registry. As shown in Table 37–2, stillbirths were more common among growth-restricted infants who were delivered at 42 weeks or beyond. Indeed, one third of the postterm stillbirths were growth restricted. During the years of these births

TABLE 37–2 Effects of Fetal Growth Restriction on Stillbirth Rates in Pregnancies Reaching 42 Weeks or More Compared with Those at 37 to 41 Weeks in Sweden (1991–1995)

Outcome	Pregnancy Duration	
	37–41 Weeks	*≥ 42 Weeks*
Births	469,056	40,973
Fetal growth restriction[a] (%)	10,312 (2)	1558 (4)
Stillbirths (per 1000)		
Appropriate growth	650 (1.4)	69 (1.8)
Fetal growth restriction	116 (11)	23 (15)

[a]Defined as birthweight below two standard deviations from the mean birthweight for fetal gender and gestational age.
From Clausson and colleagues (1999), with permission.

in Sweden, labor induction and antenatal fetal testing usually commenced at 42 weeks. Alexander and colleagues (2000d) studied infant outcomes for 355 postterm infants 42 weeks or greater whose birthweights were at or below the third percentile. They compared their outcomes with those of 14,520 infants above the third percentile delivered at Parkland Hospital and found that morbidity and mortality were significantly increased in the growth-restricted infants. Notably, one fourth of all stillbirths associated with prolonged pregnancy were in this comparatively small number of growth-restricted infants.

MANAGEMENT

It is generally accepted that antepartum interventions are indicated in management of prolonged pregnancies. The type(s) of interventions and when to use them are somewhat controversial. One major issue is whether to intervene at 41 or 42 weeks. Another is whether labor induction is warranted compared with expectant management using antepartum fetal testing. Roussis and colleagues (1993) surveyed members of the Society for Maternal–Fetal Medicine in 1990 and found that about two thirds of respondents induced labor at 41 weeks if the cervix was favorable. Antepartum fetal testing was advocated beginning at 41 weeks when the cervix was unfavorable. At 42 weeks, virtually all respondents induced labor when the cervix was favorable, and 58 percent did so even when the cervix was unfavorable. Others (42 percent) recommended antepartum testing when the cervix was unfavorable at 42 weeks. Clearly, cervical favorability has considerable impact on management (see Chap. 22, p. 537).

UNFAVORABLE CERVIX. It is difficult to precisely define an "unfavorable cervix" in prolonged pregnancies, because investigators have used different criteria. For example, Harris and colleagues (1983) reported that 92 percent of women at 42 weeks had an unfavorable cervix defined by a Bishop score of less than 7. Hannah and colleagues (1992) found that only 40 percent of 3407 women with 41-week pregnancies had an undilated cervix. Alexander and associates (2000b) evaluated 800 women induced for postterm pregnancy at Parkland Hospital. They reported that women in whom there was no cervical dilatation had a twofold increased cesarean delivery rate for "dystocia." Yang and co-workers (2004) presented preliminary findings that cervical length of 3 cm or less determined by transvaginal ultrasonography was predictive of successful induction.

A number of investigators have evaluated prostaglandin E_2 for cervical ripening in women with prolonged pregnancies and an unfavorable cervix. National Institute of Child Health and Development Network of Maternal–Fetal Medicine Units (1994) evaluated prostaglandin E_2 gel and found that it was not more effective than placebo. Alexander and associates (2000c) studied 393 women with postterm pregnancy who were given prostaglandin E_2 for cervical ripening. These women were treated even if the cervix was "favorable." The investigators reported that almost half of the 84 women with cervical dilatation of 2 to 4 cm entered labor with prostaglandin E_2 use alone. The American College of Obstetricians and Gynecologists (1997) has concluded that prostaglandin gel can be used safely in postterm pregnancies. Use of prostaglandins for cervical ripening is discussed in Chapter 22 (see p. 537).

Sweeping or stripping of the membranes, to induce labor and prevent postterm pregnancy has been studied in 15 randomized trials during the 1990s. Boulvain and co-authors (1999) performed a meta-analysis of these and found that membrane stripping at 38 to 40 weeks decreased the frequency of postterm pregnancy. Such stripping, however, did not modify the risk for cesarean delivery, and maternal and neonatal infections were not increased. The authors emphasized that membrane stripping could be painful and might provoke vaginal bleeding and irregular contractions. Wong and colleagues (2002), in a randomized trial evaluating 120 women, found that sweeping the membranes did not reduce the need to induce labor (see Chap. 22, p. 539).

Station of the vertex is likewise important in predicting successful postterm induction. Shin and colleagues (2004) studied 484 nulliparas who underwent induction after 41 weeks. The cesarean delivery rate was directly related to station. It was 6 percent if the vertex was –1, 20 percent at –2, 43 percent at –3, and 77 percent at –4.

INDUCTION VERSUS FETAL TESTING. A logical plan for reducing perinatal mortality and morbidity associated with prolonged pregnancy is to terminate pregnancy before such events occur. There have been doubts about the value of labor induction, mainly because it was feared that induction would result in more operative intervention without preventing perinatal death. As a result, many clinicians prefer to use fetal testing to avoid inductions. Major studies designed to resolve these questions have been done in both Canada and the United States.

Hannah and colleagues (1992) randomized 3407 Canadian women with pregnancies at 41 or more weeks to labor induction or fetal testing. Women assigned to fetal testing were asked to count the number of times they felt the fetus move over a 2-hour period each day, and they also underwent nonstress testing three times weekly. Amnionic fluid volume was assessed two to three times each week, and pockets less than 3 cm were considered abnormal. Labor induction resulted in a significantly lower cesarean rate (21 percent) compared with pregnancies managed with antepartum testing (24 percent). There were two stillbirths in the fetal testing group and none in the induction group. The lower cesarean rate in the induction group was due to fewer procedures for fetal distress. A cost-effectiveness analysis of the Canadian data was later reported by Goeree and colleagues (1995). The mean cost was $3132 per patient managed with fetal testing compared with $2939 for those who underwent labor induction. Thus, labor induction for postterm pregnancy resulted in more favorable outcomes than fetal testing and at a lower cost.

Menticoglou and Hall (2002) from Winnipeg have subsequently lamented that induction of labor at 41 weeks has become the standard of care in Canada. They concluded that "ritual induction at 41 weeks" had become the current practice. They opined that this practice was based on evidence that was seriously flawed, and that it constituted "an abuse of biological norms." They recommended that this *nonsensus consensus* be discontinued because it caused interference that had the potential to do more harm than good and have staggering resource implications.

The Maternal–Fetal Medicine Network trial of induction versus fetal testing was reported by Gardner and associates (1996). Nonstress tests and ultrasonic estimations of amnionic fluid volume were performed twice weekly in 175 women whose pregnancies had reached 41 weeks or more. Perinatal outcomes in these women were compared with those of 265 women randomized to induction with or without cervical ripening. There were no perinatal deaths in any study subgroup, and the rate of cesarean delivery was not different between management groups. Thus, this study supported the validity of either management scheme.

Crowley (1997) used the Oxford Database of Perinatal Trials to perform a meta-analysis of 18 studies in which management of postterm pregnancy was assessed. Routine induction after 41 weeks resulted in reduced perinatal mortality without increased risk of cesarean or instrumental delivery. Similar results were reported by Sanchez-Ramos and colleagues (2003) in their meta-analysis of 16 trials. In a study of 540,116 births, Roberts and colleagues (1999) concluded that Crowley's meta-analysis prompted routine induction after 41 weeks to be widely adopted in New South Wales, Australia. Specifically, from 1990 to 1996, there was a significant decrease in births at 42 completed weeks or more—4.6 compared with 2.8 percent, respectively. Correspondingly, there was an increased induction rate at 41 weeks, and the cesarean delivery rate also increased. Because infant outcomes were not described in this report, any beneficial neonatal effects are undetermined.

Alexander and colleagues (2001) examined the effect of labor induction at 42 weeks on rates of cesarean delivery at Parkland Hospital. Pregnancy outcomes in 638 women in whom labor was induced were compared with those of 687 women with spontaneous labor at 42 weeks. Rates of cesarean delivery were significantly increased in the induced group because of failure to progress (19 versus 14 percent). When corrected for risk factors using logistic regression, however, the researchers concluded that factors intrinsic to the patient, rather than labor induction itself, led to the increased cesarean deliveries. These factors included nulliparity, an unfavorable cervix, and epidural analgesia.

Evidence to substantiate intervention—whether induction or fetal testing—commencing at 41 versus 42 weeks is limited. Most evidence used to justify intervention at 41 weeks is from the randomized Canadian and American investigations cited earlier. No randomized studies have specifically assessed intervention at 41 weeks versus an identical intervention used at 42 weeks. Importantly, a national policy of intervention for prolonged pregnancy at 41 versus 42 weeks would mean that approximately 500,000 additional women would be subjected to interventions that have not been conclusively proved necessary or harmless.

Usher and colleagues (1988) analyzed several outcomes in 7663 pregnancies with gestational ages determined to be 40, 41, or 42 weeks confirmed by early ultrasound examinations. Perinatal death rates, corrected for malformations, were 1.5, 0.7, and 3.0 per 1000 for 40, 41, and 42 weeks, respectively. These results could be used to challenge the concept of routine intervention at 41 instead of 42 weeks. Interestingly, Divon and colleagues (1996) found that, although adverse fetal outcomes increased at 41 compared with those at 40 weeks, these were associated with growth restriction. They suggested that management strategies should be focused on fetal growth rather than simply gestational age in pregnancies reaching 41 weeks.

Based on results summarized in Table 37–1, 41-week pregnancies without other complications such as hypertension are considered normal pregnancies at Parkland Hospital. No interventions are practiced solely on the basis of fetal age until 42 completed weeks. It is our view that large, randomized studies should be performed before 41-week gestations are routinely considered pathologically prolonged.

OLIGOHYDRAMNIOS. It has been suggested that the identification of diminished amnionic fluid determined by various ultrasonic methods may help identify a postterm fetus in jeopardy. There is no doubt that when amnionic fluid is decreased in a postterm pregnancy—or for that matter in any pregnancy—the fetus is at increased risk. Many different criteria for ultrasonic diagnosis of oligohydramnios have been proposed. Fischer and colleagues (1993) attempted to determine which criteria were most predictive of normal versus abnormal outcomes in postterm pregnancies. As shown in Figure 37–10, the smaller the amnionic fluid pocket, the greater the likelihood that there was clinically significant oligohydramnios. Normal amnionic fluid volume, however, did not preclude abnormal outcomes. Alfirevic and co-authors (1997) randomized 500 women with postterm pregnancies—defined as 290 days or longer gestation—to assessment of amnionic fluid volume using either the amnionic fluid index (AFI) or the deepest vertical pocket. They concluded that the AFI overestimated the number of abnormal outcomes in postterm pregnancies.

Regardless of the criteria used to diagnose oligohydramnios in postterm pregnancies, most investigators have found an increased incidence of "fetal distress" during labor. Thus, oligohydramnios by most definitions is a clinically meaningful finding. Conversely, reassurance of continued fetal well-being in the presence of "normal" amnionic fluid volume

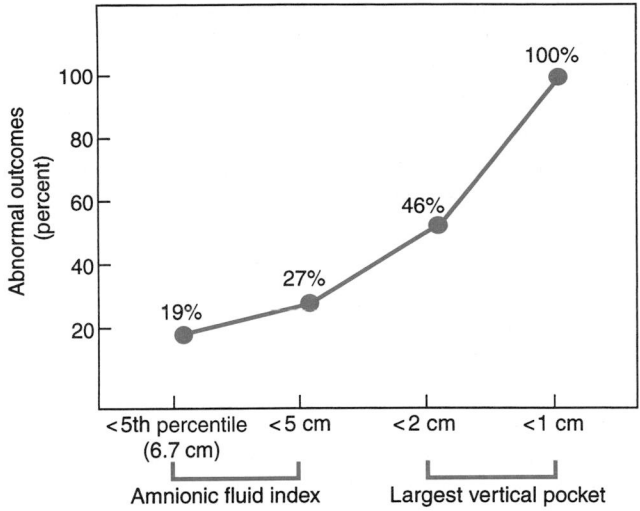

FIGURE 37–10. Comparison of the diagnostic value of various ultrasonic estimates of amnionic fluid volume in prolonged pregnancies. Abnormal outcomes include cesarean or operative vaginal delivery for fetal jeopardy, 5-minute Apgar score of 6 or less, umbilical arterial blood pH less than 7.1, or admission to the neonatal intensive care unit. (Adapted from Fischer and associates, 1993.)

is tenuous because it is unknown how quickly pathological oligohydramnios develops. Clement and co-workers (1987) reported six postterm pregnancies in which amnionic fluid volume diminished abruptly over 24 hours and one fetus died.

MACROSOMIA. The incidence of macrosomia (defined as birthweight greater than 4500 g) increases from 1.4 percent at 37 to 41 weeks to 2.2 percent at 42 weeks or more (Martin and colleagues, 2002). This raises the possibility that both the maternal and fetal morbidity associated with macrosomia might be avoidable with timely labor induction to preempt further growth. The American College of Obstetricians and Gynecologists (2000) has reviewed such interventions. It concluded that current evidence does not support a policy of early labor induction in women at term who have suspected fetal macrosomia. Moreover, in the absence of maternal diabetes, vaginal delivery is not contraindicated for women with estimated fetal weights up to 5000 g. Cesarean delivery was recommended for estimated fetal weights greater than 4500 g in the presence of a prolonged second-stage labor or a second-stage arrest of descent.

RECOMMENDATIONS OF THE AMERICAN COLLEGE OF OBSTETRICIANS AND GYNECOLOGISTS. These recommendations are summarized in Table 37–3. Although providing flexibility in the evaluation and management of pregnancies completing 42 weeks, the recommendations are that either antenatal testing or labor induction should be commenced at 42 weeks. There was insufficient evidence to recommend a management strategy between 40 and 42 completed weeks.

TABLE 37–3 Evaluation and Management of Postterm Pregnancy

1. Postterm pregnancy is defined as a pregnancy that has extended to or beyond 42 completed weeks.
2. Women with a postterm gestation who have an unfavorable cervix can either undergo labor induction or be managed expectantly.
3. Prostaglandin can be used for cervical ripening and labor induction.
4. Delivery should be effected if there is evidence of fetal compromise or oligohydramnios.
5. It is reasonable to initiate antenatal surveillance between 41 and 42 weeks despite lack of evidence that monitoring improves outcomes.
6. A nonstress test and amnionic fluid volume assessment should be adequate, although no single method has been shown to be superior.
7. Many recommend prompt delivery in a woman with a postterm pregnancy, a favorable cervix, and no other complications.

From the American College of Obstetricians and Gynecologists (2004).

Postterm pregnancy has been identified by the American College of Obstetricians and Gynecologists (1999) as a high-risk condition in which twice-weekly antepartum fetal testing may be indicated. Doppler velocimetry was not recommended. Oligohydramnios detected using ultrasound, defined as no vertical pocket of amnionic fluid greater than 2 cm or an AFI of 5 cm or less, is considered an indication for either delivery or close fetal surveillance.

MANAGEMENT AT PARKLAND HOSPITAL. In women with a *certain* gestational age, labor is induced at the completion of 42 weeks. Almost 90 percent of such women are induced successfully or enter labor within 2 days of induction. For those who do not deliver with the first induction, a second induction is performed within 3 days. Almost all women are delivered using this plan of management, but in the unusual few who are not delivered, management decisions involve a third (or more) induction versus cesarean delivery.

Women classified as having *uncertain* postterm pregnancies are followed on a weekly basis and without intervention unless fetal jeopardy is suspected. The latter is based on clinical or sonographic perception of decreased amnionic fluid volume. Equally worrisome is diminished fetal movement reported by the mother. If fetal jeopardy is suspected by either method, labor induction is carried out as described previously for the woman with a certain postterm gestation.

MEDICAL OR OBSTETRICAL COMPLICATIONS. In the event of a medical or other obstetrical complication, it is generally unwise to allow a pregnancy to continue past 42 weeks. Indeed, in many such instances *early* delivery is indicated. Timing of delivery depends on the individual complication. Common examples include hypertensive disorders due to pregnancy, prior cesarean delivery, and diabetes.

INTRAPARTUM MANAGEMENT. Labor is a particularly dangerous time for the postterm fetus. Therefore, it is important that women whose pregnancies are known or suspected to be postterm come to the hospital as soon as they suspect they are in labor. On arrival, while being observed for possible labor, we recommend that fetal heart rate and uterine contractions be monitored electronically for variations consistent with fetal distress (American College of Obstetricians and Gynecologists, 1995).

When to perform amniotomy is problematic. Further reduction in fluid volume following amniotomy can certainly enhance the possibility of cord compression. Conversely, amniotomy aids diagnosis of thick meconium, which may be dangerous to the fetus if aspirated. Moreover, once the membranes are ruptured, a scalp electrode and intrauterine pressure catheter can be placed, which usually provide more precise data concerning fetal heart rate and uterine contractions.

Identification of *thick meconium* in the amnionic fluid is particularly worrisome. The viscosity probably signifies the lack of liquid and thus oligohydramnios. Aspiration of thick meconium may cause severe pulmonary dysfunction and neonatal death (see Chap. 29, p. 675). Wenstrom and Parsons (1989) proposed *amnioinfusion* during labor as a way of diluting meconium to decrease the incidence of meconium aspiration syndrome. As discussed in Chapter 18 (see p. 462), the benefits of amnioinfusion remain controversial. In a recent randomized trial by Rathore and colleagues (2002), amnioinfusion was associated with fewer cesarean deliveries for fetal distress and fewer neonatal intensive care unit admissions for neonates with moderate to thick meconium-stained amnionic fluid. In contrast, Yoder and colleagues (2002) found that increased use of amnioinfusion—0 to 36 percent of women with moderate to thick amnionic fluid meconium—had no impact on the incidence of meconium aspiration syndrome.

The likelihood of a successful vaginal delivery is reduced appreciably for the nulliparous woman who is in early labor with thick, meconium-stained amnionic fluid. Therefore, when the woman is remote from delivery, strong consideration should be given to prompt cesarean delivery, especially when cephalopelvic disproportion is suspected or either hypotonic or hypertonic dysfunctional labor is evident. Some practitioners choose to avoid oxytocin use in these cases.

Aspiration of meconium may be minimized but not eliminated by effective suctioning of the pharynx as soon as the head is delivered but before the thorax is delivered. If meconium is identified, the trachea should be aspirated as soon as possible after delivery. Immediately thereafter, the infant should be ventilated as needed.

REFERENCES

Alexander JM, McIntire DD, Leveno KJ: Forty weeks and beyond: Pregnancy outcomes by week of gestation. Obstet Gynecol 96:291, 2000a

Alexander JM, McIntire DD, Leveno KJ: Postterm pregnancy: Does induction increase cesarean rates? J Soc Gynecol Invest 7:79A, 2000b

Alexander JM, McIntire DD, Leveno KJ: Postterm pregnancy: Is cervical "ripening" being used in the right patients? J Soc Gynecol Invest 7:247A, 2000c

Alexander JM, McIntire DD, Leveno KJ: Prolonged pregnancy: Induction of labor and cesarean births. Obstet Gynecol 97:911, 2001

Alexander JM, McIntire DD, Leveno KJ: The effect of fetal growth restriction on neonatal outcome in postterm pregnancy. Abstract No. 463. Am J Obstet Gynecol 182:S148, 2000d

Alfirevic Z, Luckas M, Walkinshaw SA, et al: A randomized comparison between amniotic fluid index and maximum pool depth in the monitoring of postterm pregnancy. Br J Obstet Gynaecol 104:207, 1997

American College of Obstetricians and Gynecologists: Management of postterm pregnancy. Practice Bulletin No. 55, September 2004

American College of Obstetricians and Gynecologists: Fetal macrosomia. Practice Bulletin No. 22, November 2000

American College of Obstetricians and Gynecologists: Antepartum fetal surveillance. Technical Bulletin No. 9, October 1999

American College of Obstetrics and Gynecologists: Fetal heart rate patterns: Monitoring, interpretation, and management. Technical Bulletin No. 207, July 1995

Amersi S, Grimes DA: The case against using ordinal numbers for gestational age. Obstet Gynecol 91:623, 1998

Bakketeig LS, Bergsjø P: Post-term pregnancy: Magnitude of the problem. In Chalmers I, Enkin M, Keirse M (eds): Effective Care in Pregnancy and Childbirth. Oxford, Oxford University Press, 1991, p 765

Ballantyne JW: The problem of the postmature infant. J Obstet Gynaecol Br Emp 2:522, 1902

Bennett KA, Crane JM, O'Shea P, et al: First trimester ultrasound screening is effective in reducing postterm labor induction rates: A randomized controlled trial. Am J Obstet Gynecol 190:1077, 2004

Blondel B, Morin I, Platt RW, et al: Algorithms for combining menstrual and ultrasound estimates of gestational age: Consequences for rates of preterm and postterm birth. Br J Obstet Gynaecol 109:718, 2002

Boulvain M, Irion O, Marcoux S, et al: Sweeping of the membranes to prevent post-term pregnancy and to induce labour: A systematic review. Br J Obstet Gynaecol 106:481, 1999

Boyce A, Magaux MJ, Schwartz D: Classical and "true" gestational post maturity. Am J Obstet Gynecol 125:911, 1976

Calkins LA: Postmaturity. Am J Obstet Gynecol 56:167, 1948

Caughey AB, Musci TJ: Complications of term pregnancies beyond 37 weeks of gestation. Obstet Gynecol 103:57, 2004

Clausson B, Cnattingus S, Axelsson O: Outcomes of postterm births: The role of fetal growth restriction and malformations. Obstet Gynecol 94:758, 1999

Clement D, Schifrin BS, Kates RB: Acute oligohydramnios in postdate pregnancy. Am J Obstet Gynecol 157:884, 1987. The Cochrane Library. The Cochrane Collaboration; Issue 4, Oxford: Update Software, 1997

Clifford SH: Postmaturity with placental dysfunction. Clinical syndromes and pathologic findings. J Pediatr 44:1, 1954

Crowley P: Interventions to prevent or improve outcome for deliveries at or beyond term. In Neilson JP, Crowther CA, Hodnett ED, Hofmeyr GJ (eds): Pregnancy and Childbirth Module of the Cochrane Database of Systematic Reviews [updated September 1997]. The Cochrane Library. The Cochrane Collaboration; Issue 4, Oxford, Update Software, 1997

Crowley P: Post-term pregnancy: Induction or surveillance? In Chalmers I, Enkin M, Keirse M (eds): Effective Care in Pregnancy and Childbirth. Oxford, Oxford University Press, 1991, p 776

Divon MY, Haglund B, Nisell H, et al: Fetal and neonatal mortality in the postterm pregnancy: The impact of gestational age and fetal growth restriction. Am J Obstet Gynecol 178:726, 1998

Divon MY, Haglund B, Nisell H, et al: Perinatal outcome in a large cohort of postdate pregnancies. Am J Obstet Gynecol 174:351, 1996

Elliott PM, Inman WH: Volume of liquor amnii in normal and abnormal pregnancy. Lancet 2:835, 1961

Fischer RL, McDonnell M, Bianculli KW, et al: Amniotic fluid volume estimation in the postdate pregnancy: A comparison of techniques. Obstet Gynecol 81:698, 1993

Gardner M, Rouse D, Goldenberg R, et al: Cost comparison of induction of labor at 41 weeks versus expectant management in the postterm pregnancy. Am J Obstet Gynecol 174:351, 1996

Goeree R, Hannah M, Hewson S: Cost-effectiveness of induction of labour versus serial antenatal monitoring in the Canadian Multicentre Postterm Pregnancy Trial. Can Med Assoc J 152:1445, 1995

Hannah ME, Hannah WJ, Hellman J, et al: Induction of labor as compared with serial antenatal monitoring in post-term pregnancy. N Engl J Med 326:1587, 1992

Harris BA Jr, Huddleston JF, Sutliff G, et al: The unfavorable cervix in prolonged pregnancy. Obstet Gynecol 62:171, 1983

Jazayeri A, Tsibris JC, Spellacy WN: Elevated umbilical cord plasma erythropoietin levels in prolonged pregnancies. Obstet Gynecol 92:61, 1998

Larsen LG, Clausen HV, Andersen B, et al: A stereologic study of postmature placentas fixed by dual perfusion. Am J Obstet Gynecol 172:500, 1995

Laursen M, Bille C, Olesen AW, et al: Genetic influence on prolonged gestation: A population-based Danish twin study. Am J Obstet Gynecol 190:489, 2004

Leveno KJ, Quirk JG, Cunningham FG, et al: Prolonged pregnancy, I. Observations concerning the causes of fetal distress. Am J Obstet Gynecol 150:465, 1984

Lindell A: Prolonged pregnancy. Acta Obstet Gynecol Scand 35:136, 1956

Lucas WE, Anefil AO, Callagan DA: The problem of postterm pregnancy. Am J Obstet Gynecol 91:241, 1965

MacDonald PC, Siiteri PK: Origin of estrogen in women pregnant with an anencephalic fetus. J Clin Invest 44:465, 1965

Martin JA, Hamilton BE, Ventura SJ, et al: Births: Final data for 2001. National Vital Statistics Reports, Vol 51, No. 2. Hyattsville, Md: National Center for Health Statistics, 2002

Menticoglou SM, Hall PF: Routine induction of labour at 41 weeks' gestation: Nonsensus consensus. Br J Obstet Gynaecol 109:485, 2002

Mogren I, Stenlund H, Högberg U: Recurrence of prolonged pregnancy. Int J Epidemiol 28:253, 1999

Munster K, Schmidt L, Helm P: Length and variation in the menstrual cycle—a cross-sectional study from a Danish county. Br J Obstet Gynaecol 99:422, 1992

Naeye RL: Causes of perinatal mortality excess in prolonged gestations. Am J Epidemiol 108:429, 1978

Nahum GG, Stanislaw H, Huffaker BJ: Fetal weight gain at term: Linear with minimal dependence on maternal obesity. Am J Obstet Gynecol 172:1387, 1995

National Institute of Child Health and Human Development Network of Maternal–Fetal Medicine Units: A clinical trial of induction of labor versus expectant management in postterm pregnancy. Am J Obstet Gynecol 170:716, 1994

Olesen AW, Westergaard JG, Olsen J: Perinatal and maternal complications related to postterm delivery: A national register-based study, 1978–1993. Am J Obstet Gynecol 189:227, 2003

Oz AU, Holub B, Mendilcioglu I, et al: Renal artery Doppler investigation of the etiology of oligohydramnios in postterm pregnancy. Obstet Gynecol 100:715, 2002

Rabe T, Hosch R, Runnebaum B: Sulfatase deficiency in the human placenta: Clinical findings. Biol Res Pregnancy Perinatol 4:95, 1983

Rathore AM, Singh R, Ramji S, et al: Randomised trial amnioinfusion during labor with meconium stained amniotic fluid. Br J Obstet Gynaecol 109:17, 2002

Roberts CL, Taylor L, Henderson-Smart D: Trends in births at and beyond term: Evidence of a change? Br J Obstet Gynaecol 106:937, 1999

Roussis P, Cox SM, Campbell BA, et al: Survey on the management of postdate pregnancy. J Matern Fetal Neonatal Med 2:155, 1993

Rushton DI: Pathology of placenta. In Wigglesworth JS, Singer DB (eds): Textbook of Fetal and Perinatal Pathology. Boston, Blackwell, 1991, p 171

Sanchez-Ramos L, Olivier F, Delke I, Kaunitz AW: Labor induction versus expectant management for postterm pregnancies: A systematic review with meta-analysis. Obstet Gynecol 101:1312, 2003

Shime J, Gare DJ, Andrews J, et al: Prolonged pregnancy: Surveillance of the fetus and the neonate and the course of labor and delivery. Am J Obstet Gynecol 148:547, 1984

Shin KS, Brubaker KL, Ackerson LM: Risk of cesarean delivery in nulliparous women at greater than 41 weeks' gestational age with an unengaged vertex. Am J Obstet Gynecol 190:129, 2004

Smith SC, Baker PN: Placental apoptosis is increased in postterm pregnancies. Br J Obstet Gynecol 106:861, 1999

Smith GC: Life-table analysis of the risk of perinatal death at term and post term in singleton pregnancies. Am J Obstet Gynecol 184:489, 2001

Trimmer KJ, Leveno KJ, Peters MT, et al: Observation on the cause of oligohydramnios in prolonged pregnancy. Am J Obstet Gynecol 163:1900, 1990

Usher RH, Boyd ME, McLean FH, et al: Assessment of fetal risk in postdate pregnancies. Am J Obstet Gynecol 158:259, 1988

Vaisanen-Tommiska M, Nuutila M, Ylikorkala O: Cervical nitric oxide release in women postterm. Obstet Gynecol 103:657, 2004

Wenstrom KD, Parsons MT: The prevention of meconium aspiration in labor using amnioinfusion. Obstet Gynecol 73:647, 1989

Wong SF, Hui SK, Choi H, et al: Does sweeping of membranes beyond 40 weeks reduce the need for formal induction of labour? Br J Obstet Gynaecol 109:632, 2002

Yang SH, Roh CR, Kim JH: Transvaginal ultrasonography for cervical assessment before induction of labor. Obstet Gynecol Surv 59:577, 2004

Yoder BA, Kirsch EA, Barth WH, et al: Changing obstetric practices associated with decreasing incidence of meconium aspiration syndrome. Obstet Gynecol 99:731, 2002

38

Fetal Growth Disorders

Each year, about 20 percent of the almost 4 million infants in the United States are born at the low and high extremes of fetal growth. Low-birthweight infants make up just less than half of these 700,000 births and include preterm infants as well as those whose growth has been impaired in utero. Although the majority of these infants are preterm, the National Institutes of Health estimated that approximately 40,000 are at term, having suffered abnormal fetal growth (Frigoletto, 1986). In 1997, 8 percent of infants weighed less than 2500 g at birth, and 10 percent weighed more than 4000 g (Ventura and colleagues, 1999). Between 1981 and 2001, the percentage of low-birthweight infants (less than 2500 g) and very-low-birthweight infants (less than 1500 g) increased by 13 percent and 24 percent, respectively (Martin and colleagues, 2002). Macrosomia, defined as birthweight of 4000 g or greater, occurred in 1 out of every 10 births in the United States in 1997. However, the incidence of macrosomia has been declining since 1991 after peaking at about 11 percent in the 1980s (Ventura and colleagues, 1999).

NORMAL FETAL GROWTH

Human fetal growth is characterized by sequential patterns of tissue and organ growth, differentiation, and maturation that are determined by maternal provision of substrate, placental transfer of these substrates, and fetal growth potential governed by the genome. Steer (1998) has summarized the potential effects of evolutionary pressures on human fetal growth. During the past 3.5 million years, the human species has become adapted to an upright posture, and the pelvis has evolved to facilitate walking. During the past 500,000 years,

human brain volume has increased from about 750 mL (*Homo erectus*) to about 1000 to 1800 mL (*Homo sapiens*). The head has to pass through the pelvis during parturition; thus, an increasing conflict between the need to walk—requiring a narrow pelvis—and the need to think—requiring a large brain—has developed. This leads to difficulty in labor because of dystocia.

The difficulty posed by a large-sized head or brain and small pelvic capacity has been resolved to some extent by an evolutionary modification known as *neoteny,* whereby humans are born increasingly early. For example, if humans were born with the same level of functional maturity as the chimpanzee, human gestation would last 17 months. The human species may be resolving this dilemma in another way— by acquiring the ability to restrict growth late in pregnancy. This characteristic "tail off" of growth from 38 weeks onward as seen in human pregnancies is not evident in other mammals. Thus, the ability to *"growth restrict"* may be adaptive rather than pathological.

Lin and Santolaya-Forgas (1998) have divided cell growth into three consecutive phases. The initial phase of hyperplasia is during the first 16 weeks and is characterized by a rapid increase in cell number. The second phase, which extends up to 32 weeks, includes both cellular hyperplasia and hypertrophy. After 32 weeks, fetal growth is by cellular hypertrophy, and it is during this phase that most fetal fat and glycogen deposition takes place. The corresponding fetal growth rates during these three phases are 5 g/day at 15 weeks, 15 to 20 g/day at 24 weeks, and 30 to 35 g/day at 34 weeks (Williams and co-authors, 1982). As shown in Figure 38–1, there is considerable biological variation in the velocity of fetal growth determined by sonography in the last half of gestation.

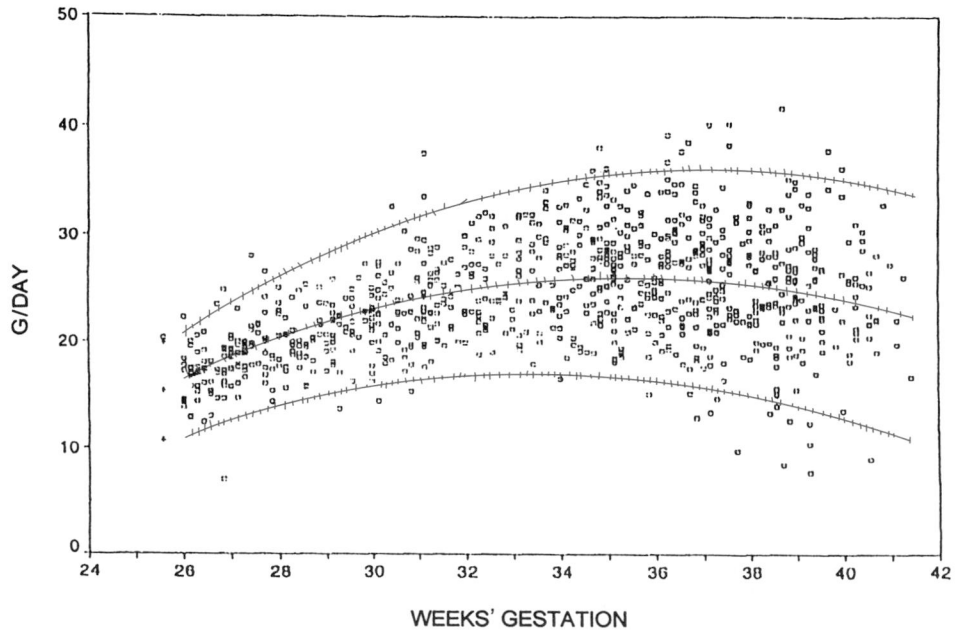

FIGURE 38–1. Increments in fetal weight in grams per day from 24 to 42 weeks' gestation. The lines represent the mean and ± 2 standard deviations. (Adapted from Owen and colleagues, 1996, with permission.)

Although many factors have been implicated in the process of fetal growth, the precise cellular and molecular mechanisms by which normal fetal growth occurs are not well understood. In early fetal life the major determinant of growth is the fetal genome, but later in pregnancy environmental, nutritional, and hormonal influences become increasingly important (Holmes and colleagues, 1998).

For example, there is considerable evidence that insulin and insulin-like growth factor-I (IGF-I) and IGF-II have a role in the regulation of fetal growth and weight gain (Verhaeghe and colleagues, 1993). Insulin is secreted by fetal pancreatic ß cells primarily during the second half of gestation and is believed to stimulate somatic growth and adiposity. The IGFs are produced by virtually all fetal organs beginning early in development. They are potent stimulators of cell division and differentiation. Verhaeghe and colleagues (1993) have found that fetal serum levels of IGF-I, IGF-II, and insulin are all related to fetal growth and weight gain. In cord serum, IGF-I correlates best with birthweight. Moreover, a polymorphism in the IGF-I gene may be associated with low birthweight (Vaessen and colleagues, 2002).

Since the discovery of the *obesity gene* and its protein product, *leptin*, which is synthesized in adipose tissue, there has been interest in maternal and fetal serum leptin levels. Fetal concentrations increase during the first two trimesters, and they correlate with birthweight (Sivan, 1998; Tamura, 1998; Tovi, 2005a,b, and all their colleagues). This relationship is controversial in growth-restricted fetuses (Grisaru-Granovsky and colleagues, 2003).

Fetal growth is also dependent on an adequate supply of nutrients. Indeed, Williams (1903) aptly commented in the first edition of this textbook that "the increase in size of the foetus affords conclusive evidence that materials in solution must, pass from the maternal to the foetal circulation...." Glucose transfer has been extensively studied during pregnancy (see Chap. 4, p. 100). Both excessive and diminished maternal glucose availability to the fetus affect fetal growth. Excessive glycemia produces macrosomia, whereas diminished glucose levels have been associated with fetal growth restriction. Indeed, the macrosomic infant of the mildly diabetic mother is the prototypical example of the effects of excessive maternal glucose supply. Characteristics of these infants include fetal hyperinsulinism and elevated umbilical cord levels of IGF-I and IGF-II (Roth and colleagues, 1996).

There is less information concerning the physiology of maternal–fetal transfer of other nutrients such as amino acids and lipids. Ronzoni and colleagues (1999) studied maternal–fetal concentrations of amino acids in 26 normal pregnancies at the time of cesarean delivery. An increase in maternal amino acid levels led to an increase in fetal levels. In growth-restricted fetuses, amino acid disturbance similar to the biochemical changes seen in postnatal protein-starvation states has been detected (Economides and colleagues, 1989b). Jones and colleagues (1999) studied 38 growth-restricted infants and found impaired utilization of circulating triglycerides consistent with peripheral adipose depletion.

FETAL GROWTH RESTRICTION

Low-birthweight infants who are small-for-gestational age are designated as suffering from *fetal growth restriction*. The term fetal growth retardation has been discarded because "retardation" implies abnormal mental function. It is estimated that 3 to 10 percent of infants are growth restricted (Divon and Hsu, 1992).

In 1961, Warkany and co-workers reported normal values for infant weights, lengths, and head circumferences that served to define fetal growth restriction. Gruenwald (1963) reported that approximately one third of infants born weighing less than 2500 g were mature and that their small size could be explained by *chronic placental insufficiency*. These observations generated the concept that birthweight was governed not only by gestational length but also by fetal growth rate.

It also has been suggested that fetal size is largely determined in the first trimester (Dickey and Gasser, 1993; Gluckman and Liggins, 1984). Smith and colleagues (1998) compared outcomes of 4229 pregnancies with the difference between measured and expected crown-rump length measured ultrasonically in the first trimester. Suboptimal first-trimester growth was associated with fetal growth restriction as well as preterm delivery between 24 and 32 weeks. It may be that a suboptimal environment in the first weeks of gestation limits fetal growth for the remainder of pregnancy and that such an environment may precipitate extremely preterm delivery.

DEFINITION. In 1963, Lubchenco and co-workers from Denver published detailed comparisons of gestational ages with birthweights in an effort to derive norms for expected fetal size at a given gestational week. Battaglia and Lubchenco (1967) then classified *small-for-gestational-age* (SGA) infants as those whose weights were below the 10th percentile for their gestational age. Such infants were shown to be at increased risk for neonatal death. For example, the neonatal mortality rate of SGA infants born at 38 weeks was 1 percent compared with that of 0.2 percent in those with appropriate birthweights.

Many infants with birthweights less than the 10th percentile are not pathologically growth restricted but are small simply because of normal biological factors. Indeed, Manning and Hohler (1991) and Gardosi and colleagues (1992) concluded that 25 to 60 percent of SGA infants were, in fact, appropriately grown when maternal ethnic group, parity, weight, and height were considered.

Because of these disparities, other classifications were proposed. Seeds (1984) suggested a definition based on birthweight below the fifth percentile. Usher and McLean (1969) proposed that fetal growth standards should be based on mean

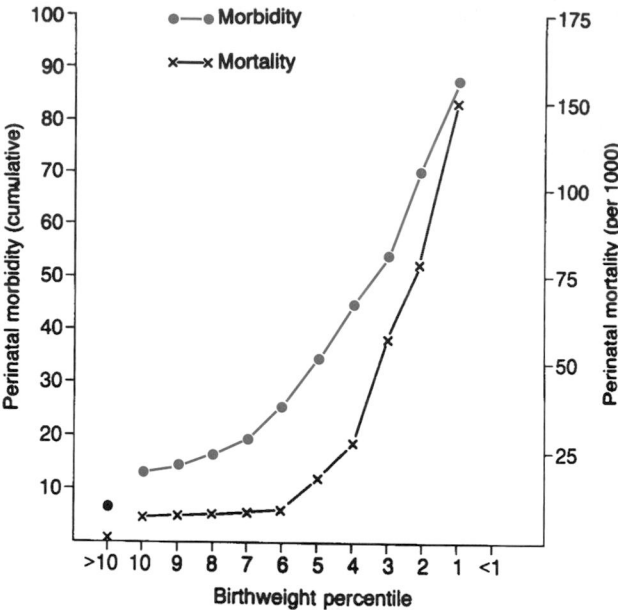

FIGURE 38–2. Relationship between birthweight percentile and perinatal mortality and morbidity in 1560 small-for-gestational-age fetuses. A progressive increase in both mortality and morbidity is observed as birthweight percentile falls. (From Manning, 1995.)

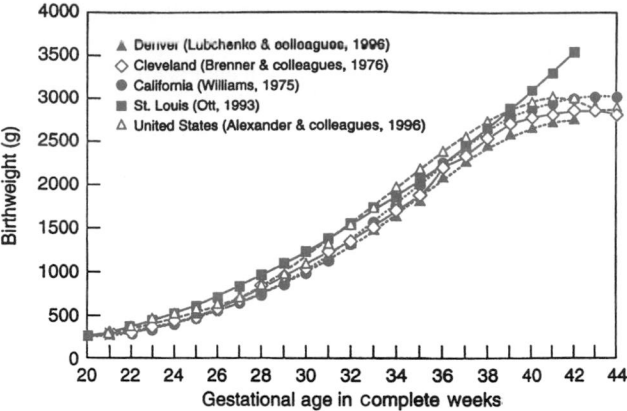

FIGURE 38–3. Comparison of fetal growth curves for infants born in different regions of the United States and compared with those of the nation at large. (Modified from Alexander and colleagues, 1996, with permission.)

weights-for-age with normal limits defined by ±2 standard deviations. This definition would limit SGA infants to 3 percent of births instead of 10 percent. Clinically, this definition is very meaningful. As shown in Figure 38–2, most poor outcomes are in infants below the third percentile. In a study of 122,754 pregnancies delivered at Parkland Hospital, McIntire and colleagues (1999) also showed that mortality and morbidity were significantly increased among term infants whose birthweights were at or below the third percentile.

Normal Infant Birthweight. Normative data for fetal growth based on birthweight have evolved considerably following the pioneering work done by Lubchenco and co-workers (1963). Their data were derived exclusively from births to white and Hispanic women who resided at high altitudes. Such infants are smaller than those born at sea level. For example, term infants average 3400 g at sea level, 3200 g at 5000 feet, and 2900 g at 10,000 feet. Other researchers have developed fetal growth curves using various populations and geographic locations throughout the United States (Brenner and colleagues, 1976; Ott, 1993; Overpeck and colleagues, 1999; Williams, 1975). Each of these curves was based on specific ethnic or regional groups; therefore, they are not representative of the entire population. To address this, fetal growth graphs were derived on a nationwide basis in both the United States (Table 38–1) and Canada (Alexander and colleagues, 1996; Arbuckle and colleagues, 1993). Data from over 3.1 million mothers with singleton liveborn infants in the United States during 1991 were used to derive the growth curve shown in Figure 38–3.

In general, the previously published fetal growth curve data underestimated birthweights when compared with national data. Importantly, there are significant ethnic or racial variations in neonatal mortality rates within the national neonatal mortality rate as well as within birthweight and gestational age categories (Alexander and colleagues, 1999, 2003).

TABLE 38–1 Smoothed Percentiles of Birthweight (g) for Gestational Age in the United States Based on 3,134,879 Single Live Births

Age (wk)	Percentile				
	5th	10th	50th	90th	95th
20	249	275	412	772	912
21	280	314	433	790	957
22	330	376	496	826	1023
23	385	440	582	882	1107
24	435	498	674	977	1223
25	480	558	779	1138	1397
26	529	625	899	1362	1640
27	591	702	1035	1635	1927
28	670	798	1196	1977	2237
29	772	925	1394	2361	2553
30	910	1085	1637	2710	2847
31	1088	1278	1918	2986	3108
32	1294	1495	2203	3200	3338
33	1513	1725	2458	3370	3536
34	1735	1950	2667	3502	3697
35	1950	2159	2831	3596	3812
36	2156	2354	2974	3668	3888
37	2357	2541	3117	3755	3956
38	2543	2714	3263	3867	4027
39	2685	2852	3400	3980	4107
40	2761	2929	3495	4060	4185
41	2777	2948	3527	4094	4217
42	2764	2935	3522	4098	4213
43	2741	2907	3505	4096	4178
44	2724	2885	3491	4096	4122

From Alexander and associates (1996), with permission.

Birthweight Versus Growth. Most of what is known about normal and abnormal human fetal growth is actually based on birthweight standards, which is the end point of fetal growth. These standards do not reveal the *rate* of fetal growth. Indeed, such birthweight curves reveal compromised growth only at the extreme of impaired growth. Thus, they cannot be used to identify the fetus who fails to achieve an expected or potential size but whose birthweight outlies the 10th percentile. Birthweight percentile is an incomplete measure of growth failure. Infants who are of apparently appropriate birthweight, but who "cross centiles," may be exhibiting signs of malnutrition because they have not achieved their full genetic potential (Owen and colleagues, 1996, 2003). The rate or velocity of human fetal growth depends on serial ultrasonic fetal anthropometry. Reports suggest that a diminished growth velocity is related to perinatal morbidity (Owen and co-workers, 1997; Owen and Khan, 1998).

Metabolic Abnormalities. Fetal blood sampling from the umbilical vein for karyotyping of severely growth-restricted fetuses has permitted remarkable insights into the pathophysiology of fetal growth (see Chap. 13, p. 330). In 38 growth-restricted fetuses, Soothill and colleagues (1987) found that the severity of hypoxia correlated significantly with hypercapnia, acidosis, lactic acidemia, hypoglycemia, and erythroblastosis. Subsequently, Economides and Nicolaides (1989a) found that the major cause of hypoglycemia in SGA fetuses was reduced supply rather than increased fetal consumption or diminished fetal glucose production. Economides and co-workers (1989c) found that these fetuses also had hypoinsulinemia and hypoglycemia. The degree of fetal growth restriction, however, did not correlate with plasma insulin, suggesting that it is not the primary determinant of poor fetal growth.

In children with *kwashiorkor,* the ratio of nonessential to essential amino acids is increased, presumably because of decreased intake of essential amino acids. Economides and colleagues (1989b) measured the glycine/valine ratio in cord blood from growth-restricted fetuses and found ratios similar to those observed in children with protein deprivation and kwashiorkor. Moreover, protein deprivation correlated with fetal hypoxemia. Economides and associates (1990) measured plasma triglyceride concentrations in small fetuses and infants and compared those with the concentrations of appropriately grown fetuses. Growth-restricted fetuses demonstrated hypertriglyceridemia that was correlated with the degree of fetal hypoxemia. They hypothesized that hypoglycemic, growth-restricted fetuses mobilize adipose tissue, and that the hypertriglyceridemia is the result of lipolysis of fetal fat stores.

Elevated plasma concentrations of interleukin-10, placental atrial natriuretic peptide, and endothelin-1, as well as a defect in epidermal growth factor function, have also been described in growth-restricted fetuses (Varner and colleagues, 1996). These findings suggest a possible role for abnormal immune activation and abnormal placentation in the genesis of growth-restricted fetuses (Gabriel, 1994; Heyborne, 1994; Kingdom, 1994; McQueen, 1993; Neerhof, 1995, and all their associates). In animals, chronic reduction in nitric oxide, an endothelium-derived, locally acting vasorelaxant, has also been shown to result in diminished fetal growth (Diket and associates, 1994).

MORBIDITY AND MORTALITY. As shown in Figure 38–2, fetal growth restriction is associated with substantive perinatal morbidity and mortality. Fetal demise, birth asphyxia, meconium aspiration, and neonatal hypoglycemia and hypothermia are all increased, as is the prevalence of abnormal neurological development (Paz and associates, 1995; Piper and colleagues, 1996). This is true for both term and preterm infants (Minior and Divon, 1998). Finally, the risk of long-term mortality in preterm growth-restricted infants is significantly increased compared with that of appropriately grown preterm infants (Kok and colleagues, 1998).

Postnatal growth and development of the growth-restricted fetus depends on the cause of restriction, nutrition in infancy, and the social environment (Kliegman, 1997). Infants with growth restriction due to congenital, viral, chromosomal, or maternal size typically remain small throughout life. If growth restriction is due to placental insufficiency, infants must often have catch-up growth to approach their inherited growth potential. Similarly, the neurodevelopmental outcome of the growth-restricted fetus is influenced by both pre- and postnatal environments. Infants born to families of higher socioeconomic status demonstrate fewer developmental problems than those born to indigent families.

ACCELERATED MATURATION. There have been numerous reports describing accelerated fetal pulmonary maturation in complicated pregnancies associated with growth restriction (Perelman and colleagues, 1985). One explanation for this phenomenon is that the fetus responds to a stressed environment by increasing adrenal glucocorticoid production, which leads to earlier or accelerated fetal lung maturation (Laatikainen and associates, 1988). Although this concept pervades modern perinatal thinking, there is scant verification for it.

Owen and associates (1990) analyzed perinatal outcomes in 178 women delivered primarily because of hypertension. They compared these with those of 159 women delivered because of spontaneous preterm labor or ruptured membranes. They concluded that a "stressed" pregnancy, which often resulted in SGA infants, did not confer an appreciable survival advantage. Similar findings were reported by Friedman and colleagues (1995) in women with severe preeclampsia. Two studies from Parkland Hospital substantiate that fetal growth restriction accrues no apparent advantages to the preterm infant (McIntire and colleagues, 1999; Tyson and colleagues, 1995). Moreover, Smulian and colleagues (2000) reported that growth-restricted infants had higher 1-year infant mortality compared with infants from normal pregnancies.

SYMMETRICAL VERSUS ASYMMETRICAL GROWTH RESTRICTION.

Campbell and Thoms (1977) described the use of the sonographically determined *head-to-abdomen circumference ratio (HC/AC)* to differentiate growth-restricted fetuses. Those that were *symmetrical* were proportionately small, and those that were *asymmetrical* had disproportionately lagging abdominal growth. These authors constructed an HC/AC ratio nomogram from approximately 500 normal fetuses. Although asymmetrical fetuses were "preferentially protected from the full effects of the growth-retarding stimulus," they more likely were associated with pregnancies complicated by severe preeclampsia, fetal distress, operative intervention, and lower Apgar scores than their symmetrical counterparts.

It is compelling to relate the type of growth restriction to the onset or etiology of a particular insult. An early insult could theoretically result in a relative decrease in cell number as well as cell size, which might be caused by chemical exposure, viral infection, or inherent cellular development abnormality due to aneuploidy. The resultant proportionate reduction in these cases of both head and body size has been termed *symmetrical growth restriction.*

On the other hand, a late pregnancy insult such as placental insufficiency from hypertension theoretically could primarily affect cell size. Placental insufficiency may result in diminished glucose transfer and hepatic storage, thus, fetal abdominal circumference—which reflects liver size—would be reduced. This sequence of events can theoretically result in *asymmetrical growth restriction.* This concept has been challenged (Roberts and co-authors, 1999). Such somatic growth restriction is proposed to result from preferential shunting of oxygen and nutrients to the brain, which allows normal brain and head growth. Because the fetal brain is normally relatively large and the liver relatively small, the ratio of brain weight to liver weight over the last 12 weeks—usually about 3 to 1—may be increased to 5 to 1 or more in severely growth-restricted infants.

Although these generalizations about the potential pathophysiology of symmetrical versus asymmetrical growth restriction are interesting from a conceptual standpoint, there is considerable evidence that fetal growth patterns are more complex. Nicolaides and co-authors (1991) found that fetuses with aneuploidy typically had disproportionately large head sizes and thus were *asymmetrically* growth restricted. Similarly, most preterm infants with growth restriction due to preeclampsia and associated uteroplacental insufficiency demonstrate symmetrical growth impairment (Salafia and co-authors, 1995).

Crane and Kopta (1980) analyzed several anthropometric measurements in growth-restricted newborns and concluded that the concept of brain sparing could not be used to identify the cause(s) of fetal growth restriction. Dashe and colleagues (2000) analyzed 8722 consecutive liveborn singletons who underwent an ultrasound examination within 4 weeks of delivery. Although only 20 percent of growth-restricted fetuses demonstrated sonographic head-to-abdomen asymmetry, these fetuses were at increased risk for intrapartum and neonatal complications. Symmetrically growth-restricted fetuses were not at increased risk for adverse outcomes when compared with those appropriately grown. The researchers concluded that asymmetrical fetal growth restriction represented significantly disordered growth, whereas symmetrical growth restriction more likely represented normal, genetically determined small stature.

RISK FACTORS

Constitutionally Small Mothers. Small women typically have smaller infants. If a woman begins pregnancy weighing less than 100 pounds, the risk of delivering an SGA infant is increased at least twofold (Simpson and colleagues, 1975). Moreover, intergenerational effects on birthweight are transmitted through the maternal line (Emanuel and associates, 1992). There is also evidence that reduced intrauterine growth of the mother is a risk factor for reduced intrauterine growth of her offspring (Klebanoff and co-authors, 1997).

Whether the phenomenon of a small mother giving birth to a small infant is nature or nurture is unclear. Brooks and co-authors (1995) analyzed 62 births after ovum donation to examine the relative influence of the donor versus the recipient on birthweight. They concluded that the environment provided by the donor mother was more important than the genetic contribution to birthweight.

Poor Maternal Nutrition. In the woman of average or low body mass index (BMI), poor weight gain throughout pregnancy may be associated with fetal growth restriction (Simpson and colleagues, 1975). Lack of weight gain in the second trimester especially correlates with decreased birthweight (Abrams and Selvin, 1995). If the mother is large and otherwise healthy, however, below-average maternal weight gain without maternal disease is unlikely to be associated with appreciable fetal growth restriction.

As discussed in Chapter 43 (see p. 1011), marked restriction of weight gain after midpregnancy should not be encouraged. Even so, it appears that caloric restriction to less than 1500 kcal/day adversely affects fetal growth only minimally (Lechtig and co-workers, 1975). The best documented effect of famine on fetal growth was in the "hunger winter" of 1944 in Holland. The German Army restricted dietary intake to 600 kcal/day for civilians, including pregnant women. The famine persisted for 28 weeks. Although this resulted in an average birthweight decrease of only 250 g, fetal mortality rates increased significantly (Stein and colleagues, 1975).

Social Deprivation. The effect of social deprivation on birthweight is interconnected to the effects of associated lifestyle factors such as smoking, alcohol or other substance abuse, and poor nutrition. In a study of 7493 British women, Wilcox and associates (1995) found that the most socially deprived mothers had the smallest infants. Similarly, Dejin-Karlsson and colleagues (2000) prospectively studied a cohort of Swedish women and found that lack of psychosocial resources increased the risk of growth-restricted infants. Indeed, more than 100 years ago, Williams (1903) wrote in the first edition of this textbook: "The social condition of the mother and the comforts by which she is surrounded also exert a marked influence on the child's weight, heavier children being more common in the upper walks of life."

Fetal Infections. Viral, bacterial, protozoan, and spirochetal infections have been implicated in up to 5 percent of cases of fetal growth restriction (Klein and Remington, 1995). The best known of these are infections caused by rubella and cytomegalovirus (Lin and Evans, 1984; Stagno and associates, 1977). Mechanisms affecting fetal growth appear to be different with these two viral infections. *Cytomegalovirus* is associated with direct cytolysis and loss of functional cells. *Rubella* infection causes vascular insufficiency by damaging the endothelium of small vessels. Rubella also reduces cell division (Pollack and Divon, 1992).

Hepatitis A and B are associated with preterm delivery but may also adversely affect fetal growth (Waterson, 1979). *Listeriosis, tuberculosis,* and *syphilis* have been reported to cause fetal growth restriction. Paradoxically, with syphilis, the placenta is almost always increased in weight and size due to edema and perivascular inflammation (Varner and Galask, 1984). *Toxoplasmosis* is the protozoan infection most often associated with compromised fetal growth, but *congenital malaria* may produce the same result (Varner and Galask, 1984).

Congenital Malformations. In a study of over 13,000 infants with major structural anomalies, 22 percent had accompanying growth restriction (Khoury and associates, 1988). In general, the more severe the malformation, the more likely the fetus is to be SGA. This is especially evident in fetuses with chromosomal abnormalities or those with serious cardiovascular malformations.

Chromosomal Aneuploidies. Placentas of fetuses with *autosomal trisomies* have a reduced number of small muscular arteries in the tertiary stem villi (Rochelson and associates, 1990). Depending on which chromosome is extra, there may be associated growth restriction.

In *trisomy 21*, fetal growth restriction is generally mild (Thelander and Pryor, 1966). Whether there is a lag in crown-rump length is controversial (Golbus 1978; Stephens and Shepard, 1980). However, after the first trimester, all long-bone growth lags behind that of normal fetuses (Fitzsimmons and colleagues, 1990). Both shortened femur length

and hypoplasia of the middle phalanx occur with increased frequency in trisomy 21.

By contrast, fetal growth in *trisomy 18* is virtually always significantly affected. In one series, 10 of 11 newborns weighed less than 2500 g (Moerman and associates, 1982). Growth failure has been documented as early as the first trimester. By the second trimester, long-bone measurements typically fall below the third percentile for age, and the upper extremity is even more severely affected (Droste and co-workers, 1990). Visceral organ growth is also abnormal (Droste, 1992).

Fetuses with *trisomy 13* have some degree of growth restriction but generally not as severely as those with trisomy 18.

Trisomy 16 is the most common trisomy in spontaneous miscarriage and is usually lethal in the nonmosaic state (Lindor and associates, 1993). As discussed in Chapter 12 (see p. 295), patches of trisomy 16 (or others) in the placenta—*confined placental mosaicism*—can cause placental insufficiency that may account for many cases of previously unexplained fetal growth restriction (Kalousek and colleagues, 1993; Towner and colleagues, 2001). It is emphasized that in these pregnancies, the chromosomal abnormality is confined to the placenta.

Significant fetal growth restriction is not seen with *Turner syndrome* (45,X) or *Klinefelter syndrome* (47,XXY) (Droste, 1992).

Disorders of Cartilage and Bone. Numerous inherited syndromes such as *osteogenesis imperfecta* and various chondrodystrophies are associated with fetal growth restriction (see Chap. 12, p. 296).

Teratogens. Any teratogen is capable of adversely affecting fetal growth. Many are considered in detail in Chapter 14. Examples include anticonvulsants and antineoplastic agents. In addition, cigarette smoking, opiates and related drugs, alcohol, and cocaine may cause growth restriction, either primarily or by decreasing maternal food intake.

Vascular Disease. Especially when complicated by superimposed preeclampsia, chronic vascular disease commonly causes growth restriction (see Chap. 34, p. 764). Preeclampsia may cause fetal growth failure and is an indicator of its severity, especially when the onset is before 37 weeks (Gainer, 2005; Odegard, 2000; Xiong, 1999, and all their colleagues).

Renal Disease. Chronic renal insufficiency is often associated with underlying hypertension and vascular disease. Chronic nephropathies are commonly accompanied by restricted fetal growth (Cunningham and colleagues, 1990; Stettler and Cunningham, 1992).

Chronic Hypoxia. When exposed to a chronically hypoxic environment, some fetuses have significantly reduced birthweight. As discussed earlier, fetuses of women who reside at high altitude usually weigh less than those born to women who live at a lower altitude (Krampl, 2002; Lichty and colleagues, 1957). As discussed in Chapter 44 (see p. 1028), severe hypoxia from maternal cyanotic heart disease frequently is associated with severely growth-restricted fetuses (Patton and co-workers, 1990).

Anemia. In most cases, maternal anemia does not cause fetal growth restriction. Exceptions include sickle cell disease and some other inherited anemias. Conversely, curtailed maternal blood volume expansion has been linked to fetal growth restriction (Duvekot and colleagues, 1995). This is further discussed in Chapter 51 (see p. 1145).

Placental and Cord Abnormalities. A number of placental abnormalities may cause fetal growth restriction (see Chap. 27). They include chronic placental abruption, extensive infarction, chorioangioma, marginal or velamentous cord insertion, circumvallate placenta, or placenta previa. Growth failure in these cases is often presumed to be due to *uteroplacental insufficiency.* Some women with otherwise unexplained fetal growth restriction and a grossly normal placenta have reduced uteroplacental blood flow when compared with normally grown fetuses (Kotini and colleagues, 2003; Lunell and Nylund, 1992; Papageorghiou and colleagues, 2001). Similar reductions have also been reported in growth-restricted fetuses with congenital malformations. These results suggest that maternal blood flow may in part be regulated by the fetus (Howard, 1987; Rankin and McLaughlin, 1979). Interestingly, there is no evidence that macrosomic infants have increased uteroplacental blood flow.

Multiple Fetuses. As shown in Figure 38–4, pregnancy with two or more fetuses is more likely to be complicated by diminished growth of one or more fetuses when compared with normal singletons (see Chap. 39, p. 922).

Antiphospholipid Antibody Syndrome. Two classes of antiphospholipid antibodies—*anticardiolipin antibodies* and *lupus anticoagulant*—have been associated with fetal growth restriction (Lockwood and Rand, 1994). These syndromes are considered in detail in Chapters 47 (p. 1078) and 54 (p. 1215). Pregnancy outcome in women with these antibodies is often poor and may involve early-onset preeclampsia and fetal demise (Levine and associates, 2002; Lockwood, 2002). Specifically, these antibodies may be found in women with repetitive second-trimester fetal loss or early-onset fetal growth restriction, especially when accompanied by early and severe hypertensive disease. Not all researchers have reported these adverse outcomes. Infante-Rivard and colleagues (2002) did not find an association between maternal or newborn thrombophilia polymorphisms and risk of fetal growth restriction. Pathophysiological mechanisms in the

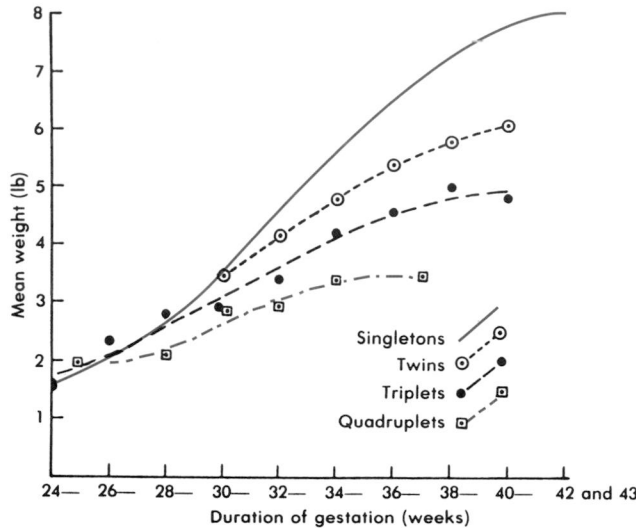

FIGURE 38–4. Birthweight and gestational age relationships in multifetal gestations. (From McKeown and Record, 1952, with permission.)

fetus appear to be caused by maternal platelet aggregation and placental thrombosis.

Extrauterine Pregnancy. If the placenta is implanted outside the uterus, the fetus is usually growth restricted (see Chap. 10, p. 265). Also, some uterine malformations have been linked to impaired fetal growth (see Chap. 40, p. 953).

IDENTIFICATION OF FETAL GROWTH RESTRICTION. *Early* establishment of gestational age, attention to maternal weight gain, and careful measurement of uterine fundal growth throughout pregnancy identify many cases of abnormal fetal growth in low-risk women. Risk factors, including a *previously growth-restricted fetus,* increases the possibility of recurrence. In women with significant risk factors, consideration should be given to serial sonography. Although frequency of examinations varies depending on clinical circumstances, an initial dating examination, ideally in the first trimester followed by a second examination at 32 to 34 weeks, or when clinically indicated, should serve to identify many cases of growth restriction. Even so, *definitive diagnosis* frequently cannot be made until delivery.

Identification of the inappropriately growing fetus remains a challenge. However, there are both simple clinical techniques and more complex technologies that may prove useful in helping to exclude and diagnose fetal growth restriction.

Uterine Fundal Height. Carefully performed serial fundal height measurements are a simple, safe, inexpensive, and reasonably accurate *screening* method to detect SGA fetuses (Gardosi and Francis, 1999). As a screening tool, its principal drawback is imprecision. For example, Jensen and Larsen (1991) and Walraven and colleagues (1995) found that this

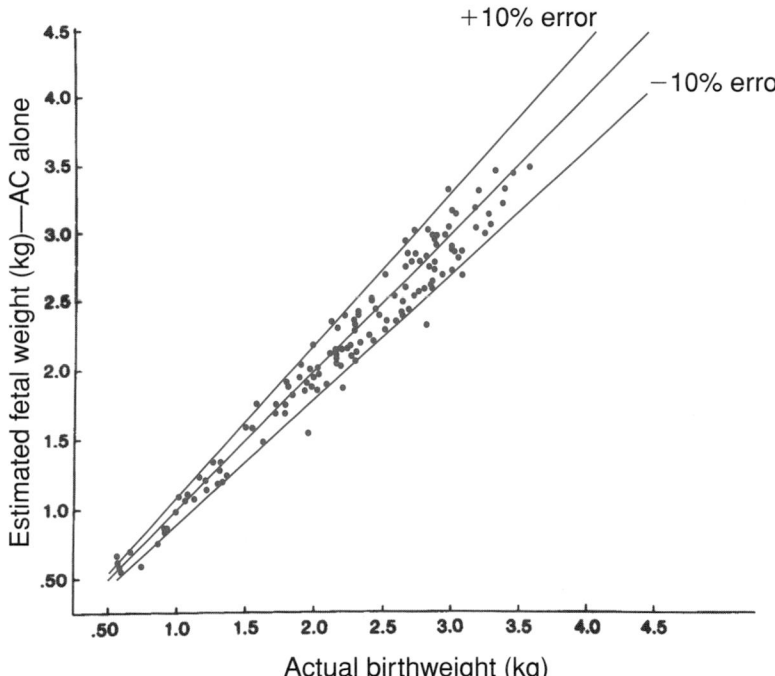

FIGURE 38–5. Correlation of fetal weight estimation using abdominal circumference (AC) with actual birthweight in 175 fetuses with birthweights ranging from 400 to 3600 g. Within this weight range, the range of error was ± 10 percent. (From Manning, 1995.)

method helped correctly identify only 40 percent of such infants. Thus, SGA fetuses were both overlooked and over-diagnosed. Despite this, these results do not diminish the importance of carefully performed fundal measurements as a simple screening method. The method used by most for fundal height measurement was described by Jimenez and colleagues (1983). Briefly, this consists of a tape calibrated in centimeters applied over the abdominal curvature from the upper edge of the symphysis to the upper edge of the uterine fundus, which is identified by palpation or percussion. The tape is applied with the markings away from the examiner to avoid bias. Between 18 and 30 weeks, the uterine fundal height in centimeters coincides with weeks of gestation. If the measurement is more than 2 to 3 cm from the expected height, inappropriate fetal growth may be suspected.

Ultrasonic Measurements. Central to the debate over whether all pregnancies should routinely undergo ultrasonic evaluation is the potential for diagnosis of growth restriction (Ewigman and colleagues, 1993). Typically, such routine screening incorporates an initial ultrasound examination at 16 to 20 weeks to establish gestational age and identify anomalies. This is repeated at 32 to 34 weeks to evaluate fetal growth (see Chap. 16, p. 392). Ironically, Gardosi and Geirsson (1998) found that accurate gestational dating at the initial examination resulted in a lower diagnosis rate of fetal growth restriction.

The optimal ultrasonic method of estimating fetal size, and therefore growth restriction, was reviewed by Manning (1995). Combining head, abdomen, and femur dimensions should in theory enhance the accuracy of predictions of fetal

size. Unfortunately, any potential improvement is apparently lost by the cumulative error inherent in measurement of each individual fetal dimension. As a result, abdominal circumference measurements have been accepted by most experts as the most reliable index of fetal size (Manning, 1995; Smith and colleagues, 1997; Snijders and Nicolaides, 1994). In these studies, the estimated fetal weight calculated with abdominal circumference measurements was almost always within 10 percent of the actual birthweight (Fig. 38–5).

Abdominal circumference measured directly in the newborn was also shown to be an important anatomical marker of growth restriction (Deter and colleagues, 1995). The elegant observations on the metabolic effects of fetal growth restriction, performed at Kings College Hospital and described earlier, were determined in fetuses whose ultrasonically determined abdominal circumference was less than the fifth percentile (Snijders and Nicolaides, 1994). As shown in Fig. 38–6, such small circumferences are linked to decreased Po_2 and pH. These observations emphasize that ultrasonic measurements of the abdominal circumference can meaningfully signify pathological growth restriction.

Unfortunately, the use of ultrasound for detection of fetal growth restriction does not preclude missed diagnoses. Dashe and colleagues (2000) studied 8400 live births at Parkland Hospital in which fetal ultrasound had been performed within 4 weeks of delivery. They reported that 30 percent of growth-restricted fetuses were not detected. In a study of 1000 high-risk fetuses, Larsen and colleagues (1992) performed serial ultrasound beginning at 28 weeks and every 3 weeks thereafter. They found that reporting the results to the clinicians significantly increased the diagnosis of SGA

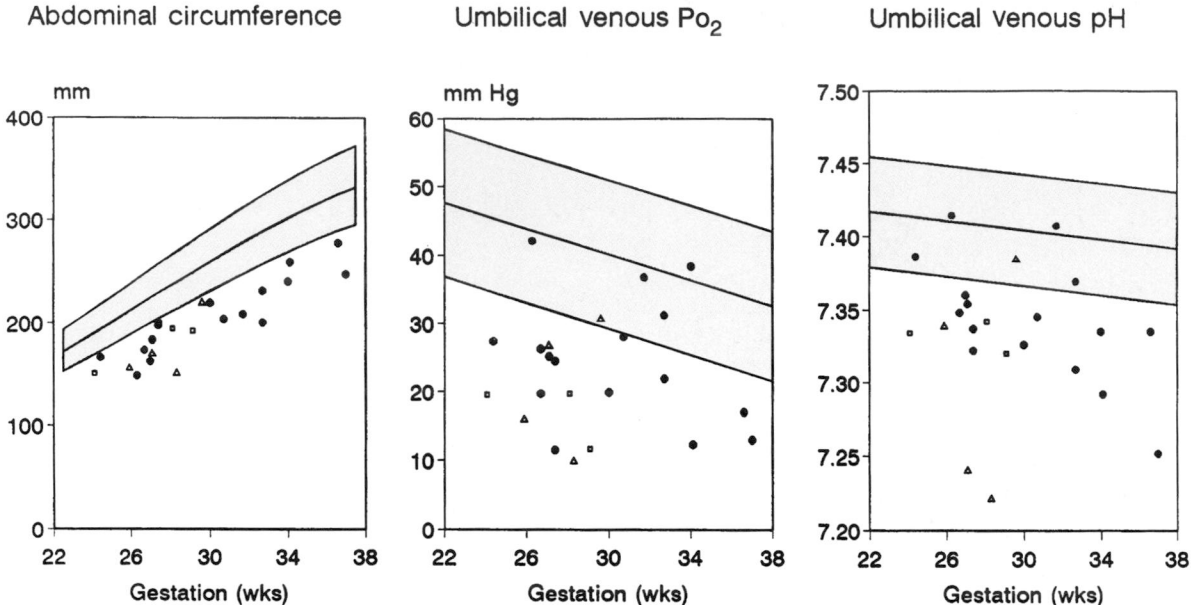

Abdominal circumference

Umbilical venous Po$_2$

Umbilical venous pH

FIGURE 38–6. Abdominal circumference and umbilical venous blood Po$_2$ and pH in growth-restricted fetuses (▲ = fetal deaths; ● = neonatal deaths). The lines within and bordering the shaded areas are the mean, 5th, and 95th percentiles for gestational age. (From Hecher and colleagues, 1995, with permission.)

fetuses. Although elective deliveries in this group were also increased, there was no overall improvement in neonatal outcome. An association between pathological fetal growth restriction and oligohydramnios has long been recognized (see Chap. 21, p. 532). As shown in Figure 38–7, the smaller the pocket of amnionic fluid, the greater the perinatal mortality. One likely explanation for oligohydramnios is diminished fetal urine production caused by hypoxia and diminished renal blood flow (Nicolaides and associates, 1990).

Doppler Velocimetry. Abnormal umbilical artery Doppler velocimetry—characterized by absent or reversed end-diastolic flow—has been uniquely associated with fetal growth restriction (see Chap. 16, p. 401). An example of this is shown in Fig. 38–8. The use of Doppler velocimetry in the management of fetal growth restriction has been recommended as a possible adjunct to techniques such as nonstress testing or a biophysical profile (American College of Obstetricians and Gynecologists, 2000b).

MANAGEMENT. Once fetal growth restriction is suspected, efforts should be made to confirm the diagnosis, assess fetal condition, and evaluate for anomalies. Although cordocentesis allows rapid karyotyping for detection of a lethal aneuploidy and thus may simplify management, the American College of Obstetricians and Gynecologists (2000b) has concluded that there are not enough data to warrant cord blood sampling in this situation. The timing of delivery is crucial, and the risks of fetal death versus the hazards of preterm delivery must be assessed as reported in the Growth Restriction Intervention Trial (GRIT) by Thornton and colleagues, 2004.

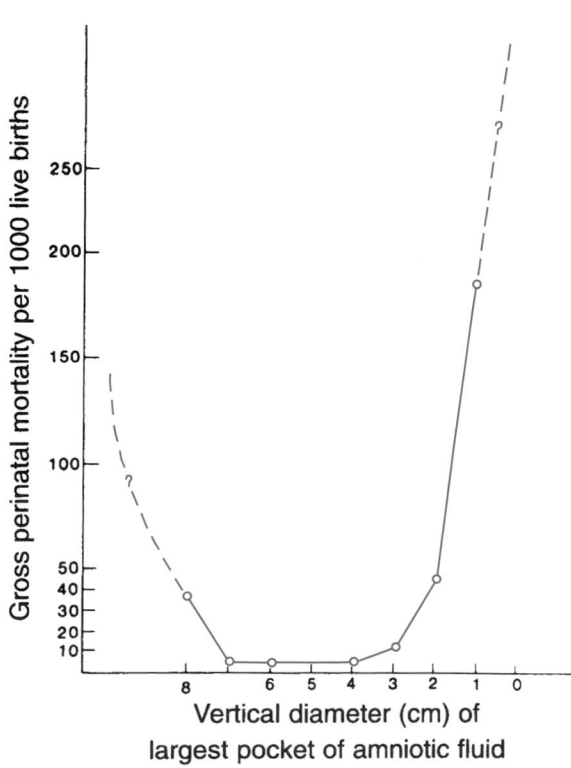

FIGURE 38–7. Relationship of amnionic fluid volume, as determined by the largest vertical pocket, to perinatal mortality. Mortality rises significantly when the largest pocket of fluid falls below 2 cm. (From Manning, 1995.)

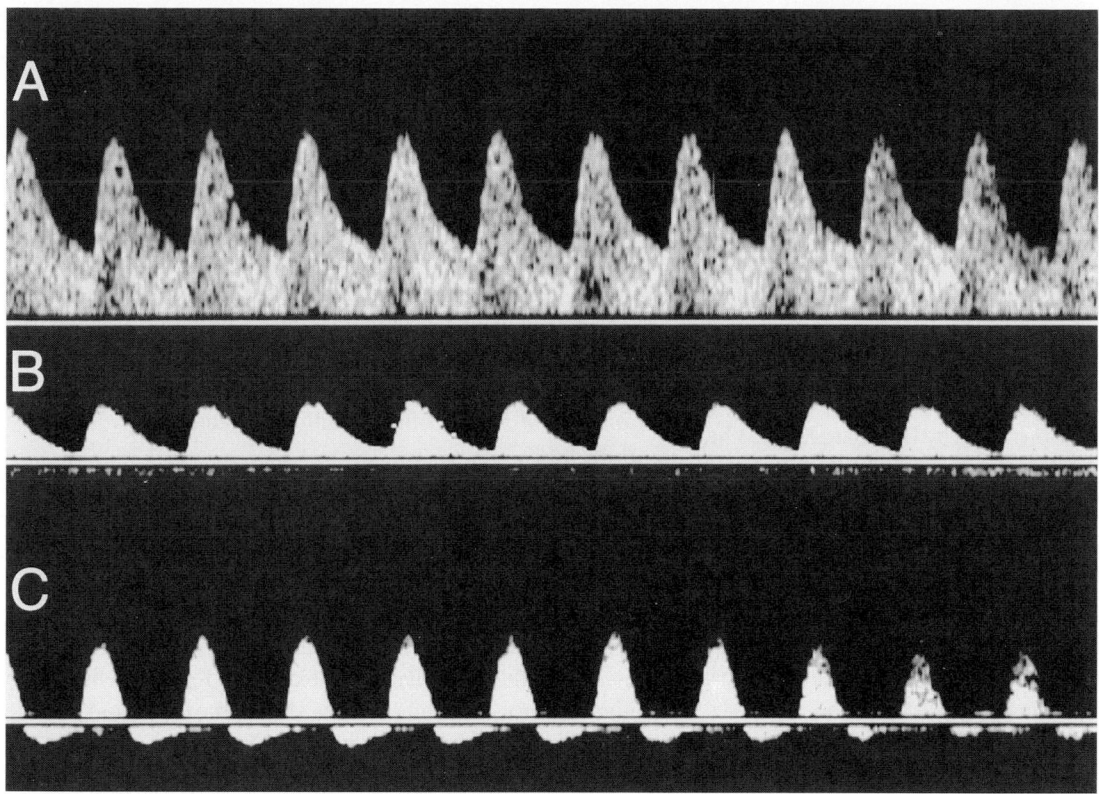

FIGURE 38–8. Umbilical arterial Doppler velocimetry studies, ranging from normal to markedly abnormal. **A.** Normal velocimetry pattern with an S/D ratio of < 30. **B.** The diastolic velocity approaching zero reflects increased placental vascular resistance. **C.** During diastole, arterial flow is reversed (negative S/D ratio), which is an ominous sign that may precede fetal demise. (Courtesy of Dr. Diane Twickler.)

Growth Restriction Near Term. Prompt delivery is likely best for the fetus at or near term who is considered growth restricted. In fact, most clinicians recommend delivery at 34 weeks or beyond if there is clinically significant oligohydramnios. With a reassuring fetal heart rate pattern, vaginal delivery may be attempted. Some of these fetuses do not tolerate labor, and cesarean delivery is necessary.

Uncertainty about the diagnosis should preclude intervention until fetal lung maturity is assured. Expectant management can be guided using antepartum fetal surveillance techniques described in Chapter 15.

Growth Restriction Remote from Term. When growth restriction is diagnosed in an anatomically normal fetus prior to 34 weeks, and amnionic fluid volume and fetal surveillance are normal, observation is recommended. Screening for toxoplasmosis, rubella, cytomegalovirus, herpes, and other infections is recommended by some clinicians, however, we have not found this to be productive.

As long as fetal growth continues and fetal evaluation remains normal, pregnancy is allowed to continue until fetal maturity. In some cases, amniocentesis may be helpful to assess pulmonary maturity. Although the onset of oligohydramnios is highly suggestive of fetal growth failure,

importantly, normal amnionic fluid volume does not preclude growth restriction. Owen and colleagues (2001) reported that 4- and 6-week evaluation intervals were superior to 2-week intervals for predicting growth restriction. Depending on the gestational age of the fetus when fetal growth restriction is first suspected, this interval may be impractical clinically, and sonography is typically repeated more frequently.

With growth restriction remote from term, no specific treatment ameliorates the condition. There is no evidence that bed rest results in accelerated growth or improved outcome. Despite this, many clinicians advise a program of modified rest. Nutrient supplementation, attempts at plasma volume expansion, oxygen therapy, antihypertensive drugs, heparin, and aspirin have all been shown to be ineffective (American College of Obstetricians and Gynecologists, 2000b).

In most cases of growth restriction diagnosed prior to term, neither a precise etiology nor a specific therapy is apparent. Management decisions hinge on an assessment of the relative risks of fetal death with expectant management versus the risks from preterm delivery. Although reassuring fetal testing may allow observation with continued maturation of the preterm growth-restricted fetus, there is concern regarding long-term neurological outcome (Blair and Stanley, 1992; Thornton and colleagues, 2004).

Some authorities challenge that various tests of fetal well-being are unnecessary to reduce risks for stillbirth. Weiner and colleagues (1996) performed nonstress tests, biophysical profiles, and umbilical artery velocimetry within 3 days of delivery in 135 fetuses confirmed at birth to have growth restriction. Other than metabolic acidosis at delivery, which was predicted by absent or reversed end-diastolic umbilical blood flow, morbidity and mortality were determined primarily by gestational age and birthweight and not by abnormal fetal testing. Importantly, there is no convincing evidence that such testing schemes reduce the risk of long-term neurological deficits (American College of Obstetricians and Gynecologists, 2000a). A review of the status of Doppler velicometry to aid in delivery timing was provided by Baschat (2004). **The optimal management of the preterm growth-restricted fetus remains problematic**.

LABOR AND DELIVERY. Fetal growth restriction is commonly the result of placental insufficiency due to faulty maternal perfusion, ablation of functional placenta, or both. If present, these conditions are likely aggravated by labor. Importantly, diminished amnionic fluid volume increases the likelihood of cord compression during labor. For these reasons, a woman with a suspected growth-restricted fetus should undergo "high-risk" intrapartum monitoring, as discussed in Chapter 18 (see p. 465). The incidence of cesarean delivery is increased.

The infant may need expert assistance in making a successful transition at birth. The risk of being born hypoxic and of having aspirated meconium is increased. Care for the newborn should be provided immediately by someone who can skillfully clear the airway below the vocal cords and ventilate the infant as needed (see Chap. 28, p. 635). The severely growth-restricted newborn is particularly susceptible to hypothermia and may also develop other metabolic derangements such as hypoglycemia, polycythemia, and hyperviscosity. In addition, low-birthweight infants are at increased risk for motor and other neurological disabilities. Risk is highest at the lowest extremes of birthweight (Nelson and Grether, 1997).

LONG-TERM SEQUELAE. In his book *Fetal and Infant Origins of Adult Disease,* Barker (1992) hypothesizes that adult mortality and morbidity are related to fetal and infant health. In the context of fetal growth restriction, there are numerous reports of a relationship between suboptimal fetal nutrition and an increased risk of subsequent adult hypertension and atherosclerosis. However, recent reports challenge this hypothesis (Hubinette and colleagues, 2001; Huxley and co-workers, 2002). In another study, Smith and colleagues (2001) found that pregnancy complications resulting in low-birthweight infants were associated with increased risk of subsequent ischemic heart disease in the mother. This suggests that common genetic risk factors might explain the link between low birthweight and risk of heart disease in both the developing fetus and the mother.

MACROSOMIA

The term *macrosomia* is used rather imprecisely to describe a very large fetus or neonate. Although there is general agreement among obstetricians that newborns weighing less than 4000 g are not excessively large, a similar consensus has not been reached for the definition of macrosomia. Indeed, the term macrosomia does not appear in the *New Shorter Oxford English Dictionary* (1993), although *Stedman's Medical Dictionary* (1995) offers the definition of "abnormally large size of the body."

The key word is "abnormal." What is the threshold for the upper limit of normal human fetal growth above which birthweight is abnormal? Which criteria should be used to define "abnormal"? Specifically, should the threshold for abnormally high birthweight be simply mathematically derived or should it include features of adverse pregnancy outcome? Given that the major hazard of excessive fetal growth is birth injury due to shoulder dystocia, should the definition include the risk of brachial plexus injury? This approach would not entirely suffice to diagnose excessive growth because shoulder dystocia would not be expected in an overgrown but preterm and thus physically small infant.

Newborn weight rarely exceeds 11 pounds (5000 g), and excessively large infants are a curiosity. The birth of a 16-pound (7300 g) infant in the United States in 1979 was widely publicized. Two of the largest newborn weights ever recorded were those of a nearly 24-pound (10,800 g) infant described by Beach in 1879 (Barnes, 1957), and a 25-pound stillborn. Among over 216,000 singleton infants who were delivered at Parkland Hospital between 1988 and 2002, only two weighed 6000 g or more for an incidence of less than 1 in 100,000 births. One infant weighed 6025 g (13 lb 4 oz) and the other 6500 g (14 lb 5 oz). The incidence of excessively large infants has increased during the 20th century. For example, according to Williams (1903), the incidence of birthweight over 5000 g was 1 to 2 per 10,000 births at the beginning of the 20th century. This compares with 15 per 10,000 at Parkland Hospital from 1988 through 2002. The latter mothers had a mean BMI of 37.8 kg/cm^2, and 20 percent were diabetic.

DEFINITION. Precise definitions of macrosomia on which all authorities agree do not exist. However, there are several definitions in general clinical use. In one scheme, macrosomia is viewed as those weights that exceed certain percentiles for populations. Another common scheme includes use of empirical birthweights.

Birthweight Distribution. Commonly, macrosomia is defined based on mathematical distributions of birthweight. Those infants exceeding the 90th percentile for a given gestational week are usually used as the threshold for macrosomia.

TABLE 38–2 **Birthweight Distribution of 216,181 Infants Born at Parkland Hospital Between 1988 and 2002.**[a]

Birthweight (g)	Births		Maternal Diabetes (percent)
	Number	Percent	
500–3999	197,540	91.4	3
4000–4249	11,087	5.1	5
4250–4499	4,734	2.2	7
4500–4749	1,805	0.8	9
4750–4999	688	0.3	11
5000–5249	214	0.1	17
5250–5499	75	—	27
5500–5749	25	—	28
5750–5999	11	—	18
6000–6249	1[b]	—	100
6250–6449	0	—	—
6500	1[c]	—	100
Total	216,181	100	2.9

[a] Also shown is the association of birthweight with maternal diabetes.
[b] 6025-g infant (13 lb 4 oz) delivered by repeat cesarean at 38 weeks to a 329-lb diabetic woman.
[c] 6500-g infant (14 lb 5 oz) delivered by repeat cesarean at 43 weeks to a 5 ft 3 in, 250-lb, class A$_1$ diabetic woman.

For example, the 90th percentile at 39 weeks is 4000 g. If, however, birthweights two standard deviations above the mean are used, the threshold would be between the 97th and 99th percentile—substantially larger infants when compared with the 90th percentile. Specifically, the birthweight threshold at 39 weeks would be approximately 4500 g for the 97th percentile rather than 4000 g for the 90th percentile.

Empirical Birthweight. Absolute birthweight exceeding a specific threshold is another commonly used definition of macrosomia. Newborn weight exceeding 4000 g, or 8 lb 13 oz, is a frequently used threshold. Others use 4250 g or even 4500 g which is almost 10 lb. As shown in Table 38–2, birthweights of 4500 g or more are rare. Over a 12-year period at Parkland Hospital, during which time there were over 216,000 singleton births, only 1.25 percent of newborns weighed 4500 g or more. We are of the view that the upper limit of fetal growth, above which growth can be deemed abnormal, is likely two standard deviations above the mean, representing perhaps 3 percent of births. At 40 weeks such a threshold would correspond to approximately 4500 g. This definition of excessive growth is clearly more restrictive than using the upper 10 percent to define macrosomia. The American College of Obstetricians and Gynecologists (2000b) concluded that the term "macrosomia" was an appropriate designation for fetuses who, at birth, weigh 4500 g or more.

RISK FACTORS. Maternal diabetes is an important risk factor for development of fetal macrosomia (see Chap. 52,

p. 1173). As shown in Table 38–2, the incidence of maternal diabetes increases as birthweight above 4000 g increases. However, it should be emphasized that maternal diabetes is associated with only a small percentage of such large infants. Of the 13,805 infants in Table 38–2 who weighed 4000 g or more, only 6 percent were born to diabetic mothers. In macrosomic fetuses of diabetic women, there is a greater shoulder circumference and a greater shoulder circumference-to-head circumference ratio. Consequent to this is a greater risk of shoulder dystocia compared with that of similar weight fetuses of nondiabetic women (Modenlau and colleagues, 1982; Neiger, 1992; Sachs, 1993). Among macrosomic fetuses of similar weight, the presence of a relatively greater proportion of body fat is associated independently with an increased risk of labor dystocia and cesarean delivery (Bernstein and Catalano, 1994). Although known risk factors for macrosomia were identified by Boyd and associates (1983) in only 40 percent of women who deliver macrosomic infants, several factors favor the likelihood of a large fetus:

1. Large size of parents, especially the mother who is obese. The risk of fetal macrosomia is 30 percent if maternal weight is *more than* 300 pounds.
2. Multiparity.
3. Prolonged gestation.
4. Increased maternal age.
5. Male fetus.
6. Previous infant weighing more than 4000 g.
7. Race and ethnicity.

These factors are additive. Among women who are simultaneously diabetic, obese, and postterm, the incidence of fetal macrosomia ranges from 5 to 15 percent (Arias, 1987; Chervenak, 1992).

DIAGNOSIS. Because there are no current methods to estimate excessive fetal size accurately, the diagnosis of macrosomia cannot be definitely made until delivery. Inaccuracy in clinical estimates of fetal weight by physical examination is often attributable, at least in part, to maternal obesity. Numerous attempts have been made to improve the accuracy of fetal weight estimations obtained by ultrasonography. A number of formulas have been proposed to estimate fetal weight using ultrasonic measurements of the head, femur, and abdomen. The estimates provided by these computations, although reasonably accurate for predicting the weight of small, preterm fetuses, are less valid in predicting the weight of very large fetuses. For example, as shown in Figure 38–9, an infant predicted to weigh 4000 g can actually weigh considerably more or less than predicted. Rouse and co-authors (1996) reviewed 13 studies completed between 1985 and 1995 to assess ultrasonic prediction of macrosomic fetuses. They found only fair sensitivity (60 percent) in the accurate diagnosis of macrosomia but higher specificity (90 percent) in excluding excessive fetal size.

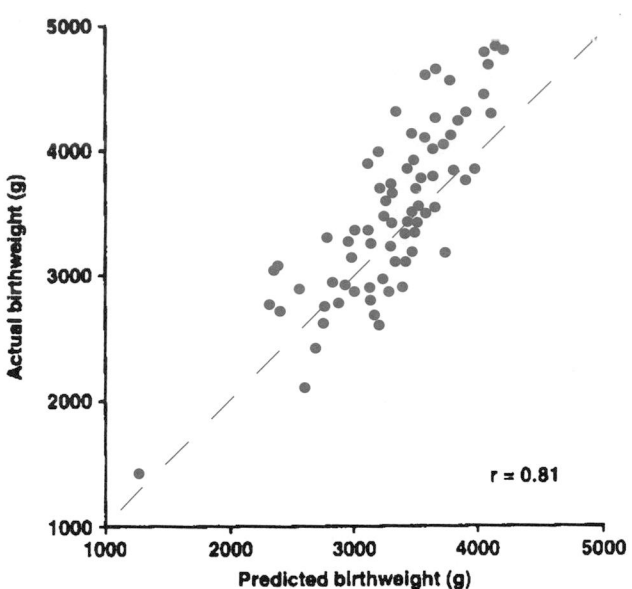

FIGURE 38-9. Relation between predicted and actual birthweight from ultrasound measurement of abdominal circumference within 7 days of delivery. (From Johnstone and colleagues, 1996, with permission.)

A formula has not been derived that gives estimates of fetal macrosomia with sufficiently accurate predictive value to be useful in constructing clinical management decisions (American College of Obstetricians and Gynecologists, 2000a). Not surprisingly, Adashek and colleagues (1996) found that women who underwent ultrasonic evaluation in the last 4 weeks of pregnancy were at significantly increased risk for cesarean delivery if the estimated fetal size exceeded 4000 g.

We can only conclude that the estimation of fetal weight from ultrasonic measurements is not reliable. Certainly its routine use to identify macrosomia cannot be recommended. Indeed, the findings of several studies are indicative that clinical estimates of fetal weight are as reliable as, or even superior to, those made from ultrasonic measurements (Sherman and colleagues, 1998).

CONTROVERSIES

"Prophylactic" Labor Induction. Some clinicians have proposed labor induction when fetal macrosomia is diagnosed in nondiabetic women. This obviates further fetal growth and thereby reduces potential delivery complications. Such prophylactic induction should theoretically reduce the risk of shoulder dystocia as well as that of cesarean delivery by preempting further fetal growth. Gonen and colleagues (1997) randomized 273 nondiabetic women with ultrasonic fetal weight estimates of 4000 to 4500 g to either induction or expectant management. Labor induction did not decrease the rate of cesarean delivery or shoulder dystocia. Similar results were reported by Leaphart and colleagues (1997)

with the added finding that induction unnecessarily increased the rate of cesarean delivery. We agree with the American College of Obstetricians and Gynecologists (2000b) that current evidence does not support a policy for early induction for suspected macrosomia.

Elective Cesarean Delivery. Rouse and colleagues (1996, 1999) analyzed the potential effects of a policy of elective cesarean delivery for ultrasonically diagnosed fetal macrosomia compared with standard obstetrical management. They concluded that for women who are not diabetic, a policy of elective cesarean delivery was medically and economically unsound. Conversely, in *diabetic* women with macrosomic fetuses, such a policy of elective cesarean delivery was tenable. Conway and Langer (1998) described a protocol of routine cesarean delivery for ultrasonic estimates of 4250 g or greater in diabetic women that significantly reduced the rate of shoulder dystocia from 2.4 to 1.1 percent.

Prevention of Shoulder Dystocia. A major concern in the delivery of macrosomic infants is shoulder dystocia and attendant risks of permanent brachial plexus palsy. Such dystocia occurs when the maternal pelvis is of sufficient size to permit delivery of the fetal head but not large enough to allow delivery of the larger-diameter fetal shoulders. In this circumstance, the anterior shoulder becomes impacted against the maternal symphysis pubis (see Chap. 20, p. 513). Even with expert obstetrical assistance at delivery, stretching and injury of the brachial plexus of the affected shoulder may be inevitable (see Chap. 29, p. 683). According to the American College of Obstetricians and Gynecologists (1997), fewer than 10 percent of all shoulder dystocia cases result in a persistent brachial plexus injury.

Planned cesarean delivery on the basis of suspected macrosomia is an unreasonable strategy in the *general population*. Ecker and colleagues (1997) analyzed 80 cases of brachial plexus injury in 77,616 consecutive infants born at Brigham and Women's Hospital. They concluded that an excessive number of otherwise unnecessary cesarean deliveries would be needed to prevent a single brachial plexus injury in infants born to women without diabetes. Conversely, planned cesarean delivery may be a reasonable strategy for diabetic women with an estimated fetal weight exceeding 4250 to 4500 g.

REFERENCES

Abrams B, Selvin S: Maternal weight gain pattern and birth weight. Obstet Gynecol 86:163, 1995

Adashek JA, Lagrew DC, Iriye BK, et al: The influence of ultrasound examination at term on the rate of cesarean section. Am J Obstet Gynecol 174:327, 1996

Alexander GR, Himes JH, Kaufman RB, et al: A United States national reference for fetal growth. Obstet Gynecol 87:163, 1996

Alexander GR, Kogan M, Bader D, et al: US birthweight/gestational age-specific neonatal mortality: 1995–1997 rates for whites, Hispanics and blacks. Pediatrics 111:e61, 2003

Alexander GR, Kogan MD, Himes JH, et al: Racial differences in birthweight for gestational age and infant mortality in extremely-low-risk US populations. Paediatr Perinat Epidemiol 13:205, 1999

American College of Obstetricians and Gynecologists: Fetal macrosomia. Practice Bulletin No. 22, November 2000a

American College of Obstetricians and Gynecologists: Intrauterine growth restriction. Practice Bulletin No. 12, January 2000b

American College of Obstetricians and Gynecologists: Shoulder dystocia. Practice Pattern No. 7, October 1997

Arbuckle TE, Wilkins R, Sherman GJ: Birth weight percentiles by gestational age in Canada. Obstet Gynecol 81:39, 1993

Arias F: Predictability of complications associated with prolongation of pregnancy. Obstet Gynecol 70:101, 1987

Barker DJP (ed): Fetal and Infant Origins of Adult Disease. London, BMJ Publishing, 1992.

Barnes AC: An obstetric record from the Medical Record. Obstet Gynecol 9:237, 1957

Baschat AA: Doppler application in the delivery timing of the preterm growth-restricted fetus: Another step in the right direction. Ultrasound Obstet Gynecol 23:111, 2004

Battaglia FC, Lubchenco LO: A practical classification of newborn infants by weight and gestational age. J Pediatr 71:159, 1967

Bernstein IM, Catalano PM: Examination of factors contributing to the risk of cesarean delivery in women with gestational diabetes. Obstet Gynecol 83:462, 1994

Blair E, Stanley F: Intrauterine growth and spastic cerebral palsy, 2. The association with morphology at birth. Early Hum Dev 28:91, 1992

Boyd ME, Usher PH, McLean FH: Fetal macrosomia: Prediction, risks and proposed management. Obstet Gynecol 61:715, 1983

Brenner WE, Edelman DA, Hendricks CH: A standard of fetal growth for the United States of America. Am J Obstet Gynecol 126:555, 1976

Brooks AA, Johnson MR, Steer PJ, et al: Birthweight: Nature or nurture? Early Hum Dev 2:29, 1995

Campbell S, Thoms A: Ultrasound measurement of the fetal head to abdomen circumference ratio in the assessment of growth retardation. Br J Obstet Gynaecol 84:165, 1977

Chervenak JL: Macrosomia in the postdates pregnancy. Clin Obstet Gynecol 35:161, 1992

Conway DL, Langer O: Elective delivery of infants with macrosomia in diabetic women: Reduced shoulder dystocia versus increased cesarean deliveries. Am J Obstet Gynecol 178:922, 1998

Crane JP, Kopta MM: Comparative newborn anthropometric data in symmetric versus asymmetric intrauterine growth retardation. Am J Obstet Gynecol 138:518, 1980

Cunningham FG, Cox SM, Harstad TW, et al: Chronic renal disease and pregnancy outcome. Am J Obstet Gynecol 163:453, 1990

Dashe JS, McIntire DD, Lucas MJ, et al: Impact of asymmetric versus symmetric fetal growth restriction on pregnancy outcomes. SGI abstract 96:321, 2000

Dejin-Karlsson E, Hanson BS, Ostergren P-O, et al: Association of a lack of psychosocial resources and the risk of giving birth to small for gestational age infants: A stress hypothesis. Br J Obstet Gynaecol 107:89, 2000

Deter RL, Nazar R, Milner LL: Modified neonatal growth assessment score: A multivariate approach to the detection of intrauterine growth retardation in the neonate. Ultrasound Obstet Gynecol 6:400, 1995

Dickey RP, Gasser RF: Ultrasound evidence of variability in the size and development of normal human embryos before the tenth post-insemination week after assisted reproductive technologies. Hum Reprod 8:331, 1993

Diket AL, Pierce MR, Munshi UK, et al: Nitric oxide inhibition causes intrauterine growth retardation and hind-limb disruptions in rats. Am J Obstet Gynecol 171:1243, 1994

Divon MY, Hsu HW: Maternal and fetal blood flow velocity waveforms in intrauterine growth retardation. Clin Obstet Gynecol 35:156, 1992

Droste S: Fetal growth in aneuploid conditions. Clin Obstet Gynecol 35:119, 1992

Droste S, Fitzsimmons J, Pascoe-Mason J, et al: Growth of linear parameters in trisomy 18 fetuses. Am J Obstet Gynecol 163:158, 1990

Duvekot JJ, Cheriex EC, Pieters FAA, et al: Maternal volume homeostasis in early pregnancy in relation to fetal growth restriction. Obstet Gynecol 85:361, 1995

Ecker JL, Greenberg JA, Norwitz ER, et al: Birthweight as a predictor of brachial plexus injury. Obstet Gynecol 89:643, 1997

Economides DL, Crook D, Nicolaides KH: Hypertriglyceridemia and hypoxemia in small-for-gestational-age fetuses. Am J Obstet Gynecol 162:387, 1990

Economides DL, Nicolaides KH: Blood glucose and oxygen tension levels in small-for-gestational-age fetuses. Am J Obstet Gynecol 160:385, 1989a

Economides DL, Nicolaides KH, Gahl WA, et al: Cordocentesis in the diagnosis of intrauterine starvation. Am J Obstet Gynecol 161:1004, 1989b

Economides DL, Proudler A, Nicolaides KH: Plasma insulin in appropriate- and small-for-gestational-age fetuses. Am J Obstet Gynecol 160:1091, 1989c

Emanuel I, Alberman HFE, Evans SJ: Intergenerational studies of human birthweight from the 1958 birth cohort, 1. Evidence for a multi-generational effect. Br J Obstet Gynaecol 99:67, 1992

Ewigman BG, Crane JP, Frigoletto FD, et al: Effect of prenatal ultrasonic screening on perinatal outcome. N Engl J Med 329:821, 1993

Fitzsimmons J, Droste S, Shepard T, et al: Growth failure in second trimester fetuses with trisomy 21. Teratology 42:337, 1990

Friedman SA, Schiff E, Kao L, et al: Neonatal outcome after preterm delivery for preeclampsia. Am J Obstet Gynecol 172:1785, 1995

Frigoletto F: Diagnostic Ultrasound Imaging in Pregnancy. Pub. No. 84667. Washington, DC, US Department of Health and Human Services, Public Health Service, National Institutes of Health, 1986

Gabriel R, Alsat E, Evion-Brion D: Alteration of epidermal growth factor receptor in placental membranes of smokers: Relationship with intrauterine growth retardation. Am J Obstet Gynecol 170:1238, 1994

Gainer J, Alexander J, Mcintire D, Leveno K: Fetal growth velocity in women who develop superimposed preeclampsia. Presented at the 25th Annual Meeting of the Society for Maternal-Fetal Medicine, Reno, Nevada, February 7–12, 2005

Gardosi J, Chang A, Kalyan B, et al: Customized antenatal growth charts. Lancet 339:283, 1992

Gardosi J, Francis A: Controlled trial of fundal height measurement plotted on customized antenatal growth charts. Br J Obstet Gynaecol 106:309, 1999

Gardosi J, Geirsson RT: Routine ultrasound is the method of choice for dating pregnancy. Br J Obstet Gynaecol 105:933, 1998

Gluckman PD, Liggins GC: Regulation of fetal growth. In Beard RW, Nathanielsz PW (eds): Fetal Physiology and Medicine: The Basis of Perinatology, 2nd ed. Rev. Vol 6 of Reproductive Medicine. New York, Marcel Dekker, 1984, p 511

Golbus MS: Development in the first half of gestation of genetically abnormal fetuses. Teratology 18:333, 1978

Gonen O, Rosen DJD, Dolfin Z, et al: Induction of labor versus expectant management in macrosomia: A randomized study. Obstet Gynecol 89:913, 1997

Grisaru-Granovsky S, Eitan R, Algur N, et al: Maternal and umbilical cord serum leptin concentrations in small-for-gestational-age and in appropriate-for-gestational-age neonates: A maternal, fetal, or placental contribution? Biol Neonate 84:67, 2003

Gruenwald P: Chronic fetal distress and placental insufficiency. Biol Neonate 5:215, 1963

Hecher K, Snijder R, Campbell S, et al: Fetal venous, intracardiac, and arterial blood flow measurements in intrauterine growth retardation: Relationship with fetal blood gases. Am J Obstet Gynecol 173:10, 1995

Heyborne KD, McGregor JA, Henry G, et al: Interleukin-10 in amniotic fluid at midtrimester: Immune activation and suppression in relation to fetal growth. Am J Obstet Gynecol 171:55, 1994

Holmes RP, Holly JMP, Soothill PW: A prospective study of maternal serum insulin-like growth factor-I in pregnancies with appropriately grown or growth restricted fetuses. Br J Obstet Gynaecol 105:1273, 1998

Howard RB: Control of human placental blood flow. Med Hypotheses 23:51, 1987

Hubinette A, Cnattingius S, Ekbom A, et al: Birthweight, early environment, and genetics: A study of twins discordant for acute myocardial infarction. Lancet 357:1997, 2001

Huxley R, Neil A, Collins R: Unraveling the fetal origins hypothesis: Is there really an inverse association between birthweight and subsequent blood pressure? Lancet 360:659, 2002

Infante-Rivard C, Rivard GE, Yotov WV, et al: Absence of association of thrombophilia polymorphisms with intrauterine growth restriction. N Engl J Med 347:19, 2002

Jensen OH, Larsen S: Evaluation of symphysis fundus measurements and weighing during pregnancy. Acta Obstet Gynecol Scand 70:13, 1991

Jimenez JM, Tyson JE, Reisch J: Clinical measurements of gestational age in normal pregnancies. Obstet Gynecol 61:438, 1983

Johnstone FD, Prescott RJ, Steel JM, et al: Clinical and ultrasound prediction of macrosomia in diabetic pregnancy. Br J Obstet Gynaecol 103:747, 1996

Jones JW, Gercel-Taylor C, Taylor DD: Altered cord serum lipid levels associated with small for gestational age infants. Obstet Gynecol 93:527, 1999

Kalousek DK, Langlois S, Barrett I, et al: Uniparental disomy for chromosome 16 in humans. Am J Hum Genet 52:8, 1993

Khoury MJ, Erickson JD, Cordero JF, et al: Congenital malformations and intrauterine growth retardation: A population study. Pediatrics 82:83, 1988

Kingdom JCP, McQueen J, Ryan G, et al: Fetal vascular atrial natriuretic peptide receptors in human placenta: Alteration in intrauterine growth retardation and preeclampsia. Am J Obstet Gynecol 170:142, 1994

Klebanoff MA, Schulsinger C, Mednick BR, et al: Preterm and small-for-gestational-age birth across generations. Am J Obstet Gynecol 176:521, 1997

Klein JO, Remington JS: Current concepts of infections of the fetus and newborn infant. In Remington JS, Klein JO (eds): Infectious Diseases of the Fetus and Newborn Infant, 4th ed. Philadelphia, Saunders, 1995, p 1

Kliegman RM: Intrauterine growth retardation. In Fanroff AA, Martin RJ (eds): Neonatal-Perinatal Medicine, 6th ed. New York, Mosby, 1997, p 203

Kok JH, den Ouden AL, Verloove-Vanhorick SP, et al: Outcome of very preterm small for gestational age infant: The first nine years of life. Br J Obstet Gynaecol 105:162, 1998

Kotini A, Avgidou K, Koutlaki N, et al: Correlation between biomagnetic and Doppler findings of umbilical artery in fetal growth restriction. Prenat Diagn 23:325, 2003

Krampl E: Pregnancy at high altitude. Ultrasound Obstet Gynecol 19:535, 2002

Laatikainen TJ, Raisanen IJ, Salminen KR: Corticotrophin-releasing hormone in amnionic fluid during gestation and labor and in relation to fetal lung maturation. Am J Obstet Gynecol 59:891, 1988

Larsen T, Larsen JF, Petersen S, et al: Detection of small-for-gestation-age fetuses by ultrasound screening in a high risk population: A randomized controlled study. Br J Obstet Gynaecol 99:469, 1992

Leaphart WL, Meyer MC, Capeless EL: Labor induction with a prenatal diagnosis of fetal macrosomia. J Matern Fetal Med 6:99, 1997

Lechtig A, Delgado H, Lasky RE, et al: Maternal nutrition and fetal growth in developing societies. Am J Dis Child 129:434, 1975

Levine JS, Branch DW, Rauch J: The antiphospholipid syndrome. N Engl J Med 346:752, 2002

Lichty JA, Ting RY, Bruns PD, et al: Studies of babies born at high altitude, 1. Relation of altitude to birth weight. Am J Dis Child 93:666, 1957

Lin CC, Evans MI: Introduction. In Lin CC, Evans MI (eds): Intrauterine Growth Retardation. New York, McGraw-Hill, 1984

Lin CC, Santolaya-Forgas J: Current concepts of fetal growth restriction: Part I. Causes, classification, and pathophysiology. Obstet Gynecol 92:1044, 1998

Lindor NM, Jalal SM, Thibedeau SM, et al: Mosaic trisomy 16 in a thriving infant: Maternal heterodisomy for chromosome 16. Clin Genet 44:185, 1993

Lockwood CJ: Inherited thrombophilias in pregnant patients: detection and treatment paradigm. Obstet Gynecol 99:333, 2002

Lockwood CJ, Rand JH: The immunobiology and obstetrical consequences of antiphospholipid antibodies. Obstet Gynecol Surv 49:432, 1994

Lubchenco LO, Hansman C, Dressler M, et al: Intrauterine growth as estimated from liveborn birth-weight data at 24 to 42 weeks of gestation. Pediatrics 32:793, 1963

Lunell NO, Nylund L: Uteroplacental blood flow. Clin Obstet Gynecol 35:108, 1992

Manning FA: Intrauterine growth retardation. In: Fetal Medicine. Principles and Practice. Norwalk, CT, Appleton & Lange, 1995, p 317

Manning FA, Hohler C: Intrauterine growth retardation: Diagnosis, prognostication, and management based on ultrasound methods. In Fleischer AC, Romero R, Manning FA, Jeanty P, James AE (eds): The Principles and Practices of Ultrasonography in Obstetrics and Gynecology, 4th ed. Norwalk, CT, Appleton & Lange, 1991, p 331

Martin JA, Hamilton BE, Ventura SJ, et al: Births: Final data for 2001. National Vital Statistics Reports Vol. 51, No. 1, 2002. Available at http://www.cdc.gov/nchs/data/nvsr/nvsr51/nvsr51_02.pdf

McIntire DD, Bloom SL, Casey BM, et al: Birthweight in relation to morbidity and mortality among newborn infants. N Engl J Med 340:1234, 1999

McKeown T, Record RG: Observations on foetal growth in multiple pregnancy in man. Endocrinology 8:386, 1952

McQueen J, Kingdom JCP, Connell JMC, et al: Fetal endothelin levels and placental vascular endothelin receptors in intrauterine growth retardation. Obstet Gynecol 82:992, 1993

Minior VK, Divon MY: Fetal growth restriction at term: Myth or reality? Obstet Gynecol 92:57, 1998

Modenlau HD, Komatsu G, Dorchester W, et al: Large for gestational age neonates: Anthropomorphic reasons for shoulder dystocia. Obstet Gynecol 60:417, 1982

Moerman P, Fryns JP, Goodeeris P, et al: Spectrum of clinical and autopsy findings in trisomy 18 syndrome. J Hum Genet 30:17, 1982

Neerhof MG: Causes of intrauterine growth restriction. Clin Perinatol 22:375, 1995

Neiger R: Fetal macrosomia in the diabetic patient. Clin Obstet Gynecol 35:138, 1992

Nelson KB, Grether JK: Cerebral palsy in low-birthweight infants: Etiology and strategies for prevention. Men Ret Dev Dis Res Rev 3:112, 1997

New Shorter Oxford English Dictionary. Brown L (ed). Oxford, Clarendon Press, 1993

Nicolaides KH, Peters MT, Vyas S, et al: Relation of rate of urine production to oxygen tension in small-for-gestational-age infants. Am J Obstet Gynecol 162:387, 1990

Nicolaides KH, Snijders RJM, Noble P: Cordocentesis in the study of growth-retarded fetuses. In Divon MY (ed): Abnormal Fetal Growth. New York, Elsevier, 1991

Odegard RA, Vatten LJ, Nilsen ST, et al: Preeclampsia and fetal growth. Obstet Gynecol 96:950, 2000

Ott W: Intrauterine growth retardation and preterm delivery. Am J Obstet Gynecol 168:710, 1993

Overpeck MD, Hediger ML, Zhang J, et al: Birthweight for gestational age of Mexican American infants born in the United States. Obstet Gynecol 93:943, 1999

Owen J, Baker SL, Hauth JC: Is indicated or spontaneous preterm delivery more advantageous for the fetus? Am J Obstet Gynecol 163:868, 1990

Owen P, Donnet ML, Ogston SA, et al: Standards for ultrasound fetal growth velocity. Br J Obstet Gynaecol 103:60, 1996

Owen P, Harrold AJ, Farrell T: Fetal size and growth velocity in the prediction of intrapartum cesarean section for fetal distress. Br J Obstet Gynaecol 104:445, 1997

Owen P, Khan KS: Fetal growth velocity in the prediction of intrauterine growth restriction in a low risk population. Br J Obstet Gynaecol 105:536, 1998

Owen P, Maharaj S, Khan KS, et al: Interval between fetal measurements in predicting growth restriction. Obstet Gynecol 97:499, 2001

Owen P, Ogah H, Bachmann LM, et al: Prediction of intrauterine growth restriction with customized estimated fetal weight centiles. Br J Obstet Gynaecol 110:411, 2003

Papageorghiou AT, Yu CKH, Bindra R, et al: Multicenter screening for pre-eclampsia and fetal growth restriction by transvaginal uterine artery Doppler at 23 weeks of gestation. Ultrasound Obstet Gynecol 18:441, 2001

Patton DE, Lee W, Cotton DB, et al: Cyanotic maternal heart disease in pregnancy. Obstet Gynecol Surv 45:594, 1990

Paz I, Gale R, Laor A, et al: The cognitive outcome of full-term small-for-gestational age infants at late adolescence. Obstet Gynecol 85:452, 1995

Perelman RH, Farrell PM, Engle MJ, et al: Development aspects of lung lipids. Annu Rev Physiol 47:803, 1985

Piper JM, Xenakis EMJ, McFarland M, et al: Do growth-retarded premature infants have different rates of perinatal morbidity and mortality than appropriate-grown premature infants? Obstet Gynecol 87:169, 1996

Pollack RN, Divon MY: Intrauterine growth retardation: Definition, classification and etiology. Clin Obstet Gynecol 35:99, 1992

Rankin JHG, McLaughlin MK: The regulation of the placental blood flows. J Dev Physiol 1:3, 1979

Roberts AB, Mitchele J, McCowan LM, et al: Ultrasonographic measurement of liver length in the small-for-gestational-age fetus. Am J Obstet Gynecol 180:634, 1999

Rochelson B, Kaplan C, Guzman E, et al: A quantitative analysis of placental vasculature in the third trimester fetus with autosomal trisomy. Obstet Gynecol 75:59, 1990

Ronzoni S, Marconi AM, Cetin I, et al: Umbilical amino acid uptake at increasing maternal amino acid concentrations: Effect of a maternal amino acid infusate. Am J Obstet Gynecol 181:477, 1999

Roth S, Abernathy MP, Lee WH, et al: Insulin-like growth factors I and II peptide and messenger RNA levels in macrosomic infants of diabetic pregnancies. J Soc Gynecol Investig 3:78, 1996

Rouse DJ, Owen J: Prophylactic cesarean delivery for fetal macrosomia diagnosed by means of ultrasonography—a Faustian bargain? Am J Obstet Gynecol 181:332, 1999

Rouse DJ, Owen J, Goldenberg RL, et al: The effectiveness and costs of elective cesarean delivery for fetal macrosomia diagnosed by ultrasound. JAMA 276:1480, 1996

Sachs DA: Fetal macrosomia and gestational diabetes: What's the problem? Obstet Gynecol 81:775, 1993

Salafia CM, Minior VK, Pezzullo JC, et al: Intrauterine growth restriction in infants of less than 32 weeks' gestation: Associated placental pathologic features. Am J Obstet Gynecol 173:1049, 1995

Seeds JW: Impaired fetal growth: Definition and clinical diagnosis. Obstet Gynecol 64:303, 1984

Sherman DJ, Arieli S, Tovbin J, et al: A comparison of clinical and ultrasonic estimations of fetal weight. Obstet Gynecol 91:212, 1998

Simpson JW, Lawless RW, Mitchell AC: Responsibility of the obstetrician to the fetus, 2. Influence of prepregnancy weight and pregnancy weight gain on birth weight. Obstet Gynecol 45:481, 1975

Sivan E, Whittaker PG, Sinha D, et al: Leptin in human pregnancy: The relationship with gestation hormones. Am J Obstet Gynecol 179:1128, 1998

Smith GCS, Pell JP, Walsh D: Pregnancy complications and maternal risk of ischaemic heart disease: A retrospective cohort study of 129,290 births. Lancet 357:2002, 2001

Smith GCS, Smith MFS, McNay MB, et al: First trimester growth and the risk of low birthweight. N Engl J Med 339:1817, 1998

Smith GCS, Smith MFS, McNay MB, et al: The relation between fetal abdominal circumference and birthweight: Findings in 3512 pregnancies. Br J Obstet Gynaecol 104:186, 1997

Smulian JC, Anauth CV, Martins ME, et al: Timing of infant death by gestational age at delivery in pregnancies complicated by intrauterine growth-restriction: A population based study. Am J Obstet Gynecol 182:S68, 2000

Snijders RJM, Nicolaides KJ: Fetal biometry at 14 to 40 weeks' gestation. Ultrasound Obstet Gynecol 4:34, 1994

Soothill PW, Nicolaides KH, Campbell S: Prenatal asphyxia, hyperlacticaemia, hypoglycaemia and erythroblastosis in growth retarded fetuses. BMJ 294:1046, 1987

Stagno S, Reynolds DW, Hwang ES: Congenital cytomegalovirus infection. N Engl J Med 296:1254, 1977

Stedman's Medical Dictionary, 26th ed. Spraycar M (ed). Baltimore, Williams & Wilkins, 1995, p 1052

Steer P: Fetal growth. Br J Obstet Gynaecol 105:1133, 1998

Stein Z, Susser M, Saenger G, et al: In Famine and Human Development: The Dutch Hunger Winter of 1944–1945. New York, Oxford University Press, 1975

Stephens TD, Shepard TH: The Down syndrome in the fetus. Teratology 22:37, 1980

Stettler RW, Cunningham FG: Natural history of chronic proteinuria complicating pregnancy. Am J Obstet Gynecol 167:1219, 1992

Tamura T, Goldenberg RL, Johnston KE, et al: Serum leptin concentrations during pregnancy and their relationship to fetal growth. Obstet Gynecol 91:389, 1998

Thelander HE, Pryor HB: Abnormal patterns of growth and development in mongolism. Clin Pediatr 5:493, 1966

Thornton JG, Hornbuckle J, Vail A, et al, GRIT study group: Infant wellbeing at 2 years of age in the Growth Restriction Intrvention Trial (GRIT): Multicentred randomised controlled trial. Lancet 364:483, 2004

Tovi SM, Kanety H, Schiff E, et al: Quantitative and qualitative changes in adiponectin during pregnancy in AGA and IUGR newborns. Presented at the 25th Annual Meeting of the Society for Maternal-Fetal Medicine, Reno, Nevada, February 7–12, 2005a

Tovi SM, Kanety H, Schiff E, et al: A putative novel biochemical marker of fetal growth. Presented at the 25th Annual Meeting of the Society for Maternal-Fetal Medicine, Reno, Nevada, February 7–12, 2005b

Towner DR, Shaffer LG, Yang SP, et al: Confined placental mosaicism for trisomy 14 and maternal uniparental disomy in association with elevated second trimester maternal serum human chorionic gonadotrophin and third trimester fetal growth restriction. Prenat Diag 21: 395, 2001

Tyson JE, Kennedy K, Broyles S, et al: The small for gestational age infant: Accelerated or delayed pulmonary maturation? Increased or decreased survival? Pediatrics 95:534, 1995

Usher R, McLean F: Intrauterine growth of live-born Caucasian infants at sea level: Standards obtained from measurements in 7 dimensions of infants born between 25 and 44 weeks' gestation. J Pediatr 74:901, 1969

Vaessen N, Janssen JA, Heutlink P, et al: Association between genetic variation in the gene for insulin-like growth factor-I and low birth weight. Lancet 359:1036, 2002

Varner MW, Dildy GA, Hunter BS, et al: Amniotic fluid epidermal growth factor levels in normal and abnormal pregnancies. J Soc Gynecol Investing 3:17, 1996

Varner MW, Galask RP: Infectious causes. In Linc CC, Evans MI (eds): Intrauterine Growth Retardation. New York, McGraw-Hill, 1984

Ventura SJ, Martin JA, Curtin SC, et al: Births: Final Data for 1997. National Vital Statistics Reports, Vol 47, No. 18. Hyattsville, MD, National Center for Health Statistics, 1999

Verhaeghe J, VanBree R, VanHerck E, et al: C-peptide, insulin-like growth factors I & II, and insulin-like growth factor binding protein-1 in umbilical cord serum: Correlations with birthweight. Am J Obstet Gynecol 169:89, 1993

Walraven GEL, Mkanje RJB, van Roosmalen J, et al: Single pre-delivery symphysis-fundal height measurement as a predictor of birthweight and multiple pregnancy. Br J Obstet Gynaecol 102:525, 1995

Warkany JB, Monroe B, Sutherland BSS: Intrauterine growth retardation. Am J Dis Child 102:24, 1961

Waterson AP: Viral infections (other than rubella) during pregnancy. BMJ 2:564, 1979

Weiner Z, Divon MY, Katz VK, et al: Multivariate analysis of antepartum fetal tests in predicting neonatal outcome of growth retarded fetus. Am J Obstet Gynecol 174:339, 1996

Wilcox MA, Smith SJ, Johnson IR, et al: The effect of social deprivation on birthweight, excluding physiological and pathological effects. Br J Obstet Gynaecol 102:918, 1995

Williams JW: Obstetrics: A Text-Book for Students and Practitioners, 1st ed. New York, Appleton, 1903, p 133

Williams RL: Intrauterine growth curves. Intra- and international comparisons with different ethnic groups in California. Prev Med 4:163, 1975

Williams RL, Creasy RK, Cunningham GC, et al: Fetal growth and perinatal viability in California. Obstet Gynecol 59:624, 1982

Xiong X, Mayes D, Demianczuk N, et al: Impact of pregnancy-induced hypertension on fetal growth. Am J Obstet Gynecol 180:207, 1999

39

Multifetal Gestation

The number and rate of twin and other higher-order multiple births have increased in the United States at an unprecedented pace over the past two decades (Martin and colleagues, 2002). This increase has been fueled largely by infertility therapy (Jewell and Yip, 1995). Between 1980 and 2001, the number of twin deliveries rose 77 percent, and the number of higher-order multiple births soared 459 percent (Fig. 39–1). The rate of twin births continues to increase, and the number of higher-order multiple births has plateaued. In contrast, the singleton birth rate rose only 11 percent during the same time period. More than 3 percent of all neonates born in the United States are now the product of a multiple gestation (Martin and colleagues, 2002).

This extraordinary increase in multiple births is a public health concern; the higher rate of preterm delivery of these neonates compromises their survival chances and increases their risk of lifelong disability. Powers and Kiely (1994)

evaluated birth and death certificates of neonates in the United States from 1985 and 1986 to measure the impact of twinning on national neonatal morbidity and mortality rates. Although twins accounted for only 1 in 94 pregnancies, they accounted for 14 percent of low-birthweight neonates and 11 percent of neonatal deaths. Similarly, at Parkland Hospital in 2002, twin neonates represented only 1 in 100 delivered neonates and yet accounted for 1 in 12 perinatal deaths (Table 39–1).

In addition to the perinatal mortality and morbidity attributable to preterm delivery, fetuses in multiple gestations are vulnerable to a variety of complications such as malformations and twin-to-twin transfusion syndrome. Maternal complications are also increased with multiple gestations. Conde-Agudelo and co-workers (2000) studied more than 15,000 twin pregnancies and found that the risks of preeclampsia, postpartum hemorrhage, and maternal death were increased twofold.

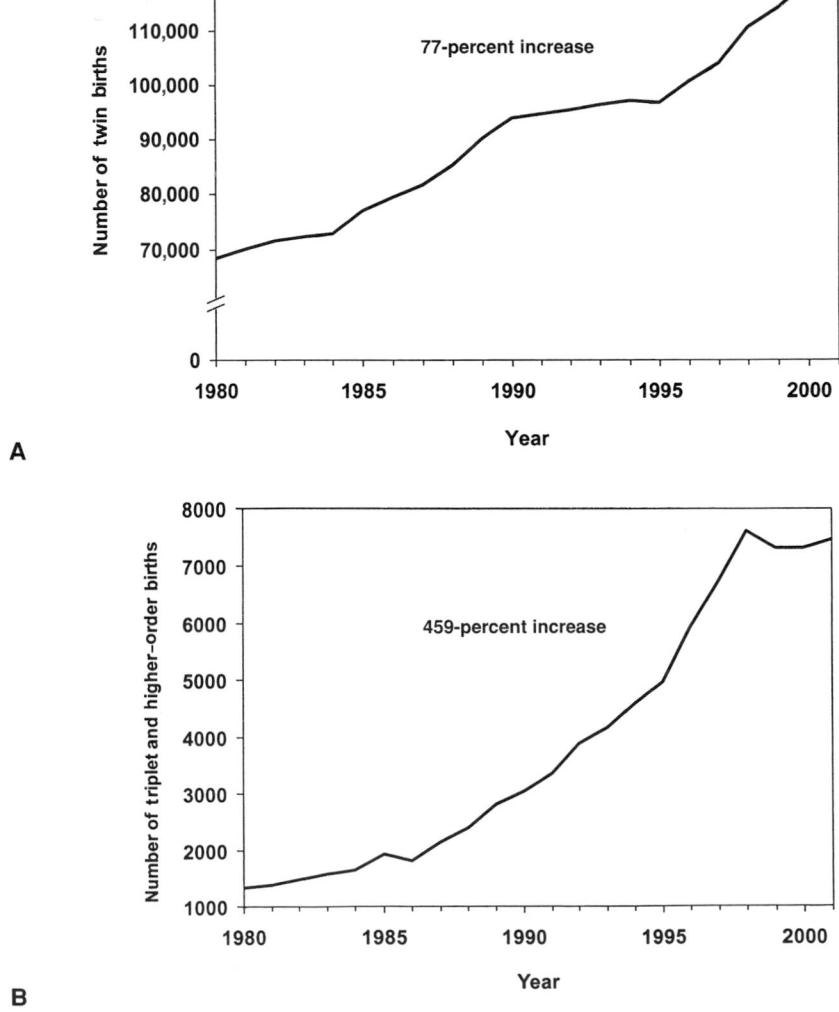

FIGURE 39–1. Number of twin **(A)** and triplet or higher-order multiple births **(B)**, United States, 1980–2001. (From Martin and colleagues, 2002; Martin and Park, 1999.)

TABLE 39–1 Selected Outcomes in Singleton and Twin Pregnancies Delivered at Parkland Hospital in 2002

Outcome	Singletons	Twins
Pregnancies delivered	15,518	155
Births	15,518	310
Stillbirths (per 1000)	82 (5.3)	5 (16.1)
Neonatal deaths (per 1000)	43 (2.8)	6 (19.7)
Perinatal deaths (per 1000)	125 (8.1)	11 (35.5)
Very-low-birthweight (< 1500 g)	1.0%	11.2%

ETIOLOGY OF MULTIPLE FETUSES

Twin fetuses commonly result from fertilization of two separate ova and are termed double-ovum, dizygotic, or fraternal twins. About a third as often, twins arise from a single fertilized ovum that subsequently divides into two similar structures, each with the potential for developing into a separate individual. These twins are termed single-ovum, monozygotic, or identical twins. Either or both processes may be involved in the formation of higher numbers of fetuses. Quadruplets, for example, may arise from as few as one to as many as four ova.

Fraternal Versus Identical Twins. Dizygotic twins are not in a strict sense true twins because they result from the maturation and fertilization of two ova during a single ovulatory cycle (Fig. 39–2). Also, monozygotic or identical twins are usually not identical. As discussed subsequently, the process of division of one fertilized zygote into two does not necessarily result in equal sharing of protoplasmic materials. Furthermore, the process of monozygotic twinning is in a sense a teratogenic event, and monozygotic twins have an increased incidence of often discordant malformations. In fact, dizygotic or fraternal twins of the same sex may appear more nearly identical at birth than monozygotic twins, and growth of monozygotic twin fetuses may be discordant, at times dramatically so.

Genesis of Monozygotic Twins. Evidence regarding the physiological basis of monozygotic twinning now suggests

that the division of the fertilized ovum may result from a delay in the timing of normal developmental events. In humans, delayed ovum transport through the fallopian tube increases the risk of twinning. Because progestational agents and combination contraceptives decrease tubal motility, delayed tubal transport and implantation are believed to increase the risk of twinning in pregnancies conceived in close temporal proximity to contraceptive use (Bressers and colleagues, 1987). Minor trauma to the blastocyst during assisted reproductive technology (ART) may possibly lead to the increased incidence of monozygotic twinning observed in pregnancies conceived in this manner (Wenstrom and co-workers, 1993).

The outcome of the twinning process depends on when the division occurs:

- If division occurs within the first 72 hours after fertilization, the inner cell mass (morula) has yet to form and the outer layer of blastocyst has not yet committed to become chorion. Two embryos, two amnions, and two chorions develop, and a monozygotic, diamnionic, dichorionic twin pregnancy evolves (Fig. 39–3). Two distinct placentas or a single fused placenta may develop (Fig. 39–4).
- If division occurs between the fourth and eighth day, the inner cell mass has formed and cells destined to become chorion have already differentiated, but those of the amnion have not. From this division, two embryos develop, each in a separate amnionic sac covered by a common chorion. This division gives rise to a monozygotic, diamnionic, monochorionic twin pregnancy (see Fig. 39–4C).
- If, however, the chorion and the amnion have already differentiated, by about 8 days after fertilization, division results in two embryos within a common amnionic sac, a monozygotic, monoamnionic, monochorionic twin pregnancy.
- If division is initiated even later, that is, after the embryonic disk has formed, cleavage is incomplete and conjoined twins result.

It has long been accepted that monochorionicity incontrovertibly indicated monozygosity. Rarely, however, monochorionic twins may in fact be dizygotic (Souter and colleagues, 2003). How this could happen is a matter of speculation, but it may result from the zygotic manipulations that accompany ART (Redline, 2003).

Superfetation and Superfecundation. In superfetation, an interval as long as or longer than a menstrual cycle intervenes between fertilizations. Superfetation requires ovulation and fertilization during the course of an established pregnancy, which would theoretically be possible until the uterine cavity is obliterated by the fusion of the decidua capsularis to the decidua vera. Although known to occur in mares, superfetation is as yet unproven to occur in humans. Most authorities believe that the alleged cases of human superfetation result from marked inequality in growth and development of twin fetuses of the same gestational age.

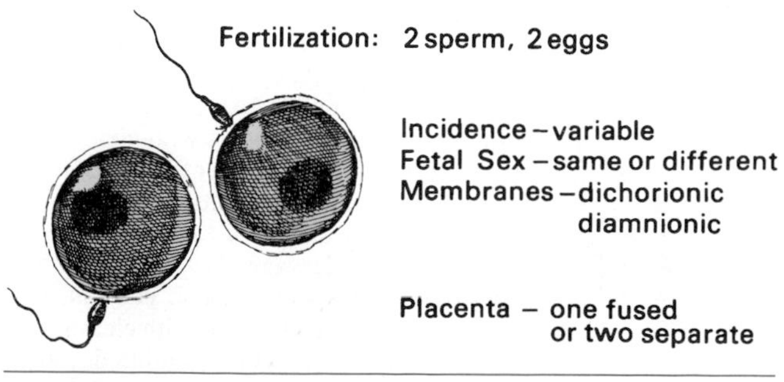

Fertilization: 2 sperm, 2 eggs

Incidence – variable
Fetal Sex – same or different
Membranes – dichorionic
             diamnionic

Placenta – one fused
         or two separate

FIGURE 39–2. Mechanism of dizygotic twinning.

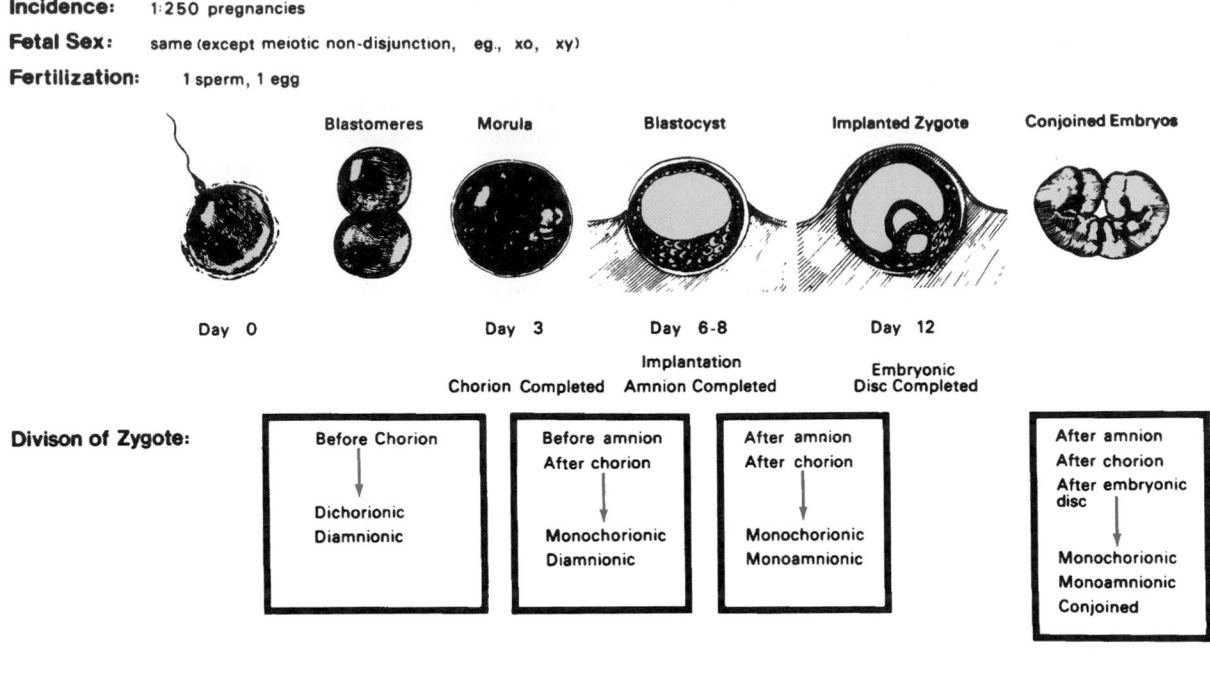

Incidence: 1:250 pregnancies

Fetal Sex: same (except meiotic non-disjunction, eg., xo, xy)

Fertilization: 1 sperm, 1 egg

FIGURE 39–3. Mechanism of monozygotic twinning.

Superfecundation refers to the fertilization of two ova within the same menstrual cycle but not at the same coitus, nor necessarily by sperm from the same male. An instance of superfecundation, documented by Harris (1982), is demonstrated in Figure 39–5. The mother was sexually assaulted on the 10th day of her menstrual cycle and had intercourse 1 week later with her husband. She was delivered of a black neonate whose blood type was A and a white neonate whose blood type was O. The blood type of both the mother and her husband was O. Terasaki and co-workers (1978) described the use of HLA typing to establish that a specific set of dizygotic twins were sired by different fathers.

Frequency of Twins. The frequency of monozygotic twin births is relatively constant worldwide, at approximately one set per 250 births, and is largely independent of race, heredity, age, and parity. The frequency was once thought to be independent of infertility therapy, however, there is now evidence that the incidence of zygotic splitting is increased following ART. The incidence of dizygotic twinning, however, is influenced remarkably by race, heredity, maternal age, parity, and especially, fertility drugs.

THE "VANISHING TWIN." Advanced technology has improved ultrasonographic studies of early gestations. These studies show that the first-trimester incidence of twins is much greater than the incidence of twins at birth. Monochorionic twins have a significantly greater risk of abortion than dichorionic twins (Sebire and colleagues, 1997). In some cases, the entire pregnancy aborts. In many cases, however, only one fetus dies, and the remaining fetus delivers as a singleton. Undoubtedly, some threatened abortions have resulted in actual

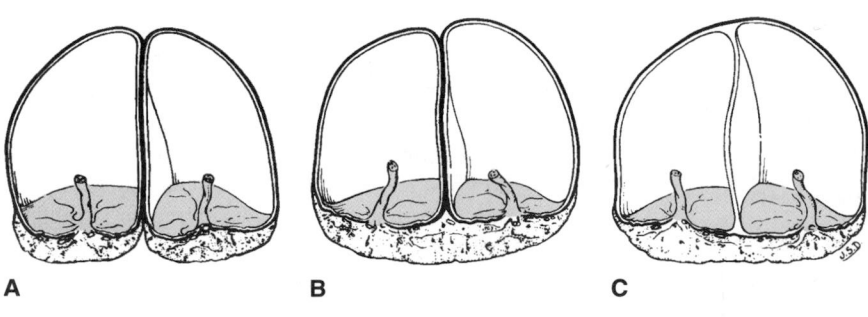

FIGURE 39–4. Placenta and membranes in twin pregnancies. **A.** Two placentas, two amnions, two chorions (from either dizygotic twins or monozygotic twins with cleavage of zygote during first 3 days after fertilization). **B.** Single placenta, two amnions, and two chorions (from either dizygotic twins or monozygotic twins with cleavage of zygote during first 3 days). **C.** One placenta, one chorion, two amnions (monozygotic twins with cleavage of zygote from the fourth to the eighth day after fertilization).

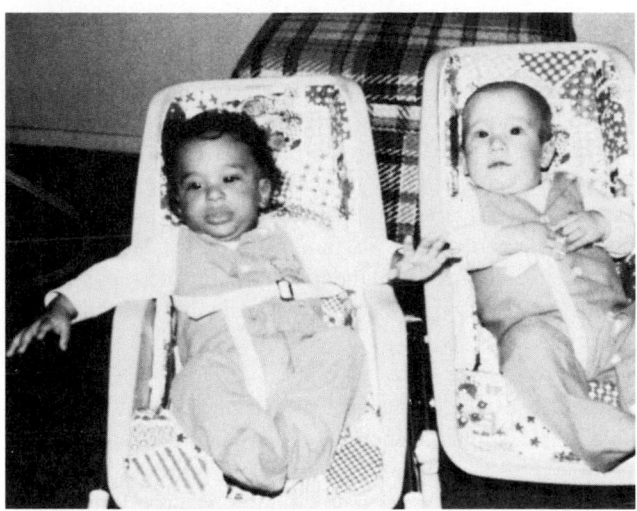

FIGURE 39–5. An example of dizygotic twin boys as the consequence of superfecundation. (Courtesy of Dr. David Harris.)

abortion of one embryo from an unrecognized twin gestation while the other embryo continued its growth and development (Jauniaux and co-workers, 1988). Studies in which fetuses were evaluated with ultrasonography in the first trimester have shown that one twin is lost or "vanishes" before the second trimester in 21 to 63 percent of spontaneous twin conceptions (Dickey, 2002; Kol, 1993; Landy, 1986; Parisi, 1983, and all their co-workers).

Dickey and colleagues (2002) described outcomes following spontaneous reduction of a multifetal pregnancy. Prior to 12 weeks, one or more embryos died in 36 percent of twin pregnancies, 53 percent of triplet pregnancies, and 65 percent of quadruplet pregnancies. Interestingly, pregnancy duration and birthweight were inversely related to the initial gestational sac number regardless of the final number of fetuses at delivery. This effect was most pronounced in twins who started as quadruplets. Others have not found this (Yaron and associates, 1999).

A vanishing twin may cause an elevated serum maternal serum alpha-fetoprotein level, an elevated amnionic fluid alpha-fetoprotein level, and a positive amnionic fluid acetylcholinesterase assay (Winsor and associates, 1987). It is important, therefore, to establish the diagnosis of vanishing twin, because this may complicate maternal serum screening for Down syndrome or for neural-tube defects. Similarly, the vanishing twin can cause a discrepancy between the karyotype established by chorionic villus sampling and the karyotype of the surviving twin when tissue from the vanished twin is inadvertently sampled. For these reasons, amniocentesis for karyotype may be preferable (Reddy and associates, 1991).

RACE. The frequency of multifetal births varies significantly among different races and ethnic groups (Table 39–2). Myrianthopoulos (1970) identified the birth of twins in 1 of every

TABLE 39–2 **Twinning Rates per 1000 Births by Zygosity**

Country	Monozygotic	Dizygotic	Total
Nigeria	5.0	49	54
United States			
Black	4.7	11.1	15.8
White	4.2	7.1	11.3
England and Wales	3.5	8.8	12.3
India (Kolkata)	3.3	8.1	11.4
Japan	3.0	1.3	4.3

From MacGillivray, 1986, with permission.

100 pregnancies among white women, compared with 1 of 80 pregnancies for black women. In some areas of Africa, the frequency of twinning is high. Knox and Morley (1960), in a survey of one rural community in Nigeria, found that twinning occurred once in every 20 births! These marked differences in twinning frequency may be the consequence of racial variations in the levels of follicle-stimulating hormone (FSH) (Nylander, 1973).

HEREDITY. As a determinant of twinning, the family history of the mother is much more important than that of the father. White and Wyshak (1964), in a study of 4000 genealogical records of the General Society of the Church of Jesus Christ of Latter-day Saints, found that women who themselves were a dizygotic twin gave birth to twins at the rate of 1 set per 58 births. Women who were not a twin, but whose husbands were a dizygotic twin, gave birth to twins at the rate of 1 set per 116 pregnancies. One explanation is that the tendency to release multiple ova is inherited. A Belgian–Dutch group has reported that dizygotic twinning may be influenced by an autosomal dominant gene carried by approximately 15 percent of the population (Meulemans and colleagues, 1996). If true, this gene may exert its effects only in women.

MATERNAL AGE AND PARITY. The rate of natural twinning rises from 0 at puberty, a time of minimal ovarian activity, to a peak at 37 years of age, when maximal hormonal stimulation increases the rate of double ovulation (Bulmer, 1959). This is in accordance with the first consistently observed sign of reproductive aging, an isolated rise in serum FSH (Klein and co-workers, 1996). The fall in incidence after 37 years of age probably reflects depletion of the Graafian follicles.

Increasing maternal age and parity have been shown to increase the incidence of twinning independently in all populations studied. Waterhouse demonstrated that twin pregnancies were a third as common in women younger than 20 years of age with no previous children, compared with women 35 to 40 years of age with four or more previous children (1950). In Sweden, Pettersson and associates (1976) determined that the frequency of multiple fetuses in first pregnancies was 1.3 percent, compared with 2.7 percent in the fourth pregnancy. In Nigeria, Azubuike (1982) showed that the frequency of twinning increased from 1 in 50 pregnancies (2 percent) among women pregnant for the first time to 1 in 15 (6.6 percent) for women pregnant six or more times!

NUTRITIONAL FACTORS. In animals, the litter size increases in proportion to nutritional sufficiency. Evidence from a variety of sources indicates that this occurs in humans as well. Nylander (1971) showed a definite increasing gradient in the twinning rate related to greater nutritional status as reflected by maternal size. Taller, heavier women had a twinning rate 25 to 30 percent greater than short, nutritionally deprived women. MacGillivray (1986) also found that dizygotic twinning is more common in large and tall women than in small women. Evidence acquired during and after World War II showed that twinning correlated more with nutrition than body size. Widespread undernourishment in Europe during those years was associated with a marked fall in the dizygotic twinning rate (Bulmer, 1959).

PITUITARY GONADOTROPIN. The common factor linking race, age, weight, and fertility to multifetal gestation may be FSH levels (Benirschke and Kim, 1973). This theory is supported by the fact that increased fecundity and a higher rate of dizygotic twinning have been reported in women who conceive within 1 month after stopping oral contraceptives, but not during subsequent months (Rothman, 1977). This may be due to the sudden release of pituitary gonadotropin in amounts greater than usual during the first spontaneous cycle after stopping hormonal contraception.

INFERTILITY THERAPY. The induction of ovulation by use of FSH plus chorionic gonadotropin or clomiphene citrate remarkably enhances the likelihood of multiple ovulations. The incidence of multifetal gestation following conventional gonadotropin therapy is 16 to 40 percent, 75 percent of which are twins (Schenker and co-workers, 1981). Tuppin and colleagues (1993) reported that in France, the incidence of twin and triplet deliveries and the sale of human menopausal gonadotropin (hMG) rose in parallel between 1972 and 1989. By 1989, half of triplet pregnancies resulted from ovulation induction. Superovulation therapy, which increases the chance of pregnancy by recruiting multiple follicles, results in multifetal gestation rates of 25 to 30 percent (Bailey-Pridham and associates, 1990).

Risk factors for multiple fetuses after ovarian stimulation with hMG include increased estradiol levels on the day of chorionic gonadotropin injection and sperm characteristics such as increased concentration and motility (Dickey and associates, 1992; Pasqualotto and colleagues, 1999). With recognition of these factors plus the ability to monitor follicular growth and size ultrasonographically, physicians may cancel cycles likely to lead to a multifetal gestation. This approach has reduced the incidence of multiple births. Previously, clomiphene therapy was associated with a lower incidence of multifetal gestation compared with hMG use.

Researchers speculate that judicious management of hMG-stimulated ovaries has decreased the incidence of these pregnancies. The majority of multifetal gestations resulting from ovulation induction are currently caused by clomiphene citrate (Rein and colleagues, 1990).

Ovulation induction increases both dizygotic and monozygotic twinning. Derom and colleagues (1987) studied the incidence of monozygotic twinning in almost 1000 pairs of twins delivered in East Flanders, Belgium, and reported that the incidence of zygotic splitting was doubled after induced ovulation.

Assisted Reproductive Technology. Techniques such as ART, which are designed to increase the probability of pregnancy, increase the probability of multifetal gestation as well. Typically, patients undergo superovulation, in vitro fertilization is attempted in all retrieved ova, and two to four embryos are transferred to the uterus. In general, the greater the number of embryos that are transferred, the greater the risk of twins and of higher-order multiple gestation.

Higher-order multiple gestation confers significant risk to both mother and fetuses and reduces the chances of both a live birth and the birth of a child without significant handicap. The only remedy is a selective reduction procedure, which also increases fetal risk. In addition, higher-order multiple gestation is financially costly. Goldfarb and colleagues (1996) estimated the combined costs of in vitro fertilization plus prenatal care and delivery totalled $39,249 for singletons or twins, and this increased to $342,788 for triplets or higher-order multiple gestation. Most of the costs for singletons or twins were attributed to in vitro fertilization, whereas most of the costs with triplets or more were due to neonatal intensive care.

Reducing Multiple Gestation. The American Society for Reproductive Medicine (1999) has initiated a concerted effort to reduce the incidence of higher-order multiple gestation because of associated morbidity and mortality. In their recent review, Jain and colleagues (2004) cited the consistent decreases in both the number of embryos transferred per cycle and the percentage of pregnancies with three or more fetuses (see Fig. 39–1B). Concurrently, there also has been a consistent increase in the percentage of live births per cycle. This has occurred for a number of reasons. For example, culturing embryos for 5 days to the blastocyst stage allowed identification of the most viable blastocysts and an acceptable chance of pregnancy implantation with a transfer of fewer embryos (Scholtes and Zeilmaker, 1996). Two-embryo transfer for women with a good prognosis for conception has been advocated as a way to maintain a high pregnancy implantation rate while decreasing the number of higher-order multiple gestations (Meldrum and Gardner, 1998). Data analyzed by Ozturk and Templeton (2002) from 27,230 ART cycles supported this approach. Two-embryo transfer was associated with a decreased rate of triplet birth but an equivalent overall live birth rate compared with the rate when more embryos were transferred. Kovacs and colleagues (2003) analyzed 2606 fresh embryo transfers and reported that transfer of only one embryo achieved a pregnancy rate similar to that with transfer of two. Conservative gonadotropin stimulation has proved of limited value (Gleicher and colleagues, 2000). These issues were reviewed recently by Adashi (2004) as well as Templeton (2004).

Sex Ratios with Multiple Fetuses. In humans, as the number of fetuses per pregnancy increases, the percentage of male conceptuses decreases. Strandskov and co-workers (1946) found the percentage of males for 31 million singleton births in the United States to be 51.6 percent. For twins, it was 50.9 percent; for triplets, 49.5 percent; and for quadruplets, 46.5 percent. An even greater number of females in twins result from late twinning events.

Seventy percent of monochorionic–monoamnionic twins and 75 percent of conjoined twins are female (Machin, 1996). Two explanations have been offered. First, there is a well-known differential fetal mortality between the sexes, which persists for the newborn, child, and adult. Generally, mortality rates are lower in females. Nutritional and space limitations associated with multiple fetuses in utero may exaggerate this biological tendency. Second, genetically female zygotes have a greater tendency to divide into twins or higher multiples.

Determination of Zygosity. The main reason to determine zygosity antenatally is that it can aid obstetrical risk assessment and guide management of multifetal gestation (Fisk and Bryan, 1993). The rate of twin-specific complications varies in relation to zygosity (Table 39–3). Clearly, monochorionic twin gestations are at increased risk for a variety of pregnancy complications, some of which may be minimized by early antepartum recognition.

Determination of zygosity frequently requires sophisticated genetic tests because dizygotic twins can look alike, whereas monozygotic twins are not always identical. Monozygotic twins may actually be discordant for genetic

mutations as the result of a postzygotic mutation, or may have the same genetic disease but with marked variability in expression. In female fetuses, skewed lyonization can produce differential expression of X-linked traits or diseases.

Most interestingly, monozygotic twins may be discordant for malformations that involve asymmetrical organs, for example, the heart (Machin, 1996).

Ultrasonographic Evaluation. Chorionicity can be determined ultrasonographically as early as the first trimester. The presence of two separate placentas and a thick—generally 2 mm or greater—dividing membrane (Fig. 39–6A) supports the presumption of the diagnosis of dichorionicity. Fetuses of opposite gender are almost always dizygotic (Mahony and co-workers, 1985).

In pregnancies in which a single placental mass is identified, it may be difficult to distinguish one large placenta from two placentas lying side by side or "fused." Examining the point of origin of the dividing membrane on the placental surface may clarify this situation. If a triangular projection of placental tissue is seen to extend beyond the chorionic surface between the layers of the dividing membrane, then two fused placentas are actually present (see Fig. 39–6). This finding is termed the "twin-peak" sign.

Monochorionic pregnancies have a dividing membrane that is so thin it may not be seen until the second trimester. The membrane is generally less than 2 mm in thickness, and magnification reveals only two layers (Scardo and associates, 1995). This right-angle relationship between the membranes and placenta with no apparent extension of placenta between the dividing membrane is called the "T" sign. Ultrasonographic evaluation of the dividing membrane is easiest and most accurate in the first half of pregnancy, because the fetuses are smaller (Stagiannis and colleagues, 1995) (Fig. 39–7).

Scardo and colleagues (1995) used the combination of placental location, dividing membrane thickness, presence or absence of the "twin-peak" sign, and fetal gender to determine

TABLE 39–3 Overview of the Incidence of Twin Pregnancy Zygosity and Corresponding Twin-Specific Complications

Type of Twinning	Twins	Twin-Specific Complication (percent)			
		Fetal Growth Restriction	Preterm Delivery[a]	Placental Vascular Anastomosis	Perinatal Mortality
Dizygotic	80	25	40	0	10–12
Monozygotic	20	40	50		15–18
Diamnionic/dichorionic	6–7	30	40	0	18–20
Diamnionic/monochorionic	13–14	50	60	100	30–40
Monoamnionic/monochorionic	< 1	40	60–70	80–90	58–60
Conjoined	0.002–0.008	—	70–80	100	70–90

[a] Delivery before 37 weeks.
Modified from Manning, 1995, with permission.

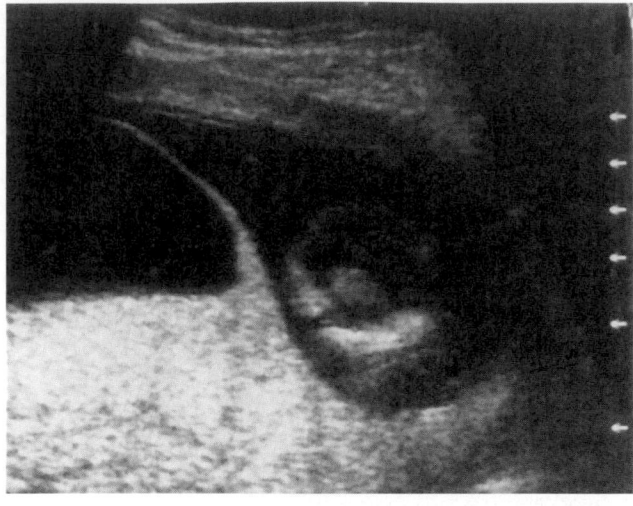

A

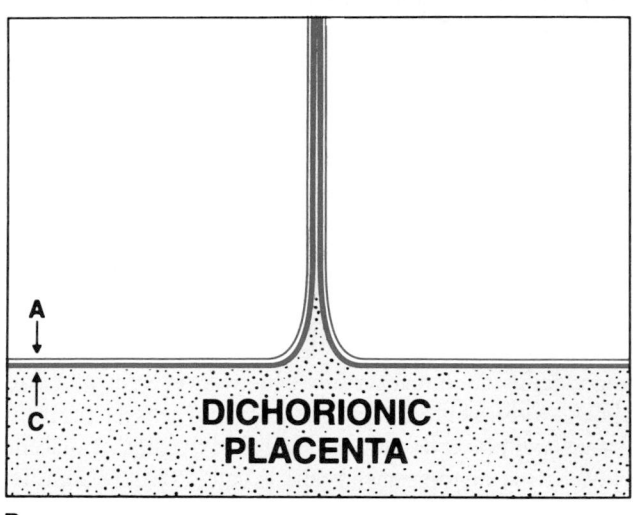

DICHORIONIC PLACENTA

B

FIGURE 39–6. A. Ultrasound image of "twin-peak" sign showing an extension of placental tissue into the intertwin membrane, confirming dichorionic twinning. **B.** Schematic diagram of the "twin-peak" sign. (From Finberg, 1992, with permission.)

the chorionicity, amnionicity, and zygosity in 110 consecutive twins at midgestation. Compared with the pathological diagnosis made by examining the placenta after delivery, the ultrasonographic determination had 91 percent sensitivity and specificity. However, zygosity could not be determined even by placental pathology in 35 percent of cases, emphasizing that determination of zygosity often requires sophisticated genetic testing. In another study of 150 twin pregnancies at 10 to 14 weeks, Carroll and colleagues (2002) used a variety of ultrasonographic signs and identified chorionicity with a high degree of accuracy. The "twin-peak" sign in combination with an assessment for separate placentas had 97 percent sensitivity and 100 percent specificity for dichorionicity. The respective values for monochorionicity using the "T" sign were 100 percent and 98 percent.

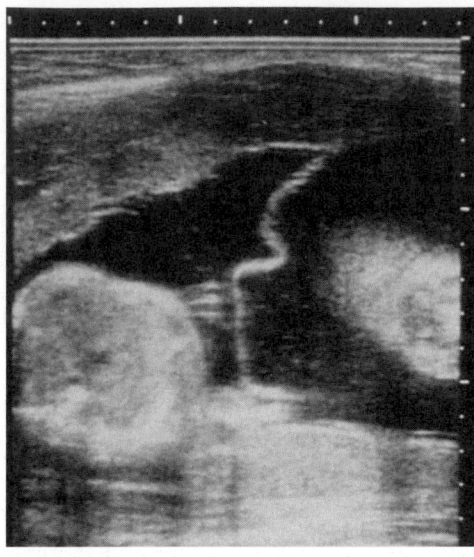

FIGURE 39–7. Sonogram of twins at 18 weeks' gestational age. Two fetal poles are separated by intervening membranes that divide the amnionic sacs. (Courtesy of Dr. R. Santos.)

Placental Examination. A carefully performed visual examination of the placenta and membranes serves to establish zygosity promptly in about two thirds of cases. The following system for examination is recommended: as the first neonate is delivered, one clamp is placed on a portion of its cord (Fig. 39–8). Cord blood is not collected until after delivery of the other twin, unless it has been clearly shown that there are two placentas. As the second neonate is delivered, two clamps are placed on that cord. Three clamps are used to mark the cord of a third neonate, and so on as necessary. Until the delivery of

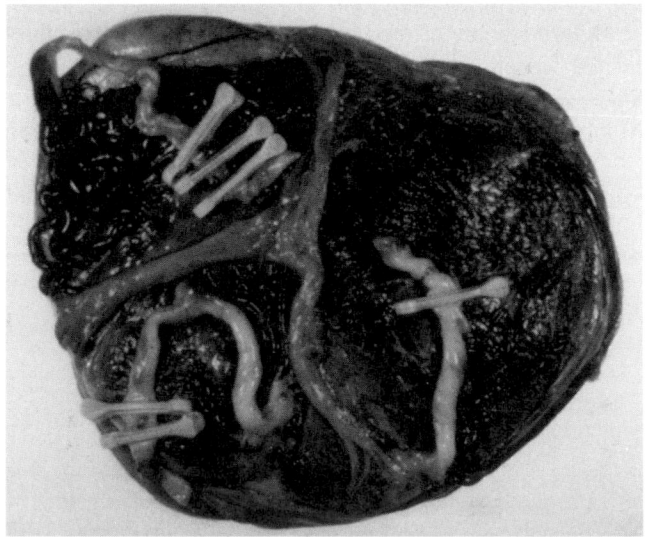

FIGURE 39–8. Placenta from a triplet gestation showing umbilical cord clamps placed in order of delivery of the infants. This identification system aids determination of zygosity.

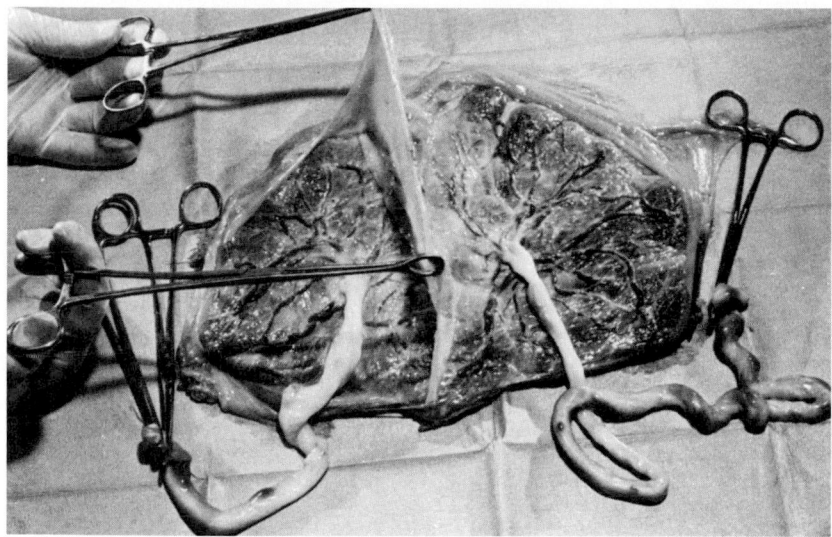

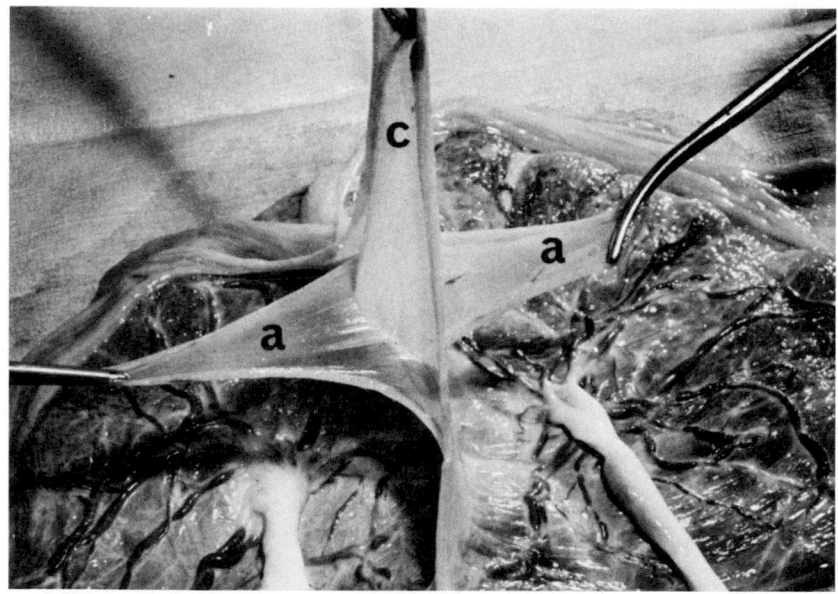

FIGURE 39–9. A. The membrane partition that separated twin fetuses is elevated. **B.** The membrane partition consists of chorion (c) between two amnions (a).

the last fetus, each cord segment must remain clamped to prevent fetal hypovolemia and anemia caused by blood leaving the placenta via anastomoses and then lost via an unclamped cord.

The placenta should be carefully delivered to preserve the attachment of the amnion and chorion to the placenta, because identification of the relationship of the membranes to each other is critical. With one common amnionic sac, or with juxtaposed amnions not separated by chorion arising between the fetuses, the fetuses are monozygotic. If adjacent amnions are separated by chorion, the fetuses could be either dizygotic or monozygotic, but dizygosity is more common (see Figs. 39–4, 39–9, and 39–10). If the neonates are of the same sex, blood typing of cord blood samples may be helpful.

Different blood types confirm dizygosity, although demonstrating the same blood type in each fetus is not enough to confirm monozygosity. For definitive diagnosis, more complicated techniques such as DNA fingerprinting can be used, but these tests are generally not performed at birth unless there is a pressing medical indication (Azuma and associates, 1989).

Infant Sex and Zygosity. Twins of opposite sex are almost always dizygotic. Rarely, monozygotic twins may be discordant for phenotypic sex. This occurs when one twin is phenotypically female due to Turner syndrome (45,X) and her sibling is 46,XY.

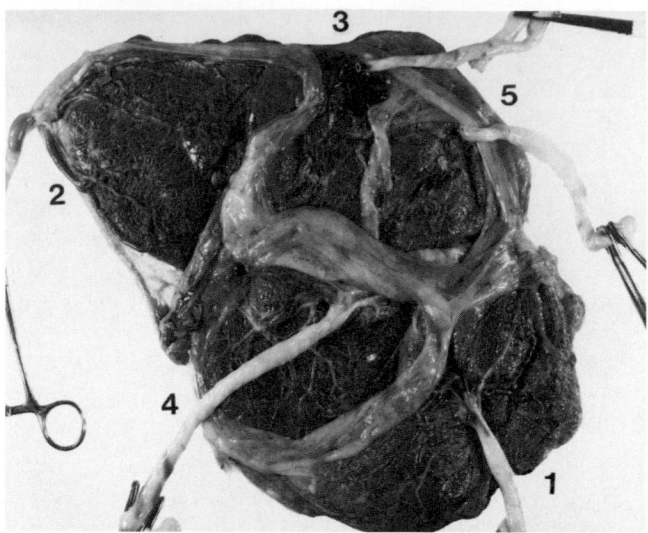

FIGURE 39–10. Quintuplet placenta with five separate amnionic sacs delivered at 32 weeks. Amnionic sacs of numbers 3 and 5 were not separated by chorion, and therefore those infants are monozygous. Infant birthweights ranged from a high of 1530 g (no. 1) to 860 g (no. 5). All of the infants survived.

DIAGNOSIS OF MULTIPLE FETUSES

HISTORY AND CLINICAL EXAMINATION.

A maternal family history of twins, advanced maternal age, high parity, large maternal size, and a personal history of twins provide weak clues to the diagnosis of multifetal gestation. Knowledge of recent administration of either clomiphene citrate or gonadotropins or pregnancy accomplished by ART provide strong ones.

Clinical examination with accurate measurement of fundal height, as described in Chapter 8 (see p. 212), is essential. During the second trimester, the uterine size is typically larger than expected for the gestational age determined from menstrual data. Rouse and co-workers (1993) reported fundal heights in 336 well-dated twin pregnancies. Between 20 and 30 weeks, fundal heights were on average about 5 cm greater than expected for singletons of the same fetal age.

In women with a uterus that appears large for gestational age, the following possibilities are considered:

1. Multiple fetuses
2. Elevation of the uterus by a distended bladder
3. Inaccurate menstrual history
4. Hydramnios
5. Hydatidiform mole
6. Uterine myomas
7. A closely attached adnexal mass
8. Fetal macrosomia (late in pregnancy)

When uterine palpation leads to the diagnosis of twins, it is most often because two fetal heads have been detected, often in different uterine quadrants. In general, however, before the third trimester it is difficult to diagnose twins by palpation of fetal parts. Even late in pregnancy it may be difficult to identify twins by abdominal palpation, especially if one twin overlies the other, if the woman is obese, or if hydramnios is present.

Late in the first trimester, fetal heart action may be detected with Doppler ultrasonic equipment. Thereafter, it becomes possible to identify two fetal heart beats if their rates are clearly distinct from each other and from that of the mother. Careful examination with an aural fetal stethoscope can identify fetal heart sounds in twins as early as 18 to 20 weeks.

ULTRASONOGRAPHY. By careful ultrasonographic examination, separate gestational sacs can be identified early in twin pregnancy (Fig. 39–11). Subsequently, each fetal head should be seen in two perpendicular planes so as not to mistake a cross section of the fetal trunk for a second fetal head. Ideally, two fetal heads or two abdomens should be seen in the same plane, to avoid scanning the same fetus twice and interpreting it as twins. Ultrasonographic examination should detect practically all sets of twins. Indeed, one argument in favor of ultrasonographic screening is earlier detection of multiple fetuses (see Chap. 16, p. 390). In a large randomized trial, LeFevre and co-workers (1993) demonstrated that routine midgestation ultrasonographic examinations detected virtually all multifetal gestations (99 percent) before 26 weeks, whereas when performed only for specific indications just 62 percent were detected before this gestational age. Higher-order multiple gestations are more difficult to evaluate. Even in the first trimester it can be difficult to determine the correct number of fetuses and their position, which is important for

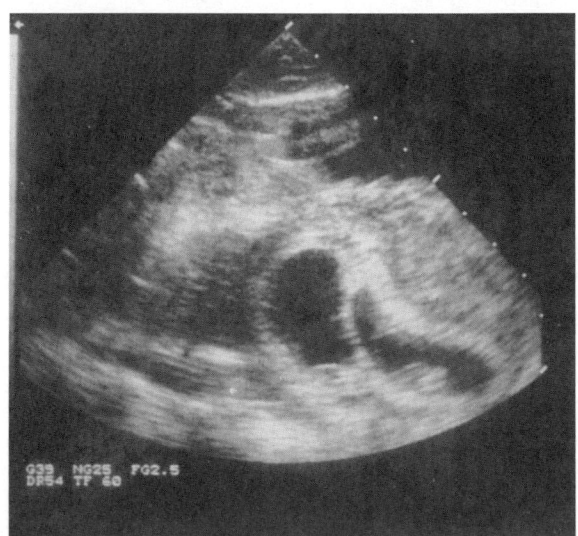

FIGURE 39–11. Longitudinal sonogram at 7 weeks' menstrual age demonstrating two gestational sacs, each containing a fetus. (Courtesy of J. and J. Ackerman and Dr. R. Santos.)

nonselective pregnancy reduction and essential for selective termination (discussed later).

OTHER DIAGNOSTIC AIDS

Radiological Examination. A radiograph of the maternal abdomen can be helpful when the number of fetuses in a higher-order multiple gestation is uncertain. Radiographs, however, are generally not useful and may lead to an incorrect diagnosis in the following circumstances:

1. The film is taken before 18 weeks, when fetal skeletons are insufficiently radiopaque.
2. The film is of poor quality from inappropriate exposure time or from malposition of the mother so that her upper abdomen and the fetus therein are excluded from the radiograph.
3. The mother is obese.
4. There is hydramnios.
5. One or more fetuses moves during the exposure.

Biochemical Tests. The amounts of chorionic gonadotropin in plasma and in urine, on average, are higher than those found with a singleton pregnancy, but not so high as to allow a definite diagnosis of multiple fetuses. Twins are frequently diagnosed during an evaluation for an elevated maternal serum alpha-fetoprotein level, although this level alone is not diagnostic (see Chap. 13, p. 320). Currently, there is no biochemical test that reliably differentiates between the presence of one and more than one fetus.

MATERNAL ADAPTATION

In general, the degree of maternal physiological change is greater with multiple fetuses than with a single fetus. Beginning in the first trimester, women with multiple gestation often have nausea and vomiting in excess of that characterizing singleton pregnancies, for reasons that are not clear. The normal maternal blood volume expansion is greater in twin pregnancies (Pritchard, 1965). Whereas the average increase in late pregnancy is about 40 to 50 percent with a single fetus, it is about 50 to 60 percent with twins (i.e., an additional 500 mL). The red cell mass increases as well, but proportionately less in twin pregnancies than in singletons, resulting in a more pronounced "physiological anemia." The average blood loss with vaginal delivery of twins is 935 mL, or nearly 500 mL more than with delivery of a single fetus. Both the remarkable increase in maternal blood volume and the increased iron and folate requirements predispose to a greater prevalence of maternal anemia.

Kametas and associates (2003) used two-dimensional and M-mode echocardiography to assess cardiac function in 119 women with twin pregnancies from 10 to 40 weeks. Cardiac output was increased 20 percent compared with that of singleton pregnancies, predominantly due to greater stroke volume, and to a much lesser degree, increased heart rate. Interestingly, formally assessed pulmonary function does not differ between women carrying twins and those carrying singletons (McAuliffe and colleagues, 2002).

Women carrying twins also have a typical pattern of arterial blood pressure change. Compared with the diastolic blood pressure of mothers carrying singletons, theirs is lower at 20 weeks but increases more by delivery. The increase is at least 15 mm Hg in 95 percent of women carrying twins compared with only 54 percent of women pregnant with singleton pregnancies (Campbell, 1986).

Uterine growth in multifetal gestation increases during pregnancy. The uterus and its nonfetal contents may achieve a volume of 10 L or more and weigh in excess of 20 pounds! Especially with monozygotic twins, rapid accumulation of excessive amounts of amnionic fluid (i.e., acute hydramnios) may develop. In these circumstances, maternal abdominal viscera and lungs may be appreciably compressed and displaced by the expanding uterus. The size and weight of the large uterus may preclude more than a sedentary existence for these women.

In multifetal gestation complicated by hydramnios, maternal renal function may become seriously impaired, most likely as the consequence of obstructive uropathy. Quigley and Cruikshank (1977) described two women each carrying twins in whom acute and severe hydramnios led to maternal oliguria and azotemia. Maternal urine output and plasma creatinine levels promptly returned to normal after delivery. In severe hydramnios, therapeutic amniocentesis may be used to provide relief for the mother, to improve obstructive uropathy, and to lower the risk of preterm delivery from preterm labor or premature rupture of membranes (see Chap. 21, p. 529). Unfortunately, the hydramnios is often characterized by acute onset remote from term and by rapid reaccumulation following amniocentesis.

The various stresses of pregnancy and the likelihood of serious maternal complications are almost invariably greater with multiple fetuses than with a singleton. This should be taken into account, especially when counseling the woman whose health is compromised and whose multifetal gestation is recognized early. The same is true for a woman who is not pregnant but is considering infertility treatment by ovulation induction or ART.

PREGNANCY OUTCOME

ABORTION. Spontaneous abortion is more likely with multiple fetuses. Detailed reviews have identified three times more twins among aborted than among term pregnancies (Livingston and Poland, 1980; Uchida and co-authors, 1983). Monochorionic abortuses greatly outnumber dichorionic abortuses (18 to 1), implicating monozygosity as a risk factor for spontaneous abortion.

MALFORMATIONS. The incidence of congenital malformations is appreciably increased in twin and higher-order multiple gestation compared with singletons. Major malformations develop in 2 percent and minor malformations in 4 percent of twins (Cameron and colleagues, 1983; Kohl and Casey, 1975). This increase is almost entirely due to the high incidence of structural defects in monozygotic twins. According to Schinzel and associates (1979), anomalies in monozygotic twins generally fall into one of three categories:

1. Defects resulting from twinning itself, which some consider to be a teratogenic event. This category includes conjoined twinning, acardiac anomaly, sirenomelia, neural-tube defects, and holoprosencephaly.
2. Defects resulting from vascular interchange between monochorionic twins. Vascular anastomoses can give rise to reverse flow with acardia in one twin. Alternatively, if one twin dies and intravascular coagulation develops, these connections can allow emboli to reach the living twin. Vascular connections may also conduct dramatic blood pressure fluctuations, causing defects such as microcephaly, hydranencephaly, intestinal atresia, aplasia cutis, or limb amputation.
3. Defects that occur as the result of crowding. Examples include talipes equinovarus (clubfoot) or congenital hip dislocation. Dizygotic twins are also subject to this.

Baldwin (1991) has comprehensively reviewed anomalies that develop in twins. Persistent hydramnios is associated with fetal anomalies of one or both twins. Hashimoto and colleagues (1986) subjectively identified increased amnionic fluid in one fourth of 75 twin pregnancies. In nine pregnancies, hydramnios was transient, and all of these fetuses were normal. In 9 of 10 pregnancies in which hydramnios persisted, fetuses had anomalies.

BIRTHWEIGHT. Multifetal gestations are more likely to be characterized by low birthweight than singleton pregnancies, due mostly to restricted fetal growth and preterm delivery (Buekens and Wilcox, 1993). In general, the larger the number of fetuses, the greater the degree of growth restriction. Two thirds of twin and even more triplet pregnancies are complicated by fetal growth restriction. However, this assessment of growth is based on growth curves established for singletons. Several authorities have made the argument that fetal growth in multiple gestation is different from that of singleton pregnancies, and that abnormal growth should be diagnosed only when fetal size is less than expected for *multifetal gestation.* Both twin and triplet growth curves have been created for this purpose (Ong and associates, 2002; Rodis and associates, 1999).

In dizygotic pregnancies, marked size discordancy usually results from unequal placentation, with one placental

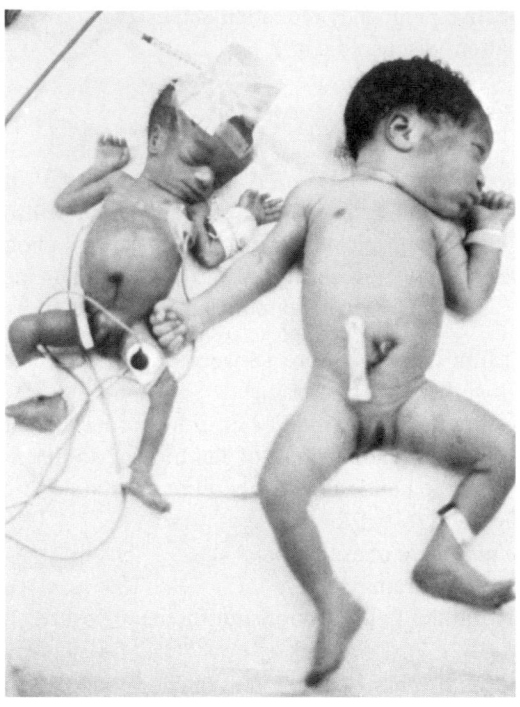

FIGURE 39–12. Marked discordance in dizygotic twins. The larger infant weighed 2300 g and was appropriate for gestational age. The markedly growth-restricted smaller infant weighed only 785 g. Both thrived.

site receiving a better blood supply than the other. However, size differences may also reflect different genetic fetal growth potentials. In the third trimester, the larger fetal mass leads to accelerated placental maturation and relative placental insufficiency. Size discordancy can also result from umbilical cord abnormalities such as velamentous insertion, marginal insertion, or vasa previa; discordancy for fetal malformations; genetic syndromes; or infection. Figure 39–12 shows dizygotic twins, one of whom weighed 2300 g and the other 785 g, delivered at Parkland Hospital. Both survived.

The degree of growth restriction in monozygotic twins is likely to be greater than that in dizygotic pairs. The allocation of blastomeres may not be equal between monochorionic embryos, vascular anastomoses within the placenta may cause unequal distribution of nutrients and oxygen, and discordant structural anomalies resulting from the twinning event itself may affect growth. For example, the quintuplets shown in Figure 39–13 represent three dizygotic and two monozygotic fetuses. When delivered at 31 weeks, the three neonates from separate ova weighed 1420, 1530, and 1440 g, whereas the two derived from the same ovum weighed 990 and 860 g.

When birthweights in more than 500,000 male singleton neonates were compared with those from more than 10,000 male twin neonates, twin birthweights closely paralleled those of singletons until about 28 to 30 weeks. Subse-

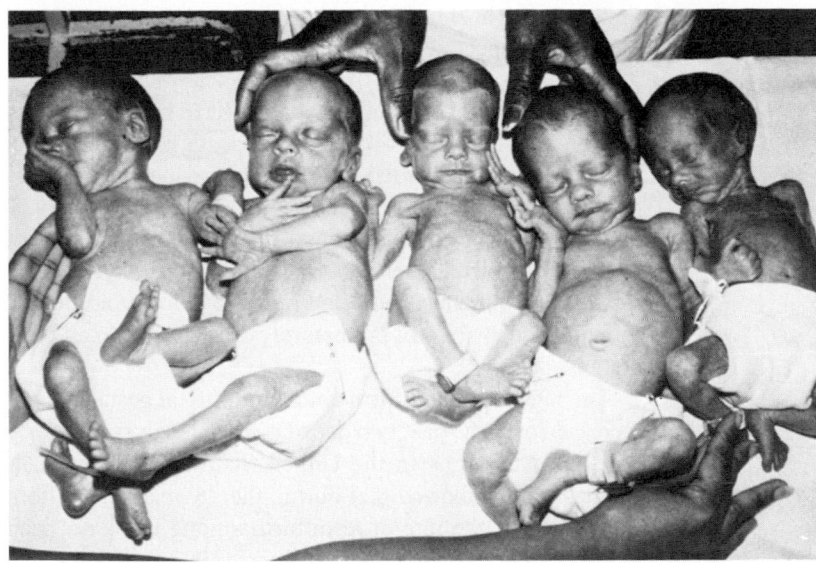

A

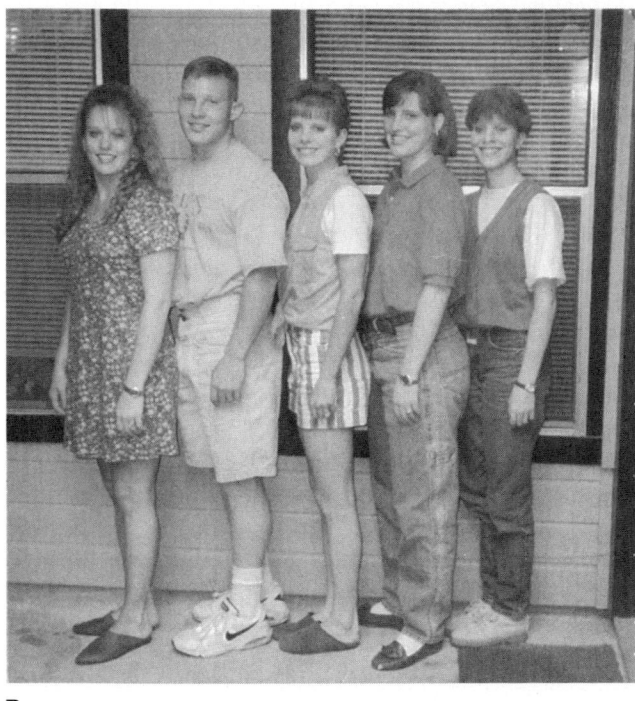

B

FIGURE 39–13. A. Davis quintuplets at 3 weeks of age. The first, second, and fourth infants from the left each arose from separate ova, whereas the third and fifth infants are from the same ovum. **B.** Davis quintuplets at 20 years of age.

quently, twin birthweights progressively lagged with advancing gestational age those of singletons (Fig. 39–14). At approximately 34 to 35 weeks and thereafter, twin birthweights clearly diverge from those of singletons. Twin growth restriction intensifies as the third trimester continues. At 38 weeks or later, the incidence of overt growth restriction quadruples to include almost half of twin births.

Other circumstantial evidence shows that in utero crowding by multiple fetuses may overtax the capacity of the mother, the uterus, or both to provide nutrients. For example, Lipitz and co-workers (1996), Smith-Levitin and colleagues

(1996), and Yaron and associates (1999) have reported that selective reduction of triplets to twins before 12 weeks results in a growth pattern typical of twins rather than triplets. Dickey and co-workers (2002) did not observe this with spontaneous reduction (see p. 941).

Casele and co-authors (1996), who studied maternal metabolic responses to eating and extended overnight fasting, provide another example that the maternal supply line is affected by the number of fetuses. Women with twins were more vulnerable to starvation ketosis after fasting compared with women with singleton pregnancies.

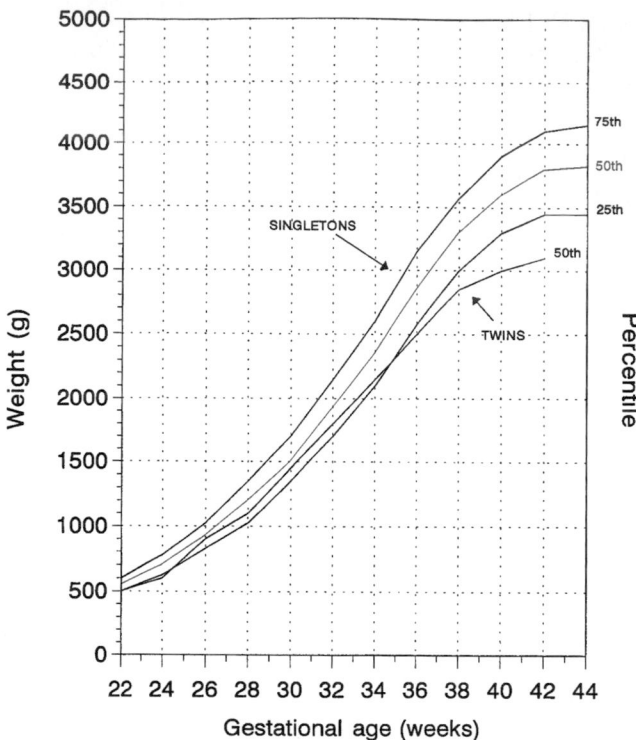

FIGURE 39–14. Birthweight percentiles (25 to 75) for singleton male infants compared with the 50th birthweight percentile for twin males, Canada, 1986–1988. (Modified from Arbuckle and colleagues, 1993, with permission.)

DURATION OF GESTATION. As the number of fetuses increases, the duration of gestation decreases (Fig. 39–15). According to Martin and colleagues (2002), 57 percent of twins born in the United States in 2001 were delivered preterm, and their mean gestational age at delivery was 35 weeks. With triplets, 92 percent were delivered preterm, and their mean gestational age at delivery was 32 weeks. Virtually all quadruplets and quintuplets were delivered

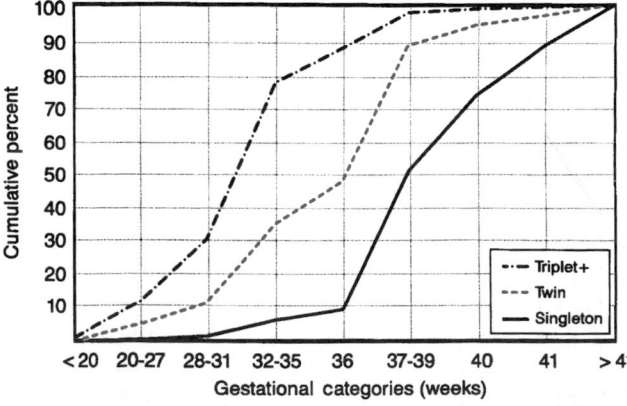

FIGURE 39–15. Cumulative percent of singleton, twin, and triplet or higher-order multiple births according to gestational age at delivery in the United States during 1990. (From Luke, 1994.)

preterm, with average gestational ages at delivery of 30 and 29 weeks, respectively.

PRETERM BIRTH. Delivery before term is the major reason for the increased risk of neonatal death and morbidity in twins. Gardner and associates (1995) found that the causes of preterm birth differed between twins and singletons. Spontaneous preterm labor accounted for a larger proportion of twin preterm birth, whereas the reverse was true for preterm ruptured membranes. Indicated preterm delivery accounted for equal proportions of prematurely delivered twins and singletons.

The rate of preterm birth among multifetal gestations has increased over the past two decades. In an analysis of nearly 350,000 twin births in the United States, Kogan and colleagues (2002) showed that during the 16-year period from 1981 to 1997, the rate of term birth among twins declined by 22 percent. Joseph and colleagues (2001) attributed this decline to an increased rate of preterm labor induction for medical indications among twins, which happily was associated with decreases in perinatal morbidity and mortality among twins that reached 34 weeks. Likewise, twin gestations in women receiving more than the recommended number of prenatal visits showed higher rates of preterm birth but lower neonatal mortality (Kogan and colleagues, 2000).

Although the causes of preterm delivery in twins and singletons may be different, once delivered, the neonatal outcome is generally the same at similar gestational ages (Gardner, 1995; Kilpatrick, 1996, and their colleagues). The primary neonatal problem with twin gestation is simply more frequent preterm delivery, not increased vulnerability to the morbidities of preterm delivery.

The previous statements apply to twins who are essentially concordant. As one would expect, the neonatal outcome for preterm twins who are markedly discordant may not be comparable to that of singletons because whatever caused the discordance may have long-lasting effects. Sonntag and co-workers (1996) compared 27 weight-discordant twin pairs with 72 pairs of concordant twins. They found that the discordant twins had a significantly higher neonatal mortality (19 versus 2 percent) and were more likely to have severe intracranial hemorrhage and persistent ductus arteriosus. Most of the increase in morbidity and mortality was due to the sequelae of chronic twin-to-twin transfusion syndrome. Nearly half of the discordant pairs in this study fulfilled the criteria for this disorder.

Population studies also reveal the harmful effects of discordancy. After analyzing matched birth and death certificates of 150,000 pairs of twins, Demissie and associates (2002) concluded that birthweight discordancy correlated directly with the risk of stillbirth. In an analysis of the same data, Blickstein and Keith (2004) demonstrated that among twins discordant by at least 25 percent, the risk of neonatal death for the smaller twin was increased only if its weight was less than the tenth percentile. Rydhström (1994) observed that adverse pregnancy outcomes and discordancy were linked only in like-sexed twin pairs. The author hypothesized that monochorionicity was responsible for the adverse outcomes.

PROLONGED PREGNANCY. More than 30 years ago, Bennett and Dunn (1969) suggested that a twin pregnancy of 40 weeks or more should be considered postterm. They based this conclusion on the observation that twin stillborn infants delivered at 40 weeks or beyond had features similar to those of postmature singletons (see Chap. 37, p. 884). Based on an analysis of almost 300,000 twin births delivered in the United States from 1995 to 1998, Kahn and colleagues (2003) calculated that at and beyond 39 weeks, the risk of subsequent stillbirth was greater than the risk of neonatal mortality. At Parkland Hospital, twin gestations have empirically been considered to be prolonged at about 40 weeks.

SUBSEQUENT DEVELOPMENT. In a study in Norway, Nilsen and associates (1984) evaluated the physical and intellectual development of male twins at 18 years of age. Compared with singletons, twice as many twins were found to be physically unfit for military service. They attributed this to sequelae of preterm delivery such as visual impairment rather than to twinning. General intelligence did not appear to differ.

At least one study has suggested that long-term physical development might be different for twins. Silva and colleagues (1982, 1985) carefully monitored 24 twins up to 11 years of age, and compared their outcomes with those of 1013 singletons who had similar gestational ages and weights at birth and who experienced similar antenatal and neonatal complications. Twins had delays in achieving developmental milestones, and at 11 years of age lagged behind singletons in intelligence quotient (IQ) scores. At each age, twins were similar in height to singletons 3 months younger, and similar in weight to singletons 6 months younger.

The pattern of subsequent development of discordant twins varies. For example, Babson and Phillips (1973) reported that in monozygotic twins whose birthweights differed on average 35 percent, the twin who was smaller at birth remained so into adulthood. Height, weight, head circumference, and intelligence often remained greater in the twin who weighed more at birth. Fujikura and Froelich (1974), however, failed to confirm a significant difference in mental and motor scores. Baigts and co-workers (1982) studied a pair of 17-year-old monozygotic twins who had similar body frames, but remarkably dissimilar weights, which had persisted since birth. The investigators documented hyperplasia of adipocytes in the heavier twin compared with those in her lower-weight sister. They suggested that intrauterine nutritional status helps determine adipocyte numbers and the way the body evolves. Others have concluded that genetic factors in twins are more influential than environment in determining body mass (Bouchard and co-workers, 1990; Stunkard and co-workers, 1990).

UNIQUE COMPLICATIONS

A number of unique complications develop in multiple fetuses. Although these have been best described in twins, they also occur in higher-order multiple gestation.

MONOAMNIONIC TWINS. Approximately 1 percent of monozygotic twins are monoamnionic (Hall, 2003). Diamnionic twins can become monoamnionic, and have all the associated morbidity and mortality, if the dividing membrane ruptures (Gilbert and colleagues, 1991). A high fetal death rate is associated with this rare variety of monozygotic twinning. Allen and colleagues (2001) in a comprehensive review reported that monoamnionic twins that are diagnosed antenatally and are still alive at 20 weeks have about a 10-percent risk of subsequent intrauterine demise. Intertwining of their umbilical cords, a common cause of death, is estimated to complicate at least half of cases (Fig. 39–16).

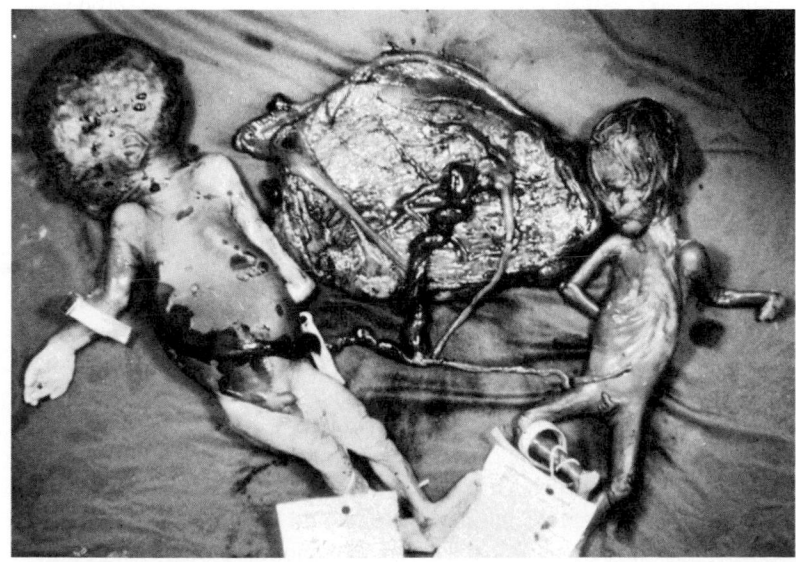

FIGURE 39–16. Monozygotic twins in a single amnionic sac. The smaller fetus apparently died first. and the second subsequently succumbed when the umbilical cords entwined.

Once diagnosed, management of monoamnionic twins is somewhat problematic due to the unpredictability of fetal death resulting from cord entanglement and to the lack of an effective means of monitoring for it. Some data suggest that morbid cord entanglement is likely to occur early, and that monoamnionic pregnancies that have successfully reached 30 to 32 weeks are at greatly reduced risk. Carr and co-authors (1990) reviewed 24 sets of monoamnionic twins in which all the fetuses were known to be alive before 18 weeks. At 30 weeks, 70 percent of the fetuses were alive and no additional fetuses died prior to delivery, at an average age of 36 weeks. The investigators concluded that the risks due to early delivery to prevent cord accidents outweighed the risks of fetal death from cord entanglement, especially after 30 weeks. Similarly, there were no fetal deaths after 32 weeks reported by Tessin and Zlatnik (1991) in their description of 20 monoamnionic twin pregnancies at the University of Iowa Hospital. Demaria and associates (2004) reported no fetal deaths in 15 women after 29 weeks.

Umbilical cords of twins frequently entangle, but the factors that lead to pathological umbilical vessel constriction during entanglement are unknown. Belfort and colleagues (1993) and Aisenbrey and co-workers (1995) used color-flow Doppler ultrasonography to diagnose umbilical cord entanglement in 10 monoamnionic twin pregnancies. The recognition of cord entanglement in seven of these pregnancies prompted hospital admission, increased fetal surveillance, or both. Interestingly, only one set of twins with entangled cords required immediate delivery. In fact, the remaining six pregnancies continued for an average of 6 weeks after the diagnosis, and one of these continued for 12 weeks!

At the University of Alabama, presumed monoamnionic twins are managed with twice-weekly fetal assessment testing starting at 28 weeks. If testing reveals fetal heart rate variability and no heart rate decelerations, amniocentesis is done to assess fetal lung maturity beginning at 34 weeks. Cesarean delivery is performed when tests indicate pulmonary maturity, or at 36 weeks. Betamethasone for fetal maturation is used on an individualized basis (see Chapter 36).

CONJOINED TWINS. In the United States, united or conjoined twins (see Fig. 39–2) are commonly referred to as Siamese twins, after Chang and Eng Bunker of Siam (Thailand), who were displayed worldwide by P.T. Barnum. When twins are conjoined, the shared body site may be:

1. Anterior (thoracopagus).
2. Posterior (pygopagus).
3. Cephalic (craniopagus).
4. Caudal (ischiopagus).

The majority are of the thoracopagus variety shown in Figures 39–17 and 39–18.

When the bodies are duplicated only partly, the attachment is usually lateral. The incomplete division of the embryonic disc may begin at either or both poles and may produce two

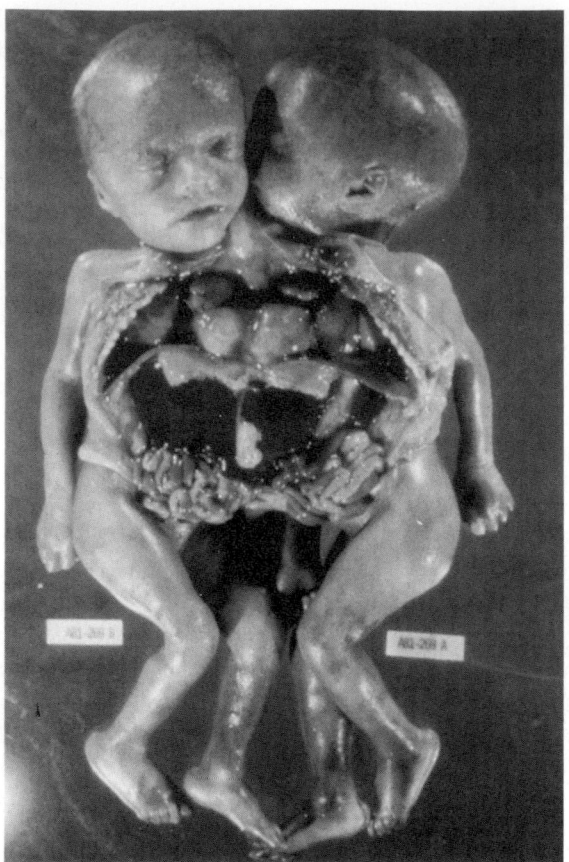

FIGURE 39–17. Conjoined twins delivered at 22 weeks and showing a shared liver.

heads; two, three, or four arms; two, three, or four legs; or some combination thereof. The frequency of conjoined twins is not well established. At Kandang Kerbau Hospital in Singapore, Tan and co-workers (1971) identified seven cases of conjoined twins among more than 400,000 deliveries (1 in 60,000).

As reviewed by van den Brand and associates (1994), the diagnosis of conjoined twins can frequently be made at midpregnancy using ultrasonography, which allows parents to decide whether to continue the pregnancy. A thorough targeted ultrasonographic examination, including a careful evaluation of the point of connection and the organs involved, is essential before counseling is provided. Surgical separation of nearly completely joined twins may be successful when organs essential for life are not shared, and when it can be performed on a planned, as opposed to an emergency basis (Spitz and Kiely, 2003). Consultation with a pediatric surgeon often assists antenatal parental decision making. Conjoined twins may have discordant structural anomalies that further complicate decisions about whether or not to continue the pregnancy. For example, one of the conjoined twins shown in Figure 39–19 was anencephalic.

Viable conjoined twins should be delivered by cesarean. However, vaginal delivery of conjoined twins for the purpose

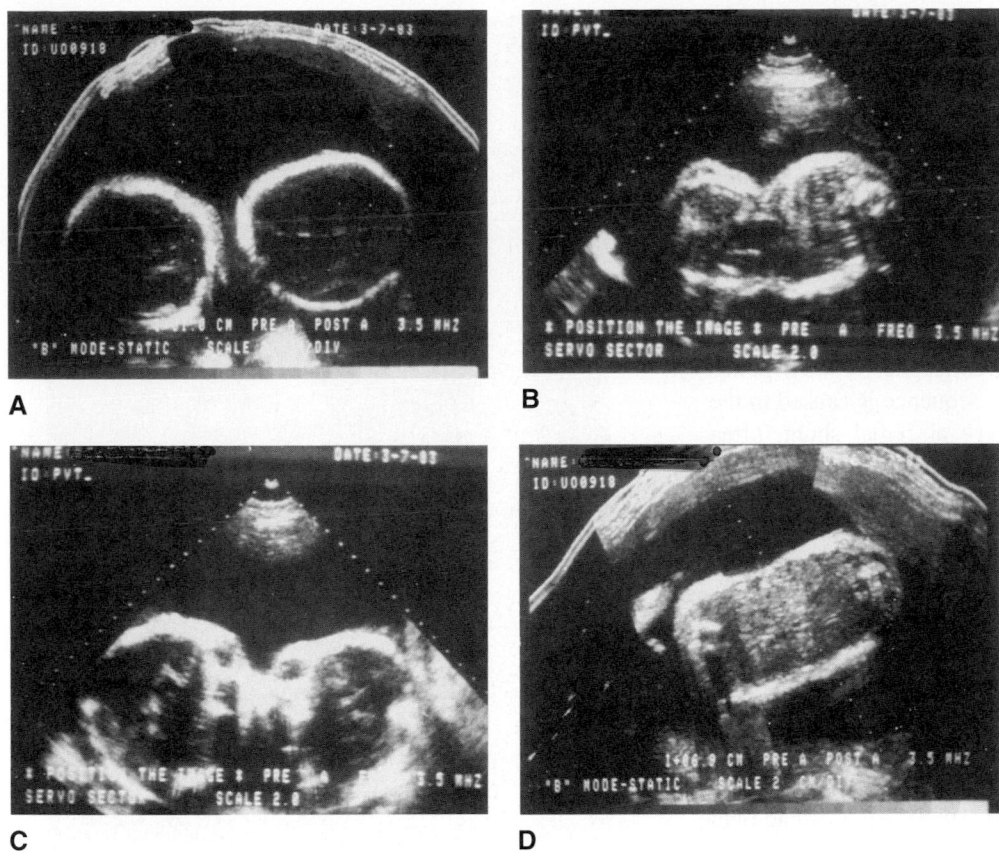

FIGURE 39–18. Transverse sonograms of thoracopagus twins at about 28 weeks' gestation. **A.** Axial view of fetal heads. **B.** Fused thorax with conjoined hearts. **C.** Oblique view of the heads showing the proximity of the two faces. **D.** Fusion of the abdomen with a common liver. (Courtesy of Dr. R. Santos.)

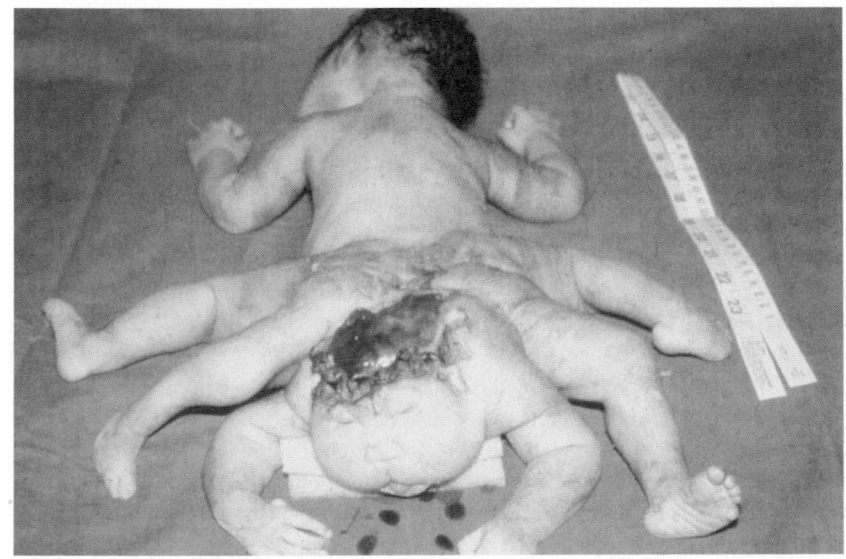

FIGURE 39–19. Conjoined twins in which one was anencephalic. (Courtesy of Dr. Craig Syrop, University of Iowa.)

of pregnancy termination is possible, because the union is most often pliable, although dystocia is common. If the fetuses are mature, vaginal delivery may be traumatic to the maternal uterus or cervix.

ACARDIAC TWIN. *Twin reversed-arterial-perfusion (TRAP) sequence* is a rare (1 in 35,000 births) but serious complication of monochorionic, monozygotic multiple gestation. In the TRAP sequence, there is usually a normally formed donor twin who has features of heart failure as well as a recipient twin who lacks a heart (acardius) and various other structures (van Allen and colleagues, 1983). It has been hypothesized that the TRAP sequence is caused in the embryo by a large artery-to-artery placental shunt, often also accompanied by a vein-to-vein shunt. The perfusion pressure of the donor twin overpowers that in the recipient twin, who thus receives reverse blood flow from its twin sibling (Jones, 1997). The "used" arterial blood reaching the recipient twin preferentially goes to the iliac vessels and thus perfuses only the lower part of the body, leading to disruption or deterioration of growth and development of the upper body. Failure or disrupted growth of the head is called *acardius acephalus*; a partially developed head with identifiable limbs is called *acardius myelacephalus*; and failure of any recognizable structure to form is *acardius amorphous* (Robie and colleagues, 1989). An acardiac twin demonstrating acephalus as well as complete malformation of the upper torso is shown in Figure 39–20.

Without treatment, the donor or "pump" twin has been reported to die in 50 to 75 percent of cases (Moore and colleagues, 1990). Quintero and colleagues (1994) have reviewed methods of in utero treatment of acardiac twinning in which the goal is interruption of the vascular communication between the donor and recipient twins. They also have described successful use of transabdominal fetoscopy to ligate the umbilical cord of 11 acardiac twins at approximately 21 weeks (Quintero and co-workers, 1996). Tsao and colleagues (2002) reported the survival of 12 of 13 donor twins when, under ultrasonographic guidance, a 14-gauge radioablation needle was used to cauterize the umbilical vessels and terminate blood flow to the recipient twin at the site of cord insertion into the umbilicus. Ablation was performed at 18 to 24 weeks.

Recently, survival was reported for 9 of 10 donor twins managed expectantly (Sullivan and associates, 2003). The authors of this report advocated that expectant management with close fetal surveillance be considered as another management option.

VASCULAR ANASTOMOSES BETWEEN FETUSES.
With rare exceptions, vascular anastomoses between twins are present only in monochorionic twin placentas (Baldwin, 1991; Hall, 2003; Robertson and Neer, 1983). Nearly 100 percent of monochorionic twin placentas have vascular anastomoses, but there are marked variations in the number,

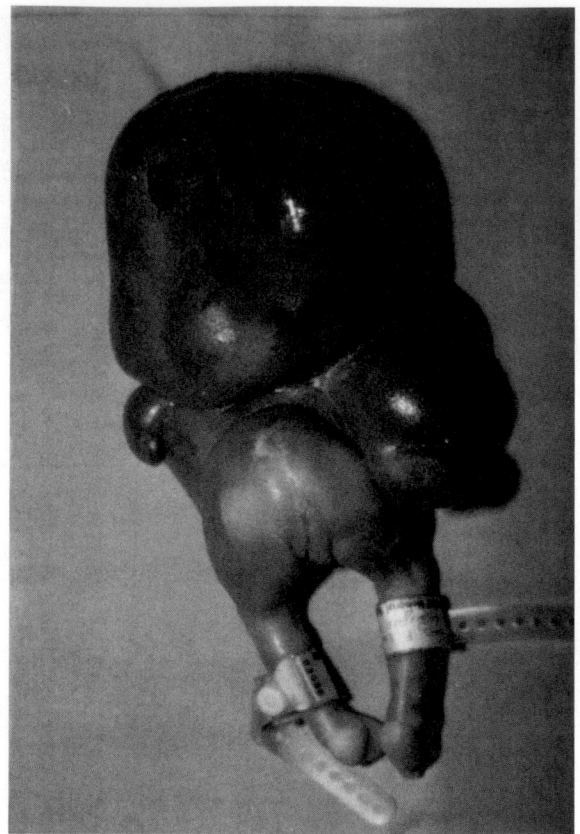

FIGURE 39–20. Acardiac twin photographed from the rear and showing acephalus with total deformity of the upper torso. (Courtesy of Dr. Paul Wendel.)

size, and direction of these seemingly haphazard connections. Artery-to-artery anastomoses on the chorionic surface of the placenta have been identified in up to 75 percent of monochorionic twin placentas and are the most common pattern (Fig. 39–21). Vein-to-vein and artery-to-vein communications are each found in approximately 50 percent of monochorionic twin placentas. One vessel may have several connections, sometimes to both arteries and veins. In contrast to these vascular connections on the surface of the chorion, artery-to-vein communications extend through the capillary bed of the villous tissue of the placenta. These deep arteriovenous anastomoses create a common villous compartment or third circulation that has been identified in approximately half of monochorionic twin placentas (Fig. 39–22).

Most of these vascular communications are hemodynamically balanced and of little fetal consequence. In others, however, they can cause hemodynamically significant shunts between fetuses. Two patterns of hemodynamically significant anastomotic circulations include acardiac twinning (described above) and the twin-to-twin transfusion syndrome. The incidence of the latter syndrome is unclear, but up to approximately a fourth of monochorionic twins have some clinical features of this syndrome (Galea and co-workers, 1982).

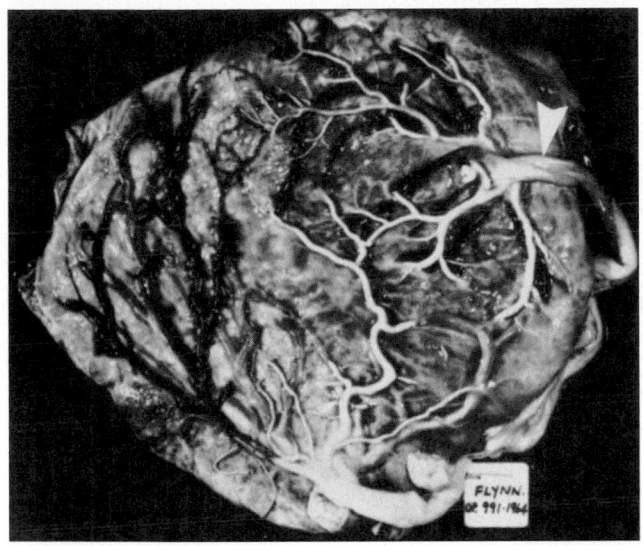

FIGURE 39–21. Monochorionic twin placenta from which the amnion has been stripped. The arteries of cord 1 (*arrow*) have been injected with barium solution and a direct communication with an artery from cord 2 (*label*) is apparent. A major artery of cord 2 was injected with India ink and a communication with veins in placenta 1 is evident, indicating a deep vascular communication. (From Fox, 1978.)

Twin-To-Twin Transfusion Syndrome. In this syndrome, blood is transfused from a donor twin to its recipient sibling such that the donor becomes anemic and its growth may be restricted, whereas the recipient becomes polycythemic and may develop circulatory overload manifest as hydrops. The donor twin is pale, and its recipient sibling is plethoric (Fig. 39–23). Similarly, one portion of the placenta often appears pale compared with the rest of the placenta.

The neonatal period may be complicated by circulatory overload with heart failure if severe hypervolemia and hyperviscosity are not identified promptly and treated. Occlusive thrombosis is also much more likely to develop in this setting. During the neonatal period, polycythemia may lead to severe hyperbilirubinemia and kernicterus (see Chap. 29, p. 672).

PATHOPHYSIOLOGY. Bajoria and colleagues (1995) perfused 30 monochorionic twin placentas with an anticoagulant solution immediately after delivery and then delineated anastomoses using dye-contrast injection. Those without twin-to-twin transfusion syndrome had multiple superficial anastomoses. In contrast, those with the twin-to-twin transfusion syndrome had solitary, deep arteriovenous channels within the capillary beds of the villous tissue. They hypothesized that multiple superficial vascular communications protected against the transfusion syndrome because this arrangement permitted bidirectional, and thus balanced, blood flow. Conversely, Bermudez and colleagues (2002) assessed 131 monochorionic twin placentas and observed that the presence of superficial anastomoses did little to mitigate the risk conferred by deep anastomoses.

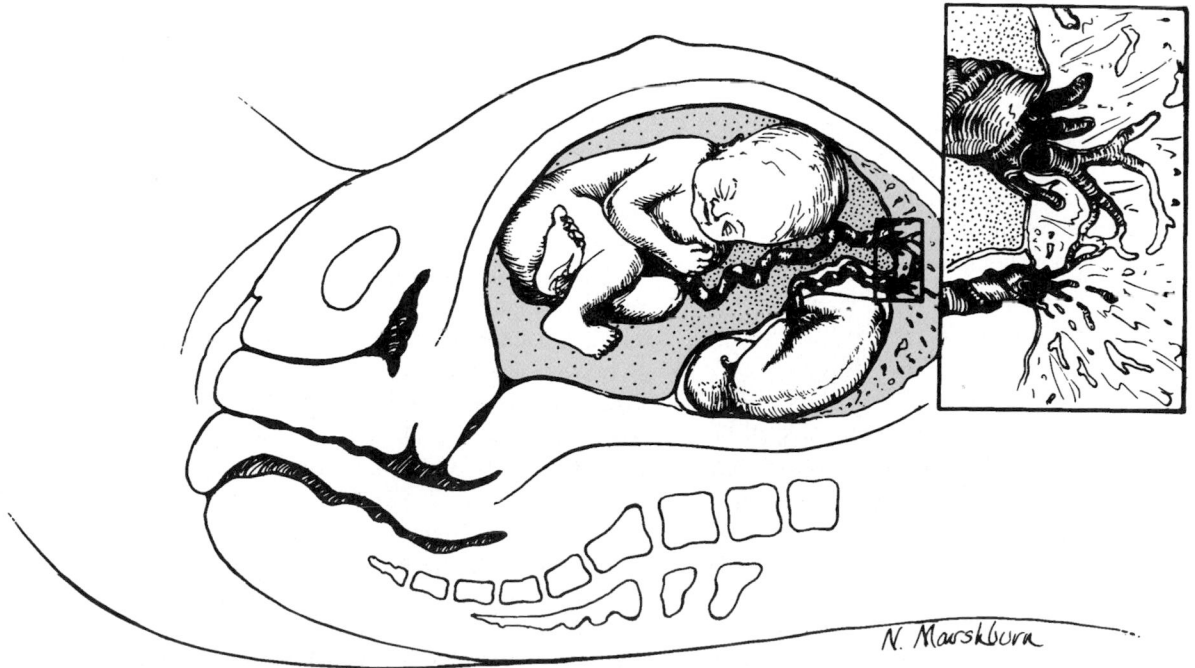

FIGURE 39–22. Schematic representation of arteriovenous anastomosis deep with the villous tissue forming a "common villous district" or "third circulation" that has been identified in monochorial placentas. Also shown is a growth-restricted discordant twin fetus with markedly reduced amnionic fluid, causing it to be "stuck."

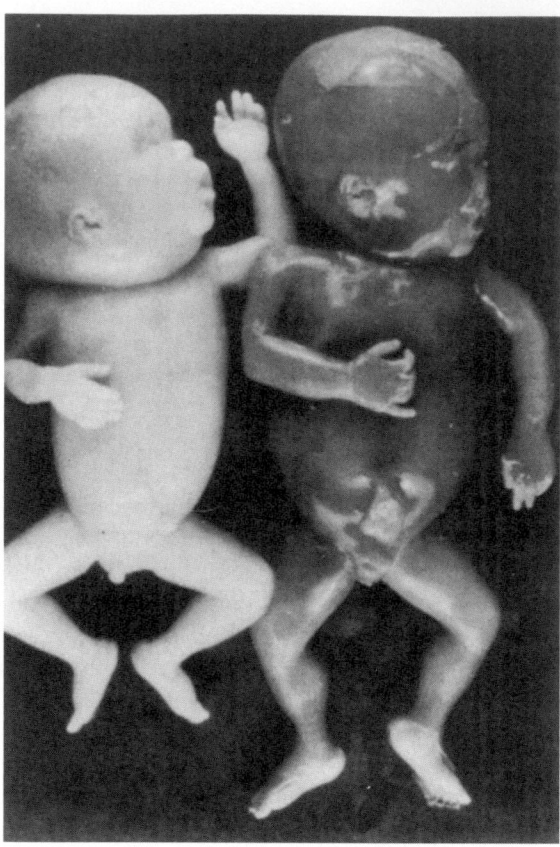

FIGURE 39–23. Twin-to-twin transfusion syndrome at 23 weeks. Pale donor twin (690 g) is shown on the left. The plethoric recipient twin (730 g) on the right also had hydramnios. The donor twin had oligohydramnios. (From Mahone and co-authors, 1993, with permission.)

Another hemodynamic explanation for twin-to-twin transfusion syndrome was offered by Fries and co-workers (1993). They postulated that a velamentous umbilical cord insertion may contribute to the development of unequal fetal blood volumes because the membranously inserted cord can be easily compressed, restricting blood flow to one twin. Talbert and colleagues (1996) used a computerized model to study the hemodynamics of unidirectional and bidirectional transfusion between twins via placental anastomoses. They determined that the net direction of blood flow is determined by the donor arterial pressure and not the number of anastomoses.

FETAL BRAIN DAMAGE. Cerebral palsy, microcephaly, porencephaly, and multicystic encephalomalacia are serious complications associated with vascular anastomoses in twin gestations. Multicystic encephalomalacia in a surviving fetus has been reported after the death at 12 weeks of its monochorionic twin (Weiss and co-workers, 2004). Whether this association was causal, however, is speculative. Neurological damage is most likely caused by ischemic necrosis leading

to cavitary brain lesions. In the donor twin, ischemia results from hypotension, anemia, or both (Fig. 39–24). In the recipient, ischemia develops from blood pressure instability and episodes of severe hypotension (Larroche and colleagues, 1990). In one study, Bejar and associates (1990) reported this in 15 percent of 89 twins and 12 triplets. Denbow and colleagues (1998) reviewed data from 17 sets of liveborn, monochorionic twins who had twin-to-twin transfusion syndrome. They found that one twin had a cerebral infarction and 10 other neonates had other antenatally acquired cerebral lesions. Both donors and recipients were affected. Sutcliffe and colleagues (2001) reported a 13-percent cerebral palsy rate for both donor and recipient twins who survived in utero laser ablation therapy for the twin-to-twin transfusion syndrome.

Cerebral pathology in the survivor most likely results from acute hypotension at the time of the death of one twin (Benirschke, 1993). A less likely cause is from emboli of thromboplastic material originating from the dead fetus. Fusi and co-workers (1990, 1991) observed that at the time of death of one twin fetus, acute twin-to-twin anastomotic transfusion from the high-pressure vessels of the living twin to the low-resistance vessels of the dead twin leads rapidly to hypovolemia and ischemic antenatal brain damage in the survivor. This group described eight monochorionic twin pregnancies in which one twin died but the pregnancy continued. Postpartum evaluation showed that none developed disseminated intravascular coagulopathy, and yet there was a high frequency of neurological damage. Pharoah and Adi (2000) surveyed 348 survivors whose twin sibling had died in utero. The prevalence of cerebral palsy was 83 per 1000 live births—a 40-fold increased risk. Okamura and colleagues (1994) performed cordocentesis on seven surviving twin fetuses within 24 hours of their sibling's death. Each surviving twin had acute anemia, and the investigators hypothesized that cerebral abnormalities were produced by hypotensive cerebral ischemia due to acute blood transfer. This result has been reported as early as 16 weeks (Anderson and co-workers, 1990).

The acute nature of the twin-to-twin transfusion and subsequent hypotension following the death of one twin makes successful intervention for the survivor nearly impossible. Even with delivery immediately after the demise is recognized, the hypotension that occurs at the moment of death has likely already caused irreversible damage (Langer and associates, 1997; Wada and co-workers, 1998).

DIAGNOSIS. The diagnosis of twin-to-twin transfusion syndrome, whether made antenatally or postnatally, is problematic. The postnatal diagnosis was classically made based on a weight discordancy between twins of 15 or 20 percent and a hemoglobin level difference of 5 g/dL or greater, with the smaller twin being anemic. It is now recognized, however, that significant weight differences between twins can have a variety of causes such as discordancy for anomalies, infection, or nutritional support.

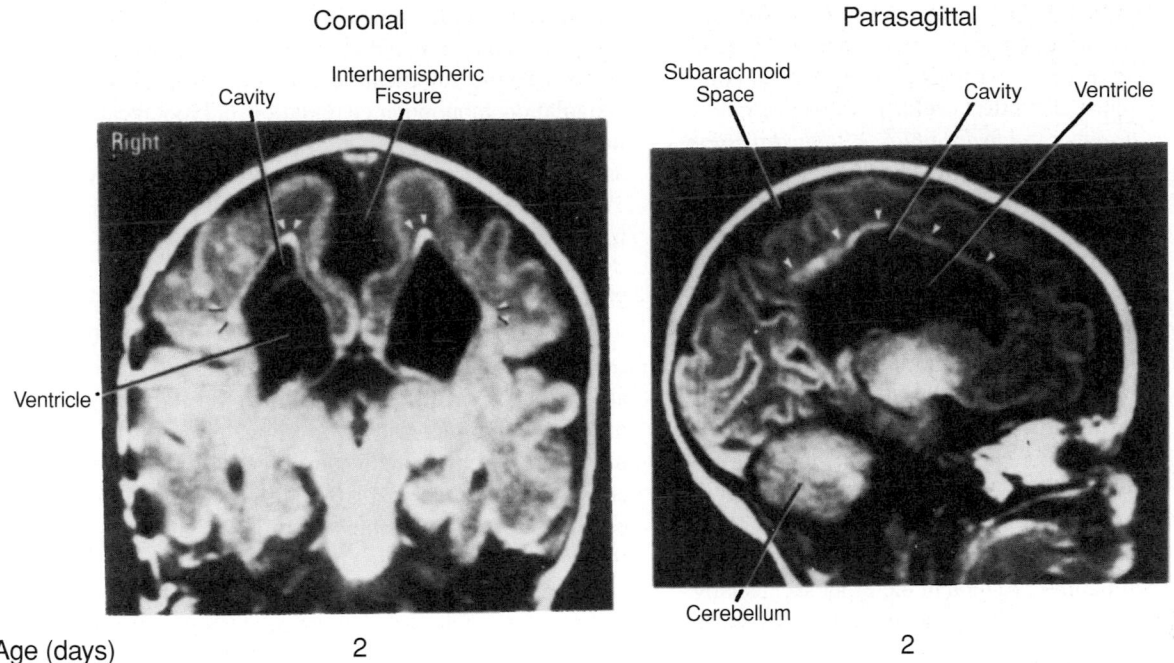

Coronal

Cavity

Interhemispheric Fissure

Right

Ventricle

Parasagittal

Subarachnoid Space

Cavity

Ventricle

Cerebellum

Age (days)   2   2

FIGURE 39–24. Cranial magnetic resonance imaging study of a diamnionic–monochorionic twin performed on day 2 of life. The subarachnoid space and lateral ventricles are markedly enlarged. There are large cavitary lesions in the white matter adjacent to the ventricles. The bright signals (*arrowheads*) in the periphery of the cavitary lesions most probably correspond to gliosis. (From Bejar and colleagues, 1990, with permission.)

In addition, hemoglobin level discordancy can develop acutely at the time of delivery. Wenstrom and colleagues (1992) illustrated this by reviewing the birthweights and hemoglobin concentrations in 97 monochorionic twin pregnancies. They found that 37 percent of weight concordant twins and 50 percent of discordant twins had a significant hemoglobin level discordancy. The twin delivered second had the higher hemoglobin value in 63 percent of pairs, including a third of the discordant twins in which this second twin was the smaller. This suggests that the hemoglobin level discordancy resulted from acute transfusion after the delivery of the first twin and before the delivery of the second twin. Although this pattern met the criteria for twin-to-twin transfusion, it was not clinically important because it was an acute phenomenon. Classic features of twin-to-twin transfusion, namely weight discordancy with the smaller twin being anemic, occurred in only 11 of these 97 twin pairs. Danskin and Neilson (1989) also concluded that this syndrome cannot be established definitively if based solely on birthweight or newborn hemoglobin level differences.

Clinically important twin-to-twin transfusion syndrome frequently is chronic and results from significant antenatal vascular volume differences between the twins. The syndrome typically presents in the midtrimester when the donor fetus becomes oliguric due to decreased renal perfusion (Mari and co-authors, 1993). This fetus develops oligohydramnios, and the recipient fetus develops severe hydramnios, presumably due to increased urine production. Virtual absence of amnionic fluid in the donor sac prevents fetal motion, giving rise to the descriptive term *stuck twin* (Berry and co-workers, 1995). This hydramnios–oligohydramnios combination can lead to growth restriction, contractures, and pulmonary hypoplasia in one twin, and premature rupture of the membranes and heart failure in the other.

The goal of antenatal diagnosis is to prevent fetal morbidity and mortality by selecting candidates for prenatal therapy or delivery. Antenatal criteria recommended for defining the twin-to-twin transfusion syndrome include the following: same sex fetuses, monochorionicity with placental vascular anastomoses, weight difference between twins greater than 20 percent, hydramnios in the larger twin, oligohydramnios or stuck twin in the smaller twin, and hemoglobin difference greater than 5 g/dL (Bruner and Rosemond, 1993). All of these criteria except hemoglobin levels can be determined ultrasonographically.

Situations in which the diagnosis must be confirmed, for example, before consideration of a high-risk therapy (see later discussion), may warrant invasive testing because the ultrasonographic diagnosis is sometimes incorrect. Saunders and co-workers (1991) used cordocentesis to show that none of four sets of monochorionic twins with all the ultrasonographic features of twin-to-twin transfusion actually had discordant hemoglobin concentrations. Bruner and Rosemond (1993) used cordocentesis and adult red blood cell infusion to show that only four of nine monochorionic twin pregnancies with ultrasonographic features of twin-to-twin transfusion actually had the syndrome. The cause of the discordant amnionic fluid volumes in these cases is unknown. When fetal hemoglobin concentrations have not been determined antenatally, it may be more accurate to refer to this situation as the *stuck twin syndrome* or the *hydramnios–oligohydramnios syndrome,* thus acknowledging that twin-to-twin transfusion has not been confirmed as the cause of the ultrasonographic findings.

THERAPY AND OUTCOME. The prognosis for multifetal gestations complicated by twin-to-twin transfusion syndrome is extremely guarded. Hazards are brain damage, antenatal death of one twin, and neonatal death due to preterm delivery. Lutfi and colleagues (2004) found the increased morbidity and mortality linked to preterm delivery rather than to weight discordancy or the effects of twin-to-twin transfusion syndrome. Unfortunately, the most serious form of twin-to-twin transfusion syndrome, with acute hydramnios in one sac and a stuck twin with anhydramnios in the other sac, usually presents between 18 and 26 weeks. The survival rate for those diagnosed before 28 weeks has been reported to vary widely, from 7 to 75 percent (Berghella and Kaufmann, 2001).

Several therapies are currently used for twin-to-twin transfusion, including amnioreduction, septostomy, laser ablation of vascular anastomoses, and selective feticide. Recently, but only in preliminary form, comparative data from randomized trials for some of these techniques have become available.

Saade and colleagues (2002) compared amnioreduction and septostomy (intentional creation of a communication in the dividing amnionic membrane) in a multicentered randomized trial. Repeated procedures were performed for symptoms or when the greatest vertical pocket of amnionic fluid exceeded 12 cm. Perinatal outcomes were the same in each group. Overall survival was 65 percent, and there was at least one survivor in 77 percent of pregnancies. The average number of procedures was two in the amnioreduction group compared with one in the septostomy group.

More recently, in a randomized trial of 142 women with severe twin-to-twin transfusion syndrome diagnosed before 26 weeks, Senat and colleagues (2004) reported increased survival of at least one twin with laser ablation of vascular anastomoses compared with serial amnioreduction (76 percent versus 51 percent). In an ongoing National Institutes of Health–sponsored multicentered trial, laser ablation is being compared with amnioreduction. Long-term evaluation of the neonates in both arms is important, because the rate of cerebral palsy in a recent cohort who survived twin-to-twin transfusion was 21 percent (Lopriore and co-workers, 2003).

Selective reduction has generally been considered when severe amnionic fluid and growth disturbances develop early (e.g., before 20 weeks), leading to the likelihood that both fetuses will die without intervention. Selection of the twin to be terminated has been based on evidence of damage to either fetus and comparison of their prognoses. Any substance injected into one twin may affect the other twin. Feticidal techniques include saline cardiac tamponade followed by intracardiac potassium chloride; injection of an occlusive substance into the umbilical vein; and fetoscopic ligation, laser coagulation, monopolar coagulation, or bipolar cautery of the umbilical cord (Challis and co-workers, 1999; Donner and associates, 1997; Weiner, 1987; Wittmann and colleagues, 1986). After these procedures, the risks to the remaining fetus are appreciable.

DISCORDANT TWINS. Size inequality of twin fetuses, which may be a sign of pathological growth restriction in one fetus, is calculated using the larger twin as the index. Generally, as the weight difference within a twin pair increases, perinatal mortality increases proportionately. Restricted growth of one twin fetus usually develops late in the second and early third trimester and is often asymmetrical (Leveno and co-workers, 1979). Earlier discordancy is usually symmetrical and indicates higher risk for fetal demise. Generally, the earlier in pregnancy discordancy develops, the more serious the sequelae. In an extreme example, Weissman and colleagues (1994) diagnosed weight discordancy between 6 and 11 weeks in five twin gestations, and all of the smaller twins had major malformations.

Pathology. The cause of birthweight inequality in twin fetuses is often unclear, but evidence indicates that the etiology in monochorionic twins differs from that in dichorionic twins. In monochorionic twins, discordancy is usually attributed to placental vascular anastomoses that cause hemodynamic imbalance between the twins. Reduced pressure and perfusion of the donor twin may result in its placenta failing to grow (Benirschke, 1993). Occasionally, monochorionic twins are discordant in size because they are discordant for structural anomalies.

A variety of factors are believed to cause discordancy in dichorionic twins. Dizygotic fetuses may have different genetic growth potential, especially if they are of opposite genders. Alternatively, because the placentas are separate and require more implantation space, one of the placentas may have a suboptimal implantation site. Mordel and colleagues (1993) observed that the incidence of discordancy is twice as great in triplets as it is in twins. This finding lends additional credence to the view that in utero crowding plays a role in fetal growth restriction.

Eberle and co-workers (1993) performed an evaluation of placental pathology in 147 twin gestations that provides important insight into the etiology of discordant twins. They quantified placental lesions that are usually associated with singleton growth restriction. Placentas from the smaller fetus in discordant dichorionic twin pairs demonstrated the lesions typical of singleton fetal growth restriction, whereas these lesions were not found in discordant monochorionic twin pairs.

Diagnosis. There are two areas of uncertainty in determination of discordancy in twins. One, which ultrasonographic anatomical measurements most reliably predict discordancy? Two, what fetal weight difference is clinically significant? Size discordancy between twins can be determined in several ways.

One common method of determining discordancy uses all fetal measurements to compute the estimated weight of each twin and then to compare the weight of the smaller twin with that of the larger twin (weight of larger twin minus weight of smaller twin, divided by weight of larger twin). Alternatively, considering that growth restriction is the primary concern and that abdominal circumference reflects fetal nutrition, some authors diagnose discordancy when abdominal circumferences differ by more than 20 mm.

Hill and colleagues (1994) evaluated the ultrasonographic assessment of twin discordancy and found that abdominal circumference was superior to head circumference, femur length, or transverse cerebellar diameter as the most useful index of size discordancy. Several different weight disparities between twins have been used to define discordancy. Accumulated data suggest that a greater than 25- to 30-percent weight discordancy, usually with growth restriction in one or both twins, most accurately predicts an adverse perinatal outcome.

Hollier and co-workers (1999) retrospectively evaluated 1370 twin pairs delivered at Parkland Hospital and stratified twin weight discordancy in 5-percent increments within a range of 15 to 40 percent. They found that the incidence of respiratory distress, intraventricular hemorrhage, seizures, periventricular leukomalacia, sepsis, and necrotizing enterocolitis increased directly with the degree of weight discordancy. These conditions increased substantially when discordancy was greater than 25 percent. The relative risk of fetal death increased significantly to 5.6 when there was more than 30-percent discordancy, and but increased to 18.9 when there was over 40-percent discordancy.

Management. Ultrasonographic monitoring of growth within a twin pair has become a mainstay in the management of twin gestations. Other ultrasonographic findings, such as oligohydramnios, may be helpful in gauging fetal risk. Depending on the degree of discordancy and the gestational age, fetal surveillance may be indicated, especially if one or both fetuses exhibit growth restriction. Delivery is usually not performed for size discordancy alone, except occasionally at advanced gestational ages.

DEATH OF ONE FETUS. On occasion, one fetus dies remote from term, but the pregnancy continues with one living fetus. Saito and co-workers (1999) reviewed 481 twin pregnancies and reported that the risk of single fetal death in a twin pregnancy was 6.2 percent. Factors influencing pregnancy loss in twins have been described by Rydhström (1994), who used the Medical Birth Registry in Stockholm to review fetal death in 15,066 twin pairs weighing 500 g or more. Same-sex twins were at highest risk. One or both twins died in 1.1

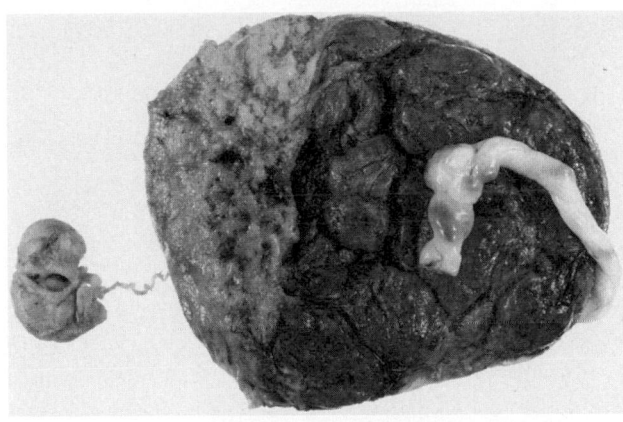

FIGURE 39–25. To the left is a fetus papyraceous that died at midpregnancy, its cord, and its pale placenta. To the right are the normal placenta and cord of the healthy 3200-g twin.

percent of opposite-sex twins and 2.6 percent of same-sex twins. Weight discordancy also increased the risk of death. In opposite-sex twins, however, the risk of death remained constant at 1.2 percent until the weight discordancy exceeded 40 to 50 percent or 1000 g. In same-sex twins, discordancy of only 20 percent or 250 g increased the risk. After the death of one twin, the risk of subsequent death in the surviving twin was sixfold greater in same-sex twins. Although chorionicity was not known in all cases, the authors estimated that the death rate for same-sex dizygotic twins was the same as for opposite-sex twins (0.8 percent), and that monochorionic twins had the greatest risk of death (3 percent).

At delivery, the dead fetus with placenta and membranes may be identifiable but may be compressed appreciably (fetus compressus) or may be flattened remarkably through loss of fluid and most of the soft tissue (fetus papyraceous). The papyraceous fetus shown in Figure 39–25 died at midpregnancy, whereas the surviving fetus and placenta thrived. The dead fetus shown in Figure 39–26 has become almost a shadow of itself compressed onto its placenta, which was separate from the placenta of the surviving twin.

The prognosis for the surviving twin depends on the gestational age at the time of the demise, the chorionicity, and the length of time between the demise and delivery of the surviving twin. Early demise such as a "vanishing twin" does not appear to increase the risk of death in the surviving fetus after the first trimester. It is intriguing that selective reduction of a higher-order multiple pregnancy (discussed subsequently) increases the risk of aborting all fetuses but does not appear to increase the risk of other maternal or fetal complications.

Later in gestation, the death of one of multiple fetuses could theoretically trigger coagulation defects in the mother. Only a few cases of maternal coagulopathy after a single fetal death in a twin pregnancy have been reported, probably because the surviving twin is usually delivered within a few weeks of the demise (see Chap. 35, p. 845).

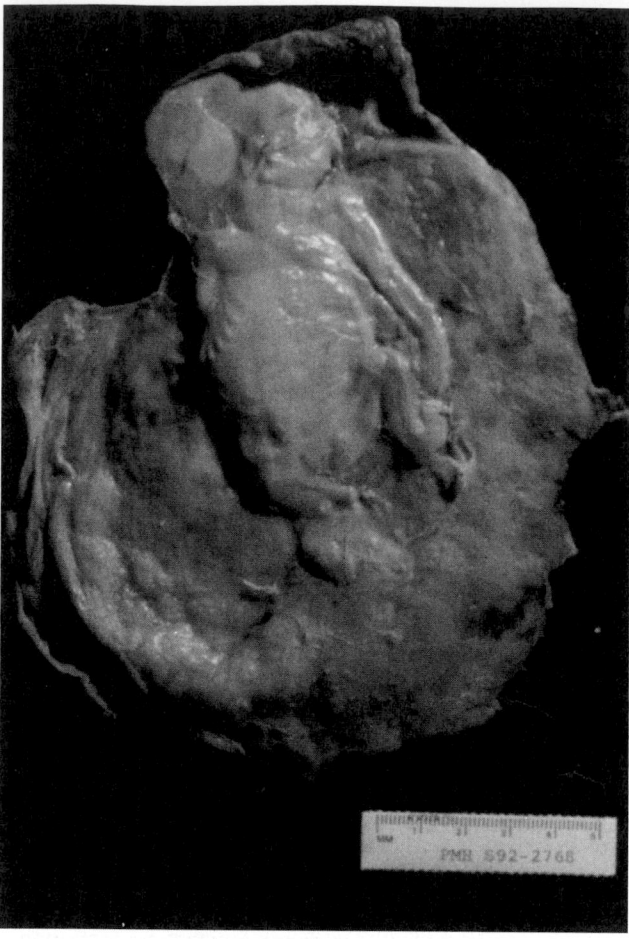

FIGURE 39–26. A long-dead twin fetus compressed onto its placenta. A separate placenta supported the surviving twin fetus.

We have observed transient, spontaneously corrected consumptive coagulopathy when one fetus died and was retained in utero along with its surviving twin. The fibrinogen concentration initially decreased but then increased spontaneously, and the level of serum fibrinogen–fibrin degradation products decreased to normal. At delivery, the portions of the placenta that supplied the living fetus appeared normal. In contrast, the part that had once provided for the dead fetus was the site of massive fibrin deposition, which may have accounted directly for the decrease in maternal fibrinogen levels and in turn, an increase in the level of fibrin degradation products. Alternatively, this site may have served to block the escape of thromboplastin from the fetus and the placenta into the maternal circulation and thereby prevented disseminated intravascular coagulation. Both mechanisms may also have been operational until extensive fibrosis was achieved. The surviving fetus continued to thrive in utero and had normal plasma fibrinogen levels, serum fibrinogen–fibrin degradation product levels, and platelet counts at birth.

Management decisions should be based on the cause of death and the risk to the surviving fetus. The majority of

cases of a single fetal death in twin pregnancy involve monochorionic placentation. Evidence indicates that morbidity in the monochorionic twin survivor is almost always due to vascular anastomoses, which first cause the demise of one twin and then produce sudden hypotension in the other. Benirschke (1993) concluded that it is implausible that degenerating material from a dead fetus could travel back to a living twin sibling. Considering that coagulopathy takes at least 5 weeks to develop, it is unlikely that there would still be shared circulation at that time.

Less frequently, fetal death results from a maternal complication such as diabetic ketoacidosis or severe preeclampsia with abruption. Pregnancy management is based on the diagnosis and the status of both mother and surviving fetus. When the death of one dichorionic twin is due to a discordant congenital anomaly, its cause of death should not affect its surviving twin. Santema and co-workers (1995b) assessed the cause and outcome of 29 consecutive twin pregnancies in which one of the fetuses died after 20 weeks. The causes of fetal death were not clear in all cases. The most common associations were monochorionic placentation and severe preeclampsia. These investigators concluded that in most cases the benefit derived from continuation of a multifetal pregnancy exceeded the risks of preterm delivery after diagnosis of fetal death. They recommended conservative management of the living fetus.

Impending Death of One Fetus. Abnormal antepartum test results of fetal health in one twin fetus but not the other pose a particular dilemma. Delivery may be the best option for the compromised fetus yet may result in death from immaturity of the second (Fig. 39–27). When fetal lung maturity is confirmed, salvage of both the healthy fetus and its jeopardized sibling is possible. Unfortunately, ideal management when twins are immature is problematic but should be based on the chances of intact survival for both fetuses. Often the compromised fetus is severely growth restricted or anomalous. An advantage of performing amniocentesis for fetal karyotyping in women of advanced maternal age carrying twin pregnancies, even for those who would continue their pregnancies regardless of the diagnosis, is that the detection of aneuploidy in one fetus allows rational decisions about intervention to be made.

Death of Both Twin Fetuses. Rydhström (1996) reported that, excluding abortions, both fetuses died in 0.5 percent of twin pregnancies. Causes implicated in these deaths were monochorionic placentation and discordant fetal growth.

COMPLETE HYDATIDIFORM MOLE AND COEXISTING FETUS. This entity is different from a partial molar pregnancy because there are two separate conceptuses, with a normal placenta supplying nutrition to one twin and a complete molar gestation supporting the other. Optimal management is uncertain, but preterm delivery is frequently required

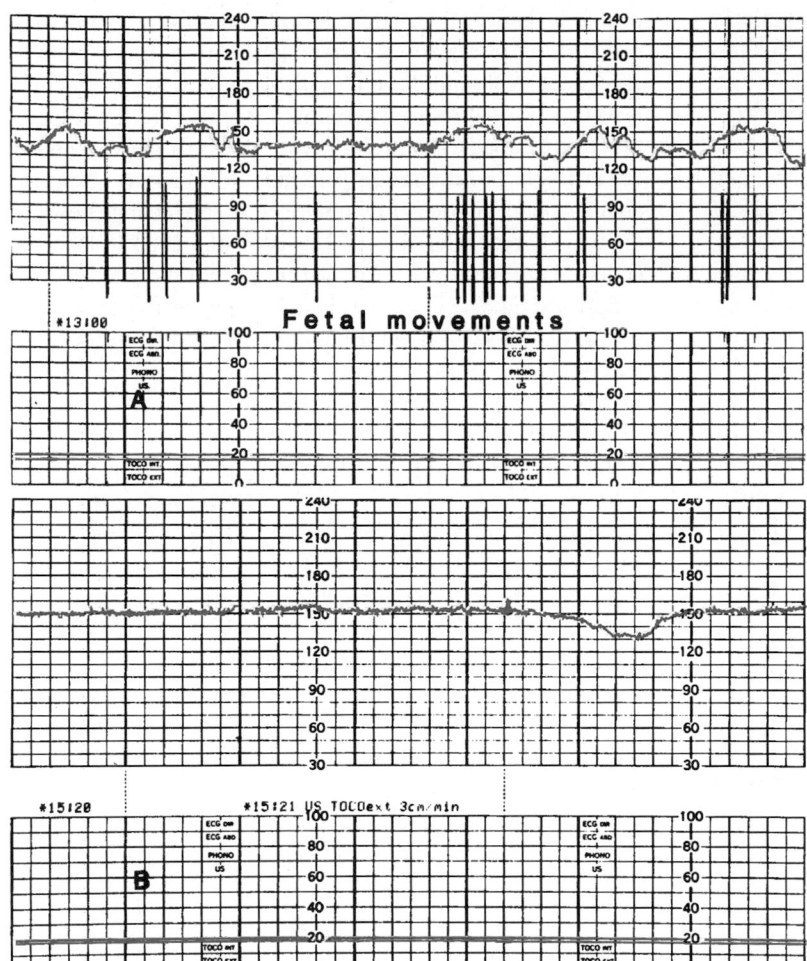

FIGURE 39–27. Antepartum fetal heart rate recordings in discordant twin fetuses at 31 weeks. **A.** Accelerations in response to movements are seen for twin A, whose birthweight was 1200 g. **B.** Spontaneous uteroplacental insufficiency–type decelerations were observed in twin B, whose birthweight was 700 g. This fetus also failed to move or accelerate its heart rate. Because of these findings, cesarean delivery was performed. Both twins died 3 days after delivery; twin A died of hyaline membrane disease and twin B died due to hypoxic encephalopathy.

because of bleeding or severe preeclampsia. Bristow and colleagues (1996) reviewed 26 cases and found that 73 percent required evacuation before the time of fetal viability, but the remainder continued without serious complications until fetal viability was reached. Sebire and colleagues (2002) reported a live birth rate of almost 40 percent in 53 such pregnancies. Any pregnancy consisting of a complete mole carries significant risk for subsequent gestational trophoblastic neoplasia (see Chap. 11, p. 279).

ANTEPARTUM MANAGEMENT OF TWIN PREGNANCY

To reduce perinatal mortality and morbidity in pregnancies complicated by twins, it is imperative that:

1. Delivery of markedly preterm infants be prevented.
2. Failure of one or both fetuses to thrive be identified and fetuses so afflicted be delivered before they become moribund.
3. Fetal trauma during labor and delivery be avoided.
4. Expert neonatal care be available.

DIET. The requirements for calories, protein, minerals, vitamins, and essential fatty acids are further increased in women with multiple fetuses. The Recommended Dietary Allowances made by the Food and Nutrition Board of the National Research Council for uncomplicated pregnancy should not only be met but in most instances exceeded (see Chap. 8, p. 213). Caloric consumption should be increased by another 300 kcal/day. Brown and Carlson (2000) have recommended that weight gain be based in part on prepregnancy weight but that women with triplet pregnancies should gain at least 50 pounds. Supplementation with 60 to 100 mg/day of iron and with 1 mg of folic acid is recommended.

MATERNAL HYPERTENSION. Hypertensive disorders due to pregnancy are more likely to develop with multiple fetuses. The exact incidence attributable to twin gestation is difficult to determine, because twin pregnancies are more likely to deliver preterm before preeclampsia can develop, and because women with twin pregnancies are often older and multiparous. For example, the incidence of pregnancy-related hypertension in women with twins is 20 percent at Parkland Hospital. Santema and co-workers (1995a) performed a case-control study in which 187 twin and 187 singleton pregnancies were matched for maternal age, parity, and gestational age at delivery. The incidence of hypertension was significantly higher in women carrying twin pregnancies (15 versus 6 percent). Coonrad and colleagues (1995) reviewed the outcomes of 3407 twin and 8287 singleton pregnancies and found that twin pregnancy carries an overall fourfold increased risk of preeclampsia independent of race and parity. Mastrobattista and colleagues (1997) compared 53 triplet with 53 twin pregnancies and observed that the rate of severe preeclampsia was significantly higher in women carrying triplets (23 versus 6 percent).

These data suggest that fetal number and placental mass are involved in the pathogenesis of preeclampsia. With multifetal gestation, hypertension not only develops more often but also tends to develop earlier and to be more severe. Interestingly, Hardardottir and colleagues (1996) have reported that women with preeclampsia due to higher-order multifetal gestations more often develop epigastric pain, hemolysis, and thrombocytopenia as a result of their disease.

ANTEPARTUM SURVEILLANCE. As discussed earlier, fetal growth is slower in multifetal pregnancies than in singleton gestations, and it also may be unequal within a twin pair. For these reasons, serial ultrasonographic examinations are usually performed throughout the third trimester. Appropriate interval growth is reassuring, and size discordancy is of greatest concern when one fetus is growth restricted.

Assessment of amnionic fluid volume is also important, because associated oligohydramnios may indicate uteroplacental pathology and should prompt further evaluation of fetal well-being. Quantifying amnionic fluid volume in multiple gestation, however, can be difficult. Some clinicians measure the deepest vertical pocket in each sac, or assess the fluid subjectively. If the sacs are side by side, as opposed to one on top of the other, measurement of the amnionic fluid index (AFI) may be helpful. Using data from 405 uncomplicated twin pregnancies, Porter and associates (1996) described a protocol for measuring the AFI in twin gestations and provided normal values. As in singletons, the deepest vertical pocket in each quadrant was measured, regardless of the location of the dividing membrane. An AFI of less than 8 cm (below the 5th percentile) or greater than 24 cm (above the 95th percentile) was considered abnormal at gestational ages from 28 to 40 weeks. If the overall AFI is abnormal, the ultrasonographer must determine which sac is involved and attempt to quantify the degree of abnormality. Subjective assessment is often required and is not always accurate. Magann and co-workers (1995) reported that oligohydramnios, defined as less than 500 mL, is poorly identified by any ultrasonographic method in twin gestations.

Tests of Fetal Well-Being. As described throughout Chapter 15, there are several methods of assessing fetal health in singleton pregnancies. The nonstress test or biophysical profile is commonly used in management of twin or higher-order multiple gestations. The complexity of complications associated with multifetal gestations as well as the potential technical difficulties in differentiating fetuses during antepartum testing appears to limit the usefulness of these methods. For example, Saacks and co-workers (1995) observed that the antepartum death rate of twin fetuses did not change between the two 10-year intervals 1952 to 1962 and 1983 to 1993 despite the availability of fetal testing during the later decade. Elliott and Finberg (1995) used the biophysical profile as the primary method for monitoring of higher-order multiple gestations. They reported that 4 of 24 monitored pregnancies had a poor outcome despite reassuring biophysical profile scores. In a randomized trial of 526 twin pregnancies, the addition of umbilical artery Doppler velocimetry to management compared with fetal testing based on fetal growth parameters alone resulted in no improvement in perinatal outcome (Giles and associates, 2003).

Whatever method is used, care must be taken to evaluate each fetus separately. Gallagher and colleagues (1992) analyzed fetal heart rate accelerations, fetal movement, and other behavioral states in 15 twin pairs. If one twin of a pair was awake or asleep so was its sibling, however, accelerations and movements were usually not coincidental (Fig. 39–28).

Doppler Velocimetry. As discussed in Chapters 15 and 16, Doppler evaluation of vascular resistance may provide a measure of fetal well-being. Increased resistance with diminished diastolic flow velocity often accompanies restricted fetal growth. Doppler values in twins and triplets are the same as in singletons and can thus be used in a similar manner (Akiyama and co-workers, 1999). As in singletons, however, the clinical utility of this technology is controversial.

Gerson and co-workers (1987) used duplex Doppler ultrasonography to measure umbilical venous blood flow and arterial systolic–diastolic velocity ratios to predict concordant and discordant growth in twins. Normal studies correctly predicted concordancy in 44 of 45 concordant twin pairs. Abnormal values, especially those from the umbilical artery, correctly predicted differences in 9 of 11 sets of discordant twins. Conversely, DiVou and co-workers (1989) reported that velocimetry alone was not consistently useful in identifying twin discordancy. Ezra and colleagues (1999) found that in triplets and quadruplets, as in singletons, absent end-diastolic blood flow in the umbilical artery was associated with low birthweight and perinatal mortality.

PREVENTION OF PRETERM DELIVERY. Several techniques have been applied in attempts to prolong multifetal gestations. These include bed rest, especially through hospitalization, prophylactic administration of beta-mimetic drugs, and prophylactic cervical cerclage.

Bed Rest. Most evidence suggests that routine hospitalization is not beneficial in prolonging multifetal pregnancy. For

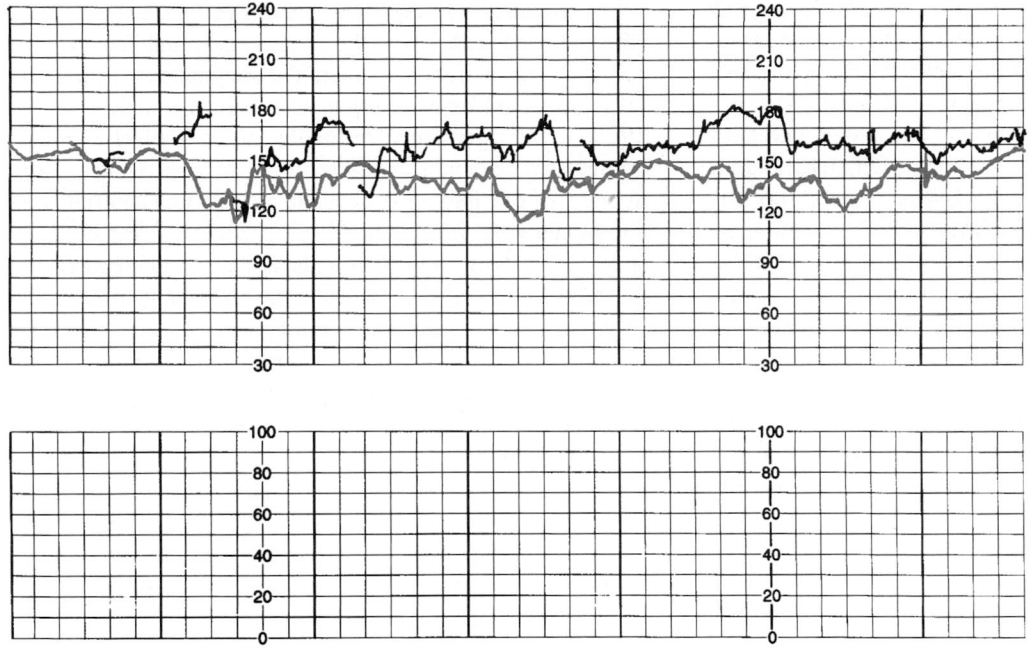

FIGURE 39–28. Simultaneous antepartum fetal heart rate recordings from twin fetuses showing that accelerations are not necessarily synchronous.

example, Crowther and co-workers (1990) randomly chose hospitalization or routine care for 139 Zimbabwean women with twin pregnancies. They found that hospitalized bed rest did not prolong pregnancy or improve neonatal survival, although it did improve fetal growth. At Parkland Hospital, elective hospitalization at 26 weeks was compared with outpatient management, and no advantages were found for routine hospitalization (Andrews and colleagues, 1991). It is worth noting, however, that almost half of the twin pregnancies studied required admission for specific indications such as hypertension or threatened preterm delivery.

Limited physical activity, early work leave, more frequent health care visits and ultrasonographic examinations, and structured maternal education on the risks of preterm delivery have been advocated to be effective in reducing preterm births in women with multiple fetuses. Unfortunately, there is little evidence that these measures substantially change outcome. For example, Pons and co-workers (1998) found virtually no difference in outcomes of 70 triplet pregnancies managed intensively from 1987 to 1993 compared with 21 triplet pregnancies managed routinely between 1975 and 1986. The only major difference between these two periods was that neonates born in the later time period group had significantly less hyaline membrane disease (13 versus 31 percent), which these investigators attributed to the use of corticosteroids.

Tocolytic Therapy. As for singleton pregnancies, there is no valid evidence that tocolytic therapy improves neonatal outcomes in multifetal gestation (Gyetvai and co-workers, 1999). Importantly, tocolytic therapy in these women entails a higher risk than in singletons. This is in part because the increased plasma volume and cardiovascular demands increase susceptibility to hydration-associated pulmonary edema. Gabriel and colleagues (1994) compared the outcomes of 26 twin and 6 triplet pregnancies with those of 51 singletons treated with a beta-mimetic for preterm labor without ruptured membranes. Women with a multifetal gestation had significantly more cardiovascular complications (43 versus 4 percent), including three cases of pulmonary edema.

Corticosteroids for Lung Maturation. Although corticosteroids are less studied in multifetal gestations than in singletons, there is no biological reason that these drugs would not benefit multiple fetuses (Crowley, 2003). Therefore, guidelines for the use of corticosteroids are not different for multifetal gestation (American College of Obstetricians and Gynecologists, 2004).

Cerclage. Prophylactic cervical cerclage has not been shown to improve perinatal outcome in multifetal pregnancies. Studies have included women who were not specially selected as well as those who were selected because of a shortened cervix as assessed by transvaginal ultrasonography (Dor and associates, 1982; Elimian and colleagues, 1999; Newman and colleagues, 2002).

PRETERM LABOR PREDICTION. Goldenberg and colleagues (1996) prospectively screened 147 twin pregnancies for more than 50 potential risk factors for preterm birth and found that only cervical length and fetal fibronectin levels predicted preterm birth. At 24 weeks, a cervical length of 25 mm or less was the best predictor of birth before 32 weeks. At 28 weeks, an elevated fetal fibronectin level was the best predictor. Similarly, Souka and co-workers (1999) ultrasonographically measured the cervices of 215 women with twin pregnancies at 23 weeks. They found that a length of 25 mm or less predicted preterm birth with a sensitivity of 100 percent at 28 weeks, 80 percent at 30 weeks, 47 percent at 32 weeks, and 35 percent at 34 weeks. Conversely, McMahon and colleagues (2002) found that women with multifetal gestation at 24 weeks who had a closed internal os on digital cervical examination, a normal cervical length by ultrasonographic examination, and a negative fetal fibronectin test result were at *low* risk to deliver before 32 weeks. Interestingly, a closed internal os by digital examination was as predictive as the combination of normal cervical length and negative fetal fibronectin test results.

PULMONARY MATURATION. As measured by determination of the lecithin-sphingomyelin ratio, pulmonary maturation is usually synchronous in twins (Leveno and associates, 1984). Moreover, although this ratio usually exceeds 2 by 36 weeks in singleton pregnancies, it often does so by about 32 weeks in multifetal pregnancy. In some cases, however, pulmonary function may be markedly different, with the smallest, most stressed fetus being more mature. We observed the lecithin–sphingomyelin ratio with quintuplets to vary from less than 2 for the largest infant, who weighed 1530 g at 32 weeks and was of appropriate size, to greater than 5 for the severely growth-restricted smallest infant, who weighed 860 g. The largest infant developed respiratory distress, whereas the smallest infant did not.

PRETERM MEMBRANE RUPTURE. Twin gestations with preterm ruptured membranes are managed expectantly much like singleton pregnancies (see Chap. 36, p. 864). Mercer and colleagues (1993) compared outcomes of twin and singleton pregnancies, both with prematurely ruptured membranes at 19 to 36 weeks. They found that labor ensued earlier in twins. Specifically, the median time from rupture to delivery was 1.1 days in twins compared with 1.7 days in singletons. More than 90 percent in both groups delivered within 7 days of membrane rupture. Similarly, Hsieh and colleagues (1999) studied 131 twin pregnancies and 48 singleton pregnancies with preterm premature membrane rupture. They found, regardless of the gestational age at rupture, that 50 percent of twins compared with 27 percent of singletons delivered within 48 hours and that 92 percent of twins and 86 percent of singletons delivered within 7 days.

DELAYED DELIVERY OF SECOND TWIN. Infrequently, after preterm birth of the presenting fetus, it may be advantageous for the undelivered fetus(es) to remain within the uterus. Trivedi and Gillett (1998) reviewed the English literature and found 45 case reports of asynchronous birth

in multifetal gestation. Most often, the first birth resulted from preterm rupture of the membranes, and the survival rate for these infants was poor. The pregnancies with a surviving retained twin or triplet continued for an average of 49 days. Management with tocolytics, prophylactic antimicrobials, and cerclage appeared to make no difference. After delivery of one fetus, Farkouh and colleagues (2000) treated 24 women with twin or triplet pregnancies with tocolytics, local and systemic antimicrobials, and cervical cerclage and reported a mean delivery delay in the remaining sibling(s) of 36 days. Whether these interventions are beneficial is a matter of speculation, because these women were not randomized. Livingston and colleagues (2004) described 14 pregnancies in which an active attempt was made to delay delivery of 19 fetuses after delivery of the twin. Only one fetus survived without major sequelae, and one mother developed sepsis syndrome with shock.

If asynchronous birth is attempted, there must be careful evaluation for infection, abruption, and congenital anomalies. The mother must be thoroughly counseled, particularly about the potential for serious, even life-threatening infection. The range of gestational age in which the benefits outweigh the risks of delayed delivery is likely narrow. Avoidance of delivery from 23 to 26 weeks would seem most beneficial. In our experience, good candidates for delayed delivery are rare.

DELIVERY OF TWIN FETUSES

LABOR. Many complications of labor and delivery, including preterm labor, uterine contractile dysfunction, abnormal presentation, prolapse of the umbilical cord, premature separation of the placenta, and immediate postpartum hemorrhage are encountered more often with multiple fetuses than with singletons. For these reasons, certain precautions and special arrangements are prudent when delivery of two or more fetuses is expected. Recommendations for intrapartum management include:

1. An appropriately trained obstetrical attendant should remain with the mother throughout labor. Continuous external electronic monitoring or, if the membranes are ruptured and the cervix dilated, simultaneous evaluation of both the presenting fetus by internal electronic monitoring and the remaining sibling(s) by external monitors, is typically used.
2. Blood transfusion products should be readily available.
3. An intravenous infusion system capable of delivering fluid rapidly should be established. In the absence of hemorrhage or metabolic disturbance during labor, lactated Ringer or an aqueous dextrose solution is infused at a rate of 60 to 120 mL/hr.
4. An obstetrician skilled in intrauterine identification of fetal parts and in intrauterine manipulation of a fetus should be present.

5. An ultrasonography machine should be readily available to help evaluate the position and status of the remaining fetus(es) after delivery of the first.

6. An experienced anesthesiologist should be immediately available in the event that intrauterine manipulation or cesarean delivery is necessary.

7. For each fetus, two people, one of whom is skilled in resuscitation and care of newborns, are appropriately informed of the case and remain immediately available.

8. The delivery area should provide adequate space for all members of the team to work effectively. Moreover, the site should be appropriately equipped to take care of any maternal problems plus resuscitation and maintenance of each neonate.

Presentation and Position. With twins, all possible combinations of fetal positions may be encountered. The most common presentations at admission for delivery are cephalic–cephalic, cephalic–breech, and cephalic–transverse (Fig. 39–29). Importantly, these presentations, especially those other than cephalic–cephalic, are unstable before and during labor and delivery. Compound, face, brow, and footling breech presentations are relatively common, especially when the fetuses are small, amnionic fluid is excessive, or maternal parity is high. Prolapse of the cord is also common in these circumstances. The presentation can often be ascertained by ultrasonography. If any confusion about the relationship of the twins to each other or to the maternal pelvis persists, a single anteroposterior radiograph of the abdomen may be helpful.

Induction or Stimulation of Labor. Although labor is generally shorter with twins, it can be desultory (Schiff and associates, 1998). If women meet all criteria for the administration of oxytocin, it may be used as described in Chapter 22 (see p. 540).

Analgesia and Anesthesia. During labor and delivery of multiple fetuses, decisions regarding analgesia and anesthesia may be complicated by the frequency of and problems imposed by preterm labor, preeclampsia, desultory labor, need for intrauterine manipulation, and development of uterine atony and hemorrhage after delivery.

Epidural analgesia is recommended by many clinicians because it provides excellent pain relief and can be rapidly extended cephalad if internal podalic version or cesarean delivery is required (Koffel, 1999). Special care must be taken in hypertensive women or those who have hemorrhaged because epidural analgesia may cause hypotension with inadequate perfusion of vital organs, especially the placenta (see Chap. 19, p. 483). Therefore, placement and maintenance of continuous epidural analgesia should be performed by health care providers knowledgeable in obstetrics, and it should be preceded by adequate hydration and administered slowly. Because women pregnant with multiple fetuses are especially vulnerable to supine hypotension during labor and delivery, they should be placed in full lateral position during and after induction of epidural analgesia. Left uterine displacement should be maintained for cesarean delivery.

When general anesthesia is used, the increased maternal oxygen demand associated with multifetal gestation increases the risk of hypoxemia, thus making adequate preoxygenation essential. Pudendal block when administered along with nitrous oxide plus oxygen can provide relief of pain for spontaneous delivery. When intrauterine manipulation is necessary, as with internal podalic version, uterine relaxation can be accomplished rapidly with the inhalation anesthetic isoflurane. Because such agents provide effective relaxation for intrauterine manipulation, they also cause an increase in blood loss during the third stage. Some clinicians use intravenous or sublingual nitroglycerin to achieve uterine relaxation yet avoid the aspiration and hypoxia risks associated with general anesthetics (Vinatier and associates, 1996).

VAGINAL DELIVERY. The presenting twin typically bears the major force of dilating the cervix and the remaining soft tissues of the birth canal. When the first twin is cephalic, delivery can usually be accomplished spontaneously or with forceps.

As in singletons, when the first fetus presents as a breech, major problems are most likely to develop if:

1. The fetus is unusually large and the aftercoming head is larger than the capacity of the birth canal.
2. The fetus is sufficiently small so that the extremities and trunk are delivered through a cervix inadequately effaced and dilated to allow the head to escape easily.
3. The umbilical cord prolapses.

When these problems are anticipated or identified, cesarean delivery is often the preferred route of delivery, except in those instances in which the fetuses are so immature that they will not survive. Fetuses with breech presentation may be delivered as described in Chapter 24.

The phenomenon of locked twins is rare. According to Cohen and co-workers (1965), it occurred only once in 817

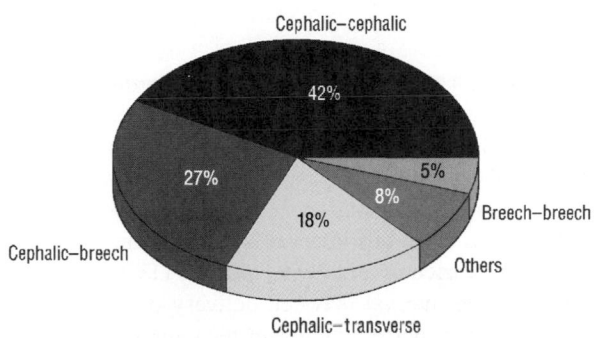

FIGURE 39–29. Presentations of twin fetuses on admission for delivery. (Data from Divon and colleagues, 1993.)

twin gestations. For twins to lock, the first fetus must present breech and the second cephalic. With descent of the breech through the birth canal, the chin of the first fetus locks between the neck and chin of the second, cephalic fetus. Cesarean delivery is recommended when the potential for locking is identified.

Hogle and colleagues (2003) performed an extensive literature review and concluded that planned cesarean delivery does not improve neonatal outcome when both twins are cephalic. The optimal delivery route for cephalic–noncephalic twins is controversial. Several reports attest to the safety of vaginal delivery of second noncephalic twins who weigh more than 1500 g (Blickstein, 1987; Chervanak, 1985; Gocke, 1989, and all their associates). According to the American College of Obstetricians and Gynecologists (1998), vaginal delivery of a nonvertex second twin is reasonable when the estimated fetal weight is greater than 1500 g. When the estimated fetal weight is less than 1500 g, the issue is less clear, although comparable or even improved fetal outcomes have been reported with vaginal relative to cesarean delivery (Caukwell and Murphy, 2002; Davidson and co-workers, 1992; Rydhström, 1990). Muleba and associates (2005) identified increased rates of respiratory distress in the second twin of preterm pairs regardless of the mode of delivery or corticosteroid use.

Mauldin and colleagues (1998) retrospectively reviewed the delivery courses of 84 cephalic–noncephalic twins. They found that vaginal delivery of the presenting twin followed by breech extraction of the second twin resulted in significantly shorter maternal and neonatal hospital stays, in part because vaginally extracted breech twins had less respiratory disease and infections.

When the first twin is breech, most physicians plan a cesarean delivery. The American College of Obstetricians and Gynecologists (1998b) has concluded that, in general, cesarean delivery is the method of choice when the first twin is noncephalic. More recently, however, Blickstein and colleagues (2000) reported the collective experience from 1990 to 1997 of 13 European centers that attempted vaginal delivery in 374 of 613 twin pairs when the presenting twin was breech. In their report, vaginal delivery did not increase the mortality of breech-presenting first twins who weighed at least 1500 g.

Vaginal Delivery of the Second Twin. As soon as the presenting twin has been delivered, the presenting part of the second twin, its size, and its relationship to the birth canal should be quickly and carefully ascertained by combined abdominal, vaginal, and at times intrauterine examination. Ultrasonography is also valuable in some cases. If the fetal head or the breech is fixed in the birth canal, moderate fundal pressure is applied and membranes are ruptured. Immediately afterward, digital examination of the cervix is repeated to exclude prolapse of the cord. Labor is allowed to resume, and the fetal heart rate is monitored. With reestablishment of labor

there is no need to hasten delivery unless a nonreassuring fetal heart rate or bleeding develops. Hemorrhage may indicate placental separation, which can be harmful to both the fetus and the mother. If contractions do not resume within approximately 10 minutes, dilute oxytocin may be used to stimulate contractions.

If the occiput or the breech presents immediately over the pelvic inlet but is not fixed in the birth canal, the presenting part can often be guided into the pelvis by one hand in the vagina while a second hand on the uterine fundus exerts moderate pressure caudally. Alternatively, an assistant can maneuver the presenting part into the pelvis using ultrasonography for guidance and to monitor heart rate. Intrapartum external version of the noncephalic second twin has also been described (Chervanak and co-workers, 1983).

A presenting shoulder may be gently converted into a cephalic presentation. If the occiput or the breech is not over the pelvic inlet and cannot be so positioned by gentle pressure, or if appreciable uterine bleeding develops, delivery of the second twin can be problematic.

It is essential to have an obstetrician skilled in intrauterine fetal manipulation and an anesthesiologist skilled in providing anesthesia to effectively relax the uterus for vaginal delivery of a noncephalic second twin to obtain a favorable outcome. To take maximum advantage of the dilated cervix before the uterus contracts and the cervix retracts, delay must be avoided. Prompt cesarean delivery of the second fetus is preferred if no one present is skilled in the performance of internal podalic version (described in the following section) or if anesthesia that will provide effective uterine relaxation is not immediately available.

INTERNAL PODALIC VERSION. With this maneuver, the fetus is turned to a breech presentation by the operator's hand placed into the uterus (Fig. 39–30). The obstetrician grasps the fetal feet to then effect delivery by breech extraction. Chauhan and colleagues (1995) compared outcomes of 23 second twins delivered by podalic version and breech extraction with those of 21 who underwent external cephalic version. Breech extraction was considered superior to external version, because less fetal distress developed. The technique of breech extraction is described in Chapter 24.

INTERVAL BETWEEN FIRST AND SECOND TWINS. In the past, the safest interval between delivery of the first and second twins was commonly cited as less than 30 minutes. Subsequently, as shown by Rayburn and colleagues (1984), as well as others, if continuous fetal monitoring is used, a good outcome is achieved even when this interval is longer. The American College of Obstetricians and Gynecologists (1998b) has determined that the interval between delivery of twins is not critical in determining the outcome of the twin delivered second. However, vigilance is required. Leung and colleagues (2002) demonstrated a direct correlation between worsening

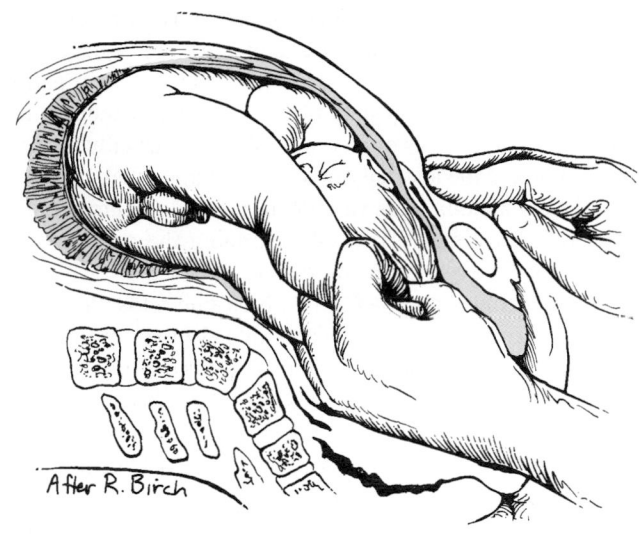

FIGURE 39–30. Internal podalic version. Upward pressure on the head is applied as downward traction is exerted on the feet.

umbilical cord blood gas values and increasing time interval between delivery of first and second twins.

CESAREAN DELIVERY. Twin fetuses create unusual intraoperative problems. Hypotension commonly develops in women carrying twins when they are placed in the supine position. Therefore, it is important to place patients in a left lateral tilt so as to deflect the uterine weight off the aorta (see Chap. 5, p. 135). The uterine incision should be large enough to allow atraumatic delivery of both fetuses. In some cases, a vertical incision in the lower uterine segment may be advantageous. For example, if a fetus is in transverse position, with the back down, and the arms are inadvertently delivered first, it is much easier and safer to extend a vertical uterine incision upward than to extend a transverse incision. If the second twin is breech and delivery of the head is obstructed, Piper forceps can be used just as for a vaginal delivery. It is important that the uterus remain well contracted during completion of the cesarean delivery and thereafter. Remarkable blood loss may be concealed within the uterus and vagina and beneath the drapes during the time taken to close the incisions.

At times, attempts to deliver the second twin vaginally after delivery of the first twin are not only unwise but also impossible, and prompt cesarean delivery is required. Cesarean delivery of the second twin may be necessary, for example, when the second fetus is much larger than the first, and is breech or transverse. Even more perplexing, cesarean delivery may be required because the cervix promptly contracts and thickens after delivery of the first infant and does not dilate subsequently or because a nonreassuring fetal heart rate pattern develops.

TRIPLET OR HIGHER-ORDER GESTATION

Fetal heart rate monitoring during labor is challenging. A scalp electrode can be attached to the presenting fetus, but it is difficult to ensure that the other two triplets are each being monitored separately. With vaginal delivery, the first infant is usually born spontaneously or with little manipulation. Subsequent fetuses, however, are delivered according to the presenting part. This often requires complicated obstetrical maneuvers such as total breech extraction with or without internal podalic version or even cesarean delivery. Associated with malposition of the fetuses is an increased incidence of cord prolapse. Moreover, reduced placental perfusion and hemorrhage from separating placentas are more likely during delivery.

For all these reasons, many clinicians believe that pregnancies complicated by three or more fetuses are best delivered by cesarean delivery. Vaginal delivery is reserved for those circumstances in which survival is not expected because the fetuses are markedly immature or maternal complications make cesarean delivery hazardous to the mother. Other clinicians believe that vaginal delivery is safe under certain circumstances. For example, Alamia and colleagues (1998) evaluated a protocol for vaginal delivery of triplet pregnancies in which the presenting fetus was cephalic. A total of 23 sets of triplets were analyzed, and a third of these were delivered vaginally. Neonatal outcomes were the same in the vaginal and cesarean groups, with no morbidity and 100 percent fetal survival. Grobman and colleagues (1998) and Alran and co-workers (2004) reported vaginal delivery completion rates of 88 and 84 percent, respectively, in women carrying triplets who underwent a trial of labor. Neonatal outcomes did not differ from those of a matched group of triplet pregnancies delivered by elective cesarean. As in any obstetrical procedure, the safety of vaginal triplet delivery depends on the skill and experience of the operator.

SELECTIVE REDUCTION OR TERMINATION

In some cases of higher-order multifetal gestation, reduction in the number of fetuses to two or three improves survival of the remaining fetuses. Selective reduction implies early pregnancy intervention, whereas selective termination is performed later.

SELECTIVE REDUCTION. Reduction of a selected fetus or fetuses in a dichorionic multifetal gestation may be chosen as a therapeutic intervention to enhance survival of the other fetuses. Multifetal pregnancy reduction was developed at Mount Sinai Medical Center in New York to improve the poor prognosis of pregnancies with three or more fetuses (Berkowitz and associates, 1988). Pregnancy reduction can be performed transcervically, transvaginally, or transabdominally, but the transabdominal route is usually easiest. Transabdominal fetal reductions are typically performed between 10 and 13 weeks. This gestational age was chosen because any spontaneous abortions have already occurred, the remaining fetuses are large enough to be evaluated ultrasonographically, the amount of devitalized fetal tissue remaining after the procedure is small, and the risk of aborting the entire pregnancy as a result of the procedure is low. The smallest fetuses and any anomalous fetuses are chosen for reduction. Potassium chloride is then injected into the heart or thorax of each selected fetus under ultrasonographic guidance, taking care not to enter or traverse the sacs of the fetuses selected for retention. In most cases, pregnancies are reduced to twins to increase the chances of delivering at least one viable fetus.

Evans and associates (2001) reported continued improvement in fetal outcomes with this procedure. They analyzed more than 1000 pregnancies managed in 11 centers from 1995 to 1998. The pregnancy loss rate varied from a low of 4.5 percent for triplets who were reduced to twins, increased with each addition to the starting number of fetuses, and peaked at 15 percent for six or more fetuses. By comparison, the respective rates in their earlier report (Evans and co-workers, 1996) were 8 and 23 percent. The investigators believed that operator skill and experience were responsible for their low and declining rates of pregnancy loss. Early preterm deliveries were more likely in pregnancies starting as higher-order gestations, reinforcing the concept that higher-order multiple gestations are hazardous to both the fetuses and the mothers (Fig. 39–31).

SELECTIVE TERMINATION. With the identification of multiple fetuses discordant for structural or genetic abnormalities, three options are available: abortion of all fetuses,

selective termination of the abnormal fetus, and continuation of the pregnancy. Because anomalies are typically not discovered until the second trimester, selective termination is performed later in gestation than selective reduction and entails more risk. This procedure is therefore usually not performed unless the anomaly is severe but not lethal, meaning that the anomalous fetus would survive and require lifetime care, or the estimated risk of continuing the pregnancy is greater than the risk of the procedure.

Thus, a triplet pregnancy in which one fetus has Down syndrome might be a candidate for selective termination, whereas a twin pregnancy in which one has trisomy 18 might not. In some cases, termination is considered because the abnormal fetus may jeopardize the normal one. For example, pathological hydramnios in a twin with esophageal atresia could lead to preterm birth of its sibling. Audibert and colleagues (2003) reported the selective termination of a severely growth-restricted twin fetus at 32 weeks, with marked improvement in the severity of maternal preeclampsia and subsequent delivery of a healthy sibling twin at 38 weeks. Prerequisites to selective termination include a precise diagnosis for the anomalous fetus and absolute certainty as to its location. Thus, when genetic amniocentesis is performed on a multifetal gestation, a map of the uterus with the locations of all the fetuses clearly labeled should be made at the time of the diagnostic procedure. Unless a special procedure such as umbilical cord interruption is used, selective termination should be performed only in dichorionic multiple gestation to avoid damaging the surviving fetus.

Evans and co-workers (1999) have provided the most comprehensive results to date on second-trimester selective termination for fetal abnormalities. A total of 402 cases were analyzed from the eight centers worldwide with the most experienced operators. Included were 345 twin, 39 triplet, and 18 quadruplet pregnancies. Selective termination using potassium chloride resulted in the delivery of a viable neonate or neonates in more than 90 percent of cases, with a mean age at delivery of 35.7 weeks. The pregnancy loss rate was 7.1 percent in pregnancies reduced to singletons and was 13 percent in those reduced to twins. The gestational age at the time of the procedure did not appear to affect pregnancy loss; the rate was 5.4 percent when the procedure was performed at 9 to 12 weeks, 8.7 percent at 13 to 18 weeks, 6.8 percent at 19 to 24 weeks, and 9.1 percent at 25 weeks. Several losses occurred because the pregnancy was actually monochorionic and potassium chloride killed the normal fetus through placental vascular anastomoses. Lynch and colleagues (1996) reported that termination of the presenting fetus or selective termination after 20 weeks significantly increased the risk of preterm premature membrane rupture and delivery.

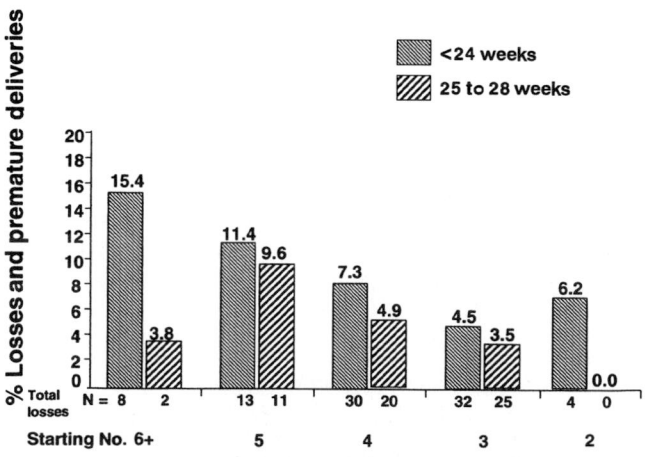

FIGURE 39–31. Histogram showing the rate of pregnancy losses at less than 24 weeks and preterm birth at 25 to 28 weeks as a function of the initial number of multiple fetuses in over 1000 women who underwent selective reduction of pregnancy from 1995 to 1998. (Modified from Evans and associates, 2001, with permission.)

ETHICS. The ethical issues associated with these techniques are almost limitless. The interested reader is referred to the excellent reviews by Evans and co-workers (1988) and Simpson and Carson (1996).

INFORMED CONSENT. Prior to selective termination or reduction, a couple should be counseled about the risks and benefits and informed consent obtained. Counseling should include a discussion of the morbidity and mortality expected if the pregnancy is continued; the morbidity and mortality expected with twins or triplets, whichever the couple would reduce to; and the risks of the procedure itself.

Ideally, the issue of selective reduction should be discussed *prior* to conception. Indeed, Ryan and colleagues (2004) reported that a minority of infertility patients expressed a preference for a multifetal gestation at their first visit. Grobman and associates (2001) documented that women seeking infertility treatment were generally unaware of the risks associated with multifetal gestation and when apprised of the risks, were less desirous of having a multifetal gestation.

Specific risks that are common to selective termination or reduction include:

1. Abortion of the remaining fetuses
2. Abortion of the wrong (normal) fetus(es)
3. Retention of genetic or structurally abnormal fetuses after a reduction in number
4. Damage without death to a fetus
5. Preterm labor
6. Development of discordancy or growth-restricted fetuses
7. Maternal infection, hemorrhage, or possible disseminated intravascular coagulopathy because of retained products of conception

The procedure should be performed by an operator skilled and experienced in ultrasonographic-guided procedures. Because selective reduction increases the maternal serum alpha-fetoprotein level, the couple should be informed that this screening test will not help them after the procedure (Lynch and Berkowitz, 1993). Instead, they are offered a second-trimester targeted ultrasonographic evaluation or possibly amniocentesis.

PSYCHOLOGICAL REACTION. Women and their spouses who elect to undergo selective termination or reduction find this decision highly stressful. Schreiner-Engel and associates (1995) retrospectively studied the emotional reactions of 100 women following selective reduction. Although 70 percent of the women mourned for their dead fetus(es), most grieved only for 1 month. Persistent depressive symptoms were mild, although moderately severe sadness and guilt continued for many for them. Fortunately, the majority were reconciled to the termination of some fetuses to preserve the lives of a remaining few. Indeed, 93 percent of the women would have made the same decision again.

REFERENCES

Adashi EY, Ekins MN, LaCoursiere Y: On the discharge of Hippocratic obligations: Challeges and opportunities. Am J Obstet Gynecol 190:885, 2004

Aisenbrey GA, Catanzarite VA, Hurley TJ, et al: Monoamniotic and pseudomonoamniotic twins: Sonographic diagnosis, detection of cord entanglement, and obstetric management. Obstet Gynecol 86:218, 1995

Akiyama M, Kuno A, Tanaka Y, et al: Comparison of alterations in fetal regional arterial vascular resistance in appropriate-for-gestational-age singleton, twin and triplet pregnancies. Hum Reprod 14:2635, 1999

Alamia V Jr, Royek AB, Jaekle RK, et al: Preliminary experience with a prospective protocol for planned vaginal delivery of triplet gestations. Am J Obstet Gynecol 179:1133, 1998

Allen VM, Windrim R, Barrett J, et al: Management of monoamniotic twin pregnancies: A case series and systematic review of the literature. Br J Obstet Gynaecol 108:931, 2001

Alran S, Sibony O, Luton D, et al: Maternal and neonatal outcome of 93 consecutive triplet pregnancies with 71% vaginal delivery. Acta Obstet Gynec Scand 83:554, 2004

American College of Obstetricians and Gynecologists: Multiple gestation: Complicated twin, triplet, and high-order multifetal pregnancy. Practice Bulletin No. 56, October 2004

American College of Obstetricians and Gynecologists: Special problems of multiple gestation. Education Bulletin No. 253, November 1998

American Society for Reproductive Medicine: A Practice Committee Report: Guidelines on number of embryos transferred. Birmingham, Alabama, November 1999

Anderson RL, Golbus MS, Curry CJ, et al: Central nervous system damage and other anomalies in surviving fetus following second trimester antenatal death of co-twin. Prenat Diagn 10:513, 1990

Andrews WW, Leveno KJ, Sherman ML, et al: Elective hospitalization in the management of twin pregnancies. Obstet Gynecol 77:826, 1991

Arbuckle TE, Wilkins R, Sherman GJ: Birthweight percentiles by gestational age in Canada. Obstet Gynecol 81:39, 1993

Audibert F, Salomon LJ, Castaigne-Meary V, et al: Selective termination of a twin pregnancy as a treatment of severe preeclampsia. Br J Obstet Gynaecol 110:68, 2003

Azubuike JC: Multiple births in Igbo women. Br J Obstet Gynaecol 89:77, 1982

Azuma C, Kamiura S, Nobunaga T, et al: Zygosity determination of multiple pregnancy by deoxyribonucleic acid finger prints. Am J Obstet Gynecol 160:734, 1989

Babson SG, Phillips DS: Growth and development of twins dissimilar in size at birth. N Engl J Med 289:937, 1973

Baigts F, Dunica S, Fumeron F, et al: Birthweight difference in monozygous twins followed by differences in development of body weight. Lancet 2:274, 1982

Bailey-Pridham DD, Reshef E, Drury K, et al: Follicular fluid lidocaine levels during transvaginal oocyte retrieval. Fertil Steril 53:171, 1990

Bajoria R, Wigglesworth J, Fisk NM: Angioarchitecture of monochorionic placentas in relation to the twin-twin transfusion syndrome. Am J Obstet Gynecol 172:856, 1995

Baldwin VJ: Pathology of multiple pregnancy. In Wigglesworth JS, Singer J (eds): Textbook of Fetal and Perinatal Pathology. Boston, Blackwell, 1991, p 238

Bejar R, Vigliocco G, Gramajo H, et al: Antenatal origin of neurological damage in newborn infants, 2. Multiple gestations. Am J Obstet Gynecol 162:1230, 1990

Belfort MA, Moise KJ, Kirshon B, et al: The use of color flow Doppler ultrasonography to diagnose umbilical cord entanglement in monoamniotic twin gestations. Am J Obstet Gynecol 168:601, 1993

Benirschke K: Intrauterine death of a twin: Mechanisms, implications for surviving twin, and placental pathology. Semin Diagn Pathol 10:222, 1993

Benirschke K, Kim CK: Multiple pregnancy. N Engl J Med 288:1276, 1973

Bennett D, Dunn LC: Genetical and embryological comparisons of semilethal t-alleles from wild mouse populations. Genetics 61:411, 1969

Berghella V, Kaufmann M: Natural history of twin-twin transfusion syndrome. J Reprod Med 46:480, 2001

Berkowitz RL, Lynch L, Chitkara U, et al: Selective reduction of multifetal pregnancies in the first trimester. N Engl J Med 318:1043, 1988

Bermudez C, Becerra CH, Bornick PW, et al: Placental types and twin-twin transfusion syndrome. Am J Obstet Gynecol 187:489, 2002

Berry SM, Puder KS, Bottoms SF, et al: Comparison of intrauterine hematologic and biochemcial values between twin pairs with and without stuck twin syndrome. Am J Obstet Gynecol 172:1403, 1995

Blickstein I, Goldman RD, Kupferminc M: Delivery of breech first twins: A multicenter retrospective study. Obstet Gynecol 95:37, 2000

Blickstein I, Keith LG: Neonatal mortality rates among growth-discordant twins, classified according to the birth weight of the smaller twin. Am J Obstet Gynecol 190:170, 2004

Blickstein I, Schwartz-Shoham Z, Lancet M, et al: Vaginal delivery of the second twin in breech presentation. Obstet Gynecol 68:774, 1987

Bouchard C, Tremblay A, Despres JP, et al: The response to long-term overfeeding in identical twins. N Engl J Med 322:1477, 1990

Bressers WM, Eriksson AW, Kostense PJ, et al: Increasing trend in the monozygotic twinning rate. Acta Genet Med Gemellol (Roma) 36:397, 1987

Bristow RE, Shumway JB, Khouzami AN, et al: Complete hydatidiform mole and surviving coexistent twin. Obstet Gynecol Surv 51:705, 1996

Brown JE, Carlson M: Nutrition and multifetal pregnancy. J Am Diet Assoc 100:343, 2000

Bruner JP, Rosemond RL: Twin-to-twin transfusion syndrome: A subset of the twin oligohydramnios–polyhydramnios sequence. Am J Obstet Gynecol 169:925, 1993

Buekens P, Wilcox A: Why do small twins have a lower mortality rate than small singletons? Am J Obstet Gynecol 168:937, 1993

Bulmer MG: The effect of parental age, parity, and duration of marriage on the twinning rate. Hum Genet 23:454, 1959

Cameron AH, Edwards JH, Derom R, et al: The value of twin surveys in the study of malformation. Eur J Obstet Gynecol Reprod Biol 14:347, 1983

Campbell DM: Maternal adaptation in twin pregnancy. Semin Perinatol 10:14, 1986

Carr SR, Aronson MP, Coustan DR: Survival rates of monoamnionic twins do not decrease after 30 weeks gestation. Am J Obstet Gynecol 163:719, 1990

Carroll SGM, Soothill PW, Abdel-Fattah SA, et al: Prediction of chorionicity in twin pregnancies at 10-14 weeks of gestation. Br J Obstet Gynaecol 109:182, 2002

Casele H, Daley S, Metzger B: Metabolic response to meal eating and extended overnight fasting in twin gestation. Am J Obstet Gynecol 174:375, 1996

Caukwell S, Murphy DJ: The effect of mode of delivery and gestational age on neonatal outcome of the non-cephalic-presenting second twin. Am J Obstet Gynecol 187:1356, 2002

Challis D, Gratacos E, Deprest JA: Cord occlusion techniques for selective termination in monochorionic twins. J Perinat Med 27:327, 1999

Chauhan SP, Roberts WE, McLaren RA, et al: Delivery of the non-vertex second twin: Breech extraction versus external cephalic version. Am J Obstet Gynecol 173:1015, 1995

Chervanak FA, Johnson RE, Berkowitz RL, et al: Intrapartum external version of the second twin. Obstet Gynecol 62:160, 1983

Chervanak FA, Johnson RE, Youcha S, et al: Intrapartum management of twin gestation. Obstet Gynecol 65:119, 1985

Cohen M, Kohl SG, Rosenthal AH: Fetal interlocking complicating twin gestation. Am J Obstet Gynecol 91:407, 1965

Conde-Agudelo A, Belizán JM, Lindmark G: Maternal morbidity and mortality associated with multiple gestations. Obstet Gynecol 95:899, 2000

Coonrad DV, Hickok DE, Zhu K, et al: Risk factors for preeclampsia in twin pregnancies: A population-based cohort study. Obstet Gynecol 85:645, 1995

Crowley P: Prophylactic corticosteroids for preterm birth. In Cochrane Pregnancy and Childbirth Group. Cochrane Database of Systematic Reviews #1, 2003

Crowther CA, Neilson JP, Ashurst HM, et al: The effects of hospitalization for rest on fetal growth, neonatal morbidity and length of gestation in twin pregnancy. Br J Obstet Gynaecol 97:872, 1990

Danskin FH, Neilson JP: Twin-to-twin transfusion syndrome: What are appropriate diagnostic criteria? Am J Obstet Gynecol 161:365, 1989

Davidson L, Easterling TR, Jackson JC, et al: Breech extraction of low-birth-weight second twins. Am J Obstet Gynecol 166:497, 1992

Demaria F, Goffinet F, Kayem G, et al: Monoamniotic twin pregnancies: Antenatal management and perinatal results of 19 consecutive cases. BJOG 111:22, 2004

Demissie K, Ananth CV, Martin J, et al: Fetal and neonatal mortality among twin gestations in the United States: The role of intrapair birth weight discordance. Obstet Gynecol 100:474, 2002

Denbow ML, Battin MR, Cowan F, et al: Neonatal cranial ultrasonographic findings in preterm twins complicated by severe fetofetal transfusion. Am J Obstet Gynecol 178:479, 1998

Derom C, Derom R, Vlietinck R, et al: Increased monozygotic twinning rate after ovulation induction. Lancet 1:1237, 1987

Dickey RP, Olar TT, Taylor SN, et al: Relationship of follicle number and other factors to fecundability and multiple pregnancy in clomiphene citrate–induced intrauterine insemination cycles. Fertil Steril 57:613, 1992

Dickey RP, Taylor SN, Lu PY, et al: Spontaneous reduction of multiple pregnancy: Incidence and effect on outcome. Am J Obstet Gynecol 186:77, 2002

Divon MY, Marin MJ, Pollack RN, et al: Twin gestation: Fetal presentation as a function of gestational age. Am J Obstet Gynecol 168:1500, 1993

DiVou MY, Girz BA, Sklar A, et al: Discordant twins—a prospective study of the diagnostic value of real time ultrasonography combined with umbilical artery velocimetry. Am J Obstet Gynecol 161:757, 1989

Donner C, Shahabi S, Thomas D, et al: Selective feticide by embolization in twin-twin transfusion syndrome. A report of two cases. J Reprod Med 42:747, 1997

Dor J, Shalev J, Mashiach S, et al: Elective cervical suture of twin pregnancies diagnosed ultrasonically in the first trimester following induced ovulation. Gynecol Obstet Invest 13:55, 1982

Eberle AM, Levesque D, Vintzileos AM, et al: Placental pathology in discordant twins. Am J Obstet Gynecol 169:931, 1993

Elimian A, Figueroa R, Nigam S, et al: Perinatal outcome of triplet gestation: Does prophylactic cerclage make a difference? J Matern Fetal Med 8:119, 1999

Elliott JP, Finberg HJ: Biophysical profile testing as an indicator of fetal well-being in high-order multiple gestations. Am J Obstet Gynecol 172:508, 1995

Evans MI, Berkowitz RL, Wapner RJ, et al: Improvement in outcomes of multifetal pregnancy reduction with increased experience. Am J Obstet Gynecol 184:97, 2001

Evans MI, Dommergues M, Wapner RJ, et al: International collaborative experience in 1798 patients having multifetal pregnancy reduction: A plateauing of risks and outcomes. J Soc Gynecol Investig 3:23, 1996

Evans MI, Fletcher JC, Zador IE, et al: Selective first-trimester termination in octuplet and quadruplet pregnancies: Clinical and ethical issues. Obstet Gynecol 71:289, 1988

Evans MI, Goldberg JD, Horenstein J, et al: Elective termination for structural, chromosomal, and mendelian anomalies: International experience. Am J Obstet Gynecol 181:893, 1999

Ezra Y, Jones J, Farine D: Umbilical artery waveforms in triplet and quadruplet pregnancies. Gynecol Obstet Invest 47:239, 1999

Farkouh LJ, Sabin ED, Heyborne KD, et al: Delayed-interval delivery: Extended series from a single maternal-fetal medicine practice. Am J Obstet Gynecol 183:1499, 2000

Finberg HJ: The "twin peak" sign: Reliable evidence of dichorionic twinning. J Ultrasound Med 11:571, 1992

Fisk NM, Bryan E: Routine prenatal determination of chorionicity in multiple gestations: A plea to the obstetrician. Br J Obstet Gynaecol 100:975, 1993

Fox H: Pathology of the Placenta. London, Saunders, 1978, p 77

Fries MH, Goldstein RB, Kilpatrick SJ, et al: The role of velamentous cord insertion in the etiology of twin-twin transfusion syndrome. Obstet Gynecol 81:569, 1993

Fujikura T, Froelich LA: Mental and motor development in monozygotic co-twins with dissimilar birth weights. Pediatrics 53:884, 1974

Fusi L, Gordon II: Twin pregnancy complicated by single intrauterine death. Problems and outcome with conservative management. Br J Obstet Gynaecol 97:511, 1990

Fusi L, McParland P, Fisk N, et al: Acute twin-twin transfusion: A possible mechanism for brain-damaged survivors after intrauterine death of a monochorionic twin. Obstet Gynecol 78:517, 1991

Gabriel R, Harika G, Saniez D, et al: Prolonged intravenous ritodrine therapy: A comparison between multiple and singleton pregnancies. Eur J Obstet Gynecol Reprod Biol 57:65, 1994

Galea P, Scott JM, Goel KM: Feto-fetal transfusion syndrome. Arch Dis Child 57:781, 1982

Gallagher MW, Costigan K, Johnson TRB: Fetal heart rate accelerations, fetal movement, and fetal behavior patterns in twin gestations. Am J Obstet Gynecol 167:1140, 1992

Gardner MO, Goldenberg RL, Cliver SP, et al: The origin and outcome of preterm twin pregnancies. Obstet Gynecol 85:553, 1995

Gerson AG, Wallace DM, Bridgens NK, et al: Duplex Doppler ultrasound in the evaluation of growth in twin pregnancies. Obstet Gynecol 70:419, 1987

Gilbert WM, Davis SE, Kaplan C, et al: Morbidity associated with prenatal disruption of the dividing membrane in twin gestations. Obstet Gynecol 78:623, 1991

Giles W, Bisits A, O'Callaghan S, et al: The Doppler assessment in multiple pregnancy randomized controlled trial of ultrasound biometry versus umbilical artery Doppler ultrasound and biometry in twin pregnancy. Br J Obstet Gynaecol 110:593, 2003

Gleicher N, Oleske DM, Tur-Kaspa I, et al: Reducing the risk of high-order multiple pregnancy after ovarian stimulation with gonadotropins. N Engl J Med 343:2, 2000

Gocke SE, Nageotte MP, Garite T, et al: Management of the non-vertex second twin: Primary cesarean section, external version, or primary breech extraction. Am J Obstet Gynecol 161:111, 1989

Goldenberg RL, Iams JD, Miodovnik M, et al: The preterm prediction study: Risk factors in twin gestations. Am J Obstet Gynecol 175:1047, 1996

Goldfarb JM, Austin C, Lisbona H, et al: Cost effectiveness of in vitro fertilization. Obstet Gynecol 87:18, 1996

Grobman WA, Milad MP, Stout J, et al: Patient perceptions of multiple gestations: An assessment of knowledge and risk aversion. Am J Obstet Gynecol 185:920, 2001

Grobman WA, Peaceman AM, Haney EI, et al: Neonatal outcomes in triplet gestations after a trial of labor. Am J Obstet Gynecol 179:942, 1998

Gyetvai K, Hannah ME, Hodnett ED, et al: Tocolytics for preterm labor: A systematic review. Obstet Gynecol 94:869, 1999

Hall JG: Twinning. Lancet 362:735, 2003

Hardardottir H, Kelly K, Bork MD, et al: Atypical presentation of preeclampsia in high order multifetal gestations. Obstet Gynecol 87:370, 1996

Harris DW: Superfecundation: Letter. J Reprod Med 27:39, 1982

Hashimoto B, Callen PW, Filly RA, et al: Ultrasound evaluation of polyhydramnios and twin pregnancy. Am J Obstet Gynecol 154:1069, 1986

Hill LM, Guzick D, Chenevey P, et al: The sonographic assessment of twin discordancy. Obstet Gynecol 84:501, 1994

Hogle KL, Hutton EK, McBrien KA, et al: Cesarean delivery for twins: A systematic review and meta-analysis. Am J Obstet Gynecol 188:220, 2003

Hollier LM, McIntire DD, Leveno KJ: Outcome of twin pregnancies according to intrapair birth weight differences. Obstet Gynecol 94:1006, 1999

Hsieh YY, Chang CC, Tsai HD, et al: Twin vs. singleton pregnancy. Clinical characteristics and latency periods in preterm premature rupture of membranes. J Reprod Med 44:616, 1999

Jain T, Missmer SA, Hornstein MD: Trends in embryo-transfer practice and in outcomes of the use of assisted reproductive technology in the United States. N Engl J Med 350:1639, 2004

Jauniaux E, Elkazen N, Leroy F, et al: Clinical and morphologic aspects of the vanishing twin phenomenon. Obstet Gynecol 72:577, 1988

Jewell SE, Yip R: Increasing trends in plural births in the United States. Obstet Gynecol 85:229, 1995

Jones KL: Smith's Recognizable Patterns of Human Malformation, 5th ed. Philadelphia, Saunders, 1997, p 658

Joseph KS, Allen AC, Dodds L, et al: Causes and consequences of recent increases in preterm birth among twins. Obstet Gynecol 98:57, 2001

Kahn B, Lumey LH, Zybert PA, et al: Prospective risk of fetal death in singleton, twin, and triplet gestations: Implications for practice. Obstet Gynecol 102:685, 2003

Kametas NA, McAuliffe F, Krampl E, et al: Maternal cardiac function in twin pregnancy. Obstet Gynecol 102:806, 2003

Kilpatrick SJ, Jackson R, Croughan-Minihane MS: Perinatal mortality in twins and singletons matched for gestational age at delivery at > or = 30 weeks. Am J Obstet Gynecol 174:66, 1996

Klein NA, Battaglia DE, Clifton DK, et al: The gonadotropin secretion pattern in normal women of advanced reproductive age in relation to the monotropic FHS rise. J Soc Gynecol Investig 3:27, 1996

Knox G, Morley D: Twinning in Yoruba women. J Obstet Gynaecol Br Emp 67:981, 1960

Koffel B: Abnormal presentation and multiple gestation. In Chestnut DH (ed): Obstetrical Anesthesia, 2nd ed. St Louis, Mosby, 1999, p 694

Kogan MD, Alexander GR, Kotelchuck M: A comparison of risk factors for twin preterm birth in the United States between 1981–82 and 1996–97. Maternal Child Health J 6:29, 2002

Kogan MD, Alexander GR, Kotelchuck M: Trends in twin birth outcomes and prenatal care utilization in the United States, 1981–1997. JAMA 283:335, 2000

Kohl SG, Casey G: Twin gestation. Mt Sinai J Med 42:523, 1975

Kol S, Levron J, Lewit N, et al: The natural history of multiple pregnancies after assisted reproduction: Is spontaneous fetal demise a clinically significant phenomenon? Fertil Steril 60:127, 1993

Kovacs G, Maclachlan V, Rombauts L, et al: Replacement of one selected embryo is just successful as two embryo transfer, without the risk of twin pregnancy. Austr NZ J Obstet Gynaecology 43:369, 2003

Landy HJ, Weiner S, Corson SL, et al: The "vanishing twin": Ultrasonographic assessment of fetal disappearance in the first trimester. Am J Obstet Gynecol 150:14, 1986

Langer B, Boudier E, Gasser B, et al: Antenatal diagnosis of brain damage in the survivor after the second trimester death of a monochorionic monoamniotic co-twin: Case report and literature review. Fetal Diagn Ther 12:286, 1997

Larroche JC, Droulle P, Delezoide AL, et al: Brain damage in monozygous twins. Biol Neonate 57:261, 1990

LeFevre ML, Bain RP, Ewigman BG, et al: A randomized trial of prenatal ultrasonographic screening: Impact on maternal management and outcome. RADIUS (Routine Antenatal Diagnostic Imaging with Ultrasound) study group. Am J Obstet Gynecol 169:483, 1993

Leung TY, Tam WH, Leung TN, et al: Effect of twin-to-twin delivery interval on umbilical cord blood gas in the second twins. Br J Obstet Gynaecol 109:63, 2002

Leveno KJ, Quirk JG, Whalley PJ, et al: Fetal lung maturation in twin gestation. Am J Obstet Gynecol 148:405, 1984

Leveno KJ, Santos-Ramos R, Duenhoelter JH, et al: Sonar cephalometry in twins: A table of biparietal diameters for normal twin fetuses and a comparison with singletons. Am J Obstet Gynecol 135:727, 1979

Lipitz S, Uval J, Achiron R, et al: Outcome of twin pregnancies reduced from triplets compared with nonreduced twin gestations. Obstet Gynecol 87:511, 1996

Livingston JC, Livingston LW, Ramsey R, et al: Second-trimester asynchronous multifetal delivery results in poor perinatal outcome. Obstet Gynecol 103:77, 2004

Livingston JE, Poland BJ: A study of spontaneously aborted twins. Teratology 21:139, 1980

Lopriore E, Nagel HT, Vanderbussche FP, Walther F: Long-term neurodevelopmental outcome in twin transfusion syndrome. Am J Obstet Gynecol 189:1314, 2003

Lutfi S, Allen VM, Fahey J, et al: Twin-twin transfusion syndrome: A population-based study. Obstet Gynecol 104:1289, 2004

Luke B: The changing patterns of multiple births in the United States: Maternal and infant characteristics, 1973 and 1990. Obstet Gynecol 84:101, 1994

Lynch L, Berkowitz RL: Maternal serum alpha-fetoprotein and coagulation profiles after multifetal pregnancy reduction. Am J Obstet Gynecol 169:987, 1993

Lynch L, Berkowitz RL, Stone J, et al: Preterm delivery after selective termination in twin pregnancies. Obstet Gynecol 87:336, 1996

MacGillivray I: Epidemiology of twin pregnancy. Semin Perinatol 10:4, 1986

Machin GA: Some causes of genotypic and phenotypic discordance in monozygotic twin pairs. Am J Med Genet 61:216, 1996

Magann EF, Chauhan SP, Martin JN, et al: Ultrasound assessment of the amniotic fluid volume in diamniotic twins. J Soc Gynecol Investig 2:609, 1995

Mahone PR, Sherer DM, Abramowicz JS, et al: Twin-twin transfusion syndrome: Rapid development of severe hydrops of the donor following selective feticide of the hydropic recipient. Am J Obstet Gynecol 169:166, 1993

Mahony BS, Filly RA, Callen PW: Amnionicity and chorionicity in twin pregnancies. Radiology 155:205, 1985

Manning FA: Fetal biophysical profile scoring. In: Fetal Medicine: Principles and Practices. Norwalk, CT, Appleton & Lange, 1995, p 288

Mari G, Kirshon B, Abuhamad A: Fetal renal artery flow velocity waveforms in normal pregnancies and pregnancies complicated by polyhydramnios and oligohydramnios. Obstet Gynecol 81:560, 1993

Martin JA, Hamilton BE, Ventura SJ, et al: Births: Final Data for 2001. Centers for Disease Control and Prevention–Natl Vital Stat Rep Vol 51, No. 2. Hyattsville, MD: National Center for Health Statistics, December 18, 2002

Martin JA, Park MM: Trends in twin and triplet births; 1980–97. Natl Vital Stat Rep Vol 47, No. 24. Hyattsville, MD, National Center for Health Statistics, 1999

Mastrobattista JM, Skupski DW, Monga M, et al: The rate of severe preeclampsia is increased in triplet as compared to twin gestations. Am J Perinatol 14:263, 1997

Mauldin JG, Newman RB, Mauldin PD: Cost-effective delivery management of the vertex and nonvertex twin gestation. Am J Obstet Gynecol 179:864, 1998

McAuliffe F, Kametas N, Costello J, et al: Respiratory function in singleton and twin pregnancy. Br J Obstet Gynaecol 109:765, 2002

McMahon KS, Neerhof MG, Haney EI, et al: Prematurity in multiple gestations: Identification of patients who are at low risk. Am J Obstet Gynecol 186:1137, 2002

Meldrum DR, Gardner DK: Two-embryo transfer—the future looks bright (editorial). N Engl J Med 339:624, 1998

Mercer B, Crocker LG, Pierce WF, et al: Clinical characteristics and outcome of twin gestation complicated by preterm premature rupture of the membranes. Am J Obstet Gynecol 168:467, 1993

Meulemans WJ, Lewis CM, Boomsma DI, et al: Genetic modelling of dizygotic twinning in pedigrees of spontaneous dizygotic twins. Am J Med Genet 61:258, 1996

Moore TR, Gale S, Benirschke K: Perinatal outcome of forty nine pregnancies complicated by acardiac twinning. Am Obstet Gynecol 163:907, 1990

Mordel N, Benshushan A, Zajicek G, et al: Discordancy in triplets. Am J Perinatol 10:224, 1993

Muleba N, Dashe N, Yost D, et al: Respiratory morbidity among second-born twins. Presented at the 25th Annual Meeting of the Society for Maternal Fetal Medicine, Reno, Nevada, 7–12 February, 2005

Myrianthopoulos NC: An epidemiologic survey of twins in a large prospectively studied population. Am J Hum Genet 22:611, 1970

Newman RB, Krombach S, Myers MC, et al: Effect of cerclage on obstetrical outcome in twin gestations with a shortened cervical length. Am J Obstet Gynecol 186:634, 2002

Nilsen ST, Bergsjo P, Nome S: Male twins at birth and 18 years later. Br J Obstet Gynaecol 91:122, 1984

Nylander PPS: Biosocial aspects of multiple births. J Biosoc Sci 3:29, 1971

Nylander PPS: Serum levels of gonadotropins in relation to multiple pregnancy in Nigeria. Br J Obstet Gynaecol 80:651, 1973

Okamura K, Murotsuki J, Tanigawara S, et al: Funipuncture for evaluation indices in the surviving twin following co-twin's death. Obstet Gynecol 83:975, 1994

Ong S, Lim MN, Fitzmaurice A, et al: The creation of twin centile curves for size. Br J Obstet Gynaecol 109:753, 2002

Ozturk O, Templeton A: In-vitro fertilization and risk of multiple pregnancy. Lancet 359:232, 2002

Parisi P, Gatti M, Prinzi G, et al: Familial incidence of twinning. Nature 304:626, 1983

Pasqualotto EB, Falcone T, Goldberg JM, et al: Risk factors for multiple gestation in women undergoing intrauterine insemination with ovarian stimulation. Fertil Steril 72:613, 1999

Pettersson F, Smedby B, Lindmark G: Outcome of twin birth: Review of 1636 children born in twin birth. Acta Paediatr Scand 64:473, 1976

Pharoah PO, Adi Y: Consequences of in-utero death in twin pregnancy. Lancet 355:1597, 2000

Pons JC, Charlemaine C, Dubreuil E, et al: Management and outcome of triplet pregnancy. Eur J Obstet Gynecol Reprod Biol 76:131, 1998

Porter TF, Dildy GA, Blanchard JR, et al: Normal values for amnionic fluid index during uncomplicated twin pregnancy. Obstet Gynecol 87:699, 1996

Powers WF, Kiely JL: The risks confronting twins: A national perspective. Am J Obstet Gynecol 170:456, 1994

Pritchard JA: Changes in blood volume during pregnancy. Anesthesiology 26:393, 1965

Quigley MM, Cruikshank DP: Polyhydramnios and acute renal failure. J Reprod Med 19:92, 1977

Quintero RA, Goncalves L, Johnson MP, et al: Percutaneous umbilical-cord ligation in complicated monochorionic multiple gestations. Am J Obstet Gynecol 174:326, 1996

Quintero RA, Reich H, Puder KS, et al: Brief report: Umbilical-cord ligation in an acardiac twin by fetoscopy at 19 weeks gestation. N Engl J Med 330:469, 1994

Rayburn WF, Lavin JP Jr, Miodovnik M, et al: Multiple gestation: Time interval between delivery of the first and second twins. Obstet Gynecol 63:502, 1984

Reddy KS, Petersen MB, Antonarakis SE, et al: The vanishing twin: An explanation for discordance between chorionic villus karyotype and fetal phenotype. Prenat Diagn 11:679, 1991

Redline RW: Nonidentical twins with a single placenta—disproving dogma in perinatal pathology. N Engl J Med 349:111, 2003

Rein MS, Barbieri RL, Greene MF: The causes of high-order multiple gestation. Int J Fertil 35:154, 1990

Robertson EG, Neer KJ: Placental injection studies in twin gestation. Am J Obstet Gynecol 147:170, 1983

Robie GF, Payne GG, Morgan MA: Selective delivery of an acardiac, acephalic twin. N Engl J Med 320:512, 1989

Rodis JF, Lawrence A, Egan JFX, et al: Comprehensive fetal ultrasonographic growth measurements in triplet gestations. Am J Obstet Gynecol 181:1128, 1999

Rothman KJ: Fetal loss, twinning and birthweight after oral contraceptive use. N Engl J Med 297:468, 1977

Rouse DJ, Skopec GS, Zlatnik FJ: Fundal height as a predictor of preterm twin delivery. Obstet Gynecol 81:211, 1993

Ryan GL, Zhang SH, Dokras A, et al: The desire of infertile patients for multiple births. Fertility & Sterility 81:500, 2004

Rydhström H: Discordant birthweight and late fetal death in like-sexed and unlike-sexed twin pairs: A population-based study. Br J Obstet Gynaecol 101:765, 1994

Rydhström H: Pregnancy with stillbirth of both twins. Br J Obstet Gynaecol 103:25, 1996

Rydhström H: Prognosis for twins with birthweight < 1,500 g: The impact of cesarean section in relation to fetal presentation. Am J Obstet Gynecol 163:528, 1990

Saacks CB, Thorp JM, Hendricks CH: Cohort study of twinning in an academic health center: Changes in management and outcome over forty years. Am J Obstet Gynecol 172:432, 1995

Saade G, Moise K, Dorman K, et al: A randomized trial of septostomy versus amnioreduction in the treatment of twin olidohydramnios polyhydramnios sequence (TOPS). Am J Obstet Gynecol 187:S54, 2002

Saito K, Ohtsu Y, Amano K, et al: Perinatal outcome and management of single fetal death in twin pregnancy: A case series and review. J Perinat Med 27:473, 1999

Santema JG, Koppelaar I, Wallenburg HC: Hypertensive disorders in twin pregnancy. Eur J Obstet Gynecol Reprod Biol 58:9, 1995a

Santema JG, Swaak AM, Wallenburg HCS: Expectant management of twin pregnancy with single fetal death. Br J Obstet Gynaecol 102:26, 1995b

Saunders NJ, Snijders RJ, Nicolaides KH: Twin-twin transfusion syndrome during the 2nd trimester is associated with small intertwin hemoglobin differences. Fetal Diagn Ther 6:34, 1991

Scardo JA, Ellings JM, Newman RB: Prospective determination of chorionicity, amnionicity, and zygosity in twin gestations. Am J Obstet Gynecol 173:1376, 1995

Schenker JG, Yarkoni S, Granat M: Multiple pregnancies following induction of ovulation. Fertil Steril 35:105, 1981

Schiff E, Cohen SB, Dulitzky M, et al: Progression of labor in twins versus singleton gestations. Am J Obstet Gynecol 179:1181, 1998

Schinzel AA, Smith DW, Miller JR: Monozygotic twinning and structural defects. J Pediatr 95:951, 1979

Scholtes MCW, Zeilmaker GH: A prospective, randomized study of embryo transfer results after 3 or 5 days of embryo culture in in vitro fertilization. Fertil Steril 65:1245, 1996

Schreiner-Engel P, Walther VN, Mindes J, et al: First-trimester multifetal pregnancy reduction: Acute and persistent psychologic reactions. Am J Obstet Gynecol 172:544, 1995

Sebire NJ, Foskett M, Paradinas FJ, et al: Outcome of twin pregnancies with complete hydatidiform mole and healthy co-twin. Lancet 359:2165, 2002

Sebire NJ, Snijders RJ, Hughes K, et al: The hidden mortality of monochorionic twin pregnancies. Br J Obstet Gynaecol 104:1203, 1997

Senat M-V, Deprest J, Boulvain M, et al: Endoscopic laser surgery versus serial amnioreduction for severe twin-to-twin transfusion syndrome. N Engl J Med 351:136, 2004

Silva PA, Crosado B: The growth and development of twins compared with singletons at ages 9 and 11. Aust Paediatr J 21:265, 1985

Silva PA, McGee RO, Powell J: Growth and development of twins compared with singletons at ages five and seven: A follow-up report from the Dunedin Multidisciplinary Child Development Study. Aust Paediatr J 18:35, 1982

Simpson JL, Carson SA: Multifetal reduction in high-order gestations: A nonelective procedure? J Soc Gynecol Invest 3:1, 1996

Smith-Levitin M, Kowalik A, Birnholz J, et al: Comparison of birthweight of twin gestations resulting from embryo reduction of higher order gestations to birthweights of twin and triplet gestations using a novel way to correct for gestational age at delivery. Am J Obstet Gynecol 174:346, 1996

Sonntag J, Waltz S, Schollmeyer T, et al: Morbidity and mortality of discordant twins up to 34 weeks of gestational age. Eur J Pediatr 155:224, 1996

Souka AP, Heath V, Flint S, et al: Cervical length at 23 weeks in twins in predicting spontaneous preterm delivery. Obstet Gynecol 94:450, 1999

Souter VL, Kapur RP, Nyholt DR, et al: A report of dizygous monochorionic twins. N Engl J Med 349:154, 2003

Spitz L, Kiely EM: Conjoined twins. JAMA 289:1307, 2003

Stagiannis KD, Sepulveda W, Southwell D, et al: Ultrasonic measurement of the dividing membrane in twin pregnancy during the second and third trimesters: A reproducibility study. Am J Obstet Gynecol 173:1546, 1995

Strandskov HH, Edelen EW, Siemens GJ: Analysis of the sex ratios among single and plural births in the total white and colored U.S. populations. Am J Phys Anthropol 4:491, 1946

Stunkard AJ, Harris JR, Pedersen NL, et al: The body-mass index of twins who have been reared apart. N Engl J Med 322:1483, 1990

Sullivan AE, Varner MW, Ball RH, et al: The management of acardiac twins: A conservative approach. Am J Obstet Gynecol 189:1310, 2003

Sutcliffe AG, Taylor B, Saunders K, et al: Outcome in the second year of life after in-vitro fertilization by intracytoplasmic sperm injection: A UK case-control study. Lancet 357:2080, 2001

Talbert DG, Bajoria R, Sepulveda W, et al: Hydrostatic and osmotic pressure gradients produce manifestations of fetofetal transfusion syndrome in a computerized model of monochorial twin pregnancy. Am J Obstet Gynecol 174:598, 1996

Tan KL, Goon SM, Salmon Y, et al: Conjoined twins. Acta Obstet Gynecol Scand 50:373, 1971

Templeton A: The multiple gestation epidemic: The role of the assisted reproductive technologies. Am J Obstet Gynecol 190:894, 2004

Terasaki PI, Gjertson D, Bernoco D, et al: Twins with two different fathers identified by HLA. N Engl J Med 299:590, 1978

Tessen JA, Zlatnik FJ: Monoamniotic twins: A retrospective controlled study. Obstet Gynecol 77:832, 1991

Trivedi AN, Gillett WR: The retained twin/triplet following a preterm delivery—an analysis of the literature. Aust N Z J Obstet Gynaecol 38:461, 1998

Tsao K, Feldstein VA, Albanese CT, et al: Selective reduction of acardiac twin by radiofrequency ablation. Am J Obstet Gynecol 187:635, 2002

Tuppin P, Blondel B, Kaminski M: Trends in multiple deliveries and infertility treatments in France. Br J Obstet Gynaecol 100:383, 1993

Uchida IA, Freeman VCP, Gedeon M, et al: Twinning rate in spontaneous abortions. Am J Hum Genet 35:987, 1983

van Allen MI, Smith DW, Shepard TH: Twin reversed atrial perfusion (TRAP) sequence: A study of 14 twin pregnancies with acardius. Semin Perinatol 7:285, 1983

van den Brand SF, Nijhuis JG, van Dongen PW: Prenatal ultrasound diagnosis of conjoined twins. Obstet Gynecol Surv 49:656, 1994

Vinatier D, Dufour P, Beard J: Utilization of intravenous nitroglycerin for obstetrical emergencies. Int J Gynecol Obstet 55:129, 1996

Wada H, Nunogami K, Wada T, et al: Diffuse brain damage caused by acute twin-twin transfusion during late pregnancy. Acta Paediatr Jpn 40:370, 1998

Waterhouse JAH: Twinning in twin pedigrees. Br J Soc Med 4:197, 1950

Weiner CP: Diagnosis and treatment of twin to twin transfusion in the mid-second trimester of pregnancy. Fetal Ther 2:71, 1987

Weiss JL, Cleary-Goldman J, Tanji K, et al: Multicystic encephalomalacia after first-trimester intrauterine fetal death in monchorionic twins. Am J Obstet Gynecol 190:563, 2003

Weissman A, Achiron R, Lipitz S, et al: The first-trimester growth-discordant twin: An ominous prenatal finding. Obstet Gynecol 84:110, 1994

Wenstrom KD, Syrop CH, Hammitt DG, et al: Increased risk of monochorionic twinning associated with assisted reproduction. Fertil Steril 60:510, 1993

Wenstrom KD, Tessen JA, Zlatnik FJ, et al: Frequency, distribution, and theoretical mechanisms of hematologic and weight discordance in monochorionic twins. Obstet Gynecol 80:257, 1992

White C, Wyshak G: Inheritance in human dizygotic twinning. N Engl J Med 271:1003, 1964

Winsor EJ, Brown BS, Luther ER, et al: Deceased co-twin as a cause of false positive amniotic fluid AFP and AChE. Prenat Diagn 7:485, 1987

Wittmann BK, Farquharson DF, Thomas WD, et al: The role of feticide in the management of severe twin transfusion syndrome. Am J Obstet Gynecol 155:1023, 1986

Yaron Y, Bryant-Greenwood PK, Dave N, et al: Multifetal pregnancy reductions of triplets to twins: Comparison with nonreduced triplets and twins. Am J Obstet Gynecol 180:1268, 1999

40

Abnormalities of the Reproductive Tract

In some cases, pregnancy is complicated by preexisting abnormalities of the reproductive tract. In general, these are developmental anomalies incurred during embryogenesis. However, they may be acquired during adulthood, sometimes during pregnancy.

DEVELOPMENTAL REPRODUCTIVE TRACT ABNORMALITIES

A number of genitourinary defects from abnormal embryogenesis occur sporadically. Serious defects often result in significant fetal and maternal hazards. In some, even minor defects may result in an increased incidence of threatened miscarriage and abnormal fetal lie.

EMBRYOGENESIS OF THE REPRODUCTIVE TRACT. To understand the etiology of developmental abnormalities of the vagina, cervix, and uterus, it is important to first understand their embryogenesis. This is discussed in Chapter 4 and summarized in Figure 40–1.

Briefly, development begins between the third and fifth gestational weeks, when the metanephric ducts emerge and connect with the cloaca. Between the fourth and fifth weeks, two ureteric buds develop distally from the mesonephric ducts and begin to grow cephalad toward the mesonephros. Müllerian (paramesonephric) ducts form bilaterally between the developing gonad and the mesonephros. The müllerian ducts extend downward and laterally to the mesonephric ducts, and they finally turn medially to meet and fuse together in the midline. The fused müllerian duct descends to the urogenital sinus to join the müllerian tubercle. **The close association between the müllerian and mesonephric ducts has clinical relevance because damage to either duct system is often associated with anomalies that involve the uterine horn, kidney, and ureter.**

The uterus is formed by the union of the two müllerian ducts at about the 10th week. Fusion begins in the middle and then extends caudally and cephalad. The characteristic uterine shape is now formed, with cellular proliferation at the upper portion and a simultaneous dissolution of cells at the lower pole, thus establishing the first uterine cavity. This cavity is at the lower pole with a thick wedge of tissue above. The upper thick wedge of tissue (septum) is dissolved slowly, creating the uterine cavity. This process is usually completed by the 20th week. Any failure to fuse the two müllerian ducts or failure to resorb the cavity between them results in separate uterine horns or some degree of persistent uterine septum.

The vagina forms between the urogenital sinus and the müllerian tubercle by a dissolution of the cell cord between the two structures. It is believed that this dissolution starts at the hymen and moves upward toward the cervix. Failure of this process is associated with persistence of the cell cord. Vaginal agenesis or lesser abnormalities of this cell cord dissolution result in varying degrees of septum formation.

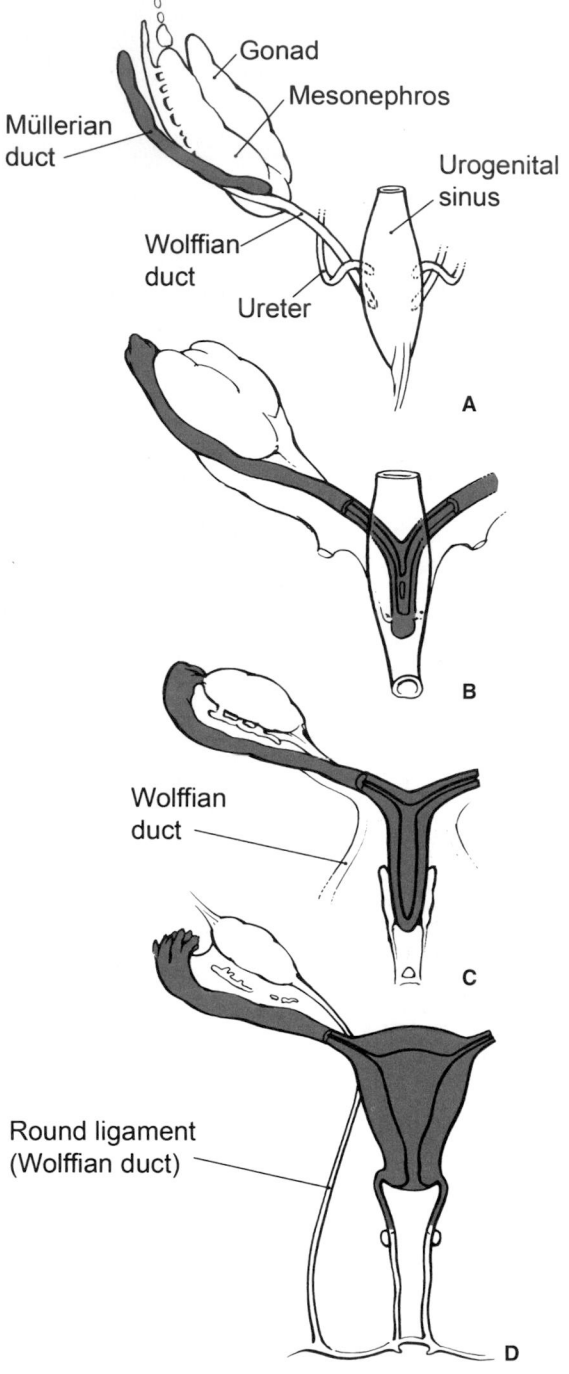

FIGURE 40–1. Development of the female reproductive systems from the genital ducts and urogenital sinus. Vestigial structures are also shown. **A.** Reproductive system at 6 weeks before differentiation. **B.** In the female, the müllerian (paramesonephric) ducts extend and enter the urogenital sinus and become fused. **C.** Uterine cavitation occurs at site of fused müllerian ducts and the uterus grows downward. **D.** Cavitation is complete and the lower segment and cervix, along with the upper vagina, are formed.

Genesis and Classification of Müllerian Abnormalities. Because fusion of the two müllerian ducts forms the upper two thirds of the vagina as well as the cervix and uterine body, the principal groups of deformities arising from three types of embryological defects can be classified as follows:

1. Defective canalization of the vagina results in a transverse septum, or in the most extreme form, vaginal agenesis.
2. Unilateral maturation of the müllerian duct with incomplete or absent development of the opposite duct results in defects associated with upper urinary tract abnormalities.
3. The most common abnormality is absent or faulty midline fusion of the müllerian ducts. Fusion anomalies are thought to be polygenic or multifactorial (see Chap. 12, p. 300). Complete lack of fusion results in two entirely separate uteri, cervices, and vaginas. Incomplete tissue resorption between the two fused müllerian ducts results in a uterine septum.

Various classifications of these anomalies have been proposed. Buttram and Gibbons (1979) suggested one based on the failure of normal development. This classification separates a diversity of anomalies into groups with similar clinical characteristics, prognosis for pregnancy, and treatment. It has been adapted by the American Society for Reproductive Medicine—formerly American Fertility Society (Table 40–1). The classification includes a category for abnormalities associated with fetal exposure to diethylstilbestrol. Vaginal anomalies have not been classified, because they are not associated with fetal loss. In this scheme, vaginal anomalies are most often associated with uterine didelphys

TABLE 40–1 American Fertility Society Classification of Müllerian Anomalies

I. Segmental müllerian hypoplasia or agenesis
   A. Vaginal
   B. Cervical
   C. Uterine fundus
   D. Tubal
   E. Combined anomalies

II. Unicornuate uterus
   A. Communicating rudimentary horn
   B. Noncommunicating horn
   C. No endometrial cavity
   D. No rudimentary horn

III. Uterine didelphys

IV. Bicornuate uterus
   A. Complete (division to internal os)
   B. Partial

V. Septate uterus
   A. Complete (septum to internal os)
   B. Partial

VI. Arcuate

VII. Diethylstilbestrol related

From the American Fertility Society, 1988.

and bicornuate anomalies. Class I segmental defects can affect the vagina, cervix, uterus, or tubes (Fig. 40–2).

VULVAR ABNORMALITIES. Complete *atresia of the vulva* includes atresia of the lower third of the vagina. Usually, vulvar atresia is incomplete and results from adhesions or scars following injury or infection. The defect may present a considerable obstacle to vaginal delivery. Although the resistance usually is overcome, deep perineal tears may result.

Labial fusion is most commonly due to congenital adrenal hyperplasia (see Chap. 4, p. 114). Other causes include fetal exogenous androgen exposure or abdominal wall defects. *Imperforate hymen* is persistence of the fusion between the sinovaginal bulbs with the urogenital sinus. Typically, it is associated with primary amenorrhea and hematocolpos and is not encountered often during pregnancy. Occasionally, *vulvar venous malformations* are encountered. These must be differentiated from both vulvar varicosities of pregnancy and tumors (Marrocco-Trischitta and colleagues, 2001).

VAGINAL ABNORMALITIES. Developmental abnormalities of the normal single vagina include:

1. *Atresia.* This may be partial or complete. Vaginal agenesis is usually due to the Rokitansky-Küster-Hauser syndrome or from androgen insensitivity syndrome (formerly testicular feminization).
2. *Double vagina.* It is often difficult to distinguish the double from the completely septate vagina. The true double vagina includes a double introitus and resembles a double-barreled shotgun, with each passage terminating in a distinct, separate cervix. At times, one passage ends blindly.
3. *Longitudinally septate vagina.* More or less complete longitudinal septum.
4. *Transversely septate vagina.* This results from faulty canalization of the fused müllerian anlage rather than faulty longitudinal fusion. The septate vagina is usually discovered during routine pelvic examination or with tampon insertion.

Obstetrical Significance. Vaginal anomalies usually present few problems. However, occasionally they obstruct vaginal delivery.

ATRESIA. *Complete vaginal atresia*, unless corrected operatively, forms an effective barrier to pregnancy (Chakravarty and colleagues, 2000). **About one third of women with vaginal atresia have associated urological abnormalities**. With complete müllerian agenesis, pregnancy is impossible, but vaginal dilatation techniques are successful in forming a functional vagina in as many as 90 percent of cases (Croak and associates, 2003; Roberts and colleagues, 2001). In some women, surgical correction is necessary (American College of Obstetricians and Gynecologists, 2002b).

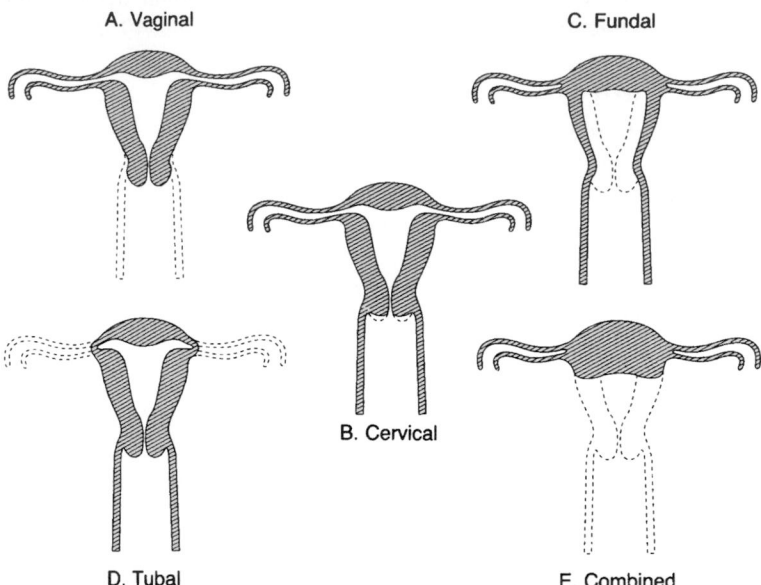

A. Vaginal

C. Fundal

B. Cervical

D. Tubal

E. Combined

FIGURE 40–2. Class I müllerian anomaly: Segmental müllerian agenesis or hypoplasia with subdivisions.

Incomplete atresia can be a manifestation of faulty development, as shown in Figure 40–2, or the result of scarring from injury or inflammation (see p. 960). In most cases of partial atresia, because of pregnancy-induced tissue softening, obstructions during labor are gradually overcome.

SEPTAE AND STRICTURES. A complete longitudinal septum usually does not cause dystocia because the half of the vagina through which the fetus descends gradually dilates satisfactorily. However, an incomplete septum occasionally interferes with descent. In these cases, the septum may become stretched around the presenting part as a band of varying thickness. Occasionally, it must be divided or cesarean delivery performed. Burgis (2001) described an obstructive septum in one vagina of a woman with uterine didelphys and a double vagina.

Sometimes the upper vagina is separated from the rest of the canal by a *transverse septum* with a small opening, as shown in Figure 40–3. Some of these are associated with in utero exposure to diethylstilbestrol (DES) (see p. 957). Such strictures may be mistaken for the upper limit of the vaginal vault. If so, at the time of labor, the septal opening is misidentified as an undilated cervical os. After the external os has dilated completely, the head impinges on the septum and causes it to bulge downward. If the septum does not yield, slight pressure on its opening usually leads to further dilatation, but occasionally cruciate incisions may be required to permit delivery (Blanton and Rouse, 2003).

CERVICAL ABNORMALITIES. There are a number of anatomical and developmental anomalies of the normal single cervix.

1. *Atresia.* The entire cervix may fail to develop. This may be combined with incomplete development of the upper vagina or lower uterus (see Fig. 40–2).
2. *Double cervix.* Each distinct cervix results from separate müllerian duct maturation. Both septate and true double cervices are frequently associated with a longitudinal vaginal septum. Many septate cervices are erroneously classified as double.
3. *Single hemicervix.* This arises from unilateral müllerian maturation.
4. *Septate cervix.* This consists of a single muscular ring partitioned by a septum. The septum may be confined to the cervix, or more often, it may be the downward continuation of a uterine septum or the upward extension of a vaginal septum.

Obstetrical Significance. Complete cervical atresia is incompatible with conception (Chakravarty and associates,

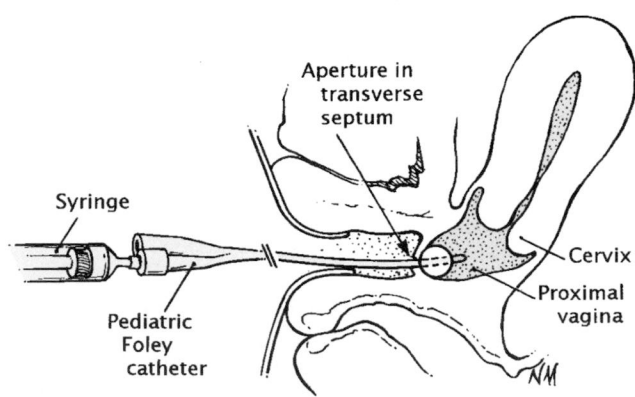

FIGURE 40–3. Sagittal view of a transverse vaginal septum with communication through a small opening into the distal vagina.

2000). Cicatricial *cervical stenosis* may follow various forms of cervical trauma (see p. 960). Because there usually is tissue softening during pregnancy, stenosis usually yields during labor, but occasionally cesarean delivery is necessary.

UTERINE MALFORMATIONS. As outlined in Table 40–1, a large variety of congenital uterine malformations may be encountered. Some of these are simply oddities to be noted, whereas others may preclude normal procreation.

Diagnosis. Some uterine anomalies are discovered by routine pelvic examination. Frequently they are discovered at cesarean delivery or during manual exploration of the uterine cavity after delivery. Fundal notching, palpated abdominally, is most often indicative of a malformed uterus. Ultrasonic screening for uterine anomalies, although 98-percent specific, is only 43-percent sensitive (Nicolini and associates, 1987). It is difficult to distinguish a septate from a bicornuate uterus without radiological examination, high-resolution sonography, or *magnetic resonance imaging* (MRI) (Raga and colleagues, 1996; Salle and co-workers, 1996). In some cases, *hysteroscopy* and *hysterography* are of value in ascertaining the configuration of the uterine cavity. Minto and colleagues (2001) reported that preoperative evaluation with MRI was helpful in determining the surgical approach in nine women with complex müllerian anomalies. Hundley and co-workers (2001) described excellent imaging of a septate uterus with a double cervix and septate vagina using three-dimensional MRI reconstruction. Laparoscopy may be necessary for confirmation of the absence or presence of an external division of the uterus or a rudimentary horn. Alborzi and associates (2002) used *sonohysterography* to differentiate septate and bicornuate uteri. Woelfer and co-workers (2001) used *three-dimensional sonography* to identify uterine anomalies in 106 women.

Incidence. Accurate figures are not available for the incidence of uterine anomalies. Green and Harris (1976) found the incidence to be about 1 in 400 for nearly 32,000 deliveries. Detection was greatest during a period when an especially interested staff member espoused routine uterine exploration at delivery. When an anomaly was suspected, they performed hysterosalpingography 6 to 8 weeks postpartum. Müllerian anomalies are more common in women with recurrent spontaneous miscarriage. Valli and associates (2001) reported that 32 percent of 344 such women were found to have an anomaly compared with 6 percent of 922 women in the control group.

Urological Defects. When asymmetrical development of the reproductive tract is found, urological evaluation should be considered because of the frequent association with urinary tract anomalies. When unilateral uterine atresia is present or when one side of a double vagina terminates blindly, an ipsilateral urological anomaly is common (Fedele

and associates, 1987; Heinonen, 1983, 1984; Wiersma and colleagues, 1976).

Auditory Defects. As many as one third of women with müllerian defects have been reported to have auditory defects (Letterie and Vauss, 1991). These are typically mild to severe sensorineural hearing deficits in the high-frequency range.

Uterine Anomalies in Wilms Tumor Survivors. Survivors of this rare malignancy appear to have an increased incidence of congenital urinary and reproductive tract anomalies (Nicholson and colleagues, 1996). This observation might partially explain the increased rate of infertility reported in female survivors.

Obstetrical Significance. Major difficulties arise from many uterine anomalies. Uterine defects that result from development of only one müllerian duct or from lack of fusion often give rise to a hemiuterus that fails to dilate and hypertrophy appropriately. This may result in miscarriage, ectopic pregnancy, rudimentary horn pregnancy, preterm delivery, fetal growth restriction, abnormal fetal lie, uterine dysfunction, or uterine rupture (Ben-Rafael and associates, 1991; Michalas, 1991). Valli and colleagues (2001) reported a five-fold increase of recurrent miscarriage in 344 women with a septate or unicornuate uterus compared with that of 922 case controls. Even in women with only a uterine septum, miscarriage is increased (Buttram and Gibbons, 1979; Raga and associates, 1997). That said, the American College of Obstetricians and Gynecologists (2001) cautions that repair of such defects may not prevent miscarriage.

UNICORNUATE UTERUS (CLASS II). Developmental anomalies that result in a unicornuate uterus are shown in Figure 40–4. The incidence of a unicornuate uterus, as diagnosed by hysterosalpingography, in a series of 1160 uterine anomalies was 14 percent (Zanetti and associates, 1978). This was likely an underestimate, because hysterosalpingography cannot be used to identify noncommunicating rudimentary horns, by far the most common anomaly. Women with a unicornuate uterus have an increased incidence of infertility, endometriosis, and dysmenorrhea (Fedele and associates, 1987, 1995; Heinonen, 1983).

As shown in Table 40–2, implantation in the normal-sized hemiuterus is associated with increased incidences of preterm delivery, fetal growth restriction, breech presentation, dysfunctional labor, and cesarean delivery. Pregnancies in the rudimentary horn are usually disastrous. Rolen and associates (1966) reported that uterine rupture occurred prior to 20 weeks in most of 70 rudimentary horn pregnancies. An example is shown in Figure 40–5. Nahum (2002) reviewed the literature from 1900 to 1999 and identified reports of 588 such pregnancies. In 419 cases, the communication status was known, half of these had uterine rupture—80 percent before the third trimester. Eighty-five percent were of the

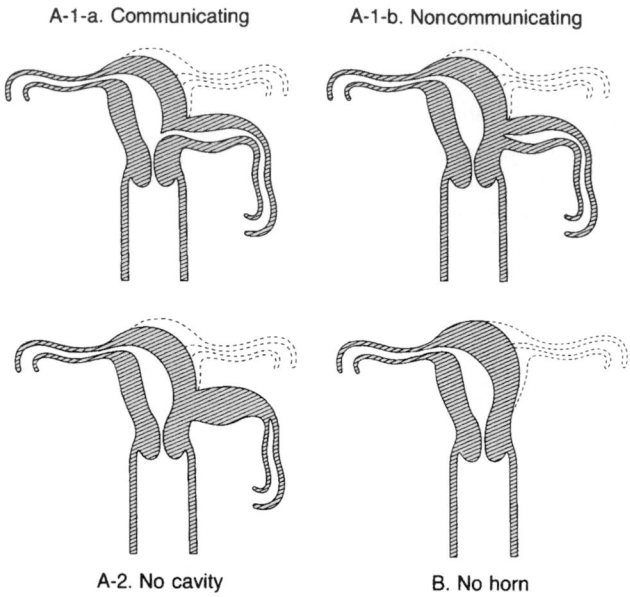

A-1-a. Communicating A-1-b. Noncommunicating

A-2. No cavity B. No horn

FIGURE 40–4. Class II müllerian anomalies: Unicornuate uterus either with rudimentary horn (**A**) or without rudimentary horn (**B**). Those with a rudimentary horn are divided into groups with an endometrial cavity (**A-1**) or without an endometrial cavity (**A-2**). Those with an endometrial cavity either have a communication with the opposite uterine horn (**A-1-a**) or do not have a communication with the opposite horn (**A-1-b**).

noncommunicating type, and the rupture rate in these was 85 percent. With a noncommunicating horn, the rupture rate was 85 percent. Fetal survival was 6 percent overall. Most of the 23 maternal deaths were before 1950. More liberal use of high-resolution ultrasound and MRI may result in an earlier diagnosis of such problems with surgical or medical therapy before the pregnancy ruptures (Edelman and associates, 2003; Vo and colleagues, 2003).

UTERINE DIDELPHYS (CLASS III). This anomaly is distinguished from bicornuate and septate uteri by the presence of complete nonfusion of the cervix and hemiuterine cavity (Fig. 40–6). Heinonen (1984) reported that all 26 women with a uterine didelphys had a longitudinal vaginal septum as well. A few cases in which there was a septate uterus instead of two hemiuteri have been reported (Hundley and associates, 2001; Wai and colleagues, 2001). Occasionally, one hemivagina is obstructed by an oblique or transverse vaginal septum (Hinckley and Milki, 2003).

Except for ectopic and rudimentary horn pregnancies, problems associated with uterine didelphys are similar to those seen with a unicornuate uterus. Heinonen (1984) reported a 70-percent successful pregnancy outcome. There was preterm delivery in 20 percent, fetal growth restriction in 10 percent, breech presentation in 43 percent, and the cesarean delivery rate was 82 percent. A trial of labor in a subsequent pregnancy following cesarean delivery resulted in a higher uterine rupture rate than expected (Ravasia and colleagues, 1999).

Multifetal gestation is unusual in women with uterine didelphys (Oláh, 2002). Mashiach and associates (1981) reported a case of triplets with a delivery interval of 72 days!

BICORNUATE AND SEPTATE UTERI (CLASSES IV AND V). In both of these types of anomalies, which are shown in Figures 40–7 and 40–8, there is a marked increase in miscarriages that is likely due to the abundant muscle tissue in the septum (Dabirashrafi and colleagues, 1995). Miscarriage with a septate uterus is more common than with a bicornuate uterus (Proctor and Haney, 2003). Pregnancy losses in the first 20 weeks were observed by Buttram and Gibbons (1979) to be 70 percent for bicornuate and 88 percent for septate uteri. Woelfer and colleagues (2001) reported a first-trimester loss rate for septate uteri of 42 percent. This extraordinarily high pregnancy wastage likely is due to partial or complete implantation on the largely avascular septum. The majority of women with müllerian anomalies have lateral placental implantation with

TABLE 40–2 Pregnancy Outcomes in Women with a Unicornuate Uterus

Outcome	Heinonen (1983)	Moutos et al. (1992)	Acien (1993)	Fedele et al. (1995)	Total
Patients	15	20	24	26	85
Pregnancies	35	36[a]	55	57	183
Spontaneous abortions (%)[b]	4 (11)	13 (36)	12 (22)	33 (58)	62 (34)
Ectopic pregnancies (%)[b]	4 (11)	1 (2.8)	1 (1.8)	3 (5.2)[c]	9 (5)
Deliveries (%)[b]	27 (77)	22 (61)	42 (76)	21 (37)	112 (61)
Breech presentations[d]	9 (33)	—	13 (31)	—	—
Cesarean deliveries[d]	8 (30)	8 (36)	—	—	—
Preterm deliveries[d]	4 (15)	3 (14)	9 (21)	5 (24)	21 (19)
Term deliveries[d]	23 (85)	19 (86)	33 (79)	16 (76)	91 (21)
Fetal survival (%)[b]	25 (71)	21 (58)	39 (71)	20 (35)	105 (57)

[a]Excludes four elective abortions.
[b]Of all pregnancies.
[c]Includes one blind horn pregnancy.
[d]Excludes abortions and ectopic pregnancies.

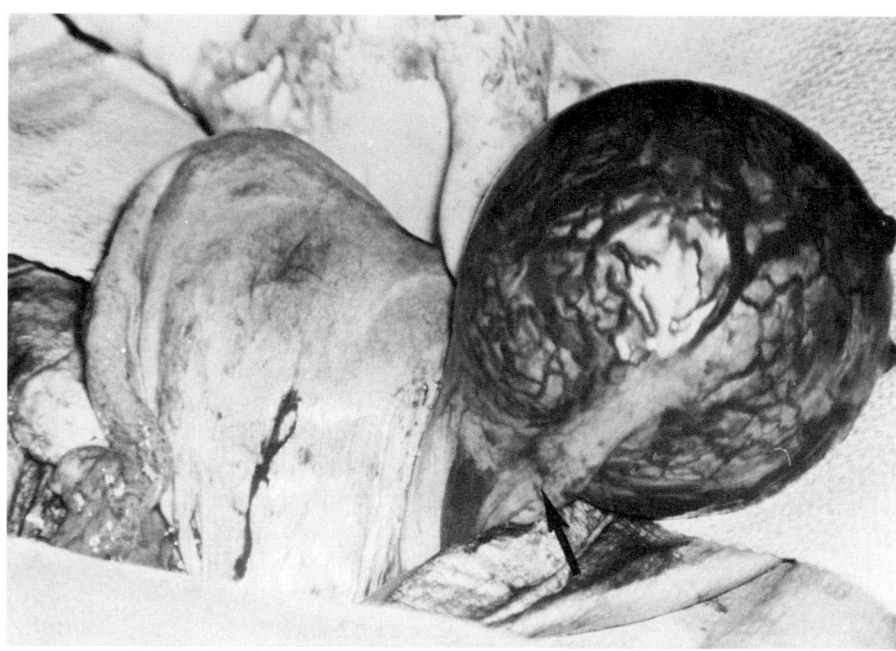

A

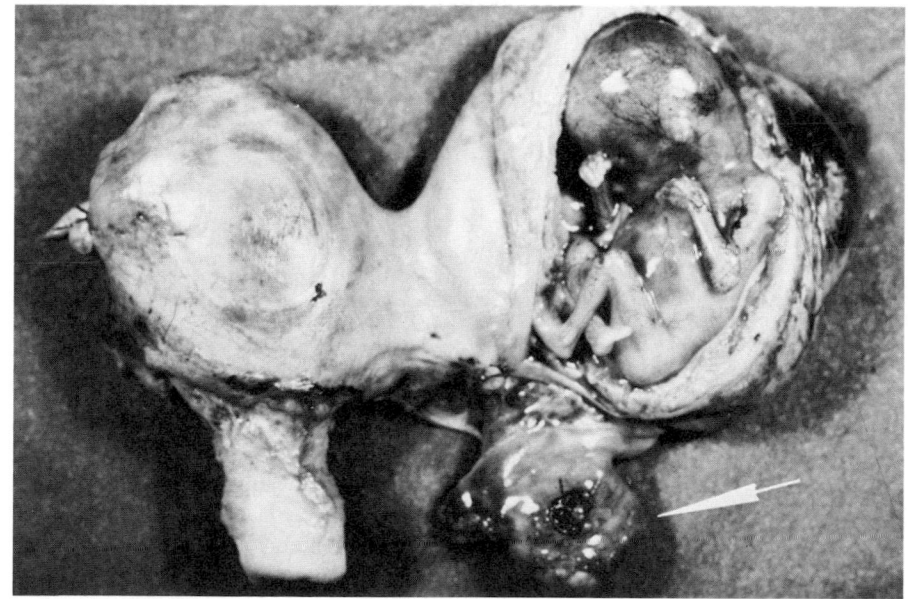

B

FIGURE 40–5. **A.** A 15-week pregnancy in a woman with three prior vaginal breech deliveries. This pregnancy is in the left noncommunicating rudimentary uterine horn as seen at laparotomy. The tense, vascular rudimentary uterus was bleeding from veins over its extremely vascular surface. The attached oviduct (*arrow*) was patent and the adjacent left ovary contained the corpus luteum of pregnancy. **B.** Hysterectomy specimen with left hemiuterus opened to display the fetus and placenta. The intact mass (*arrow*) consists of left tube and ovary.

poor perinatal outcomes (Leible and associates, 1998). There also is an increased incidence of preterm delivery, abnormal fetal lie, and cesarean delivery. Heinonen (1999) described three newborns with a limb-reduction defect born to women with a septate uterus. In one series, a subsequent trial of labor after cesarean delivery was associated with an increased risk of uterine rupture (Ravasia and associates, 1999).

ARCUATE UTERUS (CLASS VI). This malformation is only a mild deviation from the normally developed uterus. Raga and associates (1997) reported no impact on reproductive outcomes.

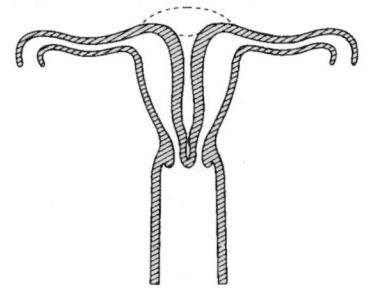

FIGURE 40–6. Class III müllerian anomaly: Uterine didelphys.

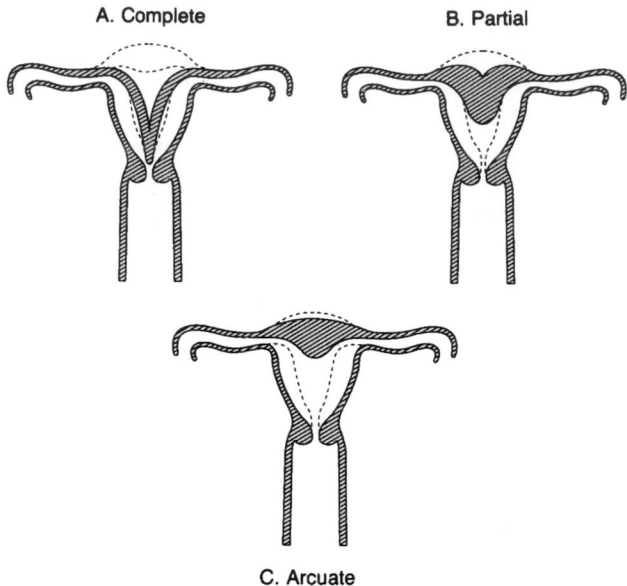

FIGURE 40–7. Class IV müllerian anomaly: Complete bicornuate uterus (**A**) and partial (**B**); Class VI arcuate uterus (**C**).

Conversely, Woelfer and colleagues (2001) found excessive second-trimester losses and preterm labor.

Management. Women with nonobstructive defects such as uterine didelphys and unicornuate uterus usually do not need surgical correction (Stenchever, 2001). Although abnormal fetal presentations are commonly seen, external cephalic version is less likely to be successful.

CERCLAGE. In women with repetitive pregnancy losses, a number of investigators have reported that cervical cerclage may lead to better outcomes (Golan, 1990b, 1992; Golan and Caspi, 1992; Maneschi, 1988; Seidman, 1991, and all their co-workers). Transabdominal cerclage may offer the best prognosis in women with partial cervical atresia or cervical hypoplasia (Hampton and colleagues, 1990; Mackey and co-workers, 2001).

Caspi and associates (1990) have described a modified Shirodkar cerclage for women with short or lacerated cer-

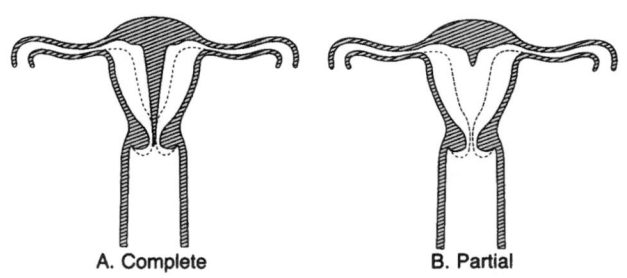

FIGURE 40–8. Class V müllerian anomaly: Septate uterus with complete septum to the cervical os (**A**) or partial septum (**B**).

vices and in women with previous McDonald cerclage failures. The results obtained were similar to those achieved with a Shirodkar cerclage. Transvaginal cervical cerclage has been used successfully in DES-exposed women with cervical hypoplasia (Ludmir and co-workers, 1991).

Cerclage should not be necessary after successful resection of a uterine septum. It probably should still be used following abdominal metroplasties for uterine didelphys and bicornuate uteri. If active labor supervenes, the cervical ligature is removed to prevent uterine rupture. Cerclage is discussed in detail in Chapter 9 (p. 237).

METROPLASTY. Women with septate or bicornuate anomalies and poor reproductive outcomes may benefit from uterine surgery (Ayhan and colleagues, 1992). Repair of a bicornuate uterus is by transabdominal metroplasty involving septal resection and recombination of the fundi (Candiani and associates, 1990; Kessler and co-workers, 1986). Following repair, uterine activity is normal if anatomically symmetrical uterine horns have been conjoined (Oliva and associates, 1992).

Repair of a septate uterus is best done by hysteroscopic resection of the septum (Daly, 1989; Grigoris, 1998; Hassiakos, 1990; Israel, 1984; Jourdain, 1998, and all their co-workers). In a review of pregnancy outcome following repair of a septate uterus, Stenchever (2001) reported that slightly over half of 351 pregnancies were liveborn. Preterm labor is common (Litta and colleagues, 2004; Pabuccu and Gomel, 2004). Despite minimal uterine wall invasion with septal resection, disastrous fundal rupture has been reported (Angell and co-workers, 2002).

DIETHYLSTILBESTROL-INDUCED REPRODUCTIVE TRACT ABNORMALITIES. From the late 1940s through the early 1960s, diethylstilbestrol (DES), a synthetic nonsteroidal estrogen, was prescribed for an estimated 3 million pregnant women in the United States. Early reports claimed the drug was useful in treating abortion, preeclampsia, diabetes, and preterm labor. It was remarkably ineffective for these indications, however, almost 20 years later, Herbst and co-workers (1971) found that DES exposure in utero was linked to the later development of vaginal clear cell adenocarcinoma. Pitkin (2003) describes this as one of the most seminal discoveries in obstetrics and gynecology of the past century. The risk of vaginal malignancy is about 1 per 1000 exposed daughters. Subsequently, it was established that daughters also had an increased risk of developing cervical intraepithelial neoplasia as well as small cell cervical carcinoma (Herbst, 2000). About one third have vaginal adenosis. In addition to carcinogenesis, several nonneoplastic abnormalities of the vagina and cervix have become apparent following DES exposure in utero.

Structural Abnormalities. As many as one fourth of women exposed to DES in utero have identifiable structural variations in the cervix and vagina (Herbst, 2000), which are in class VII of the American Fertility Society classification system (1988). These include transverse septa, circumferential ridges involving the vagina and cervix, and cervical collars. Half of all exposed women have uterine cavity anomalies evident on hysterography. Women with cervicovaginal abnormalities are more likely to have uterine anomalies. Significantly smaller uterine cavities, shortened upper uterine segments, and T-shaped and irregular cavities have been described (Barranger and associates, 2002). Finally, abnormalities of the oviduct have been described, including shortening, narrowing, and fimbrial absence. Kipersztok and colleagues (1996) believe that hysterosalpingography remains the imaging procedure of choice in the identification of these anomalies.

Structural anomalies in males have also been linked to fetal exposure to DES. These include cryptorchidism, testicular hypoplasia, microphallus, and hypospadias (Herñandez-Díaz, 2002). Klip and colleagues (2002) provided evidence suggesting a transgenerational effect in which male fetuses conceived by daughters of DES-exposed women have hypospadias.

Reproductive Performance. Women exposed to DES in utero in general have impaired conception rates (Goldberg and Falcone, 1999; Palmer and colleagues, 2001; Senekjian and co-workers, 1988). Reduced fertility in these women is poorly understood but is associated with cervical hypoplasia and atresia. Of those who conceive, the incidence of miscarriage, ectopic pregnancy, and preterm delivery are increased; the risk is greatest in women with structural abnormalities (Goldberg and Falcone, 1999; Kaufman and associates, 1984, 2000). Spontaneous uterine rupture during pregnancy is increased; Porcu and colleagues (2003) reported a woman with spontaneous rupture at 12 weeks.

ECTOPIC PREGNANCY. The incidence of ectopic pregnancy was reported to be 7 percent compared with none for controls (Herbst, 2000; Herbst and colleagues, 1989). The etiology is likely due to tubal anomalies, but decreased uterine size may also be a factor. Also, DES-exposed women with salpingitis may develop adhesions that aggravate tubal dysfunction.

PRETERM LABOR. The incidence of preterm delivery is increased, likely due to uterine and cervical anomalies (de Haas and associates, 1991; Herbst, 2000). Cervical incompetence is associated with midpregnancy losses and preterm delivery (Ludmir and colleagues, 1987). In 5 of 21 pregnancies, Michaels and co-workers (1989) documented preterm cervical effacement and dilatation using serial ultrasonic evaluation. They recommend weekly visits for these women, with serial ultrasound performed beginning at 14 weeks and continuing through 27 weeks. If there is cervical effacement and dilatation, they perform cerclage. Ayers and associates (1988) and Ludmir and co-workers (1987, 1991) also recommend cerclage for most of these women, especially those with cervical hypoplasia. Hampton and colleagues (1990) recommend abdominal cerclage for women in this latter group (see p. 956). In general, we do not perform cerclage beyond 23 weeks (see Chap. 9, p. 237).

Surgical Repair. With some uterine structural defects, surgical repair may improve reproductive performance. Katz and colleagues (1996) reported improved pregnancy outcomes with hysteroscopic resection of intrauterine tissue. Garbin and associates (1998) and Barranger and colleagues (2002) performed hysteroscopic metroplasty in a total of 54 women. Following metroplasty, they reported that over 75 percent had liveborn infants.

ACQUIRED REPRODUCTIVE TRACT ABNORMALITIES

VULVAR ABNORMALITIES. A number of acute and chronic vulvar conditions may prove vexing to both the woman and her obstetrician.

Edema. Many women have some degree of vulvar edema during pregnancy. At times it can be impressive and without an identifiable pathological cause. In women with the nephrotic syndrome and hypoproteinemia, vulvar edema may be problematic as early as midpregnancy (see Fig. 48–5, p. 1101). During labor, the vulva may become edematous, especially in women with severe preeclampsia. Venous thromboses and hematomas occasionally cause edema and significant pain. In postpartum women, edema associated with a paravaginal, vulvar, or perineal hematoma occurring from lacerations or an episiotomy may be extensive (see Chap. 35, p. 836).

Inflammatory Lesions. Extensive perineal inflammation and scarring from *hidradenitis suppurativa, lymphogranuloma venereum,* or *Crohn disease* may create difficulty with vaginal delivery, episiotomy, and repair. A mediolateral episiotomy may prevent some of these difficulties.

Bartholin Gland Lesions. Cysts of the Bartholin glands are usually sterile and need no treatment during pregnancy. If the cysts are large enough to cause difficulty at delivery, then needle aspiration as a temporary measure is sufficient. If an abscess is present, broad-spectrum antimicrobials are given and drainage is established. For a large abscess with extensive cellulitis, drainage is best performed in the operating room. The cut edges of the abscess cavity are marsupialized and packed with gauze, which is removed the next day. Alternatively, a Word catheter is used as shown in Figure 40–9. In some cases, especially in diabetic or immunocompromised women, life-threatening *necrotizing fasciitis* may develop (see Chap. 31, p. 720).

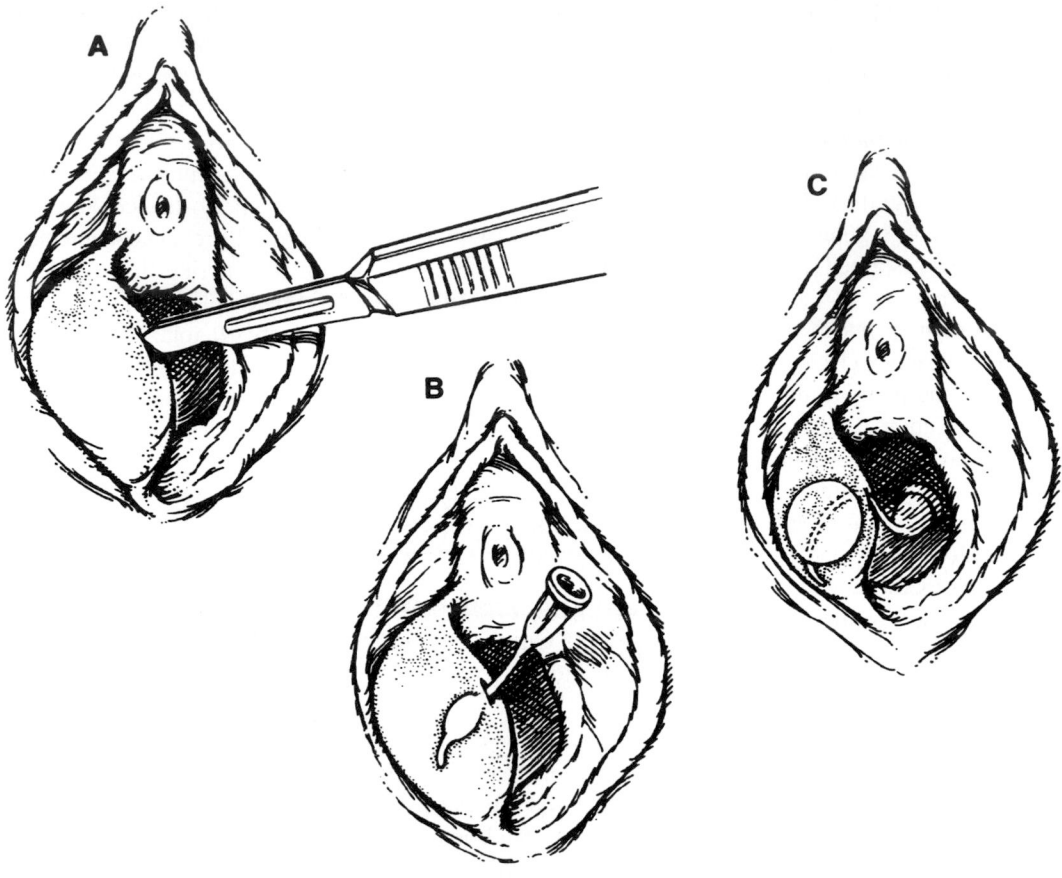

FIGURE 40–9. Management of a Bartholin gland abscess using a Word catheter. **A.** A stab wound is made into the abscess using a No. 15 scalpel blade. **B.** Insertion of catheter into cavity. **C.** Properly inflated balloon tip with external catheter tip to be tucked into the vagina. (From Wendel, 2002.)

Urethral and Bladder Lesions. Trauma to the urethra or infection of its glands may result in periurethral abscesses, cysts, and diverticula. Abscesses usually resolve spontaneously, some with asymptomatic cyst formation. A urethral diverticulum may fill with debris that intermittently empties through the urethra to give rise to proteinuria of obscure etiology. In general, surgical excision of cysts or diverticula should not be done during pregnancy.

Bladder lesions during pregnancy are uncommon. Obstruction of labor by *bladder stones* has been reported (Penning and associates, 1997; Rai and Ramesh, 1998). Hendry (1997) reviewed the literature concerning *bladder tumors* and concluded that cesarean delivery was required in some cases of bladder cancer.

Condyloma Acuminata. Genital infection with the human papillomavirus results in condyloma acuminata. These so-called *venereal warts* can be so extensive that vaginal delivery may be prohibited. These sexually transmitted lesions are discussed in Chapter 59 (see p. 1318).

Female Genital Mutilation. Inaccurately called female circumcision, mutilation refers to medically unnecessary vulvar and perineal modification. Forms of female genital mutilation are practiced in countries throughout Africa and the Middle East and in Muslim populations of Indonesia and Malaysia. Between 80 and 110 million women are affected worldwide. According to the World Health Organization (1992), mutilation is associated with poverty, illiteracy, and low social status of women. Jones and colleagues (1997) estimated that nearly 170,000 women who have had genital mutilation live in the United States. Cultural sensitivity is imperative, because many women may be offended by the suggestion that they have been mutilated (American College of Obstetricians and Gynecologists, 2002a).

The World Health Organization (1997) classifies genital mutilations into four types (Table 40–3). Other commonly used terms include *sunna* (type 1), *excision* (type 2), and *infibulation* or *pharaonic circumcision* (type 3). A type 1 procedure performed under sterile conditions (often not the case) rarely has long-term adverse physical consequences (Toubia, 1994). A type 3 procedure, an extreme form of mutilation, consists of the removal of the entire clitoris, the entire labia minora, and at least two thirds of the labia majora (Fig. 40–10). The procedure is typically performed at 7 years of age without anesthesia by midwives or village women.

TABLE 40–3 World Health Organization Classification of Female Genital Mutilation

Type 1.	Excision of the prepuce with or without excision of the clitoris.
Type 2.	Excision of the clitoris and partial or total excision of the labia minora.
Type 3.	Excision of part or all of the external genitalia and infibulation.
Type 4.	Unclassified, including pricking, piercing, incision, stretching, and introduction of corrosive substances into the vagina.

Adapted from the World Health Organization, 1997.

Commonly used instruments are razor blades, kitchen knives, scissors, glass, and in some regions, the teeth of the midwife. The two sides of the vulva are stitched together by silk or catgut or are held together by thorns. A small opening is left (usually made by the insertion of a matchstick) for the passage of menstrual blood and urine. The legs of the girl are then bound from hip to ankle for as many as 40 days so that scar tissue will form. Immediate dangers are exsanguination and severe infections. Urinary retention is common.

Long-term sequelae depend on the severity of mutilation. Okonofua and associates (2002) reported that half of women attending clinics in Nigeria had been mutilated. Of these, 70 percent had undergone type 1 procedures, and 25 percent had undergone type 2 procedures. These women had normal sexual function but a threefold risk of vaginal infection or genital ulcers. Complications of type 3 procedures include sterility, dysmenorrhea, and dyspareunia (Chen and associates, 2004; Knight and colleagues, 1999; Nour, 2004). Infibulation may also predispose to human immunodeficiency virus (HIV) infection (Kun, 1997). A case of clitoral amputation neuroma has been described by Ferñandez-Aguilar and Noël (2003).

The American College of Obstetricians and Gynecologists (2002a), along with the International Federation of Gynecology and Obstetrics, the American Medical Association, the United Nations International Children's Emergency Fund, and the World Health Organization, has supported legislation to eliminate female genital mutilation in the United States. The American Academy of Pediatrics (1998) encourages development of community educational programs for immigrant populations. Currently, it is a federal crime to perform unnecessary genital surgery on a girl younger than 18 years of age. In some countries where female genital mutilation has been routinely performed, laws are being enacted to prohibit such mutilation (Ciment, 1999; Eke and Nkanginieme, 1999). A slide lecture kit—*Female Circumcision/Female Genital Mutilation: Clinical Management of Circumcised Women*— is available to ACOG members from the ACOG Distribution Center (800-762-2264).

PREGNANCY. A number of obstetrical complications due to birth canal obstruction from scar tissue occur in women who have undergone female genital mutilation. Many of these women do not desire deinfibulation until pregnant; therefore, Nour (2004) recommends that this be done at midpregnancy using spinal analgesia. Another option is to wait and incise scarred tissue between the index and middle fingers inserted between the crowning fetal head and the scar. In our experiences, in many cases intrapartum deinfibulation allows successful vaginal delivery without major complications.

VAGINAL ABNORMALITIES. Compared with developmental anomalies, acquired vaginal abnormalities are uncommon. Even after major trauma, long-term sexual and reproductive functions are the norm (Fallat and colleagues, 1998). Vaginal stenosis may develop as a result of mucositis from graft-versus-host reaction following organ transplantation (Louis-Sylvestre and associates, 2003).

Partial Atresia. Incomplete atresia may result from infection or trauma that leads to extensive scarring. During labor, this is usually overcome by pressure from the presenting part, but occasionally incisions or even cesarean delivery are necessary.

Genital Tract Fistulas. Fistulas seen during pregnancy likely existed previously, but in rare cases they develop during pregnancy. McKay and Hanlon (2003) described a

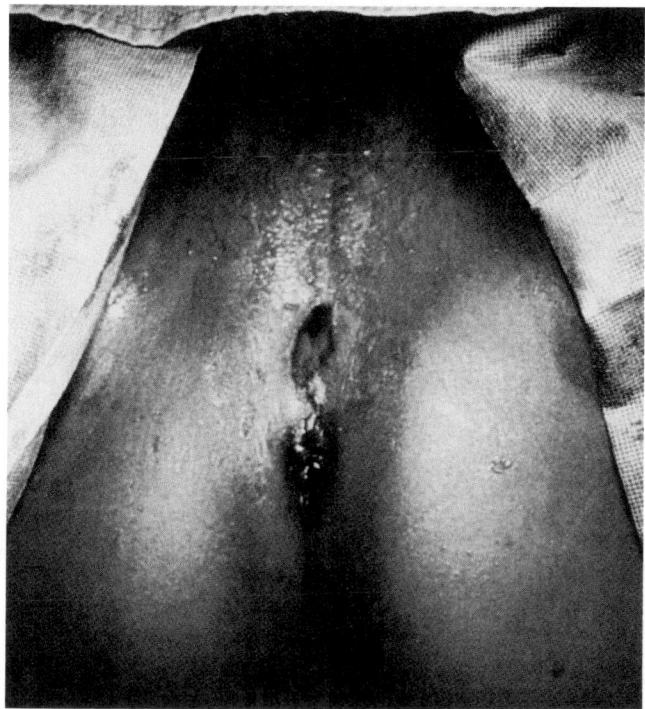

FIGURE 40–10. Sequelae of infibulation or pharaonic circumcision: This ritual mutilation procedure included clitoridectomy, excision of labia minora, and incision of labia majora. Remnant labia majora have been approximated, leaving a small neo-introitus. (From Nour, 2000, with permission.)

vesicovaginal fistula that developed following a McDonald cerclage done at 20 weeks. In prolonged obstructed labor, which is unfortunately common in developing countries, the genital tract may be compressed between the fetal head and the bony pelvis. Brief pressure is not significant, but prolonged pressure may result in necrosis with subsequent fistula formation. Miklos and colleagues (1995) described a *vesicouterine fistula* that developed following vaginal delivery after prior cesarean delivery. Rarely, the anterior cervical lip is compressed against the symphysis pubis with development of a *vesicocervical fistula.* Some of these fistulas heal spontaneously, but more often subsequent repair is necessary. Murray and associates (2002) report a high rate of successful closures performed since 1975 in over 15,000 fistulas at The Fistula Hospital in Addis Ababa, Ethiopia. Unfortunately, despite repair, urinary incontinence persists in 55 percent of cases. Wall (2002) has provided a poignant chronicle of the societal impact of these abnormalities on Nigerian culture.

CERVICAL ABNORMALITIES. Cicatricial *cervical stenosis* was once a problem (Melody, 1957). Cervical conization was a common cause (Gibbs and Moore, 1968). Cryotherapy and laser therapy occasionally produce stenosis, but large-loop excision of the transformation zone (LLETZ) usually does not (Cruickshank and associates, 1995; Spitzer and colleagues, 1995). Cervical stenosis almost always yields during labor. A so-called *conglutinated cervix* may undergo almost complete effacement, but the cervical os may not dilate. Thus, the presenting part is often separated from the

vagina by only a thin layer of cervical tissue. Ordinarily, complete dilatation promptly follows pressure with a fingertip, although in rare instances, manual dilatation or cruciate incisions may be required.

In some women, extensive *cervical carcinoma* may impair vaginal delivery. Carcinoma of the cervix complicating pregnancy is discussed in Chapter 57 (see p. 1264).

UTERINE ABNORMALITIES. A number of uterine disorders may adversely affect pregnancy as well as fertility.

Anteflexion. Exaggerated degrees of anteflexion frequently observed in early pregnancy are without significance. In later months, particularly when the abdominal wall is very lax, the uterus may fall forward. This may be so exaggerated that the fundus lies considerably below the lower margin of the symphysis pubis. Marked anteflexion of the enlarging pregnant uterus usually is associated with *diastasis recti* and a pendulous abdomen. The abnormal uterine position sometimes prevents proper transmission of contractions; this is overcome by repositioning with an abdominal binder.

Retroflexion. Occasionally during pregnancy, the growing normally retroflexed uterus remains incarcerated in the hollow of the sacrum (Fig. 40–11). Symptoms include abdominal discomfort and inability to void normally. As pressure from the full bladder increases, small amounts of urine are passed involuntarily, but the bladder never empties entirely— *paradoxical incontinence.* Acute urinary retention may also

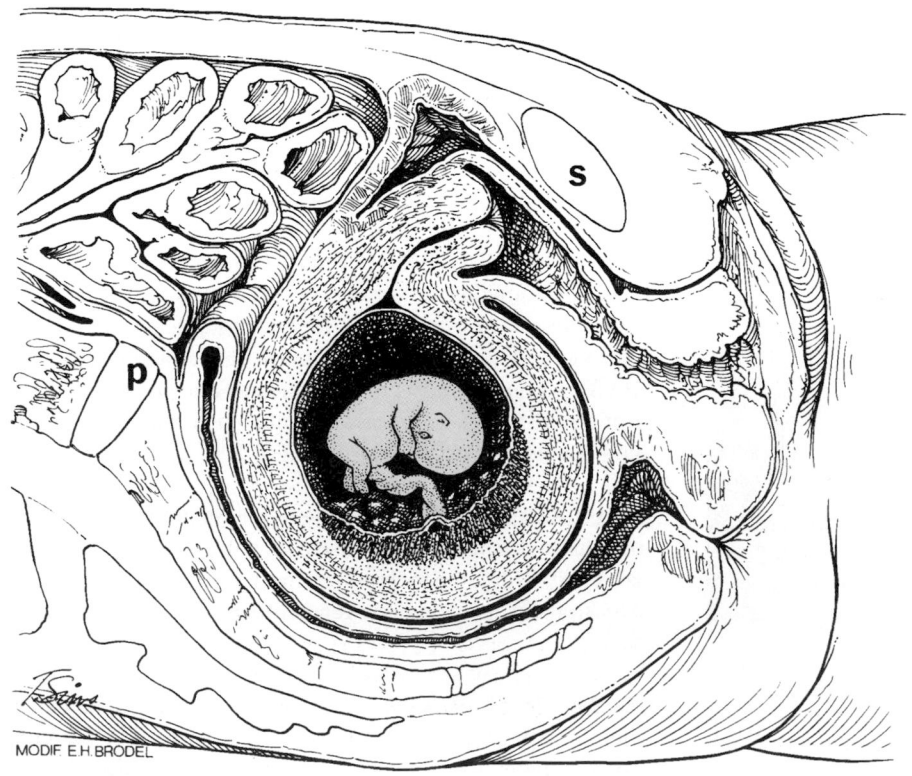

MODIF E H BRODEL

FIGURE 40–11. Incarcerated, retroflexed uterus. (p = sacral promontory; s = symphysis.)

occur (Myers and Scotti, 1995). Such blockage also can cause severe obstructive nephropathy.

Management is repositioning. After bladder catheterization, the uterus can usually be pushed out of the pelvis when the woman is placed in the knee-chest position. Occasionally spinal analgesia or general anesthesia is necessary. Following repositioning, an indwelling catheter is left in place until bladder tone returns. Insertion of a soft pessary for a few weeks usually prevents reincarceration. Lettieri and colleagues (1994) described seven cases of uterine incarceration not amenable to these simple procedures. In two women, laparoscopy was used at 13 to 14 weeks to reposition the uterus using the round ligaments for traction. Seubert and associates (1999) used colonoscopy to dislodge an incarcerated uterus in five women. Hamoda and co-workers (2002) simply observed one woman and performed cesarean delivery of a healthy infant at 36 weeks.

Sacculation. Persistent entrapment of the pregnant uterus in the pelvis may result in an anterior uterine sacculation. Extensive dilatation of the lower uterine segment takes place to accommodate the fetus (Jackson and associates, 1988; Lettieri and co-workers, 1994). Cesarean delivery is necessary. Spearing (1978) stressed the importance of identifying the distorted anatomy. An elongated vagina passing above the level of a fetal head that is deeply placed into the pelvis is suggestive of a sacculation or an abdominal pregnancy. The Foley catheter is frequently palpated above the level of the umbilicus! Spearing (1978) recommended extending the abdominal incision to above the umbilicus and delivery of the entire uterus from the abdomen before an attempt is made to incise it. **This simple procedure will restore anatomy to the correct relationships and prevent inadvertent incisions into and through the vagina and bladder.**

Friedman and associates (1986) described a rare case of posterior uterine sacculation following aggressive treatment for intrauterine adhesions, or *Asherman syndrome*. Uterine retroversion and a true uterine diverticulum have been mistaken for uterine sacculations (Engel and Rushovich, 1984; Hill and associates, 1993).

Uterine Prolapse. The cervix, and occasionally a portion of the body of the uterus, may protrude to a variable extent from the vulva during early pregnancy. With further growth, the uterus usually rises above the pelvis and may draw the cervix up with it. If the uterus persists in its prolapsed position, symptoms of incarceration may develop from 10 to 14 weeks. To prevent this, the uterus is replaced early in pregnancy and held in position with a suitable pessary. Successful vaginal deliveries have been reported following sacrospinous uterosacral fixation done before pregnancy to correct severe uterine prolapse (Kovac and Cruikshank, 1993).

Cystocele and Rectocele. Attenuation of fascial support between the vagina and the bladder can lead to prolapse of the bladder into the vagina, or cystocele. Attenuation of fascia between the vagina and the rectum results in a rectocele. A large defect may fill with feces that, at times, can only be manually evacuated. During labor, either a cystocele or a rectocele can block normal fetal descent unless they are emptied and pushed out of the way. Urinary stasis with a cystocele predisposes to infection. Pregnancy may worsen associated *urinary stress incontinence*, because urethral closing pressures do not increase sufficiently to compensate for the progressive increase in bladder pressure caused by increasing uterine weight (Iosif and Ulmsten, 1981).

Enterocele. In rare instances, an enterocele of considerable size may complicate pregnancy. If symptomatic, the protrusion should be replaced and the woman kept in a recumbent position. If the mass interferes with delivery, it should be pushed up or held out of the way.

Uterine Torsion. Rotation of the uterus, most often to the right, is common during pregnancy. Jensen (1992) has provided an extensive review of uterine torsion. Torsion of sufficient degree to arrest uterine circulation is rare. Bakos and Axelsson (1987) reported a case of severe levotorsion associated with repeated fetal heart rate decelerations that prompted cesarean delivery. Because of extreme uterine torsion, the incision inadvertently was made in the posterior wall of the uterus! The severely malpositioned uterus should be removed from the abdomen prior to hysterotomy (Spearing, 1978). Sherer and colleagues (1994) stress that torsion can be confused with an abdominal pregnancy. If suspected, antepartum diagnosis of either may be improved with MRI (Dietz and co-workers, 1998; Nicholson and associates, 1995). Although the vagina normally appears as an H-shaped structure, with torsion it appears X-shaped—the so-called "X sign." Oláh (2002) described a case in which one horn of a bicornuate uterus became ischemic from torsion.

UTERINE LEIOMYOMAS. Also known as myomas and erroneously called *fibroids*, uterine leiomyomas are benign smooth muscle tumors commonly found during pregnancy. Rice and colleagues (1989) reported that 1.4 percent of more than 6700 pregnancies were complicated by myomas. Sheiner and co-workers (2004) cited an incidence of 0.65 percent in nearly 106,000 pregnancies. Katz and associates (1989) reported that 1 in 500 of all pregnant women were admitted for a complication related to a leiomyoma.

Myomas may be located immediately beneath the endometrial or decidual surface of the uterine cavity (*submucous*), immediately beneath the uterine serosa (*subserous*), or may be confined within the myometrium (*intramural*). As an intramural myoma grows, it may develop a significant subserous component, a submucous component, or both. Submucous and subserous myomas may be pedunculated and may undergo torsion with necrosis. At times, a subserous myoma may become *parasitic*, and much or all of its blood is supplied through the highly vascularized omentum.

Myomas during pregnancy or the puerperium occasionally undergo *red* or *carneous degeneration* that is caused by hemorrhagic infarction. The symptoms and signs are focal pain, with tenderness on palpation, and sometimes low-grade fever. Moderate leukocytosis is common. On occasion, the parietal peritoneum overlying the infarcted myoma becomes inflamed, and a peritoneal friction rub develops. Myoma degeneration may be difficult to differentiate from appendicitis, placental abruption, ureteral stone, or pyelonephritis, but imaging techniques discussed subsequently will likely prove helpful (Kawakami and associates, 1994).

Treatment of symptomatic myomas consists of analgesia and observation. Most often, signs and symptoms abate within a few days, but inflammation may stimulate labor. Surgical management will be discussed (see page 964).

Infertility and Treatment. In spite of the relatively high prevalence of myomas in young women, it is not clear whether they diminish fertility, other than by possibly causing early miscarriage (Stewart, 2001). In a review of 11 studies, Pritts (2001) concluded that only submucous myomas had a significant negative impact on fertility. He also reported that hysteroscopic myomectomy improved infertility and early miscarriage rates in women with submucous tumors. **Intramural myomectomy is especially hazardous for subsequent pregnancy**. Thus, when myoma resection from the abdominal approach results in a defect into or immediately adjacent to the endometrial cavity, uterine rupture may occur remote from labor and sometimes even early in pregnancy (Golan and associates, 1990a). In these instances, cesarean delivery is recommended before active labor begins.

Arterial embolization of uterine myomas has been used to treat symptomatic leiomyoma in nonpregnant women. Many procedures are performed for uterine bleeding in perimenopausal women (Walker and Pelage, 2002). Their effect on the outcomes of subsequent pregnancies is unclear. Ravina and colleagues (2000) reported generally good outcomes. However, Goldberg and associates (2002) reviewed 50 published cases and cited increased risks for preterm birth, malpresentation, cesarean delivery, and postpartum hemorrhage. Because of the paucity of data, the American College of Obstetricians and Gynecologists (2004) considers embolization for leiomyoma investigational.

Effects of Pregnancy on Myomas. The stimulatory effects of pregnancy on the growth of uterine myomas may be impressive. It originally made sense to assume that growth was stimulated via estrogen and progesterone receptors. It now seems apparent, however, that normal rapid uterine expansion during pregnancy results from a complex mechanism mediated not only by estrogen and progesterone but also by growth factors that include *platelet-derived growth factor, epidermal growth factor, endothelin-1 (subtype ET_A),* and *insulin-like growth factor 1* (Honoré, 2000; Ichimura, 1998; Rein, 1995, and all their associates). *Angiogenic growth factors, basic fibroblast growth factor,* and at least one gene (*HMGIC*) are also involved (Stewart, 2001).

Estrogen receptors are reduced in normal myometrium during the secretory phase of the menstrual cycle and during pregnancy (Benassayag and colleagues, 1999). In myomas, estrogen receptors are present throughout the menstrual cycle, but they are suppressed during pregnancy. Progesterone receptors are present in both myometrium and myomas throughout the menstrual cycle and pregnancy. Thus, myoma growth in early pregnancy is stimulated by similar hormonal and growth factors that cause normal uterine growth.

Paradoxically, myomas respond differently in individual women, and thus, accurate prediction of their growth is not possible. For example, in the study shown in Table 40–4, only half of myomas changed significantly in size during pregnancy. During the first trimester, myomas of all sizes either remained unchanged or increased in size—a possible early response to increased estrogen. During the second trimester, smaller myomas (2 to 6 cm) usually remained unchanged or increased in size, whereas larger myomas became smaller—probably from initiation of estrogen receptor downregulation. Regardless of initial myoma size, during the third trimester, myomas usually remained unchanged or decreased, reflecting estrogen receptor downregulation.

Effects of Myomas on Pregnancy. These common tumors are associated with a number of obstetrical complications, including excessive preterm labor, placental abruption, fetal malpresentation, obstructed labor, cesarean delivery, and

TABLE 40–4 **Ultrasonically Measured Changes in Myomas During Pregnancy**

	Small Myomas (2–6 cm) (n = 111)			Large Myomas (6–12 cm) (n = 51)		
Trimester	No Change No. (%)	Increase No. (%)	Decrease No. (%)	No Change No. (%)	Increase No. (%)	Decrease No. (%)
First	7 (58)	5 (42)	0	1 (20)	4 (80)	0
Second	42 (55)	23 (30)	11 (15)	11 (38)	4 (14)	14 (48)
Third	14 (61)	1 (4)	8 (35)	5 (29)	2 (12)	10 (59)

Modified from Lev-Toaff and co-workers (1987).

TABLE 40–5 **Pregnancy Complications and Relationships of the Myoma to the Placenta**

Investigators	Complication	Myoma (Percent)	
		No Contact with Placenta No. (%)	Contact with Placenta No. (%)
Winer-Muram et al (1984)	Bleeding and pain	5/54 (9)	8/35 (23)
	Major complications		
	Abortion	1/54 (2)	9/35 (26)
	Preterm labor	0	5/35 (14)
	Postpartum hemorrhage	0	4/35 (11)
Rice et al (1989)	Major complications		
	Preterm labor	19/79 (24)	1/14 (7)
	Abruption	2/79 (3)	8/14 (57)
Total		27/133 (20)	35/49 (71)

postpartum hemorrhage (Davis, 1990; Hasan, 1990; Katz, 1989; Lev-Toaff, 1987; Rice, 1989; Sheiner, 2004; Winer-Muram, 1984, and all their colleagues). In a review of pregnancy outcomes in 2065 women with leiomyoma, Coronado and co-workers (2000) reported that placental abruption and breech presentation increased fourfold, first-trimester bleeding and dysfunctional labor increased twofold, and cesarean delivery increased sixfold. In a case-control study, Salvador and associates (2002) reported an eightfold second-trimester abortion risk. They also concluded that genetic amniocentesis did not increase the risk of midpregnancy loss in women with myomas.

The two factors most important in determining morbidity are myoma size and location. Proximity to the placental implantation site is important (Table 40–5). Specifically, abortion, placental abruption, preterm labor, and postpartum hemorrhage all are increased if the placenta is adjacent to or implanted over a myoma. Tumors in the cervix or lower uterine segment are particularly troublesome, because they may obstruct labor (Fig. 40–12). Large tumors distort anatomy and push the ureters laterally. A case of complete inferior vena caval obstruction by a large myoma at 17 weeks was described by Greene and colleagues (2002). Hemorrhage is more likely at cesarean delivery, and hysterectomy can be technically difficult (Fig. 40–13). In some cases, myomas that are contiguous with the birth canal may be carried upward as the uterus enlarges. In many cases, the route of delivery can be decided before the onset of labor.

Management of Myomas During Pregnancy. After the diagnosis is confirmed, expectant management is recommended.

IMAGING OF MYOMAS. Ultrasound is indispensable to correctly identify myomas and to follow their growth during pregnancy (see Fig. 40–12). There are limitations to sonography in evaluating myomas and other pelvic masses (Exacoustos and

Rosati, 1993; Kier and co-workers, 1990; Strobelt and associates, 1994). Specifically, myomas have been confused with ovarian masses—both benign and malignant—as well as with molar pregnancy, ectopic pregnancy, missed abortion, bowel abnormalities, and even the fetal head. In some cases the use of color Doppler may be beneficial (Kessler and colleagues, 1993; Locci and associates, 1993).

MRI serves as an adjunct to ultrasound (Hricak and associates, 1992; Karasick and colleagues, 1992; Kier and co-workers, 1990). Comparisons with ultrasonic imaging have been made in the same women, and MRI was found to be superior (Weinreb and associates, 1990; Zawin and colleagues, 1990). MRI techniques have been described which markedly improve the reliability of identifying uterine myomas (Mayer and Shipilov, 1995; Schwartz and associates, 1998; Torashima and colleagues, 1998).

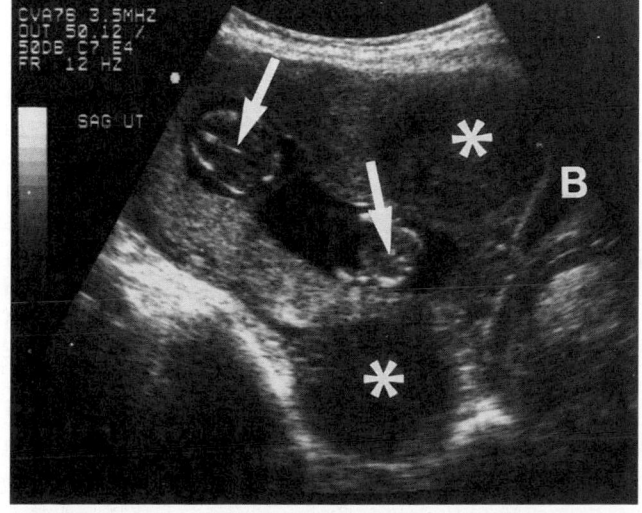

FIGURE 40–12. Two uterine myomas (*), one posterior and one anterior, are seen in this 13-week pregnancy. Arrows point to fetal head and body. (B = bladder.) (Courtesy of Dr. R. Santos.)

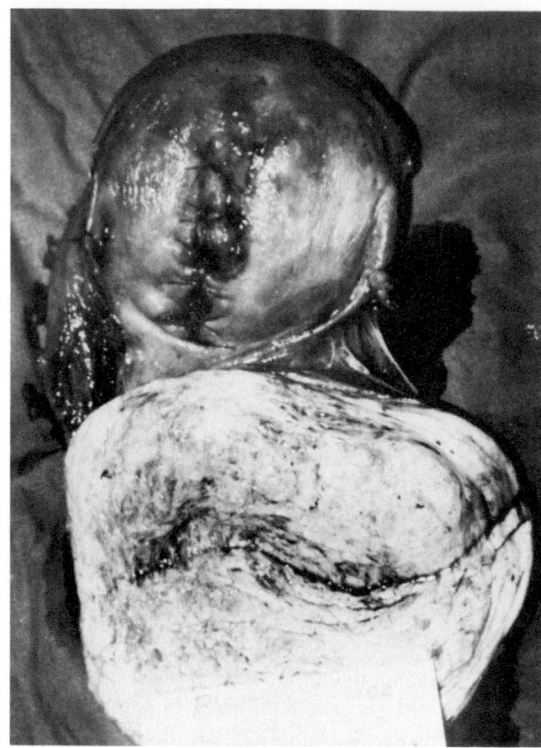

FIGURE 40–13. Cesarean hysterectomy specimen from the case shown in Figure 40–12. The upper mass is the body of the uterus which was just emptied by cesarean delivery. The lower mass is a huge myoma arising low in the uterus. The infant weighed 3250 g, and the uterus with the myoma weighed 2900 g.

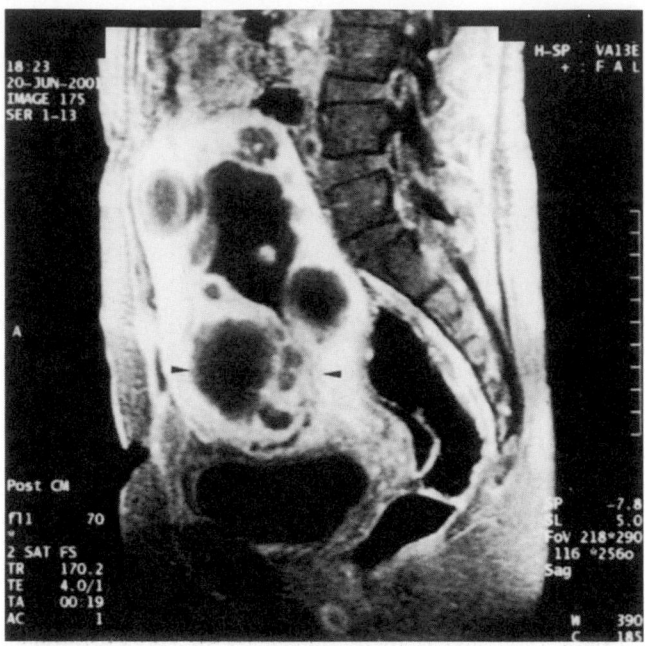

FIGURE 40–14. Infected myoma with septic shock in a woman 6 days following cesarean delivery. The sagittal T_1-weighted magnetic resonance image shows decreased signal intensity in multiple leiomyomas. The lower myoma marked with arrowheads has heterogeneous signal intensity, which represents pus. (From Lin and colleagues, 2002, with permission.)

MYOMECTOMY. Resection of myomas during pregnancy is generally contraindicated. We agree with most other authorities that surgery should be limited to tumors with a discrete pedicle that can be clamped and easily ligated (Burton and associates, 1989). Resection of intramural myomas during pregnancy, or at the time of delivery, may stimulate profuse bleeding. In some cases, unrelenting pain from infarction and degeneration prompts surgical treatment. De Carolis and colleagues (2001) and Celik and associates (2002) have described good outcomes following myomectomy in a total of 23 women. Most of the women were between 14 and 20 weeks, and in almost 50 percent of cases, the surgery was performed because of pain. In some of these cases, an intramural myoma was in contact with the implantation site. Except for one loss immediately following surgery at 19 weeks, most women had cesarean delivery at term. These investigators, as well as Mollica and associates (1996), emphasize that such management is for highly selected cases. Joó and co-workers (2001) described antepartum removal of a 940-g degenerating fundal myoma that caused fetal postural deformity and oligohydramnios at 25 weeks. Postoperatively amnionic fluid volume normalized, and a normal infant was delivered by cesarean at term.

Infection of Myomas Postpartum. Although puerperal pelvic infections and myomas are both fairly common, my-

omas rarely become infected (Genta and colleagues, 2001). Myomas may become infected postpartum when there is pelvic infection or septic abortion (Figure 40–14). They are especially likely to do so if the myoma is located immediately adjacent to the placental implantation site, or if an instrument, such as a sound or curette, perforates the myoma.

ENDOMETRIOSIS AND ADENOMYOSIS. Endometriosis and adenomyosis are rarely symptomatic during pregnancy. Rupture of an endometrioma rarely may cause bizarre and vexing clinical symptoms or labor dystocia. However, there are a number of case reports of symptoms arising from endometrial implants in cesarean delivery incisions or an episiotomy (Bumpers and associates, 2002).

Adenomyosis is common in older women. Its acquisition may be at least partially related to disruption of the endometrial-myometrial border during sharp curettage for abortion (Curtis and co-workers, 2002). Although problems during pregnancy are rare, Azziz (1986) performed an 80 year review and found that adenomyosis has been associated with uterine rupture, ectopic pregnancy, uterine atony, and placenta previa. Successful pregnancy may follow treatment of adenomyosis with gonadotropin-releasing hormone agonists (Hirata and co-workers, 1993; Silva and colleagues, 1994).

OVARIAN ABNORMALITIES. Any type of ovarian mass may complicate pregnancy. The incidence of tumors and cysts varies depending on the age group studied and the frequency with which prenatal sonography is used. From their review, Katz and colleagues (1993) found an average incidence of adnexal masses of 1 in 200 pregnancies. In a prospective population-based Italian study of almost 6650 pregnancies, Zanetta and associates (2003) found at least one mass larger than 3 cm in every 85 women. Whitecar and associates (1999) reported that masses requiring laparotomy complicated 1 in 1300 pregnancies. Koonings and co-workers (1988) reported finding one adnexal neoplasm per 200 cesarean deliveries.

The most common ovarian tumors are cystic. Whitecar and associates (1999) described 130 adnexal masses diagnosed during pregnancy at a number of military hospitals as well as University Hospital in San Antonio, Texas. About 30 percent were cystic teratomas, 28 percent were serous or mucinous cystadenomas, 13 percent were corpus luteal cysts, and 7 percent were other benign cysts. Importantly, 5 percent of all 130 masses were malignant, and 50 percent were serous carcinomas of low-malignant potential. Sherard and co-workers (2003) identified adnexal masses complicating 1 in every 600 pregnancies in Pitt County Memorial Hospital in North Carolina. About 50 percent were benign cystic teratomas, 20 percent were cystadenomas, and 13 percent were corpus luteal cysts. Likely because these cases were referred, 13 percent were malignant tumors; 5 of these 8 were of low-malignant potential. Of the 77 tumors described by Zanetta and colleagues (2003), 50 percent were simple cysts, 10 percent were benign cystic teratomas, and 4 percent were borderline malignant tumors.

Ovarian tumors unique to pregnancy are also found by ultrasound or at cesarean delivery. In addition to corpus luteal cysts, these include luteomas, which may be virilizing (Mazza and colleagues, 2002). Also, *ovarian hyperstimulation syndrome*, although usually caused by ovulation-induction therapy, may be spontaneous (Kaiser, 2003; Vasseur and associates, 2003). These are discussed further in Chapter 5 (see p. 124).

Second to malignancy, the most serious complications of ovarian cysts during pregnancy are torsion or hemorrhage. The incidence of these complications depends on tumor size and whether laparotomy is done preemptively for tumors more likely to undergo torsion. Torsion was identified in 5 percent of women reported by Whitecar (1999) and Zanetta (2003), each with their colleagues.

Management. Early in pregnancy, ovarian enlargement less than 6 cm in diameter usually is the consequence of corpus luteum formation. With the advent of high-resolution sonography, Thornton and Wells (1987) proposed a conservative approach to management based on ultrasonic characteristics. They recommend resection of all cysts suspected of rupture or torsion, those capable of obstructing labor, and measuring more than 10 cm in diameter because of the increased risk of cancer in large cysts. Cysts 5 cm or less could be left alone, and indeed, most undergo spontaneous resolution.

Management of cysts between 5 and 10 cm in diameter is controversial. Some clinicians recommend that these cysts be managed expectantly if they have a simple cystic appearance. Whitecar and co-workers (1999) caution against this approach, but most recent studies support this. Importantly, if cysts contain septae, nodules, papillary excrescences, or solid components, then resection is recommended (Caspi and co-workers, 2000; Fleischer and associates, 1990). Women with these 5- to 10-cm, intermediate-sized cysts who are observed may require emergency exploration for rupture, torsion, or infarction in as many as 50 percent of cases (Hess and colleagues, 1988; Platek and colleagues, 1995).

Laparoscopy is used with increased frequency to evaluate women with these intermediate-sized cysts as well as for surgical resection of ovarian masses (see Chap. 41, p. 975). Soriano and colleagues (1999) described comparable maternal and fetal outcomes in 39 women undergoing laparoscopic adnexal surgery in the first trimester and in 54 who had either first- or second-trimester laparotomy. Akira and associates (1999) compared gasless laparoscopy with laparotomy for ovarian cystectomy in 35 women at 12 to 16 weeks; these investigators reported advantages to the laparoscopic approach. Parker and co-workers (1996) described laparoscopy between 9 and 17 weeks for a benign cystic teratoma in 12 women. All but two of these 5- to 13-cm tumors ruptured intraoperatively, but none of the women developed evidence of peritonitis.

Thus, the major questions to be answered once a pelvic mass is discovered during pregnancy include the following:

1. What is the mass and what is the likelihood that it is malignant?
2. Is there a good possibility that the mass will regress?
3. Will the mass undergo torsion and possible rupture, or will it be an obstruction to delivery?

Only time, serial ultrasonic surveillance, and labor will provide answers to the last two questions. As for the first question, Kier and associates (1990) reported that MRI correctly identified the origin of unknown pelvic masses in 17 of 17 cases versus 12 of 17 cases using sonography. With the high-resolution sonography that is currently available, expectant management is much more common (Sherard and colleagues, 2003; Zanetta and co-workers, 2003). In some cases, transvaginal color Doppler assessment of tumor vascularity can be used for better characterization of adnexal tumors (Kurjak and Zalud, 1990).

RECOMMENDATIONS. It seems reasonable to remove all ovarian masses over 10 cm because of the substantive risk of malignancy. Tumors from 6 to 10 cm should be carefully evaluated for the possibility of neoplastic disease by ultrasound, MRI, or both. If evaluation suggests a neoplasm, then resection is indicated. If the corpus luteum is removed before 10 weeks, then 17α-OH-progesterone, 250 mg intramuscularly, is given weekly until 10 weeks. Cystic masses that are thought to be benign or are less than 6 cm are observed serially with imaging techniques, and resection is performed if they grow, begin to look suspicious, or become symptomatic. In general, we have performed elective surgery at 16 to 20 weeks. Most masses that will regress will have done so by that time.

TUMOR MARKERS. Measurement of ovarian tumor serum markers is rarely helpful during pregnancy (Zanetta and colleagues, 2003). Routine screening for neural-tube defects led to the diagnosis of an immature ovarian teratoma in two women with elevated alpha-fetoprotein levels (Frederiksen and associates, 1991; Montz and co-workers, 1989). A similar discovery of an ovarian endodermal sinus tumor was described by van der Zee and associates (1991). The role of tumor markers CA54/61, CASA, CA15-3, inhibin, macrophage colony-stimulating factor, and CA125 remains unproven even in the management of nonpregnant women (Devine and associates, 1994; Spitzer and colleagues, 1998).

Ovarian Carcinoma. Malignant ovarian neoplasms are unusual during pregnancy simply because of the young population involved. Ovarian malignancies are discussed in Chapter 57 (see p. 1266).

REFERENCES

Acien P: Reproductive performance of women with uterine malformations. Hum Reprod 8:122, 1993

Akira S, Yamanaka A, Ishihara T, et al: Gasless laparoscopic ovarian cystectomy during pregnancy: Comparison with laparotomy. Am J Obstet Gynecol 180:554, 1999

Alborzi S, Dehbashi S, Parsanezhad ME: Differential diagnosis of septate and bicornuate uterus by sonohysterography eliminates the need for laparoscopy. Fertil Steril 78:176, 2002

American Academy of Pediatrics, Committee on Bioethics: Female genital mutilation. Pediatrics 102:153, 1998

American College of Obstetricians and Gynecologists: Uterine artery embolization. Committee Opinion No. 293, February 2004

American College of Obstetricians and Gynecologists: Guidelines for Women's Health Care, 2nd ed. Washington, DC, 2002a, p 305

American College of Obstetricians and Gynecologists: Nonsurgical diagnosis and management of vaginal agenesis. Committee Opinion No. 274, July 2002b

American College of Obstetricians and Gynecologists: Management of early pregnancy loss. Practice Bulletin No. 24, February 2001

American Fertility Society: The American Fertility Society classifications of adnexal adhesions, distal tubal occlusion, tubal occlusion secondary to tubal ligation, tubal pregnancies, Müllerian anomalies and intrauterine adhesions. Fertil Steril 49:944, 1988

Angell NF, Domingo JT, Siddiqi N: Uterine rupture at term after uncomplicated hysteroscopic metroplasty. Obstet Gynecol 100:1098, 2002

Ayers JWT, DeGrood RM, Compton AA, et al: Sonographic evaluation of cervical length in pregnancy: Diagnosis and management of preterm cervical effacement in patients at risk for premature delivery. Obstet Gynecol 71:939, 1988

Ayhan A, Yucel I, Tuncer ZS, et al: Reproductive performance after conventional metroplasty: An evaluation of 102 cases. Fertil Steril 57:1194, 1992

Azziz R: Adenomyosis in pregnancy: A review. J Reprod Med 31:223, 1986

Bakos O, Axelsson O: Pathologic torsion of the pregnant uterus. Acta Obstet Gynecol Scand 66:85, 1987

Barranger E, Gervaise A, Doumerc S, et al: Reproductive performance after hysteroscopic metroplasty in the hypoplastic uterus: A study of 29 cases. Br J Obstet Gynaecol 109:1331, 2002

Benassayag C, Leroy MJ, Rigourd V, et al: Estrogen receptors (ERalpha/ERbeta) in normal and pathologic growth of the human myometrium: Pregnancy and leiomyoma. Am J Physiol 276:E1112, 1999

Ben-Rafael Z, Seidman DS, Recabi K, et al: Uterine anomalies. A retrospective, matched-control study. J Reprod Med 36:723, 1991

Blanton EN, Rouse DJ: Trial of labor in women with transverse vaginal septa. Obstet Gynecol 101:1110, 2003

Bumpers HL, Butler KL, Best IM: Endometrioma of the abdominal wall. Am J Obstet Gynecol 187:1709, 2002

Burgis J: Obstructive Müllerian anomalies: Case report, diagnosis, and management. Am J Obstet Gynecol 185:338, 2001

Burton CA, Grimes DA, March CM: Surgical management of leiomyomata during pregnancy. Obstet Gynecol 74:707, 1989

Buttram VC, Gibbons WE: Müllerian anomalies: A proposed classification (an analysis of 144 cases). Fertil Steril 32:40, 1979

Candiani GB, Fedele L, Parazzini F, et al: Reproductive prognosis after abdominal metroplasty in bicornuate or septate uterus: A life table analysis. Br J Obstet Gynaecol 97:613, 1990

Caspi B, Levi R, Appelman Z, et al: Conservative management of ovarian cystic teratoma during pregnancy and labor. Am J Obstet Gynecol 182:503, 2000

Caspi E, Schneider DF, Mor Z, et al: Cervical internal os cerclage: Description of a new technique and comparison with Shirodkar operation. Am J Perinatol 7:347, 1990

Celik C, Acar A, Cicek N, et al: Can myomectomy be performed during pregnancy? Gynecol Obstet Invest 53:79, 2002

Chakravarti S, Chin K: Rudimentary uterine horn: Management of a diagnostic enigma. Acta Obstet Gynecol Scand 82:1153, 2003

Chen G, Dharia SP, Steinkampf MP, et al: Infertility from female circumcision. Fertil Steril 81:1692, 2004

Ciment J: Senegal outlaws female genital mutilation. BMJ 318:318, 1999

Coronado GD, Marshall LM, Schwartz SM: Complications in pregnancy, labor, and delivery with uterine leiomyomas: A population-based study. Obstet Gynecol 95:764, 2000

Croak AJ, Gebhart JB, Klingele CJ, et al: Therapeutic strategies for vaginal Müllerian agenesis. J Reprod Med 48:395, 2003

Cruickshank ME, Flannelly G, Campbell DM, et al: Fertility and pregnancy outcome following large loop excision of the cervical transformation zone. Br J Obstet Gynaecol 102:467, 1995

Curtis KM, Hillis SD, Marchbanks PA, et al: Disruption of the endometrial-myometrial border during pregnancy as a risk factor for adenomyosis. Am J Obstet Gynecol 187:543, 2002

Dabirashrafi H, Bahadori M, Mohammad K, et al: Septate uterus: New idea on the histologic features of the septum in this abnormal uterus. Am J Obstet Gynecol 172:105, 1995

Daly DC, Maier D, Soto-Albors C: Hysteroscopic metroplasty: Six years' experience. Obstet Gynecol 73:201, 1989

Davis JL, Ray-Mazumder S, Hobel CJ, et al: Uterine leiomyomas in pregnancy: A prospective study. Obstet Gynecol 75:41, 1990

De Carolis S, Fatigante G, Ferrazzani S, et al: Uterine myomectomy in pregnant women. Fetal Diagn Ther 16:116, 2001 de Haas I, Harlow BL, Cramer DW, et al: Spontaneous preterm birth: A case-control study. Am J Obstet Gynecol 165:1290, 1991

Devine PL, McGuckin MA, Quin RJ, et al: Serum markers CASA and CA15-3 in ovarian cancer: All MUC1 assays are not the same. Tumour Biol 15:337, 1994

Dietz HP, Teare AJ, Wilson PD: Sacculation and retroversion of the gravid uterus in the third trimester. Aust NZ J Obstet Gynaecol 38:343, 1998

Edelman AB, Jensen JT, Lee DM, et al: Successful medical abortion of a pregnancy within a noncommunicating rudimentary uterine horn. Am J Obstet Gynecol 189:886, 2003

Eke N, Nkanginieme KE: Female genital mutilation: A global bug that should not cross the millenium bridge. World J Surg 23:1082, 1999

Engel G, Rushovich AM: True uterine diverticulum: A partial Müllerian duct duplication? Arch Pathol Lab Med 108:734, 1984

Exacoustos C, Rosati P: Ultrasound diagnosis of uterine myomas and complications in pregnancy. Obstet Gynecol 82:97, 1993

Fallat ME, Weaver JM, Hertweck SP, et al: Late follow-up and functional outcome after traumatic reproductive tract injuries in women. Am Surg 64:858, 1998

Fedele L, Bianchi S, Tozzi L, et al: Fertility in women with unicornuate uterus. Br J Obstet Gynaecol 102:1007, 1995

Fedele L, Zamberletti D, Vercellini P, et al: Reproductive performance of women with unicornuate uterus. Fertil Steril 47:416, 1987

Fernández-Aguilar S, Noël JC: Neuroma of the clitoris after female genital cutting. Obstet Gynecol 101:1053, 2003

Fleischer AC, Dinesh MS, Entman SS: Sonographic evaluation of maternal disorders during pregnancy. Radiol Clin North Am 28:51, 1990

Frederiksen MC, Casanova L, Schink JC: An elevated maternal serum alphafetoprotein leading to the diagnosis of an immature teratoma. Int J Gynaecol Obstet 35:343, 1991

Friedman A, DeFazio J, DeCherney A: Severe obstetric complications after aggressive treatment of Asherman syndrome. Obstet Gynecol 67:864, 1986

Garbin O, Ohl J, Bettahar-Lebugle K, et al: Hysteroscopic metroplasty in diethylstilbestrol-exposed and hypoplastic uterus: A report on 24 cases. Hum Reprod 13:2751, 1998

Genta PR, Dias ML, Janiszewski TA, et al: Streptococcus agalactiae endocarditis and giant pyomyoma simulating ovarian cancer. South Med J 94:508, 2001

Gibbs CE, Moore SF: The scarred cervix in pregnancy and labor. GP 37:85, 1968

Golan D, Aharoni A, Gonen R, et al: Early spontaneous rupture of the post myomectomy gravid uterus. Int J Gynaecol Obstet 31:167, 1990a

Golan A, Caspi E: Congenital anomalies of the müllerian tract. Contemp Obstet Gynecol 37:39, 1992

Golan A, Langer R, Neuman M, et al: Obstetric outcome in women with congenital uterine malformations. J Reprod Med 37:233, 1992

Golan A, Langer R, Wexler S, et al: Cervical cerclage—its role in the pregnant anomalous uterus. Int J Fertil 35:164, 1990b

Goldberg J, Pereira L, Berghella V: Pregnancy after uterine artery embolization. Obstet Gynecol 100:869, 2002

Goldberg JM, Falcone T: Effect of diethylstilbestrol on reproductive function. Fertil Steril 72:1, 1999

Green LK, Harris RE: Uterine anomalies: Frequency of diagnosis and associated obstetric complications. Obstet Gynecol 47:427, 1976

Greene JF, DeRoche ME, Ingardia C, et al: Large myomatous uterus resulting in complete obstruction of the inferior vena cava during pregnancy. Br J Obstet Gynaecol 107:1189, 2002

Grigoris G, Camus M, Clasen K, et al: Hysteroscopic septum resection in patients with recurrent abortions or infertility. Hum Reprod 13:1188, 1998

Hamoda H, Chamberlain PF, Moore NR, et al: Conservative treatment of an incarcerated gravid uterus. Br J Obstet Gynaecol 109:1074, 2002

Hampton HL, Meeks GR, Bates GW, et al: Pregnancy after successful vaginoplasty and cervical stenting for partial atresia of the cervix. Obstet Gynecol 76:900, 1990

Hasan F, Arumugam K, Sivanesaratnam V: Uterine leiomyomata in pregnancy. Int J Gynaecol Obstet 34:45, 1990

Hassiakos DK, Zourlas PA: Transcervical division of uterine septa. Obstet Gynecol Surv 45:165, 1990

Heinonen PK: Clinical implications of the unicornuate uterus with rudimentary horn. Int J Gynaecol Obstet 21:145, 1983

Heinonen PK: Limb anomalies among offspring of women with a septate uterus: Report of three cases. Early Hum Dev 56:179, 1999

Heinonen PK: Uterus didelphys: A report of 26 cases. Eur J Obstet Gynecol Reprod Biol 17:345, 1984

Hendry WF: Management of urological tumours in pregnancy. Br J Urol 1:24, 1997

Herbst AL: Behavior of estrogen-associated female genital tract cancer and relation to neoplasia following intrauterine exposure to diethylstilbestrol (DES). Gynecol Oncol 76:147, 2000

Herbst AL, Senekjian EK, Frey KW: Abortion and pregnancy loss among diethylstilbestrol-exposed women. Semin Reprod Endocrinol 7:124, 1989

Herbst AL, Ulfelder H, Poskanzer DC: Adenocarcinoma of the vagina. N Engl J Med 284:878, 1971

Hernández-Díaz S: Iatrogenic legacy from diethylstilbestrol exposure. Lancet 359:1081, 2002

Hess LW, Peaceman A, O'Brien WF, et al: Adnexal mass occurring with intrauterine pregnancy: Report of fifty-four patients requiring laparotomy for definitive management. Am J Obstet Gynecol 158:1029, 1988

Hill LM, Chenevey P, DiNofrio D: Sonographic documentation of uterine retroversion mimicking uterine sacculation. Am J Perinatol 10:398, 1993

Hinckley MD, Milki AA: Management of uterus didelphys, obstructed hemivagina and ipsilateral renal agenesis. A case report. J Reprod Med 48:649, 2003

Hirata JD, Moghissi KS, Ginsburg KA: Pregnancy after medical therapy of adenomyosis with a gonadotropin-releasing hormone agonist. Fertil Steril 59:444, 1993

Honoré JC, Robert B, Vacher-Lavenu MC, et al: Expression of endothelin receptors in human myometrium during pregnancy and in uterine leiomyomas. J Cardiovasc Pharmacol 36:S386, 2000

Hricak H, Finck S, Honda G, et al: MR imaging in the evaluation of benign uterine masses: Value of gadopentetate dimeglumine-enhanced T1-weighted images. AJR Am J Roentgenol 158:1043, 1992

Hundley AF, Fielding JR, Hoyte L: Double cervix and vagina with septate uterus: An uncommon müllerian malformation. Obstet Gynecol 98:982, 2001

Ichimura T, Kawamura N, Ito F, et al: Correlation between the growth of uterine leiomyomata and estrogen and progesterone receptor content in needle biopsy specimens. Fertil Steril 70:967, 1998

Iosif S, Ulmsten U: Comparative urodynamic studies of continent and stress incontinent women in pregnancy and in the puerperium. Am J Obstet Gynecol 140:645, 1981

Israel R, March CM: Hysteroscopic incision of the septate uterus. Am J Obstet Gynecol 149:66, 1984

Jackson D, Elliott JP, Pearson M: Asymptomatic uterine retroversion at 36 weeks' gestation. Obstet Gynecol 71:466, 1988

Jensen JG: Uterine torsion in pregnancy. Acta Obstet Gynecol Scand 71:260, 1992

Jones W, Smith J, Kieke B, et al: Female genital mutilation/female circumcision. Who is at risk in the U.S.? Public Health Rep 112:368, 1997

Joó JG, Inovay J, Silhavy M, et al: Successful enucleation of a necrotizing fibroid causing oligohydramnios and fetal postural deformity in the 25th week of gestation: A case report. J Reprod Med 46:923, 2001

Jourdain O, Dabysing F, Harle T, et al: Management of septate uterus by flexible hysteroscopy and Nd:YAG laser. Int J Gynaecol Obstet 63:159, 1998

Kaiser UB: The pathogenesis of the ovarian hyperstimulation syndrome. N Engl J Med 349:729, 2003

Karasick S, Lev-Toaff AS, Toaff ME: Imaging of uterine leiomyomas. AJR Am J Roentgenol 158:799, 1992

Katz Z, Ben-Arie A, Lurie S, et al: Beneficial effect of hysteroscopic metroplasty on the reproductive outcome in a "T-shaped" uterus. Gynecol Obstet Invest 41:41, 1996

Katz VL, Watson WJ, Hansen WF, et al: Massive ovarian tumor complicating pregnancy. A case report. J Reprod Med 38:907, 1993

Katz VL, Dotters DJ, Droegemueller W: Complications of uterine leiomyomas in pregnancy. Obstet Gynecol 73:593, 1989

Kaufman RH, Adam E, Hatch EE, et al: Continued follow-up of pregnancy outcomes in diethylstilbestrol-exposed offspring. Obstet Gynecol 96:483, 2000

Kaufman RH, Noller K, Adam E, et al: Upper genital tract abnormalities and pregnancy outcome in DES-exposed progeny. Am J Obstet Gynecol 148:973, 1984

Kawakami S, Togashi K, Konishi I, et al: Red degeneration of uterine leiomyoma: MR appearance. J Comput Assis Tomogr 18:925, 1994

Kessler A, Mitchell DG, Kuhlman K, et al: Myoma vs. contraction in pregnancy: Differentiation with color Doppler imaging. J Clin Ultrasound 21:241, 1993

Kessler I, Lancet M, Appelman Z, et al: Indications and results of metroplasty in uterine malformations. Int J Gynaecol Obstet 24:137, 1986

Kier R, McCarthy SM, Scoutt LM, et al: Pelvic masses in pregnancy: MR imaging. Radiology 176:709, 1990

Kipersztok S, Javitt M, Hill MC, et al: Comparison of magnetic resonance imaging and transvaginal ultrasonography with hysterosalpingography in the evaluation of women exposed to diethylstilbestrol. J Reprod Med 41:347, 1996

Klip H, Verloop J, Gool JD, et al: Hypospadias in sons of women exposed to diethylstilbestrol in utero: A cohort study. Lancet 359:1102, 2002

Knight R, Hotchin A, Bayly C, et al: Female genital mutilation—experience of The Royal Women's Hospital, Melbourne. Aust NZ J Obstet Gynaecol 39:50, 1999

Koonings PP, Platt LD, Wallace R: Incidental adnexal neoplasms at cesarean section. Obstet Gynecol 72:767, 1988

Kovac SR, Cruikshank SH: Successful pregnancies and vaginal deliveries after sacrospinous uterosacral fixation in five of nineteen patients. Am J Obstet Gynecol 168:1778, 1993

Kun KE: Female genital mutilation: The potential for increased risk of HIV infection. Int J Gynaecol Obstet 59:153, 1997

Kurjak A, Zalud I: Transvaginal color Doppler for evaluating gynecologic pathology of the pelvis. Ultraschall Med 11:164, 1990

Leible S, Munoz H, Walton R, et al: Uterine artery blood flow velocity waveforms in pregnant women with müllerian duct anomaly: A biologic model for uteroplacental insufficiency. Am J Obstet Gynecol 178:1048, 1998

Letterie GS, Vauss N: Müllerian tract abnormalities and associated auditory defects. J Reprod Med 36:765, 1991

Lettieri L, Rodis JF, McLean DA, et al: Incarceration of the gravid uterus. Obstet Gynecol Surv 49:642, 1994

Lev-Toaff AS, Coleman BG, Arger PH, et al: Leiomyomas in pregnancy: Sonographic study. Radiology 164:375, 1987

Lin YH, Hwang JL, Huang LW, et al: Pyomyoma after a cesarean section. Acta Obstet Gynecol Scand 81:571, 2002

Litta P, Pozzan C, Merlin F, et al: Hysteroscopic metroplasty under laparoscopic guidance in infertile women with septate uteri: Follow-up of reproductive outcome. J Reprod Med 49:274, 2004

Locci M, Nazzaro G, DePlacido G, et al: Angiogenesis: A new diagnostic aspect of obstetric and gynecologic echography. J Perinat Med 21:453, 1993

Louis-Sylvestre C, Haddad B, Paniel BJ: Treatment of vaginal outflow tract obstruction in graft-versus-host reaction. Am J Obstet Gynecol 188:943, 2003

Ludmir J, Jackson GM, Samuels P: Transvaginal cerclage under ultrasound guidance in cases of severe cervical hypoplasia. Obstet Gynecol 78:1067, 1991

Ludmir J, Landon MB, Gabbe SG, et al: Management of the diethylstilbestrol-exposed pregnant patient: A prospective study. Am J Obstet Gynecol 157:665, 1987

Mackey R, Geary M, Dornan J, et al: A successful pregnancy following transabdominal cervical cerclage for cervical hypoplasia. Br J Obstet Gynaecol 108:1111, 2001

Maneschi M, Maneschi F, Fuca G: Reproductive impairment of women with unicornuate uterus. Acta Eur Fertil 19:273, 1988

Marrocco-Trischitta MM, Nicodemi EM, Nater C, et al: Management of congenital venous malformations of the vulva. Obstet Gynecol 98:789, 2001

Mashiach S, Ben-Rafael Z, Dor J, et al: Triplet pregnancy in uterus didelphys with delivery interval of 72 days. Obstet Gynecol 58:519, 1981

Mayer DP, Shipilov V: Ultrasonography and magnetic resonance imaging of uterine fibroids. Obstet Gynecol Clin North Am 22:667, 1995

Mazza V, Di Monte I, Ceccarelli PL, et al: Prenatal diagnosis of female pseudohermaphroditism associated with bilateral luteoma of pregnancy. Hum Reprod 17:821, 2002

McKay HA, Hanlon K: Vesicovaginal fistula after cervical cerclage: Repair by transurethral suture cystorrhaphy. J Urol 169:1086, 2003

Melody GF: Obstructed cervix: A study of 100 patients. Obstet Gynecol 10:190, 1957

Michaels WH, Thompson HO, Schreiber FR, et al: Ultrasound surveillance of the cervix during pregnancy in diethylstilbestrol-exposed offspring. Obstet Gynecol 73:230, 1989

Michalas SP: Outcome of pregnancy in women with uterine malformation: Evaluation of 62 cases. Int J Gynaecol Obstet 35:215, 1991

Miklos JR, Sze E, Parobeck D, et al: Vesicouterine fistula: A rare complication of vaginal birth after cesarean. Obstet Gynecol 86:638, 1995

Minto CL, Hollings N, Hall-Craggs M, et al: Magnetic resonance imaging in the assessment of complex Müllerian anomalies. Br J Obstet Gynaecol 108:791, 2001

Mollica G, Pittini L, Minganti E, et al: Elective uterine myomectomy in pregnant women. Clin Exp Obstet Gynecol 23:168, 1996

Montz FJ, Horenstein J, Platt LD, et al: The diagnosis of immature teratoma by maternal serum alpha-fetoprotein screening. Obstet Gynecol 73:522, 1989

Moutos DM, Damewood MD, Schlaff WD, et al: A comparison of the reproductive outcome between women with a unicornuate uterus and women with a didelphic uterus. Fertil Steril 58:88, 1992

Murray C, Goh JT, Fynes M, et al: Urinary and faecal incontinence following delayed primary repair of obstetric genital fistula. Br J Obstet Gynaecol 109:828, 2002

Myers DL, Scotti RJ: Acute urinary retention and the incarcerated, retroverted, gravid uterus. A case report. J Reprod Med 40:487, 1995

Nahum GG: Rudimentary uterine horn pregnancy: The 20th-century worldwide experience of 588 cases. J Reprod Med 47:151, 2002

Nicholson HS, Blask AN, Markle BM, et al: Uterine anomalies in Wilms' tumor survivors. Cancer 78:887, 1996

Nicholson WK, Coulson CC, McCoy MC, et al: Pelvic magnetic resonance imaging in the evaluation of uterine torsion. Obstet Gynecol 85:888, 1995

Nicolini V, Bellotti M, Bannazzi B, et al: Can ultrasound be used to screen uterine malformations? Fertil Steril 47:89, 1987

Nour NM: Female genital cutting: Clinical and cultural guidelines. Obstet Gynecol Surv 59:272, 2004

Okonofua FE, Larsen U, Oronsaye F, et al: The association between female genital cutting and correlates of sexual and gynaecological morbidity in Edo State, Nigeria. Br J Obstet Gynaecol 109:1089, 2002

Oláh KS: Uterine torsion and ischaemia of one horn of a bicornute uterus: A rare cause of failed second trimester termination of pregnancy. Br J Obstet Gynaecol 109:585, 2002

Oliva GC, Fratoni A, Genova M, et al: Uterine motility in patients with bicornuate uterus. Int J Gynaecol Obstet 37:7, 1992

Pabuccu R, Gomel V: Reproductive outcome after hysteroscopic metroplasty in women with septate uterus and otherwise unexplained infertility. Fertil Steril 81:1675, 2004

Palmer JR, Hatch EE, Rao RS, et al: Infertility among women exposed prenatally to diethylstilbestrol. Am J Epidemiol 154:316, 2001

Parker WH, Childers JM, Canis M, et al: Laparoscopic management of benign cystic teratomas during pregnancy. Am J Obstet Gynecol 174:1499, 1996

Penning SR, Cohen B, Tewari D, et al: Pregnancy complicated by vesical calculus and vesicocutaneous fistula. Obstet Gynecol 176:728, 1997

Pitkin RM: Vaginal and cervical abnormalities after exposure to stilbestrol in utero. Obstet Gynecol 102:222, 2003

Platek DN, Henderson CE, Goldberg GL: The management of a persistent adnexal mass in pregnancy. Am J Obstet Gynecol 173:1236, 1995

Porcu G, Courbiere B, Sakr R, et al: Spontaneous rupture of a first-trimester gravid uterus in a woman exposed to diethylstilbestrol in utero: A case report. J Reprod Med 48:744, 2003

Pritts EA: Fibroids and infertility: A systematic review of the evidence. Obstet Gynecol Surv 56:483, 2001

Proctor JA, Haney AF: Recurrent first trimester pregnancy loss is associated with uterine septum but not with bicornuate uterus. Fertil Steril 80:1212, 2003

Raga F, Bauset C, Remohi J, et al: Reproductive impact of congenital Müllerian anomalies. Hum Reprod 12:2277, 1997

Raga F, Bonilla-Musoles F, Blanes J, et al: Congenital Müllerian anomalies: Diagnostic accuracy of three-dimensional ultrasound. Fertil Steril 65:523, 1996

Rai L, Ramesh K: Obstructed labour due to a vesical calculus. Aust NZ J Obstet Gynaecol 38:474, 1998

Ravasia DJ, Brain PH, Pollard JK: Incidence of uterine rupture among women with mullerian duct anomalies who attempt vaginal birth after cesarean delivery. Am J Obstet Gynecol 181:877, 1999

Ravina JH, Vigneron NC, Aymard A, et al: Pregnancy after embolization of uterine myoma: Report of 12 cases. Fertil Steril 73:1241, 2000

Rein MS, Barbieri RL, Friedman AJ: Progesterone: A critical role in the pathogenesis of uterine myomas. Am J Obstet Gynecol 172:14, 1995

Rice JP, Kay HH, Mahony BS: The clinical significance of uterine leiomyomas in pregnancy. Am J Obstet Gynecol 160:1212, 1989

Roberts CP, Haber MJ, Rock JA: Vaginal creation for müllerian agenesis. Am J Obstet Gynecol 185:1349, 2001

Rolen AC, Choquette AJ, Semmens JP: Rudimentary uterine horn: Obstetric and gynecologic implications. Obstet Gynecol 27:806, 1966

Salle B, Sergeant P, Gaucherand P, et al: Transvaginal hysterosonographic evaluation of septate uteri: A preliminary report. Hum Reprod 11:1004, 1996

Salvador E, Bienstock J, Blakemore KJ, et al: Leiomyomata uteri, genetic amniocentesis, and the risk of second-trimester spontaneous abortion. Am J Obstet Gynecol 186:913, 2002

Schwartz LB, Zawin M, Carcangiu ML, et al: Does pelvic magnetic resonance imaging differentiate among the histologic subtypes of uterine leiomyomata? Fertil Steril 70:580, 1998

Seidman DS, Ben-Rafael Z, Bider D, et al: The role of cervical cerclage in the management of uterine anomalies. Surg Gynecol Obstet 173:384, 1991

Senekjian EK, Potkul RK, Frey K, et al: Infertility among daughters either exposed or not exposed to diethylstilbestrol. Am J Obstet Gynecol 158:493, 1988

Seubert DE, Puder KS, Goldmeier P, et al: Colonoscopic release of the incarcerated gravid uterus. Obstet Gynecol 94:792, 1999

Sheiner E, Bashiri A, Levy A, et al: Obstetric characteristics and perinatal outcome of pregnancies with uterine leiomyomas. Obstet Gynecol Surv 59:647, 2004

Sherard GB III, Hodson CA, Williams HJ, et al: Adnexal masses and pregnancy: A 12-year experience. Am J Obstet Gynecol 189:358, 2003

Sherer DM, Smith SA, Sanko SR: Uterine sacculation sonographically mimicking an abdominal pregnancy at 20 weeks' gestation. Am J Perinatol 11:350, 1994

Silva PD, Perkins HE, Schauberger CW: Live birth after treatment of severe adenomyosis with a gonadotropin-releasing hormone agonist. Fertil Steril 61:171, 1994

Soriano D, Yefet Y, Seidman DS, et al: Laparoscopy versus laparotomy in the management of adnexal masses during pregnancy. Fertil Steril 71:955, 1999

Spearing GJ: Uterine sacculation. Obstet Gynecol 51:11S, 1978

Spitzer M, Herman J, Krumholz BA, et al: The fertility of women after cervical laser surgery. Obstet Gynecol 86:504, 1995

Spitzer M, Kaushal N, Benjamin F: Maternal CA-125 levels in pregnancy and the puerperium. J Reprod Med 43:387, 1998

Stenchever MA: Congenital abnormalities of the female reproductive tract. In Stenchever MA, Droegemueller W, Herbst AL, et al (eds): Comprehensive Gynecology, 4th ed. St. Louis, Mosby, 2001, p 253

Stewart EA: Uterine fibroids. Lancet 357:293, 2001

Strobelt N, Ghidini A, Cavallone M, et al: Natural history of uterine leiomyomas in pregnancy. J Ultrasound Med 13:399, 1994

Thornton JG, Wells M: Ovarian cysts in pregnancy: Does ultrasound make traditional management inappropriate? Obstet Gynecol 69:717, 1987

Torashima M, Yamashita Y, Matsuno Y, et al: The value of detection of flow voids between the uterus and the leiomyoma with MRI. J Magn Reson Imaging 8:427, 1998

Toubia N: Female circumcision as a public health issue. N Engl J Med 331:712, 1994

Valli E, Zupi E, Marconi D, et al: Hysteroscopic findings in 344 women with recurrent spontaneous abortion. J Am Assoc Gynecol Laparosc 8:398, 2001

van der Zee AG, de Bruijn HW, Bouma J, et al: Endodermal sinus tumor of the ovary during pregnancy: A case report. Am J Obstet Gynecol 164:504, 1991

Vasseur C, Rodien P, Beau I, et al: A chorionic gonadotropin-sensitive mutation in the follicle-stimulating hormone receptor as a cause of familial gestational spontaneous ovarian hyperstimulation syndrome. N Engl J Med 349:753, 2003

Vo CV, Dinh TV, Hankins GDV: Value of ultrasound in the early diagnosis of prerupture uterine horn pregnancy. J Reprod Med 48:471, 2003

Wai CY, Zekam N, Sanz LE: Septate uterus with double cervix and longitudinal vaginal septum: A case report. J Reprod Med 46:613, 2001

Walker WJ, Pelage JP: Uterine artery embolization for symptomatic fibroids: Clinical results in 400 women with imaging follow up. Br J Obstet Gynaecol 109:1262, 2002

Wall LL: *Fitsari'Dan Duniya*: An African (Hausa) praise song about vesicovaginal fistulas. Obstet Gynecol 100:1328, 2002

Weinreb JC, Barkoff ND, Megibow A, et al: The value of MR imaging in distinguishing leiomyomas from other solid pelvic masses when sonography is indeterminate. AJR Am J Roentgenol 154:295, 1990

Wendel GD: Surgical treatment of lower-genital-tract infections. In Gilstrap LC, Cunningham FG, VanDorsten JP (eds): Operative Obstetrics, 2nd ed. New York, McGraw-Hill, 2002, p 250

Whitecar P, Turner S, Higby K: Adnexal masses in pregnancy: A review of 130 cases undergoing surgical management. Am J Obstet Gynecol 181:19, 1999

Wiersma AF, Peterson LF, Justema EJ: Uterine anomalies associated with renal agenesis. Obstet Gynecol 47:654, 1976

Winer-Muram HT, Muram D, Gillieson MS: Uterine myomas in pregnancy. J Can Assoc Radiol 35:168, 1984

Woelfer B, Salim R, Banerjee S, et al: Reproductive outcomes in women with congenital uterine anomalies detected by three-dimensional ultrasound screening. Obstet Gynecol 98:1099, 2001

World Health Organization: Female genital mutilation: A joint WHO/UNICEF/UNFPA statement. Geneva: World Health Organization, 1997

World Health Organization, International Federation of Gynecology and Obstetrics: Female circumcision. Eur J Obstet Gynecol Reprod Biol 45:153, 1992

Zanetta G, Mariani E, Lissoni A, et al: A prospective study of the role of ultrasound in the management of adnexal masses in pregnancy. Br J Obstet Gynaecol 110:578, 2003

Zanetti E, Ferrari LR, Rossi G: Classification and radiographic features of uterine malformations: Hysterosalpingographic study. Br J Radiol 51:161, 1978

Zawin M, McCarthy S, Scoutt LM, et al: High-field MRI and US evaluation of the pelvis in women with leiomyomas. Magn Reson Imaging 8:371, 1990

VIII

Medical and Surgical Complications

41

General Considerations and Maternal Evaluation

Accurate quantification of the incidence and types of medical and surgical illnesses complicating pregnancy is difficult but can be estimated by various indices of hospitalization. In a managed-care population of over 46,000 pregnant women, Gazmararian and colleagues (2002) reported that the overall rate of antenatal hospitalization was 10.1 per 100 deliveries. About one third of these were for nonobstetrical conditions such as renal, gastrointestinal, pulmonary, and infectious diseases. Care of these women warrants a team effort between obstetricians and maternal–fetal medicine specialists, along with internists, surgeons, anesthesiologists, and others (American College of Obstetricians and Gynecologists, 2003). Obstetricians also must have a working knowledge of medical and surgical diseases common to women of childbearing age. Nonobstetricians who see these women in consultation should be familiar with the effects that various diseases have on pregnancy and vice versa, as well as pregnancy-induced physiological changes that include normal alterations in laboratory values.

A number of generalizations concern the rational approach to management of pregnancy complicated by nonobstetrical disorders. The first tenet is simple: **A woman should never be penalized because she is pregnant.** Stated differently: If a proposed medical or surgical regimen is altered because the woman is pregnant, can the alteration be justified? What therapy would be given if she was not pregnant? Such an approach should allow individualization of care for most medical and surgical disorders. Moreover, it may be especially helpful when dealing with consultants asked to see these women.

MATERNAL PHYSIOLOGY AND ALTERATIONS IN LABORATORY VALUES

Pregnancy induces profound physiological changes in most organ systems, and these may amplify or obfuscate evaluation of certain disorders. A number of standard laboratory evaluations are also altered by pregnancy. Some of these would, in the nonpregnant woman, suggest marked organ dysfunction,

or conversely, normalcy, at a time when the woman was actually quite ill. The wide ranges of pregnancy effects on normal physiology and on laboratory values are discussed in Chapter 5 as well as in the chapters that follow.

MEDICATIONS DURING PREGNANCY

Antepartum management of nonobstetrical disorders includes administration of a variety of drugs. Fortunately, the vast majority necessary to treat the most commonly encountered complications can be used with relative safety. However, there are a few notable exceptions, which are considered in detail in Chapter 14, as well as with the discussions of specific disorders for which these drugs are given.

SURGERY DURING PREGNANCY

EFFECT OF SURGERY AND ANESTHESIA ON PREGNANCY OUTCOME. The risk of an adverse pregnancy outcome does not appear to be increased in women who undergo most uncomplicated surgical procedures. However, this risk may be increased when there are complications. For example, perforative appendicitis with feculent peritonitis has significant maternal and perinatal morbidity and mortality even if surgical and anesthetic techniques are flawless. Conversely, procedure-related complications may adversely affect pregnancy outcome. For example, a woman who has uncomplicated removal of an inflamed appendix may suffer aspiration of acidic gastric contents on extubation (see Chap. 19, p. 490).

The most extensive experiences regarding anesthetic and surgical risks to pregnancy are from the Swedish Birth Registry and reported by Mazze and Källén (1989). These investigators studied the effects of 5405 nonobstetrical surgical procedures performed in 720,000 pregnant women from 1973 to 1981 (Table 41–1). Surgery was performed in the first trimester in 41 percent of women, 35 percent in the second,

TABLE 41–1 Nonobstetrical Operations in 5405 Pregnant Women

	Percent of Procedures by Trimester			Total (n = 5405) no. (%)
Type of Operation	*First* (n = 2252)	*Second* (n = 1881)	*Third* (n = 1272)	
Central nervous system	7	6	6	323 (6)
Head and neck	8	6	10	419 (8)
Heart and lung	0.7	0.8	0.6	40 (0.7)
Abdominal	20	30	23	1331 (25)
Gynecological and urological	11	23	24	1008 (19)
Laparoscopy	34	1.2	6	868 (16)
Orthopedic	9	9	14	558 (10)
Endoscopy	4	11	9	406 (8)

Adapted from Mazze and Källén (1989).

TABLE 41-2 Anesthesia for Nonobstetrical Surgery in 5405 Pregnant Women

| Type of Anesthesia | Percent by Trimester | | | Total (n = 5405) Percent |
	First (n = 2252)	Second (n = 1881)	Third (n = 1272)	
General	65	51	41	54
Spinal or epidural	3	5	6	5
Topical/local	5	8	9	7
Nerve block	1	2	3	2
Unknown	25	34	41	32

Adapted from Mazze and Källén (1989).

and 24 percent in the third. Importantly, 60 percent were abdominal or pelvic procedures—25 percent were abdominal operations, about 20 percent were gynecological and urological procedures, and about 15 percent were laparoscopic procedures. Laparoscopy was the most commonly performed first-trimester operation, and appendectomy was the most common second-trimester procedure.

The types of anesthesia administered to the 5405 women in the Swedish report are shown in Table 41-2. Over half of these procedures were performed using general anesthesia, and commonly this involved nitrous oxide supplemented by another inhalation agent or intravenous medications.

Perinatal Outcomes. Excessive perinatal morbidity associated with nonobstetrical surgery is attributable to the disease itself rather than to adverse effects of surgery and anesthesia. Mazze and Källén (1989) compared pregnancy outcomes in 5405 women undergoing surgery with those in 720,000 pregnancies without antepartum surgery. As shown in Table 41-3, rates of stillbirths and congenital malformations were similar in both groups. However, there was a significantly increased incidence of low-birthweight and preterm births as well as neonatal deaths in women who had undergone surgery. In a study from MetroHealth Medical Center in Cleveland, Stepp and associates (2002) analyzed pregnancy outcomes following abdominal surgery. Factors associated with previable or preterm delivery included first-trimester surgery, peritonitis, procedure length, and surgery after 24 weeks.

As previously stated, the Swedish researchers found that stillbirth and congenital malformation rates were not increased significantly. Czeizel and colleagues (1998) also reported that anesthetic agents are not teratogenic. However, Källén and Mazze (1990) scrutinized 572 operations performed at 4 to 5 weeks of gestation and found a possible causal relationship with neural-tube defects. Sylvester and co-workers (1994) reported similar observations from the Metropolitan Atlanta Congenital Defects Program. This case-control study documented a significantly increased risk of hydrocephaly in conjunction with other major defects—especially eye anomalies—in women exposed to general anesthesia. Thus, as Rosen (1999) concluded, we cannot state categorically that anesthetic agents are not teratogenic.

LAPAROSCOPIC SURGERY DURING PREGNANCY. Over the past decade, the use of laparoscopic techniques has become common for diagnosis and management of a number of surgical disorders complicating pregnancy. The most obvious application is management of ectopic pregnancy (see Chap. 10, p. 261). With established pregnancy, in most studies laparoscopy has been used for exploration and treatment of adnexal masses (see Chap. 40, p. 965) or for cholecystectomy or appendectomy (see Chap. 50, p. 1136, and Chap. 49, p. 1119). Lachman and colleagues (1999) reviewed 518 laparoscopic procedures performed during pregnancy—45 percent for cholecystectomy, 34 percent for adnexal surgery, and 15 percent for appendectomy. Fatum and Rojansky (2001) reported similar findings in a later review of 308 reported cases. They also concluded that gestational age of 26 to 28 weeks was the upper gestational age limit for successful laparoscopy. Al-Fozan and Tulandi (2002) have recently reviewed the safety and risks of laparoscopy in pregnancy.

Maternal and Fetal Effects. Hemodynamic changes induced by abdominal insufflation for laparoscopy are similar in pregnant and nonpregnant women. Reedy and colleagues (1995) studied these effects in baboons at the human

TABLE 41-3 Birth Outcomes in 5405 Pregnant Women Undergoing Nonobstetrical Surgery

| Birth Outcome | Trimester (Observed/Expected) | | | Total | P Value |
	First	Second	Third		
Stillborn	1.1	1.7	1.5	1.4	NS
Death by 7 days	1.4	3.2	1.9	2.1	< .05
Malformation	1.0	0.9	1.5	1.1	NS
Birthweight < 1500 g	1.7	3.2	1.5	2.2	< .05
Birthweight < 2500 g	1.4	1.8	2.2	2.0	< .05

NS = nonsignificant.
Adapted from Mazze and Källén (1989).

equivalent gestation of 22 to 26 weeks. Although there were no substantive changes at 10–mm Hg insufflation, 20 mm Hg of pressure caused significant maternal cardiovascular and respiratory changes after 20 minutes. Some of these changes were increased respiratory rate, respiratory acidosis, diminished cardiac output, and increased pulmonary artery pressure with concomitantly increased pulmonary capillary wedge pressure. Steinbrook and Bhavani-Shankar (2001) used noninvasive hemodynamic monitoring in four healthy women at 17 to 24 weeks during scheduled laparoscopic cholecystectomy. Compared with preinduction values, the cardiac index decreased 26 percent by 5 minutes of insufflation and 21 percent by 15 minutes. The mean arterial pressures, systemic vascular resistance, and heart rate did not change significantly. These changes were similar to those reported in nonpregnant women by Wahba and colleagues (1995).

The precise effects of laparoscopy in the human fetus are currently unknown. Studies of pregnant ewes have been reported by Barnard and associates (1995) and Hunter and colleagues (1995). Using carbon dioxide insufflation to establish a pneumoperitoneum, they found that uteroplacental blood flow decreases when intraperitoneal pressure exceeds 15 mm Hg. This was due to decreased perfusion pressure and increased placental vessel resistance.

To study the impact of laparoscopy on perinatal outcomes, Reedy and colleagues (1997b) used the updated Swedish Birth Registry described earlier. Between 1973 and 1993, there were slightly over 2 million deliveries. There were 2181 laparoscopies and 1522 laparotomies performed in these women. As shown in Figure 41–1, laparoscopy was performed primarily during the first trimester. Perinatal

outcomes in women undergoing surgery were compared with those of all women in the database. The investigators confirmed their previous studies and found an increased risk of low birthweight, preterm delivery, and fetal growth restriction in the operative group. There were no differences in malformations or perinatal outcome when laparoscopy and laparotomy were compared.

Technique. Preparation for laparoscopy differs little from that commonly used for laparotomy. Bowel cleansing empties the large intestine and may facilitate visualization. Nasogastric or orogastric decompression reduces the risk of injury as well as the risk of aspiration. Aorto-caval compression is avoided by a left-lateral tilt. Using this position at about 16 weeks or more maximizes uterine perfusion (Kinsella and Lohmann, 1994). Positioning of the lower extremities in boot-type stirrups maintains access to the vagina for fetal sonographic assessment or manual displacement of the uterus. Flexion at the hip should be minimal to avoid obstruction of the surgical field by the knees.

Beyond the first trimester, technical modifications of standard pelvic laparoscopic entry are required to avoid puncture or laceration of the uterus. Some clinicians recommend *open* or *gasless* laparoscopic entry techniques (Akira and co-workers, 1999) to avoid perforations of the uterus, pelvic veins, and adnexae. The abdomen is incised at or above the umbilicus. The peritoneum is incised under direct vision, and insertions of the conventional 10-mm cannula and laparoscope are directed upward. Then, under direct visual guidance, they are rotated toward the lower abdomen and pelvis. These techniques avoid the cardiovascular changes with pneumoperitoneum and decrease the risk of uterine perforation with the trocar or Veress needle. The cannula is then connected to the insufflation systems, and a 10–mm Hg pneumoperitoneum is initiated. The initial insufflation should be conducted slowly to allow for prompt assessment and reversal of any untoward pressure-related effects. Gas leakage around the cannula is managed by tightening the surrounding skin with a towel clamp.

Insertion of secondary trocars is most safely performed under direct laparoscopic visual surveillance through the primary port. The skin and fascia are incised with a scalpel, and the trocar-cannula tandem is advanced against the tension of the pneumoperitoneum with a smooth, steady motion. For lower abdominal placement, the dome of the bladder and the inferior epigastric arteries should be identified laparoscopically.

Complications. Risks inherent to laparoscopy are probably not increased during pregnancy. Reported complications are uncommon (Fatum and Rojansky, 2001; Lachman and colleagues, 1999). In a mail survey, Reedy and co-workers (1997a) surveyed 192 laparoscopic surgeons who described complications inherent to laparoscopy as well as one case of intrauterine placement of the Veress needle.

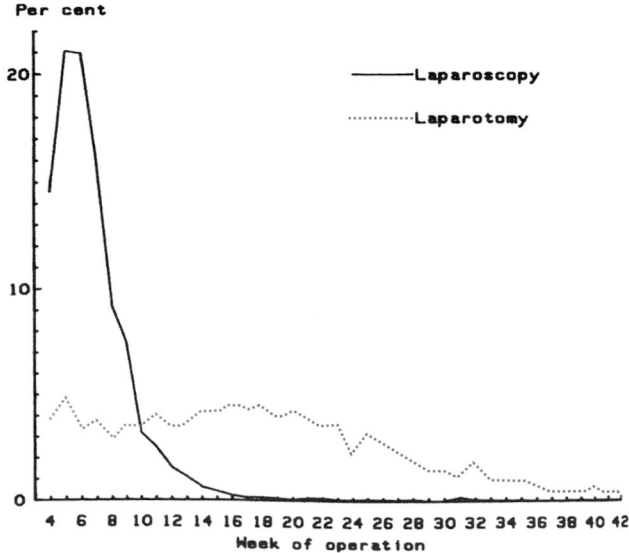

FIGURE 41–1. Distribution of laparoscopic procedures and laparotomies during pregnancy by weeks of gestation. (From Reedy and colleagues, 1997a, with permission.)

IMAGING TECHNIQUES

A number of imaging modalities are used as an adjunct for both diagnosis and therapy during pregnancy. These include radiography, ultrasound, and magnetic resonance imaging. The use of radiography is most worrisome to both the obstetrician and the patient. Inevitably, some radiographic procedures are performed prior to recognition of early pregnancy, usually because of trauma or life-threatening illness. Fortunately, most diagnostic radiographic procedures are associated with little or no known significant fetal risks. As with drugs and medications, however, radiographic procedures during pregnancy may lead to litigation if there is an adverse pregnancy outcome. Conversely, a needless therapeutic abortion may be performed because of patient or physician anxiety.

IONIZING RADIATION. The term *radiation* is poorly understood, and it often is applied not only to x-rays but also to microwaves, ultrasound, diathermy, and radio waves. Of these, x-rays and gamma rays have short wavelengths with very high energy and are forms of ionizing radiation. The other four energy forms have rather long wavelengths and low energy (Brent, 1999). The biological effects of x-rays are caused by an electrochemical reaction that can result in tissue damage. At high doses, x-rays may cause cell death, mutations, cancer, and developmental defects.

For these reasons, ionizing radiation from x-rays and gamma rays is a primary biological concern. Ionizing radiation refers to waves or particles (photons) of significant energy that can break chemical bonds, such as those in DNA, or that can create free radicals or ions capable of causing tissue damage (Hall, 1991). Methods of measuring the effects of x-rays are summarized in Table 41–4. The standard terms used are exposure (in air), dose (to tissue), and relative effective dose (to tissue). In the range of energies for diagnostic x-rays, the dose, expressed in rad, and the relative effective dose, expressed in rem, can be used interchangeably. For consistency, all doses to follow will be expressed in rad, the traditional unit, or in gray (Gy), the modern unit (1 Gy = 100 rad).

TABLE 41–4 Some Measures of Ionizing Radiation

Exposure	Number of ions produced by x-rays per kg of air Unit: roentgen (R)
Dose	Amount of energy deposited per kg of tissue Modern unit: gray (Gy) (1 Gy = 100 rad) Traditional unit: rad[a]
Relative effective dose	Amount of energy deposited per kg of tissue normalized for biological effectiveness Modern unit: sievert (Sv) (1 Sv = 100 rem) Traditional unit: rem[a]

[a]For diagnostic x-rays, 1 rad = 1 rem.

X-ray Dosimetry. When calculating the dose of ionizing radiation such as that from x-rays, several factors are considered (Wagner and colleagues, 1997). These include:

1. Type of study.
2. Type and age of equipment.
3. Distance of target organ from radiation source.
4. Thickness of the body part penetrated.
5. Method or technique used for the study.

Estimates of dose to the uterus and embryo for a variety of commonly used radiographic examinations are summarized in Table 41–5. Studies of maternal body parts farthest from the uterus (e.g., head) result in a very small dose of radiation scatter to the embryo or fetus. Because the size of the woman, radiographic technique, and equipment performance are variable factors, data in the table serve only as a guideline. When the radiation dose for a specific individual is required, a medical physicist may be consulted.

Potential Adverse Fetal Effects. The harmful effects of radiation exposure according to Brent (1999) are direct or indirect:

1. Cell death, which affects embryogenesis.
2. Growth restriction.
3. Congenital malformations.
4. Carcinogenesis (controversial).
5. Microcephaly and mental retardation.
6. Sterility.

The harmful fetal effects of ionizing radiation have been extensively studied for cell damage with resultant dysfunction of embryogenesis. These have been assessed both in animal models as well as in human studies of Japanese atomic bomb survivors.

ANIMAL STUDIES. Adverse radiation effects in animals are somewhat different from those in humans. A number of animal studies have addressed these potential embryopathological effects (Brent, 1971, 1999; Wilson and colleagues, 1953). Several conclusions can be drawn:

1. High-dose ionizing radiation is most likely to be lethal to the preblastocyst during the preimplantation stage; the embryo is very insensitive to teratogenic or other effects of radiation at this time.
2. During the period of organogenesis, high-dose radiation is more likely to cause teratogenic changes, growth restriction, or lethal effects.
3. During the fetal period, the fetus is more likely to manifest growth restriction and central nervous system effects.

In animal studies, various organs manifest teratogenic effects, whereas in humans, growth restriction and central nervous system anomalies are the most common following high-dose ionizing radiation. Most studies involved large

TABLE 41–5 Dose to the Uterus for Common Radiographical Procedures

Study	View	Dose[a] View (mrad)	Films/Study[b]	Dose/Study (mrad)
Skull[c]	AP, PA	< 0.01		
	Lat	< 0.01	4.1	< 0.05
Chest	AP, PA[c]	0.01–0.05		
	Lat[d]	0.01–0.03	1.5	0.02–0.07
Mammogram[d]	CC	0.01–0.05		
	Lat	3–5	4.0	7–20
Lumbosacral spine	AP[c,e]	92–187		
	PA[d]	40–97		
	Lat[d]	12–33	3.4	168–359
Abdomen	AP[c]	80–163		
	PA[d]	23–55		
	Lat[d]	29–82	1.7	122–245
Intravenous pyelogram[b]	AP	130–264		
	PA	43–104		
	Lat	13–37	5.5	686–1398
Hip[b] (single)	AP	72–140		
	Lat	18–51	2.0	103–213

AP = anteroposterior; PA = posteroanterior; Lat = lateral; CC = cranial-caudal.
[a] Calculated for x-ray beams with half-value layers ranging from 2- to 4-mm aluminum equivalent using the methodology of Rosenstein (1988).
[b] Based on data and methods reported by Laws and Rosenstein (1978).
[c] Entrance exposure data from Conway (1989).
[d] Authors' estimates based on compilation of above data.
[e] Based on NEXT data reported in National Council on Radiation Protection and Measurements (1989).
Table courtesy of Dr. Diane Twickler.

doses—100 to 200 rad (1 to 2 Gy)—and a threshold phenomenon has been demonstrated (Brent, 1999). Thus, it is not always possible to extrapolate animal data directly to humans.

HUMAN DATA. Possible adverse human fetal effects of high-dose ionizing radiation are principally derived from two sources. The first is from reports of large-dose radiation given to treat women for malignancy, menorrhagia, and uterine myomas (Brent, 1989). Goldstein and Murphy (1929) reported that radiation estimated to be over 100 rad caused microcephaly or hydrocephaly in 19 of 75 exposed embryos. Other adverse effects included mental retardation, abnormal genitalia, growth restriction, microphthalmia, and cataracts. Dekaban (1968) reported 22 infants with microcephaly, mental retardation, or both, following exposure to an estimated 250 rad in the first half of pregnancy. In both studies, other organ malformations were not found unless there was also microcephaly, eye abnormalities, or growth restriction (Brent, 1999).

The second and most often quoted human data of irradiation exposure are from atomic bomb survivors from Hiroshima and Nagasaki (Greskovich and Macklis, 2000; Otake and co-workers, 1987). Adverse fetal effects from exposure to fallout from the atomic bomb include an increased risk of microcephaly and severe mental retardation with high exposure beginning at certain gestational ages (Fig. 41–2). The risk is greatest at 8 to 15 weeks, and larger doses are necessary at 16 to 25 weeks to cause an equivalent proportion of

cases of mental retardation. Another important observation is the suggestion of a nonthreshold linear relationship of radiation dose at 8 to 15 weeks, so that even very low doses cause a slight increase in mental retardation incidence (Hall, 1991). There is no documented increased risk of mental retardation in humans at gestational ages less than 8 weeks or greater than

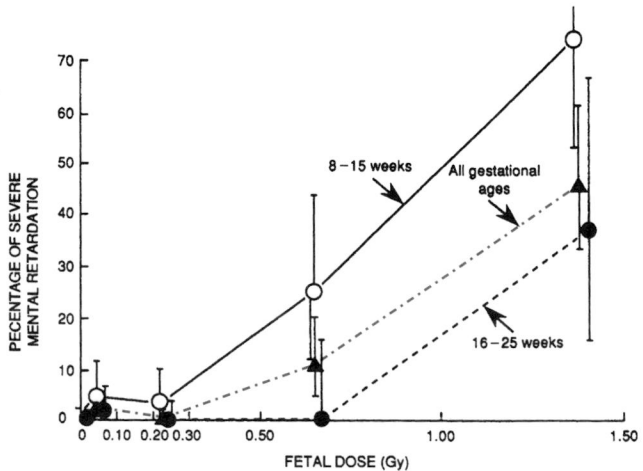

FIGURE 41–2. Severe mental retardation caused by ionizing radiation in fetuses exposed at various gestational ages to the atomic bomb in Hiroshima and Nagasaki (1 Gy = 100 rad). The bar lines represent 90-percent confidence levels. (Data from Otake and associates, 1987, with permission.)

25 weeks, even with doses exceeding 50 rad (Committee on Biological Effects, 1990).

The effect of ionizing radiation on intelligence quotient (IQ) scores in children who were exposed in utero is also dependent on gestational age as well as radiation dose. The highest risk again is at 8 to 15 weeks, followed by 16 to 25 weeks for doses greater than 50 rad.

The implications of these findings seem straightforward. At 8 to 15 weeks, the embryo is most susceptible to radiation-induced mental retardation. This risk is probably a nonthreshold linear function of dose, with the risk of severe mental retardation being as low as 4 percent for 10 rad and as high as 60 percent for 150 rad (Committee on Biological Effects, 1990). These doses are 10 to 100 times higher than those from diagnostic radiation. However, cumulative doses from multiple procedures may enter that harmful range, especially at 8 to 15 weeks. At 16 to 25 weeks, the risk is less, and there is no proven risk before 8 weeks or after 25 weeks.

Current evidence suggests that there is no increased risk of malformations, growth restriction, or abortion from a radiation dose of less than 5 rad. Indeed, Brent (1999) concluded that gross congenital malformations would not be increased in a human pregnant population exposed to less than 20 rad (0.2 Gy).

Oncogenic Effects of Ionizing Radiation. Whether there is an association between in utero diagnostic radiation exposure and increased risk of childhood cancers is controversial; supporting data are few. In older studies, some investigators reported that these cancers, and especially leukemia, were increased (Diamond and colleagues, 1973; Shu and associates, 1994; Stewart and Kneale, 1970). Conversely, Brent (1999) and others have questioned such an association, and according to the National Radiological Protection Board (1993) of the United Kingdom, the risk barely exceeds threshold for diagnostic studies. Moreover, there were only two cases of childhood cancer detected among 1630 atomic bomb survivors with high exposure (Committee on Biological Effects, 1990). Data concerning whether atomic bomb survivors are at risk for adult cancers are not yet available.

Therapeutic Radiation. According to the Radiation Therapy Committee Task Group of the American Association of Physics in Medicine, about 4000 pregnant women annually undergo cancer therapy in the United States (Stovall and colleagues, 1995). This Task Group emphasizes careful individualization of radiotherapy for the pregnant woman (see Chap. 57, p. 1258). For example, shielding of the fetus and other safeguards can be taken (Fenig and colleagues, 2001; Nuyttens and colleagues, 2002). Even then, the fetus may be exposed to unacceptable doses of radiation, and a carefully designed plan must be considered (Prado and colleagues, 2000). For example, a model to estimate fetal dosage with maternal brain radiotherapy and with tangential breast irradiation has been developed by Mazonakis and colleagues (1999, 2003).

Diagnostic Radiation. As previously discussed, therapeutic abortion is not indicated because of fetal exposure to a single diagnostic radiographic procedure (Brent, 1999). To put fetal risk into perspective, it is important to know the estimated x-ray dosimetry. According to the American College of Radiology (Hall, 1991), **no single diagnostic procedure results in a radiation dose significant enough to threaten the well-being of the developing embryo and fetus.**

Radiographs. Estimated radiation doses for standard radiographs are presented in Table 41–5. In pregnancy, the chest radiograph is the most commonly used study, and fetal exposure is exceptionally small for two views (0.07 mrad). The single abdominal radiograph has a higher dose (100 mrad), because the embryo or fetus is directly in the x-ray beam. The standard intravenous pyelogram may exceed 1 rad because of the number of films taken. For this reason, and as discussed in Chapter 48 (see p. 1099), the one-shot pyelogram may be useful when urolithiasis or other causes of urinary obstruction are suspected but unproven by ultrasound. Most "trauma series," such as radiographs of an extremity, skull, or rib series, deliver low doses because of the fetal distance from the target area.

Fetal indications for radiographic studies are limited. Perhaps the most common is pelvimetry with a breech presentation (see Chap. 24, p. 567). Another indication is for a suspected fetal skeletal anomaly where the ultrasonic diagnosis is unclear, such as with caudal regression syndrome and sirenomelia.

Fluoroscopy and Angiography. Dosimetry calculations for fluoroscopy and angiography are much more difficult because of variations in the number of radiographs obtained, fluoroscopy time, and the amount of fluoroscopy time the fetus is in the radiation field. As shown in Table 41–6, the range is quite variable. Although the Food and Drug Administration limits exposure rate for conventional fluoroscopy such as barium studies, special-purpose systems such as angiography units have potential for much higher exposure.

In nonpregnant patients, commonly performed studies involving routine fluoroscopy are the upper gastrointestinal series and barium enema. Frequently, these are done early in pregnancy, during the period of preimplantation or early organogenesis and most often before the woman realizes that she is pregnant. The upper gastrointestinal series has significantly less fetal exposure than a barium enema. Even so, endoscopy is usually preferred for evaluation during pregnancy (see Chap. 49, p. 1112).

Angiography may occasionally be necessary for serious maternal disorders. As before, the longer the distance from the embryo or fetus, the less the exposure and risk.

Computed Tomography. Imaging using computed tomography (CT) scanning involves multiple exposures of very thin x-ray beams in a 360-degree circle and their computerized

TABLE 41–6 **Estimated X-ray Doses to the Uterus or Embryo from Common Fluoroscopic Procedures**

Procedure	Total Dose to Uterus (mrad)	Fluoroscopic Exposure Time (sec)	Cinegraphic Exposure Time (sec)
Cerebral angiography[a]	<10	—	—
Cardiac angiography[b,c]	65	223 (SD = 118)	49 (SD = 9)
Single-vessel PTCA[b,c]	60	1023 (SD = 952)	32 (SD = 7)
Double-vessel PTCA[b,c]	90	1186 (SD = 593)	49 (SD = 13)
Upper gastrointestinal series[d]	56	136	—
Barium swallow[b,e]	6	192	—
Barium enema[b,f,g]	1945–3986	289–311	—

PTCA = percutaneous transluminal coronary angioplasty; SD = standard deviation.
[a]Wagner and associates (1997).
[b]Calculations based on data of Gorson and colleagues (1984).
[c]Finci and co-workers (1987).
[d]Suleiman and colleagues (1991).
[e]Based on female data from Rowley and associates (1987).
[f]Assumes embryo in radiation field for entire examination.
[g]Bednarek and co-workers (1983).
Table courtesy of Dr. Diane Twickler.

interpretations. The result is an axial (occasionally sagittal) image of a body portion, referred to as a *slice*. Multiple slices of the target are obtained.

Newer-generation tomography equipment is increasingly sensitive, however, better resolution may cause higher radiation exposure. Conversely, because there is less scatter with newer equipment, areas not directly scanned have less exposure. For example, skin exposure from a head tomographic scan is typically as high as 5 to 6 rad along the area scanned. In the body, doses typically range from approximately 5 rad at the skin surface to 2 rad in the center of the slice.

Spiral CT allows for continuous acquisition of images in a spiral with image reformatting in multiple planes compared with the conventional axial images. The exposure is dependent on the *pitch*, which is the degree of stretching or tightening of the spiral. The less the pitch, the tighter the spiral, and the greater the exposure. At the present time, a typical pitch ranges from 1.0 to 2.0 and results in radiation exposure similar to or less than that for conventional tomography (Jurik and colleagues, 1996). In a comparative study, Winer-Muram and co-workers (2002) determined body geometry for 23 pregnant women. The estimated fetal dose with helical CT was lower than that from ventilation–perfusion lung scanning during all trimesters. A note of caution—because of the ease and brevity of CT scanning, there is a tendency to increase the number of acquisitions and to increase exposure (Zoetelief and Geleijns, 1998).

Many variables in each tomographic study affect calculation of radiation doses, especially slice thickness and number of cuts obtained. If a study is performed with and without contrast, twice as many images are obtained, and the dose is doubled. Fetal radiation exposure is also dependent on factors such as the size of the mother and the size and position of the fetus (Ragossino and colleagues, 1986). Finally, the closer the

target area is to the fetus, the greater the radiation exposure. Estimated fetal doses from some CT scans are summarized in Table 41–7.

Cranial CT scanning is the most commonly requested study in pregnant women. Its use in women with eclampsia is discussed in Chapter 34 (see p. 776). Nonenhanced CT scanning is the preferred imaging technique to detect acute hemorrhage within the epidural, subdural, or subarachnoid spaces. If indicated, abdominal tomography should be performed in the pregnant woman with severe trauma (American College of Obstetricians and Gynecologists, 1998). CT pelvimetry is used in some cases before attempting breech vaginal delivery (see Chap. 24, p. 567). The fetal dose may approach 1.5 rad, but use of a low-exposure technique may reduce this to 250 mrad (see Table 41–7).

TABLE 41–7 **Estimated Maximal Fetal Doses from Computed Tomographic Scans[a]**

Trauma protocol—abdomen and pelvis
  Oral or intravenous contrast
  Slices: 65-sec delay, 8-mm slices diaphragm to chest; 10-mm iliac crest to ischium
  Dose: 2.5 to 3.2 cGy

Appendicitis
  Oral or intravenous contrast
  Slices: 5-mm slices mid-L2 to symphysis
  Dose: 2.2 to 2.5 cGy

Renal colic—ultrasonography and 1-shot intravenous pyelography inconclusive
  No contrast
  Slices: 5-mm helical from top of kidneys to symphysis
  Dose: 2.5 to 2.8 cGy

[a]Performed using Picker scanner. GE scanner has 2–3 fold increased radiation dose.
Data courtesy of Dr. Jon Anderson and Dr. Diane Twickler.

Multidetector-row CT imaging is a superior technique and allows acquisition of 16 or more slices simultaneously. Advantages are quickness; it acquires the entire thorax in 10 seconds. It results in more radiographic exposure. Goldhaber (2004) cites a detection rate of 90 percent for pulmonary emboli in nonpregnant patients. In pregnant women, however, Nuthalapaty and colleagues (2005) cite a number of quality concerns.

Nuclear Medicine Studies. These studies are performed by "tagging" a radioactive element to a chemical agent. For example, the radioisotope technetium^{99m} may be tagged to red blood cells, sulphur colloid, or pertechnetate. The method used to tag the agent determines fetal radiation exposure. Placental transfer and renal clearance, whereby fetal proximity to the maternal bladder increases exposure, are important. Measurement of radioactive technetium is based on its decay, and the units used are the curie (Ci) or the becquerel (Bq). Doses usually are expressed in millicuries (mCi).

Depending on the physical and biochemical properties of a radioisotope, an average fetal exposure can be calculated (Wagner and co-workers, 1997; Zanzonico, 2000). Commonly used radiopharmaceuticals and estimated absorbed fetal doses are given in Table 41–8. The dose of radionuclide can be kept as low as possible (Adelstein, 1999). Exposures vary with gestational age and are greatest earlier in pregnancy for most radiopharmaceuticals. One exception is the later effects of iodine^{131} on the fetal thyroid (Wagner and associates, 1997). The International Commission on Radiological Protection (2001) has compiled dose coefficients for radionuclides during pregnancy. Stather and colleagues (2002) detailed the biokinetic and dosimetric models used by the International Commission to estimate fetal radiation doses when a pregnant woman is exposed to a radionuclide.

Clinically suspected pulmonary embolism during pregnancy has been studied with *ventilation–perfusion lung* scanning (see Chap. 47, p. 1084). Perfusion is measured with injected ^{99}Tc-macroaggregated albumin, and ventilation is

TABLE 41–8 Radiopharmaceuticals Used in Nuclear Medicine Studies

Study	Estimated Activity Administered per Examination (mCi)	Weeks' Gestation[a]	Dose to Uterus/Embryo per Pharmaceutical (mrem)
Brain	20 mCi ^{99m}Tc DTPA	< 12	880
		12	700[b]
Hepatobiliary	5 mCi ^{99m}Tc sulfur colloid	12	45
	5 mCi ^{99m}Tc HIDA		150
Bone	20 mCi ^{99m}Tc phosphate	< 12	460
Pulmonary			
Perfusion	3 mCi ^{99m}Tc-macroaggregated albumin plus	Any	45–57
Ventilation	10 mCi ^{133}xenon gas		
Renal	20 mCi ^{99m}Tc DTPA	< 12	880
Abscess or tumor	3 mCi ^{67}Ga citrate	< 12	750
Cardiovascular	20 mCi ^{99m}Tc labeled red blood cells	< 12	500
	3 mCi ^{210}Tl chloride	< 12	1100
		12	640
		24	520
		36	300
Thyroid	5 mCi ^{99m}Tc O$_4$	< 8	240
	0.3 mCi ^{123}I (whole body)	1.5–6	10
	0.1 mCi ^{131}I[c]		
	Whole body	2–6	15
	Whole body	7–9	88
	Whole body	12–13	160
	Whole body	20	300
	Thyroid–fetal	11	72,000
	Thyroid–fetal	12–13	130,000
	Thyroid–fetal	20	590,000
Sentinel lymphoscintigram	5 mCi ^{99m}Tc sulfur colloid (1–3 millicuries)		500

DPTA = diethylenetriaminepentaacetic acid; HIDA = hepatobiliary iminodiacetic acid.
[a]Exposures are generally greater prior to 12 weeks compared with those at increasing gestational ages.
[b]Some measurements account for placental transfer.
[c]The uptake and exposure of ^{131}I increases with gestational age.
Compiled from data from Adelstein (1999), Schwartz (2003), Stather (2002), Wagner (1997), Zanzonico (2000), and all their colleagues.

measured with inhaled xenon[127] or xenon[133]. Fetal exposure with either is negligible (Chan and colleagues, 2002; Mountford, 1997).

Thyroid scanning with iodine[123] or iodine[131] seldom is indicated in pregnancy. With trace doses used, however, fetal risk is minimal. Therapeutic radioiodine in doses to treat Graves disease or thyroid cancer may cause fetal thyroid ablation (Green and colleagues, 1971).

The *sentinel lymphoscintigram* for detecting the axillary lymph node most likely to have metastases from breast cancer is a popular preoperative study to replace lymph node dissection (DeAngelis and co-workers, 1999). The calculated dose is approximately 500 mrad (Adelstein, 1999; Schwartz and colleagues, 2003; Steenvoorde and colleagues, 1998; Timins, 2001) and should not preclude its use during pregnancy (see Table 41–8).

ULTRASONOGRAPHY. Of all of the major advances in obstetrics, the development of ultrasonography for study of the fetus and mother certainly is one of the greater achievements. The technique has become virtually indispensable in everyday practice. The wide range of clinical uses of ultrasound in pregnancy is further discussed in Chapter 16 and in many other sections of this book.

Safety. Diagnostic ultrasonography uses sound wave transmission at certain frequencies. At very high intensities, there is a potential for human tissue damage from heat and cavitation (Callen, 2000). In the low-intensity range of real-time imaging, however, no fetal risks have been demonstrated in more than 35 years of use (Maulik, 1997; Miller and colleagues, 1998). More recently, Naumburg and associates (2000) performed a case-control study of 578 children with leukemia. When compared with healthy controls, one third of each cohort was found to have been exposed to ultrasound in utero.

Recent advances in technology have introduced Doppler-shift imaging coupled with gray-scale imaging to localize spectral waveforms and superimpose color mapping. Higher energy intensities are used with this duplex Doppler imaging. Again, however, these should have no embryo or fetal effects if low-level pulses are used (Kossoff, 1997).

Ultrasound equipment must have a video display of acoustic output to safeguard against exceeding standards set by a number of organizations (American College of Obstetricians and Gynecologists, 1996). Acoustic outputs are displayed as the *thermal index* and *mechanical index*. The thermal index is an estimate of temperature increases from acoustic output. If the index is below 1.0, then no potential risk is expected (Miller and associates, 1998). Adverse effects reflected in thermal index changes have not been demonstrated with Doppler use in clinical applications (Maulik, 1997). The mechanical index is used to estimate the potential risk of cavitation from heat generated by real-time imaging. As

long as sonographic contrast agents are not used, there is no hypothetical fetal risk.

MAGNETIC RESONANCE IMAGING. Magnetic resonance imaging (MRI) has proven extremely useful in obstetrics because it does not use ionizing radiation. Its application is cited throughout this book. Advantages include high soft tissue contrast, ability to characterize tissue, and acquisition of images in any plane—particularly axial, sagittal, and coronal. MRI uses powerful magnets to alter the state of protons temporarily. The hydrogen proton is used for imaging because of its abundance, especially in water and fat. Radio waves are then used to deflect the magnetic vector. When the radiofrequency source is turned off, hydrogen protons return to their normal state. In doing so, they emit radio waves of different frequencies, which are received by radio coils wrapped around the body part. The relative intensity of these signals is plotted on a gray scale. A series of pulse sequences in all planes can be obtained, and each acquisition includes information about the location and characteristics of the sequences. From this, an image is constructed. Technological advances have significantly reduced scan times and improved image quality.

Safety. There are no reported harmful human effects from MRI (American College of Radiology, 1998; Levine, 2000). Chew and colleagues (2001) found no differences in blastocyst formation with 1.5-T MRI use in early murine embryo development. Vadeyar and associates (2000) noted no demonstrable fetal heart rate pattern changes during MRI. Recently, Chung (2002) reviewed safety issues.

The standards of the American College of Radiology (1998) dictate that each request for an MRI of a pregnant woman be approved by the attending radiologist. Indicated imaging should be performed at any gestational age if no other imaging studies can be performed, or if MRI would provide information that would otherwise require radiation exposure. Contraindications to MRI include internal cardiac pacemakers, neurostimulators, implantable defibrillators, implantable electronic infusion pumps, cochlear implants, and some other devices. Certain intracranial aneurysm clips and any metallic foreign body in the globe of the eye contraindicate scanning.

Contrast Agents. A number of elemental *gadolinium chelates* are used to create contrast, including gadopentetate, gadodiamide, gadoteridol, and gadoterate. These cross the placenta and are found in fetal amnionic fluid. In large doses, gadopentetate causes developmental delay in animal fetuses (Briggs and colleagues, 2002). The use of contrast agents currently is not recommended unless overwhelming benefits are perceived.

Maternal Indications. The use of MRI during pregnancy has been extremely helpful. In maternal disorders unrelated to pregnancy, MRI technology has the advantage over CT because of the lack of ionizing radiation. In some cases, MRI may be complementary to CT, and in others, MRI is

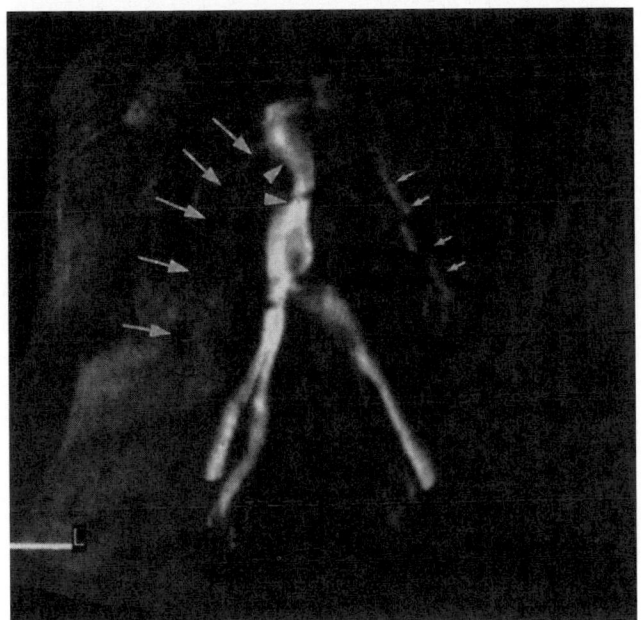

FIGURE 41–3. Reconstructed magnetic resonance venogram demonstrates normal flow in the left ovarian vein (*small arrows*). The thrombosed right ovarian vein (*large arrows*) has no flow, and the clot produces a mass effect at its confluence with the inferior vena cava (*arrowheads*). (From Nurenberg and Twickler, 1995, with permission.)

preferable. Central nervous system abnormalities, such as brain tumors or spinal trauma, are more clearly seen with MRI (Mantello and associates, 1993). As discussed in Chapter 34 (see p. 776), MRI has provided valuable insights into the pathophysiology of eclampsia (Cunningham and Twickler, 2000; Zeeman and associates, 2003). *Magnetic resonance angiography* provides imaging of the cerebral vasculature and can also be used to calculate flow of the middle and posterior cerebral arteries (Zeeman and colleagues, 2003).

MRI is a superb technique to evaluate the abdomen and retroperitoneal space in a pregnant woman. All things being equal, MRI is preferable to CT, which involves fetal radiation. MRI has been used for detection and localization of adrenal tumors, gastrointestinal lesions, intra-abdominal malignancies, and uterine and ovarian masses in pregnancy. Either CT or MRI is useful for evaluation of puerperal infections, but MRI provides better visualization of the bladder flap area following cesarean delivery (Brown and associates, 1999; Twickler and colleagues, 1997). MRI may be used to diagnose venous thrombosis of the pelvic vessels and vena cava in a pregnant woman—a decided advantage over CT. A computerized reconstructed venogram of a large ovarian vein thrombosis without extremity involvement is shown in Figure 41–3.

Fetal Indications. Specific uses of fetal MRI as a complement to ultrasonography have emerged (De Wilde and colleagues, 2005). Zaretsky and associates (2002) showed that MRI can be used to image almost all elements of the standard anatomical survey. Reichel and colleagues (2003) have validated its use for fetal central nervous system biometry. Zaretsky and co-workers (2003) also showed that fetal weight estimation was more accurate using MRI than with ultrasonography. Fast acquisition sequencing has solved problems with fetal movement to improve

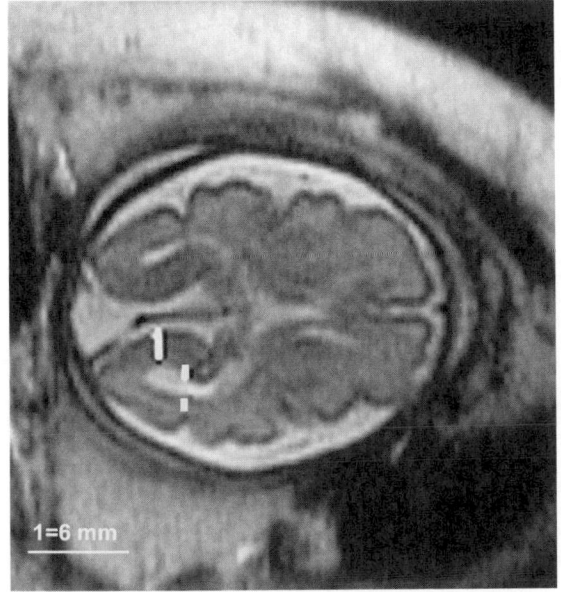

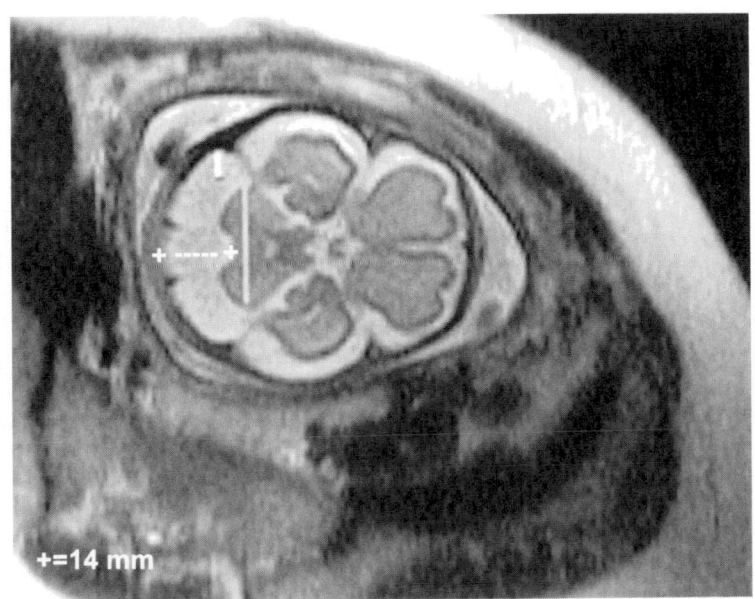

A   B

FIGURE 41–4. Magnetic resonance imaging of the fetal cranium. **A.** Cursors show atrial measurement in a 28-week normal fetus. **B.** Cursors show measurements of abnormally enlarged cisterna magna in a 29-week fetus. (From Twickler and colleagues, 2002, with permission.)

imaging; the technique is referred to as *HASTE—H*alf-*F*ourier *A*cquisition *S*ingle slow *T*urbo spin *E*cho. Levine and colleagues (2001) studied pregnant pigs and reported that HASTE protocols do not generate significant heat in the uterus or fetus.

The most common fetal indication for MRI has been with suspected brain anomalies. Levine and co-workers (1999) found that use of fast-acquisition technology altered the diagnosis in 20 of 66 (30 percent) fetuses with central nervous system abnormalities. Twickler and associates (2003) reported that fetal imaging with *single-shot fast spin echo (SSFSE)* provided additional information in 46 of 72 (64 percent) fetuses with abnormal intracranial findings by ultrasonography. Sharma and colleagues (2003) also found it helpful in further evaluating brain anomalies in fetuses aborted by dilatation and evacuation (D & E), which distorted or destroyed the anatomy. Righini and co-workers (2004) found MRI superior to ultrasound in detecting brain infarction in the surviving monochorionic twin after one fetus died from twin-to-twin transfusion syndrome. Merzoug and associates (2002) have provided a detailed review of normal and abnormal brain images. Some examples are shown in Figure 41–4.

In addition, MRI may be used to obtain very specific details of fetal anatomy and complex dysmorphology (Coakley and co-workers, 1999; Zaretsky and colleagues, 2002). In another study, Caire and co-workers (2003) showed excellent detail with MRI in fetuses with suspected genitourinary anomalies despite a high incidence of oligohydramnios,

which is common in these cases. Brody (2004) suggested using MRI to monitor fetal lung volume. Zaretsky and Twickler (2003) have provided a scholarly review of normal and abnormal fetal anatomy viewed with MRI.

Finally, Fenton and associates (2000) used *magnetic resonance spectroscopy* to analyze a lecithin peak in three term fetuses. This raises the possibility of in vivo analysis of lung maturity.

GUIDELINES FOR DIAGNOSTIC IMAGING DURING PREGNANCY. The American College of Obstetricians and Gynecologists (2004) has reviewed the effects of radiographic, ultrasonographic, and magnetic resonance exposure during pregnancy. Its suggested guidelines are shown in Table 41–9.

TABLE 41–9 Guidelines for Diagnostic Imaging During Pregnancy

1. Women should be counseled that x-ray exposure from a single diagnostic procedure does not result in harmful fetal effects. Specifically, exposure to less than 5 rad has not been associated with an increase in fetal anomalies or pregnancy loss.
2. Concern about possible effects of high-dose ionizing radiation exposure should not prevent medically indicated diagnostic radiographic procedures from being performed on the mother. During pregnancy, other imaging procedures not associated with ionizing radiation, such as ultrasonography and magnetic resonance imaging, should be considered instead of radiographs when appropriate.
3. Ultrasonography and magnetic resonance imaging are not associated with known adverse fetal effects.
4. Consultation with an expert in dosimetry calculation may be helpful in calculating estimated fetal dose when multiple diagnostic radiographs are performed on a pregnant woman.
5. The use of radioactive isotopes of iodine is contraindicated for therapeutic use during pregnancy.
6. Radiopaque and paramagnetic contrast agents are unlikely to cause harm and may be of diagnostic benefit, but these agents should be used during pregnancy only if the potential benefit justifies the potential risk to the fetus.

From the American College of Obstetricians and Gynecologists (2004), with permission.

REFERENCES

Adelstein SJ: Administered radionuclides in pregnancy. Teratology 59:236, 1999

Akira S, Yamanaka A, Ishihara T, et al: Gasless laparoscopic ovarian cystectomy during pregnancy: Comparison with laparotomy. Am J Obstet Gynecol 180:554, 1999

Al-Fozan H, Tulandi T: Safety and risks of laparoscopy in pregnancy. Cur Opin Obstet Gynecol 14:375, 2002

American College of Obstetricians and Gynecologists: Guidelines for diagnostic imaging during pregnancy. Committee Opinion No. 299, September 2004

American College of Obstetricians and Gynecologists: Nonobstetric surgery in pregnancy. Committee Opinion No. 284, August 2003

American College of Obstetricians and Gynecologists: Obstetric aspects of trauma management. Educational Bulletin No. 251, September 1998

American College of Obstetricians and Gynecologists: New ultrasound output display standard. Committee Opinion No. 180, November 1996

American College of Radiology: MR safety and sedation. American College of Radiology Standards, 1998, p 457

Barnard JM, Chaffin D, Droste S, et al: Fetal response to carbon dioxide pneumoperitoneum in the pregnant ewe. Obstet Gynecol 85:669, 1995

Bednarek DR, Rudin S, Wong, et al: Reduction of fluoroscopic exposure for the air-contrast barium enema. Br J Radiol 56:823, 1983

Brent RL: The effect of embryonic and fetal exposure to X-ray, microwaves, and ultrasound: Counseling the pregnant and nonpregnant patient about these risks. Semin Oncol 16:347, 1989

Brent RL: The response of the 91 day old rat embryo to variations in exposure rate of 150 R x-irradiation. Radiat Res 45:127, 1971

Brent RL: Utilization of developmental basic science principles in the evaluation of reproductive risks from pre- and postconception environmental radiation exposures. Teratology 59:182, 1999

Briggs GG, Freeman RK, Yaffe SJ: Drugs in pregnancy and lactation, 6th ed. Philadelphia, Lippincott Williams & Wilkins, 2002, p 606

Brody AS: How can fetal lung volume be monitored? Radiology 234:307, 2004

Brown CE, Stettler RW, Twickler D, et al. Puerperal septic pelvic thrombophlebitis: Incidence and response to heparin therapy. Am J Obstet Gynecol 181:143, 1999

Caire JT, Ramus RM, Magee KP, et al: MRI of fetal genitourinary anomalies. AJR Am J Roentgenol 181:1381, 2003

Callen PW: The obstetric ultrasound examination, Chap. 1. In Callen PW (ed): Ultrasonography in Obstetrics and Gynecology, 4th ed. Philadelphia, WB Saunders, 2000, p 1

Chan WS, Ray JG, Murray S, et al: Suspected pulmonary embolism in pregnancy. Arch Intern Med 152:1170, 2002

Chew S, Ahmadi A, Goh PS, et al: The effects of 1.5T magnetic resonance imaging on early murine in-vitro embryo development. J Magn Reson Imaging 13:417, 2001

Chung SM: Safety issues in magnetic resonance imaging. J Neuroophthalmol 22:35, 2002

Coakley FV, Hricak H, Filly RA, et al: Complex fetal disorders: Effect of MR imaging on management—preliminary experience. Radiology 213:691, 1999

Committee on Biological Effects of Ionizing Radiation, National Research Council: Other somatic and fetal effects. In Beir V: Effects of Exposure to Low Levels of Ionizing Radiation. Washington, National Academy Press, 1990

Conway BJ: Nationwide evaluation of x-ray trends: Tabulation and graphical summary of surveys 1984 through 1987. Frankfort, KY, Conference of Radiation Control Program Directors, 1989

Cunningham FG, Twickler D: Cerebral edema complicating eclampsia. Am J Obstet Gynecol 182:94, 2000

Czeizel AE, Pataki T, Rockenbauer M: Reproductive outcome after exposure to surgery under anesthesia during pregnancy. Arch Gynecol Obstet 261:193, 1998

DeAngelis GA, Gizienski T, Moore MM: Axillary sentinel node biopsy in breast cancer staging. Appl Radiol 28:8, 1999

Dekaban AS: Abnormalities in children exposed to x-irradiation during various stages of gestation: Tentative timetable of radiation injury to the human fetus. J Nucl Med 9:471, 1968

De Wilde JP, Rivers AW, Price DL: A review of the current use of magnetic resonance imaging in pregnancy and safety implications for the fetus. Prog Biophys Mol Biol 87:335, 2005

Diamond EL, Schmerler H, Lilienfeld AM: The relationship of intrauterine radiation to subsequent mortality and development of leukemia in children: A prospective study. Am J Epidemiol 97:283, 1973

Fatum M, Rojansky N: Laparoscopic surgery during pregnancy. Obstet Gynecol Surv 56:50, 2001

Fenig E, Mishaeli M, Kalish Y, et al: Pregnancy and radiation. Cancer Treat Rev 27:1, 2001

Fenton BW, Lin C-S, Ascher S, et al: Magnetic resonance spectroscopy to detect lecithin in amniotic fluid and fetal lung. Obstet Gynecol 95:457, 2000

Finci L, Meier B, Steffenino G, et al: Radiation exposure during diagnostic catheterization and single- and double-vessel percutaneous transluminal coronary angioplasty. Am J Cardiol 60:1401, 1987

Gazmararian JA, Petersen R, Jamieson DJ, et al: Hospitalizations during pregnancy among managed care enrollees. Obstet Gynecol 100:94, 2002

Goldhaber SZ: Pulmonary embolism. Lancet 263:1295, 2004

Goldstein L, Murphy DP: Etiology of the ill-health in children born after maternal pelvic irradiation, 2. Defective children born after postconception pelvic irradiation. AJR Am J Roentgenol 22:322, 1929

Gorson RO, Lassen M, Rosenstein M: Patient dosimetry in diagnostic radiology. In Waggener RG, Kereiakes JG, Shalek R (eds): Handbook of Medical Physics, Vol II. Boca Raton, FL, CRC Press, 1984.

Green HG, Gareis FJ, Shepard TH, et al: Cretinism associated with maternal sodium iodine-131 therapy during pregnancy. Am J Dis Child 122:247, 1971

Greskovich JF, Macklis RM: Radiation therapy in pregnancy: Risk calculation and risk minimization. Semin Oncol 27:633, 2000

Hall EJ: Scientific view of low-level radiation risks. Radiographics 11:509, 1991

Hunter JG, Swanstrom L, Thornburg K: Carbon dioxide pneumoperitoneum induces fetal acidosis in a pregnant ewe model. Surg Endosc 9:272, 1995

International Commission on Radiological Protection: Doses to the embryo and fetus from intakes of radionuclides by the mother. Ann ICRP 31:19, 2001

Jurik AG, Jensen LC, Hansen J: Total effective radiation dose from spiral CT and conventional radiography of the pelvis with regard to fracture classification. Acta Radiol 37:651, 1996

Källén B, Mazze RI: Neural tube defects and first trimester operations. Teratology 41:717, 1990

Kinsella SM, Lohmann G: Supine hypotensive syndrome. Obstet Gynecol 83:774, 1994

Kossoff G: Contentious issues in safety of diagnostic ultrasound. Ultrasound Obstet Gynecol 10:151, 1997

Lachman E, Schienfeld A, Voss E, et al: Pregnancy and laparoscopic surgery. J Am Assoc Gynecol Laparosc 6:347, 1999

Laws PW, Rosenstein M: A somatic index for diagnostic radiology. Health Phys. 35:629, 1978

Levine D: The role of computed tomography and magnetic resonance imaging in obstetrics, Chap. 25. In Callen PW (ed): Ultrasonography in Obstetrics and Gynecology, 4th ed. Philadelphia, WB Saunders, 2000, p 725

Levine D, Barnes PD, Madsen JR, et al: Central nervous system abnormalities assessed with prenatal magnetic resonance imaging. Obstet Gynecol 94:1011, 1999

Levine D, Zuo C, Faro CB, et al: Potential heating effect in the gravid uterus during MR HASTE imaging. J Magn Reson Imaging 13:856, 2001

Mantello MT, Schwartz RB, Jones KM, et al: Imaging of neurologic complications associated with pregnancy. Am J Roentgenol 160:843, 1993

Maulik D: Biosafety of diagnostic Doppler ultrasonography. In: Doppler Ultrasound in Obstetrics and Gynecology. New York, Springer Verlag, 1997

Mazonakis M, Damilakis J, Varveris H, et al: A method of estimating fetal dose during brain radiation therapy. Int J Radiat Oncol Biol Phys 44:455, 1999

Mazonakis M, Varveris H, Damilakis J, et al: Radiation dose to concepts resulting from tangential breast irradiation. Int J Radiat Oncol Biol Phys 55:386, 2003

Mazze RI, Källén B: Reproductive outcome after anesthesia and operation during pregnancy: A registry study of 5405 cases. Am J Obstet Gynecol 161:1178, 1989

Merzoug V, Ferey S, André CH, et al: Magnetic resonance imaging of the fetal brain. J Neuroradiol 29:76, 2002

Miller MW, Brayman AA, Abramowicz JS: Obstetric ultrasonography: A biophysical consideration of patient safety—the "rules" have changed. Am J Obstet Gynecol 179:241, 1998

Mountford PJ: Risk assessment of the nuclear medicine patient. Br J Radiol 100:671, 1997

National Council on Radiation Protection and Measurements: Exposure of the US Population from Diagnostic Medical Radiation. Bethesda, Md, National Council on Radiation Protection, Report No. 100, 1989, p 26

National Radiological Protection Board: Board statement on diagnostic medical exposures to ionizing radiation during pregnancy. Documents of the NRPB 4(4). London, HMSO, 1993

Naumburg E, Bellocco R, Cnattingius S, et al: Prenatal ultrasound examinations and risk of childhood leukaemia: Case-control study. BMJ 320:282, 2000

Nuthalapaty F, Ho M, Singh S, et al: Limitations of helical CT for the diagnosis of pulmonary thromboembolism during pregnancy and the puerperium. Presented at the 25th Annual Meeting of the Society for Maternal-Fetal Medicine, Reno, Nevada, 7–12 February, 2005

Nurenberg P, Twickler DM: Magnetic resonance imaging in obstetrics and gynecology. Williams Obstetrics, 19th ed (Suppl 11). Norwalk, CT, Appleton & Lange, February/March 1995

Nuyttens JJ, Prado KL, Jenrette JM, et al: Fetal dose during radiotherapy: Clinical implementation and review of the literature. Cancer Radiother 6:352, 2002

Otake M, Yoshimaru H, Schull WJ: Severe mental retardation among the prenatally exposed survivors of the atomic bombing of Hiroshima and Nagasaki: A comparison of the old and new dosimetry systems. Radiation Effects Research Foundation, Technical Report No. 16-87, 1987

Prado KL, Nelson SJ, Nuyttens JJ, et al: Clinical implementation of the AAPM Task Group 36 recommendations on fetal dose from radiotherapy with photon beams: A head and neck irradiation case report. J Appl Clin Med Phys 1:1-7, 2000

Ragossino MW, Breckle R, Hill LM, et al: Average fetal depth in utero: Data for estimation of fetal absorbed radiation dose. Radiology 158:513, 1986

Reedy MB, Galan HL, Bean-Lijewski JD, et al: Maternal and fetal effects of laparoscopic insufflation in the gravid baboon. J Am Assoc Gynecol Laparosc 2:399, 1995

Reedy MB, Galan HL, Richards WE, et al: Laparoscopy during pregnancy. A survey of laparoendoscopic surgeons. J Reprod Med 42:33, 1997a

Reedy MB, Källén B, Kuehl TJ: Laparoscopy during pregnancy: A study of five fetal outcome parameters with use of the Swedish Health Registry. Am J Obstet Gynecol 177:673, 1997b

Reichel TF, Ramus RM, Caire JT, et al: Fetal central nervous system biometry on MR imaging. AJR Am J Roentgenol 180:1155, 2003

Righini A, Salmona S, Bianchini E, et al: Prenatal magnetic resonance imaging evaluation of ischemic brain lesions in the survivors of monochorionic twin pregnancies: Report of 3 cases. Comput Assist Tomogr 28:87, 2004

Rosen MA: Management of anesthesia for the pregnant surgical patient. Anesthesiology 91:1159, 1999

Rosenstein M: Handbook of selected tissue doses for projections common in diagnostic radiology. Rockville, MD, Department of Health and Human Services, Food and Drug Administration. DHHS Pub No. (FDA) 89–8031, 1988

Rowley KA, Hill SJ, Watkins RA, et al: An investigation into the levels of radiation exposure in diagnostic examinations involving fluoroscopy. Br J Radiol 60:167, 1987

Schoepf UJ, Costello P: Multidetector-row CT imaging of pulmonary embolism. Semin Roentgenol 38:106, 2003

Schwartz JL, Mozurkewich EL, Johnson TM: Current management of patients with melanoma who are pregnant, want to get pregnant, or do not want to get pregnant. Cancer 97:2130, 2003

Sharma G, Heier L, Kalish RB, et al: Use of fetal magnetic resonance imaging in patients electing termination of pregnancy by dilation and evacuation. Am J Obstet Gynecol 189:990, 2003

Shu XO, Jin F, Lnet MS, et al: Diagnostic x-ray and ultrasound exposure and risk of childhood cancer. Br J Cancer 70:531, 1994

Stather JW, Phipps AW, Harrison JD, et al: Dose coefficients for the embryo and fetus following intakes of radionuclides by the mother. J Radiol Prot 22:1, 2002

Steenvoorde P, Pauwels EK, Harding LK, et al: Diagnostic nuclear medicine and risk for the fetus. Eur J Nucl Med 25:193, 1998

Steinbrook RA, Bhavani-Shankar K: Hemodynamics during laparoscopic surgery in pregnancy. Anesth Analg 93:1570, 2001

Stepp KJ, Sauchak KA, O'Malley DM, et al: Risk factors for adverse outcomes after intraabdominal surgery during pregnancy. Obstet Gynecol 99:23S, 2002

Stewart A, Kneale GW: Radiation dose effects in relation to obstetric x-rays and childhood cancers. Lancet 1:1185, 1970

Stovall M, Blackwell CR, Cundif J, et al: Fetal dose from radiotherapy with photon beams: Report of AAPM radiation therapy Committee Task Group No. 36. Med Phys 22:63, 1995

Suleiman OH, Anderson J, Jones B, et al: Tissue doses in the upper gastrointestinal examination. Radiology 178:653, 1991

Sylvester GC, Khoury MJ, Lu X, et al: First-trimester anesthesia exposure and the risk of central nervous system defects: A population-based case-control study. Am J Public Health 84: 1757, 1994

Timins JK: Radiation during pregnancy. N J Med 98:29, 2001

Twickler DM, Magee KP, Caire J, et al: Second-opinion magnetic resonance imaging for suspected fetal central nervous system abnormalities. Am J Obstet Gynecol 188:492, 2003

Twickler DM, Reichel T, McIntire DD, et al: Fetal central nervous system ventricle and cisterna magna measurements by magnetic resonance imaging. Am J Obstet Gynecol 187:927, 2002

Twickler DM, Setiawan AT, Evans R, et al: Imaging of puerperal septic thrombophlebitis: A prospective comparison of MR imaging, CT, and sonography. AJR Am J Roentgenol 169:1039, 1997

Vadeyar SH, Moore RJ, Strachan BK, et al: Effect of fetal magnetic resonance imaging on fetal heart rate patterns. Am J Obstet Gynecol 182:666, 2000

Wahba RWM, Beique F, Kleiman SJ: Cardiopulmonary function and laparoscopic cholecystectomy. Can J Anaesth 42:51-63, 1995

Wagner LK, Lester RG, Saldana LR: Exposure of the Pregnant Patient to Diagnostic Radiation. Philadelphia, Medical Physics Publishing, 1997, p 26

Wilson JG, Brent RL, Jordan HC: Differentiation as a determinant of the reaction of rat embryos on x-irradiation. Proc Soc Exp Biol Med 82:67, 1953

Winer-Muram HT, Boone JM, Brown HL, et al: Pulmonary embolism in pregnant patients: Fetal radiation dose with helical CT. Radiology 224:487, 2002

Zanzonico PB: Internal radionuclide radiation dosimetry: A review of basic concepts and recent developments. J Nucl Med 41:297, 2000

Zaretsky M, McIntire D, Twickler DM: Feasibility of the fetal anatomic and maternal pelvic survey by magnetic resonance imaging at term. Am J Obstet Gynecol 189:997, 2003

Zaretsky M, Reichel TF, McIntire DD, et al: Comparison of magnetic resonance imaging to ultrasound in the estimation of birth weight at term. Am J Obstet Gynecol 189:1017, 2003

Zaretsky MV, Twickler DM: Magnetic resonance imaging in obstetrics. Clin Obstet Gynecol 46:868, 2003

Zeeman GG, Hatab M, Twickler D: Maternal cerebral blood flow changes in pregnancy. Am J Obstet Gynecol 189:968, 2003

Zoetelief J, Geleijns J: Patient doses in spiral CT. Br J Radiol 71:584, 1998

42

Critical Care and Trauma

Women with a broad spectrum of pathophysiological conditions, some of which may have previously precluded pregnancy, may benefit from technology and expertise in *critical care obstetrics*. Examples are women with serious heart disease, acute or chronic pulmonary disorders, or trauma, or those with complications of severe preeclampsia or sepsis syndrome. Pregnancy poses unique considerations for critical care, and it is imperative that obstetricians and other members of the health care team have a working knowledge of these factors. Pregnant women are usually young and in good health, and their prognosis should be better than that of many other patients admitted to an intensive care unit (ICU). Indeed, obstetrical patients had an *actual mortality ratio* (ratio between actual and predicted mortality rate) of 0.25 to 0.42, significantly lower than the expected 1.0 ratio (Lewinsohn and colleagues, 1994; Mahutte and associates, 1999).

OBSTETRICAL INTENSIVE CARE

In most cases, obstetrical patients who need intensive care are those with complications specifically related to pregnancy. As shown in Table 42–1, Zeeman and colleagues (2003) reported that two thirds of women admitted to an obstetrical critical care unit had pregnancy-specific complications. Severe gestational hypertension and obstetrical hemorrhage were the most common reasons for admission. In some cases of life-threatening hemorrhage, such as with uterine atony or genital tract lacerations, surgical procedures are necessary to stop bleeding. In these cases, close proximity to a delivery–operating room is most advantageous. Finally, for the one third of pregnant women who have serious medical or surgical disorders, there frequently is concern for fetal well-being.

TABLE 42–1   Indications for 483 Admissions to the Obstetrical Intermediate Care Unit at Parkland Memorial Hospital Over a 2-Year Period

Diagnosis	Number
Obstetrical complications	318 (66%)
Eclampsia/severe preeclampsia	207
Hemorrhage	85
Sepsis	14
Other	12
Medical and surgical disorders	165 (34%)
Medical disorders	134
Pyelonephritis	12
Diabetes	32
Respiratory insufficiency	34
Cardiac	23
Chronic hypertension	11
Thyrotoxicosis	5
Other	30
Surgical disorders	31

From Zeeman and colleagues, 2003, with permission.

Here again, proximity to a delivery–operating room provides personnel and equipment for appropriate fetal surveillance.

Critically ill women may be managed in the obstetrical unit, and some institutions have specialized rooms with necessary equipment and experienced personnel available. Triage to a medical or surgical ICU depends on the acuity of care needed and the ability of that facility to provide it. For example, in most obstetrical units, women who require ventilatory support, invasive monitoring, or pharmacological support of circulation are transferred to a specialized ICU.

SYSTEMS FOR OBSTETRICAL CRITICAL CARE. A number of reports describe systems designed to care for critically ill pregnant women. In all, each institution has its own protocol for triage. They can be described in three categories.

1. A "full-service" obstetrical ICU, which provides all aspects of critical care that is usually given in medical or surgical ICUs (Jenkins and colleagues, 2003; Mabie and Sibai, 1990). Almost 1 percent of women delivered at the University of Tennessee were admitted to such an obstetrical ICU.
2. In most large institutions, severely ill women are transferred to a medical or surgical ICU that is operated by "intensivists." These tertiary care referral institutions show a remarkably similar proportion of obstetrical patients admitted to these ICUs: 0.4 percent at the University of California, San Francisco; 0.5 percent at the University of North Carolina; 0.3 percent at McGill University in Montreal; and 0.4 percent at Good Samaritan in Phoenix (Harris and Foley, 2002; Kilpatrick and Matthay, 1992; Mahutte and associates, 1999; Monaco and colleagues, 1993).
3. Intermediate care unit. We have developed such a unit both at Parkland Hospital as well as at the University of Alabama at Birmingham Hospital. Organization of these units is presented below, but briefly, their design permits care of most critically ill pregnant women in or near the obstetrical suite. As shown in Table 42–1, 1.7 percent of over 28,000 women delivered at Parkland Hospital over a 2-year period were admitted to this obstetrical intermediate care unit. Of these, 483 women (15 percent) were transferred to a medical or surgical ICU, usually for ventilatory support.

ORGANIZATION OF OBSTETRICAL CRITICAL CARE. The concept and development of critical care began in the 1960s. In 1983, the National Institutes of Health held the first Consensus Conference pertaining to critical care. In 1988, the Society for Critical Care Medicine promulgated definitions and established guidelines for design and staffing of ICUs. These continue to be refined by certifying organizations (Manthous, 2004). Although the evolution of critical care for obstetrical patients has generally followed these developments, there are no specific guidelines for

TABLE 42–2 Guidelines from the American College of Critical Care Medicine (1998) of Conditions That Could Qualify for Intermediate Care

Cardiac: rule out infarction, stable infarction, stable arrhythmias, mild-to-moderate congestive heart failure, hypertensive urgency without end-organ damage

Pulmonary: stable patients for weaning or chronic ventilation, patients with potential for respiratory failure who are hemodynamically stable

Neurological: stable central nervous system, neuromuscular, or neurosurgical conditions that require close monitoring

Drug overdose: hemodynamically stable

Gastrointestinal: stable bleeding, liver failure with stable vital signs

Endocrine: diabetic ketoacidosis, thyrotoxicosis that requires frequent monitoring

Surgical: postoperative major procedures or complications that require close monitoring

Miscellaneous: early sepsis, patients whose condition requires closely titrated intravenous fluids, severe preeclampsia or other medical problems in pregnant women

pregnant women. Thus, the tertiary care centers discussed above describe variations in ICU design, utilization rates, management, and outcomes.

Because of high costs incurred by ICUs, a step-down *intermediate care unit* was developed. This type of unit was designed to include patients who did not require intensive care per se but who needed a higher level of care than that provided on a general ward. In 1998, the American College of Critical Care Medicine and the Society of Critical Care Medicine published guidelines for care of critically ill patients in intermediate care units (Table 42–2). By that time, most referral centers had already incorporated these concepts of a "step-down unit," although this was not formally assessed for obstetrical patients.

At Parkland Hospital, the present system of an intermediate care unit for critically ill pregnant women has evolved over the past three decades. The two-tiered system incorporates the guidelines for intermediate and intensive care described for nonobstetrical patients. The results of an audit of this unit for 1998 to 1999 were described by Zeeman and colleagues (2003). The reasons for admission to the unit during these 2 years are listed in Table 42–1. Of these women, about 20 percent were undelivered. Because they remain in the obstetrical suite, their care is provided by specially trained obstetricians and obstetrical nurses with experience in critical care medicine. If not available, a team of physicians and nurses should be assembled that includes clinicians with special expertise sufficient to deal with all problem areas. Team members typically include obstetricians, anesthesiologists, pulmonologists, cardiologists, and other intensivists.

Institutional capabilities as well as frequency and acuity of obstetrical complications determine the need for critical care. Only a few institutions can satisfy requirements for a full-service obstetrical ICU. Most tertiary care centers have instead developed intermediate care units with selected triage to other ICUs. The vast majority of smaller hospitals are not able to fulfill the requirements for an obstetrical intermediate care unit. In these instances, transfer to a medical or surgical ICU is preferable, but there must be close collaboration between obstetricians and intensivists with other specialists.

PULMONARY ARTERY CATHETER USE. In our extensive experience, invasive hemodynamic monitoring is seldom necessary for critically ill obstetrical patients. A few women who have multiple and complex problems may sometimes be better managed with such monitoring. An example is sepsis complicated by pulmonary edema and persistent hypotension. Use of pulmonary catheter monitoring is controversial. Some studies have shown excess morbidity and mortality because of its use. Two recent randomized trials of 2670 medical and surgical patients described no benefits but no excessive morbidity (Richard and co-workers, 2003; Sandham and colleagues, 2003). Some of its uses in obstetrics and its methodology are described in detail by Clark and colleagues (1997).

Pulmonary artery catheterization has been used in a number of cardiac or pulmonary conditions complicating pregnancy. Information from these has contributed immensely to understanding of some common obstetrical conditions. These include myocardial infarction, cardiomyopathy, and mitral stenosis; acute respiratory distress syndrome (ARDS); amnionic fluid embolism; and severe preeclampsia–eclampsia (Clark, 1988, 1995, 1997; Cunningham, 1986, 1987; Hankins, 1984, 1985, and all their co-workers). The most enthusiastically perceived needs for invasive monitoring are for women with severe preeclampsia–eclampsia (Gilbert and associates, 2000). We remain unconvinced that this is justified for most cases. Ironically, with better understanding of underlying pathophysiology that has been provided by invasive monitoring, the need for its use has declined.

Measurement. The use of a pulmonary artery catheter allows measurement of pulmonary arterial pressures and filling pressures, including central venous and pulmonary capillary wedge pressures. Formulas for deriving various cardiopulmonary parameters are shown in Table 42–3. Cardiac output, stroke volume, and systemic and pulmonary vascular resistance can be corrected for body size by dividing by body surface area to obtain *index values*. Nomograms for nonpregnant adults are used.

In a landmark investigation, Clark and colleagues (1989) obtained cardiovascular measurements in healthy pregnant women and again in these same women when they were not pregnant, so that they served as their own controls (Table 42–4). These investigators showed that ventricular performance remains unchanged during pregnancy from the nonpregnant state because increased blood volume

TABLE 42–3 Formulas for Deriving Various Cardiopulmonary Parameters

MAP (mm Hg) = [SBP + 2(DBP)] ÷ 3
CO (L/min) = heart rate × stroke volume
SV (mL/beat) = CO/HR
SI (mL/beat/m²) = stroke volume/BSA
CI (L/min/m²) = CO/BSA
SVR (dynes × sec × cm⁻⁵) = [(MAP − CVP)/CO] × 80
PVR (dynes × sec × cm⁻⁵) = [(MPAP − PCWP)/CO] × 80
Lung compliance:

$$\text{Static} = \frac{\text{tidal volume}}{\text{plateau inspiratory pressure}}$$

$$\text{Dynamic} = \frac{\text{tidal volume}}{\text{peak inspiratory pressure}}$$

BSA = body surface area (m²); CI = cardiac index; CO = cardiac output (L/min); CVP = central venous pressure (mm Hg); DBP = diastolic blood pressure; HR = heart rate (beats/min); MAP = mean systemic arterial pressure (mm Hg); MPAP = mean pulmonary artery pressure (mm Hg); PCWP = pulmonary capillary wedge pressure (mm Hg); PVR = pulmonary vascular resistance; SBP = systolic blood pressure; SI = stroke index; SV = stroke volume; SVR = systemic vascular resistance.

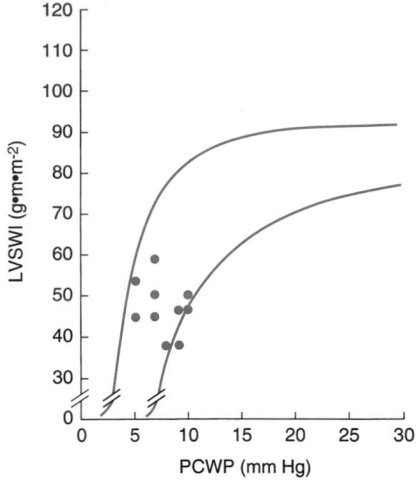

FIGURE 42–1. Ventricular function in 10 healthy pregnant women at term. Individual values are plotted and all but one fall between the lines that define normal function. (LVSWI = left ventricular stroke work index; PCWP = pulmonary capillary wedge pressure.) (Plotted data points from Clark and colleagues, 1989.)

and cardiac output are compensated by decreased vascular resistance and increased pulse rate (Fig. 42–1). A working knowledge of these changes is paramount to understanding the pathophysiology of pregnancy complications discussed throughout this book.

One important caveat regarding pulmonary artery monitoring emphasized by Van Hook and Hankins (1997): The information does not always reflect uteroplacental perfusion. Assessment of fetal status using sonography, biophysical testing, and heart rate patterns is used instead.

ACUTE PULMONARY EDEMA

The incidence of pulmonary edema complicating pregnancy averages about 1 in 500 to 1000 deliveries at tertiary referral centers. In obstetrics, the three general causes of acute pulmonary edema include:

1. Ventricular dysfunction (heart failure).
2. Permeability edema from alveolar–capillary injury or beta-mimetic tocolytic therapy.
3. Combination of these two problems.

Taken in toto, studies in pregnant women indicate that more than half who develop pulmonary edema have some degree of sepsis syndrome in conjunction with either tocolysis or vigorous fluid therapy. Cardiogenic pulmonary edema is identified in about half. In many women, obstetrical hemorrhage with resuscitation or vigorous treatment for preterm labor are common precipitating causes.

Sciscione and colleagues (2003) reported that among 51 cases of pulmonary edema, about 25 percent each were due to cardiac failure, tocolytic therapy, iatrogenic fluid overload, or preeclampsia. DiFederico and associates (1998) reported that 40 percent of 84 cases from the University of California, San Francisco, were associated with tocolytic therapy for

TABLE 42–4 Central Hemodynamic Changes in Normal Women When Nonpregnant Compared with Term Pregnancy

Measurement	Nonpregnant	Term Pregnant	Change (%)
Cardiac output (L/min)	4.3 ± 0.9	6.2 ± 1.0	+44
Heart rate (beats/min)	71.0 ± 10.0	83.0 ± 10.0	+17
Mean arterial pressure (mm Hg)	86.4 ± 7.5	90.3 ± 5.8	+4
Systemic vascular resistance (dynes/cm/sec⁻⁵)	1530 ± 520	1210 ± 266	−21
Pulmonary vascular resistance (dynes/cm/sec⁻⁵)	199.0 ± 47	78.0 ± 22	−35
Pulmonary capillary wedge pressure (mm Hg)	6.3 ± 2.1	7.5 ± 1.8	+18
Central venous pressure (mm Hg)	3.7 ± 2.6	3.6 ± 2.5	−2
Left ventricular stroke work index (g/m/m⁻²)	41.0 ± 8	48.0 ± 6	+17
Colloid oncotic pressure (mm Hg)	20.8 ± 1.0	18.0 ± 1.5	−14
Colloid oncotic/wedge pressure gradient (mm Hg)	14.5 ± 2.5	10.5 ± 2.7	−28

From Clark and colleagues, 1989, with permission.

preterm labor or fetal surgery. The importance of tocolytic therapy cannot be understated. It caused 15 percent of cases of pulmonary edema and one maternal death in 51 women who required tracheal intubation and assisted ventilation (Jenkins and colleagues, 2003).

HEART FAILURE. Most cases of cardiogenic pulmonary edema during pregnancy are due to diastolic heart failure caused by chronic hypertension and obesity leading to left ventricular hypertrophy (Jessup and Brozena, 2003; Kencha-iah and colleagues, 2002). Other cases are caused by congenital or acquired anatomical defects as discussed in Chapter 44. In many instances, heart failure is precipitated acutely by superimposed preeclampsia, excessive blood loss, anemia, and puerperal sepsis (Cunningham and associates, 1986; Sibai and colleagues, 1987).

ACUTE RESPIRATORY DISTRESS SYNDROME. The most common cause of respiratory failure in pregnancy is ARDS. This pathophysiological manifestation of acute lung injury is a continuum from mild pulmonary insufficiency to dependence on mechanical ventilation. Because there are no uniform criteria for diagnosis of ARDS, its incidence is variably reported. In a review, Catanzarite and associates (2001) computed it to be about 1 in 3000 to 6000 deliveries. Severe disease requiring ventilatory support has a mortality rate of about 50 percent for all persons. It is as high as 90 percent if caused or complicated by sepsis. Although they are younger and healthier than the overall population, pregnant women still have mortality of 25 to 40 percent (Catanzarite and co-workers, 2001; Perry and colleagues, 1996).

Definitions. Physiological criteria required for diagnosis of ARDS differ, but clinically it is important to remember that the spectrum is wide. For research purposes, most investigators define ARDS as radiographic pulmonary infiltrates, a ratio of arterial oxygen tension to the fraction of inspired oxygen (Pao_2:Fio_2) of less than 200 mm Hg, and no evidence of heart failure (Ware and Matthay, 2000; Weg and colleagues, 1998). For clinical purposes, however, a working diagnosis is used when the Pao_2:Fio_2 ratio is higher in the face of pulmonary infiltrates seen on radiograph.

Pathophysiology. Again, ARDS is a pathophysiological diagnosis. With acute lung injury from a variety of causes, there is recruitment of neutrophils to the site of inflammation by chemokines. As neutrophils accumulate, they initiate further tissue injury by their cytokine secretion. Although there is widespread injury to microvascular endothelium, including the pulmonary vasculature, there is also alveolar epithelial injury. These result in increased pulmonary capillary permeability, surfactant loss or inactivation, diminished lung volume, and vascular shunting with resultant arterial hypoxemia. The second phase of the syndrome usually begins 3 to 4 days later. It involves development of *fibrosing alveolitis* and subsequent repair. The long-term prognosis

TABLE 42–5 Some Causes of Acute Lung Injury and Respiratory Failure in Pregnant Women

• Pneumonia
   Bacterial
   Viral
   Aspiration
	• Embolism
	   Amnionic fluid
	   Trophoblastic disease
	   Air

• Sepsis
   Chorioamnionitis
   Pyelonephritis
   Puerperal infection
   Septic abortion
	• Connective tissue disease
	• Substance abuse
	• Irritant inhalation and burns

• Hemorrhage
   Shock
   Massive transfusion
   Transfusion-related acute
     lung injury (TRALI)
	• Pancreatitis
	• Pheochromocytoma
	• Drug overdose

• Preeclampsia–eclampsia	

From Bhagwanjee (2000), Catanzarite (2001), Clark (1997), Cunningham (1987), Jenkins (2003), Kopko (2002), Mattar and Sibai (2000), Perry (1996), and all of their associates.

for pulmonary function is surprisingly good (Herridge and colleagues, 2003). The subject was reviewed by Ware and Matthay (2000).

Etiology. A number of disorders have been associated with acute pulmonary injury and permeability edema during pregnancy (Table 42–5). Although many are coincidental, some are unique to pregnancy. For all patients, sepsis and diffuse infectious pneumonia are the two most common single-agent causes. In combination, they account for 60 percent of cases. Antepartum pyelonephritis, intrapartum chorioamnionitis, and puerperal pelvic infection are frequent causes of obstetrical sepsis. Severe preeclampsia, aspiration, and obstetrical hemorrhage are also commonly found (see Table 42–5). Importantly, more than half of these women have some combination of sepsis, shock, trauma, and fluid overload. The latter is exacerbated by tocolytic therapy, which Amon and associates (2000) reported to have a 5-percent incidence of pulmonary edema. Thus, multiplicity of causes is the rule with acute and severe lung injury. The contribution, if any, of *transfusion-related acute lung injury (TRALI)* as described by Kopko and colleagues (2002), is not known at this time (see Chap. 35, p. 842).

Clinical Course. With pulmonary injury, the clinical condition depends largely on the magnitude of the insult, the ability to compensate for it, and the stage of the disease. For example, if the woman presents soon after the initial injury, there commonly are no physical findings except perhaps hyperventilation. In addition, arterial oxygenation usually is adequate. Pregnancy-induced mild metabolic alkalosis may be accentuated by hyperventilation. With continuing insult, clinical and radiological evidence for pulmonary pathology becomes more obvious. Decreased lung compliance and increased intrapulmonary blood shunting are now apparent. Progressive

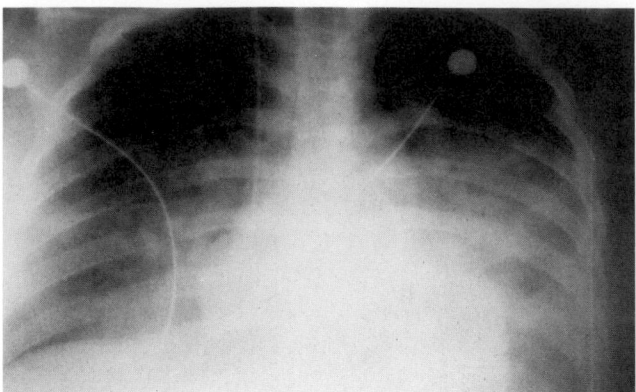

FIGURE 42–2. Severe acute respiratory distress syndrome with diffuse infiltrates. (Courtesy of Dr. Michael Landay.)

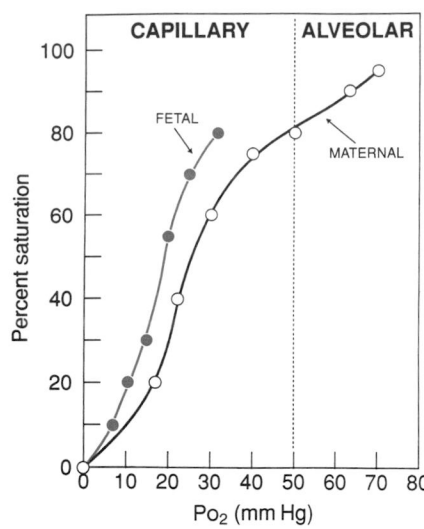

FIGURE 42–3. Oxyhemoglobin dissociation curve. With higher oxygen tension (PaO_2) in the pulmonary alveoli, adult hemoglobin is maximally saturated compared with that at the lower oxygen tension at the tissue capillary level. At any given oxygen tension, fetal hemoglobin carries more oxygen than adult hemoglobin, as indicated by percent saturation.

alveolar and interstitial edema develop along with extravasation of inflammatory cells and erythrocytes.

Ideally, pulmonary injury is identified at this early stage, with specific therapy directed at the insult if possible. Further progression may result in acute respiratory failure characterized by marked dyspnea, tachypnea, and hypoxemia. Further loss of lung volume results in worsening of pulmonary compliance and increased intrapulmonary shunting. There are now diffuse abnormalities by auscultation and the chest radiograph characteristically demonstrates bilateral lung involvement (Fig. 42–2). At this phase, injury has progressed to a point that ordinarily is lethal in the absence of high inspired-oxygen concentrations. Positive airway pressure, whether by mask or by intubation, may now also be necessary at this stage for airspace recruitment. When shunting exceeds 30 percent, severe refractory hypoxemia develops along with metabolic and respiratory acidosis that can result in myocardial irritability, dysfunction, and cardiac arrest.

Management. In acute and severe lung injury, attempts are made to provide adequate oxygenation of peripheral tissues while ensuring that therapeutic maneuvers do not further aggravate lung injury. At least intuitively, increasing oxygen delivery should produce a corresponding increase in tissue uptake, but this is difficult to measure (Evans and Smithies, 1999). Support of systemic perfusion with intravenous crystalloid and blood is imperative (see Chap. 35, p. 839). Sepsis is commonplace in lung injury, and vigorous antimicrobial therapy is given for infection. Three critical points merit emphasis:

1. Oxygen delivery is directly proportional to cardiac output.
2. The overwhelming majority of transported oxygen is bound to hemoglobin. Accordingly, oxygen delivery can be greatly improved by correction of anemia because each gram of hemoglobin carries 1.25 mL of oxygen when 90 percent saturated.

3. Increasing the arterial PO_2 from 100 to 200 mm Hg results in the transport of only 0.1 mL of additional oxygen for each 100 mL of blood.

Reasonable goals in caring for the woman with severe lung injury are to obtain a PaO_2 of 60 mm Hg or 90-percent saturation at an inspired oxygen content of less than 50 percent, along with positive end-expiratory pressures less than 15 mm Hg. It remains controversial whether delivery will improve maternal oxygenation (Jenkins and co-workers, 2003; Tomlinson and colleagues, 1998).

OXYHEMOGLOBIN DISSOCIATION CURVE. The propensity of the hemoglobin molecule to release oxygen is described by the oxyhemoglobin dissociation curve. Simplistically, the curve can be divided into an upper oxygen association curve representing the alveolar–capillary environment and a lower oxygen dissociation portion representing the tissue capillary environment (Fig. 42–3). Shifts of the curve have their greatest impact at the steep portion because they affect oxygen delivery. A rightward shift is associated with decreased hemoglobin affinity for oxygen and hence increased tissue–capillary oxygen interchange. Rightward shifts are produced by hypercapnia, metabolic acidosis, fever, and increased 2,3-diphosphoglycerate levels. During pregnancy, the erythrocyte concentration of 2,3-diphosphoglycerate is increased by approximately 30 percent. This favors oxygen delivery to both the fetus and peripheral maternal tissues (Rorth and Bille-Brahe, 1971).

Fetal hemoglobin has a higher oxygen affinity than adult hemoglobin, and its curve is positioned to the left of the adult curve (see Fig. 42–3). To achieve 50-percent hemoglobin saturation in the mother, the Pao_2 must be 27 mm Hg compared with only 19 mm Hg in the fetus. Under normal physiological conditions, the fetus is constantly on the dissociation, or tissue, portion of the curve. Even with severe maternal lung disease and very low Pao_2 levels, oxygen displacement to fetal tissues is favored. This has been confirmed by studies of pregnant women and their fetuses at high altitude, where despite a maternal Pao_2 of only 60 mm Hg, the fetal Pao_2 as is equivalent to that at sea level (Subrevilla and colleagues, 1971).

MECHANICAL VENTILATION. In some patients, positive pressure ventilation by face mask may be effective in early stages of pulmonary insufficiency (Wyncoll and Evans, 1999). In an attempt to maximize fetal environment, early intubation is preferred in the pregnant woman if respiratory failure appears to be imminent. Mechanical ventilation is adjusted to obtain a Pao_2 greater than 60 mm Hg, or a hemoglobin saturation of 90 percent and a $Paco_2$ of 35 to 45 mm Hg. Lower levels for Pao_2 should be avoided, because placental perfusion may be impaired (Levinson and co-workers, 1974).

Jenkins and associates (2003) reported their experiences with 51 women who required mechanical ventilation. Almost half had severe preeclampsia. Most were intubated postpartum, but 11 were delivered while being ventilated. Another six improved and were discharged undelivered. Of these 51 pregnancies, there were seven maternal deaths (14 percent). Importantly, one woman died as a complication of tocolytic treatment. Schneider and colleagues (2003) described 53 women who were delivered while receiving ventilatory support. The maternal mortality rate was 17 percent. In another report, Chen and co-workers (2003) reported four maternal deaths among 16 pregnant women who required mechanical ventilation. None of these investigators concluded that delivery improved maternal outcome.

POSITIVE END-EXPIRATORY PRESSURE. With severe lung injury and high intrapulmonary shunt fractions, it may not be possible to provide adequate oxygenation with usual ventilatory pressures, even with 100-percent oxygen. Positive end-expiratory pressure is usually successful in decreasing the shunt by recruiting collapsed alveoli. At low levels (e.g., 5 to 15 mm Hg), positive pressure can usually be used safely. At the higher levels, right-sided venous return can be impaired, resulting in decreased cardiac output and decreased uteroplacental circulation. High levels can also result in overdistention of alveoli, falling compliance, and barotrauma.

FLUID THERAPY. Treatment requires detailed attention to fluid balance, because fluid overload further compromises pulmonary status (Wyncoll and Evans, 1999). Intake and output records should be supplemented with daily weights. Mechanically ventilated patients retain an extra liter of fluid daily. Because respiratory distress syndrome is characterized by a pulmonary permeability defect, fluid leaks into the interstitium, even at normal pressures. Thus, it is best to maintain the lowest pulmonary capillary wedge pressure possible while avoiding decreased cardiac output.

Some pregnancy-induced physiological changes may predispose the woman to greater risk of permeability edema from fluid therapy. Colloid oncotic pressure (COP) is determined by serum albumin concentration, and 1 g/dL exerts about 6 mm Hg pressure. As discussed in Chapter 5 (see p. 140), serum albumin concentrations normally decrease in pregnancy. This results in a continuous decline in COP across normal pregnancy—from 28 mm Hg in the nonpregnant woman to 23 mm Hg at term (Robertson, 1969). There is a further decline to 17 mm Hg in the puerperium (Benedetti and Carlson, 1979). In women with preeclampsia, endothelial leakage causes extravascular albumin loss, and oncotic pressure is only 16 mm Hg antepartum and 14 mm Hg postpartum (Zinaman and co-workers, 1985). These changes have a significant clinical impact on the *colloid oncotic pressure/wedge pressure gradient*. Normally, this gradient exceeds 8 mm Hg, however, when it is 4 mm Hg or less, there is an increased risk for pulmonary edema.

OTHER THERAPY. After promising preliminary data on *artificial or replacement surfactant therapy*, Anzueto and colleagues (1996) found no benefits in 725 patients with sepsis-induced lung failure. In two subsequent studies, inhalation of *nitric oxide* caused early improvement, but mortality was unchanged (Taylor and co-workers, 2004; Wyncoll and Evans, 1999). In a small preliminary study, *prolonged methylprednisolone* therapy begun in patients with no improvement by day 7 demonstrated improved lung function and reduced mortality (Meduri and associates, 1998). Using an animal model, Imai and co-workers (2003) reported that a "protective" strategy using low tidal volumes and high end-expiratory pressure protected against end-organ epithelial apoptosis in the kidney and small intestine.

Other specific therapies under current investigation include *immunotherapy* with anti-CD blocking antibodies, *lipid mediator antagonists* to arachidonic acid, and *antioxidants* (Clark and colleagues, 1997).

SEPSIS SYNDROME

The sepsis syndrome is induced by a systemic inflammatory response to bacteria or their by-products such as endotoxins or exotoxins (Fig. 42–4). Infections that most commonly cause the sepsis syndrome in obstetrics are antepartum pyelonephritis (see Chap. 48, p. 1096), chorioamnionitis and puerperal sepsis (see Chap. 31, 712), septic abortion (see Chap. 9, p. 247), and necrotizing fasciitis (see Chap. 31, p. 720). In over 4000 nonpregnant patients, the mortality rate at 28 days was 30 to 40 percent with severe sepsis (Abraham and colleagues, 1997, 1998; Bernard and associates, 2001). When

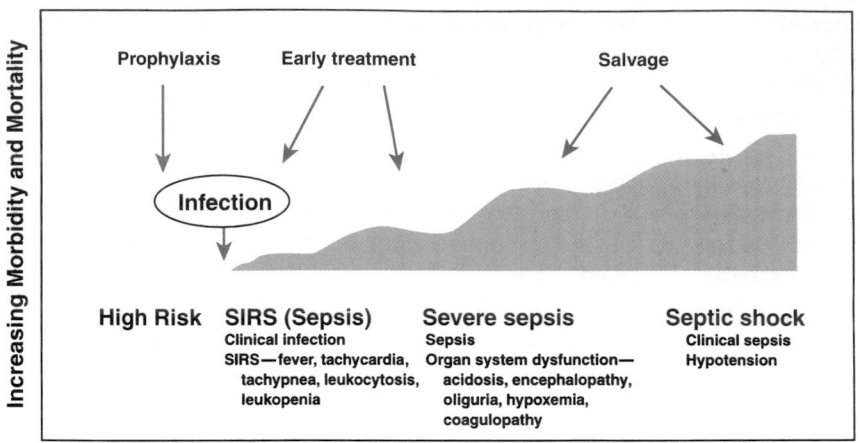

FIGURE 42–4. The sepsis syndrome begins with a systemic inflammatory response syndrome (SIRS) in response to infection that may progress to septic shock. (Courtesy Dr. Robert S. Munford.)

there is septic shock, mortality is greater regardless of the etiology. Mabie and associates (1997) reported 28-percent maternal mortality in 18 women.

ETIOPATHOGENESIS. The sepsis syndrome in obstetrics may be caused by any of a number of pathogens. Although pelvic infections are usually polymicrobial, bacteria that cause severe sepsis syndrome are frequently endotoxin-producing Enterobacteriaceae, most commonly *Escherichia coli.* Other pathogens are aerobic and anaerobic streptococci, *Bacteroides* species, and *Clostridium* species. Some group A β-hemolytic streptococci and *Staphylococcus aureus* produce virulent exotoxins that can rapidly cause all features of the sepsis syndrome (see Chap. 31, p. 713). Some virulent streptococci produce proteases that degrade IL-8 (Hidalgo-Grass and associates, 2004). In pyelonephritis, *E coli* and *Klebsiella* species commonly cause bacteremia and sepsis syndrome (Cunningham and associates, 1987; Mabie and colleagues, 1997).

Endotoxin is a lipopolysaccharide released on lysis of the cell wall of gram-negative bacteria. A number of potent bacterial *exotoxins* can also cause severe sepsis syndrome. Examples include exotoxins from *Clostridium perfringens*, toxic shock syndrome toxin from *S aureus,* and toxic shock–like exotoxin from group A β-hemolytic streptococci (Hoadley, 2002). As described by Nathan and colleagues (1993), these exotoxins cause rapid and extensive tissue necrosis and gangrene, especially of the postpartum uterus, and may cause profound cardiovascular collapse with maternal death (see Chap. 31, p. 721).

Sequelae of the sepsis syndrome begin with an inflammatory response that is directed against microbial endotoxins and exotoxins. Simply put, these and other toxins stimulate CD4 T cells to produce proinflammatory cytokines that include tumor necrosis factor-α (TNF-α) and interleukin-1 (IL-1) and IL-8. Neutrophils then adhere to endothelium and secrete a number of toxic substances such as proteases, oxidants, and cytokines. A myriad of cellular reactions follow

that include stimulation of pro- and anti-inflammatory compounds, procoagulant activity, gene activation, receptor regulation, and immune suppression (Hotchkiss and Karl, 2003; Wheeler and Bernard, 1999). It is likely that IL-6 mediates myocardial suppression (Pathan and associates, 2004).

The pathophysiological response to this cascade is selective vasodilation with maldistribution of blood flow and volume. Leukocyte and platelet aggregation cause capillary plugging. Vascular endothelial injury causes profound capillary leakage and interstitial fluid accumulation. Depending on the injury and inflammatory response, which are likely related to the virulence and dose of toxin, there is a spectrum of clinical response (see Fig. 42–4). Thus, sepsis syndrome is a clinical as well as pathophysiological continuum, the most severe result of which is *septic shock*. In its early stages, clinical shock results primarily from decreased systemic vascular resistance that is not compensated fully by increased cardiac output. Hypoperfusion results in lactic acidosis, decreased tissue oxygen extraction, and end-organ dysfunction. According to Schrier and Wang (2004), renal failure is common, and sepsis may cause *multiple organ failure* (Table 42–6).

HEMODYNAMIC CHANGES WITH SEPSIS. The pathophysiology of the sepsis syndrome has been elucidated by Parker (1987) and Parrillo (1990) and their colleagues from the National Institutes of Health. They observed that capillary leakage initially causes hypovolemia. If circulating volume is restored with intravenous crystalloid at this point, sepsis is a high cardiac output, low systemic vascular resistance condition. Concomitantly, pulmonary hypertension develops. This is often referred to as the *warm phase* of septic shock. These findings are the most common cardiovascular manifestations of early sepsis, and they often have prognostic significance. Paradoxically, despite the high cardiac output, patients with severe sepsis likely have myocardial depression (Ognibene and co-workers, 1988).

Most previously healthy pregnant women with sepsis at this stage respond well to fluid resuscitation, intensive

TABLE 42–6 Multiple Organ Effects with Sepsis and Shock

Central nervous system	
Cerebral	Confusion, somnolence, coma, combativeness
Hypothalamic	Fever, hypothermia
Cardiovascular	
Blood pressure	Hypotension (vasodilation)
Cardiac	Increased cardiac output with fluid replacement; myocardial depression with diminished cardiac output
Pulmonary	Shunting with dysoxia and hypoxemia; diffuse infiltrates from endothelial and epithelial damage
Gastrointestinal	Gastritis, toxic hepatitis, hyperglycemia
Renal	Hypoperfusion with oliguria; acute tubular necrosis
Hematological	Thrombocytopenia, leukocytosis, activation of coagulation

TABLE 42–7 Management of Obstetrical Sepsis Syndromes

Suspected sepsis
  Determine site if possible
  Rapid crystalloid infusion (2–4 L)
  Antimicrobial therapy
  Oxygen therapy
Sepsis with hypotension
  Continue crystalloid infusion
  Correct acidosis
  Excise infected tissue
    Curettage for septic abortion
    Debride wound infection
    Drain abscesses
  Monitor for organ dysfunction
    Blood pressure
    Urine output
    Mental status
    Respiratory insufficiency
    Skin perfusion
    Myocardial dysfunction
    Activation of coagulation
Severe sepsis
  Mechanical ventilation
  Support circulation
  Inotropics
  Vasopressors
  Consider pulmonary artery catheter

From Cunningham, 1998.

antimicrobial therapy, and if indicated, removal of infected tissue. Conversely, if hypotension is not corrected following vigorous fluid infusion, then the prognosis is more guarded. At this juncture, if there also is no response to β-adrenergic inotropic agents, this indicates severe and unresponsive extracellular fluid extravasation with vascular insufficiency, overwhelming myocardial depression, or both. Oliguria and continued peripheral vasoconstriction characterize a secondary, *cold phase* of septic shock, from which survival is uncommon. Another poor prognostic sign is continued renal, pulmonary, and cerebral dysfunction once hypotension has been corrected. The average risk of death increases by 15 to 20 percent with failure of each organ system (Wheeler and Bernard, 1999). If three systems are involved, mortality is 70 percent (Martin and colleagues, 2003).

DIAGNOSIS AND TREATMENT. Whenever serious bacterial infection is suspected, blood pressure and urine flow should be monitored closely. In obstetrics, whenever there is evidence of hypotension or oliguria, septicemia or hemorrhage should be immediately considered. When there is hypotension with sepsis syndrome, prompt and aggressive treatment is initiated. One treatment scheme is shown in Table 42–7. Rapid infusion with 2 L and sometimes as many as 4 to 6 L of crystalloid fluids may be required to restore renal perfusion in severely affected women. Because of the vascular leak, there is hemoconcentration. To combat this, blood is given along with crystalloid to maintain the hematocrit at about 30 percent (Rivers and colleagues, 2001). The use of colloid solution such as 5-percent human albumin is controversial (Clark and colleagues, 1997; Ware and Matthay, 2000). We do not recommend its use.

If aggressive volume replacement is not promptly followed by urinary output of at least 30 and preferably 50 mL/hr, as well as other indicators of improved perfusion, then consideration is given for vasoactive drug therapy. At this point, some clinicians opt for insertion of a pulmonary artery catheter. Mortality is high when sepsis is further complicated by respiratory or renal failure. With severe sepsis, damage to pulmonary capillary endothelium and alveolar epithelium causes alveolar flooding and pulmonary edema. This may occur even with low or normal pulmonary capillary wedge pressures. Management of *acute respiratory distress syndrome* is described on page 991.

Broad-spectrum antimicrobials are administered in maximal doses after appropriate cultures are taken. Appropriate empirical coverage results in better survival in severe sepsis (MacArthur and colleagues, 2004). Cultures of blood along with exudates that are not contaminated by normal flora are taken. For women with an infected abortion or deep fascial infections, a Gram-stained smear may be helpful in identifying *Clostridium perfringens* or group A streptococcal organisms. Generally, empirical coverage with regimens such as ampicillin plus gentamicin plus clindamycin suffices for pelvic infections (see Chap. 31, p. 714).

Surgical Treatment. Continuing sepsis may prove fatal, and debridement of necrotic tissue or drainage of purulent material is crucial. Of 18 pregnant women with septic shock, Mabie and colleagues (1997) reported that eight required surgical therapy to control the source of infection. A meticulous search is made for such foci. For women with an infected abortion, the uterine contents must be removed promptly by curettage. Hysterectomy is seldom indicated unless gangrene has resulted.

For women with pyelonephritis, continuing sepsis often is from urinary obstruction caused by calculi or a perinephric or intrarenal phlegmon or abscess. Renal sonography or "one-shot" pyelography may be used to diagnose obstruction and calculi, whereas computed tomography (CT) may be helpful to diagnose a phlegmon or abscess. With obstruction, ureteral catheterization, percutaneous nephrostomy, or flank exploration may be lifesaving (see Chap. 48, p. 1098).

Most cases of puerperal sepsis are clinically manifested in the first several days postpartum, and tissue debridement is not usually indicated this early. There are several exceptions to this:

1. Necrotizing fasciitis of the episiotomy site or abdominal surgical incision. As described by Gallup and colleagues (2002), this is a surgical emergency, and aggressive management is discussed in Chap. 31 (see p. 720).
2. Massive uterine myonecrosis caused by group A β-hemolytic streptococcal infections. The mortality rate in these women is high, and prompt hysterectomy may be lifesaving (Mabie and co-workers, 1997; Nathan and colleagues, 1993). Other virulent organisms can produce similar findings (Clad and associates, 2003).
3. Persistent or aggressive uterine infection with necrosis and dehiscence of the uterine incision with severe peritonitis. **Any woman with infection following cesarean delivery who is suspected of having peritonitis should be carefully evaluated for uterine incisional necrosis or bowel perforation.** Prompt surgical exploration, and frequently hysterectomy, must be done. CT of the pelvis is useful to characterize these infections. Overwhelming chorioamnionitis and sepsis caused by a gas-forming *E coli* and which required hysterectomy has been reported (Catanzarite and associates, 1994).
4. Peritonitis and sepsis much less commonly may result from a ruptured parametrial, intra-abdominal, or ovarian abscess (see Chap. 31, p. 718).

Adjunctive Therapy

PRESSOR AGENTS. Vasoactive drugs are not given unless aggressive fluid treatment fails to correct hypotension and perfusion abnormalities. One commonly used agent is dopamine hydrochloride, which when given in doses of 2 to 10 μg/kg/min stimulates cardiac α-receptors to increase cardiac output. Doses of 10 to 20 μg/kg/min cause β-receptor stimulation, an increase in systemic vascular resistance, and an increase in blood pressure. At doses of more than 20 μg/kg/min, α-receptor stimulation predominates, but dopamine is seldom needed at these higher doses. If there is no response to dopamine, then dobutamine, 5 to 15 μg/kg/min, or norepinephrine, 5 to 20 μg/min, may be of benefit (Wheeler and Bernard, 1999).

OXYGENATION AND VENTILATION. Oxygen is administered in an attempt to improve tissue oxygenation. As the septic shock syndrome progresses and intravascular volume is restored, there may be substantive pulmonary capillary endothelial damage with leakage into alveoli. Resultant pulmonary edema causes hypoxemia, which worsens tissue hypoxia and acidosis. When this is severe and adequate oxygenation cannot be maintained by increased oxygen delivered via a nonrebreathing mask or by a continuous positive airway pressure mask, then tracheal intubation and mechanical ventilation that delivers positive pressure may prove to be lifesaving (see p. 993).

ANTI-INFLAMMATORY AGENTS. Serum cortisol levels are typically elevated in sepsis and higher levels are associated with increased mortality (Sam and associates, 2004). Either high-dose *methylprednisolone* nor intravenous *ibuprofen* improved morbidity or mortality rates (Bernard and co-workers, 1997; Cronin and colleagues, 1995). Clinical studies of the nitric oxide synthase inhibitor, NG-methyl-L-arginine hydrochloride (546C88), indicated increased mortality rates over placebo despite improved cardiovascular status (Bakker, 2004; Lopez, 2004; Watson 2004, and all their colleagues).

ANTICOAGULANT THERAPY. Sepsis activates procoagulant production and causes microcirculatory obstruction; thus, a number of agents that block coagulation have been used for treatment. Both *antithrombin III* and *tissue factor pathway inhibitor* have been ineffective (Abraham and co-workers, 2003; Warren and colleagues, 2001). In a landmark study by Bernard and associates (2001), recombinant activated protein C was shown to improve 28-day mortality rates from sepsis. A major drawback is hemorrhage during infusion. Currently, the use of these anticoagulants seems justified with sepsis-related purpura fulminans (Dempfle, 2004).

IMMUNOTHERAPY. In general, immunotherapy for sepsis has been disappointing. Infusion of *antiendotoxin antibody* was found to have no benefits (French National Registry of HA-1A in Septic Shock, 1994). Similarly, *E5 murine monoclonal IgM antiendotoxin antibody* did not improve mortality (Angus and associates, 2000). *Anticytokine antibodies* and *competitive blockers of TNF-α binding* have also been used without benefit (Abraham and colleagues, 1997, 1998).

TRAUMA IN PREGNANCY

Trauma, homicide, and similar violent events are a leading cause of death in young women. As many as 10 to 20 percent of pregnant women suffer physical trauma (American College of Obstetricians and Gynecologists, 1998; Rickert and associates, 2003). Injury-related deaths are the most commonly identified cause of maternal morbidity in Cook County, Illinois; New York City; Maryland; Utah; and North Carolina (Dannenberg, 1995; Fildes, 1992; Harper and Parsons, 1997; Horon and Cheng, 2001; Jacob, 1998; and all their colleagues). In addition, in a California study of 4.8 million pregnancies by El Kady and co-workers (2003), almost 1 in 350 women were hospitalized for trauma.

Homicide of pregnant women is prevalent also. In a review of pregnancy-associated deaths, Frye (2001) concluded that 20 percent of maternal deaths were the result of murder. In a 10-city case-control study, McFarlane and associates (2002) found that 5 percent of female homicide victims were pregnant. By far, the most frequent form of trauma in pregnancy is from physical or sexual abuse, which commonly occurs because of domestic abuse or battering (Eisenstat and Bancroft, 1999).

BLUNT TRAUMA. Many forms of blunt trauma are encountered in pregnancy. Their common theme concerns immediate assessment of maternal effects of trauma, emergency treatment, and then evaluation of collateral effects on the fetus.

Physical Abuse. According to the U.S. Department of Justice, women who are 16 to 24 years of age have the highest per capita rates of intimate partner violence—19.4 per 1000 (Rennison and Welchans, 2000). It is estimated that 5 million women each year are physically assaulted by their male partners (American College of Obstetricians and Gynecologists, 1999). One goal in violence prevention for Healthy People 2010 is reduction of physical abuse directed at women by male partners.

Even more appalling is that pregnant women are not immune to this physical violence. Most supporting data have been accrued by public institutions. One third of injuries to pregnant women cared for at the University of Mississippi Medical Center were intentionally inflicted (Poole and colleagues, 1996). McFarlane and colleagues (1992) and Berenson and co-workers (1991) reported that almost a fourth of women attending public clinics had been physically or sexually abused during pregnancy. Cokkinides and colleagues (1999) found that 11 percent of 6000 pregnant women reported physical violence. This was linked to poverty, poor education, and use of tobacco and alcohol. Drug use is associated with half of instances in all battered women (Kyriacou and associates, 1999). Abuse during pregnancy places the woman at high risk for homicide during or after pregnancy (McFarlane and collaborators, 2002). Unfortunately, abused pregnant women tend to remain with their abusers, and 60 percent reported two or more episodes of physical assault during pregnancy (McFarlane and colleagues, 1992).

The woman who is physically abused tends to present late, if at all, for prenatal care. Occurrence of preterm labor and chorioamnionitis is increased twofold (Berenson and co-workers, 1994). There is also increased risk of low birthweight and cesarean delivery (Covington, 2001; Curry, 1998; Murphy, 2001, and all their associates). Another risk factor for adverse pregnancy outcomes is police-reported partner violence (Lipsky and colleagues, 2003).

SCREENING AND PREVENTION. Universal screening for *intimate partner violence* is not currently recommended by most researchers because its effectiveness is unknown (Wathen and MacMillan, 2003). Instead, a case-finding approach based on clinical suspicion is used. As discussed in Chapter 8 (see p. 210), the American College of Obstetricians and Gynecologists (1999) has provided screening methods for domestic violence and recommends their use at the initial prenatal visit, during each trimester, and at the time of postpartum follow-up.

Sexual Assault. According to the U.S. Department of Justice (2000), 17 percent of adult women will be sexually assaulted sometime during their lives. It is generally thought that only 10 to 20 percent of sexual assaults are reported. Satin and co-workers (1991), who reviewed over 5700 sexual assaults against women reported in Dallas County over 6 years, found that 2 percent of the victims were pregnant. Associated physical trauma occurs in about half of all women (Sugar and colleagues, 2004). In the Dallas Study, trauma was less common during pregnancy, and only one third of assaults took place after 20 weeks. From a forensic standpoint, evidence collection was not altered.

Satin and co-workers (1992) also interviewed 2404 women postpartum and found that the lifetime prevalence of forced sexual contact was 5 percent. Compared with nonvictims, rape victims had a higher incidence of sexually transmitted diseases, urinary infections, vaginitis, drug use, and multiple hospitalizations. Berenson and colleagues (1992) reported that 8 percent of pregnant adolescents had been sexually assaulted. In 46 percent of cases, the perpetrator was a member of the family and in 33 percent of cases, a spouse or boyfriend.

The importance of psychological counseling for the rape victim and her family cannot be overemphasized. In addition to attention to physical and psychological injuries, exposure to sexually transmitted diseases must be considered. The current recommendations for prophylaxis are shown in Table 42–8. If the woman is not pregnant, another very important aspect is emergency contraception as recommended by the American College of Obstetricians and Gynecologists (2001). This was recently reviewed by Westhoff (2003) and is discussed in detail in Chapter 32 (see p. 744).

Automobile Accidents. Between 1 and 3 percent of pregnant women are involved in motor vehicle accidents (Hyde and associates, 2003; Weiss and colleagues, 2002). Vehicular crashes are the most common causes of serious, life-threatening, or fatal blunt trauma during pregnancy

TABLE 42–8 Guidelines for Prophylaxis of Sexually Transmitted Disease in Victims of Sexual Assault

Prophylaxis	Regimen	Alternative
Neisseria gonorrhoeae	Ceftriaxone, 125 mg IM single dose	Cefixime, 400 mg po single dose, or Spectinomycin, 2 g IM single dose
Chlamydia trachomatis	Azithromycin, 1 g po single dose[a]	Erythromycin-base, 500 mg po qid × 7 days, or Amoxicillin, 500 mg po tid × 7 days
Trichomonas vaginalis	Metronidazole, 2 g po single dose[b]	
Hepatitis B virus	If not previously vaccinated, give first dose hepatitis vaccine, repeat at 1–2 and 4–6 months	
Human immunodeficiency virus	Consider retroviral prophylaxis if risk for HIV exposure is likely high	

[a]For nonpregnant women, doxycycline, 100 mg po for 7 days, can be given instead.
[b]Also effective for bacterial vaginosis.
From Centers for Disease Control and Prevention, 2002.

(Connolly and co-workers, 1997; Pak and colleagues, 1998). They are also the leading cause of traumatic fetal deaths (Weiss, 2001). Many of these deaths might be prevented with use of three-point restraints. Pearlman and associates (2000) found that proper seat belt use and crash severity were the best predictors of maternal–fetal outcome. Hyde and colleagues (2003) reported that fetal mortality was three times as great in women who were not wearing a seat belt. Importantly, Tyroch and associates (1999) reported that although 86 percent of pregnant women used restraints, almost 50 percent used them incorrectly.

Effects of deployment of airbags in pregnant drivers or passengers have not been widely studied. Sims and associates (1996) reported three third-trimester women whose driver-side airbag deployed in 10- to 25-mph collisions. They reported no injuries. Schultze and colleagues (1998) reported a 20-percent placental abruption that caused a stillborn 28-week fetus in a woman whose airbag deployed in a 40-mph collision. Even less is known about passenger-side bags or door bags (Moorcroft and co-workers, 2003).

Other Blunt Trauma. Some other common causes of blunt trauma are falls and aggravated assaults (Schiff and associates, 2002). In the California study by El Kady and co-workers (2004), intentionally afflicted injuries were present in about a third of pregnant women who were hospitalized for trauma. Less common are blast or crush injury (Awwad and co-workers, 1994a; Schoenfeld and colleagues, 1995). Serious intra-abdominal injuries are of particular concern. Probably related to the markedly increased pelvic and abdominal vascularity, retroperitoneal hemorrhage is encountered more commonly compared with that of nonpregnant women. Leggon and associates (2002) reviewed 101 pelvic fractures during pregnancy and found a 9-percent maternal and 35-percent fetal mortality rate. Conversely, bowel injuries are less frequent because of the protective effect of the large uterus. Diaphragmatic, splenic, liver, and kidney injuries may

also be sustained (Flick and colleagues, 1999; Icely and Chez, 1999).

Fetal Injury and Death. According to Kissinger and co-workers (1991), the risk of fetal death with trauma is significant when there is direct fetoplacental injury, maternal shock, pelvic fracture, maternal head injury, or hypoxia. In a 16-state review of fetal deaths due to trauma from 1995 through 1997, Weiss and associates (2001) found that motor vehicle crashes caused 82 percent. There was placental injury in almost 50 percent of cases and uterine rupture in 4 percent.

Although fetal injury and death are uncommon, there are many interesting case reports. Fetal skull and brain injury are most common. These injuries are more likely if the head is engaged and the maternal pelvis is fractured on impact (Palmer and Sparrow, 1994). Conversely, fetal head injuries, presumably from a *contrecoup* effect, may be sustained in unengaged vertex or nonvertex presentations. Weyerts and colleagues (1992) described a newborn with paraplegia and contractures associated with a motor vehicle accident sustained several months before birth.

Placental Abruption and Uterine Rupture. Two uniquely catastrophic events can occur with blunt trauma during pregnancy—placenta abruption and uterine rupture. These two conditions often are life-threatening to both mother and fetus. A third catastrophic event is a placental tear or "fracture" that can result in fetal hemorrhage and exsanguination, either into the amnionic sac or as fetomaternal hemorrhage.

TRAUMATIC PLACENTAL ABRUPTION. Placental separation is likely caused by deformation of the elastic myometrium around the relatively inelastic placenta (Crosby and associates, 1968). Some degree of abruption complicates 1 to 6 percent of "minor" injuries and up to 50 percent of "major" injuries (Goodwin and Breen, 1990; Pearlman and co-workers, 1990; Schiff and associates, 2002). In one study,

Reis and colleagues (2000) reported that abruption was more likely if the car was exceeding 30 mph.

Findings with traumatic abruption may be similar to those for spontaneous placental abruption discussed in Chapter 35 (see p. 811), although the causes of the two conditions are dissimilar. This is not universal, however, and Kettel and co-workers (1988) emphasized that traumatic abruption may be occult and not associated with uterine pain, tenderness, and bleeding. Stettler and associates (1992) reviewed our experiences with 13 such women at Parkland Hospital and reported that although 11 had uterine tenderness, only five had vaginal bleeding. Thus, because traumatic abruption is more likely to be concealed, the incidence of associated coagulopathy is higher than with spontaneously occurring abruption. Other common findings are uterine contractions; evidence of fetal compromise such as fetal tachycardia, late decelerations, and acidosis; and fetal death.

In women with partial separation, abruption may not be so obvious. According to Pearlman and associates (1990), detection of uterine contractile activity using electronic monitoring was suggestive of abruption. If contractions are fewer than every 10 minutes during 4 hours of monitoring, an abruption is most unlikely. Women with contractions of greater frequency, however, have a 20 percent chance of an abruption. If tocolytics are used, they may obfuscate these findings.

UTERINE RUPTURE. Blunt trauma results in uterine rupture in less than 1 percent of severe cases (American College of Obstetricians and Gynecologists, 1998). Rupture is more likely in a previously scarred uterus and is usually associated with a direct impact of substantive force. Decelerative forces following a 25-mph collision can generate up to 500 mm Hg of intrauterine pressure in a properly restrained woman (Crosby and associates, 1968). Findings may be identical to those for placental abruption with an intact uterus, and maternal and fetal deterioration are soon inevitable. Pearlman and Cunningham (1996) described uterine fundal "blow out" with fetal decapitation in a 20-week pregnancy following a high-speed collision. If the fetus is dead, it may be particularly difficult to diagnose uterine rupture, although Dash and Lupetin (1991) were able to do so in a 24-week pregnancy by using CT. In a case without rupture, Duplantier and colleagues (2002) described 180-degree uterine torsion at term.

Fetal–Maternal Hemorrhage. If there is considerable abdominal force associated with trauma, and especially if the placenta is lacerated, or "fractured," then life-threatening fetal–maternal hemorrhage may be encountered (Pritchard and associates, 1991). A small amount of fetal–maternal bleeding (less than 15 mL in 90 percent of cases) has been described in up to a third of trauma cases (Goodwin and Breen, 1990; Pearlman and associates, 1990). Massive fetal–maternal hemorrhage may coexist with traumatic abruption (Stettler and associates, 1992). Importantly, placental abruption per se is seldom associated with fetal–maternal

hemorrhage because there is no fetal bleeding into the intervillous space. Instead, fetal–maternal hemorrhage associated with trauma is caused by a placental tear or "fracture" caused by stretching of the inelastic placenta (Fig. 42–5).

PENETRATING TRAUMA. Knife and gunshot wounds are the most common penetrating injuries and may be associated with aggravated assaults, suicide attempts, or attempts to cause abortion. The incidence of maternal visceral injury with penetrating trauma is only 15 to 40 percent compared with 80 to 90 percent in nonpregnant individuals (Stone, 1999). When the uterus sustains penetrating wounds, the fetus is more likely than the mother to be seriously injured. Indeed, although the fetus sustains injury in two thirds of such cases, visceral injuries to the mother are seen in only 20 percent.

Awwad and colleagues (1994b) reported unique experiences with high-velocity penetrating wounds of the pregnant uterus collected during 16 years of civil war in Lebanon. Among 14 women, two died, but neither death was as a direct result of intra-abdominal injury. Three observations were made:

1. There were visceral injuries when the entrance wound was in either the upper abdomen or back.
2. When the entry wound site was anterior and below the uterine fundus, there were no visceral injuries in all six women.
3. Half the women had perinatal deaths due to either maternal shock, uteroplacental injury, or direct fetal injury.

MANAGEMENT OF TRAUMA. In general, the severity of injury is directly related to maternal and fetal outcomes (Schiff and colleagues, 2002). That said, severity scoring does not accurately predict significant morbidity and mortality related to placental abruption. Schiff and Holt (2002) evaluated 294 pregnant women hospitalized for injuries in Washington State from 1989 through 1997. The *injury severity score* was not accurate to predict adverse pregnancy outcomes, as relatively minor injuries were associated with placental abruption. Similarly, Biester and co-workers (1997) reported that the revised trauma score was not predictive of adverse pregnancy outcome.

With few exceptions, treatment priorities in injured pregnant women are directed as they would be in nonpregnant patients (Warner and colleagues, 2004). Primary goals are evaluation and stabilization of maternal injuries. Attention to fetal assessment during the acute evaluation may divert attention from life-threatening maternal injuries (American College of Obstetricians and Gynecologists, 1998). Basic rules are applied to resuscitation, including establishing ventilation and arrest of hemorrhage along with treatment for hypovolemia with crystalloid and blood products. **An important aspect of management is repositioning of the large uterus away from the great vessels to diminish its effect on decreased cardiac output.**

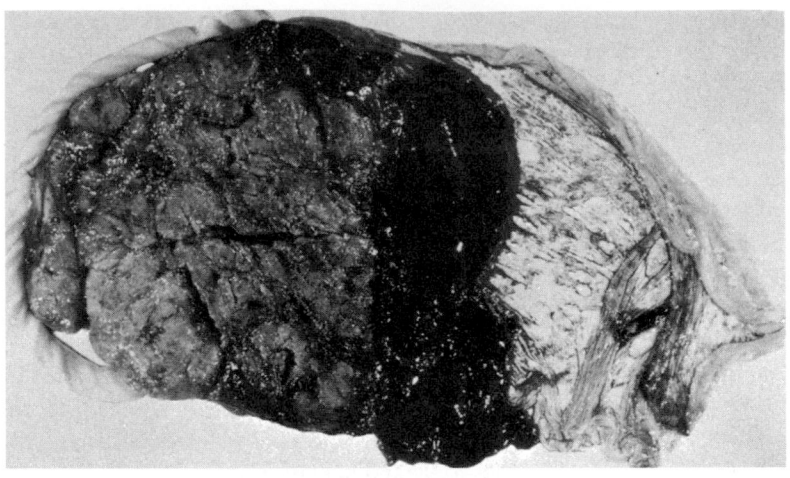

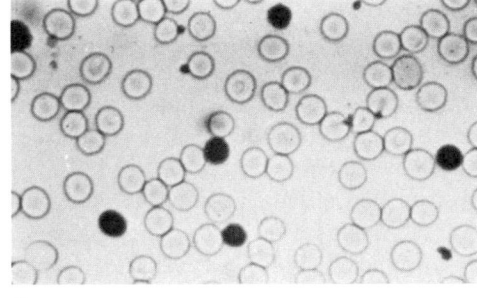

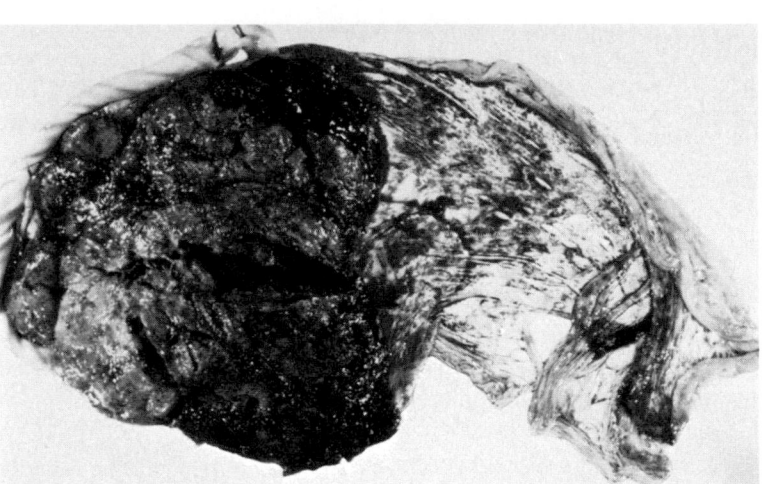

FIGURE 42–5. A. Partial placental abruption with adherent blood clot. The fetus died from massive hemorrhage, chiefly into the maternal circulation. **B.** The adherent blood clot has been removed. Note the laceration of the placenta. **C.** Kleihauer–Betke stain of a smear of maternal blood after fetal death. The dark cells that constituted 4.5 percent of peripheral cells are fetal in origin, whereas the empty cells are of maternal origin.

Following emergency resuscitation, evaluation is continued for fractures, internal injuries, bleeding sites, as well as placental, uterine, and fetal injuries. If indicated, open peritoneal lavage should be performed (Scorpio and colleagues, 1992). Penetrating injuries in most cases must be evaluated using radiography (see Chap. 41, p. 977). Because clinical response to peritoneal irritation is blunted during pregnancy, an aggressive approach to exploratory laparotomy is pursued for abdominal trauma. Whereas exploration is mandatory for abdominal gunshot wounds, some clinicians advocate close observation for selected stab wounds (Grubb, 1992).

Associated and sometimes delayed injuries can be bizarre. Hnat and colleagues (2003) described a woman who remained comatose throughout pregnancy from a closed-head injury in early gestation. Raymond and associates (2002) described a mother–fetus pair with chronic lead poisoning from an unremoved bullet lodged 15 years earlier!

Cesarean Delivery. The necessity for cesarean delivery of a live fetus depends on several factors. Laparotomy itself is not an indication for hysterotomy. Some considerations include gestational age, fetal condition, extent of uterine injury, and whether the large uterus hinders adequate treatment or evaluation of other intraabdominal injuries (Awwad and colleagues, 1994a).

Electronic Monitoring. As for many other acute or chronic maternal conditions, fetal well-being may reflect the status of the mother, and thus fetal monitoring is another "vital sign" that helps evaluate the extent of maternal injuries. Even if the mother is stable, electronic monitoring may be predictive of placental abruption. In the study cited on page 999, Pearlman and associates (1990) reported no abruptions if uterine contractions were less often than every 10 minutes within 4 hours after trauma was sustained. **Almost 20 percent of women who had contractions more frequently than every 10 minutes in the first 4 hours had an associated placental abruption.** In these cases, abnormal tracings were common and included fetal tachycardia and late decelerations. Connolly and co-workers (1997) reported no adverse outcomes in women who had normal monitor tracings.

Because placental abruption usually develops early following trauma, fetal monitoring is begun as soon as the mother is stabilized. The duration that post-trauma monitoring should be performed is not precisely known. According to Goodwin and Breen (1990), an observation period of 2 to 6 hours is sufficient if there are no other ominous signs such as contractions, uterine tenderness, or bleeding. Monitoring is continued as long as there are uterine contractions, a nonreassuring fetal heart pattern, vaginal bleeding, uterine tenderness or irritability, serious maternal injury, or ruptured membranes (American College of Obstetricians and Gynecologists, 1998). In very rare cases, abruptio placentae has developed days after trauma (Higgins and Garite, 1984).

Fetal–Maternal Hemorrhage. Routine use of the Kleihauer–Betke or an equivalent test in pregnant trauma victims is controversial (Pak and associates, 1998). It is unclear if their routine use will modify adverse outcomes associated with fetal anemia, cardiac arrhythmias, and death. In a retrospective review of 125 pregnant women with blunt injuries admitted to a level I trauma center, Towery and co-workers (1993) reported that the Kleihauer–Betke test had a sensitivity of 56 percent, a specificity of 71 percent, and an accuracy of 27 percent. The investigators concluded that the test was of little use with acute trauma management, and that electronic fetal monitoring or ultrasound, or both, are more useful in detecting fetal or pregnancy-associated complications. Dupre and associates (1993) reached similar conclusions, and although they found evidence for fetal–maternal hemorrhage in 22 percent of women studied, it was of no prognostic significance. Connolly and co-workers (1997) reached similar conclusions. In another study, however, Muench and colleagues (2003) reported that a Kleihauer-Betke test showing fetal cells of 0.1 percent or greater was predictive of preterm labor in women with blunt trauma.

For the woman who is D-negative, administration of anti-D immunoglobulin should be considered. This may be omitted if the test for fetal bleeding is negative. Isoimmunization may still develop if the fetal–maternal hemorrhage exceeds 15 mL of fetal cells.

Another important aspect of care for the pregnant trauma patient is to ensure that her tetanus immunization is current.

THERMAL INJURY. Although Parkland Hospital is a major burn center for the United States, we have not seen a large number of pregnant women with severe burns. Fetal progno-

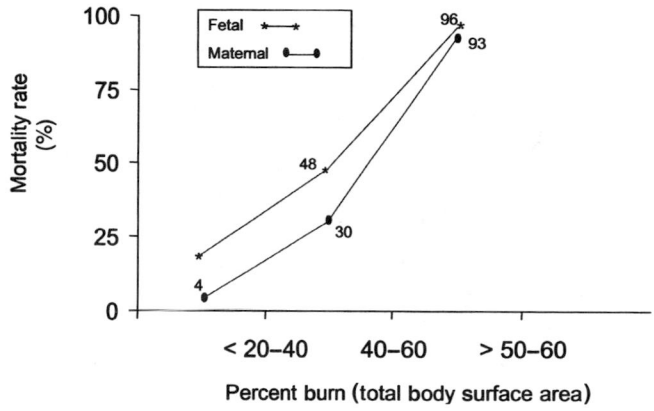

FIGURE 42–6. Maternal and fetal morbidity by burn severity in 162 women. (Data from Akhtar, 1994; Amy, 1985; Mabrouk and el-Feky, 1997; Rayburn, 1984; Rode, 1990, and all their colleagues.)

sis is poor with severe burns. Usually the woman enters labor spontaneously within a few days to a week, and often delivers a stillborn infant. Contributory factors are hypovolemia, pulmonary injury, septicemia, and the intensely catabolic state associated with burns.

Prognosis. In their review, Polko and McMahon (1998) concluded that pregnancy does not alter maternal outcome compared with that of nonpregnant women of similar age. A number of investigators have reported that maternal and fetal survival parallels the percentage of burned surface area. In the 162 pregnant burned women shown in Figure 42–6, as the burn area reaches or exceeds 50 percent, both maternal and fetal morbidity become formidable.

Skin Contractures. Following serious abdominal burns, skin contractures that develop may be painful during a subsequent pregnancy and may even necessitate surgical decompression and split skin autografts (Matthews, 1982). Widgerow and colleagues (1991) described two women in whom surgical release of contractures without covering the resulting defect was sufficient. McCauley and colleagues (1991) followed seven women with severe circumferential truncal burns sustained at a mean age of 7.7 years. All of 14 subsequent pregnancies were delivered at term without major complications. Loss or distortion of nipples may cause problems in breast feeding. Interestingly, normal abdominal tissue expansion due to pregnancy appears to be an excellent source for obtaining skin grafts postpartum to correct scar deformities at other body sites (Del Frari and colleagues, 2004).

ELECTRICAL SHOCK. Earlier case reports were suggestive of a high fetal mortality with electric shock (Fatovich, 1993). In a prospective cohort study, however, Einarson and colleagues (1997) showed similar perinatal outcomes in 31 exposed women compared with those of pregnant controls. They concluded that traditional 110-volt North American electrical current likely is less dangerous than 220-volt currents available in Europe. Sozen and Nesin (2004) described a woman with iliofemoral thrombosis at 29 weeks that *may* have been related to a mild electrical shock at 22 weeks. Koumbourlis (2002) has described the pathophysiological effects of electrical current and lightning injuries.

CARDIOPULMONARY RESUSCITATION

Cardiac arrest fortunately is rare during pregnancy. There are special considerations for cardiopulmonary resuscitation (CPR) conducted in the second half of pregnancy. In nonpregnant women, external chest compression results in a cardiac output of only 30 percent of normal (Clark and colleagues, 1997). Cardiac output may be even less in late pregnancy when uterine aortocaval compression may impede resuscitative efforts by diminishing forward flow as well as venous return. **Thus, uterine displacement is paramount to accompany other resuscitative efforts.** Left lateral displacement can be accomplished manually by a member of the team, by tilting the operating table laterally, by placing a wedge under the right hip, or by using the Cardiff resuscitation wedge. Rees and Willis (1988) showed with a manikin that resuscitation with the Cardiff wedge was as efficient as resuscitation in the supine position. If no equipment is available (e.g., in an out-of-hospital arrest), an individual kneels on the floor with the woman's back on the thighs to form a "human wedge" (Whitty, 2002).

Over the past few years, the recommendation by many authors is to perform cesarean delivery within 4 to 5 minutes of beginning CPR if the fetus is viable (Moise and Belfort, 1997). Certainly there is an inverse correlation between neurologically intact neonatal survival and the cardiac arrest-to-delivery interval in women delivered by perimortem cesarean. According to Clark and co-workers (1997), 98 percent of infants delivered within 5 minutes of arrest are neurologically intact. From 6 to 15 minutes it is 83 percent; from 16 to 25 minutes, 33 percent; and from 26 to 35 minutes, 25 percent. Based on theory and a few anecdotal case reports, delivery may also enhance maternal resuscitative efforts, which obviously must be continued throughout surgery and delivery (Finegold and colleagues, 2002). For all these reasons, the American College of Obstetricians and Gynecologists (1998) advises consideration for cesarean delivery in third-trimester pregnancy within 4 minutes of cardiac arrest. Unfortunately, as emphasized by Clark and associates (1997), and in our experiences, these goals rarely can be met in actual practice. Whitten and Irvine (2000) and Whitty (2002) have reviewed indications for postmortem and perimortem cesarean delivery.

REFERENCES

Abraham E, Anzueto A, Gutierrez G, et al: Double-blind randomised controlled trial of monoclonal antibody to human tumour necrosis factor in treatment of septic shock. Lancet 351:929, 1998

Abraham E, Glauser MP, Butler T, et al: p55 tumor necrosis factor receptor fusion protein in the treatment of patients with severe sepsis and septic shock. A randomized controlled multicenter trial. JAMA 277:1531, 1997

Abraham E, Reinhart K, Opal S, et al: Efficacy and safety of tifacogin (recombinant tissue factor pathway inhibitor) in severe sepsis: A randomized controlled trial. JAMA 290:238, 2003

Akhtar MA, Mulawkar PM, Kulkarni HR: Burns in pregnancy: Effect on maternal and fetal outcomes. Burns 20:351, 1994

American College of Critical Care Medicine and the Society of Critical Care Medicine: Guidelines on admission and discharge for adult intermediate care units. Guidelines/Practice Parameters Committee of the American College of Critical Care Medicine and the Society of Critical Care Medicine. Crit Care Med 26:607, 1998

American College of Obstetricians and Gynecologists: Emergency oral contraception. Practice Bulletin No. 25, March 2001

American College of Obstetricians and Gynecologists: Psychosocial risk factors: Perinatal screening and intervention. Educational Bulletin No. 255, November 1999

American College of Obstetricians and Gynecologists: Obstetric aspects of trauma management. Educational Bulletin No. 251, September 1998

Amon E, Midkiff C, Winn H, et al: Tocolysis with advanced cervical dilatation. Obstet Gynecol 95:358, 2000

Amy BW, McManus WF, Goodwin CW, et al: Thermal injury in the pregnant patient. Surg Gynecol Obstet 161:209, 1985

Angus DC, Birmingham MC, Balk RA, et al: E5 murine monoclonal antiendotoxin antibody in gram-negative sepsis: A randomized controlled trial. JAMA 283:1723, 2000

Anzueto A, Baughman RP, Guntupalli KK, et al: Aerosolized surfactant in adults with sepsis-induced acute respiratory distress syndrome. N Engl J Med 334:1417, 1996

Awwad JT, Azar GB, Aouad AT, et al: Postmortem cesarean section following maternal blast injury: Case report. J Trauma 36:260, 1994a

Awwad JT, Azar GB, Seoud MA, et al: High-velocity penetrating wounds of the gravid uterus: Review of 16 years of civil war. Obstet Gynecol 83:259, 1994b

Bakker J, Grover R, McLuckie A, et al: Administration of the nitric oxide synthase inhibitor NG-methyl-L-arginine hydrochloride (546C88) by intravenous infusion for up to 72 hours can promote the resolution of shock in patients with severe sepsis: Results of a randomized, double-blind, placebo-controlled multicenter study (study no. 144-002). Crit Care Med 32:1, 2004

Benedetti TJ, Carlson RW: Studies of colloid osmotic pressure in pregnancy-induced hypertension. Am J Obstet Gynecol 135:308, 1979

Berenson AB, San Miguel VV, Wilkinson GS: Prevalence of physical and sexual assault in pregnant adolescents. J Adolesc Health 13:466, 1992

Berenson AB, Stiglich NJ, Wilkinson GS, et al: Drug abuse and other risk factors for physical abuse in pregnancy among white non-Hispanic, black and Hispanic women. Am J Obstet Gynecol 164:1491, 1991

Berenson AB, Wiemann CM, Wilkinson GS, et al: Perinatal morbidity associated with violence experienced by pregnant women. Am J Obstet Gynecol 170:1760, 1994

Bernard GR, Vincent JL, Laterre PF, et al: Efficacy and safety of recombinant human activated protein C for severe sepsis. N Engl J Med 344:699, 2001

Bernard GR, Wheeler AP, Russell JA, et al: The effects of ibuprofen on the physiology and survival of patients with sepsis. N Engl J Med 336:912, 1997

Bhagwanjee S, Paruk F, Modley J, et al: Intensive care unit morbidity and mortality from eclampsia: An evaluation of the Acute

Physiology and Chronic Health Evaluation II score and the Glasgow Coma Scale score. Crit Care Med 28:120, 2000

Biester EM, Tomich PG, Esposito TJ, et al: Trauma in pregnancy: Normal Revised Trauma Score in relation to other markers of maternofetal status—a preliminary study. Am J Obstet Gynecol 176:1206, 1997

Catanzarite V, Schibanoff JM, Chinn R, et al: Overwhelming maternal sepsis due to a gas-forming *Escherichia coli* chorioamnionitis. Am J Perinatol 11:205, 1994

Catanzarite V, Willms D, Wong D, et al: Acute respiratory distress syndrome in pregnancy and the puerperium: Causes, courses, and outcomes. Obstet Gynecol 97:760, 2001

Centers for Disease Control and Prevention: Treatment guidelines. Sexually transmitted diseases. MMWR 51:1, 2002

Chen C-Y, Chen C-P, Wang K-G, et al: Factors implicated in the outcome of pregnancies complicated by acute respiratory failure. J Reprod Med 48:641, 2003

Clad A, Orlowska-Volk M, Karck U: Fatal puerperal sepsis with necrotising fasciitis due to *Streptococcus pneumoniae*. BJOG 110:213, 2003

Clark SL, Cotton DB: Clinical indications for pulmonary artery catheterization in the patient with severe preeclampsia. Am J Obstet Gynecol 158:453, 1988

Clark SL, Cotton DB, Hankins GDV, et al: Critical Care Obstetrics, 3rd ed. Boston, Blackwell Science, 1997

Clark SL, Cotton DB, Lee W, et al: Central hemodynamic assessment of normal term pregnancy. Am J Obstet Gynecol 161:1439, 1989

Clark SL, Hankins GD, Dudley DA, et al: Amniotic fluid embolism: Analysis of a national registry. Am J Obstet Gynecol 172:1158, 1995

Cokkinides VE, Coker AL, Sanderson M, et al: Physical violence during pregnancy: Maternal complications and birth outcomes. Obstet Gynecol 93:661, 1999

Connolly AM, Katz VL, Bash KL, et al: Trauma and pregnancy. Am J Perinatol 14:331, 1997

Covington DL, Hage M, Hall T, et al: Preterm delivery and the severity of violence during pregnancy. J Reprod Med 46:1031, 2001

Cronin L, Cook DJ, Carlet J, et al: Corticosteroid treatment for sepsis: A critical appraisal and meta-analysis of the literature. Crit Care Med 23:1430, 1995

Crosby WM, Snyder RG, Snow CC, et al: Impact injuries in pregnancy, 1. Experimental studies. Am J Obstet Gynecol 101:100, 1968

Cunningham FG: Sepsis syndromes. Contemp Ob/Gyn 43:13, 1998

Cunningham FG, Lucas MJ, Hankins GD: Pulmonary injury complicating antepartum pyelonephritis. Am J Obstet Gynecol 156:797, 1987

Cunningham FG, Pritchard JA, Hankins GDV, et al: Peripartum heart failure: A specific pregnancy-induced cardiomyopathy or the consequence of coincidental compounding cardiovascular events? Obstet Gynecol 67:157, 1986

Curry MA, Perrin N, Wall E: Effects of abuse on maternal complications and birth weight in adult and adolescent women. Obstet Gynecol 92:530, 1998

Dannenberg AL, Carter DM, Lawson HW, et al: Homicide and other injuries as causes of maternal death in New York City, 1987 through 1991. Am J Obstet Gynecol 172:1557, 1995

Dash N, Lupetin AR: Uterine rupture secondary to trauma: CT findings. J Comput Assist Tomogr 15:329, 1991

Del Frari B, Pulzl P, Schoeller T, et al: Pregnancy as a tissue expander in the correction of a scar deformity. Am J Obstet Gynecol 190:579, 2004

Dempfle CE: Coagulopathy of sepsis. Thromb Haemost 91:213, 2004

DiFederico EM, Burlingame JM, Kilpatrick SJ, et al: Pulmonary edema in obstetric patients is rapidly resolved except in the presence of infection or of nitroglycerine tocolysis after open fetal surgery. Am J Obstet Gynecol 179:925, 1998

Duplantier N, Begneaud W, Wood R, et al: Torsion of a gravid uterus associated with maternal trauma: A case report. J Reprod Med 47:683, 2002

Dupre AR, Morrison JC, Martin JN Jr, et al: Clinical application of the Kleihauer–Betke test. J Reprod Med 38:621, 1993

Einarson A, Bailey B, Inocencion G, et al: Accidental electric shock in pregnancy: A prospective cohort study. Am J Obstet Gynecol 176:678, 1997

Eisenstat SA, Bancroft L: Domestic violence. N Engl J Med 341:886, 1999

El Kady D, Gilbert WM, Anderson J, et al: Trauma during pregnancy: An analysis of maternal and fetal outcomes in a large population. Am J Obstet Gynecol 190:1661, 2004

Evans TW, Smithies M: ABC of intensive care. Organ dysfunction. BMJ 318:1606, 1999

Fatovich DM: Electric shock in pregnancy. J Emerg Med 11:175, 1993

Fildes J, Reed L, Jones N, et al: Trauma: The leading cause of maternal death. J Trauma 32:643, 1992

Finegold H, Darwich A, Romeo R, et al: Successful resuscitation after maternal cardiac arrest by immediate cesarean section in the labor room. Anesthesiology 96:1278, 2002

Flick RP, Bofill JA, King JC: Pregnancy complicated by traumatic diaphragmatic rupture. J Reprod Med 44:137, 1999

French National Registry of HA-1A (Centoxin) in Septic Shock: A cohort study of 600 patients. The National Committee for the Evaluation of Centoxin. Arch Intern Med 154:2393, 1994

Frye V: Examining homicide's contribution to pregnancy-associated deaths. JAMA, 285:11, 2001

Gallup DG, Freedman MA, Meguiar RV, et al: Necrotizing fasciitis in gynecologic and obstetric patients: A surgical emergency. Am J Obstet Gynecol 187:305, 2002

Gilbert WM, Towner DR, Field NT, et al: The safety and utility of pulmonary artery catheterization in severe preeclampsia and eclampsia. Am J Obstet Gynecol 182:1397, 2000

Goodwin TM, Breen MT: Pregnancy outcome and fetomaternal hemorrhage after noncatastrophic trauma. Am J Obstet Gynecol 162:665, 1990

Grubb DK: Nonsurgical management of penetrating uterine trauma in pregnancy: A case report. Am J Obstet Gynecol 166:583, 1992

Hankins GD, Wendel GD, Cunningham FG, et al: Longitudinal evaluation of hemodynamic changes in eclampsia. Am J Obstet Gynecol 150:506, 1984

Hankins GD, Wendel GD, Leveno KJ, et al: Myocardial infarction during pregnancy. A review. Obstet Gynecol 65:139, 1985

Harper M, Parsons L: Maternal deaths due to homicide and other injuries in North Carolina: 1992–1994. Obstet Gynecol 90:920, 1997

Harris CM, Foley M: Critical care obstetrics: 13 years of experience in a community practice setting. Obstet Gynecol 99:79S, 2002

Herridge MS, Cheung AM, Tansey CM, et al: One-year outcomes in survivors of the acute respiratory distress syndrome. N Engl J Med 348:683, 2003

Higgins SD, Garite TJ: Late abruptio placentae in trauma patients: Implications for monitoring. Obstet Gynecol 63:10S, 1984

Hidalgo-Grass C, Dan-Goor M, Maly A, et al: Effect of a bacterial pheromone peptide on host chemokine degradation in group A streptococcal necrotising soft-tissue infections. Lancet 363:696, 2004

Hnat MD, Sibai BM, Kovilam O: An initial Glasgow score of 4 and Apgar scores of 9 and 9: A case report of a pregnant comatose woman. Am J Obstet Gynecol 189:877, 2003

Hoadley DJ, Marck EJ: Case records of the Massachusetts General Hospital. Weekly clinicopathological exercises. Case 28-2002. A 35-year-old long-term traveler with a rapidly progressive soft-tissue infection. N Engl J Med 347:831, 2002

Horon IL, Cheng D: Enhanced surveillance for pregnancy-associated mortality—Maryland, 1993–1998. JAMA 285:1455, 2001

Hotchkiss RS, Karl IE: The pathophysiology and treatment of sepsis. N Engl J Med 348:138, 2003

Hyde LK, Cook LJ, Olson LM, et al: Effect of motor vehicle crashes on adverse fetal outcomes. Obstet Gynecol 102:279, 2003

Icely S, Chez RA: Traumatic liver rupture in pregnancy. Am J Obstet Gynecol 180:1030, 1999

Imai Y, Parodo J, Kajikawa O, et al: Injurious mechanical ventilation and end-organ epithelial cell apoptosis and organ dysfunction in an experimental model of acute respiratory distress syndrome. JAMA 289:2104, 2003

Jacob S, Bloebaum L, Shah G, et al: Maternal mortality in Utah. Obstet Gynecol 91:187, 1998

Jenkins TM, Troiano NH, Graves CR, et al: Mechanical ventilation in an obstetric population: Characteristics and delivery rates. Am J Obstet Gynecol 188:439, 2003

Jessup M, Brozena S: Heart failure. N Engl J Med 348:2007, 2003

Kenchaiah S, Evans JC, Levy D, et al: Obesity and the risk of heart failure. N Engl J Med 347:305, 2002

Kettel LM, Branch DW, Scott JR: Occult placental abruption after maternal trauma. Obstet Gynecol 71:449, 1988

Kilpatrick SJ, Matthay MA: Obstetric patients requiring critical care: A five-year review. Chest 101:1407, 1992

Kissinger DP, Rozycki GS, Morris JA Jr, et al: Trauma in pregnancy: Predicting pregnancy outcome. Arch Surg 126:1079, 1991

Kopko PM, Marshall CS, MacKenzie MR, et al: Transfusion-related acute lung injury: Report of a clinical look-back investigation. JAMA 287:1968, 2002

Koumbourlis AC: Electrical injuries. Crit Care Med 30:S424, 2002

Kyriacou DN, Anglin D, Taliaferro E, et al: Risk factors for injury to women from domestic violence. N Engl J Med 341:1892, 1999

Leggon RE, Wood GC, Indeck MC: Pelvic fractures in pregnancy: Factors influencing maternal and fetal outcomes. J Trauma 53:796, 2002

Levinson G, Shnider SM, DeLorimier AA, et al: Effects of maternal hyperventilation on uterine blood flow and fetal oxygenation and acid–base status. Anesthesiology 40:340, 1974

Lewinsohn G, Herman A, Leonov Y, et al: Critically ill obstetrical patients: Outcome and predictability. Crit Care Med 22:1412, 1994

Lipsky S, Holt VL, Easterling TR, et al: Impact of police-reported intimate partner violence during pregnancy on birth outcomes. Obstet Gynecol 102:557, 2003

Lopez A, Lorente JA, Steingrub J, et al: Multiple-center, randomized, placebo-controlled double-blind study of the nitric oxide synthase inhibitor 546C88: Effect on survival in patients with septic shock. Crit Care Med 32:21, 2004

Mabie WC, Barton JR, Sibai BM: Septic shock in pregnancy. Obstet Gynecol 90:553, 1997

Mabie WC, Sibai BM: Treatment in an obstetric intensive care unit. Am J Obstet Gynecol 162:1, 1990

Mabrouk AR, el-Feky AEH: Burns during pregnancy: A gloomy outcome. Burns 23:596, 1997

MacArthur RD, Miller M, Albertson T, et al: Adequacy of early empiric antibiotic treatment and survival in severe sepsis: Experience from the MONARCS trial. Clin Infect Dis 38:284, 2004

Mahutte NG, Murphy-Kaulback L, Le Q, et al: Obstetric admissions to the intensive care unit. Obstet Gynecol 94:263, 1999

Manthous CA: Leapfrog and critical care: Evidence- and reality-based intensive care for the 21st century. Am J Med 116:188, 2004

Martin GS, Mannino DM, Eaton S, et al: The epidemiology of sepsis in the United States from 1979 through 2000. N Engl J Med 348:1546, 2003

Mattar F, Sibai BM: Eclampsia. VIII. Risk factors for maternal morbidity. Am J Obstet Gynecol 182:307, 2000

Matthews RN: Old burns and pregnancy. Br J Obstet Gynaecol 89:610, 1982

McCauley RL, Stenberg BA, Phillips LG, et al: Long-term assessment of the effects of circumferential truncal burns in pediatric patients on subsequent pregnancies. J Burn Care Rehabil 12:51, 1991

McFarlane J, Campbell JC, Sharps P, et al: Abuse during pregnancy and femicide: Urgent implications for women's health. Obstet Gynecol 100:27, 2002

McFarlane J, Parker B, Soeken K, et al: Assessing for abuse during pregnancy. Severity and frequency of injuries and associated entry into prenatal care. JAMA 267:3176, 1992

Meduri GU, Headley AS, Golden E, et al: Effect of prolonged methylprednisolone therapy in unresolving acute respiratory distress syndrome. JAMA 280:159, 1998

Moise KJ Jr, Belfort MA: Damage control for the obstetric patient. Surg Clin North Am 77:835, 1997

Monaco TJ Jr, Spielman FJ, Katz VL: Pregnant patients in the intensive care unit: A descriptive analysis. South Med J 86:414, 1993

Moorcroft DM, Stitzel JD, Duma GG, Duma SM: Computational model of the pregnant occupant: Predicting the risk of injury in automobile crash. Am J Obstet Gynecol 189:540, 2003

Muench M, Baschat A, Kush M, et al: Maternal fetal hemorrhage of greater than or equal to 0.1 percent predicts preterm labor in blunt maternal trauma. Am J Obstet Gynecol 189:S119, 2003

Murphy CC, Schei B, Myhr TL, et al: Abuse: A risk factor for low birth weight? A systematic review and meta-analysis. CMAJ 164:1567, 2001

Nathan L, Peters MT, Ahmed AM, et al: The return of life-threatening puerperal sepsis caused by group A streptococci. Am J Obstet Gynecol 169:571, 1993

National Institutes of Health: Critical Care Medicine Consensus Conference. JAMA 250:798, 1983

Ognibene FP, Parker MM, Natanson C, et al: Depressed left ventricular performance. Response to volume infusion in patients with sepsis and septic shock. Chest 93:903, 1988

Pak LL, Reece EA, Chan L: Is adverse pregnancy outcome predictable after blunt abdominal trauma? Am J Obstet Gynecol 179:1140, 1998

Palmer JD, Sparrow OC: Extradural haematoma following intrauterine trauma. Injury 25:671, 1994

Parker MM, Shelmamer JH, Natanson C, et al: Serial cardiovascular variables in survivors and nonsurvivors of human septic shock: Heart rate as an early predictor of prognosis. Crit Care Med 15:923, 1987

Parrillo JE, Parker MM, Natanson C, et al: Septic shock in humans: Advances in the understanding of pathogenesis, cardiovascular dysfunction, and therapy. Ann Intern Med 113:227, 1990

Pathan N, Hemingway CA, Alizadeh AA, et al: Role of interleukin 6 in myocardial dysfunction of meningococcal septic shock. Lancet 363:203, 2004

Pearlman MD, Cunningham FG: Trauma in pregnancy. In Cunningham FG, MacDonald PC, Gant NF, Leveno KJ, Gilstrap LC (eds): Williams Obstetrics, 19th ed. Supplement No. 21, October/November 1996

Pearlman MD, Klinich KD, Schneider LW, et al: A comprehensive program to improve safety for pregnant women and fetuses in motor vehicle crashes: A preliminary report. Am J Obstet Gynecol 182:1554, 2000

Pearlman MD, Tintinalli JE, Lorenz RP: A prospective controlled study of outcome after trauma during pregnancy. Am J Obstet Gynecol 162:1502, 1990

Perry KG Jr, Martin RW, Blake PG, et al: Maternal outcome associated with adult respiratory distress syndrome. Am J Obstet Gynecol 174:391, 1996

Polko LE, McMahon MJ: Burns in pregnancy. Obstet Gynecol Surv 53:50, 1998

Poole GV, Martin JN, Perry KG Jr, et al: Trauma in pregnancy: The role of interpersonal violence. Am J Obstet Gynecol 174:1873, 1996

Pritchard JA, Cunningham G, Pritchard SA, et al: On reducing the frequency of severe abruptio placentae. Am J Obstet Gynecol 165:1345, 1991

Rayburn W, Smith B, Feller I, et al: Major burns during pregnancy: Effects on fetal well being. Surg Gynecol Obstet 63:392, 1984

Raymond LW, Ford MD, Porter WG, et al: Maternal-fetal lead poisoning from a 15-year old bullet. J Matern Fetal Neonatal Med 11:63, 2002

Rees GAD, Willis BA: Resuscitation in late pregnancy. Anaesthesia 43:347, 1988

Reis PM, Sander CM, Pearlman MD: Abruptio placentae after auto accidents. A case control study. J Reprod Med 45:6, 2000

Rennison CM, Welchans S: Intimate partner violence. U.S. Department of Justice, Office of Justice Programs. NCJ-178247, 2000

Richard C, Warszawski J, Anguel N, et al: Early use of the pulmonary artery catheter and outcomes in patients with shock and acute respiratory distress syndrome. JAMA 290:2713, 2003

Rickert VI, Vaughan RD, Wiemann CM: Violence against young women: Implications for clinicians. Contemp Ob/Gyn 48:30, 2003

Rivers E, Nguyen B, Havstad S, et al: Early goal-directed therapy in the treatment of severe sepsis and septic shock. N Engl J Med 345:1368, 2001

Robertson EG: Edema in normal pregnancy. J Reprod Fertil 9:27, 1969

Rode H, Millar AJW, Cywes S, et al: Thermal injury in pregnancy—the neglected tragedy. S Afr Med J 77:346, 1990

Rorth M, Bille-Brahe NE: 2,3-Diphosphoglycerate and creatine in the red cells during pregnancy. Scand J Clin Lab Invest 28:271, 1971

Sam S, Corbridge TC, Mokhlesi B: Cortisol levels and mortality in sepsis. Clin Endocrinol (Oxf) 60:29, 2004

Sandham JD, Hull RD, Brant RF, et al: A randomized, controlled trial of the use of pulmonary-artery catheters in high-risk surgical patients. N Engl J Med 348:5, 2003

Satin AJ, Hemsell DL, Stone IC Jr, et al: Sexual assault in pregnancy. Obstet Gynecol 77:710, 1991

Satin AJ, Ramin JM, Paicurich J, et al: The prevalence of sexual assault: A survey of 2404 puerperal women. Am J Obstet Gynecol 167:973, 1992

Schiff MA, Holt VL: The injury severity score in pregnant trauma patients: Predicting placental abruption and fetal death. J Trauma 53:946, 2002

Schiff MA, Holt VL, Daling JR: Maternal and infant outcomes after injury during pregnancy in Washington State from 1989 to 1997. J Trauma 53:939, 2002

Schneider MB, Ivester TS, Mabie WC, et al: Maternal and fetal outcomes in women requiring antepartum mechanical ventilation. Obstet Gynecol [abstract] 101:69S, 2003

Schoenfeld A, Warchaizer S, Royburt M, et al: Crush injury in pregnancy: An unusual experience in obstetrics. Obstet Gynecol 86:655, 1995

Schrier RW, Wang W: Acute renal failure and sepsis. N Engl J Med 351:159, 2004

Schultze PM, Stamm CA, Roger J: Placental abruption and fetal death with airbag deployment in a motor vehicle accident. Obstet Gynecol 92:719, 1998

Sciscione A, Invester T, Largoza M, et al: Acute pulmonary edema in pregnancy. Obstet Gynecol 101:511, 2003

Scorpio RJ, Esposito TJ, Smith LG, et al: Blunt trauma during pregnancy. Factors affecting fetal outcome. J Trauma 32:213, 1992

Sibai BM, Mabie BC, Harvey CJ, et al: Pulmonary edema in severe preeclampsia–eclampsia: Analysis of thirty-seven consecutive cases. Am J Obstet Gynecol 156:1174, 1987

Sims CJ, Boardman CH, Fuller SJ: Airbag deployment following a motor vehicle accident in pregnancy. Obstet Gynecol 88:726, 1996

Society of Critical Care Medicine Task Force on Guidelines: Recommendations for intensive care unit admission and discharge criteria. Crit Care Med 16:807, 1988

Sozen I, Nesin N: Accidental electric shock in pregnancy and antenatal occurrence of maternal deep vein thrombosis. A case report. J Reprod Med 49:58, 2004

Stettler RW, Lutich A, Pritchard JA, et al: Traumatic placental abruption: A separation from traditional thought. Presented at the annual clinical meeting of American College of Obstetricians and Gynecologists, Las Vegas, May 1992

Stone IK: Trauma in the obstetric patient. Obstet Gynecol Clin North Am 26:459, 1999

Subrevilla LA, Cassinelli MT, Carcelen A, et al: Human fetal and maternal oxygen tension and acid-base status during delivery at high altitude. Am J Obstet Gynecol 111:1111, 1971

Sugar NF, Fine DN, Eckert LO: Physical injury after sexual assault: findings of a large case series. Am J Obstet Gynecol 190:71, 2004

Taylor RW, Zimmerman JL, Dellinger RP, et al: Inhaled Nitric Oxide in ARDS Study Group: Low-dose inhaled nitric oxide in patients with acute lung injury: a randomized controlled trial. JAMA 291:1603, 2004

Tomlinson MW, Caruthers TJ, Whitty JE, et al: Does delivery improve maternal condition in the respiratory-compromised gravida? Obstet Gynecol 91:108, 1998

Towery R, English TP, Wisner D: Evaluation of pregnant women after blunt injury. J Trauma 35:731, 1993

Tyroch AH, Kaups KL, Rohan J, et al: Pregnant women and car restraints: Beliefs and practices. J Trauma 46:241, 1999

United States Department of Justice. Office on Violence Against Women. Full report on the prevalence, incidence, and consequences of violence against women: Findings from the National Violence Against Women Survey. Washington, DC, National Institute of Justice, July 2000

Van Hook JW, Hankins GDV: Invasive hemodynamic monitoring. Prim Care Update Ob/Gyn 4:39, 1997

Ware LB, Matthay MA: The acute respiratory distress syndrome. N Engl J Med 342:1334, 2000

Warner MW, Salfinger SG, Rao S, et al: Management of trauma during pregnancy. Aust ANZ J Surg 74:125, 2004

Warren BL, Eid A, Singer P, et al: Caring for the critically ill patient: high-dose antithrombin III in severe sepsis: a randomized controlled trial. JAMA 286:1869, 2001

Wathen CN, MacMillan HL: Interventions for violence against women: Scientific review. JAMA 289:589, 2003

Watson D, Grover R, Anzueto A, et al: Cardiovascular effects of the nitric oxide synthase inhibitor NG-methyl-L-arginine hydrochloride (546C88) in patients with septic shock: Results of a randomized, double-blind, placebo-controlled multicenter study (study no. 144-002). Crit Care Med 32:13, 2004

Weg JG, Anzueto A, Balk RA, et al: The relation of pneumothorax and other air leaks to mortality in the acute respiratory distress syndrome. N Engl J Med 338:341, 1998

Weiss HB: The epidemiology of traumatic injury-related fetal mortality in Pennsylvania, 1995–1997: The role of motor vehicle crashes. Accid Anal Prev 33:449, 2001

Weiss HB, Songer TJ, Fabio A: Fetal deaths related to maternal injury. JAMA 286:1863, 2001

Weiss HB, Strotmeyer S: Characteristics of pregnant women in motor vehicle crashes. Inj Prev 8:207, 2002

Westhoff C: Emergency contraception. N Engl J Med 349:1830, 2003

Weyerts LK, Jones MC, James HE: Paraplegia and congenital contractures as a consequence of intrauterine trauma. Am J Med Genet 43:751, 1992

Wheeler AP, Bernard GR: Treating patients with severe sepsis. N Engl J Med 340:207, 1999

Whitten M, Irvine LM: Postmortem and perimortem caesarean section: What are the indications? J R Soc Med 93:6, 2000

Whitty JE: Maternal cardiac arrest in pregnancy. Clin Obstet Gynecol 45:377, 2002

Widgerow AD, Ford TD, Botha M: Burn contracture preventing uterine expansion. Ann Plast Surg 27:269, 1991

Wyncoll DLA, Evans TW: Acute respiratory distress syndrome. Lancet 354:497, 1999

Zeeman GG, Wendel GD Jr, Cunningham FG: A blueprint for obstetric critical care. Am J Obstet Gynecol 188:532, 2003

Zinaman M, Rubin J, Lindheimer MD: Serial plasma oncotic pressure levels and echoencephalography during and after delivery in severe preeclampsia. Lancet 1:1245, 1985

43

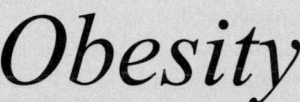

Obesity

Excessive weight has become one of the major health problems in the United States as well as in other affluent societies. Because of its medical importance and its multifaceted effects on pregnancy, it is discussed separately in this chapter. The prevalence of obesity in the United States has increased steadily as economic prosperity has increased. For a number of years, obesity has been termed *epidemic*. Strictly defined, the word *epidemic* implies a *temporary* widespread outbreak of greatly increased frequency and severity. Therefore, and unfortunately, obesity more correctly is *endemic*—a condition that is habitually present. Its prevalence continues to increase. From 1960 to 1991, the National Health and Nutrition Examination Survey (NHANES) documented an alarming increase among adults over the past decade (Kuczmarski and colleagues, 1994). By 1991, approximately one third of adults in the United States were overweight. That same year, Allison and co-workers (1999) attributed almost 300,000 deaths to obesity. Sadly, the problem is not limited to adults. Ogden and associates (2002) reported that 15 percent of children 6 through 11 years of age were overweight. The prevalence in adolescents is similar.

Public health authorities began to address the problem of obesity in the late 1980s. A stated goal of *Healthy People 2000* was to reduce the prevalence of overweight people to 20 percent or less by the end of the 20th century (Public Health Service, 1990). Unfortunately, this goal was not achieved, and in fact, more than 50 percent of the population was overweight at the beginning of 2000.

As evidence accrues, the nature and scope of morbidity due to obesity have become better elucidated. Diabetes mellitus, heart disease, hypertension, stroke, and osteoarthritis are among the many obesity-related diseases. These obesity-related diseases together result in a decreased life span. Bray (2003) aptly concluded that the worldwide obesity epidemic will be followed by a worldwide diabetes epidemic. Obese women who become pregnant—and their fetuses—are predisposed to a variety of serious pregnancy-related complications. Long-term maternal effects include significant and increased morbidity and mortality. Moreover, recent studies have suggested that the offspring of obese parents may suffer long-term morbidity. Ironically, severely growth-restricted female infants who become obese as adults are at high risk for preeclampsia (Dempsey and colleagues, 2003).

DEFINITIONS

A number of systems have been used to define and classify obesity. The *body mass index* (BMI), which is also known as the *Quetelet index,* is currently in use. The BMI is calculated as weight in kilograms divided by height in meters squared (kg/m^2). Calculated BMI values are available in various chart and graphic forms, such as the one shown in Figure 43–1. According to the National Heart, Lung, and Blood Institute (1998), a *normal* BMI is 18.5 to 24.9 kg/m^2; *overweight* is a BMI of 25 to 29.9 kg/m^2; and *obesity* is a BMI of 30 kg/m^2 or greater. According to Freedman and colleagues (2002), obesity is further categorized as class I (BMI: 30 to 34.9 kg/m^2), class II (BMI: 35 to 39.9 kg/m^2), and class III (BMI: 40-plus kg/m^2).

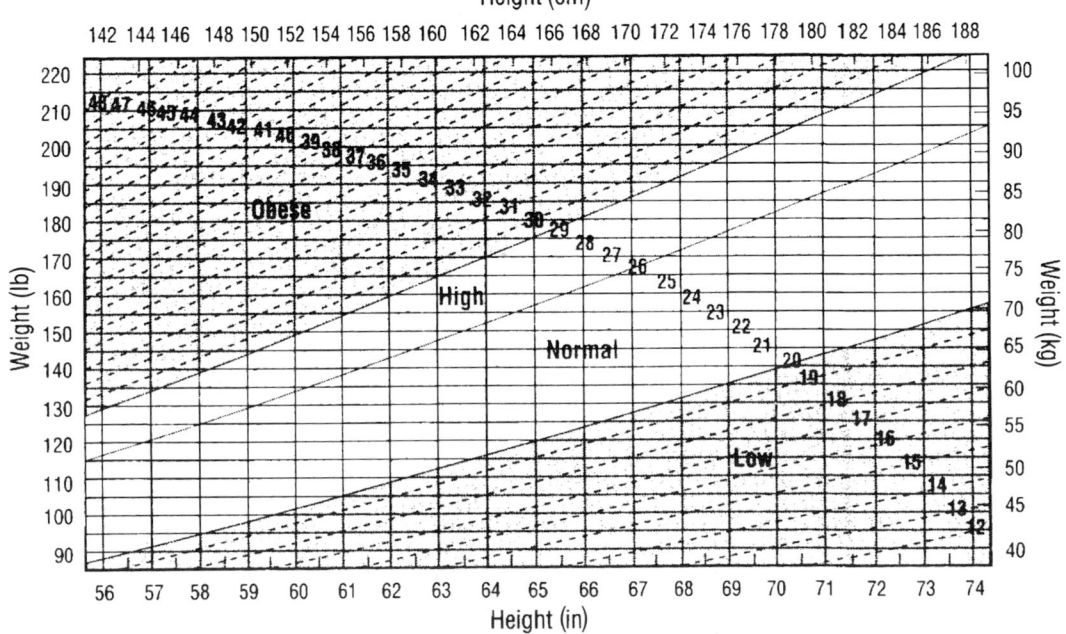

FIGURE 43–1. Chart for estimating body mass index (BMI). To find the BMI category (e.g., obese) for a particular subject, locate the point at which the height and weight intersect. The BMI is the bold number on the dashed line closest to this point. The "High" category is now termed "Overweight."

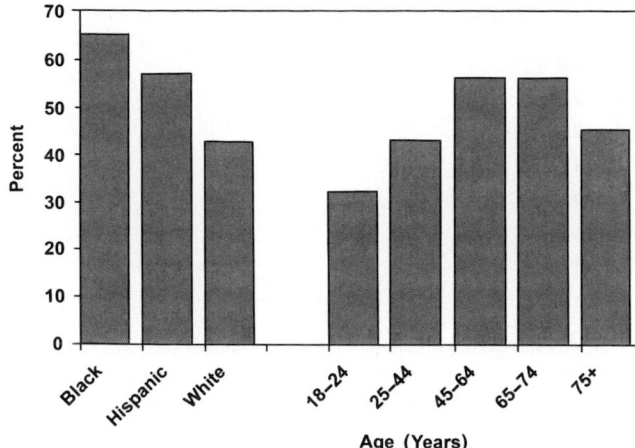

FIGURE 43–2. National Center for Health Statistics: Prevalence of overweight (BMI $\geq$ 25 k/m^2) or obese (BMI $\geq$ 30 k/m^2) women by race/ethnicity and age in the United States for 1997–1998. (BMI = body mass index.) (Data from Schoenborn and colleagues, 2002.)

PREVALENCE. By the end of 2000, Pleis and colleagues (2003) reported that 34 percent of adult American individuals were overweight. Another 27 percent were obese, an increase of 75 percent compared with 1980 statistics. **Thus, at the end of 2000, more than 50 percent of adults in the United States were either overweight or obese.** Prevalence data for women are shown in Figure 43–2. Mokdad and associates (2003) reported that 2.8 percent of women and 1.7 percent of men were extremely obese (class III), with a BMI of 40 kg/m^2 or more. There is a disparate prevalence of obesity in indigent individuals in this country (Drewnowski and Specter, 2004).

As previously stated, childhood obesity is also a serious problem. Using the definition of overweight as at or above the 95 percentile for age and ethnicity, the prevalence of obesity in children has increased two- to threefold in the United States from 1971 to 1999 (National Center for Health Statistics, 1999; Ogden and co-workers, 2002). Moreover, the problem is worldwide, even in third-world countries (Ebbeling, 2002). In adolescents, the increasing prevalence of obesity is associated with declining physical activity (Kimm and associates, 2002).

METABOLIC SYNDROME. In some people, obesity interacts with inherited factors and leads to the onset of *insulin resistance*. This metabolic abnormality in turn is responsible for altered glucose metabolism and a predisposition to type 2 diabetes mellitus. In addition, it causes a number of subclinical abnormalities that predispose to cardiovascular disease and accelerate its onset. The most important among these are type 2 diabetes, dyslipidemia, and hypertension. These conditions, when clustered together with other insulin resistance–related subclinical abnormalities, are referred to as the *metabolic syndrome* (Abate, 2000). Virtually all obese women with hypertension demonstrate elevated insulin

TABLE 43–1 Criteria for Diagnosis of the Metabolic Syndrome

Patients with three or more of the following:

- Abdominal obesity: waist circumference > 88 cm (34.7 in) in women or > 102 cm (40.2 in) in men
- Hypertriglyceridemia: $\geq$ 150 mg/dL
- High-density lipoprotein: < 50 mg/dL in women or < 40 mg/dL in men
- High blood pressure: $\geq$ 130/85 mm Hg[a]
- High fasting glucose: $\geq$ 110 mg/dL[a]

[a]Those with normal values while taking medications are considered to meet these criteria.
From the National Institutes of Health, 2001.

levels. The levels are even higher in women with excessive fat in the abdomen—an apple shape, compared with fat in the hips and thighs—a pear shape (American College of Obstetricians and Gynecologists, 2003). In fact, Gus and associates (2004) recently reported that for women, a waist circumference over 88 cm was more predictive of hypertension than a BMI greater than 30 kg/m^2.

The criteria used by the National Institutes of Health (2001) to define the metabolic syndrome are shown in Table 43–1. Drugs that increase sensitivity to insulin, such as metformin and glitazones, also cause a decrease in blood pressure levels (Chen and colleagues, 1996).

Prevalence. Because metabolic syndrome is newly defined, prevalence data have been calculated from a study in progress. Ford and colleagues (2002) did a follow-up study between 1988 and 1994 of 8814 men and women enrolled in the Third National Health and Nutrition Survey (NHANES III). Using the criteria shown in Table 43–1, there was an overall prevalence of the metabolic syndrome in 24 percent of women and 22 percent of men. As expected, prevalence increased with age. For 4549 women, prevalence was about 6 percent in those 20 to 29 years of age; 14 percent in those 30 to 39 years of age; 20 percent in those 40 to 49 years of age; and greater than 30 percent for women older than 50 years of age.

MORBIDITY AND MORTALITY ASSOCIATED WITH OBESITY

Obesity continues to be very costly, not only in morbidity and mortality, but also in health care dollars. Colditz (1999) estimated that 300,000 adults die each year from obesity-related causes. He estimated direct costs of obesity and physical inactivity to be 9.4 percent of annual health care expenditures in the United States.

Individuals who are overweight are at increased risk for an imposing number of complications (Table 43–2). The direct link between obesity and type 2 diabetes mellitus is well known (Mokdad and associates, 2001, 2003). In one study

TABLE 43–2 Long-term Complications of Obesity

Disorder	Possible Cause (s)
Type 2 diabetes mellitus	Insulin resistance
Hypertension	Increased blood volume and cardiac output
Coronary heart disease	Hypertension, dyslipidemia, type 2 diabetes mellitus
Obesity cardiomyopathy	Eccentric left ventricular hypertrophy
Sleep apnea/pulmonary dysfunction	Pharyngeal fat deposition
Ischemic stroke	Atherosclerosis, decreased cerebral blood flow
Gallbladder disease	Hyperlipidemia
Liver disease: nonalcoholic steatohepatitis	Increased visceral adiposity; elevated serum free fatty acids; hyperinsulinemia
Osteoarthritis	Stress on weight-bearing joints
Subfertility	Hyperinsulinemia
Cancer: endometrium, colon, breast	Hyperestrogenemia
Carpal tunnel syndrome	
Deep venous thrombosis	
Poor wound healing	

Compiled from Alpert, 2001; Calle, 1999, 2003; Chinali, 2004; Kenchaiah, 2002; Mokdad, 2003; Must, 1999; Ninomiya, 2004, and all of their colleagues; National Task Force on the Prevention and Treatment of Obesity, 2000.

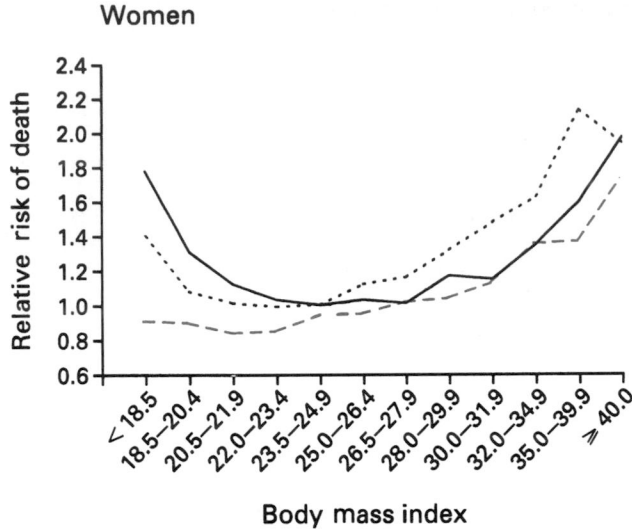

Women

Body mass index

FIGURE 43–3. Body mass index (BMI) and multivariate relative risk of death from various causes among nonsmoking women with no history of disease at enrollment. The reference category was made up of subjects with a BMI of 23.5 to 24.9 kg/m². The relative risk of death is plotted versus incremental BMI for cardiovascular disease ($\ldots$), cancer (---), and all other causes (———). (From Calle and associates, 1999, with permission.)

by Hu and co-workers (2001), 16-year follow-up data were reported from the Nurses' Health Study which began in 1974. In more than 1.3 million person-years, 3300 women developed type 2 diabetes, and the most important factor in its development was obesity.

Heart disease due to obesity (*adipositas cordis*) is caused by hypertension, hypervolemia, and dyslipidemia. Even before hypertension developed, Chinali and co-workers (2004) found evidence of abnormal left ventricular geometry and function in patients with the metabolic syndrome. Kenchaiah and colleagues (2002) reported a twofold risk for heart failure for women from the Framingham Heart Study who were either overweight or obese. Indeed, 14 percent of cases of heart failure were due to obesity alone. Ninomiya and co-workers (2004) found a twofold risk with the metabolic syndrome for myocardial infarction and stroke in the cohort from NHANES III.

Other common conditions that are increased in obesity are osteoarthritis and asthma.

Excessive weight is associated with increased early mortality, as shown by Peeters (2003) and Fontaine (2003) and their colleagues in follow-up studies from both the Framingham Heart Study and the NHANES III cohort. Results from a prospective study by Calle and associates (1999) are shown in Figure 43–3. The mortality risk from cardiovascular disease and cancer increased directly with increasing BMI. A subsequent study by Calle and co-workers (2003) confirmed that mortality from all causes combined, as well as from cancer, was increased in obese and overweight persons.

TREATMENT OF OBESITY

Weight loss is tremendously difficult for obese individuals to accomplish. If achieved, long-term maintenance poses equivalent or even more daunting difficulties. There are innumerable methods espoused to help or even directly cause weight loss. The vast majority of these are patently dishonest charlatan schemes designed to extract money from overweight individuals, and even the most legitimate methods are fraught with frequent failure. If they are successful, slow and inexorable return to preintervention weight usually follows (National Institutes of Health Technology Assessment Conference Panel, 1993). Legitimate weight loss approaches include behavioral, pharmacological, and surgical techniques, or a combination of these methods (Yanovski and Yanovski, 2002).

PREGNANCY AND OBESITY

Obesity has been associated with subfertility due to increased insulin resistance (see Table 43–2). In their review, Neill and Nelson-Piercy (2001) linked impaired fecundity in women with a BMI in excess of 30 kg/m². In the many overweight and obese women who achieve pregnancy, there are a number of increased and interrelated adverse perinatal outcomes. **Marked obesity is unequivocally hazardous to the pregnant woman and her fetus**.

PREVALENCE. Because the overall prevalence of obesity has increased over the past several decades, the prevalence of

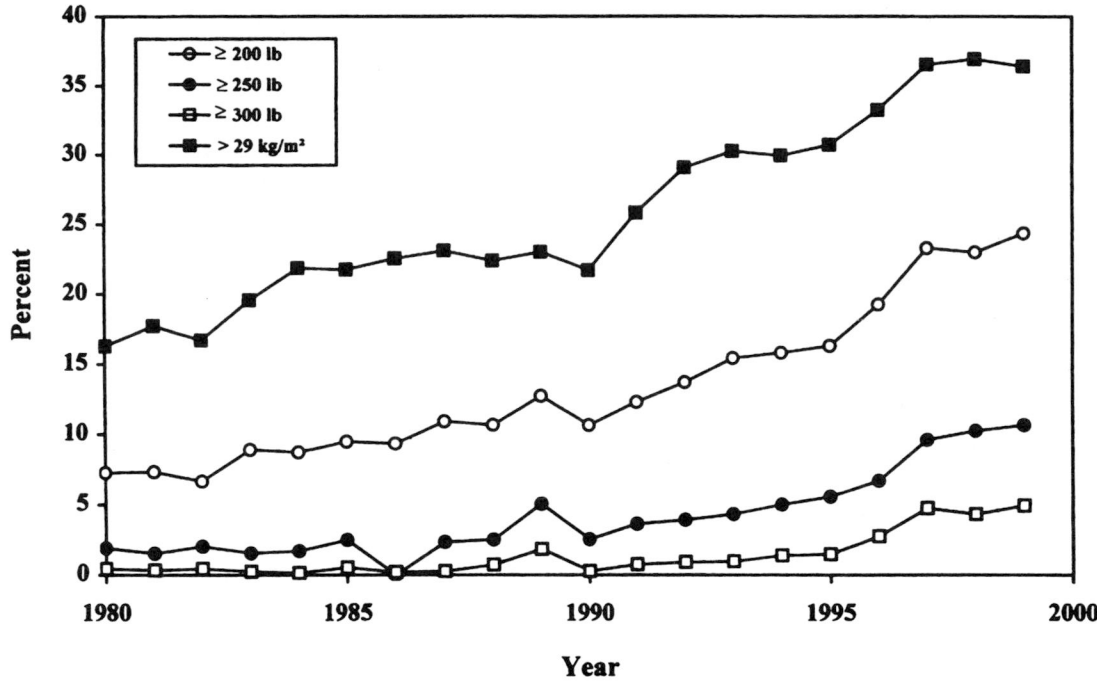

FIGURE 43–4. Increasing prevalence of obesity during 20 years in pregnant women classified at the time of their first prenatal visit at the University of Alabama at Birmingham. All women were classified into the first three categories shown on the graph. In approximately half of the women, height was available and they were classified by body mass index. (From Lu and colleagues, 2001, with permission.)

obesity complicating pregnancy has also increased. Before adoption of the BMI, investigators used a variety of definitions of obesity to assess risks during pregnancy. For example, in the study shown in Figure 43–4, four definitions were used. Regardless of how obesity was defined, all groups showed substantive increases in prevalence over the 20-year study. Ehrenberg and colleagues (2002) reported similar findings in a 15-year study in Cleveland.

WEIGHT LOSS DURING PREGNANCY. Because maternal catabolism is, intuitively, not good for fetal growth and development, the Institute of Medicine (1992) recommends that even women who are obese (BMI of 30 kg/m^2 or higher) should not attempt weight loss during pregnancy. These women should, however, limit weight gain to less than 15 pounds. This aspect of prenatal care is discussed in Chapter 8 (see p. 213).

MATERNAL MORBIDITY. Increased maternal morbidity results from obesity, defined variably as more than 150 percent of ideal body weight, BMI greater than 35 kg/m^2, BMI greater than 40 kg/m^2, and 150 pounds or more greater than ideal body weight (Bianco, 1998; Cedergren, 2004; Garbaciak, 1985; Isaacs, 1994; Kabiru and Raynor, 2004; Kumari, 2001, and all their colleagues). These investigators chronicled significantly increased incidences of a number of disorders including chronic hypertension, gestational diabetes,

preeclampsia, fetal macrosomia, as well as higher rates of cesarean delivery and postpartum complications.

In a nurse–midwife practice, women whose BMI exceeded 29 kg/m^2 had a two- to fourfold increased cesarean delivery rate (Kaiser and Kirby, 2001). Similarly, in a physician private practice, the cesarean delivery rate for dystocia was increased sixfold in obese nulliparas (Young and Woodmansee, 2002). In another study, only 15 percent of obese women with a previous cesarean delivery succeeded in having a subsequent vaginal delivery (Chauhan and colleagues, 2001). These same investigators stratified women by BMI category and reported a successful trial of labor in 82 percent of women who weighed less than 200 lb, in 57 percent of those weighing 200 to 299 lb, and in only 13 percent of those weighing more than 300 lb (Carroll and collaborators, 2003). Although Edwards and co-workers (2003) reported a success rate of greater than 50 percent, they showed that costs for a planned trial of labor and elective cesarean delivery were equivalent.

Second-trimester dilatation and evacuation was reported to take longer and be more difficult in women whose BMI was 30 kg/m^2 or greater (Dark and co-workers, 2002).

In addition, there are reports of increased adverse pregnancy outcomes in overweight women with a BMI of 25 to 29.9 kg/m^2. Sebire and collaborators (2001) studied 287,213 singleton pregnancies delivered in the North West Thames Region of London. Their results are shown in Table 43–3 according to BMI category. Cunningham and associates (1986) reported that obesity (weight greater than 200 pounds) and

TABLE 43–3 Adverse Pregnancy Effects in Overweight and Obese Women

	Normal BMI 20–24.9 (n = 176,923)	Increased Complications (Odds Ratio[a]) Overweight BMI 25–29.9 (n = 79,014)	Obese BMI > 30 (n = 31,27)
Gestational diabetes	0.8	1.7	3.6
Preeclampsia	0.7	1.5	2.1
Postterm pregnancy	0.13	1.2[b]	1.7
Emergency cesarean	7.8	1.3	1.8
Elective cesarean	4.0	1.2	1.4
Postpartum hemorrhage	10.4	1.2	1.4
Pelvic infection	0.7	1.2	1.3
Urinary tract infection	0.7	1.2	1.4
Wound infection	0.4	1.3	2.2
Macrosomia	9.0	1.6	2.4
Stillbirth	0.4	1.1[b]	1.4

BMI = body mass index.
[a]Odds ratios (99% CI) are significant except when denoted.
[b]Not significantly different.
Data from Sebire and colleagues, 2001, with permission.

hypertension were common co-factors in causing peripartum heart failure. Myles and co-workers (2002) found that obesity was an independent risk factor for postcesarean infection morbidity. Finally, obese women are less likely to breast feed (Li and colleagues, 2003).

Preeclampsia. Obesity is a consistent risk factor for preeclampsia (Cedergren, 2004; Jensen and associates, 2003; Sebire and colleagues, 2001). In a review of studies that included over 1.4 million women, O'Brien and collaborators (2003) found that the preeclampsia risk doubled with each 5 to 7 kg/m^2 increase in prepregnancy BMI. In obese, nonpregnant individuals, at least some of the long-term cardiovascular morbidity was thought to be due to obesity-mediated systemic inflammation and endothelial dysfunction (Brook and associates, 2001). According to Davi and colleagues (2002), this phenomenon was associated more with android obesity (apple shape) than gynoid obesity (pear shape)—one characteristic of the metabolic syndrome discussed on page 1009. It has become apparent that endothelial activation plays an integral role in preeclampsia (see Chap. 34, p. 769). Obesity is associated with low-grade inflammation, and Wolf and co-workers (2001) linked these two conditions by providing intriguing evidence that inflammation may explain, at least partly, the association of obesity with preeclampsia. More recently, Ramsay and collaborators (2002) confirmed that obese pregnant women had significantly elevated levels of serum interleukin-6 and C-reactive protein as well as evidence of impaired endothelial function. Specifically, 23 pregnant women with a median BMI of 31 kg/m^2 were compared with 24 with a median BMI of 22 kg/m^2. Obese women had significantly higher levels

of triglycerides, very-low-density lipoprotein cholesterol, insulin, and leptin.

Long-Term Consequences. It is intuitive that excessive prepregnancy weight can be used to predict long-term obesity with its attendant morbidity and mortality. Rooney and Schauberger (2002), however, reported that excess weight gain during pregnancy—but not prepregnancy weight—is a predictor of long-term obesity. They followed 540 women postpartum for a mean duration of 8.5 years. During this period, the average weight gain was 6.3 kg. Women who had gained less than the recommended amount of weight during pregnancy were on average 4.1 kg heavier at the end of the follow-up period. Women who gained the recommended amount were 6.5 kg heavier. Finally, women who gained more than the recommended amount were 8.4 kg heavier.

Contraception. Oral contraceptive failure is more likely in overweight women. In reviewing studies on hormonal contraceptive efficacy, it is apparent that the typical study subject is not representative of the average American woman. As discussed earlier, at least 50 percent of American women have a BMI greater than 25 kg/m^2 and thus are considered to be overweight (see Table 43–2). In contraceptive studies, however, the majority of subjects have a BMI between 18 and 28 kg/m^2 (Holt and co-workers, 2002; Zieman and collaborators, 2002). In one study, the mean serum medroxyprogesterone acetate concentration was lower in the women with a BMI greater than 28 kg/m^2 compared with that of those with a lower BMI (Rahimy and associates, 1999). Efficacy of the Ortho-Evra patch was studied by Zieman and colleagues (2002). In their analysis of the pooled data from three multicenter studies, they found a significant association between increasing body weight and contraceptive failure. Holt and colleagues (2002) studied 755 women with 2822 person-years of pill use and found that those in the highest weight quartile (70.5 kg or more) had a 1.6-fold increased risk of pregnancy. Importantly, women in this quartile who used very-low-dose oral contraceptives had a four- to fivefold increased pregnancy rate (see Chap. 32, p. 727).

PERINATAL MORBIDITY AND MORTALITY. Both fetal and neonatal complications are increased in obese women. For example, obese women, variably defined, have a two- to threefold risk for a fetus with a neural-tube defect or other anomalies (Mikhail, 1996; Waller, 1994; Werler, 1996, and all their collaborators). In another study, Shaw and colleagues (1996, 2000) reported that women with a BMI of 30 kg/m^2 or more had a twofold increased incidence of neural-tube defects compared with that of control women. In a case-control study from the Atlantic Birth Defects Risk Factor Surveillance Study, Watkins and associates (2003) reported a 3.5-fold increase in neural-tube defects in obese women. They also found a two- to threefold increased incidence in omphalocele, heart defects, and multiple anomalies. The last two were also increased twofold in overweight women whose BMI was 25 to 29.9 kg/m^2.

Two important and interrelated co-factors that contribute to excessive perinatal morbidity and mortality are chronic hypertension and diabetes mellitus, both of which are associated with obesity (Stephansson and colleagues, 2001). Chronic hypertension is a well-known cause of fetal growth restriction (see Chap. 45, p. 1047). Pregestational diabetes increases the rate of birth defects. Gestational diabetes is complicated by excessive numbers of large-for-gestational age and macrosomic infants (see Chap. 38, p. 905). Whatever the cause(s), the prevalence of macrosomic infants is increased in obese women (Bianco and co-workers, 1998; Cedergren, 2004; Isaacs and associates, 1994). There are also long-term sequelae for macrosomic infants born to these mothers. Low-birthweight infants have lower subsequent risks of type 2 diabetes, insulin resistance, and metabolic syndrome, whereas infants who weigh more than 4000 g have increased risks (Innes and colleagues, 2002). From preliminary observations, Armstrong and colleagues (2002) reported that breast feeding decreases the risk of childhood obesity in these large infants. Alternatively, Ruowei and co-workers (2003) reported that obese women were less likely to breast feed.

An increased incidence of otherwise inexplicable late-pregnancy stillbirths has been associated with obesity. Cnattingius and colleagues (1998) found a significant 1.6-fold increase in the stillbirth rate in women with a BMI of 25 to 29.9 kg/m^2. The rate was increased 2.6-fold for women with a BMI of 30 kg/m^2 or more. In addition, early neonatal death was nearly doubled in nulliparous women with a BMI of 30 kg/m^2 or higher. Stephansson and associates (2001) used the same database for a case-control study of 649 nulliparas who had stillbirths. They confirmed an almost threefold late-stillbirth rate in women with a BMI of greater than 25 kg/m^2. They attributed the increase to socioeconomic deprivation and pregnancy complications, particularly preeclampsia and diabetes. Baydock and Chari (2002) found that a prepregnancy BMI of greater than 30 kg/m^2 was an independent risk factor for stillbirth.

MANAGEMENT. A program of weight reduction is probably unrealistic during pregnancy. If such a regimen is chosen, however, it is mandatory that the quality of the diet be monitored closely and that ketosis be avoided (Rizzo and associates, 1991). Close prenatal surveillance detects most early signs of diabetes or hypertension. Standard screening tests for fetal anomalies are sufficient. Accurate assessment of fetal growth usually requires serial sonography. Wolfe and colleagues (1990) have highlighted the technical difficulties with ultrasonic fetal visualization in women with a BMI above the 90th percentile. Antepartum and intrapartum fetal heart rate monitoring are likewise made more difficult, and sometimes these are even impossible.

Evaluation by anesthesia personnel is performed at a prenatal visit or on arrival at the labor unit (American College of Obstetricians and Gynecologists, 2002). Anesthetic risks and complications faced by obese women are discussed in Chapter 19 (see p. 489). Special attention to complications that might arise during labor and delivery is mandatory. For cesarean delivery, forethought is given to optimal placement and type of abdominal incision to access the fetus and to the intervening tissue thickness. Individual differences in maternal body habitus preclude any one approach as superior (Gilstrap and colleagues, 2002). Meticulous attention to achieving a structurally secure closure is mandatory.

PREGNANCY FOLLOWING SURGICAL PROCEDURES FOR OBESITY. A number of surgical procedures have been designed to treat morbid obesity by either decreasing gastric volume or bypassing gastrointestinal absorption (Brolin, 2002; Yanovski and Yanovski, 1999). Buchwald and associates (2004) in a meta-analysis found these procedures to improve or resolve diabetes, hyperlipidemia, hypertension, and obstruction sleep apnea. Although none are recommended during pregnancy, invariably more women will become pregnant subsequent to these procedures as their popularity grows (Sheiner and associates, 2004). According to the American Society for Bariatric Surgery (2003), there were 47,000 surgeries for obesity in 2001, 63,000 in 2002, and over 100,000 for 2003 (Mitka, 2003; Steinbrook, 2004).

Jejunoileal Bypass. This was one of the earliest surgical methods that was successful for weight loss. In this procedure, the duodenum is divided and anastomosed to the terminal jejunum very near the ileocecal junction. Thus, the vast majority of the small bowel is bypassed with resultant diminished food absorption. This procedure was followed by significant long-term morbidity and mortality, and it has been abandoned by most surgeons. Older reports chronicled shorter gestations, lower mean birthweight, and more small-for-gestational-age infants after weight reduction (Knudsen and Källén, 1986).

Gastric Bypass. This older procedure excludes the lower 90 percent of the stomach by creating an upper gastrojejunostomy. Printen and Scott (1982) described 51 pregnancies in 45 morbidly obese women who had antenatal gastric bypass surgery. Complications were uncommon, and fetal growth restriction was not increased in the 46 infants delivered. Richards and colleagues (1987) reported similar experiences with 57 pregnancies at the University of Utah. These women weighed an average of 194 pounds before and 147 pounds after surgery. Compared with preprocedure pregnancies, mean birthweight decreased from 3600 to 3200 g, and the incidence of large-for-gestational-age infants decreased from 37 to 16 percent. Impressively, the incidence of pregnancy-associated hypertension fell from 46 to 9 percent.

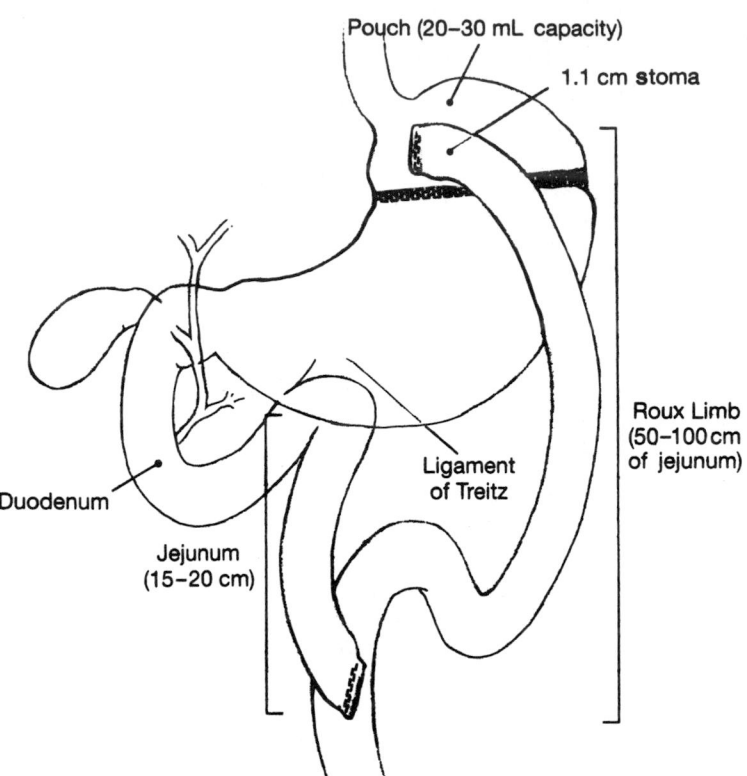

FIGURE 43–5. Roux-en-Y gastric bypass. A stapler fired across the cardia of the stomach creates a 20- to 30-mL pouch. The jejunum is divided distal to the ligament of Treitz with the distal end anastomosed to the upper stomach. (From Brolin, 2002, with permission.)

Gastroplasty. There are several variations of surgical gastroplasty in which a narrow channel is created through the stomach by using stapling devices. The *vertical-banded gastroplasty* is the most popular bariatric procedure performed currently (Brunicardi and associates, 2001). Subsequent pregnancy outcomes have been chronicled. Bilenka and colleagues (1995) described 14 pregnancies in nine women who had undergone the procedure. The mean weight loss was 80 pounds, and the women had fewer complications compared with their preprocedure pregnancies. Martin and co-workers (2000) described 23 pregnancies in women after *adjustable gastric banding.* For three women with excessive nausea and vomiting, band adjustment to decrease obstruction was successful. Dixon and associates (2001) described 22 pregnancies in 20 women who were using the Lap-Band System. In this method, the gastric band is laparoscopically placed 2 cm below the gastroesophageal junction. An internal balloon reservoir is adjusted by saline instillation into percutaneously placed tubing. The mean weight loss before pregnancy was 30 kg. Weight gain during pregnancy averaged 8.3 kg, and there were few complications. Mean birthweights of infants were similar before and after maternal banding.

Roux-en-Y Bypass. This type of bypass is the most effective bariatric procedure currently in use (Brunicardi and associates, 2001). It most often is performed laparoscopically. The procedure is depicted in Figure 43–5. The proximal stomach is transected to leave a 30-mL pouch. A gastroenterotomy is made by connecting the proximal end

of the distal jejunum which was divided 60 cm distal to the ligament of Treitz. The Roux-en-Y enteroenterostomy is completed 60 cm distal to the gastrojejunostomy. Brunicardi and colleagues (2001) summarized four series totaling almost 400 men and nonpregnant women. Mean weight loss at 1 year in the four series ranged from 21 to 43 kg. In the largest study, at 1 year, 300 patients had lost a mean of 80 percent of their excessive weight. At 5 years, 50 to 75 percent of the weight loss had been maintained, and at 14 years maintenance of lost weight still exceeded 50 percent (American Society of Bariatric Surgery, 2003). Current costs are $20,000 to $50,000 (Steinbrook, 2004).

Wittgrove and associates (1998) described 49 pregnancies in 36 women after a Roux-en-Y bypass. There were 17 who had delivered at least one child prior to surgery. When prior pregnancy outcomes were compared with those after bypass, there was a dramatic reduction in hypertension (40 versus 0 percent), diabetes (24 versus 0 percent), and infant weight greater than 4000 g (30 versus 5 percent). At least one maternal death from herniation and obstruction has been reported (Moore and colleagues, 2004).

REFERENCES

Abate N: Obesity and cardiovascular disease: Pathogenetic role of the metabolic syndrome and therapeutic implications. J Diabetes Complications 14:154, 2000

Allison DB, Fontaine KR, Manson JE, et al: Annual deaths attributable to obesity in the United States. JAMA 282:1530, 1999

Alpert MA: Obesity cardiomyopathy: Pathophysiology and evolution of the clinical syndrome. Am J Med Sci 321:225, 2001

American College of Obstetricians and Gynecologists: Weight Control: Assessment and management. Clinical updates in women's health care. Vol II, No. 3, 2003

American College of Obstetricians and Gynecologists: Obstetric analgesia and anesthesia. Practice Bulletin No. 36, July 2002

American Society for Bariatric Surgery, 2003. http://www.asbs.org/html/rationale/rationale.html.

Armstrong J, Reilly JJ; Child Health Information Team: Breastfeeding and lowering the risk of childhood obesity. Lancet 359:2003, 2002

Baydock S, Chari R: Prepregnancy obesity as an independent risk factor for unexplained stillbirth. Obstet Gynecol 99:74S, 2002

Bianco AT, Smilen SW, Davis Y, et al: Pregnancy outcome and weight gain recommendations for the morbidly obese woman. Obstet Gynecol 91:97, 1998

Bilenka B, Ben-Shlomo I, Cozacov C, et al: Fertility, miscarriage and pregnancy after vertical banded gastroplasty operation for morbid obesity. Acta Obstet Gynecol Scand 74:42, 1995

Bray GA: Low-carbohydrate diets and realities of weight loss. JAMA 289:1853, 2003

Brolin RE: Bariatric surgery and long-term control of morbid obesity. JAMA 288:2793, 2002

Brook RD, Bard RL, Rubenfire M, et al: Usefulness of visceral obesity (waist/hip ratio) in predicting vascular endothelial function in healthy overweight adults. Am J Cardiol 88:264, 2001

Brunicardi FC, Reardon PR, Matthews BD: The surgical treatment of obesity. In Townsend CM, Beauchamp RD, Evers BM, et al (eds): Sabiston Textbook of Surgery, 16th ed. Philadelphia, WB Saunders, 2001, p 247

Buchwald H, Avidor Y, Braunwald E, et al: Bariatric surgery: A systematic review and meta-analysis. JAMA 292:1724, 2004

Calle EE, Rodriguez C, Walker-Thurmond K, et al: Overweight, obesity, and mortality from cancer in a prospectively studied cohort of U.S. adults. N Engl J Med 348:1625, 2003

Calle EE, Thun MJ, Petrelli JM, et al: Body-mass index and mortality in a prospective cohort of US adults. N Engl J Med 341:1097, 1999

Carroll CS Sr, Magann EF, Chauhan SP, et al: Vaginal birth after cesarean section versus elective repeat cesarean delivery: Weight-based outcomes. Am J Obstet Gynecol 188:1516, 2003

Cedergren MI: Maternal morbid obesity and the risk of adverse pregnancy outcome. Obstet Gynecol. 103:219, 2004

Chauhan SP, Magann EF, Carroll CS, et al: Mode of delivery for the morbidly obese with prior cesarean delivery: Vaginal versus repeat cesarean section. Am J Obstet Gynecol 185:349, 2001

Chen S, Noguchi Y, Izumida T, et al: A comparison of the hypotensive and hypoglycemic actions of an angiotensin converting enzyme inhibitor, an AT1a antagonist and troglitazone. J Hypertens 14:1325, 1996

Chinali M, Devereux RB, Howard BV, et al: Comparison of cardiac structure and function in American Indians with and without the metabolic syndrome (the Strong Heart Study). Am J Cardiol 93:40, 2004

Cnattingius S, Bergstrom R, Lipworth L, et al: Prepregnancy weight and the risk of adverse pregnancy outcomes. N Engl J Med 338:147, 1998

Colditz G: Economic costs of obesity and inactivity. Med Sci Sports Exerc 31:S663, 1999

Cunningham FG, Pritchard JA, Hankins GVD, et al: Idiopathic cardiomyopathy or compounding cardiovascular events? Obstet Gynecol 67:157, 1986

Dark AC, Miller L, Kothenbeutel RL, et al: Obesity and second-trimester abortion by dilation and evacuation. J Reprod Med 47:226, 2002

Davi G, Guagnano MT, Ciabattoni G, et al: Platelet activation in obese women. Role of inflammation and oxidant stress. JAMA 288:2008, 2002

Dempsey JC, Williams MA, Luthy DA, et al: Weight at birth and subsequent risk of preeclampsia as an adult. Am J Obstet Gynecol 189:494, 2003

Dixon JB, Dixon ME, O'Brien PE: Pregnancy after Lap-Band surgery: Management of the band to achieve healthy weight outcomes. Obes Surg 11:59, 2001

Drewnowski A, Specter SE: Poverty and obesity: The role of energy density and energy costs. Am J Clin Nutr 79:6, 2004

Ebbeling CB, Pawlak DB, Ludwig DS: Childhood obesity: Public-health crisis, common sense cure. Lancet 360:473, 2002

Edwards RK, Harnsberger DS, Johnson IM, et al: Deciding on route of delivery for obese women with prior cesarean delivery. Am J Obstet Gynecol 189:385, 2003

Ehrenberg HM, Dierker L, Milluzzi C, et al: Prevalence of maternal obesity in an urban center. Am J Obstet Gynecol 187:1189, 2002

Fontaine KR, Redden DT, Wang C, et al: Years of life lost due to obesity. JAMA 289:187, 2003

Ford ES, Giles WH, Dietz WH: Prevalence of the metabolic syndrome among US adults. Findings from the Third National Health and Nutrition Examination Survey. JAMA 287:356, 2002

Freedman DS, Khan LK, Serdula MK, et al: Trends and correlates of Class 3 obesity in the United States from 1990 through 2000. JAMA 288:1758, 2002

Garbaciak JA Jr, Richter M, Miller S, et al: Maternal weight and pregnancy complications. Am J Obstet Gynecol 152:238, 1985

Gilstrap LC, Cunningham FG, VanDorsten JP (eds): Anatomy, incisions, and closures. In Operative Obstetrics, 2nd ed., New York, McGraw-Hill, 2002, p. 55

Gus M, Fuchs SC, Moreira LB, et al: Association between different measurements of obesity and the incidence of hypertension. Am J Hypertens 17:50, 2004

Holt VL, Cushing-Haugen KL, Daling J: Body weight and risk of oral contraceptive failure. Obstet Gynecol 99:820, 2002

Hu FB, Manson JE, Stampfer MJ, et al: Diet, lifestyle, and the risk of type 2 diabetes mellitus in women. N Engl J Med 345:790, 2001

Innes KE, Byers TE, Marshall JA, et al: Association of a woman's own birth weight with subsequent risk for gestational diabetes. JAMA 287:2534, 2002

Institute of Medicine: Nutrition During Pregnancy and Lactation: An Implementation Guide. Washington, DC, National Academy Press, 1992, p. 14

Isaacs JD, Magann EF, Martin RW, et al: Obstetric challenges of massive obesity complicating pregnancy. J Perinatol 14:10, 1994

Jensen DM, Damm P, Sorensen B et al: Pregnancy outcome and prepregnancy body mass index in 2459 glucose-tolerant Danish women. Am J Obstet Gynecol 189:239, 2003

Kabiru W, Raynor BD: Obstetric outcomes associated with increase in BMI category during pregnancy. Am J Obstet Gynecol 191:928, 2004

Kaiser PS, Kirby RS: Obesity as a risk factor for cesarean in a low-risk population. Obstet Gynecol 97:39, 2001

Kenchaiah S, Evans JC, Levy D, et al: Obesity and the risk of heart failure. N Engl J Med 347:305, 2002

Kimm SYS, Glynn NW, Kriska AM, et al: Decline in physical activity in black girls and white girls during adolescence. N Engl J Med 347:709, 2002

Knudsen LB, Källén B: Intestinal bypass operation and pregnancy outcome. Acta Obstet Gynecol Scand 65:831, 1986

Kuczmarski RJ, Flegal KM, Campbell SM, et al: Increasing prevalence of overweight among US adults: The National Health and Nutrition Examination Surveys, 1960 to 1991. JAMA 272:205, 1994

Kumari AS: Pregnancy outcome in women with morbid obesity. Int J Gynaecol Obstet 73:101, 2001

Li R, Jewell S, Grummer-Strawn L: Maternal obesity and breast-feeding practices. Am J Clin Nutr 77:931, 2003.

Lu GC, Rouse DJ, DuBard MA, et al: The effect of the increasing prevalence of maternal obesity on perinatal morbidity. Am J Obstet Gynecol 185:845, 2001

Martin LF, Finigan KM, Nolan TE: Pregnancy after adjustable gastric banding. Obstet Gynecol 94:927, 2000

Mikhail LN, Mittendorf R, Walker CK: The association of maternal obesity and isolated major fetal congenital cardiac anomalies in African-American women. Am J Obstet Gynecol 174:446, 1996

Mitka M: Surgery for obesity: Demand soars amid scientific, ethical questions. JAMA 289:1761, 2003

Mokdad AH, Bowman BA, Ford ES, et al: The continuing epidemics of obesity and diabetes in the United States. JAMA 286:1195, 2001

Mokdad AH, Ford ES, Bowman BA, et al: Prevalence of obesity, diabetes, and obesity-related health risk factors, 2001. JAMA 289:76, 2003

Moore KA, Ouyang DW, Whang EE: Maternal and fetal deaths after gastric bypass surgery for morbid obesity. N Engl J Med. 351:721, 2004

Must A, Spadano J, Coakley EH, et al: The disease burden associated with overweight and obesity. JAMA 282:1523, 1999

Myles TD, Gooch J, Santolaya J: Obesity as an independent risk factor for infectious morbidity in patients who undergo cesarean delivery. Obstet Gynecol 100:959, 2002

National Center for Health Statistics. Prevalence of overweight among children and adolescents: United States, 1999

National Heart, Lung, and Blood Institute. Clinical Guidelines on the Identification, Evaluation and Treatment of Overweight and Obesity in Adults: The Evidence Report. Washington, DC: Government Printing Office, 1998

National Institutes of Health Technology Assessment Conference Panel: Very low-calorie diets. National Task Force on the Prevention and Treatment of Obesity. JAMA 270: 967, 1993

National Institutes of Health. Third Report of the National Cholesterol Education Program Expert Panel on detection, evaluation, and treatment of high blood cholesterol in adults (Adult Treatment Panel III). Bethesda, MD, National Institutes of Health, NIH Publication 01-3670, 2001

National Task Force on the Prevention and Treatment of Obesity: Overweight, obesity, and health risk. Arch Intern Med 160:898, 2000

Neill AM, Nelson-Piercy C: Hazards of assisted conception in women with severe medical disease. Hum Fertil (Camb) 4:239, 2001

Ninomiya JK, L'Italien G, Criqui MH, et al: Association of the metabolic syndrome with history of myocardial infarction and stroke in the third national health and nutrition examination survey. Circulation 109:42, 2004

O'Brien TE, Ray JG, Chan WS: Maternal body mass index and the risk of preeclampsia: A systematic overview. Epidemiology 14:368, 2003

Ogden CL, Flegal KM, Carroll MD, et al: Prevalence and trends in overweight among US children and adolescents, 1999–2000. JAMA 288:1728, 2002

Peeters A, Barendregt JJ, Willekens F, et al: Obesity in adulthood and its consequences for life expectancy: A life-table analysis. Ann Intern Med 138:24, 2003

Pleis JR, Senson V, Schiller JS: Summary health statistics for US Adults: National Health Interview Survey, 2000. National Center for Health Statistics. Vital Health Stat 10, 2003

Printen KJ, Scott D: Pregnancy following gastric bypass for the treatment of morbid obesity. Am Surg 48:363, 1982

Public Health Service: Healthy People 2000: National Health Promotion and Disease Prevention Objectives. Washington, DC, US Department of Health and Human Services, Public Health Service, DHHS Publication No. (PHS) 90-50212, 1990

Rahimy MH, Cromie MA, Hopkins NK, et al: Lunelle monthly contraceptive injection (medroxyprogesterone acetate and estradiol cypionate injectable suspension): Effects of body weight and injection sites on pharmacokinetics. Contraception 60:201, 1999

Ramsay JE, Ferrell WR, Crawford L, et al: Maternal obesity is associated with dysregulation of metabolic, vascular, and inflammatory pathways. J Clin Endocrinol Metab 87:4231, 2002

Richards DS, Miller DK, Goodman GN: Pregnancy after gastric bypass for morbid obesity. J Reprod Med 32:172, 1987

Rizzo T, Metzger BE, Burns WJ, et al: Correlations between antepartum maternal metabolism and intelligence of offspring. N Engl J Med 325:911, 1991

Rooney BL, Schauberger CW: Excess pregnancy weight gain and long-term obesity: One decade later. Obstet Gynecol 100:245, 2002

Ruowei L, Jewell S, Grummer-Strawn L: Maternal obesity and breast-feeding practices. Am J Clin Nutr 77:931, 2003

Schoenborn CA, Adams PF, Barnes PM: Body weight status of adults: United States, 1997–98. Advance data from vital and health statistics, No. 330, National Center for Health Statistics, 2002

Sebire NJ, Jolly M, Harris JP, et al: Maternal obesity and pregnancy outcome: A study of 287,213 pregnancies in London. Int J Obes Relat Metab Disord 25:1175, 2001

Shaw GM, Todoroff K, Schaffer DM, et al: Maternal height and prepregnancy body mass index as risk factors for selected congenital anomalies. Paediatr Perinat Epidemiol 14:234, 2000

Shaw GM, Velie EM, Schaffer D: Risk of neural tube defect–affected pregnancies among obese women. JAMA 275:1093, 1996

Sheiner E, Levy A, Silverberg D, et al: Pregnancy after bariatric surgery is not associated with adverse perinatal outcome. Am J Obstet Gynecol 190:1335, 2004

Steinbrook R: Surgery for severe obesity. N Engl J Med 350:1075, 2004

Stephansson O, Dickman PW, Johansson A, et al: Maternal weight, pregnancy weight gain, and the risk of antepartum stillbirth. Am J Obstet Gynecol 184:463, 2001

Waller DK, Mills JL, Simpson JL, et al: Are obese women at higher risk for producing malformed offspring? Am J Obstet Gynecol 170:541, 1994

Watkins ML, Rasmussen SA, Honein MA, et al: Maternal obesity and risk for birth defects. Pediatrics 111:1152, 2003

Werler MM, Louik C, Shapiro S, et al: Prepregnant weight in relation to risk of neural tube defects. JAMA 275:1089, 1996

Wittgrove AC, Jester L, Wittgrove P, et al: Pregnancy following gastric bypass for morbid obesity. Obes Surg 8:461, 1998

Wolf M, Kettyle E, Sandler L, et al: Obesity and preeclampsia: The potential role of inflammation. Obstet Gynecol 98:757, 2001

Wolfe HM, Sokol RJ, Martier SM, et al: Maternal obesity: A potential source of error in sonographic prenatal diagnosis. Obstet Gynecol 76:339, 1990

Yanovski JA, Yanovski SZ: Recent advances in basic obesity research. JAMA 282:1504, 1999

Yanovski SZ, Yanovski JA: Obesity. N Engl J Med 346:591, 2002

Young TK, Woodmansee B: Factors that are associated with cesarean delivery in a large private practice: The importance of prepregnancy body mass index and weight gain. Am J Obstet Gynecol 187:312, 2002

Zieman M, Guillebaud J, Weisberg E, et al: Contraceptive efficacy and cycle control with the Ortho Evra/Evra transdermal system: The analysis of pooled data. Fertil Steril 77:S13, 2002

44

Cardiovascular Disease

Heart disease is the leading cause of death in women in the United States and the third leading cause in individuals who are 25 to 44 years of age (Anderson, 2002). Heart disease of varying severity complicates about 1 percent of pregnancies, and associated maternal mortality has decreased remarkably over the past 50 years. For example, Sachs and associates (1988) reported that maternal mortality from cardiac disease fell from 5.6 to 0.3 per 100,000 live births in Massachusetts from 1954 through 1985. Despite this, heart disease still contributes significantly to maternal mortality, both in the United States and throughout the world. Berg and colleagues (2003) reported that cardiomyopathy alone was responsible for 7.7 percent of 3201 pregnancy-related deaths in the United States between 1991 and 1997. Cardiac disease accounted for 40 of 105 indirect maternal deaths in the United Kingdom between 1994 and 1996 (de Swiet, 2000).

PHYSIOLOGICAL CONSIDERATIONS ASSOCIATED WITH HEART DISEASE IN PREGNANCY

As detailed in Chapter 5 (see p. 132), the marked hemodynamic changes stimulated by pregnancy have a profound effect on underlying heart disease. The most important consideration is that during pregnancy, cardiac output is increased by as much as 50 percent. Capeless and Clapp (1989) have shown that almost half of the total increase occurs by 8 weeks, and it is maximized by midpregnancy. The early increase can be attributed to augmented stroke volume that results from decreased vascular resistance. Later in pregnancy, resting pulse increases, and stroke volume increases even more, presumably because of increased diastolic filling from the expanded blood volume. These changes are even more profound in multifetal pregnancy (Kametas and colleagues, 2003).

An important study by Clark and colleagues (1989) contributed greatly to the understanding of cardiovascular physiology during pregnancy. Using right-sided heart catheterization, these investigators measured hemodynamic function in 10 healthy primigravid women. Pregnancy values were compared with values measured again 11 to 13 weeks postpartum (Table 44–1). At or near term, cardiac output in the lateral recumbent position was increased 43 percent by virtue of elevated pulse rate and stroke volume. Systemic and pulmonary vascular resistance were concomitantly decreased, and importantly, there was no change in intrinsic left ventricular contractility. As shown in Figure 5–10 (see p. 134), pregnancy is characterized by normal left ventricular function, and not hyperdynamic function as once thought. These investigators concluded that maintenance of normal left ventricular filling pressures comes about as the result of ventricular dilatation.

TABLE 44–1 Hemodynamic Changes in 10 Normal Pregnant Women at Term Compared with Postpartum Values

Parameter	Change (%)
Cardiac output	+43
Heart rate	+17
Left ventricular stroke work index	+17
Vascular resistance	
Systemic	−21
Pulmonary	−34
Mean arterial pressure	+4
Colloid osmotic pressure	−14

Data from Clark and colleagues, 1989.

Because significant hemodynamic alterations are apparent early in pregnancy, women with severe cardiac dysfunction may experience worsening of heart failure before midpregnancy. In others, heart failure develops after 28 weeks, when pregnancy-induced hypervolemia is maximal. In the majority, however, heart failure develops peripartum when the physiological capability for rapid changes in cardiac output may be overwhelmed in the presence of structural cardiac disease. In the series by Etheridge and Pepperell (1977), of 542 women whose pregnancies were complicated by heart disease, 8 of 10 maternal deaths occurred during the puerperium.

DIAGNOSIS OF HEART DISEASE

As shown in Figure 44–1, many of the physiological adaptations of normal pregnancy alter physical findings, making the diagnosis of heart disease more difficult. For example, in normal pregnancy, functional systolic heart murmurs are quite common; respiratory effort is accentuated, at times suggesting dyspnea; and edema in the lower extremities usually develops after midpregnancy. It is important not to diagnose heart disease during pregnancy when none exists, and at the same time not to fail to detect and appropriately treat heart disease when it does exist. Listed in Table 44–2 are a number of clinical findings that may suggest heart disease. Pregnant women who have none of these findings rarely have serious heart disease.

DIAGNOSTIC STUDIES. Most diagnostic cardiovascular studies are noninvasive and can be conducted safely in pregnant women. In most cases, conventional testing, including electrocardiography, echocardiography, and chest radiography, provides necessary data. Radiolabeled ^{99}Tc-albumin or red cells may be used to evaluate ventricular function. The estimated fetal radiation exposure for a 20-mCi dose is 120 mrad, well below the accepted level for significant teratogenic or oncogenic effect (see Chap. 41, p. 981). Thallium[201] is used to evaluate regional coronary perfusion. A standard

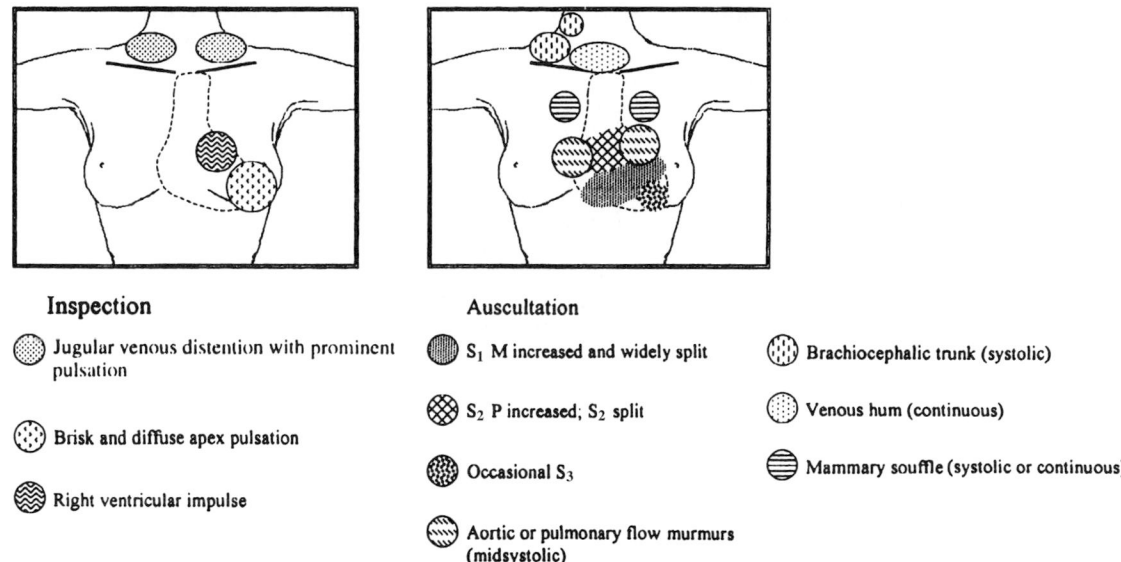

Inspection

⬤ Jugular venous distention with prominent pulsation

⬤ Brisk and diffuse apex pulsation

⬤ Right ventricular impulse

Auscultation

⬤ S₁ M increased and widely split

⬤ S₂ P increased; S₂ split

⬤ Occasional S₃

⬤ Aortic or pulmonary flow murmurs (midsystolic)

⬤ Brachiocephalic trunk (systolic)

⬤ Venous hum (continuous)

⬤ Mammary souffle (systolic or continuous)

FIGURE 44–1. Normal cardiac examination findings in the pregnant woman. Abbreviations: $S_1 =$ first sound, $S_2 =$ second sound, P = pulmonary, M = mitral. (Reproduced from Gei and Hankins, 2001, with permission.)

dose yields a fetal exposure of 300 to 1100 mrad and depends on the stage of gestation. If indicated, right-sided heart catheterization can be performed with limited fluoroscopy. On rare occasions, it may be necessary to perform left-sided heart catheterization. In women with clear indications, any minimal theoretical risk is outweighed by maternal benefits.

Electrocardiography. As the diaphragm is elevated in advancing pregnancy, there is an average 15-degree left-axis deviation in the electrocardiogram (ECG), and mild ST changes may be seen in the inferior leads. Atrial and ventricular premature contractions are relatively frequent (Carruth and colleagues, 1981). Pregnancy does not alter voltage findings.

TABLE 44–2 Clinical Indicators of Heart Disease During Pregnancy

Symptoms
Progressive dyspnea or orthopnea
Nocturnal cough
Hemoptysis
Syncope
Chest pain

Clinical Findings
Cyanosis
Clubbing of fingers
Persistent neck vein distention
Systolic murmur grade 3/6 or greater
Diastolic murmur
Cardiomegaly
Persistent arrhythmia
Persistent split second sound
Criteria for pulmonary hypertension

Chest Radiography. Anteroposterior and lateral chest radiographs may be useful when heart disease is suspected clinically. When used with a lead apron shield, fetal radiation exposure is minimized (see Chap. 41, p. 979). Slight heart enlargement cannot be detected accurately by radiography because the heart silhouette normally is larger in pregnancy. That said, gross cardiomegaly can usually be excluded.

Echocardiography. The widespread use of echocardiography has allowed accurate diagnosis of most heart diseases during pregnancy. It allows noninvasive evaluation of structural and functional cardiac factors. Some normal pregnancy-induced changes include tricuspid regurgitation as well as significantly increased left atrial size and left ventricular outflow cross-sectional area (Limacher and co-workers, 1985).

CLINICAL CLASSIFICATION. There is no clinically applicable test for accurately measuring functional cardiac capacity. A helpful clinical classification was first published in 1928 by the New York Heart Association (NYHA) and was revised for the eighth time in 1979. This classification is based on past and present disability and is uninfluenced by physical signs.

• **Class I.** *Uncompromised (no limitation of physical activity):* These women do not have symptoms of cardiac insufficiency or experience anginal pain.
• **Class II.** *Slight limitation of physical activity:* These women are comfortable at rest, but if ordinary physical

activity is undertaken, discomfort results in the form of excessive fatigue, palpitation, dyspnea, or anginal pain.

- **Class III.** *Marked limitation of physical activity:* These women are comfortable at rest, but less than ordinary activity causes excessive fatigue, palpitation, dyspnea, or anginal pain.
- **Class IV.** *Severely compromised (inability to perform any physical activity without discomfort):* Symptoms of cardiac insufficiency or angina may develop even at rest, and if any physical activity is undertaken, discomfort is increased.

Siu and associates (2001) expanded on the NYHA classification and developed a scoring system for predicting cardiac complications during pregnancy based on their prospective analysis of 562 consecutive pregnant women with heart disease in 13 Canadian teaching hospitals. Predictors of cardiac complications included the following:

1. Prior heart failure, transient ischemic attack, arrhythmia, or stroke.
2. Baseline NYHA class III or greater or cyanosis.
3. Left-sided heart obstruction defined as mitral valve area below 2 cm², aortic valve area below 1.5 cm², or peak left ventricular outflow tract gradient above 30 mm Hg by echocardiography.
4. Ejection fraction less than 40 percent.

The risk of pulmonary edema, sustained arrhythmia, stroke, cardiac arrest, or cardiac death was substantively increased with one of these factors and even more so with two or more factors.

In another study of 1000 pregnant women with heart disease from Brazil, Avila and co-workers (2003) reported that 25 percent had cardiovascular complications during pregnancy. These included heart failure (12 percent), arrhythmias (6 percent), thromboembolism, angina, hypoxemia, and infective endocarditis. Maternal mortality was 2.7 percent.

PRECONCEPTIONAL COUNSELING. Women with heart disease may benefit from counseling before deciding to become pregnant (see Chap. 7, p. 192). Maternal mortality generally varies directly with functional classification at pregnancy onset, however, this relationship may change as pregnancy progresses. In the study cited earlier, Siu and colleagues (2001) observed a 6-percent incidence of heart failure in nearly 600 women with NYHA class I or II disease. Their experiences, as well as those of McFaul and co-workers (1988), were that there were no maternal deaths in 1041 of women with class I or II disease.

In some women, life-threatening cardiac abnormalities can be reversed by corrective surgery, and subsequent pregnancy is less dangerous. In other cases, such as women with mechanical valves and those who are taking warfarin, fetal considerations predominate. The classification scheme shown in Table 44–3 stratifies the mortality risk to aid in counseling.

TABLE 44–3 Risks for Maternal Mortality Caused by Various Types of Heart Disease

Cardiac Disorder	Mortality
Group 1—Minimal Risk	0–1%
Atrial septal defect	
Ventricular septal defect	
Patent ductus arteriosus	
Pulmonic or tricuspid disease	
Fallot tetralogy, corrected	
Bioprosthetic valve	
Mitral stenosis, NYHA class I and II	
Group 2—Moderate Risk	5–15%
2A:	
Mitral stenosis, NYHA class III and IV	
Aortic stenosis	
Aortic coarctation without valvular involvement	
Fallot tetralogy, uncorrected	
Previous myocardial infarction	
Marfan syndrome, normal aorta	
2B:	
Mitral stenosis with atrial fibrillation	
Artificial valve	
Group 3—Major Risk	25–50%
Pulmonary hypertension	
Aortic coarctation with valvular involvement	
Marfan syndrome with aortic involvement	

NYHA = New York Heart Association.
From the American College of Obstetricians and Gynecologists, 1992, with permission.

Congenital Heart Disease in Offspring. Many congenital heart lesions appear to be inherited as polygenic characteristics (see Chap. 12, p. 302). Thus, it might be expected that some women with congenital lesions would give birth to similarly affected infants. In general, the risk of congenital heart disease in the offspring of a woman with a particular condition is approximately 3 to 4 percent (Lupton and colleagues, 2002). More specific estimates are presented in Table 44–4.

TABLE 44–4 Recurrence Risk of Congenital Heart Disease

Cardiac Lesion	Congenital Heart Disease in Fetus (%)		
	Previous Sibling Affected	*Father Affected*	*Mother Affected*
Marfan syndrome	NA	50	50
Aortic stenosis	2	3	15–18
Pulmonary stenosis	2	2	6–7
Ventricular septal defect	3	2	10–16
Atrial septal defect	2.5	1.5	5–11
Patent ductus arteriosus	3	2.5	4
Coarctation of the aorta	NA	NA	14
Tetralogy of Fallot	2.5	1.5	2–3

NA = not available.
Reproduced from Lupton and colleagues, 2002, with permission.

GENERAL MANAGEMENT

In most instances, management involves a team approach, including an obstetrician, cardiologist, anesthesiologist, and other specialists as needed. Cardiovascular changes likely to be poorly tolerated by an individual woman are identified, and a plan is formulated to minimize these. Four changes that affect management are emphasized by the American College of Obstetricians and Gynecologists (1992):

1. The 50-percent increase in blood volume and cardiac output by the early third trimester.
2. Further fluctuations in volume and cardiac output in the peripartum period.
3. A decline in systemic vascular resistance, reaching a nadir in the second trimester, and then rising to 20 percent below normal by late pregnancy.
4. Hypercoagulability, of special importance in women requiring anticoagulation before pregnancy with coumarin derivatives.

Within this framework, both prognosis and management are influenced by the nature and severity of the specific lesion, in addition to the functional classification.

MANAGEMENT OF CLASS I AND II DISEASE. With rare exceptions, women in NYHA class I and most in class II go through pregnancy without morbidity. Special attention should be directed toward both prevention and early recognition of heart failure. As discussed in a scholarly review by Jessup and Brozena (2003), the onset of congestive heart failure is generally gradual. The first warning sign is likely to be persistent basilar rales, frequently accompanied by a nocturnal cough. A sudden diminution in ability to carry out usual duties, increasing dyspnea on exertion, or attacks of smothering with cough are symptoms of serious heart failure. Clinical findings may include hemoptysis, progressive edema, and tachycardia.

Infection with sepsis syndrome is an important factor in precipitating cardiac failure. Moreover, bacterial endocarditis is a deadly complication of valvular heart disease. Each woman should receive instructions to avoid contact with persons who have respiratory infections, including the common cold, and to report at once any evidence for infection. Pneumococcal and influenza vaccines are recommended.

Cigarette smoking is prohibited, both because of its cardiac effects as well as the propensity to cause upper respiratory infections. Illicit drug use may be particularly harmful, given the cardiovascular effects of cocaine or amphetamines, in addition to the propensity for intravenous use of any illegal substance to cause infective endocarditis.

Labor and Delivery. In general, delivery should be accomplished vaginally unless there are obstetrical indications for cesarean delivery. Induction is generally safe (Oron and colleagues, 2004). As discussed in Chapter 42 (see p. 989), *pulmonary artery catheterization* may be indicated for continuous hemodynamic monitoring in some women with heart disease. In our experience, such monitoring is rarely indicated, especially in women who have remained in functional NYHA class I or II.

Relief from pain and apprehension is especially important. Although intravenous analgesics provide satisfactory pain relief for some women, continuous epidural analgesia is recommended in most cases. The major problem with conduction analgesia is maternal hypotension (see Chap. 19, p. 484). This is especially dangerous in women with intracardiac shunts, in whom flow may be reversed, with blood passing from right to left within the heart or aorta, thereby bypassing the lungs. Hypotension can be life-threatening with pulmonary hypertension or aortic stenosis because ventricular output is dependent on adequate preload. In women with these conditions, narcotic conduction analgesia or general anesthesia may be preferable.

During labor, the mother with significant heart disease should be kept in a semirecumbent position with lateral tilt. Vital signs should be taken frequently between contractions. Increases in pulse rate much above 100 per minute or in the respiratory rate above 24 per minute, particularly when associated with dyspnea, may suggest impending ventricular failure. If there is any evidence of cardiac decompensation, intensive medical management must be instituted immediately. It is essential to remember that delivery itself does not necessarily improve the maternal condition. Moreover, emergency operative delivery may be particularly hazardous. Clearly, both maternal and fetal conditions must be considered in the decision to hasten delivery under these circumstances.

For vaginal delivery in women with only mild cardiovascular compromise, epidural analgesia given along with intravenous sedation often suffices. This has been shown to minimize intrapartum cardiac output fluctuations and allows forceps or vacuum-assisted delivery. Subarachnoid blockade is not generally recommended in women with significant heart disease. For cesarean delivery, epidural analgesia is preferred by most clinicians with caveats for its use with pulmonary hypertension. Finally, general endotracheal anesthesia with thiopental, succinylcholine, nitrous oxide, and at least 30-percent oxygen has also proved satisfactory (see Chap. 19, p. 488).

INTRAPARTUM HEART FAILURE. Cardiovascular decompensation during labor may manifest as pulmonary edema and hypoxia, hypotension, or both. The proper therapeutic approach depends on the specific hemodynamic status and the underlying cardiac lesion. For example, decompensated mitral stenosis with pulmonary edema due to fluid overload is often best approached with aggressive diuresis, or if precipitated by tachycardia, by heart rate control with β-blocking agents. On the other hand, the same treatment in a woman suffering decompensation and hypotension due to aortic stenosis could prove fatal. **Unless the underlying pathophysiology is understood and the cause of the decompensation clear, empirical therapy is hazardous.**

Puerperium. Women who have shown little or no evidence of cardiac distress during pregnancy, labor, or delivery may still decompensate postpartum. Therefore, it is important that meticulous care be continued into the puerperium. Postpartum hemorrhage, anemia, infection, and thromboembolism are much more serious complications with heart disease. Indeed, these factors often act in concert to precipitate postpartum heart failure in women with underlying disease (Cunningham and associates, 1986).

If tubal sterilization is to be performed after vaginal delivery, it may be best to delay the procedure until it is obvious that the mother is afebrile, not anemic, and has demonstrated that she can ambulate without evidence of distress. Women who do not undergo tubal sterilization should be given detailed contraceptive advice. Special considerations for contraception in women with various cardiac disorders are discussed in some of the following sections and throughout Chapter 32.

MANAGEMENT OF CLASS III AND IV DISEASE.

These severe cases are uncommon today. In the Canadian study by Siu and associates (2001) cited earlier, only 3 percent of the women had NYHA class III heart disease, and none had class IV when first seen. The important question in these women is whether pregnancy should be undertaken. If women choose to become pregnant, they must understand the risks and cooperate fully with planned care. If seen early enough, women with some types of severe cardiac disease should consider pregnancy interruption. If the pregnancy is continued, prolonged hospitalization or bed rest is often necessary.

Epidural analgesia for labor and delivery is usually recommended. Vaginal delivery is preferred in most cases, and labor induction can usually be done safely (Oron and associates, 2004). Cesarean delivery is limited to obstetrical indications. The decision for cesarean delivery must take into account the specific cardiac lesion, overall maternal condition, availability and experience of anesthetic support, as well as physical facilities. These women often tolerate major surgical procedures poorly and should be delivered in a facility with experience with complicated cardiac disease.

SURGICALLY CORRECTED HEART DISEASE

The majority of clinically significant lesions are repaired during childhood. Examples of defects not diagnosed until adulthood include atrial septal defects, pulmonic stenosis, bicuspid aortic valve, and aortic coarctation (Brickner and colleagues, 2000). In some cases, the defect is mild and surgery is not required. In others, a significant structural anomaly is amenable to surgical correction. With successful repair, many women attempt pregnancy. In some instances, surgical corrections have been performed during pregnancy.

VALVE REPLACEMENT BEFORE PREGNANCY. A number of reproductive-aged women have had a prosthesis implanted to replace a severely damaged mitral or aortic valve. Reports of subsequent pregnancy outcomes are now quite numerous, and indeed, successful pregnancies have followed prosthetic replacement of even three heart valves (Nagorney and Field, 1981).

Effects on Pregnancy. Pregnancy is to be undertaken in these women only after serious consideration. Women with a *mechanical valve prosthesis* must be anticoagulated, and when not pregnant, warfarin is recommended. As shown in Table 44–5, a number of serious complications can develop, especially with mechanical valves. Thromboembolism involving the prosthesis and hemorrhage from anticoagulation are of extreme concern (Nassar and co-workers, 2004). There also may be deterioration in cardiac function. Overall, maternal mortality is 3 to 4 percent with mechanical valves, and fetal loss is common.

The critical issue is anticoagulation, and there is a suggestion that heparin may be less effective than warfarin in preventing thromboembolic events. Unfortunately, spontaneous abortions, stillbirths, and malformed fetuses are more common if warfarin is used (see Chap. 14, p. 349). The results shown in Table 44–5 are similar to those reported by Chan and colleagues (2000) in their review. They concluded that better maternal outcomes were achieved with continuation of warfarin throughout pregnancy, however, the embryopathy rate was 6.4 percent. Heparin substitution from 6 to 12 weeks eliminated embryopathy, but thromboembolic complications significantly increased. Cotrufo and colleagues (2002) described the outcomes of 71 pregnancies in women with mechanical valve prostheses who were anticoagulated with warfarin for the entire duration of pregnancy. Although there were no maternal deaths or thromboembolic or hemorrhagic complications, the rates of miscarriage (32 percent), stillbirth (7 percent), and embryopathy (6 percent) were all increased. The risk of complications was higher when the mean daily dose of warfarin exceeded 5 mg.

Low-dose unfractionated heparin is definitely inadequate. Iturbe-Alessio and colleagues (1986) reported that 3 of 35 women on such therapy suffered massive thrombosis of a mitral prosthesis—two of these died. Similarly, Chan and co-workers (2000) found in their review that two of five women treated solely with low-dose heparin during pregnancy died. Low-molecular-weight heparin also is problematic because of reports of valvular thrombosis in patients, especially pregnant women, who were apparently adequately anticoagulated (Leyh and colleagues, 2002, 2003; Rowan and associates, 2001). Following such reports and a warning issued by Aventis Pharmaceuticals, the American College of Obstetricians and Gynecologists (2002) advises against

TABLE 44–5 Perinatal Outcomes in Women Who Had a Heart Valve Replaced Prior to Pregnancy

Type of Valve	No.	Complications	
		Maternal	*Perinatal*
Mechanical Valves	**523**		
Iturbe-Alessio et al (1986)	72	3 thromboses 2 deaths	10/35 embryopathy 1 stillborn
Sareli et al (1989)	50	2 heart failure in labor	9 abortions; 7 stillborns; 2 neonatal deaths; 2 embryopathy
Hanania et al (1994)	108	10 thromboses with 3 emboli; 6 emboli; 4 deaths	30 abortions; 4 stillborns
Sbarouni and Oakley (1994)	151	13 thromboses; 8 emboli; 7 hemorrhage; 6 deaths	9 stillborns; 3 neonatal deaths
Suri et al (1999)	21	1 thrombosis with death; 2 hemorrhage	2 stillborns; 4 growth-restricted infants
Sadler et al (2000)	50	4/14 thromboses with heparin; 1 death	70% pregnancy loss with warfarin 25% pregnancy loss with heparin 57% preterm delivery 4 stillborns with warfarin
Cotrufo et al (2002)	71	No deaths or thromboses	23 abortions; 5 stillborns; 4 embryopathy
Porcine Xenograft	**265**		
Lee et al (1994)	95	4 valve dysfunction	—
Hanania et al (1994)	74	7 valve failure	9 abortions; 1 stillborn
Sbarouni and Oakley (1994)	63	17 valve deterioration	2 stillborns
Sadler et al (2000)	33	4 valve deterioration	1 neonatal death

use of low-molecular-weight heparins in pregnant women with prosthetic heart valves. Potential alternatives that need further evaluation include antiplatelet therapy with dipyridamole, ticlopidine, and aspirin (Ueno and collaborators, 2001). Nassar and co-workers (2003) have described the use of thrombolytic agents for a thrombosed mitral valve prosthesis during pregnancy.

Porcine tissue valves are much safer during pregnancy (see Table 44–5), primarily because anticoagulation is not required. Deviri and colleagues (1985) reported no thromboses during 22 pregnancies in 11 unanticoagulated women with a porcine xenograft. Lee and associates (1994) described generally good outcomes in 95 pregnancies in 57 women with a porcine graft. That said, valvular dysfunction with heart failure has been common (see Table 44–5). Additionally, although such bioprostheses are less thrombogenic, they are not as durable as mechanical prostheses. Their use necessitates the acceptance of another valve replacement in 10 to 15 years. Fortunately, pregnancy does not appear to shorten this interval (North and colleagues, 1999; Salazar and co-workers, 1999).

Management. For women with a mechanical heart valve, most clinicians recommend full anticoagulation throughout pregnancy (American College of Obstetricians and Gynecologists, 2000). This may be accomplished with adjusted-dose heparin to prolong the partial thromboplastin time by 1.5 to 2.5 times baseline values (see Chap. 47, p. 1082). The American Heart Association and American College of Cardiology Foundation recommend that if unfractionated heparin is used, it should be given subcutaneously twice daily, starting at a total dose of 35,000 U. Laboratory monitoring should be performed at least twice weekly (Hirsh and colleagues,

2003). Alternatively, Reimold and Rutherford (2003) recommend the use of warfarin to achieve a target international normalized ratio of 2.0 to 3.0 throughout most of pregnancy. Between 6 and 12 weeks and again after 36 weeks, they use unfractionated heparin.

Heparin is stopped just before delivery. If delivery supervenes while the anticoagulant is still effective, and extensive bleeding is encountered, *protamine sulfate* is given intravenously. Anticoagulant therapy with warfarin or heparin may be restarted 6 hours following vaginal delivery, usually with no problems. Following cesarean delivery, however, full anticoagulation should be withheld for at least 24 hours. Clark and colleagues (2000) reviewed the use of coumarin derivatives in breast feeding women and concluded that warfarin can be safely give, because transfer to milk is minimal.

CONTRACEPTION. Because of their possible thrombogenic action, estrogen–progestin oral contraceptives are relatively contraindicated in women with prosthetic valves (see Chap. 32, p. 732). Because such women are generally fully anticoagulated, however, any increased risk is speculative. Sterilization should be considered because of serious problems during pregnancy.

VALVE REPLACEMENT DURING PREGNANCY. Although usually postponed until after delivery, valve replacement during pregnancy may be lifesaving. A number of reviews all confirm that surgery on the heart or great vessels is associated with major maternal and fetal morbidity and mortality. Weiss and colleagues (1998a) reviewed cases between 1984 and 1996. In 70 women, 59 of whom had cardiopulmonary bypass, maternal mortality was 6 percent and perinatal mortality was 30 percent. With valvular surgery, maternal mortality was 9 percent. More recently, Arnoni and associates (2003) reviewed the outcomes of 58 such women from Brazil. The maternal mortality rate was 8 percent, and 18 percent of the fetuses died as a direct result of the surgery. They concluded that mortality might be reduced by performing procedures earlier in gestation, avoiding emergency operations, and minimizing bypass time.

Strickland and colleagues (1991) reported the Mayo Clinic experience in 10 women undergoing cardiopulmonary bypass with pump times ranging from 18 to 154 minutes. The fetal response to bypass was usually bradycardia, and the investigators recommended that high-flow, normothermic perfusion be used if possible. Khandelwal and associates (1996) meticulously recorded fetal and uterine blood flow velocity patterns during a 74-minute bypass procedure at 19 weeks for aortic valve replacement. Despite high peak flow rates and sustained mean arterial pressures, uterine and umbilical artery resistances increased greatly, and fetal hydrocephalus and ascites developed within 2 days.

MITRAL VALVOTOMY DURING PREGNANCY. This operation is less commonly performed because the incidence of rheumatic mitral stenosis has declined. Schenker and Polishuk (1968) described 325 pregnancies in 182 women who previously had undergone mitral valvotomy. Heart failure developed in 42 percent of these women at some point during their first pregnancy following valvular surgery. This percentage increased with successive pregnancies, and women suffering heart failure in one pregnancy inevitably had recurrence in subsequent pregnancies. Coexisting atrial fibrillation was especially ominous and commonly was associated with heart failure, thromboembolic disease, and death.

In the past, tight mitral stenosis that required intervention during pregnancy usually was treated surgically by closed mitral valvotomy (Pavankumar and associates, 1988). In the past 25 years, percutaneous transcatheter balloon dilatation of the mitral valve has largely replaced surgical valvotomy during pregnancy (Abouzied, 2001; Gupta, 1998; Malhotra, 2003, and all their associates). In one series, de Souza and colleagues (2001a) described 24 consecutive pregnant women who underwent open mitral commissurotomy between 1985 and 1990 and compared them with 21 consecutive pregnant women who underwent percutaneous balloon mitral valvuloplasty between 1990 and 1995. The one maternal death occurred in the open-repair group. The balloon procedure was over 90-percent successful, and functional outcomes between the two groups were similar. Perinatal mortality was sixfold higher in the open repair group (33 versus 5 percent). The investigators rightfully concluded that balloon valvuloplasty is the treatment of choice for refractory congestive heart failure in pregnant women.

HEART TRANSPLANTATION. By 1994, the registry of the International Society for Heart and Lung Transplantation had compiled data from more than 30,000 heart and heart–lung transplant operations (Hosenpud and associates, 1994). The procedure increasingly has become more successful, especially since more efficacious medications to prevent vasculopathy and rejection of the allograft have become available (Eisen and co-workers, 2003). It is now estimated that at least two thirds of recipients are fully functional following heart transplantation (Kapp, 2003). In a remarkable example, a 42-year-old female heart transplant recipient climbed Mount Whitney with two different hearts, and subsequently, she scaled Mount Kilimanjaro and the Matterhorn (Kapp, 2003)!

In 1988, Löwenstein and associates reported the first successful pregnancy in a heart transplant recipient. Key and associates (1989) as well as Kim and colleagues (1996) provided detailed data to show that the transplanted heart responded normally to pregnancy-induced changes. Complications are common during pregnancy. Armenti and associates (2001) analyzed 48 pregnancies in 27 heart transplant recipients entered into the National Transplantation Pregnancy Registry. Fifty percent developed hypertension, 22 percent suffered at least one rejection episode during pregnancy, and almost 50 percent delivered preterm. At followup, five women had died, all at more than 2 years postpartum. Similar results were reported by Dashe and associates (1998) in their review.

VALVULAR HEART DISEASE

Rheumatic fever is uncommon in the United States because of less crowded living conditions, availability of penicillin, and evolution of nonrheumatogenic streptococcal strains. Still, it remains the chief cause of serious mitral valvular disease.

MITRAL STENOSIS. Rheumatic endocarditis causes three fourths of cases of mitral stenosis. The contracted valve impedes blood flow from the left atrium to the ventricle. As shown in Table 44–6, with tight stenosis, the left atrium is dilated, left atrial pressure is chronically elevated, and significant passive pulmonary hypertension may develop. The increased preload of normal pregnancy, as well as other factors that require increased cardiac output, may cause ventricular failure with pulmonary edema in these women with relatively fixed cardiac output. Indeed, 25 percent of women with mitral stenosis have cardiac failure for the first time during pregnancy (Caulin-Glaser and Setaro, 1999). In some women, this may be confused with idiopathic peripartum cardiomyopathy (Cunningham and colleagues, 1986).

The normal mitral valve surface area is 4.0 cm^2. When stenosis narrows this to less than 2.5 cm^2, symptoms usually develop (Desai and colleagues, 2000). The most prominent complaint is dyspnea due to pulmonary venous hypertension and pulmonary edema. Other common symptoms are fatigue, palpitations, cough, and hemoptysis.

TABLE 44–6 Major Cardiac Valve Disorders

Type	Cause	Pathophysiology	Pregnancy
Mitral stenosis	Rheumatic	LA dilatation, pulmonary hypertension, and atrial fibrillation	Heart failure from fluid overload, tachycardia
Mitral insufficiency	Rheumatic Mitral valve prolapse LV dilatation	LV dilatation and eccentric hypertrophy	Ventricular function improves with afterload decrease
Aortic stenosis	Congenital Bicuspid valve	LV concentric hypertrophy, decreased cardiac output	Moderate stenosis tolerated; severe is life-threatening with decreased preload (e.g., hemorrhage, regional analgesia)
Aortic insufficiency	Rheumatic heart disease Connective tissue disease Congenital	LV hypertrophy and dilatation	Ventricular function improves with afterload decrease
Pulmonary stenosis	Congenital Rheumatic	Severe stenosis associated with RA and RV enlargement	Mild stenosis usually well tolerated; severe stenosis associated with right-sided heart failure and atrial arrhythmias

LA = left atrial; LV = left ventricular; RA = right atrial; RV = right ventricular.

With significant mitral stenosis, tachycardia shortens ventricular diastolic filling time and increases the mitral gradient, which raises left atrial and pulmonary venous and capillary pressures and may result in pulmonary edema. Thus, sinus tachycardia is often treated prophylactically with β-blocking agents. Atrial tachyarrhythmias, including fibrillation, are common in mitral stenosis and are treated aggressively with cardioversion if necessary. Atrial fibrillation also predisposes to mural thrombus formation and cerebrovascular embolization, causing stroke (see Chap. 55, p. 1234).

Hameed and associates (2001) described the outcomes of 66 pregnancies in 64 women with valvular heart disease managed at the University of Southern California Medical Center between 1979 and 1998. Of the 46 women with mitral stenosis, heart failure (43 percent) and arrhythmias (20 percent) were frequent complications. Fetal growth restriction was more common in those women with severe stenosis defined as a valvular area less than 1.0 cm^2. Maternal prognosis is also related to functional capacity. Among 486 pregnancies complicated by rheumatic heart disease, predominantly mitral stenosis, Sawhney and associates (2003) reported that 8 of 10 maternal deaths were in women in NYHA classes III or IV.

Management. Limited physical activity is generally recommended. If symptoms of pulmonary congestion develop, activity is further reduced, dietary sodium is restricted, and diuretic therapy is started (Siva and Shah, 2005). A β-blocker drug can be given to slow heart rate response to activity and anxiety (Al Kasab and associates, 1990). If new-onset atrial fibrillation develops, intravenous verapamil, 5 to 10 mg, is given, or electrocardioversion is performed. For chronic fibrillation, digoxin or a β-blocker or calcium channel blocker is given to slow ventricular response. Anticoagulation with heparin is also indicated.

Labor and delivery are particularly stressful for women with tight mitral stenosis. Pain, exertion, and anxiety cause tachycardia, with possible rate-related heart failure. Epidural analgesia for labor, with strict attention to avoid intravenous fluid overload, is ideal. Abrupt increases in preload may lead to increased pulmonary capillary wedge pressure and pulmonary edema. Thus, care must be taken to avoid fluid overload (Ramin and Gilstrap, 1999). As shown in Figure 44–2, pulmonary capillary wedge pressures increase even more immediately postpartum. Clark and colleagues (1985) hypothesize that this is likely due to loss of the low-resistance placental circulation as well as "autotransfusion" from the lower extremities, pelvis, and the now empty uterus.

Vaginal delivery is preferable, and some authors recommend elective induction so that labor and delivery can be monitored and attended by the most knowledgeable team. In women with severe stenosis with chronic heart failure, insertion of a pulmonary artery catheter may help guide management decisions. Intrapartum endocarditis prophylaxis, as discussed on p. 1033, may be required.

MITRAL INSUFFICIENCY. Mitral regurgitation develops when there is improper coaptation of mitral valve leaflets during systole. This is eventually followed by left ventricular dilatation and eccentric hypertrophy (see Table 44–6). Chronic mitral regurgitation may have a number of causes, including rheumatic fever, mitral valve prolapse, or left ventricular dilatation of any etiology (e.g., dilated cardiomyopathy). Less common causes include a calcified mitral annulus, possibly some appetite suppressants, and in older women, ischemic heart disease. Mitral valve vegetations, known as *Libman-Sacks endocarditis,* are relatively common in women with antiphospholipid antibodies (Roldan and colleagues, 1996). These may or may not coexist with systemic lupus erythematosus (see Chap. 54, p. 1217). Acute mitral insufficiency is caused by rupture of a chorda tendineae, infarction of papillary muscle, or leaflet perforation from infective endocarditis.

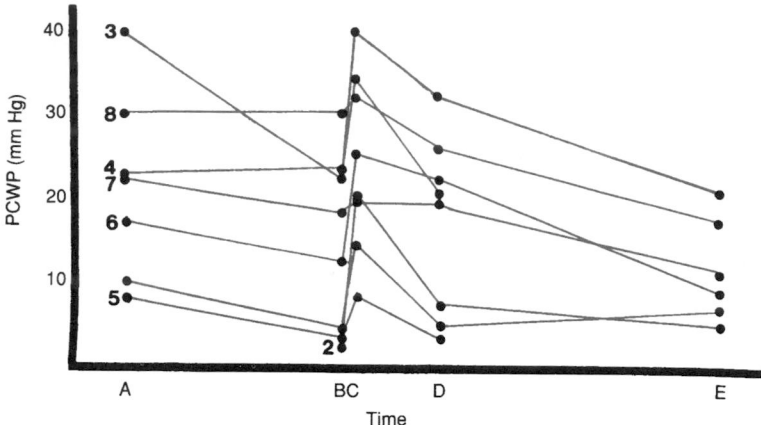

FIGURE 44–2. Intrapartum alterations in pulmonary capillary wedge pressure in eight women with mitral valve stenosis. **A.** First-stage labor. **B.** Second-stage labor, 15 to 30 minutes before delivery. **C.** Postpartum 5 to 15 minutes. **D.** Postpartum 4 to 6 hours. **E.** Postpartum 18 to 24 hours. (From Clark and colleagues, 1985, with permission.)

In nonpregnant patients, symptoms from mitral valve incompetence are rare, and valve replacement is seldom indicated, except for infective endocarditis. Likewise, mitral regurgitation is well tolerated during pregnancy, probably because of decreased systemic vascular resistance, which actually results in less regurgitation. Heart failure only rarely develops during pregnancy, and occasionally tachyarrhythmias need to be treated. Intrapartum prophylaxis against bacterial endocarditis may be indicated (see p. 1033).

AORTIC STENOSIS. Stenosis of the aortic valve is a disease of aging, and in a woman younger than 30 years of age, it is most likely due to a congenital lesion. The lesion is less common since the decline in incidence of rheumatic diseases. In the United States, the most common stenotic lesion is a bicuspid valve. Stenosis reduces the normal 2- to 3-cm^2 aortic orifice and creates resistance to ejection. Reduction in the valve area to a fourth its normal size produces severe obstruction to flow and a progressive pressure overload on the left ventricle (Carabello, 2002). Concentric left ventricular hypertrophy follows, and if severe, end-diastolic pressures become elevated, ejection fraction declines, and cardiac output is reduced (see Table 44–6). Characteristic clinical manifestations develop late and include chest pain, syncope, heart failure, and sudden death from arrhythmias. Life expectancy averages only 5 years after exertional chest pain develops, and valve replacement is indicated for symptomatic patients.

Clinically significant aortic stenosis is uncommonly encountered during pregnancy. Although mild to moderate degrees of stenosis are well tolerated, severe disease is life threatening. The principal underlying hemodynamic problem is the fixed cardiac output associated with severe stenosis. During pregnancy, a number of factors commonly decrease preload further and thus aggravate the fixed cardiac output. Some examples include blood loss, regional analgesia, and vena caval occlusion. Importantly, all of these factors decrease cardiac, cerebral, and uterine perfusion. Because of these considerations, severe aortic stenosis may be extremely dangerous during pregnancy. Indeed, reports after

1975 describe a collective mortality of 7 percent (Lao and colleagues, 1993b). In the report described earlier by Hameed and associates (2001) from Los Angeles County Medical Center, the maternal mortality rate in women with aortic stenosis was 8 percent. Patients with valve gradients exceeding 100 mm Hg appear to be at greatest risk.

Management in Pregnancy. For the asymptomatic pregnant woman, no treatment except close observation is required. Management of the symptomatic woman includes strict limitation of activity and prompt treatment of infections. If symptoms persist despite bed rest, valve replacement or valvotomy using cardiopulmonary bypass must be considered. In general, balloon valvotomy for aortic valve disease is avoided because of a serious complication rate of more than 10 percent. These complications include stroke, aortic rupture, aortic valve insufficiency, and death (Carabello and Crawford, 1997; Reich and co-workers, 2004). In rare cases, it may be preferable to perform valve replacement during pregnancy (Angel and colleagues, 1988; Lao and associates, 1993a).

For women with critical aortic stenosis, intensive monitoring during labor is important. Pulmonary artery catheterization may be helpful because of the narrow margin separating fluid overload from hypovolemia. Women with aortic stenosis are dependent on adequate end-diastolic ventricular filling pressures to maintain cardiac output and systemic perfusion. Abrupt decreases in end-diastolic volume may result in hypotension, syncope, myocardial infarction, and sudden death. Thus the key to the management of these women is the avoidance of decreased ventricular preload and maintenance of cardiac output. During labor and delivery, such women should be managed on the "wet" side, maintaining a margin of safety in intravascular volume in anticipation of possible hemorrhage. In women with a competent mitral valve, pulmonary edema is rare, even with moderate volume overload.

During labor, narcotic epidural analgesia seems ideal, thus avoiding potentially hazardous hypotension, which may be encountered with standard conduction analgesia techniques. Easterling and colleagues (1988) studied the effects of epidural analgesia for five women with severe stenosis and demonstrated immediate and profound effects of decreased filling pressures. Thus, as emphasized by Camann and Thornhill (1999), slow administration of dilute local anesthetics into the epidural space allows for a safer block. Forceps or vacuum delivery is used for standard obstetrical indications in hemodynamically stable women. Intrapartum bacterial endocarditis prophylaxis is given if bacteremia is suspected (see p. 1033).

AORTIC INSUFFICIENCY. Aortic regurgitation is the diastolic flow of blood from the aorta into the left ventricle. Common causes of aortic valvular incompetence are rheumatic fever, connective tissue abnormalities, and congenitally acquired lesions. With Marfan syndrome, the aortic root may dilate, resulting in regurgitation (see p. 1035). Acute insufficiency may develop with bacterial endocarditis or aortic dissection. Aortic as well as mitral valve insufficiency have been linked to the appetite suppressants fenfluramine and dexfenfluramine (Gardin, 2000; Jick, 2000; Khan, 1998, and all of their associates).

With chronic disease, left ventricular hypertrophy and dilatation develop (see Table 44–6). This is followed by slow-onset fatigue, dyspnea, and edema, although rapid deterioration usually follows. Aortic insufficiency is generally well tolerated during pregnancy. Like mitral valve incompetence, diminished vascular resistance is thought to improve the lesion. Symptoms necessitate therapy for heart failure, including bed rest, sodium restriction, and diuretics. Epidural analgesia is used for labor and delivery. Bacterial endocarditis prophylaxis may be required at delivery (see p. 1033).

PULMONIC STENOSIS. The pulmonic valve is affected by rheumatic fever far less often than the other valves. Instead, the lesion is usually congenital and also may be associated with Fallot tetralogy or Noonan syndrome. The clinical diagnosis is typically made by auscultating a systolic ejection murmur over the pulmonary area that is louder during inspiration. Pregnancy is usually well tolerated (Prasad and Ventura, 2001). Indeed, of the eight women with pulmonic stenosis described by Hameed and associates (2001), all had uncomplicated courses. Increased hemodynamic burdens of pregnancy can precipitate right-sided heart failure or atrial arrhythmias in women with severe stenosis. Siu and Colman (2001) recommend consideration for surgical correction before or during pregnancy if symptoms progress.

CONGENITAL HEART DISEASE

The incidence of congenital heart disease in the United States is approximately 8 per 1000 liveborn infants. About a third of these have critical disease that requires cardiac catheteriza-

tion or surgery, or they die within the first year. Others require surgery in childhood, and 85 percent survive to adulthood (Moodie, 1994). With the relative decline in rheumatic heart disease, this group now represents the majority of women with heart disease during pregnancy (Iserin, 2001).

SEPTAL DEFECTS

Atrial Septal Defects. After bicuspid aortic valve, these are the most commonly encountered congenital cardiac lesions in adults, comprising a third of cases (Brickner and colleagues, 2000). Most are asymptomatic until the third or fourth decade. The secundum-type defect accounts for 70 percent of all cases, and associated mitral valve myxomatous abnormalities with prolapse are common. Most clinicians recommend repair if discovered in adulthood. Pregnancy is well tolerated unless pulmonary hypertension has developed, but this is rare because pulmonary artery pressures are usually low (Zuber and associates, 1999). If congestive heart failure or an arrhythmia develops, treatment is given. Bacterial endocarditis prophylaxis has been recommended in certain circumstances with unrepaired defects (see p. 1033). Based on their review, Aliaga and associates (2003) concluded that the risk of endocarditis with an atrial septal defect is negligible.

Ventricular Septal Defects. These defects spontaneously close in 90 percent of patients during childhood. Almost 75 percent of defects are paramembraneous, and physiological derangements are related to the size of the defect. In general, if the defect is less than 1.25 cm^2, pulmonary hypertension and heart failure do not develop. When the effective size of the defect is greater than the aortic valve orifice, symptoms rapidly develop. For these reasons, most children undergo surgical repair before pulmonary hypertension develops. Adults with unrepaired large defects develop left ventricular failure and pulmonary hypertension, as well as a high incidence of bacterial endocarditis (Brickner and colleagues, 2000).

Pregnancy is well tolerated with small to moderate left-to-right shunts. When pulmonary arterial pressures reach systemic levels, however, there is reversal or bidirectional flow or *Eisenmenger syndrome* (see p. 1028). When this develops, maternal mortality is 30 to 50 percent. Thus, pregnancy is contraindicated, and therapeutic abortion is advised if contraception fails. Bacterial endocarditis is more common with unrepaired defects, and antimicrobial prophylaxis is often required (see p. 1033). Unless repair is associated with a residual septal defect, the risk of endocarditis is low. About 10 to 15 percent of offspring born to these women have a ventricular septal defect (see Table 44–4).

PERSISTENT DUCTUS ARTERIOSUS. Like other shunts, the physiological consequences of this lesion are related to its size. Most significant lesions are repaired in childhood. In individuals who do not undergo repair, mortality is high beginning in the fifth decade (Brickner and colleagues, 2000). Pulmonary hypertension develops in some women with an unrepaired persistent ductus. Heart failure may develop in these women, and if systemic blood pressure falls, reversal of blood flow from the pulmonary artery into the aorta causes cyanosis. Sudden drops in blood pressure at delivery, as with conduction analgesia or hemorrhage, may lead to fatal collapse. Therefore, hypotension should be avoided whenever possible and treated vigorously if it develops. Prophylaxis for bacterial endocarditis may be indicated at delivery for unrepaired defects (see p. 1033). The incidence of inheritance is about 4 percent (see Table 44–4).

CYANOTIC HEART DISEASE. When congenital heart lesions are associated with right-to-left shunting of blood past the pulmonary capillary bed, cyanosis develops. The classical and most commonly encountered lesion in pregnancy is the *Fallot tetralogy*. This is characterized by a large ventricular septal defect, pulmonary stenosis, right ventricular hypertrophy, and an overriding aorta that receives blood from both the right and left ventricles. The magnitude of the shunt varies inversely with systemic vascular resistance. Hence, during pregnancy, when peripheral resistance decreases, the shunt increases and cyanosis worsens. Women who have undergone repair, and in whom cyanosis did not reappear, do well in pregnancy.

Some women with *Ebstein anomaly* of the tricuspid valve may reach reproductive age. Right ventricular failure from volume overload and appearance or worsening of cyanosis are common during pregnancy. In the absence of cyanosis, these women usually tolerate pregnancy well.

Effects on Pregnancy. Pregnant women with cyanotic heart disease generally do poorly. With uncorrected Fallot tetralogy, for example, maternal mortality approaches 10 percent. Any disease complicated by severe maternal hypoxemia is likely to lead to miscarriage, preterm delivery, or fetal death. There is a relationship between chronic hypoxemia and the polycythemia it causes and the outcome of pregnancy. When hypoxemia is intense enough to stimulate a rise in hematocrit above 65 percent, pregnancy wastage is virtually 100 percent.

Sawhney and colleagues (1998) reported stillborn infants in 14 percent and fetal growth restriction in 36 percent of 24 pregnancies in women with cyanotic heart disease. Shime and associates (1987) reported that 13 of 23 women with cyanotic heart disease developed functional deterioration during pregnancy, and seven had cardiac failure. Three of these 23 infants died, and low birthweight was common. Zuber and co-workers (1999) reported good outcomes in 19 women with Fallot tetralogy, but they emphasized that prepregnancy functional class and systolic ventricular function were good in all the women.

PREGNANCY AFTER SURGICAL REPAIR. With satisfactory surgical correction before pregnancy, maternal risks are decreased

dramatically and fetal environment is improved. Singh and associates (1982) described 40 pregnancies in 27 women with surgically corrected tetralogy. They concluded that pregnancy is usually well tolerated in women with no major residual defects after surgery. Lao (1994), Lynch-Salamon (1993), Megerian (1994), and their colleagues described 14 pregnancies in 10 women following successful *Mustard repair* for *transposition of the great vessels.* Two women developed cardiac failure during pregnancy and two others developed worrisome arrhythmias. Connolly and co-workers (1999) reported 60 pregnancies in 22 women who had transposition corrected in childhood. Maternal complications were uncommon, however, two women developed heart failure, another had endocarditis, and a woman with a single coronary artery had a myocardial infarction. All 50 liveborn infants survived.

Hoare and Radford (2001) described four pregnancies in three women who had previously undergone a *Fontan repair* for congenital heart disease characterized by a *single functional ventricle.* Although no maternal deaths occurred, complications were frequent and included preterm birth in all pregnancies, supraventricular arrhythmias in half, and ventricular failure in half.

LABOR AND DELIVERY. Vaginal delivery is preferred unless there is an obstetrical indication for cesarean delivery. **Pulmonary artery catheter monitoring has limitations because of the sometimes bizarre anatomical abnormalities.** Care must be taken to avoid sudden blood pressure decreases. For labor pain, epidural opiates may suffice. There is controversy regarding epidural analgesia versus general anesthesia for cesarean delivery (Camann and Thornhill, 1999).

EISENMENGER SYNDROME. This is secondary pulmonary hypertension that develops with any cardiac lesion. The syndrome develops when pulmonary vascular resistance becomes greater than systemic vascular resistance and in which there is some right-to-left shunting. The most common underlying defects are atrial or ventricular septal defects and persistent ductus arteriosus. Patients are asymptomatic for years, but eventually pulmonary hypertension is severe enough to cause right-to-left shunting.

The prognosis for pregnancy depends on the severity of pulmonary hypertension. In a review of 44 cases through 1978, Gleicher and associates (1979) reported maternal and perinatal mortality rates to be about 50 percent. There has been little improvement since then. Weiss and co-workers (1998b) cited a 36-percent maternal death rate in a review of 73 pregnancies. Three of the 26 deaths were antepartum, and the remainder occurred intrapartum or within a month of delivery. Women with Eisenmenger syndrome tolerate hypotension poorly, and the cause of death usually is right ventricular failure with cardiogenic shock. Management is discussed subsequently.

OTHER CARDIOVASCULAR CONDITIONS

PULMONARY HYPERTENSION. High pulmonary blood pressure is generally secondary to cardiac or pulmonary disease, and common causes are persistent and prolonged left-to-right shunting with development of Eisenmenger syndrome. *Primary pulmonary hypertension* is a rare, usually idiopathic, condition that occurs in the absence of an intracardiac or aortopulmonary shunt. Thirty suspected risk factors include certain appetite suppressants, human immunodeficiency virus and human herpesvirus 8 infections, and sickle cell disease (Cool, 2003; Gladwin, 2004; Humbert, 2001, and all their colleagues). Pengo and associates (2004) found chronic pulmonary hypertension in 3.8 percent of nonpregnant patients 2 years after a pulmonary embolism. Some previously unexplained cases are now thought to be due to antiphospholipid antibodies (see Chap. 54, p. 1215).

The criteria for diagnosis established by a National Institutes of Health registry include a mean pulmonary artery pressure of more than 25 mm Hg at rest, or 30 mm Hg with exertion, in the absence of heart disease, chronic thromboembolic disease, underlying pulmonary disorder, or other secondary causes (Runo and Loyd, 2003). Although cardiac catheterization remains the standard criterion for the measurement of pulmonary artery pressures, noninvasive echocardiography is often used to provide an estimate. In their review of 33 pregnant women who underwent both echocardiography and cardiac catheterization, Penning and colleagues (2001) cautioned that pulmonary artery pressures were significantly overestimated by echocardiography in a third of cases.

The prognosis is poor, and the mean survival from diagnosis is about 2 years. Long-term therapy with intravenous epoprostenol (prostacyclin) or with subcutaneous trepostinil, a prostacylin analogue, significantly lowers pulmonary vascular resistance (Humbert and colleagues, 2004; Roeleveld and co-workers, 2004). Preconceptional counseling is imperative, and Easterling and associates (1999) recommend that response to nifedipine and prostacyclin be documented for at least 1 year before pregnancy.

Effects on Pregnancy. Maternal mortality is appreciable, especially with primary pulmonary hypertension. In their review, Kiss and colleagues (1995) reported maternal mortality in 7 of 11 (65 percent) women with primary disease. Weiss and associates (1998b) reviewed 27 cases reported from 1978 through 1996 and found a 30-percent mortality rate.

Although pregnancy is contraindicated with severe disease, milder degrees of secondary pulmonary hypertension probably go unnoticed. For example, with the more common use of pulmonary artery catheterization in women with heart disease, we have identified women with mild to moderate pulmonary hypertension who tolerated pregnancy, labor, and delivery quite well. Sheffield and Cunningham (2004) described an example of pulmonary hypertension that occurs with relatively long-standing thyrotoxicosis (see Chap. 53, p. 1192). Boggess and colleagues (1995) described nine women with interstitial and restrictive lung disease who ostensibly had varying degrees of pulmonary hypertension. Three women had severe disease, and all nine tolerated pregnancy reasonably well.

Treatment of symptomatic pregnant women includes limitation of activity and avoidance of the supine position in late pregnancy. Diuretics, supplemental oxygen, and vasodilator drugs are standard therapy for symptoms. Easterling and associates (1999) successfully used nifedipine and prostacyclin during pregnancy, and Badalian and co-workers (2000) described continued epoprostenol (prostacyclin) infusion throughout a twin pregnancy.

Management of labor and delivery is particularly problematic. **These women are at greatest risk when there is diminished venous return and right ventricular filling, which is associated with most maternal deaths.** To avert hypotension, careful attention is given to blood loss at delivery and avoidance of standard epidural analgesia. Pollack and colleagues (1990), as well as others, have reported successful labor analgesia without significant cardiovascular effects from morphine administered intrathecally. Camann and Thornhill (1999) argue against the use of pulmonary artery catheterization for a number of technical and safety issues, not the least of which is that data are usually not clinically useful. Lam and colleagues (2001) have described the use of intubation and inhaled nitric oxide during the labor and forceps delivery of a nullipara with severe primary pulmonary hypertension. Weiss and co-workers (2000) described a woman with severe primary pulmonary hypertension who had a successful cesarean delivery with epidural analgesia and while inhaling 20 mg of aerosolized iloprost, an analogue of prostacyclin. Successful intrapartum use of inhaled epoprostenol has also been described (Bildirici and Shumway, 2004).

MITRAL VALVE PROLAPSE. This diagnosis implies the presence of a pathological connective tissue disorder—often termed *myxomatous degeneration*—which may involve the valve leaflets themselves, the annulus, or the chordae tendineae. Until recently, this condition was thought to have a prevalence as high as 15 percent in otherwise normal young women. Community-based studies, however, indicate the incidence to be only 2 to 3 percent (Freed and colleagues, 1999). For referred cases, it is commonly associated with a wide variety of other cardiac disorders, including atrial septal defect, Marfan syndrome, Ebstein anomaly, and hypertrophic cardiomyopathy.

Most women with mitral valve prolapse are asymptomatic and are diagnosed by routine physical examination or as an incidental finding at echocardiography. The small percentage of women with symptoms have anxiety, palpitations, atypical chest pain, and syncope. Nishimura and colleagues (1985) identified only those patients with redundant mitral valve leaflets to be at increased risk of sudden death, infective endocarditis, or cerebral embolism. Looking at this another way, of 213 young women with documented ischemic strokes, only 1.9 percent had mitral valve prolapse compared with 2.7 percent of controls (Gilon and co-workers, 1999).

Diagnosis. Mitral valve prolapse implies the presence of a pathological condition and should be diagnosed with caution and precision. Reliance on strict diagnostic criteria is essential before assigning a pathological diagnosis or administration of endocarditis prophylaxis (Nishimura and McGoon, 1999).

Effects on Pregnancy. Pregnant women with mitral valve prolapse rarely have cardiac complications. In fact, pregnancy-induced hypervolemia may improve alignment of the mitral valve (Rayburn and colleagues, 1987). For women who are symptomatic, β-blocking drugs are given to decrease sympathetic tone, relieve chest pain and palpitations, and reduce the risk of life-threatening arrhythmias. In general, mitral valve prolapse is not deleterious to pregnancy. We manage these women as if not pregnant and prescribe β-blocker drugs for symptoms. Mitral valve prolapse with regurgitation or valvular damage is considered to be a significant risk factor for development of bacterial endocarditis, and antimicrobial prophylaxis should be given if bacteremia is suspected. Women without evidence of pathological myxomatous change may in general expect excellent pregnancy outcome (Chia and associates, 1994).

PERIPARTUM CARDIOMYOPATHY. This is a diagnosis of exclusion and is similar to idiopathic dilated cardiomyopathy that occurs in nonpregnant adults. Although the term peripartum cardiomyopathy has been used widely to describe women with peripartum heart failure with no readily apparent etiology, it is doubtful that there is a pregnancy-induced cardiomyopathy. In 1997, the National Heart, Lung, and Blood Institute and the Office of Rare Diseases convened a workshop that established the following diagnostic criteria (Pearson and associates, 2000):

1. Development of cardiac failure in the last month of pregnancy or within 5 months after delivery.
2. Absence of an identifiable cause for the cardiac failure.
3. Absence of recognizable heart disease prior to the last month of pregnancy.
4. Left ventricular systolic dysfunction demonstrated by classic echocardiographic criteria such as depressed shortening fraction or ejection fraction.

Although the workshop panel concluded that the disease is acute, rather than a preexisting one preceding pregnancy, our experiences do not reflect this.

Other causes of new-onset ventricular dysfunction must be excluded. Felker and colleagues (2000) performed endomyocardial biopsy in 1230 nonpregnant patients who had unexplained cardiomyopathy. In exactly half of these, a cause for cardiomyopathy was found, and the most common was myocarditis. Indeed, 26 of 51 women with peripartum cardiomyopathy had histological evidence for myocarditis. Dilated cardiomyopathy is also found in HIV infection (Barbaro and associates, 1998). We carefully evaluated 28 women at Parkland Hospital with peripartum heart failure of obscure etiology who were initially thought to have idiopathic cardiomyopathy. In 21 of these, heart failure was ultimately attributed to hypertensive heart disease, clinically silent mitral stenosis, obesity, or viral myocarditis (Cunningham and associates, 1986).

Chronic hypertension with superimposed preeclampsia is a common cause of heart failure during pregnancy (see Chap. 45, p. 1052). In some cases, mild antecedent hypertension is undiagnosed, and when superimposed preeclampsia develops, it may cause otherwise inexplicable peripartum heart failure. As discussed in Chapter 43, obesity is a common cofactor with chronic hypertension, and it can cause or contribute to underlying ventricular hypertrophy. In the Framingham Heart Study, obesity alone was associated with a doubling of the risk of heart failure in nonpregnant individuals (Kenchaiah and colleagues, 2002).

Regardless of the underlying condition that causes cardiac dysfunction, women who develop peripartum heart failure often have obstetrical complications that either contribute to or precipitate heart failure. For example, preeclampsia is common and may precipitate afterload failure. Acute anemia from blood loss magnifies the physiological effects of compromised ventricular function. Similarly, infection and accompanying fever increase cardiac output and oxygen utilization.

Idiopathic Cardiomyopathy in Pregnancy. After exclusion of an underlying cause for heart failure, idiopathic cardiomyopathy may be considered (Brown and Bertolet, 1998; Hibbard and associates, 1999). We identified this in about 1 in 15,000 deliveries, and this incidence is not different from that of idiopathic cardiomyopathy in young nonpregnant women (Cunningham and colleagues, 1986). Lampert (1993) and Mabie (1993) and their associates have implicated prolonged beta-mimetic tocolysis with terbutaline as provoking cardiomyopathy. As previously discussed, clinically undetected myocarditis is found in up to half of these women if biopsy is done. O'Connell and colleagues (1986) found that a third of pregnant women with idiopathic cardiomyopathy had biopsy evidence of myocarditis compared with only 10 percent of nonpregnant patients.

Women with cardiomyopathy present with signs and symptoms of congestive heart failure. Dyspnea is universal, and other symptoms include orthopnea, cough, palpitations, and chest pain (Sheffield and Cunningham, 1999). The

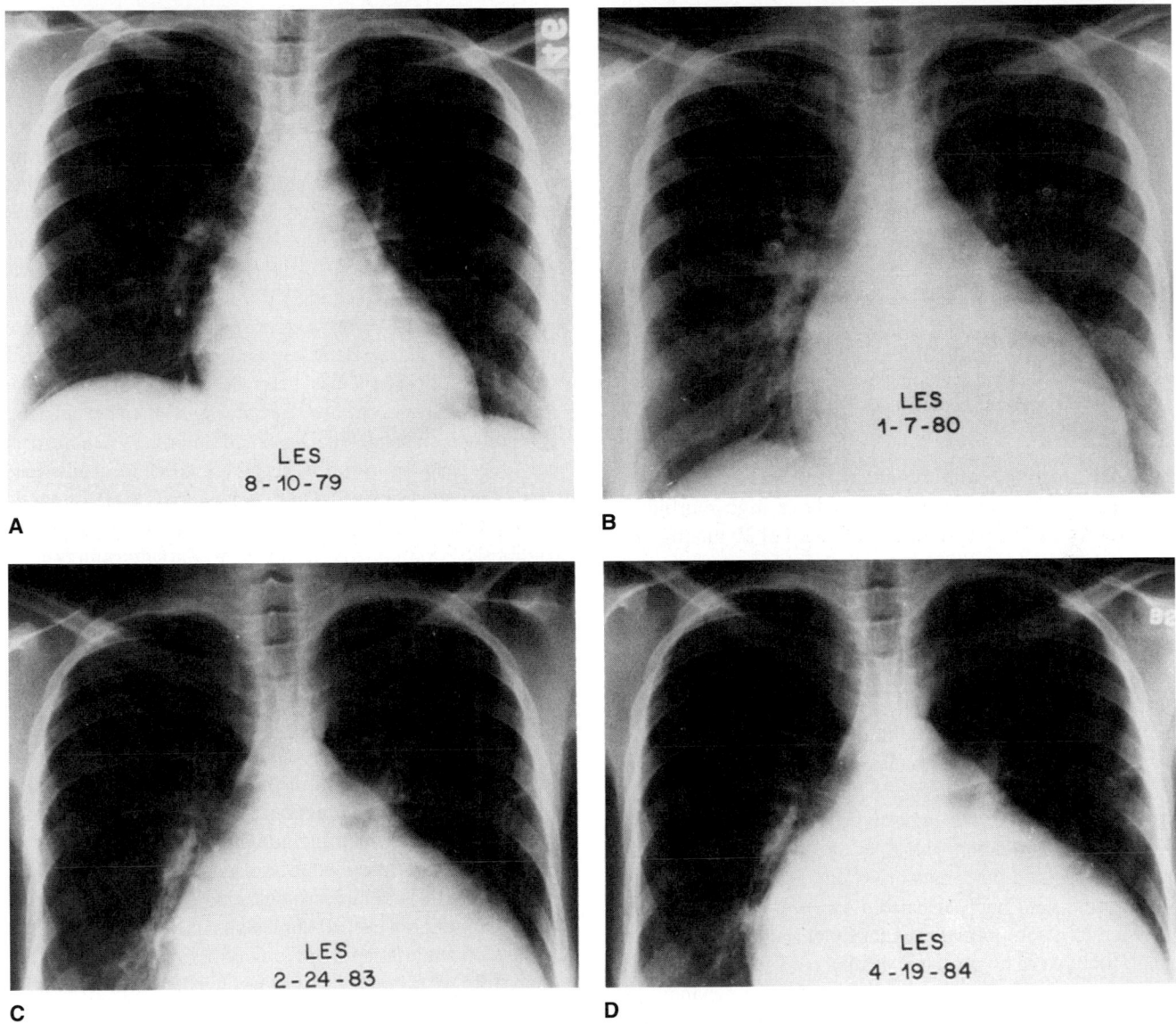

FIGURE 44–3. Idiopathic peripartum cardiomyopathy in patient L.E.S. Peripartum heart failure developed without any identifiable underlying cardiac disease. Despite an initially good symptomatic response and clearing of pulmonary edema, mild cardiomegaly persisted 3 months postpartum **(A)**. Over the ensuing 5 years **(B–D)** cardiomegaly worsened, and she died of end-stage heart failure at age 23. (From Cunningham and colleagues, 1986, with permission.)

hallmark finding usually is impressive cardiomegaly (Fig. 44–3). Echocardiographic findings include an ejection fraction less than 45 percent or a fractional shortening less than 30 percent, or both, and an end-diastolic dimension greater than 2.7 cm/m^2 (Hibbard and colleagues, 1999).

Therapy consists of treatment for heart failure. Sodium intake is limited and diuretics are given to reduce preload. Afterload reduction with hydralazine or another vasodilator is accomplished. Because of marked fetal effects discussed in Chapter 14 (see p. 349), angiotensin-converting enzyme inhibitors are avoided if the woman is undelivered. However, they are given postpartum. Digoxin is given for its inotropic effects unless complex arrhythmias are identified. Because

there is a high incidence of associated thromboembolism, prophylactic heparin is often recommended.

PROGNOSIS. The distinction between peripartum heart failure from an identifiable cause versus idiopathic cardiomyopathy is important. This distinction is somewhat artificial, recall that if biopsy is done, at least half of women with peripartum cardiomyopathy have histological myocarditis. As shown in Figure 44–4, the 5- and 10-year survival rates are substantially lower with idiopathic disease (Felker and co-workers, 2000; Pulerwitz and associates, 2004).

According to Lampert and associates (1997), half of all women with peripartum cardiomyopathy regain left

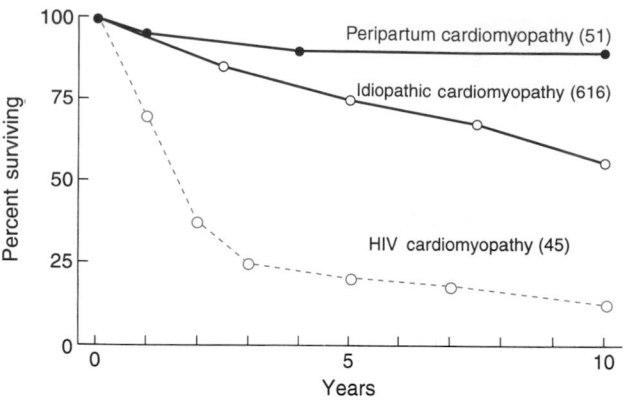

FIGURE 44–4. Survival according to underlying cause of cardiomyopathy. (HIV = human immunodeficiency virus.) (Data from Felker and colleagues, 2000.)

ventricular function within 6 months, and they have a good prognosis. Conversely, the other half have high morbidity and mortality rates. With a mean follow-up of 39 months, de Souza and colleagues (2001b) studied the longer-term outcomes of 44 such women. Eight of these (18 percent) died from end-stage heart failure. In addition, two women suffered a nonfatal pulmonary embolism, one had a cerebral ischemic stroke, and another underwent heart transplantation 14 months after the diagnosis. Of eight women with functional NYHA class IV heart failure, one woman improved to class I, four to class II, two to class III, and one remained in class IV. Seven women had a subsequent pregnancy, and all gave birth to healthy term newborns. Elkayam and co-workers (2001) surveyed members of the American College of Cardiology and obtained outcomes of 60 subsequent pregnancies in 44 women who had peripartum cardiomyopathy. Of the 28 women in whom left ventricular function had returned to normal, there were no maternal deaths. However, 20 percent developed symptoms of heart failure during pregnancy. In the remaining 16 with persistent left ventricular dysfunction, 44 percent developed heart failure and three women died between 2 and 24 months postpartum. In a prospective study, Sliwa and co-workers (2004) confirmed these findings. These studies suggest that subsequent pregnancy is inadvisable for women with an ejection fraction persistently less than 50 percent.

INFECTIVE ENDOCARDITIS. This infection involves cardiac endothelium and produces vegetations that usually deposit on a valve. Infective endocarditis can involve a native or a prosthetic valve, and it may be associated with intravenous drug abuse. Children and adults who have had corrective surgery for congenital heart disease are at greatest risk (Morris and co-workers, 1998). About half of affected adults have a known preexisting heart lesion (Hoen and colleagues, 2002).

Subacute bacterial endocarditis usually is due to a low-virulence bacterial infection superimposed on an underlying lesion. These are usually native valve infections. Organisms that cause indolent endocarditis are most commonly viridans group streptococci or *Enterococcus* species. Historically, *acute endocarditis* was usually caused by coagulase-positive staphylococci. Two large and more recent epidemiological studies, however, indicate that the most common causative organisms are streptococci—especially viridans—followed by *Staphylococcus aureus* and *Enterococcus* species (Hasbun and associates, 2003; Hoen and colleagues, 2002). *S aureus* is the predominant organism among intravenous drug abusers (Karchmer, 2001). *Staphylococcus epidermidis* commonly causes prosthetic valve infections. *Streptococcus pneumoniae* and *Neisseria gonorrhoeae* may cause acute, fulminating disease (Bataskov and colleagues, 1991). Antepartum endocarditis has been described with *Neisseria sicca* and *Neisseria mucosa*, the latter causing maternal death (Cox and associates, 1988; Deger and Ludmir, 1992). Surprisingly, few cases of group B streptococcal endocarditis have been described (Kangavari and co-workers, 2000).

Symptoms of endocarditis are variable and often develop insidiously. Fever is virtually universal, and a murmur is heard in 80 to 85 percent of cases (Karchmer, 2001). Anorexia, fatigue, and other constitutional symptoms are common, and the illness is frequently described as "flu-like." Other findings are anemia, proteinuria, and manifestations of embolic lesions, including petechiae, focal neurological manifestations, chest or abdominal pain, and ischemia in an extremity. In some cases, heart failure develops. Symptoms may persist for several weeks before the diagnosis is made, and a high index of suspicion is necessary. Diagnosis is made using the *Duke criteria*, which include positive blood cultures for typical organisms and evidence of endocardial involvement (Karchmer, 2001). Echocardiography and two-dimensional sector scanning are useful, but lesions only 3 to 4 mm in size or those on the tricuspid valve may be missed. **A negative echocardiographic study does not exclude endocarditis.**

Treatment is primarily medical with appropriate timing of surgical intervention if necessary. Knowledge of the infecting organism is imperative for sensible antimicrobial selection. Most viridans streptococci are sensitive to penicillin G given intravenously along with gentamicin for 2 weeks (Karchmer, 2001). Complicated infections are treated longer, and women allergic to penicillin are either desensitized or given intravenous ceftriaxone or vancomycin for 4 weeks. Staphylococci, enterococci, and other organisms are treated according to microbial sensitivity for 4 to 6 weeks (Darouiche, 2004). Prosthetic valve infections are treated for 6 to 8 weeks. Persistent native valve infection may require replacement, and this is even more commonly indicated with an infected prosthetic valve.

Endocarditis in Pregnancy. Infective endocarditis is uncommon during pregnancy and the puerperium. Over a 7-year period, the incidence of endocarditis at Parkland Hospital was about 1 in 16,000 deliveries (Cox and associates, 1988). Two of seven women died. Treatment is the same as that described

TABLE 44–7 American College of Cardiology/American Heart Association Recommendations for Antimicrobial Prophylaxis to Prevent Bacterial Endocarditis

Cardiac Lesion	Prophylaxis for Uncomplicated Delivery	Prophylaxis for Suspected Bacteremia[a]
High Risk		
Prosthetic cardiac valves (both homograft and bioprosthetic)	Optional	Recommended
Prior bacterial endocarditis	Optional	Recommended
Complex cyanotic congenital cardiac malformations	Optional	Recommended
Surgically constructed systemic pulmonary shunts or conduits	Optional	Recommended
Moderate Risk		
Congenital cardiac malformations (except repaired atrial septal defect, ventricular septal defect, or patent ductus arteriosus, or isolated secundum atrial septal defect)	Not Recommended	Recommended
Acquired valvular dysfunction (most commonly rheumatic heart disease)	Not Recommended	Recommended
Hypertrophic cardiomyopathy	Not Recommended	Recommended
Mitral valve prolapse with valvular regurgitation or thickened leaflets or both	Not Recommended	Recommended
Negligible Risk[b]		
Mitral valve prolapse without valvular regurgitation	Not Recommended	Not Recommended
Physiological, functional, or innocent heart murmurs	Not Recommended	Not Recommended
Previous Kawasaki disease without valvular dysfunction	Not Recommended	Not Recommended
Previous rheumatic fever without valvular dysfunction	Not Recommended	Not Recommended
Cardiac pacemakers and implanted defibrillators	Not Recommended	Not Recommended
Prior coronary bypass graft surgery	Not Recommended	Not Recommended

[a]For example, intra-amniotic infection.
[b]Risk for developing endocarditis is not higher than the general population.
Data from Bonow (1998) and Dajani (1997) and their associates. Reproduced from the American College of Obstetricians and Gynecologists (2003), with permission.

earlier. From their reviews, Seaworth and Durack (1986) and Cox and Leveno (1989) cited maternal mortality of about 25 to 35 percent.

Antimicrobial Prophylaxis. The efficacy of antimicrobial prophylaxis to prevent bacterial endocarditis is questionable. Only 13 percent of cases arising in patients with high-risk cardiac lesions do so after a procedure (Van der Meer and associates, 1992). The American Heart Association recommends prophylaxis based on risk stratification (Table 44–7). These recommendations have been endorsed by the American College of Obstetricians and Gynecologists (2003).

OBSTETRICAL PROCEDURES. The current recommendations of the American College of Cardiology and the American Heart Association suggest that prophylaxis for bacterial endocarditis be administered intrapartum to women at risk only in the presence of suspected bacteremia or active infection (see Table 44–7). They estimate that the incidence of transient bacteremia at delivery is 1 to 5 percent. Antimicrobial prophylaxis is considered optional for women undergoing an uncomplicated delivery who are at high risk for endocarditis (American College of Obstetricians and Gynecologists, 2003). Although there is meager evidence that a significant number of cases of bacterial endocarditis have been prevented with antimicrobial prophylaxis given for uncomplicated delivery, its risk and costs are not great (McFaul and associates, 1988; Seaworth and Durack, 1986). Individualization seems appropriate.

In the guidelines shown in Table 44–7, the recommended prophylaxis regimens include intravenous or intramuscular administration of 2 g of ampicillin plus 1.5 mg/kg of intravenous gentamicin (to a maximum of 120 mg), followed by 1 g of parenteral ampicillin or oral amoxicillin 6 hours later. In women who are allergic to penicillin, vancomycin, 1 g intravenously over 1 to 2 hours, is substituted for ampicillin. Ideally, prophylaxis should be completed within 30 minutes before the procedure is begun (American College of Obstetricians and Gynecologists, 2003). Obviously, accurate prediction of delivery time is problematic regarding timely administration of the first dose. In women who are at moderate risk for endocarditis, the gentamicin and the second dose of ampicillin may be eliminated.

ARRHYTHMIAS. Cardiac arrhythmias are commonly encountered during pregnancy, labor and delivery, and the puerperium. It is debated whether arrhythmias are more common during pregnancy, but in our experience, their detection is probably increased because of more frequent visits during prenatal care. Perhaps the normal but mild hypokalemia of pregnancy induces arrhythmias (see Chap. 5, p. 129). Most often, treatment is not different from that for nonpregnant patients.

Bradyarrhythmias, including complete heart block, are compatible with a successful pregnancy outcome. Some women with complete heart block have syncope during labor and delivery, and occasionally temporary cardiac pacing is necessary. Women with permanent artificial pacemakers usually tolerate pregnancy well (Jaffe and associates, 1987). With fixed-rate devices, cardiac output apparently is increased by augmented stroke volume.

Tachyarrhythmias are relatively common and should prompt consideration of underlying cardiac disease. *Wolff–Parkinson–White syndrome* may first appear during pregnancy, but some women with previously diagnosed arrhythmias have an increased incidence of tachycardia during pregnancy (Widerhorn and co-workers, 1992). *Paroxysmal supraventricular tachycardia* is encountered most frequently. Siu and associates (1997) followed 25 women who had supraventricular tachycardia diagnosed before pregnancy. Half of these women had Wolff–Parkinson–White syndrome. Three of 12 women with Wolff–Parkinson–White syndrome and 6 of 13 without the condition had supraventricular tachycardia during pregnancy. If vagal maneuvers do not stimulate conversion, treatment consists of digoxin, adenosine, or calcium-channel blocking drugs. Experience is accruing that adenosine is effective for cardioversion in hemodynamically stable pregnant women (Chakhtoura and co-workers, 1998; Robins and Lyons, 2004). Most of these drugs do not appear to do fetal harm, however, reported fetal bradycardia in response to intravenous adenosine has been described (Dunn and Brost, 2000).

Electrical cardioversion is not contraindicated in pregnancy, but vigilance is important. Barnes and associates (2002) described a case in which direct current cardioversion led directly to a sustained uterine contraction and fetal bradycardia. In some patients, accessory pathway ablation may be indicated (Pappone and colleagues, 2003). Damilakis and associates (2001) calculated that the typical fetal procedure-related radiation dose is less than 1 cGy.

Atrial flutter or fibrillation are more likely associated with underlying disease, such as thyrotoxicosis. Major complications include stroke (Ezekowitz and Levine, 1999). Thus, heparin is recommended by some if fibrillation is chronic and persists during pregnancy. If atrial fibrillation is associated with mitral stenosis, pulmonary edema may develop in late pregnancy if the ventricular rate is increased.

Ventricular tachycardia is uncommon in healthy young women without underlying heart disease. Brodsky and associates (1992) described seven pregnant women with new-onset ventricular tachycardia and reviewed 23 previously published reports. Most of these women were not found to have structural heart disease, and in 60 percent, arrhythmias were stimulated by physical exercise or psychological stress. Of those remaining, two had myocardial infarction, two had a prolonged QT interval, and anesthesia provoked tachycardia in another. In 6 of 26, no precipitating event was found. The investigators concluded that pregnancy events probably precipitated tachycardia and recommended β-blocker therapy for control. For women requiring defibrillation for ventricular arrhythmias, Nanson and associates (2001) found that standard adult energy requirements do not need to be altered solely because of pregnancy.

QT interval prolongation on the ECG may predispose individuals to a potentially fatal ventricular arrhythmia known as *torsades de pointes*. Based on their analysis of 111 pregnant women with long QT syndrome in which a significant increase in cardiac events was noted postpartum but not during pregnancy, Rashba and colleagues (1998) hypothesized that the normal increase in heart rate during pregnancy may bear a partially protective effect. Paradoxically, β-blocker therapy has been shown to decrease the risk of torsades de pointes in patients with long QT syndrome and should be continued during pregnancy and the postpartum period (Gowda and colleagues, 2003). Importantly, many medications, including some used during pregnancy such as erythromycin and clarithromycin, may predispose to QT prolongation (Al-Khatib and associates, 2003; Roden, 2004).

DISEASES OF THE AORTA. Marfan syndrome and coarctation of the aorta are two aortic diseases that place the pregnant woman at increased risk for *aortic dissection*. Half of cases of dissection in young women are related to pregnancy (O'Gara and associates, 2004). Other risk factors are bicuspid aortic valve and Turner or Noonan syndrome. Pepin and colleagues (2000) reported a high rate of aortic dissection or rupture in patients with *Ehlers–Danlos syndrome* (see Chap. 54, p. 1223). Although the mechanism(s) involved are unclear, the initiating event is an aortic intimal tear, and following medial hemorrhage, rupture may occur.

In most cases, aortic dissection presents with severe chest pain described as ripping, tearing, or stabbing in nature. Diminution or loss of peripheral pulses in conjunction with a recently acquired murmur of aortic insufficiency are important physical findings. The differential diagnosis of aortic dissection includes myocardial infarction, pulmonary embolism, pneumothorax, and aortic valve rupture. Lang and Borow (1991) rightfully add obstetrical catastrophes to the list, especially placental abruption and uterine rupture.

More than 90 percent of affected patients have an abnormal chest radiograph. Aortic angiography is the most definitive method for confirming the diagnosis, however, noninvasive imaging with sonography, computed tomography, and magnetic resonance imaging (MRI) are used more frequently. The urgency of the clinical situation frequently dictates which procedure is best. Easterling and colleagues (1991) found that aortic diameter increased significantly in normal women over the course of pregnancy. This increase was even greater for women who developed preeclampsia.

Initial medical treatment is given to lower blood pressure. Proximal dissections most often need to be resected, along with aortic valve replacement if indicated. Distal dissections are more complex, and many may be treated medically. Lederle and colleagues (2002) have shown that survival in nonpregnant patients is not improved by elective repair of abdominal aortic aneurysms smaller than 5.5 cm. Lee and associates (2001) described a successful vaginal delivery in a woman with a 4.5-cm thoracic aortic aneurysm.

Marfan Syndrome. This syndrome is usually inherited as an autosomal dominant trait with a high degree of penetrance. Prenatal diagnosis is usually possible using linkage analysis (see Chap. 12, p. 308). The syndrome is caused by abnormal *fibrillin* produced by any of nearly 50 different mutations in the *FBN1* gene, which is located on chromosome 15q21 (Biggin and co-workers, 2004). Fibrillin is a constituent of elastin. Thus, Marfan syndrome is a systemic connective tissue disorder characterized by generalized weakness that can result in dangerous cardiovascular complications. Because all tissues are involved, other defects are frequent and include joint laxity and scoliosis. Progressive aortic dilatation causes aortic valve insufficiency, and there may be infective endocarditis and mitral valve prolapse with insufficiency. Aortic dilatation and dissecting aneurysm are the most serious abnormalities. Early death is due either to valvular insufficiency and heart failure or to a dissecting aneurysm. Long-term benefits from β-blocker therapy have been described for nonpregnant adults (Shores and colleagues, 1994).

Effect of Pregnancy. In a review of published cases, Elkayam and associates (1995) found that 20 of 32 women had aortic dissection or rupture and 16 of these died. The actual mortality risk is probably lower, because these case reports likely reflect a publication bias of more severely affected pregnancies. Indeed, in a prospective longitudinal evaluation of 21 women during 45 pregnancies from the Johns Hopkins Hospital, only two had dissection and one died postpartum from graft infection (Rossiter and colleagues, 1995). Similarly, there were no maternal deaths among 14 women with Marfan syndrome followed prospectively by Rahman and co-workers (2003). Importantly, two of these women required surgical correction of an aortic aneurysm and aortic valve replacement. Both groups of investigators concluded that aortic dilatation of more than 40 mm or mitral valve dysfunction are high-risk factors for life-threatening cardiovascular complications during pregnancy. Conversely, women with minimal or no dilatation, and those with normal cardiac function by echocardiography, are counseled regarding the small but serious potential risk of aortic dissection. Elkayam and colleagues (1995) also concluded that pregnancy was safer in women with Marfan syndrome who had no cardiovascular manifestations or aortic arch dilatation. They recommended β-blocker prophylactic therapy during pregnancy.

The aortic root usually measures about 20 mm, and if dilatation reaches 40 mm, then dissection is more likely (Simpson and D'Alton, 1997). If it reaches 50 to 60 mm, then elective surgery should be considered before pregnancy (Gott and collaborators, 1999; Prêtre and Von Segesser, 1997). Williams and co-workers (2002) described a successful pregnancy following aortic root and arch replacement. Aortic root replacement during pregnancy has been associated with hypoxic–ischemic cerebral damage in a 29-week fetus (Mul and co-workers, 1998). Although Marfan syndrome itself is not an indication, the authors recommended cesarean delivery

if there is aortic involvement. Otherwise, obstetrical indications for delivery are followed.

Aortic Coarctation. This is a relatively rare lesion often accompanied by abnormalities of other large arteries. For example, a bicuspid aortic valve is seen with echocardiography in a fourth of affected patients, and another 10 percent have cerebral artery aneurysms. Other associated lesions are persistent ductus arteriosus, septal defects, and Turner syndrome. The collateral circulation arising above the level of the coarctation expands, often to a striking extent, to cause localized erosion of rib margins by hypertrophied intercostal arteries. Typical findings on physical examination are hypertension in the upper extremities but normal or reduced blood pressures in the lower extremities. Sherer (2002) and Dizon-Townson and colleagues (1995) have described diagnoses during pregnancy using MRI.

EFFECTS ON PREGNANCY. The major complications of coarctation are congestive heart failure after long-standing severe hypertension, bacterial endocarditis of the bicuspid aortic valve, and aortic rupture. Maternal mortality rates average about 3 percent (McAnulty and co-workers, 1990). Because hypertension may worsen in pregnancy, antihypertensive therapy using β-blocking drugs is usually required. Aortic rupture is more likely to occur late in pregnancy or early in the puerperium. Cerebral hemorrhage from *circle of Willis aneurysms* may also develop. Beauchesne and associates (2001) described the outcomes of 188 pregnancies in 50 women from the Mayo Clinic who had coarctation and who became pregnant. There was one maternal death due to dissection at 36 weeks. Hypertension was common (30 percent) and was related to the presence of a significant coarctation gradient.

Congestive heart failure demands vigorous efforts to improve cardiac function and may warrant pregnancy interruption. Some authors have recommended that resection of the coarctation be undertaken during pregnancy to protect against the possibility of a dissecting aneurysm and aortic rupture. This poses significant risk, especially for the fetus, because all the collaterals must be clamped for variable periods of time.

Some authors recommend cesarean delivery to prevent transient arterial blood pressure elevations that commonly accompany labor. It is feared that such blood pressure increases might lead to rupture of either the aorta or coexisting cerebral aneurysms. Available evidence, however, suggests that cesarean delivery should be limited to obstetrical indications. Intrapartum bacterial endocarditis prophylaxis is given if bacteremia is suspected.

ISCHEMIC HEART DISEASE. Coronary artery disease, which may lead to *myocardial infarction*, is a rare complication of pregnancy. Although Mendelson and Lang (1995) cite the collective incidence of myocardial infarction complicating pregnancy to be 1 in 10,000, it probably is much lower than this. Frequently, women with coronary artery disease have classical risk factors such as cigarette smoking, hyperlipidemia, obesity, or hypertension. Bagg and colleagues (1999) reviewed 22 diabetic pregnant women with ischemic heart disease or class H diabetes (see Chap. 52, p. 1180). They as well as Pombar (1995) and Reece (1986) and their colleagues documented unusually high mortality in pregnant diabetics who suffered myocardial infarction. Mousa (2000) and Sutaria (2000) and their associates each documented coronary artery occlusion in two pregnant smokers with hypercholesterolemia following a routine intramuscular injection of 0.5-mg ergometrine. Schulte-Sasse (2000) described myocardial ischemia associated with the use of prostaglandin E_1 vaginal suppositories. Karpati and co-workers (2004) reported that half of 55 women with shock from postpartum hemorrhage developed myocardial ischemia.

Diagnosis during pregnancy is not different from in the nonpregnant patient. Measurement of serum levels of the cardiac-specific contractile protein, *troponin I*, is accurate for diagnosis (Shade and associates, 2002). Shivvers and colleagues (1999) showed that troponin I was undetectable across normal pregnancy. Moreover, Koscica and colleagues (2002) found that levels do not increase following either vaginal or cesarean delivery. Myeloperoxidase, another serum marker to predict major cardiac events, has not been studied in pregnant women (Brennan and associates, 2003).

Pregnancy with Prior Ischemic Heart Disease. The advisability of pregnancy after a myocardial infarction is unclear. Ischemic heart disease is characteristically progressive, and because it is usually associated with hypertension or diabetes, pregnancy seems inadvisable.

Vinatier and associates (1994) reviewed 30 cases of pregnancy in women who had sustained an *infarction remote from pregnancy.* Although none of these women died, four had congestive heart failure and four had worsening angina during pregnancy. Pombar and co-workers (1995) reviewed outcomes of women with diabetes-associated ischemic heart disease and infarction. Three had undergone coronary artery bypass grafting before pregnancy. Of 17 women, eight died during pregnancy. Certainly, pregnancy increases cardiac workload, and all of these investigators concluded that ventricular performance should be assessed using ventriculography, radionuclide studies, echocardiography, or coronary angiography prior to conception. If there is no significant ventricular dysfunction, pregnancy will likely be tolerated. For the woman who becomes pregnant before these studies are performed, echocardiography should be done. Exercise tolerance testing may be indicated, and radionuclide ventriculography results in minimal radiation exposure for the fetus (see Chap. 41, p. 981).

Myocardial Infarction During Pregnancy. Treatment is similar to that for nonpregnant patients. Hankins and co-

workers (1985) reviewed 68 cases and reported an overall maternal mortality rate of 30 to 35 percent. Hands and colleagues (1990) found an overall mortality of 30 percent. Of 50 women who sustained infarction in the third trimester, 40 percent died, compared with 20 percent of the other 35 women who had an infarction earlier in pregnancy. Women who sustain an infarction less than 2 weeks prior to labor are at especially high risk of death (Esplin and Clark, 1999).

Acute management includes administration of nitroglycerin and morphine with close blood pressure monitoring (Esplin and Clark, 1999). Lidocaine is used to suppress malignant arrhythmias. Calcium-channel blockers or β-blockers are given if indicated. *Tissue plasminogen activator* has been used in pregnant women remote from delivery (Schumacher and associates, 1997). If the infarct has healed sufficiently, cesarean delivery is reserved for obstetrical indications, and most authors recommend epidural analgesia during labor (Esplin and Clark, 1999). Epidural analgesia or general anesthesia may be used for cesarean delivery. Camann and Thornhill (1999) recommend pulmonary artery catheter monitoring with an infarction within 6 months of delivery, or when there is ventricular dysfunction. Others, including us, recommend such monitoring only if there is cardiac dysfunction.

In some women, invasive or surgical procedures may be indicated because of unrelenting disease. Hands and associates (1990) reported successful use of percutaneous transluminal coronary angioplasty in a pregnant woman at 36 weeks. Sanchez-Ramos and co-workers (1994) and Craig and Ilton (1999) described percutaneous balloon angioplasty and transluminal intracoronary stenting. Garry and colleagues (1996) used an intra-aortic balloon pump in a woman who sustained an infarction at 25 weeks. They then performed bypass grafting at 32 weeks.

HYPERTROPHIC CARDIOMYOPATHY. Although concentric left ventricular hypertrophy commonly develops after long-standing hypertension, there is a familial as well as a sporadic form not related to hypertension termed *idiopathic hypertrophic subaortic stenosis.* Recent epidemiological studies suggest that the disorder is common, affecting approximately 1 in 500 adults (Maron, 2004). It is commonly associated with pheochromocytoma, Friedreich ataxia, Turner syndrome, and neurofibromatosis. In the half of cases that are inherited, about 50 percent are autosomally dominant disorders (Baughman, 1992). The abnormality is in the myocardial muscle, and it is characterized by idiopathic left ventricular myocardial hypertrophy that may provide a pressure gradient to left ventricular outflow (Lang and Borow, 1991). Diagnosis is confirmed by Doppler echocardiography.

The majority of affected women are asymptomatic, but dyspnea, anginal or atypical chest pain, syncope, and arrhythmias may develop. Complex arrhythmias may progress to sudden death, which is the most common form of death. Asymptomatic patients with runs of ventricular tachycardia are especially prone to sudden death. Symptoms are usually worsened by exercise. Nishimura and Holmes (2004) have provided a recent scholarly review.

Management in Pregnancy. Although limited reports suggest that pregnancy is well tolerated, congestive heart failure develops in 40 percent of cases (Benitez, 1996). Thaman and co-workers (2003) reviewed 271 pregnancies in 127 affected women. Although there were no maternal deaths, more than 25 percent experienced at least one adverse cardiac symptom including dyspnea, chest pain, or palpitations. Strenuous exercise is prohibited during pregnancy. Abrupt positional changes are avoided to prevent reflex vasodilation and decreased preload. Likewise, drugs that evoke diuresis or diminish vascular resistance are not used. If symptoms develop, especially angina, β-adrenergic or calcium-channel blocking drugs are given. The route of delivery is determined by obstetrical indications. Spinal analgesia is contraindicated, and even carefully administered epidural analgesia is controversial (Camann and Thornhill, 1999). Endocarditis prophylaxis is given if bacteremia is suspected (see Table 44–7). Infants rarely demonstrate inherited lesions at the time of birth.

REFERENCES

Abouzied AM, Abbady MA, Gendy MF, et al: Percutaneous balloon mitral commissurotomy during pregnancy. Angiology 52:205, 2001

Al Kasab SM, Sabag T, Al Zaibag M, et al: β-adrenergic receptor blockade in the management of pregnant women with mitral stenosis. Am J Obstet Gynecol 163:37, 1990

Al-Khatib SM, LaPointe NM, Kramer JM, et al: What clinicians should know about the QT interval. JAMA 289:2120, 2003

Aliaga L, Santiago FM, Marti J, et al: Right-sided endocarditis complicating an atrial septal defect. Am J Med Sci 325:282, 2003

American College of Obstetricians and Gynecologists: Prophylactic antibiotics in labor and delivery. Practice Bulletin No. 47, October 2003

American College of Obstetricians and Gynecologists: Safety of Lovenox in pregnancy. Committee Opinion No. 276, October 2002

American College of Obstetricians and Gynecologists: Thromboembolism in pregnancy. Practice Bulletin No. 19, August 2000

American College of Obstetricians and Gynecologists: Cardiac disease in pregnancy. Technical Bulletin No. 168, June 1992

Anderson RN: Deaths: Leading causes for 2000. Natl Vital Stat Health Rep Vol. 50, No. 16, September 16, 2002

Angel JL, Chapman C, Knuppel RA, et al: Percutaneous balloon aortic valvuloplasty in pregnancy. Obstet Gynecol 72:438, 1988

Armenti VT, Radomski JS, Moritz M, et al: Report from the National Transplantation Pregnancy Registry (NTPR): Outcomes of pregnancy after transplantation, Chapter 7. In Cecka JM, Terasaki PI (eds): Clinical Transplants. Los Angeles, CA, UCLA Immunogenetics Center, 2001

Arnoni RT, Arnoni AS, Bonini R, et al: Risk factors associated with cardiac surgery during pregnancy. Ann Thorac Surg 76:1605, 2003

Avila WS, Rossi EG, Ramires JA, et al: Pregnancy in patients with heart disease: Experience with 1,000 cases. Clin Cardiol 26:135, 2003

Badalian SS, Silverman RK, Aubry RH, et al: Twin pregnancy in a woman on long-term epoprostenol therapy for primary pulmonary hypertension: A case report. J Reprod Med 45:149, 2000

Bagg W, Henley PG, Macpherson P, et al: Pregnancy in women with diabetes and ischemic heart disease. Aust N Z J Obstet Gynaecol 39:99, 1999

Barbaro G, di Lorenzo G, Grisorio B, et al: Incidence of dilated cardiomyopathy and detection of HIV in myocardial cells of HIV-positive patients. N Engl J Med 339:1093, 1998

Barnes EJ, Eben F, Patterson D: Direct current cardioversion during pregnancy should be performed with facilities available for fetal monitoring and emergency caesarean section. Br J Obstet Gynaecol 109:1406, 2002

Bataskov KL, Hariharan S, Horowitz MD, et al: Gonococcal endocarditis complicating pregnancy: A case report and literature review. Obstet Gynecol 78:494, 1991

Baughman KL: Hypertrophic cardiomyopathy. JAMA 267:846, 1992

Beauchesne LM, Connolly HM, Ammash NM, et al: Coarctation of the aorta: Outcome of pregnancy. J Am Coll Cardiol 38:1728, 2001

Benitez RM: Hypertrophic cardiomyopathy and pregnancy: Maternal and fetal outcomes. J Matern Fetal Invest 6:51, 1996

Berg CJ, Chang J, Callaghan WM, et al: Pregnancy-related mortality in the United States, 1991–1997. Obstet Gynecol 101:289, 2003

Biggin A, Holman K, Brett M, et al: Detection of thirty novel FBN1 mutations in patients with Marfan syndrome or a related fibrillinopathy. Hum Mutat 23:99, 2004

Boggess KA, Easterling TR, Raghu G: Management and outcome of pregnant women with interstitial and restrictive lung disease. Am J Obstet Gynecol 173:1007, 1995

Bildirici I, Shumway JB: Intravenous and inhaled epoprostenol for primary pulmonary hypertension during pregnancy and delivery. Obstet Gynecol 103:1102, 2004

Bonow RO, Carabello B, de Leon AC Jr, et al: Guidelines for the management of patients with valvular heart disease: Executive summary. A report of the American College of Cardiology/American Heart Association Task Force on Practice Guidelines, Committee on Management of Patients with Valvular Heart Disease. Circulation 98:1949, 1998

Brennan ML, Penn MS, Van Lente F, et al: Prognostic value of myeloperoxidase in patients with chest pain. N Engl J Med 349:1595, 2003

Brickner ME, Hillis LD, Lange RA: Congenital heart disease in adults. First of two parts. N Engl J Med 342:256, 2000

Brodsky M, Doria R, Allen B, et al: New-onset ventricular tachycardia during pregnancy. Am Heart J 123:933, 1992

Brown CS, Bertolet BD: Peripartum cardiomyopathy: A comprehensive review. Am J Obstet Gynecol 178:409, 1998

Camann WR, Thornhill ML: Cardiovascular disease. In Chestnut DH (ed): Obstetric Anesthesia, 2nd ed. St. Louis, Mosby, 1999, p 776

Capeless EL, Clapp JF: Cardiovascular changes in early phase of pregnancy. Am J Obstet Gynecol 161:1449, 1989

Carabello BA: Aortic stenosis. N Engl J Med 346:677, 2002

Carabello BA, Crawford FA: Valvular heart disease. N Engl J Med 337:32, 1997

Carruth JE, Mirvis SB, Brogan DR, et al: The electrocardiogram in normal pregnancy. Am Heart J 102:1075, 1981

Caulin-Glaser T, Setaro JF: Pregnancy and cardiovascular disease. In Burrow GN, Duffy TP (eds): Medical Complications During Pregnancy, 5th ed. Philadelphia, Saunders, 1999, p 111

Chakhtoura N, Angioli R, Yasin S: Use of adenosine for pharmacological cardioversion of SVT in pregnancy. Prim Care Update Ob Gyns 5:154, 1998

Chan WS, Anand S, Ginsberg JS: Anticoagulation of pregnant women with mechanical heart valves: A systematic review of the literature. Arch Intern Med 160:191, 2000

Chia YT, Yeoh SC, Lim MCL, et al: Pregnancy outcome and mitral valve prolapse. Asia-Oceania J Obstet Gynaecol 20:383, 1994

Clark SL, Cotton DB, Lee W, et al: Central hemodynamic assessment of normal term pregnancy. Am J Obstet Gynecol 161:1439, 1989

Clark SL, Phelan JP, Greenspoon J, et al: Labor and delivery in the presence of mitral stenosis: Central hemodynamic observations. Am J Obstet Gynecol 152:984, 1985

Clark SL, Porter TF, West FG: Coumarin derivatives and breast-feeding. Obstet Gynecol 95:938, 2000

Connolly HM, Grogan M, Warnes CA: Pregnancy among women with congenitally corrected transposition of great arteries. J Am Coll Cardiol 33:1692, 1999

Cool CD, Rai PR, Yeager ME, et al: Expression of human herpesvirus 8 in primary pulmonary hypertension. N Engl J Med 349:1113, 2003

Cotrufo M, De Feo M, De Santo LS, et al: Risk of warfarin during pregnancy with mechanical valve prostheses. Obstet Gynecol 99:35, 2002

Cox SM, Hankins GDV, Leveno KJ, et al: Bacterial endocarditis: A serious pregnancy complication. J Reprod Med 33:671, 1988

Cox SM, Leveno KJ: Pregnancy complicated by bacterial endocarditis. Clin Obstet Gynecol 32:48, 1989

Craig S, Ilton M: Treatment of acute myocardial infarction in pregnancy with coronary artery balloon angioplasty and stenting. Aust N Z J Obstet Gynaecol 39:194, 1999

Cunningham FG, Pritchard JA, Hankins GDV, et al: Peripartum heart failure: Idiopathic cardiomyopathy or compounding cardiovascular events? Obstet Gynecol 67:157, 1986

Dajani AS, Taubert KA, Wilson W, et al: Prevention of bacterial endocarditis. Recommendations of the American Heart Association. JAMA 277:1794, 1997

Damilakis J, Theocharopoulos N, Perisinakis K, et al: Conceptus radiation dose and risk from cardiac catheter ablation procedures. Circulation 104:893, 2001

Darouiche RO: Treatment of infections associated with surgical implants. N Engl J Med 350:1422, 2004

Dashe JS, Ramin KD, Ramin SM: Pregnancy following cardiac transplantation. Prim Care Update Ob Gyns 5:257, 1998

Deger R, Ludmir J: Neisseria sicca endocarditis complicating pregnancy. J Reprod Med 37:473, 1992

Desai DK, Adanlawo M, Naidoo DP, et al: Mitral stenosis in pregnancy: A four-year experience at King Edward VIII Hospital, Durban, South Africa. Br J Obstet Gynaecol 107:953, 2000

de Souza JA, Martinez Jr EE, Ambrose JA, et al: Percutaneous balloon mitral valvuloplasty in comparison with open mitral valve commissurotomy for mitral stenosis during pregnancy. J Am Coll Cardiol 37:900, 2001a

de Souza JL Jr, Frimm CD, Nastari L, et al: Left ventricular function after a new pregnancy in patients with peripartum cardiomyopathy. J Card Fail 7:30, 2001b

de Swiet M: Maternal mortality: Confidential enquiries into maternal deaths in the United Kingdom. Am J Obstet Gynecol 182:760, 2000

Deviri E, Levinsky L, Yechezkel M, et al: Pregnancy after valve replacement with porcine xenograft prosthesis. Surg Gynecol Obstet 160:437, 1985

Dizon-Townson D, Magee KP, Twickler DM, et al: Coarctation of the abdominal aorta in pregnancy: Diagnosis by magnetic resonance imaging. Obstet Gynecol 85:817, 1995

Dunn JS Jr, Brost BC: Fetal bradycardia after IV adenosine for maternal PSVT. Am J Emerg Med 18:234, 2000

Easterling TR, Benedetti TJ, Schmucker BC, et al: Maternal hemodynamics and aortic diameter in normal and hypertensive pregnancies. Obstet Gynecol 78:1073, 1991

Easterling TR, Chadwick HS, Otto CM, et al: Aortic stenosis in pregnancy. Obstet Gynecol 72:113, 1988

Easterling TR, Ralph DD, Schmucker BC: Pulmonary hypertension in pregnancy: Treatment with pulmonary vasodilators. Obstet Gynecol 93:494, 1999

Eisen HJ, Tuzcu EM, Dorent R, et al: Everolimus for the prevention of allograft rejection and vasculopathy in cardiac-transplant recipients. N Engl J Med 349:847, 2003

Elkayam U, Ostrzega E, Shotan A, et al: Cardiovascular problems in pregnant women with Marfan syndrome. Ann Intern Med 123:117, 1995

Elkayam U, Tummala PP, Rao K, et al: Maternal and fetal outcomes of subsequent pregnancies in women with peripartum cardiomyopathy. N Engl J Med 344:1567, 2001

Esplin S, Clark SL: Ischemic heart disease and myocardial infarction during pregnancy. Contemp Ob/Gyn 44:27, 1999

Etheridge MJ, Pepperell RJ: Heart disease and pregnancy at the Royal Women's Hospital. Med J Aust 2:277, 1977

Ezekowitz MD, Levine JA: Preventing stroke in patients with atrial fibrillation. JAMA 281:1830, 1999

Felker GM, Thompson RE, Hare JM, et al: Underlying causes and long-term survival in patients with initially unexplained cardiomyopathy. N Engl J Med 342:1077, 2000

Freed LA, Levy D, Levine RA, et al: Prevalence and clinical outcome of mitral-valve prolapse. N Engl J Med 341:1, 1999

Gardin J, Schumacher D, Constantine G, et al: Valvular abnormalities and cardiovascular status following exposure to dexfenfluramine or phentermine/fenfluramine. JAMA 283:1703, 2000

Garry D, Leikin E, Fleisher AG, et al: Acute myocardial infarction in pregnancy with subsequent medical and surgical management. Obstet Gynecol 87:802, 1996

Gei AF, Hankins GDV: Cardiac disease and pregnancy. Obstet Gynecol Clin North Am 28:465, 2001

Gilon D, Buonanno FS, Joffe MM, et al: Lack of evidence of an association between mitral-valve prolapse and stroke in young patients. N Engl J Med 341:8, 1999

Gladwin MT, Sachdev V, Jison ML, et al: Pulmonary hypertension as a risk factor for death in patients with sickle cell disease. N Engl J Med 350:886, 2004

Gleicher N, Midwall J, Hochberger D, et al: Eisenmenger's syndrome and pregnancy. Obstet Gynecol Surv 34:721, 1979

Gott VL, Greene PS, Alejo DE, et al: Replacement of the aortic root in patients with Marfan's syndrome. N Engl J Med 340:1307, 1999

Gowda RM, Khan IA, Mehta NJ, et al: Cardiac arrhythmias in pregnancy: Clinical and therapeutic considerations. Int J Cardiol 88:129, 2003

Gupta A, Lokhandwala YY, Satoskar PR, et al: Balloon mitral valvotomy in pregnancy: Maternal and fetal outcomes. J Am Coll Surg 187:409, 1998

Hameed A, Karaalp IS, Tummala PP, et al: The effect of valvular heart disease on maternal and fetal outcome of pregnancy. J Am Coll Cardiol 37:893, 2001

Hanania G, Thomas D, Michel PL, et al: Pregnancy and prosthetic heart valves: A French cooperative retrospective study of 155 cases. Eur Heart J 15:1651, 1994

Hands ME, Johnson MD, Saltzman DH, et al: The cardiac, obstetric, and anesthetic management of pregnancy complicated by acute myocardial infarction. J Clin Anesth 2:258, 1990

Hankins GDV, Wendel GD Jr, Leveno KJ, et al: Myocardial infarction during pregnancy: A review. Obstet Gynecol 65:138, 1985

Hasbun R, Vikram HR, Barakat LA, et al: Complicated left-sided native valve endocarditis in adults: Risk classification for mortality. JAMA 289:1933, 2003

Hibbard JU, Lindheimer M, Lang RM: A modified definition for peripartum cardiomyopathy and prognosis based on echocardiography. Obstet Gynecol 94:311, 1999

Hirsh J, Fuster V, Ansell J, et al: American Heart Association/American College of Cardiology Foundation guide to warfarin therapy. J Am Coll Cardiol 41:1633, 2003

Hoare JV, Radford D: Pregnancy after Fontan repair of complex congenital heart disease. Aust N Z J Obstet Gynaecol 41:464, 2001

Hoen B, Alla F, Selton-Suty C, et al: Changing profile of infective endocarditis: Results of a 1-year survey in France. JAMA 288:75, 2002

Hosenpud JD, Novick RJ, Breen TJ, et al: The registry of the International Society for Heart and Lung Transplantation: Eleventh official report—1994. J Heart Lung Transplant 13:561, 1994

Humbert M, Sitbon O, Simonneau G: Treatment of pulmonary arterial hypertension. N Engl J Med 351:1425, 2004

Humbert M, Nunes H, Sitbon O, et al: Risk factors for pulmonary arterial hypertension. Clin Chest Med 22:459, 2001

Iserin L: Management of pregnancy in women with congenital heart disease. Heart 85:493, 2001

Iturbe-Alessio I, Fonseca MDC, Mutchinik O, et al: Risks of anticoagulant therapy in pregnant women with artificial heart valves. N Engl J Med 315:1390, 1986

Jaffe R, Gruber A, Fejgin M, et al: Pregnancy with an artificial pacemaker. Obstet Gynecol Surv 42:137, 1987

Jessup M, Brozena S: Heart failure. N Engl J Med 348:2007, 2003

Jick H: Heart valve disorders and appetite-suppressant drugs. JAMA 283:1738, 2000

Kametas NA, McAuliffe F, Krampl E, et al: Maternal cardiac function in twin pregnancy. Obstet Gynecol 102:806, 2003

Kangavari S, Collins J, Cercek B, et al: Tricuspid valve group B streptococcal endocarditis after an elective termination of pregnancy. Clin Cardiol 23:301, 2000

Kapp C: Heart transplant recipient climbs the Matterhorn. Lancet 362:880, 2003

Karchmer AW: Infective endocarditis. In Braunwald E, Fauci AS, Kasper DL, et al (eds): Harrison's Principles of Internal Medicine, 15th ed. New York, McGraw-Hill, 2001, p 809

Karpati PCJ, Rossignol M, Pirot M, et al: High incidence of myocardial ischemia during postpartum hemorrhage. Anesthesiology 100:30, 2004

Kenchaiah S, Evans JC, Levy D, et al: Obesity and the risk of heart failure. N Engl J Med 347:305, 2002

Key TC, Resnik R, Dittrich HC, et al: Successful pregnancy after cardiac transplantation. Am J Obstet Gynecol 160:367, 1989

Khan MA, Herzog CA, St. Peter JV, et al: The prevalence of cardiac valvular insufficiency assessed by transthoracic echocardiography in obese patients treated with appetite-suppressant drugs. N Engl J Med 339:713, 1998

Khandelwal M, Rasanen J, Ludormirski A, et al: Fetal and uterine hemodynamics during and after maternal cardiopulmonary bypass (CPB). Am J Obstet Gynecol 174:460, 1996

Kim K-M, Sukhani R, Slogoff S, et al: Central hemodynamic changes associated with pregnancy in a long-term cardiac transplant recipient. Am J Obstet Gynecol 174:1651, 1996

Kiss H, Egarter C, Asseryanis E, et al: Primary pulmonary hypertension in pregnancy: A case report. Am J Obstet Gynecol 172:1052, 1995

Koscica KL, Anyaogu C, Bebbington M, et al: Maternal levels of troponin I in patients undergoing vaginal and cesarean delivery. Obstet Gynecol 99:83S, 2002

Lam GK, Stafford RE, Thorp J, et al: Inhaled nitric oxide for primary pulmonary hypertension in pregnancy. Obstet Gynecol 98:895, 2001

Lampert MB, Hibbard J, Weinert L, et al: Peripartum heart failure associated with prolonged tocolytic therapy. Am J Obstet Gynecol 168:493, 1993

Lampert MB, Weinert L, Hibbard J, et al: Contractile reserve in patients with peripartum cardiomyopathy and recovered left ventricular function. Am J Obstet Gynecol 176:189, 1997

Lang RM, Borow KM: Heart disease. In Barron WM, Lindheimer MD (eds): Medical Disorders During Pregnancy. St. Louis, Mosby Yearbook, 1991, p 148

Lao TT, Adelman AG, Sermer M, et al: Balloon valvuloplasty for congenital aortic stenosis in pregnancy. Br J Obstet Gynaecol 100:1141, 1993a

Lao TT, Sermer M, Colman JM: Pregnancy following surgical correction for transposition of the great arteries. Obstet Gynecol 83:655, 1994

Lao TT, Sermer M, MaGee L, et al: Congenital aortic stenosis and pregnancy—a reappraisal. Am J Obstet Gynecol 169:540, 1993b

Lederle FA, Wilson SE, Johnson GR, et al: Immediate repair compared with surveillance of small abdominal aortic aneurysms. N Engl J Med 346:1437, 2002

Lee C-N, Wu C-C, Lin P-Y, et al: Pregnancy following cardiac prosthetic valve replacement. Obstet Gynecol 83:353, 1994

Lee M-J, Huang A, Gillen-Goldstein J, et al: Labor and vaginal delivery with maternal aortic aneurysm. Obstet Gynecol 98:935, 2001

Leyh RG, Fischer S, Ruhparwar A, et al: Anticoagulant therapy in pregnant women with mechanical heart valves. Arch Gynecol Obstet 268:1, 2003

Leyh RG, Fischer S, Ruhparwar A, et al: Anticoagulation for prosthetic heart valves during pregnancy: Is low-molecular-weight heparin an alternative? Eur J Cardiothorac Surg 21:577, 2002

Limacher MC, Ware JA, O'Meara ME, et al: Tricuspid regurgitation during pregnancy: Two-dimensional and pulsed Doppler echocardiographic observations. Am J Cardiol 55:1059, 1985

Löwenstein BR, Vain NW, Perrone SV, et al: Successful pregnancy and vaginal delivery after heart transplantation. Am J Obstet Gynecol 158:589, 1988

Lupton M, Oteng-Ntim E, Ayida G, et al: Cardiac disease in pregnancy. Curr Opin Obstet Gynecol 14:137, 2002

Lynch-Salamon DI, Maze SS, Combs CA: Pregnancy after Mustard repair for transposition of the great arteries. Obstet Gynecol 82:676, 1993

Mabie WC, Hackman BB, Sibai BM: Pulmonary edema associated with pregnancy: Echocardiographic insights and implications for treatment. Obstet Gynecol 81:227, 1993

Malhotra M, Sharma JB, Arora P, et al: Mitral valve surgery and maternal and fetal outcome in valvular heart disease. Int J Gynaecol Obstet 81:151, 2003

Maron BJ: Hypertrophic cardiomyopathy: An important global disease. Am J Med 116:63, 2004

McAnulty JH, Metcalfe J, Ueland K: Heart disease and pregnancy. In Hurst JW, Schlant RC, Rackley CE, et al (eds): The Heart, 7th ed. New York, McGraw-Hill, 1990, p 1465

McFaul PB, Dornan JC, Lamki H, et al: Pregnancy complicated by maternal heart disease. A review of 519 women. Br J Obstet Gynaecol 95:861, 1988

Megerian G, Bell JG, Huhta JC, et al: Pregnancy outcome following a Mustard procedure for transposition of the great arteries: A report of five cases and review of the literature. Obstet Gynecol 83:512, 1994

Mendelson MA, Lang RM: Pregnancy and Heart Disease. In Barron WM, Lindheimer MD (eds): Medical Disorders During Pregnancy, 2nd ed. St. Louis, Mosby Yearbook, 1995, p 129

Moodie DS: Adult congenital heart disease. Curr Opin Cardiol 9:137, 1994

Morris CD, Reller MD, Menashe VD: Thirty-year incidence of infective endocarditis after surgery for congenital heart defect. JAMA 279:599, 1998

Mousa HA, McKinley CA, Thong J: Acute postpartum myocardial infarction after ergometrine administration in a woman with familial hypercholesterolaemia. Br J Obstet Gynaecol 107:939, 2000

Mul TFM, van Herwerden LA, Cohen-Overbeek TE, et al: Hypoxic–ischemic fetal insult resulting from maternal aortic root replacement, with normal fetal heart rate at term. Am J Obstet Gynecol 179:825, 1998

Nagorney DM, Field CS: Successful pregnancy 10 years after triple cardiac valve replacement. Obstet Gynecol 57:386, 1981

Nanson J, Elcock D, Williams M, et al: Do physiological changes in pregnancy change defibrillation energy requirements? Br J Anaesth 87:237, 2001

Nassar AH, Hobeika EM, Abd Essamad HM, et al: Pregnancy outcome in women with prosthetic heart valves. Am J Obstet Gynecol 191:1009, 2004

Nassar AH, Abdallah ME, Moukarbel GV, et al: Sequential use of thrombolytic agents for thrombosed mitral valve prosthesis during pregnancy. J Perinat Med 31:257, 2003

Nishimura RA, Holmes DR, Jr: Hypertrophic obstructive cardiomyopathy. N Engl J Med 350:1320, 2004

Nishimura RA, McGoon MD: Perspectives on mitral-valve prolapse. N Engl J Med 341:48, 1999

Nishimura RA, McGoon MD, Shub C, et al: Echocardiographically documented mitral-valve prolapse: Long-term follow-up of 237 patients. N Engl J Med 313:1305, 1985

North RA, Sadler L, Stewart AW, et al: Long-term survival and valve-related complications in young women with cardiac valve replacements. Circulation 99:2669, 1999

O'Connell JB, Costanzo-Nordin MR, Subramanian R, et al: Peripartum cardiomyopathy: Clinical, hemodynamic, histologic and prognostic characteristics. J Am Coll Cardiol 8:52, 1986

O'Gara PT, Greenfield AJ, Afridi NA, Houser SL. Case 12-2004: A 38-year-old woman with acute onset of pain in the chest. N Engl J Med 350:16, 2004

Oron G, Hirsch R, Ben-Haroush A, et al: Pregnancy outcome in women with heart disease undergoing induction of labour. BJOG 111:669, 2004

Pappone C, Santinelli V, Manguso F, et al: A randomized study of prophylactic catheter ablation in asymptomatic patients with the Wolff-Parkinson-White syndrome. N Engl J Med 349:1803, 2003

Pavankumar P, Venugopal P, Kaul U, et al: Closed mitral valvotomy during pregnancy: A 20 year experience. Scand J Thorac Cardiovasc Surg 22:11, 1988

Pearson GD, Veille JC, Rahimtoola S, et al: Peripartum cardiomyopathy. National Heart, Lung, and Blood Institute and Office of Rare Diseases (National Institutes of Health) Workshop Recommendations and Review. JAMA 283:1183, 2000

Pengo V, Lensing AW, Prins MH, et al: Incidence of chronic thromboembolic pulmonary hypertension after pulmonary embolism. N Engl J Med 350:2257, 2004

Penning S, Robinson KD, Major CA, et al: A comparison of echocardiography and pulmonary artery catheterization for evaluation of pulmonary artery pressures in pregnant patients with suspected pulmonary hypertension. Am J Obstet Gynecol 184:1568, 2001

Pepin M, Schwarze U, Superti-Furga A, et al: Clinical and genetic features of Ehlers–Danlos syndrome type IV, the vascular type. N Engl J Med 342:673, 2000

Pollack KL, Chestnut DH, Wenstrom KD: Anesthetic management of a parturient with Eisenmenger's syndrome. Anesth Analg 70:212, 1990

Pombar X, Strassner HT, Fenner PC: Pregnancy in a woman with class H diabetes mellitus and previous coronary artery bypass graft: A case report and review of the literature. Obstet Gynecol 85:825, 1995

Prasad AK, Ventura HO: Valvular heart disease and pregnancy: A high index of suspicion is important to reduce risks. Postgrad Med 110:69, 2001

Prêtre R, Von Segesser LK: Aortic dissection. Lancet 349:1461, 1997

Pulerwitz TC, Cappola TP, Felker GM, et al: Mortality in primary and secondary myocarditis. Am Heart J 147:746, 2004

Rahman J, Rahman FZ, Rahman W, et al: Obstetric and gynecologic complications in women with Marfan syndrome. J Reprod Med 48:723, 2003

Ramin SM, Gilstrap LC III: Mitral-valve disease in pregnancy. Prim Care Update Ob Gyns 6:106, 1999

Rashba EJ, Zareba W, Moss AJ, et al: Influence of pregnancy on the risk for cardiac events in patients with hereditary long QT syndrome. Circulation 97:451, 1998

Rayburn WF, LeMire MS, Bird JL, et al: Mitral valve prolapse: Echocardiographic changes during pregnancy. J Reprod Med 32:185, 1987

Reece EA, Egan JFX, Coustan DR, et al: Coronary artery disease in diabetic pregnancies. Am J Obstet Gynecol 154:150, 1986

Reich O, Tax P, Marek J, et al: Long term results of percutaneous balloon valvoplasty of congenital aortic stenosis: Independent predictors of outcome. Heart 90:70, 2004

Reimold SC, Rutherford JD: Valvular heart disease in pregnancy. N Engl J Med 349:52, 2003

Robins K, Lyons G: Supraventricular tachycardia in pregnancy. Br J Anaesth 92:140, 2004

Roden DM: Drug-induced prolongation of the QT interval. N Engl J Med 350:1013, 2004

Roeleveld RJ, Vonk-Noordegraaf A, Marcus JT, et al: Effects of epoprostenol on right ventricular hypertrophy and dilatation in pulmonary hypertension. Chest 125:572, 2004

Roldan CA, Shively BK, Crawford MH: An echocardiographic study of valvular heart disease associated with systemic lupus erythematosus. N Engl J Med 335:1424, 1996

Rossiter JP, Repke JT, Morales AJ, et al: A prospective longitudinal evaluation of pregnancy in the Marfan syndrome. Am J Obstet Gynecol 173:1599, 1995

Rowan JA, McCowan LM, Raudkivi PJ, et al: Enoxaparin treatment in women with mechanical heart valves during pregnancy. Am J Obstet Gynecol 185:633, 2001

Runo JR, Loyd JE: Primary pulmonary hypertension. Lancet 361:1533, 2003

Sachs BP, Brown DAJ, Driscoll SG, et al: Hemorrhage, infection, toxemia, and cardiac disease, 1954–85: Causes for their declining role in maternal mortality. Am J Public Health 78:671, 1988

Sadler L, McCowan L, White H, et al: Pregnancy outcomes and cardiac complications in women with mechanical, bioprosthetic and homograft valves. Br J Obstet Gynaecol 107:245, 2000

Salazar E, Espinola N, Román L, et al: Effect of pregnancy on the duration of bovine pericardial bioprostheses. Am Heart J 137:714, 1999

Sanchez-Ramos L, Chami YG, Bass TA, et al: Myocardial infarction during pregnancy: Management with transluminal coronary angioplasty and metallic intracoronary stents. Am J Obstet Gynecol 171:1392, 1994

Sareli P, England MJ, Berk MR, et al: Maternal and fetal sequelae of anticoagulation during pregnancy in patients with mechanical heart valve prostheses. Am J Cardiol 63:1462, 1989

Sawhney H, Aggarwal N, Suri V, et al: Maternal and perinatal outcome in rheumatic heart disease. Int J Gynaecol Obstet 80:9, 2003

Sawhney H, Suri V, Vasishta K, et al: Pregnancy and congenital heart disease—maternal and fetal outcome. Aust N Z J Obstet Gynaecol 38:266, 1998

Sbarouni E, Oakley CM: Outcome of pregnancy in women with valve prostheses. Br Heart J 71:196, 1994

Schenker JG, Polishuk WZ: Pregnancy following mitral valvotomy —a survey of 182 patients. Obstet Gynecol 32:214, 1968

Schulte-Sasse U: Life threatening myocardial ischaemia associated with the use of prostaglandin E1 to induce abortion. Br J Obstet Gynaecol 107:700, 2000

Schumacher B, Belfort MA, Card RJ: Successful treatment of acute myocardial infarction during pregnancy with tissue plasminogen activator. Am J Obstet Gynecol 176:716, 1997

Seaworth BJ, Durack DT: Infective endocarditis in obstetric and gynecologic practice. Am J Obstet Gynecol 154:180, 1986

Shade GH Jr, Ross G, Bever FN, et al: Troponin I in the diagnosis of acute myocardial infarction in pregnancy, labor, and post partum. Am J Obstet Gynecol 187:1719, 2002

Sheffield JS, Cunningham FG: Diagnosing and managing peripartum cardiomyopathy. Contemp Ob/Gyn 44:74, 1999

Sheffield JS, Cunningham FG: Thyrotoxicosis and heart failure that complicate pregnancy. Am J Obstet Gynecol 190:211, 2004

Sherer DM: Coarctation of the descending thoracic aorta diagnosed during pregnancy. Obstet Gynecol 100:1094, 2002

Shime J, Mocarski EJM, Hastings D, et al: Congenital heart disease in pregnancy: Short- and long-term implications. Am J Obstet Gynecol 156:313, 1987

Shivvers SA, Wians FH Jr, Keffer JH, et al: Maternal cardiac troponin I levels during normal labor and delivery. Am J Obstet Gynecol 180:122, 1999

Shores J, Berger KR, Murphy EA, et al: Progression of aortic dilatation and the benefit of long-term β-adrenergic blockade in Marfan's syndrome. N Engl J Med 330:1335, 1994

Simpson LL, D'Alton ME: Marfan syndrome: An update on pregnancy. Prim Care Update Ob Gyns 4:1, 1997

Singh H, Bolton PJ, Oakley CM: Pregnancy after surgical correction of tetralogy of Fallot. BMJ 285:168, 1982

Siu SC, Colman JM: Congenital heart disease: Heart disease and pregnancy. Heart 85:710, 2001

Siu SC, Sermer M, Colman JM, et al: Prospective multicenter study of pregnancy outcomes in women with heart disease. Circulation 104:515, 2001

Siu SC, Sermer M, Harrison DA, et al: Risk and predictors for pregnancy-related complications in women with heart disease. Circulation 96:2789, 1997

Siva A, Shah AM: Moderate mitral stenosis in pregnancy: The haemodynamic impact of diuresis. Heart 91:e3, 2005

Sliwa K, Forster O, Zhanje F, et al: Outcome of subsequent pregnancy in patients with documented peripartum cardiomyopathy. Am J Cardiol 93:1441, 2004

Strickland RA, Oliver WC Jr, Chantigian RC, et al: Anesthesia, cardiopulmonary bypass, and the pregnant patient. Mayo Clin Proc 66:411, 1991

Suri V, Sawhney H, Vasishta K, et al: Pregnancy following cardiac valve replacement surgery. Int J Gynaecol Obstet 64:239, 1999

Sutaria N, O'Toole L, Northridge D: Postpartum acute MI following routine ergometrine administration treated successfully by primary PTCA. Heart 83:97, 2000

Thaman R, Varnava A, Hamid MS, et al: Pregnancy related complications in women with hypertrophic cardiomyopathy. Heart 89:752, 2003

Ueno M, Hasuda H, Nakamura K, et al: Antiplatelet therapy for a pregnant woman with a mechanical aortic valve: Report of a case. Surg Today 31:1002, 2001

Van der Meer JTM, Van Wijk W, Thompson J, et al: Efficacy of antibiotic prophylaxis for prevention of native-valve endocarditis. Lancet 339:135, 1992

Vinatier D, Virelizier S, Depret-Mosser S, et al: Pregnancy after myocardial infarction. Eur J Obstet Gynecol Reprod Biol 56:89, 1994

Weiss BM, Maggiorini M, Jenni R, et al: Pregnant patient with primary pulmonary hypertension: Inhaled pulmonary vasodilators and epidural anesthesia for cesarean delivery. Anesthesiology 92:1191, 2000

Weiss BM, von Segesser LK, Alon E, et al: Outcome of cardiovascular surgery and pregnancy: A systematic review of the period 1984–1996. Am J Obstet Gynecol 179:1643, 1998a

Weiss BM, Zemp L, Seifert B, et al: Outcome of pulmonary vascular disease in pregnancy: A systematic overview from 1978 through 1996. J Am Coll Cardiol 31:1650, 1998b

Widerhorn J, Widerhorn ALM, Rahimtoola SH, et al: WPW syndrome during pregnancy: Increased incidence of supraventricular arrhythmias. Am Heart J 123:796, 1992

Williams A, Child A, Rowntree J, et al: Marfan's syndrome: Successful pregnancy after aortic root and arch replacement. Br J Obstet Gynaecol 109:1187, 2002

Zuber M, Gautschi N, Oechslin E, et al: Outcome of pregnancy in women with congenital shunt lesions. Heart 81:271, 1999

45

Chronic Hypertension

The prevalence of chronic hypertension in American women has been chronicled for years, beginning with the 1960–1962 National Health Examination Survey (National Center for Health Statistics, 1964). Now known as the National Health and Nutrition Examination Survey (NHANES), this ongoing study is conducted by the National Center for Health Statistics and provides periodic information on the health of the United States population. In its most recent report, the average prevalence of hypertension in women 18 to 39 years of age was 7.2 percent for 1999 and 2000 (Hajjar and Kotchen, 2003). This is a substantive increase when compared with 5.1 percent for 1988 to 1991 and 6.1 percent for 1991 to 1994. Importantly, one third of all hypertensive patients in the United States are unaware of their diagnosis. The importance of hypertension in relation to women's health care was stressed in the recent review by the American College of Obstetricians and Gynecologists (2002).

Chronic hypertension is one of the most common medical complications encountered during pregnancy. Its variable incidence and severity, along with the well-known proclivity for pregnancy to induce or aggravate hypertension, has caused confusion concerning the management of hypertensive pregnant women. Most women with antecedent hypertension demonstrate improved blood pressure control during pregnancy. Some women, however, have worsening of hypertension that is frequently accompanied by proteinuria, pathological edema, and convulsions. These latter women—whose chronic hypertension antedates pregnancy—are indistinguishable from a woman who develops severe preeclampsia in her first pregnancy.

DEFINITIONS

There is a wide range of blood pressures in normal adults as well as in those with chronic hypertension. Categorization therefore relates to acute or long-term adverse effects associated with sustained levels of those blood pressures. These associations with normal or abnormal blood pressures are primarily based on morbidity and mortality in men. A useful categorization is that provided by the Joint National Committee on Prevention, Detection, Evaluation, and Treatment of High Blood Pressure. In its seventh report, the Joint National Committee (2003) used the classification and management scheme presented in Table 45–1. Within these categories, morbidity or mortality is further influenced by age, gender, race, and personal behaviors, including smoking, excessive alcohol intake, obesity, and physical activity.

In adults, proven benefits accrue with treatment of chronic hypertension at sustained diastolic blood pressures of 90 mm Hg or greater (Korotkoff phase V), systolic pressures of 160 mm Hg or more, or both. Benefits are apparent even in otherwise healthy adults. Treatment at even lower levels may benefit patients with evidence of renal or cardiac dysfunction, those who have had a cerebrovascular thrombosis or hemorrhage, elderly patients, or patients with appreciable underlying atherosclerotic disease or postmyocardial infarction. The Seventh Joint National Committee report (2003) recommends:

1. In persons older than 50 years of age, systolic pressures greater than 140 mm Hg are a more important cardiovascular disease risk factor than diastolic pressure.

TABLE 45–1 Classification and Management of Blood Pressure for Adults

| | Blood Pressure | | Management[a] | | |
| | | | | Initial Drug Therapy | |
Classification	Systolic (mm Hg)	Diastolic (mm Hg)	Lifestyle Modification	Without Compelling Indication	With Compelling Indications[b]
Normal	< 120	and < 80	Encourage	Treatment not indicated	Chronic renal disease or diabetes
Prehypertension	120–139	or 80–90	Yes		
Stage 1 hypertension	140–159	or 90–99	Yes	Thiazide-type diuretics for most May consider ACE inhibitor, ARB, β-blocker, CCB, or combination	Chronic renal disease or diabetes Other drugs as needed: diuretic, ACE inhibitor, ARB, β-blocker, CCB
Stage 2 hypertension	≥ 160	or ≥ 100	Yes	Two-drug combination[c] for most: usually thiazide-type diuretic and ACE inhibitor, or ARB, or β-blocker, or CCB	

ACE = angiotensin-converting enzyme; ARB = angiotensin-receptor blocker; CCB = calcium-channel blocker.
[a]Treatment determined by highest blood pressure category.
[b]Treat patients with chronic kidney disease or diabetes to goal of blood pressure < 130/80 mm Hg.
[c]Initial combined therapy should be used cautiously in those at risk for orthostatic hypotension.
From the Joint National Committee (2003).

2. Individuals with a systolic blood pressure of 120 to 139 mm Hg or a diastolic blood pressure of 80 to 89 mm Hg should be considered as *prehypertensive* and require health-promoting lifestyle modifications to prevent cardiovascular disease.

3. Thiazide-type diuretics should be used in drug treatment for most patients with uncomplicated hypertension, either alone or combined with drugs from other classes.

4. Most adults with hypertension require two or more medications to achieve a blood pressure less than 140/90 mm Hg (less than 130/80 mm Hg in patients with diabetes or renal disease).

Throughout middle and old age, blood pressure is strongly and directly related to vascular (and overall) mortality and with values down to at least 115/75 mm Hg (Prospective Studies Collaboration, 2002; Qureshi and colleagues, 2002).

DIAGNOSIS

Chronic hypertension precedes pregnancy or may be apparent prior to 20 weeks (see Chap. 34, p. 764). Some women without chronic hypertension have repeated pregnancies in which *transient hypertension* appears only late in pregnancy and regresses postpartum. This hypertension is evidence of latent hypertensive vascular disease and is analogous to gestational diabetes. Long-term follow-up studies of Chesley and co-workers (1976) and Sibai and colleagues (1986b, 1991, 1992) support this view.

In most women with hypertension antedating pregnancy, increased blood pressure is the only demonstrable finding. Some, however, have complications that increase the risks during pregnancy and may shorten life expectancy, including hypertensive or ischemic cardiac disease, renal insufficiency, or a prior cerebrovascular event. Such hypertensive vascular disease in pregnancy is encountered more frequently in older women.

Obesity is an important factor predisposing to chronic hypertension (see Chap. 43). Specifically, chronic hypertension may be increased as much as tenfold in obese women, and these women are more likely to develop superimposed preeclampsia. Diabetes mellitus is also prevalent in chronically hypertensive women, and its interplay with obesity is overwhelming. Heredity plays an important role, and indeed, a number of genes inherited as mendelian traits have been described to cause hypertension (Lifton and colleagues, 2001; Nabel, 2003). In some cases, candidate genes for preeclampsia and chronic hypertension have been described (Levesque and associates, 2004). Hypertension is common in African Americans and Mexican Americans, and frequently many members of the same family are hypertensive.

In most women with chronic hypertension, blood pressure falls in the second trimester and then rises during the third trimester to levels somewhat above those in early pregnancy

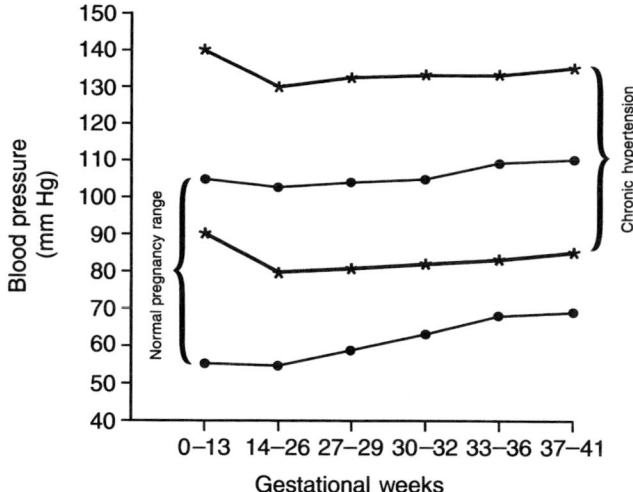

FIGURE 45–1. Systolic and diastolic blood pressures (mean ± SEM) during pregnancy in 90 untreated chronically hypertensive women (*—*). Also included are blood pressures (mean ± SD) from 22 women during normal pregnancy (●—●). (Data from MacGillivray and associates, 1969; Sibai and colleagues, 1990a.)

(Fig. 45–1). Adverse outcomes in these women are dependent largely on whether superimposed preeclampsia develops.

TREATMENT IN NONPREGNANT ADULTS

Even at the mildest end of the spectrum of abnormal blood pressures categorized in Table 45–1, interventions to reduce pressure are beneficial. Almost 30 trials involving about 162,000 participants have established that antihypertensive treatment in adults with mild to moderate hypertension decreases mortality, stroke, and major cardiac events (Blood Pressure Lowering Treatment Trialists' Collaboration, 2003; Gueyffier and collaborators, 1997; Psaty and colleagues, 2003). Antihypertensive therapy is associated with reductions in stroke that average 35 to 40 percent, myocardial infarction 20 to 25 percent, and heart failure more than 50 percent (Neal and colleagues, 2000). In patients with stage 1 hypertension (systolic pressure 140 to 159 mm Hg, diastolic pressure 90 to 99 mm Hg, or both) and additional cardiovascular risk factors, achieving a sustained 12 mm Hg-reduction in systolic pressure during 10 years in 11 patients will prevent one death (Ogden and colleagues, 2000).

Regardless of pregnancy status, women with stage 1 hypertension would likely have been placed on antihypertensive medications and lifestyle modifications, including cessation of smoking (Table 45–2). Psaty and co-workers (2003) reported that low-dose diuretics were the most effective first-line treatment. In the ALLHAT Trial (2002) of 33,357 adults 55 years of age or older, thiazide-type diuretics were superior to and less expensive than angiotensin-converting enzyme (ACE) inhibitors or calcium-channel blockers in prevention of cardiovascular disease. Results were similar for women

TABLE 45–2 Lifestyle Modifications to Manage Hypertension

Modification[a]	Recommendation	Approximate SBP Reduction (Range)
Weight reduction	Maintain normal body weight: BMI 18.5–24.9 kg/m²	5–20 mm Hg/10 kg weight loss
Adopt DASH eating plan	Consume a diet rich in fruits, vegetables, and low-fat dairy products with a reduced content of saturated and total fat	8–14 mm Hg
Dietary sodium reduction	Reduce dietary sodium intake to no more than 100 mmol/day: 2.4 g sodium or 6 g sodium chloride	2–8 mm Hg
Physical activity	Engage in regular aerobic physical activity such as brisk walking, at least 30 min per day, most days of the week	4–9 mm Hg
Moderation of alcohol consumption	Limit consumption to no more than 2 drinks/day—1 oz or 30 mL ethanol (e.g., 24 oz beer, 10 oz wine, or 3 oz 80-proof whiskey)—in most men and to no more than 1 drink/day in women and lighter weight persons	2–4 mm Hg

BMI = body mass index; DASH = dietary approaches to stop hypertension; SBP = systolic blood pressure.
[a]The effects of implementing these modifications are dose and time dependent and could be greater for some individuals.
From the Joint National Committee, 2003.

as reported by Wing and colleagues (2003) for the Second Australian National Blood Pressure Study Group.

Clearly, antihypertensive therapy in nonpregnant women of reproductive age with sustained diastolic pressures of 90 mm Hg or greater would be considered standard. In women diagnosed with presumed chronic hypertension prior to midpregnancy, however, the benefits and safety of instituting antihypertensive therapy are less clear.

PRECONCEPTIONAL AND EARLY PREGNANCY EVALUATION

Women with chronic hypertension should ideally be counseled prior to pregnancy (see Chap. 7, p. 193). The duration of hypertension, degree of blood pressure control, and current therapy is ascertained. Women with average pressures greater than 135/85 mm Hg measured at home are considered to be hypertensive. Home measurement devices should be checked for accuracy (American Heart Association, 2004). Women's general health, daily activities, diet, and adverse behaviors are also assessed. Prior adverse events such as a cerebrovascular accident or myocardial infarction, as well as cardiac or renal dysfunction, are especially pertinent. Women with these are at markedly increased risk for a recurrence or worsening during pregnancy. Those who require multiple medications for hypertension control, or those who are poorly controlled, are also at increased risk for adverse pregnancy outcomes.

Renal, hepatic, and cardiac function should be assessed. Ophthalmological evaluation is important for women with long-standing chronic hypertension. Echocardiography is indicated in women with any prior adverse outcome or in those with long-term hypertension. Gainer and co-workers (2005a) found that pregnant women with chronic hypertension requiring medication commonly have underlying heart lesions such as left ventricular hypertrophy when evaluated by echocardiography. Cardiac dysrhythmias or evidence of left ventric-

ular hypertrophy indicate long-standing or poorly controlled hypertension, or both. Women with these conditions are at increased risk for congestive heart failure during pregnancy (see Chap. 42, p. 991).

Renal function is assessed by serum creatinine and quantification of proteinuria. If either is abnormal, there is further increased risk for adverse pregnancy outcomes. The Working Group Report on High Blood Pressure in Pregnancy (2000) of the National Heart, Lung, and Blood Institute concluded that the risks of fetal loss and accelerated deterioration of renal disease are increased if serum creatinine is above 1.4 mg/dL around the time of conception. It can be difficult to separate the effects of the pregnancy from progression of renal disease (Cunningham and associates, 1990; Jones and Hayslett, 1996). Severity of renal insufficiency is inversely proportional to an increased risk of hypertensive complications during pregnancy, although the relationship is not linear (see Chap. 48, p. 1103). Most clinicians believe that pregnancy is relatively contraindicated in women who maintain persistent diastolic pressures of more than 110 mm Hg despite therapy, require multiple antihypertensives, or have a serum creatinine level of more than 2 mg/dL. Even stronger contraindications are prior cerebrovascular thrombosis or hemorrhage, myocardial infarction, or cardiac failure. Symptoms at rest and with activity should be determined. Some clinicians recommend that women with prior cardiac dysfunction undergo baseline and longitudinal vital capacity testing throughout pregnancy to identify early pulmonary congestion. We have no experience with this and prefer to assess the women clinically.

EFFECTS OF CHRONIC HYPERTENSION ON PREGNANCY

MATERNAL EFFECTS. Most women taking monotherapy and whose hypertension is well controlled prior to pregnancy do well. Even these women, however, are at increased risk for superimposed preeclampsia and placental abruption. Jain (1997) reported a maternal mortality of 230 per 100,000 live births in women with hypertension. The more severe the baseline maternal disease, especially with documented end-organ damage, the more likely these complications.

Pregnancy-aggravated hypertension manifests as a sudden increase in blood pressure. Systolic pressures greater than 200 mm Hg or diastolic pressures of 130 mm Hg or more may rapidly result in renal or cardiopulmonary dysfunction. When there is superimposed severe preeclampsia or eclampsia, the outlook for the mother is serious unless the pregnancy is terminated. Placental abruption is another common and serious complication (see Chap. 35, p. 811). Weissman-Brenner and associates (2004) have also reported aortic dissection at term (see Chap. 44, p. 1034).

Superimposed Preeclampsia. There is no precise definition of superimposed preeclampsia in women with chronic hypertension. In their review, August and Lindheimer (1999) found that superimposed preeclampsia occurred in 4 to 40 percent of these women. The incidence is higher in women with severe hypertension in early pregnancy (Sibai, 1991). The risk of superimposed preeclampsia is directly related to the severity of baseline hypertension, as well as the need for treatment to achieve control. In a Maternal–Fetal Medicine Units Network trial, Caritis and co-workers (1998) used predefined criteria for preeclampsia in 774 women with chronic hypertension. They identified superimposed preeclampsia in 25 percent. In these same women, Sibai and co-workers (1998) reported that the incidence of superimposed preeclampsia was similar whether or not the women had baseline proteinuria. The incidence significantly increased, however, in those who had hypertension for at least 4 years or who had preeclampsia during a prior pregnancy. Zeeman and colleagues (2003) found that uterine artery Doppler velocimetry showing increased impedance at 16 to 20 weeks and was predictive of superimposed preeclampsia at 28 to 32 weeks in women with chronic hypertension.

PREVENTION. Trials of low-dose aspirin to prevent preeclampsia in women with chronic hypertension have shown little benefit. In an early study, Beaufils and colleagues (1985) reported that therapy with low-dose aspirin and dipyridamole reduced the incidence of superimposed preeclampsia or fetal growth restriction. In a European multicenter trial, Uzan and co-workers (1991) found that these two drugs were associated with increased birthweight and decreased risk of fetal growth restriction when given to high-risk women. In the Network study by Caritis and associates (1998) cited above, the incidence of superimposed preeclampsia and fetal growth restriction was similar in women given low-dose aspirin or placebo. Also, reduction of thromboxane B_2 maternal serum levels was not predictive of improved pregnancy outcomes with low-dose aspirin (Hauth and colleagues, 1998).

In a summary of randomized trials of low-dose aspirin for women with chronic hypertension, Mulrow and colleagues

(2000) suggested that the only benefit may be fewer preterm deliveries. More recently, Coomarasamy and colleagues (2003) performed a meta-analysis of 14 trials involving a total of 12,416 women. The investigators concluded that low-dose aspirin therapy for women with risk factors significantly reduced the frequency of perinatal death, preeclampsia, and preterm labor.

Placental Abruption. Premature placental separation is discussed in detail in Chapter 35 (sec p. 811). From a number of reports, the incidence of placental abruption of about 1 in 150 pregnancies is increased in women with chronic hypertension. Sibai and colleagues (1998) reported this rate to be 1.5 percent of 776 women. Caritis and associates (1998) reported that 1 to 2 percent of 2539 women at high risk for preeclampsia enrolled in a low-dose aspirin trial had placental abruption. Hauth and co-workers (1995) performed a meta-analysis of low-dose aspirin trials in women at high and low risk for preeclampsia, and they identified placental abruption in about 1.4 percent of cases. Ferrer and associates (2000) reviewed nine observational trials and concluded that abruption doubled in women with chronic hypertension.

When hypertension is severe, the likelihood of abruption is concomitantly increased. Vigil-De Gracia and colleagues (2003) reported its incidence to be 8.4 percent in 154 women with severe chronic hypertension in the second half of pregnancy. Smoking further increases these risks (Ananth and colleagues, 1999).

Maternal Economic and Lifestyle Factors. There are few quantitative data to assess economic and lifestyle factors in pregnant women with chronic hypertension. These women require more time with their physicians, including office visits, fetal–maternal assessment in the third trimester, and increased hospitalization. Rest at home affects economic stability and family dynamics. Women must take more time off from work, and this is especially burdensome if women are self-employed or must care for children or other family members. These realities should be discussed during preconceptional or early pregnancy counseling (see Chap. 7, p. 193).

FETAL AND NEWBORN EFFECTS. Almost all adverse perinatal outcomes are increased in pregnancies complicated by chronic hypertension. A systematic review has been provided by Ferrer and colleagues (2000).

Fetal Growth Restriction. The incidence and severity of restricted fetal growth are directly related to the severity of hypertension. Both are also dependent on other maternal factors, on the growth chart used to arrive at this diagnosis, and on the accuracy of gestational dating. Maternal factors include age; hypertension control, including the need for additional antihypertensive medications; and the presence of end-organ damage such as renal or cardiac dysfunction. Growth restriction is further increased in women who develop superimposed preeclampsia.

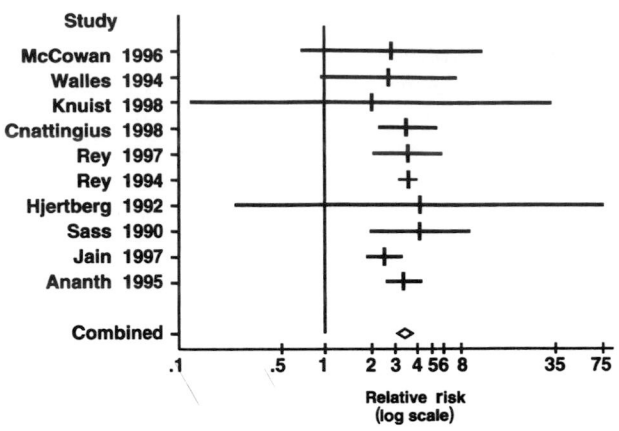

FIGURE 45–2. Perinatal death rates in women with chronic hypertension compared with that of either normotensive controls or general obstetrical populations. Outcomes are shown as odds ratio [log scale]. (Data from Ferrer and colleagues, 2000.)

In the Network trial described above, Sibai and colleagues (1998) reported that 10.7 percent of 763 women with chronic hypertension had small-for-gestational age (SGA) perinates. If these women had proteinuria early in pregnancy, 23 percent had infants with birthweights less than the 10th percentile. Although fetal growth restriction did not develop, Gainer and co-workers (2005b) found that women with chronic hypertension requiring medication who developed superimposed preeclampsia displayed sustained, slower fetal growth velocity by sonography as early as 23 weeks.

Other Adverse Perinatal Outcomes. Indicated preterm birth is increased in women with chronic hypertension (Meis and co-workers, 1998). In the Network study described earlier, Sibai and colleagues (1998) reported that 33 percent of 763 women with chronic hypertension delivered before 37 weeks and 18 percent before 35 weeks. Rey and Couturier (1994) found a 34-percent incidence of delivery before 37 weeks. The perinatal death rate is increased threefold to fourfold in women with chronic hypertension (Fig. 45–2).

MANAGEMENT DURING PREGNANCY

The goal for pregnancy complicated by chronic hypertension is to reduce adverse maternal or perinatal outcomes. Management is targeted toward prevention of moderate or severe hypertension and prevention, delay, or improvement of severe pregnancy-aggravated hypertension. To some extent, these goals can be achieved pharmacologically. Blood pressure self-monitoring is encouraged with caveats for the accuracy of automated devices (Brown and colleagues, 2004). Personal health behavioral modifications include dietary counseling and reduction of behaviors such as smoking, alcohol, cocaine, or other substance abuse (see Table 45–2).

It is accepted that pregnant women with *severe hypertension* must always be treated for maternal indications regardless of pregnancy status. This includes those with prior adverse outcomes to include cerebrovascular events, myocardial infarction, and cardiac or renal dysfunction. We agree with the philosophy of beginning antihypertensive treatment in otherwise healthy pregnant women with persistent diastolic pressures of 100 mm Hg or greater (August and Lindheimer, 1999; Working Group Report, 2000). With end-organ dysfunction, treatment of pregnant women with diastolic pressures of 90 mm Hg or higher is considered.

There are no data indicating salutary effects on pregnancy outcomes with simply lowering blood pressure. Importantly, the incidence of superimposed preeclampsia is not appreciably affected. Although there is minimal evidence that outcomes are improved by such treatment, the same evidence attests to the apparent safety of maternal antihypertensive therapy. The latter excludes angiotensin-converting enzyme (ACE) inhibitors and perhaps atenolol. Despite lack of scientific data that treatment improves maternal or perinatal outcomes, some clinicians recommend empirical antihypertensive therapy. For example, Sibai (2002) recommends therapy in women with high-risk (as opposed to low-risk) chronic hypertension. As emphasized by the Working Group Report (2000), there is a need for further trials in these women.

ANTIHYPERTENSIVE DRUGS. The following summary of antihypertensive drugs is categorized by their primary mode of action and as abstracted from several sources, including the *2004 Physicians' Desk Reference.* In nonpregnant adults with chronic hypertension, results of large trials of single-drug therapy cited earlier support conclusions of Frohlich (2003) and August (2003) that antihypertensive use should be based on proven efficacy. Moreover, this efficacy should be proven in persons with the same degree of hypertension.

Diuretics. Thiazide as well as loop-acting diuretics such as furosemide are commonly used (Brater, 1998). In nonpregnant patients, diuretics lower blood pressure in the short term by sodium and water diuresis and intravascular volume depletion. With time, there is *sodium escape,* and intravascular volume depletion is corrected. This may not be true in pregnant women. Sibai and colleagues (1984) assessed plasma volume in pregnancy in 20 chronically hypertensive women. Plasma volume expansion was only about 20 percent in the half who continued diuretic therapy throughout pregnancy compared with 50 percent in the other half who discontinued treatment early in pregnancy. Perinatal outcomes were similar in both groups.

Some aspect of lowered peripheral vascular resistance may contribute to the effectiveness of diuretics. They reduce long-term morbidity and mortality in nonpregnant individuals with chronic hypertension (Williams, 2001). Largely due to theoretical concerns regarding maternal plasma volume expansion, diuretics are usually not instituted as first-line therapy during pregnancy, particularly after 20 weeks (Working Group Report, 2000).

Adrenergic-Blocking Agents. Some of these drugs act *centrally* by reducing sympathetic outflow to effect a generalized decreased vascular tone. Central-acting agents include clonidine and α-methyldopa. *Peripherally* acting *β-adrenergic receptor blockers* also cause a generalized decrease in sympathetic tone. Examples are propranolol, metoprolol, and atenolol. Labetalol is a commonly used *α/β-adrenergic blocker*. Peripheral blockers are thought to have more potential for postural hypotension than centrally acting agents. The most commonly used drugs in pregnancy to treat hypertension are methyldopa or a *β-* or *α/β*-receptor blocker.

Vasodilators. Hydralazine relaxes arterial smooth muscle and has been used parenterally for decades to safely treat severe peripartum hypertension (see Chap. 34, p. 793). Use of oral hydralazine monotherapy for chronic hypertension is not recommended because of its weak antihypertensive effects and resultant tachycardia. It may be effective for long-term use as an adjunct to other antihypertensives, especially if chronic renal insufficiency is present.

Calcium-Channel Blockers. These agents are divided into three subclasses based on their modification of calcium entry into cells and interference with binding sites on voltage-dependent calcium channels. Common agents include the dihydropyridine, nifedipine, and the phenylalkyl amine derivative, verapamil. These agents have negative inotropic effects and thus can worsen ventricular dysfunction and congestive heart failure. Pahor and associates (2000) concluded that they are inferior to other first-line drugs in nonpregnant hypertensives. There is little published experience with these agents during pregnancy (Smith and colleagues, 2000).

Angiotensin-Converting Enzyme Inhibitors. ACE inhibitors inhibit the conversion of angiotensin-I to the potent vasoconstrictor angiotensin-II. These agents have worrisome fetal effects when used in the second and third trimesters. As discussed in Chapter 14 (see p. 349), ACE inhibitors are associated with fetal hypocalvaria and renal defects (Briggs and colleagues, 2002).

Angiotensin-receptor blockers act in a manner similar to ACE inhibitors. That is, instead of blocking the production of angiotensin-II, they inhibit binding to its receptor.

DRUG TREATMENT DURING PREGNANCY. As discussed, continuation of prepregnancy antihypertensive treatment when women become pregnant is debated. Although pressure reduction is beneficial to the mother, it at least theoretically can decrease uteroplacental perfusion to possibly jeopardize her fetus. Outcomes from the few observational reports are shown in Table 45–3. To summarize, these investigators found that most pregnancy outcomes were good without treatment. Perinatal mortality rates were low unless superimposed preeclampsia developed. Over time, neonatal care has markedly improved, with a resultant continued decline in mortality since these earlier observational reports.

Some randomized trials of drug therapy in pregnant women with mild chronic hypertension are shown in Table 45–4. Only three trials were reported during the 1990s, and only two were of appreciable size. Thus, data are not sufficient to provide a definitive answer regarding whether to treat women with mild or even moderate hypertension in pregnancy. An important observation of the two large and more contemporaneous studies was that no adverse outcomes were found in the women given treatment. Thus, it is not unreasonable to treat women with uncomplicated mild or moderate sustained chronic hypertension who would be prescribed antihypertensive therapy when not pregnant.

The concern over fetal growth restriction due to reduced placental perfusion by lowering maternal blood pressure is confounded because worsening blood pressure itself is associated with abnormal fetal growth. Breart and colleagues (1982) found that women with chronic hypertension whose diastolic pressure was less than 90 mm Hg had a 3-percent risk of fetal growth restriction, those with 90 mm Hg had a 6-percent risk, and those with 110 mm Hg or more had a 16-percent risk. Growth restriction was not increased with maternal treatment of chronic hypertension in the two most recent large randomized trials (see Table 45–4).

Results of the study of chronic hypertension in pregnant women reported by the Memphis group are summarized in Table 45–5. In this trial by Sibai and colleagues (1990a), the aim of therapy was to maintain pressure less than 140/90 mm Hg. Women treated throughout pregnancy had significantly lower blood pressures than women randomized to no treatment but, importantly, adverse outcomes were not altered by treatment. More women however, who initially were not given treatment eventually required antihypertensive therapy for serious hypertension, defined as greater than 160/110 mm Hg.

In the study by the Gruppo di Studio Ipertensione in Gravidanza (1998), 283 women were randomized to treatment with slow-release nifedipine, 10 mg twice daily, or to no treatment. After this, all women were treated with nifedipine if diastolic pressure exceeded 110 mm Hg. The investigators found neither benefits nor harm in either group. The rate of preterm delivery was 45 percent in treated women which was not significant from that of 37 percent in nontreated women. Fetal growth and birthweight were similar in both groups.

Severe Chronic Hypertension. As discussed, the prognosis for pregnancy outcomes with chronic hypertension is related to the severity of disease before pregnancy. Many women with severe hypertension often have underlying renal disease (Cunningham and colleagues, 1990). In the study by Sibai and co-workers (1986a) shown in Table 45–3, there were 44 pregnancies in women whose blood pressure at 6 to 11 weeks was 170/110 mm Hg or higher. They all were given treatment with α-methyldopa and oral hydralazine to maintain blood pressures less than 160/110 mm Hg. They were hospitalized for

TABLE 45–3 Observational Studies of the Effects of Treatment of Chronic Hypertension During Pregnancy

Study and Treatment	No.	Superimposed Preeclampsia (percent)	Perinatal Mortality (per 1000)
Chesley (1978)			
Chronic hypertension[a] (1972–1974), no antihypertensives	593	6	32
Superimposed preeclampsia[b] (1960–1974), hydralazine + α-methyldopa	196	—	214
Redman (1980)[c]			
Chronic hypertension	184	25	16
Superimposed preeclampsia	69	—	145
Sibai and associates (1983)			
Chronic hypertension, no antihypertensives	193	10	5
Superimposed preeclampsia, α-methyldopa and/or hydralazine	22	—	227
Mabie and associates (1986)			
Chronic hypertension, diastolic pressure < 90 mm Hg, no treatment	137	29	29
Chronic hypertension, diastolic pressure 90–100 mm Hg, α-methyldopa	26	46	0
Sibai and associates (1986a)			
Severe chronic hypertension, 170/100 mm Hg or greater, α-methyldopa + hydralazine	44	52	250
Rey and Couturier (1994)			
Chronic hypertension, treat if diastolic pressure > 100 mm Hg	337	21	45

[a] Three maternal deaths due to stroke, pulmonary embolus, and aspiration pneumonia.
[b] Two deaths due to stroke and postoperative infection.
[c] Data from Ounsted and associates (1983), reporting long-term follow-up of children from the original and continuing study of treatment of chronic hypertension in pregnancy by Redman (1980).

TABLE 45–4 Randomized Trials of Antihypertensive Drug Therapy in Pregnancies Complicated by Mild Chronic Hypertension

Reference	No.	Mean Gestation at Entry (weeks)	Mean DBP at Entry (mm Hg)	Treatment	Principal Findings
Leather et al (1968)	47	< 20	107	Methyldopa ± diuretics ± hydralazine versus no drug	Longer gestation and fewer perinatal deaths in treated woman
Redman et al (1976)	208	21 and 22	88–90	Methyldopa ± hydralazine versus no drug	Fewer midpregnancy losses in treated women
Arias and Zamora (1979)	58	15 and 16	90–99	Methyldopa, diuretics, or hydralazine versus no drug	Compromised infants born to mothers with severe hypertension despite treatment
Butters et al (1990)	29	16	86	Double-blind: atenolol versus placebo	Poor fetal growth in treated women
Sibai et al (1990a)	263	< 11	91–92	Methyldopa versus labetalol versus no drug	No differences in outcomes
Gruppo di Studio Ipertensione in Gravidanza (1998)	283	24	95–96	Slow-release nifedipine versus no drug	No differences in outcomes

DBP = diastolic blood pressure.
Adapted from Haddad and Sibai, 1999, with permission.

TABLE 45–5 **Maternal and Perinatal Outcomes from a Randomized Trial of 263 Chronically Hypertensive Women**

	Treatment Group[a]		
Factor	None (n = 90)	Methyldopa (n = 87)	Labetalol (n = 86)
Additional drugs for hypertension (%)	11	6	6
Superimposed preeclampsia (%)	16	18	16
Abruptio placentae (%)	2	1	2
Preterm delivery (%)	10	12	12
Fetal growth restriction (%)	9	7	8
Perinatal mortality (per 1000)	11	11	12
Gestational age at delivery (wks)	39 ± 0.2	38.6 ± 0.2	38.7 ± 0.2
Birthweight (g)	3123 ± 69	3051 ± 73	3068 ± 71
Placental weight (g)	723 ± 33	716 ± 33	755 ± 69

[a] All differences are nonsignificant.
Data from Sibai and co-workers (1990a), with permission.

treatment with parenteral hydralazine if blood pressures exceeded 180/120 mm Hg. Half of all the women developed superimposed preeclampsia, and all adverse perinatal outcomes were in this group. Specifically, all infants in the women with superimposed preeclampsia were preterm, and nearly 80 percent were growth restricted. The perinatal mortality rate was 48 percent. In the women with severe chronic hypertension who did not develop superimposed preeclampsia, only 5 percent of fetuses were growth restricted and all survived.

ANTIHYPERTENSIVE DRUG SELECTION.
Adrenergic-blocking drugs have been used extensively in England, Scotland, and Australia to treat chronically hypertensive pregnant women (Redman, 1982; Rubin and colleagues, 1983; Walker and associates, 1983). The results of treatment with labetalol are consistent with the view that the drug offers no advantages over α-methyldopa (Sibai and colleagues, 1990a). Butters and colleagues (1990) reported that atenolol treatment resulted in a higher incidence of growth-restricted neonates compared with that of untreated controls. Lydakis and colleagues (1999) studied 223 such women and concluded that atenolol treatment was associated with lower birthweight and ponderal indices (birthweight/length^3). There was also a trend toward more preterm births when compared with the effects of other antihypertensives or of no treatment. Easterling and associates (1999) also concluded that atenolol therapy was associated with reduced infant birthweight. Montan and Ingemarsson (1989) reported ominous intrapartum fetal heart rate patterns in 20 percent of women receiving β-blocker therapy for hypertension. Ominous patterns were increased even more in growth-restricted fetuses as well as in half of women given epidural analgesia. Magee and Duley (2001) concluded that it is not clear if benefits outweigh the risks when β-blockers are used to treat mild to moderate chronic hypertension.

Experiences are too meager to make recommendations about routine use of nifedipine for pregnant women with chronic hypertension. Bartolus and associates (2000) reported the effects of maternal nifedipine on child development at 18 months. Outcomes were similar in 94 infants whose mothers were treated compared with those of 161 not exposed. Malformations were identified in 5.3 percent of nifedipine-exposed women compared with 1.2 percent of controls—the number of subjects precluded any tests for significance.

Mulrow and colleagues (2000) performed a review for the Agency for Healthcare Research and Quality and summarized the risks and benefits of antihypertensive agents given during pregnancy. They found no evidence of major adverse fetal or maternal events. Cockburn and colleagues (1982) found similar outcomes in 195 children born to hypertensive women participating in a randomized trial of methyldopa treatment. (The children were followed to 7.5 years of age.)

Therapy Recommendations. The Working Group on High Blood Pressure in Pregnancy (2000) emphasizes the limited data from which to draw conclusions as to whether to treat mild chronic hypertension in pregnancy. The group did recommend empirical therapy in women whose blood pressures exceed threshold levels of 150 to 160 mm Hg systolic or 100 to 110 mm Hg diastolic or with the presence of target organ damage such as left ventricular hypertrophy or renal insufficiency. They also concluded that early treatment of hypertension would probably reduce subsequent hospitalization during pregnancy. In the study by Sibai and associates (1990a), subsequent treatment was needed for dangerous hypertension in 11 percent of women not given initial treatment. This compared with only 6 percent in women initially randomized to either α-methyldopa or labetalol earlier in pregnancy.

Methyldopa has been extensively studied during pregnancy (Montan and colleagues, 1992, 1993). In their review, Ferrer and colleagues (2000) concluded that experience with methyldopa in the first trimester is reasonably large, that no pattern of fetal anomalies has emerged, and that newer antihypertensives have not been sufficiently studied. For all of these reasons, Haddad and Sibai (1999) recommended methyldopa as the initial agent for pregnant women with chronic hypertension.

FETAL ASSESSMENT. Women with well-controlled chronic hypertension with no complicating factors can generally be expected to have a good pregnancy outcome. Because even otherwise healthy women with mild hypertension have an increased risk of superimposed preeclampsia and fetal growth restriction, serial antepartum assessment of fetal well-being as detailed in Chapter 15 (see p. 373) is recommended by the American College of Obstetricians and Gynecologists (1999). There are no data from which to assess either benefits or harm associated with various monitoring strategies for these women (Ferrer and colleagues, 2000).

PREGNANCY-AGGRAVATED HYPERTENSION OR SUPERIMPOSED PREECLAMPSIA. The cited incidence of superimposed preeclampsia for women with chronic hypertension varies depending on severity of underlying disease (see Table 45–3). In the prospective study by the Network, it was about 25 percent (Caritis and co-workers, 1998). The diagnosis may be difficult to make, especially in women with hypertension who have underlying renal disease with proteinuria (Cunningham and associates, 1990). Conditions that support the diagnosis of superimposed preeclampsia include new-onset proteinuria; neurological symptoms, including severe headaches and visual disturbances; generalized edema; oliguria; and certainly, convulsions or pulmonary edema. Laboratory abnormalities that support the diagnosis include increasing serum creatinine, thrombocytopenia, or appreciable serum hepatic transaminase elevations.

Some women with chronic hypertension have worsening during pregnancy with no other findings of superimposed preeclampsia. This is most commonly encountered near the end of the second trimester. In the absence of other supporting criteria for superimposed preeclampsia, including fetal growth restriction or decreased amnionic fluid volume, this likely represents the higher end of the normal blood pressure curve shown in Figure 45–1. In such women, it is reasonable to begin or to increase the dose of antihypertensive therapy.

DELIVERY. In women with uncomplicated and well-controlled chronic hypertension and with documented normal fetal growth and amnionic fluid volume, it is our practice to await labor at term. In women with complications or in whom fetal testing becomes abnormal, induction is considered. Superimposed severe preeclampsia prompts delivery even with markedly preterm pregnancy. Special consideration for delivery prior to term of chronically hypertensive women with a multifetal gestation also is warranted. When these women develop preeclampsia, they have an increased risk for placental abruption and poor neonatal outcomes compared with those with a singleton pregnancy (Sibai and colleagues, 2000).

Vaginal delivery is usually attempted, even in women with severe preeclampsia. Most women can be induced successfully and deliver vaginally (Alexander and colleagues, 1999; Atkinson and associates, 1995). Epidural analgesia for labor pain is appropriate in women with chronic hypertension with or without preeclampsia (see Chap. 19, p. 483).

POSTPARTUM CONSIDERATIONS. In many respects, postpartum observation and prevention and management of adverse complications are similar in women with severe chronic hypertension and in those with severe preeclampsia–eclampsia. The development of cerebral or pulmonary edema, heart failure, or renal dysfunction is especially high within 24 to 36 hours following delivery (Benedetti and colleagues, 1980, 1985; Cunningham and associates, 1986; Sibai and co-workers, 1990b). Following delivery, as maternal peripheral resistance increases, left ventricular workload also increases. This increase is further aggravated by appreciable amounts of interstitial fluid that are mobilized for excretion as endothelial damage is reversed. In these women, sudden hypertension—either moderate or severe—exacerbates diastolic dysfunction and causes pulmonary edema (Cunningham and colleagues, 1986; Gandhi and associates, 2001). Prompt hypertension control, along with diuretic therapy, usually quickly resolves pulmonary edema.

Women with chronic hypertension and superimposed severe preeclampsia most often have markedly contracted blood volumes compared with those of normal pregnant women (Silver and associates, 1998; Zeeman and colleagues, 2002). These women have marked vasoconstriction and, in general, have relatively increased blood loss, especially following cesarean delivery, which may cause appreciable postpartum prerenal oliguria. It may be difficult and hazardous to attempt to maintain intravascular volume and renal perfusion solely with intravenous crystalloid or colloid solutions. In such women, blood transfusion may be necessary to maintain intravascular volume to ensure tissue perfusion.

REFERENCES

Alexander JM, Bloom SL, McIntire DD, et al: Severe preeclampsia and the very low birth weight infant: Is induction of labor harmful? Obstet Gynecol 93:485, 1999

American College of Obstetricians and Gynecologists: Hypertension. Clinical Updates in Women's Health Care. Vol 1, No. 1, Winter 2002

American College of Obstetricians and Gynecologists: Antepartum fetal surveillance. Practice Bulletin No. 9, October 1999

American Heart Association: Home monitoring of high blood pressure. Available at: http:/www.americanheart.org/presenter.jhtml?identifier=576. Accessed January 9, 2004

Ananth CV, Smulian JC, Vintzileos AM: Incidence of placental abruption in relation to cigarette smoking and hypertensive disorders during pregnancy: A meta-analysis of observational studies. Obstet Gynecol 93:622, 1999

Antihypertensive and Lipid-Lowering Treatment to Prevent Heart Attack Trial (ALLHAT): Major outcomes in high-risk hypertensive patients randomized to angiotensin-converting enzyme inhibitor or calcium channel blocker vs. diuretic. JAMA 288:2981, 2002

Arias F, Zamora J: Antihypertensive treatment and pregnancy outcome in patients with mild chronic hypertension. Obstet Gynecol 53:489, 1979

Atkinson MW, Guinn D, Owen J, et al: Does magnesium sulfate affect the length of labor induction in women with pregnancy-associated hypertension? Am J Obstet Gynecol 173:1219, 1995

August P: Initial treatment of hypertension. N Engl J Med 348:610, 2003

August P, Lindheimer MD: Chronic hypertension in pregnancy. In Lindheimer MD, Roberts JM, Cunningham FG (eds): Chesley's Hypertensive Disorders in Pregnancy, 2nd ed. Stamford, CT, Appleton & Lange, 1999, p 605

Bartolus R, Ricci E, Chatenoud L, et al: Nifedipine administration in pregnancy: Effect on the development of children at 18 months. Br J Obstet Gynaecol 107:792, 2000

Beaufils M, Uzan S, Donsimoni R, et al: Prevention of preeclampsia by early antiplatelet therapy. Lancet 1:840, 1985

Benedetti TJ, Kates R, Williams V: Hemodynamic observations in severe preeclampsia complicated by pulmonary edema. Am J Obstet Gynecol 152:330, 1985

Benedetti TJ, Quilligan EJ: Cerebral edema in severe pregnancy-induced hypertension. Am J Obstet Gynecol 137:860, 1980

Blood Pressure Lowering Treatment Trialists' Collaboration: Effects of different blood-pressure-lowering regimens on major cardiovascular events: Results of prospectively-designed overviews of randomised trials. Lancet 362:1527, 2003

Brater DC: Diuretic therapy. N Engl J Med 339:387, 1998

Breart G, Rabarison Y, Plouin PF, et al: Risk of fetal growth retardation as a result of maternal hypertension: Preparation to a trial on antihypertensive drugs. Dev Pharmacol Ther 4:116, 1982

Briggs GG, Freeman RK, Yaffe SJ: Drugs in Pregnancy and Lactation, 6th ed. Philadelphia, Lippincott Williams & Wilkins, 2002, p 178

Brown M, McHugh L, Mangos G, et al: Automated self-initiated blood pressure or 24-hour ambulatory blood pressure monitoring in pregnancy? Br J Obstet Gynaecol 111:38, 2004

Butters L, Kennedy S, Rubin PC: Atenolol in essential hypertension during pregnancy. BMJ 301:587, 1990

Caritis S, Sibai B, Hauth J, et al: Low-dose aspirin to prevent preeclampsia in women at high risk. N Engl J Med 338:701, 1998

Chesley LC: Superimposed preeclampsia or eclampsia. In Chesley LC (ed): Hypertensive Disorders in Pregnancy. New York, Appleton-Century-Crofts, 1978, pp 14, 302, 482

Chesley LC, Annitto JE, Cosgrove RA: Long-term follow-up study of eclamptic women: Sixth periodic report. Am J Obstet Gynecol 124:446, 1976

Cockburn J, Moar VA, Ounsted M, et al: Final report of study on hypertension during pregnancy: The effects of specific treatment on the growth and development of the children. Lancet 1:647, 1982

Coomarasamy A, Honest H, Papaioannou S, et al: Aspirin for prevention of preeclampsia in women with historical risk factors: A systematic review. Obstet Gynecol 101:1319, 2003

Cunningham FG, Cox SM, Harstad TW, et al: Chronic renal disease and pregnancy outcome. Am J Obstet Gynecol 163:453, 1990

Cunningham FG, Pritchard JA, Hankins GDN, et al: Idiopathic cardiomyopathy or compounding cardiovascular events? Obstet Gynecol 67:157, 1986

Easterling TR, Brateng D, Schmuchker B, et al: Prevention of preeclampsia: A randomized trial of atenolol in hyperdynamic patients before onset of hypertension. Obstet Gynecol 93:725, 1999

Ferrer RL, Sibai BM, Mulrow CD, et al: Management of mild chronic hypertension during pregnancy: A review. Obstet Gynecol 96:849, 2000

Frohlich ED: Treating hypertension—what are we to believe? N Engl J Med 348:639, 2003

Gainer J, Alexander J, Mcintire D, Leveno K: Maternal echocardiogram findings in pregnant patients with chronic hypertension. Presented at the 25th Annual Meeting of the Society for Maternal-Fetal Medicine, Reno, Nevada, February 7–12, 2005a

Gainer J, Alexander J, Mcintire D, Leveno K: Fetal growth velocity in women who develop superimposed preeclamsia. Presented at the 25th Annual Meeting of the Society for Maternal-Fetal Medicine, Reno, Nevada, February 7–12, 2005b

Gandhi SK, Powers JC, Nomeir A, et al: The pathogenesis of acute pulmonary edema associated with hypertension. N Engl J Med 344:17, 2001

Gruppo di Studio Ipertensione in Gravidanza: Nifedipine versus expectant management in mild to moderate hypertension in pregnancy. Br J Obstet Gynaecol 105:718, 1998

Gueyffier F, Boutitie F, Boissel J, et al: Effect of antihypertensive drug treatment on cardiovascular outcomes in women and men. A meta-analysis of individual patient data from randomized controlled trials. The INDANA Investigators. Ann Intern Med 126:761, 1997

Haddad B, Sibai BM: Chronic hypertension in pregnancy. Ann Med 31:246, 1999

Hajjar I, Kotchen TA: Trends in prevalence, awareness, treatment, and control of hypertension in the United States, 1988–2000. JAMA 290:199, 2003

Hauth JC, Goldenberg RL, Parker CR Jr, et al: Low-dose aspirin: Lack of association with an increase in abruptio placentae or perinatal mortality. Obstet Gynecol 85:1055, 1995

Hauth JC, Sibai B, Caritis S, et al: Maternal serum thromboxane B_2 concentrations do not predict improved outcomes in high risk pregnancies in a low-dose aspirin trial. Am J Obstet Gynecol 179:1193, 1998

Jain L: Effect of pregnancy-induced and chronic hypertension on pregnancy outcome. J Perinatol 17:425, 1997

Joint National Committee: The seventh report of the Joint National Committee on prevention, detection, evaluation, and treatment of high blood pressure. National Institutes of Health Publication No. 03-5233, May 2003

Jones DC, Hayslett JP: Outcome of pregnancy in women with moderate or severe renal insufficiency. N Engl J Med 335:226, 1996

Leather HM, Humphreys DM, Baker P, et al: A controlled trial of hypotensive agents in hypertension in pregnancy. Lancet 2:488, 1968

Levesque S, Moutquin JM, Lindsay C, et al: Implication of an AGT haplotype in a multigene association study with pregnancy hypertension. Hypertension 43:71, 2004

Lifton RP, Gharavi AG, Geller DS: Molecular mechanisms of human hypertension. Cell 104:545, 2001

Lydakis C, Lip GYH, Beevers M, et al: Atenolol and fetal growth in pregnancies complicated by hypertension. Am J Hypertension 12:541, 1999

Mabie WC, Pernoll ML, Biswas MK: Chronic hypertension in pregnancy. Obstet Gynecol 67:197, 1986

MacGillivray I, Rose GA, Rowe B: Blood pressure survey in pregnancy. Clin Sci 37:395, 1969

Magee LA, Duley L: Oral beta-blockers for mild to moderate hypertension during pregnancy. Cochrane Database Syst Rev 4:DC002863, 2001

Meis PJ, Goldenberg RL, Mercer BM, et al: The preterm prediction study: Risk factors for indicated preterm births. Am J Obstet Gynecol 178:562, 1998

Montan S, Anandakumar C, Arulkeurnaran S, et al: Effects of methyldopa on uteroplacental and fetal hemodynamics in pregnancy-induced hypertension. Am J Obstet Gynecol 168:152, 1993

Montan S, Ingemarsson I: Intrapartum fetal heart rate patterns in pregnancies complicated by hypertension. Am J Obstet Gynecol 160, 283, 1989

Montan S, Ingemarsson I, Marsal K, et al: Randomized controlled trial of atenolol and pindolol in human pregnancy: Effects on fetal hemodynamics. BMJ 304:946, 1992

Mulrow CD, Chiquette E, Ferrer RL, et al: Evidence Report/Technology Assessment No. 14. AHRQ publication No. 00-E011. Rockville, MD: Agency for Healthcare Research and Quality. August 2000

Nabel EG: Cardiovascular disease. N Engl J Med 349:60, 2003

National Center for Health Statistics. Blood pressure of adults by age and sex, United States, 1960–1962. Vital Health Stat 11 4, 1964

Neal B, MacMahon S, Chapman N: Effects of ACE inhibitors, calcium antagonists, and other blood-pressure-lowering drugs: Results of prospectively designed overviews of randomised trials. Lancet 356:1955, 2000

Ogden LG, He J, Lydick E, et al: Long-term absolute benefit of lowering blood pressure in hypertensive patients according to the JNC VI risk stratification. Hypertension 35:539, 2000

Ounsted M, Cockburn J, Moar VA, et al: Maternal hypertension with superimposed preeclampsia: Effects on child development at 7 years. Br J Obstet Gynaecol 90:644, 1983

Pahor M, Psaty BM, Alderman MH, et al: Health outcomes associated with calcium antagonists compared with other firstline antihypertensive therapies: A meta-analysis of randomised controlled trials. Lancet 356:1949, 2000

Physicians' Desk Reference, 57th ed. Montvale, NJ: Thomson PDR, 2004

Prospective Studies Collaboration: Age-specific relevance of usual blood pressure to vascular mortality: A meta-analysis of individual data for one million adults in 61 prospective studies. Lancet 360:1903, 2002

Psaty BM, Lumley T, Furberg CD: Health outcomes associated with various antihypertensive therapies used as first-line agents. JAMA 289:2534, 2003

Qureshi AI, Suri FK, Mohammad Y, et al: Isolated and borderline isolated systolic hypertension relative to long-term risk and type of stroke: A 20-year follow-up of the National Health and Nutrition Survey. Stroke 33:2781, 2002

Redman CWG: Controlled trials of treatment of hypertension during pregnancy. Obstet Gynecol Surv 37:523, 1982

Redman CWG: Treatment of hypertension in pregnancy. Kidney Int 18:267, 1980

Redman CWG: Fetal outcome in trial of antihypertensive treatment in pregnancy. Lancet 2:753, 1976

Rubin PC, Butters L, Clark DM, et al: Placebo-controlled trial of atenolol in treatment of pregnancy-associated hypertension. Lancet 1:431, 1983

Sibai BM: Chronic hypertension in pregnancy. Obstet Gynecol 100:369, 2002

Sibai BM: Diagnosis and management of chronic hypertension in pregnancy. Obstet Gynecol 78:451, 1991

Sibai BM, Hauth J, Caritis S, et al: Hypertensive disorders in twin versus singleton pregnancies. Am J Obstet Gynecol 182:938, 2000

Sibai BM, Lindheimer M, Hauth JC, et al: Risk factors for preeclampsia, abruptio placentae, and adverse neonatal outcomes among women with chronic hypertension. N Engl J Med 339:667, 1998

Sibai BM, Sarinoglu C, Mercer BM: Eclampsia, VII. Pregnancy outcome after eclampsia and long-term prognosis. Am J Obstet Gynecol 166:1757, 1992

Sibai BM, Mercer B, Sarinoglu C: Severe preeclampsia in the second trimester: Recurrence risk and long-term prognosis. Am J Obstet Gynecol 165:1408, 1991

Sibai BM, Mabie WC, Shamsa F, et al: A comparison of no medication versus methyldopa or labetalol in chronic hypertension during pregnancy. Am J Obstet Gynecol 162:960, 1990a

Sibai BM, Villar MA, Mabie BC: Acute renal failure in hypertensive disorders of pregnancy. Pregnancy outcome and remote prognosis in thirty-one consecutive cases. Am J Obstet Gynecol 162:777, 1990b

Sibai BM, Anderson GD: Pregnancy outcome of intensive therapy in severe hypertension in first trimester. Obstet Gynecol 67:517, 1986a

Sibai BM, El-Nazer A, Gonzalez-Ruiz A: Severe preeclampsia–eclampsia in young primigravid women: Subsequent pregnancy outcome and remote prognosis. Am J Obstet Gynecol 155:1011, 1986b

Sibai BM, Grossman RA, Grossman HG: Effects of diuretics on plasma volume in pregnancies with long-term hypertension. Am J Obstet Gynecol 150:831, 1984

Sibai BM, Abdella TN, Anderson GD: Pregnancy outcome in 211 patients with mild chronic hypertension. Obstet Gynecol 61:517, 1983

Silver HM, Seebeck M, Carlson R: Comparison of total blood volume in normal, preeclamptic, and nonproteinuric gestational hypertensive pregnancy by simultaneous measurement of red blood cell and plasma volumes. Am J Obstet Gynecol 179:87, 1998

Smith P, Anthony J, Johanson R: Nifedipine in pregnancy. Br J Obstet Gynaecol 107:299, 2000

Uzan S, Beaufils M, Breart G, et al: Prevention of fetal growth retardation with low-dose aspirin: Findings of the EPREDA trial. Lancet 337:1427, 1991

Vigil-De Gracia P, Montufar-Rueda C, Smith A: Maternal outcome in patients with severe chronic hypertension during the second half of pregnancy. Obstet Gynecol (Abstract) 101:74S, 2003

Walker JJ, Bonduelle M, Greer I: Antihypertensive therapy in pregnancy. Lancet 1:932, 1983

Weissman-Brenner A, Schoen R, Divon MY: Aortic dissection in pregnancy. Obstet Gynecol 103:1110, 2004

Williams GH: Hypertensive vascular disease. In Braunwald E, Fauci AS, Kasper DL, et al (eds): Harrison's Principles of Internal Medicine, 15th ed. New York, McGraw-Hill, 2001, p 1421

Wing LMH, Reid CM, Ryan P, et al: A comparison of outcomes with angiotensin-converting-enzyme inhibitors and diuretics for hypertension in the elderly. N Engl J Med 348:583, 2003

Working Group Report on High Blood Pressure in Pregnancy. National Institutes of Health. NIH Publication No. 00-3029, 2000

Zeeman GG, Cunningham FG, Pritchard JA: Blood volumes in eclampsia. J Soc Gynecol Investig 9:112A, 2002

Zeeman GG, McIntire DD, Twickler DM: Maternal and fetal artery Doppler findings in women with chronic hypertension who subsequently develop superimposed pre-eclampsia. J Matern Fetal Neonatal Med 14:1, 2003

46

Pulmonary Disorders

To meet the increased oxygen demands of pregnancy, a number of important adaptive changes alter pulmonary physiology and function. There is no evidence that pulmonary function is impaired because of pregnancy, but inferential data suggest that advanced pregnancy may intensify the pathophysiological effects of many lung diseases. One example is the disparate number of maternal deaths during the influenza pandemics of 1918 and 1957. Another example is the poor tolerance for pregnancy of women with severe chronic lung disease.

Pulmonary disorders are common during pregnancy. As many as 4 percent of women have chronic asthma. Acute asthmatic exacerbations and pneumonia together accounted for almost 10 percent of all nonobstetrical antepartum hospitalizations in a large managed care plan (Gazmararian and colleagues, 2002). Thromboembolic disease was responsible for 10 percent of maternal deaths reported by the Pregnancy Mortality Surveillance System for 50 states from 1991 through 1997 (Berg and associates, 2003).

PULMONARY PHYSIOLOGY

The important and sometimes marked changes in the respiratory system induced by pregnancy are discussed in detail in Chapter 5 (see p. 136). Lung volumes and capacities that are commonly used to describe pulmonary physiology, except for residual volume and the values for lung capacities derived therefrom, can be measured directly. The physiological changes induced by pregnancy have been summarized by de Swiet (1991):

1. *Vital capacity* increases by 100 to 200 mL.
2. *Inspiratory capacity* increases by about 300 mL by late pregnancy.
3. *Expiratory reserve volume* decreases from a total of 1300 mL to about 1100 mL.
4. *Residual volume* decreases from a total of 1500 mL to about 1200 mL.
5. *Functional residual capacity,* the sum of expiratory reserve and residual volumes, decreases by about 500 mL.
6. *Tidal volume* increases from about 500 to 700 mL.
7. *Minute ventilation* increases 40 percent from 7.5 L/min to 10.5 L/min, primarily due to increased tidal volume because the respiratory rate is unchanged.

The sum of these changes is substantively increased ventilation due to deeper but not more frequent breathing (see Fig. 5–12, p. 136). Presumably these changes are induced because of increased basal oxygen consumption, which increases incrementally by 20 to 40 mL/min in the second half of pregnancy. As a result, arterial Po_2 falls slightly to approximately 28 mm Hg, plasma pH is slightly alkalotic at 7.45, and bicarbonate decreases to about 20 mEq/L.

PNEUMONIA

Various forms of bacterial or viral pneumonitis are relatively common during pregnancy. Gazmararian and colleges (2002) reported that pneumonia accounts for 4.2 percent of antepartum admissions for nonobstetrical complications. Mortality from community-acquired pneumonia is infrequent in young women (Lim and associates, 2001b). In pregnancy, however, pneumonitis that causes an appreciable loss of ventilatory capacity is not well tolerated. This generalization seems to hold true regardless of the etiology of the pneumonia. Severe involvement may result in hypoxemia and acidosis that is also poorly tolerated by the fetus. Moreover, acidemia frequently stimulates preterm labor after midpregnancy. Because many cases of pneumonia follow common viral upper respiratory illnesses, worsening or persistence of symptoms may represent developing pneumonia. **Any pregnant woman suspected of having pneumonia should undergo chest radiography.**

BACTERIAL PNEUMONIA. Many bacteria that cause community-acquired pneumonia, such as *Streptococcus pneumoniae,* are part of the normal resident flora (Bogaert and co-workers, 2004). A number of factors can upset the symbiotic relationship between colonizing bacteria and mucosal phagocytic defenses. Examples include acquisition of a virulent and invasive strain or bacterial infection following a viral infection. Cigarette smoking and chronic bronchitis favor colonization with *S pneumoniae, Haemophilus influenzae,* and *Legionella.* Other risk factors include asthma, binge drinking, and human immunodeficiency virus (HIV) infection (Munn and colleagues, 1999; Yost and associates, 2000).

Incidence and Causes. There is no evidence that pregnancy predisposes to pneumonia. In a recent study in the province of Alberta, Jin and colleagues (2003) reported that antepartum hospitalization occurred at a rate of 1.5 per 1000 deliveries, which did not differ from the rate of 1.47 per 1000 in nonpregnant women 18 to 49 years of age. The reported incidence of pneumonia of 1 in 660 deliveries is very similar to that of 1 in 560 for 75,000 pregnancies at Parkland Hospital from 1993 to 1997 (Yost and associates, 2000).

Over half of adult pneumonias are bacterial, and *S pneumoniae* is the most common cause. Lim and colleagues (2001a) studied 267 nonpregnant patients admitted for pneumonia. Despite intensive investigations, a causative agent was not identified in one fourth of cases. In the remaining three fourths, *S pneumoniae* caused 50 percent; influenza A virus, 19 percent; *Chlamydia pneumoniae,* 13 percent; *H influenzae,* 7 percent; *Mycoplasma pneumoniae,* 3 percent; and *Legionella pneumophila,* 3 percent.

Diagnosis. In their review, Halm and Teirstein (2002) reported that typical symptoms of pneumonia include

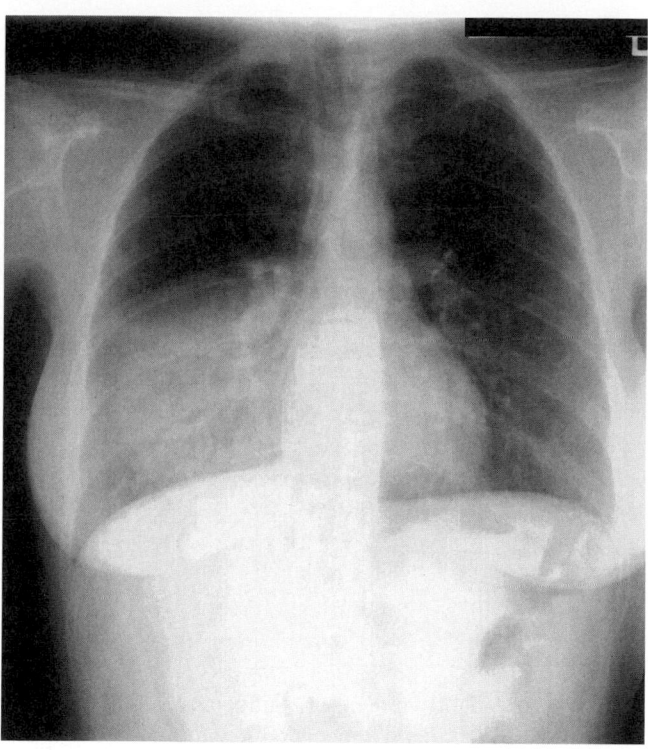

FIGURE 46–1. Chest radiograph showing right lobar pneumonia caused by pneumococcal infection. (Courtesy of Dr. Diane Twickler.)

TABLE 46–1 Factors That Increase the Risk of Death or Complications with Community-Acquired Pneumonia

Coexisting chronic conditions
Clinical findings
Respiratory rate $\geq$ 30/min, hypotension, pulse $\geq$ 125 bpm, hypothermia ($<$ 35°C), temperature $>$ 40°C, or altered mental status
Extrapulmonary disease

Laboratory findings
Leukopenia ($<$ 4000/μL) or leukocytosis $\geq$ 30,000/μL; $Po_2 \leq$ 60 mm Hg or CO_2 retention while breathing room air; elevated serum creatinine; anemia; or evidence of sepsis or organ dysfunction such as acidosis or coagulopathy

Radiological findings
More than one-lobe involvement, cavitation, or pleural effusion

Modified from the American Thoracic Society (2001).

cough (90 percent of cases), dyspnea (65 percent), sputum production (65 percent), and pleuritic chest pain (50 percent). Mild upper respiratory symptoms and malaise usually precede these symptoms, and mild leukocytosis is usually present. Chest radiography is essential for diagnosis, although radiographical appearance does not accurately predict the etiology (Fig. 46–1).

With the usual investigations, the responsible pathogen is identified in perhaps only half of cases. Examination of Gram-stained sputum for pneumococci or possibly staphylococci is controversial and the American Thoracic Society (2001) considers it optional. Routine sputum cultures, serological testing, cold agglutinin identification, and tests for bacterial antigens are also not routinely recommended.

Management. Several organizations have published guidelines (Niederman, 2004). According to the American Thoracic Society (2001), the decision for hospitalization is perhaps the single most important decision for management of pneumonia. Although many young adults are safely treated as outpatients, at Parkland Hospital we hospitalize all pregnant women. Outpatient therapy may be considered if home health care and follow-up are optimal. Risk factors shown in Table 46–1, especially if multiple, should prompt hospitalization. This can be an intermediate step to allow close observation for the first day or two to document improvement.

With severe disease, such as with some of the factors in Table 46–1, admission to an intensive care or intermediate care unit is advisable. About 20 percent of pregnant women admitted to Parkland Hospital for pneumonia require this level of care (Zeeman and associates, 2003). Severe pneumonia is a relatively common cause of acute respiratory distress syndrome during pregnancy, and mechanical ventilation may become necessary (Ware and Matthay, 2000). Indeed, of the 51 pregnant women who required mechanical ventilation in the review by Jenkins and co-workers (2003), 12 percent had pneumonia.

Antimicrobial treatment is empirical. Because the majority of adult pneumonias are caused by pneumococci, mycoplasma, or chlamydia, therapy with erythromycin or one of its newer analogues is given. Initially, it usually is given intravenously, but therapy may be administered orally. Yost and colleagues (2000) reported that erythromycin monotherapy, given intravenously and then orally, was effective in all but one of 99 pregnant women with uncomplicated pneumonia.

For women with the complications listed in Table 46–1, or in those in whom staphylococcal or *Haemophilus* pneumonia is suspected, cefotaxime or ceftriaxone is given in addition to erythromycin therapy. Monotherapy with antipneumococcal drugs such as the fluoroquinolones, including ciprofloxacin, ofloxacin, levofloxacin, and others, is also acceptable. In some areas, as many as 20 percent of pneumococcal isolates are resistant to penicillin and erythromycin (Centers for Disease Control and Prevention, 2002b). Because only 0.5 percent of these penicillin-resistant pneumococcal infections are resistant to fluoroquinolones, treatment with fluoroquinolones is recommended (Centers for Disease Control and Prevention, 2001). Little information regarding possible human teratogenicity of fluoroquinolones is available (Briggs and colleagues, 2002).

Clinical improvement is usually evident in 48 to 72 hours with resolution of fever in 2 to 4 days. Worsening disease is a poor prognostic feature and follow-up radiography is

TABLE 46–2 Maternal and Perinatal Outcomes with Pneumonia Complicating 632 Pregnancies

Series	Incidence	Adverse Maternal Outcomes	Adverse Perinatal Outcomes
Richey et al (1994) (n = 71)	1:850	5 intubations 2 deaths	1 preterm birth 4 stillbirths
Briggs et al (1996) (n = 34)	NS	7 intubations 2 deaths	1 neonatal death 1 stillbirth
Munn et al (1999) (n = 59)	1:525	6 intubations 1 death	13 preterm births 20 low-birthweight neonates
Yost et al (2000) (n = 133)	1:560	2 intubations No deaths	1 stillbirth 14 preterm births
Jin et al (2003) (n = 335)	1:660	Intubations NS No deaths	Small-for-gestational age RR 1.86 (95% CI 1.01–3.45) Perinatal mortality NS
Total (n = 632)		6.7% intubated[a] 0.8% mortality rate	2.2% perinatal mortality[a]

NS = not stated; RR = respiratory rate.
[a]Data of Jin et al (2003) excluded in calculation.
Expanded from Bloom and colleagues (1997).

recommended if fever persists. Even with improvement, however, some progression of infiltrates is not unusual, and about 20 percent of women develop a pleural effusion.

Pregnancy Outcome with Pneumonia. During the preantimicrobial era, as many as a third of pregnant women with pneumonia died (Finland and Dublin, 1939). Even now, in five recent studies, maternal and perinatal mortality both remain formidable (Table 46–2). Notably, almost 7 percent of the mothers required intubation. These outcomes serve to emphasize the need for prompt diagnosis, effective treatment, and close observation.

Prevention. Pneumococcal vaccine is 60- to 70-percent protective against its 23 included serotypes. Its use may help decrease emergence of drug-resistant pneumococci. The vaccine is not recommended for otherwise healthy pregnant women (American College of Obstetricians and Gynecologists, 2003). However, it is recommended for those who are immunocompromised, including those with HIV infection; who have diabetes or cardiac, pulmonary, or renal disease; and who have asplenia such as with sickle-cell disease.

INFLUENZA PNEUMONIA. Respiratory infection, including pneumonitis, is caused by RNA viruses of which influenza A and B form one genus (see Chap. 58, p. 1277). Influenza A infection can be serious, and it is epidemic in the winter months. The causal virus is spread by aerosolized droplets and quickly infects ciliated columnar epithelium, alveolar cells, mucus gland cells, and macrophages. In most healthy adults, infection is self-limited. Pneumonia is the most common complication, and it is difficult to distinguish from bacterial pneumonia. At Parkland Hospital during the 2003–2004 influenza season, pneumonia developed in 10

percent of pregnant women with influenza (Laibl and colleagues, 2005). Primary influenza pneumonitis is the most severe and is characterized by sparse sputum production and radiographic interstitial infiltrates (Fig. 46–2). More commonly, secondary pneumonia develops from bacterial superinfection by streptococci or staphylococci after 2 to 3 days of clinical improvement.

Management. Hospitalizations for influenza during late pregnancy are increased compared with nonpregnant women

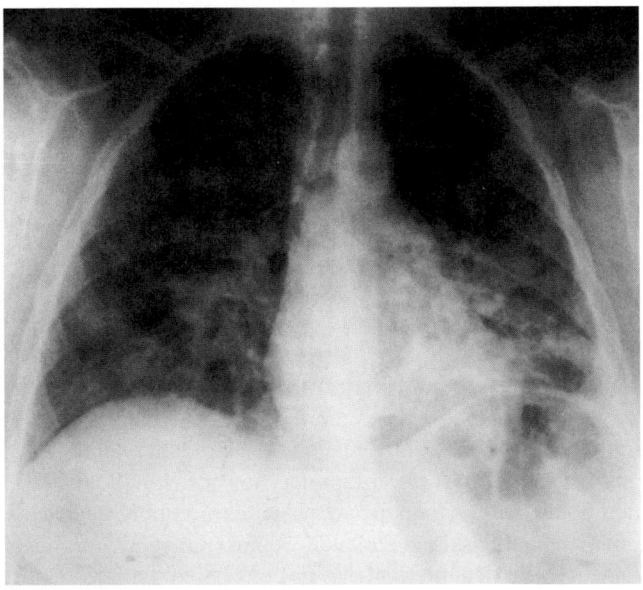

FIGURE 46–2. Chest radiograph taken at admission in a 27-week pregnant woman with presumed viral pneumonia. Diffuse infiltrates are seen. These worsened, respiratory failure developed, and she died a week later. (Richey and associates, 1994, with permission.)

(Hartert and associates, 2003; Neuzil and colleagues, 1998). Supportive treatment with antipyretics and bed rest is recommended for uncomplicated influenza. Either *amantadine* or *rimantadine*, 200 mg daily, are effective for chemoprophylaxis or treatment (Centers for Disease Control and Prevention, 2004b) (see Chap. 58, p. 1278). These drugs prevent 50 to 90 percent of clinical infections (Couch, 2000). If the drugs are begun within 48 hours of symptoms, they reduce the severity of infection. They are not routinely recommended for prophylaxis in healthy pregnant women (Hansen and Yankowitz, 2002). Both drugs are teratogenic in high doses given to animals, but it is unclear whether they are human teratogens (Briggs and colleagues, 2002).

The *neuraminidase inhibitors* are effective in the treatment of early influenza (Centers for Disease Control and Prevention, 2004b). *Oseltamivir* is given orally, 75 mg twice daily, and *zanamivir* is given by inhalation, 10 mg twice daily. When used for prophylaxis in nonpregnant patients, either is 80- to 85-percent effective in preventing symptomatic influenza (Hayden and colleagues, 1999; MIST Study Group, 1998). Neither oseltamivir nor zanamivir is approved for use in pregnant women. However, these agents were not teratogenic in animal studies (Briggs and colleagues, 2002).

Epidemiological studies provide evidence that fetal exposure to influenza A at midpregnancy increases the risks of schizophrenia, which is more common in individuals born in late winter and early spring (Limosin and co-workers, 2003). In their reviews, both McGrath and Castle (1995) and Kashyap and Gruslin (2000) concluded that the association between influenza and schizophrenia is weak (see Chap. 55, p. 1242). The perinatal effects of influenza infection are discussed in Chapter 58 (see p. 1278).

Prevention. **The Centers for Disease Control and Prevention (2004c) and the American College of Obstetricians and Gynecologists (2004) recommend attenuated influenza vaccination for all women, regardless of trimester, who will be pregnant during influenza season, which is October through mid-May.** At Parkland Hospital during the 2003–2004 influenza season, the influenza vaccine efficacy rate was greater than 99 percent, reducing the influenza rate fifteen-fold (Sheffield and colleagues, 2005). There is no evidence that inactivated influenza vaccine is teratogenic (see Chap. 8, p. 221). A recently approved live attenuated vaccine for intranasal administration (FluMist) is contraindicated in pregnant women (Centers for Disease Control and Prevention, 2003f). Vaccination is discussed in detail in Chapter 58 (p. 1277).

VARICELLA PNEUMONIA. Varicella-zoster virus is a member of the DNA herpesvirus family that causes chickenpox (see Chap. 58, p. 1276). The attack rate in seronegative individuals is 90 percent. The typical maculopapular and vesicular rash is accompanied by constitutional symptoms and fever for 3 to 5 days.

Although secondary streptococcal or staphylococcal skin infection is the most common complication, varicella pneumonitis develops in about 10 percent of adults (Nathwani and colleagues, 1998). It usually appears 3 to 5 days into the course of the illness and is characterized by tachypnea, a dry cough, dyspnea, fever, and pleuritic chest pain. Nodular infiltrates and interstitial pneumonitis seen on radiograph are similar to other viral pneumonias (see Fig. 46–2). In fatal cases, the lungs show scattered areas of necrosis and hemorrhage. Although resolution of pneumonitis parallels that of the skin lesions, fever and compromised pulmonary function may persist for weeks.

Pregnancy Outcome. There is no convincing evidence that pregnant women are more likely to develop pneumonitis (Nathwani and associates, 1998). In the Maternal–Fetal Medicine Units Network study, Harger and colleagues (2002) reported that only 5 percent of 347 pregnant women with chickenpox developed pneumonia, and none died. Risk factors for pneumonia included smoking and having more than 100 skin lesions.

Perinatal Outcome. Serious maternal infection with sepsis or pneumonia is associated with preterm delivery. Perinatal varicella infections are discussed in Chapter 58 (see p. 1277).

Management. Although the efficacy of intravenous acyclovir has not been proved, most clinicians recommend its use in the treatment of varicella pneumonitis. The dose is 10 mg/kg every 8 hours (American College of Obstetricians and Gynecologists, 2000). Treatment is also now recommended by the Infectious Disease Society of America (Mandell and colleagues, 2003). In earlier reports, maternal mortality from varicella pneumonia was 10 to 15 percent (Smego and Asperilla, 1991). This likely was biased by overreporting serious cases. In the Maternal–Fetal Medicine Units Network study, there were no deaths in 347 infected pregnant women (Harger and associates, 2002).

Prophylaxis. Administration of *varicella-zoster immunoglobulin* either prevents or attenuates varicella infection in exposed susceptible individuals if given within 96 hours of exposure. A complete discussion is found in Chapter 58 (see p. 1276).

Prevention. Attenuated live-virus vaccine (Varivax) is 87-percent effective at one year (Vázquez and colleagues, 2004). It is recommended for susceptible adults (American College of Obstetricians and Gynecologists, 2003). **The vaccine is contraindicated in pregnancy.** It is discussed in Chapter 58 (see p. 1277).

FUNGAL AND PARASITIC PNEUMONIA. Fungal and parasitic pulmonary infections are usually of greatest consequence in immunocompromised hosts, especially in women with acquired immunodeficiency syndrome (AIDS).

Pneumocystis Pneumonia. Lung infection with *Pneumocystis carinii* is a common complication in women with AIDS. *P carinii* causes interstitial pneumonia characterized by dry cough, tachypnea, and dyspnea, and characteristic radiographic findings of diffuse infiltrates. Although this organism can be identified by sputum culture, bronchoscopy with lavage or biopsy may be necessary.

In a report from the AIDS Clinical Trials Centers, Stratton and colleagues (1992) described pneumocystis pneumonia as the most common HIV-related disorder in pregnant women. Ahmad and co-workers (2001) reviewed 22 cases during pregnancy and cited a 50-percent mortality rate, which seems rather high. Treatment is with trimethoprim-sulfamethoxazole or pentamidine. Experience with dapsone or atovaquone is limited. In some cases, tracheal intubation and mechanical ventilation may be required.

For some HIV-infected pregnant women, the Centers for Disease Control and Prevention (2002a) recommend prophylaxis against pneumocystis infection with oral daily double-strength trimethoprim-sulfamethoxazole. This group includes women with CD4+ T-lymphocyte counts less than $200/\mu L$ or those with a history of oropharyngeal candidiasis. When CD4+ T lymphocytes constitute less than 14 percent of lymphocytes or if there is an AIDS-defining illness, prophylaxis should be considered.

Fungal Pneumonia. Any of a number of fungi can cause pneumonia, and in pregnancy, these are usually seen in women with HIV infection or who are otherwise immunocompromised. Infection is usually mild and self-limited. It is characterized initially by cough and fever, and dissemination is infrequent.

Histoplasmosis and *blastomycosis* do not appear to be more common or more severe during pregnancy. Data concerning *coccidioidomycosis* are conflicting. Stevens (1995) reported that it may more commonly disseminate in pregnant women than in nonpregnant women. Two recent studies differ. In a case-control study from an endemic area, Rosenstein and co-workers (2001) reported that pregnancy was a significant risk factor for disseminated disease. In another study, Caldwell and colleagues (2000) identified 32 serologically confirmed cases during pregnancy. Dissemination was documented in only three cases, treatment was given to nine women, and there were no deaths. Arsura and associates (1998) described 61 pregnant women with symptomatic infection. Half had associated *erythema nodosum,* which indicated a better overall prognosis. Specifically, disseminated infection occurred in none of the 30 women with erythema nodosum compared with 35 percent of the 31 women with no skin lesions. Caldwell and co-workers (2000) reported similar findings.

Most cases of *cryptococcosis* reported during pregnancy were manifest as meningitis. Ely and co-workers (1998) described four otherwise healthy pregnant women with cryptococcal pneumonia. Diagnosis is difficult, because clinical presentation is similar to other community-acquired pneumonias.

Pregnant women with disseminated fungal infections are given intravenous *amphotericin B* or *ketoconazole* (Caldwell and associates, 2000). Other effective antifungal drugs include *itraconazole, flucytosine,* and *fluconazole.* Of these, only amphotericin B has been used extensively in early pregnancy and has been associated with no embryofetal effects. Experience with the other four drugs is limited, and fluconazole is considered by Briggs and colleagues (2002) to be teratogenic if given for long periods in early pregnancy. *Caspofungin* is a member of the antifungal family termed echinocandins and has been proven to be as effective as amphotericin B for invasive candidiasis (Mora-Duarte and associates, 2002). It has not been used in pregnancy.

SEVERE ACUTE RESPIRATORY SYNDROME. This life-threatening disease, caused by a coronavirus, was first identified in 2002 in China. Severe acute respiratory syndrome (SARS) spread rapidly, and in March 2003, worldwide efforts to contain it were begun. Study of the virus was quick and concerted. The May 15, 2003, edition of *The New England Journal of Medicine* was devoted to SARS (Holmes, 2003; Wenzel and Edmond, 2003). Experiences in pregnant women have been described in Hong Kong (Haines, 2003; Lam and associates, 2004; Shek, 2003; Wong, 2003, 2004, and all their colleagues). Its course and management are discussed in Chapter 58 (see p. 1292). About 20 percent of infected persons develop acute lung injury and require ventilatory support (Drosten and colleagues, 2003; Ksiazek and associates, 2003). The case-fatality rate is about 5 percent (Centers for Disease Control and Prevention, 2003e).

ASTHMA

According to the Centers for Disease Control and Prevention (2004a), about 7 percent of the general population currently has asthma. In a national survey, Kwon and associates (2003) estimated current asthma prevalence in pregnant women to be 5 to 9 percent. Moreover, Namazy and Schatz (2005) reported that the prevalence of asthma in pregnant women appears to be increasing. *Status asthmaticus,* the most severe form of asthma, complicates about 0.2 percent of pregnancies (Mabie and associates, 1992).

PATHOPHYSIOLOGY. Asthma is a chronic inflammatory airway disorder with a *major hereditary component.* Increased airway responsiveness and inflammation have been linked to candidate genes on chromosomes 5, 6, 11, 12, 14, and 16 (Tattersfield and colleagues, 2002), including the

TABLE 46–3 Clinical Stages of Asthma

Stage	P_{O_2}	P_{CO_2}	pH	FEV_1 (% predicted)
Mild respiratory alkalosis	Normal	↓	↑	65–80
Respiratory alkalosis	↓	↓	↑	50–64
Danger zone	↓	Normal	Normal	35–49
Respiratory acidosis	↓	↑	↓	<35

Modified after Barth and Hankins (1991), with permission.

high-affinity IgE receptor, the cytokine gene cluster, and the T-cell antigen receptor. These conditions have also recently been linked to mutations of the *ADAM-33* gene on the short arm of chromosome 20 (Shapiro and Owen, 2002). There inevitably is an *environmental allergic stimulant* in susceptible individuals, for example, influenza or cigarette smoke (Hartert and colleagues, 2003; Sheffield, 2005).

The hallmarks of asthma are reversible airway obstruction from bronchial smooth muscle contraction, mucus hypersecretion, and mucosal edema. There is airway inflammation and responsiveness to a number of stimuli, including irritants, viral infections, aspirin, cold air, and exercise. Mast cell activation by cytokines mediates bronchoconstriction by release of histamines, prostaglandin D_2, and leukotrienes. **Because F-series prostaglandins and ergonovine exacerbate asthma, these commonly used obstetrical drugs should be avoided if possible.**

CLINICAL COURSE. Asthma represents a broad spectrum of clinical illness ranging from mild wheezing to severe bronchoconstriction. The functional result of acute bronchospasm is airway obstruction and decreased airflow. The work of breathing progressively increases, and patients present with chest tightness, wheezing, or breathlessness. Subsequent alterations in oxygenation primarily reflect ventilation–perfusion mismatching, because the distribution of airway narrowing is uneven.

The clinical stages of asthma are summarized in Table 46–3. With mild disease, hypoxia initially is well compensated by hyperventilation, as reflected by a normal arterial P_{O_2}, decreased P_{CO_2}, and resultant respiratory alkalosis. As airway narrowing worsens, ventilation–perfusion defects increase, and arterial hypoxemia ensues. With severe obstruction, ventilation becomes impaired because fatigue causes early CO_2 retention. Because of hyperventilation, this may only be seen initially as an arterial P_{CO_2} returning to the normal range. Finally, with critical obstruction, respiratory failure follows, characterized by hypercapnia and acidemia.

Although these changes are generally reversible and well tolerated in the healthy nonpregnant individual, even early stages of asthma may be dangerous for the pregnant woman and her fetus. The smaller functional residual capacity and the increased effective shunt render her more susceptible to hypoxia and hypoxemia.

EFFECTS OF PREGNANCY ON ASTHMA. There is no evidence that pregnancy has a predictable effect on underlying asthma. In two prospective studies of more than 500 pregnant women, about equal thirds of the group either improved, remained unchanged, or clearly worsened (Schatz and colleagues, 1988; Stenius-Aarniala and associates, 1988). Baseline asthma severity correlates with asthma morbidity during pregnancy (Schatz and associates, 2003). With mild disease, 13 percent of women had an exacerbation; with moderate disease, 26 percent did; and with severe asthma, about 50 percent did. In the same study, about 20 percent of women with mild or moderate asthma had an intrapartum exacerbation. Conversely, Wendel and associates (1996) observed this in only 1 percent of women. Mabie and co-workers (1992) reported an 18-fold increased risk of exacerbation following cesarean versus vaginal delivery.

PREGNANCY OUTCOME. Generally, unless there is severe disease, asthma has relatively minor effects on pregnancy outcome. Table 46–4 shows maternal and perinatal outcomes

TABLE 46–4 Maternal and Perinatal Outcomes in Pregnancies Complicated by Asthma

Study	Number (n = 9291)	Perinatal Outcomes (Percent)		
		Pregnancy Hypertension	*Growth Restriction*	*Preterm Delivery*
Alexander et al (1998)	817	~15	~5	~6
Demissie et al (1998)	2289	8	15	18
Liu et al (2001)	2193	13	12	10
Bracken et al (2003)	872	NS	8.5	8.5
Ramsey et al (2003)	1381	NS	1.7	Not ↑[a]
Dombrowski et al (2004)	1739	12.2[a]	Not ↑[a]	16[a]
Approximate average		11	12	12

NS = not stated.
[a] Incidence not significantly different compared with controls.

in more than 9000 pregnancies complicated by asthma. Most studies describe a slightly increased incidence of preeclampsia, preterm labor, low-birthweight infants, and perinatal mortality. In the observational study by the Maternal–Fetal Medicine Units Network, delivery before 37 weeks was not increased among the 1687 pregnancies complicated by asthma compared with that of 881 controls (Dombrowski and colleagues, 2004a). However, for the 52 women with severe asthma, the rate was increased about twofold. Similarly, Bracken and colleagues (2003) found that preterm delivery was only minimally increased in women with asthma and fetal growth restriction increased with asthma severity. In a prospective evaluation of 656 asthmatic pregnant women and 1052 nonasthmatic pregnant controls, Triche and co-workers (2004) found that women with moderate to severe asthma, regardless of treatment, are at increased risk of preeclampsia.

Life-threatening complications from *status asthmaticus* include muscle fatigue with respiratory arrest, pneumothorax, pneumomediastinum, acute cor pulmonale, and cardiac arrhythmias. Maternal and perinatal mortality is substantively increased when mechanical ventilation is required.

FETAL EFFECTS. In the Network study cited above, asthma was not associated with significant adverse neonatal sequelae (Dombrowski and co-workers, 2004a). Severe asthma was uncommon, and when respiratory alkalosis developed, both animal and human studies have suggested that fetal hypoxemia may occur well before maternal oxygenation is compromised (Rolston and associates, 1974). Fetal compromise is hypothesized to result from decreased uterine blood flow, decreased maternal venous return, and an alkaline-induced leftward shift of the oxyhemoglobin dissociation curve. With maternal hypoxemia, the fetus responds with decreased umbilical blood flow, increased systemic and pulmonary vascular resistance, and decreased cardiac output. Recent observations by Bracken and colleagues (2003) confirm that the incidence of fetal growth restriction increases with severity of asthma. The realization that the fetus may be seriously compromised as asthma severity increases underscores the need for aggressive management of all pregnant women with acute asthma. Monitoring the fetal response is, in effect, an indicator of maternal status.

In addition, possible teratogenic or adverse fetal effects of drugs given to control asthma are a concern. As discussed in Chapter 14 (p. 360), considerable published data indicates there is no evidence that commonly used anti-asthmatic drugs are harmful (Nelson-Piercy, 2001; Schatz, 2001; Wendel, 2001).

CLINICAL EVALUATION. The subjective severity of asthma frequently does not correlate with objective measures of airway function or ventilation. Clinical examination also is inaccurate as a predictor of severity. Useful clinical signs include labored breathing, tachycardia, pulsus paradoxus,

prolonged expiration, and use of accessory muscles. Signs of a potentially fatal attack include central cyanosis and altered consciousness.

Arterial blood gas analysis provides objective assessment of maternal oxygenation, ventilation, and acid–base status. With this information, the severity of an acute attack can be assessed (see Table 46–3). In a prospective evaluation, however, Wendel and associates (1996) found that *routine* blood gas analysis did not help direct care in most pregnant women. Importantly, the results must be interpreted in relation to normal values for pregnancy. For example, a P_{CO_2} greater than 35 mm Hg with a pH less than 7.35 is consistent with hyperventilation and CO_2 retention in a pregnant woman.

Pulmonary function testing is now routine in the management of chronic and acute asthma. Sequential measurement of the FEV_1 is the single best measure reflecting severity. An FEV_1 less than 1 L, or less than 20 percent of predicted, correlates with severe disease, defined as hypoxia, poor response to therapy, and a high relapse rate (Noble and colleagues, 1988). The *peak expiratory flow rate (PEFR)* correlates well with the FEV_1, and it can be measured reliably with inexpensive portable meters. Brancazio and associates (1997) showed that the PEFR did not change over the course of pregnancy in normal women.

MANAGEMENT OF CHRONIC ASTHMA. According to the National Asthma Education Program (1997), effective management of asthma during pregnancy includes:

1. Objective assessment of pulmonary function and fetal well-being.
2. Avoidance or control of environmental precipitating factors.
3. Pharmacological therapy.
4. Patient education.

In general, women with moderate to severe asthma are instructed to measure and record their PEFR twice daily. Predicted values range from 380 to 550 L/min. Each woman has her own baseline value, and therapeutic adjustments can be made using this.

Treatment depends on the severity of disease. Drugs recommended for home management are listed in Table 46–5. For mild asthma, inhaled *β-agonists* as needed are usually sufficient. *Inhaled corticosteroids* are the preferred treatment for persistent asthma. Inhalations are administered every 3 to 4 hours as needed. The goal is to reduce the use of *β*-agonists for symptomatic relief. A case-control study from Canada with a cohort of over 15,600 nonpregnant women with asthma showed that inhaled corticosteroids reduced hospitalizations by 80 percent (Blais and associates, 1998). In pregnant women, Wendel and colleagues (1996) reported a 55-percent reduction in readmissions for severe exacerbations in women given maintenance inhaled corticosteroids along with *β*-agonist therapy.

TABLE 46–5 Step Therapy of Chronic Asthma During Pregnancy

Severity	Step Therapy
Mild intermittent	Inhaled β-agonists—isoetharine, metaproterenol, isoproterenol, salmeterol
Mild persistent	Inhaled β-agonists—as above
	Inhaled cromolyn—continue if taking prior to pregnancy with good response
	Substitute inhaled corticosteroids if no response—beclomethasone, budesonide, triamcinolone
Moderate persistent	Inhaled β-agonists as above
	Inhaled corticosteroids as above, add oral theophylline and/or inhaled salmeterol if inhaled medium-dose steroids inadequate
Severe persistent	For moderate as above plus oral corticosteroids—burst for active symptoms, alternate-day or daily if necessary

From National Asthma Education and Prevention Program Expert Panel Report 2 (1997) and American College of Obstetricians and Gynecologists, American College of Allergy, Asthma, and Immunology (2000).

Cromolyn and *nedocromil* inhibit mast cell degranulation. They are ineffective for acute asthma and are taken chronically for prevention. They likely are not superior to inhaled corticosteroids.

Theophylline is a methylxanthine, and its various salts are bronchodilators and possibly anti-inflammatory agents. These drugs have been used less frequently since inhaled steroids became available. Some theophylline derivatives are considered useful for oral maintenance therapy if the initial response is not optimal to inhaled corticosteroids and β-agonists (see Table 46–5). Dombrowski and colleagues (2004b) conducted a randomized trial with nearly 400 pregnant women with moderate asthma. Oral theophylline was compared with inhaled beclomethasone for maintenance. In both groups, about 20 percent had exacerbations. Women taking theophylline had a significantly higher discontinuation rate because of side effects. Pregnancy outcomes were similar in both the women who received theophylline and those who received beclomethasone.

Leukotriene modifiers inhibit their synthesis and include *zileuton, zafirinkast,* and *montelukast*. These drugs are given either orally or by inhalation for prevention, but they are not effective for acute disease. For maintenance, they are used in conjunction with inhaled steroids to allow minimal dosing. Ducharme (2002) reviewed all randomized trials conducted through 2001 and concluded that these agents resulted in only slightly improved asthma control. There is little experience with their use in pregnancy.

MANAGEMENT OF ACUTE ASTHMA. Treatment of acute asthma during pregnancy is similar to that for the nonpregnant asthmatic. An exception is a significantly lowered threshold for hospitalization. Intravenous hydration may help clear pulmonary secretions, and supplemental oxygen is given by mask after a blood gas sample is obtained if indicated. The therapeutic aim is to maintain the P_{O_2} greater than 60 mm Hg, and preferably normal, along with 95-percent oxygen saturation. Baseline pulmonary function testing includes

FEV_1 or PEFR. Continuous pulse oximetry and electronic fetal monitoring may provide useful information.

First-line therapy for acute asthma includes a β-*adrenergic agonist*, either terbutaline, albuterol, isoetharine, epinephrine, isoproterenol, or metaproterenol, which is given subcutaneously, taken orally, or inhaled. These drugs bind to specific cell-surface receptors and activate adenylyl cyclase to increase intracellular cyclic AMP and modulate bronchial smooth muscle relaxation. The long-acting preparations are used for outpatient therapy.

Corticosteroids should be given early to all patients with severe acute asthma (National Heart, Lung and Blood Institute, 1993). Recommended doses, which are probably higher than necessary, are intravenous methylprednisolone, 40 to 60 mg, every 6 hours. Equipotent doses of hydrocortisone by infusion or prednisone orally can be given instead. **Because their onset of action is several hours, whether given intravenously or by aerosol, steroids are given along with β-agonists for acute asthma.** In one audit, Cydulka and associates (1999) reported that pregnant women presenting with asthma to academic medical center emergency departments were given systemic corticosteroids in only 44 percent of cases.

Further management depends on the response to therapy. If initial therapy with β-agonists is associated with improvement of FEV_1 or PEFR to above 70 percent of baseline, then discharge can be considered. Some women may benefit from 23-hour observation. Alternatively, for the woman with obvious respiratory distress, or if the FEV_1 or PEFR is less than 70 percent of predicted after three doses of β-agonist, admission is advisable. Intensive therapy includes inhaled β-agonists, intravenous corticosteroids, and close observation for worsening respiratory distress or fatigue in breathing (Wendel and colleagues, 1996).

Status Asthmaticus and Respiratory Failure. Severe asthma of any type not responding after 30 to 60 minutes of intensive therapy is termed *status asthmaticus*. Braman and Kaemmerlen (1990) have shown that management of nonpregnant patients with status asthmaticus in an intensive care setting results in a good outcome in most cases. Consideration should be given to early intubation when maternal respiratory status worsens despite aggressive treatment (see Table 46–3). Fatigue, carbon dioxide retention, and hypoxemia are indications for mechanical ventilation.

LABOR AND DELIVERY. Maintenance medications are continued through delivery. Stress-dose corticosteroids are administered to any woman given systemic steroid therapy within the preceding 4 weeks. The usual drug is 100 mg of hydrocortisone given intravenously every 8 hours. The PEFR or FEV_1 should be determined on admission and serial measurements made if symptoms develop.

A nonhistamine-releasing narcotic, such as fentanyl, may be preferable to meperidine for labor. Epidural analgesia for labor is ideal. For surgical delivery, conduction analgesia is preferred because tracheal intubation can trigger severe bronchospasm. Refractory postpartum hemorrhage is treated with prostaglandin E_2 or other uterotonics instead of prostaglandin $F_{2\alpha}$, which may cause significant bronchospasm in asthmatic patients. Oxygen desaturation following 15-methyl $PGF_{2\alpha}$ has been reported in women without reactive airway disease (Hankins and colleagues, 1988).

TUBERCULOSIS

Although tuberculosis is still a major worldwide concern, it is uncommon in the United States. Since the early 1990s, however, tuberculosis in foreign-born persons has increased by 50 percent. By 2002, almost three fourths of the 15,500 U.S. cases were in foreign-born persons (Centers for Disease Control and Prevention, 2003d). U.S.-born persons have newly acquired infection, whereas foreign-born persons have reactivation of latent infection (Geng and co-workers, 2002). In this country, tuberculosis is a disease of the elderly, the urban poor, minority groups, and patients with AIDS.

Cure rates with 6-month short-course directly observed therapy (DOT) approach 90 percent for new infections. Of special concern is the recent emergence of multidrug-resistant tuberculosis (MDR-TB). In a survey conducted by the World Health Organization, 12 percent of 12,000 isolates from the United States in 1997 were resistant to at least one drug (Espinal and colleagues, 2001). During the same year, however, only 1.2 percent of isolates were resistant to more than one drug. Drug resistance was variable worldwide but reached 14 percent in some countries. Importantly, 6-month chemotherapy with first-line drugs is inadequate in many cases caused by resistant strains. In this country, there have been documented outbreaks of MDR-TB in persons with HIV infection. In some of these cases, tuberculosis was transmitted to health care workers.

CLINICAL COURSE. Infection is via inhalation of *Mycobacterium tuberculosis,* which incites a granulomatous pulmonary reaction. In more than 90 percent of patients, infection is contained and is dormant for long periods. In some patients, especially those who are immunocompromised or who have other diseases, tuberculosis becomes reactivated to cause clinical disease. Clinical manifestations usually include cough with minimal sputum production, low-grade fever, hemoptysis, and weight loss. A variety of infiltrative patterns are seen on chest radiograph, and there may be associated cavitation or mediastinal lymphadenopathy. Acid-fast bacilli are seen on repeated stained smears of sputum in about two thirds of culture-positive patients. Extrapulmonary tuberculosis may occur in any organ, and almost 40 percent of HIV-positive patients have disseminated disease (Weinberger and Weiss, 1999).

TUBERCULOSIS AND PREGNANCY. The considerable influx of women into the United States from Asia, Africa, Mexico, and Central America has been accompanied by an increased frequency of tuberculosis in pregnant women. Symptoms are cough, fever, and weight loss. Pillay and co-workers (2004) stress the prevalence of tuberculosis in HIV-positive pregnant women. Margono and colleagues (1994) reported that for two New York City hospitals, the rate for tuberculosis during pregnancy from 1985 through 1990 was 12 cases per 100,000 deliveries. This rate rose to 95 per 100,000 in 1992, and of 16 pregnant women with active tuberculosis, 7 of 11 tested were HIV positive. At Jackson Memorial Hospital in Miami, Schulte and associates (2002) reported that 21 percent of 207 HIV-infected pregnant women had a positive skin test.

Pregnancy Outcomes. Prior to antituberculosis therapy, pregnancy was thought to have an adverse effect on the course of active tuberculosis (Anderson, 1997). Contemporaneous experiences are few, because chemotherapy has diminished severe disease. Outcomes are dependent on site of infection and timing of diagnosis in relation to delivery. Jana and colleagues (1994) reported 79 pregnancies from India complicated by active pulmonary tuberculosis. There were increased incidences of preterm delivery, low birthweight and growth-restricted infants, as well as sixfold increased perinatal mortality. Adverse outcomes correlated with late diagnosis, incomplete or irregular treatment, and advanced pulmonary lesions. Figueroa-Damian and Arrendondo-Garcia (1998) reported similar outcomes in Mexico City.

Jana and co-workers (1999) reported outcomes in 33 pregnancies complicated by extrapulmonary tuberculosis. A third of women with renal, intestinal, and skeletal infections had low-birthweight infants. In a study in London, Llewelyn and associates (2000) reported that 9 of 13 pregnant women had extrapulmonary disease concomitant with delayed diagnoses. Nanda and colleagues (2002) described paraplegia at 16 weeks from cervical spinal tuberculosis. Prevost and

Fung Kee Fung (1999) reviewed 56 cases of tuberculous meningitis in pregnancy, and there was maternal death in a third of cases.

Diagnosis. Current guidelines from the Centers for Disease Control (1990) include skin testing of pregnant women in the following high-risk groups:

- Individuals with HIV infection
- Close contacts of active cases
- Individuals with medical risk factors known to increase risk of disease if infected
- Foreign-born individuals from areas in which the prevalence of tuberculosis is high
- Individuals from medically underserved, low-income populations
- Alcoholics and intravenous drug abusers
- Residents of long-term care facilities, including mental, correctional, and nursing facilities

The preferred antigen for skin testing is purified protein derivative (PPD) in the intermediate strength of 5 tuberculin units. If the intracutaneously applied test is negative, no further evaluation is needed. A positive skin test is interpreted according to risk factors (American Thoracic Society/Centers for Disease Control and Prevention, 1990). For *very high-risk* patients—that is, those who are HIV-positive, those with abnormal chest radiography, or those who have a recent contact with an active case—5 mm or greater is considered positive. For those at *high risk*—foreign born individuals, intravenous drug users who are HIV-negative, low-income populations, or those with medical conditions that increase the risk for tuberculosis—10 mm or greater is considered positive. For persons with none of these risk factors, 15 mm or greater is defined as positive. If the chest radiograph is negative, then no treatment is necessary until after delivery, when isoniazid is given for 1 year. Patients who have been vaccinated with *bacille Calmette-Guérin* (*BCG*) pose special problems with interpretation of skin testing.

A blood test became available in 2001 to determine tuberculosis status. The assay is for quantification of interferon-γ released from sensitized lymphocytes in whole blood incubated overnight with PPD. The QuantiFERON-TB test appears to be quite promising in testing for latent infection, but it currently is not yet in widespread use (Centers for Disease Control and Prevention, 2003a).

Treatment. In nonpregnant tuberculin-positive patients who are younger than 35 years of age and who have no evidence of active disease, isoniazid, 300 mg daily, is given for 1 year. Isoniazid has been used for decades and it is considered safe in pregnancy (Briggs and colleagues, 2002). In HIV-negative women, however, most clinicians recommend that therapy be delayed until after delivery. Because of possible increased isoniazid-induced hepatitis risk in postpartum women, some clinicians recommend withholding treatment

until 3 to 6 months postpartum. Neither postpartum method is as effective as antepartum treatment to prevent active infection (Boggess and colleagues, 2000).

There are exceptions to delayed treatment in pregnancy. Known recent skin-test convertors are treated because the incidence of active infection is 3 percent in the first year. Skin-test-positive women exposed to active infection are treated because the incidence of infection is 0.5 percent per year. Finally, HIV-positive women are treated because they have an 8-percent annual risk of active disease (Brost and Newman, 1997). An alternative is to withhold therapy until after 12 weeks in these asymptomatic women. Isoniazid-induced hepatitis is more common in patients younger than 35 years of age. Although monitoring of liver enzymes indicates that 10 to 20 percent of patients have a transient elevation, therapy is not discontinued unless their increase is fivefold over normal values (Weinberger and Weiss, 1999). The Centers for Disease Control and Prevention (2003c) does not recommend routine serum transaminase monitoring.

Because of emerging drug resistance, the Centers for Disease Control and Prevention (2003c) recommends a four-drug regimen for initial empirical treatment of nonpregnant patients with symptomatic tuberculosis. These drugs are isoniazid, rifampin, pyrazinamide, and ethambutol given until susceptibility studies are performed. If the organism is fully susceptible, ethambutol is discontinued, and the remaining three-drug regimen is continued until a total of 6 months has elapsed. Drug susceptibility is performed on all first isolates.

Recommended initial treatment for pregnant patients is a three-drug regimen with isoniazid, rifampin, and ethambutol. If the organism is susceptible, the regimen is given for a total of 9 months. According to Bothamley (2001), all of these drugs are safe during pregnancy. Pyrazinamide is added if necessary. Indeed, the World Health Organization recommends initial therapy with the four-drug regimen for 6 months, as prescribed for nonpregnant adults. Reports of MDR-TB during pregnancy are few, and Lessnau and Qurah (2003) and Shin and colleagues (2003) have reviewed treatment options. Breast feeding is not prohibited during antituberculous therapy.

For HIV-infected women, the use of rifampin or rifabutin may be contraindicated if certain protease inhibitors or non-nucleoside reverse transcriptase inhibitors are being administered. Also if there is resistance to these two drugs, then pyrazinamide therapy is given. Of the many second-line antituberculous drug regimens, the aminoglycosides—streptomycin, kanamycin, amikacin, and capreomycin—are ototoxic to the fetus and are contraindicated during pregnancy (Bothamley, 2001).

Neonatal Tuberculosis. Tubercle bacillemia during pregnancy can infect the placenta. In only a few of these cases, the fetus is infected, and *congenital tuberculosis* develops. The term congenital tuberculosis also applies to newborns who are infected by aspiration of infected secretions at delivery.

Each route of infection constitutes about half of the cases of congenital infection. Neonatal tuberculosis simulates other congenital infections and includes hepatosplenomegaly, respiratory distress, fever, and lymphadenopathy (Smith, 2002).

Cantwell and associates (1994) found only 29 cases of congenital tuberculosis reported in the English literature since 1980. Only 12 of the mothers had active infection, and tuberculosis was commonly demonstrated by postpartum endometrial biopsy. Adhikari and colleagues (1997) described 11 South African pregnant women whose postpartum endometrial biopsy was culture-positive. Six of their neonates had congenital tuberculosis, and one of these died.

Neonatal infection is unlikely if the mother with active disease has been treated before delivery or if her sputum culture is negative. Because the newborn is quite susceptible to tuberculosis, most authors recommend isolation from the mother suspected of having active disease. If untreated, the risk of disease in the infant born to a woman with active infection is 50 percent in the first year (Jacobs and Abernathy, 1988).

SARCOIDOSIS

Sarcoidosis is a chronic, multisystem disease of unknown etiology characterized by an accumulation of T lymphocytes and phagocytes within noncaseating granulomas. The disease is possibly mediated by a multigene-controlled exaggerated response of helper T lymphocytes to environmental triggers (Baughman and colleagues, 2003; Thomas and Hunninghake, 2003). Pulmonary involvement is most common, followed by skin, eyes, and lymph nodes. Its prevalence in the United States is 10 to 40 per 100,000, with equal sex distribution but a 10- to 20-fold predilection for African Americans (Crystal, 2001). Most patients are between 20 and 40 years of age. Clinical presentation varies, but the most common symptoms are dyspnea and a dry cough without constitutional symptoms that develop insidiously over months. Disease onset is abrupt in about 25 percent of patients, and 10 percent are asymptomatic at discovery.

More than 90 percent of patients have an abnormal chest radiograph. *Interstitial pneumonitis* is the hallmark of pulmonary involvement. About 50 percent of affected patients develop permanent radiological changes. *Lymphadenopathy,* especially of the mediastinum, is present in 75 to 90 percent of cases; 25 percent have *uveitis*; and 25 percent have skin involvement, usually manifest as *erythema nodosum.* Any other organ system may be involved. Confirmation of diagnosis is not possible without biopsy, and because the lung may be the only obviously involved organ, tissue acquisition is often difficult.

The overall prognosis for sarcoidosis is good, and it resolves without treatment in 50 percent of patients. In the other 50 percent, permanent organ dysfunction, albeit mild and nonprogressive, persists. About 10 percent die because of their disease. Glucocorticoids are the most widely used

treatment, however, permanent organ derangement is seldom reversed by their use (Paramothayan and Jones, 2002). Thus, the decision to treat is based on symptoms, physical findings, chest radiograph, and pulmonary function tests. Unless respiratory symptoms are prominent, therapy is usually withheld for a several-month observation period. If inflammation does not subside, then prednisone, 1 mg/kg, is given daily for 4 to 6 weeks (Crystal, 2001).

SARCOIDOSIS AND PREGNANCY. Because sarcoidosis is uncommon, it is an unusual complication of pregnancy. De Regt (1987) described 14 cases of sarcoidosis in 20,000 pregnancies over a 12-year period at Downstate Medical Center. Sarcoidosis seldom affects pregnancy adversely unless there is severe preexisting disease (Selroos, 1990). However, serious complications have been described. De Regt (1987) reported two fatal cases due to extensive lung disease. Maisel and Lynam (1996) reported a maternal death at 16 weeks from granulomatous meningitis. Seballos and associates (1994) described a woman with peripartum heart failure from pulmonary and cardiac sarcoidosis. Cardonick and colleagues (2000) described a woman with painful facial palsy from neurosarcoidosis at 25 weeks.

In general, perinatal outcomes are unaffected by sarcoidosis. Selroos (1990) reviewed 655 patients with sarcoidosis referred to the Mjölbolsta Hospital District in southern Finland. Of 252 women between 18 and 50 years of age, 15 percent had sarcoidosis during pregnancy or within 1 year postpartum. There was no evidence for disease progression in the 26 pregnancies in women with active disease; three aborted spontaneously, and the other 23 women were delivered at term. In 18 pregnancies in 12 women with inactive disease, pregnancy outcome was good. Agha and colleagues (1982) reported similar experiences with 35 pregnancies at the University of Michigan.

Active sarcoidosis is treated using the same guidelines as for the woman who is not pregnant. Severe disease warrants serial determination of pulmonary function. Symptomatic uveitis, constitutional symptoms, and pulmonary symptoms are treated with prednisone, 1 mg/kg per day.

CYSTIC FIBROSIS

One of the most common fatal genetic disorders in Caucasians, cystic fibrosis is caused by one of more than 1000 mutations in a 230-kb gene on the long arm of chromosome 7 that encodes a 1480–amino acid polypeptide. This peptide functions as a chloride channel and is termed the *cystic fibrosis transmembrane conductance receptor regulator* (*CFTR*). There is a wide phenotypic variation, even among homozygotes for the common ΔF508 mutation. This is discussed in greater detail in Chapter 13, p. 325. The incidence of symptomatic homozygous cystic fibrosis is estimated to be 1 per 3300 for Caucasians, 1 per 8500 for Hispanics, 1 per

15,000 for African Americans, and 1 in 32,000 for Asian Americans (American College of Obstetricians and Gynecologists, 2001). Because of improvements in diagnosis and treatment, nearly 80 percent of females with cystic fibrosis now survive to adulthood (Gillet and associates, 2002; Ratjen and Döring, 2003). The median survival has increased from 14 years of age in 1969 to 30 to 35 years of age by 2000.

PATHOPHYSIOLOGY. The mutations in the chloride channel cause altered epithelial cell membrane transport of electrolytes, which affect all organs that express CFTR— secretory cells, sinuses, lung, pancreas, liver, and reproductive tract. Severity of the disease depends on which two alleles are inherited. Homozygosity for ΔF508 is one of the most severe (McKone and colleagues, 2003).

Exocrine gland dysfunction occurs with production of thick, viscid secretions. Eccrine sweat gland abnormalities are the basis for the diagnostic *sweat test*, characterized by elevated sodium, potassium, and chloride levels in sweat.

Lung involvement almost always occurs, and it is also the most common cause of death. Bronchial gland hypertrophy with mucous plugging and small-airway obstruction lead to subsequent infection that ultimately causes chronic bronchitis and bronchiectasis. For complex reasons that are not completely explicable, chronic inflammation from *Pseudomonas aeruginosa* occurs in more 90 percent of patients. *Staphylococcus aureus, H influenzae,* and *Stenotrophomonas maltophilia* are recovered in only a minority. More recently, it has been reported that colonization with *Burkholderia cepacia,* especially in pregnancy, signifies a worse prognosis (Gillet and colleagues, 2002). Acute and chronic parenchymal inflammation ultimately causes extensive fibrosis, and along with airway obstruction, there is a ventilation–perfusion mismatch. Pulmonary insufficiency is the end result. Lung or heart–lung transplantation has a 5-year survival rate of 33 percent (Aurora and associates, 1999). A few women have successfully undergone pregnancy following lung transplantation (Kruszka and Gherman, 2002).

PRECONCEPTIONAL COUNSELING

Infertility. Women with cystic fibrosis are subfertile because of tenacious cervical mucus. Males have oligospermia or aspermia from vas deferens obstruction, and 98 percent are infertile (Boyd and co-workers, 2004). Despite this, the North American Cystic Fibrosis Foundation estimates that 4 percent of affected women become pregnant every year (Edenborough and colleagues, 1995). The endometrium and tubes express some CFTR but are normal functionally, and the ovaries do not express the *CFTR* gene (Edenborough, 2001). Both intrauterine insemination and in vitro fertilization have been used successfully in affected women (Rodgers and colleagues, 2000). We agree with Neill and Nelson-Piercy (2001) who advise a multidisciplinary evaluation before embarking on assisted reproductive efforts.

Screening. The American Academy of Pediatrics and the American College of Obstetricians and Gynecologists (2002) recommend that carrier screening be offered to at-risk couples (see Chap. 13, p. 325).

PREGNANCY WITH CYSTIC FIBROSIS. Pregnancy outcome is inversely related to severity of lung dysfunction. Severe chronic lung disease, hypoxia, and frequent infections may prove deleterious. *Cor pulmonale* is common, and Cohen and associates (1980) reported that 13 percent of pregnant women with cystic fibrosis developed heart failure. Cameron and Skinner (2005) describe survival of both mother and neonate in a pregnancy complicated by cystic fibrosis, cor pulmonale, and end-stage respiratory failure. *Pancreatic dysfunction* may cause poor maternal nutrition.

Cystic fibrosis per se is not affected by pregnancy (Edenborough, 2001). Early reports of a deleterious effect on the course of cystic fibrosis were related to severe disease (Olson, 1997). An important factor to be considered in childbearing is the long-term prognosis for the mother. Goss and colleagues (2003) matched a cohort of pregnant and nonpregnant women by disease severity and reported that pregnancy had no deleterious effects on long-term survival.

MANAGEMENT. Prepregnancy counseling is imperative, and it is discussed further in Chapter 7, p. 193. Women who choose to become pregnant should have close surveillance for development of superimposed infection, diabetes, and heart failure. They are followed closely with serial pulmonary function testing, both for management as well as for prognosis. When the FEV_1 is at least 70 percent, women usually tolerate pregnancy well. Emphasis is placed on postural drainage and bronchodilator therapy. Inhaled recombinant human deoxyribonuclease I improves lung function by reducing sputum viscosity (Olson, 1997). Nutritional status is assessed and appropriate dietary counseling given. Pancreatic insufficiency is treated with replacement of oral pancreatic enzyme.

Currently, it is debatable whether prophylactic antistaphylococcal or antipseudomonal antimicrobials should be given. *Pseudomonas* is most problematic in adults. Inhaled tobramycin and colistin have been used successfully to cover this organism (Ratjen and Döring, 2003).

Immediate hospitalization and aggressive therapy is warranted for pulmonary infections. The threshold for hospitalization with other complications is low. For labor and delivery, epidural analgesia is recommended.

PREGNANCY OUTCOME. Cohen and colleagues (1980) conducted the first major survey of cystic fibrosis centers. At that time, severity was assessed by the *Schwachman–Kulezycki* or *Taussig* scores based on radiological and clinical criteria. Although pregnancy outcomes were not disastrous, 18 percent of 129 women died within 2 years of giving birth. In a later review of information through 1991, Kent and Farquharson (1993) described similar outcomes in 215 pregnancies in 160 women.

More recent reports describe better outcomes, but there still are serious complications. Severity of disease is now quantified by pulmonary function studies, which are the best predictor of pregnancy and long-term maternal outcome. Edenborough and colleagues (1995, 2000) reported 69 pregnancies from 11 cystic fibrosis centers in the United Kingdom. If prepregnancy FEV_1 was less than 60 percent of predicted, there was substantive risk of preterm delivery, respiratory complications, and death of the mother within a few years of childbirth.

FitzSimmons and co-workers (1996) performed a case-control study of 258 women with cystic fibrosis who had a live birth. The 889 matched controls were women with cystic fibrosis who had not been pregnant. Pregnancy had no effect on worsening of any serious complications, and 8 percent in both groups had died by 2 years. In the report by Goss and collaborators (2003) cited before, pregnancy was not harmful in matched cohorts whose FEV_1 was less than 40 percent. Gillet and co-workers (2002) reported 75 pregnancies from the French Cystic Fibrosis Registry. Almost 20 percent of infants were delivered preterm, and 30 percent had growth restriction. The one maternal death was due to pseudomonal sepsis in a woman whose FEV_1 was 60 percent prior to pregnancy. Importantly, 13 women (17 percent) had died by the end of the study, and four infants had confirmed cystic fibrosis.

CARBON MONOXIDE POISONING

Carbon monoxide is a ubiquitous gas, and most nonsmoking adults have a carbon monoxyhemoglobin saturation of 1 to 3 percent. In cigarette smokers, levels may be as high as 5 to 10 percent. Carbon monoxide causes half of all deaths from poisoning in developed countries (Greingor and associates, 2001; Raub and co-workers, 2000). Toxic levels are frequently encountered in inadequately ventilated areas warmed by space heaters.

Carbon monoxide is particularly toxic because it is odorless and tasteless and it has a high affinity for hemoglobin binding. Thus, it displaces oxygen and impedes its transfer with resultant hypoxia. Besides acute sequelae including death and anoxic encephalopathy, cognitive defects develop in as many as half of patients following loss of consciousness or with carbon monoxide levels greater than 25 percent (Weaver and colleagues, 2002).

PREGNANCY AND CARBON MONOXIDE POISONING. Through a number of physiological alterations, the rate of endogenous carbon monoxide production almost doubles in normal pregnancy (Longo, 1977). Although the pregnant woman is not more susceptible to carbon monoxide poisoning, the fetus does not tolerate excessive exposure.

With chronic exposure, maternal symptoms usually appear when the carboxyhemoglobin concentration is 5 to 20 percent. Symptoms include headache, weakness, dizziness, physical and visual impairment, palpitations, and nausea and vomiting. With acute exposure, concentrations of 30 to 50 percent produce symptoms of impending cardiovascular collapse. Levels over 50 percent may be fatal for the mother.

Because hemoglobin F has an even higher affinity for carbon monoxide, fetal carboxyhemoglobin levels are 10 to 15 percent higher than those in the mother. This may be due to facilitated diffusion (Longo, 1977). Importantly, the half-life of carboxyhemoglobin is 2 hours in the mother but 7 hours in the fetus. Because carbon monoxide is bound so tightly to hemoglobin F, the fetus may be hypoxic even before maternal carbon monoxide levels are appreciably elevated. A number of anomalies are associated with embryonic exposure, and anoxic encephalopathy is the primary sequela of later fetal exposure (Aubard and Magne, 2000).

TREATMENT. In all persons, treatment of carbon monoxide poisoning is supportive along with immediate administration of 100-percent inspired oxygen. Indications for hyperbaric oxygen treatment in nonpregnant individuals are unclear (Ernst and Zibrak, 1998). Weaver and co-workers (2002) recently reported that hyperbaric oxygen treatment minimized the incidence of cognitive defects at both 6 weeks and 1 year when compared with that of normobaric oxygen.

Hyperbaric oxygen is generally recommended in pregnancy if there has been "significant" carbon monoxide exposure (Aubard and Magne, 2000; Ernst and Zibrak, 1998). The problem is how to define significant exposure. Although maternal carbon monoxide levels are not accurately predictive of those in the fetus, some clinicians recommend hyperbaric therapy if maternal levels exceed 15 to 20 percent.

Elkharrat and colleagues (1991) reported successful hyperbaric treatments in 44 pregnant women. Silverman and Montano (1997) reported successful management of a woman whose abnormal neurological and cardiopulmonary findings abated in a parallel fashion with the associated fetal heart rate variable decelerations. Greingor and colleagues (2001) used 2.5-atm hyperbaric 100-percent oxygen for 90 minutes in a 21-week pregnant woman who was delivered of a healthy infant at term.

Locations of the nearest decompression chambers are available through the Divers Alert Network at Duke University (919-684-8111).

REFERENCES

Adhikari M, Pillay T, Pillay DG: Tuberculosis in the newborn: An emerging disease. Pediatr Infect Dis J 16:1108, 1997

Agha FP, Vade A, Amendola MA, et al: Effects of pregnancy on sarcoidosis. Surg Gynecol Obstet 155:817, 1982

Ahmad H, Mehta NJ, Manikal VM, et al: Pneumocystis carinii pneumonia in pregnancy. Chest 120:666, 2001

Alexander S, Dodds L, Armson BA: Perinatal outcomes in women with asthma during pregnancy. Obstet Gynecol 92:435, 1998

American Academy of Pediatrics and the American College of Obstetricians and Gynecologists: Guidelines for Perinatal Care, 5th ed. 2002, p 91

American College of Obstetricians and Gynecologists: Influenza vaccination and treatment during pregnancy. Committee Opinion No. 305, November 2004

American College of Obstetricians and Gynecologists: Immunization during pregnancy. Committee Opinion No. 282, January 2003

American College of Obstetricians and Gynecologists: Preconception and prenatal carrier screening for cystic fibrosis. Clinical and laboratory guidelines. Washington, DC, 2001

American College of Obstetricians and Gynecologists: Perinatal viral and parasitic infections. Practice Bulletin No. 20, September 2000

American College of Obstetricians and Gynecologists, American College of Allergy, Asthma, and Immunology: The use of newer asthma and allergy medications during pregnancy. Ann Allergy Asthma Immunol 84:475, 2000

American Thoracic Society: Guidelines for the management of adults with community-acquired pneumonia. Diagnosis, assessment of severity, initial antimicrobial therapy, and prevention. Am J Respir Crit Care Med 163:1730, 2001

American Thoracic Society/Centers for Disease Control and Prevention: Diagnostic standards and classification of tuberculosis. Am Rev Respir Dis 142:725, 1990

Anderson GD: Tuberculosis in pregnancy. Semin Perinatol 21:328, 1997

Arsura EL, Kilgore WB, Ratnayake SN: Erythema nodosum in pregnant patients with coccidioidomycosis. Clin Infect Dis 27:1201, 1998

Aubard Y, Magne I: Carbon monoxide poisoning in pregnancy. Br J Obstet Gynaecol 107:833, 2000

Aurora P, Whitehead B, Wade A, et al: Lung transplantation and life extension in children with cystic fibrosis. Lancet 354:1594, 1999

Barth WH, Hankins GDV: Severe acute asthma in pregnancy. In Clark SL, Cotton DB, Hankins GDV, Phelan JP (eds): Critical Care Obstetrics, 2nd ed. Oxford, Blackwell, 1991, p 371

Baughman RP, Lower EE, du Bois RM: Sarcoidosis. Lancet 361:1111, 2003

Berg CJ, Chang J, Callaghan WM, et al: Pregnancy-related mortality in the United States, 1991–1997. Obstet Gynecol 101:289, 2003

Blais L, Suissa S, Boivin JF, et al: First treatment with inhaled corticosteroids and the prevention of admissions to hospital for asthma. Thorax 53:1025, 1998

Bloom SL, Ramin S, Cunningham FG: A prediction rule for community-acquired pneumonia. N Engl J Med 336: 1913, 1997

Bogaert D, De Groot R, Hermans PW: Streptococcus pneumoniae colonisation: The key to pneumococcal disease. Lancet Infect Dis 4:144, 2004

Boggess KA, Myers ER, Hamilton CD: Antepartum or postpartum isoniazid treatment of latent tuberculosis infection. Obstet Gynecol 96:747, 2000

Bothamley G: Drug treatment for tuberculosis during pregnancy: Safety considerations. Drug Saf 24:553, 2001

Boyd JM, Mehta A, Murphy DJ: Fertility and pregnancy outcomes in men and women with cystic fibrosis in the United Kingdom. Hum Reprod 19:2238, 1999

Bracken MB, Triche EW, Belanger K, et al: Asthma symptoms, severity, and drug therapy: A prospective study of effects on 2205 pregnancies. Obstet Gynecol 102:739, 2003

Braman SS, Kaemmerlen JT: Intensive care of status asthmaticus. A 10-year experience. JAMA 264:366, 1990

Brancazio LR, Laifer SA, Schwartz T: Peak expiratory flow rate in normal pregnancy. Obstet Gynecol 89:383, 1997

Briggs GG, Freeman RK, Yaffe SJ (eds): Drugs in Pregnancy and Lactation, 6th ed. Baltimore, Williams & Wilkins, 2002

Briggs RG, Mabie WC, Sibai BM: Community-acquired pneumonia in pregnancy. Am J Obstet Gynecol 174:389, 1996

Brost BC, Newman RB: The maternal and fetal effects of tuberculosis therapy. Obstet Gynecol Clin North Am 24:659, 1997

Caldwell JW, Asura EL, Kilgore WB, et al: Coccidioidomycosis in pregnancy during an epidemic in California. Obstet Gynecol 95:236, 2000

Cameron AJ, Skinner TA: Management of a parturient with respiratory failure secondary to cystic fibrosis. Anaesthesia 60:77, 2005

Cantwell MF, Shehab ZM, Costello AM, et al: Congenital tuberculosis. N Engl J Med 330:1051, 1994

Cardonick EH, Naktin J, Berghella V: Neurosarcoidosis diagnosed during pregnancy by thoracoscopic lymph node biopsy. J Reprod Med 45:585, 2000

Centers for Disease Control and Prevention: Asthma prevalence and control characteristics by race/ethnicity—United States, 2002. MMWR 53:145, 2004a

Centers for Disease Control and Prevention: Influenza antiviral medications: 2004–05 interim chemoprophylaxis and treatment guidelines, 2004b http://www.cdc.gov/flu/professionals/treatment

Centers for Disease Control and Prevention: Prevention and control of influenza. Recommendations of the Advisory Committee on Immunization Practices (ACIP). MMWR 53:10, 2004c

Centers for Disease Control and Prevention: Guidelines for using the QuantiFERON®-TB Test for diagnosing latent mycobacterium tuberculosis infection. MMWR 52:(RR-2):15, 2003a

Centers for Disease Control and Prevention: Prevention and control of influenza. Recommendations of the Advisory Committee on Immunization Practices (ACIP). MMWR 32:8, 2003b

Centers for Disease Control and Prevention: Treatment of tuberculosis. American Thoracic Society, CDC, and Infection Disease Society of America. MMWR 52:RR1, 2003c

Centers for Disease Control and Prevention: Trends in tuberculosis morbidity—United States, 2003. MMWR 52:217, 2003d

Centers for Disease Control and Prevention: Update: Severe acute respiratory syndrome—United States, 2003. MMWR 52:388, 2003e

Centers for Disease Control and Prevention: Using live, attenuated influenza vaccine for prevention and control of influenza. Supplemental recommendations of the Advisory Committee on Immunization Practices (ACIP). MMWR 52:1, 2003f

Centers for Disease Control and Prevention: Guidelines for preventing opportunistic infections among HIV-infected persons—United States, 2002. MMWR 51:RR-8:4, 2002a

Centers for Disease Control and Prevention: Summary of notifiable diseases—United States, 2000. MMWR 49:IX, 2002b

Centers for Disease Control and Prevention: Resistance of Streptococcus pneumoniae to fluoroquinolones—United States, 1995–1999. MMWR 50:200, 2001

Centers for Disease Control: Screening for tuberculosis and tuberculous infection in high-risk populations. Recommendations of the Advisory Committee for Elimination of Tuberculosis. MMWR 39:1, 1990

Cohen LF, di Sant Agnese PA, Friedlander J: Cystic fibrosis and pregnancy: A national survey. Lancet 2:842, 1980

Couch RB: Prevention and treatment of influenza. N Engl J Med 343:1778, 2000

Crystal RG: Sarcoidosis. In Braunwald E, Fauci AS, Kasper DL, Hauser SL, Longo DL, Jaimeson JL (eds): Harrison's Principles of Internal Medicine, 15th ed. New York, McGraw-Hill, 2001, p 1969

Cydulka RK, Emerman CL, Schreiber D, et al: Acute asthma among pregnant women presenting to the emergency department. Am J Respir Crit Care Med 160:887, 1999

Demissie K, Breckenridge M, Rhoads G: Infant and maternal outcomes in the pregnancies of asthmatic women. Am J Respir Crit Care Med 158:1091, 1998

de Regt RH: Sarcoidosis and pregnancy. Obstet Gynecol 70:369, 1987

de Swiet M: The respiratory system. In Hytten F, Chamberlain G (eds): Clinical Physiology in Obstetrics, 2nd ed. London, Blackwell, 1991, p 83

Dombrowski MP, Schatz M, Wise R, et al: Asthma during pregnancy. Obstet Gynecol 103:5, 2004a

Dombrowski MP, Schatz M, Wise R, et al: Randomized trial of inhaled beclomethasone diprorionate versus theophylline for moderate asthma during pregnancy. Am J Obstet Gynecol 190:737, 2004b

Drosten C, Günther S, Preiser W, et al: Identification of a novel coronavirus in patients with severe acute respiratory syndrome. N Engl J Med 348:1967, 2003

Ducharme FM: Anti-leukotrienes as add-on therapy to inhaled glucocorticoids in patients with asthma: Systematic review of current evidence. BMJ 324:1545, 2002

Edenborough FP: Women with cystic fibrosis and their potential for reproduction. Thorax 56:648, 2001

Edenborough FP, Mackenzie WE, Stableforth DE: The outcome of 72 pregnancies in 55 women with cystic fibrosis in the United Kingdom 1977–1996. Br J Obstet Gynaecol 107:254, 2000

Edenborough FP, Stableforth DE, Webb AK, et al: The outcome of pregnancy in cystic fibrosis. Thorax 50:170, 1995

Elkharrat D, Raphael JC, Korach JM, et al: Acute carbon monoxide intoxication and hyperbaric oxygen in pregnancy. Intensive Care Med 17:289, 1991

Ely EW, Peacock JE, Haponik EF, et al: Cryptococcal pneumonia complicating pregnancy. Medicine 77:153, 1998

Ernst A, Zibrak JD: Carbon monoxide poisoning. N Engl J Med 339:1603, 1998

Espinal MA, Laszlo A, Simonsen L, et al: Global trends in resistance to antituberculosis drugs. N Engl J Med 344:1294, 2001

Figueroa-Damian R, Arrendondo-Garcia JL: Pregnancy and tuberculosis: Influence of treatment on perinatal outcome. Am J Perinatol 15:303, 1998

Finland M, Dublin TD: Pneumococcic pneumonias complicating pregnancy and the puerperium. JAMA 112:1027, 1939

Fitzsimmons SC, Fitzpatrick S, Thompson D, et al: A longitudinal study of the effects of pregnancy on 325 women with cystic fibrosis. Ped Pulmonol 13:99, 1996

Gazmararian JA, Petersen R, Jamieson DJ, et al: Hospitalizations during pregnancy among managed care enrollees. Obstet Gynecol 100:94, 2002

Geng E, Kreiswirth B, Driver C, et al: Changes in the transmission of tuberculosis in New York City from 1990 to 1999. N Engl J Med 346:1453, 2002

Gillet D, de Brackeleer M, Bellis G, et al: Cystic fibrosis and pregnancy. Report from French data (1980–1999). Br J Obstet Gynaecol 109:912, 2002

Gilljam M, Antoniou M, Shin J, et al: Pregnancy in cystic fibrosis: Fetal and maternal outcome. Chest 118:85, 2000

Goss CH, Rubenfeld GD, Otto K, et al: The effect of pregnancy on survival in women with cystic fibrosis. Chest 124:1460, 2003

Greingor JL, Tosi JM, Ruhlmann S, et al: Acute carbon monoxide intoxication during pregnancy. One case report and review of the literature. Emerg Med J 18:399, 2001

Haines CJ, Chu YW, Chung TK: The effect of severe acute respiratory syndrome on a hospital obstetrics and gynaecology service. Br J Obstet Gynaecol 110:643, 2003

Halm EA, Teirstein AS: Management of community-acquired pneumonia. N Engl J Med 347:2039, 2002

Hankins GDV, Berryman GK, Scott RT, et al: Maternal arterial desaturation with 15-methyl prostaglandin F2 alpha for uterine atony. Obstet Gynecol 72:367, 1988

Hansen WF, Yankowitz J: Pharmacologic therapy for medical disorders during pregnancy. Clin Obstet Gynecol 45:136, 2002

Harger JH, Ernest JM, Thurnau GR, et al: Risk factors and outcome of varicella-zoster virus pneumonia in pregnant women. J Infect Dis 185:422, 2002

Harris JW: Influenza occurring in pregnant women. JAMA 72:978, 1919

Hartert TV, Neuzil KM, Shintani AK, et al: Maternal morbidity and perinatal outcomes among pregnant women with respiratory hospitalizations during influenza season. Am J Obstet Gynecol 189:1705, 2003

Hayden FG, Atmar RL, Schilling M, et al: Use of the selective oral neuraminidase inhibitor oseltamivir to prevent influenza. N Engl J Med 341:1336, 1999

Holmes KV: SARS-associated coronavirus. N Engl J Med 348:1948, 2003

Jacobs RF, Abernathy RS: Management of tuberculosis in pregnancy and the newborn. Clin Perinatol 15:305, 1988

Jana N, Vasishta K, Jindal SK, et al: Perinatal outcome in pregnancies complicated by pulmonary tuberculosis. Int J Gynecol Obstet 44:119, 1994

Jana N, Vasishta K, Saha SC, et al: Obstetrical outcomes among women with extrapulmonary tuberculosis. N Engl J Med 341:645, 1999

Jenkins TM, Troiano NH, Grave CR, et al: Mechanical ventilation in an obstetric population: Characteristics and delivery rates. Am J Obstet Gynecol 188:549, 2003

Jin Y, Carriere KC, Marrie TJ, et al: The effects of community-acquired pneumonia during pregnancy ending with a live birth. Am J Obstet Gynecol 188:800, 2003

Kashyap S, Gruslin A: Influenza vaccination during pregnancy. Prim Care Update Ob/Gyns 7:7, 2000

Kent NE, Farquharson DF: Cystic fibrosis in pregnancy. Can Med Assoc J 149:809, 1993

Kruszka SJ, Gherman RB: Successful pregnancy outcome in a lung transplant recipient with tacrolimus immunosuppression. A case report. J Reprod Med 47:60, 2002

Ksiazek TG, Erdman D, Goldsmith CS, et al: A novel coronavirus associated with severe acute respiratory syndrome. N Engl J Med 348:1953, 2003

Kwon HL, Belanger K, Bracken MB: Asthma prevalence among pregnant and childbearing-aged women in the United States: Estimates from national health surveys. Ann Epidemiol 13:317, 2003

Laibl V, Sheffield J, Roberts S, et al: Presentation of influenza A in pregnancy during the 2003–2004 influenza season. Presented at the 25th Annual Meeting of the Society for Maternal-Fetal Medicine, Reno, Nevada, February 7–12, 2005

Lam CM, Wong SF, Leung TN, et al: A case-controlled study comparing clinical course and outcomes of pregnant and nonpregnant women with severe acute respiratory syndrome. BJOG 111:771, 2004

Lange P, Parner J, Vestbo J, et al: A 15-year follow-up study of ventilatory function in adults with asthma. N Engl J Med 339:1194, 1998

Lessnau KD, Qarah S: Multidrug-resistant tuberculosis in pregnancy: Case report and review of the literature. Chest 123:953, 2003

Lim WS, Macfarlane JT, Boswell TC, et al: Study of community acquired pneumonia etiology (SCAPA) in adults admitted to hospital: Implications for management guidelines. Thorax 56:296, 2001a

Lim WS, Macfarlane JT, Colthorpe CL: Pneumonia and pregnancy. Thorax 56:398, 2001b

Limosin F, Rouillon F, Payan C, et al: Prenatal exposure to influenza as a risk factor for adult schizophrenia. Acta Psychiatr Scand 107:331, 2003

Liu S, Wen SW, Demissie K, et al: Maternal asthma and pregnancy outcomes: A retrospective cohort study. Am J Obstet Gynecol 184:90, 2001

Llewelyn M, Cropley I, Wilkinson RJ, et al: Tuberculosis diagnosed during pregnancy: A prospective study from London. Thorax 55:129, 2000

Longo L: The biologic effects of carbon monoxide on the pregnant woman, fetus and newborn infant. Am J Obstet Gynecol 129:69, 1977

Mabie WC, Barton JR, Wasserstrum N, et al: Clinical observations on asthma in pregnancy. J Matern Fetal Med 1:45, 1992

Maisel JA, Lynam T: Unexpected sudden death in a young pregnant woman: Unusual presentation of neurosarcoidosis. Ann Emerg Med 28:94, 1996

Mandell LA, Bartlett JG, Dowell SF, et al: Update of practice guidelines for the management of community-aquired pneumonia in immunocompetent adults. Clin Infect Dis 37:1405, 2003

Margono F, Mroueh J, Garely A, et al: Resurgence of active tuberculosis among pregnant women. Obstet Gynecol 83:911, 1994

McGrath J, Castle D: Does influenza cause schizophrenia? A five year review. Aust N Z J Psychiatry 29:23, 1995

McKone EF, Emerson SS, Edwards KL, et al: Effect of genotype on phenotype and mortality in cystic fibrosis: A retrospective cohort study. Lancet 361:1671, 2003

MIST (Management of Influenza in the Southern Hemisphere Trialists) Study Group: Randomized trial of efficacy and safety of inhaled zanamivir in treatment of influenza A and B virus infections. Lancet 352:1877, 1998

Mora-Duarte J, Betts R, Rotstein C, et al: Comparison of caspofungin and amphotericin B for invasive candidiasis. N Engl J Med 347:2020, 2002

Munn MB, Groome LJ, Atterbury JL, et al: Pneumonia as a complication of pregnancy. J Matern Fetal Med 8:151, 1999

Namazy JA, Schatz M: Pregnancy and asthma: Recent developments. Curr Opin Pulm Med 11:56, 2005

Nanda S, Agarwal U, Sangwan K: Complete resolution of cervical spinal tuberculosis with paraplegia in pregnancy. Acta Obstet Gynecol Scand 81:569, 2002

Nathwani D, Maclean A, Conway S, et al: Varicella infections in pregnancy and the newborn. J Infect 36:59, 1998

National Asthma Education and Prevention Program Expert Panel Report 2: Guidelines for the diagnosis and management of asthma. NHLBI, NIH Publication No. 97-4051, April 1997

National Heart, Lung and Blood Institute: Report of the Working Group on Asthma and Pregnancy: Executive Summary: Management of Asthma During Pregnancy. National Asthma Education Program: NIH publication 93-3279A, March 1993

Neill AM, Nelson-Piercy C: Hazards of assisted conception in women with severe medical disease. Hum Fertil 4:239, 2001

Nelson-Piercy C: Asthma in pregnancy. Thorax 56:325, 2001

Neuzil KM, Reed GW, Mitchel EF, et al: Impact of influenza on acute cardiopulmonary hospitalizations in pregnant women. Am J Epidemiol 148:1094, 1998

Niederman MS: Review of treatment guidelines for community-acquired pneumonia. Am J Med 117:51S, 2004

Noble PW, Lavee AE, Jacobs NM: Respiratory diseases in pregnancy. Obstet Gynecol Clin North Am 15:391, 1988

Olson GL: Cystic fibrosis in pregnancy. Semin Perinatol 21:307, 1997

Ormerod P: Tuberculosis in pregnancy and the puerperium. Thorax 56:494, 2001

Paramothayan S, Jones PW: Corticosteroid therapy in pulmonary sarcoidosis. A systematic review. JAMA 287:1301, 2002

Pillay T, Khan M, Moodley J, et al: Perinatal tuberculosis and HIV-1: Considerations for resource-limited settings. Lancet Infect Dis 4:155, 2004

Prevost MR, Fung Kee Fung KM: Tuberculous meningitis in pregnancy—implications for mother and fetus: Case report and literature review. J Matern Fetal Med 8:289, 1999

Ramsey PS, Maddox DE, Ramin KD, et al: Asthma: Impact on maternal morbidity and adverse perinatal outcome [abstract]. Obstet Gynecol 101:40S, 2003

Ratjen F, Döring G: Cystic fibrosis. Lancet 361:681, 2003.

Raub JA, Mathieu-Nolf M, Hampson NB, et al: Carbon monoxide poisoning—a public health perspective. Toxicology 145:1, 2000

Richey SD, Roberts SW, Ramin KD, et al: Pneumonia complicating pregnancy. Obstet Gynecol 84:525, 1994

Rodgers HC, Knox AJ, Toplis PH, et al: Successful pregnancy and birth after IVF in a woman with cystic fibrosis. Human Reprod 15:2152, 2000

Rolston DH, Shnider SM, de Lorimer AA: Uterine blood flow and fetal acid–base changes after bicarbonate administration to the pregnant ewe. Anesthesiology 40:348, 1974

Rosenstein NE, Emery KW, Werner SB, et al: Risk factors for severe pulmonary and disseminated coccidioidomycosis: Kern County, California, 1995–1996. Clin Infect Dis 32:708, 2001

Schatz M: The efficacy and safety of asthma medications during pregnancy. Semin Perinatol 25:145, 2001

Schatz M, Dombrowski MP, Wise R, et al: Asthma morbidity during pregnancy can be predicted by severity classification. J Allergy Clin Immunol 112:283, 2003

Schatz M, Harden K, Forsythe A, et al: The course of asthma during pregnancy, postpartum, and with successive pregnancies: A prospective analysis. J Allergy Clin Immunol 81:509, 1988

Schulte JM, Bryan P, Dodds S, et al: Tuberculosis skin testing among HIV-infected pregnant women in Miami, 1995 to 1996. J Perinatol 22:159, 2002

Seballos RJ, Mendel SG, Mirmiran-Yazdy A, et al: Sarcoid cardiomyopathy precipitated by pregnancy with cocaine complications. Chest 105:303, 1994

Selroos O: Sarcoidosis and pregnancy: A review with results of a retrospective survey. J Intern Med 227:221, 1990

Shapiro DS, Owen CA: ADAM-33 surfaces as an asthma gene. N Engl J Med 347:936, 2002

Sheffield J: The effect of active and passive cigarette smoke on pregnant women with asthma. Presented at the 25th Annual Meeting of the Society for Maternal-Fetal Medicine, Reno, Nevada, February 7–12, 2005

Sheffield J, Laibl V, Roberts S, et al: The efficacy and safety of influenza vaccination in pregnancy. Presented at the 25th Annual Meeting of the Society for Maternal-Fetal Medicine, Reno, Nevada, February 7–12, 2005

Shek CC, Ng PC, Fung GP, et al: Infants born to mothers with severe acute respiratory syndrome. Pediatrics 112:e254, 2003

Shin S, Guerra D, Rich M, et al: Treatment of multidrug-resistant tuberculosis during pregnancy: A report of 7 cases. Clin Infect Dis 36:996, 2003

Silverman RK, Montano J: Hyperbaric oxygen treatment during pregnancy in acute carbon monoxide poisoning. A case report. J Reprod Med 42:309, 1997

Smego RA, Asperilla MO: Use of acyclovir for varicella pneumonia during pregnancy. Obstet Gynecol 78:1112, 1991

Smith KC: Congenital tuberculosis: A rare manifestation of a common infection. Curr Opin Infect Dis 15:269, 2002

Stenius-Aarniala B, Pririla P, Teramo K: Asthma and pregnancy: A prospective study of 198 pregnancies. Thorax 43:12, 1988

Stevens DA: Coccidioidomycosis. N Engl J Med 332:1077, 1995

Stratton P, Mofenson LM, Willoughby AD: Human immunodeficiency virus infection in pregnant women under care at AIDS Clinical Trials Centers in the United States. Obstet Gynecol 79:364, 1992

Tattersfield AE, Knox AJ, Britton JR, et al: Asthma. Lancet 360:1313, 2002

Thomas KW, Hunninghake GW: Sarcoidosis. JAMA 289:3300, 2003

Triche EW, Saftlas AF, Belanger K, et al: Association of asthma diagnosis, severity, symptoms, and treatment with risk of preeclampsia. Obstet Gynecol 104:585, 2004

Vázquez M, LaRussa PS, Gershon AA, et al: Effectiveness over time of varicella vaccine. JAMA 291:851, 2004

Ware LB, Matthay MA: The acute respiratory distress syndrome. N Engl J Med 342:1334, 2000

Weaver LK, Hopkins RO, Chan KJ, et al: Hyperbaric oxygen for acute carbon monoxide poisoning. N Engl J Med 347:1057, 2002

Weinberger SE, Weiss ST: Pulmonary diseases. In Duffy TP, Burrow GN (eds): Medical Complications During Pregnancy, 5th ed. Philadelphia, Saunders, 1999, p 363

Wendel PJ: Asthma in pregnancy. Obstet Gynecol Clin North Am 28:537, 2001

Wendel PJ, Ramin SM, Hamm CB, et al: Asthma treatment in pregnancy: A randomized controlled study. Am J Obstet Gynecol 175:150, 1996

Wenzel RP, Edmond MB: Managing SARS amidst uncertainty. N Engl J Med 348:1947, 2003

Wong SF, Chow KM, Leung TN, et al: Pregnancy and perinatal outcomes of women with severe acute respiratory syndrome. Am J Obsete Gynecol 191:292, 2004

Wong SF, Chow KM, de Swiet M: Severe acute respiratory syndrome and pregnancy. Br J Obstet Gynaecol 110:641, 2003

Yost NP, Bloom SL, Richey SD, et al: An appraisal of treatment guidelines for antepartum community-acquired pneumonia. Am J Obstet Gynecol 183:131, 2000

Zeeman GG, Wendel GD, Cunningham FG: A blueprint for obstetrical critical care. Am J Obstet Gynecol 188:532, 2003

47

Thromboembolic Disorders

Traditionally, the risk of venous thrombosis and pulmonary embolism in otherwise healthy women is considered highest during pregnancy and the puerperium. Indeed, the risk of venous thromboembolism has been estimated to be fivefold higher in women who are pregnant compared with those of similar age who are not (National Institutes of Health Consensus Development Conference, 1986; Melis and co-workers, 2004). Although the frequency of venous thromboembolic disease during the puerperium has decreased remarkably as early ambulation has become more widely practiced, pulmonary embolism still remains a prominent cause of maternal death in the United States (see Table 1–2, p. 8). In 2000 and 2001, thrombotic pulmonary embolism caused nearly 15 percent of the almost 800 pregnancy-related deaths in the United States (Arias and associates, 2003; Miniño and colleagues, 2002).

Shown in Table 47–1 are reported incidences of deep venous thrombosis and pulmonary embolism in more than 1.4 million pregnancies. The incidence of all thromboembolic events averages about 1 per 1000 pregnancies, and about an equal number are identified antepartum and in the puerperium. In about 15 percent of cases, pulmonary embolism either accompanies deep venous thrombosis or occurs de novo.

PATHOPHYSIOLOGY

In 1856, Rudolf Virchow postulated the conditions that predispose to the development of venous thrombosis: (1) stasis, (2) local trauma to the vessel wall, and (3) hypercoagulability. The risk for each increases during normal pregnancy. As discussed in Chapter 5 (see p. 134), compression of the pelvic veins and inferior vena cava by the enlarging uterus renders the venous system of the lower extremities particularly vulnerable to stasis. This stasis is the most constant predisposing risk factor for venous thrombosis. Venous stasis and delivery may also contribute to endothelial cell injury. In addition, there is endothelial activation with preeclampsia (see Chap. 34, p. 769). Lastly, marked increases in the synthesis of most clotting factors during pregnancy favor coagulation.

Several independent risk factors are associated with the development of thromboembolism during pregnancy. Salonen Ros and associates (2002) studied a population-based cohort of more than 1 million deliveries in Sweden. Compared with uncomplicated delivery, they calculated the relative risk of pulmonary embolism to be 4.8 with severe preeclampsia, 3.8 with cesarean delivery, 2.7 with diabetes, and 2.3 with multifetal gestation. Other risk factors include prior thromboembolism, age of 35 years or more, oral contraceptive use, orthopedic surgery, hypertension, cancer, obesity, smoking, superficial venous thrombosis, paraplegia, dehydration, infective and inflammatory illnesses, nephrotic syndrome, and immobility such as with long-distance travel or prolonged bed rest (Danilenko-Dixon and co-workers, 2001; Goldhaber and associates, 2004). A risk-scoring system to predict thromboembolism during pregnancy or postpartum has been described by Weiss and Bernstein (2000).

The risk of thrombosis during pregnancy is increased in women with associated genetic risk factors (Dilley and colleagues, 2000). It is now estimated that nearly half of—and in the future, perhaps all—patients with thrombosis have an identifiable underlying genetic disorder. Moreover, approximately 50 to 60 percent of patients with a hereditary basis for thrombosis, or a *thrombophilia*, do not experience a thrombotic event until one of the other risk factors is present (American College of Obstetricians and Gynecologists, 2000a).

THROMBOPHILIAS. Several important regulatory proteins act as inhibitors in the coagulation cascade. Inherited or acquired deficiencies of these inhibitory proteins are collectively referred to as thrombophilias, which can lead to hypercoagulability and recurrent venous thromboembolism. Although these disorders are collectively present in about 15 percent of white European populations, they are responsible for more than 50 percent of all thromboembolic events during pregnancy (Lockwood, 2002). Some aspects of the more common inherited thrombophilias and their sites of action are summarized in Table 47–2 and in Figure 47–1.

TABLE 47–1 Incidence of Thromboembolism in Pregnancy

| Study | Pregnancies | Deep Vein Thrombosis and Thromboembolism Incidence (per 1000 Pregnancies) | | | | Pulmonary Embolism | | |
		No.	Total	Antepartum	Postpartum	No.	Rate	AP/PP
Cunningham et al (1993)	35,000	20	0.57	0.48	0.09	4	1:9000	50/50
Andersen et al (1998)	63,300	78	1.23	0.75	0.50	2	1:31,000	NS
Gherman et al (1999)	268,500	165	0.61	0.35	0.26	38	1:7000	40/60
McColl et al (1999)	72,000	62	0.86	0.57	0.29	11	1:6500	50/50
Lindqvist et al (1999)	479,400	608	1.27	0.64	0.63	90	1:5300	50/50
Witlin et al (1999)	88,000	38	0.43	0.26	0.17	11	1:8000	50/50
Simpson et al (2001)	395,335	336	0.85	0.28	0.65	42	1:9400	65/35
Estimated averages	1,401,535	1307	0.93	0.48	0.37	198	1:7000	50/50

AP/PP = antepartum/postpartum incidence in percent; NS = not stated.

TABLE 47–2 Some Aspects of the More Common Inherited Thrombophilias

Thrombophilia	Genetics	Diagnosis	Prevalence (percent)	Increased Relative Risk of Venous Thromboembolism
Factor V Leiden	AD	DNA	2–15	3- to 8-fold
Prothrombin G20210A	AD	DNA	2–3	3-fold
Antithrombin	AD	Activity assay	0.02	25- to 50-fold
Protein C	AD	Activity assay	0.2–0.3	10- to 15-fold
Protein S	AD	Activity assay	0.1–2.1	2-fold
		If low, assess total and free antigen		
Hyperhomocysteinemia	AR	Fasting homocysteine level	11	2.5-fold (if > 18.5 μmol/L) 3- to 4-fold (if > 20 μmol/L)

AD = autosomal dominant; AR = autosomal recessive.
Modified from Lockwood (2002), with permission.

Information concerning these and other thrombophilias is accruing rapidly, causing some confusion in diagnosis and management. Generally, the adverse thrombogenic actions of most of these conditions are mitigated by anticoagulation with heparin or warfarin. Although thrombophilias are usually discovered in evaluation of an untoward event, their overall high incidence in healthy individuals leads to questions of the wisdom or necessity of giving anticoagulants to asymptomatic patients.

Antithrombin Deficiency. This protein, previously known as antithrombin III, is one of the most important inhibitors

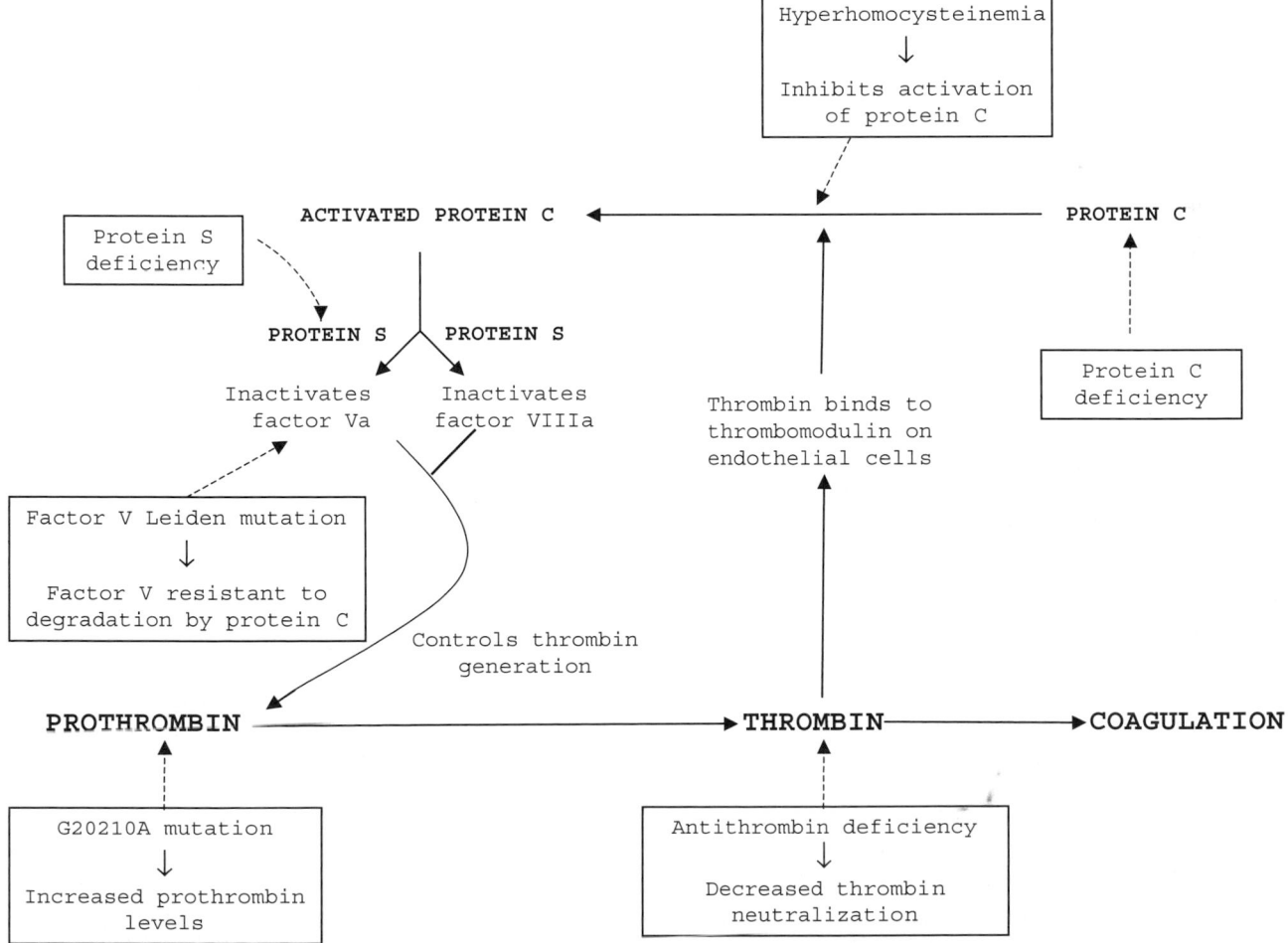

FIGURE 47–1. Overview of the inherited thrombophilias and their effect(s) on the coagulation cascade. (Adapted from Seligsohn and Lubetsky, 2001.)

of thrombin in clot formation (Weitz, 1997). Antithrombin deficiency may result from numerous mutations that are almost always autosomal dominant. Homozygous antithrombin deficiency is lethal (Katz, 2002).

Although antithrombin deficiency is rare, affecting as few as 1 in 5000 individuals, it is the most thrombogenic of the heritable coagulopathies. Indeed, the lifetime risk of thrombosis is 50 to 90 percent, with a 50- to 60-percent risk during pregnancy and a 33-percent risk during the puerperium (Eldor, 2001a; Lockwood, 2002). As shown in Table 47–3, antithrombin-deficient pregnant women are treated with adjusted-dose heparin prophylaxis regardless of whether a prior thrombosis has occurred. Heparin administration and dosing are further discussed on p. 1081.

Seguin and colleagues (1994) reviewed the outcomes of 23 newborns with antithrombin deficiency. There were 11 cases of thrombosis and 10 deaths.

Protein C Deficiency.
When thrombin is bound to thrombomodulin on endothelial cells of small vessels, its procoagulant activities are neutralized. It also activates protein C, a natural anticoagulant, that in the presence of protein S controls thrombin generation by inactivating factors Va and VIIIa (Fig. 47–1). Protein C levels are unchanged during normal pregnancy, and this itself predisposes to coagulation (Faught and colleagues, 1995).

More than 160 different protein C gene mutations have been described. The prevalence of protein C deficiency is 2 to 5 per 1000, and inheritance is autosomal dominant (Lockwood, 2002). Approximately half of heterozygotes suffer venous thrombotic episodes by adulthood. The risk of thromboembolism in pregnant women with protein C deficiency is between 3 and 20 percent, and most episodes occur during the puerperium (Eldor, 2001a; Lockwood, 2002).

Protein S Deficiency.
This circulating anticoagulant is activated by protein C to decrease thrombin generation. Protein S deficiency is measured by antigenically determined free, functional, and total S levels. All three of these levels decline substantively during normal pregnancy, in some cases by 50 percent (Lefkowitz and colleagues, 1996; Lockwood, 2002). Protein S deficiency is caused by one of several autosomal dominant mutations with an aggregate prevalence of about 0.8 per 1000 (Lockwood, 2002). There are three types of deficiency that correlate with correspondingly decreased free, functional, or total protein S levels. Because pregnancy results in a decrease in all three levels, diagnosis of protein S deficiency during pregnancy is difficult.

The lifetime risk of thromboembolism in patients with protein S deficiency is about 50 percent (Allaart and associates, 1993). The risk during pregnancy may be as high as 6 percent, and as with protein C deficiency, the risk is even higher (up to 22 percent) during the puerperium (Eldor, 2001b). Conard and colleagues (1990) described thrombosis in 5 of 29 pregnant women with this deficiency. One woman had a cerebral

vein thrombosis. Burneo and associates (2002) reported cerebral venous thrombosis at 14 weeks. Neonatal homozygous protein C or S deficiency is usually associated with a severe clinical phenotype known as *purpura fulminans*, which is characterized by extensive thromboses in the microcirculation soon after birth (Salonvaara and colleagues, 2004).

TREATMENT OF PROTEIN C OR S DEFICIENCY. According to the American College of Obstetricians and Gynecologists (2000b), it is not clear whether pregnant women with a history of thrombosis who have protein C or protein S deficiency should be given low-dose or adjusted-dose heparin prophylaxis. Toglia and Weg (1996) recommend antepartum subcutaneous heparin and warfarin given postpartum for 6 weeks.

Activated Protein C Resistance (Factor V Leiden Mutation).
The most prevalent of the known thrombophilic syndromes, this condition is characterized by resistance of plasma to the anticoagulant effects of activated protein C. The most common cause is the factor V Leiden mutation, which was named after the city where it was described. This missense mutation in the factor V gene results in a substitution of glutamine for arginine at position 506 in the factor V polypeptide, which confers resistance to degradation by activated protein C (Kalafatis and colleagues, 1994). The unimpeded abnormal factor V protein retains its procoagulant activity and predisposes to thrombosis (see Fig. 47–1).

Heterozygosity for factor V Leiden mutation is found in 20 to 40 percent of nonpregnant individuals with thromboembolic disease. Homozygous inheritance of two aberrant copies is rare and increases the risk of thrombosis by more than 100-fold (Lockwood, 2002).

Resistance to activated protein C is measured by bioassay (Bloomenthal and colleagues, 2002). As discussed in Chapter 5 (see p. 132), however, resistance is normally increased after the first trimester due to alterations in other coagulation proteins (Walker and associates, 1997). Thus, during pregnancy, DNA analysis for the factor V Leiden mutation is used instead. Activated protein C resistance can also be caused by the antiphospholipid syndrome as well as other genetic defects in the factor V molecule (Eldor, 2001b).

The Maternal–Fetal Medicine Units Network recently reported a prospective observational study of the factor V Leiden mutation in nearly 5200 pregnant women (Dizon-Townson, 2002b). The heterozygous carrier incidence was 2.7 percent. Of the three pulmonary emboli and one deep venous thrombosis (0.8 per 1000 pregnancies), none occurred among these carriers. There was no increased risk of preeclampsia, placental abruption, or fetal growth restriction in heterozygous women. The investigators concluded that universal prenatal screening for the Leiden mutation and prophylaxis for carriers without a prior venous thromboembolism are not indicated. Clark and colleagues (2002) concluded that routine screening of pregnant women was not cost effective. Women who are *homozygous* for the factor

TABLE 47–3 Recommended Options for Treatment of Venous Thromboembolism During Pregnancy and Postpartum

Clinical Scenario	Pregnancy	Postpartum
VTE develops during pregnancy	Intravenous unfractionated heparin × 5–7 days followed by subcutaneous adjusted-dose therapy for the remainder of the pregnancy.[a,b] Alternatively, after 3 months[a] or 4 months[c] of adjusted-dose treatment, low-dose therapy may be used for the remainder of the pregnancy.	Warfarin 6–18 weeks (shorter for distal leg thrombosis; longer for iliofemoral or pulmonary thrombosis)[c]
	Adjusted-dose low-molecular-weight heparin throughout pregnancy[a,b]	Warfarin for at least 6 weeks[b]
History of a thrombophilia other than AT deficiency, FVL homozygous, G20210A homozygous, or FVL/G20210A heterozygote AND		
No prior VTE	Surveillance only[b,c] or low-dose prophylaxis[b] or low-dose prophylaxis if strong family history[a]	Warfarin for 6 weeks[b]
		Warfarin for 4–6 weeks if cesarean delivery or affected first-degree relative[c]
Prior VTE	Low-dose prophylaxis[a,c]	Warfarin for 4–6 weeks[c] unless on long-term therapy[b]
	Consider adjusted-dose prophylaxis with protein C or S deficiency[a]	
	If prior VTE with history of thrombophilia in women not receiving long-term anticoagulation therapy, surveillance only or low-dose prophylaxis; use therapeutic prophylaxis with AT deficiency or more than two prior VTE episodes[b]	Low-dose heparin prophylaxis[a]
Regardless of history of VTE : AT deficiency FVL homozygous G20210A homozygous FVL/G20210A double heterozygous	Adjusted-dose prophylaxis throughout pregnancy[a,c] If no prior VTE, use surveillance only or low-dose prophylaxis; use adjusted-dose prophylaxis with AT deficiency[b]	Warfarin ≥ 6 weeks[a,b,c] Warfarin 3–6 months if prior VTE[c]
Prior VTE associated with a nonrecurring (transient) risk factor and no known thrombophilia	Surveillance only[b,c] Low-dose prophylaxis[a]	Warfarin for 6 weeks[a,b,c]
Prior idiopathic VTE related to pregnancy or OC use	Low-dose prophylaxis[a]	Low-dose heparin prophylaxis[a]
History of life-threatening thrombosis, recent thrombosis, recurrent thrombosis, or receiving chronic anticoagulation	Adjusted-dose prophylaxis[a]	Warfarin for 6 weeks[a]
Antiphospholipid syndrome:		
Prior VTE or recurrent pregnancy loss	Adjusted-dose prophylaxis[a,b]	Warfarin for 6 weeks[a]
No prior VTE, no prior recurrent pregnancy loss	Adjusted-dose[a] or low-dose prophylaxis[a,b] or surveillance only[b]	Warfarin for 6 weeks[a]
Hyperhomocysteinemia	Consider supplemental vitamin B_{12}, B_6, and folic acid. If prior VTE, consider low-dose prophylaxis if homocysteine levels are unresponsive to folic acid[c]	Warfarin for 6 weeks[a]

VTE = venous thromboembolism; AT = antithrombin; FVL = factor V Leiden; OC = oral contraceptive.

Postpartum women on adjusted-dose therapy should receive both heparin and warfarin therapy for the first 5–7 days postpartum until an INR of 2.0–3.0 has been achieved after which time the heparin may be discontinued.

Adjusted-dose subcutaneous regimens:
1. Unfractionated heparin (usually ≥ 10,000 U) given 2–3 times per day to achieve APTT prolongation of 1.5 to 2.5.[a]
2. Enoxaparin, 30–80 mg every 12 hours.[a]
3. Dalteparin, 5000–10,000 U every 12 hours.[a]
4. Weight-adjusted doses of enoxaparin (1 mg/kg every 12 hr) or dalteparin (200 U/kg every 24 hr).[b]
5. Weight-adjusted low-molecular-weight heparin wiith dose sufficient enough to achieve a peak anti–factor Xa level of 0.5–1.2 U/mL.[a]

Low-dose prophylactic subcutaneous regimens:
1. Unfractionated heparin, 5000–7500 U every 12 hr during the first trimester, 7500–10,000 U every 12 hr during the second trimester, 10,000 U every 12 hr during the third trimester unless the APTT is elevated.[a]
2. Unfractionated heparin, 5000–10,000 U every 12 hr throughout pregnancy.[a]
3. Enoxaparin, 40 mg once or twice daily.[a]
4. Dalteparin, 5000 U once or twice daily.[a]
5. Unfractionated heparin dosed twice daily to target anti–factor Xa activity 0.1–0.3 U/mL.[b]

[a] American College of Obstetricians and Gynecologists (2000b).
[b] American College of Chest Physicians (Ginsberg and colleagues, 2001).
[c] Lockwood (2002).

V Leiden mutation should be given adjusted-dose heparin prophylaxis during pregnancy (see Table 47–3).

Prothrombin G20210A Mutation.

This missense mutation in the prothrombin gene leads to excessive accumulation of prothrombin, which then may be converted to thrombin. Found in approximately 2 percent of the white population, it is extremely uncommon in nonwhites (Federman and Kirsner, 2001). The mutation is associated with a two- to threefold lifetime risk of thromboembolism (Dizon-Townson, 2002a). Case-control studies suggest that the relative risk of thromboembolism is increased 3- to 15-fold during pregnancy (Gerhardt and collaborators, 2000; Martinelli and colleagues, 2002). Homozygous women are given adjusted-dose heparin prophylaxis (see Table 47–3).

Patients who co-inherit a G20210A mutation with a factor V Leiden mutation have an increased risk of thromboembolism. Stefano and colleagues (1999) performed a retrospective cohort study of 624 nonpregnant patients with one prior episode of deep venous thrombosis. They found that those doubly heterozygous individuals had a 2.6-fold increased risk of recurrence relative to those with the Leiden mutation alone. They concluded that carriers of both mutations are candidates for lifelong anticoagulation after a first episode.

Hyperhomocysteinemia.

The thiol-containing amino acid homocysteine is produced from the demethylation of the essential amino acid methionine. Homocysteine is not used in protein synthesis; instead, it is involved in two major physiological pathways. One, it can be condensed with the amino acid serine in the presence of vitamin B_6 ultimately to form cysteine, which allows excretion of sulfur-containing compounds. Two, it can be remethylated back to methionine in a reaction requiring methyl donors from the folic acid pathway that uses vitamin B_{12} and methylenetetrahydrofolate (MTHF) as co-factors.

The most common cause of elevated homocysteine is the C667T thermolabile mutation of the enzyme 5,10-methylenetetrahydrofolate reductase, which impairs the generation of MTHF. Elevated levels of homocysteine may also result from deficiency of one of several enzymes involved in methionine metabolism and from correctible nutritional deficiencies of folic acid, vitamin B_6, or vitamin B_{12} (Hague, 2003; McDonald and Walker, 2001). Inheritance is autosomal recessive, and Kupferminc and associates (1999) found a homozygote prevalence of 8 percent in normally pregnant women.

High homocysteine concentrations activate factor V in endothelial cells, which inhibits the activation of protein C and leads to an increased risk of thrombosis (Mandel and associates, 1996). During pregnancy, the risk of thrombosis is increased two- to threefold (Villareal and colleagues, 2002). The co-inheritance of hyperhomocysteinemia with either the factor V Leiden or prothrombin G20210A mutation further increases the risk (Mandel and associates, 1996; Seligsohn and Lubetsky, 2001). Hyperhomocysteinemia also increases

the lifetime risk of premature atherosclerosis and fetal neural-tube defects (see Chap. 12, p. 302).

Hyperhomocysteinemia is diagnosed by elevated fasting homocysteine levels. During normal pregnancy, mean concentrations are decreased (López-Quesada and colleagues, 2003; McDonald and Walker, 2001). Lockwood (2002) recommends a fasting cutoff level of more than 12 μmol/L to define hyperhomocysteinemia during pregnancy. Low-dose prophylaxis is recommended in women who have had a prior venous thromboembolism (see Table 47–3).

ANTIPHOSPHOLIPID ANTIBODIES. These autoantibodies are detected in about 2 percent of patients who have nontraumatic venous thrombosis. As described in Chapter 54 (see p. 1215), they are commonly found in systemic lupus erythematosus. Patients with moderate-to-high levels of these antibodies may have *antiphospholipid syndrome,* which is associated with a number of clinical features, including venous and arterial thromboembolism. Although arterial thromboembolism most commonly involves the lower extremities, the syndrome should be considered in women with thromboses in unusual sites, such as the portal, mesenteric, splenic, subclavian, and cerebral veins (American College of Obstetricians and Gynecologists, 1998).

Antiphospholipid antibodies are also a predisposing factor for arterial thromboses. In fact, they account for up to 5 percent of arterial strokes in otherwise healthy young women (see Chap. 55, p. 1234). Thromboses may occur in relatively unusual locations, such as the retinal, subclavian, brachial, or digital arteries.

Branch and Khamashta (2003) and Levine and colleagues (2002) have reviewed a number of hypotheses proposed to explain mechanism(s) by which antiphospholipid antibodies promote thrombosis. For example, they may interfere with the normal function of phospholipids or phospholipid-binding proteins involved in coagulation regulation, including prothrombin, protein C, annexin V, and tissue factor. Many of these antibodies are directed against β_2-glycoprotein I, which may itself function as a natural anticoagulant (Chap. 54, p. 1217). Another proposed mechanism is that these antibodies promote thrombosis through endothelial cell activation or injury.

The American College of Obstetricians and Gynecologists (2000b) and Branch and Khamashta (2003) recommend that women with antiphospholipid syndrome receive adjusted-dose heparin prophylaxis. Alternatively, low-dose prophylaxis may be used if there is no history of a deep venous thrombosis. The American College of Chest Physicians (Ginsberg and colleagues, 2001) recommends that women with antiphospholipid antibodies who have not had a prior thrombosis or recurrent pregnancy loss be treated with prophylactic heparin or careful clinical surveillance (see Table 47–3).

THROMBOPHILIAS AND OTHER PREGNANCY COMPLICATIONS. Considerable attention has been

TABLE 47–4 Inherited Thrombophilias and the Approximate Relative Risk of Adverse Pregnancy Outcomes[a]

Thrombophilia	Severe Preeclampsia	Placental Infarction/ Abruption	Fetal Growth Restriction	Stillbirth	Recurrent Abortion
Factor V Leiden	1–5	0–4	1–2	1–5	1–3
Prothrombin	2–3	7–9	4–5	?	1–2
Antithrombin	3–4	3–4	?	1–5	?
Protein C	6–7	?	?	1–3	?
Protein S	7–10	1–2	7–8	3–16	1–3
Hyperhomocysteinemia	2–3	1–4	3–4	0.8–5	1–4

[a] Includes data from Alfirevic (2002); Brenner (2000); Dizon-Townson (2002b); Gerhardt (2000); Gherman (2000); Greer (1999); Kupferminc (1999, 2000); Lockwood (1999); Preston (1996); Procházka (2003); Rey (2003); Saade (2002); van der Molen (2000), and all their associates.

directed recently toward a possible relationship between certain pregnancy complications and the thrombophilias (Alfirevic, 2001; Kovalevsky, 2004; Kujovich, 2004; Kupferminc and Eldor, 2003, and all their associates). As shown in Table 47–4, many thrombophilias have been variably linked to preeclampsia and eclampsia, and especially the *HELLP syndrome* (see Chap. 34, p. 768), fetal growth restriction (see Chap. 38, p. 900), placental abruption (see Chap. 35, p. 814), recurrent abortion (see Chap. 9, p. 236), and stillbirth (see Chap. 29, p. 679). Some thrombophilias are also associated with placental findings of intervillous or spiral artery thrombosis (see Chap. 27, p. 621).

DEEP VENOUS THROMBOSIS

CLINICAL PRESENTATION. Most cases of venous thrombosis during pregnancy are confined to the deep veins of the lower extremity (Gherman and associates, 1999; Witlin and colleagues, 1999). The signs and symptoms vary greatly and depend in large measure on the degree of occlusion and the intensity of the inflammatory response. Ginsberg and colleagues (1992) reported that 58 of 60 antepartum women (97 percent) had left leg thromboses. Our experiences at Parkland Hospital are similar; 90 percent of lower extremity thromboses were in the left leg. This may result from compression of the left iliac vein by the right iliac and ovarian arteries, both of which cross the vein only on the left side (Greer, 2003).

Classical thrombosis involving the lower extremity is abrupt in onset, and there is pain and edema of the leg and thigh. The thrombus typically involves much of the deep venous system to the iliofemoral region. Occasionally, reflex arterial spasm causes a pale, cool extremity with diminished pulsations—so-called *phlegmasia alba dolens* or *milk leg*. Conversely, there may be appreciable clot, yet little pain, heat, or swelling. Importantly, calf pain, either spontaneous or in response to squeezing or to stretching the Achilles tendon (*Homans sign*), may be caused by a strained muscle or a contusion.

DIAGNOSIS. The clinical diagnosis of deep venous thrombosis is difficult, and in one study of pregnant women, the diagnosis was confirmed in only 10 percent of patients (Ginsberg and colleagues, 2001; Hull and co-workers, 1990). Given this difficulty, as well as the significant implications of either failing to diagnose venous thromboembolism or the potential hazards of unnecessary treatment, objective diagnosis is crucial. Shown in Figure 47–2 is an algorithm that may be used for evaluation of suspected thrombosis in pregnant women. With a few modifications, we follow a similar evaluation at Parkland Hospital.

Venography. Invasive contrast venography remains the standard against which all other diagnostic tests to exclude the diagnosis of lower extremity deep venous thrombosis are judged (Chunilal and Ginsberg, 2001). It has a negative predictive value of 98 percent. As discussed in Chapter 41 (see p. 979), the fetal radiation exposure associated with unilateral venography without shielding is about 300 mrad (Bates and Ginsberg, 2002). However, although venography remains the standard technique, noninvasive methods have largely replaced it to confirm the clinical diagnosis. Venography has significant complications and may even itself induce thrombosis. In addition, it is time consuming and cumbersome.

Impedance Plethysmography. This is another extremely accurate test for the assessment of thromboses in the lower iliac, femoral, and popliteal vessels. The test is based on the observation that alterations in venous return in the calf, produced by inflation and deflation of a pneumatic thigh cuff, result in changes in electrical resistance detected at the skin surface. These changes occur when the popliteal or more proximal veins are obstructed (Chunilal and Ginsberg, 2001).

Impedance plethysmography is only 50-percent sensitive for detection of clots in the small calf veins (Davis, 2001). Moreover, because of decreased venous return of the lower extremities, it is associated with increased false-positive results during pregnancy (Andres and Miles, 2001). Given

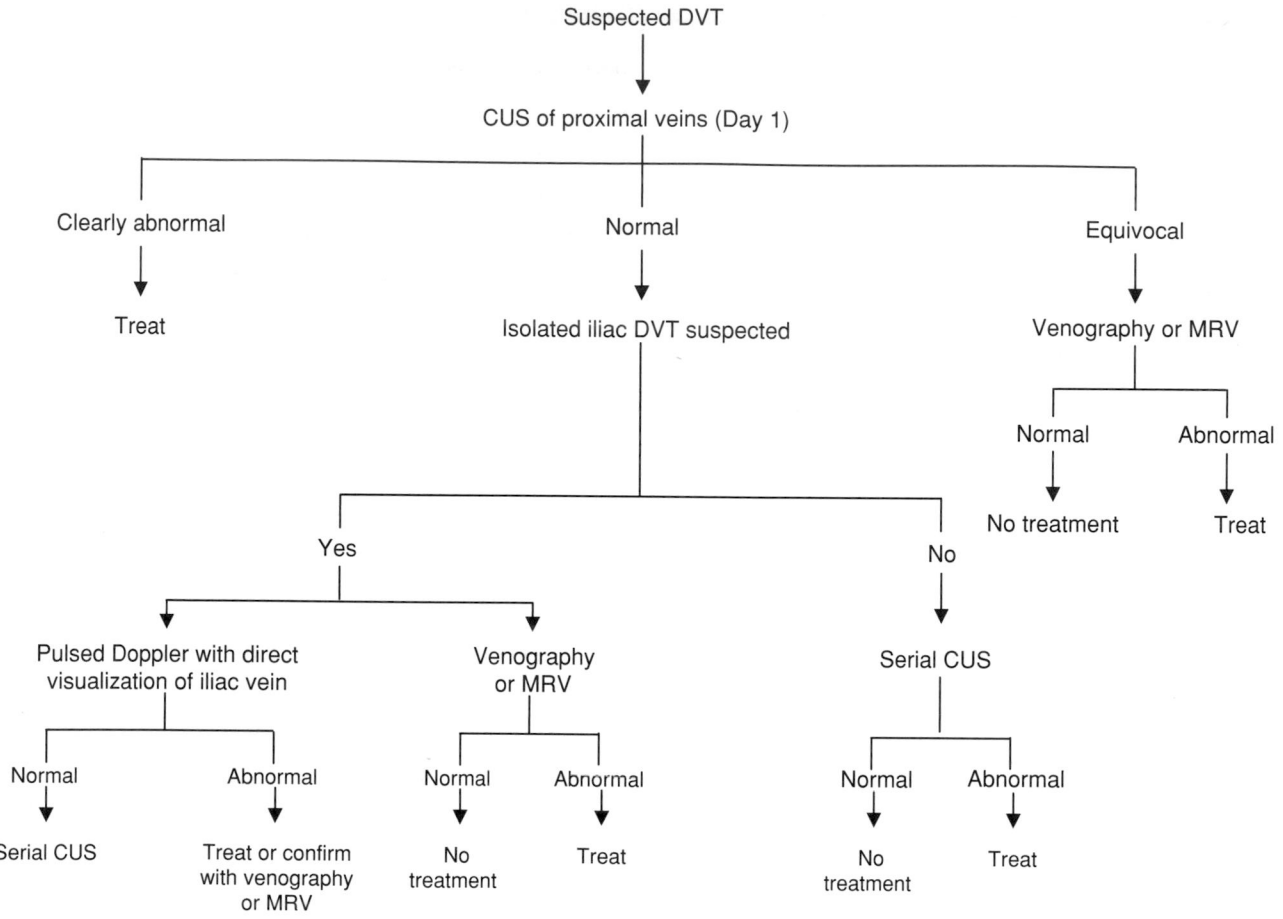

FIGURE 47–2. Algorithm for the investigation of suspected deep venous thrombosis during pregnancy. [For nonpregnant patients, if an isolated iliac DVT is suspected and if D-dimer testing is normal, further testing is withheld, and if abnormal, further investigation is done—this has not been evaluated in pregnancy.] If an isolated iliac DVT is not suspected, repeat serial compression ultrasonography (CUS) on days 2 and 3 and 6 to 8; if conditions are highly suspicious, perform magnetic resonance venography (MRV) or venography. (Reproduced from Bates and Ginsberg, 2002, with permission.)

these limitations, it is seldom used today (Chunilal and Ginsberg, 2001; Davis, 2001).

Compression Ultrasonography. This noninvasive technique is often combined with color Doppler ultrasonography. It is the primary test currently used by most clinicians to detect deep venous thrombosis (Greer, 2003). The diagnosis is based on the noncompressibility and typical echo pattern of a thrombosed vein (Davis, 2001). In symptomatic nonpregnant patients, examination of the femoral, popliteal, and calf trifurcation veins is more than 90-percent sensitive and more than 99-percent specific for proximal deep vein thrombosis. It has a negative predictive value of 98 percent (American College of Obstetricians and Gynecologists, 2000a,b). It is significantly less reliable for detecting calf vein thromboses, which as subsequently discussed may extend proximally (Bates and Ginsberg, 2004).

Lensing and colleagues (1989) compared contrast venography with real-time ultrasonography in 220 nonpregnant patients. They found that both the common femoral and popliteal veins were fully compressible—no thrombosis—in 142 of 143 patients who had a normal venogram (99-percent specific). All 66 patients with proximal vein thrombosis had noncompressible femoral or popliteal veins, or both (100-percent sensitive).

Normal venous ultrasonography results do not necessarily rule out pulmonary embolism (Goldhaber and colleagues, 2004), because the thrombosis may have already embolized or because it arose from deep pelvic veins inaccessible to ultrasound evaluation. **In pregnant women, thrombosis associated with pulmonary embolism frequently originates in the iliac veins.**

The safety of withholding anticoagulation in nonpregnant patients with suspected thrombosis who have normal serial compression examinations performed during one week has been established (Birdwell and co-workers, 1998; Heijboer and associates, 1993). Specifically, in nonpregnant patients, isolated calf thromboses extend into the proximal veins in up to 20 to 30 percent of cases. They do so within 1 to 2 weeks of presentation and are usually detected by serial ultrasonic compression. Whether the natural history of calf deep vein thrombosis is the same during pregnancy is unknown. Moreover, the safety of this strategy has not been evaluated in pregnant women who may have an isolated iliac vein thrombosis that is less accessible for imaging (Bates and Ginsberg, 2002).

D-*Dimer Tests.* These specific fibrin degradation products are generated when fibrinolysin degrades fibrin, as occurs in thromboembolism. Their measurement is frequently incorporated into diagnostic algorithms for venous thromboembolism in nonpregnant patients (Kelly and Hunt, 2002). Wells and co-workers (2003) randomly assigned nearly 1100 nonpregnant patients with suspected lower extremity thrombosis to ultrasound imaging alone or to imaging only if D-dimer testing was positive. Of 566 patients in the latter group, 40 percent had negative D-dimer tests, and only two of these were later diagnosed with a deep venous thrombosis. The investigators concluded that ultrasound testing can be safely omitted in nonpregnant patients with a negative D-dimer test.

Screening with the D-dimer test in pregnancy remains unproven. Depending on assay sensitivity, D-dimer serum levels increase with gestational age and can be high in pregnancy complications such as placental abruption, preeclampsia, and sepsis syndrome. Thus, their use during pregnancy remains uncertain (Bates and Ginsberg, 2002).

Computed Tomography. This scanning method is widely available and potentially useful for detecting lower extremity deep venous thrombosis. Computed tomography (CT) uses x-rays and requires contrast agents. Almost always, the benefits of CT outweigh any theoretical risks if lead shielding is used. Fetal radiation exposure is negligible unless the pelvic veins are imaged (see Chap. 41, p. 979).

Magnetic Resonance Imaging. This scanning technique allows excellent delineation of anatomical detail above the inguinal ligament. Thus, magnetic resonance imaging (MRI) is useful for diagnosis of pelvic vein thrombosis, including isolated iliac vein thrombosis (Fig. 47–3). The venous system can also be reconstructed using magnetic resonance venography, as discussed in Chapter 41 (see p. 982). Erdman and co-workers (1990) reported that MRI was 100-percent sensitive and 90-percent specific for detection of venographically proven deep venous thrombosis. Importantly, almost half of these nonpregnant patients without deep venous thrombosis had detectable nonthrombotic conditions to explain the clinical findings. These included cellulitis, myositis, edema, hematomas, and superficial phlebitis.

MANAGEMENT. Prevention and management of venous thromboembolism during pregnancy is a contentious area; there are no major clinical studies to support evidence-based practice (Copplestone and colleagues, 2004). That said, the mainstays of treatment consist of anticoagulation and limited

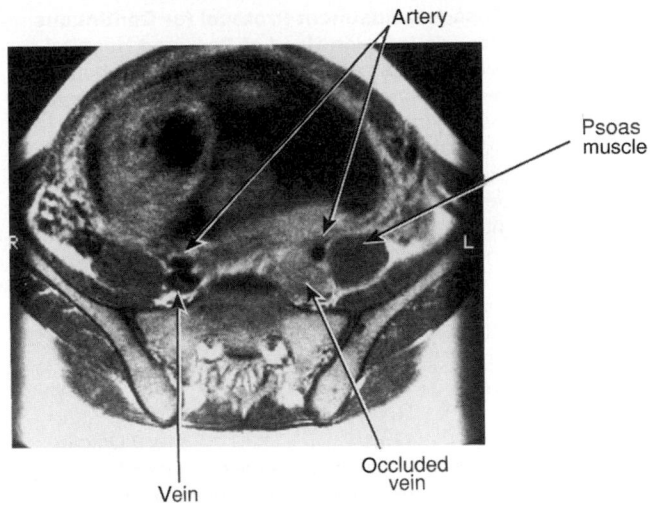

FIGURE 47–3. Magnetic resonance image through the pelvis of a 26-week pregnant woman who presented with symptoms of pulmonary embolism but without clinically apparent deep venous thrombosis of the lower extremities. The T1-weighted image shows occlusion of left common iliac vein. There is normal absence of signal in the right iliac vein and both iliac arteries. (Courtesy of Dr. Diane Twickler.)

activity. Some clinicians, but not all, recommend that thrombophilia testing be done after only one episode of thromboembolism during pregnancy. For example, the American College of Obstetricians and Gynecologists (2000b) recommends that women with a thrombosis—as well as those with a family history or a first-degree relative with a specific mutation—be tested for an underlying thrombophilia. Conversely, other practitioners have found that thrombophilia testing following a first thrombosis is not helpful for predicting recurrence (Baglin and associates, 2003). If such testing is performed, it is done before anticoagulation, because heparin induces a decline in antithrombin levels and warfarin decreases protein C and S concentrations (Lockwood, 2002).

Anticoagulation is always initiated with either unfractionated or low-molecular-weight heparin. For women who are still pregnant, heparin therapy is continued, and for those postpartum, anticoagulation is begun simultaneously with warfarin. Pulmonary embolism develops in approximately a fourth of patients with untreated deep venous thrombosis. Anticoagulation decreases this risk to less than 5 percent and the mortality rate is less than 1 percent (Douketis and co-workers, 1998; Weiss and Bernstein, 2000).

Most often, pain soon is relieved by these measures. After symptoms have completely abated, graded ambulation should be started. Elastic stockings are fitted and anticoagulation continued. Recovery to this stage usually takes about 7 to 10 days.

Heparin. Treatment of thromboembolism during pregnancy begins with an intravenous heparin bolus followed by continuous infusion titrated to achieve full anticoagulation

TABLE 47–5 Dosage Adjustment Protocol for Continuous Heparin Infusion Used at Parkland Hospital for Patients with Venous Thromboembolism

#1. Initial heparin dose:
80 U/kg IV push (maximum 10,000 U) then 18 U/kg/hr infusion (maximum 2200 U/hr).

#2. Recommended adjustments of infusion rate based on partial thromboplastin time (PTT):

PTT (sec)	Intervention	Drip Rate Change
< 33	80 U/kg bolus	↑ by 4 U/kg/hr
33–40	40 U/kg bolus	↑ by 2 U/kg/hr
41–49	None	↑ by 2 U/kg/hr
50–80	None	None
81–90	None	↓ by 2 U/kg/hr
> 90	Stop infusion, and after 60 minutes:	↓ by 3 U/kg/hr

PTT = partial thromboplastin time.

(American Academy of Pediatrics and American College of Obstetricians and Gynecologists, 2002). There are a number of protocols to accomplish this, and the one used at Parkland Hospital is shown in Table 47–5. Intravenous anticoagulation should be maintained for at least 5 to 7 days, after which treatment is converted to subcutaneous heparin. Injections are given every 8 hours to prolong the activated partial thromboplastin time (APTT) to at least 1.5 to 2.5 times control throughout the dosing interval. Treatment is continued for at least 3 months after the acute event. If the woman is still pregnant at this juncture, it is not known whether it is better to continue with a therapeutic or a lower dose of heparin for the remainder of pregnancy (American College of Obstetricians and Gynecologists, 2000b). For women with antiphospholipid syndrome, the APTT cannot assess adequacy of anticoagulation with heparin, and anti–factor Xa levels may be used instead.

Low-Molecular-Weight Heparin. This is a family of derivatives of unfractionated heparin, and their molecular weights average 4000 to 5000 daltons compared with about 12,000 to 16,000 daltons for conventional heparin. Like standard heparin, low-molecular-weight heparins do not cross the placenta (Casele and colleagues, 1999). Both types exert their anticoagulant activity by activating antithrombin. Their primary difference is in their relative inhibitory activity against factor Xa and thrombin. Specifically, unfractionated heparin has equivalent activity against factor Xa and thrombin, but low-molecular-weight heparins have greater activity against factor Xa than thrombin. They also have a more predictable anticoagulant response than unfractionated heparin. These include fewer bleeding complications that reflect their better bioavailability, longer half-life, dose-independent clearance, and decreased interference with platelets (Weitz, 1997). Using serial venograms, Breddin and co-workers (2001) observed that low-molecular-weight heparins were more effective than

the unfractionated form in reducing thrombus size without increasing mortality or major bleeding complications.

A number of studies have shown that venous thromboembolism is treated effectively with low-molecular-weight heparin (Quinlan and colleagues, 2004). Some authorities recommend that anti–factor Xa levels be periodically reevaluated during pregnancy in a woman fully anticoagulated with these agents. If used, dosing should be enough to achieve a peak anti–factor Xa level of 0.5 to 1.2 U/mL.

Casele and colleagues (1999) studied the pharmacokinetics of one low-molecular-weight heparin, enoxaparin sodium (Lovenox), during pregnancy in 13 women, who were treated with daily 40-mg enoxaparin subcutaneously. Serial measurements of anti–factor Xa activity were determined during early pregnancy, the third trimester, and then postpartum. They concluded that, likely because of increased renal clearance, twice-daily dosing may be necessary to maintain anti–factor Xa activity above 0.1 U/mL. They also suggested that optimal dosing was best achieved with periodic monitoring of peak (about 3.5 hours after a dose) and predose anti–factor Xa activity.

Rodie and co-workers (2002) studied 36 women with venous thromboembolism during pregnancy or immediately postpartum who were treated with enoxaparin. The dose was approximately 1 mg/kg given twice daily based on early pregnancy weight. Treatment was monitored by peak anti–factor Xa activity 3 hours postinjection, with a target therapeutic range of 0.4–1.0 U/mL. In 33 women, enoxaparin provided satisfactory anticoagulation. In the other three women, dose reduction was necessary. None developed recurrent thromboembolism or bleeding complications.

Other formulations of low-molecular-weight heparin have been evaluated. Sephton and associates (2003) performed a longitudinal investigation of 24 women given dalteparin. Those given once-daily dalteparin subcutaneously had mean anti–factor Xa levels that were significantly lower across pregnancy when compared with levels measured 6 weeks postpartum. Smith and co-workers (2004) reported similar results with tinzaparin given as a once-daily 50-U/kg dose. They found that a dosage of 75 to 175 U/kg/day was necessary to achieve peak anti–factor Xa levels of 0.1 to 1.0 U/mL.

Reviews by Sanson and associates (1999) and Lepercq and co-workers (2001) concluded that low-molecular-weight heparins were safe and effective. Despite this, in 2002, the manufacturer of Lovenox warned that its use in pregnancy had been associated with congenital anomalies and an increased risk of hemorrhage. After its own extensive review, the American College of Obstetricians and Gynecologists (2002) concluded that these risks were rare, that their incidence was not higher than expected, and that no cause-and-effect relationship has been established (see Chap. 14, p. 356). The committee further concluded that enoxaparin and dalteparin could be given safely during pregnancy.

One caveat is that low-molecular-weight heparins should not be used in patients with prosthetic heart valves because of reports of valvular thrombosis (see Chap. 44, p. 1022). Their use may increase the risk of spinal hematoma associated with regional analgesia (see Chap. 19, p. 486). Finally, when given within 2 hours of cesarean delivery, these agents increase the risk of wound hematoma (van Wijk and co-workers, 2002).

Warfarin. Anticoagulation with warfarin derivatives is generally contraindicated during pregnancy. These drugs readily cross the placenta and cause fetal death and malformations from hemorrhages (see Chap. 14, p. 349). They are safe, however, when ingested while breast feeding (American Academy of Pediatrics and American College of Obstetricians and Gynecologists, 2002). Postpartum venous thrombosis can be treated with intravenous heparin and oral warfarin initiated simultaneously, and heparin can usually be discontinued after 5 days. Brooks and colleagues (2002) compared anticoagulation in postpartum women with that of age-matched nonpregnant controls. Postpartum women required a significantly larger median total dose of warfarin (45 versus 24 mg), and a longer time (7 versus 4 days), to achieve the target international normalized ratio (INR). Moreover, the mean maintenance dose in the postpartum women was 4.9 mg compared with 4.3 mg in the control group.

DURATION OF THERAPY. After delivery, most women are anticoagulated with warfarin for at least 6 weeks (see Table 47–3). Actually, the optimal duration of continued anticoagulation is uncertain, and recommendations have been extrapolated from studies in nonpregnant patients. For example, two recent randomized placebo-controlled trials attempted to examine the optimal duration of warfarin following at least 3 months of anticoagulation for venous thromboembolism in nonpregnant adults (Kearon and colleagues, 1999; Ridker and co-workers, 2003). Both studies were terminated early after patients given placebo were found to be at significantly increased risk for suffering a recurrent venous thromboembolism. Ridker and co-workers (2003) concluded that long-term, low-intensity warfarin therapy (target INR of 1.5 to 2.0) is highly effective in preventing recurrent venous thromboembolism.

The results of these studies certainly suggest that patients with a first episode of thromboembolism be treated for 6 months or more (Bates and Ginsberg, 2004). It is problematic, however, to extrapolate these results to postpartum women, because most studies of warfarin for thromboembolism were in bedridden older patients with medical complications requiring prolonged confinement. The current consensus of both the American College of Obstetricians and Gynecologists (2000b) and the American College of Chest Physicians (Ginsberg and colleagues, 2001) is that postpartum anticoagulation therapy be given for at least 6 weeks.

Complications of Anticoagulation. Three significant complications associated with anticoagulation are hemorrhage, thrombocytopenia, and osteoporosis. The latter two are unique to heparin, and their risk may be reduced with low-molecular-weight heparins (American College of Obstetricians and Gynecologists, 2000b). The most serious complication is hemorrhage, which is more likely if there has been recent surgery or lacerations, such as with delivery. Troublesome bleeding also is more likely if the heparin dosage is excessive. Unfortunately, management schemes using laboratory testing to identify whether heparin dosage is sufficient to inhibit further thrombosis, yet not cause serious hemorrhage, have been discouraging.

HEPARIN-INDUCED THROMBOCYTOPENIA. There are two types of thrombocytopenia associated with heparin use. The most common type of heparin-induced thrombocytopenia (commonly referred to as *HIT*) is a *nonimmune*, benign, reversible form that occurs within the first few days of therapy and resolves in 5 days without cessation of therapy (American College of Obstetricians and Gynecologists, 2000b). The more severe form of HIT results from an *immune* reaction involving IgG antibodies directed against complexes of platelet factor 4 and heparin. When most severe, HIT paradoxically causes thrombosis, which is the most common presentation. The incidence of HIT is approximately 3 percent in nonpregnant individuals. Fausett and colleagues (2001), however, reported no cases of HIT among 244 pregnant heparin-treated women compared with 10 among 244 nonpregnant controls.

In their review of 243 nonpregnant patients with immune-mediated thrombocytopenia, Warkentin and Kelton (2001) observed that in 70 percent of patients, the platelet count decreased four or more days after the start of therapy. In 30 percent, however, a decrease in platelets began a median of 10.5 hours after the initiation of heparin therapy. The American College of Obstetricians and Gynecologists (2000a,b) recommends that platelet counts be measured on day 5 and then periodically for the first 2 weeks of heparin therapy. If unchanged, further platelet counts are not indicated because the vast majority of cases manifest within 15 days of standard heparin initiation.

If thrombocytopenia is severe, heparin therapy must be stopped and alternative anticoagulation initiated. Low-molecular-weight heparin may not be an entirely safe alternative because it has some cross reactivity with unfractionated heparin. Woo and associates (2002) successfully treated two pregnant women with *danaparoid*—a sulphated glycosaminoglycan heparinoid. Direct thrombin inhibitors, such as *hirudin*, also have been used as an alternative to heparins in these patients. However, experience with them in pregnancy is limited (Aijaz and associates, 2001; Frenkel, 2002; Prisco and colleagues, 2001). Interestingly, heparin-dependent antibodies do not invariably reappear with subsequent heparin use (Warkentin and Kelton, 2001).

HEPARIN-INDUCED OSTEOPOROSIS. Bone loss may develop with long-term heparin administration, usually 7 weeks or longer, and is more prevalent in cigarette smokers (see Chap. 53,

p. 1199). It has not been established that the process is completely reversible or that there is a clear dose-response relationship (American College of Obstetricians and Gynecologists, 2000a). In an attempt to avoid severe osteoporosis, women treated with heparin should be encouraged to take supplemental calcium and vitamin D (American College of Obstetricians and Gynecologists, 1998; von Mandach and co-workers, 2003).

Anticoagulation and Abortion. The treatment of deep venous thrombosis with heparin does not preclude termination of pregnancy by careful curettage (see Chap. 9, p. 242). After the products are removed without trauma to the reproductive tract, full-dose heparin can be restarted in several hours.

Anticoagulation and Delivery. The effects of heparin on blood loss at delivery depend on a number of variables:

1. Dose, route, and time of administration.
2. Magnitude of incisions and lacerations.
3. Intensity of postpartum myometrial contractions.
4. Presence of other coagulation defects.

Blood loss should not be greatly increased with vaginal delivery if the midline episiotomy is modest in depth, there are no lacerations, and the uterus promptly contracts. Such ideal circumstances do not always prevail. Mueller and Lebherz (1969) described 10 women with antepartum thrombophlebitis treated with heparin. Three women who continued to receive heparin during labor and delivery bled remarkably and developed large hematomas.

Thus, therapeutic heparin therapy generally is stopped during the time of labor and delivery. If the uterus is well contracted and there has been negligible trauma to the lower genital tract, it can be restarted within several hours. Otherwise, a delay of 1 or 2 days may be prudent. *Protamine sulfate* administered slowly intravenously generally reverses the effect of heparin promptly and effectively. It should not be given in excess of the amount needed to neutralize the heparin, because it also has an anticoagulant effect. Serious bleeding is likely when heparin in usual therapeutic doses is administered to a woman who has undergone cesarean delivery within the previous 24 to 48 hours.

SUPERFICIAL VENOUS THROMBOPHLEBITIS. Thrombosis limited strictly to the superficial veins of the saphenous system is treated with analgesia, elastic support, and rest. If it does not soon subside, or if deep venous involvement is suspected, appropriate diagnostic measures are performed. Heparin is given if deep vein involvement is confirmed. Superficial thrombophlebitis is typically seen in association with varicosities or as a sequela to intravenous catheterization.

PULMONARY EMBOLISM

Although it causes about 10 percent of maternal deaths, pulmonary embolism is relatively uncommon during pregnancy and the puerperium. From reports in the past 10 years of more than 1.4 million pregnancies, the incidence averages about 1 in 7000 (see Table 47–1). There is an almost equal prevalence for antepartum and postpartum embolism, but those developing postpartum have a higher mortality. In many cases, but certainly not all, clinical evidence for deep venous thrombosis of the legs precedes pulmonary embolization. In others, especially with thromboses that arise from deep pelvic veins, the woman usually is asymptomatic until embolization occurs.

CLINICAL PRESENTATION. Findings from the International Cooperative Pulmonary Embolism Registry were reported by Goldhaber and colleagues (1999). Over a 2-year period, almost 2500 nonpregnant patients with a proven pulmonary embolism were enrolled. The most common symptoms were dyspnea (82 percent), chest pain (49 percent), cough (20 percent), syncope (14 percent), and hemoptysis (7 percent). Other predominant clinical findings typically include tachypnea, apprehension, and tachycardia. In some cases, there is an accentuated pulmonic closure sound, rales, or friction rub. Right axis deviation and T-wave inversion in the anterior chest leads may be evident on the electrocardiogram. On chest radiography there may be loss of vascular markings in the region of the lungs supplied by the obstructed artery. Although most women are hypoxemic, it is emphasized that a normal arterial blood gas analysis does not rule out pulmonary embolism. Even with massive pulmonary embolism, signs, symptoms, and laboratory data to support the diagnosis may be deceivingly nonspecific.

DIAGNOSIS. As with deep venous thrombosis, the diagnosis of pulmonary embolism requires an initial high index of suspicion followed by objective testing (Chunilal and colleagues, 2003). Shown in Figure 47–4 is an algorithm for the evaluation of suspected pulmonary embolism in pregnancy. A chest radiograph should be performed if there is underlying suspicion for other diagnoses. Other imaging modalities in the diagnostic algorithm are described below. In many centers, spiral computed tomography has replaced the more cumbersome ventilation-perfusion lung scan. Fedullo and Tapson (2003) have provided an excellent review of various strategies used in the evaluation of suspected pulmonary embolism. They too recommend ultrasonography as discussed on page 1080 as an appropriate initial diagnostic approach (see Fig. 47–4).

Ventilation–Perfusion Scintigraphy—Lung Scan. Although used less commonly in the past 5 years, in some centers, women with a clinically suspected pulmonary embolism are initially evaluated with a ventilation–perfusion (V/Q) lung scan because it is the least invasive technique

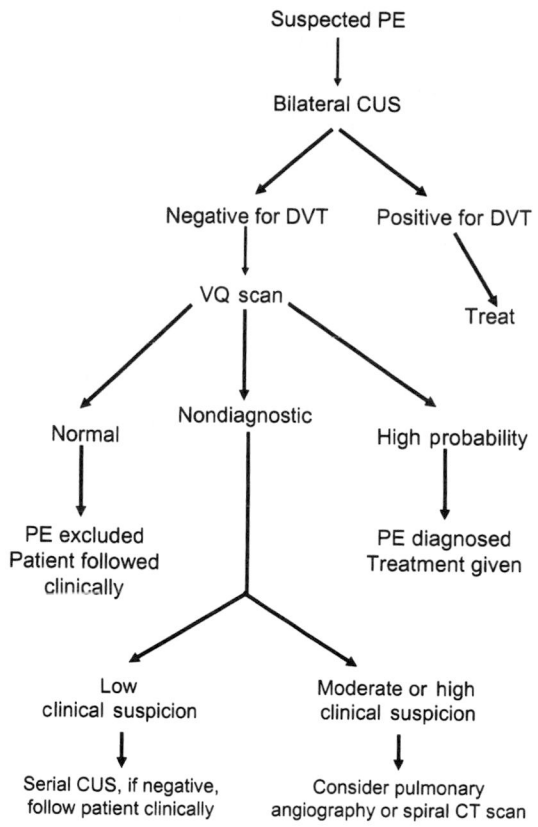

Suspected PE

↓

Bilateral CUS

Negative for DVT   Positive for DVT

↓   ↓

VQ scan   Treat

Normal   Nondiagnostic   High probability

↓   ↓

PE excluded   PE diagnosed
Patient followed   Treatment given
clinically

Low   Moderate or high
clinical suspicion   clinical suspicion

↓   ↓

Serial CUS, if negative,   Consider pulmonary
follow patient clinically   angiography or spiral CT scan

FIGURE 47–4. Evaluation of suspected pulmonary embolism during pregnancy. (CT = computed tomography; CUS = compression ultrasonography; DVT = deep vein thrombosis; PE = pulmonary embolism; VQ = ventilation–perfusion.) (Modified from Chan and Ginsberg, 2002, with permission.)

and is relatively accurately and quickly performed. V/Q scintigraphy may be used if compression ultrasound results are negative (see Fig. 47–4). These scans use a small dose of a radioactive agent, usually intravenously administered ^{99m}technetium-macroaggregated albumin, which is associated with negligible fetal radiation exposure (see Chap. 41, p. 981). The scan may not provide a definite diagnosis because many other conditions (e.g., pneumonia or local bronchospasm) can cause perfusion defects. Ventilation scans with inhaled ^{133}xenon or ^{99m}technetium were added to perfusion scans in the hope that ventilation would be abnormal, but perfusion would be normal, in areas of pneumonia or hypoventilation. Although ventilation scanning increased the probability of an accurate diagnosis in patients with large perfusion defects and ventilation mismatches, a normal V/Q scan does not rule out pulmonary embolism.

Because of these uncertainties, the National Heart, Lung and Blood Institute commissioned the Prospective Investigation of Pulmonary Embolism Diagnosis (PIOPED, 1990) to determine sensitivities and specificities of lung scans. It included 933 patients, of whom 931 underwent scintigraphy and 755 angiography. A third of those studied angiographically had a pulmonary embolism, and although almost

all of these had an abnormal scan of high, intermediate, or low probability, so did most without embolism (98-percent sensitivity and 10-percent specificity). Of 116 patients with high-probability scans, 88 percent had an embolism seen on angiography, but only a minority of those with a pulmonary embolism had a high-probability scan (41-percent sensitivity and 97-percent specificity). Of 322 with intermediate-probability scans, 33 percent had an embolism on angiography, and for those with a low-probability scan, the figure was 12 percent. **Importantly, 4 percent of patients with a near-normal to normal scan had pulmonary embolism detected by angiography.**

The PIOPED investigators concluded that a high-probability scan usually indicates pulmonary embolism, but that only a small number of patients with emboli have a high-probability scan. A low-probability scan, combined with a strong clinical impression that embolism is unlikely, makes the possibility of pulmonary embolism remote. Similarly, near-normal or normal scans make the diagnosis very unlikely. Finally, an intermediate-probability scan is of no help in establishing the diagnosis. Thus, the scan combined with clinical assessment permits a noninvasive diagnosis or exclusion of pulmonary embolism for only a minority of patients. Indeed, two thirds of nonpregnant patients with a suspected pulmonary embolism have a nondiagnostic scan and require additional testing (Raj, 2003). In our experience, this proportion is smaller in pregnant women, probably because they are younger and usually healthy and less likely to have coexisting pulmonary disease.

Chan and colleagues (2002) reported their experiences with 120 consecutive pregnant women with a suspected pulmonary embolism who underwent V/Q scanning. They reported that about 73 percent were interpreted as normal, 25 percent as nondiagnostic, and 2 percent as high probability. Anticoagulation was not given to most of the women with normal or nondiagnostic studies, and during an average 20-month follow-up period, none had thromboembolic events. They concluded that withholding anticoagulation in pregnant women with normal or nondiagnostic scans is probably safe.

Spiral Computed Tomography. Helical computed tomography (CT), or spiral CT, allows rapid imaging from the main pulmonary arteries to at least the segmental and possibly the subsegmental branches (Fig. 47–5). Fetal radiation exposure with standard single-detector spiral CT is less than with V/Q lung scanning (Winer-Muram and co-workers, 2002). Kline and colleagues (2000) calculated 86-percent sensitivity and 93-percent specificity for spiral CT scanning—an overall accuracy similar to that for V/Q scanning.

The Advances in New Technologies Evaluating the Localisation of Pulmonary Embolism (ANTELOPE) trial was a prospective evaluation of single-detector spiral CT as the initial test in 510 consecutive nonpregnant patients with suspected embolism (van Strijen and co-workers, 2003). In 24 percent, pulmonary embolism was diagnosed on the basis

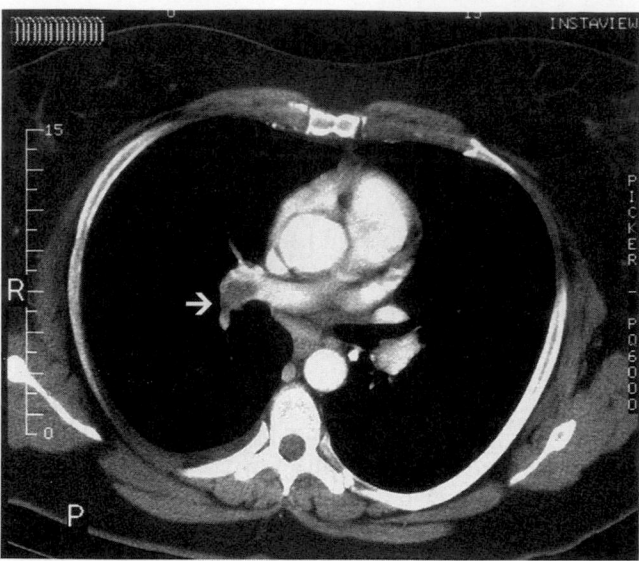

FIGURE 47–5. Axial image of the chest from a four-channel multidetector spiral computed tomography scan performed after administration of intravenous contrast. There is enhancement of the pulmonary artery with a large thrombus on the right (*arrow*) consistent with pulmonary embolism. (Courtesy of Drs. Diane Twickler and Michael Landay.)

TABLE 47–6 Comparison of Estimated Mean Fetal Radiation Dosimetry from Ventilation–Perfusion Lung Scanning Versus Four-Channel Multidetector Spiral Computed Tomographic Scanning for the Diagnosis of Pulmonary Embolism

| | V/Q Scan | | Spiral CT | |
State of Pregnancy	mGy	mrem	mGy	mrem
Early	0.46	46	0.04	4
First trimester	0.46	46	0.04	4
Second trimester	0.57	57	0.11	11
Third trimester[a]	0.45	45	0.31	31

CT = computed tomography; V/Q = ventilation–perfusion.
[a]In late pregnancy, the maximum exposure with spiral CT scanning may exceed the estimated mean by a factor of 5 to 7 due to increased proximity of the fetus to the primary beam.
Data courtesy of Dr. Jon Anderson.

of the initial CT scan, and an alternative diagnosis was made in another 26 percent without an embolism. Thus, CT was diagnostic in about half of the patients with a suspected pulmonary embolism. In the 376 patients not diagnosed with pulmonary embolism, and who were not anticoagulated, the incidence of clinical venous thromboembolism during the 3-month follow-up was only 0.8 percent. Thus, spiral CT with single-detector scanner had a negative predictive value of greater than 98 percent and appears to be a safe initial diagnostic test in nonpregnant patients (Raj, 2003).

As discussed in Chapter 41 (p. 980), the *four-channel multidetector spiral CT* will likely replace the pulmonary angiogram as the gold standard for diagnosis of pulmonary embolism (Goldhaber, 2004; Srivastava and colleagues, 2004). Except in late pregnancy, fetal x-ray exposure is less than with V/Q scanning (Table 47–6).

These new CT scanners have improved speed and resolution (Raj, 2003; Schoepf and Costello, 2004). In a prospective study of 102 consecutive nonpregnant patients with suspected pulmonary embolism who underwent multidetector spiral CT, Kavanagh and co-workers (2004) found that over a mean follow-up period of 9 months, only one patient had a false-negative scan. We now use multidetector spiral CT as first-line evaluation of pregnant women at Parkland Hospital. Although the technique has many advantages, we have found that the better resolution allows detection of previously inaccessible smaller distal emboli that have uncertain clinical significance. Alternatively, at the University of Alabama false-positive helical CT findings have been worrisome (Nuthalapaty and associates, 2005).

Magnetic Resonance Angiography. The availability of faster magnetic resonance hardware combined with intravenous gadolinium contrast allows high-resolution magnetic resonance angiography during a single suspended breath (Meaney and co-workers, 1997). In a study of 141 nonpregnant patients with suspected pulmonary embolism, Oudkerk and co-workers (2002) performed magnetic resonance angiography before conventional angiography. About a third of patients were found to have an embolus, and the sensitivity of magnetic resonance angiography for isolated subsegmental, segmental, and central or lobar pulmonary embolism was 40, 84, and 100 percent, respectively. Its sensitivity and specificity for segmental or larger pulmonary embolism are similar to those obtained with helical CT, but without radiation. Neither has been widely evaluated in pregnant women.

Pulmonary Angiography. Although currently the most definitive test for pulmonary embolism, pulmonary angiography is invasive and requires catheterization of the right side of the heart. Angiography is time consuming, uncomfortable, and associated with dye-induced allergy and renal failure. The procedure-related mortality rate is about 1 in 200 (Stein and colleagues, 1992). If less invasive tests are equivocal, then angiography should be considered. Indeed, 28 women with a suspected pulmonary embolism following cesarean delivery at a Maternal–Fetal Medicine Units Network center between 1999 and 2000 underwent pulmonary angiography (Hauth and co-workers, 2004). As discussed above, however, multidetector spiral CT can be used.

MANAGEMENT. Treatment for pulmonary embolism is similar to that for deep venous thrombosis, which is discussed on page 1081. The American College of Obstetricians and Gynecologists (2000b) recommends heparin—an intravenous loading dose of 80 U/kg followed by a continuous infusion. Other methods are acceptable, and most authors recommend starting with a dosage of 1000 U/hour after an initial bolus dose of 5000 to 10,000 U given intravenously. The dosage is maintained to produce a twofold prolongation of the APTT (see Table 47–5). Other methods include intermittent intravenous injections of either 5000 U heparin every 4 hours or 7500 U every 6 hours. The common theme in these regimens is that the total daily heparin dose is between 25,000 and 40,000 U.

In nonpregnant patients, a common cause of death is recurrent pulmonary embolism. To prevent this, most authors recommend therapeutic anticoagulation for months (Goldhaber, 2004). For women who develop thromboembolism postpartum, or for those who were given heparin antepartum and are now delivered, warfarin anticoagulation is usually substituted.

The woman who has very recently suffered a pulmonary embolism and who must undergo cesarean delivery presents a serious problem. Reversal of anticoagulation may be followed by another embolus, and surgery while fully anticoagulated frequently results in life-threatening hemorrhage or troublesome hematomas. In this situation, placement of a vena caval filter should be considered before surgery.

Vena Caval Filters. Routine placement of a filter has no added advantage to heparin given alone to prevent pulmonary embolism in patients with deep venous thrombosis (Decousus and associates, 1998). In the very infrequent circumstances in which heparin therapy fails to prevent recurrent pulmonary embolism from the pelvis or legs, or when embolism develops from these sites despite heparin treatment, then a vena caval filter may be indicated. The device is inserted through either the jugular or femoral vein. Use of the device during pregnancy has been described by Hux (1986) and Thomas (1997) and their colleagues. Greenfield and Michna (1988) recommend suprarenal placement during pregnancy. Hirano and associates (2002) described the successful use of a Greenfield filter in a pregnant woman with an internal jugular venous thrombosis.

Retrievable filters may be used as short-term protection against embolism. These may be removed before they become endothelialized by 10 days, or they can be left in place permanently. Neill and colleagues (1997) placed a *Gunther Tulip filter* at 37 weeks in a woman with recurrent embolization. She underwent cesarean delivery at 38 weeks, and the filter was removed 5 days postpartum. Deshpande and colleagues (2002) have described the successful use of a vena caval filter in six patients with severe hypoxia and tenuous cardiopulmonary status from massive pulmonary emboli who were not candidates for thrombolysis.

Thrombolysis. Compared with heparin, thrombolytic agents provide a more rapid lysis of pulmonary clots and improvement of pulmonary hypertension (Agnelli and associates, 2002). Whether these advantages result in improved outcomes has been the subject of recent research. Agnelli and associates (2002) performed a meta-analysis of nine randomized trials involving 461 patients. They reported that the risk of recurrence or death was significantly lower in patients receiving thrombolytic agents compared with that of heparin therapy (10 versus 17 percent). Of note, however, there were five (2 percent) fatal bleeding episodes in the thrombolysis group and none in the heparin group.

Konstantinides and colleagues (2002) studied 256 patients with acute submassive pulmonary embolism, defined as pulmonary hypertension or right ventricular dysfunction but without arterial hypotension. Patients were randomized to heparin with either a placebo or the recombinant tissue plasminogen activator *alteplase.* Those given the placebo had a threefold increased risk of death or treatment escalation compared with those given the alteplase. There are very few studies of thrombolysis during pregnancy. However, Ahearn and associates (2002) described a successful case and provided a detailed review.

Embolectomy. Published experience with emergency embolectomy during pregnancy is limited to case reports. Funakoshi and colleagues (2004) recently described successful emergency embolectomy performed immediately following cesarean delivery in a woman who suffered a massive pulmonary embolism at term. Based on their review, Ahearn and associates (2002) found that the operative risk to the mother may be reasonable, however, the stillbirth rate is 20 to 40 percent. They concluded that the use of vena caval filters appears to be the safest short-term method of treating massive pulmonary embolism during pregnancy.

THROMBOEMBOLISM ANTEDATING PREGNANCY. Optimal management of women with firm evidence of a prior thromboembolism is unclear. As shown in Table 47–3, surveillance only or low-dose prophylaxis may be used in women without a recurrent risk factor, including no known thrombophilia. The study by Tengborn and colleagues (1989) suggested that such prophylaxis is not effective. They reported outcomes in 87 pregnant Swedish women who had prior thromboembolic disease. Despite heparin prophylaxis, usually 5000 U twice daily, 3 of 20 (15 percent) women developed antepartum recurrence, compared with 8 of 67 (12 percent) not given heparin. These women were not tested for thrombophilia.

More recently, Brill-Edwards and associates (2000) prospectively studied 125 pregnant women with a single previous episode of venous thromboembolism. Antepartum heparin was not given, but anticoagulant therapy was given for 4 to 6 weeks postpartum. Antepartum recurrence occurred in three (2.4 percent) women, and postpartum recurrence in three others. There were no recurrences in the 44 women without a known thrombophilia or whose prior thrombosis was associated with a temporary risk factor. These findings imply that prophylactic heparin may not be required for women with a prior thrombotic event not associated with a thrombophilia or a temporary risk factor. In contrast, women whose prior thrombosis occurred in association with a thrombophilia or in the absence of a temporary risk factor should receive both antepartum and postpartum prophylaxis (see Table 47–3).

Our practice at Parkland Hospital for many years for women with a history of prior thromboembolism has been to administer subcutaneous heparin, 5000 to 7500 units two to three times daily. With this regimen, the recurrence of documented deep venous thrombosis embolization has been rare. More recently, we have successfully used 40-mg enoxaparin given subcutaneously daily.

REFERENCES

Agnelli G, Becattini C, Kirschstein T: Thrombolysis vs heparin in the treatment of pulmonary embolism. Arch Intern Med 162: 2537, 2002

Ahearn GS, Hadjiliadis D, Govert JA, et al: Massive pulmonary embolism during pregnancy successfully treated with recombinant tissue plasminogen activator. Arch Intern Med 162:1221, 2002

Aijaz A, Nelson J, Naseer N: Management of heparin allergy in pregnancy. Am J Hematol 67:268, 2001

Alfirevic Z, Mousa HA, Martlew V, et al: Postnatal screening for thrombophilia in women with severe pregnancy complications. Obstet Gynecol 97:753, 2001

Alfirevic Z, Roberts D, Martlew V: How strong is the association between maternal thrombophilia and adverse pregnancy outcome? A systematic review. Eur J Obstet Gynecol Reprod Biol 101:6, 2002

Allaart CF, Poort SR, Rosendaal FR, et al: Increased risk of venous thrombosis in carriers of hereditary protein C deficiency defect. Lancet 341:134, 1993

American Academy of Pediatrics and American College of Obstetricians and Gynecologists: Guidelines for Perinatal Care, 5th ed. 2002

American College of Obstetricians and Gynecologists: Safety of Lovenox in pregnancy. Committee Opinion No. 276, October 2002

American College of Obstetricians and Gynecologists: Prevention of deep vein thrombosis and pulmonary embolism. Practice Bulletin No. 21, October 2000a

American College of Obstetricians and Gynecologists: Thromboembolism in pregnancy. Practice Bulletin No. 19, August 2000b

American College of Obstetricians and Gynecologists: Antiphospholipid syndrome. Educational Bulletin No. 244, February 1998

Andersen BS, Steffensen FH, Sørensen HT, et al: The cumulative incidence of venous thromboembolism during pregnancy and puerperium. Acta Obstet Gynecol Scand 77:170, 1998

Andres RL, Miles A: Venous thromboembolism and pregnancy. Obstet Gynecol Clin North Am 28:613, 2001

Arias E, Anderson RN, Hsiang-Ching K, et al: Deaths: Final Data for 2001. National Vital Statistics Reports, Vol 52, No. 3. Hyattsville, MD, National Center for Health Statistics, 2003

Baglin T, Luddington R, Brown K, et al: Incidence of recurrent venous thromboembolism in relation to clinical and thrombophilic risk factors: Prospective cohort study. Lancet 362:523, 2003

Bates, SM, Ginsberg JS: Treatment of deep-vein thrombosis. N Engl J Med 351:268, 2004

Bates SM, Ginsberg JS: How we manage venous thromboembolism during pregnancy. Blood 100:3470, 2002

Birdwell BG, Raskob GE, Whitsett TL, et al: The clinical validity of normal compression ultrasonography in outpatients suspected of having deep venous thrombosis. Ann Intern Med 128:1, 1998

Bloomenthal D, Delisle MF, Tessier F, et al: Obstetric implications of the factor V Leiden mutation: A review. Am J Perinatal 19:37, 2002

Branch DW, Khamashta MA: Antiphospholipid syndrome: Obstetric diagnosis, management, and controversies. Obstet Gynecol 101:1333, 2003

Breddin HK, Hach-Wunderle V, Nakov R, et al: Effects of a low-molecular-weight heparin on thrombus regression and recurrent thromboembolism in patients with DVT. N Engl J Med 344:626, 2001

Brenner B: Inherited thrombophilia and fetal loss. Curr Opin Hematol 7:290, 2000

Brill-Edwards P, Ginsberg JS, Gent M, et al: Safety of withholding heparin in pregnant women with a history of venous thromboembolism. N Engl J Med 343:1439, 2000

Brooks C, Rutherford JM, Gould J, et al: Warfarin dosage in postpartum women: A case-control study. Br J Obstet Gynaecol 109:187, 2002

Burneo JG, Elias SB, Barkley GL: Cerebral venous thrombosis due to protein S deficiency in pregnancy. Lancet 359:892, 2002

Casele HL, Laifer SA, Woelkers DA, et al: Changes in the pharmacokinetics of the low-molecular-weight heparin enoxaparin sodium during pregnancy. Am J Obstet Gynecol 181:1113, 1999

Chan WS, Ginsberg JS: Diagnosis of deep vein thrombosis and pulmonary embolism in pregnancy. Thromb Res 107:85, 2002

Chan WS, Ray JG, Murray S, et al: Suspected pulmonary embolism in pregnancy. Arch Intern Med 162:1170, 2002

Chunilal SD, Eikelboom JW, Attia J, et al: Does this patient have pulmonary embolism? JAMA 290:2849, 2003

Chunilal SD, Ginsberg JS: Advances in the diagnosis of venous thromboembolism—a multimodal approach. J Thromb Thrombolysis 12:53, 2001

Clark P, Twaddle S, Walker ID, et al: Cost-effectiveness of screening for the factor V Leiden mutation in pregnant women. Lancet 359:1919, 2002

Conard J, Horellou MH, Van Dreden P, et al: Thrombosis and pregnancy in congenital deficiencies in AT III, protein C or protein S: Study of 78 women. Thromb Haemost 63:319, 1990

Copplestone JA, Pavord S, Hunt BJ: Anticoagulation in pregnancy: A survey of current practice [letter]. Br J Haematol 124:124, 2004

Cunningham FG, MacDonald PC, Gant NF, et al: Williams Obstetrics, 19th ed. Norwalk, CT, Appleton & Lange, 1993

Danilenko-Dixon DR, Heit JA, Silverstein MD, et al: Risk factors for deep vein thrombosis and pulmonary embolism during pregnancy or postpartum: A population-based, case-control study. Am J Obstet Gynecol 184:104, 2001

Davis JD: Prevention, diagnosis, and treatment of venous thromboembolic complications of gynecologic surgery. Am J Obstet Gynecol 184:759, 2001

Decousus H, Leizorovicz A, Parent F, et al: A clinical trial of vena caval filters in the prevention of pulmonary embolism in patients with proximal deep-vein thrombosis. N Engl J Med 338:409, 1998

Deshpande KS, Hatem C, Karwa M, et al: The use of inferior vena cava filter as a treatment modality for massive pulmonary embolism. A case series and review of pathophysiology. Respir Med 96:984, 2002

Dilley A, Austin A, El-Jamil M, et al: Genetic factors associated with thrombosis in pregnancy in a United States population. Am J Obstet Gynecol 183:1271, 2000

Dizon-Townson DS: Pregnancy-related venous thromboembolism. Clin Obstet Gynecol 45:363, 2002a

Dizon-Townson DS: The factor V Leiden mutation does not increase risk of pregnancy-related venous thromboembolism. Am J Obstet Gynecol 187:S159, 2002b

Douketis JD, Kearon C, Bates S, et al: Risk of fatal pulmonary embolism in patients with treated venous thromboembolism. JAMA 279:458, 1998

Eldor A: Thrombophilia and its treatment in pregnancy. J Thromb Thrombolysis 12:23, 2001a

Eldor A: Thrombophilia, thrombosis and pregnancy. Thromb Haemost 86:104, 2001b

Erdman WA, Jayson HT, Redman HC, et al: Deep venous thrombosis of extremities: Role of MR imaging in the diagnosis. Radiology 174:425, 1990

Faught W, Garner P, Johnes G, et al: Changes in protein C and protein S levels in normal pregnancy. Am J Obstet Gynecol 172:147, 1995

Fausett MB, Vogtlander M, Lee RM, et al: Heparin-induced thrombocytopenia is rare in pregnancy. Am J Obstet Gynecol 185:148, 2001

Federman DG, Kirsner RS: An update on hypercoagulable disorders. Arch Intern Med 161:1051, 2001

Fedullo PF, Tapson VF: The evaluation of suspected pulmonary embolism. N Engl J Med 349:1247, 2003

Frenkel EP: The direct thrombin inhibitors: Their role and use for rational anticoagulation. University of Texas Southwestern Medical Center, Department of Internal Medicine, Grand Rounds, August 15, 2002

Funakoshi Y, Kato M, Kuratani T, et al: Successful treatment of massive pulmonary embolism in the 38th week of pregnancy. Ann Thorac Surg 2004:77, 694

Gerhardt A, Scharf RE, Beckmann MW, et al: Prothrombin and factor V mutations in women with a history of thrombosis during pregnancy and the puerperium. N Engl J Med 342:374, 2000

Gherman RB, Goodwin TM: Obstetric implications of activated protein C resistance and factor V Leiden mutation. Obstet Gynecol Surv 55:117, 2000

Gherman RB, Goodwin TM, Leung B, et al: Incidence, clinical characteristics, and timing of objectively diagnosed venous thromboembolism during pregnancy. Obstet Gynecol 94:730, 1999

Ginsberg JS, Greer I, Hirsh J: Use of antithrombotic agents during pregnancy. Chest 119:122S, 2001

Ginsberg JS, Brill-Edwards P, Burrows RF, et al: Venous thrombosis during pregnancy: Leg and trimester of presentation. Thromb Haemost 67:519, 1992

Goldhaber SZ: Pulmonary embolism. Lancet 363:1295, 2004

Goldhaber SZ, Tapson VF, DVT FREE Steering Committee: A prospective registry of 5,451 patients with ultrasound-confirmed deep vein thrombosis. Am J Cardiol 93:259, 2004

Goldhaber SZ, Visani L, De Rosa M: Acute pulmonary embolism: Clinical outcomes in the International Cooperative Pulmonary Embolism Registry (ICOPER). Lancet 353:1386, 1999

Greenfield LJ, Michna BA: Twelve-year clinical experience with the Greenfield vena caval filter. Surgery 104:706, 1988

Greer IA: Prevention and management of venous thromboembolism in pregnancy. Clin Chest Med 24:123, 2003

Greer IA: Thrombosis in pregnancy: Maternal and fetal issues. Lancet 353:1258, 1999

Hague WM: Homocysteine and pregnancy. Best Prac Res Clin Obstet Gynaecol 17:459, 2003

Hauth JC for the NICHHD Maternal–Fetal Medicine Units Network: MFMU Cesarean Registry: Thromboembolism occurrence and risk factors in 39,285 cesarean births, Abstract #207. Presented at the Society for Maternal–Fetal Medicine 24th Annual Meeting, New Orleans, LA, February 5, 2004

Heijboer H, Buller HR, Lensing AW, et al: A comparison of real-time compression ultrasonography with impedance plethysmography for the diagnosis of deep-vein thrombosis in symptomatic outpatients. N Engl J Med 329:1365, 1993

Hirano Y, Kasashima F, Abe Y, et al: The use of a Greenfield filter to treat a pregnant woman for internal jugular venous thrombosis: Report of a case. Surg Today 32:635, 2002

Hull RD, Raskob GF, Carter CJ: Serial IPG in pregnancy patients with clinically suspected DVT: Clinical validity of negative findings. Ann Intern Med 112:663, 1990

Hux CH, Wapner RJ, Chayen B, et al: Use of the Greenfield filter for thromboembolic disease in pregnancy. Am J Obstet Gynecol 155:734, 1986

Kalafatis M, Rand MD, Mann KG: The mechanism of inactivation of human factor V and human factor VA by activated protein C. J Biol Chem 269:31869, 1994

Katz VL: Detecting thrombophilia in ob/gyn patients. Contemp Ob/Gyn October 2002, p 68

Kavanagh EC, O'Hare A, Hargaden G, et al: Risk of pulmonary embolism after negative MDCT pulmonary angiography findings. AJR Am J Roentgenol 182:499, 2004

Kearon C, Gent M, Hirsh J, et al: A comparison of three months of anticoagulation with extended anticoagulation for a first episode of idiopathic venous thromboembolism. N Engl J Med 340:901, 1999

Kelly J, Hunt BJ: Role of D-dimers in diagnosis of venous thromboembolism. Lancet 359:456, 2002

Kline JA, Johns KL, Colucciello SA, et al: New diagnostic tests for pulmonary embolism. Ann Emerg Med 35:168, 2000

Konstantinides S, Geibel A, Heusel G, et al: Heparin plus alteplase compared with heparin alone in patients with submassive pulmonary embolism. N Engl J Med 347:1143, 2002

Kovalevsky G, Gracia CR, Berlin JA, et al: Evaluation of the association between hereditary thrombophilias and recurrent pregnancy loss: A meta-analysis. Arch Intern Med 164:558, 2004

Kujovich JL: Thrombophilia and pregnancy complications. Am J Obstet Gynecol 191:412, 2004

Kupferminc MJ, Eldor A: Inherited thrombophilia and gestational vascular complications. Semin Thromb Hemost 29:185, 2003

Kupferminc MJ, Eldor A, Steinman N, et al: Increased frequency of genetic thrombophilia in women with complications of pregnancy. N Engl J Med 340:9, 1999

Kupferminc MJ, Fait G, Many A, et al: Severe preeclampsia and high frequency of genetic thrombophilic mutations. Obstet Gynecol 96:45, 2000

Lefkowitz JB, Clarke SH, Barbour LA: Comparison of protein S functional and antigenic assays in normal pregnancy. Am J Obstet Gynecol 175:657, 1996

Lensing AWA, Prandoni P, Brandjes D, et al: Detection of deep-vein thrombosis by real-time B-mode ultrasonography. N Engl J Med 320:342, 1989

Lepercq J, Conard J, Borel-Derlon A, et al: Venous thromboembolism during pregnancy: A retrospective study of enoxaparin safety in 624 pregnancies. Br J Obstet Gynaecol 108:1134, 2001

Levine JS, Branch DW, Rauch J: The antiphospholipid syndrome. N Engl J Med 346:752, 2002

Lindqvist P, Dahlbäck B, Maršál K: Thrombotic risk during pregnancy: A population study. Obstet Gynecol 94:595, 1999

Lockwood CJ: Heritable coagulopathies in pregnancy. Obstet Gynecol Surv 54:754, 1999

Lockwood CJ: Inherited thrombophilias in pregnant patients: Detection and treatment paradigm. Obstet Gynecol 99:333, 2002

López-Quesada E, Vilaseca MA, Lailla JM: Plasma total homocysteine in uncomplicated pregnancy and in preeclampsia. Eur J Obstet Gynecol Reprod Biol 108:45, 2003

Mandel H, Brenner B, Berant M, et al: Coexistence of hereditary homocystinuria and factor V Leiden—effect on thrombosis. N Engl J Med 334:763, 1996

Martinelli I, De Stefano V, Taioli E, et al: Inherited thrombophilia and first venous thromboembolism during pregnancy and puerperium. Thromb Haemost 87:791, 2002

McColl MD, Walker ID, Greer IA: The role of inherited thrombophilia in venous thromboembolism associated with pregnancy. Br J Obstet Gynaecol 106:756, 1999

McDonald SD, Walker MC: Homocysteine levels in pregnant women who smoke cigarettes. Med Hypotheses 57:792, 2001

Meaney JF, Weg JG, Chenevert TL, et al: Diagnosis of pulmonary embolism with magnetic resonance angiography. N Engl J Med 336:1422, 1997

Melis F, Vandenbrouke JP, Buller HR, et al: Estimates of risk of venous thrombosis during pregnancy and puerperium are not influenced by diagnostic suspicion and referral basis. Am J Obstet Gynecol 191(3):825, 2004

Miniño AM, Arias E, Kochanek KD, et al: Deaths: Final Data for 2000. National Vital Statistics Reports, Vol 50, No. 15. Hyattsville, Md: National Center for Health Statistics, 2002

Mueller MJ, Lebherz TB: Antepartum thrombophlebitis. Obstet Gynecol 34:867, 1969

National Institutes of Health Consensus Development Conference: Prevention of venous thrombosis and pulmonary embolism. JAMA 256:744, 1986

Neill AM, Appleton DS, Richards P: Retrievable inferior vena caval filter for thromboembolic disease in pregnancy. Br J Obstet Gynaecol 104:1416, 1997

Nuthalapaty F, Ho M, Singh S, et al: Limitations of helical CT for the diagnosis of pulmonary thromboembolism during pregnancy and the puerperium. Presented at the Society for Maternal–Fetal Medicine 25th Annual Meeting, Reno, Nevada, February 7, 2005

Oudkerk M, van Beek JR, Wielopolski P, et al: Comparison of contrast-enhanced magnetic resonance angiography and conventional pulmonary angiography for the diagnosis of pulmonary embolism: A prospective study. Lancet 359:1643, 2002

PIOPED Investigators: Value of the ventilation/perfusion scan in acute pulmonary embolism: Results of the Prospective Investigation of Pulmonary Embolism Diagnosis (PIOPED). JAMA 263:2753, 1990

Preston FE, Rosendaal FR, Walker ID, et al: Increased fetal loss in women with heritable thrombophilia. Lancet 348:913, 1996

Prisco D, Falciani M, Antonucci E, et al: Hirudins for prophylaxis and treatment of venous thromboembolism. Semin Thromb Hemost 27:542, 2001

Procházka M, Happach C, Maršál K, et al: Factor V Leiden in pregnancies complicated by placental abruption. Br J Obstet Gynaecol 110:462, 2003

Quinlan DJ, McQuillan A, Eikelboom JW: Low-molecular-weight heparin compared with intravenous unfractionated heparin for treatment of pulmonary embolism: A meta-analysis of randomized, controlled trials. Ann Intern Med 140:143, 2004

Raj G: Non-invasive strategies for the diagnosis of pulmonary embolism: Their role and limitations. Internal Medicine Grand Rounds, University of Texas Southwestern Medical Center, Dallas, Texas, June 12, 2003

Rey E, Kahn SR, David M, et al: Thrombophilic disorders and fetal loss: A meta-analysis. Lancet 361:901, 2003

Ridker PM, Goldhaber SZ, Danielsone E, et al: Long-term, low-intensity warfarin therapy for the prevention of recurrent venous thromboembolism. N Engl J Med 348:1425, 2003

Rodie VA, Thomson AJ, Stewart FM, et al: Low molecular weight heparin for the treatment of venous thromboembolism in pregnancy: A case series. Br J Obstet Gynaecol 109:1020, 2002

Saade GR, McLintock C: Inherited thrombophilia and stillbirth. Semin Perinatol 26:51, 2002

Salonen Ros H, Lichtenstein P, Bellocco R, et al: Pulmonary embolism and stroke in relation to pregnancy: How can high-risk women be identified? Am J Obstet Gynecol 186:198, 2002

Salonvaara M, Kuismanen K, Mononen T, et al: Diagnosis and treatment of a newborn with homozygous protein C deficiency. Acta Paediatr 93:137, 2004

Sanson BJ, Lensing AW, Prins MH, et al: Safety of low-molecular-weight heparin in pregnancy: A systematic review. Thromb Haemost 81:668, 1999

Schoepf UJ, Costello P: CT angiography for diagnosis of pulmonary embolism: State of the art. Radiology 230:329, 2004

Seguin J, Weatherstone K, Nankervis C: Inherited antithrombin III deficiency in the neonate. Arch Pediatr Adolesc Med 148:389, 1994

Seligsohn U, Lubetsky A: Genetic susceptibility to venous thrombosis. N Engl J Med 344:1222, 2001

Sephton V, Farquharson RG, Topping J, et al: A longitudinal study of maternal dose response to low molecular weight heparin in pregnancy. Obstet Gynecol 101:1307, 2003

Simpson EL, Lawrenson RA, Nightingale AL, et al: Venous thromboembolism in pregnancy and the puerperium: Incidence and additional risk factors from a London perinatal database. Br J Obstet Gynaecol 108:56, 2001

Smith MP, Norris LA, Steer PJ, et al: Tinzaparin sodium for thrombosis treatment and prevention during pregnancy. Am J Obstet Gynecol 190:495, 2004

Stefano VD, Martinelli I, Mannucci PM, et al: The risk of recurrent deep venous thrombosis among heterozygous carriers of both factor V Leiden and the G20210A prothrombin mutation. N Engl J Med 341:801, 1999

Stein PD, Athanasoulis C, Alavi A, et al: Complications and validity of pulmonary angiography in acute pulmonary embolism. Circulation 85:462, 1992

Srivastava SD, Ealeton MJ, Greenfield LJ: Diagnosis of Pulmonary embolism with various imaging modalities. Semin Vasc Surg 17:173, 2004

Tengborn L, Bergqvist D, Matzsch T, et al: Recurrent thromboembolism in pregnancy and puerperium: Is there a need for thromboprophylaxis? Am J Obstet Gynecol 160:90, 1989

Thomas LA, Summers RR, Cardwell MS: Use of Greenfield filters in pregnant women at risk for pulmonary embolism. South Med J 90:215, 1997

Toglia MR, Weg JG: Venous thromboembolism during pregnancy. N Engl J Med 335:108, 1996

van der Molen EF, Verbruggen B, Nováková I, et al: Hyperhomocysteinemia and other thrombotic risk factors in women with placental vasculopathy. Br J Obstet Gynaecol 107:785, 2000

van Strijen MJ, de Monye W, Schiereck J, et al: Single-detector helical computed tomography as the primary diagnostic test in suspected pulmonary embolism: A multicenter clinical management study of 510 patients. Ann Intern Med 138:307, 2003

van Wijk FH, Wolf H, Piek JM, et al: Administration of low molecular weight heparin within two hours before caesarean section increases the risk of wound haematoma. Br J Obstet Gynaecol 109:955, 2002

Villarreal C, Garcia-Aguirre G, Hernandez C, et al: Congenital thrombophilia associated to obstetric complications. J Thromb Thrombolysis 14:163, 2002

Virchow R: Gesammalte abhandlungen zur wissenschaftlichen medtzin. Frankfurt: Medinger Sohn & Co., 1856, p 219

von Mandach U, Aebersold F, Huch R, et al: Short-term low-dose heparin plus bedrest impairs bone metabolism in pregnant women. Eur J Obstet Gynecol Reprod Biol 106:25, 2003

Walker MC, Garner PR, Keely EJ, et al: Changes in activated protein C resistance during normal pregnancy. Am J Obstet Gynecol 177:162, 1997

Warkentin TE, Kelton JG: Temporal aspects of heparin-induced thrombocytopenia. N Engl J Med 344:1286, 2001

Weiss N, Bernstein PS: Risk factor scoring for predicting venous thromboembolism in obstetric patients. Am J Obstet Gynecol 182:1073, 2000

Weitz JI: Low-molecular-weight heparins. N Engl J Med 337:688, 1997

Wells PS, Anderson DR, Rodger M, et al: Evaluation of D-dimer in the diagnosis of suspected deep-vein thrombosis. N Engl J Med 349:1227, 2003

Winer-Muram HT, Boone JM, Brown HL, et al: Pulmonary embolism in pregnant patients: Fetal radiation dose with helical CT. Radiology 224:487, 2002

Witlin AG, Mattar FM, Saade GR, et al: Presentation of venous thromboembolism during pregnancy. Am J Obstet Gynecol 181:1118, 1999

Woo YL, Allard S, Cohen H, et al: Danaparoid thromboprophylaxis in pregnant women with heparin-induced thrombocytopenia. Br J Obstet Gynaecol 109:466, 2002

48

Renal and Urinary Tract Disorders

Although some diseases of the kidney and urinary tract may be associated with pregnancy by chance, pregnancy-induced changes may predispose to the development of renal tract disorders. One example is the markedly increased risk of pyelonephritis. Pregnancy may worsen chronic renal disease and its sequelae because of the high incidence of hypertension and preeclampsia. In the past, obstetrical dogma contraindicated pregnancy in women with significant renal disease. However, most women with these disorders go through pregnancy without serious consequences.

URINARY TRACT CHANGES DURING PREGNANCY

Significant changes in both structure and function that take place in the urinary tract during normal pregnancy are discussed in Chapter 5 (see p. 137). Dilatation of the renal calyces and ureters can be striking (Fig. 48–1). Some women have dilatation before 14 weeks, thus implicating hormonal relaxation of the muscular layers of the urinary tract. There is further dilatation beginning at midpregnancy because of ureteral compression, especially on the right side (Faúndes and associates, 1998). Interestingly, the fetal urinary tract mimics the maternal dilatation (Graif and colleagues, 1992).

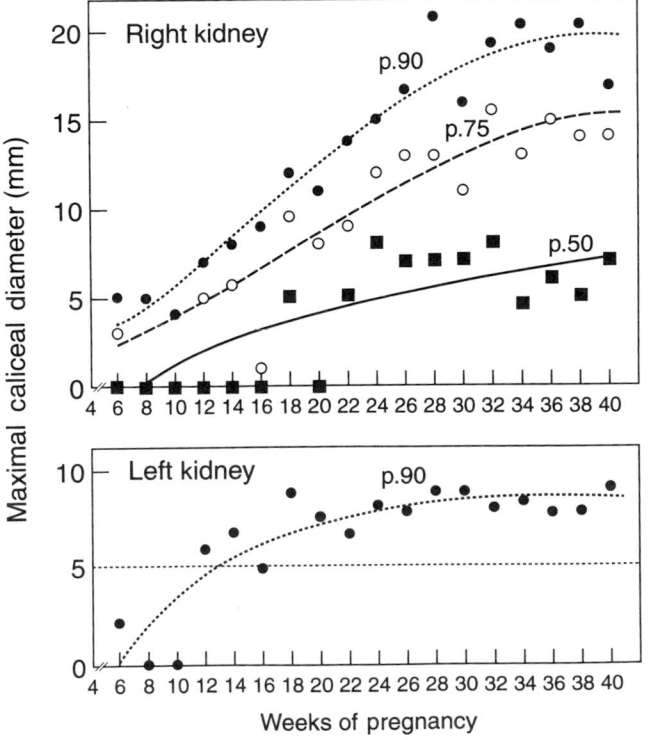

FIGURE 48–1. The 50th, 75th, and 90th percentiles for renal caliceal diameters measured using ultrasound in 1395 pregnant women from 4 to 42 weeks. (From Faúndes and co-workers, 1998, with permission.)

Increased *vesicoureteral reflux* is another change. An important consequence of these normal pregnancy-associated changes is a potentially serious upper urinary infection as well as erroneous interpretation of studies done to evaluate obstruction.

Evidence of renal function hypertrophy is apparent very soon after conception. Pregnancy-induced intrarenal vasodilatation increases effective renal plasma flow and glomerular filtration by 40 and 65 percent, respectively. By 2 weeks postpartum, the glomerular filtration rate is about 20 percent above nonpregnant normal (Hladunewich and colleagues, 2004). This has clinical relevance when interpreting renal function studies; for example, serum concentrations of creatinine and urea decrease substantively across pregnancy. Other alterations include those related to maintaining normal acid–base homeostasis, osmoregulation, and fluid and electrolyte retention.

ASSESSMENT OF RENAL DISEASE DURING PREGNANCY

The *urinalysis* is essentially unchanged during pregnancy, except for occasional glucosuria. Although *protein excretion* normally is increased, it seldom reaches levels that are detected by usual screening methods. Higby and colleagues (1994) reported 24-hour protein excretion to be 115 mg with a 95-percent confidence level at 260 mg/day. There were no significant differences by trimester. Albumin constitutes only a small part of total protein excretion and ranges from 5 to 30 mg/day. Most investigators agree that proteinuria must exceed 300 to 500 mg/day to be considered abnormal for pregnancy. Stehman-Breen and associates (2002) found that 3 percent of 4589 nulliparas had *idiopathic hematuria* when screened before 20 weeks. They also reported that these women had a twofold risk of preeclampsia.

If the serum creatinine persistently exceeds 0.9 mg/dL (75 μmol/L), then intrinsic renal disease should be suspected. A carefully collected, timed urine specimen can be used to estimate the glomerular filtration rate by creatinine clearance. *Ultrasonography* provides imaging of renal size and relative consistency, as well as elements of obstruction (see Fig. 48–1). Full-sequence *intravenous pyelography* is not done routinely, but injection of contrast media with one or two abdominal radiographs may be indicated by the clinical situation (see Chap. 41, p. 979). The usual clinical indications for *cystoscopy* are followed.

Although Packham and Fairley (1987) reported *renal biopsy* to be safe during pregnancy, biopsy usually is postponed unless it would change therapy (Lindheimer and colleagues, 2000). In a series of 15 women, Chen and co-workers (2001) found that biopsy was helpful in directing management during pregnancy. Strevens and associates (2003b) performed a renal biopsy in 12 *normal* pregnant volunteers and reported that five had slight to moderate glomerular endotheliosis. In contrast, all 27 women with proteinuric hypertension had endotheliosis and in all but one it was moderate to severe. Strevens and colleagues (2003a) showed that increasing serum levels of cystatin C correlated with glomerular swelling seen on biopsy.

Orthostatic Proteinuria. Abnormal amounts of protein are sometimes detectable in urine collected when the woman is ambulatory but not when recumbent and without other evidence of renal disease. Such *orthostatic* or *postural proteinuria* has been observed in up to 5 percent of normal young adults. The pregnant woman with orthostatic proteinuria should be evaluated for bacteriuria, abnormal urinary sediment, reduced glomerular filtration, and hypertension. In the absence of these abnormalities, orthostatic proteinuria is probably inconsequential.

Pregnancy After Unilateral Nephrectomy. In general, the excretory capacity of two kidneys exceeds ordinary needs. In addition, the surviving kidney undergoes pregnancy-induced hypertrophy of function. Therefore, women with one normal kidney most often have no difficulty in pregnancy (Baylis and Davison, 1991). Thorough functional evaluation of the remaining kidney is essential.

URINARY TRACT INFECTIONS

These are the most common bacterial infections encountered during pregnancy. Although *asymptomatic bacteriuria* is the most common, symptomatic infection may involve the lower tract and cause *cystitis*, or it may involve the renal calyces, pelvis, and parenchyma and cause *pyelonephritis*.

Organisms that cause urinary infections are those from the normal perineal flora. About 90 percent of strains of *Escherichia coli* that cause nonobstructive pyelonephritis have *adhesins* or *P-fimbriae* that enhance their virulence (Dodson and co-workers, 2001; Lügering and associates, 2003). These strains produce hemolysin and have the *PapG gene* that encodes the P-fimbriae tip (Hooton and co-workers, 2000). The *dra gene cluster* has been associated with ampicillin-resistant *E coli* (Hart and colleagues, 2001). Although pregnancy itself does not enhance these virulence factors, urinary stasis and vesicoureteral reflux predispose to symptomatic upper urinary infections.

In the puerperium, bladder sensitivity to intravesical fluid tension is often decreased as a consequence of the trauma of labor as well as epidural or spinal analgesia (see Chap. 30, p. 705). Sensations of bladder distention are also likely diminished by discomfort caused by an episiotomy, periurethral lacerations, or vaginal wall hematomas. Normal postpartum diuresis may worsen bladder overdistention. Catheterization to provide relief commonly leads to urinary infection. There appear to be no long-term sequelae from postpartum urinary retention (Yip and colleagues, 2002).

ASYMPTOMATIC BACTERIURIA. This refers to persistent, actively multiplying bacteria within the urinary tract in women who have no symptoms. The reported prevalence of bacteriuria in nonpregnant women is 5 to 6 percent (Hooton and colleagues, 2000). These are usually the same women in whom bacteriuria is discovered during prenatal care. The incidence during pregnancy varies from 2 to 7 percent and depends on parity, race, and socioeconomic status. The highest incidence is in African-American multiparas with sickle-cell trait, and the lowest incidence is in affluent white women of low parity.

Bacteriuria is typically present at the time of the first prenatal visit, and after an initial negative urine culture, fewer than 1 percent of women develop urinary infection (Whalley, 1967). A clean-voided specimen containing more than 100,000 organisms per mL is diagnostic. It may be prudent to treat when lower concentrations are identified, because pyelonephritis develops in some women with colony counts of 20,000 to 50,000 organisms/mL (Lucas and Cunningham, 1993).

Significance. If asymptomatic bacteriuria is not treated, about 25 percent of infected women subsequently develop acute symptomatic infection during that pregnancy. Eradication of bacteriuria with antimicrobial agents prevents most of these infections. The American Academy of Pediatrics and the American College of Obstetricians and Gynecologists (2002) recommend routine screening for bacteriuria at the first prenatal visit (see Chap. 8, p. 208). Screening by urine culture may not be cost effective when the prevalence is low. Because of a high prevalence (5 to 8 percent) at Parkland and the University of Alabama Hospitals, culture screening is done. Susceptibility testing is not necessary, because initial treatment is empirical. Less expensive screening tests, such as the leukocyte esterase-nitrite dipstick, are cost effective when the prevalence is about 2 percent or less (Rouse and colleagues, 1995). Millar and associates (2000) found that a method using enzymatic detection of urinary catalase activity was ineffective.

Covert bacteriuria has been associated in some studies, but not others, with preterm or low-birthweight infants (Kass, 1962). Whether eradication of bacteriuria decreases these complications is controversial. Using multivariate analysis for a perinatal registry cohort of 25,746 mother–infant pairs, Schieve and colleagues (1994) reported increased risks for low-birthweight infants, preterm delivery, hypertension or preeclampsia, and maternal anemia. These findings are at variance with those of Gilstrap and colleagues (1981b) and Whalley (1967). Thus, asymptomatic bacteriuria likely has very little, if any, impact on pregnancy outcome except for serious urinary tract infections.

Bacteriuria persists or recurs after delivery in many of these women, and symptomatic infections are common. In some, pyelographic evidence of chronic infection, obstructive lesions, or congenital urinary abnormalities is found

TABLE 48–1 Antimicrobial Agents Used for Treatment of Pregnant Women with Asymptomatic Bacteriuria

Single-dose treatment
Amoxicillin, 3 g
Ampicillin, 2 g
Cephalosporin, 2 g
Nitrofurantoin, 200 mg
Trimethoprim-sulfamethoxazole, 320/1600 mg

3-day course
Amoxicillin, 500 mg three times daily
Ampicillin, 250 mg four times daily
Cephalosporin, 250 mg four times daily
Ciprofloxacin, 250 mg twice daily
Levofloxacin, 250 mg daily
Nitrofurantoin, 50 to 100 mg four times daily; 100 mg twice daily
Trimethoprim-sulfamethoxazole, 160/800 mg two times daily

Other
Nitrofurantoin, 100 mg four times daily for 10 days
Nitrofurantoin, 100 mg at bedtime for 10 days

Treatment failures
Nitrofurantoin, 100 mg four times daily for 21 days

Suppression for bacterial persistence or recurrence
Nitrofurantoin, 100 mg at bedtime for remainder of pregnancy

(Kincaid-Smith and Bullen, 1965; Whalley and associates, 1965).

Treatment. Bacteriuria may be treated empirically with any of several antimicrobial regimens (Table 48–1). Selection can also be based on in vitro susceptibilities. In our experience, treatment for 10 days with nitrofurantoin macrocrystals, 100 mg at bedtime, is usually effective. Single-dose antimicrobial therapy has also been used with success for bacteriuria (Andriole and Patterson, 1991). The recurrence rate for all of the regimens shown in Table 48–1 is about 30 percent. Their failure to eradicate bacteriuria may indicate covert upper tract infection and the need for longer therapy. For recurrences, we have had success with nitrofurantoin, 100 mg at bedtime for 21 days (Lucas and Cunningham, 1994). For women with persistent or frequent bacteriuria recurrences, suppressive therapy for the remainder of pregnancy may be given with nitrofurantoin, 100 mg at bedtime. This regimen has been proven to be extremely safe, although nitrofurantoin may rarely cause an acute pulmonary reaction that dissipates on its withdrawal (Boggess and colleagues, 1996).

CYSTITIS AND URETHRITIS. Bladder infection during pregnancy may develop without antecedent covert bacteriuria (Harris and Gilstrap, 1981). Typically, cystitis is characterized by dysuria, urgency, and frequency. There are few associated systemic findings. Usually there is pyuria as well as bacteriuria. Microscopic hematuria is common, and occasionally there is gross hematuria from hemorrhagic cystitis

(Fakhoury and co-workers, 1994). Although cystitis is usually uncomplicated, the upper urinary tract may become involved by ascending infection. Certainly, 40 percent of pregnant women with acute pyelonephritis have preceding symptoms of lower tract infection (Gilstrap and associates, 1981a).

Treatment. Women with cystitis respond readily to any of several regimens. As with covert bacteriuria, a three-day course of therapy is usually 90-percent effective (Fihn, 2003). The three-day regimens summarized in Table 48–1 are also satisfactory for cystitis. Single-dose therapy is less effective for both nonpregnant and pregnant women, and if used, concomitant pyelonephritis must be confidently excluded.

Frequency, urgency, dysuria, and pyuria accompanied by a urine culture with no growth may be the consequence of urethritis caused by *Chlamydia trachomatis,* a common pathogen of the genitourinary tract. Mucopurulent cervicitis usually coexists, and erythromycin therapy is effective (see Chap. 59, p. 1307).

ACUTE PYELONEPHRITIS. Renal infection is the most common serious medical complication of pregnancy. In a study of the California Pregnancy Complication Surveillance System by Scott and associates (1997), genitourinary infection was the second most common reason for a nondelivery admission. The rate was 4 per 100 for nearly 150,000 pregnancies. In a recent study of more than 70,000 pregnancies in a managed care organization, Gazmararian and colleagues (2002) reported that 3.5 percent of antepartum admissions were for urinary infections. The potential seriousness is underscored by the observations of Mabie and associates (1997) that urosepsis was the leading cause of septic shock during pregnancy. Indeed, in a recent two-year audit of admissions to the Parkland Hospital Obstetrical Intensive Care Unit, 12 percent of antepartum admissions were for sepsis syndrome caused by pyelonephritis (Zeeman and co-workers, 2003). Yet another concern is that urosepsis may be related to an increased incidence of cerebral palsy in infants born preterm (Jacobsson and colleagues, 2002). There appear to be no serious long-term sequelae for the mother (Raz and collaborators, 2003).

Clinical Findings. Acute pyelonephritis develops more frequently in the second trimester and nulliparity and young age are associated risk factors (Hill and associates, 2005) It is unilateral and right-sided in more than half of cases and bilateral in a fourth. Onset is usually rather abrupt with fever, shaking chills, and aching pain in one or both lumbar regions. There may be anorexia, nausea, and vomiting. Fever of variable degrees is always present. Tenderness usually can be elicited by percussion in one or both costovertebral angles. The urinary sediment frequently contains many leukocytes, frequently in clumps, and numerous bacteria. *E coli* is isolated from urine or blood in 75 to 80 percent of infections, *Klebsiella pneumoniae* in 10 percent, and

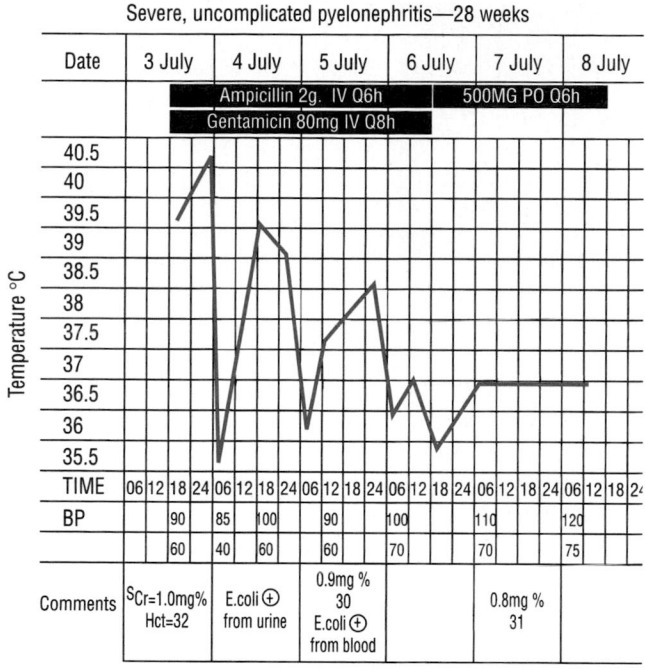

FIGURE 48–2. Vital signs graphic chart from a 28-week primigravida with acute pyelonephritis. (From Cunningham, 1988, with permission.)

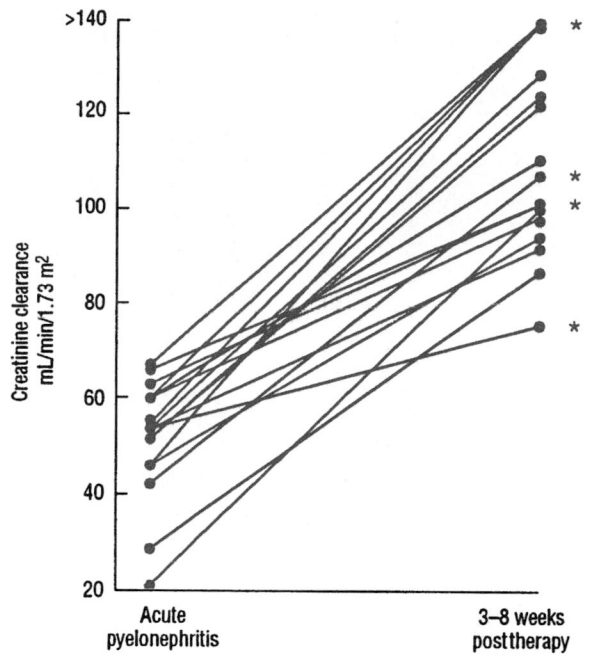

FIGURE 48–3. Endogenous creatinine clearance values in 18 pregnant women during and 3 to 8 weeks after hospitalization for acute pyelonephritis. Asterisk indicates women reevaluated while still pregnant. (From Whalley and colleagues, 1975, with permission.)

Enterobacter or *Proteus* in 10 percent (Cunningham, 1988; Wing and colleagues, 2000). **Bacteremia is demonstrated in 15 to 20 percent of women with acute pyelonephritis.** The differential diagnosis includes, among others, labor, chorioamnionitis, appendicitis, placental abruption, or infarcted myoma.

Evidence of the *sepsis syndrome* is common and is discussed in Chap. 42 (see p. 993). This includes thermoregulatory instability characterized by high spiking fever up to 42°C interspersed with hypothermia as low as 34°C (Fig. 48–2). Buhimschi and Weiner (2001) described fetal bradycardia with good reactivity in response to maternal hypothermia. Another common finding is markedly increased cardiac output from lowered systemic vascular resistance (Twickler and associates, 1994).

About 20 percent of women with pyelonephritis develop renal dysfunction; thus, plasma creatinine should be measured. As shown in Figure 48–3, any reduction in the glomerular filtration rate is reversible long term. From 1 to 2 percent of women with pyelonephritis develop varying degrees of respiratory insufficiency caused by endotoxin-induced alveolar injury and pulmonary edema (Cunningham and associates, 1987; Sanchez-Ramos and colleagues, 1995). In some cases, such as the woman whose radiographs are shown in Figure 48–4, pulmonary injury may be so severe that it causes *acute respiratory distress syndrome*.

Uterine activity from endotoxin is commonly detected (Graham and associates, 1993). This was found to be related to the severity of fever by Millar and colleagues (2003), who reported that women with pyelonephritis had an average of 5.1 contractions per hour at the time of admission. The average had decreased to 2.0 per hour within 6 hours of antimicrobial administration. As discussed in Chapter 42 (see p. 990), β-agonist therapy for tocolysis increases the likelihood of respiratory insufficiency from alveolar flooding because of its sodium- and fluid-retaining properties (Lamont, 2000). The incidence of pulmonary edema in women with pyelonephritis who were given β-agonists was reported to be 8 percent by Towers and co-workers (1991). This was a fourfold increase over the expected incidence.

Endotoxin-induced *hemolysis* is common, and about a third of these women develop acute anemia (Cox and colleagues, 1991). Hemoglobin regeneration is normal because infection does not affect erythropoietin production (Cavenee and colleagues, 1994).

Management. One scheme for management of the pregnant woman with acute pyelonephritis is shown in Table 48–2. Although we routinely obtain cultures of urine and blood, it has been shown in prospective trials that they are of limited clinical utility (Wing and co-workers, 2000). **Intravenous hydration to ensure adequate urinary output is essential.** Antimicrobials are begun promptly after diagnosis. In some cases, antimicrobials may worsen endotoxemia by causing its release from bacterial cell wall lysis. In either event, careful surveillance for worsening of sepsis syndrome is needed.

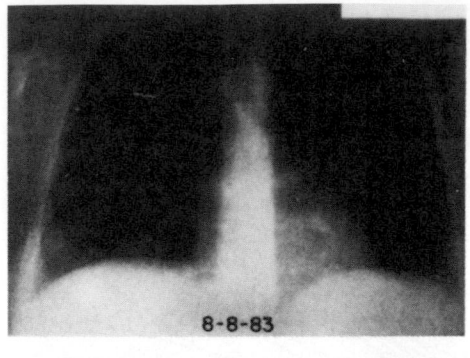
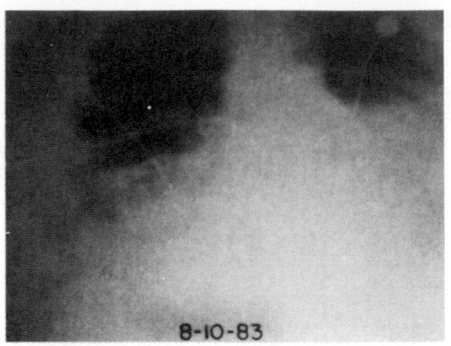
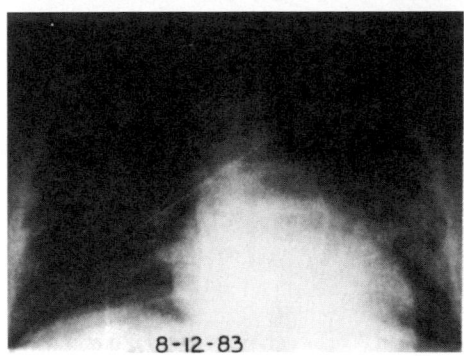
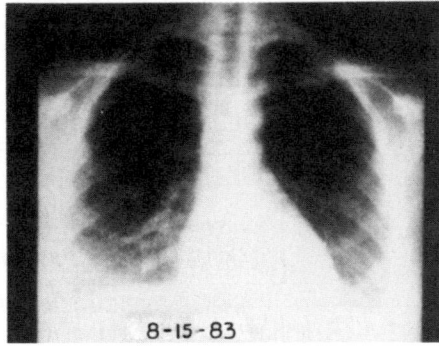

FIGURE 48–4. An 18-year-old multipara with acute pyelonephritis at 20 weeks had a normal radiograph when admitted 8-8-83. Respiratory distress 20 hours later was accompanied by a left-sided pulmonary infiltrate, which progressed to bilateral infiltrates by 8-10-83. The infiltrates improved, and she had a normal x-ray by 8-15-83. (From Cunningham and colleagues, 1987, with permission.)

Urinary output, blood pressure, and temperature are monitored closely. High fever probably should be lowered with a cooling blanket or acetaminophen. This is especially important in early pregnancy because of possible teratogenic effects of hyperthermia (see Chap. 12, p. 302).

Antimicrobial therapy is empirical, and ampicillin plus gentamicin, cefazolin, or ceftriaxone have been shown to be 95-percent effective in randomized trials (Wing and colleagues, 1998, 2000). Less than half of *E coli* strains are sensitive to ampicillin in vitro, but cephalosporins and gentamicin have excellent activity. At Parkland Hospital, our initial therapy is with gentamicin plus ampicillin. Serum

TABLE 48–2 Management of the Pregnant Woman with Acute Pyelonephritis

1. Hospitalization
2. Urine and blood cultures
3. Hemogram, serum creatinine, and electrolytes
4. Monitor vital signs frequently, including urinary output; consider indwelling catheter
5. Intravenous crystalloid to establish urinary output to ≥ 30 mL/hr
6. Intravenous antimicrobial therapy
7. Chest radiograph if there is dyspnea or tachypnea
8. Repeat hematology and chemistry studies in 48 hours
9. Change to oral antimicrobials when afebrile
10. Discharge when afebrile 24 hours; consider antimicrobial therapy for 7 to 10 days
11. Urine culture 1 to 2 weeks after antimicrobial therapy completed

Modified from Lucas and Cunningham (1994).

creatinine is monitored if these or other nephrotoxic drugs are given. Other regimens that are 95-percent effective include a cephalosporin or extended-spectrum penicillin (Sanchez-Ramos and associates, 1995). At the University of Alabama Hospital, initial treatment is with cefotetan. With any suitable regimen, response is relatively prompt in most cases, and clinical symptoms usually resolve during the first 2 days. When afebrile, the women can be discharged. Most recommend oral antimicrobial therapy for a total of 7 to 10 days.

Outpatient Management. Wing and associates (1999) described 92 women with pyelonephritis who were given in-hospital intramuscular ceftriaxone, two 1-g doses 24 hours apart. At this point, only a third were considered candidates for outpatient therapy. They were randomized to either discharge and oral antimicrobials, or continued hospitalization with intravenous therapy. Of those treated as outpatients, 30 percent were unable to adhere to their treatment regimen. Thus, outpatient management of pregnant women with pyelonephritis is applicable to very few women.

Management of Nonresponders. Almost 95 percent of women are afebrile by 72 hours (Cunningham and associates, 1973; Wing and colleagues, 2000). If there is no clinical improvement by 48 to 72 hours, then a woman should be evaluated with sonography to look for urinary tract obstruction (Seidman and co-workers, 1998). A search is made for abnormal ureteral or pyelocaliceal dilatation. Although most women with continuing infection have no evidence of obstruction, some have calculi. Renal sonography may also detect hydronephrosis, but in pregnancy, stones are not always seen (Butler and associates, 2000; Maikranz and colleagues, 1987). Occasionally, an intrarenal or perinephric abscess or phlegmon is identified (Cox and Cunningham, 1988).

If further work-up is needed for suspected renal calculi that are missed with sonography, a plain abdominal radiograph identifies nearly 90 percent of stones. Intravenous pyelography can also be performed and modified to limit the number of radiographs taken after contrast injection. The *one-shot pyelogram*, in which a single radiograph is obtained 30 minutes after contrast injection, almost always provides adequate imaging of the collecting system (Butler and colleagues, 2000). Magnetic resonance urography may be used (Spencer and associates, 2004).

Obstruction can be relieved by cystoscopic placement of a double-J ureteral stent (Rodriguez and Klein, 1988). If long-term stenting is foreseen, percutaneous nephrostomy is another option because encrusted stents are easier to replace. In some women, surgical removal of stones may be required.

Follow-up. Recurrent infection, both covert and symptomatic, is common and develops in 30 to 40 percent of women following completion of treatment for pyelonephritis (Cunningham and associates, 1973). Unless other measures are taken to ensure urine sterility, nitrofurantoin, 100 mg at bedtime, is given for the remainder of the pregnancy. Van Dorsten and co-workers (1987) reported that this regimen reduces recurrence of bacteriuria to 8 percent of cases.

REFLUX NEPHROPATHY. This is chronic interstitial nephritis that classically was thought to be due to infection, i.e., *chronic pyelonephritis.* Because radiological scarring is frequently accompanied by ureteral reflux with voiding, it is termed *reflux nephropathy.* Long-term complications include hypertension, which may be quite severe if there is demonstrable renal damage (Köhler and associates, 2003). In most cases, childhood renal infections are documented to precede these lesions. After surgical correction, half of these women have bacteriuria when pregnant (Mor and colleagues, 2003). That said, less than half of women have a clear history of preceding cystitis, acute pyelonephritis, or obstructive disease. Certainly, only a very few individuals with recurrent urinary infections develop progressive renal involvement.

Maternal and fetal prognosis depends on the extent of renal destruction. El-Khatib (1994), Jungers (1996), Köhler (2003) and their associates reported outcomes of 939 pregnancies in 379 women with reflux nephropathy. Impaired renal function and bilateral renal scarring were associated with increased maternal complications.

NEPHROLITHIASIS

Urinary stones are more common in men than in women, and the average age of onset is in the third decade. Calcium salts make up about 80 percent of renal stones, and in half of these, *familial idiopathic hypercalciuria* is the most common

predisposing cause (Asplin and colleagues, 2001). Hyperparathyroidism should be excluded. Calcium oxalate stones are the most commonly found during pregnancy (Maikranz and colleagues, 1994). Because of heritable associations, patients who have a stone typically form another stone every 2 to 3 years. Struvite stones are associated with staghorn calculi and infection, and often *Proteus* or *Klebsiella* are cultured from the urine (Bihl and Meyers, 2001).

Patients with calcium stones caused by hypercalciuria can prevent recurrences with hydration and a diet low in sodium, calcium, and protein. Thiazide diuretics also diminish stone formation. In general, obstruction, infection, intractable pain, or heavy bleeding are indications for stone removal. Removal by a flexible basket via cystoscopy to ensnare the calculus is used less often than before, however, this method is still reasonable for pregnant women. In nonpregnant patients, stone destruction by *lithotripsy* has replaced surgical therapy in most cases. Extracorporeal means, such as percutaneous ultrasonic lithotripsy or ureteroscopic laser lithotripsy, may be used. There is little information concerning these procedures during pregnancy.

STONE DISEASE DURING PREGNANCY. There is no evidence that pregnancy increases the risk of stone formation (Maikranz and associates, 1994). Moreover, stone disease does not appear to have any adverse effects on pregnancy outcome except for increased urinary infections. Pregnant women may even have fewer symptoms with stone passage because of urinary tract dilatation (Hendricks and colleagues, 1991). Symptomatic disease has a variably reported incidence, and in their review, Hendricks and co-workers (1991) cited an average incidence of 1 per 2000 pregnancies. Butler and colleagues (2000) found a 1 per 3300 incidence in more than 186,000 deliveries at Parkland Hospital. Lewis and associates (2003) reported an unprecedented incidence of 1 in 244 that they attributed to their geographic location and predominantly Caucasian population.

Diagnosis. More than 90 percent of pregnant women with nephrolithiasis present with pain. Gross hematuria was a presenting symptom in 23 percent of women described by Butler and associates (2000). However, only 2 percent of women had hematuria in the series described by Lewis and co-workers (2003). As discussed, sonography may confirm a suspected stone, but pregnancy hydronephrosis may obscure these findings (Butler and colleagues, 2000; McAleer and Loughlin, 2004). If there is abnormal dilatation without stone visualization, then the one-shot pyelogram may be useful. Transabdominal color Doppler ultrasonography to detect *absence* of ureteral "jets" of urine into the bladder has been used to exclude obstruction (Asrat and colleagues, 1998). Teichman (2004) considers the helical CT-scan as the initial imaging study in nonpregnant patients.

Management. Treatment depends on the symptoms and the duration of pregnancy. Intravenous hydration and analgesics are always given. As many as 50 percent of pregnant women with symptomatic stones have associated infection, which is treated vigorously. **Although urinary calculi infrequently cause symptomatic obstruction during pregnancy, persistent pyelonephritis despite adequate therapy should prompt a search for obstruction, which most frequently is due to nephrolithiasis.**

In about two thirds of women with symptomatic stones, there is improvement with conservative therapy and the stone usually passes spontaneously. The other third require an invasive procedure such as ureteral stenting, percutaneous nephrostomy, laser lithotripsy, basket extraction, or occasionally surgical exploration (Butler and colleagues, 2000; Lewis and co-workers, 2003). Transurethral laser lithotripsy has been used satisfactorily for stone fragmentation (Carlan and co-workers, 1995; Scarpa and associates, 1996). In the study by Watterson and colleagues (2002), holmium:YAG laser lithotripsy was successful in 9 of 10 women. Because stents for obstruction have to be changed every 4 to 6 weeks, these authors preferred lithotripsy in early pregnancy.

GLOMERULOPATHIES

The kidney, especially the glomerulus and its capillaries, is subject to a large number and variety of acute and chronic diseases. They may result from a single stimulus such as poststreptococcal glomerulonephritis, or from a multisystem disease such as systemic lupus erythematosus or diabetes. Many first become apparent because of chronic renal insufficiency. According to Brady and colleagues (2001), there are five major clinical glomerulopathic syndromes: acute nephritic syndrome, rapidly progressive glomerulonephritis, nephrotic syndrome, asymptomatic abnormalities of the urinary sediment, and chronic glomerulonephritis. The majority of these diseases are encountered in young women of childbearing age and thus are encountered during pregnancy.

ACUTE NEPHRITIC SYNDROME. Acute glomerulonephritis may result from any of several causes as shown in Table 48–3. All are characterized by an abrupt onset of hematuria and proteinuria accompanied by varying degrees of renal insufficiency and salt and water retention, causing edema, hypertension, and circulatory congestion.

Acute poststreptococcal glomerulonephritis is prototypical of these syndromes. It is of historical interest because it was confused with the renal involvement of eclampsia up until the mid-19th century. In 1843, Lever discovered that the proteinuria of eclampsia was different from that due to *Bright's disease* because it disappeared after delivery (Purkerson and Vekerdy, 1999). Currently, acute poststreptococcal glomerulonephritis rarely develops during pregnancy.

The prognosis and treatment of the other causes of the acute nephritic syndrome listed in Table 48–3 depend on their etiology. Renal biopsy may be necessary in determining

TABLE 48–3 Causes of Acute Nephritic Syndrome or Rapidly Progressive Glomerulonephritis

Immune complex disease (~ 70%)
Idiopathic
Postinfectious (streptococcal, viral)
Lupus
Bacterial endocarditis
IgA nephropathy (uncommon)
Visceral abscesses
Pauci-immune disease (~ 30%)
Wegener granulomatosis
Polyarteritis nodosa
Antiglomerular basement membrane disease (< 1%)
Anti-GBM disease (ANCA negative)
Goodpasture syndrome (pulmonary hemorrhage)
Mimickers
Malignant hypertension
Thrombotic microangiopathies (HUS/TTP)
Interstitial nephritis
Scleroderma
Preeclampsia–eclampsia

ANCA = antineutrophil cytoplasmic antibodies; GBM = glomerular basement membrane; HUS/TTP = hemolytic uremic syndrome/thrombotic thrombocytopenic purpura.
From Brady and colleagues (2001).

etiology as well as to direct management (Lindheimer and Cunningham, 1994). For example, Yankowitz and colleagues (1992) reported successful management of a pregnancy complicated by *Goodpasture syndrome,* characterized by anti–basement membrane autoantibodies, pulmonary hemorrhage, and glomerulonephritis. In some patients, *rapidly progressive glomerulonephritis* leads to end-stage renal failure. In others, *chronic glomerulonephritis* develops with slowly progressive renal disease.

IgA Nephropathy. This condition, which is also known as *Berger disease*, is the most common form of acute glomerulonephritis worldwide. Its primary form is an immune-complex disease. *Henoch-Schönlein purpura* may be a systemic form of the disease (Donadio and Grande, 2002). In a review of over 300 pregnancies complicated by IgA nephropathy, Lindheimer and colleagues (2000) concluded that pregnancy outcome depended on the degree of renal insufficiency and hypertension.

Effect of Glomerulonephritis on Pregnancy. Although the underlying etiology is not always found, acute glomerulonephritis has a profound effect on pregnancy outcome. Packham and colleagues (1989) described 395 pregnancies in 238 women previously diagnosed with *primary* glomerulonephritis. The most common lesions on biopsy were membranous glomerulonephritis, IgA glomerulonephritis, and diffuse mesangial glomerulonephritis. Despite that most of these women had normal renal function before pregnancy, overall fetal loss was 25 percent and perinatal mortality after

28 weeks was 80 per 1000. A fourth were delivered preterm and 15 percent of fetuses were growth restricted. Overall, about half of these women developed hypertension; a fourth did so before 32 weeks, and it was severe in three fourths who did. Proteinuria worsened in 60 percent of these women. Factors that portended the worst perinatal prognosis included impaired renal function, early or severe hypertension, and nephrotic-range proteinuria.

RAPIDLY PROGRESSIVE GLOMERULONEPHRITIS. In some cases, acute glomerulonephritis does not resolve, and rapidly progressive glomerulonephritis leads to end-stage renal failure within weeks to months. Patients with this form of disease may have a positive test for antineutrophil cytoplasmic antibody. Because extensive extracapillary *crescenteric glomerulonephritis* is commonly identified, the two terms are often used interchangeably.

CHRONIC GLOMERULONEPHRITIS. In many cases the cause of chronic nephritis is unknown, but it may follow any of the primary lesions in Table 48–3. Chronic glomerulonephritis is characterized by progressive renal destruction over a period of years or decades, eventually producing *end-stage renal disease (ESRD)*. Persistent proteinuria and hematuria commonly accompany a gradual decline in renal function. Microscopically, the renal lesions are categorized as proliferative, sclerosing, or membranous.

In most cases, the patient is asymptomatic, and proteinuria, anemia, or elevated creatinine are detected by screening. In others it is found during evaluation for chronic hypertension. In some women, "typical" preeclampsia–eclampsia does not resolve postpartum, and they are found to have chronic glomerulonephritis. The evolution, management, and prognosis of chronic glomerulonephritis depends on its etiology. In some patients, 10 to 20 years may elapse before end-stage renal failure supervenes. Renal biopsy may be helpful to establish prognosis.

NEPHROTIC SYNDROME. This is a spectrum of renal disorders in which proteinuria is the hallmark. It has many causes (Table 48–4), and their overlap with acute nephritic syndrome is obvious (see Table 48–3). Nephrotic syndrome is characterized by proteinuria in excess of 3 g/day, hypoalbuminemia, hyperlipidemia, and edema. There may be accompanying evidence of renal dysfunction. Most patients who undergo biopsy have microscopic renal abnormalities. The defects in the barriers of the glomerular capillary wall that allow excessive filtration of plasma proteins are caused by primary glomerular disease. These lesions may follow immunological or toxic injury, or they are from diabetes or vascular diseases.

Management of the nephrotic syndrome depends on its etiology. Edema is managed cautiously, especially during pregnancy. Jakobi and associates (1995) have described problems associated with massive vulvar edema that may complicate the nephrotic syndrome (Fig. 48–5). Normal

TABLE 48–4 Causes of the Nephrotic Syndrome in Adults

Minimal change disease (20%)
  Idiopathic (majority)
  Drug-induced (NSAIDs, rifampin)
  HIV infection
  Lymphoproliferative disorders

Focal and segmental glomerulosclerosis (33%)
  Idiopathic (majority)
  HIV infection
  Diabetes mellitus
  Reflux nephropathy
  Sickle-cell disease
  Obesity

Membranous glomerulopathy (30–40%)
  Idiopathic (majority)
  Hepatitis B, C; syphilis; malaria; endocarditis
  Amnioimmune disease (connective tissue diseases, Graves
    and Hashimoto thyroiditis)
  Cancer
  Drugs

Membranoproliferative glomerulonephritis
  Autoimmune disease (systemic lupus erythematosus)
  Chronic hepatitis B, C; HIV infection; endocarditis
  Leukemias, lymphomas

Diabetic nephropathy

Amyloidosis

HIV = human immunodeficiency virus; NSAID = nonsteroidal anti-inflammatory drug.
From Brady and colleagues (2001).

amounts of dietary protein of high biological value are encouraged, however, high-protein diets only increase proteinuria. Thromboembolism occurs with some frequency and includes arterial as well as venous thromboses. Renal vein thrombosis is particularly worrisome. The value, if any, of prophylactic anticoagulation is unclear. Some cases of

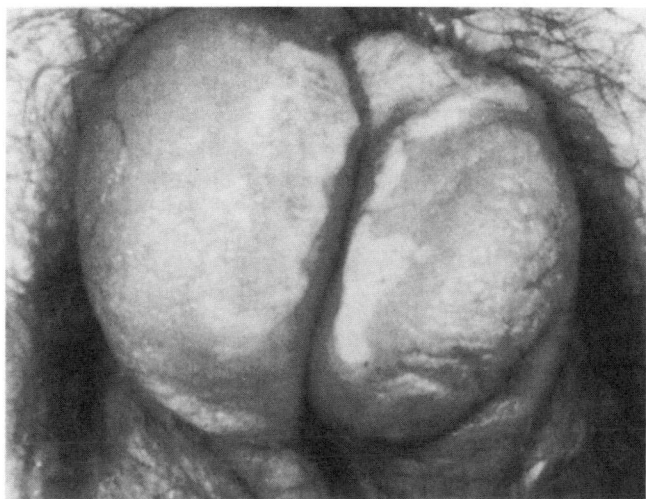

FIGURE 48–5. Massive vulvar edema at 32 weeks in a woman with the nephrotic syndrome secondary to diabetic nephropathy. (From Jakobi and colleagues, 1995, with permission.)

nephrosis from primary glomerular disease respond to corticosteroid or cytotoxic drug therapy. In most of those cases caused by infection or drugs, proteinuria recedes when the underlying cause is corrected.

Nephrotic Syndrome Complicating Pregnancy. When the nephrotic syndrome complicates pregnancy, the maternal and fetal prognosis, as well as appropriate treatment, depend on the underlying cause of the disease and the extent of renal insufficiency. Whenever possible, the specific cause should be ascertained. In this regard, when the etiology is not apparent, renal biopsy may be of value (see p. 1094).

About half of women with the nephrotic syndrome have increased protein excretion during pregnancy (Katz and associates, 1980; Packham and colleagues, 1989). In two thirds of women, protein excretion exceeds 3 g/day (Stettler and Cunningham, 1992). Despite this, women without appreciably diminished renal function usually have an increased glomerular filtration rate (Cunningham and colleagues, 1990).

The majority of women with the nephrotic syndrome who do not have severe hypertension or renal insufficiency have a successful pregnancy outcome. With renal insufficiency, moderate to severe hypertension, or both, the prognosis for mother and fetus is poor. Our experience from Parkland Hospital indicates that women with proteinuria before pregnancy frequently develop a number of complications during pregnancy (Stettler and Cunningham, 1992). Protein excretion in 65 pregnancies averaged 4 g/day, and 33 percent of these women had classical nephrotic syndrome. Some degree of renal insufficiency was found in 75 percent, chronic hypertension in 40 percent, and persistent anemia in 25 percent. Importantly, preeclampsia developed in 60 percent, and 45 percent had preterm deliveries. Excluding abortions, however, 53 of 57 infants were born alive. In the 21 women who subsequently underwent renal biopsy, histological evidence of renal disease was found. Long-term follow-up indicated that at least 20 percent of women had progressed to ESRD. Chen and colleagues (2001) reported that 8 of 15 women undergoing biopsy during pregnancy for the nephrotic syndrome either had died (3), had developed chronic renal failure (3), or had ESRD (2) by 2 years following delivery.

POLYCYSTIC KIDNEY DISEASE

This usually autosomally dominant systemic disease primarily affects the kidneys. The disease is found in 1 in 800 live births and causes about 10 percent of the ESRD in the United States (Wilson, 2004). Although genetically heterogeneous, almost 85 percent of cases are due to *PKD1* gene mutations on chromosome 16 and the other 15 percent to *PKD2* mutations on chromosome 4 (Chauvet and associates, 2002). Genetic and environmental influences on disease progression were reviewed by Peters and Breuning (2001). Prenatal diagnosis

is available if the mutation has been identified in a family member or if linkage has been established in the family.

Renal complications are more common in men than in women. Symptoms usually appear in the third or fourth decade. Flank pain, hematuria, nocturia, proteinuria, and associated calculi and infection are common findings. Hypertension develops in three fourths of patients, and progression to ESRD is a major problem. Superimposed acute renal failure results from infection or obstruction from ureteral angulation by cyst displacement.

Other organs are commonly involved. Hepatic involvement is more common and more aggressive in women than in men (Chapman, 2003). Asymptomatic *hepatic cysts* coexist in a third of patients with polycystic kidneys. Hossack and colleagues (1988) studied 163 nonpregnant patients and reported substantively increased *cardiac valvular lesions* with excessive mitral, aortic, and tricuspid incompetence. The incidence of *mitral valve prolapse* was increased 13-fold. Importantly, about 10 percent die from rupture of an associated *intracranial berry aneurysm.*

POLYCYSTIC KIDNEY DISEASE AND PREGNANCY. Fertility in men and women is not impaired. Pregnancy outcome depends on the degree of associated hypertension and renal insufficiency. Upper urinary tract infections are common. Chapman and co-workers (1994) studied 235 affected women who had 605 pregnancies. These outcomes were compared with those of 108 unaffected family members who had 244 pregnancies. Composite perinatal complication rates were similar (33 versus 26 percent), but hypertension, including preeclampsia, was more common in women with polycystic kidneys. Pregnancy does not seem to accelerate the natural disease course (Lindheimer and colleagues, 2000).

CHRONIC RENAL DISEASE

A number of kidney diseases listed in Tables 48–3 and 48–4 may become chronic. In some, there is subclinical loss of function and the serum creatinine is within a normal range. In others, there is intrinsic renal disease and proteinuria with preserved renal function. Fortunately, very few young women have ESRD that requires dialysis or renal transplantation. According to Skorecki and colleagues (2001), the most common causes of ESRD are diabetes (33 percent), hypertension (24 percent), glomerulonephritis (17 percent), and polycystic kidney disease (5 percent).

In most young women with one of these diseases, there is usually some renal insufficiency, proteinuria, or both. For counseling regarding fertility and pregnancy outcome, it is important to determine the degree of renal functional impairment as well as any associated hypertension (see Chap. 7, p. 197). Successful pregnancy outcome in general may be more related to these two factors than to the specific underlying disorder. A general prognosis can be estimated by considering women in arbitrary categories of renal function (Lindheimer and associates, 2000). These include normal or *mild impairment,* defined as a serum creatinine of less than 1.5 mg/dL; *moderate impairment,* defined as a serum creatinine of 1.5 to 3.0 mg/dL; and *severe renal insufficiency,* defined as a serum creatinine greater than 3.0 mg/dL.

PREGNANCY AND CHRONIC RENAL DISEASE. As stated, most of these women have mild renal dysfunction, and the degree of hypertension and renal insufficiency are predictive of pregnancy outcome. Other co-morbidities that contribute to adverse outcomes are diabetes and cardiopulmonary disease (Fischer and colleagues, 2004). **Even when preserved renal function is normal and the woman is normotensive, pregnancy outcome is still not always good.** Despite the high incidence of hypertension and preeclampsia, preterm and growth-restricted infants, as well as other problems, the National High Blood Pressure Education Working Group (2000) concluded that the prognosis has substantively improved over the past decades.

Physiological Changes. With mild renal insufficiency, pregnancy is accompanied by increased renal plasma flow and glomerular filtration rate (Baylis, 2003). These changes are thought to be induced by intrarenal vasodilation. With advanced renal disease, however, this vasodilation is already maximal and augmented flow is diminished to absent. In one study, only half of pregnant women with moderate renal insufficiency demonstrated augmented glomerular filtration, and none of those with severe disease had an increase (Cunningham and colleagues, 1990).

Nonpregnant women with chronic renal insufficiency have blood volumes similar to healthy women. Blood volume expansion during pregnancy is dependent on disease severity, and it correlates inversely with serum creatinine concentration (Fig. 48–6). In women with mild to moderate dysfunction, there is normal pregnancy-induced hypervolemia that averages 50 percent (Cunningham and associates, 1990). In women with severe renal insufficiency, however, volume expansion averages only 25 percent. Finally, because there is only minimal pregnancy-induced erythropoiesis in these women, preexisting anemia is intensified.

Chronic Renal Disease with Preserved Function. A number of studies allow an estimation of risk of pregnancy for the woman with preserved renal function. Surian and colleagues (1984) described 123 pregnancies in 86 women with biopsy-proven glomerular disease. Although only a few had renal dysfunction, 40 percent developed obstetrical or renal complications, or both. Hypertension developed in 20 percent, and it persisted in 50 percent of these postpartum. In 8 percent of the women, renal function deteriorated, and in half, it did not return to normal.

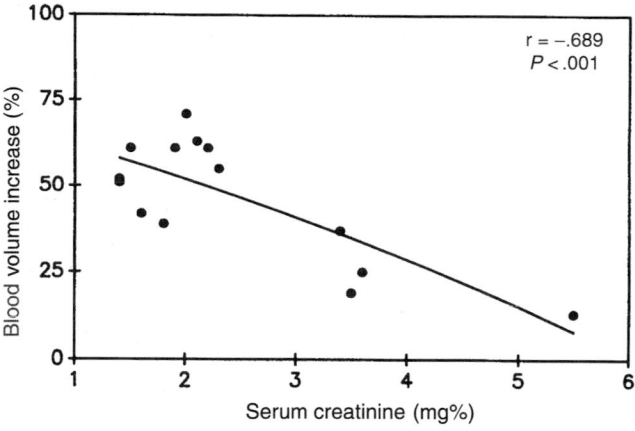

FIGURE 48–6. Blood volume expansion during pregnancy plotted as a function of serum creatinine concentration. As renal insufficiency worsens and serum creatinine increases, the degree of hypervolemia of pregnancy is diminished. (From Cunningham and colleagues, 1990, with permission.)

Packham and co-workers (1989) described their experiences from Melbourne with 238 women and 395 pregnancies. All had biopsy-proven preexisting primary glomerulonephritis, but only a few had renal insufficiency. Diffuse mesangial proliferative disease and IgA nephritis composed 70 percent of the lesions. During pregnancy, 15 percent of these women developed impaired renal function and 60 percent had worsening proteinuria. Although only 12 percent had hypertension antedating pregnancy, more than 50 percent of all women developed gestational hypertension, and in 20 percent it was severe. Importantly, hypertension developed before 20 weeks in a fourth of these pregnancies. In about 5 percent, there was irreversible worsening of renal function during pregnancy. The overall perinatal mortality rate was 140 per 1000, and after 28 weeks it was 80 per 1000. Factors associated with increased perinatal mortality and preterm delivery were impaired renal function, early or severe hypertension, and nephrotic-range proteinuria. In the absence of these three factors, however, perinatal mortality was still 50 per 1000.

Other retrospective studies from Japan and France of large numbers of pregnancies in women with chronic primary glomerulonephritis have substantiated these conclusions (Abe, 1991; Jungers and colleagues, 1991).

Chronic Renal Insufficiency. Perinatal outcome in these women is directly related to the degree of renal impairment. Hou and colleagues (1985) described 25 pregnancies complicated by moderate renal insufficiency and serum creatinines ranging from 1.2 to 1.7 mg/dL. Pregnancy-induced or aggravated hypertension developed in slightly more than 50 percent of pregnancies, and primarily because of hypertension, 60 percent were delivered preterm.

Cunningham and associates (1990) described 37 pregnancies complicated by moderate (creatinine 1.4 to 2.5 mg/dL) or severe (creatinine greater than 2.5 mg/dL) renal insufficiency.

TABLE 48–5 Renal Disease and Pregnancy Outcomes: Improvements in Perinatal Mortality over Five Decades[a]

Renal Disease	Pregnancy Outcome	Incidence (%)				
		1950s	1960s	1970s	1980s	1990s
Mild	Preterm delivery	8	10	19	25	25
	Perinatal mortality	18	15	7	< 5	< 3
Moderate	Preterm delivery	15	21	40	52	57
	Perinatal mortality	58	45	23	10	10
Severe	Preterm delivery	100	100	100	100	100
	Perinatal mortality	100	91	58	53	10

[a]Estimates are based on 3049 women with 4136 pregnancies reported from 1954 to 1997. Does not include connective tissue disorders.
Modified from Davison and Lindheimer (1999), with permission.

Complications included chronic hypertension (70 percent), anemia (75 percent), preeclampsia (60 percent), preterm delivery (35 percent), and fetal growth restriction (30 percent). Despite this, perinatal outcomes were good, and 30 of 31 infants reaching 26 weeks survived. Birthweight correlated inversely with serum creatinine concentration. Jones and Hayslett (1996) and Trevisan and colleagues (2004) described similar outcomes in pregnancies complicated by moderate to severe chronic renal insufficiency.

Shown in Table 48–5 is a summary of perinatal outcomes in over 4100 pregnancies complicated by renal disease and reported from 1954 to 1997. There is obvious marked improvement in perinatal mortality over the five decades.

Management. Frequent prenatal visits are scheduled to monitor blood pressure. Serial renal function is estimated with serum creatinine levels, and protein excretion is quantified if indicated. Women are screened and treated for bacteriuria to decrease the risk of pyelonephritis. Protein-restricted diets are not recommended (Lindheimer and colleagues, 2000; Ruggenenti and associates, 2001). Anemia from chronic renal insufficiency responds to recombinant erythropoietin, however, hypertension is a well-documented side effect. Suspected fetal growth restriction is managed as discussed in Chapter 38. If hypertension develops, it is managed as described in Chapter 34.

Follow-up. A long-standing unresolved issue is whether pregnancy accelerates chronic renal disease. Theoretically, renal hyperperfusion and increased glomerular blood pressure could accelerate nephrosclerosis (Baylis, 2003). Despite this, Jungers and associates (1995) found no adverse effect of pregnancy on survival in 360 women with chronic glomerulonephritis who mostly had normal renal function. In women with antecedent disease, however, Abe (1991) concluded that pregnancy may accelerate moderate dysfunction. **In most women, in the absence of superimposed preeclampsia or severe obstetrical hemorrhage and hypovolemia, it** **appears that pregnancy does not appreciably accelerate renal insufficiency.**

Even if pregnancy has no ill effects on renal function in the short term, there is still the likelihood that the natural history is one of long-term progression of chronic disease. Thus, the ultimate maternal prognosis can be serious. For example, Cunningham and associates (1990) reported that at least 20 percent of women with moderate to severe disease had developed end-stage renal failure by a mean of 4 years. Similarly, Stettler and Cunningham (1992) reported that at least 20 percent of women with chronic proteinuria discovered during pregnancy developed end-stage renal failure within several years. In the series reported by Chen and colleagues (2001), more than half of women who had disease prompting renal biopsy during pregnancy had end-stage renal failure by 2 years.

PREGNANCY AFTER RENAL TRANSPLANTATION

In early 2003, there were about 66,000 registrants on the waiting list for renal transplantations through the United Network for Organ Sharing (Harper and co-workers, 2002). The half-life for grafts from living donors is now 36 years and that for cadaveric grants is 20 years (Hariharan and co-workers, 2000). These survival rates approximately doubled between 1988 and 1996, due in large part to the introduction of cyclosporine for the prevention of acute and chronic rejection and the introduction of muromonab-CD3 (OKT3 monoclonal antibody) for the treatment of acute rejection. In recent years, use of newer immunosuppressive drugs such as mycophenolate mofetil and tacrolimus has been associated with further reduction of acute rejection episodes. Experience with these newer drugs during pregnancy is very limited (Alston and colleagues, 2001; Hou, 2003; Le Ray and associates, 2004). Importantly, resumption of renal function after transplantation promptly restores fertility in reproductive-age women (Lessan-Pezeshki and associates, 2004).

Davison (1994) reviewed the outcomes in 3382 pregnancies in 2409 women, 80 percent of whom had had cadaveric transplants. Most were treated with azathioprine and prednisone. The incidence of spontaneous and therapeutic abortion was 35 percent. Of pregnancies that continued beyond the first trimester, the outcome was successful in more than 90 percent of cases. Beginning early in pregnancy, the glomerular filtration rate in these women usually increased in proportion to that seen in normal women. Although proteinuria developed in 40 percent, it was not significant in the absence of hypertension.

In pregnancies reviewed by Davison (1994), preeclampsia developed in 30 percent, and signs of kidney rejection were observed in about 10 percent. Without renal biopsy, however, rejection may be difficult to distinguish from acute pyelonephritis, recurrent glomerulopathy, or severe preeclampsia. Serious infections, most likely related to immunosuppressive therapy, complicated some pregnancies. Urinary infections were diagnosed in 40 percent and the incidence of viral infections was increased. Prematurely ruptured membranes and preterm labor were common, and about half of liveborn infants were delivered preterm. Fetal growth restriction averaged 20 percent. Fortunately, although respiratory distress syndrome was common among the preterm infants, it was seldom fatal. Fetal malformations were not increased. The newborns, as well as the mothers, were at increased risk of infection because of maternal immunosuppressive therapy.

Armenti and colleagues (2000) periodically update observations from the National Transplantation Pregnancy Registry. They describe an excess of preterm and low-birthweight infants, as well as hypertension and cesarean deliveries, although fetal outcomes are generally satisfactory. Lindheimer and colleagues (2000) recommend that women who have undergone transplantation satisfy the following requisites before attempting pregnancy:

1. They should be in good general health for at least 2 years after transplantation.
2. There should be stable renal function without severe renal insufficiency (serum creatinine < 2 mg/dL and preferably < 1.5 mg/dL), none to minimal proteinuria, no evidence of graft rejection, and absence of pyelocalyceal distention by urography.
3. Absent or easily controlled hypertension.
4. Drug therapy is reduced to maintenance levels (i.e., prednisone dosage to 15 mg/day or less, azathioprine at 2 mg/kg/day or less, and cyclosporine at 5 mg/kg/day or less).

Cyclosporine or tacrolimus are given routinely to renal transplantation recipients (Jain and associates, 2004). Unfortunately, these agents are nephrotoxic and also may cause hypertension. In fact, they likely contribute substantively to ESRD that develops in 10 to 20 percent of nonrenal organ transplanted patients (Ojo and colleagues, 2003). Thomas and associates (1997) reported that cyclosporine blood levels declined during pregnancy, although this was not associated with rejection episodes. Concern persists over the possibility of late effects in offspring subjected to immunosuppressive therapy in utero. These include malignancy, germ cell dysfunction, and malformations in the children of the *offspring*. In addition, cyclosporine is secreted in breast milk, and in one instance, it produced therapeutic serum levels in the nursing child (Moretti and associates, 2003).

Finally, although pregnancy-induced renal hyperfiltration theoretically may impair long-term graft survival, Sturgiss and Davison (1995) found no evidence for this in a case-control study of 34 allograft recipients followed for a mean of 15 years.

Management. Close surveillance is necessary. Covert bacteriuria is treated, and if recurrent, suppressive treatment

for the remainder of pregnancy is given. Serial hepatic enzyme concentrations and blood counts are monitored for toxic effects of azathioprine and cyclosporine. Hou (2003) recommends measurement of serum cyclosporine levels. Gestational diabetes is more common if corticosteroids are taken. Therefore, glucose tolerance testing is done at about 26 weeks. Overt diabetes must be excluded. Opportunistic infections with herpesvirus, cytomegalovirus, and toxoplasmosis are more common.

Renal function is monitored, at first with serum creatinine determinations, but if abnormal, determination of glomerular filtration rate. If a significant decline is detected, then its cause must be determined. Possibilities include acute rejection, cyclosporine toxicity, preeclampsia, and urinary tract obstruction. Imaging studies and kidney biopsy may be indicated.

Throughout pregnancy, the woman is carefully monitored for development or worsening of underlying hypertension, and especially superimposed preeclampsia. Management of hypertension during pregnancy is the same as for nontransplanted patients. The kidney dilates minimally to moderately as do normal kidneys (Levine and colleagues, 1995). Evidence of pyelonephritis or graft rejection should prompt admission for aggressive management. Because of the significantly increased incidences of fetal growth restriction and preterm delivery, vigilant fetal surveillance is indicated. Although cesarean delivery is reserved for obstetrical indications, occasionally the transplanted kidney obstructs labor. The cesarean delivery rate approaches 50 percent (Armenti and co-workers, 2000).

DIALYSIS DURING PREGNANCY

Most often, significantly impaired renal function is accompanied by infertility. With chronic hemodialysis or peritoneal dialysis, however, fertility may be restored. As perhaps expected, pregnancies in these women are quite complicated. Okundaye and associates (1998) surveyed dialysis units listed by the Health Care Financing Administration to determine the frequency and course of pregnancies during dialysis between 1992 and 1995. A total of 241 women were identified and hemodialysis was used in 60 percent, and 40 percent received peritoneal dialysis. Almost 80 percent of the women had some degree of hypertension. In more than 95 percent of cases, the hematocrit was less than 30 percent. Pregnancy outcomes included 42 percent early losses, 26 percent preterm births, and 8 percent stillbirths. There were 11 infants with congenital malformations. Infant survival was only 40 percent in women who conceived during dialysis compared with 75 percent in those who commenced dialysis after becoming pregnant. The type of dialysis did not influence pregnancy outcome.

In a single-center study, Chao and associates (2003) described 17 pregnancies in 14 women maintained on hemodialysis for a mean of 5.3 years before conception. Of 13 pregnancies that these women chose to continue, all were delivered preterm at a mean of 32 weeks. There were four perinatal deaths. Growth restriction occurred in seven of nine infant survivors. Hydramnios developed in six of nine survivors and it was partially relieved by hemodialysis. In another report of five women, Luciani and colleagues (2002) described hydramnios in all cases.

Indications for Dialysis. Either dialysis route is feasible, and if peritoneal dialysis is ongoing, this can be continued during pregnancy. Lindheimer and colleagues (2000) recommend initiation of dialysis when serum creatinine levels are between 5 and 7 mg/dL. Abrupt volume changes that cause hypotension are avoided. To do this, dialysis time likely will be extended, and Bagon and colleagues (1998) suggest that this improves pregnancy outcome. Calciferol and erythropoietin doses may have to be increased. Complications are common and include severe hypertension, heart failure, and sepsis.

ACUTE RENAL FAILURE

The incidence of renal failure associated with pregnancy has decreased substantively over the past 30 years. Associated mortality depends on its severity and whether dialysis is needed (Singri and colleagues, 2003). Data from four studies in pregnancy are shown in Table 48–6. Except for a decreased incidence of abortion-related renal failure, the etiology has not changed dramatically over the past several decades. Turney and colleagues (1989) described findings from the Renal Unit in Leeds, England. Whereas in earlier years obstetrical cases composed 33 percent of all patients requiring dialysis, more recently these accounted for only 10 percent.

Today, renal failure is most often associated with severe preeclampsia–eclampsia. Frangieh and co-workers (1996) reported that 3.8 percent of eclamptic women from the University of Tennessee had acute renal failure. From the same institution, Audibert and colleagues (1996) reported that 3

percent of 69 women with hemolysis, elevated liver enzymes, and low platelets (*HELLP syndrome*) developed renal failure. Obstetrical hemorrhage, notably placental abruption, when it develops either alone or in concert with severe preeclampsia, is strongly linked to severe renal failure (Drakeley and coworkers, 2002). Hill and associates (2002) reported a woman managed at Parkland Hospital whose acute renal failure was accompanied by a serum creatinine level of 10.7 mg/dL. This was caused by hyperemesis at 15 weeks and required five days of hemodialysis.

Management. Identification of acute renal failure and its cause(s) is important. In most women, renal failure develops postpartum so management is not complicated by fetal considerations. Oliguria is an important sign of acutely impaired renal function. In obstetrical cases, both prerenal and intrarenal factors are commonly operative. For example, with total placental abruption, severe hypovolemia is common from massive hemorrhage. Superimposed preeclampsia may cause oliguria. Intense consumptive coagulopathy commonly triggered by an abruption might impede intrarenal microcirculation. More likely, however, consumptive coagulopathy intensifies hemorrhage due to blood loss from lacerations and surgical incisions.

When azotemia is evident and severe oliguria persists, hemodialysis should be initiated before marked deterioration of general well-being occurs. Medication dose adjustments are imperative (Singri and associates, 2003). Early dialysis appears to reduce appreciably the mortality and may enhance the extent of recovery of renal function. With time, renal function usually returns to normal or near normal.

Prevention. Acute tubular necrosis may often be prevented by the following means:

1. Prompt and vigorous replacement of blood in instances of massive hemorrhage, such as in placental abruption, placental previa, uterine rupture, and postpartum uterine atony.

TABLE 48–6 Causes and Outcomes of Obstetrical Acute Renal Failure

Study	No.	Preeclampsia–Eclampsia	Obstetrical Hemorrhage	Abortion	Others	Dialysis	Maternal Mortality (%)
Turney (1989) Leeds, United Kingdom	142	50	35	25	–		20
Sibai (1987)[a] Memphis, TN	31	100	Abruption (50) Postpartum (90)			15/31	10
Nzerue (1998) Atlanta, GA	21	38 HELLP (50%)	14	14		2/21	16
Drakeley (2002) Cape Town, South Africa	72	93	32 Abruption (10%)			10/72	0

HELLP = hemolysis, elevated liver enzymes, low platelets.
[a]Review was limited to women with hypertension.

2. Termination of pregnancies complicated by severe pre-eclampsia and eclampsia with careful blood replacement if loss is excessive.
3. Close observation for early signs of sepsis syndrome and shock in women with pyelonephritis, septic abortion, amnionitis, or sepsis from other pelvic infections.
4. Avoidance of potent diuretics to treat oliguria before initiating appropriate efforts to ensure that cardiac output is adequate for renal perfusion.
5. Avoidance of vasoconstrictors to treat hypotension, unless pathological vasodilation is unequivocally the cause of the hypotension.

Renal cortical necrosis has become exceedingly uncommon. In the not so distant past, it complicated between 15 and 30 percent of all cases of obstetrical renal failure (Grünfeld and Pertuiset, 1987; Turney and colleagues, 1989). Most cases followed placental abruption, preeclampsia–eclampsia, and endotoxin-induced shock. Histologically, the lesion appears to result from thrombosis of segments of the renal vascular system. The lesions may be focal, patchy, confluent, or gross. Clinically, renal cortical necrosis follows the course of acute renal failure and its differentiation from acute tubular necrosis is not possible during the early phase. The prognosis depends on the extent of the necrosis, and there is variable recovery of function with stable renal insufficiency (Lindheimer and colleagues, 2000).

OBSTRUCTIVE RENAL FAILURE. Rarely, bilateral ureteral compression by a very large pregnant uterus is greatly exaggerated, causing ureteral obstruction and, in turn, severe oliguria and azotemia. Brandes and Fritsche (1991) reviewed 13 cases that were the consequence of a markedly overdistended gravid uterus. They described a woman with twins who developed anuria and a serum creatinine level of 12.2 mg/dL at 34 weeks. After amniotomy, urine flow at 500 mL/hr was followed by rapid return to normal of the serum creatinine. Eckford and Gingell (1991) described 10 women in whom ureteral obstruction was relieved by stenting. The stents were left in place for a mean of 15.5 weeks and removed 4 to 6 weeks postpartum. Sadan and associates (1994) reported a similar experience in eight women who underwent ureteral stent placement during pregnancy for moderate to severe hydronephrosis. Mean gestational age at insertion was 29 weeks, and the stents remained in situ for a mean of 9 weeks. Renal function remained normal.

We have observed this phenomenon on several occasions (Satin and colleagues, 1993). Partial ureteral obstruction may be accompanied by fluid retention and significant hypertension. When the obstructive uropathy is relieved, diuresis ensues and hypertension dissipates. In one woman with massive hydramnios (9.4 L) and an anencephalic fetus, amniocentesis and removal of some of the amnionic fluid was followed promptly by diuresis, lowering of the plasma creatinine concentration, and improvement of hypertension. In our experience, women with previous urinary tract surgery are more likely to have such obstructions. Even so, the phenomenon appears uncommon. Vordermark and associates (1990) reviewed pregnancy following major urinary reconstruction and found minimal complications.

IDIOPATHIC POSTPARTUM RENAL FAILURE. In 1968, Robson and associates described what they believed to be a new syndrome of *acute irreversible renal failure* that developed within the first 6 weeks postpartum. Pregnancy and delivery were otherwise normal in the seven cases reported, and none of the known causes of renal failure was found. The pathological changes identified by renal biopsy were necrosis and endothelial proliferation in glomeruli, plus necrosis, thrombosis, and intimal thickening of the arterioles. No vascular abnormalities were demonstrated in the other visceral organs in the four cases in which autopsy was performed. Morphological changes in the erythrocytes consistent with microangiopathic hemolysis and thrombocytopenia were usually present. These findings are similar to those reported for either the *hemolytic uremic syndrome* or *thrombotic thrombocytopenic purpura*. These syndromes are collectively termed *thrombotic microangiopathies* and are considered in detail in Chapter 51 (see p. 1159).

REFERENCES

Abe S: An overview of pregnancy in women with underlying renal disease. Am J Kidney Dis 17:112, 1991

Alston PK, Kuller JA, McMahon MJ: Pregnancy in transplant recipients. Obstet Gynecol Surv 56:289, 2001

American Academy of Pediatrics and American College of Obstetricians and Gynecologists: Guidelines for perinatal care, 5th ed. Washington, DC, 2002, p 90

Andriole VT, Patterson TF: Epidemiology, natural history, and management of urinary tract infections in pregnancy. Med Clin North Am 75:359, 1991

Armenti VT, Radomski JS, Moritz MJ, et al: Report from the National Transplantation Pregnancy Registry (NTPR): Outcomes of pregnancy after transplantation. Clin Transpl 123, 2000

Asplin JR, Coe FL, Favus MJ: Nephrolithiasis. In Braunwald E, Fauci AS, Kasper DL, et al (eds): Harrison's Principles of Internal Medicine, 15th ed. New York, McGraw-Hill, 2001, p 1615

Asrat T, Roossin M, Miller EI: Ultrasonographic detection of ureteral jets in normal pregnancy. Am J Obstet Gynecol 178:1194, 1998

Audibert F, Friedman SA, Frangieh AY, et al: Diagnostic criteria for HELLP syndrome: Tedious or "helpful"? Am J Obstet Gynecol 174:454, 1996

Bagon JA, Vernaeve H, DeMuylder X, et al: Pregnancy and dialysis. Am J Kidney Dis 31:756, 1998

Baylis C, Davison J: The urinary system. In Hytten F, Chamberlain G (eds): Clinical Physiology in Obstetrics, 2nd ed. London, Blackwell, 1991, p 245

Baylis C: Impact of pregnancy on underlying renal disease. Adv Ren Replace Ther 10:31, 2003

Bihl G, Meyers A: Recurrent renal stone disease—advances in pathogenesis and clinical management. Lancet 358:651, 2001

Boggess KA, Benedetti TJ, Raghu G: Nitrofurantoin-induced pulmonary toxicity during pregnancy: A report of a case and review of the literature. Obstet Gynecol Surv 41:367, 1996

Brady HR, O'Meara YM, Brenner BM: The major glomerulopathies. In Braunwald E, Fauci AS, Kasper DL, et al (eds): Harrison's Principles of Internal Medicine, 15th ed. New York, McGraw-Hill, 2001, p 1580

Brandes JC, Fritsche C: Obstructive acute renal failure by a gravid uterus: A case report and review. Am J Kidney Dis 18:398, 1991

Buhimschi C, Weiner CP: Endotoxemia causing fetal bradycardia during urosepsis. Obstet Gynecol 97:818, 2001

Butler EL, Cox SM, Eberts E, et al: Symptomatic nephrolithiasis complicating pregnancy. Obstet Gynecol 96:753, 2000

Carlan SJ, Schorr SJ, Ebenger MF, et al: Laser lithotripsy in pregnancy. A case report. J Reprod Med 40:74, 1995

Cavenee MR, Cox SM, Mason R, et al: Erythropoietin in pregnancies complicated by pyelonephritis. Obstet Gynecol 84:252, 1994

Chao AS, Huang JY, Lien R, et al: Pregnancy in women who undergo long-term hemodialysis. Am J Obstet Gynecol 188:597, 2003

Chapman AB: Cystic disease in women: Clinical characteristics and medical management. Adv Ren Replace Ther 10:24, 2003

Chapman AB, Johnson AM, Gabow PA: Pregnancy outcome and its relationship to progression of renal failure in autosomal dominant polycystic kidney disease. J Am Soc Nephrol 5:1178, 1994

Chauvet V, Qian F, Boute N, et al: Expression of PKD1 and PKD2 transcripts and proteins in human embryo and during normal kidney development. Am J Pathol 160:973, 2002

Chen HH, Lin HC, Yeh JC, et al: Renal biopsy in pregnancies complicated by undetermined renal disease. Acta Obstet Gynecol Scand 80:888, 2001

Cox SM, Cunningham FG: Acute focal pyelonephritis (lobar nephronia) complicating pregnancy. Obstet Gynecol 71:510, 1988

Cox SM, Shelburne P, Mason R, et al: Mechanisms of hemolysis and anemia associated with acute antepartum pyelonephritis. Am J Obstet Gynecol 164:587, 1991

Cunningham FG: Urinary tract infections complicating pregnancy. Clin Obstet Gynecol 1:891, 1988

Cunningham FG, Cox SM, Harstad TW, et al: Chronic renal disease and pregnancy outcome. Am J Obstet Gynecol 163:453, 1990

Cunningham FG, Lucas MJ, Hankins GDV: Pulmonary injury complicating antepartum pyelonephritis. Am J Obstet Gynecol 156:797, 1987

Cunningham FG, Morris GB, Mickal A: Acute pyelonephritis of pregnancy: A clinical review. Obstet Gynecol 42:112, 1973

Davison JM, Lindheimer MD: Renal disorders. In Creasy RK, Resnick R (eds): Maternal–Fetal Medicine, 4th ed. Philadelphia, Saunders, 1999, p 873

Davison JM: Pregnancy in renal allograft recipients: Problems, prognosis, and practicalities. Baillieres Clin Obstet Gynecol 8:501, 1994

Dodson KW, Pinkner JS, Rose T, et al: Structural basis of the interaction of the pyelonephritic E. coli adhesin to its human kidney receptor. Cell 105:733, 2001

Donadio JV, Grande JP: IgA nephropathy. N Engl J Med 347:738, 2002

Drakeley AJ, Le Roux PA, Anthony J, et al: Acute renal failure complicating severe preeclampsia requiring admission to an obstetric intensive care unit. Am J Obstet Gynecol 186:253, 2002

Eckford SD, Gingell JC: Ureteric obstruction in pregnancy—diagnosis and management. Br J Obstet Gynaecol 98:1137, 1991

El-Khatib M, Packham DK, Becker GJ, et al: Pregnancy-related complications in women with reflux nephropathy. Clin Nephrol 41:50, 1994

Fakhoury GF, Daikoku NH, Parikh AR: Management of severe hemorrhagic cystitis in pregnancy. A report of two cases. J Reprod Med 39:485, 1994

Faúndes A, Bricola-Filho M, Pinto e Silva JC: Dilatation of the urinary tract during pregnancy: Proposal of a curve of maximal caliceal diameter by gestational age. Am J Obstet Gynecol 178:1082, 1998

Fihn SD: Acute uncomplicated urinary tract infection in women. N Engl J Med 349:259, 2003

Fischer MJ, Lehnerz SD, Hebert JR, et al: Kidney disease is an independent risk factor for adverse fetal and maternal outcomes in pregnancy. Am J Kidney Dis 43:415, 2004

Frangieh SA, Friedman SA, Audibert F, et al: Maternal outcome in women with eclampsia. Am J Obstet Gynecol 174:453, 1996

Gazmararian JA, Petersen R, Jamieson DJ, et al: Hospitalizations during pregnancy among managed care enrollees. Obstet Gynecol 100:94, 2002

Gilstrap LC III, Cunningham FG, Whalley PJ: Acute pyelonephritis in pregnancy: An anterospective study. Obstet Gynecol 57:409, 1981a

Gilstrap LC III, Leveno KJ, Cunningham FG, et al: Renal infection and pregnancy outcome. Am J Obstet Gynecol 141:708, 1981b

Graham JM, Oshiro BT, Blanco JD, et al: Uterine contractions after antibiotic therapy for pyelonephritis in pregnancy. Am J Obstet Gynecol 168:577, 1993

Graif M, Kessler A, Hart S, et al: Renal pyelectasis in pregnancy: Correlative evaluation of fetal and maternal collecting systems. Am J Obstet Gynecol 167:1304, 1992

Grünfeld JP, Pertuiset N: Acute renal failure in pregnancy: 1987. Am J Kidney Dis 9:359, 1987

Hariharan S, Johnson CP, Bresnahan BA, et al: Improved graft survival after renal transplantation in the United States, 1988 to 1996. N Engl J Med 342:605, 2000

Harper AM, Taranto SE, Edwards EB: The OPTN waiting list, 1988–2001. Clin Transpl 79, 2002

Harris RE, Gilstrap LC III: Cystitis during pregnancy: A distinct clinical entity. Obstet Gynecol 57:578, 1981

Hart A, Nowicki BJ, Reisner B, et al: Ampicillin-resistant Escherichia coli in gestational pyelonephritis: Increased occurrence and association with the colonization factor Dr adhesin. J Infect Dis 183:1526, 2001

Hendricks SK, Ross SO, Krieger JN: An algorithm for diagnosis and therapy of management and complications of urolithiasis during pregnancy. Surg Gynecol Obstet 172:49, 1991

Higby K, Suiter CR, Phelps JY, et al: Normal values of urinary albumin and total protein excretion during pregnancy. Am J Obstet Gynecol 171:984, 1994

Hill JB, Sheffield JS, McIntire DD, et al: Acute pyelonephritis in pregnancy. Obstet Gynecol 105:38, 2005

Hill JB, Yost NP, Wendel GD Jr: Acute renal failure in association with severe hyperemesis gravidarum. Obstet Gynecol 100:1119, 2002

Hladunewich MA, Lafayette RA, Derby GC, et al: The dynamics of glomerular filtration in the puerperium. Am J Physiol Renal Physiol 286:F496, 2004

Hooton TM, Scholes D, Stapleton AE, et al: A prospective study of asymptomatic bacteriuria in sexually active young women. N Engl J Med 343:992, 2000

Hossack KF, Leddy CL, Johnson AM, et al: Echocardiographic findings in autosomal dominant polycystic kidney disease. N Engl J Med 319:907, 1988

Hou S: Pregnancy in renal transplant recipients. Adv Ren Replace Ther 10:40, 2003

Hou SH, Grossman SD, Madias NE: Pregnancy in women with renal disease and moderate renal insufficiency. Am J Med 78:185, 1985

Jacobsson B, Hagberg G, Hagberg B, et al: Cerebral palsy in preterm infants: A population-based case-control study of antenatal and intrapartal risk factors. Acta Paediatr 91:946, 2002

Jain AB, Shapiro R, Scantlebury VP, et al: Pregnancy after kidney and kidney-pancreas transplantation under tacrolimus: a single center's experience. Transplantation 77:897, 2004

Jakobi P, Friedman M, Goldstein I, et al: Massive vulvar edema in pregnancy: A case report. J Reprod Med 40:479, 1995

Jones DC, Hayslett JP: Outcome of pregnancy in women with moderate or severe renal insufficiency. N Engl J Med 335:226, 1996

Jungers P, Houillier P, Chauveau D, et al: Pregnancy in women with reflux nephropathy. Kidney Int 50:593, 1996

Jungers P, Houillier P, Forget D, et al: Influence of pregnancy on the course of primary chronic glomerulonephritis. Lancet 346:1122, 1995

Jungers P, Houillier P, Forget D, et al: Specific controversies concerning the natural history of renal disease in pregnancy. Am J Kidney Dis 17:116, 1991

Kass EH: Pyelonephritis and bacteriuria. Ann Intern Med 56:46, 1962

Katz AI, Davison JM, Hayslett JP, et al: Pregnancy in women with kidney disease. Kidney Int 18:192, 1980

Kincaid-Smith P, Bullen M: Bacteriuria in pregnancy. Lancet 1:395, 1965

Köhler JR, Tencer J, Thysell H, et al: Long-term effects of reflux nephropathy on blood pressure and renal function in adults. Nephron Clin Pract 93:c35, 2003

Lamont RF: The pathophysiology of pulmonary edema with the use of beta-agonists. Br J Obstet Gynaecol 107:439, 2000

Le Ray C, Coulomb A, Elefant E, et al: Mycophenolate mofetil in pregnancy after renal transplantation: a case of major fetal malformations. Obstet Gynecol 103:1091, 2004

Lessan-Pezeshki M, Ghazizadeh S, Khatami MR, et al: Fertility and contraceptive issues after kidney transplantation in women. Transplant Proc 36:1405, 2004

Levine D, Filly RA, Graber M: The sonographic appearance of renal transplants during pregnancy. J Ultrasound Med 14:291, 1995

Lewis DF, Robichaux AG III, Jaekle RK, et al: Urolithiasis in pregnancy: Diagnosis, management and pregnancy outcome. J Reprod Med 48:28, 2003

Lindheimer MD, Cunningham FG: Renal disease complicating pregnancy. Williams Obstetrics, 19th ed (Suppl 6). Norwalk, CT, Appleton & Lange, April/May 1994

Lindheimer MD, Grünfeld JP, Davison JM: Renal disorders. In Barron WM, Lindheimer MD (eds): Medical Disorders During Pregnancy, 3rd ed. St. Louis, Mosby, 2000, p 39

Lucas MJ, Cunningham FG: Urinary infection in pregnancy. Clin Obstet Gynecol 36:855, 1993

Lucas MJ, Cunningham FG: Urinary tract infections complicating pregnancy. Williams Obstetrics, 19th ed (Suppl 5). Norwalk, CT, Appleton & Lange, February/March 1994

Luciani G, Bossola M, Tazza L, et al: Pregnancy during chronic hemodialysis: A single dialysis-unit experience with five cases. Ren Fail 24:853, 2002

Lügering A, Benz I, Knochenhauer S, et al: The Pix pilus adhesin of the uropathogenic Escherichia coli strain X2194 (O2:K(-): H6) is related to Pap pili but exhibits a truncated regulatory region. Microbiology 149:1387, 2003

Mabie WC, Barton JR, Sibai B: Septic shock in pregnancy. Obstet Gynecol 90:553, 1997

Maikranz P, Coe FL, Parks J, et al: Nephrolithiasis in pregnancy. Am J Kidney Dis 9:354, 1987

Maikranz P, Lindheimer MD, Coe FL: Nephrolithiasis in pregnancy. Baillieres Clin Obstet Gynecol 8:375, 1994

McAleer SJ, Loughlin KR: Nephrolithiasis and pregnancy. Curr Opin Urol 14:123, 2004

Millar L, DeBuque L, Leialoha C, et al: Rapid enzymatic urine screening test to detect bacteriuria in pregnancy. Obstet Gynecol 95:601, 2000

Millar LK, DeBuque L, Wing DA: Uterine contraction frequency during treatment of pyelonephritis in pregnancy and subsequent risk of preterm birth. J Perinat Med 31:41, 2003

Mor Y, Leibovitch I, Zalts R, et al: Analysis of the long-term outcome of surgically corrected vesico ureteric reflux. BJU Int 92:97, 2003

Moretti ME, Sgro M, Johnson DW, et al: Cyclosporine excretion into breast milk. Transplantation 75:2144, 2003

National High Blood Pressure Education Program Working Group on High Blood Pressure in Pregnancy: Report of the National High Blood Pressure Education Program Working Group on High Blood Pressure in Pregnancy. Am J Obstet Gynecol 183:S1, 2000

Nzerue CM, Hewan-Lowe K, Nwawka C: Acute renal failure in pregnancy: A review of clinical outcomes at an inner city hospital from 1986–1996. J Natl Med Assoc 90:486, 1998

Ojo AO, Held PJ, Port FK, et al: Chronic renal failure after transplantation of a nonrenal organ. N Engl J Med 349:931, 2003

Okundaye I, Abrinko P, Hou S: Registry of pregnancy in dialysis patients. Am J Kidney Dis 31:766, 1998

Packham D, Fairley KF: Renal biopsy: Indications and complications in pregnancy. Br J Obstet Gynaecol 94:935, 1987

Packham DK, North RA, Fairley KF, et al: Primary glomerulonephritis and pregnancy. Q J Med 71:537, 1989

Peters DJM, Breuning MH: Autosomal dominant polycystic kidney disease: Modification of disease progression. Lancet 358:1439, 2001

Purkerson ML, Vekerdy L: The history of eclampsia, toxemia and the kidney in pregnancy. Am J Nephrol 19:313, 1999

Raz R, Sakran W, Chazan B, et al: Long-term follow-up of women hospitalized for acute pyelonephritis. Clin Infect Dis 37:1014, 2003

Robson JS, Martin AM, Ruckley VA, et al: Irreversible postpartum renal failure. Q J Med 37:423, 1968

Rodriguez PN, Klein AS: Management of urolithiasis during pregnancy. Surg Gynecol Obstet 166:103, 1988

Rouse DJ, Andrews WW, Goldenberg RL, et al: Screening and treatment of asymptomatic bacteriuria of pregnancy to prevent pyelonephritis. A cost-effectiveness and cost benefit analysis. Obstet Gynecol 86:119, 1995

Ruggenenti P, Schieppati A, Remuzzi G: Progression, remission, regression of chronic renal diseases. Lancet 357:1601, 2001

Sadan O, Berar M, Sagiv R, et al: Ureteric stent in severe hydronephrosis of pregnancy. Eur J Obstet Gynecol Reprod Biol 56:79, 1994

Sanchez-Ramos L, McAlpine KJ, Adair CD, et al: Pyelonephritis in pregnancy: Once a day ceftriaxone versus multiple doses of cefazolin. A randomized double-blind trial. Am J Obstet Gynecol 172:129, 1995

Satin AJ, Seiken GL, Cunningham FG: Reversible hypertension in pregnancy caused by obstructive uropathy. Obstet Gynecol 81:823, 1993

Scarpa RM, de Lisa A, Usai E: Diagnosis and treatment of ureteral calculi during pregnancy with rigid ureteroscopes. J Urol 155:875, 1996

Schieve LA, Handler A, Hershow R, et al: Urinary tract infection during pregnancy: Its association with maternal morbidity and perinatal outcome. Am J Public Health 84:405, 1994

Scott CL, Chavez GF, Atrash HK, et al: Hospitalizations for severe complications of pregnancy 1987–1992. Obstet Gynecol 90:225, 1997

Seidman DS, Soriano D, Dulitzki M, et al: Role of renal ultrasonography in the management of pyelonephritis in pregnant women. J Perinatol 18:98, 1998

Sibai BM, Villar MA, Mabie BC: Acute renal failure in hypertensive disorders of pregnancy. Pregnancy outcome and remote prognosis in thirty-one consecutive cases. J Infect Dis 156:870, 1987

Singri N, Ahya SN, Levin ML: Acute renal failure. JAMA 289:747, 2003

Skorecki K, Green J, Brenner BM: Chronic renal failure. In Braunwald E, Fauci AS, Martin JB, et al (eds): Harrison's Principles of Internal Medicine, 15th ed. New York, McGraw-Hill, 2001, p 1551

Spencer JA, Chahal R, Kelly A, et al: Evaluation of painful hydronephrosis in pregnancy: Magnetic resonance urographic patterns in physiological dilatation versus calculous obstruction. J Urol 171:256, 2004

Stehman-Breen CO, Levine RJ, Qian C, et al: Increased risk of preeclampsia among nulliparous pregnant women with idiopathic hematuria. Am J Obstet Gynecol 187:703, 2002

Stettler RW, Cunningham FG: Natural history of chronic proteinuria complicating pregnancy. Am J Obstet Gynecol 167:1219, 1992

Strevens H, Wide-Swensson D, Grubb A, et al: Serum cystatin C reflects glomerular endotheliosis in normal, hypertensive and pre-eclamptic pregnancies. Br J Obstet Gynaecol 110:825, 2003a

Strevens H, Wide-Swensson D, Hansen A, et al: Glomerular endotheliosis in normal pregnancy and pre-eclampsia. Br J Obstet Gynaecol 110:831, 2003b

Sturgiss SN, Davison JM: Effect of pregnancy on long-term function of renal allografts. Am J Kidney Dis 26:54, 1995

Surian M, Imbasciati E, Cosci P, et al: Glomerular disease and pregnancy: A study of 123 pregnancies in patients with primary and secondary glomerular diseases. Nephron 36:101, 1984

Teichman JM: Clinical practice. Acute renal colic from ureteral calculus. N Engl J Med 350:684, 2004

Thomas AG, Burrows L, Knight R, et al: The effect of pregnancy on cyclosporine levels in renal allograft patients. Obstet Gynecol 90:916, 1997

Towers CV, Kaminskas CM, Garite TJ, et al: Pulmonary injury associated with antepartum pyelonephritis: Can patients at risk be identified? Am J Obstet Gynecol 164:974, 1991

Trevisan G, Ramos JG, Martins-Costa S, et al: Pregnancy in patients with chronic renal insufficiency at Hospital de Clinicas of Porto Alegre, Brazil. Ren Fail 26:29, 2004

Turney JH, Ellis CM, Parsons FM: Obstetric acute renal failure 1956–1987. Br J Obstet Gynaecol 96:679, 1989

Twickler DM, Lucas MJ, Bowe L, et al: Ultrasonographic evaluation of central and end-organ hemodynamics in antepartum pyelonephritis. Am J Obstet Gynecol 170:814, 1994

Van Dorsten JP, Lenke RR, Schifrin BS: Pyelonephritis in pregnancy: The role of in-hospital management and nitrofurantoin suppression. J Reprod Med 32:897, 1987

Vordermark JS, Deshon GE, Agee RE: Management of pregnancy after major urinary reconstruction. Obstet Gynecol 75:564, 1990

Watterson JD, Girvan AR, Beiko DT, et al: Management strategy for ureteral calculi in pregnancy. Urology 60:383, 2002

Whalley PJ: Bacteriuria of pregnancy. Am J Obstet Gynecol 97:723, 1967

Whalley PJ, Cunningham FG, Martin FG: Transient renal dysfunction associated with acute pyelonephritis of pregnancy. Obstet Gynecol 46:174, 1975

Whalley PJ, Martin FG, Peters PC: Significance of asymptomatic bacteriuria detected during pregnancy. JAMA 198:879, 1965

Wilson PD: Polycystic kidney disease. N Engl J Med 350:151, 2004

Wing DA, Hendershott CM, Debuque L, et al: A randomized trial of three antibiotic regimens for the treatment of pyelonephritis in pregnancy. Am J Obstet Gynecol 92:249, 1998

Wing DA, Hendershott CM, Debuque L, et al: Outpatient treatment of acute pyelonephritis in pregnancy after 24 weeks. Obstet Gynecol 94:683, 1999

Wing DA, Park AS, DeBuque L, et al: Limited clinical utility of blood and urine cultures in the treatment of acute pyelonephritis during pregnancy. Am J Obstet Gynecol 182:1437, 2000

Yankowitz J, Kuller JA, Thomas RL: Pregnancy complicated by Goodpasture syndrome. Obstet Gynecol 79:806, 1992

Yip S-K, Sahota D, Chang AMZ, et al: Four-year follow-up of women who were diagnosed to have postpartum urinary retention. Am J Obstet Gynecol 187:648, 2002

Zeeman GG, Wendel GD Jr, Cunningham FG: A blueprint for obstetric critical care. Am J Obstet Gynecol 188:532, 2003

49

Gastrointestinal Disorders

During normal pregnancy, the gastrointestinal tract and its appendages undergo significant anatomical, physiological, and functional changes. These changes can appreciably alter the criteria for diagnosis and treatment of a number of disorders. For example, nausea and vomiting are frequent early in normal pregnancy, but if these symptoms are erroneously attributed to normal physiological changes, then a surgical disorder may be overlooked. Conversely, persistent nausea and vomiting in late pregnancy should always prompt a search for underlying pathology. In another example, most obstetricians, but not most internists or gastroenterologists, are aware that epigastric or right upper quadrant pain can be an ominous sign of severe preeclampsia. As pregnancy progresses, gastrointestinal symptoms become more difficult to assess, and physical findings are often obscured by the large uterus, which displaces abdominal organs and can alter the location and intensity of pain and tenderness.

DIAGNOSTIC TECHNIQUES

Fiber-optic endoscopic instruments have revolutionized the diagnosis and management of most gastrointestinal conditions. These instruments are particularly well suited for use during pregnancy. Cappell (2003) estimates that annually 12,000 pregnant women have indications for gastrointestinal endoscopy, which permits evaluation of the esophagus, stomach, and duodenum (Van Dam and Brugge, 1999). With specialized instruments, the proximal jejunum can be studied, and the ampulla of Vater can be cannulated to perform *endoscopic retrograde cholangiopancreatography*. Cappell and Sidhom (1993) described endoscopy in 20 pregnant women. A diagnosis was made in 14 (70 percent); seven had esophagitis, two had duodenal ulcers, three had gastritis, and two had Mallory–Weiss tears. Cappell and colleagues (1996) described successful use of *flexible sigmoidoscopy* in 48 pregnant women. *Colonoscopy* is used to view the entire colon and the distal ileum in diagnosis and management of inflammatory bowel disease. Its use in pregnancy is limited, but preliminary results are encouraging (Cappell, 2003).

Of noninvasive imaging techniques, abdominal ultrasonography has a crucial role in evaluation of some gastrointestinal disorders. The use of computed tomography (CT) is limited because of radiation exposure. Magnetic resonance imaging (MRI) commonly is used instead for evaluating the abdomen and retroperitoneal space during pregnancy. Imaging modalities are considered in detail in Chapter 41 (see p. 977).

LAPAROTOMY AND LAPAROSCOPY

Abdominal surgery may be lifesaving for certain gastrointestinal conditions, acute appendicitis being the most common. In their first study using the Swedish Registry database through 1981, Mazze and Källén (1989) reported that abdominal exploration by laparotomy or laparoscopy was performed in 1331 of 720,000 pregnancies—about 1 in every 500 pregnancies. Kort and associates (1993) reported a similar incidence of 1 in 635 in over 49,500 births. In both studies, the most common indications for surgery were appendicitis, adnexal masses, and cholecystitis.

In nonpregnant patients, laparoscopic procedures have replaced traditional techniques for many abdominal disorders. During the past decade, laparoscopy has also been used more often during pregnancy (Carter and Soper, 2004). Reedy and associates (1997) updated the Swedish Registry database, which through 1993 included 2 million pregnancies. Of these, 2181 pregnant women underwent laparoscopy and 1522 laparotomy for nonobstetrical indications—about 1 in every 800 pregnancies. As expected, laparoscopic procedures were mostly performed before 20 weeks, and importantly, the technique was shown to be safe. Moreover, long-term follow-up studies suggest no deleterious effects for either mother or child (Rizzo, 2003). The most commonly reported nongynecological procedures are cholecystectomy and appendectomy (Fatum and Rojansky, 2001; Rollins and associates, 2004). For more details and for descriptions of surgical technique, see Chapter 41 (see p. 976) and *Operative Obstetrics* (Gilstrap and colleagues, 2002).

NUTRITIONAL SUPPORT

Specialized nutritional support can be delivered by *enteral* feedings, usually via a nasogastric tube, or parenterally, by peripheral or central venous access. When possible, enteral alimentation is preferable because it has fewer dangerous complications, the most dreaded being aspiration pneumonia (Fischer, 2001; Hamaoui and Hamaoui, 2003). In obstetrical patients, very few conditions prohibit enteral nutrition as a first effort to prevent catabolism.

The purpose of *parenteral* feeding, or *hyperalimentation*, is to provide nutrition when the intestinal tract must be kept quiescent. Peripheral venous access may be adequate for short-term supplemental nutrition, which derives calories from isotonic fat solutions. Jugular or subclavian venous catheterization is necessary for total parenteral nutrition, because its hyperosmolarity requires rapid dilution in a high-flow system. These solutions provide up to 24 to 40 kcal/kg, principally as a hypertonic glucose solution. Heyland and colleagues (1998) reviewed 26 randomized trials involving more than 2200 critically ill nonpregnant patients and reported that overall mortality was not influenced by parenteral nutrition.

Parenteral Nutrition during Pregnancy. Shown in Table 49–1 are some reported uses of total parenteral nutrition during pregnancy. Gastrointestinal disorders were the most common indication, and the duration of parenteral feeding averaged 33 days. Unfortunately, complications are frequent

TABLE 49–1 Some Conditions in Which Parenteral Nutrition Has Been Used During 81 Pregnancies

Anorexia nervosa	Intracranial hemorrhage
Appendiceal rupture	Jejunoileal bypass
Bowel obstruction	Leukemia
Burns	Pancreatic cancer
Cholecystitis	Preeclampsia
Diabetic complications	Preterm labor/ruptured membranes
Esophageal injury	Short bowel syndrome
Inflammatory bowel disease	Small bowel obstruction
Hyperemesis gravidarum	

Data from Kirby (1988), Ogura (2003), and Russo-Stieglitz (1999) and their colleagues.

and may be severe. Russo-Stieglitz and associates (1999) described a 50-percent complication rate with central catheters used during 26 pregnancies. Major mechanical complications include pneumothorax, hemothorax, and brachial plexus injury. The major serious complication is catheter sepsis, however, with an experienced nutritional support team this should be less than 1 percent (Fischer, 2001). The Centers for Disease Control and Prevention (2002) has published detailed guidelines for management to prevent catheter-related sepsis. Fetal subdural hematoma from vitamin K deficiency has also been described (Sakai and colleagues, 2003).

There is also appreciable morbidity from a *peripherally inserted central catheter* during pregnancy. Ogura and colleagues (2003) described its use for long-term access in 52 pregnant women. Proven or presumed infection affected 60 percent.

DISORDERS OF THE UPPER GASTROINTESTINAL TRACT

HYPEREMESIS GRAVIDARUM. Nausea and vomiting of moderate intensity are especially common until about 16 weeks (see Chap. 8, p. 224). In some women it is severe and unresponsive to simple dietary modification and antiemetics. Thus, *hyperemesis gravidarum* is defined variably as vomiting sufficiently severe to produce weight loss, dehydration, acidosis from starvation, alkalosis from loss of hydrochloric acid in vomitus, and hypokalemia. There is partial starvation (Chihara and co-workers, 2003). In some women, transient hepatic dysfunction develops (see Chap. 50, p. 1126). The incidence of hyperemesis severe enough to require hospitalization varies with populations studied. Borowski and associates (2003) found it to be 1.6 percent in over 9500 deliveries at the Mayo Clinic. Gazmararian and colleagues (2002) studied over 46,000 women and 0.8 percent required antepartum hospitalization for hyperemesis.

Hyperemesis appears to be related to high or rapidly rising serum levels of either chorionic gonadotropin, estrogens, or both (Goodwin and associates, 1994; van de Ven, 1997).

Recently, Schiff and colleagues (2004) reported that women with severe disease have a 1.5-fold increased chance of having a female fetus, thus lending support to the estrogen hypothesis. The most severe cases may have an interrelated psychological component (Buckwalter and Simpson, 2002). Finally, an association with seropositivity to *Helicobacter pylori,* the causative agent of peptic ulcer disease, has been convincingly disproved by several groups (Jacobson, 2003; McKenna, 2003; Yost, 2003, and all their co-workers).

Complications. Unrelenting hyperemesis can be vexing to all concerned. Godsey and Newman (1991) reported that 27 percent of 140 affected women required multiple admissions. In a prospective randomized trial of 110 women given antiemetic therapy with and without dexamethasone, Yost and associates (2003) found that 35 percent in each treatment group required rehospitalization.

Vomiting may be prolonged, frequent, and severe. Various degrees of acute renal failure from prerenal causes are encountered. We have cared for a number of women with markedly impaired renal function. The extreme is one woman who had a serum creatinine of 10.7 mg/dL and who required 5 days of dialysis (Hill and colleagues, 2002). Other life-threatening complications of continuous retching include *Mallory–Weiss tears* and *esophageal rupture, pneumothoraces,* and *pneumomediastinum* (Schwartz and Rossoff, 1994; Yamamoto and colleagues, 2001).

At least two vitamin deficiencies associated with hyperemesis are known to be serious. *Wernicke encephalopathy* from thiamine deficiency is accompanied by signs of central nervous system involvement, including confusion, visual symptoms, ataxia, and nystagmus. Usually, there are MRI findings. Complications include blindness, convulsions, and coma (Hillbom, 1999; Kim, 2002; Rees, 1997; Spruill and Kuller, 2002; Tesfaye, 1998, and all their associates). We are aware of one maternal death at midpregnancy from Wernicke encephalopathy in a woman with delayed diagnosis.

Another complication of prolonged vomiting is *vitamin K deficiency.* Robinson and colleagues (1998) have described coagulopathy with epistaxis. Plasma zinc levels are increased, copper levels decreased, and magnesium levels unchanged (Dokmeci and associates, 2004).

Management. Methods of dietary modification are discussed in Chapter 8 (see p. 224). Treatment of nausea and vomiting pregnancy with vitamin B_6 or vitamin B_6 plus doxylamine is safe and effective and should be considered first-line pharmacotherapy (American College of Obstetricians and Gynecologists, 2004). Jewell and Young (2000) surveyed the Cochrane Database System and confirmed a salutary effect with many antiemetics administered orally or by rectal suppository. When these fail, intravenous crystalloid solutions are given to correct dehydration, ketonemia, electrolyte deficits, and acid–base imbalances. Thiamine, 100 mg, is added to the first liter. Intravenous fluids are given until vomiting is controlled.

After rehydration, most women can be discharged, but if vomiting is persistent, they are usually admitted. Antiemetics such as promethazine, prochlorperazine, chlorpromazine, or metoclopramide are given parenterally. There is little evidence that treatment with corticosteroids is effective (Magee and colleagues, 2002; Ziaei and associates, 2004). In two small randomized trials, there were no benefits from *methylprednisolone* or placebo, but the steroid group had significantly fewer readmissions (Duggar and Carlan, 2001; Safari and co-workers, 1998). In another study, Yost and colleagues (2003) randomized 110 women to receive placebo or intravenous methylprednisolone followed by tapered oral steroids. An equal proportion of women in each group (35 percent) required readmission. *Serotonin antagonists* are used by some clinicians to treat severe nausea in nonpregnant patients. In one trial, *ondansetron* was not superior to promethazine (Sullivan and associates, 1996). Use of these type of drugs in pregnancy has been limited (Hansen and Yankowitz, 2002).

With persistent vomiting, appropriate steps should be taken to diagnose and treat possible underlying diseases such as gastroenteritis, cholecystitis, pancreatitis, hepatitis, peptic ulcer, pyelonephritis, and fatty liver of pregnancy. Although clinical thyrotoxicosis has been implicated as a cause of hyperemesis, it is likely that elevated serum thyroxine levels are a surrogate for elevated serum chorionic gonadotropin levels (see Chap. 3, p. 72). Tan and colleagues (2002) have described this as "chemical hyperthyroidism" without clinical symptoms. There often is associated psychiatric morbidity with hyperemesis (Swallow and co-workers, 2004). If social and psychological factors contribute to the illness, the woman usually improves remarkably while hospitalized, only to relapse after discharge (Deuchar, 1995). Thus, positive assistance with psychosocial problems is beneficial.

By this juncture, most women have had a salutary response. If there is still prolonged vomiting, consideration is given for enteral nutrition as discussed on page 1112. Vaisman and co-workers (2004) recently described successful use of nasojejunal feeding for 4 to 21 days in 11 women with refractory disease. In a very few women, parenteral nutrition may be necessary (van de Ven, 1997).

Scholarly monographs on hyperemesis gravidarum have been published (Association of Professors of Obstetrics and Gynecology, 2001; Goodwin and Romero, 2002).

REFLUX ESOPHAGITIS. Heartburn, also called pyrosis, is a common symptom in late pregnancy. The retrosternal burning sensation is caused by esophagitis from gastroesophageal reflux related to relaxation of the lower esophageal sphincter (Hytten, 1991). Raising the head of the bed and treatment with oral antacids usually relieves symptoms. If severe symptoms persist, an H_2-receptor antagonist is prescribed. Both cimetidine and ranitidine are considered safe, but misoprostol is contraindicated (Briggs and associates, 2002; Hansen and Yankowitz, 2002). One of the proton pump inhibitors, omeprazole, also appears safe for use in pregnancy (Nikfar and colleagues, 2002). If there is then no relief, endoscopy should be considered. Women who had antireflux fundoplication before pregnancy had few complications (Gonzalez and associates, 2004).

HIATAL HERNIA. Rigler and Eneboe (1935) performed upper gastrointestinal radiographic series in 195 women in late pregnancy. Almost 20 percent of 116 multiparas and 5 percent of 79 nulliparas had a hiatal hernia. Notably, in only 3 of 10 women, a hernia persisted 1 to 18 months postpartum. The relationship of hiatal hernia with reflux esophagitis, and thus symptoms, is not clear. Cohen and Harris (1971) demonstrated no relationship between reflux and hernia and showed that the lower esophageal sphincter functioned effectively even when displaced intrathoracically. Nevertheless, during pregnancy these hernias may cause vomiting, epigastric pain, and bleeding from ulceration. Curran and colleagues (1999) described a 30-week pregnancy complicated by gastric outlet obstruction from a paraesophageal hernia, which they subsequently successfully repaired.

DIAPHRAGMATIC HERNIA. Symptomatic diaphragmatic hernias are herniations of abdominal contents through either the foramen of Bochdalek or the foramen of Morgagni which rarely complicate pregnancy. Kurzel and associates (1988) reviewed the outcomes of 18 pregnant women with a hernia who developed acute obstruction. Maternal mortality was 45 percent. They recommend repair during pregnancy even if the woman is asymptomatic. Flick and co-workers (1999) reported a 23-week pregnancy complicated by bowel herniation into the chest through an old traumatic diaphragmatic defect. There have also been case reports of spontaneous diaphragmatic rupture from increased intra-abdominal pressure during delivery (Ortega-Carnicer, 1998; Sharifah, 2003; Watkin, 1993, and all their colleagues).

ACHALASIA. This is a motility disorder of esophageal smooth muscle. Achalasia means "failure to relax," viz., the lower esophageal sphincter does not relax properly with swallowing, and there are abnormal esophageal contractions (Richter, 2001). The cause is inflammatory destruction of the myenteric (Auerbach) plexus of smooth muscle of the lower esophagus and its sphincter. Postganglionic cholinergic neurons are unaffected, thus, there is unopposed sphincter stimulation. Symptoms are dysphagia, chest pain, and regurgitation. Diagnosis is by barium esophagogram demonstrating "bird beak" narrowing at the distal esophagus. Endoscopy is used to exclude gastric carcinoma. There also may be esophageal dilatation, and manometry is confirmatory.

Although pregnancy normally relaxes the lower esophageal sphincter, this theoretically should not occur with achalasia. In either case, pregnancy does not seem to worsen achalasia. Mayberry and Atkinson (1987) reported no excessive reflux esophagitis in 20 pregnant women compared with that of nonpregnant women with achalasia. Of 16 women who became pregnant after symptoms developed, 11 had no change in symptomatology, two improved, and three worsened.

If symptoms persist despite soft foods and anticholinergic drugs, balloon dilatation is used; 85 percent of nonpregnant patients respond to this mode of therapy. Esophageal perforation is a serious complication of dilatation. Satin and colleagues (1992) and Fiest and associates (1993) reported successful use of pneumatic dilatation in two pregnant women with achalasia.

PEPTIC ULCER. In young women, peptic ulcer disease more often involves the duodenum rather than the stomach. Gastroduodenal ulcers in nonpregnant women may be caused by chronic gastritis induced by *H pylori,* or they develop from use of aspirin and other nonsteroidal anti-inflammatory drugs. Ulcer disease is uncommon in pregnancy, and there have been no links of dyspepsia in pregnancy associated with *H pylori* infection (McKenna and colleagues, 2003; Weyermann and associates, 2003). Acid secretion is also important, thus explaining the temporary efficacy of antisecretory agents (Chan and Leung, 2002; Suerbaum and Michetti, 2002).

During pregnancy, gastric acid secretion is reduced, motility is decreased, and there is considerably increased mucus secretion (Hytten, 1991). Presumably this explains why active peptic ulcer disease is uncommon during pregnancy. Cappell and Garcia (1998), however, conclude that ulcer disease may be underdiagnosed because of frequent treatment for reflux esophagitis. In the past 35 years at Parkland Hospital, during which time we have cared for over 350,000 pregnant women, we have encountered very few who had symptomatic peptic ulcer disease. Before appropriate therapy was available, Clark (1953) studied 313 pregnancies in 118 women with proven ulcer disease and reported a clear remission in almost 90 percent. Benefits were short lived, however, and symptoms recurred in over half by 3 months postpartum and in almost all by 2 years.

Antacids are first-line therapy, and H_2-receptor blockers are prescribed for those who do not respond. Proton pump inhibitors have been avoided during pregnancy (Briggs and colleagues, 2002). Recently, however, Nikfar and associates (2002) studied 600 fetuses exposed to omeprazole and did not find a significant teratogenic risk. Sucralfate is the aluminum salt of sulfated sucrose that provides a protective coating at the ulcer base. Only about 10 percent of the aluminum salt is absorbed, and it is considered safe for pregnant women. With active ulcers, a search for *H pylori* is considered. Diagnostic aids include the urea breath test, serological testing, or endoscopic biopsy. If any of these are positive, antimicrobial therapy is indicated. There are a number of effective treatment regimens that do not include tetracycline (Suerbaum and Michetti, 2002).

UPPER GASTROINTESTINAL BLEEDING. Occasionally, persistent vomiting may be accompanied by worrisome upper gastrointestinal bleeding. The obvious concern is that there is a bleeding peptic ulceration, however, most of these women have minute linear mucosal tears near the gastroesophageal junction. Women with these so-called *Mallory–Weiss tears* usually respond promptly to conservative measures, including iced saline irrigations, topical antacids, and intravenously administered H_2-blockers. Blood transfusions may be needed. With persistent bleeding, endoscopy is used for diagnosis and perhaps hemostasis (Cappell and Garcia, 1998; Van Dam and Brugge, 1999). With severe persistent retching, esophageal rupture may be caused by greatly increased esophageal pressure—*Boerhaave syndrome.*

DISORDERS OF THE SMALL BOWEL AND COLON

The small bowel has diminished motility during pregnancy. Using a nonabsorbable carbohydrate, Lawson and colleagues (1985) showed that small bowel transit time was prolonged beginning early in pregnancy. They reported mean transit times were 99, 125, and 137 minutes in each trimester, respectively, compared with 75 minutes when nonpregnant. In a study cited by Everson (1992), mean transit time for a mercury-filled balloon from the stomach to the cecum was 58 hours in pregnant women at term compared with 52 hours in nonpregnant controls.

Muscular relaxation of the colon is accompanied by increased absorption of water and sodium that predisposes to *constipation,* which is common during pregnancy (see Chap. 8, p. 221). Constipation at some time during pregnancy is reported by almost 40 percent of women with low-fiber diets (Everson, 1992). Such symptoms are usually only mildly bothersome, and preventive measures include a high-fiber diet along with bulk-forming laxatives. Treatment options have been reviewed by Wald (2003). We have encountered several pregnant women who developed megacolon from impacted stool. These women almost invariably had chronically abused stimulatory laxatives.

INFLAMMATORY BOWEL DISEASE. There are at least two forms of intestinal inflammation—*ulcerative colitis* and *Crohn disease.* The latter also is known as regional enteritis, Crohn ileitis, and granulomatous colitis. Differentiation between the two is important because treatment is different in some major aspects. That said, they both share common factors, and sometimes it is impossible to distinguish between them when Crohn disease involves the colon. The salient clinical and laboratory features shown in Table 49–2 permit a confident diagnostic differentiation in most. The etiopathogenesis of both is enigmatic, but there appears to be a genetic predisposition toward both diseases. Inflammation

TABLE 49–2 Some Differentiating Characteristics of Ulcerative Colitis and Crohn Disease

Characteristic	Ulcerative Colitis	Crohn Disease
Genetic factors		
Twin concordance	10–20% (monozygous)	~50% (monozygous)
Family history	~25%	~25%
HLA association	Bw35, B27, DR2	A2, B27, DR5, DQ1
Genomic linkage	Chromosomes 3, 5, 7, 12	Chromosomes 16 (IBD1)
Natural history		
Bowel involvement	Large bowel mucosa and submucosa Continuous involvement beginning at rectum (40% ulcerative proctitis only)	Small and large bowel mucosa and deeper layers; transmural involvement common Small or large bowel only, or both; discontinuous and segmental involvement Strictures or fistulas common
Colonoscopy	Mucosal granularity and friability with superficial ulceration Rectal involvement very common	Patchy involvement Perianal disease Rectal involvement common
Symptoms	Bloody diarrhea, tenesmus	Cramping abdominal pain and watery diarrhea, vomiting, malnutrition, weight loss
Clinical course	Exacerbations and remission (60–75% acute intermittent; 15–20% continuous chronic unremitting)	Exacerbations and remission; surgery commonly required
Extraintestinal manifestations	Arthritis, pyoderma, erythema nodosum (about 10%)	Same
Serum antibodies	pANCA ~70%	Anti–Saccharomyces cerevisiae ~50%
Complications	Toxic megacolon (2%) Reactive arthritis Sclerosing cholangitis Cancer (3–5%)	Fistula formation Reactive arthritis Toxic megacolon Cancer risk less
Management	Medical Proctocolectomy curative	Medical Segmental resection if indicated

pANCA = perinuclear antineutrophil cytoplasmic antibody.
From Farrell and Peppercorn (2002), Friedman and Blumberg (2001), and Podolsky (2002).

is thought to result from inappropriate and continuous activation of the mucosal immune system driven by normal flora (Podolsky, 2002).

Ulcerative Colitis. This is confined to the superficial layers of the colon, typically beginning at the rectum and extending proximally for a variable distance. Sigmoidoscopic or colonoscopic findings include mucosal granularity and friability interspersed with mucosal ulcerations and a mucopurulent exudate. The extent of inflammation is proportional to symptoms, and bloody diarrhea is the cardinal presenting finding. The disease is characterized by exacerbations and remissions. *Toxic megacolon* is a particularly dangerous complication that necessitates colectomy in half of cases (Sheth and LaMont, 1998). For unknown reasons, prior appendectomy protects against development of ulcerative colitis (Selby and colleagues, 2002). *Extraintestinal manifestations* include arthritis, uveitis, and erythema nodosum. The risk of cancer approaches 1 percent per year.

MANAGEMENT. Ulcerative colitis is primarily a medical disease. Sulfasalazine is used for maintenance therapy as well as treatment for active colitis (Podolsky, 2002). One of its active metabolites is 5-aminosalicylic acid (5-ASA), which inhibits prostaglandin synthase. Prednisone is used for more severe disease that does not respond. Immunosuppressive drugs, including azathioprine and cyclosporine, have been used in conjunction with prednisone in nonpregnant patients with success. Finally, high-dose cyclosporine is beneficial for severely ill patients (Farrell and Peppercorn, 2002). Proctocolectomy is performed for recalcitrant disease, with permanent ileostomy or an ileoanal anastomosis with a continent ileal pouch.

Crohn Disease. This inflammatory disease has more protean manifestations than ulcerative colitis. It involves not only the bowel mucosa but also the deeper layers, and sometimes there is transmural involvement (see Table 49–2). The disease is typically segmental. About 30 percent of patients have small bowel involvement, 25 percent have isolated colon involvement, and 40 percent have both, usually with the terminal ileum and colon involved.

Complaints include abdominal pain and diarrhea, and obstructive symptoms are common. The disease is chronic and marked by exacerbations and remissions. Almost 30 percent of patients require surgery during the first year after the diagnosis is made; thereafter, 5 percent per year require surgery. Indeed, Crohn disease is the most common surgical disease of the small bowel (Evers and associates, 1999). Complications include fistula formation and perineal communications that interfere with vaginal delivery (Forsnes and co-workers, 1999; Ilnyckyji and colleagues, 1999). Reactive arthritis is common, and the risk of cancer, although not as great as with ulcerative colitis, is increased substantively.

MANAGEMENT. There is no regimen that is universally effective for maintenance of asymptomatic periods. Sulfasalazine is effective for symptomatic disease in some patients. The newer 5-aminosalicylate formulations are better tolerated (Rampton, 1999). Prednisone therapy controls active disease but is less effective for small bowel involvement. Immunosuppressive drugs, including azathioprine and 6-mercaptopurine, are used more successfully than with ulcerative colitis. Oral cyclosporine is effective to control corticosteroid-resistant disease. Methotrexate is used in steroid-dependent cases, and low-dose methotrexate maintains a remission. All of these drugs appear safe (Moskovitz and associates, 2004).

A number of regimens are currently being tested that include fish oil, monoclonal tumor necrosis factor antibodies, probiotics, and unfractionated heparin (Farrell and Peppercorn, 2002; Feagan and colleagues, 2000; Present and associates, 1999). In a recent study, Ghosh and co-workers (2003) compared infusions of natalizumab, a selective inhibitor of leukocyte adhesion, and reported it superior to placebo in decreasing remissions.

Because cure is unlikely with resection of affected bowel, conservative surgery is indicated for complications, including no response to medical therapy. Unfortunately, resection is associated with a 50-percent recurrence requiring further surgery within 10 years (Rampton, 1999).

Inflammatory Bowel Disease and Fertility. Subfertility is linked to that of any chronic medical disease (Bradley and Rosen, 2004). According to Alstead and Nelson-Piercy (2003), decreased female fertility from active Crohn disease returned to normal with remission. This is not so after ileal pouch–anal anastomosis (Johnson and associates, 2004). Subfertility may also be partially due to sulfasalazine, which causes reversible sperm abnormalities.

Inflammatory Bowel Disease and Pregnancy. Both forms of chronic inflammatory bowel disease are relatively common in women of childbearing age. Donaldson (1985) concluded the following:

1. Pregnancy does not increase the likelihood of an attack of inflammatory bowel disease. If the disease is quiescent in early pregnancy, then flares are uncommon, but if they develop, they may be severe.

2. Active disease at conception increases the likelihood of poor pregnancy outcome.
3. Diagnostic evaluations should not be postponed if their results are likely to affect management.
4. Many of the usual treatment regimens may be continued during pregnancy, and if indicated, surgery should be performed.

When all studies are taken together, it is likely that adverse perinatal outcomes are increased in women with inflammatory bowel disease. Kornfeld and co-workers (1997) described outcomes in a population-based cohort study of 756 Swedish women with preexisting ulcerative colitis or Crohn disease. Preterm birth, low birthweight, fetal growth restriction, and cesarean delivery were all increased 1.5- to 2-fold. Importantly, despite these results, perinatal mortality was not increased. Fedorkow and colleagues (1989) and Baird and associates (1990) reported similar findings earlier from retrospective case-control studies. It now appears that much of this excessive morbidity is caused by Crohn disease (Dominitz and associates, 2002; Fonager and co-workers, 1998).

ULCERATIVE COLITIS AND PREGNANCY. In a meta-analysis of 755 pregnancies, Fonager and colleagues (1998) reported that ulcerative colitis quiescent at conception worsened during pregnancy in about a third of cases. In women with active disease at the time of conception, 45 percent worsened, 25 percent remained unchanged, and only 25 percent improved. These observations were similar to those previously described in an extensive review by Miller (1986).

Therapy for colitis is the same as for nonpregnant patients. *Calcium supplementation* is important because osteoporosis is common. Maintenance is continued with 5-ASA derivatives, and flares can be treated with corticosteroids. Habal and associates (1993) described the successful use of 5-ASA during 19 pregnancies. Nørgård and co-workers (2003) found an increased risk of stillbirth, but could not separate 5-ASA use from disease activity. Flares may be caused by psychogenic stress, and reassurance is important (Farrell and Peppercorn, 2002). Parenteral nutrition can be used in women with severe and prolonged exacerbations (see p. 1112).

If indicated, colorectal endoscopy should be performed (Katz, 2002). In some cases, colectomy is indicated, and it has been performed during the third trimester for severe disease (Boulton and colleagues, 1994; Watson and Gaines, 1987). Decompression colostomy with ileostomy—Turnbull-Blowhole colostomy—was described by Ooi and co-workers (2003) in a 10- and a 16-week pregnancy. In women who have had a colectomy, long-term function of an ileal pouch–anal anastomosis is not impaired by childbirth (Farouk and colleagues, 2000; Ravid and associates, 2002). In at least one case, however, adhesions to the growing uterus led to pouch perforation (Aouthmany and Horattas, 2004).

By most accounts, ulcerative colitis has minimal adverse effects on pregnancy outcome. Modigliani (2000) reviewed

2398 pregnancy outcomes in women with colitis. Perinatal outcomes were not substantively different from the general obstetrical population. The incidences of spontaneous abortion, preterm delivery, and stillbirths were remarkably low. In a population-based cohort study from Washington State, Dominitz and co-workers (2002) described pregnancy outcomes in 107 women with ulcerative colitis. Except for an inexplicably increased incidence of congenital malformations, perinatal outcomes were similar to those of 1308 normal controls. The other exception was that cesarean delivery was increased compared with that of controls (29 versus 20 percent).

CROHN DISEASE AND PREGNANCY. Disease activity is related to its status at the time of conception. In their cohort study, Fonager and associates (1998) studied 279 pregnancies and analyzed outcomes based on disease activity at conception. For 186 women whose disease was inactive at conception, only a fourth relapsed during pregnancy. In contrast, each of a third of the remaining 93 either worsened, had no change, or they improved. Miller (1986) described similar findings in his review. Woolfson and colleagues (1990) reported that abdominal surgery was required during 5 percent of pregnancies. Forsnes and associates (1999) described an enterovesical fistula diagnosed in a 15-week pregnant woman.

Maintenance therapy is similar to that for nonpregnant women. *Calcium supplementation* is given to combat osteoporosis. Parenteral hyperalimentation has been used successfully for severe recurrences (Russo-Stieglitz and colleagues, 1999). Endoscopy is performed if indicated (Katz, 2002).

Crohn disease is associated with increased adverse perinatal outcomes. Based on a 20-year review, Korelitz (1998) found that perinatal outcomes were generally good with quiescent disease. In a large case-controlled Danish study, Fonager and colleagues (1998) reported a twofold risk of low-birthweight and preterm infants. More recently, Dominitz and co-workers (2002) reported a two- to threefold increase in preterm delivery, low-birthweight, and fetal growth restriction in 149 women with Crohn disease. Cesarean delivery was also increased compared with that of normal controls (28 versus 20 percent).

OSTOMY AND PREGNANCY. A colostomy or an ileostomy is problematic during pregnancy because of its location. Gopal and colleagues (1985) described 82 pregnancies in 66 women with an ostomy that usually was created as a result of inflammatory bowel disease. Stomal dysfunction was common, but it responded to conservative management in all cases. Bowel obstruction developed in six women, and in three of these, surgery was necessary. Ileostomy prolapse was surgically corrected in four women during pregnancy, at cesarean delivery, or in the puerperium. The cesarean delivery rate was 37 percent, and a third of these were done because of prior abdominoperineal resection.

Colectomy with mucosal proctectomy and ileal pouch–anal anastomosis is the surgical procedure of choice for ulcerative colitis and familial colonic polyposis. Disadvantages include frequent bowel movements, nocturnal fecal soilage in almost half of patients, and *pouchitis*. Juhasz (1995), Hahnloser (2004), and Ravid (2002) and all their colleagues have described subsequent pregnancies in women with this anastomosis. Although stool frequency, pad soilage, and incontinence temporarily worsened during pregnancy, these abated postpartum. Importantly, Farouk and associates (2000) reported that childbirth did not worsen long-term function. These investigators as well as others have concluded that vaginal delivery is acceptable in these women.

INTESTINAL OBSTRUCTION. Bowel obstruction during pregnancy is not more common than in the general population, although it is more difficult to diagnose. Meyerson and colleagues (1995) reported an incidence of 1 in 17,000 deliveries over a 20-year period at two Detroit hospitals. As shown in Table 49–3, about 50 percent of the cases of intestinal obstruction are due to adhesions from previous pelvic surgery, including cesarean deliveries. Volvulus causes another 25 percent. Volvulus of the cecum and small bowel has been reported in late pregnancy or early in the puerperium (Carral and colleagues, 1998; Ranjan and Boulton, 1993). Cesarean delivery may be necessary to obtain proper exposure (Harer and Harer, 1958). Small bowel obstruction without a discernible cause can develop during pregnancy (Ventura-Braswell and associates, 1998; Wax and Christie, 1993). A case of sigmoid obstruction with perforation, sepsis, and death was described in a woman with severe geophagia (Woywodt and Kiss, 1999).

Most cases of intestinal obstruction during pregnancy result from pressure of the growing uterus on intestinal adhesions. According to Davis and Bohon (1983), this is more likely around midpregnancy, when the uterus becomes an

TABLE 49–3 Causes of Intestinal Obstruction During Pregnancy and the Puerperium in 216 Women

Cause of Obstruction	Number (%)
Adhesions by trimester	118 (55)
First (8)	
Second (32)	
Third (53)	
Postpartum (25)	
Volvulus	53 (25)
Midgut (6)	
Cecal (19)	
Sigmoid (23)	
Other (5)	
Intussusception	11 (5)
Hernia, carcinoma, appendicitis	12 (5)
Other	22 (10)

Adapted from Connolly and colleagues (1995).

abdominal organ; in the third trimester, when the fetal head descends; and immediately postpartum, when there is an acute change in the uterine size. In their review, Perdue and colleagues (1992) found that 80 percent of pregnant women had nausea and vomiting. Importantly, abdominal pain, either continuous or colicky, affected 98 percent. Abdominal tenderness occurred in 70 percent and abnormal bowel sounds in only 55 percent. Limited radiographic examinations, including plain abdominal radiographs, and those following administration of soluble contrast showed evidence of obstruction in 38 of 42 women described by these investigators.

The mortality rate with obstruction during pregnancy can be very high because of delayed diagnosis, reluctance to operate during pregnancy, and the emergency nature of the surgery (Firstenberg and Malangoni, 1998). Of 66 pregnancies, Perdue and associates (1992) described 6-percent maternal mortality and 26-percent fetal mortality. Two of the four women who died had sigmoid or cecal volvulus caused by adhesions late in pregnancy.

Colonic pseudo-obstruction, or *Ogilvie syndrome,* is caused by adynamic colonic ileus, and about 10 percent of all reported cases follow delivery. The syndrome is characterized by massive abdominal distention with cecal dilatation. In most cases, intravenous infusion of 2-mg neostigmine results in prompt decompression (Amaro and Rogers, 2000; Ponec and associates, 1999). Although unusual, the large bowel may rupture, therefore decompression is recommended when the bowel becomes dangerously distended. We have had success with colonoscopic decompression as reported by Moore and associates (1986). If peritonitis is suspected, however, laparotomy must be considered.

APPENDICITIS. Suspected appendicitis is one of the most common indications for surgical abdominal exploration during pregnancy. Mazze and Källén (1991) found that an appendectomy was done in about 1 in 1000 pregnancies in the Swedish registry of 720,000 pregnancies. Appendicitis was confirmed in 65 percent, or about 1 in 1500 pregnancies. From the Danish registry of over 320,000 pregnancies, Hée and Viktrup (1999) reported an appendectomy rate of 1 in 2800 pregnancies with a 50-percent verification of appendicitis (1 in 5500). Reason(s) for this disparity are unknown.

Appendicitis may be less common during pregnancy compared with that in nonpregnant women of similar age. Andersson and Lambe (2001) performed a case-control study in more than 53,000 women who had undergone appendectomy in Sweden. These women were less likely to have been pregnant than their age-matched controls. This "protection" was most apparent in the third trimester.

Pregnancy often makes the diagnosis of appendicitis more difficult for the following reasons:

1. Anorexia, nausea, and vomiting that accompany normal pregnancy are also common symptoms of appendicitis.

2. As the uterus enlarges, the appendix commonly moves upward and outward toward the flank, so that pain and tenderness may not be prominent in the right lower quadrant (Baer and colleagues, 1932).

3. Some degree of leukocytosis is the rule during normal pregnancy.

4. Appendicitis may be confused with preterm labor, pyelonephritis, renal colic, placental abruption, or degeneration of a uterine myoma.

5. Pregnant women, especially those late in gestation, frequently do not have symptoms considered "typical" for appendicitis.

As the appendix is pushed progressively higher by the growing uterus, containment of infection by the omentum becomes increasingly unlikely, and appendiceal rupture and generalized peritonitis are more common during later pregnancy. In the Swedish study by Andersson and Lambe (2001), the incidence of perforation was 6, 10, and 13 percent in each trimester, respectively.

Diagnosis. Persistent abdominal pain and tenderness are the most reproducible findings. Although most investigators have reported that pain migrates upward with appendiceal displacement, Mourad and associates (2000) and Eryilmaz and colleagues (2002) did not find this.

Graded compression ultrasonography during pregnancy is difficult, because cecal displacement with uterine imposition makes precise examination difficult. Despite this, Landwehr and associates (1996) and Eryilmaz and co-workers (2002) found it fairly accurate. *Appendiceal computed tomography* is more sensitive and accurate than ultrasound in nonpregnant patients with suspected appendicitis (Paulson and associates, 2003). An example is shown in Figure 49–1. Specific views decrease fetal radiation exposure (see Chap. 41, p. 980.) Experiences in pregnancy are limited, but the preliminary observations of Castro and associates (2001) are promising.

Management. If appendicitis is suspected, treatment is prompt surgical exploration. Even though diagnostic errors sometimes lead to removal of a normal appendix, it is better to operate than to postpone intervention until generalized peritonitis has developed. In most reports, the diagnosis is verified in about 60 to 70 percent of pregnant women who undergo surgical exploration. Accuracy of diagnosis is inversely proportional to gestational age. In the Swedish study by Mazze and Källén (1991), 77 percent of first-trimester diagnoses were correct. In the latter two trimesters, however, only 57 percent were confirmed. Importantly, and related, as diagnosis becomes more difficult, so does surgical delay and an increased risk of perforation.

In nonpregnant patients, laparoscopy is done routinely for suspected appendicitis (Hellberg and colleagues, 1999). During the first half of pregnancy, laparoscopy for suspected

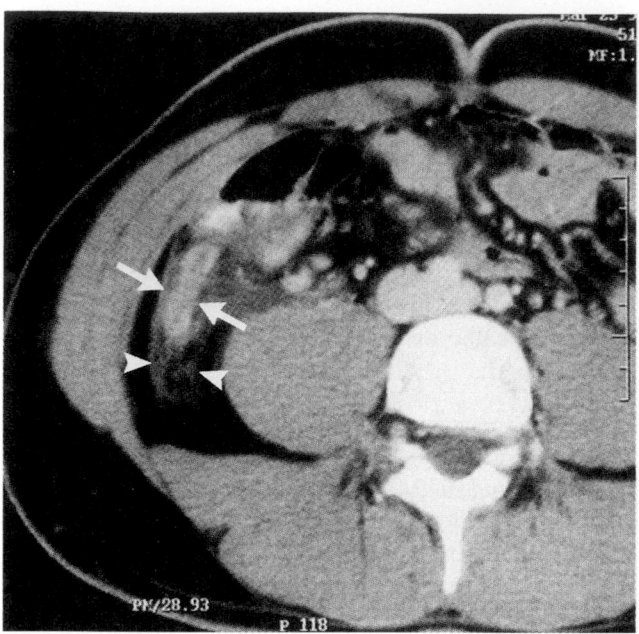

FIGURE 49–1. Computed tomographic scan with contrast showing inflamed appendix. The dilated fluid-filled appendix with a thickened wall (*arrows*) has inflammatory changes in the adjacent fat tissue (*arrowheads*). (From Paulson and colleagues, 2003, with permission.)

appendicitis has become the norm. Although some clinicians have questioned the possibility of a CO_2 pneumoperitoneum causing fetal acidosis and hypoperfusion, physiological responses as well as experience with its use are reassuring (see Chap. 41, p. 975). From the Swedish database, Reedy and colleagues (1997) reported similar perinatal outcomes in nearly 2000 laparoscopic procedures compared with those of over 1500 laparotomies done before 20 weeks. If laparotomy is chosen, most practitioners prefer an incision over the McBurney point (Popkin and colleagues, 2002).

Before exploration, intravenous antimicrobial therapy is begun, usually with a second-generation cephalosporin or third-generation penicillin. Unless there is gangrene, perforation, or a periappendiceal phlegmon, antimicrobial therapy can usually be discontinued after surgery. Without generalized peritonitis, the prognosis is quite good. Seldom is cesarean delivery indicated at the time of appendectomy. Uterine contractions are common, and although some clinicians recommend tocolytic agents, we do not. De Veciana and colleagues (1994) reported that increased intravenous fluid administration with tocolytic use increased the risk for pulmonary permeability edema from the sepsis syndrome (see Chap. 42, p. 993).

If appendicitis is undiagnosed before delivery, often when the large uterus rapidly empties, walled-off infection is disrupted causing an acute surgical abdomen. New-onset appendicitis during the immediate puerperium is very uncommon simply because of chance. It is important to remember that **puerperal pelvic infections typically do not cause peritonitis.**

Effects on Pregnancy. Appendicitis increases the likelihood of abortion or preterm labor, especially if there is peritonitis. Mazze and Källén (1991) found that spontaneous labor ensued with greater frequency if surgery for appendicitis was performed after 23 weeks. In the 45 cases described by Mourad and associates (2000), uterine contractions were reported in 19 of 23 women who were 24 weeks or greater. Fetal loss overall is about 15 percent. In the Swedish study, fetal loss was 22 percent if surgery was performed after 23 weeks. Mays and colleagues (1995) have suggested a link between maternal–fetal sepsis and neonatal neurological injury with antepartum appendicitis. Viktrup and Hée (1998) found that appendicitis during pregnancy was not associated with subsequent infertility.

REFERENCES

Alstead EM, Nelson-Piercy C: Inflammatory bowel disease in pregnancy. Gut 52:159, 2003

Amaro R, Rogers AI: Neostigmine infusion: New standard of care for acute colonic pseudo-obstruction? Am J Gastroenterol 95:304, 2000

American College of Obstetricians and Gynecologists: Nausea and vomiting of pregnancy. Practice Bulletin No. 52, April 2004

Andersson RE, Lambe M: Incidence of appendicitis during pregnancy. Int J Epidemol 30:1281, 2001

Aouthmany A, Horattas MC: Ileal pouch perforation in pregnancy: Report of a case and review of the literature. Dis Colon Rectum 47(2):243, 2004

Association of Professors of Gynecology and Obstetrics: Nausea and vomiting of pregnancy. APGO Educational Series. Washington, DC, 2001

Baer JL, Reis RA, Arens RA: Appendicitis in pregnancy with changes in position and axis of normal appendix in pregnancy. JAMA 98:1359, 1932

Baird DD, Narendranathan M, Sandler RS: Increased risk of preterm birth for women with inflammatory bowel disease. Gastroenterology 99:987, 1990

Borowski KS, Ramsey PS, Williams L, et al: The impact of hyperemesis gravidarum on pregnancy outcome [abstract]. Obstet Gynecol 101:86S, 2003

Boulton R, Hamilton M, Lewis A, et al: Fulminant ulcerative colitis in pregnancy. Am J Gastroenterol 89:931, 1994

Bradley RJ, Rosen MP: Subfertility and gastrointestinal disease: "Unexplained" is often undiagnosed. Obstet Gynecol Surv 59:108, 2004

Briggs GG, Freeman RK, Yaffee SJ: Drugs in Pregnancy and Lactation, 6th ed. Baltimore, Williams & Wilkins, 2002

Buckwalter JG, Simpson SW: Psychological factors in the etiology and treatment of severe nausea and vomiting in pregnancy. Am J Obstet Gynecol 186:S210, 2002

Cappell MS: The fetal safety and clinical efficacy of gastrointestinal endoscopy during pregnancy. Gastroenterol Clin North Am 32:123, 2003

Cappell MS, Garcia A: Gastric and duodenal ulcers during pregnancy. Gastroenterol Clin North Am 27:169, 1998

Cappell MS, Sidhom O: A multicenter, multiyear study of the safety and clinical utility of esophagogastroduodenoscopy in 20 consecutive pregnant females with follow-up of fetal outcome. Am J Gastroenterol 88:1900, 1993

Cappell MS, Colon VJ, Sidhom OA: A study at 10 medical centers of the safety and efficacy of 48 flexible sigmoidoscopies and 8 colonoscopies during pregnancy with follow-up of fetal outcome and with comparison to control groups. Dig Dis Sci 41:2353, 1996

Carral JML, Chandrashekar MV, Rogers IM, et al: Volvulus of the right colon in pregnancy. Int J Clin Prac 52:270, 1998

Carter JF, Soper DE: Operative laparoscopy in pregnancy. JSLS 8:57, 2004

Castro MA, Shipp TD, Castro EE, et al: The use of helical computed tomography in pregnancy for the diagnosis of acute appendicitis. Am J Obstet Gynecol 184:954, 2001

Centers for Disease Control and Prevention: Guidelines for the prevention of intravascular catheter-related infections. MMWR 51:RR-10, 2002

Chan FKL, Leung WK: Peptic-ulcer disease. Lancet 360:933, 2002

Chihara H, Otsubo Y, Yoneyama Y, et al: Basal metabolic rate in hyperemesis gravidarum: Comparison to normal pregnancy and response to treatment. Am J Obstet Gynecol 188:434, 2003

Clark DH: Peptic ulcer in women. BMJ 2:1254, 1953

Cohen S, Harris LD: Does hiatus hernia affect competence of the gastroesophageal sphincter? N Engl J Med 284A:1053, 1971

Connolly MM, Unti JA, Nora PF: Bowel obstruction in pregnancy. Surg Clin North Am 75:101, 1995

Curran D, Lorenz R, Czako P: Gastric outlet obstruction at 30 weeks' gestation. Obstet Gynecol 93:851, 1999

Davis MR, Bohon CJ: Intestinal obstruction in pregnancy. Clin Obstet Gynecol 26:832, 1983

Deuchar N: Nausea and vomiting in pregnancy: A review of the problem with particular regard to psychological and social aspects. Br J Obstet Gynaecol 102:6, 1995

De Veciana M, Towers CV, Major CA, et al: Pulmonary injury associated with appendicitis in pregnancy: Who is at risk? Am J Obstet Gynecol 171:1008, 1994

Dokmeci F, Engin-Ustun Y, Ustun Y, et al: Trace element status in plasma and erythrocytes in hyperemesis gravidarum. J Reprod Med 49:200, 2004

Dominitz JA, Young JC, Boyko EJ: Outcomes of infants born to mothers with inflammatory bowel disease: A population-based cohort study. Am J Gastroenterol 97:641, 2002

Donaldson RM: Management of medical problems in pregnancy—inflammatory bowel disease. N Engl J Med 312:1618, 1985

Duggar CR, Carlan SJ: The efficacy of methylprednisolone in the treatment of hyperemesis gravidarum: A randomized double-blind controlled study [abstract]. Obstet Gynecol 97:45S, 2001

Eryilmaz R, Sahin M, Bas G, et al: Acute appendicitis during pregnancy. Dig Surg 19:40, 2002

Evers BM, Townsend CM, Thompson JC: Small intestine. In Schwartz SI, Shires GT, Spencer FC, et al (eds): Principles of Surgery. New York, McGraw-Hill, 1999, p 1229

Everson GT: Gastrointestinal motility in pregnancy. Gastroenterol Clin North Am 21:751, 1992

Farouk R, Pemberton JH, Wolff BG, et al: Functional outcomes after ileal pouch–anal anastomosis for chronic ulcerative colitis. Ann Surg 231:919, 2000

Farrell RJ, Peppercorn MA: Ulcerative colitis. Lancet 359:331, 2002

Fatum M, Rojansky N: Laparoscopic surgery during pregnancy. Obstet Gynecol Surv 56:50, 2001

Feagan BG, Fedorak RN, Irvine EJ, et al: A comparison of methotrexate with placebo for the maintenance of remission in Crohn's disease. N Engl J Med 342:1627, 2000

Fedorkow DM, Persaud D, Nimrod CA: Inflammatory bowel disease: A controlled study of late pregnancy outcome. Am J Obstet Gynecol 160:998, 1989

Fiest TC, Foong A, Chokhavatia S: Successful balloon dilation of achalasia during pregnancy. Gastrointest Endosc 39:810, 1993

Firstenberg MS, Malangoni MA: Gastrointestinal surgery during pregnancy. Gastroenterol Clin North Am 27(1):73, 1998

Fischer JE: Metabolism in surgical patients: Protein, carbohydrate, and fat utilization by oral and parenteral routes, Chapter 5. In Townsend CM, Beauchap RD, Evers BM, et al (eds): Sabiston Textbook of Surgery. Philadelphia, Saunders, 2001, p 101

Flick RP, Bofill JA, King JC: Pregnancy complicated by traumatic diaphragmatic rupture. A case report. J Reprod Med 44:127, 1999

Fonager K, Sorensen HT, Olsen J, et al: Pregnancy outcome for women with Crohn's disease: A follow-up study based on linkage between national registries. Am J Gastroenterol 93:2426, 1998

Forsnes EV, Eggleston MK, Heaton JO: Enterovesical fistula complicating pregnancy: A case report. J Reprod Med 44:297, 1999

Friedman S, Blumberg RS: Inflammatory bowel disease: Ulcerative colitis and Crohn's disease. In Braunwald E, Fauci AS, Kasper DL, Hauser SL, Longo DL, Jameson JL (eds): Harrison's Principles of Internal Medicine, 15th ed. New York, McGraw-Hill, 2001, p 1679

Gazmararian JA, Petersen R, Jamieson DJ, et al: Hospitalizations during pregnancy among managed care enrollees. Obstet Gynecol 100:94, 2002

Ghosh S, Goldin E, Gordon FH, et al: Natalizumab for active Crohn's disease. N Engl J Med 348:24, 2003

Gilstrap LC, Van Dorsten PV, Cunningham FG (eds): Diagnostic and operative laparoscopy. In Operative Obstetrics, 2nd ed. New York, McGraw-Hill, 2002

Godsey RK, Newman RB: Hyperemesis gravidarum: A comparison of single and multiple admissions. J Reprod Med 36:287, 1991

Gonzalez R, Bowers SP, Swafford V, et al: Pregnancy and delivery after antireflux surgery. Am J Surg 188:34, 2004

Goodwin TM, Romero R: Understanding and treating nausea and vomiting of pregnancy. Am J Obstet Gynecol 186:181, 2002

Goodwin TM, Hershman JM, Cole L: Increased concentration of the free β-subunit of human chorionic gonadotropin in hyperemesis gravidarum. Acta Obstet Gynecol Scand 73:770, 1994

Gopal KA, Amshel AL, Shonberg IL, et al: Ostomy and pregnancy. Dis Colon Rectum 28:912, 1985

Habal FM, Hui G, Greenberg GR: Oral 5-aminosalicylic acid for inflammatory bowel disease in pregnancy: Safety and clinical course. Gastroenterology 105:1057, 1993

Hahnloser D, Pemberton JH, Wolff BG, et al: Pregnancy and delivery before and after ileal pouch-anal anastomosis for inflammatory bowel disease: immediate and long-term consequences and outcomes. Dis Colon Rectum 47:1127, 2004

Hamaoui E, Hamaoui M: Nutritional assessment and support during pregnancy. Gastroenterol Clin North Am 32:59, 2003

Hansen WF, Yankowitz J: Pharmacologic therapy for medical disorders during pregnancy. Clin Obstet Gynecol 45:136, 2002

Harer WB Jr, Harer WB Sr: Volvulus complicating pregnancy and the puerperium: A report of three cases and review of the literature. Obstet Gynecol 12:399, 1958

Hée P, Viktrup L: The diagnosis of appendicitis during pregnancy and maternal and fetal outcome after appendectomy. Int J Gynaecol Obstet 65:129, 1999

Hellberg A, Rudberg C, Kullman E, et al: Prospective randomized multicentre study of laparoscopic versus open appendicectomy. Br J Surg 86:48, 1999

Heyland DK, MacDonald S, Keefe L, et al: Total parenteral nutrition in the critically ill patient. JAMA 280:2013, 1998

Hill JB, Yost NP, Wendel GW Jr: Acute renal failure in association with severe hyperemesis gravidarum. Obstet Gynecol 100:1119, 2002

Hillbom M, Pyhtinen J, Pylvänen V, et al: Pregnant, vomiting, and coma: A case report. Lancet 353:1584, 1999

Hytten FE: The alimentary system. In Hytten F, Chamberlain G (eds): Clinical Physiology in Obstetrics. London, Blackwell, 1991, p 137

Ilnyckyji A, Blanchard JF, Rawsthorne P, et al: Perianal Crohn's disease and pregnancy: Role of the mode of delivery. Am J Gastroenterol 94:3274, 1999

Jacobson GF, Autry AM, Somer-Shely TL, et al: *Helicobacter pylori* seropositivity and hyperemesis gravidarum. J Reprod Med 48:578, 2003

Jewell D, Young G: Interventions for nausea and vomiting in early pregnancy. Cochrane Database System Review 2: CD000145, 2000

Johnson P, Richard C, Ravid A, et al: Female infertility after ileal pouch-anal anastomosis for ulcerative colitis. Dis Colon Rectum 47:1119, 2004

Juhasz ES, Fozard B, Dozois RR, et al: Ileal pouch–anal anastomosis function following childbirth: An extended evaluation. Dis Colon Rectum 38:159, 1995

Katz JA: Endoscopy in the pregnant patient with inflammatory bowel disease. Gastrointest Endosc Clin North Am 12:635, 2002

Kim YH, Lee SJ, Rah SH, et al: Wernicke's encephalopathy in hyperemesis gravidarum. Can J Ophthalmol 37:37, 2002

Kirby DF, Fiorenza V, Craig RM: Intravenous nutritional support during pregnancy. JPEN J Parenter Enteral Nutr 12:72, 1988

Korelitz BI: Inflammatory bowel disease and pregnancy. Gastroenterol Clin North Am 27:214, 1998

Kornfeld D, Cnattingius S, Ekbom A: Pregnancy outcomes in women with inflammatory bowel disease—a population based cohort study. Am J Obstet Gynecol 177:942, 1997

Kort B, Katz VL, Watson MJ: The effect of nonobstetric operation during pregnancy. Surg Gynecol Obstet 177:371, 1993

Kurzel RB, Naunheim KS, Schwartz RA: Repair of symptomatic diaphragmatic hernia during pregnancy. Obstet Gynecol 71:869, 1988

Landwehr JG, Leonardi MR, Bryant DR, et al: Graded-compression ultrasound (GCUS) for early recognition of appendicitis in pregnancy. Am J Obstet Gynecol 147:389, 1996

Lawson M, Kern F, Everson GT: Gastrointestinal transit time in human pregnancy: Prolongation in the second and third trimesters followed by postpartum normalization. Gastroenterology 89:996, 1985

Magee LA, Mazzotta P, Koren G: Evidence-based view of safety and effectiveness of pharmacologic therapy for nausea and vomiting of pregnancy (NVP). Obstet Gynecol 186:S256, 2002

Mayberry JF, Atkinson M: Achalasia and pregnancy. Br J Obstet Gynaecol 94:855, 1987

Mays J, Verma U, Klein S, et al: Acute appendicitis in pregnancy and the occurrence of major intraventricular hemorrhage and periventricular leukomalacia. Obstet Gynecol 86:650, 1995

Mazze RI, Källén B: Appendectomy during pregnancy: A Swedish registry study of 778 cases. Obstet Gynecol 77:835, 1991

Mazze RI, Källén B: Reproductive outcome after anesthesia and operation during pregnancy: A registry study of 5405 cases. Am J Obstet Gynecol 161:1178, 1989

McKenna D, Watson P, Dornan J: *Helicobacter pylori* infection and dyspepsia in pregnancy. Obstet Gynecol 102:845, 2003

Meyerson S, Holtz T, Ehrinpresis M, et al: Small bowel obstruction in pregnancy. Am J Gastroenterol 90:299, 1995

Miller JP: Inflammatory bowel disease in pregnancy: A review. J R Soc Med 79:221, 1986

Modigliani RM: Gastrointestinal and pancreatic disease. In Barron WM, Lindheimer MD, Davison JM (eds): Medical Disorders of Pregnancy, 3rd ed. St. Louis, Mosby, 2000, p 316

Moore JG, Gladstone NS, Lucas GW, et al: Successful management of post-cesarean-section acute pseudo obstruction of the colon

(Ogilvie's syndrome) with colonoscopic decompression. A case report. J Reprod Med 31:1001, 1986

Moskovitz DN, Bodian C, Chapman ML, et al: The effect on the fetus of medications used to treat pregnant inflammatory bowel-disease patients. Am J Gastroenterol 99:656, 2004

Mourad J, Elliott JP, Erickson L, et al: Appendicitis in pregnancy: New information that contradicts long-held clinical beliefs. Am J Obstet Gynecol 185:1027, 2000

Nikfar S, Abdollahi M, Moretti ME, et al: Use of proton pump inhibitors during pregnancy and rates of major malformations: A meta-analysis. Dig Dis Sci 47:1526, 2002

Nørgård B, Fonager K, Pedersen L, et al: Birth outcome in women exposed to 5-amniosalicyclic acid during pregnancy: A Danish cohort study. Gut 52:243, 2003

Ogura JM, Francois KE, Perlow JH, et al: Complications associated with peripherally inserted central catheter use during pregnancy. Am J Obstet Gynecol 188:1223, 2003

Ooi BS, Remzi FH, Fazio VW: Turnbull-blowhole colostomy for toxic ulcerative colitis in pregnancy: Report of two cases. Dis Colon Rectum 46:111, 2003

Ortega-Carnicer J, Ambrós A, Alcazar R: Obstructive shock due to labor-related diaphragmatic hernia. Crit Care Med 26:616, 1998

Paulson EK, Kalady MF, Pappas TN: Suspected appendicitis. N Engl J Med 348:236, 2003

Perdue PW, Johnson HW Jr, Stafford PW: Intestinal obstruction complicating pregnancy. Am J Surg 164:384, 1992

Podolsky DK: Inflammatory bowel disease. N Engl J Med 347:417, 2002

Ponec RJ, Saunders MD, Kimmey MB: Neostigmine for the treatment of acute colonic pseudo-obstruction. N Engl J Med 341:137, 1999

Popkin CA, Lopez PP, Cohn SM, et al: The incision of choice for pregnant women with appendicitis is through McBurney's point. Am J Surg 183:20, 2002

Present DH, Rutgeerts P, Targan S, et al: Infliximab for the treatment of fistulas in patients with Crohn's disease. N Engl J Med 340:1398, 1999

Rampton DS: Management of Crohn's disease. BMJ 319:1480, 1999

Ranjan V, Boulton JM: Primary volvulus of the small bowel following normal delivery. Br J Obstet Gynaecol 100:860, 1993

Ravid A, Richard CS, Spencer LM, et al: Pregnancy, delivery, and pouch function after ileal pouch-anal anastomosis for ulcerative colitis. Dis Colon Rectum 45:1283, 2002

Reedy MB, Källén B, Kuehl TJ: Laparoscopy during pregnancy: A study of five fetal outcome parameters with use of the Swedish Health Registry. Am J Obstet Gynecol 177:673, 1997

Rees JH, Ginsberg L, Schapira AHV: Two pregnant women with vomiting and fits. Am J Obstet Gynecol 177:1539, 1997

Richter JE: Oesophageal motility disorders. Lancet 358:823, 2001

Rigler LG, Eneboe JB: Incidence of hiatus hernia in pregnant women and its significance. J Thorac Surg 4:262, 1935

Rizzo AG: Laparoscopic surgery in pregnancy: Long-term follow-up. J Laparoendosco Adv Surg Tech A 13:11, 2003

Robinson JN, Banerjee R, Thiet MP: Coagulopathy secondary to vitamin K deficiency in hyperemesis gravidarum. Obstet Gynecol 92:673, 1998

Rollins MD, Chan KJ, Price RR: Laparoscopy for appendicitis and cholelithiasis during pregnancy: A new standard of care. Surg Endosc 18:237, 2004

Russo-Stieglitz KE, Levine AB, Wagner BA, et al: Pregnancy outcome in patients requiring parenteral nutrition. J Matern Fetal Med 8:164, 1999

Safari HR, Fassett MJ, Souter IC, et al: The efficacy of methylprednisolone in the treatment of hyperemesis gravidarum: A randomized, double-blind, controlled study. Am J Obstet Gynecol 179:921, 1998

Sakai M, Yoneda S, Sasaki Y, et al: Maternal total parenteral nutrition and fetal subdural hematoma. Obstet Gynecol 101:1142, 2003

Satin AJ, Twickler D, Gilstrap LC: Esophageal achalasia in late pregnancy. Obstet Gynecol 79:812, 1992

Schiff MA, Reed SD, Daling JR: The sex ratio of pregnancies complicated by hospitalisation for hyperemesis gravidarum. Br J Obstet Gynaecol 111:27, 2004

Schwartz M, Rossoff L: Pneumomediastinum and bilateral pneumothoraces in a patient with hyperemesis gravidarum. Chest 106:1904, 1994

Selby WS, Griffin S, Abraham N, et al: Appendectomy protects against the development of ulcerative colitis but does not affect its course. Am J Gastroenterol 97:2834, 2002

Sharifah H, Naidu A, Vimal K: Diaphragmatic hernia: An unusual cause of postpartum collapse. Br J Obstet Gynaecol 110:701, 2003

Sheth SG, LaMont JT: Toxic megacolon. Lancet 351:509, 1998

Spruill SC, Kuller JA: Hyperemesis gravidarum complicated by Wernicke's encephalopathy. Obstet Gynecol 99:875, 2002

Suerbaum S, Michetti P: *Helicobacter pylori* infection. N Engl J Med 347:1175, 2002

Sullivan CA, Johnson CA, Roach H, et al: A pilot study of intravenous ondansetron for hyperemesis gravidarum. Am J Obstet Gynecol 174:1565, 1996

Swallow BL, Lindow SW, Masson EA, et al: Psychological health in early pregnancy: Relationship with nausea and vomiting. J Obstet Gynaecol 24:28, 2004

Tan JY, Loh KC, Yeo GS, et al: Transient hyperthyroidism of hyperemesis gravidarum. Br J Obstet Gynaecol 109:683, 2002

Tesfaye S, Achari V, Yang YC, et al: Pregnant, vomiting, and going blind: A case report. Lancet 352:1594, 1998

Vaisman N, Kaidar R, Levin I, et al: Nasojejunal feeding in hyperemesis gravidarum—a preliminary study. Clin Nutr 23:53, 2004

Van Dam J, Brugge WR: Endoscopy of the upper gastrointestinal tract. N Engl J Med 341:1738, 1999

van de Ven CJM: Nasogastric enteral feeding in hyperemesis gravidarum. Lancet 349:445, 1997

Ventura-Braswell AM, Satin AJ, Higby K: Delayed diagnosis of bowel infarction secondary to maternal midgut volvulus at term. Obstet Gynecol 91:808, 1998

Viktrup L, Heé P: Fertility and long-term complications four to nine years after appendectomy during pregnancy. Acta Obstet Gynecol Scand 77:746, 1998

Wald A: Constipation, diarrhea, and symptomatic hemorrhoids during pregnancy. Gastroenterol Clin North Am 32:309, 2003

Watkin DS, Hughes S, Thompson MH: Herniation of colon through the right diaphragm complicating the puerperium. J Laparoendosc Surg 3:583, 1993

Watson WJ, Gaines TE: Third-trimester colectomy for severe ulcerative colitis. J Reprod Med 32:869, 1987

Wax JR, Christie TL: Complete small-bowel volvulus complicating the second trimester. Obstet Gynecol 82:689, 1993

Weyermann M, Brenner H, Adler G, et al: *Helicobacter pylori* infection and the occurrence and severity of gastrointestinal symptoms during pregnancy. Am J Obstet Gynecol 189:526, 2003

Woolfson K, Cohen Z, McLeod RS: Crohn's disease and pregnancy. Dis Colon Rectum 33:869, 1990

Woywodt A, Kiss A: Perforation of the sigmoid colon due to geophagia. Arch Surg 134:88, 1999

Yamamoto T, Suzuki Y, Kojima K, et al: Pneumomediastinum secondary to hyperemesis gravidarum during early pregnancy. Acta Obstet Gynecol Scand 80:1143, 2001

Yost NP, McIntire DD, Wians FH Jr, et al: A randomized, placebo-controlled trial of corticosteroids for hyperemesis due to pregnancy. Obstet Gynecol 102:1250, 2003

Ziaei S, Hosseiney FS, Faghihzadeh S: The efficacy low dose of prednisolone in the treatment of hyperemesis gravidarum. Acta Obstet Gynecol Scand 83(3):272, 2004

50

Hepatic, Biliary Tract, and Pancreatic Disorders

Disorders of the liver, biliary tract, and pancreas together comprise a formidable list of complications that may affect the pregnant woman and her fetus. In some of these disorders, the interrelationships with pregnancy are fascinating and intriguing.

Hepatic Physiology in Pregnancy. Pregnancy may normally induce appreciable changes in some of the tests to assess liver function (see Chap. 5, p. 140). Physical findings such as palmar erythema and spider angiomas, which may suggest liver disease, may be found during normal pregnancy. Histological liver findings from normal pregnant women are unchanged compared with those of nonpregnant subjects (Ingerslev and Teilum, 1945). Postpartum, there is a significant rise in serum bilirubin and transaminase, however, only 10 percent are in the abnormal range (David and colleagues, 2000; Girling and co-workers, 1997).

DISEASES OF THE LIVER

It is customary to divide liver diseases into those specifically related to pregnancy, those coincidental to pregnancy, and those that are chronic and antedate pregnancy. Pregnancy-induced disorders that resolve spontaneously or following delivery include hepatic dysfunction from hyperemesis gravidarum, intrahepatic cholestasis, acute fatty liver, and hepatocellular damage with severe preeclampsia. Most acute hepatic disorders complicating pregnancy are coincidental (e.g., acute viral hepatitis, drug-induced hepatic failure). Finally, pregnancy may be superimposed on chronic liver disease such as hepatitis, cirrhosis, or esophageal varices, and after liver transplantation.

HYPEREMESIS GRAVIDARUM. Pernicious nausea and vomiting is discussed in Chapter 49 (see p. 1113). The liver may be involved, and biopsy findings either are normal or show some fatty changes (Knox and Olans, 1996). There may be mild hyperbilirubinemia, and serum transaminase levels are elevated in up to half of women hospitalized. Enzyme levels seldom exceed 200 U/L.

INTRAHEPATIC CHOLESTASIS OF PREGNANCY. Cholestasis of pregnancy also has been referred to as recurrent jaundice of pregnancy, cholestatic hepatosis, and icterus gravidarum. It is characterized clinically by pruritus, icterus, or both. Because of genetic influences, the incidence of cholestasis varies by population. It is uncommon in North America, with an incidence of about 1 in 500 to 1000 pregnancies. The incidence is 1 percent in Italy, and as many as 4 percent of pregnancies are affected in Sweden and Chile (Paternoster and colleagues, 2002; Reyes, 1997).

Pathogenesis. The cause of obstetrical cholestasis is unknown, although it was thought to be caused by high estrogen concentrations in susceptible women. Leslie and colleagues (2000), however, reported that maternal plasma estrogens are *decreased* in affected women. Defects in secretion of sulfated progesterone metabolites may play a role (Mullally and Hansen, 2001; Reyes and Sjovall, 2000). At least some cases are related to the many gene mutations that control hepatocellular transport systems (Germain and associates, 2002; Trauner and associates, 1998). One example is mutation of the *multidrug resistance 3 (MDR3)* gene found with *progressive familial intrahepatic cholestasis.* Some drugs that similarly decrease the canalicular transport maximum for bile acids aggravate the disorder. For example, we have encountered cholestatic jaundice in several pregnant women taking azathioprine following renal transplantation.

Whatever the inciting cause(s), bile acids are cleared incompletely and accumulate in plasma. Total bile acid concentration may be elevated 10- to 100-fold (Lunzer and associates, 1986). Hyperbilirubinemia results from retention of conjugated pigment, and total plasma concentrations rarely exceed 4 to 5 mg/dL. Alkaline phosphatase is usually elevated even more than in normal pregnancy. Serum transaminase levels are normal to moderately elevated but seldom exceed 250 U/L. Liver biopsy shows mild cholestasis with bile plugs in the hepatocytes and canaliculi of the centrilobular regions without inflammation or necrosis. These changes disappear after delivery but often recur in subsequent pregnancies or with estrogen-containing contraceptives.

Clinical Presentation. Most women with cholestasis develop pruritus in late pregnancy, although the syndrome occasionally occurs late in the second trimester. In an unusual case, Kirkinen and Ryynänen (1995) described a woman at 13 weeks with cholestasis associated with hyperplacentosis and a triploid fetus. There are no constitutional symptoms. Generalized pruritus develops, and there is a predilection for the soles of the feet. Skin changes are limited to excoriations from scratching. Biochemical tests may be abnormal at presentation, but pruritus usually precedes laboratory findings by a mean of 3 weeks and sometimes by months (Kenyon and colleagues, 2001, 2002). About 10 percent of women develop jaundice.

With normal liver enzymes, the differential diagnosis includes other skin disorders (see Chap. 56, p. 1251). Normal blood pressure without proteinuria militates against preeclamptic liver disease. Ultrasound may be warranted to exclude cholelithiasis and biliary obstruction. *Acute* viral hepatitis is not likely with such low serum transaminase levels. As discussed subsequently, however, otherwise asymptomatic *chronic* hepatitis C is associated with a 20-fold increased incidence of cholestasis (Locatelli and colleagues, 1999; Paternoster and associates, 2002).

Management. Pruritus is thought to be caused by elevated serum bile salts, and it may be quite troublesome. *Antihistamines* and *topical emollients* may provide some relief.

Based on their review of several small uncontrolled studies, Kroumpouzos and Cohen (2003) estimated that *cholestyramine* may be effective in 50 to 70 percent of patients. This compound also causes decreased absorption of fat-soluble vitamins, which is already impaired, and vitamin K deficiency may develop. Fetal coagulopathy with intracranial hemorrhage as well as stillbirth have been reported (Matos and colleagues, 1997; Sadler and associates, 1995). Some reports suggest that *ursodeoxycholic acid* quickly relieves pruritus and lowers serum enzyme levels (Germain and co-workers, 2002; Mazzella and associates, 2001). The addition of S-adenosylmethionine (SAMe) to ursodeoxycholic acid improved its effects (Nicastri and co-workers, 1998). In a randomized trial comparing ursodeoxycholic acid and SAMe, Roncaglia and associates (2004) reported equally significant relief of pruritus. In a Cochrane Database Systematic Review, Burrows and colleagues (2001) concluded that data were inadequate to confirm any significant benefits.

Other agents have been evaluated in small randomized trials. Hirvioja and colleagues (1992) reported prompt relief of pruritus in 10 women given *dexamethasone*, however, Kretowicz and co-workers (1994) reported worsening of symptoms after dexamethasone. Terg and colleagues (2002) reported that the opioid antagonist *naltrexone* was superior to placebo to relieve itching.

Cholestasis and Pregnancy Outcomes. Most earlier reports described excessive adverse pregnancy outcomes in women with cholestatic jaundice (Germain and associates, 2002). Rioseco and co-workers (1994) compared outcomes in 320 affected pregnancies with normal controls and attributed equivalent perinatal mortality to close pregnancy surveillance. Despite this, meconium-stained amnionic fluid (25 versus 16 percent) and preterm delivery (12 versus 4 percent) were significantly increased with cholestasis. Williamson and colleagues (2004) reviewed 352 affected pregnancies and 7 percent ended in stillbirths, the majority after 37 weeks. In a case-control study of 79 affected women, Alsulyman and associates (1996) reported that those with cholestasis had an excessive number of antepartum fetal tests performed which more often prompted delivery. Fetuses of affected women had more frequent meconium passage (44 versus 8 percent), with two associated fetal deaths. In a prospective investigation of 70 women with cholestasis, Kenyon and co-workers (2002) found that weekly amnionic fluid assessment, every-other-day antepartum fetal testing, and elective delivery at 37 to 38 weeks resulted in zero perinatal mortality, but again this management was associated with increased interventions.

ACUTE FATTY LIVER OF PREGNANCY. Acute liver failure during pregnancy may be caused by fulminant viral hepatitis, drug-induced hepatic toxicity, or acute fatty liver of pregnancy. The latter is also called *acute fatty metamorphosis* or *acute yellow atrophy*, and it is an uncommon complication that often has proved fatal for both mother and fetus. In its worst form, the incidence is probably about 1 in 10,000 pregnancies. Reyes and associates (1994) reported the incidence to be 1 in 15,000 in Santiago, Chile, whereas Castro and colleagues (1996a) found it to be 1 in 7000 in Los Angeles.

Fatty liver is characterized by accumulation of microvesicular fat that literally "crowds out" normal hepatocytic function. Gross examination shows a small, soft, yellow, and greasy liver. Prominent histological abnormalities are swollen hepatocytes with central nuclei and cytoplasm filled with microvesicular fat, periportal sparing, and minimal hepatocellular necrosis (Fig. 50-1).

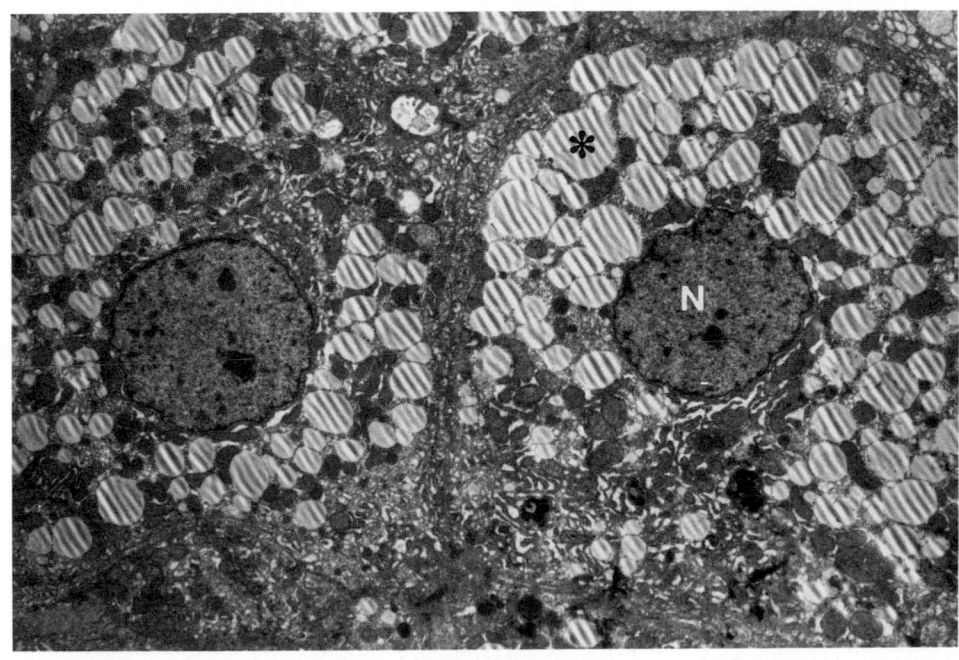

FIGURE 50-1. Fatty liver of pregnancy. Electron photomicrograph of two hepatocytes containing numerous microvesicular fat droplets (*). The nuclei (N) remain centered within the cells, unlike with the case of macrovesicular fat deposition. (Courtesy of Dr. Don Wheeler.)

Etiology and Pathogenesis. Some, if not all, cases of maternal fatty liver are due to recessively inherited mitochondrial abnormalities of fatty acid oxidation. These defects were first studied in children with Reye-like syndromes and were later found to be associated with microvesicular liver disease in pregnancy. At least 17 mutations have been described for the mitochondrial trifunctional protein enzyme complex that catalyzes the last oxidative steps in the pathway (Rakheja and colleagues, 2002; Yang and co-workers, 2002b). The most common thus far is the G1528C (E474Q) mutation of the gene coding for long-chain-3-hydroxyacyl-CoA-dehydrogenase—known as LCHAD (Ibdah and associates, 1999). There are other enzyme mutations for medium- and short-chain dehydrogenase—MCHAD and SCHAD (Maitra and colleagues, 2002).

Sims and co-workers (1995) reported that while homozygous LCHAD-deficient children had Reye-like syndromes, some of their heterozygous mothers had fatty liver. This was also described with a compound heterozygous fetus and heterozygous mother (Isaacs and colleagues, 1996). Shekhawat and associates (2003) found that the placenta of the LCHAD-deficient fetus may produce metabolites toxic to the maternal liver. Some conclude that heterozygous LCHAD-deficient mothers are at risk for obstetrical complications *only* if their fetus is homozygous (Tyni and colleagues, 1998). Blish and Ibdah (2005), however, identified a genotypically normal fetus born to a mother heterozygous for a LCHAD mutation and who developed HELLP syndrome.

There is a much weaker association between fatty acid β-oxidation enzyme defects and severe preeclampsia, or especially with the HELLP syndrome—hemolysis, elevated liver enzymes, low platelets (Minakami and co-workers, 1988; Yang and colleagues, 2002c). In the study by Tyni and associates (1998), 29 of 63 pregnancies with a clinically affected, presumably homozygous, fetus had increased incidences of preeclampsia, HELLP syndrome, acute fatty liver, and cholestasis. Clinically and biochemically, however, severe preeclampsia/HELLP syndrome and fatty liver are distinct syndromes (Rahman and Weldon, 2002; Vigil-De Gracia, 2001).

Recurrence. Fatty liver recurring in subsequent pregnancy is uncommon, but a few cases have been described (MacLean and co-workers, 1994; Reyes and associates, 1994; Usta and colleagues, 1994). Recurrence appears to be more likely if the woman has a homozygous enzyme-deficient fetus (Treem and associates, 1994; Tyni and colleagues, 1998).

Clinical Findings. Acute fatty liver almost always manifests late in pregnancy. Castro and colleagues (1996a) reported a mean gestational age of 37.5 weeks (range 31 to 42) in 28 women. A few case reports describe onset at midpregnancy (Monga and Katz, 1999; Suzuki and colleagues, 2001). Fatty liver is more common in nulliparas with a male fetus, and in 15 percent of cases there is a multifetal gestation (Davidson and associates, 1998).

Symptoms usually develop over several days to weeks and include malaise, anorexia, nausea and vomiting, epigastric pain, and progressive jaundice. **In many women, persistent vomiting in late pregnancy is the major symptom.** About half of all women have hypertension, proteinuria, and edema—signs suggestive of preeclampsia. There is usually severe liver dysfunction with hypofibrinogenemia, hypoalbuminemia, hypocholesterolemia, and prolonged clotting times. Hyperbilirubinemia usually is less than 10 mg/dL, and there are modestly elevated serum transaminase levels (Table 50–1). Endothelial cell activation and exudation cause hemoconcentration, leukocytosis, and thrombocytopenia. Hemolysis can be severe, and it is likely caused by impaired cholesterol synthesis, with resultant effects on erythrocyte membranes (Cunningham and colleagues, 1985). Markedly reduced antithrombin III levels

TABLE 50–1 Laboratory Findings in 72 Women with Acute Fatty Liver of Pregnancy

Series	No.	Most Abnormal Laboratory Values Mean ± 1 SD (range)				
		Fibrinogen (mg/dL)	FSP (μg/mL)	Platelets ($10^3/\mu L$)	Creatinine (mg/dL)	AST (U/L)
Usta et al (1994)	14	139 ± 79 (37–110)	ND	126 ± 96	2.4 ± 1.0 (1.1–3.6)	1067 ± 1098 (200–3670)
Castro et al (1996a)	28	125 (32–446)	ND	113 (11–186)	2.5 (1.1–5.2)	210 (45–1200)
Pereira et al (1997)	32	ND	ND	123 (26–262)	2.7 (1.1–8.4)	99 (25–911)
Vigil-De Gracia (2001)	10	136 ± 120 (0 to > 300)	ND	76 ± 50	ND	444 ± 358
Parkland Hospital[a]	35	166 ± 112 (35–515)	50 (16–256)	160 ± 86 (9–385)	1.7 ± 0.7 (0.7–4.3)	381 ± 292 (25–1166)

AST = aspartate aminotransferase; FSP = fibrin/fibrinogen split products; ND = not done.
[a] Data courtesy of Dr. Nicole Yost.

have also been described (Castro and associates, 1996a; Vigil-De Gracia, 2001).

Various imaging techniques have been purported to confirm the clinical diagnosis, however, this has not been our experience. Castro and associates (1996b) also reported poor sensitivity with sonography (3 of 11 patients), computed tomography (5/10), and magnetic resonance imaging (0/5).

The syndrome continues to progressively worsen. Marked hypoglycemia is common, and obvious hepatic encephalopathy develops in 60 percent, severe coagulopathy in 55 percent, and some degree of renal failure in about 50 percent. Fetal death is common with severe disease. Fortunately, delivery arrests rapid deterioration of liver function. During recovery, over the next week to 10 days, evidence of *transient diabetes insipidus* is common and presumably due to elevated vasopressinase concentrations. When *acute pancreatitis* develops, the prognosis is more ominous (Moldenhayer and colleagues, 2004). Ascites is almost universal (Kennedy and co-workers, 1994). With supportive care, recovery usually is complete.

We have encountered a number of women with what appears to be a *forme fruste* of this disorder. Clinical involvement is relatively minor and laboratory aberrations—usually hemolysis and decreased plasma fibrinogen—call attention to the abnormality. Thus, there is a spectrum of liver involvement, and hepatic failure varies in intensity, with encephalopathy as the most extensive involvement. Many milder cases go unnoticed or are attributed to preeclampsia.

Coagulopathy. This can be a dramatic component of fatty liver of pregnancy. Primarily caused by diminished hepatic synthesis, there is also increased procoagulant consumption. Of women shown in Table 50–1, almost all had hypofibrinogenemia, elevations of fibrin split products and D-dimers, and occasionally profound thrombocytopenia.

Maternal and Perinatal Outcomes. Although maternal mortality in the past approached 75 percent, the contemporaneous outlook is much better. Even so, 4 of 72 women shown in Table 50–1 died. Fetal mortality in the past was nearly 90 percent, but now is about 15 to 20 percent.

Management. Spontaneous resolution usually follows delivery. Presumably because of maternal acidosis and hemoconcentration in severe cases, some fetuses are dead when the diagnosis is made. Importantly, many others tolerate labor poorly. Significant procrastination in effecting delivery may increase the maternal risk of coma, hypoglycemia, renal failure, worsening acidosis, and severe hemorrhage. We prefer to begin a trial of labor induction with close fetal surveillance. Other clinicians recommend cesarean delivery to hasten hepatic healing. With a severe coagulopathy, however, this increases maternal risk. Transfusions with variable amounts of fresh-frozen plasma, cryoprecipitate, whole blood, packed red cells, and platelets are usually necessary if surgery is

performed or if lacerations complicate vaginal delivery (see Chap. 35, p. 840).

Hepatic dysfunction begins to resolve postpartum. Liver function usually normalizes within a week, and in the interim, intensive medical support may be required. Maternal deaths are caused by sepsis, hemorrhage, aspiration, renal failure, pancreatitis, and gastrointestinal bleeding. Only rarely is liver transplantation necessary (Franco and colleagues, 2000; Gill and co-workers, 2002). In our experience, *diabetes insipidus,* as described above as presumably due to elevated vasopressinase concentrations, is common and some of these women have prodigious urine output.

THE LIVER IN PREECLAMPSIA–ECLAMPSIA. Hepatic involvement is relatively common in women with severe preeclampsia and eclampsia and is discussed in detail in Chapter 34 (see p. 775).

VIRAL HEPATITIS. Symptomatic hepatitis has become less common in pregnant women over the past 15 years (Centers for Disease Control and Prevention, 2002). There are at least five distinct types of viral hepatitis: hepatitis A, hepatitis B, hepatitis D caused by the hepatitis B–associated delta agent, hepatitis C, and hepatitis E. Other agents such as hepatitis G virus (GBV-C) and TT virus do not cause hepatitis. All hepatitis viruses except hepatitis B are RNA viruses. During their acute phases, these are often clinically similar. The viruses themselves probably are not hepatotoxic; rather the immune response to them causes hepatocellular necrosis (Dienstag and Isselbacher, 2001a).

Infections are most often subclinical. When clinically apparent, nausea and vomiting, headache, and malaise may precede jaundice by 1 to 2 weeks. Low-grade fever is more common with hepatitis A. When jaundice develops, symptoms usually improve. Serum transaminase levels vary, and their peaks do not correspond with disease severity. Peak levels that range from 400 to 4000 U/L are usually reached by the time jaundice develops. Serum bilirubin typically continues to rise despite falling aminotransferase levels and peaks at 5 to 20 mg/dL. There usually is complete clinical and biochemical recovery within 1 to 2 months in all cases of hepatitis A and most cases of hepatitis B.

Guidelines to minimize infectivity of patients hospitalized for viral hepatitis have been established. Feces, secretions, bedpans, and other articles in contact with the intestinal tract should be handled with glove-protected hands. Extra precautions, such as double gloving during delivery and surgical procedures, are recommended with hepatitis B and C. Due to significant exposure of health care personnel to hepatitis B, the Centers for Disease Control and Prevention (2001) recommend active and passive vaccination. There is no vaccine for hepatitis C, so recommendations are for postexposure serosurveillance only.

Complications. The case-fatality rate for nonpregnant patients with acute hepatitis is 0.1 percent. For those ill enough to be hospitalized, it is as high as 1 percent. Most fatalities are due to *fulminant hepatic necrosis,* which in later pregnancy may resemble acute fatty liver. About 50 percent of patients with fulminant disease have hepatitis B infection, and co-infection with the delta agent is common. Hepatic encephalopathy is the usual presentation with fulminant hepatitis, and mortality is 80 percent.

Chronic hepatitis is by far the most common complication of hepatitis B and C. Chronic infection follows acute hepatitis B in about 10 percent of cases. Most become asymptomatic carriers, but others have low-grade chronic persistent hepatitis or chronic active hepatitis with or without cirrhosis. Chronic hepatitis follows acute hepatitis C in the *majority* of patients. It causes persistently abnormal biochemical tests. Biopsy usually discloses chronic active hepatitis and cirrhosis.

Hepatitis A. This 27-nm RNA picornavirus is transmitted by the fecal–oral route. The infection is usually spread by ingestion of contaminated blood or water, and the incubation period is about 4 weeks. Individuals shed virus in their feces, and during the relatively brief period of viremia their blood is also infectious. Signs and symptoms are nonspecific, and the majority of cases are anicteric and usually mild. Early serological detection is by identification of IgM antibody that may persist for several months (Table 50–2). During convalescence, IgG antibody predominates, and it persists and provides subsequent immunity.

IMMUNIZATION. Active immunization using formalin-inactivated viral vaccine is more than 90-percent effective. The Centers for Disease Control and Prevention (1999) recommend vaccination of susceptible persons traveling to high-risk countries, illicit drug users, food handlers, and those with chronic liver disease or clotting-factor disorders. Passive immunization for the pregnant woman recently exposed by close personal or sexual contact with a person with hepatitis A is with 0.02 mL/kg immune globulin.

TABLE 50–2 Simplified Diagnostic Approach in Patients with Hepatitis

Diagnosis	HBsAg	Serological Test		
		IgM Anti-HAV	IgM Anti-HBc	Anti-HCV
Acute hepatitis A	−	+	−	−
Acute hepatitis B	+	−	+	−
Chronic hepatitis B	+[a]	−	−	−
Acute hepatitis A with chronic B	+[a]	+	−	−
Acute hepatitis A and B	+	+	+	−
Acute hepatitis C	−	−	−	+

HAV = hepatitis A virus; HBc = hepatitis B core; HBsAg = hepatitis B surface antigen; HCV = hepatitis C virus.
[a] HBsAg may be below detection threshold and thus negative.
Modified from Dienstag and Isselbacher (2001a).

PERINATAL OUTCOME. The effects of hepatitis A on pregnancy are not dramatic in developed countries. However, both perinatal and maternal mortality are substantively increased in underprivileged populations. Treatment consists of a balanced diet and diminished activity. Women with less severe illness may be managed as outpatients (American College of Obstetricians and Gynecologists, 1998). There is no evidence that hepatitis A virus is teratogenic, and transmission to the fetus is negligible. Even so, preterm birth may be increased and neonatal cholestasis has been reported (Urganci and co-workers, 2003). Vertical transmission may occur in neonatal intensive care units (Watson and colleagues, 1993).

Hepatitis B. This infection is found worldwide but is endemic in some regions, especially in Asia and Africa. Hepatitis B is caused by a DNA hepadnavirus that is a major cause of acute hepatitis with its serious sequelae of chronic hepatitis, cirrhosis, and hepatocellular carcinoma. The latter is so common that the World Health Organization considers hepatitis B to be second only to tobacco among human carcinogens. Chronic infection follows in 5 to 10 percent of acutely infected adults and 70 to 90 percent of infants. Although its prevalence has decreased because of vaccination, there are an estimated 1.2 million chronic carriers in the United States and 350 million worldwide.

Half of initial cases are icteric and symptomatic. A variety of immunological serum markers have been identified in those with acute or chronic hepatitis B, in those previously infected but now immune, and in chronic carriers. The hepatitis B virus (Dane particle), hepatitis B core antigen (HBcAg), hepatitis B surface antigen (HBsAg), hepatitis B e antigen (HBeAg), and their corresponding antibodies are all detectable by various techniques. Concentrations of viral antigen and particles in serum and other body fluids may reach 10^{12}/mL.

Hepatitis B infection occurs most often among intravenous drug abusers, homosexuals, health care personnel, and those requiring frequent blood products, such as hemophiliacs. It is transmitted by infected blood or blood products, and it is sexually transmitted by saliva, vaginal secretions, and semen. Because of similar modes of transmission, co-infection with human immunodeficiency virus type 1 (HIV-1) is common and has increased liver-related morbidity (Thio and colleagues, 2002).

After infection, the first serological marker is HBsAg (Fig. 50–2). The HBeAg antigen signifies intact viral particles that invariably are present during early acute hepatitis, however, its persistence indicates chronic infection. After acute hepatitis, approximately 90 percent of persons recover completely. The 10 percent who remain chronically infected are considered to have chronic hepatitis, and about a fourth develop chronic liver disease (see p. 1132). Those seropositive for HBeAg are at greatest risk for hepatocellular carcinoma (Yang and co-workers, 2002a).

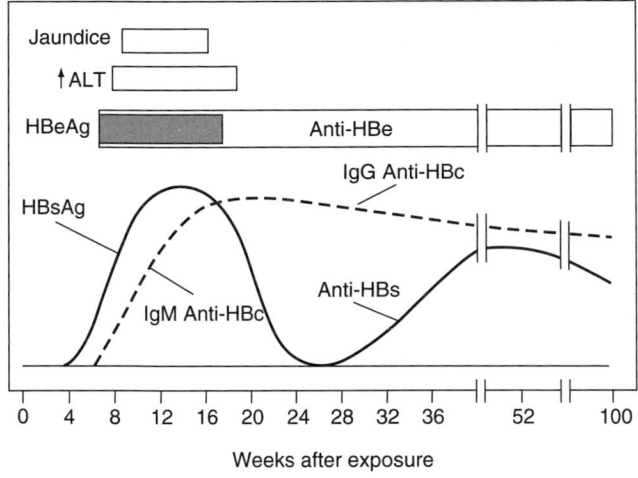

FIGURE 50–2. Appearance of various antigens and antibodies in acute hepatitis B. (ALT = alanine aminotransferase; anti-HBc = antibody to hepatitis B core antigen; anti-HBe = antibody to hepatitis B e antigen; anti-HBs = antibody to hepatitis B surface antigen; HBeAg = hepatitis B e antigen; HBsAg = hepatitis B surface antigen.) (From Dienstag and Isselbacher, 2001a, with permission.)

PREGNANCY OUTCOME. As with hepatitis A, the clinical course of acute hepatitis B is not altered by pregnancy in developed countries. Treatment is supportive, and the likelihood of preterm delivery is increased. Most infections are chronic, asymptomatic, and diagnosed at prenatal screening (see Chap. 8, p. 208). These women are considered to have chronic hepatitis, however, antiviral treatment is generally not given during pregnancy (see p. 1133). The prevalence of seropositivity in inner-city groups is about 1 percent. It is somewhat lower for military populations and private patients.

Transplacental viral infection of the fetus is not as common as once thought. Indeed, Towers and associates (2001) reported that viral DNA is rarely found in amnionic fluid or cord blood. Thus, most neonatal infection is vertically transmitted by peripartum ingestion of infected maternal fluids including breast milk. Mothers with hepatitis B surface and e antigens are more likely to transmit the disease to their infants, whereas those positive for anti-HBe antibody are not infective. **Infants infected with hepatitis B are generally asymptomatic, but an astounding 85 percent become chronically infected.**

PREVENTION OF NEONATAL INFECTION. The Centers for Disease Control and Prevention (2002) estimate that from 1987 to 2000, perinatal infection in the United States was reduced by 75 percent. Neonatal infection can usually be prevented by prenatal screening, with infants of seropositive mothers given hepatitis B immune globulin very soon after birth. This is accompanied by the first dose of a three-dose hepatitis B recombinant vaccine. Hill and colleagues (2002) applied this strategy in 369 infants born to seropositive mothers, and found

that the 2.4-percent transmission rate was not increased with breast feeding if vaccination was completed. As discussed in Chapter 8 (see p. 222), concern for adverse vaccine effects are unfounded according to the Institute of Medicine as well as the Food and Drug Administration (Niu and colleagues, 1999).

For high-risk mothers who are seronegative, vaccine can be given during pregnancy. Ingardia and colleagues (1999) observed that seroprotection in pregnant women was only 45 percent. This is lower than the 60 to 70 percent cited for nonpregnant individuals and the 96-percent rate reported by Jurema and associates (2001) for postpartum women given all three doses. Duration following immunization is a factor. Ingardia and co-workers (2004) later demonstrated that women immunized during one pregnancy had an 85-percent seropositivity rate in a subsequent pregnancy.

Hepatitis D. Also called *delta hepatitis*, this is a defective RNA virus that is a hybrid particle with a HBsAg coat and a delta core. The virus must co-infect with hepatitis B and cannot persist in serum longer than hepatitis B virus. Transmission is similar to hepatitis B. Chronic infection with B and D hepatitis is more severe than B alone, and up to 75 percent of co-infected patients develop cirrhosis. Neonatal transmission is unusual because neonatal hepatitis B vaccination usually prevents delta hepatitis.

Hepatitis C. This is a single-stranded RNA virus of the family Flaviviridae. Transmission of hepatitis C infection appears to be identical to that of hepatitis B. Although more prevalent in intravenous drug abusers, hemophiliacs, and those with high-risk sexual behavior, only half of anti-HCV–positive persons have risk factors (Alter and co-workers, 1999). The Centers for Disease Control and Prevention (1998) cite a seroprevalence of 1.8 percent, or 4 million infected Americans. After acute infection, anti-C antibody is not detected for an average of 15 weeks, and in some cases it is not detectable for a year. Antibody usually does not prohibit transmission. Conry-Cantilena and colleagues (1996) found that 86 percent of 213 anti-HCV–positive persons also had hepatitis C virus RNA and thus were infective.

Patients who are seropositive for anti-HCV antibody are considered to have chronic hepatitis (see p. 1132). The incidence of persistent disease is common after initial infection. Nearly 75 percent of patients have chronic viremia, and 50 percent of these have abnormal liver tests for more than a year (Lauer and Walker, 2001). In 67 percent of patients with transaminase elevations, biopsy shows chronic active hepatitis, and in 20 to 30 percent, this progresses to cirrhosis within 20 to 30 years. Despite this, long-term mortality is not appreciably increased (Dienstag and Isselbacher, 2001b). Chronic hepatitis C does not worsen the prognosis of patients who have HIV co-infection (Sulkowski and colleagues, 2002).

Screening of blood donors for hepatitis C virus has markedly decreased the incidence of posttransfusion hepatitis.

Lauer and Walker (2001) cite a risk of transfusion-related hepatitis C of 1 in 103,000 transfused units that tested seronegative.

PREVALENCE IN PREGNANCY. The incidence of prenatal infection varies with the population studied. Bohman and colleagues (1992) reported a 2.3-percent prenatal seroprevalence rate at Parkland Hospital. Risk factors included intravenous drug use, sexually transmitted diseases, increased age and parity, history of transfusions, multiple sex partners, and sex partners who used intravenous drugs. In over 500 HIV-infected pregnancies at Parkland Hospital, Santiago and associates (2005) found that 10 percent were co-infected with hepatitis B or C. Silverman and colleagues (1993) reported a 5.2-percent incidence in women attending public clinics in Philadelphia compared with only 1.5 percent in private patients. In another high-risk population, Leikin and co-workers (1994) reported a seroprevalence of 4.6 percent.

PREGNANCY OUTCOME. There is no evidence that hepatitis C infection is modified during pregnancy. For example, serum transaminase levels are not different from those in infected nonpregnant individuals. There are conflicting reports concerning changes in RNA viral load in pregnancy (Gervais and associates, 2000; Paternoster and co-workers, 2001). As discussed on page 1129, Locatelli and co-workers (1999) observed a 16-percent incidence of cholestatic jaundice in seropositive women compared with only 0.8 percent in controls. Recall that almost 75 percent of anti-HCV–positive individuals have chronic liver disease. Still, antiviral treatment is usually not given during pregnancy (see p. 1133).

Perinatal outcome also is not adversely affected in HCV-positive women, even when the viral load exceeds 500,000 copies/mL (Laibl and associates, 2005). The primary concern is that hepatitis C infection is transmitted vertically to the fetus–infant, and the rate varies between 3 and 6 percent (Conte, 2000; Hillemanns, 2000; Paternoster, 2001; Resti, 1998, and all their colleagues). The risk appears to be greater when the mother is co-infected with HIV (Ferrero and associates, 2003). Transmission may be limited to those who have HCV RNA detected in serum (Dal Molin and associates, 2002). As in adults, antibody is not protective, and Floreani and co-workers (1996) found that 65 percent of anti-HCV–positive mothers also had hepatitis C viral RNA.

Currently, there are no methods to prevent transmission at birth (American College of Obstetricians and Gynecologists, 1998). Because of this, the Centers for Disease Control and Prevention (1998) do not recommend prenatal screening. However, neonates of known HCV-positive mothers should be tested and provided follow-up. Burns and Minkoff (1999) recommend selective screening based on risk factors.

Hepatitis E. This waterborne RNA virus usually is enterically transmitted by contaminated water supplies. It is not easily communicable by person-to-person contact. Epidemi-ologically it has features resembling hepatitis A; for example, it causes epidemic outbreaks in undeveloped countries. Serological confirmation using IgM and IgG anti-HEV is not routinely available. There is some evidence that during pregnancy there is a high incidence of vertical transmission, including transplacentally (Khuroo and colleagues, 1995). In addition, Baker (2000) has cited evidence that hepatitis E is more severe in pregnancy.

Hepatitis G. Bloodborne infection with this flavivirus-like RNA virus is usually with hepatitis C co-infection. It does not cause hepatitis (Dienstag and Isselbacher, 2001a). In a Scottish study, 0.08 percent of over 180,000 volunteer nonpaid blood donors were seropositive (Jarvis and associates, 1996). Infant transmission has been described by Feucht (1996), Inaba (1997), and all their colleagues.

CHRONIC HEPATITIS. This disorder of varying etiology is characterized by continuing hepatic necrosis, active inflammation, and fibrosis that may lead to cirrhosis and ultimately liver failure. Disease is classified by cause; grade, defined by histological activity; and stage, that is, degree of progression (Dienstag and Isselbacher, 2001b). As previously discussed, it has only been in the last decade that the extent of chronic liver disease due to acute viral hepatitis has been appreciated. By far, most cases are due to chronic infection with either hepatitis B or C viruses. Another cause is autoimmune chronic hepatitis, characterized by high serum titers of homogeneous antinuclear antibodies. In both forms, there is evidence that a cellular immune reaction is interactive with a genetic predisposition.

Most cases of acute viral hepatitis B and C are anicteric and are clinically unnoticed. Similarly, most cases of chronic hepatitis are asymptomatic and are diagnosed by elevated serum transaminase levels obtained for screening (e.g., during blood donation). When present, symptoms are nonspecific and usually include fatigue. Diagnosis can be confirmed by liver biopsy. However, treatment is given in most patients after serological or virological diagnosis. In some patients, cirrhosis with liver failure or bleeding varices may be the presenting findings.

Treatment. There is now considerable experience with treatment of chronic viral hepatitis in nonpregnant patients, and a third of patients can be cured (Gow and Mutimer, 2001).

Chronic hepatitis B treatment includes one of the *interferons* given with ribavirin. Interferons are cytokines with antiviral, antiproliferative, and immunoregulatory effects. Treatment for 6 months has been shown to decrease viremia and improve histological findings in about 20 percent of patients per year with a cure rate of 30 to 40 percent. The nucleoside analogue *lamivudine* also has been found effective in about half of patients (Dienstag and colleagues, 1999; Lai and associates, 1998). It is better tolerated than interferon, however, a major problem is viral resistance of 15 to 30 percent per year. More recently, the nucleotide analogue *adefovir dipivoxil* has been used successfully for both e antigen–negative as well as antigen-positive hepatitis B (Hadziyannis and colleagues, 2003; Marcellin and associates, 2003). Surveillance is important; Hill and co-workers (2001) described two pregnant women who had hepatotoxicity caused by antiretroviral therapy that included lamivudine.

Chronic hepatitis C is treated with interferon alfa-2a or -2b in combination with the synthetic nucleoside *ribavirin* (Davis and associates, 1998; Flamm, 2003). Interferon alfa 2a is combined with polyethylene glycol and the resulting *pegylated interferon* can be given weekly along with daily ribavirin (Fried and associates, 2002).

In women with *autoimmune chronic hepatitis,* corticosteroids, alone or combined with azathioprine, have increased fertility and survival. Pregnancy outcomes of these women are also related to severity of disease (Levine, 2000).

Chronic Hepatitis and Pregnancy. Most young women with chronic hepatitis either are asymptomatic or have only mild liver disease. For seropositive, asymptomatic women, there usually is no problem with pregnancy. With symptomatic chronic active hepatitis, pregnancy outcome depends primarily on the intensity of the disease and whether there is portal hypertension (Lee, 1992). The few women whom we have managed have done well, but because their long-term prognosis is poor, they should be counseled regarding possible liver transplantation as well as abortion and sterilization options.

TREATMENT DURING PREGNANCY. There are currently no firm guidelines for treatment of pregnant women, and antiviral agents are usually not given.

NONALCOHOLIC FATTY LIVER DISEASE. This is an increasingly recognized condition that may progress to end-stage liver disease (Angulo, 2002). Although it resembles alcohol-induced liver injury, it is seen in patients without alcohol abuse. It is known by several names: *fatty liver hepatitis, nonalcoholic Laënnec disease, diabetes hepatitis, alcohol-like liver disease,* and *nonalcoholic steatohepatitis ("NASH").* All of these describe a wide spectrum of liver damage ranging from simple steatosis to steatohepatitis, advanced fibrosis, and cirrhosis. Nonalcoholic steatohepatitis is but one entity in the spectrum of nonalcoholic fatty liver disease.

Obesity, type 2 diabetes mellitus, and hyperlipidemia are coexisting conditions. Specifically, steatohepatitis affects 20 percent of obese persons and 50 percent of those who are morbidly obese (see Chap. 43, p. 1009). Moreover, 50 percent of persons with type 2 diabetes mellitus have steatohepatitis. The disease is usually asymptomatic and is a common explanation for elevated transaminase levels in blood donors. Indeed, it is the cause of elevated asymptomatic aminotransferase levels in up to 90 percent of cases in which other liver disease is excluded. It also is the most common cause of abnormal liver tests among adults in this country.

The natural history of nonalcoholic fatty liver disease has not been well defined, but is related to severity of liver damage. Some cases progress to cirrhosis. Currently, weight loss along with diabetes and dyslipidemia control are the only recommended treatment.

CIRRHOSIS. Hepatic cirrhosis is characterized by irreversible chronic liver injury with extensive fibrosis and regenerative nodules. In all patients, *Laënnec cirrhosis* from chronic exposure to alcohol is the most common cause. In young women, however, and thus most pregnant women, *postnecrotic cirrhosis* from chronic B or C viral hepatitis is the most common cause. Cryptogenic cirrhosis is most often caused by nonalcoholic fatty liver disease (Clark and Diehl, 2003). The clinical manifestations of cirrhosis include jaundice, edema, coagulopathy, metabolic abnormalities, and portal hypertension with gastroesophageal varices and splenomegaly.

Cirrhosis and Pregnancy. Although usually infertile, women with symptomatic cirrhosis who do become pregnant generally have poor outcomes. Common complications include transient hepatic failure, variceal hemorrhage, preterm delivery and fetal growth restriction, as well as maternal death (Aggarwal and associates, 1999; Pajor and Lehoczky, 1994). In older studies, outcome generally was worse if there were esophageal varices. Schreyer and associates (1982) reviewed 69 pregnancies in 60 women with cirrhosis without hepatic shunts and 28 pregnancies in another 23 women who had undergone portal decompression shunting. Severe variceal hemorrhage was increased sevenfold in nonshunted women compared with those who had undergone such procedures (24 versus 3 percent).

PORTAL HYPERTENSION AND ESOPHAGEAL VARICES. Portal venous hypertension with resultant esophageal varices may result either from cirrhosis or from extrahepatic portal vein obstruction. In young women, esophageal varices are caused by equal numbers of each. About half of cases of extrahepatic portal hypertension are idiopathic, although some follow thrombosis from umbilical vein catheterization when the woman was a neonate. This may be more common than realized. For example, Kim and colleagues (2001) performed serial ultrasonic examinations in 100 such neonates. They documented silent portal venous thrombosis in 43 percent, and it resolved spontaneously in only 50 percent.

With either intrahepatic or extrahepatic resistance to flow, portal vein pressure rises from its normal value of 10 to 15 mm Hg to exceed 30 mm Hg. A collateral circulation develops that carries portal blood to the systemic circulation. Drainage is via the gastric, intercostal, and other veins to the esophageal system, where varices develop. Bleeding is usually from varices near the gastroesophageal junction, and hemorrhage can be torrential. About a third of all patients with varices bleed, and the 1-year mortality is 30 to 80 percent (Sharara and Rockey, 2001).

Acute management for bleeding varices consists of endoscopy for diagnosis with *band ligation* to control hemorrhage (Patch and colleagues, 2002). In some cases, *sclerotherapy* may facilitate banding. *Balloon tamponade* of severe bleeding using a triple-lumen tube can be lifesaving. Emergency shunting is used in 10 to 20 percent of patients in whom hemorrhage cannot be controlled by endoscopy. The interventional radiology procedure, known as *transjugular intrahepatic portosystemic stent shunting (TIPSS)*, can also control bleeding from gastric varices. Bleeding recurrence by one year is over 60 percent and this rate is lowered substantively by β-blocker treatment (Bosch and García-Pagán, 2003).

Varices and Pregnancy. In pregnant women, as in young nonpregnant women, esophageal varices are caused equally by either cirrhosis or extrahepatic portal hypertension. Prognosis is largely dependent on whether there is variceal hemorrhage. Bleeding during pregnancy from varices occurs in a third to half and is the major cause of maternal mortality (Aggarwal and colleagues, 2001; Britton, 1982). Mortality is higher if varices are associated with cirrhosis (18 percent in women with cirrhosis compared with only 2 percent in women without cirrhosis).

Perinatal mortality is high in these women with esophageal varices. Outcomes are even worse if cirrhosis causes the varices (Aggarwal and colleagues, 1999, 2001; Britton, 1982).

Management. Treatment for pregnant women is the same as for nonpregnant women. Beta-blocking drugs such as propranolol are given to reduce portal pressure and hence the risk of bleeding. Some practitioners prefer endoscopic band ligation for acute bleeding (Patch and co-workers, 2002; Starkel and associates, 1998). Banding also can be done prophylactically, and Zeeman and Moise (1999) described a woman who underwent banding at 15, 26, and 31 weeks to prevent bleeding. Sclerotherapy is recommended by other clinicians (Aggarwal and co-workers, 2001; Pauzner and associates, 1991). Even though experience is limited, *TIPSS* is preferred by some for emergency shunting (Sharara and Rockey, 2001). This can also be done electively in patients with previous variceal hemorrhage.

ACUTE ACETAMINOPHEN OVERDOSE. Nonsteroidal anti-inflammatory drugs are commonly used in suicide attempts. In a recent study from Denmark, Flint and associates (2002) reported that over half of such attempts in 122 pregnancies were with either acetaminophen or aspirin. In the United States, acetaminophen is much more commonly used during pregnancy, and overdose may lead to acute liver

failure. Early symptoms of overdose are nausea, vomiting, diaphoresis, malaise, and pallor. After a latent period of 24 to 48 hours, liver failure begins to develop and usually begins to resolve in 5 days.

The antidote is *N-acetylcysteine,* which must be given promptly. The drug is thought to act by increasing glutathione levels that facilitate metabolism of the toxic metabolite, *N*-acetyl-para-benzoquinoneimine. The need for treatment is based on projections of possible plasma hepatotoxic levels as a function of the time from acute ingestion. Many clinicians use the nomogram established by Rumack and Matthew (1975). Plasma levels are obtained 4 hours after ingestion, and if greater than 120 μg/mL, treatment is given. If plasma determinations are not available, empirical treatment is given if the dose exceeded 7.5 g. An oral loading dose of 140 mg/kg of *N*-acetylcysteine is followed by 17 maintenance doses of 70 mg/kg every 4 hours for 72 hours of total treatment time. The drug reaches therapeutic concentrations in the fetus, but its protective effects are unknown (Horowitz and colleagues, 1997).

Effects on Pregnancy. After 14 weeks, the fetus has some cytochrome P_{450} activity necessary for metabolism of acetaminophen to the toxic metabolite. Riggs and colleagues (1989) reported data from the Rocky Mountain Poison and Drug Center and described follow-up experiences in 60 such women. The likelihood of maternal and fetal survival was better if the antidote was given soon after overdose. At least one 33-week fetus appears to have died as a direct result of hepatotoxicity 2 days after ingestion. In another case, Wang and associates (1997) confirmed acetaminophen placental transfer with maternal and cord blood levels of 41 μg/mL. Both mother and infant died from hepatorenal failure.

LIVER TRANSPLANTATION. The first successful pregnancy in a liver transplantation recipient was reported by Walcott and associates (1978). A number of successful pregnancies were then described by the Pittsburgh group (Laifer and colleagues, 1990). In the most recent update from the National Transplantation Pregnancy Registry, Armenti and associates (2001) described outcomes in 158 pregnancies in 92 liver recipients. More than 33 percent of pregnancies were complicated by hypertension, 33 percent had an infection, and about 10 percent had a rejection episode. Preeclampsia developed in 25 percent of women, and excluding early pregnancy losses and terminations, 5 percent of 110 infants were stillborn. Although 33 percent were born before 37 weeks, there were no neonatal deaths. Very similar outcomes have been described for 29 women who underwent liver transplantation at Mount Sinai Medical Center (Nagy and colleagues, 2003).

At least two women have had a successful outcome following a combined liver–kidney transplant (Armenti and colleagues, 2001). Eguchi and co-workers (2002) performed a successful right-lobe liver transplant in a woman at 15 weeks with fulminant hepatic failure.

In pregnant women who have undergone transplantation, close surveillance is mandatory to detect hypertension, renal dysfunction, preeclampsia, and graft rejection. The use of immunosuppressive drugs during pregnancy was recently reviewed by Alston and colleagues (2001).

Briceno and co-workers (2004) recently described successful transplantation with the liver donor being a pregnant woman who died from complications of HELLP syndrome.

DISEASES OF THE GALLBLADDER AND PANCREAS

CHOLELITHIASIS AND CHOLECYSTITIS. In the United States, 20 percent of women older than 40 years of age have gallstones. Most stones contain cholesterol, and its oversecretion into bile is thought to be a major factor in stone formation. Biliary sludge, which may increase during pregnancy, is an important precursor to gallstone formation. The cumulative risk of all patients with silent gallstones to require surgery for symptoms or complications is 10 percent at 5 years, 15 percent at 10 years, and 18 percent at 15 years (Greenberger and Paumgartner, 2001). For these reasons, prophylactic cholecystectomy is not warranted for asymptomatic stones.

Nonsurgical approaches that have been used for symptomatic gallstone disease include oral bile acid therapy with ursodeoxycholic acid and extracorporeal shock wave lithotripsy. There is no experience with these during pregnancy.

Acute cholecystitis usually develops when there is obstruction of the cystic duct. Bacterial infection plays a role in 50 to 85 percent of cases. In more than 50 percent of patients with acute cholecystitis, a history of previous right upper quadrant pain from cholelithiasis is elicited. With acute disease, pain is accompanied by anorexia, nausea and vomiting, low-grade fever, and mild leukocytosis. Ultrasonography can be used to visualize stones as small as 2 mm, and false-positive and false-negative rates are about 2 to 4 percent (Greenberger and Paumgartner, 2001). Ultrasonic examination confirms gallstones in up to 90 percent of patients (Fig. 50–3).

Symptomatic gallbladder diseases include acute cholecystitis, biliary colic, and acute pancreatitis. Rarely, gallbladder torsion occurs (Kleiss and co-workers, 2003). In most of these cases, cholecystectomy is warranted. Although acute cholecystitis responds to medical therapy, contemporary consensus is that early cholecystectomy is indicated (Greenberger and Paumgartner, 2001). In acute cases, medical therapy consisting of nasogastric suction, intravenous fluids and antimicrobials, and analgesics is instituted before surgical therapy. Laparoscopic cholecystectomy has become the treatment of choice for most patients. Data from most centers indicate a twofold increased incidence of major biliary, vascular, and bowel complications when the laparoscopic technique is compared with open cholecystectomy (Fletcher and co-workers, 1999).

Gallbladder Disease During Pregnancy. During pregnancy, about 1 in 1000 women develops cholecystitis. There is no doubt that pregnancy is "lithogenic" and increases the risk of gallstones. After the first trimester, both gallbladder volume during fasting and residual volume after contracting in response to a test meal are doubled (Braverman and colleagues, 1980). Incomplete emptying may result in retention of cholesterol crystals, a prerequisite for cholesterol gallstones. Biliary sludge, which can be a forerunner to gallstones, develops in 30 percent of women during pregnancy (Maringhini and co-workers, 1987). In many cases this resolves within a year.

Management. Acute cholecystitis during pregnancy or the puerperium is usually associated with gallstones or biliary sludge. Symptomatic cholecystitis is initially managed in a manner similar to that for nonpregnant women. In the past, most favored medical therapy, however, 25 to 50 percent of women ultimately require cholecystectomy for persistent symptoms (Cosenza and associates, 1999; Glasgow and co-workers, 1998). In an observational study of 44 women, Dixon and colleagues (1987) performed cholecystectomies in 18 with symptomatic acute cholecystitis or cholelithiasis. Although these women did well, 15 of the 26 managed

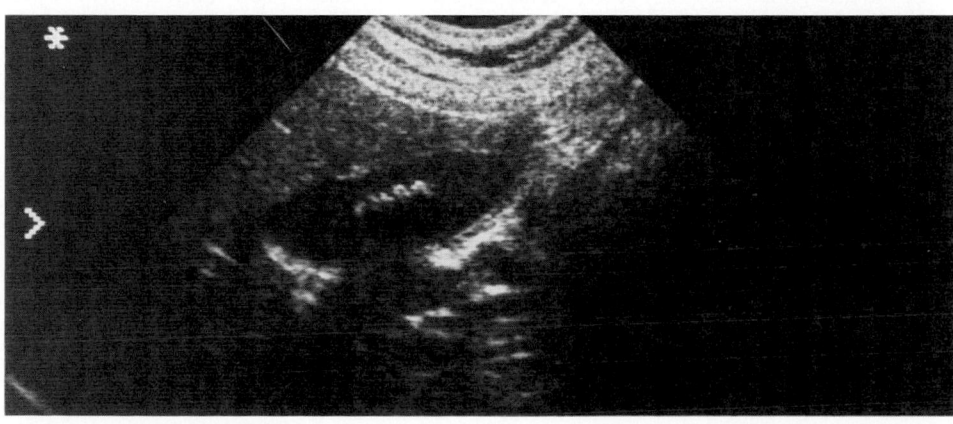

FIGURE 50–3. Multiple floating gallstones visualized in a 26-week pregnant woman. (Courtesy of Dr. Diane Twickler.)

medically had recurrent symptoms during pregnancy. Multiple hospitalizations were common in this latter group, and two women required prolonged parenteral nutrition. Davis and co-workers (1995) and Lee and associates (2000) described a total of 77 cases of cholecystitis and cited better outcomes with primary surgical management.

All of these factors have been associated with a trend favoring surgical therapy during pregnancy. If treated conservatively, there is a high recurrence rate during the same pregnancy. Moreover, if cholecystitis recurs later in gestation, preterm labor is more likely and cholecystectomy technically more difficult. Management at Parkland Hospital has evolved to a more aggressive surgical approach, especially if there is concomitant biliary pancreatitis as subsequently discussed.

LAPAROSCOPIC CHOLECYSTECTOMY. Reasonable experiences have been reported from several centers to indicate that laparoscopic surgery is as equally acceptable as open cholecystectomy in pregnant women (Barone, 1999; Cosenza, 1999; Glasgow, 1998, and all their colleagues). After their review of 213 cases, Lachman and co-workers (1999) concluded that laparoscopic cholecystectomy was safe throughout pregnancy. This procedure is discussed in Chapter 41 (see p. 975).

ENDOSCOPIC RETROGRADE CHOLANGIOPANCREATOGRAPHY. Relief of biliary duct gallstones during pregnancy has been greatly facilitated by use of endoscopic retrograde cholangiopancreatography (ERCP) (Nesbitt and co-workers, 1996). ERCP is performed if there is suspected common duct obstruction. Approximately 10 percent of patients with symptomatic stone disease have common duct stones (Ahrendt and Pitt, 2001). It has become commonplace to perform endoscopic sphincterotomy and gallstone extraction to be followed in a few days by laparoscopic cholecystectomy, especially with associated biliary pancreatitis. Boerma and colleagues (2002) randomized 120 nonpregnant patients to a wait-and-see approach versus laparoscopic cholecystectomy following endoscopic common duct stone removal. Half of those in the nonsurgical group had recurrent symptoms.

Asymptomatic Gallstones During Pregnancy. The incidence of ultrasonically visualized asymptomatic gallstones in over 1500 pregnant or postpartum women was 2.5 to 10 percent (Maringhini and colleagues, 1987; Valdivieso and co-workers, 1993). Cholecystectomy is not indicated for silent stones.

PANCREATITIS. Acute pancreatic inflammation is triggered by activation of pancreatic trypsinogen followed by autodigestion. It is characterized by cellular membrane disruption and proteolysis, edema, hemorrhage, and necrosis (Mitchell and colleagues, 2003). About 20 percent have severe pancreatitis with mortality rates up to 25 percent (Swaroop and associates, 2004). In nonpregnant patients, acute pancreatitis is almost equally associated with gallstones

(45 percent) and alcohol abuse (35 percent). During pregnancy, however, cholelithiasis is almost always the predisposing condition.

Nonbiliary pancreatitis occasionally develops postoperatively, or it is associated with trauma, drugs, or some viral infections. Certain metabolic conditions, including acute fatty liver of pregnancy and familial hypertriglyceridemia, also predispose to pancreatitis. Acute and chronic pancreatitis have been linked to the more than 1000 mutations of the cystic fibrosis transmembrane conductance regulator gene (Mitchell and co-workers, 2003; Rowntree and Harris, 2003).

Acute pancreatitis is characterized by mild to incapacitating epigastric pain, nausea and vomiting, and abdominal distention. Patients are usually in distress and have low-grade fever and tachycardia, hypotension, and abdominal tenderness. As many as 10 percent of patients have systemic inflammatory response syndrome, causing endothelial activation that can lead to *acute respiratory distress syndrome* (see Chap. 42, p. 991).

Laboratory confirmation is from serum amylase levels three times upper normal values, however, there is no correlation of their degree of elevation and disease severity. Indeed, usually by 48 to 72 hours amylase levels return to normal despite other evidence for continuing pancreatitis. Measurement of serum lipase activity increases the diagnostic yield. There is usually leukocytosis, and 25 percent of patients have hypocalcemia. Serum bilirubin and aspartate aminotransferase levels are usually somewhat elevated.

A number of prognostic factors may be used to predict severity of the disease (Mitchell and co-workers, 2003). Some of these are respiratory failure, shock, need for massive colloid replacement, hypocalcemia of less than 8 mg/dL, and dark hemorrhagic fluid on paracentesis. If three of the first four features are documented, survival is only 30 percent.

Management. Therapy is medical and includes analgesics for pain, intravenous hydration, and measures to decrease pancreatic secretion by interdiction of oral intake. Nasogastric suction has not been shown to improve the outcome of mild to moderate disease. Antimicrobials may improve survival in necrotizing pancreatitis (Mitchell and associates, 2003). Acute pancreatitis is usually self-limited, and in 90 percent of cases, inflammation subsides within 3 to 7 days.

For patients with severe necrotizing pancreatitis, ERCP and papillotomy are usually done along with intensive supportive therapy. Laparotomy with debridement and drainage may be lifesaving in some cases.

Pancreatitis During Pregnancy. The predisposition of pregnancy for biliary stasis and gallstone formation likely also links pregnancy with pancreatitis. At Parkland Hospital, with a predominate Mexican-American population, pancreatitis complicated about 1 in 3300 pregnancies (Ramin and colleagues, 1995). Swisher and associates (1994) reported an incidence of 1 in 1500 at the UCLA Medical Center. Legro

TABLE 50–3 Laboratory Values in 43 Pregnant Women with Pancreatitis

Test	Mean	Range	Normal
Serum amylase (IU/L)	1,392	111–4,560	30–110
Serum lipase (IU/L)	6,929	36–41,824	23–208
Total bilirubin (mg/dL)	1.7	0.1–4.9	0.2–1.3
Aspartate transferase (U/L)	120	11–498	3–35
Leukocytes (per μL)	12,000	7,000–14,600	4,100–10,900

From Ramin and colleagues (1995), with permission.

and Laifer (1995) found an incidence of 1 in 4000 at Magee Women's Hospital.

In most pregnant women, cholelithiasis coexists, but some have an associated hyperlipidemic syndrome, usually hypertriglyceridemia (Bildirici, 2002; Choy, 2002; Loo, 2002, and all their colleagues). As discussed in Chapter 46 (see p. 1066), it may complicate cystic fibrosis (Virgilis and co-workers, 2003). At least two pregnant women have been described with hypertriglyceridemia due to *familial lipoprotein lipase deficiency* (Watts and associates, 1992). Finally, as discussed in Chapter 53 (see p. 1198), pancreatitis may also be associated with hyperparathyroidism (Dahan and Chang, 2001).

DIAGNOSIS. The same criteria apply to nonpregnant and pregnant patients. Ramin and colleagues (1995) reported that all but 1 of 43 pregnant women with pancreatitis presented with nausea, vomiting, and abdominal pain. Serial determinations of amylase and lipase activity remain the best methods to confirm the clinical diagnosis, and their baseline levels are not changed during pregnancy (Ordorica and associates, 1991). As shown in Table 50–3, the mean amylase value in 43 pregnant women with pancreatitis was about 1400 IU/L, and the mean lipase value about 7000 IU/L. Again, amylase values did not correlate with the severity of disease.

MANAGEMENT. Therapy is the same as for nonpregnant patients. Mild inflammation usually subsides with conservative therapy. In the series by Ramin and colleagues (1995), all 43 women responded to conservative treatment and were hospitalized for a mean of 8.5 days. ERCP as discussed above for removal of common duct stones and sphincterotomy has been used successfully in pregnancy (Nesbitt and colleagues, 1996; Simmons and co-workers, 2004). Cholecystectomy should be considered after inflammation subsides. Severe necrotizing pancreatitis can be life threatening (Gosnell and colleagues, 2001). This concern prompted Swisher and associates (1994) to undertake laparotomy in 3 of 30 women who had unrelenting pain.

Pregnancy outcome usually is good. In women with severe disease, however, fetal loss is high because of associated hypovolemia, hypoxia, and acidosis.

PANCREATIC TRANSPLANTATION. According to the United Network for Organ Sharing, the 3-year graft survival for pancreatic transplantation is almost 70 percent (Lin and associates, 1998). Because there is improved survival when a combined pancreas and kidney are grafted, most operations include both organs. At least two successful pregnancies have followed pancreatic islet autotransplantation (Teuscher and colleagues, 1994; Wahoff and associates, 1995).

Tydén and colleagues (1989) described four women in whom pancreas–kidney transplantation was followed in 1 to 2 years by pregnancy. Pelvic placement of the graft was not problematic. Glucose homeostasis was well maintained throughout pregnancy. Successful vaginal deliveries have been described by Allenby and colleagues (1998). Armenti and co-workers (2001) recently updated results reported to the National Transplantation Pregnancy Registry. Of 44 pregnancies in 31 women following pancreas–kidney transplantation, outcomes have been encouraging. Although the incidence of hypertension, preeclampsia, preterm delivery, and fetal growth restriction was high, there was only one perinatal death. There were three rejection episodes during pregnancy, which were treated successfully.

REFERENCES

Aggarwal SH, Suril V, Vasishta K, et al: Pregnancy and cirrhosis of the liver. Aust N Z J Obstet Gynaecol 39:503, 1999

Aggarwal N, Sawhney H, Vasishta K, et al: Non-cirrhotic portal hypertension in pregnancy. Int J Gynaecol Obstet 72:1, 2001

Ahrendt SA, Pitt HA: Biliary tract. In Townsend CM, Beauchamp RD, Evers MB, et al (eds): Sabiston Textbook of Surgery, 16th ed. Philadelphia, Saunders, 2001, p. 1076

Allenby K, Campbell DJ, Lodge JPA: Vaginal delivery following combined pelvic renal and pancreatic transplant. Br J Obstet Gynaecol 105:1036, 1998

Alston PK, Kuller JA, McMahon MJ: Pregnancy in transplant recipients. Obstet Gynecol Surv 56:289, 2001

Alsulyman OM, Ouzounian JG, Ames-Castro M, et al: Intrahepatic cholestasis of pregnancy: Perinatal outcome associated with expectant management. Am J Obstet Gynecol 175:957, 1996

Alter MJ, Kruszon-Moran D, Nainan OV, et al: The prevalence of hepatitis C virus infection in the United States, 1988 through 1994. N Engl J Med 341:556, 1999

American College of Obstetricians and Gynecologists: Viral hepatitis in pregnancy. Educational Bulletin No. 248, July 1998

Angulo P: Nonalcoholic fatty liver disease. N Engl J Med 346:16, 2002

Armenti VT, Radomski JS, Moritz MJ, et al: Report from the National Transplantation Pregnancy Registry (NTPR): Outcomes of pregnancy after transplantation, Chapter 7. In Cecka JM, Terasaki PI (eds): Clinical Transplants 2001. Los Angeles, UCLA Immunogenetics Center, 2001, p 97

Baker AL: Liver and biliary tract diseases. In Barron WM, Lindheimer MD (eds): Medical Disorders During Pregnancy, 3rd ed. St. Louis, Mosby, 2000, p 330

Barone JE, Bears S, Chen S, et al: Outcome study of cholecystectomy during pregnancy. Am J Surg 177:232, 1999

Bildirici I, Esinler I, Deren O, et al: Hyperlipidemic pancreatitis during pregnancy. Acta Obstet Gynecol Scand 81:468, 2002

Blish KR, Ibdah JA: Maternal heterozygosity for a mitochondrial trifunctional protein mutation as a cause for liver disease in pregnancy. Med Hypotheses 64:96, 2005

Boerma D, Rauws EA, Keulemans YC, et al: Wait-and-see policy or laparoscopic cholecystectomy after endoscopic sphincterotomy for bile-duct stones: A randomized trial. Lancet 360:761, 2002

Bohman V, Stettler RW, Little BB, et al: Seroprevalence and risk factors for hepatitis C virus antibody in pregnant women. Obstet Gynecol 80:609, 1992

Bosch J, García-Pagán JC: Prevention of variceal rebleeding. Lancet 361:952, 2003

Braverman DZ, Johnson ML, Kern F Jr: Effects of pregnancy and contraceptive steroids on gallbladder function. N Engl J Med 302:362, 1980

Briceno PJ, Ortiz JA, Manzarbeitia C, et al: Liver transplantation using an organ donor with HELLP syndrome. Transplantation 77:137, 2004

Britton RC: Pregnancy and esophageal varices. Am J Surg 143:421, 1982

Burns DN, Minkoff H: Hepatitis C: Screening in pregnancy. Obstet Gynecol 94:1044, 1999

Burrows RF, Clavisi O, Burrows E: Interventions for treating cholestasis in pregnancy. Cochrane Database System Review (4):CD000493, 2001

Castro MA, Goodwin TM, Shaw KJ, et al: Disseminated intravascular coagulation and antithrombin III depression in acute fatty liver of pregnancy. Am J Obstet Gynecol 174:211, 1996a

Castro MA, Ouzounian JG, Colletti PM, et al: Radiologic studies in acute fatty liver of pregnancy. A review of the literature and 19 new cases. J Reprod Med 41:839, 1996b

Centers for Disease Control and Prevention: Hepatitis B vaccination—United States, 1982–2002. MMWR 51:549, 2002

Centers for Disease Control and Prevention: Update US Public Health Service guidelines for the management of occupational exposures to HBV, HCV, and HIV and recommnendations for postexposure prophylaxis. MMWR 50:21, 2001

Centers for Disease Control and Prevention: Prevention of hepatitis A through active or passive immunization. MMWR 48:1, 1999

Centers for Disease Control and Prevention: Recommendations for prevention and control of hepatitis C virus (HCV) infection and HCV-related chronic disease. MMWR 47:1, 1998

Choy CM, Tam WH, Leung TN: Gestational hyperlipidaemic pancreatitis. Br J Obstet Gynaecol 109:847, 2002

Clark JM, Diehl AM: Nonalcoholic fatty liver disease: An underrecognized cause of cryptogenic cirrhosis. JAMA 289:3000, 2003

Conry-Cantilena C, VanRaden M, Gibble J, et al: Routes of infection, viremia, and liver disease in blood donors found to have hepatitis C virus infection. N Engl J Med 334:1691, 1996

Conte D, Fraquelli M, Prati D, et al: Prevalence and clinical course of chronic hepatitis C virus (HVC) infection and rate of HCV vertical transmission in a cohort of 15,250 pregnant women. Hepatology 31:751, 2000

Cosenza CA, Saffari B, Jabbour N, et al: Surgical management of biliary gallstone disease during pregnancy. Am J Surg 178:545, 1999

Cunningham FG, Lowe TW, Guss S, et al: Erythrocyte morphology in women with severe preeclampsia and eclampsia. Am J Obstet Gynecol 153:358, 1985

Dahan M, Chang RJ: Pancreatitis secondary to hyperparathyroidism during pregnancy. Obstet Gynecol 98:923, 2001

Dal Molin G, D'Agaro P, Ansaldi F, et al: Mother-to-infant transmission of hepatitis C virus: Rate of infection and assessment of viral load and IgM anti-HCV as risk factors. J Med Virol 67:137, 2002

David AL, Kotecha M, Girling JC: Factors influencing postnatal liver function tests. Br J Obstet Gynaecol 107:1421, 2000

Davidson KM, Simpson LL, Knox TA, et al: Acute fatty liver of pregnancy in triplet gestation. Obstet Gynecol 91:806, 1998

Davis A, Katz VL, Cox R: Gallbladder disease in pregnancy. J Reprod Med 40:759, 1995

Davis GL, Esteban-Mur R, Rustgi V, et al: Interferon alfa-2b alone or in combination with ribavirin for the treatment of relapse of chronic hepatitis C. N Engl J Med 339:1493, 1998

Dienstag JL, Isselbacher KJ: Acute viral hepatitis. In Braunwald E, Fauci AS, Kasper DL, et al (eds): Harrison's Principles of Internal Medicine, 15th ed. New York, McGraw-Hill, 2001a, p 1721

Dienstag JL, Isselbacher KJ: Chronic hepatitis. In Braunwald E, Fauci AS, Kasper DL, et al (eds): Harrison's Principles of Internal Medicine, 15th ed. New York, McGraw-Hill, 2001b, p 1742

Dienstag JL, Schiff ER, Wright TL, et al: Lamivudine as initial treatment for chronic hepatitis B in the United States. N Engl J Med 341:1256, 1999

Dixon NP, Faddis DM, Silberman H: Aggressive management of cholecystitis during pregnancy. Am J Surg 154:294, 1987

Eguchi S, Yanaga K, Fujita F, et al: Living-related right lobe liver transplantation for a patient with fulminant hepatic failure during the second trimester of pregnancy. Transplantation 73:1970, 2002

Ferrero S, Lungaro P, Bruzzone BM, et al: Prospective study of mother-to-infant transmission of hepatitis C virus: A 10-year survey (1990–2000). Acta Obstet Gynecol Scand 82:229, 2003

Feucht HH, Zollner B, Polywka S, et al: Vertical transmission of hepatitis G. Lancet 347:615, 1996

Flamm SL: Chronic hepatitic C virus infection. JAMA 289:18, 2003

Fletcher DR, Hobbs MST, Tan P, et al: Complications of cholecystectomy: Risks of the laparoscopic approach and protective effects of operative cholangiography. Ann Surg 229:449, 1999

Flint C, Larsen H, Nielsen GL, et al: Pregnancy outcome after suicide attempt by drug use: A Danish population-based study. Acta Obstet Gynecol Scand 81:516, 2002

Floreani A, Paternoster D, Zappalá F, et al: Hepatitis C virus infection in pregnancy. Br J Obstet Gynaecol 103:325, 1996

Franco J, Newcomer J, Adams M, et al: Auxiliary liver transplant in acute fatty liver of pregnancy. Obstet Gynecol 95:1042, 2000

Fried MW, Shiffman ML, Reddy KR, et al: Peginterferon alfa-2a plus ribavirin for chronic hepatitis C virus infection. N Engl J Med 347:975, 2002

Germain AM, Carvajal JA, Glasinovic JC, et al: Intrahepatic cholestasis of pregnancy: An intriguing pregnancy-specific disorder. J Soc Gynecol Investig 9:10, 2002

Gervais A, Bacq Y, Bernuau J, et al: Decrease in serum ALT and increase in serum HCV RNA during pregnancy in women with chronic hepatitis C. J Hepatol 32:293, 2000

Gill EJ, Contos MJ, Peng TCC: Acute fatty liver of pregnancy and acetaminophen toxicity leading to liver failure and postpartum liver transplantation: A case report. J Reprod Med 47:584, 2002

Girling JC, Dow E, Smith JH: Liver function tests in pre-eclampsia: Importance of comparison with a reference range derived for normal pregnancy. Br J Obstet Gynaecol 104:246, 1997

Glasgow RE, Visser BC, Harris HW, et al: Changing management of gallstone disease during pregnancy. Surg Endosc 12:241, 1998

Gosnell FE, O'Neill BB, Harris HW: Necrotizing pancreatitis during pregnancy: A rare cause and review of the literature. J Gastrointest Surg 5:371, 2001

Gow PJ, Mutimer D: Treatment of chronic hepatitis. BMJ 323:1164, 2001

Greenberger NJ, Paumgartner G: Diseases of the gallbladder and bile ducts. In Braunwald E, Fauci AS, Kasper DL, et al (eds): Harrison's Principles of Internal Medicine, 15th ed. New York, McGraw-Hill, 2001, p 1776

Hadziyannis SJ, Tassopoulos NC, Heathcote EJ, et al: Adefovir dipivoxil for the treatment of hepatitis B e antigen-negative chronic hepatitis B. N Engl J Med 348:800, 2003

Hill JB, Sheffield JS, Kim MJ, et al: Risk of hepatitis B transmission in breast-fed infants of chronic hepatitis B carriers. Obstet Gynecol 99;1049, 2002

Hill JB, Sheffield JS, Zeeman GG, Wendel GD: Hepatotoxicity with antiretroviral treatment of pregnant women. Obstet Gynecol 98:909, 2001

Hillemanns P, Dannecker C, Kimmig R, et al: Obstetric risks and vertical transmission of hepatitis C virus infection in pregnancy. Acta Obstet Gynecol Scand 79:543, 2000

Hirvioja ML, Tuimala R, Vuori J: The treatment of intrahepatic cholestasis of pregnancy by dexamethasone. Br J Obstet Gynaecol 99:109, 1992

Horowitz RS, Dart RC, Jarvie DR, et al: Placental transfer of N-acetylcysteine following human maternal acetaminophen toxicity. Clin Toxicol 35:447, 1997

Ibdah JA, Bennett MJ, Rinaldo P, et al: A fetal fatty-acid oxidation disorder as a cause of liver disease in pregnant women. N Engl J Med 340:1723, 1999

Inaba N, Okajima Y, Kang XS, et al: Maternal–infant transmission of hepatitis G virus. Am J Obstet Gynecol 177:1537, 1997

Ingardia CJ, Kelley L, Steinfeld JD, et al: Hepatitis B vaccination in pregnancy: Factors influencing efficacy. Obstet Gynecol 93:983, 1999

Ingardia C, Morgan M, Feldman D, et al: Hepatitis B vaccination in pregnancy—factors associated with immunity in subsequent pregnancy. Abstract 137. Presented at the 24th Annual Meeting of the Society for Maternal–Fetal Medicine, 2–7 February 2004

Ingerslev M, Teilum G: Biopsy studies on the liver in pregnancy, 2. Liver biopsy on normal pregnant women. Acta Obstet Gynecol Scand 25:352, 1945

Isaacs JD, Sims HF, Powell CK, et al: Maternal acute fatty liver of pregnancy associated with fetal trifunctional protein deficiency: Molecular characterization of a novel maternal mutant allele. Pediatr Res 40:393, 1996

Jarvis LM, Davidson F, Hanley JP, et al: Infection with hepatitis G virus among recipients of plasma products. Lancet 348:1352, 1996

Jurema MW, Polaneczky M, Ledger WJ: Hepatitis B immunization in postpartum women. Am J Obstet Gynecol 185:355, 2001

Kennedy S, Hall PM, Seymour AE, et al: Transient diabetes insipidus and acute fatty liver of pregnancy. Br J Obstet Gynaecol 101:387, 1994

Kenyon AP, Piercy CN, Girling J, et al: Obstetric cholestasis, outcome with active management: A series of 70 cases. Br J Obstet Gynaecol 109:282, 2002

Kenyon AP, Piercy CN, Girling J, et al: Pruritus may precede abnormal liver function tests in pregnant women with obstetric cholestasis: A longitudinal analysis. Br J Obstet Gynaecol 108:1190, 2001

Khuroo MS, Kamili S, Jameel S: Vertical transmission of hepatitis E virus. Lancet 345:1025, 1995

Kim JH, Lee YS, Kim SH, et al: Does umbilical vein catheterization lead to portal venous thrombosis? Prospective US evaluation in 100 neonates. Radiology 219:645, 2001

Kirkinen P, Ryynänen M: First-trimester manifestation of intrahepatic cholestasis of pregnancy and high fetoplacental hormone production in a triploid fetus. J Reprod Med 40:471, 1995

Kleiss K, Choy-Hee L, Fogle R, et al: Torsion of the gallbladder in pregnancy: A case report. J Reprod Med 48:206, 2003

Knox TA, Olans LB: Liver disease in pregnancy. N Engl J Med 335:568, 1996

Kretowicz E, McIntyre HD: Intrahepatic cholestasis of pregnancy, worsening after dexamethasone. Aust N Z J Obstet Gynaecol 34:211, 1994

Kroumpouzos G, Cohen LM: Specific dermatoses of pregnancy: An evidence-based systematic review. Am J Obstet Gynecol 188:1083, 2003

Lachman E, Schienfeld A, Voss E, et al: Pregnancy and laparoscopic surgery. J Am Assoc Gynecol Laparosc 6:347, 1999

Lai CL, Chien RN, Leung NWY, et al: A one-year trial of lamivudine for chronic hepatitis B. N Engl J Med 339:61, 1998

Laibl V, Sheffield J, Robert S, et al: Hepatitis C quantitative viral load as a predictor of pregnancy outcome. Presented at the 25th Annual Meeting of the Society for Maternal–Fetal Medicine, Reno, Nevada, February 7, 2005

Laifer SA, Darby MJ, Scantlebury VP, et al: Pregnancy and liver transplantation. Obstet Gynecol 76:1083, 1990

Lauer GM, Walker BD: Hepatitis C virus infection. N Engl J Med 345:41, 2001

Lee S, Bradley JP, Mele MM, et al: Cholelithiasis in pregnancy: Surgical versus medical management. Obstet Gynecol 95:S70, 2000

Lee WM: Pregnancy in patients with chronic liver disease. Gastroenterol Clin North Am 21:889, 1992

Legro RS, Laifer SA: First trimester pancreatitis: Maternal and neonatal outcome. J Reprod Med 40:689, 1995

Leikin EL, Reinus JF, Schmell E, et al: Epidemiologic predictors of hepatitis C virus infection in pregnant women. Obstet Gynecol 84:529, 1994

Leslie KK, Reznikov L, Simon FR, et al: Estrogens in intrahepatic cholestasis of pregnancy. Obstet Gynecol 95:372, 2000

Levine AB: Autoimmune hepatitis in pregnancy. Obstet Gynecol 95:1033, 2000

Lin HM, Kauffman HM, McBride MA, et al: Center-specific graft and patient survival rates. 1997 United Network for Organ Sharing (UNOS) report. JAMA 280:1153, 1998

Locatelli A, Roncaglia N, Arreghini A, et al: Hepatitis C virus infection is associated with a higher incidence of cholestasis of pregnancy. Br J Obstet Gynaecol 106:498, 1999

Loo CC, Tan JYL: Decreasing the plasma triglyceride level in hypertriglyceridemia-induced pancreatitis in pregnancy: A case report. Am J Obstet Gynecol 187:241, 2002

Lunzer M, Barnes P, Byth K, et al: Serum bile acid concentrations during pregnancy and their relationship to obstetric cholestasis. Gastroenterology 91:825, 1986

MacLean MA, Cameron AD, Cumming GP, et al: Recurrence of acute fatty liver of pregnancy. Br J Obstet Gynaecol 101:453, 1994

Maitra A, Domiati-Saad R, Yost N, et al: Absence of the G1528C (E474Q) mutation in the α-subunit of the mitochondrial trifunctional protein in women with acute fatty liver of pregnancy. Pediatr Res 51:658, 2002

Marcellin P, Chang TT, Lim SG, et al: Adefovir dipivoxil for the treatment of hepatitis B e antigen-positive chronic hepatitis B. N Engl J Med 348:808, 2003

Maringhini A, Marcenó MP, Lanzarone F, et al: Sludge and stones in gallbladder after pregnancy: Prevalence and risk factors. J Hepatol 5:218, 1987

Matos A, Bernardes J, Ayres-de-Campos D, et al: Antepartum fetal cerebral hemorrhage not predicted by current surveillance methods in cholestasis of pregnancy. Obstet Gynecol 89:803, 1997

Mazzella G, Nicola R, Francesco A, et al: Ursodeoxycholic acid administration in patients with cholestasis of pregnancy: Effects on primary bile acids in babies and mothers. Hepatology 33:504, 2001

Minakami H, Oka N, Sato T, et al: Preeclampsia: A microvesicular fat disease of the liver? Am J Obstet Gynecol 159:1043, 1988

Mitchell RMS, Byrne MF, Baillie J: Pancreatitis. Lancet 361:1447, 2003

Moldenhauer JS, O'brien JM, Barton JR, et al: Acute fatty liver of pregnancy associated with pancreatitis: A life-threatening complication. Am J Obstet Gynecol 190:502, 2004

Monga M, Katz AR: Acute fatty liver in the second trimester. Obstet Gynecol 93:811, 1999

Mullally B, Hansen W: Intrahepatic cholestasis of pregnancy: Review of the literature. Obstet Gynecol Surv 57:47, 2001

Nagy S, Bush MC, Berkowitz R, et al: Pregnancy outcome in liver transplant recipients. Obstet Gynecol 102:121, 2003

Nesbitt TH, Kay HH, McCoy MC, et al: Endoscopic management of biliary disease during pregnancy. Obstet Gynecol 87:806, 1996

Nicastri PL, Diaferia A, Tartagni M, et al: A randomised placebo-controlled trial of ursodeoxycholic acid and S-adenosylmethionine in the treatment of intrahepatic cholestasis of pregnancy. Br J Obstet Gynaecol 105:1205, 1998

Niu MT, Salive ME, Ellenberg SS: Neonatal deaths after hepatitis B vaccine: The vaccine adverse event reporting system, 1991–1998. Arch Pediatr Adolesc Med 153:1279, 1999

Ordorica SA, Frieden FJ, Marks F, et al: Pancreatic enzyme activity in pregnancy. J Reprod Med 36:359, 1991

Pajor A, Lehoczky D: Pregnancy in liver cirrhosis—assessment of maternal and fetal risks in eleven patients and review of the management. Gynecol Obstet Invest 38:45, 1994

Patch D, Sabin CA, Goulis J, et al: A randomized, controlled trial of medical therapy versus endoscopic ligation for the prevention of variceal rebleeding in patients with cirrhosis. Gastroenterology 123:1013, 2002

Paternoster DM, Fabris F, Palù G, et al: Intra-hepatic cholestasis of pregnancy in hepatitis C virus infection. Acta Obstet Gynecol Scand 81:99, 2002

Paternoster DM, Santarossa C, Grella P, et al: Viral load in HCV RNA-positive pregnant women. Am J Gastroenterol 96:2751, 2001

Pauzner D, Wolman I, Niv D, et al: Endoscopic sclerotherapy in extrahepatic portal hypertension in pregnancy. Am J Obstet Gynecol 164:152, 1991

Pereira SP, O'Donohue J, Wendon J, et al: Maternal and perinatal outcome in severe pregnancy-related liver disease. Hepatology 26:1258, 1997

Rahman TM, Wendon J: Severe hepatic dysfunction in pregnancy. Q J Med 95:343, 2002

Rakheja D, Bennett MJ, Rogers BB: Long-chain L-3-hydroxyacyl-coenzyme A dehydrogenase deficiency: A molecular and biochemical review. Lab Invest 82:815, 2002

Ramin KD, Ramin SM, Richey SD, et al: Acute pancreatitis in pregnancy. Am J Obstet Gynecol 173:187, 1995

Resti M, Azzari C, Mannelli F, et al: Tuscany Study Group on Hepatitis C virus infection in children: Mother to child transmission of hepatitis C virus: Prospective study of risk factors and timing of infection in children born to women seronegative for HIV-1. BMJ 317:437, 1998

Reyes H: Intrahepatic cholestasis. A puzzling disorder of pregnancy [review]. J Gastroenterol Hepatol 12:211, 1997

Reyes H, Sandoval L, Wainstein A, et al: Acute fatty liver of pregnancy: A clinical study of 12 episodes in 11 patients. Gut 35:101, 1994

Reyes H, Sjovall J: Bile acids and progesterone metabolites in intrahepatic cholestasis of pregnancy. Ann Med 32:94, 2000

Riggs BS, Bronstein AC, Kulig K, et al: Acute acetaminophen overdose during pregnancy. Obstet Gynecol 74:247, 1989

Rioseco AJ, Ivankovic MB, Manzur A, et al: Intrahepatic cholestasis of pregnancy: A retrospective case-control study of perinatal outcome. Am J Obstet Gynecol 170:890, 1994

Roncaglia N, Locatelli A, Arreghini A, et al: A randomised controlled trial of urodeoxycholic acid and S-adenosyl-l-methionine in the treatment of gestational cholestasis. Br J Obstet Gynaecol 111:17, 2004

Rowntree RK, Harris A: The phenotypic consequences of CFTR mutations. Ann Hum Genet 67:471, 2003

Rumack BH, Matthew H: Acetaminophen poisoning and toxicity. Pediatrics 55:871, 1975

Sadler LC, Lane M, North R: Severe fetal intracranial haemorrhage during treatment with cholestyramine for intrahepatic cholestasis of pregnancy. Br J Obstet Gynaecol 102:169, 1995

Santiago P, Roberts S, Sheffield J, et al: Prevalence of hepatitis B and C in HIV infected women. Presented at the 25th Annual Meeting of the Society for Maternal-Fetal Medicine, Reno, Nevada, February 7–12, 2005

Schreyer P, Caspi E, El-Hindi JM, et al: Cirrhosis—pregnancy and delivery: A review. Obstet Gynecol Surv 37:304, 1982

Sharara AI, Rockey DC: Gastroesophageal variceal hemorrhage. N Engl J Med 345:669, 2001

Shekhawat P, Bennett MJ, Sadovsky Y, et al: Human placenta metabolizes fatty acids: Implications for fetal fatty acid oxidation disorders and maternal liver diseases. Am J Physiol Endocrinol Metab 284:E1098, 2003

Silverman NS, Jenkin BK, Wu C, et al: Hepatitis C virus in pregnancy: Seroprevalence and risk factors for infection. Am J Obstet Gynecol 169:583, 1993

Simmons DC, Tarnasky PR, Rivera-Alsina ME, et al: Endoscopic retrograde cholangiopancreatography (ERCP) in pregnancy without the use of radiation. Am J Obstet Gynecol 190:1467, 2004

Sims HF, Brackett JC, Powell CK, et al: The molecular basis of pediatric long chain 3-hydroxyacyl-CoA dehydrogenase deficiency associated with maternal acute fatty liver of pregnancy. Proc Natl Acad Sci USA 92:841, 1995

Starkel P, Horsman Y, Geubel A: Endoscopic band ligation: A safe technique to control bleeding esophageal varices in pregnancy. Gastrointest Endosc 48:212, 1998

Sulkowski MS, Moore RD, Mehta SH, et al: Hepatitis C and progression of HIV disease. JAMA 288:199, 2002

Suzuki S, Watanabe S, Araki T: Acute fatty liver of pregnancy at 23 weeks of gestation. Br J Obstet Gynaecol 108:223, 2001

Swaroop VS, Chari ST, Clain JE: Severe acute pancreatitis. JAMA 291:2865, 2004

Swisher SG, Hunt KK, Schmit PJ, et al: Management of pancreatitis complicating pregnancy. Am Surg 60:759, 1994

Terg R, Coronel E, Sorda J, et al: Efficacy and safety of oral naltrexone treatment for pruritus of cholestasis, a crossover, double blind, placebo-controlled study. J Hepatol 37:717, 2002

Teuscher AU, Sutherland DER, Robertson RP: Successful pregnancy after pancreatic islet autotransplantation. Transplant Proc 26:3520, 1994

Thio CL, Seaberg EC, Skolasky R, et al: HIV-1, hepatitis B virus, and risk of liver-related mortality in the multicenter cohort study (MACS). Lancet 360:1921, 2002

Towers CV, Asrat T, Rumney P: The presence of hepatitis B surface antigen and deoxyribonucleic acid in amniotic fluid and cord blood. Am J Obstet Gynecol 184:1514, 2001

Trauner M, Meier PJ, Boyer JL: Molecular pathogenesis of cholestasis. N Engl J Med 339:1217, 1998

Treem WR, Rinaldo P, Hale DE, et al: Acute fatty liver of pregnancy and long-chain 3-hydroxyacyl-coenzyme A dehydrogenase deficiency. Hepatology 19:339, 1994

Tyden G, Brattstrom C, Bjorkman U, et al: Pregnancy after combined pancreas-kidney transplantation. Diabetes 38 Suppl 1:43, 1989

Tyni T, Ekholm E, Pihko H: Pregnancy complications are frequent in long-chain 3-hydroxyacyl-coenzyme A dehydrogenase deficiency. Am J Obstet Gynecol 178:603, 1998

Urganci N, Arapoglu M, Akyildiz B, et al: Neonatal cholestasis resulting from vertical transmission of hepatitis A infection. Pediatr Infect Dis J 22(4):381, 2003

Usta IM, Barton JR, Amon EA, et al: Acute fatty liver of pregnancy: An experience in the diagnosis and management of fourteen cases. Am J Obstet Gynecol 171:1342, 1994

Valdivieso V, Covarrubias C, Siegel F, et al: Pregnancy and cholelithiasis: Pathogenesis and natural course of gallstones diagnosed in early puerperium. Hepatology 17:1, 1993

Vigil-De Gracia P: Acute fatty liver and HELLP syndrome: Two distinct pregnancy disorders. Int J Gynaecol Obstet 73:215, 2001

Virgilis D, Rivkin L, Samueloff A, et al: Cystic fibrosis, pregnancy, and recurrent, acute pancreatitis. J Pediatr Gastroenterol Nutr 36:486, 2003

Wahoff DC, Leone JP, Farney AC, et al: Pregnancy after total pancreatectomy and autologous islet transplantation. Surgery 117:353, 1995

Walcott WO, Derick DE, Jolley JJ, et al: Successful pregnancy in a liver transplant patient. Am J Obstet Gynecol 132:340, 1978

Wang PH, Yang MJ, Lee WL, et al: Acetaminophen poisoning in late pregnancy. A case report. J Reprod Med 42:367, 1997

Watson JC, Fleming DW, Borella AJ, et al: Vertical transmission of hepatitis A resulting in an outbreak in a neonatal intensive care unit. J Infect Dis 167:567, 1993

Watts GF, Morton K, Jackson P, et al: Management of patients with severe hypertriglyceridaemia during pregnancy: Report of two cases with familial lipoprotein lipase deficiency. Br J Obstet Gynaecol 99:163, 1992

Williamson C, Hems LM, Goulis DG, et al: Clinical outcome in a series of cases of obstetric cholestasis identified via a patient support group. BJOG 111:676, 2004

Yang HI, Lu SN, Liaw YF, et al: Hepatitis B e antigen and the risk of hepatocellular carcinoma. N Engl J Med 347:168, 2002a

Yang Z, Yamada J, Zhao Y, et al: Prospective screening for pediatric mitochondrial trifunctional protein defects in pregnancies complicated by liver disease. JAMA 288:2163, 2002b

Yang Z, Zhao Y, Bennett MJ, et al: Fetal genotypes and pregnancy outcomes in 35 families with mitochondrial trifunctional protein mutations. Am J Obstet Gynecol 187:715, 2002c

Zeeman GG, Moise KJ: Prophylactic banding of severe esophageal varices associated with liver cirrhosis in pregnancy. Obstet Gynecol 94:842, 1999

51

Hematological Disorders

Pregnancy induces physiological changes that often confuse the diagnosis of hematological disorders and assessment of their treatment. This is especially true for anemia. A number of pregnancy-induced hematological changes are discussed in detail in Chapter 5 (see p. 129). One of the most significant changes is blood volume expansion with a disproportionate plasma volume increase, resulting in a normally decreased hematocrit.

Pregnant women are susceptible to hematological abnormalities that may affect any woman of childbearing age. These include chronic disorders such as hereditary anemias; immunological thrombocytopenia; and malignancies, including leukemias and lymphomas. Other disorders arise during pregnancy because of pregnancy-induced demands, such as iron-deficiency and megaloblastic anemias. Pregnancy may also unmask underlying hematological disorders such as compensated hemolytic anemias caused by hemoglobinopathies or red cell membrane defects. Finally, any hematological disease may first arise during pregnancy, such as autoimmune hemolysis or aplastic anemia.

ANEMIAS

Extensive hematological measurements have been made in healthy nonpregnant women. As shown in Table 51–1, anemia is defined as hemoglobin concentration less than 12 g/dL in nonpregnant women and less than 10 g/dL during pregnancy or the puerperium. The Centers for Disease Control and Prevention (1990) defined anemia as less than 11 g/dL in the first and third trimesters and less than 10.5 g/dL in the second trimester (Fig. 51–1).

The modest fall in hemoglobin levels during pregnancy is caused by a relatively greater expansion of plasma volume compared with the increase in red cell volume. The disproportion between the rates at which plasma and erythrocytes are added to the maternal circulation is greatest during the second trimester. The long-used term *physiological anemia* to describe this process is an oxymoron and should be discarded. Late in pregnancy, plasma expansion essentially ceases while hemoglobin mass continues to increase.

After delivery, the hemoglobin level typically fluctuates to a modest degree and then rises to and usually exceeds the

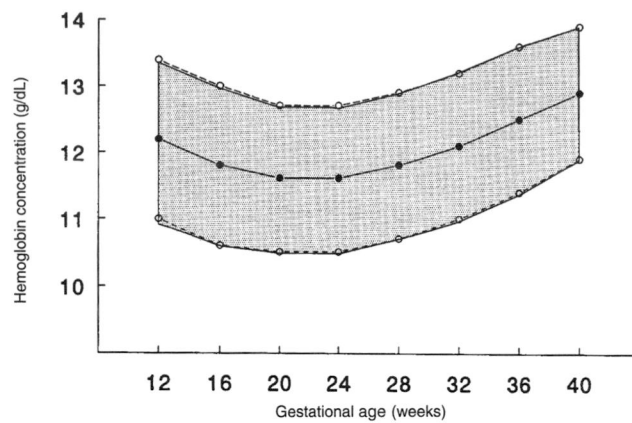

FIGURE 51–1. Mean hemoglobin concentrations (●—●) and 5th and 95th (○—○) percentiles for healthy pregnant women taking iron supplements. (Data from Centers for Disease Control and Prevention, 1989.)

nonpregnant level. The rate and magnitude of increase early in the puerperium result from the amount of hemoglobin added during pregnancy and the amount of blood loss at delivery modified by a puerperal decrease in plasma volume.

Frequency of Anemia. The frequency of anemia during pregnancy depends primarily on iron supplementation. It is more common among indigent women. Taylor and associates (1982) reported that hemoglobin levels at term averaged 12.7 g/dL among women who took supplemental iron compared with 11.2 g/dL for women who did not. Bodnar and associates (2001) studied a cohort of 59,248 pregnancies and found a prevalence of 27 percent for postpartum anemia. Although this was strongly correlated with prenatal anemia, it was found in 21 percent of women with normal prenatal hemoglobin levels.

Effects of Anemia on Pregnancy. The etiology of the more common anemias encountered in pregnancy are listed in Table 51–2. The specific cause of anemia is important when evaluating effects on pregnancy outcome. For example,

TABLE 51–1 Hemoglobin Concentrations in 85 Healthy Women with Proven Iron Stores

Hemoglobin (g/dL)	Nonpregnant	Midpregnancy	Late Pregnancy
Mean	13.7	11.5	12.3
Less than 12.0	1%	72%	36%
Less than 11.0	None	29%	6%
Less than 10.0	None	4%	1%
Lowest	11.7	9.7	9.8

From Scott and Pritchard (1967), with permission.

TABLE 51–2 Causes of Anemia During Pregnancy

Acquired
Iron-deficiency anemia
Anemia caused by acute blood loss
Anemia of inflammation or malignancy
Megaloblastic anemia
Acquired hemolytic anemia
Aplastic or hypoplastic anemia

Hereditary
Thalassemias
Sickle-cell hemoglobinopathies
Other hemoglobinopathies
Hereditary hemolytic anemias

maternal and perinatal outcomes are altered markedly in women with sickle-cell anemia.

Most studies of the effects of anemia on pregnancy, such as those discussed in Chapter 8 (see p. 216), describe large populations. These likely deal with nutritional anemias and specifically those due to iron deficiency. Klebanoff and co-workers (1991) studied nearly 27,000 women and found a slightly increased risk of preterm birth with midtrimester anemia. Lieberman and colleagues (1987) found an association with low hematocrit and preterm birth in black women. Anemia may be associated with fetal growth restriction that, according to Barker and associates (1990), may lead to adult cardiovascular disease (see Chap. 38, p. 1028). Kadyrov and co-workers (1998) have provided evidence that maternal anemia influences placental vascularization by altering angiogenesis during early pregnancy.

According to the World Health Organization, anemia contributes to 40 percent of maternal deaths in third world countries (Viteri, 1994). The at-first paradoxical finding was that ironically, healthy women with higher hemoglobin concentrations are also at increased risk for adverse pregnancy outcome. These latter findings may result from the curtailment of normal blood volume expansion of pregnancy. For example, Murphy and colleagues (1986) described over 54,000 singleton pregnancies in the Cardiff Birth Survey and reported excessive perinatal morbidity with *high* maternal hemoglobin concentrations. Scanlon and associates (2000) studied the relationship between maternal hemoglobin levels and preterm or growth-restricted infants in 173,031 pregnancies. Women whose hemoglobin concentration was three standard deviations *below* the mean at 12 weeks had a 1.7-fold risk of preterm birth. Conversely, those women whose levels were three standard deviations *above* the mean at 12 or 18 weeks had 1.3- to 1.8-fold increases in fetal growth restriction.

IRON-DEFICIENCY ANEMIA. The two most common causes of anemia during pregnancy and the puerperium are iron deficiency and acute blood loss. The Centers for Disease Control and Prevention (1989) estimated that about 8 million American women of childbearing age were iron deficient. In a typical singleton gestation, the maternal need for iron averages close to 800 mg—300 mg for the fetus and placenta and 500 mg, if available, for maternal hemoglobin mass expansion. Approximately 200 mg more are shed through the gut, urine, and skin. The total amount (1000 mg) considerably exceeds the iron stores of most women and results in iron-deficiency anemia.

With the rather rapid expansion of blood volume during the second trimester, iron deficiency is often manifested by an appreciable drop in hemoglobin concentration. In the third trimester, additional iron is needed to augment maternal hemoglobin and for transport to the fetus. Because the amount of iron diverted to the fetus is similar in a normal and in an iron-deficient mother, the newborn infant of a severely anemic mother does not suffer from iron-deficiency anemia.

As discussed in Chapter 17 (see p. 431), neonatal iron stores are related to maternal iron status and to cord clamping.

Diagnosis. Classical morphological evidence of iron-deficiency anemia—erythrocyte hypochromia and microcytosis—is less prominent in the pregnant woman compared with that in the nonpregnant woman. Moderate iron-deficiency anemia during pregnancy usually is not accompanied by obvious morphological changes in erythrocytes. Serum ferritin levels, however, are lower than normal, and there is no stainable bone marrow iron. **Iron-deficiency anemia during pregnancy is the consequence primarily of expansion of plasma volume without normal expansion of maternal hemoglobin mass.**

The initial evaluation of a pregnant woman with moderate anemia should include measurements of hemoglobin, hematocrit, and red cell indices; careful examination of a peripheral blood smear; a sickle-cell preparation if the woman is of African origin; and measurement of serum iron, ferritin, or both. Serum ferritin levels normally decline during pregnancy (Goldenberg and colleagues, 1996). Levels less than 15 μg/L confirm iron-deficiency anemia (Centers for Disease Control and Prevention, 1989). Van den Broek and colleagues (1998) found that a cutoff point of 30 μg/L has an 85-percent positive and a 90-percent negative predictive value. Pragmatically, the diagnosis of iron deficiency in moderately anemic pregnant women usually is presumptive and based largely on exclusion.

When pregnant women with moderate iron-deficiency anemia are given adequate iron therapy, a hematological response is detected by an elevated reticulocyte count. The rate of increase of hemoglobin concentration or hematocrit is typically slower than in nonpregnant women due to the differences in blood volumes.

Treatment. Correction of anemia and restitution of iron stores can be accomplished with simple iron compounds—ferrous sulfate, fumarate, or gluconate—that provide about 200 mg daily of *elemental iron*. If the woman cannot or will not take oral iron preparations, then parenteral therapy is given (Andrews, 1999; Hallak and associates, 1997). There are equivalent increases in hemoglobin levels in women given either oral or parenteral iron therapy (Bayouneu and colleagues, 2002; Sharma and co-workers, 2004).

Transfusions of red cells or whole blood seldom are indicated unless hypovolemia from blood loss coexists or an emergency operative procedure must be performed on a *severely* anemic woman. To replenish iron stores, oral therapy should be continued for 3 months after anemia has been corrected.

ANEMIA FROM ACUTE BLOOD LOSS. In early pregnancy, anemia caused by acute blood loss is common in instances of abortion, ectopic pregnancy, and hydatidiform mole. More commonly, anemia from obstetrical hemorrhage is encountered postpartum. Massive hemorrhage demands immediate treatment as described in Chapter 35 (see p. 839). After hypovolemia has been overcome and hemostasis achieved, residual anemia is treated with iron. In a moderately anemic woman (hemoglobin greater than 7 g/dL) who is hemodynamically stable, can ambulate without adverse symptoms, and is not septic, iron therapy is given for at least 3 months.

ANEMIA ASSOCIATED WITH CHRONIC DISEASE.

Weakness, weight loss, and pallor have been recognized since antiquity as characteristics of chronic disease. A wide variety of disorders, such as chronic infections and neoplasms, result in moderate and sometimes severe anemia, usually with slightly hypochromic and microcytic erythrocytes. Chronic renal failure, cancer and chemotherapy, human immunodeficiency virus (HIV) infection, and chronic inflammation are the most common causes.

In nonpregnant patients with chronic inflammatory diseases, the hemoglobin concentration is rarely less than 7 g/dL, bone marrow cellular morphology is not altered, serum iron concentration is decreased, and serum ferritin levels usually are elevated. Thus, although slightly different from each other mechanistically, these anemias share similar features that include varying degrees and combinations of alterations in reticuloendothelial function, iron metabolism, and decreased erythropoiesis (Andrews, 1999).

During pregnancy, a number of chronic diseases may cause anemia, including chronic renal disease, suppuration, inflammatory bowel disease, systemic lupus erythematosus, granulomatous infections, malignant neoplasms, and rheumatoid arthritis. Chronic anemia is typically intensified as plasma volume expands out of proportion to red cell mass expansion.

Chronic Renal Disease. Any type of chronic renal insufficiency can be accompanied by anemia, usually due to erythropoietin deficiency with an element of anemia of chronic disease. During pregnancy, the degree of red cell mass expansion is inversely related to renal impairment. However, total blood volume expansion usually is normal and anemia is intensified (Cunningham and associates, 1990).

Pyelonephritis. Women who have acute *pyelonephritis* with sepsis syndrome often develop overt anemia. This is caused by acute red cell destruction from endotoxin-mediated sepsis, but with normal erythropoietin production (Cavenee and colleagues, 1994).

Treatment. Treatment with *recombinant erythropoietin* has been used successfully to treat anemia of chronic renal insufficiency, chronic inflammation, and malignancy (Goodnough and associates, 1997). Reports of its use during pregnancy are limited (Braga and colleagues, 1996; Vora and Gruslin, 1998). One worrisome side effect is hypertension, which is already prevalent in women with renal disease. In the study by

Braga and co-workers (1996), one of the five treated pregnant women developed a placental abruption associated with hypertension. In addition, Casadevall and colleagues (2002) reported pure red cell aplasia and anti-erythropoietin antibodies in 13 nonpregnant patients given erythropoietin.

MEGALOBLASTIC ANEMIA.

These anemias are characterized by blood and bone marrow abnormalities from impaired DNA synthesis. Worldwide, the prevalence of megaloblastic anemia during pregnancy varies considerably, and in the United States, it is rare.

Folic Acid Deficiency. In the United States, megaloblastic anemia beginning during pregnancy almost always results from folic acid deficiency. In the past, this condition was referred to as *pernicious anemia of pregnancy*. It usually is found in women who do not consume fresh green leafy vegetables, legumes, or animal protein. As folate deficiency and anemia worsen, anorexia often becomes intense, further aggravating the dietary deficiency. In some instances, excessive ethanol ingestion either is the cause or contributes to folate deficiency.

In nonpregnant women, folic acid requirement is 50 to 100 μg/day. During pregnancy, requirements are increased, and 400 μg/day are recommended (see Chap. 8, p. 218). The earliest biochemical evidence is low plasma folic acid concentrations. The earliest morphological evidence usually is hypersegmentation of neutrophils, and newly formed erythrocytes are macrocytic. With preexisting iron deficiency, macrocytic erythrocytes cannot be detected by measurement of the mean corpuscular volume. Careful examination of a smear of peripheral blood, however, usually demonstrates some macrocytes. As the anemia becomes more intense, peripheral nucleated erythrocytes appear. At the same time, examination of the bone marrow discloses megaloblastic erythropoiesis. Anemia may then become severe, and thrombocytopenia, leukopenia, or both may develop. The fetus and placenta extract folate from maternal circulation so effectively that the fetus is not anemic despite severe maternal anemia. There have been instances in which newborn hemoglobin levels were 18 g/dL or more, whereas maternal values were as low as 3.6 g/dL (Pritchard and Scott, 1970).

TREATMENT. The treatment of pregnancy-induced megaloblastic anemia should include folic acid, a nutritious diet, and iron. As little as 1 mg of folic acid administered orally once daily produces a striking hematological response. By 4 to 7 days after beginning treatment, the reticulocyte count is increased, and leukopenia and thrombocytopenia are corrected.

PREVENTION. A diet sufficient in folic acid prevents megaloblastic anemia. A great deal of attention has been devoted to the role of folate deficiency in the genesis of neural-tube defects (see Chap. 8, p. 218; see Chap. 12, p. 302). The

Centers for Disease Control and Prevention (1992) and the American College of Obstetricians and Gynecologists (1996) recommended that all women of childbearing age consume at least 0.4 mg of folic acid daily. Additional folic acid is given in circumstances in which folate requirements are increased, such as in multifetal pregnancy, hemolytic anemia, Crohn disease, alcoholism, and inflammatory skin disorders. There is evidence that women who previously have had infants with neural-tube defects have a lower recurrence rate if daily 4-mg folic acid is given prior to and throughout early pregnancy.

Vitamin B₁₂ Deficiency. Megaloblastic anemia caused by lack of vitamin B_{12}, that is, cyanocobalamin, during pregnancy is exceedingly rare. In *Addisonian pernicious anemia,* a lack of intrinsic factor results in failure to absorb vitamin B_{12}. It is an extremely uncommon autoimmune disease in women of reproductive age and typically has its onset in women older than 40 years. Unless treated with vitamin B_{12}, infertility may be a complication. In our limited experience, vitamin B_{12} deficiency in pregnant women is more likely encountered following partial or total gastric resection. Other causes are Crohn disease, ileal resection, and bacterial overgrowth in the small bowel.

During pregnancy, vitamin B_{12} levels are lower than nonpregnant values because of decreased serum concentrations of carrier proteins, the *transcobalamins* (Zamorano and colleagues, 1985). Women who have had a total gastrectomy require 1000 μg of vitamin B_{12} intramuscularly at monthly intervals. Those with a partial gastrectomy usually do not need such therapy, but vitamin B_{12} levels during pregnancy should be measured.

ACQUIRED HEMOLYTIC ANEMIAS

Autoimmune Hemolytic Anemia. This is an uncommon condition, and the cause of aberrant antibody production is unknown. Typically both the direct and indirect antiglobulin (Coombs) tests are positive. Anemias caused by these factors may be due to warm-active autoantibodies (80 to 90 percent), cold-active antibodies, or a combination. These syndromes also may be classified as primary (idiopathic) or secondary due to underlying diseases or other factors. Examples of the latter include lymphomas and leukemias, connective tissue diseases, infections, chronic inflammatory diseases, or drug-induced (Provan and Weatherall, 2000). *Cold-agglutinin disease* may be induced by *Mycoplasma pneumoniae* or infectious mononucleosis.

Hemolysis and positive antiglobulin tests may be the consequence of either IgM or IgG anti-erythrocyte antibodies. Spherocytosis and reticulocytosis are characteristic of the peripheral blood smear. IgM antibodies do not cross the placenta, and thus fetal red cells are not affected.

There may be marked acceleration of hemolysis during pregnancy. Glucocorticoids usually are effective, and

treatment is with prednisone, 1 mg/kg per day, or its equivalent. Coincidental thrombocytopenia usually is corrected by therapy. Transfusion of red cells is complicated by the presence of circulating anti-erythrocyte antibodies. Warming the donor cells to body temperature decreases their destruction by cold agglutinins.

Drug-Induced Hemolytic Anemia. This must be differentiated from other forms of autoimmune hemolytic anemia. Hemolysis typically is mild, resolves on withdrawing the drug, and can be prevented by avoidance of the drug. Mechanisms of action generally are through drug-mediated immunological injury to red cells. The drug may act as a high-affinity hapten with a red cell protein to which antidrug antibodies attach (e.g., IgM antipenicillin or anticephalosporin antibodies). Other drugs become low-affinity haptens and adhere to cell membrane proteins. Examples include probenecid, quinidine, rifampin, and thiopental. In other cases, the mechanism of antibody induction is unknown.

The severity of symptoms depends on the degree of hemolysis. Usually there is mild to moderate chronic hemolysis, but some drugs that act as low-affinity haptens may precipitate severe acute hemolysis. Garratty and associates (1999) described seven cases of severe direct Coombs-positive hemolytic anemia caused by cefotetan prophylaxis for obstetrical procedures. In most cases, withdrawing the offending drug results in reversal of symptoms. Corticosteroids are of questionable efficacy. Drug-induced hemolysis is much more often related to a congenital erythrocyte enzymatic defect, such as *glucose-6-phosphate dehydrogenase (G6PD) deficiency,* especially in African-American women (see p. 1149).

Pregnancy-Induced Hemolytic Anemia. Unexplained hemolytic anemia during pregnancy is a rare but distinct entity in which severe hemolysis develops early in pregnancy and resolves within months after delivery. There is no evidence of an immune mechanism or for any intraerythrocytic or extraerythrocytic defects (Starksen and associates, 1983). Because the fetus-infant also may demonstrate transient hemolysis, an immunological cause is suspected. Maternal corticosteroid treatment usually is effective. We have observed one woman with recurrent hemolysis during several pregnancies, and in each instance, intense severe hemolytic anemia was controlled by prednisone given until delivery.

Paroxysmal Nocturnal Hemoglobinuria. Although commonly regarded as a hemolytic anemia, this hemopoietic stem cell disorder is characterized by formation of defective platelets, granulocytes, and erythrocytes. Paroxysmal nocturnal hemoglobinuria is acquired and arises from one abnormal clone of cells, much like a neoplasm (Packham, 1998). One mutated X-linked gene responsible for this condition is termed *PIG-A* because it codes for phosphatidylinositol glycan protein A. Resultant abnormal anchor proteins of the erythrocyte and granulocyte membrane make them unusually susceptible to lysis by complement (Provan and Weatherall, 2000).

This is an acquired chronic hemolytic anemia with insidious onset. The severity ranges from mild to lethal. Hemoglobinuria develops at irregular intervals and is not necessarily nocturnal. Hemolysis may be initiated by transfusions, infections, or surgery. Almost 40 percent of patients suffer venous thromboses, as well as renal dysfunction, hypertension, and Budd-Chiari syndrome. Median survival after diagnosis is 10 years, but spontaneous long-term remission occurs in 15 percent of cases (Hillmen and colleagues, 1995). Hillmen and associates (2004) reported decreased hemolysis from treatment with eculizumab, an antibody that inhibits complement activation. Bone marrow transplantation is the definitive treatment.

EFFECTS ON PREGNANCY. Paroxysmal nocturnal hemoglobinuria is a serious and unpredictable disease and pregnancy may be dangerous. Greene and colleagues (1983) reviewed 31 cases in pregnancy and found that complications developed in over 75 percent. Maternal mortality was 10 percent, and postpartum venous thrombosis occurred in almost 50 percent of the women. Solal-Céligny and co-workers (1988) reported eight pregnancies with only four surviving infants. In a multicenter study, De Gramont and colleagues (1987) reported complications in two thirds of 38 pregnancies. Although there were no maternal deaths, there was life-threatening hemolysis and hemorrhage.

Other Acquired Anemias. Fragmentation (microangiopathic) hemolysis with visible hemoglobinemia is seen with severe preeclampsia and eclampsia (Pritchard and associates, 1976). Mild degrees are likely present in most cases of severe disease and may be referred to as *HELLP syndrome—h*emolysis, *e*levated *l*iver enzymes, and *l*ow *p*latelets (see Chap. 34, p. 773). The most fulminant acquired hemolytic anemia encountered during pregnancy is caused by the exotoxin of *Clostridium perfringens* (see Chap. 42, p. 994) or by group A β-hemolytic streptococcus (see Chap. 31, p. 721). Gram-negative bacterial endotoxin, that is, lipopolysaccharide, especially with severe pyelonephritis, may be accompanied by hemolysis and mild to moderate anemia (Cox and colleagues, 1991).

HEMOLYTIC ANEMIAS CAUSED BY INHERITED ERYTHROCYTE DEFECTS.

The normal erythrocyte is shaped like a biconcave disc, and there is a redundancy of membrane surface area relative to volume. This allows numerous cycles of reversible deformations as the erythrocyte withstands shearing forces within arteries and negotiates through splenic slits half the width of its cross-sectional diameter. Several inherited red cell membrane defects or enzyme deficiencies result in destabilization of the membrane

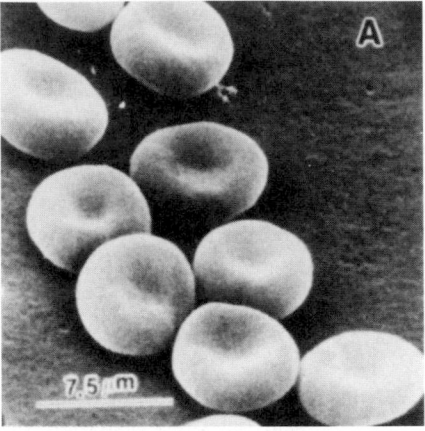

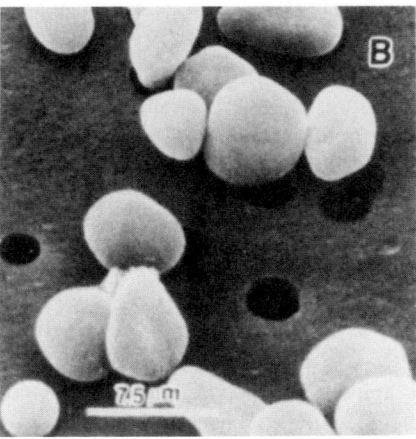

FIGURE 51–2. Scanning electron micrograph showing **(A)** normal-appearing erythrocytes from a heterozygous carrier of recessive spherocytosis, and **(B)** her daughter, a homozygote with severe anemia. (From Agre, 1989, with permission.)

lipid bilayer. The loss of lipids from the erythrocyte membrane causes a surface area deficiency and poorly deformable cells that undergo hemolysis (Fig. 51–2). There are varying degrees of anemia. Examples of these inherited membrane defects that cause accelerated destruction are *hereditary spherocytosis, pyropoikilocytosis*, and *ovalocytosis*.

Hereditary Spherocytosis. Several inherited molecular deficits in erythrocyte membrane proteins give rise to the syndrome of hereditary spherocytosis. Although most are due to an autosomally dominant, variably penetrant *spectrin* deficiency. Others are autosomally recessive or de novo gene mutations and may be caused by deficiency of *ankyrin, protein 4.2, moderate band 3,* or combinations thereof (Bunn and Rosse, 2001, Yawata and colleagues, 2000). These disorders are characterized by varying degrees of anemia and jaundice as the consequence of hemolysis. Confirmation of the diagnosis is by documentation of spherocytes on peripheral smear, reticulocytosis, and increased osmotic fragility.

Hemolysis with corresponding anemia is dependent on an intact spleen, which is usually enlarged. Splenectomy, although not correcting the membrane defect, does greatly reduce hemolysis, anemia, and jaundice. So-called *crisis*, characterized by severe anemia from accelerated red cell destruction or more likely failure of production, or both, may develop in the woman with a functioning spleen. Infection must be detected and vigorously treated. In some cases, red cell hypoplasia develops concomitantly with B19 parvovirus infection (see Chap. 58, p. 1279).

PREGNANCY. In general, women with hereditary spherocytosis do well during pregnancy. Folic acid supplementation is recommended. Maberry and associates (1992) reported the Parkland Hospital experience with 50 pregnancies in 23 women with spherocytosis. In late pregnancy, the mean hematocrit was 31 percent (range 23 to 41) and reticulocyte counts ranged from 1 to 23 percent. There were eight abortions, and four of 42 infants were born preterm, but none were growth restricted. Infection in four women intensified hemolysis, and three required transfusions. Similar results were reported by Pajor and colleagues (1993) in 19 pregnancies in eight women. The newborn who has inherited hereditary spherocytosis may have hyperbilirubinemia and anemia. We observed the hemoglobin level to fall to as low as 5.0 g/dL by 5 weeks of age in one infant.

Red Cell Enzyme Deficiencies. A deficiency of erythrocyte enzymes used for anaerobic glucose utilization may cause *hereditary nonspherocytic anemia*. Most cases are inherited as autosomal recessive traits. *G6PD deficiency*, by far the most common, a well-known exception, is X-linked. There are more than 400 variants of G6PD, predominantly due to a base substitution leading to an amino acid replacement and a broad range of clinical severity (Beutler, 1991). In the A (homozygous) variant, both X chromosomes are affected, and erythrocytes are markedly deficient in normal enzyme activity. This condition is inherited by about 2 percent of African-American women. In the heterozygous variant, only one X chromosome is deficient. This condition occurs in 10 to 15 percent of African-American women and may confer some degree of protection against malaria (Mockenhaupt and colleagues, 2003). Random X-chromosome inactivation, or *lyonization,* results in a variable deficiency of enzyme activity. Infections or drugs may induce hemolysis in both heterozygous as well as homozygous women. Anemia is usually episodic, although some variants induce chronic nonspherocytic hemolysis. Because young erythrocytes contain more enzyme activity than older erythrocytes, in the absence of bone marrow depression, anemia ultimately stabilizes and is corrected soon after the drug is discontinued.

Pyruvate kinase deficiency, although uncommon, is probably the next most common enzyme deficiency. It is inherited as an autosomal recessive trait. Due to recurrent transfusions in homozygous carriers, iron overload is common, and associated myocardial dysfunction should be monitored (Dolan and colleagues, 2002). Conservative management without

transfusions can usually be accomplished (Ghidini and Korker, 1998). Recurrent hydrops fetalis due to homozygously affected fetuses has been described, and fetal anemia and pyruvate kinase deficiency were confirmed using funipuncture (Gilsanz and colleagues, 1993).

Other very rare enzyme abnormalities may cause hemolysis. Although the degree of chronic hemolysis varies, most episodes of severe anemia with enzyme deficiencies are induced by drugs or infections. During pregnancy, iron and folic acid are given, oxidant drugs are avoided, and bacterial infections are treated promptly.

APLASTIC AND HYPOPLASTIC ANEMIA. Although rarely encountered during pregnancy, aplastic anemia is a grave complication. The diagnosis includes anemia, usually with thrombocytopenia, leukopenia, and markedly hypocellular bone marrow (Marsh and colleagues, 1999). The etiology can be identified in about a third of cases, and these are due to drugs and other chemicals, infection, irradiation, leukemia, immunological disorders, or inherited conditions such as *Fanconi anemia* and *Diamond–Blackfan syndrome* (Provan and Weatherall, 2000). The functional defect appears to be a marked decrease in committed marrow stem cells. The condition is likely immunologically mediated (Young and Maciejewski, 1997).

With immunosuppressive therapy and bone marrow transplantation, the 5-year survival rate is 75 percent. About half of patients have a good response and long-term survival when treated with antithymocyte globulin and cyclosporine (Marsh and associates, 1999; Rosenfeld and colleagues, 2003). Immunosuppressive therapy is also given for some months after transplantation. Previous blood transfusions, and even pregnancy, enhance the risk of graft rejection. This is the most common serious complication and causes two thirds of deaths within the first 2 years (Socié and co-workers, 1999).

Aplastic Anemia During Pregnancy. In most cases, aplastic anemia and pregnancy simultaneously occur by chance. It has been postulated that pregnancy induces erythroid hypoplasia (Aitchison and colleagues, 1989). Certainly, in a few women, hypoplastic anemia has been identified first during a pregnancy and then improved or even resolved when the pregnancy terminated, only to recur with a subsequent pregnancy (Bourantas and associates, 1997; Snyder and colleagues, 1991).

Rijhsinghani and Wiechert (1994) described two pregnancies in a woman with *Diamond–Blackfan anemia.* This rare form of pure red cell aplasia may be inherited in an autosomal recessive pattern. Some patients respond to glucocorticoid therapy, but most are transfusion-dependent. *Gaucher disease* is an autosomally recessive lysosomal enzyme deficiency that has multisystem involvement. When these women are pregnant, anemia and thrombocytopenia become worse (Granovsky-Grisaru and associates, 1995). In another report, *alglucerase* enzyme replacement improved pregnancy outcomes in six affected women (Elstein and colleagues, 1997).

The major risks to the pregnant woman with aplastic anemia are hemorrhage and infection (Ascarelli and co-workers, 1998). In cases reported since 1960, mortality during or after pregnancy has been 50 percent, and almost invariably, this is due to bleeding or sepsis. *Fanconi anemia* appears to be associated with a better prognosis (Alter and colleagues, 1991).

Management depends on gestational age, severity of disease, and whether treatment has been given. Supportive care includes continuous infection surveillance and prompt antimicrobial therapy. Granulocyte transfusions are given only during infections. Red cell transfusions are given for symptomatic anemia, and routinely to maintain the hematocrit at about 20. Platelet transfusions may be needed to control hemorrhage. Even when thrombocytopenia is intense, the risk of severe hemorrhage can be minimized using vaginal delivery.

There have been several case reports of successful pregnancies in women with bone marrow transplantation (Borgna-Pignatti and associates, 1996; Eliyahu and Shalev, 1994). We have followed two women with prior transplantation, and both demonstrated a normal pregnancy-induced hematological response, including red cell and plasma volume expansion. Sanders and colleagues (1996) reviewed outcomes in 41 women with 72 pregnancies following bone marrow transplantation. Excluding spontaneous and induced abortions, 52 resulted in liveborn infants, however, almost half of these pregnancies were complicated by preterm delivery or hypertension.

HEMOGLOBINOPATHIES

SICKLE-CELL HEMOGLOBINOPATHIES. Sickle hemoglobin (hemoglobin S) results from a single β-chain substitution of glutamic acid by valine because of an A for T substitution at codon 6 of the β-globin gene. Sickle-cell anemia (SS disease), sickle cell–hemoglobin C disease (SC disease), and sickle cell–β-thalassemia disease (S–β-thalassemia disease) are the most common sickle hemoglobinopathies and are associated with increased maternal and perinatal morbidity and mortality.

Pathophysiology. Red cells with hemoglobin S undergo sickling when deoxygenated and the hemoglobin aggregates. Constant sickling and de-sickling cause membrane damage, and the cell may become irreversibly sickled. Clinically, the hallmark of sickling episodes are periods during which there is ischemia and infarction in various organs. These produce clinical symptoms, predominately pain, which is often severe, and are called *sickle-cell crises*. There may be aplastic, megaloblastic, sequestration, and hemolytic crises.

Chronic and acute changes from sickling include bony abnormalities such as osteonecrosis of femoral and humeral heads; renal medullary damage; autosplenectomy in homozygous SS patients and splenomegaly in other variants; hepatomegaly; ventricular hypertrophy; pulmonary infarctions; pulmonary hypertension; cerebrovascular accidents; leg ulcers; and a propensity to infection and sepsis (Driscoll and colleagues, 2003; Gladwin and associates, 2004; Serjeant, 1997; Weatherall and Provan, 2000). The median age at death for women is 48 years.

Inheritance of Sickling Syndromes. The inheritance of the gene for S hemoglobin from each parent results in sickle-cell anemia. In the United States, 1 of 12 African-Americans has the sickle-cell trait, which results from inheritance of one gene for hemoglobin S and one for normal hemoglobin A. The computed incidence of sickle-cell anemia among African Americans is 1 in 576 ($1/12 \times 1/12 \times 1/4 = 576$), but the disease is less common during pregnancy because of earlier mortality, especially during early childhood.

About 1 in 40 African Americans has the gene for hemoglobin C. The theoretical incidence for co-inheritance of the gene for hemoglobin S and an allelic gene for hemoglobin C in an African-American child is about 1 in 2000 ($1/12 \times 1/40 \times 1/4$). Similarly, because the incidence of β-thalassemia minor is about 1 in 40 to 50, S–β-thalassemia occurs about 1 in 2000 ($1/12 \times 1/40 \times 1/4$).

Pregnancy and Sickle-Cell Syndrome. Pregnancy is a serious burden to women with any of the three major sickle hemoglobinopathies, especially hemoglobin SS disease. Ischemic necrosis of multiple organs, especially bone marrow, causes severe pain which usually becomes more frequent in pregnancy. Infections and pulmonary complications are common. Powars and colleagues (1986) compared maternal and perinatal outcomes from before and after 1972 and found that maternal mortality decreased from 6 to 1 percent. Poddar and colleagues (1986) reported a maternal mortality rate of 1.1 percent in 644 pregnancies complicated by hemoglobin SS disease. In addition to horrifically excessive maternal mortality, more than a third of pregnancies in women with sickle syndromes end in abortion, stillbirth, or neonatal death.

HEMOGLOBIN SC. In nonpregnant women, morbidity and mortality from SC disease are appreciably lower than from sickle-cell anemia. Indeed, fewer than half of women with SC disease have ever been symptomatic prior to pregnancy. During pregnancy and the puerperium, however, attacks of severe bone pain and episodes of pulmonary infarction and embolization become more common (Cunningham and associates, 1983). A particularly worrisome pulmonary complication is the *acute chest syndrome* discussed subsequently. In an 18-year prospective observational study from Parkland Hospital, the maternal mortality rate for women with hemoglobin SC disease was close to 2 percent (Pritchard

TABLE 51–3 Pregnancy Outcomes Reported Since 1956 for Women with Sickle-Cell Anemia and Hemoglobin SC Disease

	Sickle-Cell (SS) Disease	Hemoglobin SC Disease
Women	1213	351
Pregnancies	2214	798
Maternal deaths (per 100,000)	~2500	~2300
Perinatal mortality (per 1000)	~175	~75

Data from Carache (1980); El-Shafei (1992); Howard (1995); Milner (1980); Morris (1994); Poddar (1986); Powars (1986); Seoud (1994); Smith (1996); Sun (2001), and all their colleagues.

and co-workers, 1973). As shown in Table 51–3, maternal deaths with hemoglobin SC disease were as common as with SS disease. The perinatal mortality rate is somewhat greater than that of the general population but nowhere as great as with sickle-cell anemia.

Management During Pregnancy. Adequate management of pregnant women with sickle-cell hemoglobinopathies necessitates close observation. These women maintain hemoglobin mass by intense hemopoiesis to compensate for the markedly shortened erythrocyte life span. Thus, any factor that impairs erythropoiesis or increases red cell destruction, or both, aggravates the anemia. The folic acid requirements during pregnancy are considerable and supplementary folic acid is given.

One rather common danger is that the symptomatic woman may categorically be considered to be suffering from a sickle-cell crisis. As a result, serious obstetrical or medical problems that cause pain, anemia, or both, may be overlooked. Some examples are ectopic pregnancy, placental abruption, pyelonephritis, or appendicitis. **The term "sickle-cell crisis" should be applied only after all other possible causes of pain or fever or worsening anemia have been excluded.**

Pain is from intense sequestration of sickled erythrocytes with infarction in various organs. These episodes may develop acutely, especially late in pregnancy, during labor and delivery, and early in the puerperium. Acute infarction is usually accompanied by severe pain, and because the bone marrow is frequently involved, intense bone pain is common. A system for care of these women has been appropriately stressed by Rees and colleagues (2003). Intravenous hydration is given, along with opioids administered promptly for severe pain. Oxygen given via nasal cannula may decrease the intensity of sickling at the capillary level. We have found that red cell transfusions after the onset of severe pain do not dramatically improve the intensity of the pain and may not shorten its duration. Conversely, as discussed later, prophylactic transfusions almost always prevent vaso-occlusive episodes.

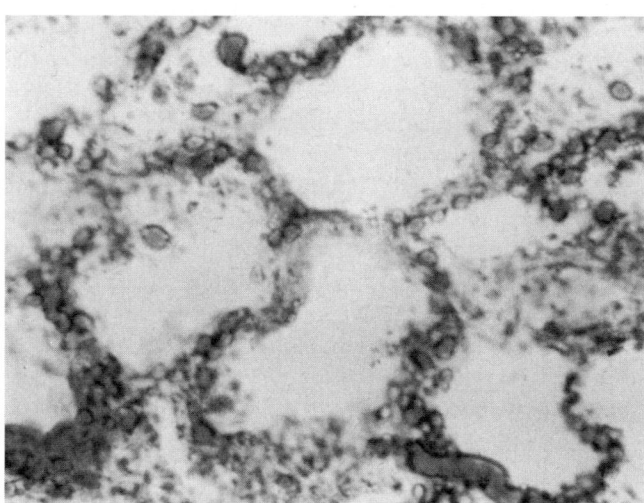

FIGURE 51–3. Photomicrograph of a section of lung from a 21-year-old primipara with hemoglobin SC who died 36 hours postpartum after developing acute dyspnea. There was massive amounts of fat and bone marrow embolized to both lungs. (From Maberry and Cunningham, 1993.)

Covert bacteriuria and acute pyelonephritis are increased substantively, and screening and treatment for bacteriuria is essential. If pyelonephritis develops, sickle cells are extremely susceptible to endotoxin, which can cause dramatic and rapid red cell destruction while simultaneously suppressing erythropoiesis. Pneumonia, especially due to *Streptococcus pneumoniae,* is common. The Advisory Committee on Immunization Practices (1997) recommends polyvalent pneumococcal vaccine for these women. Influenza vaccine should be given annually. In addition, vaccination against *Haemophilus influenzae* type B is recommended for asplenic patients.

As many as 40 percent of patients suffer from *acute chest syndrome,* which is characterized by pleuritic chest pain, fever, cough, lung infiltrates, and hypoxia (Vichinsky and colleagues, 2000). The spectrum of pathology includes infection, infarction, pulmonary sequestration, and fat embolization from bone marrow (Fig. 51–3). Recurrent episodes may lead to restrictive chronic lung disease associated with arteriolar vasculopathy (Powars and co-workers, 1988). Pregnant women with sickle-cell anemia usually have some degree of *cardiac dysfunction* from ventricular hypertrophy. There is increased preload and decreased afterload with a normal ejection fraction and a high cardiac output. Chronic hypertension worsens this (Gandhi and colleagues, 2000). During pregnancy, the basal hemodynamic state characterized by high cardiac output and increased blood volume is augmented (Veille and Hanson, 1994). Although most women tolerate pregnancy without problems, complications such as severe preeclampsia or serious infections may result in ventricular failure (Cunningham and associates, 1986). With heart failure in these patients, pulmonary hypertension must be considered (Castro and associates, 2003; Stuart and Nagel, 2004).

Assessment of Fetal Health. Because of the high incidence of fetal growth restriction and perinatal mortality, serial fetal assessment is necessary. The American College of Obstetricians and Gynecologists (1999) recommends weekly antepartum fetal surveillance beginning at 32 to 34 weeks with serial ultrasonography to monitor fetal growth and amnionic fluid. Anyaegbunam and colleagues (1991) evaluated fetal well-being during 39 sickling crises in 24 women. Almost 60 percent had nonreactive stress tests, which became reactive with crisis resolution, and all had an increased uterine artery systolic–diastolic (S/D) ratio. At the same time, they found no changes in the umbilical artery S/D ratios. They concluded that transient effects of sickle-cell crisis do not compromise umbilical and hence fetal blood flow. At Parkland Hospital, we serially assess these women with ultrasound for fetal growth and amnionic fluid volume. Nonstress or contraction stress tests are not done routinely unless complications develop or fetal movement is reported to be diminished.

Labor and Delivery. Management is essentially identical to that for women with cardiac disease (see Chap. 44, p. 1021). Women should be kept comfortable but not oversedated. Epidural analgesia is ideal. Compatible blood should be available. If a difficult vaginal or cesarean delivery is contemplated, and the hematocrit is less than 20 percent, packed erythrocyte transfusions are administered. Care must be taken to prevent circulatory overload and pulmonary edema from ventricular failure.

Prophylactic Red Cell Transfusions. These have been shown to decrease morbidity in sickle-cell syndromes when given perioperatively and during pregnancy or to prevent strokes in high-risk children (Adams and co-workers, 1998). The use of routine prophylactic transfusions during pregnancy remains controversial (American College of Obstetricians and Gynecologists, 2000a). Their most dramatic impact has been on maternal morbidity. In a 10-year study at Parkland Hospital, we offered prophylactic transfusions to all pregnant women with sickle-cell syndromes. Red cell transfusions were given throughout pregnancy to maintain the hematocrit greater than 25 percent and hemoglobin S no greater than 60 percent (Cunningham and Pritchard, 1979). There was minimal maternal morbidity such as pain, fever, and suppression of erythropoiesis. In a later study, these women were compared with historical controls not given blood, and there was a significant reduction in maternal morbidity and hospitalizations (Cunningham and associates, 1983). A comparative study by Howard and colleagues (1995) produced similar data.

In a multicenter trial, Koshy and colleagues (1988) randomized 72 pregnant women with sickle-cell disease to prophylactic or indicated transfusions. They reported a significant decrease in the incidence of painful sickle-cell crises with prophylactic transfusions but no differences in perinatal outcomes. Because of risks inherent with blood administration, they concluded that prophylactic transfusions were not necessary.

Current consensus is that management should be individualized. Some clinicians choose prophylactic transfusions in women with a history of multiple vaso-occlusive episodes and poor obstetrical outcomes (Castro and colleagues, 2003).

Complications. Morbidity from multiple transfusions is significant. Delayed hemolytic transfusion reactions occur in as many as 10 percent of patients (Garratty, 1997). Hepatitis is a major concern. At Parkland Hospital, the incidence of red cell isoimmunization was 3 percent per unit of blood transfused (Cox and associates, 1988). In 12 studies reviewed by Garratty (1997), a mean of 25 percent of chronically transfused sickle-cell patients had become isoimmunized. Although the specter of iron overload and transfusion hemochromatosis is worrisome, we found no evidence for this or for chronic hepatitis in liver biopsies from 40 women transfused during pregnancy (Yeomans and co-workers, 1990).

Other Therapy. There are several therapeutic schemes for sickle-cell patients, some of which are still experimental (Stuart and Nagel, 2004). Recently, Raff and colleagues (2002) reported that if compatible blood is not available because of red cell alloantibodies, a polymerized human hemoglobin solution in combination with erythropoietin may be considered for a sickling crisis. With erythropoietin, however, increasing hemoglobin S may be potentially harmful. Hemoglobin F induction has been studied for sickling and thalassemia syndromes. Some drugs stimulate gamma-chain synthesis and thus hemoglobin F, which inhibits polymerization of hemoglobin S and resultant sickling. Regimens of *hydroxyurea* along with either *5-azacytidine* or *recombinant erythropoietin* increase fetal hemoglobin production with fewer clinical sickling episodes (Schechter and Rodgers, 1995). Hydroxyurea also reduces sickle erythrocyte adherence to endothelium (Steinberg, 1999). In a follow-up study of patients in a randomized trial of hydroxyurea from 1992 to 1995, Steinberg and colleagues (2003) found that hydroxyurea reduced mortality. Experience with hydroxyurea in pregnancy is limited, but it is teratogenic in animals (Briggs and colleagues, 1998). Another cancer drug, *decitabine*, has been used in patients who are unresponsive to hydroxyurea (DeSimone and colleagues, 2002). Findings from a placebo-controlled trial of inhaled nitric oxide versus placebo suggested benefit for acute vaso-occlusive crises (Weiner and colleagues, 2003).

Bone marrow transplantation, as discussed on page 1149, has been used to provide normal hemoglobin A erythrocyte precursors (Walters and associates, 1996). According to Steinberg (1999), about 100 patients with sickle-cell anemia—mostly children—have undergone transplantation. Mortality is about 10 percent. Of 26 patients with at least 2-year follow-up, 22 had a stable donor engraftment and resolution of complications (Walters and colleagues, 2000). Pilot data from matched unrelated bone marrow transplantation indicates a 70-percent success rate with a 20-percent mortality rate (Vichinsky, 2002) Prenatal diagnosis of sickle-cell disease may allow for in utero *stem cell therapy* with hemoglobin A cells (Eddleman, 1998; Shaaban and Flake, 1999).

Experimental projects include a gene therapy technique using a modified β-globin gene that encodes a sickling resistant protein, which corrected the globin chain in transgenic hemoglobin SS "knock-out" mice (Pawliuk and colleagues, 2001). Orringer and colleagues (2001) reported preliminary success using purified poloxamer 188 (PP188) in nonpregnant sickle patients. This copolymer surfactant with antithrombotic properties improves microvascular blood flow by reducing blood viscosity and reducing adhesive frictional forces.

Contraception and Sterilization. Because of chronic debility, complications caused by pregnancy, and the predictably shortened life span of women with sickle-cell anemia, contraception and possibly sterilization are important considerations. According to the American College of Obstetricians and Gynecologists (2000b), estrogen–progesterone oral contraceptives have not been assessed well in women with sickle hemoglobinopathies. Many clinicians do not recommend their use because of potential adverse vascular and thrombotic effects (see Chap. 32, p. 732).

Progesterone has been long known to prevent painful sickle-cell crises. Because of this, low-dose oral progesterone, progesterone injections, or implants seem ideal. In one study, de Abood and associates (1997) reported significantly fewer and less intense pain crises in women given depot medroxyprogesterone intramuscularly. Intrauterine devices probably should not be used routinely because of increased risk of infection. The safest contraceptives are unfortunately those with the highest failure rates—condoms with foam and diaphragms. Permanent sterilization is also an option (see Chap. 33, p. 751).

Sickle-Cell Trait. The heterozygous inheritance of the gene for hemoglobin S results in sickle-cell trait, or AS hemoglobin. The amount of S hemoglobin averages only about 30 percent. The frequency of sickle-cell trait among African-Americans is about 8 percent. The trait is not associated with increased abortion, perinatal mortality, low birthweight, or pregnancy-induced hypertension (Pritchard and associates, 1973; Tuck and co-workers, 1983). One unquestioned complication, however, is the twofold increased incidence of asymptomatic bacteriuria and urinary infection. **Sickle-cell trait therefore should not be considered a deterrent to pregnancy on the basis of increased maternal risks.**

Inheritance is a concern for the infant of a mother with sickle trait whenever the father carries a gene for some abnormal hemoglobins (S, C, D) or for β-thalassemia. Prenatal diagnosis through amniocentesis or chorionic villus sampling is now available (see Chap. 12, p. 328). Xu and colleagues

TABLE 51–4 Outcomes in 72 Pregnancies Complicated by Hemoglobin CC and C-β-Thalassemia

	Hemoglobin CC	C-β-thalassemia
Women	15	5
Pregnancies	49	23
Hematocrit (range)	27 (21–23)	30 (28–33)
Birthweight (g)		
Mean	2990	2960
Range	1145–4770	2320–3980
Perinatal deaths	1	2
Surviving infants	42	20

Data from Maberry and colleagues (1990).

(1999) described single-blastomere DNA analysis, successful in vitro fertilization, and delivery of an unaffected neonate to parents both carrying sickle-cell trait.

OTHER HEMOGLOBINOPATHIES

Hemoglobin C and C–β-Thalassemia. The single β-chain substitution of glutamic acid by lysine at position 6 results in production of hemoglobin C. It is quite common in West Africa, but only about 2 percent of African-Americans have hemoglobin C trait, which does not cause anemia or adverse pregnancy outcomes. When co-inherited with sickle-cell trait, hemoglobin SC causes the problems previously discussed on page 1150.

Pregnancy and homozygous hemoglobin C or hemoglobin C–β-thalassemia are relatively benign associations. Maberry and colleagues (1990) reported our experiences from Parkland Hospital as shown in Table 51–4. Other than mild to moderate anemia, pregnancy outcomes were not different compared with that of the general obstetrical population. When severe anemia is identified, iron or folic acid deficiency or some other superimposed cause should be suspected. Supplementation with folic acid and iron is indicated.

Hemoglobin E. This is the second most common hemoglobin variant worldwide. Hemoglobin E results from a single β-chain substitution of lysine for glutamic acid at codon 26. The hemoglobin is susceptible particularly to oxidative stress. The heterozygous E trait is common in Southeast Asia. Hurst and co-workers (1983) identified homozygous hemoglobin E, hemoglobin E plus β-thalassemia, or hemoglobin E trait in 36 percent of Cambodians and 25 percent of Laotians. In addition, α- and β-thalassemia traits were prevalent in all groups.

Homozygous hemoglobin EE is associated with little or no anemia, hypochromia, marked microcytosis, and erythrocyte targeting. In our limited experience, pregnant women do not appear to be at increased risk. Iron-deficiency anemia as the consequence of intestinal parasites, repeated pregnancies, or both may co-exist. Conversely, doubly heterozygous *hemoglobin E–β-thalassemia* is a common cause of childhood anemia in Southeast Asia (Fucharoen and Winichagoon, 2000). It may cause severe anemia requiring transfusions during pregnancy (Hsia, 1991). Doubly heterozygous *hemoglobin SE* is usually benign, but Eichhorn and colleagues (1999) reported a sickle-like crisis in a patient with B19 parvovirus infection. It is not clear if hemoglobin SE disease is as ominous during pregnancy as hemoglobin SC or S–β-thalassemia disease (Ramahi and colleagues, 1988).

Hemoglobinopathy in the Newborn. Infants with homozygous SS, SC, and CC disease can be identified accurately at birth by cord blood electrophoresis. The Agency for Health Care Policy and Research (1993) of the U.S. Public Health Service has recommended that all newborn infants be tested for sickle-cell disease. In most states, such screening is performed routinely on blood submitted for phenylketonuria and hypothyroidism testing. The benefit of screening for sickle hemoglobinopathies is that there is clearly decreased mortality in children with sickle-cell disease identified at birth. They are given monthly prophylactic injections of penicillin G and assessed closely for risk factors for strokes (Adams and colleagues, 1998; Centers for Disease Control and Prevention, 2000).

Prenatal Diagnosis. Using polymerase chain reaction, prenatal diagnosis of sickle-cell anemia is simple, accurate, and rapid (see Chap. 12, p. 308). The DNA is obtained by amniocentesis or chorionic villus sampling. Hemoglobin C and most instances of β-thalassemia can be identified by analysis of DNA polymorphism or by identifying in vitro the kinds of globin chains synthesized by fetal red cells.

THALASSEMIAS. The genetically determined hemoglobinopathies termed thalassemias are characterized by impaired production of one or more of the normal globin peptide chains. Abnormal synthesis rates may result in ineffective erythropoiesis, hemolysis, and varying degrees of anemia. Thalassemias are classified according to the globin chain that is deficient. Several hundred syndromes have been identified. The two major forms involve impaired production or stability either of α-peptide chains, causing α-thalassemia, or of β-chains, causing β-thalassemia. The incidence of these traits during pregnancy for all races is 1 in 300 to 500 (Gehlbach and Morgenstern, 1988).

Alpha-Thalassemias. Because there are four α-globin genes, the inheritance of α-thalassemia is more complicated than for β-thalassemia. Four clinical syndromes, the consequence of impaired α-globin chain synthesis, have been identified. For each syndrome, a close correlation has been established between clinical severity and the degree of impairment of synthesis of α-globin chains. In most populations, the α-globin chain "cluster" or gene loci are duplicated on chromosome 16. Thus, the normal genotype for diploid cells can be expressed as $\alpha\alpha/\alpha\alpha$. There are two main groups of

α-thalassemia determinants: α^0-thalassemia is characterized by the deletion of both loci from one chromosome ($-/\alpha\alpha$), whereas α^+-thalassemia is characterized by the loss of a single locus from one chromosome ($-\alpha/\alpha\alpha$ heterozygote) or both ($-\alpha/-\alpha$ homozygote).

There are two major phenotypes. The deletion of all four α-globin chain genes ($-/-$) characterizes *homozygous α-thalassemia.* Because α chains make up fetal hemoglobin, the fetus is affected. Without α-globin chains, hemoglobin Bart (γ_4) and hemoglobin H (β_4) are formed as abnormal tetramers.

Hemoglobin Bart has an appreciably increased affinity for oxygen, and *hemoglobin Bart disease* is a common cause of stillbirths in Southeast Asia. Hsieh and associates (1989) studied 20 such hydropic fetuses by funipuncture and reported that blood contained 65 to 98 percent Bart hemoglobin. The fetus dies either in utero or very soon after birth and demonstrates the typical features of nonimmune hydrops fetalis as shown in Figure 51–4 (see Chap. 29, p. 672). Lam and associates (1999) reported that sonography at 12 to 13 weeks was 100-percent sensitive and specific for identifying affected fetuses by measuring the cardiothoracic ratio. Carr and colleagues (1995) transfused a fetus with α-thalassemia at 25, 26, and 32 weeks and reversed its ascites. The transfusion-dependent infant was delivered at 34 weeks.

The compound heterozygous state for α^0- and α^+-thalassemia results in the deletion of three of four genes ($-/-\alpha$). There is only one functional α-globin gene per diploid genome. This is referred to as *hemoglobin H disease* (β_4) and is compatible with extrauterine life. The abnormal red cells at birth contain a mixture of hemoglobin Bart (γ_4), hemoglobin H (β_4), and hemoglobin A. The neonate appears well at birth but soon develops hemolytic anemia. Most hemoglobin Bart present at birth is replaced postnatally by hemoglobin H. The disease is characterized by hemolytic anemia, which may be severe and similar to β-thalassemia major. Anemia in these women usually is worsened during pregnancy.

A deletion of two genes results clinically in *α-thalassemia minor*, which is characterized by minimal to moderate hypochromic microcytic anemia. This may be due to α^0- or α^+-thalassemia traits. Thus, genotypes may be $-\alpha/-\alpha$ or $-/\alpha\alpha$. Differentiation is only by DNA analysis (Weatherall and Provan, 2000). Because there is no associated clinical abnormality with α-thalassemia minor, it often goes unrecognized. Hemoglobin Bart is present at birth, but as its levels drop, it is not replaced by hemoglobin H. Red cells are hypochromic and microcytic, and the hemoglobin concentration is normal to slightly depressed. Women with α-thalassemia minor tolerate pregnancy quite well.

The single gene deletion ($-\alpha/\alpha\alpha$) is the silent carrier state. No clinical abnormality is evident in the individual with a single gene deletion.

FREQUENCY. The relative frequency of α-thalassemia minor, hemoglobin H disease, and hemoglobin Bart disease varies

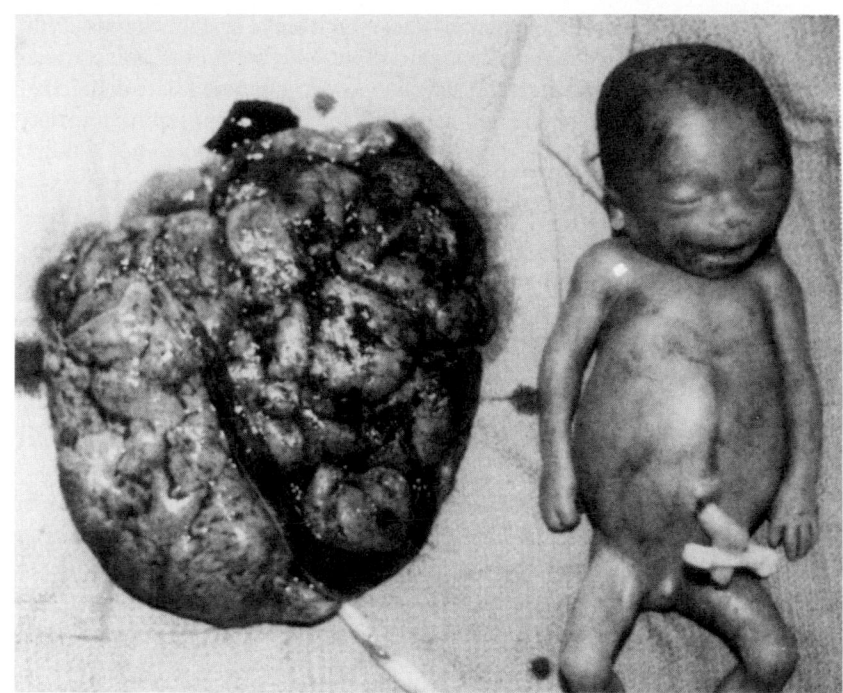

FIGURE 51–4. Stillborn hydropic fetus with extremely large placenta caused by homozygous α-thalassemia. (From Hsia, 1991, with permission.)

remarkably among racial groups. All of these variants are encountered in Asians. In individuals of African descent, however, even though α-thalassemia minor is demonstrated in about 2 percent, hemoglobin H disease is extremely rare and hemoglobin Bart disease is unreported. Asians usually have α^0-thalassemia minor with both gene deletions typically from the same chromosome ($-/\alpha\alpha$), whereas in blacks with α^+-thalassemia minor, one gene is deleted from each chromosome ($-\alpha/-\alpha$). The α-thalassemia syndromes appear sporadically in other racial and ethnic groups. Diagnosis of α-thalassemia minor as well as α-thalassemia major in the fetus can be accomplished by DNA analysis using molecular techniques (American College of Obstetricians and Gynecologists, 2000c).

Beta-Thalassemias. These are the consequence of impaired production of β-globin chains or impaired stability of α chains. More than 150 point mutations in the β-globin gene have been described (Weatherall, 2000). Most are single-nucleotide substitutions that produce transcription or translation defects, RNA splicing or modification, or frameshifts which result in highly unstable hemoglobins. Thus, deletional and nondeletional mutations affect β-globin RNA. The $\delta\gamma\beta$-gene "cluster" is on chromosome 11.

In β-thalassemia, there is decreased β-chain production, and excess α chains precipitate to cause cell membrane damage. In addition, β-thalassemia may be due to impaired α-chain stability. Kihm and colleagues (2002) recently identified a molecular chaperone that regulates α-globin subunit stability, α-hemoglobin–stabilizing protein (AHSP), which forms a stable complex with free α-globin and prevents

precipitation. Mutations in AHSP may modify the clinical picture of β-thalassemia. For example, an overexpression of AHSP may convert β-thalassemia major to β-thalassemia intermedia. These basic defects lead to the panorama of pathology that characterizes homozygous β-thalassemia, so-called β-thalassemia major or *Cooley anemia*. With heterozygous β-thalassemia minor, hypochromia, microcytosis, and slight to moderate anemia develop without the intense hemolysis that characterizes the homozygous state. The hallmark of the common β-thalassemias is an elevated hemoglobin A_2 level.

In the typical case of *thalassemia major*, the neonate is healthy at birth, but as the hemoglobin F level falls, the infant becomes severely anemic and fails to thrive. A child who is entered into an adequate transfusion program develops normally until the end of the first decade, when effects of iron loading become apparent. Prognosis is improved by iron chelation therapy with deferoxamine (Olivieri and associates, 1998). A female who survives beyond childhood usually is sterile, and life expectancy even with transfusion therapy is shortened. Prior to the standardization of iron chelation and transfusions, pregnancy in women with severe thalassemia was rare. Aessopos (1999), Daskalakis (1998), and Kumar (1997) and their colleagues reported a total of 63 pregnancies without severe complications. All these investigators stressed the need for intensive surveillance and exclusion of women with underlying cardiomyopathy.

With β-*thalassemia minor*, hemoglobin A_2, which is composed of two α- and two δ-globin chains, is increased to more than 3.5 percent. Simultaneously, hemoglobin F, which is composed of two α- and two γ-globin chains, is usually increased to more than 2 percent. Anemia is mild, and the red cells are hypochromic and microcytic. There is usually pregnancy-induced augmentation of erythropoiesis and, using ^{51}chromium-tagged erythrocytes, we have documented normal blood volume expansion with slightly subnormal red cell mass expansion.

There is no specific therapy for β-thalassemia minor during pregnancy. Prophylactic iron and folic acid are given. Sheiner and associates (2004) reported that fetal growth restriction and oligohydramnios were increased twofold in 261 affected women.

Prenatal diagnosis of β-thalassemia using chorionic villus sampling can be carried out at 9 to 13 weeks (Weatherall and Provan, 2000). This analysis may be difficult and is not always successful. Techniques include a combination of site-specific restriction endonuclease analysis, restriction fragment polymorphism linkage analysis, polymerase chain reaction, and oligonucleotide probes (Monni and co-workers, 1993). Preimplantation blastomere biopsy has been described by Galvani (2000) and Kanavakis (1999) and their associates. In addition, fetal human leukocyte antigen typing has been described (Orofino and colleagues, 2003).

POLYCYTHEMIA. Excessive erythrocytosis during pregnancy is usually related to chronic hypoxia due to congenital cardiac disease or a pulmonary disorder (see Chap. 44, p. 1028). Occasionally, it is from heavy cigarette smoking. We have encountered otherwise healthy young pregnant women who were heavy smokers with chronic bronchitis and hematocrits of 55 to 60 percent! Brewer and colleagues (1992) described a woman with persistent erythrocytosis associated with a placental site tumor. If polycythemia is severe, the probability of a successful pregnancy outcome is low.

Polycythemia vera is a myeloproliferative hemopoietic stem cell disorder characterized by excessive proliferation of erythroid, myeloid, and megakaryocytic precursors. It likely is an acquired genetic disorder of stem cells and is seen in older patients (Provan and Weatherall, 2000). Measurement of serum erythropoietin by radioimmunoassay differentiates polycythemia vera (low values) from secondary polycythemia (high values). Symptoms are related to increased blood viscosity, and thrombotic complications are common. Ruch and Klein (1964) described a woman whose nonpregnant hematocrit was as high as 63. During her pregnancies her hematocrit ranged from a low of 35 during the second trimester to 44 at term. Fetal loss has been reported to be high in women with polycythemia vera (Tefferi and associates, 2000).

PLATELET DISORDERS

Thrombocytopenia in pregnant women may be inherited or idiopathic. More often, it is associated with the following disorders: acquired hemolytic anemia, severe preeclampsia or eclampsia, severe hemorrhage with blood transfusions, consumptive coagulopathy from placental abruption or similar

hypofibrinogenemic states, septicemia, systemic lupus erythematosus, antiphospholipid antibody syndrome, aplastic anemia, and megaloblastic anemia from severe folate deficiency. It also may result from viral infection, exposure to a variety of drugs, allergic reaction, and irradiation (George, 2000).

GESTATIONAL THROMBOCYTOPENIA. Normal pregnancy may be accompanied by a physiological decrease in platelet concentration. This is usually evident in the third trimester and is due predominantly to hemodilution. At least until recently, there was no evidence that platelet life span is decreased or that there is excessive platelet activation in normal pregnancy (Baker and Cunningham, 1999; Star and colleagues, 1997). In studies of platelet activation in preeclampsia, Holthe and associates (2004) demonstrated that platelets from normally pregnant women expressed higher basal CD63 levels, indicating platelet activation, and that platelet counts were significantly lower than in nonpregnant women.

Thus, *gestational thrombocytopenia* is considered normal, and it is a diagnosis of exclusion. Obviously, the definition used for thrombocytopenia is important. In their review, Rouse and associates (1998) cite an incidence of 4 to 7 percent for gestational thrombocytopenia, defined by platelet counts of less than 150,000/μL. Burrows and Kelton (1993a) reported that 6.6 percent of 15,471 pregnant women had platelet counts of less than 150,000/μL, and in 1.2 percent they were less than 100,000/μL. They reported that almost 75 percent of 1027 women whose platelet counts were less than 150,000/μL were found to have normal-variant incidental thrombocytopenia. The others had either a hypertensive disorder of pregnancy (21 percent) or an immunological disorder (4 percent). In another study, Boehlen and associates (2000) found that 11.6 percent of 6770 pregnant women had platelet counts of less than 150,000/μL. In this study, 116,000/μL was 2.5 standard deviations below the mean. Al-Kouatly and colleagues (2003) found a much higher rate of thrombocytopenia in triplet gestations, affecting nearly a third of cases. In contrast to thrombocytopenia in singletons, more than 70 percent of cases were due to hypertensive disorders.

INHERITED THROMBOCYTOPENIAS. The *Bernard–Soulier syndrome* is characterized by lack of platelet membrane glycoprotein (GPIb/IX), which causes severe dysfunction. Maternal antibodies against fetal GPIb/IX antigen can cause isoimmune fetal thrombocytopenia. Peng and colleagues (1991) described an affected woman who during four pregnancies had episodes of postpartum hemorrhage, gastrointestinal hemorrhage, and fetal thrombocytopenia. Fujimori and associates (1999) described a similarly affected woman whose neonate died from thrombocytopenic intracranial hemorrhage.

Chatwani and associates (1992) reported a woman with autosomally dominant *May–Hegglin anomaly* but whose infant was not affected. Urato and Repke (1998) also described such a woman who was delivered vaginally, yet despite a platelet count of 16,000/μL, she did not bleed excessively. The neonate inherited the anomaly, but also had no bleeding despite a platelet count of 35,000/μL. Fayyad and colleagues (2002) managed three pregnancies in a woman with May–Hegglin anomaly. In the first, the mother had a term cesarean delivery of an unaffected infant; in the second, she had a fetal demise with multiple placental infarcts; and in the third, she received low-dose aspirin (75 mg/d) and gave birth to an unaffected infant.

IMMUNE THROMBOCYTOPENIC PURPURA. This is also called *idiopathic thrombocytopenic purpura (ITP)* and is usually the consequence of antibodies directed against platelets. Antibody-coated platelets are destroyed prematurely in the reticuloendothelial system, especially the spleen. The mechanism of production of these platelet-associated immunoglobulins—PAIgG, PAIgM, and PAIgA—is not known, but most investigators consider them to be autoantibodies.

The American Society of Hematology convened a panel to formulate guidelines for diagnosis and management of ITP (George and colleagues, 1996). Acute ITP is most often a childhood disease that follows a viral infection. Most cases resolve spontaneously, although perhaps 10 percent become chronic. Conversely, in adults, immune thrombocytopenia is primarily a chronic disease of young women and rarely resolves spontaneously.

Secondary forms of chronic thrombocytopenia appear in association with systemic lupus erythematosus, lymphomas, leukemias, and a number of systemic diseases. For example, about 2 percent of patients with thrombocytopenia have positive serological tests for lupus, and in some cases there are high levels of anticardiolipin antibodies. As many as 10 percent of HIV-positive patients have associated thrombocytopenia (Glantz and Roberts, 1994; Scaradavou, 2002).

Outcomes for adults with primary ITP are shown in Table 51–5. Only a small number recover spontaneously, and

TABLE 51–5 Outcome of Immunological Thrombocytopenic Purpura in 1761 Adults from 12 Studies

Outcome	Number	%
Complete remission		
Spontaneous (no therapy)	27	1.5
Following therapy	1027	64
Hemorrhagic complications		
Acute deaths		
Intracerebral hemorrhage	36	2
Other hemorrhage	7	<1
Other deaths	35	2
Persistent thrombocytopenia	465	26
Later spontaneous recovery	22	5
Later hemorrhagic death	25	5

Data from George and colleagues (1996).

for those who do not, platelet counts usually range from 10,000 to 100,000/μL. In those whose platelet counts remain less than 30,000/μL, or those with significant bleeding at higher levels, treatment with prednisone, 1 to 2 mg/kg, raises the platelet count in about two thirds of cases, but relapse is exceedingly common (George and associates, 1996). Glucocorticoids suppress phagocytic activity of the splenic monocyte–macrophage system. Godeau and colleagues (2002) reported results of a randomized trial of intravenous immunoglobulin or high-dose methylprednisolone given for three days. These were followed by oral prednisone or placebo. Intravenous immunoglobulin plus oral prednisone was most effective, although methylprednisolone with prednisone was effective and well tolerated. Recently, Cheng and colleagues (2003) found that 85 percent of adults with ITP responded to high-dose dexamethasone. Half had a sustained response at 6 months.

For patients with no response to corticosteroid therapy in 2 to 3 weeks, those in whom massive doses are needed to sustain remission, or those with frequent recurrences, splenectomy is indicated. In about 60 percent, there is substantive improvement as the consequence of decreased splenic removal of platelets and reduced antibody production. Massive doses (400 mg/kg) of gamma globulin given intravenously over 5 days result in satisfactory platelet count elevation in two thirds of patients. Such therapy may be useful in patients with life-threatening thrombocytopenia refractive to other therapy, or preoperatively before splenectomy.

Therapy is problematic for the 30 percent of adults who do not respond to corticosteroids or splenectomy. Immunosuppressive drugs, including azathioprine, cyclophosphamide, and cyclosporine, have been used with some success. Danazol, vinca alkaloids, plasma exchange, and high-dose dexamethasone pulse therapy have been described.

Immune Thrombocytopenia and Pregnancy. There is no evidence that pregnancy increases the risk of relapse in women with previously diagnosed immune thrombocytopenia. Nor does it make the condition worse in women with active disease. It is certainly not unusual for women who have been in clinical remission for several years to have recurrent thrombocytopenia during pregnancy. Although this may be from closer surveillance, hyperestrogenemia has also been suggested as a cause.

Treatment is considered if the platelet count is less than 50,000/μL (George and associates, 1996). Prednisone in a dose of 1 mg/kg per day may be required for improvement, and most likely treatment will have to be continued throughout pregnancy. Corticosteroid therapy usually produces amelioration, but in refractory disease, high-dose immunoglobulin is given intravenously. Clark and Gall (1997) reviewed 16 case reports of 21 pregnancies in which ITP was treated with immunoglobulin. All but four responded with posttreatment platelet counts greater than 50,000/μL, and in 11 cases, counts exceeded 100,000/μL. Such therapy is expensive, and in 2003, hospital costs for a 5-day course of treatment ranged from $5500 to $8000 for a 70-kg person. In addition, shortages of immunoglobulin for high-dose infusion are not uncommon (Centers for Disease Control and Prevention, 1999).

In pregnant women with no response to steroid or immunoglobulin therapy, splenectomy may be effective. In late pregnancy, surgery technically is more difficult, and cesarean delivery may be necessary for exposure.

FETAL AND NEONATAL EFFECTS. Platelet-associated IgG antibodies cross the placenta and may cause thrombocytopenia in the fetus-neonate. Fetal death from hemorrhage occurs occasionally (Webert and associates, 2003). The severely thrombocytopenic fetus is at increased risk for intracranial hemorrhage with labor and delivery. This fortunately is unusual. Payne and colleagues (1997) reviewed studies of maternal ITP published since 1973 and added their experiences with 55 cases. Of a total of 601 newborns, 12 percent had severe thrombocytopenia defined as less than 50,000/μL. Six infants had intracranial hemorrhage, and in three the initial platelet count was greater than 50,000/μL.

Considerable attention has been directed at identifying the fetus with potentially dangerous thrombocytopenia. All investigators have concurred that there is not a strong correlation between fetal and maternal platelet counts (George and associates, 1996; Payne and co-workers, 1997). Because of this, there have been attempts to quantify the relationship between maternal IgG free platelet antibody, platelet-associated antibody, and fetal platelet count. Again, there is little concurrence. Kaplan and associates (1990) and Samuels and colleagues (1990) reported conflicting results in using indirect platelet immunoglobulin for identification of high-risk neonates. They both found, however, that a history of ITP remote from pregnancy increased the likelihood of neonatal thrombocytopenia.

Burrows and Kelton (1993a) detected neonatal umbilical cord platelets of less than 50,000/μL in 19 of 15,932 consecutive newborns (0.12 percent). But only 1 of 756 mothers with gestational thrombocytopenia had an affected infant. Of 1414 hypertensive women with thrombocytopenia, five infants had thrombocytopenia. Conversely, of 46 mothers with immune thrombocytopenic purpura, four infants had thrombocytopenia. Importantly, isoimmune thrombocytopenia was associated with profound thrombocytopenia with cord platelet counts less than 20,000/μL. One of these fetuses died, and two others had intracranial hemorrhage (see later discussion). In a similar population study, Boehlen and associates (1999) determined antiplatelet antibodies in 430 pregnant women whose platelet counts were less than 150,000/μL. Antibodies were detected in 9 percent but had no predictive value. Sainio and co-workers (2000) performed cord platelet counts in almost 4500 neonates. About 2 percent were less than 150,000/μL, and only 0.2 percent (1 in 410) were less than 50,000/μL. All cases with bleeding were due to isoimmune thrombocytopenia.

Detection of Fetal Thrombocytopenia. There are no clinical characteristics or laboratory tests that accurately predict fetal platelet count. This led Scott and associates (1983) to recommend intrapartum fetal scalp platelet determinations once the cervix was 2 cm dilated and the membranes ruptured. Cesarean delivery was performed for fetuses with platelet counts less than 50,000/μL. Daffos and colleagues (1985) subsequently reported percutaneous umbilical cord blood sampling for platelet quantification with a high complication rate (see Chap. 13, p. 330). Berry and associates (1997) reported no complications but found only a high negative predictive value. Payne and colleagues (1997) summarized six such studies reported since 1988. Of 195 cases, severe neonatal thrombocytopenia of less than 50,000/μL was found in 7 percent, however, serious complications from cordocentesis were identified in 4.6 percent.

Because of the low incidence of severe neonatal thrombocytopenia and morbidity, Burrows and Kelton (1993b), Silver and colleagues (1995), Payne and associates (1997) and the American Society of Hematology (George and co-workers, 1996) all concluded that fetal platelet determinations and cesarean delivery are not necessary. Peleg and Hunter (1999) surveyed members of the Society of Maternal–Fetal Medicine and received a 60-percent response. Only a third of respondents recommended fetal testing with chronic ITP, and a fourth would perform fetal testing in women with new-onset ITP during pregnancy.

ISOIMMUNE THROMBOCYTOPENIA. Platelet isoimmunization can develop in a manner identical to erythrocyte antigen isoimmunization. Its incidence may be as high as 1 in 1000 to 5000 births (Richmond and colleagues, 2003). If fetal platelet antigens for which maternal platelets are negative gain access to the mother's circulation, she then may produce antibodies that are manifest in subsequent pregnancies. The most common antibody is against PL^{A1} platelet-specific antigen. About 2 percent of Caucasians are homozygous for PL^{B1} antigen and thus are exposed to isoimmunization by PL^{A1} antigens (Jaegtvik and associates, 2000). The first pregnancy is affected in about half of cases. This disorder is discussed in Chapter 29 (see p. 677).

THROMBOCYTOSIS. Also called *thrombocythemia*, thrombocytosis generally is defined as platelets persisting in numbers greater than 450,000/μL. Common causes of *secondary* or *reactive thrombocytosis* are malignant tumors, iron deficiency, hemorrhage, inflammatory diseases, and connective tissue disorders. Platelet counts seldom exceed 800,000/μL in these secondary disorders, and prognosis depends on the underlying disease. On the other hand, *essential thrombocytosis* is a myeloproliferative disorder that accounts for most cases in which platelet counts exceed 1 million/μL. Thrombocytosis usually is asymptomatic, but arterial and venous thromboses may develop. Cortelazzo and colleagues (1995) reported that myelosuppression with hydroxyurea for nonpregnant patients with essential thrombocytosis decreased thrombotic episodes from 24 to 4 percent compared with those of untreated controls.

Pregnancy. Although reports indicate that pregnancies associated with thrombocytosis have excessive spontaneous abortions, placental infarctions, and preterm delivery, this likely is not the case. Beard and co-workers (1991) and Randi and colleagues (1994) described essentially normal pregnancies in women whose mean platelet counts were greater than 1.25 million/μL. Treatment that has been suggested during pregnancy includes aspirin, dipyridamole, heparin, plateletpheresis, or combinations thereof (Griesshammer and associates, 2003). Delage and co-workers (1996) reviewed 11 cases in which interferon-α was given during pregnancy with successful outcomes. They also described a woman at midpregnancy who had platelets of 2.3 million/μL and transient blindness. Thrombocytapheresis and interferon-α were used to keep the platelets at around 1 million/μL until delivery.

THROMBOTIC MICROANGIOPATHIES. Although not proven a primary platelet disorder, there almost always is some degree of thrombocytopenia. Moschcowitz (1925) described *thrombotic thrombocytopenic purpura* by the pentad of thrombocytopenia, fever, neurological abnormalities, renal impairment, and hemolytic anemia. Gasser and colleagues (1955) later described the similar *hemolytic uremic syndrome*, which had more profound renal involvement and fewer neurological aberrations. The British Committee for Standards in Haematology has recently published guidelines on diagnosis and management of thrombotic microangiopathic hemolytic anemias (Allford and associates, 2003). The syndromes have an incidence of 2 to 6 per million per year (Miller and colleagues, 2004).

Although it is likely that different causes account for the variable findings within these syndromes, they currently are clinically indistinguishable in adults (Moake, 1998). There is, however, a pure form of the hemolytic uremic syndrome in children, incited by viral or bacterial infection with severe prothrombin disturbance in which thrombin generation and inhibition of fibrinolysis precede the renal injury (Chandler and colleagues, 2002). There is no evidence that postpartum renal failure is a separate syndrome (Robson and associates, 1968). This probably accounts for the unusual case of severe preeclampsia with hemolysis and thrombocytopenia that does not respond to delivery (Kahra and associates, 1998; Magann and colleagues, 1994).

Pathogenesis. Microthrombi, consisting of hyaline material made up of platelets and small amounts of fibrin, develop within arterioles and capillaries. These aggregates produce ischemia or infarctions in various organs. The general consensus is that intravascular platelet aggregation stimulates the cascade of events leading to end-organ failure. Although there is endothelial activation and damage, it is unclear whether this is a consequence or a cause. Unusually large multimers of von Willebrand factor have been identified with active disease. Later, it was shown that the endothelial-derived metalloproteinase responsible for cleaving von Willebrand factor is neutralized by antibodies during an acute episode (Furlan and colleagues, 1998; Tsai and associates, 1998). More recently, Levy and colleagues (2001) identified the *ADAMTS13 gene* that encodes the protease. They found that defects in this gene result in various clinical presentations of thrombotic microangiopathy (Moake, 2002; 2004).

Clinical Presentation. Thrombotic microangiopathies are characterized by thrombocytopenia, fragmentation hemolysis, and variable organ dysfunction. A viral prodrome may precede up to 40 percent of cases. Neurological symptoms develop in up to 90 percent of patients and include headache, altered consciousness, convulsions, fever, or stroke. Because renal involvement is common, the two syndromes are difficult to separate (Moake, 1998). Renal failure is thought to be more severe with the hemolytic uremic syndrome, and in half of the cases, dialysis is required.

Hematological Abnormalities. Thrombocytopenia is usually severe. Fortunately, even with very low platelet counts, spontaneous severe hemorrhage is uncommon. Microangiopathic hemolysis is associated with moderate to marked anemia, and transfusions are frequently necessary. The blood smear is characterized by erythrocyte fragmentation with schizocytosis. The reticulocyte count is high, and nucleated red blood cells are numerous. Consumptive coagulopathy, although common, is usually subtle and clinically insignificant.

Treatment. Plasmapheresis and exchange transfusion with normal plasma have remarkably improved the outcome for patients with these formerly commonly fatal diseases. Red cell transfusions are imperative for life-threatening anemia. Rock and colleagues (1991) found plasma exchange to be superior to plasma infusion in nonpregnant patients, but overall mortality was still 30 percent. Bell and co-workers (1991) reported their experiences with 108 patients treated at Johns Hopkins Hospital, and 10 percent of these patients were pregnant. Those with minimal neurological symptoms were given prednisone, 200 mg daily. If there were neurological abnormalities or rapid clinical deterioration, plasmapheresis and plasma exchange were performed daily. About a fourth of patients with mild disease responded to prednisone alone. Of those requiring plasmapheresis, relapses were common, but overall survival was 91 percent. As emphasized by Hayward (1994) and Shumak (1995) and their associates, relapses develop in 20 to 30 percent and include long-term sequelae such as renal impairment.

Pregnancy and Thrombotic Microangiopathy. Evidence is lacking that pregnancy predisposes women to develop thrombotic microangiopathies. Over a 25-year period, Dashe and co-workers (1998) encountered 11 pregnancies complicated by these syndromes or their presumed variants among nearly 275,000 obstetrical patients within our well-defined catchment area for Parkland Hospital. This frequency of 1 in 25,000 is about the same as in our general nonobstetrical hospital population.

It is not surprising that severe preeclampsia and eclampsia complicated further by thrombocytopenia and overt hemolysis have been confused with thrombotic thrombocytopenic purpura and vice versa (Hsu and colleagues, 1995; Magann and co-workers, 1994). One constant feature of thrombotic microangiopathies is hemolytic anemia, which is rarely severe with preeclampsia, even with the *HELLP syndrome*. Although deposition of hyaline microthrombi within the liver is seen with thrombotic microangiopathy, hepatocellular necrosis characteristic of preeclampsia has not been described. In addition, whereas delivery is imperative to treat preeclampsia in women with the HELLP syndrome, there is no evidence that thrombotic microangiopathy is improved by delivery (Letsky, 2000). Finally, microangiopathy syndromes are usually recurrent and unassociated with pregnancy. For example, 7 of 11 women described by Dashe and colleagues (1998) had recurrent disease either when not pregnant or within the first trimester of a subsequent pregnancy.

Unless the diagnosis is unequivocally one of these thrombotic microangiopathies, rather than severe preeclampsia, the response to pregnancy termination should be evaluated before resorting to plasmapheresis and exchange transfusion, massive-dose glucocorticoid therapy, or other therapy. **Plasmapheresis is not indicated for preeclampsia–eclampsia complicated by hemolysis and thrombocytopenia.**

In the past, maternal and perinatal mortality was as high as 70 to 80 percent (Weiner, 1987). With plasma therapy, maternal survival is now excellent. Egerman and co-workers (1996) described 11 pregnant women whom they treated with plasmapheresis. There were two maternal and three fetal deaths. In our experiences at Parkland Hospital, five of eight women treated by plasmapheresis had a dramatic salutary response (Dashe and associates, 1998).

LONG-TERM PROGNOSIS. Pregnant women with thrombotic microangiopathy have a number of long-term complications. In the study by Dashe and associates (1998), 9-year followup disclosed multiple recurrences; renal disease requiring dialysis, transplantation, or both; severe hypertension; and transfusion-acquired infectious diseases. Two women died remote from pregnancy—one from dialysis complications and one from HIV infection transmitted by blood or plasma transfusions. Egerman and colleagues (1996) reported similar observations. Although it is not possible to ascertain if the guarded prognosis in these women is different from the nonpregnant course, clearly, development of thrombotic microangiopathy during pregnancy has severe immediate and long-term mortality.

INHERITED COAGULATION DEFECTS

Obstetrical hemorrhage, a common event, is rarely the consequence of an inherited defect in the coagulation mechanism. Several syndromes, however, are particularly important.

HEMOPHILIAS. There are two types of hemophilias, which are seen in varying degrees. They are considered mild, moderate, or severe, corresponding to plasma factor levels of 6 to 30, 2 to 5, or less than 1 percent, respectively (Mannucci and Tuddenham, 2001).

Hemophilia A is an X-linked recessively transmitted disease characterized by a marked deficiency of *small component* antihemophilic factor (factor VIII:C). It is rare among women compared with men, in whom the heterozygous state is responsible for the disease. Although heterozygous women have diminished factor VIII levels, almost invariably the homozygous state is the requisite for hemophilia A. In a few instances, it appears in women spontaneously as a newly mutant gene.

The genetic and clinical features of severe deficiency of factor IX—*Christmas disease* or *hemophilia B*—are quite similar to those of hemophilia A. Guy and associates (1992) reviewed five cases in pregnancy, all with a favorable outcome. They recommended administration of factor IX where levels are below 10 percent.

The degree of risk for each of these hemophilias is influenced markedly by the level of circulating factor VIII:C or factor IX. If the level is at or very close to zero, the risk is major. In female carriers, activity is expected to average 50 percent, but there is a range due to lyonization (Letsky, 2000). If levels fall below 10 to 20 percent, hemorrhage may occur. These clotting factors increase appreciably during normal pregnancy and in carriers of hemophilia A and B. Desmopressin may also stimulate factor VIII:C release. The risk of hemorrhage is reduced by avoiding lacerations, minimizing episiotomy, and maximizing postpartum myometrial contractions and retraction. Kadir and co-workers (1997) reported that 20 percent of carriers had postpartum hemorrhage, and in two, it was massive.

An affected male fetus may develop hematomas with either vaginal or cesarean delivery (Kadir and associates, 1997). After delivery, the risk of hemorrhage in the neonate increases, especially if circumcision is attempted.

Whenever the mother has hemophilia A or B, all of her sons will have the disease, and all of her daughters will be carriers. If she is a carrier, half of her sons will inherit the disease and half of her daughters will be carriers. Prenatal diagnosis of hemophilia is possible in some families using chorionic villus biopsy (see Chap. 13, p. 329). The confirmation of a male fetus also identifies a 50-percent risk of inheriting hemophilia.

FACTOR VIII OR IX INHIBITORS. Rarely, antibodies directed against factor VIII or IX are acquired and may lead to life-threatening hemorrhage. These antibodies may be troublesome in patients with hemophilia A or B. This phenomenon has also been identified rarely in women during the puerperium. The prominent clinical feature is severe, protracted, repetitive hemorrhage from the reproductive tract starting a week or so after an apparently uncomplicated delivery (Reece and associates, 1988). The activated partial thromboplastin time is markedly prolonged. Treatment has included multiple transfusions of whole blood and plasma; huge doses of cryoprecipitate; large volumes of an admixture of activated coagulation factors, including porcine factor VIII; immunosuppressive therapy; and attempts at various surgical procedures, especially curettage and hysterectomy. Another treatment involves bypassing factor VIII or IX by the use of activated forms of factors VII, IX, and X. A recombinant activated factor VII (NovoSeven) stops bleeding in up to 75 percent of patients with inhibitors (Mannucci and Tuddenham, 2001). It has also been used in cases of intractable obstetrical hemorrhage caused by uterine atony as well as multiple transfusions in nonhemophilic patients (Bouwmeester and colleagues, 2003; Danilou and associates, 2003).

VON WILLEBRAND DISEASE. Clinically, von Willebrand disease is actually a heterogenous group of about 20 functional disorders involving aberrations of factor VIII complex and platelet dysfunction. These abnormalities are the most commonly inherited bleeding disorders, and their prevalence is as high as 1 to 2 percent (Mannucci, 2004). Most of von Willebrand variants are inherited as autosomal dominant traits. Examples are types I and II which are the most common variants. Type III, which is the most severe, is phenotypically recessive.

The *von Willebrand factor* (vWF) is a series of large plasma multimeric glycoproteins that form part of the factor VIII complex. It essential for normal platelet adhesion to subendothelial collagen and formation of a primary hemostatic plug at the site of blood vessel injury. It also plays a major role in the stabilization of the coagulant properties of factor VIII. The procoagulant component is the antihemophilic factor or factor VIII:C, which is a glycoprotein synthesized by the liver. Conversely, von Willebrand precursor, which is present in platelets as well as plasma, is synthesized by endothelium and megakaryocytes under the control of autosomal genes on chromosome 12. The von Willebrand factor antigen (vWF:Ag) is the antigenic determinant measured by immunoassays. Von Willebrand disease rarely is acquired when antibodies to vWF develop in autoimmune or lymphoproliferative disorders (Handin, 2001).

Clinical Presentation. Symptomatic patients usually present with evidence of a platelet defect. The possibility of von Willebrand disease is usually considered in women with bleeding suggestive of a chronic disorder of coagulation. The classical autosomal dominant form usually is symptomatic in the heterozygous state. The less common but clinically more severe autosomal recessive form is manifest when inherited from both parents, both of whom typically demonstrate little or no disease. Type I, which accounts for 75 percent of von Willebrand variants, is characterized clinically by easy bruising; epistaxis; mucosal hemorrhage; and excessive bleeding with trauma, including surgery. Its laboratory features are usually a prolonged bleeding time, prolonged partial thromboplastin time, decreased vWF antigen, decreased factor VIII immunological as well as coagulation-promoting activity, and inability of platelets in plasma from an affected person to react to a variety of stimuli.

Effect of Pregnancy. Pregnant women with von Willebrand disease often develop normal levels of factor VIII coagulant activity as well as vWF antigen, although the bleeding time still may be prolonged. These levels may double or triple by term. If factor VIII activity is very low, or if there is bleeding, treatment is recommended. Desmopressin by infusion may transiently increase factor VIII and vWF factor levels (Mannucci, 2004). With significant bleeding, 15 or 20 units or "bags" of cryoprecipitate are given every 12 hours. Alternatively, factor VIII concentrates may be given that contain high-molecular-weight vWF multimers (Alfanate, Hemate-P). These concentrates are highly purified and are heat treated to destroy HIV. Lubetsky and associates (1999) have described continuous infusion with Hemate-P in nonpregnant patients during nine surgical procedures and in another woman during a vaginal delivery.

Pregnancy outcomes in women with von Willebrand disease are generally good but postpartum hemorrhage is encountered in up to 50 percent of cases. Conti and associates (1986) summarized 38 cases, and in a fourth, bleeding was reported with abortion, delivery, or the puerperium. Greer and colleagues (1991) reported that eight of 14 pregnancies were complicated by postpartum hemorrhage. Kadir and coworkers (1998) reported their experiences from the Royal Free Hospital in London with 84 pregnancies and described a 20-percent incidence of immediate postpartum hemorrhage and another 20 percent had late hemorrhage. Most cases were associated with low vWF levels in untreated women, and none given treatment peripartum had hemorrhage.

Inheritance. Although most patients with von Willebrand disease have heterozygous variants with a mild bleeding disorder, the disease can be severe. Certainly when both parents have the disorder, their homozygous offspring develop a serious bleeding disorder. Mullaart and colleagues (1991) reported periventricular hemorrhage in a 32-week fetus who inherited type IIa von Willebrand disease from her father. Chorionic villus biopsy with DNA analysis to detect the missing genes has been accomplished (see Chap. 13, p. 329). Some authorities recommend cesarean delivery to avoid trauma to a possibly affected fetus if the mother has severe disease.

OTHER INHERITED COAGULATION FACTOR DEFICIENCIES. A number of rare coagulopathies may be inherited in a manner similar to the hemophilias. *Factor*

VII deficiency is a rare autosomal recessive disorder. The gene that codes for factor VII is on chromosome 13. Normally, factor VII increases during pregnancy, but it may do so only mildly in women with factor VII deficiency (Fadel and Krauss, 1989). Treatment with factor VIIa has been reported during labor, delivery and the puerperium (Eskandari and associates, 2002).

Factor X or *Stuart–Prower factor* deficiency is extremely rare and is inherited as an autosomal recessive trait. Factor X levels typically rise by 50 percent during normal pregnancy. Konje and colleagues (1994) described a woman with 2-percent activity who was given prophylactic treatment with plasma-derived factor X, which raised plasma levels to 37 percent. Despite this, she suffered an intrapartum placental abruption. Bofill and co-workers (1996) gave intrapartum fresh-frozen plasma to a woman with less than 1-percent factor X activity, and she delivered spontaneously without incident.

Factor XI (plasma thromboplastin antecedent) deficiency probably is the consequence of an autosomal trait that is manifest as severe disease in homozygotes but a minor defect in heterozygotes. This deficiency state is most prevalent in Ashkenazi Jews, and it is rarely seen in pregnancy. Musclow and colleagues (1987) described 41 deliveries in 17 women with factor XI deficiency, none of whom required transfusions. They also described a woman who developed a spontaneous hemarthrosis at 39 weeks. Kadir and associates (1998) described 29 pregnancies in 11 women. In none of these did factor XI levels increase; 15 percent had immediate postpartum hemorrhage, and another 25 percent had delayed hemorrhage. David and colleagues (2002) reported three cases in which factor XI deficiency was first diagnosed after obstetrical hemorrhage. Peripartum treatment with factor XI concentrate at the time of delivery prevents hemorrhage (Letsky, 2000).

Factor XII deficiency is another autosomal recessive disorder that rarely complicates pregnancy. An increased incidence of thromboembolism is encountered in nonpregnant patients with this deficiency. Lao and colleagues (1991) reported an affected pregnant woman in whom placental abruption developed at 26 weeks.

Factor XIII deficiency is autosomal recessive and may be associated with maternal intracranial hemorrhage (Letsky, 2000). Treatment is given with fresh frozen plasma.

Autosomally inherited abnormalities of fibrinogen usually involve the formation of a functionally defective fibrinogen, and are commonly referred to as *dysfibrinogenemias* (Edwards and Rijhsinghani, 2000). Familial *hypofibrinogenemia,* and sometimes *afibrinogenemia*, are infrequent recessive disorders. In some cases, both conditions occur—*hypodysfibrinogenemia* (Deering and colleagues, 2003). Our experience suggests that hypofibrinogenemia represents a heterozygous autosomal dominant state with 50 percent of the offspring affected. Typically, thrombin-clottable protein level in these patients has ranged from 800 to 110 mg/dL when nonpregnant, and this increases by 40 or 50 percent in normal pregnancy. Those pregnancy complications that give rise to acquired hypofibrinogenemia (i.e., placental abruption) are more common with fibrinogen deficiency. Trehan and Fergusson (1991) and Funai and associates (1997) described successful outcomes in two women in whom fibrinogen or plasma infusions were given weekly or biweekly throughout pregnancy.

THROMBOPHILIAS. Several important regulatory proteins inhibit clotting. There are physiological antithrombotic proteins that act as inhibitors at strategic sites in the coagulation cascade to maintain blood fluidity under normal circumstances. Inherited deficiencies of these inhibitory proteins are caused by mutations of genes influencing their control. Because they may be associated with recurrent thromboembolism, they are collectively referred to as *thrombophilias*. Examples include *antithrombin III; protein C* and its cofactor, *protein S; activated protein C resistance* from factor V single-gene mutations; a function-enhancing mutation in the *prothrombin gene (G20210A);* and *hyperhomocystinemia*. Because these deficiencies are typically associated with thromboembolism, they are discussed in detail in Chapter 47 (see p. 1074).

REFERENCES

Adams RJ, McKie VC, Hsu L, et al: Prevention of a first stroke by transfusions in children with sickle-cell anemia and abnormal results on transcranial Doppler ultrasonography. N Engl J Med 339:5, 1998

Advisory Committee on Immunization Practices: Prevention of pneumococcal diseases. MMWR 46:1, 1997

Aessopos A, Karabatsos F, Farmakis D, et al: Pregnancy in patients with well-treated β-thalassemia: Outcome for mothers and newborn infants. Am J Obstet Gynecol 180:360, 1999

Agency for Health Care Policy and Research, Sickle Disease Guideline Panel: Sickle Cell Disease: Comprehensive Screening and Management in Newborns and Infants. Rockville, MD, US Public Health Service, Department of Health and Human Services, April 1993

Agre P: Hereditary spherocytosis. JAMA 262:2887, 1989

Aitchison RGM, Marsh JCW, Hows JM, et al: Pregnancy associated aplastic anaemia: A report of five cases and review of current management. Br J Haematol 73:541, 1989

Al-Kouatly HB, Chasen ST, Kalish RB, et al: Causes of thrombocytopenia in triplet gestations. Am J Obstet Gynecol 189:177, 2003

Allford SL, Hunt BJ, Rose P, et al: Guidelines on the diagnosis and management of the thrombotic microangiopathic haemolytic anaemias. Br J Haematol 120:556, 2003

Alter BP, Frissora CL, Halpérin DS, et al: Fanconi's anaemia and pregnancy. Br J Haematol 77:410, 1991

American College of Obstetricians and Gynecologists: Precis: An update in obstetrics and gynecology. Obstetrics, 2nd ed. Washington, DC, American College of Obstetricians and Gynecologists, 2000a, p 82

American College of Obstetricians and Gynecologists: The use of hormonal contraception in women with coexisting medical conditions. Practice Bulletin No. 18, July 2000b

American College of Obstetricians and Gynecologists: Genetic screening for hemoglobinopathies. Committee on Genetics. Committee Opinion No. 238, July 2000c

American College of Obstetricians and Gynecologists: Antepartum fetal surveillance. Practice Bulletin No. 9, October 1999

American College of Obstetricians and Gynecologists: Nutrition and women. Educational Bulletin No. 229, October 1996

Andrews NC: Disorders of iron metabolism. N Engl J Med 341:1986, 1999

Anyaegbunam A, Morel MIG, Merkatz IR: Antepartum fetal surveillance tests during sickle cell crisis. Am J Obstet Gynecol 165:1081, 1991

Ascarelli MH, Emerson ES, Bigelow CL, et al: Aplastic anemia and immune-mediated thrombocytopenia: Concurrent complications encountered in the third trimester of pregnancy. Obstet Gynecol 91:803, 1998

Baker PN, Cunningham FG: Platelet and coagulation abnormalities. In Lindheimer MD, Roberts JM, Cunningham FG (eds): Chesley's Hypertensive Disorders in Pregnancy, 2nd ed. Stamford, CT, Appleton & Lange, 1999, p 349

Barker DJP, Bull AR, Osmond C, et al: Fetal and placental size and risk of hypertension in adult life. BMJ 301:259, 1990

Bayouneu F, Subiran-Buisset C, Baka NE, et al: Iron therapy in iron deficiency anemia in pregnancy: Intravenous route versus oral route. Am J Obstet Gynecol 186:518, 2002

Beard J, Hillmen P, Anderson CC, et al: Primary thrombocythaemia in pregnancy. Br J Haematol 77:371, 1991

Bell WR, Braine HG, Ness PM, et al: Improved survival in thrombotic thrombocytopenic purpura–hemolytic uremic syndrome. Clinical experience in 108 patients. N Engl J Med 325:398, 1991

Berry SM, Leonardi MR, Wolfe HM, et al: Maternal thrombocytopenia. Predicting neonatal thrombocytopenia with cordocentesis. J Reprod Med 42:276, 1997

Beutler E: Glucose-6-phosphate dehydrogenase deficiency. N Engl J Med 324:169, 1991

Bodnar LM, Scanlon KS, Freedman DS, et al: High prevalence of postpartum anemia among low-income women in the United States. Am J Obstet Gynecol 185:438, 2001

Boehlen F, Hohlfeld P, Extermann P, et al: Maternal antiplatelet antibodies in predicting risk of neonatal thrombocytopenia. Obstet Gynecol 93:169, 1999

Boehlen F, Hohlfeld P, Extermann P, et al: Platelet count at term pregnancy: A reappraisal of the threshold. Obstet Gynecol 95:29, 2000

Bofill JA, Young RA, Perry KG Jr: Successful pregnancy in a woman with severe factor X deficiency. Obstet Gynecol 88:723, 1996

Borgna-Pignatti C, Marradi P, Rugolotto S, et al: Successful pregnancy after bone marrow transplantation for thalassaemia. Bone Marrow Transplant 18:235, 1996

Bourantas K, Makrydimas G, Georgiou I, et al: Aplastic anemia: Report of a case with recurrent episodes in consecutive pregnancies. J Reprod Med 42:672, 1997

Bouwmeester FW, Jonkhoff AR, Verheijen RHM, et al: Successful treatment of life-threatening postpartum hemorrhage with recombinant activated factor VII. Obstet Gynecol 101:1174, 2003

Braga J, Marques R, Branco A, et al: Maternal and perinatal implications of the use of human recombinant erythropoietin. Acta Obstet Gynecol Scand 75:449, 1996

Brewer CA, Adelson MD, Elder RC: Erythrocytosis associated with a placental-site trophoblastic tumor. Obstet Gynecol 79:846, 1992

Briggs GG, Freeman RK, Yaffe SJ: Drugs in Pregnancy and Lactation, 5th ed. Baltimore, Williams & Wilkins, 1998, p 517

Bunn HF, Rosse W: Hemolytic anemias and acute blood loss. In Braunwald E, Fauci AS, Kasper DL, et al (eds): Harrison's Principles of Internal Medicine, 15th ed. New York, McGraw-Hill, 2001, p 681

Burrows RF, Kelton JG: Fetal thrombocytopenia and its relation to maternal thrombocytopenia. N Engl J Med 329:1463, 1993a

Burrows RF, Kelton JG: Pregnancy in patients with idiopathic thrombocytopenic purpura: Assessing the risks for the infant at delivery. Obstet Gynecol Surv 48:781, 1993b

Carache S, Scott J, Niebyl J, et al: Management of sickle cell disease in pregnant patients. Obstet Gynecol 55:407, 1980

Carr S, Dixon D, Star J, et al: Intrauterine therapy for homozygous α-thalassemia. Obstet Gynecol 85:876, 1995

Casadevall N, Natataf J, Viron B, et al: Pure red-cell aplasia and antierythropoietin antibodies in patients treated with recombinant erythropoietin. N Engl J Med 346:469, 2002

Castro O, Hogue M, Brown BD: Pulmonary hypertension in sickle cell disease: Cardiac catheterization results and survival. Blood 101:4, 2003

Cavenee MR, Cox SM, Mason R, et al: Erythropoietin in pregnancies complicated by pyelonephritis. Obstet Gynecol 84:252, 1994

Centers for Disease Control and Prevention: Update: Newborn screening for sickle cell disease—California, Illinois, and New York, 1998. MMWR 49:729, 2000

Centers for Disease Control and Prevention: Availability of immune globulin intravenous for treatment of immune deficient patients—United States, 1997–1998. MMWR 48:159, 1999

Centers for Disease Control and Prevention: Recommendations for the use of folic acid to reduce the number of cases of spina bifida and other neural tube defects. MMWR 41 (RR-14), 1992

Centers for Disease Control and Prevention: Anemia during pregnancy in low income women—United States, 1987. MMWR 39:73, 1990

Centers for Disease Control and Prevention: CDC criteria for anemia in children and childbearing-aged women. MMWR 38:400, 1989

Chandler WL, Jelacic S, Boster DR, et al: Prothrombotic coagulation abnormalities preceding the hemolytic-uremic syndrome. N Engl J Med 346:23, 2002

Chatwani A, Bruder N, Shapiro T, et al: May–Hegglin anomaly: A rare case of maternal thrombocytopenia in pregnancy. Am J Obstet Gynecol 166:143, 1992

Cheng Y, Wong RSM, Soo YOY, et al: Initial treatment of immune thrombocytopenic purpura with high-dose dexamethasone. N Engl J Med 349:831, 2003

Clark AL, Gall SA: Clinical uses of intravenous immunoglobulin in pregnancy. Am J Obstet Gynecol 176:241, 1997

Conti M, Mari D, Conti E, et al: Pregnancy in women with different types of von Willebrand disease. Obstet Gynecol 68:282, 1986

Cortelazzo S, Finazzi G, Ruggeri M, et al: Hydroxyurea for patients with essential thrombocythemia and a high risk of thrombosis. N Engl J Med 332:1132, 1995

Cox JV, Steane E, Cunningham G, et al: Risk of alloimmunization and delayed hemolytic transfusion reactions in patients with sickle cell disease. Arch Intern Med 148:2485, 1988

Cox SM, Shelburne P, Mason R, et al: Mechanisms of hemolysis and anemia associated with acute antepartum pyelonephritis. Am J Obstet Gynecol 164:587, 1991

Cunningham FG, Pritchard JA: Prophylactic transfusions of normal red blood cells during pregnancies complicated by sickle cell hemoglobinopathies. Am J Obstet Gynecol 135:994, 1979

Cunningham FG, Cox SM, Harstad TW, et al: Chronic renal disease and pregnancy outcome. Am J Obstet Gynecol 163:453, 1990

Cunningham FG, Pritchard JA, Hankins GDV, et al: Idiopathic cardiomyopathy or compounding cardiovascular events. Obstet Gynecol 67:157, 1986

Cunningham FG, Pritchard JA, Mason R: Pregnancy and sickle hemoglobinopathy: Results with and without prophylactic transfusions. Obstet Gynecol 62:419, 1983

Daffos F, Capella-Pavlovsky M, Forestier F: Fetal blood sampling during pregnancy with the use of a needle guided by ultrasound: A study of 606 consecutive cases. Am J Obstet Gynecol 153:655, 1985

Daniloú J, Goral A, Paluszkiewicz P, et al: Successful treatment with recombinant factor VIIa for intractable bleeding at pelvic surgery. Obstet Gynecol 101:1172, 2003

Dashe JS, Ramin SM, Cunningham FG: The long-term consequences of thrombotic microangiopathy (thrombotic thrombocytopenic purpura and hemolytic uremic syndrome) in pregnancy. Obstet Gynecol 91:662, 1998

Daskalakis GJ, Papageorgiou IS, Antsaklis AJ, et al: Pregnancy and homozygous beta thalassaemia major. Br J Obstet Gynaecol 105:1028, 1998

David AL, Paterson-Brown S, Letsky EA: Factor XI deficiency presenting in pregnancy: Diagnosis and management. Br J Obstet Gynaecol 109:840, 2002

de Abood M, de Castillo Z, Guerrero F, et al: Effect of Depo-Provera® or Microgynon® on the painful crises of sickle cell anemia patients. Contraception 56:313, 1997

Deering SH, Landy HL, Tchabo N, et al: Hypodysfibrinogenemia during pregnancy, labor, and delivery. Obstet Gynecol 101:1092, 2003

De Gramont A, Krulik M, Debray J: Paroxymal nocturnal haemoglobinuria and pregnancy. Lancet 1:868, 1987

Delage R, Demers C, Cantin G, et al: Treatment of essential thrombocythemia during pregnancy with interferon-α. Obstet Gynecol 87:814, 1996

DeSimone J, Koshy M, Dorn L, et al: Maintenance of elevated fetal hemoglobin levels by decitabine during dose interval treatment of sickle cell anemia. Blood 99:3905, 2002

Dolan LM, Ryan M, Moohan J: Pyruvate kinase deficiency in pregnancy complicated by iron overload. Br J Obstet Gynaecol 109:844, 2002

Driscoll MC, Hurlet A, Styles L, et al: Stroke risk in siblings with sickle cell anemia. Blood 101:2401, 2003

Eddleman KA: Stem cells: What the obstetrician needs to know. Contemp Ob/Gyn 43:141, 1998

Edwards RZ, Rijhsinghani A: Dysfibrinogenemia and placental abruption. Obstet Gynecol 95:1043, 2000

Egerman RS, Witlin AG, Friedman SA, et al: Thrombotic thrombocytopenic purpura and hemolytic uremic syndrome in pregnancy: Review of 11 cases. Am J Obstet Gynecol 195:950, 1996

Eichhorn RF, Buurke EJ, Blok P, et al: Sickle cell-like crisis and bone marrow necrosis associated with parvovirus B19 infection and heterozygosity for haemoglobins S and E. J Intern Med 245:103, 1999

Eliyahu S, Shalev E: A successful pregnancy after bone marrow transplantation for severe aplastic anaemia with pretransplant conditioning of total lymph-node irradiation and cyclophosphamide. Br J Haematol 86:649, 1994

El-Shafei AM, Dhaliwal JK, Sandhu AK: Pregnancy in sickle cell disease in Bahrain. Br J Obstet Gynaecol 99:101, 1992

Elstein D, Granovsky-Grisaru S, Rabinowitz R, et al: Use of enzyme replacement therapy for Gaucher disease during pregnancy. Am J Obstet Gynecol 177:1509, 1997

Eskandari N, Feldman N, Greenspoon JS: Factor VII deficiency in pregnancy treated with recombinant factor VIIa. Obstet Gynecol 99:935, 2002

Fadel HE, Krauss JS: Factor VII deficiency and pregnancy. Obstet Gynecol 73:453, 1989

Fayyad AM, Brummitt DR, Barker HF, et al: May-Hegglin anomaly: The role of aspirin in the treatment of this rare platelet disorder in pregnancy. Br J Obstet Gynaecol 109:223, 2002

Fucharoen S, Winichagoon P: Clinical and hematologic aspects of hemoglobin E beta-thalassemia. Curr Opin Hematol 7:106, 2000

Fujimori K, Ohto H, Honda S, et al: Antepartum diagnosis of fetal intracranial hemorrhage due to maternal Bernard–Soulier syndrome. Obstet Gynecol 94:817, 1999

Funai EF, Klein SA, Lockwood CJ: Successful pregnancy outcome in a patient with both congenital hypofibrinogenemia and protein S deficiency. Obstet Gynecol 90:858, 1997

Furlan M, Robles R, Galbusera M, et al: Von Willebrand factor–cleaving protease in thrombotic thrombocytopenic purpura and the hemolytic-uremic syndrome. N Engl J Med 339:1578, 1998

Galvani DW, Jayakumar KS, Jordan A, et al: Antenatal testing for haemoglobinopathies [letter]. Br J Haematol 108:198, 2000

Gandhi SK, Powers JC, Nomeir A-M, et al: The pathogenesis of acute pulmonary edema associated with hypertension. N Engl J Med 344:17, 2000

Garratty G, Leger RM, Arndt PA: Severe immune hemolytic anemia associated with prophylactic use of cefotetan in obstetric and gynecologic procedures. Am J Obstet Gynecol 181:103, 1999

Garratty G: Severe reactions associated with transfusion of patients with sickle cell disease. Transfusion 37:357, 1997

Gasser C, Gautier E, Steck A, et al: Haemolytisch-uramisch Syndrome: Bilaterale Nierenrindennekrosen bei akuten erworbenin haemolytischen Anamien. Schweiz Med Wochenschr 85:905, 1955

Gehlbach DL, Morgenstern LL: Antenatal screening for thalassemia minor. Obstet Gynecol 71:801, 1988

George JN, Woolf SH, Raskob GE, et al: Idiopathic thrombocytopenic purpura: A practice guideline developed by explicit methods for The American Society of Hematology. Blood 88:3, 1996

George JV: Platelets. Lancet 355:1531, 2000

Ghidini A, Korker VL: Severe pyruvate kinase deficiency anemia. A case report. J Reprod Med 43:713, 1998

Gilsanz F, Vega MA, Gomez-Castillo E, et al: Fetal anaemia due to pyruvate kinase deficiency. Arch Dis Child 69:523, 1993

Gladwin MT, Sachdev V, Jison ML, et al: Pulmonary hypertension as a risk factor for death in patients with sickle cell disease. N Engl J Med 350:886, 2004

Glantz JC, Roberts DJ: Pregnancy complicated by thrombocytopenia secondary to human immunodeficiency virus infection. Obstet Gynecol 83:825, 1994

Godeau B, Chevret S, Varet B, et al: Intravenous immunoglobulin or high-dose methylprednisolone, with or without oral prednisone, for adults with untreated severe autoimmune thrombocytopenic purpura: A randomized, multicenter trial. Lancet 359:23, 2002

Goldenberg RL, Tamura T, DuBard M, et al: Plasma ferritin and pregnancy outcome. Am J Obstet Gynecol 175:1356, 1996

Goodnough LT, Monk TG, Andriole GL: Erythropoietin therapy. N Engl J Med 336:933, 1997

Granovsky-Grisaru S, Aboulafia Y, Diamant YZ, et al: Gynecologic and obstetric aspects of Gaucher's disease: A survey of 53 patients. Am J Obstet Gynecol 172:1284, 1995

Greene MF, Frigoletto FD Jr, Claster SZ, et al: Pregnancy and paroxysmal nocturnal hemoglobinuria: Report of a case and review of the literature. Obstet Gynecol Surv 38:591, 1983

Greer IA, Lowe GDO, Walker JJ, et al: Haemorrhagic problems in obstetrics and gynaecology in patients with congenital coagulopathies. Br J Obstet Gynaecol 98:909, 1991

Griesshammer M, Grunewald M, Michiels JJ: Acquired thrombophilia in pregnancy: essential thrombocythemia. Semin Thromb Hemost 29:205, 2003

Guy GP, Baxi LV, Hurlet-Jensen A, et al: An unusual complication in a gravida with factor IX deficiency: Case report with review of the literature. Obstet Gynecol 80:502, 1992

Hallak M, Sharon A-S, Diukman R, et al: Supplementing iron intravenously in pregnancy: A way to avoid blood transfusions. J Reprod Med 42:99, 1997

Handin RI: Disorders of the platelet and vessel wall. In Braunwald E, Fauci AS, Kasper DL, et al (eds): Harrison's Principles of Internal Medicine, 15th ed. New York, McGraw-Hill, 2001, p 747

Hayward CPM, Sutton DMC, Carter WH, et al: Treatment outcomes in patients with adult thrombotic thrombocytopenic purpura–hemolytic uremic syndrome. Arch Intern Med 154:982, 1994

Hillmen P, Hall C, Marsh JC, et al: Effect of eculizumab on hemolysis and transfusion requirements in patients with paroxysmal nocturnal hemoglobinuria. N Engl J Med 350:552, 2004

Hillmen P, Lewis SM, Bessler M, et al: Natural history of paroxysmal nocturnal hemoglobinuria. N Engl J Med 333:1253, 1995

Holthe MR, Staff AC, Berge LN, et al: Differences in platelet activation between preeclamptic, normotensive pregnant and nonpregnant women. Am J Obstet Gynecol 190:1128, 2004

Howard RJ, Tuck SM, Pearson TC: Pregnancy in sickle cell disease in the UK: Results of a multicentre survey of the effect of prophylactic blood transfusion on maternal and fetal outcome. Br J Obstet Gynaecol 102:947, 1995

Hsia YE: Detection and prevention of important α-thalassemia variants. Semin Perinatol 15:35, 1991

Hsieh FJ, Chang FM, Ko TM, et al: The antenatal blood gas and acid–base status of normal fetuses and hydropic fetuses with Bart hemoglobinopathy. Obstet Gynecol 74:722, 1989

Hsu HW, Belfort MA, Vernino S, et al: Postpartum thrombotic thrombocytopenic purpura complicated by Budd–Chiari syndrome. Obstet Gynecol 85:839, 1995

Hurst D, Little B, Kleman KM, et al: Anemia and hemoglobinopathies in Southeast Asian refugee children. J Pediatr 102:692, 1983

Jaegtvik S, Husebekk A, Aune B, et al: Neonatal alloimmune thrombocytopenia due to anti-HPA 1a antibodies; the level of maternal antibodies predicts the severity of thrombocytopenia in the newborn. Br J Obstet Gynaecol 107:691, 2000

Kadir RA, Economides DL, Braithwaite J, et al: The obstetric experience of carriers of haemophilia. Br J Obstet Gynaecol 104:803, 1997

Kadir RA, Lee CA, Sabin CA, et al: Pregnancy in women with von Willebrand's disease or factor XI deficiency. Br J Obstet Gynaecol 105:314, 1998

Kadyrov M, Kosanke G, Kingdom J, et al: Increased fetoplacental angiogenesis during first trimester in anaemic women. Lancet 352:1747, 1998

Kahra K, Draganov B, Sund S, et al: Postpartum renal failure: A complex case with probable coexistence of hemolysis, elevated liver enzymes, low platelet count, and hemolytic uremic syndrome. Obstet Gynecol 92:698, 1998

Kanavakis E, Vrettou C, Palmer G, et al: Preimplantation genetic diagnosis in 10 couples at risk for transmitting beta-thalassaemia major: Clinical experience including the initiation of six singleton pregnancies. Prenat Diagn 19:1217, 1999

Kaplan C, Daffos F, Forestier F, et al: Fetal platelet counts in thrombocytopenic pregnancy. Lancet 336:979, 1990

Kihm AJ, Kong Y, Hong W, et al: An abundant erythroid protein that stabilizes free a haemoglobin. Nature 417:758, 2002

Klebanoff MA, Shiono PH, Selby JV, et al: Anemia and spontaneous preterm birth. Am J Obstet Gynecol 164:59, 1991

Konje JC, Murphy P, de Chazal R, et al: Severe factor X deficiency and successful pregnancy. Br J Obstet Gynaecol 101:910, 1994

Koshy M, Burd L, Wallace D, et al: Prophylactic red-cell transfusions in pregnant patients with sickle cell disease: A randomized cooperative study. N Engl J Med 319:1447, 1988

Kumar RM, Rizk DEE, Khuranna A: β-thalassemia major and successful pregnancy. J Reprod Med 42:294, 1997

Lam YH, Tang MHY, Lee CP, et al: Prenatal ultrasonographic prediction of homozygous type 1 α-thalassemia at 12 to 13 weeks of gestation. Am J Obstet Gynecol 180:148, 1999

Lao TT, Lewinsky RM, Ohlsson A, et al: Factor XII deficiency and pregnancy. Obstet Gynecol 78:491, 1991

Letsky EA: Hematologic disorders. In Barron WM, Lindheimer MD (eds): Medical Disorders During Pregnancy, 3rd ed. St. Louis, Mosby, 2000, p 267

Levy GG, Nichols WC, Lian EC, et al: Mutations in a member of the ADAMTS gene family cause thrombotic thrombocytopenic purpura. Nature 413:488, 2001

Lieberman E, Ryan KJ, Monson RR, et al: Risk factors accounting for racial differences in the rate of premature birth. N Engl J Med 317:743, 1987

Lubetsky A, Schulman S, Varon D, et al: Safety and efficacy of continuous infusion of a combined factor VIII–von Willebrand factor (vWF) concentrate (Haemate-P) in patients with von Willebrand disease. Thromb Haemost 81:229, 1999

Maberry MC, Cunningham FG: Sickle cell hemoglobinopathies complicating pregnancy. In Williams Obstetrics, 19th ed. Norwalk, CT, Appleton & Lange, Suppl 2, August/September, 1993

Maberry MC, Mason RA, Cunningham FG, et al: Pregnancy complicated by hemoglobin CC and C–β-thalassemia disease. Obstet Gynecol 76:324, 1990

Maberry MC, Mason RA, Cunningham FG, et al: Pregnancy complicated by hereditary spherocytosis. Obstet Gynecol 79:735, 1992

Magann EF, Bass D, Chauhan SP, et al: Antepartum corticosteroids: Disease stabilization in patients with the syndrome of hemolysis, elevated liver enzymes, and low platelets (HELLP). Am J Obstet Gynecol 171:1148, 1994

Mannucci PM: Treatment of von Willebrand's Disease. N Engl J Med 351:683, 2004

Mannucci PM, Tuddenham EGD: The hemophilias—from royal genes to gene therapy. N Engl J Med 344:1773, 2001

Marsh J, Schrezenmeier H, Marin P, et al: Prospective randomized multicenter study comparing cyclosporin alone versus the combination of antithymocyte globulin and cyclosporin for treatment of patients with non-severe aplastic anemia: A report from the European Blood and Marrow Transplant (EBMT) Severe Aplastic Anaemia Working Party. Blood 93:2191, 1999

Miller DP, Kaye JA, Shea K, et al: Incidence of thrombotic thrombocytopenic purpura/hemolytic uremic syndrome. Epidemiology 15:208, 2004

Milner PF, Jones BR, Döbler J: Outcome of pregnancy in sickle cell anemia and sickle cell–hemoglobin C disease. Am J Obstet Gynecol 138:239, 1980

Moake JL: von Willebrand factor, ADAMTS-13, and thrombotic thrombocytopenic purpura. Semin Hematol 41:4, 2004

Moake JL: Moschcowitz, multimers, and metalloprotease. N Engl J Med 339:1629, 1998

Moake JL: Thrombotic microangiopathies. N Engl J Med 347:589, 2002

Mockenhaupt FP, Mandelkow J, Till H, et al: Reduced prevalence of *Plasmodium falciparum* infection and of concomitant anaemia in pregnant women with heterozygous G6PD deficiency. Trop Med Int Health 8:118, 2003

Monni G, Ibba RM, Lai R, et al: Early transabdominal chorionic villus sampling in couples at high genetic risk. Am J Obstet Gynecol 168:170, 1993

Moschcowitz E: An acute febrile pleiochromic anemia with hyaline thrombosis of the terminal arterioles and capillaries. Arch Intern Med 36:89, 1925

Mullaart RA, Van Dongen P, Gabreëls FJM, et al: Fetal periventricular hemorrhage in von Willebrand's disease: Short review and first case presentation. Am J Perinatol 8:190, 1991

Murphy JF, O'Riordan J, Newcombe RG, et al: Relation of haemoglobin levels in first and second trimester to outcome of pregnancy. Lancet 1:992, 1986

Musclow CE, Goldenberg H, Bernstein EP, et al: Factor XI deficiency presenting as hemarthrosis during pregnancy. Am J Obstet Gynecol 157:178, 1987

Olivieri NF, Brittenham GM, McLaren CE, et al: Long-term safety and effectiveness of iron-chelation therapy with deferiprone for thalassemia major. N Engl J Med 339:417, 1998

Orofino MG, Argiolu F, Sanna MA, et al: Fetal HLA typing in β thalassaemia: Implications for haemopoietic stem-cell transplantation. Lancet 362:41, 2003

Orringer EP, Casella JF, Ataga KI, et al: Purified poloxamer 188 for treatment of acute vaso-occlusive crisis of sickle cell disease. JAMA 286:2099, 2001

Packham CH: Pathogenesis and management of paroxysmal nocturnal haemoglobinuria. Blood Rev 12:1, 1998

Pajor A, Lehoczky D, Szakács Z: Pregnancy and hereditary spherocytosis. Arch Gynecol Obstet 253:37, 1993

Pawliuk R, Westerman KA, Fabry ME, et al: Correction of sickle cell disease in transgenic mouse models by gene therapy. Science 294:2368, 2001

Payne SD, Resnik R, Moore TR, et al: Maternal characteristics and risk of severe neonatal thrombocytopenia and intracranial hemorrhage in pregnancies complicated by autoimmune thrombocytopenia. Am J Obstet Gynecol 177:149, 1997

Peleg D, Hunter SK: Perinatal management of women with immune thrombocytopenic purpura: Survey of United States perinatologists. Am J Obstet Gynecol 180:645, 1999

Peng TC, Kickler TS, Bell WR, et al: Obstetric complications in a patient with Bernard–Soulier syndrome. Am J Obstet Gynecol 165:425, 1991

Platt OS, Brambilla DJ, Rosse WF, et al: Mortality in sickle cell disease—life expectancy and risk factors for early death. N Engl J Med 330:1639, 1994

Poddar D, Maude GH, Plant MJ, et al: Pregnancy in Jamaican women with homozygous sickle cell disease: Fetal and maternal outcome. Br J Obstet Gynaecol 93:927, 1986

Powars DR, Sandhu M, Niland-Weiss J, et al: Pregnancy in sickle cell disease. Obstet Gynecol 67:217, 1986

Powars D, Weidman JA, Odom-Maryon T, et al: Sickle cell chronic lung disease: Prior morbidity and the risk of pulmonary failure. Medicine 67:66, 1988

Pritchard JA, Cunningham FG, Mason RA: Coagulation changes in eclampsia: Their frequency and pathogenesis. Am J Obstet Gynecol 124:855, 1976

Pritchard JA, Scott DE: Iron demands in pregnancy. In Hallberg L, Harwerth HG, Vanotti A (eds): Iron Deficiency Pathogenesis, Clinical Aspects, Therapy. New York, Academic Press, 1970

Pritchard JA, Scott DE, Whalley PJ, et al: The effects of maternal sickle cell hemoglobinopathies and sickle cell trait on reproductive performance. Am J Obstet Gynecol 117:662, 1973

Provan D, Weatherall D: Red cells II: Acquired anaemias and polycythaemia. Lancet 355:1260, 2000

Raff JP, Dobson CE, Tsai HM: Transfusion of polymerized human haemoglobin in a patient with severe sickle cell anemia. Lancet 360:464, 2002

Ramahi AJ, Lewkow LM, Dombrowski MP, et al: Sickle cell E hemoglobinopathy and pregnancy. Obstet Gynecol 71:493, 1988

Randi ML, Barbone E, Rossi C, et al: Essential thrombocythemia and pregnancy. A report of six normal pregnancies in five untreated patients. Obstet Gynecol 83:915, 1994

Reece EA, Coustan DR, Hayslett JP, et al: Diabetic nephropathy: Pregnancy performance and fetomaternal outcome. Am J Obstet Gynecol 159:56, 1988

Rees DC, Olujohungbe AD, Parker NE, et al: Guidelines for the management of the acute painful crisis in sickle cell disease. Br J Haematol 120:744, 2003

Richmond JR, Koufogianis V, Benjamin A, et al: A case of thrombotic thrombocytopenic purpura and neonatal alloimmune thrombocytopenia in the same pregnancy. Br J Obstet Gynaecol 110:533, 2003

Rijhsinghani A, Wiechert RJ: Diamond–Blackfan anemia in pregnancy. Obstet Gynecol 83:827, 1994

Robson JS, Martin AM, Ruckley VA, et al: Irreversible postpartum renal failure. Q J Med 37:423, 1968

Rock GA, Shumak KH, Buskard NA, et al: Comparison of plasma exchange with plasma infusion in the treatment of thrombotic thrombocytopenic purpura. N Engl J Med 325:393, 1991

Rosenfeld S, Follmann D, Nunez O, et al: Antithymocyte globulin and cyclosporine for severe aplastic anemia: Association between hematologic response and long-term outcome. JAMA 289:1130, 2003

Rouse DJ, Owen J, Goldenberg RL: Routine maternal platelet count: An assessment of a technologically driven screening practice. Am J Obstet Gynecol 179:573, 1998

Ruch WA, Klein RL: Polycythemia vera and pregnancy. Obstet Gynecol 23:107, 1964

Sainio S, Järvenpää AL, Renlund M, et al: Thrombocytopenia in term infants: A population-based study. Obstet Gynecol 95:441, 2000

Samuels P, Bussel JB, Braitman LE, et al: Estimation of the risk of thrombocytopenia in the offspring of pregnant women with presumed immune thrombocytopenic purpura. N Engl J Med 323:229, 1990

Sanders JE, Hawley J, Levy W, et al: Pregnancies following high-dose cyclophosphamide with or without high-dose busulfan or total body irradiation and bone marrow transplantation. Blood 87:3045, 1996

Scanlon KS, Yip R, Schieve LA, et al: High and low hemoglobin levels during pregnancy: Differential risk for preterm birth and small for gestational age. Obstet Gynecol 96:741, 2000

Scaradavou A: HIV-related thrombocytopenia. Blood Rev 16:73, 2002

Schechter AN, Rodgers GP: Sickle cell anemia—basic research reaches the clinic. N Engl J Med 332:1372, 1995

Scott DE, Pritchard JA: Iron deficiency in healthy young college women. JAMA 199:147, 1967

Scott JR, Rote NS, Cruikshank DP: Antiplatelet antibodies and platelet counts in pregnancies complicated by autoimmune thrombocytopenic purpura. Am J Obstet Gynecol 145:932, 1983

Serjeant GR: Sickle-cell disease. Lancet 350:725, 1997

Shaaban AF, Flake AW: Fetal hematopoietic stem cell transplantation. Semin Perinatol 23:515, 1999

Sharma JB, Jain S, Mallika V, et al: A prospective, partially randomized study of pregnancy outcomes and hematologic responses to oral and intramuscular iron treatment in moderately anemic pregnant women. Am J Clin Nutr 79:116, 2004

Sheiner E, Levy A, Yerushalmi R, et al: Beta-thalassemia minor during pregnancy. Obstet Gynecol 103:1273, 2004

Shumak KH, Rock GA, Nair RC: Late relapses in patients successfully treated for thrombotic thrombocytopenic purpura. Ann Intern Med 122:569, 1995

Silver RM, Branch W, Scott JR: Maternal thrombocytopenia in pregnancy: Time for a reassessment. Am J Obstet Gynecol 173:479, 1995

Smith JA, Espeland M, Bellevue R, et al: Pregnancy in sickle cell disease: Experience of the cooperative study of sickle cell disease. Obstet Gynecol 87:199, 1996

Snyder TE, Lee LP, Lynch S: Pregnancy-associated hypoplastic anemia: A review. Obstet Gynecol Surv 46:264, 1991

Socié G, Stone JV, Wingard JR, et al: Long-term survival and late deaths after allogeneic bone marrow transplantation. N Engl J Med 341:14, 1999

Solal-Céligny P, Tertian G, Fernandez H, et al: Pregnancy and paroxysmal nocturnal hemoglobinuria. Arch Intern Med 148:593, 1988

Star J, Rosene K, Ferland J, et al: Flow cytometric analysis of platelet activation throughout normal gestation. Obstet Gynecol 90:562, 1997

Starksen NF, Bell WR, Kickler TS: Unexplained hemolytic anemia associated with pregnancy. Am J Obstet Gynecol 146:617, 1983

Steinberg MH: Management of sickle cell disease. N Engl J Med 340:1021, 1999

Steinberg MH, Barton F, Castro O, et al: Effect of hydroxyurea on mortality and morbidity in adult sickle cell anemia. JAMA 289:1645, 2003

Stuart MJ, Nagel RL: Sickle-cell disease. Lancet 364:1343, 2004

Sun PM, Wilburn W, Raynor D, et al: Sickle cell disease in pregnancy: Twenty years of experience at Grady Memorial Hospital, Atlanta, Georgia. Am J Obstet Gynecol 184:1127, 2001

Taylor DJ, Mallen C, McDougal N, et al: Effect of iron supplementation on serum ferritin levels during and after pregnancy. Br J Obstet Gynaecol 89:1011, 1982

Tefferi A, Soldberg LA, Silverstein MN: A clinical update in polycythemia vera and essential thrombocythemia. Am J Med 109:141, 2000

Trehan AK, Fergusson ILC: Congenital a fibrinogenaemia and successful pregnancy outcome. Case report. Br J Obstet Gynaecol 98:722, 1991

Tsai HM, Lian ECY: Antibodies to Von Willebrand factor–cleaving protease in acute thrombotic thrombocytopenic purpura. N Engl J Med 339:1585, 1998

Tuck SM, Studd JWW, White JM: Pregnancy in women with sickle cell trait. Br J Obstet Gynaecol 90:108, 1983

Urato AC, Repke JT: May–Hegglin anomaly: A case of vaginal delivery when both mother and fetus are affected. Am J Obstet Gynecol 179:260, 1998

van den Broek NR, Letsky EA, White SA, et al: Iron status in pregnant women: Which measurements are valid? Br J Haematol 103:817, 1998

Veille J, Hanson R: Left ventricular systolic and diastolic function in pregnant patients with sickle cell disease. Am J Obstet Gynecol 170:107, 1994

Vichinsky E: New therapies in sickle cell disease. Lancet 360:629, 2002

Vichinsky EP, Neumayr LD, Earles AN, et al: Causes and outcomes of the acute chest syndrome in sickle cell disease. N Engl J Med 342:1855, 2000

Viteri FE: The consequences of iron deficiency and anemia in pregnancy. Adv Exp Med Biol 352:127, 1994

Vora M, Gruslin A: Erythropoietin in obstetrics. Obstet Gynecol Surv 53:500, 1998

Walters MC, Patience M, Leisenring W, et al: Bone marrow transplantation for sickle-cell disease. N Engl J Med 335:369, 1996

Walters MC, Storb R, Patience M, et al: Impact of bone marrow transplantation for symptomatic sickle cell disease: An interim report. Blood 95:1918, 2000

Weatherall DJ: Single gene disorders or complex traits: Lessons from the thalassaemias and other monogenic diseases. BMJ 321:1117, 2000

Weatherall DJ, Provan AB: Red cell I: Inherited anaemias. Lancet 355:1169, 2000

Webert KE, Mittal R, Sigouin C, et al: A retrospective 11-year analysis of obstetric patients with idiopathic thrombocytopenic purpura. Blood 102:4306, 2003

Weiner CP: Thrombotic microangiopathy in pregnancy and the postpartum period. Semin Hematol 24:119, 1987

Weiner DL, Hibberd PL, Betit P, et al: Preliminary assessment of inhaled nitric oxide for acute vaso-occlusive crisis in pediatric patients with sickle cell disease. JAMA 289:1136, 2003

Xu K, Shi ZM, Veeck LL, et al: First unaffected pregnancy using preimplantation genetic diagnosis of sickle cell anemia. JAMA 281:1701, 1999

Yawata Y, Kanzaki A, Yawata A, et al: Characteristic features of the genotype and phenotype of hereditary spherocytosis in the Japanese population. Int J Hematol 71:118, 2000

Yeomans E, Lowe TW, Eigenbrodt EH, et al: Liver histopathologic findings in women with sickle cell disease given prophylactic transfusion during pregnancy. Am J Obstet Gynecol 163:958, 1990

Young NS, Maciejewski J: The pathophysiology of acquired aplastic anemia. N Engl J Med 336, 1365, 1997

Zamorano AF, Arnalich F, Sánchez-Casas E, et al: Levels of iron, vitamin B_{12}, folic acid and their binding proteins during pregnancy. Acta Haematol 74:92, 1985

52

Diabetes

The prevalence of diagnosed diabetes among American adults has increased by 40 percent in 10 years from 4.9 percent in 1990 to 6.9 percent in 1999 (Narayon and colleagues, 2003). Even worse is that it is estimated that this incidence will increase another 165 percent by 2050. To put this into perspective, the lifetime risk of diabetes in individuals born in 2000 is 33 percent for males and 39 percent for females! This increase primarily is due to type 2 diabetes, which is also referred to as *diabesity*, because of the strong relationship with the current epidemic of obesity in the United States and other countries (Gale, 2003; Mokdad and colleagues, 2003). Other aspects of adverse effects of obesity on health and pregnancy outcome are discussed in Chapter 43.

The increasing prevalence of type 2 diabetes in general, and in younger people in particular, has led to an increasing number of pregnancies with this complication (Feig and Palda, 2002; Ferrara and colleagues, 2004). Many women found to have gestational diabetes are likely to have type 2 diabetes that has previously gone undiagnosed (Feig and Palda, 2002). Indeed, the incidence of diabetes complicating pregnancy has increased about 40 percent between 1989 and 2002 (Martin and colleagues, 2003).

There is keen interest in events that precede diabetes, which includes the *mini-environment of the uterus,* where it is believed that early imprinting can have effects later in life (Saudek, 2002). For example, in utero exposure to maternal hyperglycemia leads to fetal hyperinsulinemia, causing an increase in fetal fat cells, which leads to obesity and insulin resistance in childhood (Feig and Palda, 2002). This in turn leads to impaired glucose tolerance and diabetes in adulthood. Thus, a cycle of fetal exposure to diabetes leading to childhood obesity and glucose intolerance is set in motion. This sequence has been reported in Pima Indians as well as a heterogeneous Chicago population (Silverman and colleagues, 1995).

CLASSIFICATION

Diabetes is now classified based on the pathogenic processes involved (Powers, 2001). Absolute insulin deficiency characterizes type 1 diabetes, whereas defective insulin secretion or insulin resistance characterizes type 2 diabetes (Table 52–1). The terms insulin-dependent diabetes mellitus (IDDM) and noninsulin-dependent diabetes mellitus (NIDDM) are no longer used. Age is also no longer used in classification, because β-cell destruction can occur at any age; most commonly, onset is before age 30, but in 5 to 10 percent of affected individuals, onset is after 30 years of age. Type 2 diabetes, although most typical with increasing age, also occurs in obese adolescents.

Diabetes is the most common medical complication of pregnancy. Women can be separated into those who were known to have diabetes before pregnancy—*pregestational* or *overt*, and those diagnosed during pregnancy—*gestational*. In 2002, slightly more than 131,000 American women had pregnancies complicated by diabetes, representing 3.3 percent of all live births (Martin and colleagues, 2003). More than 90 percent of these women had gestational diabetes.

CLASSIFICATION DURING PREGNANCY. Table 52–2 shows a classification recommended by the American College of Obstetricians and Gynecologists in 1986. This was replaced in 1994 because, according to the College, "a single classification based on the presence or absence of good maternal metabolic control and the presence or absence of maternal diabetic vasculopathy is more helpful." In the 1986 classification, women diagnosed with gestational diabetes are subdivided according to their degree of glycemia. Specifically, those with fasting hyperglycemia, which is defined as 105 mg/dL or greater, are placed into class A_2. About 15 percent of women with gestational diabetes exhibit fasting hyperglycemia (Sheffield and co-workers, 1999). Women in classes B to H, corresponding to the White classification (1978), have overt diabetes antedating pregnancy. The White system emphasizes that end-organ derangements, especially involving the eyes, kidneys, and heart, have significant effects on pregnancy outcome.

DIAGNOSIS OF OVERT DIABETES DURING PREGNANCY. Women with high plasma glucose levels, glucosuria, and ketoacidosis present no problem in diagnosis.

TABLE 52–1 Etiological Classification of Diabetes Mellitus

Type 1 A	Immune-mediated β-cell destruction
Type 1 B	Idiopathic β-cell destruction
Type 2	May range from predominantly insulin resistance to predominantly an insulin secretory defect with insulin resistance
Genetic mutations in β-cell function	
Genetic defects in insulin action	
Genetic syndromes—Down, Klinefelter, Turner	
Diseases of the exocrine pancreas—e.g., pancreatitis, cystic fibrosis	
Endocrinopathies—e.g., Cushing syndrome, pheochromocytoma, others	
Drug or chemical induced—e.g., glucocorticosteroids, thiazides, β-adrenergic agonists, others	
Infections—e.g., congenital rubella, cytomegalovirus, coxsackievirus	

Adapted from Powers, 2001.

TABLE 52–2 Classification of Diabetes Complicating Pregnancy

Class	Onset	Fasting Plasma Glucose	2-hour Postprandial Glucose	Therapy
A₁	Gestational	< 105 mg/dL	< 120 mg/dL	Diet
A₂	Gestational	> 105 mg/dL	> 120 mg/dL	Insulin

Class	Age of Onset (yr)	Duration (yr)	Vascular Disease	Therapy
B	Over 20	< 10	None	Insulin
C	10 to 19	10 to 19	None	Insulin
D	Before 10	> 20	Benign retinopathy	Insulin
F	Any	Any	Nephropathy[a]	Insulin
R	Any	Any	Proliferative retinopathy	Insulin
H	Any	Any	Heart	Insulin

[a]When diagnosed during pregnancy: 500 mg or more proteinuria per 24 hours measured before 20 weeks' gestation.

Similarly, women with a random plasma glucose level greater than 200 mg/dL plus classic signs and symptoms such as polydipsia, polyuria, and unexplained weight loss or a fasting glucose exceeding 125 mg/dL are considered to have overt diabetes by the American Diabetes Association (2004). The new diagnostic cutoff value for overt diabetes of a fasting plasma glucose of 126 mg/dL or higher is used because data indicate the risk of retinopathy rises dramatically at that fasting level. Women at the opposite end of the spectrum, or those with only minimal metabolic derangement, may be difficult to identify. The likelihood of impaired carbohydrate metabolism is increased appreciably in women who have a strong familial history of diabetes, have given birth to large infants, demonstrate persistent glucosuria, or have unexplained fetal losses.

Reducing substances are commonly found in the urine of pregnant women. Commercially available dipsticks may be used to identify glucosuria while avoiding a positive reaction from lactose. Even then, glucosuria most often does not reflect impaired glucose tolerance, but rather augmented glomerular filtration (see Chap. 5, p. 138). Nonetheless, the detection of glucosuria during pregnancy warrants further investigation (Gribble and coauthors, 1995).

DETECTION OF GESTATIONAL DIABETES. Gestational diabetes is defined as carbohydrate intolerance of variable severity with onset or first recognition during pregnancy. This definition applies whether or not insulin is used for treatment. Undoubtedly, some women with gestational diabetes have previously unrecognized overt diabetes. Sheffield and co-workers (1999) studied outcomes in 1190 diabetic women delivered at Parkland Hospital between 1991 and 1995. They found that women with fasting hyperglycemia diagnosed before 24 weeks had pregnancy outcomes similar to those for women in classes B through FR. Thus, fasting hyperglycemia early in pregnancy likely represents overt diabetes. Bartha and colleagues (2000) also found that women diagnosed to have gestational diabetes early in pregnancy are a high-risk subgroup.

Screening. Despite more than 30 years of research, there is no consensus regarding the optimal approach to screening for gestational diabetes. The major issues include whether universal or selective screening should be used and which plasma glucose level after a 50-g glucose test threshold is best to identify women at risk for gestational diabetes (Bonomo and colleagues, 1998; Danilenko-Dixon and colleagues, 1999).

Since 1980, there have been four international workshop–conferences on gestational diabetes, and participants have attempted to provide consensus statements on screening (Metzger and Coustan, 1998). At the most recent 1997 workshop, prior recommendations for *universal screening* were changed to *selective screening* using the guidelines shown in Table 52–3. It was recommended that screening for gestational diabetes should be performed between 24 and 28 weeks in those women not known to have glucose intolerance earlier in pregnancy. This evaluation is usually done in two steps. In the two-step procedure, a 50-g oral glucose challenge test is followed by a diagnostic 100-g oral glucose tolerance test if results exceed a predetermined plasma glucose concentration.

Plasma glucose level is measured 1 hour after a 50-g glucose load without regard to the time of day or time of last meal. A value of 140 mg/dL (7.8 mmol/L) or higher identifies 80 percent of all women with gestational diabetes. Using a value of 130 mg/dL (7.2 mmol/L) or higher increases the yield to more than 90 percent; however, 20 to 25 percent of women have positive test results compared with 14 to 18 percent when the 140 mg/dL or greater cutoff value is used. Recommended criteria for interpretation of the 100-g diagnostic glucose tolerance test are shown in Table 52–4. Pennison and Egerman (2001) compared perinatal outcomes in 130 women with gestational diabetes diagnosed using the National Diabetes Data Group Criteria with those of 43 women diagnosed using the Carpenter and Coustan criteria and concluded that the benefits of the latter were unclear.

In two different surveys, more than 95 percent of obstetricians and residency programs were found to screen all pregnant women for gestational diabetes, usually between 25

TABLE 52-3 **Fourth International Workshop–Conference on Gestational Diabetes: Recommended Screening Strategy Based on Risk Assessment for Detecting Gestational Diabetes**

Low Risk
    Blood glucose testing not routinely required if all of the following characteristics are present:
        Member of an ethnic group with a low prevalence of gestational diabetes
        No known diabetes in first-degree relatives
        Age less than 25 years
        Weight normal before pregnancy
        No history of abnormal glucose metabolism
        No history of poor obstetrical outcome

Average Risk
    Perform blood glucose testing at 24–28 weeks using one of the following:
        Average risk—women of Hispanic, African, Native American, South or East Asian origins
        High risk—women with marked obesity, strong family history of type 2 diabetes, prior
            gestational diabetes, or glucosuria

High Risk
    Perform blood glucose testing as soon as feasible. If gestational diabetes is not diagnosed,
        blood glucose testing should be repeated at 24–28 weeks or at any time a patient has
        symptoms or signs suggestive of hyperglycemia

From Metzger and Coustan (1998), with permission.

and 29 weeks (Gabbe and co-workers, 1998; Owen and colleagues, 1995). The American College of Obstetricians and Gynecologists (2001) has concluded that it may be appropriate to use selective screening in some clinical settings and universal screening in others. Brody and colleagues (2003) reviewed the evidence and concluded that it is insufficient to recommend for or against routine screening.

The day-to-day reproducibility of the 50-g screening test has also been tested (Espinosa de los Monteros and co-workers, 1993). Although 90 percent of normal results were reproducible the next day, only 83 percent of abnormal test results were reproducible. Murphy and colleagues (1994) studied the accuracy and precision of reflectance photometers (Accu-Check III) for screening. Use of this glucometer required redefining the circumstances for testing as well as threshold values for abnormal results. It seems best to avoid these devices for screening.

TABLE 52-4 **American College of Obstetricians and Gynecologists 2001 Criteria for Diagnosis of Gestational Diabetes Using the 100-g Oral Glucose Tolerance Test**

	Plasma/Serum Carpenter and Coustan		National Diabetes Plasma Data Group	
Status	mg/dL	mmol/L	mg/dL	mmol/L
Fasting	95	5.3	105	5.8
1 hr	180	10.0	190	10.6
2 hr	155	8.6	165	9.2
3 hr	140	7.8	145	8.0

Adapted from the American College of Obstetricians and Gynecologists (2001), with permission.

Diagnosis. There is not international agreement as to the optimal glucose tolerance test for the definitive diagnosis of gestational diabetes. The World Health Organization (1985) has recommended the 75-g 2-hour oral glucose tolerance test, and this approach is often used in Europe (Weiss and colleagues, 1998). In the United States, the *100-g 3-hour oral glucose tolerance test* performed after an overnight fast remains the standard (American College of Obstetricians and Gynecologists, 2001). Even so, Catalano and co-workers (1993) found that the 100-g 3-hour test was not reproducible in 25 percent of women when repeated 1 week after the initial test. They attributed this to increased norepinephrine-mediated gluconeogenesis from maternal stress at initial testing.

GESTATIONAL DIABETES

Use of the word *gestational* implies that diabetes is induced by pregnancy, perhaps from exaggerated physiological changes in glucose metabolism (see Chap. 5, p. 127). An alternative explanation is that gestational diabetes is type 2 diabetes unmasked or discovered during pregnancy. For example, Harris (1988) found that the prevalence of undiagnosed glucose intolerance in nonpregnant women between the ages of 20 and 44 years was virtually identical to the prevalence of gestational diabetes. Catalano and colleagues (1999) compared longitudinal changes in insulin sensitivity, insulin response, and endogenous glucose production in women with normal glucose tolerance with those in women with gestational diabetes. They found that women with gestational diabetes had abnormalities in glucose metabolism that are hallmarks of type 2 diabetes.

Use of the diagnostic term *gestational diabetes* has been encouraged to communicate the need for increased surveillance and to convince women of the need for further testing postpartum. The likelihood of fetal death with appropriately treated gestational diabetes has been found no different than in the general population (Metzger and Coustan, 1998). The most important perinatal concern is excessive fetal growth, which may result in birth trauma. **More than half of women with gestational diabetes ultimately develop overt diabetes in the ensuing 20 years, and there is mounting evidence for long-range complications that include obesity and diabetes in their offspring.**

MATERNAL AND FETAL EFFECTS. There has been an important shift in focus concerning adverse fetal consequences of gestational diabetes. Importantly, unlike in women with overt diabetes, fetal anomalies are not increased (Sheffield and colleagues, 2002). Similarly, whereas pregnancies in women with overt diabetes are at greater risk for fetal death, this danger is not apparent for those who have only postprandial hyperglycemia (namely, class A_1 gestational diabetes) (Lucas and co-workers, 1993; Sheffield and colleagues, 2002).

In contrast, gestational diabetes with elevated fasting glucose class A_2 has been associated with unexplained stillbirth similar to overt diabetes (Johnstone and colleagues, 1990). The American Diabetes Association (1999a) has concluded that fasting hyperglycemia defined as more than 105 mg/dL may be associated with an increased risk of fetal death during the last 4 to 8 weeks of gestation. Adverse maternal effects include an increased frequency of hypertension and cesarean delivery.

Macrosomia. Fetal macrosomia is defined by the American College of Obstetricians and Gynecologists (2000) as infants whose birthweight exceeds 4500 g. The perinatal focal point is avoidance of difficult delivery due to macrosomia, with concomitant birth trauma associated with shoulder dystocia. Except for the brain, most fetal organs are affected by the macrosomia that commonly characterizes the fetus of a diabetic woman. Macrosomic infants of diabetic mothers are described as anthropometrically different from other large-for-gestational age infants (McFarland and associates, 2000; Modanlou and colleagues, 1982). Specifically, those whose mothers are diabetic have excessive fat deposition on the shoulders and trunk, which predisposes to shoulder dystocia (Fig. 52–1). Similarly, Bernstein and Catalano (1994) reported that fat infants of diabetic women more often required cesarean delivery for cephalopelvic disproportion. Fortunately, shoulder dystocia is uncommon, even in women with gestational diabetes. For example, Magee and colleagues (1993) diagnosed shoulder dystocia in 3 percent of women with class A_1 diabetes. None of their infants sustained brachial plexus injuries.

Macrosomia is compatible with the long-recognized association between fetal hyperinsulinemia resulting from maternal hyperglycemia, which in turn stimulates excessive

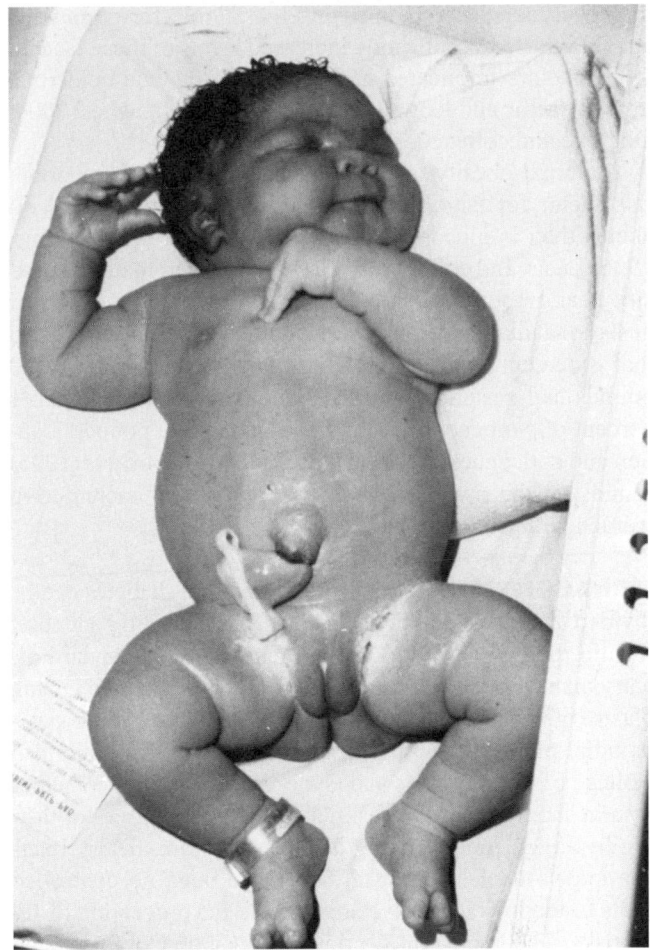

FIGURE 52–1. This macrosomic infant who weighed 6050 g was born to a woman with gestational diabetes.

somatic growth. Similarly, neonatal hyperinsulinemia may provoke hypoglycemia within minutes of birth. The incidence varies greatly depending on the threshold used to define significant neonatal hypoglycemia. According to the American Diabetes Association (1995), values less than 35 mg/dL at term are abnormal. A lower value is considered abnormal in preterm infants, because glycogen stores have not reached term levels. Magee and co-workers (1993) reported that 4 percent of infants of women with gestational diabetes required intravenous glucose therapy for hypoglycemia.

There is extensive evidence that insulin and the insulin-like growth factors I (IGF-I) and II (IGF-II) play a role in the regulation of fetal growth (see Chap. 38, p. 895). Insulin is secreted by fetal pancreatic β-cells primarily during the second half of gestation and is believed to stimulate somatic growth and adiposity. These growth factors, which structurally are proinsulin-like polypeptides, are produced by virtually all fetal organs and are potent stimulators of cell differentiation and division. Verhaeghe and co-workers (1993) measured cord IGFs and insulin (C-peptide) concentrations throughout gestation in women without diabetes and found that levels correlated with birthweight. Large-for-gestational age infants had significantly increased levels of these factors. Other factors implicated in macrosomia include epidermal growth factor and leptin (Loukovaara and colleagues, 2004; Okereke and colleagues, 2002).

Maternal obesity is an independent and more important risk factor for large infants in women with gestational diabetes than is glucose intolerance (Leonardi and Bottoms, 1996; Lucas and colleagues, 1993). Moreover, maternal obesity is an important confounding factor in the diagnosis of gestational diabetes. Johnson and colleagues (1987) reported that 8 percent of 588 women who weighed more than 250 pounds had gestational diabetes compared with less than 1 percent of women who weighed less than 200 pounds. Landon and colleagues (1994) and Zhang and co-workers (1995) found that the risk of gestational diabetes was increased in women with truncal obesity.

MANAGEMENT. Women with gestational diabetes can be divided into two functional classes using fasting glucose. Insulin therapy is usually recommended when standard dietary management does not consistently maintain the fasting plasma glucose at less than 95 mg/dL or the 2-hour postprandial plasma glucose at less than 120 mg/dL (American College of Obstetricians and Gynecologists, 2001). Whether insulin should be used in women with lesser degrees of fasting hyperglycemia (105 mg/dL or less before dietary intervention) is unclear because there have been no controlled trials to identify ideal glycemia targets for prevention of fetal risks. The Fourth International Workshop Conference on Gestational Diabetes (Metzger and Coustan, 1998), however, recommended that maternal capillary glucose levels be kept at 95 mg/dL or less in the fasting state.

Diet. There are no available data comparing diet therapy alone with no treatment in women with gestational diabetes (American College of Obstetricians and Gynecologists, 2001). The American Diabetes Association (2000) has recommended nutritional counseling with individualization based on height and weight and a diet that provides an average of 30 kcal/kg/d based on prepregnant body weight for nonobese women. Although the association acknowledges that the most appropriate diet for women with gestational diabetes has not been established, it has suggested that obese women with a body mass index greater than 30 kg/m² may benefit from a 30- to 33-percent caloric restriction. This should be monitored with weekly tests for ketonuria, because maternal ketonemia has been linked with impaired psychomotor development in the offspring (Rizzo and colleagues, 1995).

Exercise. This is known to be important in nonpregnant patients. The American College of Obstetricians and Gynecologists (2001) reviewed three randomized trials of exercise in women with gestational diabetes (Avery, 1997; Bung, 1993;

Jovanovic-Peterson, 1989, and all their colleagues). They suggested that exercise improved cardiorespiratory fitness without improving pregnancy outcome. Dempsey and colleagues (2004) found that physical activity during pregnancy reduced the risk of gestational diabetes. Brankston and associates (2004) reported that resistance exercise helped avoid insulin therapy in overweight women with gestational diabetes.

Plasma Glucose Control. Postprandial surveillance for gestational diabetes has been shown to be superior to preprandial surveillance, and because glycemic control is significantly improved, less neonatal hypoglycemia, less macrosomia, and fewer cesarean deliveries for dystocia result. These conclusions have been challenged, however, because women in these studies had fasting glucose values that were consistent with overt diabetes.

Prophylactic insulin given to decrease complications related to macrosomia in class A₁ diabetic women with fasting euglycemia has not been proved beneficial. Langer and co-authors (1994) reviewed 23 reports from 1979 through 1993 and found that none demonstrated improved perinatal outcomes related to any management approach, including prophylactic insulin treatment. There have been only three randomized studies to date (Garner, 1997; Nordlander, 1989; Thompson, 1990, and all their colleagues). Intensive therapy had little effect on birthweight, birth trauma, operative delivery, or neonatal complications.

Langer and colleagues (1994) managed 1145 women with gestational diabetes using an "intensified" approach guided by glucometer measurements seven times each day. Goals included fasting glucose levels between 60 and 90 mg/dL and postprandial levels less than 120 mg/dL. In contrast, another 1316 women in the "conventional" management group had the same glucose control goals, but used blood glucose test strips in place of glucometers. Women in both groups underwent glucose surveillance for an average of 12 weeks, and a similar number of glucose measurements were performed in each study group—approximately 350 per patient. Although mean glucose values were not different between the two management groups, macrosomia, cesarean delivery, and shoulder dystocia were significantly reduced in women managed intensively.

Kjos and colleagues (2001) randomized 98 women with gestational diabetes and fasting plasma glucose levels between 105 and 120 mg/dL to empirical insulin therapy versus insulin given only if the fetal abdominal circumference measured with ultrasonography indicated macrosomia. This allowed 93 percent of the women in the ultrasound group to be managed without insulin. There were no differences in macrosomia or birth trauma between the two groups.

INSULIN. Most practitioners—93 percent according to Owen and colleagues (1995)—initiate insulin therapy in women with gestational diabetes if fasting glucose levels exceeding 105 mg/dL persist despite diet therapy. At Parkland Hospital, this is accomplished in a specialized outpatient clinic, but occasionally hospitalization is necessary.

Experts differ in their approach to insulin therapy in gestational diabetes. A total dose of 20 to 30 units given once daily, before breakfast, is commonly used to initiate therapy. The total dose is usually divided into two thirds intermediate-acting insulin and a third short-acting insulin. Once therapy has been initiated, it must be recognized that the level of glycemia control to reduce fetal and neonatal complications has not been established. DeVeciana and colleagues (1995) studied 66 pregnant women with class A_2 diabetes in whom insulin was initiated for fasting hyperglycemia. The women were randomized to glucose surveillance using either preprandial or 1-hour postprandial capillary blood glucose concentrations measured by glucometer. Postprandial surveillance was shown to be superior in that blood glucose control was significantly improved and was associated with fewer cases of neonatal hypoglycemia (3 versus 21 percent), less macrosomia (12 versus 42 percent), and fewer cesarean deliveries for dystocia (24 versus 39 percent).

ORAL HYPOGLYCEMIC AGENTS. The American College of Obstetricians and Gynecologists (2001) has not recommended these agents during pregnancy. Langer and colleagues (2000) randomized 257 women with gestational diabetes to insulin or *glyburide* therapy. Near normoglycemic levels were achieved equally well with either regimen. There were no apparent neonatal complications attributable to the glyburide. In a follow-up report, Conway and co-workers (2004) found that women with fasting glucose levels greater than 110 mg/dL did not adequately respond to glyburide therapy.

Metformin, which has been used as a treatment for infertility due to polycystic ovarian disease, also has been reported to reduce the incidence of gestational diabetes in women who use the drug throughout pregnancy (Glueck and colleagues, 2004). Even so, it is usually recommended that metformin be discontinued once pregnancy is diagnosed (Harborne and colleagues, 2003).

OBSTETRICAL MANAGEMENT. In general, women with gestational diabetes who do not require insulin seldom require early delivery or other interventions. Whether elective cesarean delivery is used to avoid brachial plexus injuries in macrosomic infants is an important issue. The American College of Obstetricians and Gynecologists (2001) has suggested that cesarean delivery should be considered in women with a sonographically estimated fetal weight of 4500 grams or more. Gonen and colleagues (2000) retrospectively analyzed the effects of a policy of elective cesarean delivery when estimated fetal weight exceeded 4500 grams in a general obstetrical population of more than 16,000 deliveries. **Elective cesarean delivery had no significant effect on the incidence of brachial plexus injury.**

Elective induction to prevent shoulder dystocia in women with sonographically diagnosed fetal macrosomia, compared with spontaneous labor, is also controversial. Conway and Langer (1996) found that elective delivery reduced the rate of shoulder dystocia from 2.2 to 0.7 percent. In contrast, Combs and colleagues (1993b) and Adasheck and associates (1996) found no advantages.

There is no consensus regarding whether antepartum fetal testing is necessary, and if so, when to begin such testing in women without severe hyperglycemia (American College of Obstetricians and Gynecologists, 2001; Metzger and Coustan, 1998). This is based on the low risk of fetal death. Women who require insulin therapy for fasting hyperglycemia, however, typically undergo fetal testing and are managed as if they had overt diabetes.

POSTPARTUM CONSEQUENCES. The Fourth International Workshop–Conference on Gestational Diabetes recommended that women diagnosed with gestational diabetes undergo evaluation with a 75-g oral glucose tolerance test at 6 to 12 weeks after delivery (Table 52–5). Women whose 75-g test is normal should be reassessed at a minimum of 3-year intervals (American Diabetes Association, 2003). Although postpartum follow-up of women diagnosed with gestational diabetes was recommended throughout the 1990s, reports on compliance have only recently become available. Kaufmann and colleagues (1999) measured physician and patient compliance rates during a 5-year postpartum follow-up period in 66 such women. Compliance was poor, and only 30 percent of the women reported receiving a yearly 2-hour glucose tolerance test, although the risk of developing diabetes was 60 percent in others tested on an annual basis.

TABLE 52–5 Postpartum Evaluation for Glucose Intolerance in Women with Gestational Diabetes

Normal	Impaired Fasting Glucose or Impaired Glucose Tolerance	Diabetes Mellitus
Fasting < 110 mg/dL 2 hr < 140 mg/dL[a]	110–125 mg/dL 2 hr ≥ 140–199 mg/dL[a]	≥ 126 mg/dL 2 hr ≥ 200 mg/dL[a]

[a] Requires a 75-g oral glucose load.
From the American Diabetes Association (2003), with permission.

These recommendations for postpartum follow-up are based on the 50-percent likelihood of women with gestational diabetes developing overt diabetes within 20 years (O'Sullivan, 1982). If fasting hyperglycemia develops during pregnancy, diabetes is more likely to persist postpartum. For example, in women with fasting glucose levels of 105 to 130 mg/mL, 43 percent were found to be overtly diabetic (Metzger and colleagues, 1985). When fasting glucose exceeded 130 mg/dL during pregnancy, 86 percent of women became overtly diabetic. Insulin therapy during pregnancy, and especially before 24 weeks, is a powerful predictor of diabetes after the pregnancy (Dacus and co-workers, 1994; Greenberg and colleagues, 1995).

Women with gestational diabetes are also at risk for cardiovascular complications associated with abnormal serum lipids, hypertension, and abdominal obesity—the *metabolic syndrome* (see Chapter 43, p. 1009). Pallardo and colleagues (1999) evaluated cardiovascular disease risk factors in 788 women with gestational diabetes 3 to 6 months postpartum. They found that the degree of postpartum glucose intolerance was significantly associated with these risk factors.

Recurrence of gestational diabetes in subsequent pregnancies was documented in 20 of 30 women reported by Philipson and Super (1989). Obese women were more likely to have impaired glucose intolerance in subsequent pregnancies. Thus, lifestyle behavioral changes, including weight control and exercise between pregnancies, likely would prevent recurrence of gestational diabetes as well as modify onset and severity of type 2 diabetes later in life (Pan and associates, 1997). Interestingly, perinatal outcomes in women with previous gestational diabetes but with normal glucose tolerance tests during a subsequent pregnancy were not improved with regard to birthweight, macrosomia, route of delivery, and neonatal complications (Danilenko-Dixon and colleagues, 2000). Finally, Lu and colleagues (2002) found that women *without* gestational diabetes in their first pregnancy were unlikely to have gestational diabetes when screened in a second pregnancy.

Contraception. Low-dose hormonal contraceptives may be used safely by women with recent gestational diabetes (see Chap. 32, p. 731). The rate of subsequent diabetes in oral contraceptive users is not significantly different than in those who did not use hormonal contraception (Kjos and colleagues, 1990a).

GESTATIONAL DIABETES AT PARKLAND HOSPITAL. Universal glucose screening was not performed at Parkland until 1997. Selective screening was instead based on many of the risk factors previously enumerated. For these women, a standard 50-g oral glucose tolerance test was performed between 24 and 28 weeks without regard to recent meal status. The criteria shown in Table 52–4 were used. Women diagnosed to have class A_1 gestational diabetes were seen weekly in a specific clinic designed to provide dietary

counseling. Fasting plasma glucose measurements were obtained at each visit. Women without other complications such as hypertension or postterm gestation were permitted to enter spontaneous labor, and antepartum testing was not used. Women diagnosed to have class A_2 gestational diabetes were managed as overt diabetics, as described later.

In January 1997, universal screening for gestational diabetes was performed between 24 and 28 weeks using a standard 1-hour, 50-g oral glucose challenge test. All obstetrical management practices previously used during selective screening were continued. The practice of universal screening doubled the number of women tested in one year from approximately 4300 to 8200. Importantly, universal screening for gestational diabetes did not increase or decrease obstetrical outcomes attributable to this diagnosis (Casey and colleagues, 1999).

PREGESTATIONAL (OVERT) DIABETES

Unlike gestational diabetes, it is unquestioned that overt diabetes has a significant impact on pregnancy outcome. The embryo, the fetus, and the mother can experience serious complications directly attributable to diabetes. The likelihood of successful outcomes with overt diabetes is related somewhat to the degree of glycemic control, but more importantly, to the degree of any underlying cardiovascular or renal disease. Therefore, as the alphabetic classification shown in Table 52–2 worsens, the likelihood of good pregnancy outcomes lessen.

Hanson and Persson (1993) prospectively chronicled the effects of overt diabetes on pregnancy outcomes in Sweden. Their unique analysis included all deliveries between 1983 and 1985, during which period 491 insulin-dependent women in classes B or worse were identified. Their outcomes were compared with those of 279,000 pregnancies in women without diabetes (Table 52–6). Pregnant women with diabetes experienced significantly worse pregnancy outcomes. As shown in Table 52–7, women in the more advanced classes of overt diabetes increasingly developed preeclampsia. Indeed,

TABLE 52–6 Outcomes in Percent of Pregnancies Complicated by Type 1 Diabetes Compared with National Data in Sweden (1983–1985)

Factor	Type 1 Diabetes (n = 491)	National Data (n = 279,000)	P value
Preeclampsia	21	5	< .001
Preterm birth	25	6	< .001
Macrosomia	20	4	< .001
Growth restriction	1	3	< .05
Stillbirths	2	0.4	< .01
Perinatal mortality	3	0.7	< .0001

Adapted from Hanson and Persson (1993), with permission.

TABLE 52–7 Frequency of Preeclampsia in Pregnancies Complicated by Type 1 Diabetes in Sweden (1983–1985)

White Classification	Pregnancies n (%)	Preeclampsia %
B	164 (33)	12
C	129 (26)	22
D	172 (35)	23
F	26 (5)	54
Total	491 (100)	21

From Hanson and Persson (1993), with permission.

54 percent of those in class F with diabetic nephropathy developed this complication. Similar results have been reported for France and the Netherlands (Diabetes Pregnancy Group, France, 2004; Evers and co-workers, 2004).

FETAL EFFECTS. Improved fetal surveillance, neonatal intensive care, and maternal metabolic control have reduced perinatal losses with overt diabetes to 2 to 4 percent. These rates have seemingly plateaued because the two major causes of fetal death—congenital malformations and unexplained fetal death—remain unchanged by medical intervention (Garner, 1995b).

Abortion. Several studies have shown that first-trimester abortion is associated with poor glycemic control (Greene and colleagues, 1989; Mills and associates, 1988a). In 215 women with type 1 diabetes enrolled for prenatal care by Rosenn and colleagues (1994) before 9 weeks, 24 percent had miscarriages. Only women with type 1 diabetes and initial glycohemoglobin A_1 concentrations greater than 12 percent or persistent preprandial glucose concentrations greater than 120 mg/dL were at increased risk for abortion.

Preterm Delivery. Pregestational diabetes is a risk factor for preterm birth. The Maternal–Fetal Medicine Units Network of the National Institute of Child Health and Human Development analyzed pregnancy outcomes in 461 women with pregestational diabetes (Sibai and colleagues, 2000). Investigators reported that 9 percent of these women spontaneously delivered before 35 weeks compared with 4.5 percent of nondiabetic women. Moreover, 7 percent of diabetic women compared with 2 percent of normal women underwent indicated preterm delivery.

Malformations. The incidence of major malformations in women with type 1 diabetes is about 5 percent (Sheffield and co-workers, 2002). Fetal anomalies account for almost half of perinatal deaths in diabetic pregnancies. Importantly, diabetes is not associated with increased risk for fetal chromosomal abnormalities. Specific types of anomalies linked to maternal diabetes and their relative incidence are summarized in Table 52–8.

TABLE 52–8 Congenital Malformations in Infants of Women with Overt Diabetes

Anomaly	Ratios of Incidence[a]
Caudal regression	252
Situs inversus	84
Spina bifida, hydrocephaly, or other central nervous system defect	2
Anencephaly	3
Heart anomalies	4
Anal/rectal atresia	3
Renal anomalies	5
Agenesis	4
Cystic kidney	4
Duplex ureter	23

[a]Ratio of incidence is in comparison with the general population. Heart anomalies include transposition of the great vessels, ventricular septal defect, and atrial septal defect.
Adapted from Mills and colleagues (1979) and the American Diabetes Association (1995), with permission.

It is generally believed that the increased risk of severe malformations is the consequence of poorly controlled diabetes both preconceptionally as well as early in pregnancy. Miller and co-workers (1981) suggested that women with lower glycosylated hemoglobin values at conception had fewer fetuses with anomalies compared with women with abnormally high values. Mills and colleagues (1988b) from the Diabetes in Early Pregnancy Study did not totally corroborate these findings. More than 600 women with diabetes were enrolled in this investigation, and the investigators concluded that a normal glycosylated hemoglobin distribution did not guarantee that diabetes-associated anomalies would be avoided. Conversely, not all women with an elevated level had poor outcomes. Investigators observed that women in whom periconceptional glucose control was optimized had a 5-percent fetal malformation rate compared with 9 percent in the group who presented after organogenesis was complete. Ray and colleagues (2001) performed a meta-analysis of seven studies addressing preconceptional care published between 1970 and 2000. They concluded that such care was associated with a lower risk of congenital anomalies and this was associated with lower glycosylated hemoglobin values.

Unexplained Fetal Demise. Stillbirths without identifiable causes are a phenomenon found in pregnancies complicated by pregestational diabetes. They are declared "unexplained" because no factors such as obvious placental insufficiency, abruption, fetal growth restriction, or oligohydramnios are apparent. These infants are typically large-for-gestational age and die before labor, usually at 35 weeks or later (Garner, 1995a). In the Swedish study shown in Table 52–6, the incidence of unexplained stillbirths was 1 percent.

Investigations using cordocentesis have provided new insights into acid–base metabolism in fetuses of diabetic mothers. Salvesen and colleagues (1992, 1993) reported decreased fetal pH and increased P_{CO_2}, lactate, and erythropoietin in diabetic pregnancies. Such findings lend credence to the long-held hypothesis that hyperglycemia-mediated chronic aberrations in transport of oxygen and fetal metabolites may account for unexplained fetal deaths (Pedersen, 1977).

Between 1984 and 1993, Richey and co-workers (1995) were at the bedside in two pregnancies at Parkland Hospital where otherwise unexplained fetal deaths were seemingly in progress. In both of these rare clinical instances, the fetus was macrosomic and there was excessive amnionic fluid. Both fetuses were acidemic before labor, and both placentae were hydropic due to edema of the chorionic villi. These features were linked to maternal hyperglycemia, and it was hypothesized that osmotically induced villous edema led to impaired fetal oxygen transport.

Explicable stillbirths due to placental insufficiency also occur with increased frequency in women with overt diabetes, usually in association with severe preeclampsia. This, in turn, is increased in women with advanced diabetes and vascular complications. Similarly, ketoacidosis can cause fetal death.

Hydramnios. Although diabetic pregnancies are often complicated by hydramnios, the cause is unclear. A likely, although unproven explanation is fetal polyuria resulting from fetal hyperglycemia (see Chap. 21, p. 528). In a study from Parkland Hospital, Dashe and co-authors (2000) found that the amnionic fluid index parallels the amnionic fluid glucose level among women with diabetes. This finding suggests that the hydramnios associated with diabetes is a result of increased amnionic fluid glucose concentration.

NEONATAL EFFECTS. Before tests of fetal health and maturity became available, preterm delivery was deliberately effected to avoid unexplained fetal deaths. Although this practice has been abandoned, there is still an increased frequency of preterm delivery in women with diabetes (Sibai and co-workers, 2000). Most preterm births are associated with advanced diabetes and superimposed preeclampsia.

Modern neonatal care has largely eliminated neonatal deaths due to immaturity. Cnattingius and colleagues (1994) reported only one infant death due to immaturity in 914 singleton births to B to F diabetic women. Conversely, neonatal *morbidity* due to preterm birth continues to be a serious consequence. Indeed, some of the morbidities in these infants are considered to be uniquely related to aberrations in maternal glucose metabolism.

Respiratory Distress. Conventional obstetrical teaching through the late 1980s generally held that fetal lung maturation was delayed in diabetic pregnancies. Thus, these infants were at increased risk for respiratory distress (Gluck and Kulovich, 1973). Subsequent observations have challenged this concept, and gestational age rather than overt diabetes is likely the most significant factor associated with neonatal

respiratory distress (Berkowitz and colleagues, 1996; Kjos and colleagues, 1990b).

Hypoglycemia. A rapid decrease in plasma glucose concentration after delivery is characteristic of the infant of a diabetic mother. This is attributed to hyperplasia of the fetal β-islet cells induced by chronic maternal hyperglycemia. Taylor and associates (2002) found that neonatal hypoglycemia (blood glucose less than 45 mg/dL before the second feeding) was related to maternal blood glucose exceeding 145 mg/dL during labor. Prompt recognition and treatment of the hypoglycemic infant has minimized sequelae.

Hypocalcemia. Defined as serum calcium concentration less than 7 mg/dL, hypocalcemia is one of the major metabolic derangements in infants of diabetic mothers. Its cause has not been explained. Theories include aberrations in magnesium–calcium economy, asphyxia, and preterm birth (Cruikshank and co-workers, 1980). In the randomized study by DeMarini and colleagues (1994), 137 pregnant women with type 1 diabetes were managed with strict versus customary glucose control to ascertain the effect of maternal glucose levels on neonatal hypocalcemia. Almost a third of infants in the customary control group developed hypocalcemia compared with only 18 percent of those in the strict control group. Gestational age and preeclampsia were also implicated.

Hyperbilirubinemia. The pathogenesis of hyperbilirubinemia in infants of diabetic mothers is uncertain. Factors implicated have included preterm birth and polycythemia with hemolysis. Venous hematocrits of 65 to 70 volume percent have been observed in as many as 40 percent of these infants (Salvesen and associates, 1992). Renal vein thrombosis is also reported to result from polycythemia.

Cardiac Hypertrophy. Infants of diabetic pregnancies may have hypertrophic cardiomyopathy that occasionally progresses to congestive heart failure (Gandhi and co-authors, 1995; Reller and Kaplan, 1988). These infants typically have macrosomia, and fetal hyperinsulinemia has been implicated in the pathogenesis of heart disease. Way (1979) reported that the cardiomyopathy generally disappears by 6 months of age.

Long-Term Cognitive Development. Rizzo and colleagues (1995) used multiple tests of intelligence and psychomotor development to assess 196 children of diabetic women up to 9 years of age. They concluded that maternal diabetes had a negligible impact on cognitive development.

Inheritance of Diabetes. Offspring born to women with overt diabetes have a low risk of developing type 1 diabetes; the incidence ranges from 1 to 3 percent (Garner, 1995b). The risk is 6 percent if only the father has overt diabetes. If both parents have type 1 diabetes, the risk is 20 percent. McKinney and colleagues (1999) studied 196 children with

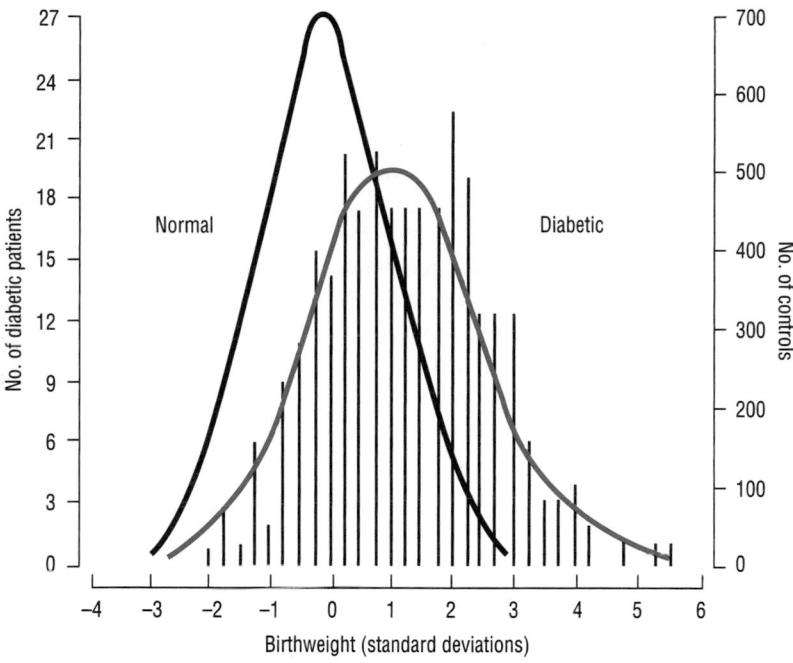

FIGURE 52–2. Distribution of birthweights (standard deviation from the normal mean for gestational age) for 280 infants of diabetic mothers and 3959 infants of normal mothers. (From Bradley and coworkers, 1988, with permission.)

type 1 diabetes and found that older maternal age and maternal type 1 diabetes are important risk factors. Plagemann and colleagues (2002) have implicated breast feeding by diabetic mothers in the genesis of childhood diabetes.

Altered Fetal Growth. The incidence of macrosomia rises significantly when mean maternal blood glucose concentrations exceed 130 mg/dL (Willman and co-authors, 1986). Some authors have objected to classification of these infants as either "macrosomic" or "nonmacrosomic," because this ignores the observation that virtually all are *growth promoted*

(Bradley and associates, 1988). This is discussed in Chapter 38 (see p. 904). As shown in Figure 52–2, the birthweight distribution of infants of diabetic mothers is skewed toward consistently heavier birthweights compared with that of normal pregnancies.

Landon and co-workers (1989) performed serial ultrasound examinations during the third trimester in 79 women with diabetes and observed that excessive fetal abdominal circumference growth was detectable by 32 weeks (Fig. 52–3). This suggests that excessive weight accrues primarily during the third trimester. Keller and colleagues (1990), however,

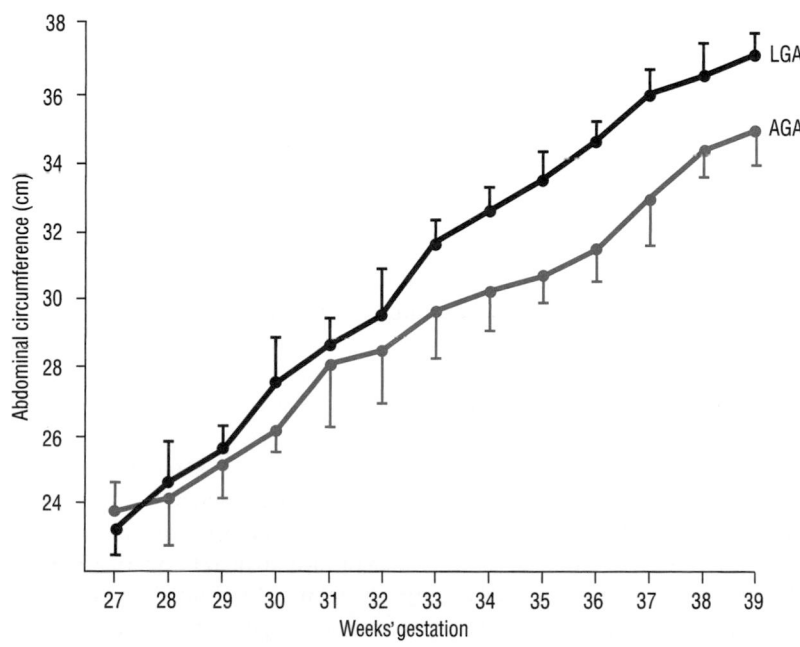

FIGURE 52–3. Comparison of abdominal circumference growth curve for appropriate-for-gestational age (AGA) and large-for-gestational age (LGA) fetuses of diabetic mothers. Growth is accelerated at 32 weeks in the LGA group. (From Landon and co-workers, 1989, with permission.)

reported that some macrosomic fetuses can be recognized before 24 weeks. Similarly, Rey and co-authors (1999) and Raychaudhuri and Maresh (2000) concluded that macrosomia was determined primarily by early pregnancy diabetes control.

MATERNAL EFFECTS. Diabetes and pregnancy interact significantly such that maternal welfare can be seriously jeopardized. With the possible exception of diabetic retinopathy, however, the long-term course of diabetes is not affected by pregnancy.

Even though uncommon, maternal deaths in women with diabetes are still increased 10-fold (Cousins, 1987). They most often result from ketoacidosis, hypertension, preeclampsia, and pyelonephritis. The rare woman with coronary artery disease (class H diabetes) is at particular risk. Pombar and colleagues (1995) reviewed 17 such women and reported that only half survived pregnancy (see Chapter 44, p. 1036).

Diabetic Nephropathy. This is the leading cause of end-stage renal disease in the United States (see Chapter 48, p. 1102). The incidence of renal failure is nearly 30 percent in individuals with type 1 diabetes and ranges from 4 to 20 percent in those with type 2 diabetes. Importantly, the incidence of nephropathy in individuals with type 1 diabetes declined during the 1980s, presumably from improved glucose control. The Diabetes Control and Complications Trial (2002) found that there was a 25-percent decrease in nephropathy for each 10-percent decrease in hemoglobin A_{1C} levels.

Clinically detectable nephropathy in type 1 disease begins with microalbuminuria—30 to 300 mg/24 h of albumin. This may manifest as early as 5 years after the onset of diabetes (Nathan, 1993). After another 5 to 10 years, overt proteinuria (more than 300 mg/24 h of albumin) develops in patients destined to have end-stage renal disease. Hypertension invariably develops during this period, and renal failure ensues typically in the next 5 to 10 years.

Approximately 5 percent of pregnant women with diabetes are class F (Hanson and Persson, 1993; Siddiqi and associates, 1991). These women have significantly increased preeclampsia and indicated preterm delivery. As shown in Table 52–7, approximately 50 percent develop preeclampsia. Combs and associates (1993a) measured urinary protein excretion before 20 weeks in 311 diabetic women. In those with proteinuria that exceeded 500 mg/day, 38 percent developed preeclampsia. They also found that women with microproteinuria defined as 190 to 500 mg/day had an increased risk of preeclampsia. Conversely, in an analysis of 460 women with classes B through F-R diabetes, How and colleagues (2004) did not find an increased rate of preeclampsia in women with microproteinuria. Chronic hypertension with diabetic nephropathy increased the risk of preeclampsia to 60 percent. Gordon and associates (1996) reported that

chronic renal insufficiency as well as heavy proteinuria before 20 weeks were predictive of preeclampsia.

There appear to be no long-term sequelae of pregnancy on diabetic nephropathy. Chaturvedi and associates (1995) studied long-term complications in 1358 European women with type 1 diabetes, of whom 582 had been pregnant. The incidence of either micro- or microalbuminuria was not increased in women with prior pregnancies compared with that of nulliparas. Still, renal involvement carries a guarded long-term prognosis for these women. Miodovnik and colleagues (1996) found that a fourth of 46 women with class F diabetes developed end-stage renal failure at a mean of 6 years after pregnancy. This is not dissimilar from women with other severe nephropathies (see Chapter 48, p. 1104).

Diabetic Retinopathy. Retinal vasculopathy is a highly specific complication of both type 1 and type 2 diabetes. Its prevalence is related to duration of diabetes. After 20 years, nearly all patients with type 1 diabetes and more than 60 percent of those with type 2 diabetes have some degree of retinopathy (American Diabetes Association, 1999b). In the United States, diabetic retinopathy is the most important cause of visual impairment in persons younger than 60 years of age. Frank (2004) has recently reviewed this complication of diabetes.

The first and most common visible lesions are small microaneurysms followed by blot hemorrhages when erythrocytes escape from the aneurysms. These areas leak serous fluid that forms hard exudates. These features are termed *benign* or *background* or *nonproliferative retinopathy* and would place a pregnant woman in class D regardless of the duration of diabetes (see Table 52–2). With increasingly severe retinopathy, the abnormal vessels of background eye disease become occluded, leading to retinal ischemia with infarctions that appear as *cotton wool exudates*. These are considered *preproliferative retinopathy*. In response to ischemia, there is neovascularization on the retinal surface and out into the vitreous cavity, and these obscure vision when there is hemorrhage. Laser photo coagulation as shown in Figure 52–4 before hemorrhage reduces the rate of progression of visual loss and blindness by half. The procedure is done as indicated during pregnancy for affected women. Siddiqi and colleagues (1991) reported that almost a third of 175 insulin-dependent pregnant women examined by 10 weeks had background retinal changes (class D) or proliferative retinopathy (class R).

The effects of pregnancy on proliferative retinopathy are controversial (Garner, 1995b). It has been long taught that this complication is a rare example of pregnancy having long-term adverse effects. Klein and co-workers (1990) concluded that pregnancy worsened proliferative retinopathy. Conversely, Chaturvedi and co-authors (1995) found an equivalent prevalence of background and proliferative retinopathy in multiparas and nulliparous women. Most authors agree that laser photocoagulation and good glycemic control during

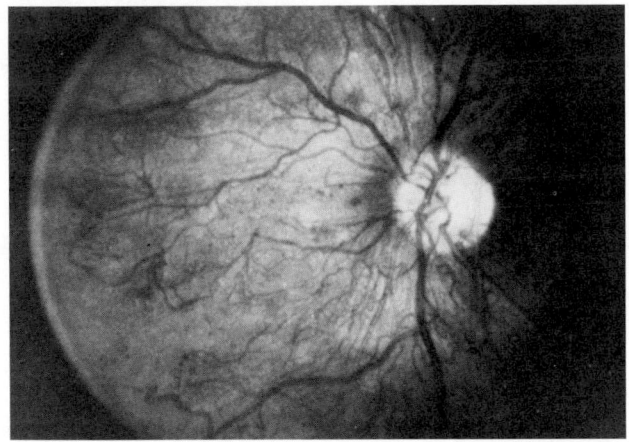

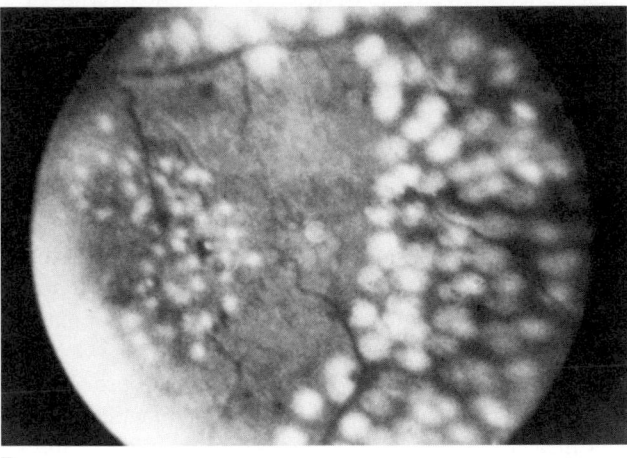

FIGURE 52–4. Retinal photographs from a 30-year-old diabetic woman. **A.** Optic nerve head showing severe proliferative retinopathy characterized by extensive networks of new vessels surrounding the optic disc. **B.** A portion of the acute photocoagulation full "scatter" pattern following argon laser treatment. (From Elman and colleagues, 1990, with permission.)

pregnancy minimize the potential for deleterious effects of pregnancy (Garner, 1995b).

Ironically, there are case reports that link "acute" rigorous metabolic control during pregnancy to acute worsening of retinopathy (Dahl-Jørgensen and colleagues, 1985; Van Ballegooie and associates, 1984). In a study of 201 women with retinopathy, McElvy and colleagues (2001) found that almost 30 percent suffered progression of eye disease during pregnancy despite intensive glucose control. That said, Wang and co-workers (1993) have observed that retinopathy worsened during the critical months of rigorous glucose control, but in the longer term, deterioration of eye disease slowed. In the report by McElvy and co-workers (2001), progression of retinopathy was associated with reduced fetal growth. Lauszus and colleagues (1998), however, reported that proliferative retinopathy, per se, did not worsen perinatal outcome.

In a preliminary report, Kitzmiller and colleagues (1999) implicated insulin lispro in the development of proliferative retinopathy during pregnancy. Conversely, Buchbinder and associates (2000) found no evidence that such therapy was linked to the development or progression of diabetic retinopathy in a study of 13 treated pregnant women.

Diabetic Neuropathy. Although uncommon, some pregnant women have peripheral symmetrical sensorimotor diabetic neuropathy. A form of this, known as *diabetic gastropathy*, is very troublesome in pregnancy because it causes nausea and vomiting, nutritional problems, and difficulty with glucose control. Treatment with metoclopramide and H_2-receptor antagonists is sometimes successful. *Hyperemesis gravidarum* is further discussed in Chapter 49 (see p. 1113).

Preeclampsia. Hypertension induced or exacerbated by pregnancy is the major complication that most often forces preterm delivery in diabetic women. According to Garner (1995b), the perinatal mortality rate is increased 20-fold for preeclamptic women with diabetes compared with those who remain normotensive. Special risk factors for preeclampsia include any vascular complications and preexisting proteinuria, with or without chronic hypertension. Sibai and colleagues (2000) reported the risk of preeclampsia to be 11 percent in class B, 22 percent in class C, 21 percent in class D, and 36 percent in classes F-R. Savvidou and colleagues (2002) described impaired vascular reactivity in pregnant women with type 1 diabetes that may make them more susceptible to the development of preeclampsia. Interestingly, the incidence of preeclampsia does not seem to be related to glucose control (Garner and co-authors, 1990). Management of preeclampsia is discussed in Chapter 34.

Ketoacidosis. Although ketoacidosis affects only about 1 percent of diabetic pregnancies, it remains one of the most serious complications (Garner, 1995b). Diabetic ketoacidosis may occur as a result of hyperemesis gravidarum, use of β-sympathomimetic drugs for tocolysis, infections, and use of corticosteroids to induce fetal lung maturation. The incidence of fetal loss is about 20 percent with ketoacidosis.

Kent and colleagues (1994) found that only half of young women with recurrent ketoacidosis had successful pregnancies compared with 95 percent of women without ketoacidosis. Noncompliance is a prominent factor, and ketoacidosis and poor compliance have long been considered prognostically bad signs in pregnancy (Pedersen and colleagues, 1974).

Infections. Almost all types of infections are increased in diabetic pregnancies. Stamler and co-authors (1990) reported that almost 80 percent of women with type 1 diabetes develop at least one episode of infection during pregnancy compared with 25 percent in those without diabetes. Common infections include candida vulvovaginitis, urinary infections, respiratory tract infections, and puerperal pelvic infections. Cousins

(1987) observed that antepartum pyelonephritis developed in 4 percent of women with type 1 diabetes compared with 1 percent in those without diabetes. Cousins also reported that renal infection was associated with increased preterm delivery. Fortunately, these latter infections can be minimized by screening for asymptomatic bacteriuria (see Chap. 48, p. 1095).

MANAGEMENT. The goals of management are tailored somewhat uniquely for pregnant women. Management preferably should begin before pregnancy and include specific goals during each trimester.

Preconception. To prevent early pregnancy loss as well as congenital malformations in infants of diabetic mothers, optimal medical care and patient education are recommended before conception. This is also discussed in Chapter 7. Unfortunately, unplanned pregnancies, thus preempting preconceptional care, continue to occur in approximately 60 percent of these women (Holing and co-authors, 1998). Thus, diabetic women frequently begin pregnancy with suboptimal glucose control (Casele and Laifer, 1998).

The American Diabetes Association (1999a) has defined optimal preconceptional glucose control using insulin to include self-monitored preprandial glucose levels of 70 to 100 mg/dL and postprandial values of less than 140 mg/dL and less than 120 mg/dL at 1 and 2 hours, respectively. Hemoglobin A_1 or A_{1c} measurement, which expresses an average of circulating glucose for the past 4 to 8 weeks, is useful to assess early metabolic control. Optimal preconceptional glycated hemoglobin values have been defined as those within or near the upper limit of normal for a specific laboratory or within three standard deviations of the normal mean (American Diabetes Association, 1999a). The most significant risk for malformations is with levels exceeding 10 percent (American College of Obstetricians and Gynecologists, 1994). Folate, 400 μg/day, is given periconceptionally and during early pregnancy to decrease the risk of neural-tube defects (Milunsky and co-workers, 1989).

First Trimester. Careful monitoring of glucose control is essential. For this reason, many clinicians hospitalize these women during early pregnancy to institute an individualized glucose control program and to provide education concerning the ensuing months of pregnancy. It also provides an opportunity to assess the extent of vascular complications of diabetes and to precisely establish gestational age.

Maternal glycemic control can usually be achieved with *multiple daily insulin injections* and adjustment of dietary intake. Oral hypoglycemic agents are not usually used because they may cause fetal hyperinsulinemia. Piacquadio and colleagues (1991) demonstrated increased rates of congenital malformations, especially ear defects, in infants of women treated during early pregnancy with oral hypoglycemic drugs (see p. 1175).

TABLE 52–9 Patient-Monitored Capillary Blood Glucose Goals During Pregnancy in Diabetic Women

Specimen	Blood Glucose (mg/dL)
Fasting	60–90 (3.3–5.0 mmol)
Premeal	60–105 (3.3–5.8 mmol)
Postprandial 1 hr	100–120 (5.5–6.7 mmol)
0200–0600 hr	60–120 (3.3–6.7 mmol)

Adapted from the American Diabetes Association (1995).

Subcutaneous insulin infusion by a calibrated pump may be used during pregnancy. It has both advantages and disadvantages, and as emphasized by Kitzmiller and associates (1985) and Leveno and colleagues (1988), any salutary pregnancy effects have yet to be determined. Patients who use an insulin pump must be highly motivated and compliant so as to minimize the risk of nocturnal hypoglycemia (Gabbe and Graves, 2003).

The goals of self-monitored capillary blood glucose control recommended during pregnancy are shown in Table 52–9. Self-monitoring of capillary glucose levels using glucometers is strongly recommended as this involves the woman in her own care. Parretti and colleagues (2001) measured maternal capillary glucose responses to meals throughout normal pregnancies to better characterize glucose goals for management of diabetic women (Table 52–10).

New technology under development may provide noninvasive glucose monitoring. Such an automatic and painless means to obtain blood glucose information would undoubtedly greatly facilitate patient compliance. Tamada and colleagues (1999) reported clinical results in nonpregnant diabetics with such a monitoring device (Cygnus, Inc., Redwood City, California). It extracts glucose through the skin using electrical potentials—a process known as iontophoresis.

TABLE 52–10 Diurnal Capillary Blood Glucose Values During the Third Trimester in 51 Normal Women

Time of Day	Blood Glucose Range of Values (mg/dL)
0800 hr	51–65
← Breakfast	
0900 hr	87–112
1000 hr	73–100
1200 hr	58–75
← Lunch	
1400 hr	77–102
2000 hr	59–73
← Dinner	
0400 hr	57–70

Approximate glucose levels based on the range of mean values ± SD between 28 and 38 weeks' gestation.
Adapted from Parretti and colleagues (2001), with permission.

It then measures glucose concentrations in the extracted sample. The device provides up to three glucose readings per hour and causes only transient mild skin irritation at the sensor site. These investigators found close agreement between noninvasive glucose measurements and those obtained by standard fingersticks.

The Committee on Maternal Nutrition of the National Research Council has recommended a total caloric intake of 30 to 35 kcal/kg of ideal body weight, given as three meals and three snacks daily (Garner, 1995b). An ideal dietary composition is 55 percent carbohydrate, 20 percent protein, and 25 percent fat with less than 10 percent saturated fat. There are no studies to support or refute these guidelines. Obese women may be managed with lower caloric intake as long as weight loss and ketonuria are avoided.

Euglycemia based on normal pregnancy blood glucose values is the goal in management of women with overt diabetes, but achieving this goal is not always possible. Thus, individualized programs are often necessary to avoid both excessive hyperglycemia as well as frequent episodes of hypoglycemia. Diabetes tends to be unstable in the first trimester, followed by a stable period, and then by an increase in insulin requirement after about 24 weeks (Steel and co-workers, 1994). This rise is due to the increased production of pregnancy hormones, which are insulin antagonists (see Chap. 3, p. 74 and Chap. 5, p. 127). The absolute increase in mean insulin requirement was 52 units in 237 women with type 1 diabetes, but there was wide variation (Steel and associates, 1994). The magnitude of increase was directly related to maternal weight and inversely related to the duration of diabetes.

Rosenn and colleagues (1995) assessed the impact of maternal hypoglycemia in 84 pregnant women with overt diabetes. Clinically significant hypoglycemia with glucometer values less than 35 mg/dL was documented in 70 percent of the women, with a peak incidence between 10 and 15 weeks. Almost 25 percent of these 84 women experienced unconsciousness, and 15 percent developed seizures as a result of hypoglycemia. These investigators recommended caution in attempting euglycemia in women with recurrent episodes of hypoglycemia.

We have reported that good pregnancy outcomes can be achieved in women with mean preprandial plasma glucose values up to 143 mg/dL (Leveno and associates, 1979). Interestingly, in women with diabetes who are not pregnant, the Diabetes Control and Complications Trial Research Group (1993) found that similar glucose values—intensive control was defined as mean values less than 155 mg/dL—delayed and slowed diabetic retinopathy, nephropathy, and neuropathy. Thus, women with overt diabetes who have glucose values considerably above those defined as normal both during and after pregnancy can expect good outcomes.

Second Trimester. Maternal serum alpha-fetoprotein concentration at 16 to 20 weeks is used in association with targeted ultrasound at 18 to 20 weeks in an attempt to detect neural-tube defects and other anomalies (American College of Obstetricians and Gynecologists, 1994). The program and its details are discussed in Chapter 12 (see p. 319). Maternal alpha-fetoprotein levels may be lower in diabetic pregnancies, and interpretation is altered accordingly (Martin and associates, 1990). Adjunctive ultrasonography is important; Albert and colleagues (1996) identified 72 percent of 29 fetal anomalies in 289 diabetic pregnancies.

Third Trimester and Delivery. In the woman with overt diabetes in the class B or C White classification, cesarean delivery has commonly been used to avoid traumatic birth of a large infant at or near term. In women with more advanced diabetes, especially those with vascular disease, the reduced likelihood of successfully inducing labor remote from term has also contributed appreciably to an increased cesarean rate. Labor induction may be attempted when the fetus is not excessively large and the cervix is considered favorable (see Chap. 22, p. 536). In the reports cited earlier with low perinatal mortality, the cesarean rate ranged from 50 to 80 percent (Gabbe, 1977; Kitzmiller, 1978; Leveno, 1979; Martin, 1987; Schneider, 1980, and all their associates). The cesarean delivery rate for women with overt diabetes has remained at about 80 percent for the past 25 years at Parkland Hospital.

It is important to considerably reduce or delete the dose of long-acting insulin given on the day of delivery. Regular insulin should be used to meet most or all of the insulin needs of the mother at this time, because insulin requirements typically drop markedly after delivery. We have found that constant insulin infusion by calibrated pump is most satisfactory (Table 52–11). During labor and after either cesarean or vaginal delivery, the woman should be hydrated adequately intravenously as well as given glucose in sufficient amounts to maintain normoglycemia. Capillary or plasma glucose levels should be checked frequently, and regular insulin should be administered accordingly. It is not unusual for the woman to require virtually no insulin for the first 24 hours or so and then for insulin requirements to fluctuate markedly during the next few days. Infection must be promptly detected and treated.

TABLE 52–11 **Low-Dose Insulin Infusion for the Diabetic Woman During the Intrapartum Period**

Blood Glucose (mg/dL)	Insulin Dosage[a] (U/hr)	Intravenous Fluids (125 mL/hr)
< 100	0	D$_5$ lactated Ringer
100–140	1.0	D$_5$ lactated Ringer
141–180	1.5	Normal saline
181–220	2.0	Normal saline
> 220	2.5	Normal saline

[a] Dilution is 25 U of regular insulin in 250 mL of normal saline with 25 mL flushed through line administrated intravenously. A fingerstick glucose test is performed every 1 to 2 hours. The insulin pump and intravenous solution are adjusted accordingly.

CONTRACEPTION

There is no single contraceptive method appropriate for all women with diabetes. Because of the risk of vascular disease, hormonal contraceptives may be problematic. Many clinicians are reluctant to recommend intrauterine devices in women with diabetes, primarily because of a possible increased risk of pelvic infections. All of these concerns, along with available options, are discussed in Chapter 32. For many of these reasons, and because of frequent associated morbidity with chronic diseases, many overtly diabetic women elect puerperal sterilization as discussed in Chapter 33. This option should be made readily available.

REFERENCES

Adashek JA, Lagrew DC, Iriye BK, et al: The influence of ultrasound examination at term on the rate of cesarean section. Am J Obstet Gynecol 174:328, 1996

Albert TJ, Landon MB, Wheller JJ, et al: Prenatal detection of fetal anomalies in pregnancies complicated by insulin-dependent diabetes mellitus. Am J Obstet Gynecol 174:1424, 1996

American College of Obstetricians and Gynecologists: Gestational diabetes. Practice Bulletin No. 30, September 2001

American College of Obstetricians and Gynecologists: Fetal macrosomia. Practice Bulletin No. 22, November 2000

American College of Obstetricians and Gynecologists: Diabetes and pregnancy. Technical Bulletin No. 200, December 1994

American College of Obstetricians and Gynecologists: Management of diabetes mellitus in pregnancy. Technical Bulletin No. 92, May 1986

American Diabetes Association: Report of the Expert Committee on the Diagnosis and Classification of Diabetes Mellitus. Diabetes Care 27(Suppl):5, 2004

American Diabetes Association: Gestational diabetes mellitus. Diabetes Care 26:S103, 2003

American Diabetes Association: Nutritional management during pregnancy in preexisting diabetes. In Medical Management of Pregnancy Complicated by Diabetes, 3rd ed. Alexandria, VA, American Diabetes Association, 2000, p 70

American Diabetes Association: Clinical practice recommendations, 1999. Diabetes Care 23:S10, 1999a

American Diabetes Association: Report of the Expert Committee on the Diagnosis and Classification of Diabetes Mellitus. Diabetes Care 22(Suppl 1):512, 1999b

American Diabetes Association: Medical Management of Pregnancy Complicated by Diabetes, 2nd ed. Jovanovic-Peterson L (ed). Alexandria, VA, American Diabetes Association, 1995

Avery MD, Leon AS, Kopher RA: Effects of a partially home-based exercise program for women with gestational diabetes. Obstet Gynecol 89:10, 1997

Bartha JL, Martinez-Del-Fresno P, Comino-Delgado R: Gestational diabetes mellitus diagnosed during early pregnancy. Am J Obstet Gynecol 182:346, 2000

Berkowitz K, Reyes C, Sadaat P, et al: Comparison of fetal lung maturation in well dated diabetic and non-diabetic pregnancies. Am J Obstet Gynecol 174:373, 1996

Bernstein IM, Catalano PM: Examination of factors contributing to the risk of cesarean delivery in women with gestational diabetes. Obstet Gynecol 83:462, 1994

Bonomo M, Gandini ML, Mastropasqua A, et al: Which cutoff level should be used in screening for glucose intolerance in pregnancy? Am J Obstet Gynecol 179:179, 1998

Bradley RJ, Nicolaides KH, Brudenell JM: Are all infants of diabetic mothers "macrosomic"? BMJ 297:1583, 1988

Brankston GH, Mitchell BF, Ryan EA, et al: Resistance exercise decreases the need for insulin in overweight women with gestational diabetes mellitus. Am J Obstet Gynecol 190:188, 2004

Brody SC, Harris R, Lohr K: Screening for gestational diabetes: A summary of the evidence for the U.S. Preventive Services Task Force. Obstet Gynecol 101:380, 2003

Buchbinder A, Miodovnik M, McElvy S, et al: Is insulin lispro associated with the development or progression of diabetic retinopathy during pregnancy? Am J Obstet Gynecol 183:1162, 2000

Bung P, Bung C, Artal R, et al: Therapeutic exercise for insulin-requiring gestational diabetes: Effects on the fetus—results of a randomized prospective longitudinal study. J Perinat Med 21:125, 1993

Casele HL, Laifer SA: Factors influencing preconception control of glycemia in diabetic women. Arch Intern Med 158:1321, 1998

Casey BM, Lucas MJ, McIntire DD, et al: Population impact of universal screening for gestational diabetes. Am J Obstet Gynecol 180:536, 1999

Catalano PM, Avallone DA, Drago BS, et al: Reproducibility of the oral glucose tolerance test in pregnant women. Am J Obstet Gynecol 169:874, 1993

Catalano PM, Huston L, Amini SB, et al: Longitudinal changes in glucose metabolism during pregnancy in obese women with normal glucose tolerance and gestational diabetes mellitus. Am J Obstet Gynecol 180:903, 1999

Chaturvedi N, Stephenson JM, Fuller JH: The relationship between pregnancy and long-term maternal complications in the EURO-DIAB IDDM complications study. Diabetic Med 12:494, 1995

Cnattingius C, Berne C, Nordstrom ML: Pregnancy outcome and infant mortality in diabetic patients in Sweden. Diabetic Med 11:696, 1994

Combs CA, Rosenn B, Kitzmiller JL, et al: Early-pregnancy proteinuria in diabetes related to preeclampsia. Obstet Gynecol 82:802, 1993a

Combs CA, Singh NB, Khoury JC: Elective induction versus spontaneous labor after sonographic diagnosis of fetal macrosomia. Obstet Gynecol 81:492, 1993b

Conway D, Langer O: Elective delivery for macrosomia in the diabetic pregnancy: A clinical cost-benefit analysis. Am J Obstet Gynecol 174:331, 1996

Conway DL, Gonzales O, Skiver D: Use of glyburide for the treatment of gestational diabetes: The San Antonio experience. J Matern Fetal Neonatal Med 15:51, 2004

Cousins L: Pregnancy complications among diabetic women: Review 1965–1985. Obstet Gynecol Surv 42:140, 1987

Cruikshank DP, Pitkin RM, Reynolds WA, et al: Altered maternal calcium homeostasis in diabetic pregnancy. J Clin Endocrinol Metab 50:264, 1980

Dacus JV, Meyer NL, Muram D, et al: Gestational diabetes: Postpartum glucose tolerance testing. Am J Obstet Gynecol 171:927, 1994

Dahl-Jørgensen K, Brinchmann-Hansen O, Hanssen KF, et al: Rapid tightening of blood glucose control leads to transient deterioration of retinopathy in insulin-dependent diabetes mellitus: The Oslo study. BMJ 290:811, 1985

Danilenko-Dixon D, Annamalai A, Mattson L, et al: Perinatal outcomes in consecutive pregnancies discordant for gestational diabetes. Am J Obstet Gynecol 182:S80, 2000

Danilenko-Dixon DR, Van Winter JT, Nelson RL, et al: Universal versus selective gestational diabetes screening: Application of 1997 American Diabetes Association recommendations. Am J Obstet Gynecol 181:798, 1999

Dashe JS, Nathan L, McIntire DD, et al: Correlation between amniotic fluid glucose concentration and amniotic fluid volume in pregnancy complicated by diabetes. Am J Obstet Gynecol 182:901, 2000

DeMarini S, Mimouni F, Tsang RC, et al: Impact of metabolic control of diabetes during pregnancy on neonatal hypocalcemia: A randomized study. Obstet Gynecol 83:918, 1994

Dempsey JC, Sorensen TK, Williams MA, et al: Prospective study of gestational diabetes mellitus in relation to maternal recreational physical activity before and during pregnancy. Am J Epidemiol 159:663, 2004

DeVeciana M, Major CA, Morgan M, et al: Postprandial versus preprandial blood glucose monitoring in women with gestational diabetes mellitus requiring insulin therapy. N Engl J Med 333:1237, 1995

Diabetes Control and Complications Trial/Epidemiology of Diabetes Interventions and Complications Research Group: Effects of intensive therapy on the microvascular complications of type 1 diabetes mellitus. JAMA 287:2563, 2002

Diabetes Control and Complications Trial Research Group: The effect of intensive treatment of diabetes on the development and progression of long-term complications in insulin-dependent diabetes mellitus. N Engl J Med 329:977, 1993

Diabetes Pregnancy Group (France): French multicentric survey of outcome of pregnancy in women with pregestational diabetes and pregnancy group. Obstet Gynecol Surv 59:323, 2004

Elman KD, Welch RA, Frank RN, et al: Diabetic retinopathy in pregnancy: A review. Obstet Gynecol 75:119, 1990

Espinosa de los Monteros A, Parra A, Carino N, et al: The reproducibility of the 50-g, 1-hour glucose screen for diabetes in pregnancy. Obstet Gynecol 82:515, 1993

Evers IM, de Valk HW, Visser GH: Risk of complications of pregnancy in women with type 1 diabetes: Nationwide prospective study in Netherlands. BMJ 328:915, 2004

Feig DS, Palda VA: Type 2 diabetes in pregnancy: A growing concern. Lancet 359:1690, 2002

Ferrara A, Kahn HS, Quesenberry CP, et al: An increase in the incidence of gestational diabetes mellitus: Northern California, 1991–2000. Obstet Gynecol 103:526, 2004

Frank RN: Diabetic retinopathy. N Engl J Med 350:48, 2004

Gabbe SG, Graves CR: Management of diabetes mellitus complicating pregnancy. Obstet Gynecol 102:857, 2003

Gabbe SG, Hill L, Schmidt L, et al: Management of diabetes by obstetrician-gynecologists. Obstet Gynecol 91:643, 1998

Gabbe SG, Mestman JH, Freeman RK, et al: Management and outcome of diabetes mellitus, classes B–R. Am J Obstet Gynecol 129:723, 1977

Gale EAM: Is there really an epidemic of type 2 diabetes? Lancet 362:503, 2003

Gandhi JA, Zhang Y, Maidman JE: Fetal cardiac hypertrophy and cardiac function in diabetic pregnancies. Am J Obstet Gynecol 173:1132, 1995

Garner PR: Type 1 diabetes and pregnancy. Correspondence. Lancet 346:966, 1995a

Garner P: Type 1 diabetes mellitus and pregnancy. Lancet 346:157, 1995b

Garner P, Okun N, Keely E, et al: A randomized controlled trial of strict glycemic control and tertiary level obstetric care versus routine obstetric care in the management of gestational diabetes: A pilot study. Am J Obstet Gynecol 177:190, 1997

Garner PR, D'Alton ME, Dudley DK, et al: Preeclampsia in diabetic pregnancies. Am J Obstet Gynecol 163:505, 1990

Gluck L, Kulovich MV: Lecithin:sphingomyelin ratios in amniotic fluid in normal and abnormal pregnancy. Am J Obstet Gynecol 115:539, 1973

Glueck CJ, Goldenberg N, Wang P, et al: Metformin during pregnancy reduces insulin, insulin resistance, insulin secretion,

weight, testosterone and development of gestational diabetes: Prospective longitudinal assessment of women with polycystic ovary syndrome from preconception throughout pregnancy. Hum Reprod 19:510, 2004

Gonen R, Bader D, Ajami M: Effects of policy of elective cesarean delivery in cases of suspected fetal macrosomia on the incidence of brachial plexus injury and the rate of cesarean delivery. Am J Obstet Gynecol 183:1296, 2000

Gordon M, Lawdon MB, Samuels P, et al: Perinatal outcome and long-term follow-up associated with modern management of diabetic nephropathy. Obstet Gynecol 87:401, 1996

Greenberg LR, Moore TR, Murphy H: Gestational diabetes mellitus: Antenatal variables as predictors of postpartum glucose intolerance. Obstet Gynecol 86:97, 1995

Greene MF, Hare JW, Cloherty JP, et al: First-trimester hemoglobin A_1 and risk for major malformation and spontaneous abortion in diabetic pregnancy. Teratology 39:225, 1989

Gribble RK, Meier PR, Berg RL: The value of urine screening for glucose at each prenatal visit. Obstet Gynecol 86:405, 1995

Hanson U, Persson B: Outcome of pregnancies complicated by type 1 insulin-dependent diabetes in Sweden: Acute pregnancy complications, neonatal mortality and morbidity. Am J Perinatol 10:330, 1993

Harborne L, Fleming R, Lyall H, et al: Descriptive review of the evidence for the use of metformin in polycystic ovary syndrome. Lancet 361:1894, 2003

Harris MI: Gestational diabetes may represent discovery of preexisting glucose intolerance. Diabetes Care 11:402, 1988

Holing EV, Brown ZA, Beyer CS, et al: Why don't women with diabetes plan their pregnancies? Diabetes Care 21:889, 1998

How HY, Sibai B, Lindheimer M, et al: Is early-pregnancy proteinuria associated with an increased rate of preeclampsia in women with pregestational diabetes mellitus? Am J Obstet Gynecol 190:775, 2004

Innes KE, Byers TE, Marshall JA, et al: Association of a woman's own birthweight with subsequent risk for gestational diabetes. JAMA 287:2534, 2002

Johnson SR, Kolberg BH, Vance MW, et al: Maternal obesity and pregnancy. Surg Gynecol Obstet 164:431, 1987

Johnstone FD, Nasrat AA, Prescott RJ: The effect of established and gestational diabetes on pregnancy outcome. Br J Obstet Gynaecol 97:1009, 1990

Jovanovic-Peterson L, Durak EP, Peterson CM: Randomized trial of diet versus diet plus cardiovascular conditioning on glucose levels in gestational diabetes. Am J Obstet Gynecol 161:415, 1989

Kaufmann RC, Smith T, Bochantin T, et al: Failure to obtain follow-up testing for gestational diabetic patients in a rural population. Obstet Gynecol 93:734, 1999

Keller JD, Metzger BE, Dooley SL, et al: Infants of diabetic mothers with accelerated fetal growth by ultrasonography: Are they all alike? Am J Obstet Gynecol 163:893, 1990

Kent LA, Gill GV, Williams G: Mortality and outcome of patients with brittle diabetes and recurrent acidosis. Lancet 344:778, 1994

Kitzmiller JL, Main E, Ward B, et al: Insulin lispro and the development of proliferative diabetic retinopathy during pregnancy [letter]. Diabetes Care 22:874, 1999

Kitzmiller JL, Younger MD, Hare JW, et al: Continuous subcutaneous insulin therapy during early pregnancy. Obstet Gynecol 65:606, 1985

Kitzmiller JL, Cloherty JP, Younger MD, et al: Diabetic pregnancy and perinatal outcome. Am J Obstet Gynecol 131:560, 1978

Kjos SL, Schaefer-Grae U, Sardesi S, et al: A randomized controlled trial using glycemic plus fetal ultrasound parameters versus glycemic parameters to determine insulin therapy in gestational diabetes with fasting hyperglycemia. Diabetes Care 24:1904, 2001

Kjos SL, Shoupe D, Donyou S, et al: Effect of low-dose oral contraceptives on carbohydrate and lipid metabolism in women with recent gestational diabetes: Results of a controlled, randomized, prospective study. Am J Obstet Gynecol 163:1822, 1990a

Kjos SL, Walther FJ, Montoro M, et al: Prevalence and etiology of respiratory distress in infants of diabetic mothers: Predictive value of fetal lung maturation tests. Am J Obstet Gynecol 163:898, 1990b

Klein BEK, Moss SE, Klein R: Effect of pregnancy on progression of diabetic retinopathy. Diabetes Care 13:34, 1990

Landon MB, Mintz MC, Gabbe SG: Sonographic evaluation of fetal abdominal growth: Predictor of the large-for-gestational-age infant in pregnancies complicated by diabetes mellitus. Am J Obstet Gynecol 160:115, 1989

Landon MB, Osei K, Platt M, et al: The differential effects of body fat distribution on insulin and glucose metabolism during pregnancy. Am J Obstet Gynecol 171:875, 1994

Langer O, Conway DL, Berkus MD, et al: A comparison of glyburide and insulin in women with gestational diabetes mellitus. New Engl J Med 343:1134, 2000

Langer O, Rodriquez DA, Xenakis EMJ, et al: Intensified versus conventional management of gestational diabetes. Am J Obstet Gynecol 170:1036, 1994

Lauszus FF, Gron PL, Klebe JG: Pregnancies complicated by diabetic retinopathy. Acta Obstet Gynecol Scand 77:814, 1998

Leonardi MR, Bottoms SF: Increased incidence of large for gestational age infants not attributable to gestational diabetes. Am J Obstet Gynecol 174:393, 1996

Leveno KJ, Fortunato SJ, Raskin P, et al: Continuous subcutaneous insulin infusion during pregnancy. Diabetes Res Clin Pract 4:257, 1988

Leveno KJ, Hauth JC, Gilstrap LC III, et al: Appraisal of "rigid" blood glucose control during pregnancy in the overtly diabetic woman. Am J Obstet Gynecol 135:853, 1979

Loukovaara M, Leinonen P, Teramo K, et al: Diabetic pregnancy associated with increased epidermal growth factor in cord serum at term. Obstet Gynecol 103:240, 2004

Lu GC, Lucheese A, Chapman V, et al: Screening for gestational diabetes in the subsequent pregnancy: Is it worthwhile? Am J Obstet Gynecol 187:918, 2002

Lucas MJ, Lowe TW, Bowe L, et al: Class A1 gestational diabetes: A meaningful diagnosis? Obstet Gynecol 82:260, 1993

Magee MS, Walden CE, Benedetti TJ, et al: Influence of diagnostic criteria on the incidence of gestational diabetes and perinatal mortality. JAMA 26:609, 1993

Martin AO, Dempsey LM, Minogue J, et al: Maternal serum α-fetoprotein levels in pregnancies complicated by diabetes: Implications for screening programs. Am J Obstet Gynecol 163:1209, 1990

Martin FR, Health P, Mountain KR: Pregnancy in women with diabetes. Fifteen years' experience: 1973–1985. Med J Aust 146:187, 1987

Martin JA, Hamilton BE, Sutton PD, et al: Births: Final data for 2002. National Vital Statistics Reports, Vol 52, No. 10. Hyattsville, MD, National Center for Health Statistics, 2003

McElvy SS, Demarini S, Miodovnik M, et al: Fetal weight and progression of diabetic retinopathy. Obstet Gynecol 97:587, 2001

McFarland MB, Langer O, Fazioni E, et al: Anthropometric and body composition differences in large-for-gestational age, but not appropriate-for-gestational age infants of mothers with and without diabetes mellitus. J Soc Gynecol Investig 7:231, 2000

McKinney PA, Parslow R, Gurney KA, et al: Perinatal and neonatal determinants of childhood type 1 diabetes: A case-control study in Yorkshire, U.K. Diabetes Care 22:928, 1999

Metzger BE, Bybee DE, Freinkel N, et al: Gestational diabetes mellitus: Correlations between the phenotypic and genotypic characteristics of the mother and abnormal glucose tolerance during the first year postpartum. Diabetes 34:111, 1985

Metzger BE, Coustan DR: Summary and recommendations of the fourth international workshop-conference on gestational diabetes mellitus. Diabetes Care 21:B161, 1998

Miller E, Hare JW, Cloherty JP, et al: Elevated maternal hemoglobin A_{1c} in early pregnancy and major congenital anomalies in infants of diabetic mothers. N Engl J Med 304:1331, 1981

Mills JL, Baker L, Goldman AS: Malformations in infants of diabetic mothers occur before the seventh gestational week. Implications for treatment. Diabetes 28:292, 1979

Mills JL, Knopp RH, Simpson JL, et al: Incidence of spontaneous abortion among normal women and insulin-dependent diabetic women whose pregnancies were identified within 21 days of conception. N Engl J Med 319:1617, 1988a

Mills JL, Knopp RH, Simpson JL: Lack of relation of increased malformation rates in infants of diabetic mothers to glycemic control during organogenesis. N Engl J Med 318:671, 1988b

Milunsky A, Jick H, Bruell CL, et al: Multivitamin/folic acid supplementation in early pregnancy reduces the prevalence of neural tube defects. JAMA 262:2847, 1989

Miodovnik M, Rosenn BM, Khoury JC, et al: Does pregnancy increase the risk for development and progression of diabetic nephropathy? Am J Obstet Gynecol 174:1180, 1996

Modanlou HD, Komatsu G, Dorchester W, et al: Large-for-gestational-age neonates: Anthropometric reasons for shoulder dystocia. Obstet Gynecol 60:417, 1982

Mokdad AH, Ford ES, Bowman BA, et al: Prevalence of obesity, diabetes and obesity-related health risk factors. JAMA 289:76, 2003

Murphy NJ, Meyer BA, O'Kell RT, et al: Screening for gestational diabetes mellitus with a reflectance photometer: Accuracy and precision of a single-operator model. Obstet Gynecol 83:1038, 1994

Narayan KM, Boyle JP, Thompson TJ, et al: Lifetime risk for diabetes mellitus in the United States. JAMA 290:1884, 2003

Nathan DM: Long-term complications of diabetes mellitus. N Engl J Med 328:1676, 1993

Nordlander E, Hanson U, Persson B: Factors influencing neonatal morbidity in gestational diabetic pregnancy. Br J Obstet Gynaecol 96:671, 1989

Okereke NC, Uvena-Celebrezze J, Hutson-Presley L, et al: The effect of gender and gestational diabetes mellitus on cord leptin concentration. Am J Obstet Gynecol 187:798, 2002

O'Sullivan JB: Body weight and subsequent diabetes mellitus. JAMA 248:949, 1982

Owen J, Phelan ST, Landon MP, et al: Gestational diabetes survey. Am J Obstet Gynecol 172:615, 1995

Pallardo F, Herranz L, Garcia-Ingelmo T, et al: Early postpartum metabolic assessment in women with prior gestational diabetes. Diabetes Care 22:1053, 1999

Pan XR, Li GW, Hu YH, et al: Effects of diet and exercise in preventing NIDDM in people with impaired glucose tolerance. The Da Qing IGT and Diabetes Study. Diabetes Care 20:537, 1997

Parretti E, Mecacci F, Papini M, et al: Third-trimester maternal glucose levels from diurnal profiles in nondiabetic pregnancies: Correlation with sonographic parameters of fetal growth. Diabetes Care 24:1319, 2001

Pedersen J: The Pregnant Diabetic and Her Newborn, 2nd ed. Baltimore, Williams & Wilkins, 1977, p 211

Pedersen J, Mølsted-Pedersen L, Andersen B: Assessors of fetal perinatal mortality in diabetic pregnancy. Analysis of 1332 pregnancies in the Copenhagen series, 1946–1972. Diabetes 23:302, 1974

Pennison EH, Egerman RS: Perinatal outcomes in gestational diabetes: A comparison of criteria for diagnosis. Am J Obstet Gynecol 184:1118, 2001

Philipson EH, Super DM: Gestational diabetes mellitus: Does it recur in subsequent pregnancy? Am J Obstet Gynecol 160:1324, 1989

Piacquadio K, Hollingsworth DR, Murphy H: Effects of in utero exposure to oral hypoglycemic drugs. Lancet 338:866, 1991

Plagemann A, Franke K, Harder T, et al: Long-term impact of neonatal breast-feeding on bodyweight and glucose tolerance in children of diabetic mothers. Diabetes Care 25:16, 2002

Pombar X, Strassner HT, Fenner PC: Pregnancy in a woman with class H diabetes mellitus and previous coronary artery bypass graft: A case report and review of the literature. Obstet Gynecol 85:825, 1995

Powers AC: Diabetes mellitus. In Braunwald E, Fauci AS, Kasper DL, et al (eds): Harrison's Principles of Internal Medicine, 15th ed. New York, McGraw-Hill, 2001, p 2109

Ray JG, O'Brien TE, Chan WS: Preconception care and the risk of congenital anomalies in the offspring of women with diabetes mellitus: A meta-analysis. Q J Med 94:435, 2001

Raychaudhuri K, Maresh MJ: Glycemic control throughout pregnancy and fetal growth in insulin-dependent diabetes. Obstet Gynecol 95:190, 2000

Reller MD, Kaplan S: Hypertrophic cardiomyopathy in infants of diabetic mothers: An update. Am J Perinatol 5:353, 1988

Rey E, Attie C, Bonin A: The effects of first-trimester diabetes control on the incidence of macrosomia. Am J Obstet Gynecol 181:202, 1999

Richey SD, Sandstad JS, Leveno KJ: Observations concerning "unexplained" fetal demise in pregnancy complicated by diabetes mellitus. J Matern Fetal Med 4:169, 1995

Rizzo TA, Dooley SL, Metzger BE, et al: Prenatal and perinatal influences on long-term psychomotor development in offspring of diabetic mothers. Am J Obstet Gynecol 173:1753, 1995

Rosenn B, Miodovnik M, Combs CA, et al: Glycemic thresholds for spontaneous abortion and congenital malformations in insulin-dependent diabetes mellitus. Obstet Gynecol 84:515, 1994

Rosenn BM, Miodovnik M, Holcberg G, et al: Hyperglycemia: The price of intensive insulin therapy for pregnant women with insulin-dependent diabetes mellitus. Obstet Gynecol 85:417, 1995

Salvesen DR, Brudenell MJ, Nicolaides KH: Fetal polycythemia and thrombocytopenia in pregnancies complicated by maternal diabetes mellitus. Am J Obstet Gynecol 166:1287, 1992

Salvesen DR, Brudenell MJ, Snijders JM, et al: Fetal plasma erythropoietin in pregnancies complicated by maternal diabetes mellitus. Am J Obstet Gynecol 168:88, 1993

Saudek CD: Progress and promise of diabetes research. JAMA 287:2582, 2002

Savvidou MD, Geerts L, Nicolaides KH: Impaired vascular reactivity in pregnant women with insulin-dependent diabetes mellitus. Am J Obstet Gynecol 186:84, 2002

Schneider JM, Curet LB, Olson RW, et al: Ambulatory care of the pregnant diabetic. Obstet Gynecol 56:144, 1980

Sheffield JS, Butler-Koster EL, Casey BM, et al: Maternal diabetes mellitus and infant malformations. Obstet Gynecol 100:925, 2002

Sheffield JS, Casey BM, Lucas MJ, et al: Gestational diabetes: Effects of the degree of hyperglycemia and the gestational age at diagnosis. Soc Gynecol Invest 6:6A, 1999

Sibai BM, Caritis S, Hauth J, et al: Risks of preeclampsia and adverse neonatal outcomes among women with pregestational diabetes mellitus. Am J Obstet Gynecol 182:364, 2000

Siddiqi T, Rosenn B, Mimouni F, et al: Hypertension during pregnancy in insulin-dependent diabetic women. Obstet Gynecol 77:514, 1991

Silverman BL, Metzger BI, Cho NH, et al: Fetal hyperinsulinism and impaired glucose intolerance in adolescent offspring of diabetic mothers. Diabetes Care 18:611, 1995

Stamler EF, Cruz ML, Mimouni F, et al: High infectious morbidity in pregnant women with insulin-dependent diabetes: An understated complication. Am J Obstet Gynecol 163:1217, 1990

Steel JM, Johnstone FD, Hume R, et al: Insulin requirements during pregnancy in women with type 1 diabetes. Obstet Gynecol 83:253, 1994

Tamada JA, Garg S, Jovanovic L, et al: Non-invasive glucose monitoring: Comprehensive clinical results. JAMA 282:1839, 1999

Taylor R, Lee C, Kyne-Grzebalski D, et al: Clinical outcome of pregnancy in women with type 1 diabetes. Obstet Gynecol 99:537, 2002

Thompson DJ, Porter KB, Gunnells DJ, et al: Prophylactic insulin in the management of gestational diabetes. Obstet Gynecol 75:960, 1990

Van Ballegooie E, Hooymans JMM, Timmerman Z, et al: Rapid deterioration of diabetic retinopathy during treatment with continuous subcutaneous insulin infusion. Diabetes Care 7:236, 1984

Verhaeghe J, Van Bree B, Van Herck E, et al: C-peptide, insulin-like growth factor I and II, and insulin-like growth factor binding protein-1 in umbilical cord serum: Correlations with birthweight. Am J Obstet Gynecol 169:89, 1993

Wang PH, Lau J, Chalmers TC: Meta-analysis of effects of intensive blood-glucose control on late complications of type 1 diabetes. Lancet 341:1306, 1993

Way GL: The natural history of hypertrophic cardiomyopathy in infants of diabetic mothers. J Pediatr 95:1020, 1979

Weiss PAM, Haeusler M, Kainer F, et al: Toward universal criteria for gestational diabetes: Relationships between seventy-five and one hundred gram glucose loads and between capillary and venous concentrations. Am J Obstet Gynecol 178:830, 1998

White P: Classification of obstetric diabetes. Am J Obstet Gynecol 130:228, 1978

Willman SP, Leveno KJ, Guzick DS, et al: Glucose threshold for macrosomia in pregnancy complicated by diabetes. Am J Obstet Gynecol 154:470, 1986

World Health Organization: Diabetes Mellitus: Report of a WHO Study Group. Geneva, WHO, 1985. Technical Report Series No. 727

Zhang S, Folsom AR, Flack JM, et al: Body fat distribution before pregnancy and gestational diabetes: Findings from coronary artery risk development in young adults (CARDIA) study. BMJ 311:1139, 1995

53

Thyroid and Other Endocrine Disorders

A variety of endocrine disorders can complicate pregnancy and vice versa. Diabetes mellitus is the most common and is discussed in Chapter 52. Thyroid disorders are also common in young women, and thus they are frequently encountered during pregnancy. In addition, there are a number of less common endocrinopathies that may have devastating effects on pregnancy outcome (e.g., pheochromocytoma).

The pathogenic basis of most endocrinopathies is disordered autoimmunity. A number of autoantigens, autoantibodies, and cellular immune elements have been identified to cause destruction or stimulation of thyroid, pancreatic, or adrenal glandular tissue (Baker, 1997). In many cases, a nonspecific event (e.g., viral infection) initiates an antigen and organ-specific response with subsequent immune-mediated glandular destruction. Frequently, a genetic predisposition may also be involved, such as inheritance of major histocompatibility complex antigens. Certain environmental factors may predispose to development of some autoimmune endocrinopathies. Finally, intriguing evidence has accrued that fetal lymphocytes, stem cells, DNA, or both may take up residence in maternal organs during pregnancy and form the basis for some autoimmune diseases.

Thyroid Physiology. The impact of pregnancy on maternal thyroid physiology is substantial. Changes in the structure and function of the gland sometimes cause confusion in the diagnosis of thyroid abnormalities. These are discussed in detail in Chapter 5 (see p. 141) and are discussed below.

Moderate thyroid enlargement occurs due to glandular hyperplasia, and thyroid volume determined ultrasonographically increases, although its echostructure and echogenicity remain unchanged (Rasmussen and colleagues, 1989). Iodide uptake by the maternal gland is increased, and daily thyroxine secretion is probably increased. In early pregnancy at least, thyroxine is transferred from mother to fetus, and with fetal hypothyroidism, transfer continues throughout pregnancy (Calvo and associates, 2002; Vulsma and colleagues, 1989). Thyroid hormone is necessary for normal development of the brain and mental function (Forrest, 2004). Maternal serum concentration of *thyroid-binding globulin* is increased considerably along with total or bound hormone levels.

Thyrotropin, or *thyroid-stimulating hormone (TSH),* currently plays a central role in screening and diagnosis of many thyroid disorders. In early pregnancy, thyrotropin activity decreases because of thyroid stimulation from the weak crossover activity of chorionic gonadotropin (Grossman and associates, 1997). The hormone does not cross the placenta. In the first 12 weeks when chorionic gonadotropin levels are maximal, free thyroxine levels increase, and these suppress thyrotropin levels (Fig. 53–1). Accordingly, *thyrotropin-releasing hormone (TRH)* is undetectable in maternal serum. Beginning at midpregnancy, fetal serum TRH is detectable but does not increase, and there is only minimal placental transfer (Bajoria and co-workers, 1998).

THYROID DISEASES

Taken in aggregate, thyroid disorders are common in young women. The incidence of hyperthyroidism, hypothyroidism, and thyroiditis is each approximately 1 percent. There is an intimate relationship between maternal and fetal thyroid function. The fetus is dependent on maternal thyroxine, and drugs that affect the maternal thyroid also affect the fetal gland. Clinical thyrotoxicosis may be stimulated by gestational trophoblastic disease. Thyroid autoantibodies have been associated with increased early pregnancy wastage, and uncontrolled thyrotoxicosis and untreated hypothyroidism are both associated with adverse pregnancy outcomes. Finally, there is evidence that the severity of autoimmune thyroid disorders is ameliorated during pregnancy, only to be exacerbated postpartum.

AUTOIMMUNE THYROID DISEASE. Most thyroid disorders are inextricably linked to the presence of autoantibodies to various cell components. Several antibodies variably

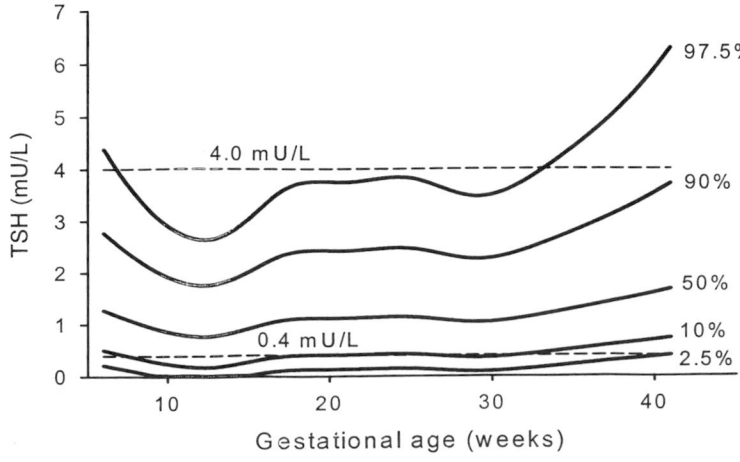

FIGURE 53–1. Maternal serum thyrotropin levels across pregnancy in 13,851 women. (From Dashe and colleagues, 2003, with permission.)

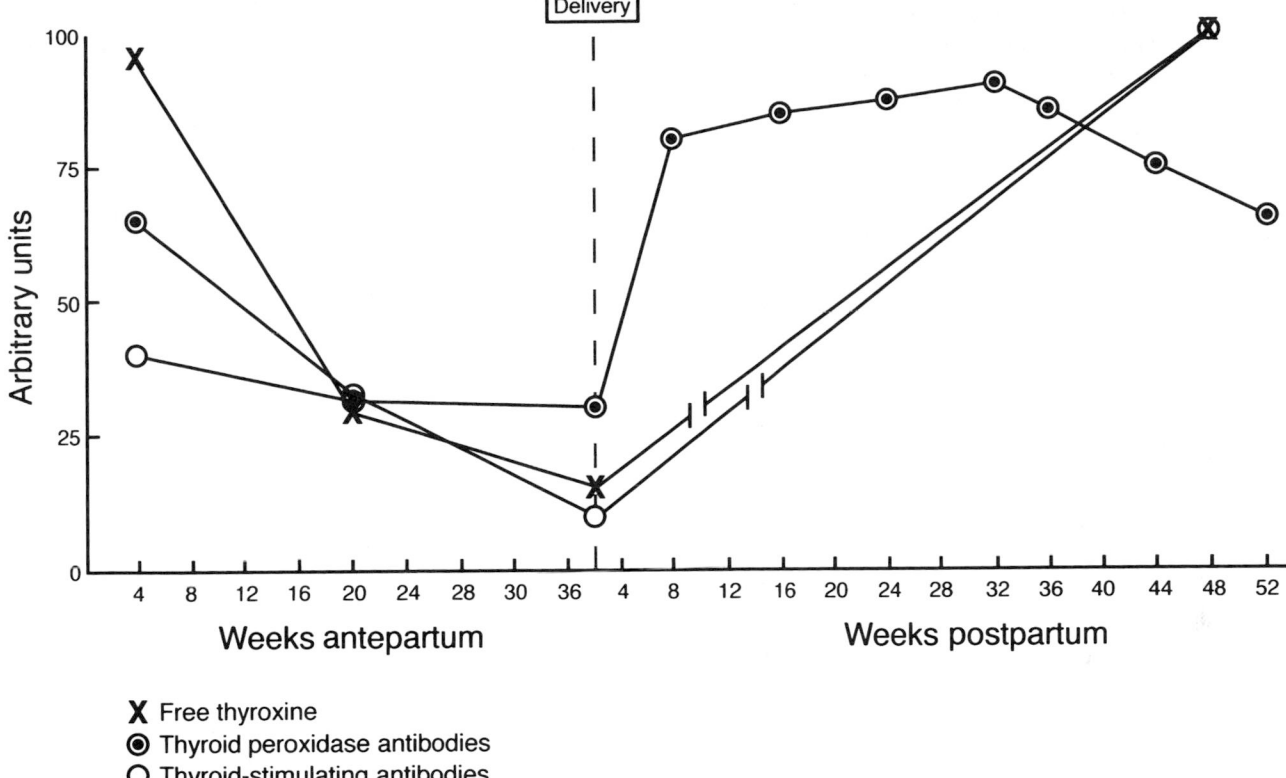

X Free thyroxine
⊙ Thyroid peroxidase antibodies
○ Thyroid-stimulating antibodies

FIGURE 53–2. Schematic change across pregnancy and up to 1-year postpartum of serum levels of free thyroxine and various antithyroid antibodies. Arbitrary units are used to depict reciprocal relationships. From early pregnancy until delivery, levels of thyroid-stimulating antibodies (O—O) and thyroid peroxidase antibodies (⊙—⊙) decrease. At the same time, levels of serum free thyroxine (X—X) also decrease. Postpartum, the trend is reversed. (Data from Amino and associates, 2003; Fung and colleagues, 1988; Kung and Jones, 1998.)

stimulate thyroid function, block function, or cause thyroid inflammation that may lead to destruction. These not uncommonly coexist.

Thyroid-stimulating autoantibodies, also called *thyroid-stimulating immunoglobulins,* attach to the thyrotropin receptor and activate it, causing thyroid hyperfunction and growth. These antibodies are identified in the majority of patients with classic Graves disease. Simultaneous production of *thyroid-stimulating blocking antibodies* may blunt this effect (Weetman, 2000).

Thyroid peroxidase antibodies, previously called thyroid *microsomal autoantibodies,* have been identified in 10 to 20 percent of pregnant women (Jansson and associates, 1988; Kuijpens and co-workers, 2001). Up to half develop *autoimmune thyroiditis* that may be transient, but thyroid failure occurs in a significant number of women (Amino and colleagues, 2000). These antibodies are also associated with miscarriage and Down syndrome (Abramson and Stagnaro-Green, 2001; Cuckle and colleagues, 1988). As with other autoimmune endocrinopathies, there usually is a precipitating event such as a viral illness that interacts with genetic and other factors. For example, Pacini and associates (1998) found serum thyroid antibodies in 30 percent of preadolescent girls exposed to radioactive fallout from the Chernobyl disaster, compared with 3 percent of nonexposed controls. Some investigators regard pregnancy as an inciting event (Amino and colleagues, 2000).

As shown in Figure 53–2, all of these antibodies have a characteristic pattern during pregnancy and the first year postpartum. In many cases, these patterns parallel clinical disease activity. Detection of peroxidase antibodies in early pregnancy or postpartum identifies women at high risk for postpartum thyroid dysfunction and at lifelong risk for permanent thyroid failure (Hidaka and associates, 1994; Premawardhana and co-workers, 2000).

Autoimmune thyroid disease is much more common in women than in men. One intriguing explanation for this disparity is fetal-to-maternal cell trafficking. When fetal lymphocytes enter the maternal circulation, they may live for more than 20 years. Stem cell interchange likely occurs also, and these can reside in a number of maternal tissues, including the thyroid gland (Bianchi and Romero, 2003; Khosrotehrani and associates, 2004). Maternal *microchimerism* with male fetuses has been demonstrated using the *SRY* sex-determining

TABLE 53–1 Incidence of Hyper- and Hypothyroidism in 17,298 Women Undergoing Serum Thyrotropin Screening Before 20 Weeks at Parkland Hospital

Thyroid Activity	Rate
Hyperthyroidism	1.9%
Overt	3.9 per 1000
Subclinical	15 per 1000
Hypothyroidism	2.5%
Overt	1.8 per 1000
Subclinical	23 per 1000

From Casey and colleagues (2003), with permission.

gene for foreign cell identification. About a third of women who have borne a male fetus have *SRY*-positive lymphocytes in their peripheral blood. Specimens from women with thyroiditis or Graves disease have *SRY*-positive thyrocyte microchimerism with greater frequency and intensity than controls (Ando and associates, 2002; Klintschar and colleagues, 2001). These are presumed to have arisen from stem cells transferred from the male fetus.

HYPERTHYROIDISM. Symptomatic thyrotoxicosis, or hyperthyroidism, complicates about 1 in 1000 to 2000 pregnancies (Mestman and colleagues, 1995). The incidence cited by Casey and associates (2003) was 3.9 per 1000, including women identified before pregnancy (Table 53–1). Because normal pregnancy simulates some clinical findings similar to thyroxine (T_4) excess, mild thyrotoxicosis may be difficult to diagnose. Some suggestive findings include tachycardia that exceeds that with normal pregnancy, elevated sleeping pulse rate, thyromegaly, exophthalmos, and failure to gain weight despite adequate food intake. Laboratory confirmation is an elevated serum free T_4 level along with a markedly depressed thyrotropin level. The thyrotropin assay is sensitive to less than 0.1 mU/L, and this has led to discovery of *subclinical* hyperthyroidism, which Casey and co-workers (2003) identified in 1.5 percent of pregnant women. Rarely, hyperthyroidism is caused by abnormally high serum triiodothyronine (T_3) levels—so-called T_3-*toxicosis*.

SUBCLINICAL HYPERTHYROIDISM. This relatively new clinical entity was defined when sensitive thyrotropin assays became available. It is encountered in about 1 percent of patients and is characterized by an abnormally low serum thyrotropin concentration in concert with normal thyroid hormone levels (Roberts and Ladenson, 2004). When not due to exogenous thyroxine intake, about half of these eventually developed normal thyrotropin concentrations. Long-term effects in those with persistent subclinical thyrotoxicosis are for the most part currently unclear. Because the condition may cause cardiac arrhythmias, ventricular hypertrophy, and osteopenia, affected patients should be periodically monitored.

Thyrotoxicosis and Pregnancy. The overwhelming cause of thyrotoxicosis in pregnancy is *Graves disease*, an organ-specific autoimmune process usually associated with thyroid-stimulating antibodies as discussed previously. As shown in Figure 53–2, thyroid-stimulating antibody activity declines during pregnancy, leading to chemical remission in many women (Amino and co-workers, 1982; Kung and Jones, 1998). Amino and colleagues (2003) have found that blocking antibodies are also decreased during pregnancy.

TREATMENT. Thyrotoxicosis during pregnancy can nearly always be controlled by thioamide drugs. Some clinicians prefer *propylthiouracil* because it partially inhibits the conversion of T_4 to T_3 and it crosses the placenta less readily than *methimazole.* Although not definitely proven, methimazole use in early pregnancy has been associated with otherwise rarely encountered *esophageal* and *choanal atresia* as well as *aplasia cutis* (Diav-Citrin and Ornoy, 2002). Wing and co-workers (1994) studied 185 pregnant thyrotoxic women and showed that both drugs are effective and safe. Transient leukopenia manifests in about 10 percent, but this does not require cessation of therapy. In about 0.2 percent, *agranulocytosis* develops suddenly and mandates discontinuance of the drug. It is not dose related, and because of its acute onset, serial leukocyte counts during therapy are not helpful (Cooper, 2003; Mestman and colleagues, 1995). If fever or sore throat develop, patients are instructed to discontinue medication immediately and to report for a complete blood count (Vanderpump and associates, 1996). About 20 percent of all patients treated with propylthiouracil *develop antineutrophil cytoplasmic antibodies,* but only a small percentage of these develop serious vasculitis (Helfgott, 2002). Finally, although thioamides have the potential to cause fetal complications, these are uncommon. In some cases, thioamides may even be therapeutic, because thyrotropin-blocking antibodies also cross the placenta and stimulate the fetal thyroid gland to cause thyrotoxicosis.

The dose of propylthiouracil is empirical, and for nonpregnant patients, the American Thyroid Association recommends an initial daily dose of 100 to 600 mg for propylthiouracil or 10 to 40 mg for methimazole (Singer and colleagues, 1995). In a study of 509 nonpregnant thyrotoxic patients, Reinwein and associates (1993) randomized therapy with either 10 or 40 mg of methimazole. At 6 weeks, 85 and 92 percent respectively, were euthyroid. In pregnant women given either thioamide, Wing and colleagues (1994) reported the median time to normalization of thyroid function tests to be 7 to 8 weeks.

In our experience, overt thyrotoxicosis in pregnant women requires higher doses (Davis and colleagues, 1989). With a propylthiouracil dose that averaged 600 mg daily, only half of women had a remission, and in these the dose was decreased to less than 300 mg daily within 8 weeks. In a third, however, it was necessary to increase the dose. Kriplani and colleagues (1994) reported similar findings.

Other therapy includes *thyroidectomy* after thyrotoxicosis is medically controlled. However, this seldom is done during pregnancy. It may be appropriate for the very few women who cannot adhere to medical treatment or in whom drug therapy proves toxic (Davison and co-workers, 2001).

Ablation with therapeutic radioactive iodine is contraindicated. Therapeutic doses given to treat maternal thyroid disease may also cause fetal thyroid gland destruction. If given unintentionally, most clinicians recommend abortion. Any exposed infant must be carefully evaluated for hypothyroidism (Berg and colleagues, 1998). The incidence of fetal hypothyroidism depends on gestational age and dose of radioiodine given (Berlin, 2001). There is no evidence that therapeutic radioiodine given before pregnancy causes fetal anomalies if enough time has passed to allow radiation effects to dissipate and the woman is euthyroid (Ayala and associates, 1998; Casara and colleagues, 1993).

Thyroid Storm and Heart Failure. Thyroid storm is an acute, life-threatening, hypermetabolic state in patients with thyrotoxicosis. Storm is rare in pregnancy. In contrast, heart failure from cardiomyopathy caused by the profound myocardial effects of thyroxine is quite common in pregnant women (Sheffield and Cunningham, 2004). As shown in Table 53–2, heart failure developed in 8 percent of 90 women with uncontrolled thyrotoxicosis. In these women, cardiomyopathy is characterized by a high-output state (Klein and Kaie, 1998). Similar changes during normal pregnancy are additive or synergistic. Thus, the pregnant woman with thyrotoxicosis has minimal cardiac reserve, and decompensation is usually precipitated by preeclampsia, anemia, sepsis, or a combination of these. Fortunately, thyroxine-induced cardiomyopathy is ultimately reversible (Sheffield and Cunningham, 2004).

TABLE 53–2 Pregnancy Outcomes in 239 Women with Overt Thyrotoxicosis

Factor	Treated and Euthyroid (n = 149)	Uncontrolled Thyrotoxicosis (n = 90)
Maternal Outcome		
Preeclampsia	17 (11%)	15 (17%)
Heart failure	1	7 (8%)
Death	0	1
Perinatal Outcome		
Preterm delivery	12 (8%)	29 (32%)
Growth restriction	11 (7%)	15 (17%)
Stillborn	0/59	6/33 (18%)
Thyrotoxicosis	1	2
Hypothyroid	4	0
Goiter	2	0

Data from Davis (1989), Kriplani (1994), Millar (1994), and all their colleagues.

MANAGEMENT. Treatment of thyrotoxic storm or heart failure is similar and should be carried out in an intensive care unit (Zeeman and colleagues, 2003). Specific treatment consists of 1 g of propylthiouracil given orally or crushed and placed through a nasogastric tube. This drug is continued in 200-mg doses every 6 hours. An hour after initial propylthiouracil dosing, iodide is given to inhibit thyroidal release of T_3 and T_4. It is given intravenously as 500 to 1000 mg of sodium iodide every 8 hours; orally as 5 drops of supersaturated solution of potassium iodide (SSKI) every 8 hours; or as Lugol solution, 10 drops orally every 8 hours. With a history of iodine-induced anaphylaxis, lithium carbonate, 300 mg every 6 hours, is given instead (Burch and Wartofsky, 1993). Some investigators recommend maintenance of serum lithium levels of 0.5 to 1.5 mmol/L. Most authorities recommend dexamethasone, 2 mg intravenously every 6 hours for four doses, to further block peripheral conversion of T_4 to T_3. If a β-blocker drug is given to control tachycardia, its effect on heart failure must be considered. Propranolol, labetalol, and esmolol have all been used successfully intrapartum (Bowman and colleagues, 1998). Concurrent, severe preeclampsia, infection, or anemia should be aggressively managed.

Pregnancy Outcome. Perinatal outcomes in neonates of women with thyrotoxicosis depend on whether metabolic control is achieved. Excess thyroxine may cause spontaneous miscarriage (Anselmo and associates, 2004). In untreated women, or in those who remain hyperthyroid despite therapy, there is a higher incidence of preeclampsia, heart failure, and adverse perinatal outcomes (see Table 53–2). Perinatal mortality varied from 6 to 12 percent in several studies.

FETAL AND NEONATAL EFFECTS. In most cases, the perinate is euthyroid. In some cases, however, hyper- or hypothyroidism may occur. Either condition can develop with or without a goiter. If fetal thyroid disease is suspected, nomograms are available for sonographic measurement of the thyroid (Ranzini and co-workers, 2001). Newborns exposed to excessive maternal thyroxine may have any of several clinical presentations.

1. The fetus or newborn may manifest goitrous thyrotoxicosis caused by placental transfer of thyroid-stimulating immunoglobulins. This is related to maternal serum antibody levels and may be predicted in the fetus whose thyromegaly does not respond to maternal thioamide treatment (Cohen and colleagues, 2003; Peleg and associates, 2002). *Nonimmune hydrops* and fetal demise have been reported with fetal thyrotoxicosis (Nachum and co-workers, 2003; Stulberg and Davies, 2000). If thyrotoxic, the fetus is treated with maternal administration of thioamide drugs (Duncombe and Dickerson, 2001). If hypothyroid, it is treated with injection of intra-amnionic thyroxine. In some cases, neonatal thyrotoxicosis may require short-course antithyroid drug treatment.

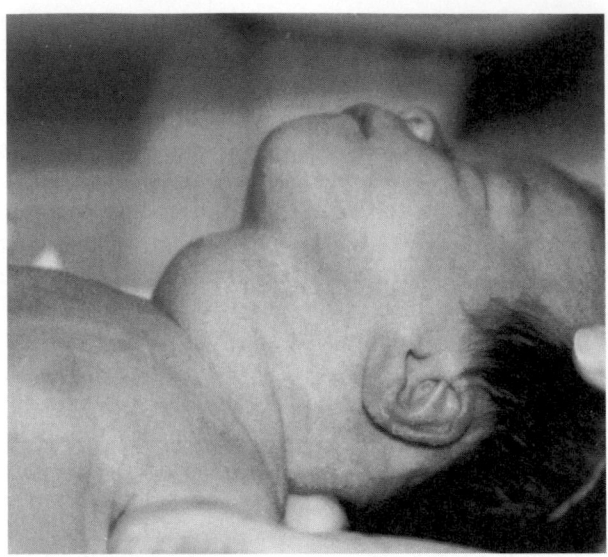

FIGURE 53–3. Term neonate delivered of a woman with a 3-year history of thyrotoxicosis that recurred at 26 weeks' gestation. The mother was given methimazole, 30 mg daily and was euthyroid at delivery. Laboratory studies showed that the infant was hypothyroid.

2. Fetal exposure to maternally administered thioamides may cause goitrous hypothyroidism (Fig. 53–3). In some cases, a fetal goiter is detected ultrasonographically, and cord blood sampling can be used to diagnose hypothyroidism, which can be treated with intra-amnionic thyroxine (Davidson and colleagues, 1991). Amnionic fluid total and free T_4 levels have also been studied (Singh and co-workers, 2003). Reports of adverse fetal effects have been exaggerated, and current data indicate that thioamides carry an extremely small risk (Momotani and associates, 1997; O'Doherty and colleagues, 1999). Of the 239 treated thyrotoxic women shown in Table 53–1, there was evidence of hypothyroidism in only four infants despite relatively high doses of propylthiouracil. At least four long-term studies have found no abnormal intellectual and physical development of these children (Mestman, 1998).

3. The fetus may develop nongoitrous hypothyroidism from transplacental passage of maternal thyrotropin-receptor blocking antibodies (Gallagher and associates, 2001).

4. Even after maternal thyroid gland ablation, usually with ^{131}I radioiodine, fetal thyrotoxicosis may result from transplacental thyroid-stimulating antibodies.

FETAL DIAGNOSIS. Fetal evaluation is somewhat controversial. For example, Nachum and colleagues (2003) recommend fetal blood sampling if maternal thyroid-stimulating antibodies are abnormal, or if there is evidence in the fetus of growth restriction, heart failure, or goiter, with or without tachycardia. Antibody testing is not standard, and Kilpatrick (2003) recommends its use only if the mother has previously undergone ^{131}I ablation. Because fetal hyper- or hypothyroidism

may cause hydrops, growth restriction, goiter, or tachycardia, fetal blood sampling seems appropriate if these conditions develop in pregnancy complicated by Graves disease (Brand and co-workers, 2005).

Hyperemesis Gravidarum. Many women with hyperemesis gravidarum have abnormally high serum thyroxine levels and low thyrotropin levels (see Chap. 49, p. 1113). This results from thyrotropin receptor stimulation from massive—but normal for pregnancy—concentrations of chorionic gonadotropin. Rarely do these women have clinical thyrotoxicosis, and thyroxine and serum thyrotropin values become more normal by midpregnancy (see Fig. 53–1). This condition is also termed *gestational thyrotoxicosis.* Even if it is associated with hyperemesis, treatment is not warranted (American College of Obstetricians and Gynecologists, 2002).

Gestational Trophoblastic Disease. Thyroxine levels in women with molar pregnancy usually are appreciably elevated. Because these tumors are usually now diagnosed early, clinically apparent hyperthyroidism has become less common (Goodwin and Hershman, 1997). This is discussed further in Chapter 11 (see p. 277).

HYPOTHYROIDISM. Most adult hypothyroidism results from glandular destruction by autoantibodies, particularly antithyroid peroxidase antibodies. Hypothyroid disorders are thus related to Graves thyrotoxicosis. As discussed on page 1191, both disorders are possibly related to bidirectional fetal cell transfer during a prior pregnancy.

In most patients, hypothyroidism is difficult to diagnose clinically. The distinction of overt from subclinical hypothyroidism frequently is made by laboratory assessment. *Clinical* or *overt hypothyroidism* is diagnosed when an abnormally high serum thyrotropin level is accompanied by an abnormally low thyroxine level. *Subclinical hypothyroidism* is defined by an elevated serum thyrotropin level with *normal* serum thyroxine (Surks and associates, 2004). *Severe* hypothyroidism with pregnancy is uncommon, probably because it is often associated with infertility and increased miscarriage rates (Abalovich and colleagues, 2002).

Incidence in Pregnancy. In the study by Casey and colleagues (2003), the overall incidence of hypothyroidism was 2.5 percent (see Table 53–1). Overt thyroid deficiency was found in 1.3 per 1000 and subclinical disease in 23 per 1000.

SUBCLINICAL HYPOTHYROIDISM. The incidence of subclinical hypothyroidism in all women between 18 and 45 years of age is about 5 percent (Canaris and colleagues, 2000). Of these, 2 to 5 percent per year progress to overt thyroid failure. Heredity is a potent risk factor. Other risk factors for thyroid failure include type 1 diabetes and antimicrosomal antibodies. At this time, evidence that subclinical hypothyroidism is associated with hypertension, cardiac dysfunction,

TABLE 53-3 Pregnancy Complications in 112 Women with Hypothyroidism

Complications	Hypothyroidism (%)	
	Overt (n = 49)	Subclinical (n = 63)
Preeclampsia	31	16
Abruptio placentae	8	0
Cardiac dysfunction	3	2
Birthweight less than 2000 g[a]	31	19
Stillbirths	8	2[b]

[a]Preterm or term delivery were the only outcomes reported by Abalovich and colleagues (2002).
[b]One infant died from syphilis.
Modified from Abalovich (2002), Davis (1988), and Leung (1993), and all their associates.

and dyslipidemia is not conclusive enough to warrant thyroxine replacement (Surks and associates, 2004). These authors went on to say that if the serum thyrotropin levels exceed 10 mU/L, some physicians choose to give thyroxine therapy but that there is no evidence of its beneficial effects. Possible effects of subclinical hypothyroidism on pregnancy outcome are subsequently discussed.

Pregnancy Outcome with Overt Hypothyroidism. A few studies, although limited, indicate that *overt hypothyroidism* is associated with excessive adverse perinatal outcomes (Table 53-3). If thyroid deficiency is reversed before pregnancy, there usually are normal perinatal outcomes (Matalon and associates, 2003; Wolfberg and collaborators, 2003). Replacement therapy is with thyroxine, 50 to 100 μg daily. Serum thyrotropin levels are measured at 4- to 6-week intervals and thyroxine adjusted by 25- to 50-μg increments until they reach normal values.

Pregnancy is associated with an increase in thyroxine requirements of about a third (Alexander and associates, 2004; Mandel and colleagues, 1990). In a study of 259 mothers with hypothyroidism given thyroxine replacement throughout pregnancy, Blazer and associates (2003) reported slightly higher thyrotropin levels in their newborns compared with those of normal control women. This suggests that the nonpregnant thyroxine replacement dose was insufficient for pregnancy. Because a similar increased requirement is seen in postmenopausal women with hypothyroidism who are given estrogen replacement, this increased demand in pregnancy may be caused by increased estrogen production (Arafah, 2001).

There is no doubt that maternal and fetal thyroid abnormalities are related. In both, thyroid function is dependent on adequate iodide ingestion, and deficiency early in pregnancy can cause maternal hypothyroidism. In addition, maternal antithyroid antibodies that cause thyroiditis may result in hypothyroidism in both mother and infant. Dussault and Fisher (1999) studied mothers of 259 hypothyroid newborns

detected by the Quebec screening program and found a 20-percent incidence of thyroid dysfunction.

Subclinical Hypothyroidism and Pregnancy. Two studies published in 1999 suggested that maternal hypothyroidism may impair fetal neuropsychological development. In one study, Pop and associates (1999) studied a group of women beginning at 12 weeks' gestation. Children born to women with free T_4 levels below the 10th percentile were at increased risk for impaired psychomotor development. In the other study, Haddow and colleagues (1999) retrospectively evaluated children born to 48 untreated women whose serum thyrotropin values exceeded the 98th percentile. Some offspring of these women had diminished school performance, reading recognition, and IQ scores. Importantly, while described as "subclinically hypothyroid," these women had significantly lower mean serum free thyroxine levels, and thus had overt hypothyroidism. Subsequently, Casey and co-workers (2003) identified subclinical hypothyroidism in 2.3 percent of 17,298 women screened before midpregnancy. These women had significantly higher incidences of preterm birth, placental abruption, and admission of infants to the intensive care nursery (Table 53-4).

SCREENING IN PREGNANCY. Because of the 1999 studies indicating possible long-term neuropsychological effects in children born to women with asymptomatic hypothyroidism, some organizations recommended development of prenatal screening and treatment programs. Others emphasized the unknowns concerned with population screening (Davies, 2000). Specifically, the American College of Obstetricians and Gynecologists (2002) concluded that observational data from the Haddow study were consistent with the *possibility* that subclinical hypothyroidism was associated with adverse neuropsychological development. The College thus recommended against implementation of screening until further studies were done to validate or refute these findings. One major concern is that it seems unlikely that treatment given *after* the period of early cerebral development would be totally efficacious to prevent neurological damage (Utiger, 1999).

Because of all the uncertainties, at least two consensus conferences have been held to help elucidate these findings. One was arranged by the American Thyroid Association, the American Association of Clinical Endocrinologists, and the Endocrine Society (Surks and associates, 2004). The other was held in 2004 by the Centers for Disease Control and Prevention in conjunction with the American Thyroid Association. Both groups recommended against routine prenatal thyrotropin screening at this time. The American Thyroid Association (2004) has since recommended randomized placebo-controlled trials to determine any risks or benefits of detecting and treating subclinical hypothyroidism in pregnancy. It is again emphasized that the 1999 Haddow study included pregnant women with *overt*, albeit mild, *hypothyroidism*.

TABLE 53–4 Pregnancy Outcomes in Women with Untreated Subclinical Hypothyroidism

Outcome	Euthyroid Controls (n = 15,689)	Subclinical Hypothyroidism (n = 404)	P Value
Hypertension (%)	9	11	.39
Placental abruption (%)	0.3	1.0	.026
Gestational age delivered (%)			
≤ 36 weeks	6.0	7.0	.390
≤ 34 weeks	2.5	4.0	.011
≤ 32 weeks	1.0	2.5	.068
Mean birthweight (g)	3367 ± 567	3317 ± 599	.081
RDS–ventilator (%)	1.5	3.0	.048
Neonatal intensive care (%)	2.0	4.0	.019

RDS = Respiratory distress syndrome.
Data from Casey and colleagues (2005).

Iodine Deficiency. In the United States over the past 25 years, iodide fortification of table salt and bread products has diminished, and iodide deficiency has been identified in some of the population (Hollowell and associates 1998; Malee and co-workers, 2004). Adequate iodide is requisite for normal fetal neurological development beginning soon after conception. The recommended daily intake during pregnancy is at least 220 μg/day (American Thyroid Association, 2004).

The World Health Organization (WHO) estimated in 1990 that 20 million people worldwide have varying degrees of preventable brain damage due to fetal iodide deficiency (Hetzel, 1994). Neurodevelopmental abnormalities are dependent on the degree of deficiency. Although it is doubtful that *mild deficiency* causes intellectual impairment, supplementation prevents fetal goiter (Fadeyev and colleagues, 2003). Conversely, *severe deficiency* is associated with frequent and severe damage such as encountered with *endemic cretinism* (Delange, 2001). Although not quantified, it is presumed that *moderate deficiency* has intermediate and variable effects on intellectual and psychomotor function (Glinoer, 2001).

Iodide supplementation before pregnancy prevents neurological morbidity from severe deficiency and apparently does so partially even if given after pregnancy is established. Cao and co-workers (1994) studied pregnancies in a severely iodine-deficient region of China. Women given supplementation before 28 weeks had infants with a 2-percent incidence of moderate or severe neurological abnormalities. The incidence was 9 percent in women who did not receive supplements until the last trimester. The WHO has ongoing programs of universal salt iodization in areas of endemic iodine deficiency (Delange, 2001). Addition of supplemental iodine to prenatal vitamins has been proposed (Malee and associates, 2004).

Congenital Hypothyroidism. Because the clinical diagnosis of hypothyroidism in neonates is usually missed, newborn mass screening was introduced in 1974 and is now required by law. Congenital hypothyroidism is found in about 1 in 4000 to 7000 infants by these programs. For example, in the first 20 years of screening in Texas, 1 in 2500 of 6 million newborns had confirmed hypothyroidism (Drummond-Borg and colleagues, 2003).

About 75 percent of hypothyroid infants have thyroid agenesis or dyshormonogenesis, and another 10 percent have transient hypothyroidism (Lindsay and Toft, 1997). Early and aggressive thyroxine replacement is critical for these infants. Follow-up data from infants identified by screening programs who were treated promptly and adequately are encouraging. Except in those with severe congenital hypothyroidism, sequelae including intellectual impairment are typically preventable (Burrow and colleagues, 1994). Unfortunately, Grant and colleagues (1992) reported that 8 percent of 449 infants with congenital hypothyroidism also had other major associated anomalies.

PRETERM INFANTS. Transient hypothyroxinemia is common in preterm infants, and it had been assumed that treatment with thyroxine is not necessary. Van Wassenaer and colleagues (1997) randomized 157 infants born before 30 weeks to daily thyroxine or placebo. There were no differences in the groups when evaluated at 2 years with psychomotor and neurological testing. In another randomized trial, Briët and co-workers (2001) supplemented neonates and reported better mental outcomes at 2 years in those born before 29 weeks compared with those born after 29 weeks.

POSTPARTUM THYROIDITIS. Transient autoimmune thyroiditis has consistently been found in 5 to 10 percent of women during the first year after childbirth (Amino and colleagues, 2000; Dayan and Daniels, 1996). The propensity for thyroiditis antedates pregnancy and is directly related to increasing serum levels of thyroid autoantibodies. Women with high antibody titers in early pregnancy commonly are affected (Pearce and co-workers, 2003). Up to 25 percent of women with type 1 diabetes develop postpartum thyroid dysfunction (Alvarez-Marfany and associates, 1994). In some women with quiescent Graves disease, a recurrence of hyperthyroxinemia may be stimulated by thyroid destruction (Iitaka and co-workers, 2004).

In clinical practice, thyroiditis is diagnosed infrequently because it typically develops months after delivery and has vague and nonspecific symptoms. These include depression, carelessness, and memory impairment (Hayslip and colleagues, 1988). Looked at another way, Kuijpens and associates (2001) found that peroxidase antibodies were a high-risk marker for postpartum depression. Not all studies are consistent, and Lucas and co-workers (2001) found a 1.7-percent incidence of postpartum depression at 6 months in women with thyroiditis as well as in controls.

Pathogenesis. Most women with postpartum thyroiditis have a positive assay result for microsomal autoantibodies. Histologically, there is a destructive lymphocytic thyroiditis. Affected women usually have antibodies throughout pregnancy, but as shown in Figure 53–2, their production is suppressed. Other risk factors are previous thyroid dysfunction or a family history of thyroid or other autoimmune disease. As discussed on page 1190, fetal cell microchimerism may be linked causally to thyroiditis (Ando and Davies, 2003).

Clinical Manifestations. The two recognized clinical phases of postpartum thyroiditis are summarized in Table 53–5. Between 1 and 4 months after delivery, approximately 4 percent of all women develop transient *destruction-induced thyrotoxicosis* from excessive release of hormone from glandular disruption (Lucas and colleagues, 2000). The onset is abrupt, and a small, painless goiter is commonly found. Although there may be many symptoms, only fatigue and palpitations are more frequent in thyrotoxic women compared with that in controls. Antithyroid medications such as thioamides are ineffective. If symptoms are severe, a β-blocker may be given. Approximately two thirds of these women return to a euthyroid state, but the other third develop transient or permanent hypothyroidism.

Between 4 and 8 months postpartum, 2 to 5 percent of all women develop *hypothyroidism* from thyroiditis (Amino and associates, 2000; Jansson and co-workers, 1988). From thyroiditis onset, hypothyroidism can develop within one month. About a third will have gone through the thyrotoxic phase. Thyromegaly and other symptoms are common and more prominent than during the thyrotoxic phase. Thyroxine replacement is given for 6 to 12 months.

Women who experience either type of postpartum thyroiditis have about a 30-percent risk of developing permanent hypothyroidism (Muller and colleagues, 2001; Premawardhana and associates, 2000). Others may develop subclinical disease. Half of these women with thyroiditis who are positive for peroxidase antibodies develop permanent hypothyroidism by 6 to 7 years.

NODULAR THYROID DISEASE. Management of a palpable thyroid nodule during pregnancy depends on the stage of gestation. Small nodules detected by sensitive ultrasonic methods are common during pregnancy in some populations. Kung and associates (2002) used high-resolution sonography to study 221 Chinese women and found that 15 percent had nodules larger than 2 mm. Almost half of these were multiple. These small nodules usually enlarged modestly across pregnancy and did not regress postpartum. Nodules over 5 mm^3 that persisted at 3 months postpartum were biopsied, and most showed nodular hyperplasia. None was malignant. In these same 221 women, eight (3.6 percent) had clinically palpable nodules larger than 1 cm. Although none of these was malignant, previous studies have reported that up to 40 percent of solitary nodules are malignant (Doherty and co-workers, 1995; Rosen and Walfish, 1986). Even so, the majority are low-grade neoplasms.

Most authorities recommend against radioiodine scanning in pregnancy, although tracer doses used are associated

TABLE 53–5 Clinical Phases of Postpartum Thyroiditis

| Characteristics | Postpartum Thyroiditis | |
	Thyrotoxicosis	*Hypothyroidism*
Onset	1–4 months postpartum	4–8 months postpartum
Incidence	4%	2–5%
Mechanism	Destruction-induced hormone release	Thyroid insufficiency
Symptoms	Small, painless goiter; fatigue; palpitations	Goiter, fatigue, inability to concentrate
Treatment	β-blockers for symptoms	Thyroxine for 6–12 months
Sequelae	2/3 become euthyroid 1/3 develop hypothyroidism	1/3 permanent hypothyroidism

with minimal fetal irradiation (see Chap. 41, p. 981). *Ultrasound* examination reliably detects nodules greater than 0.5 cm, and their solid or cystic nature also can be determined. *Fine-needle aspiration* is an excellent method for assessment, and tumor markers and immunostaining are reliable to evaluate for malignancy (Bartolazzi and associates, 2001; Hegedüs, 2004). Mestman (1999) has recommended biopsy for nonfunctional solitary nodules, before midpregnancy for solid lesions over 2 cm and cystic lesions over 4 cm.

Because most thyroid carcinomas are well differentiated and pursue an indolent course, some practitioners recommend that surgery be postponed until after delivery. In either case, there should be a multidisciplinary approach (American College of Obstetricians and Gynecologists, 2002). Moosa and Mazzaferri (1997) studied 61 women with thyroid cancer diagnosed during pregnancy. In 75 percent, thyroidectomy was delayed until after delivery and outcomes were similar to those in nonpregnant controls. In their reviews, Driggers and co-workers (1998) and Morris (1998) found minimal fetal loss attributed to thyroid cancer surgery. We are of the view that thyroid surgery can be safely performed before 24 to 26 weeks (i.e., the time before surgery *might* stimulate preterm labor).

PARATHYROID DISEASES

The function of *parathyroid hormone (PTH)* is to maintain extracellular fluid calcium concentration. This 115–amino acid hormone acts directly on bone and kidney and indirectly on small intestine through its effects on synthesis of vitamin D (1,25(OH$_2$)D) to increase serum calcium. Secretion is regulated by serum ionized calcium concentration through a negative feedback system. *Calcitonin* is a potent hypocalcemic parathyroid hormone that acts in many ways as a physiological parathyroid hormone antagonist. The interrelationships between these hormones and calcium metabolism, as well as *PTH-related protein* produced by fetal tissue, are discussed in Chapter 5 (see p. 142).

Because of substantive fetal calcium needs—300 mg/day in late pregnancy and a total of 30 g—as well as increased renal calcium loss from augmented glomerular filtration, PTH levels were assumed to be increased in pregnant women. With newer assay methods, however, Seely and co-workers (1997) as well as others have reported a significant decrease in intact 1-84 PTH level longitudinally during pregnancy. At the same time, they showed a twofold increase in serum concentrations of 1,25-dihydroxyvitamin D, which is probably of placental and decidual origin. Presumably this latter hormone increases gastrointestinal absorption to meet the needs of pregnancy. At the same time, total serum calcium levels decline to parallel the decreased serum albumin concentration (Power and associates, 1999). Importantly, however, ionized calcium levels are unchanged in pregnancy (Dahlman and colleagues, 1994). According to Molitch (2000), even if immunoreactive

hormone levels are decreased, the biological activity on the kidney is normal.

HYPERPARATHYROIDISM. Hypercalcemia is caused by hyperparathyroidism or cancer in 90 percent of cases. Primary hyperparathyroidism from elevated levels of PTH is relatively common, and its incidence peaks between the third and fifth decades (Potts, 2001). Because many automated laboratory systems include measurement of serum calcium, more cases are being detected (Mestman, 2002). Almost 80 percent are caused by a solitary adenoma and another 15 percent by hyperfunction of all four glands. In most tumor-related cases, the malignancy and the cause of increased serum calcium are obvious. PTH produced by tumors is similar but not identical to the natural hormone, and therefore it is usually not detected by routine assays. In most patients, the serum calcium is elevated to within only 1 mg/dL over the upper normal limit. This may help to explain why only 20 percent of those who have abnormally elevated levels are symptomatic. In most of these patients, serum levels are stable over a 10-year period (Bilezikian and Silverberg, 2004). In a fourth, however, symptoms become apparent when the serum calcium continues to rise. *Hypercalcemic crisis* manifests as stupor, nausea, vomiting, weakness, fatigue, and dehydration.

Management of hyperparathyroidism in nonpregnant patients is controversial. Silverberg and colleagues (1999) compared surgical excision with observation in 121 patients with primary hyperparathyroidism. Half were cured by parathyroidectomy and their bone density improved. Of the half observed, about a fourth had progression of disease, and six of eight who had nephrolithiasis had a recurrence. The second National Institutes of Health Consensus Development Conference recently updated its recommendations, which include parathyroid surgery when the serum calcium exceeds 1.0 mg/dL of the upper normal range (Bilezikian and colleagues, 2002).

Hyperparathyroidism in Pregnancy. In a recent review, Schnatz (2002) found fewer than 200 reported cases. It is presumed that many hypercalcemic pregnant women with hyperparathyroidism are either not detected or not reported. As in nonpregnant patients, hyperparathyroidism is usually caused by a parathyroid adenoma. Cases have been described as due to ectopic parathyroid hormone production, or even more rarely to parathyroid carcinoma (Montoro and colleagues, 2000). Symptoms include hyperemesis, generalized weakness, renal calculi, and psychiatric disorders. Occasionally pancreatitis is the presenting finding (Dahan and Chang, 2001).

Pregnancy theoretically improves hyperparathyroidism because of significant calcium shunting to the fetus as well as augmented renal excretion (Power and colleagues, 1999). When the "protective effects" of pregnancy are withdrawn, however, there is significant danger of postpartum hypercalcemic crisis. Early reports described excessive stillbirths, preterm deliveries, and neonatal tetany in pregnancy complicated by hyperparathyroidism (Shangold and associates, 1982). Currently, with earlier detection and management, adverse effects are much less common (Schnatz, 2002).

MANAGEMENT. If pregnant women are symptomatic, surgical removal of the parathyroid adenoma is preferable (Mestman, 2002). Elective neck exploration during pregnancy is usually well tolerated (Graham and associates, 1998; Kort and colleagues, 1999). In one woman, a mediastinal adenoma was removed at 23 weeks (Rooney and co-workers, 1998). If pregnant women are asymptomatic, they may be given oral phosphate, 1 to 1.5 g daily in divided doses. Serum calcium may decrease so that parathyroidectomy can be postponed until after delivery.

For women with dangerously elevated serum calcium levels, or in those who are mentally obtunded (*hypercalcemic crisis*), emergency treatment is instituted. Diuresis with intravenous normal saline is begun so that urine flow exceeds 150 mL/hr. *Furosemide* is given in conventional doses to block tubular calcium reabsorption. Careful attention to prevent hypokalemia and hypomagnesemia is important. Adjunctive therapy includes *mithramycin,* which inhibits bone resorption; *calcitonin,* which decreases skeletal calcium release; and oral phosphorus.

NEONATAL EFFECTS. In normal infants, cord blood calcium levels are higher than maternal levels. With maternal hyperparathyroidism, abnormally elevated maternal and thence fetal levels further suppress fetal parathyroid function. Thus, at birth there is a rapidly decreasing newborn calcium level, which reaches a nadir at 24 to 48 hours. About 15 to 25 percent of these infants develop severe hypocalcemia with or without tetany (Molitch, 2000). In some cases, neonatal tetany alone has stimulated a search to diagnose maternal parathyroid adenoma (Beattie and co-workers, 2000).

HYPOPARATHYROIDISM. The most common cause of hypocalcemia is hypoparathyroidism that usually follows parathyroid or thyroid surgery. Chronically hypocalcemic pregnant women may have a fetus with skeletal demineralization. Treatment usually prevents symptomatic hypocalcemia. The woman is given 1,25-dihydroxyvitamin D_3 (calcitriol), dihydrotachysterol, or large doses of vitamin D (50,000 to 150,000 U/day); calcium gluconate or calcium lactate (3 to 5 g/day); and a diet low in phosphates. The fetal risks from large doses of vitamin D have not been established. Caplan and Beguin (1990) observed that whereas the calcitriol dose had to be increased in five women during the second half of pregnancy, it could be reduced during lactation.

PREGNANCY-ASSOCIATED OSTEOPOROSIS. It is unlikely that normal pregnancy causes osteopenia in most women (Kaur and associates, 2003; To and co-workers, 2003). That said, some women develop idiopathic osteoporo-

sis while pregnant or lactating. The cause of this is controversial, but most authorities believe that pregnancy unmasks preexisting bone disease (Black and co-workers, 2000; Henderson and colleagues, 2000). For example, Rizzoli and Bonjour (1996) suggested that accentuated lordosis in pregnancy leads to pain and fractures in the already osteopenic woman. The most common symptom of osteoporosis is back pain in late pregnancy or postpartum. Other symptoms are hip pain, either unilateral or bilateral, and difficulty in weight bearing (Dunne and colleagues, 1993; Smith and associates, 1995). In more than half of women, no apparent reason for osteopenia is found. Some known causes include heparin, prolonged bed rest, and corticosteroid therapy (von Mandach and co-workers, 2003). In a few cases, overt hyperparathyroidism or thyrotoxicosis eventually develops.

Idiopathic osteonecrosis of the femoral head during normal pregnancy has been described (Chang and associates, 1993; Gribble and Berres, 2001). We have seen osteonecrosis only as a known complication of sickle-cell disease, prolonged heparin therapy, or corticosteroid therapy (Spencer and colleagues, 1999).

Treatment is problematical, but most clinicians recommend calcium and vitamin D supplementation. Long-term follow-up indicates that although bone density improves, these women, as well as their offspring, may have chronic osteopenia (Blanch and co-workers, 1994; Carbone and colleagues, 1995).

ADRENAL GLAND DISORDERS

Pregnancy has profound effects on adrenal cortical secretion and its control or stimulation. These interrelationships are discussed in detail in Chapter 5 (see p. 143). Serum corticotropin levels increase after a marked reduction in early pregnancy, undoubtedly related to corticotropin-releasing hormone synthesized by the placenta (Carr and Rainey, 1994). The considerable increase in plasma cortisol is explained by increased transcortin production and binding. In addition, plasma renin increases, which increases angiotensin II and in turn aldosterone secretion. Baseline adrenal medullary hormone secretion is probably unaffected. Although there is no evidence that pregnancy causes any specific adrenal disorders, a number may coexist with pregnancy.

PHEOCHROMOCYTOMA. These are chromaffin tumors that secrete catecholamines. Most are located in the adrenal medulla, but 10 percent are located in the sympathetic ganglia. In adults, they are called the *10-percent tumor* because 10 percent are bilateral, 10 percent are extra-adrenal, and about 10 percent are malignant. There is an association with medullary thyroid carcinoma and hyperparathyroidism in some of the autosomally dominant or recessive *multiple endocrine neoplasia syndromes* as well as in neurofibromatosis and von Hippel–Lindau disease. Pheochromocytomas are common findings at autopsy but are frequently not diagnosed. Only 0.1 percent of hypertensive patients have a pheochromocytoma.

Symptoms are usually paroxysmal and manifest as hypertensive crisis, seizure disorders, or anxiety attacks. Hypertension is sustained in 60 percent of patients, but half of these also have paroxysmal crises. Other symptoms during paroxysmal attacks are headaches, profuse sweating, palpitations, and apprehension. Chest pain, tachycardia, nausea and vomiting, and pallor or flushing are also common.

The standard screening test is quantification of catecholamine metabolites in a 24-hour urine specimen (Keely, 1998). Diagnosis is established by measurement of a 24-hour urine collection with at least two of three assays for free catecholamines, metanephrines, or vanillylmandelic acid (VMA). Determination of plasma catecholamine levels is accurate but is associated with technical difficulties (Conlin, 2001; Lenders and associates, 2002). In nonpregnant women, adrenal localization is usually successful with either computed tomography (CT) or magnetic resonance imaging (MRI). Extra-adrenal tumors may also be localized using these, but occasionally ^{131}I-metaiodobenzylguanidine (MIBG) scanning is necessary for localization.

In most cases today, preferred treatment is laparoscopic adrenalectomy (Lal and Duh, 2003).

Pheochromocytoma Complicating Pregnancy. These tumors are rare but dangerous complications of pregnancy. Geelhoed (1983) cited an earlier review of 89 cases in which 43 mothers died. Maternal death was much more common if the tumor was not diagnosed antepartum (58 versus 18 percent). With modern diagnostic methods and management, maternal survival has improved. Shown in Table 53–6 are results from two reviews done during two contiguous eras. Maternal mortality decreased from 16 to 4 percent. **There were no maternal deaths when the diagnosis was made antepartum.** Fortunately, antepartum diagnosis has now become common.

TABLE 53–6 Outcomes of Pregnancies Complicated by Pheochromocytoma and Reported in Two Contiguous Epochs

Factor	Incidence in %	
	1980–1987[a] (n = 48)	1988–1997[b] (n = 42)
Diagnosis		
Antepartum	51	83
Postpartum	36	14
Autopsy	12	2
Maternal mortality	16	4
Fetal wastage	26	11

[a]Data from Harper and colleagues (1989).
[b]Data from Ahlawat and associates (1999).

There are several methods for tumor localization during pregnancy. Ahlawat and colleagues (1999) reported that 21 of 22 tumors were found using sonography, 10 of 11 using CT, and 10 of 10 using MRI (Fig. 53–4).

In some cases, the principal challenge is to differentiate preeclampsia from the hypertensive crisis caused by pheochromocytoma. Combs and colleagues (1989) have shown that cardiac output falls during paroxysmal hypertension; thus, adverse fetal effects must be considered. In one instance, a postpartum woman presented with dilated cardiomyopathy (Ahn and associates, 2003).

As in nonpregnant patients, there are individual considerations. For example, Grimbert and colleagues (1999) diagnosed two pheochromocytomas during 56 pregnancies in 30 women with *von Hippel–Lindau disease.* Bassoon-Zaltzman and associates (1995) described a normotensive 20-week pregnant woman with intermittent ventricular tachycardia caused by a bladder pheochromocytoma.

MANAGEMENT. Immediate control of hypertension and symptoms with an α-adrenergic blocker such as *phenoxybenzamine* is imperative. The dose is 10 to 30 mg, two to four times daily. After α-blockade is achieved, β-blockers may be given for tachycardia if necessary. In selected cases, surgical exploration and tumor removal may be performed during pregnancy. Successful laparoscopic removal of an adrenal pheochromocytoma has been described in 16- and 20-week pregnancies (Janetschek and associates, 1998). Favorable outcomes were described for 10 of 26 women in whom the diagnosis was made in pregnancy. Blood pressure was controlled pharmacologically during cesarean delivery that was accompanied by tumor resection (Ahlawat and colleagues, 1999). Recurrent tumors are troublesome, and even with good blood pressure control, dangerous peripartum hypertension may develop. We have cared for three women in whom recurrent pheochromocytoma was identified during pregnancy. Hypertension was managed with phenoxybenzamine in all three. Two infants were healthy, but a third was stillborn in a mother with a massive tumor burden who was receiving phenoxybenzamine, 100 mg daily. In all three women, tumor resection was done postpartum. One woman died of persistent metastases several years later.

CUSHING SYNDROME. Long-term exposure to glucocorticoids leads to Cushing syndrome, which is either corticotropin-dependent or -independent (Williams and Dluhy, 2001). **The most common cause of Cushing syndrome is iatrogenic corticosteroid treatment.** The cause of endogenous Cushing syndrome is increased adrenal cortisol production. Most cases are due to *Cushing disease*, bilateral adrenal hyperplasia that is, stimulated by corticotropin-producing pituitary adenomas. Most of these are microadenomas less than 1 cm, and half are 5 mm or less. Occasionally, abnormal secretion of hypothalamic corticotropin-releasing factor may cause corticotropic hyperplasia. Hyperplasia may

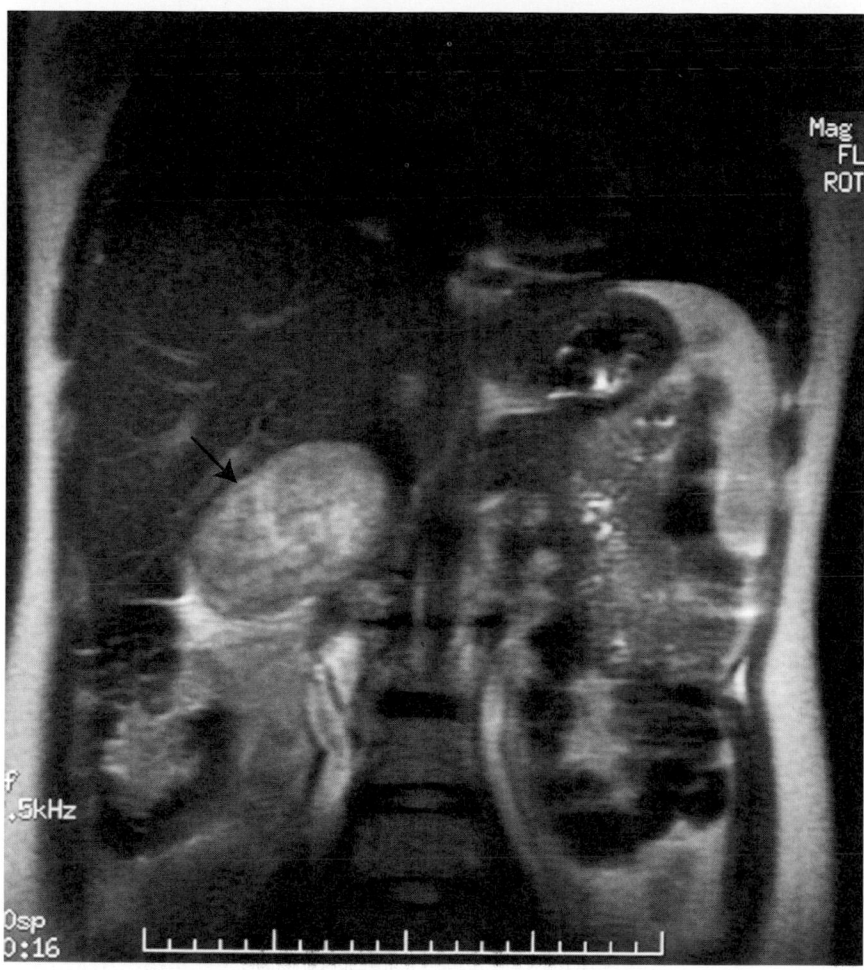

FIGURE 53–4. Coronal magnetic resonance image taken in a 32-week pregnant woman shows a right-sided pheochromocytoma (arrow) and its position in relation to the liver. (Courtesy of Dr. Diane Twickler.)

also be caused by nonendocrine tumors that produce polypeptides similar to either corticotropin-releasing factor or corticotropin. About a fourth of cases of Cushing syndrome are corticotropin-independent. Most are caused by an adrenal adenoma, which is usually bilateral, and half are malignant. Occasionally, androgens may cause rather severe virilization (Danilowicz and colleagues, 2002).

The typical body habitus is caused by adipose tissue deposition, which characteristically results in *moon facies,* a *buffalo hump,* and *truncal obesity.* Fatigability and weakness, hypertension, hirsutism, and amenorrhea are each encountered in 75 to 85 percent of nonpregnant patients (Williams and Dluhy, 2001). Personality changes, cutaneous striae, and easy bruisability are common. Up to 20 percent have nephrolithiasis. Confirmation is by elevated plasma cortisol that cannot be suppressed by dexamethasone or by elevated 24-hour urine free cortisol excretion (Boscaro and colleagues, 2001). Neither test is totally accurate, and both are harder to interpret in obese patients. CT and MRI are used to localize pituitary and adrenal tumors or hyperplasia.

Pregnancy and Cushing Syndrome. Because most women with Cushing syndrome have amenorrhea, associated pregnancy is rare. Otherwise, pregnant women usually have classic clinical findings. Buescher and co-workers (1992) found only about 70 reported cases, and Kamiya and colleagues (1998) summarized 97 cases from the Japanese literature. The distribution of causes of the syndrome is different in pregnant women. For example, most cases were caused by adrenal tumors, of which 80 percent were benign. These reports stressed difficulties in diagnosis because of pregnancy-induced increases in plasma cortisol, corticotropin, and corticotropin-releasing factor. Measurement of 24-hour urinary free cortisol excretion is recommended, with consideration for the elevation in normal pregnancy. Molitch (2000) emphasizes that in normal pregnancy the diurnal variation is unchanged.

Maternal complications include hypertension in 60 to 90 percent and gestational diabetes in about 50 percent. Heart failure is common during pregnancy, and Buescher and associates (1992) reported three maternal deaths in 65 pregnancies. Perinatal morbidity and mortality are correspondingly high. Preterm delivery was reported in 60 percent and perinatal mortality in about 25 percent.

MANAGEMENT. Long-term medical therapy for Cushing syndrome usually is ineffective. Ketoconazole blocks steroid production, and it has been used successfully. Definitive therapy is resection of the pituitary or adrenal adenoma or bilateral adrenalectomy for hyperplasia. During pregnancy, management of hypertension in mild cases may suffice until delivery. Otherwise, pituitary adenomas causing Cushing disease are treated by transsphenoidal resection (Boscaro and colleagues, 2001; Mellor and associates, 1998). Removal of an adrenal adenoma in pregnancy can be curative (Kamiya and colleagues, 1998; Keely, 1998).

Antepartum treatment of 16 pregnant women with Cushing syndrome was summarized by Aron and associates (1990). In six women, unilateral adrenalectomy was performed for an adenoma; in five, bilateral resection was done for hyperplasia; four were treated with either *metyrapone, aminoglutethimide,* or *cyproheptadine;* and one underwent pituitary irradiation. A few cases during pregnancy have been successfully treated with oral *ketoconazole* (Berwaerts and co-workers, 1999). Because it also blocks testicular steroidogenesis, treatment during pregnancy with a male fetus is worrisome. *Mifepristone,* the norethindrone derivative used for abortion and labor induction, has shown promise for treating Cushing disease. However, it cannot be used in pregnancy.

ADRENAL DEFICIENCY. Primary adrenocortical insufficiency, or *Addison disease,* is rare. More than 90 percent of the glands must be destroyed for symptoms to develop. In the majority of cases, it is caused by *idiopathic autoimmune adrenalitis,* which has surpassed tuberculosis and histoplasmosis as common causes. There is an increased incidence of concurrent Hashimoto thyroiditis, premature ovarian failure, type 1 diabetes, and Graves disease. These *polyglandular autoimmune syndromes* also include pernicious anemia, vitiligo, alopecia, nontropical sprue, and myasthenia gravis.

Adrenal Insufficiency and Pregnancy. Untreated adrenal hypofunction frequently causes infertility, but with replacement therapy, ovulation is restored. If untreated, common symptoms include weakness, fatigue, nausea and vomiting, and weight loss (Mestman, 2002). Because serum cortisol levels are increased during pregnancy, initial diagnostic evaluation should include documentation of a lack of response to infused corticotropin (O'Shaughnessy and Hackett, 1984).

Seaward and colleagues (1989) found only five cases of Addison disease during pregnancy published since 1972. They reported a woman with unrecognized Addison disease who suffered a placental abruption and fetal death associated with Addisonian crisis. Albert and associates (1989) reported successful pregnancy outcomes in six women in whom adrenal insufficiency had been diagnosed before conception.

Most pregnant women with Addison disease are already taking cortisone-like drugs and these are continued. With treatment, the pregnant woman is observed for evidence of either inadequate or excessive steroid replacement. During labor, delivery, and postpartum, or after a surgical procedure, steroid replacement must be increased appreciably to approximate the normal adrenal response—so-called *stress doses.* Hydrocortisone, 100 mg, is usually given intravenously every 8 hours. It is important that shock from causes other than adrenocortical insufficiency (e.g., hemorrhage or sepsis) be recognized and treated promptly.

PRIMARY ALDOSTERONISM. Hyperaldosteronism is caused by an adrenal aldosteronoma in about 75 percent of cases, and idiopathic bilateral adrenal hyperplasia in the remainder (Ganguly, 1998). Findings include hypertension, hypokalemia, and muscle weakness. High serum or urine levels of aldosterone confirm the diagnosis.

Pregnancy and Hyperaldosteronism. Progesterone blocks aldosterone action, thus, there are very high levels of aldosterone in normal pregnancy (see Chap. 5, p. 143). It therefore is not surprising that there may be amelioration of symptoms and electrolyte abnormalities during pregnancy (Biglieri and Slaton, 1967; Murakami and associates, 2000). Unless an unequivocal adrenal adenoma is localized by CT or MRI for resection, medical therapy is given. In many cases, hypertension responds to *spironolactone,* but β-blockers or calcium-channel blockers also may be required. Tumor resection is curative, and laparoscopic adrenalectomy should prove useful during pregnancy (Ganguly, 1998).

Webb and Bayliss (1997) reviewed 15 cases of primary aldosteronism associated with pregnancy. Most presented with hypertension and hypokalemia, and in 10, an adrenal adenoma was identified. Baron and associates (1995) reported curative adrenalectomy at 17 weeks for an adenoma. Nezu and co-workers (2000) described two women found to have an aldosteronoma postpartum. They were normotensive throughout pregnancy, but developed severe hypertension several weeks postpartum.

PITUITARY DISEASES

The normal pituitary enlarges in pregnancy, predominately from lactotrophic cellular hyperplasia. These effects are from estrogen stimulation as discussed in Chapter 5 (see p. 141).

PROLACTINOMAS. These adenomas have been found to be relatively common since the advent of widely available assays for serum prolactin. Symptoms include amenorrhea, galactorrhea, and hyperprolactinemia. Tumors are classified arbitrarily by their size, determined by imaging: a microadenoma is 10 mm or less, and a macroadenoma is greater than 10 mm. Treatment for microadenomas is usually with bromocriptine, which is a dopamine agonist and powerful prolactin inhibitor. Treatment frequently restores ovulation. For suprasellar macroadenomas, most recommend surgical therapy before pregnancy is attempted (Schlechte, 2003).

Prolactinomas and Pregnancy. Molitch (1985) analyzed outcomes in almost 250 pregnant women with previously untreated *microadenomas*. Only four women developed symptomatic enlargement during pregnancy, and another 11 who remained asymptomatic had radiographic evidence of enlargement. Albrecht and Betz (1986) reviewed 352 pregnancies in women with microadenomas and reported incidences of 2.3 percent for visual disturbances, 4.8 percent for headaches, and 0.6 for percent diabetes insipidus. Conversely, symptomatic enlargement of *macroadenomas* during pregnancy is more common. When the tumor has extended into the suprasellar region, 15 to 35 percent of women have tumor enlargement during pregnancy that cause visual disturbances, headaches, and diabetes insipidus (Schlechte, 2003). Kupersmith and colleagues (1994) described visual loss during pregnancy in six of eight women with macroadenomas.

Molitch (2000) recommends that pregnant women with microadenomas be queried regularly for headaches and visual symptoms. Those with macroadenomas should also have visual field testing during each trimester. Serial serum prolactin levels are not recommended because of normal increases during pregnancy. CT or MRI is recommended only if symptoms develop. Symptomatic tumor enlargement is treated immediately with bromocriptine, however, relative resistance of macroprolactinomas has been described (Shanis and Check, 1996). More than 6000 pregnant women have taken bromocriptine at some time during pregnancy, and there have been no adverse effects (Molitch, 2001). Surgery is undertaken for women with no response. Gondim and colleagues (2003) have described transnasal transseptal minimally invasive endoscopic resection.

ACROMEGALY. This is caused by excessive growth hormone, usually from an acidophilic or a chromophobic pituitary adenoma. In normal pregnancy, pituitary growth hormone levels decrease as placental epitopes are secreted. Conventional radioimmunoassays cannot differentiate between the two causal adenomas. Diagnosis is confirmed by the failure of an oral glucose tolerance test to suppress pituitary growth hormone (Molitch, 2000). Pregnancy is rare in women with acromegaly, possibly because half are hyperprolactinemic.

Management is similar to that for prolactinomas, with close monitoring for symptoms of tumor enlargement. Bromocriptine is not as effective as it is for prolactinomas, and surgery may be necessary for symptomatic tumor enlargement during pregnancy (Prager and Braunstein, 1995). Herman-Bonert and associates (1998) and Neal (2000) have reported successful treatment of pregnant women with *octreotide.*

DIABETES INSIPIDUS. Vasopressin deficiency is usually due to a hypothalamic or pituitary stalk disorder rather than to a pituitary lesion (Lamberts and associates, 1998). True diabetes insipidus is a rare complication of pregnancy (Hime and Richardson, 1978). Only a few cases have been cared for in the last 45 years at Parkland Hospital, during which time there were over 350,000 deliveries.

Preferable therapy is intranasal administration of *desmopressin,* the synthetic analogue of vasopressin, which is 1-deamino-8-D-arginine vasopressin (DDAVP). Ray (1998) reviewed 53 cases in which DDAVP was used during pregnancy with no adverse sequelae. Most women require increased doses during pregnancy, likely because of an increased metabolic clearance rate stimulated by placental vasopressinase (Lindheimer and Barron, 1994). By this same mechanism, *subclinical diabetes insipidus* may become symptomatic during an otherwise normal pregnancy (Iwasaki and colleagues, 1991). Krege and associates (1989) reviewed 17 such cases. A case of diabetes insipidus during pregnancy has been described as arising from a hemorrhage into a macroadenoma and another following an occluded ventriculoperitoneal shunt (Freeman and co-workers, 1992; Goolsby and Harlass, 1996). Another case was described that manifested during pregnancy as oligohydramnios and diabetes insipidus that did not resolve postpartum (Hanson and colleagues, 1997). Another cause is pituitary infarction with severe obstetrical hemorrhage (see below). In our experience, transient secondary diabetes insipidus is more likely encountered with *acute fatty liver of pregnancy* (see Chap. 50, p. 1127). This likely is due to altered vasopressinase clearance because of hepatic dysfunction. Harper and associates (1987) described transient disease in a 38-week pregnant woman with biopsy-proven viral hepatitis.

SHEEHAN SYNDROME. In 1937, Sheehan reported that pituitary ischemia and necrosis associated with obstetrical blood loss may cause hypopituitarism. Contemporaneously, these events are rare (Vaphiades and colleagues, 2003). One woman who was undelivered developed hemorrhage and necrosis with lymphocytic hypophysitis (Lee and Pless, 2003). When it occurs acutely, affected women may have persistent hypotension, tachycardia, hypoglycemia, and failure of lactation. Subsequent deficiencies of some or all pituitary responsive hormones may develop. For example, as discussed above, diabetes insipidus with or without anterior pituitary deficiency has been described following massive obstetrical hemorrhage and prolonged shock (Kan and Calligerous, 1998). Ammini and Mathur (1994) described 12 cases of Sheehan syndrome encountered in New Delhi. The average duration of onset of symptoms was 5 years. Pituitary apoplexy can also occur with infarction of a macroadenoma (Kaiser, 2001).

LYMPHOCYTIC HYPOPHYSITIS. This autoimmune pituitary disorder is characterized by massive infiltration by lymphocytes and plasma cells with parenchymal destruction of the gland. The majority of cases have been associated with pregnancy (Madsen, 2000; Patel and associates, 1995; Thodou and colleagues, 1995). There are varying degrees of hypopituitarism or symptoms of mass effect, including headaches and visual field defects. A sellar mass is seen on CT or MRI. A mass accompanied by a modestly elevated serum prolactin level (less than 100 pg/mL) suggests lymphocytic hypophysitis, whereas levels exceeding 200 pg/mL are encountered with a prolactinoma. Associated hypothyroidism is common. Pressman and colleagues (1995) reviewed 44 cases and found that 25 percent had other autoimmune diseases. Treatment is with hormone replacement, but the disease may be self-limited (Gagneja and associates, 1999). Surgery during pregnancy is warranted only in cases of severe chiasmal compression unresponsive to corticosteroid therapy (Lee and Pless, 2003). With infertility, both spontaneous and ovulation-induced pregnancies have been successful (Verdú and colleagues, 1998).

REFERENCES

Abalovich M, Gutierrez S, Alcaraz G, et al: Overt and subclinical hypothyroidism complicating pregnancy. Thyroid 12:63, 2002

Abramson J, Stagnaro-Green A: Thyroid antibodies and fetal loss: An evolving story. Thyroid 11:57, 2001

Ahlawat SK, Jain S, Kumari S, et al: Pheochromocytoma associated with pregnancy: Case report and review of the literature. Obstet Gynecol Surv 54:728, 1999

Ahn JT, Hibbard JU, Chapa JB: Atypical presentation of pheochromocytoma as part of multiple endocrine neoplasia IIa in pregnancy. Obset Gynecol 102:1202, 2003

Albert E, Dalaker K, Jorde R, et al: Addison's disease and pregnancy. Acta Obstet Gynecol Scand 68:185, 1989

Albrecht BH, Betz G: Prolactin-secreting pituitary tumors and pregnancy. In Olefshy JM, Robinson RJ (eds): Contemporary Issues in Endocrinology and Metabolism: Prolactinomas, Vol II. New York, Churchill Livingstone, 1986, p 195

Alexander EK, Marqusee E, Lawrence J, et al:Timing and magnitude of increases in levothyroxine requirements during pregnancy in women with hypothyroidism. N Engl J Med 351:241, 2004

Alvarez-Marfany M, Roman SH, Drexler AJ, et al: Long-term prospective study of postpartum thyroid dysfunction in women with insulin dependent diabetes mellitus. J Clin Endocrinol Metab 79:10, 1994

American College of Obstetricians and Gynecologists: Thyroid disease in pregnancy. Practice Bulletin No. 37, August 2002

American Thyroid Association: Statement on early maternal thyroidal insufficiency: Recognition, clinical management and research directions. Available at: www.thyroid.org. Accessed April 29, 2004

Amino N, Izumi Y, Hidaka Y, et al: No increase of blocking type antithyrotropin receptor antibodies during pregnancy in patients with Graves' disease. J Clin Endocrinol Metab 88(12):5871, 2003

Amino N, Tada H, Hidaka Y, et al: Postpartum autoimmune thyroid syndrome. Endocr J 47:645, 2000

Amino N, Tanizawa O, Mori H, et al: Aggravation of thyrotoxicosis in early pregnancy and after delivery in Graves' disease. J Clin Endocrinol Metab 55:108, 1982

Ammini AC, Mathur SK: Sheehan syndrome: An analysis of possible aetiological factors. Aust N Z J Obstet Gynaecol 34:534, 1994

Ando T, Davies TF: Postpartum autoimmune thyroid disease: The potential role of fetal microchimerism. J Clin Endocrinol Metab 88:2965, 2003

Ando T, Imaizumi M, Graves PN, et al: Intrathyroidal fetal microchimerism in Graves' disease. J Clin Endocrinol Metab 87:3315, 2002

Anselmo J, Cao D, Karrison T, et al: Fetal loss associated with excess thyroid hormone exposure. JAMA 292:691, 2004

Arafah BM: Increased need for thyroxine in women with hypothyroidism during estrogen therapy. N Engl J Med 344:1743, 2001

Aron DC, Schnall AM, Sheeler LR: Cushing's syndrome and pregnancy. Am J Obstet Gynecol 162:244, 1990

Ayala C, Navarro E, Rodríguez JR, et al: Conception after iodine-131 therapy for differentiated thyroid cancer. Thyroid 8:1009, 1998

Bajoria R, Peek MJ, Fisk NM: Maternal-to-fetal transfer of thyrotropin-releasing hormone in vivo. Am J Obstet Gynecol 178:264, 1998

Baker JR Jr: Autoimmune endocrine disease. JAMA 278:1931, 1997

Baron F, Sprauve ME, Huddleston JF, et al: Diagnosis and surgical treatment of primary aldosteronism in pregnancy: A case report. Obstet Gynecol 86:644, 1995

Bartolazzi A, Gasbarri A, Papotti M, et al: Application of an immunodiagnostic method for improving reoperative diagnosis of nodular thyroid lesions. Lancet 357:1644, 2001

Bassoon-Zaltzman C, Sermer M, Lao TT, et al: Bladder pheochromocytoma in pregnancy without hypertension. J Reprod Med 40:149, 1995

Beattie GC, Ravi NR, Lewis M, et al: Rare presentation of maternal primary hyperparathyroidism. BMJ 321:223, 2000

Berg GEB, Nyström EH, Jacobsson L, et al: Radioiodine treatment of hyperthyroidism in a pregnant woman. J Nucl Med 39:357, 1998

Berlin L: Malpractice issues in radiology: Iodine-131 and the pregnant patient. AJR Am J Roentgenol 176:869, 2001

Berwaerts J, Verhelst J, Mahler C, et al: Cushing's syndrome in pregnancy treated by ketoconazole: Case report and review of the literature. Gynecol Endocrinol 13:175, 1999

Bianchi DW, Romero R: Biological implications of bi-directional fetomaternal cell trafficking summary of a National Institute of Child Health and Human Development-sponsored conference. J Matern Fetal Neonatal Med 14:123, 2003

Biglieri EG, Slaton PE Jr: Pregnancy and primary aldosteronism. J Clin Endocrinol Metab 27:1628, 1967

Bilezikian JP, Potts JT Jr, Fuleihan Gel-H, et al: Summary statement from a workshop on asymptomatic primary hyperparathyroidism: A perspective for the 21st century. J Bone Miner Res 17:Suppl 2:N2, 2002

Bilezikian JP, Silverberg SJ: Asymptomatic primary hyperparathyroidism. N Engl J Med 350:1746, 2004

Black AJ, Topping J, Durham B, et al: A detailed assessment of alterations in bone turnover, calcium homeostasis, and bone density in normal pregnancy. J Bone Miner Res 15:557, 2000

Blanch J, Pacifici R, Chines A: Pregnancy-associated osteoporosis: Report of two cases with long-term bone density follow-up. Br J Rheumatol 33:269, 1994

Blazer S, Moreh-Waterman Y, Miller-Lotan R, et al: Maternal hypothyroidism may affect fetal growth and neonatal thyroid function. Obstet Gynecol 102:232, 2003

Boscaro M, Barzon L, Fallo F, et al: Cushing's syndrome. Lancet 357:783, 2001

Bowman ML, Bergmann M, Smith JF: Intrapartum labetalol for the treatment of maternal and fetal thyrotoxicosis. Thyroid 8:795, 1998

Brand F, Liegeois P, Langer B: One case of fetal and neonatal variable thyroid dysfunction in the context of Graves' disease. Fetal Diagn Ther 20:12, 2005

Briët JM, van Wassenaer AG, Dekker FW, et al: Neonatal thyroxine supplementation in very preterm children: Developmental outcome evaluated at early school age. Pediatrics 107:712, 2001

Buescher MA, McClamrock HD, Adashi EY: Cushing syndrome in pregnancy. Obstet Gynecol 79:130, 1992

Burch HB, Wartofsky L: Life-threatening thyrotoxicosis. Endocrinol Metab Clin North Am 22:263, 1993

Burrow GN, Fisher DA, Larsen PR: Maternal and fetal thyroid function. N Engl J Med 331:1072, 1994

Calvo RM, Jauniaux E, Gulbis B, et al: Fetal tissues are exposed to biologically relevant free thyroxine concentrations during early phases of development. J Clin Endocrinol Metab 87:1768, 2002

Canaris GJ, Manowitz NR, Mayor G, et al: The Colorado Thyroid Disease Prevalence Study. Arch Intern Med 160:526, 2000

Cao XY, Jiang XM, Dou ZH, et al: Timing of vulnerability of the brain to iodine deficiency in endemic cretinism. N Engl J Med 331:1739, 1994

Caplan RH, Beguin EA: Hypercalcemia in a calcitriol-treated hypoparathyroid woman during lactation. Obstet Gynecol 76:485, 1990

Carbone LD, Palmieri GMA, Graves SC, et al: Osteoporosis of pregnancy: Long-term follow-up of patient, and their offspring. Obstet Gynecol 86:664, 1995

Carr BR, Rainey WE: The adrenal. Infert Reprod Med Clin North Am 5:749, 1994

Casara D, Rubello D, Saladini G, et al: Pregnancy after high therapeutic doses of iodine 131 in differentiated thyroid cancer: Potential risks and recommendations. Eur J Nucl Med 20:192, 1993

Casey BM, Dashe JS, Wells CE, et al: Subclinical hypothyroidism pregnancy outcomes. Obstet Gynecol 105:38, 2005

Chang CC, Greenspan A, Gershwin ME: Osteonecrosis: Current perspectives on pathogenesis and treatment. Semin Arthritis Rheum 23:47, 1993

Cohen O, Pinhas-Hamiel O, Sivian E, et al: Serial in utero ultrasonographic measurements of the fetal thyroid: A new complimentary tool in the management of maternal hyperthyroidism in pregnancy. Prenat Diagn 23:740, 2003

Combs CA, Easterling TR, Schmucker BC, et al: Hemodynamic observations during paroxysmal hypertension in a pregnancy with pheochromocytoma. Obstet Gynecol 74:439, 1989

Conlin PR: Case records of the Massachusetts General Hospital: Case 13-2001. N Engl J Med 344:1314, 2001

Cooper DS: Hyperthyroidism. Lancet 362:459, 2003

Cuckle H, Wald N, Stone R, et al: Maternal serum thyroid antibodies in early pregnancy and fetal Down's syndrome. Prenat Diagn 8:439, 1988

Dahan M, Chang RJ: Pancreatitis secondary to hyperparathyroidism during pregnancy. Obstet Gynecol 98:923, 2001

Dahlman T, Sjoberg HE, Bucht E: Calcium homeostasis in normal pregnancy and puerperium. Acta Obstet Gynecol Scand 73:393, 1994

Danilowicz K, Albiger N, Vanegas M, et al: Androgen-secreting adrenal adenomas. Obstet Gynecol 100:1099, 2002

Dashe J, Casey B, McIntire D, et al: Use of a pregnancy-specific nomogram for thyroid stimulating hormone (TSH) to improve screening for thyroid disease [abstract]. Am J Obstet Gynecol 189:S188, 2003

Davidson KM, Richards DS, Schatz DA, et al: Successful in utero treatment of fetal goiter and hypothyroidism. N Engl J Med 324:543, 1991

Davies TF: The ATA, the Endocrine Society, and AACE confuse endocrinologists on thyroid disease in pregnancy. Thyroid 10:107, 2000

Davis LE, Leveno KL, Cunningham FG: Hypothyroidism complicating pregnancy. Obstet Gynecol 72:108, 1988

Davis LE, Lucas MJ, Hankins GDV, et al: Thyrotoxicosis complicating pregnancy. Am J Obstet Gynecol 160:63, 1989

Davison S, Lennard TWJ, Davison J, et al: Management of a pregnant patient with Graves' disease complicated by thionamide-induced neutropenia in the first trimester. Clin Endocrinol 54:559, 2001

Dayan CM, Daniels GH: Chronic autoimmune thyroiditis. N Engl J Med 335:99, 1996

Delange F: Iodine deficiency as a cause of brain damage. Postgrad Med J 77:217, 2001

Diav-Citrin O, Ornoy A: Teratogen update: Antithyroid drugs—methimazole, carbimazole, and propylthiouracil. Teratology 65:38, 2002

Doherty CM, Shindo ML, Rice DH, et al: Management of thyroid nodules during pregnancy. Laryngoscope 105:251, 1995

Driggers RW, Kopelman JN, Satin AJ: Delaying surgery for thyroid cancer in pregnancy. A case report. J Reprod Med 43:909, 1998

Drummond-Borg M, Johnson D, Aldis B, et al: Newborn screening for congenital hypothyroidism: The Texas experience. Tex Med September: 50, 2003

Duncombe GJ, Dickinson JE: Fetal thyrotoxicosis after maternal thyroidectomy. Aust N Z J Obstet Gynaecol 41:224, 2001

Dunne F, Walters B, Marshall T, et al: Pregnancy associated osteoporosis. Clin Endocrinol 39:487, 1993

Dussault JH, Fisher DA: Thyroid function in mothers of hypothyroid newborns. Obstet Gynecol 93:15, 1999

Fadeyev V, Lesnikova S, Melnichenko G: Prevalence of thyroid disorders in pregnant women with mild iodine deficiency. Gynecol Endocrinol 17:413, 2003

Forrest D: The developing brain and maternal thyroid hormone: finding the links. Endocrinology 145:4034, 2004

Freeman R, Wezenter B, Silverstein M, et al: Pregnancy-associated subacute hemorrhage into a prolactinoma resulting in diabetes insipidus. Fertil Steril 58:427, 1992

Fung HY, Kologln M, Collison K, et al: Postpartum thyroid dysfunction in Mid Glamorgan. BMJ 296:241, 1988

Gagneja H, Arafah B, Taylor HC: Histologically proven lymphocytic hypophysitis: Spontaneous resolution and subsequent pregnancy. Mayo Clin Proc 74:150, 1999

Gallagher MP, Schachner HC, Levine LS, et al: Neonatal thyroid enlargement associated with propylthiouracil therapy of Graves' disease during pregnancy: A problem revisited. J Pediatr 139:896, 2001

Ganguly A: Primary aldosteronism. N Engl J Med 339:1828, 1998

Geelhoed GW: Surgery of the endocrine glands in pregnancy. Clin Obstet Gynecol 26:865, 1983

Glinoer D: Pregnancy and iodine. Thyroid 11:471, 2001

Gondim J, Ramos JF, Pinheiro I, et al: Minimally invasive pituitary surgery in a hemorrhagic necrosis adenoma during pregnancy. Minim Invasive Neurosurg 46(3):173, 2003

Goodwin TM, Hershman JM: Hyperthyroidism due to inappropriate production of human chorionic gonadotropin. Clin Obstet Gynecol 40:32, 1997

Goolsby L, Harlass F: Central diabetes insipidus: A complication of ventriculoperitoneal shunt malfunction during pregnancy. Am J Obstet Gynecol 174:1655, 1996

Graham EM, Freedman LJ, Forouzan I: Intrauterine growth retardation in a woman with primary hyperparathyroidism. J Reprod Med 43:451, 1998

Grant DB, Smith I, Fuggle PW, et al: Congenital hypothyroidism detected by neonatal screening: Relationship between biochemical severity and early clinical features. Arch Dis Child 67:87, 1992

Gribble RK, Berres LE: Idiopathic osteonecrosis of the hip during pregnancy: Outcome in a subsequent gestation. Obstet Gynecol 98:911, 2001

Grimbert P, Chauveau D, Richard S, et al: Pregnancy in von Hippel–Lindau disease. Am J Obstet Gynecol 180:110, 1999

Grossman M, Weintraub BD, Szkudlinski MW: Novel insights into the molecular mechanisms of human thyrotropin action: Structural, physiological, and therapeutic implications for the glycoprotein hormone family. Endocr Rev 18:476, 1997

Haddow JE, Palomaki GE, Allan WC, et al: Maternal thyroid deficiency during pregnancy and subsequent neuropsychological development of the child. N Engl J Med 341:549, 1999

Hanson RS, Powrie RO, Larson L: Diabetes insipidus in pregnancy: Treatable cause of oligohydramnios. Obstet Gynecol 89:816, 1997

Harper MA, Murnaghan GA, Kennedy L, et al: Pheochromocytoma in pregnancy. Five cases and a review of the literature. Br J Obstet Gynaecol 96:594, 1989

Harper M, Hatjis CG, Appel RG, et al: Vasopressin resistant diabetes insipidus, liver dysfunction, and hyperuricemia and decreased renal function. J Reprod Med 32:862, 1987

Hayslip CC, Fein HG, O'Donnell VM, et al: The value of serum antimicrosomal antibody testing in screening for symptomatic postpartum thyroid dysfunction. Am J Obstet Gynecol 159:203, 1988

Hegedüs L: The thyroid nodule. N Eng J Med 351:1764, 2004

Helfgott SM: Weekly clinicopathological exercises: Case 21-2002. N Engl J Med 347:122, 2002

Henderson PH, Sowers MF, Kutzko KE, et al: Bone mineral density in grand multiparous women with extended lactation. Am J Obstet Gynecol 182:1371, 2000

Herman-Bonert V, Seliverstov M, Melmed S: Pregnancy in acromegaly: Successful therapeutic outcome. J Clin Endocrinol Metab 83:727, 1998

Hetzel BS: Iodine deficiency and fetal brain damage. N Engl J Med 331:1770, 1994

Hidaka Y, Tamaki H, Iwatani Y, et al: Prediction of postpartum Graves thyrotoxicosis by measurement of thyroid stimulating antibody in early pregnancy. Clin Endocrinol 41:15, 1994

Hime MC, Richardson JA: Diabetes insipidus and pregnancy: Case report, incidence, and review of literature. Obstet Gynecol Surv 3:375, 1978

Hollowell JG, Staehling NW, Hannon WH, et al: Iodine nutrition in the United States. Trends and public health implications: Iodine excretion data from National Health and Nutrition Examination Surveys I and III (1971–1974 and 1988–1994). J Clin Endocrinol Metab 83:3401, 1998

Iitaka M, Morgenthaler NG, Momotani N, et al: Stimulation of thyroid-stimulating hormone (TSH) receptor antibody production following painless thyroiditis. Clin Endocrinol 60:49, 2004

Iwasaki Y, Oiso Y, Kondo K, et al: Aggravation of subclinical diabetes insipidus during pregnancy. N Engl J Med 324:522, 1991

Janetschek G, Finkenstedt G, Gasser R, et al: Laparoscopic surgery for pheochromocytoma: Adrenalectomy, partial resection, excision of paragangliomas. J Urol 150:330, 1998

Jansson R, Dahlberg PA, Karlsson FA: Postpartum thyroiditis. Baillieres Clin Endocrinol Metab 2:619, 1988

Kaiser UB: Weekly clinicopathological exercises: Case 15-2001. N Engl J Med 344:1536, 2001

Kamiya Y, Okada M, Yoneyama A, et al: Surgical successful treatment of Cushing's syndrome in a pregnant patient complicated with severe cardiac involvement. Endocr J 45:499, 1998

Kan AKS, Calligerous D: A case report of Sheehan syndrome presenting with diabetes insipidus. Aust N Z J Obstet Gynaecol 38:224, 1998

Kaur M, Pearson D, Godber I, et al: Longitudinal changes in bone mineral density during normal pregnancy. Bone 32:449, 2003

Keely E: Endocrine causes of hypertension in pregnancy—when to start looking for zebras. Semin Perinatol 22:471, 1998

Khosrotehrani K, Johnson KL, Cha DH, et al: Transfer of fetal cells with multilineage potential to maternal tissue. JAMA 292:75, 2004

Kilpatrick S: Umbilical blood sampling in women with thyroid disease in pregnancy: Is it necessary? Am J Obstet Gynecol 189:1, 2003

Klein I, Kaie O: Thyrotoxicosis and the heart. Endocrinol Metab Clin North Am 27:51, 1998

Klintschar M, Schwaiger P, Mannweiler S, et al: Evidence of fetal microchimerism in Hashimoto's thyroiditis. J Clin Endocrinol Metab 86:2494, 2001

Kort KC, Schiller HJ, Numann PJ: Hyperparathyroidism and pregnancy. Am J Surg 177:66, 1999

Krege J, Katz VL, Bowes WA Jr: Transient diabetes insipidus of pregnancy. Obstet Gynecol Surv 44:789, 1989

Kriplani A, Buckshee K, Bhargava VL, et al: Maternal and perinatal outcome in thyrotoxicosis complicating pregnancy. Eur J Obstet Gynecol Reprod Biol 54:159, 1994

Kuijpens JL, Vader HL, Drexhage HA, et al: Thyroid peroxidase antibodies during gestation are a marker for subsequent depression postpartum. Eur J Endocrinol 145:579, 2001

Kung AWC, Chau MT, Lao TT, et al: The effect of pregnancy on thyroid nodule formation. J Clin Endocrinol Metab 87:1010, 2002

Kung AWC, Jones BM: A change from stimulatory to blocking antibody activity in Graves' disease during pregnancy. J Clin Endocrinol Metab 83:514, 1998

Kupersmith MJ, Rosenberg C, Kleinberg D: Visual loss in pregnant women with pituitary adenomas. Ann Intern Med 121:473, 1994

Lal G, Duh QY: Laparoscopic adrenalectomy—indications and technique. Surg Oncol 12:105, 2003

Lamberts SWJ, de Herder WW, van der Lely AJ: Pituitary insufficiency. Lancet 352:127, 1998

Lee MS, Pless M: Apoplectic lymphocytic hypophysitis: Case report. J Neurosurg 98:183, 2003

Lenders JWM, Pacak K, Walther MM, et al: Biochemical diagnosis of pheochromocytoma: Which test is best? JAMA 287:1427, 2002

Leung AS, Millar LE, Koonings PP, et al: Perinatal outcome in hypothyroid pregnancies. Obstet Gynecol 81:349, 1993

Lindheimer MD, Barron WM: Water metabolism and vasopressin secretion during pregnancy. Baillieres Clin Obstet Gynaecol 8:311, 1994

Lindsay RS, Toft AD: Hypothyroidism. Lancet 349:413, 1997

Lucas A, Pizzaro E, Granada ML, et al: Postpartum thyroid dysfunction and postpartum depression: Are they two linked disorders? Clin Endocrinol 55:809, 2001

Lucas A, Pizarro E, Granada ML, et al: Postpartum thyroiditis: Epidemiology and clinical evolution in a nonselected population. Thyroid 10:71, 2000

Madsen JR: Case records of the Massachusetts General Hospital: Case 34-2000. N Engl J Med 343:1399, 2000

Mandel SJ, Larsen PR, Seely EW, et al: Increased need for thyroxine during pregnancy in women with primary hypothyroidism. N Engl J Med 323:91, 1990

Matalon S, Sherner E, Levy A, et al: Maternal hypothyroidism is not associated with adverse perinatal outcome [abstract]. Obstet Gynecol 189:S190, 2003

Mellor A, Harvey RD, Pobereskin LH, et al: Cushing's disease treated by transsphenoidal selective adenomectomy in mid-pregnancy. Br J Anaesth 80:850, 1998

Mestman JH: Endocrine diseases in pregnancy. In Gabbe S, Niebyl JR, Simpson JL (eds): Obstetrics: Normal and Problem Pregnancies, 4th ed. New York, Churchill Livingstone, 2002, p 1117

Mestman JH: Hyperthyroidism in pregnancy. Endocrinol Metab Clin North Am 27:127, 1998

Mestman JH: Management of thyroid nodules in pregnancy. Contemp Obstet Gynecol 43:27, 1999

Mestman JH, Goodwin TM, Montoro MM: Thyroid disorders of pregnancy. Endocrinol Metab Clin North Am 24:41, 1995

Millar LK, Wing DA, Leung AS, et al: Low birth weight and preeclampsia in pregnancies complicated by hyperthyroidism. Obstet Gynccol 84:946, 1994

Molitch ME: Disorders of prolactin secretions. Endocrinol Metab Clin North Am 30:585, 2001

Molitch ME: Pituitary, thyroid, adrenal, and parathyroid disorders. In Barron WM, Lindheimer MD (eds): Medical Disorders During Pregnancy, 3rd ed. St. Louis, Mosby, 2000, p 101

Molitch ME: Pregnancy and the hyperprolactinemic woman. N Engl J Med 312:1364, 1985

Momotani N, Noh JH, Ishikawa N, et al: Effects of propylthiouracil and methimazole on fetal thyroid status in mothers with Graves' hyperthyroidism. J Clin Endocrinol Metab 82:3633, 1997

Montoro MN, Paler RJ, Goodwin TM, et al: Parathyroid carcinoma during pregnancy. Obstet Gynecol 96: 841, 2000

Moosa M, Mazzaferri EL: Outcome of differentiated thyroid cancer diagnosed in pregnant women. J Clin Endocrinol Metab 82:2862, 1997

Morris PC: Thyroid cancer complicating pregnancy. Obstet Gynecol Clin North Am 25:401, 1998

Muller AF, Drexhage HA, Berghout A: Postpartum thyroiditis and autoimmune thyroiditis in women of childbearing age: Recent insights and consequences for antenatal and postnatal care. Endocr Rev 22:605, 2001

Murakami T, Ogura EW, Tanaka Y, et al: High blood pressure lowered by pregnancy. Lancet 356:1980, 2000

Nachum Z, Rakover Y, Weiner E, Shalev E: Graves' disease in pregnancy: Prospective evaluation of a selective invasive treatment protocol. Am J Obstet Gynecol 189:159, 2003

Neal JM: Successful pregnancy in a woman with acromegaly treated with octreotide: Case report. Endocr Pract 6:148, 2000

Nezu M, Miura Y, Noshiro T, et al: Primary aldosteronism as a cause of severe postpartum hypertension in two women. Am J Obstet Gynecol 182:745, 2000

O'Doherty MJ, McElhatton PR, Thomas SHL: Treating thyrotoxicosis in pregnant or potentially pregnant women. BMJ 318:5, 1999

O'Shaughnessy RW, Hackett KJ: Maternal Addison's disease and fetal growth retardation. J Reprod Mcd 29:752, 1984

Pacini F, Vorontsova T, Molinaro E, et al: Prevalence of thyroid autoantibodies in children and adolescents from Belarus exposed to the Chernobyl radioactive fallout. Lancet 352:763, 1998

Patel MC, Guneratne N, Haq N, et al: Peripartum hypopituitarism and lymphocytic hypophysitis. Q J Med 88:571, 1995

Pearce EN, Farwell AP, Braverman LE: Thyroiditis. N Engl J Med 348:2646, 2003

Peleg D, Cada S, Peleg A, et al: The relationship between maternal serum thyroid-stimulating immunoglobulin and fetal and neonatal thyrotoxicosis. Obstet Gynecol 99:1040, 2002

Pop VJ, Kujipens JL, van Baar AL, et al: Low maternal free thyroxine concentrations during early pregnancy are associated with impaired psychomotor development in infancy. Clin Endocrinol 50:149, 1999

Potts JT: Disease of the parathyroid gland and other hyper- and hypocalcemic disorders. In Braunwald E, Fauci AS, Kasper DL,

et al (eds): Harrison's Principles of Internal Medicine, 15th ed. New York, McGraw-Hill, 2001, p 2205

Power ML, Heaney RP, Kalkwarf HJ, et al: The role of calcium in health and disease. Am J Obstet Gynecol 181:1560, 1999

Prager D, Braunstein GD: Pituitary disorders during pregnancy. Endocrinol Metab Clin North Am 24:1, 1995

Premawardhana LD, Parkes AB, Ammari F, et al: Postpartum thyroiditis and longterm thyroid status: Prognostic influence of thyroid peroxidase antibodies and ultrasound echogenicity. J Clin Endocrinol Metab 85:71, 2000

Pressman EK, Zeidman SM, Reddy UM, et al: Differentiating lymphocytic adenohypophysitis from pituitary adenoma in the peripartum patient. J Reprod Med 40:251, 1995

Ranzini AC, Ananth CV, Smulian JC, et al: Ultrasonography of the fetal thyroid: Nomograms based on biparietal diameter and gestational age. J Ultrasound Med 20:613, 2001

Rasmussen NG, Hornnes PJ, Hegedüs L: Ultrasonographically determined thyroid size in pregnancy and postpartum: The goitrogenic effect of pregnancy. Am J Obstet Gynecol 160:1216, 1989

Ray JG: DDAVP use during pregnancy: An analysis of its safety for mother and child. Obstet Gynecol Surv 53:450, 1998

Reinwein D, Benker G, Lazarus JH, et al: A prospective randomized trial of antithyroid drug doses in Graves' disease therapy. J Clin Endocrinol Metab 76:1516, 1993

Rizzoli R, Bonjour JP: Pregnancy-associated osteoporosis. Lancet 347:1274, 1996

Roberts CG, Ladenson PW. Hypothyroidism.: Lancet 363:793, 2004

Rooney DP, Traub AI, Russell CFJ, et al: Cure of hyperparathyroidism in pregnancy by sternotomy and removal of a mediastinal parathyroid adenoma. Postgrad Med J 74:233, 1998

Rosen IB, Walfish PG: Pregnancy as a predisposing factor in thyroid neoplasia. Arch Surg 121:1287, 1986

Schlechte JA: Prolactinoma. N Engl J Med 349:2035, 2003

Schnatz PF: Surgical treatment of primary hyperparathyroidism during the third trimester. Obstet Gynecol 99:961, 2002

Seaward PGR, Guidozzi F, Sonnendecker EWW: Addisonian crisis in pregnancy: Case report. Br J Obstet Gynaecol 96:1348, 1989

Seely EW, Brown EM, DeMaggio DM, et al: A prospective study of calciotropic hormones in pregnancy and postpartum: Reciprocal changes in serum intact parathyroid hormone and 1,25-dihydroxyvitamin D. Am J Obstet Gynecol 176:214, 1997

Shangold MM, Dor N, Welt SI, et al: Hyperparathyroidism and pregnancy: A review. Obstet Gynecol Surv 37:217, 1982

Shanis BS, Check JH: Relative resistance of a macroprolactinoma to bromocriptine therapy during pregnancy. Gynecol Endocrinol 10:91, 1996

Sheehan HL: Post-partum necrosis of the anterior pituitary. J Path Bact 45:189, 1937

Sheffield JS, Cunningham FG: Thyrotoxicosis and heart failure that complicate pregnancy. Am J Obstet Gynecol 190:211, 2004

Sherif IH, Oyan WT, Bosairi S, et al: Treatment of hyperthyroidism in pregnancy. Acta Obstet Gynecol Scand 70:461, 1991

Silverberg SJ, Shane E, Jacobs TP, et al: A 10-year prospective study of primary hyperparathyroidism with or without parathyroid surgery. N Engl J Med 341:1249, 1999

Singer PA, Cooper DS, Levy EG, et al: Treatment guidelines for patients with hyperthyroidism and hypothyroidism. JAMA 273:808, 1995

Singh PK, Parvin CA, Gronowski AM: Establishment of reference intervals for markers of fetal thyroid status in amniotic fluid. J Clin Endocrinol Metab 88:4175, 2003

Smith R, Athanasou NA, Ostlere SJ, et al: Pregnancy associated osteoporosis. Q J Med 88:865, 1995

Spencer C, Smith P, Rafla N, et al: Corticosteroids in pregnancy and osteonecrosis of the femoral head. Obstet Gynecol 94:848, 1999

Srivatsa B, Srivatsa S, Johnson KL, et al: Microchimerism of presumed fetal origin in thyroid specimens from women: A case-control study. Lancet 358:2034, 2001

Stulberg RA, Davies GAL: Maternal thyrotoxicosis and fetal nonimmune hydrops. Obstet Gynecol 95:1036, 2000

Surks MI, Ortiz E, Daniels GH, et al: Subclinical thyroid disease: Scientific review and guidelines for diagnosis and management. JAMA 291:228, 2004

Thodou E, Asa SL, Kontogeorgos G, et al: Clinical case seminar: Lymphocytic hypophysitis: Clinicopathological findings. J Clin Endocrinol Metab 80:2302, 1995

To WW, Wong MW, Leung TW: Relationship between bone mineral density changes in pregnancy and maternal and pregnancy characteristics: A longitudinal study. Acta Obstet Gynecol Scand 82:820, 2003

Utiger RD: Maternal hypothyroidism and fetal development. N Engl J Med 341:601, 1999

Vanderpump MPJ, Ahlquist JAO, Franklyn JA, et al: Consensus statement for good practice and audit measures in the management of hypothyroidism and hyperthyroidism. BMJ 313:539, 1996

Vaphiades MS, Simmons D, Archer RL, et al: Sheehan syndrome: A splinter of the mind. Surv Ophthalmol 48(2):230, 2003

Van Wassenaer AG, Kok JH, de Vijlder JJM, et al: Effects of thyroxine supplementation on neurologic development in infants born at less than 30 weeks' gestation. N Engl J Med 336:21, 1997

Verdú LI, Marin-Caballero C, García-López G, et al: Ovulation induction and normal pregnancy after panhypopituitarism due to lymphocytic hypophysitis. Obstet Gynecol 91:850, 1998

von Mandach U, Aebersold F, Huch R, et al: Short-term low-dose heparin plus bedrest impairs bone metabolism in pregnant women. Eur J Obstet Gynecol Reprod Biol 106:25, 2003

Vulsma T, Gons M, De Vijilder JJM: Maternal–fetal transfer of thyroxine in congenital hypothyroidism due to a total organification defect or thyroid agenesis. N Engl J Med 321:13, 1989

Webb JC, Bayliss MP: Pregnancy complicated by primary aldosteronism. South Med J 90:243, 1997

Weetman AP: Graves' disease. N Engl J Med 343:1236, 2000

Williams DH, Dluhy RG: Diseases of the adrenal cortex. In Braunwald E, Fauci AS, Kasper DL, et al (eds): Harrison's Principles of Internal Medicine, 15th ed. New York, McGraw-Hill, 2001, p 2084

Wing DA, Millar LK, Koonings PP, et al: A comparison of propylthiouracil versus methimazole in the treatment of hyperthyroidism in pregnancy. Am J Obstet Gynecol 170:90, 1994

Wolfberg A, Lee-Parritz A, Cohen A, et al: Maternal hypothyroid disease is not associated with poor obstetric or neonatal outcomes [abstract]. Am J Obstet Gynecol 189:S187, 2003

Zeeman GG, Wendel G, Cunningham FG: A blueprint for obstetric critical care. Am J Obstet Gynecol 188:532, 2003

54

Connective Tissue Disorders

IMMUNE-MEDIATED CONNECTIVE TISSUE DISEASES

Systemic Lupus Erythematosus
Antiphospholipid Antibodies
Rheumatoid Arthritis
Systemic Sclerosis (Scleroderma)
Vasculitis Syndromes
Dermatomyositis and Polymyositis

INHERITED CONNECTIVE TISSUE DISORDERS

Marfan Syndrome
Ehlers–Danlos Syndrome

REFERENCES

Connective tissue disorders, also referred to as *collagen-vascular disorders,* cause generalized clinical findings and are principally characterized by connective tissue abnormalities that are mediated by a variety of autoantibodies. These are also called *immune-complex diseases* because many are mediated by deposition of immune complexes in specific organ or tissue sites. Some disorders that are characterized by sterile inflammation, especially of the skin, joints, blood vessels, and kidney, are referred to as *rheumatic diseases.* For inexplicable reasons, many of these rheumatic diseases primarily affect women. Another major category of connective tissue diseases includes inherited disorders of bone, skin, cartilage, blood vessels, and basement membranes. Examples of these are Marfan syndrome, osteogenesis imperfecta, and Ehlers–Danlos syndrome.

IMMUNE-MEDIATED CONNECTIVE TISSUE DISEASES

Although the pathogenesis has not been elucidated, immune-mediated disorders can be separated into those clearly associated with autoantibody formation and those without evidence of the rheumatoid factor, the so-called seronegative spondyloarthropathies (Hahn, 1997). The former category includes systemic lupus erythematosus, rheumatoid arthritis, systemic sclerosis (scleroderma), mixed connective tissue disease, dermatomyositis, polymyositis, and a variety of vasculitis syndromes. The seronegative spondyloarthropathies are strongly associated with the presence of the HLA-B27 antigen but not the rheumatoid factor (Benjamin and Parham, 1992; Moll, 1994). These include ankylosing spondylitis, psoriatic arthritis, Reiter disease, and likely the arthritis syndromes associated with ulcerative colitis and Crohn disease.

Because renal involvement is common and often adversely affects pregnancy, a search for coexisting renal involvement is paramount. Hypertension likewise is common, and exacerbation during pregnancy frequently forces early delivery (Wolfberg and colleagues, 2004). In some of these immune-mediated diseases, *antiphospholipid antibodies* are formed that can cause injury to maternal vasculature and to the placenta.

Immunological Aspects. The immune system is designed to protect cells, tissues, and organs perceived as *self* and to attack and destroy foreign or *nonself* antigenic material by the production of antibodies. This protection has two phases. The first is the *innate phase,* which is broad and rapid and is mediated through neutrophils, macrophages, and complement. The second is the *adaptive phase,* which is precise and is caused by antigen-specific reactions through T and B lymphocytes that result in memory for future exposures (Parkin and Cohen, 2001).

For some as yet unknown reason, the immune system may be stimulated to begin producing antibodies directed against self or normal tissues. These "misdirected" antibodies are called *autoantibodies.* The stimulus responsible for their production is unknown, but a variety of inciting reasons are suspected that include bacterial or viral injury to genetically susceptible tissues.

Autoantibodies induce destruction in susceptible tissues by at least two mechanisms. The *cytotoxic mechanism* involves direct antibody attachment to a specific surface antigen, which results in cell injury or destruction. The *immune-complex mechanism* results in tissue damage when the antigen–antibody complex attaches to a susceptible tissue. The complex may then incite a complement response or *cascade,* resulting in the release of chemotactic substances that attract polymorphonuclear cells.

The *major histocompatibility complex (MHC)* is a series of 40 to 50 genes located on the short arm of chromosome 6, and is known as the *human leukocyte antigen (HLA)* complex. These genetic loci code for distinct cell-surface glycoproteins, including transplantation antigens, and are involved in self and nonself recognition. Class I antigens include HLA-A, -B, and -C. Class II antigens include HLA-DR, -DQ, and -DP. Through a variety of complex interactions, including T- and B-cell stimulation and interaction with immunoglobulins and the complement system, nonself antigens or, in the abnormal state, self antigens (normal tissue), are destroyed.

Immune-Mediated Disease and Pregnancy. Very few immune disorders appear to arise only during pregnancy. Maternal isoimmunization from fetal red cell or platelet antigens is the most common (see Chap. 29, p. 663). Some theories of the cause of preeclampsia–eclampsia (see Chap 34, p. 766) and recurrent abortion (see Chap 9, p. 235) implicate an immunological basis.

Some pregnancy-induced immune alterations may modulate connective tissue disorders (see Chap. 5, p. 130). Although it is generally thought that these immunological changes have negligible effects on immune-mediated collagen-vascular disorders, the effects of large amounts of estrogen, progesterone, and prolactin must be considered. For example, estrogens upregulate and androgens downregulate T-cell response, and a number of cytokines are regulated by sex hormones (Lockshin and Druzin, 1995; Refojo and colleagues, 2003). In addition, recall that autoimmune rheumatic diseases mostly affect women. Lockshin (2002) postulates a modulating effect of hormones rather than a causative role.

Fetal Cell Microchimerism. Fetal cells are present in maternal blood starting in the first trimester (Sitar and associates, 2005). An intriguing phenomenon has been used to explain the predilection of autoimmune disorders for women. For example, there have been many observations on the role of *fetal cell microchimerism* to explain immune-mediated diseases (Adams and Nelson, 2004). By this putative mechanism, persistent fetal cells in the maternal circulation stimulate the production of autoantibodies and underlie autoimmune conditions. In this scheme, fetal cells such as thymocytes become engrafted in maternal tissues, or "immortal" long-lived lymphocytes circulate. Lupus may therefore represent a chronic graft-versus-host response to transplacentally acquired fetal cells, as suggested for some thyroid diseases and systemic sclerosis (Artlett and associates, 1998; Jimenez and Artlett, 2005; Srivatsa and associates, 2001). Women with lupus have also been found to have male cells in every histologically abnormal tissue type, but not in normal tissue. Although this suggests that fetal cells may be associated with lupus, it is unclear if this causes disease or is an effect of disease progression, or even unrelated (Johnson and colleagues, 2001). Interestingly, microchimeric cells may also be beneficial by helping repair damaged or diseased tissue, suggesting these fetal cells may have a beneficial role (Barinaga, 2002).

SYSTEMIC LUPUS ERYTHEMATOSUS.

Lupus is a heterogeneous syndrome with a complex pathogenesis, and its genetic contribution is clustered on the 1q and 6p chromosomes (Tsokos, 2001). Immune system abnormalities include overactive B lymphocytes that are responsible for autoantibody production. These result in tissue and cellular damage when autoantibodies or immune complexes are directed at one or more cellular nuclear components (Mills, 1994). Almost 90 percent of cases are in women. The prevalence in women of childbearing age is about 1 in 500 (Lockshin and Sammaritano, 2000). The 10- and 20-year survival rates are 75 and 50 percent (Jacobsen and colleagues, 1999). Infection, lupus flares, end-organ failure, and cardiovascular disease account for most deaths.

Some autoantibodies produced in patients with lupus are shown in Table 54–1. Genetic influences are implicated by a higher concordance with monozygotic compared with dizygotic twins and a 10-percent frequency in patients with one affected family member. The relative risk of disease is increased threefold if HLA-DR2 or -DR3 genes are found (Arnett, 1997). Under the influence of multiple genes, often triggered by environmental stimuli and highly influenced by gender, a number of clinical syndromes may develop, fulfilling diagnostic criteria for lupus.

Clinical Findings. Lupus is notoriously variable in its presentation, course, and outcome (Gladman and Urowitz, 1997). Clinical manifestations may be confined initially to one organ system, with others becoming involved as the disease progresses (Table 54–2). Alternatively, the disease may initially manifest by multisystem involvement. Common findings are malaise, fever, arthritis, rash, pleuropericarditis, photosensitivity, anemia, and cognitive dysfunction. At least half of patients have renal involvement. *Libman–Sacks endocarditis* was described with lupus but likely is due to anticardiolipin antibodies (Hojnik and associates, 1996). Associated hemodynamic dysfunction is uncommon, but it has been reported (Moyssakis and colleagues, 2002). In addition, these valvular lesions may cause thromboembolic seeding.

Laboratory Findings. Identification of antinuclear antibodies (ANA) is the best screening test, however, a positive test result is not specific for lupus. For example, low titers are found in normal individuals, other autoimmune diseases, acute viral infections, and chronic inflammatory processes. Several drugs can also cause a positive reaction. Antibodies to double-stranded DNA (dsDNA) and to Smith (Sm) antigens are relatively specific for lupus, whereas other antibodies are not (see Table 54–1).

Anemia is common, and there may be leukopenia and thrombocytopenia. Proteinuria and casts are found in the half of patients with glomerular lesions, and there may be renal insufficiency. Other laboratory findings include false-positive syphilis serology, prolonged partial thromboplastin time, and positive serum rheumatoid factor assay.

TABLE 54–1 Some Autoantibodies Produced in Patients with Systemic Lupus Erythematosus

Antibody	Incidence (%)	Clinical Associations
Antinuclear	84–98	Multiple antibodies; repeat negative test makes lupus unlikely
Anti-dsDNA	62–70	Specific for systemic lupus erythematosus—associated with nephritis and lupus activity
Anti-Sm	30–38	Specific for lupus
Anti-RNP	33–40	Present in lupus; correlates with myositis, esophageal dysmotility; defining antibody for mixed connective tissue disease
Anti-Ro (SS-A)	30–49	Sjögren syndrome, cutaneous lupus, antinuclear antibody–negative lupus, neonatal lupus with heart block
Anti-La (SS-B)	10–35	Present in lupus—possibly decreased risk of nephritis; Sjögren syndrome
Antihistone	70	Common in drug-induced lupus (95%)
Antiphospholipid	21–50	Lupus anticoagulant and anticardiolipin antibodies associated with thrombosis, fetal loss, thrombocytopenia, valvular heart disease; false-positive test for syphilis
Anti-erythrocyte	60	Overt hemolysis uncommon
Antiplatelet	30	Thrombocytopenia (15%)

Data from Arbuckle and colleagues (2003), Hahn (2001), Shmerling (2003).

TABLE 54–2 Clinical Manifestations of Systemic Lupus Erythematosus

Organ System or Process	Clinical Manifestations	Percent[a]
Systemic	Fatigue, malaise, fever, weight loss	95
Musculoskeletal	Arthralgias, myalgias, polyarthritis, myopathy	95
Hematological	Anemia, hemolysis, leukopenia, thrombocytopenia, lupus anticoagulant	85
Cutaneous	Malar (butterfly) rash, discoid rash, photosensitivity, oral ulcers, alopecia, skin rashes	80
Neurological	Cognitive dysfunction, mood disorder, headache, seizures	60
Cardiopulmonary	Pleuritis, pericarditis, myocarditis, Libman–Sacks endocarditis	60
Renal	Proteinuria, casts, nephrotic syndrome, renal failure	60
Gastrointestinal	Anorexia, nausea, pain, diarrhea	45
Thrombosis	Venous (10%), arterial (5%)	15
Ocular	Conjunctivitis	15
Pregnancy	Recurrent abortion, early preeclampsia, stillbirths	30

[a] Percent of patients who have the manifestation sometime during the course of illness.
Modified from Hahn (2001).

Diagnosis. The revised criteria of the American Rheumatism Association for diagnosis of systemic lupus are in Table 54–3. If any four or more of these 11 criteria are present, serially or simultaneously, the diagnosis of lupus is made.

Drug-Induced Lupus. Numerous drugs have been reported to induce a lupus-like syndrome. These include procainamide, quinidine, hydralazine, α-methyldopa, phenytoin, and phenobarbital. Drug-induced lupus is rarely associated with glomerulonephritis, and it usually regresses when the medication is discontinued (Rubin, 1997).

Lupus and Maternal Outcome. Important factors for pregnancy outcome include whether disease is active at the beginning of pregnancy, age and parity, coexistence of other medical or obstetrical disorders, and whether there are antiphospholipid antibodies.

During pregnancy, lupus improves in a third of women, remains unchanged in a third, and worsens in the remaining third. Thus, in any given pregnancy, the clinical condition can worsen or *flare* without warning (Khamashta and colleagues, 1997; Ruiz-Irastorza and co-workers, 1996). Petri (1998) reported a 7-percent risk of major morbidity during pregnancy and estimated a 1 in 20 chance of a life-threatening event. Generally, these are due to renal impairment, myocarditis, or serositis.

Interestingly, Leong and colleagues (1994) reported that serum lipid levels in nonpregnant patients reflect intensity of lupus activity, particularly renal disease. Women with lupus are at increased risk for accelerated atherogenesis and premature cardiac disease. Certain medications have been shown to improve lupus symptoms as well as lower serum lipid levels. Because there are increased serum lipid levels in normal pregnancy, these associations may be related to disease severity only in some cases. This deserves further evaluation.

In studies in which women served as their own nonpregnant controls, investigators have universally reported increased disease activity during pregnancy (Petri, 1991;

TABLE 54–3 The 1997 Revised Criteria of American Rheumatism Association for Systemic Lupus Erythematosus

Criteria[a]	Comments
Malar rash	Malar erythema
Discoid rash	Erythematous patches, scaling, follicular plugging
Photosensitivity	
Oral ulcers	Usually painless
Arthritis	Nonerosive involving two or more peripheral joints
Serositis	Pleuritis or pericarditis
Renal disorder	Proteinuria greater than 0.5 g/day or > 3+ dipstick, or cellular casts
Neurological disorders	Seizures or psychosis without other cause
Hematological disorders	Hemolytic anemia, leukopenia, lymphopenia, or thrombocytopenia
Immunological disorders	Anti-dsDNA or anti-Sm antibodies, or false-positive VDRL, IgM or IgG anticardiolipin antibodies, or lupus anticoagulant
Antinuclear antibodies	Abnormal titer of ANAs

VDRL = Venereal Disease Research Laboratory.
[a] If four criteria are present at any time during course of disease, systemic lupus can be diagnosed with 98-percent specificity and 97-percent sensitivity.
From Hochberg (1997), with permission.

Ruiz-Irastorza, 1996; Zulman, 1980, and all their co-workers). For example, Petri (1998) reported an increased incidence of renal and hematological flares, but no change in overall severity. **One fact is certain: lupus can be life threatening to both the mother and her fetus-infant.** The clinician must remain vigilant about the development of such life-threatening dangers.

In general, pregnancy outcome is better if:

1. Lupus activity has been quiescent for at least 6 months before conception.
2. There is no active renal involvement manifest by proteinuria or renal dysfunction.
3. Superimposed preeclampsia does not develop.
4. There is no evidence of antiphospholipid antibody activity.

Lupus Nephropathy. Renal disease is more common if antiphospholipid antibodies are detected (Moroni and co-workers, 2004). Women with nephropathy whose disease stays in remission usually have a good pregnancy outcome. Packham and associates (1992) found similar outcomes in 64 pregnancies before and after nephritis was diagnosed. Hypertension developed and proteinuria worsened in half of these women during pregnancy. Huong (2001), Julkunen (1993b), Moroni (2002), and all their colleagues reported similar findings. Of the 125 pregnancies reported by Lockshin (1989), 63 percent of women with preexisting renal disease developed preeclampsia compared with only 14 percent of those without underlying renal disease.

Although most authorities recommend continuation of immunosuppressive therapy during pregnancy in women with nephritis, it is not clear whether the dosage should be increased peripartum. Although it is often stated that this is the time that activation or exacerbations are most likely to develop, firm evidence is not conclusive.

LUPUS VERSUS PREECLAMPSIA–ECLAMPSIA. Preeclampsia is common in all women with lupus, and superimposed preeclampsia is encountered even more often in those with nephropathy. It may be difficult, if not impossible, to differentiate lupus nephropathy from severe preeclampsia (Repke, 1998). It has not been proven if decreased complement values or increased anti-DNA titers are useful to identify worsening lupus activity. If identified, these laboratory features support the diagnosis of a reactivation of lupus nephritis, termed *renal flare.* According to Petri (1998), most women with renal flares during pregnancy do not develop hypertension. Central nervous system involvement with lupus may culminate in convulsions similar to those of eclampsia. Thrombocytopenia, with or without hemolysis, may further confuse the diagnosis. Management is identical to that for preeclampsia–eclampsia, described in Chapter 34. Corticosteroid therapy is continued. The most common causes of death in these women when not pregnant are malignant hypertension with glomerulonephritis and neurological catastrophes such as seizures, strokes, and coma.

Management During Pregnancy. Management consists primarily of monitoring the clinical conditions of both maternal and fetal patients and maternal laboratory values. Pregnancy-induced thrombocytopenia and proteinuria resemble lupus disease activity, and the identification of a lupus flare is confounded by the increase in facial and palmar erythema of normal pregnancy (Lockshin and Sammaritano, 2003). Some authorities have advocated a number of numerical scales to emphasize ongoing disease activity. Components are weighted for severity, including the SLE-Pregnancy Disease Activity Index (SLEPDAI) and the Lupus Activity Index (Buyon and colleagues, 1999; Ruiz-Irasforza and associates, 2004).

Monitoring of lupus activity and identification of pending lupus flares by a variety of laboratory techniques has been recommended. The sedimentation rate is uninterpretable because of pregnancy-induced hyperfibrinogenemia. Although falling or low levels of complement components C_3, C_4, and CH_{50} are more likely to be associated with active disease, higher levels provide no insurance against disease activation. Varner and co-workers (1983) found no correlation between clinical manifestations of disease and complement levels. Our experiences, as well as those of Lockshin and Druzin (1995), have been similar. Buyon and colleagues (1999) recommended that hypocomplementemia should be attributed to disease activity in pregnant women in the following circumstances: (1) when there is decreased C_3, C_4, or CH_{50} levels without evidence of a synthetic defect; (2) when levels of C_3, C_4, or CH_{50} fall by 25 percent as pregnancy progresses; or (3) when there are normal levels of C_3, C_4, or CH_{50} but other evidence of complement activation such as abnormal levels of C_{3a}.

Serial hematological studies may detect changes in disease activity. Hemolysis is characterized by a positive Coombs test, anemia, reticulocytosis, and unconjugated hyperbilirubinemia. Thrombocytopenia, leukopenia, or both may develop. According to Lockshin and Druzin (1995), chronic thrombocytopenia in early pregnancy may be due to *antiphospholipid antibodies.* Later, thrombocytopenia may indicate the onset of preeclampsia.

Serum transaminase activity reflects hepatic involvement, as does a rise in serum bilirubin. Azathioprine therapy also may induce enzyme elevations. Urine is tested frequently to detect new-onset or worsening proteinuria. Overt proteinuria that persists is an ominous sign, even more so if accompanied by other evidence of the nephrotic syndrome or abnormal serum creatinine levels.

The fetus should be closely observed for adverse effects. Fetal growth is monitored closely and careful attention is given to the development of hypertension. Singsen and colleagues (1985) and Petri (1998) recommend screening for anti-SS-A and anti-SS-B antibodies, and if found, fetal cardiac function should be evaluated (see p. 1215). Although we routinely evaluate the fetus for an arrhythmia, we do not screen for these antibodies. As discussed in Chapter 15 (see

p. 383), antepartum fetal surveillance is done as outlined by the American College of Obstetricians and Gynecologists (1999). Farine and associates (1998) reported an 11-percent incidence of absent end-diastolic umbilical artery velocity in 56 fetuses.

Unless hypertension develops, or there is evidence of fetal compromise or growth restriction, pregnancy is allowed to progress to term. Peripartum corticosteroids in "stress doses" are given to women who are taking these drugs or who recently have done so.

PHARMACOLOGICAL TREATMENT. There is no cure, and complete remissions are rare. Approximately a fourth of patients have mild disease, which is not life threatening, but may be disabling because of pain and fatigue. Arthralgia and serositis are managed by *nonsteroidal anti-inflammatory drugs,* including aspirin. Because of the risk of premature closure of the fetal ductus arteriosus, therapeutic doses probably should not be used after 24 weeks (Briggs and colleagues, 2002). Low-dose aspirin, however, can be used safely throughout gestation (see p. 1218). Severe disease is managed with *corticosteroids* such as prednisone, 1 to 2 mg/kg per day. After the disease is controlled, this is tapered to a daily dose of 10 to 15 mg each morning. Corticosteroid therapy can result in the development of gestational or even type 1 diabetes. Long-term antibody-based immunoadsorption has been used in pregnancy for removal of autoantibodies and lipoproteins in women with serious complications who did not respond to conventional therapy (Dittrich and colleagues, 2002).

Immunosuppressive and *cytotoxic agents* such as *azathioprine* and *cyclophosphamide* are beneficial in controlling active disease (Contreras and colleagues, 2004; Hahn, 2001). In nonpregnant patients, they are usually reserved for lupus nephritis or disease that is steroid resistant. Azathioprine is less toxic, and recommended daily oral doses are 2 to 3 mg/kg. It is avoided during pregnancy unless life-threatening complications develop. Although Ramsey-Goldman and associates (1993) found that women exposed to either drug did not have more adverse pregnancy outcomes, Enns and associates (1999) reported that cyclophosphamide is teratogenic.

Antimalarials help control skin disease. Although these agents cross the placenta, *hydroxychloroquine* has not been associated with congenital malformations (Østensen, 1998). Because of the long half life of antimalarials, and because discontinuing therapy can precipitate a lupus flare, most authors recommend their continuation if in use (Borden and Parke, 2001; Harris, 2002). Levy and colleagues (2001) randomized 20 pregnant women to hydroxychloroquine or placebo and reported improvement in SLEPDAI scores when the drug was compared with placebo.

When severe disease supervenes, usually with a lupus flare, high-dose glucocorticoid therapy is given. Petri (1998) recommends pulse therapy consisting of methylprednisolone, 1000 mg per 24 hours for 3 days, then a return to maintenance doses if possible.

Long-term Prognosis and Contraception. In general, women with lupus and chronic vascular or renal disease should limit family size because of morbidity associated with the disease as well as increased adverse perinatal outcomes. Tubal sterilization may be advantageous. It is performed with greatest safety postpartum or whenever the disease is quiescent. Oral contraceptives must be used with caution in women with lupus because vascular disease is relatively common. Progestin-only implants and injections provide effective contraception with no known effects on lupus flares. Intrauterine devices probably should not be prescribed if the woman is receiving immunosuppressive therapy (see Chap. 32, p. 739).

Effects of Lupus on the Fetus and Neonate. Fetal growth restriction and perinatal mortality and morbidity are increased significantly in pregnancies complicated by lupus (Table 54–4). Prognosis is worsened with a lupus flare;

TABLE 54–4 Maternal and Perinatal Effects of Systemic Lupus Erythematosus

Outcome	Description
Maternal	
Lupus flare	Overall a third flare during pregnancy
	Flare can be life threatening (1 in 20 chance)
	Flares associated with worse perinatal outcomes
	Prognosis worse if antiphospholipid antibodies present
	Increased incidence common with nephritis
Preeclampsia	Controversial if incidence is increased
Preterm labor	Increased
Perinatal	
Preterm delivery	Increased with preeclampsia
Growth restriction	Increased
Stillbirth	Increased, especially with antiphospholipid antibodies
Neonatal lupus	About 10% incidence (transient except for heart block)

Data from Lockshin and Sammaritano (2000); Petri and Albritton (1993); Yasmeen and co-workers (2001).

significant proteinuria; renal impairment; and with associated hypertension, development of preeclampsia, or both (Aggarwal, 1999; Carmona, 1999; Rahman, 1998; Scott, 2002, and all their associates). The reasons at least partially responsible for adverse fetal consequences include decidual vasculopathy with placental infarction and decreased perfusion (Hanly and colleagues, 1988; Lubbe and Liggins, 1984). Anti-SS-A (Ro) and anti-SS-B (La) antibodies may damage the fetal heart and conduction system, causing neonatal death (Alexander and co-workers, 1992; Tseng and Buyon, 1997). For example, women with livedo reticularis and lupus or a lupus-like illness, but who do not produce antiphospholipid antibodies, display increased rates of pregnancy complications (Sangle and associates, 2005). The recurrence risk in subsequent offspring for cutaneous lupus is 25 percent, and for congenital heart block it is 10 to 15 percent (Julkunen and colleagues, 1993a).

NEONATAL LUPUS. This unusual syndrome is characterized by skin lesions, or *lupus dermatitis*; a variable number of hematological and systemic derangements; and occasionally congenital heart block (Boh, 2004; Tseng and Buyon, 1997). Thrombocytopenia and hepatic involvement may also manifest (Weston and colleagues, 1999). The incidence is about 5 to 10 percent. One report suggests that neonatal lupus may appear up to 4 weeks after birth (Stirnemann and associates, 2002). Lockshin and co-workers (1988) prospectively followed 91 infants born to women with lupus; four had definite neonatal lupus and four had possible disease. Cutaneous lupus, thrombocytopenia, and autoimmune hemolysis are transient and clear within a few months (Lee and Weston, 1984).

CONGENITAL HEART BLOCK. This is the consequence of diffuse myocarditis and fibrosis in the region between the atrioventricular node and bundle of His. Buyon and colleagues (1993) reported that congenital heart block occurred almost exclusively in infants of women with antibodies to the SS-A or SS-B antigens. They may cause otherwise unexplained stillbirths (Ottaviani and co-workers, 2004). Even in the presence of such antibodies, however, the incidence of arrhythmia is only 3 percent (Lockshin and associates, 1988). The cardiac lesion is permanent, and a pacemaker is generally necessary. Long-term prognosis is not good, and a third of affected infants die within 3 years (Waltuck and Buyon, 1994).

Maternal corticosteroid administration to treat fetal heart block is controversial. Richards and associates (1990) described such a fetus whose ascites cleared promptly with maternal therapy even though heart block and bradycardia persisted. Shinohara and colleagues (1999) reported no heart block in 26 neonates whose mothers received corticosteroid maintenance therapy before 16 weeks. By contrast, 15 of 61 neonates with heart block were born to women in whom corticosteroid therapy was begun after 16 weeks. Saleeb and colleagues (1999) recommend fluorinated steroids.

ANTIPHOSPHOLIPID ANTIBODIES. Several antibodies directed against negatively charged phospholipids have been described and studied in detail over the past 25 years. These antiphospholipid antibodies include *lupus anticoagulant (LAC)* and *anticardiolipin antibodies (ACAs)*. They may be of IgG, IgM, and IgA classes, alone or in combination. Although they may be found in normal persons, they also are associated with the *antiphospholipid antibody syndrome (APS)*. This is characterized by recurrent arterial or venous thromboses, thrombocytopenia, and fetal losses—especially stillbirths—during the second half of pregnancy (Branch and Khamashta, 2003; Oshiro and associates, 1996; Warren and colleagues, 2004).

APS may occur alone or in association with lupus or other autoimmune disorders. Central nervous system involvement is one of the most prominent clinical manifestations and includes arterial and venous thrombotic events, psychiatric features, and other nonthrombotic neurological syndromes (Sanna and co-workers, 2003). Interestingly, APS may mimic the presentation of multiple sclerosis (Ruiz-Irastorza and associates, 2001).

Feinstein and Rapaport (1972) introduced the term *lupus anticoagulant* in a review of acquired inhibitors of coagulation. This was based on the early recognition that certain patients with lupus had some coagulation tests that were prolonged and thus suggested anticoagulant activity. Paradoxically, the so-called anticoagulant is powerfully thrombotic in vivo, although the LAC prolongs all phospholipid-dependent coagulation tests, including the prothrombin time, partial thromboplastin time, and Russell viper venom time. Each of these tests requires a phospholipid surface to which other clotting factors attach and combine (Fig. 54–1).

Thus, detection of the LAC is based indirectly on the prolongation of in vitro tests by this circulating antiphospholipid antibody. ACA usually is detected serologically using enzyme-linked immunoabsorbent assay (ELISA). Most often IgM anticardiolipin antibodies that are found alone are stimulated by infections or drugs and are innocuous (Silver and colleagues, 1996).

Pathophysiology. Many patients with lupus have circulating antibodies specifically directed either against cardiolipin(s) or against phospholipid-binding proteins such as β_2-glycoprotein I (apolipoprotein H). The latter are associated with arterial thrombosis (Lopez and associates, 2004). ACAs apparently bind directly to β_2-glycoprotein I, and these proteins act as a co-factor in this antigen–antibody reaction (Chamley and co-workers, 1999).

The major activity of β_2-glycoprotein I appears to be its phospholipid-dependent anticoagulant inhibition of prothrombinase activity of platelets and ADP–induced platelet aggregation (Shi and colleagues, 1993). β_2-glycoprotein I competitively inhibits the binding of coagulation factors, especially factor XII and the prothrombinase complex to negatively charged phospholipid surfaces, and prevents activation

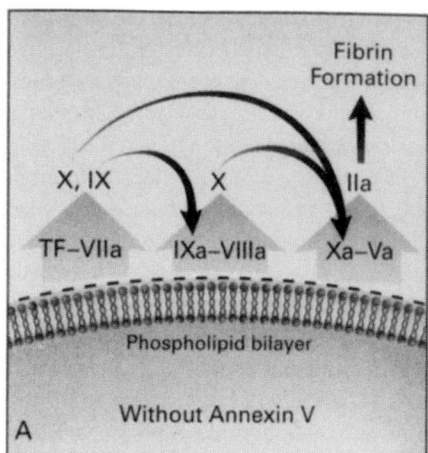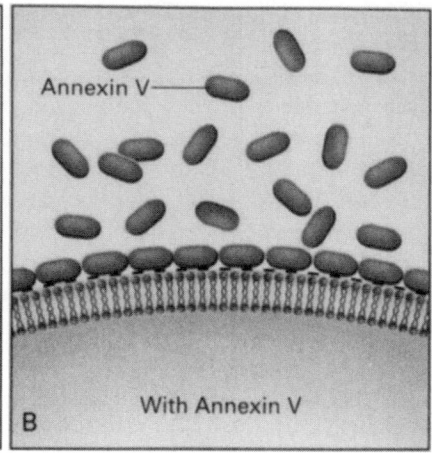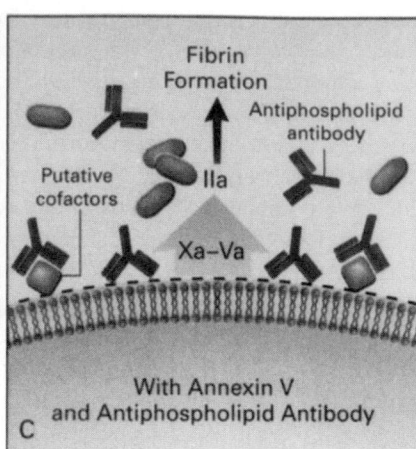

FIGURE 54–1. Mechanisms of reduction of annexin V levels and acceleration of coagulation associated with antiphospholipid antibodies. **A.** Anionic phospholipids (–) on the surface of the cell-membrane bilayer serve as potent co-factors for assembly of three coagulation complexes: tissue factor–VIIa (TF-VIIa) complex, IXa-VIIIa complex, and Xa-Va complex. The phospholipids thus accelerate blood coagulation by generating factors IXa and Xa. Factor Xa yields factor IIa (thrombin), which in turn cleaves fibrinogen to form fibrin. **B.** When antiphospholipid antibodies are absent, annexin V forms clusters that bind to the surface of anionic phospholipids and inhibit coagulation. **C.** Directly or through an interaction with protein-phospholipid co-factors, antiphospholipid antibodies disrupt the ability of annexin V to cluster on the phospholipid surface. This reduces binding affinity of annexin V, which permits more anionic phospholipid to be available to form complexes with coagulation proteins. Coagulation is thus accelerated and thrombosis promoted. (From Rand and colleagues, 1997a, with permission.)

of the coagulation cascade (Schousboe and Rasmussen, 1995). An antibody directed against β_2-glycoprotein I would bind and prevent it from acting as a phospholipid-dependent anticoagulant. β_2-glycoprotein I is found in high concentrations on the surface of the syncytiotrophoblast (see Chap. 3, p. 54). This might be expected, because it is a critical area to ensure that coagulation does not occur. In addition, β_2-glycoprotein I may be involved in implantation, because it is known that this protein binds heparin. Moreover, trophoblastic cells have heparin-like binding sites. Thus, a local loss of β_2-glycoprotein I by an antibody directed against it might prevent implantation or result in intervillous space thrombosis, or both (Chamley and associates, 1999).

LAC appears to require a co-factor for its in vitro anticoagulant function. Specifically, it does not bind directly to negatively charged phospholipids, but instead, it binds to phospholipid-bound prothrombin (Galli and Bevers, 1994). Other phospholipid-binding proteins may be involved in the pathophysiology of the APS. These include *protein C* and *protein S,* both endogenous anticoagulants, and *annexin V.* The latter is also known as placental anticoagulant protein I or lipocortin V, and it coats the syncytiotrophoblast in high concentration (Chamley, 1999). Thus, an antibody that binds protein C or S would result in venous, arterial, or decidual thrombosis, while binding of annexin V would result in coagulation and thrombosis in the intervillous space (see Fig. 54–1).

Rand and co-workers (1997b) reported that placental tissue from pregnancy complicated by the APS had significantly

less apical membrane-associated annexin V than normal placenta. Exposure of placental villous cultures to five antiphospholipid IgGs also resulted in a significant reduction in apical membrane annexin V. In another study, there was a reduction in annexin V in endothelial cell tissue cultures exposed to antiphospholipid antibodies (Rand and colleagues, 1997a). The pathophysiology of this sequence of events is illustrated in Figure 54–1.

These discoveries led to the development of direct assays to measure antibodies against β_2-glycoprotein I and prothrombin. The latter are increased in and associated with pregnancies complicated by the APS (Faden, 1997; Falcón, 1997; Forastiero, 1997; Ogasawara, 1996, and all their co-workers). Conversely, others have not observed a clinically significant association with these antibodies (Lee, 1999; Lynch, 1999; Tinahones, 1998, and all their associates).

Association of Antiphospholipid Antibodies with Lupus. Patients with clinical lupus frequently are found to have LAC and ACAs. Love and Santoro (1990) reviewed 29 series that included more than 1000 patients with lupus and reported an average frequency of 34 percent for LAC and 44 percent for ACAs. In nearly half, both antibodies were found.

In general, patients with LAC have higher levels of ACAs, and about a third of those with biological false-positive tests for syphilis have ACAs (Branch, 1991). Conversely, only about 20 percent of patients with identifiable ACAs have LAC. Importantly, in patients with lupus, documentation of either ACA or LAC is a risk factor for thrombosis, neurological disorders, and thrombocytopenia (Love and Santoro, 1990). As discussed in Chapter 9 (see p. 235), these antibodies have also been associated with excessive pregnancy loss (Kutteh and colleagues, 1999). Hojnik and colleagues (1996) reported that *Libman–Sacks endocarditis* is much more prevalent in patients with lupus who have antiphospholipid antibodies. These antibodies have been associated with the development of "primary" vaso-occlusive disease involving different organs. In the kidney, this has been documented by renal biopsy (Nochy and colleagues, 1999).

Antiphospholipid Antibodies in Normal Pregnancy. About 5 percent of all otherwise healthy nonpregnant populations screened have nonspecific antiphospholipid antibodies in low titers. This has been documented also during pregnancy. Lockwood and colleagues (1989) studied 737 normally pregnant women and found that two (0.3 percent) had lupus anticoagulant and 16 (2.2 percent) had elevated concentrations of either IgM- or IgG-ACAs. Harris and Spinnato (1991) studied 1449 consecutive pregnant women and found 1.8 percent positive for IgG-anticardiolipin and 4.3 percent for IgM-anticardiolipin antibodies. Pattison and co-workers (1993) studied 933 consecutive prenatal patients and found nine (0.1 percent) with ACAs, 11 (1.2 percent) with LACs, and two women with both. Yasuda and associates (1995) found that 7 percent of 860 pregnant Japanese women had ACAs.

Diagnosis of Antiphospholipid Antibody Syndrome. By international consensus, APS is diagnosed on the basis of clinical and laboratory criteria (Levine and co-workers, 2002). One of two clinical criteria that include vascular thrombosis or certain pregnancy morbidity must be present. In addition, at least two laboratory criteria that include LAC activity, or medium- to high-positive specific IgG- or IgM-ACAs must be confirmed on two occasions 6 weeks apart.

Several indications for testing are listed in Table 54–5. Branch and Khamashta (2003) recommend conservative interpretation of results based on repeated tests from a reliable laboratory that are consistent with each clinical case. Be-

TABLE 54–5 Indications to Identify Lupus Anticoagulant and Antiphospholipid Antibodies

Recurrent pregnancy loss
Unexplained second- or third-trimester loss
Early-onset severe preeclampsia
Venous or arterial thrombosis
Unexplained fetal growth restriction
Autoimmune or connective tissue disease
False-positive serological test for syphilis
Prolonged coagulation studies
Positive autoantibody tests

From Kutteh (1995).

cause only approximately 20 percent of patients with APS have a positive LAC reaction alone, both the clotting test to identify the LAC and the anticardiolipin ELISA test must be performed.

Efforts have been made to standardize ACA assays by using ELISA, and values are reported in units and expressed as either *negative* or *low, medium,* or *high positive* (Harris and colleagues, 1987). Despite this, there still is no totally accurate standardization for these assays (Branch and Khamashta, 2003). Interlaboratory variation can be large, and agreement between commercial kits is also poor.

Tests for the LAC are nonspecific coagulation tests. The *partial thromboplastin time* is generally prolonged because the anticoagulant interferes with conversion of prothrombin to thrombin in vitro. Tests considered most specific are the *dilute Russell viper venom test (dRVVT)* and the *platelet neutralization procedure.* There is currently disagreement as to which of these is best for screening. However, if any are positive after adding normal plasma, the diagnosis is confirmed.

Pathophysiology of Antiphospholipid Antibodies in Pregnancy. There is a strong association between the LAC and high levels of ACAs with decidual vasculopathy, placental infarction, fetal growth restriction, early-onset preeclampsia, and recurrent fetal death. Some of these women, like those with lupus, also have a high incidence of venous and arterial thromboses, cerebral thrombosis, hemolytic anemia, thrombocytopenia, and pulmonary hypertension (Khamashta and colleagues, 1997; Silver and associates, 1994).

MECHANISM OF ACTION. It is not precisely known how these antibodies act, but it is likely that their actions are multifactorial. According to Chamley (1999), platelets may be damaged directly by antiphospholipid antibody or indirectly by binding β_2-glycoprotein I, which causes platelets to be susceptible to aggregation. Rand and colleagues (1997a, 1997b, 1998) propose that phospholipid-containing endothelial cell or syncytiotrophoblast membranes may be damaged directly by the antiphospholipid antibody or indirectly by antibody binding to either β_2-glycoprotein I or annexin V (see Fig. 54–1). This prevents the cell membranes from protecting the syncytiotrophoblast and endothelium and results in exposure of basement membrane. It is known that damaged platelets adhere to exposed basement membrane of endothelium and syncytiotrophoblast and result in thrombus formation (Lubbe and colleagues, 1983).

There are other proposed mechanisms. Pierro and co-workers (1999) reported that antiphospholipid antibodies decreased decidual production of the vasodilating prostaglandin E_2. Decreased protein C or S activity as well as increased prothrombin activation have been reported (Ogunyemi and associates, 2002; Zangari and colleagues, 1997). Amengual and co-workers (2003) presented evidence that thrombosis with APS is due to activation of the tissue factor pathway. Recent studies suggest that uncontrolled placental complement activation by antiphospholipid antibodies may play a role in fetal loss and growth restriction (Holers and colleagues, 2002).

ADVERSE PREGNANCY OUTCOMES. There is no doubt that antiphospholipid antibodies are associated with increased fetal wastage (see Chap. 9, p. 235). In most early reports, however, women were usually included because they had repeated adverse outcomes. Moreover, as previously discussed, the incidence of antiphospholipid antibodies in the general obstetrical population is about 5 percent. Currently, data are too limited to draw precise conclusions concerning the impact of these antibodies on adverse pregnancy outcomes. According to the Utah group, fetal deaths are more characteristic than first-trimester miscarriages (Oshiro and co-workers, 1996; Roque and colleagues, 2001).

Looking at the issue another way, the incidence of these antibodies may be increased in adverse obstetrical outcomes associated with the syndromes. Polzin and colleagues (1991) identified antiphospholipid antibodies in a fourth of 37 women with growth-restricted fetuses. None had evidence of LAC. Branch and co-workers (1989) found a 16-percent incidence of antiphospholipid antibodies in 43 women with severe preeclampsia before 34 weeks. Six of the seven women with antibodies also had LAC, and one woman had multiple cerebral infarctions. Similarly, Moodley and associates (1995) found antibodies in 11 percent of 34 women with severe preeclampsia before 30 weeks.

When otherwise unexplained fetal deaths are examined, ACAs do not appear to play a significant role. Haddow and co-workers (1991) measured ACAs in 309 pregnancies with fetal death and found no differences when compared with 618 normal pregnancies. Despite a worse pregnancy outcome, there was no evidence of greater endothelial cell activation during pregnancy in women who were receiving treatment for APS (Stone and colleagues, 2003).

Treatment Guidelines. As aptly stated by Branch and Khamashta (2003), because of the heterogeneity of studies, current treatment recommendations may be confusing to the clinician. As discussed in Chapter 47 (see p. 1078), women with prior thromboembolic events who have antiphospholipid antibodies should be given heparin in subsequent pregnancies (American College of Obstetricians and Gynecologists, 2000). Women with high-titer ACA or with LAC activity and a previous second- or third trimester fetal death not attributable to other causes should be treated (Dizon-Townson and Branch, 1998; Lockshin and Druzin, 1995). Similarly, women with recurrent early pregnancy loss and high titers of antibodies may benefit from therapy (Kutteh, 1996). A number of treatments for women with antiphospholipid antibodies have been evaluated, including low-dose aspirin, prednisone, heparin, and immunoglobulin (Levine and colleagues, 2002). These are thought to counteract the adverse action of

antiphospholipid antibodies by affecting both the immune and coagulation systems.

Low-dose aspirin, 60 to 80 mg given daily, blocks the conversion of arachidonic acid to thromboxane A_2 while allegedly sparing prostacyclin production (Kaaja and co-workers, 1993; Lellouche and colleagues, 1991). This results in reduced thromboxane A_2, which aggregates platelets and causes vasoconstriction, while sparing prostacyclin, which has the opposite effect. There appear to be no major side effects from low-dose aspirin other than a slight risk of small vessel bleeding during surgical procedures.

Heparin is used in doses of 5000 to 10,000 units administered subcutaneously every 12 hours. Some authors recommend measurement of heparin levels because clotting tests may be altered by LAC. According to Cowchock (1998), preinjection heparin levels are monitored to ensure protection of patients most at risk of thromboembolism. The rationale for heparin therapy is to prevent venous and arterial thrombotic episodes. Heparin therapy also prevents thrombosis in the microcirculation, including the decidual–trophoblastic interface (Toglia and Weg, 1996). As discussed, heparin binds to β_2-glycoprotein I, which coats the syncytiotrophoblast. This prevents binding of anticardiolipin and anti–β_2-glycoprotein I antibodies to their surfaces, which likely prevents cellular damage (Chamley, 1999; Schousboe and Rasmussen, 1995). Heparin also binds to antiphospholipid antibodies in vitro, and likely in vivo (Ermel and associates, 1995). Heparin therapy is associated with a number of complications. These are discussed in detail in Chapter 47 (see p. 1083) and include bleeding, thrombocytopenia, osteopenia, and osteoporosis. Most consider *low-molecular-weight heparin* preparations as a reasonable substitute.

Glucocorticoids likely should not be used with "primary" APS (i.e., without an associated connective tissue disorder). Even so, some patients with these conditions can be expected to develop an associated disorder such as lupus over time (Carbone and colleagues, 1999). In instances of "secondary" APS, the dose of prednisone should be maintained at the lowest effective level to prevent flares. Steroid therapy has significant adverse effects, including osteopenia, osteoporosis, and pathological fractures. Steroids also impede wound healing, and they induce gestational and overt diabetes (Laskin and co-workers, 1997).

Immunoglobulin therapy has usually been reserved for women with overt disease, heparin-induced thrombocytopenia, or both. It is used when other first-line therapies have failed, especially in the setting of preeclampsia and fetal growth restriction (Cowchock, 1996, 1998; Heilmann and colleagues, 2003; Petri, 1997; Silver and Branch, 1997). Immunoglobulin is administered intravenously in doses of 0.4 g/kg daily for 5 days (total dose of 2 g/kg). This is repeated monthly, or it is given as a single dose of 1 g/kg each month. Immunoglobulin has been evaluated in a preliminary placebo-controlled study by Branch and colleagues (2000). The drug may cause anaphylactic reactions, especially in women who have IgA deficiency due to anti-IgA antibodies.

Immunosuppressive therapy has also not been well evaluated, but azathioprine and cyclosporine do not appear to improve standard therapies (Silver and Branch, 1997). Methotrexate and cyclophosphamide are contraindicated because of teratogenic potential (Enns and associates, 1999).

RESULTS OF TREATMENT. Although improved outcomes are reported with some of the preceding treatments, Branch and Khamashta (2003) cautioned that recurrent fetal loss is still 20 to 30 percent. Thus, low-dose aspirin and corticosteroid therapy are not universally successful. In one study, Lockshin and co-workers (1989) reported that 23 of 32 women with a prior fetal death and antiphospholipid antibody greater than 40 IgG units had a recurrent fetal death despite treatment with prednisone, aspirin, or both. Conversely, some women with lupus and antiphospholipid antibodies have normal pregnancy outcomes without treatment. In addition, women with LAC and prior bad pregnancy outcomes have had liveborn infants without treatment (Trudinger and associates, 1988).

Current data suggest the most efficacious therapy to be low-dose heparin—7500 to 10,000 units administered subcutaneously, twice daily—given along with low-dose aspirin, 60 to 80 mg once daily. If active lupus also is present, then prednisone is usually also given.

RHEUMATOID ARTHRITIS.

This is a chronic multisystem disease of unknown cause with an immunologically mediated pathogenesis. Infiltrating T cells secrete cytokines that mediate inflammation and systemic symptoms. Its prevalence is about 0.8 percent, and women are affected three times more often than men (Lipsky, 2001). The cardinal feature is inflammatory synovitis that usually involves the peripheral joints. The disease has a propensity for cartilage destruction, bony erosions, and joint deformities. Onset is generally between 35 and 50 years of age.

There is a genetic predisposition, and the results of several studies have shown a higher disease concordance among monozygotic than dizygotic twins (15 versus 4 percent) (Lee and Weinblatt, 2001). There is also an association with the class II major histocompatibility complex molecule HLA-DR4 as well as HLA-DRB1 alleles (Harney and colleagues, 2003). A prolonged duration of cigarette smoking also appears to increase the risk of rheumatoid arthritis in women (Karlson and colleagues, 1999). Hazes and colleagues (1990) reported a protective effect of pregnancy in the development of rheumatoid arthritis. Conversely, van Dunne and associates (2004) found that miscarriage is associated with accelerated joint destruction.

Clinical Manifestations. Rheumatoid arthritis is a chronic polyarthritis with symptoms of synovitis, fatigue, anorexia, weakness, weight loss, depression, and vague musculoskeletal symptoms. The hands, wrists, knees, and feet are commonly involved. Pain, aggravated by movement, is accompanied by swelling and tenderness. Extra-articular manifestations include rheumatoid nodules, vasculitis, and pleuropulmonary symptoms. The 1987 revised criteria of the American Rheumatism Association have approximately a 90-percent specificity and sensitivity for the diagnosis (Arnett and colleagues, 1988).

Management. Treatment is directed at pain relief, reduction of inflammation, protection of articular structures, and preservation of function. Physical and occupational therapy and self-management instructions are essential. Aspirin or nonsteroidal anti-inflammatory drugs are the cornerstone of symptomatic therapy. The relatively new cyclooxygenase-2 (COX-2) inhibitors are used widely because of decreased gastrointestinal ulceration. Glucocorticoid therapy may be added, and 7.5 mg of prednisone daily for the first 2 years of active disease substantively reduces progressive joint erosions (Kirwan and colleagues, 1995). Otherwise, corticosteroids are avoided if possible, but low-dose therapy is used by some clinicians, along with salicylates.

More recently, Lee and Weinblatt (2001) described a paradigm shift in treatment of rheumatoid arthritis. In this scheme, *disease-modifying antirheumatic drugs (DMARDs)* are given early. There are a variety of DMARDs, and most have considerable toxicity. These include hydroxychloroquine, sulfasalazine, azathioprine, cyclosporine, methotrexate, and gold compounds. More recently, the tumor necrosis factor biological-response modifiers etanercept and infliximab have been approved for use. Orthopedic surgery for joint deformities, including replacement, is commonly performed.

Effects of Pregnancy. In 1938, Hench reported marked improvement in the inflammatory component of rheumatoid arthritis during pregnancy. Conversely, postpartum exacerbation is common (Lockshin and Druzin, 1995). As discussed on page 1210, sex hormones supposedly interfere with a number of putative processes involved in arthritis pathogenesis, including immunoregulation and interactions with the cytokine system (Masi and associates, 1999; Østensen, 1999; Wilder and Elenkov, 1999).

Unger and associates (1983) reported that amelioration of rheumatoid arthritis correlated with serum levels of *pregnancy-associated α_2-glycoprotein*. This compound has immunosuppressive properties and may suppress at least one mediator of an inflammatory response, interleukin-2 (Nicholas and colleagues, 1985). Nelson and co-workers (1993) reported that amelioration of disease was associated with a disparity in HLA class II antigens between mother and fetus. They suggested that the maternal immune response to paternal HLA antigens may play a role in pregnancy-induced remission of arthritis.

Silman and associates (1992) performed a case-control study of 88 women with rheumatoid arthritis and reported that pregnancy had a "protective effect" for disease onset.

Conversely, there was a sixfold increased likelihood of new-disease onset in the first 3 months postpartum. Iijima and associates (1998) observed only two new cases in 2547 post-partum women. Barrett and co-workers (2000a) reported that a flare was more common if women were breast feeding.

In a prospective study, Østensen and Husby (1983) confirmed the amelioration of symptoms during early pregnancy in women with rheumatoid arthritis. They also described exacerbations within 3 months postpartum in 11 of 12 women. In a study from Leiden, van der Horst-Bruinsma and colleagues (1998) found that a favorable outcome was related to maternal–fetal MHC class II incompatibility. Conversely, Barrett and co-workers (2000b) performed a prospective study in the United Kingdom, and 140 women recruited during the last trimester were seen at 1 and 6 months postpartum. There was only a modest fall in objective disease activity. Only 16 percent had complete remission. At least 25 percent had substantive levels of disability. Thus, although overall disease actually did not exacerbate postpartum, the mean number of inflamed joints increased significantly. Thus, most women with rheumatoid arthritis improve during pregnancy, some women develop disease during pregnancy, and others become worse (Nelson and Østensen, 1997).

Østensen (1991) reviewed outcomes of 76 pregnancies in 51 women with *juvenile rheumatoid arthritis*. Pregnancy had no effects on presentation of disease, but disease activity became quiescent or remained so during pregnancy. Postpartum flares were common, as discussed for rheumatoid arthritis. Joint deformities were common in these women, and 15 of 20 cesarean deliveries were done for contracted pelves or joint prostheses. These observations are supported by the summary of similar results in 39 Polish women with a history of juvenile rheumatoid arthritis (Musiej-Nowakowska and Ploski, 1999).

Perinatal Outcome. There are no obvious adverse effects of rheumatoid arthritis on pregnancy outcome, including preterm labor (Klipple and Cecere, 1989). Although Kaplan (1986) reported that women who later develop the disease have had a higher-than-expected incidence of spontaneous abortion, Nelson and colleagues (1992) did not observe this.

Management During Pregnancy. In a national population-based cohort study in Norway, Skomsvoll and colleagues (2002) found that women with rheumatic disease were at high risk for adverse pregnancy outcome. It may be that large doses of aspirin or other nonsteroidal anti-inflammatory drugs typically used to treat these diseases might adversely affect the fetus and neonate (see Chap. 14, p. 355). Concerns include impaired hemostasis, prolonged gestation, and premature closure of the ductus arteriosus (Briggs and colleagues, 2002). Nonetheless, these drugs remain appropriate for treatment of symptomatic women during pregnancy. Corticosteroids are also used as indicated. Gold compounds have been used in pregnancy, but their fetal effects are largely unknown. Immunosuppressive therapy with azathioprine, cyclophosphamide, or methotrexate is not routinely used during pregnancy. Of these, only azathioprine should be considered for use during early pregnancy because the other agents are teratogenic (Buckley and co-workers, 1997; Enns and associates, 1999; Ramsey-Goldman and Shilling, 1997). As discussed on page 1219, a number of newer agents have been used in nonpregnant patients.

If cervical spine involvement exists, particular attention is warranted during pregnancy. Subluxation is common, and pregnancy, at least theoretically, predisposes to this because of joint laxity, as discussed in Chapter 5 (see p. 144).

Contraception. Combination oral contraceptives are a logical choice because of their effectiveness and the possibility they might improve rheumatoid arthritis (Bijlsma and Van Den Brink, 1992). In fact, all reversible methods of contraception discussed in Chapter 32 are appropriate except intrauterine devices, which should not be used in immunosuppressed women.

SYSTEMIC SCLEROSIS (SCLERODERMA). This is a multisystem disorder of unknown etiology characterized by fibrosis and thickening of the skin resulting from accumulation of connective tissue and by involvement of visceral organs. Its prevalence averages 1 in 10,000, with a 3-to-1 female dominance. This strong prevalence for women and the increased incidence in the years following childbirth has led to the hypothesis that *microchimerism* may be involved in the pathogenesis of systemic sclerosis (Maloney and associates, 1999; Nelson and colleagues, 1998). As discussed on page 1210, small amounts of fetal cells or DNA are found in maternal blood or tissues (Lambert and collaborators, 2004). Artlett and co-workers (1998) demonstrated Y-chromosomal DNA in 32 of 69 women (46 percent) with systemic sclerosis compared with that in only 4 percent of controls. Fetal cells are likely present long before fibrosis develops (Sawaya and associates, 2004). Also, low concentrations of male DNA may normally remain in the maternal circulation for decades after birth of a male infant (see Chap. 13, p. 331). Lambert and colleagues (2002) used quantitative methods and found that higher degrees of microchimerisms are due to intact cells and not free DNA. Maloney and colleagues (1999) have shown persistent maternal microchimerism in six of nine immunocompetent women with systemic sclerosis. Whether this contributes to the development of systemic sclerosis currently is unresolved (Ichinohe and colleagues, 2002; Russo-Stieglitz and associates, 2001).

Clinical Course. Symptoms with systemic sclerosis involve its attacks on the gastrointestinal tract, heart, lungs, and kidneys. *Overlap syndrome* refers to the presence of systemic sclerosis with features of other connective tissue disorders. *Mixed connective tissue disease* is a term used for the syndrome involving features of lupus, systemic sclerosis, polymyositis, rheumatoid arthritis, and high titers of anti-RNP antibodies (see Table 54–1).

The hallmark of the disease is overproduction of normal collagen. This results in fibrosis of skin and the gastrointestinal tract, especially the distal esophagus. Pulmonary interstitial fibrosis along with vascular changes may cause pulmonary hypertension. Antinuclear antibodies are found in 95 percent of patients, and immunoincompetence is common. Common symptoms are Raynaud phenomenon (95 percent) and swelling of the distal extremities and face. Half of patients have symptoms from esophageal involvement, especially fullness and epigastric burning pain. Pulmonary involvement is common and causes dyspnea. Mortality is high with renal or pulmonary involvement, and 10-year survival is less than 50 percent. Renal failure causes half of the deaths. Women with limited cutaneous disease such as the *CREST syndrome—calcinosis, Raynaud phenomenon, esophageal involvement, sclerodactyly, and telangiectasia—* have milder disease.

Even though systemic sclerosis cannot be cured, treatment directed at end-organ involvement can relieve symptoms and improve function. Corticosteroids are helpful only for inflammatory myositis, pericarditis, and hemolytic anemia. *Angiotensin-converting enzyme (ACE) inhibitors* are most effective for hypertension and progressive renal failure (Gilliland, 2001). Although Steen (1999) reported the use of ACE inhibitors under such conditions during pregnancy without fetal effects, these agents have been associated with severe fetal consequences (see Chap. 14, p. 349).

There has been one multicenter randomized trial of *recombinant human relaxin* in nonpregnant patients with systemic sclerosis. In this study, Seibold and co-workers (2000) reported improvement of skin thickening and mobility after 24 weeks of use.

Effects on Pregnancy. Pregnancy outcome with scleroderma is related to the severity of underlying disease. In the past, a high cited incidence of maternal deaths was due to case reports that did not accurately reflect the risks involved. In a review of 94 pregnancies, Maymon and Fejgin (1989) found that a third of women had exacerbations of symptoms during pregnancy. The maternal mortality rate was 15 percent and was due to hypertension, renal failure, or cardiopulmonary complications. The fetal mortality rate was 20 percent.

Steen and colleagues (1989, 1999) reported more optimistic outcomes in 214 women with systemic sclerosis, 45 percent of whom had had diffuse disease. Major complications included *renal crisis* in three women, characterized by malignant hypertension and renal failure that was not considered different from that of nonpregnant women with systemic sclerosis during the same period. They reported that the risks of preterm delivery, fetal growth restriction, and perinatal mortality were increased but not dramatically so. A higher incidence of prediagnosis early pregnancy wastage was observed in one case-control study (Silman and Black, 1988).

As perhaps expected, dysphagia and reflux esophagitis are aggravated by pregnancy (Steen, 1999). Dysphagia results from loss of esophageal motility due to neuromuscular dysfunction. A decrease in amplitude or disappearance of peristaltic waves in the lower two thirds of the esophagus is seen with manometry. Symptomatic treatment for reflux is described in Chapter 49 (see p. 1114). Chin and colleagues (1995) described a woman with scleroderma who developed a Mallory–Weiss tear from persistent vomiting.

Women with renal insufficiency and malignant hypertension have an increased incidence of superimposed preeclampsia. In the presence of rapidly worsening renal or cardiac disease, pregnancy termination should be considered.

Vaginal delivery may be anticipated, unless the soft tissue thickening wrought by scleroderma produces dystocia requiring abdominal delivery. Tracheal intubation for general anesthesia has special concerns because of limited ability of these women to open their mouths widely (Black and Stevens, 1989). Because of esophageal dysfunction, aspiration is also more likely, and epidural analgesia is preferable.

Contraception. Scleroderma may be associated with subfertility (Lambe and colleagues, 2004). For those who do not choose pregnancy, several reversible contraceptive methods are acceptable. That said, hormonal agents, especially combination oral contraceptives, probably should not be used, especially in women with pulmonary, cardiac, or renal involvement (see Chap. 32, p. 731). Due to the progressive and often unrelenting nature of progressive systemic sclerosis, permanent sterilization should also be considered (see Chap. 33, p. 751).

VASCULITIS SYNDROMES. Inflammation and damage to blood vessels may be primary or due to another disease. Most cases are presumed to be caused by immunopathogenetic mechanisms, specifically, immune-complex deposition. These syndromes are difficult to classify because of overlap. One classification includes systemic necrotizing vasculitis such as polyarteritis nodosa, Wegener granulomatosis, temporal or giant cell arteritis, Takayasu arteritis, Henoch–Schönlein purpura, and cutaneous or hypersensitivity arteritis.

Polyarteritis Nodosa. This type of systemic necrotizing vasculitis is an uncommon disease with protean manifestations. The pathological lesion is necrotizing vasculitis of small and medium-sized arteries. The classic variety is one of the progressive vasculitis syndromes characterized clinically by myalgia, neuropathy, gastrointestinal disorders, hypertension, and renal disease. About a fourth of cases are associated with hepatitis B antigenemia.

Symptoms are nonspecific and vague. Fever, weight loss, and malaise are present in over half of cases. Renal failure, hypertension, and arthralgias are common (Rao and associates, 1998). The diagnosis of polyarteritis nodosa is made on biopsy. Treatment consists of high-dose prednisone plus cyclophosphamide. Using this regimen, a 90-percent long-term remission is expected. Vasculitis due to hepatitis B antigenemia responds to lamivudine (see Chap. 50, p. 1132).

PREGNANCY. Only a few documented cases of polyarteritis nodosa in association with pregnancy have been reported. Although definitive conclusions are unclear, certainly if active arteritis is identified during pregnancy, mortality is high. Owen and Hauth (1989) reviewed the courses of 12 pregnant women. In seven, polyarteritis first manifested during pregnancy, and it was rapidly fatal by 6 weeks postpartum. The diagnosis was not made until autopsy in six of the seven women. Four women continued pregnancy, resulting in one stillborn and three successful outcomes.

Wegener Granulomatosis.

This is a necrotizing granulomatous vasculitis of the upper and lower respiratory tract and kidney. According to Sneller (1995), common lesions include sinusitis and nasal disease (90 percent), pulmonary infiltrates or nodules (85 percent), glomerulonephritis (75 percent), and musculoskeletal lesions (65 percent). It is uncommon and usually encountered after 50 years of age. Only a few cases have been reported in association with pregnancy (Fields and colleagues, 1991; Luisiri and associates, 1997; Palit and Clague, 1990; Pauzner and co-workers, 1994).

Takayasu Arteritis.

So-called *pulseless disease,* this syndrome is most prevalent in young women. It is a chronic inflammatory arteritis affecting large vessels. Unlike *temporal arteritis,* which occurs almost exclusively after 55 years of age, the onset of Takayasu arteritis is almost exclusively in patients before age 40. It is associated with abnormal angiography of the upper aorta and its main branches, resulting in upper extremity vascular impairment. Noninvasive methods such as computed tomography or magnetic resonance angiography can be used to detect this disorder prior to the development of severe vascular compromise (Numano and Kobayashi, 1999).

Takayasu arteritis may respond symptomatically to corticosteroid therapy, however, it is not curative. Surgical bypass or angioplasty have improved survival.

Severe renovascular hypertension, cardiac involvement, or pulmonary hypertension worsen pregnancy prognosis. Despite this, from their review of 14 cases, Nagey and colleagues (1983) reported good pregnancy outcomes. Subsequent reports and reviews support this (Johnston and colleagues, 2002; Langford and Kerr, 2002). When the abdominal aorta is involved, however, pregnancy outcome is disastrous (Sharma and associates, 2000).

Most authors advise that blood pressure be taken in the lower extremity. Epidural analgesia has been advocated for labor and delivery (Langford and Kerr, 2002).

DERMATOMYOSITIS AND POLYMYOSITIS. These are uncommon acute, subacute, or chronic inflammatory diseases of unknown cause involving mainly skin and muscle. Prevailing theories are that the syndromes are caused by viral infections, autoimmune disorders, or both. Polymyositis is a subacute inflammatory myopathy that is frequently associated with one of the autoimmune connective tissue disorders. Dermatomyositis is manifest as a characteristic rash accompanying or preceding weakness. Laboratory manifestations include elevated muscle enzyme levels in serum and an abnormal electromyogram. Confirmation is by biopsy. It usually occurs alone but can overlap with scleroderma or mixed connective tissue disease. The disease usually responds to high-dose corticosteroid therapy, and immunosuppressive drugs such as azathioprine or methotrexate are usually also required (Dalakas and Hohlfeld, 2003).

About 15 percent of adults who develop dermatomyositis have an associated malignant tumor. The time of appearance of the two diseases may be separated by several years. The most common sites of associated cancer are breast, lung, stomach, and ovary. There are only a few reports of dermatomyositis complicating pregnancy. King and Chow (1985) reported five uneventful pregnancies in three women with dermatomyositis. Gutierrez and colleagues (1984) reviewed outcomes in 10 pregnancies among seven women with active disease and found three abortions, three perinatal deaths, and five preterm deliveries. Rosenzweig and colleagues (1989) reviewed 24 pregnancy outcomes in 18 women with primary polymyositis-dermatomyositis. In half, the diagnosis preceded pregnancy. Of these, a fourth had an exacerbation in the second or third trimester. Excluding abortions, there were two perinatal deaths and two growth-restricted neonates. In the other half in whom disease became manifest first during pregnancy, outcomes were less favorable. One woman died 6 weeks postpartum. Excluding abortions, half of the eight pregnancies resulted in perinatal death. Ohno and associates (1992) and Papapetropoulos and co-workers (1998) described similar cases.

The best form of contraception for these women is not known. Contraceptives containing hormones probably should not be used, unfortunately, little data are available. Although sterilization might seem at first to be an obvious choice, some women have mild chronic disease, and others may experience a permanent remission if an associated malignancy is identified and cured.

INHERITED CONNECTIVE TISSUE DISORDERS

MARFAN SYNDROME. This autosomal dominant connective tissue disorder affects both sexes equally with a prevalence of 2 to 3 per 10,000. There appears to be no racial or ethnic basis for the syndrome. The *FBN1* gene that mutates is on the long arm of chromosome 15 (Dietz and colleagues,

2002; Loeys and colleagues, 2002). The *FBN1* gene has a high mutation rate, and there are many mild cases in which the intrinsic connective tissue lesion is subclinical with no effect on longevity.

In severe disease, there is degeneration of the elastic lamina in the media of the aorta, which predisposes to aortic dilatation or dissecting aneurysm. Early death in Marfan syndrome is ultimately caused by either valvular insufficiency and congestive heart failure or rupture of a dissecting aneurysm. Mor-Yosef and colleagues (1988) report an increased frequency of dissecting and ruptured aneurysms during pregnancy, especially in the last trimester. The syndrome was reviewed by Elkayam and associates (1995) and is discussed in detail in Chapter 44 (p. 1034).

EHLERS–DANLOS SYNDROME. This disease is characterized by a variety of changes in connective tissue, including hyperelasticity of the skin. In the more severe types, there is a strong tendency for fatal rupture of any of several arteries to cause either strokes or bleeding. Rupture of the colon or uterus has been described. There are at least 11 types of disease based on skin, joint, or other tissue involvement; some are autosomal dominant, some recessive, and some X-linked. The estimated aggregate prevalence is about 1 in 5000 (Prockop and colleagues, 2001). Types I, II, and III are autosomally dominant, and each accounts for about 30 percent of cases. There is overlap between these types, and in most, the underlying molecular defect of collagen or procollagen is unknown.

Women with Ehlers–Danlos syndrome have an increased frequency of preterm rupture of membranes, preterm delivery, and antepartum and postpartum hemorrhage. Tissue fragility makes episiotomy repair and cesarean delivery difficult. Sorokin and colleagues (1994) surveyed women members of the Ehlers–Danlos National Foundation. They reported a stillbirth rate of 3 percent, a preterm delivery rate of 23 percent, a cesarean delivery rate of 8 percent, and problematic postpartum bleeding in 15 percent. Case reports and literature reviews have been provided by Hordnes (1994) and Sakala and Harding (1991).

REFERENCES

Adams KM, Nelson JL: Microchimerism: An investigative frontier in autoimmunity and transplantation. JAMA 291:1127, 2004

Aggarwal N, Sawhney H, Vasishta K, et al: Pregnancy in patients with systemic lupus erythematosus. Aust N Z J Obstet Gynaecol 39:28, 1999

Alexander E, Buyon JP, Provost TT, et al: Anti-Ro/SSA antibodies in the pathophysiology of congenital heart block in neonatal lupus syndrome: An experimental model. Arthritis Rheum 35:176, 1992

Amengual O, Atsumi T, Khamashta MA: Tissue factor in antiphospholipid syndrome: Shifting the focus from coagulation to endothelium. Rheumatology 42: 1029, 2003

American College of Obstetricians and Gynecologists: Thromboembolism in pregnancy. Practice Bulletin No. 19, August 2000

American College of Obstetricians and Gynecologists: Antepartum fetal surveillance. Practice Bulletin No. 9, October 1999

Arbuckle MF, McClain MT, Rubertone MV, et al: Development of autoantibodies before the clinical onset of systemic lupus erythematosus. N Engl J Med 349:1526, 2003

Arnett FC: The genetics of human lupus. In Wallace DJ, Hahn BH (eds): Dubois' Lupus Erythematosus, 5th ed. Baltimore, Williams & Wilkins, 1997, p 77

Arnett FC, Edworthy SM, Bloch DA, et al: The American Rheumatism Association 1987 revised criteria for the classification of rheumatoid arthritis. Arthritis Rheum 31:315, 1988

Artlett CM, Smith B, Jimenez SA: Identification of fetal DNA and cells in skin lesions from women with systemic sclerosis. N Engl J Med 338:1186, 1998

Barinaga M: Cells exchanged during pregnancy live on. Science 296:2169, 2002

Barrett JH, Brennan P, Fiddler M, et al: Breast-feeding and postpartum relapse in women with rheumatoid and inflammatory arthritis. Arthritis Rheum 43:1010, 2000a

Barrett JH, Brennan P, Fiddler M, et al: Does rheumatoid arthritis remit during pregnancy and relapse postpartum? Results from a nationwide study in the United Kingdom performed prospectively from late pregnancy. Arthritis Rheum 42:1219, 2000b

Benjamin R, Parham P: HLA-B27 and diseases: A consequence of inadvertent antigen presentation? Rheum Dis Clin North Am 18:11, 1992

Bijlsma JWJ, Van Den Brink HR: Estrogens and rheumatoid arthritis. Am J Reprod Immunol 28:231, 1992

Black CM, Stevens WM: Scleroderma. Rheum Dis Clin North Am 15:193, 1989

Boh EE: Neonatal lupus erythematosus. Clin Dermatol 22:125, 2004

Borden M, Parke A: Antimalarial drugs in systemic lupus erythematosus. Drug Saf 24:1055, 2001

Branch DW, Andres R, Digre KB, et al: The association of antiphospholipid antibodies with severe preeclampsia. Obstet Gynecol 73:541, 1989

Branch DW: Antiphospholipid syndrome—laboratory concerns, fetal loss, and pregnancy management. Semin Perinatol 15:230, 1991

Branch DW, Khamashta M: Antiphospholipid syndrome: Obstetric diagnosis, management, and controversies. Obstet Gynecol 101:1333, 2003

Branch DW, Peaceman AM, Druzin M, et al: A multicenter, placebo-controlled pilot study of intravenous immune globulin treatment of antiphospholipid syndrome during pregnancy. Am J Obstet Gynecol 182:122, 2000

Briggs GG, Freeman RK, Yaffee SJ: Drugs in Pregnancy and Lactation, 6th ed. Baltimore, Williams & Wilkins, 2002

Buckley LM, Bullaboy CA, Leichtman L, et al: Multiple congenital anomalies associated with weekly low-dose methotrexate treatment of the mother. Arthritis Rheum 40:971, 1997

Buyon J, Kalunian K, Ramsey-Goldman R, et al: Assessing disease activity in SLE patients during pregnancy. Lupus 8:677, 1999

Buyon JP, Winchester RJ, Slade SG, et al: Identification of mothers at risk for congenital heart block and other neonatal lupus syndromes in their children. Comparison of enzyme-linked immunoabsorbent assay and immunoblot for measurement of anti SSA/Ro and anti SSB/La antibodies. Arthritis Rheum 36:1263, 1993

Carbone J, Sanchez-Ramon S, Cobo-Soriano R: Antiphospholipid antibodies: A risk factor for occlusive retinal vascular disorders. Comparison with ocular inflammatory diseases. J Rheumatol 28:2437, 2001

Carbone J, Orera M, Rodriguez-Mahou M, et al: Immunological abnormalities in primary APS evolving into SLE:6 years' follow-up in women with repeated pregnancy loss. Lupus 8:274, 1999

Carmona F, Font J, Cervera R, et al: Obstetrical outcome of pregnancy in patients with systemic lupus erythematosus. A study of 60 cases. Eur J Obstet Gynecol Reprod Biol 83:137, 1999

Chamley LW, Duncalf AM, Konarkowska B, et al: Conformationally altered beta(2)-glycoprotein I is the antigen for anti-cardiolipin autoantibodies. Clin Exp Immunol 115:571, 1999

Chin KAJ, Kaseba CM, Weaver JB: Mallory–Weiss syndrome complicating pregnancy in a patient with scleroderma: Diagnosis and management. Br J Obstet Gynaecol 102:498, 1995

Contreras G, Pardo V, Leclercq B, et al: Sequential therapies for proliferative lupus nephritis. N Engl J Med 350:971, 2004

Cowchock S: Prevention of fetal death in the antiphospholipid antibody syndrome. Lupus 5:467, 1996

Cowchock S: Treatment of antiphospholipid syndrome in pregnancy. Lupus 7:S95, 1998

Dalakas MC, Hohlfeld R: Polymyositis and dermatomyositis. Lancet 362:971, 2003

Dietz HC, Cutting GR, Pyeritz RE, et al: Marfan syndrome caused by a recurrent de novo missense mutation in the fibrillin gene. Nature 352:337, 1991

Dittrich E, Schamaldienst S, Langer M, et al: Immunoadsorption and plasma exchange in pregnancy. Kidney Blood Press Res 25:232, 2002

Dizon-Townson D, Branch DW: Anticoagulant treatment during pregnancy: An update. Semin Thromb Hemost 24: 55S, 1998

Elkayam U, Ostrzega E, Shotan A, et al: Cardiovascular problems in pregnant women with the Marfan syndrome. Ann Intern Med 123:117, 1995

Enns GM, Roeder E, Chan RT, et al: Apparent cyclophosphamide (Cytoxan) embryopathy: A distinct phenotype? Am J Med Genet 86:237, 1999

Ermel LD, Marshburn PB, Kutteh WH: Interaction of heparin with antiphospholipid antibodies (APA) from the sera of women with recurrent pregnancy loss (RPL). Am J Reprod Immunol 33:14, 1995

Faden D, Tincani A, Tanzi P, et al: Anti-beta 2 glycoprotein I antibodies in a general obstetric population: Preliminary results on the prevalence and correlation with pregnancy outcome. Anti-beta 2 glycoprotein I antibodies are associated with some obstetrical complications, mainly preeclampsia-eclampsia. Eur J Obstet Gynecol Reprod Biol 73: 37, 1997

Falcón CR, Martinuzzo ME, Forastiero RR, et al: Pregnancy loss and autoantibodies against phospholipid-binding proteins. Obstet Gynecol 89:975, 1997

Farine D, Granovsky-Grisaru S, Ryan G, et al: Umbilical artery blood flow velocity in pregnancies complicated by systemic lupus erythematosus. J Clin Ultrasound 26:379, 1998

Feinstein DI, Rapaport SI: Acquired inhibitors of blood coagulation. In Spaet TH (ed): Progress in Hemostasis and Thrombosis, Vol 1. New York, Grune & Stratton, 1972, p 75

Fields GL, Ossorio MA, Roy TM, et al: Wegener's granulomatosis complicated by pregnancy: A case report. J Reprod Med 36:463, 1991

Forastiero RR, Martinuzzo ME, Carreras LO, et al: Enhanced thromboxane biosynthesis in patients with antiphospholipid antibodies is related to the presence of antibodies to beta(2) glycoprotein. Thromb Haemost 78:1008, 1997

Galli M, Bevers EM: Inhibition of phospholipid-dependent coagulation reactions by antiphospholipid antibodies—possible modes of action. Lupus 3:223, 1994

Gilliland BC: Systemic sclerosis (scleroderma). In Braunwald E, Fauci AS, Kasper DL, et al (eds): Harrison's Principles of Internal Medicine, 15th ed. New York, McGraw-Hill, 2001, p 1937

Gladman DD, Urowitz MB: Systemic lupus erythematosus—clinical features. In Klippel JH, Dieppe PA (eds): Rheumatology. St. Louis, Mosby, 1997, p 7.1

Gutierrez G, Dagnino R, Mintz G: Polymyositis/dermatomyositis and pregnancy. Arthritis Rheum 27:291, 1984

Haddow JE, Rote NS, Dostaljohnson D, et al: Lack of an association between late fetal death and antiphospholipid antibody measurements in the 2nd trimester. Am J Obstet Gynecol 165:1308, 1991

Hahn BH: Pathogenesis of systemic lupus erythematosus. In Kelley WN, Harris ED, Ruddy S, et al (eds): Textbook of Rheumatology, Vol 2, 5th ed. Philadelphia, Saunders, 1997, p 1015

Hahn BH: Systemic lupus erythematosus. In Braunwald E, Fauci AS, Kasper DL, et al (eds). Harrison's Principles of Internal Medicine, 15th ed. New York, McGraw-Hill, 2001, p 1922

Hanly JG, Gladman DD, Rose TH, et al: Lupus pregnancy: A prospective study of placental changes. Arthritis Rheum 31:358, 1988

Harney S, Newton J, Milicic A, et al: Non-inherited maternal HLA alleles are associated with rheumatoid arthritis. Rheumatology 42:171, 2003

Harris EN: Antirheumatic drugs in pregnancy. Lupus 11:683, 2002

Harris EN, Hughes GRV: Standardizing the anticardiolipin antibody-test. Lancet 1:277, 1987

Harris EN, Spinnato JA: Should anticardiolipin tests be performed in otherwise healthy pregnant women? Am J Obstet Gynecol 165:1272, 1991

Harris EN, Gharavi AE, Patel SP, Hughes GVR: Evaluation of the anti-cardiolipin antibody test: Report of an international workshop. Clin Exp Immunol 68:215, 1987

Hazes JMW, Dijkmans BAC, Vandenbroucke JP, et al: Pregnancy and the risk of developing rheumatoid arthritis. Arthritis Rheum 33:1770, 1990

Heilmann L, von Tempelhoff GF, Pollow K: Antiphospholipid syndrome in obstetrics. Clin Appl Thromb Hemost 9:143, 2003

Hench PG: Ameliorating effect of pregnancy on chronic atrophic (infectious rheumatoid) arthritis, fibrositis and intermittent hydrarthrosis. Proc Mayo Clin 13:161, 1938

Hochberg MC: Updating the American College of Rheumatology revised criteria for the classification of systemic lupus erythematosus. Arthritis Rheum 40:1725, 1997

Hojnik M, George J, Ziporen L, et al: Heart valve involvement (Libman–Sacks endocarditis) in the antiphospholipid syndrome. Circulation 93:1579, 1996

Holers VM, Girardi G, Mo L, et al: Complement C3 activation is required for antiphospholipid antibody-induced fetal loss. J Exp Med 195:211, 2002

Hordnes K: Ehlers–Danlos syndrome and delivery. Acta Obstet Gynecol Scand 73:671, 1994

Huong DLT, Wechsler B, Vauthier-Brouzes D, et al: Pregnancy in past or present lupus nephritis: A study of 32 pregnancies from a single centre. Ann Rheum Dis 60:599, 2001

Ichinohe T, Maruya E, Saji H: Long-term feto-maternal microchimerism: Nature's hidden clue for alternative donor hematopoietic cell transplantation? Int J Hematol 76:229, 2002

Iijima T, Tada H, Hidaka Y, et al: Prediction of postpartum onset of rheumatoid arthritis. Ann Rheum Dis 57:460, 1998

Jacobsen S, Petersen J, Ullman S, et al: Mortality and causes of death of 513 Danish patients with systemic lupus erythematosus. Scand J Rheumatol 28:75, 1999

Jimenez SA, Artlett CM: Microchimerism and systemic sclerosis. Curr Opin Rheumatol 17:86, 2005

Johnson KL, McAlindon TE, Mulcahy E, et al: Microchimerism in a female patient with systemic lupus erythematosus. Arthritis Rheum 44:2107, 2001

Johnston SL, Lock RJ, Gompels MM: Takayasu arteritis: A review. J Clin Pathol 55:481, 2002

Julkunen H, Jouhikainen T, Kaaja R, et al: Fetal outcomes in lupus pregnancy: A retrospective case control study of 242 pregnancies in 112 patients. Lupus 2:125, 1993a

Julkunen H, Kaaja R, Palosuo T, et al: Pregnancy in lupus nephropathy. Acta Obstet Gynecol Scand 72:258, 1993b

Kaaja R, Julkunen H, Viinikka L, et al: Production of prostacyclin and thromboxane in lupus pregnancies—effect of small dose of aspirin. Obstet Gynecol 81:327, 1993

Kaplan D: Fetal wastage in patients with rheumatoid arthritis. J Rheumatol 13:875, 1986

Karlson EW, Lee I-M, Cook NR, et al: A retrospective cohort study of cigarette smoking and risk of rheumatoid arthritis in female health professionals. Arthritis Rheum 42:910, 1999

Khamashta MA, Ruiz-Irastorza G, Hughes GRV: Systemic lupus erythematosus flares during pregnancy. Rheum Dis Clin North Am 23:15, 1997

King CR, Chow S: Dermatomyositis and pregnancy. Obstet Gynecol 66:589, 1985

Kirwan JR, the Arthritis and Rheumatism Council Low-Dose Glucocorticoid Study Group: The effect of glucocorticoids on joint destruction in rheumatoid arthritis. N Engl J Med 333:142, 1995

Klipple GL, Cecere FA: Rheumatoid arthritis and pregnancy. Rheum Dis Clin North Am 15:213, 1989

Kutteh WH: Antiphospholipid antibody-associated recurrent pregnancy loss: Treatment with heparin and low-dose aspirin is superior to low-dose aspirin alone. Am J Obstet Gynecol 174:1584, 1996

Kutteh WH: Recurrent pregnancy loss. In Williams Obstetrics, 19th ed (Suppl 15). Stamford, CT, Appleton & Lange, October/November 1995

Kutteh WH, Rote NS, Silver R: Antiphospholipid antibodies and reproduction: The antiphospholipid antibody syndrome. Am J Reprod Immunol 41:133, 1999

Lambe M, Bjornadal L, Neregard P, et al: Childbearing and the risk of scleroderma: A population-based study in Sweden. Am J Epidemiol 159:162, 2004

Lambert NC, Erickson TD, Yan Z, et al: Quantification of maternal microchimerism by HLA-specific real-time polymerase chain reaction: studies of healthy women and women with scleroderma. Arthritis Rheum 50:906, 2004

Lambert NC, Lo TMD, Erickson TD, et al: Male microchimerism in healthy women and women with scleroderma: Cells or circulating DNA? A quantitative answer. Blood 100:2845, 2002

Langford C, Kerr G: Pregnancy in vasculitis. Curr Opin Rheumatol 14:36, 2002

Laskin CA, Bombardier C, Hannah ME, et al: Prednisone and aspirin in women with autoantibodies and unexplained recurrent fetal loss. New Engl J Med 337:148, 1997

Lee DM, Weinblatt ME: Rheumatoid arthritis. Lancet 358:903, 2001

Lee LA, Weston WL: New findings in neonatal lupus syndrome. Am J Dis Child 138:233, 1984

Lee RM, Emlen W, Scott JR, et al: Anti-β_2 glycoprotein I antibodies in women with recurrent spontaneous abortion, unexplained fetal death, and antiphospholipid syndrome. Am J Obstet Gynecol 181:642, 1999

Lellouche F, Falcon C, Carreras L, et al: Selective inhibition of platelet-derived thromboxane A2 in patients with lupus anticoagulant using low doses aspirin as assessed by enzyme-immunoassay. Adv Prostaglandin Thromboxane Leukot Res 21:611, 1991

Leong KH, Koh ET, Feng PH, et al: Lipid profiles in patients with systemic lupus erythematosus. J Rheumatol 21:1264, 1994

Levine JS, Branch W, Rauch J: The antiphospholipid syndrome. N Engl J Med 346:752, 2002

Levy RA, Vilela VS, Cataldo MJ, et al: Hydroxychloroquine (HCQ) in lupus pregnancy: Double-blind and placebo-controlled study. Lupus 10:401, 2001

Lipsky PE: Rheumatoid arthritis. In Braunwald E, Fauci AS, Kasper DL, et al (eds): Harrison's Principles of Internal Medicine, 15th ed. New York, McGraw-Hill, 2001, p 1880

Lockshin MD: Sex ratio and rheumatic disease: Excerpts from an Institute of Medicine reports. Lupus 11:662, 2002

Lockshin MD: Pregnancy does not cause systemic lupus erythematosus to worsen. Arthritis Rheum 32:665, 1989

Lockshin MD, Druzin ML: Rheumatic disease. In Barron WM, Lindheimer JD (eds): Medical Disorders During Pregnancy, 2nd ed. St. Louis, Mosby, 1995, p 307

Lockshin M, Sammaritano L: Lupus pregnancy. Autoimmunity 36:33, 2003

Lockshin MD, Sammaritano LR: Rheumatic disease. In Barron WM, Lindheimer MD (eds): Medical Disorders During Pregnancy, 3rd ed. St. Louis, Mosby, 2000, p 355

Lockshin MD, Druzin ML, Qamar T: Prednisone does not prevent recurrent fetal death in women with antiphospholipid antibody. Am J Obstet Gynecol 160:439, 1989

Lockshin MD, Bonfa E, Elkon K, et al: Neonatal lupus risk to newborns of mothers with systemic lupus erythematosus. Arthritis Rheum 31:697, 1988

Lockwood CJ, Romero R, Feinberg RF, et al: The prevalence and biologic significance of lupus anticoagulant and anticardiolipin antibodies in a general obstetric population. Am J Obstet Gynecol 161:369, 1989

Loeys B, Nuytinck L, Van Acker P, et al: Strategies for prenatal and preimplantation genetic diagnosis in Marfan syndrome (MFS). Prenat Diagn 22:22, 2002

Lopez LR, Dier KJ, Lopez D, et al: Anti-β_2 glycoprotein I and antiphosphatidylserine antibodies are predictors of arterial thrombosis in patients with antiphospholipid syndrome. Am J Clin Pathol 121:142, 2004

Love PE, Santoro SA: Antiphospholipid antibodies: Anticardiolipin and the lupus anticoagulant in systemic lupus erythematosus (SLE) and in non-SLE disorders. Ann Intern Med 112:682, 1990

Lubbe WF, Liggins GC: The lupus-anticoagulant: Clinical and obstetric complications. N Z Med J 97:398, 1984

Lubbe WFF, Palmer SJ, Butler WS, Liggins GC: Fetal survival after prednisone suppression of maternal lupus anticoagulant. Lancet 2:1361, 2002

Luisiri P, Lance NJ, Curran JJ: Wegener's granulomatosis: Time to change the standard of care. Arthritis Rheum 40:2099, 1997

Lynch A, Byers T, Emlen W, et al: Association of antibodies to beta$_2$-glycoprotein 1 with pregnancy loss and pregnancy-induced hypertension: A prospective study in low-risk pregnancy. Obstet Gynecol 93:193, 1999

Maloney S, Smith A, Furst DE, et al: Microchimerism of maternal origin persists into adult life. J Clin Invest 104:41, 1999

Masi AT, Chatterton RT, Aldag JC: Perturbations of hypothalamic–pituitary–gonadal axis and adrenal androgen functions in rheumatoid arthritis: An odyssey of hormonal relationships to the disease. Ann N Y Acad Sci 876:53, 1999

Maymon R, Fejgin M: Scleroderma in pregnancy. Obstet Gynecol Surv 44:530, 1989

Mills JA: Systemic lupus erythematosus. N Engl J Med 330:1871, 1994

Miyagawa S, Shinohara K, Kidoguchi K, et al: Neonatal lupus erythematosus: HLA-DR and -DQ distributions are different among the groups of anti-Ro/SSA-positive mothers with different neonatal outcomes. J Invest Dermatol 108:881, 1997

Moll JMH: The place of psoriatic arthritis in the spondarthritides. Baillières Clin Rheumatol 8:395, 1994

Moodley J, Ramphal SR, Duursma J, et al: Antiphospholipid antibodies in eclampsia. Hypertens Preg 14:179, 1995

Moroni G, Quaglini S, Banfi G, et al: Pregnancy in lupus nephritis. Am J Kidney Dis 40:713, 2002

Moroni G, Ventura D, Riva P, et al: Antiphospholipid antibodies are associated with an increased risk for chronic renal insufficiency in patients with lupus nephritis. Am J Kidney Dis 43:28, 2004

Mor-Yosef S, Younis J, Granat M, et al: Marfan's syndrome in pregnancy. Obstet Gynecol Surv 43:382, 1988

Moyssakis I, Tzioufas A, Triposkiadis F, et al: Severe aortic stenosis and mitral regurgitation in a woman with systemic lupus erythematosus. Clin Cardiol 25:194, 2002

Musiej-Nowakowska E, Ploski R: Pregnancy and early onset pauciarticular juvenile chronic arthritis. Ann Rheum Dis 58:475, 1999

Nagey DA, Fortier KJ, Hayes BA, et al: Takayasu's arteritis in pregnancy: A case presentation demonstrating the absence of placental pathology. Am J Obstet Gynecol 147:463, 1983

Nelson JL, Furst DE, Maloney S, et al: Microchimerism and HLA-compatible relationships of pregnancy in scleroderma. Lancet 351:559, 1998

Nelson JL, Hughes KA, Smith AG, et al: Maternal–fetal disparity in HLA class II alloantigens and the pregnancy-induced amelioration of rheumatoid arthritis. N Engl J Med 329:466, 1993

Nelson JL, Østensen M: Pregnancy and rheumatoid arthritis. Rheum Dis Clin North Am 23:195, 1997

Nelson JL, Voigt LF, Koepsell TD, et al: Pregnancy outcome in women with rheumatoid arthritis before disease onset. J Rheumatol 19:18, 1992

Nicholas NS, Panayi GS, Nouri AME: Human pregnancy serum inhibits interleukin-2 production. Clin Exp Immunol 58:587, 1985

Nochy D, Daugas E, Droz D, et al: The intrarenal vascular lesions associated with primary antiphospholipid syndrome. J Am Soc Nephrol 10: 507, 1999

Numano F, Kobayashi Y: Takayasu arteritis—beyond pulselessness. Intern Med 38:226, 1999

Ogasawara M, Aoki K, Matsuura E, et al: Anti β_2 glycoprotein I antibodies and lupus anticoagulant in patients with recurrent pregnancy loss: Prevalence and clinical significance. Lupus 5:587, 1996

Ogunyemi D, Ku W, Arkel Y: The association between inherited thrombophilia, antiphospholipid antibodies and lipoprotein A levels with obstetrical complications in pregnancy. J Thromb Thrombolysis 14:157, 2002

Ohno T, Imai A, Tamaya T: Successful outcomes of pregnancy complicated with dermatomyositis. Gynecol Obstet Invest 33:187, 1992

Østensen M: Sex hormones and pregnancy in rheumatoid arthritis and systemic lupus erythematosus. Ann N Y Acad Sci 876:131, 1999

Østensen M: Pregnancy in patients with a history of juvenile rheumatoid arthritis. Arthritis Rheum 34:881, 1991

Østensen M, Husby G: A prospective clinical study of the effect of pregnancy on rheumatoid arthritis and ankylosing spondylitis. Arthritis Rheum 26:1155, 1983

Østensen M, Ramsey-Goldman R: Treatment of inflammatory rheumatic disorders in pregnancy—what are the safest treament options? Drug Saf 19:389, 1998

Oshiro BT, Silver RM, Scott JR, et al: Antiphospholipid antibodies and fetal death. Obstet Gynecol 87:489, 1996

Ottaviani G, Lavezzi AM, Rossi L, et al. Sudden unexpected death of a term fetus in an anticardiolipin-positive mother. Am J Perinatol 21:79, 2004

Owen J, Hauth JC: Polyarteritis nodosa in pregnancy: A case report and brief literature review. Am J Obstet Gynecol 160:606, 1989

Packham DK, Lam SS, Nicholls K, et al: Lupus nephritis and pregnancy. QJM 83:315, 1992

Palit J, Clague RB: Wegener's granulomatosis presenting during first trimester of pregnancy. Br J Rheumatol 29:389, 1990

Papapetropoulos T, Kanellakopoulou N, Tsibri E, et al: Polymyositis and pregnancy: Report of a case with three pregnancies. J Neurol Neurosurg Psychiatry 64:406, 1998

Parkin J, Cohen B: An overview of the immune system. Lancet 357:1777, 2001

Pattison NS, Chamley LW, Mckay EJ, et al: Antiphospholipid antibodies in pregnancy—prevalence and clinical associations. Br J Obstet Gynecol 100:909, 1993

Pauzner R, Mayan H, Hershko E, et al: Exacerbation of Wegener's granulomatosis during pregnancy: Report of a case with tracheal stenosis and literature review. J Rheumatol 21:1153, 1994

Petri M: Pregnancy in SLE. Baillières Clin Rheumatol 12:449, 1998

Petri M: Pathogenesis and treatment of the antiphospholipid antibody syndrome. Adv Rheumatol 81:151, 1997

Petri M, Albritton J: Fetal outcome of lupus pregnancy: A retrospective case-control study of the Hopkins Lupus Cohort. J Rheumatol 20:650, 1993

Petri M, Howard D, Repke J: Frequency of lupus flare in pregnancy: The Hopkins lupus pregnancy center experience. Arthritis Rheum 34:1538, 1991

Pierro E, Cirino G, Bucci MR, et al: Antiphospholipid antibodies inhibit prostaglandin release by decidual cells of early pregnancy: Possible involvement of extracellular secretory phospholipase A$_2$. Fertil Steril 71:342, 1999

Polzin WJ, Kopelman JN, Robinson RD, et al: The association of antiphospholipid antibodies with pregnancies complicated by fetal growth restriction. Obstet Gynecol 78:1108, 1991

Prockop DJ, Kuivaniemi H, Tromp G, et al: Inherited disorders of connective tissue. In Braunwald E, Fauci AS, Kasper DL, et al (eds): Harrison's Principles of Internal Medicine, 15th ed. New York, McGraw-Hill, 2001, p 2290

Rahman P, Gladman DD, Urowitz MB: Clinical predictors of fetal outcome in systemic lupus erythematosus. J Rheumatol 25:1526, 1998

Ramsey-Goldman R, Mientus MJ, Kutzer JE, et al: Pregnancy outcome in women with systemic lupus erythematosus treated with immunosuppressive drugs. J Rheumatol 20:1152, 1993

Ramscy-Goldman R, Schilling E: Immunosuppressive drug use during pregnancy. Rheum Dis Clin North Am 23:149, 1997

Rand JH, Wu XX, Andree HAM, et al: Antiphospholipid antibodies accelerate plasma coagulation by inhibiting annexin-V binding to phospholipids: A "lupus procoagulant" phenomenon. Blood 92:1652, 1998

Rand JH, Wu XX, Andree HAM, et al: Pregnancy loss in the antiphospholipid antibody syndrome—a possible thrombogenic mechanism. N Engl J Med 337:154, 1997a

Rand JH, Wu XX, Guller S, et al: Antiphospholipid immunoglobulin G antibodies reduce annexin-V levels on syncytiotrophoblast apical membranes and in culture media of placental villi. Am J Obstet Gynecol 177:918, 1997b

Rao JK, Allen NB, Pincus T: Limitations of the 1990 American College of Rheumatology classification criteria in the diagnosis of vasculitis. Ann Intern Med 129:345, 1998

Refojo D, Liberman AC, Giacomini D: Integrating systemic information at the molecular level. Ann N Y Acad Sci 922:196, 2003

Repke JT: Hypertensive disorders of pregnancy: Differentiating preeclampsia from active systemic lupus erythematosus. J Reprod Med 43:350, 1998

Richards DS, Wagman AJ, Cabaniss ML: Ascites not due to congestive heart failure in a fetus with lupus-induced heart block. Obstet Gynecol 76:957, 1990

Roque H, Paidas M, Rebarber A, et al: Maternal thrombophilia is associated with second- and third-trimester fetal death. Am J Obstet Gynecol 184: S27, 2001

Rosenzweig BA, Rotmensch S, Binette SP, et al: Primary idiopathic polymyositis and dermatomyositis complicating pregnancy: Diagnosis and management. Obstet Gynecol Surv 44:162, 1989

Rubin RL: Drug induced lupus. In Wallace DJ, Hahn BH (eds): Dubois' Lupus Erythematosus, 5th ed. Baltimore, Williams & Wilkins, 1997, p 871

Ruiz-Irastorza G, Khamashta MA, Gordon C, et al: Measuring systemic lupus erythematosus activity during pregnancy: Validation of the lupus activity index in pregnancy scale. Arthritis Rheum 51:78, 2004

Ruiz-Irastorza G, Khamashta MA, Hughes G: Systemic lupus erythematosus. Lancet 358:586, 2001

Ruiz-Irastorza G, Lima F, Alves J, et al: Increased rate of lupus flare during pregnancy and the puerperium: A prospective study of 78 pregnancies. Br J Rheumatol 35:133, 1996

Russo-Stieglitz K, Rasheed M, Artlett C, et al: Influence of prior pregnancies on disease course and mortality in systemic sclerosis. Am J Obstet Gynecol 184:S190, 2001

Sakala EP, Harding MD: Ehlers–Danlos syndrome type III and pregnancy. J Reprod Med 36:622, 1991

Saleeb S, Copel J, Friedman D, et al: Comparison of treatment with fluorinated glucocorticoids to the natural history of autoantibody-associated congenital heart block. Arthritis Rheum 42:2335, 1999

Sangle S, D'Cruz DP, Hughes GR: Livedo reticularis and pregnancy morbidity in patients negative for antiphospholipid antibodies. Ann Rheum Dis 64:147, 2005

Sanna G, Bertolaccini ML, Cuadrado MJ. Central nervous system involvement in the antiphospholipid (Hughes) syndrome. Rheumatology 42:200, 2003

Sawaya HH, Jimenez SA, Artlett CM. Quantification of fetal microchimeric cells in clinically affected and unaffected skin of patients with systemic sclerosis. Rheumatology 43:965, 2004

Schousboe I, Rasmussen MS: Synchronized inhibition of the phospholipid mediated autoactivation of factor XII in plasma by β_2 glycoprotein I and anti-β_2 glycoprotein I. Thromb Haemost 73:798, 1995

Scott JR: Risks to the children born to mothers with autoimmune diseases. Lupus 11:655, 2002

Seibold JR, Korn JH, Simms R, et al: Recombinant human relaxin in the treatment of scleroderma—a randomized, double-blind, placebo-controlled trial. Ann Intern Med 132:871, 2000

Sharma BK, Jain S, Vasishta K: Outcome of pregnancy in Takayasu arteritis. Int J Cardiol 75:S159, 2000

Shi W, Chong BH, Hogg PJ, et al: Anticardiolipin antibodies block the inhibition by β_2 glycoprotein I of the factor Xa generating activity of platelets. Thromb Haemost 70:342, 1993

Shinohara K, Miyagawa S, Fujita T, et al: Neonatal lupus erythematosus: Results of maternal corticosteroid therapy. Obstet Gynecol 93:952, 1999

Shmerling RH: Autoantibodies in systemic lupus erythematosus—there before you know it. N Engl J Med 349:1499, 2003

Silman A, Black CM: Increased incidence of spontaneous abortion and infertility in women with scleroderma before disease onset: A controlled study. Ann Rheum Dis 47:441, 1988

Silman A, Kay A, Brennan P: Timing of pregnancy in relation to the onset of rheumatoid arthritis. Arthritis Rheum 35:152, 1992

Silver RM, Branch DW: Autoimmune diseases in pregnancy: Systemic lupus erthematosus and antiphospholipid syndrome. Clin Perinatol 24:91, 1997

Silver RM, Draper ML, Scott JR, et al: Clinical consequences of antiphospholipid antibodies: An historic cohort study. Obstet Gynecol 83:372, 1994

Silver RM, Porter TF, Van Leeuween I, et al: Anticardiolipin antibodies: Clinical consequences of "low titers." Obstet Gynecol 87:494, 1996

Singsen BH, Akhter JE, Weinstein MM, et al: Congenital complete heart block and SSA antibodies: Obstetric implications. Am J Obstet Gynecol 153:495, 1985

Sitar G, Brambati B, Baldi M, et al: The use of non-physiological conditions to isolate fetal cells from maternal blood. Exp Cell Res 302:153, 2005

Skomsvoll JF, Baste V, Irgens LM, et al: The recurrence risk of adverse outcome in the second pregnancy in women with rheumatic disease. Obstet Gynecol 100:1196, 2002

Sneller MC: Wegener's granulomatosis. JAMA 273:1288, 1995

Sorokin Y, Johnson MP, Rogowski N, et al: Obstetric and gynecologic dysfunction in the Ehlers–Danlos syndrome. J Reprod Med 39:281, 1994

Srivatsa B, Srivatsa S, Johnson K, et al: Microchimerism of presumed fetal origin in thyroid specimens from women: A case-control study. Lancet 358:2034, 2001

Steen VD: Pregnancy in women with systemic sclerosis. Obstet Gynecol 94:15, 1999

Steen VD, Conte C, Day N, et al: Pregnancy in women with systemic sclerosis. Arthritis Rheum 32:151, 1989

Stirnemann J, Fain O, Lachassinne E, et al: Neonatal lupus erythematosus. Presse Med 31:1407, 2002

Stone S, Hunt BJ, Seed PT: Longitudinal evaluation of markers of endothelial cell dysfunction and hemostasis in treated antiphospholipid syndrome and in healthy pregnancy. Am J Obstet Gynecol 188:454, 2003

Tinahones FJ, Cuadrado MJ, Khamashta MA, et al: Lack of cross-reaction between antibodies to beta2-glycoprotein-I and oxidized low-density lipoprotein in patients with antiphospholipid syndrome. Br J Rheumatol 37:746, 1998

Toglia MR, Weg JG: Venous thromboembolism during pregnancy. N Engl J Med 335:108, 1996

Trudinger BJ, Stewart GJ, Cook C, et al: Monitoring lupus anticoagulant-positive pregnancies with umbilical artery flow velocity waveforms. Obstet Gynecol 72:215, 1988

Tseng CE, Buyon JP: Neonatal lupus syndrome. Rheum Dis Clin North Am 23:31, 1997

Tsokos G: A disease with a complex pathogenesis. Lancet 358:S65, 2001

Unger A, Kay A, Griffin AJ, et al: Disease activity and pregnancy associated β_2-glycoprotein in rheumatoid arthritis. BMJ 286:750, 1983

van der Horst-Bruinsma IE, de Vries RRP, de Buch PDM, et al: Influence of HLA-class II incompatibility between mother and fetus on the development and course of rheumatoid arthritis of the mother. Ann Rheum Dis 57:286, 1998

van Dunne FM, Lard LR, Rook D, et al: Miscarriage but not fecundity is associated with progression of joint destruction in rheumatoid arthritis. Ann Rheum Dis 63:956, 2004

Varner MW, Meehan RT, Syrop CH, et al: Pregnancy in patients with systemic lupus erythematosus. Am J Obstet Gynecol 145:1025, 1983

Waltuck J, Buyon JP: Autoantibody-associated congenital heart block: Outcome in mothers and children. Ann Intern Med 120:544, 1994

Warren JB, Silver RM: Autoimmune disease in pregnancy: systemic lupus erythematosus and antiphospholipid syndrome. Obstet Gynecol Clin North Am 31:345, 2004

Weston WL, Morelli JG, Lee LA: The clinical spectrum of anti-Ro-positive cutaneous neonatal lupus erythematosus. J Am Acad Dermatol 40:675, 1999

Wilder RL, Elenkov IJ: Hormonal regulation of tumor necrosis factor-α, interleukin-12 and interleukin-10 production by activated macrophages. Ann N Y Acad Sci 876:14, 1999

Wilson WA, Gharavi AE, Koike TL: International consensus statement on preliminary classification criteria for definite antiphospholipid syndrome. Arthritis Rheum 42:1309, 1999

Wolfberg AJ, Lee-Parritz A, Peller AJ, et al: Association of rheumatologic disease with preeclampsia. Obstet Gynecol. 103:1190, 2004

Yasuda M, Takakuwa K, Okinaga A, et al: Prospective studies of the association between anticardiolipin antibody and outcome of pregnancy. Obstet Gynecol 86:555, 1995

Yasmeen S, Wilkins EE, Field NT, et al: Pregnancy outcomes in women with systemic lupus erythematosus. J Matern Fetal Med 10:91, 2001

Zangari M, Lockwood CJ, Scher J, et al: Prothrombin activation fragment (F1.2) is increased in pregnant patients with antiphospholipid antibodies. Thromb Res 85:177, 1997

Zulman JI, Talal N, Hoffman GS, et al: Problems associated with the management of pregnancies in patients with systemic lupus erythematosus. J Rheumatol 7:37, 1980

55

Neurological and Psychiatric Disorders

Neurological and psychiatric disorders during pregnancy are as common as they are in all women of reproductive age, if not more so. In some cases, pregnancy may predispose to some of these disorders, or it may act to worsen them. For example, Bell palsy and benign intracranial hypertension appear to be more common during pregnancy. Depression, a common affliction of young women, is definitely linked to pregnancy and the puerperium.

NEUROLOGICAL DISORDERS

Neurological diseases are relatively common in women of childbearing age. Many of these disorders once precluded childbearing, but therapeutic advances have changed this. Currently, many women with chronic neurological disease become pregnant, and most of these conditions are compatible with a successful pregnancy outcome. Neurological diseases do contribute to maternal mortality (Shehata and Okosun, 2004), however, and most affected pregnant women require special therapy and entail specific risks with which the clinician should be familiar.

Diagnosis of Neurological Disease During Pregnancy. Most women with chronic neurological disease have been diagnosed before pregnancy. Occasionally, however, new neurological symptoms arise during gestation and must be distinguished from complications of pregnancy. Because neurological symptoms may involve cognitive as well as neuromuscular functions, they must also be distinguished from psychiatric disorders. In general, pregnant women should receive the same evaluation as other patients, and if indicated, the techniques discussed subsequently should not be withheld.

Central Nervous System Imaging. Various imaging techniques have been developed during the past 30 years that have revolutionized the visualization of anatomical lesions responsible for neurological disease.

Computed tomography (CT) and *magnetic resonance imaging (MRI)* have opened new vistas for the diagnosis, classification, and management of many neurological and psychiatric disorders. As discussed in Chapter 41 (see p. 979), both are safe during pregnancy (see Table 41–7). In some diseases (e.g., hemorrhagic lesions), cranial CT is preferable to MRI, whereas in others, it is complementary. CT is commonly used whenever rapid diagnosis is necessary to decide between medical and surgical management of an acute neurological catastrophe.

In less acute situations, MRI is often the imaging modality of choice during pregnancy because of its low radiation exposure. It is helpful in diagnosing demyelinating diseases, screening for arteriovenous malformations, evaluating congenital and developmental nervous system abnormalities, identifying posterior fossa lesions, and diagnosing spinal cord

TABLE 55–1 Prevalence of Neurological Disorders

Disorder	Prevalence (per 100,000)
Migraine	2000
Epilepsy	650
Cerebral palsy	250
Multiple sclerosis	100
Spinal cord injury	50
Subarachnoid hemorrhage	50
Myasthenia gravis	4
Genetic disorders (excluding malformations)	< 10

From Kurtzke (1982), with permission.

diseases. A relative disadvantage is the limited space available to a patient within the scanner, which may hinder monitoring critically ill patients. In addition, the claustrophobic conditions of the scanner may not be tolerated by some pregnant women. Premedication may be beneficial. Alternatively, an open MRI scanner may be used to accommodate claustrophobic patients. Scanning times are longer, however, and image quality may be lower than with standard MRI (Schnitker and Light, 2001). For both MRI and CT, women should be positioned in a left lateral tilt with a wedge under their right hips to avoid hypotension and to diminish aortic pulsations, which may degrade the image.

Cerebral angiography with contrast injection, usually via the femoral artery, is a valuable adjunct to the diagnosis and treatment of some cerebrovascular diseases. *Fluoroscopy* involves more radiation than most radiographic procedures but can be performed if necessary during pregnancy with careful abdominal shielding.

HEADACHE. The most common neurological complaint during pregnancy is headache (Table 55–1). There are several causes, and their classification was recently updated by the International Headache Society (2004). More than 90 percent of headaches are tension or migraine headaches (Paulson, 1995).

Tension Headache. Characteristic features of tension headaches include muscle tightness and pain that can persist for hours in the back of the neck and head. There are no associated neurological disturbances. The pain usually responds to rest, massage, application of heat or ice, anti-inflammatory medications, or mild tranquilizers. Patients with recurrent tension headaches may benefit from counseling about stress management, including biofeedback techniques. Headaches may also be a symptom of depression.

Migraine Headache. The term *migraine* describes a periodic, incapacitating neurovascular disorder. It is characterized by episodic attacks of severe headache and autonomic nervous system dysfunction (Goadsby and colleagues, 2002). The International Headache Society (2004) classifies three migraine types based on the presence or absence of an aura and chronicity. Migraine without aura is characterized by a unilateral throbbing headache, nausea and vomiting, or photophobia. About a third of patients have migraine with an aura (classic migraine) with similar symptoms preceded by premonitory neurological phenomena such as visual scotoma or hallucinations. This type of migraine can sometimes be averted if medication is taken at the first premonitory sign. Chronic migraine is defined as migraine headache occurring at least 15 days each month for more than 3 months without obvious cause.

Migraines may begin in childhood, peak in adolescence, and tend to diminish in both frequency and severity with advancing years. Stewart and colleagues (1992) reported that 18 percent of women and 6 percent of men suffer from migraine headaches at some time. Migraines are especially common in young women and have been linked to hormone levels in an as yet unclear relationship. The exact pathophysiology of migraines is uncertain, but they occur when neuronal dysfunction leads to decreased cortical blood flow, activation of vascular and meningeal nociceptors, and stimulation of the trigeminal sensory neurons (Silberstein, 2004). Kruit and co-workers (2004) recently described a predilection for the posterior circulation. In some cases, migraine is associated with stroke (Tietjen, 2000). Tzourio and colleagues (1995) reported a three- to sixfold increase in ischemic stroke in young women with migraines, although the absolute risk was small; it increased from 10 to 20 per 100,000. Migraineurs who smoked or used oral contraceptives, however, were particularly vulnerable and had a 10- to 14-fold increased risk.

EFFECTS OF PREGNANCY. From studies with a total of more than 1500 pregnant women, approximately 70 percent of women with migraines experience a dramatic improvement during pregnancy (Uknis and Silberstein, 1991; Welch, 1994). Menstrual migraine typically improves, most likely because it is provoked by the drop in estrogen levels just before menstruation and is thus relieved by the high estrogen levels of pregnancy (Aube, 1999; Fettes, 1997). Women with menstrual migraines can expect a relapse postpartum.

For nonmenstrual migraine headaches, pregnant women perceive either no change or worsening of symptoms. About 15 percent of migraine headaches appear for the first time during pregnancy and often develop in the first trimester, when hormone levels are rising (Aube, 1999). These migraines are more likely to be preceded by an aura. Because migraine symptoms are similar to those of other more serious disorders, the new onset of neurological symptoms should prompt a complete evaluation, including neuroimaging as needed.

MANAGEMENT. Most migraine headaches respond to simple analgesics such as aspirin, ibuprofen, or acetaminophen, especially if given early. Butalbital-containing products are no more effective than placebo (Wenzel and Sarvis, 2002). Severe headaches should be treated aggressively with in-

travenous hydration, parenteral antiemetics, and opioids if necessary (American College of Obstetricians and Gynecologists, 2002c). Antiemetics, such as promethazine, are frequently needed and are commonly given in combination with meperidine. One randomized trial involving 179 migraineurs showed that acupuncture is as effective as sumatriptan for early treatment of migraine (Melchart and colleagues, 2003).

Almost half of migraines with aura can be aborted by ergotamine. These potent vasoconstrictors should be avoided in pregnancy (Au and colleagues, 1985). Anomalies in exposed fetuses have been reported (Graham, 1983; Hughes, 1988; Verloes, 1990, and all their colleagues). Importantly, when given parenterally to the peripartum woman, ergotamine may be associated with myocardial infarction, pulmonary edema, bronchospasm, bowel infarction, and stroke (Reprotox, 2003a).

Triptans are serotonin 5-$HT_{1B/2D}$-receptor agonists found in the cranial arteries and dura mater. They relieve headaches by causing intracranial vasoconstriction and are highly effective in the treatment of migraine headaches (Silberstein, 2004). The drugs also relieve nausea and vomiting and greatly reduce the need for analgesics. At least five are available to be given orally, by injection, as rectal suppository, or as a nasal spray. Sumatriptan has not been studied extensively in pregnancy, but it appears to be safe (Reprotox, 2003b). Three series totaling 768 exposures have shown no adverse pregnancy effects (Kallen, 2001; Olesen, 2000; O'Quinn, 1999, and all their colleagues). The manufacturer's Sumatriptan and Naratriptan Registry (2002) of 348 cases has also failed to identify any teratogenic effects.

For women with frequent migraine headaches, prophylactic therapy is indicated (American College of Obstetricians and Gynecologists, 2002c). Amitriptyline, 10 to 150 mg/day; propranolol, 20 to 80 mg three times daily; atenolol, 50 to 100 mg/day; or labetalol, 50 to 150 mg two times daily, are safe in pregnancy and have been used with success (Dey and associates, 2002; Kaniecki, 2003).

SEIZURE DISORDERS. Approximately 0.5 to 2.0 percent of the population, including as many as 1.1 million American women of childbearing age, have epilepsy, which complicates 1 in 200 pregnancies (Brodie and Dichter, 1996; Yerby, 1994). Convulsive disorders are the second most prevalent and certainly the most serious common neurological condition encountered in pregnant women. Epilepsy itself can alter fetal development and can affect the course of pregnancy, labor, and delivery. In addition, the teratogenic effects of several anticonvulsant medications are unquestioned. On the other hand, pregnancy can exacerbate epilepsy by altering the metabolism of these anticonvulsant medications.

Pathophysiology. A seizure is defined as a paroxysmal disorder of the central nervous system characterized by an abnormal neuronal discharge with or without loss of consciousness. Epilepsy encompasses a number of different syndromes whose cardinal feature is a predisposition to recurrent unprovoked seizures (Chang and Lowenstein, 2003). This definition excludes seizures due to acute metabolic derangement or an acute central nervous system insult. Epileptic syndromes fit into two broad categories, which are subsequently discussed.

Partial seizures originate in one localized area of the brain and affect a correspondingly localized area of neurological function. They are believed to result from trauma, abscess, tumor, or perinatal factors, although a specific lesion is rarely demonstrated. *Simple motor seizures* start in one region of the body and progress toward other areas on the same side of the body, producing tonic and then clonic movements. Simple seizures can affect sensory function or produce autonomic dysfunction or psychological changes. Consciousness is usually not lost, and recovery is rapid. *Partial seizures* can secondarily generalize, producing loss of consciousness and convulsions. *Complex partial seizures,* also called *temporal lobe* or *psychomotor seizures*, usually involve clouding of the consciousness.

Generalized seizures involve both hemispheres of the brain simultaneously and may be preceded by an aura before an abrupt loss of consciousness. There is a strong hereditary component. In grand mal seizures, loss of consciousness is followed by tonic contraction of the muscles and rigid posturing, and then by clonic contractions of all extremities while the muscles gradually relax. Return to consciousness is gradual, and the patient may remain confused and disoriented for several hours. *Absence* seizures, also called *petit mal seizures*, are a form of generalized epilepsy that involve a brief loss of consciousness without muscle activity and are characterized by immediate recovery of consciousness and orientation.

Accurate seizure classification and consideration of the risks and benefits specific to each medication must factor into the appropriate selection of any anticonvulsant (see Chap. 14, p. 347 and Table 14–4).

Causes of Seizures. Some identifiable causes of convulsive disorders in adolescents and young adults include trauma, alcohol and other drug-induced withdrawals, brain tumors, biochemical abnormalities, or arteriovenous malformations. A search for all of these is necessary when a new-onset seizure disorder is encountered in a pregnant woman. The diagnosis of idiopathic epilepsy is one of exclusion. Lumbar puncture, skull radiography, and arteriography have been largely replaced by CT, MRI, or both.

Epilepsy During Pregnancy. The major pregnancy-related threats to women with epilepsy are an increase in seizure frequency and risk of congenital malformations in their fetuses. Hollingsworth and Resnik (1988) reviewed studies involving 2385 pregnancies and found increased seizure frequency in 35 percent of women, decreased frequency in 15 percent, and no change in 50 percent. Increased seizure frequency is often associated with subtherapeutic anticonvulsant levels or a lower seizure threshold, or both. Subtherapeutic levels are caused by a variety of factors, some of which are amenable to therapeutic intervention. Nausea and vomiting lead to missed doses; decreased gastrointestinal motility and the use of antacids reduces drug absorption; expanded intravascular volume lowers serum drug levels; induction of hepatic, plasma, and placental enzymes increases drug metabolism; and increased glomerular filtration hastens drug clearance. These changes are minimized in part by the fact that decreased protein binding during pregnancy increases free drug levels. In addition, women often self-discontinue medication because of teratogenicity concerns. Appropriate counseling can often avert this pitfall.

The seizure threshold can be affected by a variety of pregnancy-related factors, including exhaustion from sleep deprivation and hyperventilation and pain during labor. Women with the most recalcitrant disease are susceptible to minor changes and are at greatest risk of increased seizure frequency during pregnancy.

Women with epilepsy who take anticonvulsant medications have an increased risk of congenital malformations in the fetus (see Chap. 14, p. 347). Recent evidence suggests that untreated epilepsy is not associated with increased malformations (Holmes and colleagues, 2001). Almost 10 percent of the offspring of individuals with epilepsy develop a seizure disorder later in life.

Early studies suggested that women with epilepsy have an increased risk of a variety of pregnancy complications other than seizures, but much of these data were flawed by ascertainment bias and failure to address the confounding effects of alcohol and drug abuse and of socioeconomic factors. More recent data indicate only a small increase in risk. For example, Olafsson and colleagues (1998) performed a population-based study of all women with epilepsy who gave birth in Iceland during a 19-year period. Although these women had a twofold increased cesarean delivery rate, the risk of other adverse obstetrical events was similar to that for the general population. The risk of major congenital malformations was increased 2.7-fold in the neonates of women with epilepsy, but the mean birthweight and perinatal mortality were not different. In a cohort study in Montreal, Richmond and coworkers (2004) found that women with epilepsy had an increased incidence of nonproteinuric hypertension and labor induction as well as increased cardiovascular anomalies in their children.

Management

PRECONCEPTIONAL COUNSELING. For a number of reasons, women with epilepsy may benefit from preconceptional counseling (see Chap. 7, p. 191). This discussion should address the optimal anticonvulsant management, including a switch to the least teratogenic drug if possible or a reduction in the number of anticonvulsant types prescribed.

Although some clinicians recommend that medications be limited if possible to the older, more traditional anticonvulsants, namely, phenytoin, carbamazepine, and phenobarbital, some newer drugs may actually have less teratogenic potential. Eight newer anticonvulsant drugs that are available were recently reviewed by LaRoche and Helmers (2004a, b).

Other topics should include diet; activity, including refraining from driving during the first trimester if pregnancy-associated vomiting prevents therapeutic drug levels; prenatal fetal evaluation; and optimal labor and delivery management. Folic acid supplementation should also be given.

Postpartum contraception should be discussed. Anticonvulsants such as phenobarbital, primidone, phenytoin, and carbamazepine may cause breakthrough bleeding and oral contraceptive failure because they induce hepatic P_{450} microsomal enzyme systems, which in turn increase estrogen metabolism. Although an increased failure rate is speculative, the American College of Obstetricians and Gynecologists (1990) has recommended that oral contraceptives containing 50 μg of estrogen be used in women with epilepsy who take anticonvulsants. Oral contraceptives are not associated with exacerbation of seizures.

PRENATAL CARE. The major goal of pregnancy management is seizure prevention. To accomplish this, treatment for nausea and vomiting should be provided, seizure-provoking stimuli should be avoided, and medication compliance should be emphasized. In general, anticonvulsant medication should be maintained at the lowest dosage associated with seizure control. Although some clinicians routinely monitor serum drug levels during pregnancy, antenatal serum drug levels may be unreliable because of altered protein binding. Free or unbound drug levels, although more helpful, are not widely available. Lander and Eadie (1991) reported that seizure control is not improved by routine drug level monitoring. For these reasons, drug levels may be measured only following seizures or if noncompliance is suspected.

Some investigators recommend vitamin K for women taking phenytoin because it has been implicated in functionally defective neonatal vitamin K–dependent clotting factors II, VII, IX, and X. Cornelissen and associates (1993) demonstrated diminished vitamin K levels in 50 percent of cord blood samples from women taking anticonvulsants compared with 20 percent of those from women in a control group. It is not clear, however, that vitamin K crosses the placenta, and hemorrhage in the newborn is usually prevented by prompt parenteral administration of vitamin K (see Chap. 29, p. 676). For these reasons, many clinicians do not administer vitamin K to pregnant women with epilepsy.

A midpregnancy specialized ultrasonographic examination may aid in identifying anomalies (see Chap. 16, p. 392). Tests of fetal well-being are generally not performed for epilepsy alone but may be indicated if there is poor fetal growth, inadequate seizure control, or co-morbid maternal conditions.

TABLE 55–2 **Types of Strokes During Pregnancy or the Puerperium in 127 Women**

Type	Number
Ischemic Strokes (74)	
Preeclampsia–eclampsia	11
Arterial thrombosis	17
Venous thrombosis	18
Arterial embolism	8
Vasculopathy	5
Arterial dissection	2
Other and unknown	13
Hemorrhagic Strokes (53)	
Hypertensive	12
Arteriovenous malformation	12
Saccular aneurysm	6
Cocaine	3
Cavernous angioma	2
Vasculopathy	2
Unknown or other	13

From Jaigobin (2000); Kittner (1996); Sharshar (1995); Witlin (2000), and all their colleagues.

CEREBROVASCULAR DISEASES. These diseases refer to abnormalities of one or more blood vessels of the brain, with the majority involving the arterial system. The resultant pathology is termed *stroke*, which is defined as acute ischemic neurological damage caused by embolization or occlusion—*ischemic stroke*—or rupture of a cerebral vessel—*hemorrhagic stroke* (Warlow and colleagues, 2003). Some causes of stroke are shown in Table 55–2.

The Pregnancy Mortality Surveillance System, initiated in 1987 by the Centers for Disease Control and Prevention (2003) to monitor maternal deaths in all 50 states, reported that stroke caused 5 percent of maternal deaths from 1991 to 1999 and accounted for approximately 23 deaths per year. Analyses of several large data bases in the United States have shown that there are approximately 13 to 18 cases of stroke per 100,000 deliveries (Lanska and Kryscio, 1998, 2000). In Toronto, Jaigobin and Silver (2000) identified 34 cases of stroke among 50,700 women delivered at one hospital—an incidence of 67 per 100,000. In another study that included more than 1.4 million deliveries, the co-variates most significantly associated with peripartum stroke included cesarean delivery; hypertension; and fluid, electrolyte, and acid–base disorders (Lanska and Kryscio, 2000). In a population-based cohort of more than 1 million Swedish pregnant women, severe preeclampsia was associated with a sixfold increased risk of stroke, and there was almost a 100-fold risk of stroke around the time of delivery (Ros and associates, 2002).

The postpartum period is the time of greatest risk, especially for hemorrhagic stroke. Kittner and colleagues (1996) reviewed the records of all women from 15 to 44 years of age in the Central Maryland and Washington, D.C., area who were diagnosed with stroke between 1988 and 1991. Among 254 cases, 31 were associated with pregnancy. The relative risk of stroke was 0.7 during pregnancy but increased to 8.7 postpartum. The relative risk of intracerebral hemorrhage was 2.5 during pregnancy and increased to 28-fold postpartum.

Ischemic Stroke. These may result from thrombosis or thromboembolism of an artery or from venous thrombosis.

CEREBRAL ARTERY THROMBOSIS. The vast majority of thrombotic strokes are caused by atherosclerosis and thus typically affect older individuals. The internal carotid artery is the most commonly affected site, and the majority of cases are preceded by one or more transient ischemic attacks. At the time of stroke, a patient may present with sudden onset of severe headache, hemiplegia or other neurological deficits, or seizures. A thorough evaluation should be performed, including serum lipid profile, echocardiography, and cranial CT or angiography as necessary. The patient should also be evaluated for antiphospholipid antibody syndrome (see Chap. 54, p. 1215). Cerebral thrombosis and other thrombotic complications develop more frequently in women who have antiphospholipid antibodies. These may cause as many as a third of ischemic strokes in otherwise healthy patients younger than 50 years (Branch, 1990).

Therapy for thrombotic stroke includes rest, analgesia, and aspirin. Although there is evidence that prompt treatment with low-molecular-weight heparin or recombinant tissue plasminogen activator (t-PA or alteplase) may improve outcome with acute ischemic stroke, this is not without risk (Warlow and colleagues, 2003). To be effective, t-PA must be administered without delay, and this can result in it being given before radiological evaluation confirms arterial occlusion. Caplan and colleagues (1997) estimated that among every 100 patients who are eligible for thrombolysis according to current guidelines, 25 or more do not have arterial occlusions. These individuals have a 5- to 10-percent risk of intracerebral hemorrhage from the therapy.

The recurrence risk for ischemic stroke in association with pregnancy is low, unless a specific, persistent cause is identified. Lamy and colleagues (2000) studied 489 consecutive women of reproductive age with stroke, of which 373 were ischemic. There were 37 women with an ischemic stroke during pregnancy or the puerperium, and none of their 24 subsequent pregnancies was complicated by recurrent stroke. In another report by Coppage and associates (2004), 23 women with strokes before pregnancy due to a variety of causes had 35 subsequent pregnancies without a recurrent stroke. In the report from the Antiphospholipid Antibodies and Stroke Study Investigators (APASS Investigators, 2004), there was no difference in the risk of recurrent ischemic stroke in 1770 nonpregnant patients with or without anticardiolipin or antiphospholipid antibodies if preventative treatment was given with warfarin or aspirin.

CEREBRAL EMBOLISM. This usually involves the middle cerebral artery and is more common during the latter half of pregnancy or early puerperium (Lynch and Nelson, 2001). The diagnosis can be made with confidence only after thrombosis and hemorrhage have been excluded, which may be difficult. Because cerebral artery embolization and thrombosis are both followed by infarction, they can be difficult to distinguish. The diagnosis of thromboembolism is more certain if an embolic source is identified. The most common origin of emboli is a cardiac arrhythmia, especially atrial fibrillation associated with rheumatic valvular disease. Emboli also may arise from rheumatic heart disease without arrhythmia or from mitral valve prolapse. Finally, emboli from infective endocarditis must be considered (Cox and associates, 1988). Management of embolic stroke consists of supportive measures and consideration of anticoagulation.

CEREBRAL VENOUS THROMBOSIS. Lateral or superior sagittal venous sinus thrombosis usually occurs in the puerperium, and often in association with preeclampsia, sepsis, or thrombophilias. Venous thrombosis is more common in patients with inherited thrombophilias, lupus anticoagulant, or antiphospholipid antibodies (see Chap. 54, p. 1215). It has also been reported in association with thyrotoxicosis (Ra and co-workers, 2001).

Cerebral venous thrombosis is rare in developed countries, with reported incidences ranging from 1 in 11,000 to 1 in 45,000 (Cross, 1968; Lanska and Kryscio, 1997; Simolke, 1991, and all their colleagues). In contrast, because of the link with sepsis and preeclampsia, cerebral venous thrombosis remains common in undeveloped countries. Srinivasan (1984) reported its incidence in Madurai, India, to be 1 in 250 deliveries.

Headache is the most common presenting symptom (73 percent) and 10 percent of these women have convulsions (Cantú and Barinagarrementeria, 1993). MRI is the procedure of choice (Cartlidge, 2000). Management includes anticonvulsants to control seizures and antimicrobials if septic thrombophlebitis is suspected. Heparin anticoagulation is controversial, because spontaneous bleeding may develop. Donaldson and Lee (1994) recommend that the consequences of heparin be risked, especially if there is no hemorrhagic infarction demonstrated by tomography. In a small randomized study, Einhäupl and associates (1991) described improved outcomes in nonpregnant patients given heparin therapy. In all cases the prognosis is guarded, but survivors can expect to have a recurrence rate of only 1 to 2 percent, including during subsequent pregnancy (Mehraein and colleagues, 2003; Pathan and Kittner, 2003; Preter and co-workers, 1996).

Hemorrhagic Stroke. Two distinct categories of hemorrhagic stroke are recognized.

INTRACEREBRAL HEMORRHAGE. Bleeding into the substance of the brain most commonly is caused by spontaneous rupture of small vessels damaged by chronic hypertension (Qureshi and colleagues, 2001; Takebayashi and Kaneko, 1983).

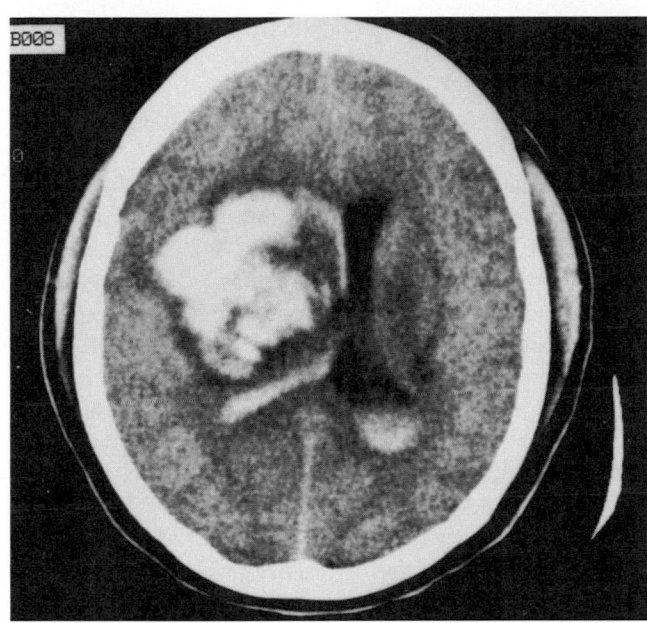

FIGURE 55–1. Cranial computed tomography showing a massive, ultimately fatal, right-sided intracerebral hemorrhage with associated contralateral hydrocephaly. The 23-year-old primigravid woman refused hospitalization for gestational hypertension, and she next was seen comatose with blood pressures as high as 260/160 mm Hg.

In pregnancy, there often is hypertension with superimposed preeclampsia, or occasionally pure preeclampsia (Fig. 55–1). Hemorrhage can also be precipitated by crack cocaine abuse (Witlin and associates, 2000). Intracerebral hemorrhage has a higher mortality rate than subarachnoid hemorrhage because of its location (Cartlidge, 2000). In the series reported by Jaigobin and Silver (2000), 3 of 13 pregnant women with hemorrhagic stroke died. These experiences underscore the importance of proper management for acute hypertension to prevent cerebrovascular pathology (see Chap. 34, p. 776).

SUBARACHNOID HEMORRHAGE. These bleeds are more likely caused by an underlying cerebrovascular malformation in an otherwise normal patient. Ruptured aneurysms cause 80 percent of all subarachnoid hemorrhages, and ruptured arteriovenous malformations (AVMs), coagulopathies, angiopathies, venous thromboses, infections, drug abuse, tumors, and trauma cause the remainder. Rupture of a cerebral aneurysm or angioma or bleeding from an AVM occurs in 1 in 75,000 pregnancies. This incidence does not differ from that in the general nonobstetrical population, but the mortality rate during pregnancy is reported to be as high as 35 percent (Dias and Sekhar, 1990; Minielly and associates, 1979). Case-control studies from Japan and New Zealand found that nulligravidity significantly increased the risk of subarachnoid hemorrhage (Mhurchu and co-workers, 2001; Okamoto and colleagues, 2001).

Intracerebral Aneurysm. According to Bendok and colleagues (1998), ruptured intracerebral aneurysms cause 25

percent of all cerebrovascular deaths and 8 percent of all strokes. During pregnancy, bleeding from aneurysms is three times more common than bleeding from AVMs (Dias and Sekhar, 1990). Although aneurysms are more likely to bleed during the second half of pregnancy, about 20 percent bleed during the first half (Dias and Sekhar, 1990). As in the nonpregnant population, most aneurysms identified during pregnancy are in the circle of Willis and 20 percent are multiple (Stoodley and co-workers, 1998). The cardinal symptom is sudden severe headache, accompanied by visual changes, cranial nerve abnormalities, focal neurological deficits, or altered consciousness. Patients typically have signs of meningeal irritation, tachycardia, hypertension, low-grade fever, leukocytosis, and proteinuria.

Prompt diagnosis and treatment may prevent potentially lethal complications. Noncontrast CT of the head is the preferred test initially, because MRI may not show the changes of acute hemorrhage until several hours into its evolution (Warlow and colleagues, 2003). If the CT scan is normal but the clinical picture strongly suggests subarachnoid hemorrhage, the cerebrospinal fluid should be examined to confirm the presence of blood. If found, angiography is done to locate the lesion (Roman and associates, 2004).

Treatment includes bed rest, analgesia, and sedation, with neurological monitoring and strict control of blood pressure, usually best accomplished in an intensive care unit. The decision to attempt repair of a potentially accessible aneurysm during pregnancy depends in part on the risk of recurrent hemorrhage and the risks of surgery. With conservative treatment only, the risk of subsequent bleeding from the aneurysm is 20 to 30 percent for the first month and then 3 percent per year. Recurrent hemorrhage leads to death in 70 percent of these patients (Bendok and colleagues, 1998). Surgical excision may be recommended for accessible aneurysms. For women near term, cesarean delivery followed by craniotomy is a consideration. If neurosurgery is performed remote from term, fetal conditions should be optimized. Although fetuses generally tolerate hypothermia well, hypotension is problematic and should be avoided. There appears to be no advantage to pregnancy termination unless there is associated preeclampsia.

Some authorities allow vaginal delivery if labor occurs at least at 2 months after hemorrhage and subsequent repair of an aneurysm. A major obstetrical problem concerns the management of delivery in women who survive subarachnoid hemorrhage, but in whom surgical repair is not done. Some authorities, but certainly not all, recommend against bearing down and thus favor cesarean delivery (Cartlidge, 2000). Others recommend cesarean delivery only if the aneurysm bled in the third trimester (Wiebers, 1988).

Arteriovenous Malformations. The incidence of bleeding from cerebral AVMs is not increased during pregnancy (Finnerty and co-workers, 1999). In a study from Parkland Hospital, Simolke and associates (1991) encountered only

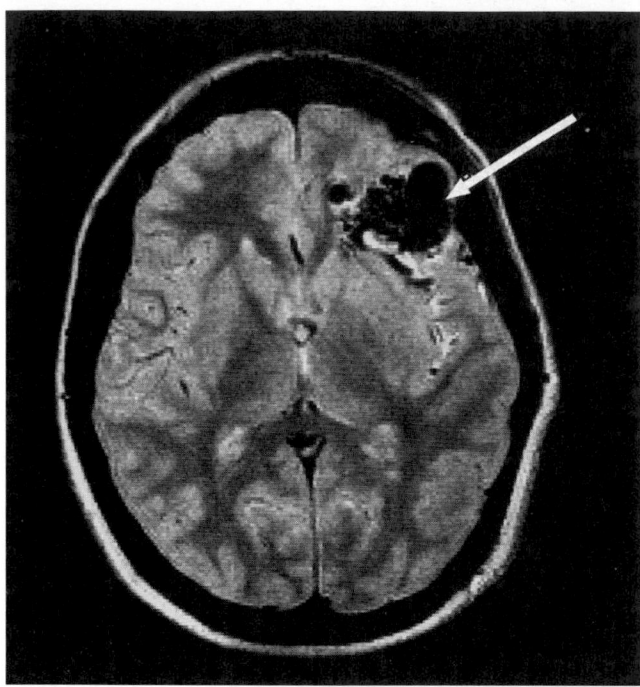

FIGURE 55–2. Magnetic resonance imaging of a left-sided frontal lobe atriovenous malformation. The lesion caused subarachnoid bleeding at 29 weeks in a 24-year-old primigravida who presented with severe headache, nausea, and vomiting. (From Simolke and colleagues, 1991, with permission.)

one case in nearly 90,000 deliveries (Fig. 55–2). Although some data suggest that AVMs bleed with similar frequency throughout gestation, Dias and Sekhar (1990) reported increased frequency with advancing gestational age. Data also show that the risk of bleeding from an AVM increases with maternal age (Karlsson and colleagues, 1997).

In nonpregnant patients, there is no consensus on whether all of these lesions should be resected, even when they are accessible. The risk of recurrent hemorrhage in unoperated lesions is high. Without surgery 5 to 7 percent will bleed again within the first year and 2 to 3 percent per year thereafter (Itoyama and associates, 1989). The mortality rate in nonpregnant patients is 10 percent after the first hemorrhage, 13 percent after the second hemorrhage, and approximately 20 percent after subsequent hemorrhages (Wilkins, 1985). The mortality rate is reported to be even higher during pregnancy. Indeed, 28 percent of pregnant women die after the first bleeding event (Dias and Sekhar, 1990).

The decision to operate should be based on neurosurgical considerations (Finnerty and associates, 1999). Because of the high risk of recurrent hemorrhage from an unresected or inoperable lesion, the route of delivery following a bleeding episode during pregnancy is critical. As for ruptured aneurysm, it seems best to avoid vaginal delivery if the malformation was not surgically excised.

DEMYELINATING OR DEGENERATIVE DISEASES.

Demyelinating diseases compose a group of neurological disorders that involve focal or patchy destruction of central nervous system myelin sheaths accompanied by an inflammatory response. The degenerative diseases are multifactorial and are characterized by progressive neuronal death.

Multiple Sclerosis. The yearly incidence of multiple sclerosis (MS) is 7 per 100,000, and the prevalence of MS is 120 per 100,000 (Compston and Coles, 2002). Because MS affects women twice as often as men and usually begins in the 20s and 30s, women of reproductive age are most susceptible. Susceptibility appears to be genetic. Most disease sufferers are of northern European descent, and the familial recurrence rate is 15 percent (Compston and Coles, 2002). The incidence of MS in offspring is increased 15-fold. Genes conferring susceptibility include the major histocompatibility complex and TNFα.

MS results from the autoimmune destruction of oligodendrocytes, the cells that synthesize myelin. It is theorized that this abnormal immune response is triggered in susceptible individuals by exposure to certain bacteria and viruses, possibly *Chlamydia pneumoniae,* human herpesvirus 6, or Epstein-Barr virus (Derfuss and colleagues, 2001; Levin and associates, 2003).

There are four forms of MS (Confavreux and colleagues, 2000; Lublin and Reingold, 1996). As many as 85 percent of affected individuals present with *relapsing-remitting MS,* characterized by unpredictable recurrent episodes of focal or multifocal neurological dysfunction followed by full recovery. Some relapses appear to be triggered by infection, and over time, relapses lead to persistent deficits. Eventually there is *secondary progression,* when the disease pursues a progressive downhill course after each relapse. A small number of patients present initially with *primary progressive MS,* which is characterized by gradual progression of disability from the time of initial diagnosis. *Progressive-relapsing MS* refers to primary progressive MS with apparent relapses.

Classic symptoms include loss of vision or diplopia, and more than 40 percent of patients have optic neuritis during the course of disease. In fact, 75 percent of women who are diagnosed with isolated optic neuritis develop multiple sclerosis within 15 years. Other common symptoms are dysarthria, muscle weakness, hyperreflexia, spasticity, paresthesia, ataxia and intention tremor, nystagmus, diminished vibratory sense, and bladder dysfunction. The diagnosis is one of exclusion and is confirmed by cerebrospinal fluid analysis and MRI. The characteristic multifocal white matter lesions, termed plaques, are present in more than 95 percent of patients and represent discrete areas of demyelination (Compston and Coles, 2002).

The goal of treatment is to arrest the disease and also to provide symptomatic relief. Several studies have shown that decreasing the amount of inflammation during the initial episode improves the disease course, in part by reducing the number and extent of white matter lesions. For example, weekly treatment with *interferon-β 1a* for 2 years significantly reduces progression of MS (Comi and colleagues, 2001). Because depression, thrombotic thrombocytopenic purpura, and various autoimmune reactions are side effects of treatment, patients receiving interferon should be closely monitored (Walther and Hohlfeld, 1999).

Natalizumab is an α_4-integrin antagonist that reduced the development of brain lesions and lowered the frequency of relapses in patients with relapsing MS during a 6-month trial (Miller and colleagues, 2003). Other medications used to diminish inflammation include *glatiramer acetate*, a mixture of synthetic polypeptides that interferes with T-cell function; *azathioprine*, which inhibits lymphocyte proliferation; and *mitoxantrone*, which prevents DNA synthesis and repair in rapidly dividing cells (Edan, 1997; Johnson, 1995; Palace, 1997, and all their co-workers). Data concerning the safety of these drugs in pregnancy are limited, but none of the drugs appears to be teratogenic (Reprotox, 2002).

Corticosteroids may diminish the severity of acute flares, but they have no effect on permanent disability. Although several investigators have found positive effects with the use of intravenous immunoglobulin for the treatment of relapsing-remitting MS, Hommes and associates (2004) found no clinical benefit in patients with secondary progressive MS. Symptomatic relief can be provided by analgesics; carbamazepine, phenytoin, or amitriptyline for neurogenic pain; baclofen for spasticity; α_2-adrenergic blockade to relax the bladder neck; and cholinergic and anticholinergic drugs to stimulate or inhibit bladder contractions.

EFFECTS OF PREGNANCY. Pregnancy appears neither to precipitate MS nor, in most cases, to have a deleterious effect on its course. Several studies indicate that women who have been pregnant have less deterioration than those who have not (Damek and Shuster, 1997). Acute exacerbation of MS during the first few months postpartum is common, possibly because of the reversal of the relative immune suppression of pregnancy (Cartlidge, 2000; Schneider and associates, 1996). In a review of eight observational studies of more than 1000 pregnancies, Abramsky (1994) found that the disease worsened during pregnancy in only 10 percent of women, but relapsed in a third in the puerperium. Roullet and colleagues (1993) reported a 43 percent postpartum exacerbation rate. Conversely, Sadovnick and co-workers (1994) found that postpartum relapses were no more common than in nonpregnant controls.

Uncomplicated MS usually has no adverse effects on pregnancy outcome. Women may become fatigued more easily, and those with bladder dysfunction are prone to urinary infection. Labor is unaffected, and the indications for cesarean delivery are obstetrical. Women with spinal lesions at or above T6 are at risk for autonomic dysreflexia (see p. 1240). Because of this, epidural analgesia is recommended (Weinreb, 1994). The incidence of postpartum exacerbation is not altered by epidural analgesia (Bader, 1994).

Postpartum exacerbations may prevent women from breast feeding. These may also inhibit the ability to provide general newborn care, and the need for assistance during this period should be anticipated (Nelson and colleagues, 1988).

Huntington Disease. This degenerative disease of the cerebral cortex and basal ganglia is characterized by a combination of choreoathetotic movements and progressive dementia. Because the mean age of onset is 40 years, Huntington disease rarely complicates pregnancy. It is inherited as an autosomal dominant trait, and prenatal diagnosis is now possible (see Chap. 12, p. 299). Prenatal screening is controversial because pregnancy termination is rarely considered for a late-onset adult disease.

MYASTHENIA GRAVIS. This immune-mediated neuromuscular disorder affects about 1 in 10,000 persons and has a predilection for women of childbearing age. The etiology is unknown, but genetic factors likely play a role; for example, it is more common in those with the HLA-B8 antigen. The pathological basis of the disease is IgG-mediated destruction of postsynaptic striated muscle acetylcholine receptors. Without adequate receptors, acetylcholine produces diminished end plate action potentials that inconsistently trigger muscle action potentials, resulting in weakened muscle contractions. Accordingly, myasthenia gravis is characterized by easy fatigability of facial, oropharyngeal, extraocular, and limb muscles. Cranial muscles are involved early and disparately, and diplopia and ptosis are common. Facial muscle weakness causes difficulty in smiling, chewing, and speaking. In 85 percent of patients, the weakness becomes generalized.

The disease course is marked by exacerbations and remissions, especially when it first becomes clinically apparent. Unfortunately, remissions are not always complete and are seldom permanent. Systemic diseases, concurrent infections, and even emotional upset may precipitate exacerbations or crises, of which there are three types: *myasthenic crises,* characterized by severe muscle weakness, inability to swallow, and respiratory muscle paralysis; *refractory crises,* characterized by the same symptoms but unresponsive to the usual therapy; and *cholinergic crises,* in which excessive cholinergic medication leads to nausea, vomiting, muscle weakness, abdominal pain, and diarrhea. All three can be life threatening, but a refractory crisis is a medical emergency. Women with bulbar myasthenia are at particular risk during a crisis because they may be unable to swallow or even ask for help.

Myasthenia is manageable but not curable. About 75 percent of patients have thymic hyperplasia or a thymoma, and some patients, especially young women, respond to thymectomy with remission (Cartlidge, 2000). Anticholinesterase medications such as *pyridostigmine*, an analogue of neostigmine, bring about improvement by impeding degradation of acetylcholine but seldom produce normal muscle function. Ironically, the side effects of overdose are increased weakness, which is sometimes difficult to differentiate from myasthenic symptoms. Nearly all patients respond to immunosuppressive therapy with corticosteroids, azathioprine, and cyclosporine (Cartlidge, 2000). Cyclophosphamide is used for refractory cases. Short-term clinical improvement has been reported following intravenously administered immunoglobulin or plasmapheresis.

Effects of Pregnancy. Because the greatest period of risk is within the first year following diagnosis, it is preferable to postpone pregnancy until there is sustained symptomatic improvement (Cartlidge, 2000). Antepartum management includes close observation with liberal bed rest and prompt treatment of any infections. Most patients respond well to pyridostigmine administered every 3 to 4 hours. Those in remission who become pregnant while taking corticosteroids or azathioprine should continue these. Acute onset of myasthenia or its exacerbation demands prompt hospitalization and supportive care. *Plasmapheresis* should be used for emergency situations, taking care not to provoke maternal hypotension or hypovolemia (Drachman, 1994). *Thymectomy* has been performed during pregnancy in cases refractory to medical management (Ip and colleagues, 1986).

Pregnancy does not appear to affect the course of myasthenia gravis. The enlarging uterus may compromise respiration, and the fatigue common to most pregnancies may be tolerated poorly. The disease course during pregnancy is unpredictable. In two observational studies of 123 women, about 20 percent worsened during pregnancy (Batocchi and associates, 1999; Djelmis and co-workers, 2002). Maternal deaths are usually due to complications of myasthenia or its treatment (Plauché, 1991).

Myasthenia gravis does not affect smooth muscle, and most women with the disease have normal labor, which they tolerate well. Oxytocin can be administered as necessary. Close observation and prompt respiratory support are essential. Narcotics must be used with care to avoid respiratory depression. In addition, any drug with a curare-like effect must be avoided; examples include magnesium sulfate, muscle relaxants used with general anesthesia, and aminoglycoside antimicrobials. Amide-type local anesthetic agents should be used for epidural analgesia for labor (Bader, 1994). Cesarean delivery is for obstetrical indications, and regional analgesia is preferred unless there is significant bulbar involvement or respiratory compromise. During second-stage labor, some women may have impairment of voluntary expulsive efforts, and forceps delivery may be necessary.

Neonatal Effects. In most patients with myasthenia, acetylcholine-receptor IgG antibodies have been detected, which can cross the placenta and affect the fetus. About 10 to 20 percent of exposed neonates develop symptoms, and in most of these, antibodies are detected (Batocchi and associates, 1999). Neonatal symptoms are most likely if the mother produces autoantibodies directed against embryonic rather than adult acetylcholine receptors (Vernet-der Garabe-

dian and colleagues, 1994). Transient symptomatic myasthenia gravis in an affected neonate typically results in a feeble cry, poor suckling, and respiratory distress. All of these can be corrected by parenteral neostigmine or small doses of edrophonium. Although symptoms usually resolve within 2 to 6 weeks as the antibodies are cleared, the perinatal death rate among neonates of mothers with myasthenia was considerably higher (68 per 1000) than the background rate (Plauché, 1991).

NEUROPATHIES. Peripheral neuropathy is a general term used to describe a disorder of peripheral nerve(s). Because neuropathy can result from a variety of causes, its discovery should prompt a search for an etiology. Polyneuropathies are often associated with systemic diseases such as diabetes, with drug or environmental toxin exposure, or with genetic diseases. Mononeuropathies signify focal involvement of a single nerve trunk and imply local causation such as trauma, compression, or entrapment (England and Asbury, 2004).

Guillain–Barré Syndrome. This syndrome is an acute demyelinating polyradiculoneuropathy. In more than 67 percent of cases of Guillain–Barré syndrome, there is clinical or serological evidence of a viral infection, such as cytomegalovirus or Epstein-Barr virus. Approximately 10 percent of cases develop within weeks following a surgical procedure (Kuwabara, 2004). In 1977, an outbreak of the disease occurred following immunization against swine influenza. The syndrome is thought to be immune-mediated, but its pathogenesis is unclear. The main pathological finding is a primary T-cell lymphocytic infiltration of cranial nerves, ventral and dorsal roots, dorsal root ganglia, peripheral nerves, lymph nodes, liver, heart, spleen, and other organs, apparently occurring aberrantly in response to a precipitating infection (Ropper, 1992).

Clinical features include areflexic paralysis with mild sensory disturbances and at times, evidence of autonomic dysfunction. The full syndrome develops after 1 to 3 weeks. Management is supportive, but patients should be hospitalized because about 25 percent need ventilatory assistance and the mortality rate for this complication is high. Corticosteroids have not been effective, although plasmapheresis or intravenous high-dose immunoglobulin (0.4 g/kg per day for 5 days) has been shown to be beneficial if begun within 1 to 2 weeks of symptom onset (van der Meché and colleagues, 1992). Almost 85 percent of patients recover fully, but about 3 percent die from complications of the acute condition.

EFFECTS OF PREGNANCY. Pregnancy does not appear to increase the incidence of Guillain–Barré syndrome. It is, however, increased threefold postpartum, with the first 2 weeks being a time of particularly increased risk (Cheng and co-workers, 1998). When the syndrome does develop during pregnancy, the course of the disease does not seem to be changed. After an insidious onset, paresis and paralysis most often continue to ascend, and respiratory insufficiency can then become a common and serious problem. In a series reported by Hurley and colleagues (1991), about a third of affected pregnant women ultimately required ventilatory support, and the overall maternal mortality rate was 13 percent. Kuller and associates (1995) and Rockel and co-workers (1994) described successful outcomes in pregnant women in whom plasmapheresis was performed. High-dose immunoglobulin may also be administered safely in pregnancy (Chan and colleagues, 2004).

Bell Palsy. This acute idiopathic peripheral facial paralysis of unknown etiology is relatively common, especially in women of reproductive age. Women are affected two to four times more often than men of the same age, and pregnant women are affected three to four times more often than nonpregnant women (Cohen and colleagues, 2000). The onset is usually abrupt and painful, with maximum weakness within 48 hours. In some cases, hyperacusis and loss of taste accompany varying degrees of facial muscle paralysis.

Increased extracellular fluid, viral inflammation, and the relative immune suppression of pregnancy are thought to be predisposing factors. In addition, many cases are associated with or herald the development of preeclampsia (Shapiro and associates, 1999). One study described the experience of five Canadian centers during 11 years and found that women who developed Bell palsy had an incidence of preeclampsia or pregnancy-induced hypertension fivefold higher than the national average (Shmorgun and colleagues, 2002).

EFFECTS OF PREGNANCY. It is not known if pregnancy alters the prognosis for spontaneous recovery from Bell palsy. Gillman and colleagues (2002) found that only 50 percent of pregnant women recovered to a satisfactory level after 1 year, compared with about 80 percent of nonpregnant women and men. Bilateral disease and recurrence in a subsequent pregnancy are prognostic markers for incomplete recovery (Cohen and associates, 2000). Electroneurography may also be helpful in determining prognosis. It is best used in those with complete paralysis and performed after the third day of loss but within the first 2 weeks. A greater percentage of nerve function loss and faster rate of loss predict a worse prognosis (Gilden, 2004).

No specific treatment improves prognosis (Peitersen, 2002). The bulk of evidence suggests that corticosteroids do not hasten resolution, and surgical decompression is seldom indicated. Supportive care includes prevention of injury to the constantly exposed cornea, facial muscle massage, and reassurance. Regional analgesia does not exacerbate the neuropathy (Dorsey and Camann, 1993).

Carpal Tunnel Syndrome. Characteristics of this syndrome include burning, numbness, or tingling in the inner half of one or both hands, and wrist pain and numbness extending into the forearm and sometimes into the shoulder. A variety of conditions, including pregnancy, are associated with it. It is caused by increased pressure in the carpal tunnel, leading to ischemia of the median or (less frequently) ulnar nerves (Katz and Simmons, 2002). Seror (1998) reported that 67 percent of pregnant women with carpal tunnel syndrome had evidence of an acute median nerve lesion at the wrist with a motor or sensory conduction block (or both) and that approximately 10 percent had signs of severe denervation. Symptoms are bilateral in 80 percent of cases and often exhibit a diurnal pattern (Seror, 1998).

Carpal tunnel syndrome should be distinguished from De Quervain tendonitis, which is caused by swelling of the conjoined tendons and sheaths near the distal radius. Nerve conduction studies may be helpful in distinguishing these entities.

The incidence of carpal tunnel syndrome seems to vary according to how vigilantly the diagnosis is sought. Researchers in one large Italian study determined the incidence of carpal tunnel syndrome during the third trimester of pregnancy, when tissue edema is greatest. They found that carpal tunnel syndrome was diagnosed clinically in more than 50 percent and confirmed by neurophysiological evaluation in 42 percent (Padua and colleagues, 2001). In a follow-up study by the same group, 54 percent of women who experienced carpal tunnel syndrome during pregnancy still had some symptoms 1 year later (Padua and co-workers, 2002). In contrast, Stolp-Smith and colleagues (1998) made the diagnosis in fewer than 1 percent of nearly 11,000 pregnant women and found that virtually all cases resolved satisfactorily after pregnancy.

Carpal tunnel syndrome is usually self-limited, and in most cases symptomatic treatment is sufficient. A splint applied to a slightly flexed wrist and worn during sleep keeps the carpal bones in the optimal position to relieve pressure on the nerves and thus provides relief for the majority of sufferers (Courts, 1995). Most symptoms regress after delivery, although surgical decompression and corticosteroid injections may become necessary (Dammers and associates, 1999; Gerritsen and co-workers, 2002). In rare instances, symptoms persist or recur long after pregnancy, and surgical release is required (al Qattan and colleagues, 1994).

SPINAL CORD INJURY. Of the 11,000 spinal cord injuries each year, at least 50 percent are in patients of reproductive age, and 18 percent of these are women (American College of Obstetricians and Gynecologists, 2002b). Fertility is not impaired, and in a survey of 472 women of reproductive age with spinal cord injury, Jackson and Wadley (1999) found that approximately 67 percent resumed intercourse after the injury, and almost 14 percent became pregnant.

Women with spinal cord injury have lower-birthweight neonates and experience more pregnancy complications than unaffected women. The majority of women have either asymptomatic bacteriuria or symptomatic urinary infection. Serum creatinine levels are used to detect renal compromise caused by repeated infection and in predicting pregnancy outcome (see Chap. 7, p. 197). Significant bowel dysfunction and aggravation of constipation develop in more than half of women. Anemia and pressure necrosis of the skin are also common (Baker and associates, 1992; Glickman and Kamm, 1996).

Two serious and life-threatening complications can develop. If the spine is transected above T10, the cough reflex is impaired, and respiratory function may be compromised. Pulmonary function tests may be indicated, and some women with high lesions may need ventilatory support in late pregnancy or in labor. In women with lesions above T5–T6, *autonomic dysreflexia* can develop. With this complication, stimuli from structures innervated below the level of the lesion—usually the bowel, bladder, or uterus—lead to massive disordered sympathetic stimulation. Vasoconstriction and sudden catecholamine release follow with severe hypertension and a range of symptoms, including a throbbing headache, facial flushing, sweating, bradycardia, tachycardia, arrhythmia, and respiratory distress. Dysreflexia can be precipitated by a variety of stimuli, including urethral, bladder, rectal, or cervical distention; catheterization; cervical dilatation; uterine contractions; or manipulation of pelvic structures (American College of Obstetricians and Gynecologists, 2002b). In a report by Westgren and colleagues (1993), 12 of 15 women at risk for dysreflexia suffered at least one episode during pregnancy.

Spinal or epidural analgesia extending to T10 prevents dysreflexia and should be instituted at the start of labor. If severe symptoms present before the epidural has been placed, the first step is to stop whatever stimulus provoked the episode. Then an antihypertensive agent or a peripheral vasodilator should be given.

Uterine contractions are not affected by cord lesions, and labor is usually easy, even precipitous, and comparatively painless. If the lesion is below T12, uterine contractions are felt normally. For lesions above T12, the risk of delivery at home can be minimized by teaching women to palpate for uterine contractions. Some practitioners recommend tocodynamometry and weekly cervical examinations beginning at about 28 weeks. Hughes and associates (1991) recommend elective hospitalization between 36 and 37 weeks. Up to 20 percent of women deliver preterm (Westgren and co-workers, 1993).

Vaginal delivery is preferred, with epidural or spinal analgesia used to minimize autonomic dysreflexia. Prolonged second-stage labor may be expedited with forceps or vacuum.

SHUNTS FOR MATERNAL HYDROCEPHALUS.

Pregnancies in women with ventriculoperitoneal, ventriculoatrial, or ventriculopleural shunts for hydrocephalus have been described, and outcomes have usually been satisfactory (Landwehr and colleagues, 1994). In some cases, the shunts become obstructed typically late in pregnancy. Wisoff and associates (1991) reported that neurological complications developed in 13 of 17 pregnancies in women with preexisting shunts, including headaches (60 percent), nausea and

vomiting (35 percent), lethargy (30 percent), ataxia (20 percent), and gaze paresis (20 percent). Most responded to conservative management. If CT discloses acute hydrocephaly, the shunt can be tapped or pumped several times daily. However, surgical revision is sometimes necessary.

Vaginal delivery is preferred, and unless there is a meningomyelocele, epidural analgesia is permitted (Bader, 1994). Some authorities believe that subarachnoid block is contraindicated, but others support its use (Littleford and colleagues, 1999). Antimicrobial prophylaxis is indicated if the peritoneal cavity is entered for cesarean delivery or tubal sterilization.

BRAIN DEATH. Cases of maternal brain death during pregnancy have been described in which life-support systems and parenteral alimentation were used for extended periods of time while the fetus achieved maturity (Bernstein, 1989; Dillon, 1982; Field, 1988, and all their co-workers). Aggressive tocolysis and antimicrobial therapy also have been used (Catanzarite and colleagues, 1997). Although not always successful, such therapy occasionally is attempted (Feldman and colleagues, 2000). The ethical, financial, and legal implications, both civil and criminal, that arise from attempting or not attempting such care are profound.

BENIGN INTRACRANIAL HYPERTENSION (PSEUDOTUMOR CEREBRI). This condition is characterized by increased intracranial pressure without hydrocephalus, possibly as the result of either overproduction or underabsorption of cerebrospinal fluid. Symptoms include headache in at least 90 percent of cases and visual disturbance, such as loss of a visual field or central visual acuity, in 70 percent (Evans and Friedman, 2000). Other complaints are stiff neck, back pain, pulsatile tinnitus, facial palsy, ataxia, or paresthesias. The syndrome is commonly found in young women, especially those who are obese or who recently have gained weight. Criteria for diagnosis include elevated cerebrospinal fluid pressure and normal composition, along with normal cranial CT or MRI findings. Cerebrospinal fluid prolactin concentration usually is significantly increased even in men and nonpregnant women (Bates and associates, 1982).

Benign intracranial hypertension is usually self-limited. If needed, treatment aims to prevent visual defects by lowering the elevated pressure. Repeated lumbar punctures to remove cerebrospinal fluid lower pressure and can be performed safely without brainstem herniation if there is no ventriculomegaly. Drugs given during pregnancy to lower pressure include acetazolamide, furosemide, or dexamethasone. In rare cases, lumboperitoneal shunting of spinal fluid is necessary.

Effects of Pregnancy. Benign intracranial hypertension is probably not more prevalent during pregnancy. Pregnancy, however, may be coincident with the new onset of symptoms, and women who already have the diagnosis may become symptomatic during pregnancy (Huna-Baron and

Kupersmith, 2002). It is usually detected by midpregnancy, is self-limited, and resolves postpartum.

Pregnancy does not alter treatment. Medication as described above, repeated lumbar punctures, and a salt-restricted diet are generally successful in reducing symptoms. Lumboperitoneal shunting is also an option (Landwehr and colleagues, 1994). Some authorities have recommended that these women be followed with serial visual field testing during pregnancy because visual loss can become permanent (Evans and Friedman, 2000). Huna-Baron and Kupersmith (2002) followed 16 pregnancies in 240 women with benign intracranial hypertension. Visual field loss occurred in four women and was permanent in one. Visual field loss is often coincident with the development of papilledema.

Pregnancy complications are likely due to the associated obesity, not to pseudotumor. In their review of 54 pregnancies, Katz and associates (1989) did not report increased adverse perinatal outcomes. Labor is permitted, the route of delivery is decided by obstetrical indications, and epidural analgesia is not contraindicated.

CHOREA GRAVIDARUM. Involuntary writhing of the limbs or facial muscles, called chorea, may develop during pregnancy and is known as chorea gravidarum (Golbe, 1994). Because most cases in the past were linked to rheumatic fever, chorea is now rare. It can still develop in association with streptococcus A infection, but more often may be caused by collagen-vascular disease (Prasher and Barrett, 1993). According to Branch (1990), up to 2 percent of patients with systemic lupus erythematosus exhibit chorea, and most of these have antiphospholipid antibodies (see Chap. 54, p. 1215). Omdal and Roalsø (1992) described a woman with chorea gravidarum who had a recurrence while taking steroidal contraceptives 20 years later.

PSYCHIATRIC DISORDERS

Pregnancy and the puerperium are at times sufficiently stressful to provoke mental illness. Such illness may represent recurrence or exacerbation of a preexisting psychiatric disorder, or may be the onset of a new disorder. In a Swedish population-based study, Andersson and associates (2003) found that the point prevalence of psychiatric disorders during pregnancy is 14 percent.

ADJUSTMENT TO PREGNANCY. Women respond in a variety of ways psychologically to the stressors of pregnancy. They may express persistent concerns about fetal health, postpartum child care and lifestyle changes, or fear of childbirth pain. Anxiety and functional impairment are common (Morewitz, 2003). The level of perceived stress is significantly higher for women whose fetus is at high risk for a congenital malformation and for those who have

medical and obstetrical complications (Josefsson and colleagues, 2002).

Because psychological stress often increases in the puerperium, this is a time of increased risk for mental illness. For example, 10 to 20 percent of women develop a nonpsychotic postpartum depressive disorder within 6 months of delivery (Josefsson and colleagues, 2002). Others have a severe, psychotic illness following delivery that usually is manic-depressive (Wisner and associates, 2002). Data of Evans and co-workers (2001) indicate that depressive disorders are just as common during pregnancy as in the puerperium.

PRENATAL EVALUATION. Many mental illnesses, especially depression, develop during the reproductive years. According to Andersson and associates (2003), the point prevalence of psychiatric disorders is 3.3 percent for major depression, 6.9 percent for minor depression, and 6.6 percent for anxiety disorders. Screening for mental illness is done during the first prenatal examination to ascertain psychiatric disorders, including hospitalizations, outpatient care, prior or current use of psychoactive medications, and current symptoms (Table 55–3).

Risk factors should be evaluated. A prior personal or family history of depression is a significant risk for recurrent depression. Women with a history of sexual abuse also are more likely to have depressive symptomatology, negative life events, and physical and verbal abuse before and during pregnancy (Benedict and co-workers, 1999). Substance abuse, violence, and depression are also linked (Horrigan and

TABLE 55–3 Helpful Questions in Assessing Depression

Depressed mood
- How has your mood been lately?

Loss of feelings of pleasure
- What have you enjoyed doing lately?
- Have you been getting less pleasure from the things you typically enjoy?

Physical symptoms
- How have you been sleeping?
- Has your appetite or your weight changed?
- How is your energy?
- Have you been feeling slowed down or agitated?

Psychological symptoms
- How is your concentration?
- Have you been feeling down on yourself?
- How does the future look to you?
- Do you ever feel like life is not worth living?

Effects of symptoms on function
- How are things at home and at work?
- How have (the symptoms) affected your home or work life?

From American College of Obstetricians and Gynecologists (2002a), with permission.

colleagues, 2000). Women who report one of these factors should be carefully monitored for evidence of the other two (see Chaps. 7, p. 193 and 42, p. 997). In addition, because eating disorders may be exacerbated by pregnancy, affected women should be followed closely.

CLASSIFICATION OF MENTAL DISORDERS. The Diagnostic and Statistical Manual (DSM-IV) is written and periodically updated by the American Psychiatric Association (1994). Its purpose is to assist in the classification of mental disorders, and it specifies criteria required for each diagnosis.

Major Mood Disorders. These include major depression—a unipolar disorder—and manic-depression—a bipolar disorder that includes both manic and depressive episodes.

MAJOR DEPRESSION. The National Mental Health Association (2004) estimates that each year 12 million women in the United States have a depressive disorder. The lifetime incidence is 12 percent. Even worse, only half ever seek care.

Major depression is multifactorial, prompted by both genetic and environmental factors. First-degree relatives of individuals with depression have a 25-percent risk of being similarly affected, and female relatives may be at even higher risk (Tsuang and Faraone, 1996). The families of affected individuals often include members with alcohol abuse and anxiety disorders, suggesting a link between these three diagnoses (Doris and associates, 1999). Provocative conditions leading to depression include life events that prompt grief reactions, substance abuse, use of certain medications, and other medical disorders. Although life events can trigger depression, genes influence the liability to life events, making the distinction between genetic and environmental factors difficult.

BIPOLAR DISORDER. Manic-depressive illness also has a strong genetic component. The risk that monozygotic twins are both affected is 40 to 70 percent, and the risk that first-degree relatives of individuals with manic-depression have a similar illness is 5 to 10 percent (Muller-Oerlinghausen and colleagues, 2002). Periods of depression last at least 2 weeks. In addition, affected individuals have manic episodes, defined as distinct periods during which there is an abnormally raised, expansive, or irritable mood. Potential causes of mania or manic symptoms include substance abuse such as cocaine, hyperthyroidism, and central nervous system tumors. About 10 to 20 percent of patients with manic-depression commit suicide, and major mood disorders as a group contribute to two thirds of all suicides in the United States.

Schizophrenia. This common major form of mental illness affects 1 percent of the population (Harvard Medical School, 1999a). Four major subtypes of schizophrenia are recognized: catatonic, disorganized, paranoid, and undifferentiated. The hallmarks of paranoid schizophrenia are delusions, hallucinations, flat or blunted affect, and confused or impoverished speech.

Research using brain scanning techniques such as positron emission tomography and functional magnetic resonance imaging have shown that schizophrenia is a degenerative brain disorder. Subtle anatomical brain abnormalities are present early in life and worsen with time. They include atrophy in and around the limbic region, thalamus, and cerebral cortex; abnormally low blood flow in the frontal lobes; and abnormal brain wave responses (Harvard Medical School, 1999b).

Schizophrenia has a major genetic component, with 50-percent concordance in monozygotic twins. If one parent has schizophrenia, the risk to offspring is 5 to 10 percent. Some data, including a strong association between schizophrenia and the velocardiofacial syndrome, suggest that genes influencing disease development are located on chromosome 22q11 (Murphy, 2002).

Signs of illness begin approximately at 20 years of age, and commonly, work and psychosocial functioning deteriorate over time. Because women have a slightly later onset than men and are less susceptible to autism and other neurodevelopmental abnormalities, many investigators theorize that estrogen has a protective effect. Affected women may marry and become pregnant before symptoms manifest. With appropriate treatment, patients may experience a decrease or cessation of symptoms. Within 5 years from the first signs of illness, 60 percent have social recovery, 50 percent are employed, 30 percent are mentally handicapped, and 10 percent require continued hospitalization (American Psychiatric Association, 1994).

Patients with *schizoaffective disorder* have a chronic deteriorating psychotic disorder similar to schizophrenia but combined with prominent mood symptoms. Although the psychosis rarely abates, the mood symptoms often improve with therapy.

Anxiety Disorders. Examples of these relatively common disorders include panic attack, panic disorder, social phobia, specific phobia, obsessive-compulsive disorder, posttraumatic stress disorder, and generalized anxiety disorder. All are characterized by irrational fear, tension, and worry, accompanied by physiological changes such as trembling, nausea, hot or cold flashes, dizziness, dyspnea, insomnia, and frequent urination (Mufson, 2002). These disorders are treated with psychotherapy and medication, including selective serotonin-reuptake inhibitors, tricyclic antidepressants, monoamine oxide inhibitors, and others.

Personality Disorders. These disorders are characterized by the chronic use of certain coping mechanisms in an inappropriate, stereotyped, and maladaptive manner. The American Psychiatric Association (1994) recognizes three clusters of personality disorders:

1. Paranoid, schizoid, and schizotypal personality disorders, which are characterized by oddness or eccentricity.
2. Histrionic, narcissistic, antisocial, and borderline disorders, which are all characterized by dramatic presentations along with self-centeredness and erratic behavior.
3. Avoidant, dependent, compulsive, and passive-aggressive personalities, which are characterized by underlying fear and anxiety.

Genetic and environmental factors are important in the genesis of these disorders, whose prevalence may be as high as 20 percent. Although management is through psychotherapy, the majority of affected individuals do not recognize that they have a problem and only about 20 percent seek help.

EFFECTS OF PREGNANCY ON MENTAL ILLNESS. It is likely that both biochemical factors and life stressors influence the onset of mental illness in pregnancy. Hormones are known to affect mood, as evidenced by premenstrual syndrome and menopausal depression. Estrogen modulates serotonergic function and has been used therapeutically to treat depression; it may be a factor in the mood elevation experienced by many women during pregnancy (Joffe and Cohen, 1998). Corticotropin-releasing hormone, which is usually elevated in pregnancy, is present at lower levels in women with pregnancy-related depression (Schmeelk and colleagues, 1999). The absolute hormone levels and their rate of change also appear to be influential. Women who experience postpartum depression often have higher predelivery estrogen and progesterone levels and experience a greater drop to lower levels postpartum (Ahokas and co-workers, 1999).

Pregnancy is also a major life stressor that can unmask or exacerbate depressive tendencies. Depression is more likely to occur with marital problems, unwanted pregnancy, a personal or family history of depression, and low socioeconomic status (Smith and colleagues, 2004). Depression may be linked to increased risk for preeclampsia (Dawes, 2005).

PREGNANCY OUTCOMES. There are only a few reports of psychiatric disorders and their effects on pregnancy outcomes. In a population-based, retrospective cohort analysis of over 500,000 California births in 1995, Kelly and colleagues (2002) assessed the perinatal effects of a maternal psychiatric diagnosis. The latter included all ICD-9-CM diagnostic codes recorded in the discharge summary. Women with these diagnoses had a 1.5- to 3-fold increased incidence of very-low- or low-birthweight neonates or preterm delivery. More specifically, conditions such as eating disorders may cause low-birthweight infants (Sollid and associates, 2004).

POSTPARTUM DISORDERS

Maternity Blues. Also called *postpartum blues*, this is a transient state of heightened emotional reactivity experienced by half of women within approximately the first week after parturition (Miller, 2002). The predominant mood is happiness, but they are more emotionally labile with insomnia, weepiness, depression, anxiety, poor concentration, irritability, and affective lability. They may be transiently tearful for several hours and then recover completely, only to be tearful again the next day. Symptoms are mild and usually last only between a few hours to a few days. Supportive treatment is indicated, and sufferers can be reassured that the dysphoria is transient and most likely due to biochemical changes. They should be monitored for development of more severe psychiatric disturbances, including postpartum disorders.

Postpartum Depression. In nearly all respects, postpartum depression is similar to other major and minor depressions. Symptoms must be present for most of the day, every day, for at least 2 weeks. Postpartum depression is defined as beginning within 4 weeks of delivery, although researchers often include cases that begin within 3 months.

According to the National Mental Health Association (2004), postpartum depression develops in 10 to 15 percent of women following delivery. This incidence is only slightly higher than the usual 6-month prevalence for depression among women in the general population. Postpartum depression has been associated with antenatal depression, young maternal age, single marital status, cigarette smoking or illegal drug use during pregnancy, hyperemesis gravidarum, high utilization of emergency services and sick leave during pregnancy, and previous affective disorder (Bryan, 1999; Evans, 2001; Josefsson, 2002, and all their colleagues).

Up to 70 percent of women with previous postpartum depression have a subsequent episode. Women with both a previous puerperal depression and a current episode of blues have their chances of developing a major depression increase to 85 percent (Hannah and associates, 1992).

COURSE. Without treatment, the natural course is one of gradual improvement in the 6 months after delivery (Fleming and colleagues, 1992). As the duration of depression increases, however, so do the number of sequelae and their severity. In addition, maternal depression during the first weeks and months after delivery can lead to insecure attachment and later behavioral problems in the child.

TREATMENT. Accordingly, most authorities recommend treatment with an antidepressant drug (Table 55–4). A selective serotonin-reuptake inhibitor should be tried initially. If depressive symptoms improve during a 6-week trial, the medication should be continued for a minimum of 6 months to prevent relapse (Wisner and associates, 2002). If the response is suboptimal or a relapse occurs, patients should be referred to a psychiatrist.

Recurrence of depression develops in 50 to 85 percent of women with an initial postpartum depression some time after medication is stopped. Women with a history of more

TABLE 55–4 Pharmacotherapy for Postpartum Depression

Drug	Dosage (mg/day)[a]	Use During Breast Feeding
Selective serotonin-reuptake inhibitors		
Sertraline	50–200	No reports of adverse events.
Paroxetine	20–60	No reports of adverse events.
Fluvoxamine	50–200	No reports of adverse events.
Citalopram	20–40	One infant with a measurable level had colic.
Fluoxetine	20–60	Drug and active metabolite have comparatively long half-lives; serum levels similar to those in adults reported in some symptomatic infants.
Tricyclic antidepressants		
Nortriptyline[b,c]	50–150	No reports of adverse events.
Desipramine[b,c]	100–300	No adverse effects.
Serotonin-norepinephrine reuptake inhibitor		
Venlafaxine	75–300	Undectable or low serum levels of drug; metabolite usually measurable and levels similar to those in adults observed in some infants; drug level greater in breast milk than in maternal serum.
Other		
Bupropion[b]	300–450	Unknown
Nefazodone	300–600	No published data on serum levels in infants; sedation and poor feeding in a premature infant described.
Mirtazapine	15–45	Unknown

[a] Treatment with any of these agents should be initiated at half of the lowest recommended therapeutic dose. Dosages are from the *Physician's Desk Reference*, 55th ed.
[b] Drug interactions are possible because of inhibition of the following cytochrome P450 (CYP) enzyme systems: sertraline, 2D6, 2C, and 3A4; paroxetine, nortriptyline, desipramine, and bupropion, 2D6; fluvoxamine, 1A2, 2C, and 3A4; fluoxetine, 2D6, 2C, and 3A4; and nefazodone, 3A4.
[c] If the electrocardiogram (ECG) shows conduction defects, consider a non–tricyclic antidepressant.

than one depressive episode are at greater risk for recurrence (American Psychiatric Association, 2000). Surveillance should also include monitoring for thoughts of suicide or infanticide, emergence of psychosis, and response to therapy. For some women, the course of illness is severe enough to warrant hospitalization.

Although some psychotropic medications pass into breast milk, in most cases the levels are very low or undetectable (see Chap. 14, p. 363). There have been no reports of adverse events in breast feeding mothers who took the drugs listed in Table 55–4. Therefore, most women so treated can breast feed, with close observation of the infant.

Postpartum Psychosis. The most severe puerperal mental disorder, this condition usually manifests within 2 weeks of delivery and is usually evidence of a bipolar disorder (Wisner and colleagues, 2002). Affected women have signs of confusion and disorientation but may also have episodes of lucidity. Women with preexisting psychotic illness are at highest risk, as well as those with prior episodes of postpartum depression. In one study, Marks and co-workers (1991) followed 88 women at high risk for psychiatric disorders. A fourth developed postpartum psychosis, either a bipolar or a schizoaffective disorder, and another fourth had a nonpsychotic postpartum depression.

Because women with underlying disease have a 10- to 15-fold risk for recurrence postpartum, close monitoring is imperative. In addition, postpartum psychosis has a high risk of recurrence in the next pregnancy. In most instances, these women ultimately develop relapsing, chronic psychotic illness.

The course of postpartum psychosis is variable and depends on the type of underlying illness. The clinical course of bipolar illness or schizoaffective disorder in puerperal women is comparable to that for nonpregnant women. They usually require hospitalization, pharmacological treatment, and long-term psychiatric care. Psychotic women may have delusions leading to thoughts of self-harm or harm to their infants. Unlike women with nonpsychotic depression, these women commit infanticide, albeit uncommonly.

TREATMENT OF MENTAL DISORDERS

Pharmacological Therapy. A large number of psychotropic medications are now available for management of mental disorders (Kuller and colleagues, 1996). Women taking psychotropic medication should also be informed of likely side effects at the start of therapy (see Chap. 14, p. 363). Dell and O'Brien (2003) advocate a risk-benefit model of drug selection that factors the health and well-being of both mother and fetus.

Electroconvulsive Therapy. Treatment of depression with electroconvulsive therapy (ECT) during pregnancy is occasionally necessary for women with major mood disorders unresponsive to pharmacological therapy. With proper preparation, the risks to both mother and fetus are few. Women undergoing ECT should be treated as if they have a full stomach. They should be given a rapid-acting antacid before the procedure, and the airway should be protected to decrease the likelihood of aspiration. A wedge should be placed under the right hip to prevent sudden maternal hypotension from aortocaval compression. Other important preparatory steps include cervical assessment, discontinuation of nonessential anticholinergic medication, uterine and fetal heart rate monitoring, and intravenous hydration. During the procedure, excessive hyperventilation should be avoided.

In most cases, maternal and fetal heart rate and maternal blood pressure and oxygen saturation remain normal throughout the procedure. Miller (1994) reviewed 300 published case reports of ECT during pregnancy and found that complications occurred in about 10 percent, including transient benign fetal arrhythmias, mild vaginal bleeding, abdominal pain, and self-limited uterine contractions. Women who were not adequately prepared had an increased risk of aspiration, aortocaval compression, and respiratory alkalosis.

REFERENCES

Abramsky O: Pregnancy and multiple sclerosis. Ann Neurol 36:S38, 1994

Ahokas A, Kaukoranta J, Aito M: Effect of oestradiol on postpartum depression. Psychopharmacology 146:108, 1999

al Qattan MM, Manktelow RT, Bowen CVA: Pregnancy induced carpal tunnel syndrome requiring surgical release longer than 2 years after delivery. Obstet Gynecol 84:249, 1994

American College of Obstetricians and Gynecologists: Depression in women. Clinical Updates in Women's Health Care, Vol I, No. 2, Spring 2002a

American College of Obstetricians and Gynecologists: Obstetric management of patients with spinal cord injuries. Committee Opinion No. 275, September 2002b

American College of Obstetricians and Gynecologists: Migraine and other headache disorders. Clinical Updates in Women's Health Care, Vol I, No. 3, Summer 2002c

American College of Obstetricians and Gynecologists: Precis IV. Fertility Control. Washington, DC: American College of Obstetricians and Gynecologists, 1990, p 8

American Psychiatric Association: Guidelines for the treatment of patients with major depressive disorder (Revision). Am J Psychiatry 157:1, 2000

American Psychiatric Association: The Diagnostic and Statistical Manual of Mental Disorders, 4th ed (DSM-IV). Washington, DC, 1994

Andersson L, Sundström-Poromaa I, Bixo M, et al: Point prevalence of psychiatric disorders during the second trimester of pregnancy: A population-based study. Am J Obstet Gynecol 189:148, 2003

APASS Investigators: Antiphospholipid antibodies and subsequent thrombo-occlusive events in patients with ischemic stroke. JAMA 291:576, 2004

Au KL, Woo JS, Wong VC: Intrauterine death from ergotamine overdosage. Eur J Obstet Gynecol Reprod Biol 19:313, 1985

Aube M: Migraine in pregnancy. Neurology 53:S26, 1999

Bader AM: Neurological and neuromuscular disease. In Chestnut DH (eds): Obstetric Anesthesia: Principles and Practice. St. Louis, Mosby, 1994, p 920

Baker ER, Cardenas DD, Benedetti TJ: Risks associated with pregnancy in spinal cord-injured women. Obstet Gynecol 80:428, 1992

Bates GW, Whitworth NS, Parker JL, et al: Elevated cerebrospinal fluid prolactin concentration in women with pseudotumor cerebri. South Med J 75:807, 1982

Batocchi AP, Majolini L, Evoli A, et al: Course and treatment of myasthenia gravis during pregnancy. Neurology 52:447, 1999

Bendok BR, Getch CC, Malisch TW, et al: Treatment of aneurismal subarachnoid hemorrhage. Semin Neurol 18:521, 1998

Benedict MI, Paine LL, Paine LA, et al: The association of childhood sexual abuse with depressive symptoms during pregnancy, and selected pregnancy outcomes. Child Abuse Negl 23:659, 1999

Bernstein IM, Watson M, Simmons GM, et al: Maternal brain death and prolonged fetal survival. Obstet Gynecol 74:434, 1989

Branch DW: Antiphospholipid antibodies and pregnancy: Maternal implications. Semin Perinatol 14:139, 1990

Brodie MJ, Dichter MA: Antiepileptic drugs. N Engl J Med 334:168, 1996

Bryan TL, Georgiopoulos AM, Harms RW, et al: Incidence of postpartum depression in Olmsted County, Minnesota. A population-based, retrospective study. J Reprod Med 44:352, 1999

Cantú C, Barinagarrementeria F: Cerebral venous thrombosis associated with pregnancy and puerperium. Stroke 24:1880, 1993

Caplan LR, Mohr JP, Kistler JP, et al: Should thrombolytic therapy be the first-line treatment for acute ischemic stroke? N Engl J Med 337:1309, 1997

Cartlidge NEF: Neurologic disorders. In Barron WM, Lindheimer MD (eds): Medical Disorders During Pregnancy, 3rd ed. St. Louis, Mosby, 2000, p 516

Catanzarite VA, Willms DC, Holdy KE, et al: Brain death during pregnancy: Tocolytic therapy and aggressive maternal support on behalf of the fetus. Am J Perinatol 14:431, 1997

Centers for Disease Control and Prevention: Pregnancy-related mortality surveillance—United States, 1991–1999. MMWR Surveillance Summaries 52:1, Feb 21, 2003

Chan LY, Tsui MH, Leung TN: Guillain-Barre syndrome in pregnancy. Acta Obstet Gynecol Scand 83:319, 2004

Chang BS, Lowenstein DH: Epilepsy. N Engl J Med 349:1257, 2003

Cheng Q, Jiang GX, Fredrikson S, et al: Increased incidence of Guillain–Barre syndrome postpartum. Epidemiology 9:601, 1998

Cohen Y, Lavie O, Granoxsky-Grisaru S, et al: Bell palsy complicating pregnancy: A review. Obstet Gynecol Surv 55:184, 2000

Comi G, Fillippi M, Barkhof F, et al: Effect of early interferon treatment on conversion to definite multiple sclerosis: A randomized study. Lancet 357:1576, 2001

Compston A, Coles A: Multiple sclerosis. Lancet 359:1221, 2002

Confavreux C, Vukusic S, Moreau T, et al: Relapses and progression of disability in multiple sclerosis. N Engl J Med 343:1430, 2000

Coppage KH, Hinton AC, Moldenhauer J, et al: Maternal and perinatal outcome in women with a history of stroke. Am J Obstet Gynecol 190:1331, 2004

Cornelissen M, Steegers-Theunissen R, Kollée L, et al: Increased incidence of neonatal vitamin K deficiency resulting from maternal anticonvulsant therapy. Am J Obstet Gynecol 168:923, 1993

Courts RB: Splinting for symptoms of carpal tunnel syndrome during pregnancy. J Hand Ther 8:31, 1995

Cox SM, Hankins GDV, Leveno KJ, et al: Bacterial endocarditis: A serious pregnancy complication. J Reprod Med 33:671, 1988

Cross JN, Castro PO, Jennett WB: Cerebral strokes associated with pregnancy and the puerperium. BMJ 3:214, 1968

Damek DM, Shuster EA: Pregnancy and multiple sclerosis. Mayo Clin Proc 72:977, 1997

Dammers JWHH, Veering MM, Vermeulen M: Injection with methylprednisolone proximal to the carpal tunnel: Randomised double blind trial. BMJ 319:884, 1999

Dawes SD: Can SSRIs reduce the risk of preeclampsia in pregnant, depressed patients? Med Hypotheses 64:33, 2005

Dell DL, O'Brien BW: Suicide in pregnancy. Obstet Gynecol 102:1306, 2003

Depression Guideline Panel: Depression in Primary Care, Vol I. Detection and Diagnosis. Clinical Practice Guideline No. 5. Rockville, MD, US Department of Health and Human Services, Public Health Service, Agency for Health Care Policy and Research (AHCPR Pub. No. 93-0550), April 1993

Derfuss T, Gurkov R, Then Bergh F, et al: Intrathecal antibody production against *Chlamydia pneumoniae* in multiple sclerosis is part of a polyspecific immune response. Brain 124:1325, 2001

Dey R, Khan S, Akhouri V, et al: Labetalol for prophylactic treatment of intractable migraine during pregnancy. Headache 42:642, 2002

Dias MS, Sekhar LN: Intracranial hemorrhage from aneurysms and arteriovenous malformations during pregnancy and the puerperium. Neurosurgery 27:855, 1990

Dillon WP, Lee RV, Tronolone MJ, et al: Life support and maternal death during pregnancy. JAMA 248:1089, 1982

Djelmis J, Sostarko M, Mayer D, et al: Myasthenia gravis in pregnancy: Report on 69 cases. Eur J Obstet Gynecol Reprod Biol 104:21, 2002

Donaldson JO, Lee NS: Arterial and venous stroke associated with pregnancy. Neurol Clin 12:583, 1994

Doris A, Ebmeier K, Shajahan P: Depressive illness. Lancet 354:1369, 1999

Dorsey DL, Camann WR: Obstetric anesthesia in patients with idiopathic facial paralysis (Bell's palsy): A 10-year survey. Anesth Analg 77:81, 1993

Drachman DB: Myasthenia gravis. N Engl J Med 330:1797, 1994

Edan G, Miller D, Clanet M, et al: Therapeutic effect of mitoxantrone combined with methylprednisolone in multiple sclerosis: A randomized multicenter study of active disease using MRI and clinical criteria. J Neurol Neurosurg Psychiatry 62:112, 1997

Einhäupl KM, Villringer A, Meister W, et al: Heparin treatment in sinus venous thrombosis. Lancet 338:597, 1991

England JD, Asbury AK: Peripheral neuropathy. Lancet 363:2151, 2004

Evans J, Heron J, Francomb H, et al: Cohort study of depressed mood during pregnancy and after childbirth. BMJ 323:257, 2001

Evans RW, Friedman DI: The management of pseudotumor cerebri during pregnancy. Headache 40:495, 2000

Feldman DM, Borgida AF, Rodis JF, et al: Irreversible maternal brain injury during pregnancy: A case report and review of the literature. Obstet Gynecol Surv 44:708, 2000

Fettes I: Menstrual migraine. Methods of prevention and control. Postgrad Med 101:67, 1997

Field DR, Gates EA, Creasy RK, et al: Maternal brain death during pregnancy. JAMA 260:816, 1988

Finnerty JJ, Chisholm CA, Chapple H, et al: Cerebral arteriovenous malformation in pregnancy: Presentation and neurologic, obstetric, and ethical significance. Am J Obstet Gynecol 181:296, 1999

Fleming AS, Klein E, Corter C: The effects of a social support group on depression, maternal attitudes and behavior in new mothers. J Child Psychol Psychiatry 33:685, 1992

Gerritsen AAM, de Vet HCW, Scholten RJPM, et al: Splinting vs surgery in the treatment of carpal tunnel syndrome. JAMA 288:1245, 2002

Gilden DH: Bell's palsy. N Engl J Med 351:1323, 2004

Gillman GS, Schaitkin BM, May M, et al: Bell's palsy in pregnancy: A study of recovery outcomes. Otolaryngol Head Neck Surg 126:26, 2002

Glickman S, Kamm MA: Bowel dysfunction in spinal-cord injury patients. Lancet 347:1651, 1996

Goadsby PJ, Lipton RB, Ferrari MD: Migraine—current understanding and treatment. N Engl J Med 346:257, 2002

Golbe LI: Pregnancy and movement disorders. Neurol Clin 12:497, 1994

Graham JM Jr, Marin-Padilla M, Hoefnagel D: Jejunal atresia associated with Cafergot ingestion during pregnancy. Clin Pediatr 22:226, 1983

Hannah P, Adams D, Lee A, et al: Links between early postpartum mood and post-natal depression. Br J Psychiatry 160:777, 1992

Harvard Medical School: Schizophrenia and the Brain—Part I. Harvard Mental Health Letter 15(11), May 1999a

Harvard Medical School: Schizophrenia and the Brain—Part II. Harvard Mental Health Letter 15(11), June 1999b

Hollingsworth DR, Resnik R (eds): Medical Counseling Before Pregnancy. New York, Churchill Livingstone, 1988, p 415

Holmes LB, Harvey EA, Coull BA, et al: The teratogenicity of anticonvulsant drugs. N Engl J Med 344:1132, 2001

Hommes OR, Sørensen PS, Fazekas F, et al: Intravenous immunoglobulin in secondary progressive multiple sclerosis: Randomised placebo-controlled trial. Lancet 364:1149, 2004

Horrigan TJ, Schroeder AV, Schaffer RM: The triad of substance abuse, violence, and depression are interrelated in pregnancy. J Subst Abuse Treat 18:55, 2000

Hughes HE, Goldstein DA: Birth defects following maternal exposure to ergotamine, beta-blockers, and caffeine. J Med Genet 25:396, 1988

Hughes SJ, Short DJ, Usherwood MM, et al: Management of the pregnant women with spinal cord injuries. Br J Obstet Gynaecol 98:513, 1991

Huna-Baron R, Kupersmith MJ: Idiopathic intracranial hypertension in pregnancy. J Neurol 249:1078, 2002

Hurley TJ, Brunson AD, Archer RL, et al: Landry Guillain–Barré Strohl syndrome in pregnancy: Report of three cases treated with plasmapheresis. Obstet Gynecol 78:482, 1991

International Headache Society: Headache Classification Committee. The International Classification of Headache Disorders, 2nd ed. Cephalgia 24:1, 2004

Ip MSM, So SY, Lam WK, et al: Thymectomy in myasthenia gravis during pregnancy. Postgrad Med J 62:473, 1986

Itoyama Y, Uemura S, Ushio Y, et al: Natural course of unoperated intracranial arteriovenous malformation: Study of 50 cases. J Neurosurg 71:805, 1989

Jackson AB, Wadley V: A multicenter study of women's self reported reproductive health after spinal cord injury. Arch Phys Med Rehabil 80:1420, 1999

Jaigobin C, Silver FL: Stroke and pregnancy. Stroke 31:2948, 2000

Joffe H, Cohen LS: Estrogen, serotonin, and mood disturbance: Where is the therapeutic bridge? Biol Psychiatry 44:798, 1998

Johnson KP, Brooks BR, Cohen JA, et al: Copolymer 1 reduces relapse rate and improves disability in relapsing-remitting multiple sclerosis: Results of a phase III multicenter, double-blind, placebo-controlled trial. Neurology 45:1268, 1995

Josefsson A, Angelsiöö L, Berg G, et al: Obstetric, somatic and demographic risk factors for postpartum depressive symptoms. Obstet Gynecol 99:223, 2002

Kallen B, Lygner PE: Delivery outcome in women who used drugs for migraine during pregnancy with special reference to suma-triptan. Headache 41:351, 2001

Kaniecki R: Headache assessment and management. JAMA 289:1430, 2003

Karlsson B, Lindquist C, Johansson A, et al: Annual risk for the first hemorrhage from untreated cerebral arteriovenous malfor-mations. Minim Invasive Neurosurg 40:40, 1997

Katz JN, Simmons BP: Carpal tunnel syndrome. N Engl J Med 346:1807, 2002

Katz VL, Peterson R, Cefalo RC: Pseudotumor cerebri and preg-nancy. Am J Perinatol 6:442, 1989

Kelly RH, Russo J, Holt VL, et al: Psychiatric and substance use dis-orders as risk factors for low birth weight and preterm delivery. Obstet Gynecol 100:297, 2002

Kittner SJ, Stern BJ, Feeser BR, et al: Pregnancy and the risk of stroke. N Engl J Med 335:768, 1996

Kruit MC, van Buchem MA, Hofman PA, et al: Migraine as a risk factor for subclinical brain lesions. JAMA 291:427, 2004

Kuller JA, Katz VL, McCoy MC, et al: Pregnancy complicated by Guillain Barré syndrome. South Med J 88:987, 1995

Kuller JA, Katz VL, McMahon MJ, et al: Pharmacologic treatment of psychiatric disease in pregnancy and lactation: Fetal and neonatal effects. Obstet Gynecol 87:789, 1996

Kurtzke JF: The current neurologic burden of illness and injury in the United States. Neurology 32:1207, 1982

Kuwabara S: Guillain-Barre syndrome: Epidemiology, pathophysi-ology and management. Drugs 64:597, 2004

Lamy C, Hamon JB, Coste J, et al: Ischemic stroke in young women. Neurology 55:269, 2000

Lander CM, Eadie MJ: Plasma antiepileptic drug concentrations during pregnancy. Epilepsia 32:257, 1991

Landwehr JB, Isada NB, Pryde PG, et al: Maternal neurosurgical shunts and pregnancy outcome. Obstet Gynecol 83:134, 1994

Lanska DJ, Kryscio RJ: Peripartum stroke and intracranial venous thrombosis in the National Hospital Discharge Survey. Obstet Gynecol 89:413, 1997

Lanska DJ, Kryscio RJ: Risk factors for peripartum and postpartum stroke and intracranial venous thrombosis. Stroke 31:1274, 2000

Lanska DJ, Kryscio RJ: Stroke and intracranial venous thrombosis during pregnancy and puerperium. Neurology 53:1162, 1998

LaRoche SM, Helmers SL: The new antiepileptic drugs. Clinical applications. JAMA 291:615, 2004a

LaRoche SM, Helmers SL: The new antiepileptic drugs. Scientific review. JAMA 291:605, 2004b

Levin LI, Munger KL, Rubertone MV, et al: Multiple sclerosis and Epstein-Barr virus. JAMA 289:1533, 2003

Littleford JA, Brockhurst NJ, Bernstein EP, et al: Obstetrical anes-thesia for a parturient with a ventriculoperitoneal shunt and third ventriculostomy. Can J Anaesth 46:1057, 1999

Lublin FD, Reingold SC: Defining the course of multiple sclerosis: Results of an international survey. National Multiple Sclerosis Society (USA) Advisory Committee on Clinical Trials of New Agents for Multiple Sclerosis. Neurology 46:907, 1996

Lynch JK, Nelson KB: Epidemiology of perinatal stroke. Curr Opin Pediatr 13:499, 2001

Marks MN, Wieck A, Checkley SA, et al: Life stress and post-partum psychosis: A preliminary report. Br J Psychiatry Suppl 10:45, 1991

Mehraein S, Ortwein H, Busch M, et al: Risk of recurrence of cere-bral venous and sinus thrombosis during subsequent pregnancy and puerperium. J Neurol Neurosurg Psychiatry 74:814, 2003

Melchart D, Thormaehlen J, Hager S, et al: Acupuncture versus placebo versus sumatriptan for early treatment of migraine at-tacks: A randomized controlled trial. J Intern Med 253:181, 2003

Mhurchu CN, Anderson C, Jamrozik K, et al: Hormonal factors and risk of aneurysmal subarachnoid hemorrhage: An international population-based, case-control study. Stroke 32:606, 2001

Miller DH, Khan OA, Sheremata WA, et al: A controlled trial of na-talizumab for relapsing multiple sclerosis. N Engl J Med 348:15, 2003

Miller LJ: Postpartum depression. JAMA 287:762, 2002

Miller LJ: Use of electroconvulsive therapy during pregnancy. Hosp Community Psychiatry 45:444, 1994

Minielly R, Yuzpe AA, Drake CG: Subarachnoid hemorrhage secondary to ruptured cerebral aneurysm in pregnancy. Obstet Gynecol 53:64, 1979

Morewitz SJ: Feelings of anxiety and functional impairment during pregnancy. Obstet Gynecol 101:109S, 2003

Mufson M: Coping with Anxiety and Phobias. Harvard Medical School Special Health Report. Harvard Health Publications. Boston, MA, 2002

Muller-Oerlinghausen B, Berghofer A, Bauer M: Bipolar disorder. Lancet 359:241, 2002

Murphy KC: Schizophrenia and velocardiofacial syndrome. Lancet 359:426, 2002

National Mental Health Association: Depression in women. Available at: http://www.nmha.org/infoctr. Accessed April 15, 2004

Nelson LM, Franklin GM, Jones MC, et al: Risk of multiple scle-rosis exacerbation during pregnancy and breast-feeding. JAMA 259:3441, 1988

Okamoto K, Horisawa R, Kawamura T, et al: Menstrual and reproductive factors for subarachnoid hemorrhage risk in women: A case-control study in Nagoya, Japan. Stroke 32:2841, 2001

Olafsson E, Hallgrimsson JT, Hauser WA, et al: Pregnancies of women with epilepsy: A population-based study in Iceland. Epilepsia 39:887, 1998

Olesen C, Steffensen FH, Sorensen HT, et al: Pregnancy outcome following prescription for sumatriptan. Headache 40:20, 2000

Omdal R, Roalsø S: Chorea gravidarum and chorea associated with oral contraceptives—diseases due to antiphospholipid antibod-ies? Acta Neurol Scand 86:219, 1992

O'Quinn S, Ephross SA, Williams V, et al: Pregnancy and perinatal outcomes in migraineurs using sumatriptan: A prospective study. Arch Gynecol Obstet 263:7, 1999

Padua L, Aprile I, Caliandro P, et al: Carpal tunnel syndrome in pregnancy: Multiperspective follow-up of untreated cases. Neurology 59:1643, 2002

Padua L, Aprile I, Caliandro P, et al: Symptoms and neurophysi-ological picture of carpal tunnel syndrome in pregnancy. Clin Neurophysiol 112:1946, 2001

Palace J, Rothwell P: New treatments and azathioprine in multiple sclerosis. Lancet 350:261, 1997

Pathan M, Kittner SJ: Pregnancy and stroke. Curr Neurol Neurosci Rep 3:27, 2003

Paulson GW: Headaches in women, including women who are preg-nant. Am J Obstet Gynecol 173:1734, 1995

Peitersen E: Bell's palsy: The spontaneous course of 2,500 periph-eral facial nerve palsies of different etiologies. Acta Otolaryngol Suppl 549:4, 2002

Plauché WC: Myasthenia gravis in mothers and their newborns. Clin Obstet Gynecol 34:82, 1991

Prasher VP, Barrett K: Neuropsychiatric aspects of Sydenham's chorea: A case report. J Psychosom Obstet Gynaecol 14:159, 1993

Preter M, Tzourio C, Ameri A, et al: Long-term prognosis in cerebral venous thrombosis. Follow-up of 77 patients. Stroke 27:243, 1996

PRISMS Study Group: Randomised double-blind placebo-controlled study of interferon beta-1a in relapsing/remitting multiple sclerosis. Lancet 352:1498, 1998

Qureshi AI, Tuhrim S, Broderick JP, et al: Spontaneous intracerebral hemorrhage. N Engl J Med 344:1450, 2001

Ra CS, Lui CC, Liang CL, et al: Superior sagittal sinus thrombosis induced by thyrotoxicosis. Case report. J Neurosurg 94:130, 2001

Reprotox Database: Ergotamine. RTC: 1396; CAS Registry: 113-15-5; 2003a

Reprotox Database: Interferons. RTC: 1418; CAS Registry: 9008-11-1; May 2002

Reprotox Database: Sumatriptan. RTC: 3147; CAS Registry: 103628-46-2; March 2003b

Richmond JR, Krishnamoorthy P, Andermann E, et al: Epilepsy and pregnancy: An obstetric perspective. Am J Obstet Gynecol 190:371, 2004

Rockel A, Wissel J, Rolfs A: Guillain–Barré syndrome in pregnancy: An indication for caesarean section? J Perinat Med 22:393, 1994

Roman H, Descargues G, Lopes M, et al: Subarachnoid hemorrhage due to cerebral aneurysmal rupture during pregnancy. Acta Obstet Gynecol Scand 83:330, 2004

Ropper AH: The Guillain–Barré syndrome. N Engl J Med 326:1130, 1992

Ros HS, Lichtenstein P, Bellocco R, et al: Pulmonary embolism and stroke in relation to pregnancy: How can high-risk women be identified? Am J Obstet Gynecol 186:198, 2002

Roullet E, Verdier-Taillefer MH, Amarenco P, et al: Pregnancy and multiple sclerosis: A longitudinal study of 125 remittent patients. J Neurol Neurosurg Psychiatry 56:299, 1993

Sadovnick AD, Eisen K, Hashimoto SA, et al: Pregnancy and multiple sclerosis. A prospective study. Arch Neurol 51:1120, 1994

Schmeelk KH, Granger DA, Susman EJ, et al: Maternal depression and risk for postpartum complications: Role of prenatal corticotropin-releasing hormone and interleukin-1 receptor antagonist. Behav Med 25:88, 1999

Schneider J, Blea C, Hendricks SK: Increased familial incidence of multiple sclerosis: Genetics and epidemiology in pregnancy. Am J Obstet Gynecol 174:445, 1996

Schnitker JB, Light DW: Nonneurologic indications for MRI: Technological advances have broadened applications. Postgrad Med 109:81, 2001

Séguin L, Potvin L, St. Denis M, et al: Chronic stressors, social support, and depression during pregnancy. Obstet Gynecol 85:583, 1995

Seror P: Pregnancy-related carpal tunnel syndrome. J Hand Surg [Br] 23:98, 1998

Shapiro JL, Yudin MH, Ray JG: Bell's palsy and tinnitus during pregnancy: Predictors of pre-eclampsia? Three cases and a detailed review of the literature. Acta Otolaryngol 119:647, 1999

Sharshar T, Lamy C, Mas JL: Incidence and causes of strokes associated with pregnancy and puerperium. A study in public hospitals of Île de France. Stroke 26:930, 1995

Shehata HA, Okosun H: Neurological disorders in pregnancy. Curr Opin Obstet Gynecol 16:117, 2004

Shmorgun D, Chan WS, Ray JG: Association between Bell's palsy in pregnancy and pre-eclampsia. QJM 95:359, 2002

Silberstein SD: Migraine. Lancet 363:381, 2004

Simolke GA, Cox SM, Cunningham FG: Accidents complicating pregnancy and the puerperium. Obstet Gynecol 78:37, 1991

Smith MV, Brunetto WL, Yonkers KA: Identifying perinatal depression—sooner is better. Contemp Ob/Gyn 44:58, 2004

Sollid CP, Wisborg K, Hjort J, et al: Eating disorder that was diagnosed before pregnancy and pregnancy outcome. Am J Obstet Gynecol 190:206, 2004

Srinivasan K: Ischemic cerebral vascular disease in the young. Two common causes in India. Stroke 15:733, 1984

Stewart WF, Lipton RB, Celentano DD, et al: Prevalence of migraine headache in the United States: Relation to age, income, race and other sociodemographic factors. JAMA 267:64, 1992

Stolp-Smith KA, Pascoe MK, Ogburn PL Jr: Carpal tunnel syndrome in pregnancy: Frequency, severity, and prognosis. Arch Phys Med Rehabil 79:1285, 1998

Stoodley MA, Macdonald RL, Weir BK: Pregnancy and intracranial aneurysms. Neurosurg Clin N Am 9:549, 1998

Sumatriptan and Naratriptan Pregnancy Registries: Sumatriptan and naratriptan pregnancy registries. International Interim Report: 1 January 1996–30 April 2002. Wilmington, NC, Pharma Research Corporation, July 2002

Takebayashi S, Kaneko M: Electron microscopic studies of ruptured arteries in hypertensive intracerebral hemorrhage. Stroke 14:28, 1983

Tietjen GE: The relationship of migraine and stroke. Neuroepidemiology 19:13, 2000

Tsuang MT, Faraone SV: The inheritance of mood disorders. In Hall LL (ed): Genetics and Mental Illness: Evolving Issues for Research and Society. New York, Plenum Press, 1996, p 79

Tzourio C, Tehindrazanarivelo A, Iglésias S, et al: Case control study of migraine and risk of ischemic stroke in young women. BMJ 310:830, 1995

Uknis A, Silberstein SD: Migraine and pregnancy. Headache 31:372, 1991

van der Meché FGA, Schmitz PIM, The Dutch Guillain–Barré Study Group: A randomized trial comparing intravenous immune globulin and plasma exchange in Guillain–Barré syndrome. N Engl J Med 326:1123, 1992

Verloes A, Emonts P, Dubois M, et al: Paraplegia and arthrogryposis multiplex of the lower extremities after intrauterine exposure to ergotamine. J Med Genet 27:213, 1990

Vernet-der Garabedian B, Lacokova M, Eymard B, et al: Association of neonatal myasthenia gravis with antibodies against the fetal acetylcholine receptor. J Clin Invest 94:555, 1994

Walther EU, Hohlfeld R: Multiple sclerosis: Side effects of interferon beta therapy and their management. Neurology 53:1622, 1999

Warlow C, Sudlow C, Dennis M, et al: Stroke. Lancet 362:1211, 2003

Weinreb HJ: Demyelinating and neoplastic diseases in pregnancy. Neurol Clin 12:509, 1994

Welch KMA: Migraine and pregnancy. Adv Neurol 64:77, 1994

Wenzel RG, Sarvis CA: Do butalbital-containing products have a role in the management of migraine? Pharmacotherapy 22:1029, 2002

Westgren N, Hultling C, Levi R, Westgren M: Pregnancy and delivery in women with a trauma spinal cord injury in Sweden, 1980–1991. Obstet Gynecol 81:926, 1993

Wiebers DO: Subarachnoid hemorrhage in pregnancy. Semin Neurol 8:226, 1988

Wilkins RH: Natural history of intracranial vascular malformations: A review. Neurosurgery 16:421, 1985

Wisner KL, Parry BL, Piontek CM: Postpartum depression. N Engl J Med 347:194, 2002

Wisoff JH, Kratzert KJ, Handwerker SM, et al: Pregnancy in patients with cerebrospinal fluid shunts: Report of a series and review of the literature. Neurosurgery 29:827, 1991

Witlin AG, Mattar F, Sibai BM: Postpartum stroke: A twenty year experience. Am J Obstet Gynecol 183:83, 2000

Yerby MS: Pregnancy, teratogenesis, and epilepsy. Neurol Clin 12:749, 1994

56

Dermatological Disorders

In addition to some recognized pregnancy-specific dermatoses, any skin disease that affects women of childbearing age may be encountered in pregnancy. Importantly, some skin changes caused by the hormonal influences of pregnancy may be worrisome. For example, some cases of generalized pruritus during late pregnancy are caused by intrahepatic cholestasis and bile salt retention; this condition is commonly known as *pruritus gravidarum* (see Chap. 50, p. 1126).

PHYSIOLOGICAL SKIN CHANGES IN PREGNANCY

Normal pregnancy-induced hormonal changes may have rather remarkable influences on the skin. As discussed in Chapters 3 and 5, fetoplacental hormone production, stimulation, or alteration of clearance may increase the plasma availability of estrogens, progesterone, and a variety of androgens. Similarly, there are profound changes in the availability or concentrations of some adrenal steroids, including cortisol, aldosterone, and deoxycorticosterone. Paus and Cotsarelis (1999) have described hair-growth modulation by estrogens, androgens, thyroid hormones, glucocorticoids, and prolactin.

Presumably as a result of enlargement of the intermediate lobe of the pituitary gland, plasma levels of melanocyte-stimulating hormone (MSH) become remarkably elevated by 8 weeks' gestation. Production of pro-opiomelanocortin has been demonstrated in placental extracts, and this ultimately is a source of α- and β-MSH.

HYPERPIGMENTATION. Some degree of skin darkening resulting from melanin deposition into epidermal and dermal macrophages occurs in 90 percent of pregnant women. Pigmentation is more pronounced in brunettes and in women with dark complexions, especially those of Hispanic descent (Aronson and Bass, 2000). Its exact cause is not known, but it is doubtful that elevated serum levels of MSH are responsible. Estrogens play a role in melanogenesis and may be the inciting factor.

Hyperpigmentation is evident beginning early in pregnancy and is more pronounced in naturally hyperpigmented areas such as the areolae, perineum, and umbilicus. Areas prone to friction, including the axillae and inner thighs, also may become darkened. When the *linea alba* becomes pigmented, it is renamed the *linea nigra.*

In rare cases, *acquired dermal melanocytosis* first appears during pregnancy (Rubin and colleagues, 2001). The lesions are nonpalpable, brown to blue-gray patches of skin that contain spindle-shaped melanocytes.

Pigmentation of the face, referred to as the mask of pregnancy, is also called *chloasma* or *melasma.* This is seen in about half of pregnant women. Ultraviolet (UV) light exacerbates melasma, because it too stimulates melanogenesis.

Thus, the severity of pigmentation may be mitigated by avoiding excessive sun exposure and by using sunscreens.

Although hyperpigmentation usually regresses postpartum, dermal melanosis may persist up to 10 years in a third of affected women. Oral contraceptives may aggravate melasma and should be avoided in susceptible women. If particularly disfiguring, topical application of 2- to 5-percent hydroxyquinone, 0.1-percent tretinoin gel or cream, or 20-percent azelaic acid cream may provide some improvement (Griffiths and colleagues, 1993; Kimbrough-Green and co-workers, 1994). Sunscreen use should be continued.

NEVI. All persons have some form of benign or melanocytic nevi. Although it was traditionally taught that these pigmented cutaneous tumors commonly enlarge and darken during pregnancy, leading to their confusion with malignant melanomas, this is not the case. Pennoyer and colleagues (1997) performed a careful observational study and found that only 6 percent of 129 nevi changed in diameter over pregnancy. Of the eight that changed, four increased by 1 mm, and four *decreased* by 1 mm.

Thus, although nevi can be shown histologically to have enlarged melanocytes and increased melanin deposition during pregnancy, there is no evidence that they undergo malignant transformation as a result of pregnancy. Malignant melanoma is discussed in Chapter 57 (see p. 1263).

CHANGES IN HAIR GROWTH. During pregnancy, the *anagen* phase, or the growing hair phase, is increased relative to the *telogen* phase, or the resting hair phase (Lynfield, 1960; Randall, 1994). Estrogens prolong the anagen state, and androgens cause enlargement of follicles in dependent areas such as the face (Paus and Cotsarelis, 1999). Postpartum, these effects are lost, and shedding of hair becomes prominent. *Telogen effluvium* describes the rather abrupt hair loss that is seen beginning approximately 1 to 4 months postpartum. This process is sometimes characterized by alarming amounts of hair shedding, usually associated with brushing or washing. Fortunately, the process is self limited, and women may be reassured that normal hair growth is usually restored in 6 to 12 months (Headington, 1993; Kois and Phelan, 1994).

Mild *hirsutism* is common during pregnancy, and this may be most noticeable on the face. Women who are predisposed genetically to coarse hair growth are affected most profoundly. Hirsutism typically regresses within several months after delivery. More severe hirsutism is unusual, and if accompanied by other evidence of masculinization, this should prompt consideration of another androgen source. For example, there are reports of pregnant women who had virilization caused by adrenal tumors or pregnancy luteomas (Choi and colleagues, 2000; Danilowicz and co-workers, 2002).

VASCULAR CHANGES. Augmented cutaneous blood flow in pregnancy is due to a marked decrease in peripheral vascular resistance (Spetz, 1964). One salutary effect of this is dissipation of excess heat generated by increased metabolism. In addition to augmented cutaneous blood flow, pregnancy incites a number of common estrogen-induced changes in small blood vessels. *Spider angiomas* are found in two thirds of white women and about 10 percent of African Americans during pregnancy (Wong and Ellis, 1984). Most of these vascular lesions regress postpartum. *Palmar erythema* is noticed in two thirds of white women and a third of black women. *Capillary hemangiomas*, especially of the head and neck, are seen in about 5 percent of women during pregnancy.

One vascular condition that may be distressing is *pregnancy gingivitis,* which is caused by growth of the gum capillaries. This so-called *epulis of pregnancy* may become more severe, but it may be controlled by proper dental hygiene and avoidance of trauma. Epulis should not be confused with *pyogenic granuloma of pregnancy,* which is also called *granuloma gravidarum.* These lesions are typical pyogenic granulomas, which are found in the oral cavity and often arise from the gingival papillae. They are associated with extensive gingivitis. Sheehan and Lesher (2004) described such a lesion arising in a port-wine stain. Treatment is usually unnecessary, but Powell and colleagues (1994) described laser excision of a large granuloma.

DERMATOSES OF PREGNANCY

A number of dermatological conditions have been identified as either unique to pregnancy or encountered with a greater frequency during gestation. Their terminology can be quite confusing. Shornick (1998) concluded that only three conditions arc universally accepted as unique to pregnancy: *cholestasis* with its attendant pruritus, *pruritic urticarial papules and plaques of pregnancy*, and herpes gestationis (Table 56–1). Their gross appearance may be similar to the two other skin disorders in Table 56–1.

Pruritus during pregnancy is common, and its incidence varies directly with the vigilance for which it is searched. The best data are from nearly 3200 pregnant women carefully studied over one year by Roger and colleagues (1994). **By a uniform definition, 1.6 percent of women had significant pruritus at some time during pregnancy.**

PRURITUS GRAVIDARUM. This common pregnancy-related skin condition is not primarily a dermatological disorder. In the study by Roger and associates (1994), almost half of women with pruritus during pregnancy (0.6 percent) had pruritus gravidarum. This condition is considered to be a mild variant of *intrahepatic cholestasis of* pregnancy, discussed in Chapter 50 (see p. 1126). There is associated bile salt retention, and as serum levels increase, bile salts are deposited in the dermis. This in turn causes pruritus and although skin lesions develop, they are secondary to scratching and excoriation. The condition is associated with pregnancy

hormones, genetics, and environmental factors (Germain and colleagues, 2002; Sherard and Atkinson, 2001).

PRURITIC URTICARIAL PAPULES AND PLAQUES OF PREGNANCY. This is the most common pruritic pregnancy-specific dermatosis. It is called *PUPPP* in the United States and referred to as *polymorphic eruption of pregnancy (PEP)* in the United Kingdom. In the study by Roger and co-workers (1994), almost half of 3200 pregnant women with pruritus had this dermatosis. Although the incidence is about 1 in 200 singleton pregnancies, it is 8 in 200 for twin gestation (Kroumpouzos and Cohen, 2003). It is characterized by an intensely pruritic cutaneous eruption that usually appears late in pregnancy (see Table 56–1). Shown in Figure 56–1 are the erythematous urticarial papules and plaques that first develop on the abdomen, usually around striae. The lesions then are likely to spread to the buttocks, thighs, and extremities (Aronson and colleagues, 1998).

Pruritus may be severe with these lesions. In about 40 percent of women, the urticarial component predominates; in 45 percent, the erythematous pattern is prominent; and in 15 percent, a combination is seen (Aronson and associates, 1998). The erythematous patches are widespread. The face is usually spared, and seldom is there excoriation. The disease is more common in nulliparas and seldom recurs in subsequent pregnancies. It may resemble herpes gestationis, but there usually are no vesicles or bullae (Sherard and Atkinson, 2001). There is no evidence that perinatal morbidity is increased (Kroumpouzos and Cohen, 2003).

Pathophysiology. The etiopathogenesis is unknown. Because of diverse clinical findings, classification can be confusing. On biopsy, there is a mild, nonspecific lymphohistiocytic perivasculitis with an eosinophilic component. Importantly, there is no immunoglobulin or complement deposition seen using immunofluorescent staining of dermis (Aronson and colleagues, 1998). The absence of a linear band of C3 in the basement membrane differentiates this dermatosis from herpes gestationis. Aractingi and associates (1998) have reported provocative evidence that this disorder may be stimulated by fetal cells that have invaded maternal skin. Similar observations have been made for progressive systemic sclerosis (see Chap. 54, p. 1220) and postpartum thyroiditis (see Chap. 53, p. 1191). Recently, the reverse phenomenon has been described, and maternal cells have been linked to some autoimmune childhood disorders (Barinaga, 2002; Srivatsa and colleagues, 2003). Bidirectional maternal–fetal cell trafficking was the subject of a 2000 National Institutes of Health–sponsored conference (Bianchi and Romero, 2003).

Treatment. Some women obtain relief from oral antihistamines and skin emollients, but most require topical corticosteroid creams or ointments. Oral corticosteroids are given if these fail to relieve severe itching. In most cases,

TABLE 56–1 Dermatosis Unique to Pregnancy

Disorder	Frequency	Clinical Characteristics	Histopathology	Perinatal Outcome	Treatment	Comments
Pruritus gravidarum (cholestasis of pregnancy)	Common (1–2%)	Onset in third trimester; intense pruritus; generalized; excoriations common	Nonspecific; no primary lesions, but excoriations common	Perinatal morbidity increased	Antipruritics, cholestyramine, ursodeoxycholic acid	Mild form of cholestatic jaundice; recurs in subsequent pregnancies
Pruritic urticarial papules and plaques of pregnancy (PUPPP) (polymorphic eruption of pregnancy)	Common (0.25–1%)	Onset usually in third trimester; intense pruritus; patchy or generalized on abdomen, thighs, arms, buttocks; erythematous papules, urticarial papules, plaques	Lymphocytic perivascular infiltrate; negative immunofluorescence	No adverse effects	Antipruritics, emollients, topical steroids, oral steroids if severe	Common in nulliparas and twins; seldom recurs in subsequent pregnancies
Prurigo of pregnancy (prurigo gestationis, papular dermatitis)	Uncommon (1:300–1:2400)	Onset in late second or early third trimester; localized or generalized; 1–5 mm pruritic papules; excoriations common	Lymphocytic perivascular infiltrate, parakeratosis; acanthosis; negative immunofluorescence	Probably unaffected	Antipruritics, topical steroids, oral steroids if severe	Prurigo gestationis localized to forearms and trunk; papular dermatitis is generalized; does not recur in subsequent pregnancies
Herpes gestationis (pemphigoid gestationis)	Rare (1:10,000)	Onset in second or third trimester, sometimes 1–2 weeks postpartum; severe pruritus; abdomen, extremities, or generalized; urticarial papules and plaques, erythema, vesicles, and bullae	Edema; infiltrate of lymphocytes, histiocytes, and eosinophils; C3 and IgG deposition at basement membrane	Possibly increased preterm birth; transient neonatal lesions (5–10%)	Antipruritics, topical steroids, oral steroids if severe	Autoimmune HLA-related; seen with trophoblastic disease; exacerbations and remissions during pregnancy and postpartum common; recurrence common; neonatal skin lesions in 10%
Pruritic folliculitis of pregnancy (impetigo herpetiformis)	Rare	Onset in third trimester; local, then generalized; erythema with marginal sterile pustules; mucous membranes involved; systemic symptoms	Microabscesses; spongiform pustules of Kogoj; neutrophils	Maternal sepsis common	Antimicrobials, oral steroids	Possibly pustular psoriasis; persists for weeks to months postpartum; usually does not recur with subsequent pregnancies

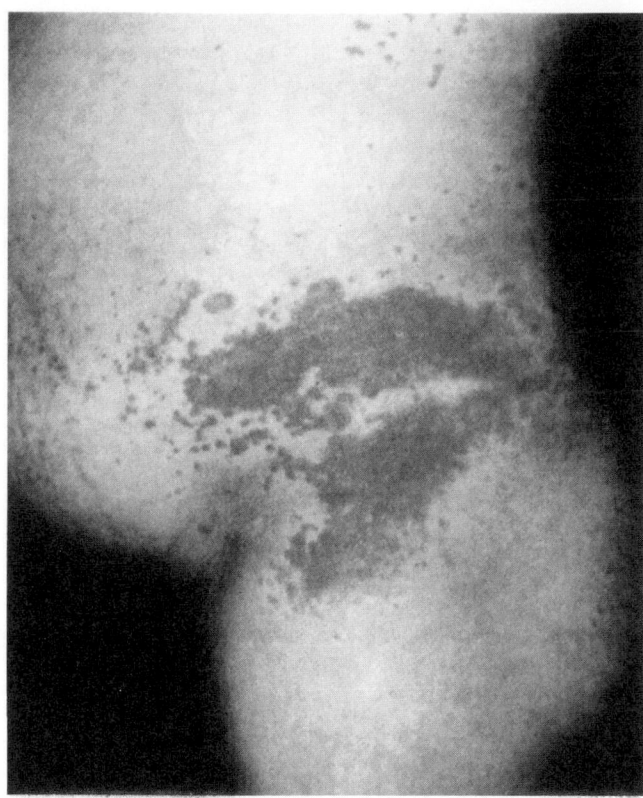

FIGURE 56–1. Pruritic urticarial papules and plaques of pregnancy. (From Aractingi and colleagues, 1998, with permission.)

the rash disappears quickly either before or within several days following delivery. In 15 to 20 percent of women, symptoms persist for 2 to 4 weeks postpartum (Vaughan Jones and co-workers, 1999). One biopsy-proven case beginning 4 weeks postpartum lasted 4 weeks (Kirkup and Dunnill, 2002).

PRURIGO OF PREGNANCY. These lesions, also called *papular eruptions of pregnancy*, have been described by a multitude of names. According to Shornick (1998), the disorder includes *prurigo gestationis* and *papular dermatitis,* which likely are variants of the same disease and are not specific to pregnancy (see Table 56–1). The mild and more common variant, prurigo gestationis, is characterized by small, pruritic, rapidly excoriated lesions on the forearms and trunk. The bitelike papules may resemble scabies or other insect bites. Vesicles or bullae do not develop. The course is protracted; lesions typically have their onset at 25 to 30 weeks and may persist for 3 months after delivery. Recurrence in subsequent pregnancy is common.

Pruritus is usually controlled with oral antihistamines and topical corticosteroid creams. Perinatal outcome does not appear to be adversely affected (Vaughan Jones and Black, 1999).

HERPES GESTATIONIS. Although this noninfectious skin disorder shares the name of the more common viral infection, the connection is etymological and not biological. The names of both conditions are derived from the Greek herpes (*to creep*). This autoimmune pruritic blistering skin eruption usually affects multiparous women in late pregnancy, but it may begin early in pregnancy or within a week or so postpartum (see Table 56–1). It occasionally may accompany gestational trophoblastic disease. It is also called *pemphigoid gestationis* because it is immunologically similar to *bullous pemphigoid* seen in elderly patients (van den Bergh and Giudice, 2003). Thus, it is an autoimmune blistering skin disease (Engineer and associates, 2000; Kolanko and colleagues, 2004).

Severe herpes gestationis can be serious. Fortunately, it is rare, even though the commonly cited incidence of about 1 in 50,000 pregnancies may be an underestimate.

Herpes gestationis is characterized by an extremely pruritic widespread eruption with lesions that vary from erythematous and edematous papules to large, tense vesicles and bullae (Figs. 56–2 and 56–3). Before bullae form, these findings may resemble PUPPP, which is described above. Common sites of involvement are the abdomen and the extremities. Morphological changes may develop in the small intestinal mucosa similar to those of adult celiac disease. Exacerbations and remissions throughout pregnancy are common, and up to 75 percent of women suffer intrapartum flares (Shornick, 1998). In subsequent pregnancies, the disease invariably recurs, and it usually does so earlier and is more severe. Baxi and colleagues (1991) reported a woman in whom recurrence was documented in five pregnancies.

Etiopathogenesis. This autoimmune disease is caused by development of an immunoglobulin G_1 antibody to the basement membrane in the epidermis. There is an inherited predisposition with a markedly increased rate among women with HLA-DR3 and HLA-DR4 antigens. Over half of women with herpes gestationis have these antigens, but they are found in only 3 percent of unaffected women. These maternal HLA-DR antigens are associated with other autoimmune disorders, including Addison disease, type 1 diabetes mellitus, systemic lupus erythematosus, Graves disease, and Hashimoto thyroiditis. In one study, Shornick and Black (1992) found that 10 percent of 75 women with herpes gestationis also had Graves disease. Paternal HLA-DR2 is also commonly found in these pregnancies (Shimanovich and colleagues, 2002a).

Shornick and associates (1993) demonstrated anti-HLA antibodies in all 39 women with biopsy-proven disease. This antibody is a thermostable immunoglobulin G (IgG) that reacts with the bullous pemphigoid 180-kD (BP180) antigen in the epidermis. Autoantibodies can be quantified using immunoblotting or ELISA (Sitaru and associates, 2004). BP180, a glycoprotein, is integral to adhesion structures that anchor basal cells to their basement membrane (Shimanovich and colleagues, 2002b). It is also called *herpes gestationis serum factor,* and it reacts with amnionic tissue, and is passively transferred to the fetus.

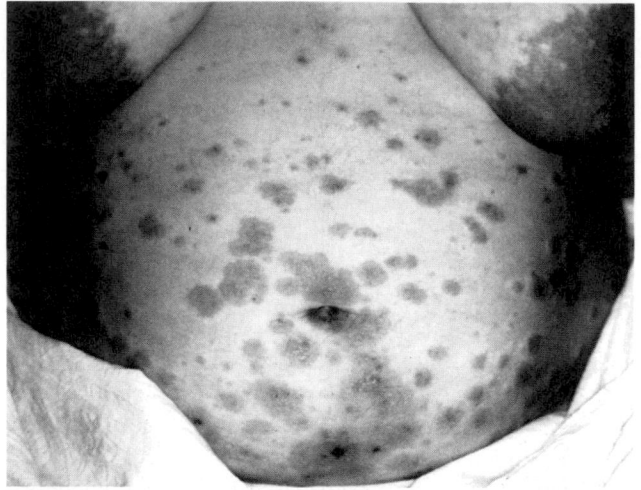

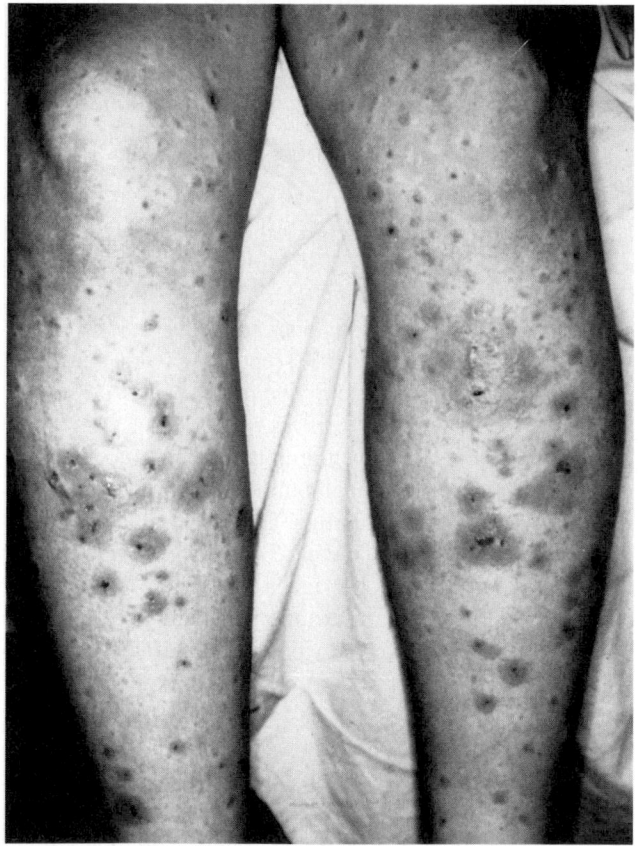

FIGURE 56–2. Herpes gestationis at 30 weeks' gestation. Corticosteroid treatment provided remarkable relief from the intense pruritus and considerable decrease in the intensity of the skin reaction.

Histologically, the classical finding in herpes gestationis is subepidermal edema with perivascular infiltrates of lymphocytes, histocytes, and eosinophils. Immunofluorescent techniques applied to a skin biopsy are of value for confirming the diagnosis. As shown in Figure 56–4, C3 complement and sometimes IgG are deposited along the basement membrane zone between the epidermis and the dermis (Kroumpouzos and Cohen, 2003).

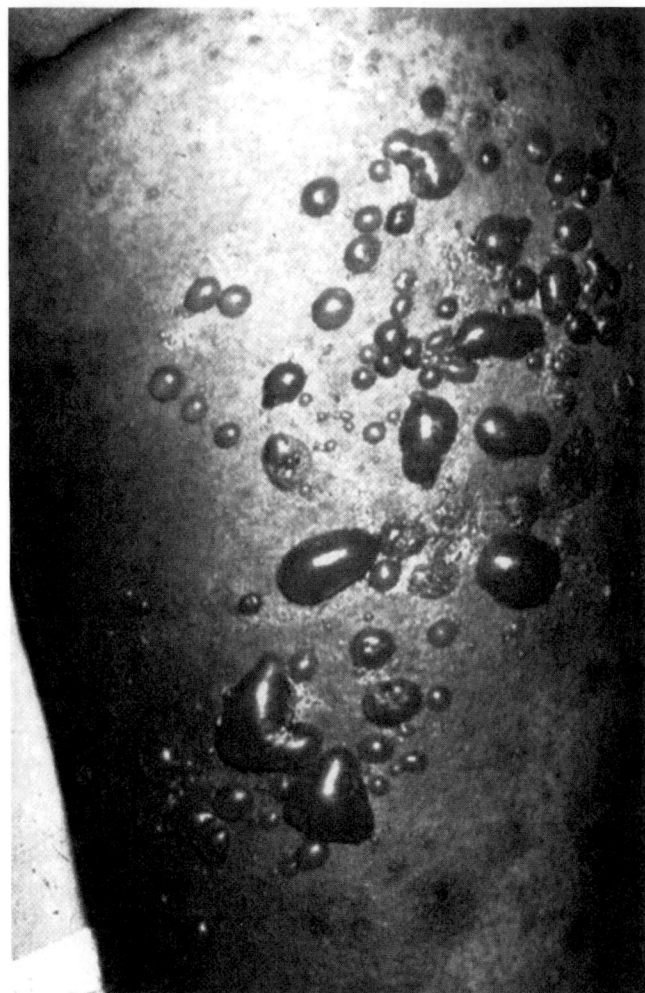

FIGURE 56–3. Herpes gestationis with large, tense bullae located on the thigh. (From Black, 2001, with permission.)

Treatment. Pruritus may be quite severe. Topical corticosteroids and oral antihistamines effect relief in only a few women. Orally administered prednisone, 0.5 to 1 mg/kg daily, usually brings relief promptly and inhibits formation of new lesions. The healed sites usually are not scarred but frequently are hyperpigmented. Refractory cases that persist postpartum have been treated with immunosuppressives such as cyclophosphamide, methotrexate, and cyclosporine (Wallengren, 2004). Some women develop chronic disease, which may be bullous pemphigoid (Amato and associates, 2003). In some intractable cases, plasmapheresis and high-dose intravenous immunoglobulin therapy have been used (Kroumpouzos and Cohen, 2003; Mazzi and colleagues, 2003).

Effect on Pregnancy. Although there are reports of an association with preterm birth, stillbirths, and growth restriction, these are from small studies (Aronson and Bass, 2000). Nevertheless, increased antepartum surveillance is recommended. Lesions similar to those of the mother develop

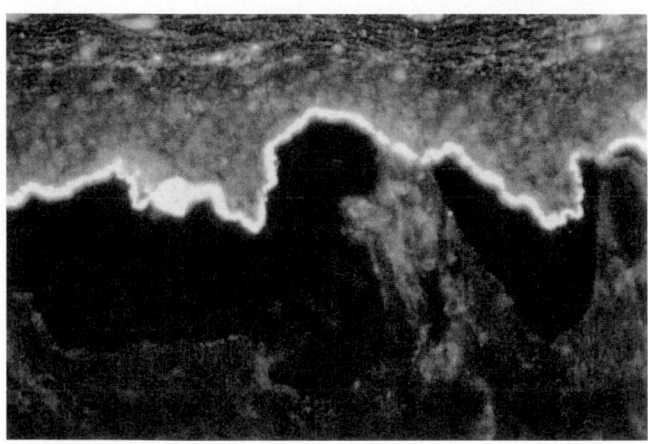

FIGURE 56–4. Herpes gestationis: indirect immunofluorescence microscopy of skin biopsy showing linear deposition of C3 along the epidermal basement membrane. (From Shimanovich and colleagues, 2002a, with permission.)

in up to 10 percent of neonates (Chen and colleagues, 1999; Erickson and Ellis, 2002). They have the same histological characteristics and usually clear spontaneously within a few weeks.

PRURITIC FOLLICULITIS OF PREGNANCY. This rare pustular eruption, which is also called *impetigo herpetiformis,* is seen in late pregnancy. It is uncertain if it is unique to pregnancy, or if it is a form of pustular psoriasis that occurs coincidental to pregnancy. Only 24 cases have been reported (Kroumpouzos and Cohen, 2003). In one intriguing report, Oumeish and associates (1982) described a woman in whom this dermatosis recurred in nine successive pregnancies and also when taking estrogen–progesterone oral contraceptives.

The hallmark lesions of pruritic folliculitis are sterile pustules that form around the margin of erythematous patches that characteristically begin at flexures and extend peripherally. Mucous membranes are usually involved. The characteristic histological lesion is a spongelike epidermal cavity filled with neutrophils, which is referred to as the *spongiform pustule of Kogoj.*

Pruritus is not severe, but constitutional symptoms are common. In addition to nausea, vomiting, diarrhea, and chills and fever, hypoalbuminemia and hypocalcemia are common. Although the pustules are initially sterile, they may become secondarily infected after rupture, and sepsis is a serious concern. Treatment is systemic corticosteroids along with antimicrobials to treat secondary infection and sepsis. The disease may persist for several weeks to months after delivery.

PREEXISTING SKIN DISEASE

A number of chronic dermatological disorders may complicate pregnancy. These may antedate pregnancy or manifest for the first time during pregnancy. Like other chronic disorders, many of these skin diseases usually have no predictable course during pregnancy.

Acne is usually unaffected by pregnancy. For nonpregnant women, treatment may include some of the highly teratogenic cogeners of retinoic acid (see Chap. 14, p. 350). **Isotretinoin, etretinate, and tretinoin are strictly contradicted in pregnancy.** For the pregnant woman with severe acne, topically applied benzoyl peroxide appears to be safe. Severe disease can usually be controlled when it is applied along with either clindamycin or erythromycin gel. *Topical tretinoin* is thought to pose no significant teratogenic risk (Akhavan and Bershad, 2003).

There is evidence that *psoriasis* improves in up to 50 percent of women during pregnancy. It also may worsen in up to 20 percent. A number of regimens used in nonpregnant individuals are contraindicated during pregnancy. Tauscher and co-workers (2002) provided a learned and detailed review of the disorder during pregnancy. They recommended topical corticosteroids for localized disease, and if nonresponsive, stepwise therapy with topical calcipotriene, anthralin, and then tacrolimus. For generalized mild disease, they recommended UV-B phototherapy. If unresponsive, psoralens with UV-B phototherapy are used, followed by oral cyclosporine if unsuccessful. Topical or oral corticosteroids may also be given for moderate or severe disease. Coal tar derivatives, as well as oral and systemic immunosuppressives (e.g., methotrexate, cyclosporine, tacrolimus), are avoided.

Hidradenitis suppurativa is a chronic, progressive, inflammatory and suppurative disorder of skin and supporting structures. It is characterized by apocrine gland plugging that leads to anhidrosis and bacterial infection (von der Werth and Jemec, 2001). The disease is hormonally responsive and thus not seen until puberty. It has been said to be improved by pregnancy, but in our experiences, it is not appreciably changed. Treatment is control of acute infections with either systemic antimicrobials or clindamycin ointment (Boer and van Gemert, 1999).

If *pemphigus* appears during pregnancy for the first time, it may be confused with herpes gestationis (Vaughan Jones and Black, 1999). Even with corticosteroid therapy, mortality is 10 percent secondary to sepsis caused by infection of denuded skin. Lesions of *neurofibromatosis* may increase in size and number as a result of pregnancy. *Hansen disease* primarily affects the skin, and it likely worsens during pregnancy (Aronson and Bass, 2000). Its treatment is discussed in Chapter 58 (see p. 1289).

REFERENCES

Akhavan A, Bershad S: Topical acne drugs: Review of clinical properties, systemic exposure, and safety. Am J Clin Dermatol 4:473, 2003

Amato L, Mei S, Gallerani I, et al: A case of chronic herpes gestationis: Persistent disease or conversion to bullous pemphigoid? J Am Acad Dermatol 49:302, 2003

Aractingi S, Berkane N, Bertheau P, et al: Fetal DNA in skin of polymorphic eruptions of pregnancy. Lancet 352:1898, 1998

Aronson IK, Bass BN: Dermatologic disease. In Barron WM, Lindheimer MD (eds): Medical Disorders During Pregnancy, 3rd ed. St Louis, Mosby, 2000, p 540

Aronson IK, Bond S, Fiedler VC, et al: Pruritic urticarial papules and plaques of pregnancy: Clinical and immunopathologic observations in 57 patients. J Am Acad Dermatol 39:933, 1998

Barinaga M: Cells exchanged during pregnancy live on. Science 296:2169, 2002

Baxi LV, Kovilam OP, Collins MH, et al: Recurrent herpes gestationis with postpartum flare: A case report. Am J Obstet Gynecol 164:778, 1991

Bianchi DW, Romero R: Biological implications of bi-directional fetomaternal cell traffic: A summary of a National Institute of Child Health and Human Development-sponsored conference. J Matern Fetal Neonatal Med 14:123, 2003

Black MM: Dermatoses of pregnancy: New developments. J Dermatol 28:635, 2001

Boer J, van Gemert MJ: Long-term results of isotretinoin in the treatment of 68 patients with hidradenitis suppurativa. J Am Acad Dermatol 40:73, 1999

Chen SH, Chopra K, Evans TY, et al: Herpes gestationis in a mother and child. J Am Acad Dermatol 40:847, 1999

Choi JR, Levine D, Finberg H: Luteoma of pregnancy: Sonographic findings in two cases. J Ultrasound Med 19:877, 2000

Danilowicz K, Albiger N, Vanegas M, et al: Androgen-secreting adrenal adenomas. Obstet Gynecol 100:1099, 2002

Engineer L, Bhol K, Ahmed AR: Pemphigoid gestationis: A review. Am J Obstet Gynecol 183:483, 2000

Erickson NI, Ellis RL: Neonatal rash due to herpes gestationis. N Engl J Med 347:660, 2002

Germain AM, Carvajal JA, Glasinovic JC, et al: Intrahepatic cholestasis of pregnancy: An intriguing pregnancy-specific disorder. J Soc Gynecol Investig 9:10, 2002

Griffiths CEM, Finkel LJ, Ditre CM, et al: Topical tretinoin (retinoic acid) improves melasma. A vehicle-controlled, clinical trial. Br J Dermatol 129:415, 1993

Headington JT: Telogen effluvium: New concepts and review. Arch Dermatol 129:356, 1993

Kimbrough-Green CK, Griffiths CEM, Finkel LJ, et al: Topical retinoic acid (tretinoin) for melasma in black patients. A vehicle-controlled clinical trial. Arch Dermatol 130:727, 1994

Kirkup ME, Dunnill MG: Polymorphic eruption of pregnancy developing in the puerperium. Clin Exp Dermatol 27:657, 2002

Kois JM, Phelan ST: Hair loss in women. Prim Care Update Ob Gyns 1:130, 1994

Kolanko E, Bickle K, Keehn C, et al: Subepidermal blistering disorders: A clinical and histopathologic review. Semin Cutan Med Surg 23:10, 2004

Kroumpouzos G, Cohen LM: Specific dermatoses of pregnancy: An evidence-based systematic review. Am J Obstet Gynecol 188:1083, 2003

Lynfield VL: Effect of pregnancy on the human hair cycle. J Invest Dermatol 35:323, 1960

Mazzi G, Raineri A, Zanolli FA, et al: Plasmapheresis therapy in pemphigus vulgaris and bullous pemphigoid. Transfus Apheresis Sci 28:13, 2003

Oumeish OY, Farraj SE, Bataineh AS: Some aspects of impetigo herpetiformis. Arch Dermatol 118:103, 1982

Paus R, Cotsarelis G: The biology of hair follicles. N Engl J Med 341:491, 1999

Pennoyer JW, Grin CM, Driscoll MS, et al: Changes in size of melanocytic nevi during pregnancy. J Am Acad Dermatol 36:378, 1997

Powell JL, Bailey CL, Coopland AT, et al: Nd:YAG laser excision of a giant gingival pyogenic granuloma of pregnancy. Lasers Surg Med 14:178, 1994

Randall VA: Androgens and human hair growth. Clin Endocrinol 40:439, 1994

Roger D, Vaillant L, Fignon A, et al: Specific pruritic diseases of pregnancy: A prospective study of 3192 pregnant women. Arch Dermatol 130:734, 1994

Rubin AI, Laborde SV, Stiller MJ: Acquired dermal melanocytosis: Appearance during pregnancy. J Am Acad Dermatol 45:609, 2001

Sheehan DJ, Lesher JL Jr. Pyogenic granuloma arising within a port-wine stain. Cutis 73:175, 2004

Sherard GB III, Atkinson SM Jr: Focus on primary care: Pruritic dermatological conditions in pregnancy. Obstet Gynecol Surv 56:427, 2001

Shimanovich I, Bröcker EB, Zillikens D: Pemphigoid gestationis: New insights into the pathogenesis lead to novel diagnostic tools. Br J Obstet Gynaecol 109:970, 2002a

Shimanovich I, Skrobek C, Rose C, et al: Pemphigoid gestationis with predominant involvement of oral mucous membranes and IgA autoantibodies targeting the C-terminus of BP180. J Am Acad Dermatol 47:780, 2002b

Shornick JK: Dermatoses of pregnancy. Semin Cutan Med Surg 17:172, 1998

Shornick JK, Black MM: Fetal risks in herpes gestationis. J Am Acad Dermatol 26:63, 1992

Shornick JK, Jenkins RE, Briggs DC, et al: Anti-HLA antibodies in pemphigoid gestationis (herpes gestationis). Br J Dermatol 129:257, 1993

Sitaru C, Powell J, Messer G, et al: Immunoblotting and enzyme-linked immunosorbent assay for the diagnosis of pemphigoid gestationis. Obstet Gynecol 103:757, 2004

Spetz S: Peripheral circulation during normal pregnancy. Acta Obstet Gynecol Scand 43:309, 1964

Srivatsa B, Srivatsa S, Johnson KL, et al: Maternal cell microchimerism in newborn tissues. J Pediatr 142:31, 2003

Tauscher AE, Fleischer AB Jr, Phelps KC, Feldman SR: Psoriasis and pregnancy. J Cutan Med Surg 6:561, 2002

Van den Bergh F, Giudice GJ: BP180 (type XVII collagen) and its role in cutaneous biology and disease. Adv Dermatol 19:37, 2003

Vaughan Jones SA, Black MM: Pregnancy dermatoses. J Am Acad Dermatol 40:233, 1999

Vaughan Jones SA, Hern S, Nelson-Piercy C, et al: A prospective study of 200 women with dermatoses of pregnancy correlating clinical findings with hormonal and immunopathological profiles. Br J Dermatol 141:71, 1999

von der Werth JM, Jemec GB: Morbidity in patients with hidradenitis suppurativa. Br J Dermatol 144:809, 2001

Wallengren J: Prurigo: Diagnosis and management. Am J Clin Dermatol 5:85, 2004

Wong RC, Ellis CN: Physiologic skin changes in pregnancy. J Am Acad Dermatol 10:929, 1984

57

Neoplastic Diseases

Cancer during pregnancy is uncommon but not rare. Reported rates for most cancers vary widely, reflecting not only differences in populations, but also differing methods of ascertainment and inconsistency of reporting. In a review of more than 4.8 million deliveries in California during a 9-year period, Smith and colleagues (2003) reported the overall incidence of malignant neoplasms to be 0.94 per 1000 live births. The incidence of cancer within 12 months of delivery was 0.6 per 1000; in the prenatal period, 0.27 per 1000; and when diagnosed at the time of delivery, 0.07 per 1000.

According to the National Vital Statistics Report for 2001, malignancies are the second leading cause of death in women 25 to 44 years of age (Arias and associates, 2003). The most common cancers are melanoma and cancers of the hemopoietic and lymphatic systems, thyroid, breast, cervix, ovary, and colon. In their extensive review, Dinh and Warshal (2001) reported that the most frequent cancers in pregnant women were melanoma (1:350), cervical cancer (1:2250), Hodgkin lymphoma (1:3000), breast cancer (1:7500), ovarian cancer (1:18,000), and leukemia (1:75,000). A number of others have reached similar conclusions (Kaiser and associates, 2000; Smith and colleagues, 2003).

Although management of the pregnant woman with cancer is problematic, one basic tenet should be followed: **A woman should not be penalized for being pregnant**. Treatment should be individualized and should include consideration of factors such as type and stage of cancer, the woman's desire to continue the pregnancy, and the risks of modifying or delaying treatment.

PRINCIPLES OF CANCER THERAPY DURING PREGNANCY

SURGERY. Surgical intervention for cancer may be indicated for diagnostic, staging, or therapeutic purposes. Most procedures that do not interfere with the reproductive tract are well tolerated by both mother and fetus. If indicated, the ovaries may be removed without affect to the pregnancy after about 8 weeks. Progesterone should be administered if oophorectomy is performed prior to this (see Chap. 40, p. 966).

Although diagnostic and staging operations have classically been deferred until the second trimester to minimize abortion risks, this probably is not necessary. Specifically, documenting a live fetus with ultrasound between 9 and 11 weeks indicates a 95-percent chance that it will reach viability. In all cases, therapeutic surgery should be performed regardless of gestational age if maternal well-being is imperiled.

RADIATION THERAPY. It is important to emphasize that *diagnostic* radiographic procedures have very low exposure and should not be delayed if they would directly affect therapy (American College of Obstetricians and Gynecologists, 2004). *Therapeutic* radiation, however, can result in significant fetal exposure to ionizing radiation. The amount depends on the dose, tissue being treated, and field size. Potential adverse effects of diagnostic radiation include cell death, carcinogenesis, and genetic effects on future generations (Brent, 1989, 1999; Hall, 1991). As discussed in Chapter 41 (see p. 978), exposure of the embryo to less than 5 cGy (5 rad) has negligible risk of major malformations. In fact, it is likely that the threshold for radiation effects is 15 to 20 cGy (Brent, 1999).

Although the most susceptible period is during organogenesis, no gestational age is considered safe for therapeutic radiation exposure. Characteristic adverse fetal effects are microcephaly and mental retardation. In some cases, even late exposure can cause fetal growth restriction and brain damage. These dangers raise very practical issues. For example, therapeutic radiation doses to the abdomen are contraindicated because of a high risk of fetal death or damage, unless of course abortion induction is one of its purposes. In some cases, such as head and neck cancers, radiotherapy to supradiaphragmatic areas can be given relatively safely with abdominal shielding. In others, such as breast cancer, significant scatter doses can accrue to the fetus.

CHEMOTHERAPY

Effect on Pregnancy Outcome. Chemotherapy is recommended for treatment or as adjunctive therapy along with surgery or radiation in an increasing number of malignancies. Although chemotherapy is often associated with improved long-term maternal outcome, there still is a general reluctance to use these potent agents during pregnancy. Fetal concerns include malformations, growth restriction, mental retardation, and the risk of future malignancies.

The risk for adverse fetal effects is dependent primarily on gestational age during chemotherapy. Most antineoplastic drugs should be considered potentially harmful to the fetus, especially if given during organogenesis. Indeed, embryonic exposure to cytotoxic drugs causes major malformations in 10 to 20 percent of cases (Muslin and colleagues, 2001). After the first trimester, most antineoplastic drugs are without obvious adverse sequelae, although long-term effects have not been evaluated thoroughly (Partridge and Garber, 2000; Nulman and associates, 2001).

In a review of the reproductive toxicology of alkylating agents, Glantz (1994) concluded that these agents could be used after the first trimester if indicated. Doll and colleagues (1988) reached similar conclusions. These observations also apparently apply to the two potent teratogens *all-*trans-*retinoic acid* and *methotrexate,* both of which have few adverse effects after the first trimester (Briggs and coworkers, 2002).

Because the magnitude of secretion of chemotherapeutic agents into breast milk has not been established, breast feeding is not recommended. There is also concern for exposure of health care workers to chemotherapeutic agents. Selevan and colleagues (1985) and Stucker and co-workers (1990) reported a twofold increased risk of fetal loss in nurses exposed during the first trimester. They recommend caution during mixing and administration of antineoplastic drugs (see Chap. 14, p. 353).

Late mutagenic effects on offspring of women treated during pregnancy have also been of concern. Data are limited, but in one study, Li and associates (1979) found only two childhood malignancies in offspring of 146 women treated during 286 pregnancies. In another study, Avilés and Neri (2001) found no adverse sequelae in 84 children exposed to antineoplastic drugs in utero.

Fertility and Pregnancy After Cancer Therapy. In both men and women, subsequent fertility may be diminished after chemotherapy. For example, treatment of advanced Hodgkin lymphoma with multiple-drug regimens may result in azoospermia in men and in decreased follicular maturation with destruction and ovarian fibrosis in women (Waxman, 1985). Gershenson (1988) reviewed subsequent outcomes in women successfully treated with chemotherapy for germ cell ovarian tumors. A third had total or partial ablation of ovarian function. Tangir and associates (2003) reviewed women who had fertility-sparing surgery, usually with chemotherapy, for ovarian germ cell malignancies. More than 75 percent who attempted pregnancy were successful at least once. Falconer and Ferns (2002) presented similar findings. The likelihood of fertility effects is both age- and dose-related. Interestingly, the prepubertal ovary is more resistant to effects of chemotherapy.

With subsequent conception, even with subfertility, there does not appear to be an increased incidence of abortion, fetal chromosomal damage, or fetal anomalies (Rustin and colleagues, 1984). Green and colleagues (2002) reported an analysis of 4029 pregnancies subsequent to treatment for childhood or adolescent cancer. Prior chemotherapy was with most agents not associated with an increased risk of adverse pregnancy outcomes. However, prior therapy with daunorubicin or doxorubicin as well as prior pelvic radiation therapy were associated with an approximately twofold increased risk of delivering an infant who weighed less than 2500 g at birth. Chiarelli and associates (2000) reported similar results.

BREAST CARCINOMA

Likely the most feared cancer by women, breast cancer is the most common malignancy of women of all age groups. Indeed, almost 1 of every 8 women will eventually be afflicted (American College of Obstetricians and Gynecologists, 2003c). Breast cancer is also one of the more common malignancies encountered during pregnancy (Berry and colleagues, 1999; Sorosky and Scott-Conner, 1998). Its

incidence in pregnancy varies with the age of the population studied and averages perhaps 1 in 25,000 to 50,000 pregnancies (Dinh and Warshal, 2001; Shah and Saunders, 2001). As more women choose to delay childbearing until a later age, the frequency of associated breast cancer is expected to increase (Woo and associates, 2003).

According to some studies, women with *BRCA1* and *BRCA2* breast cancer genes, as well as those with a family history of breast cancer, are more likely to develop the malignancy during pregnancy (Johannsson and co-workers, 1998; Shen and colleagues, 1999). Women undergoing induced abortions or those who breast feed do not have an increased risk of breast cancer (Beral and associates, 2004; Michels and colleagues, 1996).

PREGNANCY AND BREAST CANCER. The effects of pregnancy on the course of breast cancer and its prognosis are complex. There are massively increased levels of both estrogens and progestins during pregnancy, and some data suggest that higher estrogen levels cause excess cancer later in life, whereas progesterone may be protective (Ward and Bristow, 2002). Chorionic gonadotropin and relaxin, also produced in prodigious amounts, may inhibit tumor growth (Shah and Saunders, 2001). There is intriguing evidence that higher serum levels of alpha-fetoprotein are associated with a decreased incidence of breast cancer (Melbye and colleagues, 2000). Finally, it appears that interruption of pregnancy has no influence on the course or prognosis of breast cancer.

Most clinical reports maintain that when breast cancer is diagnosed during pregnancy, the regional lymph nodes are more likely to contain microscopic metastases. This is important, because the 5-year survival rate with pregnancy-associated breast cancer is primarily dependent on its stage at diagnosis (Hochman and Schreiber, 1953). Still, survival in pregnant women is comparable stage-for-stage with that in nonpregnant women (King and colleagues, 1985; Nugent and O'Connell, 1985; Zemlickis and associates, 1992). According to Jacob and Stringer (1990), about 30 percent of pregnant women with breast cancer have stage I disease, 30 percent have stage II, and 40 percent stages III or IV. Studies published after 1990 indicate that about 60 percent of pregnant women have concomitant axillary node involvement (Table 57–1).

Other findings support more advanced breast cancer in pregnant women. Zemlickis and associates (1992) found that pregnant women had a 2.5-fold increased risk of metastatic disease compared with that of nonpregnant women. Bonnier and associates (1997) found an inordinately higher incidence of *inflammatory cancer* in 154 pregnant women compared with that of 308 age-matched nonpregnant controls (26 versus 9 percent).

There are usually slight delays in clinical assessment, diagnostic procedures, and treatment of pregnant women with breast tumors (Berry and colleagues, 1999). The mean delay was reported to be 1 to 2 months in recent studies (Woo and associates, 2003). Part of the delay can be attributed to

TABLE 57–1 **Axillary Node Involvement in Pregnancy-Associated Breast Cancer in Reports After 1990**

Investigators	Number	Positive Nodes	
		No.	*(%)*
Petrek et al (1991)	56	34	(61)
Ishida et al (1992)	192	111	(58)
Souadka et al (1994)	43	34	(80)
Bonnier et al (1997)	114	64	(56)
Berry et al (1999)	22	14	(67)
Total	427	257	(60)[a]

[a]Compared with 80 percent reported before 1980.

pregnancy-induced breast changes that tend to obscure breast masses. These are even more magnified during lactation when there is lobular hyperplasia and galactostasis. An important concern is that excessive nodal involvement may be related to delayed diagnosis. This seems unlikely, considering the biology of breast cancer. Nettleton and colleagues (1996) used mathematical modeling to conclude that even a 6-month delay increases the chance of axillary metastasis by only 5 percent. Thus, a delay of a few months to treatment would seem clinically insignificant.

There is no doubt that breast cancer is more aggressive in younger women. Whether it is more aggressive during pregnancy in these same women is debatable. It is reasonable to conclude that later disease stages seem to be more prevalent, and thus overall survival is adversely affected. In the Swedish Cancer Registry, Bladstrom and associates (2003) reported a 5-year survival rate of 52 percent if breast cancer was diagnosed in pregnant women compared with that of 80 percent if it was detected in nonpregnant women.

Placental Metastases. Occasionally, malignant breast cells are found on placental microscopic examination (Dunn and co-workers, 1999). These have been confined to the intervillous space, and fetal disease has not been reported (see Chap. 27, p. 624).

DIAGNOSIS. The diagnostic approach in pregnant women with a breast tumor should not differ significantly from that for nonpregnant women. **Any suspicious breast mass found during pregnancy should prompt an aggressive plan to determine its cause, whether this involves ultrasound, fine-needle aspiration, or biopsy.**

At the University of Alabama, ultrasound is the initial diagnostic study performed on pregnant women with a palpable breast mass. An oval or elongated lesion with smooth borders and no shadowing is highly suggestive of a benign mass. Most masses in pregnancy have these reassuring features, and definitive diagnosis can often await the conclusion of pregnancy.

Mammography should be performed if indicated. The fetal radiation risk is negligible with appropriate shielding, and the exposure is only 0.004 cGy for the typical two-view test (Nicklas and Baker, 2000). Importantly, breast tissue is denser in pregnancy, and mammography is associated with a false-negative rate of 35 to 40 percent (Samuels and colleagues, 1998; Woo and associates, 2003).

In all women in whom ultrasound or mammography of a suspicious mass is still nondiagnostic, or with worrisome clinical features such as skin changes or immobility of the mass, then biopsy is indicated. Although there are no large studies in pregnant women, *core biopsy* may be an ideal diagnostic technique. Fine needle aspiration for cytology is an alternative technique, but it requires a pathologist experienced with pregnancy-associated breast cancer (Woo and associates, 2003).

Once malignancy is diagnosed, a chest radiograph and a limited metastatic search are performed. Although routine computed tomography (CT) scans of bone and liver are both sensitive and specific, they are usually avoided during pregnancy because of excessive radiation (Pelsang, 1998). Magnetic resonance imaging (MRI) is a reasonable alternative to assess liver involvement. It is sensitive and has excellent contrast resolution.

TREATMENT. Breast conservation surgery for small tumors, with or without adjunctive chemo- or radiotherapy, is preferable in nonpregnant women (Fisher and colleagues, 2002; Veronesi and co-workers, 2002). *Surgical treatment* may be definitive for breast carcinoma during pregnancy (Woo and colleagues, 2003). In the absence of metastatic disease, either wide excision, modified radical mastectomy, or total mastectomy with axillary node staging can be performed (Isaacs, 1995). In 22 women treated with modified radical mastectomy followed in most by chemotherapy, Berry and colleagues (1999) reported minimal risks. In nonpregnant women, *adjunctive radiotherapy* is usually given with breast-conserving surgery. However, this is not recommended during pregnancy (Sorosky and Scott-Conner, 1998). Abdominal scatter is considerable; when the maternal radiation dose is 5000 cGy, the fetus receives at least 100 to 150 cGy (Sorosky and Scott-Conner, 1998).

Chemotherapy is recommended for node-positive disease if proximate delivery is not anticipated. It is given for advanced disease, and termination should be considered if pregnancy is early (Shah and Saunders, 2001). Cyclophosphamide, doxorubicin, and 5-fluorouracil are currently recommended by most clinicians. After the first trimester, methotrexate can be substituted for doxorubicin (Sorosky and Scott-Conner, 1998). Because survival is improved with chemotherapy in premenopausal women, it should be considered even if the nodes are cancer free.

PREGNANCY FOLLOWING BREAST CANCER. Some women are rendered infertile by chemotherapy, as discussed previously (see p. 1259). For those who can choose pregnancy, there is little evidence to suggest that pregnancy adversely affects survival in women who have undergone prior breast cancer treatment (Averette and colleagues, 1999). Dow and colleagues (1994) found no differences in rates of recurrences or distant metastases with or without subsequent pregnancies. Reports by Kroman (1997) and Velentgas (1999) and their colleagues have since confirmed these findings.

No data suggest that lactation adversely affects the course of breast cancer. Successful lactation and breast feeding are possible after conservative surgery and radiation for breast cancer, even from the treated side (Higgins and Haffty, 1994).

Recommendations for future pregnancies in women successfully treated for breast malignancy are based on several factors, including consideration for chances of recurrence. It seems reasonable to advise a delay of 2 to 3 years, which is the most critical observation period.

LYMPHOMAS

HODGKIN DISEASE. This is the most common malignant lymphoma encountered in women of childbearing age. It is usually B-cell derived and distinguished from other lymphomas by *Reed–Sternberg cells*. It has a bimodal peak incidence at 18 to 30 years of age and again after 50 years of age. Prognosis is good, and survival is greater than 70 percent.

In more than 70 percent of cases of Hodgkin disease, patients present with painless enlargement of lymph nodes above the diaphragm—the axillary, cervical, or submaxillary chains (Peleg and Ben-Ami, 1998). Other symptoms include fever, night sweats, malaise, weight loss, and pruritus. The most common finding is peripheral adenopathy, and neck and supraclavicular nodes are commonly involved. Diagnosis is established by histological examination of involved nodes.

Pregnancy and Hodgkin Disease. Over the past 30 years at Parkland Hospital, with more than 250,000 pregnancies, Hodgkin disease has been encountered uncommonly. Similarly, in a population-based review of more than 3 million deliveries, Smith and associates (2003) reported this lymphoma to complicate only 1 per 20,000 live births. In their review, however, Pavlidis and colleagues (2002) reported an incidence of Hodgkin disease in pregnancy of 1 in 1000 to 1 in 6000.

Pregnant women with Hodgkin disease present special management considerations. A tenet of treatment is that careful staging is essential, and either local radiotherapy or systemic chemotherapy is indicated. The *Ann Arbor staging system,* shown in Table 57–2, was designed for Hodgkin lymphomas but is also used for other lymphomas. Although pregnancy limits the widespread application of some radiographic studies, at minimum, work-up includes chest radiography, bone marrow biopsy, and abdominal imaging (Williams and Schilsky, 2000). Spiral CT can be used with the "pitch" set so that radiation dose approaches that of conventional scanning

TABLE 57–2 Ann Arbor Staging System for Lymphomas

Stage	Findings
I	Involvement in a single lymph node region or single extralymphatic site.
II	Involvement of two or more lymph node groups on the same side of the diaphragm.
III	Involvement of lymph nodes on both sides of the diaphragm.
IV	Diffuse or disseminated involvement.
V	Extranodal involvement.

Substage A = no symptoms; substage B = fever, sweats, or weight loss.

(see Chap. 41, p. 980). MRI is an excellent alternative for evaluating thoracic and abdominal para-aortic lymph nodes. Radionuclide gallium scanning, which is being used more frequently in nonpregnant patients, emits 0.75 to 1.0 cGy. Staging is considered essential for those patients in whom radiotherapy alone is chosen, because the presence of abdominal disease would significantly alter treatment.

Treatment is individualized depending on stage and pregnancy duration. Radiotherapy is given for stage I disease (isolated lymph node involvement), and the cure rate approaches 90 percent. In pregnancy, radiotherapy is preferable for isolated neck adenopathy, but it is not recommended for areas that deliver significant radiation scatter to the fetus. Nisce and colleagues (1986) temporarily modified their regimen to deliver only 15 to 20 Gy to supradiaphragmatic sites in seven women after the first trimester. Despite this reduction to what were considered subcurative doses, fetal radiation exposure ranged from 2 to 50 cGy and averaged about 20 cGy. When evaluated at 6 to 11 years of age, all seven children were normal, but two mothers had died.

As discussed on page 1258, chemotherapy is probably best avoided during the first trimester. With obvious widespread disease, however, we recommend that chemotherapy be given. Postponement of therapy until fetal maturity is achieved seems justifiable only when the diagnosis is made late in pregnancy and maternal health would not be jeopardized.

Pregnancy does not adversely affect the course or survival of women with Hodgkin lymphoma (Pavlidis, 2002). Moreover, pregnancy wastage is not increased. Because aggressive radiation and chemotherapy are often necessary for cure, pregnancy termination is reasonable when the diagnosis is made in the first half of pregnancy. Jacobs and associates (1981) reported their experiences from Stanford University and found that neither chemotherapy during the second and third trimesters nor irradiation to the mediastinum and neck adversely affected the fetus or neonate. **Pregnant women with Hodgkin disease are inordinately susceptible to infections and sepsis, and both radiotherapy and chemotherapy increase this susceptibility.**

Long-Term Prognosis. Horning and co-workers (1981) reported that 55 percent of women resumed normal menses after chemotherapy. There were no birth defects in 24 infants subsequently born to these women. The risk of second cancers, especially leukemia, is substantively increased after cure of Hodgkin disease. Tucker and colleagues (1988) reported a secondary cancer rate of almost 20 percent within 15 years. Kaldor and associates (1990) reported that the risk of leukemia was increased almost ninefold following chemotherapy when compared with that of radiotherapy given alone. Travis and co-workers (2003) recently presented follow-up data from 3817 female survivors who were treated for Hodgkin disease before 30 years of age. Women treated with radiation had an overall 3.2-fold increased risk of breast cancer. When given chemotherapy alone, the risk was significantly decreased below baseline. Other complications of therapy for Hodgkin disease include myocardial damage and infarction, pulmonary fibrosis, hypothyroidism, and marrow suppression (Peleg and Ben-Ami, 1998).

NON-HODGKIN LYMPHOMAS. Usually B-cell lymphomas, these can also be T-cell or natural killer–cell neoplasms. They are further classified as indolent, aggressive, or highly aggressive (Williams and Schilsky, 2000). Their biology, classification, and treatment were recently reviewed by Evans and Hancock (2003). Non-Hodgkin lymphomas are more aggressive than Hodgkin lymphomas, and survival is perhaps 50 percent. The incidence of non-Hodgkin lymphomas has risen sharply because of their relationship to human immunodeficiency virus (HIV) infection. Indeed, 5 to 10 percent of persons infected with HIV develop a lymphoma.

Reported concurrence of non-Hodgkin lymphoma with pregnancy is limited. In an earlier review, Ward and Weiss (1989) described only 75 cases associated with pregnancy. Avilés and colleagues (1990) reported their experiences with 16 pregnant women with non-Hodgkin lymphomas, half of whom were in the first trimester. They were treated with cytotoxic drugs and there were no fetal malformations. All but one offspring were healthy at 3 to 11 years. Half of the mothers who had remissions were alive 4 to 9 years later. In another study, Avilés and Neri (2001) described long-term follow-up of 55 children whose mothers had received chemotherapy for lymphomas during pregnancy. They found no congenital, neurological, or psychological abnormalities at 6 to 29 years and observed that there were also no cancers, including leukemia.

Burkitt lymphoma is an aggressive B-cell tumor. Barnes and associates (1998) reviewed 19 pregnancies complicated by this lymphoma and 17 women did not survive for one year. Pollack and colleagues (1993) described an HIV-infected woman with a B-cell lymphoma that metastasized to the placenta. Catlin and co-workers (1999) described a fascinating case in which a maternal T-cell/natural killer–cell lymphoma metastasized transplacentally and engrafted the fetus. Both mother and infant succumbed from the malignancy.

Management. Staging for non-Hodgkin lymphomas is also with the Ann Arbor system (see Table 57–2). Radiotherapy typically is used for stage I disease, whereas chemotherapy is recommended for most stage II and all stage III and IV tumors. Unfortunately, the disease is often widespread when the peripheral nodes are involved, and staging laparotomy is of little or no benefit (Peleg and Ben-Ami, 1998).

LEUKEMIAS

Adult leukemias are more prevalent after 40 years of age. Despite this, acute leukemias are among the most common malignancies of young women. Paradoxically, their incidence complicating pregnancy is only about 1 case per 100,000 (Harrison and colleagues, 1994; Pavlidis, 2002). Our experiences at Parkland Hospital indicate that it is more common, and we have managed about 15 women with leukemia in nearly 350,000 pregnancies. Caligiuri and Mayer (1989) reviewed 350 reports of pregnancy complicated by leukemia. Of 72 newly diagnosed cases during pregnancy and reported since 1975, 44 had acute myelogenous leukemia, 20 had acute lymphocytic leukemia, and eight had one of the chronic leukemias.

PREGNANCY AND LEUKEMIA. Before 1970, maternal mortality in 256 women was reported to be 100 percent and perinatal mortality was 34 percent (McLain, 1974). According to Lewis and Laros (1986), maternal death since 1970 has been negligible, although ultimate survival is poor. With contemporaneous therapy, remission during pregnancy is almost 75 percent. Unfortunately, acute leukemias commonly relapse within a year (Pejovic and colleagues, 2001).

Greenlund and associates (2001) reviewed experiences with 17 cases of acute leukemia during pregnancy. There were 13 women with newly diagnosed acute myeloid leukemia, and the remission rate was 70 percent. Importantly, three of four women who elected to delay chemotherapy until after delivery died within days of delivery and just after beginning such therapy. Survival has also improved for women with *chronic myelogenous* and *chronic lymphocytic leukemias*. The rare, chronic *hairy-cell leukemia* has been reported in only six pregnancies (Stiles and colleagues, 1998).

Perinatal Outcome. Although perinatal survival has improved somewhat, morbidity is still substantial. Reynoso and colleagues (1987) reviewed 58 cases of acute leukemia in pregnant women. Nearly 75 percent were diagnosed during the second and third trimesters. About 50 percent were acute myelogenous leukemia, and most cases were treated with chemotherapy and had a remission rate of 75 percent. Only 40 percent of these pregnancies resulted in liveborn infants. Caligiuri and Mayer (1989) reported preterm delivery in about half of women diagnosed during pregnancy. The stillbirth rate was also increased. Leukemia cells may be seen in the placenta, however, these are usually in the intervillous space, and maternal-to-fetal transmission has never been authenticated (see Chap. 27, p. 624).

Management. Manifestations of leukemia include anemia, neutropenia, and thrombocytopenia. Thus significant complications in pregnancy, including infection and hemorrhage, should be anticipated at the time of delivery in women with active disease.

In general, aggressive multi-agent chemotherapy is given as soon as leukemia is diagnosed, even in the first trimester. There is no evidence that pregnancy has a deleterious effect on leukemia, thus, termination will not improve the prognosis. Abortion is a consideration in early pregnancy to avoid potential teratogenesis from chemotherapy and to simplify management of an acutely ill woman.

Treatment given for acute promyelocytic leukemia in pregnancy has included all-*trans*-retinoic-acid (or tretinoin) (Carradice, 2002; Celo, 1994; Harrison, 1994, and all their associates). As discussed in Chapter 14 (see p. 351), this is a potent teratogen. Although outcomes have been generally good, Siu and colleagues (2002) described transient dilated cardiomyopathy in a newborn exposed to tretinoin in the second trimester. Hansen and colleagues (2001) reported transient oligohydramnios in each of three cycles of intensive multi-agent chemotherapy for leukemia.

MALIGNANT MELANOMA

Melanomas are relatively common in women of childbearing age, and many may have the diagnosis made during pregnancy (MacKie, 1999). The general incidence of melanomas has been increasing over the last several decades at a rate faster than other malignancies (Katz and associates, 2002; MacKie and co-workers, 2002). The incidence in pregnancy has been estimated to range from 0.14 to 2.8 per 1000 live births (Wong and Strassner, 1990). As emphasized by Salopek and colleagues (1995), however, melanomas are underreported because many are treated on an outpatient basis and are not entered into a tumor registry.

Melanomas are most common in light-skinned Caucasians. More than 90 percent originate in the skin from pigment-producing melanocytes, usually arising from a preexisting nevus. Any suspicious "behavior" in a pigmented cutaneous lesion such as changes in contour, surface elevation, discoloration, itching, bleeding, or ulceration warrants a biopsy.

Melanomas are staged clinically. In stage I, there are no palpable lymph nodes; in stage II, there are palpable nodes; and in stage III, there are distant metastases. According to Squatrito and Harlow (1998), approximately 85 percent of cases are stage I disease. In contrast, Daryanani and colleagues (2003) reported that only about 50 percent of 610 consecutive women of childbearing age with melanoma had stage I disease. Tumor thickness is the single most important predictor of survival in stage I patients. The *Clark classification* is most widely used and includes five levels of involvement by depth into the epidermis, dermis, and subcutaneous fat. Tumor thickness is also measured using the *Breslow scale.*

PREGNANCY AND MELANOMA. In a recent review, Katz and associates (2002) explored the "myths of melanoma in pregnancy." For example, for many years it was widely held that the prognosis was worse during pregnancy and that future pregnancies increased the recurrence risk. In a review of 11 studies, however, Holly (1986) concluded that there was no adverse effect on survival if melanoma was diagnosed during pregnancy, or if pregnancy developed in a woman with previously recognized melanoma. Pregnancy is, however, associated with a later stage at diagnosis. MacKie and colleagues (1999) described findings from the World Health Organization Melanoma Programme indicating that women diagnosed during pregnancy had significantly greater tumor thickness.

Primary surgical treatment for melanoma is determined by the stage of the disease and includes wide local resection, sometimes with extensive regional lymph node dissection. Schwartz and associates (2003) have recommended sentinel lymph node mapping and biopsy using ^{99m}Tc-sulfur colloid that has a fetal dose of less than 100 mGy (see Chap. 41, p. 981). Cascinelli and co-workers (1998) reported that routine regional node dissection improved survival in nonpregnant patients with microscopic metastases. Prophylactic chemotherapy or immunotherapy is usually avoided during pregnancy. However, chemotherapy for active disease is given if indicated by tumor stage and maternal prognosis. In most cases of distant metastatic melanoma, treatment is at best palliative.

Therapeutic abortion does not appear to improve survival in women with melanoma (Dipaola and colleagues, 1997). Prognosis is determined by the stage, and deep cutaneous invasion or regional node involvement confers a much poorer prognosis. As discussed, women who are pregnant when melanoma is diagnosed typically have thicker skin tumors. These women have a correspondingly higher mortality rate when compared with women whose melanoma was diagnosed before or after pregnancy (Fig. 57–1). Survival is equivalent, however, stage-for-stage, when pregnancy is compared with nonpregnancy. Kjems and Krag (1993) summarized the survival rate from five studies of 338 pregnant and 1360 nonpregnant women with stage I melanoma. They found no significant differences in 5-year survival rates between the two groups. Recurrences manifest by 2 years in 60 percent and 5 years in 90 percent, thus, most clinicians recommend that pregnancy be avoided for 3 to 5 years after treatment. There does not appear to be an adverse effect of oral contraceptives in these women (Katz and associates, 2002; Schwartz and colleagues, 2003).

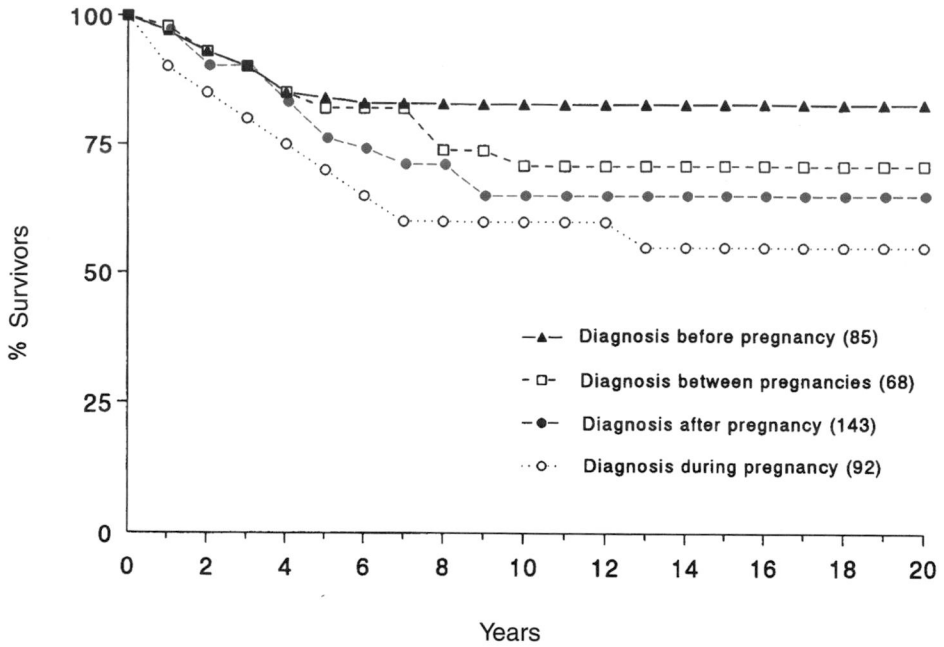

FIGURE 57–1. Disease-free survival in 388 women with malignant melanoma enrolled in the World Health Organization Melanoma Programme. Decreased survival in women diagnosed during pregnancy is due to increased thickness of tumors. (Modified from MacKie and colleagues, 1991, with permission.)

Placental Metastases. Metastasis of any tumor type to the placenta or fetus is uncommon. However, a third of reported cases have been malignant melanoma. In an extensive review, Alexander and colleagues (2003) found that placental metastasis had been reported in 27 cases of melanoma. The infants were affected in six of these cases and died in five.

GENITAL CANCER

Combined together, genital tract cancers are the most common malignancies encountered during pregnancy. Their distribution is summarized in Table 57–3.

CERVICAL NEOPLASIA. Pregnancy provides an opportune time for screening for cervical neoplasia and premalig-

nant disease, especially in women who do not seek or have access to routine health care (American College of Obstetricians and Gynecologists, 2002). Incidence data for cervical neoplasia complicating pregnancy varies widely. As expected, cervical dysplasia is quite common; Jolles (1989) cited an incidence in women of reproductive age of 26 per 1000. The incidence of carcinoma in situ was about 5 per 1000 women. According to Hacker and associates (1982), the average incidence of carcinoma in situ in pregnancy is about 1.3 per 1000. The incidence of invasive carcinoma is usually cited at about 1 per 2000 pregnancies (Anderson and colleagues, 2001). In our experiences with a high-risk population both from Parkland Hospital and from the University of Alabama, invasive cervical cancer is not nearly so common.

There is very limited experience with pregnancy following *radical trachelectomy* for fertility preservation in stage IB$_1$ and IB$_2$ cervical cancer. Del Priore and colleagues (2003) presented preliminary results in 20 women treated in this manner.

INTRAEPITHELIAL NEOPLASIA. The effects of pregnancy and delivery on premalignant and malignant epithelial cervical lesions are not understood completely. In the study by Kiguchi and co-workers (1981), progression from dysplasia to invasive carcinoma after delivery was 0.4 percent compared with that of 1 percent for nonpregnant women. The regression rates of moderate and marked dysplasia within 6 months after delivery were also higher than for the general population. It is well known that certain types of human papillomavirus (HPV) are associated with high-grade intraepithelial lesions as well as invasive cancer. Fife and colleagues (1996) found an increased incidence of high-cancer-risk viruses—HPV types 16, 18, 31, 35, 45, 51, 52, and 56—when they compared pregnant with nonpregnant women.

TABLE 57–3 Frequency of Genital Malignancies Associated with Pregnancy

	Primary Site (%)			
	Cervix	*Ovary*	*Corpus*	*Vulva/Vagina*
Barber and Brunschwig (1963) (n = 62)	76	16	3	5
Phelan (1968) (n = 27)	96	4	—	—
Lutz et al (1977) (n = 40)	75	10	—	15
Haas (1984) (n = 261)	88	8	1	—
Total (n = 390)	85	9	1	3

Adapted from Nevin and associates (1995).

The incidence of abnormal cervical cytology during pregnancy is at least as high as that reported for nonpregnant women. Evaluation of the Papanicolaou smear can, however, be more difficult during pregnancy (Connor, 1998). According to the 2001 Consensus Guidelines for the Management of Women with Cervical Cytological Abnormalities, evaluation of a smear with atypical squamous cells of undetermined significance (ASCUS) is the same as for nonpregnant women (Wright and colleagues, 2002). For pregnant women with high-grade squamous intraepithelial lesions, it is recommended that colposcopic examination be performed by clinicians with experience in pregnancy-induced cytological changes. They further recommend that lesions suspicious of high-grade disease or malignancy be biopsied. In the event of unsatisfactory colposcopy, repeat examination should be performed in 6 to 12 weeks. After delivery, repeat cytology and colposcopy should generally be delayed for at least 6 weeks (Wright and associates, 2002).

During pregnancy, colposcopic evaluation is easier to perform because the transformation zone is better exposed due to physiological eversion. Colposcopically directed biopsies are used liberally to assess any suspicious lesions (Palle and co-workers, 2000; Wright and associates, 2002). Multiple biopsies need not all be taken on one occasion but rather may be obtained over time. The diagnostic accuracy of colposcopy is 99 percent, and complications occur in less than 1 percent of cases (Economos and associates, 1993). Biopsy sites may actively bleed because of hyperemia, but this can be stopped with Monsel solution, silver nitrate, vaginal packing, or occasionally a suture.

For obvious reasons, *endocervical curettage* should **not** be performed during pregnancy (Wright and associates, 2002).

Loop electrosurgical excision procedure (LEEP) and *cone biopsy* usually are reserved to exclude invasive cancer. If possible, conization is avoided in pregnant women because of an increased incidence of hemorrhage, abortion, and preterm labor. Indeed, conization during pregnancy is less than satisfactory for at least three reasons:

1. The epithelium and underlying stroma within the cervical canal cannot be excised extensively because of the risk of membrane rupture. Of 376 conizations during pregnancy reviewed by Hacker and colleagues (1982), residual neoplasia was found in 43 percent of subsequent specimens.
2. Blood loss is common. Averette and colleagues (1970) reported that nearly 10 percent of 180 pregnant women required transfusion.
3. There is a 1.6-fold relative risk of preterm delivery (El-Bastawissi and colleagues, 1999).

If cytological changes of mild cervical intraepithelial neoplasia are identified and subsequently confirmed, further follow-up during pregnancy may consist of colposcopic evaluation. In the absence of lesions detected by a satisfactory colposcopy, simply repeating the cervical smears later in pregnancy is usually adequate. Cytological changes suggestive of moderate or severe dysplasia or invasive disease require colposcopically directed biopsies.

Women with histologically confirmed intraepithelial neoplasia may be followed with cytology and colposcopically directed biopsies, allowed to deliver vaginally, and provided definitive treatment after delivery. In a study by Yost and colleagues (1999), there was regression postpartum in 68 percent of women with grade II and 70 percent of those with grade III neoplasia. Although 7 percent of women with grade II lesions progressed to grade III lesions, no lesion progressed to invasive carcinoma.

Invasive Cervical Cancer. Pregnancy coexisting with cervical carcinoma complicates both staging and treatment. Accurate determination of the extent of cancer is more difficult during pregnancy because induration of the base of the broad ligaments may be less prominent during pregnancy. Such induration in nonpregnant women characterizes tumor spread beyond the cervix. Thus, the extent of the tumor is more likely to be underestimated in pregnant women.

Limited CT of the pelvis is acceptable. During pregnancy, MRI is a useful adjunct to ascertain disease extent, including urinary tract involvement (Gilstrap and colleagues, 2001; Hannigan, 1990). Cystoscopy and sigmoidoscopy can be performed as necessary to rule out mucosal involvement.

Because cervical carcinoma is relatively uncommon during pregnancy, only a few institutions have had extensive experience with its management. Some generalizations, however, can be made. Stage-for-stage, the survival rate for invasive carcinoma has not been profoundly different for pregnant and nonpregnant women. Van der Vange and colleagues (1995) performed a case-control study of 44 women with pregnancy-associated cervical cancer. The overall 5-year survival rate was 80 percent among pregnant women and 82 percent among nonpregnant controls.

The mode of delivery has not been shown to affect maternal survival significantly. Experiences are limited, however, and most women have undergone hysterotomy (Hacker and colleagues, 1982). In general, when frankly invasive carcinoma is identified, most clinicians favor abdominal delivery, if for no other reason than to prevent cervical laceration during labor and delivery.

MANAGEMENT. Treatment of cervical cancer varies for each individual patient, depending on the stage and pregnancy duration as well as the woman's desire to continue the pregnancy. Counseling and treatment include a multidisciplinary approach (American College of Obstetricians and Gynecologists, 2002). Treatment for microinvasive disease diagnosed by cone biopsy follows guidelines similar to those for intraepithelial disease. In general, continuation of pregnancy and vaginal delivery are considered safe, and definitive therapy is provided postpartum.

Invasive cancer demands relatively prompt therapy. During the first half of pregnancy, immediate treatment may be advisable. This of course depends on the decision to continue the pregnancy. During the latter half of pregnancy, a reasonable option is to await not only fetal viability but also fetal maturity (Greer and colleagues, 1989). In a review of 12 pregnant women with invasive cervical carcinoma, van Vliet and colleagues (1998) concluded that delayed treatment was reasonable in women with nonbulky lesions. These included women past 20 weeks with lesions less than stage IIB. Takushi and associates (2002) described outcomes in 28 pregnant women, 22 with stage I disease, and reached similar conclusions. The bulk of other studies of women with early stages of cervical cancer indicate that intentional delay in treatment did not appear to increase the recurrence risk (American College of Obstetricians and Gynecologists, 2002; Goff and associates, 2000).

Preferred treatment for invasive carcinoma in most women with stage I and early stage IIA lesions less than 3 cm is *radical hysterectomy plus pelvic lymphadenectomy*. This said, both radical surgery and radiation result in similar cure rates for early cervical cancer during pregnancy (American College of Obstetricians and Gynecologists, 2002). Surgical treatment is favored because it preserves ovarian and sexual function as well as avoids exposure of the intestinal and urinary tracts to radiation and its adverse effects. Nisker and Shubat (1983) described 49 cases of stage IB cervical cancer complicating pregnancy and reported a 30-percent severe complication rate from radiotherapy compared with only a 7-percent with radical surgery. Before 20 weeks, hysterectomy is usually performed with the fetus in situ. In later pregnancy, however, hysterotomy may first be necessary.

Radiotherapy is given for more extensive cancer. If the woman chooses treatment early in pregnancy, external irradiation is given and if spontaneous abortion does not ensue, then curettage is performed. During the second trimester, spontaneous abortion may be delayed, and hysterotomy may be necessary in up to a fourth of cases. About a week following abortion, external radiation is begun, followed by intracavitary radium application. After 24 weeks, the risk of delay to allow fetal maturity is unknown, but allowing pulmonary maturity seems reasonable, especially for early lesions.

DELIVERY. The mode of delivery remains controversial, especially for small, early-stage lesions. It is not clear if vaginal delivery through a cancerous cervix worsens the prognosis (American College of Obstetricians and Gynecologists, 2002). Most gynecological oncologists, however, favor abdominal delivery based on theoretical considerations. Large bulky and friable lesions may cause significant hemorrhage with vaginal delivery. Finally, recurrences in the episiotomy scar after vaginal delivery have been reported (Cliby and colleagues, 1994). In their review, Goldman and Goldberg (2003) described 12 cases. Although most recurrent lesions manifest by 6 months postpartum, one woman was asymptomatic until 5 years after delivery.

TABLE 57–4 Five-Year Survival Rates of Pregnant and Nonpregnant Women Treated for Cervical Cancer

Study	Pregnant		Nonpregnant	
	No.	(%)	No.	(%)
Sablinska et al (1977)				
Stage I	114	(72)	208	(76)
Stage II	116	(54)	270	(56)
Lee et al (1981)				
Stage IA	3	(100)	30	(100)
Stage IB–surgery	17	(93)	156	(91)
Stage IB–radiation	4	(80)	32	(88)
Nisker and Shubat (1983)				
Stage IB	49	(70)	NS	(87)
van der Vange et al (1995)				
Stages IA, IB, IIA	21	(85)	18	(85)

NS = not stated.

PROGNOSIS. The overall prognosis for all stages of cervical cancer during pregnancy is probably similar to that for nonpregnant women (Sood and Sorosky, 1998). The results from several reports suggest no difference in survival when pregnant women are compared with nonpregnant women (Table 57–4).

ENDOMETRIAL CARCINOMA. Because endometrial carcinoma characteristically develops in women past reproductive age, it is seen only rarely with pregnancy. Schammel and colleagues (1998) reviewed 14 reported cases and described an additional five. The majority of cases described have been well-differentiated adenocarcinomas. Treatment usually consists primarily of abdominal hysterectomy and bilateral salpingo-oophorectomy. Schammel and colleagues (1998) have described conservative therapy with curettage with or without progestational therapy in nonpregnant women. At least four viable infants subsequently were delivered to these 19 women. Gotlieb and associates (2003) reported 13 women treated with progestins for adenocarcinoma. Four of six women with a recurrence were re-treated and responded. At least nine infants have been delivered to these 13 women. Anderson and associates (2001) emphasized that this approach should not be encouraged as standard therapy.

OVARIAN CARCINOMA. Malignant ovarian neoplasms are the fourth most common cause of death from cancer in women and the leading cause of death from genital tract cancers. The incidence of death from ovarian cancer is higher than from both cervical and uterine cancer combined (American College of Obstetricians and Gynecologists, 2003a). The incidence of ovarian malignancy during pregnancy is not accurately known, but it averages about 1 per 20,000 deliveries (Rahman and co-workers, 2002). According to the American

College of Obstetricians and Gynecologists (1990), about 1 of every 1000 pregnant women undergoes surgical exploration for an adnexal mass. As discussed in Chapter 40 (see p. 965), most adnexal masses encountered during pregnancy are either mature teratomas or cystadenomas (Boulay and Podczaski, 1998). According to several reviews, perhaps 5 percent of adnexal neoplasms diagnosed during pregnancy are malignant, compared with 15 to 20 percent in nonpregnant women (Jacob and Stringer, 1990; Whitecar and associates, 1999). This is likely due to the younger age of pregnant women and because of the disparate number of corpus luteum cysts.

Pregnancy apparently does not alter the prognosis of most ovarian malignancies, but complications such as torsion and rupture may develop. Occasionally, primary or metastatic ovarian tumors cause virilization during pregnancy (Powell and associates, 2002; Tinkanen and Kuoppala, 2001). Because most women undergo sonography during pregnancy, the detection of adnexal masses has increased concomitantly. Certainly, sonography is indicated for women in whom there is a palpable adnexal mass. Sonography is also helpful to differentiate cystic masses from solid or multiseptated masses. With the former, expectant management is acceptable, but the latter require surgery for diagnosis (see Chap. 40, p. 965).

Management. Treatment of ovarian cancer in pregnant women is similar to that for nonpregnant women. It also depends on gestational age as well as the stage, histological type, and grade of the tumor.

After frozen section verifies malignancy, complete surgical staging with careful inspection of all peritoneal and visceral surfaces is performed (Yazigi and associates, 1988). **Even malignant ovarian tumors apparently confined to one ovary require complete surgical staging, as do tumors of low malignant potential.** Procedures include peritoneal washings for cytological examination, multiple biopsies of the diaphragmatic undersurface and pelvic and parietal peritoneum, wedge resection of the opposite ovary, partial omentectomy, and excisional biopsies of pelvic and aortic lymph nodes. Whereas in most advanced stages, hysterectomy and bilateral adnexectomy are indicated, in certain circumstances it may be justified to remove the tumor and await fetal maturity. In some cases, chemotherapy can be given while awaiting pulmonary maturation. Maternal CA-125 serum levels are too variable during pregnancy to monitor response to therapy (Aslam and associates, 2000; Spitzer and colleagues, 1998).

Prognosis. Two thirds of ovarian cancers found during pregnancy are of the common epithelial types (Jolles, 1989). The remainder are germ cell tumors, and occasionally a stromal cell tumor. There have been about 80 or 90 cases of invasive *epithelial cell tumors* reported coexistent with pregnancy (Dgani and colleagues, 1989; Rahman and associates, 2002). Because of the relatively young age of the pregnant population, there is a higher proportion of less-advanced tumors.

Thus, tumors with low malignant potential and stage IA disease are seen more often in pregnant women than in nonpregnant women.

Karlen and associates (1979) reviewed 27 cases of *dysgerminomas* during pregnancy. They found significant obstetrical complications in nearly half and reported a 30-percent recurrence with apparent stage IA cases. Since then, a number of reports have been more encouraging. Tangir and colleagues (2003) described their 20-year experiences with 64 women with *malignant germ cell ovarian tumors* treated with fertility-sparing surgery and usually chemotherapy. Of 38 who attempted pregnancy, 29 had a total of 39 children. They also reviewed a number of studies with similar successes.

Young and associates (1984) reviewed 36 cases of stage I *gonadal stromal tumors* that had an excellent prognosis. An *endodermal sinus tumor* has been diagnosed because of persistently elevated maternal serum alpha-fetoprotein levels (van der Zee and colleagues, 1991). This tumor has an overall bad prognosis (Malhotra and Sood, 2000). Maymon and co-workers (1998) described a woman with primary ovarian *hepatoid carcinoma* who also had elevated maternal serum alpha-fetoprotein levels. Kalir and Friedman (1998) have described a *gynandroblastoma*—sex cord and stromal cells of both ovarian and testicular types—in a 32-year-old pregnant woman.

VULVAR CANCER. Invasive *squamous cell carcinoma* of the vulva is primarily a disease of postmenopausal women and thus is only rarely associated with pregnancy (Regan and Rosenzweig, 1993). In their review, Heller and associates (2000) found 23 cases and described a 28-year-old woman with a 4-cm vulvar lesion noted near term. They concluded that radical surgery for stage I disease was feasible during pregnancy, even in the last trimester. Anderson and colleagues (2001) are of the opinion that definitive therapy can often be delayed because of the slow rate of progression of vulvar carcinoma. Treatment is individualized according to the clinical stage and depth of invasion. Vaginal delivery is not contraindicated if the vulvar and inguinal incisions are well healed.

Vulvar intraepithelial neoplasia is seen more often in young women, and it is often associated with HPV. It may progress to invasive disease, the rate of which seems to have risen in younger women (Messing and Gallup, 1995).

Kuller and colleagues (1990) reviewed five cases of *vulvar sarcoma* discovered during pregnancy. In four of these, cure was obtained by a variety of therapies. **Any suspicious vulvar lesion detected during pregnancy should be biopsied.**

UTERINE LEIOMYOMAS. Benign uterine leiomyomas are common in older pregnant women, especially in black women. Because they are seldom malignant, leiomyomas complicating pregnancy are considered in detail in Chapter 40 (see p. 962).

Leiomyomatosis Peritonealis Disseminata. Rarely at cesarean section or puerperal tubal ligation, numerous subperitoneal smooth muscle tumors are found that at first appear to be disseminated carcinomatosis. This is termed *leiomyomatosis peritonealis disseminata* and it results from stimulation, probably by estrogen, of multicentric subcoelomic mesenchymal cells to become smooth muscle cells. According to the review by Lashgari and colleagues (1994), about half of the 45 reported cases were discovered during pregnancy. Although surgical excision has been recommended, there is evidence that these tumors regress after pregnancy. Marom and associates (1998) as well as Ling and colleagues (2000) have described women who had tumors extending up the vena cava into the heart. Bekkers and colleagues (1999) have reported a rare malignant *leiomyoblastoma* during pregnancy.

GASTROINTESTINAL TRACT CANCER

COLORECTAL CARCINOMA. Cancers of the colon and rectum are the second most frequent malignancies in women of all age groups in the United States. These tumors seldom complicate pregnancy because they are uncommon before 40 years of age. Accordingly, fewer than 250 cases of colon cancer have been reported in pregnant women (Walsh and Fazio, 1998). The majority (80 percent or more) of colorectal carcinomas in pregnant women arise from the rectum (Skilling, 1998).

The most common symptoms of colorectal cancer are abdominal pain, distention, nausea and vomiting, constipation, and rectal bleeding. The diagnosis may be delayed because these symptoms may be ascribed to the pregnancy. Certainly, if symptoms suggestive of colon disease persist, digital rectal examination, tests for occult blood, and flexible sigmoidoscopy or colonoscopy are done. Tumors above the peritoneal reflection are uncommon in pregnancy, and Chan and associates (1999a) described only 41 cases in their review. Van Voorhis and Cruikshank (1989) reported two women with colon cancer who had persistent microcytic, hypochromic anemia from occult bleeding.

Treatment of colorectal cancer in pregnant women follows the same general guidelines as for nonpregnant women. When there is no evidence of metastatic disease, surgery is performed. Unfortunately, pregnant women usually present with advanced disease (Walsh and Fazio, 1998). During the first half of the pregnancy, hysterectomy is not necessary to perform colon or rectal resection, and thus therapeutic abortion is not mandated. During later pregnancy, as well as in the presence of metastatic disease, delaying therapy to allow fetal maturation is considered. Vaginal delivery is usually permitted if obstetrical conditions are favorable, but rectal lesions below the pelvic brim may cause dystocia. Hemorrhage, obstruction, or perforation may force surgical intervention (Donegan, 1983).

There is no evidence that pregnancy influences the usual course of colorectal cancer. Thus, prognosis is similar to that for identical stages in nonpregnant patients. Carcinoembryonic antigen (CEA), a useful tumor marker for colon cancer, may be elevated during normal pregnancy and therefore is of little value.

OTHER GASTROINTESTINAL NEOPLASMS. *Gastric cancer* is rarely associated with pregnancy, and most reported cases are from Japan. Hirabayashi and collaborators (1987) reviewed outcomes in 60 pregnant women with this malignancy seen over a 70-year period from 1916 to 1985. Unfortunately, delay in diagnosis during pregnancy was common, and the prognosis was consistently poor; 88 percent of women were dead within 1 year of diagnosis. Persistent upper gastrointestinal symptoms should be evaluated by endoscopy. Davis and Chen (1991) and Chan and colleagues (1999b) each described a woman with gastric cancer who attributed her continued epigastric pain during pregnancy to preexisting peptic ulcer disease.

Stewart and colleagues (1997) reviewed their experiences with seven pregnancies in five women with *Zollinger–Ellison syndrome*. They advise surgical resection of the tumor before pregnancy is undertaken, but in women with metastatic disease or in those with previously undiagnosed tumors, antacid and antisecretory treatment usually suffices.

At least 21 cases of *carcinoid tumors* complicating pregnancy have been reported. In his review, Durkin (1983) found that most cases were of gastrointestinal origin, and some were incidentally diagnosed at cesarean delivery. *Pancreatic cancer* is rare during pregnancy (Gamberdella, 1984; Levy and colleagues, 2004). Primary *hepatocellular carcinoma* during pregnancy also is rare (Gisi and Floyd, 1999; Hsieh and associates, 1996). Balderston and co-workers (1998) described a 23-year-old woman at 26 weeks who had a massive intrahepatic cholangiocarcinoma masquerading as HELLP syndrome (hemolysis, elevated liver enzymes, low platelet count). She died 3 weeks postpartum. Hsu and colleagues (2001) reported a case of spontaneous rupture of hepatocellular carcinoma at 25 weeks that was treated by packing. The pregnancy continued until 41 weeks.

RENAL TUMORS

Walker and Knight (1986) reviewed 71 cases of primary renal neoplasms associated with pregnancy. Half were *renal cell carcinoma*, and a palpable abdominal mass was the presenting finding in almost 90 percent of these women. In half, pain was the presenting symptom, and hematuria was also found in half. Only a fourth of these women had the classical triad of hematuria, pain, and palpable mass. Diagnosis of these and other intra-abdominal or retroperitoneal tumors has been improved by CT and MRI studies such as the one shown in Figure 57–2. Smith and co-workers (1994) added nine new

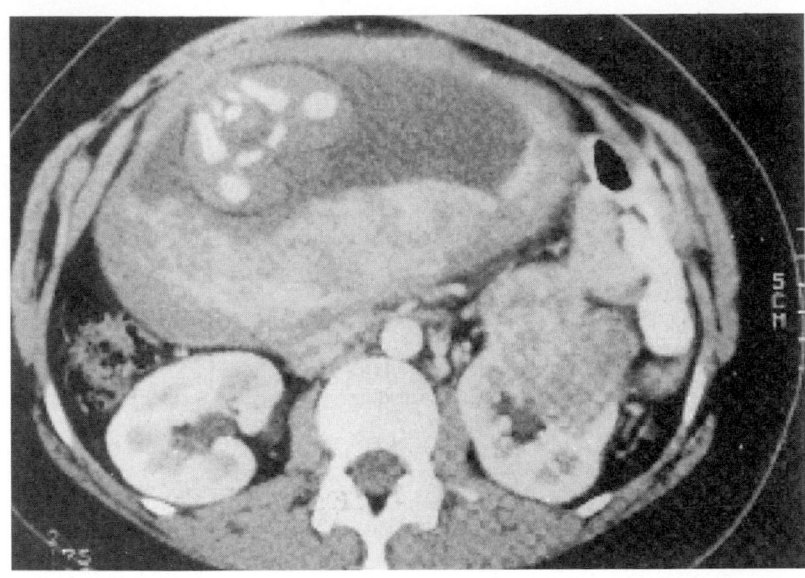

FIGURE 57–2. Computed tomography scan of a pregnant woman with large renal mass on left side. (From Gross and associates, 1995, with permission.)

cases since 1986 in their updated review. They suggest that earlier diagnosis is common now because of ultrasonography. Fazeli-Matin and co-workers (1998) described partial nephrectomy in a woman with renal carcinoma at 14 weeks.

We have encountered only six pregnant women with this malignancy during the past 30 years at Parkland Hospital. Either they presented because of painless hematuria, or the tumor was found by abdominal palpation done routinely in conjunction with cesarean delivery.

OTHER TUMORS

Thyroid cancers are the most common endocrine malignancies. Morris (1998) has estimated that approximately 10 percent occurring during the reproductive years are diagnosed during pregnancy or within the first year after birth. Most thyroid cancers are well-differentiated and follow an indolent course. Tewari and associates (1998) described a woman with Graves thyrotoxicosis and thyroid storm who was subsequently found to also have papillary adenocarcinoma. Rossing and colleagues (2000) have presented intriguing findings suggesting that thyroid stimulation during pregnancy and lactation may result in a transient increase in growth of papillary thyroid cancer. Diagnosis is usually by fine-needle aspiration. Treatment consists primarily of surgery performed during the second trimester or after delivery (see Chap. 53, p. 1198).

Soft-tissue and *bone tumors*, although rare in pregnancy, in most cases, can be successfully managed with surgery during gestation (Maxwell and associates, 2004).

Brain tumors are uncommon during pregnancy. Isla and colleagues (1997) described seven cases in more than 126,000 deliveries from Hospital La Paz in Madrid. According to Finfer (1991), the types of tumors are the same as for identically aged nonpregnant women, and about a third each are gliomas or meningiomas. Tewari and co-workers (2000) described eight women with malignant brain tumors associated with pregnancy. Another two women had postpartum gestational choriocarcinoma metastatic to the brain. These cases were from a 20-year survey of five California hospitals with about 312,000 deliveries during the 20-year study period. Maternal outcomes were horrific—five women died, two survived with significant neurological defects, and only three attained remission.

REFERENCES

Alexander A, Samlowski WE, Grossman D, et al: Metastatic melanoma in pregnancy: Risk of transplacental metastases in the infant. J Clin Oncol 21:2179, 2003

American College of Obstetricians and Gynecologists: Guidelines for diagnostic imaging during pregnancy. Committee Opinion No. 299, September 2004

American College of Obstetricians and Gynecologists: Cancer of the ovary. Technical Bulletin No. 141, August 2003a

American College of Obstetricians and Gynecologists: Induced abortion and breast cancer risk. Committee Opinion No. 285, August 2003b

American College of Obstetricians and Gynecologists: Breast cancer screening. Practice Bulletin No. 42, April 2003c

American College of Obstetricians and Gynecologists: Diagnosis and treatment of cervical carcinomas. Practice Bulletin No. 35, October 2002

American College of Obstetricians and Gynecologists: Cancer of the ovary. Technical Bulletin No. 141, May 1990

Anderson ML, Mari G, Schwartz PE: Gynecologic malignancies in pregnancy. In Barnea ER, Jauniaux E, Schwartz PE (eds): Cancer and Pregnancy. London, Springer, 2001, p 33

Arias E, Anderson RN, Hsiang-Ching K, et al: Deaths: Final data for 2001. National Vital Statistics Report, Vol 52, No. 3. Hyattsville, Md, National Center for Health Statistics, 2003

Aslam N, Ong C, Woelfer B, et al: Serum CA125 at 11–14 weeks of gestation in women with morphologically normal ovaries. Br J Obstet Gynaecol 107:689, 2000

Averette HE, Mirhashemi R, Moffat FL: Pregnancy after breast carcinoma: The ultimate medical challenge. Cancer 85:2301, 1999

Averette HE, Nasser N, Yankow SL, et al: Cervical conization in pregnancy: Analysis of 180 operations. Am J Obstet Gynecol 106:543, 1970

Avilés A, Diaz-Maqueo JC, Torras V, et al: Non-Hodgkin lymphomas and pregnancy: Presentation of 16 cases. Gynecol Oncol 37:355, 1990

Avilés A, Neri N: Hermatological malignancies and pregnancy: A final report of 84 children who received chemotherapy in utero. Clin Lymphoma 2:173, 2001

Baldstrom A, Anderson H, Olsson H: Worse survival in breast cancer among women with recent childbirth: Results from a Swedish population-based register study. Clin Breast Cancer 4:280, 2003

Barber HRK, Brunschwig A: Gynecologic cancer complicating pregnancy. Am J Obstet Gynecol 85:156, 1963

Barnes MN, Barrett JC, Kimberlin DF, et al: Burkitt lymphoma in pregnancy. Obstet Gynecol 92:675, 1998

Bekkers RL, Massuger LF, Berg PP, et al: Uterine malignant leiomyoblastoma (epithelioid leiomyosarcoma) during pregnancy. Gynecol Oncol 72:433, 1999

Beral V, Bull D, Doll R, et al: Breast cancer and abortion: collaborative reanalysis of data from 53 epidemiological studies, including 83,000 women with breast cancer from 16 countries. Lancet 363:1007, 2004

Berry DL, Theriault RL, Holmes FA, et al: Management of breast cancer during pregnancy using a standardized protocol. J Clin Oncol 17:855, 1999

Bladerston KD, Tewari K, Azizi F, et al: Intrahepatic cholangiocarcinoma masquerading as the HELLP syndrome (hemolysis, elevated liver enzymes, and low platelet count) in pregnancy: Case report. Am J Obstet Gynecol 179:823, 1998

Blakely LJ, Buzdar AU, Lozada JA, et al: Effects of pregnancy after treatment for breast carcinoma on survival and risk of recurrence. Cancer 100:465, 2004

Bonnier P, Romain S, Dilhuydy JM, et al: Influence of pregnancy on the outcome of breast cancer: A case-control study. Int J Cancer 72:720, 1997

Boulay R, Podczaski E: Ovarian cancer complicating pregnancy. Obstet Gynecol Clin North Am 25:3856, 1998

Brent RL: The effect of embryonic and fetal exposure to x-ray, microwaves, and ultrasound: Counseling the pregnant and nonpregnant patient about these risks. Semin Oncol 16:347, 1989

Brent RL: Utilization of developmental basic science principles in the evaluation of reproductive risks from pre- and postconception environmental radiation exposures. Teratology 59:182, 1999

Briggs GG, Freeman RK, Yaffe SJ: Drugs in Pregnancy and Lactation, 6th ed. Philadelphia, Lippincott Williams & Wilkins, 2002

Caligiuri MA, Mayer RJ: Pregnancy and leukemia. Semin Oncol 16:388, 1989

Carradice D, Austin N, Bayston K, et al: Successful treatment of acute promyelocytic leukaemia during pregnancy. Clin Lab Haematol 24:307, 2002

Cascinelli N, Morabito A, Santinami M, et al: Immediate or delayed dissection of regional nodes in patients with melanoma of the trunk: A randomised trial. Lancet 351:793, 1998

Catlin EA, Roberts JD Jr, Erana R, et al: Transplacental transmission of natural-killer-cell lymphoma. N Engl J Med 341:85, 1999

Celo JS, Kim HC, Houlihan C, et al: Acute promyelocytic leukemia in pregnancy: All-trans retinoic acid as a newer therapeutic option. Obstet Gynecol 83:808, 1994

Chan YM, Ngai SW, Lao TT: Colon cancer in pregnancy. A case report. J Reprod Med 44:733, 1999a

Chan YM, Ngai SW, Lao TT: Gastric adenocarcinoma presenting with persistent, mild gastrointestinal symptoms in pregnancy: A case report. J Reprod Med 44:986, 1999b

Chiarelli AM, Marrett LD, Darlington GA: Pregnancy outcomes in females after treatment for childhood cancer. Epidemiology 11:161, 2000

Cliby WA, Dodson MK, Podratz KC: Cervical cancer complicated by pregnancy: Episiotomy site recurrences following vaginal delivery. Obstet Gynecol 84:179, 1994

Connor JP: Noninvasive cervical cancer complicating pregnancy. Obstet Gynecol Clin North Am 25:331, 1998

Daryanani D, Plukker JT, De Hullu JA, et al: Pregnancy and early-stage melanoma. Cancer 97:2248, 2003

Davis JL, Chen MD: Gastric carcinoma presenting as an exacerbation of ulcers during pregnancy: A case report. J Reprod Med 36:450, 1991

Del Priore G, Unger L, Boyle D, et al: Abdominal radical trachelectomy for fertility preservation in cervical cancer. Obstet Gynecol, April 2003, p 2S

Dgani R, Shoham Z, Atar E, et al: Ovarian carcinoma during pregnancy: A study of 23 cases in Israel between the years 1960 and 1984. Gynecol Oncol 33:326, 1989

Dinh TA, Warshal DP: The epidemiology of cancer in pregnancy. In Barnea ER, Jauniaux E, Schwartz PE (eds): Cancer and Pregnancy. London, Springer, 2001, p 1

Dipaola RS, Goodin S, Ratzell M, et al: Chemotherapy for metastatic melanoma during pregnancy. Gynecol Oncol 66:526, 1997

Doll DC, Ringenberg QS, Yarbro JW: Management of cancer during pregnancy. Arch Intern Med 148:2058, 1988

Donegan WL: Cancer and pregnancy. CA Cancer J Clin 33:194, 1983

Dow KH, Harris JR, Roy C: Pregnancy after breast-conserving surgery and radiation therapy for breast cancer. J Natl Cancer Inst Monogr 16:131, 1994

Dunn JS Jr, Anderson CD, Brost BC: Breast carcinoma metastatic to the placenta. Obstet Gynecol 94:846, 1999

Durkin JW Jr: Carcinoid tumor and pregnancy. Am J Obstet Gynecol 145:757, 1983

Economos K, Perez-Veridiano N, Delke I, et al: Abnormal cervical cytology in pregnancy: A 17-year experience. Obstet Gynecol 81:915, 1993

El-Bastawissi AY, Becker TM, Daling JR: Effect of cervical carcinoma in situ and its management on pregnancy outcome. Obstet Gynecol 93:207, 1999

Evans LS, Hancock BW: Non-Hodgkin lymphoma. Lancet 362:139, 2003

Falconer AD, Ferns P: Pregnancy outcomes following treatment of cancer. J Obstet Gynaecol 22:43, 2002

Fazeli-Matin S, Goldfarb DA, Novick AC: Renal and adrenal surgery during pregnancy. Urology 52:510, 1998

Fife KH, Katz BP, Roush J, et al: Cancer-associated human papillomavirus types are selectively increased in the cervix of women in the first trimester of pregnancy. Am J Obstet Gynecol 174:1487, 1996

Finfer SR: Management of labour and delivery in patients with intracranial neoplasms. Br J Anaesth 67:784, 1991

Fisher B, Anderson S, Bryant J, et al: Twenty-year follow-up of a randomized trial comparing total mastectomy, lumpectomy, and lumpectomy plus irradiation for the treatment of invasive breast cancer. N Engl J Med 347:1233, 2002

Gamberdella FR: Pancreatic carcinoma in pregnancy: A case report. Am J Obstet Gynecol 149:15, 1984

Gershenson DM: Menstrual and reproductive function after treatment with combination chemotherapy for malignant ovarian germ cell tumors. J Clin Oncol 6:270, 1988

Gilstrap LG, Van Dorsten PV, Cunningham FG (eds): Cancer in pregnancy. In Operative Obstetrics, 2nd ed. New York, McGraw-Hill, 2001

Gisi P, Floyd R: Hepatocellular carcinoma in pregnancy: A case report. J Reprod Med 44:65, 1999

Glantz JC: Reproductive toxicology of alkylating agents. Obstet Gynecol Surv 49:709, 1994

Goff BA, Paley PJ, Koh WJ, et al: Cancer in the pregnant patient. In Hoskins WJ, Perez CA, Young RC (eds): Principles and Practice of Gynecologic Oncology. Philadelphia: Lippincott Williams & Wilkins, 2000

Goldman NA, Goldberg GL: Late recurrence of squamous cell cervical cancer in an episiotomy site after vaginal delivery. Obstet Gynecol 101:1127, 2003

Gotlieb WH, Beiner ME, Shalmon B, et al: Outcome of fertility-sparing treatment with progestins in young patients with endometrial cancer. Obstet Gynecol 102:718, 2003

Green DM, Whitton JA, Stovall M, et al: Pregnancy outcome of female survivors of childhood cancer: A report from the Childhood Cancer Survivor Study. Am J Obstet Gynecol 187:1070, 2002

Greenlund LJ, Letendre L, Tefferi A: Acute leukemia during pregnancy: A single institutional experience in 17 cases. Leuk Lymphoma 41:571, 2001

Greer BE, Easterling TR, McLennan DA, et al: Fetal and maternal considerations in the management of stage I-B cervical cancer during pregnancy. Gynecol Oncol 34:61, 1989

Gross AJ, Zoller G, Hermanns M, et al: Renal cell carcinoma during pregnancy. Br J Urol 75:254, 1995

Haas JF: Pregnancy in association with newly diagnosed cancer: A population-based epidemiologic assessment. Int J Cancer 34:229, 1984

Hacker NF, Berek JS, Lagasse LD, et al: Carcinoma of the cervix associated with pregnancy. Obstet Gynecol 59:735, 1982

Hall EJ: Scientific view of low-level radiation risks. Radiographics 11:509, 1991

Hannigan EV: Cervical cancer in pregnancy. Clin Obstet Gynecol 33:837, 1990

Hansen WF, Fretz P, Hunter SK, et al: Leukemia in pregnancy and fetal response to multiagent chemotherapy. Obstet Gynecol 97:809, 2001

Harrison P, Chipping P, Fothergill GA: Successful use of all-trans retinoic acid in acute promyelocytic leukemia presenting during the second trimester of pregnancy. Br J Haematol 86:681, 1994

Heller DS, Cracchiolo B, Hameed M, et al: Pregnancy-associated invasive squamous cell carcinoma of the vulva in a 28-year-old, HIV-negative woman: A case report. J Reprod Med 45:659, 2000

Higgins S, Haffty BG: Pregnancy and lactation after breast-conserving therapy for early stage breast cancer. Cancer 73:2175, 1994

Hirabayashi M, Ueo H, Okudaira Y, et al: Early gastric cancer and a concomitant pregnancy. Am Surg 53:730, 1987

Hochman A, Schreiber H: Pregnancy and cancer of the breast. Obstet Gynecol 2:268, 1953

Holly EA: Melanoma and pregnancy. Recent Results Cancer Res 102:118, 1986

Horning SJ, Hoppe RT, Kaplan HS, et al: Female reproductive potential after treatment for Hodgkin's disease. N Engl J Med 304:1377, 1981

Hsieh TT, Hou HC, Hsu JJ, et al: Term delivery after hepatocellular carcinoma resection in previous pregnancy. Acta Obstet Gynecol Scand 75:77, 1996

Hsu KL, Ko SF, Cheng YF, et al: Spontaneous rupture of hepatocellular carcinoma during pregnancy. Obstet Gynecol 98:913, 2001

Isaacs JH: Cancer of the breast in pregnancy. Surg Clin North Am 75:47, 1995

Ishida T, Yoko T, Kasumi F: Clinical pathological characteristics and progess of breast cancer patients associated with pregnancy and lactation. Analysis of case-control study in Japan. Jpn J Cancer Res 83:1143, 1992

Isla A, Alvarez F, Gonzalez A, et al: Brain tumor and pregnancy. Obstet Gynecol 89:19, 1997

Jacob JH, Stringer CA: Diagnosis and management of cancer during pregnancy. Semin Perinatol 14:79, 1990

Jacobs C, Donaldson SS, Rosenberg SA, et al: Management of the pregnant patient with Hodgkin's disease. Ann Intern Med 95:669, 1981

Johannsson O, Loman N, Borg A, et al: Pregnancy-associated breast cancer in BRCA1 and BRCA2 germ-line mutation carriers. Lancet 352:1359, 1998

Jolles CJ: Gynecologic cancer associated with pregnancy. Semin Oncol 16:417, 1989

Kaiser HE, Nawab E, Nasir A, et al: Neoplasms during the progression of pregnancy. In Vivo 14:277, 2000

Kaldor JM, Day NE, Clarke EA, et al: Leukemia following Hodgkin's disease. N Engl J Med 322:7, 1990

Kalir T, Friedman F Jr: Gynandroblastoma in pregnancy: Case report and review of literature. Mt Sinai J Med 65:292, 1998

Karlen JR, Akbari A, Cook WA: Dysgerminoma associated with pregnancy. Obstet Gynecol 53:330, 1979

Katz VL, Farmer RM, Dotters D: Focus on primary care: From nevus to neoplasm: Myths of melanoma in pregnancy. Obstet Gynecol Surv 57:112, 2002

Kiguchi K, Bibbo M, Hasegawa T, et al: Dysplasia during pregnancy: A cytologic follow-up study. J Reprod Med 26:66, 1981

King RM, Welch JS, Martin JK Jr, et al: Carcinoma of the breast associated with pregnancy. Surg Gynecol Obstet 160:228, 1985

Kjems E, Krag C: Melanoma and pregnancy. Acta Oncol 32:371, 1993

Kroman N, Jensen MB, Melbye M, et al: Should women be advised against pregnancy after breast-cancer treatment? Lancet 350:319, 1997

Kuller JA, Zucker PK, Peng TC: Vulvar leiomyosarcoma in pregnancy. Am J Obstet Gynecol 162:164, 1990

Lashgari M, Behmaram B, Ellis M: Leiomyomatosis peritonealis disseminata: A report of two cases. J Reprod Med 39:652, 1994

Lee RB, Neglia W, Park RC: Cervical carcarcino ma in pregnancy. Obstet Gynecol 58:584, 1981

Levy C, Pereira L, Dardarian T, et al: Solid pseudopapillary pancreatic tumor in pregnancy. A case report. J Reprod Med 49:61, 2004

Lewis BJ, Laros RK Jr: Leukemia and lymphoma. In Laros RK Jr (ed): Blood Disorders in Pregnancy. Philadelphia, Lea & Febiger, 1986, p 85

Li FP, Fine W, Jaffe N, et al: Offspring of patients treated for cancer in childhood. J Natl Cancer Inst 62:1193, 1979

Ling FT, David TE, Merchant N, et al: Intracardiac extension of intravenous leiomyomatosis in a pregnant woman: A case report and review of the literature. Can J Cardiol 16:73, 2000

Lutz MH, Underwood PB Jr, Rozier JC, et al: Genital malignancy in pregnancy. Am J Obstet Gynecol 129:536, 1977

MacKie RM: Pregnancy and exogenous hormones in patients with cutaneous malignant melanoma. Curr Opin Oncol 11:129, 1999

MacKie RM, Bray CA, Hole DJ, et al: Incidence of and survival from malignant melanoma in Scotland: An epidemiological study. Lancet 360:587, 2002

Malhotra N, Sood M: Endodermal sinus tumor in pregnancy. Gynecol Oncol 78:265, 2000

Marom D, Pitlik S, Sagie A, et al: Intravenous leiomyomatosis with cardiac involvement in a pregnant woman. Am J Obstet Gynecol 178:620, 1998

Maxwell C, Barzilay B, Shah V, et al: Maternal and neonatal outcomes in pregnancies complicated by bone and soft-tissue tumors. Obstet Gynecol 104:344, 2004

Maymon E, Piura B, Mazor M, et al: Primary hepatoid carcinoma of ovary in pregnancy. Am J Obstet Gynecol 179:820, 1998

McLain CR Jr: Leukemia in pregnancy. Clin Obstet Gynecol 17:185, 1974

Melbye M, Wohlfahrt J, Lei U, et al: Alpha-fetoprotein levels in maternal serum during pregnancy and maternal breast cancer incidence. J Natl Cancer Inst 92:1001, 2000

Messing MJ, Gallup DG: Carcinoma of the vulva in young women. Obstet Gynecol 86:51, 1995

Michels KB, Willett WC, Rosner BA, et al: Prospective assessment of breastfeeding and breast cancer incidence among 89,887 women. Lancet 347:431, 1996

Morris PC: Thyroid cancer complicating pregnancy. Obstet Gynecol Clin North Am 25:401, 1998

Muslin M, Goldberg J, Hageboutros A: Chemo and radiation therapy during pregnancy. In Barnea ER, Jauniaux E, Schwartz PE (eds): Cancer and Pregnancy. London, Springer, 2001, p 108

Nettleton J, Long J, Kuban D, et al: Breast cancer during pregnancy: Quantifying the risk of treatment delay. Obstet Gynecol 87:414, 1996

Nevin J, Soefers R, Dahaeck K, et al: Cervical carcinoma associated with pregnancy. Obstet Gynecol Surv 50:228, 1995

Nicklas A, Baker M: Imaging strategies in pregnant cancer patients. Semin Oncol 27:623, 2000

Nisce LZ, Tome MA, He S, et al: Management of coexisting Hodgkin's disease and pregnancy. Am J Clin Oncol 9:146, 1986

Nisker JA, Shubat M: Stage IB cervical carcinoma and pregnancy: Report of 49 cases. Am J Obstet Gynecol 145:203, 1983

Nugent P, O'Connell TX: Breast cancer and pregnancy. Arch Surg 120:1221, 1985

Nulman I, Laslo D, Fried S, et al: Neurodevelopment of children exposed in utero to treatment of maternal malignancy. Br J Cancer 85:1611, 2001

Palle C, Bangsboll S, Andreasson B: Cervical intraepithelial neoplasia in pregnancy. Acta Obstet Gynecol Scand 79:306, 2000

Partridge AH, Garber JE: Long-term outcomes of children exposed to antineoplastic agents in utero. Semin Oncol 27:712, 2000

Pavlidis NA: Coexistence of pregnancy and malignancy. Oncologist 7:279, 2002

Pejovic T, Schwartz PE, Mari G: Hematologic malignancies in pregnancy. In Barnea ER, Jauniaux E, Schwartz EP (eds): Cancer and Pregnancy. London, Springer, 2001, p 50

Peleg D, Ben-Ami M: Lymphoma and leukemia complicating pregnancy. Obstet Gynecol Clin North Am 25:365, 1998

Pelsang RE: Diagnostic imaging modalities during pregnancy. Obstet Gynecol Clin North Am 25:287, 1998

Petrek JA, Dukoff R, Rogatko A: Prognosis of pregnancy-associated breast cancer. Cancer 67:869, 1991

Phelan JT: Cancer and pregnancy. N Y State J Med 68:3011, 1968

Pollack RN, Sklarin NT, Rao S, et al: Metastatic placental lymphoma associated with maternal human immunodeficiency virus infection. Obstet Gynecol 81:856, 1993

Powell JL, Bock KA, Gentry JK, et al: Metastatic endocervical adenocarcinoma presenting as a virilizing ovarian mass during pregnancy. Obstet Gynecol 100:1129, 2002

Rahman MS, Al-Sibai MH, Rahman J, et al: Ovarian carcinoma associated with pregnancy: A review of 9 cases. Acta Obstet Gynecol Scand 81:260, 2002

Regan MA, Rosenzweig BA: Vulvar carcinoma in pregnancy: A case report and literature review. Am J Perinatol 10:334, 1993

Reynoso EE, Shepherd FA, Messner HA, et al: Acute leukemia during pregnancy: The Toronto Leukemia Study Group experience with long-term follow-up of children exposed in utero to chemotherapeutic agents. J Clin Oncol 5:1098, 1987

Rossing MA, Voigt LF, Wicklund KG, et al: Reproductive factors and risk of papillary thyroid cancer in women. Am J Epidemiol 151:765, 2000

Rustin GJ, Booth M, Dent J, et al: Pregnancy after cytotoxic chemotherapy for gestational trophoblastic tumours. Br Med J 288:103, 1984

Sablinska R, Tarlowska L, Stelmachow J: Invasive carcinoma of the cervix associated with pregnancy: Correlation between patient age, advancement of cancer and gestation, and result of treatment. Gynecol Oncol 5:363, 1977

Salopek TG, Marghoob AA, Slade JM, et al: An estimate of the incidence of malignant melanoma in the United States: Based on a survey of members of the American Academy of Dermatology. Dermatol Surg 21:301, 1995

Samuels TH, Liu FF, Yaffe M, et al: Gestational breast cancer. Can Assoc Radiol J 49:172, 1998

Schammel DP, Mittal KR, Kaplan K, et al: Endometrial adenocarcinoma associated with intrauterine pregnancy: A report of five cases and a review of the literature. Int J Gynecol Pathol 17:327, 1998

Schwartz JL, Mozurkewich EL, Johnson TM: Current management of patients with melanoma who are pregnant, want to get pregnant, or do not want to get pregnant. Cancer 97:2130, 2003

Selevan SG, Lindbohm ML, Hornung RW, et al: A study of occupational exposure to antineoplastic drugs and fetal loss in nurses. N Engl J Med 313:1173, 1985

Shah E, Saunders C: Breast cancer in pregnancy. In Barnea ER, Jauniaux E, Schwartz PE (eds): Cancer and Pregnancy. London, Springer, 2001, p 21

Shen T, Vortmeyer AO, Zhuang Z, et al: High frequency of allelic loss of BRCA2 gene in pregnancy-associated breast carcinoma. J Natl Cancer Inst 91:1686, 1999

Siu BL, Alonzo MR, Vargo TA, et al: Transient dilated cardiomyopathy in a newborn exposed to idarubicin and all-trans-retinoic acid (ATRA) early in the second trimester of pregnancy. Int J Gynecol Cancer 12:399, 2002

Skilling JS: Colorectal cancer complicating pregnancy. Obstet Gynecol Clin North Am 25:417, 1998

Smith DP, Goldman SM, Beggs DS, et al: Renal cell carcinoma in pregnancy: Report of three cases and review of the literature. Obstet Gynecol 83:818, 1994

Smith LH, Danielsen B, Allen ME, et al: Cancer associated with obstetric delivery: Results of linkage with the California cancer registry. Am J Obstet Gynecol 189:1128, 2003

Sood AK, Sorosky JI: Invasive cervical cancer complicating pregnancy: How to manage the dilemma. Obstet Gynecol Clin North Am 25:343, 1998

Sorosky JI, Scott-Conner CE: Breast disease complicating pregnancy. Obstet Gynecol Clin North Am 25:353, 1998

Souadka A, Zouhal A, Souadka F, et al: Breast cancer and pregnancy: Forty-three cases reported in the National Oncology Institute between 1985 and 1988. Rev Fr Gynecol Obstet 89:67, 1994

Spitzer M, Kaushal N, Benjamin F: Maternal CA-125 levels in pregnancy and the puerperium. J Reprod Med 43:387, 1998

Squatrito RC, Harlow SP: Melanoma complicating pregnancy. Obstet Gynecol Clin North Am 25:407, 1998

Stewart CA, Termanini B, Sutliff VE, et al: Management of the Zollinger–Ellison syndrome in pregnancy. Am J Obstet Gynecol 176:224, 1997

Stiles GM, Stanco LM, Saven A, et al: Splenectomy for hairy cell leukemia in pregnancy. J Perinatol 18:200, 1998

Stucker I, Caillard JF, Collin R, et al: Risk of spontaneous abortion among nurses handling antineoplastic drugs. Scand J Work Environ Health 16:102, 1990

Takushi M, Moromizato H, Sakumoto K, et al: Management of invasive carcinoma of the uterine cervix associated with pregnancy: Outcome of intentional delay in treatment. Gynecol Oncol 87:185, 2002

Tangir J, Zelterman D, Ma W, et al: Reproductive function after conservative surgery and chemotherapy for malignant germ cell tumors of the ovary. Obstet Gynecol 101:251, 2003

Tewari K, Balderston KD, Carpenter SE, et al: Papillary thyroid carcinoma manifesting as thyroid storm of pregnancy: Case report. Am J Obstet Gynecol 179:818, 1998

Tewari KS, Cappuccini F, Asrat T, et al: Obstetric emergencies precipitated by malignant brain tumors. Am J Obstet Gynecol 182:1215, 2000

Tinkanen H, Kuoppala T: Virilization during pregnancy caused by ovarian mucinous cystadenocarcinoma. Acta Obstet Gynecol Scand 80:476, 2001

Travis LB, Hill DA, Dores GM, et al: Breast cancer following radiotherapy and chemotherapy among young women with Hodgkin disease. JAMA 290:465, 2003

Tucker MA, Coleman CN, Cox RS, et al: Risk of second cancers after treatment for Hodgkin's disease. N Engl J Med 318:76, 1988

van der Vange N, Weverling GJ, Ketting BW, et al: The prognosis of cervical cancer associated with pregnancy: A matched cohort study. Obstet Gynecol 85:1022, 1995

van der Zee AGJ, de Bruijn HWA, Bouma J, et al: Endodermal sinus tumor of the ovary during pregnancy: A case report. Am J Obstet Gynecol 164:504, 1991

van Vliet W, van Loon AJ, ten Hoor KA, et al: Cervical carcinoma during pregnancy: Outcome of planned delay in treatment. Eur J Obstet Gynecol Reprod Biol 79:153, 1998

Van Voorhis B, Cruikshank DP: Colon carcinoma complicating pregnancy: A report of two cases. J Reprod Med 34:923, 1989

Velentgas P, Daling JR, Malone KE, et al: Pregnancy after breast carcinoma: Outcomes and influence on mortality. Cancer 85:2424, 1999

Veronesi U, Cascinelli N, Mariani L, et al: Twenty-year follow-up of a randomized study comparing breast-conserving surgery with radical mastectomy for early breast cancer. N Engl J Med 347:1227, 2002

Walker JL, Knight EL: Renal cell carcinoma in pregnancy. Cancer 58:2343, 1986

Walsh C, Fazio VW: Cancer of the colon, rectum, and anus during pregnancy. The surgeon's perspective. Gastroenterol Clin North Am 27:257, 1998

Ward FT, Weiss RB: Lymphoma and pregnancy. Semin Oncol 16:397, 1989

Ward RM, Bristow RE: Cancer and pregnancy: Recent developments. Curr Opin Obstet Gynecol 14:613, 2002

Waxman J: Cancer, chemotherapy and fertility. Br Med J 290:1096, 1985

Whitecar MP, Turner S, Higby MK: Adnexal masses in pregnancy: A review of 130 cases undergoing surgical management. Am J Obstet Gynecol 181:19, 1999

Williams SF, Schilsky RL: Neoplastic disorders. In Barron WM, Lindheimer MD (eds): Medical Disorders during Pregnancy, 3rd ed. St. Louis, Mosby, 2000, p 392

Wong DJ, Strassner HT: Melanoma in pregnancy: A literature review. Clin Obstet Gynecol 33:782, 1990

Woo JC, Yu T, Hurd TC: Breast cancer in pregnancy. Arch Surg 138:91, 2003

Wright TC Jr, Cox JT, Massad LS, et al: 2001 Consensus guidelines for the management of women with cervical cytological abnormalities. JAMA 287:2120, 2002

Yazigi R, Sandstad J, Munoz AK: Primary staging in ovarian tumors of low malignant potential. Gynecol Oncol 31:402, 1988

Yost NP, Santoso JT, McIntire DD, et al: Postpartum regression rates of antepartum cervical intraepithelial neoplasia II and III lesions. Obstet Gynecol 93:359, 1999

Young RH, Dudley AG, Scully RE: Granulosa cell, Sertoli–Leydig cell, and unclassified sex cord-stromal tumors associated with pregnancy: A clinicopathological analysis of thirty-six cases. Gynecol Oncol 18:181, 1984

Zemlickis D, Lishner M, Degendorfer P, et al: Maternal and fetal outcome after breast cancer in pregnancy. Am J Obstet Gynecol 166:781, 1992

58

Infections

The pregnant woman and her fetus are susceptible to many infectious diseases that may be serious and life-threatening.

IMMUNOLOGICAL CHANGES OF PREGNANCY

There is much speculation concerning possible effects of decreased immune surveillance during pregnancy. These effects are brought about by maternal tolerance of the foreign-tissue antigens of the semiallogeneic fetal "graft" (see Chap 3, p. 64). Although there are subtle changes in circulating immunoglobulin levels in pregnancy, these appear to be of no clinical consequence (Stirrat, 1991).

Fetal and Newborn Immunology. The active immunological capacity of the fetus and neonate is compromised compared with that of older children and adults. According to Stirrat (1991), fetal cell-mediated and humoral immunity begin to develop by 9 to 15 weeks. The primary fetal response to infection is immunoglobulin M (IgM). Passive immunity is provided by IgG transferred across the placenta. By 16 weeks, this transfer begins to increase rapidly, and by 26 weeks, fetal concentrations are equivalent to those of the mother. After birth, breast feeding is protective against some infections. But this begins to decline at 2 months of age (World Health Organization Collaborative Study Team, 2000).

Neonatal infection, especially in its early stages, may be difficult to diagnose because neonates may fail to express classical clinical signs. If the fetus was infected in utero, there may be depression and acidosis at birth for no apparent reason. The neonate may suck poorly, vomit, or develop abdominal distention. Respiratory insufficiency may develop, which may present similarly to idiopathic respiratory distress syndrome. The neonate may be lethargic or jittery. The response to sepsis may be hypothermia rather than hyperthermia, and the total leukocyte and neutrophil counts may be depressed.

Bacteria, viruses, or parasites may gain access transplacentally during the viremic, bacteremic, or parasitemic stage of maternal infection (Newton, 1999). They may also cross intact amnionic membranes. Fetal infections may develop early in pregnancy to produce obvious stigmata at birth. Alternatively, organisms may colonize and infect the fetus during labor and delivery. Thus, preterm rupture of membranes, prolonged labor, and manipulations may increase the risk of neonatal infection (Yancey and colleagues, 1996). Infections occurring in neonates who are less than 72 hours after delivery usually are caused by bacteria acquired in utero or during delivery, whereas infections after that time most likely have been acquired after birth.

Hospital-acquired infections are dangerous for preterm neonates, and the individuals who care for them are a major source for postnatal infection (Stoll and Hansen, 2003). Ventilatory systems and indwelling venous and arterial umbilical catheters may be the source of life-threatening infection.

The very-low-birthweight infant who survives the first few days is still at considerable risk of dying from infection acquired in the intensive care nursery.

Ascending infection by bacteria (e.g., *Escherichia coli,* group B streptococci, *Ureaplasma urealyticum*) is the most common infectious cause of neonatal sepsis and stillbirth. In developed countries, 10 to 25 percent of stillbirths may be caused by infectious pathogens, and in developing countries, the percentage may be much greater (Goldenberg and Thompson, 2003). In high-prevalence areas, syphilis and malaria in nonimmune women in pregnancy are also major causes of stillbirths.

VIRAL INFECTIONS

VARICELLA-ZOSTER. This DNA herpesvirus remains latent in the dorsal root ganglia after primary infection. Most adults acquire varicella infection, namely chickenpox, during childhood, and 95 percent have serological evidence of immunity (Wharton, 1996). Varicella infection tends to be more severe in adults than in children. Approximately half of all varicella deaths occur in the 5 percent of the adult population that are susceptible (Centers for Disease Control and Prevention, 1999a).

Although disputed, there is evidence that varicella infection may be more severe during pregnancy. Harger and associates (2002b) reported that 18 of 347 (5 percent) infected pregnant women developed pneumonitis. Despite this, successful pregnancy outcomes can follow complicated varicella pneumonia (Chandra and colleagues, 1998). Its treatment is described in Chapter 46 (see p. 1059).

Primary varicella infection may be reactivated years later, causing herpes zoster or shingles (Gilden and co-workers, 2000). Maternal herpes zoster infection is more common in older or immunocompromised patients. There is no evidence, however, that zoster is more frequent or more severe in pregnant women. In addition, in a review of 366 cases of zoster during pregnancy, Enders and associates (1994) concluded that there was little evidence that zoster caused congenital malformations.

Prevention. Administration of *varicella-zoster immunoglobulin* (*VZIG*) prevents or attenuates varicella infection in exposed susceptible individuals if given within 96 hours of viral exposure. The dose is 125 U per 10 kg given intramuscularly, with a maximum dose of 625 units or five vials. VZIG is recommended by the Centers for Disease Control and Prevention (1996) for immunocompromised susceptible adults who are exposed to varicella, and it should be strongly considered for all susceptible pregnant women. Despite this recommendation, Enders and colleagues (1994) and Harger and associates (2002a) both found that only 7 to 11 percent of more than 1700 pregnant women with varicella infection had received VZIG.

A new intravenous form of VZIG has been developed and was found to have higher initial anti-varicella antibody levels and comparable efficacy and safety in a preliminary study of 57 gravidas (Koren and associates, 2002). This new form of VZIG is not approved for use in the United States.

Up to 80 to 90 percent of adults are immune because of prior symptomatic or asymptomatic infection. Thus, antibody testing with enzyme-linked immunosorbent assay (ELISA) or fluorescent antibody to membrane antigen (FAMA) should precede, if possible, use of VZIG.

An attenuated live-virus vaccine (Varivax) was approved for use in 1995 (American College of Obstetricians and Gynecologists, 2000). Two doses, given 4 to 8 weeks apart, are recommended for adolescents and adults with no history of varicella. This successfully results in 97-percent seroconversion (American College of Obstetricians and Gynecologists, 2003). **The vaccine is not recommended for pregnant women.** However, a pregnancy registry listing 362 vaccine-exposed pregnancies has reported no cases of congenital varicella syndrome or other congenital malformations (Shields and colleagues, 2001). Vaccine virus is not secreted in breast milk, so postpartum vaccination should not be delayed because of breast feeding (Bohlke and associates, 2003).

Fetal Effects. Maternal varicella during the first half of pregnancy may cause congenital malformations by transplacental infection. Some of these include chorioretinitis, cerebral cortical atrophy, hydronephrosis, and cutaneous and bony leg defects (Fig. 58–1). In a prospective study, Enders and co-workers (1994) evaluated 1373 women who had varicella infection during pregnancy. When maternal infection developed before 13 weeks, only 2 of 472 pregnancies (0.4 percent) had neonates with congenital varicella. The highest risk

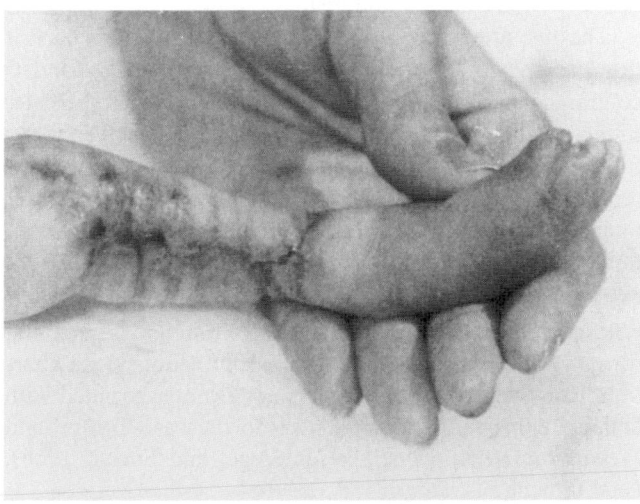

FIGURE 58–1. Atrophy of the lower extremity with bony defects and scarring in a fetus infected during the first trimester by varicella. (From Paryani and Arvin, 1986, with permission.)

was between 13 and 20 weeks, during which time 7 of 351 exposed fetuses (2 percent) had evidence of congenital varicella. There was no clinical evidence of congenital varicella infection after 20 weeks gestation. Other evidence shows that fetal exposure later in pregnancy is associated with only congenital varicella lesions (Chiang and colleagues, 1995). Similarly, Harger and colleagues (2002a) evaluated a prospective cohort of 347 women with primary varicella infection and found only one case (0.4 percent) of congenital varicella syndrome.

Fetal exposure to the virus just before or during delivery, and therefore before maternal antibody has been formed, poses a serious threat to newborns. The incubation period for varicella infection is short, usually less than 2 weeks. In some instances, neonates develop disseminated visceral and central nervous system disease, which is commonly fatal. For this reason, VZIG or zoster immunoglobulin (ZIG) should be administered to neonates whenever the onset of maternal disease is within about 5 days before or after delivery. Neonates exposed earlier or later are protected by maternal antibody, and perinatal mortality is minimal. Despite VZIG administration, however, Miller and associates (1998) reported that 30 to 40 percent of newborns still developed infection, but the number of complications and fatal outcomes was substantially reduced (Centers for Disease Control and Prevention, 1996).

INFLUENZA. These infections are caused by members of the family *Orthomyxoviridae*. *Influenza A* and *B* form one genus of these RNA viruses. Influenza A viruses are subclassified further by hemagglutinin (H) and neuraminidase (N) antigenic makeup. Symptoms include fever, dry cough, and systemic symptoms, and infection can be confirmed with rapid enzyme immunoassay or immunofluorescence assay (Salgado and co-workers, 2002). Influenza A is more serious than influenza B and usually develops during winter.

Infection usually is not life-threatening in otherwise healthy adults, but pregnant women do not tolerate serious pulmonary involvement (Neuzil and colleagues, 1998). For example, in early 2003, widespread influenza A was associated with extensive infection among pregnant women. At Parkland Hospital, more than 100 women were hospitalized for infection. Pulmonary infiltrates complicated approximately 20 percent of cases.

Prevention. Vaccination against influenza, optimally in October or November, is recommended by the Centers for Disease Control and Prevention (2004b) and the American College of Obstetricians and Gynecologists (2003) for all women who will be pregnant during the influenza season (from November through February) at any gestational age. This is most important for women who have chronic underlying medical disorders such as diabetes, heart disease, asthma, or human immunodeficiency virus (HIV) infection. The inactivated vaccine prevents clinical illness in 70 to 90 percent

TABLE 58–1 Antiviral Agents for Prevention and Treatment of Influenza in Pregnancy

Drug	Influenza Virus Type	Approved Use	FDA Pregnancy Category	Dosage
Amantadine	A	Treatment/prophylaxis	C_M	100 mg twice daily
Rimantadine[a]	A	Treatment/prophylaxis	C_M	100 mg twice daily
Zanamivir[b]	A and B	Treatment	C	10 mg twice daily
Oseltamivir[c]	A and B	Treatment	C	75 mg twice daily
		Prophylaxis		75 mg daily

FDA = Food and Drug Administration.
[a]Reduced dosage is recommended with severe hepatic or renal dysfunction.
[b]Breath-activated plastic inhaler device. Not generally recommended for women with asthma or chronic obstructive pulmonary disease.
[c]Reduced dosage is recommended for persons with creatinine clearance less than 30 mL/min.

of healthy adults, and there is no evidence of teratogenicity (see Chap. 8, p. 221). A recent survey of obstetricians found that only 44 percent provided influenza vaccination in pregnancy. Many did not offer vaccine because of reimbursement issues or availability of vaccination elsewhere (Schrag and co-workers, 2003). There was a shortage of the 2004–2005 vaccine because of manufacturing problems.

An intranasal, trivalent, cold-adapted, live attenuated-virus vaccine was approved for use in healthy adults in 2003. It is not recommended for pregnant women (Centers for Disease Control and Prevention, 2003c).

Treatment. Amantadine and *rimantadine* are antiviral agents with specific activity against influenza A viruses (Table 58–1). Given as chemoprophylaxis, both antivirals are 70 to 90 percent effective in preventing influenza (Centers for Disease Control and Prevention, 2004b). They are especially recommended for prophylaxis for nonimmunized women at high risk for influenza complications (see Chap. 46, p. 1059). If influenza develops, amantadine or rimantadine, begun within 48 hours of the onset of symptoms, reduces the duration of fever and systemic symptoms.

Another class of antiviral drugs—*neuraminidase inhibitors*—is highly effective for the treatment of early influenza A and B in adults (Centers for Disease Control and Prevention, 2004b). *Oseltamivir* is taken orally and is approved for both treatment and chemoprophylaxis in adults. *Zanamivir* is inhaled and is approved for treatment in adults. They are discussed further in Chapter 46 (see p. 1059). Both agents reduce the odds of developing influenza by 70 to 90 percent and reduce the duration of uncomplicated illness by about 1 day (Cooper and colleagues, 2003).

There is limited experience with the use of any of these four antiviral agents in pregnant women. All the agents are Food and Drug Administration category C drugs, and they should be used when the potential benefits outweigh the risks. Unfortunately, none of the agents has been demonstrated to be effective in preventing serious influenza-related complications such as pneumonia.

Fetal Effects. There is no firm evidence that influenza A virus causes congenital malformations (Irving and co-workers, 2000; Korones, 1988). Specifically, Saxén and associates (1990) found no association with first-trimester influenza in 248 mothers of anencephalic fetuses. Irving and colleagues (2000) identified no specific fetal or maternal complications in 182 pregnancies with serological evidence of second- or third-trimester influenza. Conversely, Lynberg and co-workers (1994) reported increased neural-tube defects in neonates born to women with influenza early in pregnancy. In addition, there is controversial evidence that fetal exposure to influenza A may predispose to schizophrenia in later life (Kunugi and associates, 1995; McGrath and Castle, 1995).

MUMPS. This uncommon adult infectious disease is caused by an RNA paramyxovirus. As a result of childhood immunization, as many as 80 to 90 percent of adults are seropositive. The virus primarily infects the salivary glands but may involve the gonads, meninges, pancreas, and other organs. Treatment is symptomatic, and mumps during pregnancy is no more severe than in nonpregnant adults.

The live attenuated Jeryl–Lynn vaccine strain is part of the *MMR vaccine*—measles, mumps, and rubella—and is contraindicated in pregnancy (American College of Obstetricians and Gynecologists, 2003). No malformations attributable to MMR vaccination in pregnancy have been reported, but pregnancy should be avoided for 30 days after mumps vaccination (Centers for Disease Control and Prevention, 1998b, 2002a).

Fetal Effects. Women who develop mumps in the first trimester may have an increased risk of spontaneous abortion. However, infection in pregnancy is not associated with congenital malformations (Centers for Disease Control and Prevention, 1998; Siegel, 1973; Siegel and Fuerst, 1966). Fetal infection is rare.

RUBEOLA (MEASLES). Most adults are immune to measles due to childhood immunization. Unfortunately, when measles becomes epidemic, unvaccinated women may develop measles, and if pregnant, they have an increased risk of pneumonia with adverse maternal and perinatal outcomes (Ali and Alber, 1997; Chiba and co-workers, 2003; Eberhart-Phillips and colleagues, 1993).

Passive maternal immunization can be achieved by administering immune serum globulin (0.25 mL/kg, maximum dose 15 mL), given intramuscularly within 6 days of exposure. Active vaccination is not done during pregnancy, but susceptible women can be vaccinated routinely postpartum (American College of Obstetricians and Gynecologists, 2003; Centers for Disease Control and Prevention, 1998).

Fetal Effects. The virus does not appear to be teratogenic (Siegel, 1973), but there is an increased frequency of abortion, prematurity, and low-birthweight neonates with maternal measles (Siegel and Fuerst, 1966). If a woman develops measles shortly before birth, there is considerable risk of serious infection developing in the neonate, especially in a preterm neonate.

RESPIRATORY VIRUSES.
More than 200 antigenically distinct respiratory viruses cause the common cold, pharyngitis, laryngotracheobronchitis, bronchitis, and pneumonia. Rhinovirus, coronavirus, and adenovirus are major causes of the common cold. The RNA-containing rhinovirus and coronavirus usually produce a trivial, self-limited illness characterized by rhinorrhea, sneezing, and congestion. The DNA-containing adenovirus is more likely to produce cough and lower respiratory tract involvement, including pneumonia.

Fetal Effects. Mothers suffering from the common cold had a four- to fivefold increased risk of fetal anencephaly when a 393-woman cohort of the Finnish Register of Congenital Malformations was analyzed (Kurppa and associates, 1991). Shaw and co-workers (1998), however, examined births in California from 1989 to 1991 and concluded that the attributable risk for neural-tube defects associated with many illnesses and medications used in early pregnancy is low.

Adenoviral infection is a common cause of childhood myocarditis. Towbin and colleagues (1994) and Forsnes and associates (1998) used polymerase chain reaction (PCR) to identify and link adenovirus to fetal myocarditis and nonimmune hydrops.

HANTAVIRUSES.
These RNA viruses are members of the family *Bunyaviridae*. They are associated with a rodent reservoir, and transmission involves inhalation of virus excreted in rodent urine and feces. An outbreak in the Western United States occurred in 1993 due to Sin Nombre virus. The resulting hantavirus pulmonary syndrome was characterized by severe noncardiogenic pulmonary edema resembling adult respiratory distress syndrome and carried a case-fatality rate of 45 percent. Hantaviruses are a heterogenous group of viruses with low and variable rates of transplacental transmission.

Howard and co-workers (1999) reported the syndrome to cause maternal death, fetal demise, and preterm birth. They found no evidence of vertical transmission of the Sin Nombre virus. Vertical transmission, however, occurred inconsistently in association with hemorrhagic fever with renal syndrome caused by another hantavirus species, the Hantaan virus.

Clinical management should be individualized in cases of noncardiogenic pulmonary edema in women from endemic areas who have a history of possible exposure. Prevention focuses on lowering exposure to infected rodents (Centers for Disease Control and Prevention, 2002b).

ENTEROVIRUS INFECTIONS.
These viruses are a major subgroup of RNA picornaviruses that include poliovirus, coxsackievirus, and echovirus. They are trophic for intestinal epithelium but can also cause widespread maternal, fetal, and neonatal infections that may include the central nervous system, skin, heart, and lungs. Most maternal infections, however, are subclinical, yet can be fatal to the fetus-neonate (Goldenberg and Thompson, 2003). Garcia and associates (1991) reported that histological placentitis was common following maternal enteroviral infection. Hepatitis A is an enterovirus that is discussed in Chapter 50 (see p. 1130).

Coxsackievirus. Infections with coxsackievirus are usually asymptomatic. However, the virus can cause aseptic meningitis, a polio-like illness, rashes, respiratory disease, or pleuritis, pericarditis, and myocarditis. Brown and Karunas (1972) reported that congenital malformations were increased slightly in pregnant women who had serological evidence of coxsackievirus but not echovirus infections. In addition, viremia with coxsackievirus can cause fetal hepatitis, myocarditis, and encephalomyelitis, all of which may be fatal.

Poliovirus. Most of these rare infections are subclinical or mild. The virus is trophic for the central nervous system, and symptomatic infections can cause paralytic disease—poliomyelitis. Siegel and Goldberg (1955) demonstrated that pregnant women not only were more susceptible to polio but also had a higher death rate. Inactivated subcutaneous polio vaccine is recommended for susceptible pregnant women who must travel to endemic areas or are placed in other high-risk situations. Live oral polio vaccine has been used for mass vaccination during pregnancy without harmful fetal effects (Harjulehto and associates, 1989).

PARVOVIRUS.
Human parvovirus B19 causes *erythema infectiosum*, or *fifth disease*. This is a mild maternal infection that occasionally causes fetal death. The B19 virus is a small, single-stranded DNA virus that replicates in rapidly proliferating cells such as erythroblast precursors (Young and Brown, 2004). Only individuals with the erythrocyte membrane P antigen are susceptible. In women with hemolytic anemia (e.g., sickle-cell disease), parvovirus infection may cause an aplastic crisis.

The main mode of parvovirus transmission is respiratory or hand-to-mouth contact, and the infection is common in spring months. The maternal infection rate is highest in women with school-aged children and in day-care workers, but not usually schoolteachers. Viremia develops 4 to 14 days after exposure. Fever, headache, and flulike symptoms may begin in the last few days of the viremic phase. Several days later, a bright red rash with erythroderma affects the face, giving a *slapped cheek* appearance. The rash becomes lace-like and spreads to the trunk and extremities. Adults often have milder rashes and develop a symmetrical polyarthralgia that may persist several weeks. In 20 to 30 percent of adults, however, the infection is asymptomatic.

There is no evidence that parvovirus infection is altered by pregnancy (Valeur-Jensen and colleagues, 1999). Recovery includes production of IgM antibody 10 to 12 days postinfection. IgM usually persists for 3 months but may last for up to 6 months. IgG antibody is detectable several days after IgM appears. IgG persists for life and confers natural immunity against subsequent infections. Roughly half of pregnant women are immune. The attack rate of susceptible adults in school outbreaks is 20 to 30 percent (Young, 1995).

Fetal Effects. Maternal infection may be associated with abortion, nonimmune hydrops, and fetal death (Goldenberg and Thompson, 2003). Parvovirus DNA was found by Nyman and co-workers (2002) in 3 percent of first-trimester miscarriages. Shilleto and associates (1996) found evidence of fetal myocardial damage by measuring creatine kinase levels obtained by cordocentesis. Crane (2002) reviewed 1089 cases of maternal B19 infection from nine studies and reported an overall fetal loss rate of 10 percent. It was 15 percent for infection between 19 to 20 weeks but only 2.3 percent after 20 weeks. The role of parvovirus B19 infection in late second-trimester and third-trimester unexplained stillbirths is unclear, because most derived data are from retrospective cohorts with incomplete maternal and fetal histological evaluations (Norbeck, 2002; Skjöldebrand-Sparre, 2000; Tolfvenstam, 2001, and all their colleagues). As a result, at present there are inadequate data to support evaluating asymptomatic mothers and their stillborn fetuses for parvovirus infection.

Parvovirus is the most common infectious cause of nonimmune hydrops in autopsied fetuses (Rogers, 1999). This complication, however, develops only in approximately 1 percent of infected women and is largely confined to infection in the first 20 weeks of gestation (Crane, 2002; Enders and co-workers, 2004). Considering that concomitant fetal infection follows maternal infection in about a fourth of cases, infection resolves in most fetuses without sequelae (Dembinski and colleagues, 2003).

Yaegashi (2000) has extensively investigated the development and pathophysiology of parvovirus B19 fetal hydrops. At least 85 percent of cases of fetal infection developed within 10 weeks of maternal infection, and the mean interval was 6 to 7 weeks. More than 80 percent of hydrops cases were found in the second trimester, with a mean gestational age of 22 to 23 weeks. Yaegashi estimated that the critical period for maternal infection leading to fetal hydrops was between 13 and 16 weeks—coincident with the period in which fetal hepatic hemopoiesis is greatest.

Rodis and colleagues (1998) and Miller and associates (1998) described long-term outcomes of children following maternal parvovirus infection. They concluded that developmental delay was not increased in these children.

Management. The diagnosis of maternal infection is generally made by serological testing for specific IgG and IgM antibodies (Fig. 58–2). Viral DNA may be detectable by PCR in maternal serum during the prodrome but not after the rash develops. Fetal infection can be identified by detecting viral DNA in amnionic fluid or fetal parvoviral IgM using cordocentesis (Schild and colleagues, 1999).

For women with a positive IgM serology, ultrasonographic fetal evaluation for hydrops is indicated. Delle Chiaie and colleagues (2001) and Cosmi and co-workers (2002) have shown that elevated peak systolic velocity values in the fetal middle cerebral artery accurately predict fetal anemia. Fetal blood sampling is warranted in the presence of hydrops to assess the degree of fetal anemia. Fetal myocarditis may induce hydrops with less severe anemia.

Fetal management is dependent on gestational age, but transfusion for hydrops may improve outcome in some cases (Enders and co-workers, 2004; Schild and colleagues, 1999; von Kaisenberg and Jonat, 2001). The technique for fetal transfusion is described in Chapter 13 (see p. 332).

Prevention. There is no vaccine for human parvovirus B19, and there is no evidence that antiviral treatment prevents maternal or fetal infection. Decisions to leave higher-risk work settings are complex and require assessment of exposure risks. Pregnant patients should be counseled that risks of infection are approximately 5 percent for casual, infrequent contact; 20 percent for intense, prolonged work exposure (e.g., teachers); and 50 percent for close, frequent interaction (e.g., in the home). Workers at day-care centers and schools need not avoid infected children, because infectivity is greatest before any clinical illness. Ill children do not require isolation.

RUBELLA (GERMAN MEASLES). This virus typically causes infections of minor import in the absence of pregnancy. During pregnancy, however, it has been directly responsible for abortion and severe congenital malformations.

Prevention. Although large epidemics of rubella have virtually disappeared in the United States because of immunization, the disease, with its significant teratogenic potential, persists. Up to 25 percent of women in the United States are susceptible (McElhaney and associates, 1999), and cluster outbreaks during the 1990s mainly involved persons born

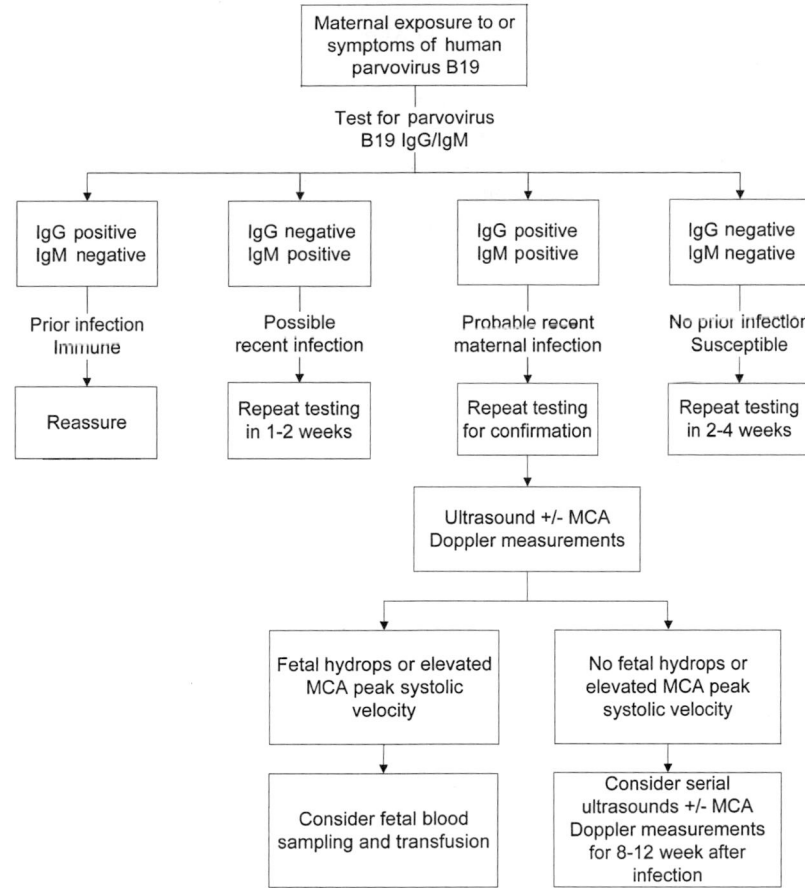

FIGURE 58–2. Algorithm for evaluation and management of human parvovirus B19 infection in pregnancy. (MCA = middle cerebral artery.)

outside the United States (Reef and co-workers, 2002). Congenital rubella is still common in developing nations (Banatvala and Brown, 2004).

To eradicate rubella and prevent congenital rubella syndrome completely, a comprehensive approach is recommended for immunizing the adult population (Centers for Disease Control and Prevention, 1998). The MMR vaccine should be offered to women of childbearing age who do not have evidence of immunity whenever they make contact with the health care system. Vaccination of susceptible women should:

1. Be part of routine general medical and gynecological care, including college health services.
2. Take place in all family planning settings.
3. Be provided routinely to unimmunized women immediately after hospitalization, childbirth, or abortion, unless there are specific contraindications.

Vaccination of all susceptible hospital personnel who might be exposed to patients with rubella or who might have contact with pregnant women is recommended. Rubella vaccination should be avoided 1 month before or during pregnancy because the vaccine contains attenuated live virus (Centers for Disease Control and Prevention, 2002a,e).

Although there is a small overall theoretical risk of 0.5 percent, fortunately, according to pooled data from the Centers for Disease Control and Prevention, there is no evidence that the vaccine induces malformations. If maternal antibody is demonstrated at the time of exposure to rubella or before, it is exceedingly unlikely that the fetus will be affected.

Despite native or vaccine-induced immunity, subclinical rubella *reinfection* may develop during outbreaks. Although asymptomatic reinfection in early pregnancy has been described without fetal effects, fetal infection can rarely occur.

Diagnosis. Rubella is usually a mild, febrile illness in adults with a generalized maculopapular rash. Other symptoms may include arthralgias or arthritis, lymphadenopathy (usually suboccipital, postauricular, and cervical), or conjunctivitis. The incubation period is 12 to 23 days, and 20 to 50 percent of infections may be asymptomatic. Viremia usually precedes clinical signs by about a week, and adults are infectious during viremia through 5 to 7 days of the rash.

Confirmation of rubella infection is often difficult. Not only are the clinical features of other illnesses similar, but about a fourth of rubella infections are subclinical despite viremia that may infect the embryo and fetus.

Specific IgM antibody can be detected using enzyme-linked immunoassay from 4 to 5 days after onset of clinical disease, but it can persist for 6 weeks after appearance of the rash (American College of Obstetricians and Gynecologists, 1992). Importantly, rubella reinfection can give rise to transient low levels of IgM. Best and associates (2002) reviewed the low rubella-specific IgM antibody levels in gravidas without a rash in locales where rubella seldom occurs. They were able to exclude recent maternal infection by detecting high rubella IgG avidity in most cases.

Nonimmune persons demonstrate peak IgG antibody titers 1 to 2 weeks after the onset of the rash or 2 to 3 weeks after the onset of viremia. This rapid antibody response, therefore, may complicate serodiagnosis unless serum is initially collected within a few days after the onset of the rash. If, for example, the first specimen was obtained 10 days after the rash, detection of IgG antibodies would fail to differentiate between very recent disease and preexisting immunity to rubella.

Congenital Rubella Syndrome. Rubella is one of the most teratogenic agents known (see Chap. 14, p. 342). With rubella, as with any fetal infection, the concept of an *infected* versus an *affected* neonate must be understood. Only about half of women with affected neonates give a history of a rash during pregnancy.

Sequelae of fetal infection are worse during organogenesis. Miller and colleagues (1982) have shown that 80 percent of pregnant women with rubella infection and a rash during the first 12 weeks have a fetus with congenital infection. At 13 to 14 weeks, this incidence was 54 percent, and by the end of the second trimester, it was 25 percent. As the duration of pregnancy increases, fetal infections are less likely to cause congenital malformations. According to Reef and colleagues (2000), congenital rubella syndrome includes one or more of the following:

- Eye defects, including cataracts and congenital glaucoma
- Heart disease, including patent ductus arteriosus and peripheral pulmonary artery stenosis
- Sensorineural deafness—the most common single defect
- Central nervous system defects, including microcephaly, developmental delay, mental retardation, and meningoencephalitis
- Pigmentary retinopathy
- Purpura
- Hepatosplenomegaly and jaundice
- Radiolucent bone disease

Neonates born with congenital rubella may shed the virus for many months and thus be a threat to other infants, as well as to susceptible adults who come in contact with them.

The *extended rubella syndrome*, with progressive panencephalitis and type 1 diabetes, may not develop clinically until the second or third decade of life. Perhaps as many as a third of neonates who are asymptomatic at birth may manifest such developmental injury (Webster, 1998).

Prenatal Diagnosis. Confirmation of fetal infection is possible in confirmed cases of maternal rubella in the first half of pregnancy. Tanemura and associates (1996) found rubella RNA in chorionic villi, amnionic fluid, or fetal blood in 23 percent of 34 suspected cases. Detection of second-trimester fetal rubella infection using fetal blood has been described by Tang and colleagues (2003).

CYTOMEGALOVIRUS. This ubiquitous DNA herpesvirus eventually infects most humans. Cytomegalovirus (CMV) is the most common cause of perinatal infection in the developed world, and evidence of fetal infection is found in from 0.2 to 2 percent of all neonates (Revello and Gerna, 2002, 2004). CMV is present in body fluids, and person-to-person transmission usually occurs through sexual or close and intimate contact. There may be fetal intrauterine infection, intrapartum infection, or postpartum infection from breast feeding. Day-care centers are a common source of infection. Usually by 2 to 3 years of age, children acquire the infection from one another and may transmit it to their parents (Demmler, 1991; Pass, 1991).

The public health importance concerning morbidity of perinatal CMV infection was first emphasized in 1971. In the ensuing 20 years, according to Yow and Demmler (1992), more than 800,000 fetuses were infected and 50,000 were born with symptomatic disease. Many have died, and most of the survivors have severe handicaps, including mental retardation, blindness, and deafness. Collectively, the annual cost for their care is nearly $2 billion (American College of Obstetricians and Gynecologists, 2000). Another 120,000 infected children who were asymptomatic at birth have neurological impairments.

Maternal Infection. There is no evidence that pregnancy increases the risk or clinical severity of maternal CMV infection. Most infections are asymptomatic, but about 15 percent of adults have a mononucleosis-like syndrome characterized by fever, pharyngitis, lymphadenopathy, and polyarthritis. Nigro and associates (2003) reported that the majority of women in a cohort with primary infection had elevated serum aminotransferases or lymphocytosis.

Following primary infection, the virus becomes latent, and as in other herpesvirus infections, there is periodic reactivation with viral shedding despite serum IgG antibody. Maternal immunity to CMV does not prevent recurrence–reactivation or exogenous reinfection, nor unfortunately does it prevent congenital infection. The risk of seroconversion among susceptible women during pregnancy is 1 to 4 percent. Immunity from previous infection can be demonstrated in up to 85 percent of pregnant women from lower socioeconomic backgrounds, whereas only half of women in higher income groups are seropositive.

Primary CMV infection, which is transmitted to the fetus in approximately 40 percent of cases, can cause severe morbidity (Fowler and co-workers, 1992; Liesnard and associates, 2000). Although transplacental infection is not universal, an infected fetus is more likely with maternal infection during the first half of pregnancy. Fowler and colleagues (2003a) calculated that naturally acquired immunity results in a 70-percent reduction of risk of congenital CMV infection in future pregnancies. Boppana and associates (2001) observed that women who are seropositive for CMV can also be reinfected with a different strain of virus that can cause fetal infection and symptomatic congenital disease. Congenital infections from recurrent maternal infection reactivation are less often associated with clinically apparent sequelae than with primary infections.

Congenital Infection. Symptomatic congenital CMV infection is a syndrome that includes low birthweight, microcephaly, intracranial calcifications, chorioretinitis, mental and motor retardation, sensorineural deficits, hepatosplenomegaly, jaundice, hemolytic anemia, and thrombocytopenic purpura. Of the estimated 40,000 infected neonates born each year, only 5 to 6 percent demonstrate this syndrome (Fowler and associates, 1992).

Treatment. There is no treatment for maternal primary CMV infection, nor is there fetal prophylaxis or treatment.

Management. Maternal serological screening is not recommended for the following reasons (American College of Obstetricians and Gynecologists, 2000; Peckham and associates, 2001):

1. There is no accurate prediction of the sequelae of primary infection.
2. Some cases of fetal infection are due to maternal reinfection with a different CMV strain.
3. There is no vaccine or treatment.
4. About 2 percent of all neonates excrete CMV, and attempts to identify and isolate them are expensive and impractical.

The predictive value of a positive maternal genitourinary culture or of cervical cytology results in assessing fetal risk of infection is likewise minimal. Asymptomatic CMV excretion can be shown in up to 10 percent of pregnant women, and the majority have recurrent infections with low fetal risk.

Primary infection is diagnosed by seroconversion of CMV-specific IgG in paired acute and convalescent sera, which are assayed simultaneously. It is preferable to document maternal CMV IgM antibody. Unfortunately, specific IgM antibody may be present with primary infection, recurrent infection, or reactivation of infection, limiting its utility for serological diagnosis.

As shown in Figure 58–3, when maternal CMV-specific IgG and IgM are detected, complimentary tests are used to date the infection (Grangeot-Keros and Cointe, 2001). The measurement of specific IgG avidity is valuable in confirming primary CMV infection (Lazzarotto and associates, 2004). The IgG antibody response matures from low-avidity to high-avidity production over several weeks to months (Revello and Gerna, 2002, 2004).

Management is directed to identification of women with recent primary infection who should be offered invasive prenatal diagnosis with ultrasonography and amniocentesis. In utero infection can be identified, and serial ultrasonography can identify fetuses with symptomatic infection and damage. The use of quantitative CMV measurements in amnionic fluid may correlate with outcome, but its interpretation may also be dependent on the gestational age at amniocentesis and the interval since maternal infection. Pregnancy termination may be an option in some settings or delivery followed by early neonatal treatment (Kimberlin and associates, 2003).

Counseling regarding fetal outcome depends on the stage of gestation during which primary infection is documented. Even with the high infection rate with primary infection in the first half of pregnancy, the majority of fetuses develop normally. Kimberlin and co-workers (2003) have shown that intravenous ganciclovir administered for 6 weeks to neonates symptomatic with central nervous system disease prevents hearing deterioration at 6 months and possibly at greater than or equal to one year.

Prenatal Diagnosis. In some cases, effects of fetal infection are detected by ultrasonography, computed tomography (CT), or magnetic resonance imaging. Microcephaly, ventriculomegaly, or cerebral calcifications may be seen (Malinger and colleagues, 2003). Ascites, hepatomegaly, splenomegaly, hydrops, hyperechoic bowel, and oligohydramnios have also been described. Enders and co-workers (2001) observed that an abnormal ultrasonographic examination in combination with positive findings in fetal blood or amnionic fluid predicted an approximate 75-percent risk of symptomatic congenital infection.

Currently, PCR is used to detect and quantify viral DNA in amnionic fluid and fetal blood (Revello and Gerna, 2002, 2004). Bodéus and colleagues (1999) and Antsaklis and associates (2000) both emphasized that a negative culture or PCR result from amnionic fluid does not always exclude fetal infection. In another study, Liesnard and co-workers (2000) showed that combined culture and PCR results allowed diagnosis in 44 of 55 infected fetuses (80 percent).

Recently, other investigators have extended these observations in an attempt to increase the specificity and sensitivity of amnionic fluid testing for CMV to predict both the risk of fetal infection and of symptomatic neonates (Gouarin and co-workers, 2001, 2002; Guerra and associates, 2000; Lazzarotto and colleagues, 2000).

Prevention. There is neither an available CMV vaccine nor an effective mode of passive prophylaxis. Prevention of congenital infection relies on the prevention of maternal primary

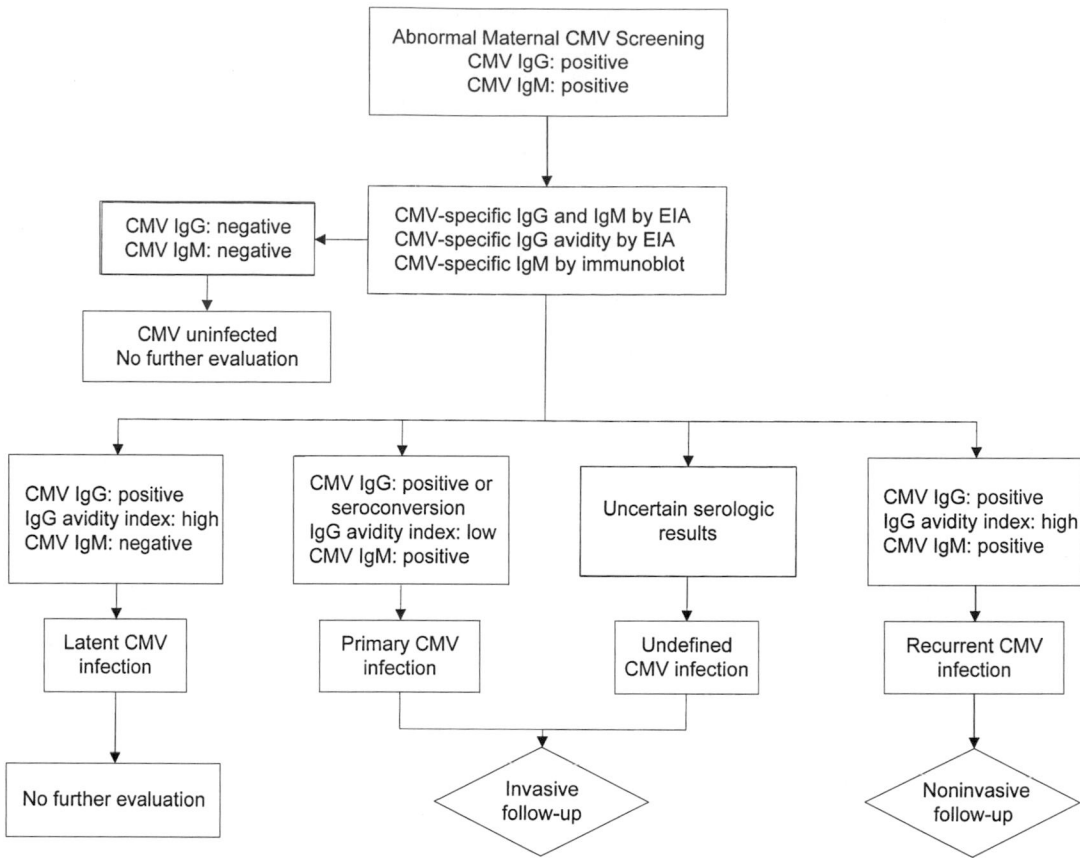

FIGURE 58–3. Algorithm for evaluation of suspected maternal primary cytomegalovirus (CMV) infection in pregnancy. (EIA = enzyme immunoassay.)

infection, especially in early pregnancy. Basic measures such as good hygiene and handwashing have been promoted, particularly for women with toddlers in day-care settings (Fowler, 2000). Sexual transmission from infected partners can also occur, but there is no data on the efficacy of any preventive strategy (Nigro and co-workers, 2003).

BACTERIAL INFECTIONS

GROUP A STREPTOCOCCUS. Infections caused by *Streptococcus pyogenes* are rarely encountered today (O'Brien and colleagues, 2002). Only 0.06 cases per 1000 births, that is, 220 cases are reported annually (Chuang and associates, 2002). *S pyogenes* produces a number of toxins and enzymes, and infections especially with M3 strains are particularly severe (Beres and collaborators, 2004). As discussed in Chapter 31 (see p. 713), the most common presentations for invasive postpartum group A streptococcal infection are bacteremia without a septic focus (46 percent), metritis (28 percent), peritonitis (8 percent), and septic abortion (7 percent).

Maternal colonization may also play a role in postpartum infection (Barnham and Weightman, 2001; Davies and

co-workers, 1996). Puerperal sepsis following identification of group A streptococci during group B surveillance testing has been reported (Stefonek and colleagues, 2001).

S pyogenes causes a *toxic shock-like syndrome* that is often fatal (Brown, 2004). The case-fatality rate for postpartum group A streptococcal infection is 3 to 4 percent (Chuang and associates, 2002). In one series, it was 73 percent (Udagawa and co-workers, 1999). Of three cases at Parkland Hospital in 1992, there were two maternal deaths (Nathan and colleagues, 1993). Prompt penicillin treatment, sometimes combined with surgical debridement, may be lifesaving (see Chapter 31, p. 721).

A less virulent exotoxin causes *scarlet fever*, which is also treated with penicillin. *Erysipelas* is an acute streptococcal skin infection, and bacteremia is common (Bisno and Stevens, 1996).

GROUP B STREPTOCOCCUS. Asymptomatic carriage of group B streptococcus (GBS)—*S agalactiae*—is common, especially in the vagina and rectum. Schrag and associates (2002, 2003) reported a colonization rate of 20 to 30 percent in a nationwide cohort sampled at a mean of 35 weeks. In a study done at Parkland Hospital in 1995 by Wendel and co-workers (2002), group B streptococcal carriage was detected in 15 percent of 8536 women in labor. Throughout pregnancy, colonization can be transient, intermittent, or chronic.

There is a spectrum of maternal and fetal GBS infections ranging from asymptomatic colonization to sepsis. *S agalactiae* has been implicated in adverse pregnancy outcomes, including preterm labor, prematurely ruptured membranes, clinical and subclinical chorioamnionitis, and fetal and neonatal infections. The bacterium can also cause bacteriuria, pyelonephritis, and postpartum metritis. Postpartum maternal osteomyelitis and mastitis caused by GBS infection have also been described (Barbosa-Cesnik and associates, 2003; Berkowitz and McCaffrey, 1990).

Neonatal Sepsis. Infection in neonates less than 7 days after birth is defined as *early-onset disease* (Schrag and colleagues, 2000). Many investigators use a threshold of less than 72 hours of life as most compatible with intrapartum acquisition of disease (Stoll and associates, 2002a; Wendel and co-workers, 2002). We have encountered a number of unexpected intrapartum stillbirths from GBS infections. In many neonates, septicemia involves signs of serious illness that usually develop within 6 to 12 hours of birth, including respiratory distress, apnea, and shock. At the outset, therefore, the neonatal infection must be differentiated from idiopathic respiratory distress syndrome. The mortality rate with early-onset disease has declined to about 4 percent. Preterm newborns do not fare as well.

Late-onset disease usually manifests as meningitis 1 week to 3 months after birth. These cases are most often caused by serotype III organisms. The mortality rate, although appreciable, is less for late-onset meningitis than for early-onset sepsis. Unfortunately, it is not uncommon for surviving infants of both early- and late-onset disease to exhibit neurological sequelae.

Epidemiology. Intrapartum fetal transmission from the colonized mother may lead to severe neonatal sepsis soon after birth. Reported rates of early-onset sepsis historically ranged from 2 to 3 per 1000 live births before widespread intrapartum chemoprophylaxis was implemented. Currently most centers and countries have experienced a decline in early-onset neonatal sepsis to rates of less than 1 to 2 per 1000 live births. Most reports, however, indicate no change or variable increases in rates of non-GBS organisms, such as *E coli* and other Enterobacteriaceae (Baltimore, 2001; Hyde, 2002; Levine, 1999; Moore, 2003; Towers and Briggs, 2002, and all their colleagues).

There is worrisome evidence that the major association with current intrapartum antimicrobial prophylaxis has been an increase in non-GBS early-onset sepsis in preterm, low-birthweight neonates, and especially very-low-birthweight neonates. (Eschenbach, 2002; Towers and Briggs, 2002). For example, while Stoll and Hansen (2003) and Stoll and associates (2002a) observed a marked reduction in group B streptococcal sepsis in these preterm neonates, this was offset by an increase in *E coli* sepsis. Very-low-birthweight neonates with early-onset sepsis have higher rates of respiratory distress, intraventricular hemorrhage with periventricular leukomalacia, and bronchopulmonary dysplasia. The death rate in newborns with early-onset infection was 37 percent, compared with 13 percent in uninfected newborns. The death rate for gram-negative infections was 36 percent, compared with 11 percent for gram-positive ones.

Late-onset neonatal GBS sepsis is less well understood. Cited rates vary from 0.5 to 2 cases per 1000 live births and account for about 50 percent of GBS disease in newborns (Lin and colleagues, 2003). The incidence of late-onset disease has remained stable despite widespread use of intrapartum antimicrobials, suggesting that GBS screening and chemoprophylaxis intervention may not affect late-onset disease. Lin and co-workers (2003) reported that preterm birth before 34 weeks was the major risk factor. Stoll and associates (2002b) found that late-onset sepsis was identified in a fourth of very-low-birthweight newborns; there was a preponderance of gram-positive organisms, mainly coagulase-negative staphylococci.

Recommended Prevention Strategies. Lacking randomized trials, consensus opinions and guidelines on prevention strategies have been promulgated by the American College of Obstetricians and Gynecologists (2002a) and the Centers for Disease Control and Prevention (2002d). These guidelines advocate a culture-based screening approach to identify women who should receive intrapartum prophylaxis (Fig. 58–4). This recommendation was derived from a multistate, retrospective cohort study of live births in 1998 and 1999 from the Active Bacterial Surveillance/Emerging Infections Program network, which suggested that the culture-based approach was superior to a risk-based approach.

The recommendations also describe management of imminent preterm delivery in the setting of preterm labor or preterm prematurely ruptured membranes (Fig. 58–5). Data suggesting a single course of management or recommending a specific treatment duration for GBS-positive women with arrested preterm labor or preterm prematurely ruptured membranes are insufficient (American College of Obstetricians and Gynecologists, 2002a).

With the culture-based approach, women are screened for GBS colonization at 35 to 37 weeks, and intrapartum antimicrobials are given to rectovaginal carriers. Previous siblings with GBS invasive disease and prior identification of GBS bacteriuria are also considered indications for prophylaxis. A risk-based approach is recommended for women with unknown group B streptococcal culture results at the time of labor (see Fig. 58–4).

The choice of antimicrobials may be important in terms of allergic reaction; selection of resistant GBS strains; and emergence of other pathogens, including antimicrobial-resistant strains, as agents of neonatal sepsis. Treatments are shown

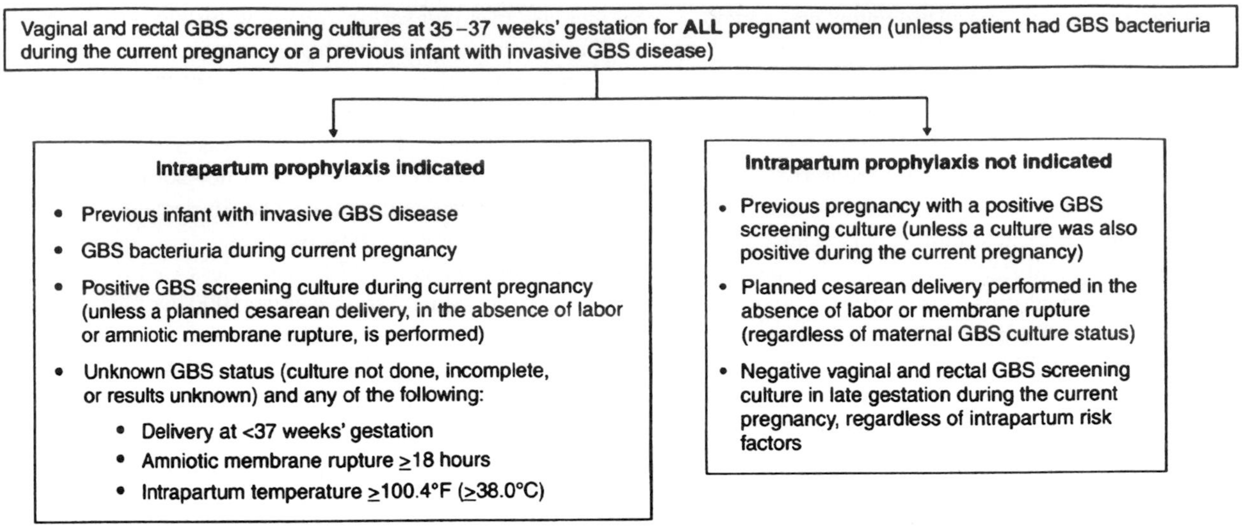

Vaginal and rectal GBS screening cultures at 35–37 weeks' gestation for ALL pregnant women (unless patient had GBS bacteriuria during the current pregnancy or a previous infant with invasive GBS disease)
Intrapartum prophylaxis indicated
• Previous infant with invasive GBS disease
• GBS bacteriuria during current pregnancy
• Positive GBS screening culture during current pregnancy (unless a planned cesarean delivery, in the absence of labor or amniotic membrane rupture, is performed)
• Unknown GBS status (culture not done, incomplete, or results unknown) and any of the following:
• Delivery at <37 weeks' gestation
• Amniotic membrane rupture ≥18 hours
• Intrapartum temperature ≥100.4°F (≥38.0°C)
Intrapartum prophylaxis not indicated
• Previous pregnancy with a positive GBS screening culture (unless a culture was also positive during the current pregnancy)
• Planned cesarean delivery performed in the absence of labor or membrane rupture (regardless of maternal GBS culture status)
• Negative vaginal and rectal GBS screening culture in late gestation during the current pregnancy, regardless of intrapartum risk factors

FIGURE 58–4. Indications for intrapartum prophylaxis to prevent perinatal group B streptococcal (GBS) disease under a universal prenatal screening strategy based on combined vaginal and rectal cultures taken at 35 to 37 weeks' gestation. (From Centers for Disease Control and Prevention, 2002d.)

in Table 58–2. The Centers for Disease Control and Prevention recommendations specify penicillin as a first-line agent (Johnson and colleagues, 2001). Ampicillin is an acceptable alternative (Bloom and co-workers, 1996). For women with penicillin allergy, if the risk of anaphylaxis is low, cefazolin is recommended (Mitchell and associates, 2001). If the risk of anaphylaxis is high, selection of a prophylactic agent is dependent on GBS susceptibility testing. Patients with isolates susceptible to clindamycin or erythromycin may be given either drug. Antimicrobial-resistant strains require vancomycin prophylaxis. This treatment scheme is dependent on laboratory capability to perform susceptibility testing.

Importantly, there have been no randomized controlled trials comparing antenatal screening, whether culture-based or risk-based, with no antenatal screening. In addition, there have been no randomized trials comparing the different

Onset of labor or rupture of membranes at < 37 weeks' gestation with significant risk for imminent preterm delivery
No GBS culture
GBS positive
GBS negative
Obtain vaginal and rectal GBS culture and initiate IV antimicrobials
GBS positive
IV antimicrobials for ≥ 48 hours (during tocolysis)
No GBS prophylaxis
No growth at 48 hours
Stop antimicrobials
Intrapartum antimicrobial prophylaxis at delivery

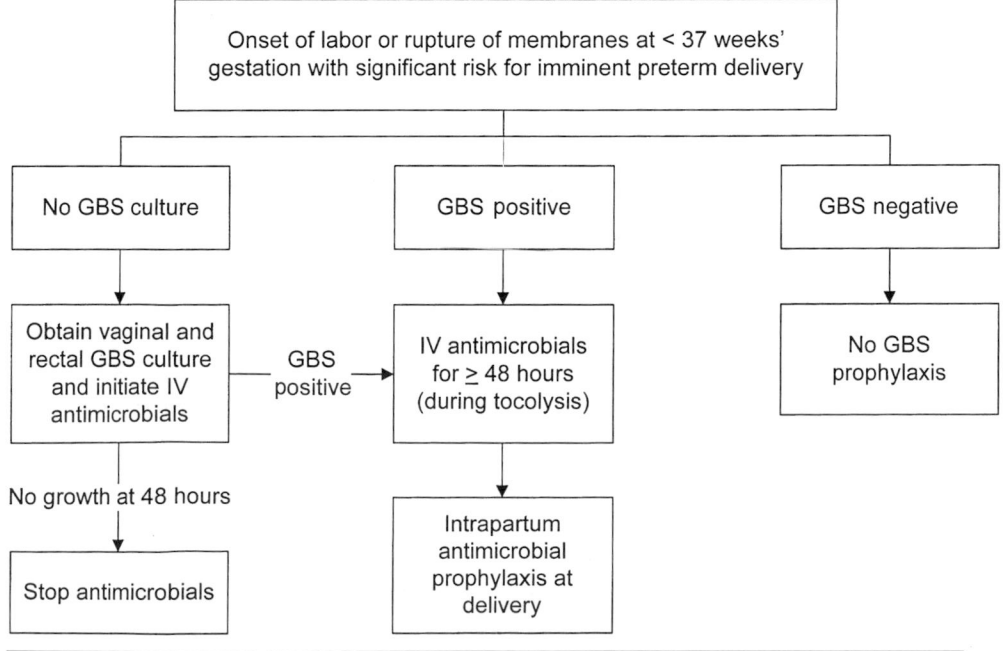

FIGURE 58–5. Sample algorithm for prophylaxis for women with group B streptococcal (GBS) disease and threatened preterm delivery. This algorithm is not an exclusive course of management and variations that incorporate individual circumstances or institutional preferences may be appropriate. (Adapted from Centers for Disease Control and Prevention, 2002d.)

TABLE 58–2 Regimens for Intrapartum Antimicrobial Prophylaxis for Perinatal Prevention of Group B Streptococcal Disease

Regimen	Treatment
Recommended	Penicillin G, 5 million units IV initial dose, then 2.5 million units IV every 4 hours until delivery
Alternative	Ampicillin, 2 g IV initial dose, then 1 g IV every 4 hours or 2 g every 6 hours until delivery
If penicillin allergic[a]	
Patients **not** at high risk for anaphylaxis	Cefazolin, 2 g IV initial dose, then 1 g IV every 8 hours until delivery
Patients at high risk for anaphylaxis and with GBS susceptible to clindamycin and erythromycin	Clindamycin, 900 mg IV every 8 hours until delivery **OR** Erythromycin, 500 mg IV every 6 hours until delivery
GBS resistant to clindamycin or erythromycin or susceptibility unknown	Vancomycin, 1 g IV every 12 hours until delivery

GBS = group B streptococcus.
[a] History of penicillin allergy should be assessed to determine whether a high risk for anaphylaxis is present. Penicillin-allergic patients at high risk for anaphylaxis are those who have experienced immediate hypersensitivity to penicillin including a history of penicillin-related anaphylaxis. Other high-risk patients are those with asthma or other diseases that would make anaphylaxis more dangerous or difficult to treat, such as persons being treated with β-adrenergic blocking agents.
Adapted from the Centers for Disease Control and Prevention (2002d).

screening strategies and whether prenatal GBS screening has a significant impact on overall neonatal sepsis. For these reasons, clinicians in other countries state that there is insufficient evidence to recommended screening for GBS carriage (Canadian Task Force on Preventive Health Care, 2002; Jakobi and colleagues, 2003; Royal College of Obstetricians and Gynaecologists, 2003).

Alternative prevention strategies have been described with limited evidence to recommend them. These include intramuscular benzathine penicillin G and chlorhexidine vaginal lavage (Bland and associates, 2000; Rouse and co-workers, 2003). In another study, Haberland and colleagues (2002) reported that intrapartum rapid PCR screening for GBS may be superior to current strategies, however, this must be proven effective in clinical trials. In GBS-positive women, appropriate vaginal examinations or indicated intrauterine fetal monitoring should not be avoided as their avoidance could actually prolong labor and thus increase the risk of infection (Gibbs and associates, 2004).

In 1995, prior to the consensus guidelines, we adopted the risk-based approach at Parkland Hospital for intrapartum treatment of women at high risk for GBS infection. In addition, all term neonates born to women at high risk for GBS infection who were not given intrapartum prophylaxis were treated in the delivery room with aqueous penicillin G, 50 to 60,000 units intramuscularly. Early-onset GBS infection and sepsis, as well as non-GBS sepsis, all decreased during the study (Wendel and associates, 2002). Almost 80 percent of failures (i.e., neonatal infections) were caused by chorioamnionitis (Velaphi and associates, 2003).

Implementation of several protocols is associated with diminished GBS sepsis. There are, however, still ma-

jor concerns about antimicrobial resistance, particularly among very-low-birthweight neonates. Ongoing surveillance is necessary to monitor protocol efficacy for prevention of early-onset GBS sepsis as well as for any effects on maternal morbidity, overall neonatal sepsis, and resistant infections.

Vaccination. Some protection against serious neonatal infection is conferred by maternal antibodies. Indeed, Lin and colleagues (2001) have confirmed that the susceptibility to invasive GBS disease correlates with deficiency in maternal type-specific antibody levels. Baker and co-workers (1988, 1999, 2000) reported that maternal immunization to type III antigen produces antibody in about 60 percent of women. Monovalent tetanus toxoid conjugate vaccines are immunogenic for common GBS disease-associated serotypes. Paoletti and Madoff (2002) have reviewed the progress toward development of a multivalent vaccine.

LISTERIOSIS. *Listeria monocytogenes* is an uncommon but probably underdiagnosed cause of neonatal sepsis. The Centers for Disease Control and Prevention (2001a) estimate that nearly 2500 individuals in the United States annually are ill with listeriosis, and more than 500 die. This Gram-positive, aerobic, motile bacillus can be isolated from the feces of 1 to 5 percent of adults. Food-borne transmission is important. Outbreaks of listeriosis have been reported from raw vegetables; coleslaw; apple cider; milk; fresh Mexican-style cheese; smoked fish; and processed foods, such as paté, hot dogs, and sliced delicatessen meat.

Listerial infections are more common in very old or young, pregnant, or immunocompromised patients. Some authors have speculated that pregnant women are susceptible because

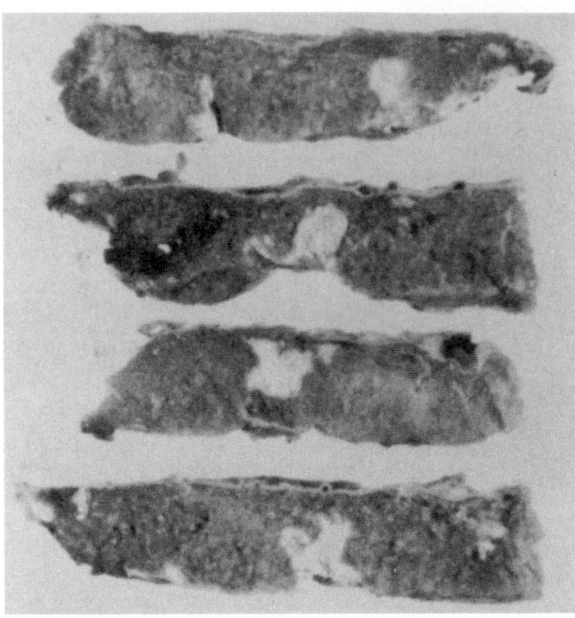

FIGURE 58–6. Listeriosis: multiple cut surfaces of placenta show several well-demarcated, grayish-white macroabscesses that appear solid and are indistinguishable from ischemic infarcts. (From Topalovski and colleagues, 1993, with permission.)

of decreased cell-mediated immunity (Wing and Gregory, 2002).

Listeriosis during pregnancy may be asymptomatic or cause a febrile illness that is confused with influenza, pyelonephritis, or meningitis (Mylonakis and colleagues, 2002; Silver, 1998). The diagnosis usually is not apparent until blood cultures are reported as positive. Alvarez and associates (2004) described a 13-week pregnant woman with *S typhimurium* isolated from blood and urine cultures. Occult or clinical infection also may stimulate labor (Boucher and Yonekura, 1986). Discolored, brownish, or meconium-stained amnionic fluid is common with fetal infection, even with preterm gestations.

Maternal listeremia causes fetal infection that characteristically produces disseminated granulomatous lesions with microabscesses (Topalovski and colleagues, 1993). Chorioamnionitis is common with maternal infection and placental lesions may develop (Fig. 58–6). In a review of 222 cases by Mylonakis and associates (2002), infection resulted in abortion or stillbirth in 20 percent, and neonatal sepsis developed in 68 percent of surviving newborns. There are two types of neonatal infection, very similar to GBS sepsis. *Early-onset infection* develops within 5 to 7 days, is usually associated with maternal illness, and presents with respiratory distress and with fever or neurological abnormalities or both. Most neonates are preterm and symptomatic at birth. *Late-onset infection* after 5 to 7 days of life usually presents as meningitis, and it may be associated with nosocomial transmission. The overall neonatal mortality from listeriosis is about 25 percent in reported cases (Mylonakis and associates, 2002).

Treatment. There are no clinical trials, but an ampicillin-gentamicin combination is usually recommended because of its synergism. Trimethoprim-sulfamethoxazole is given to penicillin-allergic women. Maternal outcome is excellent, and there is evidence that maternal treatment may also be effective for fetal infection.

Prevention. There is no vaccine for listeriosis. Pregnant women may choose to avoid the implicated foods listed previously.

SALMONELLA AND SHIGELLA

Salmonellosis. Infections from *Salmonella* and *Shigella* species continue to be a major cause of food-borne illness. There are 800,000 to 4 million cases of salmonella infections each year in the United States, which result in 500 deaths (Centers for Disease Control and Prevention, 1999b). Gastroenteritis is contracted through contaminated food, and symptoms include diarrhea, abdominal pain, fever, chills, nausea, and vomiting. Management is usually intravenous fluid rehydration. Antimicrobials do not shorten illness and may prolong the convalescent carrier state. They are not given in uncomplicated infections.

Typhoid Fever. Uncommonly seen in the United States, this disease is caused by *Salmonella enterica* serotype typhi, which is spread by oral ingestion of contaminated food, water, or milk. In pregnant women, the disease is more likely to be encountered during epidemics or in those who are infected with HIV (Hedriana and colleagues, 1995). In their review, Dildy and associates (1990) reported that antepartum typhoid fever in former years resulted in abortion, preterm labor, and maternal or fetal death.

Fluoroquinolones are the most effective treatment, but clinicians may choose to use intravenous third-generation cephalosporins or azithromycin in pregnant women (Parry and co-workers, 2002). Typhoid vaccines appear to exert no harmful effects when administered to pregnant women and should be given in an epidemic or before travel to endemic areas (Centers for Disease Control and Prevention, 2003a).

Shigellosis. Bacillary dysentery caused from *Shigella* infection is a relatively common, highly contagious cause in adults of inflammatory exudative diarrhea, frequently with bloody stools. Shigellosis is more common in children attending day-care centers, and it is highly contagious. Clinical manifestations range from mild diarrhea to severe dysentery, abdominal cramping, tenesmus, fever, and systemic toxicity.

Although shigellosis may be self-limited, careful attention to treatment of dehydration is essential in severe cases. We have cared for pregnant women in whom secretory diarrhea exceeded 10 L/day! Effective treatments during pregnancy include fluoroquinolones, ceftriaxone, azithromycin, and trimethoprim-sulfamethoxazole (Bhattacharya and Sur, 2003).

HANSEN DISEASE. This chronic infection, also known as leprosy, is caused by *Mycobacterium leprae*. Dapsone, rifampin, and clofazimine for treatment appear to be safe for use during pregnancy (Britton and Lockwood, 2004; Farb and associates, 1982). Rifampin therapy is also effective. Duncan (1980) reported an excessive incidence of low-birthweight newborns born to infected women. The placenta is not involved, and neonatal infection apparently is acquired from skin-to-skin or droplet transmission (Duncan and colleagues, 1984).

LYME DISEASE. This disease is caused by the spirochete *Borrelia burgdorferi*. It is the most commonly reported vector-borne illness in the United States. Lyme borreliosis results from the bite of ticks of the genus *Ixodes*. Early infection causes a distinctive local skin lesion, *erythema migrans*, which may be accompanied by a flulike syndrome and regional adenopathy. If untreated, disseminated infection follows in days to weeks. Multisystem involvement is common, but skin lesions, arthralgia and myalgia, carditis, and meningitis predominate. If still untreated after several weeks to months, late or persistent infection manifests in perhaps half of patients. Native immunity is acquired, and the disease enters a chronic phase. Although some patients remain asymptomatic, others in the chronic phase develop a variety of dermatological, rheumatic, or neurological manifestations (Steere, 2001).

Serological diagnosis has pitfalls, and clinical diagnosis is important. Although positive in only about half of patients with early disease, most with late, untreated Lyme disease have a positive ELISA result.

Treatment. Optimal treatment has not been established. In early infection, treatment with doxycycline or amoxicillin is recommended. Pregnant women are given oral amoxicillin or penicillin V for 3 weeks (Steere, 2001). Cefuroxime is preferred, but erythromycin can be used for penicillin-allergic women. For later infection manifested by meningitis or carditis, intravenous ceftriaxone, cefotaxime, or penicillin G is recommended. Chronic arthritis and post–Lyme disease syndrome are treated with prolonged oral or intravenous regimens, however, symptoms respond poorly to treatment (Klempner and colleagues, 2001).

Neonatal Infection. Literature regarding the reproductive effects of Lyme disease has failed to define a teratogenic effect or an association with fetal death, preterm delivery, or malformations (Elliott, 2001; Maraspin, 1999; Strobino, 1999, and all their colleagues).

Prevention. A vaccine was withdrawn from the market in 2002 due to low sales. Avoidance of areas where Lyme disease is endemic and improved tick control in those areas may be beneficial. Personal tick checks and removal of unengorged ticks within 36 hours of attachment reduce risks of infection (Hayes and Piesman, 2003). For tick bites recognized within 72 hours, a single 200-mg dose of doxycycline reduces the risk of erythema migrans by 87 percent (Nadelman and associates, 2001). Prompt treatment of maternal early infection should prevent most adverse pregnancy outcomes.

TUBERCULOSIS. Diagnosis and management of tuberculosis is discussed in detail in Chapter 46 (see p. 1065).

PROTOZOAL INFECTIONS

TOXOPLASMOSIS. *Toxoplasma gondii* has a complex life cycle and may exist in one of three forms: (1) as a *tachyzoite* invading and replicating intracellularly during infection, (2) as a *bradyzoite* forming tissue cysts during latent infection, and (3) as a *sporozoite* found in oocysts that can be environmentally resistant (Jones and associates, 2001b). Maternal infection is transmitted by eating raw or undercooked meat infected with tissue cysts or through contact with oocysts from infected cat feces in contaminated litter, soil, or water.

Adults rarely develop symptoms, but they do have tachyzoite parasitemia temporarily. In pregnant women, focal lesions then develop in the placenta, and the fetus may become infected. The fetus initially has generalized infection that is then cleared from visceral organs, but may localize in the central nervous system (Hill and Dubey, 2002).

According to the Third National Health and Nutrition Examination Survey cohort from 1988 to 1994, the seroprevalence of toxoplasmosis was only 15 percent in women 15 to 44 years of age. This suggests that 85 percent of pregnant women are susceptible to *T gondii* infection. Literature reviews indicate that the incidence of new infection ranges from 0.5 to 8.1 per 1000 in susceptible pregnancies (Gilbert and Peckham, 2002).

The incidence of congenital toxoplasmosis varies from 0.8 per 10,000 live births in the United States to 10 per 10,000 in France (Dubey, 2000). The Centers for Disease Control and Prevention (Lopez and colleagues, 2000) estimate that there are between 400 and 4000 cases of congenital toxoplasmosis each year in the United States. The incidence and severity of congenital infection depend on the gestational age of the fetus at the time of maternal primary infection. The risk of fetal infection increases with duration of pregnancy, with the risk of fetal infection rising from 6 percent at 13 weeks to 72 percent at 36 weeks (Fig. 58–7). Fetuses infected in early pregnancy, however, are much more likely to show signs of infection (Dunn and associates, 1999).

Most acute infections in mothers and neonates are asymptomatic and can be detected only by prenatal or newborn serological screening. Maternal symptoms may include fatigue, muscle pain, and sometimes lymphadenopathy, but most often infection is subclinical. In immunocompetent adults, initial infection confers immunity, and prepregnancy infection nearly eliminates any risk of vertical transmission. Infection

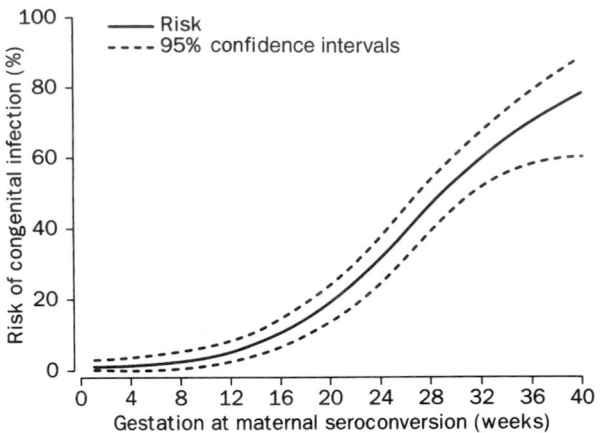

FIGURE 58–7. Risk of congenital toxoplasmosis infection by gestational age at maternal seroconversion. (From Dunn and colleagues, 1999, with permission.)

in immunocompromised women, however, may be severe, with reactivation involving encephalitis or mass lesions.

The majority of infected fetuses are born without obvious signs of toxoplasmosis on routine examination. Clinically affected neonates at birth usually have generalized disease with low birthweight, hepatosplenomegaly, icterus, and anemia. Some primarily have neurological disease, intracranial calcifications (Fig. 58–8), and hydrocephaly or microcephaly. Many eventually develop chorioretinitis and exhibit learning disabilities. These findings make up the classic triad

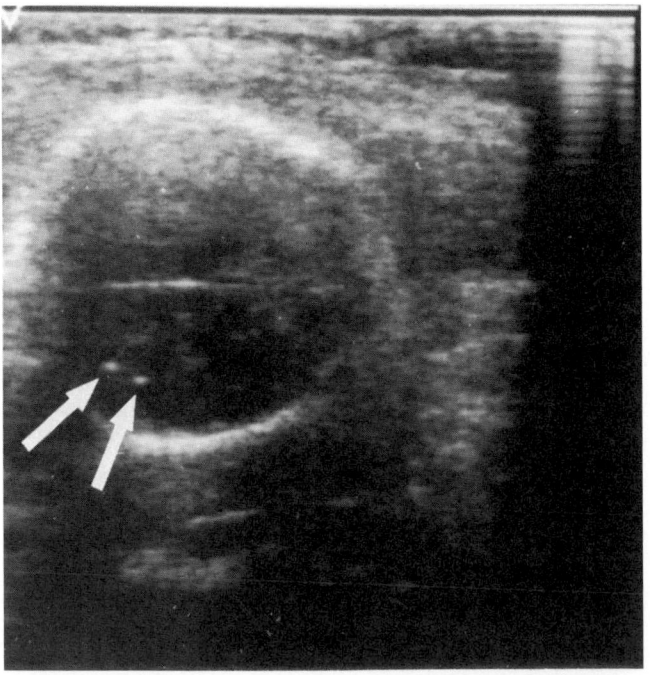

FIGURE 58–8. Intracranial calcifications (*arrows*) seen by ultrasonography in a microcephalic fetus at about 30 weeks. (Courtesy of Dr. R. Santos.)

described for this congenital infection—chorioretinitis, intracranial calcifications, and hydrocephalus. It often is accompanied by convulsions. Infected neonates with clinical signs are at risk for long-term complications.

Management. There is no consensus on the most appropriate screening or treatment strategy. In some European countries, *prenatal screening* is done routinely. However, the United Kingdom National Screening Committee recommended against universal prenatal or neonatal screening in the United Kingdom (Gilbert and Peckham, 2002). The American College of Obstetricians and Gynecologists (2000) does not recommend screening except for pregnant women with HIV infection. If anti-toxoplasma IgG antibody is confirmed before pregnancy, then a woman is not at risk for a congenitally infected fetus (Montoya, 2002).

Acute infection may be documented by seroconversion of IgG and IgM antibodies or by a greater than fourfold rise in paired specimens. Unfortunately, no single test accomplishes the goal of timing maternal seroconversion, because IgG may persist in high titer for years and IgM may also be detectable for more than 1 year. A panel of tests, however, performed in reference laboratories is often used (Roberts and associates, 2001). For many, the best resource is the Toxoplasma Serology Laboratory at the Palo Alto Medical Foundation Research Institute, which uses a Toxoplasma Serologic Profile consisting of the Sabin Feldman dye test, a double-sandwich IgM ELISA, an IgA ELISA, an IgG ELISA, and a differential agglutination test (AC/HS test) (Montoya and Liesenfeld, 2004).

Recently, an avidity test for toxoplasma IgG antibody has been added to maternal serum panel testing (Beghetto, 2003; Liesenfeld, 2001; Montoya, 2002, 2004, and all their coworkers). The functional avidity of IgG antibody is low with primary infection and increases during weeks and months. When high-avidity IgG is determined, infection within the preceding 3 to 5 months is excluded. Maternal antibody panel testing, combined with IgG avidity testing, aids diagnosis and dating of maternal toxoplasma infection with a single serum specimen. In addition, a PCR assay with high specificity (96 percent) and sensitivity (81 percent) for *T gondii* has been developed to permit prenatal testing of amnionic fluid (Hohlfeld and colleagues, 1994). A high PCR quantitative parasite load before 20 weeks has the greatest risk for a poor fetal outcome (Romand and colleagues, 2004).

Treatment. Treatment of pregnant women is thought to prevent and reduce, but not eliminate, the risk of congenital infection (American College of Obstetricians and Gynecologists, 2000). *Spiramycin*, used alone, is thought to reduce the risk of congenital infection but not to treat established fetal infection. Presumptive treatment with pyrimethamine and sulfonamides has been suggested for primary maternal infection in late pregnancy with negative amnionic fluid testing (Romand and associates, 2001). When fetal infection is diagnosed by prenatal testing, pyrimethamine, sulfonamides, and folinic acid are added to spiramycin to eradicate parasites in the placenta and fetus.

Three large, recent trials in Europe, however, have questioned the therapeutic value of maternal treatment and found no effect from the type of medication or by a delay in treatment of up to 8 weeks (European Multicentre Study on Congenital Toxoplasmosis, 2003; Gilbert and associates, 2001; Gras and co-workers, 2001). Randomized controlled trials likely are required to measure the true effect of prenatal treatment on mother-to-child transmission.

Prevention. There is no vaccine for toxoplasmosis, but many cases of congenital infection could be prevented by the following specific recommendations (Lopez and colleagues, 2000):

- Cook meat to safe temperatures
- Peel or thoroughly wash fruits and vegetables before consumption
- Clean cooking surfaces and utensils that contain raw meat, poultry, seafood, or unwashed fruits and vegetables
- Wear gloves when changing cat litter or delegate this duty
- Avoid feeding cats raw or undercooked meat and keep cats indoors

Unfortunately, the effectiveness of these measures is uncertain (Jones and co-workers, 2001a).

MALARIA. There are four species of *Plasmodium* that cause human malaria: *vivax, ovale, malariae,* and *falciparum.* Nearly 300 to 500 million persons worldwide are infected at any given time, and the disease causes 1 to 3 million deaths annually (Murray and colleagues, 2000). Almost 48 percent of the world population—3 billion people—are at risk of contracting the disease (Hay and associates, 2004). Malaria has been effectively eradicated in Europe and most of North America except for parts of Mexico.

The disease is characterized by fever and flulike symptoms, including chills, headaches, myalgia, and malaise, which may occur at intervals. Symptoms are less severe with recurrences. Malaria may be associated with anemia and jaundice, and falciparum infections may cause kidney failure, coma, and death.

Effects on Pregnancy. Malarial episodes increase significantly by three- to fourfold during the latter two trimesters of pregnancy and 2 months postpartum (Diagne and associates, 2000). Pregnancy enhances the severity of falciparum malaria, especially in nonimmune primiparas (Nathwani and colleagues, 1992; Robier and co-workers, 1999). The incidence of abortion and preterm labor is increased with malaria (Menendez and associates, 2000). Increased fetal loss may be related to placental and fetal infection (Goldenberg and Thompson, 2003). In an earlier study, however, Jones (1950) observed that parasites have an affinity for decidual vessels and may involve the placenta extensively without

affecting the fetus. According to McGready and co-workers (2004), malarial parasites are more common with falciparum than with vivax infections. Covell (1950) studied this extensively in Africa and cited an incidence of neonatal malaria of only 0.3 percent. In nonimmune women, congenital malaria may develop in up to 7 percent of neonates (Hulbert, 1992).

Treatment. Commonly used antimalarial drugs are not contraindicated during pregnancy. Some of the newer antimalarial agents have antifolic acid activity and may theoretically contribute to the development of megaloblastic anemia. In actual practice, this does not appear to be the case.

Chloroquine is the treatment of choice for malaria caused by *Plasmodium* species sensitive to the drug (Taylor and White, 2004). For the woman with chloroquine-resistant infection, *mefloquine* is given orally. At high doses, mefloquine is teratogenic and embryotoxic in some laboratory animals. Despite this, limited data indicate the drug to be safe and effective in pregnancy (Newman and colleagues, 2003).

The severity of malaria, especially with *P falciparum* infection, may be underestimated on initial clinical presentation. A thorough assessment of the severity of infection should precede but not delay treatment in pregnant women (Moore and associates, 2003; World Health Organization, 2000). For severe or complicated malaria, quinine is given parenterally. Its major side effect is hypoglycemia. Artemisinin and its derivatives have been used in a limited number of cases in the second half of pregnancy with success and without apparent complications (Alecrim and co-workers, 2000).

Prophylaxis. Pregnant women in areas in which malaria is endemic are primary candidates for chemoprophylaxis to prevent the adverse consequences of infection during pregnancy. Cot and colleagues (1992) showed that chloroquine chemoprophylaxis decreased placental infection in asymptomatic infected women to 4 percent compared with 19 percent of untreated controls. Alternatively, a simple control strategy of intermittent presumptive treatment with sulfadoxine-pyrimethamine at the start of the second and third trimesters significantly reduces maternal anemia, placental parasitemia, and low-birthweight, although HIV-infected women may require additional doses (Parise and co-workers, 1998; Verhoeff and associates, 1998). The World Health Organization has recommended this preventive regimen in areas where *P falciparum* is chloroquine resistant yet sensitive to sulfadoxine-pyrimethamine (Nahlen, 2000). There are limited data about the safety of newer agents such as amodiaquine and the artemisinins in pregnancy to recommend their routine use (McGready and colleagues, 2001). Pregnant women should not take doxycycline or the combination of atovaquone and proguanil for chemoprophylaxis.

Chemoprophylaxis is recommended for travel to endemic areas. If chloroquine-resistant falciparum or vivax malaria has not been reported, prophylaxis is initiated 1 to 2 weeks before the endemic area is entered. Chloroquine, 500 mg of base, is given orally once a week, and this is continued until 4 weeks after return to nonendemic areas (Bradley and Warhurst, 1995; Centers for Disease Control and Prevention, 2003b; Wyler, 1993). Travel to areas endemic for chloroquine-resistant strains is discouraged during early pregnancy, after which mefloquine prophylaxis is given (Centers for Disease Control and Prevention, 2003a).

Schwartz and associates (2003) emphasized the complexity of contemporary malaria prophylaxis due to drug resistance and the limitations of common regimens to protect against subsequent relapses from the liver stages of *P vivax* and *P ovale*. Providers and travelers can obtain the latest chemoprophylaxis regimens for pregnancy from the Centers for Disease Control and Prevention *Travelers Health* web site at http://www.cdc.gov/travel/. The Centers for Disease Control and Prevention (2003b) also publish *Health Information for International Travel*, also called *The Yellow Book*, with detailed information.

Several malaria vaccines are currently under evaluation that target different stages of the parasitic cycle (Guerin and co-workers, 2002).

AMEBIASIS. Most persons infected with *Entamoeba histolytica* are asymptomatic. Amebic dysentery, however, may take a fulminant course during pregnancy. Prognosis is worse if complicated by a hepatic abscess, which may be serious, and rupture has been reported (Constantine and colleagues, 1987). Therapy is similar to that for the nonpregnant woman, and metronidazole is the drug of choice for amebic colitis and invasive disease. Noninvasive infections may be treated with paromomycin (Haque and associates, 2003).

MYCOTIC INFECTIONS

Disseminated infection during pregnancy is uncommon with coccidiomycosis, blastomycosis, cryptococcosis, or histoplasmosis. Their identification and management are considered in Chapter 46 (see p. 1060).

EMERGING INFECTIONS

WEST NILE VIRUS. This mosquito-borne flavivirus is a human neuropathogen. Since 1999, reported numbers of human and animal infections have increased, and the geographical range of disease activity has expanded (Morse, 2003). Infection may be acquired through mosquito bites, typically in late summer. The incubation period is 3 to 14 days, and most persons have mild or no symptoms. Less than 1 percent of adults develop meningoencephalitis. In pregnant women,

presenting symptoms are fever, mental status changes, muscle weakness, and coma (Centers for Disease Control and Prevention, 2002c; Chapa and colleagues, 2003).

The diagnosis is made based on clinical symptoms and the detection of West Nile virus IgG and IgM in serum and IgM in cerebrospinal fluid. There is no known effective antiviral treatment, and management is supportive. Fetal infection has been described at 27 weeks, and the term neonate had chorioretinitis along with severe temporal and occipital lobe white matter loss and temporal lobe cystic changes (Alpert and co-workers, 2003; Centers for Disease Control and Prevention, 2002c). Currently, the fetal risks are not quantified. The Centers for Disease Control and Prevention (2004a) have established a registry for birth outcomes of infected women. Breast feeding is not proscribed (Centers for Disease Control and Prevention, 2002c).

SEVERE ACUTE RESPIRATORY SYNDROME (SARS). Starting in 2002, several outbreaks of this infection have been reported in Asia and North America. The disease is associated with a novel *coronavirus* that is transmitted through droplets, close contact with infected secretions, fluids, and waste (Drosten and associates, 2003; Ksiazek and co-workers, 2003). The clinical picture is very similar to community-acquired pneumonia, and a history of SARS exposure or travel to an affected area increases the likelihood of diagnosis (Wenzel and Edmond, 2003).

There appears to be a triphasic pattern to the clinical progression of SARS. The first week is characterized by the viral replication and cytolysis with fever and myalgias. During the second week, patients may suffer recurrent fever, diarrhea, and hypoxemia coincident with IgG seroconversion and a declining viral load. Progression at this stage is thought to be due to an overexuberant host immune response. The third phase is seen in about 20 percent of patients. These individuals develop acute respiratory distress syndrome and require ventilatory support (Fowler and colleagues, 2003b; Peiris and associates, 2003a,b). Much of the mortality from SARS is related to acute lung injury (Lew and co-workers, 2003; Rubenfeld, 2003).

Radiographic and CT manifestations of SARS include ground-glass opacities and unilateral and bilateral airspace consolidations in the lungs that can rapidly progress to extensive bilateral consolidation within 1 to 2 days. Patients also may have lymphopenia, thrombocytopenia, and elevated lactate dehydrogenase (Lew and colleagues, 2003; Tsang and co-workers, 2003).

At this time, treatment choices are unproven (Peiris and associates, 2003a). Most patients have been treated with broad-spectrum antimicrobials. In pregnancy, oral therapy is with clarithromycin, 500 mg twice daily, plus amoxicillin with clavulanate, 375 mg three times daily (So and colleagues, 2003; Wong and co-workers, 2003). Ribavirin and corticosteroids have been used to decrease viral replication and to modulate the immune response, respectively. Their use is controversial and should be reserved for those with severe illness (Mandell and associates, 2003).

Fetal Effects. The effect of SARS on pregnancy is unclear because of the small number of reported cases (Haines and colleagues, 2003; Wong and co-workers, 2003, 2004). In a small case-control study, Lam and collaborators (2004) provided evidence that SARS had a worse clinical outcome in pregnant compared with nonpregnant women. No fetal transmission has been documented in five neonates born to mothers with SARS (Peiris and colleagues, 2003a; Shek and associates, 2003). Gastrointestinal complications were described in two preterm neonates who had small bowel perforation.

METHICILLIN-RESISTANT *Staphylococcus au-reus.* Strains of *Staphylococcus aureus* acquire resistance to methicillin, which confers resistance to all penicillinase-resistant penicillins and cephalosporins. Community-acquired methicillin-resistant *Staphylococcus aureus* (MRSA) infections sometimes occur in clusters but often develop sporadically. We have observed an increased frequency of community-acquired MRSA in pregnant women over the last few years. Most infections tend to involve skin and soft tissues, forming abscesses or cellulitis, especially in HIV-infected women, injection drug users, and diabetics. We have also encountered community-acquired MRSA in postoperative wound infections and with puerperal mastitis.

Community-acquired MRSA strains are usually not resistant to other antimicrobials. Erythromycin and clindamycin resistance is variable, but most strains are sensitive to either fluoroquinolones, trimethoprim-sulfamethoxazole, gentamicin, rifampin, or vancomycin (Eady and Cove, 2003; Laibl and associates, 2005; Naimi and colleagues, 2003). Parenteral vancomycin therapy can be reserved for more serious, community-acquired MRSA infections such as wound infections and mastitis. Most uncomplicated, noninvasive skin and soft tissue infections should still be managed by draining any abscess, culturing and ordering susceptibility testing of any skin or abscess drainage, and empirically prescribing β-lactam oral agents.

There are unique issues related to pregnancy and the puerperium regarding MRSA. No data suggest that community-acquired MRSA patients or their families require decolonization. However, careful follow-up examination must ensure resolution of infection. The frequency and significance of intrapartum transmission are unclear, and there are no current recommendations regarding prophylaxis to prevent neonatal or surgical site infections. We have substituted vancomycin for β-lactam drugs in perioperative prophylaxis for cesarean deliveries and fourth-degree perineal injury repair and in treatment of chorioamnionitis in women with prior antepartum community-acquired MRSA infections. We do not discourage breast feeding in women with prior community-acquired MRSA but stress good hygiene and attention to minor nipple skin breaks.

TRAVEL IN PREGNANCY

Pregnant travelers face obstetrical risks, general medical risks, and potentially hazardous destination risks. These may include high altitudes, areas with serious food- or insect-borne infections, areas of drug-resistant *Plasmodium falciparum*, and areas where live-virus vaccines are recommended or required. Precautions may include dietary advice, malaria chemoprophylaxis, and avoidance of insect bites. The International Society for Tropical Medicine has comprehensive information at http://www.istm.org. The Centers for Disease Control and Prevention have extensive travel information regarding pregnancy and breast feeding at its *Travelers' Health* home page at http://www.cdc.gov/travel/index.htm and *The Yellow Book* (Centers for Disease Control and Prevention, 2003b). The American College of Obstetricians and Gynecologists (2003) has updated its recommendations on active and passive immunization in pregnancy, include some vaccination issues pertinent to travel.

Travel medicine has become a specialized field and informed consultations require a knowledge of global infectious disease and current recommendations. Frequently these can be provided by specialists in maternal–fetal medicine, travel or tropical medicine, or infectious diseases (Ryan and colleagues, 2002; Ryan and Kain, 2000).

BIOTERRORISM

Bioterrorism threats have heightened awareness that chemical, nuclear, radiological, or infectious emergencies may affect individual persons or countries. Clinicians should be alert for significant increases in the number of persons with febrile illnesses accompanied by respiratory symptoms or with rashes not easily associated with common illnesses. These cases, if due to biological weapon use, need an infrastructure that includes reporting, treatment, prophylaxis, infection control, and public health measures. Clinicians are urged to contact their state health department or bioterrorism web sites of the Centers for Disease Control and Prevention for contemporary information and recommendations.

SMALLPOX. The variola virus is considered a serious weapon due to its high transmission and case-fatality rate of 30 percent. The last case of smallpox in this country was reported to the Centers for Disease Control and Prevention in 1968 (2003e). Suarez and Hankins (2002) reviewed the severe perinatal and maternal morbidity and mortality caused by smallpox. Because the only vaccine is made with live vaccinia virus, pregnancy should be delayed for 4 weeks in recipients. It is generally not given to pregnant women because of the risk of fetal vaccinia, a rare but serious complication. The Centers for Disease Control and Prevention (2003d) recommends smallpox vaccination in pregnant women with emergency exposure, and it maintains a registry for those exposed. Vaccination is not ordinarily an indication for pregnancy termination.

ANTHRAX. The causative agent is *Bacillus anthracis*, a gram-positive, spore-forming, aerobic bacterium. There are three main types of clinical anthrax: inhalational, cutaneous, and gastrointestinal (Swartz, 2001). The bioterrorist anthrax attacks of 2001 reaffirmed the effectiveness and high mortality of inhalational anthrax as a biological weapon (Inglesby and colleagues, 2002).

Maternal naturally occurring cutaneous anthrax is usually associated with preterm birth and may be treated with penicillin (Kadanali and associates, 2003). Most authorities, however, presume a resistant strain would be used in a terrorist attack. Postexposure prophylaxis after documented environmental contamination is with ciprofloxacin, 500 mg twice daily for 60 days. This can be changed to amoxicillin, 500 mg three times daily, if the strain is proven sensitive (Centers for Disease Control and Prevention, 2001b). In this situation, doxycycline or ciprofloxacin may be given, and combination therapy for inhalational anthrax may be warranted.

The anthrax vaccine is an inactivated, cell-free product that requires six injections during 18 months. Vaccination is generally avoided in pregnancy due to a lack of safety data (Centers for Disease Control and Prevention, 2002f). That said, anthrax vaccine is an essential adjunct to postexposure antimicrobial prophylaxis, even in pregnancy (American College of Obstetricians and Gynecologist, 2002b). There appear to be no effects on fertility or pregnancy loss rates (Wiesen and Littell, 2002).

OTHER AGENTS. There are consensus statements regarding the management of mass exposure and treatment of *tularemia* (Dennis and associates, 2001). Recommended postexposure prophylaxis for *Francisella tularensis* is ciprofloxacin or doxycycline for 14 days. Effective prophylaxis following exposure to *hemorrhagic fever viruses* is hampered by the absence of effective vaccines and antiviral agents for *Ebola* and *Marburg viruses* (Borio and co-workers, 2002). Ribavirin may be of use for arenaviruses, such as *Lassa fever virus* or *bunyavirus*.

The guidelines for all biological weapons are continually evolving. The most current information is available at the Centers for Disease Control and Prevention *Emergency Preparedness and Response* web site at http://www.bt.cdc.gov.

REFERENCES

Alecrim WD, Espinosa FE, Alecrim MG: *Plasmodium falciparum* infection in the pregnant patient. Infect Dis Clin North Am 14:83, 2000

Ali ME, Alber HM: Measles in pregnancy: Maternal morbidity and perinatal outcome. Int J Gynaecol Obstet 59:109, 1997

Alpert SG, Fergerson J, Noël L-P: Intrauterine West Nile Virus: Ocular and systemic findings. Am J Ophthalmol 136:722, 2003

American College of Obstetricians and Gynecologists: Immunization during pregnancy. Committee Opinion No. 282, January 2003

American College of Obstetricians and Gynecologists: Prevention of early-onset group B streptococcal disease in newborns. Committee Opinion No. 279, December 2002a

American College of Obstetricians and Gynecologists: Management of asymptomatic pregnant or lactating women exposed to anthrax. Committee Opinion No. 268, February 2002b

American College of Obstetricians and Gynecologists: Perinatal viral and parasitic infections. Practice Bulletin No. 20, September 2000

American College of Obstetricians and Gynecologists: Rubella and pregnancy. Technical Bulletin No. 171, August 1992

Antsaklis AJ, Daskalakis GJ, Mesogitis SA, et al: Prenatal diagnosis of fetal primary cytomegalovirus infection. Br J Obstet Gynaecol 107:84, 2000

Alvarez JA, Al-Khan A, Ganesh V, et al: Salmonella as a causative organism of acute pyelonephritis during pregnancy. Am J Obstet Gynecol 190:1482, 2004

Baker CJ, Paoletti LC, Rench MA, et al: Use of capsular polysaccharide-tetanus toxoid conjugate vaccine for Type II group B streptococcus in healthy women. J Infect Dis 182:1129, 2000

Baker CJ, Paoletti LC, Wessels MR, et al: Safety and immunogenicity of capsular polysaccharide-tetanus toxoid conjugate vaccines for group B streptococcal types Ia and Ib. J Infect Dis 179:142, 1999

Baker CJ, Rench MA, Edwards MS, et al: Immunization of pregnant women with a polysaccharide vaccine of group B streptococcus. N Engl J Med 319:1180, 1988

Baltimore RS, Huie SM, Meek JI, et al: Early-onset neonatal sepsis in the era of group B streptococcal prevention. Pediatrics 108:1094, 2001

Banatvala JE, Brown DW: Rubella. Lancet 363:1127, 2004

Barbosa-Cesnik C, Schwartz K, Foxman B: Lactation mastitis. JAMA 289:1609, 2003

Barnham MRD, Weightman NC: Bacteraemic *Streptococcus pyogenes* infections in the peripartum period: Now a rare disease and prior carriage by the patient may be important. J Infect 43:173, 2001

Beghetto E, Buffolano W, Spadoni A, et al: Use of an immunoglobulin G avidity assay based on recombinant antigens for diagnosis of primary *Toxoplasma gondii* infection during pregnancy. J Clin Microbiol 41:5414, 2003

Beres SB, Sylva GL, Sturdevant DE, et al: Genome-wide molecular dissection of serotype M3 group A Streptococcus strains causing two epidemics of invasive infections. Proc Natl Acad Sci USA 101:11833, 2004

Berkowitz K, McCaffrey R: Postpartum osteomyelitis caused by group B streptococcus. Am J Obstet Gynecol 163:1200, 1990

Best JM, O'Shea S, Tipples G, et al: Interpretation of rubella serology in pregnancy—pitfalls and problems. BMJ 325:147, 2002

Bhattacharya SK, Sur D: An evaluation of current shigellosis treatment. Expert Opin Pharmacother 4:1315, 2003

Bisno AL, Stevens DL: Streptococcal infections of skin and soft tissues. N Engl J Med 334:240, 1996

Bland MI, Vermillion ST, Soper DE: Late third-trimester treatment of rectovaginal group B streptococci with benzathine penicillin G. Am J Obstet Gynecol 183:372, 2000

Bloom SL, Leveno KJ, Gilstrap LC, et al: Timing of intrapartum ampicillin infusion for group B streptococcus (GBS) prophylaxis. Am J Obstet Gynecol 174:407, 1996

Bodéus M, Hubinont C, Bernard P, et al: Prenatal diagnosis of human cytomegalovirus by culture and polymerase chain reaction: 98 pregnancies leading to congenital infection. Prenat Diagn 19:314, 1999

Bohlke K, Galil K, Jackson LA, et al: Postpartum varicella vaccination: Is the vaccination virus excreted in breast milk? Obstet Gynecol 102:970, 2003

Boppana SB, Rivera LB, Fowler KB, et al: Intrauterine transmission of cytomegalovirus to infants of women with preconceptional immunity. N Engl J Med 344:1366, 2001

Borio L, Inglesby T, Peters CJ, et al: Hemorrhagic fever viruses as biological weapons. JAMA 287:2391, 2002

Boucher M, Yonekura ML: Perinatal listeriosis (early onset): Correlation of antenatal manifestations and neonatal outcome. Obstet Gynecol 68:593, 1986

Bradley DJ, Warhurst DC: Malaria prophylaxis: Guidelines for travelers from Britain. BMJ 310:709, 1995

Britton WJ, Lockwood DN: Leprosy. Lancet. 363(9416):1209, 2004

Brown EJ: The molecular basis of streptococcal toxic shock syndrome. N Engl J Med 350:2093, 2004

Brown GC, Karunas RS: Relationship of congenital anomalies and maternal infection with selected enteroviruses. Am J Epidemiol 95:207, 1972

Canadian Task Force on Preventive Health Care: Prevention of early-onset group B streptococcal (GBS) infection in the newborn. Systematic review and recommendations. CMAJ 166:928, 2002

Centers for Disease Control and Prevention: Prevention and control of influenza. Recommendations of the Advisory Committee on Immunization Practices (ACIP). MMWR 53(RR-6):1, 2004a

Centers for Disease Control and Prevention: Interim guidelines for the evaluation of infants born to mothers infected with West Nile Virus during pregnancy. MMWR 53:154, 2004b

Centers for Disease Control and Prevention: Decline in annual incidence of varicella—selected states, 1990–2001. MMWR 52:884, 2003a

Centers for Disease Control and Prevention: Health Information for International Travel 2003–2004. Atlanta, GA, US Department of Health and Human Services, 2003b

Centers for Disease Control and Prevention: Using live, attenuated influenza vaccine for prevention and control of influenza. MMWR 52(RR-13):1, 2003c

Centers for Disease Control and Prevention: Women with smallpox vaccine exposure during pregnancy reported to the National Smallpox Vaccine in Pregnancy Registry—United States, 2003. MMWR 52:386, 2003d

Centers for Disease Control and Prevention: General recommendations on immunization. MMWR 51(RR-1):1, 2002a

Centers for Disease Control and Prevention: Hantavirus pulmonary syndrome—United States: Updated recommendations for risk reduction. MMWR 51(RR-9):1 2002b

Centers for Disease Control and Prevention: Intrauterine West Nile Virus Infection—New York, 2002. MMWR 51:1135, 2002c

Centers for Disease Control and Prevention: Prevention of perinatal group B streptococci disease. Revised guidelines from the CDC. MMWR 51(RR-11):1, 2002d

Centers for Disease Control and Prevention: Recommended adult immunization schedule—United States, 2002–2003. MMWR 51:904, 2002e

Centers for Disease Control and Prevention: Status of US Department of Defense preliminary evaluation of the association of anthrax vaccination and congenital anomalies. MMWR 51:127, 2002f

Centers for Disease Control and Prevention: Multistate outbreak of listeriosis—United States, 2000. MMWR 49:1129, 2001a

Centers for Disease Control and Prevention: Updated recommendations for antimicrobial prophylaxis among asymptomatic pregnant women after exposure to Bacillus anthracis. MMWR 50:960, 2001b

Centers for Disease Control and Prevention: Evaluation of varicella reporting to the National Notifiable Disease Surveillance System—United States, 1972–1997. MMWR 48:55, 1999a

Centers for Disease Control and Prevention: Salmonella: Fact Sheets. July 16, 1999b

Centers for Disease Control and Prevention: Measles, mumps, and rubella—vaccine use and strategies for elimination of measles, rubella, and congenital rubella syndrome and control of mumps. MMWR 47(RR-8):1, 1998

Centers for Disease Control and Prevention: Prevention of varicella: Recommendations of the Advisory Committee on Immunization Practices (ACIP). MMWR 45(RR-11):1, 1996

Chandra PC, Patel H, Schiavello HJ, et al: Successful pregnancy outcome after complicated varicella pneumonia. Obstet Gynecol 92:680, 1998

Chapa JB, Ahn JT, DiGiovanni LM, et al: West Nile virus encephalitis during pregnancy. Obstet Gynecol 102:229, 2003

Chiang CP, Chiu CH, Huang YC, et al: Two cases of disseminated cutaneous herpes zoster in infants after intrauterine exposure to varicella-zoster virus. Pediatr Infect Dis J 14:395, 1995

Chiba ME, Saito M, Suzuki N, et al: Measles infection in pregnancy. J Infect 47:40, 2003

Chuang I, Beneden CV, Beall B, et al: Population-based surveillance for postpartum invasive group A streptococcus infections, 1995–2000. Clin Infect Dis 35:665, 2002

Constantine G, Menon V, Luesley D: Amoebic peritonitis in pregnancy in the United Kingdom. Postgrad Med J 63:495, 1987

Cooper NJ, Sutton AJ, Abrams KR, et al: Effectiveness of neuraminidase inhibitors in treatment and prevention and treatment of influenza A and B: Systematic review and meta-analyses of randomised controlled trials. BMJ 326:1235, 2003

Cosmi E, Mari G, Delle Chiaie L, et al: Noninvasive diagnosis by Doppler ultrasonography of fetal anemia resulting from parvovirus infection. Am J Obstet Gynecol 187:1290, 2002

Cot M, Roisin A, Barro D, et al: Effect of chloroquine chemoprophylaxis during pregnancy on birth weight: Results of a randomized trial. Am J Trop Med Hyg 46:21, 1992

Covell G: Congenital malaria. Trop Dis Bull 47:1174, 1950

Crane J: Parvovirus B19 infection in pregnancy. J Obstet Gynaecol Can 24:727, 2002

Davies HD, McGeer A, Schwartz B, et al: Invasive group A streptococcal infections in Ontario, Canada. N Engl J Med 335:547, 1996

Delle Chiaie L, Buck G, Grab D, et al: Prediction of fetal anemia with Doppler measurement of the middle cerebral artery peak systolic velocity in pregnancies complicated by maternal blood group alloimmunization or parvovirus B19 infection. Ultrasound Obstet Gynecol 18:232, 2001

Dembinski J, Eis-Hübinger AM, Maar J, et al: Long term follow up of serostatus after maternofetal parvovirus B19 infection. Arch Dis Child 88:219, 2003

Demmler GJ: Summary of a workshop on surveillance for congenital cytomegalovirus disease. Rev Infect Dis 13:315, 1991

Dennis DT, Inglesby TV, Henderson DA, et al: Tularemia as a biological weapon: Medical and public health management. JAMA 285:2763, 2001

Diagne N, Rogier C, Sokhna CS, et al: Increased susceptibility to malaria during the early postpartum period. N Engl J Med 343:598, 2000

Dildy GA III, Martens MG, Faro S, et al: Typhoid fever in pregnancy: A case report. J Reprod Med 35:273, 1990

Drosten C, Günther S, Preiser W, et al: Identification of a novel coronavirus in patients with severe acute respiratory syndrome. N Engl J Med 348:1967, 2003

Dubey JP: Sources of *Toxoplasma gondii* infection in pregnancy. Until rates of congenital toxoplasmosis fall, control measures are essential. BMJ 321:127, 2000

Duncan ME: Babies of mothers with leprosy have small placentae, low birth weights and grow slowly. Br J Obstet Gynaecol 87:461, 1980

Duncan ME, Fox H, Harkness RA, et al: The placenta in leprosy. Placenta 5:189, 1984

Dunn D, Wallon M, Peyron F, et al: Mother-to-child transmission of toxoplasmosis: Risk estimates for clinical counseling. Lancet 353:1829, 1999

Eady EA, Cove JH: Staphylococcal resistance revisited: Community-acquired methicillin resistant *Staphylococcus aureus*—an emerging problem for the management of skin and soft tissue infections. Curr Opin Infect Dis 16:103, 2003

Eberhart-Phillips JE, Frederick PD, Baron RC, et al: Measles in pregnancy: A descriptive study of 58 cases. Obstet Gynecol 82:797, 1993

Elliott DJ, Eppes SC, Klein JD: Teratogen update: Lyme disease. Teratology 64:276, 2001

Enders M, Weidner A, Zoellner I, et al: Fetal morbidity and mortality after acute human parvovirus B19 infection in pregnancy: prospective evaluation of 1018 cases. Prenat Diagn 24:513, 2004

Enders G, Bäder U, Lindemann L, et al: Prenatal diagnosis of congenital cytomegalovirus infection in 189 pregnancies with known outcome. Prenat Diagn 21:362, 2001

Enders G, Miller E, Cradock-Watson J, et al: Consequences of varicella and herpes zoster in pregnancy: Prospective study of 1739 cases. Lancet 343:1548, 1994

Eschenbach DA: Prevention of neonatal group B streptococcal infection. N Engl J Med 347:280, 2002

European Multicentre Study on Congenital Toxoplasmosis: Effect of timing and type of treatment on the risk of mother to child transmission of *Toxoplasma gondii*. Br J Obstet Gynaecol 110:112, 2003

Farb H, West DP, Pedvis-Leftick A: Clofazimine in pregnancy complicated by leprosy. Obstet Gynecol 59:122, 1982

Forsnes EV, Eggleston MK, Wax JR: Differential transmission of adenovirus in a twin pregnancy. Obstet Gynecol 91:817, 1998

Fowler KB, Stagno S, Pass RF: Maternal immunity and prevention of congenital cytomegalovirus infection. JAMA 289:1008, 2003a

Fowler KB, Stagno S, Pass RF, et al: The outcome of congenital cytomegalovirus infection in relation to maternal antibody status. N Engl J Med 326:663, 1992

Fowler RA, Lapinsky SE, Hallett D, et al: Critically ill patients with severe acute respiratory syndrome. JAMA 290:367, 2003b

Fowler SL: A light in the darkness: Predicting outcomes for congenital cytomegalovirus infections. J Pediatr 137:4, 2000

Garcia AGP, Basso NG, Fonseca MEF, et al: Enterovirus associated placental morphology: A light, virological, electron microscopic and immunohistologic study. Placenta 12:53, 1991

Gibbs RS, Schrag S, Schuchat A: Perinatal infections due to group B streptococci. Obstet Gynecol 104:1062, 2004

Gilbert RE, Gras L, Wallon M, et al: Effect of prenatal treatment on mother to child transmission of *Toxoplasma gondii*: Retrospective cohort study of 554 mother-child pairs in Lyon, France. Int J Epidemiol 30:1303, 2001

Gilbert RE, Peckham CS: Congenital toxoplasmosis in the United Kingdom: To screen or not to screen? J Med Screen 9:135, 2002

Gilden DH, Kleinschmidt-DeMasters BK, LaGuardia JJ, et al: Neurologic complications of the reactivation of varicella-zoster virus. N Engl J Med 342:635, 2000

Goldenberg RL, Thompson C: The infectious origins of stillbirth. Am J Obstet Gynecol 189:861, 2003

Gourarin S, Gault E, Vabret A, et al: Real-time PCR quantification of human cytomegalovirus DNA in amniotic fluid samples from mothers with primary infection. J Clin Microbiol 40:1767, 2002

Gouarin S, Palmer P, Cointe D, et al: Congenital HCMV infection: A collaborative and comparative study of virus detection in amniotic fluid by culture and by PCR. J Clin Virol 21:47, 2001

Grangeot-Keros L, Cointe D: Diagnosis and prognostic markers of HCMV infection. J Clin Virol 21:213, 2001

Gras L, Gilbert RE, Ades AE, et al: Effect of prenatal treatment on the risk of intracranial and ocular lesions in children with congenital toxoplasmosis. Int J Epidemiol 30:1309, 2001

Guerin PJ, Olliaro P, Nosten F, et al: Malaria: Current status of control, diagnosis, treatment and a proposed agenda for research and development. Lancet Infect Dis: 2:564, 2002

Guerra B, Lazzarotto T, Quarta S, et al: Prenatal diagnosis of symptomatic congenital cytomegalovirus infection. Am J Obstet Gynecol 183:476, 2000

Haberland CA, Benitz WE, Sanders GD, et al: Perinatal screening for group B streptococci: Cost-benefit analysis of rapid polymerase chain reaction. Pediatrics 110:471, 2002

Hagay ZJ, Biran G, Ornoy A, et al: Congenital cytomegalovirus infection: A long-standing problem still seeking a solution. Am J Obstet Gynecol 174:241, 1996

Haines CJ, Chu YW, Chung TKH: The effect of severe acute respiratory syndrome on a hospital obstetrics and gynaecology service. Br J Obstet Gynaecol 110:643, 2003

Haque R, Huston CD, Hughes M, et al: Amebiasis. N Engl J Med 348:1565, 2003

Harger JH, Ernest JM, Thurnau GR, et al: Frequency of congenital varicella syndrome in a prospective cohort of 347 pregnant women. Obstet Gynecol 100:260, 2002a

Harger JH, Ernest JM, Thurnau GR, et al: Risk factors and outcome of varicella-zoster virus pneumonia. J Infect Dis 185:422, 2002b

Harjulehto T, Aro T, Hovi T, et al: Congenital malformations and oral poliovirus vaccination during pregnancy. Lancet 1:771, 1989

Hay SI, Guerra CA, Tatem AJ, et al: The global distribution and population at risk of malaria: Past, present, and future. Lancet Infect Dis 4:327, 2004

Hayes EB, Piesman J: How can we prevent Lyme disease? N Engl J Med 348:2424, 2003

Hedriana HL, Mitchell JL, Williams SB: Salmonella typhi chorioamnionitis in a human immunodeficiency virus–infected pregnant woman. J Reprod Med 40:157, 1995

Hill D, Dubey JP: *Toxoplasma gondii*: Transmission, diagnosis and prevention. Clin Microbiol Infect 8:634, 2002

Hohlfeld P, Daffos F, Costa JM, et al: Prenatal diagnosis of congenital toxoplasmosis with a polymerase-chain reaction test on amniotic fluid. N Engl J Med 331:695, 1994

Howard MJ, Doyle TJ, Koster FT, et al: Hantavirus pulmonary syndrome in pregnancy. Clin Infect Dis 29:1538, 1999

Hulbert TV: Congenital malaria in the United States: Report of a case and review. Clin Infect Dis 14:922, 1992

Hyde TB, Hilger TM, Reingold A, et al: Trends in incidence and antimicrobial resistance of early-onset sepsis: Population-based surveillance in San Francisco and Atlanta. Pediatrics 110:690, 2002

Inglesby TV, O'Toole T, Henderson DA, et al: Anthrax as a biological weapon, 2002. JAMA 287:2236, 2002

Irving WL, James DK, Stephenson T, et al: Influenza virus infection in the second and third trimesters of pregnancy: A clinical and seroepidemiological study. Br J Obstet Gynaecol 107:1282, 2000

Jakobi P, Goldstick O, Sujov P, et al: New CDC guidelines for prevention of perinatal group B streptococcal disease. Lancet 361:351, 2003

Johnson JR, Colombo F, Gardner D, et al: Optimal dosing of penicillin G in the third trimester of pregnancy for prophylaxis against group B streptococcus. Am J Obstet Gynecol 185:850, 2001

Jones BS: Congenital malaria: 3 cases. BMJ 2:439, 1950

Jones JL, Dietz VJ, Power M, et al: Survey of obstetrician-gynecologists in the United States about toxoplasmosis. Infect Dis Obstet Gynecol 9:23, 2001a

Jones JL, Lopez A, Wilson M, et al: Congenital toxoplasmosis: A review. Obstet Gynecol Surv 56:296, 2001b

Kadanali A, Tasyaran MA, Kadanali S: Anthrax during pregnancy: Case reports and review. Clin Infect Dis 36:1343, 2003

Kimberlin DW, Lin CY, Sanchez PJ, et al: Effect of ganciclovir therapy on hearing in symptomatic congenital cytomegalovirus disease involving the central nervous system: A randomized, controlled trial. J Pediatr 143:16, 2003

Klempner MS, Hu LT, Evans J, et al: Two controlled trials of antibiotic treatment in patients with persistent symptoms and a history of Lyme disease. N Engl J Med 345:85, 2001

Koren G, Money D, Boucher M, et al: Serum concentrations, efficacy, and safety of a new intravenously administered varicella zoster immune globulin in pregnant women. J Clin Pharmacol 42:267, 2002

Korones SB: Uncommon virus infections of the mother, fetus, and newborn: Influenza, mumps and measles. Clin Perinatol 15:259, 1988

Ksiazek TG, Erdman D, Goldsmith CS, et al. A novel coronavirus associated with severe acute respiratory syndrome. N Engl J Med 348:1953, 2003

Kunugi H, Nanko S, Takei N, et al: Schizophrenia following in utero exposure to the 1957 influenza epidemics in Japan. Am J Psychiatry 152:450, 1995

Kurppa K, Holmberg PC, Kuosma E, et al: Anencephaly and maternal common cold. Teratology 44:51, 1991

Laibl V, Sheffield J, Roberts S, et al: Clinical presentation of community-acquired methicillin-resistant *Staphylococcus aureus* in pregnancy. Presented at the 25th Annual Meeting of the Society for Maternal–Fetal Medicine, Reno, Nevada, 7–12 February, 2005

Lam CM, Wong SF, Leung TN, et al: A case-controlled study comparing clinical course and outcomes of pregnant and non-pregnant women with severe acute respiratory syndrome. BJOG 111:771, 2004

Lazzarotto T, Gabrielli L, Lanari M, et al: Congenital cytomegalovirus infection: recent advances in the diagnosis of maternal infection. Hum Immunol 65:410, 2004

Lazzarotto T, Varani S, Guerra B, et al: Prenatal indicators of congenital cytomegalovirus infection. J Pediatr 137:90, 2000

Levine EM, Ghai V, Barton JJ, et al: Intrapartum antibiotic prophylaxis increases the incidence of gram-negative neonatal sepsis. Infect Dis Obstet Gynecol 7:210, 1999

Lew TWK, Kwek T-K, Tai D, et al: Acute respiratory distress syndrome in critically ill patients with severe acute respiratory syndrome. JAMA 290:374, 2003

Liesenfeld O, Montoya JG, Kinney S, et al: Effect of testing for IgG avidity in the diagnosis of *Toxoplasma gondii* infection in pregnant women: Experience in a US reference laboratory. J Infect Dis 183:1248, 2001

Liesnard C, Donner C, Brancart F, et al: Prenatal diagnosis of congenital cytomegalovirus infection: Prospective study of 237 pregnancies at risk. Obstet Gynecol 95:881, 2000

Lin FYC, Philips JB III, Azimi PH, et al: Level of maternal antibody required to protect neonates against early-onset disease caused by group B streptococcus type Ia: A multicenter, seroepidemiology study. J Infect Dis 184:1022, 2001

Lin FYC, Weisman LE, Troendle J, et al: Prematurity is the major risk factor for late-onset group B streptococcus disease. J Infect Dis 188:267, 2003

Lopez A, Dietz VJ, Wilson M, et al: Preventing congenital toxoplasmosis. MMWR 49(RR02):57, 2000

Lynberg MC, Khoury MJ, Lu X, et al: Maternal flu, fever, and the risk of neural tube defects: A population-based case-control study. Am J Epidemiol 140:244, 1994

Malinger G, Lev D, Zahalka N, et al: Fetal cytomegalovirus infection of the brain: The spectrum of sonographic findings. AJNR Am J Neuroradiol 24:28, 2003

Mandell LA, Bartlett JG, Dowell SF, et al: Update of practice guidelines for the management of community acquired pneumonia in immunocompetent adults. Clin Infect Dis 37:1405, 2003

Maraspin V, Cimperman J, Lotric-Furlan S, et al: Erythema migrans in pregnancy. Wien Klin Wochenschr 111:933, 1999

McElhaney RD Jr, Ringer M, DeHart DJ, et al: Rubella immunity in a cohort of pregnant women. Infect Control Host Epidemiol 20:64, 1999

McGrath J, Castle D: Does influenza cause schizophrenia? A five year review. Aust N Z J Psychiatry 29:23, 1995

McGready R, Cho T, Keo NK, et al: Artemisinin antimalarials in pregnancy: A prospective treatment study of 539 episodes of multidrug-resistant *Plasmodium falciparum*. Clin Infect Dis 33:2009, 2001

McGready R, Davison BB, Stepniewska K, et al: The effects of *Plasmodium falciparum* and *P. vivax* infections on placental histopathology in an area of low malaria transmission. Am J Trop Med Hyg 70:398, 2004

Menendez C, Ordi J, Ismail MR, et al: The impact of placental malaria on gestational age and birthweight. J Infect Dis 181:1740, 2000

Miller E, Cradock-Watson JE, Pollock TM: Consequences of confirmed maternal rubella at successive stages of pregnancy. Lancet 2:781, 1982

Miller E, Fairley CK, Cohen BJ, et al: Immediate and long term outcome of human parvovirus B19 infection in pregnancy. Br J Obstet Gynaecol 105:174, 1998

Mitchell TF, Pearlman MD, Chapman RL, et al: Maternal and transplacental pharmacokinetics of cefazolin. Obstet Gynecol 98:1075, 2001

Montoya JG: Laboratory diagnosis of *Toxoplasma gondii* infection and toxoplasmosis. J Infect Dis 185 Suppl 1:S73, 2002

Montoya JG, Liesenfeld O: Toxoplasmosis. Lancet 363:1965, 2004

Montoya JG, Liesenfeld O, Kinney S, et al: VIDAS test for avidity of *Toxoplasma*-specific immunoglobulin G for confirmatory testing of pregnant women. J Clin Microbiol 40:2504, 2002

Moore MR, Schrag SJ, Schuchat A: Effects of intrapartum antimicrobial prophylaxis for prevention of group B streptococcal disease on the incidence and ecology of early-onset neonatal sepsis. Lancet Infect Dis 3:201, 2003

Morse DL: West Nile Virus—not a passing phenomenon. N Engl J Med 348:22, 2003

Murray HW, Pépin J, Nutman TB, et al: Tropical medicine. BMJ 320:490, 2000

Mylonakis E, Paliou M, Hohmann EL, et al: Listeriosis during pregnancy. Medicine 81:260, 2002

Nadelman RB, Nowakowski J, Fish D, et al: Prophylaxis with single-dose doxycycline for the prevention of Lyme disease after an *Ixodes scapularis* tick bite. N Engl J Med 345:79, 2001

Nahlen BL: Rolling back malaria in pregnancy. N Engl J Med 343: 651, 2000

Naimi TS, LeDell KH, Como-Sabetti K, et al: Comparison of community- and health-care associated methicillin-resistant *Staphylococcus aureus* infection. JAMA 290:2976, 2003

Nathan L, Peters MT, Ahmed AM, et al: The return of life-threatening puerperal sepsis caused by group A streptococci. Am J Obstet Gynecol 169:571, 1993

Nathwani D, Currie PF, Douglas JG, et al: *Plasmodium falciparum* malaria in pregnancy: A review. Br J Obstet Gynaecol 99:118, 1992

Neuzil KM, Reed GW, Mitchel EF, et al: Impact of influenza on acute cardiopulmonary hospitalizations in pregnant women. Am J Epidemiol 148:1094, 1998

Newman RD, Parise ME, Slutsker L, et al: Safety, efficacy and determinants of effectiveness of antimalarial drugs during pregnancy: Implications for prevention programmes in *Plasmodium falciparum*-endemic sub-Saharan Africa. Trop Med Int Health 8:488, 2003

Newton ER: Diagnosis of perinatal TORCH infections. Clin Obstet Gynecol 42:59, 1999

Nigro G, Anceschi MM, Cosmi EV, et al: Clinical manifestations and abnormal laboratory findings in pregnant women with primary cytomegalovirus infection. Br J Obstet Gynaecol 110:572, 2003

Norbeck O, Papadogiannakis N, Petersson K, et al: Revised clinical presentation of parvovirus B19–associated intrauterine fetal death. Clin Infect Dis 35:1032, 2002

Nyman M, Tolfvenstam T, Petersson K, et al: Detection of human parvovirus B19 infection in first-trimester fetal loss. Obstet Gynecol 99:795, 2002

O'Brien KL, Beall B, Barrett NL, et al: Epidemiology of invasive group A streptococcus disease in the United States, 1995–1999. Clin Infect Dis 35:268, 2002

Paoletti LC, Madoff LC: Vaccines to prevent neonatal GBS infection. Semin Neonatol 7:315, 2002

Parise ME, Ayisi JG, Nahlen BL, et al: Efficacy of sulfadoxine-pyrimethamine for prevention of placental malaria in an area of Kenya with a high prevalence of malaria and human immunodeficiency virus infection. Am J Trop Med Hyg 59:813, 1998

Parry CM, Hien TT, Dougan G, et al: Typhoid fever. N Engl J Med 347:1770, 2002

Paryani SG, Arvin AM: Intrauterine infection with varicella zoster virus after maternal varicella. N Engl J Med 314:1542, 1986

Pass RF: Day-care centers and the spread of cytomegalovirus and parvovirus B19. Pediatr Ann 20:419, 1991

Peckham C, Tookey P, Logan S, et al: Screening options for prevention of congenital cytomegalovirus infection. J Med Screen 8:119, 2001

Peiris JSM, Chu CM, Cheng VCC, et al: Clinical progression and viral load in a community outbreak of coronavirus-associated SARS pneumonia: A prospective study. Lancet 361:1767, 2003a

Peiris JSM, Yeun KY, Osterhaus ADME, et al: The severe acute respiratory syndrome. N Engl J Med 349:2431, 2003b

Reef SE, Frey TK, Theal K, et al: The changing epidemiology of rubella in the 1990s: On the verge of elimination and new challenges for control and prevention. JAMA 287:464, 2002

Reef SE, Plotkin S, Cordero JS, et al: Preparing for elimination of congenital rubella syndrome (CRS): Summary of a workshop on CRS elimination in the United States. Clin Infect Dis 31:85, 2000

Revello MG, Gerna G: Pathogenesis and prenatal diagnosis of human cytomegalovirus infection. J Clin Virol 29:71, 2004

Revello MG, Gerna G: Diagnosis and management of human cytomegalovirus infection in the mother, fetus and newborn infant. Clin Microbiol Rev 15:680, 2002

Roberts A, Hedman K, Luyasu V, et al: Multicenter evaluation of strategies for serodiagnosis of primary infection with *Toxoplasma gondii*. Eur J Clin Microbiol Infect Dis 20:467, 2001

Robier C, Tall A, Diagne N, et al: *Plasmodium falciparum* clinical malaria: Lessons from longitudinal studies in Senegal. Parassitologia 41:255, 1999

Rodis JF, Rodner C, Hansen AA, et al: Long-term outcome of children following maternal human parvovirus B19 infection. Obstet Gynecol 91:125, 1998

Rogers BB: Parvovirus B19: Twenty-five years in perspective. Pediatr Develop Pathol 2:296, 1999

Romand S, Chosson M, Franck J, et al: Usefulness of quantitative polymerase chain reaction in amniotic fluid as early prognostic marker of fetal infection with *Toxoplasma gondii*. Am J Obstet Gynecol 190:797, 2004

Romand S, Wallon M, Franck J, et al: Prenatal diagnosis using polymerase chain reaction on amniotic fluid for congenital toxoplasmosis. Obstet Gynecol 97:296, 2001

Rouse DJ, Lincoln T, Cilver S, et al: Intrapartum chlorhexidine vaginal irrigation and chorioamnion and placental microbial colonization. Int J Gynaecol Obstet 83:165, 2003

Royal College of Obstetricians and Gynaecologists: Prevention of early onset neonatal group B streptococcal disease. Guideline No. 36, November 2003

Rubenfeld GD: Is SARS just ARDS? JAMA 290:397, 2003

Ryan ET, Kain KC: Health advice and immunizations for travelers. N Engl J Med 342:1716, 2000

Ryan ET, Wilson ME, Kain KC: Illness after international travel. N Engl J Med 347:505, 2002

Salgado CD, Farr BM, Hall KK, et al: Influenza in the acute hospital setting. Lancet Infect Dis 2:145, 2002

Saxén L, Holmberg PC, Kurppa K, et al: Influenza epidemics and anencephaly. Am J Public Health 80:473, 1990

Schild RL, Bald R, Plath H, et al: Intrauterine management of fetal parvovirus B19 infection. Ultrasound Obstet Gynecol 13:151, 1999

Schrag SJ, Arnold KE, Mohle-Boetani JC, et al: Prenatal screening for infectious diseases and opportunities for prevention. Obstet Gynecol 102:753, 2003

Schrag SJ, Zell ER, Lynfield R, et al: A population-based comparison of strategies to prevent early-onset group B streptococcal disease in neonates. N Engl J Med 347:233, 2002

Schrag SJ, Zywicki S, Farley MM, et al: Group B streptococcal disease in the era of intrapartum antibiotic prophylaxis. N Engl J Med 342:15, 2000

Schwartz E, Parise M, Kozarsky P, et al: Delayed onset of malaria—implications for chemoprophylaxis in travelers. N Engl J Med 349:1510, 2003

Shaw GM, Todoroff K, Velie EM, et al: Maternal illness, including fever, and medication use as risk factors for neural tube defects. Teratology 57:1, 1998

Shek CC, Ng PC, Fung GPG, et al: Infants born to mothers with severe acute respiratory syndrome. Pediatrics 112:254, 2003

Shields KE, Galil K, Seward J, et al: Varicella vaccine exposure during pregnancy: Data from the first 5 years of the Pregnancy Registry. Obstet Gynecol 98:14, 2001

Shilleto N, Barrett JR, Allen L, et al: Human parvovirus B19 related hydrops and elevated fetal creatine kinase. Am J Obstet Gynecol 174:403, 1996

Siegel M: Congenital malformations following chickenpox, measles, mumps, and hepatitis: Results of a cohort study. JAMA 226:1521, 1973

Siegel M, Fuerst HT: Low birth weight and maternal virus diseases: A prospective study of rubella, measles, mumps, chickenpox, and hepatitis. JAMA 197:88, 1966

Siegel M, Goldberg M: Incidence of poliomyelitis in pregnancy. N Engl J Med 253:841, 1955

Silver HM: Listeriosis during pregnancy. Obstet Gynecol Surv 53:737, 1998

Skjöldebrand-Sparre L, Tolfvenstam T, Papadogiannakis N, et al: Parvovirus B19 infection: Association of third-trimester intrauterine fetal death. Br J Obstet Gynaecol 107:476, 2000

So LK, Lau AC, Yam LY, et al: Development of a standard treatment protocol for severe acute respiratory syndrome. Lancet 361:1615, 2003

Steere AC: Lyme disease. N Engl J Med 345:115, 2001

Stefonek KR, Maerz LL, Nielsen MP, et al: Group A streptococcal puerperal sepsis preceded by positive surveillance cultures. Obstet Gynecol 98:846, 2001

Stirrat G: The immune system. In Hytten F, Chamberlain G (eds): Clinical Physiology in Obstetrics. London, Blackwell, 1991, p 101

Stoll BJ, Hansen N: Infections in VLBW infants: Studies from the NICHD Neonatal Research Network. Semin Perinatol 27:293, 2003

Stoll BJ, Hansen N, Fanaroff AA, et al: Changes in pathogens causing early-onset sepsis in very-low-birth-weight infants. N Engl J Med 347:240, 2002a

Stoll BJ, Hansen N, Fanaroff AA, et al: Late-onset sepsis in very low birth weight neonates: The experience of the NICHD Neonatal Research Network. Pediatrics 110:285, 2002b

Strobino B, Abid S, Gewitz M: Maternal Lyme disease and congenital heart disease: A case-control study in an endemic area. Am J Obstet Gynecol 180:711, 1999

Suarez VR, Hankins GDV: Smallpox and pregnancy: From eradicated disease to bioterrorist threat. Obstet Gynecol 100:87, 2002

Swartz MN: Recognition and management of anthrax—an update. N Engl J Med 345:1621, 2001

Tanemura M, Suzumori K, Yagami Y, et al: Diagnosis of fetal rubella infection with reverse transcription and nested polymerase chain reaction: A study of 34 cases diagnosed in fetuses. Am J Obstet Gynecol 174:578, 1996

Tang JW, Aarons E, Hesketh LM, et al: Prenatal diagnosis of congenital rubella infection in the second trimester of pregnancy. Prenat Diagn 6:509, 2003

Taylor WR, White NJ: Antimalarial drug toxicity: A review. Drug Saf 27:25, 2004

Tolfvenstam T, Papadogiannakis N, Norbeck O, et al: Frequency of human parvovirus B19 infection in intrauterine fetal death. Lancet 357:1494, 2001

Topalovski M, Yang SS, Boonpasat Y: Listeriosis of the placenta: Clinicopathologic study of seven cases. Am J Obstet Gynecol 169:616, 1993

Towbin JA, Griffin LD, Martin AB, et al: Intrauterine adenoviral myocarditis presenting as nonimmune hydrops fetalis: Diagnosis by polymerase chain reaction. Pediatr Infect Dis J 13:144, 1994

Towers CV, Briggs GG: Antepartum use of antibiotics and early-onset neonatal sepsis: The next four years. Am J Obstet Gynecol 187:495, 2002

Tsang KW, Ho PL, Ooi CG, et al: A cluster of cases of severe acute respiratory syndrome in Hong Kong. N Engl J Med 348:1977, 2003

Udagawa H, Oshio Y, Shimizu Y: Serious group A streptococcal infection around delivery. Obstet Gynecol 94:153, 1999

Valeur-Jensen AK, Pedersen CB, Westergaard T, et al: Risk factors for parvovirus B19 infection in pregnancy. JAMA 281:1099, 1999

Velaphi S, Siegel JD, Wendel GD Jr, et al: Early-onset group B streptococcal infection after a combined maternal and neonatal group B streptococcal chemoprophylaxis strategy. Pediatrics 111:541, 2003

Verhocff FH, Brabin BJ, Chimsuku L, et al: An evaluation of the effects of intermittent sulfadoxine pyrimethamine treatment in pregnancy on parasite clearance and risk of low birthweight in rural Malawi. Ann Trop Med Parasitol 92:141, 1998

von Kaisenberg CS, Jonat W: Fetal parvovirus B19 infection. Ultrasound Obstet Gynecol 18:280, 2001

Webster WS: Teratogen update: Congenital rubella. Teratology 58:13, 1998

Wendel GD Jr, Leveno KJ, Sánchez PJ, et al: Prevention of neonatal group B streptococcal disease: A combined intrapartum and neonatal protocol. Am J Obstet Gynecol 186:618, 2002

Wenzel RP, Edmond MB: Managing SARS amidst uncertainty. N Engl J Med 348:1947, 2003

Wharton M: The epidemiology of varicella-zoster virus infections. Infect Dis Clin North Am 10:571, 1996

Wiesen AR, Littell CT: Relationship between prepregnancy anthrax vaccination and pregnancy and birth outcomes among US Army women. JAMA 287:1556, 2002

Wing EJ, Gregory SH: Listeria monocytogenes: Clinical and experimental update. J Infect Dis 185:S18, 2002

Wong SF, Chow KM, Leung TN, et al: Pregnancy and perinatal outcomes of women with severe acute respiratory syndrome. Am J Obstet Gynecol 191:292, 2004

Wong SF, Chow KM, de Swiet M: Severe acute respiratory syndrome and pregnancy. Br J Obstet Gynaecol 110:641, 2003

World Health Organization Collaborative Study Team on the Role of Breastfeeding on the Prevention of Infant Mortality: Effect of breastfeeding on infant and child mortality due to infectious diseases in less developed countries: A pooled analysis. Lancet 355:451, 2000

Wyler DJ: Malaria chemoprophylaxis for the traveler. N Engl J Med 329:31, 1993

Yaegashi N: Pathogenesis of nonimmune hydrops fetalis caused by intrauterine B19 infection. Tohoku J Exp Med 190:65, 2000

Yancey MK, Duff P, Kubilis P, et al: Risk factors for neonatal sepsis. Obstet Gynecol 87:188, 1996

Young NS: B19 parvovirus. Ballieres Clin Haematol 8:25, 1995

Young NS, Brown KE: Mechanisms of disease: Parvovirus B19. N Engl J Med 350:586, 2004

Yow MD, Demmler GJ: Congenital cytomegalovirus disease—20 years is long enough. N Engl J Med 326:703, 1992

59

Sexually Transmitted Diseases

Sexually transmitted diseases (STDs) are relatively common during pregnancy. Education, screening, treatment, and prevention are important components of prenatal care for women at increased risk for these infections (Piper and colleagues, 2003). As a part of routine prenatal care, common STDs that are often sought include syphilis, gonorrhea, chlamydia, hepatitis B, human immunodeficiency virus (HIV), and human papillomavirus infections (HPV) (Schrag and associates, 2003). The recommended treatment protocols adhere to the intensive and frequently updated schedules provided by the Centers for Disease Control and Prevention (2002d). Treatment of most STDs is clearly associated with improved pregnancy outcome and prevention of perinatal mortality (Goldenberg and Thompson, 2003; Gray and colleagues, 2001).

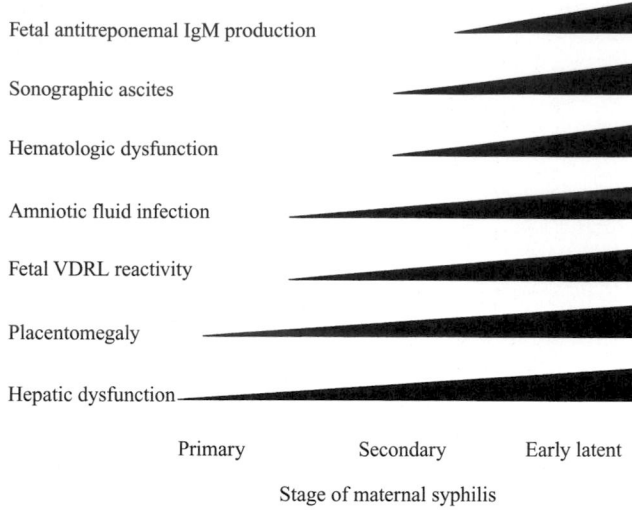

FIGURE 59–1. Hypothesized continuum of fetal syphilis infection. (VDRL = Venereal Disease Research Laboratory.) (From Hollier and colleagues, 2001, with permission.)

SYPHILIS

The incidence of syphilis increased in the United States through the 1980s peaked in 1990, and then subsequently declined (Centers for Disease Control and Prevention, 2003a). The rate of syphilis in the United States in 2002 was 2.4 cases per 100,000 persons, and the rate among neonates was even lower at 1.1 cases per 100,000 population. The Centers for Disease Control and Prevention created a National Syphilis Elimination Plan with a goal of fewer than 1000 cases of primary and secondary syphilis in the country by 2005 (Mitka, 2000).

Increased rates of maternal syphilis have been linked to substance abuse, especially crack cocaine, and to inadequate prenatal care (Lago, 2004; Minkoff, 1990; Warner, 2001, and all their colleagues). Klass and associates (1994), in a study of prenatal syphilis at the Boston City Hospital during four decades, concluded that the continued prevalence of syphilis at delivery was associated with substance abuse, HIV infection, lack of prenatal care, treatment failures, and reinfection.

Antepartum syphilis can profoundly affect pregnancy outcome by causing preterm labor, fetal death, and neonatal infection by transplacental or perinatal infection (Genc and Ledger, 2000; Watson-Jones and co-workers, 2002). Fortunately, of the many congenital infections, syphilis is the most readily prevented and the most susceptible to therapy.

FETAL AND NEONATAL INFECTIONS. In the past, syphilis accounted for nearly a third of stillbirths. Today it plays a smaller but persistent role in fetal death, especially before 30 weeks (Goldenberg and Thompson, 2003; Gust and associates, 2002). Spirochetes readily cross the placenta and can result in congenital infection. Because of fetal immunocompetence prior to about 18 weeks, the fetus generally does not manifest the immunological inflammatory response characteristic of clinical disease before this time (Silverstein, 1962). Once fetal syphilis develops, there appears to be a

continuum of involvement (Fig. 59–1). Hepatic involvement is followed by anemia and thrombocytopenia and then ascites and hydrops (Hollier and colleagues, 2001).

The frequency of congenital syphilis varies with both the stage and duration of maternal infection. McFarlin and associates (1994) reported that high serological titers and unknown duration of infection were major predictors of congenital syphilis. Thus, the highest incidence is in neonates born to mothers with early syphilis—primary, secondary, and early latent—and the lowest incidence with late latent disease of greater than 1-year duration (Fiumara and colleagues, 1952; Golden and co-workers, 2003). **Importantly, any stage of infectious maternal syphilis may result in fetal infection.**

PATHOLOGY. The newborn may have jaundice with petechiae or purpuric skin lesions, lymphadenopathy, rhinitis, pneumonia, myocarditis, or nephrosis. With syphilitic infection, the placenta becomes large and pale. Microscopically, villi appear to have lost their characteristic arborescent appearance and to have become thicker and club shaped. Sheffield and colleagues (2002c) described large villi in 64 percent of placentas from 33 pregnancies with stillborn fetuses from syphilis. More than 60 percent of placentas from 18 liveborn neonates also had large villi. Blood vessels markedly diminish in number, and in advanced cases, they almost entirely disappear as a result of endarteritis and proliferation of stromal cells. Perhaps related to this, Lucas and co-workers (1991) demonstrated increased vascular resistance in uterine and umbilical arteries of infected pregnancies. In a study of 25 untreated women, Schwartz and associates (1995) reported that necrotizing funisitis was present in a third of cases. Spirochetes were detected in almost 90 percent using silver and immunofluorescent staining.

SEROLOGICAL DIAGNOSIS. A suitable serological screening test such as the *Venereal Disease Research Laboratory* (*VDRL*) *slide test* or the *rapid plasma reagin* (*RPR*) *test* should be performed at the first prenatal visit. Testing is required by law in many states and is probably cost-effective even if the prevalence is low (Connor and colleagues, 2000; Hollier and associates, 2003). Serological tests yield positive results in the majority of women with primary syphilis and in all of those with secondary and latent syphilis. Because such reagin tests lack specificity, a treponemal test is used to confirm a positive result (Pope and Fears, 2000; Young, 2000). These include the *fluorescent treponemal antibody absorption test* (*FTA-ABS*), the *microhemagglutination assay for antibodies to* Treponema pallidum (*MHA-TP*), or the Treponema pallidum *passive particle agglutination* (*TP-PA*) *test*.

Cord blood screening is an insensitive test to detect early congenital syphilis. For women at high risk for syphilis, a nontreponemal screening test should be repeated in the third trimester and at the time of delivery (Centers for Disease Control and Prevention, 2002d; Lumbiganon and co-workers, 2002).

FETAL DIAGNOSIS. Polymerase chain reaction (PCR) is specific for detection of *Treponema pallidum* in amnionic fluid, and treponemal DNA has been found in 40 percent of pregnancies infected before 20 weeks (Nathan and colleagues, 1997; Wendel and associates, 1991). Fetal syphilis has also been verified by amnionic fluid darkfield examination or rabbit infectivity testing in 64 percent of a cohort of women with untreated syphilis (Hollier and co-workers, 2001). Although prenatal diagnosis can be made by funipuncture or amniocentesis, its clinical utility is not yet clear.

Because of a myriad of pathological changes in the fetus, ultrasonographic examination may be suggestive or even diagnostic of congenital infection. For example, the neonate shown in Figure 59–2 has a large abdomen due to marked hepatosplenomegaly from congenital syphilis. The placenta

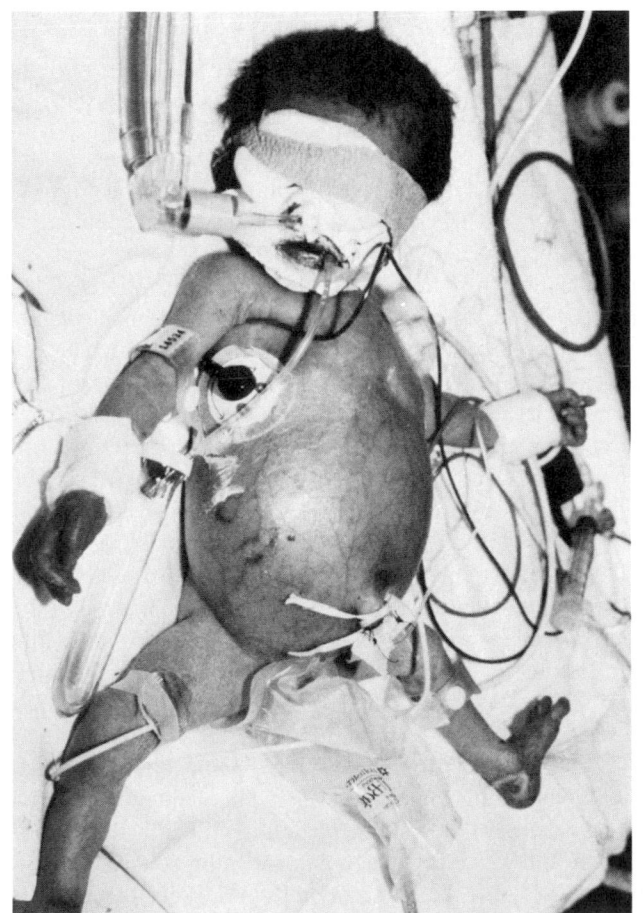

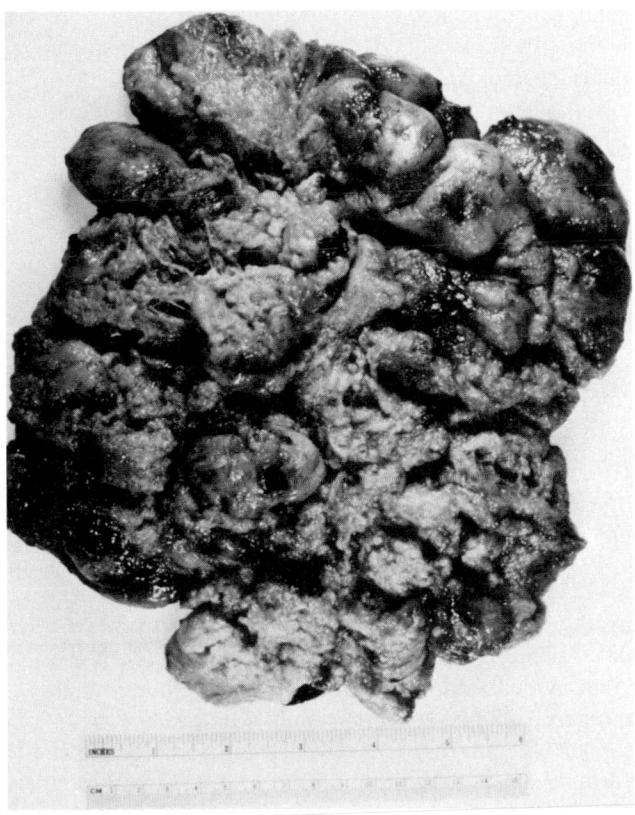

A **B**

FIGURE 59–2. Congenital syphilis. **A.** A 29-week-old, severely ill neonate with an enlarged abdomen caused by marked hepatosplenomegaly plus ascites. **B.** The large syphilitic placenta of the same neonate weighed 1200 g, almost the birthweight of the newborn.

was thickened and weighed almost as much as the neonate. The fetus may also have edema, ascites, or hydrops. Whenever possible, fetal evaluation for signs of syphilis should precede, but not delay, treatment after 20 weeks' gestation. Barton and colleagues (1992) found, however, that delivery followed by neonatal treatment may be the best option for near-term hydropic fetuses with congenital syphilis.

TREATMENT. Syphilis therapy during pregnancy is given to eradicate maternal infection and to prevent congenital syphilis. Penicillin is the treatment of choice even though it has not been evaluated rigorously. Rolfs (1995), Walker (2001), and Wendel and co-workers (2002) concluded that there are few useful comparative data available for ascertaining optimal therapy.

In retrospective analyses, benzathine penicillin G has been shown to cure early maternal infection and prevent neonatal syphilis in 98 percent of cases (Wendel and colleagues, 2002; Zenker and Rolfs, 1990). In a study of 340 pregnant women so treated, Alexander and associates (1999) reported six cases (1.8 percent) of congenital syphilis. Four of these six neonates were from a group of 75 women with secondary syphilis. The other two were identified in those delivered from a group of 102 women with early latent syphilis. Congenital syphilis was generally confined to neonates of women treated after 26 weeks and is likely related to the duration and severity of fetal infection. Sheffield and co-workers (2002b) reported that high maternal serological titers, preterm delivery, and delivery shortly after antepartum therapy are all risks of maternal treatment failing to prevent neonatal infection.

The currently recommended treatment guidelines for syphilis in pregnancy shown in Table 59–1 are the same as for nonpregnant adults. As indicated, some authorities recommend a second dose of benzathine penicillin 1 week after the initial dose, especially for women in the third trimester or for those with secondary syphilis. Women with a history of penicillin allergy can be skin tested to confirm the risk of immunoglobulin E (IgE)–mediated anaphylaxis. If skin tests are reactive, penicillin desensitization is recommended and is followed by benzathine penicillin G treatment (Chisholm and associates, 1997; Wendel and co-workers, 1985).

There are no proven alternatives to penicillin therapy during pregnancy. Erythromycin may be curative for the mother, but it does not prevent all congenital syphilis, and it is not currently recommended as a penicillin alternative (Wendel, 1988). The cephalosporins, such as ceftriaxone, and the newer macrolide, azithromycin, may prove useful in adults (Augenbraun, 2002; Augenbraun and Workowski, 1999). Azithromycin therapy results in significant maternal and fetal serum drug levels (Ramsey and colleagues, 2003). Its efficacy in pregnancy, however, has not been adequately evaluated, and both resistance and treatment failures have been reported in adults (Centers for Disease Control and Prevention, 2004a; Lukehart and colleagues, 2004; Wendel and associates, 2002). Tetracyclines, including doxycycline, are effective

TABLE 59–1 Recommended Treatment for Pregnant Women with Syphilis

Category	Treatment
Early syphilis[a]	Benzathine penicillin G, 2.4 million units intramuscularly as a single injection—some recommend a second dose 1 week later
More than 1 year duration[b]	Benzathine penicillin G, 2.4 million units intramuscularly weekly for 3 doses
Neurosyphilis[c]	Aqueous crystalline penicillin G, 3–4 million units intravenously every 4 hours for 10–14 days
	or
	Aqueous procaine penicillin, 2.4 million units intramuscularly daily, plus probenecid 500 mg orally four times daily, both for 10–14 days

[a] Primary, secondary, and latent syphilis of less than 1 year duration.
[b] Latent syphilis of unknown or more than 1 year duration; tertiary syphilis.
[c] Some recommend benzathine penicillin, 2.4 million units intramuscularly after completion of the neurosyphilis treatment regimens.
From the Centers for Disease Control and Prevention (2002d).

for treatment of syphilis in the nonpregnant woman but are generally not recommended during pregnancy because of the risk of yellow-brown discoloration of fetal deciduous teeth.

In most women with primary syphilis and about half with secondary infection, penicillin treatment is followed by the *Jarisch–Herxheimer reaction.* Uterine contractions frequently develop with this reaction, and they may be accompanied by late fetal heart rate decelerations (Klein and co-workers, 1990). In a study of 50 pregnant women who received benzathine penicillin for syphilis, Myles and colleagues (1998) reported a 40-percent incidence of Jarisch–Herxheimer reaction. Of the 31 women monitored electronically, 42 percent developed regular uterine contractions with a median onset of 10 hours, and 39 percent developed variable decelerations with a median onset of 8 hours. All contractions resolved within 24 hours of therapy. Lucas and associates (1991) used Doppler velocimetry and demonstrated acutely increased vascular resistance during this time.

All women with syphilis should be offered counseling and testing for HIV (Koumans and co-workers, 2000). For women with concomitant HIV infection, the Centers for Disease Control and Prevention (2002d) recommended the same treatment as for HIV-negative persons (Augenbraun, 2002). Some authorities, however, recommend two additional weekly doses of benzathine penicillin G. Clinical and serological follow-up to detect treatment failures is also recommended at 3, 6, 9, 12, and 24 months in HIV-positive patients.

Lumbar Puncture. Whether to routinely analyze cerebrospinal fluid has been controversial. Many asymptomatic patients have abnormalities with primary, secondary, and early latent syphilis, but most do not develop neurosyphilis if appropriately treated. The Centers for Disease Control and Prevention (2002d) recommended lumbar puncture for latent syphilis of more than 1-year duration if there are neurological or ophthalmological symptoms, for treatment failures, for evidence of active tertiary syphilis (aortitis, gummas, or iritis), or for concomitant HIV infection.

Follow-Up. Any patient treated for syphilis needs conscientious follow-up. Sexual contacts within the last 3 months should be evaluated for syphilis and treated presumptively, even if seronegative. Maternal serological titers should be repeated in the third trimester and at delivery to confirm a serological response to treatment or to document reinfection in this high-risk group.

Treatment of Congenital Syphilis. Every newborn with suspected or proven congenital syphilis should undergo cerebrospinal fluid examination prior to treatment. After therapy, they should be followed at 2- to 3-month intervals until nontreponemal serological tests become negative or serofast. **Infants born to mothers treated with erythromycin or a nonpenicillin regimen for syphilis during pregnancy should be retreated as though they have congenital syphilis.**

GONORRHEA

The incidence of gonorrhea in the United States for 2002 was 125 cases per 100,000 persons (Centers for Disease Control and Prevention, 2003b). The highest rates in women of any ethnicity were in the 15- to 24-year age groups. The prevalence of gonorrhea in sentinel, study prenatal clinics in 2002 was 0.9 percent. Risk factors included single marital status, adolescence, poverty, drug abuse, prostitution, other STDs, and lack of prenatal care. Gonococcal infection is also a marker for concomitant chlamydial infection in about 40 percent of infected pregnant women (Christmas and colleagues, 1989). In most pregnant women, gonococcal infection is limited to the lower genital tract—the cervix, urethra, and periurethral and vestibular glands. Acute salpingitis is rare in pregnancy, but pregnant women account for a disproportionate number of disseminated gonococcal infections (Ross, 1996; Yip and associates, 1993). A screening test for gonorrhea is recommended at the first prenatal visit or prior to an induced abortion. In high-risk populations, the Centers for Disease Control and Prevention (2002d) and Miller and co-workerss (2003) have recommended that a repeat culture be obtained after 28 weeks' gestation. Ickovics and associates (2003) and Mahon and associates (2002) also recommend postpartum screening in the at-risk teenage population. For women who test positive, screening for syphilis and *Chlamydia trachomatis* should precede treatment, if possible. If chlamydial testing is unavailable, presumptive therapy is given. In addition, offering HIV testing is wise.

EFFECT ON PREGNANCY. Gonococcal infection may have deleterious effects in any trimester. There is an association between untreated gonococcal cervicitis and septic abortion as well as infection after voluntary abortion (Burkman and co-workers, 1976). Preterm delivery, prematurely ruptured membranes, chorioamnionitis, and postpartum infection are more common in women infected with *Neisseria gonorrhoeae* at delivery (Alger and associates, 1988). Expectant management of culture-positive women is reasonable even with prematurely ruptured membranes as long as antimicrobial treatment is given promptly (Maxwell and Watson, 1992).

Sheffield and colleagues (1999) reviewed clinical outcomes of 25 pregnant women admitted to Parkland Hospital for disseminated gonococcal infection. Their mean gestational age at presentation was 25 weeks, and all of the women promptly responded to appropriate antimicrobial therapy. One stillborn neonate and one spontaneous abortion, however, were attributed to gonococcal sepsis.

TREATMENT. Antimicrobial resistance of *N gonorrhoeae,* particularly to penicillin, tetracycline, and quinolones, has rendered most β-lactam drugs ineffective (Centers for Disease Control and Prevention, 2002d). As shown in Table 59–2, ceftriaxone and cefixime are recommended for uncomplicated infection during pregnancy, although cefixime may not be available in 2004 (Brocklehurst, 2003). Ramus and associates (2001), in a study of 62 pregnant women with probable endocervical gonorrhea, reported that intramuscular ceftriaxone (125 mg) and oral cefixime (400 mg) resulted in a cure rate of 95 percent and 96 percent, respectively. Spectinomycin is recommended for women allergic to penicillin or β-lactam antimicrobials. Treatment is recommended for sexual contacts. A test-of-cure is unnecessary if symptoms resolve, but because gonococcal reinfection is common, a second screening in late pregnancy should be considered for women treated earlier during pregnancy (Centers for Disease Control and Prevention, 2002d; Miller and co-workers, 2003).

Disseminated Gonococcal Infections. Gonococcal bacteremia may lead to petechial or pustular skin lesions, arthralgias, septic arthritis, or tenosynovitis. The Centers for Disease

TABLE 59–2 Treatment of Uncomplicated Gonococcal Infections During Pregnancy

Ceftriaxone, 125 mg intramuscularly as a single dose
or
Cefixime, 400 mg orally[a] in a single dose
or
Spectinomycin, 2 g intramuscularly as a single dose
plus
Treatment for chlamydial infection unless it is ruled out[b]

[a]Limited availability after 2003.
[b]See Table 59–3.
From the Centers for Disease Control and Prevention (2002d).

Control and Prevention (2002d) have recommended ceftri-axone, 1000 mg intramuscularly or intravenously every 24 hours. Treatment should be continued for 24 to 48 hours after improvement and then therapy changed to an oral agent to complete a week of therapy.

For gonococcal *endocarditis,* antimicrobials should be continued for at least 4 weeks, and for *meningitis,* 10 to 14 days (Centers for Disease Control and Prevention, 2002d). Endocarditis rarely complicates pregnancy, but it may be fatal (Bataskov and colleagues, 1991).

Treatment of Neonates. Gonococcal conjunctivitis is frequently severe in the neonates. *N gonorrhoeae* can penetrate intact corneal epithelium and cause keratitis, ulceration, perforation, and blindness. All newborns are given prophylaxis against conjunctivitis (see Chap. 28, p. 641). Neonates born to untreated infected women are given ceftriaxone, 25 to 50 mg/kg, either intravenously or intramuscularly for one dose. Mortality results from systemic involvement, and those who develop gonococcal ophthalmia should be hospitalized and evaluated for disseminated infection. Both parents also should be treated for gonorrhea and evaluated for chlamydial infection.

CHLAMYDIAL INFECTIONS

Chlamydia trachomatis is an obligate intracellular bacterium that has several serotypes, including those that cause *lymphogranuloma venereum (LGV).* The most commonly encountered strains are those that attach only to columnar or transitional cell epithelium and cause cervical infection.

MATERNAL INFECTIONS. Genital infection with *C trachomatis* is one of the most common sexually transmitted bacterial diseases in women of reproductive age (Miller and colleagues, 2004). They are also common in pregnant women, and their incidence depends on the demographical makeup of the population. In 2002, the median chlamydial infection rate among young women screened at prenatal clinics in 28 states was 10.1 percent (Centers for Disease Control and Prevention, 2003b). Risk factors for infection in pregnant women include age younger than 25 years, presence or history of other STD(s), multiple sexual partners, and a new sexual partner within 3 months (Centers for Disease Control and Prevention, 2002d).

Diagnosis. Cultures are expensive and less accurate than newer nucleic acid amplification tests, including PCR. Andrews and associates (1997) reported that a ligase chain reaction assay was both sensitive and specific for genitourinary infection in pregnant women.

Symptomatic Infection. Most pregnant women have asymptomatic infection, but some present with urethral syndrome, urethritis, or Bartholin gland infection (Peipert,

2003). Although mucopurulent cervicitis may be due to either chlamydial or gonococcal infection, or both, it may also result from the normal, hormonally stimulated endocervical glands with abundant mucus production. Other chlamydial infections not usually seen in pregnancy are endometritis, salpingitis, peritonitis, reactive arthritis, and Reiter syndrome.

Asymptomatic Infection and Pregnancy Outcome. Many investigators have examined the effects of asymptomatic chlamydial infection on pregnancy outcome, and its role remains controversial. Sozio and Ness (1998) found no association with increased abortion. Some investigators, but not all, have found that untreated cervical infection increases the risk of preterm delivery, prematurely ruptured membranes, and perinatal mortality.

Chlamydial infection appears to be associated neither with an increased risk of chorioamnionitis nor with pelvic infection after cesarean delivery (Blanco and colleagues, 1985; Gibbs and Schachter, 1987). Conversely, delayed postpartum uterine infection with *C trachomatis* has been described by Hoyme and associates (1986). The syndrome, which develops 2 to 3 weeks postpartum, is distinct from early postoperative metritis. It is characterized by vaginal bleeding or discharge, low-grade fever, lower abdominal pain, and uterine tenderness.

NEONATAL INFECTIONS. There is vertical transmission to 30 to 50 percent of neonates delivered vaginally from infected women. Perinatal transmission to neonates can cause pneumonia, and *C trachomatis* is the most common identifiable infectious cause of ophthalmia neonatorum (see Chap. 28, p. 641).

Conjunctivitis. Chlamydial eye infections are one of the most common causes of preventable blindness in developing countries. Symptomatic conjunctivitis tends to appear later (5 to 12 days) than disease caused by *N gonorrhoeae* (2 to 5 days). Tissue culture, direct fluorescent antibody tests, enzyme immunoassays, and nucleic amplification tests are sensitive and specific. None of the neonatal conjunctivitis prophylaxis regimens for gonococcal infection (e.g., silver nitrate, erythromycin, or tetracycline) is effective in the prevention of chlamydial conjunctivitis or pneumonia (Centers for Disease Control and Prevention, 2002d). When eye infection is identified, oral erythromycin, 50 mg/kg/day in four divided doses, is given for 10 to 14 days.

Pneumonitis. *C trachomatis* is a relatively common cause of afebrile pneumonia in infants at 1 to 3 months of age (Centers for Disease Control and Prevention, 2002d). Bilateral pulmonary infiltrates and chronic cough are often associated with poor weight gain.

PRENATAL SCREENING. Routine antepartum screening for *C trachomatis* is a complex issue, although there is little evidence of its effectiveness in asymptomatic women who are not in high-risk groups (Kohl and colleagues, 2003; Peipert, 2003). Identification and treatment of infected pregnant women may prevent neonatal infections, but evidence of prevention of adverse pregnancy outcome is lacking. Therefore, neither the American College of Obstetricians and Gynecologists (2002), the American Academy of Pediatrics, nor the U.S. Preventive Services Task Force (2001) recommend routine screening of all pregnant women. However, these organizations do suggest routine screening for young women at increased risk. The Centers for Disease Control and Prevention (2002d) have recommended screening at the first prenatal visit and again in the third trimester for women younger than 25 years of age or for those who have new or multiple sex partners. In a study of 149 pregnant women with lower genital tract chlamydia, Miller (1998) found that 17 percent had recurrent chlamydial colonization after treatment. Accordingly, a second culture in the third trimester would seem reasonable in women with positive initial culture results or for those at high risk.

TREATMENT. Currently recommended regimens for the treatment of chlamydial infection in pregnant women are shown in Table 59–3. Erythromycin base, 500 mg orally four times daily for 7 days, is the primarily recommended regimen. For women who cannot tolerate erythromycin, the dose can be reduced by half and the duration of therapy doubled. Alternatively, the amoxicillin regimen may be given. In a randomized trial of treatment of *C trachomatis* in pregnancy, Silverman and associates (1994) reported cure rates of 82 percent for amoxicillin and 85 percent for erythromycin.

There have been a number of trials demonstrating the efficacy of azithromycin for chlamydial infection in pregnancy (Jacobson, 2001; Kacmar, 2001; Wehbeh, 1998, and all their colleagues). Comparable efficacy was reported by Adair and associates (1998) in a group of 106 women treated

TABLE 59–3 Treatment of *Chlamydia trachomatis* During Pregnancy

Regimen	Drug and Dosage
First choice	Erythromycin base, 500 mg orally four times daily for 7 days *or* Amoxicillin, 500 mg orally three times daily for 7 days
Alternatives	Erythromycin base, 250 mg orally four times daily for 14 days *or* Erythromycin ethylsuccinate, 800 mg orally four times daily for 7 days *or* Erythromycin ethylsuccinate, 400 mg orally four times daily for 14 days *or* Azithromycin, 1 g orally as a single dose

From the Centers for Disease Control and Prevention (2002d).

with erythromycin (93-percent cure) or azithromycin (88-percent cure). Of concern, Cooper and co-workers (2002b) noted an increased incidence of hypertrophic pyloric stenosis in neonates of mothers treated with nonerythromycin macrolides, however, there was no similar association with erythromycin exposure (see Chap. 14, p. 358). These data are very limited, and azithromycin currently remains an alternative regimen (Adimora, 2002). Tetracyclines are avoided because of concerns regarding fetal dental discoloration. Erythromycin estolate is also avoided because of risks for maternal hepatic toxicity.

LYMPHOGRANULOMA VENEREUM

Several serovars of *C trachomatis* cause lymphogranuloma venereum (LGV). The primary genital infection is transient and seldom recognized. Inguinal adenitis may develop, and at times lead to suppuration. It may be confused with chancroid. Ultimately, the lymphatics of the lower genital tract and perirectal tissues may be involved, with sclerosis and fibrosis, which can cause vulvar elephantiasis and severe rectal stricture. Fistula formation involving the rectum, perineum, and vulva also may evolve.

For treatment during pregnancy, erythromycin, 500 mg four times daily, is given for 21 days (Centers for Disease Control and Prevention, 2002d). Although data regarding efficacy are scarce, some authorities recommend azithromycin given in multiple doses for 3 weeks.

HERPES SIMPLEX VIRUS INFECTION

Management of pregnancy complicated by maternal herpesvirus genital infection remains problematic. There are currently no available rapid diagnostic tests that reliably document contemporary infection. Moreover, there are few data to estimate risks for the neonate exposed to recurrent maternal infection.

VIROLOGY. Two types of herpes simplex virus (HSV) have been distinguished based on immunological as well as clinical differences. Type 1 HSV is responsible for most nongenital herpetic infections, although genital HSV-1 occasionally recurs in adults (Engelberg and colleagues, 2003). In many adolescents and young adults, however, HSV-1 infection causes more than half of new cases of genital herpes (Mertz and associates, 2003). Type 2 HSV is recovered almost exclusively from the genital tract and is usually transmitted by sexual contact. It has been estimated that approximately 22 percent of adults in the United States have HSV-2 infection. There have been projections that the seroprevalence in women may rise to nearly 50 percent by 2025 without intervention (Fisman and co-workers, 2002).

Antibodies. Several serological assay systems are available commercially and in research settings to detect antibody to HSV glycoproteins G-1 and G-2, which evoke type-specific antibody responses to HSV-1 and HSV-2 infection, respectively (Ashley, 2001). These tests have the potential to reliably differentiate HSV-1 from HSV-2 antibody and permit confirmation of clinical infection and identification of asymptomatic carriers.

Brown (2000) and Wald and Ashley-Morrow (2002) have proposed that serological screening of couples for HSV-2 antibodies during pregnancy would stimulate the need for safer sex practices and for antiviral suppression precautions if there is a discordancy (i.e., one seronegative and one seropositive partner). This is controversial, and there is no clinical evidence in pregnancy of its efficacy to prevent HSV transmission and neonatal infection (Scoular, 2002; Wilkinson and associates, 2000). The financial cost of prenatal type-specific antibody testing and of suppressive therapy for partners was judged excessive by Rouse and Stringer (2000) and Barnabas and co-workers (2002), but potentially cost-effective by Baker and associates (2004).

CLINICAL INFECTION. Symptoms vary depending on whether there has been previous infection. Prior HSV-1 infection may modify a primary HSV-2 genital infection because of cross-reacting antibodies. According to the American College of Obstetricians and Gynecologists (1999a), HSV-2 infections clinically may be divided into three groups:

1. *Primary infection* is indicated by no prior antibodies to HSV-1 or HSV-2.
2. *Nonprimary first episode* defines newly acquired HSV-2 infection with preexisting HSV-1 cross-reacting antibodies.
3. *Recurrent infection* is reactivation of prior HSV-1 or HSV-2 infection in the presence of antibodies to the same type of HSV.

Primary Infection. Only a third of newly acquired HSV-2 genital infections are symptomatic (Langenberg and colleagues, 1999). The typical incubation period of 3 to 6 days is followed by a papular eruption with itching or tingling, which then becomes painful and vesicular, with multiple vulvar and perineal lesions that may coalesce (Fig. 59–3). Inguinal adenopathy may be severe. Transient systemic influenza-like symptoms are common and are presumably caused by viremia. Occasionally, hepatitis, encephalitis, or pneumonia may develop. Cervical involvement is common, but it may be inapparent clinically. Some cases are severe enough to require hospitalization. In 2 to 4 weeks, all signs and symptoms of infection disappear.

Nonprimary First Episode. In general, these infections are characterized by fewer lesions, less systemic manifestations, less pain, and briefer duration of lesions and viral shedding.

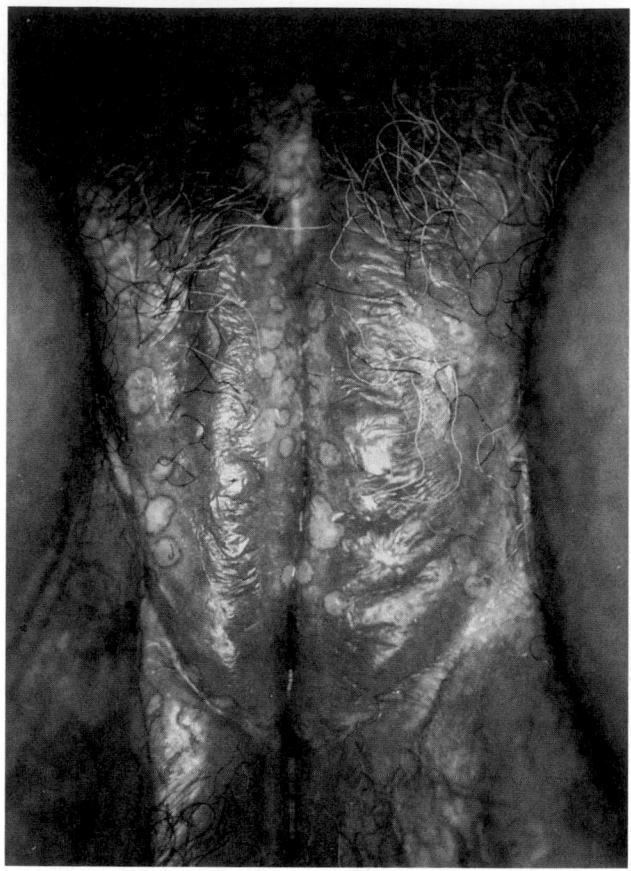

FIGURE 59–3. First-episode primary genital herpes simplex virus infection. (From Wendel and Cunningham, 1991.)

This is likely because of some immunity from cross-reacting antibodies from childhood-acquired type 1 infection. In some cases, it may be impossible to differentiate clinically between the two types of first infection (Hensleigh and associates, 1997). Serological diagnosis is beneficial in this setting.

Recurrent Infections. During the latency period in which viral particles reside in nerve ganglia, reactivation is common and mediated through variable but poorly understood stimuli. Reactivation is termed recurrent infection and results in herpesvirus shedding. Most recurrent genital herpes is caused by type 2 virus (Centers for Disease Control and Prevention, 2002d). These lesions generally are fewer in number, are less tender, and shed virus for shorter periods (2 to 5 days) than those of primary infection. Typically, they recur at the same sites. Finally, although commonly involved in primary disease, cervical involvement is less frequent with recurrent infections (Brown and co-workers, 1985).

In a study of 110 women with genital herpes infection, Wald and associates (1995) reported that 55 percent had subclinical shedding of HSV-2 at some time during a mean follow-up of 105 days. Shedding averaged 1.5 days and often followed symptomatic recurrence. Wald and colleagues (2000) reported that 3 percent of HSV-2 seropositive patients had subclinical shedding whether or not they had a history of genital infection.

DIAGNOSIS. Recovery of virus by *tissue culture* is optimal for confirmation of clinically apparent infection and asymptomatic recurrences. The sensitivity of culture is nearly 95 percent before the lesions undergo crusting. There are virtually no false positives. About half of cultures are positive 48 hours following the onset of a symptomatic recurrence.

Cytological examination after alcohol fixation and Papanicolaou staining—the *Tzanck smear*—has a maximum sensitivity of 70 percent. False-positive cervical smears commonly may be due to cytomegalovirus infection. Use of *PCR* increases HSV detection by four- to eightfold (Cone and associates, 1994; Wald and co-workers, 2003).

TREATMENT. Antiviral therapy with acyclovir, famciclovir, and valacyclovir has been used for treatment of first-episode genital herpes in nonpregnant women. Oral or parenteral preparations attenuate clinical infection as well as the duration of viral shedding. Suppressive therapy with these agents has also been given to limit recurrent infections and to reduce heterosexual transmissions (Corey and colleagues, 2004). For intense discomfort, analgesics and topical anesthetics may provide some relief, and severe urinary retention is treated with an indwelling bladder catheter.

Acyclovir appears to be safe for use in pregnant women (Ratanajamit and associates, 2003). The manufacturer of acyclovir and valacyclovir, in cooperation with the Centers for Disease Control and Prevention, maintained a registry for exposure to these drugs during pregnancy through 1999. More than 700 neonates have been exposed to acyclovir during the first trimester, and there do not appear to be increased adverse fetal or neonatal effects (Reiff-Eldridge and co-workers, 2000; Scott, 1999). There are theoretical concerns about potential neutropenia in the newborn, which is similar to that seen in infants given long-term suppressive acyclovir therapy (Kimberlin, 2004). Valacyclovir results in higher plasma drug levels than acyclovir when given in late pregnancy (Kimberlin and colleagues, 1998). There are insufficient data on valacyclovir and famciclovir exposure in pregnancy for analyses.

Many women with HIV infection also have genital herpes, and treatment failures with recommended doses of acyclovir have been reported. Higher doses of acyclovir may be beneficial for immunoincompetent women with HIV infection and severe recurrent genital herpes (Centers for Disease Control and Prevention, 2002d). In addition, reactivation of genital herpes in labor is common among HIV co-infected women; it was 8 percent in a cohort study from Washington (Hitti and associates, 1997).

Recurrent Infection. Other than suppression, acyclovir is of little benefit in recurrent genital herpes. It has been evaluated as suppressive therapy during pregnancy to prevent recur-

rences near term in several studies (Brocklehurst, 1998; Scott, 1996, 2001, 2002; Watts, 2004, and all their colleagues). In a meta-analysis of five randomized trials, Sheffield and associates (2003) reported that suppressive therapy after 36 weeks reduced the risk of a clinical or asymptomatic recurrence at delivery and of cesarean delivery for recurrent infection. The incidence of asymptomatic viral shedding was reduced but not eliminated. Scott and Alexander (1998) reported that acyclovir suppression in late pregnancy was cost effective.

Vaccine. In their recent review, Kimberlin and Rouse (2004) cite studies done with an HSV-2 glycoprotein-D subunit vaccine. In women seronegative for HSV-1 and -2, the vaccine prevented 75 percent of clinically apparent genital infection. The vaccine was not effective in women with anti–HSV-1 antibodies or in men.

CLINICAL COURSE DURING PREGNANCY. Approximately 80 percent of women with recently acquired genital herpes infection have an average of 2 to 4 *symptomatic* recurrences during pregnancy (Brown and co-workers, 1985; Harger and associates, 1989). Concomitant cervical viral shedding is identified in about 15 percent of pregnant women with clinically evident vulvar recurrences. In addition, *remote recurrences*—those on the buttocks, back, thigh, and anus— have low rates of concomitant cervical virus shedding, and this allows consideration for vaginal delivery (Harger and colleagues, 1989; Wittek and co-workers, 1984).

Viral Shedding at Delivery. The reported prevalence rates for recovery of genital tract herpesvirus at delivery vary considerably depending on the population studied. Equally important is whether women were included or excluded because of prior symptomatic infection. Studies of viral shedding at delivery without regard to maternal history of genital herpes report positive culture results in 0.2 to 0.35 percent (Brown and associates, 1991; Prober and colleagues, 1988).

FETAL AND NEONATAL DISEASE. Most primary and first-episode infections in early pregnancy are probably not associated with an increased rate of spontaneous abortion or stillbirth (Eskild and co-workers, 2002). In their review, Fagnant and Monif (1989) found only 15 cases of congenital herpetic infection that were acquired during early pregnancy. Brown and Baker (1989) reported that late-pregnancy primary infection results in an increased incidence of preterm labor. Fortunately, HSV acquisition in pregnancy is uncommon (0.34 percent) in most settings, and therefore neonatal herpes is rare (Mindel and associates, 2000).

According to Kimberlin (2004), neonatal infection is acquired in three ways: intrauterine (5 percent), peripartum (85 percent), or postnatal (10 percent). The fetus becomes infected by virus shed from the cervix or lower genital tract. The virus either invades the uterus following membrane rupture

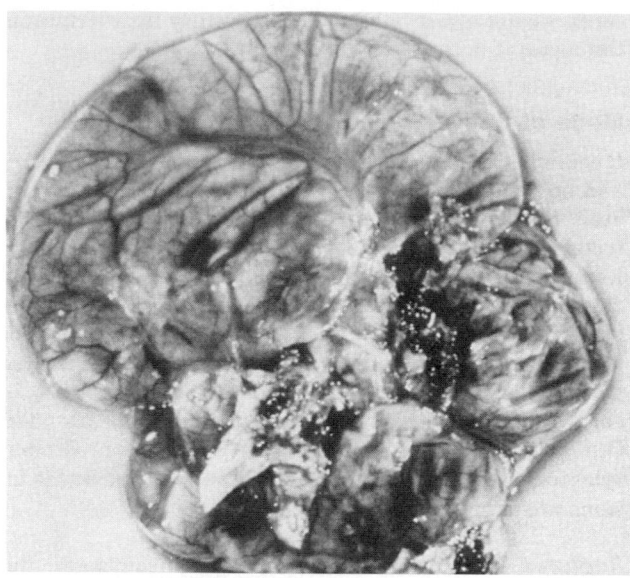

FIGURE 59–4. Cross-section showing necrotic brain tissue in a newborn who died from disseminated herpesvirus infection.

or contacts the fetus at delivery. Newborn infection has three forms:

1. Skin, eye, or mouth disease with localized involvement (45 percent of cases).
2. Central nervous system disease with encephalitis, with or without above involvement (30 percent of cases).
3. Disseminated disease with involvement of multiple major organs (25 percent of cases) (Fig. 59–4).

The risk of neonatal infection correlates with whether there is primary or recurrent maternal infection. Nahmias and colleagues (1971) reported a 50-percent risk of neonatal infection with primary maternal infection but only 4 to 5 percent with recurrent infection. Prober and associates (1987) reported that none of 34 neonates exposed to recurrent viral shedding at delivery became infected, which is thought to be due to a smaller viral load in maternal secretions with recurrent infection. It also likely is related to transplacentally acquired antibody, which decreases the incidence and severity of neonatal disease. An additional risk is prematurity, and nearly half of infected neonates are born preterm.

Localized infection is usually associated with a good outcome. Conversely, even with treatment with acyclovir, disseminated neonatal infection is associated with a mortality rate of nearly 30 percent (Kimberlin and co-workers, 2001a,b). Importantly, serious developmental and central nervous system morbidity still occurs in 20 to 50 percent of survivors with disseminated or cerebral infection (see Fig. 59–4).

Antepartum Management. Virological monitoring is not recommended. Because of the severity of neonatal infection, cesarean delivery has been used widely in instances when active genital herpetic recurrences are suspected. It seems reasonable to give acyclovir suppressive therapy beginning at 36 weeks for women with recurrent genital herpes who have had clinical recurrences during pregnancy (American College of Obstetricians and Gynecologists, 1999a; Centers for Disease Control and Prevention, 2002d; Sheffield and colleagues, 2003).

According to the American College of Obstetricians and Gynecologists (1999a), cesarean delivery is indicated in women with an active genital lesion or in those with a typical prodrome of an impending outbreak. Thus, cesarean delivery is performed only if primary or recurrent lesions are visualized near the time of labor or when the membranes are ruptured. Roberts and associates (1995) reported a decrease in the cesarean delivery rate in women with herpes during pregnancy from 59 percent to 37 percent after adoption of these guidelines, which succinctly stated are "no lesions, no cesarean." Brown and colleagues (2003) confirmed this viewpoint by showing a reduced risk of neonatal HSV with cesarean delivery (85 percent) among women with symptomatic and asymptomatic HSV shedding at delivery.

Ruptured Membranes. There is no evidence that external lesions cause ascending fetal infection in the presence of preterm ruptured membranes. Major and associates (2003) described expectant management of preterm ruptured membranes in a cohort of 29 women at less than 31 weeks. There were no cases of neonatal HSV, and the maximum risk of infection was calculated to be 10 percent. The use of antivirals in this setting is reasonable, but of unproven efficacy.

For women with a clinical recurrence at delivery, there is not an absolute duration of membrane rupture beyond which the fetus would not benefit from cesarean delivery (American College of Obstetricians and Gynecologists, 1999a). Unless there are other contradictory factors (e.g., extreme immaturity), then cesarean delivery is performed.

CARE OF THE NEONATE. An exposed infant born to a mother known to have or suspected of having genital herpes initially should be isolated from other neonates and cultures performed for herpes. It is not necessary to separate the pair. Instead, the woman should wash her hands thoroughly and avoid contact between her lesions, her hands, and the infant. Breast feeding is allowed, including if the woman is taking antiviral therapy. Acyclovir does not reach appreciable levels in breast milk (Sheffield and colleagues, 2002a). Family members with oral herpetic lesions should avoid kissing the newborn and should use careful hand-washing techniques.

HUMAN IMMUNODEFICIENCY VIRUS INFECTION

Acquired immunodeficiency syndrome (AIDS) was first described in 1981 when a cluster of patients was found to have defective cellular immunity and *Pneumocystis carinii*

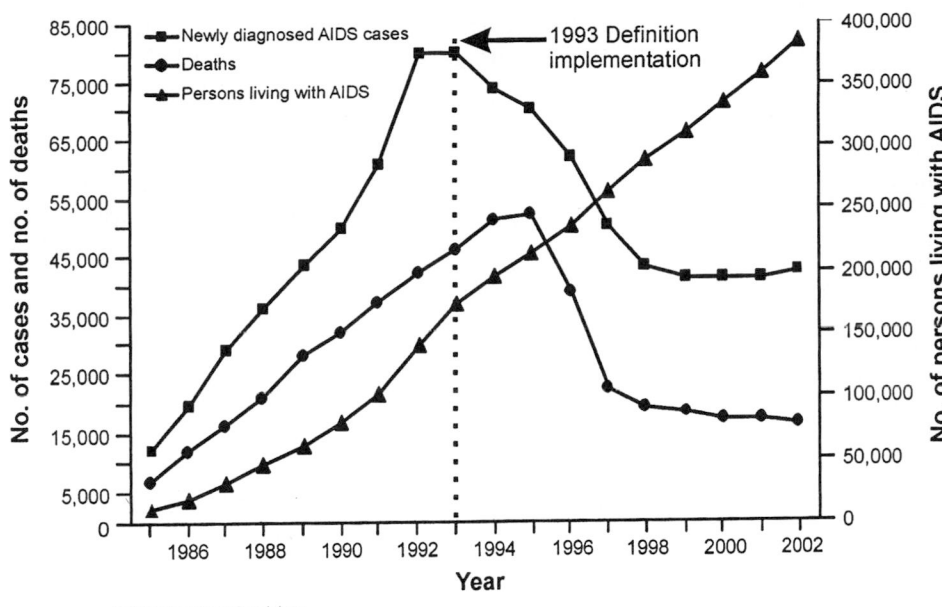

FIGURE 59–5. AIDS cases, deaths, and persons living with acquired immunodeficiency syndrome (AIDS) in the United States from 1985 through 2002. (From Centers for Disease Control and Prevention, 2002b.)

pneumonia (Gallo and Montagnier, 2003). Worldwide, it was estimated in 2003 that there were 40 million infected persons with HIV/AIDS, 5 million new cases of HIV, and 3 million HIV-related deaths (Clinton, 2003; Gayle, 2003; Steinbrook, 2004).

In the United States through 2001, the Centers for Disease Control and Prevention (2002b) estimated that there were 1.3 to 1.4 million infected individuals and almost a half million deaths. In 2002, HIV infection was the fifth leading cause of death in persons 25 to 44 years of age (Kochanek and Smith, 2004). Currently, a third of new cases result from heterosexual transmission, and two thirds of these are in women (Centers for Disease Control and Prevention, 2004b). Fortunately, the number of children with AIDS attributed to perinatal transmission has decreased by more than 90 percent in the past 10 years (Centers for Disease Control and Prevention, 2002b). In addition, during this time, highly active antiretroviral therapy has led to an increasing number of people living with chronic HIV infection (Fig. 59–5).

ETIOLOGY. Causative agents of AIDS are DNA retroviruses termed *human immunodeficiency viruses*, HIV-1 and HIV-2. Most cases worldwide are caused by HIV-1 infection. Transmission of these viruses is similar to hepatitis B virus, and sexual intercourse is the major mode of transmission. The virus also is transmitted by blood or blood-contaminated products, and mothers may infect their fetuses.

PATHOGENESIS. The common denominator of clinical illness with AIDS is profound immunosuppression that gives rise to a variety of opportunistic infections and neoplasms. Thymus-derived lymphocytes, or *T lymphocytes,* defined phenotypically by the CD4 surface antigen, are the principal targets. The CD4 site serves as a receptor for the virus. Co-receptors are necessary for infection, and two chemokine

receptors—CCR5 and CXCR4—have been identified to fill this role (Kahn and Walker, 1998; Sheffield and colleagues, 2005). After initial infection, the level of viremia usually decreases to a *set-point,* and patients with the highest viral burden at this time progress more rapidly to AIDS and death (Kahn and Walker, 1998).

Over time the number of T cells drops insidiously and progressively, resulting eventually in profound immunosuppression. Although it is thought that pregnancy has minimal effects on CD4$^+$ T-cell counts and HIV RNA levels, the latter are often higher 6 months postpartum than during pregnancy (U.S. Public Health Service, 2003). Monocyte-macrophages may also be infected, and microglial brain cell infection may cause neuropsychiatric abnormalities. HIV-infected persons also have an increased incidence of neoplasms, notably Kaposi sarcoma, B-cell and non-Hodgkin lymphomas, and some carcinomas (see Chap. 57, p. 1262).

CLINICAL MANIFESTATIONS. The incubation period from exposure to clinical disease is days to weeks. Acute illness is similar to many other viral syndromes and usually lasts less than 10 days. Common symptoms include fever and night sweats, fatigue, rash, headache, lymphadenopathy, pharyngitis, myalgias, arthralgias, nausea, vomiting, and diarrhea. After symptoms abate, the set-point of chronic viremia is established. Stimuli that cause further progression from asymptomatic viremia to AIDS are presently unclear, but the median time is about 10 years (Fauci, 2003).

When HIV-positive assay results are associated with any number of clinical findings, then AIDS is diagnosed. Generalized lymphadenopathy, oral hairy leukoplakia, aphthous ulcers, and thrombocytopenia are common. A number of opportunistic infections that may herald AIDS include esophageal or pulmonary candidiasis; persistent herpes simplex or zoster lesions; condyloma acuminata; tuberculosis; cytomegaloviral pneumonia, retinitis, or gastrointestinal disease; molluscum contagiosum; pneumocystis pneumonia; toxoplasmosis; and others. Neurological disease is common, and about half of patients have central nervous system symptoms. A CD4$^+$ count of less than 200/mm^3 is also considered definitive for the diagnosis of AIDS.

There are unique gynecological issues for women with HIV, such as menstrual abnormalities, genital neoplasia, other STDs, and contraceptive needs that overlap into pregnancy (Cejtin, 2003; Stuart and Castaño, 2003). Repeated pregnancy does not have significant effect on the clinical or immunological course of viral infection (Minkoff and colleagues, 2003).

SEROLOGICAL TESTING. The enzyme immunoassay (EIA) is used as a screening test for HIV antibodies as a part of a *standard testing protocol.* A repeatedly positive screening test has a sensitivity of more than 99.5 percent. A positive test is confirmed with either the Western blot or immunofluorescence assay (IFA). Results typically are available in several days.

Although highly specific, the Western blot is less sensitive than immunoassay because more antibody is required for a positive result. Thus, IFA can be used to resolve an EIA-positive, Western blot–indeterminate sample. According to the Centers for Disease Control and Prevention (2001a,b), antibody can be detected in most patients within 1 month of infection, and thus, antibody serotesting may not exclude early infection. For acute primary HIV infection, identification of viral p24 core antigen or viral RNA or DNA is possible. False-positive confirmatory results are rare (Centers for Disease Control and Prevention, 2001a).

In some cases, the first opportunity for HIV testing may occur when women present late for prenatal care or when they are in labor. *Rapid tests* can detect HIV antibody in 10 to 60 minutes at the point-of-care, and they have sensitivity and specificity comparable with EIAs (Branson, 2003; Centers for Disease Control and Prevention, 2004c,d). A reactive rapid screening test result should be supplemented with a confirmatory Western blot or IFA test. Peripartum and neonatal interventions to reduce perinatal transmission, however, may be based on the initial rapid testing results.

The Mother–Infant Rapid Intervention at Delivery (MIRIAD) multicenter study indicated that rapid HIV testing can be used to identify infected women and their neonates so that peripartum antiretroviral prophylaxis can be administered (Bulterys and colleagues, 2004). A set of practical guidelines for rapid HIV testing in labor and delivery is available from the Centers for Disease Control and Prevention (2004d).

SCREENING. In 1991, universal, but voluntary, prenatal screening was recommended by the Institute of Medicine, the Centers for Disease Control and Prevention (2002c), the American Academy of Pediatrics, and the American College of Obstetricians and Gynecologists (1999b, 2002, 2004).

A study conducted from 1998 to 2001 in the United States and Canada reported that the rates of acceptance of HIV prenatal testing depend on the approach used (Centers for Disease Control and Prevention, 2002c). Under an *opt-in approach,* women receive pretest counseling and must specifically consent to HIV testing. In the *opt-out approach,* women are notified that an HIV test is part of a comprehensive set of antenatal tests and procedures, and they may decline testing (Stringer and colleagues, 2001). Areas that used or switched to the opt-out approach had much higher rates of prenatal serotesting. The Centers for Disease Control and Prevention (2004e) recommended adoption of the opt-out protocol into routine prenatal care. Sansom and associates (2003) suggest that it may be cost effective to repeat HIV testing in the third trimester in areas with a prevalence of 1 per 1000 person years or higher. Several states also recommend or require a second HIV test at delivery.

MATERNAL AND FETAL-NEONATAL INFECTION. Mother-to-child transmission accounts for most pediatric HIV infections. Transplacental transmission can occur early, and the virus has been identified in specimens from elective abortion (Lewis and co-workers, 1990). According to Blair and associates (2004), pregnancy rates among women with HIV infection increased significantly in the current era of antiretroviral therapy compared with rates before 1996. In most cases, however, the virus is transmitted peripartum, and 15 to 40 percent of neonates born to nonbreast feeding, untreated, HIV-infected mothers are infected. Kourtis and colleagues (2001) have proposed a model for estimation of the temporal distribution of vertical transmission. They estimate that 20 percent of transmission occurs before 36 weeks, 50 percent in the days before delivery, and 30 percent intrapartum (Fig. 59–6). Transmission rates for breast feeding may be as high as 30 to 40 percent.

Vertical transmission is more common in preterm births, especially those associated with prolonged membrane rupture. Analyzing data from the Perinatal AIDS Collaborative Transmission Study, Kuhn and associates (1999) reported a 3.7 relative risk for intrapartum viral transmission with preterm delivery. Landesman and co-workers (1996) reported that HIV-1 transmission at birth was increased from 15 to 25 percent in women whose membranes were ruptured for more than 4 hours.

Concurrent syphilis infection is common and is also associated with vertical perinatal HIV transmission (Koumans and colleagues, 2000; Schulte and associates, 2001). Finally, there is evidence that placental inflammation and chorioamnionitis may increase HIV-1 transmission by 3 percent, but it is unclear if antimicrobials decrease this risk (Mwanyumba and co-workers, 2002).

Perinatal HIV transmission can be most accurately correlated with measurement of maternal plasma HIV RNA burden

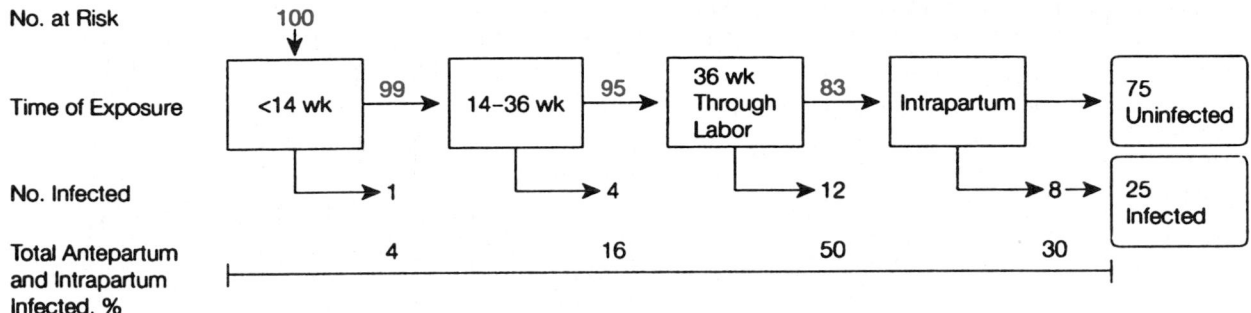

FIGURE 59-6. Estimated rates of perinatal human immunodeficiency virus (HIV) transmission for different times of gestation and delivery in nonbreast feeding populations. Estimates are based on a hypothetical cohort of 100 children born to HIV-infected women without any interventions. Numbers in blue indicated number of children at risk for infection. (From Kourtis and colleagues, 2001.)

(U.S. Public Health Service 2004b, 2003; Watts, 2002). As shown in Figure 59–7, cohort neonatal infection was 1 percent with less than 400 copies/mL, and it was more than 30 percent when viral RNA exceeded 100,000 copies/mL (Cooper and colleagues, 2002a). Importantly, zidovudine therapy that reduced these levels to less than 500 copies/mL also minimized the risk of transmission. The investigators also reported that maternal infusions of HIV-1 hyperimmune globulin did not alter the risk of transmission.

According to the U.S. Public Health Service Guidelines (2003), maternal morbidity and mortality are not increased by pregnancy in seropositive asymptomatic women. Conversely, adverse fetal outcomes may be increased in these cases. In a review of 634 women delivered after 24 weeks, Stratton and associates (1999) reported that adverse pregnancy outcomes were common in HIV-infected women. Moreover, they reported that adverse outcomes were associated with a CD4$^+$ cell proportion of less than 15 percent. In these otherwise asymptomatic women, the rate of preterm birth was 20 percent and fetal growth restriction was identified in 24 percent. Watts (2002) emphasized that these adverse outcomes were even more prevalent in developing countries.

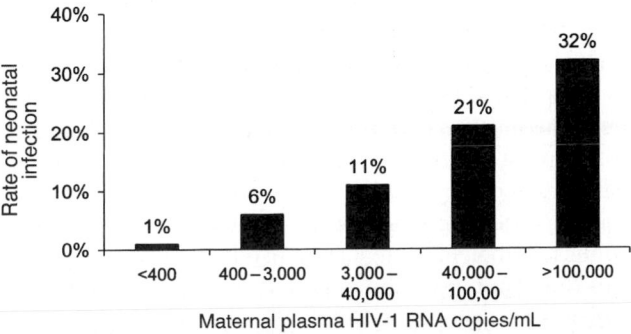

FIGURE 59-7. Incidence of perinatal human immunodeficiency virus (HIV) infection plotted against plasma HIV-1 RNA levels in 1542 neonates born to mothers in the Women and Infants Transmission Study. (Data from Cooper and colleagues, 2002a.)

MANAGEMENT DURING PREGNANCY. Counseling is mandatory for HIV-positive women. This is preferable early in pregnancy, and if the woman chooses to continue pregnancy, ongoing counseling for psychological support is important.

The availability of an increasing number of antiretroviral agents and the rapid evolution of new information has introduced substantial complexity into HIV therapy. In addition, separate strategies are used for pregnant and nonpregnant adults. Therapeutic goals are a maximal and enduring suppression of viral load and restoration and preservation of immunological function.

For nonpregnant patients, treatment is generally offered to adults with less than 350 CD4$^+$ T cells/mm^3 or plasma HIV RNA levels exceeding 55,000 copies/mL (Table 59–4). A more aggressive strategy has evolved for the management of HIV infection in pregnancy, because RNA level reduction is paramount to reduce perinatal transmission. **Antiretroviral therapy should be offered to all HIV-infected pregnant women to begin maternal treatment as well as to reduce the risk of perinatal transmission regardless of CD4$^+$ T-cell count or HIV RNA level.**

The many approved antiretroviral agents can be grouped into several classes and used to design antiretroviral regimens (Table 59–5). Antiretroviral agents may be combined into non-nucleoside reverse transcriptase inhibitor (NNRTI)–based, protease inhibitor (PI)–based, triple nucleoside reverse transcriptase inhibitor (NRTI)–based, or fusion inhibitor (FI)–based regimens (Table 59–6). The new FI agents—*cell membrane fusion inhibitors*—block HIV-1 cell membrane binding and cell entry. One member of this class, enfuvirtide, has been used in salvage regimens with resistant HIV-1 in settings in which therapeutic options are limited (Kilby and Eron, 2003). Its efficacy and safety in pregnancy are unclear. Information on the safety and toxicity of antiretroviral agents has been reviewed by Money (2003) and also is available as a supplement to the U.S. Public Health Services guidelines (2004a,b, 2003) and through the web site http://AIDSinfo.nih.gov, which is frequently updated.

TABLE 59–4 Indications for Initiating Antiretroviral Therapy for HIV-1 Infections

Clinical Category	CD4+ T-Cell Count	Plasma HIV RNA	Adult and Postpartum Recommendation	Pregnancy Recommendation
Symptomatic (AIDS or severe symptoms)	Any value	Any value	Treat	Treat
Asymptomatic AIDS	< 200/mm³	Any value	Treat	Treat
Asymptomatic	200–350/mm³	Any value	Treatment should be offered, although controversial	Treat
Asymptomatic	> 350/mm³	> 100,000/mL	Some recommend initiating therapy, recognizing that the 3-year risk for untreated patients to develop AIDS is > 30%; in the absence of increased levels of plasma HIV RNA, others recommend deferring therapy and monitoring the CD4+ T-cell count and HIV RNA level more frequently; outcome data with therapy are lacking	Treat
Asymptomatic	> 350/mm³	< 100,000/mL	Most recommend deferring therapy and monitoring CD4+ T-cell count, recognizing that the 3-year risk for untreated patients to develop symptomatic AIDS is < 15%	Treat

AIDS = acquired immunodeficiency syndrome; HIV = human immunodeficiency virus.
From U.S. Public Health Service (2004a, 2003); updated from http://AIDSinfo.nih.gov; accessed October 29, 2004.

The perinatal guidelines (U.S. Public Health Service, 2003) recommend measurement of CD4+ T-lymphocyte counts approximately each trimester, or about every 3 to 4 months. HIV RNA levels should be monitored 4 weeks after

TABLE 59–5 Classes of Antiretroviral Drugs

Drug Class	Category[a]
Nucleoside reverse transcriptase inhibitors	
Abacavir	C
Didanosine	B
Emtricitabine	B
Lamivudine	C
Stavudine	C
Tenofovir	B
Zalcitabine	C
Zidovudine	C
Non-nucleoside reverse transcriptase inhibitors	
Delavirdine	C
Efavirenz	C
Nevirapine	C
Protease inhibitors	
Amprenavir	C
Atazanavir	B
Fosaprenavir	C
Indinavir	C
Lopinavir/ritonavir	C
Nelfinavir	B
Ritonavir	B
Saquinavir	B
Fusion inhibitors	
Enfuvirtide	B

[a]FDA pregnancy category classification—see Chapter 14 (p. 344).
From U.S. Public Health Service (2004a).

initiation of a change in treatment, then monthly until undetectable, then every 3 months, and finally near term for planning delivery. These results are used to make decisions to alter therapy, to decide route of delivery, or to begin prophylaxis for opportunistic infections such as *P carinii* pneumonia.

Even with treatment, the incidence of perinatal complications is increased. Lorenzi and colleagues (1998) reported that 78 percent of women treated with two reverse transcriptase inhibitors had one or more adverse events, especially preterm delivery. Half of the neonates in this study had adverse events. Newer drug regimens may diminish these complications. For example, Tuomala and associates (2002) found no association with preterm birth, low birthweight, or stillbirths when combination antiretroviral therapy was used. They did, however, show that women given combination PI regimens had an increased risk of very-low-birthweight infants. Despite this, combined therapy should not be withheld if indicated (Watts, 2002).

At least two follow-up studies of children from the Pediatric AIDS Clinical Trial Group (PACTG) 076 Study found no adverse effects in children at 18 months and up to a mean of 5.6 years after zidovudine exposure (Culnane and associates, 1999; Sperling and colleagues, 1998).

Treatment failures may be due to nonadherence, inadequate drug potency, suboptimal levels of antiretrovirals, or viral resistance. Poor adherence to therapy appears to be a significant problem in pregnancy. In one study of 549 women from New York, poor compliance was reported in a third of women (Laine and associates, 2000).

Most HIV-infected women require additional medical care during pregnancy (Minkoff, 2003; Watts, 2002). They are given hepatitis B, influenza, and pneumococcal vaccines, ideally after viral suppression is achieved. Frequent monitoring

TABLE 59–6 Antiretroviral Regimens Recommended for HIV-1 Treatment in Drug-Naive Pregnant Women

Regimen	Combination Treatment	Possible Advantages	Possible Disadvantages	Drug Interaction	Impact
Protease inhibitor-based HAART regimen (NNRTI- and FI-sparing)	Lopinavir/ritonavir + lamivudine + (zidovudine or stavudine[a]) (Atazanavir or fosamprenavir or fosamprenavir/ritonavir or indinavir/ritonavir or lopinavir/ritonavir or nelfinavir or saquinavir/ritonavir) + (lamivudine or emtricitabine) + (zidovudine or stavudine[a] or abacavir)	Efficacy documented. Resistance requires multiple mutations. Spares NNRTI and FI side effects. Targets HIV at two steps of viral replication (RT and PI)	Some regimens are difficult to use, especially long term. Long-term side effects often include lipodystrophy, hyperlipidemia, and insulin resistance	Mild to severe inhibition of cytochrome P_{450} pathway—ritonavir is most potent, but this can be exploited to boost levels of other PIs	Preserves NNRTIs and FIs for use in treatment failure. Resistance primes for cross-resistance with other PIs
Non-nucleoside reverse transcriptase inhibitor-based HAART regimen (PI- and FI-sparing)	Efavirenz + lamivudine + (zidovudine or tenofovir DF or stavudine[a]). Efavirenz + emtricitabine + (zidovudine or tenofovir DF or stavudine[a]). Efavirenz + (lamivudine or emtricitabine) + (didanosine or abacavir). Nevirapine + (lamivudine or emtricitabine) + (zidovudine or stavudine* or didanosine or abacavir)	Virological and immunological efficacy well-documented. Spares PI and FI side effects. Easier use, including long-term, compared with PIs	Those with CD4+ counts > 250/mm^3 have increased risk of symptomatic nevirapine hepatotoxicity. Efavirenz should be avoided in the first trimester. Resistance conferred by single or limited number of mutations	Fewer drug interactions compared with PIs	Preserves PIs and FIs for use in treatment failure. Resistance usually leads to cross-resistance across entire NNRTI class
Triple nucleoside reverse transcriptase inhibitor regimen (NNRTI-, PI-, and FI-sparing)	Abacavir + lamivudine + zidovudine (or stavudine[a])	Generally easier use and greater adherence compared with PIs. Spares NNRTI, PI, and FI side effects	Only when an NNRTI- or a PI-based regimen cannot or should not be used as first-line therapy. Efficacy inferior to efavirenz-based regimen	No cytochrome P_{450} interaction	Preserves NNRTI, PI, and FI classes for use in treatment failure

NNRTI = non-nucleoside reverse transcriptase inhibitor; NRTI = nucleoside reverse transcriptase inhibitor; PI = protease inhibitor; HAART = highly active antiretroviral treatment; FI = fusion inhibitor; HIV = human immunodefiency virus.

Lopinavir and ritonavir is formulated as Kaletra, and zidovudine and lamivudine are formulated as Combivir.

[a]Higher incidence of lipoatrophy, hyperlipidemia, and mitochondrial toxicities reported with stavudine than with other NRTIs.

Modified from the U.S. Public Health Services (2004a, 2003) from http://AIDSinfo.nih.gov; accessed March 23, 2004.

is necessary for antiretroviral clinical and laboratory toxicities during the initial 1 to 2 months of treatment; this is particularly important with nevirapine regimens. Thereafter, surveillance for hepatic toxicity and lactic acidosis may be decreased. Reviewing a variety of regimens in the PACTG Protocol 316, Watts and co-workers (2004) found moderate-grade toxicity in 5 percent of women. Gestational diabetes varied by treatment regimen and was highest with early combination PI treatment. These latter women should have early glucose intolerance screening. Careful surveillance is important for antiretroviral drug interactions with other antiretrovirals, as well as therapies for opportunistic infection, methadone, and tuberculosis (Piscitelli and Gallicano, 2001). Information about this issue in pregnancy has been reviewed by Minkoff (2003) and Watts (2002). More detailed updates are available at the previously cited web site (http://AIDSinfo.nih.gov).

The management of some HIV complications can be altered by pregnancy. If the CD4$^+$ T-cell count is below 200/mm^3, primary prophylaxis for *P carinii* pneumonia is recommended with sulfamethoxazole-trimethoprim or dapsone. Pneumonia is treated with oral or intravenous sulfamethoxazole-trimethoprim or dapsone-trimethoprim. Other symptomatic opportunistic infections that may develop include toxoplasmosis, herpesvirus, mycobacteria, and candida. The U.S. Public Health Service, the Infectious Diseases Society of America, and the American Thoracic Society have published guidelines for prevention and treatment of opportunistic infections in persons infected with HIV (Centers for Disease Control and Prevention, 2002a,d, 2004f).

Prevention of Transmission. Precautions for antepartum, peripartum, and pediatric care of infected mothers and newborns are similar to those for hepatitis B, with avoidance of exposure to blood and body fluids. Antepartum antiretroviral therapy can be continued intrapartum. Optimal management of labor is uncertain, but if labor is progressing with intact membranes, artificial rupture and invasive fetal monitoring are avoided. Labor augmentation is used whenever needed to shorten the interval to delivery.

Pooled data from several prospective studies of health care workers suggest that the average risk of HIV transmission is 0.3 percent after percutaneous exposure to infected blood and 0.09 percent after mucous membrane exposure (Gerberding, 2003). Important for obstetricians, suture needles have not been implicated as a source of infection in prospective studies. However, occupational infection has occurred among surgical personnel. For health care workers with significant percutaneous or mucosal HIV exposure, postexposure prophylaxis is recommended (Centers for Disease Control and Prevention, 2001c; Gerberding, 2003).

Prevention of Vertical Transmission. The two principal approaches suggested for prevention of maternal–neonatal transmission of HIV infection are antiretroviral therapy and cesarean delivery. When standard treatment regimens are combined with zidovudine perinatal prophylaxis shown in Table 59–7, vertical transmission is substantively lowered (Minkoff, 2003; Watts, 2002). The lowest transmission rates are achieved using prenatal combination therapy; they were 1 and 2 percent in two prospective studies reported by Cooper (2002a), Dorenbaum (2002), and all their colleagues. Short-term toxicity appears to be minimal for most women and newborns.

The main long-term problem is development of resistance. This is associated most commonly with prenatal combination therapy with lamivudine and with peripartum nevirapine (Clavel and Hance, 2004; Mandelbrot and associates, 2001; Moodley and co-workers, 2003). At present the known risks are clearly outweighed by the potential benefits of prophylaxis.

Indications for resistance testing for pregnant women are the same as for nonpregnant adults and include acute HIV-1 infection, virological failure, suboptimal viral suppression after initiation of antiretroviral therapy, and high likelihood of exposure to resistant virus based on community prevalence. Women who have presumed or documented zidovudine resistance and are on regimens that do not include zidovudine should still be given intravenous zidovudine intrapartum, and their neonates are given oral zidovudine (see Table 59–7).

TABLE 59–7 Pediatric AIDS Clinical Trials Group (PATCG) 076 Zidovudine Regimen

Time of Administration	Zidovudine Regimen
Antepartum	100 mg orally five times daily, initiated at 14 to 34 weeks and continued throughout the pregnancy.[a]
Intrapartum	During labor, intravenous zidovudine in a 1-hour initial dose of 2 mg/kg, followed by a continuous infusion of 1 mg/kg/hr until delivery.[b]
Neonate	Begin at 8 to 12 hours after birth, and give syrup at 2 mg/kg every 6 hours for 6 weeks.[c]

[a]Acceptable alternative regimens include 200 mg three times daily or 300 mg twice daily.
[b]For elective cesarean delivery, intravenous zidovudine is begun at least 3 hours prior to surgery. For premature rupture of membranes or labor with a planned operative delivery, the loading dose may be given during 30 minutes prior to surgery.
[c]Intravenous dosage for infants who cannot tolerate oral intake is 1.5 mg/kg intravenously every 6 hours.
From U.S. Public Health Service, 2003.

If women on combination therapy temporarily discontinue treatment during pregnancy, all drugs should be stopped and restarted simultaneously to reduce the potential for emergence of resistance.

A number of clinical scenarios have been anticipated by the U.S. Public Health Service perinatal guidelines (2003):

1. If maternal HIV RNA level is more than 1000 copies/mL, then combination antiretroviral therapy is indicated.
2. When the maternal HIV RNA level is less than 1000 copies/mL, either combination antiretroviral therapy or zidovudine monotherapy can be given.
3. For women with no treatment prior to labor, intrapartum prophylaxis is appropriate with zidovudine, zidovudine with lamivudine, zidovudine with nevirapine, or nevirapine alone.
4. If delivery occurs before treatment is given, the newborn can receive prophylaxis for 6 weeks with zidovudine, or in some cases combination antiretroviral treatment.

A multistate surveillance program determined that by 1996, 80 percent of HIV-infected women were identified before delivery and that most received antepartum and intrapartum prophylaxis (Wortley and colleagues, 2001). By 2001, nearly 60 percent of American women were aware of effective intervention strategies to prevent perinatal HIV transmission (Anderson and associates, 2004). This rapid adoption of clinical practices clearly has resulted in the dramatic reductions in perinatal transmission to the current levels of 1 to 2 percent.

Cesarean Delivery. A meta-analysis of 15 prospective cohort studies by the International Perinatal HIV Group (1999) included 8533 mother–neonate pairs. Vertical HIV transmission was reduced by about one half when cesarean was compared with vaginal delivery. When antiretroviral therapy was given in the prenatal, intrapartum, and neonatal periods along with cesarean delivery, the likelihood of neonatal transmission was reduced by 87 percent compared with that of other modes of delivery and without antiretroviral therapy. The European Mode of Delivery Collaboration (1999) as well as others had similar findings. Based on these, the American College of Obstetricians and Gynecologists (2000) concluded that scheduled cesarean delivery should be discussed and recommended for HIV-infected women whose HIV-1 RNA load exceeds 1000 copies/mL. Scheduled delivery was recommended as early as 38 weeks to lessen the chances of premature membrane rupture. Data are insufficient to estimate any benefits of cesarean delivery for women whose HIV RNA levels were below 1000 copies/mL. Given their lower rate of transmission, it is unlikely that scheduled cesarean delivery would confer additional risk reduction.

Others have expressed concern that morbidity may be significantly increased in HIV-infected women undergoing cesarean delivery (Read and co-workers, 2001). Stringer and

colleagues (1999) as well as Star and associates (1999) made a plea for restraint regarding routine cesarean delivery for prevention of vertical transmission. They concluded that combination antiretroviral therapy alone may reduce the risk to less than 2 percent. Our experiences at Parkland Hospital are similar, and perinatal transmission in women taking combination antiretroviral therapy has been 1 to 2 percent.

Breast Feeding. Vertical transmission is increased by breast feeding which generally is not recommended in HIV-positive women in this country (Read and co-workers, 2003). The probability of HIV transmission per liter of breast milk ingested is estimated to be similar in magnitude to heterosexual transmission with unsafe sex in adults (Richardson and colleagues, 2003). The risk is related to the maternal HIV RNA level, HIV disease status, breast health, and duration of breast feeding (De Cock and associates, 2000; John-Stewart and co-workers, 2004). Most transmission occurs in the first 6 months, and as many as two thirds of infections in breast-fed infants are from breast milk. In the Petra study (2002) from Africa, the prophylactic benefits of short-course perinatal antiviral regimens were diminished considerably by 18 months of age due to breast feeding. The World Health Organization (2001) has recommended continuing breast feeding promotion with early weaning by 6 months for women living in developing countries in which infectious diseases and malnutrition are the primary causes of infant deaths.

Postpartum. Many otherwise healthy women with normal CD4$^+$ T-cell counts and low HIV RNA levels may discontinue treatment after delivery and be closely monitored according to adult guidelines. Psychosocial support is essential during this time, especially while awaiting diagnostic testing for pediatric infection. Contraceptive needs are complex and also may entail condoms in discordantly infected couples. There are effects on hormone levels with oral contraceptives and possibly with injectable agents (Stuart and Castaño, 2003). Intrauterine devices may be an acceptable choice in some women with normal immunocompetence and a low risk for STDs. Gynecological care is complex in HIV-infected women and has been comprehensively reviewed recently by Cejtin (2003).

HUMAN PAPILLOMAVIRUS INFECTION

Genital human papillomavirus infection (HPV), either symptomatic or asymptomatic, is common. Of 2597 high-risk pregnant women enrolled in the New Orleans Center of the Vaginal Infections and Prematurity Study, 28 percent were seropositive for HPV-16 capsid antibodies (Hagensee and colleagues, 1999). The most important sequelae of HPV infection are cervical, vaginal, vulvar, and anal neoplasia (see Chap. 57, p. 1264). Mucocutaneous external genital warts are usually caused by HPV types 6 and 11 but may also

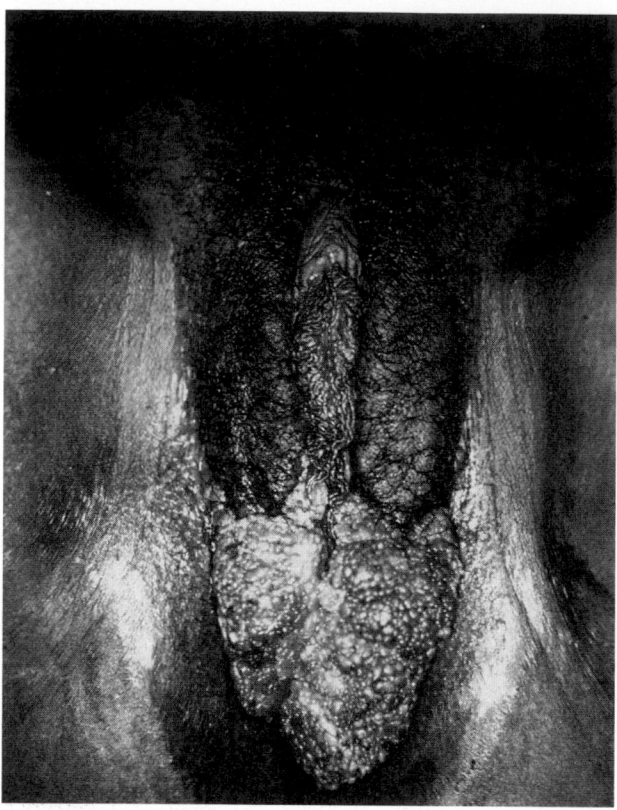

FIGURE 59–8. Extensive external genital warts in a woman near term. (From Wendel and Cunningham, 1991.)

be caused by intermediate- and high-oncogenic–risk HPV (Centers for Disease Control and Prevention, 1999; Wiley and associates, 2002).

EXTERNAL GENITAL WARTS. For unknown reasons, genital warts frequently increase in number and size during pregnancy. Accelerated viral replication by the physiological changes of pregnancy might explain the growth of perineal lesions and progression of some to cervical neoplasm (Fife and co-workers, 1999; Rando and colleagues, 1989). High-risk HPV types are cleared more slowly during pregnancy, and clearance increases postpartum (Nobbenhuis and associates, 2002). These lesions may grow to fill the vagina or cover the perineum, making it difficult to perform vaginal delivery or episiotomy and prompting cesarean delivery (Fig. 59–8). In women without grossly visible lesions, Snyder and co-workers (1990), but not Goldaber and colleagues (1993), found an association between papillomavirus infection and episiotomy breakdown. Because HPV infection may be sub-clinical and multifocal, most women with vulvar lesions also have cervical HPV infection, and vice versa (Ault, 2003; Spitzer and associates, 1989).

TREATMENT. Although there may be an incomplete response to treatment during pregnancy, these lesions com-monly improve or regress rapidly following delivery. Conse-quently, eradication of warts during pregnancy is not always necessary. Therapy is directed toward minimizing treatment toxicity to the mother and fetus and debulking symptomatic genital warts. There are several agents employed in adults, but pregnancy limits their use. There is no definitive evidence that any one of the subsequently discussed treatments is superior to any other (Centers for Disease Control and Prevention, 2002d; Wiley and co-workers, 2002).

Trichloroacetic or *bichloracetic acid,* 80- to 90-percent solution, applied topically once a week, is an effective reg-imen for external warts. Some prefer *cryotherapy* or *laser ablation* of these lesions (Arena and colleagues, 2001). In one study, Schwartz and associates (1988) reported good re-sults in 31 of 32 women treated with combination laser and 85-percent trichloroacetic acid therapy. *Podophyllin resin, podofilox* 0.5-percent solution or gel, *5-fluorouracil* cream, *imiquimod* 5-percent cream, and *interferon* therapy are not recommended in pregnancy because of concerns for maternal and fetal safety (Centers for Disease Control and Prevention, 2002d).

NEONATAL INFECTION. Juvenile-onset recurrent res-piratory papillomatosis is a rare, benign neoplasm of the larynx. It can cause hoarseness and respiratory distress in children and is often due to HPV types 6 or 11. In some cases, maternal genital HPV infection is associated with laryngeal papillomatosis, and studies differ in their findings of neona-tal transmission rates. A Danish population-based study in-dicated a risk of neonatal transmission of 7 in 1000 infected women (Silverberg and co-workers, 2003). In this study, pro-longed ruptured membranes was associated with a twofold increased risk, but was not associated with the method of delivery. Tseng and colleagues (1998), in a study of 301 in-fected women, reported a transmission rate of 40 percent for HPV 16 and 18. The rate was higher for vaginal compared with that of cesarean delivery (51 versus 27 percent). Tenti and associates (1999) reported a 30-percent neonatal trans-mission rate. Watts and co-workers (1998) found HPV DNA in 5 percent of samples from the oral or nasopharynx, anus, and genital areas of newborns. Surprisingly, the rates were higher in mothers without HPV detected during pregnancy (Winer and Koutsky, 2004).

Because these reports cite very few clinical infections when these children are followed, there is a question of transient HPV infection versus contamination. Smith and col-leagues (2004) studied oral and genital samples from mother–newborn pairs to identify HPV DNA using PCR sequencing and found virus in only 9 of 574 (1.6 percent) newborns. The transmission rate was 3.7 percent among HPV-positive women. Importantly, they found no HPV DNA in any of the infants who returned for follow-up. In another study, Manns and associates (1999) measured the seropositive rates for HPV-16 in children at 1 to 2 years and confirmed this low rate of vertical transmission. These data support the rarity of perinatal HPV transmission. Given our limited understanding of the development of laryngeal papillomatosis and current obstetrical data, cesarean delivery cannot be recommended to reduce the risk of this disease.

CHANCROID

Haemophilus ducreyi can cause painful, nonindurated genital ulcers, termed soft chancres, at times accompanied by painful inguinal lymphadenopathy. Although common in some developing countries, it had become rare in the United States. In 1987, however, its incidence had increased tenfold during the previous 10 years, and drug use and sex-for-drugs were shown to be important risk factors (Schmid and co-workers, 1987). Importantly, the infection is a high-risk co-factor for HIV and syphilis transmission (Centers for Disease Control and Prevention, 2002d).

Diagnosis by culture is difficult because appropriate media are not widely available. Instead, clinical diagnosis is made when typical painful genital ulcer(s) are darkfield negative and herpesvirus tests are negative. Recommended treatment in pregnancy is azithromycin, 1 g orally as a single dose; erythromycin base, 500 mg orally four times daily for 7 days; or ceftriaxone, 250 mg in a single intramuscular dose (Centers for Disease Control and Prevention, 2002d).

TRICHOMONIASIS

This protozoal infection was previously considered a common but minor sexually transmitted disease. Lately, however, its importance has been reassessed in light of its associations with other STDs, particularly HIV, and with possible preterm birth (Soper, 2004). *Trichomonas vaginalis* was identified in 13 percent of nearly 14,000 women cultured at midpregnancy by the Vaginal Infections and Prematurity Study Group (Cotch and colleagues, 1991). Ethnic-specific prevalence was 23 percent for blacks and about 6 percent for Hispanic and white women.

Symptomatic vaginitis is less common and is characterized by a yellow discharge, abnormal odor, and vulvar pruritus. These women usually have a purulent vaginal discharge, vulvovaginal erythema, and *colpitis macularis* or *strawberry cervix*. Trichomonads are demonstrated readily in a wet mount of vaginal secretions as flagellated, ovoid, motile organisms that are somewhat larger than leukocytes. The sensitivity of this technique depends on the concentration of organisms, the degree of dilution, and the experience of the examiner, but it is generally considered to be 60 to 85 percent. Trichomonads are identified most accurately by culture using Diamond medium. PCR techniques under development have had variable results (Schwebke, 2002).

The Vaginal Infections and Prematurity Study Group reported significant associations between trichomoniasis and preterm prematurely ruptured membranes, preterm delivery, and low-birthweight neonates (Cotch and associates, 1997). According to Goldenberg and co-workers (1997), however, the association with preterm delivery is difficult to assess because of commonly associated risk factors. Prenatal screening for asymptomatic infection and treatment of carriers was unexpectedly associated with an *increased* rate of preterm births (Klebanoff and colleagues, 2001). Similarly, Kigozi and associates (2003) also reported an increased rate of low-birthweight neonates in a cohort of women treated for trichomoniasis. It is currently recommended that only symptomatic infections be treated. This association is considered further in Chapter 36 (see p. 863).

TREATMENT. Metronidazole is the only trichomonacidal drug available in the United States, and it is quite effective. Oral administration is preferred. Lossick (1990) reviewed clinical experiences with metronidazole and found that 250 mg given three times daily for 7 days, or 2 g as a single dose, had median cure rates of 92 and 96 percent, respectively. There are few data regarding efficacy of any regimen in pregnancy. According to the Centers for Disease Control and Prevention (2002d), pregnant women can be treated with either a single 2-g oral dose, or 500 mg twice a day for 7 days. Several studies and meta-analyses have not detected association with teratogenic or mutagenic effects in fetuses (see Chap. 14, p. 360).

Men have a transient infection with *T vaginalis*. Although the need for concomitant treatment is uncertain, most investigators have found higher relapse rates in women whose partners were not treated. Thus, the Centers for Disease Control and Prevention (2002d) recommend that all partners be treated.

BACTERIAL VAGINOSIS

This is not an actual vaginal infection but rather a clinical syndrome resulting from replacement of the normal H_2O_2-producing *Lactobacillus* species with high concentrations of anaerobic bacteria (e.g., *Prevotella* and *Mobiluncus* species), *Gardnerella vaginalis*, and *Mycoplasma hominis*. Bacterial vaginosis (BV) is a common cause of vaginal discharge or malodor, however, as many as half of women are asymptomatic. The pathophysiology of the microbial interactions is not fully understood, particularly in pregnancy (Nelson and Macones, 2002). Diagnosis, treatment, and possible associations of asymptomatic BV with preterm birth are discussed in Chapter 36 (see p. 862).

It is unclear whether BV is a sexually transmitted syndrome, but it is rare among women who have never been sexually active. Treatment of the male sex partner has not been beneficial in preventing the recurrence of BV.

DIAGNOSIS. BV can be diagnosed by clinical criteria or by Gram stain. The clinical criteria of Amsel require at least three of the following symptoms or signs:

1. Homogeneous, white, noninflammatory discharge that smoothly coats the vaginal walls.
2. Presence of clue cells on microscopic examination.
3. Vaginal fluid pH greater than 4.5.
4. Fishy odor of discharge before or after addition of 10-percent potassium hydroxide—the *whiff test.*

When a Gram stain is applied to the discharge, assessment of the relative concentration of bacterial morphotypes characteristic of the altered flora is an acceptable laboratory method for diagnosing BV—the *Nugent criteria.* Cervical Papanicolaou tests have limited clinical usefulness for the diagnosis of BV because of low sensitivity.

TREATMENT. All symptomatic pregnant women should be tested and treated. A number of studies discussed in Chapter 36 (see p. 862) have shown that BV is associated with adverse pregnancy outcomes. These include prematurely ruptured membranes, preterm labor, preterm birth, chorioamnionitis, and postabortion and postpartum pelvic infection. Unfortunately, prospective studies have shown no improvement of perinatal outcomes with treatment.

Therapy for symptomatic BV in pregnant women may have other benefits such as reduction of the risk for sexually transmitted infections. The optimal regimen for women during pregnancy is not known, but the oral metronidazole regimens shown in Table 59–8 probably are equally effective. Cure rates with these are about 70 percent (Koumans and associates, 2002). The clindamycin and topical regimens are less effective. There have been no consistent association between metronidazole and teratogenic or mutagenic effects in newborns (see Chap. 14, p. 360).

FOLLOW-UP. If symptoms resolve, no further evaluation is needed. Recurrence of symptomatic BV is not unusual,

TABLE 59–8 Recommended Regimens for Symptomatic Bacterial Vaginosis

Metronidazole, 250 mg orally three times a day for 7 days
Metronidazole, 500 mg orally twice daily for 7 days
Clindamycin, 300 mg orally twice a day for 7 days
Metronidazole gel, 0.75%, one applicatorful (5 g) intravaginally, once daily for 5 days
Clindamycin cream, 2%, one applicatorful (5 g) intravaginally at bedtime for 7 days

Adapted from Centers for Disease Control and Prevention (2002d).

and additional therapy is given with another listed regimen. Routine treatment of sex partners is not recommended.

OTHER SEXUALLY TRANSMITTED DISEASES

There are many more infections and infestations that can be acquired as the consequence of sexual intercourse. These include hepatitis B and C, *Candida vulvovaginitis, scabies,* and *pediculosis pubis.* These infections are discussed elsewhere in the text.

REFERENCES

Adair CD, Gunter M, Stovall TG, et al: Chlamydia in pregnancy: A randomized trial of azithromycin and erythromycin. Obstet Gynecol 91:165, 1998

Adimora AA: Treatment of uncomplicated genital *Chlamydia trachomatis* infections in adults. Clin Infect Dis 35:S183, 2002

Alexander JM, Sheffield JS, Sanchez PJ, et al: Efficacy of treatment for syphilis in pregnancy. Obstet Gynecol 93:5, 1999

Alger LS, Lovchik JC, Hebel JR, et al: The association of *Chlamydia trachomatis, Neisseria gonorrhoeae,* and group B streptococci with preterm rupture of the membranes and pregnancy outcome. Am J Obstet Gynecol 159:397, 1988

American Academy of Pediatrics and American College of Obstetricians and Gynecologists: Guidelines for Perinatal Care, 5th ed. Washington, DC, AAP and ACOG, 2002

American College of Obstetricians and Gynecologists: Prenatal and perinatal human immunodeficiency virus testing: expanded recommendations. Committee Opinion No. 304, November 2004

American College of Obstetricians and Gynecologists: Scheduled cesarean delivery and the prevention of vertical transmission of HIV infection. Committee Opinion No. 234, May 2000

American College of Obstetricians and Gynecologists: Management of herpes in pregnancy. Practice Bulletin No. 8, October 1999a

American College of Obstetricians and Gynecologists: Joint Statement on human immunodeficiency virus screening. Policy Statements, Compendium of Selected Publications, May 1999b

Anderson JE, Ebrahim SH, Sansom S: Women's knowledge about treatment to prevent mother-to-child human immunodeficiency virus transmission. Obstet Gynecol 103:165, 2004

Andrews WW, Lee H, Roden WJ, et al: Detection of genitourinary tract *Chlamydia trachomatis* infection in pregnant women by ligase chain reaction assay. Obstet Gynecol 89:556, 1997

Arena S, Marconi M, Frega A, et al: Pregnancy and condyloma. Evaluation about therapeutic effectiveness of laser CO_2 on 115 pregnant women. Minerva Ginecol 53:389, 2001

Ashley RL: Sorting out the new HSV type specific antibody tests. Sex Trans Infect 77:232, 2001

Augenbraun MH: Treatment of syphilis 2001: Nonpregnant adults. Clin Infect Dis 35:S187, 2002

Augenbraun M, Workowski K: Ceftriaxone therapy for syphilis: Report from the Emerging Infections Network. Clin Infect Dis 29:1337, 1999

Ault K: Human papillomavirus infections: Diagnosis, treatment and hope for a vaccine. Obstet Gynecol Clin North Am 30:809, 2003

Baker D, Brown Z, Hollier LM, et al: Cost-effectiveness of herpes simplex virus type 2 serologic testing and antiviral therapy in pregnancy. Am J Obstet Gynecol 191:2074, 2004

Barnabas RV, Carabin H, Garnett GP: The potential role of suppressive therapy for sex partners in the prevention of neonatal herpes: A health economic analysis. Sex Transm Infect 78:425, 2002

Barton JR, Thorpe EM Jr, Shaver DC, et al: Nonimmune hydrops fetalis associated with maternal infection with syphilis. Am J Obstet Gynecol 167:56, 1992

Bataskov KL, Hariharan S, Horowitz MD, et al: Gonococcal endocarditis complicating pregnancy: A case report and literature review. Obstet Gynecol 78:494, 1991

Blair JM, Hanson DL, Jones JL, et al: Trends in pregnancy rates among women with human immunodeficiency virus. Obstet Gynecol 103:663, 2004

Blanco JD, Diaz KC, Lipscomb KA, et al: *Chlamydia trachomatis* isolation in patients with endometritis after cesarean section. Am J Obstet Gynecol 152:278, 1985

Branson BM: Point-of-care rapid tests for HIV antibodies. J Lab Med 27:288, 2003

Brocklehurst P: Antibiotics for gonorrhoea in pregnancy (Cochrane Review). In The Cochrane Library. Chichester, UK, John Wiley & Sons, Issue 4, 2003

Brocklehurst P, Kinghorn G, Carney O, et al: A randomized placebo controlled trial of suppressive acyclovir in late pregnancy in women with recurrent genital herpes infection. Br J Obstet Gynaecol 105:275, 1998

Brown ZA: HSV-2 specific serology should be offered routinely to antenatal patients. Rev Med Virol 10:145, 2000

Brown ZA, Baker DA: Acyclovir therapy during pregnancy. Obstet Gynecol 73:526, 1989

Brown ZA, Benedetti J, Ashley R, et al: Neonatal herpes simplex virus infection in relation to asymptomatic maternal infection at the time of labor. N Engl J Med 324:1247, 1991

Brown ZA, Vontver LA, Benedetti J, et al: Genital herpes in pregnancy: Risk factors associated with recurrences and asymptomatic shedding. Am J Obstet Gynecol 153:24, 1985

Brown ZA, Wald A, Morrow A, et al: Effect of serologic status and cesarean delivery on transmission rates of herpes simplex virus from mother to infant. JAMA 289:203, 2003

Bulterys M, Jamieson DJ, O'Sullivan MJ, et al: Rapid HIV-1 testing during labor: A multicenter study. JAMA 292:219, 2004

Burkman RT, Tonascia JA, Atienza MF, et al: Untreated endocervical gonorrhea and endometritis following elective abortion. Am J Obstet Gynecol 126:648, 1976

Cejtin HE: Gynecologic issues in the HIV-infected woman. Obstet Gynecol Clin North Am 30:711, 2003

Centers for Disease Control and Prevention: Azithromycin treatment failures in syphilis infections—San Francisco, California, 2002–2003. MMWR 53:197, 2004a

Centers for Disease Control and Prevention: Heterosexual transmission of HIV—29 states. MMWR 53:125, 2004b

Centers for Disease Control and Prevention: Protocols for confirmation of reactive rapid HIV tests. MMWR 53:221, 2004c

Centers for Disease Control and Prevention: Rapid HIV antibody testing during labor and delivery for women of unknown HIV status. A practical guide and model protocol. Available at: http://www.cdc.gov/hiv/projects/perinatal. Accessed March 2004d

Centers for Disease Control and Prevention: Routine prenatal testing—the opt-out approach. Available at: http://www.cdc.gov/hiv/PROJECTS/perinatal/OptOutNews32.pdf. Accessed February 24, 2004e

Centers for Disease Control and Prevention: Updated guidelines for the use of rifamycins for the treatment of tuberculosis among HIV-infected patients taking protease inhibitors or nonnucleoside reverse transcriptase inhibitors. MMWR 53:37, 2004f

Centers for Disease Control and Prevention: Primary and secondary syphilis—United States, 2002. MMWR 52:1117, 2003a

Centers for Disease Control and Prevention: Sexually transmitted disease surveillance, 2002. Atlanta, GA: U.S. Department of Health and Human Services, September 2003b

Centers for Disease Control and Prevention: 2002 IDSA guidelines for preventing opportunistic infections among HIV-infected persons—2002. Recommendations of the U.S. Public Health Service and the Infectious Diseases Society of America. MMWR 51:RR-9, 2002a

Centers for Disease Control and Prevention: Cases of HIV infection and AIDS in the United States, 2002. HIV/AIDS Surveillance Report (Addendum) 14:1, 2002b

Centers for Disease Control and Prevention: HIV testing among pregnant women—United States and Canada, 1998–2001. MMWR 51:1013, 2002c

Centers for Disease Control and Prevention: Sexually transmitted diseases treatment guidelines 2002. MMWR 51:RR-6, 2002d

Centers for Disease Control and Prevention: Revised guidelines for HIV counseling and testing. MMWR 50:1, 2001a

Centers for Disease Control and Prevention: Revised recommendations for HIV screening of pregnant women. MMWR 50:RR-19, 2001b

Centers for Disease Control and Prevention: Updated U.S. Public Health Service guidelines for the management of occupational exposures to HBV, HCV, and HIV and recommendations for postexposure prophylaxis. MMWR 50:RR-11, 2001c

Centers for Disease Control and Prevention: Prevention of genital HPV infection and sequelae: Report of an external consultants' meeting. Atlanta, Centers for Disease Control and Prevention, December 1999

Chisholm CA, Katz VL, McDonald TL, et al: Penicillin desensitization in the treatment of syphilis during pregnancy. Am J Perinatol 14:553, 1997

Christmas JT, Wendel GD, Bawdon RE, et al: Concomitant infection with *Neisseria gonorrhoeae* and *Chlamydia trachomatis* in pregnancy. Obstet Gynecol 74:295, 1989

Clavel F, Hance AJ: HIV drug resistance. N Engl J Med 350:1023, 2004

Clinton WJ: Turning the tide on the AIDS pandemic. N Engl J Med 348:1800, 2003

Cone RW, Hobson AC, Brown Z, et al: Frequent detection of genital herpes simplex virus DNA by polymerase chain reaction among pregnant women. JAMA 272:792, 1994

Connor N, Roberts J, Nicoll A: Strategic options for antenatal screening for syphilis in the United Kingdom: A cost effectiveness analysis. J Med Screen 7:7, 2000

Cooper ER, Charurat M, Mofenson L, et al: Combination antiretroviral strategies for the treatment of pregnant HIV-1-infected women and prevention of perinatal HIV-1 transmission. J Acquir Immune Defic Syndr 29:484, 2002a

Cooper WO, Ray WA, Griffin MR: Prenatal prescription of macrolide antibiotics and infantile hypertrophic pyloric stenosis. Obstet Gynecol 100:101, 2002b

Corey L, Wald A, Patel R, et al: Once-daily valacyclovir to reduce the risk of transmission of genital herpes. N Engl J Med 350:11, 2004

Cotch MF, Pastorek JG II, Nugent RP, et al: Demographic and behavioral predictors of *Trichomonas vaginalis* infection among pregnant women. Obstet Gynecol 78:1087, 1991

Cotch MF, Pastorek JG II, Nugent RP, et al: *Trichomonas vaginalis* associated with low birth weight and preterm delivery. Sex Transm Dis 24:353, 1997

Culnane M, Fowler M, Lee SS, et al: Lack of long-term effects of in utero exposure to zidovudine among uninfected children born to HIV-infected women. Pediatric AIDS Clinical Trials Group Protocol 219/076 Teams. JAMA 13:281, 1999

De Cock KM, Fowler MG, Mercier E, et al: Prevention of mother-to-child HIV transmission in resource-poor countries. JAMA 283:1175, 2000

Dorenbaum A, Cunningham CK, Gelber RD, et al: Two-dose intrapartum/newborn nevirapine and standard antiretroviral therapy to reduce perinatal HIV transmission. JAMA 288:189, 2002

Engelberg R, Carrell D, Krantz E, et al: Natural history of genital herpes simplex virus type 1 infection. Sex Transm Dis 30:174, 2003

Eskild A, Jeansson S, Stray-Pedersen B, et al: Herpes simplex virus type-2 infection in pregnancy. No risk of fetal death: Results from a nested case-control study within 35,940 women. Br J Obstet Gynaecol 109:1030, 2002

European Mode of Delivery Collaboration: Elective caesarean-section versus vaginal delivery in prevention of vertical HIV-1 transmission: A randomized clinical trial. Lancet 353:1035, 1999

Fagnant RJ, Monif GRG: How rare is congenital herpes simplex? A literature review. J Reprod Med 34:417, 1989

Fauci AS: HIV and AIDS: 20 years of science. Nat Med 9:839, 2003

Fife KH, Katz BP, Brizendine EJ, et al: Cervical human papillomavirus deoxyribonucleic acid persists throughout pregnancy and decreases in the postpartum period. Am J Obstet Gynecol 180:1110, 1999

Fisman DN, Lipsitch M, Hook EW III, et al: Projection of the future dimensions and costs of the genital herpes simplex type 2 epidemic in the United States. Sex Transm Dis 29:608, 2002

Fiumara NJ, Fleming WL, Downing JG, et al: The incidence of prenatal syphilis at the Boston City Hospital. N Engl J Med 247:48, 1952

Gallo RC, Montagnier L: The discovery of HIV as the cause of AIDS. N Engl J Med 349:2283, 2003

Gayle HD: Curbing the global AIDS epidemic. N Engl J Med 348:1802, 2003

Genc M, Ledger WJ: Syphilis in pregnancy. Sex Transm Infect 76:73, 2000

Gerberding JL: Occupational exposure to HIV in health care settings. N Engl J Med 348:826, 2003

Gibbs RS, Schachter J: Chlamydial serology in patients with intraamniotic infection and controls. Sex Transm Dis 14:213, 1987

Goldaber KG, Wendel PJ, McIntire DD, et al: Postpartum perineal morbidity after fourth degree perineal repair. Am J Obstet Gynecol 168:489, 1993

Golden MR, Marra CM, Holmes KK: Update on syphilis: Resurgence of an old problem. JAMA 290:1510, 2003

Goldenberg RL, Andrews WW, Yuan AC, et al: Sexually transmitted disease and adverse outcomes of pregnancy. Clin Perinatol 24:23, 1997

Goldenberg RL, Thompson C: The infectious origins of stillbirth. Am J Obstet Gynecol 189:861, 2003

Gray RH, Wabwire-Mangen F, Kigozi G, et al: Randomized trial of presumptive sexually transmitted disease therapy during pregnancy in Rakai, Uganda. Am J Obstet Gynecol 185:1209, 2001

Gust DA, Levine WC, St. Louis ME, et al: Mortality associated with congenital syphilis in the United States, 1992–1998. Pediatrics 109:E79, 2002

Hagensee ME, Slavinsky J 3rd, Gaffga CM, et al: Seroprevalence of human papillomavirus type 16 in pregnant women. Obstet Gynecol 94:653, 1999

Harger JH, Amortegui AJ, Meyer MP, et al: Characteristics of recurrent genital herpes simplex infections in pregnant women. Obstet Gynecol 73:367, 1989

Hensleigh PA, Andrews WW, Brown Z, et al: Genital herpes during pregnancy: Inability to distinguish primary and recurrent infections clinically. Obstet Gynecol 89:891, 1997

Hitti J, Watts DH, Burchett SK, et al: Herpes simplex virus seropositivity and reactivation at delivery among pregnant women infected with human immunodeficiency virus-1. Am J Obstet Gynecol 177:450, 1997

Hollier LM, Harstat TW, Sanchez PJ, et al: Fetal syphilis: Clinical and laboratory characteristics. Obstet Gynecol 97:947, 2001

Hollier LM, Hill J, Sheffield JS, et al: State laws regarding prenatal syphilis screening in the United States. Am J Obstet Gynecol 189:1178, 2003

Hoyme UB, Kiviat N, Eschenbach DA: The microbiology and treatment of late postpartum endometritis. Obstet Gynecol 68:226, 1986

Ickovics JR, Niccolai LM, Lewis JB, et al: High postpartum rates of sexually transmitted infections among teens: Pregnancy as a window of opportunity for prevention. Sex Transm Infect 79:469, 2003

Institute of Medicine, Committee on Prenatal and Newborn Screening for HIV Infection: HIV Screening of Pregnant Women and Newborns. Washington, DC, National Academy Press, 1991

International Perinatal HIV Group: The mode of delivery and the risk of vertical transmission of human immunodeficiency virus type 1: A meta-analysis of 15 prospective cohort studies. N Engl J Med 340:977, 1999

Jacobson GF, Autry AM, Kirby RS, et al: A randomized controlled trial comparing amoxicillin and azithromycin for the treatment of Chlamydia trachomatis in pregnancy. Am J Obstet Gynecol 184:1352, 2001

John-Stewart G, Mbori-Ngacha D, Ekpini R, et al: Breastfeeding and transmission of HIV-1. J Acquir Immune Defic Syndr 35:196, 2004

Kacmar J, Cheh E, Montagno A, et al: A randomized trial of azithromycin versus amoxicillin for the treatment of Chlamydia trachomatis in pregnancy. Infect Dis Obstet Gynecol 9:197, 2001

Kahn JO, Walker BD: Acute human immunodeficiency virus type 1 infection. N Engl J Med 339:33, 1998

Kigozi GG, Brahmbhatt H, Wabwire-Mangen F, et al: Treatment of trichomonas in pregnancy and adverse outcomes of pregnancy: A subanalysis of a randomized trial in Rakai, Uganda. Am J Obstet Gynecol 189:1398, 2003

Kilby JM, Eron JJ: Novel therapies based on mechanisms of HIV-1 cell entry. N Engl J Med 348:2228, 2003

Kimberlin DW: Neonatal herpes simplex infection. Clin Microbiol Rev 17:1, 2004

Kimberlin DW, Rouse DJ: Genital herpes. N Engl J Med 350:1970, 2004

Kimberlin DW, Lin CY, Jacobs RF, et al: Natural history of neonatal herpes simplex virus infections in the acyclovir era. Pediatrics 108:223, 2001a

Kimberlin DW, Lin CY, Jacobs RF, et al: Safety and efficacy of high-dose intravenous acyclovir in the management of neonatal herpes simplex virus infections. Pediatrics 108:230, 2001b

Kimberlin DF, Weller S, Whitley RJ, et al: Pharmacokinetics of oral valacyclovir and acyclovir in late pregnancy. Am J Obstet Gynecol 179:846, 1998

Klass PE, Brown ER, Pelton SI: The incidence of prenatal syphilis at the Boston City Hospital: A comparison across four decades. Pediatrics 94:24, 1994

Klebanoff MA, Carey JC, Hauth JC, et al: Failure of metronidazole to prevent preterm delivery among pregnant women with asymptomatic Trichomonas vaginalis infection. N Engl J Med 345:487, 2001

Klein VR, Cox SM, Mitchell MD, et al: The Jarisch–Herxheimer reaction complicating syphilotherapy in pregnancy. Obstet Gynecol 75:375, 1990

Kochanek KD, Smith BL: Deaths: Preliminary data for 2002. National Vital Statistics Reports, Vol 52, No. 27. Hyattsville, MD, National Center for Health Statistics, 2004

Kohl KS, Markowitz LE, Koumans EH: Developments in the screening for *Chlamydia trachomatis*: A review. Obstet Gynecol Clin North Am 30:637, 2003

Koumans EH, Markowitz LE, Hogan V: Indications for therapy and treatment recommendations for bacterial vaginosis in nonpregnant and pregnant women: A synthesis of data. Clin Infect Dis 35:S152, 2002

Koumans EH, Sternberg M, Gwinn M, et al: Geographic variation of HIV infection in childbearing women with syphilis in the United States. AIDS 14:279, 2000

Kourtis AP, Bulterys M, Nesheim SR: Understanding the timing of HIV transmission from mother to infant. JAMA 285:709, 2001

Kuhn L, Steketee RW, Weedon J, et al: Distinct risk factors for intrauterine and intrapartum human immunodeficiency virus transmission and consequences for disease progression in infected children. Perinatal AIDS Collaborative Transmission Study. J Infect Dis 179:52, 1999

Lago EG, Rodrigues LC, Fiori RM, et al: Identification of two distinct profiles of maternal characteristics associated with risk. Sex Transm Dis 31:33, 2004

Laine C, Newschaffer CJ, Zhang D, et al: Adherence to antiretroviral therapy by pregnant women infected with human immunodeficiency virus: A pharmacy claims-based analysis. Obstet Gynecol 95:167, 2000

Landesman SH, Kalish LA, Burns DN, et al: Obstetrical factors and the transmission of human immunodeficiency virus type 1 from mother to child. N Engl J Med 334:1617, 1996

Langenberg AGM, Corey L, Ashley RL, et al: A prospective study of new infections with herpes simplex virus type 1 and type 2. N Engl J Med 341:1432, 1999

Lewis SH, Reynolds-Kohler C, Fox HE, et al: HIV-1 in trophoblastic and villous Hofbauer cells, and haematological precursors in eight-week fetuses. Lancet 335:565, 1990

Lorenzi P, Spicher VM, Laubereau B, et al: Antiretroviral therapies in pregnancy: Maternal, fetal and neonatal effects. Swiss HIV Cohort Study, the Swiss Collaborative HIV and Pregnancy Study, and the Swiss Neonatal HIV Study. AIDS 12:F241, 1998

Lossick JG: Treatment of sexually transmitted vaginosis/vaginitis. Rev Infect Dis 12:S665, 1990

Lucas MJ, Theriot SK, Wendel GD: Doppler systolic–diastolic ratios in pregnancies complicated by syphilis. Obstet Gynecol 77:217, 1991

Lukehart SA, Godornes C, Molini BJ, et al: Macrolide resistance in *Treponema pallidum* in the United States and Ireland. N Engl J Med 351:154, 2004

Lumbiganon P, Piaggio G, Villar J, et al: The epidemiology of syphilis in pregnancy. Int J STD AIDS 13:486, 2002

Mahon BE, Rosenman MB, Graham MF, et al: Postpartum *Chlamydia trachomatis* and *Neisseria gonorrhoeae* infections. Am J Obstet Gynecol 186:1320, 2002

Major CA, Towers CV, Lewis DF, et al: Expectant management of preterm rupture of membranes complicated by active recurrent genital herpes. Am J Obstet Gynecol 188:1551, 2003

Mandelbrot L, Landreau-Mascaro A, Rekacewicz C, et al: Lamivudine-zidovudine combination for prevention of maternal-infant transmission of HIV-1. JAMA 285:2083, 2001

Manns A, Strickler HD, Wiktor SZ, et al: Low incidence of human papillomavirus type 16 antibody seroconversion in young children. Pediatr Infect Dis J 18:833, 1999

Maxwell GL, Watson WJ: Preterm premature rupture of membranes: Results of expectant management in patients with

cervical cultures positive for group B streptococcus or *Neisseria gonorrhoeae*. Am J Obstet Gynecol 166:945, 1992

McFarlin BL, Bottoms SF, Dock BS, et al: Epidemic syphilis: Maternal factors associated with congenital infection. Am J Obstet Gynecol 170:535, 1994

Mertz GJ, Rosenthal SL, Stanberry LR: Is herpes simplex virus type 1 (HSV-1) now more common than HSV-2 in first episodes of genital herpes? Sex Transm Dis 30:801, 2003

Miller JM Jr: Recurrent chlamydial colonization during pregnancy. Am J Perinatol 15:307, 1998

Miller WC, Ford CA, Morris M, et al: Prevalence of chlamydial and gonococcal infections among young adults in the United States. JAMA 291:2229, 2004

Miller JM Jr, Maupin RT, Mestad RE, et al: Initial and repeated screening for gonorrhea during pregnancy. Sex Transm Dis 30:728, 2003

Mindel A, Taylor J, Tideman RL, et al: Neonatal herpes prevention: A minor public health problem in some communities. Sex Transm Infect 76:287, 2000

Minkoff HL: Human immunodeficiency virus infection in pregnancy. Obstet Gynecol 101:797, 2003

Minkoff HL, Hershow R, Watts H, et al: The relationship of pregnancy to human immunodeficiency virus disease progression. Am J Obstet Gynecol 189:552, 2003

Minkoff HL, McCalla S, Delke I, et al: The relationship of cocaine use to syphilis and human immunodeficiency virus infections among inner-city parturient women. Am J Obstet Gynecol 163:521, 1990

Mitka M: US effort to eliminate syphilis moving forward. JAMA 283:1555, 2000

Money DM: Antiviral and antiretroviral use in pregnancy. Obstet Gynecol Clin North Am 30:731, 2003

Moodley D, Moodley J, Coovadia H, et al: A multicenter randomized controlled trial of nevirapine versus a combination of zidovudine and lamivudine to reduce intrapartum and early postpartum mother-to-child transmission of human immunodeficiency virus type 1. J Infect Dis 187:725, 2003

Mwanyumba F, Galillard P, Inion I, et al: Placental inflammation and perinatal transmission of HIV-1. J Acquir Immune Defic Syndr 29:262, 2002

Myles TD, Elam G, Park-Hwang E, et al: The Jarisch–Herxheimer reaction and fetal monitoring changes in pregnant women treated for syphilis. Obstet Gynecol 92:859, 1998

Nahmias AJ, Josey WE, Naib ZM, et al: Perinatal risk associated with maternal genital herpes simplex virus infection. Am J Obstet Gynecol 110:825, 1971

Nathan L, Bohman VR, Sanchez PJ, et al: In utero infection with *Treponema pallidum* in early pregnancy. Prenat Diagn 17:119, 1997

Nelson DB, Macones G: Bacterial vaginosis in pregnancy: Current findings and future directions. Epidemiol Rev 24:102, 2002

Nobbenhuis MAE, Helmerhorst TJM, van den Brule AJC, et al: High-risk human papillomavirus clearance in pregnant women: Trends for lower clearance during pregnancy with a catch-up postpartum. Br J Cancer 87:75, 2002

Peipert JF: Clinical practice: Genital chlamydial infections. N Engl J Med 18:349, 2003

Petra Study Team: Efficacy of three short-course regimens of zidovudine and lamivudine in preventing early and late transmission of HIV-1 from mother to child in Tanzania, South Africa and Uganda (Petra study): A randomized, double-blind, placebo-controlled trial. Lancet 359:1178, 2002

Piper JM, Shain RN, Korte JE, et al: Behavioral interventions for prevention of sexually transmitted diseases in women: A physician's perspective. Obstet Gynecol Clin North Am 30:659, 2003

Piscitelli SC, Gallicano KD: Interactions among drugs for HIV and opportunistic infections. N Engl J Med 344:984, 2001

Pope V, Fears MB: Serodia *Treponema pallidum* passive particle agglutination (TP-PA) test. In Larsen SA, Pope V, Jonnson RE, et al (eds): Supplement to A Manual of Tests for Syphilis, 9th ed. Washington, DC, American Public Health Association, 2000, p 365

Prober CG, Hensleigh PA, Boucher FD, et al: Use of routine viral cultures at delivery to identify neonates exposed to herpes simplex virus. N Engl J Med 318:887, 1988

Prober CG, Sullender WM, Yasukawa LL, et al: Low risk of herpes simplex virus infections in neonates exposed to the virus at the time of vaginal delivery to mothers with recurrent genital herpes simplex virus infections. N Engl J Med 316:240, 1987

Ramsey PS, Vaules MB, Vasdev GM, et al: Maternal and transplacental pharmacokinetics of azithromycin. Am J Obstet Gynecol 188:714, 2003

Ramus R, Sheffield JS, Mayfield JA, et al: A randomized trial that compared oral cefixime and intramuscular ceftriaxone for the treatment of gonorrhea in pregnancy. Am J Obstet Gynecol 185:629, 2001

Rando RF, Lindheim S, Hasty L, et al: Increased frequency of detection of human papillomavirus deoxyribonucleic acid in exfoliated cervical cells during pregnancy. Am J Obstet Gynecol 161:50, 1989

Ratanajamit C, Skriver MV, Jepsen P, et al: Adverse pregnancy outcome in women exposed to acyclovir during pregnancy: A population-based observational study. Scand J Infect Dis 35:255, 2003

Read JS and the Committee on Pediatric AIDS: Human milk, breast-feeding, and transmission of human immunodeficiency virus type 1 in the United States. Pediatrics 112:1196, 2003

Read JS, Tuomala R, Kpamegan E, et al: Mode of delivery and postpartum morbidity among HIV-infected women: The women and infants transmission study. J Acquir Immune Defic Syndr 26:236, 2001

Reiff-Eldridge R, Heffner CR, Ephross SA, et al: Monitoring pregnancy outcomes after prenatal drug exposure through prospective pregnancy registries: A pharmaceutical company commitment. Am J Obstet Gynecol 182:159, 2000

Richardson BA, John-Stewart GC, Hughes JP, et al: Breast milk infectivity in human immunodeficiency virus type 1-infected mothers. J Infect Dis 187:736, 2003

Roberts SW, Cox SM, Dax J, et al: Genital herpes during pregnancy: No lesions, no cesarean. Obstet Gynecol 85:261, 1995

Rolfs RT: Treatment of syphilis in 1993. Clin Infect Dis 20:23, 1995

Ross JDC: Systemic gonococcal infection. Genitourin Med 72:404, 1996

Rouse DJ, Stringer JS: An appraisal of screening for maternal type-specific herpes simplex virus antibodies to prevent neonatal herpes. Am J Obstet Gynecol 183:400, 2000

Sansom SL, Jamieson DJ, Farnham PG: Human immunodeficiency virus retesting during pregnancy: Costs and effectiveness in preventing perinatal transmission. Obstet Gynecol 102:782, 2003

Schmid GP, Sanders LL, Blount JH, et al: Chancroid in the United States: Reestablishment of an old disease. JAMA 258:3265, 1987

Schrag SJ, Arnold KE, Mohle-Boetani JC, et al: Prenatal screening for infectious diseases and opportunities for prevention. Obstet Gynecol 102:753, 2003

Schulte JM, Burkham S, Hamaker D, et al: Syphilis among HIV-infected mothers and their infants in Texas from 1988 to 1994. Sex Transm Dis 28:316, 2001

Schwartz DA, Larsen SA, Beck-Sague C, et al: Pathology of the umbilical cord in congenital syphilis: Analysis of 25 specimens using histochemistry and immunofluorescent antibody to *Treponema pallidum*. Hum Pathol 26:784, 1995

Schwartz DB, Greenberg MD, Daoud Y, et al: Genital condylomas in pregnancy: Use of trichloroacetic acid and laser therapy. Am J Obstet Gynecol 158:1407, 1988

Schwebke JR: Update of trichomoniasis. Sex Transm Infect 78:378, 2002

Scott LL: Prevention of perinatal herpes: Prophylactic antiviral therapy? Clin Obstet Gynecol 42:134, 1999

Scott LL, Alexander J: Cost-effectiveness of acyclovir suppression to prevent recurrent genital herpes in term pregnancy. Am J Perinatol 15:57, 1998

Scott LL, Hollier LM, McIntire D, et al: Acyclovir suppression to prevent clinical recurrences at delivery after first episode genital herpes in pregnancy: An open-label trial. Infect Dis Obstet Gynecol 9:75, 2001

Scott LL, Hollier LM, McIntire D, et al: Acyclovir suppression to prevent recurrent genital herpes at delivery. Infect Dis Obstet Gynecol 10:71, 2002

Scott LL, Sanchez PJ, Jackson GL, et al: Acyclovir suppression to prevent cesarean section after first episode genital herpes in pregnancy. Obstet Gynecol 87:69, 1996

Scoular A: Using the evidence base on genital herpes: Optimizing the use of diagnostic tests and information provision. Sex Transm Infect 78:160, 2002

Sheffield J, Pybus C, Wendel G, et al: The effect of progesterone and pregnancy on HIV-1 co-receptor expression. Presented at the 25th Annual Meeting of the Society for Maternal–Fetal Medicine, Reno, Nevada, 7–12 February 2005

Sheffield JS, Fish DN, Hollier LM, et al: Acyclovir concentrations in human breast milk after valacyclovir administration. Am J Obstet Gynecol 186:100, 2002a

Sheffield JS, Hollier LM, Hill JB, et al: Acyclovir prophylaxis to prevent herpes simplex virus recurrence at delivery: A systematic review. Obstet Gynecol 102:1396, 2003

Sheffield JS, Sanchez PJ, Morris G, et al: Congenital syphilis after maternal treatment for syphilis during pregnancy. Am J Obstet Gynecol 186:569, 2002b

Sheffield JS, Sanchez PJ, Wendel GD Jr, et al: Placental histopathology of congenital syphilis. Obstet Gynecol 100:126, 2002c

Sheffield JS, Sigman A, McIntire D, et al: Disseminated gonococcal infection in women: A 24-year experience (Abstract No. 522). Presented at the Thirteenth Annual Meeting of the International Society for Sexually Transmitted Diseases Research, Denver, July 11–14, 1999

Silverberg MJ, Thorsen P, Lindeberg H, et al: Condyloma in pregnancy is strongly predictive of juvenile-onset recurrent respiratory papillomatosis. Obstet Gynecol 101:645, 2003

Silverman NS, Sullivan M, Hochman M, et al: A randomized, prospective trial comparing amoxicillin and erythromycin for the treatment of *Chlamydia trachomatis* in pregnancy. Am J Obstet Gynecol 170:829, 1994

Silverstein AM: Congenital syphilis and the timing of immunogenesis in the human fetus. Nature 194:196, 1962

Smith EM, Ritchie JM, Yankowitz J, et al: Human papillomavirus prevalence and types in newborns and parents. Sex Transm Dis 31:1:57, 2004

Snyder RR, Hammond TL, Hankins GDV: Human papillomavirus associated with poor healing of episiotomy repairs. Obstet Gynecol 76:664, 1990

Soper D: Trichomoniasis: Under control or undercontrolled? Am J Obstet Gynecol 190:281, 2004

Sozio J, Ness RB: Chlamydial lower genital tract infection and spontaneous abortion. Infect Dis Obstet Gynecol 6:8, 1998

Sperling RS, Shapiro DE, McSherry GD, et al: Safety of the maternal–infant zidovudine regimen utilized in the

Pediatric AIDS Clinical Trial Group 076 Study. AIDS 12:1805, 1998

Spitzer M, Krumholz BA, Seltzer VL: The multicentric nature of disease related to human papillomavirus infection of the female lower genital tract. Obstet Gynecol 73:303, 1989

Star J, Powrie R, Cu-Uvin S, et al: Should women with human immunodeficiency virus be delivered by cesarean? Obstet Gynecol 94:799, 1999

Steinbrook R: The AIDS epidemic in 2004. N Engl J Med. 351:115, 2004

Stratton P, Tuomala RE, Abboud R, et al: Obstetric and newborn outcomes in a cohort of HIV-infected pregnant women: A report of the women and infants transmission study. J Acquir Immune Defic Syndr Hum Retrovirol 20:179, 1999

Stringer EM, Stringer JS, Cliver SP, et al: Evaluation of a new testing policy for human immunodeficiency virus to improve screening rates. Obstet Gynecol 96:1004, 2001

Stringer JSA, Rouse DJ, Goldenberg RL: Prophylactic cesarean delivery for the prevention of perinatal human immunodeficiency virus transmission. JAMA 281:1946, 1999

Stuart GS, Castaño PM: Sexually transmitted infections and contraceptives: Selective issues. Obstet Gynecol Clin North Am 30:795, 2003

Tenti P, Zappatore R, Migliora P, et al: Perinatal transmission of human papillomavirus from gravidas with latent infections. Obstet Gynecol 93:475, 1999

Tseng CJ, Liang CC, Soong YK, et al: Perinatal transmission of human papillomavirus in infants: Relationship between infection rate and mode of delivery. Obstet Gynecol 91:92, 1998

Tuomala RE, Shapiro DE, Mofenson LM: Antiretroviral therapy during pregnancy and the risk of an adverse outcome. N Engl J Med 346:1863, 2002

U.S. Preventive Services Task Force: Screening for chlamydial infection: Recommendations and rationale. Am J Prev Med 20:90, 2001

U.S. Public Health Services Panel on Clinical Practices for Treatment of HIV Infection: Guidelines for the use of antiretroviral agents in HIV-1-infected adults and adolescents. March 23, 2004. Available at: http://AIDSinfo.nih.gov. Accessed March 2004a

U.S. Public Health Services Panel on Clinical Practices for Treatment of HIV Infection: Considerations for antiretroviral therapy in women. Supplement to guidelines for the use of antiretroviral agents in HIV-1-infected adults and adolescents. March 23, 2004. Available at: http://AIDSinfo.nih.gov. Accessed March 2004b

U.S. Public Health Service Task Force Perinatal HIV Guidelines Working Group: Recommendations for use of antiretroviral drugs in pregnant HIV-1-infected women for maternal health and interventions to reduce perinatal HIV-1 transmission in the United States. November 26, 2003. Available at: http://AIDSinfo.nih.gov. Accessed March 2004

Wald A, Ashley-Morrow R: Serological testing for herpes simplex virus (HSV)-1 and HSV-2 infection. Clin Infect Dis 35:S173, 2002

Wald A, Huang M-L, Carrell D, et al: Polymerase chain reaction for detection of herpes simplex virus (HSV) DNA on mucosal surfaces: Comparison with HSV isolation in cell culture. J Infect Dis 188:1345, 2003

Wald A, Zeh J, Selke S, et al: Reactivation of genital herpes simplex virus type 2 infection in asymptomatic seropositive persons. N Engl J Med 342:844, 2000

Wald A, Zeh J, Selke S, et al: Virologic characteristics of subclinical and symptomatic genital herpes infections. N Engl J Med 333:770, 1995

Walker GJ: Antibiotics for syphilis diagnosed during pregnancy. Cochrane Database Syst Rev 3:CD001143, 2001

Warner L, Rohcat RW, Fichtner RR, et al: Missed opportunities for congenital syphilis prevention in an urban southeastern hospital. Sex Transm Dis 28:92, 2001

Watson-Jones D, Changalucha J, Gumodoka B, et al: Syphilis in pregnancy in Tanzania. I. Impact of maternal syphilis on outcome of pregnancy. J Infect Dis 186:940, 2002a

Watts DH: Management of human immunodeficiency virus infection in pregnancy. N Engl J Med 346:1879, 2002

Watts DH, Balasubramanian R, Maupin RT Jr, et al: Maternal toxicity and pregnancy complications in human immunodeficiency virus-infected women receiving antiretroviral therapy: PACTG 316. Am J Obstet Gynecol 190:506, 2004

Watts DH, Koutsky LA, Holmes KK, et al: Low risk of perinatal transmission of human papillomavirus: Results from a prospective cohort study. Am J Obstet Gynecol 178:365, 1998

Wehbeh HA, Ruggeirio RM, Shahem SR, et al: Single-dose azithromycin for Chlamydia in pregnant women. J Reprod Med 43:509, 1998

Wendel GD: Gestational and congenital syphilis. Clin Perinatol 15:287, 1988

Wendel GD, Cunningham FG: Sexually transmitted diseases in pregnancy. In Williams Obstetrics, 18th ed. (Suppl 13). Norwalk, CT, Appleton & Lange, August/September 1991

Wendel GD Jr, Sanchez PJ, Peters MT, et al: Identification of Treponema pallidum in amniotic fluid and fetal blood from pregnancies complicated by congenital syphilis. Obstet Gynecol 78:890, 1991

Wendel GD Jr, Sheffield JS, Hollier LM, et al: Treatment of syphilis in pregnancy and prevention of congenital syphilis. Clin Infect Dis 35:S200, 2002

Wendel GD Jr, Stark BJ, Jamison RB, et al: Penicillin allergy and desensitization in serious infections during pregnancy. N Engl J Med 312:1229, 1985

Wiley DJ, Douglas J, Beutner K, et al: External genital warts: Diagnosis, treatment and prevention. Clin Infect Dis 35:S210, 2002

Wilkinson D, Barton S, Cowan F: HSV-2 specific serology should not be offered routinely to antenatal patients. Rev Med Virol 10:145, 2000

Winer RL, Koutsky LA: Delivering reassurance to parents: Perinatal human papillomavirus transmission is rare. Sex Transm Dis 31:63, 2004

Wittek AE, Yeager AS, Au DS, et al: Asymptomatic shedding of herpes simplex virus from the cervix and lesion site during pregnancy: Correlation of antepartum shedding with shedding at delivery. Am J Dis Child 138:439, 1984

World Health Organization: Effect of breastfeeding on mortality among HIV-infected women. WHO Statement, June 7, 2001. Available at: http://www.who.int/reproductive-health/rtis/MTCT/WHO_Statement_on_breast_feeding_June_2001.html. Accessed March, 2004

Wortley PM, Lindegren ML, Fleming PL: Successful implementation of perinatal HIV prevention guidelines. MMWR 50:17, 2001

Yip L, Sweeny PJ, Bock BF: Acute suppurative salpingitis with concomitant intrauterine pregnancy. Am J Emerg Med 11:476, 1993

Young H: Guidelines for serological testing for syphilis. Sex Transm Infect 75:403, 2000

Zenker PN, Rolfs RT: Treatment of syphilis, 1989. Rev Infect Dis 12:S590, 1990

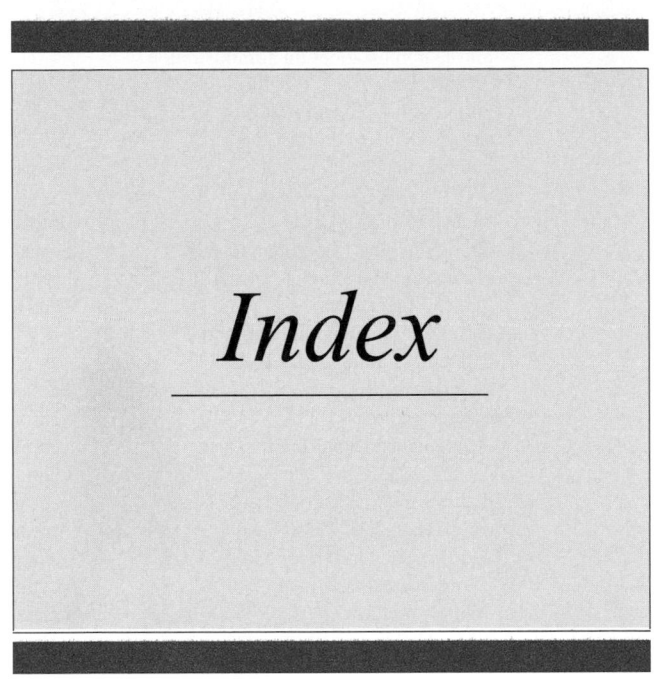

Index

Note: Page numbers followed by *f* and *t* indicate figures and tables, respectively.